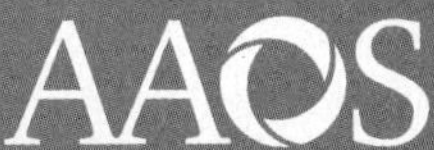

Advanced Emergency

Care and Transportation of the Sick and Injured

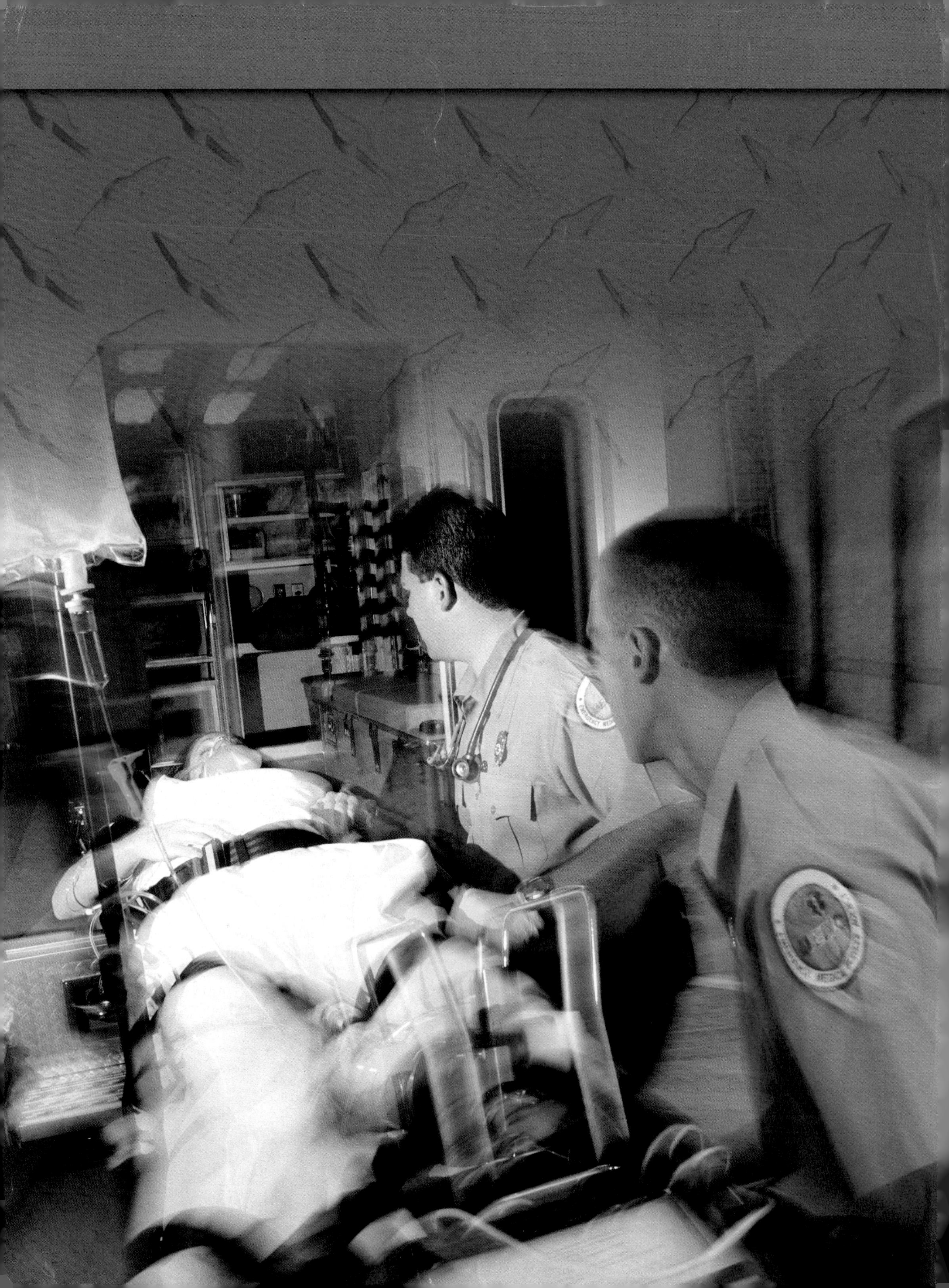

Third Edition

Advanced Emergency

Care and Transportation of the Sick and Injured

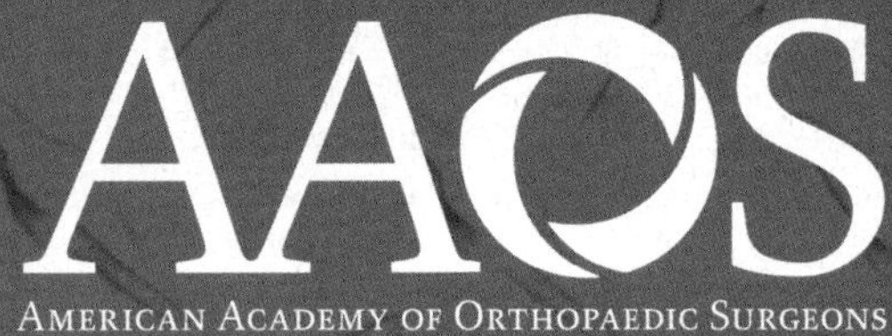

Series Editor:
Andrew N. Pollak, MD, FAAOS

Coeditor:
Alfonso Mejia, MD, MPH

Author:
Rhonda J. Hunt, BAS, NRP

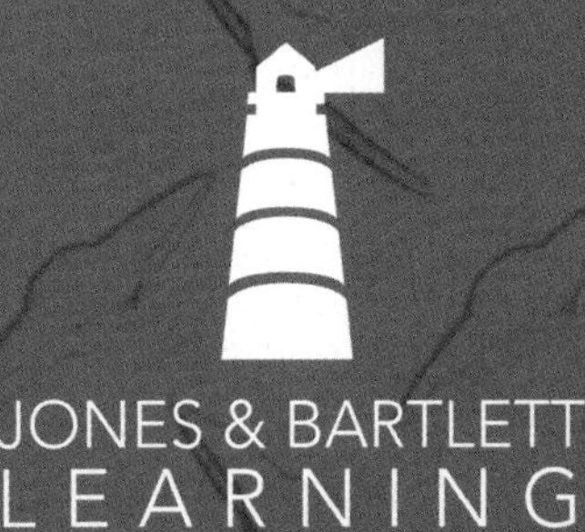

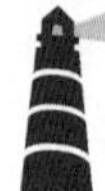

World Headquarters
Jones & Bartlett Learning
5 Wall Street
Burlington, MA 01803
978-443-5000
info@jblearning.com
www.jblearning.com
www.psglearning.com

Jones & Bartlett Learning books and products are available through most bookstores and online booksellers. To contact the Jones & Bartlett Learning Public Safety Group directly, call 800-832-0034, fax 978-443-8000, or visit our website, www.psglearning.com.

Substantial discounts on bulk quantities of Jones & Bartlett Learning publications are available to corporations, professional associations, and other qualified organizations. For details and specific discount information, contact the special sales department at Jones & Bartlett Learning via the above contact information or send an email to specialsales@jblearning.com.

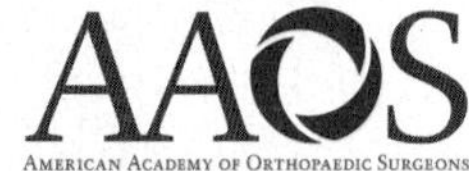

Editorial Credits:
Chief Education Strategist: Anna Salt Troise, MBA
Director, Publishing Partner Relationships: Hans J. Koelsch, PhD
Senior Manager, Publishing Operations: Joan Golembiewski
Senior Manager, Editorial: Lisa Claxton Moore
Senior Editor, Publications: Steven Kellert

13643-2

Production Credits
General Manager and Executive Publisher: Kimberly Brophy
VP, Product Development: Christine Emerton
Product Manager: Tiffany Sliter
Senior Editor: Carol B. Guerrero
Senior Editor: Amanda Mitchell
Editorial Assistant: Jessica Sturtevant
Editorial Assistant: Ashley Procum
VP, Sales, Public Safety Group: Matthew Maniscalco
Production Editor: Kristen Rogers
Director of Marketing Operations: Brian Rooney
Production Services Manager: Colleen Lamy
VP, Manufacturing and Inventory Control: Therese Connell
Composition: S4Carlisle Publishing Services
Cover Design: Kristin E. Parker
Text Design: Kristin E. Parker
Director of Rights & Media: Joanna Gallant
Rights & Media Specialist: Robert Boder
Media Development Editor: Troy Liston
Cover and Title Page Image: © Thinkstock/Stockbyte/Getty
Printing and Binding: LSC Communications
Cover Printing: LSC Communications

Library of Congress Cataloging-in-Publication Data
Names: Hunt, Rhonda J., editor. | American Academy of Orthopaedic Surgeons, author.
Title: Advanced emergency care and transportation of the sick and injured / American Academy of Orthopaedic Surgeons ; series editor, Andrew N. Pollak; editor, Rhonda J. Hunt.
Other titles: Orange book series.
Description: Third edition. | Burlington, MA : Jones & Bartlett Learning, [2019] | Series: Orange book series | Includes bibliographical references and index.
Identifiers: LCCN 2018003083 | ISBN 9781284121100 (paperback)
Subjects: | MESH: Emergency Treatment--methods | Transportation of Patients--methods | Emergency Medical Technicians--education
Classification: LCC RC86.7 | NLM WB 105 | DDC 362.18--dc23
LC record available at https://lccn.loc.gov/2018003083

6048

Printed in the United States of America
22 21 20 19 18 10 9 8 7 6 5 4 3 2

Brief Contents

Contents

Skill Drills

Prepare for Class with Navigate 2 Digital Curriculum Solution Packages

Navigate 2 resources offer unbeatable value with mobile-ready course materials to help you prepare for your AEMT class.

ADVANTAGE PACKAGE

Navigate 2 Advantage Access Includes:

- eBook
- Audiobook
- Study Center
- Assessments
- Analytics
- Fisdap Internship Scheduler
- Fisdap Skills Tracker

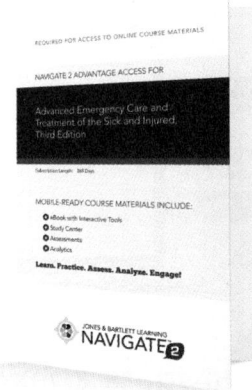

ISBN: 978-1-284-13639-5

PREFERRED PACKAGE

Navigate 2 Preferred Access Includes:

- eBook
- Audiobook
- Study Center
- Assessments
- Analytics
- TestPrep
- Fisdap Internship Scheduler
- Fisdap Skills Tracker

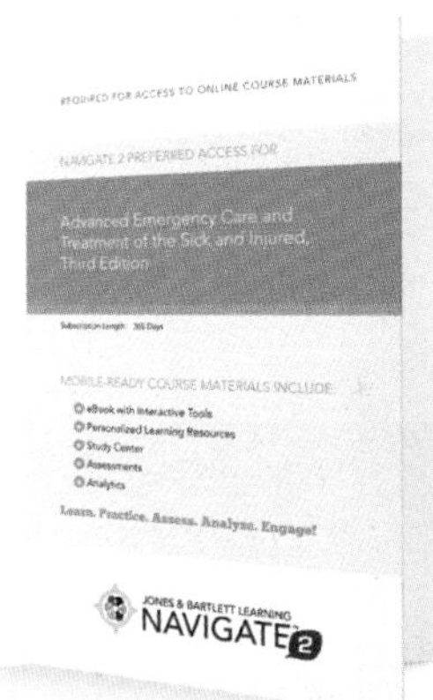

ISBN: 978-1-284-12287-9

PREMIER PACKAGE

Navigate 2 Premier Access Includes:

- eBook
- Audiobook
- Study Center
- Assessments
- Analytics
- TestPrep
- Lectures
- Simulations
- Fisdap Internship Scheduler
- Fisdap Skills Tracker

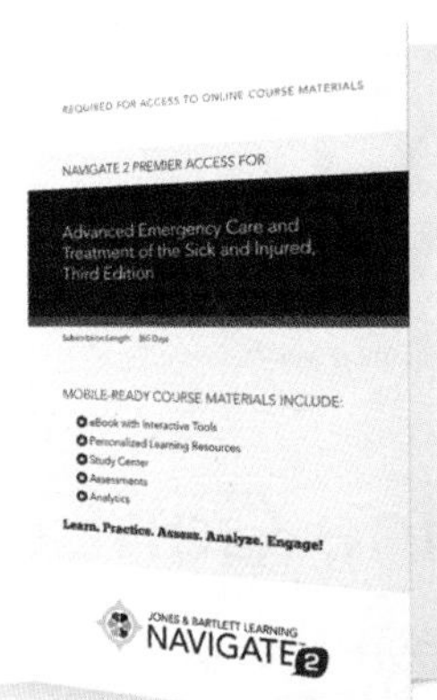

ISBN: 978-1-284-12300-5

Order today at www.psglearning.com

Acknowledgments

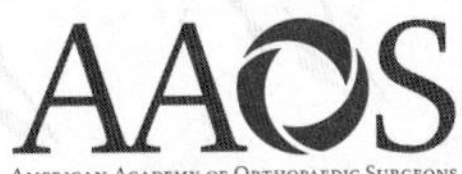

The American Academy of Orthopaedic Surgeons would like to acknowledge the contributors and reviewers of previous editions of *Advanced Emergency Care and Transportation of the Sick and Injured, Third Edition*, and those involved in the development of this edition.

Series Editor

Andrew N. Pollak, MD, FAAOS
The James Lawrence Kernan Professor and Chairman
Department of Orthopaedics
University of Maryland School of Medicine
Senior Vice President for Clinical Transformation and Chief of Orthopaedics
University of Maryland Medical System
Medical Director
Baltimore County Fire Department
Director, Shock Trauma Go Team
Special Deputy US Marshal

Coeditor

Alfonso Mejia, MD, MPH
Program Director, Orthopedic Surgery Residency Program
Vice Head, Department of Orthopedic Surgery
University of Illinois College of Medicine
Medical Director
Tactical Emergency Medical Support Physician
South Suburban Emergency Response Team
Chicago, Illinois

Author

Rhonda J. Hunt, BAS, NRP
Albany State University
Darton College of Health Professions
Albany, Georgia

Reviewers

J. Adam Alford, BS, NRP
Piedmont Virginia Community College
Charlottesville, Virginia

Gary Rex Anderson
Layton, Utah

Jeffrey Asher
Education Manager
Grady EMS Academy
Atlanta, Georgia

Kenneth E. Ashley, MS, LAT, ATC, AEMT
Prince Edward County Public Schools & Longwood University
Farmville, Virginia

Charles Avery, BA, NRP
EMS Programs Coordinator
Bainbridge State College
Bainbridge, Georgia

Ken Bartz, AEMT, I/C
Southwest Wisconsin Technical College
Fennimore, Wisconsin

Dana Baumgartner, NRP, BS
Nicolet College
Rhinelander, Wisconsin

Jason Baumgartner, NRP/CCEMTP
Nicolet College
Rhinelander, Wisconsin

Roger Beckman, MS, CEM, EMT-P
Utah Valley University
Orem, Utah

Shawn Bjarnson, AEMT, Law Enforcement Officer
Utah State Department of Corrections
Gunnison Valley Police Department
Gunnison Valley Hospital
Gunnison, Utah

James Blivin, NRP, NCEE
Training 911
Dumfires, Virginia

Michael Bolack, Paramedic, RN
Bevill State Community College
Sumiton, Alabama

Nick Bourdeau, RN, Paramedic I/C
Huron Valley Ambulance
Ann Arbor, Michigan

Deb Branden, ACP
Community Paramedic
Lethbridge, Alberta
Canada

Wayne D. Burdette Jr, MS, NR-P
Gwinnett County Fire Academy
Dacula, Georgia

Karen Burns
Captain
Clovis Fire Department
Clovis Community College
Clovis, New Mexico

Rebecca Carmody
College of Southern Nevada
Las Vegas, Nevada

Ginger Castle
G&E Training
Saint Charles, Virginia

Leon Charpentier
Harker Heights Fire Chief (retired)
CEO, Integrated Training Services
Harker Heights, Texas

Julie Chase, MSEd, FAWM, TP-C
Berryville, Virginia

David M. Claborn, DrPH, CDR, USN (ret.)
Missouri State University, Master of Public Health Program
Springfield, Missouri

Channing Clymer
EMS Program Coordinator
Delta-Montrose Technical College
Delta, Colorado

Kevin T. Collopy, BA, FP-C, CCEMT-P, NR-P, CMTE
Clinical Outcomes Manager
NHRMC AirLink/VitaLink Critical Care Transport
Wilmington, North Carolina

Helen T. Compton, NRP
Mecklenburg County Lifesaving & Rescue Squad
Clarksville, Virginia

Kevin Curry, AS, NRP, CCEMTP
United Training Center
Lewiston, Maine

Lyndal M. Curry, MS, NRP
Southern Union State Community College
Wadley, Alabama

H. Joel Dishroon, PM, IC
EMS Coordinator
Chattanooga State Community College
Children's Hospital at Erlanger
Chattanooga, Tennessee

Jeannett Edwards, NR, BS, MEd
James City County Fire Department
Williamsburg, Virginia

Steve Erwin
Baton Rouge, Louisiana

Darrell Wayne Fixler Jr, AAS, RRT, AEMT
Fort Rucker Fire & Emergency Services
Fort Rucker, Alabama

Jeffrey L. Foster, EMD, NRP, CCEMTP, IC
CarolinaEast Health Systems
New Bern, North Carolina

Alton Fowler Jr, EMT-P
Coliseum Medical Center
Macon, Georgia

Rodney Geilenfeldt II, BS, EMT-P
Paramedic Coordinator
EMSTA College
Santee, California

John Gloede
Moraine Park Technical College
Fond du Lac, Wisconsin

Shane Grier
Chocowinity EMS
Chocowinity, North Carolina

Ronald Grimstead
Houston, Texas

Kevin M. Gurney, MS, CCEMT-P, I/C
Delta Ambulance
Waterville, Maine

Jennifer Hannigan, MEd, Paramedic, CLI
Fire Department of the City of New York
Emergency Medical Services Bureau of Training
New York, New York

Anthony S. Harbour, BSN, MEd, RN, NRP
Southern Virginia EMS
Roanoke, Virginia

Keith B. Hermiz, NREMT-A, I/C
Grafton Rescue Squad, Inc.
Grafton, Vermont

Thomas R. Herron Jr, AAS, NRP
Roane State Community College
Harriman, Tennessee

Rick Hilinski, BA, EMT-P
Director, Fire/Public Safety
Community College of Allegheny County—Allegheny Campus
Oakdale, Pennsylvania

Gregory Hogan, BA, NREMT-P
Lyons Ambulance Service
Danvers, Massachusetts
Boston Medical Education Center
Boston, Massachusetts
Smugglers' Notch EMS
Smugglers' Notch, Vermont

Connie Holder, MS, AEMT
University of Utah
Salt Lake City, Utah

Joseph Hurlburt, BS, NREMT-P, EMT-P I/C
Instructor Coordinator/Training Officer
Rapid Response EMS
Romulus, Michigan

Amanda M. Jackson, NRP, RN
Level II Instructor
Darton State College
Albany, Georgia

Craig H. Jacobus, BA, BS, NRP, EMSI, DC
Metropolitan Community College—Fremont Center
Fremont, Nebraska

Beth Moody Jones, PT, DPT, MS, OCS
University of New Mexico School of Medicine
Department of Orthopedics
Albuquerque, New Mexico

Kristina Jordan
Blackhawk Technical College
Jamesville, Wisconsin

Thomas M. Kamplain Jr
Georgia Institute of EMS
Covington, Georgia

Timothy M. Kimble, AAS, NRP
Carilion Clinic Life Support Training Center
Roanoke, Virginia
Craig County Emergency Services
New Castle, Virginia

Mark A. King
Kennebec Valley Community College
Fairfield, Maine

Christopher Kroboth, MS, NR-P, CCEMT-P
Fairfax County Fire and Rescue
Fairfax, Virginia

William LaCost
Louisiana Department of Corrections
St. Gabriel, Louisiana

James Larsen, BS/BA, NR-P
Mitchell Community College
Statesville, North Carolina

William Leggio, EdD, NRP
Creighton University EMS Education
Omaha, Nebraska

Tyler McCardell, NRAEMT
Chief
Wakefield EMS
Peach Bottom, Pennsylvania

Randy McCartney
Moraine Park Technical College
Fond du Lac, Wisconsin

Eric McCullough, MEd, NRP
Columbia State Community College
Clifton, Tennessee

Amanda McDonald, MA, NRP
University of South Alabama
Mobile, Alabama

Dennis McMillin, NREMT I/99
Pro-Board Fire & EMS Instructor
Western Dakota Vo-Tech EMS
Oglala Lakota Nation EMS
Hermosa, South Dakota

Terry Mendez, EdM, CCEMT-P
Truckee Meadows Community College
Reno, Nevada

Lucian Mirra, MEd, NRP
University of Virginia
Charlottesville, Virginia

David Mixter, EMT-P
Central Georgia Technical College
Macon, Georgia

Robert Wayne Morgan, Paramedic
Obsidian Training Solutions
Valencia, California

David R. Murack, FF/CCP, I/C
Lakeshore Technical College
Cleveland, Wisconsin

Jessica Musselman, AEMT
EMS Division Training Captain
Nye County Emergency Management
Pahrump, Nevada

Gregory S. Neiman, MS, NRP, NCEE, CEMA (VA)
Virginia Office of EMS
Richmond, Virginia

Jim O'Connor
Columbus Division of Fire
Columbus, Ohio
Hocking College
Nelsonville, Ohio

Joseph J. Ogershok Jr, BS, NRAEMT
Ft. Detrick Medical University
Frederick, Maryland
8-koi.com
Melbourne, Florida

Heath S. Ormord, EMT-P/FF
Ford County Fire and EMS
Dodge City, Kansas

Nancy Peifer, PhD, MSN, RN
Palm Beach State College
Lake Worth, Florida

Glenn D. Phillips, AS, EMT-P
Mercer County EMS
Salvisa, Kentucky

Mark Podgwaite, NRAEMT NECEMS I/C
VT EMS District 5
Lyndonville, Vermont

Valerie Quick, MSN, RN, EMT-I, NCEE
University of Virginia Health System
Charlottesville, Virginia

Holly A. Scribner AAS, AS, BAS, MSEd, FF/Paramedic
Cushing Rescue Squad
Cushing, Maine

Douglas P. Skinner, MPA, NRP, NCEE
Prince Georges Community College
SCS Safety Health and Security Associates LLC
Leesburg, Virginia

Jennifer TeWinkel Smith, BA, AEMT
Regions Hospital EMS
St. Paul, Minnesota

Captain Katharine R. Smith, AS, NRP
Professional Standards and Training Officer
Florence County EMS
Florence, South Carolina

Donna Spink
Finger Lakes Regional EMS
Geneva, New York

Tynell N. Stackhouse, MTh, NRP
Marion County EMS, FTO
Marion, South Carolina

Bruce Swanson, Paramedic
Huntsville Fire & Rescue
Huntsville, Alabama

Antoinette Tharrett, BSN, RN-BC, NREMT-P, CCEMT-P
Zack's Superior Services
Russell Springs, Kentucky

Stephen Trala, MPH, BSN, RN, NRP, CHS-IV
University of Vermont HealthNet Critical Care Transport
Burlington, Vermont

Brian J. Turner, CCEMT-P, RN
Genesis Medical Center
Davenport, Iowa

Cynthia Turnmire, NREMTP
AEMT Program Director
Walters State Community College
Morristown, Tennessee

Robert K. (Bob) Waddell II, EMT-P (ret), BS
SAM Medical, Inc.
Wilsonville, Oregon

Jon W. Walker
Upper Valley Ambulance, Inc—Retired
Fairlee, Vermont

Tom Watson, AS, AAS, Paramedic
Adjunct Instructor
Texas A&M University System
Texas Engineering Extension Service
Emergency Services Training Institute
EMS/Public Health Program
College Station, Texas

Timothy L. Weir, Paramedic
Wisconsin Technical College System
Madison, Wisconsin

James Welch, BS, FP-C
Fort Greely Fire & Emergency Services
USAG Fort Greely, Alaska

William M. Wells Sr, MEd, NRP
Instructor
Technical College High School—Brandywine Campus
Downingtown, Pennsylvania

Gregory West, EdD, JD, NRP
Waukesha County Technical College
Pewaukee, Wisconsin

Kelly R. Whitacre, NRP, NCEE
Frederick County Fire and Rescue Department
Winchester, Virginia

Ken Whittaker NRP, CCEMTP
Humboldt General Hospital
Winnemucca, Nevada

Michael H. Wilhelm, CRNA, APRN
Integrated Anesthesia Associates School of Nurse Anesthesia
Hartford, Connecticut

Marla Williams, BS, NRP
EMS/Fire Science Program Coordinator
Hawkeye Community College
Waterloo, Iowa

Earl M. Wilson III, BIS, NRP
Nunez Community College
Chalmette, Louisiana

Photoshoot Acknowledgments

We would like to thank the following people and institutions for their collaboration on the photoshoots for this project. Their assistance was greatly appreciated.

Technical Consultants and Institutions

UMass Memorial Paramedics—Worcester EMS
Worcester, Massachusetts

Richard A. Nydam, AS, NREMT-P
Training and Education Specialist, EMS
UMass Memorial Paramedics—Worcester EMS
Worcester, Massachusetts

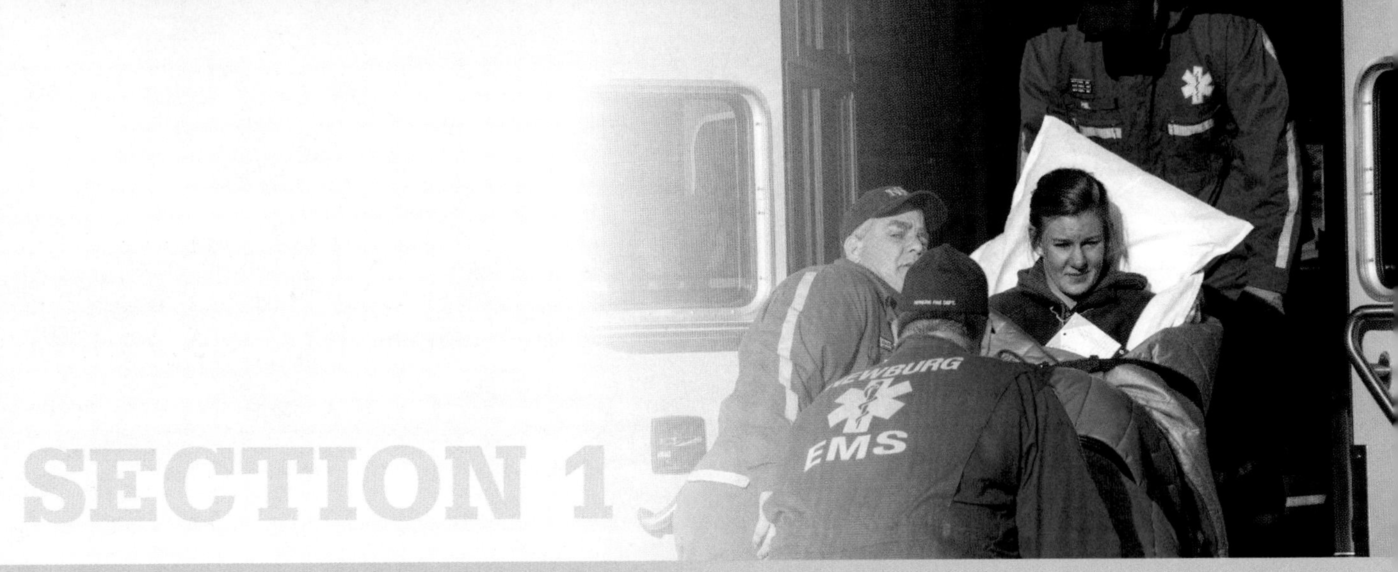

SECTION 1

Preparatory

CHAPTER 1

EMS Systems

National EMS Education Standard Competencies

Preparatory

Applies fundamental knowledge of the EMS system, safety/well-being of the AEMT, medical/legal and ethical issues to the provision of emergency care.

EMS Systems

- EMS systems (pp 11-18)
- History of EMS (pp 5-6)
- Roles/responsibilities/professionalism of EMS personnel (pp 20-21)
- Quality improvement (p 14)
- Patient safety (pp 20-21)

Research

- Impact of research on emergency medical responder (EMR) care (p 18)
- Data collection (pp 15, 17-18)
- Evidence-based decision making (p 18)

Public Health

Uses simple knowledge of the principles of the role of EMS during public health emergencies.

Knowledge Objectives

1. Define emergency medical services (EMS). (p 3)
2. Discuss the four levels of EMS training and licensure. (pp 3-4)
3. Describe licensure criteria for advanced emergency medical technicians (AEMTs). (p 5)
4. Describe how the Americans with Disabilities Act (ADA) applies to employment as an AEMT. (p 5)
5. Discuss the history of the development of the EMS system. (pp 5-6)
6. Describe the levels of EMS training in terms of skill sets needed for each of the following: emergency medical responder (EMR), emergency medical technician (EMT), AEMT, and paramedic. (pp 6-9)
7. Discuss the possible presence of other responders at a scene with EMR training, some knowledge of first aid, or merely good intentions, and their need for direction. (p 10)
8. Describe the components of the EMS system. (pp 11-18)
9. Describe how medical direction of an EMS system works and your role in the process. (pp 12-13)
10. Describe the goals of Mobile Integrated Healthcare (MIH) and community paramedicine. (p 14)
11. Discuss the purpose of the EMS continuous quality improvement (CQI) process. (p 14)
12. Characterize the EMS system's role in prevention and public education in the community. (pp 17-18)
13. Describe situations in which transport to a specialty center is warranted. (pp 18-19)
14. Describe your roles and responsibilities as an AEMT. (pp 20-21)
15. Describe the attributes you are expected to possess. (pp 20-21)
16. Discuss the impact of the Health Insurance Portability and Accountability Act (HIPAA) on patient privacy. (p 21)

Skills Objectives

There are no skills objectives for this chapter.

Introduction

This textbook is designed to serve as the text and primary resource for the advanced emergency medical technician (AEMT) course. This chapter describes the content and objectives of the AEMT course. It discusses what is expected of you during the course and what other requirements you need to meet to be licensed or certified as an AEMT in most states. The differences in basic first aid training, emergency medical responder (EMR) training, and the training for emergency medical technicians (EMTs), AEMTs, and paramedics are described.

Emergency medical services is a system. The key components of this system and how these components influence and affect your delivery of prehospital emergency care are carefully discussed. Discussions on administration, medical direction, quality control, and regulation of EMS systems are also presented. The chapter concludes with a detailed discussion of the roles and responsibilities of AEMTs as health care professionals.

Course Description

Emergency medical services (EMS) consists of a team of health care professionals who, in each area or jurisdiction, are responsible for and provide prehospital emergency care and transportation for sick and injured people **Figure 1-1**. Each emergency medical service is part of a local or regional EMS system that provides the prehospital and hospital components required for the delivery of proper emergency medical care. The standards for prehospital emergency care and the people who provide it are governed by the laws in each state served and are typically regulated by a state office of EMS.

The people who provide emergency medical care in the field are trained and, except for licensed physicians, must be either certified EMS personnel or state-licensed. A **certification** exam is used to ensure all health care providers have at least the same basic level of knowledge and skill. After you pass this exam, you are eligible to apply for state licensure. **Licensure** is the process by which states ensure applicant competency in an examination setting. This allows states to manage who can function as a health care provider. The ways in which these terms are used may vary by state. For the purpose of this textbook, the term *licensure* will be used.

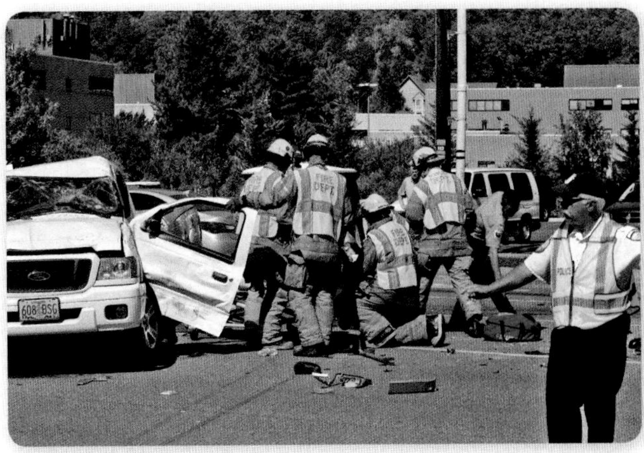

Figure 1-1 As an AEMT, you will be part of a larger team that responds to a variety of calls and provides a wide range of prehospital emergency care.

In most states, providers are categorized into four different training and licensure levels: **emergency medical responder (EMR)**, **emergency medical technician (EMT)**, **advanced EMT (AEMT)**, and **paramedic**. **Table 1-1** shows some of the responsibilities and requirements of these roles.

> **Words of Wisdom**
>
> In some states, AEMT is the introductory level and may not require prerequisites.

Although the specific training and licensure requirements vary from one state to another, almost every state's requirements follow or exceed the guidelines recommended in the current National Highway Traffic Safety Administration (NHTSA) EMS Education Standards. In the United States, NHTSA is the federal administrative source for education standards and related documents.

This textbook covers the practice and skills identified in the 2009 *National EMS Education Standards*. It also covers the information required for AEMTs to perform the skills outlined in the 2005 *National EMS Scope of Practice Model*.

YOU are the Provider — PART 1

You were just hired as an AEMT and report to your first day on the job with the local ambulance service. As you begin your orientation, the EMS director asks you two initial questions:

1. What is emergency medical services (EMS)?
2. Why was the National Registry of Emergency Medical Technicians (NREMT) established?

Table 1-1 EMS Responsibilities and Requirements

Training/Licensure Level	Responsibilities and Requirements[a]
EMR	First medically trained professional to arrive on scene; provides initial care before the ambulance arrives; assistant role
EMT	Trained in BLS including the use of AEDs and airway adjuncts; assists with administering certain medications
AEMT	Advanced training in specific aspects of **advanced life support (ALS)** (eg, **intravenous (IV) therapy**); administers certain emergency medications and certain types of advanced airway management
Paramedic	Trained in ALS, endotracheal intubation, emergency pharmacology, cardiac monitoring, and other advanced assessment and emergency medical treatment skills

[a]Responsibilities and requirements vary by state.
Abbreviations: AEDs, automatic external defibrillators; ALS, advanced life support; BLS, basic life support

In addition to the required core content, this textbook includes additional information to help you understand and apply the material and skills included in the AEMT course.

Words of Wisdom

Study Tips for Using This Textbook

Complete each assignment diligently and carefully.

Read the textbook like a textbook, not like a blog, magazine, or novel.

Read each chapter several times, and underline key points. Take notes!

Note the chapter's objectives so you can effectively measure your knowledge.

Ask your instructor to clarify any questions you have.

Take additional notes when the assigned material is expanded upon in class.

Use supporting materials (eg, assessments, animations, videos, and workbooks) to enhance your learning experience.

Remember: The only dumb question is the one you fail to ask.

AEMT Training: Focus and Requirements

As an AEMT, some of the patients you treat will have life-threatening conditions, whereas others require only supportive care. The skills needed to safely deliver this care are found within this text. Some of the main subjects that will be discussed include the following:

- **Scene size-up.** During scene size-up, you must gain a big-picture perspective of the call, determine if it is safe to proceed, determine whether additional resources are needed, and identify the initial approach to mitigate the emergency scene. EMS operates in a wide variety of environments that can create situations where EMS personnel can be injured. A primary role of any EMS provider is to ensure he or she is as safe as possible.
- **Patient assessment.** Patient assessment is the foundation of any EMS call. You must determine what is wrong with the patient. Patients can have many complaints, and you will learn to determine which complaints are life threatening.
- **Treatment.** As an AEMT, ensure the patient is oxygenated, administer certain medications, and administer IV therapy if needed. Control bleeding and assist patients during childbirth. In addition to hands-on skills, you will learn how to manage patients who are in emotional crisis and to calm patients and relieve some of their anxieties.
- **Packaging.** In EMS, **packaging** refers to the act of preparing a patient for movement as a unit by means of a backboard or similar stabilization device. Most patients need to be transported to a facility. This could mean a hospital, clinic, or other medical care facility. You will learn how to transport patients with a wide variety of illnesses and injuries.
- **EMS as a career.** Many of you are taking this course because you want to help people. To ensure all EMS providers have a long, healthy

career, it is important for you to learn how to take care of yourself. We will discuss job stressors and successful ways to cope with stress.

Licensure Requirements

To be recognized and to function as an AEMT, you must meet certain requirements. The specific requirements differ from state to state. Ask your instructor or learning institute, or contact your state EMS official to find out about the requirements in your state. Generally, the criteria to be licensed and employed as an AEMT will include the following:

- High school diploma or equivalent
- Proof of immunization against certain communicable diseases
- Successful completion of a background check and drug screening
- Valid driver's license
- Successful completion of a recognized health care provider's basic life support (BLS)/cardiopulmonary resuscitation (CPR) course
- Successful completion of a state-recognized AEMT course
- Successful completion of a state-recognized written certification examination
- Successful completion of a state-recognized practical certification examination
- Demonstration that you can meet the psychological and physical criteria necessary to perform safely and properly all the tasks and functions described in the defined role of an AEMT
- Compliance with other state, local, and employer provisions

The state-recognized written and practical examination may be the National Registry of Emergency Medical Technician's (NREMT) Exam based on the individual state. The NREMT was established in 1970 to certify and register EMS professionals through a valid and uniform process that assesses their knowledge and skills to ensure competent practice. The NREMT requires recertification every 2 years to ensure continued competence. Because most states now recognize NREMT certification, it is easy for an AEMT to move to another state and continue to work without attending another course and taking another certification exam for that area. If you move to a different state, you may be allowed to apply for reciprocity rather than starting your training all over or taking the new state's certification exam. **Reciprocity** is the recognition by one state of another state's licensure, allowing a health care professional from another state to practice in the new state.

The **Americans with Disabilities Act (ADA)** of 1990 protects people who have a disability from being denied access to programs and services that are provided by state or local governments and prohibits employers from failing to provide full and equal employment to people with disabilities. In addition, Title I of the ADA protects those with disabilities seeking gainful employment under many circumstances. Employers with 15 or more employees are required to adjust processes so a candidate with a disability can be considered for the position and, when possible, to modify the work environment or how the job is normally performed.[1] This allows many people who can perform the functional job skills the opportunity to pursue a career in EMS. To obtain further information about the Americans with Disabilities Act and employment as an AEMT, contact your state EMS office.

One of the primary responsibilities of each state is to ensure the safety of its residents. As such, states have requirements prohibiting people with certain legal infractions from becoming EMS providers. The specific legal exclusions vary from state to state. States may exclude from certification persons with a history of a health problem that could make their performance of AEMT tasks dangerous to themselves or others. Contact your state EMS official for more information.

Overview of the EMS System

History of EMS

As an AEMT, you will join a long tradition of people who have provided emergency medical care to their fellow human beings. With the early use of motor vehicles in warfare, volunteer ambulance squads were organized and went overseas to provide care for the wounded in World War I. In World War II, the military trained special corpsmen to provide care in the field and bring the casualties to aid stations staffed by nurses and physicians. In the Korean conflict, the care system evolved to the field medic and rapid helicopter evacuation to nearby Mobile Army Surgical Hospital units, where immediate surgical intervention was provided. Many advances in the immediate care of trauma patients resulted from the casualty experiences in the Korean and Vietnam conflicts.

Unfortunately, emergency medical care of people injured and ill at home or elsewhere outside a hospital had not progressed to a similar level. As late as the early 1970s, emergency ambulance service and care across the United States varied widely. In some places, care was provided by well-trained, advanced first aid squads that had well-equipped, modern ambulances. In a few urban areas, it was provided by hospital-based ambulance services that were staffed with interns and early forms of prehospital care providers. In many places, the only emergency medical care and ambulance service was provided by the local funeral home using a hearse that could be converted to carry a cot and serve as an ambulance. In other places, the police or fire department used a station wagon that carried a cot and a first aid kit.

In most cases, both of these were staffed by a driver and an attendant who had some first aid training. In the few areas where a commercial ambulance was available to transport ill and injured people, it was usually similarly staffed and served primarily as a means to transport the patient to the hospital.

Words of Wisdom

As an AEMT, you will continue a long tradition of people who have provided emergency medical care to their fellow human beings. The AEMT is an important contributor to the overall health care community and ultimately helps reduce mortality and morbidity.

Many communities had no formal provision for prehospital emergency care or transportation. Injured people were given first aid by police or fire personnel at the scene and were transported to the hospital in a police or fire officer's car. Customarily, patients with an acute illness were transported to the hospital by a relative or neighbor and were met by their family physician or an on-call hospital physician who assessed them and then summoned any specialists and operating room staff who were needed. Except in large urban centers, most hospitals did not have the staffed emergency departments (EDs) that we are accustomed to today.

EMS as we know it today had its origins in 1966 with the publication of *Accidental Death and Disability: The Neglected Disease of Modern Society*. This report, known more commonly as The White Paper, prepared jointly by the Committees on Trauma and Shock of the National Academy of Sciences/National Research Council, revealed to the public and Congress the serious inadequacy of prehospital emergency care and transportation in many areas.

As a result, Congress mandated that two federal agencies address these issues. The NHTSA of the Department of Transportation (DOT), through the Highway Safety Act of 1966, and the Department of Health, Education, and Welfare (now known as the Department of Health and Human Services), through the Emergency Medical Services Development Act of 1973, created funding sources and programs to develop improved systems of prehospital emergency care.[2] They also required states to focus on EMS personnel training and the legislation and regulation of EMS personnel levels.

In the early 1970s, the DOT developed and published the first National Standard Curriculum to serve as the guideline for the training of EMTs.[3] To support the EMT course, the American Academy of Orthopaedic Surgeons prepared and published the first EMT textbook—*Emergency Care and Transportation of the Sick and Injured*—in 1971. This textbook is the AEMT adaptation of that publication. Through the 1970s, following the recommended guidelines, each state developed the necessary legislation, and the EMS system was developed throughout the United States. During this same period, emergency medicine became a recognized emergency medical specialty, and fully staffed EDs became the accepted standard of care.

In the late 1970s, the DOT developed a recommended National Standard Curriculum for the training of paramedics and identified a part of the course to serve as training for AEMTs.

During the 1980s, many areas enhanced the EMS National Standard Curriculum by adding providers with higher levels of training who could provide key components of ALS care. The availability of paramedics and ALS-level care on calls that require or benefit from advanced care has grown steadily in recent years. In addition, with the evolution in training and technology, EMTs and AEMTs can now perform a number of important advanced skills in the field that were formerly reserved for paramedics.

This growth and sophistication of the EMS system did not come without drawbacks. As each state sought to create a system that would meet the needs of its citizens, the roles and responsibilities of EMS providers began to vary from state to state. For example, in some states EMTs were allowed to administer medications, while in other states they were not.

In the 1990s, NHTSA began an examination of EMS from a national perspective. With the counsel of EMS providers, physicians, fire chiefs, nurses, state administrators, educators, and other interested professionals, NHTSA created the *EMS Agenda for the Future*. This important document creates a plan to standardize the levels of EMS education and EMS providers in an effort to ensure a more seamless delivery of EMS care across the United States.

The skills you learn and the scope of practice that AEMTs now enjoy are part of this national movement toward an EMS system that meets the needs of an ever-changing health care industry and meets those needs through a safe and efficient method.

Levels of Training

As discussed earlier, licensure of AEMTs is a state function, subject to the laws and regulations of the state in which the AEMT practices. Each state is granted the ability to control the functions of its licensed providers. For this reason, there remains some variation from state to state on the scope of AEMT practice, as well as training and recertification requirements. Here is how the system is supposed to work from the federal level down to the local level.

At the federal level, NHTSA brought in experts from around the United States to create the ***National EMS Scope of Practice Model***. This document provides overarching guidelines for the minimum skills each level of EMS providers should be able to perform. Table 1-2 shows the guidelines from that model. Some items in the table are flagged, and corresponding notes are provided to show areas where current practice has evolved. For example, certain skills listed in the table are no longer practiced or have been aligned with a different skill level. Because licensure is a state function, at the state level laws are enacted to regulate how EMS providers will operate and are then executed by the state-level EMS administrative offices that control licensure. Finally, the local medical director decides the day-to-day limits of EMS personnel. For example, the medications that will be carried on an ambulance or where patients are transported are the day-to-day operational concerns about which the medical director will have direct input.

The national guidelines are intended to create more consistent delivery of EMS across the United States. A medical director can allow an AEMT to perform a skill

Table 1-2 The Interpretive Guidelines: *National EMS Scope of Practice Model*

An EMT also provides the skills listed in the EMR level.
An AEMT also provides the skills listed in the EMR and EMT levels.
A paramedic also provides the skills listed in the EMR, EMT, and AEMT levels.

Airway and Breathing Minimum Psychomotor Skill Set			
EMR	**EMT**	**AEMT**	**Paramedic**
Oral airway	Humidifiers	Supraglottic airway	BPAP/CPAP
Bag-mask device	Partial rebreathing mask		Needle chest decompression
Sellick maneuver[a]	Venturi mask		Chest tube monitoring
Head tilt–chin lift	Manually triggered ventilators		Percutaneous cricothyrotomy
Jaw-thrust maneuver	Automatic transport ventilators		$ETCO_2$/capnography
Modified chin lift	Oral and nasal airways		NG/OG tube
Obstruction, manual			Nasal and oral endotracheal intubation
Oxygen therapy			Airway obstruction removal by direct laryngoscopy
Nasal cannula			Positive end-expiratory pressure
Nonrebreathing mask			
Upper airway suctioning			
Assessment Minimum Psychomotor Skill Set			
Manual BP	Pulse oximetry	Blood glucose monitoring[b]	ECG interpretation
	Manual and automatic BP		Interpretive 12-lead
			Blood chemistry analysis
Pharmacologic Intervention Minimum Psychomotor Skill Set			
Medication Administration Routes ▪ Unit dose auto-injector for self or peer care (MARK 1)[c]	*Assisted Medications* ▪ Assisting a patient in administering his/her own prescribed medications, including auto-injector	▪ Peripheral IV insertion ▪ IV fluid infusion ▪ Pediatric IO insertion	▪ Central line monitoring ▪ IO insertion ▪ Venous blood sampling

(continued)

Table 1-2 The Interpretive Guidelines: *National EMS Scope of Practice Model* (continued)

EMR	EMT	AEMT	Paramedic
Pharmacologic Intervention Minimum Psychomotor Skill Set			
	Medication Administration Routes ▪ Buccal ▪ Oral	*Medication Administration Routes* ▪ Aerosolized ▪ Subcutaneous ▪ IM ▪ Nebulized ▪ SL ▪ IN ▪ IV push for D_{50} and narcotic antagonist only	*Medication Administration Routes* ▪ Endotracheal ▪ IV (push and infusion) ▪ NG ▪ Rectal ▪ IO ▪ Topical ▪ Accessing implanted central IV port
	Medications to Be Administered ▪ Physician-approved over-the-counter medications (oral glucose, aspirin for chest pain or suspected ischemic origin)	*Medications to Be Administered* ▪ SL nitroglycerin for chest pain of suspected ischemic origin ▪ Subcutaneous[d] and IM epinephrine for anaphylaxis ▪ Glucagon and IV D_{50} for hypoglycemia ▪ Inhaled beta agonist for dyspnea and wheezing ▪ Narcotic antagonist ▪ Nitrous oxide for pain relief	*Medications to Be Administered* ▪ Physician-approved medications ▪ Maintenance of blood administration ▪ Initiation of thrombolytics
Emergency Trauma Care Minimum Psychomotor Skill Set			
Manual cervical stabilization	Spinal immobilization		Morgan lens
Manual extremity stabilization	Seated spinal immobilization		
Eye irrigation	Long backboard		
Direct pressure	Extremity splinting		
Hemorrhage control	Traction splinting		
Emergency moves for endangered patients	Mechanical patient restraint		
	Tourniquet[e]		
	MAST/PASG[f]		
	Cervical collar		
	Rapid extrication		

Medical/Cardiac Care Minimum Psychomotor Skill Set			
CPR	Mechanical CPR		Cardioversion
AED	Assisted complicated delivery of an infant		Carotid massage
Assisted normal delivery of an infant			Manual defibrillation
			TC pacing

Abbreviations: AED, automated external defibrillator; AEMT, advanced emergency medical technician; BPAP, bilevel positive airway pressure; BP, blood pressure; CPAP, continuous positive airway pressure; CPR, cardiopulmonary resuscitation; D50, 50% dextrose; ECG, electrocardiogram; EMR, emergency medical responder; EMT, emergency medical technician; $ETCO_2$, end-tidal carbon dioxide; IM, intramuscular; IN, intranasal; IO, intraosseous; IV, intravenous; MAST, military antishock trousers; NG, nasogastric, OG, orogastric; PASG, pneumatic antishock garments; SL, sublingual; TC, transcutaneous

Note: The 2005 *National EMS Scope of Practice Model* serves as a foundation for states to build their own model. It is intended to illustrate the operation of each level of EMS provider and the progression from one level to another. It is not inclusive of every skill a state may allow.

[a]The Sellick maneuver is no longer recommended.
[b]Blood glucose monitoring is now considered an EMT-level skill.
[c]Mark 1 has been replaced by the DuoDote and the Antidote Treatment Nerve Agent Auto-Injector (ATNAA).
[d]Subcutaneous epinephrine administration is typically considered a paramedic-level skill now.
[e]Tourniquet use has evolved to be practiced by all providers including the EMR level.
[f]MAST/PASG has very specific indications including stabilizing bilateral femur fractures or pelvic fractures. See Chapter 27, *Bleeding,* for further information.

only if the state has already approved performance of that skill. The medical director can limit the scope of practice but cannot expand it beyond state law. Expanding the scope of practice requires state approval.

The EMT, AEMT, and paramedic education standards and instructional guidelines can be downloaded from www.ems.gov. In addition, the NREMT is a nongovernmental agency that provides national standardized testing for EMS testing and certification in much of the United States. Many states use the National Registry standards to certify their AEMTs and grant licensing reciprocity to NREMT-certified AEMTs. However, it is important to remember EMS is regulated entirely by the state in which you are licensed.

Public Basic Life Support and Immediate Aid

With the development of EMS and increased awareness of the need for immediate emergency medical care, millions of laypeople have been trained in BLS/CPR. In addition to CPR, many people have taken short basic first aid courses that include control of bleeding and other simple skills that may be required to provide immediate essential care. These courses are designed to train people so that people in the workplace, such as teachers, coaches, baby-sitters, and others, can provide the necessary critical care in the minutes before AEMTs or other responders arrive at the scene.

In addition, many people, such as people who regularly accompany groups on camping trips or are in other situations in which the arrival of EMS may be delayed because of a remote location, are trained in advanced first aid. This course includes BLS and the essential additional care and packaging that may be necessary until the help of rescuers and providers can be obtained at a remote location.

One of the most dramatic recent developments in prehospital emergency care is the use of an **automated external defibrillator (AED)**. These remarkable devices,

YOU are the Provider PART 2

The director continues to explain that the service uses the *National EMS Scope of Practice Model* as the framework for what its providers can do in the field. He also mentions that the local 9-1-1 center hires only dispatchers who have completed the Emergency Medical Dispatch (EMD) course.

3. What is the *National EMS Scope of Practice Model*?
4. How does the EMD system work?

some no larger than a cell phone, detect treatable life-threatening cardiac dysrhythmias (ventricular fibrillation and ventricular tachycardia) and deliver the appropriate electrical shock to the patient. Designed to be used by an untrained layperson, they are now included at every level of prehospital emergency training.

▶ Emergency Medical Responder

Because the presence of a person who is trained and able to initiate BLS and other urgent care cannot be ensured, the EMS system includes immediate care by EMRs, such as law enforcement officers, firefighters, park rangers, ski patrollers, or other organized rescuers who often arrive at the scene before the ambulance and providers **Figure 1-2**. EMR training provides these people with the skills necessary to initiate immediate care and then assist other EMS providers on their arrival. The course focuses on providing immediate BLS and urgent care with limited equipment. It also familiarizes students with the additional procedures, equipment, and packaging techniques that other EMS providers may use and with which the EMR may be called on to assist.

In addition to professional EMRs, AEMTs often encounter a variety of people on the scene eager to help. You will encounter Good Samaritans trained in first aid and CPR, physicians and nurses, and other well-meaning people with or without prior training and experience. If identified and used properly, these people can provide valuable assistance when you are shorthanded. At other times, they can interfere with operations and even create problems or a danger to themselves or others. It will be your task in your initial scene size-up to identify the various people on the scene and orchestrate well-meaning attempts to assist.

▶ Emergency Medical Technician

The EMT course requires approximately 150 hours (more in some states) and provides the essential knowledge and skills required to provide basic emergency medical care in the field. The course serves as the foundation on which additional knowledge and skills are built in AEMT training. On arrival at the scene, you and the other providers who have responded with the ambulance should assume responsibility for the assessment and care of the patient, followed by proper packaging and transport of the patient to the ED if appropriate.

▶ Advanced Emergency Medical Technician

The AEMT course and training are designed to add knowledge and skills in specific aspects of ALS to providers who have been trained and have experience in providing emergency medical care as EMTs. Additional skills above the EMT level include IV therapy, use of advanced airway adjuncts, and the knowledge and skills necessary for the administration of a limited number of medications **Figure 1-3**. The AEMT course range is approximately 200 to 400 hours. The purpose of this level of EMS provider is to deliver an expanded range of skills beyond the EMT. In some parts of the United States, the availability of paramedics is limited. AEMTs help to fill the gap by providing limited ALS care to regions where paramedics are not available.

▶ Paramedic

The paramedic has completed an extensive course of training that significantly increases knowledge and mastery of basic skills and covers a wide range of ALS skills. This course ranges from 1,000 to more than 1,300

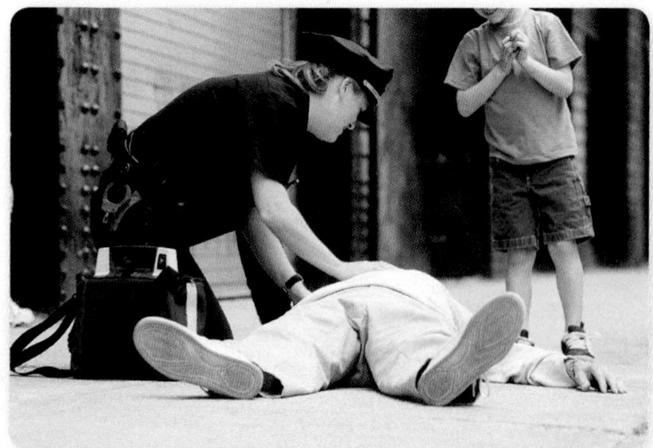

Figure 1-2 Emergency medical responders, such as law enforcement officers, are trained to provide immediate basic life support until providers arrive on the scene.

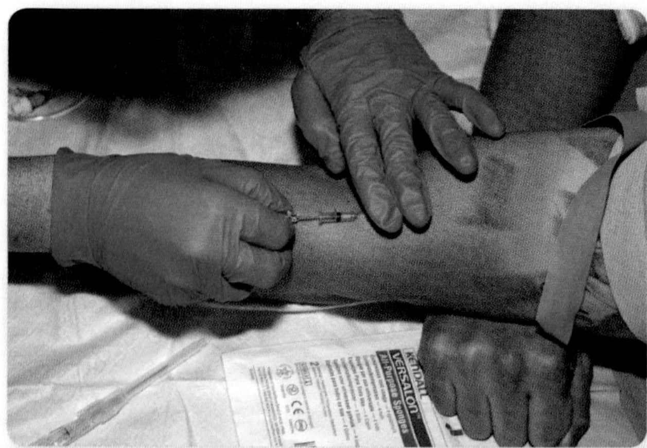

Figure 1-3 AEMTs have EMT training and various advanced skills such as performing intravenous therapy.

hours, usually equally divided between classroom and internship training. Increasingly, this training is offered within the context of an associate degree or bachelor degree college program.

Components of the EMS System

The *EMS Agenda for the Future,* which was first published by the NHTSA in 1996, is a multidisciplinary, national review outlining all aspects of EMS delivery. The intent of the agenda is to develop a more cohesive and consistent system across the United States. There are 14 EMS attributes described in this document, which are the guiding principles for the continued evolution of EMS. The following sections provide a description of these attributes, as well as a discussion about the new care delivery model known as Mobile Integrated Healthcare.

In 1999, the NHTSA and the Maternal and Child Health Bureau, Health Resources Services Administration developed the *EMS Agenda for the Future: Implementation Guide.*[4] The guide proposes 10 priority objectives aimed at leading us closer to achieving all of the components outlined in the *EMS Agenda for the Future*. The objectives correspond to three priority areas in particular:

1. **Build bridges** to strengthen partnerships and relationships with agencies, organizations, and individuals.
2. **Create tools and resources** to increase efficiency and standardize activities across widespread areas.
3. **Develop infrastructure** to increase the capacity of EMS.

In the past 20 years, we have seen vast changes to the health care system, and EMS providers are facing new challenges every day. The *EMS Agenda for the Future* revision process is data-driven and includes a broad representation of stakeholders, including private, governmental, academic, professional, and public interest groups and other interested parties.[5]

Public Access

Easy access to help in an emergency is essential. In most of the United States, an emergency communications center that dispatches fire, police, rescue, and EMS units can be reached by dialing 9-1-1. At the communications center, trained dispatchers obtain the necessary information from the caller and, following dispatch protocols, dispatch the ambulance crew and other equipment and responders who might be needed. This communications center is called a **public safety access point**.

In an enhanced 9-1-1 system, the address of the caller is displayed on a screen. The address remains on the screen until the dispatcher releases it so that if the caller is unable to speak or hangs up, his or her location remains displayed. Most emergency communications centers also include special equipment that allows people with speech or hearing disabilities to communicate with the dispatcher via a keyboard and printed messages. In some areas, rather than 9-1-1, a different special published emergency number may be used to call for EMS. Social media may play an evolving role in allowing laypeople trained in CPR to be alerted of a cardiac arrest in their area. Training the public in how to summon an EMS unit is an important part of the public education responsibility of each EMS service.

Enhanced 9-1-1 systems for cell phones are now available that identify not only the cellular phone number from which an emergency call is being placed, but also the exact geographic coordinates of the phone at the time the call is made. Such systems use GPS (global positioning system) technology. Because cell phones capable of transmitting a GPS signal and a system capable of receiving that signal are both required, the technology will require additional time and resources to implement.

A system called **emergency medical dispatch (EMD)** was developed to assist dispatchers in providing callers with vital instructions to help them manage medical emergencies until EMS crews arrive. Dispatchers are trained and provided with scripts to help them relay relevant instructions to callers. The system helps dispatchers select appropriately resourced units to respond to a request for assistance. It is the dispatcher's duty to relay all relevant and available information to the responding crews in a timely manner. Keep in mind, however, current technology does not allow the dispatcher to see what is actually going on at the scene and that it is not uncommon for you to find the reality of the call quite different from the dispatch information. The dispatchers can relay only the information provided to them by the caller.

Communication Systems

With the information provided by the caller, the dispatcher will select the appropriate parts of the emergency system that need to be activated. According to the National Fire Protection Association, 46% of fire departments nationwide provide BLS care and 16% of fire departments provide ALS care. Nationwide, 39% of fire departments do not provide emergency medical services.[6]

In most municipalities, EMS is a part of the fire department. In others, it is a part of the police department or is an independent public or private safety service. In some areas, a contractor may provide BLS or ALS service, whereas in other areas, a hospital-based program, possibly covering several towns, may provide the ambulance services.

New technologies are constantly being developed that can assist responders in locating their patients. As previously described, cellular telephones can be linked to GPS units to display their location. Responding units can transmit their position to dispatch, and dispatch can transmit the location of a call to a moving digital map in the unit, complete with turn-by-turn directions. Medical databases can be queried and patient information can be directly downloaded to your computer or uploaded from your laptop to the database. The pace of technological developments in communications makes the latest device soon obsolete, so constant training and education are required to keep your knowledge up-to-date.

Being active in your community will keep you abreast of the best local resources. When you are developing a potential care plan, ask yourself, "Does the receiving facility have the resources needed for this patient?" When you are active in your community, you will know the answer. If the answer is no, the next question, "Is there an appropriate facility within a reasonable distance?" will also be a part of your community knowledge. And of course, remember, your patients have the ultimate decision regarding where they go, as long as they are in stable condition, alert, and oriented.

▶ Clinical Care

As an AEMT, you will use a wide range of emergency equipment. During the AEMT course, you will learn how to use a variety of the appliances and devices that you may need to use on a call. Clinical care describes the various pieces of equipment and scope of practice for using that equipment. You will learn when the use of the equipment or practice is indicated and when it is contraindicated because it will not be of benefit or may cause harm. Although the use of different models and brands of a given device will follow the same generic principles and methods, some variations and peculiarities exist from one model to another. When you join a service, check each key piece of equipment before going on duty to ensure it is in its assigned place, it works properly, and you are familiar with the specific model carried on your ambulance.

Words of Wisdom

An *indication* is a reason for performing an action or giving a medication. A *contraindication* is a reason not to. For example, a fall is an indication for cervical spine immobilization, and hypersensitivity to a medication is a contraindication to giving that medication.

Each AEMT may be called on to drive the ambulance. Therefore, you must familiarize yourself with the roads in your **primary service area (PSA)** or sector. The PSA is the main area in which an EMS agency operates. Before you go on duty, check all the equipment and supplies and communications equipment that the ambulance carries and ensure it is fully fueled, that it has sufficient oil and other key fluids, and that the tires are in good condition and inflated properly. You should test each of the driver's controls and each built-in unit and control in the patient compartment. If you have not driven the specific ambulance before, it is a good idea to take it out and become familiar with it before you respond to a call. Maintenance and safe driving of the ambulance are discussed in detail in Chapter 39, *Transport Operations*.

▶ Human Resources

This component of EMS examines the profession. Human resources deals with the people within EMS systems. Who delivers the care? How are these people compensated for their time and energy? How do other members of the medical community interact and participate within the EMS world? These are some of the questions discussed within the component of human resources. The overarching concept is to encourage the creation of EMS systems that provide an environment where talented people want to work and can turn their passion into a rewarding career.

Several objectives need to be accomplished to help make a career in EMS a lasting one. As discussed, efforts are being made to ensure EMS providers can relocate from one state to another more seamlessly. From a global point of view, one of the core functions of a state is to provide for and protect its citizens. This obligation has led to the creation of EMS levels that are unique to a particular state. Though effective for any one state, these idiosyncratic EMS levels make movement from one state to another complicated. One of the functions of the *National EMS Scope of Practice Model* is to create stable foundations on which each level of EMS provider is grounded. The net effect is to encourage a more consistent definition of "what is an EMT" so providers can serve more freely throughout the United States.

The *EMS Agenda for the Future* encourages the creation of systems that help to protect the well-being of EMS providers. It also encourages systems to develop career ladders, allowing talented EMS providers ways to use their talent for many years.

▶ Medical Direction and Control

Each EMS system has a physician **medical director** who authorizes the providers in the service to provide medical care in the field. The appropriate care for each injury, condition, or illness that you will encounter in the field is determined by the medical director and is described in a set of written standing orders and protocols. Protocols are described in a comprehensive guide delineating the scope of practice for AEMTs. Standing orders are part of protocols and designate what an AEMT is required to do for a specific complaint or condition. Providers are not required to consult medical control before implementing standing orders.

The medical director is the ongoing working liaison among the medical community, hospitals, and the AEMTs in the service. If treatment problems arise or different procedures should be considered, these are referred to the medical director for decision and action. To ensure the proper training standards are met, the medical director determines and approves the continuing education and training that are required of each AEMT in the service and approves any obtained elsewhere.

Medical control is off-line (indirect) or online (direct), as authorized by the medical director. Online medical control consists of direction given over the phone or radio directly from the medical director or designated physician. The medical direction can be communicated by the physician's designee; it does not have to be communicated personally by the physician. Off-line medical control consists of standing orders, training, and supervision authorized by the medical director. You must know and follow the protocols developed by your medical director.

The service's protocols will identify an EMS physician who can be reached by radio or telephone for medical control during a call **Figure 1-4**. This is a type of direct online medical control. On some calls, once the squad has initiated any immediate urgent care and given its radio report, the online medical control physician may confirm or modify the proposed treatment plan or may prescribe additional special orders that you are to follow for that patient. The point at which you should give your radio report or obtain online medical direction will vary based on the patient's condition.

For example, once the patient has been assessed and you believe that the patient needs a treatment that requires medical control's permission, you would contact medical control.

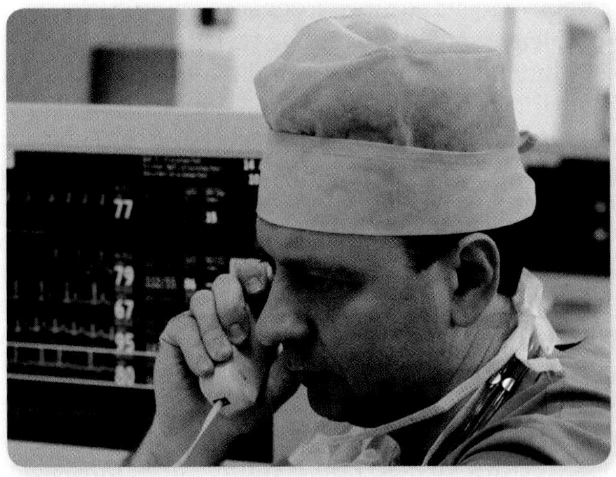

Figure 1-4 Online or direct medical control is provided by a physician.

Legislation and Regulation

Although each EMS system, medical director, and training program has vast latitude, their training, protocols, and practices must conform to the EMS legislation, rules, regulations, and guidelines adopted by each state. Medical directors, along with EMS supervisors and others, develop protocols for individual service areas based on the training levels of the EMS providers in that area. The state EMS office is responsible for authorizing, auditing, and regulating all EMS systems, training institutions, courses, instructors, and providers within the state. In most states, the state EMS office obtains input from an advisory committee made up of representatives of the services, service medical directors, medical associations, hospitals, training programs, instructors' associations, EMT associations, and the public in that state.

EMS is usually administered by a senior EMS official. Daily operational and overall direction of the service is provided by an appointed chief executive officer and several other officers who serve under him or her. When the EMS unit is a part of a fire or police department, the department chief will usually delegate the responsibility for directing EMS to an assistant chief or other officer whose sole responsibility is to manage the EMS activities of the department. To provide clear guidelines, most services have written standard operating procedures and policies. When you join a service, you will be expected to learn and follow its protocols.

The chief executive of the service is in charge of the necessary administrative tasks (such as scheduling, personnel, budgets, purchasing, and vehicle maintenance) and the daily operations of the ambulances and crews. Except for medical matters, he or she operates as the chief (similar to a fire chief or police chief) of EMS for the service and the PSA that it covers.

YOU are the Provider — PART 3

Midway through your first day of orientation, you are introduced to the medical director. He explains to you his roles and responsibilities as medical director of the service. He further tells you specific rules and regulations that you, as an AEMT, must follow on every call to maintain your certification.

5. What dictates the skills that you, as an AEMT, may perform in the course of your duties?
6. What are the two types of medical control?

Integration of Health Services

EMS does not work in a vacuum. EMS personnel travel to people's homes and to incident locations. Once on scene, they deliver care and transport the patient to a care facility. Integration of health services means the prehospital care you administer is coordinated with the care administered at the hospital. When you deliver a patient to the ED, you are simply transferring that patient to another care provider. The excellent care that you began should be continued in the ED. This component helps to decrease errors, to increase efficiencies, and, most of all, to ensure the patient receives comprehensive continuity of care.

Words of Wisdom

Accurate, comprehensive documentation is a must for the integration of health services to work effectively. Each component of the system must know what care the previous component provided (eg, medications given) to offer optimal care for the patient. Failure to document a medication that was provided could result in a repeat dosage by the next provider resulting in an overdose to the patient.

Some EMS systems have collaborated with local hospitals to improve patient outcomes associated with time sensitive treatment like heart attacks, trauma, and stroke. This is accomplished through special training in the EMS system and certain hospital departments. For example, when paramedics determine a patient is having a heart attack, they alert the ED. In turn, the personnel in the ED notify the cardiac catheterization team, or you may be directed to transport the patient to a cardiac specialty center. As a result, the key personnel are ready to begin critical treatments as soon as the patient arrives at the hospital. Similar activities take place for stroke and trauma patients.

Mobile Integrated Healthcare

Mobile Integrated Healthcare (MIH) is a new system of delivering health care that utilizes the prehospital spectrum. It has evolved as a result of the Patient Protection and Affordable Care Act (more commonly known as the Affordable Care Act), with the goal to facilitate improved access to health care at an affordable price. In the MIH model, health care is provided within the community, rather than at a physician's office or hospital. An integrated team of health care professionals, including EMS providers, delivers health care services in the community and connects patients with other valuable resources such as social services. An advantage of this model is that it offers access to care to patients who live in communities with limited medical resources and leads to better service for those who are homebound or disabled.

This new branch of health care is causing the evolution of additional training levels for EMS providers. One new training aspect is **community paramedicine**, in which experienced paramedics receive advanced training to equip them to provide services within a community. In addition to the patient care services a paramedic would typically provide, services provided by community paramedics may include performing health evaluations, monitoring chronic illnesses or conditions, obtaining laboratory samples, administering immunizations, and serving as a patient advocate.

Evaluation

The medical director is responsible for maintaining **quality control** to ensure all staff members who are involved in caring for patients meet appropriate medical care standards on each call. To provide the necessary quality control, the medical director and other involved staff review patient care reports (PCR), audit administrative records, and survey patients.

Continuous quality improvement (CQI), which may also be known as quality assurance (QA), is a dynamic circular system of continuous internal and external reviews and audits of all aspects of an EMS call. To provide CQI, periodic run review meetings are held in which all staff involved in patient care review the run reports and discuss any areas of care that seem to need change or improvement. Positive feedback is also discussed. If a problem seems to be repeated by a specific AEMT or crew, the medical director will discuss the details with the providers involved and, if necessary, assign remedial training or some other educational activity. The medical director also ensures the appropriate continuing education and training are available.

Information and skills in emergency medical care change constantly. You need refresher training or continuing education as new modalities of care, equipment, and understanding of critical illnesses and trauma develop. In addition, when you have not done a particular procedure for some time, skill decay may occur. Therefore, your medical director might establish a CQI process to correct the deficit. For example, an ED physician noted that despite their assessments, many AEMTs were missing a high number of closed long bone fractures, resulting in inadequate prehospital care. A subsequent audit of calls led to a review and retraining session for assessment and care of fractures. This same process can apply to CPR or any other type of skill that you do not use often. You may also choose to follow up on specific patients delivered to the hospital. By doing so, you have the opportunity to critique your prehospital care and, in turn, improve any weak areas. As an AEMT, you have an ongoing commitment to ensure your skills and knowledge are current.

Another function of the evaluation process is to determine ways to limit or eliminate human error. During the delivery of EMS, as with any occupation, there are times when errors can occur. Communicating with other AEMTs or transferring the patient to the ED presents circumstances where errors can happen. Driving to the scene can be hazardous. A patient can be dropped during lifting and moving. Remember, errors can occur at any point during the call that can result in harm to the patient, public, and you.

It is important that you strive to eliminate errors as much as possible. Understanding the circumstances of the errors helps to minimize them. There are three main sources of errors. Errors can occur as a result of a *rules-based failure*, a *knowledge-based failure*, or a *skills-based failure* (or any combination of these). For example, does an AEMT have the legal right to administer the particular medication needed by the patient? If not, a rules-based failure has occurred if an AEMT assists with the administration. Does an AEMT know all of the pertinent information about the medication being administered? If not, a breakdown at this point, such as the administration of the wrong medication, would be referred to as a knowledge-based failure. Finally, is the equipment operating and being used properly? If not, a skills-based error has occurred. Any error can come from multiple sources.

Agencies need to have clear protocols, which are detailed plans that describe how certain patient issues, such as chest pain or shortness of breath, are to be managed. These protocols need to be understood by all AEMTs within the service.

The environment can also contribute to errors. Are there ways to limit distractions and minimize interruptions? Can you find what you need in a timely manner? Sometimes the solution is as easy as ensuring flashlights are available on all ambulances. Make sure all medications and equipment are properly labeled and organized.

When you are about to perform a skill, ask yourself, "Why am I doing this?" Consider the reason for your actions, and allow yourself time to reflect and make an informed decision. If you have considered what to do and cannot come up with a solution, ask for help. Talk with your partner, contact medical control, or call your EMS supervisor.

Another way to help limit medical errors is to use "cheat sheets." Have a copy of your protocol book with you. Emergency physicians have many reference materials available to them. Physicians recognize they cannot memorize everything, so referencing a book or a reliable Internet resource helps ensure the use of accurate information.

Use down time to refresh the skills used less often. Use decision-making aids, such as algorithms, and reflect on what has been done as an informal critique for future improvement of performance. Finally, after a troublesome call, sit down and talk. Talk with your partner and/or your supervisor. Discussing the events that just happened provides an excellent avenue for learning. Your discussions can help lead to changes in protocol, how equipment is stocked, or even the purchase of new equipment.

▶ Information Systems

EMS is not unlike any other profession in today's world. Without computers, the job would be much more difficult. An information system allows EMS providers to efficiently document the emergency medical care that has been delivered. Once that information is stored electronically, it can be used to improve care. For example, how many times has a department seen patients with chest pain? What is the average on-scene time for major trauma patients? How many AED runs has the department had? These questions and many more can be answered using the information gathered from computerized medical records.

This information is used for a variety of purposes. It is used to construct educational sessions for the department. Data from ambulance activity logs are used to justify hiring more personnel. Examining the types of patients and their frequency can provide the foundation for the purchase of new equipment and guide continuing education sessions. This information can also be combined with other database resources, such as from a hospital, to determine patient outcome. Departments from around the United States are sending information to Washington, DC, so a national snapshot of EMS activities can be obtained. Information gathered by the National EMS Information System (NEMSIS) can be found at www.nemsis.org.[7] This information will be used to better plan for the needs of EMS systems today and in the future.

▶ System Finance

All EMS departments need a funding system that allows them to continue to provide care; however, the type of system needed depends on many variables. There are several types of EMS departments in the United States. The *Journal of Emergency Medical Services* reports annually on how EMS is delivered in the 200 largest cities within the United States. The 2013 survey included more participation from the 15 largest cities, so the results may vary from previous years. Table 1-3 provides the breakdown of types of EMS services within the United States for the year 2013.

These departments may have paid or volunteer personnel, or a mix of both. Financial resources are available for EMS departments through taxation, fee for service, paid subscription, donations, federal/state/local grants, fund-raisers, or combinations of same. Which financial system is used depends on the needs and makeup of each EMS department.

How are AEMTs involved with the financial side of EMS? You may be asked to gather insurance information from patients, secure signatures on certain documents such as HIPAA (Health Insurance Portability and Accountability Act; discussed later in the chapter) notifications, or obtain written permission from patients to bill their health insurance companies. These steps are important to the health care process. When you do not provide needed information, the patient may be billed, rather than the insurance company.

Table 1-3 Types of EMS Services That Transport Patients in the 200 Largest Cities Within the United States

Organization Type	Percent of Service Provided
EMS	28.1%
Fire department	44.9%
Hospital/private/ volunteer	27.0%

Abbreviation: EMS, emergency medical services

AEMTs are also involved in helping with fund-raisers, stuffing envelopes, or just making calls to potential subscribers to the service. Regardless of the type of system you work in, you will help the department secure its financial resources.

▶ Education Systems

Your training will be conducted by many knowledgeable EMS educators. In most states, the instructors who are responsible for coordinating and teaching the AEMT course and continuing education courses are approved and licensed by the state EMS office or agency. Most EMS training programs must adhere to national standards established by the accrediting organizations CoAEMSP (Committee on Accreditation of Educational Programs for the Emergency Medical Services Professions) and CAAHEP (Commission on Accreditation of Allied Health Education Programs).[8] To be licensed in some states, an instructor must have extensive emergency medical and educational training and teach for a designated period while being observed and supervised by an experienced instructor. ALS-level instructors and directors must hold a four-year degree.

Generally, ALS training is provided either in a college/university, adult career center, or hospital setting. In most states, educational programs that provide ALS training must be approved by the state and have their own medical director. In these courses, many of the lectures and small group sessions are presented by the medical director or other physicians, nurses, and EMS instructors. In clinical sessions in which supervised practice is obtained in the ED or other in-hospital settings, students are supervised directly by physicians and nurses.

The quality of care you provide depends on your ability and the quality of your training. Therefore, your instructor and the many others who develop and participate in your training program are key members of the emergency care team.

When you no longer have the structured learning environment that is provided in your initial training course, you must assume responsibility for directing your own study and learning. As an AEMT, you are required to attend a certain number of hours of continuing education approved for AEMTs each year to maintain, update, and expand your knowledge and skills. In many services, the required hours are provided by the training officer and medical director. In addition, most EMS education programs and hospitals offer a number of regular continuing education opportunities in each region. You may also attend state and national EMS conferences to help you stay current about local, state, and national issues affecting EMS. Because there are many levels of licensing, you should ensure the continuing education you receive is approved for AEMTs. Whether you take advantage of these opportunities depends on you. You may decide to remain an AEMT or you may want to achieve a higher level of training and certification, but whatever you choose, the key to being a good AEMT and providing high-quality care is your commitment to continual learning and increasing your knowledge and skills.

AEMTs possess special knowledge and skills that are directed to the care of patients in emergency situations. The authority that is delegated to you to care for patients is a very special one. Maintaining your knowledge and skills is a substantial responsibility. Knowledge and skills that

YOU are the Provider — PART 4

The final speaker for your first day of orientation was the service's quality assurance/continuous quality improvement (QA/CQI) officer. He explains to you the required format for documenting your calls, as well as what can be expected of him.

7. What is the purpose of a QA/CQI meeting?
8. How can a QA/CQI review make you a better provider?

are learned in any profession weaken when they are not used on a continual basis. Consider the steps involved in CPR, for example. If you have not used these skills since your original training, it is unlikely you will perform CPR proficiently. Frequent continuing education, refresher courses, and computer-based or manikin-based self-education exercises are measures you can take to maintain your skills and knowledge.

▶ Prevention and Public Education

Prevention and public education are often closely associated with each other. They are components of the EMS system where the focus is on public health. **Public health** examines the health needs of entire populations with the goal of preventing health problems and works to prevent illness and injury by being proactive. Significant accomplishments of the public health systems include vaccination programs, helmet and seat belts laws, tobacco use laws, prenatal screenings, and the formation of the Food and Drug Administration.

Health care in the United States is currently in a state of flux. The high-tech, on-demand style of care that is prevalent has two major drawbacks. One, it is very expensive. In the United States, more than 17.14% of the gross domestic product is accounted for by health care.[9] Two, it may not deliver a better product. The Centers for Disease Control and Prevention (CDC) reports people born in the United States have an average life expectancy of 79 years.[10] There are 35 other countries where people are living longer.

Words of Wisdom

A good example of public health at work is the common product, salt. The next time you buy salt, look at the contents. In the United States, salt is sold with the additive iodine. It was discovered years ago that certain thyroid diseases, such as goiter (abnormally large thyroid gland), are caused by a decrease in iodine levels within people's diets. The solution was to add this important element into a commonly used food source. Today, goiter is rare within the United States.

EMS is able to work with public health agencies on both primary and secondary prevention strategies. **Primary prevention** focuses on strategies that will prevent the event from ever happening. For example, in the early 1900s polio was a devastating disease causing death and disability for thousands of Americans. It was discovered that a vaccine could be developed to prevent the disease. In the span of one generation, the disease was virtually eliminated. Vaccinations are a good example of primary prevention within public health.

In June 2009, the World Health Organization (WHO) declared the swine flu (H1N1) virus to be at pandemic levels, which meant the virus had spread throughout the world. The CDC estimated between April 2009 and April 2010, there were approximately 60.8 million cases and 12,469 deaths in the United States.[11] By August 2010, the WHO declared an end to the pandemic. The CDC has classified H1N1 as a regular human flu virus, treatable with the flu vaccine.[12] If another major outbreak of a virus were to occur in the United States, EMS providers may be called on to assist in the administration of vaccinations. Other examples of primary prevention include ensuring people know the dangers of drinking and driving, and the harmful effects of using tobacco and other drugs. There are several ways you can contribute to primary prevention strategies. Become involved in programs that educate the community. Small actions can lead to big differences.

In a **secondary prevention** strategy, the event has already happened. The question is, how can we decrease the effects of the event? Helmets and seat belts do not prevent the accident from happening, yet they prevent serious injuries from occurring due to the accident. The next time you drive down a major roadway, take note of the construction of the guardrails. There have been significant changes in guardrail construction over the years as more information has become available on what happens during a vehicle collision.

You may also be involved in the surveillance of illnesses and injuries. The PCRs that are generated by EMS personnel can be used to determine if a serious, widespread condition exists. For example, EMS is in a perfect position to provide statistical information to the local government about collisions. Injury surveillance data can be used to determine ways to improve a dangerous intersection, to prevent crashes from ever happening, or to limit the severity of injuries to drivers.

As discussed, you can help educate the public. People may not understand why an incident has happened. A parent allows her 15-month-old child to play outside with other children unsupervised. The child falls and cuts her hand. EMS arrives and determines the cause of the injury is obvious. You can work professionally, respectfully, and kindly with the parents to help educate them on how to prevent this injury from occurring in the future.

The public may not understand the education that EMS providers have and what services they can provide. You can go to local schools and teach children to call 9-1-1 when there is a medical emergency. EMS personnel can work with local health care institutions to inform local residents when to call for an ambulance and when other transportation methods are more appropriate. Efforts to use social media to alert the public of a cardiac arrest are also developing. Consider advocating for social-media-directed or mobile phone dispatch systems that encourage laypeople trained in CPR to respond to episodes of cardiac arrest that occur in close proximity to them.

Teaching people how to perform CPR, how to help a choking victim, and even how to assist in the delivery of a baby are all aspects of public education. Educating the public on the benefits of compression-only CPR is another example. One of the important effects of public education is an increase in public respect for EMS. When people understand what it means to work on an ambulance and provide care to the sick and injured, they are more likely to consider EMS a vital part of the public health care system. This change in attitude can be powerful and lead to increased EMS funding and greater respect for EMS as a profession.

▶ EMS Research

Traditional medical practice is based on medical knowledge, intuition, and judgment. In the early years of EMS, many standards relating to professionalism, protocols, training, and equipment were developed from EMS providers' direct experience. Now, ongoing EMS research provides a scientific basis for standards, in a way similar to research in any other health care profession.

In the early days of EMS, it was believed major trauma patients needed to be stabilized on the scene before they were transported. Paramedics would start IV lines and use advanced airways. There was no foundation to support this behavior; it was assumed that this care needed to be done. After compiling significant amounts of prehospital EMS research, it was determined major trauma patients needed to be transported to an operating room more than they needed IV fluids. This is the power of EMS research.

Applying evidence-based practice is becoming an integral part of functioning as an EMS provider. Patient care should be focused on the procedures that have proven useful in improving patient outcomes. There is a limited amount of prehospital EMS research relative to other areas of medical research; however, as EMS research continues, evidence-based decision making will have a correspondingly greater role in EMS.

EMS research may be performed by EMS providers or other people who are studying a particular branch of medicine. AEMTs will be involved in research typically through gathering data. You may be part of a study to determine how much oxygen should be given to patients with shortness of breath. You may be involved in a study to track the time it takes to transport serious trauma patients to the ED. Your job is to ensure all of the information about patients is recorded carefully. The information gathered is analyzed by others to answer these questions, and the results are shared with the rest of the EMS community to improve patient care practices. Traditional medical practice is based on such research.

Research can also be done at each EMS facility. EMS personnel can examine patient care records to determine where the department can improve. This information can be used to generate educational sessions for AEMTs or can be used to plan public education/public prevention strategies. High-quality patient care should focus on procedures useful in improving patient outcomes through sound research. It is important for EMS providers to stay current on the latest advances in health care. In the past, the American Heart Association (AHA), in concert with the International Liaison Committee on Resuscitation (ILCOR), revised the *Guidelines for Cardiopulmonary Resuscitation and Emergency Cardiac Care* every 5 years. As of 2015, it was determined a 5-year cycle is insufficient to keep pace with the rapidly evolving research in resuscitation science, so it is planned for the guidelines to be updated on a more regular basis.[13] The ILCOR guidelines are an excellent example of evidence-based medical decision making in progress. These changes occur because more information is known.

One word of caution: When reading new research results, make sure you understand what the results mean. Research information can be powerful, but it is often powerful within a very limited setting. A manufacturer of a defibrillator boasts its new machine will terminate ventricular fibrillation on the first shock 95% of the time. On the basis of this information, you may immediately want to buy this new product. Terminating ventricular fibrillation is certainly a positive result, but does this defibrillator save more lives than other defibrillators? In this example, the manufacturer is reporting the defibrillator is able to terminate ventricular fibrillation, not that the defibrillator is able to save more lives. People who do not examine the research will often make that hasty conclusion.

Be skeptical when reading research. Ask questions and conduct your own research. Conclusions that seem too good to be true are usually not true.

Words of Wisdom

Remember, each patient is unique and has different needs. An algorithm, or treatment plan, should be altered to meet the needs of each individual patient as opposed to using an "across-the-board" approach.

Transport Considerations and Communication

▶ Transport to Specialty Centers

In addition to hospital EDs, many EMS systems include specialty centers that focus on specific types of care (such as trauma, burns, poisoning, or psychiatric conditions) or specific types of patients (for example, children). Specialty centers require in-house staffs of surgeons and other specialists; other facilities must page operating teams, surgeons, or other specialists from outside the hospital. Typically, only a few hospitals in a region are designated as specialty centers. Transport time to a specialty center may be slightly longer than the time to an ED, but patients will receive definitive care more quickly at a specialty center. You must know the location of the centers in your area and when, according to your protocol, you must transport the patient directly to one. Sometimes, air medical transport will be necessary. Local, regional, and state protocols will guide your decision in these instances.

▶ Interfacility Transports

Many EMS systems provide interfacility transportation for nonambulatory patients or patients with acute and chronic medical conditions requiring medical monitoring Figure 1-5. This transportation may include transferring patients to and from hospitals, skilled nursing facilities, board and care homes, or even their home residence.

During ambulance transportation, the health and well-being of the patient is the responsibility of AEMTs. You should obtain the patient's medical history, chief complaint, and latest vital signs and provide ongoing patient assessment. In certain circumstances, depending on local protocols, a nurse, physician, respiratory therapist, or medical team will accompany the patient, especially when the patient requires care that extends beyond the scope of practice of AEMTs.

▶ Working With Hospital Staff

You should become familiar with the hospital by observing hospital equipment and how it is used, the functions of staff members, and the policies and procedures in all emergency areas of the hospital. You will also learn about advances in emergency medical care and how to interact with hospital personnel. This experience helps you understand how your care influences a patient's recovery and will emphasize the importance and benefits of proper prehospital care. It will also show you the consequences of delayed care, inadequate care, or poor judgment.

Physicians are not likely to be in the field with you to provide personal, on-the-spot instructions. However, you may consult with appropriate medical staff by using the radio through established medical control procedures.

A physician or nurse may serve as an instructor for medical subjects in your training program. Through these experiences, you will become more comfortable using medical terms, interpreting patient signs and symptoms, and developing patient management skills. The best patient care occurs when all emergency care providers have close rapport. This rapport allows you and hospital staff the opportunity to discuss mutual problems and to benefit from each other's experiences.

▶ Working With Public Safety Agencies

Some public safety workers have EMS training. As an AEMT, you must become familiar with all the roles and responsibilities of these workers. Personnel from certain agencies are better prepared than you are to perform certain functions. For example, employees of a utility company are better equipped to control downed power lines. Law enforcement personnel are better able to handle violent scenes and traffic control Figure 1-6. Recognize that each person has special training and a job to do at the

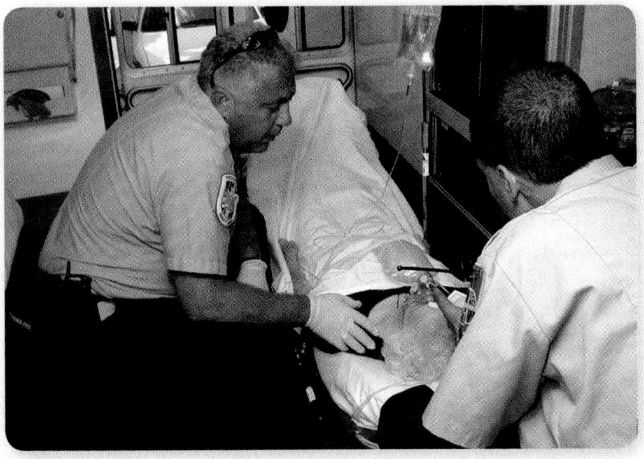

Figure 1-5 As an AEMT, part of your job may be transporting patients from one facility to another.

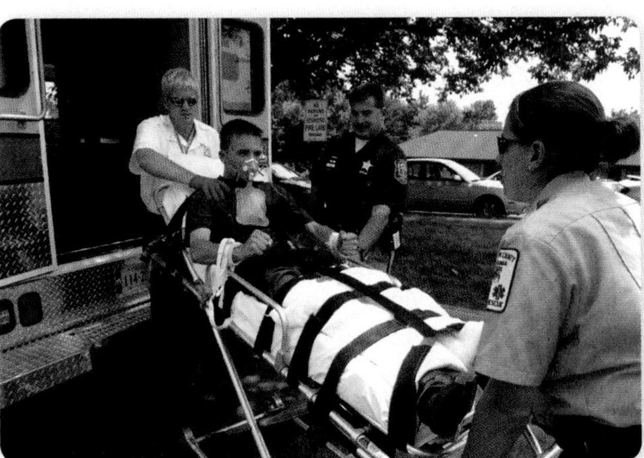

Figure 1-6 As an AEMT, you will work with law enforcement personnel when dealing with violent patients.

scene. Remember, the best, most efficient patient care is achieved through cooperation among agencies.

Roles and Responsibilities of AEMTs

You will be one of the first health care professionals to assess and treat the patient; as such, you have certain roles and responsibilities Table 1-4. Often, patient outcomes are determined by the care that you provide in the field and your identification of patients who need prompt transport. You are responsible for all aspects of EMS, from the preparation of the equipment to the delivery of care to providing a good example for others within the community.

Professional Attributes

As an AEMT, you are expected to have certain professional attributes Table 1-5. Whether you are paid or a volunteer, you are a health care professional. A professional is skilled and trained for work by extended study or practice. Part of your responsibility is to ensure patient care is given a high priority without endangering your own safety or the safety of others. Another part of your responsibility to yourself, other emergency care providers, the patient, and other health care professionals is to maintain a professional appearance and manner at all times Figure 1-7.

Appearance, including uniforms, hair length, and tattoos, are usually regulated by the policies of your department. Your attitude and behavior must reflect your knowledge, proficiency, and sincere dedication to serving anyone who is injured or experiencing an acute medical emergency. A professional appearance and manner help to build confidence and ease the patient's anxiety. You will be expected to perform under pressure with composure and self-confidence. Patients and families who are under stress need to be treated with understanding, respect, and compassion.

Table 1-4 Roles and Responsibilities of AEMTs

- Keep vehicles and equipment ready for an emergency.
- Ensure the safety of yourself, your partner, the patient, and bystanders.
- Properly and safely operate the emergency vehicle.
- Be an on-scene leader.
- Perform an evaluation of the scene.
- Call for additional resources as needed.
- Gain patient access.
- Perform a patient assessment.
- Give emergency medical care to the patient.
- Properly and safely move patients.
- Communicate effectively with the patient and advise him or her of any procedures you will perform.
- Give emotional support to the patient, the patient's family, and other responders.
- Maintain continuity of care by working with other health care professionals.
- Resolve emergency incidents.
- Uphold medical and legal standards.
- Ensure and protect patient privacy.
- Give administrative support.
- Constantly continue your professional development.
- Cultivate and sustain community relations.
- Give back to the profession.

Words of Wisdom

It is imperative that you treat all patients with respect and compassion. This extends to concerned relatives on scene as well. Taking a few moments to reassure a distraught spouse or anxious parent goes a long way and requires little effort on your part.

Most patients will treat you with respect and appreciation, but some will not. Some patients are uncooperative, demanding, unpleasant, ungrateful, and verbally abusive. You must be nonjudgmental and overcome your instincts to react poorly to such behavior. Remember, when people are hurt, ill, under stress, frightened, despondent, under the influence of alcohol or drugs, or feel threatened, they will often react with inappropriate behavior, even toward the people who are trying to help and care for them. Every patient, regardless of his or her attitude or beliefs, is entitled to compassion, respect, and the best care that you can provide, including patients with special needs, alternative lifestyles, and culturally diverse backgrounds. Personal prejudices should not interfere with appropriate medical care.

Many people in the United States can obtain proper routine medical care when they are ill and are surrounded by relatives and friends who will help to take care of them. However, when you are called to a home for a medical problem that is clearly not an emergency, remember, for some people, calling an ambulance and being transported to the ED is their only way to obtain medical care. You may find yourself in the role of patient advocate in these cases. The issue may arise from lack of funds, special needs, or other problems. If there is an issue that is not addressed, your job as a professional is to bring it to the attention of the professionals who are designated to find

Table 1-5 Professional Attributes of AEMTs

Attribute	Description
Integrity	Consistent actions, adheres firmly to a code of honest behavior
Empathy	Shows awareness and consideration about the needs of others
Self-motivation	Discovers problems and solves them without direction
Appearance and hygiene	Uses persona to project a sense of trust, professionalism, knowledge, and compassion
Self-confidence	Knows what you know *and* what you do not know; asks for help when needed
Time management	Performs or delegates multiple tasks while ensuring efficiency and safety
Communication	Understands others and ensures they understand you
Teamwork and diplomacy	Works with others; knows your place within a team; communicates while giving respect to the listener
Respect	Places others in high regard or importance; understands others are more important than you
Patient advocacy	Constantly keeps the needs of the patient at the center of care; supports patients' rights
Careful delivery of care	Pays attention to detail; ensures what is being done for the patient is done as safely as possible

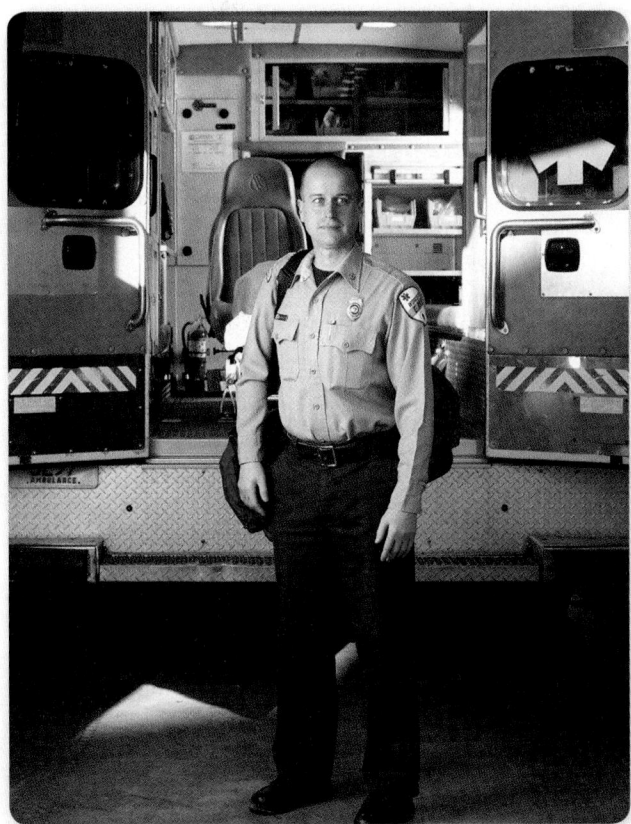

Figure 1-7 A professional appearance and manner help to build confidence and ease patient anxiety.

assistance for patients in need. It may be as simple as providing transportation or as complex as investigating a possible abuse or neglect case.

As a new AEMT, you will be given a lot of advice and training from the more experienced providers with whom you serve. Some may voice a callous disregard for some patients. You should not be influenced by this unprofessional attitude, regardless of how experienced or skilled they appear.

As a health care professional and an extension of physician care, you are bound by patient confidentiality. Do not discuss your findings or any disclosures made by the patient with anyone but other providers who are treating the patient or, as required by law, the police or other social agencies. If you must discuss a call with other providers, you should be careful to avoid any information that might disclose the name or identity of patients you have treated. Do not gossip about calls and patients with others, even in your own home. The protection of patient privacy has drawn national attention with the passage of the **Health Insurance Portability and Accountability Act (HIPAA)**, which was enacted in 1996 to limit the availability of patients' health care information and penalize violations of patient privacy. You should be familiar with the requirements of this legislation, especially as it applies to your particular practice. For more information on the HIPAA, see Chapter 3, *Medical, Legal, and Ethical Issues*.

YOU are the Provider SUMMARY

1. What is emergency medical services (EMS)?

EMS consists of a team of health care professionals who are responsible for and provide prehospital emergency care and transportation for sick and injured people. Each EMS agency is part of a local or regional EMS system that provides the prehospital components required to delivery proper emergency medical care.

2. Why was the National Registry of Emergency Medical Technicians (NREMT) established?

The NREMT was established to certify and register EMS professionals through a valid and uniform process that assesses their knowledge and skills to ensure competent practice. The NREMT requires a reregistration process every 2 years to ensure continued competence.

3. What is the *National EMS Scope of Practice Model?*

At the federal level, NHTSA brought in experts from around the country to create the *National EMS Scope of Practice Model*. This document provides overarching guidelines for the minimum skills each level of EMS provider should be able to accomplish. Because licensure is a state function, at the state level laws are enacted to regulate how EMS providers will operate and are then executed by the state-level EMS administrative offices that control licensure. Finally, the local medical director decides the day-to-day limits of EMS personnel. For example, the medications that will be carried on an ambulance or where patients are transported are both day-to-day operational concerns in which the medical director will have direct input.

The national guidelines are intended to create more consistent delivery of EMS across the country. The only way a medical director can allow an AEMT to perform a skill is if the state has already approved performance of that skill. The medical director can limit the scope of practice but cannot expand it beyond state law. Expanding the scope of practice requires state approval.

4. How does the EMD system work?

Emergency medical dispatch was developed to assist dispatchers in providing callers with vital instructions to help them deal with an emergency until the arrival of EMS crews. Dispatchers are trained and provided with scripts to help them relay relevant instructions to the callers. The system helps the dispatchers select appropriately resourced units to respond to a request for assistance. It is the dispatcher's duty to relay all relevant and available information to the responding crews in a timely manner. Keep in mind, however, that current technology does not allow the dispatcher to see what is actually going on at the scene and that it is not uncommon for you to find the reality of the call quite different from the dispatch information. A dispatcher can only relay the information provided by the caller.

5. What dictates the skills that you, as an AEMT, may perform in the course of your duties?

Each EMS system has a physician medical director who authorizes the providers in the service to provide emergency medical care in the field. The appropriate care for each injury, condition, or illness that you will encounter in the field is determined by the medical director and is described in a set of written standing orders and protocols. Protocols are described in a comprehensive guide delineating the scope of practice of AEMTs. Standing orders are part of protocols and designate what AEMTs are required to do for a specific complaint or condition.

6. What are the two types of medical control?

Medical control is off-line (indirect) or online (direct), as authorized by the medical director. Online medical control consists of direction given over the phone or radio directly from the medical director or designated physician. Off-line medical control consists of standing orders, training, and supervision authorized by the medical director.

7. What is the purpose of a QA/CQI meeting?

A QA/CQI meeting is part of a circular system of continuous internal and external reviews and audits of all aspects of an EMS call. Periodic run review meetings are held in which all involved in patient care review the run reports and discuss any areas of care that seem to need change or improvement.

8. How can a QA/CQI review make you a better provider?

A QA/CQI review can identify overall problems within a service or EMS system and individual or team performance problems. The review helps to identify the source of the problem and possible solutions. The potential solutions can be evaluated by discussing their potential benefits and risks and by trying the most likely beneficial solutions in a "safe" setting, such as role playing, and/or in practice, depending on the nature of the problem and solution. You can learn about how to clearly identify problems and to propose and evaluate solutions by participating in QA/CQI meetings. You can also learn new information and techniques by participation in the meetings and by receiving feedback from the meetings.

Prep Kit

▶ Ready for Review

- Emergency medical services (EMS) is the system that provides the emergency medical care needed by people who have been injured or have an acute medical emergency.
- The standards for prehospital emergency care and the people who provide it are governed by the laws in each state and are typically regulated by a state office of EMS.
- The advanced emergency medical technician (AEMT) course you are now taking provides the information and skills you need to pass the examination required to become a licensed AEMT.
- The EMS ambulance is staffed by providers who have been trained to the emergency medical technician (EMT), AEMT, or paramedic level according to recommended national standards and have been licensed by the state.
- An EMT has training in basic emergency medical care skills, including automated external defibrillation, use of airway adjuncts, and assisting patients with certain medications.
- An AEMT has training in specific aspects of advanced life support, such as intravenous therapy and the administration of certain emergency medications.
- A paramedic has extensive training in advanced life support, including endotracheal intubation, emergency pharmacology, cardiac monitoring, and other advanced assessment and treatment skills.
- Key components of an AEMT's job include scene size-up, patient assessment, treatment, and packaging. After assessing the scene and the patient, you will provide the emergency care and transport that is indicated by your findings and ordered by your medical director in the service's standing order protocols or the physician who is providing online medical direction.
- The *National EMS Scope of Practice Model* provides overarching guidelines for the minimum skills each level of EMS provider should be able to accomplish.
- The *EMS Agenda for the Future* is a multidisciplinary, national review outlining the aspects of EMS delivery. There are 14 EMS attributes described in this document.
- When the dispatcher at the 9-1-1 emergency communications center receives a call for emergency medical care, he or she dispatches to the scene the designated EMS ambulance squad and any fire, rescue, or police units that may be needed.
- As an AEMT, you will work in a primary service area and be responsible for ensuring all equipment and supplies are functional and ready for use.
- Each EMS system has a physician medical director who authorizes the providers in the service to provide emergency medical care in the field. Medical control is off-line (indirect) or online (direct).
- In the Mobile Integrated Healthcare model, health care is provided within the community, rather than at a physician's office or hospital.
- Community paramedicine allows experienced paramedics to receive advanced training to equip them to provide services within a community.
- Continuous quality improvement is a circular system of continuous internal and external reviews and audits of all aspects of an EMS call.
- It is important to determine ways to reduce human error by ensuring you understand your protocols, ensuring your environment is organized and functional, and acting as a patient advocate.
- EMS research and evidence-based decision making are beginning to have a role in functioning as an EMS provider. Stay aware of research, and focus patient care on procedures that have proven effective in improving patient outcomes.
- As an AEMT, you will work with many other professionals, including hospital staff and public safety personnel. Remember, the best, most efficient patient care is achieved through cooperation among agencies.
- AEMT attributes include compassion and motivation to reduce suffering, pain, and death in patients who are injured or acutely ill; a desire to provide each patient with the best possible care; commitment to obtain the knowledge and skills that this requires; and the drive to continually increase your knowledge, skills, and ability.
- As a health care professional and an extension of physician care, you are bound by patient confidentiality.

▶ Vital Vocabulary

advanced emergency medical technician (AEMT) An individual trained in specific aspects of advanced life support, such as intravenous therapy and administration of certain emergency medications.

advanced life support (ALS) Advanced lifesaving procedures, some of which are now being provided by emergency medical technicians and advanced emergency medical technicians.

Americans with Disabilities Act Comprehensive legislation that is designed to protect people with disabilities against discrimination.

Prep Kit *(continued)*

automated external defibrillator A device that detects treatable life-threatening cardiac dysrhythmias (ventricular fibrillation and ventricular tachycardia) and delivers the appropriate electrical shock to the patient.

certification A process in which a person, an institution, or a program is evaluated and recognized as meeting certain predetermined standards to provide safe and ethical care.

community paramedicine A health care model in which experienced paramedics receive advanced training to allow them to provide additional services in the prehospital environment, such as health evaluations, monitoring of chronic illnesses or conditions, and patient advocacy.

continuous quality improvement (CQI) A system of internal and external reviews and audits of all aspects of an emergency medical services system.

emergency medical dispatch (EMD) A system that assists dispatchers in selecting appropriate units to respond to a particular call for assistance and provides callers with vital instructions until the arrival of emergency medical services crews.

emergency medical responder (EMR) The first trained person, such as a police officer, firefighter, lifeguard, or other rescuer, to arrive at the scene of an emergency to provide initial medical assistance.

emergency medical services (EMS) A multidisciplinary system that represents the combined efforts of several professionals and agencies to provide prehospital emergency care to sick and injured people.

emergency medical technician (EMT) An individual trained in basic emergency medical care skills, including automated external defibrillation, use of a definitive airway adjunct, and assisting patients with certain medications.

Health Insurance Portability and Accountability Act (HIPAA) Federal legislation enacted in 1996. Its main effect in emergency medical services is in limiting availability of patients' health care information and penalizing violations of patient privacy.

intravenous (IV) therapy The delivery of a medication directly into a vein.

licensure The process whereby a competent authority, usually the state, allows people to perform a regulated act.

medical control Physician instructions given directly by radio or cell phone (online/direct) or indirectly by protocol/guidelines (off-line or indirect), as authorized by the medical director of the service program.

medical director The physician who authorizes or delegates to the provider the authority to perform health care in the field.

Mobile Integrated Healthcare (MIH) A system of delivering health care services within the community, rather than at a physician's office or a hospital, with an integrated team of health care professionals.

National EMS Scope of Practice Model A document created by the National Highway Traffic Safety Administration that outlines the skills performed by various emergency medical services providers.

packaging The act of preparing a patient for movement as a unit by means of a backboard or similar stabilization device.

paramedic An individual extensively trained in advanced life support, including endotracheal intubation, emergency pharmacology, cardiac monitoring, and other advanced assessment and treatment skills.

primary prevention Efforts to prevent an injury or illness from ever occurring.

primary service area (PSA) The designated area in which an emergency medical services agency is responsible for the provision of prehospital emergency care and transportation to the hospital.

public health Focused on examining the health needs of entire populations with the goal of preventing health problems.

public safety access point A call center staffed by trained personnel who are responsible for managing requests for police, firefighting, and ambulance services.

quality control The responsibility of the medical director to ensure the appropriate medical care standards are met by providers on each call.

Prep Kit *(continued)*

reciprocity The recognition by one state of another state's licensure, allowing a health care professional from another state to practice in the new state.

secondary prevention Efforts to limit the effects of an injury or illness that you cannot completely prevent.

▶ References

1. Employers' responsibilities. United States Department of Labor website. https://www.dol.gov/general/topic/disability/employersresponsibilities. Accessed July 20, 2016.
2. Shah MN. The formation of the emergency medical services system. *Am J Public Health*. 2006;96(3): 414-423. http://www.ncbi.nlm.nih.gov/pmc/articles/PMC1470509/. Accessed July 20, 2016.
3. History of the NREMT and EMS in the United States. National Registry of Emergency Medical Technicians website. https://www.nremt.org/nremt/about/nremt_history.asp#1970s. Accessed July 20, 2016.
4. The National Highway Traffic Safety Administration. *EMS Agenda for the Future: Implementation Guide.* https://www.ems.gov/pdf/advancing-ems-systems/Provider-Resources/EMS_Agenda_Imp_Guide.pdf. Accessed July 5, 2017.
5. *Journal of Emergency Medical Services (JEMS). NHTSA: Public Comment Requested on Revision of the EMS Agenda for the Future.* http://www.jems.com/articles/2016/04/nhtsa-public-comment-requested-on-revision-of-the-ems-agenda-for-the-future.html. Accessed November 1, 2016.
6. U.S. fire department profile. National Fire Protection Association website. http://www.nfpa.org/news-and-research/fire-statistics-and-reports/fire-statistics/the-fire-service/administration/us-fire-department-profile. Accessed July 26, 2016.
7. National Reporting. National EMS Information System (NEMSIS) website. www.nemsis.org. Accessed March 1, 2017.
8. Emergency medical technician-paramedic. Commission on Accreditation of Allied Health Education Programs website. http://www.caahep.org/Content.aspx?ID=39. Accessed July 20, 2016.
9. Health expenditure ratios, by country, 1995–2014 United States of America. World Health Organization website. http://apps.who.int/gho/data/view.main.HEALTHEXPRATIOUSA?lang=en. Updated July 11, 2016. Accessed July 26, 2016.
10. Life expectancy. Centers for Disease Control and Prevention website. http://www.cdc.gov/nchs/fastats/life-expectancy.htm. Updated October 7, 2016. Accessed July 26, 2016.
11. CDC estimates of 2009 H1N1 influenza cases, hospitalizations and deaths in the United States. Centers for Disease Control and Prevention website. https://www.cdc.gov/h1n1flu/estimates_2009_h1n1.htm. Updated May 14, 2010. Accessed July 26, 2016.
12. The 2009 H1N1 pandemic: summary highlights, April 2009-April 2010. Centers for Disease Control and Prevention website. https://www.cdc.gov/h1n1flu/cdcresponse.htm. Accessed July 26, 2016.
13. American Heart Association. Web-based Integrated Guidelines for Cardiopulmonary Resuscitation and Emergency Cardiovascular Care – Part 1: Executive Summary. ECCguidelines.heart.org. Accessed October 10, 2016.

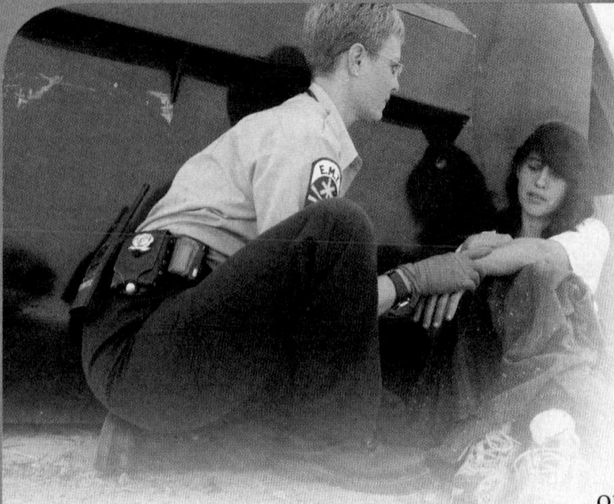

Assessment *in Action*

A call comes in to the 9-1-1 center for a child who is not breathing. The caller, the mother of the patient, states she found her 4-year-old son facedown in the pool. He is not breathing, but has a carotid pulse. The 9-1-1 dispatcher ascertains the nature of the call and the address. She assures the mother help is on the way and asks her to please remain on the line for further instructions.

1. What is the name of the system that allows the 9-1-1 call taker to immediately see vital information such as the location and call-back number from which the call originated?

- **A.** 9-1-1
- **B.** Enhanced 9-1-1 (E-911)
- **C.** Geographic 9-1-1 (G-911)
- **D.** Computer Automated Dispatch (CAD)

2. Which system was developed to assist dispatchers in providing callers with vital instructions to help them deal with a medical emergency until EMS crews arrive?

- **A.** Priority dispatch
- **B.** Emergency call dispatch
- **C.** Emergency monitoring dispatch
- **D.** Emergency medical dispatch

3. Each EMS ambulance service operates in a designated __________ in which it is responsible for the provision of prehospital emergency care and the transportation of sick and injured people to the hospital.

- **A.** principal service area
- **B.** primary service area
- **C.** geographic boundary area
- **D.** service territory

4. According to the *National EMS Scope of Practice*, AEMTs are able to use which of the following airway adjuncts?

- **A.** Multilumen airways
- **B.** Nasal endotracheal tubes
- **C.** Oral endotracheal tubes
- **D.** Needle cricothyroidotomies

5. Which of the following is an example of online medical control?

- **A.** Written protocols
- **B.** Standing orders
- **C.** Radio communication with the hospital
- **D.** Training exercises

6. Protocols are approved by:

- **A.** the EMS director.
- **B.** medical control.
- **C.** the medical director.
- **D.** the State Office of EMS.

7. Which of the following agencies is the federal source for the AEMT national standards?

- **A.** Department of Health and Human Services
- **B.** National Highway Traffic Safety Administration
- **C.** Federal Emergency Management Agency
- **D.** Department of Transportation

Assessment ***in Action*** *(continued)*

8. This incident may have been avoided if the mother had practiced *primary prevention strategies*. Explain what this means.

9. Explain what is meant by *integration of health services*.

10. Mobile Integrated Healthcare (MIH) is a new method of delivering health care that utilizes the prehospital spectrum. One new aspect of MIH is community paramedicine. What is *community paramedicine*?

CHAPTER 2

Workforce Safety and Wellness

National EMS Education Standard Competencies

Preparatory

Applies fundamental knowledge of the EMS system, safety/well-being of the AEMT, medical/legal, and ethical issues to the provision of emergency care.

Workforce Safety and Wellness

- Standard safety precautions (pp 31-39)
- Personal protective equipment (pp 31-36)
- Stress management (pp 52-54)
  - Dealing with death and dying (pp 60-64)
- Prevention of response-related injuries (pp 42-50)
- Lifting and moving patients (Chapter 6, *Lifting and Moving Patients*)
- Prevention of work-related injuries (pp 42-50)
- Disease transmission (pp 29-31)
- Wellness principles (pp 55-58)

Knowledge Objectives

1. Define infectious disease and communicable disease. (p 29)
2. Describe the routes of disease transmission. (pp 29-31)
3. Explain the mode of transmission and the steps to prevent and/or manage an exposure to hepatitis, tuberculosis, and human immunodeficiency virus/acquired immunodeficiency syndrome (HIV/AIDS). (pp 29-41)
4. Describe the steps to take for personal protection from airborne and bloodborne pathogens. (pp 30-39)
5. Know the standard precautions that are used in treating patients to prevent infection. (pp 31-39)
6. Explain proper handwashing techniques. (pp 31, 33)
7. Explain proper glove removal techniques. (pp 33-34)
8. Describe components of an infection control plan. (pp 36-37)
9. Describe the steps to prevent a potential exposure. (pp 36-39)
10. List the ways immunity to infectious diseases is acquired. (pp 39-40)
11. Explain postexposure management of exposure to patient blood or body fluids, including completing a postexposure report. (p 41)
12. Describe the steps necessary to determine scene safety and to prevent work-related injuries at the scene. (pp 42-47)
13. Describe the various hazards that may be encountered and how to prepare for them. (pp 42-46)
14. Explain how to recognize possibly violent situations and which steps to take to deal with them. (pp 46-47)
15. Describe how to handle behavioral emergencies. (pp 46-47)
16. Describe the protective clothing and gear that is available to protect you. (pp 47-50)
17. Explain the physiologic, physical, and psychological responses to stress. (pp 51-52)
18. Describe posttraumatic stress disorder (PTSD) and steps that can be taken to decrease the likelihood that PTSD will develop, including critical incident stress management. (pp 52-53)
19. Describe components that can contribute to stress, such as burnout. (pp 53-55)
20. Identify the steps that contribute to wellness and their importance in managing stress. (pp 55-58)
21. Discuss workplace issues such as diversity, sexual harassment, and substance abuse. (pp 58-60)
22. Describe issues concerning care of the dying patient, death, and the grieving process of family members. (pp 60-64)
23. Describe reactions to expect from critically ill and injured patients and how you can effectively work with patients exhibiting a range of behaviors. (pp 64-65)

Skills Objectives

1. Demonstrate proper handwashing techniques. (p 33, Skill Drill 2-1)
2. Demonstrate how to properly remove gloves. (p 34, Skill Drill 2-2)
3. Demonstrate the necessary steps to take to prevent a potential exposure situation. (pp 36-39, Skill Drill 2-3)

Introduction

There is an ancient proverb, "Physician, heal thyself." As providers of health care, physicians need to look after themselves—in all respects—so that they can minister to others. Ill physicians are in no position to provide care as they were trained to do. That dictum applies to all health care providers and goes well beyond just physical issues. When caring for critically ill and injured patients, many factors and situations can interfere with the ability of the advanced emergency medical technician (AEMT) to treat the patient.

Your personal health, safety, and well-being are vital to an emergency medical services (EMS) operation. As a part of your training, you will learn how to recognize possible hazards and protect yourself from them. These hazards vary greatly, ranging from personal neglect to environmental and human-created threats to your health and safety. You will also learn about the mental and physical stress that you must cope with as a result of caring for the sick and injured. Death and dying challenge you to deal with the realities of human weaknesses and the emotions of the survivors.

It is important to remain calm so that you can perform effectively when you are confronted with horrifying events, life-threatening illness, or injury. A special kind of self-control is needed to respond efficiently and effectively to the suffering of others. This self-control is developed through the following:

- Proper training
- Ongoing experience in dealing with all types of physical and mental distress
- A dedication to serve humanity

Protection From Infectious Diseases

As an AEMT, you will be called on to treat and transport patients with a variety of communicable or infectious diseases. An **infectious disease** is a medical condition caused by the growth and spread of small, harmful organisms within the body. A **communicable disease** is a disease that can be spread from one person or species to another. Chapter 16, *Medical Overview*, covers recognition and care of patients with infectious diseases, while this chapter covers protection of the AEMT against such diseases.

Immunizations, protective techniques, and simple handwashing can dramatically reduce the health care provider's risk of **infection** (the abnormal invasion of a host or host tissues by organisms such as bacteria, viruses, or parasites). When these protective measures are used, the risk of the health care provider contracting a serious communicable disease is negligible. Proper cleaning and disinfecting of the ambulance and equipment will also help to prevent transfer of illnesses to other patients.

Along with personal protection, it is necessary to inform other health care workers who may come in contact with the patient of the potential risk. Discretion is imperative when communicating with other providers. Sensitive patient history should not be given out over the radio during your patient report. However, during your transfer of care, you should provide a complete patient history for the receiving facility. In addition, you should include all patient history in your written documentation.

Routes of Transmission

Many people confuse the terms *infectious* and *contagious*. In fact, all contagious diseases are infectious, but only some infectious diseases are contagious. For example, pneumonia caused by pneumococcal bacteria is an infectious process, but it is not contagious. In other words, the bacteria will not be transmitted from one person to another. However, other infectious agents, such as the **hepatitis** B virus, are contagious because they can be transmitted from one person to another.

A **pathogen** is a microorganism that is capable of causing disease in a host. A **host** is simply the organism or person invaded by the pathogen. An infectious disease, then, is a disease that is caused by an infection. For example, Lyme disease is an infectious disease caused by the *Borrelia burgdorferi* bacterium, which lives in deer ticks. However, Lyme disease is not contagious. Again, a contagious or communicable disease can be transmitted

YOU are the Provider — PART 1

You and your partner are returning to your station after dropping off a patient at the hospital in a neighboring county when you witness a vehicle in front of you lose control and roll multiple times. You activate your emergency lighting and stop at the scene. As you approach the vehicle, you find one occupant restrained in the driver's seat and note copious amounts of blood. The patient appears to have minor wounds despite the bleeding; he immediately states that he is human immunodeficiency virus (HIV) positive.

1. Do you have a duty to provide care to this patient?
2. What is the minimal amount of personal protective equipment (PPE) you would want to have on prior to exiting the ambulance?
3. What is the minimal amount of PPE you would want to have on prior to initiating care?

from one person to another. The only way to get Lyme disease is to be bitten by a deer tick.

While all infections result from an invasion of body spaces and tissues by germs, different germs use different means of attack. These means are known as the mechanisms of transmission. **Transmission** is the way an infectious disease is spread. Infectious diseases can be transmitted in several ways—contact (direct or indirect), airborne, foodborne, and vector-borne (transmitted through insects or parasitic worms) transmission.

Contact transmission is the movement of an organism from one person to another through physical touch. There are two types of contact transmission: direct and indirect. **Direct contact** occurs when an organism is moved from one person to another through touching without any intermediary.

Words of Wisdom

Routes of Transmission

- Contact (direct or indirect)
- Airborne
- Foodborne
- Vector-borne

The scenario of a vehicle crash can help you understand how transmission occurs through direct contact. Suppose the driver of the vehicle has hepatitis B and is bleeding from an arm injury. The AEMT caring for the patient is not wearing gloves and has a small unnoticed cut on his hand. As the AEMT handles a bloody dressing, the hepatitis virus moves from the victim's blood on the dressing into the AEMT's body through the cut on the hand, thereby infecting the AEMT Figure 2-1. This is an example of direct contact, where blood is the vehicle for transmission of the pathogen. **Bloodborne pathogens** are microorganisms that are present in human blood and can cause disease in humans. Another example of direct contact is sexual transmission. Patients who are infected with the **human immunodeficiency virus (HIV)** can transfer the virus to their partners during sex. Likewise, hepatitis C—an infection that is caused by a different viral strain than hepatitis B—is another example of an infectious disease that is transmitted through blood or sexual contact.

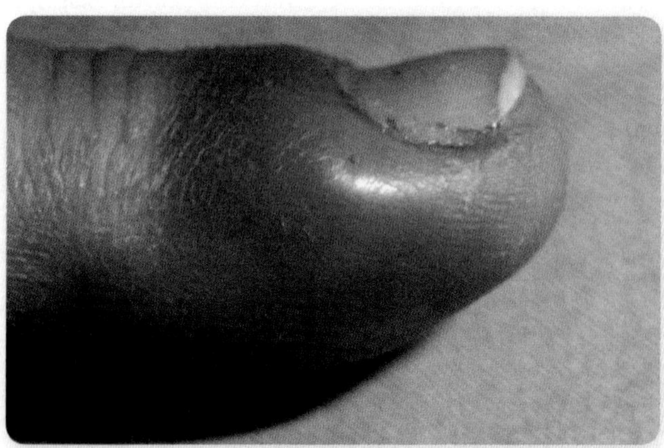

Figure 2-1 Finger infection resulting from not wearing gloves during patient contact.

Indirect contact involves the spread of infection between the patient with an infection to another person through an inanimate object. The object that transmits the infection is called a fomite. Suppose that, when caring for the same patient from the previous example, the AEMT wore gloves. As the AEMT was caring for the patient, blood got onto the ambulance stretcher. If the stretcher is not correctly cleaned afterward, the virus might remain on the stretcher and be transmitted to someone else days later. Needlesticks are another example of the spread of infection through indirect contact. In this case, the virus moves from the patient to the needle to the health care provider. This route of transmission was common many years ago before the advent of safety equipment such as needleless intravenous (IV) systems.

Airborne transmission involves spreading an infectious agent through mechanisms such as droplets or dust. The common cold, for example, moves from person to person by coughing and sneezing. Interestingly, when a person sneezes, the moisture from the airway moves forcefully and quickly through a narrow opening. If the moisture droplets are large, they travel short distances and can be involved in direct contact transmission. If the droplets are very small, they are turned into an aerosol and can float in the air for long distances. Sneezing can actually transmit disease through direct contact and airborne routes.

Because of airborne transmission, it is unsanitary to use your hands to cover a cough or sneeze because the organism travels onto your hands. If you then touch a telephone, doorknob, or a patient, the organisms will travel to that point as well. Using a tissue when coughing or sneezing is better for controlling the spread of organisms, but you then have a piece of paper full of organisms. One of the best techniques to avoid contaminating your hands is to cough or sneeze into your arm/sleeve. Since you do not touch objects with your inner arms, the risk of moving the organism to an object or person is reduced Figure 2-2. The organisms are trapped in the fabric and will eventually die.

Foodborne transmission involves the contamination of food or water with an organism that can cause disease. When food is prepared, it is important to ensure that raw meats do not come into contact with other foods to prevent the spread of bacteria. It is also important that food is prepared and stored properly at all times to minimize the possibility of illness. Proper cleaning of food preparation surfaces, as well as good handwashing techniques, before and after use also helps to decrease the likelihood of transmitting foodborne bacteria.

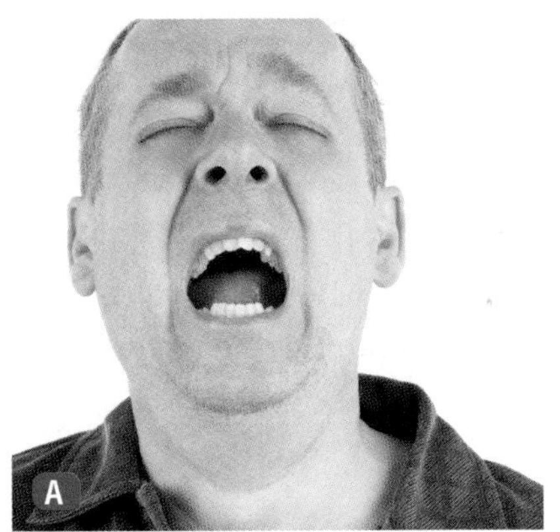
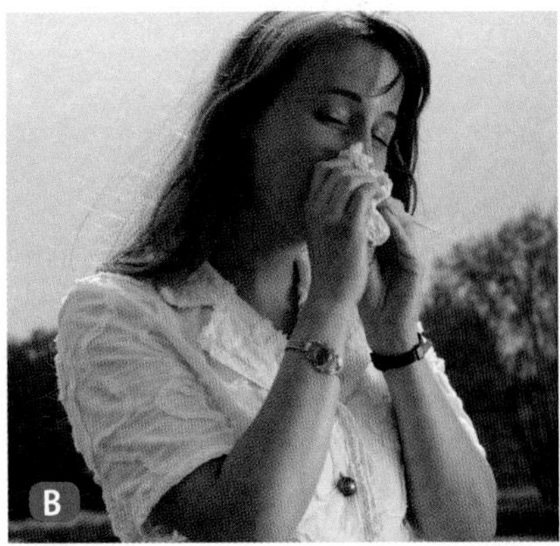
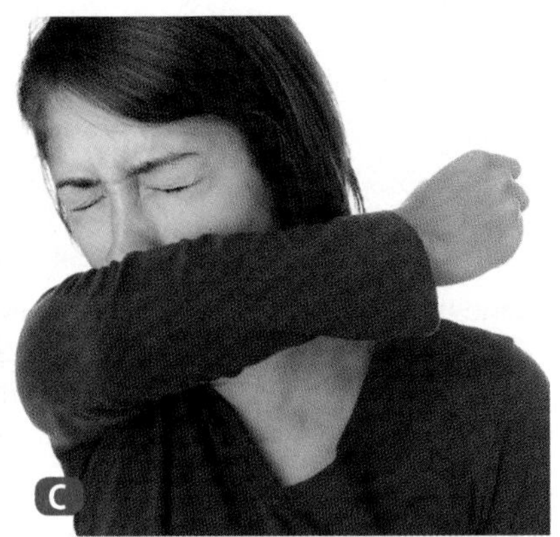

Figure 2-2 Coughing/sneezing techniques. **A.** Poor coughing/sneezing technique. **B.** Acceptable coughing/sneezing technique. **C.** Best coughing/sneezing technique.

Transmission of some illnesses occurs via the fecal–oral route, when there is ingestion of food or water that has been contaminated by infected feces. One example of contamination is the use of human waste as fertilizer.

Vector-borne transmission involves the spread of infection by animals or insects that carry an organism from one person or place to another. In the Middle Ages, the Black Death (bubonic plague) killed more than 25 million people in Europe and Asia. This disease is thought to have been transmitted by a flea that lived on rats. The vector—the fleas—was unaffected by disease, as were the rats (the hosts). As the rats moved, so did their fleas. When the fleas bit humans, they infected them with the disease, which proved deadly to the humans. Lyme disease is spread in much the same way, with ticks (vector) being carried on deer (unaffected hosts) and then biting humans to transmit the pathogen. In the vector-borne disease of rabies, however, the vector (raccoon, skunk, or other species) may also develop the disease; it transmits the rabies virus to humans through its saliva (biting or drooling).

Safety

Other potentially infectious materials include cerebrospinal fluid, pericardial fluid, amniotic fluid, synovial fluid, peritoneal fluid, and any fluid containing visible blood.

Risk Reduction and Prevention

Although the risk of contracting a communicable disease is real, it should not be exaggerated and certainly should not be a source of fear and stress. Fear comes from lack of proper education and training, and there is no reason an AEMT should not be properly educated about disease issues.

Standard Precautions

The **Occupational Safety and Health Administration (OSHA)** is the federal regulatory compliance agency that develops, publishes, and enforces guidelines concerning reducing risk in the workplace. All EMS personnel are required by OSHA to be trained in handling bloodborne pathogens and in approaching the patient who may have a communicable or infectious disease. Training must also be provided for issues including blood and body fluid precautions and **contamination** precautions.

Because health care workers are exposed to so many different kinds of infections, the **Centers for Disease Control and Prevention (CDC)** developed a set of **standard precautions** for health care workers to use when providing patient care. These protective measures are designed to prevent workers from coming in direct contact with germs carried by patients. The CDC recommendation is to assume that every person is potentially infected or can spread an organism that could be transmitted in the health care setting; therefore, you must apply infection control procedures to reduce infection in patients and health care personnel.[1] Table 2-1 summarizes the CDC recommendations.[1,2] You must also notify your **designated officer** if you are exposed.

Safety

One of the most effective ways to control disease transmission is by washing your hands thoroughly with soap and water after any patient contact.

Proper Hand Hygiene

Proper handwashing is perhaps one of the simplest, yet most effective, ways of controlling disease transmission. You should always wash your hands before and after contact with a patient, regardless of whether you wore gloves. The longer the germs remain with you, the greater their chance

Table 2-1 Standard Precautions for the Care of All Patients in All Health Care Settings, Centers for Disease Control and Prevention 2015

Component	Recommendation
Hand hygiene	▪ Before, after, and between patient contacts ▪ After touching blood, body fluids, secretions, excretions, or contaminated items ▪ Immediately after removing gloves or other PPE
Personal Protective Equipment	
Gloves	▪ For touching blood, body fluids, secretions, excretions, or contaminated items ▪ For touching mucous membranes and nonintact skin
Gown	▪ During procedures and patient care activities when contact of the AEMT's clothing/exposed skin to blood, body fluids, secretions, excretions, or contaminated items is anticipated
Mask, eye protection, face shield	▪ During procedures and patient care activities likely to generate splashes or sprays of blood, body fluids, secretions, or excretions; examples include suctioning or endotracheal intubation
HEPA respirator	▪ Use when working with a patient with tuberculosis
Patient Care Environment	
Soiled patient care equipment	▪ Handle in a manner that prevents transfer of microorganisms to others and to the environment ▪ Wear gloves if visibly contaminated ▪ Hand hygiene
Environmental controls	▪ Have procedures for the routine care, cleaning, and disinfection of environmental surfaces ▪ Special attention to frequently touched surfaces within the ambulance (handrails, seats, cabinets, doors) ▪ Have patients with tuberculosis wear a surgical mask
Textiles and laundry	▪ Handle in a manner that prevents transfer of microorganisms to others and to the environment
Needles and other sharp objects	▪ Do not recap, bend, break, or hand-manipulate used needles ▪ Use safety features when available (needleless IV systems) ▪ Place sharps in puncture-resistant containers
Special Circumstances	
Patient resuscitation	▪ Use a mouthpiece, resuscitation bag, or other ventilation device to prevent contact with mouth and oral secretions
Respiratory hygiene/cough etiquette	▪ Instruct symptomatic patients to cover the mouth/nose when sneezing or coughing ▪ Use tissues and dispose of them in a no-touch receptacle ▪ Perform hand hygiene after touching tissues ▪ Place surgical mask(s) on the patient/provider ▪ If a mask cannot be used, maintain special separation (more than 3 inches) if possible

Abbreviations: AEMT, advanced emergency medical technician; HEPA, high-efficiency particulate air; IV, intravenous; PPE, personal protective equipment

of getting through your barriers. Although soap and water are not protective in all cases, in certain cases their use provides excellent protection against further transmission from your skin to others (cross-contamination).

If no running water is available, you may use waterless handwashing substitutes Figure 2-3. If you use a waterless substitute in the field, make sure that you wash your hands as soon as possible.

Follow the steps shown in Skill Drill 2-1 for proper hand-washing.[3]

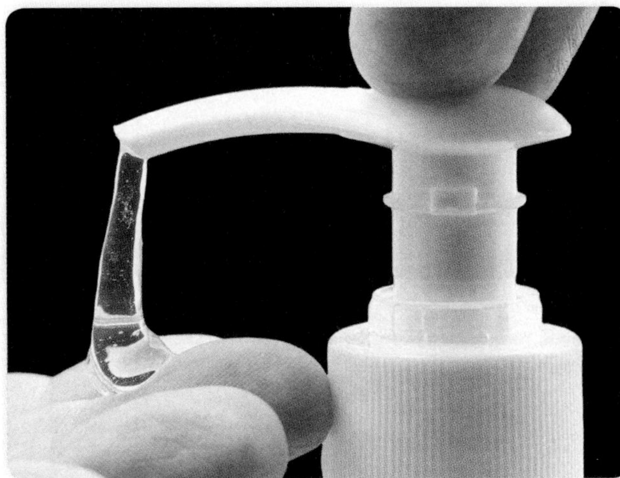

Figure 2-3 Use a waterless handwashing solution if there is no running water available. Be sure to wash your hands with soap once you arrive at the hospital.

Gloves

Gloves and eye protection are the minimum standard for all EMS personnel. Both vinyl and latex gloves provide adequate protection, though latex gloves are falling out of favor in many agencies. Your department may prefer one type of glove over the other, or you may choose the glove. You should evaluate each situation and choose the glove that works best. Some people are allergic to latex. If you suspect that you are, consult your supervisor for options. Vinyl gloves may be best for routine procedures, and latex gloves may be best for invasive procedures.

In some cases you may be exposed to large volumes of blood or body fluids. Wearing double gloves may reduce your chance of exposure. In the course of routine care, gloves may receive minor punctures or tears without your knowledge. In these instances, wearing a second pair provides an additional layer of protection.[4] Also, if the outer gloves become visibly contaminated, you can remove the outer gloves before continuing with patient care or before donning and doffing personal protective equipment (PPE).[5] Be sure to change gloves as you move from one patient to another. For cleaning and disinfecting the unit, you should use heavy-duty utility gloves Figure 2-4. You should never use lightweight latex or vinyl gloves for cleaning.

Change latex gloves if they have been exposed to motor oil, gasoline, or any petroleum-based product. Do not perform tasks such as using a radio, driving, writing a patient care report, or using any monitoring device such as a cardiac monitor or pulse oximeter when wearing contaminated gloves.

Skill Drill 2-1 Handwashing

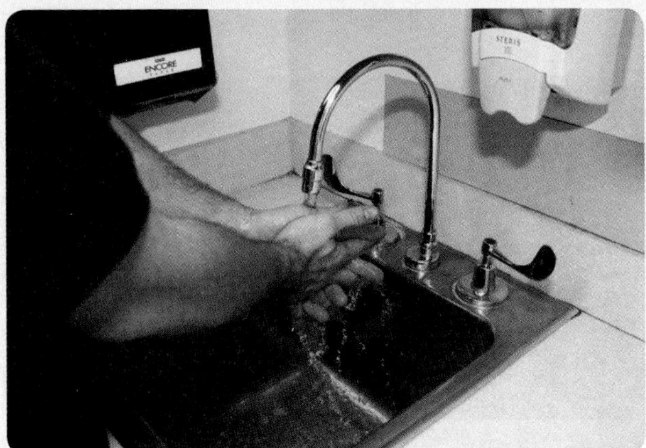

Step 1 Apply soap to hands. Rub hands together for at least 15 seconds to work up a lather. Pay particular attention to your fingernails. Rinse both hands using warm water.

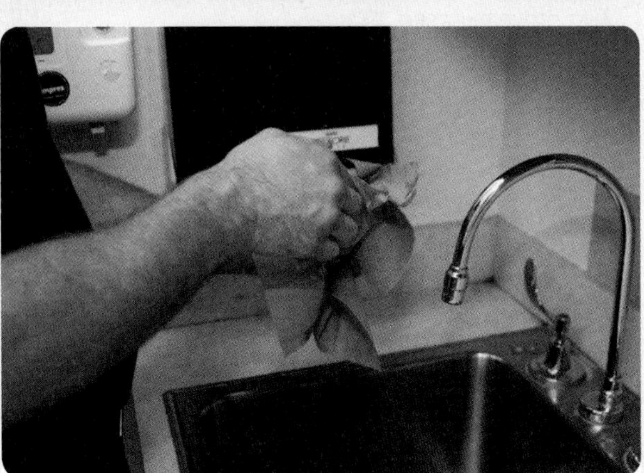

Step 2 Dry your hands with a paper towel and use the paper towel to turn off the faucet.

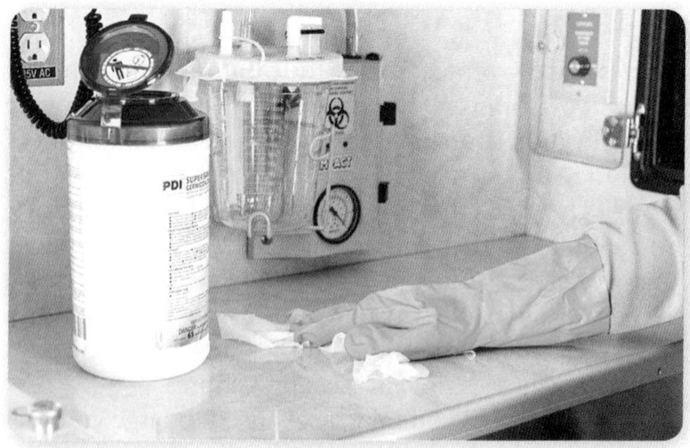

Figure 2-4 Use heavy-duty utility gloves to clean the unit. You should never use lightweight latex or vinyl gloves for cleaning.

Removing used latex or vinyl gloves requires a methodical technique to avoid contaminating yourself with the materials from which the gloves have protected you Skill Drill 2-2.

Gloves are the most common type of **personal protective equipment (PPE)**. In many EMS rescue operations, you must also protect your hands and wrists from injury. You may wear puncture-proof leather gloves, with latex gloves underneath. This combination will allow you free use of your hands with added protection from blood and body fluids. Remember that latex or vinyl gloves are considered medical waste and must be disposed of properly. Leather gloves must be treated as contaminated material until they can be properly decontaminated.

Skill Drill 2-2 Proper Glove Removal Technique

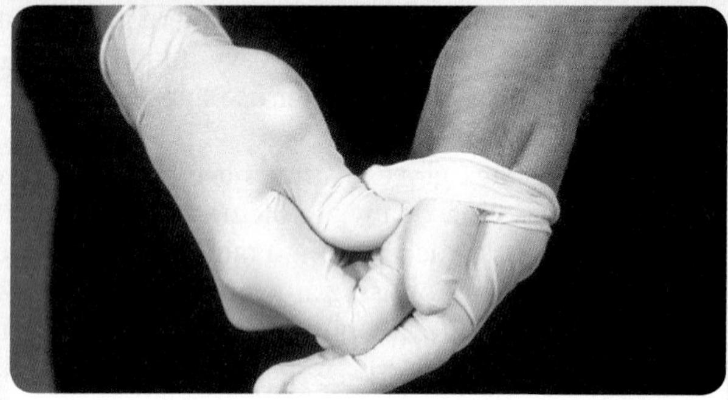

Step 1 Begin by partially removing one glove. With the other gloved hand, pinch the first glove at the wrist—being certain to touch only the outside of the first glove—and start to roll it back off the hand, inside out. Leave the exterior of the fingers on the first glove exposed.

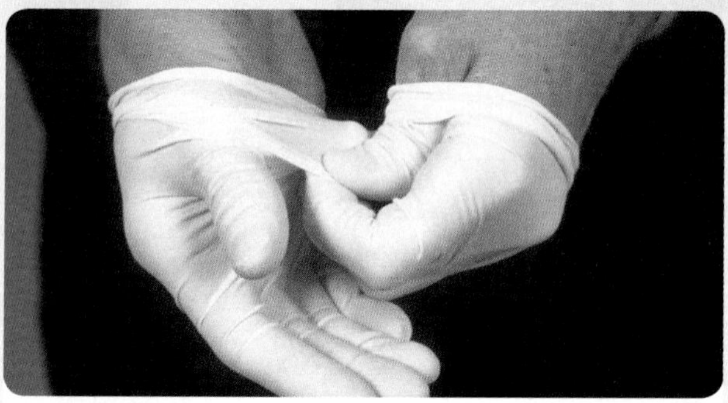

Step 2 Use the partially gloved fingers to pinch the wrist of the second glove and begin to pull it off, rolling it inside-out toward the fingertips as you did with the first glove.

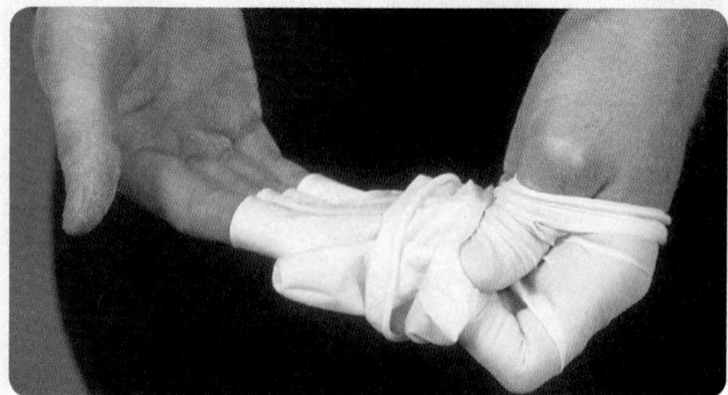

Step 3 Continue pulling the second glove off until you can pull the second hand free.

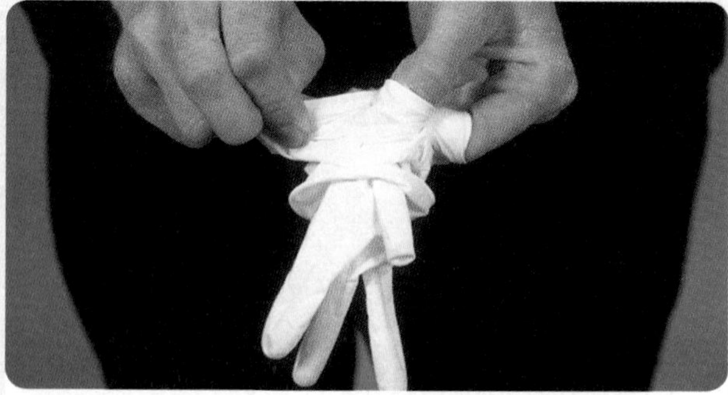

Step 4 With your now-ungloved second hand, grasp the exposed inside of the first glove and pull it free of your first hand and over the now-loose second glove. Be sure that you touch only clean, interior surfaces with your ungloved hand.

▶ Eye Protection

Eye protection is important in case blood splatters toward your eyes Figure 2-5. If this is a possibility, wearing goggles is your best protection. People who wear prescription eyeglasses will also need additional protection for their eyes, as prescription eyeglasses offer little side protection. Obviously, contact lenses offer no added protection from splashing. Face shields will also provide good eye protection Figure 2-6.

▶ Gowns

Occasionally, you may need to wear a gown. When used together with other PPE, a gown provides good protection from extensive blood splatter. Gowns may be worn in situations such as field delivery of an infant or major trauma. However, wearing a gown may not be practical in many situations. Your department will likely have a policy regarding gowns. Be sure you know your local policy. There are times when a change of uniform is preferred because trying to clean off contaminants is difficult and sometimes impossible without professional cleaning and disinfection or disposing of the uniform entirely.

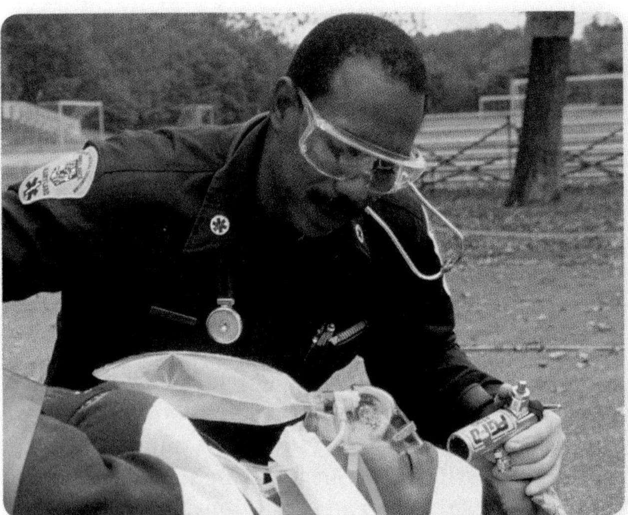

Figure 2-5 Wear eye protection to prevent blood splatter into your eyes.

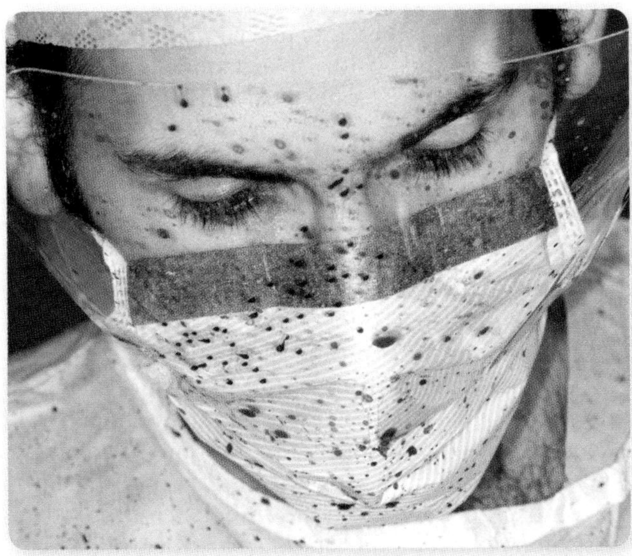

Figure 2-6 The surgical mask/face shield combination.

▶ Masks, Respirators, and Barrier Devices

The use of masks is a complex issue, especially in light of OSHA and CDC requirements regarding protection from **tuberculosis**. You should wear a standard surgical mask if blood or body fluid splatter is a possibility. If you suspect that a patient has an airborne disease, you should place a surgical mask on the patient. However, if you suspect that the patient has tuberculosis, place a surgical mask on the patient and a high-efficiency particulate air (HEPA) respirator on yourself Figure 2-7. If the patient needs oxygen, apply a nonrebreathing mask with an oxygen flow rate of 10 to 15 L/min instead of a surgical mask. Do not place a HEPA respirator on the patient; it is unnecessary and uncomfortable. A simple surgical mask will reduce the risk of transmission of germs from the patient into the air. Use of a HEPA respirator should comply with OSHA standards, which state that facial hair, such as long sideburns or a mustache, will prevent a proper fit.[6]

Although there are no documented cases of disease transmission to rescuers as a result of performing unprotected mouth-to-mouth resuscitation on a patient with an infection, you should use a pocket mask with a one-way valve or bag-mask device Figure 2-8. Mouth-to-mouth resuscitation is rarely necessary in a work situation.

Remember that the outside surfaces of these items are considered contaminated after they have been exposed to the patient. You must ensure that gloves, masks, gowns, and all other items that have been exposed to infectious processes or blood are properly disposed of according to local guidelines. If you are stuck by a

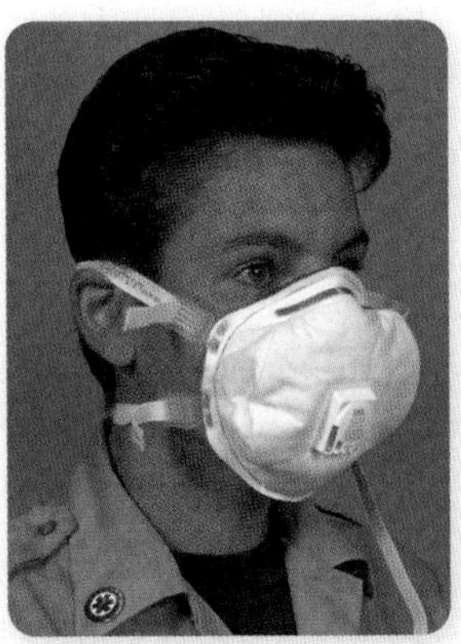

Figure 2-7 Wear a high-efficiency particulate air respirator if you treat a patient whom you suspect has tuberculosis.

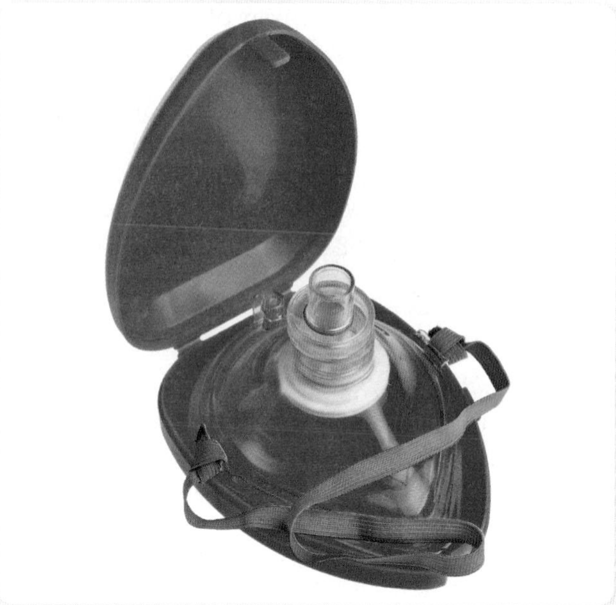

Figure 2-8 Barrier devices such as a pocket mask are necessary when providing artificial ventilations.

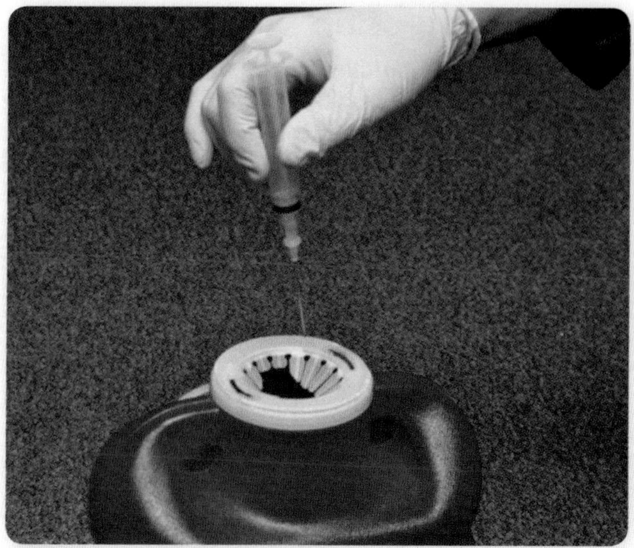

Figure 2-9 Properly dispose of sharps in a closed, rigid, marked container.

needle, get blood or other body fluid in your eye, or have contact with any body fluid from the patient, seek medical care as soon as it is feasible and report the incident to your supervisor.

▶ Proper Disposal of Sharps

Be careful when handling needles, scalpels, and other sharp items. The spread of HIV and hepatitis in the health care setting can usually be traced to careless handling of sharps. Preventive measures to help you reduce the number of needlestick and sharps injuries include the following:[7]

- Do not recap, break, or bend needles. Even the most careful people may stick themselves accidentally.
- Use needleless systems and IV catheters with safety systems when available.
- Ensure that sharps containers are within easy reach.
- Dispose of all sharp items that have been in contact with human secretions in approved, closed, puncture-proof containers **Figure 2-9**. Such containers are labeled with a biohazard insignia.

▶ Employer Responsibilities

Your employer cannot guarantee a 100% risk-free environment. Taking the risk of **exposure** to a communicable disease is a part of your job. You have a right to know about diseases that may pose a risk to you. Remember, though, that your risk for infection is not high; however, OSHA regulations, especially for private and federal agencies, require that all employees be offered a workplace environment that reduces the risk for exposure.[8] Note that in some states that have their own OSHA plans, state and municipal employees must also be covered.

In addition to OSHA guidelines, other national guidelines and standards, including those from the CDC and National Fire Protection Association (NFPA) 1581, *Standard on Fire Department Infection Control Program*, address reducing the risk for exposure to bloodborne pathogens (disease-causing organisms) and airborne diseases.[9] These agencies set a standard of care for all fire and EMS personnel and apply whether you are a full-time paid employee or a volunteer. It is your responsibility to know your department's infection control plan and to use it **Table 2-2**.

▶ Establishing an Infection Control Routine

Infection control, or the use of procedures to reduce infection in patients and health care personnel, should be an important part of your daily routine. For example, good hand hygiene is always necessary. Typically, gloves will be used for all patient contacts.

Remember to change gloves and wash hands between patients. If you or your partner is exposed while providing care, try to relieve each other as soon as possible so that you can seek care and notify the designated officer to report the incident. Follow the steps in **Skill Drill 2-3** to prevent potential exposure situations.

Be sure to routinely clean the ambulance after each run and on a daily basis. Cleaning is an essential part of the prevention and control of communicable diseases and will remove surface organisms that may remain in the unit. You should clean the ambulance as quickly as possible so that it can be returned to service. Address the high-contact areas, including surfaces that were in direct contact with the patient's blood or body fluids or surfaces

Table 2-2 Components of an Infection Control Plan

Determination of exposure	▪ Determines who is at risk for ongoing contact with blood and other body fluids ▪ Creates a list of tasks that pose a risk for contact with blood or other body fluids ▪ Includes PPE required by OSHA
Education and training	▪ Explains why a qualified person is required to answer questions about communicable diseases and infection control, rather than relying on packaged training materials ▪ Includes availability of an instructor able to train AEMTs regarding bloodborne and airborne pathogens, such as hepatitis B and C viruses, HIV, and the bacteria that cause diseases such as syphilis and tuberculosis ▪ Ensures that the instructor provides appropriate education, which is the best means for correcting many myths surrounding these issues
Hepatitis B vaccine program	▪ Describes the vaccine offered, its safety and efficacy, record keeping, and tracking ▪ Addresses the need for postvaccine antibody titers to identify people who do not respond to the initial three-dose vaccination series
Personal protective equipment	▪ Lists the PPE offered and why it was selected ▪ Lists how much equipment is available and where to obtain additional PPE ▪ States when each type of PPE is to be used for each risk procedure
Cleaning and disinfection practices	▪ Describes how to care for and maintain vehicles and equipment ▪ Identifies where and when cleaning should be performed, how it is to be done, what PPE to use, and which cleaning solution to use ▪ Addresses medical waste collection, storage, and disposal
Tuberculin skin testing/fit testing	▪ Addresses how often employees should undergo tuberculin skin testing (PPD) ▪ Addresses how often fit testing should be done to determine the proper size HEPA mask to protect the AEMT from tuberculosis ▪ Addresses all issues dealing with HEPA respirator masks
Postexposure management	▪ Identifies who to notify when exposure may have occurred, forms to be filled out, where to go for treatment, and which treatment is to be administered
Compliance monitoring	▪ Addresses how the service or department evaluates employee compliance with each aspect of the plan ▪ Ensures that employees understand what they are to do and why it is important ▪ States that noncompliance should be documented ▪ Indicates what disciplinary action should be taken in the face of noncompliance
Record keeping	▪ Outlines all records to keep, how confidentiality will be maintained, and how, when, and by whom records can be accessed

Abbreviations: AEMT, advanced emergency medical technician; HEPA, high-efficiency particulate air; HIV, human immunodeficiency virus; OSHA, Occupational Safety and Health Administration; PPD, purified protein derivative; PPE, personal protective equipment

that you touched while caring for the patient after having contact with the patient's blood or body fluids.

Whenever possible, cleaning should be done at the hospital. If you clean the unit back at the station, make sure you have a designated area with good ventilation and a floor drain. Any medical waste should be put in a red bag and disposed of at the hospital whenever possible. Any contaminated equipment that is left with the patient at the hospital should be cleaned by hospital staff or bagged for transport and cleaned at the station.

You can use a bleach and water solution at a 1:100 dilution to clean the unit.[10] This equates to approximately $^{1}/_{10}$ cup of bleach in 1 gallon of water. The solution you mix should not have a strong odor of bleach if mixed correctly. A hospital-approved disinfectant that is effective against *Mycobacterium tuberculosis* can also be used. Use the cleaning solution in a bucket or pistol-handled spray container. When using commercially prepared disinfectants, pay attention to manufacturer directions.

Skill Drill 2-3 Preventing a Potential Exposure

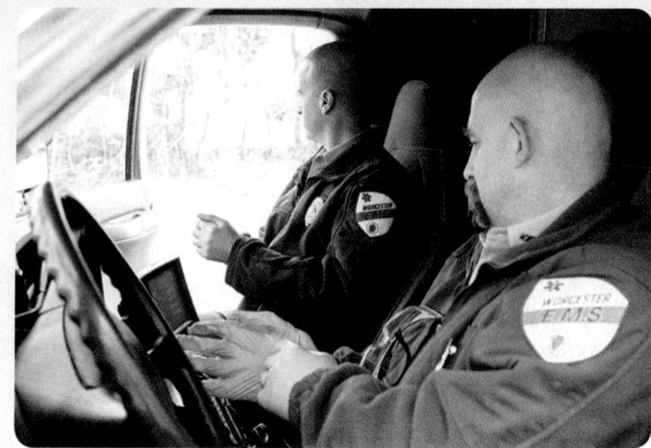

Step 1 En route to the scene, make sure that PPE is out and available.

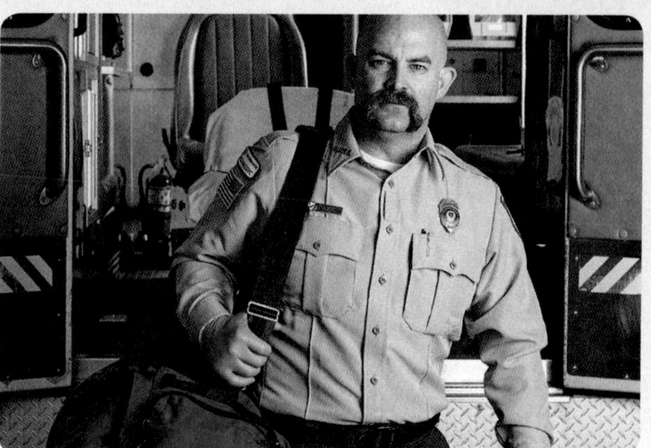

Step 2 Upon arrival, make sure the scene is safe to enter, and perform a 60-90 second rapid exam of the patient, noting whether any blood or body fluids are present. Select the proper PPE according to the tasks you are likely to perform. Limit the number of people who are involved in patient care.

Remove contaminated linen and place it into an appropriate bag for handling. Each hospital may have a different system for handling contaminated linen; you should learn hospital or department protocols Figure 2-10.

Any reusable medical equipment should be properly cleaned and sanitized or sterilized per your department's standard operating procedures. Keep in mind that in hospitals entire departments are devoted to sterilizing medical instruments. Proper sterilization requires the right tools and the right skills; follow your department's procedures. Discard all disposable equipment in an appropriate receptacle that was used in the care of the patient and meets the definition of medical waste as dictated by your state.

YOU are the Provider PART 2

After you ensure that you and your partner have on the appropriate PPE, your partner performs a rapid exam of the patient and finds only lacerations to each arm as a result of broken glass. You do a 360-degree survey of the vehicle and find that it is leaking unknown fluids onto the ground. You proceed to contact your dispatch to have the local fire department and law enforcement respond to the scene.

Recording Time: 1 Minute	
Appearance	Calm
Level of consciousness	Alert and oriented to person, place, time, and event
Airway	Patent
Breathing	Nonlabored
Circulation	Strong radial pulses; skin warm, dry, and pink

4. Does the fire department need to be informed of the patient's HIV-positive status?

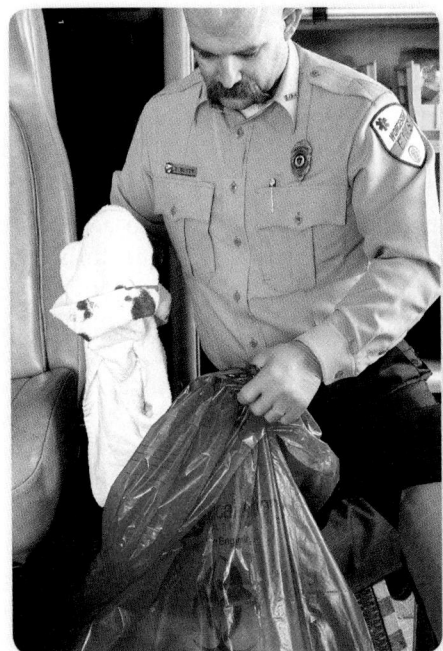

Figure 2-10 Contaminated linen should be bagged appropriately and disposed of according to your local protocols.

Learn the regulations defining medical waste in your area. The procedures for disposal of infectious waste such as needles and heavily soiled dressings may vary from hospital to hospital and from state to state. More information about the steps to take, including how to decontaminate your ambulance and equipment during the postrun phase, can be found in Chapter 39, *Transport Operations*.

Words of Wisdom

In order to avoid unnecessary delays in treatment, ensure that you are wearing proper PPE when you reach the patient.

Immunity

Even if germs do reach you, they may not infect you because you may be **immune**, or resistant, to those particular germs. Immunity is a major factor in determining which hosts become ill from which germs Table 2-3. One way to gain immunity from many diseases today is to be immunized, or vaccinated, against them. Vaccinations

Table 2-3 Immunity to Infectious Diseases

Type of Immunity	Characteristics	Examples	Comments
Lifelong	The illness will not recur.	Measles Mumps Polio Rubella Hepatitis A Hepatitis B	Infection or vaccination provides long-term immunity to new infection. A live vaccine is required for measles only.
Partial	The person who has recovered from a first infection is unlikely to get a new infection from another person, but may experience illness from germs that lie dormant from the initial infection.	Chickenpox Tuberculosis	Infection provides lifelong immunity to the patient from acquiring a new infection, but the original illness may recur, or it may recur in a different way. In the case of chickenpox, which is caused by the herpes zoster virus, an infection may recur years later in the form of shingles.
None	Exposure confers no protection from reinfection. The infection may wear down the patient's resistance.	Gonorrhea Syphilis HIV infection	No vaccine is available. Repeated infections are common. For example, there is effective immediate treatment for gonorrhea, and the germs may be eradicated; however, reinfection is likely if the high-risk practices continue (eg, unprotected sex). For syphilis and HIV infection, the lack of immunity allows the germs to continue to cause damage within the host.

Abbreviation: HIV, human immunodeficiency virus

have almost eliminated some childhood diseases, such as measles and polio.

Another way in which the body becomes immune to a disease is to recover from an infection from that germ. Afterward, the body will recognize and repel that germ when it shows up again. Once exposed, healthy people will develop lifelong immunity to many common pathogens. For example, a person who contracts and becomes infected with the hepatitis A virus may be ill for several weeks, but because immunity will develop, he or she will not have to worry about getting the illness again. Sometimes, however, the immunity is only partial. Partial immunity protects against new infections, but germs that remain in the body from the first illness may still be able to cause the same disease again when the body is stressed or has some impairment in its immune system. For example, tuberculosis can cause a mild, unnoticeable infection before the body builds up a partial immunity. If the infection is never treated, it may be reactivated when immunity is weakened; however, people with partial immunity are protected against a new infection from another person.

Humans seem unable to mount an effective immune response to some infections, such as HIV infection, which is infection with the human immunodeficiency virus that can progress to acquired immunodeficiency syndrome (AIDS). HIV is a virus that attacks the immune system and weakens the body's ability to fight infections. Since the immune system is our natural defense, the body is unable to fight off disease if it is not strong.

Although OSHA does not require hepatitis A immunization, you may want to be vaccinated as a preventive measure. Hepatitis A vaccination is not necessary if you have had hepatitis A in the past. All these vaccines are effective and rarely cause side effects. Many EMS systems require you to show proof that you are up-to-date with your immunizations.

Remember, germs that cause no symptoms in one person may cause serious illness in another.

▶ Immunizations

As an AEMT, you are at risk for acquiring an infectious or communicable disease. Using basic protective measures can minimize the risk. You are responsible for protecting yourself.

Prevention begins by maintaining your personal health. EMS personnel should receive annual health examinations. A history of all your childhood infectious diseases should be recorded and kept on file. Childhood infectious diseases include chickenpox, mumps, measles, rubella, and whooping cough. If you have not had one of these diseases, you must be immunized.

The CDC and OSHA have developed requirements for protection from bloodborne pathogens such as the hepatitis B virus.[11] An immunization program should be in place in your EMS system. Immunizations should be kept up-to-date and recorded in your file. Recommended immunizations include the following:[12]

- Tetanus, diphtheria, pertussis (Tdap) boosters (every 10 years)
- Measles, mumps, and rubella (MMR) vaccine (typically a one-time vaccination)
- Influenza vaccine (yearly)
- Hepatitis B vaccine (as required by OSHA)
- Varicella (chickenpox) vaccine or having had chickenpox

Note that pregnant AEMTs need to get a dose of the tetanus/diphtheria/pertussis vaccine during each pregnancy. Health care workers who are routinely exposed to meningitis should receive one dose of meningococcal vaccine.[13]

You should also have a skin test for tuberculosis before you begin working as an AEMT. The purpose of this test is to identify anyone who has been exposed to tuberculosis in the past. Testing should be repeated every year. It is important to know that testing positive for a tuberculosis skin test does not mean that you contracted the disease; rather, it simply indicates that you have been exposed. Additional follow-up will be needed to determine whether the disease is active. Another vaccine being investigated is *Staphylococcus aureus*. This vaccine is not currently recommended, but may be soon.

If you know that you will be transporting a patient who has a communicable disease, you have a definite advantage. This is when your health record will be valuable. If you have already had the disease or been vaccinated, you are not at risk. However, you will not always know whether a patient has a communicable

Special Populations

Infants and small children, because of their relatively immature immune systems, are especially susceptible to infectious diseases. Pediatric immunizations prevent disease in children who receive them and protect those who come into contact with unvaccinated people. Although vaccine-preventable diseases have decreased in the United States, the viruses and bacteria that cause them still exist. According to the Centers for Disease Control and Prevention, all children should be immunized against the following diseases:[14,15]

- Measles, mumps, and rubella (MMR)
- Diphtheria, pertussis, and tetanus (DTaP)
- Chickenpox (varicella)
- Hepatitis A virus (HAV)
- Hepatitis B virus (HBV)
- Polio (inactivated polio vaccine; IPV)
- Haemophilus influenzae type b (Hib)
- Pneumococcal virus (PCV)
- Rotavirus (RT)
- Human papillomavirus (HPV)
- Flu (annual vaccine)
- Meningococcal virus
- Human papillomavirus (HPV)

Refer to the CDC website (www.cdc.gov) for the most current pediatric immunization schedule.

disease. Therefore, always take standard precautions if there is the possibility of exposure to blood or other body fluids.

General Postexposure Management

The likelihood of becoming infected during your performance of routine patient care is low. In the event that you are exposed to blood or other body substances despite all of your precautions, there are still preventive measures that you can take to protect your health. If you are exposed to a patient's blood or body fluids, first turn over patient care to another EMS provider. When it is safe to do so, clean the exposed area with soap and water. If your eyes were exposed, rinse them with water for at least 20 minutes as soon as possible.

> **Safety**
>
> In the event of exposure involving the eyes, immediately flush with sterile water or saline for at least 20 minutes.

Next, activate your department's infection control plan. This usually involves contacting a supervisor or your department's infection control officer to assist you. This person will help you to navigate the infection control process.

You will need to be screened to determine if there was a significant exposure to possible bloodborne pathogens. Just because you were exposed to a patient's blood or body fluids does not mean that there is a risk of infection. Typically, you will need a follow-up evaluation by a physician to determine if a significant exposure occurred. If the exposure was significant, blood may need to be drawn from both you and the patient to determine if any infectious agents were present.

You will have to complete a postexposure report. Questions in the report may include: When did the event happen? What were you doing when you were exposed? What did you do after you were exposed? Completion of this paperwork will help relay critical information to the right people, resulting in help for you and possibly new protocols in the future to help prevent another incident.

Time is important! If you are exposed, let your supervisor or infection control officer know immediately. Some diseases will act quickly whereas others may lie dormant for a long time. The best way to reduce your risk of contracting a work-related disease is through early activation of your department's infection control plan.

> **Words of Wisdom**
>
> The ability of your EMS system to support you in case of exposure to a communicable disease depends on your understanding of how exposure can occur and your immediate report of exposure to potentially infectious materials. Document the event as soon as possible to ensure that you remember all pertinent information, and make a report immediately after the exposure, following your service's guidelines.

YOU are the Provider PART 3

The patient denies having any head, neck, or back pain, stating that his cell phone rang and as he answered it, he swerved and rolled his vehicle. You inform the patient that he will require full spinal immobilization, which he promptly refuses. The patient states that he just wants to be "bandaged up" and left on scene.

Recording Time: 4 Minutes	
Respirations	18 breaths/min, normal
Pulse	Strong and regular, 82 beats/min
Skin	Warm, dry, and pink
Blood pressure	124/86 mm Hg
Oxygen saturation (Spo_2)	100% on room air
Pupils	Pupils Equal, Round, and Reactive to Light and Accommodation (PERRLA)

5. Does this patient have the right to refuse care?

Illness and Injury Prevention

Grouping injuries into common health problems makes it possible to consider the breadth and depth of the problem and has enabled public health officials and other health care providers to call attention to important problems and target more effective interventions. Intentional injuries, such as assault or suicide, is one group of injuries. EMS can play a role in preventing intentional injuries, but can usually have a greater impact in preventing unintentional injuries.

How big of a problem are injuries in the United States? To many health experts, they are the largest public health problem facing the country today. Table 2-4 shows the top 10 causes of death in the United States in 2015.[16] This information is important in understanding how injury has an impact on different age groups. From ages 1 to 44 years, unintentional injuries are the leading cause of death. For all ages combined, unintentional injuries are the fourth leading killer behind heart disease, cancer, and the effects of bronchitis, emphysema, and asthma.[17]

It is easier to measure death rates than to measure nonfatal injury rates because visits to clinics, emergency departments, physicians' offices, and other places for treatment are scattered in a number of agencies and professional groups. According to the CDC, each year more than 136 million people will judge their medical condition to be severe enough to seek treatment in an emergency department; more than 40 million of those visits are for injuries.[18]

Another factor to consider is the early release of patients from hospitals. Whether the reason is insurance restrictions or physician discretion, the outcome is the same—an increased number of at-risk patients for EMS providers to manage.

In most areas, EMS providers are considered high-profile role models. They generally reflect the composition of the community and, in a rural setting, may be the most medically educated people. EMS providers are often considered advocates of the injured or ill and, as such, are welcomed into schools and other environments. They are considered authorities on injury and prevention.

Table 2-4 Top 10 Causes of Death in 2015

1. Heart disease
2. Cancer
3. Chronic, lower respiratory disease
4. Unintentional injuries
5. Stroke
6. Alzheimer disease
7. Diabetes
8. Influenza and pneumonia
9. Kidney disease/renal disease
10. Suicide

Data from: 10 Leading Causes of Death by Age Group, United States—2015. Centers for Disease Control and Prevention. https://www.cdc.gov/injury/wisqars/LeadingCauses.html. Accessed September 22, 2017.

Words of Wisdom

There are many prevention strategies that an AEMT can be involved in. Patient education can help prevent injuries from occurring. EMS providers are in a good position to recognize signs and symptoms of suspected abuse and abusive situations. When an EMS provider recognizes such signs, he or she can report these suspicions to local law enforcement or other appropriate authorities. EMS providers can also refer patients to care and rehabilitation services, to help prevent further problems as a result of an event that has already occurred. Such services may include child protective services; shelters for sexual, spousal, or elder abuse; food; clothing; counseling; alternative sources of health care such as free clinics; grief support; and numerous others. Keeping a list of resources or a few pamphlets from a local shelter in your ambulance can be very beneficial in a time of crisis.

Special Populations

With a growing geriatric population, a good fall prevention program may be one of the keys to preventing an overload of the health care system. Evaluate all community options available to the older population in your area and bridge any gaps with programs to meet their needs and prevent injuries related to falls.

Scene Safety and Personal Protection

The personal safety of all people involved in an emergency situation is very important. In fact, it is so important that the steps you take to preserve personal safety must become automatic. Anticipate danger based on the type of scene you are about to enter. Drivers who gawk at the scene of a crash may run into you or another vehicle. A second accident at the scene or an injury to you or your partner creates more problems, delays emergency medical care for patients, increases the burden on the other AEMTs, and may result in unnecessary injury or death.

You should begin protecting yourself as soon as you are dispatched. Before you leave for the scene, begin preparing yourself both mentally and physically. Make sure you wear seat belts and shoulder harnesses en route to the scene. Also be sure to wear seat belts and shoulder harnesses at all times during transport unless patient care makes it impossible Figure 2-11. It is also important to ensure that all equipment is restrained so it does not become a hazard to you or the patient during transport. Finally, remember to don the appropriate PPE prior to departing the ambulance when you arrive on scene.

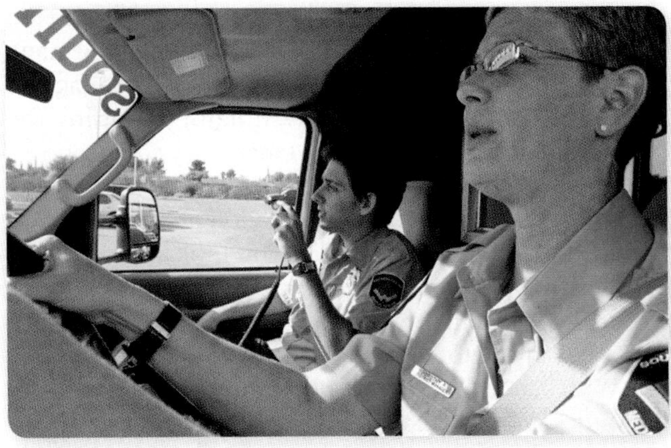

Figure 2-11 Wear seat belts and shoulder harnesses en route to the scene.

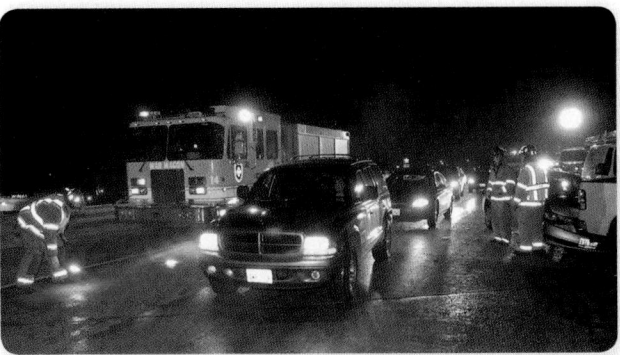

Figure 2-12 Wear reflective emblems or clothing to help make you more visible at night and improve your safety in the dark.

Protecting yourself at the scene is also very important. A second accident may damage the ambulance and may result in injury to you or your partner or additional injury to the patient. To prevent this kind of event, crash scenes must be well marked. If law enforcement has not already done so, you should make sure that proper warning devices are placed at a sufficient distance from the scene. This will alert motorists coming from both directions that a crash has occurred. You should park the ambulance at a safe but convenient distance from the scene. Before attempting to access patients trapped in a vehicle, check the vehicle's stability, and then take any necessary measures to secure it. Do not rock or push on a vehicle to find out whether it will move: this can overturn the vehicle or send it crashing into a ditch. If you are uncertain about the safety of a crash scene, wait for appropriately trained personnel to arrive before approaching.

When working at night, you must have plenty of light. Poor lighting increases the risk of further injury to you and the patient. It also results in poor emergency medical care. The ANSI (American National Standards Institute) and the ISEA (International Safety Equipment Association) require EMS personnel to wear reflective vests or clothing that meet Class 2 or 3 standards on roadways. You can also wear emblems or clothing to help make you more visible at night and decrease your risk of injury **Figure 2-12**.

Scene Hazards

During your career, you will be exposed to many hazards. Some situations will be life threatening. In these cases, you must be properly protected, or you must avoid the hazard completely.

Hazardous Materials

Your safety is the most important consideration at a hazardous materials incident. On arrival, you should look at the scene and try to read any labels, placards, and identification numbers from a distance, perhaps using binoculars. Placards are used on transportation vehicles and buildings, and labels are used on individual packages

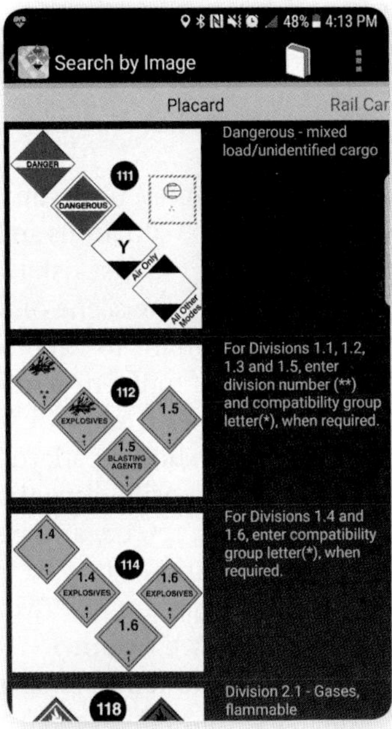

Figure 2-13 The Department of Transportation's *Emergency Response Guidebook* is available as a mobile app that lists many hazardous materials and the proper procedures for scene control and emergency care of patients.

containing hazardous materials (hazmat). The placards are colored and diamond-shaped. The Department of Transportation's (DOT's) *Emergency Response Guidebook* is an important resource.[19] It lists most hazardous materials and the proper procedures for scene control and emergency care of patients. Several similar resources are also available. In addition, some state and local government agencies may have information about the hazardous materials in their areas. A copy of the guidebook (which is now also available as a mobile app) and other information relevant to your area should be available in your unit or at the dispatch center **Figure 2-13**.[20]

Always maintain a high index of suspicion when approaching a scene with a placard or label. Remember, some hazardous materials may not be marked properly. A specially trained and equipped hazardous materials team will be called to handle disposal of materials and removal of patients. You should not begin caring for patients until they have been moved away from the scene or the scene is safe for you to enter. For more information on recognizing a hazmat situation, see Chapter 40, *Vehicle Extrication, Special Rescue, and Hazardous Materials*.

Safety

AEMTs should be aware of the potential hazards that may be present when responding to the scene. The best protection when hazards are present is early recognition that a hazard may exist. Remember that scenes are dynamic and have the potential to become dangerous at any time, even though they may appear safe initially.

Vehicle Crashes

The site of a vehicle collision can pose some of the most unstable and potentially lethal situations an EMS provider will face. Traffic hazards are the first risk to consider. As you drive your ambulance to the scene of a motor vehicle crash (MVC), it is important to keep several things in mind: What is the flow of traffic near and around the crash? How will you be able to safely leave and move about the scene? Ideally, you should park your ambulance in a manner where you can easily leave the scene. Keep in mind that additional fire, rescue, and police vehicles may be parked in the same area or may be blocking your exit. Hydraulic and hose lines are just two examples of common blockages you may encounter.

If you are the first to arrive at the scene, use the ambulance itself as a shield to protect the scene. The ambulance can be relocated for easier exit once additional help arrives. Park at least 100 feet (30 m) away from all crash sites.

As you approach the scene, be very conscious about the flow of traffic. If needed, request police assistance to shut down the roadway. This will ensure a safe scene as you work with patients.

When you are approaching damaged vehicles, look for signs of fluid leakage. Leaking fluids can be flammable, but a more common problem is slipping and sliding on the roadway.

Also look for signs of vehicle instability. How is the vehicle positioned? Is it stable? Motor vehicles can come to rest in a wide array of positions. As the center of gravity of the vehicle is raised, its ability to fall onto you increases. The standard approach for all MVCs should be for firefighters to first stabilize the vehicles to ensure safety for the passengers and any EMS providers.

Are there other hazards such as power lines? Downed lines can generate lethal electrical charges many feet away from MVCs. If there are lines down, you should assume they are power lines and not approach them. Call for additional resources to manage this hazard. Be aware that most electric companies will not shut power down to the grid. Though this seems like a logical solution, how many injuries are caused by the unscheduled power outage? If people in their homes are on ventilators, shutting the power off could create another emergency situation.

Look closely at the scene. Where are the occupants of the vehicle? Does it appear that violence is present? Is there a good risk of violence? As you look at the vehicle, are there weapons inside? Do the passengers look suspicious? If you feel that there may be violence or if violence is obvious, have the police dispatched to assist you.

With proper equipment and training, you may enter the vehicle itself. In the interior of the vehicle, airbags can be another hazard. If the airbag has not deployed, there is a risk that it may accidentally activate while you are in the vehicle, potentially injuring you and the patients. Airbags are typically rendered inoperable by the fire department when the power from the car battery is cut.

Your protective clothing will help you to remain safe while working in and around the MVC. The risk of injuries from glass and sharp metal objects cannot be underestimated. Make sure if you are working inside the vehicle you have sufficient protective gear.

Electricity

Electrical shock can be produced by human-made sources (power lines) or natural sources (lightning). No matter what the source, you must evaluate the risk to yourself and to the patient before you begin patient care.

Power Lines. You should not touch downed power lines. Dealing with power lines is beyond the scope of AEMT training. However, you should mark off a danger zone around the downed lines. Energized, or "live" power lines, especially high-voltage lines, behave in unpredictable ways. You need in-depth training to be able to handle the equipment that is used in an electrical emergency. The equipment also has specific storage needs and requires careful cleaning. Dirt or other contaminants can make this equipment useless or dangerous.

At the scene of an MVC, above-ground and below-ground power lines may become hazards. Disrupted overhead wires may or may not be a visible hazard. You must be careful even if you do not see sparks coming from the lines. Visible sparks are not always present in charged wires. The area around downed power lines is always a danger zone—this danger zone extends well beyond the immediate accident scene.

Use the utility poles as landmarks for establishing the perimeter of the danger zone. The danger zone must be a restricted area. Remember, the safety zone is generally one span of the power pole's distance. Only emergency personnel, equipment, and vehicles are allowed inside this area.

Do not approach downed wires or touch anything that downed wires have come in contact with until qualified personnel have concluded that no risk of electrical injury exists. This may mean that you are unable to access a severely injured victim of an MVC even though you can see and talk to him or her.

Lightning. Lightning is a complex natural phenomenon. You are unwise to think "lightning never strikes in the same place twice." If the right conditions remain, a repeated strike in the same area can occur.

Lightning is a threat in two ways: through a direct hit and through ground current. After the lightning bolt strikes, the current drains along the earth, following the most conductive pathway. To avoid being injured by a ground current, stay away from drainage ditches, moist areas, small depressions, and wet ropes. If you are involved in a rescue operation, you may need to delay it until the storm has passed. Recognize the warning signs just before a lightning strike. As your surroundings become charged, you may feel a slight tingling sensation on your skin, or your hair may even stand on end. In this situation, a strike may be imminent. Move immediately to the lowest possible area.

If you are caught in an open area, try to make yourself the smallest possible target for a direct hit or for ground current. To keep from being hit by the initial strike, stay away from projections from the ground, such as a single tree. Drop all equipment, particularly metal objects that project above your body. Avoid fences and other metal objects, as they can transmit current from the initial strike over a long distance. Position yourself in a low crouch. This position exposes only your feet to the ground current. By comparison, if you sit, both your feet and your buttocks are exposed. Place an object made of nonconductive material, such as a blanket, under your feet. Get inside a vehicle or your unit, if possible, as vehicles will protect you from lightning.

Safety

Recognize the warning signs before a lightning strike. You may feel a tingling sensation on your skin, or your hair may stand on end. Move immediately to a low-lying area. If caught in an open area, make yourself the smallest possible target.

Fire

You will often be called to the scene of a fire to care for victims or to stand by in anticipation of possible injuries to fire personnel on the scene. Therefore, you should understand some basic information about fire. There are seven common hazards in a fire:

1. Smoke
2. Oxygen deficiency
3. High ambient temperatures
4. Toxic gases
5. Building collapse
6. Equipment
7. Explosions

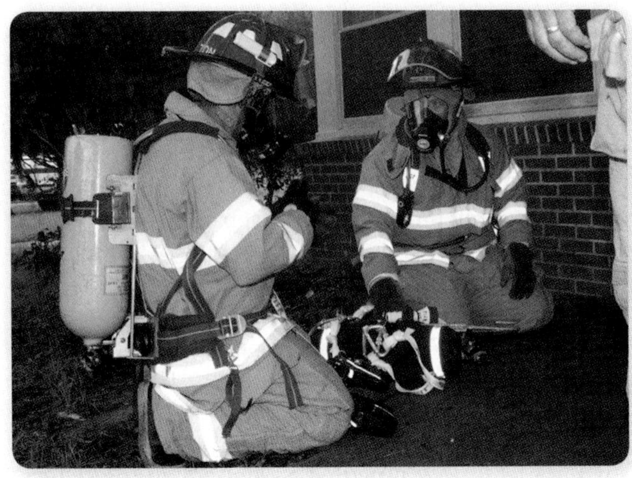

Figure 2-14 AEMTs who are also firefighters should be trained in the use of a self-contained breathing apparatus and have it available if they may be working near fire scenes.

Courtesy of Lance Cpl. Brian Kester/US Marines.

Smoke is made up of a variety of particles and gases, many of which are highly toxic. The particles irritate the respiratory system on contact. Most smoke particles become trapped in the upper respiratory system, but many smaller particles enter the lungs. In addition to causing airway irritation, some smoke particles may be deadly. Notably, many modern building materials contain nitrogen or halogens, and their burning results in the release of hydrogen cyanide and inorganic acids in fire smoke; these toxic by-products are major threats to health.[21] You must be trained in the use of appropriate airway protection, such as a disposable short-term device, or, if you are a firefighter, a self-contained breathing apparatus, and have it available at all fire scenes Figure 2-14.

Fire consumes oxygen, particularly in an enclosed space, making breathing difficult for anyone in that space. The high ambient temperatures in a fire can result in thermal burns and damage to the respiratory system. Breathing air that is heated to more than 120°F (49°C) can damage the respiratory system.

A typical building fire emits a number of toxic gases, including carbon monoxide, cyanide, and carbon dioxide. Carbon monoxide is a colorless, odorless gas that is responsible for more fire deaths each year than any other by-product of combustion. Carbon monoxide has an affinity for hemoglobin that is 200 times greater than that of oxygen, so it blocks the ability of the hemoglobin to transport oxygen to your body tissues. Cyanide is a product of the combustion of many materials that burn. Inhaling cyanide prevents cells from using oxygen. In sufficiently high concentrations, it causes signs and symptoms of shock and severe hypoxia leading to death. Carbon dioxide is also a colorless, odorless gas. Exposure to this gas causes increased respirations, dizziness, and sweating. Breathing concentrations of carbon dioxide greater than 10% to 12% will result in death within a few minutes.

During and after a fire, there is always a possibility that all or part of the burned structure will collapse. Often, there are no warning signs that collapse is imminent. Thus, you must be extremely cautious whenever you are near a burning structure or one in which a fire has just been put out. As an EMS provider, you should never enter a burning building without proper breathing apparatus and approval. At any fire scene, follow the instructions of the incident commander and safety officer and never undertake any task (ie, enter a burning structure or initiate search and rescue) unless you have been properly trained to do so.

Fuel and fuel systems of vehicles that have been involved in crashes are also a fire hazard. A vehicle leaking fuel may ignite under the right conditions. If you see or smell a fuel leak or if people are trapped in the vehicle, you must coordinate the use of appropriate fire protection equipment.

Make sure that you are properly protected if there is or has been a fire in the vehicle. Wear appropriate respiratory protection and thermal protection because the smoke from a vehicle fire contains many toxic by-products. The use of appropriate protective gear at a crash scene can reduce your risk of injury. Avoid using oxygen in or near a vehicle that is smoking, smoldering, or leaking fuel.

Violence

The safety of you and your team should always be your primary concern. Civil disturbances, domestic disputes, and crime scenes, especially those involving gangs, can create many hazards for EMS personnel. Large gatherings of hostile or potentially hostile people pose an even greater threat. Several agencies will respond to large civil disturbances. In these instances, it is important for you to know who is in command and will be issuing orders. However, you and your partner may initially be present at a scene at which a group of people subsequently grows larger and becomes increasingly hostile. In these cases, you should call law enforcement personnel immediately if they are not already at the scene. You may need to remove yourself from the scene and wait for law enforcement personnel to arrive and secure the scene before you can begin treatment or safely approach the patient.

A crime scene often poses potential problems for EMS personnel. A perpetrator who is still at the scene could reappear and threaten you and your partner or attempt to further injure the patient you are treating. Bystanders who are trying to be helpful may interfere with your emergency medical care. Family members may be distraught and not understand what you are doing when you attempt to splint an injured extremity and the patient cries out in pain. Be sure that you have adequate assistance from the appropriate public safety agency in these cases.

Remember that anytime you are on someone else's turf, that person has a clear advantage. You can expect that person to know everything about the environment while you know nothing (including the location of any weapons). Hostile patients in their home environment are much more dangerous there than anywhere else—especially in poor lighting.

Remember that your personal safety is of utmost importance. You must thoroughly understand the risks of each environment you enter. Whenever you are in doubt about your safety, do not put yourself at risk. Never enter an unstable environment, such as a shooting, a brawl, a hostage situation, or a riot. Therefore, as part of sizing up the scene, evaluate it for the potential for violence. If possible, call for additional resources. Failure to do so may put you and your partner at serious risk. Rely on the advice of law enforcement personnel because they have more experience and expertise in handling these situations.

If you believe that an event is a crime scene, you must attempt to maintain the chain of evidence. Make sure that you do not disturb the scene unless it is absolutely necessary in caring for the patient.

Words of Wisdom

Always keep loose hair pulled back and do not wear any loose jewelry. Loose hair, necklaces, and dangling earrings not only have the potential to get caught during the course of patient care, but also offer a hazard that allows for grabbing or pulling when dealing with a violent patient or one with an altered mental status.

Behavioral Emergencies

There are many potential causes of a behavioral emergency, ranging from physical causes (hypoglycemia, head injury) to psychiatric diseases. Although most behavioral emergencies do not pose a threat to you, the potential of threat to either the patient or yourself exists, and you should use caution. Consider these questions as you evaluate the patient in terms of a behavioral or psychiatric emergency that may lead to a violent patient reaction:

- How does this patient relate to you? Are your questions answered appropriately? Are the patient's vocabulary and expressions what you would expect under the circumstances?
- Is the patient withdrawn or detached? Is the patient hostile or friendly?
- Does the patient understand why you are there?
- How is the patient dressed? Is the dress appropriate for the time of the year and occasion? Are the clothes clean? Dirty?
- Does the patient appear relaxed, stiff, or guarded? Are the patient's movements coordinated? Does the patient make sudden movements? Is the patient hyperactive?
- Are the patient's movements purposeful—for example, in putting his or her clothes on? Are the actions aimless, such as sitting and rocking back and forth in a chair?

Words of Wisdom

Determinants of Violence

The following principal determinants of violence, although not intended to be all-inclusive, are of value to the AEMT:

- **Past history.** Has the patient previously exhibited hostile, overly aggressive, or violent behavior? This information should be solicited by EMS personnel at the scene or requested from law enforcement personnel, family, or previous EMS records.
- **Posture.** How is the patient sitting or standing? Does the patient appear to be tense or rigid, or is the patient sitting on the edge of the bed, chair, or wherever he or she is positioned? The observation of increased tension as shown by physical posture is often a warning signal of hostile behavior.
- **Vocal activity.** What is the nature of the patient's speech? Loud, obscene, erratic, and bizarre speech patterns usually indicate emotional distress. The patient who is conversing in quiet, ordered speech is not as likely to strike out against others as is the patient who is yelling and screaming.
- **Physical activity.** Perhaps one of the most demonstrative factors to look for is the motor activity of a person who is undergoing a behavioral crisis. The patient who is pacing, cannot sit still, or is displaying protection of his or her boundaries of personal space needs careful watching. Agitation is a prognostic sign to be observed with great care and scrutiny.

Other factors to take into consideration for potential violence include the following:

- Poor impulse control
- The behavior triad of truancy, fighting, and uncontrollable temper
- Instability of family structure
- Inability to keep a steady job
- Tattoos, such as those with gang identification or statements like "born to kill" or "born to lose"
- Substance abuse
- Functional disorder (If the patient says that he or she is hearing voices that say to kill, believe it!)
- Depression
- Diagnosed illness such as bipolar disease

- Has the patient harmed himself or herself? Is there damage to the surroundings?
- Does the patient appear physically rigid, or is there waxy flexibility?
- What are the patient's facial expressions? Are they bland or flat, or are they expressive? Does the patient show joy, fear, or anger to appropriate stimuli? If so, to what degree?

It might not be possible for you to obtain answers to all of these questions. Sometimes a patient who is experiencing a behavioral emergency will not respond at all. In those cases, the patient's facial expressions, pulse and respirations, tears, sweating, and blushing may be significant indicators of his or her emotional state.

Protective Clothing: Preventing Injury

Wearing protective clothing and other appropriate gear is crucial to your personal safety. It is essential that you become familiar with the protective equipment that is available to you, so that you will know which clothing and gear are needed for the job. You should also be able to adapt or change items as the situation and environment change. Remember that protective clothing and gear are safe only when they are in good condition. It is your responsibility to inspect your clothing and gear. Learn to recognize how wear and tear can make your equipment unsafe. Be sure to inspect equipment before you use it; ideally, this is done before reaching the scene so care is not delayed.

Clothing that is worn for rescue must be appropriate for the activity and the environmental conditions in which the activity will take place. For example, turnout gear worn for firefighting may be too restrictive for working in a confined space. In every situation involving blood and/or other body fluids, take standard precautions. You must protect yourself and the patient by wearing gloves and eye protection and any additional protective clothing that may be needed.

Words of Wisdom

NFPA 1999, *Standard on Protective Clothing for Emergency Medical Operations,* outlines criteria for single-use and multi-use protective clothing. Prior to the 2008 revision of this standard, the same physical strength criteria were being used for single- and multiuse garments. With the revision of the standard, criteria is established for barrier protection, breathability, penetration, flammability, and visibility.[22]

Cold Weather Clothing

When dressing for cold weather, you should wear several layers of clothing. Multiple layers provide much better protection than a single thick cover. You have more flexibility to control your body temperature by adding or removing a layer. Cold weather protection should consist of at least the following three layers:

1. A thin inner layer (sometimes called the transport layer) next to your skin. This layer pulls moisture away from your skin, keeping you dry and warm. Underwear made of polypropylene or polyester material works well.
2. A thermal middle layer of bulkier material for insulation. Wool has been the material of choice for warmth, but newer materials, such as polyester pile, are also commonly used.
3. An outer layer that will resist chilling winds and wet conditions, such as rain, sleet, or snow. The two top layers should have zippers to allow you to vent some body heat if you become too warm.

When choosing clothing to protect yourself from the weather, pay attention to the type of material used. Cotton should be avoided in cold, wet environments. Cotton tends to absorb moisture, causing chilling from wetness. For example, if you wear cotton trousers and walk through wet grass, the cotton soaks up the moisture from the grass. However, cotton is appropriate in warm, dry weather because it absorbs moisture and pulls heat away from the body.

As an outer layer in cold weather, you might consider plastic-coated nylon because it provides good waterproof protection. However, it can also hold in body heat and perspiration. Newer, less airtight materials allow perspiration and some heat to escape while the material retains its water resistance. Avoid flammable or meltable synthetic material anytime there is a possibility of fire.

▶ Turnout Gear

Turnout or bunker gear is a fire service term for protective clothing designed for use in structural firefighting environments Figure 2-15. Turnout gear provides some protection by using different layers of fabric or other material to provide protection from the heat of fire, to reduce trauma from impact or cuts, and to keep water away from the body. Like most protective clothing, however, turnout gear adds weight and reduces range of motion to some degree. Also, turnout gear is hard to clean; avoid using it in situations that will likely expose you to a patient's blood or body fluids.

The exterior fabrics provide increased protection from cuts and abrasions. They also act as a barrier to high external temperatures. In cold weather, an insulated thermal inner layer of material that helps to retain body heat is recommended.

Turnout gear or a bunker jacket provides minimal protection from electrical shock, but it does protect you from heat, fire, possible flashover, and flying sparks. The front opening of the jacket should be fastened, and the jacket should be worn with the collar up and closed in front to protect your neck and upper part of the chest. Proper fit is important so that you can move freely.

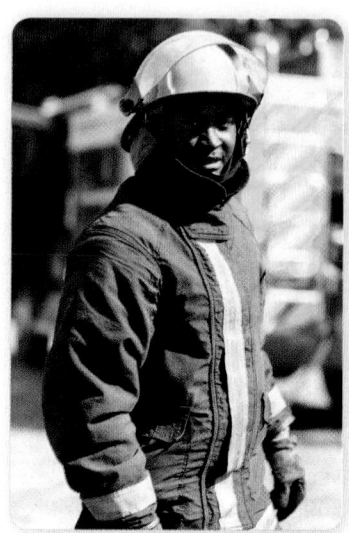

Figure 2-15 Turnout or bunker gear is protective clothing designed for use in structural firefighting.

Safety

The American National Standards Institute (ANSI) requires that all EMS providers use an approved high-visibility public safety vest while on or near the road way.[23]

▶ Gloves

Firefighting gloves provide the best protection from heat, cold, and cuts, but these gloves reduce manual dexterity Figure 2-16. In addition, firefighting gloves will not protect you from electrical hazards. In rescue situations, you must be able to use your hands freely to operate rescue tools, provide patient care, and perform other duties. Puncture-proof leather gloves, with latex gloves underneath, will permit free use of your hands with added protection from injury and body fluids.

▶ Helmets

You should wear a helmet any time you are working in a fall zone. A fall zone is an area where you are likely to encounter falling objects. The helmet should provide top and side impact protection Figure 2-17. It should also have a secure chin strap. Objects will often fall one after another: If the strap is not secure, the first falling object may knock off your helmet. This leaves your head unprotected as the remaining objects fall.

Construction-type helmets are not well suited for rescue situations. They offer minimal impact protection and have inadequate chin straps. Modern fire helmets afford the best thermal and impact protection.

In cold weather, you can lose a significant amount of body heat if you are not wearing a hat or helmet. An insulated hat made from wool or a synthetic material can

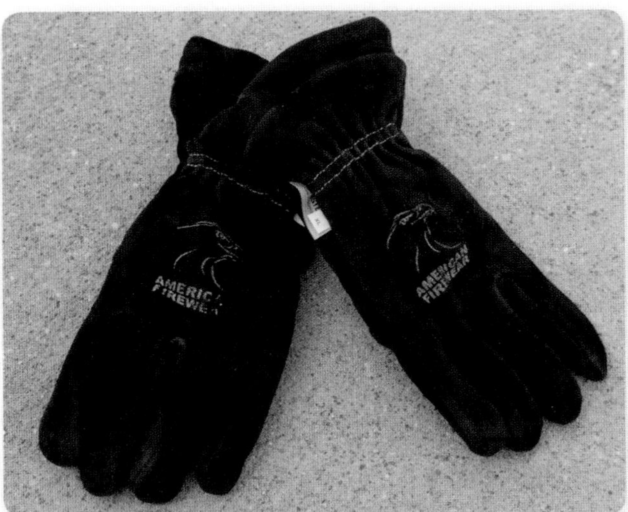

Figure 2-16 Firefighting gloves protect your hands and wrists from heat, cold, and injury.

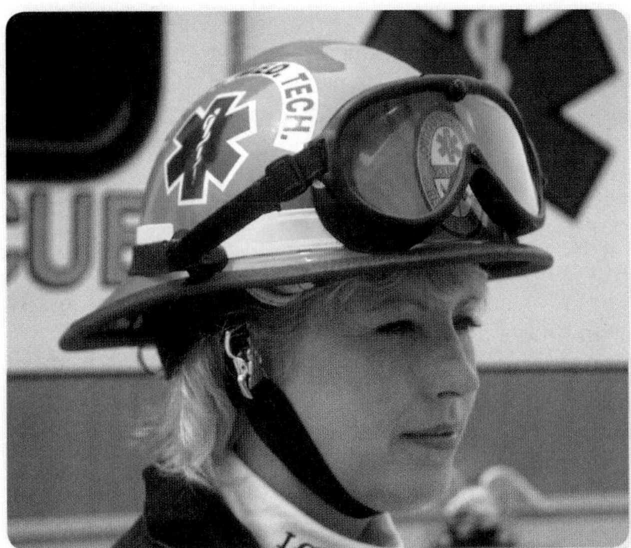

Figure 2-17 A helmet with top and side impact protection.

be pulled down over the face and the base of the skull to reduce heat loss in extremely cold weather.

In situations that may involve an electrical hazard, you should always wear a helmet with a chin strap and face shield. The shell of the helmet should be made of a certified electrical nonconductor. The chin strap should not stretch, but rather should fasten securely so that the helmet will stay in place if you are knocked down or a power line hits your head. You should also be able to lock the face shield on the helmet; this will protect your face and eyes from power lines and flying sparks. A standard fire turnout helmet should meet all of these needs.

▶ Boots

Boots should be water resistant, well fitting, and flexible so that you can walk long distances comfortably. If you will be working outdoors, you should choose boots that cover and protect your ankles, keeping out stones, debris, and snow. Steel-toed boots are preferred **Figure 2-18**. In cold weather, your boots must also protect you from the cold. Leather is one of the best materials for boots. However, boots made of other materials, such as waterproof, windproof, and breathable fabrics, are also very good. The soles of your boots must provide traction. Lug-type soles may grip well in snow, but they become very slippery when caked with mud.

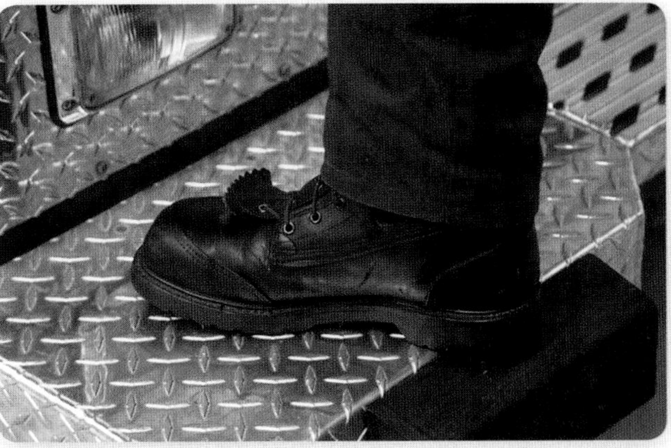

Figure 2-18 Boots should cover and protect your ankles, keeping out stones, debris, and snow. Steel-toed boots are preferred.

Properly fitted boots and shoes are extremely important, because a minor annoyance can progress to become a disabling injury. You may develop painful blisters if your feet slip around inside your boots. However, make sure you have enough room to wiggle your toes.

Boots should be puncture-resistant, protect the toes, and provide foot and ankle support. It may be difficult to obtain a good fit with firefighting boots; shoe inserts or sock layering may be needed for a comfortable fit. Make sure the tops of your boots are sealed off to prevent entry of rain, snow, glass, or other materials. Moisture increases blistering—wool or wicking socks help prevent feet from becoming wet.

Socks will keep your feet warm and provide some cushioning for you as you walk. In cold weather, two pairs of socks are generally preferable to one thick pair. A thin sock next to the foot helps to wick perspiration away to a thicker, outer sock. This tends to keep your feet warmer, drier, and generally more comfortable. When you purchase new shoes or boots, keep these points in mind.

▶ Eye Protection

The human eye is fragile, and permanent loss of sight can occur from even very minor injuries. You need to protect your eyes from blood and other body fluids, foreign objects, plants, insects, and debris from extrication. You may wear eyeglasses with side shields during routine patient care.

In contrast, when tools are being used during extrication, you should wear a face shield or goggles. In these instances, prescription eyeglasses do not provide adequate protection.

In snow or white sand, particularly at higher altitudes, you must also protect your eyes from ultraviolet exposure. Specially designed eyeglasses or goggles can provide this protection. In addition, your eye protection must be adaptable to the weather and the physical demands of the task. It is crucial that you have clear vision at all times.

▶ Ear Protection

Exposure to loud noises for long periods can cause permanent hearing loss. Certain equipment, such as helicopters, some extrication tools, and sirens, produces high levels of noise. Wearing soft foam industrial-type earplugs usually provides adequate protection.

▶ Skin Protection

Your skin needs protection against sunburn while you are working outdoors. Long-term exposure to the sun increases the possibility of skin cancer. It might be considered an annoyance, but sunburn is a type of thermal burn. In reflective areas such as sand, water, and snow, your risk of sunburn increases. Protect your skin by applying a sunscreen with a minimum sun protection factor (SPF) of 15.

In addition, because of the need for frequent handwashing, your hands may begin cracking, as the natural oils are also washed off your skin during this procedure. Use hand lotion several times a day, both on and off duty. Your skin is a very effective barrier to pathogens, as long as it has not been breached by the drying effects of frequent washing.

▶ Body Armor

Although you are trained to avoid any situation that may involve violence, scenes are dynamic and a situation that appears safe initially may quickly deteriorate and become dangerous. For this reason, EMS responders sometimes wear ballistic-resistant or stab-resistant armor for personal protection.

Safety

Remember, ballistic protection is not fail-proof and has the potential to provide a sense of false security.

The National Institute of Justice (NIJ) developed a scale for the global minimum for performance requirements and testing methods for personal body armor.[24] The resulting scale is known as the NIJ threat level and is found on the product's label. An expiration date can also be found on the product label. There are five general classifications of protection ranging from extremely lightweight and flexible to heavy and bulky Table 2-5.[25] The lighter vests do not stop large-caliber bullets, but they offer more flexibility and are preferred by most EMS and law enforcement personnel. Lighter vests are commonly worn under a uniform shirt or jacket.

Table 2-5 National Institute of Justice (NIJ) Threat Levels

Threat Level	Protection Offered
Type IIA	Higher velocity and mass ammunition. Examples: 9 mm and .40 Smith & Wesson
Type II	High velocity and those that travel up to 1400 feet/second. Examples: 9 mm and .357 Magnum
Type IIIA	Better protection from jacketed hollow point rounds. Examples: .44 Magnum and high-velocity 9 mm
Type III	Often used in tactical situations. Examples: Protection from rifles and other high-velocity rounds
Type IV	Highest protection level made with heavy ceramic plates. Example: Armor-piercing bullets

Data from: National Institute of Justice.

The larger, heavier vests are worn on the outside of your uniform and may be bulky and difficult to wear in hot temperatures and high humidity. They are also costly and require replacement at various intervals.

While body armor may protect underlying organs from penetrating injury, the blunt force trauma may still be significant, especially from high-powered gunfire rounds. Vests also offer little or no protection from fragments that occur during an explosion or against stabbing attacks. While body armor may not be practical in all circumstances, it still offers a measure of protection that is better than nothing at all.

Familiarize yourself with the type of body armor used by your department and remember that scene safety is always your first concern. The body armor is there for additional protection; it does not take the place of surveying the scene and avoiding dangerous conditions. Like all EMS equipment, training should be done while wearing your vest to ensure ease of use in real-life situations.

Stress

EMS is a high-stress job. Many situations—such as mass-casualty scenes; serious MVCs; excavation cave-ins; house fires; infant and child trauma; amputations; abuse of an infant, child, spouse, or older adult; or death of a coworker or other public safety personnel—will be stressful for everyone involved. Understanding the causes of stress and knowing how to deal with them are crucial to your job performance, health, and interpersonal relationships. To prevent stress from affecting your life negatively, you need to understand what stress is, what its physiologic effects are, how to minimize these effects, and how to deal with stress on an emotional level.

Stress is the impact of stressors on your physical and mental well-being. Stressors include emotional, physical, and environmental situations or conditions that may cause a variety of physiologic, physical, and psychological responses. The body's response to stress begins with an alarm response, which is followed by a stage of reaction and resistance, and then recovery or, if the stress is prolonged, exhaustion. This three-stage response is referred to as the **general adaptation syndrome**.

Physiologic responses to stress involve the interaction of the endocrine and nervous systems, which result in chemical and physical responses. This is commonly known as the fight-or-flight response. Positive stressors, such as exercise, and negative stressors, such as shift work, long hours, or the frustration of losing a patient, may all result in the same physiologic manifestations:

- Increased respirations and heart rate
- Increased blood pressure
- Dilated venous vessels near the skin surface (causes cool, clammy skin)
- Dilated pupils
- Muscle tension
- Increased blood glucose levels
- Perspiration
- Decreased blood flow to the gastrointestinal tract

Reactions to stress can be categorized as acute, delayed, or cumulative. **Acute stress reactions** occur during a stressful situation. During this stage, you may feel nervous and excited, and your ability to focus increases. If the stress of the situation becomes too great, however, you may experience emotional and physical reactions to stress.

Delayed stress reactions manifest after the stressful event. During the crisis, you are able to focus and function, but after things have calmed down, you may be left with nervous, excited energy that continues to build and becomes a distraction. Learn certain stress-management techniques to improve your chance of effectively managing this kind of delayed stress when it occurs.

Cumulative stress reactions occur when you are exposed to prolonged or excessive stress. After the stressful event is over, are you able to shake off the effects? Inevitably, another stressful situation occurs, and the cycle repeats. Each time, the AEMT finds it harder and harder to recover and becomes more and more exhausted.

Cumulative stress can have physical symptoms such as fatigue, changes in appetite, gastrointestinal problems, or headaches. Stress may cause insomnia or hypersomnia, irritability, inability to concentrate, and hyperactivity or

YOU are the Provider — PART 4

You inform the patient that you would like to clean and bandage his wounds in the back of the ambulance where the lighting is better, and he agrees. Once inside of the ambulance, you examine the injuries and find no arterial sources of bleeding. You then cover the wounds with the appropriate dressings. Finding the patient competent to refuse care, you have the patient sign an EMS Refusal of Care form. As the patient exits the ambulance, you notice blood on the bench seat where the patient was sitting, as well as on the door handles.

Recording Time: 12 Minutes	
Respirations	18 breaths/min, normal
Pulse	Strong and regular, 80 beats/min
Skin	Warm, dry, and pink
Blood pressure	126/82 mm Hg
Oxygen saturation (Spo_2)	100% on room air
Pupils	PERRLA

6. How would you decontaminate your ambulance?
7. Should the ambulance be decontaminated alongside the road before you depart the scene, or should you wait to decontaminate until your arrival at the station?

underactivity. In addition, stress may manifest itself in psychological reactions such as fear, dull or nonresponsive behavior, depression, oversensitivity, anger, guilt, irritability, frustration, isolation, inability to concentrate, alcohol or drug abuse, and loss of interest in work or sexual activity. Often, today's fast-paced lifestyles compound these effects by not allowing a person to rest and recover after periods of stress. Prolonged or excessive stress has been proven to be a strong contributor to heart disease, hypertension, cancer, alcoholism, and depression.

Many people are subject to cumulative stress. In the emergency services environment (EMS personnel, police, firefighters), stressors may also be sudden and severe. Some events are unusually stressful or emotional, even by emergency services standards. These acute severe stressors result in the phenomenon referred to as critical incident stress. Events that can trigger critical incident stress include the following:

- Mass-casualty incidents
- Serious injury or traumatic death of a child
- Crashes with injuries, caused by an emergency services provider while responding to or from a call
- Death or serious injury of a coworker in the line of duty

Posttraumatic stress disorder (PTSD) may develop after a person has experienced one or more psychologically distressing events. PTSD is characterized by reexperiencing the event and over-responding to stimuli that recall the event. In PTSD, social and psychological problems resulting from a failure to resolve traumatic stress or grief can result in delayed reactions classified as "delayed stress syndrome." Stressful events in EMS are sometimes psychologically overwhelming. Some of the symptoms of PTSD include depression, startle reactions, flashback phenomena, and dissociative episodes (such as amnesia of the event).

Supporting patients in emergency situations is stressful both for them and for you. It is crucial that you recognize the signs of stress so that it does not interfere with your work and your personal life. The signs and symptoms of chronic stress may not be obvious at first, but rather may be subtle and not present continuously Table 2-6.

Table 2-6 Warning Signs of Stress
Irritability toward coworkers, family, and friends
Inability to concentrate
Difficulty sleeping, increased sleeping, or nightmares
Feelings of sadness, anxiety, guilt, or hopelessness
Indecisiveness
Loss of appetite (gastrointestinal disturbances)
Loss of interest in sexual activities
Isolation
Loss of interest in work
Increased use of alcohol
Recreational drug use
Physical symptoms such as chronic pain (headache, backache)

▶ Stress Management

Many methods must be used to manage stress. Some are positive and healthy; others are harmful or destructive. For example, many people take medications—either prescription or over-the-counter agents—to address the symptoms of stress. While the medications may provide temporary relief, they do not eliminate the root causes of stress or represent ways to manage it effectively.

The term *stress management* refers to the tactics that have been shown to alleviate or eliminate stress reactions. These may involve changing a few habits, changing your attitude, and demonstrating perseverance Table 2-7. Ultimately, dealing with stress as an AEMT requires the ability to emotionally distance yourself from the situation, and accept the limits of what you can personally do.

A clue to the best management approach for stress comes from the fact that it is not the event itself but rather the person's reaction to the event that determines how much the stress will tax the body's resources. Remember that stress results from anything that you perceive as a threat to your equilibrium. Stress is an undeniable and unavoidable part of our everyday life. Understanding how it affects you physiologically, physically, and psychologically can help you manage it more successfully.

A process called **critical incident stress management (CISM)** was developed to address acute stress situations and potentially decrease the likelihood that PTSD will develop after such an incident Figure 2-19. This process theoretically confronts the responses to critical incidents and defuses them, directing the emergency services responder toward physical and emotional equilibrium. CISM can occur formally, as a debriefing for those who were present at a scene. In such situations, trained CISM teams of peers and mental health professionals may facilitate this debriefing. Additionally, CISM can occur at an ongoing scene in the following circumstances:

- When personnel are assessed for signs and symptoms of distress while resting
- Before reentering the scene
- During a scene demobilization in which personnel are educated about the signs of critical incident stress and given a buffer period to collect themselves before leaving

Table 2-7 Strategies to Manage Stress
Minimize or eliminate stressors.
Change partners to avoid a negative or hostile personality.
Change work hours.
Change the work environment.
Cut back on overtime.
Change your attitude about the stressor.
Talk about your feelings with people you trust.
Seek professional counseling if needed.
Do not obsess over frustrating situations that you are unable to change, such as relapsing alcoholics and nursing home transfers; focus on delivering high-quality care.
Try to adopt a more relaxed, philosophical outlook.
Expand your social support system beyond your coworkers.
Sustain friends and interests outside emergency services.
Minimize the physical response to stress by using a variety of techniques, including: ▪ A deep breath to settle an anger response ▪ Periodic stretching ▪ Slow, deep breathing ▪ Regular physical exercise ▪ Progressive muscle relaxation and/or meditation ▪ Limit intake of caffeine, alcohol, and tobacco use

Defusing sessions are the first to occur. These sessions are held during the event or immediately afterward. The participants informally discuss events that they experienced together. Defusing sessions are designed to educate the participants as to the expectations over the next few days and to give guidance on proper techniques to manage the feelings they may be experiencing. One example is to discourage drinking alcohol during this stressful time.

Debriefing sessions are held within 24 to 72 hours of a major incident. These meetings involve a CISM team consisting of peers and mental health professionals. At the debriefing session, pent-up emotions can be properly expressed. It is more likely you will be ready to express your emotions more freely a few days following the event.

One of the important rules associated with the debriefing session is to not turn it into an operational critique. No one is right. No one is wrong. No one is to blame. Only emotions about the specific event are to be relayed. These debriefing sessions may also have to be repeated at a later time.

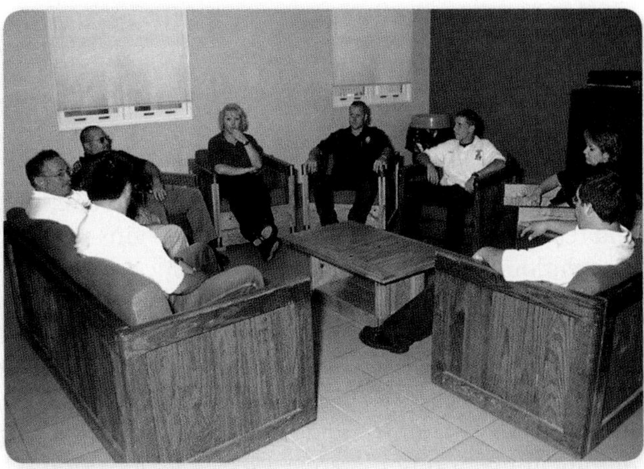

Figure 2-19 Critical incident stress management is sometimes used to help providers to relieve stress.

CISM programs have been established throughout the United States. CISM teams usually can be found via the Internet, by calling telephone directory assistance in your area and asking for CISM, or they can be requested through your employer. An especially helpful organization is the International Critical Incident Stress Foundation (www.icisf.org), which is dedicated to limiting the effects of stress on EMS providers through education and support services.

▶ Burnout

Why should EMS providers start worrying now about something that may (or may not) happen? Burnout needs to be considered now—at an early stage of training—because now is the time for you to start developing attitudes and habits that will help prevent burnout.

The dictionary defines **burnout** as the exhaustion of physical or emotional strength. Burnout, in fact, may be a consequence of chronic, unrelieved stress. Your job, by its very nature, is full of potential stresses. But burnout does not occur solely because of stress. There are more subtle stresses associated with interpersonal relations, pay, prestige, fringe benefits, and other issues. These complaints and stresses are, no doubt, legitimate. Burnout develops because of the way a person reacts to stress.

One person's eustress (beneficial stress, which may lead to greater motivation or alertness) may be another's distress (harmful stress). The reason is that distress is a learned reaction, based on the way a person perceives and interprets the world around him or her. In other words, distress is nearly always the result of what a person believes. Here are some beliefs that are common among EMS personnel:

- I have to be perfect all the time.
- My safety depends on being able to anticipate every possible danger.

- I am totally responsible for what happens to patients; if they die, it is wholly my fault.
- If there is something I do not know, people will think less of me.
- A good AEMT never makes mistakes.

These are all false beliefs and can lead to burnout. Prevention and relief of stress among EMS providers begins with the recognition that such beliefs are unrealistic and invalid.

Like many of the conditions you will study in this text in regard to patients, burnout is a type of illness and has its own set of signs and symptoms. These signs and symptoms may be trivial at first, but when ignored the illness grows in nature until it debilitates you. Symptoms of impending burnout include the following:

- Chronic fatigue and irritability
- Cynical, negative attitudes
- Lack of desire to report to work
- Emotional instability (crying easily, flying off the handle without provocation, laughing inappropriately)
- Changes in sleep patterns (insomnia or sleeping more than usual), and waking without feeling refreshed
- Feelings of being overwhelmed or being helpless or hopeless
- Loss of interest in hobbies
- Decreased ability to concentrate
- Declining health—having frequent colds, stomach upsets, and muscle aches and pains (especially headaches or backaches)
- Constant tightness in your muscles
- Overeating, smoking, or abusing drugs or alcohol

Some AEMTs have been in the field for 20 years and show no signs of burnout, reporting to work every day with the same enthusiasm they did as rookies. What is their secret? In general, the ones who do not experience burnout are those who have learned to respect and value themselves. That is not as easy as it sounds. Practically speaking, what does it mean to respect and value yourself? How can you translate that attitude into concrete actions? Some of the steps you can take to protect yourself from burnout are summarized in Table 2-8. Notably, one of the best ways of dealing with the stress of working as an AEMT is to invest in relationships and activities outside of work that are meaningful to you.

Table 2-8 Guidelines for Preventing Burnout

1. AEMT, heal thyself! Take care of your own health.
   - Get enough rest.
   - Eat a balanced diet.
   - Get regular physical exercise—at least 30 minutes of aerobic activity (walking, running, or swimming) three to four times a week.
   - Do not abuse your body. Smoking, overindulgence in alcohol, taking recreational drugs, or self-prescribing any other drugs are all forms of self-abuse.
2. Give yourself some "me" time every day. Some of the most stress-resistant providers are those who have learned the techniques of meditation and can use them to escape. Try different methods of meditation or relaxation and see which one works best for you.
3. Learn how to relax.
   - Take time for hobbies.
   - Engage in social activities with people not involved in EMS.
   - Leave your job behind when your shift is over.
4. Do not make unreasonable demands on yourself.
   - Forget the idea that you have to be perfect. No one is perfect. If you do the best job you can, that is good enough.
   - You do not have to be right all the time. Accept the fact that now and then you will make a mistake—and that the world will not come to an end on account of it.
5. Do not make unreasonable demands on others.
6. Stay in touch with your feelings.
   - Find someone you can talk to. Share the stress.
   - Cry when you need to. There is no shame in being sad sometimes.
7. Learn techniques for shedding stress while on duty. Do not let stress accumulate.
8. Debrief after tough calls.

Abbreviation: AEMT, advanced emergency medical technician

Peer Support and Suicide Prevention

Like all people, EMS providers are not immune to thoughts of suicide or suicide attempts. Because prolonged stress is a risk factor for suicide, prevention starts with recognizing that you or your colleagues are becoming overwhelmed. Even if you do not identify suicidal tendencies in yourself, you may receive input from colleagues. Do not disregard what you recognize or what others note to you. A survey of over 4,000 respondents showed that 37% of EMS respondents contemplated suicide and 6.6% attempted it.[26] Although the attempt number may seem relatively low, in comparison, the CDC showed levels for the general population to be 3.9% and 0.6%, respectively.[27] The study suggests that emergency workers are at higher risk for suicidal thoughts and attempts than nonemergency workers.

A combination of cumulative stress and acute, intense stress can weigh heavily on EMS providers. While awareness of EMS provider suicide has grown over the years, you should understand and select strategies to deal with stress in a constructive manner. It is important for you to be aware of the signs of stress and burnout in yourself as well as in coworkers. Any suicidal thoughts or attempts must be taken seriously. If you encounter any suicidal ideations or if a colleague expresses such ideations, you should seek help, including professional counseling.

Wellness

Wellness is not simply prevention of disease, but rather a state of complete mental, physical, and social well-being. As a health care provider, you should model a lifestyle of health and wellness.

You will be called upon to work in less than ideal circumstances and situations, which can challenge your ability to maintain your wellness. Anyone can respond to a sudden physical stress for a short time. If stress is prolonged, however, and especially if physical action is not a permitted response, the body can quickly be drained of its reserves. This can leave it depleted of key nutrients, weakened, and more susceptible to illness.

Nutrition

Your body's three sources of fuel—carbohydrates, fat, and protein—are consumed in increased quantities during stress, particularly if physical activity is involved. The quickest source of energy is glucose, taken from stored glycogen in the liver. However, this supply will last less than a day. Protein, drawn primarily from muscle, is a long-term source of glucose. Tissues can use fat for energy. The body also conserves water during periods of stress. To do so, it retains sodium by exchanging and losing potassium from the kidneys. Other nutrients that are susceptible to depletion are the vitamins and minerals that are not stored by the body in substantial quantities. These include water-soluble B and C vitamins and most minerals.

As an AEMT, you have little control over which stressors you will face on any given day. Consequently, stress in one form or another will be an unavoidable part of your life as an AEMT. Just as you would study for a test, dress properly for a day of snow skiing, or train for a sporting event, so you should physically prepare your body for stress. Physical conditioning and proper nutrition are the two variables over which you have absolute control. Muscles will grow and retain protein only with sufficient activity. Bones will not passively accumulate calcium. In response to the physical stress of exercise, bones will store calcium and become denser and stronger. Regular, well-balanced meals are essential to provide the nutrients that are necessary to keep your body fueled Figure 2-20.[28] Vitamin–mineral preparations that provide a balanced mix of all the nutrients may be necessary to supplement a less than perfectly balanced diet.

To perform efficiently, you must eat nutritious food. Food is the fuel that makes the body run. The physical exertion and stress that are a part of your job require a high-energy output. If you do not have a readily available source of fuel, your performance may be less than optimal. This can be dangerous for you, your partner, and your patient. Therefore, it is important for you to learn about and follow the rules of good nutrition.

In general, you should limit your consumption of sugar, fats, sodium, and alcohol. Candy and soft drinks contain sugar. These foods are quickly absorbed and converted to fuel by the body. But simple sugars also stimulate the body's production of insulin, which reduces blood glucose levels. For some people, eating a lot of sugar can actually result in lower energy levels.

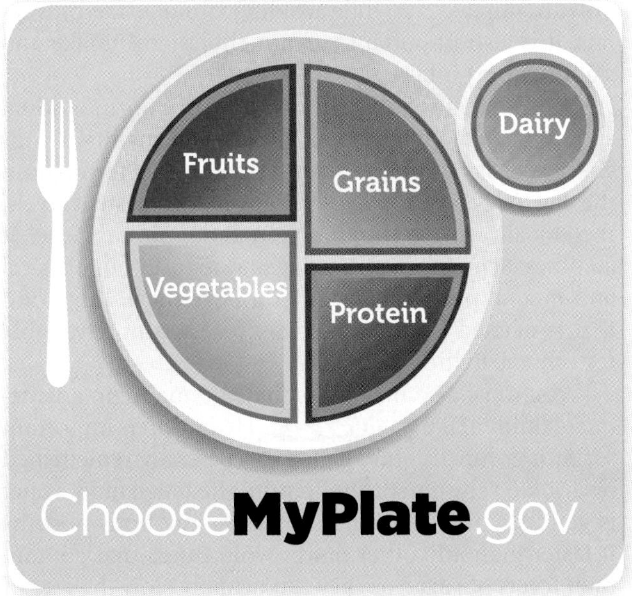

Figure 2-20 The United States Department of Agriculture's MyPlate icon emphasizes healthy portions of vegetables, fruits, grains, proteins, and dairy.

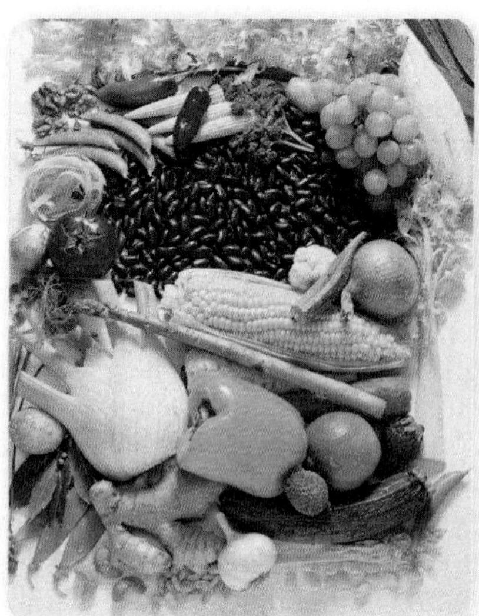

Figure 2-21 Complex carbohydrates are a good source of long-term energy.

Complex carbohydrates rank next to simple sugars in their ability to produce energy. Complex carbohydrates such as pasta, rice, and vegetables are among the safest, most reliable sources for long-term energy production Figure 2-21. However, some carbohydrates take hours to be converted into usable body fuel.

Fats are also easily converted to energy, but eating too much fat can lead to obesity, cardiac disease, and other long-term health problems. The proteins in meat, fish, chicken, beans, and cheese take several hours to convert to energy. Consumption of fats should be limited to 10% of calories and should focus on monounsaturated and polyunsaturated fats while avoiding saturated fats or trans fats. It is also important to limit cholesterol intake and salt (sodium) intake.

While on the job, you should carry an individual supply of high-energy food to help you maintain your energy levels. Try eating several small meals throughout the day to keep your energy resources at consistent levels, thereby allowing you to function at the optimal level at all times. Remember, overeating may reduce your physical and mental performance. After a large meal, the blood that is needed for the digestive process is not available for other activities.

You must also make sure that you maintain an adequate fluid intake Figure 2-22. Hydration is important for proper functioning. Fluids can be easily replenished by drinking any nonalcoholic, noncaffeinated fluid. Water is generally the best fluid available—the body absorbs it faster than any other fluid. Avoid fluids that contain high levels of sugar, as they can actually slow the rate of fluid absorption by the body. These beverages can also cause abdominal discomfort. One indication of adequate hydration is frequent urination. Infrequent urination or urine that is dark yellow indicates dehydration.

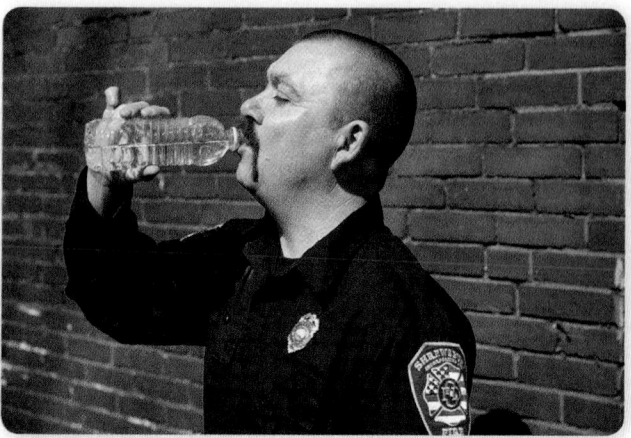

Figure 2-22 Maintain an adequate fluid intake by drinking plenty of water or other nonalcoholic, caffeine-free fluids.

Exercise and Relaxation

A regular program of exercise will enhance the benefits attained through maintaining good nutrition and adequate hydration. When you are in good physical condition, you can handle job stress more effectively. A regular program of exercise will increase your strength and endurance Figure 2-23. Exercise should be moderate or vigorous to have good health benefits. To maintain good health, you should engage in at least 30 minutes of physical activity at least 5 days per week.[29] You may also want to practice relaxation techniques, meditation, and visual imagery.

Your exercise routine should involve aspects of cardiovascular endurance, muscular strength building, and muscle flexibility. Endurance will ensure that your cardiovascular system is able to provide your muscles and brain with needed oxygen. Strength and flexibility building ensures that the body is able to handle the requirements that you will place on it by lifting patients, performing cardiopulmonary resuscitation (CPR), and moving heavy equipment. Exercise is crucial to maintaining a healthy body.

> **Words of Wisdom**
>
> If you don't use it, you lose it! Plan your exercise routine ahead of time, and use strategies that make your session convenient.

Smoking Avoidance or Cessation

In your career as an AEMT, you will routinely see the effects of smoking in your patients—and they are quite sobering. The lesson you should learn from them is simple: If you do not smoke, do not start. In addition, smoking by AEMTs sets an awful example for the public—especially

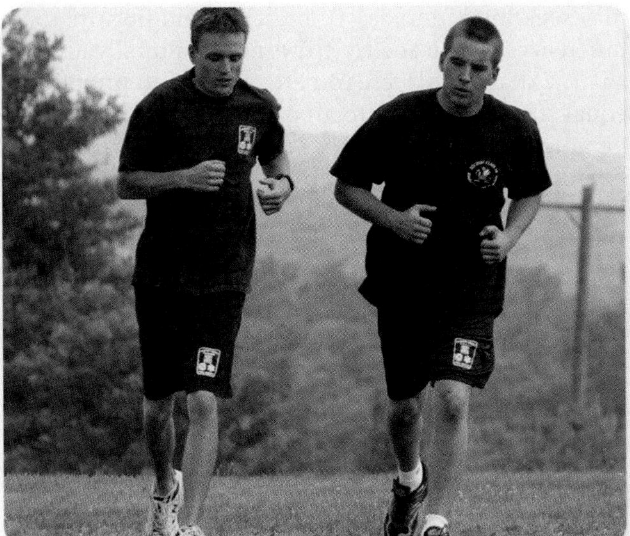

Figure 2-23 A regular program of exercise will increase strength and endurance.

to people who have breathing disorders such as asthma. Finally, it makes you look and smell like anything but a professional caregiver.

You must also understand that everyone responds differently to smoke, and some of your patients may be highly sensitive to it. If you smoke right before a call, the smell on your uniform may be enough to cause serious effects in an already sick patient.

If you are a smoker who is trying to quit, first understand that smoking is truly an addiction and quitting may not be easy. Try to cultivate a relationship with a mentor who was once truly addicted to smoking but who has successfully quit. Use that person as a support, and draw on his or her advice and encouragement. Talk to your primary care physician. A variety of programs are available that can help reduce a smoker's psychological dependency. These programs may include instructions, audiotapes, medications, and counseling to provide ongoing support. Other options that have been known to help some people are psychotherapy, hypnotism, and acupuncture.

▶ Sleep

Good productive sleep is as important as eating well and exercising to maintain good health. Sleep should be regular and uninterrupted. The number of hours is not nearly as important as the quality of sleep. Unfortunately, as an AEMT, you may not have the luxury of sleeping throughout the night.

Working in EMS systems often imposes schedules on AEMTs that conflict with the body's circadian rhythms, or natural timing system. These rhythms are controlled by special areas of the brain, called the suprachiasmatic nuclei, which govern a person's "internal clock." Ignoring your circadian rhythms can cause you to experience consistent difficulty with sleep, thought functions, physical coordination, and even social functions. Signs that your sleep pattern is ineffective include the following:

- You fall asleep within seconds of lying down.
- Within an hour or so after an EMS call, you find yourself routinely fatigued. The excitement is over and now your adrenaline rush crashes.
- You are unable to make it through an entire day without severe fatigue.
- You are unable to concentrate on repetitive tasks such as driving or completing paperwork.

Try to determine what your natural rhythms are, and design a schedule that is best for you. Research on circadian rhythms is only beginning to appear in medical journals, suggesting that someday a person might be able to alter his or her internal clock.

The most important point for all AEMTs is this: Do not overlook the need for rest, whatever your rhythms. Impacts of sleep deprivation may become evident when there is an increase of errors and accidents in the workplace and a decrease in production. As the body becomes deprived of sleep, deficits will be noticed in varying tasks that require logical reasoning or complex thought. Mood may also be affected.[30]

Actions that you can take to improve your sleep include limiting your caffeine intake and tobacco use. Both agents have stimulating effects that can interrupt sleep. Also limit your alcohol use. Alcohol is a depressant and encourages sleep, but routine or excessive use of alcohol can change your sleep pattern, preventing deep sleep from occurring. Try to create as consistent a sleep cycle as possible. This may require naps. Many EMS providers are able to change their sleep pattern into several sleep episodes throughout the day.

Do not worry if you are unable to get 8 straight hours of sleep. Three sleep episodes of 2 to 3 hours each will provide similar effects. Each sleep episode needs to be more than 1 hour in length to encourage deep sleep.

Finally, do not forget the effects of exercise and sleep. Routine exercise will promote the needed fatigue to slip into a restful sleep.

▶ Disease Prevention

Besides sleep, diet, exercise, hydration, and all the other things that make up a healthy lifestyle, you need to be aware of the hereditary factors that may influence your wellness. Consider what you might know about your immediate family's and your ancestors' health. Alzheimer disease, chemical addiction, cancer, cardiac illness, hypertension, migraine, mental illness, and stroke all feature prominent hereditary factors. The most common of all hereditary health factors are those affecting the risk for heart disease and cancer.

Share this information with your personal physician. Your physician is bound by the same oath of confidentiality that you are. Work with him or her to set up a schedule for health assessments, building them into your routine physical check-ups. Your physician should be your ally in screening for these diseases and in assessing your lifestyle as well as your hereditary factors.

Knowing your hereditary factors will help you adjust your lifestyle to help prevent disease. For example, if diabetes runs in your family, exercise and diet are crucial to your well-being. Maintaining a healthy weight and sustaining a consistent exercise routine will help minimize your risk of developing this disease.

One of the most important ways to prevent disease is quite simple: If you don't already smoke, don't start! If you do, please stop! Not only does this habit fly in the face of everything that EMS stands for, but it also produces many of the worst cardiovascular and lung disasters that you will confront during your career.

▶ Balancing Work, Family, and Health

As an AEMT, you will often be called to assist the sick and injured at all times of the day and night. Unfortunately, there is no rhyme or reason to the timing of illness, injury, or interfacility transfers. Volunteer AEMTs may often be called away from family or friends during social activities. Shift workers may be required to be apart from loved ones for long periods. Even so, you should never let the job interfere excessively with your own needs. Find a balance between work and family: You owe it to yourself and to them. It is important to make sure that you have the time that you need to relax with family and friends.

It is also important to realize that coworkers, family, and friends often may not understand the stress caused by responding to EMS calls. As a result of a "bad call," you might not feel like going out to a movie or attending a family event that has been planned for some time. In these situations, help from a critical incident stress debriefing team or information sessions conducted by the EMS unit's employee assistance program may assist you in resolving these problems.

When possible, rotate your schedule to give yourself time off. If your EMS system allows you to move from station to station, rotate to reduce or vary your call volume. Take vacations to provide for your good health so that you will be able to better respond the next time you are needed.

If at any point you feel that the stress of work is more than you can handle, seek help. You may want to discuss your stress informally with your family or coworkers. Help from more experienced team members can be invaluable. You may also want to get help from peer counselors or other professionals. Seeking this help does not make you weak in the eyes of others, but rather demonstrates that you are in control of your life.

Workplace Issues

As our society continues to grow more culturally diverse, some groups that may have been satisfied in the past to accept and participate in American cultural traditions may seek instead to assert, preserve, and nurture their differences. As our society grows more culturally diverse, so do EMS workplaces. You are required to provide an equal standard of care to all patients. You also need to be able to work efficiently and effectively with other health care professionals from a variety of different backgrounds.

▶ Diversity on the Job

Each person is different, and you should communicate with coworkers and patients in a way that is sensitive to everyone's needs. Look at cultural diversity as a resource, and make the most of the differences among people in EMS, thereby enabling them to provide optimal patient care. It is possible to build the strength of your workgroup through the use of diversity. Be respectful toward others who differ from you in terms of culture, race/ethnicity, religion, and other bases, and be sensitive to their needs when communicating with them.

> **Words of Wisdom**
>
> When you are working with patients or calling the hospital on the radio, other AEMTs may be sensitive to how you treat patients from their cultural group. Therefore, when referring to patients, you should use the appropriate terminology. Avoid using terms such as *crippled*, *deformed*, *deaf*, *dumb*, *crazy*, and *retarded* when referring to patients. Instead, use the term *disabled*, and describe the specific disability.

For many years, EMS and public safety services in many regions of the United States have been dominated by white men. This trend is falling by the wayside, as more women and minorities begin working in public safety. The proactive AEMT understands the benefits of using cultural diversity to improve patient care and expects to work alongside workers with different backgrounds and to accept their differences.

Cultural diversity in EMS allows you to enjoy the benefits from fully realizing the skills of a broad range of people. When you accept coworkers as individuals, the need to fit them into rigid roles is eliminated. To be more sensitive to cultural diversity issues, you must first be aware of your own cultural background. Ask yourself, "What are my own issues relative to race, color, religion, and ethnicity?" Since culture is not restricted to different nationalities, you should also consider age, disability, handicap, gender/gender identity, sexual orientation, marital status, work experience, and education.

Remember that your patients and their families will likely span a wide range of cultures. Although it is unrealistic to become a cross-cultural expert with knowledge about all ethnicities, you should learn how to relate and communicate effectively with coworkers and patients from various backgrounds. Even the perception of discrimination can weaken morale and motivation and negatively affect the goal of EMS; be aware of how your words or actions could be interpreted by a person from another culture.

As a health care professional, you should try to be a role model for new AEMTs by showing them the value of diversity. If you are working with a coworker or patient from a particular cultural group, be careful about any opinion you may have formed about that group. Do not assume that there is a language barrier, and do not seem patronizing by saying, "Some of my best friends are . . . ." Recognize that there are legitimate differences in how various cultures respond to stress. For example, you should be prepared to accept that people of different cultures might respond differently to the death of a loved one.

You might want to consider taking multilingual training classes. This training not only will be useful in communicating with your coworkers, but also will improve your ability to communicate with your patients and will help you become accustomed to the culture of the people who are using the language.

▶ Sexual Harassment

Sexual harassment is any unwelcome sexual advance, unwelcome request for sexual favors, or other unwelcome verbal or physical conduct of a sexual nature when submitting is a condition of employment, submitting or rejecting is a basis for an employment decision, or such conduct substantially interferes with performance and/or creates a hostile or offensive work environment.[31] Remember that even an overheard conversation can be construed as sexual harassment.

There are two types of sexual harassment: quid pro quo (the harasser requests sexual favors in exchange for something else, such as a promotion) and hostile work environment (jokes, touching, leering, requests for a date, talking about body parts). Sexual harassment complaints include complaints of a hostile work environment. Remember, it does not matter what the intent or who the harasser was; what matters are the other person's perceptions and what impact the behavior had on that person. For many years, it was not uncommon to walk into a fire station and see sexually suggestive posters, calendars, or cartoons and to hear sexual jokes or comments. This situation is changing because it is not acceptable professional practice.

Because AEMTs and other public safety professionals depend on each other for their own safety, it is especially important to try to develop nonadversarial relationships with coworkers. Most EMS facilities and fire stations make arrangements for different bunkrooms for men and women. If this is not the case at your facility, you should discuss this with your supervisor and talk openly with coworkers of the opposite gender to allow for their privacy.

If you are concerned about a particular behavior, it may be helpful to ask yourself these questions: "Would I do or say this in front of my spouse, significant other, or parents?" "Would I want my family members to be exposed to this behavior?" "Would I want my behavior videotaped and shown on the evening news?"

If you have been harassed, you should report it to your supervisor immediately according to your local policy and procedure. Keep factual documentation of what happened and what was said. You should confront the harasser only if you feel comfortable doing so. If you are asked for a date, say, "I'm not interested." If remarks or touching offends you, say, "Please don't say/do that to me; it offends me."

If your employer's complaint mechanism does not resolve your grievance regarding sexual harassment, then you may need to file a complaint with the Equal Employment Opportunity Commission (EEOC). When investigating allegations of sexual harassment, EEOC looks at the whole record: the circumstances, such as the nature of the sexual advances, and the context in which the alleged incidents occurred. Its decision about the sexual harassment allegations is then made from those facts, on a case-by-case basis.[31]

The best way to deal with sexual harassment is to prevent it from occurring at all. Each agency must develop—and then enforce—a policy on sexual harassment. Training on this issue should also be provided, if necessary. In addition to hurting morale and potentially leading to ineffective performance by employees, sexual harassment can have dire consequences for the EMS system as a whole: If it must defend itself in a sexual harassment case, it runs the risk of a large financial loss if found culpable.

▶ Substance Abuse

In the past, part of the fire service ritual was to go back to the fire station after the fire, clean and maintain the equipment, and discuss the call. At some locations, having a few beers was not uncommon. EMS today is very different from the ambulance service of 20 years ago.

Drugs and alcohol use in the workplace causes an increase in accidents and tension among workers, but most important, it can lead to poor treatment decisions. The EMS personnel who abuse substances such as alcohol or marijuana are more likely to have problems with their work habits, and their drivers' licenses may be revoked as a result. They may be absent from work more often than other workers. If the abuse has occurred within hours before the start of their shift, their ability to provide safe and effective emergency medical care may be lessened because of mental or physical impairment. Because of the seriousness of substance abuse, many EMS systems now require their personnel to undergo periodic random tests for illegal drug use. Since public safety workers depend so much on coworkers for their own safety, it is even more important that ways be found to manage this problem.

As an AEMT, you will witness firsthand the tremendous effects of violence, trauma, and disease. Beyond CISM, members of the public safety community have a way of covering for each other. It is important to understand that the problem behavior will usually get worse before it gets better. Unfortunately, the stereotypical image of the alcoholic or addict lying in the gutter in an urban area often blinds EMS personnel to the existence of a coworker's drug or alcohol problem. People with substance abuse problems often do not fit the stereotype.

If you or one of the members of your team has an alcohol or other drug problem, the risks associated with working in EMS increase significantly. Drug use that occurs off the job also increases the risk. Although laws and rules vary from state to state, a drug- or alcohol-related arrest may result in the revocation of some or all driving privileges and even loss of EMS certification.

If you suspect your partner or a coworker is abusing drugs or alcohol, it is critical that this problem be addressed. When confronting a coworker, make it clear to the coworker that if the problem is personal, he or she needs to take care of it. You have the power to assist this person. In many workplaces, coworkers are often in a position to notice a change in a coworker's behavior or their ability to do the job before a supervisor does. It is helpful to be knowledgeable of the agency's resources and policies for handling such issues. Policies vary widely based on the guidance agencies receive from their legal advisors and human resources departments; you should be aware of your employer's policies.

To help reduce the potential for drug and alcohol use in the EMS workplace, AEMTs can learn about alcohol and other drugs. Management sets the tone on these issues, but senior AEMTs can also emphasize to new personnel that drug and alcohol abuse will not be tolerated. Employee assistance programs (EAPs) are often available for EMS personnel. These agencies are contracted with the EMS department to provide a wide array of mental health, substance abuse, crisis management, and counseling services. Talk with your supervisor to see which resources are available at your EMS department. Early intervention is the best bet to ensure a safe, alcohol- and drug-free workplace.

Safety

Substance abuse does not just reduce EMS personnel's ability to provide safe and effective patient care—it also compromises the safety of that responder and other members of the team. Ignoring a substance abuse problem puts you and those you work with at increased risk.

Death and Dying

According to the Centers for Disease Control and Prevention (CDC), life expectancy has dramatically increased to nearly 79 years, although most deaths continue to occur among people age 65 years and older. Of all deaths today, 24% are attributed to heart disease, followed closely by deaths from cancer (23% of all deaths).[32] For people from the age of 1 year to the age of 44 years, trauma and unintentional injuries are the leading cause of death.[33]

Today, death is likely to occur somewhere other than the home—such as in the hospital, in a convalescent home, at work, or on the highway, and death is likely to occur quite suddenly or after a prolonged terminal illness. Life-support systems and impersonal care remove the whole experience of death from most people's awareness. The mobility of families also makes it less likely that there will be extended family support when death occurs. For these reasons, we are less familiar with death than our ancestors were.

No matter what the frequency of response to emergency calls, death is something that every AEMT will face. During these situations, you must exercise extreme caution in your words and your actions. For some AEMTs, it may be an infrequent occurrence. Others, especially in urban settings, may see death many times in responding to MVCs, drug overdoses, suicides, or homicides. Some EMS personnel will deal with the mass-casualty incident of an airplane crash or a hazardous materials accident. In all of these cases, coming to grips with your thoughts, understandings, and adjustment to death is not only important personally, but also a function of providing emergency medical care.

Words of Wisdom

In the event of a death, you must handle the body with respect and dignity. It must be exposed as little as possible. Learn your local regulations and protocols about moving the body or changing its position, especially if you are at a possible crime scene. Even in these situations, CPR and appropriate treatment must be given unless there are obvious signs of death.

▶ The Grieving Process

The death of a human being is one of the most difficult events for another human being to accept. If the survivor is a relative or close friend of the deceased, it is even more difficult. Emotional responses to the loss of a loved one or friend are appropriate and should be expected. In fact, it is expected that you will feel emotional about the death of a patient. Feelings and emotions are part of the grieving process. All of us experience these feelings after a stressful situation that causes us personal pain.

In 1969, Elisabeth Kübler-Ross published *On Death and Dying*, revealing that people go through several stages of grief:[34]

1. **Denial.** Refusal to accept diagnosis or care, unrealistic demands for miracles, or persistent failure to understand why there is no improvement.
2. **Anger and hostility.** Projection of bad news onto the environment and commonly in all

directions, at times almost at random. The person lashes out. Someone must be blamed, and those who are responsible must be punished. This is typically an unpleasant phase.

3. **Bargaining.** An attempt to secure a prize for good behavior or a promise to change lifestyle. "I promise to be a 'perfect patient' if only I can live until 'x' event."
4. **Depression.** Open expression of grief, internalized anger, hopelessness, or the desire to die. It sometimes involves suicidal threats, complete withdrawal, or giving up long before the illness seems terminal. The patient is usually silent.
5. **Acceptance.** The simple "yes." Acceptance grows out of a person's conviction that all has been done and the person is ready to die. While the acceptance phase is usually the most peaceful for the patient, it is often the most traumatic for the family.

These stages may follow each other in sequence, occur simultaneously, or a person may jump back and forth between stages. The stages may last for different spans of time. Family members may experience similar phases.

▶ Working With Family Members

While you must treat all patients with respect and dignity, use special care with dying patients and their families Table 2-9. Be concerned about their privacy and their wishes, and let them know that you take their concerns seriously. However, it is best to be honest with patients and their families; do not give them false hope.

When working with the family of a patient who has died, ask whether there is anything you can do that will be of help, such as calling a relative or a religious advisor. Provide gentle and caring support. Reinforcing the reality of the situation is important. This can be accomplished by merely saying to a grieving person, "I am so sorry for your loss." It is not important that you have a well-rehearsed script, as it is not likely that your exact words or consolations will be remembered. Rather, the important thing is to be honest and sincere.

Some statements of consolation may sound trite, and some suggest a kind of silver lining behind the clouds. Although they may be intended to make the person feel better about a situation, they also can be viewed as an attempt to diminish the person's grief. The grieving person needs to grieve. Statements like these can also indicate our inability to comprehend the profound sadness of grief because we have not experienced that kind of loss.

Each person will experience grief and respond to it in his or her own way. Attempts to take grief away too quickly are not good. If you do not know how the person really feels, you should not say that you do. People may be offended by responses that give advice or explanations about the death. Statements such as "Oh, you shouldn't feel that way" are judgmental. If you judge what the grieving person is feeling, it is likely that he or she will stop talking with you. There is no right or wrong way to grieve.

Remember that anger is a stage of grieving. Patients or family members may express rage, anger, and despair, and their anger may be directed at you. This anger seems irrational to everyone but the person grieving. A professional attitude is a necessity, and you must not take this anger as a personal attack. The patient's or family's concerns will usually be relieved by your calm, efficient manner.

Statements and comments that suggest action on your part are generally helpful. These statements imply a sense of understanding; they focus on the grieving person's feelings. It is not necessary to go into an extensive discussion. You may say, "I am so sorry. I just want you to know that I am thinking about you." What people really appreciate is somebody who will listen to them. Simply ask, "Would you like to talk about how or what you are feeling?" Then accept the response.

Table 2-9 Responding to Grief

Don't Say...	Try Instead...
Give it time. Things will get better.	I'm sorry for your loss.
You should not question God's will.	It is okay to be angry.
You have to get on with your life.	It must be hard to accept.
You have to keep going.	That must be painful for you.
You can always have another child.	Tell me how you are feeling.
You're not the only one who suffers.	If you want to cry, it's okay.
Life goes on.	People really cared for...
I know how you feel.	I can only imagine how terrible this must be for you...

Words of Wisdom

Be compassionate, but remember that patient care always takes precedence in emergency situations. It would be inappropriate to prioritize a screaming, frightened child with minor injuries over another patient who actually has life-threatening injuries.

▶ Working With the Patient

Even though the event (death) has not yet happened, the dying patient knows that it will happen. The patient has no control over this process. The patient will die whether or not he or she is ready. Furthermore, being ready to die does not mean that the patient will be happy about dying. You may encounter situations in which the patient is close to death, and you may need to provide reassurance and emotional care.

People who are in the process of dying as a result of trauma, an acute medical condition, or a terminal disease will feel threatened. That threat may be related to their concern about survival. These concerns may involve feelings of helplessness, disability, pain, and separation Table 2-10.

Words of Wisdom

Many factors influence how a patient reacts to the stress of an emergency incident. Among these factors are the following:

- Personality
- Socioeconomic background
- Fear of health care personnel
- Alcohol or substance abuse
- History of chronic disease
- Mental disorders
- Reaction to medication
- Age
- Nutritional status
- Feelings of guilt
- Past experience with illness or injury

Table 2-10	Concerns of the Dying, Critically Ill, or Injured Patient
Anxiety	
Pain and fear	
Anger and hostility	
Depression	
Dependency	
Guilt	
Mental health problems	
Receiving unrelated bad news	

Do not make light of a patient's pain and fear. Instead, you might say, "I'm sure you are really scared right now, but you should know that I am doing everything I can to help you." Making a connection with your patient through eye contact and the squeeze of a hand can often do more to allay fear than the most eloquent words. The following sections discuss some of the responses you may receive from critical patients.

Anxiety

Anxiety is a response to the anticipation of danger. The source of the anxiety is often unknown, but in the case of seriously injured or ill patients, the source is usually recognizable. What may increase the anxiety are the unknowns of the current situation. Patients may ask the following:

- What will happen to me?
- What are you doing?
- Will I make it?
- What will my disabilities be?

Patients who are anxious may have the following signs and symptoms:

- Emotionally upset
- Sweaty and cool skin (diaphoretic)
- Rapid breathing (hyperventilating)
- Fast pulse (tachycardic)
- Restlessness
- Tension
- Fear
- Shakiness (tremulous)

For the anxious patient, time seems to be extended: Seconds can seem like minutes and minutes can seem like hours. It is your job to do everything you can to reduce the patient's anxiety and help the patient cope and minimize the physiologic harm caused by anxiety.

Pain and Fear

Pain and fear are interrelated. Pain often is associated with illness or trauma. Fear is generally thought of in relation to the oncoming pain and the outcome of the damage. It is often helpful to encourage patients to express their pains and fears; this expression begins the process of adjusting to the pain and accepting the emergency medical care that may be necessary. Some people have difficulty openly admitting their fear. The fear may be expressed as bad dreams, withdrawal, tension, restlessness, "butterflies" in the stomach, or nervousness. In some cases, it may be expressed as anger.

Anger and Hostility

Anger may be expressed by very demanding and complaining behavior. Often this may be related to the fear and anxiety caused by the emergency itself or by the medical care that is being given. Sometimes the fear is so acute that the patient may want to express anger toward you or others but is unable to do so because of the dependency factor. If you find that you are the target of the patient's anger, make sure that you are safe; do not take the anger or insults personally. Be tolerant, and do not become defensive.

Anger may also be expressed physically, and you may be the target of the displaced aggression. If the patient or a relative becomes so emotionally upset that you are physically assaulted or you believe that this could happen, retreat from the situation. Such hostility must be contained. If emergency medical care is not possible under these circumstances, law enforcement intervention is required.

Depression

Depression is a natural physiologic and psychological response to illness, especially if the illness is prolonged, debilitating, or terminal. Whether the depression is a temporary sadness or clinical depression that has a long history, there is, of course, little you can do to alleviate the pain of depression during the brief time the patient is being treated and transported. The best you can do in treating and transporting a patient experiencing depression is to be compassionate, supportive, and nonjudgmental.

Dependency

Dependency usually takes longer to develop than is possible with the very brief relationships developed in EMS. However, when medical care is given to any individual, a sense of dependency may develop. People who are placed in this position may feel helpless and become resentful. The resentfulness may arouse feelings of inferiority, shame, or weakness. Make every attempt to remain supportive and compassionate.

Guilt

Many patients who are dying, their families, or the caregivers of the patients may feel guilty about what has happened. Occasionally family members and long-term caregivers may feel a degree of relief when an extended illness is finally over. That relief may later turn into guilt. Most of the time, however, no one can explain these feelings. The magnitude of the guilt may be great. Sometimes, feelings of guilt can result in a delay in seeking emergency medical care. Again, understanding the complex emotions that often surface during times of emergency may help you cope with some of the intense behavior you will encounter as an AEMT.

Mental Health Problems

Mental health problems such as disorientation, confusion, or delusions may develop in the dying patient. In these instances, the patient may display behavior inconsistent with normal patterns of thinking, feeling, or acting. Common characteristics of such behavior may include the following:

- Loss of contact with reality
- Distortion of perception
- Regression
- Diminished control of basic impulses and desires
- Abnormal mental content, including delusions and hallucinations

In some long-term situations, generalized personality deterioration may occur. See Chapter 24, *Psychiatric Emergencies*, for a discussion on mental health.

Receiving Unrelated Bad News

A patient who is in critical condition or is dying may not want to hear unrelated bad news, such as a message about the death of a close relative or friend. Such news may depress the patient or cause the patient to give up hope.

▶ Dealing With the Death of a Child

The death of a child is a tragic and dreaded event. It is not unusual to think about the fact that a dead or dying child is missing out on a lot more of life. In our society, we assume that only older people are supposed to die. Children die less frequently now than they did in earlier times, so most people are unprepared for what they will feel when a child dies. You may think about your own children and those whom you know: nephews, nieces, grandchildren, and children of close friends. And you may think, "Why should this child, who is only 5 years old, die?"

Answering the difficult questions about your own mortality will be of help when dealing with the death of a child. Even so, the death of a child will not be an easy subject to discuss. This will be especially true for the family. As an AEMT involved in a call that involves the death of a child, you will also likely experience stress.

One of your responsibilities is to help the family through the initial period after the death. Until more definitive and professional help can be available, you may be in the best position to help family members begin to cope with their loss. How family members deal with the death of a child will affect their stability and endurance. You can help family members through the initial period of grief and alert them to the follow-up counseling and support services that are available.

If the child is dead, acknowledging the fact of the death is important. This should be done in a private place, even if that is inside an ambulance. Often, the parents cannot believe that the death is real, even if they have been preparing for it, as in the case of a child with a terminal illness. Reactions vary, but shock, disbelief, and denial are common. Some parents show little emotion at the initial news.

If possible and appropriate, find a place where the mother and father can hold the child. This is important in the parents' grieving process; it helps to lessen the sense of disbelief and makes the death real. Even if the parents do not ask, you should tell them that they can see the child. Your decision in permitting the parents to see the child may need some discretion. For example, in the case of a traumatic death in which there is significant disfigurement, that decision might have to be delayed. The delay may involve having support services available or contacting the family physician or others who can help the parents through this difficult situation. This may involve preparing the parents for what they will see and the changes brought on by rigor mortis or asphyxiation, for example.

Sometimes you do not need to say much. Alternatively, you may choose to express your own sorrow. Do not overload grieving parents with a lot of information; at this point, they cannot handle it. Nonverbal communication, such as holding a hand or touching a shoulder, may also be valuable. Let the family's actions be your guide regarding what is appropriate. It is important to encourage parents to talk about their feelings.

Caring for Critically Ill and Injured Patients

When you are caring for a critically ill or injured patient, the patient needs to know who you are and what you are doing. Let the patient know that you are attending to his or her immediate needs and that these are your primary concerns at that particular moment Figure 2-24. As soon as possible, explain to the patient what is going on. Confusion, anxiety, and other feelings of helplessness will be decreased if you keep the patient consistently informed. For example, patients may be concerned about the safety or well-being of others who are involved in the accident and about the damage or loss of personal property. Your responses must be discreet and diplomatic, giving reassurance when appropriate. If a loved one has been killed or critically injured, you should wait, if possible, until clergy or emergency department staff can inform the patient. They can then provide the psychological support the patient needs.

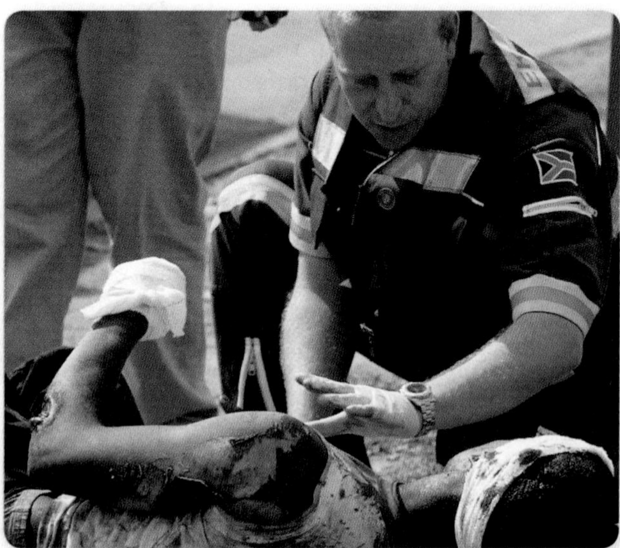

Figure 2-24 Let the patient know immediately that you are there to help.

Some patients, especially children and older adults, may be terrified or feel rejected when separated from family members by the uniformed EMS provider team. Other patients may not want family members to share their stress, see their injury, or witness their pain. It is usually best if parents go with their children and relatives accompany older patients.

Religious customs or needs of the patient must also be respected. Some people will cling to religious medals or charms, especially if any attempt is made to remove them. Others will express a strong desire for religious counsel, baptism, or last rites if death is near. You must try to accommodate these requests if it is practical. Some people have religious convictions that strongly oppose the use of drugs and blood products. If you obtain such information, it is imperative that you report it to the personnel who will be responsible for the next level of care. The following sections provide effective techniques for communicating with a critical patient.

Avoid Sad and Grim Comments

AEMTs, other safety personnel, family, and bystanders must avoid grim comments about a patient's condition. Remarks such as "This is a bad one" or "The leg is badly damaged, and I think he will lose it," are inappropriate. These remarks may upset or increase anxiety in the patient and compromise possible recovery outcomes. This is especially true for the patient who may be able to hear but not respond.

Orient the Patient

You should expect a patient to be disoriented in an emergency situation. The aura of the emergency situation—lights, sirens, smells, and strangers—is intense. The impact and effect of injuries or acute illness may cause the patient to be confused or unsettled. It is important to orient the patient to his or her surroundings Figure 2-25. Use brief, concise statements, such as "Mr. Smith, you have had an accident, and I am now splinting your arm. I am John Foxworth of the New Britain EMS; I will be caring for you."

Be Honest

When approaching any patient, you must determine the patient's ability to understand and accept. You should be honest without further shocking the patient or giving information that is unnecessary or that may not be understood. Simply explain what you are doing and allow the patient to be part of the care being given; this can relieve feelings of helplessness and some of the fear.

Initial Refusal of Care

On occasion a patient may refuse emergency medical care, insisting that you do nothing and leave him or her alone. In these cases, it is important to impress upon the

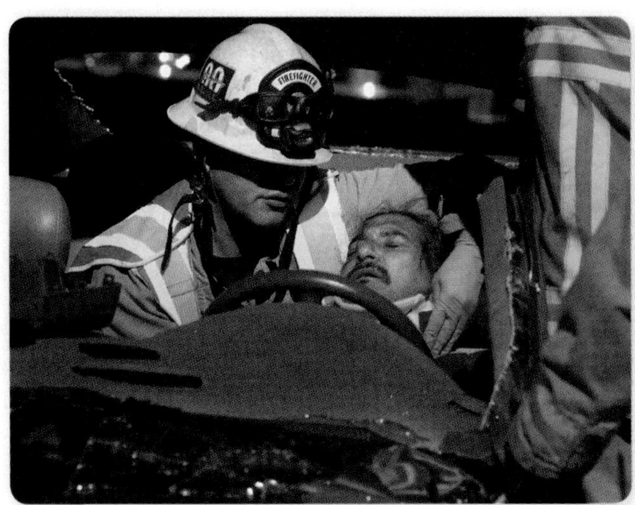

Figure 2-25 The aura of an emergency situation can be confusing and frightening to the patient. Make sure you explain to the patient what has happened and what you are doing.

patient the seriousness of the condition without causing undue alarm. Saying, "Everything will be okay," when it is obvious that it will not be, makes you appear dishonest. Generally, seriously ill or injured patients know that they are in trouble; however, many people refuse care because of their inability to pay the medical expenses. It is imperative to stress to patients that their inability to pay should in no way have a bearing on whether they seek care. If there is a need, EMS should be called and the patient will receive appropriate care regardless of his or her financial situation.

▶ Allow for Hope

In trauma and acute medical conditions, patients may ask you whether they are going to die. You may feel at a loss for words. You may also know, on the basis of experience or in view of the seriousness of the present situation, that the prognosis is poor. Even so, it is not your responsibility to tell the patient that he or she is dying. Statements such as "I don't know when you are going to die; let's deal with the current problem," or "I'm not going to give up on you, so don't give up on yourself," are helpful. These statements transmit a sense of trust and hope, and they let the patient know that you are doing everything possible to save his or her life. If there is the slightest chance of hope remaining, you want that message transmitted in your attitude and in the statements you make to the patient.

▶ Locate and Notify Family Members

Many patients will be concerned and ask you to notify their family or others close to them. The patient may or may not be able to assist you in doing this. You should ensure that an appropriate and responsible person makes an effort to locate the desired people. Assuring the patient that someone is going to do this is a significant part of the patient's care because it will help to calm the patient.

Words of Wisdom

When you are transporting an older adult who lives with a spouse or other older relative or friend, try to transport that person along with the patient if time permits. Many older adults cannot drive.

▶ Injured and Critically Ill Children

Children who are critically ill or injured should be cared for as any patient would be, insofar as an assessment of airway, breathing, circulation, disability, and exposure (the ABCDEs) and immediate life threats are concerned. Due regard should be given to variations in height, weight, and size in providing emergency medical care to pediatric patients.

When children are seriously ill or injured, family members and other people at the scene may become frantic. You need to remain calm and confident in your skills—this may be all that is needed to provide reassurance to everyone at the scene. Children will often respond better to a person who is calm, even if their illness or injury is significant. Because of the increased excitement and extraordinary nature of the emergency scene for a child, it is important that a relative or responsible adult accompany the child to relieve anxiety and assist in care as appropriate.

▶ Uncertain Situations

There will be times when you are unsure whether a true medical emergency exists. If you are unsure, contact medical control about the need to transport. If you cannot reach medical control, it is always best to err on the side of caution and transport the patient. For ethical and medicolegal reasons, a physician must examine all patients who are transported and determine the degree of medical need.

Many minor signs or symptoms may be early indicators of severe illness or injury. Symptoms of many illnesses can be similar to those of substance abuse, hysteria, or other conditions. You must accept the patient's complaints and provide appropriate care until you are able to transfer care of the patient to a higher level (such as a paramedic, nurse, or physician). Your local protocols will direct your actions in these situations. When in doubt, err on the side of caution, and acquire the patient's consent and transport to the medical facility.

YOU are the Provider SUMMARY

1. Do you have a duty to provide care to this patient?

Yes, you have a duty to provide care to this patient. Because this crash occurred in your presence, and you are available for service, you have the responsibility to evaluate the patient and provide any needed care and treatment. Depending on jurisdictional requirements, you may or may not have to notify the local ambulance service and have its personnel respond as well. Regardless of this patient's HIV status, he has a right to receive appropriate medical care.

2. What is the minimal amount of personal protective equipment (PPE) you would want to have on prior to exiting the ambulance?

At a minimum, both you and your partner should be wearing some type of American National Standards Institute (ANSI) II high-visibility compliance clothing (vest, jacket), eye protection, safety-toed boots, and, if applicable to your jurisdiction, firefighting-type turnout gear.

3. What is the minimal amount of PPE you would want to have on prior to initiating care?

As with any patient, the appropriate PPE should be based on the anticipated exposures. With the amount of blood present, you should have on eye protection, gloves, and possibly a face shield and gown. The patient's HIV status does not require any additional PPE other than standard precautions.

4. Does the fire department need to be informed of the patient's HIV-positive status?

The patient has a right to have his health status remain private. Because of Health Insurance Portability and Accountability Act (HIPAA) regulations, the firefighters would need to be informed of his status only if they might come in contact with potentially biohazardous substances.

5. Does this patient have the right to refuse care?

As with all patients, as long as he is competent to refuse care (not under the influence of intoxicating substances) and understands the risks and consequences of refusing care, this patient has every right to refuse care.

6. How would you decontaminate your ambulance?

The substance that should be used to decontaminate your ambulance will vary depending on departmental policies, but you can use a bleach and water solution at a dilution between 1:10 and 1:100 to clean the unit. The solution you mix should not have a strong odor of bleach if mixed correctly. A hospital-approved disinfectant that is effective against *Mycobacterium tuberculosis* can also be used. Use the cleaning solution in a bucket or pistol-handled spray container, making sure to thoroughly clean all surfaces, especially common areas, such as door handles.

7. Should the ambulance be decontaminated alongside the road before you depart the scene, or should you wait to decontaminate until your arrival at the station?

The location where you clean your ambulance will again depend on local policies. It is recommended that you clean the ambulance as soon as practical upon contamination. Regardless, the ambulance should be placed out of service until it can be completely decontaminated.

YOU are the Provider SUMMARY (continued)

EMS Patient Care Report (PCR)					
Date: 1-12-18	**Incident No.:** 20107913557		**Nature of Call:** Witnessed MVC		**Location:** I-29 SB MM214
Dispatched: 1233	**En Route:** 1233	**At Scene:** 1233	**Transport:**	**At Hospital:**	**In Service:** 1257

Patient Information	
Age: 54 **Sex:** M **Weight (in kg [lb]):** 101 kg (222 lb)	**Allergies:** NSAIDs **Medications:** Enfuvirtide **Past Medical History:** HIV+ **Chief Complaint:** Multiple lacerations

Vital Signs				
Time: 1237	**BP:** 124/86	**Pulse:** 82	**Respirations:** 18	**Spo$_2$:** 100%
Time: 1244	**BP:** 126/82	**Pulse:** 80	**Respirations:** 18	**Spo$_2$:** 100%
Time:	**BP:**	**Pulse:**	**Respirations:**	**Spo$_2$:**

EMS Treatment (circle all that apply)				
Oxygen @ ______ L/min via (circle one): **NC NRM Bag-mask device**		**Assisted Ventilation**	**Airway Adjunct**	**CPR**
Defibrillation	**Bleeding Control:** Yes (circled)	**Bandaging:** Yes (circled)	**Splinting**	**Other:**

Narrative

While returning from Altru Hospital, Medic 6284 witnessed a single vehicle rollover MVC on I-29. Vehicle appeared to be traveling at approximately 55 mph when it swerved, lost control, and rolled 3-4 times. Patient was restrained, no airbag deployment, passenger compartment intact. Patient presents with copious amounts of blood on his arms, states he is HIV+. Proper PPE in place. Manual immobilization to cervical spine established. Patient denies any loss of consciousness or head, neck, or back pain. He states his only complaint is arm pain from the lacerations. Patient further refuses to be secured to long backboard, and only wishes to be treated and not transported. Assisted patient to back of ambulance, where wounds were examined. No arterial bleeding noted. Bleeding controlled with pressure and dressings applied. Advised patient of need to be evaluated in emergency department for possible sutures. Also advised patient of risks and consequences of refusing EMS, up to and including death. Patient verbalized understanding of refusing EMS, and appeared competent to refuse. Appropriate forms signed. Patient left in care of law enforcement on scene. Medic 6284 returned to service.**End of report**

Prep Kit

▶ Ready for Review

- As an AEMT, you will arrive at scenes where potential danger to you is easily apparent. Every patient encounter should be considered potentially dangerous. Therefore, it is essential that you take all available precautions to minimize exposure and risk. Potential risks include scene hazards and infectious and communicable diseases.
- A communicable disease is any disease that can be spread from person to person or from animal to person.
- Infectious diseases can be transmitted by contact (direct or indirect); they are spread by airborne, foodborne, or vector-borne means.
- Even if you are exposed to an infectious disease, your risk of becoming ill is low. Whether or not an acute infection occurs depends on several factors, including the amount and type of infectious organism and your resistance to that infection.
- You can take several steps to protect yourself against exposure to infectious diseases, including remaining up-to-date with recommended vaccinations, following standard precautions at all times, and handling all needles and other sharp objects with great care.
- Because it is often impossible to tell which patients have infectious diseases, you should avoid direct contact with the blood and body fluids of all patients.
- Standard precautions are protective measures designed to prevent health care workers from coming into contact with germs carried by patients. One extremely effective step is properly washing your hands. You must also use the proper personal protective equipment for the situation, including gloves, gowns, eye protection, masks, and possibly other specialized equipment.
- Keep up-to-date immunizations. Recommended immunizations include tetanus and diphtheria boosters (every 10 years); measles, mumps, and rubella (MMR) vaccine; influenza vaccine (yearly); hepatitis B vaccine; and varicella (chickenpox) vaccine if you have not had chickenpox. You should also have a skin test for tuberculosis before you begin working as an AEMT and ensure that you receive appropriate regular testing as dictated by your employee health department.
- Infection control should be an important part of your daily routine. Be sure to follow the proper steps when dealing with potential exposure situations.
- You should know what to do if you are exposed to an airborne or bloodborne disease. Your department's designated officer will be able to help you follow the protocol set up in your area.
- If you think you may have been exposed to an infectious disease, see your physician (or your employer's designated physician) immediately.
- Cleaning and disinfecting the ambulance is an important part of protecting yourself and patients. Use cleaning solutions that are appropriate for the equipment category.
- During your career as an AEMT, you will be exposed to many hazards. In a life-threatening situation, you should be properly protected, or you must avoid the situation altogether.
- Scene hazards may include traffic hazards, unstable vehicles, potential exposure to hazardous materials, electricity, and fire. Your safety is the most important consideration. Never approach a scene without first observing it from a safe distance.
- Hazards associated with a vehicle crash are some of the most unstable and lethal. Be very conscious about the flow of traffic. When approaching damaged vehicles, look for signs of fluid leakage. Look for signs of vehicle instability. Other rescuers may need to work at the scene before you can safely provide patient care.
- If a hazardous material may be present, do not begin caring for patients until they have been moved away from the scene by the hazardous materials team and properly decontaminated, or until the scene has been made safe for you to enter.
- Electrical shock can be produced by power lines or by lightning. If you encounter a downed power line, do not touch it. Mark off a danger zone around the downed lines and contact the power company. If a lightning strike is possible, move immediately to the lowest area possible. If you are in an open area, position yourself in a low crouch. If possible, get inside a vehicle or your unit, as it may provide some measure of protection.
- Five common hazards in a fire include smoke, oxygen deficiency, high ambient temperatures, toxic gases, and building collapse. You must be trained in the use of appropriate protective equipment and have it available at all fire scenes. Follow the instructions of the incident commander while on scene.
- Wearing protective clothing and other appropriate gear is crucial to your personal safety. Protective clothing and gear must be in good condition, and may include cold weather clothing, turnout gear, firefighting gloves, helmets, boots, eye protection, ear protection, skin protection, and possibly body

Prep Kit *(continued)*

armor. A high-visibility public safety vest must be worn while on or near a roadway.

- Violent situations such as civil disturbances, domestic disputes, and crime scenes can create many hazards for EMS personnel. Whenever you are in doubt about your safety, do not put yourself at risk. If you see the potential for violence when you are sizing up the scene, call for the appropriate resources. Rely on the advice of law enforcement.
- Stress reactions can be acute, delayed, or cumulative. Posttraumatic stress disorder is a syndrome with onset following a traumatic, usually life-threatening event. Critical incident stress management is a process developed to address acute stress situations. AEMTs may also seek help through an employee assistance program.
- When signs of stress such as fatigue; anxiety; anger; feelings of hopelessness, worthlessness, or guilt; and other such indicators manifest themselves, behavioral problems can develop. Recognizing the signs of stress is important for all AEMTs.
- An important part of ensuring your own optimal functioning is to nurture your own wellness through proper nutrition, exercise and relaxation, smoking cessation, sleep, and disease prevention.
- AEMTs will encounter death, dying patients, and the families and friends of those who have died. Understanding the concerns of the dying patient, assisting a family following the death of a loved one, and dealing with your own feelings about death are personally and professionally important. Make appropriate statements such as "I am sorry for your loss."
- Patients who are critically ill or injured may be anxious, afraid, angry, hostile, or depressed. They may be concerned about becoming dependent, may feel guilty, or may experience a behavioral emergency. Behave professionally, have compassion, and remain nonjudgmental.
- Critically ill or injured patients need to know who you are and what you are doing. Be sure to communicate with them, avoiding sad and grim comments and allowing for hope. Always be honest. You can often help calm a patient by locating and notifying family members.

▶ Vital Vocabulary

acute stress reactions Reactions to stress that occur during a stressful situation.

airborne transmission The spread of an infectious agent via droplets or dust.

bloodborne pathogens Pathogenic microorganisms that are present in human blood and can cause disease in humans. These pathogens include, but are not limited to, hepatitis B virus and human immunodeficiency virus (HIV).

burnout A state of exhaustion of physical or emotional strength, which may be a consequence of chronic, unrelieved stress.

Centers for Disease Control and Prevention (CDC) The primary federal agency that conducts and supports public health activities in the United States. The CDC is part of the US Department of Health and Human Services.

communicable disease A disease that can be spread from one person or species to another.

contamination The presence of infectious organisms on or in objects such as dressings, water, food, needles, wounds, or a patient's body.

cover The tactical use of an impenetrable barrier for protection.

critical incident stress management (CISM) A process that confronts the responses to critical incidents and defuses them, directing the emergency services personnel toward physical and emotional equilibrium.

cumulative stress reactions Exposure to prolonged or excessive stress.

delayed stress reactions Reactions to stress that occur after a stressful situation.

designated officer The person in the department who is charged with the responsibility of managing exposures and infection control issues.

direct contact Exposure to or transmission of a communicable disease from one person to another by physical contact.

exposure A situation in which a person has had contact with blood, body fluids, tissues, or airborne particles in a manner that suggests disease transmission may occur.

foodborne transmission The contamination of food or water with an organism that can cause disease.

general adaptation syndrome The body's response to stress that begins with an alarm response, followed by a stage of reaction and resistance, and then recovery or, if the stress is prolonged, exhaustion.

hepatitis Inflammation of the liver, usually caused by a viral infection, that causes fever, loss of appetite, jaundice, fatigue, and altered liver function.

host The organism or person that is attacked by the infecting agent.

Prep Kit *(continued)*

human immunodeficiency virus (HIV) Acquired immunodeficiency syndrome (AIDS) is caused by HIV, which damages the cells in the body's immune system so that the body is unable to fight infection or certain cancers.

immune The body's ability to protect itself from acquiring a disease.

indirect contact Exposure to or transmission of infection from one person to another by contact with a contaminated object.

infection The abnormal invasion of a host or host tissues by organisms such as bacteria, viruses, or parasites, with or without signs or symptoms of disease.

infection control Procedures to reduce transmission of infection among patients and health care personnel.

infectious disease A medical condition that is caused by the growth and spread of small, harmful organisms within the body.

Occupational Safety and Health Administration (OSHA) The federal regulatory compliance agency that develops, publishes, and enforces guidelines concerning safety in the workplace.

pathogen A microorganism that is capable of causing disease in a susceptible host.

personal protective equipment (PPE) Protective equipment that blocks exposure to a pathogen or a hazardous material.

posttraumatic stress disorder (PTSD) A delayed stress reaction to a prior incident. Often the result of one or more unresolved issues concerning the incident, and may relate to an incident that involved physical harm or the threat of physical harm.

standard precautions Protective measures that have traditionally been developed by the Centers for Disease Control and Prevention for use in dealing with objects, blood, body fluids, or other potential exposure risks of communicable disease.

transmission The way in which an infectious disease is spread: contact, airborne, by vehicles, or by vectors.

tuberculosis A chronic bacterial disease, caused by *Mycobacterium tuberculosis,* that usually affects the lungs but also can affect other organs such as the brain and kidneys; it is spread by cough and can lie dormant in a person's lungs for decades and then reactivate.

vector-borne transmission The use of an animal or insects to spread an organism from one person or place to another.

▶ References

1. Centers for Disease Control and Prevention. *Guide to infection prevention for outpatient settings: minimum expectations for safe care.* Version 2.3. September 2016. https://www.cdc.gov/infectioncontrol/pdf/outpatient/guide.pdf. Accessed December 27, 2016.
2. Centers for Disease Control and Prevention. *2007 Guideline for Isolation Precautions: Preventing Transmission of Infectious Agents in Healthcare Settings.* https://www.cdc.gov/hicpac/pdf/isolation/Isolation2007.pdf. Accessed December 27, 2016.
3. Centers for Disease Control and Prevention. *Clean hands count for healthcare providers.* https://www.cdc.gov/handhygiene/providers/index.html. Accessed December 5, 2016.
4. Robbins SL, Cotran RS, Kumar V, eds. *Robbins Basic Pathology*. 7th ed. Philadelphia: WB Saunders, 2003. http://www.medical.ansell.com.au/resources/double-gloving. Accessed December 27, 2016.
5. Centers for Disease Control and Prevention. *Ebola Virus Disease, Personal Protective Equipment.* http://www.cdc.gov/vhf/ebola/healthcare-us/ppe/guidance.html. Accessed December 27, 2016.
6. Occupational Safety and Health Administration. *Healthcare wide hazards: tuberculosis.* https://www.osha.gov/SLTC/etools/hospital/hazards/tb/tb.html. Accessed December 5, 2016.
7. Centers for Disease Control and Prevention. *How to Prevent Needlestick and Sharps Injuries.* http://www.cdc.gov/niosh/docs/2012-123/pdfs/2012-123.pdf. Accessed December 27, 2016.
8. Occupational Safety and Health Administration. *Healthcare wide hazards.* https://www.osha.gov/as/opa/worker/employer-responsibility.html. Accessed December 5, 2016.
9. National Fire Protection Association (NFPA). NFPA 1581: Standard on Fire Department Infection Control Program. http://www.nfpa.org/codes-and-standards/all-codes-and-standards/list-of-codes-and-standards?mode=code&code=1581. Accessed December 5, 2016.
10. McCallion T. How clean is your ambulance? *J Emerg Med Serv.* April 30, 2012. http://www.jems.com/articles/2012/04/how-clean-your-ambulance.html. Accessed December 5, 2016.
11. Centers for Disease Control and Prevention, National Institute for Occupational Safety and Health. *Bloodborne infectious diseases: HIV/AIDS, hepatitis B, hepatitis C.* http://www.cdc.gov/niosh/topics/bbp/genres.html. Accessed December 6, 2016.
12. Occupational Safety and Health Administration. *OSHA fact sheet: hepatitis B vaccination protection.* https://www.osha.gov/OshDoc/data_BloodborneFacts/bbfact05.pdf. Accessed December 6, 2016.

Prep Kit *(continued)*

13. Centers for Disease Control and Prevention. *Recommended Vaccines for Healthcare Workers.* http://www.cdc.gov/vaccines/adults/rec-vac/hcw.html. Accessed December 6, 2016.
14. Centers for Disease Control and Prevention. *2016 Recommended Immunizations for Children From Birth Through 6 Years Old.* https://www.cdc.gov/vaccines/parents/downloads/parent-ver-sch-0-6yrs.pdf. Accessed December 1, 2016.
15. Centers for Disease Control and Prevention. *2016 Recommended Immunizations for Children 7-18 Years Old.* https://www.cdc.gov/vaccines/who/teens/downloads/parent-version-schedule-7-18yrs.pdf. Accessed December 1, 2016.
16. Centers for Disease Control and Prevention. *10 Leading Causes of Death by Age Group, United States—2015.* https://www.cdc.gov/injury/wisqars/LeadingCauses.html. Accessed September 22, 2017.
17. Centers for Disease Control and Prevention. *Injury prevention and control: data and statistics: key injury and violence data.* http://www.cdc.gov/injury/wisqars/overview/key_data.html. Accessed October 28, 2016.
18. Centers for Disease Control and Prevention. *Emergency department visits.* http://www.cdc.gov/nchs/fastats/emergency-department.htm. Accessed October 31, 2016.
19. Department of Transportation, Pipeline and Hazardous Materials Safety Administration. *Emergency response guidebook.* http://www.phmsa.dot.gov/hazmat/library/erg. Accessed October 28, 2016.
20. Department of Transportation, Pipeline and Hazardous Materials Safety Administration. *ERG 2016 mobile app.* http://www.phmsa.dot.gov/hazmat/erg-mobile-app. Accessed October 28, 2016.
21. Alarie Y. Toxicity of fire smoke. *Crit Rev Toxicol.* 2002;32(4):259-289. https://www.ncbi.nlm.nih.gov/pubmed/12184505/. Accessed December 5, 2016.
22. Stull JO, Grace G. *New revised requirements for emergency medical protective clothing.* FireRescue1.com. https://www.firerescue1.com/fire-products/apparel/boots/articles/333642-New-Revised-Requirements-for-Emergency-Medical-Protective-Clothing/. Accessed December 27, 2016.
23. American National Standards Institute. *Z96-15: High-visibility safety apparel. 2015.* http://webstore.ansi.org/RecordDetail.aspx?sku=CSA+Z96-2015. Accessed October 28, 2016.
24. National Institute of Justice. *Body Armor.* https://www.nij.gov/topics/technology/body-armor/pages/welcome.aspx. Accessed December 27, 2016.
25. National Institute of Justice. Ballistic Resistance of Body Armor, NIJ Standard 0101.06. https://www.ncjrs.gov/pdffiles1/nij/223054.pdf#page=17. Accessed December 27, 2016.
26. Newland C, Barber E, Rose M, Young A. Survey reveals alarming rates of EMS provider stress and thoughts of suicide. *J Emerg Med Serv.* September 28, 2015. http://www.jems.com/articles/print/volume-40/issue-10/features/survey-reveals-alarming-rates-of-ems-provider-stress-and-thoughts-of-suicide.html. Accessed November 1, 2016.
27. Centers for Disease Control and Prevention. Facts at a glance: suicide. 2015. http://www.cdc.gov/violenceprevention/pdf/suicide-datasheet-a.pdf. Accessed November 1, 2016.
28. United States Department of Agriculture. *My Plate.* https://www.cnpp.usda.gov/MyPlate. Accessed December 5, 2016.
29. American Heart Association. *American Heart Association Recommendations for Physical Activity in Adults.* http://www.heart.org/HEARTORG/HealthyLiving/PhysicalActivity/FitnessBasics/American-Heart-Association-Recommendations-for-Physical-Activity-in-Adults_UCM_307976_Article.jsp#. Accessed December 5, 2016.
30. Division of Sleep Medicine, Harvard Medical School. *Why Sleep Matters: Sleep, Performance, and Public Safety.* http://healthysleep.med.harvard.edu/healthy/matters/consequences/sleep-performance-and-public-safety. Accessed December 27, 2016.
31. Equal Employment Opportunity Commission. Facts about sexual harassment. June 27, 2002. https://www.eeoc.gov/facts/fs-sex.html. Accessed October 28, 2016.
32. Kochanek KD, Murphy SL, Xu J, Tejada-Vera B. Deaths: final data for 2014. *Natl Vital Stat Rep.* 2016;65(4). http://www.cdc.gov/nchs/data/nvsr/nvsr65/nvsr65_04.pdf. Accessed October 31, 2016.
33. Centers for Disease Control and Prevention. *10 Leading Causes of Death by Age Group, 2014.* http://www.cdc.gov/injury/wisqars/pdf/leading_causes_of_death_by_age_group_2014-a.pdf. Accessed December 5, 2016.
34. Kübler-Ross E. *On Death and Dying.* New York, NY: Macmillan; 1969.

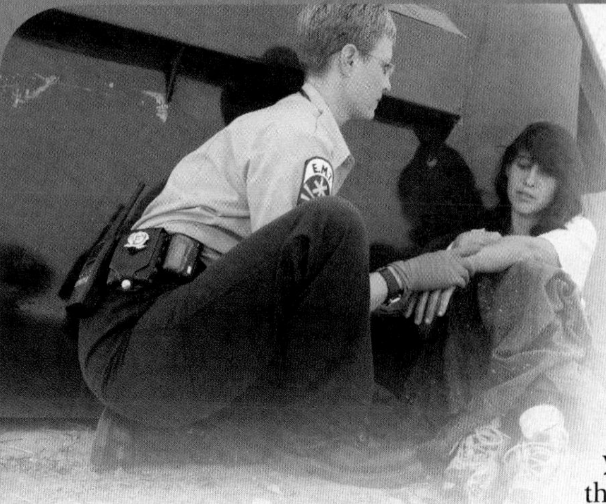

Assessment *in Action*

You are transporting a 43-year-old woman with a complaint of abdominal pain to the local emergency department for evaluation. En route, you elect to establish IV access. Just as you are withdrawing the IV catheter from the patient, your partner hits a pothole in the road, and you accidently stick yourself with a dirty needle. As you mumble under your breath, the patient looks at you and states that she has hepatitis C.

1. This type of transmission is a result of which of the following?

A. Indirect contact
B. Direct contact
C. Airborne transmission
D. Foodborne transmission

2. To reduce the risk of needlestick injuries, you should do all of the following EXCEPT:

A. inform your partner that you are starting an IV line.
B. inform the patient that he or she should hold as still as possible while you attempt the IV line.
C. recap the needle as soon as it is removed from the patient.
D. use IV catheters with a protective mechanism.

3. Hepatitis C is transmitted via sexual contact and:

A. cerebrospinal fluid.
B. urine.
C. saliva.
D. blood.

4. When you have been exposed to a patient's blood or other body fluids, what is the first action you should take, if possible?

A. Go to the emergency department.
B. Wash your hands with soap and water.
C. Activate your agency's infection control plan.
D. Turn over care to another provider.

5. In this case, ______________ is the vehicle for transmission of the pathogen.

A. blood
B. sexual contact
C. saliva
D. urine

6. How often should EMS providers receive a tuberculosis skin test?

A. Once
B. Every 6 months
C. Every year
D. Every 5 years

7. ______________ involves spreading an infectious agent through mechanisms such as droplets or dust.

A. Indirect contact
B. Direct contact
C. Airborne transmission
D. Foodborne transmission

Assessment *in Action* *(continued)*

8. Lyme disease is spread by which route of transmission?

A. Direct
B. Foodborne
C. Airborne
D. Vector-borne

9. What are the warning signs of a lightning strike, and what should you do to protect yourself if such an event is imminent?

10. Patients, family members, friends, and others may all go through the grieving process during a time of death or other serious incident. List the five stages of grief.

CHAPTER 3

Medical, Legal, and Ethical Issues

National EMS Education Standard Competencies

Preparatory

Applies fundamental knowledge of the EMS system, safety/well-being of the AEMT, medical/legal and ethical issues to the provision of emergency care.

Medical/Legal and Ethics

- Consent/refusal of care (pp 83-88)
- Confidentiality (p 91)
- Advance directives (pp 88-89)
- Tort and criminal actions (pp 79-82)
- Evidence preservation (p 93)
- Statutory responsibilities (pp 75-79)
- Mandatory reporting (pp 92-93)
- Ethical principles/moral obligations (pp 89-91)
- End-of-life issues (pp 83-84, 88-89, 93-95)

Knowledge Objectives

1. Discuss the scope of practice and standards of care that are imposed on you as an advanced emergency medical technician (AEMT). (pp 75-79)
2. Differentiate between licensure and certification as they apply to your practice as an AEMT. (p 79)
3. Discuss the four factors that determine negligence. (pp 80-81)
4. Describe your legal duty to act. (p 80)
5. Discuss the issues of abandonment, assault, battery, kidnapping, and false imprisonment, including the implications for you as an AEMT. (pp 81-82)
6. Compare defamation, slander, and libel. (p 82)
7. Describe situations in which Good Samaritan laws or immunity would apply. (pp 82-83)
8. Define consent, including how it relates to decision-making capacity. (p 83)
9. Compare expressed consent, informed consent, implied consent, and involuntary consent. (pp 84-86)
10. Discuss consent by minors for treatment or transport. (pp 85-86)
11. Describe local emergency medical services (EMS) system protocols for using forcible restraint. (pp 86-87)
12. Explain your role and obligations if a patient refuses treatment or transport. (pp 87-88)
13. Discuss the importance of do not resuscitate orders and local protocols as they relate to the EMS environment. (pp 88-89)
14. Describe ethics and morality, including the implications for you as an AEMT. (pp 89-91)
15. Describe the relationship between patient communications, confidentiality, and the Health Insurance Portability and Accountability Act (HIPAA). (p 91)
16. Explain the mandatory reporting requirements for special situations, including abuse or neglect, drug- or felony-related injuries, childbirth, and crime scenes. (pp 92-93)
17. Describe the presumptive and definitive signs of death. (pp 93-94)
18. Explain how to manage patients who are identified as organ donors. (p 95)
19. Explain the importance of medical identification devices in treating the patient. (p 95)

Skills Objectives

There are no skills objectives for this chapter.

Introduction

A basic principle of emergency care is to do no harm. **Emergency medical care**, or immediate care or treatment, is often provided by emergency medical services (EMS) personnel, who may be the first link in the chain of prehospital care. As the scope and nature of emergency medical care becomes more complex and EMS becomes more widely available, litigation involving EMS systems will no doubt increase. All medical professionals provide care under laws. As an advanced emergency medical technician (AEMT), you too will be governed by a set of laws affecting how you treat patients. Providing competent emergency medical care that conforms with the standards of care taught to you will help you to avoid civil and criminal actions.

You must also consider ethical issues. Ethics are principles, either personal or societal, that determine what is right and wrong (discussed in more detail later in this chapter). For example, as an AEMT, should you stop and treat patients who were involved in a motor vehicle crash while you are en route to another emergency call? Should you begin cardiopulmonary resuscitation (CPR) on a patient who, according to the family, has terminal cancer? Should you release patient information to a patient's attorney over the telephone?

One of the major differences between laws and ethics is that laws have sanctions for violations that are enforceable. Laws define your obligations and protect your rights and the rights of others. It is essential, therefore, that you have a basic understanding of laws and ethics applicable to prehospital emergency care. Failure to perform your job within the law can result in civil or even criminal liability (responsibility). Practicing outside the law may also result in regulatory action within your state—for example, a disciplinary hearing or action by your EMS agency and medical director.

Consider the following situations:

- You are transporting a patient, and while the stretcher is being loaded into the ambulance, your partner slips, the stretcher crashes to the ground, and the patient is injured.
- You are about to begin treating a child, and the father commands you to stop.

What should you do? Even when you properly render emergency medical care, at times you may be sued by a patient who seeks to obtain relief, often in the form of a monetary award, for loss of income or pain and suffering. Or, administrative action, such as suspension of your state license or AEMT certificate, may be brought against you for failure to abide by the regulations of your state EMS agency. For these reasons, you must understand the various legal aspects of emergency medical care.

This chapter reviews important legal and ethical concepts affecting your practice as an AEMT and provides the framework to help you understand these issues. However, this text cannot substitute for competent legal advice because many laws and legal obligations differ from state to state. Contact an attorney who specializes in the representation of medical professionals if you need legal advice related to your practice.

Scope of Practice

The **scope of practice** for AEMTs, which is most commonly defined by state law, outlines the boundaries for the emergency medical care you are permitted to provide for the patient. This care is based on generally accepted standards. Your medical director further defines the scope of practice by developing **protocols** (precise and detailed plans for a regimen of therapy) and **standing orders** (local protocols, usually pertaining to a particular service or area). The medical director gives you the legal authorization to provide patient care through telephone or radio communication (online medical control) or standing orders and protocols (off-line medical control). It is your responsibility as an AEMT to know your scope of practice and follow it.

Words of Wisdom

Treat all your patients in a kind and professional manner—the way you would like members of your own family to be treated. This courtesy is important to the patient, and it can also decrease the chance of a lawsuit being brought against you.

YOU are the Provider — PART 1

You respond to a patient who has fallen. On arrival, you find an older man who states that he tripped over a lamp cord, striking his head on the corner of a table. The patient denies any pain or loss of consciousness. You note a laceration to his forehead, which you believe will require stitches. When you inform the patient of the need for medical treatment and transport, he advises you that he does not want to go to the hospital because he cannot afford the ambulance ride.

1. Can this patient refuse treatment when it is obvious that he needs stitches?
2. What can you and your partner do to attempt to persuade this patient to consent to treatment and transport?

If you carry out a procedure for which you are not authorized, then you are practicing outside your scope of practice. This action may be considered negligence (discussed later in this chapter) or, in some states, even a criminal offense (considered practicing medicine without a license). Do not confuse the scope of practice with the standard of care (discussed next).

You and other EMS providers have a legal responsibility to provide proper, consistent patient care and to report problems—such as possible liability or exposure to airborne or bloodborne pathogens or infectious disease—to your medical director immediately.

Standards of Care

The law requires you to act or behave toward other people in a certain, definable way, regardless of the activity involved. Under given circumstances, you have a legal duty to act or not (discussed later in this chapter). Generally, you must be concerned about the safety and welfare of others when your behavior or activities have the potential for causing others injury or harm **Figure 3-1**. The manner in which you are required to act or behave as an AEMT is called the **standard of care**.

The standard of care is established in many ways, among them published medical literature, local customs, statutes, ordinances, administrative regulations, protocols, and case law. In addition, professional and institutional standards have a bearing on determining the adequacy of your conduct.

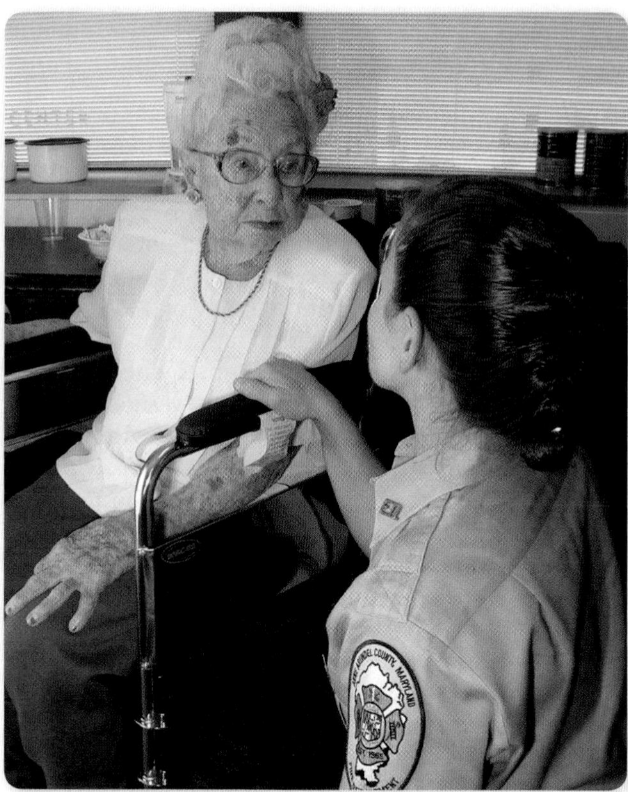

Figure 3-1 Act or behave toward others in a way that shows your concern for their safety and welfare.

Words of Wisdom

If you must deviate from the standard of care due to extenuating circumstances, then your best protection against legal action is good documentation. For example, if you place a patient with severe respiratory distress on a nasal cannula because he will not tolerate a nonrebreathing mask or bag-mask device, then provide a detailed explanation in the narrative portion of your patient care report (PCR).

Standards Imposed by Local Custom

The standard of care is how a reasonably prudent person with similar training and experience would act under similar circumstances (that is, with similar equipment and in the same or a similar place). For example, the conduct of an AEMT who is employed by an ambulance service would be judged in comparison with the expected conduct of other AEMTs from comparable ambulance services in the same geographic area. These standards are often based on locally accepted protocols. The prevailing custom of the community is an important element in determining the standard of emergency medical care required. Examples of prevailing customs include determining when EMS helicopters are used, how hospital destinations are selected, and protocols for spinal immobilization.

As an AEMT, you will not be held to the same standard of care as physicians or other more highly trained professionals. In addition, your conduct must be judged in the context of the given emergency situation, taking into consideration the following factors:

- Any issues concerning the safety of the patient or rescuer
- General confusion at the scene of the emergency
- The needs of other patients
- The type of equipment available

In this context, an **emergency** is a serious situation, such as injury or illness that arises suddenly, threatens the life or welfare of a person or group of people, and requires immediate intervention **Figure 3-2**.

Standards Imposed by Law

In addition to local customs, standards of emergency medical care may be imposed by statutes, ordinances, administrative regulation, or case law. In many jurisdictions, violating one of these standards is said to create *presumptive negligence*. Therefore, become familiar with the particular legal standards that may exist in your state. In many states, the standards may take the form of treatment protocols published by a state agency.

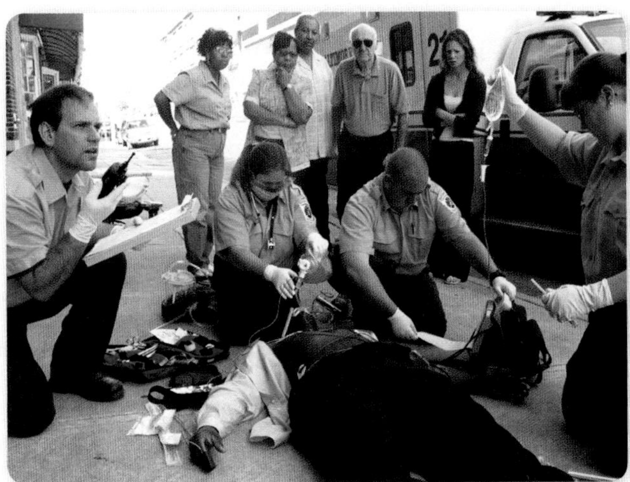

Figure 3-2 An emergency is a serious situation that arises suddenly, threatens the life or welfare of one or more people, and requires immediate intervention.

Emergency Medical Treatment and Active Labor Act (EMTALA)

The **Emergency Medical Treatment and Active Labor Act (EMTALA)** was enacted in 1986 to combat the practice of so-called patient dumping and pays particular attention to the practice of sending women in labor to distant hospitals. Patient dumping occurs when hospital emergency department (ED) staff deny medical screening or stabilizing treatment, or when staff inappropriately transfer a person whose condition is unstable. Historically, most patient dumping occurred when hospital staff discovered that the patient did not have health insurance or was otherwise unable to pay. In recent years, *economic triage* has been introduced. This term refers to the practice of making health care decisions based on the ability of the patient or the insurance carrier to provide payment for services. Although such considerations may have a place in certain aspects of the health care field, an EMS provider should never make a decision to treat or transport based on financial considerations, regardless of the current financial state of the EMS employer. As an AEMT, your only consideration should be the needs of the patient; reimbursement issues should be addressed by billing personnel. EMS providers have occasionally been accused of providing a lower standard of care for indigent people or those on public assistance; therefore, make sure that financial status never becomes a deciding factor in your practice. Always provide the highest possible quality of emergency medical care to all patients regardless of their financial status.

As an AEMT, it is also important that you have a clear understanding of local protocols regarding the choice of hospitals to which you may transfer your patient. In some rural areas, only one hospital may be available, but in other places several options may be available. Some EMS systems simply require you to transfer the patient to the nearest hospital. In other systems, however, protocols dictate that hospital selection must be based on the specific needs of the patient. For example, some patients may require the services of a trauma center, a children's hospital, or a hospital with cardiac catheterization capabilities. Depending on local protocols, you may be able to make the choice of destination alone, whereas in others you may be required to consult with medical control in making such decisions. It is important to become familiar with the protocols in your area of practice.

EMTALA issues are regulated by the Centers for Medicare and Medicaid Services (CMS) and carry severe monetary penalties—up to and including loss of Medicare funding—for hospitals that fail to comply.[1] The CMS also issues severe fines for hospitals and physicians who violate EMTALA provisions. In addition, EMTALA further allows private citizens to sue for violations of the act. Under most circumstances, neither an ambulance service nor an AEMT can be sued or charged with a violation under EMTALA. An ambulance service that is owned by a hospital, however, may be subject to a claim under EMTALA in certain cases.

EMTALA guarantees a medical screening exam, and treatment to stabilize any emergency medical conditions found, to any patient presenting to a hospital that has an ED. It prohibits discrimination for any reason, including the ability to pay. Some urgent care centers may also be covered by EMTALA. Although EMTALA does not directly regulate EMS providers, EMS is often the vehicle—both figuratively and literally—by which patient dumping takes place.

Words of Wisdom

EMTALA legislation requires that every patient must receive emergency medical treatment—regardless of his or her ability to pay for medical treatment when it is received.

EMTALA also regulates patient transfers and applies to both the sending and receiving facilities. Never transfer a patient who needs emergency medical care that falls outside your scope of practice. You must feel comfortable that the patient is stable enough to transfer. A transferring hospital staff has an obligation to ensure the transferring ambulance and crew are capable of meeting the needs of the patient during transfer, and should request an ambulance that is appropriately staffed and equipped. It would be a potential EMTALA violation if hospital staff requested a basic life support (BLS) ambulance and crew to transport a patient with a serious cardiac condition who required cardiac monitoring and the administration of medication during the transport. Should a patient need a higher level of care, it is the responsibility of the transferring hospital to provide someone to ride along (a nurse, respiratory therapist, or even a physician). Make sure you have received all appropriate paperwork before leaving on a patient transfer, including all pertinent medical records, laboratory results, radiographs, and other documents. When you arrive at the receiving hospital, that hospital staff should have a bed ready for the patient, after agreeing to accept the patient.

▶ Professional or Institutional Standards

In addition to standards imposed by law, professional or institutional standards may be used as evidence in determining the adequacy of your conduct as an AEMT. Professional standards include recommendations published by organizations and societies that are involved in emergency medical care. For example, consider the standard of care for BLS and CPR Figure 3-3. In the past, the American Heart Association (AHA), in concert with the International Liaison Committee on Resuscitation, came together to revise the *Guidelines for Cardiopulmonary Resuscitation and Emergency Cardiac Care* every 5 years. However, it was recognized in the 2015 guidelines that a 5-year cycle is insufficient to keep pace with the rapidly evolving research in resuscitation science, and you should expect to see updates released more frequently in the future.

Institutional standards include specific rules and procedures of the EMS system, ambulance service, or organization with which you are affiliated. Be familiar with the standards of your organization. The standards formulated for a particular agency should be reasonable and realistic so that they do not impose an unreasonable burden on EMS providers. Providing the best emergency medical care should be your goal as an AEMT, but it is unrealistic to have institutional standards that demand the best care.

Ordinary care is a minimum standard of care. In general, it is expected that anyone who offers assistance during an emergency will exercise reasonable care and act prudently. If you act reasonably, according to the standard practices you have been trained to use, then you can likely avoid liability. If you deviate from these standards, then you may be liable for civil action and possibly criminal prosecution (discussed later in this chapter). In addition, state regulatory agencies that oversee EMS operations can sanction you for deviating from the standard of care.

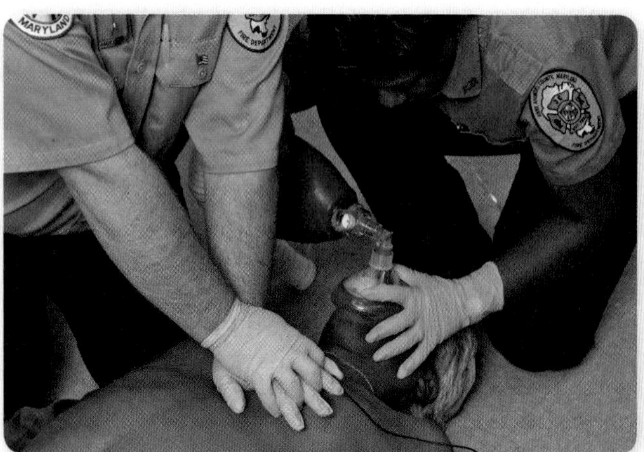

Figure 3-3 Many standards of care are imposed on you as an AEMT, such as those for performing cardiopulmonary resuscitation. Learn the standards of care for your level of training and organization.

▶ Standards Imposed by Textbooks

In the course of a lawsuit, an attorney will often ask an AEMT if he or she recognizes various textbooks as being authoritative works in the field of EMS. Because virtually all EMS textbooks follow standards established by the National Highway Transportation Safety Administration, these textbooks are often recognized as contributing to the standard of care that is followed by AEMTs. Local protocols or state standards may differ from material presented in textbooks. When such differences occur, you are bound to follow local protocols.

▶ EMS-Enabling Legislation

Most states now have what is called EMS-enabling legislation, which defines how EMS is structured and designates responsibilities to government agencies. These laws also provide the state-based framework for the AEMT's actual practice—what you are permitted to do in the field. For example, EMS legislation may define the need for a medical director and may also define the scope of practice for the different levels of EMS personnel. Familiarize yourself with the EMS legislation in your state and any regulations that flow from those statutes.

▶ Standards Imposed by States

Individual states have their own requirements for licensure or certification (discussed next). Most states now recognize the National Registry of Emergency Medical Technicians as their certifying agency; however, check with the state in which you work to learn its specifications. An overview of this process follows.

Medical Practices Act

The practice of medicine is defined as the diagnosis and treatment of disease or illness. In some states, EMS personnel are exempt from the licensure requirements of the Medical Practices Act because an AEMT is regarded as a nonmedical professional. This act usually defines the minimum qualifications of those who may perform various health services, defines the skills that each type of practitioner is legally permitted to use, and establishes a means of licensure or certification for different categories of health care professionals. Requirements for relicensure or recertification based on continuing education and other factors may also be included in the Medical Practice Act.[2] As an AEMT, you must be aware of the standards established by legislation in your state so that you can provide emergency medical care that is consistent with those standards.

When you are unsure of the proper care, always contact medical control for orders. Question any order that is unclear or seems inappropriate. Do not blindly follow an order that is incorrect or does not make sense to you. The physician may have misunderstood or may have missed part of the report. In that case, he or she may not be able to respond appropriately to the patient's needs.

Certification and Licensure

Some states provide certification or licensure of people who perform emergency medical care. These terms are often confused. **Certification** is the process by which an individual, institution, or program is evaluated and recognized as meeting certain predetermined standards to ensure safe and ethical patient care. It generally refers to a certain level of credentials based on hours of training and assessment exams and addresses criteria met for a minimum competency. Certification may be granted by a government agency or by a private organization such as the AHA or the American Red Cross. The fact that you have received a certification from a private organization does not necessarily mean that you have authority to practice the skills included in that certification. **Licensure** is the process by which a competent authority, usually the state, grants permission to practice a job, trade, or profession. A license itself is a privilege granted by a government authority on certain conditions. You must comply with the government's requirements for professional behavior, continuing education, and licensure renewal, or risk losing that privilege. The rights and privileges conferred by licensing in one state may not be conferred in other states.

Another concept that you may encounter is that of **credentialing**. Credentialing is an established process to determine the qualifications necessary to be allowed to practice a particular profession or to function as an organization. Credentialing may be adopted by a specific EMS agency as part of its employment requirements. For example, although you may be licensed as an AEMT by your state, the agency for which you are seeking work may impose additional requirements as part of its eligibility standards. Common examples include certification in CPR or trauma.

Words of Wisdom

Medical control consists of the physician at the receiving facility who answers your call and provides guidance for patient care or allows you to administer certain medications that are within your scope of practice. Always echo (repeat) orders back to ensure complete understanding on both parts and do not blindly follow orders that seem inappropriate for your patient.

Negligence

Negligence is the failure to provide the same care that a person with similar training would provide in the same or similar situation. It is a deviation from the accepted standard of care that may result in further injury to the patient. Some states differentiate between ordinary negligence and gross negligence. **Gross negligence** is defined as conduct that constitutes a willful or reckless disregard for a duty or standard of care.

Negligence is commonly divided into three categories: (1) malfeasance, (2) misfeasance, and (3) nonfeasance. **Malfeasance** occurs if you perform an act that you are not authorized to do, such as a medical intervention that is outside of the scope of practice. **Misfeasance** occurs if you perform an act that you are legally permitted to do, but you do so in an improper manner. For example, you administer a medication that is clearly within the scope of practice, but you accidentally calculate an incorrect dose. **Nonfeasance** occurs if you fail to perform an act that you are required or expected to perform. Failure to perform CPR when a patient goes into cardiac arrest would be an example of nonfeasance.

In some cases, negligence may be so obvious that it does not require extensive proof. **Res ipsa loquitur** is Latin for "the thing speaks for itself." Under this theory, the injury could only have been caused by negligence. For example, if you drop the stretcher while the patient is unresponsive and the patient sustains an injury, then the patient may prevail in a lawsuit against you by showing that he was under your care, that he sustained an injury, and that his injury would not have occurred unless negligence was present.

In rare cases, the theory of **negligence per se** may be used if the conduct of the person being sued is alleged to have occurred in clear violation of a statute. For example, if you were to perform a paramedic skill, such as endotracheal intubation, the plaintiff might allege that this act was negligence per se. In that case, the plaintiff would not have to establish the circumstances surrounding your conduct. He or she would not need to show that the procedure was inappropriate because you clearly exceeded your scope of practice as an AEMT.

A legal action of that sort is called a **civil lawsuit**—that is, an action instituted by a private person or entity (the **plaintiff**) against another private person or entity (the **defendant**)—and the wrongful act that gives rise to a civil lawsuit is called a **tort**. All forms of negligence come under this general category of law. The law recognizes two classifications of torts: unintentional torts (commonly referred to as negligence) and intentional torts (those that describe an intent to cause harm). Torts are simply defined as civil wrongs and are not within the jurisdiction of the criminal courts. Examples of tort actions other than negligence are lawsuits for defamation of character and invasion of privacy (discussed later in this chapter).

> **Words of Wisdom**
>
> Contributory negligence is a legal defense that may be raised when the defendant feels that the plaintiff has done something that contributed to his or her own injuries. For example, you are treating a patient with chest pain and you feel that the administration of aspirin is indicated. You ask the patient if he is allergic to aspirin and he says no. Shortly after you administer the aspirin, the patient develops the signs and symptoms of a severe allergic reaction. Later in the hospital, the physician advises you that the patient's medical history indicates that the patient has an allergy to aspirin. The patient states that he forgot he was allergic to aspirin. In this case, the defense of contributory negligence might be raised because it was the patient's forgetfulness and his denial of an aspirin allergy that contributed to his allergic reaction.

Determination of negligence is based on the following four factors:

1. Duty
2. Breach of duty
3. Damages
4. Proximate cause

All four elements must be present for the legal doctrine of negligence to apply and for the plaintiff to prevail in a lawsuit against an EMS system or provider. These elements are discussed in more detail in the following sections.

▶ Duty

Duty is prescribed by law. It is an obligation to provide patient care in a manner that is consistent with the standard of care established by training and local protocols. Responsibility comes from either statute or function. A bystander is under no obligation to assist a stranger in distress and therefore has no legal duty to act. Instances in which you have a legal duty to act may include the following:

- You are dispatched to or witness an emergency situation while on duty.
- The policy of your service or department states that you must assist in any emergency.

After your ambulance responds to a call or treatment is initiated, you have a legal duty to act. In most cases, if you are off duty and come upon a crash, then you are not legally obligated to stop and assist patients. However, laws vary from state to state. Be familiar with the laws and policies that apply in your service area. If you choose to intervene while off duty, then continue to provide competent care until a medical professional with an equal or higher level of training assumes care of the patient.

Most services have a policy addressing the discovery of another incident while en route to a call or en route to the hospital with a patient. The key to legal duty is to make sure the appropriate personnel are dispatched if you cannot stop to render assistance due to the severity of the patient you are currently treating.

▶ Breach of Duty

The second element a patient must prove for a lawsuit to be successful is that the AEMT failed to perform within the standard of care. A **breach of duty** occurs when the person accused of negligence failed to act as another person with similar training would have acted under the same or similar circumstances. Breach of duty may involve doing less than the person was trained to do (an error of omission; ie, an AEMT who fails to splint an injured extremity) or doing more than the person was trained to do (an error of commission; ie, an AEMT who sutures a laceration when doing so is not within the scope of practice).

In a lawsuit, a jury will listen to the testimony of expert witnesses on both sides and ultimately decide whether your care was reasonable or not. These expert witnesses will provide a number of sources on which to base their testimony about whether your care was reasonable. Those sources will include their own training and experience; your training, experience, and continuing education; textbooks; protocols; national standards; standard operating procedures; and the patient care report (PCR). Good documentation will go a long way to prove your high standards of care.

▶ Damages

The objective of a civil lawsuit is usually some sort of compensation (**damages**) when a patient is physically or psychologically harmed in some noticeable way. Although physical injury is usually part of any lawsuit for medical negligence, patients may also claim damages for emotional distress, loss of income, loss of enjoyment of life, loss of spousal consortium, loss of household services, and loss of future earning capacity. Patients will have to show that your actions were proximate causes of each of these losses.

▶ Proximate Cause

A reasonable cause-and-effect relationship must exist between the breach of duty and the injury sustained by the patient. **Proximate cause** is a legal term that, in the sense of medical malpractice, essentially considers whether the alleged harm to the patient would have occurred "but for" the negligent act. If the injury would have still occurred regardless of the alleged act of malpractice, then no valid claim exists.[3]

If you have a legal duty to act and abuse it, causing harm to another individual, then you, your EMS agency, and/or medical director may be sued for negligence. Even in cases in which the AEMT had a legal duty to the patient, and the AEMT breached the standard of care, a plaintiff must still link the act that fell below the standard of care directly to his or her injury by showing that the act (or failure to act) proximately caused the harm. Proving that an act or a failure to act caused an injury is the most difficult part of a lawsuit. For example, imagine that you are treating a patient from a motor vehicle crash who has a spinal cord injury and you drop the stretcher during patient care. The patient may try to show that his or her spinal cord injury resulted from the dropped stretcher and not from the crash itself. In such a case, careful documentation of the patient's neurologic status at the time you first encountered the patient would be essential to your defense.

Abandonment

Abandonment is a form of negligence that involves the termination of emergency medical care without the patient's consent. (Consent is discussed later in this chapter.) The term also implies that the patient had a continuing need for medical treatment and that the abrupt termination of treatment was the cause of subsequent injury or death. Therefore, after you have initiated patient care, you have assumed a duty that must not cease until an equally competent person with an equal or higher level of training assumes responsibility (that is, another AEMT, a paramedic, nurse, or physician). Abandonment is a legally and ethically serious matter that exposes the patient to harm and can result in civil action against you.

For example, suppose you arrive at the scene of a single-car crash and begin emergency medical care of two injured patients. A passerby tells you of a two-car collision farther down the road in which five people are injured. You turn over care of the two injured patients from the first crash to the passerby and leave to go to the other collision site. Abandonment has occurred because you did not turn over the care of the patients to a person with a level of training equal to or higher than yours. Consider the following general questions when you are faced with making a decision such as this one:

- What consequences may develop from your actions?
- How might the patient's condition worsen if you leave?
- Does the patient need emergency medical care?
- Are you neglecting your duty to your patient?
- Is the person assuming care capable of providing the level of care needed by the patient?
- Are you abandoning the patient if you leave the scene?
- Are you violating a standard of care?
- Are you acting prudently?

Surprisingly, abandonment may also take place in the ED where you drop off your patient. A part of your obligation as an AEMT is to provide hospital personnel with a report of your assessment findings, the emergency medical care you provided, and any changes in patient status that occurred during transport to the hospital. The failure to file a PCR could result in a delay in treatment or a misdiagnosis. In such a case, a claim for abandonment could be filed against you. It is always a good idea to obtain a signature on your PCR from the person accepting transfer of care at the hospital. This step will help protect you from allegations of abandonment.

Words of Wisdom

A mass-casualty incident during which you perform triage does not constitute abandonment. The nature of triage is to do the most good for the greatest number of people, accomplished by a simple, rapid evaluation and categorization. Triage is discussed further in Chapter 41, *Incident Management.*

Assault, Battery, Kidnapping, and False Imprisonment

Sometimes the same allegedly wrongful or harmful act that gave rise to a lawsuit may also result in criminal prosecution. A **criminal prosecution** is an action taken by the government against a person the prosecutors feel has violated criminal laws. In a criminal case, the government must prove guilt beyond all reasonable doubt to a jury. If the government succeeds, then the defendant can be fined, imprisoned, or both.

The criminal laws most likely to apply to prehospital care include assault, battery, kidnapping, and false imprisonment. Examples of these actions include using improper restraining methods, making physical contact with a patient before asking for permission from the patient, or transporting a patient without his or her consent.

- **Assault** is defined as threatening a person or causing a person fear of immediate bodily harm without the person's consent—regardless of whether the threat of harm is actually carried out. Threatening to start an intravenous (IV) line on a patient using a large needle, or threatening to restrain a patient who does not want to be transported, may be considered assault.
- **Battery** is unlawfully touching another person. Making physical contact with a patient before asking if you may touch him or her may be considered battery. Just about any act of medical treatment performed without consent may be considered assault or battery or both, because such acts constitute a threat to the patient's bodily security ("Now I'm going to stick you with this needle . . .") and an unsanctioned contact with the patient's body. Assault and battery can be either civil or criminal in nature. To prosecute a criminal charge of assault or battery, the prosecution generally needs to prove the intent to cause harm. In a civil case, the plaintiff need only establish that the conduct took place without his or her consent.

- **Kidnapping** is the seizing, confining, abducting, or carrying away of a person by force. In theory, this might include a situation where a patient is transported against his or her will. Criminal charges of false imprisonment or kidnapping are rarely filed against EMS providers. Civil lawsuits alleging false imprisonment or kidnapping are more common and usually arise out of circumstances in which the patient claims to have been transported or restrained against his or her will. In reality, criminal charges of kidnapping are almost unheard of in EMS because the EMS provider is almost always acting in a good faith effort to provide care to the patient. It is far more likely that an EMS provider could be the target of a civil lawsuit for false imprisonment.
- **False imprisonment** is defined as the unauthorized confinement of a person that lasts for an appreciable period. Consider a patient who withdraws consent during transport and demands to be let out of the ambulance. If you refuse, then you may be accused of false imprisonment. Your best protection against these charges is to obtain informed consent for almost everything you do (discussed later in this chapter). Consult your medical director if you have questions or doubts about a specific situation.

Defamation, Slander, and Libel

As an AEMT, you may also be sued for **defamation**, which is intentionally making a false statement through written or verbal communication that injures a person's good name or reputation. **Libel** is making a false statement in the written form that injures a person's good name (reputation or standing in the community). When you write your PCR, avoid using terms that may be considered judgmental or offensive, such as "The patient appears to be drunk." Instead, use descriptions such as "The patient walks with an unsteady gait," or "The patient's words were slurred." Whatever your personal views, think about the way in which your PCR would read in court. Do not let thoughtless comments become evidence against you.

Slander is making a false verbal statement that injures a person's good name. Once again, avoid using terms that could be considered judgmental or offensive to the patient when you are passing along prehospital care information to ED personnel. Always keep in mind that your patient is someone's son or daughter, husband or wife, brother or sister, or father or mother. Consider how you would like information about members of your own family to be presented to the hospital staff.

Good Samaritan Laws and Immunity

All states have **Good Samaritan laws**, which are based on the common law principle that when you reasonably help another person, you should not be liable for errors and omissions that are made while giving good faith emergency medical care. However, Good Samaritan laws do not necessarily protect you from a lawsuit. Good Samaritan provisions vary significantly from state to state. For example, some laws provide Good Samaritan protection for anyone who stops to render aid during an emergency, whereas other laws only provide protection for those with no medical training. Good Samaritan statutes in some jurisdictions provide **immunity** from a lawsuit, whereas others provide an affirmative defense if you are sued for rendering care. In most cases, Good Samaritan laws do not prohibit the filing of a lawsuit, nor do they pertain to acts that could be considered wanton, gross, or willful negligence, or if care is provided for remuneration (any sort of payment, monetary or otherwise).

Words of Wisdom

To be protected by the provisions of a Good Samaritan law, you must meet several conditions:

1. You acted in good faith in rendering care.
2. You rendered care without expectation of compensation.
3. You acted within your scope of practice.
4. You did not act in a grossly negligent manner.

Another group of laws grants immunity from liability to official EMS providers in specific circumstances. These laws, which vary from state to state, do not provide immunity when injury or damage is caused by gross negligence or willful misconduct. In most cases, immunity statutes apply to EMS systems that are considered government agencies.

An abiding principle of English law is that you cannot sue the queen (or king) because "the queen can do no wrong." In the United States, this concept, called sovereign immunity, has taken the form of legislation that identifies only limited types of lawsuits that can be filed against government agencies. EMS personnel working for government agencies, such as a fire department, also have some **governmental immunity** for their actions. Governmental immunity generally applies only to EMS systems that are operated by municipalities or other government entities. If your service is covered by immunity, then it may mean that you cannot be sued at all, or it may limit the amount of the monetary judgment that the plaintiff may recover. State laws vary significantly. Understand the laws that apply in your state.

The **statute of limitations**, which limits the number of years after an incident during which a lawsuit can be filed, may also aid in protecting you from litigation. It is set by law, may differ for cases involving adults and children, and varies from state to state.

Most states have also adopted specific laws granting special privileges to EMS personnel, authorizing them to perform certain medical procedures. Many states also grant partial immunity to EMS providers, physicians, and nurses who give emergency instructions to EMS personnel via radio or other forms of communication. Consult your medical director or state EMS agency for more information about the laws in your area.

Words of Wisdom

The AEMT in Court

The **discovery** phase of a legal case is an opportunity for both sides to obtain information that will enable the attorneys to have a better understanding of the case, which will assist in negotiating a possible settlement or in preparing for a trial. Discovery may include interrogatories, depositions, requests for documents, and physical exams. **Interrogatories** are written questions that each side sends to the other, and **depositions** are statements from parties and witnesses taken under oath.

At trial, each side will have an opportunity to present evidence. After both sides have concluded, a judge or jury will render a decision or verdict. If a judgment is rendered against you or your service, then the plaintiff may be awarded compensatory or punitive damages. **Compensatory damages** are intended to compensate the plaintiff for the injuries he or she sustained, such as medical bills, damages to personal property, lost earnings, and physical or emotional pain and suffering. **Punitive damages** are not commonly awarded in cases of negligence and are reserved for those cases in which the defendant acted intentionally or with a reckless disregard for the safety of the public.

Consent

Under most circumstances, consent is required from every responsive, mentally **competent** adult before emergency medical care can be started. Remember, any touching of a patient's body without consent may give rise to charges of assault and battery. A person receiving emergency medical care must first give permission, or **consent**, for treatment. If a person is alert, rational, and capable of making informed decisions, then he or she has a legal right to refuse emergency medical care, even though ill or injured. A patient may also consent to some aspects of emergency medical care and deny consent to others. If a patient refuses emergency medical care, then you may not care for the patient. In fact, doing so may be grounds for criminal and civil action. Consent can be either expressed (actual) or implied.

The foundation of consent is **decision-making capacity**, the ability of a patient to understand the information you are providing, coupled with the ability to process that information and make an informed choice regarding medical care that is appropriate for him or her. You have a number of tools that you can use to evaluate a patient's decision-making capacity, but the best one is your ability to talk to the patient to find out whether the patient understands what is happening to him or her. In addition, if pulse oximetry and blood glucose measurements are outside normal ranges, then these readings can provide measurable information regarding your patient's ability to understand and communicate. Detailed documentation of decision-making capacity is important to include in your PCR to show that the patient was able to understand your proposed treatment plan.

Keep in mind that the law allows the patient to make choices that may seem medically unsound and that might endanger the patient's life. The right of patients to make decisions concerning their care and to decide how they want their end-of-life medical care provided to them is known as **patient autonomy**. Because the assistance of

Words of Wisdom

The terms decision-making capacity and competence are often used interchangeably, but *competence* is generally regarded as a legal term, and determinations regarding competence are typically made by a court of law. *Decision-making capacity* is more commonly used in health care to determine whether or not a patient is capable of making health care decisions. Consider the following factors when determining a patient's decision-making capacity:

- Is the patient's intellectual capacity impaired by a mental limitation or any type of dementia?
- Is the patient of legal age (age 18 years in most states)?
- Is the patient impaired by alcohol or drug intoxication or serious injury or illness?
- Does the patient appear to be experiencing significant pain?
- Does the patient have a significant injury that could distract him or her from a more serious injury? (For example, a significant non–life-threatening injury can cause extreme pain and distract the patient from neck pain, which could indicate a more serious injury.)
- Does the patient exhibit any hearing or visual problems?
- Is a language barrier present? Do you and your patient speak the same language?
- Does the patient appear to understand what you are saying? Does he or she ask rational questions that demonstrate an understanding of the information you are trying to share?

medical technology has made the distinction between life and death more imprecise, a number of high-profile cases have brought the issue of patient autonomy to the forefront of the medical ethics debate in the past 20 years. For example, the legal case involving Terri Schiavo from 1990 to 2005 demonstrated that the courts will ultimately support the right of the patient, or the patient's closest relative, to make end-of-life decisions **Figure 3-4**. Terri Schiavo did not prepare a written advance directive about her end-of-life care, which ultimately put the case in the hands of the state and federal courts. Advance directives are discussed later in this chapter.

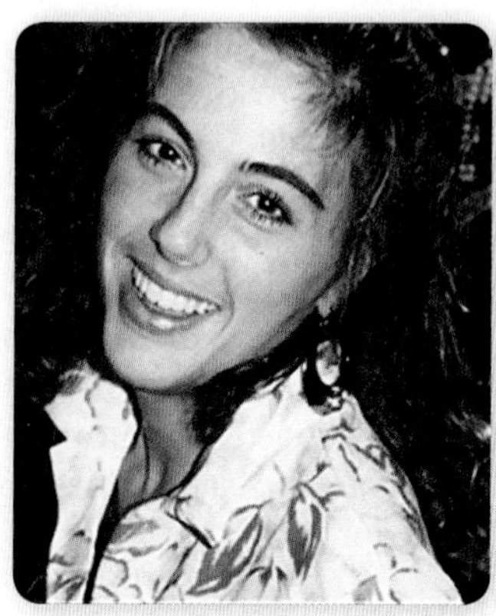

Figure 3-4 Because Terri Schiavo did not prepare an advance directive specifying the end-of-life care she wanted to receive, her case became a battleground between family members who held different viewpoints about care of the terminally ill.

▶ Expressed Consent

Expressed consent (or actual consent) is a type of consent that occurs when the patient acknowledges that he or she wants you to provide emergency medical care or transport. Expressed consent may be either verbal or nonverbal. For example, if you ask a patient if you can check his or her blood pressure and the patient extends an arm to you, then the patient is expressing nonverbal consent.

You must obtain **informed consent** from every adult patient who has decision-making-capacity. To obtain informed consent, use the following steps:

1. Describe the suspected illness or injury to the patient.
2. Describe the treatment you would like to administer, and list the potential risks associated with the proposed treatment.
3. Discuss any alternative types of treatment available.
4. Advise the patient regarding any potential consequences of refusing treatment.

Often, the prehospital environment requires that consent be obtained more quickly than in the hospital setting. The key is to ensure that your patient understands what you are trying to do and grants you permission to treat. Informed consent is valid if given verbally, but it may be difficult to prove at a later point in time. It is important to document how you obtained informed consent in the event that legal issues arise later. The legal basis for this doctrine rests on the assumption that the patient has a right to determine what is to be done with his or her body (patient autonomy). The patient must be of legal age (age 18 years in most states) and able to make a rational decision. Paramedics will often

YOU are the Provider — PART 2

Your primary survey reveals the following:

Recording Time: 1 Minute	
Appearance	Calm; seated on chair with laceration noted to forehead; minimal bleeding
Level of consciousness	Alert and oriented to person, place, time, and event
Airway	Patent
Breathing	Within normal limits
Circulation	Strong radial pulses; skin warm, dry, and pink

3. What concerns do you have regarding the patient's mechanism of injury?
4. What alternative options do you have regarding transport to the ED?

provide additional information if advanced life support (ALS) interventions are necessary. In such cases, a greater potential exists for adverse effects and other responses associated with drug administration and other forms of advanced care.

Words of Wisdom

A number of challenges can get in the way of giving a patient the information he or she needs to make a decision, such as a language barrier, his or her emotional state, and mental ability.

A patient might agree to only certain types of emergency medical care. For example, a patient might agree to receive oxygen and transport but might refuse insertion of an IV line. An injured person might agree to emergency medical care at home but might refuse to be transported to a medical facility.

▶ Implied Consent

When a person is unresponsive or otherwise unable to make a rational, informed decision about his or her medical care, and is therefore unable to give consent, the law assumes that the patient would consent to care and transport to a medical facility if he or she were able to do so **Figure 3-5**. This principle is called **implied consent**. Implied consent is limited to true emergency situations and is appropriate when the patient is unresponsive, delusional, exhibiting an altered mental status as a result of drug or alcohol use, or is otherwise physically unable to give expressed consent. Do not rely on implied consent unless a threat to life or limb exists. For this reason, the principle of implied consent is also known as the **emergency doctrine**, which allows EMS personnel to act in critical situations without danger of recrimination. However, the exact situations or conditions that represent a "serious threat to life" may be unclear, and it may become a legal question. Use of the emergency doctrine may result in legal proceedings and a **medicolegal** judgment against you, which should be defended by your best efforts to obtain consent and a thoroughly documented PCR. Medicolegal is a term that relates to medical jurisprudence (law) or forensic medicine. In most instances, the law allows the spouse, a close relative, or next of kin to give consent for a person who is unable to do so, and you should make every effort to obtain consent from an available relative before treating based on implied consent. However, never delay treatment if the patient has imminently life-threatening injuries. A patient's refusal of your offer to provide emergency medical care may also be implied. For example, if a patient pulls his or her arm from your splint, then this action may be an indication of refusal of consent. Finally, it is important to understand that if a patient being treated based on implied consent were to regain consciousness and appear capable of making an informed decision, then the emergency doctrine of implied consent would no longer apply. This situation is commonly seen with patients with hyperglycemia who are initially unresponsive and then regain complete use of their mental faculties when their glucose levels are returned to normal.

▶ Minors and Consent

Because a minor might not have the wisdom, maturity, or judgment to give valid consent, the law requires that a parent or legal guardian give consent for treatment or transport when available **Figure 3-6**. In every state, if

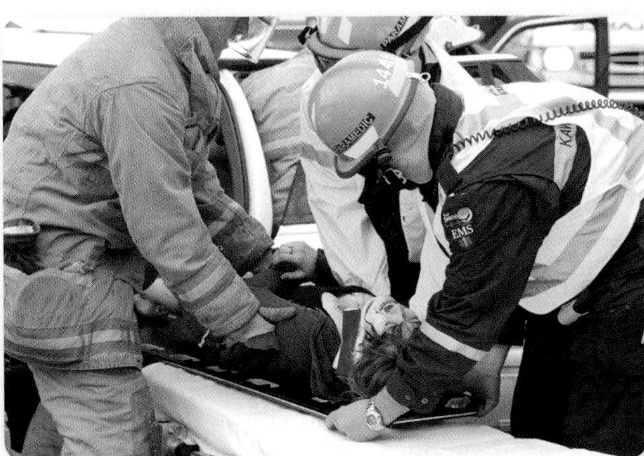

Figure 3-5 When a serious threat to life exists and the patient is unresponsive or otherwise unable to give consent, the law assumes that the patient would give consent to emergency medical care and transport to the hospital.

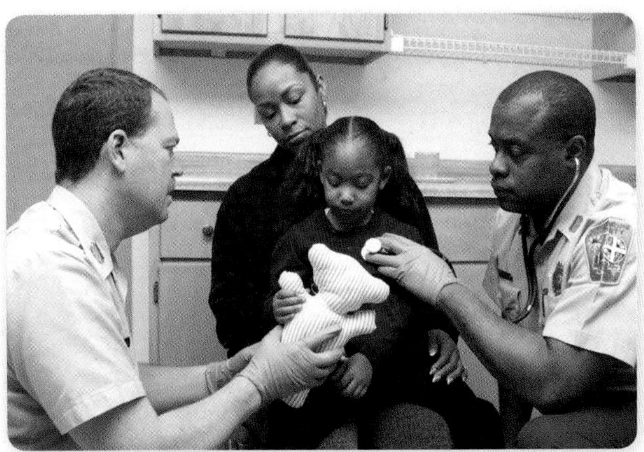

Figure 3-6 The law requires that a parent or legal guardian give consent for treatment or transport of a minor. However, never withhold life-saving emergency medical care.

a parent cannot be reached to provide consent, then health care providers are allowed to give emergency medical care to a child. However, in some states, a minor can give valid consent to receive emergency medical care, depending on the minor's age and maturity level. An **emancipated minor** is a person who, despite being under the legal age in a given state (in most cases, age 18 years), can be legally treated as an adult based on certain circumstances. For example, many states consider minors to be emancipated if they are married, if they are members of the armed services, or if they are parents. A minor may also be considered emancipated if he or she is living away from and no longer relying on his or her parents for support. A minor who is a parent may also give consent for his or her own child. A court may issue an order declaring a minor to be emancipated, but such a situation is uncommon. Know the laws of your state concerning the issues surrounding emancipation.

Also be aware of the legal principle known as **in loco parentis**. This term literally means "in the place of the parent." This principle may apply in school, day care, or summer camp if a parent is unavailable. The school administrator or day care director may make treatment and transportation decisions on behalf of the minor. Make every effort to immediately contact the parent or legal guardian, but do not withhold life-saving emergency medical care for a minor because a person authorized to give consent is unavailable.

A particularly difficult circumstance can arise if a parent or legal guardian refuses to grant consent to treat a minor who clearly requires life-saving or limb-saving treatment. Although adults clearly have the right to refuse treatment for themselves, state laws generally do not permit a parent or guardian to deny treatment to a minor. In fact, the failure of a parent or guardian to allow such treatment may constitute neglect. If confronted with such a circumstance, then notify law enforcement and medical control. State law may permit the state to assume custody of the minor for the purposes of ensuring that necessary emergency treatment be provided.

Special Populations

In the absence of a parent or legal guardian, minors are treated under implied consent in critical situations. You must never withhold life-saving care. However, if the child does not have a life-threatening illness or injury, then proper consent for treatment must be obtained prior to providing emergency medical care.

Words of Wisdom

Every report should be as detailed and accurate as possible, especially reports of patient refusals. When a patient, parent, or legal guardian refuses treatment or transport, a thorough PCR and an official refusal form will help to protect you from legal action. Have the patient or other refusing party sign the form, and ask an impartial observer (eg, a police officer, if available) to witness the signature if possible. Document in the PCR what you have done to ensure an informed refusal, and note the involvement of medical control in the situation. Be sure to submit the refusal form with your PCR. Reporting requirements are discussed in detail later in this chapter.

▶ Involuntary Consent

Some EMS personnel incorrectly use the term involuntary consent to refer to situations in which a law enforcement officer or a legal guardian grants permission to treat someone who is under arrest (or otherwise in custody), mentally ill, developmentally delayed, incapacitated, a minor, or for other reasons. Involuntary consent is an oxymoron because consent can never be involuntary. People under arrest or in prison do not necessarily lose their right to be involved in medical treatment decisions. It is not uncommon for a law enforcement officer to direct EMS personnel to treat a person under arrest, but you should continue to follow informed consent guidelines. If a prisoner refuses treatment, then involve medical control. Remember that when a true emergency exists, you can assume that implied consent exists.

▶ Forcible Restraint

Forcible restraint is the act of physically subduing a patient to prevent harm. Forcible restraint may be necessary if you are confronted with patients who are in need of medical treatment and transportation but are physically violent and present a significant risk to others. This behavior may result from an underlying psychiatric or behavioral condition, the effects of drugs or alcohol, or a medical condition such as a head injury or hypoxia. Forcible restraint of a patient may be required before you can give emergency medical care. If you believe that a patient will injure himself, herself, or others, then you can legally restrain the patient. However, you must consult medical control (either online or off-line, depending on local protocol) for authorization to restrain, or contact law enforcement personnel who have authority to restrain people. In some states, only a law enforcement officer may forcibly restrain a person Figure 3-7. Understand the local laws. Restraint without authority exposes you to civil and criminal penalties. Restraint may be used only in circumstances of risk to the patient, yourself, or others.

Your service should have clearly defined protocols pertaining to situations involving restraint. After restraints are applied, they must not be removed en route—even if the patient promises to act calmly. It is also important to monitor the restrained patient closely for any signs of breathing difficulty. It is possible to suffocate the patient if he or she is facedown (creating positional asphyxia), or if a mask placed over the patient's face blocks airflow.

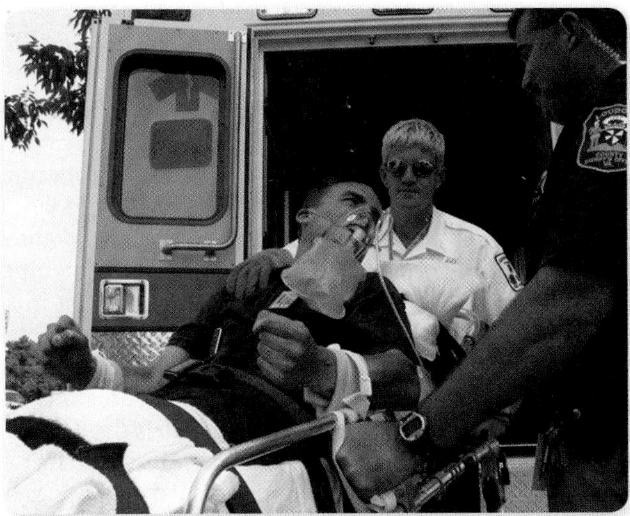

Figure 3-7 Know the local laws about forcible restraint of a patient. In some states, only a law enforcement officer has the authority to restrain a patient.

Remember that if the patient is responsive and the situation is not urgent, then consent is required.

> **Safety Tips**
>
> If you are faced with a potentially violent patient, then ensure the scene is safe and law enforcement is present before proceeding.

The Right to Refuse Treatment

As discussed previously, adults who are alert, rational, and appear to have decision-making capacity have the right to refuse treatment or withdraw from treatment at any time, even if doing so may result in death or serious injury. Such patients present you with an ethical dilemma. Should you provide emergency medical care against their will? Should you leave them alone? Calls involving refusal of treatment are commonly litigated in EMS and require you to proceed cautiously. If you leave a patient alone, then you risk being accused of negligence or abandonment if his or her condition becomes worse. You may also face charges of false imprisonment if you transport a patient against his or her wishes.

If a patient refuses treatment or transport, then you must ensure that he or she understands, or is informed about, the potential risks, benefits, treatments, and alternative treatments (due diligence). To refuse, the patient must be alert and oriented to person, place, time, and event. Ensure the patient does not have an altered mental status, and extensively document your assessment findings. If you have any doubts, then consult medical control for direction. The most prudent approach is to inform the patient in a calm and sympathetic manner of the possible consequences of refusing treatment. Keep in mind that many people who refuse medical treatment do so out of fear and emotional distress, and you need to recognize and manage the patient's stress in an understanding way. It is not uncommon for patients to refuse treatment and transport to the hospital because of concern for the costs associated with the ambulance and hospital treatment. Patients may also refuse treatment and transport because of denial that something is wrong. Addressing these concerns can be challenging for you and may require all of your "people skills." Remember the phrase: "It never hurts to have these things checked out."

Let patients know that your chief concern is their well-being, and tell them that it is all right to change their mind. Urge patients to seek further medical evaluation from the physician of their choice. Help them make concrete plans for follow-up. As discussed previously, some patients will consent to treatment but refuse transport. If patients refuse transport, then try to make sure someone will be with them after you leave.

> **Words of Wisdom**
>
> In general, any patient with an altered mental status or unstable vital signs probably cannot be considered able to refuse transport to the hospital. Become proficient in quickly establishing whether a patient has decision-making capacity. The criteria for determining mental competence should be clearly spelled out in the protocols of every ambulance service. As a rule, such criteria will include the following:
>
> - The patient is oriented to person, place, time, and event.
> - The patient responds to questions appropriately.
> - The patient does not exhibit significant mental impairment from alcohol or drug intoxication, head injury, or organic illness. (Ask the family or bystanders, if present, if this behavior is considered normal for the patient.) What constitutes significant mental impairment is a subjective judgment call.
> - The patient demonstrates to you that he or she understands the nature of his or her condition and the risks of refusing treatment and transport. This demonstration can take place only after the patient has been thoroughly informed of your assessment findings and the risks associated with refusal.
> - The patient can describe a reasonable plan for follow-up care.
> - The patient's oxygen saturation levels are within normal limits.
> - The patient's blood glucose levels are within normal limits.
> - The patient does not appear to have serious, distracting injuries that might impair his or her decision-making capacity.

As discussed, although adults have the right to refuse treatment for themselves, state laws generally do not permit a parent or legal guardian to deny treatment to a minor. In this situation, consider the emotional impact of the emergency on the parent or guardian's judgment. You can usually resolve the situation with patience and calm persuasion. A resolution may require the help of others, such as medical control or law enforcement officials. In most states, consent to treat a minor is required from only one parent or guardian.

If you are unable to obtain consent, then carefully document all your assessment findings, including the patient's history, the reasons for refusing emergency medical care, and all of the information provided to the patient, parent, or legal guardian. Note how much time you spent attempting to provide emergency medical care. Remember, the report and patient signature should be witnessed by an impartial observer. If the patient refuses to sign the release form, then the best you can do is inform your medical director and thoroughly document the situation and the refusal. Report to medical control and follow your local protocols with regard to this situation. Always advise the patient and family members to call 9-1-1 again for help if needed, and document this exchange on your PCR.

Words of Wisdom

If a patient refuses treatment and transport, but agrees to go to the hospital in a personal vehicle, then offer to assist the patient with getting into the vehicle to ensure he or she does seek medical care.

Advance Directives

Imagine that you and your partner respond to a call in which a patient is dying of an illness. When you arrive at the scene, you find that family members do not want you to try to resuscitate the patient. Without valid written documentation from a physician, such as a **do not resuscitate (DNR) order** (also known as a do not attempt resuscitation order), this type of request places you in a difficult position. Recall that a competent patient is able to make rational decisions about his or her well-being. An **advance directive** is usually a written document (but can also be a verbal statement) that specifies the desired medical treatment for a competent patient, should he or she become unable to make decisions. An advance directive is also commonly called a living will, but may also be referred to as a **health care directive**. Advance directives specify what is to be done in specific situations and are most commonly used when a patient becomes comatose. Living wills, DNR orders, and organ donation orders are all examples of advance directives.

DNR orders give you permission not to attempt resuscitation. Although laws might differ from state to state, generally speaking, DNR orders must meet the following requirements to be valid:

- Clearly state the patient's medical condition(s)
- Signature of the patient or legal guardian
- Signature of one or more physicians (or other licensed health care providers)
- In some states, DNR orders contain expiration dates. DNR orders with expiration dates must be dated in the preceding 12 months to be valid.

YOU are the Provider — PART 3

Through effective communication, you are able to persuade your patient to agree to transport by ambulance. After securing your patient to the stretcher and initiating nonemergent transport to the hospital, you obtain the following vital signs.

Recording Time: 5 Minutes	
Respirations	22 breaths/min; clear bilaterally
Pulse	Strong and irregular; 92 beats/min
Skin	Warm, dry, and pink
Blood pressure	146/92 mm Hg
Oxygen saturation (Spo_2)	96% on room air
Pupils	Pupils Equal, Round, and Reactive to Light and Accommodation (PERRLA)

5. Does this patient's irregular heart rate concern you?
6. Is any evidence of a head injury present?

However, even in the presence of a DNR order, you are still obligated to provide supportive measures (oxygen, pain relief, and comfort) to a patient who is not in cardiac or respiratory arrest, whenever possible. Each EMS agency, in consultation with its medical director and legal counsel, must develop a protocol to follow in these circumstances.

In the absence of an advance directive or DNR, some patients may have a **durable power of attorney for health care** or a **health care proxy**, a named surrogate to make decisions for them regarding their health care in the event they are incapacitated and unable to make decisions themselves. Many different types of powers of attorney exist, and not all authorize the exercise of medical decision making. Some powers of attorney simply authorize someone to handle the financial affairs of the person executing the power, and others will apply only if the person executing the power is still competent. Also, remember that a patient who remains responsive and competent has the right to make medical decisions; the person named in the power of attorney or health care proxy is only authorized to make decisions when the patient is no longer capable of doing so. When presented with a power of attorney at the scene of a medical emergency, read it carefully to ascertain its meaning and validity. If you have any questions, then contact online medical control for assistance. Do not delay emergency medical care while efforts to interpret the power of attorney are made.

Because of placement in nursing homes, hospice programs, and home health programs, you may often be faced with this situation. Specific guidelines vary from state to state, but the following four statements may be considered general guidelines:

1. Patients have the right to refuse treatment, including resuscitative efforts, provided that they are able to communicate their wishes in a competent manner. Patients also have the right to withdraw a DNR for themselves and request emergency medical care.
2. A written order from a physician is required for DNR orders to be valid in a health care facility.
3. You should periodically review state and local protocols and legislation regarding advance directives.
4. If you are in doubt or the written orders are not present, then begin BLS and contact medical control for guidance.

If little chance of patient survival exists, then resuscitation is considered to be medically futile. Futile resuscitation efforts include situations where death is imminent, such as resuscitative efforts for patients who are terminally ill, life-sustaining interventions for patients in a persistent vegetative state, or use of chemotherapy in patients with cancer in advanced stages. This area is controversial because it often places the physician in opposition to the patient's family. The physician may feel that it is unethical to provide futile treatment and give false hope, yet the family may not be ready to let go.

Words of Wisdom

An advance directive specifically states what type of medical care the patient wishes to receive in a given situation—for example, the desire to have BLS performed, but no ALS procedures or equipment.

Words of Wisdom

DNR orders typically state that if the patient is apneic and pulseless, then no resuscitative measures are to be taken.

Physician Orders for Life-Sustaining Treatment

You may also encounter an end-of-life document that emerged in the early 1990s known as Physician Orders for Life-Sustaining Treatment (POLST). POLST is also known as Medical Orders for Life-Sustaining Treatment, Medical Orders on Scope of Treatment, and Physician's Orders on Scope of Treatment, depending on the state or geographic location. Although similar to a DNR in many respects, the POLST is more expansive and encourages physicians to speak with patients with a terminal illness and create specific medical orders to be followed at the end of life. It is intended to be followed by all health care providers, not just EMS personnel. A DNR generally applies to patients who are in cardiac arrest, whereas POLST may apply to patients with impending pulmonary failure who are not in cardiac arrest. POLST typically contains provisions that address the initiation of CPR, intubation, feeding tubes, the use of antibiotics, and comfort care or palliative care (intended to provide comfort and relief from pain during the dying process). POLST applies only when the patient has lost decision-making capacity. Be familiar with which documents are recognized in your state, and always contact medical control in complex situations involving resuscitation or end-of-life care.

Ethical Principles and Moral Obligations

In addition to legal duties, you have certain ethical responsibilities as a health care provider. These responsibilities are to yourself, your coworkers, the public, and the patient. As mentioned previously, ethics are related to action, conduct, motive, character, and responsibility. **Ethics** is the philosophy of right and wrong, of moral duties, and of ideal professional behavior. It is often referred to as the study of morality. **Morality** is a code of conduct that can be defined by society, religion, or a person, affecting character, conduct, and conscience. From an EMS standpoint, ethics are associated with what the EMS profession deems right or fitting conduct. An entire field of ethics known as **bioethics** has evolved over the past several decades that addresses issues that arise in the practice of health care. Many such issues have drawn national attention, such as those dealing with the termination of life support, rationing of medical resources, and physician-assisted suicide. Ethical issues are present in nearly every EMS incident. Treating a patient ethically means doing so in a manner that conforms to professional standards of conduct and keeps the patient's best interests at the forefront of decision making. The manner in which principles of ethics are incorporated into professional conduct is known as **applied ethics**.

How can you make sure that you are acting ethically, especially with all the decisions you have to make in the field? Table 3-1 lists guidelines to assist you in ethical decision making.

You must meet your legal and ethical responsibilities while caring for your patients' physical and emotional needs. Patient needs vary depending on the situation. In most cases, an existing rule, law, or policy will guide your decision making and your actions. As a professional, you are bound to follow all such rules, laws, and policies, even in those rare circumstances where your own personal sense of ethics might lead you to a different result.

One unquestionable responsibility you have is honest reporting. Absolute honesty in reporting is essential. You must provide a complete account of the events and the details of all patient care and professional duties. Accurate records are also important for quality improvement activities.

To provide the best level of emergency medical care, it is necessary to maintain mastery of skills. Participating in continuing education and refresher training not only provides updates on changes and new procedures in EMS, but also keeps you current in the areas that are dealt with infrequently (such as obstetrics and pediatrics). As an AEMT, you have a moral obligation to make sure that you are knowledgeable in all areas of emergency medical care to ensure that you care for patients to the best of your ability. Critically reviewing your performance and seeking improvement are ethical concerns.

Ethical conflicts may arise during your work as an AEMT, causing distress. As mentioned previously, medical futility becomes an issue when faced with a situation in which attempts to provide life support may be futile due to location. An example would be the case of a cardiac arrest in the wilderness in which time to definitive care makes the attempt at resuscitation futile. Allocation of resources becomes an ethical decision-making process in the event of a triage situation in which the demand for emergency medical care exceeds your resources. Recall that triage is the practice of doing the most good for the greatest number of patients. This practice means making the decision to leave patients who, under other circumstances, may have been viable. Professional misconduct presents yet another conflict when evidence of patient abuse by EMS professionals exists. Finally, consider the practice of economic triage or patient dumping, where patients are left because they may not generate as much income as another or a patient is denied medical treatment because of the inability to pay.

Words of Wisdom

Regardless of the ethical circumstances you may encounter, you should always apply three basic ethical concepts, considered an inherent part of health care for centuries, when making a decision:

1. Do no harm.
2. Act in good faith.
3. Always act in the patient's best interest.

Failure to meet legal or ethical standards may result in you being charged civilly, criminally, or both. The best legal protection is performing an appropriate assessment

Table 3-1 Guidelines for Ethical Decision Making

1. Have you considered all options available to you and the consequence of each option?
2. What decisions have been made regarding a similar situation? Is this a type of problem that reflects a rule or policy? Can an existing policy or rule be applied? This guideline uses the concept of **precedence**, defined as basing current action on lessons, rules, or guidelines derived from previous similar experiences.
3. How would this action affect you if you were in your patient's position, or his or her family's position? What action is in the patient's best interest?
4. Would you feel comfortable having all prehospital care providers apply this action in all similar circumstances?
5. Can you justify your action(s) to:
   - Your peers?
   - The public?
   - Your supervisor?
   - Your medical director?
6. How will the consequences of your decision provide the greatest benefit in view of all of the alternatives?
7. Have you involved online medical control in your decision making?

and providing emergency medical care that is safe, effective, and competent, coupled with accurate and complete documentation. Laws differ from state to state and area to area, so be sure to seek legal advice if needed. By staying up-to-date on skills and information and treating patients with the same consideration and respect that you would give one of your close family members, you may limit possible complications that can have legal ramifications.

Confidentiality

Communication between you and the patient is considered confidential and generally cannot be disclosed without permission from the patient or a court order. Confidential information includes the patient history, assessment findings, and treatment provided. You cannot disclose information regarding a patient's diagnosis, treatment, or mental or physical condition without consent; if you do, you may find yourself liable for **breach of confidentiality**. In certain situations, you may release confidential information to designated people. In most states, patient records may be released when a legal subpoena is presented or the patient signs a written release form. The patient must be mentally competent and fully understand the nature of the release. In some situations, confidential information may be released for other purposes, which are not considered a breach of confidentiality. These situations include sharing patient information with third-party billing personnel, disclosure to state or local health agencies concerning certain diseases that may affect a population, and also events such as seizure activity that may be reported to the Department of Motor Vehicles. In many states, you do not need a written release to report information about cases of rape or abuse to proper authorities.

Another means for disclosing confidential information is through automatic release, which does not require a written form. This type of release allows you to share information with other health care providers so that they may continue the patient's care.

Improper release of confidential information or release of inaccurate information can result in liability. *Invasion of privacy* is the release, without legal justification, of information about a patient's private life that might reasonably expose the patient to ridicule, notoriety, or embarrassment. The fact that the information is true is not a defense. These statements, whether verbal or written, are made with malicious intent or reckless disregard for the accuracy of the statements. Breaches of confidentiality may also result in charges of libel or slander.

To protect yourself, be sure to document only objective findings and omit personal opinions. Do not give information to anyone other than other health care professionals directly involved in the patient's continuing care. Briefly, but politely, explain to others such as family members and concerned friends that you cannot give out information regarding the patient's condition. Instead, suggest that they follow up with immediate family members after the patient has been seen in the ED.

Health Insurance Portability and Accountability Act

The **Health Insurance Portability and Accountability Act (HIPAA)**, enacted in 1996, provides for criminal sanctions as well as civil penalties for releasing a patient's confidential medical information in an unauthorized manner. Although this act had many aims, including improving the portability and continuity of health insurance coverage and combating waste and fraud in health insurance and the provision of health care, the section of the act that most affects EMS relates to patient privacy. The aim of the HIPAA Privacy Rule was to strengthen laws for the protection of the privacy of health care information and to safeguard patient confidentiality. As such, it provides guidance on what types of information are protected, the responsibility of health care providers regarding that protection, and penalties for breaching that protection. Medical information can be disclosed only if it is necessary for a patient's treatment, billing, or operations. As mentioned previously, this practice means you are permitted to report your assessment findings and treatment to other health care providers directly involved in the care of the patient. You may also release medical information for third-party billing.

HIPAA considers all patient information that you obtain in the course of providing medical treatment to a patient to be **protected health information (PHI)**. This PHI includes not only medical information, but also any information that can be used to identify the patient. As an AEMT, you have an obligation to safeguard all PHI from unlawful disclosure, either written or verbal.

If you are unsure, then do not give any information to anyone other than those directly involved in the care of the patient. For specific policies, each EMS agency is required to have a manual and a designated privacy officer who can answer questions. You can expect to receive further training on how HIPAA has an impact on your specific response agency.

Records and Reports

Certain people and agencies, such as the EMS system, are in a position to obtain information about diseases, injuries, and emergency events, and they may be required by statute or regulation to compile the information and report it to regulatory or accreditation agencies. Even if no such requirement exists, you should compile a complete and accurate record of all incidents in which you come into contact with sick or injured patients. A complete and accurate record of an emergency medical incident is an important safeguard against legal action. The absence of a record or a substantially incomplete record may mean that you have to testify about the events, your findings, and your actions by relying on memory alone, which can prove to be inadequate and embarrassing in the face of aggressive cross-examination.

The courts often consider the following two rules of thumb regarding reports and records:

- If an action or procedure is not recorded on the written report, then it was not performed.
- An incomplete or untidy report is evidence of incomplete or inexpert emergency medical care.

You can avoid both of these potentially dangerous presumptions by compiling and maintaining accurate PCRs and records of all events and patients. PCRs also help the EMS system evaluate individual and service provider performance. PCRs are an integral part of most quality assurance programs. Data extraction from PCRs is also used to conduct prehospital emergency care research, which may improve patient outcomes.

The National EMS Information System (NEMSIS) is a tool for the EMS profession. NEMSIS provides the ability to collect, store, share, and analyze standardized EMS data throughout the United States. This useful database can be used to improve the speed and accuracy of data collection. NEMSIS could, for example, provide early warning of a disease outbreak. According to NEMSIS, although more than 90% of the United States and its territories have the NEMSIS system in place, many states are still working to ensure full compliance with the system.[4]

Words of Wisdom

Remember: If you did not document it, then you did not do it! Ensure your documentation is accurate and thorough.

Mandatory Reporting Requirements

All states and the District of Columbia have enacted laws to protect children who have been abused, and some have added other protected groups such as the older population and at-risk adults. Most states have a reporting obligation for certain people, ranging from physicians to any person. Be aware of the requirements of the law in your state. Failure to report child abuse or neglect is usually classified as a misdemeanor and may result in a fine or imprisonment, and in subsequent cases, it may become a felony. Failure to report most of the situations listed below may result in disciplinary action, suspension of your privileges to practice as an AEMT, a fine, and even criminal prosecution.

The obligation to report is most frequently applied to the following categories of cases:

- Neglect or abuse of children
- Neglect or abuse of older people
- Domestic violence
- Injury sustained during the commission of a felony or specific injuries considered to be of suspicious origin (such as gunshot wounds or stab wounds)
- Drug-related injuries
- Childbirth occurring outside a licensed medical facility
- Rape
- Animal bites
- Certain communicable diseases

YOU are the Provider PART 4

Per your protocols, any patient being transported to the ED with a possible head injury requires IV access. As you prepare your equipment, the patient looks at you and states, "I do not like needles, and I do not want an IV line."

Recording Time: 12 Minutes	
Respirations	21 breaths/min; clear bilaterally
Pulse	Strong and irregular; 87 beats/min
Skin	Warm, dry, and pink
Blood pressure	142/88 mm Hg
Oxygen saturation (Spo_2)	96% on room air
Pupils	PERRLA

7. Because your protocols state that all patients with possible head injuries require an IV line, can you force the patient to receive one?
8. What are the possible consequences of placing an IV line in this patient against his wishes?

As noted, reporting requirements vary widely from state to state. Learn the laws of your state and observe the reporting obligations that apply to you.

▶ Scene of a Crime

If evidence is present at an emergency scene that indicates a crime may have been committed, then notify the dispatcher immediately so that law enforcement authorities can respond. Such circumstances should not stop you from providing necessary emergency medical care to the patient; however, your safety is a priority, so first ensure that the scene is safe to enter. If the patient shows signs of obvious death (such as decapitation), then take necessary precautions not to disturb the crime scene because this may interfere with the subsequent investigation.

Special Populations

EMS personnel are often the best source to recognize abuse or neglect of those patients unable to speak for themselves. It is your responsibility to be an advocate for these populations when the need arises. Always look for injuries that are inconsistent with explanations, as well as other signs of abuse or neglect. Always report suspicious behavior, suspicious circumstances, or poor living conditions to the appropriate authorities for investigation. Removing a patient from an unhealthy environment may be the best course of action; however, this step may require convincing a caregiver to allow that patient to be transported. Remain professional and explain the need for treatment and transport based on physical findings.

Words of Wisdom

When you obtain the medical history from a patient you suspect has been abused, you may get more accurate information if your partner interviews the parents or other caregivers separately. Patients who have been abused may be reluctant to speak openly in front of their abusers.

At times, you may have to transport the patient to the hospital before the authorities arrive. While you provide emergency medical care, be careful not to disturb the scene of the crime any more than absolutely necessary. Make notes and drawings of the position of the patient and of the presence and position of any weapon or other objects that may be valuable to the investigating officers. If possible, do not cut through holes in clothing from knife or gunshot wounds. Confer periodically with local authorities and be aware of the actions they want you to take at the scene of a crime. It is best if these guidelines can be established by protocol.

▶ The Deceased

In most states, AEMTs do not have the authority to pronounce a patient dead. If there is any chance that life exists or that the patient can be resuscitated, then initiate resuscitative efforts at the scene and during transport. However, at times death is obvious. In such instances, no urgent reason exists to move the body. The only immediate action that is required of you is to cover the body and prevent its disturbance. Local protocol will determine your ultimate action in these instances.

Physical Signs of Death

Determination of the cause of death is the medical responsibility of a physician. There are both definitive and presumptive signs of death. In many states, death is defined as the absence of circulatory and respiratory function. Many states have also adopted "brain death" provisions; these provisions refer to irreversible cessation of all functions of the brain and brainstem. Questions often arise as to whether to begin BLS. In the absence of physician orders such as DNR orders, the general rule is as follows: if the body is still intact and no definitive signs of death are present, then initiate emergency medical care. An exception to this rule is cold temperature (hypothermia) emergencies. Hypothermia is a general cooling of the body in which the core body temperature becomes abnormally low: 95°F (35°C). It is a serious condition and is often fatal. At 86°F (30°C), the brain can survive without perfusion for about 10 minutes. When the core body temperature drops to 82.4°F (28°C), the patient is in grave danger; however, people have survived a hypothermia incident with a body temperature of 64°F (18°C). In cases of hypothermia, the patient should not be considered dead until he or she is warm and dead. If the patient's condition is unclear, or if you are unsure whether to initiate care, then it is best to begin CPR immediately and contact medical control for guidance. Remember, not all incidents of hypothermia occur outdoors; for example, an older patient in a home without heat or who has been lying on a cold floor could have hypothermia.

Words of Wisdom

Clinical death is the absence of respirations and a pulse. *Biologic death* begins within 4 to 6 minutes of clinical death as cells start to die. This process can be slowed in cold environments.

▶ Presumptive Signs of Death

Most medicolegal authorities will consider the presumptive signs of death that are listed in Table 3-2 adequate, particularly when the signs follow a severe trauma or occur at the end stages of a long-term illness such as cancer. These signs alone would not be adequate in cases of sudden

Table 3-2 Presumptive Signs of Death

- Unresponsiveness to painful stimuli
- Lack of a carotid pulse or heartbeat
- Absence of chest rise and fall
- No deep tendon or corneal reflexes
- Absence of pupillary reactivity
- No systolic blood pressure
- Profound cyanosis
- Lowered or decreased body temperature

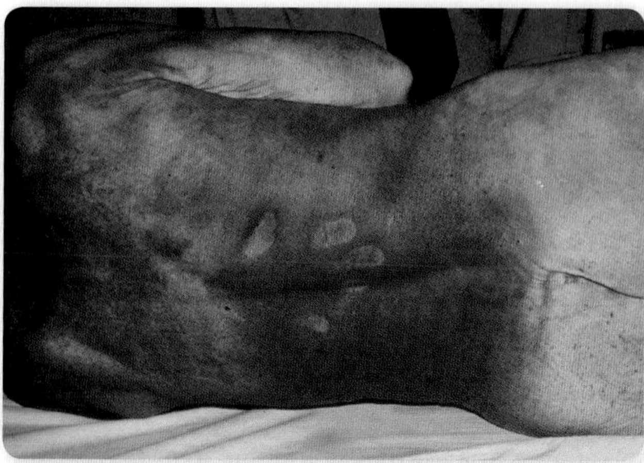

Figure 3-8 Dependent lividity is an obvious sign of death caused by discoloration of the body from pooling of the blood to the lower parts of the body.

death as a result of hypothermia, acute poisoning, or cardiac arrest. Usually, in these cases, some combination of the presumptive signs is needed to declare death, not only one of them.

Definitive Signs of Death

Definitive or conclusive signs of death that are obvious and clear to even nonmedical people include the following:

- Obvious mortal damage, such as dismemberment at the waist or neck (decapitation)
- **Dependent lividity:** blood settling to the lowest point of the body, causing discoloration of the skin **Figure 3-8**
- **Rigor mortis**: the stiffening of body muscles caused by chemical changes within muscle tissue. It develops first in the face and jaw, gradually extending downward until the body is in full rigor. The rate of onset is affected by the body's loss of heat to its surroundings. A thin person experiences heat loss faster than a person with obesity. A person on a tile floor experiences heat loss faster than a person wrapped up in a blanket in a bed. Rigor mortis occurs sometime between 2 and 12 hours after death.
- **Putrefaction**: the decomposition of body tissues. Depending on temperature conditions, this sign occurs sometime between 40 and 96 hours after death.

Coroner and Medical Examiner Cases

Involvement of the medical examiner, or the coroner in some states, depends on the nature and scene of the death. In most states, when trauma is a factor or the death involves suspected criminal or unusual situations such as hanging or poisoning, the medical examiner must be notified **Figure 3-9**. When the medical examiner or coroner assumes responsibility for the scene, that responsibility supersedes all others at the scene, including that of the family's. The following are a few examples of deaths that may be considered medical examiner cases:

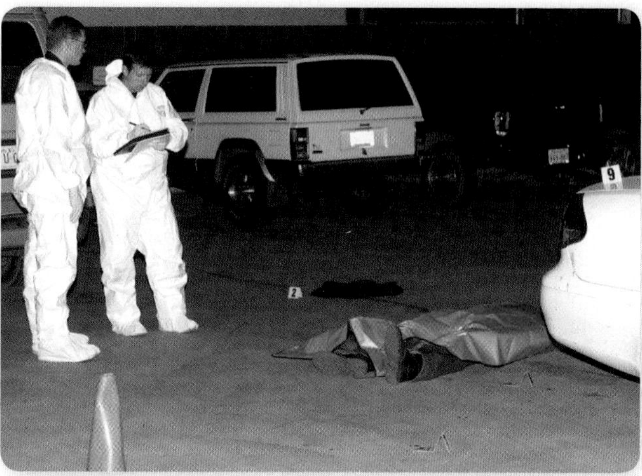

Figure 3-9 When trauma is a factor or the death involves an unusual or suspected criminal situation, the medical examiner is required to investigate.

- When the person is dead on arrival
- Death without previous medical care or when the physician is unable to state the cause of death
- Suicide (self-destruction)
- Violent death
- Poisoning, known or suspected
- Death resulting from accidents
- Suspicion of a criminal act
- Death of an infant or child

As mentioned previously, make every attempt to limit your disturbance of a scene involving a death. After you have adequately determined death based on local protocols, remove yourself from the scene. This practice is especially important if the cause of death is potentially suspicious.

If emergency medical care has been initiated, then keep thorough notes of what was done or found. These records may be important during a subsequent investigation.

Organ/Tissue Donor Card

DONATE LIFE

I wish to donate my organs and tissues. I wish to give:

☐ any needed organs and tissues ☐ only the following organs and tissues:

____

Donor Signature _______________ Date _______________

Witness _______________

Witness _______________

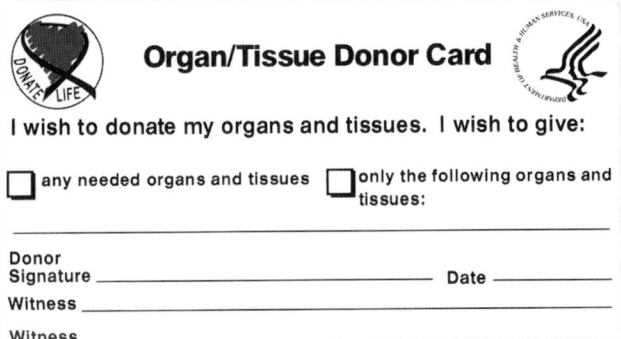

Figure 3-10 The patient may be carrying a donor card or driver's license indicating that he or she wishes to be an organ donor.

These records should include the position in which the patient was found; any weapons, medication bottles, or other important objects; and anything else relating to the scene that you witnessed.

Special Situations

▶ Organ Donors

You may be called to a scene involving a potential organ donor, a person who has expressed a wish to donate organs. Consent to organ donation is voluntary and informed. Consent is evidenced by either a donor card or a driver's license indicating that the person wants to be a donor Figure 3-10. You may need to consult with medical control when you encounter this situation.

In specific circumstances, a patient who is not successfully resuscitated may be a potential organ donor. Certain centers can procure organs, including the kidneys and liver, in certain situations. These situations typically occur after in-hospital cardiac arrest, but may be associated with certain specific out-of-hospital cardiac arrest situations that occur in close proximity to specialized centers. Be aware of your local centers and the respective protocols and capabilities.

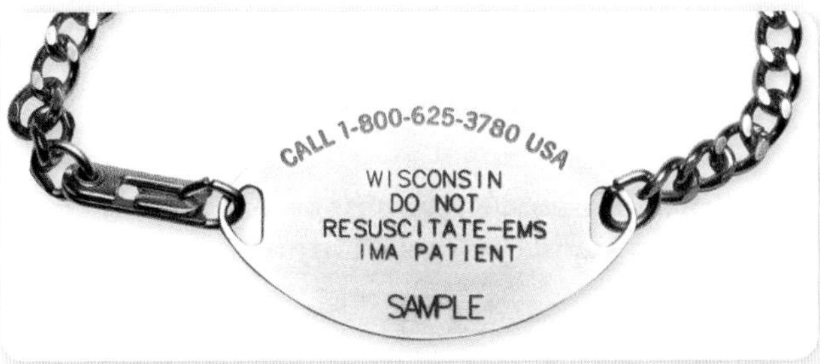

Figure 3-11 The patient may carry a medical identification card or wear a bracelet or necklace that indicates important medical information and a possible do not resuscitate order. In the case of a MedicAlert bracelet, the EMS provider can obtain stored patient information from the MedicAlert Foundation.

Treat a potential organ donor in the same way that you would treat any other patient. The fact that a patient is a possible donor does not mean that you should not use all means necessary to keep that patient alive. Organs that are often donated, such as a kidney, heart, or liver, need oxygen at all times; you must give the possible donor oxygen, or the organs will be damaged and become useless.

Remember that your priority is to save the patient's life. Learn the specific protocols in your area for these situations.

▶ Medical Identification Insignia

Many patients will carry important medical identification and information, often in the form of a bracelet, necklace, keychain, or wallet card Figure 3-11. This patient history information may include a DNR order, or specify whether the patient has allergies, diabetes, epilepsy, or some other serious condition. This information is helpful to you in assessing and treating the patient. Be sure to check any jewelry that the patient may be wearing because identification comes in many different forms. Some patients wear medical bracelets with USB flash drives that contain important medical information.

YOU are the Provider — SUMMARY

1. Can this patient refuse treatment when it is obvious that he needs stitches?

This patient is fully within his rights to refuse treatment because he is alert and oriented, and competent to refuse treatment (not under the influence of mind-altering substances). The fact that he requires stitches does not deny any of his rights to patient autonomy.

2. What can you and your partner do to attempt to persuade this patient to consent to treatment and transport?

Calmly and clearly explain to the patient that his condition requires treatment that you are currently unable to provide. Further explain to the patient the potential risks of not obtaining treatment, as well as the complications of not seeking immediate treatment.

YOU are the Provider SUMMARY *(continued)*

3. What concerns do you have regarding the patient's mechanism of injury?

It is obvious, both by visual clues and the patient's own explanation, that he struck his head on a table. Because of this evidence, the potential for a closed head injury exists. However, the patient is showing no signs of a head injury and is able to recount all of the events prior to and after the incident—minimizing, but not totally removing, the possibility of a head injury.

4. What alternative options do you have regarding transport to the ED?

Because this patient does not want to go to the hospital in an ambulance, it may be possible to persuade the patient to go to the hospital by alternative means, such as a taxi or in the personal vehicle of a friend or family member. If possible, and if the patient agrees to alternate transportation, then attempt to secure another means of transportation for him.

5. Does this patient's irregular heart rate concern you?

It may. However, your level of concern depends on the history that the patient is able to provide to you. Does this patient have a history of an irregular heartbeat? Was he feeling any heart palpitations prior to falling? Did he experience any other abnormal feeling prior to falling? If, after careful questioning, the patient's history points to a new primary cardiac event, then strongly urge ambulance transport so that cardiac monitoring may be initiated en route to the ED. Medical emergencies will be covered fully in later chapters.

6. Is any evidence of a head injury present?

No evidence of a head injury is present, other than the laceration to the forehead. The patient does not exhibit any signs of Cushing triad (hypertension, bradycardia, or abnormal respiratory pattern), which you will learn about in Chapter 19, *Neurologic Emergencies.* Although an underlying problem that you cannot see may exist, the patient is not experiencing any of the classic signs or symptoms of a head injury.

7. Because your protocols state that all patients with possible head injuries require an IV line, can you force the patient to receive one?

No. As long as the patient is conscious, alert and oriented, and competent to refuse treatment, the patient has the right to refuse any portion of treatment.

8. What are the possible consequences of placing an IV line in this patient against his wishes?

The possible consequences of placing an IV line in a patient who has stated that he does not want one are charges of assault and battery. The patient has stated that he does not like needles, and by threatening him with an IV line, you could be found guilty of assault. Battery is unlawfully touching a person, as in the case of physically starting the IV line.

EMS Patient Care Report (PCR)					
Date: 12-16-18	**Incident No.:** 20090508431		**Nature of Call:** Fall		**Location:** 176 South Cavalier St
Dispatched: 1825	**En Route:** 1828	**At Scene:** 1832	**Transport:** 1854	**At Hospital:** 1902	**In Service:** 1915
Patient Information					
Age: 84 **Sex:** M **Weight (in kg [lb]):** 57 kg (125.4 lb)			**Allergies:** No known drug allergies **Medications:** Coumadin **Past Medical History:** Irregular heartbeat **Chief Complaint:** Head laceration		
Vital Signs					
Time: 1837	**BP:** 146/92	**Pulse:** 92, Irregular	**Respirations:** 22	**Spo_2:** 96%	
Time: 1844	**BP:** 142/88	**Pulse:** 87, Irregular	**Respirations:** 21	**Spo_2:** 96%	
Time:	**BP:**	**Pulse:**	**Respirations:**	**Spo_2:**	
EMS Treatment (circle all that apply)					
Oxygen @ ______ L/min via (circle one): **NC NRM Bag-mask device**		**Assisted Ventilation**	**Airway Adjunct**	**CPR**	
Defibrillation	**Bleeding Control**	**Bandaging**	**Splinting**	**Other:**	

YOU are the Provider SUMMARY *(continued)*

Narrative
EMS called to above location for a man who fell. On arrival, met by above patient with an obvious laceration to his forehead approximately 1 inch (2.5 cm) in length, jagged in appearance. Patient states he was walking to the sofa and tripped over a lamp cord. Patient states that he struck his head on the corner of the coffee table, but denies a loss of consciousness or any pain. Bleeding stopped spontaneously. Advised patient of the need to be transported to the ED for possible stitches. Patient states that he does not want to go to the hospital via ambulance because he cannot afford the bill because he is on a fixed income. Reiterated to the patient the need for evaluation at the ED. Patient reluctantly consented for treatment and transport. Assisted the patient to the stretcher, where he was secured, and transported nonemergent to Marias Medical Center. En route—vital signs obtained. Pulse noted to be irregular; however, patient states that he has a history of atrial fibrillation and that an irregular heartbeat was normal for him. While setting up equipment for IV line insertion, patient stated that he did not want an IV line because he does not like needles. Informed the patient of the purpose for the IV line, and the risks and consequences of refusing such treatment. Patient verbalized understanding of the risks and benefits, and still refused. Report called to ED with condition and ETA. On arrival, care and report given to RN without incident.**End of report**

Prep Kit

▶ Ready for Review

- The scope of practice outlines the emergency medical care you are able to provide to the patient and is most commonly defined by law. The medical director further defines the scope of practice.
- Standards of care are established in many ways, among them local customs, statutes, ordinances, protocols, textbooks, administrative regulations, and case law.
- Determination of negligence is based on the following four factors: (1) duty, (2) breach of duty, (3) damages, and (4) proximate cause. All four elements must be present for the legal doctrine of negligence to apply and for a plaintiff to prevail in a lawsuit against an EMS system or provider.
- After your ambulance responds to a call or treatment is begun, you have a legal duty to act. In most cases, if you are off duty and encounter a motor vehicle crash, you are not legally obligated to stop and assist patients.
- Abandonment is the termination of emergency medical care without the patient's consent and without making provisions for the transfer of care to a health care professional with skills at the same level or a higher level than yours. Abandonment is a legally and ethically serious matter that exposes the patient to harm and can result in civil action against you. Always try to obtain a signature on your patient care report from the person accepting transfer of care.
- To protect yourself from charges of assault, battery, kidnapping, or false imprisonment, be sure to obtain expressed consent whenever possible.
- Defamation is intentionally making a false statement through written communication (libel) or verbal communication (slander) that injures a person's good name. Only communicate information about your patients to authorized people and ensure that the information contained in your patient care reports and other documentation is accurate and relevant.
- Good Samaritan laws are based on the common law principle that when you reasonably help another person, you should not be liable for errors and omissions that are made in giving good faith emergency care. Whereas some laws provide Good Samaritan protection for anyone who stops to render aid during an emergency, others only provide protection for those with medical training.
- Under most circumstances, you are required to obtain consent from every responsive adult before starting emergency medical care. The foundation of consent is decision-making capacity. To protect yourself from legal action, be sure to obtain expressed consent (either verbal or nonverbal) whenever possible.

Prep Kit *(continued)*

- When a patient is unresponsive and unable to give consent, the law assumes implied consent (also known as the emergency doctrine); therefore, you should proceed with treatment.
- Never withhold life-saving emergency medical care unless a valid do-not-resuscitate order or advance directive is present.
- Try to obtain consent from a parent or legal guardian of a minor (younger than age 18 years in most states) whenever possible. Again, never withhold life-saving emergency medical care.
- Mentally competent patients have the right to refuse treatment. In these instances, have the patient sign a refusal form, and make sure your department keeps a copy.
- Advance directives, living wills, or health care directives are most commonly used when a patient becomes comatose.
- As an AEMT, you have ethical responsibilities. Treating a patient ethically means doing so in a manner that conforms to professional standards of conduct and keeps the patient's best interests at the forefront of decision making.
- Communication between you and the patient is confidential; do not disclose private medical information without permission from the patient or a court order. In some situations, confidential information may be released for other purposes, which include sharing patient information with third-party billing personnel.
- Records and reports are important; ensure that you compile a complete and accurate record of each incident. You may need to testify about certain events, and the courts often consider the following two rules of thumb:
  - If an action or procedure is not recorded on the written report, then it was not performed.
  - An incomplete or untidy report is evidence of incomplete or inexpert emergency medical care.
- Understand the mandatory reporting requirements involving abuse or neglect of children, older adults, and other at-risk populations; injuries related to crimes; drug-related injuries; and childbirths occurring outside a licensed medical facility.
- There are both definitive and presumptive signs of death. In many states, death is defined as the absence of circulatory and respiratory function. Many states have also adopted "brain death" provisions; these provisions refer to irreversible cessation of all functions of the brain and brainstem.
- Be sure to note whether the patient is carrying some type of medical identification information (eg, in the form of a bracelet, necklace, keychain, or wallet card). If you fail to take this information into account, then you may harm the patient.

▶ Vital Vocabulary

abandonment Unilateral termination of emergency medical care by the advanced emergency medical technician without the patient's consent and without making provisions for transferring care to another medical professional with the skills and training necessary to meet the needs of the patient.

advance directive Written documentation that specifies medical treatment for a competent patient should the patient become unable to make decisions; also see *health care directive*.

applied ethics The manner in which principles of ethics are incorporated into professional conduct.

assault Unlawfully placing a patient in fear of immediate bodily harm.

battery Unlawfully touching a patient or providing emergency medical care without consent.

bioethics The study of ethics related to issues that arise in health care.

breach of confidentiality Disclosure of medical information without proper authorization.

breach of duty Occurs when a person accused of negligence fails to act as another person with similar training would act under the same or similar circumstances.

certification A process in which a person, an institution, or a program is evaluated and recognized as meeting certain predetermined standards to provide safe and ethical patient care.

civil lawsuit An action instituted by a person or entity against another person or entity.

compensatory damages Compensation awarded in a civil lawsuit that is intended to restore the plaintiff to the same condition that he or she was in prior to the incident.

competent Able to make rational decisions about personal well-being.

consent Permission to render emergency medical care.

credentialing An established process to determine the qualifications necessary to be allowed to practice a particular profession, or to function as an organization.

criminal prosecution An action instituted by the government against a person for violation of criminal law.

damages Compensation for injury; awarded by a court.

decision-making capacity The ability to understand and process information and make a choice regarding appropriate medical care.

Prep Kit *(continued)*

defamation The communication of false information about a person that is damaging to that person's reputation or standing in the community.

defendant In a civil lawsuit, the person against whom a legal action is brought.

dependent lividity Blood settling to the lowest point of the body, causing discoloration of the skin; a definitive sign of death.

depositions Verbal statements from parties and witnesses taken under oath.

discovery The phase of a civil lawsuit where the plaintiff and defense obtain information from each other that will enable the attorneys to have a better understanding of the case and that will assist them in negotiating a possible settlement or in preparing for trial; includes depositions, interrogatories, and demands for production of records.

do not resuscitate (DNR) order Written documentation by a physician giving permission to medical personnel not to attempt resuscitation in the event of cardiac arrest.

durable power of attorney for health care A type of advance directive executed by a competent adult that appoints another individual to make medical treatment decisions on his or her behalf in the event that the person making the appointment has a loss of decision-making capacity; also see *health care proxy*.

duty A medicolegal term relating to certain personnel who either by statute or by function have a responsibility to provide patient care.

emancipated minor A person who is under the legal age in a given state (age 18 years in most cases) but, because of other circumstances, is legally considered an adult.

emergency A serious situation, such as injury or illness, that threatens the life or welfare of a person or group of people and requires immediate intervention.

emergency doctrine The principle of law that permits a health care provider to treat a patient in an emergency situation when the patient is incapable of granting consent because he or she is unresponsive, delusional, exhibiting an altered mental status as a result of drug or alcohol use, or is otherwise physically unable to give expressed consent; also see *implied consent*.

emergency medical care Immediate care or treatment.

Emergency Medical Treatment and Active Labor Act (EMTALA) A federal law enacted to combat the practice of patient dumping and that pays particular attention to the practice of sending women in labor to distant hospitals; prevents emergency department staff from denying medical screening or stabilizing treatment, or inappropriately transferring a patient whose condition is not stable to another hospital.

ethics The philosophy of right and wrong, of moral duties, and of ideal professional behavior.

expressed consent A type of consent in which a patient gives verbal or nonverbal authorization for provision of emergency medical care or transport.

false imprisonment The confinement of a person without legal authority or the person's consent that lasts for an appreciable period.

forcible restraint The act of physically subduing a patient to prevent harm.

Good Samaritan laws Statutory provisions enacted by many states to protect citizens from liability for errors and omissions in giving good faith emergency medical care, unless there is wanton, gross, or willful negligence.

governmental immunity Legal doctrine that can protect an emergency medical services provider from being sued or that may limit the amount of the monetary judgment that the plaintiff may recover; generally applies only to emergency medical services systems that are operated by municipalities or other government entities.

gross negligence Conduct that constitutes a willful or reckless disregard for a duty or standard of care.

health care directive A written document that specifies medical treatment for a competent patient, should he or she become unable to make decisions; also see *advance directive*.

health care proxy A type of advance directive executed by a competent adult that appoints another individual to make medical treatment decisions on his or her behalf in the event that the person making the appointment loses decision-making capacity; also see *durable power of attorney for health care*.

Health Insurance Portability and Accountability Act (HIPAA) The law enacted in 1996 that provides for criminal sanctions as well as for civil penalties for releasing a patient's protected health information in a way not authorized by the patient.

immunity Legal protection from penalties that could normally be incurred under the law.

implied consent A type of consent in which a patient who is unable to give consent (because he or she is unresponsive, delusional, exhibiting an altered mental status as a result of drug or alcohol use, or is otherwise physically unable to give expressed consent) is given treatment under the legal assumption

Prep Kit *(continued)*

that he or she would want treatment; also see *emergency doctrine*.

in loco parentis Latin phrase meaning "in the place of the parent" that refers to the legal responsibility of a person or organization to take on some of the functions and responsibilities of a parent or legal guardian on the behalf of a minor.

informed consent Permission for treatment given by a competent patient after the potential risks, benefits, and alternatives to treatment have been explained.

interrogatories Written questions that the defense and plaintiff send to one other.

kidnapping The seizing, confining, abducting, or carrying away of a person by force, including transporting a competent adult for medical treatment without his or her consent.

libel False and damaging information about a person that is communicated in writing.

licensure The process whereby a competent authority, usually the state, allows people to perform a regulated job, trade, or profession.

malfeasance An unauthorized act committed outside the scope of medical practice as defined by law.

medicolegal A term relating to medical jurisprudence (law) or forensic medicine.

misfeasance Appropriate act performed in an improper manner, such as a medication administered at the wrong dose.

morality A code of conduct that can be defined by society, religion, or a person, affecting character, conduct, and conscience.

negligence Failure to provide the same care that a person with similar training would provide.

negligence per se A theory that may be used when the conduct of the person being sued is alleged to have occurred in clear violation of a statute.

nonfeasance Failure to perform a required or expected act.

patient autonomy The right of a patient to make informed choices regarding his or her health care.

plaintiff In a civil lawsuit, the person who brings a legal action against another person.

precedence Basing current action on lessons, rules, or guidelines derived from previous similar experiences.

protected health information (PHI) Any information about health status, provision of health care, or payment for health care that can be linked to an individual. This information is interpreted rather broadly and includes any part of a patient's medical record or payment history.

protocols Precise and detailed plans for a regimen of therapy (for example, advanced cardiac life support algorithms).

proximate cause The specific reason that an injury occurred; one of the items that must be proven in order for an advanced emergency medical technician to be held liable for negligence.

punitive damages Compensation that is sometimes awarded in a civil lawsuit when the conduct of the defendant was intentional or constituted a reckless disregard for the safety of the public.

putrefaction Decomposition of body tissues; a definitive sign of death.

res ipsa loquitur Theory of negligence that assumes an injury can only occur when a negligent act occurs.

rigor mortis Stiffening of the body muscles caused by chemical changes within muscle tissue; a definitive sign of death.

scope of practice Most commonly defined by state law; outlines the emergency medical care that the advanced emergency medical technician is able to provide to the patient.

slander False and damaging information about a person that is communicated by the spoken word.

standard of care Written, accepted levels of emergency medical care expected by reason of training and profession; written by legal or professional organizations so that patients are not exposed to unreasonable risk or harm.

standing orders Local protocols, usually pertaining to a particular service or area.

statute of limitations The number of years after an incident during which a lawsuit can be filed.

tort A wrongful act that gives rise to a civil lawsuit.

▶ References

1. Emergency Medical Treatment and Labor Act (EMTALA). Centers for Medicare and Medicaid Services website. https://www.cms.gov/Regulations-and-Guidance/Legislation/EMTALA/. Updated March 26, 2012. Accessed September 16, 2016.
2. Medical practice act summary. Illinois State Medical Society website. https://www.isms.org/uploadedFiles/Main_Site/Content/Advocacy/Legislative_Action_Hub/Past_Issues/MedicalPracticeActSummaryPrimer.pdf. Accessed September 15, 2016.
3. Medical malpractice overview. FindLaw website. http://injury.findlaw.com/medical-malpractice/medical-malpractice-overview.html. Accessed October 27, 2016.
4. Goals and objectives. National EMS Information System (NEMSIS) website. http://www.nemsis.org/theProject/whatIsNEMSIS/goalsAndObjectives.html. Updated March 15, 2013. Accessed September 16, 2016.

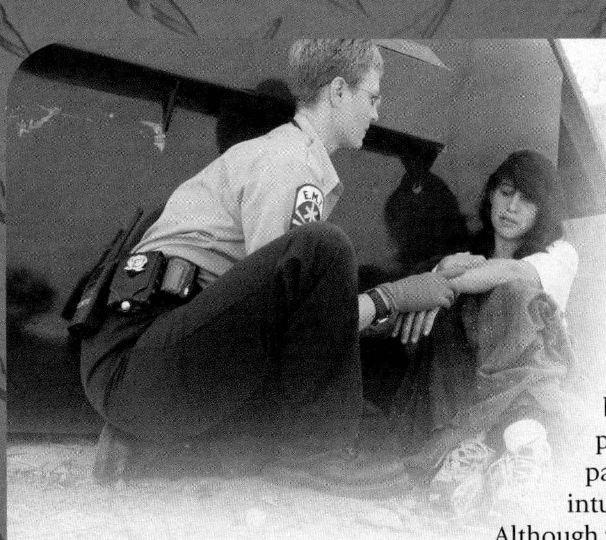

Assessment *in Action*

Your volunteer ambulance is dispatched to a call involving a patient in cardiac arrest at an interstate rest area. On arrival, you find the patient pulseless and apneic. As your partner begins CPR, you contact your dispatch and request that ALS personnel respond to the scene. You are almost finished with paramedic training and you know that you can successfully intubate the patient and begin advanced cardiac life support. Although paramedic backup is just minutes away, you elect to perform endotracheal (ET) intubation on the patient. While you are securing the ET tube, backup arrives, and you see your supervisor getting out of the ambulance.

1. Which of the following terms describes the boundaries of emergency medical care you are permitted to provide for the patient?

- **A.** Scope of practice
- **B.** Standard of care
- **C.** Duty to act
- **D.** Standing orders

2. In this scenario, you may be found negligent for working outside of your scope of practice. The determination of negligence is based on the following factors EXCEPT:

- **A.** duty.
- **B.** breach of duty.
- **C.** damages.
- **D.** believed cause.

3. Who is responsible for establishing the written protocols and standing orders for your service?

- **A.** Medical Director
- **B.** EMS Supervisor
- **C.** Department of Transportation
- **D.** The National Registry of EMTs

4. __________ occurs if you perform an act that you are legally permitted to do, but you do so in an improper manner.

- **A.** Malfeasance
- **B.** Nonfeasance
- **C.** Misfeasance
- **D.** Defamation

5. Which of the following terms describes the unilateral termination of emergency medical care without the patient's consent and without making any provisions for continuing care by a medical professional with skills at the same level or higher?

- **A.** Negligence
- **B.** Abandonment
- **C.** Malfeasance
- **D.** Restraint

6. Which of the following events does NOT require mandatory reporting?

- **A.** Neglect or abuse of children
- **B.** Drug-related injuries
- **C.** Childbirth occurring outside a licensed medical facility
- **D.** Extreme sports injuries

7. Which type of consent is used to treat the patient in this scenario?

- **A.** Informed
- **B.** Expressed
- **C.** Implied
- **D.** Involuntary

8. What is the difference between assault and battery?

9. What is a *Physician Orders for Life-Sustaining Treatment* and when is it used?

10. The Emergency Medical Treatment and Active Labor Act (EMTALA) was enacted in 1986 to combat the practice of so-called patient dumping and pays particular attention to the practice of sending women in labor to distant hospitals. What is patient dumping?

CHAPTER 4

Communications and Documentation

National EMS Education Standard Competencies

Preparatory

Applies fundamental knowledge of the EMS system, safety/well-being of the advanced emergency medical technician (AEMT), medical/legal, and ethical issues to the provision of emergency care.

Therapeutic Communication

Principles of communicating with patients in a manner that achieves a positive relationship

- Adjusting communication strategies for age, stage of development, patients with special needs, and differing cultures (pp 104-105, 111-114)
- Interviewing techniques (pp 105-111)
- Verbal defusing strategies (p 111)
- Family presence issues (p 109)
- Dealing with difficult patients (p 111)

EMS System Communication

Communication needed to

- Call for resources (pp 123-124)
- Transfer care of the patient (pp 114-115, 125-126, 127-128)
- Interact within the team structure (pp 114-115, 123-128, 133-134)
- EMS communication system (pp 115-123)
- Communication with other health care professionals (pp 114-115, 125-128)
- Team communication and dynamics (pp 114-115, 123-128, 133-134)

Documentation

- Recording patient findings (pp 129-133)
- Principles of medical documentation and report writing (pp 129-133)

Knowledge Objectives

1. Describe factors and strategies to consider for therapeutic communication with patients. (pp 103-111)
2. Discuss the techniques of effective nonverbal communication. (pp 105-106)
3. Discuss the techniques of effective verbal communication. (pp 106-111)
4. Understand special considerations in communicating with difficult patients, older adults, children, hard-of-hearing patients, visually impaired patients, non–English-speaking patients, and special needs patients. (pp 111-114)
5. Describe how to effectively communicate transfer of care, including delivery of the oral report on arrival at the hospital. (pp 114-115, 125-126, 127-128)
6. Understand the basic principles of the various types of communications equipment used in emergency medical services (EMS). (pp 115-123)
7. Describe EMS communication procedures during the following phases of a typical call: notification or initial receipt of call, communication with dispatch en route to call, on scene, during transport, and on arrival at hospital (or point of transfer), and return to service. (pp 123-125)
8. List the proper sequence of information to communicate in radio delivery of a patient report. (pp 125-126)
9. Describe the use of radio communications, including the proper methods of initiating and terminating a radio call. (p 128)
10. Describe the use of written communication and documentation. (pp 129-131)
11. Explain the legal implications of the patient care report (PCR). (p 131)
12. Identify the information required in a PCR and how to report errors. (pp 131-134)
13. Understand how to document refusal of care, including the legal implications of the patient's decision. (pp 135-138)
14. Discuss state and/or local special reporting requirements, such as for gunshot wounds, dog bites, and abuse. (p 138)

Skills Objectives

1. Demonstrate the techniques of successful cross-cultural communication. (pp 104-105, 114)
2. Demonstrate delivery of a formal oral report during transfer of care. (pp 114-115)
3. Demonstrate how to provide a verbal radio report to the receiving facility. (pp 125-126)
4. Demonstrate a simulated, concise radio transmission with dispatch. (pp 127-128)
5. Demonstrate completion of a PCR. (pp 131-134)

Introduction

Effective communication is an essential component of prehospital care. **Communication** is the transmission of information to another person—whether it is verbal or nonverbal. A fully functional emergency medical services (EMS) communications system links you with other members of your team as well as with responders from other involved EMS, fire, and law enforcement agencies. Timely, clear communication allows a team to work together efficiently and safely. Excellent communication is also an integral part of organizing, summarizing, and transferring information about the patient's care to the nurses and physicians at a receiving hospital. You must know the capabilities of your teams' communication system to make the most of the tools available to you and your teammates.

Verbal communication skills are vital for advanced emergency medical technicians (AEMTs). Your verbal skills will enable you to gather information from the patient and bystanders at an emergency scene. They will also make it possible for you to effectively coordinate with and present instructions to the variety of responders who are often present at the scene. Part of verbal communication is having good listening skills that allow you to fully understand the nature of the scene and the patient's problem.

Documentation is the written or electronically recorded portion of the AEMT's patient care interaction that becomes part of the patient's permanent medical record. Documentation such as a **patient care report (PCR)**, also known as a prehospital care report, provides you with an opportunity to communicate the patient's story to others who may participate in the patient's future medical care. This form should be completed only after the patient's condition has been stabilized; actual patient care is always the priority. Adequate reporting and accurate records ensure the continuity of patient care. Complete patient records also guarantee proper transfer of responsibility, comply with the requirements of health departments and law enforcement agencies, and fulfill your organization's administrative policies.

Radio and telephone communications link you and your team with other members of the EMS, fire, and law enforcement communities. This link helps the entire team to work together more effectively and provides an important layer of safety and protection for each member of the team. You must know what your communications system can and cannot do, and you must be able to use your system efficiently and effectively.

This chapter describes the skills and knowledge you need to be an effective communicator and discusses a variety of effective methods of verbal and nonverbal communication. The various types of communications systems and equipment are discussed, along with an overview of the EMS communication process, including standard radio operating procedures and protocols. The roles of the Federal Communications Commission (FCC) in EMS are also described. The chapter concludes with a discussion about written communication and documentation.

Therapeutic Communication

Communicating with the dispatcher and fellow health care professionals is certainly important for the AEMT—but so is communicating with the patient. The latter, which is called **therapeutic communication**, involves the art and skill of communicating with people on what may be one of the worst days of their lives. Therapeutic communication uses various communication techniques and strategies, both verbal and nonverbal, to encourage patients to express how they are feeling and to achieve a positive relationship with the patient. A professional demeanor and skilled communication techniques are key components of a successful patient–AEMT interaction. This section discusses the factors and strategies that are necessary for therapeutic communication.

How do we communicate? This simple question can be surprisingly complex, as a number of things must be considered during communication Table 4-1.

People communicate in a variety of ways, such as through eye contact, body position, and facial expressions. Factors such as culture and age need to be taken into consideration during communication. Patients with special needs may require you to consider alternative forms of communication. For example, if the patient is deaf and you cannot communicate using sign language, you may need to communicate by having the patient write down his or her messages.

If you want people to tell you about their problems, then convince them you want to hear what they have to

YOU are the Provider — PART 1

At 1623 hours, your ambulance is dispatched to a reported laceration. Three minutes later, you and your partner are en route to the scene, arriving in about 8 minutes. At the scene, law enforcement officers direct you to the backyard, where you find a 23-year-old woman seated at a picnic table. The patient states her drunken boyfriend threw a bottle at her, and it broke on her forearm. You see a minor laceration, with no active bleeding on her right forearm. The patient denies having any other injuries.

1. What are some nonverbal forms of communication you can use to perform an effective interview?
2. As a general rule, how close should you be to the patient while you are interviewing?

Table 4-1 Factors and Strategies to Consider During Communication

Age	Eye contact
Body language	Facial expression
Clothing	Gender
Culture	Posture
Educational background	Voice tempo
Environment	Volume

say. Give patients your full attention; do not treat them like they are a bother. There is nothing worse than talking about someone as if they are not there—or worse, as though the person does not even exist. It is unforgivable to ask someone a question that you will just have to repeat later because you did not pay attention to the answer the first time. Jot down the answer. When it is time to communicate, *communicate*. That means you must listen, not just talk. Listening is part of communicating, too—it is part of the two-way exchange that transmits information.

Words of Wisdom

The Shannon–Weaver communication model was developed to assist in the development of the mathematical theory of communication for Bell Telephone Labs in the late 1940s[1] **Figure 4-1**. Shannon and Weaver were trying to figure out the math involved in sending information through telephone lines. After its creation, it quickly became apparent that this model had application in areas other than math. Social scientists picked up this model, and it remains a valuable tool in understanding the variables involved in human communication. In the communication model, the sender must take a thought, encode it into a message, and send the message to the receiver. The receiver then decodes the message and sends feedback to the sender.

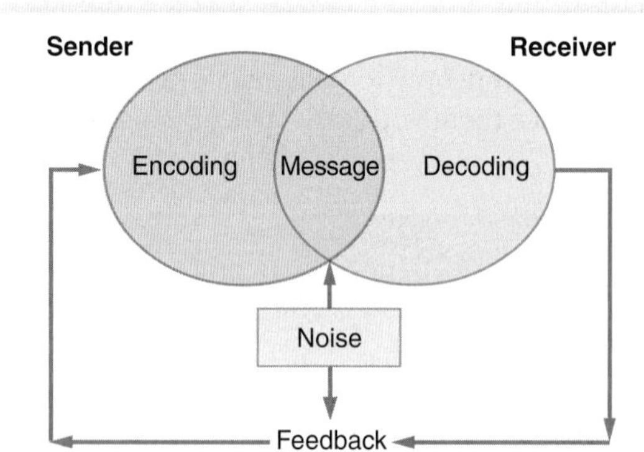

Figure 4-1 Shannon–Weaver communication model.

▶ Age, Culture, and Personal Experience

The thoughts of people are greatly influenced by their personal experiences. For example, an older adult who often experiences great pain may view pain as more of an inconvenience than a problem. A child who has limited experience with pain would likely react much differently. People are also taught to handle pain differently. Some cultures encourage people to express their emotions about illness and injury; others see this kind of expression as a sign of weakness and prefer to remain unemotional in the face of a health issue. Thus, both social and personal influences will shape a person's thoughts.

Patients may talk, make gestures, or write a note to express how they are feeling. Again, culture and personal experience will shape how people communicate. Consider the difference between the following examples of communication: "I am so sorry to bother you, but my chest hurts a little" versus "Hey! What took you so long? My chest is killing me! Are you going to help me or what?" Both of these messages talk about pain, but they also contain much more information about the people sending them.

The tone, pace, and volume of a person's language tell us about the mood of the person who is communicating. They also provide some insight into the perceived importance of the message. For example, the patient who is yelling at you may be angry, scared, or both. Take note of not only the words being spoken but also of how the words are said.

You need to recognize that these concepts of body language and eye contact are often greatly affected by culture. In some cultures, direct eye contact is viewed as impolite, while in other cultures, it is impolite to look away while speaking. Consider the following differences in nonverbal communication:[2]

- **Hands on hips.** This stance is considered a sign of hostility in Mexico and Argentina.
- **Touching with the left hand.** Islamic and Hindu cultures avoid touching with the left hand, because traditionally this hand was used for unclean functions. It is considered rude and offensive to offer the left hand in greeting.
- **Eye contact.** Avoid direct eye contact to show respect in most Asian, African, Latin American, and Caribbean cultures. Exceptions to this rule include Somalian and Brazilian cultures, in which prolonged eye contact is acceptable; these cultures believe it communicates honesty and interest in the recipient.
- **Slouching.** This practice is considered rude in Japan and in Northern European areas.

Another American usage that may be looked on with disfavor is use of hand gestures. The thumbs-up sign that Americans use to indicate "everything is okay" or "ready to go" is actually the equivalent of an extended middle finger in many Arabic and some Latin countries.

The okay sign—made with thumb and index finger circled, and the other three fingers extended—is a standard American gesture meaning "good to go." In Latin countries, Germany, Italy, and Russia, it is a reference to the anus. In France, the gesture means zero and can be used to indicate something is worthless. In other cultures, it represents the evil eye. In Japan, it indicates that money is needed, or that coins are preferred.

The extended middle finger is probably the rudest American gesture. In Japan, the middle digit is used as the index finger and has the same significance as pointing. Please remember this fact when providing care to a Japanese family if they seem to "flip you off" when you ask to be shown where it hurts.

Words of Wisdom

Many people fall short of giving even basic respect in everyday interactions, let alone in a health care environment. In the United States, emphasis is often placed on getting the job done, and many people seem to be too hurried and busy to seem concerned about how they appear to others. We can offend with the abruptness of our behavior. In other cultures, appearance and manners mean everything, and lack of respect is unforgivable. Such an offense can have greater implications in the health care field, where a patient's impression of his or her care is partly based on the demeanor of the provider.

People tend to translate the messages they receive using their own worldviews. **Ethnocentrism** occurs when you consider your own cultural values as more important when you are interacting with people of a different culture. If you are North American, for example, then you might suspect that a patient is hiding something, afraid, or untrustworthy if the patient looks away from you while you are talking. These conclusions may be true if the two people communicating are from the same culture—but they may not be valid if the partners in the communication exchange come from different backgrounds. Remember, all aspects of communication—eye contact, social distances, body language, and even touching—have a cultural foundation. In Thailand, for example, the touching of the head is reserved for those who are very intimate. This cultural belief can present a problem for you if the patient's head is bleeding.

Cultural imposition takes ethnocentrism to an extreme. Some health care providers may consciously or subconsciously force their cultural values onto their patient because they believe their values are better. For example, consider a child who is brought to the emergency department (ED) with red marks on his back from a traditional Asian healing practice called coining—rubbing hot coins on the child's back as a treatment for medical illness. The parents explain to the physician that the coining helped for a short time, but now the child seems to be getting sicker. The physician responds angrily to the parents, accusing them of poor parenting and insisting that their practices are harmful (although they are not). This accusation reflects cultural imposition.

Nonverbal Communication

Facial Expressions, Body Language, and Eye Contact

Eye contact and body language are powerful aspects of communication. Consider how dogs interact. When two dogs meet for the first time, they look at each other. The position of the head, shoulders, tail, and back all help to communicate to the other dog. Before they get any closer, the dogs need to understand their new relationship. Who is dominant? Will you hurt me? These questions must be answered quickly.

People communicate using a similar technique. The body language we consciously or subconsciously choose provides more information than words alone. Consider the images in Figure 4-2. Without any words, it should be clear what each person's mood is.

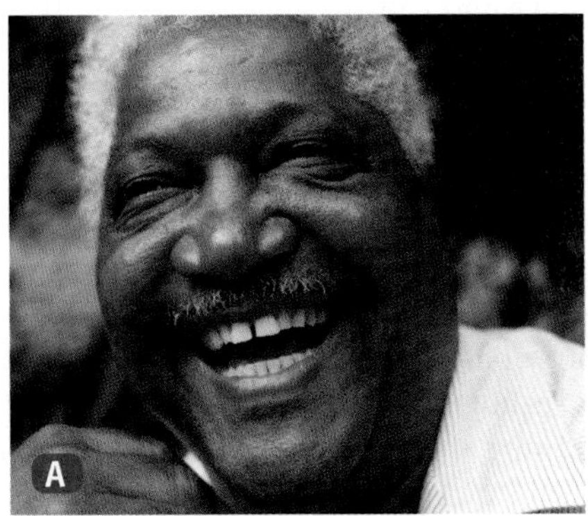

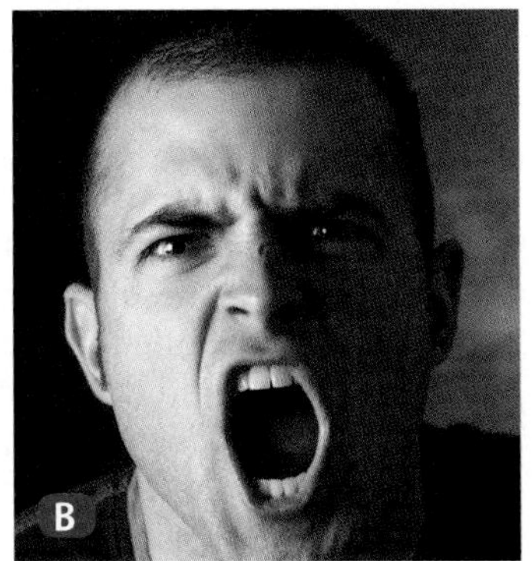

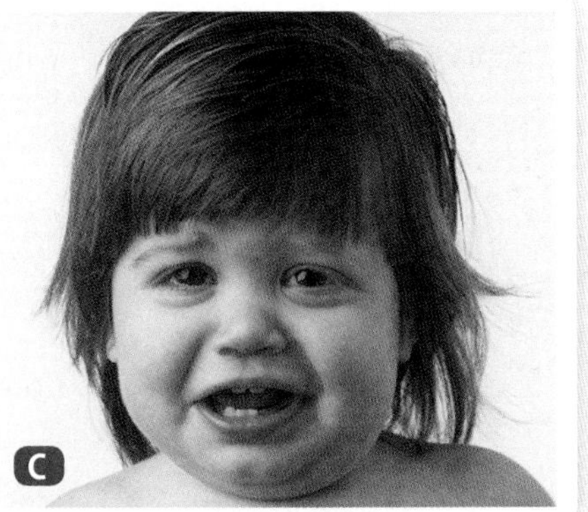

Figure 4-2 Examples of body language. **A.** Happy. **B.** Angry. **C.** Sad.

Patients may initially be hostile toward EMS providers, or a calm situation may escalate into a hostile situation. When you are treating a potentially hostile patient, it is important that you understand and be aware of your own body language. People tend to react to anger with anger. If you are dealing with an angry patient, then the last thing you want to do is become angry. Be aware of your body language. Do not assume an aggressive posture. Make good eye contact, but do not stare. Speak calmly, confidently, and slowly. Give the patient choices, but limit those choices to ones you can live with. Do not be drawn into the verbal violence your patient may be projecting. Remember, your patient cannot make you angry if you do not allow it to happen.

It is important for you to be attentive to facial expressions, body language, and eye contact—your own and your patient's. These physical cues will help you and your patient to truly understand the message being sent.

Physical Factors

Various physical factors affect communication, which are collectively referred to as noise. **Noise** is anything that dampens or obscures the true meaning of the message. Literal noise, or sounds in the environment, can make it difficult to understand the patient or for the patient to understand you. Lighting, distance, or obstacles are other factors that may affect your communication.

Proxemics is the study of space and how the distance between people affects communication **Table 4-2**. The appropriate distance depends on the levels of trust and intimacy between the two parties. As a person gets closer, a greater and greater sense of trust must be established. When you finally enter someone's intimate space, there must be a high sense of trust.

Understanding how communication works and the importance of effective communication is important when gathering information from the patient. Your communication skills will be put to the test when you communicate with patients and/or families in emergency situations. Remember, someone who is sick or injured is scared and might not understand what you are doing or saying. Therefore, your gestures, body movements, and attitude toward the patient are critically important in gaining the trust of both the patient and family.

Table 4-2 Proxemics for American Culture

Space	Distance	Description
Intimate	Less than 18 in. (46 cm)	Whispering, touching; must be invited
Personal	18 in. to 4 ft (46 cm to 1 m)	Conversations with close friends or family
Social	4 to 10 ft (1 to 3 m)	Conversations with acquaintances
Public	10 to 25 ft (3 to 8 m)	Interacting with strangers

Words of Wisdom

Anyone who has dealt with people experiencing a crisis can tell you that a smile can greatly help relieve stress. Think back to a time when you were troubled by something and someone's smile told you that everything was going to be okay. Your ability to smile can be just as valuable when you are communicating with patients, especially to those who are hard of hearing or who speak a different language.

▶ Verbal Communication

As an AEMT, you must master many communication skills, including those associated with radio operations and written communications. Skilled verbal communication with the patient and family, bystanders, and the rest of the health care team is an essential part of high-quality patient care. It will make it possible for you to effectively coordinate the variety of responders who are often present at the scene, transfer the patient's care to nurses and physicians at the hospital, and allow you to listen to fully understand the nature of the scene and the patient's problem. You must also be able to organize your thoughts quickly and accurately to verbalize instructions to the patient, bystanders, and other health care professionals.

One of the most fundamental aspects of what AEMTs do is to ask patients questions **Table 4-3**. There are two types of questions: **open-ended questions**, which require the patient to provide an answer with some level of detail, and **closed-ended questions**, which can be answered in very short or single-word responses. When you first approach your patient, you should use open-ended questions: "Good day. My name is Chuck and I am an AEMT. What seems to be bothering you today?" Open-ended questions allow a free flow of conversation. They let the patient direct you to what is bothering him or her.

Closed-ended questions are important to use when patients are unable to provide long or complete answers to questions. Perhaps the patient is having severe breathing difficulties, or maybe the patient is a child who is scared and does not know what to say. In situations for which thoughtful answers are not possible, closed-ended questions are appropriate and are particularly useful when assessing a patient's condition. "Are you having trouble breathing? Do you take medications for your heart?"

However, with closed-ended questions it is possible for you to miss important information if pertinent

questions are not asked. Imagine how many ways a person can be sick or injured. Now imagine trying to come up with a single yes/no question for each sickness or injury. Closed-ended questions typically provide limited information, and you should consider the answers to these questions as only a starting point toward understanding the patient's condition.

Other types of questions that can reveal underlying issues include the following payoff questions. These were developed by AEMTs based on field experience:

- Have you ever felt like this before?
- Have you been upset about anything lately?
- Are you afraid of someone? (Save this one for the privacy of the ambulance.)
- Have you been thinking about hurting yourself?
- What happened the last time you felt this way?

When you are asking questions of the patient, be conscious of how many questions you are asking: "How are you doing today? Have you been feeling ill?" This common approach asks the patient two kinds of questions, one open-ended and one closed-ended. Often the patient will respond with a simple "yes." To avoid this situation, it is best to ask a single question, wait for an answer, and then ask another question.

Many powerful communication tools can be used when trying to obtain information from patients. Sometimes patients will hide information, either consciously or unconsciously. Patients may be afraid or they may be confused. Children are easily distracted, so a toy may distract them and facilitate communication. The techniques in Table 4-4 are tools that can assist you in gathering patient information. They can be helpful to use not only in patients who are willing to share but also in those who are resistant to sharing information.

Table 4-3 Types of Patient Interview Questions

Open-ended questions	Questions without a definitive, "yes" or "no" answer. Let patients describe their pain in their own words because those will probably be more accurate. The following are some examples of open-ended questions: ▪ How have you been feeling lately? ▪ Do you have an idea of what is causing this? ▪ Do you have any other concerns about your health? ▪ Is there anything else you would like to discuss?
Closed-ended questions	Questions with a definitive answer. Develop a standard set of questions concerning medical history that you ask almost all patients, using words that people without medical training can understand. Your standard questions may include the following: ▪ Have you ever had any heart problems? ▪ Any lung problems? ▪ Any high or low blood pressure? ▪ Diabetes? ▪ Seizures? ▪ Fainting spells? ▪ Any prior head injury? ▪ Do you have both lungs and both kidneys?

Table 4-4 Communication Tools

Communication Tool	Meaning	Example
Facilitation	Encourage the patient to talk more or provide more information.	AEMT: "Can you tell me more about that? I am listening to you."
Silence	Do not speak.	Giving the patient space and time to think and respond.
Reflection	Restate a patient's statement made to you to confirm your understanding.	Patient: "I am so depressed that I could die." AEMT: "I understand that you are feeling sad."

(continued)

Table 4-4 Communication Tools *(continued)*

Communication Tool	Meaning	Example
Empathy	Be sensitive to the patient's feelings and thoughts.	Use eye contact and touch to reinforce your communication; adjust your tone of voice and pace to allow for open communication.
Clarification	Ask the patient to explain what he or she meant by an answer.	Patient: "I just feel sick." AEMT: "Please tell me what you mean by 'feeling sick'? Help me to understand what is going on."
Confrontation	Make the patient who is in denial or in a mental state of shock focus on urgent and life-critical issues.	Patient: "I am having pain in my chest, my back has been hurting me, I feel nauseated, and I ran out of my blood pressure medication." AEMT: "Please tell me about your chest pain. We will talk about your other concerns in a moment."
Interpretation	Sum up the patient's complaint to confirm your understanding.	AEMT: "If I understand correctly, you have been feeling pain for the past 3 days, and it has gotten worse today." Patient: "That's right."
Explanation	Provide factual information to support a conversation.	Patient: "I do not understand what is happening." AEMT: "We have checked your blood sugar and blood pressure and both appear to be normal."
Summary	Provide the patient with an overview of the conversation and the steps you will take.	AEMT: "We will be taking you to the emergency department to care for your chest pain. I will give you some medication that should make you feel better."

Abbreviation: AEMT, advanced emergency medical technician

When you are interviewing the patient, you can consider using touch as a means to communicate caring and compassion. Touch is a powerful tool, so it should be used both consciously and sparingly **Figure 4-3**. Many people will be uncomfortable with a stranger suddenly touching them. If you are going to touch the patient, then approach slowly and touch the patient's shoulder or arm respectfully. You may hold the patient's hand. This allows you to touch the patient, showing you care about what he or she is telling you, yet also allows you to remain at a slight distance.

Avoid touching the patient's torso, chest, or face simply as a means of communication, because these areas are often viewed as intimate. Also, to touch these areas, you will need to get closer to the patient, potentially invading the patient's intimate space. **Table 4-5** provides other tips on what to avoid when communicating with patients.

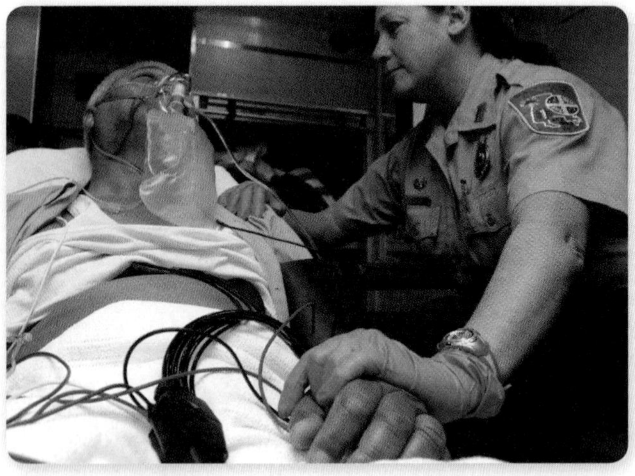

Figure 4-3 Using touch can portray care and compassion.

Table 4-5 Interview Techniques to Avoid

Improper Technique	Example	Reason
Providing false assurance or reassurance	AEMT: "It will be okay." "This is nothing to worry about."	You really do not know that everything will be okay.
Giving unsolicited advice	AEMT: "Well, if I were you, I wouldn't have called the ambulance at all."	This demeans the patient and makes you seem arrogant rather than helpful. It is inappropriate to suggest that an ambulance was not needed, even if that is what you believe.
Asking leading or biased questions	AEMT: "Are you telling me that this cut is the only reason you called the ambulance?"	Your patient deserves respectful communication. It is inappropriate to suggest that an ambulance was not needed, even if that is what you believe.
Talking too much	The AEMT talks to the patient without really listening to the patient, simply going through the motions.	Guide the patient through the conversation. When the patient provides you information, you need to consider the information and move the conversation toward a goal.
Interrupting the patient	Patient: "Well, I was having trouble breathing the past month and . . . " AEMT: "Can we move on to how you are feeling now?"	You may seem bored or annoyed that the patient is taking up your time.
Using "why" questions	AEMT: "Why did you call the ambulance today?"	"Why" questions often appear to accuse the listener. You may seem annoyed that the patient called 9-1-1.
Using authoritative language	AEMT: "Tell me what is wrong with you." "Just give me the details."	This language does not encourage open communication.
Speaking in professional jargon	AEMT: "I think we will need to take you to the ED stat. We will give you ASA and NTG en route. Any questions?"	This type of communication confuses the patient. Most patients do not understand medical jargon. It is also abrupt and may deter open communication.

Abbreviation: AEMT, advanced emergency medical technician

The presence of family, friends, and bystanders during your interview of the patient can be valuable. Sometimes, however, well-meaning family members will speak for the patient, and, at times, you may need to ask the family member to allow the patient to answer. Ultimately, you will need to assess the situation and determine whether the additional people are helping you care for the patient or hindering your efforts. Do not be afraid to ask others to step outside or step aside for a moment while you talk with the patient. Take into account how the patient will feel without his or her loved ones nearby. Removing them may make the patient more anxious.

These 10 Golden Rules will help you to calm and reassure the patient and provide a therapeutic rapport:

1. **Make and keep eye contact with the patient at all times.** Give the patient your undivided attention. This will let the patient know that he or she is your top priority. Look the patient straight in the eye to establish a **rapport**. Establishing a rapport means building a trusting relationship with your patient. This will make caring for the patient much easier. Use the following techniques to develop rapport:
   - Watch your inflection. Use a calm and steady tone of reassurance to reinforce your interest in and concern for the patient.
   - Respond to the patient. Acknowledge what the patient is telling you. If you are not

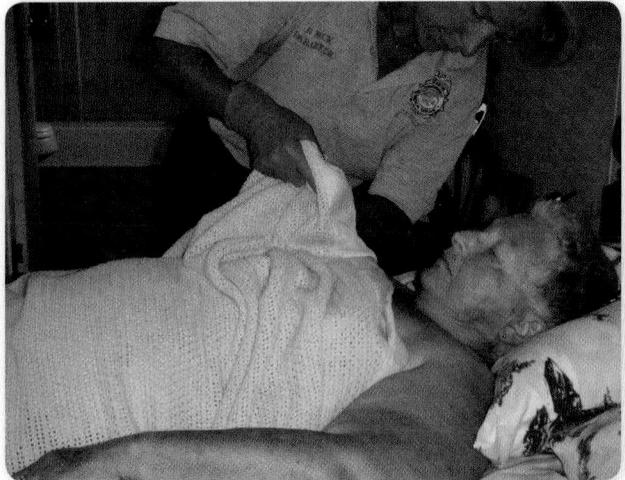

Figure 4-4 Show your patient the same respect you would want others to show your family. Protect modesty with a blanket or towel.

Courtesy of Rhonda J. Hunt.

comfortable responding, then simply nod or restate what the patient said, without providing a definitive answer right away.

- Anticipate and deal with fear. Reassurance may be one of the most important treatments you can provide.
- Respect the importance of pain. People deserve to have their pain relieved to the extent that it is safe and feasible—with a medical consultation if necessary.
- Respect and protect people's modesty. This is especially important when treating the very old, adolescents, and, sometimes, the very young Figure 4-4.

2. **Provide your name and use the patient's proper name.** Introduce yourself and your partner. If your department provides you with a name tag, then wear it. Ask the patient what he or she wishes to be called. Avoid using terms such as "honey" or "dear." Use only a patient's first name if the patient is a child or the patient asks you to use his or her first name. Rather, use a courtesy title, such as "Mr. Peters," "Mrs. Smith," or "Ms. Butler." If you do not know the patient's name, then refer to him or her as "sir" or "ma'am."
3. **Tell the patient the truth.** Even if you have to say something very unpleasant, telling the truth is better than lying. Lying will destroy the patient's trust in you and decrease your own confidence. You might not always tell the patient everything, but if the patient or a family member asks a specific question, you should answer truthfully. A direct question deserves a direct answer. If you do not know the answer to a patient's question, then say so. For example, a patient may ask, "Am I having a heart attack?" You might then answer, "I don't know, but we will certainly get more information at the hospital. Right now, I am providing you with all the care needed for a person who may be having a heart attack."
4. **Use language that the patient can understand.** Do not talk up or down to the patient in any way. Avoid technical medical terms that the patient might not understand. For example, ask the patient whether he or she has a history of "heart problems." This will usually result in more accurate information than if you ask about "previous episodes of myocardial infarction" or a "history of cardiomyopathy."
5. **Be careful what you say about the patient to others.** You need to understand the relationship between the person you are talking with and the patient. Does the patient want you talking with this person? Ask the patient if it is okay to talk with this person. While speaking to others, ensure you leave the general area of the patient if you must have a confidential conversation. Be mindful that sharing patient information may be a violation of the Health Insurance Portability and Accountability Act (HIPAA).
6. **Be aware of your body language.** Nonverbal communication is extremely important in dealing with patients. In stressful situations, patients may misinterpret your gestures and movements. Be particularly careful not to appear frustrated or threatening. Instead, position yourself at the same level or at a lower level than the patient when practical. Remember, always conduct yourself in a calm, professional manner.
7. **Always speak slowly, clearly, and distinctly.** Pay close attention to your tone of voice.
8. **If the patient is hard of hearing, then face the person so he or she can read your lips.** Do not shout at a person who is hard of hearing; shouting will not make it any easier for the patient to hear you. Shouting may also frighten the patient and can end up making communication with the patient even more difficult. Never assume an older adult patient is hard of hearing or otherwise unable to understand you. Also, never use "baby talk" with older adult patients or with anyone other than infants.
9. **Allow time for the patient to answer or respond to your questions.** Do not rush a patient unless there is immediate danger. Sick and injured people may not be thinking clearly and may need time to answer even simple questions. This is especially true when treating older adult patients.
10. **Act and speak in a calm, confident manner while caring for the patient.** Ensure you attend to the patient's pains and needs. Try to make the

patient physically comfortable and relaxed. Find out whether the patient is more comfortable sitting or lying down. Is the patient cold or hot? Does the patient want a friend or relative nearby?

Patients place their lives in your hands. They deserve to know that you can provide medical care and that you are concerned about their well-being. These 10 Golden Rules will help provide a good foundation and will make it easier to gather information when the patient wants to talk.

▶ Communicating With Specific Types of Patients

Difficult Patients

Sometimes, you need to gather information from a reluctant patient. For example, some patients may be defensive about their problems and may not want to talk about them because they are embarrassed. They may direct the conversation away from the true problem. With these patients, start the conversation as usual. Introduce yourself. Be open and compassionate. If you find yourself not getting any real answers, then consider using one of the techniques discussed later in this section.

On some occasions, patients may become hostile toward EMS providers. To help defuse these potentially escalating circumstances, stay calm. Talk to the patient openly and honestly. You will find that meeting hostility with calmness and confidence defuses a situation. Use open-ended questions, provide positive feedback, ensure the patient understands the questions, and continue to calmly ask questions. At the same time, consider the safety of the scene. Decide whether you need law enforcement. Ensure you have sufficient backup to provide safety for the patient and the crew. Then, with your backup clearly visible, calmly advise the patient what needs to be done: "Sir, I need you to sit on the ambulance stretcher now. You may proceed to the stretcher or we can help you to the stretcher." No one should threaten the patient, and no one should move toward the patient. In this rare circumstance, you are providing the patient with choices, while at the same time limiting those choices to ones you can accept.

You are guaranteed to receive some unpleasant insults from people who are in crisis, especially from patients who are chemically impaired or under the influence of street drugs or alcohol. Discipline yourself never to respond in kind. Nothing escalates a situation faster than trading insults. Very often, there are plenty of witnesses and you could experience legal ramifications from your disrespectful behavior. Nevertheless, you should consider the possibility that you may not be able to defuse someone's anger. If the situation gets out of control, then you may have to defer to law enforcement.

Your primary responsibility is to yourself and your partner—that is, to ensure scene safety. It is imperative to recognize the potential for violence and to react accordingly. Call for law enforcement as soon as you have reason to believe you may be encountering a difficult patient. This assistance may be sought en route to the call based on information obtained by the dispatcher. Remember, it is better to have law enforcement and not need them than to wait until the situation escalates before calling for help.

You may also encounter patients who are sexually aggressive. In this instance, simply changing caregivers may solve the problem. If not, then firmly explain to the patient that this is not an option and that the individual will be turned over to law enforcement if the behavior continues. In most situations, simply rebuking the advancement is enough to stop the aggression. However, if drugs or alcohol are involved, bringing in law enforcement for restraint may be necessary.

Older Adult Patients

You should not assume communicating with older adults will be harder than communicating with anyone else just because they are older. Older adults' illnesses often tend to be more complex than the illnesses of younger people, however, because they may have more than one disease or disorder and they may be taking more kinds of medicines concurrently. You may note individual differences among members of the geriatric population related to hearing, eyesight, mental status, and mobility; you need to adapt to them. Table 4-6 lists techniques to employ

Table 4-6	Interviewing Older Adult Patients
Identify yourself. Do not assume the older adult patient knows who you are.	
Be aware of how you present yourself. Frustration and impatience can be portrayed through body language.	
Look directly at the patient.	
Speak slowly and distinctly.	
Explain what you are going to do before you do it. Use simple terms to explain the use of medical equipment and procedures. Avoid medical jargon or slang.	
Listen to the answer the patient gives you.	
Show the patient respect. Refer to the patient as Mr., Mrs., or Miss.	
Do not discuss the patient in front of him or her; doing so gives the impression that the patient has no choice in his or her medical care. This point is easy to forget when the patient has impaired cognitive (thought) processes or has difficulty communicating.	
Be patient!	

when interviewing an older adult; note that these same techniques actually apply to most any patient.

Generally speaking, older adults think clearly, can give you a clear medical history, and are able to answer your questions appropriately. Do not assume an older adult is senile or confused. Also, do not assume that hostility, irritability, and confusion are normal behavior for older adults: these signs may be caused by a simple lack of oxygen (hypoxia), brain injury including a cerebrovascular accident, unintentional drug overdose, or even hypovolemia. Never attribute altered mental status to old age. Some older adult patients may have difficulty hearing or seeing you, so exercise great patience and compassion when you are called on to care for these patients. Think of the patient as someone's grandmother or grandfather—or even as yourself when you reach that age. Approach an older adult slowly and calmly. Allow plenty of time for the patient to respond to your questions.

Older adult patients often do not feel much pain. In fact, an older adult who has fallen or been injured may report no pain. Likewise, older adult patients might not be fully aware of important changes in their body systems. Therefore, be especially vigilant for objective changes—no matter how subtle—in their conditions. Objective changes are those that any observer would be able to witness. For example, respiratory rate, heart rate, sweating, or vomiting are all objective findings. Subjective findings are those that only the patient can experience, such as pain or nausea. Even minor changes in breathing or mental state may signal major problems.

Special Populations

When possible, give the patient time to pack a few personal items before leaving for the hospital. Document on the PCR that these items accompanied the patient and the person to whom they were given in the ED.

Children

Children can be difficult patients because they pose communication challenges and will likely be very frightened. They tend to protest pain vigorously, they may be afraid of strangers (including you), they may panic when separated from their parents, and their bodies may not be as familiar to many of us as are the bodies of adults. However, with a little practice, you can become comfortable treating children.

Equipment (such as stethoscopes or needles) is not as important early in your contact with children as are friendly eye contact, smiles, and calm, subdued explanations, geared to match each child's age. Discipline yourself to minimize your movements, lower your voice, and touch as gently as you can. Try placing yourself at or below the child's eye level, for instance, by sitting on the floor and placing the child on the cot or on a parent's lap **Figure 4-5**. If possible, then involve a parent in the hands-on care of an alert small child (for instance, by holding an extremity while you insert an intravenous [IV] line). This is much less effective when treating older children but is more important with infants and toddlers. If you are caring for a noncritical pediatric patient, then demonstrating the assessment procedure (eg, taking blood pressure) on a sibling or parent can often put the child at ease and facilitate assessment.

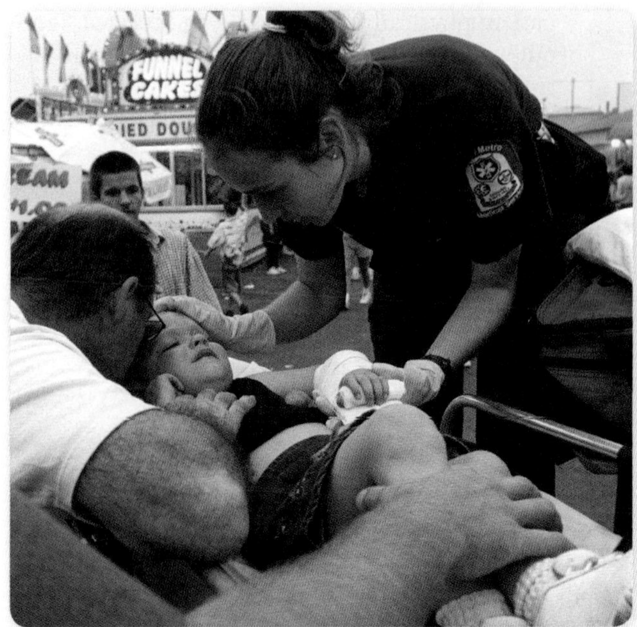

Figure 4-5 When you are examining a very young child, involve the parents. Have the father hold the child on his lap, or ask the mother to keep the child occupied while you examine the child.

Toys are useful for bridging the emotional gap between AEMTs and some children. Many crews stock their ambulances with teddy bears for toddlers. If those kinds of toys are not available, then you can make a serviceable chicken out of an exam glove by inflating the glove and marking its eyes with a felt marker; however, these can pose a choking hazard and cannot be left with the child at the end of the encounter. You are more likely to connect with the child if you do this right in front of the child rather than if you ask someone else to do it.

Children can easily see through lies or deceptions, so you must always be honest with them. Ensure you explain to the child over and over again what and why certain things are happening. If treatment will hurt, such as applying a splint, then tell the child ahead of time.

Respect a child's modesty. Children are often embarrassed if they have to undress or be undressed in front of strangers. This anxiety often intensifies during adolescence. When a wound or site of injury has to be exposed, try to do so out of the sight of strangers, and when appropriate ensure a parent or guardian is present. Again, it is extremely important to tell the child what you are doing and why you are doing it.

Special Populations

When you are assessing children, it is important to give choices so that they feel involved in their care. However, do not give yes or no choices:

- Do not ask: "Can I touch you?"
- Instead ask: "I need to listen to your heart and touch your tummy. Which would you like me to do first?"

While still involving the child in the decision process, you are not limiting your assessment.

Hard-of-Hearing Patients

Patients who are hard of hearing or deaf are usually not ashamed or embarrassed by their disability. Often, it is the people around a deaf or hard-of-hearing person who have difficulty coping. Remember, you must be able to communicate with hard-of-hearing patients so you can provide necessary or even life-saving care.

Hard-of-hearing patients have normal intelligence. They can usually understand what is going on around them, provided that you can successfully communicate with them. Most patients who are hard of hearing can read lips to some extent. Therefore, you should place yourself in a position so that the patient can see your lips.

Many hard-of-hearing patients have hearing aids to help them communicate. Be careful that hearing aids are not lost during an accident or fall. Hearing aids may also be forgotten if the patient is confused or ill. Look around, or ask the patient or the family about a hearing aid.

Remember the following five steps to help you efficiently communicate with patients who are hard of hearing:

1. **Have paper and a pen available.** This way, you can write down questions and the patient can write down answers, if necessary. Be sure to print clearly so your handwriting is not a communication barrier.
2. **If the patient can read lips, then face the patient and speak slowly and distinctly.** Do not cover your mouth or mumble. If it is night or dark, then consider moving to a lighted area or shining a light on your face.
3. **Never shout.** This will not help the patient hear you and may frighten him or her.
4. **Listen carefully, ask short questions, and give short answers.** Remember, although many hard-of-hearing patients can speak distinctly, some cannot.
5. **Learn some simple phrases in sign language.** For example, knowing the signs for "sick," "hurt," and "help" may be useful if you cannot communicate in any other way **Figure 4-6**.

Visually Impaired Patients

Like patients who are hard of hearing, visually impaired and blind patients have usually accepted and learned to deal with their disabilities. Of course, not all visually impaired patients are completely blind. Many can perceive light and dark or can see shadows or movement. Ask the patient whether he or she has any vision. Also, remember, as with other patients who have disabilities, you should expect visually impaired patients to have normal intelligence.

As you begin caring for a visually impaired patient, explain everything that you are doing in detail as you are doing it. Stay in physical contact with the patient as you begin your care. Hold your hand lightly on the patient's shoulder or arm. Try to avoid sudden movements. If the patient can walk to the ambulance, then place his or her hand on your arm, taking care not to rush. Transport any mobility aids, such as a cane, with the patient to the hospital.

Some visually impaired people may have a guide dog. Guide dogs are easily identified by their special harnesses. They are trained to not leave their owners and to not respond to strangers. A visually impaired patient who is conscious can tell you about the dog and give instructions

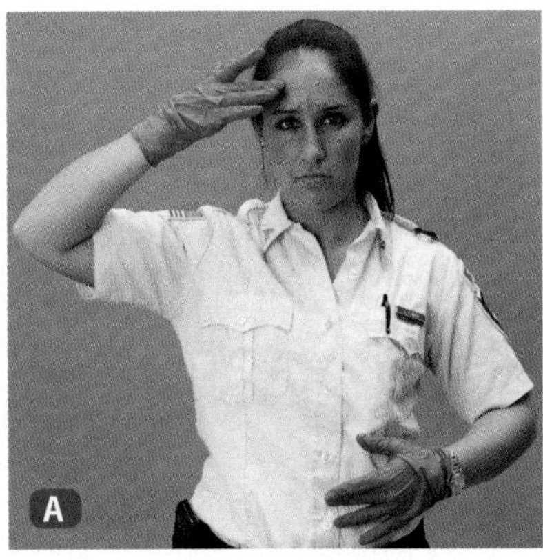

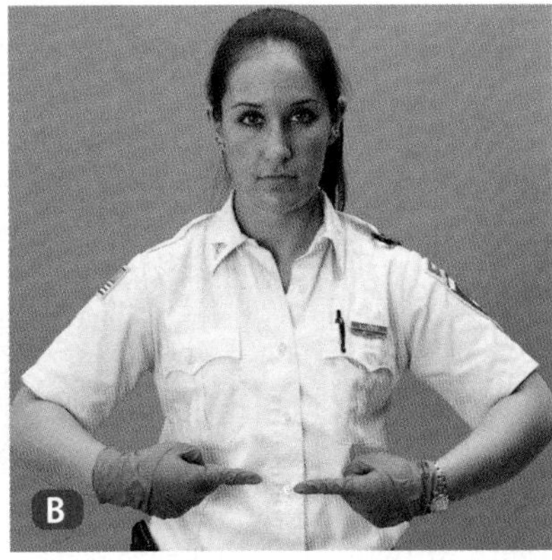

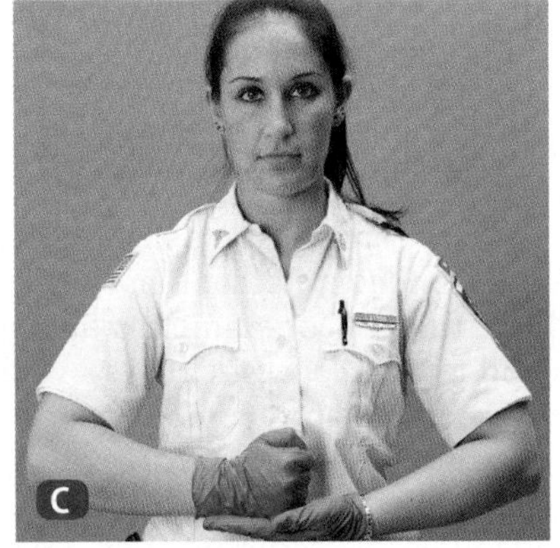

Figure 4-6 Learn simple phrases in sign language. **A.** Sick. **B.** Hurt. **C.** Help.

for its care. If circumstances permit, then bring the guide dog to the hospital with the patient. If the dog has to be left behind, then you should arrange for its care.

Non–English-Speaking Patients

Part of patient care includes obtaining a medical history from the patient. You cannot skip this step simply because the patient does not speak English. Most patients who do not speak English fluently will still know certain important words or phrases.

Your first step is to find out how much English the patient can speak. Use short, simple questions and simple words whenever possible and avoid difficult medical terms. You can help patients better understand if you point to specific parts of the body as you ask questions. Speaking louder will not increase a patient's ability to understand you.

In many areas, particularly large urban centers, major segments of the population do not speak English. Your job will be much easier if you learn some common words and phrases in their language, especially common medical terms. Pocket cards that show the pronunciation of these terms are available. If the patient does not speak any English, then use a smartphone app or website to help you translate or find an interpreter. In an emergency, it may be necessary to have a family member or friend translate until a professional interpreter is located. Also, remember to request a translator at the hospital while providing the radio report if the patient's language is known.

It is your responsibility to research which languages are spoken in your area of practice and learn how to deal with members of each culture accordingly. You may not get everything right when you encounter a representative from one of these groups, but your efforts at communicating will translate the idea of respect and that makes all the difference.

Special Needs Patients

It would be a mistake to overlook the needs of people who have speech or other kinds of communication disorders. When you encounter a patient who has trouble communicating, remember that family members or primary caregivers who know these patients well can facilitate your efforts. Just as importantly, they can also help you to alleviate fear.

Many caregivers find that touch and eye contact are helpful bridging mechanisms when dealing with some of these patients. For example, a light touch on a patient's shoulder can convey kindness, while a firm grasp can express reassurance. Some patients respond well to brief, one-armed hugging.

Another group of patients that providers are beginning to encounter more often are those with autism.[3] Children with autism may have difficulty developing language skills and understanding what others say to them. They may also have difficulty communicating nonverbally, such as through hand gestures, eye contact, and facial expressions. However, not every person with an autism spectrum disorder will have a language problem. A person's ability to communicate will vary depending on his or her intellectual and social development. If you encounter difficulty when communicating with a patient with autism, then it may be best to address questions to the caregiver. Most caregivers have developed knowledge of the patient's needs through years of working with the patient. They are your best resource for communicating with the patient with an autism spectrum disorder.

▶ Communicating With Other Health Care Professionals

Effective communication with other health care professionals in the receiving facility is a cornerstone of efficient, effective, and appropriate patient care. Your reporting responsibilities do not end when you arrive at the hospital—in fact, they have just begun. The transfer of care officially occurs during your oral report at the hospital, not during your radio report en route.

Once you arrive at the hospital, a hospital staff member will take responsibility for the patient from you **Figure 4-7**. Depending on the hospital and the condition of the patient, the training of the person who takes over the care of the patient will vary. However, you may transfer the care of your patient only to someone with at least your level of training. Once a hospital staff member is ready to take responsibility for the patient, you must provide that person with a formal oral report of the patient's condition.

Giving a report is a crucial part of transferring the patient's care from one provider to another. Your oral

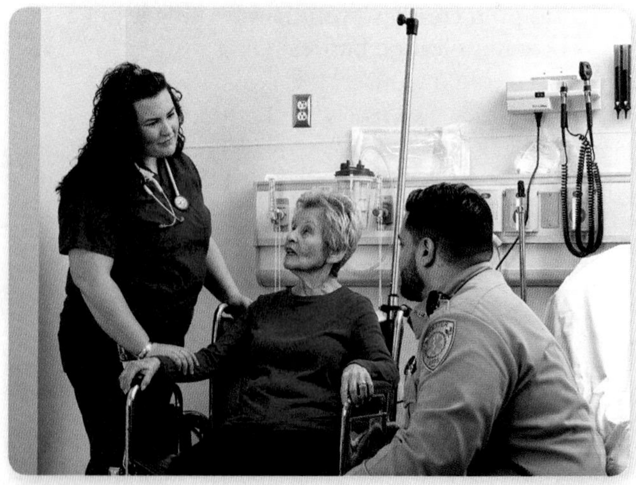

Figure 4-7 Once you arrive at the hospital, staff members will take responsibility for the patient from you.

report is usually given at the same time that the staff member is doing something for the patient. For example, a nurse or physician may be looking at the patient, beginning assessment, or helping you to move the patient from the stretcher to an examination table. Therefore, you must report important information in a complete, precise way. The following components must be included in your oral report:

1. **Opening information.** This includes the patient's name (if you know it) and the chief complaint, nature of illness, or mechanism of injury (MOI). For example: "Good morning. This is Mrs. McCarty. She is 65 years old and is reporting back pain. She woke up around 0300 hours, tripped, and fell into the bathtub after using the restroom."
2. **Detailed information.** This may include information that was not provided during the radio report. For example: "She denies losing consciousness; states she has no history of stroke, transient ischemic attacks, or cardiac compromise; but has been feeling a little light-headed when she stands."
3. **Any important history.** This includes information that was not already provided. For example: "Mrs. McCarty lives by herself. She was unable to get out of the tub and was found by a hospice worker at 1000 hours this morning. We suspect hypothermia because she had a core temperature of 94°."
4. **Pertinent findings of the physical exam.** Relay any pertinent findings of the physical exam. For example: "We noted two wounds: a small one on the patient's abdomen and a larger one on the patient's back."
5. **The patient's response to treatment.** It is especially important to report any changes in the patient or the treatment provided since your radio report. Include treatments given en route. For example: "Oxygen was initiated by nonrebreathing face mask at 15 L/min. Although we suspected that her midback pain was a result of her leaning against the faucet of the bathtub for 7 hours, we put her in the Kendrick extrication device for both precautionary and extrication reasons. Hot packs wrapped in hand towels were used to help warm her up."
6. **Vital signs.** Vital signs must also be assessed during transport and after the radio report. For example: "Her vitals include a blood pressure of 112/84 mm Hg, a pulse of 72 beats/min, respirations of 14 breaths/min, and core body temperature of 94° at the time of transport. They are generally unchanged since then, except that her last temperature was 96°."
7. **Other information.** Include any other information that you may have gathered but was not important enough to report sooner. Information that was gathered during transport, any patient medications you have brought with you, and any other details about the patient that were provided by family members or friends may be included. For example: "Mrs. Woods, the home hospice worker, has contacted Mrs. McCarty's family and followed us here to answer any questions."

You can use the same process described for giving an oral report if you need to transfer care during an EMS event. For example, if there are many patients present at the scene (eg, mass-casualty event), you may need to remain on the scene while someone else continues the assessment you began. Begin the oral report with a quick introduction, letting the other EMS provider know who you are and what your level of licensure is. You should then continue to transfer care to someone of an equal or higher level of training just as you would inside the hospital.

As an AEMT, you will also need to communicate routinely with many other professionals—law enforcement, social service personnel, fire personnel, and other EMS providers. Ensure your language and general demeanor are professional. Remember, federal laws protect a patient's right to privacy and that you should not give any health information about your patient to anyone other than those directly involved in the care of the patient.

As an AEMT, you must be able to quickly and accurately find out what the patient needs and be able to tell others. Never forget that you are the vital link between the patient and the health care team.

Words of Wisdom

In 1996, HIPAA established mandatory patient privacy rules and regulations to safeguard patient confidentiality.[4] The act provides guidance on the types of information that are protected, the responsibility of health care providers regarding that protection, and penalties for breaching that protection.

Communications Systems and Equipment

Communication during an emergency call will require the use of specialized equipment. Although the digital revolution is improving communications, most EMS communications systems today are based on the use of radios, so it is important for you to learn about radio signals and to know which equipment is available for sending and receiving those messages.

A key aspect of EMS communications is a reliable method of sending and receiving information back and forth to medical direction. Although this communication has mainly been accomplished by radio in the past, cellular devices and mobile data terminals (MDTs) are becoming more popular ways to share this kind of information. The EMS system must be configured to allow 24-hour methods of contact with medical direction at local and regional facilities.

Although these communications systems are relatively dependable, a backup communications system is also needed. For example, if the primary method of communication is digital radio, a secondary means might include the use of cell phones, a satellite phone, or an MDT. Having backup communications systems in place ensures there will always be a method to access medical direction, in any circumstance, 24 hours per day.

Backup communications are even more critical in times of disaster or mass-casualty incidents (MCIs). In these situations, primary methods of communications may be disabled. Cell towers may be damaged, cell sites may be disabled, and computer data servers may be crippled. In these circumstances, disaster communications are often established by amateur radio groups. Most of the equipment for this type of communication is available after a major incident through your local emergency management office.

No matter which type of system you are using for EMS communications, you must know what that system can and cannot do, and you must be able to use your system efficiently and effectively. You must be able to send precise, accurate reports about the scene, the patient's condition, and the treatment that you provide. Thus, you must know when to use your communications equipment and what to say when you are transmitting (effective radio communications is discussed later in this chapter).

At the same time, you must recognize that the information shared through EMS communications systems is subject to some constraints. Under the HIPAA regulations, most personal health information is considered protected and should not be released without the patient's permission. These regulations apply to all forms of communication—written and verbal. To ensure that you are protecting your patient's right to confidentiality, do not give any information to anyone other than those directly involved in the care of the patient. When sharing information verbally (eg, by radio or cell phone), ensure unauthorized people nearby cannot overhear the content of that communication. Finally, become familiar with all policies and procedures governing communication established by your particular agency.

A **scanner** is a radio receiver that searches or "scans" across several frequencies until the message is completed. These devices may be used by their owners to eavesdrop on nearby radio traffic. Although cell/satellite telephones are more private than most other forms of radio communications (because they use digital communication,

YOU are the Provider — PART 2

While you are interviewing the patient, bystanders come out of the house and start raising their voices, stating, "He didn't throw anything at you, you did that to yourself!" Recognizing that her friends are intoxicated and that this scene could easily escalate, you request that law enforcement officers remove the disruptive parties.

Recording Time: 1 Minute	
Appearance	Anxious
Level of consciousness	Alert and oriented
Airway	Patent
Breathing	16 breaths/min
Circulation	Strong radial pulse; skin is warm, dry, and pink

3. What are two types of questions that are asked during a patient interview?
4. Which techniques can be used to deescalate difficult situations?

rather than radio frequencies), they can still be overheard. Given that the risk of someone overhearing your messages is essentially omnipresent, you must always be careful to appropriately respect patient privacy and to speak in a professional manner every time you use any form of an EMS communications system.

▶ Regulation of Radio and Telephone Communications

All radio operations in the United States, including those used in EMS systems, are regulated by the **Federal Communications Commission (FCC)**.[5] The FCC has jurisdiction over interstate and international telephone and telegraph services and satellite communications—all of which may involve EMS activity.

The FCC has five principal EMS-related responsibilities:

1. **Allocating specific radio frequencies for use by EMS providers.** Modern EMS communications began in 1974. At that time, the FCC assigned 10 MED channels in the 460- to 470-MHz (UHF) band to be used by EMS providers. These UHF channels were added to the several VHF frequencies that were already available for EMS systems. However, these VHF frequencies had to be shared with other "special emergencies" uses, including school buses and veterinarians. In 1993, the FCC created an EMS-only block of frequencies in the 220-MHz portion of the radio spectrum.
2. **Licensing base stations and assigning appropriate radio call signs for those stations.** An FCC license is usually issued for 5 years, after which time it must be renewed. Each FCC license is granted only for a specific operating group. Often, the longitude and latitude (locations) of the antenna and the address of the base station determine the call signs.
3. **Establishing licensing standards and operating specifications for radio equipment used by EMS providers.** Before it can be licensed, each piece of radio equipment must be submitted to the FCC by its manufacturer for type acceptance, based on established operating specifications and regulations.
4. **Establishing limitations for transmitter power output.** The FCC regulates broadcasting power to reduce radio interference between neighboring communications systems.
5. **Monitoring radio operations.** This includes making spot field checks to help ensure compliance with FCC rules and regulations.

The FCC's rules and regulations fill many volumes and are written in technical and legal language. Only a small section (part 90, subpart B) deals with EMS communications issues. You are not responsible for reading these detailed and often complex documents. For appropriate guidance on technical issues, contact your EMS systems' supervisor. In fact, many EMS systems look to radio and telephone communications experts for advice on technical issues.

▶ Radio Communications

As an AEMT, you must be familiar with two-way radio communications and have a working knowledge of the mobile and handheld portable radios that are used in your unit. A two-way radio consists of two units: a transmitter and a receiver. Some base stations may have more than one transmitter and/or more than one receiver. They may also be equipped with one multichannel transmitter and several single-channel receivers. A **channel** is an assigned frequency or frequencies used to carry voice and/or data communications. A **frequency** is the number of cycles (oscillations) per second of a radio signal.

Base Station Radios

The dispatcher usually communicates with field units by transmitting through a fixed radio base station that is controlled by the dispatch center. The **base station** is any radio hardware containing a transmitter and a receiver that is located in a fixed place. The base station may be used in a single place by an operator speaking into a microphone that is connected directly to the equipment. It also works remotely through telephone lines or by radio from a communications center. Base station locations may include dispatch centers, fire stations, ambulance bases, or hospitals.

Base station radios usually have more power (often 100 watts or more) and higher, more efficient antenna systems than mobile or portable radios. The increased broadcasting range allows the base station operator to communicate with field units and other stations at much greater distances.

The base station radio must be physically close to its antenna. Therefore, the actual base system cabinet and hardware are commonly found on the roof of a tall building or at the bottom of an antenna tower. The antenna system has a vital part in transmission and reception efficiency. The base station operator may be miles away in a dispatch center or hospital, communicating with the base station radio by dedicated lines or special radio links.

A **dedicated line**, also known as a hotline, is used for specific point-to-point contact within a base station system. This type of phone, which is typically located within an ED, is not on the main switchboard. EMS personnel are able to call the number directly without being placed on hold or transferred. Generally, once the handset is lifted, the phone on the opposite end rings. This type of line makes contacting and recording medical command conversations much easier.

Mobile and Portable Radios

Once you leave the station, you will use both mobile and portable radios to communicate with the dispatcher and/or medical control. A **mobile radio** is mounted inside a vehicle. An ambulance will often have more than one mobile radio, each on a different frequency. One radio may be used to communicate with the dispatcher or other public safety agencies, while a second radio, mounted in the patient compartment, is often used for communicating patient information to medical control. A mobile radio usually operates at lower power than a base station (20 to 50 watts). It is also assigned to a specific radio frequency band. Certain frequency bands are more suitable for use under specific conditions.

Mobile transmitters/receivers, or transceivers, come in a variety of power ranges. The power output largely determines the distance over which the signal can be effectively transmitted. A transmitter in the 7.5-watt range, for example, will transmit for distances of 10 to 12 miles (16 to 19 km) over slightly hilly terrain. Transmission distances are greater over water or flat terrain and reduced in mountainous areas or where there are many tall buildings. Mobile transmitters with higher outputs have proportionally greater transmission ranges, making them useful, for example, in disaster situations where mobile units are in use. Today, the typical mobile transmitter operates at between 20 and 50 watts of power output.

Frequency bands are portions of the radio frequency spectrum assigned for specific uses. The most commonly used bands for medical communications are the **very high-frequency (VHF) band** and the **ultrahigh-frequency (UHF) band**. The VHF band extends from roughly 30 to 300 MHz. VHF has been arbitrarily divided into a low band (30 to 50 MHz) and a high band (132 to 174 MHz).

Words of Wisdom

VHF low-band frequencies may have ranges up to 2,000 miles (3,219 km) but are unpredictable because changes in ionospheric (about 30 miles [about 50 km] into the atmosphere) conditions may cause "skip interference," with patchy losses in communication. The high-band frequencies are almost wholly free of skip interference, but have a much shorter transmission range. The most commonly used of the VHF high-band frequencies for emergency medical purposes are in the 150- to 160-MHz range. This has historically been the main radio band assigned by the FCC.[6]

In the late 1970s, the UHF band was assigned to EMS in the form of the MED channels. The UHF band extends from 300 to 3,000 MHz, with most medical communications occurring around 450 to 470 MHz. At these frequencies, communications are entirely free of skip interference and have minimal noise (ie, signal distortion). The UHF band has better penetration in dense metropolitan areas, and UHF reception is usually quite adequate inside buildings. The UHF band, however, has a shorter range than the VHF band, and energy at UHF frequencies is more readily absorbed by rain and environmental objects, such as trees and brush.

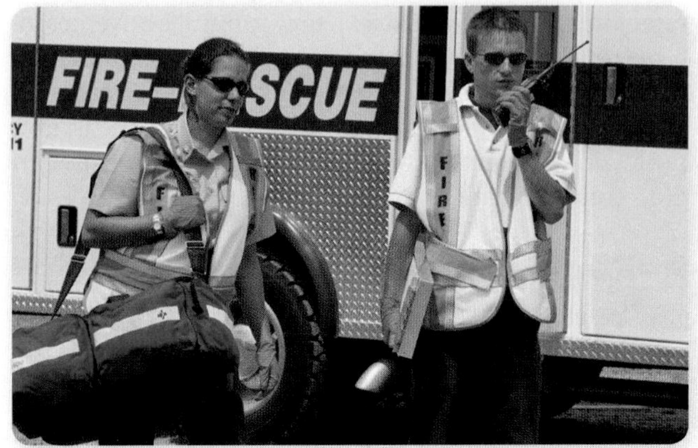

Figure 4-8 A portable radio is essential if you need to communicate with the dispatcher or medical control when you are away from the ambulance.

A **portable radio** is a handheld, two-way radio with a limited range and low power (1 to 5 watts), although the signal of a handheld transmitter can be boosted by retransmission through the vehicle. These radios are carried by EMS providers when they are away from the vehicle **Figure 4-8**. Portable units may also be used by physician consultants when not stationed at the hospital.

Radios that operate at 800 MHz (also known as trunked systems, discussed later) are also becoming increasingly common in EMS systems. This frequency offers excellent penetration of buildings and has minimal interference and reduced channel noise. What was once accomplished with 30 separate frequencies can be done with less than 10. Mobile antennas are much closer to the ground than base station antennas, so communications from the unit are typically limited to 10 to 15 miles over average terrain.

Assigned radio frequencies may be used in a variety of systems. In a **simplex** (push to talk, release to listen) system, or half-duplex system, portable units can transmit in either direction but not simultaneously in both. When one party transmits, the other can only receive. A simplex system requires only a single radio frequency. A network that uses two different frequencies at the same time to permit simultaneous transmission (talk) and reception (listen) (like a telephone) is referred to as **duplex**. In the full duplex mode, radios can simultaneously transmit and receive communications on one channel—an approach sometimes called a pair of frequencies. **Multiplex** communications (combining both analog and digital signals) can simultaneously transmit two or more different types of information, such as voice and telemetry, in either or both directions over the same frequency. As noted earlier, a number of VHF and UHF channels, commonly called **MED channels**, are reserved exclusively for EMS use.

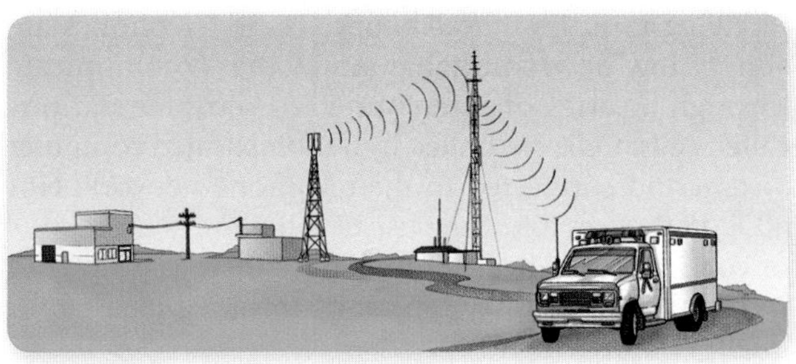

Figure 4-9 A message is sent from the control center to the transmitter by a landline. The radio carrier wave is picked up by the repeater for rebroadcast to outlying units. Return radio traffic is picked up by the repeater and rebroadcast to the control center.

However, hundreds of other commercial, local government, and fire services frequencies are also used for EMS communications.

Repeater-Based Systems

A **repeater** is a special base station that receives messages and signals on one frequency and then automatically retransmits them on a second frequency **Figure 4-9**. A repeater is a base station (with a large antenna) that is able to receive lower-power signals, such as those from a portable radio, from a long distance away. The signal is then rebroadcast with all the power of the base station. EMS systems that use repeaters usually have outstanding systemwide communications and are able to get the best signal from portable radios. Mobile repeaters may also be found in ambulances or placed in various areas around an EMS system area.

At times, you may be able to communicate with a base station radio, but you will not be able to hear or transmit to another mobile unit that is also communicating with that base. Repeater base stations eliminate such problems. They allow two mobile or portable units that cannot reach each other directly to communicate through the repeater, using its greater power and antenna.

Digital Radio and Trunked Systems

Digital radio may help clear up distorted or lost transmissions, which are always possible with base station, mobile, and portable radio communications. **Digital radio** systems allow the transmission of digital signals (computer) or analog (voice) signals that have been digitized and compressed by a computer. Digital signals are clearer and allow the transmission of a greater volume of data in the same bandwidth. Digital radios can communicate with other digital radios and with analog radios. Conventional radios operate on fixed radio frequency channels. When radios have multiple channels, they operate on one channel at a time and the proper channel is selected by a user. That is, the user picks the channel by using a channel selector or pressing a button on the radio control panel.

With digital **trunked radios**, either 800- or 900-MHz systems, instead of being assigned to one or two frequencies, many frequencies are assigned to a group. These groups can be thought of as virtual channels that appear and disappear as conversations occur. As a radio conversation begins, a computer selects or *scans* for the next open frequency and you can begin talking. When you speak a second time, you will likely be speaking on a different frequency because the computer is constantly monitoring for frequency load and reassigning transmissions to unused frequencies. These systems allow for greater traffic without greater numbers of frequencies. Therefore, you do not need to worry about being able to transmit or receive. In a trunking system, the computer will switch you to another channel without your knowledge and you will operate the radio as you normally do.

Concerns Related to Radio Communication

Your ability to effectively communicate with other units or medical control via radio depends on how well the weaker radio can "talk back." Base and repeater station radios often have higher antennas and much greater power than mobile or portable units do. This increased power ensures that signals are generally heard and understood from a far greater distance than the signal produced from a mobile unit. Remember, when you are at the scene, you may be able to clearly hear the dispatcher or hospital on your radio, but you may not be heard or understood when you transmit.

Even small changes in your location can significantly affect the quality of your transmission. Also remember that the location of the antenna is critically important for clear transmission. Commercial aircraft flying at an altitude of 37,000 feet (11 km) can transmit and receive signals over hundreds of miles, yet their radios have only a few watts of power. The "power" comes from their antenna positioned at 37,000 feet.

The success of communications depends on the efficiency of your equipment. A damaged antenna or microphone often prevents high-quality communications. Check the condition and status of your equipment at the start of each shift, and then correct or report any problems.

Maintenance of Radio Equipment

Like all other EMS equipment, radio equipment must be serviced by properly trained and equipped personnel. Remember, the radio is your lifeline to other public safety agencies (which function to protect you), as well as medical control, and it must perform under emergency conditions. Radio equipment that is operating properly should be serviced at least once a year. Any equipment that is not working properly should be immediately removed from service and sent for repair. Outdated equipment should be immediately removed from service as new equipment becomes available.

When you are beginning your shift, it is typical to check the ambulance to ensure it is ready to go. You cannot assume the crew before you left the ambulance well stocked and in operational readiness. The radio is also an important component that needs to be checked to ensure that it is operating correctly and using the correct frequency.

Maintaining radio equipment will also help to ensure efficient, effective communication and ensure the radio is not drifting from its assigned frequency. If possible, do not subject radio equipment to dusty, damp, or wet environments. Frequent cleaning of radio equipment will improve its appearance as well as life expectancy. Use only a slightly damp rag with very mild detergent (no cleaning solvents on the exterior surfaces of radio equipment).

Properly used, rechargeable batteries in portable radios and other equipment (including monitor/defibrillators) will maximize life and power output. Ensure you recharge batteries as needed. Finally, familiarize yourself with the manufacturer's instructions for each piece of equipment you are using.

▶ Cell/Satellite Telephones

While it is common for dispatchers to communicate with field units by transmitting through a fixed radio base station, it is common for providers to communicate to receiving facilities by **cell phone**. These telephones are simply low-power portable radios that communicate through a series of interconnected repeater stations called cells. Cells are linked by a sophisticated computer system and connected to the telephone network. Not all EMS services allow the use of cell phones for reports or contacting medical control; since there is no way to record these calls, they cannot be reviewed or used for quality improvement.

Another option is a satphone, or satellite phone. These phones use a satellite, which receives and relays the signals, instead of a cellular system. Satellite telephones and messaging devices can be valuable in rural and remote areas with spotty or absent radio and cell phone coverage. They are also an invaluable resource in disaster situations. However, this technology is expensive, compared to the alternatives that exist, which can limit its accessibility.

Many cellular systems make equipment and air time available to EMS at little or no cost as a public service. The public is often able to call 9-1-1 or other emergency numbers on a cell phone free of charge. However, this easy access may result in overloading and jamming of cellular systems in MCIs and disaster situations, and you should have a backup communications plan in your service to circumvent these overloads.

As with all repeater-based systems, a cell/satellite telephone is useless if the equipment fails, loses power, or is damaged by severe weather or other circumstances. Because these telephones use digital signals, eavesdropping on communication shared through these devices is difficult—but not impossible.

Words of Wisdom

Since the introduction of smartphones, EMS communication has been greatly enhanced. Not only is a cell phone convenient for calling medical control or a supervisor, but it also provides a wealth of knowledge at the touch of a button. Global positioning system (GPS) receivers and mapping software are excellent resources in unfamiliar territories. Translating apps are available for almost any language you may encounter; written or verbal translations make it much easier to care for a non–English-speaking patient. There are also many apps created especially for medical personnel and EMS personnel, such as pharmaceutical references and EMS field guides at every level. Many services have even created apps or internet links to local protocols.

Remember the saying "A picture is worth a thousand words"? Think how valuable a quick photo of the extensive damage to a vehicle and the resulting size of the patient compartment may be to a trauma surgeon who is receiving a patient from that particular crash. Photos of injuries might also be sent ahead to the ED in preparation for patient arrival. Video conferences (such as telemedicine or the use of video conferencing apps) between medical control and the reluctant patient may be the push needed to convince him or her to accept treatment and transport. However, you must never infringe on a patient's privacy. Any photos or videos taken should be shown or sent only to those personnel who are providing care for the patient.

▶ Digital Equipment

The term *biotelemetry* in emergency medical care is usually shortened to *telemetry*. **Telemetry** is the capability of measuring vital life signs and transmitting these data to a distant terminal. Telemetry started with electrocardiograms (ECGs), but now often includes other measurements. Even the US space program uses telemetry to send pulse and respiratory rate data for astronauts from space to a receiving station on earth.[7]

Most often, telemetry is a short way of saying that you are transmitting an ECG signal from the patient to a distant receiving station. The standard ECG is composed of low-frequency signals (100 Hz or less), which would be filtered out by a voice communications system. To ensure voice communication does not filter out the ECG, the ECG signal must be **encoded** if it is to be sent over the same radio channels used to transmit voice. ECG telemetry over UHF frequencies is confined to one lead of a 12-lead ECG, so it can be used to interpret cardiac rhythms. For a more complete diagnosis of an ECG, such as in the case of examining the ECG of a patient with suspected acute coronary syndrome, the information from all 12 leads of the ECG must be examined.

New technology also allows for digital telemetry. For example, data from cardiac monitors can be transmitted via Bluetooth-enabled mobile devices to a monitoring center, where physicians can review the data quickly and give further orders if needed. The majority of cardiac monitors used on ambulances today have the technology to transmit 12-lead ECGs directly to the ED where the patient is being transported. Digital signals are also used in some kinds of paging and tone alerting systems because they transmit faster than spoken words and allow more choices and flexibility.

Distortion of the ECG signal by extraneous spikes and waves (noise) may arise from a variety of sources:

- Muscle tremor
- Loose ECG electrodes
- Sources of 60-cycle alternating current (AC), such as transformers, power lines, and electric equipment
- Attenuation (reduction) of transmitter power, caused by weak batteries or transmission beyond the range of the transmitter

Other Communications Equipment

Interoperability

Any large-scale emergency requires cooperative efforts from several agencies such as law enforcement, fire departments, and EMS. At times, more than one jurisdiction is involved and effective communication among all of those involved becomes challenging. Due to difficulties arising from incompatible communications systems, there is a push for interoperability—compatibility of an agency's communications system with that of another agency. An **interoperable communications system** allows all of the agencies involved to share valuable information with each other in real time. This system utilizes voice-over-Internet-protocol (VoIP) technology to connect landlines, cell phones, and computers to create a seamless, reliable exchange of information among all parties.

The US Department of Homeland Security developed the SAFECOM communications program, a set of national interoperability standards intended to develop compatibility across communications systems, whether local, state, or federal, etc. An important part of these interoperability standards is the use of nationally standardized frequencies for disasters and other communications. Each state has also established its own internal standards for interoperability between local jurisdictions.

In addition, the Association of Public-Safety Communications Officials-International has established digital radio hardware standards, known as the Project 25 (P25) standards, to ensure digital radio equipment manufacturers develop systems that are compatible with each other, and with older systems that may still be in use.

Words of Wisdom

Public safety agencies must place greater importance on how they use technology and how it enhances the ability to protect and serve.[8] Public safety communications channels are available for listening on the Internet or are openly broadcast, giving the public, media, criminals, and potential terrorists immediate access to information. While public safety agencies must work together to enhance interoperability, they must also respect the need to protect critical communications from compromise. Failure to do so may result in a delay in emergency response, an impedance of investigations or surveillance, and endangerment to the public.

Encryption (scrambling of data so that only those with a "key" can understand it) of information transmitted via public safety radios may be the best way to protect critical information transmitted over the airwaves. However, encryption can be an issue if responding agencies do not have the key and therefore cannot hear the broadcast. While encryption is common for federal agencies, state and local governments must consider the costs of implementation, the associated complex legal issues, and the question of who will have access. Then they must weigh these costs against the risks associated with exposure of sensitive information.

Computer-Aided Dispatch

Digital systems may also communicate text from **computer-aided dispatch (CAD)**. Ambulances are equipped with vehicle locators that allow the computer to "see" the location of each ambulance. A CAD system is a computerized method of call handling in which a computer collects and manages the call information and makes recommendations for which EMS unit is closest based on existing dispatch policy. As it does this, the data for dispatch can be sent directly to the individual EMS unit by data transfer. The result is that the EMS unit will see what is seen on the CAD terminal. For example, a display in an ambulance might give a textual location for a call and any related details, including mapping and directions to a call. When the driver presses an acknowledge button, data are sent in the opposite direction and the call is flagged as having been received by the driver. The entire dispatch and call response information exchange is visible on the mobile display.

In addition to managing call dispatch and location information, the CAD can recommend emergency actions to the dispatcher for relay to the patient or bystanders at the emergency scene. Such **prearrival instructions** allow care to begin even before the ambulance arrives on the scene. The CAD operator has access to emergency aid information relating to almost every possible EMS-related emergency. These protocols are typically developed by a major supplier and then reviewed by a physician. On installation, the

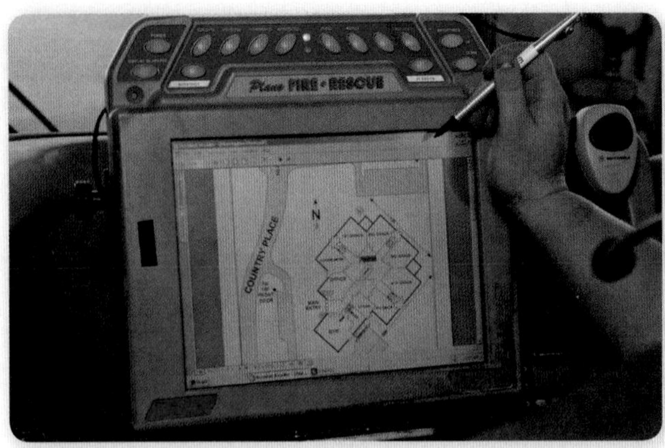

Figure 4-10 A mobile data terminal.

protocols must then be reviewed and approved by local medical direction and the EMS system.

Mobile Data Terminals

Another type of communications system becoming popular is **mobile data terminals (MDTs)** Figure 4-10. An MDT is a small computer terminal inside an ambulance that directly receives data from the dispatch center. An MDT allows for greatly expanded communication capabilities. Instead of having to listen to the dispatcher and determine whether he said 11345 Main Street or 11354 Main Street, you look at the terminal where the address is displayed and obtain directions. An MDT may also allow for communication without the use of the radio. For example, providers can press a button on the MDT that corresponds with *en route* or *on scene*, to communicate their acknowledgment to dispatch. Satellite communications can track your progress to the scene via GPS mapping and can provide important scene information, such as known violent calls to this address, the nature of those calls, and the number of times the ambulance has been called.

Backup Communications Strategies

Sometimes, radio equipment will stop working during a run. Your EMS system must have several backup plans and options. The goal of a backup plan is to ensure you can maintain contact when the usual procedures do not work. There are quite a few options.

The simplest backup plan relies on written standing orders. **Standing orders** are written documents that have been signed by the EMS system's medical director. These orders outline specific directions, permissions, and sometimes prohibitions regarding patient care. By their very nature, standing orders do not require prior communication with medical control. When properly followed, standing orders or formal protocols have the same authority and legal status as orders given over the radio. They exist in every EMS system and can be applied to all levels of EMS providers.

In addition to radio communications, most EMS systems use **landline** (telephone) backup to link various fixed components of their communications system, such

YOU are the Provider PART 3

Using verbal techniques, you and the officers are able to calm the friends, and the officers walk the friends to the opposite side of the yard in an attempt to keep them away from the patient. You ask her if she would like to be transported to the ED. She replies, "I guess it's not that bad; I would just like to stay here." On the basis of local protocols requiring medical control approval for any patient refusals, you contact your medical control for permission to obtain a refusal of care. Next, you ask the patient to wash the injury and apply a bandage to the laceration on the patient's arm.

Recording Time: 8 Minutes	
Respirations	16 breaths/min
Pulse	Strong and regular, at 74 beats/min
Skin	Warm, dry, and pink
Blood pressure	112/84 mm Hg
Oxygen saturation (Spo_2)	100% on room air
Pupils	Pupils Equal, Round, and Reactive to Light and Accommodation (PERRLA)

5. What is the main thing to remember when communicating with medical control?
6. Does this patient have the right to refuse transport to the hospital?

as hospitals, public safety services, and poison control. Telephones may also be patched into radio transmissions through the base station, enabling, for example, communication between paramedics using radios in the field and a physician using his or her telephone at home.

Moreover, as mentioned earlier, cell phones are becoming an increasingly important part of EMS communications, overcoming many of the problems associated with the overcrowded EMS radio frequencies. Cell phones are less expensive than radios and generally give a much clearer signal. Furthermore, they enable an AEMT in the field to communicate with anyone who has a telephone—for example, the patient's family physician, an injured child's parent, or an expert in another state who can advise on a hazardous materials situation. However, the limitations of using cellular communications as a backup become apparent in disasters. If a disaster affects your primary communications system (eg, through widespread power outages or tower damage), then the cell towers may be affected as well. In addition, the cell sites may be overwhelmed with civilian traffic. The cellular computer that assigns channels will not recognize an AEMT's phone and give it priority over another user's phone, so you may face delays in getting a channel.

In these situations, older low-band and high-band simplex systems that are still licensed and maintained just for redundancy may prove invaluable. In the case of disasters or power failures, older systems can still transmit and receive because most base stations have generators and EMS units operate off batteries. Because no power supply is necessary at a cell site or repeater site miles away, the older radios continue to allow communication.

The EMS Communication Process

The verb "to dispatch" means "to send out on a mission," but the **emergency medical dispatcher (EMD)** does a lot more than just send ambulances out to emergencies. The EMD functions as a vital part of the AEMT team who obtains as much information as possible about the emergency, then directs the appropriate vehicle to the scene, and provides the caller with whatever advice may be needed to manage the situation until help arrives. The EMD also monitors and coordinates communication with the field and maintains written records pertaining to the response to the call.

Notification

The first stage of EMS response is notification; that is, someone has to tell EMS that an emergency exists. Usually, notification is carried out by telephone or cell phone, and the person requesting help communicates with the EMD **Figure 4-11**. A universal emergency telephone number—9-1-1 in the United States—and the availability of telephones and cell phones in most places has greatly helped notification. Notification may, less frequently, come by radio, when the emergency is detected by a law enforcement or other public vehicle.

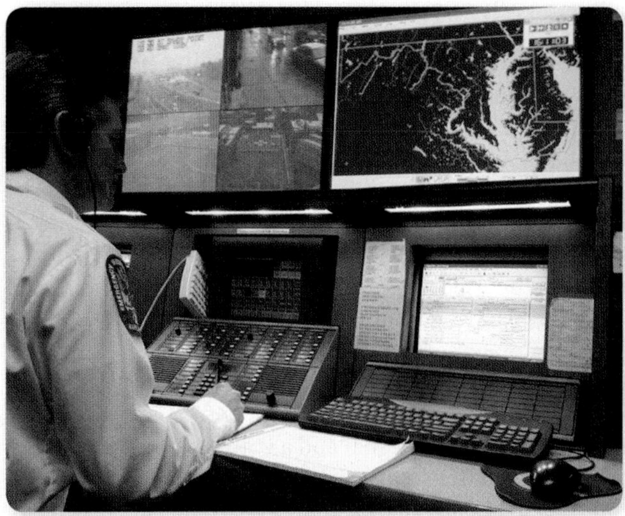

Figure 4-11 The dispatcher receives the first call to 9-1-1.

When the first call to 9-1-1 comes in, the dispatcher must judge its relative importance to begin the appropriate EMS response using emergency medical dispatch protocols. First, the dispatcher must find out the exact location of the patient and the nature and severity of the problem. The dispatcher asks for the caller's telephone number, the patient's name and age, and other information, as directed by local protocol. Next, the dispatcher asks for some description of the scene, such as the number of patients or special environmental hazards.

From this information, the dispatcher will assign the appropriate EMS response unit or units on the basis of local protocols to determine the level and type of response and the following factors:

- The dispatcher's determination of the nature and severity of the problem (Many emergency medical dispatch systems will determine this automatically based on a caller's answers to a defined series of questions.)
- Anticipated response time to the scene
- Level of training (emergency medical responder, emergency medical technician, AEMT, Paramedic) of available EMS response unit or units
- Need for additional EMS units, fire suppression, rescue, a hazardous materials team, air medical support, or law enforcement

Information about such hazards enables the EMD to contact other agencies that may have to be involved, such as utility workers to take care of downed wires. In most modern dispatch centers, the EMD has visual prompts with the key questions to ask on the computer screen. In services equipped with **enhanced 9-1-1**, much of the call information—such as the phone number and location of the caller—is recorded automatically, and the EMD just needs to confirm the information on the screen.

Dispatch

The next step is dispatch, communicating from the service headquarters with the responding EMS team. The appropriate crew is contacted and informed of the nature of the call and its exact location. The dispatcher may use the dispatch radio system to contact units that are already in service and monitoring the channel. Dedicated lines (hotlines) between the control center and the EMS station may also be used.

The dispatcher may also page EMS personnel. Pagers are commonly used in EMS operations to alert on-duty and off-duty personnel, and in many cases are simulcast with radio transmissions. **Paging** involves the use of a coded tone or digital radio signal and a voice or display message that is transmitted to pagers (beepers) or desktop monitor radios. Paging signals may be sent to alert only certain personnel, or they may be blanket signals that will activate all the pagers in the EMS service. Pagers and monitor radios are convenient because they are usually silent until their specific paging code is received. Alerted personnel contact the dispatcher to confirm the message and receive details of their assignments. This step is eliminated when pages and radio transmissions are simultaneous. For example, personnel may acknowledge the transmission via radio without the need to verbally verify addresses (because they are available on the pager). Additional information may also be sent to the pager instead of over the radio. This is especially helpful when information is sensitive or radio traffic is particularly heavy.

Once EMS personnel have been alerted, they must be properly dispatched and sent to the incident. Every EMS system should use a standard dispatching procedure. The dispatcher should give the responding unit or units the following information:

- Nature and severity of the injury, illness, or incident
- Exact location of the incident
- Number of patients
- Responses by other public safety agencies
- Special directions or advisories, such as adverse road or traffic conditions, severe weather reports, or potential scene hazards
- Time at which the unit or units are dispatched
- Any additional pertinent information gathered, such as the potential for exposure to infectious diseases

Your unit must confirm with the dispatcher that you have received the information and are en route to the scene. Local protocol will dictate whether it is the job of the dispatcher or your unit to notify other public safety agencies that you are responding to an emergency. In some areas, the ED is also notified when an ambulance responds to an emergency.

While en route to and from the scene, you should report to the dispatcher any special hazards or road conditions that might affect other responding units. Report any unusual delay, such as roadblocks, traffic, or construction.

You should inform the dispatcher when you have arrived at the scene. The arrival report to the dispatcher should include any obvious details that you see during scene size-up. For example, you might say, "Dispatcher, BLS Unit Two is on scene at 381 Mitchell Street. It is a blue house with long driveway." This information is particularly useful if additional units are responding to the same scene. You should also report to the dispatcher any problems during your response.

Words of Wisdom

Some agencies use a *tiered response system.* Initially, a basic life support (BLS) unit responds to a scene and makes the determination of which resources are needed. If a higher level of training is required, then the dispatcher sends the appropriate unit or units. This frees up resources and ensures advanced units respond only to advanced life support (ALS) calls.

En Route Communications

Once the ambulance is dispatched, the EMD may return to the telephone to obtain further information from the original caller. Further questioning may reveal special conditions that might affect your team's travel to a scene or actions at the scene. The EMD will relay that information to you while you are en route, to prepare you to respond effectively. Conversely, you may need to contact the dispatcher to request additional resources.

If the dispatcher suspects the patient has a life-threatening emergency, then he or she should also use simple terms to provide prearrival instructions to the caller. These prearrival instructions include explaining to the caller how to perform procedures such as bleeding control and cardiopulmonary resuscitation (CPR) until help arrives. Some dispatch centers have trained EMS providers to relay basic medical instructions to callers when needed. The caller is likely to be in an agitated state, so instructions must be clear and simple. Such prearrival instructions give your service what many in EMS call "zero response time," providing immediate aid and assistance, which can be vital in saving a life. Simple but life-saving acts such as clearing an obstructed airway, performing chest compressions, or reassuring the patient can be performed by a layperson under the instructions of a good dispatcher. In many cases, these prearrival instructions may bring a sense of emotional support to a caller in a time of great need, reassuring people close to the patient that everything that can be done is being done.

Once the patient is ready to be moved, you must communicate with the receiving facility to let the hospital know what to expect. During transport, you must periodically

Table 4-7 Typical EMS Communications With Dispatch	
Phase of EMS Call	**EMS Unit Communication**
Initial receipt of call	Acknowledge call. Respond to the call.
En route to call	Request assistance with directions, when needed. Request additional resources, when needed.
On scene	Report arrival at scene. Check in; EMS systems will often require units to transmit every 20 minutes as a safety measure. Request additional resources, when needed. Report when leaving the scene.
Arrival at hospital (or point of transfer)	Notify dispatch of arrival at point of transfer.
Return to service	Notify dispatch when the unit is available for another call.
Others	Some systems require EMS units to notify dispatch any time they are not in the station.

Abbreviation: EMS, emergency medical services

reassess the patient's overall condition, vital signs, and response to care provided. You should immediately report any significant changes in the patient's condition, especially if the patient seems worse. This allows medical control to issue new orders and to prepare to receive the patient.

Some services have wireless systems that transmit the data in the PCR to the ED as the ambulance is pulling into the hospital's parking lot. Once back at their stations, the AEMTs can transmit the PCR, and any additional documents specific to their department, to the service's computer system.

Table 4-7 summarizes instances when EMS providers communicate with dispatch.

▶ Communicating With Medical Control and Hospitals

The principal reason for radio communication is to facilitate communication between you and medical control (and the hospital). Medical control may be located at the receiving hospital, another facility, or sometimes even in another city or state. You must, however, consult with medical control to notify the hospital of an incoming patient, to request advice or orders from medical control, or to advise the hospital of special situations.

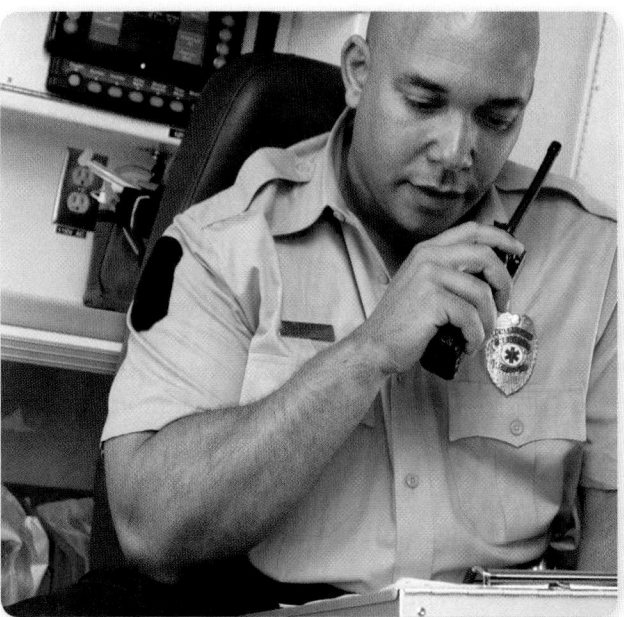

Figure 4-12 The patient report should be given in an objective, accurate, professional manner.

It is important to plan and organize your radio communication before you push the transmit button. Remember, a concise, well-organized report demonstrates your competence and professionalism in the eyes of all who hear your report. Well-organized radio communications with the hospital will engender confidence in the receiving facility's physicians and nurses, as well as others who are listening. In addition, the patient and family will be comforted by your organization and ability to communicate clearly. A well-delivered radio report puts you in control of the information, which is where you need to be.

Hospital notification is the most common type of communication between you and the hospital. The purpose of these calls is to notify the receiving facility of the patient's complaint and condition Figure 4-12. On the basis of this information, the ED is able to appropriately prepare staff and equipment to receive the patient.

The Verbal Radio Report

The verbal radio report or patient report should follow the standard format established by your EMS system. It commonly includes the following elements:

1. The receiving hospital, your unit identification, level of certification, and status of transport. Example: "Columbus Community Hospital, this is Med 2, AEMT Smythe and AEMT Jennings, en route to your emergency status."
2. The patient's age, sex, and approximate weight (if needed for drug orders). Example: "We are

en route to your facility with a 15-year-old male, approximately 50 kg." The patient's name should not be given over the radio because it may be overheard. This could be a violation of the patient's confidentiality.

3. Description of the scene. Example: "Patient was playing on a neighbor's trampoline when he jumped off the one-story garage onto the trampoline. From there he bounced off and landed on his head and shoulders."
4. The patient's level of consciousness, chief complaint or your perception of the problem, and its severity and associated symptoms. Example: "The patient is alert and oriented times three, denies any loss of consciousness, but stated he had the wind knocked out of him. Complains of numbness and tingling in all four extremities."
5. A brief, pertinent history of the patient's present illness or injury. Example: "The patient has a history of epilepsy and takes Dilantin. He says he takes it daily, but forgot to take it today."
6. A brief report of physical findings. This report should include the patient's general appearance, degree of distress, pertinent abnormalities noted, and baseline vital signs. Example: "The patient is pale, cool, and diaphoretic. Complains of numbness and tingling in all four extremities. BP is 78/32, pulse is 116, and respirations are 20."
7. A brief summary of the care given and any patient response. Example: "We have immobilized him on a long backboard. PMS in the extremities are intact. We initiated an IV bolus of normal saline and patient is on oxygen via nonrebreathing mask at 15 L/min."
8. Any other pertinent information and the estimated time of arrival (ETA). Example: "Patient physician is Kip Anderson. ETA is 4 minutes."
9. Determine whether the receiving facility has any additional questions or orders.

Ensure you report all patient information in an objective, accurate, and professional manner Table 4-8. Keep in mind that scanners may be used to monitor radio traffic. Stick to the pertinent facts of the report to avoid HIPAA violations as well as an invasion of patient privacy.

Table 4-8 Verbal Radio Report
▪ Identify destination facility ▪ Unit name and number ▪ Crew and level of certification ▪ Status of transport (emergency/nonemergency)
▪ Patient's age ▪ Patient's sex ▪ Level of consciousness
▪ Chief complaint or primary problem
▪ Description of scene ▪ General appearance
▪ Brief history of present illness/injury
▪ Associated signs/symptoms ▪ Pertinent negatives ▪ Degree of distress
▪ Vital signs • Blood pressure • Pulse • Respirations • Skin • Glucose level • Pulse oximetry
▪ Neurologic exam • Pulse, motor, sensation in extremities • Pupillary response
▪ Past pertinent medical history
▪ Secondary assessment findings
▪ Any treatment provided ▪ Response to treatment (favorable/unfavorable)
▪ Any request for treatment
▪ Name of personal physician (if appropriate)
▪ Estimated time of arrival

The Role of Medical Control

The delivery of EMS involves an impressive array of assessments, stabilization, and treatments. AEMTs may initiate medication therapy based on the patient's presenting signs. For logical, ethical, and legal reasons, the delivery of such sophisticated care must be done in association with physicians. For this reason, every EMS system needs input and involvement from physicians. One or more physicians, including your system or department medical director, will provide medical direction (medical control) for your EMS system. Medical control is either off-line (indirect) or online (direct), as authorized by the medical director. Medical control guides the treatment of patients in the system through protocols, direct orders and advice, and postcall review.

Depending on how your system's protocols are written, you may need to call medical control for direct orders (permission) to administer certain treatments, to determine the transport destination of patients, or to be allowed to stop treatment and/or transport of a patient. In these cases, the radio or cell phone provides a vital link between you and the expertise available through the base physician.

To maintain this link 24 hours a day, 7 days a week, medical control must be readily available on the radio at the hospital or on a mobile or portable unit when you call. In most areas, medical control is provided by the physicians who work at the receiving hospital. However, many variations have developed across the country. For example, some EMS units receive medical direction from one hospital even though they are taking the patient to another hospital. In other areas, medical direction may come from a free-standing center or even from an individual physician. Regardless of your system's design, your link to medical control is vital to maintain the high quality of care that your patient requires and deserves.

Calling Medical Control

You can use the radio in your unit or a portable radio to call medical control. A cell phone can also be used for this purpose. Regardless of the type of communication, you should use a channel that is relatively free of other radio traffic and interference and one that will be recorded. Medical command communications create medical legal requirements that such conversations should be recorded. There are a number of ways to control access on ambulance-to-hospital channels. In some EMS systems, the dispatcher monitors and assigns appropriate, clear medical control channels. Other EMS systems rely on special communications operations, such as a CMED (Centralized Medical Emergency Dispatch) or resource coordination centers, to monitor and allocate the medical control channels.

Because of the large number of EMS calls to medical control, your radio report must be well organized, be precise, and contain only pertinent information. In addition, if you are requesting orders for patient care, the information that you provide to medical control must be accurate. Remember, the physician on the other end bases his or her instructions on the information that you provide.

You should never use codes when communicating with medical control unless you are directed by local protocol to do so. Instead, use proper medical terminology when giving your report. Never assume medical control will know what a "10-50" or "Signal 70" means. Most medical control systems handle many different EMS agencies and will most likely not know your unit's special codes or signals.

To ensure complete understanding, once you receive an order from medical control, you must repeat the order back, word for word, and then receive confirmation that your understanding is correct. This "echo" exchange helps to eliminate confusion and the possibility of poor patient care. Orders that are unclear or seem inappropriate or incorrect should be questioned. Do not blindly follow an order that does not make sense to you. The physician may have misunderstood or may have missed part of your report. In that case, he or she may not be able to respond appropriately to the patient's needs.

> **Words of Wisdom**
>
> When contacting medical control for orders, always "echo" the orders back to the physician to avoid misunderstandings. If an order is not clear or seems inappropriate, then ask for clarification, repeating vital signs and other information as needed.

Information About Special Situations

Depending on your system's procedures, you may initiate communication with one or more hospitals to advise them of an extraordinary call or special situation. For example, a small rural hospital may be better able to respond to multiple victims of a highway crash if it is notified when the ambulance is first responding. At the other extreme, an entire hospital system must be notified of any disaster, such as a plane or train crash, as early as possible to enable activation of its staff call-in system. These situations might also include hazardous materials (hazmat) scenes, rescues in progress, MCIs, or any other situation that might require special preparation on the part of the hospital. In some areas, mutual aid frequencies may be designated in MCIs so that responding agencies can communicate with one another on a common frequency.

It is also important to notify the receiving hospital of the need for specialty items. For example, if you are transporting a ventilator-dependent patient from home and providing bag-mask ventilations, then call the hospital prior to disconnecting the patient from his or her own ventilator to ensure the receiving facility has a ventilator available on your arrival.

When notifying the hospital or hospitals of any special situations, keep the following in mind: the earlier the notification, the better. You should ask to speak to the charge nurse or physician in charge, as he or she is best able to mobilize the resources necessary to respond. Also, whenever possible, provide an estimate of the number of people who may be transported to the facility. Ensure you identify any conditions the patient or patients might have that require special resources, such as burns or hazmat exposure, to assist the hospital in preparation. In many cases, hospital notification is part of a larger disaster or hazmat plan. Follow the plan for your system.

▶ Effective Radio Communications

You must use your radio communications system effectively from the time you acknowledge a call until you complete your run. Standard radio operating procedures are designed to reduce the number of misunderstood messages, to keep transmissions brief, and to develop effective radio discipline.

Table 4-9 Guidelines for Effective Radio Communication

Guidelines for Effective Radio Communication
Turn on the radio and adjust the volume.
Ensure a clear frequency and minimal noise before speaking.
Monitor background noise. If you are in transit, then shut off the siren when possible. Plan your message to keep your transmissions brief and precise.
Use the standard format for transmission of information.
To speak, use the "press-to-talk" (PTT) button, and wait for 1 second before speaking.
Hold the microphone 2 to 3 inches (5 to 7 cm) from your mouth.
Address the unit or hospital you are calling, and provide the name of your unit.
Wait for the signal that you can begin your transmission.
Use a clear, calm, monotone voice and speak at a reasonable pace.
Keep the transmission brief.
Use clear text.
Avoid the use of codes or agency-specific terms.
Use the words *affirmative* and *negative* instead of *yes* and *no*.
Limit saying "please," "thank you," and "you're welcome."
Do not use vague phrases such as *be advised*.
Do not use slang.
Never use profanity; always be professional.
When you are transmitting a number, such as an address, provide both the number and the individual digits. For example, "Respond to 381, 3-8-1, Main Street."
Remember that the airwaves are public and the use of scanners is popular.
Use EMS frequencies only for EMS communications.
Ensure other radios on the same frequency are turned down to avoid feedback.
Remain objective and impartial in describing patients.
Do not provide a diagnosis of the patient's problem.
Do not use names; protect the privacy of patients.
When you are finished transmitting, indicate this by saying an accepted phrase such as *over*.

Abbreviation: EMS, emergency medical services

Standard radio communications protocols help both you and the dispatcher to communicate properly (Table 4-9). Protocols should include guidelines specifying a preferred format for transmitting messages, definitions of key words and phrases, and procedures for troubleshooting common radio communications problems.

Words of Wisdom

Question any orders you did not hear clearly or did not understand.

Written Communications and Documentation

The PCR is the legal document used to record all aspects of the care the patient received, from initial dispatch to arrival at the hospital. This report may be used as a record of transfer of care until the primary PCR can be completed. It should contain a minimum data set as well as a transfer signature.

You may be able to complete the written report en route to the hospital if the trip is long enough and the patient needs minimal care. Your goal should be to provide a report prior to departing from the hospital. Usually, you will finish the written report after you have transferred the care of the patient to an ED staff member. There are two types of PCRs: written and electronic (ePCRs), which will be discussed later in this chapter.

The information you collect during a call becomes part of the PCR, and that information is ultimately entered into a data pool. The National Emergency Medical Services Information System (NEMSIS; nemsis.org) has been collecting patient care information for research purposes since the early 1970s. NEMSIS has identified specific data points (uniform components) needed to enable communication and comparison of EMS runs between agencies, regions, and states. The minimum data set includes both narrative components and check-off boxes **Figure 4-13**. You can see the national data set and discover interesting facts about the delivery of EMS within the United States at ems.gov.

Because EMS systems track their own time, ensure your watch is set with dispatch time at the beginning of the shift, if that is your system's procedure. Another way you can manage this information is to contact the dispatcher and have him or her provide you with the time. Either way, it is important to be able to keep close track of time. Accurate documentation will depend on it.

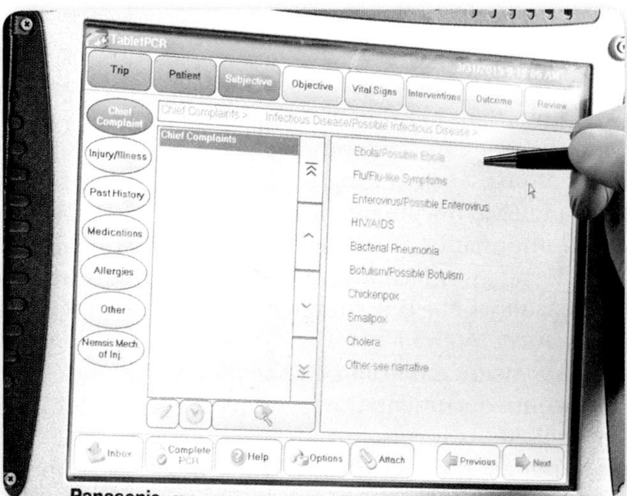

Figure 4-13 The minimum data set includes both patient information and administrative information.

It is standard procedure to use 24-hour (military) time in EMS documentation. This ensures that each time is unique; for example, 1:00 AM cannot be confused with 1:00 PM. Military times are shown in **Table 4-10**.

You will begin gathering the patient information as soon as you reach the patient. Continue collecting information as you provide care until you arrive at the ED.

You need to understand what constitutes documentation of a PCR, which information must be included, who might read the report, when the report must be completed, and which terminology may be used. Learning to write effectively and accurately is an important AEMT skill.

Information may be categorized as objective or subjective. **Objective information** includes the measurable signs that you observe and record, such as blood pressure. **Subjective information** includes information that is told to you, but that cannot be seen, such as the patient's description of his or her symptoms—the degree of pain, for example. You must record objective *and* subjective information and the details of patient care for every call in a written or computer-based report.

Every report needs to be complete, accurate, and legible, for numerous reasons. Your report should "paint a picture" of the entire call that is accurate and clear to the reader. It provides the basis for continuity of care by describing the initial presentation of the patient, treatment provided, and any changes. It can also provide the basis of defense in legal proceedings. It is of vital importance

Table 4-10 Military Times

Standard Time	Military Time	Standard Time	Military Time
Midnight	0000	Noon	1200
1:00 AM	0100	1:00 PM	1300
2:00 AM	0200	2:00 PM	1400
3:00 AM	0300	3:00 PM	1500
4:00 AM	0400	4:00 PM	1600
5:00 AM	0500	5:00 PM	1700
6:00 AM	0600	6:00 PM	1800
7:00 AM	0700	7:00 PM	1900
8:00 AM	0800	8:00 PM	2000
9:00 AM	0900	9:00 PM	2100
10:00 AM	1000	10:00 PM	2200
11:00 AM	1100	11:00 PM	2300

to your service or agency for many other reasons as well, such as for facilitation of quality care, development of protocols, and billing insurance.

▶ Types of PCRs

EMS has entered an age in which electronic documentation has become the standard. Although some services still use paper documentation, you will most likely document your emergency calls and other reports electronically. The many benefits of electronic documentation are discussed later in this section. Perhaps the most significant benefit is the ability for electronic data to be shared—not only between the facilities and personnel involved in a patient's care, thereby improving continuity and efficiency, but also among state and national databases to improve national data collection and further the advancement of evidence-based practice.

A multitude of PCR designs exist throughout the United States and range from half-page notes to complete and thorough reports. EMS patient care reporting has evolved over the years because the field of medicine has recognized the necessity for information about the patient's condition and interventions performed in the field. Some services have developed PCRs that nearly eliminate the narrative section and replace the space with either check boxes or dropdown menus with predetermined terms. You may encounter some reports that have hundreds of check boxes, allowing for you to mark every action you took. The problem with these types of reports is that the format increases the risk of errors that may occur when your eyes become overwhelmed by so many check boxes and you accidentally select the wrong box. Regardless of what form of patient reporting your service may use, it is important that you obtain the proper information.

Paper reporting is becoming a thing of the past because it duplicates work done in other parts of the health care system. To fulfill EMS data collection requirements, handwritten reports must be entered into an electronic system, either by health care agencies or by separate companies to which this task has been outsourced. Along with the additional data entry needs, a paper system requires space to store the records, possibly for a lengthy period of time depending on state laws.

The final reason there has been a major shift away from paper reporting systems is the drive to reduce errors in documentation. Often, penmanship and spelling errors lead to medical mistakes when it comes to medication doses and orders; an electronic system minimizes these issues.

With today's technology, a multitude of companies have created a variety of electronic PCRs. These services range from scanning of paper forms to computer-based programs for desktops, tablets, laptops, and smartphones, allowing for a more accurate and legible report **Figure 4-14**.

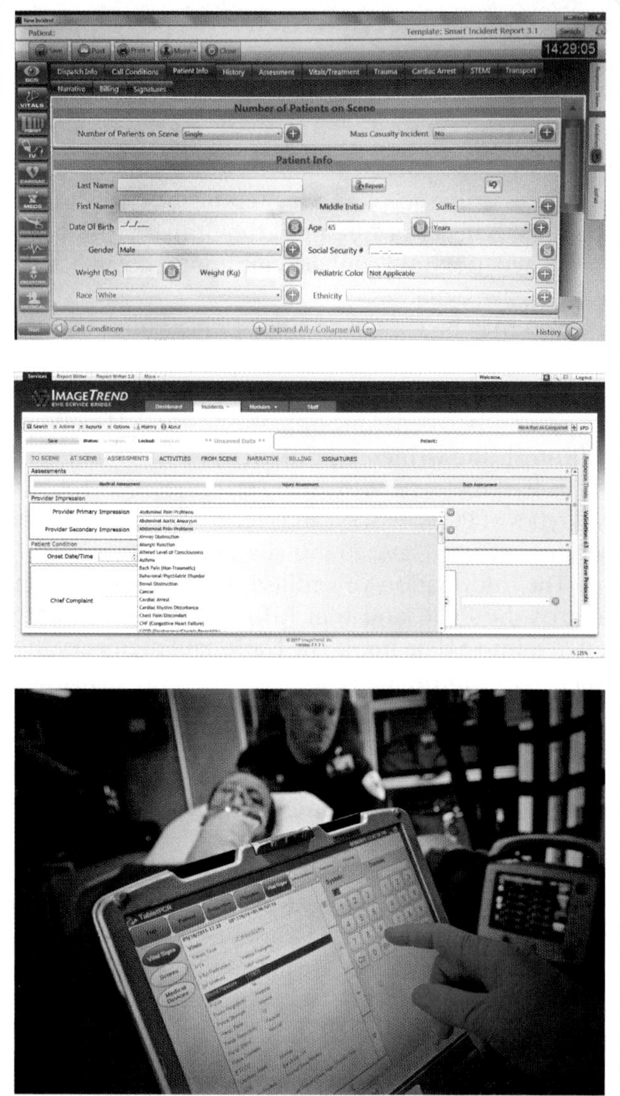

Figure 4-14 A variety of software programs exist for creating electronic patient care reports, allowing EMS personnel to clearly document details of the call.

Courtesy of Rhonda Hunt; Courtesy of Jim Emerton; Provided with permission by Zoll Medical.

Modern data systems can incorporate data from various sources, such as multiple facilities. This feature is in line with the major effort on the part of hospitals and physicians to improve the quality of cardiac, stroke, and diabetic care, and improve the success of resuscitation efforts. Such cutting-edge systems will ultimately include EMS documentation so that the PCR contains both information from the field and further data from the hospitals or facilities where the patient was treated. The result will be one comprehensive record of the care the patient received.

To ensure data can be shared on a national level, electronic documentation systems should be NEMSIS compliant. As mentioned, data submission to NEMSIS is important for EMS research and to assess and improve EMS care throughout the country. The goal of NEMSIS is to facilitate submission of EMS data from all states, and part of that process is to implement electronic documentation systems in all states. Today, the majority of states and territories of the United States are either submitting electronic data to NEMSIS or are actively working toward achieving this goal in the near future.

▶ Legal Issues of a PCR

Although you may include subjective information from the patient, such as statements from him or her about symptoms, no bias or personal opinions (subjectivity) of your own should appear in your report. For example, rather than stating "the patient was drunk and out of control," your documentation might say, "the patient presented with an altered mental status and stated he had eight beers today." Poorly written, inappropriately documented PCRs could have adverse implications both for patient care and for your career. Omissions or errors in your report could lead to further errors in care. Improper and inadequate reports can also result in legal action, cause loss of job or position, have a negative impact on your reputation as an EMS professional, and have other unfortunate consequences.

No matter what your particular writing style is, your report should be complete, well written, legible, and professional, and it should be your sole source of information about the call, because it may be used in legal proceedings against you or someone else. In some cases, it may be your only defense against a complaint about a call: if you document what happened, then you will have solid evidence of your conduct and what transpired on the call. Your memory may not serve you well 5 to 7 years from now, but your written report will remain as a record. If it is well written, then it will jog your memory and should clearly recall the events of the call for all who read it.

As a health care professional, it is important that you use proper spelling, proper grammar, and accurate terminology in your report. Do not attempt to use medical terms and abbreviations if you do not fully understand their meanings. Never make up your own abbreviations, because they will be meaningful only to you and could confuse others.

▶ Components of a PCR

As discussed, a PCR helps ensure efficient continuity of patient care. This report describes the nature of the patient's injuries or illness at the scene and the treatment you provide. Although this report might not be read immediately at the hospital, it may very well be referred to later for important information. The report serves the following six functions:

1. Continuity of care
2. Legal documentation
3. Education
4. Administrative information
5. Essential research record
6. Evaluation and continuous quality improvement

Besides reporting the patient's condition on arrival at the scene and the care that was provided, a good PCR documents any changes in the patient's condition en route and on arrival at the hospital. It is critical that you document everything as clearly as possible, because the report serves multiple purposes. The information in the report will help to prove that you have provided a standard of care and, in some instances, shows you have properly handled unusual or uncommon situations.

The following are examples of patient information collected on a PCR:

- Chief complaint
- Level of consciousness (according to the AVPU [Awake and alert, responsive to Verbal stimuli, responsive to Pain, Unresponsive] scale) or mental status
- Vital signs
- Assessment findings
- Patient demographics (age, sex, ethnic background)

Typically, the person who completes the form is the one who goes to court. Should you ever be called to provide testimony concerning patient care, you and your PCR will be used to present evidence. As with your personal appearance, your PCR will reflect a professional or a nonprofessional image. A neat, concise, well-written document—including correct spelling and grammar—will reflect good patient care.

These reports also provide valuable administrative information. For example, the report provides information for patient billing. It can also be used to evaluate response times, equipment usage, and other areas of administrative responsibility. In addition, information gathered may be used to improve different components of the EMS system and prevent problems from occurring. The following are examples of administrative information gathered from a PCR:

- The time the incident was reported
- The time the EMS unit was notified
- The time the EMS unit arrived at the scene
- The time the EMS unit left the scene
- The time the EMS unit arrived at the receiving facility
- The time the patient care was transferred

Data may be obtained from the PCR to analyze causes, severity, and types of illness or injury requiring emergency medical care. These reports may also be used in an ongoing program for evaluation of the quality of patient care. Reports are periodically reviewed by your system. The purpose of these reviews is to ensure trauma triage and/or other prehospital care criteria have been met. They may also be used to review an individual's performance. Finally, the administrative data may be used by the billing department to complete the billing process.

Data Collected via PCR

There are many required components of a PCR Table 4-11. Often, these requirements vary from jurisdiction to jurisdiction, mainly because different agencies

Table 4-11 Sample Uniform Components of a PCR

Patient's name, sex, date of birth, and address
Dispatched as (When was the ambulance called? What was the nature of the call as reported by the dispatcher?)
Chief complaint
Location of the patient when first seen (including specific details, especially if the incident is a motor vehicle crash or when criminal activity is suspected)
Rescue and treatment given before your arrival
Signs and symptoms found during your patient assessment
Care and treatment given by you at the site and during transport
Response to treatment
Vital signs
SAMPLE history
Changes in vital signs and condition
Additional orders received from the hospital
Name of person receiving the patient report
Date of the call
Time of the call
Location of the call
Time of dispatch
Time of arrival at the scene
Time of leaving the scene
Time of arrival at the hospital
Patient's insurance information
Names and/or certification numbers of the AEMTs who responded to the call
Name of the transport destination
Type of run to the scene: emergency or routine

Abbreviations: AEMT, advanced emergency medical technician; PCR, patient care report; SAMPLE, Signs and symptoms, Allergies, Medications, Pertinent past history, Last oral intake, Events leading to the injury or illness

obtain information from them. Although no universally accepted form exists, certain data points (uniform components of a PCR) are common in all areas. The benefits of collecting such information are significant, including the fact that national trends can be detected if all agencies collect and report the same information. For example, approximately 10% of the nation's EMS calls involve pediatric and adolescent patients. Such information is invaluable and, when collected, forms uniform data points.[9] In addition, PCRs are used by individual agencies to determine patterns of EMS responses. Busy times and high-call volume areas can be predicted to some extent by reviewing PCR data, and a thorough review of PCRs can set the stage for scheduling shifts and for system status management, including where units are placed.

Words of Wisdom

When you are quoting a patient, place quotation marks around the exact words stated. For example: Patient states his chest pain "feels like an elephant sitting on my chest."

Narrative Section

The narrative section of the PCR is arguably the most important portion of this report. Here you will describe all of the facts related to the EMS call. Be sure to include negative findings and important observations about the scene. Negative findings include those findings that warrant no medical care or intervention, but that, by seeking them, show evidence of the thoroughness of the AEMT's examination and history of the event. Do not record your conclusions or opinions about the incident. For example, you may write, "The patient admits to drinking today." This is a clear description that does not make any judgments about the patient's condition. You may also write that the patient's breath smelled of alcohol, but saying "The patient was drunk" is a judgment that may not be able to be supported. Choose your words carefully and thoughtfully. Ensure what you write is not an opinion, but is fact based on findings. Your job is to reproduce the important facts of the EMS call in writing.

Words of Wisdom

The time from the event until it goes to court may vary from very short to a couple of years. It is imperative that you document thoroughly because memories may become distorted after a long period of time.

When information is of a sensitive nature, note the source of the information. Be sure to spell words correctly, especially medical terms. If you do not know how to spell a particular word, then find out how to spell it, or use another word. Also be sure to record the time with all assessment findings. Table 4-12 provides guidelines on points to be covered in the narrative portion of your report. Remember to follow any state reporting requirements.

Words of Wisdom

Some examples of narrative writing styles for PCRs are as follows:

- **Chronological order.** This method allows you to explain the call in a story format from start (time of the initial dispatch) to finish (completion of the call).
- **SOAP method: Subjective information, Objective information, Assessment, and Plan (for treatment).** This simple and logical method allows you to document various aspects of the patient care encounter.
- **CHARTE method: Chief complaint, History, Assessment, Treatment, Transport, and Exceptions.** This method is similar to the SOAP method, but allows you to break down the narrative into logical sections similar to that of your patient assessment.
- **Body systems/parts approach.** In this format, your assessment of each body system is documented from head to toe. This method of report writing may be difficult to apply in EMS and may be too time consuming.

Although the CHARTE and SOAP methods are widely used in health care, the chronological method might better fit the EMS intervention.

▶ Medical Terminology

Medical terms are mainly derived from Latin. Many new EMS providers are confused as to why they need to learn this language: "If a person has a sour stomach, why can we not simply write 'Patient complains of a sour stomach' and be done with it?"

The reason to learn medical terms is to ensure accurate understanding by all people involved in the patient's care. What does "sour stomach" mean? Is there pain? Does the patient feel like he or she will vomit? Is the patient feeling as if he or she does not want to eat? There are many possible options. Through medical terminology, all readers—no matter where they are located in the chain of care—will understand the patient's complaint. Gastritis, an inflammation of the stomach, is understood equally in Ohio, Florida, England, and Thailand. Medical personnel around the globe speak the same language—Latin.

Medical terminology uses a system that combines prefixes, root words, and suffixes to describe complaints or diseases. If a patient has a headache, then this can be

Table 4-12 Components of the Narrative Portion of a PCR

The following general information should be included for *every* call:

- Why you were called
- Scene size-up
- The patient's primary complaint
- Any secondary complaints
- Pertinent bystander or family information and the identity of the people who provide the information
- Pertinent history, medications, and allergies, or the lack thereof
- Position/location of the patient and your general impression of the patient on your arrival
- Any unusual circumstances of the call
- All assessment findings and pertinent negatives
- OPQRST-I for any complaint of pain
- MOI with any pertinent details
- At least two sets of vital signs, including breath sounds and glucose level
- Mental status
- Individual body system assessments
- Indications for any treatment given
- Description and time of treatment given
- Response, or lack of, to treatment given
- Any changes in the patient's condition
- Any treatment that should have been provided but was not and *why*
- Patient demographic information: age, sex, ethnic background
- Whether or not the patient was ambulatory, and how he or she got to the stretcher/ambulance
- Patient's condition when turned over to other health care personnel

Additional information pertinent to the specific nature of the call should be included *in addition* to the information listed previously. For example, a PCR for a motor vehicle crash should include all of the information listed previously, as well as other findings, such as the following:

- Whether or not the patient was restrained
- Position of the patient in the vehicle
- Any ejection or death in the passenger compartment
- Location and extent of damage to the vehicle
- Whether or not the patient was ambulatory at the scene
- Approximate velocity of the crash, if known
- Any extrication or other delay
- Any loss of consciousness
- Any other pertinent details

Abbreviations: MOI, mechanism of injury; OPQRST-I, Onset, Provocation/palliation, Quality, Region/radiation, Severity, Timing, and any Interventions; PCR, patient care report

described in medical terms as *cephalgia*. This term combines the Latin roots *ceph* (head) and *algia* (pain). When you are talking about medical issues with other health care providers, using appropriate medical language will help ensure accurate understanding.

In Chapter 7, *The Human Body*, it is clear that Latin prevails. There may be slight spelling changes, but the meaning of the Latin roots, prefixes, and suffixes remains. Common directional terms such as *superior* (toward the head), *lateral* (toward the side), and *distal* (away from the midline) are also found in the anatomy and physiology chapter. Taking a medical terminology course can certainly be helpful when working in medicine. Chapter 5, *Medical Terminology*, provides a full list of prefixes, suffixes, root words, abbreviations, and their meanings.

Words of Wisdom

If you are unsure of an abbreviation, then always spell out the word completely.

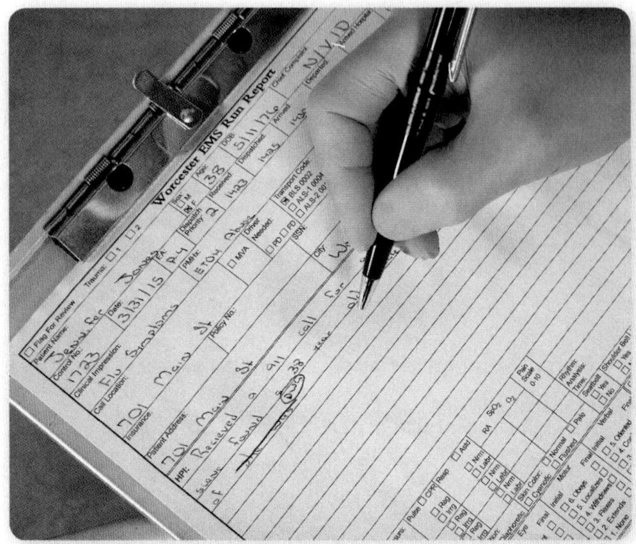

Figure 4-15 If you make a mistake in writing your report, then the proper way to correct it is to draw a single horizontal line through the error, initial it, and write the correct information next to it.

▶ Reporting Errors

Everyone makes mistakes. If you leave something out of a report or incorrectly record information, then do not try to cover it up. Rather, write down what did or did not happen and the steps that were taken to correct the situation. Falsifying information on the PCR may result in suspension and/or revocation of your certification or license. More important, falsifying information may result in poor patient care, because other health care providers have the wrong impression of assessment findings or the treatment given. Document only the vital signs that were actually obtained. If you did not administer oxygen to the patient, then do not document that the patient was given oxygen.

What if the wrong drug or the wrong dose was given to a patient? What if the patient is accidentally dropped? Unfortunately, these things can and do happen. It is important that you document the event. Do not lie or cover it up. In your narrative, provide a factual account of what happened. For example, you might record the following information: "Medical control ordered one sublingual nitroglycerin. Two sublingual nitroglycerin were given. Patient's blood pressure was checked following administration and at subsequent intervals with no changes noted." Or, "While loading the patient into the ambulance, the stretcher fell a total of 4 feet (1 m). Stretcher landed upright and the patient was not thrown from the stretcher. Patient was assessed and complained of being scared and having neck pain. Hospital advised."

If you discover an error as you are writing your report, then draw a single horizontal line through the error, initial it, and write the correct information next to it **Figure 4-15**. Do not try to erase or alter the error. This may be interpreted as an attempt to cover up a mistake.

If you discover you made an error after you submit your written report, then follow the same process of error correction by drawing a single line through the error, preferably in a different color ink, initial it, and date it. Ensure you add a note with the correct information. If you accidently left out information, then begin a new section with the word "addendum," add the new information, and then add the date and your initials. Know your own agency's policies regarding modification or addendums to medical records that you make after the fact.

If you discover you made an error after you submit an electronic report, then most systems will allow for amendments but will prevent erasure in a completed document. Refer to the system's direction as to how to make an amendment to the original document. In the event that there is no way to electronically change the report, the same procedure should be followed as for a written document. Simply follow the correction method used for a handwritten report on a printout of the electronic report.

Only the person who wrote the original report can revise it. Additions or notations added by others after the completion of the report may raise questions about the authenticity of the report and the confidentiality practices of your agency. Additions or notations by others can be submitted on a separate report.

▶ Minimum Requirements and Billing

Billing and administration are significant reasons why PCR writing needs to be accurate and complete. Most EMS agencies now need to bill for services to recover the costs of providing patient care. For complete and accurate revenue recovery, you must ensure all procedures performed are documented, insurance codes obtained, and the appropriate **medical necessity** signature obtained (where required).

To ensure your service's billing information will result in payment from the responsible insurer, agency, or private payer, the PCR should indicate why a patient may have needed emergency care, especially in the case of private or scheduled transports. It is imperative that your documentation be accurate and complete so time is not spent correcting the documentation, thereby delaying the billing processing. You will often be trained by your agency and its billing company about which additional forms you need to complete as a part of each EMS response. EMS providers must understand that completing billing paperwork and supplying the most accurate and defensible information to the EMS agency are necessary portions of the call.

Medicare sets the standard for medical necessity. Table 4-13 gives some of the significant findings that are required to show the patient needed to be transported by an ambulance rather than by other means.

Words of Wisdom

Document the use of any support services, such as helicopter or rescue services, and also the use of any mutual aid services in the PCR.

▶ Documenting Refusal of Care

Refusal of care is a common source of litigation in EMS; therefore, thorough documentation is crucial. As discussed in Chapter 3, *Medical, Legal, and Ethical Issues*, competent adult patients have the right to refuse treatment and, in fact, must specifically provide permission for treatment to be initiated. If you are not able to persuade the patient to proceed with treatment, then document any assessment findings, emergency medical care given, your efforts to obtain consent, and the patient's response to your efforts. Have the patient sign a refusal form Figure 4-16. You should also have a family member, law enforcement officer, or bystander sign the form as a witness. If the patient refuses to sign the refusal form, then have a family member, law enforcement officer, or bystander sign the form verifying that the patient refused to sign. Depending on local protocols, you may be required to inform online medical control when a patient refuses care.

Table 4-13 Significant Findings That Indicate Medical Necessity for Ambulance Transport

- Patient is transported in an emergency fashion (with lights and siren)
- Patient is in shock
- Patient needs to be restrained
- Patient requires emergency treatment while being transported (eg, oxygen therapy, IV therapy)
- Patient must be immobilized for transport or fracture management
- Patient is experiencing an AMI or stroke
- Patient has uncontrollable hemorrhage
- Patient is able to be moved only by a stretcher due to condition

Abbreviations: AMI, acute myocardial infarction; IV, intravenous

Words of Wisdom

Contact medical control for direction if you are unsure of what to do with a patient who is refusing care. A physician may be able to offer a different perspective that convinces the patient to agree to treatment and/or transport. If the patient still refuses, then you must document that you tried everything possible to provide care for the patient.

Even if a patient refuses care, you must complete the PCR. If the patient refuses care or will not allow for a complete assessment, then document that a proper assessment was not performed because of patient refusal. You will need to document the advice you gave as to the risks associated with refusal of care. Report clinical information, such as the level of consciousness, showing the competency of the person refusing care. Note pertinent patient comments and any medical advice given to the patient by the physician or medical control through phone or radio. Include a description of the care that you wished to provide for the patient.

There are many local variations of requirements for patient refusals. Table 4-14 provides a reasonable list of items that should be included within the PCR of a patient refusal.

Refusal of care concerns arise not only with patients who do not wish to be transported to the hospital but also with those who refuse a certain aspect of care. For example, a victim of a motor vehicle crash may wish to be treated and transported but refuses to be fully immobilized. It is appropriate to carry out all other medical care and document the patient's refusal of spinal immobilization. Just

Words of Wisdom

Regardless of the method you choose for documentation, consistency is the key. If you repeatedly use the same format, then you are less likely to leave out pertinent information.

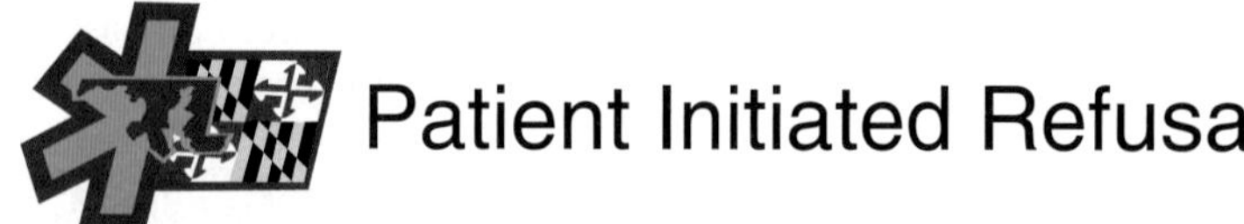

Patient Initiated Refusal of EMS

Patient Name: Doe, John | Primary Care Giver: John Smith, NREMT-P

Agency: BALTIMORE COUNTY FIRE DEPARTMENT | Incident#: 1122141 | eMEDS#: 00314105399

Unit #: Medic 14 | Inc Date Entered: 11/22/2016 | Inc Time Entered: 1824 hrs

I (or my guardian) have been informed regarding the state of my present physical condition to the extent I allowed an examination, and I (or my guardian) hereby refuse to accept such medical care and/or transportation as recommended by representatives of the EMS System above.

I (or my guardian) do hereby for myself, my heirs, executors, and administrators and assigns forever release and fully discharge said EMS system, its officers, employees, medical consultants, hospitals, borrowed servants or agents from any and all conceivable liability that might arise from this refusal of care and/or transportation, and I (and my guardian) therefore agree to hold them completely harmless. I (or my guardian) have been informed that a refusal of care and/or transportation for an evaluation may cause me to suffer PAIN, DISABILITY, LOSS of FUNCTION, WORSENING of my CONDITION, or even DEATH as a result of my illness/injury. As a competent adult, I (or my guardian) fully understand all of the above, and am/is capable of determining a rational decision on my own behalf.

Providers: When encountering a patient who is attempting to refuse EMS treatment or transport, access his or her condition, and record whether the patient screening reveals any lack of medical decision-making capability (1-3,4a or b) or high risk criteria (5-8).

1) Medical Capacity: Was the patient disoriented to person? If yes, transport	☐ Yes ☑ No
2) Medical Capacity: Was the patient disoriented to place? If yes, transport	☐ Yes ☑ No
3) Medical Capacity: Was the patient disoriented to time? If yes, transport	☐ Yes ☑ No
4) Medical Capacity: Was the patient disoriented to situation? If yes, transport	☐ Yes ☑ No
5) Medical Capacity: Did the patient show altered level of consciousness? If yes, transport	☐ Yes ☑ No
6) Medical Capacity: Alcohol or drug ingestion by history or exam with slurred speech? If yes, transport	☐ Yes ☑ No
7) Medical Capacity: Alcohol or drug ingestion by history or exam with unsteady gait? If yes, transport	☐ Yes ☑ No
8) Medical Capacity: Patient does not understand the nature of illness and potential for bad outcome? If yes, transport	☐ Yes ☑ No
9) At Risk Criteria (Abnormal vital signs): For adults. Pulse greater than 120 or less than 60? If yes, consult	☐ Yes ☑ No
10) At Risk Criteria (Abnormal vital signs): For adults. Systolic BP less than 90? If yes, consult	☐ Yes ☑ No
11) At Risk Criteria (Abnormal vital signs): For adults. Respirations greater than 30 or less than 10? If yes, consult	☐ Yes ☑ No
12) At Risk Criteria (Abnormal vital signs): For minor/pediatric patients. Age inappropriate HR? If yes, consult	☐ Yes ☑ No
13) At Risk Criteria (Abnormal vital signs): For minor/pediatric patients. Age inappropriate RR? If yes, consult	☐ Yes ☑ No
14) At Risk Criteria (Abnormal vital signs): For minor/pediatric patients. Age inappropriate BP? If yes, consult	☐ Yes ☑ No
15) At Risk Criteria: Serious chief complaint (chest pain, SOB, syncope)? If yes, consult	☐ Yes ☑ No
16) At Risk Criteria: Head injury with history of loss of consciousness? If yes, consult	☐ Yes ☑ No
17) At Risk Criteria: Significant MOI or high suspicion of injury? If yes, consult	☐ Yes ☑ No

Inc. Date: 11/22/2016 | Patient Name: Doe, John | BALTIMORE COUNTY FIRE DEPARTMENT | Page: 1

Incident #: 1122141 | Date Printed: 11/24/2016 18:24

18) At Risk Criteria: For minor/pediatric patients. ALTE, significant past medical history, or suspected intentional injury? If yes, consult	☐ Yes ☑ No
19) At Risk Criteria: Provider impression is that the patient requires hospital evaluation? If yes, consult	☐ Yes ☑ No
20) Providers: Did you perform an assessment (including exam) on this patient? If yes to # 20, skip to # 22	☐ Yes ☑ No
21) Providers: If unable to examine, did you attempt vital signs?	☐ Yes ☑ No
22) Providers: Did you attempt to convince the patient or guardian to accept transport?	☐ Yes ☑ No
23) Providers: Did you contact medical direction for patient still refusing service?	☐ Yes ☑ No
24) Patient: The patient or his or her representative refuses EMS examination.	☐ Yes ☑ No
25) Patient: The patient or his or her representative refuses EMS treatment.	☐ Yes ☑ No
26) Patient: The patient or his or her representative refuses EMS transport.	☐ Yes ☑ No

Patient Signature: **Printed Name:**

Patient Phone: **Date:** 18:24 11/24/2016

Patient Address:

Initial Disposition

Patient Refused Exam ☑	Patient Refused Treatment ☑	Patient Refused Transport ☑
Patient Accepted Exam ☐	Patient Accepted Treatment ☐	Patient Accepted Transport ☐
Auth. Decision Maker (ADM) Refused Exam ☐	Auth. Decision Maker (ADM) Refused Treatment ☐	Auth. Decision Maker (ADM) Refused Transport ☐

Intervention

Attempt to Convince Patient ☑ Attempt to Convince Family Member/Auth. Decision Maker (ADM) ☐ Contact Medical Direction ☑ Contact Law Enforcement ☐ None of the Above Available ☐

AMA Contact Medical Direction Facility St Elsewhere Hospital

Final Disposition

Patient Refused Exam ☐	Patient Refused Treatment ☐	Patient Refused Transport ☑
Patient Accepted Exam ☑	Patient Accepted Treatment ☑	Patient Accepted Transport ☐
Auth. Decision Maker (ADM) Refused Exam ☐	Auth. Decision Maker (ADM) Refused Treatment ☐	Auth. Decision Maker (ADM) Refused Transport ☐

Provide in the patient's own words why he/she refused the above care/service:

"Patient reports that despite the damage to his vehicle, he has only a small laceration on his finger and no other symptoms. He eventually agreed to allow EMS to evaluate him and provide a bandage for a small finger laceration (index finger, right hand). He agreed to follow-up with his primary care MD later today. When offered transport to the hospital he indicated, "No. thanks. I will be fine." Discussed plan with Dr Smith at St Elsewhere ED who agreed with plan and recommended reiterating to Mr Smith the importance of close follow-up with his primary care MD for tetanus prophylaxis and consideration of laceration care to include sutures.

Inc. Date: 11/22/2016 Patient Name: Doe, John BALTIMORE COUNTY FIRE DEPARTMENT Page: 2

Incident #: 1122141 Date Printed: 11/24/2016 18:24

Figure 4-16 A competent adult patient has the right to refuse medical treatment and must sign a refusal form.

Table 4-14 Components of a Thorough Patient Refusal Document
Complete assessment.
Evidence that the patient is able to make a rational, informed decision.
Documentation of complete assessment. If the patient refused care or did not allow a complete assessment, then document that the patient did not allow for proper assessment and document whatever assessments were completed.
Discussion with the patient as to which care/transportation the AEMT feels is in the best interest of the patient.
Discussion with the patient as to what may happen if he or she does not allow care or transportation. Typically, these consequences should be listed clearly and should include the possibility of severe illness/injury or death if care or transportation is refused.
Discussion with family/friend/bystanders to try to encourage the patient to allow care.
Discussion with medical direction according to local protocol.
Providing the patient with other alternatives: going to see his or her family doctor, having a family member drive him or her to the hospital.
Willingness of EMS to return if the patient changes his or her mind.
Signatures: Have a family member, law enforcement officer, or bystander sign the form as a witness. If the patient refuses to sign the refusal form, have a family member, law enforcement officer, or bystander sign the form verifying that the patient refused to sign.

Abbreviations: AEMT, advanced emergency medical technician; EMS, emergency medical services

because the patient refuses a cervical collar is no reason to deny oxygen. The same is true for the patient who wishes to use a local hospital when the injuries dictate transport to a trauma facility. Anytime a patient refuses any part of the standard treatment, it needs to be documented in the PCR and the patient needs to sign for the care he or she is refusing.

▶ Special Reporting Situations

In some situations, you may be required to file special reports with appropriate authorities. These may include incidents involving gunshot wounds, dog bites, certain infectious diseases, or suspected physical or sexual abuse. In case of suspected abuse, for example, you must document your objective findings and allow the legal system to investigate and make the ultimate determination of abuse or neglect. Other special situations include exposure or injury of the AEMT. If you treat and/or transport a coworker for an occupational exposure, then you should complete a full PCR along with the occupational exposure form. Learn your local requirements for reporting these incidents. Failure to report them may have legal consequences. It is important that the report be accurate and objective; it should be descriptive without making conclusions. It should be submitted in a timely manner and should include the names of all agencies, people, and facilities involved in the response.

You should also document the use of mutual aid services such as helicopters, specialized rescue teams, and other agencies called in to assist. Unusual occurrences should be documented as well, including having to secure the patient with restraining devices for safe transport or other unusual circumstances that arise.

Another special reporting situation is an MCI. The local MCI plan should have some means of recording important medical information temporarily (such as a triage tag that can be used later to complete the form). The standard for completing documentation in an MCI is not the same as for a typical call. In some areas, one trip report may be completed for the entire incident instead of individual reports for each patient.[10] Your local protocols should have specific guidelines.

▶ Submitting the Report

The PCR form itself and all the information on it are considered confidential documents, so ensure you are familiar with your state and local laws concerning confidentiality. All prehospital forms must be handled with care and stored in an appropriate manner once you have completed them. After you have completed a report, distribute the copies to the appropriate locations, according to state and local protocol. In most instances, a copy of the report will remain at the hospital and will become a part of the patient's record.

Depending on the requirements of the EMS system in which you work, you may not have the time to complete the full PCR while at the hospital. Even in these circumstances, however, a written record should be left with the patient. In these cases, most systems will have a "drop report" or "transfer report" Figure 4-17. These single-page, abbreviated forms are used as a memory aid during an EMS call. If you are unable to remain at the hospital to complete the PCR, then copy these documents and leave them with the nurse or physician.

Maryland Institute For Emergency Medical Services Systems

Short Form Patient Information Sheet 2017

Jurisdiction: ______ **Date:** ______
Incident # ______ **Time Arrived at Hospital:** ______
Unit #: ______
Age: ______ **DOB:** ______ **Wt:** ____ **Kg** **Gender:** ❑M ❑F
Priority: ❑1 ❑2 ❑3 ❑4 **Trauma Category:** ❑A ❑B ❑C ❑D
Patient's Name: ______
Patient's Address: ______
City: ______ **State:** ______
Point of Contact: ______ **Phone Number:** ______
Chief Complaint: ______
Time of Onset: ______ **Past Medical History: (DNR/MOLST ❑A1 ❑A2 ❑B)**
Cardiac ❑ CHF ❑ Hypertension ❑ Seizure ❑ Diabetes ❑ COPD ❑ Asthma ❑
Other: ______
Current Meds: ______
Allergies: Latex ❑ Penicillin/Ceph ❑ Sulfa ❑ Other: ______

Assessments

Vitals	Respiration (Left / Right)	Skin	GCS
Time: ______	❑ Clear ❑	❑ Warm	Eyes (4): ______
B/P: ____ / ____	❑ Rales ❑	❑ Hot	Verbal (5): ______
Pulse: ______	❑ Labored ❑	❑ Cool	Motor (6): ______
Respirations: ______	❑ Stridor ❑	❑ Dry	TOTAL: ______
SAO2: ______%	❑ Rhonchi ❑	❑ Clammy	**Pupils**
Capnography: ______	❑ Wheezes ❑	❑ Diaphoretic	❑ PERRL
Carbon Monoxide: ______	❑ Decreased ❑	❑ Cyanotic	❑ Unequal
Repeat Vitals	❑ Agonal ❑		❑ Fixed/Dilated
Time: ______	❑ Absent ❑		**Neuro**
B/P: ____ / ____	**Pulse**		❑ A ❑ V
Pulse: ______	❑ Regular ❑ Irregular		❑ P ❑ U
Respirations: ______	❑ JVD ❑ Peripheral Edema		
SAO2: ______%	Cap Refill: ______ seconds		
Capnography: ______			
Carbon Monoxide: ______			

Assessment

Procedures

Cardiac Rhythm:	Cincinnati Stroke Scale
______	*Normal/Abnormal*
12 Lead Transmit Yes ❑ No ❑	Facial Droop Normal ❑ Abnormal ❑
Perform 12 Lead Yes ❑ No ❑	Arm Drift Normal ❑ Abnormal ❑
Glucometer:	Speech Normal ❑ Abnormal ❑
______	Last Known Well Time/Date: ______
❑IV1 ❑IV2	**Oxygen**
❑IO ❑EJ	❑ NRB Mask ❑ King Airway
Amount Infused:	❑ Nasal Cannula ❑ CPAP
______	❑ NPA/OPA ❑ NDT
CPR Performed Yes ❑ No ❑	❑ BVM ❑ Ventilator
ROSC Yes ❑ No ❑	❑ ET ❑ NT ❑ NGT
Induced Hypothermia Yes ❑ No ❑	❑ Easy Tube

Treatment:

Jurisdictional Additions:

Print Provider Name: ______

Figure 4-17 Prehospital notepad/drop report (transfer report).

YOU are the Provider PART 4

Medical control authorizes a patient refusal. Echoing back the authorization, you proceed to have the patient sign the appropriate forms. You emphasize that you would be happy to return, and advise her to call 9-1-1 again if she requires further treatment or transport. As you return to your ambulance, you see several people in handcuffs being placed into the patrol vehicle.

Recording Time: 10 Minutes	
Respirations	14 breaths/min
Pulse	Strong and regular, 71 beats/min
Skin	Warm, dry, and pink
Blood pressure	112/80 mm Hg
Oxygen saturation (Spo_2)	100% on room air
Pupils	PERRLA

7. This patient refused care. Are you required to complete a PCR?

YOU are the Provider SUMMARY

1. What are some nonverbal forms of communication you can use to perform an effective interview?

The three main forms of nonverbal communication are eye contact, body language, and facial expression. When you are treating a patient, it is important that you understand and are aware of your own body language. Do not assume an aggressive posture. Make good eye contact, but do not stare. Speak calmly, confidently, and slowly. It is important for you to be attentive to facial expressions, body language, and eye contact—your own and your patient's. These physical cues will help you and your patient to truly understand the message being sent.

2. As a general rule, how close should you be to the patient while you are interviewing?

Proxemics is the study of space and how the distance between people affects communication. The degree to which people feel comfortable depends on with whom they are communicating. As trust is established between two people, a smaller distance between the two people becomes comfortable. When you finally enter someone's intimate space, there must be a high sense of trust. On the basis of American culture, when you are interviewing a patient, you should use social distancing and remain between 4 and 10 feet (1 to 3 m) from the patient.

3. What are two types of questions that are asked during a patient interview?

Open-ended and closed-ended questions are commonly used during a patient interview. Open-ended questions require a patient to provide some level of detail in an answer, whereas closed-ended questions can be answered in very short or single-word responses. Closed-ended questions are important to use when patients are unable to provide long or complete answers to questions. Open-ended questions allow a free flow of conversation; they let the patient direct you to what is bothering him or her.

4. Which techniques can be used to deescalate difficult situations?

To help defuse potentially escalating circumstances, stay calm. Talk to the patient openly and honestly. You will find that meeting hostility with calmness and confidence defuses a situation. Use open-ended questions, provide positive feedback, ensure the patient understands the questions, and continue to calmly ask questions. Consider the safety of the scene. If law enforcement officers are not present and a scene could escalate, then immediately request law enforcement backup. Ensure you have sufficient backup to provide safety for the patient, the crew, and yourself.

5. What is the main thing to remember when communicating with medical control?

It is important to plan and organize your radio communication before you push the transmit button. A concise, well-organized report demonstrates your competence and professionalism to all people who hear your report. Well-organized radio communications with the hospital will engender confidence in the receiving facility's physicians and nurses, as well as others who are listening. In addition, the patient and family will be comforted by your organization and ability to communicate clearly. A well-delivered radio report puts you in control of the information, which is where you need to be.

6. Does this patient have the right to refuse transport to the hospital?

Competent adult patients have the right to refuse treatment and, in fact, must specifically provide permission for treatment to be provided by EMS or any other health care provider. Consult medical control as directed by local protocol. Also, ensure the patient is an adult or an emancipated minor; is able to make a rational, informed decision; and is not under the influence of alcohol or other drugs or the effects of an illness or injury. If a patient still refuses care after you have explained potential outcomes, then ensure he or she understands that you would be happy to return, and that he or she should not hesitate to call 9-1-1 again.

7. This patient refused care. Are you required to complete a PCR?

There are many local variations to document patient refusals, but generally, all patients that you come in contact with will require you to complete a PCR. Ensure you complete the PCR, including the patient assessment findings. If the patient refuses care or will not allow for a complete assessment, then document that a proper assessment was not performed because of patient refusal. You will need to document the advice you gave as to the risks associated with refusal of care. Report clinical information, such as the level of consciousness, showing the competency of the person refusing care. Note pertinent patient comments and any medical advice given to the patient by the physician or medical control through phone or radio. Include a description of the care that you wished to provide for the patient.

YOU are the Provider SUMMARY *(continued)*

EMS Patient Care Report (PCR)					
Date: 6-5-18	**Incident No.:** 20108547		**Nature of Call:** Trauma	**Location:** 152 W Rollette Street	
Dispatched: 1623	**En Route:** 1626	**At Scene:** 1634	**Transport:** N/A	**At Hospital:** N/A	**In Service:** 1702
Patient Information					
Age: 23 **Sex:** F **Weight (in kg [lb]):** 149 kg (328 lb)			**Allergies:** None **Medications:** None **Past Medical History:** None **Chief Complaint:** Laceration to right forearm		
Vital Signs					
Time: 1635	**BP:** Not obtained	**Pulse:** Not obtained	**Respirations:** 16	**Spo_2:** Not obtained	
Time: 1642	**BP:** 112/84	**Pulse:** 74	**Respirations:** 16	**Spo_2:** 100% on room air	
Time: 1644	**BP:** 112/80	**Pulse:** 71	**Respirations:** 14	**Spo_2:** 100% on room air	
EMS Treatment (circle all that apply)					
Oxygen @ ______ L/min via (circle one): **NC NRM Bag-mask device**		**Assisted Ventilation**	**Airway Adjunct**	**CPR**	
Defibrillation	**Bleeding Control**	**Bandaging** (circled)	**Splinting**	**Other:**	
Narrative					

EMS dispatched to above location for woman with a laceration. On arrival, Greenville County Sheriff's Office (GCSO) law enforcement officers are present. Patient found seated on picnic bench in backyard. Patient states that her "drunk friend threw a bottle at me," subsequently breaking on her right forearm. Minor laceration approximately 1 inch in length, with no active bleeding. Bandage applied. Friends come out of house, appear intoxicated, aggressive, and belligerent. Request that law enforcement remove friends. Parties separated by officers. Remainder of physical exam is unremarkable. Patient offered transport to ED, which she refused. Per protocol, contacted online medical control, spoke with Dr. Helland, who granted refusal of services. AEMT explained the risks and consequences of refusing EMS to patient. The patient was asked to wash the injury with soap and water before bandaging. Advised that the patient should call EMS back if needed and seek further medical attention if any redness or swelling develops. Patient verbalized understanding and appeared competent to refuse. Documentation completed and refusal of treatment/transport form signed. Patient left in care of self and GCSO deputy on scene.**End of report**

Prep Kit

▶ Ready for Review

- Excellent communication skills are crucial in gathering and relaying pertinent information.
- AEMTs must have excellent person-to-person communication skills. You should be able to interact with the patient, family members, friends, bystanders, and other health care professionals.
- It is important for you to remember that people who are sick or injured may not understand what

Prep Kit (continued)

you are doing or saying. Therefore, your body language and attitude are very important in gaining the trust of both the patient and family.

- You may need to adjust your body language to account for different cultures. It is especially important to be aware of eye contact; direct eye contact is viewed as impolite or aggressive in some cultures.
- There are specific communication techniques you can learn to facilitate working with patients. You may opt to use open-ended questions in some instances and closed-ended questions in others. Other techniques include using the patient's proper name; speaking in a steady, calm tone; allowing the patient time to answer; listening to and acknowledging what the patient says; reassuring the patient; and protecting his or her modesty. It is also important to tell the patient the truth, even if it is unpleasant.
- The presence of family, friends, and bystanders can be valuable or problematic. If someone is hindering your efforts to care for the patient, then ask him or her to step outside for a moment, but remember to consider whether this will make the patient more anxious.
- Be careful what you say about the patient to others. Sharing patient information may be inappropriate and can be a Health Insurance Portability and Accountability Act violation.
- You must also take special care with people such as difficult patients, older adult patients, children, hard-of-hearing patients, visually impaired patients, non–English-speaking patients, and patients with other special needs.
- When you are working with difficult patients, use the same techniques, but make extra effort to be open and compassionate. Use open-ended questions, provide positive feedback, ensure the patient understands the questions, and continue to calmly ask questions. Consider the safety of the scene and request additional resources if needed.
- Verbal radio reports and in-person oral reports are crucial parts of transferring the patient's care; it is essential to report important information in a complete, precise way.
- Reporting and record-keeping duties are essential, but they should never come before the care of a patient.
- Radio and telephone communication links you and your team to other members of the EMS, fire, and law enforcement communities. You must know what your communications system can and cannot handle.
- The lines of communication are not always exclusive, so you should speak in a professional manner at all times.
- Components of an EMS communications system include a base station, from which a dispatcher communicates with field units. A repeater may be used; this special base station receives messages and signals on one frequency and then automatically retransmits them on a second frequency.
- In the ambulance, you will use both mobile and portable radios to communicate with the dispatcher and/or medical control. Cell phones and satellite phones are also commonly used.
- Digital radio may help clear up distorted or lost transmissions; digital trunked systems may carry simultaneous conversations on one physical channel.
- Telemetry is the capability of measuring vital life signs and transmitting these data to a distant terminal—specifically, transmitting an electrocardiogram signal from the patient to a distant receiving station.
- At a large-scale incident, an interoperable communications system allows all of the agencies involved to share valuable information with each other in real time. This system utilizes a voice-over-Internet-protocol format to connect landlines, cell phones, and computers to create a seamless, reliable exchange of information.
- You will communicate with dispatch at many points during an emergency call. Communication begins when you are dispatched. You will also communicate with the dispatcher to report any special information en route, to confirm that you have arrived at the scene, and to request any additional needed resources.
- Once you are transporting the patient, you will communicate with the receiving facility to let it know what to expect. You must also report any significant changes in the patient's condition, especially if the patient seems worse. Medical control can then give new orders and prepare to receive the patient.
- You must also be able to communicate effectively by sending precise, accurate reports about the scene, the patient's condition, and the treatment that you provide.
- Along with your radio report and oral report, you must complete a formal written report about the patient before you leave the hospital. This is a vital part of providing emergency medical care and ensuring the continuity of patient care. This information guarantees the proper transfer of responsibility, complies with the requirements of health departments and law enforcement agencies, and fulfills your administrative needs.
- The patient care report (PCR) may be handwritten or electronic. Either way, it will include a checklist and a narrative portion. The report should be objective, accurate, and neat; this reflects good

Prep Kit (continued)

patient care and may be a valuable resource if a legal complaint is made.

- When you are talking about medical issues with other health care providers, use appropriate medical language to help ensure accurate understanding.
- If you make an error or omission in writing a report, then correct it and initial it. If you make an error in patient care, then write down what did or did not happen and the steps that were taken to correct the situation. Falsifying information on the PCR may result in suspension and/or revocation of your certification/license.
- Competent adult patients have the right to refuse treatment and, in fact, must specifically provide permission for treatment to be provided by EMS or any other health care provider. If they refuse care, then thorough documentation of that decision is crucial.

▶ Vital Vocabulary

base station Any radio hardware containing a transmitter and receiver that is located in a fixed place.

cell phone A low-power portable radio that communicates through an interconnected series of repeater stations called cells.

channel An assigned frequency or frequencies that are used to carry voice and/or data communications.

closed-ended questions Questions that can be answered in short or single-word responses.

communication The transmission of information to another person—verbally or through body language.

computer-aided dispatch (CAD) Linked dispatch center computer consoles and vehicle-mounted mobile data terminals in which a computer collects and manages the call information and makes recommendations for which emergency medical services unit is closest based on existing dispatch policy.

cultural imposition When one person imposes his or her beliefs, values, and practices on another because he or she believes his or her ideals are superior.

dedicated line A special telephone line that is used for specific point-to-point communications; also known as a hotline.

digital radio The transmission of information via radio waves using native digital (computer) data or analog (voice) signals that have been converted to a digital signal and compressed.

documentation The recorded portion of the AEMT's patient interaction, either written or electronic; it becomes part of the patient's permanent medical record.

duplex The ability to transmit and receive simultaneously.

emergency medical dispatcher (EMD) A specially trained member of the emergency medical services team who receives information, makes decisions about resource allocation, and relays that information in an organized manner during the emergency.

encoded A message is put into a code before it is transmitted.

enhanced 9-1-1 An emergency communications system that collects information about 9-1-1 calls from the telephone network, such as the telephone number and location of the caller, and displays this information on the dispatcher's computer terminal.

ethnocentrism When a person considers his or her own cultural values as more important when interacting with people of a different culture.

Federal Communications Commission (FCC) The federal agency that has jurisdiction over interstate and international telephone and telegraph services and satellite communications, all of which may involve EMS activity.

frequency The number of cycles (oscillations) per second of a radio signal.

interoperable communications system A communications system that uses a voice-over-Internet-protocol (VoIP) technology to allow multiple agencies to communicate and transmit data.

landline Communications system linked by wires, usually in reference to a conventional telephone system.

MED channels Very high-frequency and ultra high-frequency channels that the Federal Communications Commission has designated exclusively for EMS use.

medical necessity A standard used by Medicare to determine whether a patient's condition requires ambulance transport in a particular situation.

mobile data terminal (MDT) A small computer terminal inside an ambulance that directly receives data from the dispatch center.

mobile radio A radio that is mounted inside a vehicle and used to communicate with dispatch or medical control; it operates at lower power than a base station (20 to 50 watts) and is assigned to a specific radio frequency band.

multiplex Simultaneous transmission of multiple data streams, most often voice and electrocardiographic signals, in either or both directions over the same frequency.

noise Anything that dampens or obscures the true meaning of a message.

objective information Information that you observe and that is measurable, such as a patient's blood pressure.

Prep Kit (continued)

open-ended questions Questions for which the patient must provide detail to give an answer.

paging The use of a radio signal and a voice or digital message that is transmitted to pagers ("beepers") or desktop monitor radios.

patient care report (PCR) The legal document used to record all patient care activities. This report has direct patient care functions as well as administrative and quality control functions. PCRs are also known as prehospital care reports.

portable radio A handheld two-way radio with a limited range and low power (1 to 5 watts).

prearrival instructions Instructions provided by the emergency medical dispatcher to an emergency caller to care for life-threatening emergencies until help arrives.

proxemics The study of space between people and its effects on communication.

rapport A trusting relationship that you build with your patient.

repeater A special base station radio that receives messages and signals on one frequency and then automatically retransmits them on a second frequency.

scanner A radio receiver that searches or "scans" across several frequencies until the message is completed; the process is then repeated.

simplex Single-frequency radio; transmissions can occur in either direction but not simultaneously in both; when one party transmits, the other can only receive, and the party that is transmitting is unable to receive.

standing orders Written documents, signed by the EMS system's medical director, that outline specific directions, permissions, and sometimes prohibitions regarding patient care; also called protocols.

subjective information Information that is told to you but that cannot be seen, such as the symptoms a patient describes.

telemetry A process in which electronic signals are converted into coded, audible signals; these signals can then be transmitted by radio or telephone to a receiver with a decoder at the hospital.

therapeutic communication Verbal and nonverbal communication techniques that encourage patients to express their feelings and to achieve a positive relationship.

trunked radios Computerized sharing of radio frequencies by multiple units, agencies, or systems.

ultrahigh-frequency (UHF) band Radio frequencies between 300 and 3,000 MHz.

very high-frequency (VHF) band Radio frequencies between 30 and 300 MHz; the VHF spectrum is further divided into high and low bands.

▶ References

1. Weaver W, Shannon CE. *The mathematical theory of communication*. Champaign, IL: University of Illinois Press; 1963.
2. Carteret M. *Cross-cultural communication for EMS*. American Ambulance Association. https://the-aaa.org/2015/06/25/cross-cultural-communication-for-ems/. Published June 25, 2015. Accessed November 11, 2016.
3. Bechtel T. Considerations for EMS response to autistic patients. *EMS World*. March 28, 2014. http://www.emsworld.com/article/11362588/considerations-for-ems-response-to-autistic-patients-and-undertanding-autism-challenges-in-emergency-situations. Accessed November 11, 2016.
4. U.S. Department of Health and Human Services. HIPAA for professionals. http://www.hhs.gov/hipaa/for-professionals/index.html. Accessed November 6, 2016.
5. Code of Federal Regulations. CFR Title 47, Chapter 1, Subchapter D, Part 90, Subpart B, §90.15. http://www.ecfr.gov/cgi-bin/text-idx?SID=b41258b0691d3b0b98a9ff13931e8597&mc=true&node=pt47.5.90&rgn=div5#se47.5.90_115. Accessed December 14, 2016.
6. International Association of Fire Chiefs, National Volunteer Fire Council, Congressional Fire Services Institute, National Fallen Firefighters Foundation. *Radio communications for the fire service: a planning guide for obtaining the communications system you need for enhanced safety and emergency preparedness.* https://www.iafc.org/topics-and-tools/resources/resource/radio-communications-for-the-fire-service. Accessed November 11, 2016.
7. National Aeronautics and Space Administration. *A brief history of NASA's contributions to telemedicine.* http://www.nasa.gov/content/a-brief-history-of-nasa-s-contributions-to-telemedicine/. Accessed November 6, 2016.
8. Federal Partnership for Interoperable Communications. *Considerations for encryption in public service radio systems.* https://www.dhs.gov/publication/encryption. Published September 2016. Accessed December 28, 2016.
9. Winters G, Brazelton T. (2003). Safe transport of children. *EMS Professionals.* 2003;(Jul/Aug):13–21.
10. Federal Emergency Management Agency. *Operational templates and guidance for EMS mass incident deployment.* https://www.usfa.fema.gov/downloads/pdf/publications/templates_guidance_ems_mass_incident_deployment.pdf. Published June 2012. Accessed November 10, 2016.

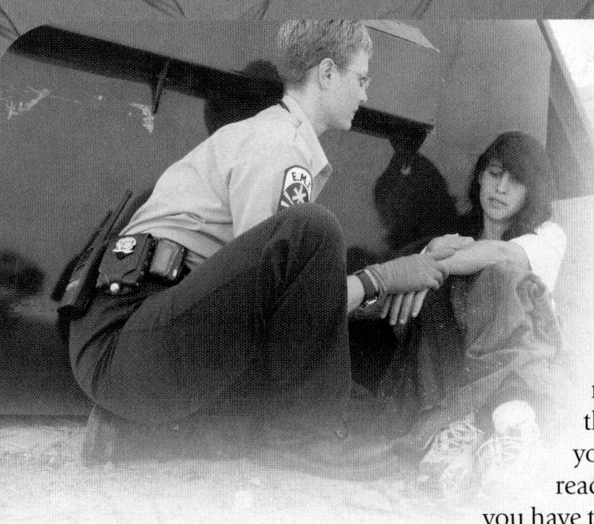

Assessment in Action

Your ambulance is dispatched to a reported motor vehicle crash in a wooded area in the country. As you get into the ambulance, your partner acknowledges the dispatcher on the radio and states that you are en route to the location. Along the way you and your partner discuss the various complications you may encounter in this type of area. Will it be difficult to reach the patient? Will there be adequate access by radio? Will you have the option of using a portable radio or be forced to return to the mounted radio in the ambulance for communication?

1. Which organization regulates radio communications?

A. Federal Communications Commission (FCC)
B. Mobile radio network (MRN)
C. Amateur Radio Relay League (ARRL)
D. Mobile Data Network (MDN)

2. A two-way radio consists of two parts, a transmitter and:

A. an operator.
B. a power supply.
C. an interrogator.
D. a receiver.

3. You will likely need to work at a distance from your vehicle in this incident. Which device should you take with you to stay in communication with the base or with other providers?

A. Pager
B. Portable radio
C. Cell phone
D. Computer

4. If necessary, how will you transmit vital signs data to the receiving facility?

A. By acquisition
B. By transmission
C. By technology
D. By telemetry

5. Which name is given to the small computer terminals inside ambulances that directly receive data from the dispatch center?

A. Mobile relay terminals (MRTs)
B. Mobile data terminals (MDTs)
C. Mobile computer terminals (MCTs)
D. Mobile portable terminals (MPTs)

6. What is the first stage of an EMS response?

A. Dispatch
B. Notification
C. En route communications
D. Transport communications

7. When you contact medical control for orders, you should do all of the following EXCEPT:

A. echo the order.
B. receive confirmation.
C. be precise and accurate.
D. use appropriate codes.

8. List five significant findings that indicate a medical necessity for ambulance transport.

9. What is the difference between *objective* and *subjective* information?

10. List the five principal EMS-related responsibilities of the FCC.

CHAPTER 5

Medical Terminology

National EMS Education Standard Competencies

Medical Terminology

Uses foundational anatomic and medical terms and abbreviations in written and oral communication with colleagues and other health care professionals.

Knowledge Objectives

1. Explain the purpose and the importance of being familiar with medical terminology. (p 147)
2. Explain the Greek and Latin origins of medical terms. (pp 147-148)
3. Define medical eponyms, homonyms, antonyms, and synonyms; include examples for each. (pp 148-149)
4. Name the four word parts or components used to build medical terms; include examples of each. (pp 149-152)
5. Describe how compound words are created and how the plural is formed when using medical terminology; include examples of each. (pp 152-153)
6. Describe the anatomic position and why it is used. (p 153)
7. List the three planes of the human body. (pp 153-155)
8. List medical terms associated with regional anatomy. (pp 155-156)
9. Explain the importance of using accurate medical terminology for direction, movement, and position in your documentation and other communication. (pp 157, 159-160)
10. Describe the topography of the abdominal region, including the four abdominal quadrants and the nine abdominal regions. (pp 160-161)
11. Identify specialized prefixes used to indicate position, direction, and location. (pp 160-162)
12. Define specific terms used to indicate the patient's position on the scene or prior to transport: prone, supine, Fowler position, and recovery (left lateral recumbent) position. (pp 162-163)
13. Interpret standardly accepted medical abbreviations, acronyms, and symbols. (pp 162-164)
14. Identify error-prone medical abbreviations, acronyms, and symbols. (pp 163-164)
15. Know appropriate terminology related to pharmacology. (pp 164-165)

Skills Objectives

There are no skills objectives for this chapter.

Introduction

As an AEMT, it is imperative that you develop a strong working knowledge of medical terminology, the language of medicine and health care. Medical terminology is used to describe and record every aspect of patient care, including medical history, assessment results, treatment, and outcomes. The language of medicine is derived primarily from Greek and Latin terms. If you understand the origin of medical terms (words), then the components (parts), and the guidelines for forming words, you will be able to identify and use medical terminology correctly and communicate effectively with other health care providers.

Consider what could happen if you, as an AEMT, used medical terminology incorrectly:

- A term used incorrectly in a radio report or documented improperly in the patient care report could lead to the patient being given an ineffective or even harmful treatment at the hospital.
- The patient could lose trust in your ability to care appropriately for him or her.

Your comprehension of key terms, acronyms, symbols, and abbreviations is important for effective communication and documentation. Understanding medical terminology requires you to break down each word into its separate components—prefix, suffix, and root—and to have a good working knowledge of those parts. Learn the established and accepted medical terms and abbreviations for your local area. Some emergency medical services (EMS) systems have specific lists of approved medical abbreviations and terms you must use.

In addition to accepted terminology, you will undoubtedly hear some common slang terms used in EMS, such as "boarding a patient" for transport or "bagging" or "tubing" the patient during airway management. The more extensive your vocabulary is, the more competent you will seem to be by the rest of the medical community and the better the patient care you will be able to deliver. Download a medical terminology app or carry a field guide or documentation handbook, so you can look up quickly and easily any unfamiliar terms without memorizing page after page of terms Figure 5-1.

Words of Wisdom

Never use a medical term if you're uncertain of its meaning. If you can't remember *femur*, then it is better to say "thigh bone" than to risk using an incorrect term.

Origins

Understanding the origins of medical terms helps you decipher the meanings of terms. Most medical terms have Greek or Latin origins Table 5-1. In general, medical terms that refer to disease are derived from Greek words. Words that refer to anatomic structures are usually derived from Latin words. The original word and the meaning are

YOU are the Provider PART 1

You and your partner are dispatched to a local elementary school to evaluate a child who has fallen. Upon arrival, you are directed to the playground, where a young boy is lying beneath a set of monkey bars on his left side, curled into a fetal position, sniffling and holding his abdomen. His first-grade teacher, Miss Jennings, tells you he fell from the top, approximately 6 feet (2 m), and has a lump on the right side of his head just above his eye. She says she's been trying to keep him still and has not let him try to get up.

Recording Time: 0 Minutes	
Appearance	Awake
Level of consciousness	Alert
Airway	Open
Breathing	Adequate
Circulation	Appears normal

1. What is the correct medical term for the position in which the child is lying?
2. How can knowledge of medical terminology assist in your documentation of care for this patient?

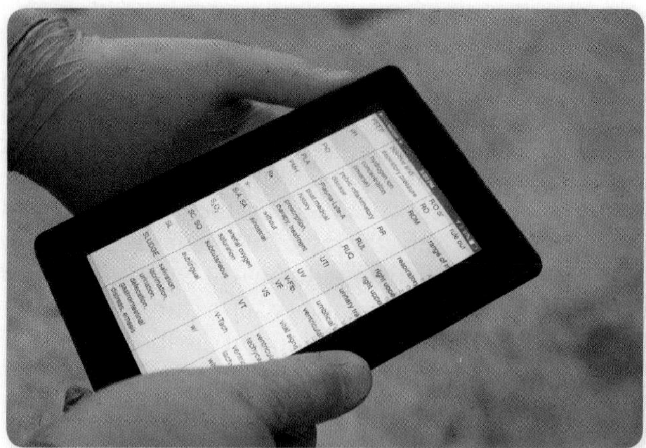

Figure 5-1 Medical terminology apps are excellent resources to use to reference terms while working in the field.

often interesting. For example, the word *muscle* comes from a Latin word for mouse, because the movement of a muscle under the skin was thought to resemble the scampering of a mouse. The word *coccyx*, the lower end of the spine, originated from the Greek word for cuckoo because it resembles a cuckoo's bill.

▶ Eponyms

The language used in medicine also comes from eponyms and terms that have resulted from advances in modern medicine, such as *fiberoptic* and *pacemaker*. An **eponym** is the name of a disease, device, procedure, or drug that is based on the person who invented, discovered, or first described it. You use eponyms every day and may not even be aware of where they originated. For example, the diesel engine is named for its German inventor, Rudolf Diesel. The word *denim* is derived from the French *serge de Nîmes*, a serge fabric from the town of Nîmes in France.

Medical eponyms sometimes appear in the possessive form (such as Hodgkin's disease) and sometimes not (Hodgkin disease). (Note: This text does not include the possessive form.) As in this example, they often include the name of the physician or surgeon who discovered, described, developed, identified, or invented a particular anatomic part or region, physiologic function or process, disease or syndrome, diagnostic or surgical procedure, treatment protocol, or instrument:

- McBurney point
- Foley catheter
- Babinski reflex
- Crohn disease
- Cesarean section
- Levine sign
- Apgar score

In medical terminology, we can often use a single word to express a concept that might otherwise require many words of explanation. For example, you can say "arthritis" faster than you can say "painful inflammation of the joint." In the next section, we will take a more in-depth look at commonly used medical terms and their meanings.

▶ Homonyms

Incorrect pronunciation of medical terms can lead to misdiagnosis or other serious medical errors. Correct pronunciation and spelling are especially important with certain words known as **homonyms**—pairs of words that are pronounced almost the same way but are spelled differently and have different meanings. For instance, *ileum* (il'e-um) is the third portion of the small intestine, while *ilium* is the largest bone of the pelvis. Or compare *dysphagia* with *dysphasia*. These two words may be spelled similarly and sound almost identical, but they have very different meanings. The word root *-phasia* means speaking, whereas *-phagia* means eating or swallowing. The prefix *dys* -means difficult or painful. *Dysphasia*, then, means difficulty speaking, while *dysphagia* means difficulty eating or swallowing.

Table 5-1 Selected Medical Terms With Greek or Latin Origins

Greek	Medical Term	Latin	Anatomic Structure
burs/o	bursitis	dors/o, dors/i	back/dorsal
cholecyst/o	cholecystitis	faci/o	face/facioplegic
gloss/o	glossitis	lingua	tongue/linguistic
hepat/ic	hepatitis	mamm/o	breast/mammogram
nephr/o	nephritis	ren	kidney/renal

Safety Tips

One type of medication error involves prescribing and dispensing "look alike, sound alike" (LASA) medications (eg, magnesium sulfate and morphine [MS and MS04]). The Joint Commission recommends focusing on prescription legibility through improved handwriting or the use of electronic prescriptions. Other solutions include physically separating LASA medications into different storages areas and using "tall man" or mixed-case lettering to emphasize the differences in drug names (eg, DOPamine versus DoBUTamine).

Words of Wisdom

A thorough knowledge of anatomy and an understanding of the context in which each term is typically used can help you determine (and spell) which word is the correct one to use in a given situation.

▶ Antonyms

Different word parts perform different functions. **Antonyms** are pairs of word roots, prefixes, or suffixes that have the opposite meaning of another word Table 5-2.

▶ Synonyms

Synonyms are pairs of word roots, prefixes, or suffixes that have the same or almost the same meaning. For example, the prefixes of the words pneumonologist and pulmonologist both mean lung, yet these words are not interchangeable. The reasons why are more historical than logical; the term *pneumonologist* simply has not gained acceptance, but the term *pulmonologist* has. Table 5-3 shows more synonyms you're likely to encounter in your work.

Components of a Medical Term

When you encounter a new word, break it up into its component parts. Some medical terms are quite long, consisting of three or four parts. If you know the meaning

Table 5-2 Selected Antonyms Used in Medical Terminology

		Examples			
		Word part and meaning		Opposite word part and meaning	
Antonyms	Pairs of word roots, prefixes, or suffixes that have opposite meanings	eu-	good	mal-	bad
		dextro-	right	sinistr/o	left
		ad-	toward	ab-	away from

Table 5-3 Selected Synonyms Used in Medical Terminology

		Examples			
		Word part and meaning		Similar word part and meaning	
Synonyms	Pairs of word roots, prefixes, or suffixes that have the same or almost the same meaning	pulmon/o	lung (as in pulmonologist)	pneum/o	lung (as in pneumonia)
		mamm/o	breast (as in mammogram)	mast/o	breast (as in mastectomy)
		cardi/o	heart (as in cardiology)	coron/o	heart (as in coronary)
		nephr/o	kidney (as in nephritis)	ren/o	kidney (as in renal)
		angi/o	vessel (as in angiogram)	vas/o	vessel (as in vascular)

of each part, then you can combine the definitions to determine the broader meaning of the word. Medical terms are composed of distinct parts that perform specific functions:

- **Prefix.** The portion that appears before the word root
- **Suffix.** The portion that appears after the word root
- **Word root.** The foundation of the term
- **Combining vowel.** Vowel that links one or more word roots to another component of a term

The way in which the parts of a word are combined determines its meaning. Changing or deleting any portion of a term can significantly alter its content. For example, hyperglycemia (hi′per-gli-se′me-ah) is too much blood glucose, and hypoglycemia (hi′po-gli-se′me-ah) is too little blood glucose. Thus, accurate spelling is essential in medical terminology.

▶ Prefixes

Prefixes are often found in general language (for instance, *auto*pilot, *sub*marine, *tri*cycle), and they are common in medical and scientific terminology. A prefix appears at the beginning of a word and generally describes the location or intensity of the word root that follows. Of course, not all medical terms have prefixes. A prefix does not change the meaning of the word root—*cutaneous,* for example, means skin regardless of what precedes it. However, the prefix does change the meaning of the medical term as a whole by describing the what, how, why, or when of the root. To expand on our previous example, the prefix *sub-* means below; therefore, *subcutaneous* means "below the skin." Another word, *atypical,* which means "not typical," can easily be understood when you know it is formed from the prefix *a-*, which means not, and the word root *typical.*

By learning to recognize a few commonly used medical prefixes, you can determine the meaning of terms that may not be immediately familiar to you. *Hypo-*, for instance, is a prefix that means low. We can add it to the word root *volumen,* meaning "volume," and the suffix *-emia,* meaning "blood," to figure out what hypovolemia means:

- Hypovolemia = Low blood volume

Likewise, we can add *hypo-* to the word root *glyc/o,* meaning glucose, and the suffix *-emia*:

- Hypoglycemia = Low blood glucose

Sometimes, we have just two word parts to work with. In the following example, we can define "hypotension" by adding *hypo-* to the word root *tensio,* which means "to stretch":

- Hypotension = Low blood pressure

YOU are the Provider — PART 2

After briefly speaking with the teacher, you kneel down to get eye level with the child. "Hi, I'm an AEMT, and we're here to take care of you. My partner, Matt, is going to hold your head really still while we talk for a minute. Does your head or your tummy hurt?"

He says his name is Kevin and his stomach hurts more than his head does. He is alert and oriented to person, place, time, and event. His respiratory rate is 22 breaths/min and normal, and his radial pulse is strong and regular, with a rate of 104 beats/min. He says he has felt dizzy all morning, and it made him fall. Miss Jennings tells you Kevin has type 1 diabetes. The school nurse has arrived and indicates that his mother reported his glucose level was 183 mg/dL when he arrived at school this morning. The nurse also states he is not allergic to any medications and that she normally checks his glucose level just before lunch each day.

Recording Time: 3 Minutes	
Respirations	22 breaths/min
Pulse	104 beats/min
Skin	Cool and dry
Oxygen saturation (Spo_2)	98%
Pupils	Pupils Equal, Round, and Reactive to Light and Accommodation (PERRLA)

3. Why would you want to avoid using medical terminology when talking to this patient?
4. What are the correct medical terms to describe Kevin's mental status and blood glucose level?
5. How would you document that the patient has no medication allergies?

Master tables at the end of this chapter list medical terminology, including prefixes, suffixes, word roots, and abbreviations, you will use most every day in your work.

▶ Numerical Prefixes

Many prefixes are used to indicate the number of sides, limbs, or sensory organs affected ("monocular vision," for example). Other numerical prefixes are used to specify time, such as "octogenarian" (a person between 80 and 89 years of age) or to indicate quantities that are uncountable (semicomatose, for instance). Common numerical prefixes are listed in Table 5-4.

▶ Suffixes

A *suffix* is a component added to the end of a word root. It changes or adds to the word's meaning or provides further definition. In medical terminology, a suffix usually specifies a procedure, condition, disease, or part of speech. For example, the suffix *-ase* indicates an enzyme. Lipase (*lip-*, which means fat, plus *-ase*) is an enzyme that digests fats. Gastritis, which means inflammation of the stomach, is a combination of the word root *gastr-*, which means stomach, and the suffix *-itis*, which means inflammation. Suffixes are able to change the medical term to a noun or adjective as needed.

Table 5-4 Common Numerical Prefixes

Prefix	Meaning	Example	Definition
un-	one	unilateral	affecting one side of the body
dipl-	double or in pairs	diplopia	double vision
null-	none	nullipara	a woman who has never given birth
primi-	first	primigravida	a woman pregnant for the first time
multi-	many	multipara	a woman who has given birth to more than one child
bi-	two	bilateral	pertaining to both sides of the body
tri-	three	trigeminy	irregular heart rhythm consisting of two normal beats followed by one premature beat
quad-	four	quadriplegia	paralysis of all four extremities
tetra-	four	tetralogy of Fallot	a congenital anomaly involving four anatomic abnormalities of the heart
quint-	five	quintipara	a woman who has had five pregnancies resulting in five live births
sexti-	six	sextuplets	six offspring of the same pregnancy
septi-	seven	septuplets	seven offspring of the same pregnancy
octo- or octi-	eight	octigravida	a woman pregnant for the eighth time
nona-	nine	nonan	occurring on the ninth day
deca-	ten	decagram	measurement of ten grams
semi-	half; part	semiconscious	partially conscious
hemi-	half; one sided	hemiplegia	weakness on one side of the body
ambi-	both	ambidextrous	able to use right and left hands equally
pan-	all, entire	pandemic	an epidemic over a wide area

Word Roots

The *word root* establishes the basic meaning of the word and frequently indicates a body part. Some books use the term *word root*; others use *root word*. The terms are synonymous. (Note: This textbook uses the term word root.) Prefixes are added to the beginning of a word root, and suffixes are added to the end of a word root. Changing the prefix or suffix will change the meaning of the term. Some word roots are complete words by themselves, but not all are. Furthermore, the same word root may have different meanings in different fields of study. You may have to consider the context of a word before assigning its meaning.

Colors

Several word roots are used to describe color. The most common include those listed in Table 5-5.

Combining Forms and Vowels

Some word roots, prefixes, and suffixes cannot combine with other word forms without help Table 5-6. To make pronunciation easier, sometimes it is necessary to change the last letter or the last few letters of a word root or prefix when a suffix is added. These letters, called combining vowels, facilitate the formation of new, more complex terms. They often consist of a vowel, most commonly *o*, added to a word root to create a combining form. A **combining form** is a word root, prefix, or suffix with an added vowel, known as a *combining vowel*. For example, in *osteopathic*, the first word root is *osteon* (Greek for bone). The *n* is dropped and the combining vowel *o* is added to create the combining form *oste/o*. Thus, adding the *o* facilitates the addition of a second combining form, *-pathy* (from the word root *patho-*, meaning disease).

Let's take another example. The word root *gastr-*, which means stomach, cannot combine gracefully with *megaly*, which means enlargement. The resulting term "gastrmegaly" would be awkward to pronounce and would have an odd spelling. A hyphen at the end of a word root indicates that *gastr-* is not a complete word. Adding a vowel to it, in this case an *o*, solves the problem. The result, *gastr/o*, is referred to as a combining form because it is used when combining the root with other roots or suffixes. *Gastr/o* + *megaly* makes *gastromegaly*, or enlargement of the stomach. If the suffix begins with a vowel, then a combining vowel is unnecessary. For example, *gastr-* + *-ic* = *gastric*. No additional letters are needed to form the word.

When adding combining vowels to word roots, use the following guidelines:

- Use a combining vowel before a suffix that begins with a consonant (eg, cyt/o + logy).
- Use a combining vowel to join other word roots (eg, gastr/o/enteritis).
- Do not use a combining vowel before a suffix that begins with a vowel (eg, *gastritis*, not *gastroitis*).

Some other examples of combining forms and vowels are:

- *cardi/o* + *logy* = cardiology (study of the heart)
- *neur/o* + *logy* = neurology (study of the nervous system)

Compound Words

Some medical terms contain more than a one-word root. These words are called **compound words**. In compound words, each word root retains its basic meaning. Simple

Table 5-5 Word Roots That Describe Color

Root	Meaning	Example	Definition
cyan/o	blue	cyanosis	Blue discoloration of the skin
leuk/o	white	leukocyte	White blood cell that fights infection
erythr/o	red	erythrocyte	Red blood cell that contains hemoglobin to carry oxygen
cirrh/o	yellow-orange	cirrhosis	Inflammation of an organ, such as cirrhosis of the liver, which causes yellow-orange pigmentation of the skin
melan/o	black	melena	Black, tarry stool caused by upper GI bleeding
poli/o	gray	poliomyelitis	An acute viral disease that attacks the gray matter of the brain
alb-	white	albinism	A condition in which a person's skin, hair, and eyes lack pigmentation (white hair, very pale skin, and a nonpigmented iris)
chlor/o	green	chlorophyll	A green pigment in leaves that is necessary for the plant to carry out photosynthesis

Abbreviation: GI, gastrointestinal

Table 5-6 Selected Combining Forms

Combining Form	Meaning	Combining Form	Meaning
brachi/o	arm	pil/o	hair
cardi/o	heart	steth/o	chest
carp/o	wrist	thorac/o	chest, thorax
cephal/o	head	thyr/o	thyroid gland
cervic/o	neck	trache/o	trachea
encephal/o-	brain	ureter/o	ureter
faci/o	face	vas/o	vessel
gloss/o	tongue	vesic/o	bladder, blister
nas/o	nose	viscer/o	viscera
ot/o	ear		

examples of compound words containing two word roots are *electrocardiogram* and *thermometer*. A more complicated example is *osteoarthritis*. The combining form *oste/o* comes from the word root *ost-*, meaning bone. The word root *arthr-* means joint or joints. The suffix *-itis* means inflammation. Therefore, the combined word *osteoarthritis* means inflammation of the bone joints.

Plural Endings

To change a medical term from singular to plural, certain rules apply. In most cases, as with other words in English, the plural is formed simply by adding an *-s* to the singular word. *Lung* becomes *lungs*, for instance. However, for some medical terms forming the plural is more complicated:

Singular words ending in *-a* change to *-ae* in the plural.
- Example: *vertebra* becomes *vertebrae*

Singular words ending in *-is* change to *-es* in the plural.
- Example: *diagnosis* becomes *diagnoses*

Singular words ending in *-ex* or *-ix* change to *-ices*.
- Example: *apex* becomes *apices*

Singular words ending in *-on* or *-um* change to *-a*.
- Examples: *ganglion* becomes *ganglia; ovum* becomes *ova*

Singular words ending in *-us* change to *-i*.
- Example: *bronchus* becomes *bronchi*

Topographic Anatomy

The surface of the body has many superficial visible features that serve as guides or landmarks indicating the structures that lie beneath them. Taken together, these features make up the body's topography (from the Greek word *topos*, meaning place, and *-graphy*, meaning description). Familiarize yourself with these living landmarks—the body's **topographic anatomy**—to perform a thorough assessment.

To describe topography accurately, you must imagine the body in a fixed position, known as the **anatomic position**: the person is standing, facing you, arms at his or her sides, with the palms of the hands facing forward, so the thumbs point away from the body. This position serves as a shared reference point, so the meaning of various directional terms stays constant, regardless of body position or movement. For example, let's say a person reports pain in his arm and you need to document it. Whose left or right do you use? To be consistent, the reference point health care providers should use is the patient's left and right in the anatomic position.

Words of Wisdom

There is only one anatomic position. Don't confuse this with the patient's position—prone or supine, for instance—or with patient positioning, such as the Fowler or Trendelenburg position.

Anatomic Planes and Axes of the Body

An anatomic plane of the body is an imaginary flat surface—imagine sheets of glass slicing through the body, dividing it horizontally and vertically into sections Figure 5-2. An *axis* is an imaginary line that divides the body equally and creates a point of rotation. Think of a skewer or pole through the middle of an object. The body can be divided along three main axes, to create the following planes:

1. **Coronal plane.** Imagine a sheet of glass (the plane) slicing the body vertically, from ear to ear, dividing it into front (ventral) and back (dorsal) portions. We call this the frontal or **coronal plane**—easy to remember, since "corona" means head.
2. **Transverse plane.** Now imagine a plane passing horizontally through the body at the waist, creating top and bottom portions. This slice is referred to as the **transverse (axial) plane**.
3. **Sagittal (lateral) plane.** Finally, let's divide the body vertically again, but this time slicing it from front to back. This is the **sagittal (lateral) plane**. *Sagitta*, Latin for arrow, describes the way in which the straight line of this plane divides the body into two sides. A sagittal plane might not go through the midline of the body. If it does, then it is called the **midsagittal plane (midline)**, which divides the body into equal left and right halves. Your nose and navel are found along this imaginary line. Other sagittal planes lie parallel to the midline.

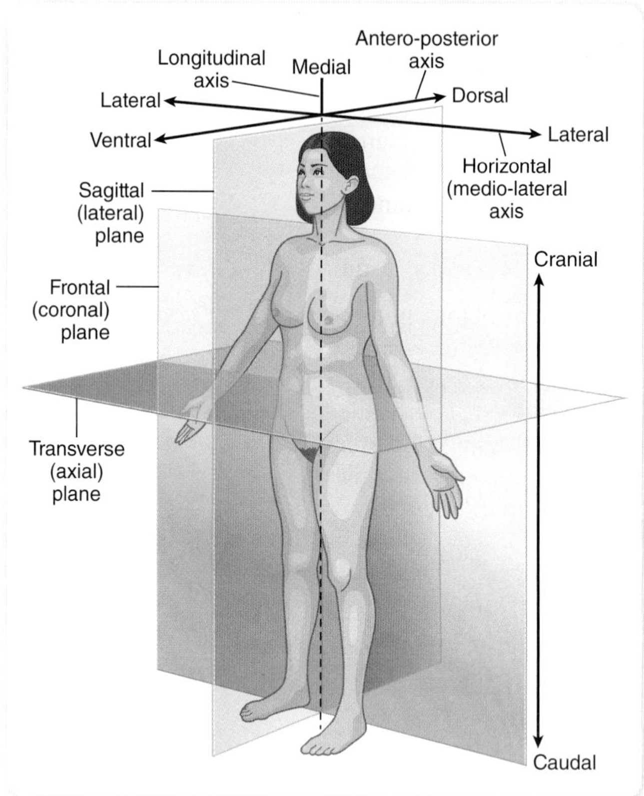

Figure 5-2 Planes and axes of the body.

YOU are the Provider PART 3

You explain to Kevin that your partner is going to hold his head still and you are going to roll him over onto his back so you can check where it hurts. He presents with a golf ball size hematoma and a small laceration just above his right eye. There is no active bleeding, and his pupils are equal and reactive. His abdomen is very tender on the right side just below his ribs, and you note bruising in the area. He denies pain in any other area. He tells you he took his insulin this morning and ate breakfast before school.

Recording Time: 8 Minutes	
Respirations	22 breaths/min
Pulse	108 beats/min
Skin	Cool and dry
Oxygen saturation (Spo_2)	99%
Pupils	PERRLA

6. Describe the position of the patient's head injury.
7. What is the abbreviation for the abdominal quadrant that is tender to the touch?

The three axes along which the body can be divided are as follows, and are also shown in Figure 5-2:

1. The **anteroposterior axis** runs perpendicular to the coronal plane.
2. The **longitudinal axis** runs perpendicular to the transverse plane.
3. The **horizontal axis**, also called the medio-lateral axis, runs perpendicular to the sagittal plane.

These planes help you to identify the location of internal structures and understand the relationships between and among the organs Table 5-7.

A **cross section** is taken by slicing across an object, perpendicular to its long axis, as you would do if you wanted to count the rings in a tree trunk. A **longitudinal section**, in contrast, is a view of an object cut along its long axis. In medicine, this slicing, of course, is often imaginary, or can be accomplished with, say, a camera or a beam of radiation, rather than a scalpel.

Table 5-7 Anatomic Planes of the Body

Plane of the Body	Description
Coronal	Front and back
Transverse	Top and bottom
Sagittal ▪ Midsagittal (midline)	Left and right (divides the body at any point on or parallel to the midline) ▪ Left and right (divides the body into equal left and right halves)

▶ Specific Areas of the Body

In addition to using planes and topographic landmarks, many body areas have specific names. When a person is injured, AEMTs rely on anatomic planes, body surfaces, and imaginary lines to describe the location of the injury. Familiarizing yourself with these body regions will not only help you communicate with other professionals, but it will also help you break down other terms, because many of them are used as word roots. For example, "sternocleidomastoid" is a combination of *sterno-*, *cleido-*, and *-mastoid*, which refers to the sternum, clavicle, and mastoid process, respectively. If you understand those roots, then you will be able to locate the origin and insertion of this large neck muscle. The most common body regions are described in Table 5-8.

Table 5-8 Terminology Associated With Specific Body Regions

Term	Word Parts	Definition
Abdominal	abdomin/o = abdomen -al = pertaining to	Pertaining to the abdomen
Axillary	axill- = armpit -ary = pertaining to	Pertaining to the armpit
Brachial	brachi/o = arm between the shoulder and elbow -al = pertaining to	Pertaining to the upper arm
Buccal	bucc/o = cheek -al = pertaining to	Pertaining to the cheek
Cardiac	cardi/o = heart -ac = pertaining to	Pertaining to the heart
Cervical	cervic/o = neck -al = pertaining to	Pertaining to the neck
Cranial	crani/o- = cranium or skull -al = pertaining to	Pertaining to the skull or cranium
Cutaneous	cutane/o = skin -ous = pertaining to	Pertaining to the skin
Deltoid	N/A – word root	Pertaining to the shoulder muscle

(continued)

Table 5-8 Terminology Associated With Specific Body Regions *(continued)*

Term	Word Parts	Definition
Femoral	femor/o = femur -al = pertaining to	Pertaining to the thigh
Gastric	gastr/o = stomach -ic = pertaining to	Pertaining to the stomach
Gluteal	glute/o = buttocks -al = pertaining to	Pertaining to the buttocks
Hepatic	hepat/ic = liver -ic = pertaining to	Pertaining to the liver
Inguinal	inguin- = groin -al = pertaining to	Pertaining to the groin (depressions in the abdominal wall near the thighs)
Lumbar	lumb/o = loin -ar = pertaining to	Pertaining to the loin (the lower back between the ribs and pelvis)
Mammary	mamm/o = breast -ary = pertaining to	Pertaining to the breast
Nasal	nas/o = nose -al = pertaining to	Pertaining to the nose
Occipital	occiput = the back of the head or skull -al = pertaining to	Pertaining to the inferior posterior region of the head
Orbital	orbit = the bones surrounding the eye -al = pertaining to	Pertaining to the bones surrounding the eye
Pectoral	pector- = breast or chest -al = pertaining to	Pertaining to the chest
Perineal	perineo/o = around -eal = pertaining to	Pertaining to the perineum, the area between the sacrum and pubis
Plantar	plant/o- = sole of the foot -ar = pertaining to	Pertaining to the sole of the foot
Popliteal	poplit- = posterior knee -al = pertaining to	Pertaining to the posterior knee
Pulmonary	pulm/o, pulmon/o = lungs -ary = pertaining to	Pertaining to the lungs
Renal	ren/o = kidney -al = pertaining to	Pertaining to the kidneys
Sacral	sacr/o = the lowest portion of the spine -al = pertaining to	Pertaining to the lowest portion of the spine
Temporal	temp/o, tempor/o = temples -al = pertaining to	Pertaining to the temples of the head
Umbilical	umbilic- = navel -al = pertaining to	Pertaining to the navel
Volar	vol- = palm of hand or sole of foot -ar = pertaining to	Pertaining to the sole of the foot or palm of the hand

▶ Body Cavities

The human body contains several cavities, each containing various organs and other structures. These cavities can be grouped into dorsal cavities, which are more posterior, and ventral cavities, which are anterior. The dorsal cavities include the cranial cavity, which contains the brain, and the spinal cavity, which surrounds the spinal cord. The ventral cavities include the thoracic cavity, which encloses the heart, lungs, and great vessels; the abdominal cavity, which holds several digestive and endocrine organs; and the pelvic cavity, which contains many digestive organs as well as the female reproductive organs. The abdominal and pelvic cavities can be referred to together as the abdominopelvic cavity **Figure 5-3**. Another cavity is the retroperitoneal cavity, which is separate from and lies posterior (dorsal) to the abdominal cavity and contains different organs, most notably the kidneys.

▶ Directional Terms

Directional terms used in the study of anatomy describe relative positions of body parts as well as imaginary anatomic divisions. When you discuss, describe, or document the location of pain or injury, use the correct directional terms **Figure 5-4**. **Table 5-9** provides the basic terms used in medicine. Since every direction has an opposite—above and below, front and behind, and so on—directional terms in medicine tend to occur in pairs.

Superior and Inferior

The **superior** portion of any body part is the portion above or closest to the head from a specific reference point. The body part closest to the feet is the **inferior** portion. These terms are used to describe the relationship of one structure to another. For example, the knee is superior to the foot and inferior to the pelvis.

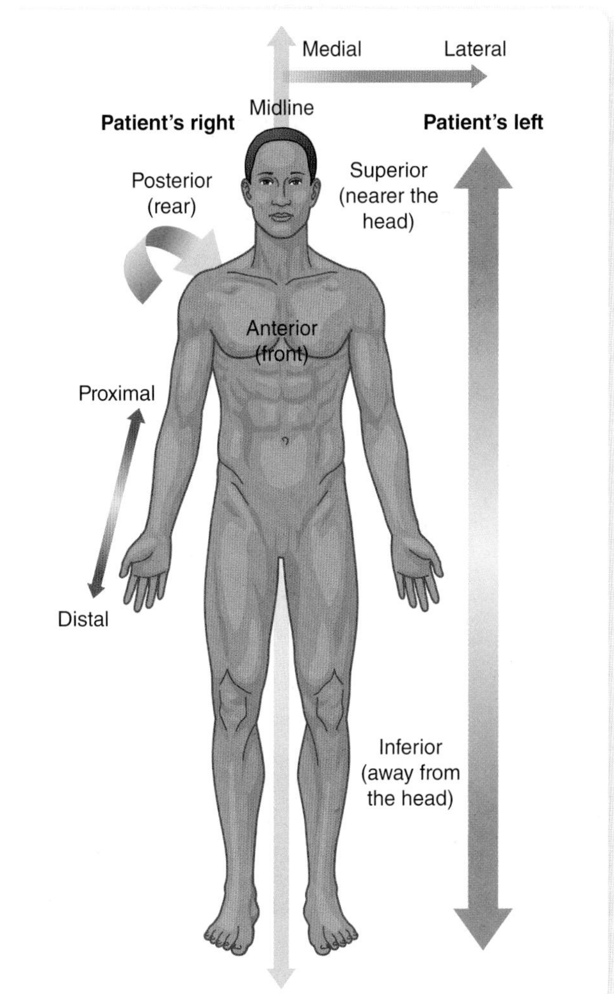

Figure 5-4 Directional terms indicate distance and direction from the midline.

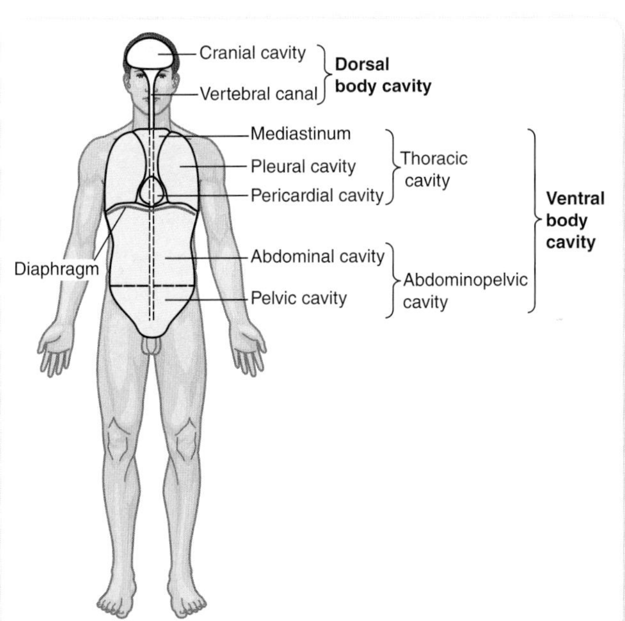

Figure 5-3 Body cavities.

Lateral and Medial

Parts of the body that lie farther from the midline are described as **lateral** (outer). The parts that lie closer to the midline are described as **medial** (inner). For example, the knee has medial (inner) and lateral (outer) aspects (surfaces).

Proximal and Distal

It is sometimes useful to describe a portion of an extremity relative to its distance from the midline of the body. **Proximal** describes structures that are closer to the body. For example, a fracture of the proximal humerus would involve the end of the bone that is closest to the shoulder. **Distal** indicates structures that are farther from the trunk—that is, nearer to the free end of the extremity. Using our previous example, a fracture of the distal humerus is one that involves the end of the bone farther from the

Table 5-9 Common Directional Terms

Common Term	Directional Term	Definition
Right and left	Right Left	The patient's right The patient's left
Top and bottom	Superior Inferior	Closest to the head Closest to the feet
Middle and side	Medial Lateral	Closest to the midline Farthest from the midline
Closest and farthest	Proximal Distal	Closest to the point of attachment Farthest from the point of attachment
In and out	Superficial Deep	Closest to the surface of the skin Farther inside the body
Front and back	Anterior (ventral) Posterior (dorsal)	The front of the body The back of the body

YOU are the Provider PART 4

"Well, Kevin, we need to take you to the hospital so they can check that bump on your head and find out why your tummy hurts. Matt and I are going to put you on a board with some seat belts and fix it so your head doesn't move. Don't worry, it won't hurt, and we will be right here with you. Miss Jennings called your mom and dad, and they're going to meet us at the hospital."

After applying a cervical collar and securing the patient on a backboard with straps and a cervical immobilization device, the child is loaded onto the stretcher and into the ambulance. His heart rate is regular and 98 beats/min. His blood pressure is 96/54 mm Hg and respirations are 18 breaths/min and normal, but his skin is a little cool and clammy to touch. He has good, equal breath sounds. His oxygen saturation (Spo_2) is 96%. You apply a small bandage to his forehead and reassess his abdomen. You note that it is still very tender to the touch and appears a little more discolored than it was initially.

Recording Time: 13 Minutes	
Respirations	18 breaths/min, normal
Pulse	98 beats/min
Skin	Cool, clammy
Blood pressure	96/54 mm Hg
Oxygen saturation (Spo_2)	96%
Pupils	PERRLA

8. Why is knowledge of anatomy pertinent when assessing and treating this patient?
9. What is the medical term for clammy skin?
10. What is the medical term for a phenomenon (such as pain, swelling, or a rash) affecting both sides of the body?

body (adjacent to the elbow). You can use these terms to describe the relationship of one structure to another. For example, the elbow is distal to the shoulder and proximal to the wrist and hand.

Superficial and Deep

Superficial means closer to or on the surface of the skin. **Deep** means farther inside the body and away from the skin.

Anterior and Posterior

Anterior refers to the belly side of the body. Another term for anterior is **ventral**. **Posterior** refers to the spinal side of the body, including the back of the hand (recall, the palms face forward when the body is in the anatomic position). Another term for posterior is **dorsal**. In human medicine, the terms anterior and posterior are used more frequently than the terms ventral and dorsal, which are more common in the veterinary and zoologic sciences.

Palmar and Plantar

The front region of the hand is referred to as the palm or **palmar** or volar surface. The bottom of the foot is referred to as the **plantar** or volar surface.

Apex

The **apex** (the plural is *apices* or *apexes*) is the tip of a structure. For example, the apex of the heart is the bottom (inferior portion) of the ventricles in the left side of the chest.

▶ Movement and Positional Terms

All body movement, from the simplest grasp to the most graceful ballet step, can be broken down into a series of simple components and described with specific terms. As with the terms describing anatomic location and direction, an accepted set of terms describes body movement. These are particularly useful in explaining mechanism of injury.

Range of motion is the full distance that a joint can be moved. In the anatomic position, moving the distal point of an extremity toward the trunk is usually called **flexion**. For example, flexion of the elbow brings the hand closer to the shoulder, flexion of the knee brings the foot up to the buttocks, and flexion of the fingers forms the hand into a fist.

In certain cases, specific terms are used to clarify movement, such as in the foot. Dorsiflexion is movement of the foot toward the dorsal aspect, while plantar flexion describes movement toward the sole. **Extension** is the return of a body part from a flexed position to the anatomic position. In the anatomic position, all extremities are in extension. **Abduction** of an extremity moves it away from the midline. **Adduction** moves the extremity toward the midline **Figure 5-5**. A patient's neck can be in one of several positions when the patient is lying supine **Figure 5-6**.

The prefix *hyper-* is often added to the terms *flexion* or *extension* to indicate a mechanism of injury. Hyper- indicates excess, for example, when a joint moves beyond its physiologic range of motion, possibly resulting in injury. The term **hyperflexion** refers to a body part that was flexed beyond its normal range of motion. **Hyperextension** refers to extension of a body part beyond its normal range of motion. An example of a hyperextension injury is one that occurs when a person falls on an outstretched hand, resulting in a distal radius fracture. A hyperflexion injury of the back can occur while bending. Wrist injuries can also be described using the terms **supination** and **pronation**. Turning the palms upward (toward the sky) constitutes supination of the forearm. Turning the palms downward (toward the ground) pronates the forearm.

Internal rotation means turning the anterior portion of an extremity toward the midline. The lower extremity is internally rotated when the toes are turned inward. **External rotation** means turning an extremity away from the midline. Often, when you are comparing an injured extremity with the uninjured extremity, you will note rotational deformities. A hip can be dislocated anteriorly or posteriorly. In an anterior hip dislocation, the

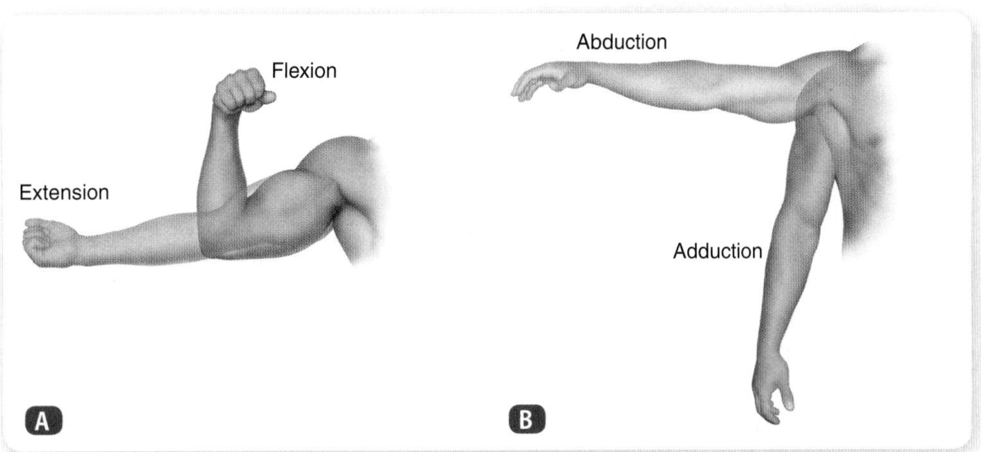

Figure 5-5 A. Elbow flexion and extension. **B.** Shoulder abduction and adduction.

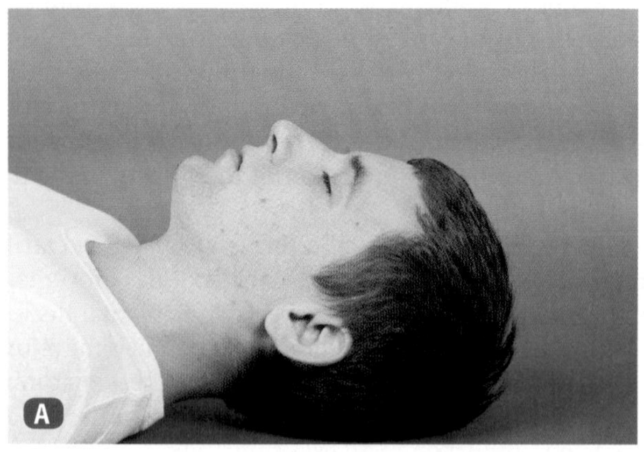

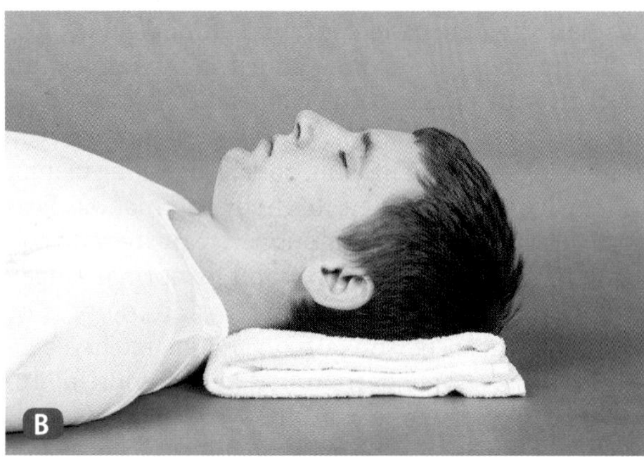

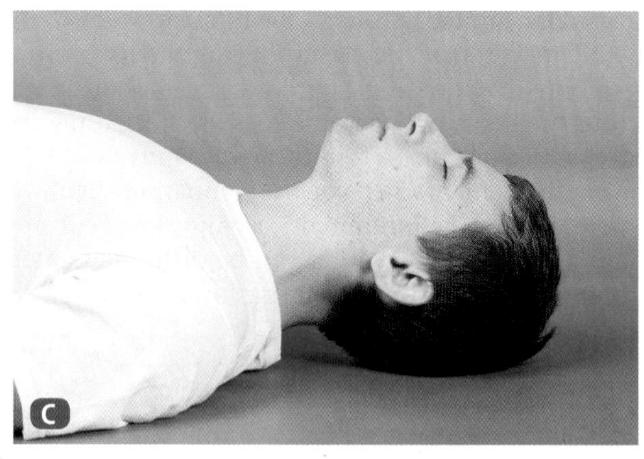

Figure 5-6 Positions of the neck in a patient found in a supine position. **A.** Neutral. **B.** Flexed. **C.** Extended.

foot is externally rotated and the head of the femur is palpable in the inguinal area (the lower lateral regions of the abdomen and the groin). In the more common posterior hip dislocation, the knee and foot are usually flexed and internally rotated. The term *rotation* can also be applied to the spine. The spine is rotated when it twists on its axis. Placing the chin on the shoulder rotates the cervical spine.

Words of Wisdom

Use the correct anatomic terminology in your patient care report (PCR). It makes the report more useful to hospital personnel and enhances your professional image as an AEMT.

▶ Other Directional Terms

A body part or condition that appears on both sides of the midline is said to be **bilateral**. For example, the eyes, ears, hands, and feet are bilateral structures. This is also true of structures inside the body, such as the lungs and kidneys. Structures that appear on only one side of the body are said to be **unilateral**. For example, the spleen is only on the left side of the body, and the liver is predominantly on the right side. The terms *unilateral* and *bilateral* can also describe the location of pain, numbness, itching, or other phenomena; for example, pain on only one side of the body is unilateral pain. You may also use the terms *ipsilateral* and *contralateral*. The term **ipsilateral** refers to the same side of the body. A patient having a stroke in the right hemisphere of the brain will usually have facial drooping ipsilaterally, in this case on the right side. **Contralateral** refers to the opposite side of the body. The same patient would have hemiplegia on the contralateral, or the opposite, side from the area of brain injury.

As part of your assessment process, you will palpate the abdomen and report your findings. Therefore, you must be able to describe the exact location of areas of the abdomen. The abdominal cavity is divided into four equal parts called **quadrants**: the right upper quadrant (RUQ), left upper quadrant (LUQ), right lower quadrant (RLQ), and left lower quadrant (LLQ). The quadrants are formed from two lines intersecting at the umbilicus **Figure 5-7**. Pain or injury in a given quadrant usually arises from or involves the organs that lie in that quadrant. Again, remember right and left refer to the patient's right and left, not yours.

To describe location even more specifically, the abdomen can also be divided into nine regions **Figure 5-8**.

▶ Prefixes Indicating Position, Direction, and Location

Specialized prefixes are used to specify position, direction, or location. Such terms describe, for instance, movement of the body or something within it, such as a blood clot or tumor metastasis. These prefixes indicate the location of an organ, foreign body, or mass, describe a surgical procedure and the medical instrument used to perform it, or refer to the direction of radiation or ultrasound waves used in diagnosis or treatment. Of course, these are just a few examples of how these versatile prefixes are used in medicine. Which words come to mind as you study **Table 5-10**?

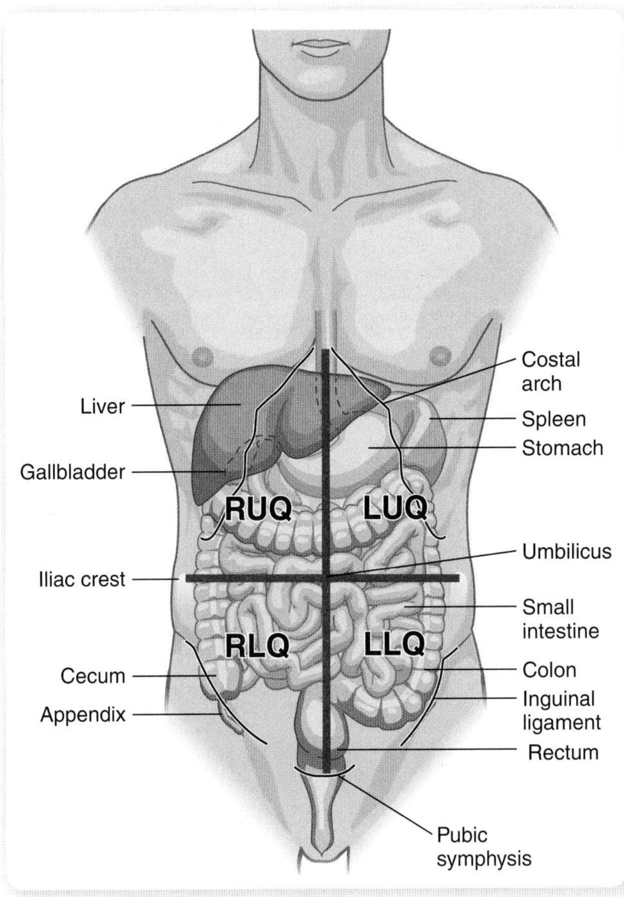

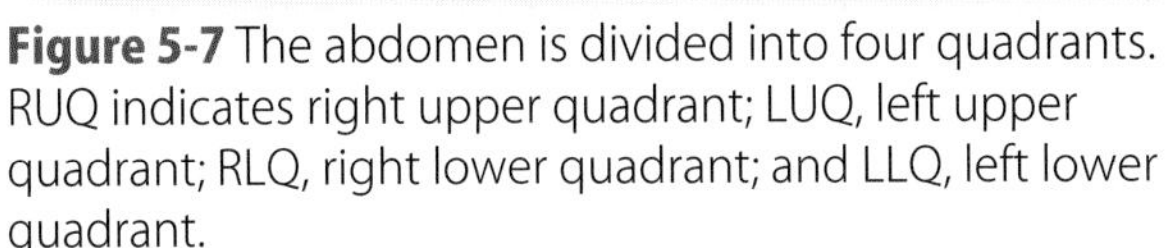
Figure 5-7 The abdomen is divided into four quadrants. RUQ indicates right upper quadrant; LUQ, left upper quadrant; RLQ, right lower quadrant; and LLQ, left lower quadrant.

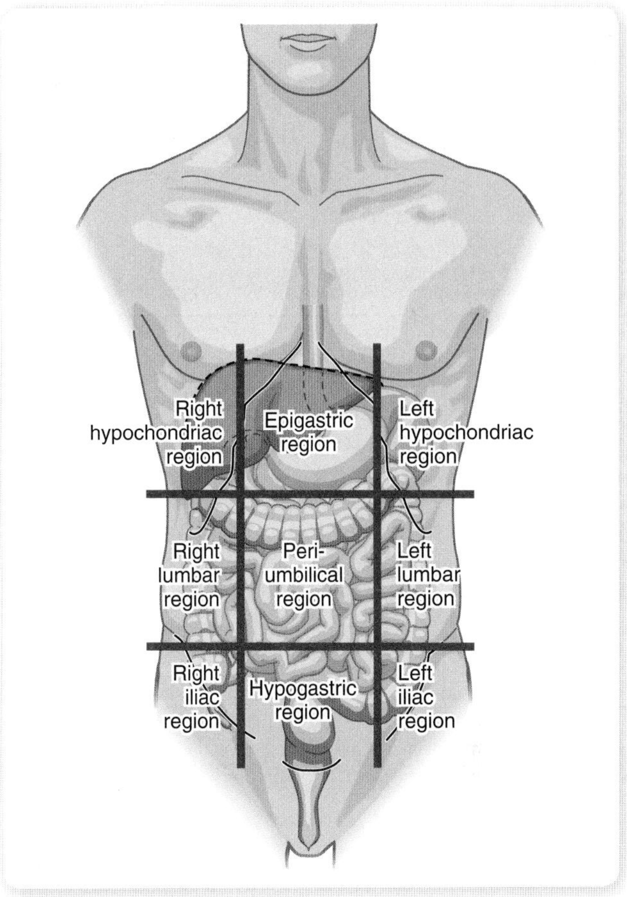

Figure 5-8 Abdominal regions.

Table 5-10 Prefixes Specifying Position, Direction, or Location

Prefix	Meaning	Example	Description
To/From			
ab-	away from	abduction	Away from the midline of the body, or a specified point of reference
ad-	to, toward	adduction	Toward the midline of the body
Above/Below/Around			
de-	down from, away	decay	To waste away
circum-	around, about	circumferential burn	A burn around an entire area (arm, chest, abdomen, etc)
peri-	around	pericardium	The sac around the heart
trans-	across, through, beyond	transvaginal	Across or through the vagina
epi-	above, upon, on	epigastric	Above or over the stomach
supra-	above, upper	suprasternal notch	Top of the sternum

(continued)

Table 5-10 Prefixes Specifying Position, Direction, or Location *(continued)*

Prefix	Meaning	Example	Description
Above/Below/Around			
retro-	behind	retroperitoneal	The area behind the peritoneum
sub-	under, below	subcutaneous	Under the skin
infra-	below, under	infrathoracic	Below or at the bottom of the thorax
para-	near, beside, beyond, apart from	parasternal	Near the sternum
contra-	against, opposite	contraindicated	Something that is not indicated
Outside/Inside			
ecto-	out, outside	ectopic pregnancy	Pregnancy where the embryo develops outside of the uterus
endo-	within	endoscopy	View inside the body (with an endoscope)
extra-	outside, in addition	extraneous	Existing or belonging outside the organism
intra-	inside, within	intrauterine	Within the uterus
ipsi-	same	ipsilateral	On or affecting the same side
Within			
inter-	between	intercostal	Between the ribs

Position of the Patient

You will use specific terms to describe the patient's position as you find him or her on the scene or when you are ready to transport the patient to the emergency department Figure 5-9.

Prone and Supine

The body is in the **prone** position when lying face down; it is **supine** when lying face up.

Fowler Position

The **Fowler position** was named after an American surgeon, George R. Fowler, at the end of the nineteenth century. Dr. Fowler placed his patients in a sitting position with their heads elevated to a 90° angle to help them breathe easier and to control their airways. A patient who is sitting straight up, with the knees either bent or straight, is described as being in the Fowler position. A patient in the semi-Fowler position is sitting with his or her back at a 45° angle. This position is generally a position of comfort for those who do not need spinal immobilization.

Recovery Position

The recovery position helps maintain a clear airway in an unresponsive patient. In this position, the patient is lying on his or her left side, with the head resting on the bottom arm. The top knee is bent, angling the front of the patient's body slightly toward the floor or ground. This position, also referred to as the *left lateral recumbent position,* helps prevent aspiration of vomitus. This is discussed in greater detail in Chapter 11, *Airway Management.*

Abbreviations, Acronyms, and Symbols

Medical abbreviations, acronyms, and symbols are types of shorthand used to communicate in the medical world. They evolve for the same reason we abbreviate words in text messages and chats—they allow us to communicate faster. However, in patient care, it is important not to trade speed for accuracy. To minimize misinterpretation and errors, use only commonly understood acronyms and other abbreviations

All acronyms are abbreviations, but not all abbreviations are acronyms. When you shorten a word using an abbreviation, you pronounce each letter of the abbreviation separately. For example, emergency medical technician is abbreviated "EMT," pronounced E–M–T. Acronyms form shortened words from the initials of several words to produce a new word. Acronyms and other abbreviations are sometimes combined to shorten a phrase. For example, the acronym for Urban Search and Rescue, USAR, is pronounced "U-sar."

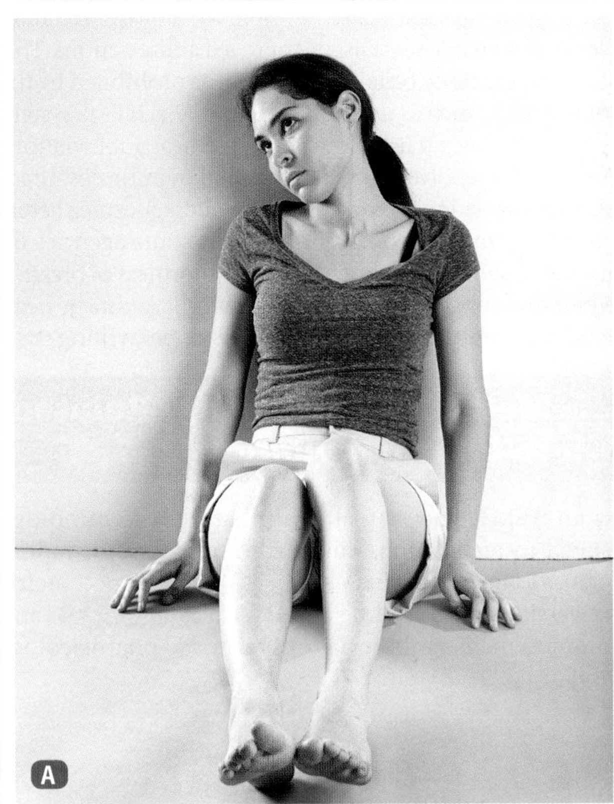

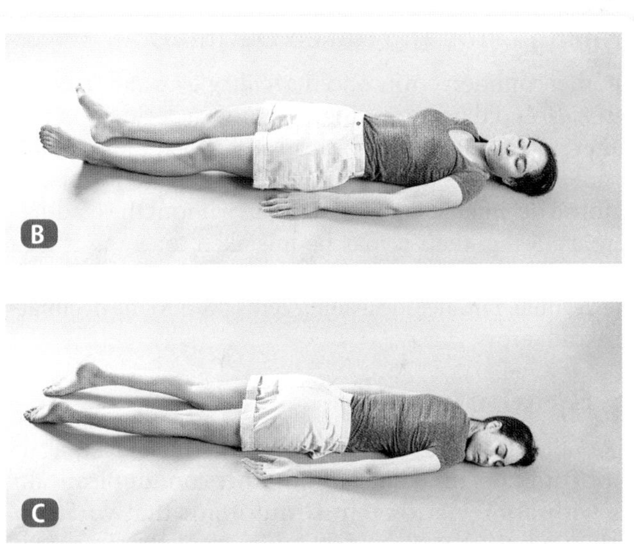

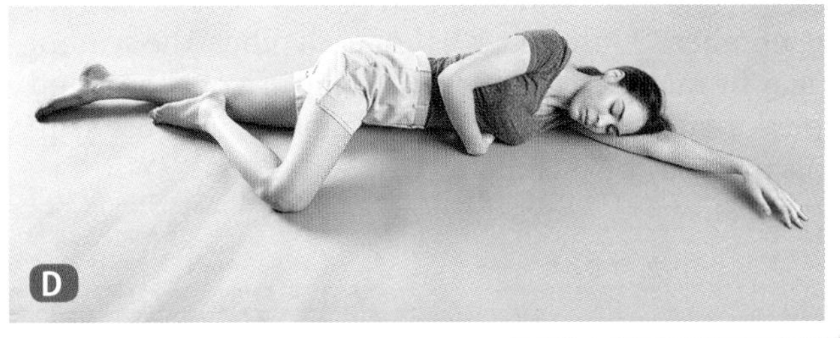

Figure 5-9 Anatomic positions. **A.** Fowler position. **B.** Supine. **C.** Prone. **D.** Recovery (left lateral recumbent) position.

An abbreviation is still considered an acronym if it is pronounced as a word, even if the word formed is not part of the English language. An example is HIPAA, short for the Health Insurance Portability and Accountability Act, a law that protects patients' privacy. This abbreviation is classified as an acronym because it is pronounced "hippa," not spelled out letter by letter. DEA, on the other hand, is not considered an acronym because it is spelled out as "D-E-A," rather than pronounced like "dia."

Words of Wisdom

In addition to medical terminology, the population of a specific geographic area can have its own slang or regional jargon. Familiarize yourself with this language to improve your communication when responding to calls in these locations. For example, in the south most older adults refer to diabetes as "the sugars" and hypertension as "high blood."

▶ Medical Abbreviations

Abbreviations take the place of the words they represent, to shorten patient care notes or other documentation. Some acronyms have become a common part of the English language. ASAP, for example, stands for "as soon as possible," but is commonly spoken as its own word. Medical abbreviations can be very useful for documentation purposes, but you must ensure they are consistent with those approved for use in your EMS system.

▶ Error-Prone Abbreviations

The Joint Commission and the Institute for Safe Medication Practices (ISMP) have each published a "do not use" list of abbreviations they believe to be especially prone to misinterpretation.[1,2] Serious errors can occur when an abbreviation is not interpreted as intended. For example, "HS" on a prescription can mean either "hour of sleep" (take at bedtime) or "half strength." To avoid such errors, some agencies limit the use of abbreviations or do not allow abbreviations at all.

Safety Tips

Be very careful with *look-alike, sound-alike* drug names. Pay close attention to labels to ensure you accurately write down the names. Some common mistakes are listed below. Each drug is different, yet each can be confused because of similar spelling and/or pronunciation:

- Zantac – Xanax
- Toradol – Tegretol
- Clonazepam – Lorazepam
- Alprazolam – Lorazepam
- Amiodarone – Amrinone
- Celebrex – Celexa
- Sinequan – Singulair
- Prozac – Prilosec

Trailing Zeros and Naked Decimals

Another common error concerns *trailing zeros* and *"naked" decimals*. Avoid using trailing zeros after a decimal point. For example, 5.0 mg may be read as 50 mg if the decimal is not seen. The same is true if a leading zero is left off before a decimal. If 0.5 mg is written without the leading zero as .5 mg, then it may be mistaken for 5 mg if the decimal is not seen. Always leave off trailing zeros after the decimal, but include leading zeros prior to the decimal to avoid errors.

To protect patients' safety, The Joint Commission requires every hospital to issue a list of approved abbreviations. This list cannot include certain abbreviations prohibited by the commission, such as *μm* for micrograms. Each EMS system should also keep a list of approved medical abbreviations available for reporting and documentation purposes. Learn which abbreviations are acceptable in your service area before you use them in a report. For example, some agencies do not use "SOB" as an abbreviation for "shortness of breath." When in doubt, write out the term in full. Accuracy, neatness, and completeness reflect a professional writing style.

▶ Symbols

Like abbreviations, symbols are sometimes used as a shortcut in documentation and other communication. As with abbreviations, it is important that you use only symbols that are widely understood and accepted Table 5-11. The symbols > or < may be mistaken for the number "7," the letter "L," or each other. The symbol μ may be mistaken for "mg," resulting in a one thousand times overdose. It is better to spell it out than to use symbols that may be misinterpreted.

Medical Terminology Related to Pharmacology

As an AEMT, you must be familiar with terminology related to medications and medication administration, such as common prefixes Table 5-12, common metric conversions used in drug calculation Table 5-13, and common medical abbreviations related to pharmacology Table 5-14.

Table 5-11 Commonly Used Symbols

°	degrees	/	per
1°	primary, first, first degree	±	plus or minus
2°	secondary, second degree	≠	not equal
↑	increase(d)	>	greater than
↓	decrease(d)	<	less than
α	alpha	≥	greater than or equal to
β	beta	≤	less than or equal to
#	number, pound	?	questionable, possible
Ø	null or none	Δ	change
~, ≈	approximately	—	negative
N	normal	♀	female
×2	times two	♂	male

Table 5-12 Prefixes Commonly Used in Medication Administration

Prefix Name	Prefix Symbol	Prefix Value
micr/o	mc	1/1,000,000 or 0.000001
milli-	m	1/1,000 or 0.001
centi-	c	10 or 0.01
kil/o	k	1,000
mega-	M	1 million or 1,000,000

Table 5-13 Metric Conversions Used in Drug Calculation

Weight	
1 kilogram (kg)	1,000 grams (g) 2.2 pounds (lb)
1 gram (g)	1,000 milligrams (mg)
1 milligram (mg)	1,000 micrograms (mcg)
Volume	
1 liter (L)	1,000 milliliters (mL)
Temperature	
37° Celsius (°C)	98.6° Fahrenheit (°F)
Length	
1 centimeter (cm)	0.39 inches (in.) 10 millimeters (mm)
100 centimeters (cm)	1 meter (m)

Master Tables

Table 5-15 through Table 5-18 provide a reference list of prefixes, suffixes, common word roots, and abbreviations.

YOU are the Provider PART 5

You cover Kevin with a blanket and start an IV line in the back of his left hand, using a 20-gauge catheter to infuse normal saline at a rate of 10 drops per minute. You also assess the patient's blood glucose level, which is now 147 mg/dL.

You and your crew transport the patient to a pediatric trauma center, where the child's parents are waiting, and give a verbal report to the receiving staff. Then you sit down in the EMS office to write your report while Matt cleans and restocks the ambulance.

Recording Time: 18 Minutes	
Respirations	20 breaths/min
Pulse	98 beats/min
Skin	Cool and clammy
Blood pressure	98/60 mm Hg
Oxygen saturation (Spo_2)	99%
Pupils	PERRLA
Blood glucose level	147 mg/dL

Table 5-14 Selected Medical Abbreviations Associated With Pharmacology

Abbreviation	Meaning	Abbreviation	Meaning
amp	ampule	MAX	maximum
caps	capsules	MDI	metered-dose inhaler
Elix	elixir	mEq	milliequivalents
gtt	drop(s)	MS or MSO_4	morphine sulfate
HHN	handheld nebulizer	pr	per rectus (by rectum)
IC	intracardiac	RL	Ringer's lactate (solution)
IVP	intravenous push	SVN	small-volume nebulizer
IVPB	intravenous piggyback	tid	ter in die (three times a day)
KO	keep open	TKO	to keep open
KVO	keep vein open	ut dict	ut dictum (as directed)
LR	lactated Ringer's (solution)		

Table 5-15 Selected Prefixes Used in Medical Terminology

Prefix	Meaning	Prefix	Meaning	Prefix	Meaning
a-	without, lack of	anti-	against, opposed to	calc-	stone; also heel
ab-	away from	arteri/o	artery	cardi/o	pertaining to the heart
abdomin/o	abdomen	arthro-	pertaining to a joint	cephal/o	pertaining to the head
acr/o	to, toward	auto-	self	cerebr/o	pertaining to the cerebrum, a part of the brain
aden/o	pertaining to a gland	bi-	two	cervic/o	pertaining to the neck or the uterine cervix
an-	without, lack of	bio-	pertaining to life	chole-	pertaining to bile
ana-	up, back, again	blast/o	germ or cell	chondr/o	pertaining to cartilage
angio-	vessel	blephar/o	pertaining to an eyelid	circum-	around, about
ante-	before, forward	brady-	slow	contra-	against, opposite

Prefix	Meaning	Prefix	Meaning	Prefix	Meaning
cost/o	pertaining to a rib	ex-	outside	inter-	between
cyan/o	blue	extra-	outside, in addition	intra-	within
cyst/o	pertaining to the bladder or any fluid–containing sac	gastr/o	pertaining to the stomach	iso-	equal
cyt/o	pertaining to a cell	glyc/o	sugar	latero-	side
de-	down from	gynec/o	pertaining to females or the female reproductive organs	leuk/o	pertaining to anything white or to leukocytes (white blood cells)
dermat/o	pertaining to the skin	hemat/o	pertaining to blood	lith/o	pertaining to a stone
di-	twice, double	hemi-	half	macro-	large
dia-	through, across	hem/o	pertaining to blood	mal-	bad or abnormal
dys-	difficult, painful, abnormal	hepat/o	pertaining to the liver	medi-	middle
ect/o	out, out from	hetero-	other, different	mega-	large
electro-	pertaining to electricity	homo-	same or like	melan-	black
endo-	within	hydr/o	water	mening/o	pertaining to a membrane, particularly the meninges
enter/o	pertaining to the intestines or gut	hyper-	over, excessive	micro-	small
epi-	upon, on, above	hypo-	under, deficient	mono-	one
erythr/o	pertaining to anything red or to erythrocytes (red blood cells)	hyster/o	pertaining to the uterus	myel/o	pertaining to the spinal cord, the bone marrow, or myelin
eu-	easy, good, normal	infra-	below	my/o	pertaining to muscle

(continued)

Table 5-15 Selected Prefixes Used in Medical Terminology *(continued)*

Prefix	Meaning	Prefix	Meaning	Prefix	Meaning
nas/o	pertaining to the nose	peri-	around	quart-	fourth, four
neo-	new	phag/o	pertaining to eating, ingesting, or engulfing	quat-	four
nephr/o	pertaining to the kidney	pharyng/o	pertaining to the throat, or pharynx	retr/o	backward or behind
neur/o	pertaining to nerves or the nervous system	phleb/o	pertaining to a vein	rhin/o	pertaining to the nose
noct-	night	pneum/o	pertaining to respiration, the lungs, or air	salping/o	pertaining to a tube
olig/o	little, deficient	poly-	many	scler/o	hard; also means pertaining to the sclera of the eye
oophor/o	pertaining to the ovary	post-	after, behind	semi-	half or partial
ophthalm/o	pertaining to the eye	pre-	before	sub-	under, moderately
orchid/o	pertaining to the testicles	pro-	before, in front of	supra-	above
orchi/o	pertaining to the testicles	proct/o	pertaining to the rectum	tachy-	fast
oro-	pertaining to the mouth	pseudo-	false	therm-	pertaining to temperature
ortho-	straight or normal	psych/o	pertaining to the mind	thorac/o	pertaining to the chest
oste/o	pertaining to bone	pulm/o	pertaining to the lung	trans-	across
ot/o	pertaining to the ear	pur-	pertaining to pus	tri-	three
para-	by the side of	pyel/o	pertaining to the kidney or pelvis	uni-	one
path/o	pertaining to disease	py/o	pertaining to pus	vas/o	vessel
per-	through	quadr/i	four		

Table 5-16 Selected Suffixes Used in Medical Terminology

Suffix	Meaning	Suffix	Meaning	Suffix	Meaning
-algia	pertaining to pain	-logy	science of	-ptosis	drooping
-asthen/o	weakness	-lysis	decline, disintegration, or destruction	-rrhage or -rrhagia	abnormal or excessive flow or discharge
-blast	immature cell	-megaly	enlargement of	-rrhaphy	suture of; repair of
-cele	a tumor or swelling	-oma	tumor	-rrhea	flow or discharge
-centesis	a procedure in which an organ or body cavity is punctured, often to drain excess fluid or obtain a sample for laboratory analysis	-osis	a disease process (see also -sis)	-scope	instrument for examination
-cyte	cell	-ostomy	surgical creation of an opening, or hole	-scopy	examination with an instrument
-ectomy	surgical removal of	-otomy	surgical incision	-sis	a process, action, or condition
-emia	pertaining to the presence of a substance in the blood	-pathy	pertaining to disease or a system for treating disease	-taxis	order, arrangement of
-genic	causing	-phobia	an irrational fear	-trophic	nutrition
-gram	record (as in written documentation or results of a study)	-plasty	plastic or reconstructive surgery	-uria	pertaining to a substance in the urine or the condition so indicated
-graph	a record or the instrument used to create the record	-plegia	pertaining to paralysis		
-itis	inflammation	-pnea	pertaining to breathing		

Table 5-17 Selected Word Roots and Combining Forms Used in Medical Terminology

Word Root	Meaning	Word Root	Meaning	Word Root	Meaning
acou-	pertaining to hearing	callus	hard, thick skin; also a lattice of connective tissue that forms during the healing process after a fracture	febr-	fever
adip-	fat	carcin/o	cancer	flex	bend
alb-	white	carotid	pertaining to the great arteries of the neck	foramen	opening
alges-	pertaining to pain	carp/o	pertaining to the carpus, or wrist	fract-	break
andr-	male	cent/i	a fraction in the metric system; one hundredth or 100	gest-	carry, produce, congestion
aort/o	pertaining to the aorta, the large artery exiting from the left ventricle of the heart	cent/e	to puncture (a body cavity)	gno-	know
aqua-	water	cili-	eyelid	-gram	something written or recorded
asphyxia	lack of oxygen or excess of carbon dioxide in the body that results in unconsciousness	cleid/o	clavicle	graph-	write, record
asthen-	weak	cubitus	elbow	humer/o	pertaining to the humerus, the long bone of the upper arm
audi-	to hear	cycl-	circle or cycle	idi-, idi/o	separate, distinct or pertaining to the self
bronch-	windpipe	digit-	finger or toe	iod/o	iodine
bucc-	cheek	edema-	swelling	lact/o	milk
bursa	pouch or sac	esthesi/o	pertaining to sensation or perception	lingu/o	tongue

Word Root	Meaning	Word Root	Meaning	Word Root	Meaning
men-	month	pod-	foot	seps-	literally means "decay"; refers to the presence of microorganisms or toxins in the blood, or to the toxic condition that their presence causes in the body
ocul/o	eye	pto-	fall	sept-	wall, divider; also refers to the number seven
ov-	egg	ptyal-	saliva	ser/o	pertaining to serum, the clear portion of body fluids, including blood
palpate	to examine by touch	pyr-	fire	sin/o	pertaining to a cavity, channel, or hollow space
ped-	child or foot	radius	the forearm bone on the thumb side; also a line from the center of a circle or sphere to the edge	som/a or somat/o	body or soma
percuss	to examine by striking	ren-	kidney	spir-	coil
phagia	pertaining to eating or swallowing	retina	inner nerve–containing layer of the eye	stasis	slowing or stopping of the normal flow of a fluid, such as blood
phasia	pertaining to speech	sangu/i	blood	stature	height
phot/o	light	seb/o	pertaining to sebum, a fatty secretion of the sebaceous glands	stern/o	sternum (breastbone)
pleur-	rib, side	sect-	cut	stoma	any small opening on the surface of the body, such as a pore; also, the opening created in the abdominal wall for the passage of urine or feces

(continued)

Table 5-17 Selected Word Roots and Combining Forms Used in Medical Terminology *(continued)*

Word Root	Meaning	Word Root	Meaning	Word Root	Meaning
tact-	touch	trich-	hair	viscer-	internal organs
tetra-	four	ur-	urine	viscum	sticky
tom/o	cut	varic-	varicose vein	xen/o	foreign (material)
toxic	poisonous	vertigo	a disordered sensation in which one's own body or the surroundings are perceived as moving	xer-	dry

Table 5-18 Common Abbreviations in Medical Terminology[a]

Abbreviation	Meaning	Abbreviation	Meaning
A&P	anatomy and physiology	AICD	automatic implantable cardioverter-defibrillator
ā	before	AIDS	acquired immunodeficiency syndrome
AAA	abdominal aortic aneurysm	AK	above the knee
abd	abdomen	AKA	above the knee amputation
ABCDE	airway, breathing, circulation, disability, and exposure	AMA	against medical advice
ac	before meals	amb	ambulatory
ACLS	advanced cardiac life support	AMI	acute myocardial infarction
ACS	acute coronary syndrome	AMS	altered mental status
ADL	activities of daily living	ant	anterior
ad lib	as desired	AO × 4, A/O × 4, A&O × 4	alert and oriented to person, place, time, and event
AED	automated external defibrillator	AP	anteroposterior, front-to-back, action potential, angina pectoris, anterior pituitary, arterial pressure
AF, A-fib, A fib, AFib	atrial fibrillation	ARDS	adult respiratory distress syndrome or acute respiratory distress syndrome

Abbreviation	Meaning	Abbreviation	Meaning
ASA	aspirin (acetylsalicylic acid)	CCU	coronary care unit or critical care unit
ASHD	arteriosclerotic or atherosclerotic heart disease	C diff	*Clostridium difficile*
AV	atrioventricular	cm	centimeter
BBB	bundle branch block	CNS	central nervous system
BGL	blood glucose level	c/o	complains of
bid/b.i.d./BID	twice daily	CO	cardiac output, carbon monoxide
BKA	below the knee amputation	CO_2	carbon dioxide
BM	bowel movement	COLD	chronic obstructive lung disease
BMD	bag-mask device	COPD	chronic obstructive pulmonary disease
BMV	bag-mask ventilation	CP	chest pain, chemically pure, cerebral palsy
BP, B/P	blood pressure	CPAP	continuous positive airway pressure
BPM	beats per minute	CPR	cardiopulmonary resuscitation
BS	blood sugar, breath sounds, bowel sounds, bachelor of science (degree)	CR	capillary refill
BSA	body surface area	CRNA	certified registered nurse anesthetist
BVM	bag-valve mask	CRT	capillary refill time, cathode ray tube
bx, Bx	biopsy	CSF	cerebrospinal fluid
c̄	with	CVA	cerebrovascular accident
°C	degrees Celsius (centigrade)	DM	diabetes mellitus
CA	cancer, carcinoma, cardiac arrest, chronologic age, coronary artery, cold agglutinin	DNR	do not resuscitate
CABDE	circulation, airway, breathing, disability, and exposure	DOA	dead on arrival
CABG	coronary artery bypass graft	DOB	date of birth
CAD	coronary artery disease	DOD	date of death
CBC	complete blood cell count	DOE	dyspnea on exertion
CC or C/C	chief complaint	DON	director of nursing

(continued)

Table 5-18	Common Abbreviations in Medical Terminology[a] *(continued)*		
Abbreviation	**Meaning**	**Abbreviation**	**Meaning**
DPT	diphtheria and tetanus toxoids and pertussis vaccine, Doctor of Physical Therapy	°F	degrees Fahrenheit
DSD	dry sterile dressing	FIO_2	fraction of inspired oxygen
DtaP	diphtheria and tetanus toxoids and acellular pertussis vaccine	FBS	fasting blood sugar
DTP	diphtheria and tetanus toxoids and pertussis vaccine	Fe	iron
DTs	delirium tremens	FHR	fetal heart rate
DVT	deep venous thrombosis	FHx	family history
Dx	diagnosis	fl or fld	fluid
EBL	estimated blood loss	fx	fracture
ECG	electrocardiogram	GB	gallbladder
ED	emergency department, erectile dysfunction	GCS	Glasgow Coma Scale
EDC	estimated date of confinement	GERD	gastroesophageal reflux disease
EDD	expected (estimated) date of delivery	GI	gastrointestinal
EEG	electroencephalogram	GSW	gunshot wound
EKG	electrocardiogram (the "k" comes from the German word "Elektrokardiogramm")	GTT	glucose tolerance test
ENT	ears, nose, and throat	GYN, gyn	gynecology
EOC	Emergency Operations Center	GU	genitourinary
ER	emergency room	h	hour, hours
ET, ETT	endotracheal, endotracheal tube	H&P	history and physical exam
ETA	estimated time of arrival	HA	headache
$ETCO_2$	end-tidal carbon dioxide	Hb, Hgb	hemoglobin
ETOH	ethyl alcohol	HBV	hepatitis B virus

Abbreviation	Meaning	Abbreviation	Meaning
HCV	hepatitis C virus	IV	intravenous
HCVD	hypertensive cardiovascular disease	JVD	jugular venous distention
HF	heart failure	kg	kilogram
HH	hiatus hernia	KVO	keep vein open
HIV	human immunodeficiency virus	L	liter
H_2O	water	lac, LAC	laceration
HPI	history of present illness	lb	pound, pounds
HPV	human papilloma virus	LE	lower extremity, left eye, lupus erythematosus
HR	heart rate	LLL	left lower lobe (of the lung)
hr	hour, hours	LLQ	left lower quadrant (of the abdomen)
HTN	hypertension	L/M, LPM	liters per minute
Hx	history	LMP	last menstrual period
I&O	intake and output	LOC	level of consciousness, loss of consciousness
ICP	intracranial pressure	LOM	loss of motion
ICS	incident command system, intercostal space	LUL	left upper lobe (of the lung)
ICU	intensive care unit	LUQ	left upper quadrant (of the abdomen)
IDDM	insulin-dependent diabetes mellitus	LVAD	left ventricular assist device
IHD	ischemic heart disease	MAE	moves all extremities
IM	intramuscular	MAEW	moves all extremities well
IMS	incident management system	mcg	microgram
IO	intraosseous	mg	milligram
IPPB, IPPV	intermittent positive pressure breathing, intermittent positive pressure ventilation	MI	myocardial infarction
IUD	intrauterine (contraceptive) device	MICU	mobile intensive care unit; medical intensive care unit

(continued)

Table 5-18 Common Abbreviations in Medical Terminology[a] *(continued)*

Abbreviation	Meaning	Abbreviation	Meaning
min	minute	N/V, N&V	nausea and vomiting
mL	milliliter	N/V/D	nausea, vomiting, and diarrhea
mm	millimeter	O_2	oxygen
mm Hg	millimeters of mercury	OB	obstetrics
MOI	mechanism of injury	OBS	organic brain syndrome
MRI	magnetic resonance imaging	OD	overdose, right eye, optical density, outside diameter, doctor of optometry
MRSA	methicillin-resistant *Staphylococcus aureus*	OP	outpatient
MVA	motor vehicle accident	OPA	oropharyngeal airway
MVC	motor vehicle crash	OR	operating room
MVP	mitral valve prolapse	oz	ounce
NA, N/A	not applicable	p̄	after
NAD	no apparent distress, no appreciable disease	pc	after meals
NC	nasal cannula	PCI	percutaneous coronary intervention
NG	nasogastric (tube)	Pco_2	partial pressure of carbon dioxide
NICU	neonatal intensive care unit	*PDR*	*Physicians' Desk Reference*
NIDDM	non–insulin-dependent diabetes mellitus	PE	pulmonary embolism, physical examination
NKA	no known allergies	PEARL or PERL	pupils equal and reactive to light
NKDA	no known drug allergies	PEARLA	pupils equal and reactive to light and accommodation
NPA	nasopharyngeal airway	PEARRL	pupils equal and round, regular in size, react to light
NPO	nil per os (nothing by mouth)	ped or peds	pediatric
NRB, NRBM	nonrebreathing mask	PEEP	positive end-expiratory pressure
NS	normal saline	PERRL	pupils equal, round, and reactive to light
NSR	normal sinus rhythm	PERRLA	pupils equal, round, and reactive to light and accommodation
NTG	nitroglycerin	PID	pelvic inflammatory disease

Abbreviation	Meaning	Abbreviation	Meaning
PMH	past medical history	RUL	right upper lobe (of the lung)
PND	paroxysmal nocturnal dyspnea	RUQ	right upper quadrant (of the abdomen)
po	per os (by mouth)	Rx	prescription
PO	postoperative, "post op"	$\bar{s}$	without
PRN	pro re nata (as needed)	SAH	subarachnoid hemorrhage
psi	pounds per square inch	Sao_2	oxygen saturation
PSVT	paroxysmal supraventricular tachycardia	SARS	severe acute respiratory syndrome
PT	physical therapy, prothrombin time	SICU	surgical intensive care unit
pt	patient	SIDS	sudden infant death syndrome
PTA	prior to admission, plasma thromboplastin antecedent	SL	sublingual
PTT	partial thromboplastin time	SOB	shortness of breath
PVC	premature ventricular complex, polyvinyl chloride	Spo_2	saturation of peripheral oxygen
PVD	peripheral vascular disease	S/S, S&S	signs and symptoms
$\bar{q}$	every	stat	immediately
RA	rheumatoid arthritis, right atrium	STEMI	ST-segment elevation myocardial infarction
RAD	reactive airway disease, right axis deviation	STI	sexually transmitted infection
RBC	red blood cell	SUID	sudden unexpected infant death
Rh	Rhesus blood factor, rhodium	SVN	small-volume nebulizer
RLL	right lower lobe (of the lung)	SVT	supraventricular tachycardia
RLQ	right lower quadrant (of the abdomen)	sym or Sx	symptoms
RML	right middle lobe (of the lung)	T	temperature
RN	registered nurse	tab	tablet
R/O	rule out	TB	tuberculosis
ROM	range of motion, rupture of membranes	TBA	to be admitted, to be announced

(continued)

Table 5-18 Common Abbreviations in Medical Terminology[a] *(continued)*

Abbreviation	Meaning	Abbreviation	Meaning
tech	technician, technologist	VS	vital signs
TIA	transient ischemic attack	VT/V tach	ventricular tachycardia
tid/t.i.d./TID	three times a day	W/	with
Tx	treatment	WBC	white blood cell
UA, U/A	urinalysis	WMD	weapon of mass destruction
UE	upper extremity	WNL	within normal limits
URI	upper respiratory infection	W/O	without
UTI	urinary tract infection	wt	weight
VF/V fib/VFib	ventricular fibrillation	x̄	except
VRE	vancomycin-resistant enterococcus	yo; y.o.; y/o	years old

[a] Sometimes abbreviations are written with periods (for example, abd. and a.c.), and sometimes different capitalization might be used and might convey a different meaning. Not all possible meanings for each abbreviation are given in this table. Unless you are certain about the meaning, ask the person who used the abbreviation and do not use it yourself.

YOU are the Provider SUMMARY

1. What is the correct medical term for the position in which the child is lying?

He is lying on his left side, which is the recovery position, also called the *left lateral recumbent* position.

2. How can knowledge of medical terminology assist in your documentation of care for this patient?

Medical terminology is the language of medicine and health care. As an AEMT, you should have a good understanding of medical terminology and be able to identify and use terms correctly. This not only allows you to communicate effectively with other health care providers, but also ensures you use accurate and concise documentation, resulting in better continuity of care.

3. Why would you want to avoid using medical terminology when talking to this patient?

Patients, especially children, are rarely familiar with medical terminology. Therefore, using medical terms during a patient interview will probably lead to misunderstanding and a lack of pertinent information. When you talk with patients, use everyday terms to help improve the likelihood of communicating clearly. As an AEMT, you must also be familiar with terms and phrases that are common in the geographic area in which you work.

4. What are the correct medical terms to describe Kevin's mental status and blood glucose level?

His mental status is documented as AOx4 because he is alert to person, place, time, and event. The appropriate term for a high blood glucose level is *hyperglycemia.* It is formed from the prefix *hyper–* (excessive) + the word root *glyc/o* (glucose) + the suffix *–emia* (pertaining to the blood).

5. How would you document that the patient has no medication allergies?

The correct abbreviation for "no known drug allergies" is *NKDA.*

YOU are the Provider SUMMARY *(continued)*

6. Describe the position of the patient's head injury.

His injury is on the right side of his forehead, just above his eye. Since *superior* is the term for above and *orbit* is the eye socket, it would be documented as *superior to the right orbit.*

7. What is the abbreviation for the abdominal quadrant that is tender to the touch?

The abdomen is divided into quadrants by two imaginary lines intersecting at the umbilicus. The area where Kevin reports having pain is the upper quadrant on the right side. The abbreviation is *RUQ.*

8. Why is knowledge of anatomy pertinent when assessing and treating this patient?

Familiarity with the structures and functions of the body systems will allow you to better assess a patient as well as predict potential complications resulting from occult injuries (those not visible to the eye). In this instance, if you know what organs are located in the RUQ, you can predict possible injuries, which allows for a greater index of suspicion resulting in more appropriate treatment and transport to the proper facility.

9. What is the medical term for clammy skin?

The term for clammy skin associated with signs of shock is *diaphoresis.*

10. What is the medical term for a phenomenon (such as pain, swelling, or a rash) affecting both sides of the body?

Many body structures are bilateral, and certain medical conditions tend to occur either unilaterally or bilaterally. A phenomenon affecting or appearing on both sides of the midline is said to be *bilateral.*

EMS Patient Care Report (PCR)					
Date: 4-20-18	**Incident No.:** 050124		**Nature of Call:** Fall	**Location:** 184 Elementary Way	
Dispatched: 0935	**En Route:** 0936	**At Scene:** 0942	**Transport:** 0957	**At Hospital:** 1009	**In Service:** 1027
Patient Information					
Age: 7 **Sex:** M **Weight (in kg [lb]):** 25 kg (56 lb)			**Allergies:** NKDA **Medications:** Insulin **Past Medical History:** IDDM **Chief Complaint:** Fall		

Vital Signs				
Time: 0945	**BP:**	**Pulse:** 104	**Respirations:** 22	**Spo_2:** 98%
Time: 0950	**BP:**	**Pulse:** 108	**Respirations:** 22	**Spo_2:** 99%
Time: 0955	**BP:** 96/54	**Pulse:** 98	**Respirations:** 18	**Spo_2:** 96%
Time: 1000	**BP:** 98/60	**Pulse:** 98	**Respirations:** 20	**Spo_2:** 99%

EMS Treatment (circle all that apply)				
Oxygen @ ______ L/min via (circle one): **NC NRM Bag-mask device**		**Assisted Ventilation**	**Airway Adjunct**	**CPR**
Defibrillation	**Bleeding Control**	**Bandaging:** Hematoma, right forehead (circled)	**Splinting**	**Other:** Spinal immobilization (circled)

YOU are the Provider SUMMARY (continued)

Narrative
9-1-1 dispatch for a male patient who fell. On arrival at the scene, found the patient, a 7-y/o male, lying left lateral recumbent in fetal position and holding abdomen; comforted by teacher. Teacher states pt fell approximately 6 feet from top of playground equipment and has not been moved. Patient AOx4, c/o pain in right upper quadrant. Presents with a golf ball–size hematoma superior to the right orbit with small laceration—bleeding controlled. Patient states he has been "dizzy" this morning, causing his fall. PERRLA, slightly tachycardic and tachypneic. Hx—IDDM, for which he takes insulin and has NKDA. Teacher states blood glucose level was 183 mg/dL upon arrival this a.m. Pt states he ate and took insulin this a.m. Further assessment of patient's abdomen revealed that it was soft, but very tender to palpation of the RUQ, with discoloration of the area. Patient fully c-spine immobilized on LSB with c-collar and CID and loaded into ambulance for transport to the pediatric trauma center. En route, vital signs reassessed and noted above, breath sounds clear and equal bilaterally, skin cool and diaphoretic, glucose 147 mg/dL. Pt covered to maintain warmth, head wound bandaged, and 20 g IV left dorsal hand with normal saline at TKO rate. Reassessment of abdomen finds increased tenderness and darker discoloration. Met patient's parents and transferred care of patient to receiving hospital without incident. Written report completed and ambulance cleaned and restocked. Departed the hospital and returned to service.**End of report**

Prep Kit

▶ Ready for Review

- Knowledge of medical terminology is essential for health care team members to communicate effectively and document calls.
- You must be able to identify superficial landmarks of the body. These landmarks indicate which structures lie underneath the skin, so you can perform an accurate patient assessment.
- Understanding how terms are formed, and the definitions for the various parts of a medical term, will help you determine the meaning of an unknown term.
- To strengthen your grasp of medical terminology, become familiar with commonly used medical eponyms, homonyms, and antonyms, as well as symbols and terms used in pharmacology.
- A prefix is the part of a term that appears at the beginning of a word. It generally describes location and intensity of the word root that follows.
- A suffix is placed at the end of a word to change the original meaning. In medical terminology, a suffix usually indicates a procedure, condition, disease, or part of speech.
- The word root is the foundation of the term. It establishes the basic meaning of the word.
- A combining vowel is the part of a term that connects a word root to a suffix or other word root to make it easier to pronounce.
- Prefixes can also indicate numbers or direction. Word roots can also describe color.
- Compound words are words that contain more than one word root.
- To make some terms plural, an *s* is added to the term. Other terms use other plural forms.
- Anatomic position refers to the body in a standing position, facing you, with arms at the sides and palms facing forward. Patient position is the position in which the patient is found when you arrive on scene.
- Anatomic planes of the body include coronal, transverse, and sagittal (lateral).
- Directional terms indicate distance and direction from the midline. These include right, left, superior, inferior, lateral, medial, proximal, distal, superficial, deep, ventral, dorsal, anterior, posterior, palmar, plantar, and apex.

Prep Kit (continued)

- Terms related to movement and position include flexion, extension, adduction, abduction, supination, pronation, and rotation.
- Other directional terms relate to a position on one or both sides of the body. Such terms include bilateral, unilateral, ipsilateral, and contralateral.
- The concept of quadrants is useful in medical terminology. The abdomen is commonly categorized into quadrants to help specify an area of pain or injury.
- Abbreviations, acronyms, and symbols are used as shorthand to communicate and document in a concise manner. To avoid potentially dangerous misinterpretation of your documentation, ensure you use only abbreviations that are commonly understood in your system; avoid using abbreviations that are not recommended.

▶ Vital Vocabulary

abduction Movement of a limb away from the midline.

adduction Movement of a limb toward the midline.

anatomic position The position of reference, in which the patient stands facing you, arms at the side, with the palms of the hands facing forward.

anterior The front surface of the body; the side facing you in the anatomic position.

anteroposterior axis The axis that runs perpendicular to the coronal plane.

antonyms Pairs of word roots, prefixes, or suffixes that have opposite meanings.

apex (plural *apices* or *apexes*) The pointed extremity of a conical structure.

bilateral In anatomy, a body part or condition that appears on both sides of the midline.

combining form A word root followed by a vowel.

combining vowel The vowel used to combine two word roots or a word root and a prefix or suffix.

compound word A word containing more than one word root.

contralateral On the opposite side of the body.

coronal plane An imaginary plane in which the body is cut into front and back portions.

cross section The product of slicing an object crosswise, perpendicular to its long axis.

deep Farther inside the body and away from the skin.

distal Farther from the trunk and nearer to the free end of the extremity.

dorsal The posterior surface of the body, including the back of the hand.

eponym The name of a disease, device, procedure, or drug that is based on the person who invented, discovered, or first described it.

extension The straightening of a joint.

external rotation Rotating an extremity at its joint away from the midline.

flexion The bending of a joint.

Fowler position A sitting position, with the head elevated at a 90° angle (sitting straight upright).

homonyms Words that sound alike but are spelled differently and have different meanings.

horizontal axis The axis that runs perpendicular to the sagittal plane; also called the medio-lateral axis.

hyperextension Extension beyond the normal range of motion.

hyperflexion Flexion beyond the normal range of motion.

inferior Below what is indicated; closer to the feet.

internal rotation Rotating the anterior surface of an extremity toward the midline.

ipsilateral On the same side of the body.

lateral In anatomy, parts of the body that lie farther from the midline.

longitudinal axis The axis that runs perpendicular to the transverse plane.

longitudinal section The view of an object cut along its long axis.

medial In anatomy, parts of the body that lie closer to the midline.

midsagittal plane (midline) An imaginary vertical line drawn from the middle of the forehead through the nose and the umbilicus (navel) to the floor.

palmar The position in which the palm of the hand is facing forward when in the anatomic position.

plantar The sole or bottom surface of the foot.

posterior In anatomy, the back surface of the body; the side away from you in the standard anatomic position.

prefix The word part that appears before a word root, changing the meaning of the term.

pronation Turning the palms downward (toward the ground).

prone Lying flat, face down.

proximal Closer to the trunk.

quadrants The four sections of the abdominal cavity shown by two imaginary lines intersecting at the umbilicus, dividing the abdomen into four equal areas.

range of motion The full distance that a joint can be moved.

Prep Kit *(continued)*

sagittal (lateral) plane A plane of the body that passes vertically from front to back, dividing the body into left and right portions.

suffix The word part that comes after the word root, at the end of the term.

superficial Closer to or on the surface of the skin.

superior Above what is indicated; closer to the head.

supination Turning the palms upward (toward the sky).

supine Lying face up.

synonyms Pairs of word roots, prefixes, or suffixes that have the same or almost the same meaning.

topographic anatomy Superficial landmarks of the body that serve as guides to the structures that lie beneath them.

transverse (axial) plane An imaginary plane passing horizontally through the body at the waist, dividing it into top and bottom halves.

unilateral Occurring or appearing on only one side of the body.

ventral The anterior surface of the body.

word root The foundation of a word; establishes the basic meaning of a word.

▶ References

1. ISMP's list of error-prone abbreviations, symbols, and designations. Institute for Safe Medication Practices website. http://www.ismp.org/Tools/errorproneabbreviations.pdf. Accessed February 5, 2016.
2. Facts about the official "do not use" list of abbreviations. The Joint Commission website. http://www.jointcommission.org/facts_about_the_of cial_/default.aspx. Updated June 30, 2016. Accessed February 5, 2016.

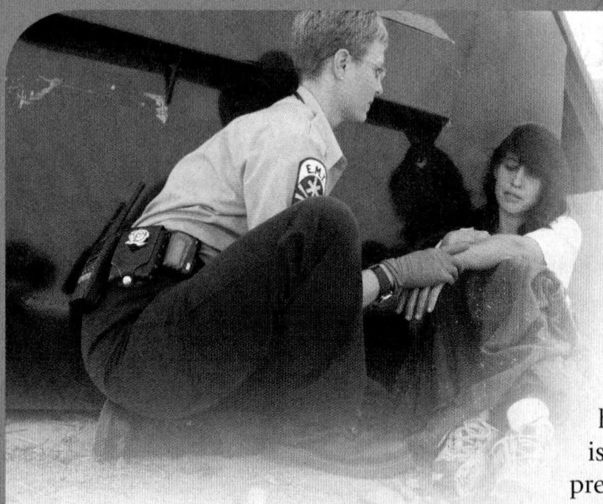

Assessment *in Action*

You respond to a call for a stabbing outside a local bar. Upon arrival, you find a 37-year-old man lying on his back on the sidewalk, bleeding from his abdomen and right upper arm. He is screaming in pain and holding the right side of his abdomen. During your assessment, you note his breathing is 24 breaths/min, his pulse rate is 132 beat/min, his blood pressure is 92/60 mm Hg, he is diaphoretic, his skin is pale, and his pupils are equal and reactive bilaterally. He presents with a 1-inch (3-cm) puncture just above and to the right of his umbilicus and a slashing wound approximately 2 inches (5 cm) in length on his right upper arm, just above the elbow. He tells you he is not allergic to any medications and takes lisinopril for high blood pressure. You place him on oxygen; put him in a position of comfort, with his legs drawn up and the head of the stretcher elevated to a 45° angle; gain intravenous access; and provide rapid transport. Just prior to arrival at the trauma center you notice that his mental status has deteriorated and he is now responsive only to pain.

Assessment *in Action* *(continued)*

1. The medical term for high blood pressure is *hypertension*. What is the abbreviation?
   - **A.** HBP
   - **B.** HYP
   - **C.** HTN
   - **D.** HYN
2. The patient has been stabbed in which abdominal quadrant?
   - **A.** RUQ
   - **B.** LUQ
   - **C.** RLQ
   - **D.** LLQ
3. The patient was initially found in what position?
   - **A.** Prone
   - **B.** Supine
   - **C.** Fowler
   - **D.** Recovery
4. The wound to his right arm is in what position relative to his right elbow?
   - **A.** Medial
   - **B.** Lateral
   - **C.** Distal
   - **D.** Proximal
5. The patient has an elevated respiratory rate and an elevated heart rate. What is the prefix for "fast"?
   - **A.** brady-
   - **B.** tachy-
   - **C.** hyper-
   - **D.** supra-
6. The patient's blood pressure is 92/60 mm Hg. What is the appropriate term for this reading?
   - **A.** Hypotensive
   - **B.** Normotensive
   - **C.** Hypertensive
   - **D.** Hemotensive
7. What is the appropriate abbreviation for the patient's pupillary response?
   - **A.** PEEP
   - **B.** PMH
   - **C.** PERRLA
   - **D.** PRRLL
8. What is the term for the position in which the patient is transported?
   - **A.** Recumbent
   - **B.** Lateral
   - **C.** Fowler
   - **D.** Semi-Fowler
9. What are some possible misunderstandings that could occur if an AEMT uses incorrect medical terminology on the job?
10. Rewrite the scenario using medical terminology and abbreviations.

CHAPTER 6

Lifting and Moving Patients

National EMS Education Standard Competencies

Preparatory

Applies fundamental knowledge of the EMS system, safety/well-being of the AEMT, medical/legal and ethical issues to the provision of emergency care.

Workforce Safety and Wellness

› Lifting and moving patients (pp 185-218)

Knowledge Objectives

1. Describe the technical skills and general considerations that are required of the advanced emergency medical technician (AEMT) during patient packaging and patient handling. (p 185)
2. Describe how following proper patient lifting and moving techniques helps prevent work-related injuries. (p 186)
3. Describe the guidelines for properly lifting a patient, using a power grip, a draw sheet, or blanket. (pp 187-188)
4. Summarize the general considerations required to safely move patients without causing them further harm while simultaneously protecting the AEMT from injury. (p 190)
5. Describe the guidelines and safety precautions AEMTs should follow when lifting and carrying a patient on a stretcher or backboard, and how to avoid common mistakes. (pp 192-196)
6. Describe specific situations in which emergency moves or urgent moves (rapid extrication) may be necessary for moving a patient; include how each move is performed. (pp 196-201)
7. Describe specific situations in which nonurgent moves may be necessary for moving a patient; include how each move is performed. (pp 201-206)
8. Discuss special considerations when moving and transporting geriatric patients and the guidelines to follow when lifting and moving geriatric patients. (pp 207-208)
9. Define the term bariatrics; include the guidelines for lifting and moving bariatric patients. (p 208)
10. Name 11 patient-moving devices; include how each one is used to move a patient. (pp 209-215)
11. Explain the importance of equipment decontamination in the prevention of disease transmission. (p 217)
12. Describe proper patient positioning with the following medical conditions: (pp 217-218)
    - Unresponsive patients without suspected spine injury
    - Patients with chest pain, discomfort, or difficulty breathing
    - Patients with suspected spine injury
    - Pregnant patients with hypotension
    - Patients who are nauseated or vomiting
13. Discuss situations that may require the use of medical restraints on a patient; include the guidelines and safety considerations regarding use. (p 218)

Skills Objectives

1. Demonstrate the body mechanics and principles required for safe reaching and pulling, including the safe reaching technique used for performing log rolling. (pp 186-192)
2. Demonstrate a power lift to lift a patient. (pp 186-188, Skill Drill 6-1)
3. Demonstrate using a power grip. (pp 187-189)
4. Demonstrate the two-person body drag. (p 191, Skill Drill 6-2)
5. Demonstrate how to log roll a patient. (pp 191-192)
6. Demonstrate the diamond carry to move a patient. (pp 194-195, Skill Drill 6-3)
7. Demonstrate the one-handed carrying technique to move a patient. (pp 194-195, Skill Drill 6-4)
8. Demonstrate how to perform an emergency or urgent move such as a one-person technique for removing an unresponsive patient from a vehicle. (p 197, Skill Drill 6-5)
9. Demonstrate the rapid extrication technique to move a patient from a vehicle. (pp 197-201, Skill Drill 6-6)

10. Demonstrate the direct ground lift to lift a patient. (pp 201-202, Skill Drill 6-7)
11. Demonstrate the extremity lift to move a patient. (pp 202-203, Skill Drill 6-8)
12. Demonstrate the direct carry to move a patient. (pp 202-204, Skill Drill 6-9)
13. Demonstrate how to use the draw sheet method to transfer a patient onto a stretcher. (pp 202, 204, Skill Drill 6-10)
14. Demonstrate the use of a scoop stretcher to move a patient. (p 205, Skill Drill 6-11)
15. Demonstrate how to lift a patient from the ground. (p 206, Skill Drill 6-12)
16. Demonstrate how to move a patient from a chair to a stair chair. (p 206, Skill Drill 6-13)
17. Demonstrate how to load a stretcher into an ambulance. (pp 211-212, Skill Drill 6-14)
18. Demonstrate how to carry a patient on stairs using a stair chair. (pp 215-216, Skill Drill 6-15)
19. Demonstrate a patient carry to move a patient up or down stairs. (pp 216-217, Skill Drill 6-16)
20. Demonstrate the correct use of medical restraints on a patient. (p 218)

Introduction

In the course of a call, you will have to move the patient several times when assessing, treating, and transporting the patient to the emergency department (ED). Often, you will have to move the patient into a different position or location. These moves will likely involve the use of a stretcher, backboard, or other devices. Once you have assessed the patient and provided emergency medical care, you and your team will have to move the patient from the scene to the ambulance and from the ambulance to the ED bed. To avoid injury to the patient, yourself, and your partners, you need to learn how to lift and carry the patient properly and safely, using proper body mechanics and a power grip.

To be able to move a patient safely and properly in the various situations that you will encounter in the field, you need to learn how to perform emergency body drags and lifts, rapidly move a patient from a vehicle onto the stretcher, assist a patient from a chair or bed onto the stretcher, and lift a patient from the floor onto the stretcher. In addition, you may need to carry a patient up or down stairs. You and your team need to know how to place a patient with a suspected spinal injury onto an immobilization device and package patients with and without suspected spinal injury. At times, you and your team will need to move a patient who is very heavy or carry a patient on a trail or across rugged terrain. You and your team should be familiar with the special techniques for lifting and moving patients, and should practice them often.

Lifting and carrying are dynamic processes. To ensure no person suddenly bears unexpected, dangerous weight and to reduce the risk of injury to a provider or a patient, you must know where all providers should be positioned and how to give and receive lifting commands so all parties act simultaneously. You need to know how to prepare patient-moving devices, such as a wheeled ambulance stretcher, stair chair, backboard, scoop stretcher, folding ambulance stretcher, basket stretcher, flexible stretcher, and any other equipment your service may carry. Most important, you need to know how and when to use them.

Training and practice are required to use all the equipment that is described in this chapter. You must master the skills necessary to use each device and understand its advantages and limitations. Practice each technique with your team often so you can perform the move quickly, safely, and efficiently. After each patient transfer, you and your team should evaluate the appropriateness of the technique that you used and your technical skill in completing the transfer. You must also ensure you maintain your equipment according to the manufacturer's instructions. Using clean, well-maintained equipment is a critical part of providing high-quality patient care. This chapter covers a review of body mechanics, lifting, carrying, and reaching techniques and the principles of moving patients, including emergency, urgent, and nonurgent moves. In addition, different types of patient-moving equipment and patient positioning are discussed in detail.

YOU are the Provider — PART 1

Your ambulance is requested for a direct admittance from a private residence to the local hospital's surgical unit. Your patient is a bedridden older adult male who weighs approximately 325 pounds (147 kg). He is alert and oriented, but he is unable to assist in being moved to the stretcher. He has an indwelling catheter in place.

1. What additional resources may be needed to move this patient?
2. How will you move this patient from his bed to the stretcher?

Words of Wisdom

Patient packaging and handling are technical skills that you will learn and perfect through practice and training. Every year, a significant number of emergency medical services (EMS) personnel are injured when they attempt to lift and move patients. Even when you are lifting, moving, or transferring relatively light-weight patients, the need for proper body mechanics should remain paramount.

Body Mechanics

Anatomy Review

When you are lifting, moving, or transferring patients, the need for proper body mechanics should remain paramount. When the person is standing upright, the individual weight-bearing vertebrae are stacked on top of each other and aligned over the sacrum. The sacrum is the mechanical weight-bearing base of the spinal column and the fused central posterior section of the pelvic girdle. The shoulder girdle rests on the rib cage and is supported by the vertebrae that lie inferior to it. The arms are connected to and hang from the shoulder girdle.

When a person is standing upright, the weight of anything being lifted and carried in the hands is reflected onto the shoulder girdle, the rib cage, the spinal column inferior to it, the pelvis, and then the legs **Figure 6-1**. In lifting, if the shoulder girdle is aligned over the pelvis and the hands are held close to the legs, the force that is exerted against the spine occurs in an essentially straight line down the strong, stacked vertebrae in the spinal column. Therefore, with the back properly maintained in an upright position, very little strain occurs against the muscles and ligaments that keep the spinal column in alignment, and significant weight can be lifted and carried without injury to the back **Figure 6-2**. However, you may injure your back if you lift while leaning forward, or even if straight, bent significantly forward at the hips **Figure 6-3**. With the back in either of these positions, the shoulder girdle lies significantly anterior to the pelvis, and the force of lifting is exerted primarily across, rather than down, the spinal column. When this occurs, the weight is supported by the muscles of the back and ligaments that run from the base of the skull to the pelvis, keeping the spinal column in alignment, rather than by each vertebral body and disk resting on those aligned below it. In addition, the upper spine and torso serve as a lever so that the force that is exerted against the muscles and ligaments in the lumbar and sacral regions, as a result of the mechanical advantage produced, is many times that of the combined weight of your upper body and the object you are lifting. Therefore, the first key rule of lifting is to always keep the back in a straight, upright (vertical) position and to lift without twisting or bending. Always face the patient and point your feet in the same direction. After lifting the patient, change the direction of your feet as opposed to twisting or turning from the waist.

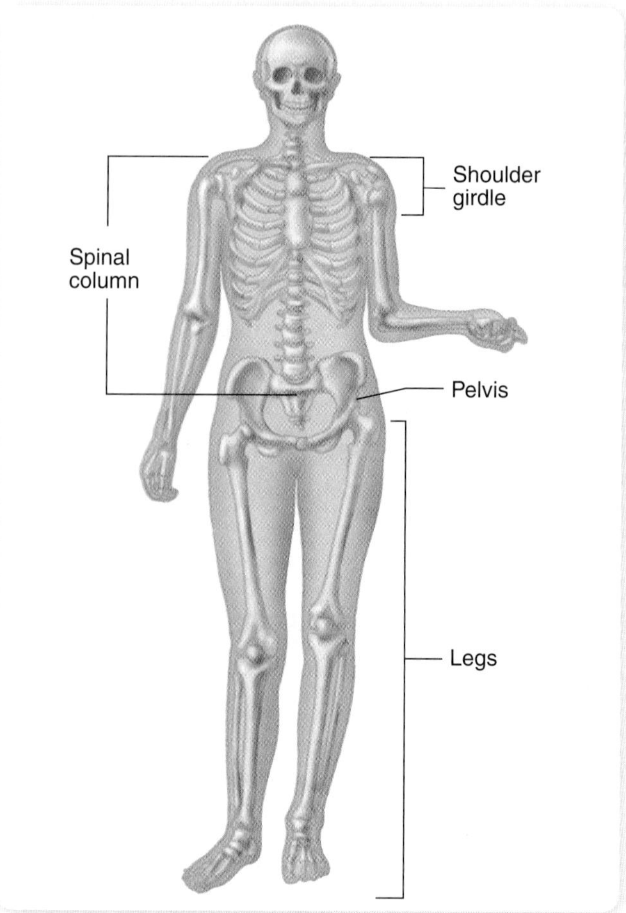

Figure 6-1 When you are standing upright, the weight of anything that you lift and carry in your hands is borne by the shoulder girdle, the spinal column, the pelvis, and the legs.

Proper Lifting Technique

When you are lifting, spread your legs about 15 inches (38 cm) apart (shoulder width) and place your feet so your center of gravity is properly balanced between them. Then, with the back held upright, bring your upper body down by bending the legs into a squat. Once you have properly grasped the patient or stretcher and made any necessary adjustments in the location of your feet, lift the patient by straightening your legs and raising your upper body until you are again standing. Your arms should still be extended. You can then *curl* your forearms if you need to lift higher. This is the same technique used when performing a bicep curl with weights. Because the leg muscles are regularly exercised by walking, climbing stairs, or running, they are well developed and extremely strong. Therefore, as well as being the safest way to lift, lifting by extending the properly placed flexed legs is also the most powerful way to lift. This method is appropriately called a **power lift**. The power lift position is also useful for people who have weak knees or thighs.

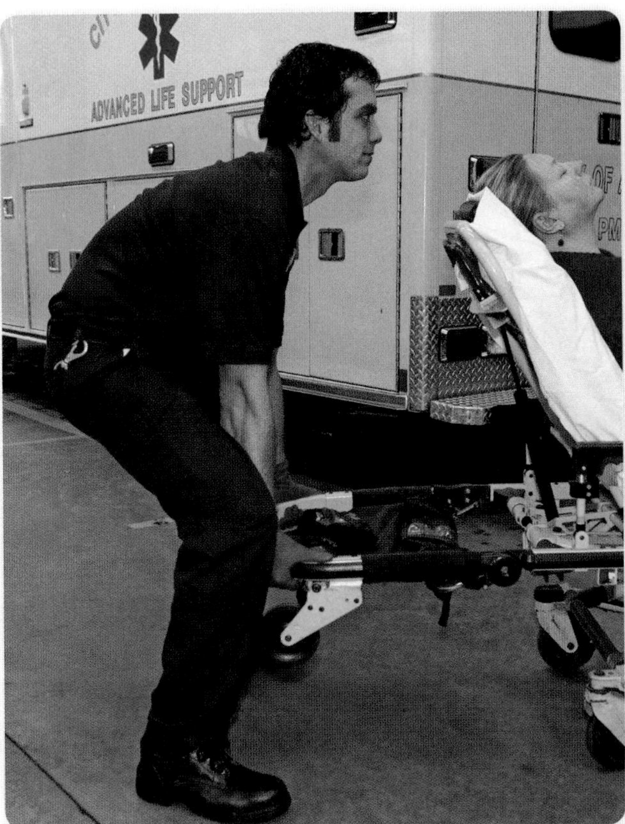

Figure 6-2 If your body is properly aligned when you lift, the line of force exerted against the spine occurs in an essentially straight line down the vertebrae. In this way, the vertebrae support the lift.

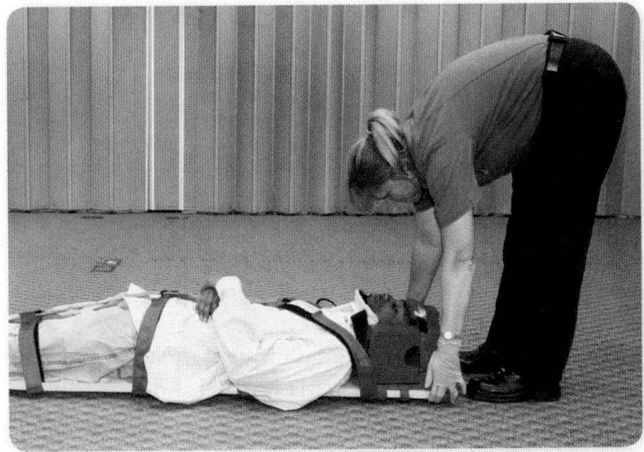

Figure 6-3 This photo demonstrates an incorrect method of lifting. When this occurs, the muscles of the back, not the vertebrae, are supporting the lift.

One mistake you can make while performing a patient lift is to lift a patient or other heavy object with your arms outstretched. Even if the back is held properly upright, the same adverse force across the spinal column and leverage against the lower back will occur if you lift a heavy object with your arms significantly outstretched. Whenever you are lifting or carrying a patient, hold your arms so your elbows are aligned with the sides of your body. Always keep the weight that you are lifting as close to your body as possible.

Another rule to remember when lifting is to avoid placing lateral force across the spine and sideways leverage against the lower back. If you lift with only one arm or with the arms extended more to one side than the other, more force will be exerted against one side of the shoulder girdle than the other, causing lateral force to be exerted across the spinal column. To prevent this, keep your arms approximately the same distance apart as when hanging at each side of the body, with the weight distributed equally and properly centered between them. If the weight is not balanced between both arms or properly centered between the shoulders when you are preparing to lift, turn your body and/or move to the left or right until the weight is properly balanced and centered. To lift safely and produce the maximal power lift, take the steps shown in **Skill Drill 6-1**.

Reverse these steps whenever you are lowering the stretcher. Always remember to avoid bending at the waist.

> **Safety Tips**
>
> The safety of advanced emergency medical technicians (AEMTs) and patients depends on proper lifting techniques and maintaining a proper hold while lifting and carrying. Loss of grasp by one AEMT may cause injury to another team member and to the patient.

▶ Proper Hold

Your safety, as well as that of the other AEMTs and the patient, depends on the use of proper lifting techniques, having and maintaining a proper hold when lifting or carrying a patient, and being in good physical health. If you do not have proper hold of the stretcher or of the patient in a body lift, you will not be able to bear a proper share of the weight, and there is an increased chance that you can suddenly lose your grasp with one or both hands. If you temporarily lose your grasp with one or both hands, the position and weight distribution of the stretcher changes suddenly, and the other members of the team must quickly reach beyond a safe distance to avoid dropping the patient. As a result, sudden excessive force may be placed across each one's spine, causing lower back injury.

Use the **power grip** to get the maximum force from your hands whenever you are lifting a patient **Figure 6-4**. The arm and hand have their greatest lifting strength when facing palm up. Whenever you grasp a stretcher or backboard, your hands should be at least 10 inches (25 cm) apart. Each hand should be inserted under the handle with the palm facing up and the thumb extended upward. Then, advance the hand until the thumb prevents further insertion and the cylindrical handle lies firmly in the crease of the curved palm. Curl your fingers and

Skill Drill 6-1 Performing the Power Lift

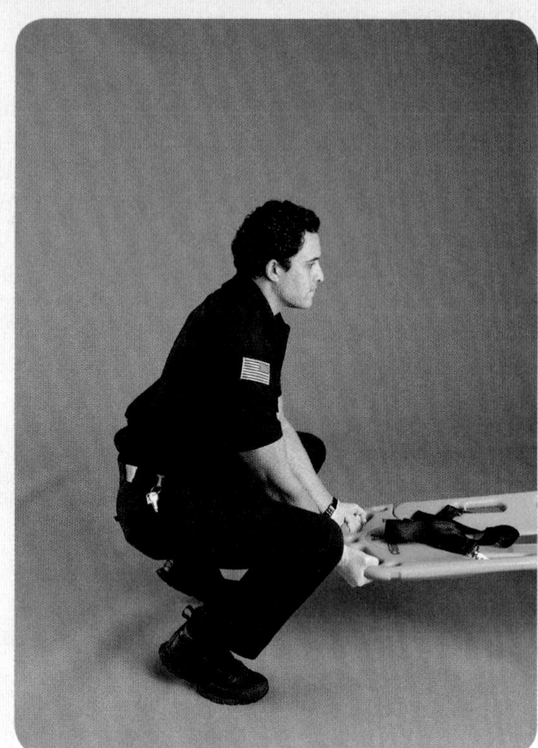

Step 1 Tighten your back in a normal upright position and lock it in a slight inward curve at the lumbar area. Spread your legs about 15 inches (38 cm) apart, and bend your legs to lower your torso and arms. With your arms extended down, grasp the stretcher or backboard with your hands held palm up and just in front of you. Balance and center the weight between your arms.

Step 2 Reposition your feet as necessary so they are about 15 inches (38 cm) apart with one slightly farther forward and rotated so your center of gravity is properly balanced between your legs. Straddle the object and distribute your weight. Do not bend your knees more than 90°, nor extend your knees past your toes. With your arms extended downward, lift by straightening your legs until you are fully standing. Hold your back upright and ensure your upper body comes up before your hips.

thumb tightly over the top of the handle. All your fingers should be at the same angle. To have the proper power grip, make sure the underside of the handle is fully supported on your curved palm with only the fingers and thumb preventing it from being pulled sideways or upward out of the palm.

If you must lift the object higher once you have lifted by extending your legs, you will be able to "curl" the object higher by using your biceps to flex the arms while maintaining the power grip and weight supported in the palms.

Never grasp a stretcher or backboard with your hand placed palm down over the handle. Doing so will cause the weight to be supported by your fingers rather than your palm. This hand orientation places the tips of the fingers and thumb under the handle. If the weight forces them apart, or if the stretcher is pushed suddenly downward in the process of moving, you will lose your grasp on the handle.

If at all possible, use a draw sheet or other approved lifting device so you are not pulling directly on the patient's skin (discussed later in the chapter). This is especially important when lifting patients who are heavy and/or older. When you are lifting a patient by a sheet or blanket, center the patient on the sheet and tightly roll up the excess fabric on each side. This produces a cylindrical handle that provides a strong, secure way to grasp the fabric. It is crucial that there is no "give" in the sheet and that it is kept as taut as possible because a sudden shift of weight as the fabric gives can injure providers.

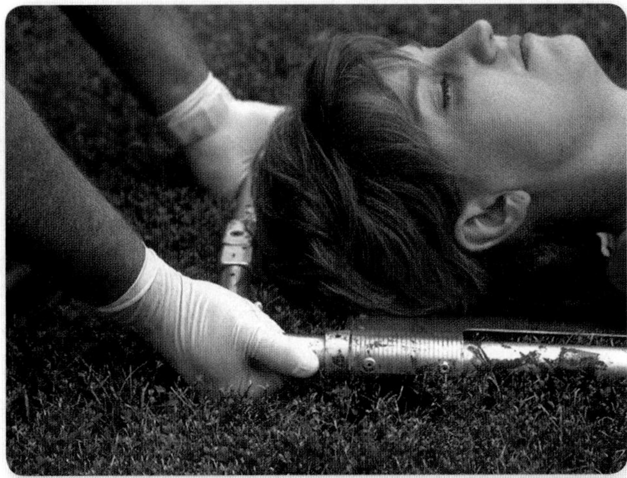

Figure 6-4 To perform the power grip, grasp the handle of the stretcher or backboard with your palms up and your thumbs extending up. Make sure your hands are about 10 inches (25 cm) apart and that your fingers are all at the same angle. The underside of the handle should be fully supported by the palms of your hands.

Words of Wisdom

Ensure you are lifting in tandem to prevent injury to the patient or providers. The person calling the move should always announce "We are going to lift on 3" or "We are going to count to 3 and then lift."

Directions and Commands

To safely lift and carry a patient, you and your team must anticipate and understand every move, and each move must be executed in a coordinated manner. The team leader should indicate where each team member is to be located and rapidly describe the sequence of steps that will be performed to ensure team members know what is expected of them before they initiate any lifting. If you must lift and move a patient through a number of separate steps, the team leader should first give an abbreviated overview of the steps, followed by a more detailed explanation of each step just before it will occur.

Orders that will initiate the actual lifting or moving or any significant changes in movement should be given in two parts: a preparatory command and a command of execution. For example, if the team leader says "All ready to stop. STOP!" the "All ready to stop" will get your attention, identify who should act, and prepare you to act; the declarative "STOP!" will indicate the exact moment for execution. Commands of execution should be delivered in a louder voice. Often, a countdown is helpful when you need to lift a patient. To avoid confusion when you countdown, always clarify whether "three" is to be a part of the preparatory command or whether it is to serve as the order to execute. In other words, say "We're going to lift on three. One-two-THREE!" or "I'm going to count to three and then we're going to lift. One-two-three-LIFT!"

YOU are the Provider — PART 2

You request additional lifting assistance and clear a path for the stretcher to travel through the living room. The patient states he has several small wounds on his back and buttocks and asks you to be careful when moving him. An engine crew arrives and you decide that the best way to move him is to use the draw sheet method.

Recording Time: 1 Minute	
Appearance	Alert
Level of consciousness	Alert and oriented
Airway	Patent
Breathing	Nonlabored
Circulation	Skin warm, pink, and dry

3. What are some potential complications when patients are moved improperly?
4. Should you use an emergency, urgent, or nonurgent move?
5. What are some of the differences between a normal stretcher and a bariatric stretcher?

Principles of Safe Reaching and Pulling

When you use a body drag to move a patient, the same basic body mechanics and principles apply as when you move, lift, and carry a patient. Your back should always be locked in a slight curve created by tightening your abdominal muscles, not curved laterally or bent laterally. It should be held in a normal upright position. Avoid any twisting so your vertebrae remain in normal alignment. When you are reaching overhead, avoid hyperextending your back. When you are pulling a patient who is on the ground, always kneel to minimize the distance that you will have to lean over Figure 6-5A. To keep your reach within the recommended distance, reach forward and grasp the patient so your elbows are just beyond the anterior part of the torso Figure 6-5B. When you are pulling a patient who is at a different height from you, bend your knees until your hips are just below the height of the plane across which you will be pulling the patient. When you are pulling, do not extend your arms more than about 15 to 20 inches (38 to 50 cm) in front of your torso. Reposition your feet (or knees, if kneeling) so the force of pull will be balanced equally between both arms and the line of pull will be centered between them Figure 6-5C. Pull the patient by slowly flexing your arms. When you cannot pull further because your hands have reached the front of your torso, stop and move back another 15 to 20 inches (38 to 50 cm). Then, when properly positioned, repeat the steps. Alternate between pulling the patient by flexing your arms and then repositioning yourself so your arms are again extended with your hands about 15 inches (38 cm) in front of your torso. By not moving simultaneously with the patient, you prevent an undesirable jostling of the patient and the chance that sudden unscheduled force will occur across your spine. You may prevent injury to yourself by avoiding situations that involve strenuous effort lasting more than 1 minute.

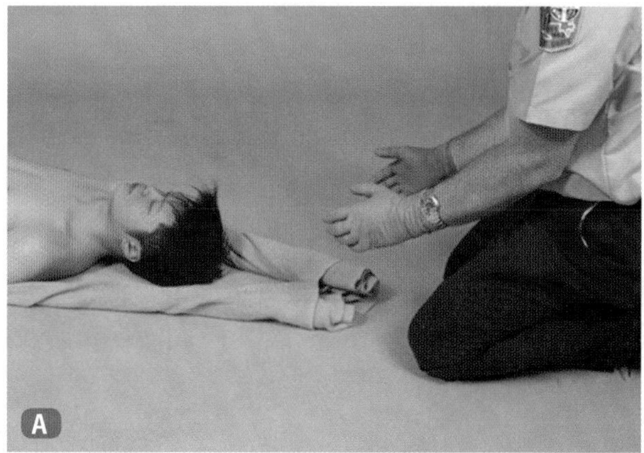

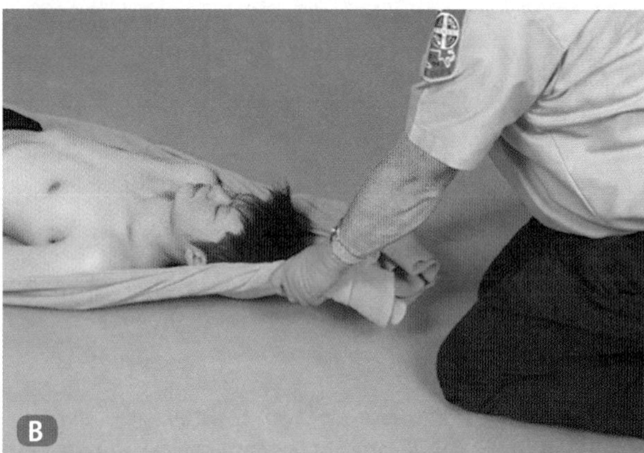

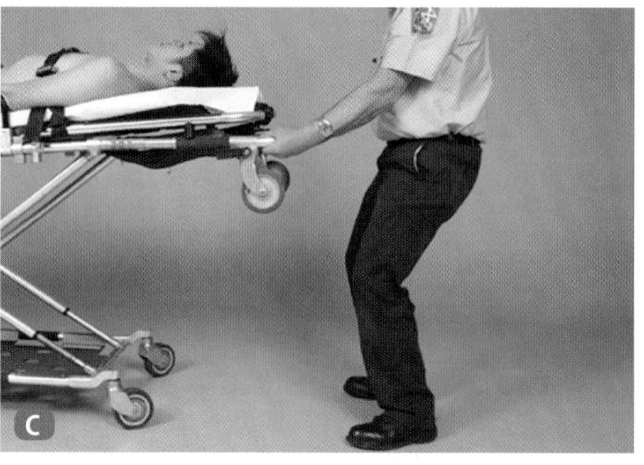

Figure 6-5 Reaching and pulling safely. **A.** Kneel to pull a patient who is on the ground. **B.** When pulling, your elbows should only extend just beyond the anterior torso. **C.** Bend your knees to pull a patient who is at a different height than you are. Position your feet or knees to balance the force of pull.

Words of Wisdom

It is acceptable to use a belt to assist in moving a patient; however, NEVER rely on belt loops or pockets to attach the belt to. They may rip or tear and result in injury to the patient or providers.

▶ Moving a Patient Across a Bed

If you must drag a patient across a bed, kneel on the bed to avoid reaching beyond the recommended distance. Follow the steps described previously until the patient is within 15 to 20 inches (38 to 50 cm) of the bed's edge. Complete the drag while standing at the side of the bed. Rather than dragging the patient by his or her clothing, use the sheet or blanket under the patient for this purpose. Roll the bedding under the patient until it is about 6 inches (15 cm) wider than the patient. Pull on the rolled bedding smoothly and evenly to glide the patient to the bedside. Watch out for soiled sheets. Wear proper protective equipment as needed.

Unless the patient is on a backboard, transfer the patient from the stretcher to a bed in the ED or the patient's

Skill Drill 6-2 Performing a Two-Person Body Drag

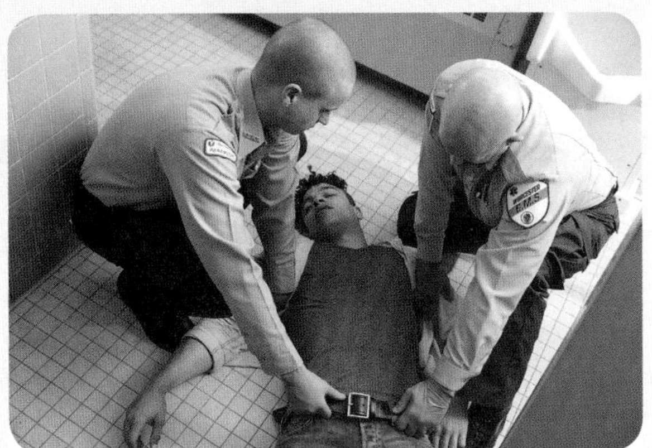

Step 1 Position yourself by kneeling on either side of the patient, just beyond the patient's shoulders, facing his or her groin. You and your lifting partner will each extend one arm across and in front of your chests and grasp the patient's armpit closest to you. With the other arm extended in front and to the side of the patient's torso, you and your partner will grasp the patient's clothing at the beltline.

Step 2 As a unit, raise your elbows and flex your arms to pull the patient lengthwise, as close to the floor as possible.

hospital room with a body drag. With the stretcher at the same height as the bed or slightly higher and held firmly against its side, you and another provider should kneel on the hospital bed and, in the manner previously described, drag the patient in increments until he or she is properly centered on the bed. When transferring the patient onto a narrow examining table, rather than kneel on the table, drag the patient while you stand against the opposite side. A third person may need to take both sides of the draw sheet at the head to move the patient safely.

▶ The Two-Person Body Drag

Sometimes during a body drag, you and another provider may have to pull the patient with one of you on each side of the patient. You will have to alter the usual pulling technique to prevent pulling sideways and producing adverse lateral leverage against your lower back. Follow the steps in Skill Drill 6-2 to perform a two-person body drag.

▶ Log Rolling a Patient

Generally, when log rolling a patient onto his or her side, you will initially have to reach farther than 18 inches (46 cm) Figure 6-6. To minimize this distance, kneel as close to the patient's side as possible, leaving only enough room so your knees will not prevent the patient from being rolled. When you lean forward, keep your back straight, and lean solely from the hips. Use your shoulder muscles to help with the roll. To minimize the amount of time you are extended like this and to support the patient's weight, roll the patient without stopping until the patient is resting on his or her side and braced against your thighs. During a log roll, some EMS experts recommend pulling rather than pushing the patient. This

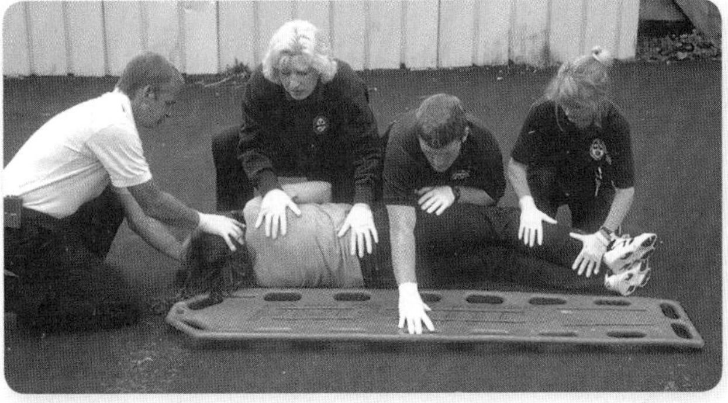

Figure 6-6 When placing a patient onto a backboard, log roll the patient onto his or her side. Kneel as close to the patient's side as possible, leaving only enough room so your knees will not prevent the patient from being rolled. Lean forward, keep your back straight and lean solely from the hips. Use your shoulder muscles to help with the roll.

gives you more control. Local protocols will guide your training in this area. Pulling toward you allows your legs to prevent the patient from rolling over completely and from rolling beyond the intended distance.

Rolling a Wheeled Ambulance Stretcher

The wheeled ambulance stretcher is the most commonly used device to move and transport patients. When you are rolling the wheeled ambulance stretcher, ensure it is in the fully elevated position. If you are guiding the stretcher from the foot end, hold your arms close to your body, and avoid reaching significantly behind you or hyperextending your back Figure 6-7. Your back should be locked, straight, and untwisted. While you are walking and pulling the stretcher, bend slightly forward at your hips. As you walk, your legs are pulled back with the feet on the ground, your pelvis is moved forward, and the movement of the pelvis is transferred to the stretcher through your straight torso and firmly held arms. Keep the line of the pull through the center of your body by bending your knees.

A second AEMT should guide the head end and assist you by pushing with his or her arms positioned so the elbows are bent and the hands are about 12 to 15 inches (30 to 38 cm) in front of the torso. To protect your elbows from injury, never push an object with your arms fully extended in a straight line and the elbows locked. When you push with the elbow bent but firmly held from bending further, the strong muscles of the arm serve as a shock absorber if the wheels or foot end of the stretcher strikes an obstacle that causes its progress to be suddenly slowed or stopped. Push from the area of your body that is between the waist and shoulder. If the weight you are pushing is lower than your waist, push from a kneeling position, and move forward little by little as needed to stay close to the patient. Do not push or pull from an overhead position.

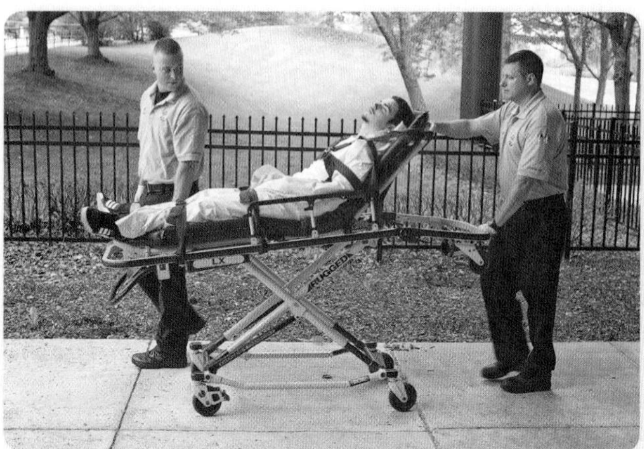

Figure 6-7 Push the stretcher from the head end. If you are guiding the stretcher from the foot end, hold your arms close to your body, and avoid reaching significantly behind you or hyperextending your back. Your back should be locked, straight, and untwisted.

Words of Wisdom

It is far safer to push the stretcher from the ends than to move it sideways. Avoid moving a stretcher sideways if possible.

Lifting and Carrying a Patient on a Backboard or Stretcher

Whenever possible, use a device that can be rolled to move a patient. When moving a wheeled stretcher, pull the foot end of the stretcher while your partner guides it from the head end.

If a wheeled device is not available, make sure you understand and follow certain guidelines for carrying a patient on a stretcher. Table 6-1 shows the guidelines.

When a stretcher must be carried, it is best if four providers are available to carry it. There is more stability with a four-person carry, and the carry requires less strength. One AEMT should be positioned at each corner of the stretcher to provide an even lift. A four-person carry is much safer if the stretcher must be moved over rough ground. If only two AEMTs are available, or if limited space will allow room for only two AEMTs to carry the stretcher, there is a risk that the stretcher will become unbalanced. In a two-person carry, the two AEMTs should stand facing each other, with one person at the head end of the stretcher and the other at the foot end. With this type of carry, one AEMT will have to walk backward.

If a patient is supine on a backboard or is lying or in a semi-Fowler position on the stretcher, his or her weight is not equally distributed between the two ends of the device. Between 68% and 78% of the body weight of a patient in a horizontal position is in the torso. Therefore, more of the patient's weight rests on the head half of the device than on the foot half. It is important that you and your team use the correct lifting techniques to lift the stretcher. If possible, all team members should be of the same approximate height and strength.

Weight and Distribution

You should estimate how much the patient weighs before attempting to lift him or her. Commonly, adult patients weigh between 120 and 220 pounds (54 and 100 kg). If you use the correct technique, you and one other AEMT should be able to safely lift this weight. Depending on your individual strength, you and another provider may be able to safely lift an even heavier patient. However, because it is safer to have four providers lift, use four providers whenever the available resources allow. You should know how much you can comfortably and safely lift and should not attempt to lift a proportional weight (the share of the weight that you will bear) that exceeds this weight. If lifting the patient places a strain on you, call for the lifting

Table 6-1 Guidelines for Carrying a Patient on a Stretcher

Estimate the weight of both the patient and the associated equipment to be lifted and gauge the limitations of your team's abilities.
Coordinate your movements with those of the other team members while constantly communicating with them.
Do not twist your body as you are carrying the patient.
Keep the weight that you are carrying as close to your body as possible while keeping your back in a locked-in position.
Do not bend at the waist; this could hyperextend your back. Instead, flex at the hips, and bend at the knees.

to be stopped and the patient to be lowered. Then obtain additional help before again attempting to lift the patient. Communicate clearly and frequently with your partner and other providers whenever you are lifting a patient.

Do not attempt to lift a patient who weighs more than 250 pounds (114 kg) with fewer than four providers, regardless of your strength. Protocols should include a method to rapidly summon additional help to lift and carry a patient of such weight or, as in the case of a cardiac arrest, provide and maintain the necessary care in the field and when moving and transporting the patient. In addition, you must know, or be able to find out, the weight limitations of the equipment you are using and how to handle patients who exceed the weight limitations. Special bariatric techniques, equipment, and resources are generally required to move any patient who weighs more than 350 pounds (159 kg) to the ambulance. These resources should be summoned when you arrive on scene and have assessed the situation.

As discussed, more than one-half of a patient's weight is distributed to the head end of the backboard or stretcher. Therefore, the strongest of the available AEMTs should be located at the head end of the device. Even with four or more AEMTs carrying a patient, the strain on the AEMT carrying the head end of the device will be increased when you must negotiate a narrow area or flight of stairs.

In carrying a patient up a flight of stairs, however, proportionally greater weight will be distributed to the AEMT who is carrying the foot end when the backboard or stretcher becomes angled on the incline. You should anticipate this and, in such cases, ensure the two strongest AEMTs are positioned at the head end and foot end of the device. Because of the incline of the stairway, if one AEMT is considerably taller than the other, it will be easier if the shorter one is at the head end and the taller one is at the foot end.

The dynamics that are involved in carrying a patient down a flight of stairs or for any significant distance will not allow you to carry as much proportional weight to safely lift or support the patient during a move onto a nearby backboard or stretcher. Therefore, if you believe you are approaching your maximum lifting capacity as you are moving the patient onto a backboard or stretcher, do not attempt to lift and carry the patient for any significant distance or down a flight of stairs. Make another attempt to lift and carry the patient after you have decreased the amount of proportional weight you will be carrying by changing your position on the device or the position of the others on the team, or after you have obtained additional help.

Safety Tips

Know your limits! Always call for assistance as soon as you realize the patient's weight exceeds your lifting capabilities.

▶ Planning the Move

Move a patient in an orderly, planned, directed, and unhurried manner. This approach will protect you and the patient from further injury and reduce the risk of worsening the patient's condition when he or she is moved.

At a minimum, on most calls you will have to lift and carry the patient to the wheeled ambulance stretcher, move the stretcher and patient to the ambulance, load and unload the stretcher from the patient compartment, and move the patient from the ambulance to the ED bed. You will often have to include several additional steps to place the patient onto a backboard and/or carry him or her down a flight of stairs. You will also have to add a stop at the top of the stairway so everyone can reposition to carry the patient down the stairs. Repositioning usually requires lowering the backboard to the ground and lifting it again when all providers are in their proper places. If you are carrying the patient in a stair chair, the additional step occurs after you have descended the stairs and reached the stretcher. At that point, you will have to assist or lift the patient from the stair chair onto the stretcher.

Plan ahead and carefully select the methods that will involve the least lifting and carrying. Always consider whether there is an option that will cause less strain to you and the other providers.

In addition, it is the responsibility of every team member to share with the leader any issue that may result in injury to anyone involved in the move.

Safety Tips

Follow these rules to keep yourself and your patient safe:

- Minimize the number of total body lifts you have to perform.
- Coordinate every lift in advance.
- Minimize the total amount of weight you have to lift.
- *Never* lift with your back.
- Do not carry what you can put on wheels.
- Ask for help any time.

▶ The Diamond Carry

A patient on a backboard or stretcher can be lifted and carried by four providers in a **diamond carry**, with one provider at the head end of the device, one at the foot end, and one at each side of the patient's torso. Follow the steps in Skill Drill 6-3 to perform the diamond carry.

If you must carry a patient through a narrow doorway or hallway using a diamond carry, modify your positions Figure 6-8A. Simply stop and have all the providers turn until each is again facing in toward the patient. Then, take small, slow steps to move through the doorway. If the doorway is still too narrow for the AEMTs at the sides of the backboard to fit through, one provider may need to let go of the backboard and move through the doorway first. The remaining three providers can carry the backboard but may need to alter their positions before the fourth provider lets go, to properly balance the weight among three providers Figure 6-8B. The fourth provider then steadies and guides the first AEMT as he or she moves through the passage.

A patient on a backboard or stretcher should be carried feet first to place the lightest load on the provider at the patient's feet, who, to walk forward, must turn and grasp the handles with his or her back to the device. Carrying the patient feet first allows a conscious patient to see in the direction of movement.

▶ The One-Handed Carrying Technique

One method of lifting and carrying a patient on a backboard is the one-handed carrying technique. With this method, four or more providers each use one hand to support the backboard so they are able to face forward as they are walking. To perform the one-handed carrying technique, follow the steps in Skill Drill 6-4.

Pick up and carry the backboard with your back in the locked-in position. If you need to lean to either side

Skill Drill 6-3 Performing the Diamond Carry

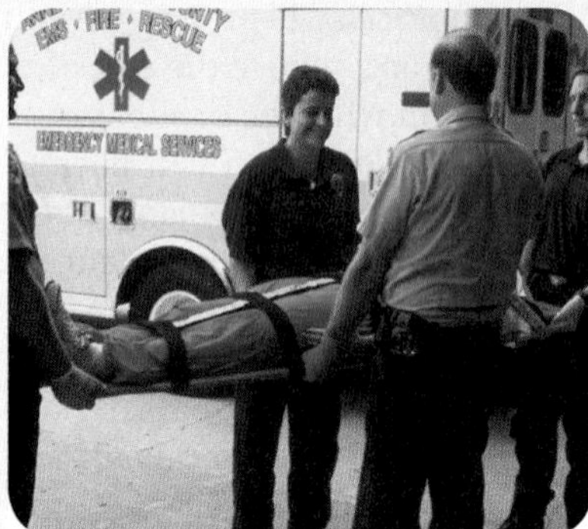

Step 1 To best balance the weight, four providers should be positioned at each side and end while facing the patient. Providers grasp the backboard or stretcher with one hand adjacent to the distal edge of the patient's pelvis and the other midthorax. When the command is given, all four providers lift the device while facing toward the patient.

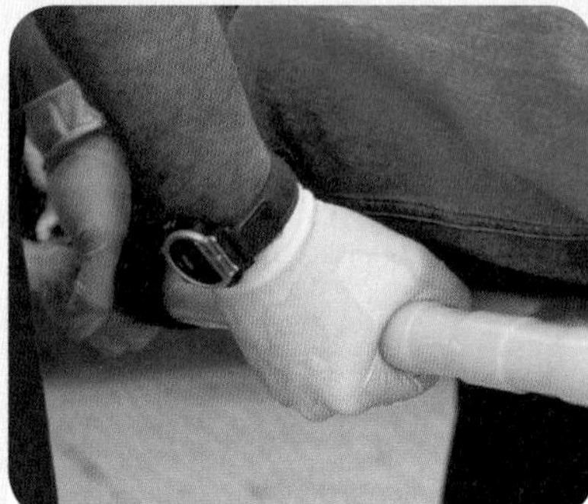

Step 2 The provider at each side grasps the backboard or stretcher with the head-end hand.

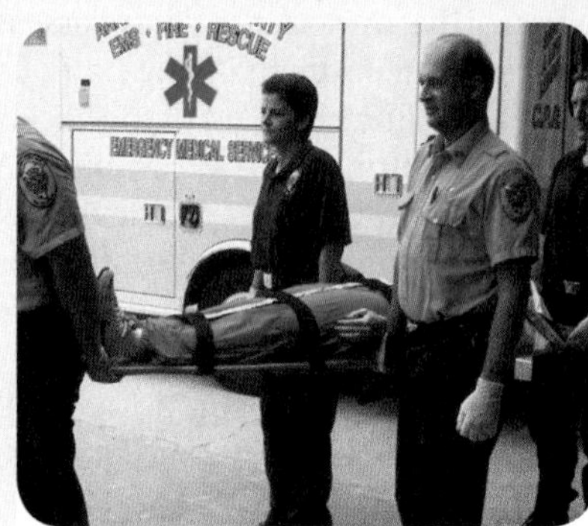

Step 3 The providers at each side turn toward the patient's feet. The provider at the foot end turns to face forward. All four providers face the same direction and walk forward when carrying the patient.

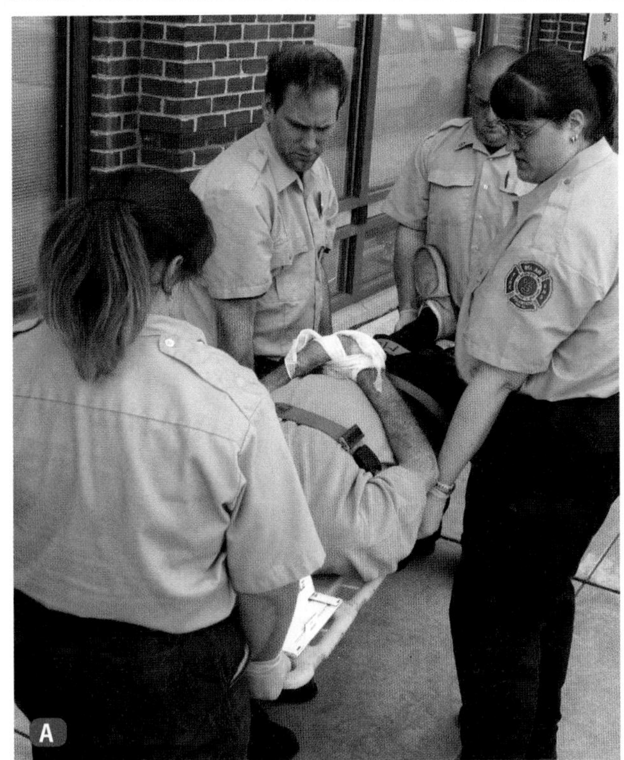

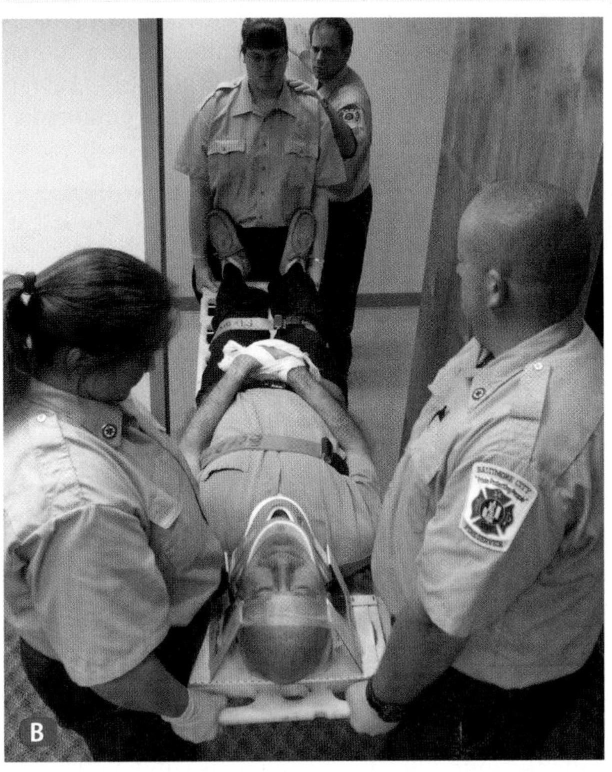

Figure 6-8 Options for moving a patient through a narrow doorway or hallway while performing the diamond carry. **A.** Stop and turn in to face the patient until you move through the passage. **B.** If the doorway or hallway is very narrow, a provider on one side may move to the foot end and out of the way, and then steady and guide the other providers through the passage.

Skill Drill 6-4 Performing the One-Handed Carry

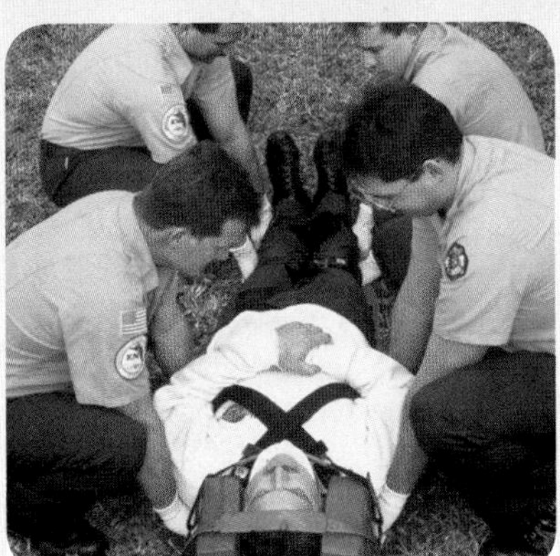

Step 1 Before lifting the backboard, ensure at least two providers are positioned on each side of the backboard facing each other and using both hands.

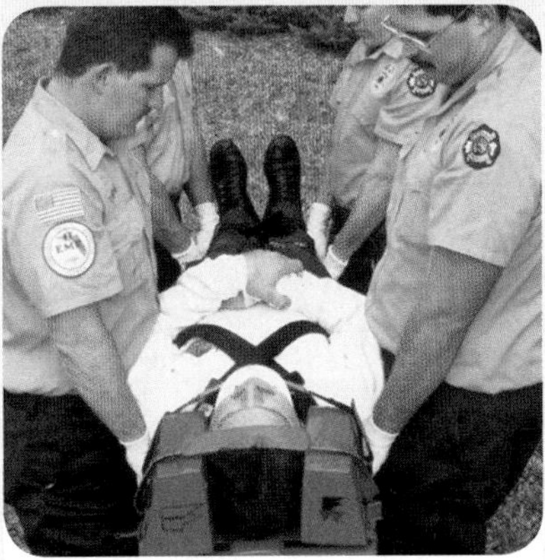

Step 2 Lift the backboard to carrying height using correct lifting techniques, including a locked-in back.

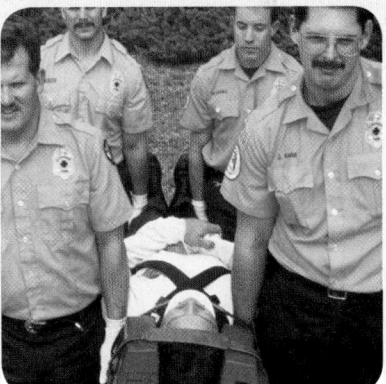

Step 3 After you lifted the backboard to a carrying height, you and your partners turn in the direction you will be walking and switch to using one hand.

to compensate for a weight imbalance, you have probably exceeded your weight limitation. If this occurs, you may need additional assistance or you may need to reevaluate the carry; otherwise you or others might be injured or drop the patient.

Emergency Moves

When there is a potential for danger, use an **emergency move** to move a patient before assessment and care are provided. The presence of fire, explosives, or hazardous materials and your inability to protect the patient from other hazards or gain access to others in a vehicle who need life-saving care are all situations in which you should use an emergency move.

The only other time you should use an emergency move is if you cannot properly assess the patient or provide immediate potentially critical emergency medical care (for example, a patient in cardiac arrest) because of the patient's location or position.

If you are alone and danger at the scene makes it necessary for you to use an emergency move, regardless of a patient's injuries, use a drag to pull the patient along the long axis of the body. This will help to keep the spinal column in line as much as possible. When performing an emergency move, one of your primary concerns is the danger of aggravating an existing spinal injury. Remember, it is impossible to remove a patient quickly from a vehicle while providing as much protection to the spine as you would give by using an immobilization device. However, if you follow certain guidelines during the move, you can usually move a patient from a life-threatening situation without causing further injury to the patient.

You can move a patient on his or her back along the floor or ground by using one of the following methods.

- Pull on the patient's clothing in the neck and shoulder area Figure 6-9A. If the shirt has buttons, the top two should be undone to prevent choking the patient.
- If possible, place the patient onto a blanket, coat, or other item that can be pulled Figure 6-9B.
- Rotate the patient's arms so they are extended straight on the ground beyond his or her head, grasp the wrists, and, with the arms elevated above the ground, drag the patient Figure 6-9C.
- Place your arms under the patient's shoulders and through the armpits, and, while grasping the patient's arms, drag the patient backward Figure 6-9D.

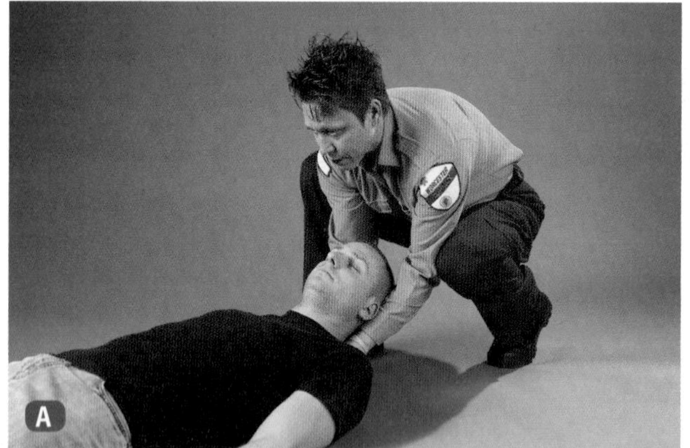

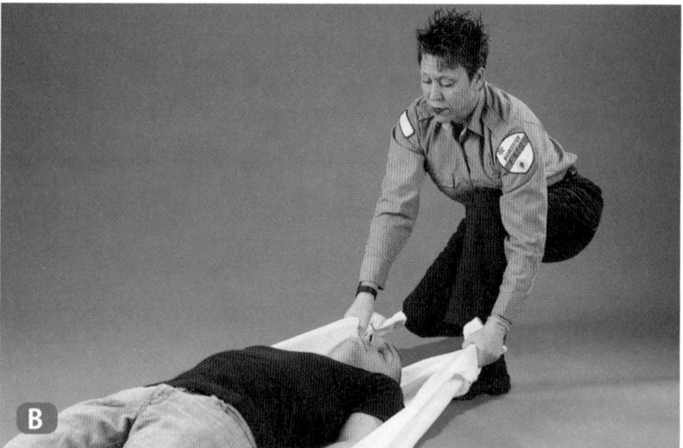

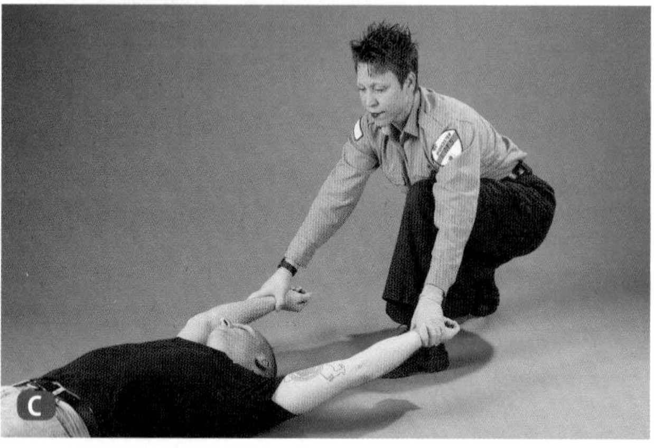

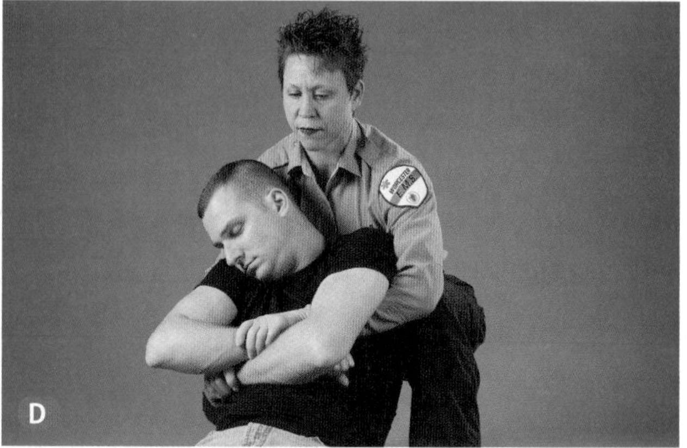

Figure 6-9 Dragging methods. **A.** Emergency clothes drag. **B.** Blanket drag. **C.** Arm drag. **D.** Arm-to-arm drag.

Skill Drill 6-5 One-Person Technique for Removing an Unresponsive Patient From a Vehicle

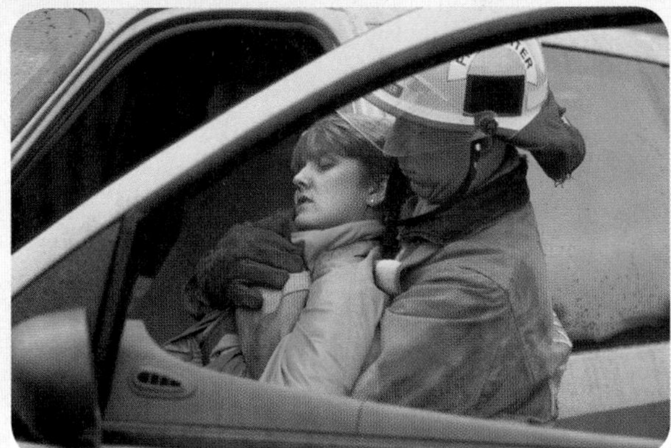

Step 1 Move the patient's legs against the seat so they are clear of the gas and brake pedals. Rotate the patient so his or her back is positioned facing the open vehicle door. Place your arms through the patient's armpits and support the patient's head against your body.

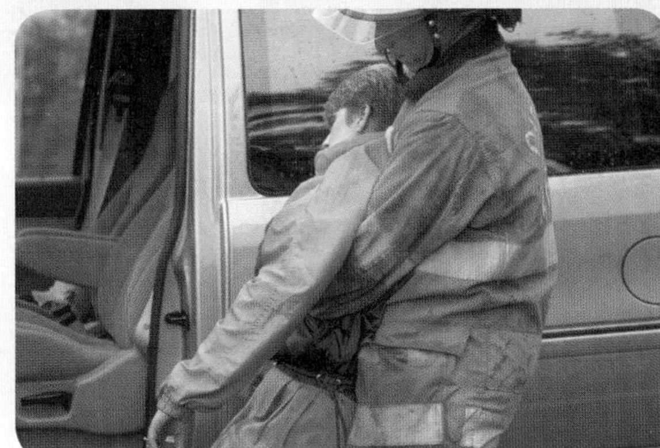

Step 2 Support the patient's weight while lowering the patient down into a supine position.

If you are alone and must remove an unresponsive patient from a vehicle, follow the steps in Skill Drill 6-5.

If the legs and feet do not clear the vehicle easily, slowly lower the patient until he or she is lying on his or her back next to the vehicle, clear the legs from the vehicle, and, as previously described, use a long-axis body drag to move the patient a safe distance from the vehicle.

Use one-person techniques to move a patient only if a potentially life-threatening danger exists and you are alone or, because of the pressing nature of the danger, your partner is moving a second patient simultaneously. Additional one person drags, carries, and lifts are shown in Figure 6-10.

Urgent Moves

An urgent move is necessary when a patient requires immediate life-saving care, yet is in an unsafe environment. For example, an urgent move may be necessary for moving a patient with an altered level of consciousness, inadequate ventilation, or shock (hypoperfusion) but the needed care cannot be rendered where the patient is currently located. An extreme weather condition may also make an urgent move necessary. In some cases, patients must be urgently moved from the location or position in which they are found. When you need to urgently move a patient who is sitting in a car or truck, use the rapid extrication technique.

▶ Rapid Extrication Technique

The backboard, short backboard, and vest-type devices are known as spinal immobilization devices. You usually use an extrication-type vest or short backboard device to immobilize a seated patient with a suspected spinal injury before removing the patient from the vehicle (see Chapter 40, *Vehicle Extrication, Special Rescue, and Hazardous Materials*). However, proper placement of either of these devices on the patient usually requires between 6 and 8 minutes, and in some cases even longer. By using the **rapid extrication technique** instead, the patient can be moved from sitting in the vehicle to lying supine on a backboard in 1 minute or less. Table 6-2 describes the situations in which you should use the rapid extrication technique.

In such cases, the delay that occurs in applying immobilization devices is contraindicated. However, the manual support and immobilization that you provide when using the rapid extrication technique produce a greater risk of spine movement. You should use the rapid extrication technique only if extreme urgency exists.

The rapid extrication technique requires a team of three providers who are knowledgeable and practiced in the procedure. The first provider is usually positioned in the backseat and applies in-line support and stabilization of the patient's head and neck. At some point, either because the doorpost is in the way or because he or she cannot reach farther from the backseat, the first provider

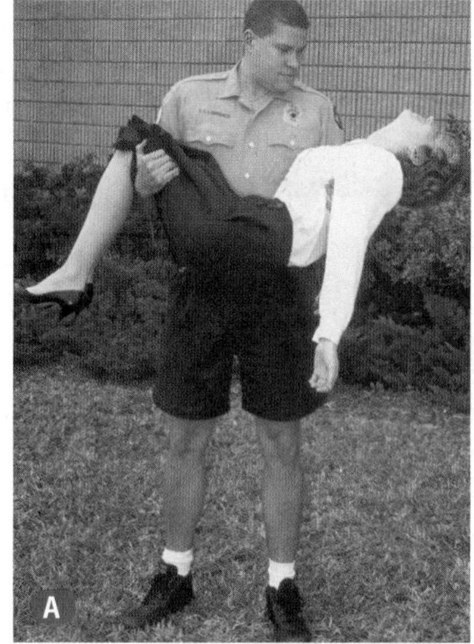

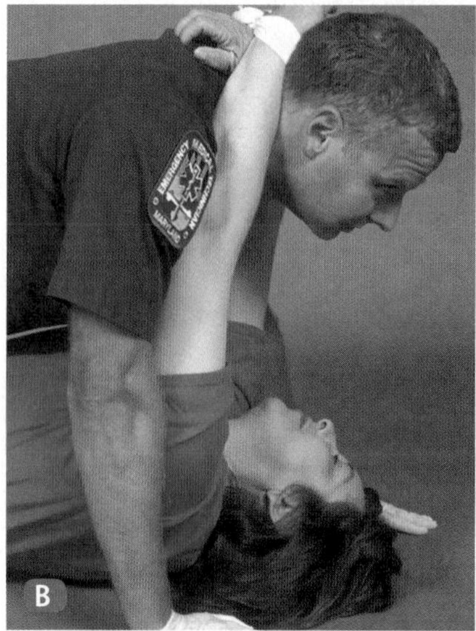

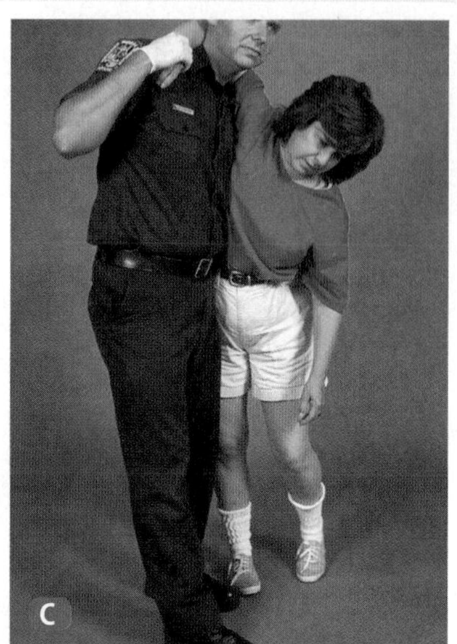

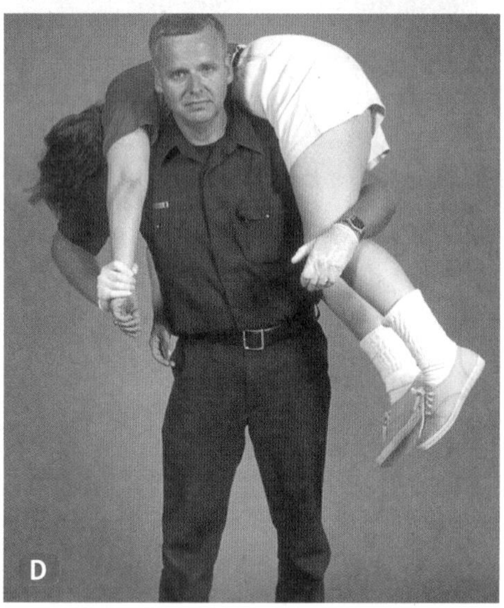

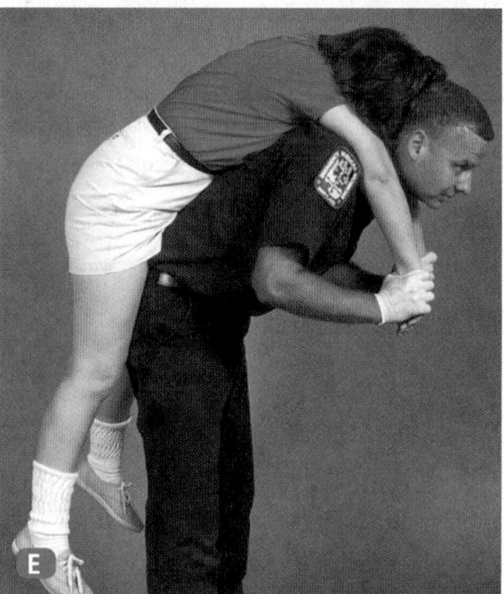

Figure 6-10 One-person drags, carries, and lifts. **A.** Front cradle. **B.** Firefighter's drag. **C.** One-person walking assist. **D.** Firefighter's carry. **E.** Pack-strap carry.

Table 6-2 Situations in Which to Use the Rapid Extrication Technique
The vehicle or scene is unsafe.
Explosives or other hazardous materials are on the scene.
There is a fire or a danger of fire.
The patient cannot be assessed properly before being removed from the vehicle.
The patient needs immediate intervention that requires a supine position.
The patient has a life-threatening condition that requires rapid transport to the hospital.
The patient is hemodynamically unstable.
The patient blocks your access to another seriously injured patient.

will be unable to follow the torso rotation. At that time, the third (or even a fourth) provider assumes temporary in-line support of the head and neck. The provider at the patient's head always calls the moves. The second provider gives orders and supports the torso. Because the second provider lifts and turns the patient's torso, he or she must be physically capable of moving the patient. The third provider moves and supports the patient's legs. Take the steps shown in Skill Drill 6-6 when using the rapid extrication technique.

Skill Drill 6-6 Performing the Rapid Extrication Technique

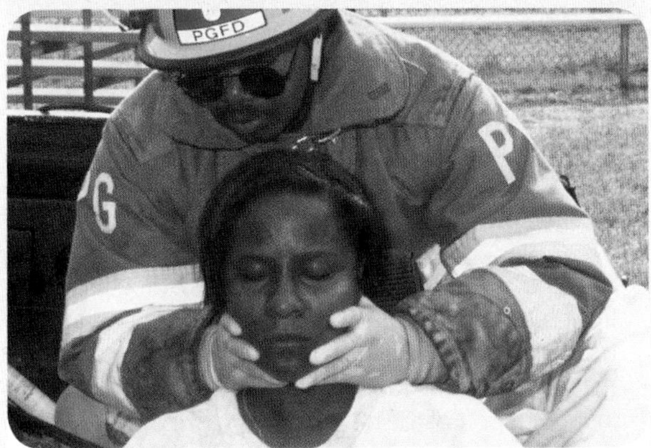

Step 1 The first provider applies manual in-line support of the patient's head and cervical spine from behind the patient, usually from the backseat. Support may be applied from the side, if necessary, by reaching through the driver's side doorway.

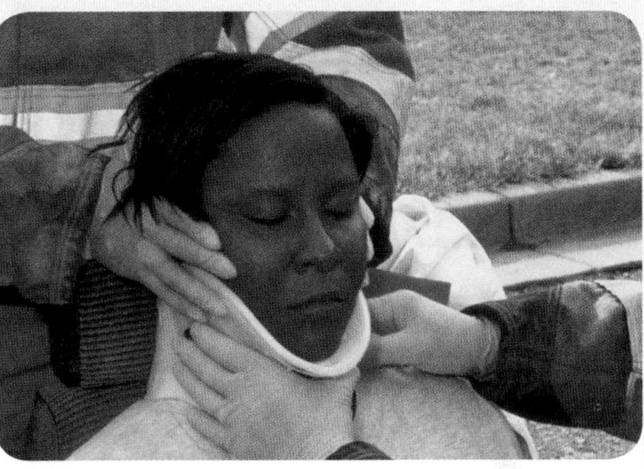

Step 2 The provider holding in-line stabilization gives commands, applies a cervical collar, and performs the primary survey from the driver's side doorway. If the first provider is also working from that doorway, the second provider should stand closer to the door hinges toward the front of the vehicle.

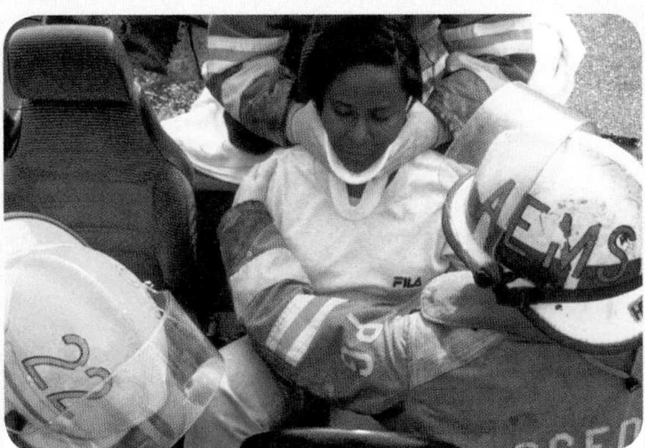

Step 3 The second provider provides continuous support of the patient's torso until the patient is supine on the backboard. The third provider works from the front passenger's seat and frees the patient's legs from the gas and brake pedals and moves the legs together, without moving the pelvis or spine. After the third provider moves the legs together, the legs should be moved as a unit.

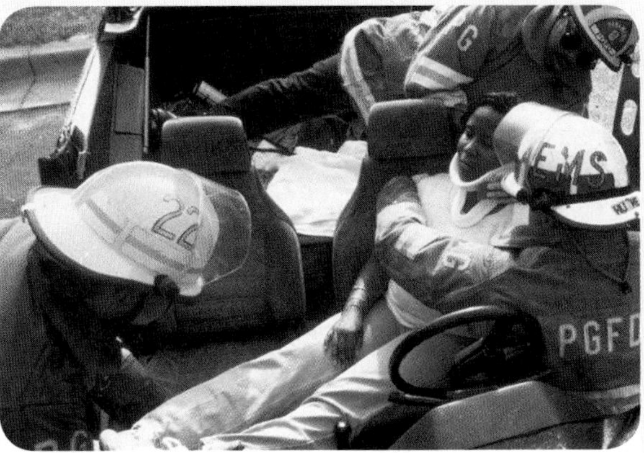

Step 4 The second provider and the third provider rotate the patient as a unit in three or four short, quick "eighth turns" until the patient's back is facing out the driver's door and the legs are on the front passenger's seat. The first provider directs each quick turn by saying, "Ready, turn" or "Ready, move." Make hand position changes between moves. The first provider (relieved by the fourth provider or a bystander as needed) supports the patient's head and neck during rotation (and later steps).

(continued)

Skill Drill 6-6 Performing the Rapid Extrication Technique *(continued)*

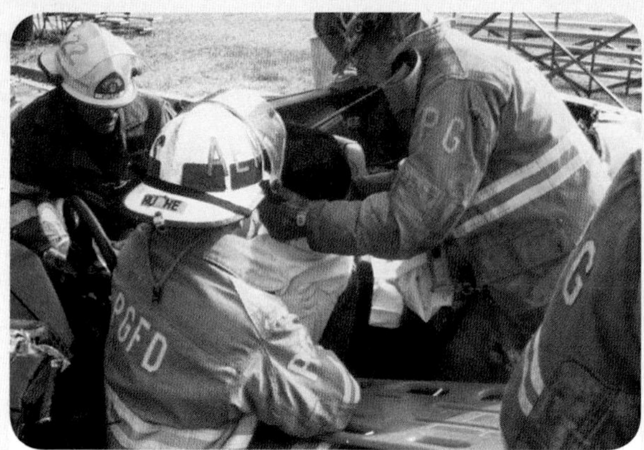

Step 5 Once the patient has been rotated fully, place the backboard on the seat against the patient's buttocks. The second provider and the third provider lower the patient onto the board while supporting the head and torso to maintain neutral alignment. The first provider holds the backboard until the patient is secured. (Use of a backboard may depend on local protocols.)

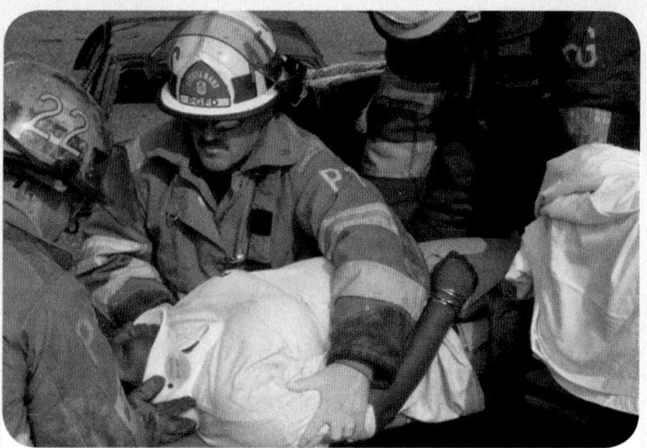

Step 6 The third provider moves across the front seat to be in position at the patient's hips. The backboard should be immediately in front of the third provider. The fourth provider maintains manual in-line support of the head and now takes over giving the commands. If a fourth provider is not present, direct a volunteer to assist you. The second provider maintains the direction of the extrication and stands with his or her back to the door, facing the rear of the vehicle. The second provider grasps the patient's shoulders or armpits. On command, the second provider and third provider slide the patient along the backboard in 8- to 12-inch (20- to 30-cm) moves, repeating this slide until the patient's hips are firmly on the backboard.

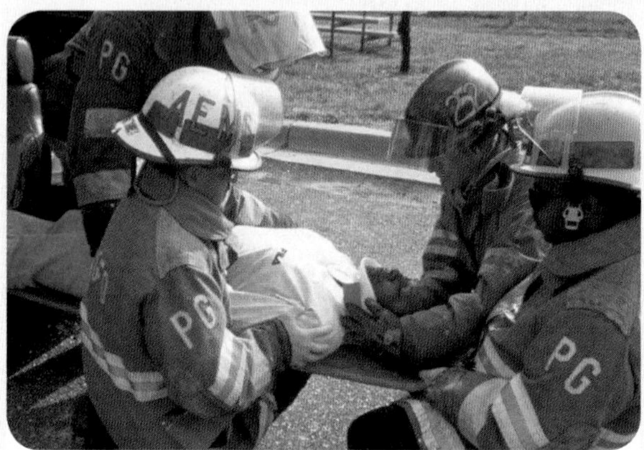

Step 7 The third provider exits the vehicle and moves to the opposite side of the backboard opposite the second provider. On command, they continue to slide the patient along the backboard in 8- to 12-inch (20- to 30-cm) slides until the patient is placed fully on the backboard.

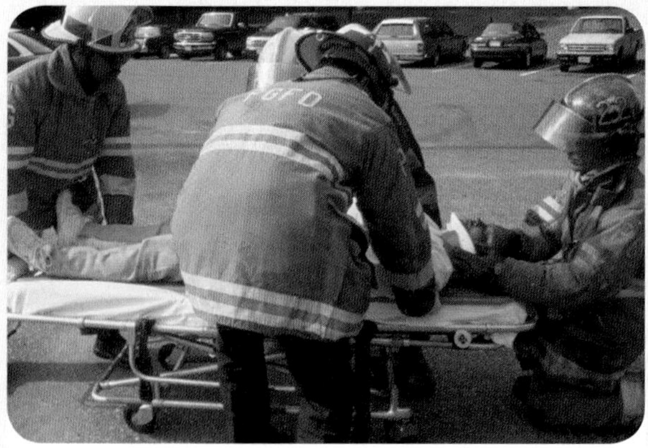

Step 8 The first (or fourth) provider continues to stabilize the patient's head and neck while the second provider and the third provider carry the patient away from the vehicle and onto the prepared stretcher.

In some cases, you can rest the head end of the backboard on the stretcher while the patient is moved onto the backboard. In other cases, you will not be able to do this. Once the backboard and patient have been placed on the stretcher, you should begin life-saving treatment immediately. If you used the rapid extrication technique because the scene was dangerous, you and your team should immediately move the stretcher a safe distance away from the vehicle before you assess or treat the patient.

Words of Wisdom

The person holding the cervical spine always calls the move.

The steps of the rapid extrication technique must be considered a general procedure to be adapted as needed. For example, two-door vehicles differ from four-door models. Larger vehicles differ from smaller compact models, pickup trucks, and full-size sedans and four-wheel-drive vehicles. You will handle a large, heavy adult differently from a small adult or child. Every situation will be different—a different vehicle, a different patient, and a different crew. Your resourcefulness and ability to adapt are necessary elements to successfully perform the rapid extrication technique.

Nonurgent Moves

When the scene is stable and the patient is in stable condition, carefully plan how to move the patient. If your patient move is rushed or not well planned, it may result in discomfort or injury to the patient, you, and your team. Before you attempt any move, the team leader must ensure there are enough personnel, identify and remove any obstacles, ensure the proper equipment is available, and clearly identify and discuss the procedure and path to be followed. In addition, remember, it is every team member's responsibility to share with the leader any issue that may result in injury to anyone involved in the move.

In nonurgent situations, you and your team may choose one of several methods for lifting and carrying a patient. Three general methods are presented here, which may serve as a basis for your plan. Adapt these procedures to meet your needs on a case-by-case basis.

Direct Ground Lift

The **direct ground lift** is used for patients with no suspected spinal injury who are found lying supine on the ground. Use this lift technique when you have to lift and carry the patient some distance to be placed on the stretcher. If you find the patient semiprone or lying on his or her side, roll the patient onto his or her back. Ideally, the direct ground lift should be performed by three providers; however, it can be done with only two. To perform the direct ground lift, follow the steps in Skill Drill 6-7. Reverse the steps to lower the patient onto the stretcher.

YOU are the Provider PART 3

As you form your plan for moving the patient, your partner obtains vital signs and the engine crew positions the bariatric stretcher. You tell the patient and your crew that the safest way to get him onto the stretcher is to roll him onto his side and hold him in position long enough to position a draw sheet underneath him. He reminds you to be careful with his sore back and bottom. After everyone voices understanding of the plan, you are able to get the patient onto the draw sheet and move to the stretcher where he is secured for transport.

Recording Time: 8 Minutes	
Respirations	18 breaths/min; clear
Pulse	102 beats/min
Skin	Warm, dry, and pink
Blood pressure	146/88 mm Hg
Oxygen saturation (Spo_2)	97% on room air
Pupils	Pupils Equal, Round, and Reactive to Light and Accommodation (PERRLA)

6. Why is it important to have only one person issuing commands when moving patients?
7. What are some advantages and disadvantages of a hydraulic stretcher?

Skill Drill 6-7 The Direct Ground Lift

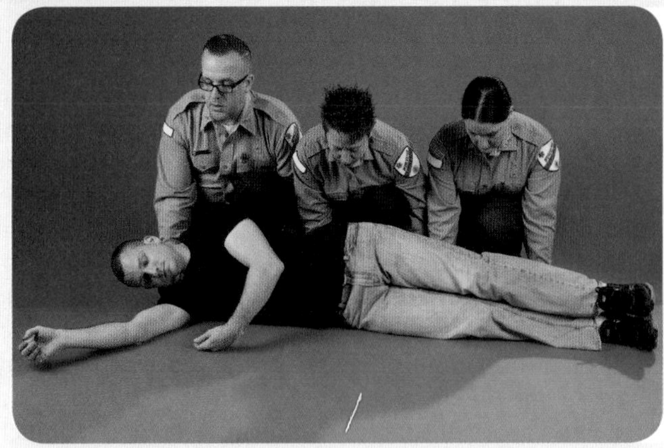

Step 1 Line up on one side of the patient, with the first provider at the head, the second provider at the waist, and the third provider at the patient's knees. All providers kneel on one knee, preferably the same knee. Place the patient's arms on his or her chest, if possible. The first provider places one arm under the patient's neck and shoulders and cradles the patient's head. The first provider then places the other arm under the patient's lower back. The second provider places one hand under the patient's waist, and the other under the knees. The third provider places one arm under the patient's knees and the other under the ankles.

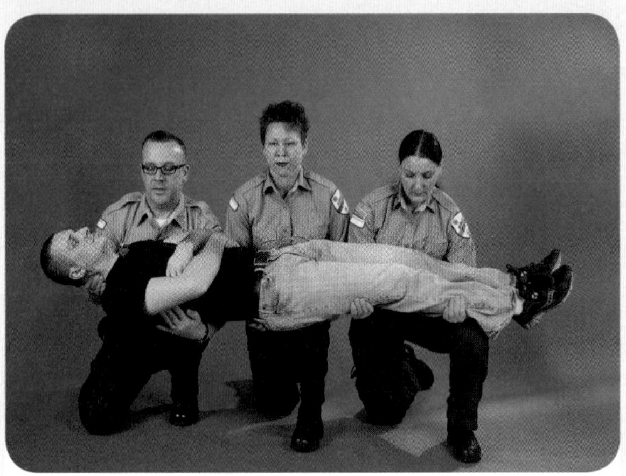

Step 2 On command, the providers lift up the patient to knee level as each provider rests an arm on his or her knee.

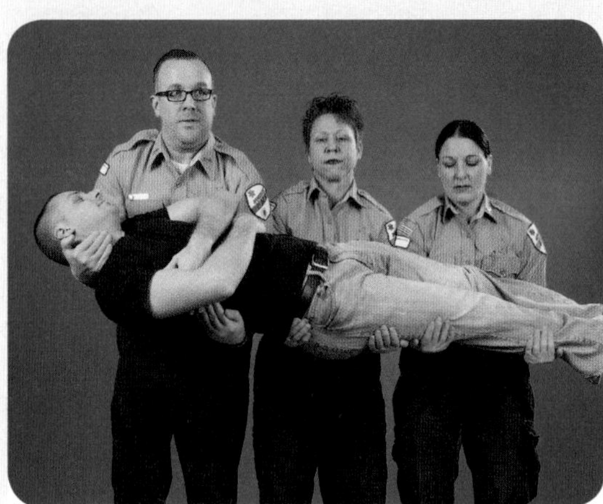

Step 3 Together and on command, each provider rolls the patient in toward his or her chest. Again on command, providers stand and carry the patient to the stretcher.

▶ Extremity Lift

The **extremity lift** may also be used for patients with no suspected extremity or spinal injuries who are supine or in a sitting position on the ground. The extremity lift may be especially helpful when the patient is in a very narrow space or there is not enough room for the patient and a team of AEMTs to stand side by side.

Communication is the key to success with this lift. You and your partner must coordinate your movements through direct verbal commands. Perform the extremity lift as seen in Skill Drill 6-8.

You are less likely to injure yourself if you bend at the hips and knees and use your legs for lifting. However, this lift and carry method increases the pressure on the patient's chest, so the patient may be uncomfortable in this position.

▶ Transfer Moves

There are several ways to transfer the patient from a bed onto the stretcher.

Direct Carry

Transfer a supine patient from a bed to the stretcher using the **direct carry method** Skill Drill 6-9.

Draw Sheet Method

To move the patient from a bed onto a stretcher, use the draw sheet method. Follow the steps in Skill Drill 6-10.

To avoid the strain of unnecessary lifting and carrying, you should use the draw sheet method to move an unable patient whenever possible. This method is not only easier on providers, but also easier on the patient. For example,

Skill Drill 6-8 Extremity Lift

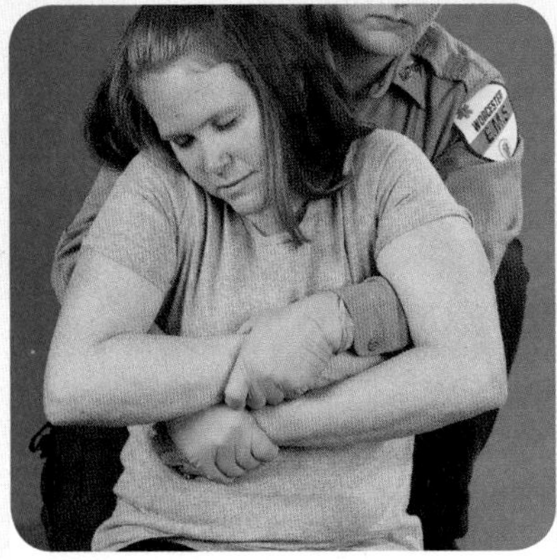

Step 1 Kneel behind the patient's head as your partner kneels at the patient's feet. The patient's hands should be crossed over his or her chest. Place one hand under each of the patient's armpits. Grasp the patient's wrists or forearms and pull the upper torso until the patient is in a sitting position.

Step 2 Your partner moves to a position between the patient's legs, faces the same direction as the patient, and slips his or her hands under the patient's knees.

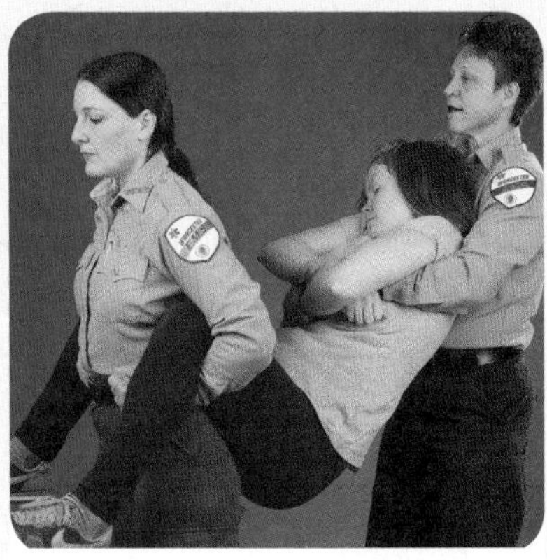

Step 3 Rise to a crouching position. As you give the command, stand fully upright and move the patient to the stretcher.

Skill Drill 6-9 Direct Carry

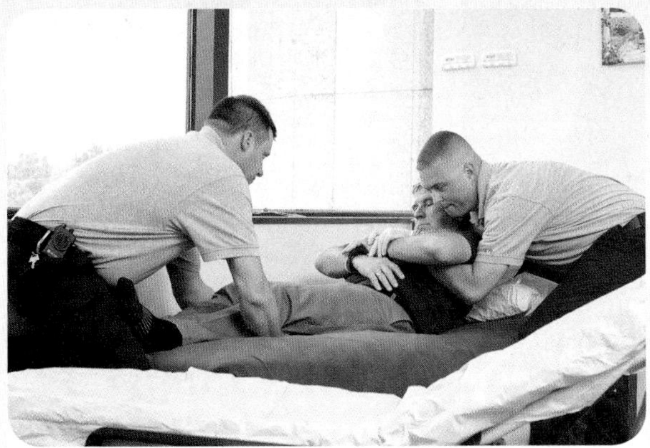

Step 1 Position the stretcher parallel to the bed. Secure the stretcher to prevent movement. Position yourself at the head end of the bed facing toward the patient. Your partner positions himself or herself between the bed and the stretcher and faces you and the patient. Place your arms under the patient's armpits. Your partner positions his or her hands under the patient's knees.

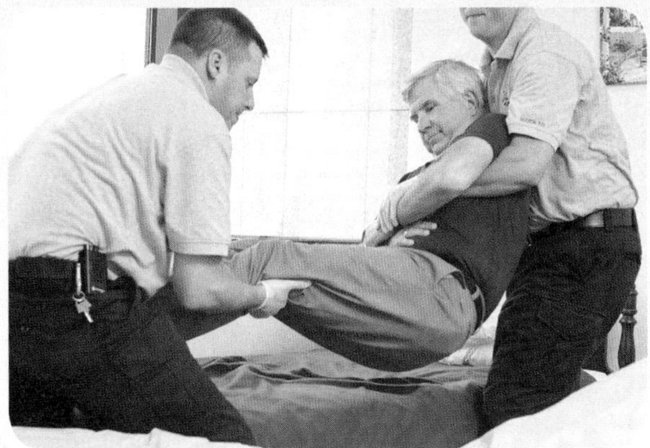

Step 2 Slowly and smoothly lift the patient in a smooth, coordinated fashion.

(continued)

Skill Drill 6-9 Direct Carry *(continued)*

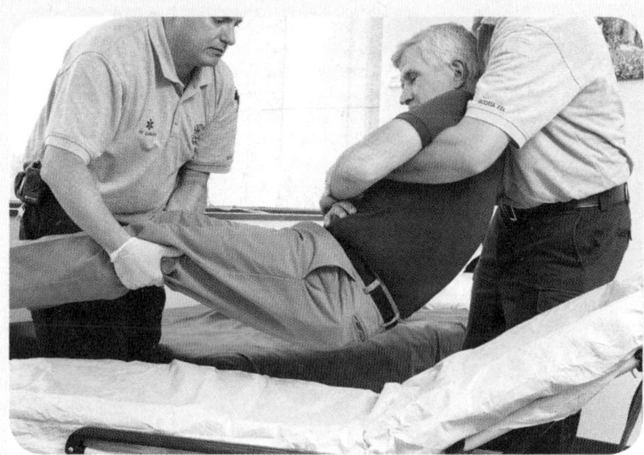

Step 3 Slowly carry the patient from the bed to the stretcher.

Step 4 Gently lower the patient onto the stretcher and secure with straps.

Skill Drill 6-10 Draw Sheet Method

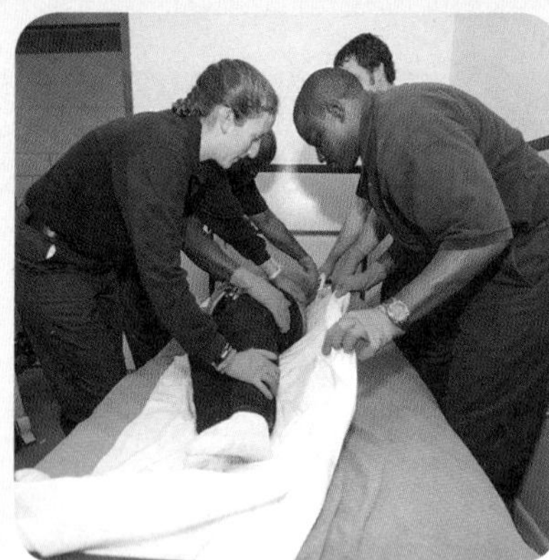

Step 1 Loosen the bottom sheet under the patient, or log roll the patient onto a blanket.

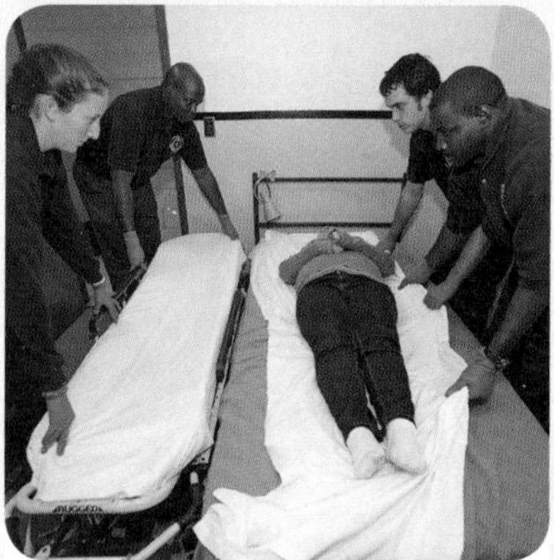

Step 2 Place the stretcher next to the bed, ensure it is at the same height, or slightly lower than the bed. Hold or secure the stretcher to keep it from moving. Reach across the stretcher, and grasp the sheet or blanket firmly at the patient's head, chest, hips, and knees.

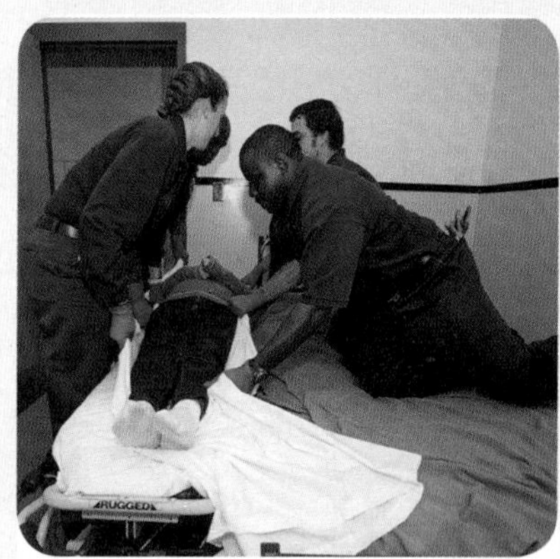

Step 3 Gently slide the patient onto the stretcher.

if you try to help a heavy person to his or her feet, you could injure your shoulder or bruise the patient. In older patients, you could cause a skin tear because their skin is more fragile. The draw sheet method is less likely to cause these problems.

Other Carries

Other carries are performed in the following manner:

- Place a backboard next to the patient, and, after using a log roll or slide to move the patient onto the backboard, secure the patient and lift and carry the backboard to the nearby prepared stretcher.
- Insert the halves of a scoop stretcher under each side of the patient, and fasten the two sides together. Lift and carry the patient to the nearby prepared stretcher. (Note: You can also log roll a patient onto a scoop stretcher that is already locked together.)
- Assist an able patient to the edge of the bed. Place the patient's legs over the side and help the patient to sit up. Move the stretcher so its foot end touches the bed near the patient. Help the patient to stand and rotate so he or she can sit down on the center of the stretcher. Lift the patient's legs, and rotate them onto the stretcher while your partner lowers the patient's torso onto the stretcher.

If a patient is able, you should always assist him or her to the stretcher to avoid the strain of unnecessary lifting and carrying.

Follow the steps in Skill Drill 6-11 to use a scoop stretcher.

Skill Drill 6-11 Using a Scoop Stretcher

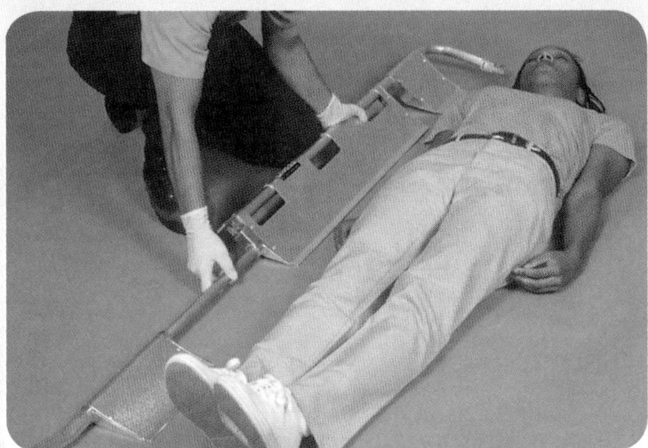

Step 1 With the scoop stretcher separated, measure the length of the scoop and adjust to the proper length.

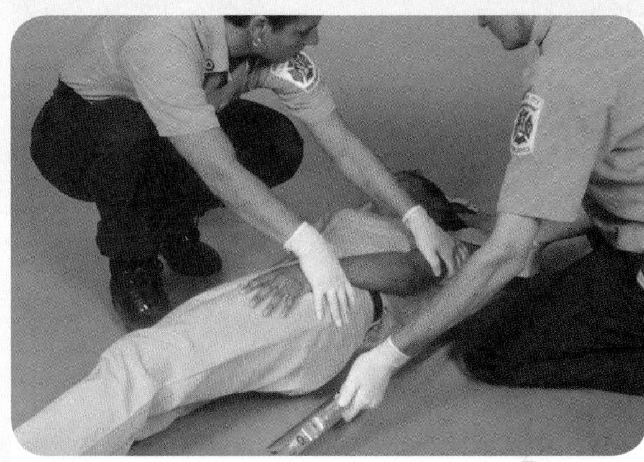

Step 2 Position the stretcher, one side at a time. Slightly lift the patient's side by pulling on the far hip and upper arm, while your partner slides the stretcher into place.

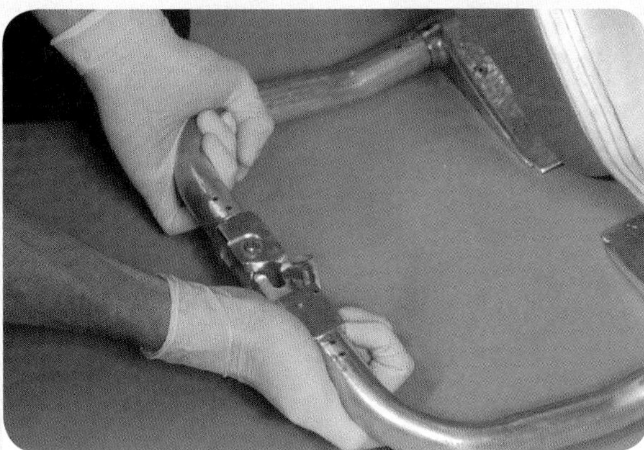

Step 3 Lock the stretcher ends together by engaging its locking mechanisms one at a time and continue to slightly lift the patient as needed to avoid pinching.

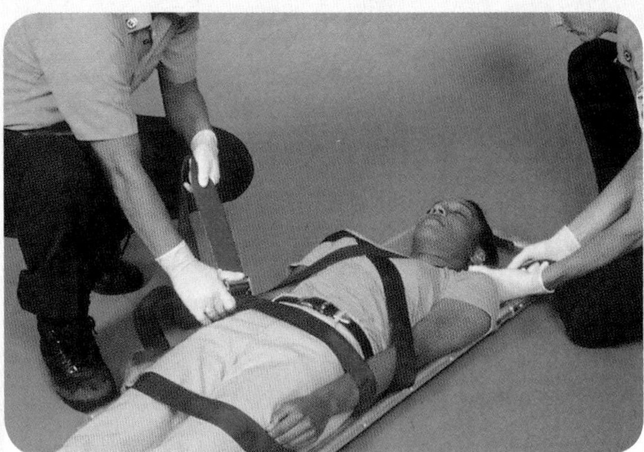

Step 4 Secure the patient to the scoop stretcher, and transfer it to the stretcher.

Use one of the following methods to move a patient from the ground or the floor onto the stretcher:

- Lift and carry the patient to the nearby prepared stretcher using a direct ground lift.
- Use a log roll or long-axis drag to place the patient onto a backboard, and then lift and carry the backboard to the stretcher. Place both the backboard and the patient onto the stretcher.
- Use a scoop stretcher.
- Log roll the patient onto a blanket.

Follow the steps in Skill Drill 6-12 to lift a patient from the ground using a blanket:

If the patient is sitting in a chair and cannot assist you, transfer the patient from the chair to a stair chair Skill Drill 6-13 .

Skill Drill 6-12 Lifting a Patient From the Ground

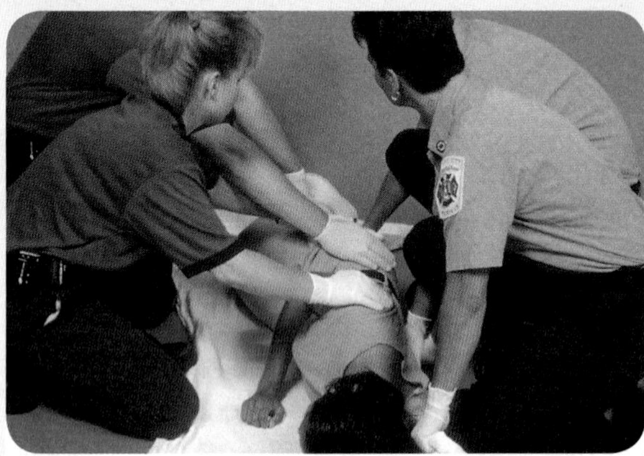

Step 1 Log roll the patient onto a blanket.

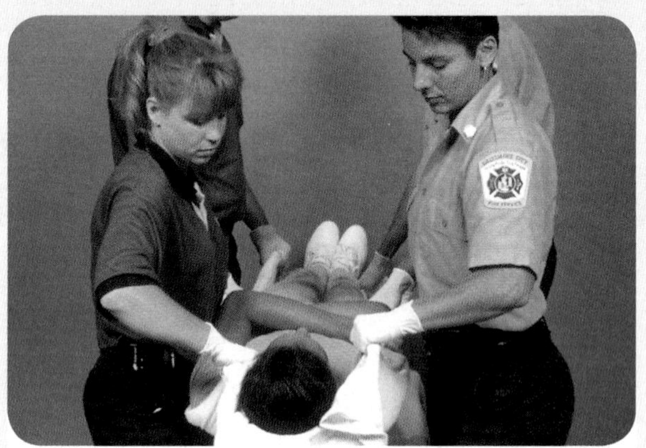

Step 2 Lift the patient by the blanket, and carry the patient to the nearby stretcher.

Skill Drill 6-13 Moving a Patient From a Chair to a Stair Chair

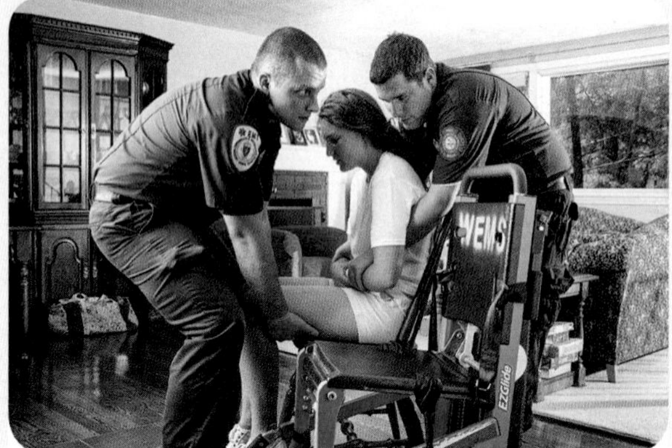

Step 1 Remove any removable side pieces on the chair or move the side pieces to a position so as to not interfere. Slide your arms through the patient's armpits, and grasp the patient's crossed forearms. Your partner grasps the patient's legs at the knees.

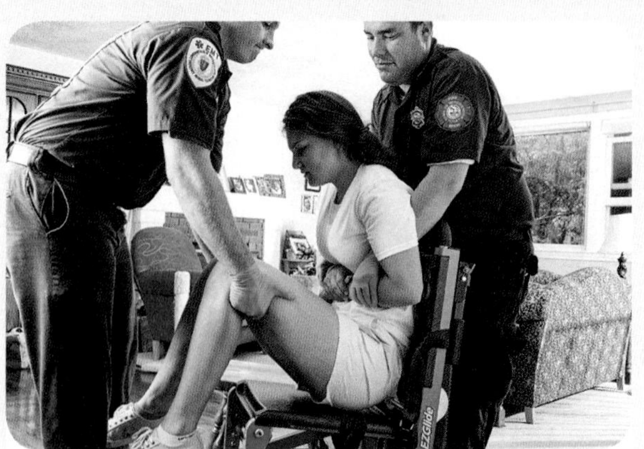

Step 2 Gently lift the patient into the locked stair chair.

Special Populations

Geriatric patients often fear the loss of their independence. What constitutes a minor injury for the average individual can be debilitating for an older person. Unless there is a true emergency, take the time to talk to geriatric patients and reassure them often.

Geriatrics

Most patients transported by EMS are geriatric patients. For many older patients, the fear of illness and disability is ever present, and an emergency trip to the hospital can be a terrifying and disorienting experience. In addition, there are physiologic changes that occur with aging that require special attention on your part as an AEMT.

- **Skeletal changes:** Brittle bones (osteoporosis), rigidity, and spinal curvatures (kyphosis and scoliosis) Figure 6-11 present special challenges in packaging and moving older patients. Many patients cannot lie supine on a backboard or scoop stretcher without causing additional injury, such as fractures, pressure sores, and skin breakdown. Special care and creativity must be taken in immobilizing patients with such conditions. For example, a patient with spinal curvature may have to be placed on his or her side and immobilized in place with towel and blanket rolls to prevent exacerbating his or her injuries. Consult your local protocols and medical director about alternative ways of immobilizing the patient, and be familiar with effective methods for padding voids.
- **Skin changes:** Geriatric patients have delicate skin and are prone to significant skin tears and bruises during even the simplest moves. Protect their elbows when carrying or moving through hallways.
- **Fear:** A sympathetic and compassionate approach can go a long way in allaying the natural fears many older patients experience when interacting with caregivers. Slow down, explain, and anticipate: these actions can help you gain an older patient's cooperation and take some of the anxiety out of the process of packaging and transportation. Imagine how frightening being strapped to a stretcher and carried down a flight of stairs can be to a person who lives in constant fear of falls and broken bones.

Special Populations

Cover the patient with a blanket to protect privacy and keep the patient warm.

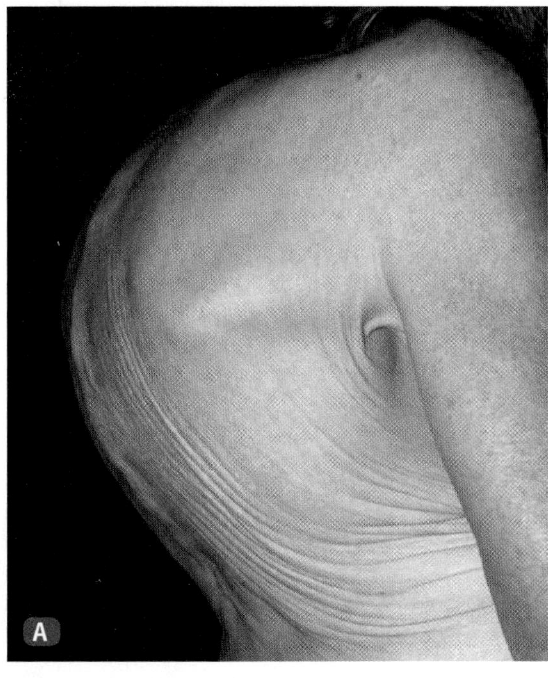

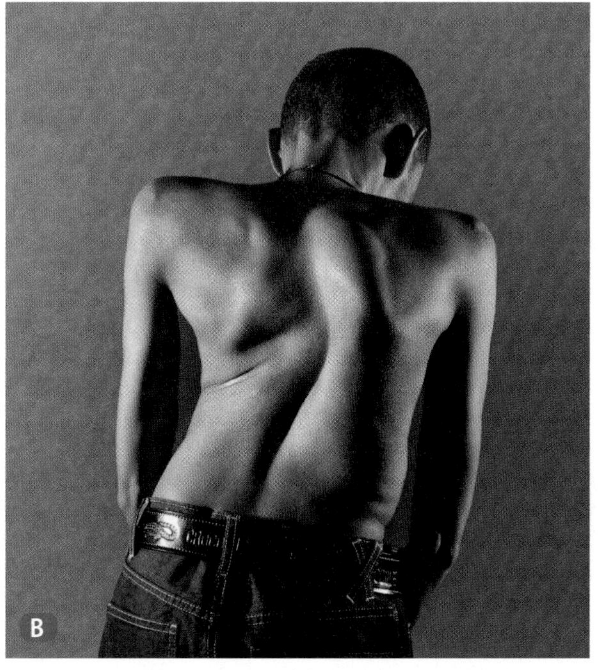

Figure 6-11 Skeletal changes. **A.** Kyphosis. **B.** Scoliosis.

Words of Wisdom

Whenever possible, use a draw sheet to move geriatric or bariatric patients rather than lifting them by their arms. Geriatric patients have thin skin that may bruise or tear easily, and the sheer weight of a bariatric patient exerts a tremendous amount of pressure on the patient's extremities. Pulling on the arms of these patients may result in pain, dislocation, or skin tears.

Bariatrics

From 2011 through 2014, over one-third of the adults in the United States (36.5%) were considered obese, according to the US Centers for Disease Control and Prevention.[1] The incidence of obesity is higher among adults aged 40 to 59 years (40.2%) than among adults aged 20 to 39 (32.3%), or adults aged 60 years or above (37%). The numbers among children are also alarming; approximately 17% of all children aged 2 to 19 years in the United States are classified in the obese category. The obesity rate has tripled compared to just one generation ago. In 2008, the estimated annual cost of medical care for obese patients in the United States was $147 billion annually, or approximately $1,429 higher per obese person than a person of normal weight.[2] Obesity has reached epidemic proportions in the United States, and many programs are now aimed at teaching people from a young age the importance of exercise and a healthy diet.

Obesity has become such a significant issue that a new field of medicine has emerged to provide specialty care for obese patients. **Bariatrics** is the branch of medicine concerned with the management (prevention or control) of obesity and allied diseases. It comes from the Greek words *baros*, weight, and *iatreia*, medical treatment. Because there is a direct correlation between the degree of obesity and the frequency and severity of health problems, the larger the patient the more likely he or she is to need emergency medical treatment and transportation. This problem is taking an increasing toll on the health and functioning of AEMTs because back injuries account for the highest number of missed days of work and for temporary and permanent disability.

Although equipment manufacturers are producing equipment with ever higher capacities, this does not address the danger to the users of that equipment. European ambulance manufacturers regularly install mechanical lifts on their units, but these are not as common in the United States.

YOU are the Provider — PART 4

After you ensure your patient is properly secured and in a position of comfort, you wheel him out to your awaiting ambulance. As you arrive at the rear of the ambulance, you instruct your partner to take one corner of the stretcher, while you take the corner with the controls. On the count of three, you take pressure off of the wheels, activate the controls to raise the undercarriage, and secure the patient into the back of the ambulance. You thank the engine crew for their assistance and inform your partner that this patient requires a smooth trip to the local ED. While en route, you obtain another set of vital signs and perform a more detailed examination. The patient explains he is being admitted to the hospital for treatment for his decubitus ulcers. Other than the pain, he has no other complaints. Once you arrive at the ED, you and your partner use the same process to take the patient out of the ambulance and safely move him to his room. You ask for additional assistance in moving the patient to his bed, and once he is positioned comfortably, you give your report to the nurse and return to service.

Recording Time: 52 Minutes	
Respirations	18 breaths/min; clear
Pulse	96 beats/min
Skin	Warm, dry, and pink
Blood pressure	142/82 mm Hg
Oxygen saturation (Spo_2)	98% on room air
Pupils	PERRLA

8. What steps should you take to safely roll the stretcher into the hospital?
9. How should this patient be moved onto the hospital bed?

Patient-Moving Equipment

▶ The Wheeled Ambulance Stretcher

The **wheeled ambulance stretcher** (also called an ambulance stretcher, gurney, or simply "the stretcher") can be rolled along the ground and weighs between 40 and 145 pounds (18 and 66 kg), depending on its design and features Figure 6-12. Because its weight must be added to that of the patient's, it is generally not taken up or down stairs or to other locations where the patient must be carried rather than rolled for any significant distance. When the patient is upstairs, take the wheeled ambulance stretcher to the ground floor landing and prepare it for the patient. Then, take a wheeled stair chair, scoop stretcher, or backboard upstairs. These devices are considerably lighter than a wheeled stretcher and may be used to carry the patient to the waiting stretcher.

Follow the manufacturer's directions for maintenance, inspection, weight limitations, repair, and upkeep for any device that you use as patient-handling equipment.

Stretchers are available in a number of different models, which may include different features. Before going on a call, familiarize yourself with all the specific features of the stretcher that your ambulance carries. Know the location of the controls that adjust and lock each feature and how each feature works.

The stretcher has a specific head end and foot end. The stretcher has a strong horizontal rectangular tubular metal main frame to which all of its other parts are attached.

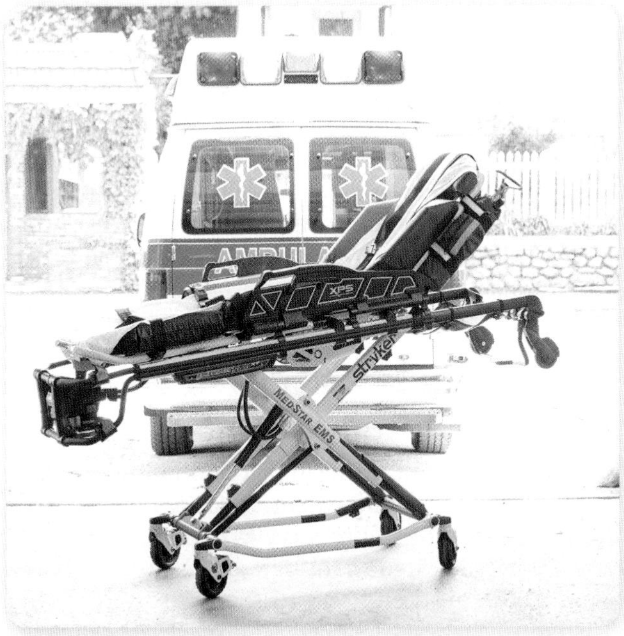

Figure 6-12 The wheeled ambulance stretcher is specially designed to roll along the ground.

The stretcher should be pulled, pushed, and lifted only by its main frame or handles, which are attached to the main frame specifically for this purpose.

On most models, a second tubular frame made up of three sections is attached within or above the main frame. A metal plate is fastened to each of the three sections between its sides. This plate serves as the platform on which the stretcher mattress and patient are supported. The head section runs from the head end of the stretcher to near the center of the stretcher, where the patient's hips will be. Hinges at the area where the hips will be allow the head end to be elevated and the patient's back to be positioned at any desired angle from flat to fully upright. The head end of the stretcher is designed to be elevated or moved down only when a tilt control is purposely released. At all other times, the back will remain locked at the position in which it was placed. The frame and plates that lie from the hips to the foot end of the stretcher are divided into two hinged sections. These sections may be connected so the foot end can be drawn in toward the knees, causing the frame and plates to hinge upward under the patient's knees to elevate them as desired. This feature is not found in all models.

A retractable guardrail is attached along the central portion of the main frame of the stretcher at each side and is lowered out of the way when a patient is being loaded onto the stretcher. Once the patient has been properly placed on the stretcher, the handle is drawn up and locked in an elevated position perpendicular to the surface of the stretcher. The patient cannot roll off either side of the stretcher even if a securing strap becomes released. The guardrail at each side can be lowered only if its locking handle is released.

The underside of the main frame of the stretcher is supported on a folding undercarriage that has a smaller horizontal rectangular frame and four large rubber casters at its bottom end. The folding undercarriage is designed to allow the stretcher to be adjusted to any height from about 12 inches (30 cm) above the ground, which is the desired height when the stretcher is secured in the ambulance, to 32 to 36 inches (81 to 91 cm) above the ground, which is the desired height when the stretcher is being rolled. Because you are able to lock the stretcher at any height between its lowest height and its fully extended height, it can be locked at the same height as any bed or examining table to allow the patient to be slid from one to the other. This permits you to transfer the patient without the need for any additional lifting. The controls for folding the undercarriage allow the stretcher to remain locked at its present height when the controls are not being activated. As an additional safety feature on most stretchers, the main frame must be lifted slightly so the undercarriage becomes unweighted before it will fold, even if the control is pulled. Therefore, if the handle is accidentally pulled, the elevated stretcher will not suddenly drop. Controls for elevating and lowering most stretchers are located at the foot end and at one or both sides. You and your partner must use the proper lifting mechanics to lift the wheeled ambulance stretcher.

The mattress on a stretcher must be fluid resistant so it does not absorb any type of potentially infectious material, including water, blood, or other body fluid.

Most patients are placed directly on the stretcher. However, patients with possible spinal injuries or multiple systems trauma should be placed and secured onto a backboard before placing them on the stretcher. Patients who may need cardiopulmonary resuscitation or must be carried down (or up) a flight of stairs while supine should also be placed on a backboard. The backboard and patient are then secured onto the stretcher.

Always secure patients with the straps on the stretcher. In the event of a crash while en route to the hospital, the straps help prevent further injury to the patient.

Words of Wisdom

Ensure a thorough patient care report by including details of how you moved the patient. For example "Moved patient to stretcher with draw sheet method."

▶ Bariatric Stretchers

Because of their large girth, bariatric patients may not fit comfortably on the standard wheeled stretcher. As a result, a specialized type of wheeled stretcher has been developed, called the bariatric stretcher Figure 6-13. This type of stretcher is similar in design to the common wheeled stretcher; however, it has several differences. Bariatric stretchers typically have a wider patient surface area to allow for increased comfort and increased dignity for the patient. Bariatric stretchers also have a wider wheelbase, allowing for increased stability when rolling the patient over uneven terrain. Bariatric stretchers are also sometimes equipped with optional features such as a tow package, which allows an ambulance-mounted winch to assist in loading the patient into the ambulance, decreasing the potential for AEMTs to have back injuries. Another optional feature is telescoping side lift handles, which allow for increased leverage when lifting with multiple providers. However, the most important feature of the bariatric stretcher is the increased weight-lifting capacity. Typical wheeled ambulance stretchers, depending on manufacturer ratings, are rated to a maximum weight of 650 pounds (295 kg). Bariatric stretchers are usually rated between 850 and 900 pounds (386 and 408 kg).

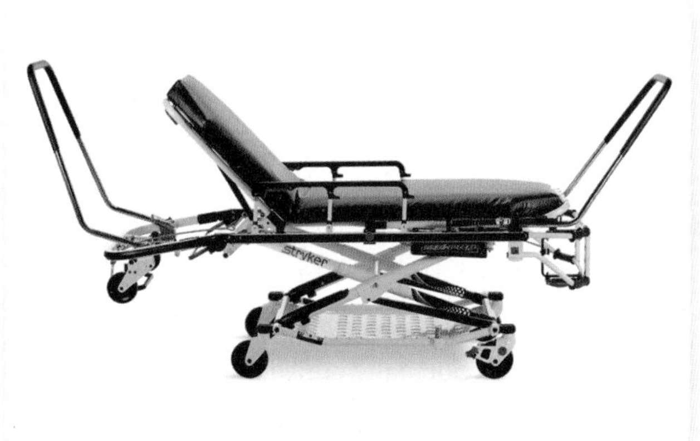

Figure 6-13 A bariatric stretcher.
Courtesy of Stryker Medical, a division of Stryker Corporation.

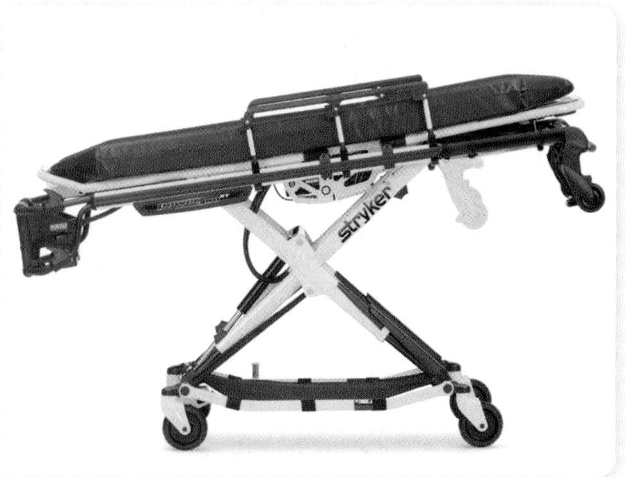

Figure 6-14 An electronic stretcher.
Courtesy of Stryker Medical, a division of Stryker Corporation.

▶ Pneumatic and Electronic Powered Wheeled Stretchers

In an effort to decrease the potential for back injuries to EMS providers, manufacturers have developed pneumatic and electronic stretchers. Similar in appearance to conventional wheeled stretchers, electronic stretchers are battery operated and have electronic controls to facilitate raising and lowering of the undercarriage at the touch of a button Figure 6-14. A drawback to the powered wheeled stretcher is that by adding the electronic controls, as well as the associated equipment, the weight of the stretcher is increased, typically by 75 to 100 pounds (34 to 45 kg). Combined with the weight of the patient on the loaded stretcher, this creates a potential hazard when transporting the patient over uneven terrain or down one or two steps in the front of a residence.

▶ Loading the Wheeled Stretcher Into an Ambulance

Whenever a patient has been placed onto the stretcher, one AEMT must hold the main frame to ensure it does not roll. When the stretcher is elevated, the main frame and the patient extend considerably beyond the wheels at both the head end and foot end of the stretcher. Therefore, whenever a patient is on an elevated stretcher, ensure it is held firmly between two hands at all times so even if the patient moves, the stretcher cannot tip Figure 6-15.

If the loaded stretcher must be carried down a short flight of stairs, first, retract the undercarriage; however, this is not necessary when the stretcher must be lifted over a curb, a single step, or an obstacle of a similar height Figure 6-16. Remember, if the patient must be carried up or down a full flight or several flights of stairs, prepare the stretcher and leave it on the ground floor at the bottom (or top) of the stairs. Use a backboard or stair chair to carry the patient up or down the stairs to the waiting stretcher.

Follow the steps shown in Skill Drill 6-14 to load the stretcher into an ambulance.

The clamps will hold the stretcher in place until they are released at the hospital. You can control and release the clamps with a single handle that is positioned so that you can activate it when standing on the ground at the open back doors of the ambulance when the stretcher is to be unloaded. The stretcher is designed to be rolled on

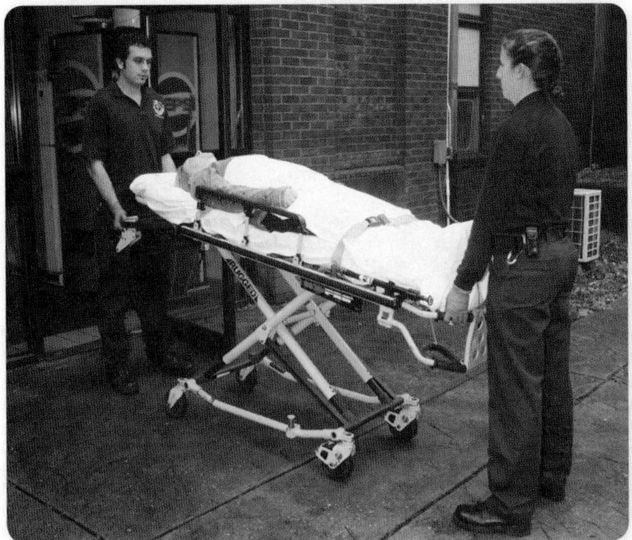

Figure 6-15 Always hold the main frame of the stretcher when it is elevated so that even when the patient moves, the stretcher does not tip.

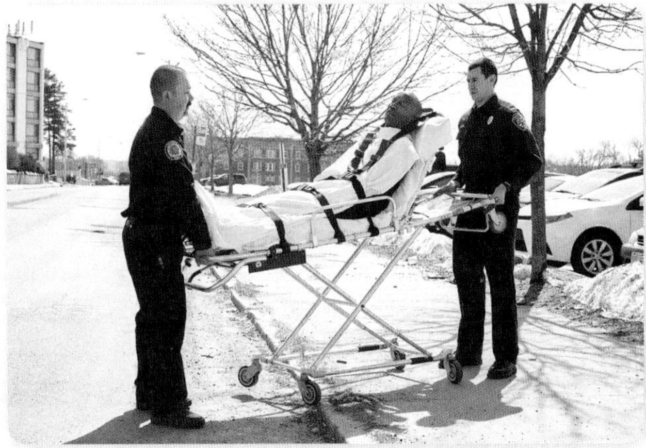

Figure 6-16 Retract the undercarriage of the stretcher when lifting it over a curb, a single step, or an obstacle of similar height.

Skill Drill 6-14 Loading a Stretcher Into an Ambulance

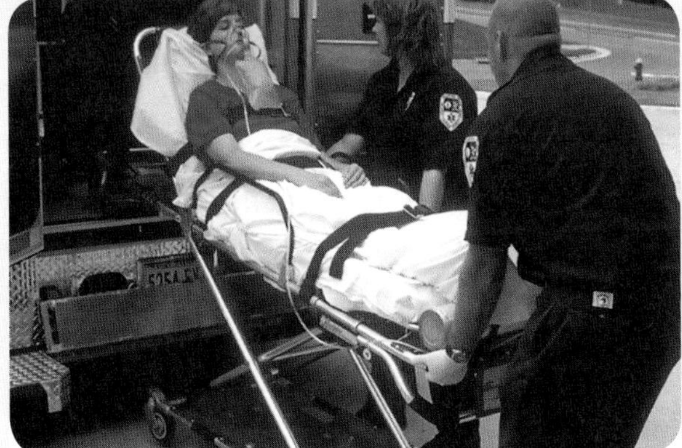

Step 1 Tilt the head end of the stretcher upward, and place it into the patient compartment with the wheels on the floor. Ensure the safety bar under the head of the stretcher catches on the hook prior to lifting the stretcher.

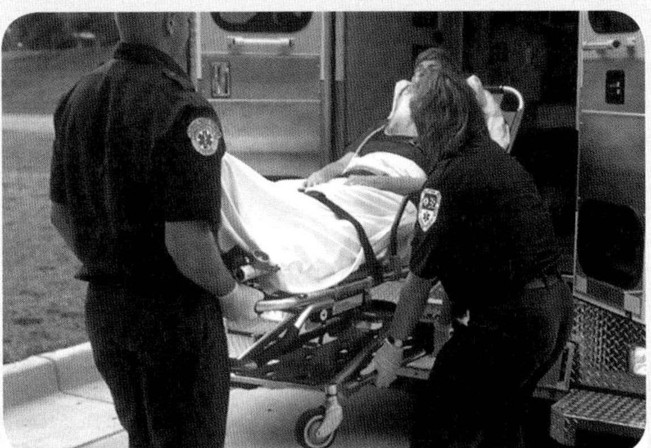

Step 2 With the patient's weight supported by the two head-end wheels and the provider at the foot end of the stretcher, move to the side of the main frame and release the undercarriage lock to lift the undercarriage up to its fully retracted position.

(continued)

Skill Drill 6-14 Loading a Stretcher Into an Ambulance *(continued)*

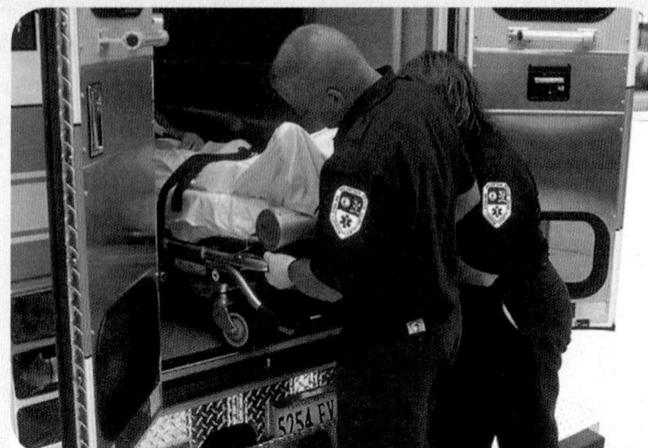

Step 3 Roll the stretcher the rest of the way into the back of the ambulance, where it will rest on all six wheels.

Step 4 Secure the stretcher to the clamps mounted in the ambulance.

regular flat surfaces. If the patient must be moved over a lawn or other irregular surface, lift and carry the stretcher over the terrain.

An intravenous (IV) pole is attached to many stretchers. The IV pole can be unfolded or extended above the main frame to hold an IV bag above the patient while you move the stretcher to the ambulance. Some wheeled ambulance stretchers even include a carrier to hold an electrocardiographic monitor or automated external defibrillator and portable oxygen unit. If the model you use does not include these features, secure the portable oxygen unit and cardiac monitor and automated external defibrillator to the top surface of the stretcher mattress at the patient's legs; however, remember, when you attempt to lift the stretcher these items will add more weight.

The extra wheels below the head end of the main frame of the stretcher are not featured on some older or less expensive wheeled ambulance stretchers. These stretchers are not self-loading. When you reach the back of the ambulance with such a stretcher, you must lower it until the undercarriage is in its lowest retracted position and then, with you and your partner at each side of the stretcher, lift it to the height of the floor of the ambulance and roll it into the track that locks it into place. Table 6-3 shows the guidelines that you must follow to load the stretcher into the ambulance.

Table 6-3 Guidelines for Loading the Stretcher Into the Ambulance
Make sure there is sufficient lifting power.
Follow the manufacturer's directions for safe and proper use of the stretcher.
Make sure that all stretchers and patients are fully secured before the ambulance is moved.

▶ Portable/Folding Stretchers

A **portable stretcher** is a stretcher with a strong, rectangular, tubular metal frame and rigid fabric stretched across it Figure 6-17. Portable stretchers do not have a second multipositioning frame or adjustable undercarriage. Some models have two wheels that fold down about 4 inches (10 cm) underneath the foot end of the frame and legs of a similar length that fold down from the head end at each side. The wheels make it easier to move the loaded stretcher. The legs should not be used as handles.

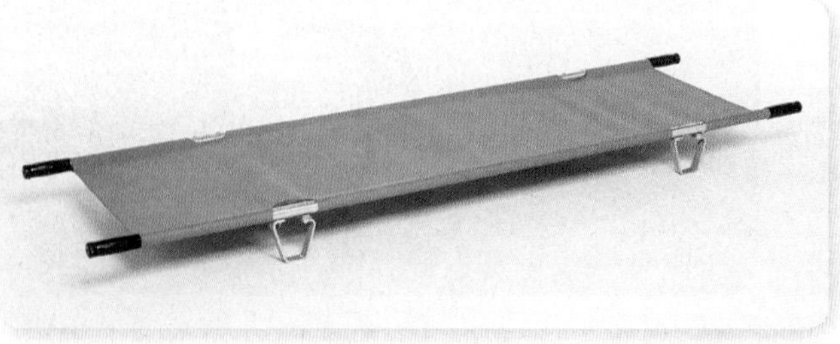

Figure 6-17 A portable stretcher.

Some portable stretchers can be folded in half across the center of each side so the stretcher is only one-half its usual length during storage. Many ambulances carry a portable stretcher to use if a patient is in an area that is difficult to reach with a wheeled ambulance stretcher or a second patient must be transported on the squad bench of the ambulance.

A portable stretcher weighs much less than a wheeled stretcher and does not have a bulky undercarriage. However, because most models do not have wheels, you and your team must support all of the patient's weight and any equipment along with the weight of the stretcher.

Flexible Stretchers

Several types of flexible stretchers, such as the Sked, Reeves, and Navy stretcher, are available and can be rolled up across either the stretcher's width or, in the case of the Sked, its length, so the stretcher becomes a smaller tubular package for storage and carrying Figure 6-18. This is an important consideration when you must carry the equipment a considerable distance from the nearest place that the ambulance can be located. A **flexible stretcher** forms a rigid stretcher that conforms around the patient's sides and does not extend beyond them. When these stretchers are extended, they are particularly useful when you must remove a patient from or through a confined space. Certain flexible stretchers can also be used if the patient must be belayed or rappelled by ropes.

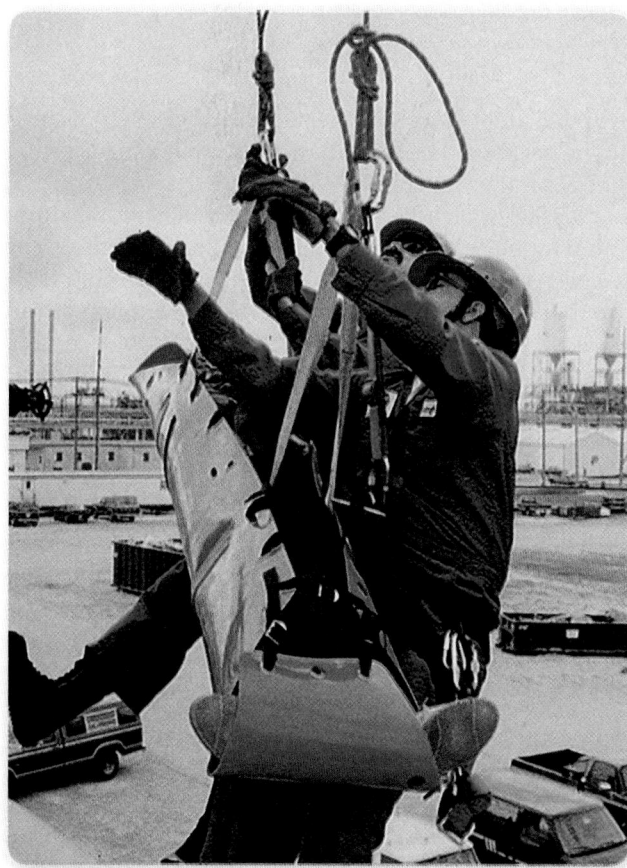

Figure 6-18 A flexible stretcher.

The flexible stretcher is the most uncomfortable of all the various devices and it provides excellent support. When the stretcher is wrapped around the patient and the straps are secured, the patient is completely immobilized. The stretcher can then be lowered by rope or slid down a flight of stairs by resting it on the front edge of each step.

Backboards

When a patient is unresponsive, in cardiac arrest, must be moved in a lying position, or must be immobilized, secure the patient onto a backboard. A **backboard** is a device used to carry patients and to immobilize supine patients with suspected hip, pelvic, spinal, and lower extremity injuries or other multiple trauma Figure 6-19. Backboards can also be used to move patients out of awkward places and to provide a rigid surface for patients in cardiac arrest. They are also called long backboards, spine boards, trauma boards, or longboards.

Backboards are long, flat, rectangular boards made of rigid material. They are 6 to 7 feet long (approximately 2 m) and are commonly used for patients who are found lying down. Parallel to the sides and ends of the backboard are a number of long holes that are about 0.5 to 1 inch (1 to 3 cm) from the outer edge. These holes form handles and handholds so the board can be easily grasped, lifted, and carried. The handles and adjacent holes also allow straps to be used to secure and immobilize the patient to the backboard to be secured to each side and end of the backboard at any needed location.

Backboards are usually made of plastic nowadays. For many years, backboards were made of thick marine plywood whose surface was sealed with polyurethane or another marine varnish. Wooden backboards are still used in some places. If you use wooden backboards, follow infection control procedures before you reuse the backboards. Where wooden backboards are no longer used, they have generally been stored so they will be available in the event of a mass-casualty incident. Newer backboards are made of lighter plastic materials that will not absorb blood or other infectious substances.

Use a short backboard to immobilize the torso, head, and neck of a seated patient with a suspected spinal injury until you can immobilize the patient on a backboard.

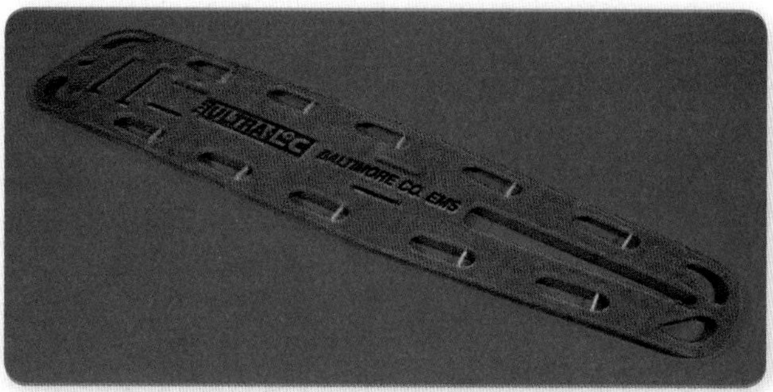

Figure 6-19 A backboard is used to transfer patients who must be moved in a supine or immobilized position.

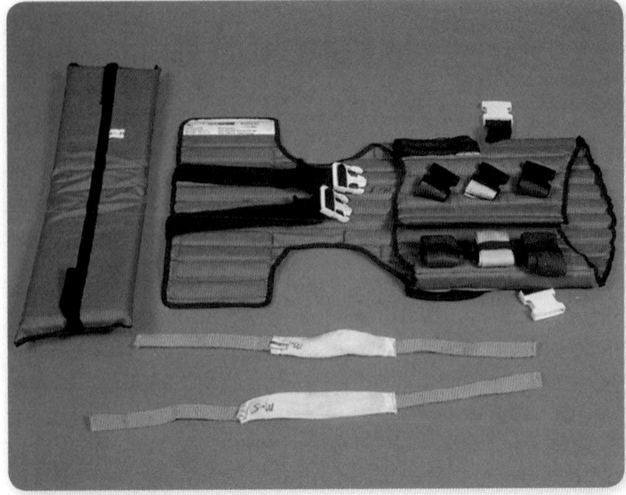

Figure 6-20 The Kendrick Extrication Device is a vest-type immobilization device.

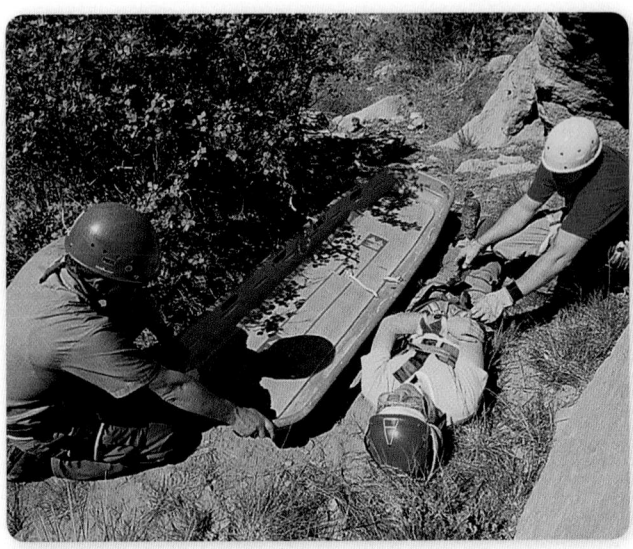

Figure 6-21 A basket stretcher.

Short backboards are 3 to 4 feet long (approximately 1 m). The original short wooden backboard has generally been replaced with a vest-type device that is specifically designed to immobilize the patient until he or she is moved from a sitting position to supine on a backboard **Figure 6-20**. The vest-type devices are easier to use than the wooden short backboard.

▶ Vacuum Mattresses

Another alternative to the backboard, especially for immobilizing geriatric and pediatric patients, is the vacuum mattress. With this device, the patient is placed on the mattress and the air is removed from the device, allowing it to mold around the patient. It fits snugly to the curvatures and contours of the body and limits pressure point tenderness. As the mattress molds to the body, it provides a high degree of immobilization and comfort. It also provides thermal insulation, thereby reducing the risk of hypothermia. Padding may be used for tender areas, but is not required for most patients.

It is imperative to maintain spinal immobilization while placing the patient on the device and to secure the patient properly once he or she is placed on the mattress. The vacuum mattress cannot be used on patients weighing 350 pounds (159 kg) or more. See Chapter 30, *Head and Spine Injuries*, for more information about the vacuum mattress.

▶ Basket Stretchers

Use a rigid **basket stretcher**, often called a Stokes litter or Stokes basket, to carry a patient across uneven terrain from a remote location that is inaccessible by ambulance or other vehicle **Figure 6-21**. If you suspect the patient has a spinal injury, first immobilize him or her on a backboard and then place the backboard into the basket stretcher. Once you have reached the ambulance and wheeled ambulance stretcher, remove the patient secured to the backboard from the basket stretcher and place him or her on the stretcher.

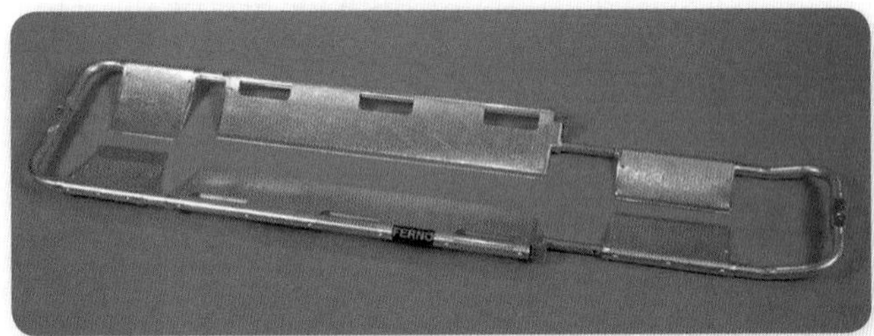

Figure 6-22 A scoop stretcher.

Basket stretchers are made of plastic with an aluminum frame or have a full steel frame that is connected by a woven wire mesh. The wire basket is very uncomfortable for the patient unless the wire is padded. Either type can be used to carry a patient across fields, rough terrain, or trails or on a toboggan, boat, or all-terrain vehicle. Basket stretchers surround and support the patient, yet their design allows water to drain through holes in the bottom. Basket stretchers are also used for technical rope rescues and some water rescues. Not all basket stretchers are rated or appropriate for each of these specialized rescue uses. The types of basket stretchers that are acceptable for specialized rescue must be determined by people with additional special training.

▶ Scoop Stretchers

The **scoop stretcher**, also referred to as an orthopaedic stretcher, is designed to be split into two or four sections **Figure 6-22**. These sections are fitted around a patient who is lying on the ground or another relatively flat surface. The parts are reconnected, and the patient is lifted and placed on a long backboard or stretcher. A scoop stretcher may be used for patients who have been struck by a motor vehicle.

A scoop stretcher is efficient; however, both sides of the patient must be accessible. You must pay special attention to the closure area beneath the patient so clothing, skin, and other objects are not trapped or pinched. As with the long backboard, you must fully immobilize and secure the patient before moving him or her; however, do not slip a scoop stretcher under the long axis of the patient's body. Scoop stretchers are narrow, well constructed, and compact and have excellent body support features but are not adequate when used alone for standard immobilization of a spinal injury. You and your team should practice often with a scoop stretcher, so you are ready to use it with a patient. It is important to remember a scoop stretcher has internal supports running throughout its length; this feature prohibits hospitals from being able to obtain a radiograph while the patient is secured to it, often mandating another move to a standard backboard before obtaining the radiograph.

Stair Chairs

Words of Wisdom

To use a stair chair, the patient must be alert and oriented and able to remain in an upright seated position. Otherwise, you must adopt another method for moving the patient.

A **stair chair** is a lightweight folding chair with a molded seat, adjustable safety straps, and fold-out handles at both the head end and foot end Figure 6-23. Stair chairs serve as an adjunct for moving a conscious patient up or down stairs to the ground floor, to the waiting wheeled ambulance stretcher. Use a stair chair if the patient's condition allows him or her to be placed in a sitting position.

Most models have rubber wheels in the back with casters in front so they can roll and make turns along the floor. Some have a specially designed track to facilitate movement down steps with little lifting required. Roll the stair chair on the floor until you reach the stairwell, then both providers carry it (rather than roll and bump it) up or down the stairs. Once you reach the ground floor, roll the stair chair to the waiting stretcher and assist or lift the patient onto the stretcher.

Ensure the wheeled ambulance stretcher is at the proper height, lower the side rails, turn down the cover sheet, and remove any equipment that you may have secured on the top.

Follow the steps shown in Skill Drill 6-15 to use a stair chair.

As with other carries, always remember to keep your back in a locked-in position and to flex at the hips, not the waist. Bend at the knees and keep the patient's weight and your arms as close to your body as possible. Twisting while carrying or moving a patient will increase your risk

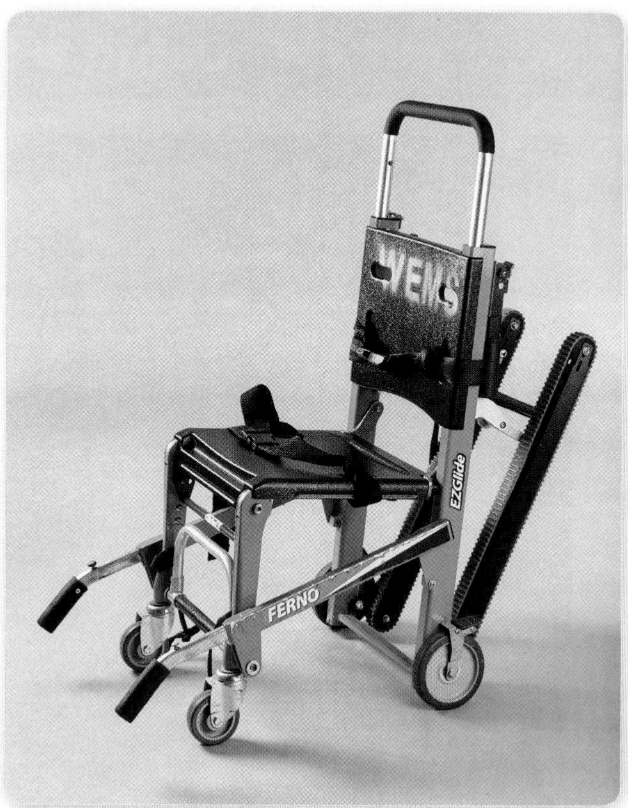

Figure 6-23 A wheeled stair chair can be used to transfer a conscious patient up or down a flight of stairs.

of injury. Avoid lifting and carrying the patient unnecessarily. A log roll or a body drag may aid you in moving your patient onto the backboard or the stretcher. Use one of these moves, if these techniques will not harm or jeopardize your patient's condition.

Moving a Patient on Stairs With a Backboard

Do not use a stair chair if a patient is unresponsive, in cardiac arrest, must be moved in a supine position, or must be immobilized; instead, secure the patient onto a backboard. Ensure the patient is anatomically secured to the device so he or she cannot slide significantly when the stretcher is at an angle. Carry the patient on the backboard down the stairs to the prepared stretcher. More than one-half of a patient's weight is distributed to the head end of the backboard when moving on stairs, so ensure the strongest provider is positioned at the head end. (Even with four or more providers carrying the patient, the strain on the provider at the head end will be increased when you must negotiate a narrow flight of stairs.) In carrying a patient up or down a flight of stairs, proportionally greater weight will also be distributed to the provider who carries the foot end when the device becomes angled because of the incline or decline. You should anticipate this and, in such cases, ensure the two strongest providers are positioned at the head and foot ends of the board. Because of the incline

Skill Drill 6-15 Using a Stair Chair

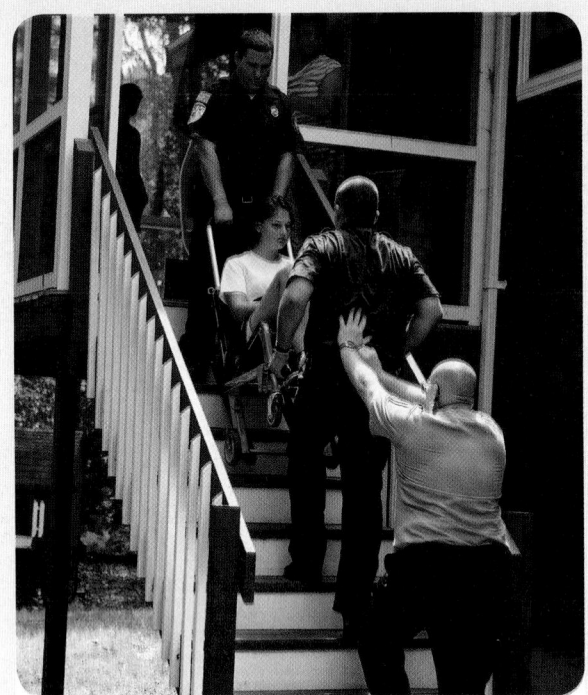

Step 1 Secure the patient to the stair chair with straps. One provider should be positioned at the head end and one provider at the foot end. The provider at the head will coordinate lifts and movement. If a third provider is on scene, the third provider keeps his or her hand on the back of the second provider who is at the patient's feet. The third provider will open doors and provide guidance and support.

Step 2 When you reach landings and other flat intervals in the move, lower the chair to the ground and roll the chair to the next position. When you reach the ground level where the stretcher awaits, roll the chair into position next to the stretcher in preparation for transferring the patient.

of the stairway, if one of the two strongest providers is considerably taller than the other, it will be easier if the shorter provider is at the head end and the taller provider is at the foot end. This minimizes bending while lifting and moving the patient. Once you reach the stretcher, place both the backboard and the patient on the stretcher; then secure both to the stretcher with additional straps.

To carry a patient on stairs on a backboard, follow the steps in Skill Drill 6-16.

Words of Wisdom

Make sure the stretcher is prepared prior to lifting the patient. Ensure the side rail is down, the stretcher is at a height that will not require you to lift the board any higher, the straps are unfastened and out of the way, and the head and foot ends are positioned appropriately to allow a smooth transition without having to rotate the stretcher or move around it.

▶ Neonatal Isolettes

When you are requested to transport a neonatal patient from one hospital to another, the common wheeled ambulance stretcher will not suffice. To safely transport a neonatal patient, the patient must be placed inside an **isolette**, sometimes referred to as an incubator. The isolette keeps the neonatal patient warm with moistened air in a clean environment and helps to protect the infant from noise, drafts, infection, and excess handling. The specialized transport devices come in two forms: the Isolette that is placed directly on top of the wheeled stretcher and secured with seat belts, and the

Skill Drill 6-16 Carrying a Patient on Stairs

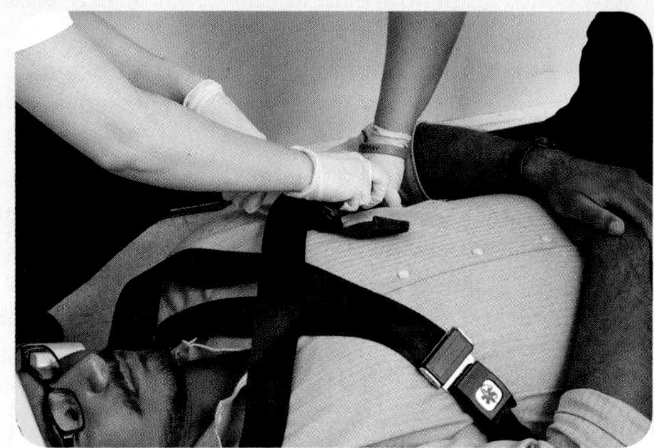

Step 1 Strap the patient securely. Ensure one strap is tight across the patient's upper torso, under the arms, and secured to the handles to prevent the patient from sliding.

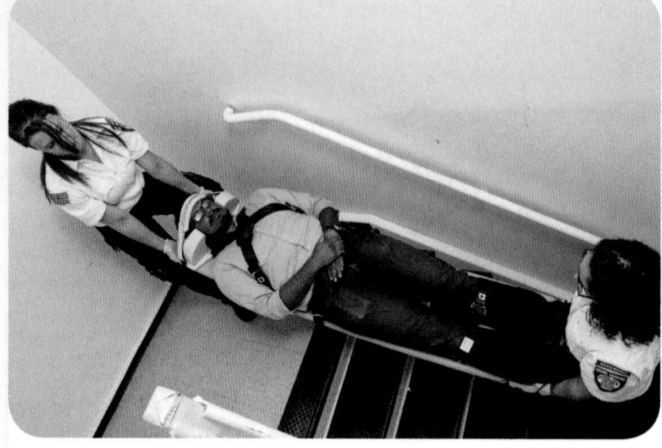

Step 2 When you carry the patient down stairs or an incline, ensure the backboard or stretcher is carried with the foot end first so the head end is elevated higher than the foot end.

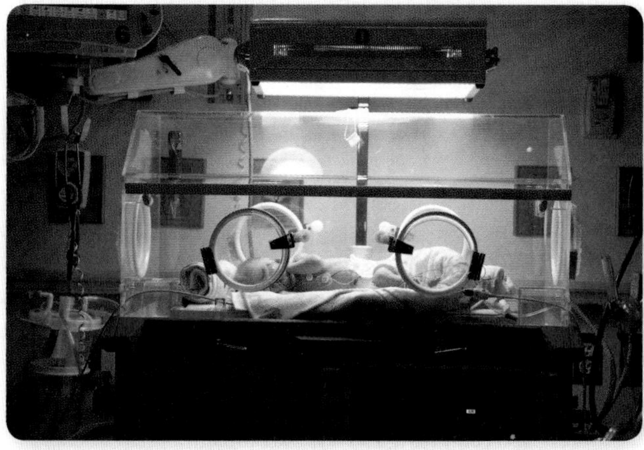

Figure 6-24 Neonatal isolette.

freestanding isolette that is secured into the back of the ambulance, taking the place of the standard stretcher Figure 6-24. Isolettes are often utilized by advanced practice personnel. Carefully follow their directions when assisting with the isolette.

Decontamination

It is essential that you decontaminate your equipment after each use, for your safety, the safety of the crew using the equipment after you, and the safety of your patients. Decontamination prevents the spread of disease. Just as we expect a hospital bed to be disinfected after the last patient, your stretcher and other transport equipment must be disinfected too. Know and follow your local standard operating procedures for disinfecting equipment after each call.

Patient Positioning

While you are treating a patient, you must ensure he or she is properly positioned based on the chief complaint. Certain patient conditions, such as head injury, shock, spinal injury, pregnancy, and obese patients call for special lifting and moving techniques. While a patient with a potential spinal injury should be fully immobilized, a patient with no suspected injury who reports chest pain or respiratory distress should be placed in a position of comfort—typically a Fowler or semi-Fowler position—unless he or she is hypotensive. Patients who are in shock should be packaged and placed in a supine position. Patients in the third trimester of pregnancy should be positioned and transported on their left side if they are uncomfortable or hypotensive when supine. Place an unresponsive patient with no suspected spinal, hip, or pelvic injury into the recovery position by rolling the patient onto his or her side without twisting the body. Transport a patient who is nauseated or vomiting in a position of comfort, but ensure you are positioned appropriately to manage and maintain a patent airway. Obese patients should be positioned the same as other patients with a similar conditions; however, pay particular attention to ensure you maintain their dignity.

Special Populations

Certain patient conditions, such as head injury, shock, spinal injury, and pregnancy, call for special lifting and moving techniques. Patients with chest pain or difficulty breathing should sit in a position of comfort, as long as they are not hypotensive. Those with suspected spinal injuries must be immobilized on a long backboard. Patients who are in shock should be packaged and moved in the position dictated by local protocol for shock. Pregnant patients who are hypotensive should be positioned and transported on their left sides. Move an unresponsive patient with no suspected spinal injury into the recovery position by rolling the patient onto his or her side without twisting the body. Transport a patient who is nauseated or vomiting in a position of comfort, but be sure you are positioned appropriately to manage the airway. Obese patients should be positioned the same as other patients; however, pay particular attention to ensure you maintain their dignity.

Medical Restraints

While not a common occurrence, there may be a time when you are called on to physically restrain a patient. After you evaluate the patient for correctible causes of combativeness, such as head injury, hypoxia, and hypoglycemia, the decision needs to be made as to whether to restrain your patient. There may be legal consequences for applying the restraints or failing to restrain a patient who should have been restrained. Contact law enforcement and consult local protocols before applying restraints; in some jurisdictions, medical control authorization is needed before an AEMT may apply restraints. See Chapter 24, *Psychiatric Emergencies*, for more detail about managing patients having psychiatric emergencies, including the use of restraints.

The decision to restrain a patient is not one you should take lightly; however, if the patient is posing a danger to you, your crew, himself or herself, or to bystanders, consider applying physical restraints. Before you take action to restrain the patient, attempt to speak to the patient in a calm manner, but remain firm in your requests. If that does not work and the patient continues to be combative, all providers present should develop a plan as to who will do what, when it will happen, and how you will accomplish the restraint.

There should be a minimum of five providers present to assist in the restraint of a combative patient, one for each extremity and one for the head. One AEMT should be established as the team leader, the one who will give commands. A plan to restrain the patient should be developed and agreed on by all providers. A patient who is caught off guard and is unsuspecting allows for a decreased likelihood of injury to the providers.

When you prepare to secure the patient on the stretcher, it is very important to have the patient in the supine position. If the patient is placed in a prone position, a condition called positional asphyxia could develop. In the prone position, the increased weight on the patient's lungs and his or her inability to fully expand the thoracic cavity could render the patient unable to breathe, creating a preventable, life-threatening emergency.

If a patient for whom use of medical restraints is indicated is in the supine position, some type of humane restraint should be applied to each extremity, such as triangle bandages, roller gauze, soft commercially available disposable restraints, or leather restraints. Preferably the patient should be restrained onto a backboard, which allows for easy movement should the patient begin to vomit. However, if it is impractical or inadvisable to secure the patient to the backboard, then secure the patient to the stretcher. Regardless of whether the patient is secured to a backboard or the stretcher, one arm should be secured above the patient's head and one arm should be secured at the patient's side. This technique will not give the patient the leverage to break free from the restraints. After the upper extremities are secured, each leg should be secured as well. Ensure you will be able to quickly remove the restraints during transport if necessary. Patients should not be transported in handcuffs unless a police officer rides in the ambulance with you during transport.

After you apply the restraints, assess and continually reassess the patient's ABCDEs (airway, breathing, circulation, disability, and exposure), mental status, and distal circulation (pulse and motor and sensory function). Document your findings on the patient care report. Include what types of restraints were used and why.

Personnel Considerations

In an effort to minimize personnel injuries, before moving any patient, a complete plan needs to be developed and discussed among the team members. One question to ask is: Am I physically strong enough to lift or move this patient? Many back injuries are the result of poor physical condition. As an AEMT, you will be required to assist in moving patients. Do your best to maintain a level of physical fitness. Other questions may include: Is there adequate room to get the proper stance to lift the patient? Do I need additional providers for lifting assistance? Evaluate the answers to these questions before you move your patient. Remember, injured providers cannot help anyone.

Words of Wisdom

After you deliver the patient to the ED, you and your team must begin preparing for your next call. Review the positive points about the transport. Discuss changes that would improve the next run. Review and evaluate the process to identify the following:

- Procedures that need more practice
- Equipment that needs to be cleaned or serviced
- Skills that you need to review or acquire

Most important, a critical review helps you and your team to become more confident and better-skilled AEMTs.

YOU are the Provider SUMMARY

1. What additional resources may be needed to move this patient?

When you attempt to move patients who weigh more than 250 pounds (113 kg), it is recommended you use at least four people to assist you in the move. Always know your limits and do not attempt to lift more than you are physically capable of lifting; otherwise, you may injure yourself, your partner, and the patient.

2. How will you move this patient from his bed to the stretcher?

Use the draw sheet method to move this patient from his bed to the EMS stretcher. Ensure the sheet is durable and all of the slack has been taken up prior to the move. The stretcher should be positioned next to the patient's bed with the mattress of the stretcher slightly lower than the mattress of the patient's bed. This will prevent the EMS mattress from rolling onto itself during the transition.

3. What are some potential complications when patients are moved improperly?

Your safety, as well as the safety of the other AEMTs and the patient, depends on using proper lifting techniques and having and maintaining a proper hold when lifting or carrying a patient. If you do not have proper hold of the stretcher or the patient in a body lift, you will not be able to bear a proper share of the weight, which may increase the chance you could suddenly lose your grasp with one or both hands. If you temporarily lose your grasp, the position and weight distribution of the stretcher changes suddenly, and the other members of the team must quickly reach beyond a safe distance to avoid dropping the patient. As a result, sudden excessive force may be placed across each one's spine, causing lower back injury.

4. Should you use an emergency, urgent, or nonurgent move?

In this scenario, use a nonurgent move. When the scene is stable and the patient is in stable condition, carefully plan how to move the patient. If the move is rushed or not well planned, it may result in discomfort or injury to the patient, you, and your team. Before you attempt any move, the team leader must ensure there are enough personnel, identify and remove any obstacles, ensure the proper equipment is available, and clearly identify and discuss the procedure and path to be followed. In nonurgent situations, you and your team may choose one of several methods for lifting and carrying a patient.

5. What are some of the differences between a normal stretcher and a bariatric stretcher?

Bariatric stretchers typically have a wider patient surface area to allow for increased comfort and increased dignity for patients. Bariatric stretchers also have a wider wheelbase, allowing for increased stability when rolling the patient over uneven terrain. Bariatric stretchers are also sometimes equipped with optional features such as a tow package, which allows an ambulance-mounted winch to assist in loading the patient into the ambulance, decreasing the potential for back injuries. Another optional feature is telescoping side lift handles, which allow for increased leverage when lifting with multiple providers. However, the most important feature of the bariatric stretcher is the increased weight-lifting capacity. Typical wheeled ambulance stretchers, depending on manufacturer ratings, are rated to a maximum weight of 650 pounds (295 kg). Bariatric stretchers are usually rated to 850 to 900 pounds (386 to 408 kg).

6. Why is it important to have only one person issuing commands when moving patients?

To safely lift and carry a patient, you and your team must anticipate and understand every move, and each move must be executed in a coordinated manner. The team leader should indicate where each team member is to be located and rapidly describe the sequence of steps that will be performed to ensure team members know what is expected before they initiate any lifting. If you must lift and move the patient through a number of separate steps, the team leader should first give an abbreviated overview of the steps, followed by a more detailed explanation of each step just before it will occur. By having an identified team leader issuing commands, everyone involved in the move will know who is in charge and who will be issuing the commands.

7. What are some advantages and disadvantages of a hydraulic stretcher?

In an effort to decrease the potential for back injuries to EMS providers, manufacturers have developed pneumatic and electronic stretchers. Similar in appearance to conventional wheeled stretchers, electronic stretchers are battery operated and have electronic controls to facilitate raising and lowering the undercarriage at the touch of a button. A drawback to the powered wheeled stretcher is that by adding the electronic controls, as well as the associated equipment, the weight of the stretcher is increased, typically by 75 to 100 pounds (34 to 45 kg). Combined with the weight of the patient on the loaded stretcher, this creates a potential hazard when transporting the patient over uneven terrain or down one to two steps in the front of a residence.

8. What steps should you take to safely roll the stretcher into the hospital?

When you are rolling the wheeled ambulance stretcher, make sure you elevate it. Pull the stretcher from the foot end. Make sure your arms are held close to your body, and

YOU are the Provider SUMMARY *(continued)*

avoid reaching significantly behind you or hyperextending your back. Your back should be locked, straight, and untwisted. While you are walking and pulling the stretcher, bend slightly forward at the hips. Keep the line of the pull through the center of your body by bending your knees.

9. How should this patient be moved onto the hospital bed?

In this scenario, the stretcher should be placed directly next to the hospital bed. The draw sheet that was used to move the patient initially should be used to move him to the hospital bed. Ensure the stretcher is at the same height as the bed and held firmly against its side. Then, you and another AEMT should kneel on the hospital bed and pull on the draw sheet smoothly and evenly to glide the patient in increments until he is properly centered on the bed. Request additional help to assist in lessening the strain on you and your partner. When you transfer the patient onto a narrow examining table, rather than kneel on the table, drag the patient while standing against the opposite side. A third person may need to take both sides of the head to safely move the patient. Some hospitals use a sliding board that helps to facilitate the move from bed to bed.

EMS Patient Care Report (PCR)					
Date: 9-12-18	**Incident No.:** 9-8712	**Nature of Call:** Fall		**Location:** 169 S Sulfur Lane	
Dispatched: 0944	**En Route:** 0948	**At Scene:** 0956	**Transport:** 1056	**At Hospital:** 1105	**In Service:** 1130
Patient Information					
Age: 69 **Sex:** M **Weight (in kg [lb]):** 147 kg (325 lb)			**Allergies:** Sulfa **Medications:** Lisinopril, atenolol, metformin **Past Medical History:** Hypertension, diabetes mellitus, cardiac **Chief Complaint:** Transfer for treatment of decubitus ulcers		
Vital Signs					
Time: 0958	**BP:** Not obtained	**Pulse:** Not obtained	**Respirations:** Nonlabored	**Spo_2:** Not obtained	
Time: 1004	**BP:** 146/88	**Pulse:** 102	**Respirations:** 18	**Spo_2:** 97% on room air	
Time: 1048	**BP:** 142/82	**Pulse:** 96	**Respirations:** 18	**Spo_2:** 98% on room air	
EMS Treatment (circle all that apply)					
Oxygen @ ______ L/min via (circle one): **NC NRM Bag-mask device**		**Assisted Ventilation**	**Airway Adjunct**	**CPR**	
Defibrillation	**Bleeding Control**	**Bandaging**	**Splinting**	**Other:**	
Narrative					
EMS dispatched to above location for transport to the hospital for a direct admittance. On arrival, patient found supine in bed, alert and oriented × 4, ABCs intact; weight 325 lb (147 kg), per the patient. Chief complaint is pain from decubitus ulcers for which patient is being transported. Additional lifting assistance requested and engine crew utilized to assist in moving patient via the draw sheet method from his bed onto a bariatric stretcher. Patient placed in a position of comfort, secured to stretcher, and loaded into the ambulance for transport. Nonemergency transport initiated. En route: Vitals as above. Detailed assessment is unremarkable. Patient was transported to Room 223 on the surgical floor where additional assistance was requested to move patient into bed. Patient moved without incident, report given to attending nurse, and unit returned to service.**End of report**					

Prep Kit

▶ Ready for Review

- The first key rule of lifting is to always keep your back in an upright position and lift without twisting or bending. You can lift and carry significant weight without injury as long as your back is in the proper upright position.
- The power lift is the safest and most powerful way to lift.
- The safety of you, your team, and the patient depend on the use of proper lifting techniques and maintaining a proper hold when lifting or carrying a patient.
- Pushing is better than pulling.
- If you do not have a proper hold in a body lift, you will not be able to bear your share of the weight, and you may lose your grasp with one or both hands and possibly cause a lower back injury to one or more AEMTs.
- Use the power grip to get the maximum force from your hands whenever you are lifting a patient.
- Directions and commands are an important part of safe lifting and carrying. You and your team must anticipate and understand every move and execute it in a coordinated manner. The team leader is responsible for coordinating the moves.
- The same basic body mechanics apply for safe reaching and pulling as for lifting and carrying. Keep your back locked and straight, and avoid twisting. Do not hyperextend your back when reaching overhead.
- It is always best to move a patient on a device that can be rolled. However, if a wheeled device is not available, you must understand and follow certain guidelines for carrying a patient on a stretcher.
- When lifting a stretcher, ensure you and your team use correct lifting techniques. Ideally, members of the lifting team should be of similar height and strength.
- Use four providers whenever resources allow. Also, know how much you can comfortably and safely lift, and do not attempt to lift more than this weight. Rapidly summon additional help to lift and carry a weight that is greater than you are able to lift.
- If you must carry a loaded backboard or stretcher up or down stairs or other inclines, ensure the patient is secured tightly to the device to prevent sliding.
- Ensure the patient's head is elevated higher than his or her feet.
- Whenever there is a potential for danger, use an emergency move to move a patient before providing a primary survey and care. The presence of fire, explosives, or hazardous materials may prompt an emergency move.
- Perform an urgent move when the patient requires immediate life-saving care, yet is in an unsafe environment. An urgent move may be necessary for moving a patient with an altered level of consciousness, with inadequate ventilation, or who is in shock, or in extreme weather conditions.
- Move a patient in an orderly, planned, and unhurried manner, selecting methods that involve the least amount of lifting and carrying.
- Transfer moves are used to transfer patients from a bed to a stretcher. Two examples of transfer moves are the direct carry method and the draw sheet method.
- Special equipment and protocols are needed when lifting or moving geriatric, bariatric, and neonatal patients.
- The wheeled ambulance stretcher is the most commonly used device to move and transport patients. Other devices that are used to lift and carry patients include portable stretchers, flexible stretchers, backboards, basket stretchers (Stokes litter or Stokes basket), scoop stretchers, and stair chairs.
- It is essential to decontaminate patient-moving equipment after each use to prevent the spread of disease.
- While you are treating a patient, you must ensure he or she is properly positioned based on the chief complaint.
- Apply medical restraints when they are indicated according to your local protocols and, depending on your jurisdiction, after receiving authorization from medical control.
- Whenever you are moving a patient, you must take special care to ensure no one is injured. You will learn the technical skills of patient packaging and handling through practice and training.
- Training and practice are also required to use all the equipment that is available to you. Practice each technique with your team often so you are able to perform the move quickly, safely, and efficiently.

Prep Kit (continued)

Vital Vocabulary

backboard A long, flat board made of rigid rectangular material that is used to provide support to a patient who is suspected of having a hip, pelvic, spinal, or lower extremity injury; also called a long backboard, spine board, trauma board, and longboard.

bariatrics A branch of medicine concerned with the management (prevention or control) of obesity and allied diseases.

basket stretcher A rigid stretcher commonly used in technical and water rescues that surrounds and supports the patient yet allows water to drain through holes in the bottom; also called a Stokes litter.

diamond carry A carrying technique in which one provider is located at the head end of the stretcher or backboard, one at the foot end, and one at each side of the patient; each of the two providers at the sides uses one hand to support the stretcher or backboard so that all are able to face forward as they walk.

direct carry method A nonurgent move that is a method for moving a patient from a bed to a stretcher, in which a stretcher is positioned next to the bed and two providers move the patient.

direct ground lift A lifting technique that is used for patients who are found lying supine on the ground with no suspected spinal injury.

draw sheet method A nonurgent move that is a method for moving a patient from a bed onto a stretcher using a sheet on which the patient is lying.

emergency move A move in which the patient is dragged or pulled from a dangerous scene before a primary survey and care are provided.

extremity lift A lifting technique that is used for patients who are supine or in a sitting position on the ground with no suspected extremity or spinal injuries.

flexible stretcher A stretcher that is a rigid carrying device when secured around a patient but can be folded or rolled when not in use.

isolette A device used to transport a neonate in an ambulance; also called an incubator.

portable stretcher A stretcher with a strong, rectangular, tubular metal frame and rigid fabric stretched across it.

power grip A technique in which the stretcher or backboard is gripped by inserting each hand under the handle with the palm facing up and the thumb extended, fully supporting the underside of the handle on the curved palm with the fingers and thumb.

power lift A lifting technique in which the AEMT's back is held upright, with legs bent, and the patient is lifted when the AEMT straightens the legs to raise the upper body and arms.

rapid extrication technique A technique to move a patient from a sitting position inside a vehicle to supine on a backboard in less than 1 minute when conditions do not allow for standard immobilization.

scoop stretcher A stretcher that is designed to be split into two or four sections that can be fitted around a patient who is lying on the ground or other relatively flat surface; also called an orthopaedic stretcher.

stair chair A lightweight folding device that is used to carry a conscious, seated patient up or down stairs.

wheeled ambulance stretcher A specially designed stretcher that can be rolled along the ground. A collapsible undercarriage allows it to be loaded into the ambulance; also called an ambulance stretcher.

References

1. Centers for Disease Control and Prevention. *Adult Obesity Facts, 2015.* http://www.cdc.gov/nchs/fastats/obesity-overweight.htm. Accessed October 11, 2016.
2. Centers for Disease Control and Prevention. *Childhood Obesity Facts: Prevention of Childhood Obesity in the United States 2011–2012.* http://www.cdc.gov/obesity/childhood/index.html. Accessed June 23, 2016.

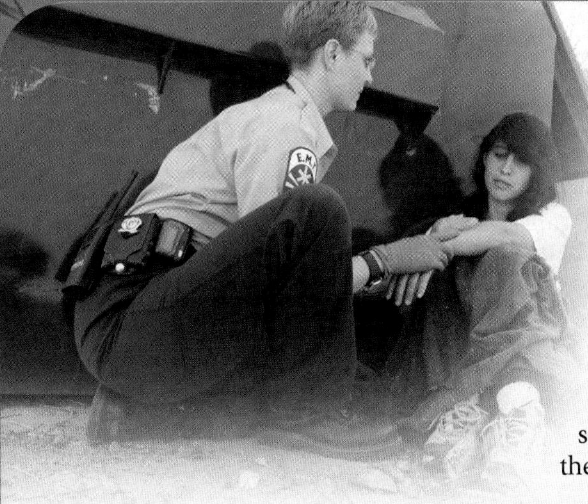

Assessment *in Action*

Your ambulance is dispatched to a reported motor vehicle crash on the local interstate highway. As you arrive on the scene, you find one vehicle that appears to have driven off the roadway and hit a bridge abutment. You have one patient, an older adult man, who appears unresponsive in the driver's seat. As you are assessing the patient, your partner states that there is a large amount of fuel spilling from the vehicle's gas tank.

1. How should this patient be moved?

A. Urgent move
B. Emergency move
C. Nonurgent move
D. Nonemergency move

2. To remove the patient from the vehicle, you should first:

A. rotate your patient so his back is positioned facing the open car door.
B. drag the patient from the seat.
C. apply a cervical collar, and prepare a spinal immobilization device.
D. move the patient's legs so they are clear of the pedals.

3. Once you get the patient out of the vehicle and secured onto a long backboard, what grip should you use to lift the patient?

A. Diamond grip
B. Vice grip
C. Power grip
D. Overhand grip

4. When lifting, you should have your feet approximately __________ inches apart.

A. 12
B. 15
C. 18
D. 24

5. You should use a __________ to carry a patient across uneven terrain from a remote location that is inaccessible by ambulance or other vehicle.

A. long backboard
B. stair chair
C. basket stretcher
D. flexible stretcher

6. There should be a minimum of __________ personnel present to assist in the restraint of a combative patient.

A. 3
B. 4
C. 6
D. 8

Assessment in Action (continued)

7. More than one-half of the patient's weight is distributed to the __________ of the backboard or stretcher.

   A. head end
   B. foot end
   C. middle
   D. Depends on the patient

8. When transporting a geriatric patient, it is important to remember that there are physiologic changes that occur with aging that require special attention on your part as an AEMT. Discuss those changes.

9. To safely lift and carry a patient, each move must be executed in a coordinated manner. How should this be accomplished?

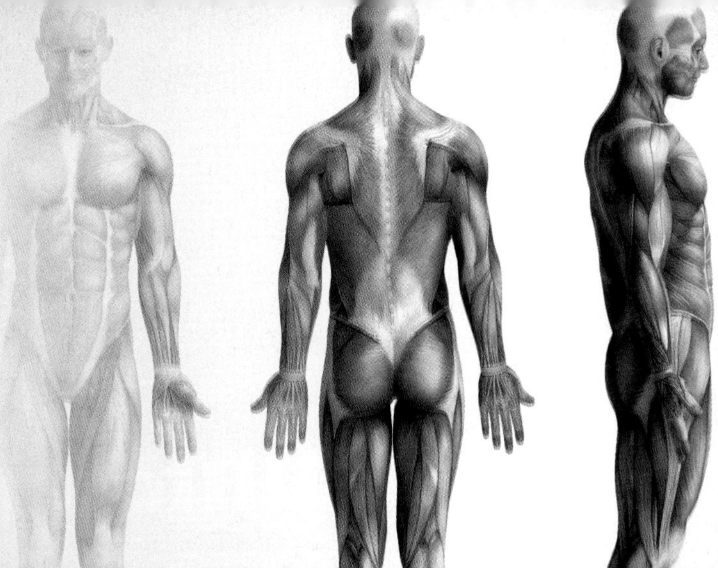

SECTION 2

The Human Body and Human Systems

CHAPTER 7

The Human Body

National EMS Education Standard Competencies

Preparatory

Applies fundamental knowledge of the EMS system, safety/well-being of the AEMT, medical/legal and ethical issues to the provision of emergency care.

Anatomy and Physiology

Integrates complex knowledge of the anatomy and physiology of the airway, respiratory, and circulatory systems to the practice of EMS.

Pathophysiology

Applies comprehensive knowledge of the pathophysiology of respiration and perfusion to patient assessment and management.

Knowledge Objectives

1. Describe the structure of a cell. (p 227)
2. Describe how the structure of a cell membrane relates to movement into and out of the cell. (p 228)
3. Discuss the four steps that make up the life cycle of the cell. (p 230)
4. Describe the process of cellular respiration. (pp 231-232)
5. Compare aerobic to anaerobic processes. (pp 231-232)
6. Discuss cell transport mechanisms, including diffusion, osmosis, facilitated diffusion, active transport, endocytosis, and exocytosis. (pp 232-235)
7. Explain the concept of fluid balance, as well as the purpose and mechanisms for maintaining homeostasis. (pp 235-236)
8. Identify the anatomy and describe the physiology of the skeletal and musculoskeletal systems. (pp 236, 238-252)
9. Discuss the anatomy and physiology of the respiratory system. (pp 253-257)
10. Discuss the concepts of respiration and ventilation. (p 258)
11. Describe the process of gas exchange in the alveoli. (pp 258-259)
12. Explain the brainstem's role in regulating respiration. (pp 258-259)
13. Describe the concept of hypoxic drive. (p 259)
14. Explain how the level of carbon dioxide in the blood and the blood's pH relate to ventilation. (p 261)
15. Discuss the anatomy and physiology of the circulatory system. (pp 263-280)
16. Discuss the concepts of afterload, stroke volume, and cardiac output. (p 268)
17. Discuss the Starling law of the heart. (p 268)
18. Discuss the anatomy and physiology of the nervous system. (pp 280-287)
19. Describe the anatomy and physiology of the integumentary system. (pp 287-289)
20. Explain the anatomy and physiology of the digestive system. (pp 290-293)
21. Discuss the anatomy and physiology of the endocrine system. (pp 293-296)
22. Describe the anatomy and physiology of the urinary system. (p 296)
23. Discuss the anatomy and physiology of the genital system. (pp 297-298)

Skills Objectives

There are no skills objectives for this chapter.

Introduction

The study of **anatomy** is concerned with the structure of an organism and the components that make up the organism, in this case, the human body. Gross anatomy includes body parts that are generally visible to the naked eye—the bones, the muscles, and the organs. Microscopic anatomy involves components of the body that are small, often visible only through a microscope. **Physiology** examines the body functions of the living organism. With general knowledge of the structures and function of the body's systems, you will be able to better assess a patient as well as predict potential complications resulting from occult injuries (those not visible to the eye).

Cells

Cells are the basic functional unit of the body. The cells of the body are extremely varied in their shape and function. Over time cells mature, or differentiate. Through this process of differentiation, cells become specialized to perform a specific function. Cells with a common function are grouped closely together and are called tissues. Groups of tissues that all perform interrelated jobs form organs. A series of organs working together make up the body systems discussed in this chapter.

There are many types of cells (for example, muscle, nerve, kidney, and mucous gland cells) that perform specific functions. All cells, regardless of the type, perform excretion and respiration as part of their cellular functions. Cells communicate electrochemically within themselves, and externally with other cells. This is referred to as cellular signaling.

Cell Structure

The human body contains two general classes of cells. Sex cells (also called germ cells or reproductive cells) are discussed in more detail later in this chapter. Somatic cells (derived from the term *soma*, meaning body) include all the other cells in the human body. This section focuses on somatic cells.

Cells have a cell membrane, a nucleus, and cytoplasm **Figure 7-1**. Structures within the cell organelles are specialized to perform specific functions. The nucleus contains genetic material and controls the activities of the cell.

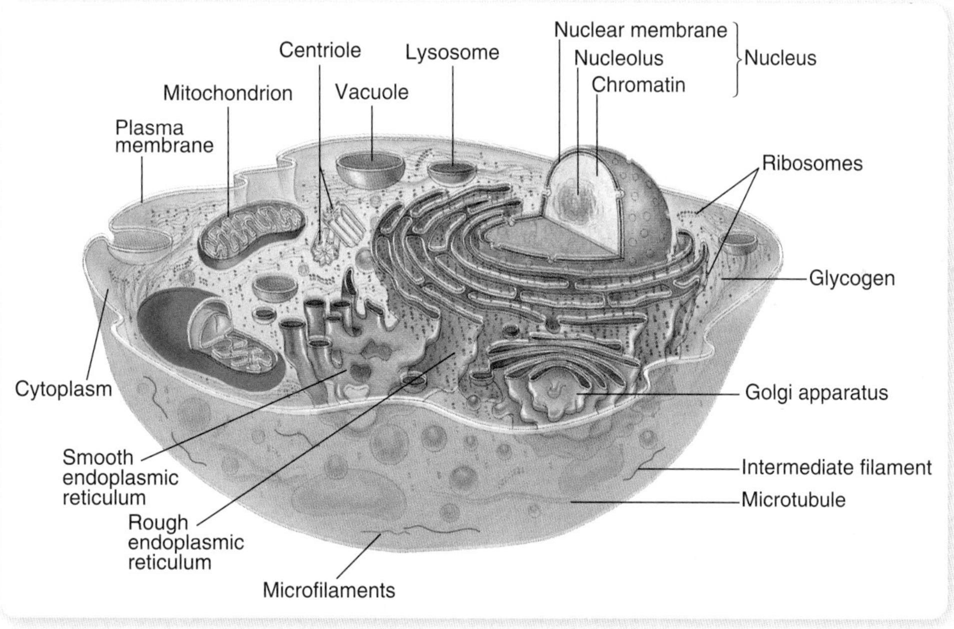

Figure 7-1 Cell structure. The cell is divided into nuclear and cytoplasmic compartments. The cytoplasm is packed with organelles.

YOU are the Provider PART 1

Your ambulance is notified about a shooting at a local apartment complex. As you inform dispatch that you are responding, you are advised that law enforcement is at the scene and the scene is secured. The dispatcher further states that you will have one patient, with multiple gunshot wounds in the chest and abdomen. As you arrive on scene, you find your patient lying left lateral on the ground, covered in blood.

1. How can knowledge of anatomy and physiology help you care for patients?
2. How can knowledge of medical terminology help you care for patients?

▶ Cell Membrane

The **cell membrane**, also called the plasma membrane, contains molecules that form pathways that allow movement into and out of the cell. These pathways allow signals from outside the cell to be detected and transmitted inside. When cells form tissues, the cell membrane assists by adhering the cell to other cells. The terms *intracellular* and *extracellular* refer to inside and outside the membrane, respectively.

The cell membrane is extremely thin and delicate, able to stretch to differing degrees. Tiny folds on the surface help the cell to increase its surface area. The cell membrane is composed of a bilayer (two layers), containing phosphate and fat molecules called phospholipids. This double layer of phospholipid molecules allows substances such as oxygen and carbon dioxide to easily pass through, while other substances cannot Figure 7-2. This means it is **semipermeable**; it allows certain elements to pass through while not allowing others to do so. In some instances, and often depending on various factors, only certain substances can enter or leave each cell (a condition known as selective permeability).

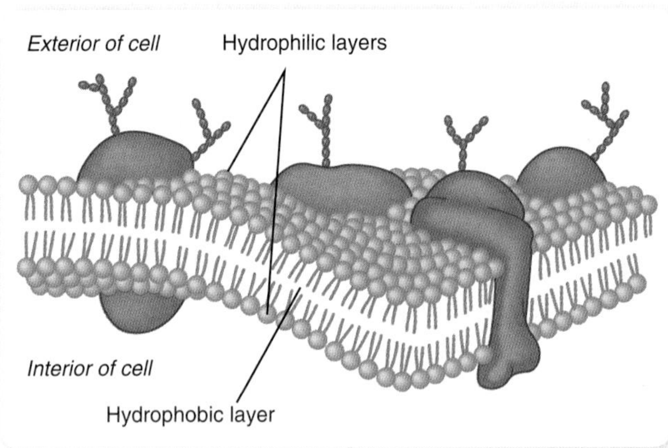

Figure 7-2 The phospholipid bilayer.

The cell membrane also has several proteins, classified as shown in Table 7-1.

▶ Cytoplasm

The cytoplasm is the fluid-like material in which the contents of the cell are contained. Cytoplasm usually appears clear with scattered specks, although more powerful magnification reveals that it contains membranous networks, protein frameworks, and a cytoskeleton (cell skeleton).

Cytosol, which is the fluid portion of cytoplasm, contains mostly water, as well as glucose, amino acids, fatty acids, ions, lipids, proteins, **adenosine triphosphate (ATP)**, and waste products. Many of the chemical reactions necessary for life, including glycolysis, take place within the cytoplasm.

▶ Organelles

The organelles within the cytoplasm perform specific functions. Each organelle accomplishes tasks related to cell structure, growth, maintenance, and metabolism. The following organelles have specific actions that help the cell to carry out its activities:

- **Centrioles.** Cell division requires a pair of centrioles, which are cylindrical structures made up of short microtubules. During cell division, the centrioles form the spindle-shaped structure needed for movement of deoxyribonucleic acid (DNA) strands. Cardiac muscle cells, skeletal muscle cells, mature red blood cells (RBCs), and typical neurons (nerve cells) have no centrioles; therefore, these cells are incapable of dividing. The centrosome is the cytoplasm surrounding the centrioles. Microtubules of the cytoskeleton usually begin at the centrosome and radiate through the cytoplasm.
- **Cilia and flagella.** These structures extend from certain cell surfaces. Cilia are hairlike structures, moving in a coordinated sweeping motion to

Table 7-1 Cell Membrane Proteins

Type of Membrane Protein	Description
Channel proteins	Allow passive passage into intracellular compartment. Some are gated ion channels, which open and close at specific times and only allow specific substances to pass.
Enzyme receptors	Act as sites where enzymes can bind (occurs inside the cell); enzyme acts as a catalyst for a reaction.
Proteins that act as receptor sites	Binding site on outside of cell membrane; specific to certain molecules; binding causes a change in cellular function.
Identifier proteins	Identify cell as part of a particular organism; used by the immune system to determine "self" from "nonself."
Carrier proteins	Bind to substances and transport them across the cell membrane.

move fluids over the surface of tissues. They are found on cells lining both the respiratory and reproductive tracts. The cells that line the respiratory tract have many cilia to move particles out of the airway. Flagella, which are longer than cilia, propel the cells to which they are attached. In humans, a flagellum appears as the tail of a sperm cell.

- **Ribosomes.** Ribosomes are composed of protein and ribonucleic acid (RNA). Ribosomes may be found either floating freely within the cytoplasm or attached to the endoplasmic reticulum (ER). Because their functions involve the formation of proteins, they are called the protein factories of the cell.
- **Endoplasmic reticulum.** The ER is a network of paths through which substances and proteins move. It is connected to the nuclear membrane and to the cell membrane. There are two types of ER: smooth and rough **Figure 7-3**. The smooth ER lacks ribosomes and it can synthesize phospholipids and cholesterol, which are needed for the growth and maintenance of the cell membrane. The rough ER has ribosomes on its surface. Both free and fixed ribosomes synthesize proteins via instructions from messenger RNA.

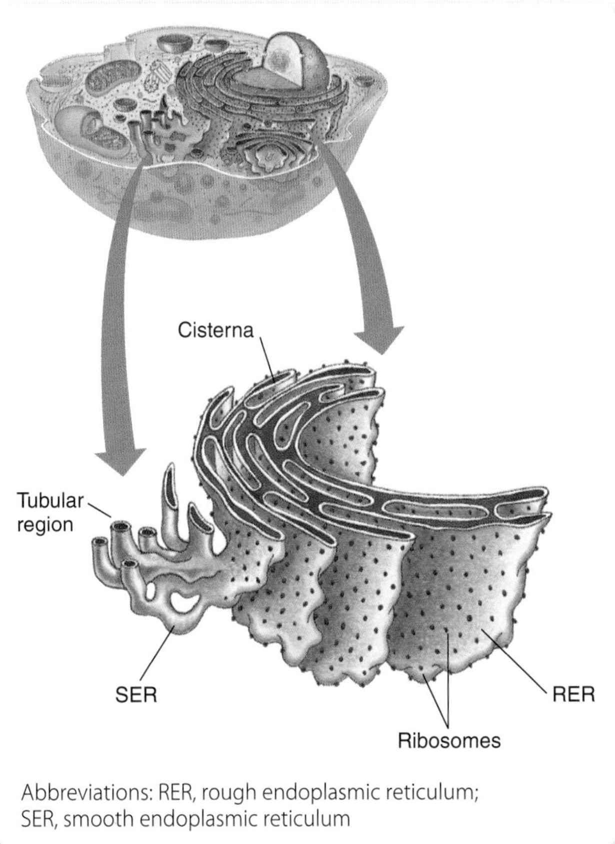

Figure 7-3 Rough endoplasmic reticulum with fixed ribosomes on its outer surface.

- **Golgi apparatus.** This organelle, also called the Golgi complex, consists of a stack of several flattened sacs. These pancakelike structures are hollow, with cavities called cisternae inside them. The Golgi apparatus deals primarily with proteins synthesized on the ribosomes. The end of the Golgi apparatus is specialized to receive glycoproteins, modifying them by removing or adding sugar molecules. The Golgi apparatus has three main functions: (1) concentrating and packaging secretions (such as hormones or enzymes) that are released for secretion out of the cell, (2) packaging special enzymes inside vesicles for use in the cytosol, and (3) renewing or modifying the cell membrane.
- **Lysosomes.** These tiny sacs dispose of cell wastes using enzymes to break down nutrients and foreign particles (such as bacteria). They also destroy older, worn-out parts of the cell. This breakdown process requires the use of powerful enzymes. It often generates toxic chemicals capable of damaging or killing the cell. Lysosomes are specialized vesicles that provide an isolated environment for potentially dangerous chemical reactions. They are produced close to the Golgi apparatus and contain digestive enzymes.
- **Microfilaments.** The smallest of the cytoskeletal elements, microfilaments are composed of the proteins actin and myosin. They are typically found in muscle cells. Microfilaments provide cell movement and contraction via interaction with actin and myosin. This process can also change the shape of the entire cell.
- **Mitochondria.** All cells in the body, except for mature RBCs, have between 100 and a few thousand organelles called mitochondria (singularly called a mitochondrion). Mitochondria have double membranes that play the central role in the production of energy (via ATP). The number of mitochondria in a particular cell varies, based on the cell's energy demands; mitochondria are the "powerhouses" of cells. The liver, kidneys, and muscles have a large number of mitochondria in their cells because they use ATP at a high rate.

  A mitochondrion is surrounded by two membranes similar in structure to the plasma membrane. The outer mitochondrial membrane is smooth. The inner mitochondrial membrane has a series of folds called cristae. The central fluid-filled cavity is called the matrix and is enclosed by the inner membrane and cristae.

  Mitochondria can migrate through the cytoplasm of a cell and are able to reproduce themselves. Mitochondria contain their own DNA, but in a more primitive form than that found within the cell nucleus.

- **Peroxisomes.** These sacs have enzymes that speed up many biochemical reactions. They are abundant in the liver and kidney cells, and their diverse actions include the synthesis of bile acids, detoxification of hydrogen peroxide or alcohol, and breakdown of lipids and biochemicals.
- **Thick filaments.** These organelles are relatively massive bundles of subunits composed of the protein myosin. Thick filaments appear in muscle cells only, where they interact with actin filaments to produce powerful contractions.
- **Vesicles.** Also known as vacuoles, these sacs are formed when a part of a cell membrane folds inward, establishing a bubble-like structure within the cytoplasm. Vesicles contain various liquid or solid materials that formerly existed outside of the cell membrane.

Nucleus

The nucleus is the largest structure in the cell. It serves as the control center and is located in the middle. It contains DNA, or genetic material, that controls cell activities. A single nucleus stores all required information that directs the synthesis of the 100,000 proteins in the human body. A cell without a nucleus cannot repair itself. It will disintegrate within 3 to 4 months. The nucleus contains the genetic instructions needed to synthesize the proteins that determine cell structures and functions. These instructions are stored in the **chromosomes**. These structures consist of DNA and various proteins that control and access genetic information. Most cells contain a single nucleus, with the exception of skeletal muscle cells (with numerous nuclei) and mature RBCs (with no nuclei).

The nucleus of a cell is usually round and is enclosed in a double nuclear envelope, with inner and outer lipid membranes. This envelope also has a protein lining, allowing certain molecules to exit the nucleus. Inside the nucleus is a fluid called nucleoplasm that suspends the following structures:

- **Nucleolus.** A "mini nucleus" made up mostly of RNA and protein molecules, with no surrounding membrane. Ribosomes form in the nucleolus and migrate out to the cell's cytoplasm.
- **Chromatin.** Loosely coiled DNA and protein fibers that condense, forming chromosomes. The DNA controls protein synthesis, and when the cell starts to divide, the chromatin fibers coil tightly to form the chromosomes.

Life Cycle of the Cell

The life cycle of the cell is regulated via stimulation from hormones or growth factors. Disruption of the cycle can affect the health of the body. Most human cells divide between 40 to 60 times before they die. The life cycle of a cell includes the following four steps:

1. **Interphase.** The cell obtains nutrients to grow and duplicate.
2. **Cell division (mitosis).** The nucleus divides.
3. **Cytoplasmic division (cytokinesis).** The cytoplasm divides.
4. **Differentiation.** The cell becomes specialized.

Interphase

A cell must grow and duplicate most of its contents before it can actively divide. *Interphase* describes this period of preparation to divide. During interphase, the cell manufactures new living material by duplicating membranes, lysosomes, mitochondria, and ribosomes. The cell also replicates its own genetic material.

Cell Division and Cytoplasmic Division

The two types of cell division are meiosis and mitosis/cytokinesis. **Meiosis**, which occurs in the production of eggs (oocytes) and sperm, reduces the number of chromosomes by one-half, from 46 to 23. When a sperm and egg unite, the resulting fertilized egg will have a total of 46 chromosomes.

In the rest of the body, cell numbers are increased by mitosis, the division of the nucleus of a cell, and cytokinesis, the division of the cytoplasm of a cell. During mitosis, a cell duplicates itself into daughter cells—identical copies of the original cell. The nucleus must divide precisely so an accurate copy of the DNA can be made by the new cell. Most of the cells of the human body, except for sex cells and RBCs, reproduce by mitosis.

Cytoplasmic division (cytokinesis) begins during the second phase of mitosis, when the cell membrane constricts down the middle portion of the cell. This process continues through the fourth phase to divide the cytoplasm. The two newly formed nuclei are then separated and nearly one-half of the organelles are distributed into each new cell.

Differentiation

Differentiation, the process of specialization of a cell, makes each cell unique. New cells must be generated for growth and tissue repair to occur. A **stem cell** can divide repeatedly without specializing. Stem cells can either divide into two identical daughter cells or divide so that one daughter cell becomes partially specialized (progenitor cells). In the human body, all differentiated cell types are created because of the variance of stem and progenitor cells. Researchers are exploring the use of stem cells in the treatment of disease.

Cell Division and Cancer

Cell division and growth normally occur at approximately the same rate as cell death. However, when cell division and growth occur at a higher rate than the cell death rate, tissues enlarge. A **neoplasm** (tumor) is a mass of tissue produced by abnormal cell growth and division. A tumor is *benign* when it remains within the epithelium (a capsule made of connective tissue). A benign tumor seldom becomes life threatening and can usually be surgically removed if it affects tissue function.

In contrast, a *malignant* tumor spreads into surrounding tissues in a process called invasion. The tumor of origin (the primary tumor or primary neoplasm) may result in malignant cells traveling to other organs or tissue to establish secondary tumors. This process, called metastasis, is not easily controlled: cancer develops and exhibits mutations disrupting normal cell growth. Usually, all tumor cells are daughter cells of just one malignant cell. Malignancy often occurs when a normal gene mutates. These modified genes are called oncogenes. Cancer often begins where stem cells divide. This is because there is a greater chance of error the more frequently that chromosomes are copied for cell division.

Cancer cells change shape as they grow and gradually resemble normal cells less and less. If tumor cells penetrate blood vessels, then they circulate throughout the body. If tumor cells enter the lymphatic system, then they build up in lymph nodes. The presence of tumor cells stimulates the growth of new blood vessels where the cells situate themselves, which supplies them with more nutrients and accelerates their growth and further metastasis.

As metastasis increases, organ function changes. Cancer cells grow and multiply by taking nutrients and space from normal cells, causing weight loss in most patients with cancer as the normal cells deteriorate. Death may occur when cancer cells compress vital organs or replace healthy cells in vital organs.

Cellular Respiration

Cells use glucose and oxygen to release energy from organic compounds in a process called **cellular respiration**. This process requires three types of reactions: glycolysis, the Krebs cycle, and the electron transport chain. The result of cellular respiration is carbon dioxide (co_2), water (H_2O), and the high-energy molecule ATP. Energy is released from ATP when bonds between phosphate molecules (that are part of the ATP molecule) break to release their stored energy.

Glycolysis

Glycolysis, which occurs in the cytosol of the cytoplasm, is a process that involves a series of enzymatically catalyzed reactions in which glucose is broken down to yield lactic acid and pyruvic acid Figure 7-4. Glucose is broken down into 2 three-carbon pyruvic acid molecules, gaining two ATP molecules and releasing high-energy electrons. Glycolysis does not require oxygen and therefore is referred to as an **anaerobic** process.

If oxygen is present in the right amounts, pyruvic acid can enter the more energy-efficient pathways of aerobic

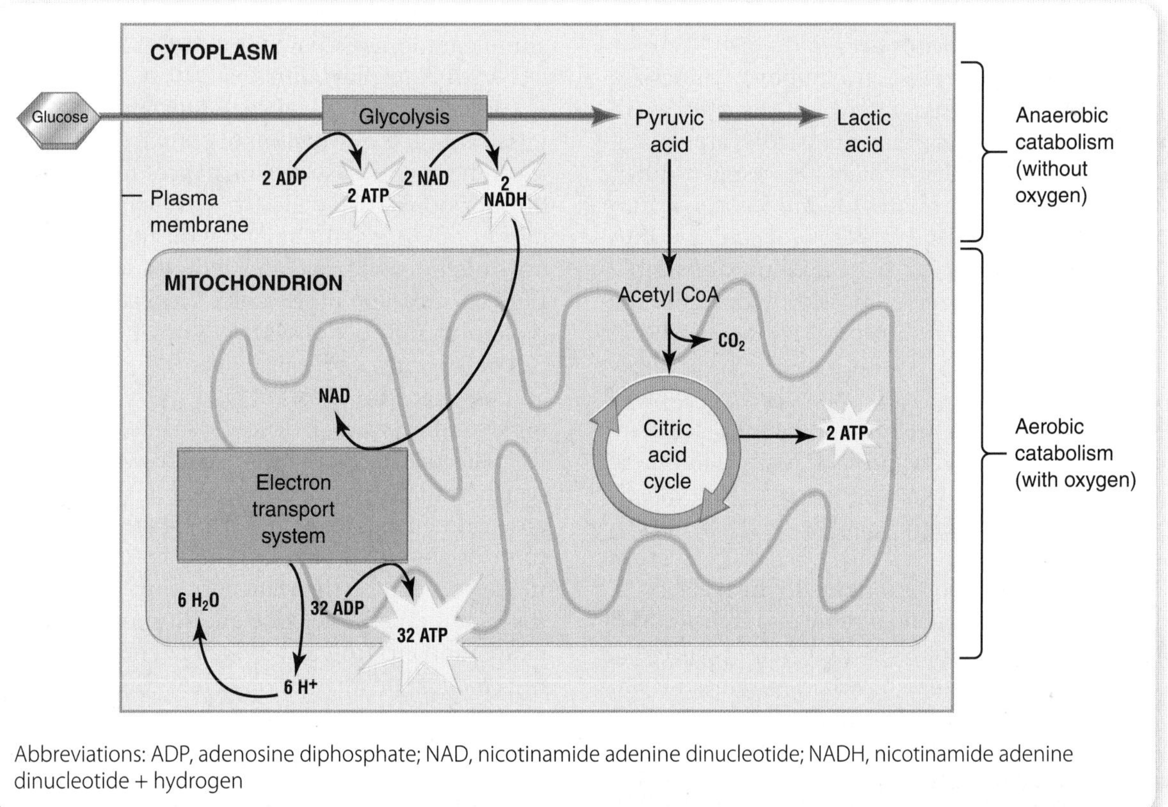

Abbreviations: ADP, adenosine diphosphate; NAD, nicotinamide adenine dinucleotide; NADH, nicotinamide adenine dinucleotide + hydrogen

Figure 7-4 During anaerobic metabolism, which occurs in the cytoplasm, the breakdown of glucose results in lactic acid. During aerobic metabolism, which occurs in the mitochondrion, the breakdown of glucose results in carbon dioxide, water, and adenosine triphosphate.

respiration. These pathways are located in the mitochondria. Aerobic reactions yield as many as 36 ATP molecules per glucose molecule. Most result from the aerobic phase, with only two resulting from glycolysis. Approximately one-half of the released energy is used for ATP synthesis, while the rest becomes heat.

Words of Wisdom

When not enough oxygen is available, respiration can occur in the form of anaerobic respiration. In this scenario, pyruvic acid converts to lactic acid. This can result in lactic acidosis. Pyruvic acid is created from lactic acid when oxygen is present.

▶ Krebs Cycle

The Krebs cycle, also called the citric acid cycle or tricarboxylic acid cycle is an **aerobic** process. It is a sequence of enzymatic reactions involving the metabolism of carbon chains of glucose, fatty acids, and amino acids to yield carbon dioxide, water, and high-energy phosphate bonds (ATP). It is important to note that this stage is an aerobic process; the Krebs cycle occurs in the presence of oxygen. The three-carbon pyruvic acids enter the mitochondria, each losing a carbon atom. The molecules then combine with a coenzyme to form a two-carbon acetyl coenzyme A and release more high-energy electrons. Each acetyl coenzyme A combines with a four-carbon oxaloacetic acid to form a six-carbon citric acid.

A series of reactions removes two carbons, synthesizes one ATP molecule, and releases more high-energy electrons. When food is ingested, large macromolecules are broken down to simple molecules. Proteins are broken down into amino acids, carbohydrates are broken down into simple sugars (glucose), and fats are broken down into both glycerol and fatty acids. The breakdown of simple molecules to acetyl coenzyme A is accompanied by the production of limited amounts of ATP (via glycolysis) and high-energy electrons.

As already discussed, glucose was converted to pyruvic acid during glycolysis. Glycerol and amino acids are also broken down into pyruvic acid. Actually, all of these processes result, in differing ways, in acetyl coenzyme A. Complete oxidation of acetyl coenzyme A to H_2O and CO_2 produces high-energy electrons, which yield greater amounts of ATP via the electron transport chain. In the Krebs cycle, the process of oxidation provides more molecules of ATP.

After glycolysis and the Krebs cycle have occurred, a total of four molecules of ATP have been produced—two from glycolysis and two from the Krebs cycle.

When oxygen is absent, respiration can still occur via an anaerobic process. In this case, glycolysis occurs, but since oxygen is absent, pyruvic acid converts to lactic acid. Anaerobic processes can ultimately lead to lactic acidosis if they occur in excess. Lactic acidosis can develop with shock due to insufficient oxygen.

▶ Electron Transport Chain

In this last step, 34 molecules of ATP are produced in an aerobic process. High-energy electrons still contain most of the chemical energy of the original glucose molecule. Special carrier molecules bring them to enzymes that store most of the remaining energy in more ATP molecules; heat and water are also produced. Oxygen is the final electron acceptor in this step; therefore, the overall process is termed aerobic respiration.

For cellular respiration, glucose and oxygen are required. This process produces carbon dioxide, water, and energy. Nearly one-half of the energy is recaptured as high-energy electrons stored in the cells through the synthesis of ATP.

Each ATP molecule has a chain of three chemical groups. These groups are called phosphates. Some of the energy is recaptured in the bond of the end phosphate. When energy is later needed, the terminal phosphate bond breaks to release the stored energy. Cells use ATP for many functions, including active transport and the synthesis of needed compounds.

The end result of glycolysis, the Krebs cycle, and the electron transport chain is 38 molecules of ATP.

Cellular Transport Mechanisms

Cellular transport mechanisms refer to how materials enter and exit the cell. Such movement relates to fluid administration, discussed in Chapter 13, *Vascular Access and Medication Administration*.

Each body compartment is separated by a membrane. Recall that the cell membrane is selectively permeable, meaning it allows some substances to pass through it, but not others. This selective permeability helps maintain homeostasis, the maintenance of a stable internal physiologic environment including a stable temperature, fluid balance, and pH balance. Various enzymes, glucose molecules, and electrolytes freely pass in and out of the cell. **Electrolytes** are chemicals that are dissolved in the blood and are made up of salt or acid substances that become ionic conductors when dissolved in a solvent such as water.

Selective permeability also allows for differences in concentrations between intracellular and extracellular environments. (Normally, if there are unequal concentrations on either side of a cell membrane, they will move to balance the concentration on both sides of the membrane.) The concentration of the compounds (water and electrolytes) as well as the concentration of the charges (positive or negative) carried on the atoms determines movement, and the natural tendency is to move from an area of higher concentration to an area of lower concentration. The difference in concentrations of a substance on either side of the cell membrane is called the **concentration gradient**. The cell membrane plays an important role in the flow down a concentration gradient; it determines whether materials are allowed to pass through. Several mechanisms, such as diffusion, osmosis, facilitated diffusion, active transport, endocytosis, and exocytosis, allow material to pass through the cell wall.

▶ Diffusion

Diffusion is the passive movement of a **solute** (a particle such as salt that is dissolved in a solvent) moving from an area of higher concentration to an area of lower concentration until an even distribution of particles is achieved Figure 7-5. Small molecules diffuse more easily than large ones. Watery solutions diffuse more rapidly than thicker, viscous solutions. Many of the cell's nutrients enter the cell by diffusion. Oxygen and carbon dioxide are examples of substances that can move by diffusion.

To visualize diffusion, imagine that too many people show up for a theater performance. The theater manager decides to open another seating area to accommodate the crowd. Patrons (charges or compounds) are concentrated in a small area (the cell) outside the door (the cell membrane) leading to the new seating area. When the theater manager opens the door, patrons can move through it (selective cell membrane permeability) from the congested area (down a concentration gradient). The patrons spread themselves out evenly (diffuse) throughout the total area, with some choosing to stay behind in the original seating area as others move into the new area, until all patrons have an equal amount of room.

Diffusion in the lungs and pulmonary vasculature occurs as the capillaries that surround the alveoli, which contain a high content of oxygen, circulate blood that is high in carbon dioxide. Carbon dioxide leaves the blood and moves into the alveoli while oxygen moves in the opposite direction, from the alveoli into the blood, until the concentrations of each are equal on either side of the membrane. For this reason, the amount of carbon dioxide that remains in the arterial blood is almost equal to the amount of carbon dioxide that is exhaled.

▶ Filtration

Another method for moving substances is **filtration**. The kidneys essentially filter compounds from the blood; water containing dissolved compounds enters the tubules of the kidney and then continues on while the dissolved compounds remain behind. The end result is that wastes have been removed from the blood (and thereby, from the body) and are excreted in the urine.

▶ Facilitated Diffusion

Facilitated diffusion is the process in which a carrier molecule moves substances in or out of cells from areas of high concentration to areas of lower concentration Figure 7-6. Energy is not required; the number of molecules transported is directly proportional to the amount of concentration. An example of a substance that enters the cell by facilitated diffusion is glucose. The hormone insulin is required to move glucose into the cells.

Active transport is the movement of a substance against a concentration or gradient such as the cell membrane, opposite the normal movement of diffusion; substances move toward the side with a higher concentration. Active transport requires energy as well as some type of carrier mechanism. At times, the active transport mechanism may exchange one substance for another.

Endocytosis and exocytosis are processes that use energy from the cell to move substances into or out of the cell without crossing the cell membrane. In endocytosis, a secretion from the cell membrane moves particles too large to enter the cell by other processes within a vesicle of the cell. The three forms of endocytosis are pinocytosis, phagocytosis, and receptor-mediated endocytosis. Pinocytosis ("cell drinking") involves cells taking in small liquid droplets from the surrounding cell environment with a small indentation of the cell membrane. Phagocytosis ("cell eating") involves cells taking in solids instead of liquids, by engulfing the foreign particle. Receptor-mediated endocytosis involves the movement of specific kinds of particles into the cell, with protein molecules extending through part of the cell membrane to the outer surface. The opposite process to endocytosis is exocytosis, in which a substance stored in a vesicle is secreted from the cell.

An example is the cell's transport of sodium and potassium across the membrane. The cell allows two potassium ions to enter the cell while three sodium ions exit (this is called the sodium/potassium pump). If there is an inadequate amount of potassium present, sodium will not be transported as needed, leading to swelling and potential rupture.

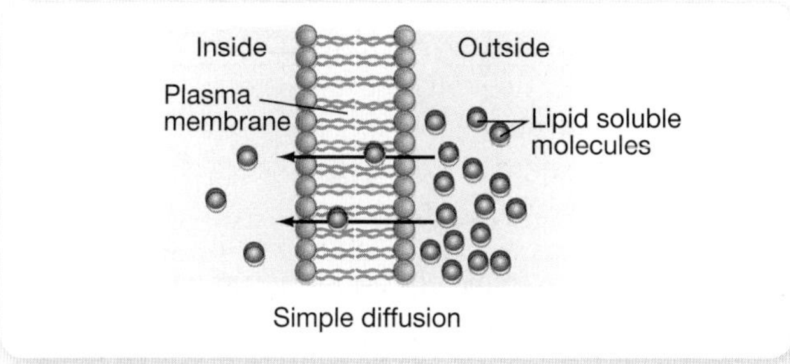

Figure 7-5 Diffusion.

Words of Wisdom

Think of sitting in a rowboat in a strong current. As long as you wish to go in the direction the current is flowing, no energy is exerted. If you wish to go against the current, you must expend energy to row against the current. This energy expenditure is similar to active transport—you must expend energy to move against the concentration gradient.

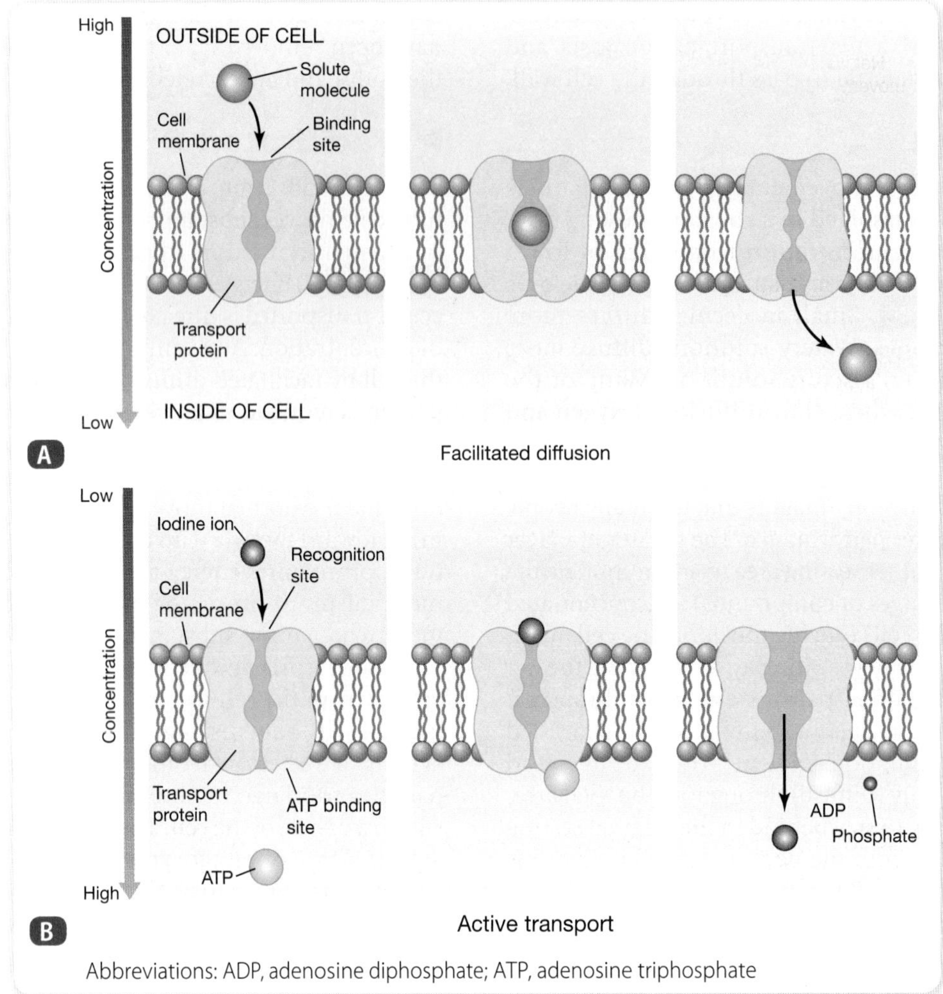

Figure 7-6 A. Facilitated diffusion involves particles moving from an area of higher concentration toward an area of lower concentration with the assistance of a protein. **B.** Active transport uses energy from adenosine triphosphate to open a pathway for compounds to move against a concentration gradient.

▶ Osmosis

Osmosis is the passive movement of a solvent, or liquid, from an area of low solute concentration to one of high concentration through a selectively permeable membrane. The membrane is permeable to the solvent but not to the solute. Movement generally continues until the concentrations of the solute equalize on both sides of the membrane **Figure 7-7**. **Osmotic pressure** is a measure of the tendency of water to move by osmosis across a membrane. The osmotic pressure of a solution, or the ability to affect the movement of water, is osmolality.

The concentration of a solution, or ability to draw or give water, is its *tonicity* **Figure 7-8**. A solution with a higher solute concentration compared with another solution is **hypertonic**, and a solution with a lower solute concentration is **hypotonic**. An **isotonic** solution is one in which there is an equal concentration of solutes and liquid on either side of the membrane. If too much water moves out of a cell, then the cell shrinks abnormally, a process known as **crenation**. If too much water enters a cell, then it will swell and burst, a process known as **lysis**.

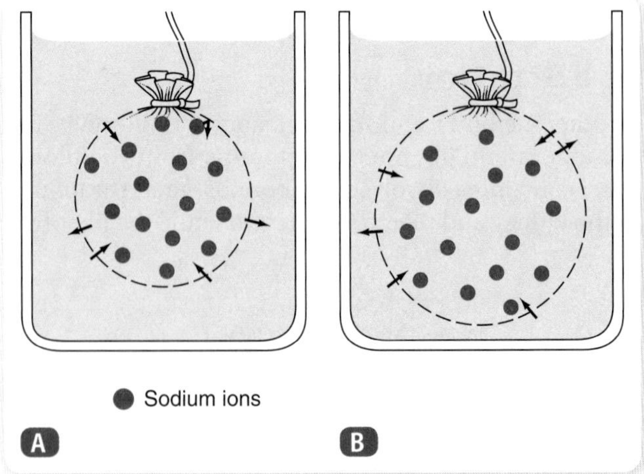

Figure 7-7 A. An example of osmosis occurs when a permeable bag of salt water is immersed in a solution of pure water. **B.** Water moves into the bag (toward the area with lower water concentration) equalizing the concentrations on each side of the membrane.

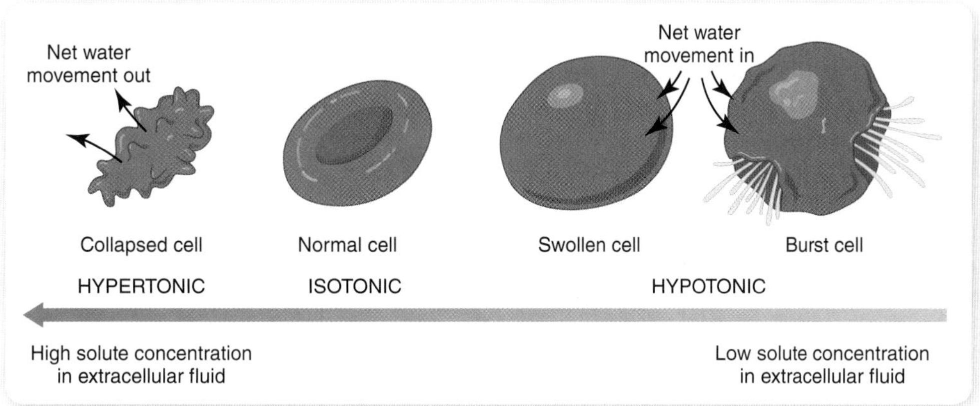

Figure 7-8 Tonicity.

Body Fluid Balance

The total body water content of the average adult ranges from 50% to 70% of total body weight, depending on age and sex. A newborn's total body water content may be as high as 75% to 80% of total body weight.

Body fluid is divided into two main compartments: intracellular fluid and extracellular fluid. **Intracellular fluid (ICF)** exists within individual cells and equals approximately 40% to 45% of total body weight. The ICF makes up approximately 75% of all body fluid. **Extracellular fluid (ECF)** exists outside of the cell membranes. It equals approximately 15% to 20% of the total body weight, or 25% of all body fluid. ECF is further divided into intravascular fluid and interstitial fluid. **Intravascular fluid (plasma)**, the fluid portion of blood, is found within the blood vessels and accounts for approximately 4.5% of total body weight. **Interstitial fluid** is located outside of the blood vessels, in the spaces between the body's cells. It accounts for approximately 10.5% of total body weight. There is a delicate balance among the various fluid compartments of the body that is essential to maintain homeostasis.

If fluid is lost from anywhere in the body, there can be serious ramifications because this disturbs the balance among various fluid compartments (homeostasis). The result can be shock. Under normal conditions, the total volume of water in the body and its distribution in the body compartments remain relatively constant, even though there are fluctuations in the amount of water that enters and is excreted from the body each day. **Fluid balance** is the process of maintaining homeostasis through equal intake (water taken into the body) and output (water excreted from the body) of fluids.

There are mechanisms in the body that maintain the balance between what is taken in and what is excreted **Table 7-2**. For example, when the fluid volume drops, the pituitary gland secretes antidiuretic hormone (ADH) **Figure 7-9**. ADH causes the kidney tubules to reabsorb more water into the blood and excrete less urine, allowing

Table 7-2 Major Mechanisms for Fluid Homeostasis
• Antidiuretic hormone
• Thirst
• Kidneys
• Water shifts

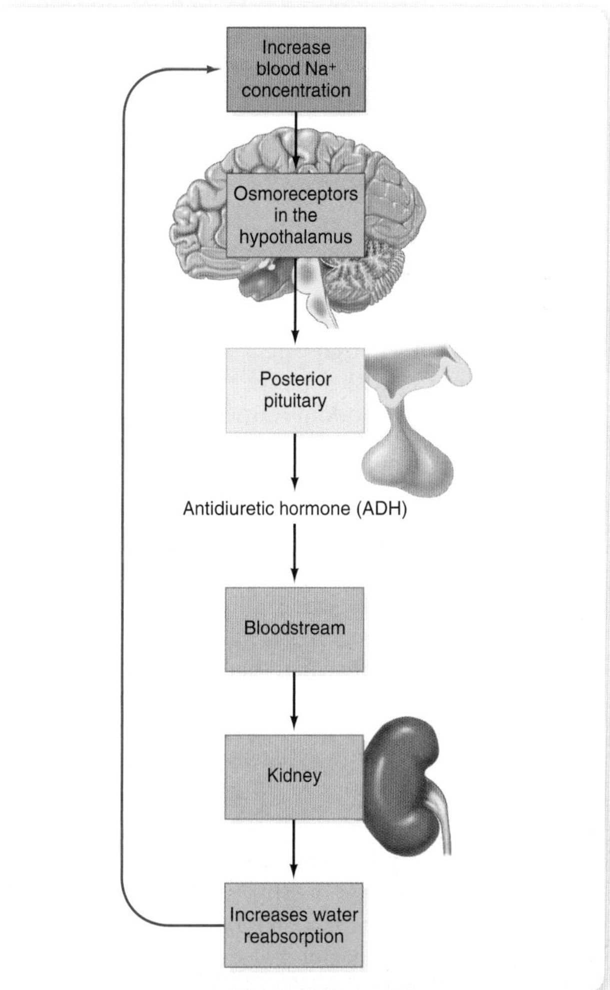

Figure 7-9 The role of antidiuretic hormone in regulating fluid levels.

fluid volume in the body to build up. Thirst also regulates fluid intake. The sensation of thirst occurs when body fluids become decreased, stimulating a person to take in more fluids. Conversely, when too many fluids enter the body, thirst decreases, the kidneys are activated, and more urine is excreted, eliminating the excess fluid.

It is important to maintain the proper balance of fluids and electrolytes within the body, because this is necessary for life. A person's body can become depleted of fluids and electrolytes for several reasons, including severe burns or dehydration. The body can maintain fluid balance by shifting water from one compartment to another. Water moves in response to osmotic forces as well as hormonal stimuli such as ADH. For a patient whose fluids or electrolytes are depleted, rapid restoration of fluid balance may mean the difference between life and death.

Organ Systems

An organ is composed of at least two kinds of tissue that are organized to perform a more complex task than a single tissue can. An organ system is composed of at least two kinds of organs that, again, are organized to perform a more complex task than a single organ can. The 12 major organ systems of the body include the integumentary, skeletal, muscular, nervous, endocrine, circulatory, lymphatic, immune, respiratory, digestive, urinary, and reproductive systems Figure 7-10. All of these except the lymphatic system are shown in the figure.

The Skeletal System: Anatomy

The **skeleton** gives us our recognizable human form and protects our vital internal organs. Bones constitute the major structure of the skeletal system. Cartilage, tendons, and ligaments are important connective tissues that work with bones to provide the support framework of the skeleton Table 7-3.

A **tendon** is a specialized tough cord or band of dense white connective tissue that connects muscle to bone. A **ligament** is a tough white band of tissue that connects bones to each other. Tendons and ligaments are composed of densely packed fibers of collagen, a twisted ropelike protein. A sprain occurs when the bone ends partially or temporarily dislocates and the supporting ligaments are partially stretched or torn.

When a muscle contracts, tendon pulls on bone, resulting in motion at the joint, the point where two or more bones come together, allowing movement to occur. A strain, or muscle pull, occurs when a muscle is stretched or torn. A strain results in pain, swelling, and bruising of surrounding soft tissues. No ligament or joint damage occurs with a strain. Sprains and strains are graded based on their severity and physical findings during examination.

Shiny connective tissue called **cartilage** is lubricated by a transparent viscous (thick) joint fluid (synovial fluid). It receives nutrients through diffusion from the outer covering of the cartilage or from the synovial fluid.

Bones

Bones are classified according to their shape, as long bones, short bones, or flat bones. Long bones include the femur, tibia, fibula, ulna, radius, and humerus. Short bones include the bones of the wrist and of the ankle. Flat bones include certain skull bones, ribs, the sternum, and the scapulae. There are also irregular bones, which have unique shapes and are designed to perform a specific function. These bones include the mandible, many facial bones, and those that make up the vertebrae in the spine and pelvis.

Long bones consist of a shaft, the diaphysis; the ends, or **epiphyses**; and the growth plate or epiphyseal plate (the physis), which is the major site of bone elongation Figure 7-11. The epiphyseal plate is located just proximal to the epiphysis. The **periosteum**, which consists of a double layer of connective tissue, lines the outer surface of the bone, and the inner surfaces are lined with **endosteum**.

Special Populations

Fractures are more common in older people because of a decrease in bone mineral density. The result is weaker bones.

Words of Wisdom

Dysfunction or suppression of the bone marrow may develop in people who have adverse reactions to certain drugs, such as nonsteroidal anti-inflammatory drugs (NSAIDs), or who receive chemotherapy treatments for cancer. Use of chemotherapy and NSAIDs can result in anemia caused by a decrease in the number of RBCs produced by the marrow, increased susceptibility to infection caused by a decrease in the number of infection-fighting white blood cells (WBCs), and a tendency for internal or external bleeding caused by a decrease in the number of platelets (blood-clotting cells).

The diaphysis of many bones includes the **medullary cavity**, an internal cavity that contains a substance known as **bone marrow**. In adults, most bone marrow in the long bones in the extremities contains adipose (fat) tissue and is, therefore, called yellow marrow. The bones of the axial skeleton and girdles contain red marrow, where most RBCs are manufactured.

The two main types of bone are compact bone and cancellous bone. Compact bone is mostly solid, with few spaces; **cancellous bone** consists of a lacy network of bony rods called **trabeculae**. The trabeculae are oriented along the lines of stress to increase the weight-bearing capacity of the long bones.

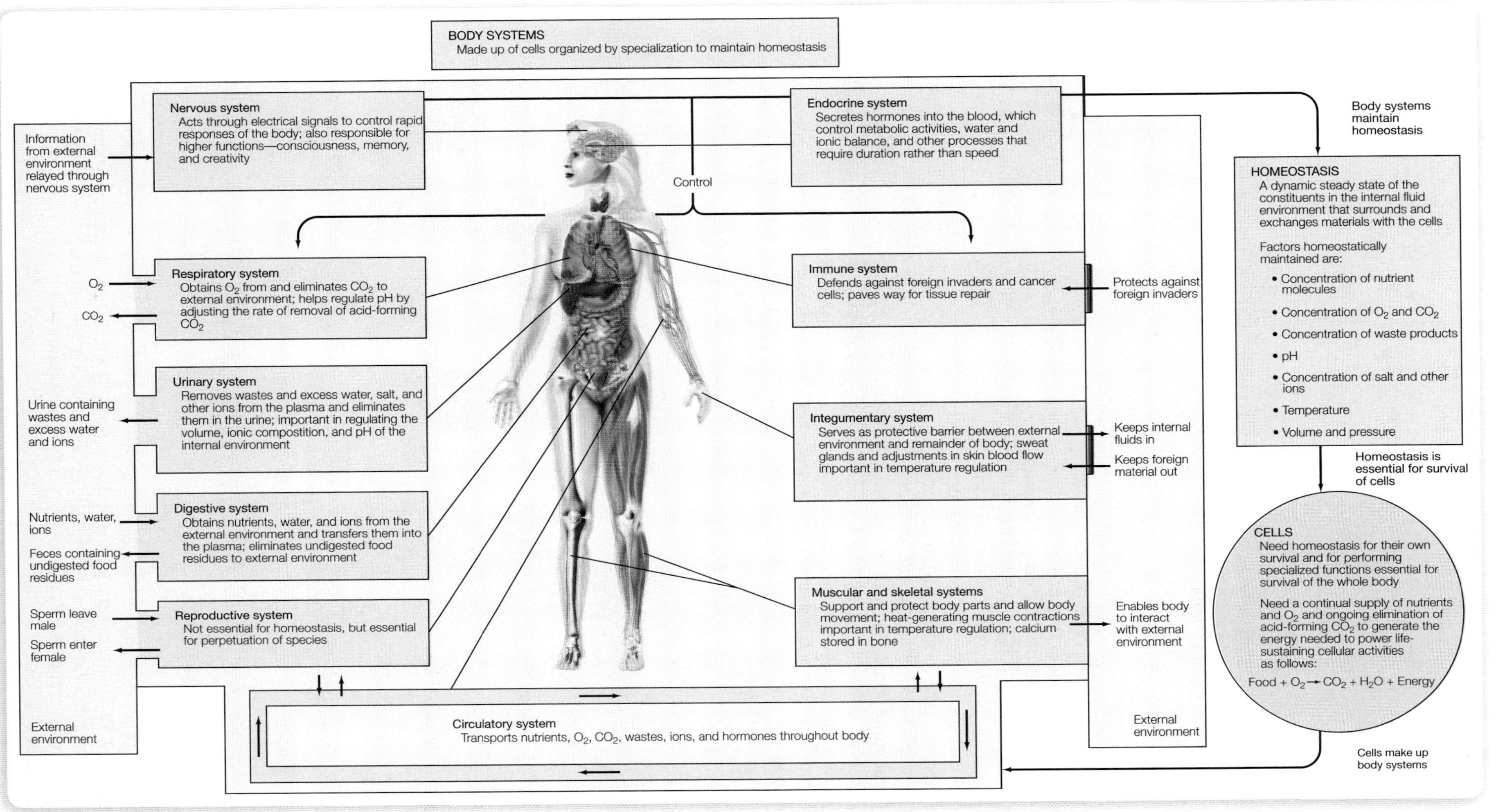

Figure 7-10 Systems of the body.

Table 7-3 Support Structures Within the Skeletal System

Name	Function
Ligament	Connects bone to bone
Tendon	Connects muscle to bone
Cartilage	Cushion between bones

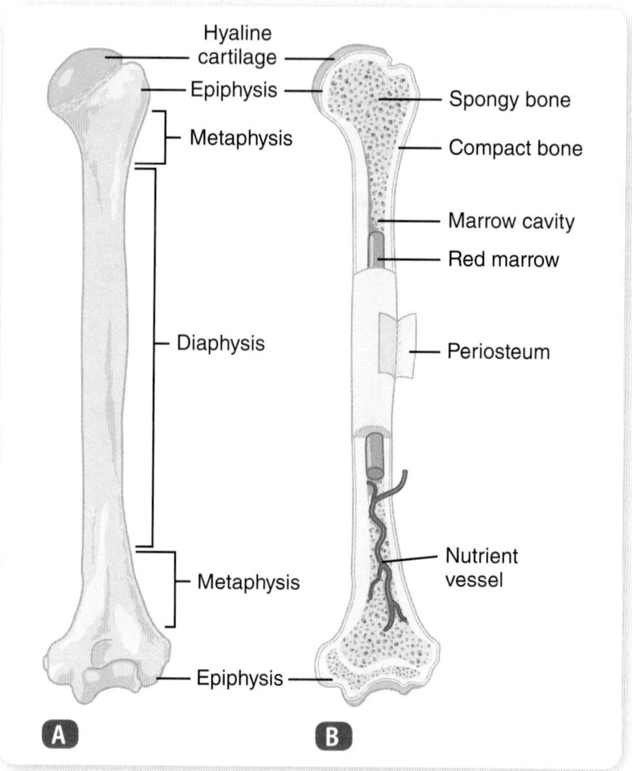

Figure 7-11 The components of the long bone. **A.** Drawing of the humerus. Notice the long shaft and dilated ends. **B.** Longitudinal section of the humerus showing compact bone, spongy bone, and marrow.

▶ Joints

Wherever two long bones come in contact, a **joint (articulation)** is formed. A joint consists of the ends of the bones that make up the joint and the surrounding connecting and supporting tissue Figure 7-12. Many joints in the body are named by combining the names of the two bones that form that joint. For example, the sternoclavicular joint is the articulation between the sternum and the clavicle. Most joints allow motion—for example, the knee, hip, and elbow—whereas some bones fuse with one another at joints to form a solid, immobile, bony structure. For example, the skull is composed of several bones that fuse as a child grows. Some joints have slight, limited motion in which the bone ends are held together by fibrous tissue. Such a joint is called a **symphysis**.

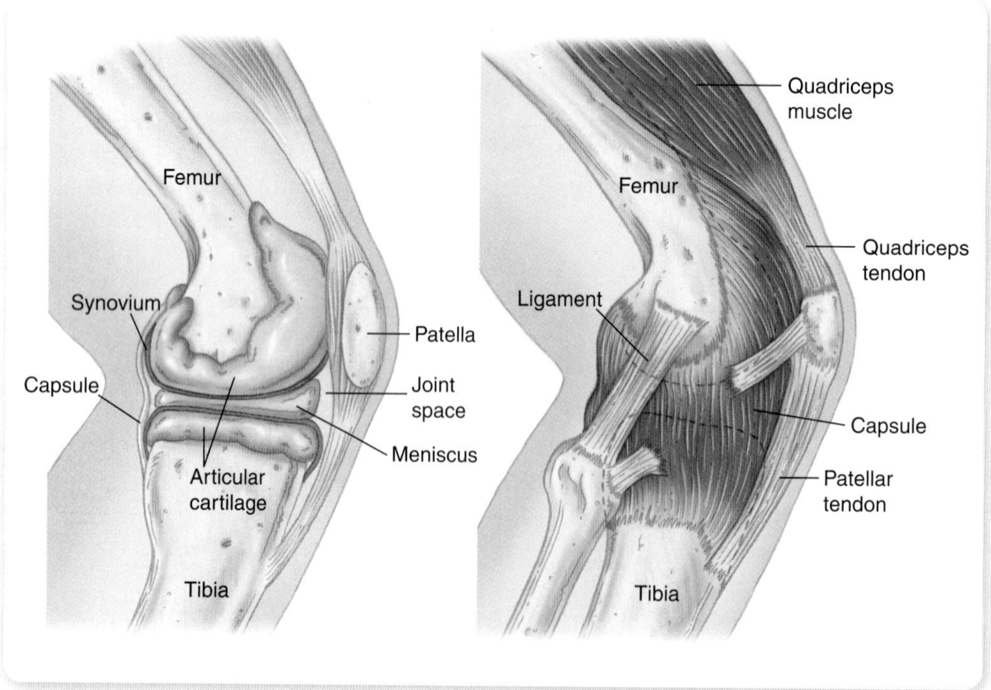

Figure 7-12 A joint consists of bone ends, the fibrous joint capsule, the synovial membrane, and ligaments. The degree to which a joint can move is determined by how the ligaments hold the bone ends and by the configuration of the bones themselves.

The bone ends of a joint are held together by a fibrous sac called the **joint capsule**. This sac is composed of tissue called ligaments (which connect bone to bone). At certain points around the circumference of the joint, the capsule is lax and thin so motion can occur. In other areas, it is quite thick and resists stretching or bending. A joint such as the sacroiliac joint that is virtually surrounded by tough, thick ligaments will have little motion, whereas a joint such as the shoulder, with fewer ligaments, will be free to move in almost any direction (and will, as a result, be more susceptible to dislocation). On the inner lining of the joint capsule is the **synovial membrane**. This special tissue makes a thick lubricant called **synovial fluid**. This "oil" allows the ends of the bones to glide over each other as opposed to rubbing and grating over each other. Synovial fluid contains WBCs to fight infections and provides nourishment to the cartilage covering the bone.

The degree to which a joint can move is determined by the extent to which the ligaments hold the bone ends together and also by the configuration of the bone ends themselves. The shoulder joint is a **ball-and-socket joint** Figure 7-13. Possible motions at a ball-and-socket joint include flexion, extension, abduction, adduction, rotation, and circumduction (a circular movement such as "windmilling" the arms). The finger joints, elbow, and knee are **hinge joints**, with motion largely restricted to one plane Figure 7-14. They primarily flex (bend) and extend (straighten).

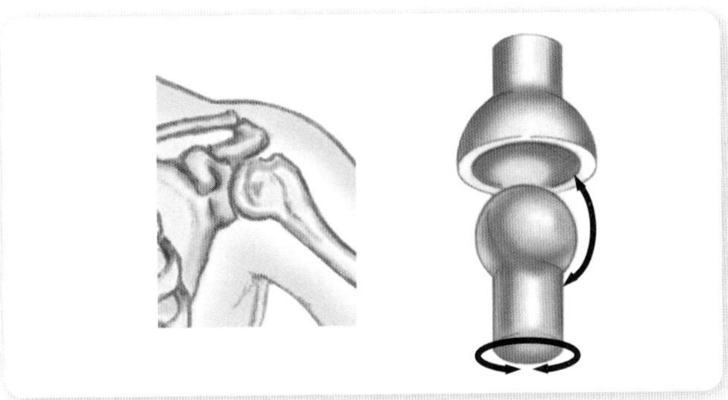

Figure 7-13 The shoulder is an example of a ball-and-socket joint.

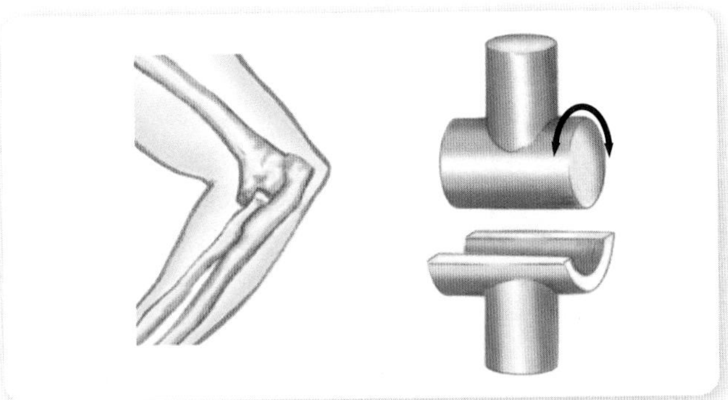

Figure 7-14 The elbow joints are hinge joints, which allow motion primarily in one plane (flexion and extension).

The biceps muscle, for example, has its origin on the scapula; the biceps tendon passes over the head of the humerus, where it fuses with the body of the biceps muscle; at the distal end of the biceps, a tendon passes over the anterior surface of the elbow and inserts on the radius. Thus, when the biceps muscle contracts, the force causes the elbow to bend (flex).

Rotation is not possible because of the shape of the joint surfaces and the strong restraining ligaments on both sides of the joint. Although the amount of motion varies from joint to joint, all joints have a limit beyond which motion cannot occur. When a joint is forced beyond this limit, damage to some structure (bones, joints, or ligaments) occurs.

▶ The Axial Skeleton

The skeletal system is divided into two main portions: the **axial skeleton** and the **appendicular skeleton**. The axial skeleton forms the foundation on which the arms and legs are hung. The axial skeleton is composed of the skull, thoracic cage, and vertebral column. The arms and legs, their connection points, and the pelvis make up the appendicular skeleton Figure 7-15. The brain lies within the skull. The heart, lungs, and great vessels are enclosed in the **thorax**, also called the thoracic cavity, which is part of the torso. Much of the liver and spleen are protected by the lower ribs. The spinal cord is contained within and protected by a bony spinal canal formed by the vertebrae.

The 206 bones of the skeleton provide a framework for the attachment of muscles. The skeleton is also designed to allow motion of the body. Bones come into contact with one another at joints where, with the help of muscles, the body is able to bend and move.

The Skull

At the top of the axial skeleton is the **skull**, which consists of 28 bones in three anatomic groups: the auditory ossicles, the **cranium**, and the face Figure 7-16. The six **auditory ossicles** function in hearing and are located, three on each side of the head, deep within cavities of the temporal bone. The remaining 22 bones comprise the cranium and the face.

At the base of the temporal bone is a cone-shaped section of bone known as the **mastoid process**. This area is an important site for attachment of various muscles.

The **cranial vault** consists of the eight bones that encase and protect the brain: the parietal, temporal, frontal, occipital, sphenoid, and ethmoid bones. The brain and the spinal cord are connected through a large opening at the base of the skull called the **foramen magnum**.

The bones of the skull are connected together at special joints known as **sutures** Figure 7-17. The paired parietal bones join together at the sagittal suture. The parietal bones abut the frontal bone at the coronal suture. The occipital bone attaches to the parietal bones at the lambdoid suture. Fibrous tissues called **fontanelles**, which soften and expand during childbirth, link the sutures.

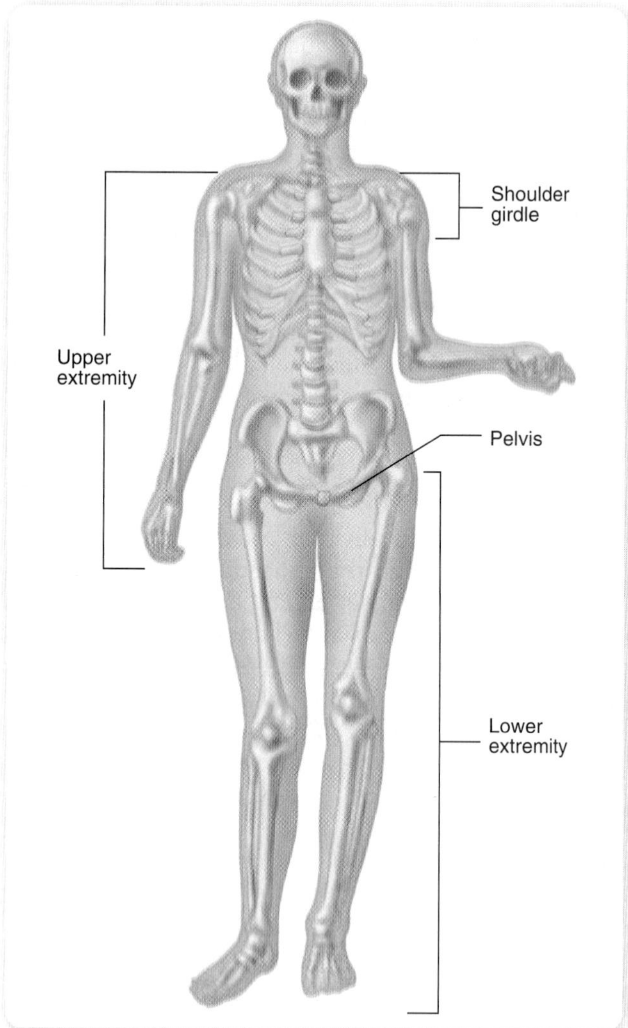

Figure 7-15 The 206 bones of the skeleton give us our form, protect our vital organs, and allow us to move. The axial skeleton runs in a straight line from the head to the pelvis. The appendicular skeleton is made up of the arms and legs and the pelvis.

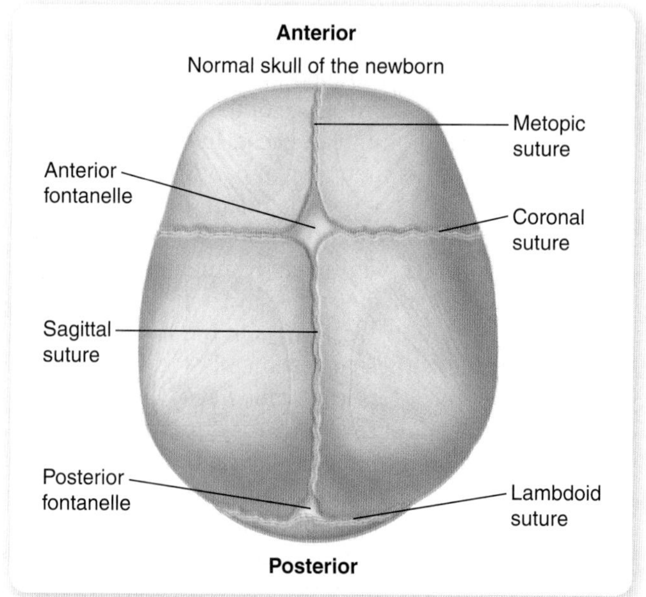

Figure 7-17 The sutures of the skull.

The tissues felt through the fontanelles are layers of the scalp and thick membranes overlying the brain. Under normal conditions, the brain may not be felt through the fontanelles. By the time a child reaches age 2 years, the sutures should have solidified and the fontanelles closed.

The Floor of the Cranial Vault. Viewed from above, the floor of the interior of the skull, or cranial vault, is divided into three compartments: the anterior fossa, middle fossa, and posterior fossa **Figure 7-18**.

The **crista galli** forms a prominent bony ridge in the center of the anterior fossa and is the point of attachment of the meninges, the three layers of membranes—the dura mater, arachnoid, and pia mater—that surround the brain. On either side of the crista galli is the **cribriform plate** of the ethmoid bone, the horizontal bone that is perforated

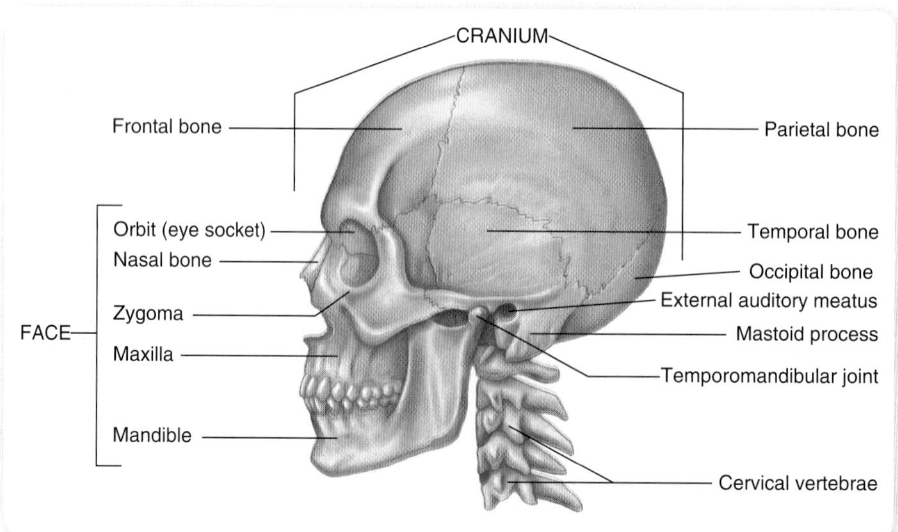

Figure 7-16 The skull consists of 28 bones in three anatomic regions: the auditory ossicles, the cranium, and the face.

with numerous openings (**foramina**) for the passage of the olfactory nerve filaments from the nasal cavity. The **olfactory nerve**, the cranial nerve for smell, sends projections through the foramina in the cribriform plate and into the **nasal cavity**, the chamber inside the nose that lies between the floor of the cranium and the roof of the mouth.

The Facial Bones. The frontal and ethmoid bones are part of both the cranial vault and the face. The 14 facial bones form the structure of the face, without contributing to the cranial vault. These bones include the **maxillae**, mandible, **zygoma**, palatine, nasal, lacrimal, vomer, and inferior nasal concha bones **Figure 7-19**.

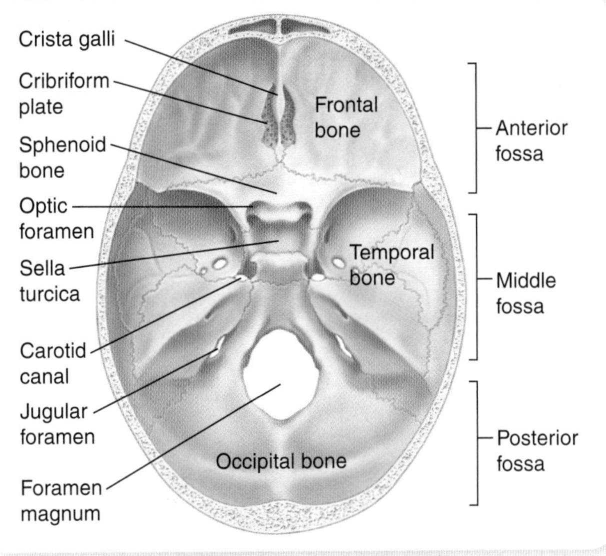

Figure 7-18 The floor of the cranial vault and its anatomy.

Words of Wisdom

Fractures of the cribriform plate result in leakage of cerebrospinal fluid (CSF) from the nose. CSF is the fluid that bathes and provides hydraulic cushioning to the brain and spinal cord. Leakage of clear, watery fluid from the nose following head trauma suggests leakage of CSF.

The facial bones protect the eyes, nose, and tongue and provide attachment points for the muscles that allow chewing. The zygomatic process of the temporal bone and the temporal process of the zygomatic bone form the zygomatic arch **Figure 7-20**. The zygomatic arch lends shape to the cheeks.

Bones of the Orbit. The **orbit** is the cone-shaped fossa that encloses and protects each eye. In addition to the eyeball and muscles that move it, the orbit contains blood vessels, nerves, and fat. The frontal, sphenoid, zygomatic, maxilla, lacrimal, ethmoid, and palatine bones each form portions of the orbits.

A blow to the eye may result in fracture of the floor of the orbit. This bone is extremely thin and breaks easily. The result is transmission of forces away from the eyeball itself to the bone. Blood and fat then leak into the maxillary sinus below. This type of fracture is called a blowout fracture.

Bones of the Nose. The nasal cavity comprises portions of several of the facial bones, including the frontal, nasal, sphenoid, ethmoid, inferior nasal concha, maxilla, palatine, and vomer bones. The **nasal septum** is the separation

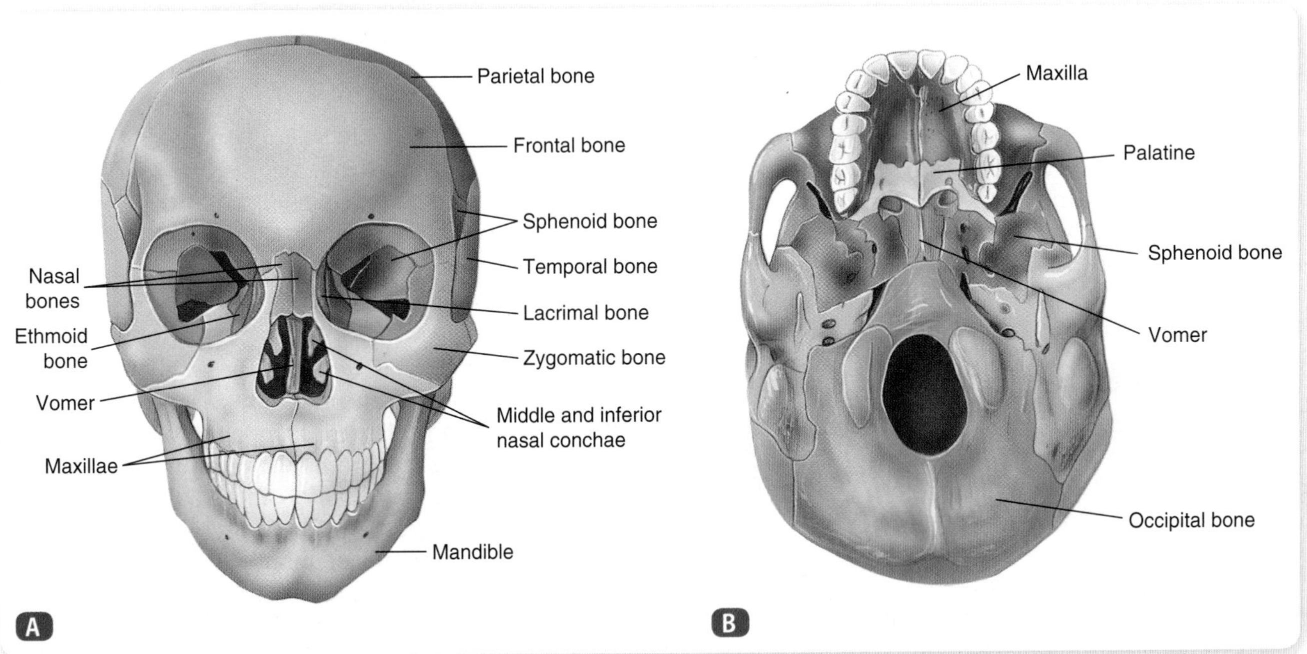

Figure 7-19 The skull and its components. **A.** Front view. **B.** Bottom view.

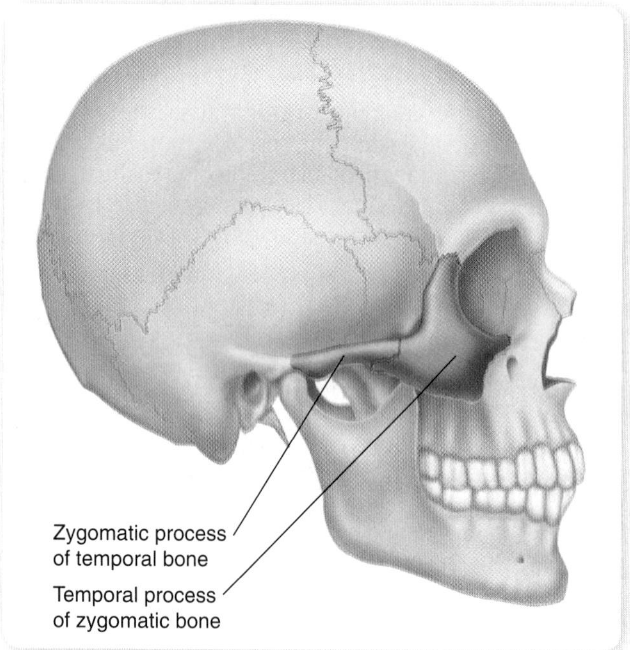

Figure 7-20 The zygomatic arch.

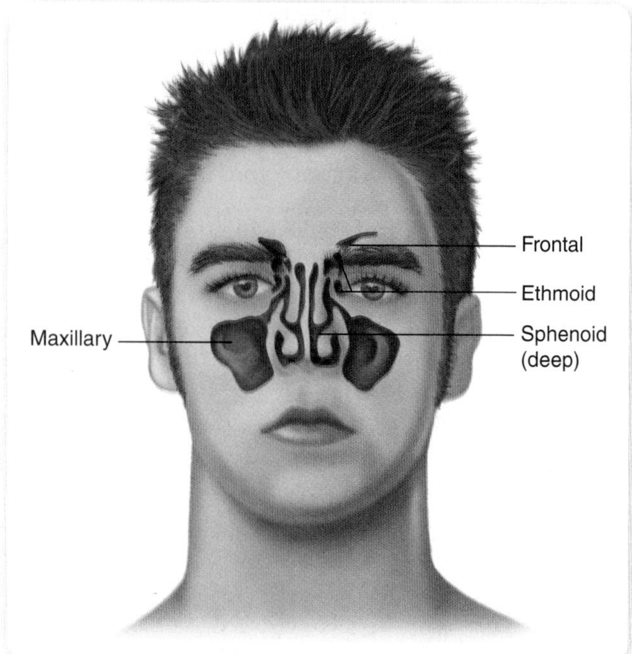

Figure 7-21 The paranasal sinuses.

between the nostrils and is located in the midline. Often, it bulges slightly to one side or the other. The external portion of the nose is formed mostly of cartilage.

Several of the bones associated with the nose contain cavities known as the **paranasal sinuses**, or sinuses **Figure 7-21**. These hollowed sections of bone are lined with mucous membrane and decrease the weight of the skull as well as provide resonance for the voice. The contents of the sinuses drain into the nasal cavity. **Sinusitis** is an inflammation of the paranasal sinuses that is relatively common. Sinusitis may range in severity from a simple upper respiratory tract infection consisting of headache and nasal drainage to a potentially life-threatening brain infection, depending on the extent of the infection and which sinuses are affected.

The Mandible and Temporomandibular Joint. The **mandible** is the large movable bone comprising the lower jaw and containing the lower teeth. Numerous muscles of chewing attach to the mandible. The posterior condyle of the mandible articulates with the temporal bone at the **temporomandibular joint (TMJ)**, allowing movement of the mandible.

The Hyoid Bone. The **hyoid bone** "floats" in the superior aspect of the neck just below the mandible. It is not actually part of the skull, but it supports the tongue and serves as a point of attachment for many important neck and tongue muscles.

▶ The Neck

The neck is supported by the cervical spine, or the first seven vertebrae in the spinal column (C1 through C7). The spinal cord exits from the foramen magnum and lies within the spinal canal formed by the vertebrae. The upper part of the esophagus and the **trachea** lie in the midline of the neck. The carotid arteries are found on either side of the trachea, along with the jugular veins and several nerves.

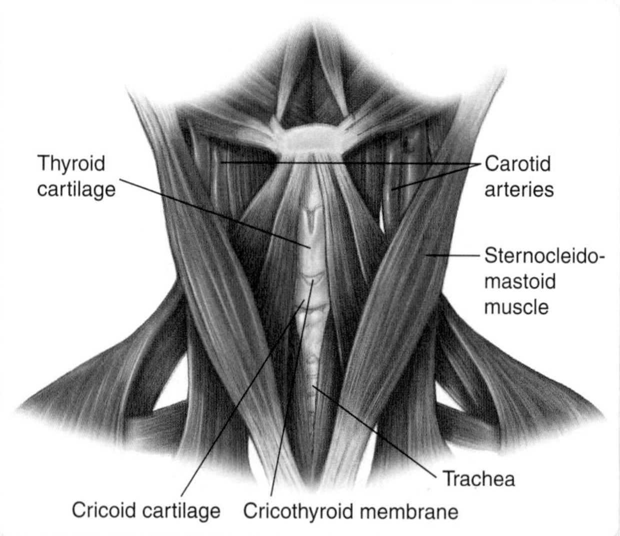

Figure 7-22 The principal structures of the neck include the trachea, along with many blood vessels, muscles, and nerves.

Several useful landmarks can be palpated and seen in the neck **Figure 7-22**. The most obvious is the firm prominence in the center of the anterior surface commonly known as the Adam's apple. This prominence is the upper part of the **thyroid cartilage** and is more prominent in men than in women. The lower portion is the **cricoid cartilage**, a firm ridge of cartilage inferior to the thyroid cartilage, which is somewhat more difficult to palpate. Between the thyroid cartilage and the cricoid cartilage in the midline of the neck is a soft depression, the **cricothyroid membrane**. This is a thin sheet of connective tissue (**fascia**) that joins the two cartilages. The cricothyroid membrane is covered at this point only by skin.

Inferior to the larynx, several additional firm ridges are palpable in the anterior midline. These ridges are the cartilage rings of the trachea. The trachea connects the larynx with the main air passages of the lungs (the bronchi). On either side of the lower larynx and the upper trachea lies the thyroid gland. Unless it is enlarged, this gland is usually not palpable.

Pulsations of the carotid arteries are easily palpable in a groove approximately one-half inch (1 cm) lateral to the larynx. Lying immediately adjacent to these arteries, but not palpable, are the internal jugular veins and several important nerves. Lateral to these vessels and nerves lie the **sternocleidomastoid muscles**, which allow movement of the head. These muscles originate from the mastoid process of the cranium and insert into the medial border of each collarbone and the **sternum** (breastbone) at the base of the neck.

▶ The Spinal Column

The spinal column, or **vertebral column**, is the central supporting structure of the body and is composed of 33 bones, each called a vertebra (7 cervical, 12 thoracic, 5 lumbar, 5 sacral, and 4 coccygeal), and protects the spinal cord. The **vertebrae** are named according to the section of the spine in which they lie and are numbered from top to bottom **Figure 7-23**. From the top down, the spine is divided into five sections:

- **Cervical spine**. The first seven vertebrae (C1 through C7) in the neck form the cervical spine. In addition to protecting the vital cervical spinal cord, the cervical spine supports the weight of the head and permits a high degree of mobility in multiple planes. The atlas (C1) and axis (C2) are uniquely suited to allow for rotational movement of the skull.
- **Thoracic spine**. The next 12 vertebrae (T1 through T12) in addition to the supporting muscles and ligaments found in the vertebral column make up the thoracic spine. One pair of ribs is attached to each of the thoracic vertebrae and further stabilizes the thoracic spine. The spinous processes are slightly larger, reflecting their role as attachment points for muscles that hold the upper body erect and assist with the movement of the thoracic cavity during respiration.
- **Lumbar spine**. The next five vertebrae form the lumbar spine. These are the largest bones in the vertebral column and they are integral in carrying a large portion of the upper body weight. The lumbar spine is especially susceptible to injury because of this weight-bearing capacity.

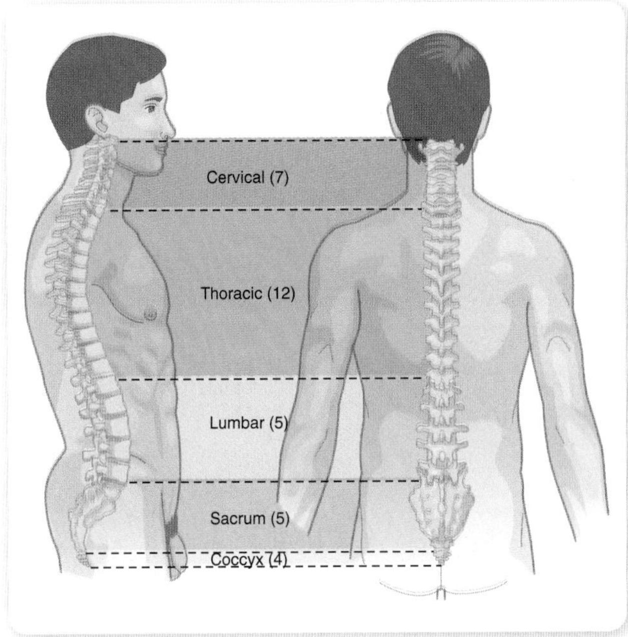

Figure 7-23 The spinal column is composed of 33 bones divided into five sections. Each vertebra is numbered and referred to by a letter corresponding to the section of the spine where it is located. For example, the fifth thoracic vertebra is referred to as T5.

- **Sacrum**. The sacrum is composed of five fused vertebrae that form the posterior plate of the pelvis. The sacrum is joined to the iliac bones of the pelvis with strong ligaments at the sacroiliac joints to form the pelvis.
- **Coccyx**. The last small three to five vertebrae, also fused together, form the coccyx, or tailbone. Coccyx injuries, although often extremely painful, are typically neurologically insignificant.

The first cervical vertebra (C1) is called the **atlas**. The atlas is located directly beneath the skull and provides support for the head. The atlas articulates with the occipital condyles at the base of the skull at the **atlanto-occipital joint**. The only motions of this joint are flexion and extension and lateral bending.

The second cervical vertebra (C2) is known as the **axis** and is the point at which the head rotates, such as when moving the head from left to right. A large offshoot of C2 is the dens, or odontoid process, which fits into the enlarged vertebral foramen of the atlas. The atlas rotates around the axis at the dens. The cervical vertebrae numbered C3 through C6 form the cervical curve. C7, called the vertebra prominens, is different. It has a large spinous process that may be seen and felt at the base of the neck **Figure 7-24**.

The spinal cord is an extension of the brain, composed of virtually all the nerves that carry messages between the brain and the rest of the body. It exits through a large hole in the base of the skull called the foramen magnum and

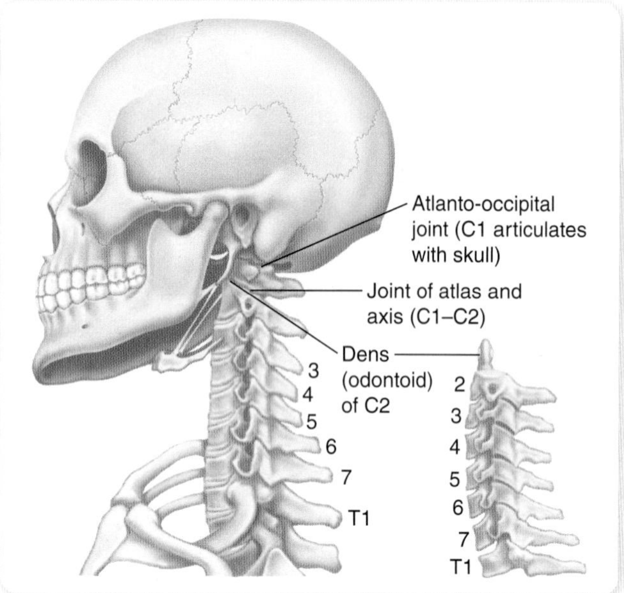

Figure 7-24 The cervical vertebrae.

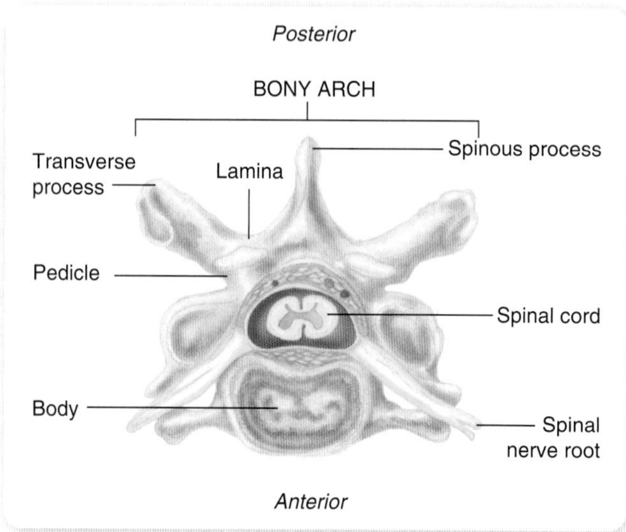

Figure 7-25 The bones of the spinal column encase and protect the spinal cord. The vertebrae are shaped to accommodate space for the spinal cord and nerve roots, which pass through.

is contained within and protected by the vertebrae of the spinal column. The spinal column is virtually surrounded by muscles. However, the posterior spinous process of each vertebra can be felt as it lies just under the skin in the midline of the back.

The anterior part of each vertebra consists of a round, solid block of bone called the body. The posterior part of each vertebra forms a bony arch. This series of arches from one vertebra to the next forms a tunnel that runs the length of the spine called the spinal canal. The bones of the spinal canal encase and protect the spinal cord Figure 7-25. Nerves branch from the spinal cord and exit from the spinal canal between each two vertebrae to form the motor and sensory nerves of the body.

The vertebrae are connected by ligaments, and between each vertebra is a cushion called the intervertebral disk. These ligaments and disks allow some motion so the trunk can bend forward (flex) and back (extend), and they allow for rotation and lateral movement. However, they also limit motion of the vertebrae so that the spinal cord will not be injured. An injury to the spine may damage part of the spinal cord and its nerves that may not be protected by the vertebrae. Therefore, until the injury is stabilized, you must use extreme caution in caring for the patient to prevent injury to the spinal cord.

▶ The Thorax

The thorax (chest) is formed by the 12 thoracic vertebrae (T1 through T12) and their 12 pairs of ribs. The boundaries of the thorax are the rib cage anteriorly, superiorly, and posteriorly and the diaphragm inferiorly.

Anteriorly, in the midline of the chest is the sternum. The superior border of the sternum forms the easily palpable jugular, or sternal, notch. This is the location where the trachea enters the chest. The sternum has three

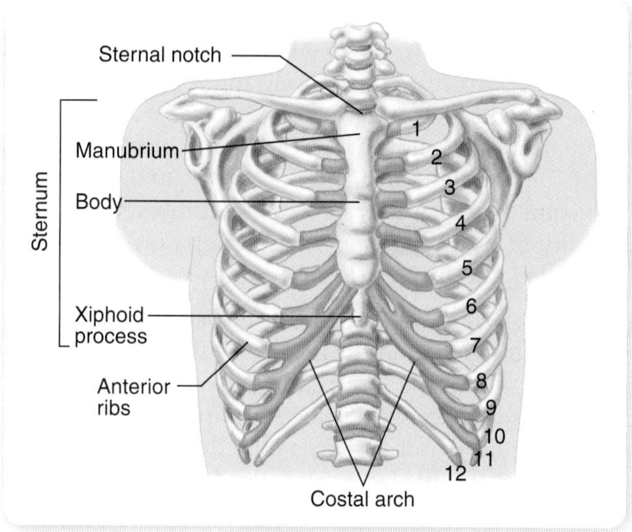

Figure 7-26 Thoracic cavity.

components: the manubrium, the body, and the xiphoid process. The upper section of the sternum is called the **manubrium**. The body comprises the rest of the sternum except for a narrow, cartilaginous tip inferiorly, which is called the **xiphoid process** Figure 7-26.

Within the thoracic cage, the largest structures are the heart, lungs, and great vessels Figure 7-27. The heart lies immediately behind the sternum (retrosternal). It extends from the second to the sixth ribs anteriorly and from the fifth to the eighth thoracic vertebrae posteriorly. The inferior border of the heart extends into the left side of the chest. Diseased hearts may be larger or smaller. The major blood vessels that travel to and from the heart also lie in the chest cavity. On the right side of the spinal column, the superior and inferior venae cavae carry blood to the heart.

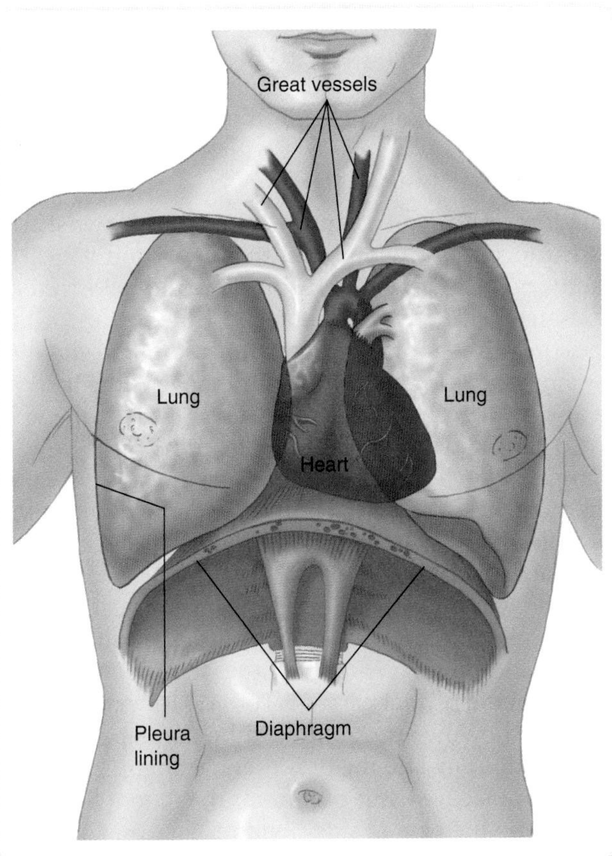

Figure 7-27 The anterior aspect of the thorax shows the relative positions of the principal organs beneath the surface.

Just beneath the manubrium of the sternum, the arch of the **aorta** (the body's largest artery) and the **pulmonary artery** exit the heart. The arch of the aorta passes to the left and lies along the left side of the spinal column as it descends into the abdomen. The **esophagus** lies behind the great vessels and directly on the anterior aspect of the spinal column as it passes through the chest into the abdominal cavity.

All space within the chest that is not occupied by the heart, great vessels, and esophagus is occupied by the lungs. Anteriorly, the lungs extend down to the surface of the diaphragm at the level of the xiphoid process. Posteriorly, the lungs extend farther inferiorly to the surface of the diaphragm at the level of the 12th thoracic vertebra.

▶ The Appendicular Skeleton

The appendicular skeleton includes the bones of the shoulder and pelvic girdles, the upper extremities (arms [more commonly thought of as the upper arms], forearms, wrist, hands, and fingers), and the lower extremities (thighs, legs, ankles, instep, and toes).

The Shoulder Girdle

The **shoulder girdle** attaches the upper extremity to the body at the glenohumeral joint. The two major components of the shoulder girdle are the **scapula** (shoulder blade) and the **clavicle** (collarbone). The scapula is a flat, triangular bone held to the rib cage posteriorly by powerful muscles that buffer it against injury.

The clavicle is a slender, S-shaped bone that is easily felt on either side of the sternal notch. The lateral end of the clavicle articulates with the acromion and the medial end with the manubrium.

The raised tip of the scapula is called the **acromion process**. It protects the shoulder joint and provides a site of attachment for both the clavicle and various shoulder muscles **Figure 7-28A**. Important muscles of the shoulder, including those of the rotator cuff, originate here.

The Shoulder Joint

The shoulder joint is a ball-and-socket joint in which the head of the humerus articulates with the **glenoid fossa**, which is part of the scapula **Figure 7-28B**. The hip and shoulder are typical ball-and-socket joints.

Four ligaments attach the humeral head to the glenoid fossa. A fibrocartilage ring surrounds the glenoid rim and provides a point of attachment for the capsule, which is made up of fibrous connective tissue. A **bursa** is a padlike sac situated between a tendon and a bone that cushions

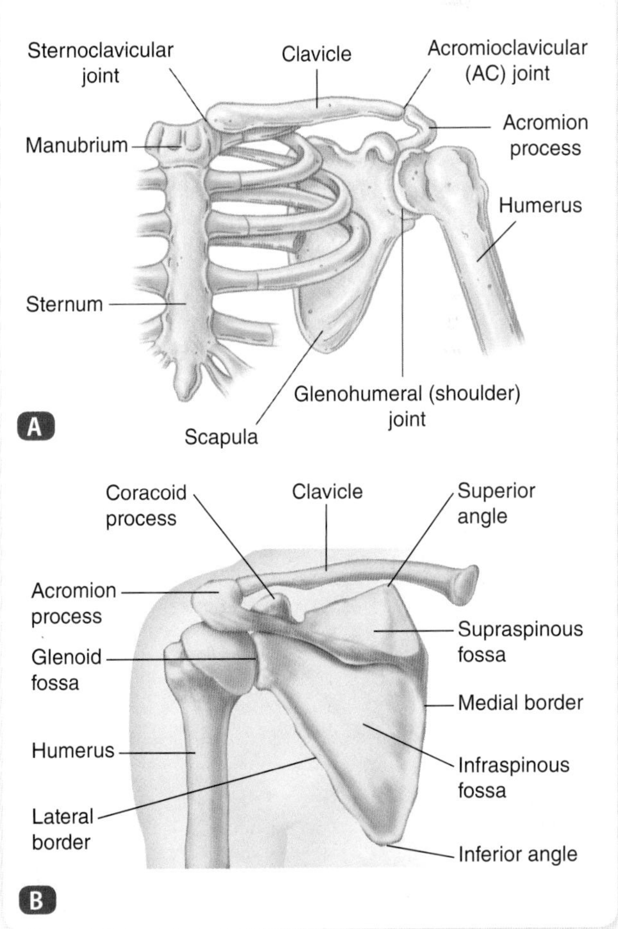

Figure 7-28 A. Anterior view of the shoulder girdle, including the clavicle. **B.** Posterior view of the shoulder girdle, including the scapula.

and protects joints such as the shoulder, hip, or knee. It may be lined with a synovial membrane and typically contains fluid that helps reduce the amount of friction between a tendon and a bone or between a tendon and a ligament. Examples include the olecranon bursa of the elbow and the prepatellar bursa of the knee. Bursitis is inflammation of a bursa.

> **Words of Wisdom**
>
> **Acromioclavicular (AC) separation**, also called a separated shoulder, occurs when any of the four ligaments of the AC joint are partially or completely torn. In partial tears, no deformity is noted unless the patient attempts to hold a weight with the arm directed downward. In this case, the weakened joint is transiently widened, a finding visible on radiographs. In patients with complete separation, in which all four ligaments are severely damaged, the clavicle essentially lies above the acromion, causing a visible deformity in the patient's shoulder area.

The Upper Extremity

The upper extremity consists of the arm (commonly described as the upper arm), forearm, wrist, hand, and fingers.

The **humerus** is the bone of the upper arm Figure 7-29. It articulates proximally with the glenoid fossa and distally with the radius and ulna at the elbow joint. The elbow joint is a hinge joint, permitting motion in one plane only. Several ligaments connect the humerus, radius, and ulna at the elbow joint, and a fluid-filled bursa cushions and protects the joint posteriorly.

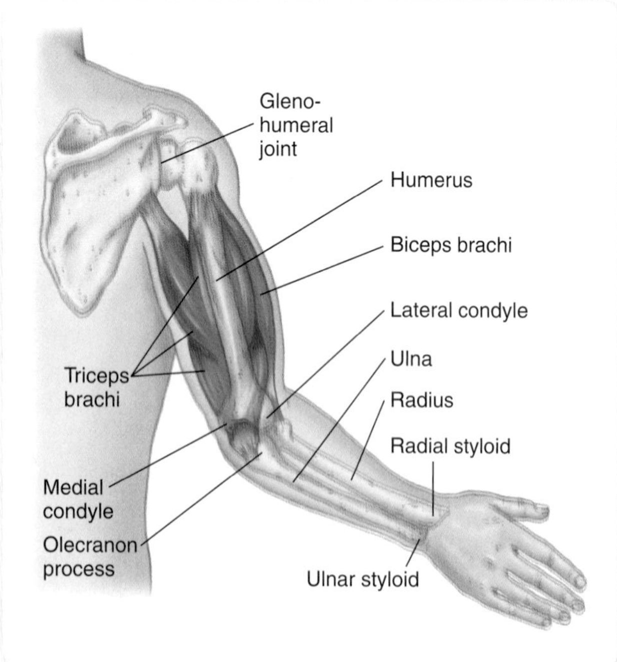

Figure 7-29 The (upper) arm contains the humerus; the forearm contains the radius and ulna.

The Forearm and Wrist

The forearm extends from the elbow to the wrist. The forearm contains two bones, the **radius** and **ulna**. The radius is the larger of the two bones and is located on the lateral side (the thumb side) of the forearm when the forearm is in the anatomic position, and the ulna is narrow and located on the little finger side. It serves as the pivot around which the radius turns at the wrist to rotate the palm upward (supination) or downward (pronation). The proximal portion of the radius is called the radial head. The distal portion contains a small bony protrusion, the styloid process, to which ligaments of the wrist are attached.

The wrist is made of a group of eight irregularly shaped bones, called the carpals. The carpals include the triquetrum, pisiform, capitate, lunate, hamate, trapezoid, trapezium, and scaphoid (carpal navicular) bones. The carpal tunnel is formed by the space bounded by the trapezium and hamate dorsally and the flexor retinaculum, a sheath of tough connective tissue that forms the roof of the carpal tunnel, on the palmar side. Tendons, nerves, and blood vessels lie within the carpal tunnel. Structures within the carpal tunnel include the long flexor tendons to the fingers and the median nerve, which supplies sensory and motor function to the radial half of the palm of the hand.

The Hand

The **metacarpal bones** are the bones that form the hand. The **phalanges** (singularly called a phalanx) are a series of small bones that exist in each finger. The phalanges in the fingers form hinge joints. Each finger has three phalanges, except the thumb, which has only two Figure 7-30. The **carpometacarpal joint** of the thumb is a **saddle joint**, consisting of two saddle-shaped articulating surfaces that are oriented at right angles to one another so that the complementary surfaces articulate with each other. Movement in these joints can occur in two planes. Arthritis commonly affects the carpometacarpal joint, resulting in stiffness and deformity.

▶ The Pelvic Girdle

The **pelvis**, or pelvic girdle, is where the lower extremity attaches to the body Figure 7-31. The pelvis contains a ring of bones formed by the sacrum and the coxal, or pelvic, bones; the sacrum is posterior and the coxal bones are on each side. Each coxa consists of three fused bones: the **ilium**, **ischium**, and **pubis**. The pelvis contains three joints: the two posterior **sacroiliac joints** and the interior midline **pubic symphysis**. The location where the ilium connects with the sacrum is the sacroiliac joint. The pubic symphysis is the lower midportion of the pelvic ring where the left and right sides fuse together. The superior portion

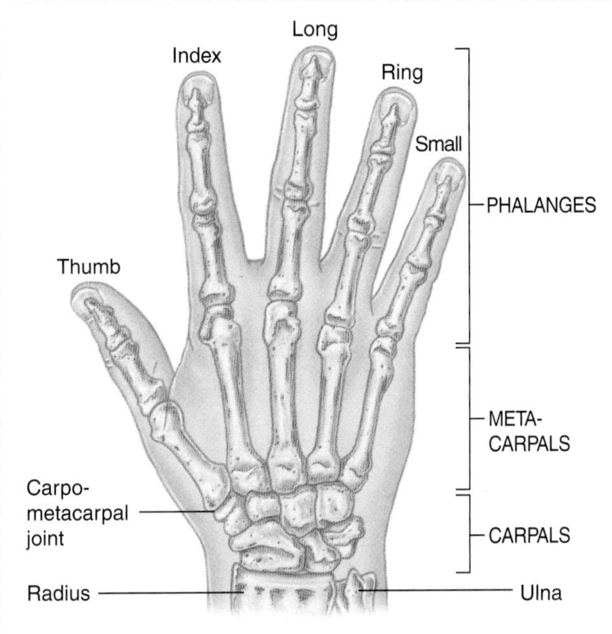

Figure 7-30 The principal bones in the wrist and hand include the carpals, the metacarpals, and the phalanges.

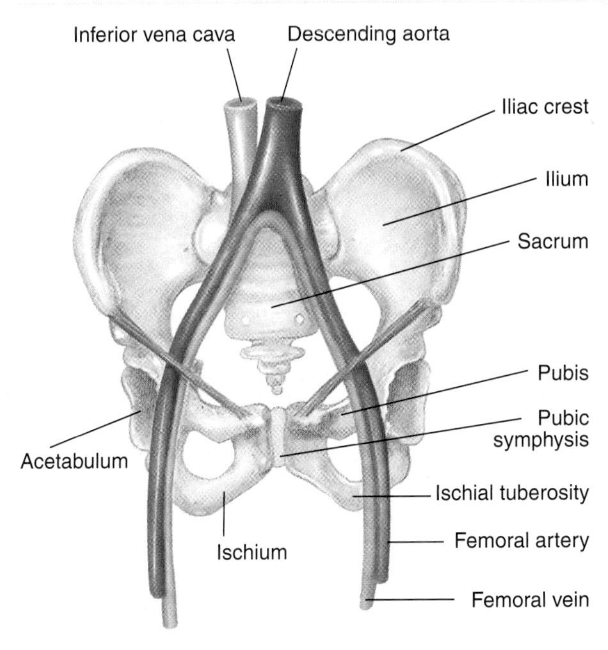

Figure 7-31 The pelvis is a closed bony ring that consists of the sacrum, ilium, ischium, pubis, acetabulum, and pubic symphysis.

of the ilium is the iliac crest. The obturator foramen is an opening between the ischium and pubis that contains several important nerves and muscles. The pelvic girdle supports the body weight and protects the internal organs. In a pregnant woman, the bones protect the developing fetus and provide a passageway through which the infant passes during delivery.

Words of Wisdom

Pay attention to spelling to prevent misunderstandings. Although *ilium* and *ileum* are pronounced the same, they refer to two different parts of the body.

- Ilium = the bony prominences of the pelvis
- Ileum = the lower $\frac{3}{5}$ of the small intestine

▶ The Lower Extremity

The lower extremity is made of the hip, thigh, knee, leg, ankle, foot, and toes **Figure 7-32**. The **acetabulum** is the socket of the ball-and-socket joint that connects the pelvic girdle with the lower extremity. The thigh is the part of the lower extremity that extends from the hip to the knee and contains the **femur**, which is the longest and strongest bone in the body. The uppermost portion of the femur, the **femoral head**, articulates with the pelvic girdle at the acetabulum. In addition to the femoral head, the proximal femur consists of the neck, **greater trochanter** (upper part of the femur), and lesser trochanter (lower part of the femur). The greater trochanter arises lateral to the juncture of the neck and shaft and is part of the femur. Several ligaments

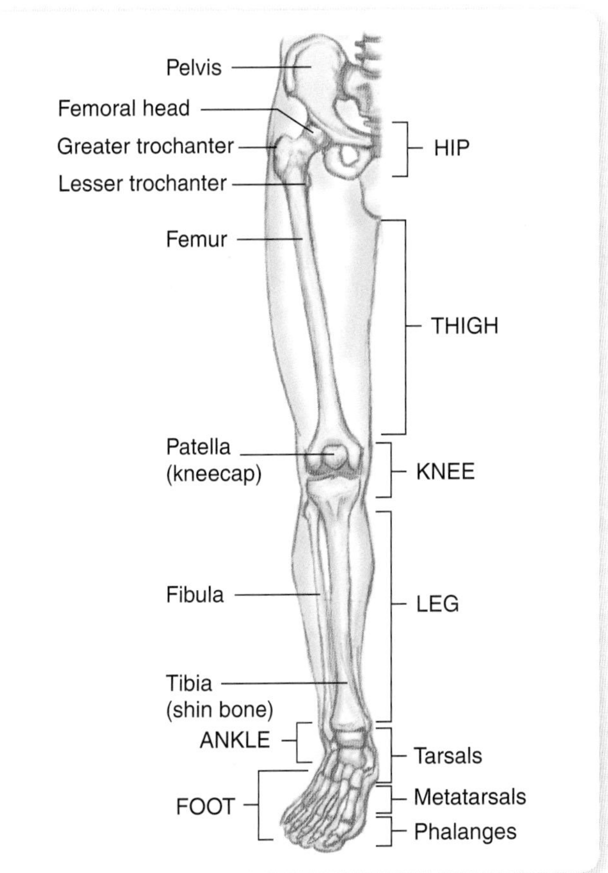

Figure 7-32 The principal parts of the lower extremity, including the femur, femoral head, greater and lesser trochanters, patella, tibia, and fibula.

and tendons provide integrity to the hip joint. The articular capsule is supported by three ligaments that are quite strong; they support much of the body's weight.

The Leg

At the distal end of the femur, the lateral and medial condyles articulate with the proximal tibia at the knee Figure 7-33. These are important sites of muscle and ligament attachment. The **patella**, or kneecap, lies within the major anterior tendon of the thigh muscles and articulates with the femur.

The leg is made of the tibia and fibula, and extends from the knee to the ankle. The **tibia** is the longer and thicker of the two bones and is situated on the anterior surface of the leg. The anterior portion of the tibia, covered only by skin, is commonly called the shin. The flat medial and lateral condyles of the proximal tibia articulate with the femoral condyles at the knee. The **medial malleolus**, which forms the medial side of the ankle joint, lies at the distal end of the tibia.

The second of the two leg bones, the **fibula**, runs behind and beside the tibia. It does not articulate directly with the femur, but rather with the tibia at the head. An enlargement of the distal end of the fibula forms the lateral wall of the ankle joint, the **lateral malleolus**.

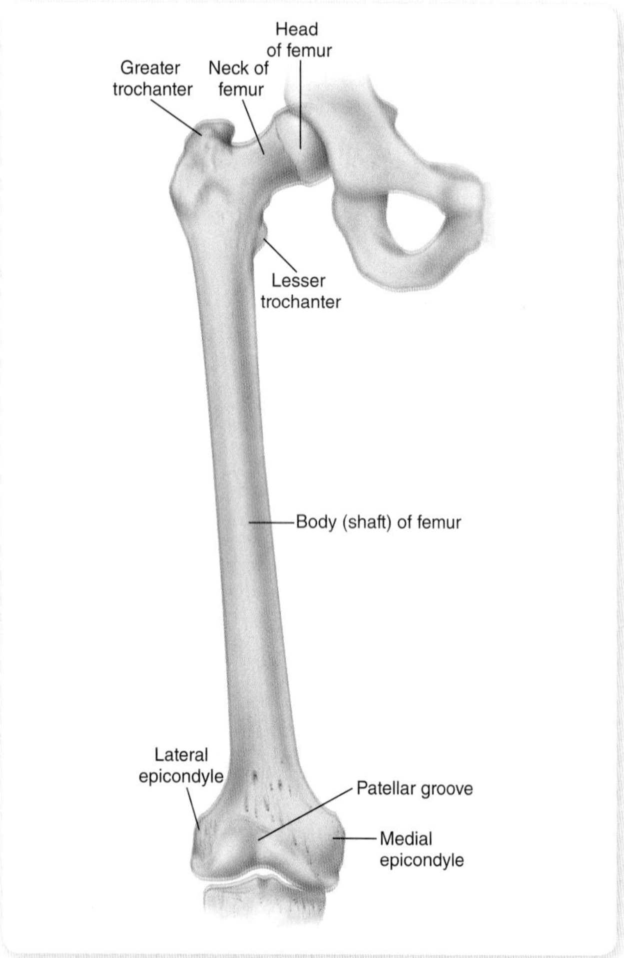

Figure 7-33 The femur.

The Knee

The knee joint is traditionally classified as a hinge joint and is unusual because it contains ligaments within the joint. Thick crescent-shaped articular disks, menisci, cover the margins of the tibia to cushion the articular surface. The anterior cruciate ligament, which extends between the tibia and femur, prevents abnormal anterior movement (**hyperextension**) of the tibia. The posterior cruciate ligament prevents abnormal posterior displacement of the tibia. Several tendons, as well as collateral ligaments, lend additional strength to the knee joint. The knee is surrounded by several fluid-filled bursae Figure 7-34.

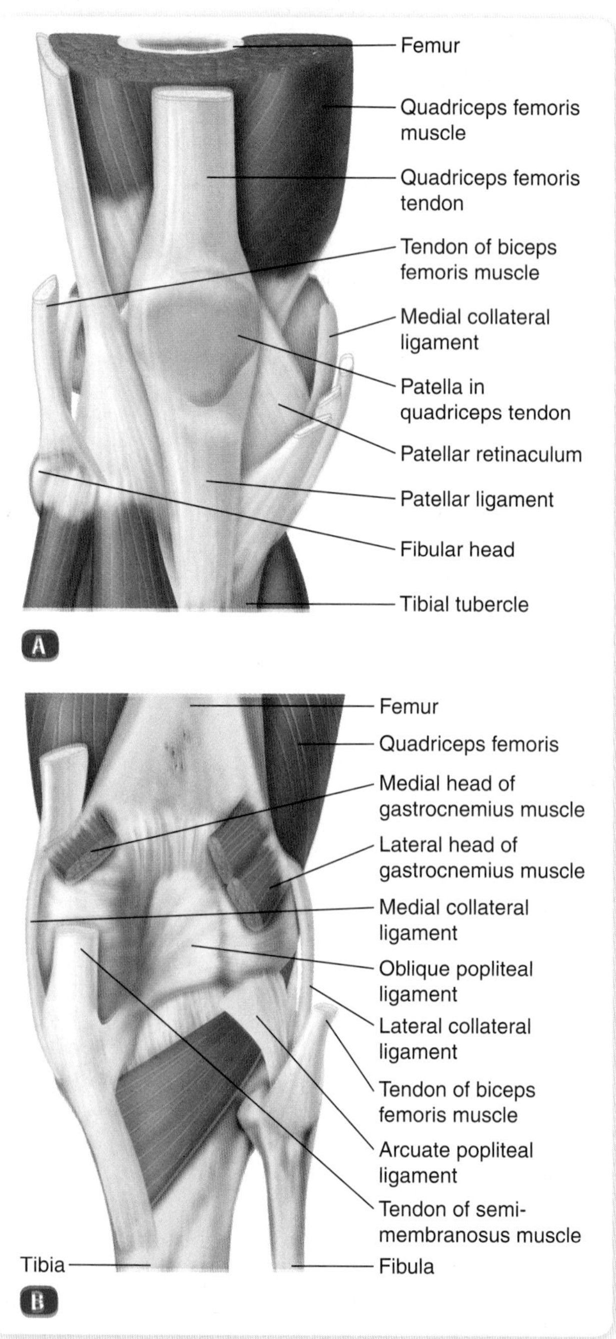

Figure 7-34 A. Anterior view of the knee. **B.** Posterior view of the knee.

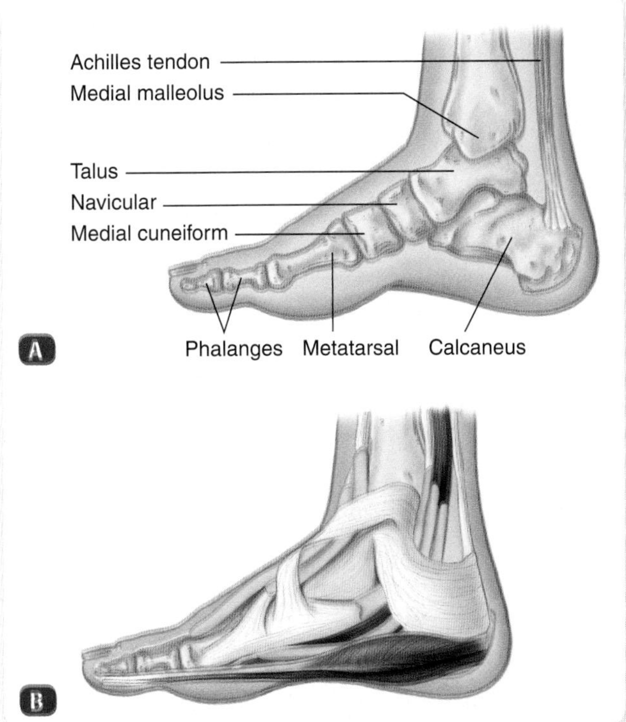

Figure 7-35 **A.** The surface landmarks of the foot, including the talus, the calcaneus, and the phalanges. **B.** Soft tissue of the ankle.

The Ankle

The talus articulates with the tibia and fibula to form the ankle Figure 7-35. The calcaneus, or heel bone, lies inferior and lateral to the talus, providing additional support. A fibrous capsule surrounds the ankle joint; the medial and lateral portions are thickened to form ligaments. Movements include dorsiflexion and plantar flexion, as well as limited inversion and eversion.

The metatarsals and phalanges of the foot are arranged similarly to the bones of the hand. The toes have three phalanges each, except the big toe, which has two phalanges. The ball of the foot is the junction between the metatarsals and the phalanges.

The Skeletal System: Physiology

The skeletal system is responsible for several functions. Bones protect internal organs and, with muscles, enable movement. Bone also serves as a storage site for minerals, particularly calcium, and has a role in the formation of blood cells and platelets. Calcium is the main element the various bone cells use to create a structure that is hard and resilient. Bones store and release calcium, which is important for other body systems.

Bones consist of collagen and the mineral hydroxyapatite, a compound that contains calcium and phosphate.

Special Populations

Hip fractures are actually fractures of the proximal portion of the femur near or at the site of articulation with the acetabulum. These fractures are classified based on the structures of the femur involved Figure 7-36.

Dislocations of the hip joint commonly occur from a fall or during a motor vehicle crash in which the knee impacts the dashboard. The force of the impact is transmitted posteriorly to the hip, resulting in posterior dislocation. Anterior hip dislocations are less common.

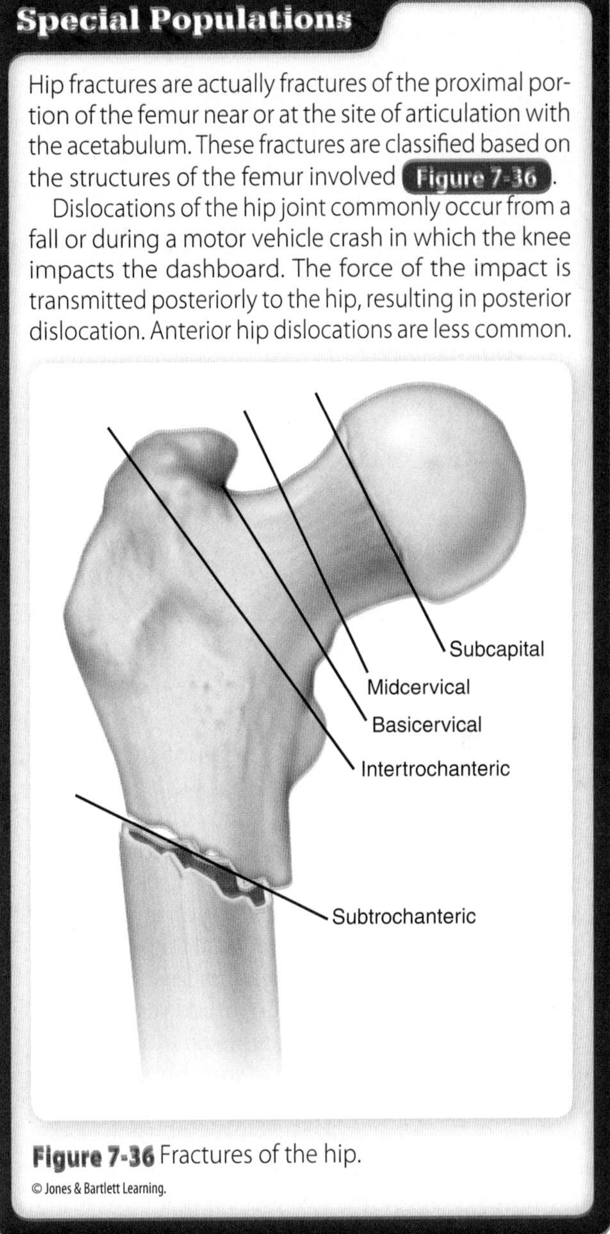

Figure 7-36 Fractures of the hip.

The collagen fibers in bone act much like reinforcing rods in a concrete structure, lending flexibility and strength to the bone. The mineral components of the bone supply strength for bearing weight, much like concrete does in a structure. Bone without the necessary amount of mineral is excessively flexible; bone without enough collagen is extremely brittle.

The skeletal system also helps with the creation of various types of blood cells. In the marrow of certain types of bones, special cells are present that can transform themselves into RBCs, WBCs, and platelets. The cells, when stimulated, help replace worn out cells in the blood.

Bones are a living substance with cells requiring a blood supply. During a person's life, bones are constantly remodeled to meet the stresses that are placed on them. The level of a person's activity directly affects how the bones are remodeled.

Words of Wisdom

As you gain a better understanding of the anatomy and physiology of the body, it is important to remember that body systems work together and not in isolation. A person who falls and breaks a leg has a very isolated injury. It may appear to you that the skeletal system is the only system that is involved. But then ask yourself the following questions: Is there bleeding inside the leg? Is there damage to the nerves, tendons, or ligaments? Has the injury broken the skin and is there now a risk of infection? A seemingly simple illness or injury can involve several body systems. Give each patient a thorough assessment.

The Musculoskeletal System: Anatomy

The human body is a well-designed system whose form, upright posture, and movement are provided by the **musculoskeletal system**. The term *musculoskeletal* refers to the bones and voluntary muscles of the body. The musculoskeletal system also protects the vital internal organs of the body. Muscles are a form of tissue that allows body movement. There are more than 600 muscles in the musculoskeletal system. The type of muscle found here is called skeletal muscle. Other types of muscle outside of the musculoskeletal system include smooth muscle (**involuntary muscle**) and cardiac muscle.

Smooth muscle is found within blood vessels, bronchi, the intestines, and other places. Smooth muscle responds only to primitive stimuli such as stretching, heat, or the need to relieve waste. A person cannot exert any voluntary control over this type of muscle. For example, when you hear your stomach growling, you really are hearing the rhythmic contractions of the smooth muscles of your intestines.

Cardiac muscle contributes to the functioning of the cardiovascular system and is found only within the heart Figure 7-37. The heart is a large muscle composed of a pair of pumps of unequal force: one of lower pressure and one of higher pressure. The heart must function continuously from birth to death. It is a specifically adapted involuntary muscle with a rich blood supply and its own electrical system, which makes it different from both skeletal and smooth muscle. Another difference is that cardiac muscle has the property of "automaticity," which means that the heart muscle can generate and conduct electricity without influence from the brain. This property is unique to heart muscle. Cardiac muscle can tolerate an interruption of its blood supply for only a few seconds. It requires a continuous supply of oxygen and glucose for normal function. Because of its special structure and function, cardiac muscle is placed in a separate category.

Skeletal muscle includes all of the muscles attached to the skeleton. It forms the bulk of the tissue of the arms and legs, and the major muscle mass of the body. It is also called **striated muscle**, because striations can be seen in it during microscopic examination, or **voluntary muscle**, because all skeletal muscle is under direct voluntary control of the brain and can be stimulated to contract or relax at will. Movement of the body, like waving or walking, results from skeletal muscle contraction or relaxation. Usually, a specific motion is the result of several muscles contracting and relaxing simultaneously.

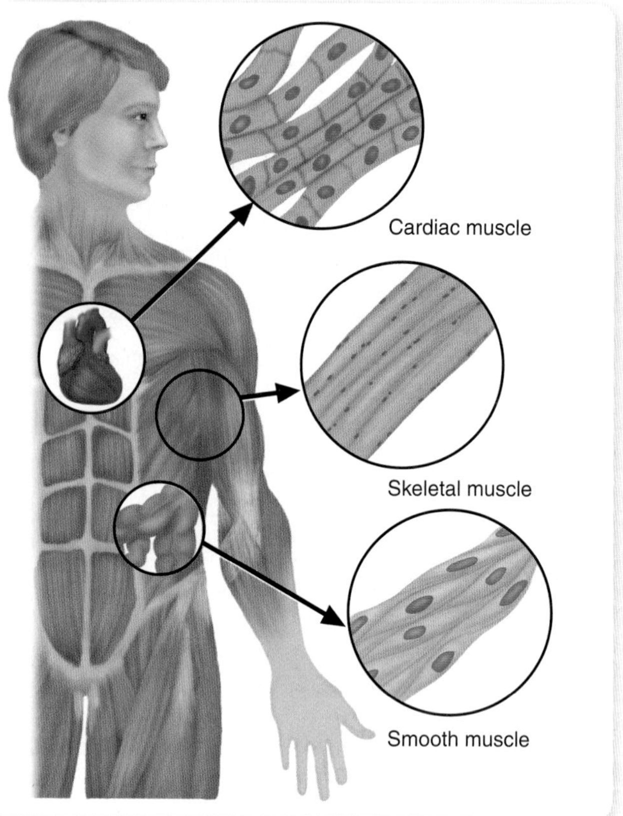

Figure 7-37 The three types of muscle are skeletal, smooth, and cardiac.

Skeletal muscle varies greatly in size and shape, from thin strands to the large muscles of the thigh and back. It is also found along the spine and buttocks, and comprises the muscles of the tongue, soft palate, scalp, pharynx, upper esophagus, and eye. Approximately 40% to 50% of normal body weight is skeletal muscle because it has a high water content.

Skeletal muscles are profoundly affected by the amount of training and work to which they are subjected. Unused muscles tend to **atrophy** (shrink or waste away), whereas physical training promotes **hypertrophy** (increase in size).

Most muscles within the body operate on the principle of antagonistic pairs. The muscles of the upper arm include the **biceps** muscle, which is located on the anterior aspect of the humerus. This muscle moves the lower part of the arm toward the head. If the muscle were working alone, the person would have little control over the speed of that movement. The way the body achieves control and fine movement is to have the biceps compete against another muscle group. The biceps competes with the **triceps** muscle. Without the triceps, you would slap yourself in the face every time you bend your arm. The biceps works to slow the movement of the triceps as the arm is extended.

There are some important muscle groups to know. Figure 7-38 and Table 7-4 show the major muscles, their locations, and their functions.

The Musculoskeletal System: Physiology

The musculoskeletal system has several functions. A person's ability to move and to manipulate his or her environment is made possible by the contraction and relaxation of this system. A by-product of this movement is heat. When you get cold, you involuntarily shake your muscles, or shiver, to produce heat. Shivering is an essential function. Another function of muscles is to protect the structures under them, such as the intestines, which are protected by the rectus abdominus muscles.

▶ Energy Sources

Muscular contraction requires an energy source—ATP—and continues as long as a certain neurotransmitter, acetylcholine (ACh), is released. Muscle fibers have just enough ATP for short-term contraction. ATP must be regenerated when fibers are active, using existing ATP molecules in the cells. ATP is regenerated from adenosine diphosphate (ADP) and phosphate. Creatine phosphate is an organic compound in muscle tissue that can store and provide energy for muscle contraction with high-energy phosphate bonds. Creatine phosphate is between four and six times more abundant in muscle fibers than ATP; however, it does not directly supply energy. Rather, it stores excess energy from the mitochondria in the phosphate bonds.

When ATP breaks down, energy from creatine phosphate is transferred to ADP molecules to convert them back into ATP. Creatine phosphate stores are exhausted rapidly when muscles are active; therefore, the muscles use cellular respiration of glucose as energy to synthesize ATP.

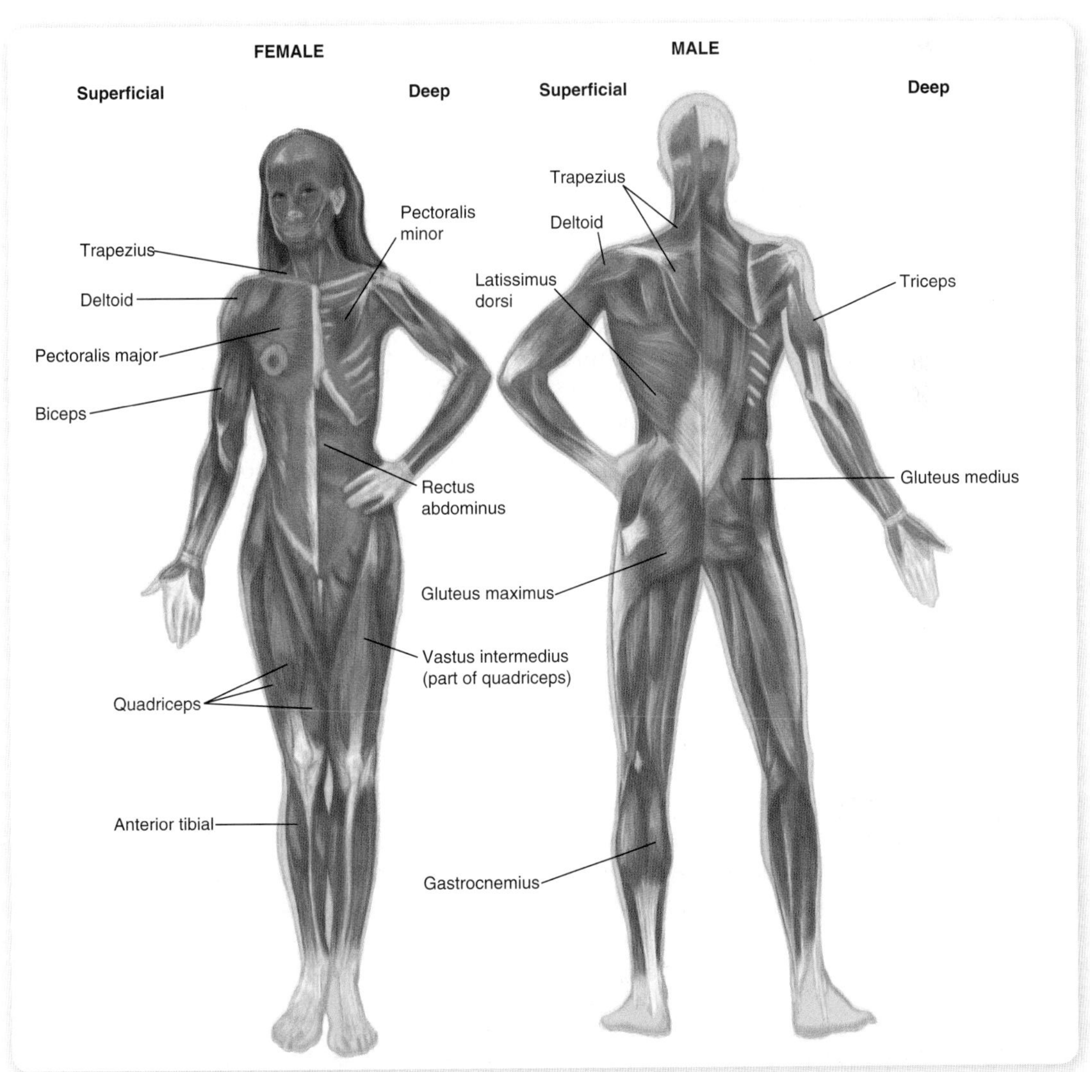

Figure 7-38 The major muscle groups.

Table 7-4 Muscles: Locations and Functions

Name of Muscle	Location	Function
Biceps	Anterior, humerus	Flexes lower arm
Triceps	Posterior, humerus	Extends lower arm
Pectoralis	Anterior, thorax	Flexes and rotates arm
Latissimus dorsi	Posterior, thorax	Extends and rotates arm
Rectus abdominis	Anterior, abdomen	Flexes and rotates spine
Tibialis anterior	Anterior, tibia	Flexes foot toward head
Gastrocnemius	Posterior, tibia	Points foot away from head
Quadriceps (four separate muscles)	Anterior, femur	Extends lower leg
Biceps femoris	Posterior, femur	Flexes lower leg
Gluteus (three separate muscles)	Posterior, pelvis	Extends and rotates leg

Oxygen Use and Debt

Oxygen is required for the breakdown of glucose in the mitochondria. RBCs carry oxygen bound to hemoglobin molecules. **Hemoglobin** is the pigment that makes blood appear red. One hemoglobin molecule reversibly binds with four oxygen molecules. The pigment **myoglobin** is synthesized in the muscles to give skeletal muscles their red-brown color. Myoglobin can also combine with oxygen and temporarily store it to reduce muscular requirements for continuous blood supply during contraction.

When skeletal muscles are used for 1 minute or longer, anaerobic respiration is required for energy. In one type of anaerobic respiration, glucose is broken down via glycolysis to yield pyruvic acid, which reacts by producing lactic acid. Recall that **lactic acid** can accumulate in muscles but diffuses in the bloodstream, reaching the liver, where it is synthesized into glucose.

When a person exercises strenuously, oxygen is used mostly to synthesize ATP. As lactic acid increases, an oxygen debt develops. Oxygen debt is equivalent to the amount of oxygen that liver cells require to convert the lactic acid into glucose, as well as the amount needed by muscle cells to restore ATP and creatine phosphate levels.

The sensation of muscle fatigue occurs when the energy supply to the muscle is inadequate to meet the energy demands. If muscle fatigue occurs as a result of excessive muscular activity, rest produces quick recovery. If it occurs from a lack of oxygen or essential nutrients or electrolytes (such as sodium or calcium), however, rest will not result in such a quick recovery.

It may take several hours for the body to convert lactic acid back into glucose. Muscles may experience a change in their metabolic activity as exercise levels change. Increased exercise raises the capacity of the muscles for glycolysis. Aerobic exercise increases the capacity of the muscles for aerobic respiration. This process is summarized in Table 7-5.

Table 7-5 Changes in Muscular Metabolism

Type of Exercise	Pathway Needed	Production of ATP	Result
Low to moderate intensity: blood flow provides enough oxygen for the needs of the cell	Glycolysis, which results in formation of pyruvic acid and aerobic respiration	For skeletal muscle, 36 molecules of ATP per glucose	Exhalation of carbon dioxide
High intensity: oxygen supply is not enough for the needs of the cell	Glycolysis, which results in formation of lactic acid	Two molecules of ATP per glucose	Buildup of lactic acid

Abbreviation: ATP, adenosine triphosphate

The Respiratory System: Anatomy

The **respiratory system** consists of all the structures of the body that contribute to respiration, or the process of breathing **Figure 7-39**. It includes the nose, mouth, throat, larynx, trachea, bronchi, and bronchioles, which are all air passages or airways. The system also includes the lungs, where oxygen passes into the blood and carbon dioxide escapes. Finally, the respiratory system includes the diaphragm, the muscles of the chest wall, and accessory muscles of breathing, which permit normal respiratory movement. In this text, the term *airway* usually refers to the upper airway or the passage above the larynx (voice box).

> **Safety**
>
> A cough is the perfect mechanism for aerosolizing infectious materials. Whenever possible, minimize the risk of exposure by placing an oxygen mask on a patient with a cough.

The Upper Airway

The structures of the upper airway are located anteriorly and at the midline. The upper airway includes the nose, mouth, tongue, jaw, oral cavity, larynx, and pharynx.

The tongue is a large muscle attached at the mandible and hyoid bone. The hyoid bone is a small bone located between the chin and the mandibular angle. The jaw, tongue, epiglottis, and thyroid cartilage attach at this point. The palate forms the roof of the mouth and separates the oropharynx and nasopharynx. The anterior portion is the hard palate, and the posterior portion, beyond the teeth, is the soft palate. The adenoids are located on the posterior nasopharyngeal wall. Adenoids are lymph tissues that filter bacteria and viruses.

The lateral borders of the glottis are the vocal cords, which are white bands of tough, fibrous tissue. Voice is generated by air passing through the vibrating vocal cords. The arytenoid cartilage is a pyramidlike cartilaginous structure that forms the posterior attachment of the vocal cords. The pyriform fossae are hollow "pockets" along the lateral borders of the larynx.

The larynx is typically considered the dividing line between the upper and lower airway. The larynx is a rather complex arrangement of tiny bones, cartilage, muscles, and two vocal cords. The larynx does not

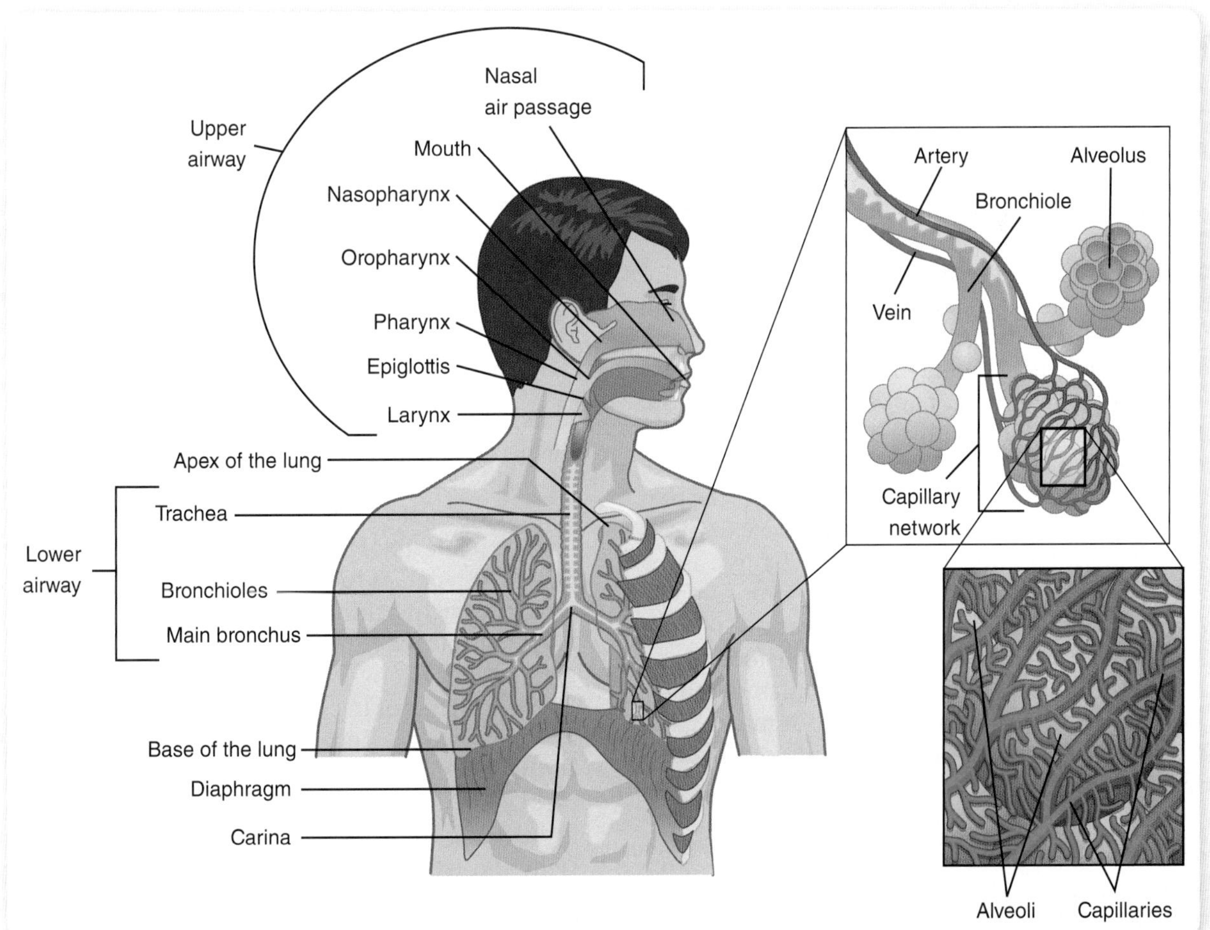

Figure 7-39 The respiratory system consists of all structures of the body that contribute to the process of breathing.

tolerate any foreign solid or liquid material. A violent episode of coughing and spasm of the vocal cords will result from contact with solids or liquids. The nose and mouth lead to the oropharynx, the upper part of the throat that lies at the back of the mouth, behind the oral cavity. The pharynx is composed of the nasopharynx, oropharynx, and the laryngopharynx. The nostrils lead to the **nasopharynx** (above the roof of the mouth, or soft palate), and the mouth leads to the oropharynx. The nasopharynx and the nasal passages, which include the turbinates (three curved bone shelves inside each nasal passage that force inhaled air to flow in a steady pattern across the largest possible surface of the cilia and tissue), warm, filter, and humidify air as a person breathes. The nasal mucosa is the mucous membrane that lines the nasal cavity. Olfactory receptors located in the epithelium in the nasal cavity are responsible for recognizing odors. Air enters through the mouth more rapidly and directly. As a result, it is less moist than air that enters through the nose.

Two passageways are located at the bottom of the pharynx: the esophagus behind and the trachea (windpipe) in front. The trachea is a tubular structure approximately 10 to 12 cm in length and consists of C-shaped cartilaginous rings. Food and liquids enter the pharynx and pass into the esophagus, which carries them to the stomach. Air enters the trachea and goes to the lungs.

Protecting the opening of the trachea is a thin, leaf-shaped valve called the **epiglottis**. This valve allows air to pass into the trachea but prevents food and liquid from entering the airway under normal circumstances. Air moves past the epiglottis into the larynx and the trachea. The glottis or glottic opening is the space between the vocal cords where air enters the trachea.

The shield-shaped thyroid cartilage is the major laryngeal structure and is formed by two plates that join in a "V" shape anteriorly to form the laryngeal prominence known as the Adam's apple. This is easily seen in the middle of the front of the neck. The thyroid cartilage is actually the anterior part of the larynx. Tiny muscles open and close the vocal cords and control tension on them. Sounds are created as air is forced past the vocal cords, making them vibrate. These vibrations make the sound. The pitch of the sound changes as the cords open and close. You can feel the vibrations if you place your fingers lightly on the larynx as you speak or sing. The vibrations of air are shaped by the tongue and muscles of the mouth to form understandable sounds. The posterior portion is made of smooth muscle. The thyroid cartilage is suspended from the hyoid bone by the thyroid ligament.

The Lower Airway

The lower airway contains the trachea, bronchial tree, alveoli, and lungs. The lower airway is where gas exchange occurs; oxygen diffuses into the pulmonary capillaries and carbon dioxide diffuses in the opposite direction.

Words of Wisdom

Asthma is a recurring condition of reversible acute airflow obstruction in the lower airway. It is the most common chronic disease of childhood. Four distinct events occur in an asthma attack. First, a muscle spasm occurs when the smooth muscle layers around the airways constrict (**bronchospasm**), resulting in narrowing of the airway diameter. Second, increased secretion of mucus causes a mucus plug, further decreasing the airway diameter. Third, inflammatory cell proliferation causes swelling of the lining of the airways, also decreasing airway diameter. Finally, WBCs accumulate in the airway and secrete substances that worsen the muscle spasm and increase mucus production.

The most common cause of an asthma attack is an upper respiratory infection, such as bronchitis or a cold. Other causes include changes in environmental conditions; emotions, especially stress; allergic reactions to pollens, foods (chocolate, shellfish, milk, nuts), or drugs (penicillin, local anesthetics); and occupational exposures.

The severity of asthma attacks varies among patients. In severe cases (status asthmaticus), the patient may die as a result of respiratory failure. In other cases, treatment may produce rapid improvement and resolution of the asthmatic crisis.

As mentioned earlier, immediately below the thyroid cartilage is the palpable cricoid cartilage. The inferior aspect of the thyroid cartilage articulates with the cricoid cartilage or cricoid ring. The cricoid cartilage is the only upper airway structure that forms a complete ring. It is the first tracheal ring and is completely cartilaginous. The anterior portion of the cricoid ring is the narrowest and is separated from the thyroid cartilage by the cricothyroid membrane—a thin, fibrous membrane located between the cricoid ring and the thyroid cartilage. The cricothyroid membrane can be felt as a depression in the midline of the neck just inferior to the thyroid cartilage.

Below the cricoid cartilage is the trachea. The trachea is approximately 5 inches long and is a semirigid, enclosed air tube made up of rings of cartilage that are open in the back. This enables food to pass through the esophagus, which lies right behind the trachea. The rings of cartilage keep the trachea from collapsing when air moves into and out of the lungs.

At the level of the fifth thoracic vertebra, the trachea branches into the right and left mainstem bronchi at the carina, a projection of the lowest portion of the tracheal cartilage.

Beyond the carina, air enters the lungs through the right and left **mainstem bronchi**. The point of entry for the bronchi, blood vessels, and nerves into each lung is called the **hilum**. The mainstem bronchi divide into the smaller **secondary bronchi**, each one going to a separate lobe of the lung **Figure 7-40**.

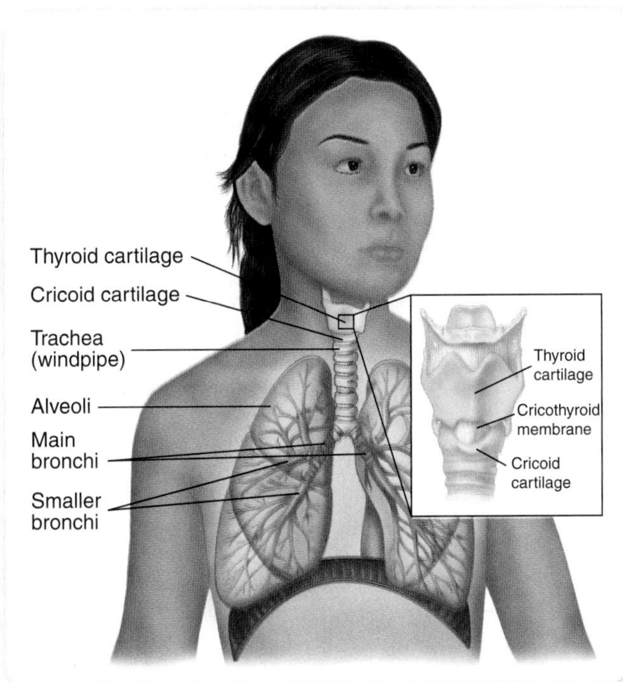

Figure 7-40 The mainstem bronchi and related structures.

Secondary bronchi branch into the even smaller **tertiary bronchi**, which continue to branch several times. After several generations of successive branching, **bronchioles**, extremely small subdivisions of the bronchi, are formed. Each bronchiole divides to form **alveolar ducts**. Each alveolar duct ends in clusters known as **alveoli**, tiny sacs of lung tissue in which gas exchange takes place. Pulmonary **surfactant** found in the alveoli reduces surface tension to increase pulmonary compliance and prevent atelectasis (alveolar collapse) at the end of expiration. The lung contains approximately 300 million alveoli; each alveolus is approximately 0.33 mm in diameter. Capillaries cover the alveoli. The **alveolocapillary membrane** (better known as the pulmonary-capillary membrane) lies between the alveolus and the capillary and is extremely thin, consisting of only one cell layer. Respiratory exchange between the lung and blood vessels occurs in the alveoli at the alveolocapillary membrane.

Lungs

The **lungs** are the primary organs of breathing. The right lung contains three lobes (the upper, middle, and lower lobes); the left lung contains only two (the upper and lower lobes). The lungs are surrounded by a membrane of connective tissue known as **pleura**. Another pleural membrane lines the inner borders of the rib cage, or **pleural cavity**.

The connective tissue, small airways, and alveoli are collectively referred to as the lung parenchyma. The lung parenchyma is composed of two lobes on the left and three lobes on the right. It is surrounded by the pleurae, or pleural membranes. The pleural membrane that lines the pleural cavity is the **parietal pleura**. The parietal pleura covers the thoracic wall and superior face of the diaphragm. The pleural membrane that covers the external surface of the lungs is referred to as the **visceral pleura**. The pleurae produce a pleural or serous lubricating fluid that allows

YOU are the Provider — PART 2

As you approach the patient, a police officer stops you and states that the patient was an innocent bystander in an apparent drive-by shooting. Officers have searched the scene and have found no other patients. Your patient presents as conscious, alert, and oriented, and in a substantial amount of pain. He states that he heard five or six gunshots; but he is unsure of how many times he was hit. You direct your partner to manually stabilize the neck as you roll the patient onto his back. As you remove the blood-soaked shirt, you find three gunshot wounds: one in his left chest, one on his left arm, and one to his left upper abdominal quadrant. His chief complaint is that it is becoming increasingly difficult to breathe and that it feels like his stomach is on fire.

Recording Time: 1 Minute	
Appearance	Severe pain
Level of consciousness	Alert and oriented
Airway	Patent
Breathing	12 breaths/min, shallow
Circulation	Cool, pale, and clammy

3. What are the components of the respiratory system?
4. On the basis of your knowledge of anatomy, what possible organs may be damaged as a result of the gunshot wound to the abdomen?

Special Populations

The anatomy of the respiratory system in children is proportionally smaller and less rigid than that in an adult Figure 7-41. A child's nose and mouth are much smaller than those of an adult. The larynx, cricoid cartilage, and trachea are smaller, softer, and more flexible as well. This makes the mechanics of breathing much more delicate. A child's pharynx is also smaller and less deeply curved. The tongue takes up proportionally more space in a child's mouth than in an adult's mouth.

These anatomic differences are important for your assessment. For example, the smaller larynx of a child becomes obstructed more easily. The chest wall in children is softer. Therefore, children depend more heavily on the diaphragm for breathing. You will notice that the abdomen moves in and out considerably with each breath, especially in an infant. Young infants do not know how to breathe through the mouth. Therefore, as you assess an infant or a child, you must carefully consider these differences.

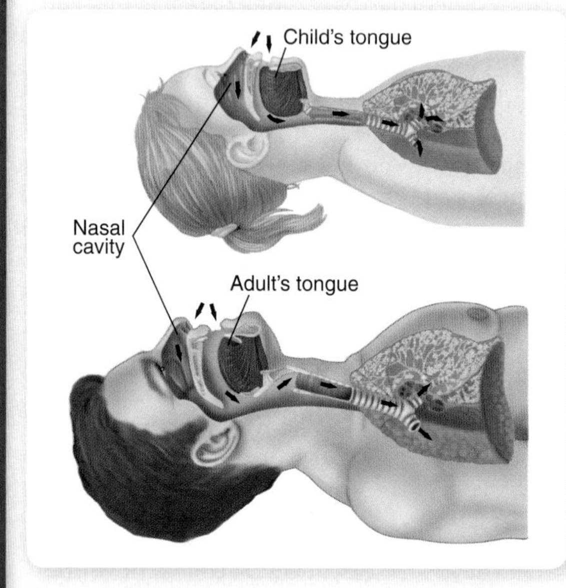

Figure 7-41 The respiratory system of a child is proportionally smaller and less rigid than that of an adult.

the lungs to glide easily over the intrathoracic wall during breathing. Both layers of pleura work together to help maintain normal expansion and contraction of the lung.

A potential space known as the **pleural space** exists between the visceral and parietal pleura. Normally, the two membranes are close together and an actual space does not exist. Under certain disease conditions or following trauma, blood, excess pleural fluid, and/or air may accumulate in the pleural space, potentially causing respiratory problems Figure 7-42.

The lungs receive blood in two ways. Deoxygenated blood flows from the right ventricle via the pulmonary

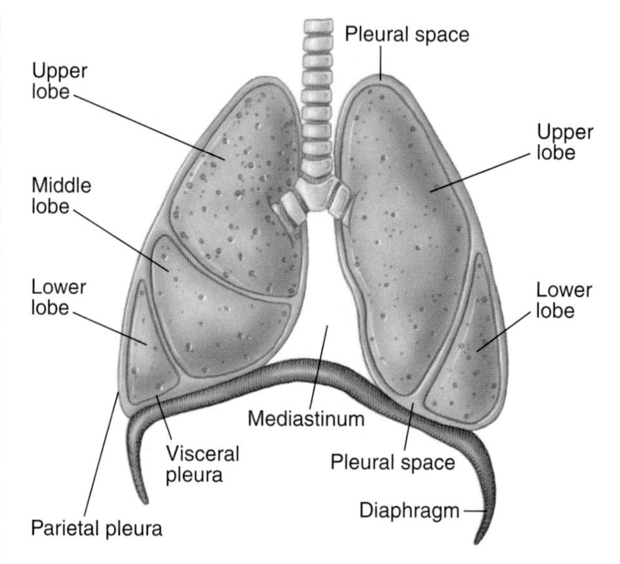

Figure 7-42 The pleura lining the chest wall and covering the lungs is an essential part of the breathing mechanism. The pleural space is not an actual space until blood or air leaks into it, causing the pleural surfaces to separate.

arteries. This blood flows through pulmonary capillaries, is reoxygenated at the alveoli, and then returns to the heart via the pulmonary veins.

In addition, bronchial arteries branch off of the thoracic aorta and supply the lung tissues themselves with blood. Deoxygenated blood returns to the heart via the bronchial veins. Peripherally in the lungs, venous blood from the bronchi enters the pulmonary veins, returning with oxygenated blood from the alveoli.

▶ Muscles of Breathing

There are several muscles involved in making the lungs expand and contract. The primary muscle is called the **diaphragm**. Contraction of the diaphragm, along with that of the chest wall muscles, allows air to be drawn into the lungs. Anteriorly, it attaches to the costal arch; posteriorly, it attaches to the lumbar vertebrae. The diaphragm cannot be seen or palpated without opening the chest or abdomen.

The diaphragm is unique because it has characteristics of voluntary (skeletal) and involuntary (smooth) muscle. It is a dome-shaped muscle that divides the thorax from the abdomen and is pierced by the great vessels and the esophagus Figure 7-43. It acts like a voluntary muscle when you take a deep breath, cough, or hold your breath. You control these variations in the way you breathe.

However, unlike other skeletal or voluntary muscles, the diaphragm performs an automatic function. Breathing continues during sleep and at all other times. Although you can hold your breath or temporarily breathe faster or slower, you cannot continue these variations in the breathing pattern indefinitely. When the concentration of carbon dioxide becomes too high, automatic regulation of breathing resumes. Therefore, although the diaphragm looks like

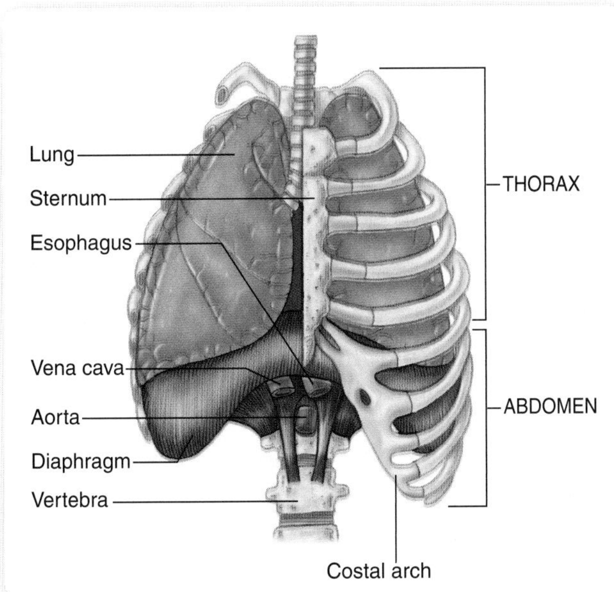

Figure 7-43 The dome-shaped diaphragm divides the thorax from the abdomen. It is pierced by the great vessels and the esophagus.

voluntary skeletal muscle and is attached to the skeleton, it behaves, for the most part, like an involuntary muscle.

The other muscles involved in breathing are the intercostal muscles, the abdominal muscles, and the pectoral muscles. Muscles of the chest wall are innervated by the intercostal nerves, causing them to expand and contract, along with the diaphragm, to facilitate breathing. During inhalation, the diaphragm and intercostal muscles contract. When the diaphragm contracts, it moves down slightly, enlarging the thoracic cage from top to bottom. When the intercostal muscles contract, they move the ribs up and out. These actions combine to enlarge the chest cavity in all dimensions. Pressure in the thoracic cavity then falls, making it lower than atmospheric pressure, causing air to flow into the lungs. This is referred to as negative pressure breathing because air is essentially sucked into the lungs. This part of the cycle is active, requiring the muscles to contract.

Words of Wisdom

Each intercostal muscle is actually made up of a muscle group (muscle layers) that works together to move the ribs and facilitate breathing.

- External intercostal muscles are the inspiratory breathing muscles. They help move the ribs up and out during inhalation.
- Internal intercostal muscles are the expiratory breathing muscles. They pull the ribs down and in during forced exhalation.
- Innermost intercostal muscles are deep to the plane of the internal and external intercostal muscles and work in conjunction with internal intercostal muscles during exhalation.

During exhalation, the diaphragm and the intercostal muscles relax. Unlike inhalation, exhalation does not normally require muscular effort. As these muscles relax, all dimensions of the thorax decrease, and the ribs and muscles assume a normal resting position. When the volume of the thoracic cavity decreases, air in the lungs is compressed into a smaller space and pressure is greater than atmospheric pressure. Intrapulmonary pressure is increased, and air is pushed out through the trachea. This phase of the cycle is passive.

The process of breathing is typically easy and requires little muscular effort. But, now imagine breathing through a straw and suddenly the diameter of the straw decreases. The smaller the diameter of the straw, the more effort you will now have to exert to move air. As the resistance in the airway increases, you will begin to use more muscle groups, namely your abdominal and pectoral muscles, to assist the diaphragm in moving that air.

Words of Wisdom

Chronic obstructive pulmonary disease (COPD) is a progressive, irreversible disease of the airway marked by decreased inspiratory and expiratory capacity of the lungs. COPD may result from chronic bronchitis (excess mucus production) or emphysema (lung tissue damage with loss of elastic recoil of the lungs). Patients with COPD usually have a combination of both problems and generally function at a certain baseline level until an event occurs that causes an acute episode.

Chronic bronchitis results from overgrowth of the airway mucous glands and excess secretion of mucus, which blocks the airway. Patients have a chronic productive cough. Emphysema results from destruction of the alveolar walls, which creates resistance to expiratory airflow. The major cause of COPD is cigarette smoking.[1] Industrial inhalants (such as asbestos and coal dust), air pollution, and tuberculosis also can result in COPD. The patient who is experiencing an acute COPD episode will report shortness of breath with gradually increasing symptoms over a period of days. This concept is discussed in greater detail in Chapter 17, *Respiratory Emergencies*.

The Respiratory System: Physiology

The primary function of the respiratory system is to exchange gases at the alveolocapillary membrane, or to conduct **respiration**. Oxygen is essential for the body to function. The amount of oxygen in inspired air is approximately 21%. The blood does not use all inhaled oxygen as it passes through the body. Exhaled air contains 16% oxygen and 3% to 5% carbon dioxide; the rest is nitrogen. This 16% concentration of oxygen is adequate to support artificial ventilation.

Ventilation is the process of moving air in and out of the lungs. Therefore, as you provide mouth-to-mouth artificial ventilations to a patient who is not breathing, the patient is receiving a 16% concentration of oxygen with each ventilation.

▶ Respiration

At the alveolocapillary exchange surface, the alveolus and the RBCs are located very close together. Diffusion is the process by which a gas dissolves in a liquid. Through the process of diffusion, the gases move from a higher concentration to a lower concentration. Therefore, oxygen moves across the membrane into the capillaries where it attaches to the hemoglobin. Likewise, carbon dioxide moves into the alveoli where the concentration is lower. Oxygenated blood enters the left side of the heart and is pumped to the tissues. Oxygen is "offloaded" from the RBCs to the tissues as carbon dioxide and waste products from the tissues are "loaded" into the bloodstream. Venous blood returns to the right side of the heart and the pulmonary capillary bed (via the pulmonary arteries). The carbon dioxide diffuses into the alveoli and is released into the atmosphere as the person exhales Figure 7-44. The primary waste product of metabolism is carbon dioxide, which is carried in the blood to the lungs.

Because there are so many alveoli, a fairly large surface area exists for respiratory exchange to occur in the context of the relatively limited size of the thoracic cavity. The total surface area created around the alveoli is more than 85 m^2. This is substantially more than would exist if each lung consisted of only a single sphere, like a large balloon. In that case, the surface area would be only 0.01 m^2 (1 m = 39.37 inches).

The Chemical Control of Breathing

The brain—or more specifically, the respiratory center in the brainstem—controls breathing. This area is in one of the best-protected parts of the nervous system—deep within the skull. The nerves in this area act as sensors for the level of carbon dioxide in the blood and subsequently the spinal fluid. The brain automatically controls breathing if the level of carbon dioxide or oxygen in the arterial blood is too high or too low. In fact, adjustments can be made in just one breath. For these reasons, you cannot hold your breath indefinitely or breathe rapidly and deeply indefinitely.

Words of Wisdom

Measurements of oxygen and carbon dioxide levels in the blood are called the **partial pressure of oxygen (Pao_2)** and the **partial pressure of carbon dioxide ($Paco_2$)**. These values are not obtained directly by AEMTs, but are useful for AEMTs to understand. **pH** is the degree of acidity or alkalinity. Deviations from normal Pao_2, $Paco_2$, and pH values occur in many different disease states.

A complicated interaction of signals provides feedback to the respiratory center, allowing it to continuously control respiration. The main respiratory stimulus is accumulation of carbon dioxide in the blood. Typically, this is measured as the $Paco_2$ on the arterial blood gases. Increases in the $Paco_2$ result in decreased pH levels in the respiratory center, which triggers an increase in ventilation. Decreases in the $Paco_2$ result in increased pH levels in the respiratory center and a decrease in ventilation. Low blood oxygen

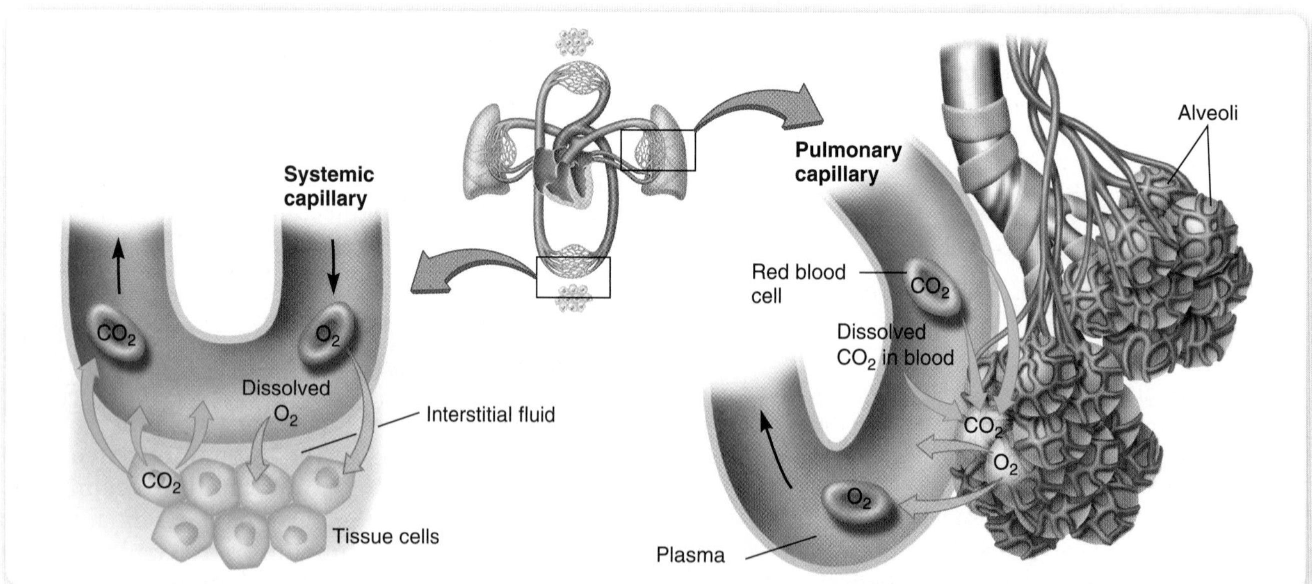

Figure 7-44 In the capillaries of the lungs, oxygen (O_2) passes from the blood to the tissue cells, and carbon dioxide (CO_2) and waste pass from the tissue cells to the blood.

levels also stimulate breathing, but normally have much less of an effect than does the $Paco_2$.

Essentially, $Paco_2$ acts as "respiratory acid." Changes in the $Paco_2$ value rapidly change the pH levels, either making it more basic (increased) or more acidic (decreased). Changes in the $Paco_2$ can result from diseases such as asthma or COPD exacerbation, from drug overdose, or can be a response to a change in the blood pH because of a metabolic problem. A decrease in the pH of the arterial blood that is caused by an elevation in the $Paco_2$ is called a primary **respiratory acidosis**, whereas an increase in the pH of the blood that is caused by excessive exhalation of CO_2 is called a primary **respiratory alkalosis**. Conversely, changes in the $Paco_2$ may occur in response to primary metabolic problems (**metabolic alkalosis** or **metabolic acidosis**); these are called compensatory changes.

The body also has a "backup system" to control respiration called the **hypoxic drive**. When the oxygen level falls, this system will also stimulate breathing. There are areas in the brain, the walls of the aorta, and the carotid arteries that act as oxygen sensors. These sensors are easily satisfied by minimal levels of oxygen in the arterial blood. Therefore, the backup system, the hypoxic drive, is much less sensitive and less powerful than the carbon dioxide sensors in the brainstem.

Acid-Base Balance

An **acid** is a substance that increases the concentration of hydrogen ions in a water solution. A **base** is a substance that decreases the concentration of hydrogen ions.

Whether the blood or body fluid is acidic, basic, or neutral depends on the concentration of dissolved hydrogen (H^+). Hydrogen is an acid. This means that the higher the concentration, the more acidic the blood will be; conversely, the lower the H^+ concentration, the more basic (less acidic) the blood will be. Normal homeostatic functions keep the concentration of H^+ within a fairly narrow range.

The most common expression of acidity is pH, which is a value calculated from H^+ concentration:

$$pH = \text{Concentration of hydrogen ions}$$

Therefore, the lower the hydrogen ion concentration, the greater the pH (more basic) will be, and the higher the hydrogen ion concentration, the lower the pH (more acidic) will be. pH ranges from 0 (most acidic) to 14 (most basic), with 7.0 being neutral. (The pH of pure water, which is considered neutral, is 7.0.) The pH of the human body is normally slightly basic, or alkaline, ranging approximately from 7.35 to 7.45. Normal body functions work best within this narrow range of pH. When pH is higher than this, the blood is too basic, or *alkalotic*. When pH is lower, the blood is too acidic, or *acidotic* Figure 7-45. Cellular function deteriorates and death occurs when the pH drops below 6.9 or rises above 7.8.

Buffer Systems. A **buffer** is a compound that can repeatedly neutralize excess acids or bases to prevent the pH from going beyond an acceptable level. A buffer can absorb or donate H^+. Buffers absorb hydrogen ions when they are in excess and donate hydrogen ions when they are depleted. Therefore, a **buffer system** acts as a fast defense for acid-base changes, providing almost immediate protection against changes in the hydrogen ion concentration of the ECF. The generic reaction between a hydrogen ion and a buffer is expressed as follows:

$$H^+ + \text{Buffer} \leftrightarrow \text{H-Buffer}$$

Free H^+ (acid) binds with the buffer to form a weak acid (H-Buffer). This reaction can shift to the right or left depending on the hydrogen ion concentration. When the H^+ concentration increases and buffer is available, the reaction is forced to the right and more H-Buffer is formed. When the H^+ concentration decreases, the reaction shifts toward the left, and H^+ disassociates from the buffer, leaving H^+ and buffer.

An analogy for understanding a buffer system is to imagine it as a bucket Figure 7-46. Like a bucket, the buffer system can hold only a certain amount of acid before it reaches the point at which it is saturated (the bucket is full) and overflows. The body responds to shifts in the pH level by absorbing or releasing small amounts of acid into the blood. Problems begin when the amount

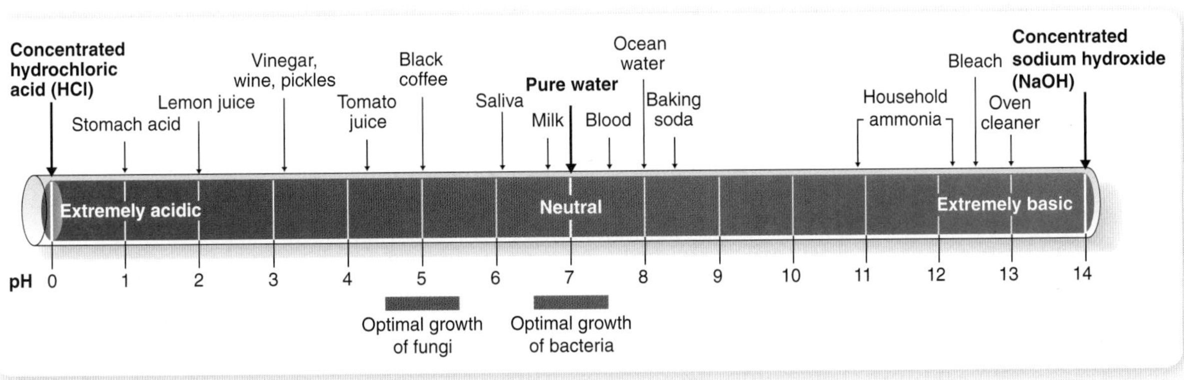

Figure 7-45 The pH scale.

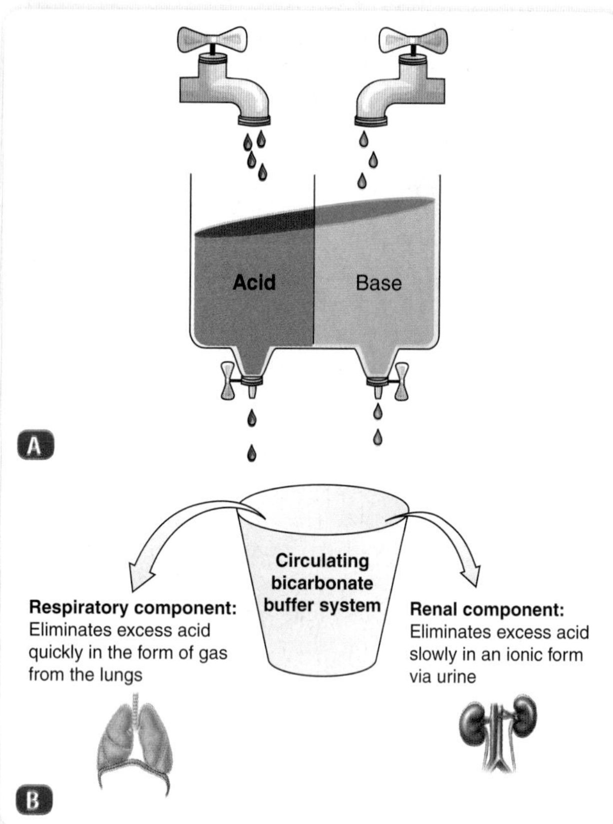

Figure 7-46 Bucket analogy of the body's buffer system. **A.** Acid and base levels in the body fluctuate. **B.** The respiratory and renal systems eliminate excess acid.

of acid in circulation is too great and the buffer system becomes overwhelmed.

Ion Shifts. Concentrations of H+ ions can be increased by adding more H+ ions to a solution or by removing OH−. To make a **solution** more acidic, that is decrease its pH, a higher concentration of H+ and a lower concentration of OH− are needed. If the solution needs to be more basic, meaning increasing the pH level, there are two options:

1. Decrease the amount of H^+.
2. Increase the amount of OH^-.

Acids can be classified as strong or weak, depending on how completely they dissociate (how easily they lose a hydrogen atom) in water. It is the ability of weak acids to bond weakly to hydrogen ions that makes them ideal buffers because they can accept or donate hydrogen ions, depending on the needs of the body.

To function properly, acid-base balance, or a balance of charges, must exist on both sides of the cell. If intracellular pH is low, excess H^+ ions exist in the ECF (fluid outside the cells), and H^+ ions move into the cell. This causes the cell to have an overall positive charge. To return its overall charge to neutral, the cell begins to shift cations (ions with a positive charge) into the interstitial fluid. Potassium shifts out into the ECF until no more potassium can safely be shifted out. This shift has significant consequences and can lead to hyperkalemia, a serious medical emergency.

Calcium ions also shift out of the cell in response to the influx of hydrogen. A high serum calcium level (hypercalcemia) decreases neural transmissions (the speed at which an impulse travels through the nerve cell), whereas a low serum calcium level (hypocalcemia) leads to hypersensitive nerve cells and increased neural transmissions. An increase in extracellular H^+ ions results in **acidosis**; a decrease in extracellular H^+ ions results in **alkalosis**.

$\downarrow$ pH means $\uparrow$ H^+ ion concentration = Acidosis
$\uparrow$ pH means $\downarrow$ H^+ ion concentration = Alkalosis

Types of acid-base imbalance are discussed in Chapter 8, *Pathophysiology*.

The respiratory system and the renal system work in conjunction with the bicarbonate buffer to maintain homeostasis. The fastest way the body can get rid of excess acid is through the respiratory system. Excess acid can be expelled as CO_2 from the lungs. Conversely, slowing respirations will increase CO_2 in alkalotic states. The renal system regulates pH by filtering out more hydrogen and retaining bicarbonate in acidotic states, and doing just the reverse in alkalotic states.

Also, bone acts as a buffer by absorbing excess acids and bases and by releasing calcium into the circulation.

There are three main components to the buffer system in the body:

- The circulating bicarbonate buffer component
- The respiratory component
- The renal component

The following equation illustrates the balance among these three components:

$CO_2 + H_2O$	$\leftrightarrow$	H_2CO_3	$\leftrightarrow$	$HCO_3^- + H^+$
Respiratory component		Circulating bicarbonate buffer component		Renal component

The Circulating Bicarbonate Buffer Component. The circulating bicarbonate buffer component is the "bucket" that holds and neutralizes excess acid. The circulating bicarbonate buffer system is found in the ICF and ECF and is the fastest acting segment of the buffer system.

$$H_2CO_3 \leftrightarrow H^+ + HCO_3^-$$

Carbonic acid (H_2CO_3) is a weak acid that can give up an extra H^+ ion to reform as the bicarbonate ion (HCO_3^-). Through metabolic processes, the extra H^+ ion is then converted into compounds that are easily expelled from the body, eliminating the extra acid.

The Respiratory Component. The fastest way the body can get rid of the excess H+ ions is to create water and carbon dioxide, which can be expelled as gases from the lungs. The following equation illustrates this process, which occurs in the lungs:

$$H_2CO_3 \leftrightarrow CO_2 + H_2O$$

The main reason for breathing is to bring oxygen in for aerobic metabolism and to remove excess carbon dioxide in the blood. Carbon dioxide combines with the circulating water of the blood to create carbonic acid. Chemoreceptors in the brain sense the rising level of carbonic acid and signal the respiratory center to increase respirations and to reduce the available amount of circulating carbon dioxide. Although the respiratory component reacts within minutes, it is much slower to respond than the circulating buffer system. Consider the buffer bucket example again; the respiratory component can be thought of as a large faucet that allows acid to spill out of the buffer bucket, returning the pH to a normal level.

Anything that limits respirations can lead to acid retention and acidosis. Any time a patient is in respiratory distress or is unable to breathe, acidosis quickly develops:

$$\uparrow H^+ \rightarrow \uparrow H_2CO_3 \rightarrow \uparrow CO_2 \rightarrow \text{Tachypnea}$$

A patient can develop acidosis as a result of respiratory difficulty. The following equation demonstrates this:

$$\downarrow \text{Respirations} \rightarrow \uparrow CO_2 \rightarrow \uparrow H_2CO_3 \rightarrow \text{Acidosis}$$

Alkalosis can also develop if the respiratory rate is too high (or the volume too much), as shown in the following equation:

$$\uparrow \text{Respirations} \rightarrow \downarrow CO_2 \rightarrow \downarrow H_2CO_3 \rightarrow \text{Alkalosis}$$

The Renal Component. Another smaller faucet connected to the buffer bucket is the renal component. The smaller faucet represents the slower nature by which the kidneys respond to the increasing acid level. The renal response could take from hours to days to restore the body's pH to normal. Kidneys account for every molecule, ion, and electrolyte found in the circulation; they maintain homeostasis by retaining certain products and filtering out others.

As with the respiratory system, the renal system can control the increasing acid level in the blood by excreting the acid. The kidneys excrete acid in an ionic form, unlike the respiratory system, which excretes acid as a gas.

$$H_2CO_3 \leftrightarrow H^+ + HCO_3^-$$

If the patient experiences decreased urine output, excess acid cannot be removed from the blood, and acidosis can develop.

$$\downarrow \text{Output} \rightarrow \uparrow H^+ \rightarrow \text{Acidosis}$$

If urine output becomes excessive, alkalosis can develop.

$$\uparrow \text{Output} \rightarrow \downarrow H^+ \rightarrow \text{Alkalosis}$$

The Nervous System Control of Breathing

The exact way breathing occurs is complicated and also poorly understood by science. It is known that the medulla oblongata—the lower half of the brainstem that, among others, controls those autonomic functions such as breathing, heart rate, and blood pressure—is primarily responsible for initiating the ventilation cycle and is primarily stimulated by high carbon dioxide levels. The function of the medulla is to keep you breathing so you do not have to think about it. The medulla has two main portions that control breathing: the **dorsal respiratory group (DRG)** and the **ventral respiratory group (VRG)**. The DRG is the main pacemaker for breathing and is responsible for initiating inspiration. It sets the base pattern for respirations. The DRG sends signals down the phrenic nerves to the diaphragm. (Originating from the cervical plexus of nerves in the neck, the phrenic nerves are among the most important nervous structures in the body.) The diaphragm contracts, and inspiration begins. The DRG shuts off, the diaphragm relaxes, and expiration begins. The VRG helps facilitate forced inspiration or expiration as needed.

The pons, another area within the brainstem, helps regulate the DRG activities. The pons has two areas. The **pneumotaxic (pontine) center**, located in the superior portion of the pons, helps shut off the DRG, resulting in shorter, faster respirations. The apneustic center, located in the inferior portion of the pons, stimulates the DRG, resulting in longer, slower respirations. Both areas of the pons are used to help augment respirations during emotional or physical stress. The two areas of the medulla and the two areas of the pons work together to help you get the right amount of air when you need it.

The VRG, pneumotaxic center, and apneustic center are involved in changing the depth of inspiration, expiration, or both. How does the body know when to stop breathing in or out? When the VRG is causing you to take a forced inspiration, what prevents you from taking in so much air that you pop your lungs like a balloon? The answer is the **Hering-Breuer reflex**. Special stretch receptors in the chest wall are able to detect if the lungs are too full or too empty. The Hering-Breuer reflex stops the VRG, pneumotaxic center, and apneustic centers from accidentally causing lung trauma. Because this reflex also increases ventilatory frequency, it maintains a constant alveolar ventilation.[2]

Table 7-6 Nervous System Control of Breathing

Name	Location	Function	Timing
Dorsal respiratory group	Medulla	Causes inspiration when stimulated	Normal, resting respirations Rhythmic, mechanical pattern
Ventral respiratory group	Medulla	Causes forced expiration or inspiration	Speech, increased emotional or physical stress
Pneumotaxic (pontine) center	Pons	Inhibits the DRG; increases speed and depth of respirations	Increased emotional or physical stress
Apneustic center	Pons	Excites the DRG; prolongs inspiration, decreases rate	Increased emotional or physical stress
Hering-Breuer inflation reflex (stretch reflex)	Chest	Detects lung expansion to a point and then tells VRG and pneumotaxic and apneustic centers to stop	Increased emotional or physical stress
Hering-Breuer deflation reflex	Chest	Detects potential lung collapse and then tells VRG and pneumotaxic and apneustic centers to stop	Increased emotional or physical stress

Abbreviations: DRG, dorsal respiratory group; VRG, ventral respiratory group

Table 7-6 summarizes the nervous system functions regarding respirations.

▶ Lung Volumes

A substantial amount of air can be moved within the respiratory system. Figure 7-47 shows the typical volumes. An adult male has a total lung capacity of 6,000 mL (equivalent to three 2-liter bottles of soda). An adult female has approximately one-third less total capacity because the lung size is smaller.

As you are reading this book, unless you just finished exercising, the amount of your air movement is approximately 500 mL. This is called **tidal volume**. Tidal volume is the amount of air that is moved into or out of the lungs during a single breath. **Inspiratory reserve volume** is the deepest breath you can take after a normal breath. Conversely, **expiratory reserve volume** is the maximum amount of air that you can forcibly breathe out after a normal breath. Gas remains in the lungs simply to keep the lungs open. This is called the **residual volume**. This gas does not move during ventilation. Some residual volume is lost when a person is hit in the chest and has the "wind knocked out of him." **Vital capacity** is the amount of air moved in and out of the lungs with maximum inspiration and expiration.

When you assist a patient's breathing, you move air in and out of the lungs. You will use a bag-mask device—a large bag filled with air that, when squeezed, pushes air out one end. The typical bag-mask device holds approximately 1,000 to 1,200 mL of air. Note that although a person's resting tidal volume is 500 mL, you need to use a bag-mask device that provides more than twice that volume. This is because of dead space.

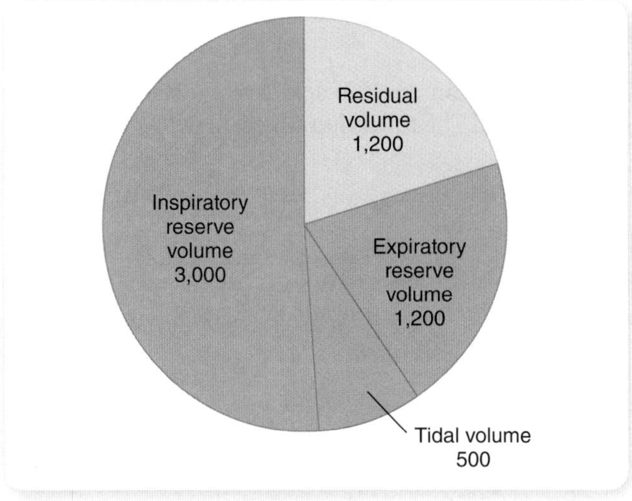

Figure 7-47 Lung volumes (mL).

Dead space is the portion of the respiratory system that has no alveoli, and, therefore, little or no exchange of gas between air and blood occurs. The mouth, trachea, bronchi, and bronchioles are all considered dead space. When you ventilate a patient with any device, you create more dead space. Gas must first fill the device before it can be moved into the patient.

When you are assessing your patient, you need to accurately determine whether he or she is having trouble breathing. Often, AEMTs will look at the patient's respiratory rate; however, this rate provides only part of the information that is needed. The depth of each breath is critical information to know when assessing ventilation. Another measurement called minute volume provides you with a more accurate determination of effective ventilation. **Minute volume**, also referred to as minute ventilation, is easy to understand; it is the amount of air that moves in and out of the lungs in 1 minute minus the dead space.

$$\text{Minute volume} = \text{Respiratory rate} \times \text{Tidal volume}$$

This calculation helps you to determine how deeply a patient is breathing. While riding in the ambulance, it will be difficult to determine the patient's exact tidal volume, but you will be able to estimate it. Consider the scenario of a patient who is breathing at a normal rate of 20 breaths/min. Yet, when you look at the patient's chest, it is barely moving. When you feel for air movement out of the mouth, you find very little movement. The patient is in trouble and needs your assistance now! Even though the patient's respiratory rate is normal, the amount of air being moved is inadequate. The minute volume is too low, and the patient needs ventilatory assistance. You will need to always evaluate the amount of air being moved with each breath when assessing a patient's respirations.

Characteristics of Normal Breathing

You can think of a normal breathing pattern as a bellows system. Normal breathing (eupnea) should appear easy, not labored. As with a bellows that is used to move air to start a fire, breathing should be a smooth flow of air moving into and out of the lungs.

Normal breathing has the following characteristics:

- A normal rate and depth (tidal volume)
- A regular rhythm or pattern of inhalation and exhalation
- Good audible breath sounds on both sides of the chest
- Regular rise and fall movement on both sides of the chest
- Movement of the abdomen

The Circulatory System: Anatomy

The **circulatory system** is a complex arrangement of tubes connected to one another and to a pump, including the heart and the arteries, arterioles, capillaries, venules, and veins Figure 7-48. Another name for this system is the cardiovascular (heart/blood vessels) system. The circulatory system is entirely closed, and through arterial and venous anastomosis (connections), vessels are able to branch off to deliver blood with capillaries connecting arterioles and venules. There are two circuits in the body: the **systemic circulation** in the body and the **pulmonary circulation** in the lungs. The systemic circulation, the circuit in the body, carries oxygen-rich blood from the left ventricle through the body and back to the right atrium. In the systemic circulation, as blood passes through the tissues and organs, it gives up oxygen and nutrients and absorbs cellular wastes and carbon dioxide. The cellular wastes are eliminated in passages through the liver and kidneys. The pulmonary circulation, the circuit in the lungs, carries oxygen-poor blood from the right ventricle through the lungs and back to the left atrium. In the pulmonary circulation, as blood passes through the lungs, it is refreshed with oxygen and gives up carbon dioxide.

The Heart

Location and Major Structures of the Heart

The **heart** is a muscular organ that pumps blood throughout the body Figure 7-49. The heart is located behind the sternum and is about the size of the closed fist of the person it belongs to, roughly 5 inches long, 3 inches wide, and 2 inches thick. It weighs 10 to 12 oz in male adults

> **Special Populations**
>
> Normal breathing patterns in infants and children are essentially the same as those in adults. However, infants and children breathe faster than adults. An infant who is breathing normally will have respirations of 30 to 53 breaths/min. A child will have respirations of 12 to 37 breaths/min. Like adults, infants and children who are breathing normally will have smooth, regular inhalation and exhalation, equal breath sounds, and regular rise and fall movements on both sides of the chest.
>
> Breathing problems in infants and children often appear the same as breathing problems in adults. Signs such as increased respirations, an irregular breathing pattern, unequal breath sounds, unequal chest expansion, and muscle retractions (accessory muscle use) indicate breathing problems in adults and children. Other signs that an infant or child is not breathing normally include the following:
>
> - Nasal flaring, in which the nostrils flare out as the child breathes
> - Seesaw respirations in infants, in which the chest and abdominal muscles alternately contract to look like a seesaw
>
> Exhalation becomes active when infants and children have trouble breathing. Normally, inhalation alone is the active, muscular part of breathing, as described earlier. However, with **labored breathing**, both inhalation and exhalation are hard work. With labored breathing, exhalation is not passive. Instead, air is forced out of the lungs during exhalation, and the child will often begin to wheeze. This type of labored breathing involves the use of the accessory muscles of breathing.

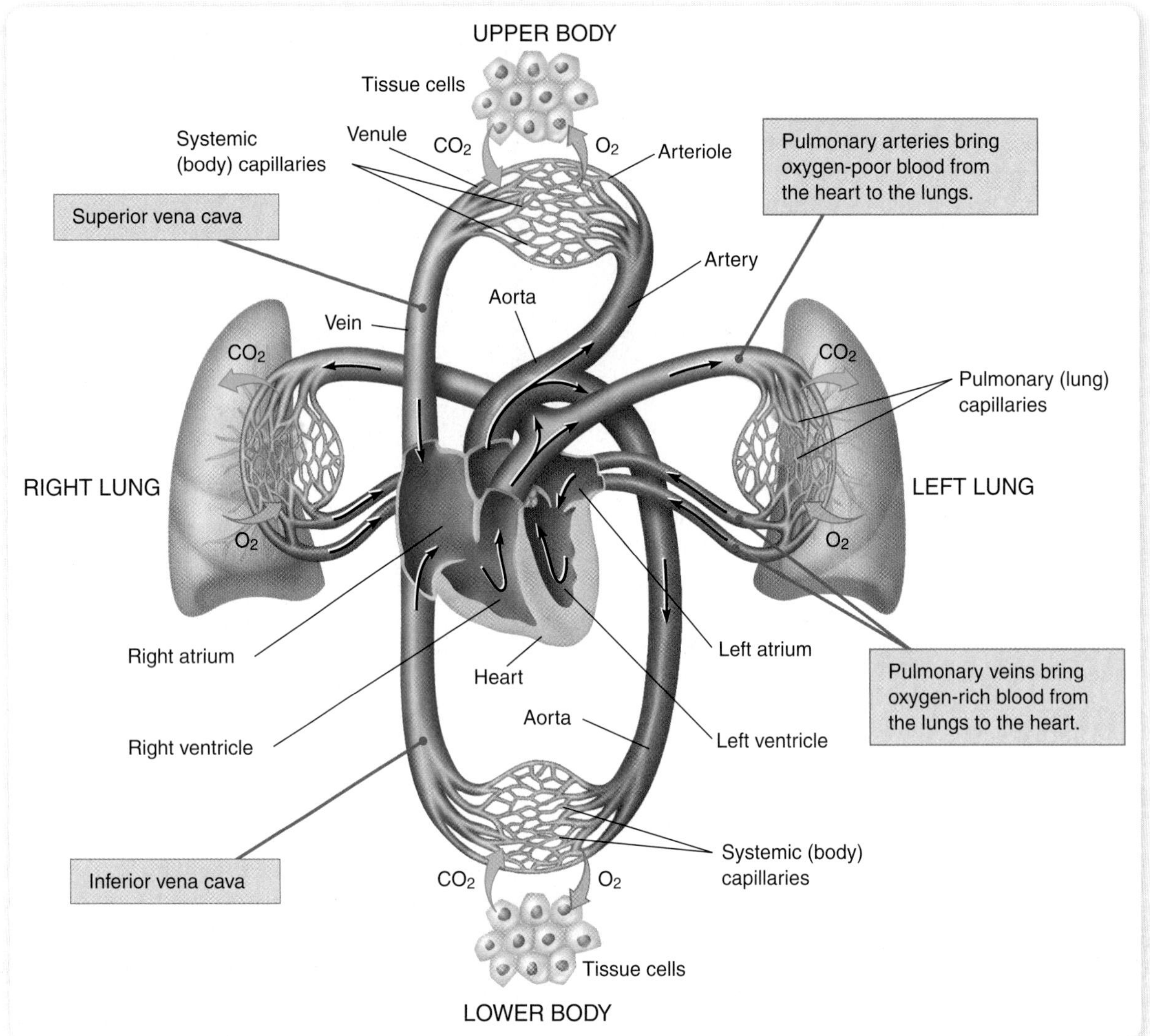

Figure 7-48 The circulatory system includes the heart, arteries, veins, and interconnecting capillaries. The capillaries are the smallest vessels and connect venules and arterioles. At the center of the system, and providing its driving force, is the heart. Blood circulates through the body under pressure generated by the two sides of the heart.

and 8 to 10 oz in female adults. Approximately two-thirds of the heart lies in the left part of the **mediastinum**, the area between the lungs that also contains the great vessels.

Heart muscle is called **myocardium**. The term *myo* means muscle and the word root *cardium* means heart. The **pericardium**, also called the pericardial sac, is a thick, fibrous membrane that surrounds the heart and the bases of the great vessels. The pericardium anchors the heart within the mediastinum and prevents overdistention of the heart. The inner membrane of the pericardium is the serous pericardium. This inner membrane contains two layers: the visceral and the parietal pericardium. The visceral layer of the pericardium lies closely against the heart and is also called the **epicardium**. The second layer of the pericardium, the parietal pericardium, is separated from the visceral layer by a small amount of **pericardial fluid** that reduces friction within the pericardial sac. The **endocardium** is the interior lining of the heart.

The normal human heart consists of four chambers: two atria and two ventricles. The upper chambers are the atria and the lower chambers are the ventricles. Each side of the heart contains one atrium and one ventricle. A membrane, the **interatrial septum**, separates the two atria; a thicker wall, the **interventricular septum**, separates the right and left ventricles. Each **atrium** receives blood that is returned to the heart from other parts of the body; each **ventricle** pumps blood out of the heart. The upper and lower portions of the heart are separated by the atrioventricular valves, which prevent blood from flowing backward. There are also valves located between the ventricles and the arteries into which they pump blood. These are called the **semilunar valves**.

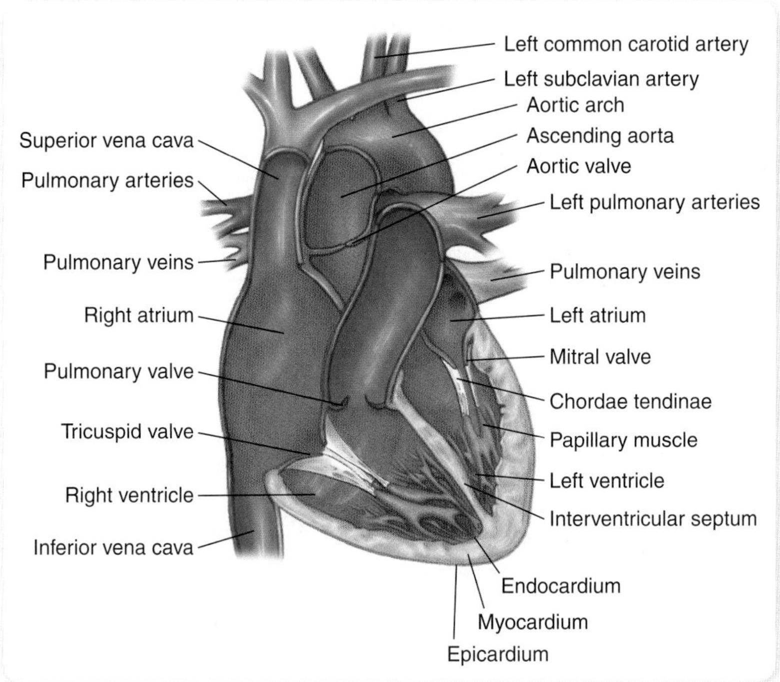

Figure 7-49 Anatomy of the heart.

> **Words of Wisdom**
>
> Complete blockage of an artery that supplies oxygen to the heart results in death to a portion of the myocardium; this event is called a **myocardial infarction**.

Blood enters the right atrium via the superior and inferior venae cavae and the **coronary sinus**, which consists of veins that collect blood that is returning from the walls of the heart. Blood from four **pulmonary veins** enters the left atrium. Between the right and left atria is a depression, the **fossa ovalis**, which represents the former location of the **foramen ovale**, an opening between the two atria that is present in the fetus.

Valves of the Heart

Blood passing from the atria to the ventricles flows through one of two **atrioventricular valves**. The **tricuspid valve** separates the right atrium from the right ventricle, and the **mitral valve**, a bicuspid valve, separates the left atrium from the left ventricle. The valves consist of flaps called cusps. **Papillary muscles** attach to the ventricles and send small muscular strands called **chordae tendineae** to the cusps. When the papillary muscle contracts, these strands tighten, preventing regurgitation of blood through the valves from the ventricles to the atria.

The two semilunar valves, the aortic valve and the pulmonic valve, divide the heart from the aorta and the pulmonary artery. The **pulmonic valve** regulates blood flow from the right ventricle to the pulmonary artery. The **aortic valve** regulates blood flow from the left ventricle to the aorta. The semilunar valves are not attached to papillary muscles. When these valves close, they prevent backflow from the aorta and pulmonary artery into the left and right ventricles, respectively.

Blood Flow Within the Heart

Two large veins, the **superior vena cava** and the **inferior vena cava**, join together to return deoxygenated blood from the body to the right atrium. Blood from the upper part of the body returns to the heart through the superior vena cava, and blood from the lower part of the body returns through the inferior vena cava. The inferior vena cava is the larger of the two veins. From the right atrium, blood passes through the tricuspid valve into the right ventricle. Blood is then pumped by the right ventricle through the pulmonic valve into the pulmonary artery and to the lungs. In the lungs, as mentioned, various processes take place that return oxygen to the blood and, at the same time, remove carbon dioxide and other waste products.

Freshly oxygenated blood is returned to the left atrium through the pulmonary veins. Blood then flows through the mitral valve into the left ventricle, which pumps the oxygenated blood through the aortic valve, into the aorta and then to the entire body. The left ventricle is the strongest and largest of the four cardiac chambers because it is responsible for pumping blood through blood vessels throughout the body.

Heart Sounds

Heart sounds are created by the contraction and relaxation of the heart and flow of blood. These sounds can be heard during auscultation with a stethoscope. Normal heart sounds are often described as sounding like "lub-DUB, lub-DUB, lub-DUB. . . ." The "lub" is called the first heart sound or S_1, and the "DUB" is called the second heart sound or S_2 Figure 7-50. S_2 ("DUB") is often louder than S_1 ("lub"). The sudden closure of the mitral and tricuspid valves at the start of ventricular contraction causes S_1. The closure of both the aortic and pulmonic valves at the end of a ventricular contraction causes S_2.

Two other heart sounds, S_3 and S_4, are not usually heard in people with normal heart function Figure 7-51. The S_3 or third heart sound is a soft, low-pitched heart sound that occurs about one-third of the way through diastole (the period during which the ventricles are relaxed). When an S_3 sound is present, the heart beat cycle is described as sounding like "lub-DUB-da." This sound may correlate to a period of rapid ventricular filling. Although the S_3 sound sometimes is present in healthy young people, it most commonly is associated with abnormally increased filling pressures in the atria secondary to moderate to severe heart failure.

The S_4 heart sound is a medium-pitched sound that occurs immediately before the normal S_1 sound. When an S_4 sound is present, the heart contraction cycle sounds like "bla-lub-DUB." The S_4 sound represents either decreased stretching (compliance) of the left ventricle or increased pressure in the atria. An S_4 heart sound is almost always abnormal.

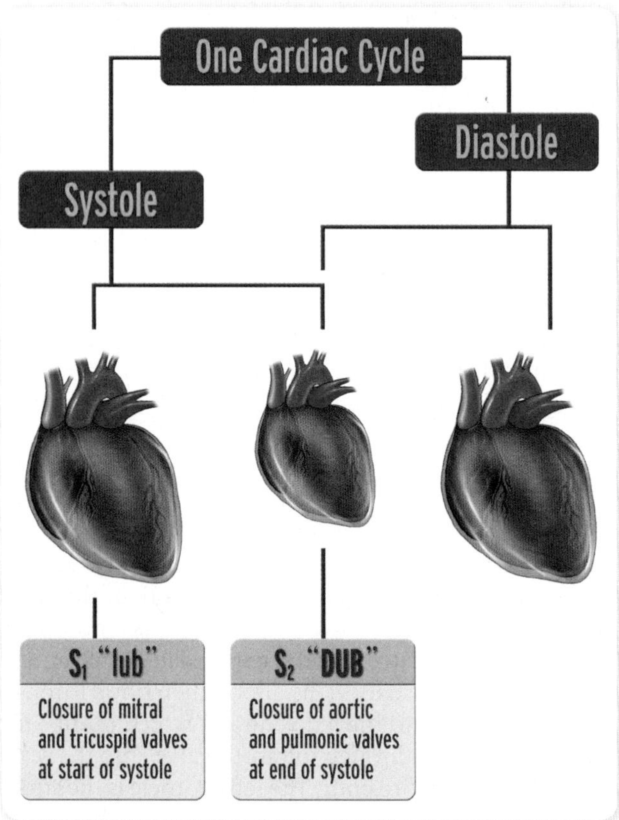

Figure 7-50 The normal S_1 and S_2 heart sounds.

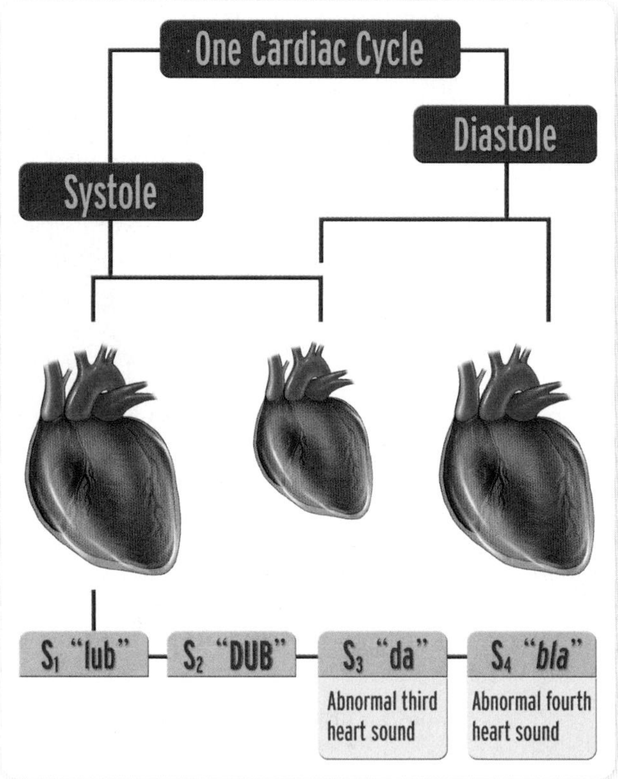

Figure 7-51 The abnormal S_3 and S_4 heart sounds.

Four other sounds, all abnormal, may be heard when auscultating the heart and great vessels. Some of these sounds are very easy to hear; others may require years of experience to identify. These additional abnormal sounds include murmurs, bruits, clicks, and snaps. A **murmur** is an abnormal "whooshinglike" sound heard over the heart that indicates turbulent blood flow within the heart. Although many murmurs are "functional" (benign) and often go away, several are characteristic of heart disease. A **bruit** is an abnormal "whooshinglike" sound heard over a main blood vessel that indicates turbulent blood flow within the blood vessel. A bruit often indicates localized atherosclerotic disease (plaque formation in the arteries). Both clicks and snaps indicate abnormal cardiac valve function. They occur at different times in the cardiac cycle, depending on which valve is diseased. Although these sounds are important, most are fleeting and difficult to hear.

The Electrical Conduction System

The mechanical pumping action of the heart occurs in response to an electrical stimulus. This impulse causes the heart to beat via a set of complex chemical changes within the myocardial cells. The brain partially controls the heart's rate and strength of contraction via the autonomic nervous system. The myocardium is the only muscle that has the property of automaticity, or the ability to generate its own electrical impulses. Therefore, the contractions are initiated within the heart itself, in a group of complex electrical tissues that are part of a **conduction system**. The cardiac conduction system consists of six parts **Figure 7-52**:

- The sinoatrial (SA) node
- The atrioventricular (AV) node
- The bundle of His
- The right and left bundle branches
- The Purkinje fibers

The **sinoatrial (SA) node** is located high in the right atrium and is the normal site of origin of the electrical impulse. It is the heart's natural pacemaker. Impulses originating in the SA node travel through the right and left atria, resulting in atrial contraction. The impulse then travels to the **atrioventricular (AV) node**, located in the right atrium adjacent to the septum, where it transiently slows. Electrical stimulation of the heart muscle then continues toward the **bundle of His**, which is a continuation of the AV node. From here, it proceeds rapidly to the right and left bundle branches, stimulating the intraventricular septum. The impulse then spreads out, via the Purkinje fibers, to the left and then to the right ventricular myocardium, resulting in ventricular contraction or systole.

Regulation of Heart Function

The heart's **chronotropic state** (control of the rate of contraction), **dromotropic state** (control of the rate of electrical conduction), and **inotropic state** (control of the strength of contraction) are provided by the brain via the autonomic nervous system, the hormones of the endocrine system, and the heart tissue. Receptors in the blood vessels, kidneys, brain, and heart constantly monitor body functions to help maintain homeostasis. Baroreceptors and chemoreceptors are also involved in regulation of heart function. **Baroreceptors** respond to changes in pressure, usually within the heart or the main arteries. **Chemoreceptors** sense changes in the chemical composition of the blood. If either of these types of receptors sense abnormalities, they transmit nerve signals to the appropriate organs. As a result, hormones or neurotransmitters are released to correct the situation. The transmission of nerve signals stops when conditions return to normal.

Stimulation of receptors often causes activation of either the parasympathetic or sympathetic branches of the autonomic nervous system, affecting both the heart rate and the strength of heart muscle contraction (**contractility**). Parasympathetic stimulation slows the heart rate, primarily by affecting the AV node. Sympathetic

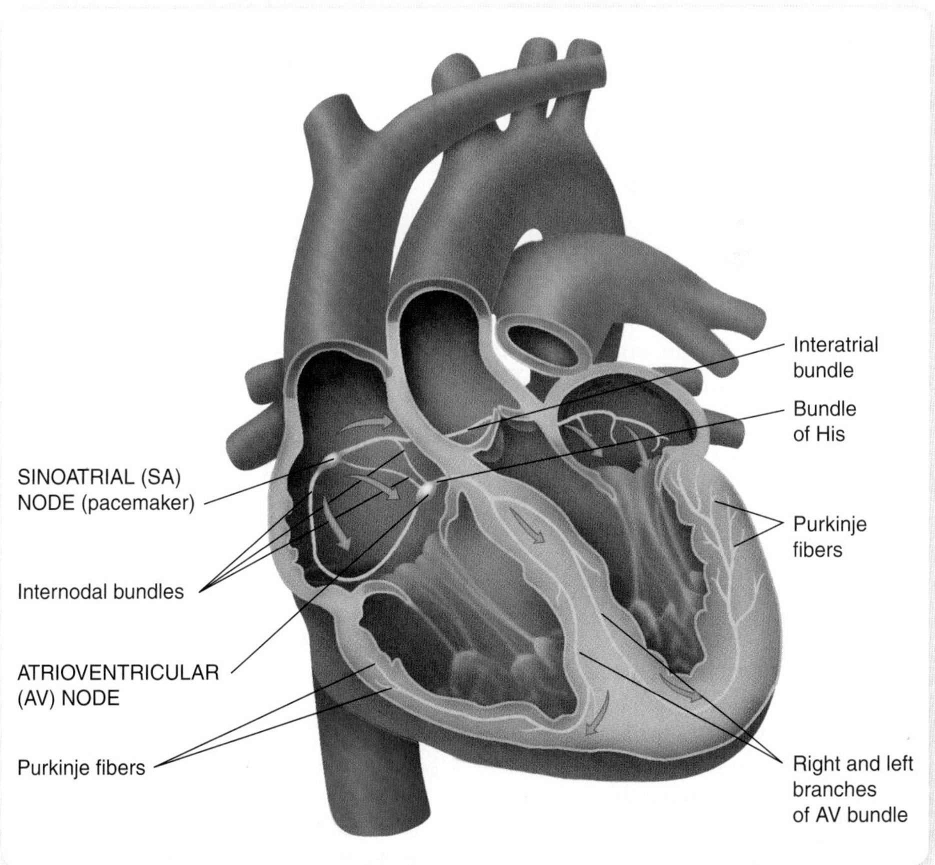

Figure 7-52 The cardiac conduction system. Specialized groups of cardiac muscle cells initiate an electrical impulse throughout the heart. The conduction pathway travels through the six parts of the cardiac conduction system, starting at the sinoatrial node.

stimulation has two potential effects, alpha effects or beta effects, depending on which nerve receptor is stimulated. **Alpha effects** occur when alpha receptors are stimulated, resulting in vasoconstriction. **Beta effects** occur when beta receptors are stimulated, resulting in increased inotropic, dromotropic, and chronotropic states.

Epinephrine and norepinephrine, also referred to as catecholamines, are naturally occurring hormones that also may be given as cardiac drugs. Epinephrine has a greater stimulatory effect on beta receptors, and norepinephrine has predominant stimulatory actions on alpha receptors.

The Cardiac Cycle

The process that creates the pumping of the heart is known as the **cardiac cycle**. This cycle begins with myocardial contraction and concludes at the beginning of the next contraction. The heart's contraction results in pressure changes within the cardiac chambers, resulting in the movement of blood from areas of high pressure to areas of low pressure.

Systole is a term that refers to the contraction of the ventricular mass and the pumping of blood into the systemic circulation. During systole, a pressure is created within the arteries that can be recorded and is known as the systolic blood pressure. A normal systolic blood pressure in an adult is between 110 and 140 mm Hg. A pressure also exists in the vessels during **diastole**, the relaxation phase of the heart cycle, and is called the diastolic blood pressure. A normal diastolic blood pressure in an adult is between 70 and 90 mm Hg. The **pulse pressure** is the difference between the systolic and diastolic pressures:

$$\text{Pulse pressure} = \text{Systolic pressure} - \text{Diastolic pressure}$$

Blood pressure is noted as a fraction, and the systolic reading is placed above the diastolic reading (for example, a systolic reading of 140 and a diastolic reading of 70 would be noted as 140/70 mm Hg). The unit of measure mm Hg refers to millimeters of mercury and describes the height, in millimeters, to which the blood pressure elevates a column of liquid mercury in a glass tube. Although most blood pressure measurement devices now use dials or other non–mercury dependent sensors, blood pressure is still described in millimeters of mercury.

The pressure in the aorta against which the left ventricle must pump blood is called the **afterload**. The greater the afterload, the harder it is for the ventricle to eject blood into the aorta, reducing the **stroke volume (SV)**, or the amount of blood ejected per contraction. To a large degree, afterload is governed by arterial blood pressure. Afterload is greater with vasoconstriction and less with vasodilation.

Cardiac output is the amount of blood pumped through the circulatory system in 1 minute. Cardiac output is expressed in liters per minute (L/min). The cardiac output equals the heart rate multiplied by the stroke volume:

$$\text{Cardiac output} = \text{Stroke volume} \times \text{Heart rate}$$

Factors that influence the heart rate, the stroke volume, or both will affect cardiac output and, thus, oxygen delivery (perfusion) to tissue.

Starling Law. Increased venous return to the heart stretches the ventricles, resulting in increased cardiac contractility. This relationship has become known as the **Starling law** of the heart.

In a mechanical piston pump, the stroke volume is a fixed quantity related to the distance traveled by the piston. The heart, by contrast, has several ways of increasing stroke volume. To begin with, one of the characteristics of cardiac muscle is that when it is stretched, it contracts with greater force. That property is called the Frank-Starling mechanism, or the Starling law, after the men who first described it. If for any reason an increased volume of blood is returned from the systemic veins to the right heart, or from the pulmonary veins to the left heart, the muscle surrounding the cardiac chambers will have to stretch to accommodate the larger volume. The more the cardiac muscle stretches, the greater will be the force of its contraction, the more completely it will empty, and therefore the greater the stroke volume will be. The amount of blood returning to the right atrium may vary somewhat from minute to minute, but the normal heart continues to pump out the same percentage of blood returned. This is called the **ejection fraction**.

If we recall our equation:

$$\text{Cardiac output} = \text{Stroke volume} \times \text{Heart rate}$$

it is clear that any increase in stroke volume, with the heart rate held constant, will cause an increase in the overall cardiac output. The pressure under which a ventricle fills is called the **preload** and is influenced by the volume of blood returned by the veins to the heart.[3] In situations of increased oxygen demand, the body returns more blood to the heart (preload increases), and cardiac output therefore increases as described in the Starling law. In the diseased heart, the same mechanism is used to achieve a normal resting cardiac output (that is why some diseased hearts become enlarged).

Words of Wisdom

The Starling law states that primarily the length of fibers constituting the heart's muscular wall determines the force of the heartbeat. In other words, an increase in diastolic filling increases the force of the contraction.

Think of stretching a rubber band: the further it is stretched, the greater the strength of the recoil.

▶ The Vascular System

Blood is transported through the body in the **arteries**, which carry blood away from the heart, and **veins**, which carry blood back to the heart. Arteries become smaller as they get farther from the heart. Eventually, they branch into many small **arterioles** that divide even further into **capillaries**, which are microscopic, thin-walled blood vessels. Oxygen and nutrients pass out of the capillaries into the cells, and carbon dioxide and waste products such as lactic acid pass from the cells into the capillaries by diffusion **Figure 7-53**.

After oxygenated blood has been delivered in the capillaries, deoxygenated blood is returned to the heart, starting from the capillaries. The capillaries eventually enlarge to form venules, which merge together and form veins. Eventually the veins empty into the superior and inferior vena cava and, finally, the heart, where blood is reoxygenated and the process begins again.

The walls of the blood vessels are composed of three layers of tissue **Figure 7-54**. The smooth, thin, inner lining is called the **tunica intima**, or endothelium. The middle layer, the **tunica media**, is composed of elastic tissue and smooth muscle cells that allow the vessels to expand or contract in response to changes in blood pressure and tissue demand. It is the thickest of the three tissue layers. The outer layer of tissue is called the **tunica adventitia** and consists of elastic and fibrous connective tissue.

Circulation to the Heart

The heart, like any other muscle, requires oxygen and nutrients. These are supplied via the **coronary arteries**, which arise from the aorta shortly after it leaves the left ventricle. Coronary arteries receive their blood supply during the diastolic phase. The coronary circulation emanates from the left and right coronary arteries **Figure 7-55**.

The right coronary artery divides into nine important branches. Not all branches are always present in all people. These branches supply blood to the walls of the right atrium and ventricle, a portion of the inferior part of the left ventricle, and portions of the conduction system (the sinus and AV nodes). When vessels to the conduction system fail to arise from the right coronary artery, they originate from the left side instead.

The left main coronary artery is the largest and shortest of the myocardial blood vessels. It rapidly divides into two branches, the **left anterior descending (LAD) artery** and the **circumflex coronary arteries**. These arteries subdivide further, supplying blood to most of the left ventricle, the intraventricular septum, and, at times, the AV node.

Pulmonary Circulation

As discussed previously, the pulmonary circulation carries blood within the body from the right side of the heart to the lungs and back to the left side of the heart, and the systemic circulation is responsible for blood flow throughout the body. Deoxygenated blood from the right ventricle is pumped through the pulmonic valve into the pulmonary artery. This artery rapidly divides into the right and left pulmonary arteries. These arteries transport the blood to the right and left lungs. Inside the lungs, the arteries branch, becoming smaller and smaller. At the level of the capillary, waste products are exchanged and the blood is reoxygenated. The reoxygenated blood travels through venules into the pulmonary veins.

YOU are the Provider PART 3

You apply direct pressure and a dressing over the abdominal wound and the arm wound, and an occlusive dressing on the chest wound. You instruct a police officer to assist in placing the patient on a nonrebreathing mask at 15 L/min. As you and your partner place the patient on the stretcher, you examine his back and find no wounds. You then quickly move him into the back of the ambulance. You obtain the following vital signs:

Recording Time: 4 Minutes	
Respirations	12 breaths/min, shallow
Pulse	Unobtainable L radial, 126 via R radial
Skin	Cool, pale, and clammy
Blood pressure	86/54 mm Hg
Oxygen saturation (Spo_2)	95% on 15 L/min
Pupils	Pupils Equal, Round, and Reactive to Light and Accommodation (PERRLA)

5. What are the possible results of respiratory compromise in this patient?
6. What type of shock is this patient most likely experiencing?

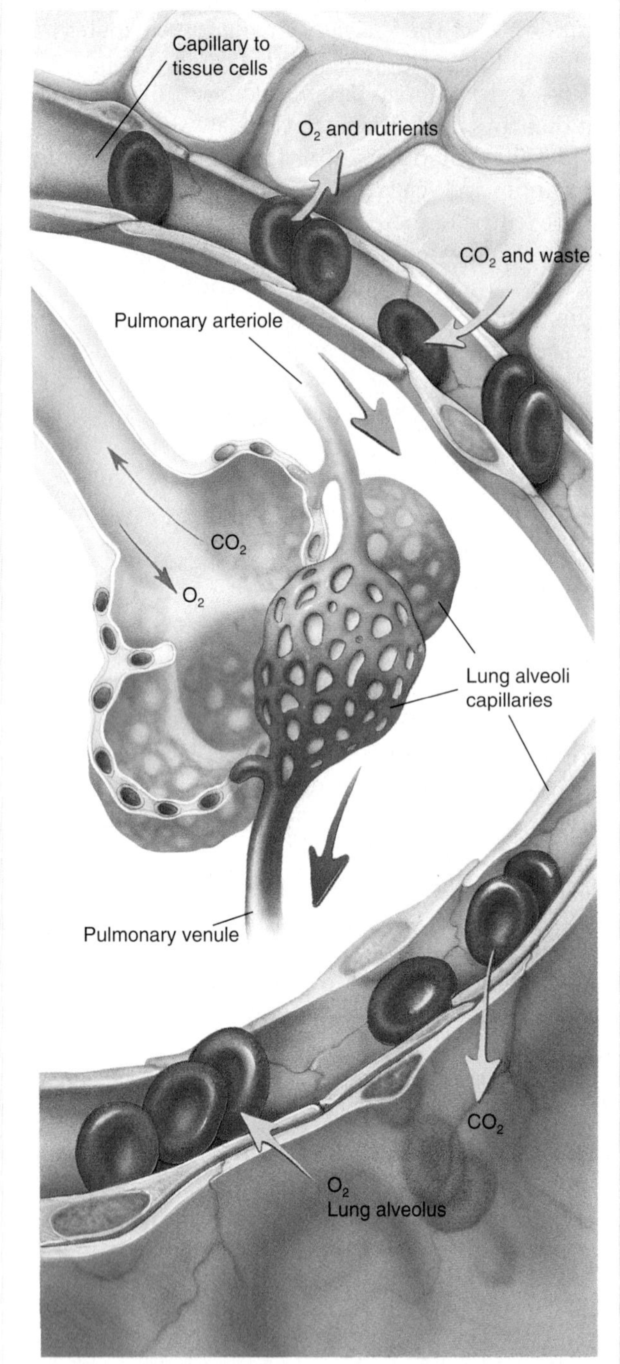

Figure 7-53 Diffusion. Oxygen and nutrients pass easily from the capillaries into the cells, and waste and carbon dioxide pass from the cells into the capillaries.

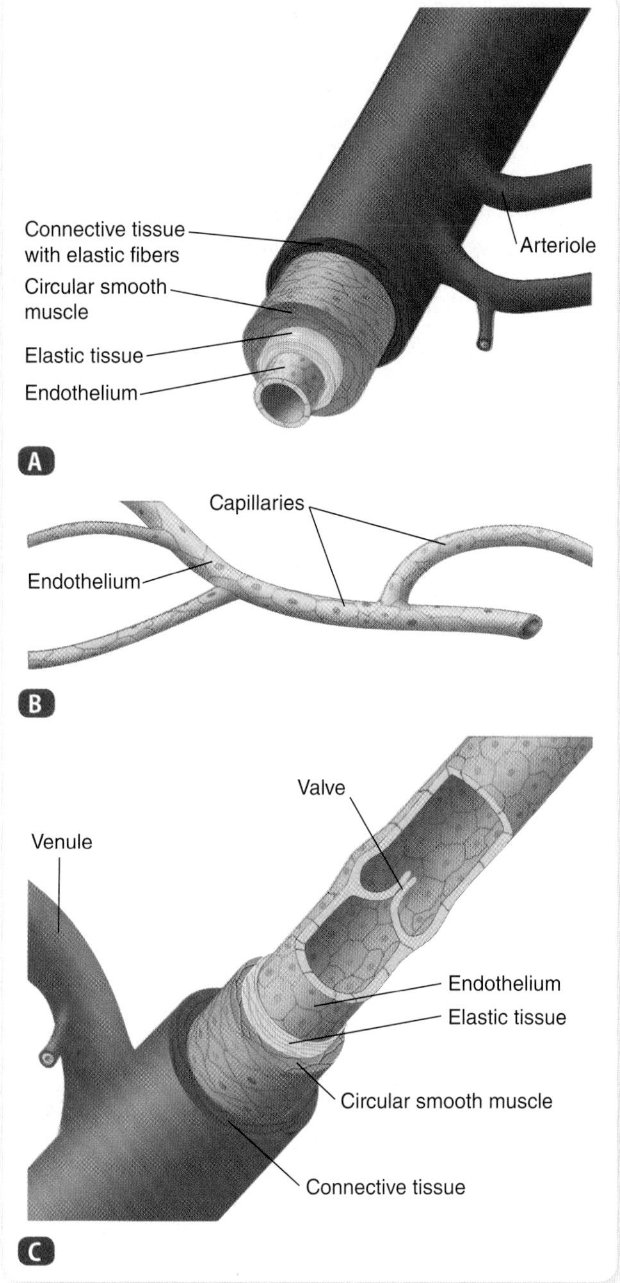

Figure 7-54 The walls of the blood vessels are composed of three layers of tissue: the endothelium, elastic tissue, and connective tissue. **A.** Artery. **B.** Capillary. **C.** Vein.

The four pulmonary veins empty into the left atrium, two from each lung (see Figure 7-47).

Systemic Arterial Circulation

Oxygenated blood leaves the heart through the aortic valve and passes into the aorta. From the aorta, blood is distributed to all parts of the body **Figure 7-56**. All arteries of the body are derived from the aorta. The aorta is divided into three portions: the ascending aorta, the aortic arch, and the descending aorta.

The **ascending aorta** arises from the left ventricle and consists of only two branches, the right and left main coronary arteries. The aorta then arches posteriorly and to the left, forming the aortic arch. Three major arteries arise from the **aortic arch**: the brachiocephalic (innominate) artery, the left common **carotid artery**, and the left subclavian artery.

The **descending aorta** is the longest portion of the aorta and is subdivided into the thoracic aorta and the abdominal aorta. The descending aorta extends through the thorax and abdomen into the pelvis. In the pelvis,

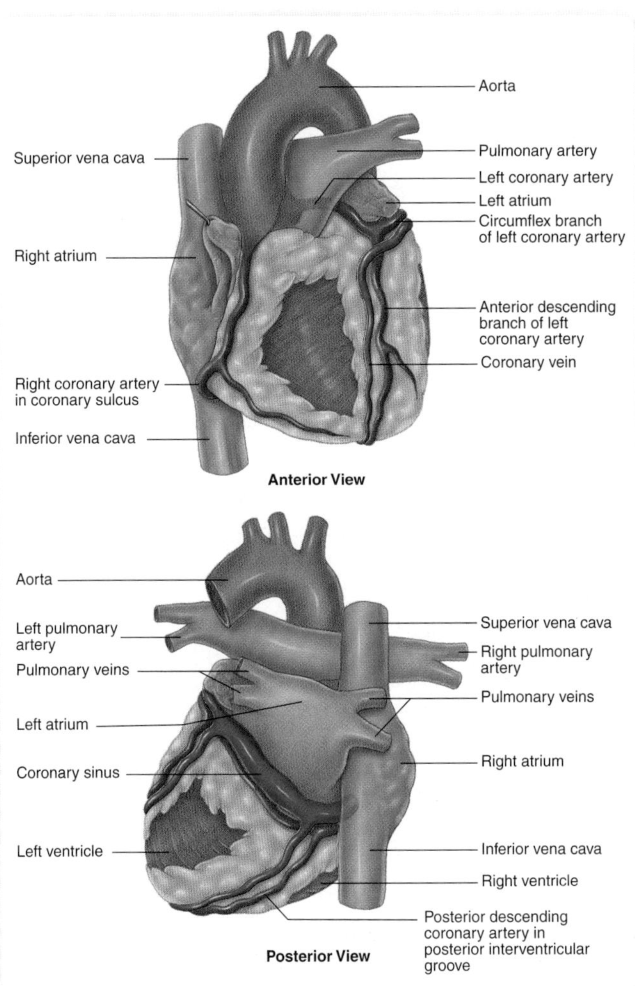

Figure 7-55 The two main coronary arteries supply the myocardium with blood.

the descending aorta divides into the two common iliac arteries, which further divide into the internal and external iliac arteries.

The Head and Neck. The brachiocephalic artery is the first vessel to branch from the aortic arch. It is relatively short and rapidly divides into the right common carotid artery and the right subclavian artery. The carotid arteries transport blood to the head and neck, whereas the subclavian arteries transport blood to the upper extremities.

Each common carotid artery branches at the angle of the mandible into the internal and external carotid arteries. This point of division is called the carotid bifurcation. Here, a slight dilation, the carotid sinus, contains the baroreceptors mentioned earlier—structures that are important in regulating blood pressure (these are also found in the aortic arch). Branches of the external carotid artery supply blood to the face, nose, and mouth. The internal carotid arteries, together with the vertebral arteries (branches of the subclavian arteries), supply blood to the brain Figure 7-57.

The Upper Extremity. The **subclavian artery** supplies blood to the brain, neck, anterior chest wall, and shoulder. Shortly after its point of origin, the subclavian artery gives rise to the vertebral arteries. The subclavian system then continues from the thorax into the upper extremity. At the shoulder joint, it becomes the axillary artery, and then the **brachial artery** below the head of the humerus. The brachial artery eventually divides into the ulnar and radial arteries at the level of the forearm Figure 7-58.

The Thoracic Aorta. Two types of branches of arteries make up the thoracic aorta: the visceral arteries and the parietal arteries. Visceral arteries supply blood to the thoracic organs, and parietal arteries supply blood to the thoracic wall.

The right brachiocephalic and left subclavian arteries and their branches, the internal thoracic arteries (also known as the mammary arteries), the carotid arteries, and the anterior and posterior intercostal arteries, branch off the aorta and provide the blood supply to the thoracic cavity. Intercostal arteries run along the ribs and provide circulation to the chest wall. Intercostal arteries branch into anterior and posterior intercostal arteries. The anterior intercostal arteries originate as branches of the subclavian system. The posterior intercostal arteries arise directly from the aorta. Visceral branches of the thoracic aorta supply the bronchial arteries in the lungs and the esophageal arteries.

The Abdominal Aorta. Like their thoracic counterpart, branches of the abdominal aorta are divided into visceral and parietal portions. The visceral arteries are subdivided into paired and nonpaired arteries. The three major unpaired branches of the abdominal aorta's visceral arteries include the celiac trunk, the superior mesenteric, and the inferior mesenteric arteries Figure 7-59. The celiac trunk supplies blood to the esophagus, stomach, duodenum, spleen, liver, and pancreas Figure 7-60. The superior mesenteric artery and its branches supply blood to the pancreas, small intestine, and colon. The inferior mesenteric artery and its branches supply blood to the descending colon and rectum. Paired branches of the visceral abdominal aorta supply blood to the kidneys, adrenal gland, and gonads. The parietal branches supply blood to the diaphragm and abdominal wall.

The Pelvis and Lower Extremity. At the level of the fifth lumbar vertebra, the aorta divides into the two common iliac arteries. These arteries further divide into the internal iliac arteries, which supply blood to the pelvis, and the external iliac arteries, which enter the lower extremity Figure 7-61. The internal iliac artery sends out visceral branches to the rectum, vagina, uterus, and ovary. Parietal branches supply blood to the sacrum, gluteal muscles of the buttocks region, the pubic region, rectum, external genitalia, and proximal thigh.

Similar to the upper extremity, the vessels of the lower extremity form a continuum. The external iliac arteries become the **femoral arteries**. Each femoral artery supplies blood to the thigh, external genitalia, anterior abdominal wall, and knee. The femoral artery becomes the **popliteal artery** in the lower thigh. Each popliteal artery

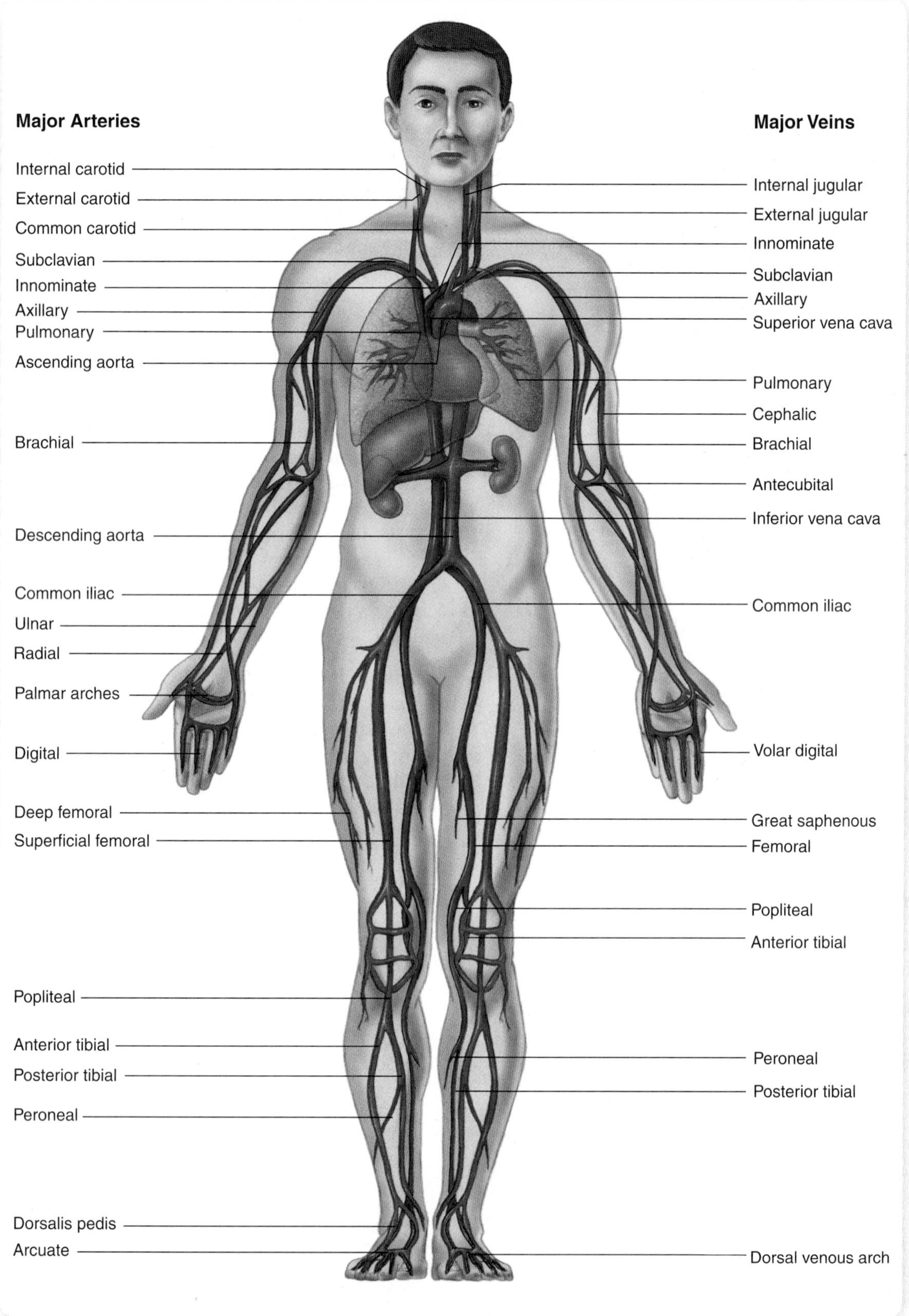

Figure 7-56 The principal arteries supply blood to a vast network of smaller arteries and arterioles. Venules deliver oxygen-poor blood to the veins that return blood to the heart.

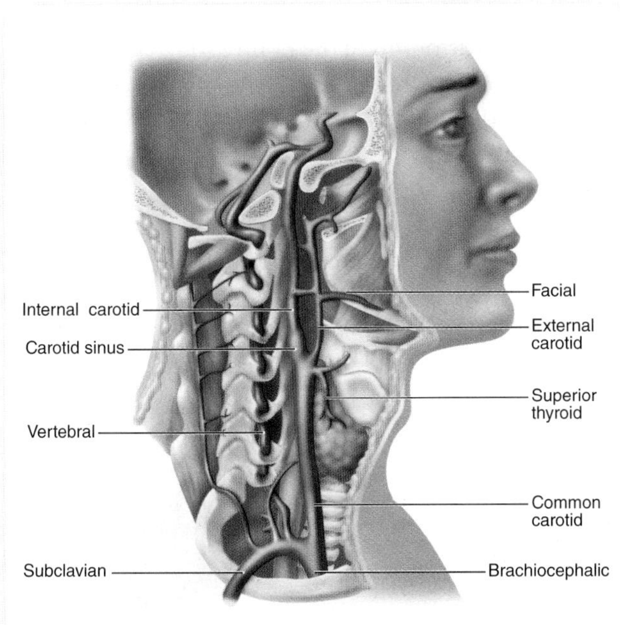

Figure 7-57 The arteries of the head and neck.

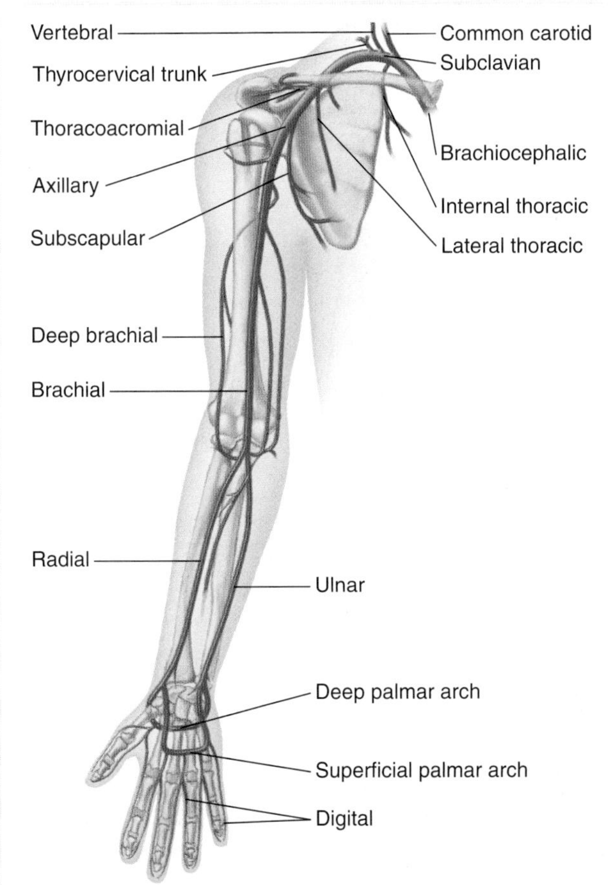

Figure 7-58 The arteries of the upper extremity.

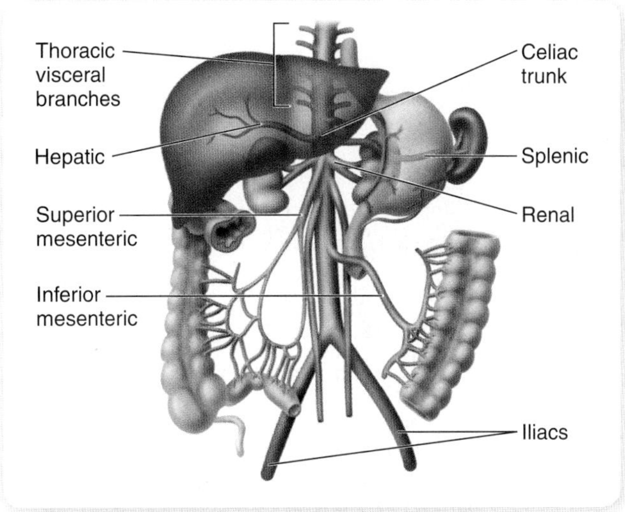

Figure 7-59 The branches of the abdominal aorta.

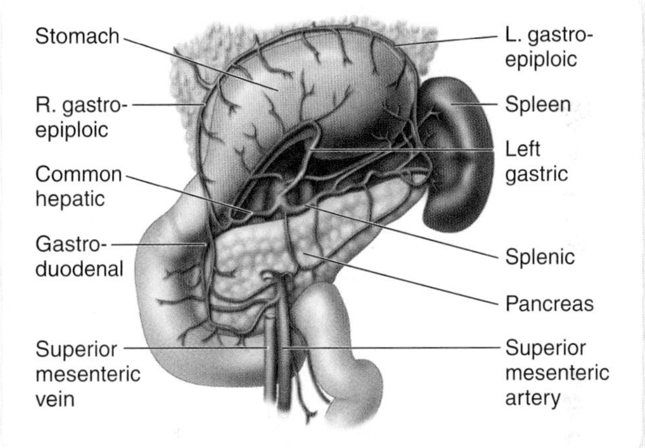

Figure 7-60 The celiac trunk and superior mesenteric vessels.

then branches into the anterior tibial, posterior tibial, and peroneal arteries. At the foot, the anterior tibial artery becomes the **dorsalis pedis artery**. Plantar arteries arise from the **posterior tibial artery** and subdivide into digital branches that supply blood to the toes **Figure 7-62**.

The Systemic Venous Circulation

As a rule, veins accompany the major arteries. Many veins generally have the same names as the arteries they accompany.

The Head and Neck. The two major veins that drain the head and neck are called the external and internal **jugular veins**. The external jugular vein is more superficial and often is visible immediately beneath the skin. The external jugular vein primarily drains the posterior head and neck. The internal jugular vein drains the cranial vault as well as the anterior portion of the head, face, and neck. Spaces between membranes surrounding the brain form **venous sinuses**. These sinuses are the primary means of venous drainage from the brain and feed into the internal jugular vein.

The external and internal jugular veins join the **subclavian veins** (the proximal part of the main vein of the arm) **Figure 7-63** to form the brachiocephalic veins, which drain into the superior vena cava.

The Upper Extremity. The veins of the upper extremity vary somewhat from person to person **Figure 7-64**.

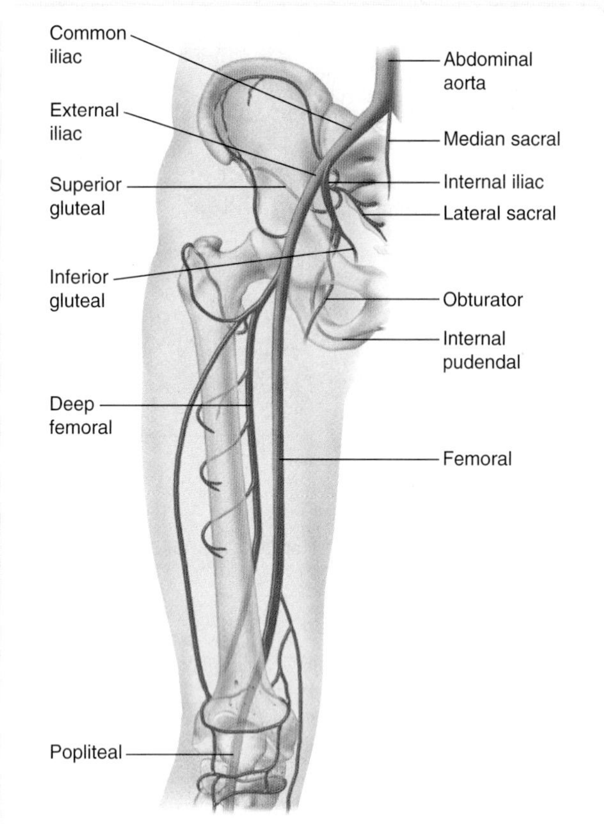

Figure 7-61 The arteries of the pelvis and thigh.

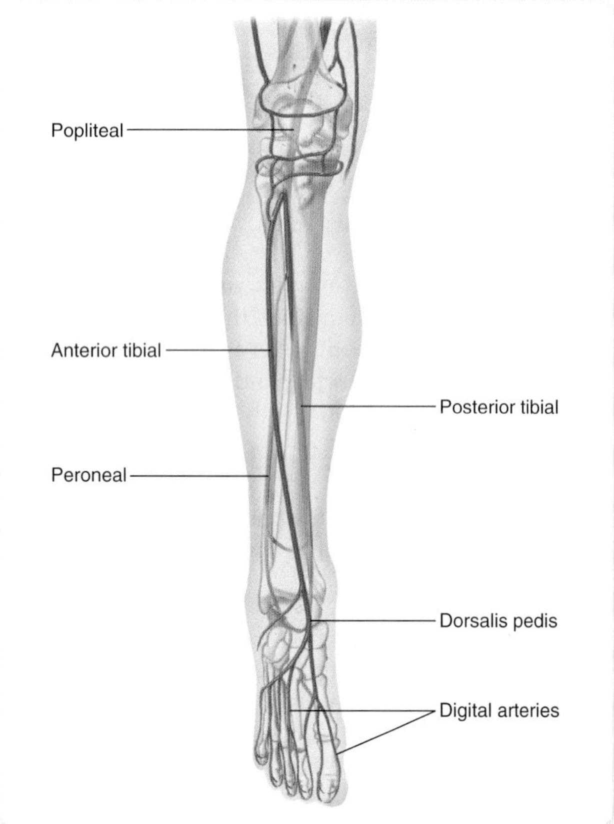

Figure 7-62 The arteries of the lower extremity.

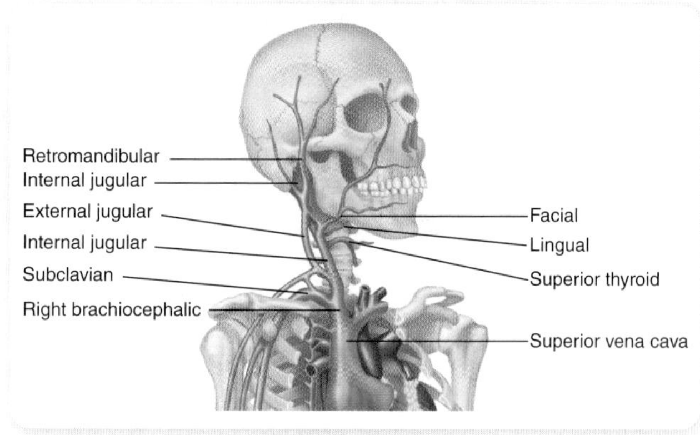

Figure 7-63 The veins of the head and neck.

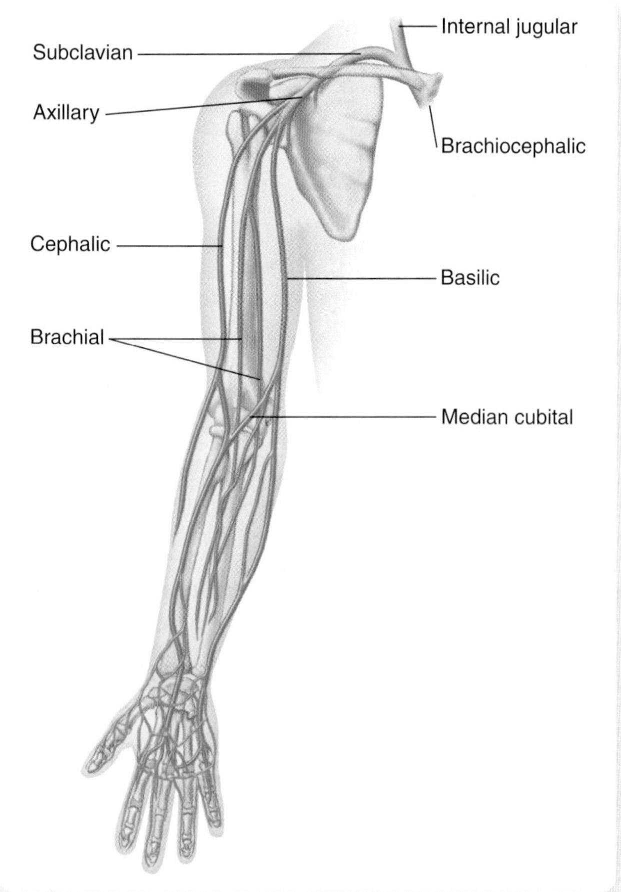

Figure 7-64 The veins of the upper extremity.

The names of the veins of the hands, wrists, and forearm follow the arteries of the same name. In the upper forearm, these veins combine to form the **basilic vein** and the cephalic vein, the major veins of the arm. The basilic and cephalic veins combine to form the **axillary vein**, which drains into the subclavian vein.

The Thorax. In the thorax, venous drainage begins at the anterior and posterior intercostal veins. The intercostal veins empty into the azygos vein on the right side of the thorax and the hemiazygos vein on the left side. These veins, along with the right and left brachiocephalic veins, provide the major source of flow into the superior vena cava.

The Abdomen and Pelvis. Ultimately, all venous drainage from the lower part of the body passes through the inferior vena cava. The inferior vena cava returns deoxygenated blood from the lower parts of the body to the right atrium for oxygenation. Within the abdominal and pelvic cavities, veins of the same name accompany the major arteries, providing venous drainage from structures including the kidney, adrenal glands, gonads, and diaphragm. The internal iliac veins drain the pelvis, and the external iliac veins drain the lower limbs. The internal and external iliac veins combine together in the pelvis, forming the common iliac veins, which combine to form the inferior vena cava.

The **hepatic portal system** is a specialized part of the venous system that drains blood from the liver, stomach, intestines, and spleen **Figure 7-65**. Blood from the system flows first through the liver, where blood collects in sinusoids. In the sinusoids, the liver extracts nutrients, filters the blood, and metabolizes various drugs. The blood then empties into the **hepatic veins**, which join the inferior vena cava.

The Lower Extremity. The longest vein in the body is the great **saphenous vein**. It drains the foot, leg, and thigh. The saphenous vein originates over the dorsal and medial side of the foot, ascends along the medial side of the leg and thigh, and empties into the **femoral vein**, which then drains into the external iliac vein. Laterally, the small saphenous vein helps drain the leg and lateral side of the foot. The veins of the feet also drain into the anterior and posterior tibial veins, which accompany their respective arteries, uniting at the knee to form the popliteal vein. The popliteal vein ascends through the thigh, becoming the femoral vein **Figure 7-66**.

▶ Blood Composition

Blood is the substance that is pumped by the heart through the arteries, veins, and capillaries. Blood consists of plasma (55%) and formed elements or cells that are suspended in the plasma (45%). These cells include RBCs, WBCs, and platelets. The purpose of blood is to transport oxygen and nutrients to the tissues and carry cell waste products away from the tissues. In addition, the formed elements are the mainstay of numerous other body functions such as fighting infection and controlling bleeding. Human adult male bodies contain approximately 70 mL/kg (approximately 5 L) of blood, whereas female bodies contain approximately 65 mL/kg.

Plasma is a watery, straw-colored fluid that accounts for more than one-half of the total blood volume. Plasma is made up of 92% water and 8% dissolved substances

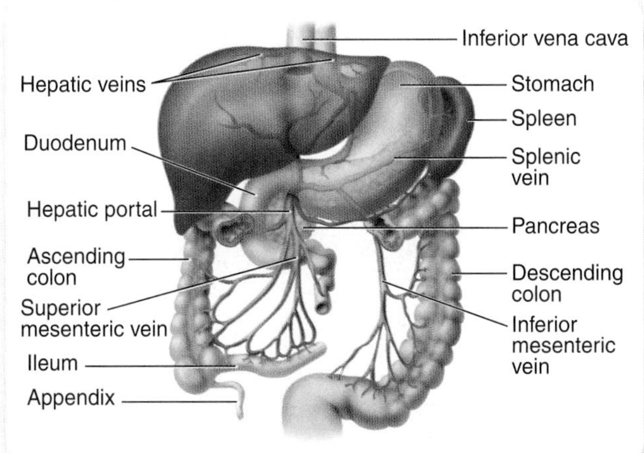

Figure 7-65 The hepatic portal system.

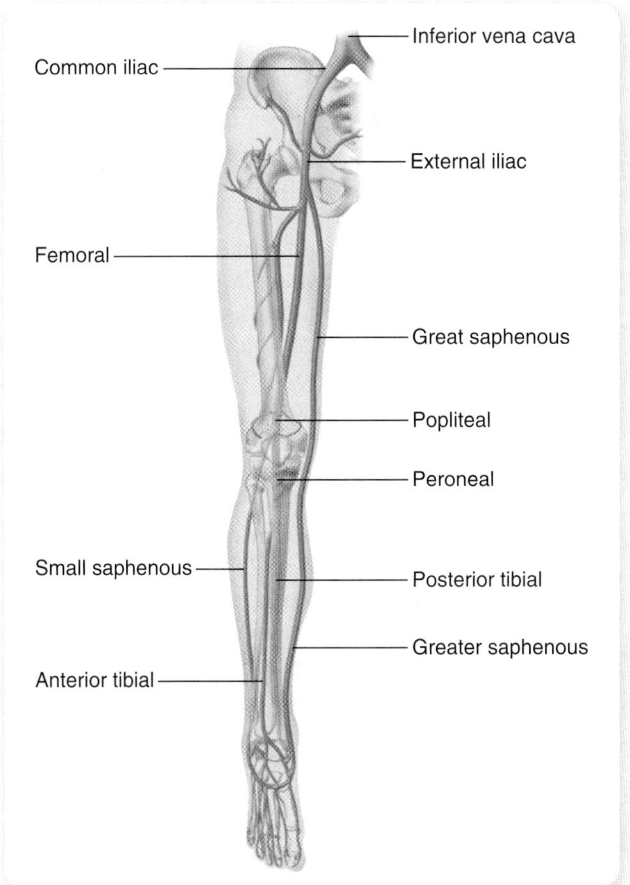

Figure 7-66 The veins of the lower extremity.

such as proteins, electrolytes, and nutrients. All other components together make up 1% of the plasma:

- **Water.** Constitutes 92% of plasma
- **Proteins.** Constitute 7% of the plasma. Most of this protein is albumin, which functions mainly to regulate oncotic pressure, and thereby controls the movement of water into and out of the circulation. Also includes clotting factors, enzymes, and some hormones
- **Oxygen.** Little oxygen is dissolved in the plasma; almost all oxygen is bound to hemoglobin.
- **Carbon dioxide.** Transported as bicarbonate in the plasma
- **Nitrogen.** The air that we breathe is mostly nitrogen; therefore, this gas is dissolved within the plasma.
- **Nutrients.** Fuel for the cells
- **Cellular wastes.** Lactic acid, carbon dioxide, etc
- **Others.** Hormones, other cellular products

Water enters the plasma from the digestive tract, from fluids between cells, and as a by-product of metabolism.

In adults, blood cells are most commonly manufactured in the red bone marrow of the sternum, ribs, vertebral bodies, pelvis, and proximal portions of the femur and humerus. Each day, the body produces billions of new RBCs, WBCs, and platelets from the stem cells that are present in the bone marrow, thereby replacing those that have been lost or are no longer functional.[4]

Red Blood Cells

Red blood cells (RBCs) carry oxygen to the tissues. They are disk-shaped and are also known as erythrocytes. These are the most numerous of the formed elements in the blood. An average human has between 4.2 and 5.8 million erythrocytes per cubic millimeter of blood. RBCs are unable to move on their own; the flowing plasma passively propels them. RBCs contain a protein known as hemoglobin, which gives them their reddish color. Hemoglobin carries oxygen from the lungs and to the tissues by binding to it.

Erythropoiesis is the ongoing process by which RBCs are made. In hypoxic states (such as anemia), RBC production is increased.[5] Approximately 25 trillion RBCs are contained in the normal adult circulation; of these, 2.5 million erythrocytes are destroyed every second.

RBCs have a finite life span of 120 days. Those cells destined for destruction decompose in the spleen and other tissues rich in cells known as **macrophages**. Macrophages protect the body against infection. The body "recycles" some components of hemoglobin, such as the protein, globin, and iron. The part of hemoglobin that is not recycled is converted to **bilirubin**, which is a waste product that undergoes further metabolism in the liver. Normally, a chemical derivative of bilirubin, urobilinogen, is excreted in the stool and in the urine.

ABO and Rh Blood Groups. RBCs contain **antigens** on their surface. Antigens are substances that, when taken into the body, stimulate the formation of specific protective proteins called **antibodies**. After antibodies are formed and exist within the plasma, they react with antigens. To ensure compatibility and prevent medical complications during blood component replacement, people are classified as having one of four blood types based on the presence or absence of these specific antigens. This process of classification is referred to as blood typing, or determining the ABO blood group. In the ABO system, the RBC classification types are O, A, B, and AB Table 7-7.

Type A blood contains RBCs with type A surface antigens and plasma containing type B antibodies; type B blood contains type B surface antigens and plasma containing type A antibodies. Type AB blood contains both types of antigens but the plasma contains no ABO antibodies. Type O contains neither A nor B antigens but contains both A and B plasma antibodies. A person's blood type determines which type of blood he or she may receive in a blood transfusion. A person with type O blood is called a *universal donor*, because type O blood can be given to anyone, no matter their blood type, without an adverse reaction occurring. Also, a person with type AB blood can accept any type of blood—A, B, AB, or O—without an adverse reaction occurring; therefore, a person with type AB blood is called a *universal recipient*.

Another antigen, called Rh antigen, can exist in the blood as well. A person can have **Rh factor**, a specific type of Rh antigen, present in their blood or not; they can be Rh-positive if the antigen exists or Rh-negative if it does not. This can be very problematic in pregnancy. The fetus inherits the father's Rh factor, so when a woman who is Rh-negative is pregnant with a child who is Rh-positive, the woman's body will produce antibodies if exposed to the Rh factor. Those antibodies can attack future pregnancies, if the fetus is Rh-positive. Treatment can be initiated to prevent this situation.

The presence of Rh factor must also be considered during blood administration. If a person develops antibodies to Rh antigen (after first being exposed to it), then he or she can have a severe hemolytic reaction the next time he or she is exposed to it.

Table 7-7 ABO Blood Groups

Blood Type	Antigen	Antibody	Potential Donor
A	A	Anti-B	A, O
B	B	Anti-A	B, O
AB	A and B	Neither antibody	AB, A, B, O
O	Neither antigen	Anti-A and Anti-B	O

Words of Wisdom

Any decrease in the number of RBCs in the body is called anemia. Causes of anemia include inadequate nutrition (such as iron deficiency), inadequate production of RBCs by bone marrow, increased destruction of RBCs by the body (hemolysis), or bleeding.

White Blood Cells

White blood cells (WBCs) are also known as leukocytes. There are several different types of WBCs and each has a different function. The primary function of all WBCs is to fight infection. Antibodies to fight infection may be produced, or WBCs may directly attack and kill bacterial invaders. WBCs are larger than RBCs. Most WBCs are motile and leave the blood vessels by a process known as **diapedesis** to move toward the tissue where they are needed most.

WBCs are named according to their appearance in a stained preparation of blood. In general, **granulocytes** have large cytoplasmic granules that are easily seen with a simple light microscope; **agranulocytes** are WBCs that lack these granules. There are three types of granulocytes (neutrophils, eosinophils, and basophils) and two types of agranulocytes (monocytes and lymphocytes).

Neutrophils are normally the most common type of granulocyte in the blood. Neutrophils destroy bacteria, antigen-antibody complexes, and foreign matter. **Eosinophils** are granulocytes that contain granules that stain bright red with the acidic stain eosin. Eosinophils function in the body's allergic response and are, thus, increased in people with allergies. Certain parasitic infections, such as trichinosis, also result in an increase in the number of eosinophils present. **Basophils** are the least common of all granulocytes and play a role in both allergic and inflammatory reactions. Basophils contain large amounts of **histamine**, a substance that increases tissue inflammation, and **heparin**, a substance that inhibits blood clotting.

Lymphocytes are the smallest of the agranulocytes. Lymphocytes originate in the bone marrow but migrate through the blood to the lymphatic tissues. Most lymphocytes are located in the lymph nodes, spleen, tonsils, lymph nodules, and thymus.

Monocytes and macrophages are among the first lines of defense in the inflammatory process. Monocytes migrate out of the blood and into the tissues in response to an infection. They engulf microbes and digest them in a process called phagocytosis. Unlike their counterparts, the neutrophils, which are short-lived, monocytes mature into long-lived macrophages when in the tissues.

Platelets and Blood Clotting

Platelets are small cells in the blood that are necessary for the series of chemical reactions that occur to form a clot. The blood clotting or coagulation process is a complex set of events involving platelets, clotting proteins in the plasma (clotting factors), other proteins, and calcium. The process begins with platelets clumping together. Clotting proteins produced by the liver then solidify the remainder of the clot, which eventually includes RBCs and WBCs.

Following injury to a blood vessel wall, a predictable series of events takes place, resulting in **hemostasis** (cessation of bleeding) and formation of the final blood clot. Chemicals released from the vessel wall cause local vasoconstriction, as well as activation of the platelets. The combination of vessel contraction and loose platelet aggregation forms a temporary "plug." Other factors released by the tissues, known as tissue thromboplastin, activate a cascade of clotting proteins. Eventually, **thrombin** is formed. This causes the conversion of fibrinogen to **fibrin**, which binds to the platelet plug, forming the final mature clot.

The body also has two systems to counterbalance the clotting system. One, the fibrinolytic system, lyses or disrupts clots that already have formed. The main steps in the fibrinolytic system are the activation of **tissue plasminogen activator (t-PA)**, which converts plasminogen to **plasmin**.

Together, the fibrinolytic system and the body's own anticoagulants attempt to provide a balance between clotting and bleeding; however, neither system is completely effective (for example, in patients where formation of clots is creating problems, such as myocardial infarction or stroke, as well as in patients with spontaneous bleeding, such as subarachnoid hemorrhage).

The Circulatory System: Physiology

The **pulse**, which is palpated most easily at the neck, wrist, or groin, is created by the forceful pumping of blood out of the left ventricle and into the major arteries. It is present throughout the entire arterial system. It can be felt most easily where the larger arteries are near the skin. The central pulses are the carotid artery pulse, which can be felt at the upper portion of the neck, and the femoral artery pulse, which is felt in the groin. The peripheral pulses include the radial pulse, which is felt at the wrist at the base of the thumb; the brachial artery pulse, which is felt on the medial aspect of the arm, midway between the elbow and shoulder; the posterior tibial artery pulse, which is felt posterior to the medial malleolus; and the dorsalis pedis artery pulse, which is felt on the top of the foot Figure 7-67.

Blood pressure is the pressure that the blood exerts against the walls of the arteries as it passes through them. As mentioned earlier, systole and diastole are the phases that occur when the left ventricle contracts and when the ventricle relaxes, respectively. The pulsed forceful ejection of blood from the left ventricle of the heart into the aorta is transmitted through the arteries as a pulsatile pressure wave. This pressure wave keeps the blood moving through the body. The high and low points of the wave can be

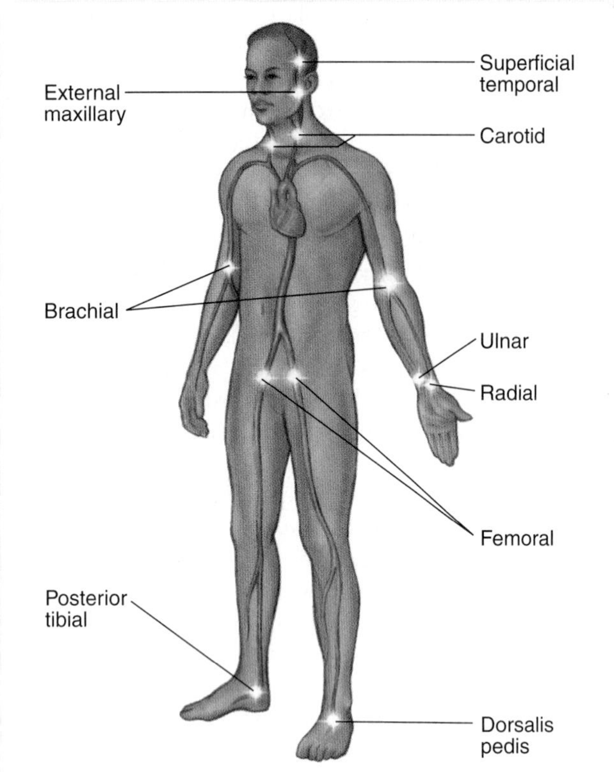

Figure 7-67 The central and peripheral pulses can be felt where the large arteries are near the skin.

measured with a **sphygmomanometer** (blood pressure cuff) and are expressed numerically in millimeters of mercury (mm Hg).

The state of the blood vessels, how dilated or constricted they are, is referred to as the **systemic vascular resistance (SVR)**. SVR is the resistance to blood flow within all blood vessels except the pulmonary vessels. The relationship between the size of the vessels and shock is important to understand. In some types of shock, blood vessels dilate and the patient's blood pressure falls dramatically (Table 7-8).

Table 7-8 Effects of Blood Vessel Diameter on Blood

State	Effects
Constricted blood vessel	Decreased size of container Increased pressure within container
Normal diameter	Balance of size and pressure
Dilated blood vessel	Increased size of container Decreased pressure within container

The typical adult has approximately 5 L of blood in the vascular system. Children have less, 2 to 3 L, depending on their age and size. Infants have only approximately 300 mL. The loss of an amount of blood that may be negligible for an adult could be fatal for an infant.

▶ Normal Circulation in Adults

In all healthy people, the circulatory system is automatically adjusted and readjusted constantly so 100% of the capacity of the arteries, veins, and capillaries holds 100% of the blood at that moment. All vessels are never fully dilated or constricted. The size of arteries and veins is controlled by the nervous system, according to the amount of blood that is available and many other factors, to keep blood pressure normal constantly. Under the condition of normal pressure, with a system that can hold just 100% of the blood available, all parts of the system will have adequate blood supply all the time.

Perfusion is the circulation of blood in an organ or tissue in adequate amounts to meet the tissue's current needs. Blood enters an organ or tissue through the arteries and leaves it through the veins (Figure 7-68). Loss of normal blood pressure is an indication that blood is no longer circulating efficiently to every organ in the body. (However, a "good blood pressure" does not indicate that it is reaching all parts of the body.) There are many

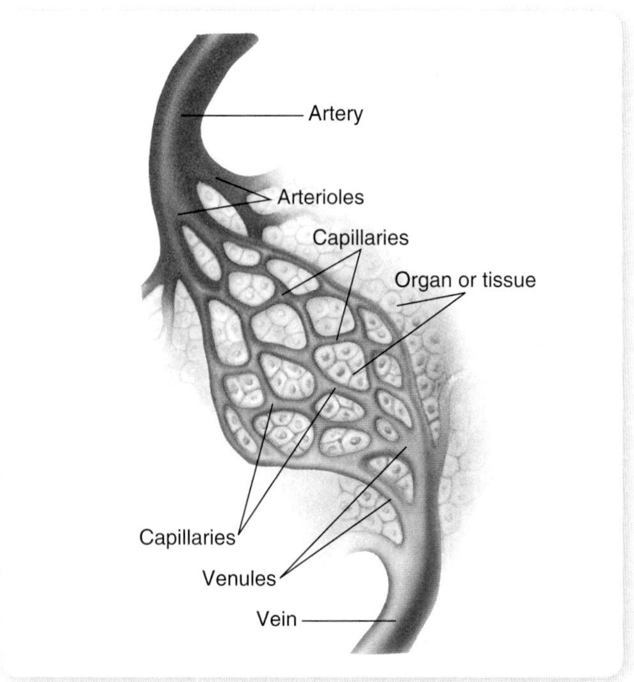

Figure 7-68 Blood enters an organ or tissue through the arteries and leaves through the veins. This process, called perfusion, results in the blood flow to the tissue that is necessary to meet the cells' needs.

reasons for loss of blood pressure. The result in each case is the same: organs, tissues, and cells are no longer adequately perfused or supplied with oxygen and food, and wastes can accumulate. Under these conditions, cells, tissues, and whole organs may die. The state of inadequate circulation, when it involves the entire body, is called **shock**, or hypoperfusion.

▶ Inadequate Circulation in Adults

When a patient loses a small amount of blood, the arteries, veins, and heart automatically adjust to the smaller new volume. The adjustment occurs to maintain adequate pressure throughout the circulatory system and maintain circulation for every organ. The adjustment occurs rapidly after the loss, usually within minutes. Specifically, the vessels constrict to provide a smaller bed for the reduced volume of blood to fill. The heart then pumps more rapidly to circulate the remaining blood more efficiently. As the blood pressure decreases, the pulse increases in an attempt to keep the cardiac output constant at 5 to 6 L/min. If the loss of blood is too great, the adjustment fails, and the patient goes into shock.

Words of Wisdom

If a patient is bleeding or severely dehydrated, baroreceptors sense the abnormally low volume of blood in the circulatory system. Although several different body responses occur at once, a major response is the release of epinephrine and norepinephrine from the adrenal glands, causing sympathetic (adrenergic) stimulation, resulting in an increased heart rate, as well as increased myocardial contractility.

▶ The Function of Blood

Blood under pressure will gush or spurt intermittently from an artery and is bright red. When blood comes from a vein, it flows in a steady stream and is dark bluish red. From capillaries, blood will ooze at many tiny individual points. Clotting normally takes from 6 to 10 minutes.

Where is all of this blood distributed? This concept involves blood reservoirs. Most blood is unevenly distributed throughout the body. Approximately 30% of blood is found within the heart, arteries, and capillaries. Seventy percent of blood is found within the veins and venules. This may seem confusing, but if you remember that the heart and arteries are high-pressure systems and veins are low-pressure systems, it becomes clearer. As blood pressure falls, blood flow slows down and there is more blood in the veins.

Consider the movement of blood and its ultimate function of perfusion. Recall that capillaries are the smallest portions of the circulatory system where materials are able to exit and enter the bloodstream. Nutrients move from the capillaries into the interstitial space and into the cells. (The **interstitial space** is the space between the cells.) Wastes move from the cells through the interstitial space and into the capillaries.

Here is a simplified version of what is happening inside the capillary: the two main forces at work inside the capillary are **hydrostatic pressure** and **oncotic pressure**. Hydrostatic pressure is pressure exerted by a liquid and occurs when blood is moved through the artery at relatively high pressures. When that blood meets the capillary walls, the pressure of the fluid pushes against the walls to force fluid out of the capillary. The opposing force is oncotic pressure. Oncotic pressure is a form of osmotic pressure exerted by proteins in the blood plasma that usually tends to pull water into the circulatory system. These proteins tend to make the blood thicker. This thickness means that relative to the interstitial space, there is more water outside the capillary than inside. Diffusion occurs, and water seeks to move into the capillary.

Here is the entire process Figure 7-69. Blood flows into the arterial side of the capillary. Plasma is trying to enter the capillary from the interstitial space, but hydrostatic pressure on the arterial side of the capillary is higher, so plasma, carrying nutrients, leaves the capillary and enters the interstitial space. The hydrostatic pressure is greatly diminished by the time the fluid reaches the venous side of the capillary because the effort of pushing the fluid out of the capillary decreased its force. This decrease in pressure is beneficial because now oncotic pressure can push fluid into the capillary; plasma, with all wastes from the cells, enters the venous side of the capillary. These wastes are then carried away.

As mentioned, another function of blood is the ability to clot. Coagulation, or clotting, occurs as the result of a complex chemical process that creates small fibers near the injured blood vessel, trapping RBCs. This chemical process involves platelets and clotting factors that are in the bloodstream. Table 7-9 outlines the major functions of the blood.

The Lymphatic System

The **lymphatic system** transports lymph by passive circulation. **Lymph** is a thin plasmalike fluid formed from interstitial or ECF that bathes the tissues of the body. Lymphatic capillaries pick up the lymph and drain it into larger vessels. Lymph circulates through the body in thin-walled **lymph vessels** that travel close to the major arteries and veins Figure 7-70. Similar to veins, lymphatic vessels contain valves that limit backflow. Foreign material such as debris or bacteria is filtered from the lymph in the **lymph nodes**, round or bean-shaped structures that are interspersed along the course of the lymph vessels, and returns to the main circulatory system via the **thoracic duct**, one of two great lymph vessels, which empties into the junction of the left subclavian vein and the left internal jugular vein. The lymphatic system helps absorb fat from the digestive tract, maintain fluid balance in the body, and fight infection.

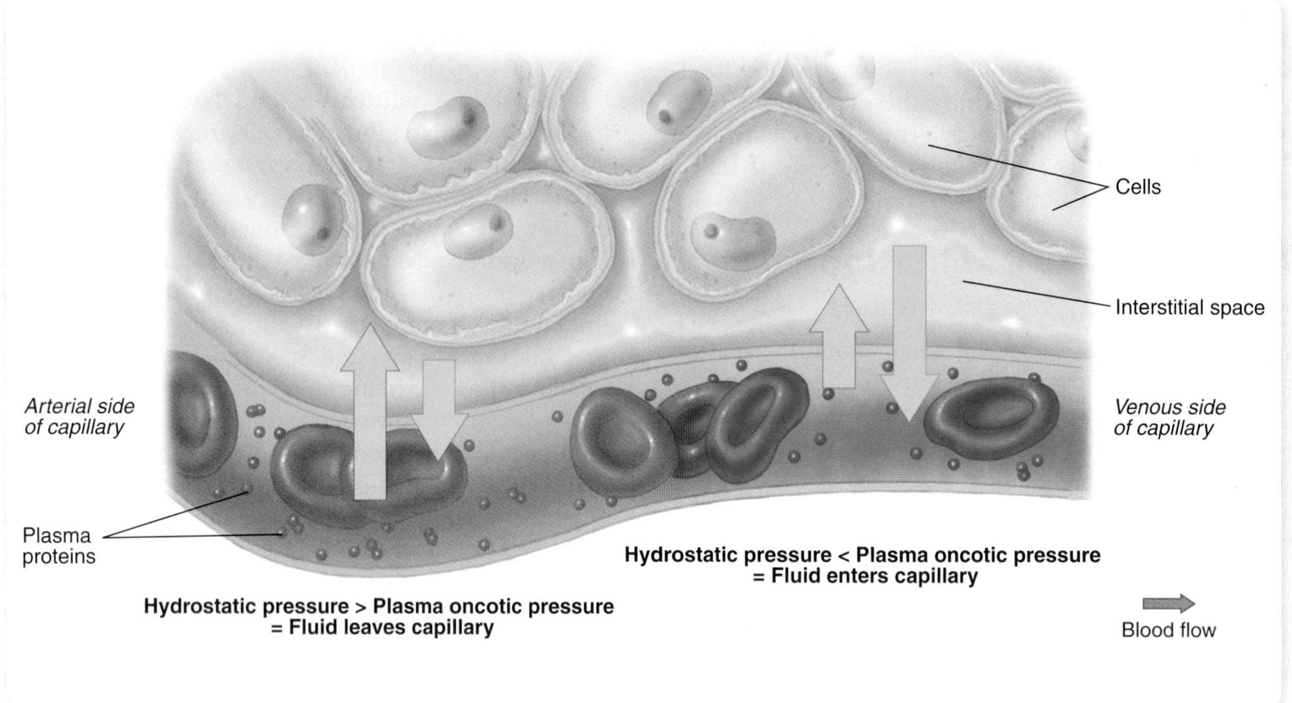

Figure 7-69 Fluid movement from capillaries to interstitial space and back.

Table 7-9 Functions of the Blood and the Components of Blood in Use

Function	Component of the Blood in Use
Fighting infection	White blood cells
Transporting oxygen	Red blood cells (hemoglobin)
Transporting carbon dioxide	Plasma
Controlling (buffering) pH	Chemicals within the plasma
Transporting wastes and nutrients	Plasma (water)
Clotting (coagulation)	Platelets and clotting factors in the plasma

▶ Lymphatic Vessels

Lymphatic vessels only carry fluid away from the tissues. In the lymphatic capillaries, the epithelial cells contain one-way valves that allow fluid to enter the vessel but prevent it from flowing back into the tissues. Lymphatic capillaries are present in all tissues except the central nervous system, bone marrow, cartilage, epidermis, and **cornea**. Generally, fluid flows from the blood capillaries to the tissues, then out of the tissue spaces into lymph capillaries. In the major blood capillary beds of the body, the internal hydrostatic pressure allows a normal, continuous leak of a total of 3 to 4 mL/min of fluid into the interstitial spaces. To prevent the tissues from becoming edematous, the lymphatic vessel must absorb this excess fluid and return it to the central venous circulation.

The Nervous System: Anatomy and Physiology

The **nervous system** is perhaps the most complex organ system within the human body. It is composed of two major structures, the brain and the spinal cord, and thousands of nerves that allow every part of the body to communicate. This system is responsible for fundamental functions such as controlling breathing, heart rate, and blood pressure. However, what makes the nervous system so special is that it allows the performance of higher level activity, such as memory, understanding, and thought.

The nervous system is divided into two main portions: the **central nervous system (CNS)** and the peripheral nervous system. The **somatic nervous system** is the part of the peripheral nervous system that regulates activities over which there is voluntary control, such as walking, talking, and writing. The **autonomic nervous system** controls the many body functions that occur without voluntary control. These activities include body functions such as digestion,

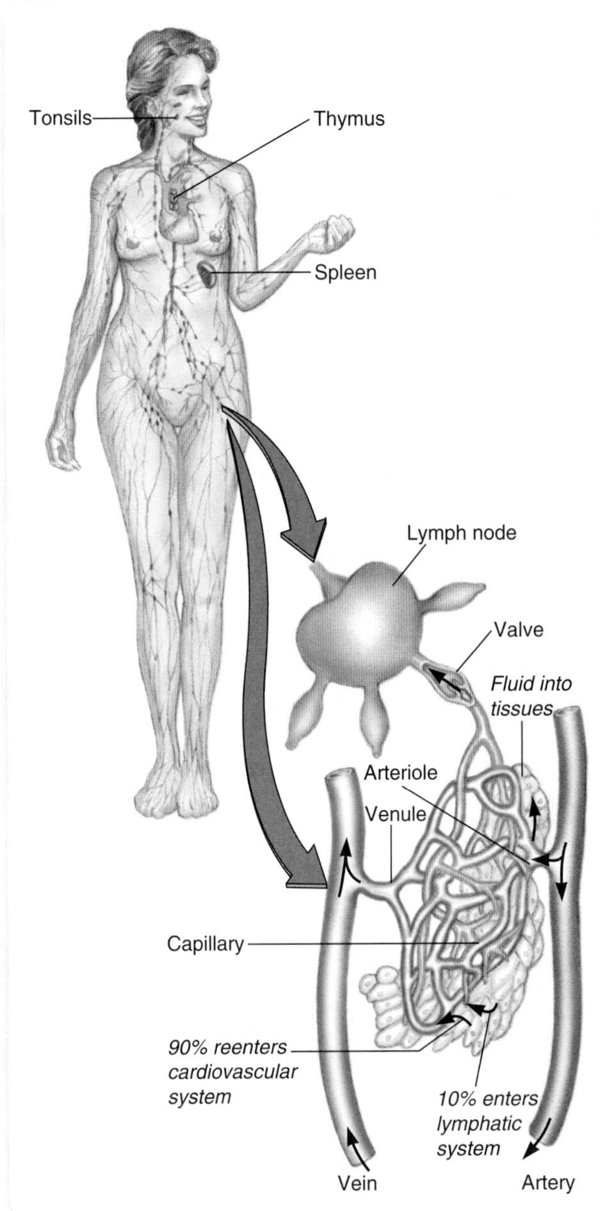

Figure 7-70 The lymphatic vessel. The enlarged diagram of a lymph node and vessels shows the path of the excess fluid that leaves the capillary, enters the adjacent tissue spaces, and is absorbed by lymphatic capillaries.

dilation and constriction of blood vessels, sweating, and all other involuntary actions that are necessary for basic body functions. Thus, the nervous system as a whole can be divided anatomically into the central and peripheral nervous systems and functionally into somatic (voluntary) and autonomic (involuntary) components Figure 7-71.

▶ The Central Nervous System

Brain

The **brain** is the controlling organ of the body. It is the center of consciousness. It is responsible for all of your voluntary body activities, your perception of your surroundings, and the control of your reactions to the environment. In addition, the brain enables you to experience all the fine shadings of thought and feeling that make each of us an individual. The brain is subdivided into several areas, all of which have specific functions. Three major subdivisions of the brain are the cerebrum, the cerebellum, and the brainstem Figure 7-72.

The **cerebrum**, which is the largest part of the brain and is sometimes called the gray matter, makes up approximately three-fourths of the volume of the brain and is composed of four lobes: frontal, parietal, temporal, and occipital. The cerebrum on one side of the brain controls activities on the opposite side of the body. Each lobe of the cerebrum is responsible for a specific function. For example, one group of brain cells in the frontal lobe is responsible for the activity of all the voluntary muscles of the body. Brain cells in this area generate impulses that are sent along nerve fibers that extend from each cell into the spinal cord. An area in the parietal lobe has cells that receive sensory impulses from the peripheral nerves of the body. Other parts of the cerebrum are responsible for other body functions. For example, the occipital region, in the back of the cerebrum, receives visual impulses from the eyes; other areas control hearing, balance, and speech. Still other parts of the cerebrum are responsible for emotions and other characteristics of a person's personality Figure 7-73.

The **cerebellum**, which is located underneath the great mass of cerebral tissue, is sometimes called the little brain. The major function of this area is to coordinate the various activities of the body, particularly body movements. Without the cerebellum, specialized muscular activities such as writing would be impossible.

The **brainstem** is named such because the brain appears to be sitting on this portion of the CNS as a plant sits on its stem. The brainstem is the most primitive part of the CNS. It lies deep within the cranium and is the best-protected part of the CNS. The brainstem is the controlling center for virtually all body functions that are absolutely necessary for life. Cells in this part of the brain control cardiac, respiratory, and other basic body functions. The brainstem comprises three areas: the **midbrain**, the **pons**, and the **medulla oblongata**. One of the interesting operations of the brainstem is the regulation of consciousness. The **reticular activating system** in the midbrain keeps you conscious.

The brain has many other anatomic areas, all of which have specific and important functions. The brain receives a vast amount of information from the environment, sorts it all out, and directs the body to respond appropriately. Many of the responses involve voluntary muscle action; others are automatic and involuntary. Table 7-10 summarizes the major portions of the nervous system and their functions.

Spinal Cord

The **spinal cord** is an extension of the brainstem Figure 7-74. As with the brain, the spinal cord contains nerve cell bodies, but the major portion of the spinal cord

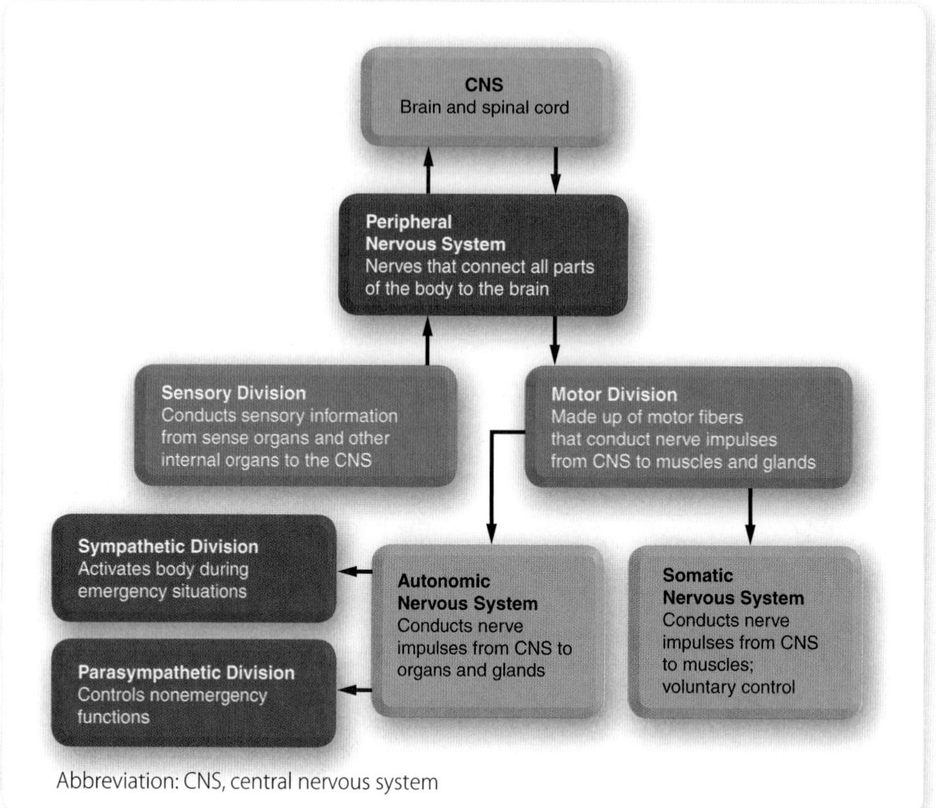

Figure 7-71 The basic configuration of the nervous system.

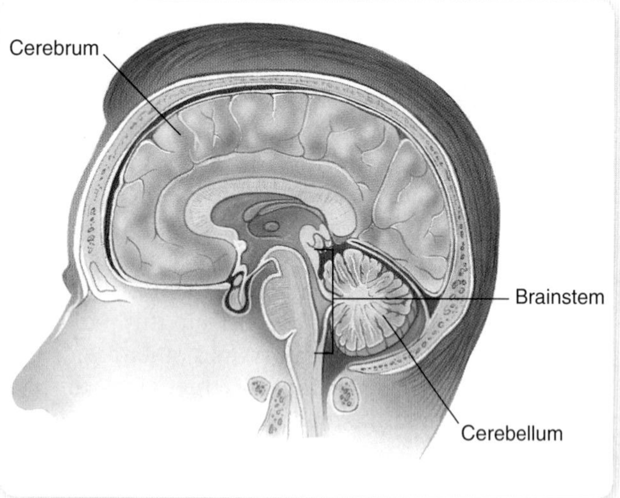

Figure 7-72 The brain lies well protected within the skull. Its principal subdivisions are the cerebrum, the cerebellum, and the brainstem.

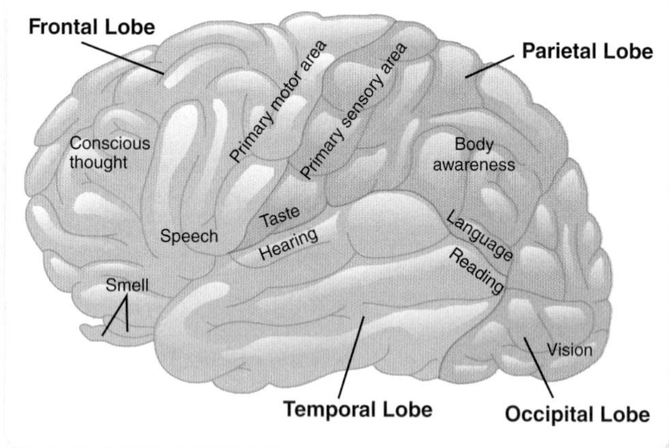

Figure 7-73 The cerebral cortex.

is made up of nerve fibers that extend from the cells of the brain. These nerve fibers transmit information to and from the brain. All fibers join together just below the brainstem to form the spinal cord. The spinal cord exits through a large opening at the base of the skull called the foramen magnum. It is encased within the spinal canal down to the level of the second lumbar vertebra. The spinal canal is created by an opening through the vertebrae, stacked one on another. Each vertebra surrounds the cord, and together the vertebrae form the bony spinal canal.

The principal function of the spinal cord is to transmit messages between the brain and the body. These messages are passed along the nerve fibers as electrical impulses, just as messages are passed along a telephone cable. The nerve fibers are arranged in specific bundles within the spinal cord to carry the messages from one specific area of the body to the brain and back.

Table 7-10 Structures of the Nervous System and General Functions

System	Major Structure	Subdivision	General Function
Central nervous system	Brain	Occipital lobe	Vision and storage of visual memories
		Parietal lobe	Sense of touch and texture; storage of those memories
		Temporal lobe	Hearing, smell, and language; storage of sound and odor memories
		Frontal lobe	Voluntary muscle control and storage of those memories
		Prefrontal area	Judgment and predicting consequences of actions, abstract intellectual functions
		Limbic system	Basic emotions, basic reflexes (chewing, swallowing, etc)
		Diencephalon (thalamus)	Relay center; filters important signals from routine signals
		Diencephalon (hypothalamus)	Emotions, temperature control, interface with endocrine system (hormone control)
	Brainstem	Midbrain	Level of consciousness, reticular activating system, muscle tone, and posture
		Pons	Respiratory patterning and depth
		Medulla oblongata	Heart rate, blood pressure, respiratory rate
	Spinal cord		Reflexes, relays information to and from body
Peripheral nervous system	Cranial nerves		Brain to body part; special peripheral nerves that connect directly to body parts
	Peripheral nerves		Brain to spinal cord to body part; receive stimulus from body, send commands to body

Safety

CSF is a clear body fluid that can carry the same infectious diseases as blood. The risk of exposure to infectious agents from CSF can be even greater than from blood because its presence is not as obvious as blood at first sight. To avoid exposure to infectious agents, ALWAYS wear gloves when making patient contact.

The Meninges

The entire CNS is enclosed by a set of three tough membranes known as the **meninges**. The outer membrane is the **dura mater** and is the toughest membrane. The second layer is called the **arachnoid** because the blood vessels it contains have the appearance of a spider web. The innermost layer, resting directly on the brain or spinal cord, is the **pia mater**.

When a hematoma develops, it can be classified according to its location in respect to the meninges (an epidural or a subdural hematoma). The meninges float in **cerebrospinal fluid (CSF)**, which is manufactured by cells within the **choroid plexus** in the ventricles, hollow storage areas in the brain. These areas normally are interconnected, and CSF flows freely within the **subarachnoid space**. The subarachnoid space is located between the pia mater and the arachnoid membrane. CSF is similar in composition to plasma. The meninges and CSF form a fluid-filled sac that cushions and protects the brain and spinal cord.

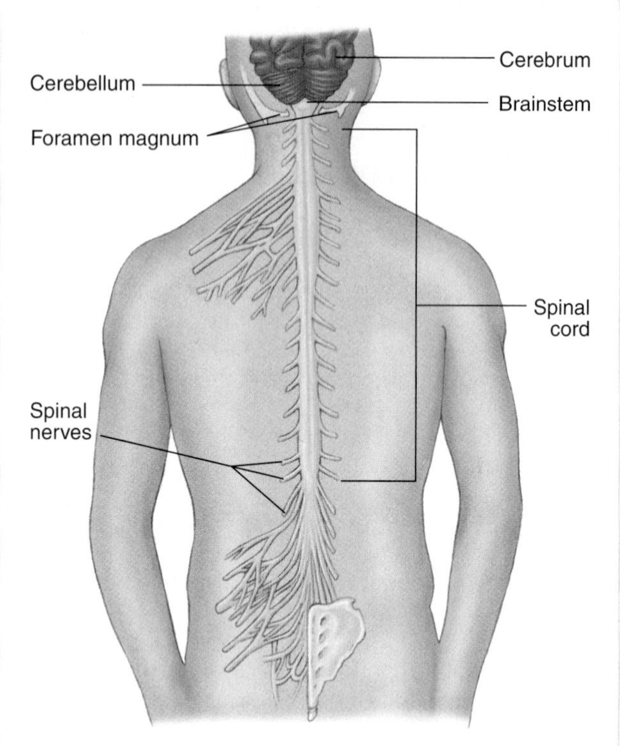

Figure 7-74 The spinal cord is a continuation of the brainstem. It exits the skull at the foramen magnum and extends down to the level of the second lumbar vertebra in most adults.

Words of Wisdom

Bleeding can occur between the meninges and the brain, usually as a result of trauma. The most common type of bleeding occurs with a **subarachnoid hemorrhage**, in which the blood lies between the arachnoid and the pia mater.

Words of Wisdom

In patients with a fracture at the base of the skull, CSF can leak into the eustachian tubes, past the eardrums, and out through the ears. Because CSF does not mix well with blood, it sometimes appears as a halo of clear fluid around drops of blood when it leaks onto a gauze pad. CSF that leaks into the back of a patient's throat is often described as having a "salty" taste.

▶ The Diencephalon

The **diencephalon**, which is located between the brainstem and the cerebrum, includes the thalamus, subthalamus, hypothalamus, and epithalamus. The **thalamus** processes most sensory input and influences mood and general body movements, especially those associated with fear and rage. The subthalamus controls motor functions. The functions of the epithalamus include regulation of circadian rhythms, mood, and motor pathways. The most inferior portion of the diencephalon, the **hypothalamus**, is vital in the control of many body functions, including heart rate, digestion, sexual development, temperature regulation, emotion, hunger, thirst, vomiting, and regulation of the sleep cycle. Portions of the cerebrum and diencephalon constitute the limbic system.

The Limbic System

The **limbic system** is the so-called emotional brain, or the feeling and reacting brain. It influences emotions, motivation, mood, and sensations of pain and pleasure Figure 7-75. The limbic system also has roles in learning and short- and long-term memory.

▶ The Peripheral Nervous System

Many of the cells in the CNS have long fibers that extend from the cell body out through openings in the bony covering of the spinal canal to form a cable of nerve fibers that link the CNS to the various organs of the body. These cables of nerve fibers make up the **peripheral nervous system (PNS)**. The PNS is divided into two portions. The first is the somatic nervous system that transmits signals from the brain to the voluntary muscles. As you turn the page of this text, you are accessing your somatic nervous system.

The other portion of the PNS is the autonomic nervous system, which, in turn, is split into two areas. The **sympathetic nervous system** is responsible for the "fight-or-flight" response, enabling you to fight if you find yourself in a dangerous situation or to run away. This fight-or-flight

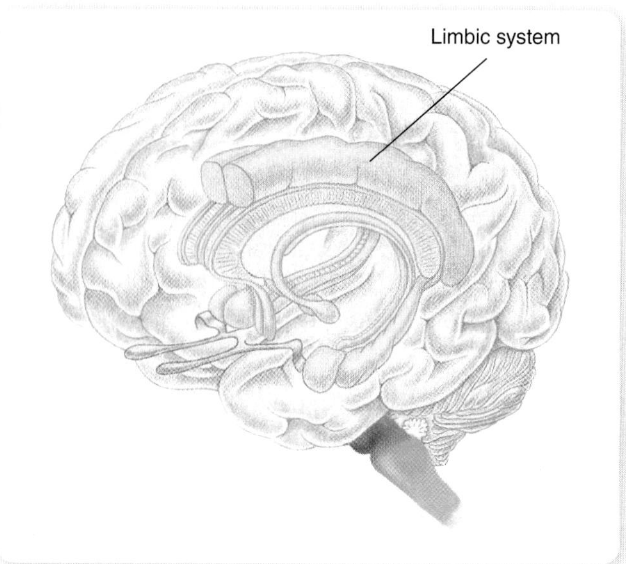

Figure 7-75 The limbic system.

response generally increases the activity within your body so that your muscles are able to perform more effectively. Sympathetic responses include the shunting of blood from the extremities to the vital core organs, increasing the heart rate and respirations, increasing blood pressure, dilation of the pupils, and reduction of digestive system activity.

The **parasympathetic nervous system**, the other half of the autonomic nervous system, generally slows down the body. When you are eating, your blood supply needs to move to your stomach and intestines so the food you eat can be processed. The parasympathetic responses include slowing the heart and respiratory rates, lowering the blood pressure, constricting the pupils, and increasing digestive system activity.

There are two types of nerves within the peripheral nervous system. **Sensory nerves** carry information from the body to the CNS. **Motor nerves** carry information from the CNS to the muscles of the body.

Sensory Nerves

Sensory nerves of the body are quite complex. There are many types of sensory cells in the nervous system. One type forms the retina of the eye; others are responsible for the hearing and balancing mechanisms in the ear. Other sensory cells are located in the skin, muscles, joints, lungs, and other organs of the body. When a sensory cell is stimulated, it transmits its own special message to the brain. There are special sensory nerves to detect heat, cold, position, motion, pressure, pain, balance, light, taste, and smell, as well as other sensations. Specialized nerve endings are adapted for each cell so it perceives only one type of sensation and transmits only that message.

The sensory impulses constantly provide information to the brain about what the different parts of our body are doing in relation to our surroundings. Thus, the brain is continuously made aware of its surroundings. The cranial nerves supply sensations directly to the brain. Visual sensations (what we see) reach the brain directly by way of the optic nerve (the second cranial nerve) in each eye. The nerve endings for the optic nerve lie in the retina of the eye. The nerve endings are stimulated by light, and the impulses travel along the nerve that passes through a hole in the back of the eye socket and carries impulses to the occipital portion of the brain.

When sensory nerve endings in the extremities are stimulated, the impulses are transmitted along a peripheral nerve to the spinal cord. The cell body of the peripheral nerve lies in the spinal cord. The impulse is then transmitted from that cell body to another nerve ending in the spinal cord and from there up the spinal cord to the sensory area in the parietal lobe of the brain, where the sensory information can be interpreted and acted on by the brain.

Motor Nerves

Each muscle in the body has its own motor nerve. The cell body for each motor nerve lies in the spinal cord, and a fiber from the cell body extends as part of the peripheral nerve to its specific muscle. Electrical impulses that are produced by the cell body in the spinal cord are transmitted along the motor nerve to the muscle and cause it to contract. The cell body in the spinal cord is stimulated by an impulse produced in the motor strip of the cerebral cortex. This impulse is transmitted along the spinal cord to the cell body of the motor nerve.

Spinal Reflexes

Within the spinal cord are cells with short fibers that connect the sensory nerves with the motor nerves. These are direct connections bypassing the brain. These cells are where spinal reflexes occur. In addition, these cells allow sensory and motor impulses to transmit from one nerve to another within the CNS.

Words of Wisdom

In the brainstem, most nerves cross from one side to the other. Motor and sensory nerves on the left side of the brain, for example, serve the right side of the body. This is why a person who has had a stroke or sustained trauma in one hemisphere has nerve deficits on the opposite side of the body. Because the cranial nerves are above this crossover point, their function will be affected on the same side of the face as the injury or stroke.

An irritating stimulus to the sensory nerve, such as heat, will be transmitted from the sensory nerve along the connecting nerve directly to the motor nerve. This will stimulate the motor nerve. The muscle responds promptly, withdrawing the limb from the irritating stimulus even before this information can be transmitted to the brain. Technically, you do not "feel" the heat of the fire before you move your hand away. This process is in place to limit damage to the body. When a physician taps your knee with a rubber hammer, he or she is testing to see whether your reflex arc is intact.

Cranial Nerves

Twelve pairs of **cranial nerves** arise from the base of the brain. All but two pairs, the olfactory nerves and the optic nerves, exit from the brainstem **Figure 7-76**.

Some of the cranial nerves carry only sensory fibers (I, II, and VIII), and others carry only motor fibers (III, IV, VI, XI, and XII). Many are mixed nerves, carrying a combination of sensory fibers and motor fibers (V, VII, IX, and X). Some cranial nerves also carry nerves of the parasympathetic nervous system in combination with motor, sensory, or both types of nerves (III, VII, IX, and X). Each nerve passes from the brain through a foramen in the skull to reach its end point.

The olfactory nerve (I) provides the sense of smell. The optic nerve (II) provides the sense of vision.

The **oculomotor nerve** (III) innervates the muscles that cause motion of the eyeballs and upper lid.

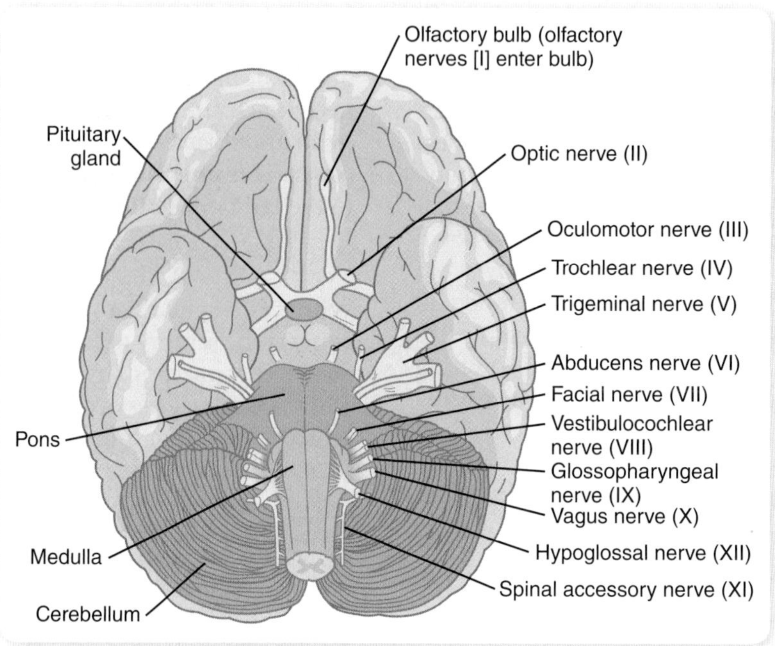

Figure 7-76 The cranial nerves.

The oculomotor nerve also carries parasympathetic nerve fibers that cause constriction of the pupil (sphincter muscle) and accommodation of the lens (ciliary muscle).

The trochlear nerve (IV) innervates the superior oblique muscle of the eyeball, which allows a downward gaze. The trigeminal nerve (V) supplies sensation to the scalp, forehead, face, and lower jaw via three branches: the ophthalmic, maxillary, and mandibular divisions. The trigeminal nerve also provides motor innervation to the muscles of mastication (chewing), the throat, and the inner ear.

The abducens nerve (VI) supplies the lateral rectus muscle of the eyeball (lateral movement). The facial nerve (VII) supplies motor activity to all muscles of facial expression, the sense of taste to the anterior two-thirds of the tongue, and cutaneous sensation to the external ear, tongue, and palate. The facial nerve also carries parasympathetic stimulation to the salivary glands, lacrimal gland, and the glands of the nasal cavity and palate.

The vestibulocochlear nerve (VIII) passes through the internal auditory meatus and provides the senses of hearing and balance. The glossopharyngeal nerve (IX) supplies motor fibers to the pharyngeal muscles. It provides taste sensation to the posterior portion of the tongue and carries parasympathetic fibers to the salivary glands (parotid glands) located on each side of the face.

The **vagus nerve** (X) provides motor functions to the soft palate, pharynx, and larynx (voice). The vagus nerve carries sensory fibers from the inferior pharynx, larynx, thoracic, and abdominal organs, taste bud fibers from the posterior tongue, and parasympathetic fibers to thoracic and abdominal organs.

The spinal accessory nerve (XI) provides motor innervation to the muscles of the soft palate and the pharynx and to the sternocleidomastoid and trapezius muscles. The spinal accessory nerve controls swallowing, speech, and head and shoulder movements. The hypoglossal nerve (XII) provides motor function to the muscles of the tongue and throat.

Dermatomes. A **dermatome** is an area of the skin that corresponds to certain spinal nerves **Figure 7-77**. It is helpful to be familiar with dermatomes when assessing for potential spinal cord injury. When a spinal cord injury has occurred, the patient may have impairment in a specific dermatome that translates to impairment distal to a certain nerve or vertebra.

▶ The Eye

The cranial nerves connect the body's senses to the brain. The eye and other senses provide a multitude of information to the brain for it to process in an effort to understand the world around us.

The eyeball is called the globe. The inner surface of the eyelids and the exposed surface of the eye itself, which are covered by a delicate membrane, the **conjunctiva**, are kept moist by fluid produced by the **lacrimal glands**, often called tear glands. Humans blink unconsciously many times per minute. This action sweeps fluid from the lacrimal glands over the surface of the eye, cleaning it. The tears drain on the inner side of the eye through two lacrimal (tear) ducts into the nasal cavity. This is why, when people cry, they sometimes need to blow their nose.

Behind the **iris** is the **lens**. Like the lens of a camera, this lens focuses images on the light-sensitive area at the back of the globe, called the **retina**. Within the retina are numerous nerve endings, which respond to light by transmitting nerve impulses through the **optic nerve**

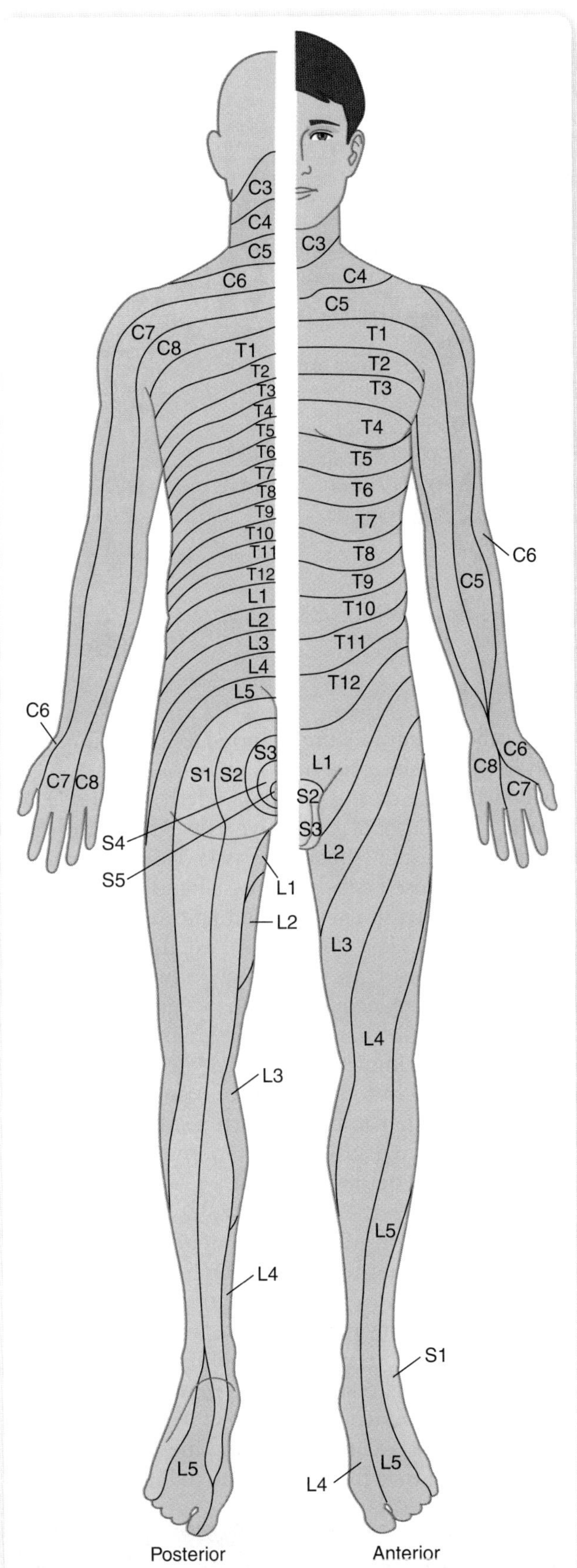

Figure 7-77 Dermatome map showing the association of the spinal nerves and the cutaneous areas of the body.

to the brain. In the brain, the impulses are interpreted as vision. There are two types of vision. **Central vision** facilitates visualization of objects directly in front of you and is processed by the macula, the central portion of the retina. The remainder of the retina processes **peripheral vision**, which allows visualization of lateral objects while you are looking forward.

The retina is nourished by a layer of blood vessels (the choroid) between it and the sclera at the back of the globe. If the retina becomes detached from the underlying choroid and sclera, the nerve endings are not nourished, and the patient experiences blindness. The extent of the blindness (partial versus complete) depends on how much of the retina is separated. A detached retina is sometimes surgically treatable.

The Integumentary System (Skin): Anatomy

The **integumentary system** is the largest system in the human body and serves as the interface between the body and the outside world. Human skin is a complex organ that plays a crucial role in maintaining the constancy of the internal environment (homeostasis). It protects tissue from injury, helps regulate body temperature, prevents excessive water loss, and serves as a sense organ. Substantial damage to the skin may leave the body vulnerable to bacterial invasion, temperature instability, and major disturbances of fluid balance.

The skin is divided into two parts: the superficial **epidermis**, which is composed of several layers of cells and is the body's first line of defense, and the deeper **dermis**, which is a tough, highly elastic layer of connective tissues. Below the skin lies the **subcutaneous tissue** layer, which consists mainly of fat Figure 7-78.

The cells of the epidermis are sealed to form a watertight protective covering for the body. The epidermis varies in thickness in different areas of the body. On the soles of the feet, the back, and the **scalp**, it is quite thick, but in some areas of the body, the epidermis is only two or three cell layers thick. The epidermis is actually composed of several layers of cells. These layers can be separated into two regions. At the base of the epidermis is the **germinal layer**, which continuously produces new cells that gradually rise to the surface. On the way to the surface, these cells die and enter the **stratum corneal layer**. This is the dead layer of skin. Whereas the germinal layer has a blood supply, the stratum corneal layer does not. The journey from the germinal layer to the surface takes approximately 4 weeks. The outermost cells of the epidermis are constantly rubbed away and replaced by new cells produced by the germinal layer. Deeper cells in the germinal layer contain pigment (melanin) granules. Along with blood vessels in the dermis, these granules produce skin color.

Below the germinal layer is the dermis. It is composed chiefly of collagen fibers, elastic fibers, and a

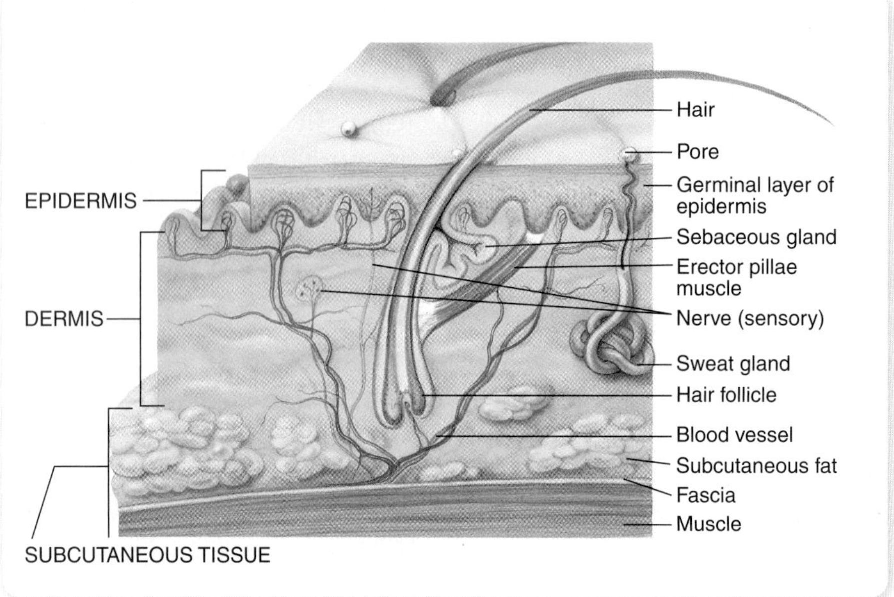

Figure 7-78 The skin has two principal layers: the epidermis and the dermis. Below the skin is a layer of subcutaneous tissue.

mucopolysaccharide gel. Numerous fibroblasts—cells that secrete collagen, elastin, and ground substance—are found within the dermis. These substances provide resistance to skin breakage and elasticity. Within the dermis lie many of the special structures of the skin: sweat glands, sebaceous (oil) glands, hair follicles, blood vessels, lymph vessels, and specialized nerve endings.

Dilation of vessels in the dermis assists with thermoregulation by increasing blood flow to the skin, allowing heat to dissipate. Conversely, blood vessel constriction results in retention of heat. Macrophages and lymphocytes are also found within the dermal layer. They are responsible for combating microorganisms that breach the epidermal layer.

Sweat glands produce sweat for cooling the body. The sweat is discharged onto the surface of the skin through small pores, or ducts, that pass through the epidermis. The sebaceous glands produce sebum, the oily material that seals the surface epidermal cells. The **sebaceous glands** lie next to hair follicles and secrete sebum along the hair follicle to the skin surface. In addition to providing waterproofing for the skin, sebum keeps the skin soft so it does not crack.

Hair follicles are the small organs that produce hair. The hair grows from the follicle along a shaft until it reaches the epidermal surface. A sebaceous gland is located along the hair shaft. Connected to the hair is a small muscle. The muscle pulls the hair into an erect position when a person is cold or frightened. Hair goes through stages of growth and rest. Blood vessels provide nutrients and oxygen to the skin. The blood vessels lie in the dermis. Small branches extend up to the germinal layer. A complex array of nerve endings also lies in the dermis. These specialized nerve endings are sensitive to environmental stimuli; they respond to these stimuli and send impulses along the nerves to the brain.

Between the dermis and the underlying muscle and bone is a thick layer of connective tissue known as subcutaneous tissue, or the superficial fascia. This subcutaneous tissue is composed of adipose tissue and areolar tissue. Blood vessels, lymph vessels, and hair follicle roots are also found in this layer (as well as the dermis). The subcutaneous tissue insulates, protects, and stores energy in the form of fat. Subcutaneous injections are given in this layer.

Below the subcutaneous tissue is a thick, dense layer of fibrous tissue known as the **deep fascia**. The deep fascia is composed of tough bands of tissue that surround muscles and other internal structures. It supports and protects underlying structures from injury. Muscles and bones are found below this layer.

The skin covers the entire external surface of the body. The various orifices—including the mouth, nose, anus, and vagina—are not covered by skin. Orifices are lined with mucous membranes. **Mucous membranes** are similar to skin in that they provide a protective barrier against bacterial invasion. Mucous membranes differ from skin in that they secrete **mucus**, a sticky substance that lubricates the openings. Thus, mucous membranes are moist, whereas the skin is dry. For example, a mucous membrane lines the entire digestive tract from the mouth to the anus.

The Integumentary System (Skin): Physiology

The integumentary system serves three major functions: to protect the body in the environment, to regulate the temperature of the body, and to transmit information from the environment to the brain. The protective functions of the skin are numerous. Water makes up a large portion of the body. This water contains a delicate balance of chemical substances in solution. The skin is watertight and helps keep this balanced internal solution intact. The skin also protects the body from the invasion of infectious organisms: bacteria, viruses, and fungi. These organisms are everywhere and are routinely found lying on the skin surface. However, they never penetrate the skin unless it is broken by injury; thus, the skin provides a constant protection against outside invaders.

The major organ for regulation of body temperature is the skin. Blood vessels in the skin constrict when the body is in a cold environment and dilate when the body is in a warm environment. In a cold environment, constriction of the blood vessels shunts the blood away from the skin to decrease the amount of heat radiated from the body surface. When the outside environment is hot, the vessels in the skin dilate, the skin becomes flushed or red, and heat radiates from the body surface.

Also, in a hot environment, sweat is secreted to the skin surface from the sweat glands. Evaporation of the sweat requires energy. This energy, as body heat, is taken from the body during the evaporation process, which causes the body temperature to fall. Sweating alone will not reduce body temperature; evaporation of the sweat must also occur.

Information from the environment is carried to the brain through a rich supply of sensory nerves that originate in the skin. Nerve endings that lie in the skin are adapted to perceive and transmit information about heat, cold, external pressure, pain, and the position of the body in space. The skin thus recognizes any changes in the environment. The skin also reacts to pressure, pain, and pleasurable stimuli.

The integument responds to injuries and wounds with inflammation, which causes redness, increased warmth, and painful swelling. The blood vessels of the wounded area dilate and allow fluids to leak into the damaged tissues. This provides more nutrients and oxygen to the tissues, aiding in healing.

Words of Wisdom

Considerable damage to the skin may make the body vulnerable to bacterial invasion, temperature instability, and major disturbances of fluid balance, which is precisely what happens when an injury results in an opening in the skin.

Words of Wisdom

The skin, the largest single organ in the body, serves three major functions: to protect the body in the environment, to regulate the temperature of the body, and to transmit information from the environment to the brain.

YOU are the Provider — PART 4

Knowing that time is of the essence in patients such as these, you direct your partner to drive emergently to the local Level 1 trauma center. Prior to transport you establish an 18-gauge intravenous line to the uninjured arm and infuse fluid at a to-keep-open rate since the systolic blood pressure is above 90 mm Hg, per your local protocols. The patient denies any medical problems or having any known allergies. While en route, you reevaluate your treatments and find that bleeding remains controlled, and the patient's breathing, while still shallow, seems to be improving with the administration of oxygen. You remove the remainder of the patient's clothing and find no additional injuries. On arriving at the trauma center, you turn over care of the patient to the awaiting trauma team.

Recording Time: 14 Minutes	
Respirations	14 breaths/min, shallow
Pulse	Weak L radial, 126 via R radial
Skin	Cool, pale, and clammy
Blood pressure	98/58 mm Hg
Oxygen saturation (Spo$_2$)	97% on 15 L/min
Pupils	PERRLA

7. What could be causing the difference in left and right radial pulses in this patient?
8. Body fluid is divided into two main compartments. What are they and where are they found?

The Digestive System: Anatomy

The digestive system, also called the gastrointestinal system, is composed of the gastrointestinal tract (stomach and intestines), mouth, salivary glands, pharynx, esophagus, liver, gallbladder, pancreas, rectum, and anus. The function of this system is **digestion**: the processing of food that nourishes the individual cells of the body. The major organs of this system are found within the abdomen.

The Abdomen

The **abdomen** is the second major body cavity; it contains the major organs of digestion and excretion. The diaphragm separates the thoracic cavity from the abdominal cavity. Anteriorly and posteriorly, thick muscular abdominal walls create the boundaries of this space. Inferiorly, the abdomen is separated from the pelvis by an imaginary plane that extends from the pubic symphysis through the sacrum **Figure 7-79**. Some organs lie in the abdomen and the pelvis, depending on the posture of the patient.

The simplest and most common method of describing the portions of the abdomen is by **quadrants**, the four equal areas formed by two imaginary lines that intersect at right angles at the umbilicus. On the anterior abdominal wall, the quadrants thus formed are the right upper, right lower, left upper, and left lower. The terms *right quadrant* and *left quadrant* refer to the patient's right and left. Pain or injury in a given quadrant usually arises from or involves the organs that lie in that quadrant. This simple means of designation will allow you to identify injured or diseased organs that require emergency attention.

In the right upper quadrant (RUQ), the major organs are the liver, the gallbladder, and a portion of the colon and small intestine. Most of the liver lies in this quadrant, almost entirely under the protection of the 8th to 12th ribs. The liver fills the entire anteroposterior depth of the abdomen in this quadrant. Therefore, injuries in this area are frequently associated with injuries of the liver.

In the left upper quadrant (LUQ), the principal organs are the stomach, the spleen, and a portion of the colon and small intestine. The spleen is almost entirely under the protection of the left rib cage, whereas the stomach may sag well down into the left lower quadrant (LLQ) when full. The spleen lies in the lateral and posterior portion of this quadrant, under the diaphragm and immediately in front of the posterior portion of the 9th to 11th ribs. The spleen is frequently injured, especially when these ribs are fractured.

The right lower quadrant (RLQ) contains two portions of the large intestine: the **cecum**, the first portion into which the small intestine (ileum) opens, and the ascending colon. The **appendix** is a small tubular structure that is attached to the lower border of the cecum. Appendicitis is the most frequent cause of tenderness and pain in this region. In the LLQ lie the descending and the sigmoid portions of the colon.

As mentioned early in this chapter, several organs lie in more than one quadrant. The small intestine, for example, occupies the central part of the abdomen around the umbilicus, and parts of it lie in all four quadrants. The pancreas lies just behind the abdominal cavity on the posterior abdominal wall in both upper quadrants. The large intestine also traverses the abdomen, beginning in the RLQ and ending in the LLQ as it

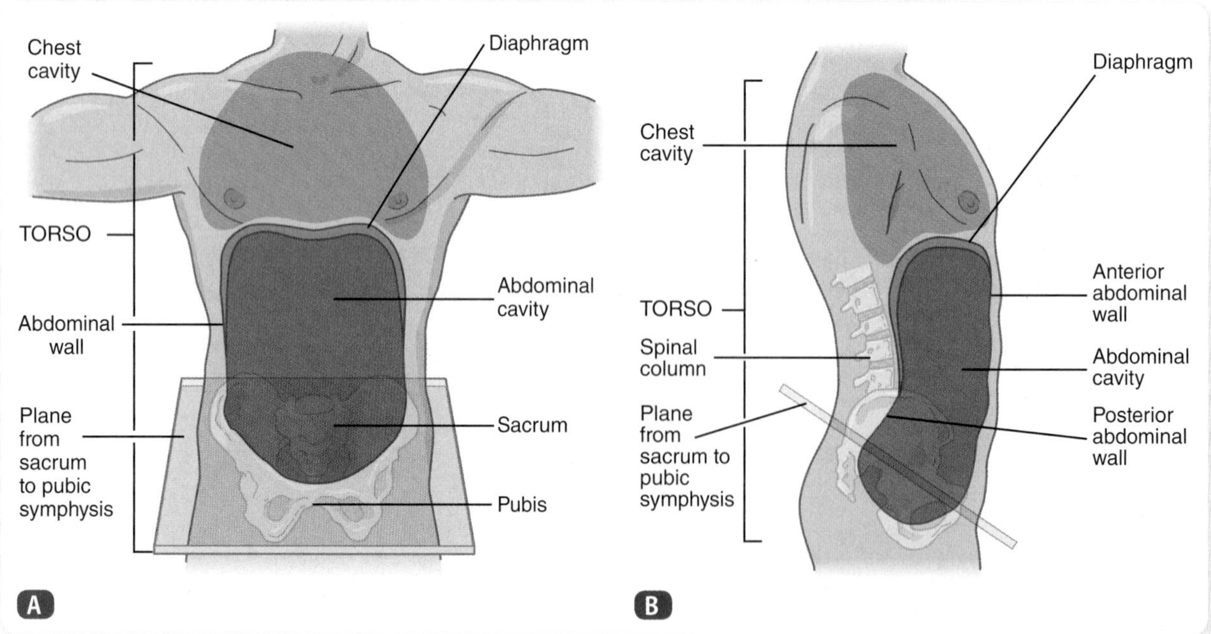

Figure 7-79 The boundaries of the abdomen are the anterior and posterior abdominal cavity walls, the diaphragm, and an imaginary plane from the pubic symphysis to the sacrum. **A.** Anterior view. **B.** Lateral view.

passes through all four quadrants. The urinary bladder lies just behind the pubic symphysis in the middle of the abdomen and therefore lies in both lower quadrants and also in the pelvis.

The kidneys are called retroperitoneal organs because they lie behind the abdominal cavity Figure 7-80. They are above the level of the umbilicus, extending from the 11th rib to the 3rd lumbar vertebra on each side. The kidneys are approximately 5 inches (13 cm) long and lie just anterior to the costovertebral angle.

▶ Mouth

The mouth consists of the lips, cheeks, gums, teeth, and tongue. A mucous membrane lines the mouth. The roof of the mouth is formed by the hard and soft palates. The hard palate is a bony plate lying anteriorly; the soft palate is a fold of mucous membrane and muscle that extends posteriorly from the hard palate into the throat. The soft palate is designed to hold food that is being chewed within the mouth and to help initiate swallowing.

Salivary Glands

There are two **salivary glands** located under the tongue, one on each side of the lower jaw, and one inside each cheek. These six glands combined produce nearly 1.5 L of saliva daily. Saliva is approximately 98% water. The remaining 2% is composed of mucus, salts, and organic compounds. Saliva serves as a binder for the chewed food that is being swallowed and as a lubricant within the mouth. Saliva also contains certain digestive enzymes.

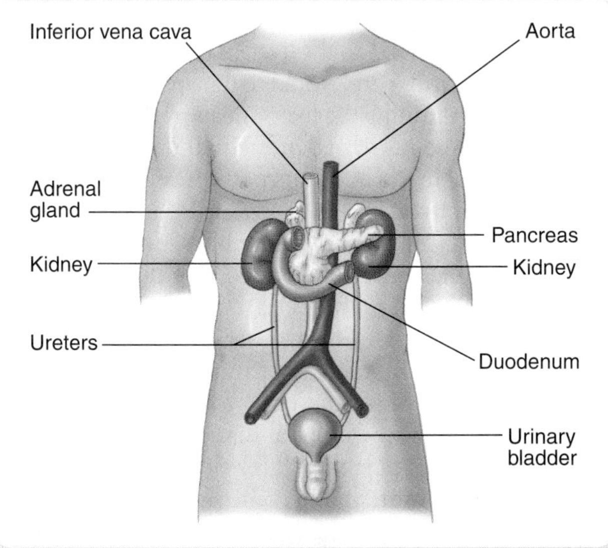

Figure 7-80 The major organs of the retroperitoneal space lie behind the abdominal cavity, above the level of the umbilicus, and extend from the 11th rib to the 3rd lumbar vertebra. Note that the bladder, inferior vena cava, and aorta also lie in this plane.

▶ Oropharynx

The **oropharynx** is a tubular structure that extends vertically from the back of the mouth to the esophagus and trachea. An automatic movement of the pharynx during swallowing lifts the larynx to permit the epiglottis to close over it so that liquids and solids are moved into the esophagus and away from the larynx and trachea.

▶ Esophagus

The esophagus is a collapsible tube about 10 inches (25 cm) long that extends from the end of the pharynx to the stomach and lies just anterior to the spinal column in the chest. Contractions of the muscle in the wall of the esophagus propel food through it to the stomach. Liquids pass with minimal assistance.

▶ Stomach

The stomach is a hollow organ located in the LUQ of the abdominal cavity, largely protected by the lower left ribs. Muscular contractions in the wall of the stomach and gastric juice, which contains a lot of mucus, convert ingested food to a thoroughly mixed semisolid mass, called **chyme**. The stomach produces approximately 1.5 L of gastric juice daily for this process. The principal function of the stomach is to receive food in large quantities intermittently, store it, and provide for its movement into the small bowel in regular, small amounts. In 1 to 3 hours, the semisolid food mass derived from one meal is propelled by muscular contraction into the duodenum, the first part of the small intestine.

▶ Pancreas

The **pancreas**, a flat, solid organ, lies below and behind the liver and stomach and behind the peritoneum. It is firmly fixed in position, deep within the abdomen, and is not easily damaged. It contains two kinds of glands, and the two portions of the pancreas are intertwined. One portion is exocrine, and it secretes nearly 2 L of pancreatic juice daily. This juice contains many enzymes that aid in the digestion of fat, starch, and protein. Pancreatic juice flows directly into the duodenum through the pancreatic ducts. The other portion of the gland is endocrine. It is called the islets of Langerhans, and this is where insulin is produced. Insulin regulates the amount of glucose in the blood.

▶ Liver

The **liver** is a large, solid organ that takes up most of the area immediately beneath the diaphragm in the RUQ and also extends into the LUQ. It is the largest solid organ in the abdomen and has several functions. Poisonous substances produced by digestion are brought to the liver and rendered harmless. Factors that are necessary for blood clotting and for the production of normal plasma are formed here. Between 0.5 and 1 L of bile is made by the liver daily to assist in the normal digestion of fat. The liver is the principal organ for the storage of sugar or starch for immediate use by the body for energy. It also produces many of the factors that aid in the proper regulation of immune responses. Anatomically, the liver is a large mass of blood vessels and cells, packed tightly together. It is fragile and, because of its size, relatively easily injured. Blood flow in the liver is high, because all of the blood that is pumped to the gastrointestinal tract passes into the liver, through the portal vein, before it returns to the heart. In addition, the liver has a generous arterial blood supply of its own. Ordinarily, approximately 25% of the cardiac output of blood (1.5 L) passes through the liver each minute.

Bile Ducts

The liver is connected to the intestine by the **bile ducts**. The **gallbladder** is an outpouching from the bile ducts that serves as a reservoir and concentrating organ for bile produced in the liver. Together, the bile ducts and the gallbladder form the biliary system. The gallbladder discharges stored concentrated bile into the duodenum through the common bile duct. The presence of food in the duodenum triggers a contraction of the gallbladder to empty it. The gallbladder usually contains approximately 60 to 90 mL of bile.

▶ Small Intestine

The **small intestine** is the major hollow organ of the abdomen. The cells lining the small intestine produce enzymes and mucus to aid in digestion. Enzymes from the pancreas and the small intestine carry out the final processes of digestion. More than 90% of the products of digestion (amino acids, fatty acids, and simple sugars), together with water, ingested vitamins, and minerals, are absorbed across the wall of the lower end of the small intestine into veins to be transported to the liver. The small intestine is composed of the duodenum, the jejunum, and the ileum. The duodenum, which is approximately 12 inches (30 cm) long, is the part of the small intestine that receives food from the stomach. Here, food is mixed with secretions from the pancreas and liver for further digestion. Bile, produced by the liver and stored in the gallbladder, is emptied as needed into the duodenum. It is greenish black, but through changes during digestion, it gives feces its typical brown color. Its major function is in the digestion of fat. The jejunum and ileum together measure more than 20 feet (6 m) on average to make up the rest of the small intestine.

▶ Large Intestine

The **large intestine**, another major hollow organ, consists of the cecum, the colon, and the rectum. Approximately 5 feet (1.5 m) long, it encircles the outer border of the abdomen around the small bowel. The major function of the colon, the portion of the large intestine that extends from the cecum to the rectum, is to absorb the final 5% to 10% of digested food and water from the intestine to form solid stool, which is stored in the rectum and passed out of the body through the anus.

▶ Appendix

The appendix is a tube 3 to 4 inches (8 to 10 cm) long that opens into the cecum (the first part of the large intestine) in the RLQ of the abdomen. It may easily become obstructed and, as a result, inflamed and infected. Appendicitis, which is the term for this inflammation, is one of the major causes of severe abdominal distress.

▶ Rectum

The lowermost end of the colon is the **rectum**. It is a large, hollow organ that is adapted to store quantities of feces until it is expelled. At its terminal end is the anus, a 2-inch (5-cm) canal lined with skin. The rectum and anus are supplied with a complex series of circular muscles called **sphincters** that control, voluntarily and automatically, the escape of liquids, gases, and solids from the digestive tract. Table 7-11 provides a summary of the organs and functions of the digestive system.

The Digestive System: Physiology

Digestion of food, from the time it is taken into the mouth until essential compounds are extracted and delivered by the circulatory system to nourish all cells in the body, is a complicated chemical process. In succession, different secretions, primarily **enzymes**, are added to the food by the salivary glands, the stomach, the liver, the pancreas, and the small intestine to convert the food into basic sugars, fatty acids, and amino acids. These basic products of digestion are carried across the wall of the intestine and transported through the portal vein to the liver. In the liver, the products are processed further and stored or transported to the heart through veins draining the liver. The heart then pumps the blood with these nutrients throughout the arteries to the capillaries, where the nutrients pass through the capillary walls to nourish the body's individual cells.

In normal routine activity, without any food or fluid ingestion at all, between 8 and 10 L of fluid is secreted daily into the gastrointestinal tract. This fluid comes from the salivary glands, stomach, liver, pancreas, and small intestine. In a healthy adult, approximately 7% of the body weight is delivered as fluid daily to the gastrointestinal tract. If substantial vomiting or diarrhea occurs for more than 2 or 3 days, a person will lose a substantial portion of body composition and become severely ill.

The Endocrine System: Anatomy and Physiology

The **endocrine system** is a complex message and control system that integrates many body functions. This system is made up of various glands located throughout the body. **Glands** are

Table 7-11 Digestive Organs and Functions

Organ/Structure	Function
Mouth	Mechanically breaks down food; begins chemical breakdown with saliva
Esophagus	Moves food from the mouth to the stomach; muscular and vascular structure
Stomach	Performs mechanical and chemical breakdown of food: food in, chyme out
Small intestine: duodenum, jejunum, and ileum	Major site for chemical breakdown of food; major absorption of water, fats, proteins, carbohydrates, and vitamins
Large intestine	Water absorption; formation of feces; bacterial digestion of food
Anus/rectum	Last portion of large intestine; sphincter to control release of feces
Liver	Production of bile; assists with carbohydrate, protein, and fat metabolism of nutrients within the bloodstream; vitamin storage and manufacture; detoxification of blood; elimination of waste
Pancreas	Exocrine: enzymes for protein, carbohydrate, and fat breakdown within the duodenum Endocrine: insulin and glucagon
Gallbladder	Storage of bile

cells or organs that remove, concentrate, or alter materials in the blood and then secrete them back into the body.

Exocrine glands (*exo* means "outside") excrete chemicals for elimination. These glands have ducts that carry their secretions to the surface of the skin or into a body cavity. Sweat glands, salivary glands, and the liver are examples of exocrine glands.

Endocrine glands (*endo* means "inside") secrete or release chemicals that are used inside the body. These glands lack ducts, so they release hormones directly into the surrounding tissue and blood.

Glands secrete proteins called **hormones** that regulate many body functions, including growth, reproduction, temperature, metabolism, and blood pressure. Endocrine cells and neurosecretory cells manufacture and secrete hormones that are released into the bloodstream and move to their target tissue **Figure 7-81**.

Hormones act on the body's cells by increasing or decreasing the rate of cellular metabolism. They transfer information from one set of cells to another to coordinate bodily functions, such as the regulation of mood, growth and development, metabolism, tissue function, and sexual development and function.

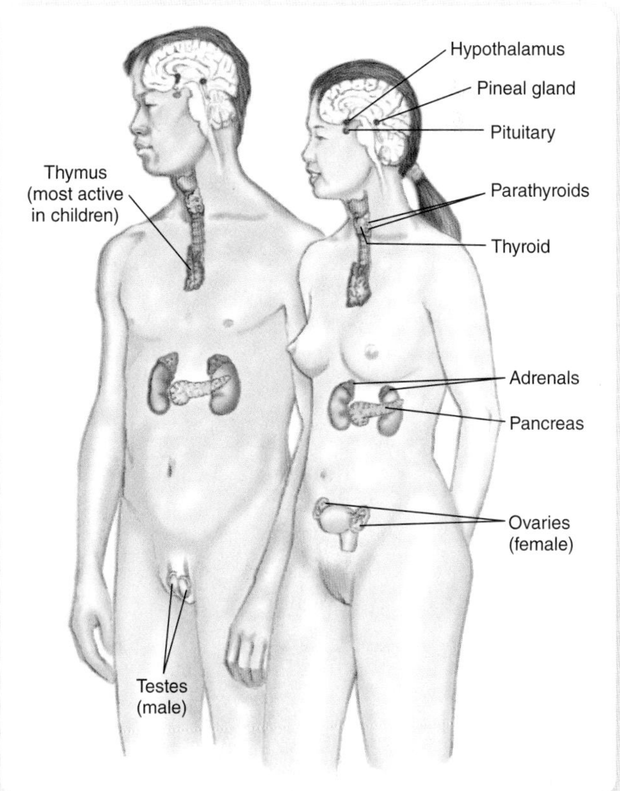

Figure 7-81 The endocrine system controls the release of hormones in the body.

Hormones, regardless of their source, act by binding to receptors. The nervous system regulates hormone release via nerve impulses. When released into the bloodstream, hormones travel to target tissues. Each target cell has specific receptor sites on the cell membrane, or inside the cell, to which the specific hormone can attach or bind. These receptors have two main functions: to recognize and bind to their particular hormones and to initiate an appropriate signal. Once the hormone has attached to the receptor site of the cell, the "message" to alter the cellular function is delivered.

Many cells contain multiple receptors and act as targets for several hormones—or for molecules introduced into the body as therapy. An **agonist** is a molecule that binds to a cell's receptor and triggers a response by that cell; agonists produce some kind of action or biologic effect. An **antagonist** is a molecule that binds to a cell's receptor and blocks the action of an agonist. Hormone antagonists are widely used as drugs.

Steroids and thyroid hormones bind to receptors located within cells. All other hormones, as a rule, bind to receptors located on the surface of cells. Hormones stimulate the production of intracellular proteins and other substances that carry out the next task in whichever body process the particular hormone is involved.

The Pituitary Gland and the Hypothalamus

The **pituitary gland** is often referred to as the master gland because its secretions control the secretions of other endocrine glands. It is located at the base of the brain and is about the size of a grape. The hypothalamus is a small region of the brain (not a gland) that regulates the function of the pituitary gland. The hypothalamus is the primary link between the endocrine system and the nervous system. The pituitary is attached to the hypothalamus by a very thin piece of tissue.

The pituitary gland is divided into two portions: the anterior pituitary, which produces and secretes six hormones (growth hormone, thyroid-stimulating hormone, adrenocorticotropin hormone, and three gonadotropic hormones), and the posterior pituitary, which secretes two hormones (ADH and oxytocin) but does not produce them Figure 7-82. ADH and oxytocin are synthesized in hypothalamic neurons but are stored in the posterior pituitary gland until the hypothalamus sends nerve signals to the pituitary to release them.

During times of stress, the hypothalamus secretes a hormone that stimulates the anterior pituitary to release **adrenocorticotropic hormone (ACTH)**. ACTH targets the adrenal cortex and causes it to secrete **cortisol** (a glucocorticoid). Cortisol stimulates most body cells to increase their energy production.

The Thyroid Gland

The large gland at the base of the neck is called the **thyroid gland**. It consists of two lobes that are connected by a narrow band of tissue. The thyroid gland manufactures and secretes hormones that have a role in growth, development, and metabolism.

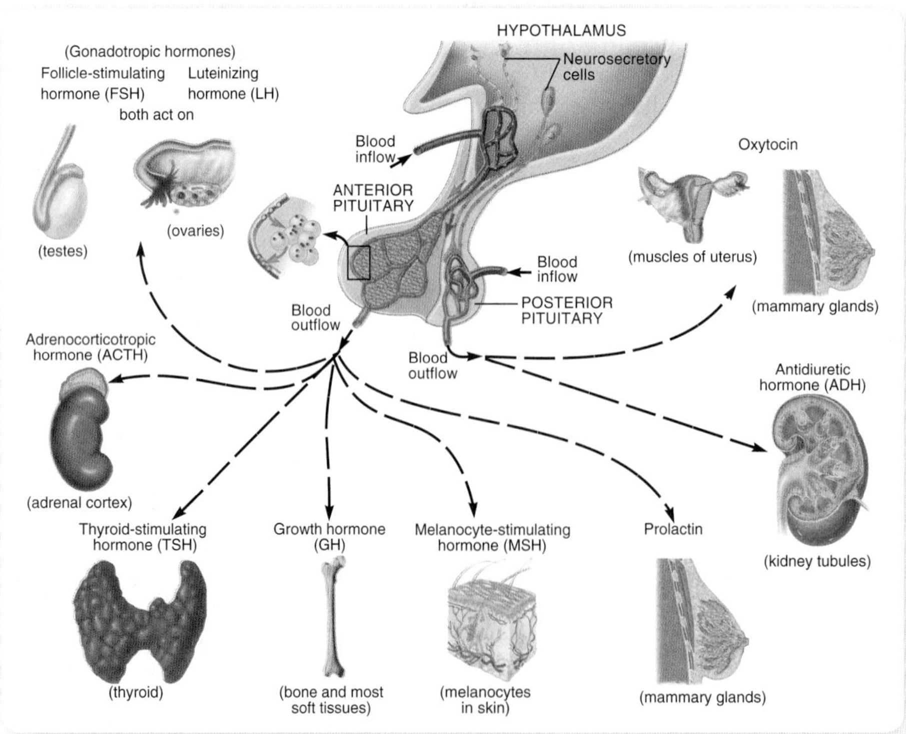

Figure 7-82 The pituitary gland secretes hormones from its two regions: the anterior pituitary lobe and the posterior pituitary lobe.

The thyroid gland secretes **calcitonin**, which helps maintain normal calcium levels in the blood. This hormone is secreted directly into the bloodstream when the thyroid detects high levels of calcium. Calcitonin travels to the bones, where it stimulates the bone-building cells to absorb the excess calcium. It also stimulates the kidneys to absorb and excrete excess calcium.

▶ The Parathyroid Glands

The **parathyroid glands** are embedded in the posterior portion of each lobe of the thyroid. They produce and secrete **parathyroid hormone**, which maintains normal levels of calcium in the blood and normal neuromuscular function. Parathyroid hormone effects are opposite to those of calcitonin.

▶ The Pancreas

The pancreas is an organ of both the endocrine and digestive systems. It produces two hormones, insulin and glucagon, as well as digestive enzymes. The pancreas lies between the greater curvature of the stomach and the duodenum in the **retroperitoneum**, or space behind the peritoneum. The head of the pancreas rests near the duodenum; the body and tail of the pancreas project toward the spleen.

In the pancreas, within each islet of Langerhans are **alpha cells** that secrete glucagon, **beta cells** that secrete insulin, and delta cells that secrete somatostatin. Insulin and glucagon perform opposite functions. Insulin causes substances such as sugar, fatty acids, and amino acids to be taken up and metabolized by cells. Insulin also stimulates the storage of unmetabolized food and the conversion of glucose into **glycogen**. Somatostatin is responsible for the inhibition of insulin and glucagon secretion.

Glucagon stimulates the breakdown of glycogen to glucose by a process known as **glycogenolysis**. In addition, glucagon stimulates both the liver and the kidneys to produce glucose from noncarbohydrate molecules by a process known as **gluconeogenesis**. In addition, glucagon activates the breakdown of triglycerides into free fatty acids and glycerol. Depending on the metabolic needs of the body, the free fatty acids and glycerol may be metabolized directly or converted to ketones. In small amounts, ketone production is normal. In disease states, such as diabetic ketoacidosis, increased plasma glucagon concentrations and unopposed glucagon activity result in excessive production, resulting in possible harm to the patient.

▶ The Adrenal Glands

The **adrenal glands** are located on top of each kidney. The adrenal gland manufactures and secretes certain sex hormones, as well as other hormones that are vital in maintaining the body's water and salt balance. The inner portion of the adrenal glands (the medulla) produces **adrenaline** (also called **epinephrine**), which mediates the "fight-or-flight" response of the sympathetic nervous system when the body is under stress. The medulla also produces **norepinephrine**. Epinephrine and norepinephrine are vital in the function of the sympathetic nervous system. The remainder of adrenal tissue is known as the **adrenal cortex** Figure 7-83.

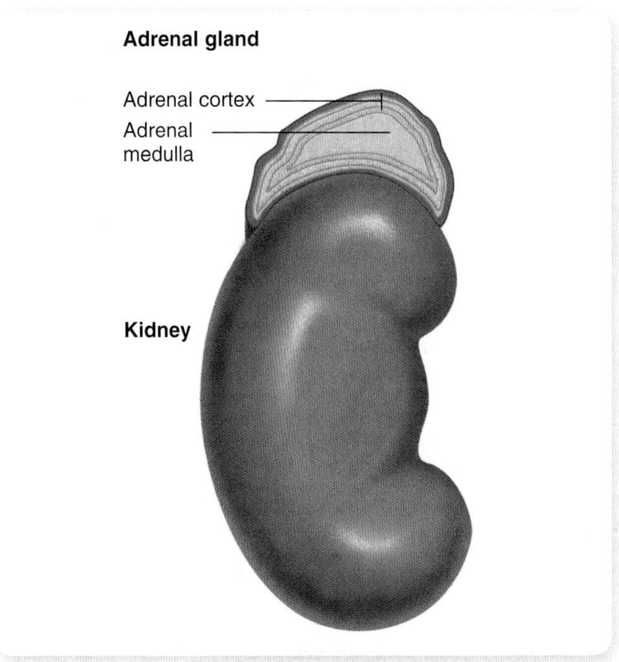

Figure 7-83 The adrenal glands sit on top of the kidney and consist of the adrenal medulla and adrenal cortex.

The adrenal cortex produces hormones called **corticosteroids**, which regulate the body's metabolism, its balance of salt and water, the immune system, and sexual function. The adrenal medulla produces hormones called **catecholamines** (epinephrine and norepinephrine), which assist the body in coping with physical and emotional stress by increasing the heart and respiratory rates and the blood pressure.

▶ The Reproductive Glands and Hormones

Finally, the endocrine system includes reproductive glands. The **gonads** are the reproductive glands and consist of the **ovaries** in women and the **testes** in men. Testosterone is the major androgen manufactured by the testes. Testosterone also is produced in small amounts in the adrenal glands and in the ovaries. Testosterone is responsible for the development of male secondary sex characteristics, such as a deep voice and facial hair.

The three major female hormones are **estrogen**, **progesterone**, and **human chorionic gonadotropin (hCG)**. The developing embryo in the uterus manufactures hCG if conception takes place to keep the lining of the uterus (endometrium) thick and able to sustain the pregnancy. The ovaries produce estrogen and progesterone. Estrogen functions in the menstrual cycle and in the development of secondary sex characteristics, such as breast development in adolescence. Progesterone, which is produced by the corpus luteum of the ovary, prepares the uterus for implantation of a fertilized egg. In men, small amounts of estrogen and progesterone also are produced in the testes and adrenal glands.

Excesses or deficiencies in hormone levels cause various diseases. With endocrine diseases, specific body functions are increased, decreased, or absent. Diabetes mellitus is a common problem. Because production of the hormone insulin is deficient, the body is unable to use glucose normally. Insulin is responsible for rapidly moving glucose into cells. Without insulin, glucose moves slowly. This creates a series of complications as the body struggles to find a more readily available fuel for its cells. People with diabetes begin to burn fats and proteins to create the glucose that cells are craving. Interestingly, this results in higher and higher blood glucose levels as glucose accumulates, unable to be moved efficiently into the cells. Chapter 21, *Endocrine and Hematologic Emergencies,* discusses how high blood glucose levels affect the body.

Finally, the pineal gland is an endocrine gland that lies deep in the brain and produces melatonin, which has a role in maintaining circadian rhythm and regulating reproductive hormones.[6]

The Urinary System: Anatomy and Physiology

The **urinary system** controls the discharge of **certain** waste materials filtered from the blood by the kidneys. In the urinary system, the kidneys are solid organs; the ureters, bladder, and urethra are hollow organs **Figure 7-84**. The main functions of the urinary system are: (1) to control fluid balance in the body, (2) to filter and eliminate wastes, and (3) to control pH balance.

The body has two **kidneys** that lie on the posterior muscular wall of the abdomen behind the peritoneum in the retroperitoneal space. These organs rid the blood of toxic waste products and control its balance of water and salt. Blood flow in the kidneys is high. Nearly 20% of the output of blood from the heart passes through the kidneys each minute. Large vessels attach the kidneys directly to the aorta and the inferior vena cava. Waste products and water are constantly filtered from the blood to form urine. The kidneys continuously concentrate this filtered urine by reabsorbing the water as it passes through a system of specialized tubes within them. The tubes finally unite to form the **renal pelvis**, a cone-shaped collecting area that connects the ureter and the kidney. Normally, each kidney drains its urine into one ureter through which the urine passes to the bladder.

A **ureter** passes from the renal pelvis of each kidney along the surface of the posterior abdominal wall behind the peritoneum to drain into the urinary bladder. The ureters are small (0.2 inch in diameter), hollow, muscular tubes. **Peristalsis**, a wavelike contraction of smooth muscle, occurs in these tubes to move the urine to the bladder.

The **urinary bladder** is located immediately behind the pubic symphysis in the pelvic cavity and is composed of smooth muscle with a specialized lining membrane. The two ureters enter posteriorly at its base on either side. The bladder empties to the outside of the body through the **urethra**. In the male, the urethra passes from the anterior base of the bladder through the penis. In the female, the urethra opens in front of the vagina. A healthy adult forms 1.5 to 2 L of urine every day. This waste is extracted and concentrated from the 1,500 L of blood that circulates through the kidneys daily.

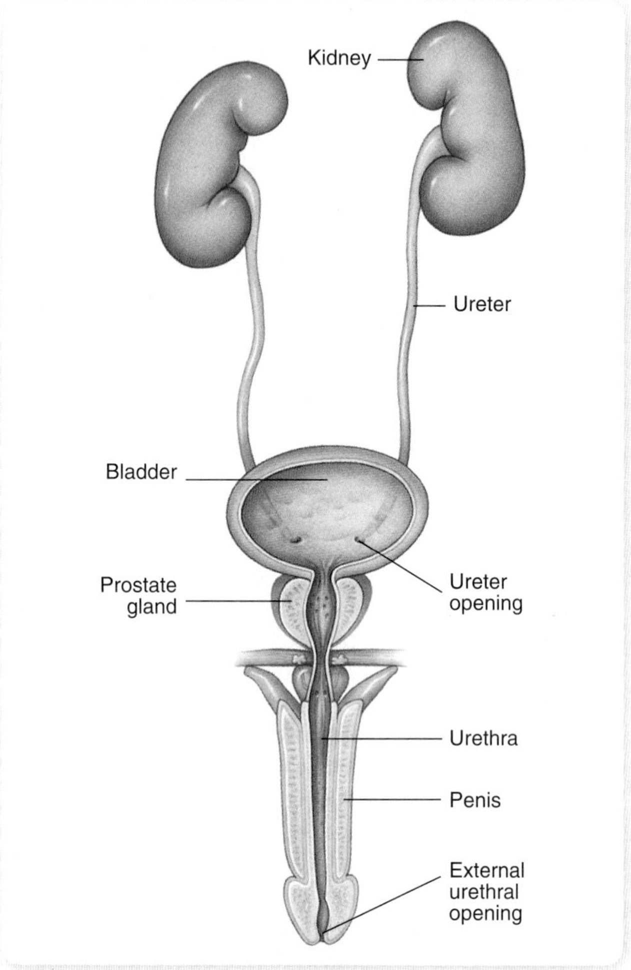

Figure 7-84 The urinary system lies in the retroperitoneal (behind the peritoneum) space behind the organs of the digestive system. The urinary system in males and females includes the kidneys, ureters, bladder, and urethra. This diagram shows the male urinary system.

Words of Wisdom

The kidneys also are important in the regulation of the body's fluid balance and blood pressure. They perform these vital functions in conjunction with complex hormone-driven mechanisms. Fluid balance is controlled by the effects of ADH on the kidney. The blood pressure effects are influenced by the **renin-angiotensin system**, of which the kidneys are an important part.

The Genital System: Anatomy and Physiology

The **genital system** controls the reproductive processes by which life is created. The male genitalia, except for the **prostate gland** and the **seminal vesicles**, lie outside the pelvic cavity. The female genitalia, except for the clitoris and labia, are contained entirely within the pelvis. The male and female reproductive organs have certain similarities and, of course, basic differences. They produce sperm and egg cells and reproductive hormones and play an important role in sexual intercourse and reproduction.

The Male Reproductive System and Organs

The male reproductive system consists of the scrotum, testicles, epididymis, vasa deferentia, ejaculatory ducts, urethra, and penis Figure 7-85. Each testicle contains specialized cells and ducts; some of these produce male hormones, and others develop sperm. The hormones are absorbed directly into the bloodstream from the testicles. The sperm are immature and are moved from the testicles to the epididymis so they can develop. During ejaculation, the sperm are carried through **vasa deferentia** (or vas deferens) to the urethra. Finally, the sperm are deposited by the penis.

The function of the reproductive system is to reproduce. Sperm are able to join with an egg to begin the process of life. In addition to reproduction, this system is also responsible for the production of sex hormones. Many of the physical characteristics of men, such as increased muscle mass, body hair, and deep voice, are attributed to the powerful effects of the hormones released by the testes. Finally, the penis, although part of the reproductive system, is also part of the urinary system. Any damage or infection to the penis can cause problems within the urinary bladder and/or the kidneys.

The Female Reproductive System and Organs

The female reproductive organs include the ovaries, fallopian tubes, uterus, cervix, and vagina Figure 7-86. The ovaries (the female reproductive organs) are usually located one on each side of the lower abdominal quadrants. The ovaries, like the testicles, produce sex hormones and specialized cells for reproduction. These hormones regulate female reproductive function and secondary sexual characteristics such as pubic hair and breast development. The female sex hormones are absorbed directly into the bloodstream.

The ovaries also produce the precursors to mature eggs, the **oocytes**. Within the ovaries, oocytes undergo a maturation process, called **oogenesis**, resulting in production of a specialized **ovum**, a mature egg cell. During the reproductive years of a woman's life, the pituitary gland releases hormones at roughly monthly intervals. These hormones, **follicle-stimulating hormone** and **luteinizing hormone**, stimulate one oocyte to undergo cell division that results in the formation of a mature ovum. A mature ovum is released into one of the fallopian tubes during **ovulation** and is then ready for fertilization by a sperm.

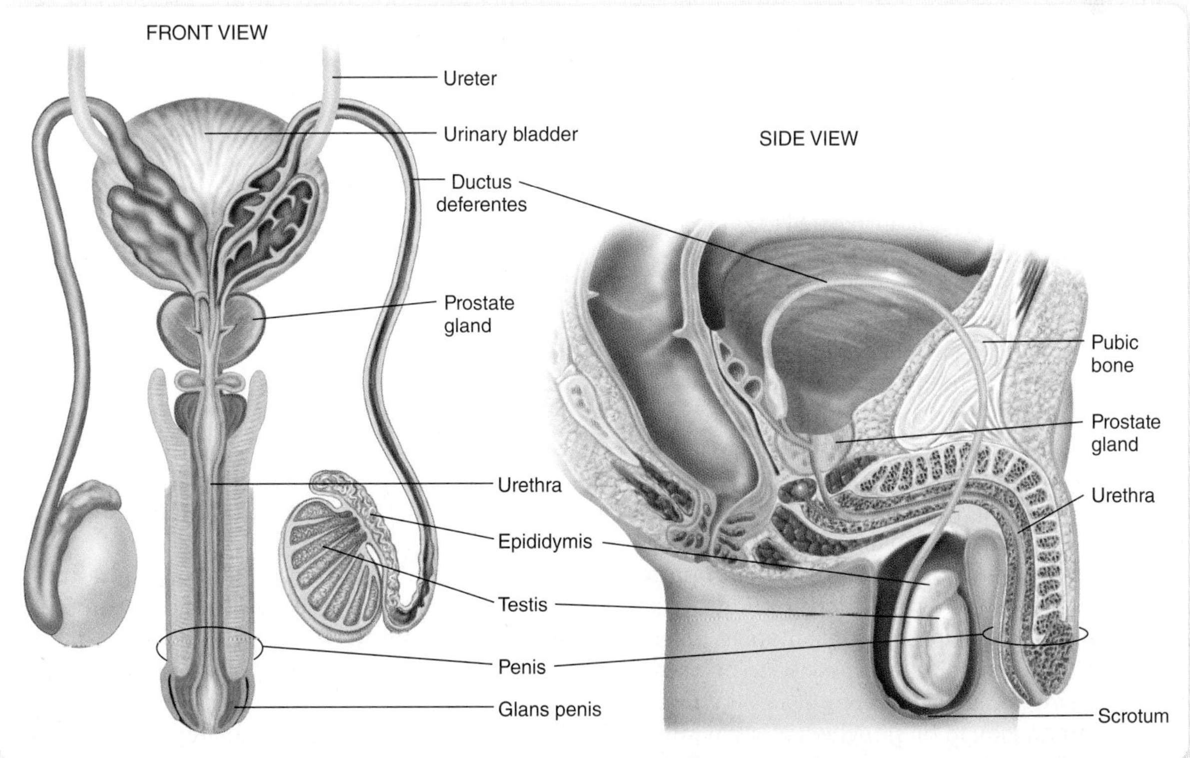

Figure 7-85 The male reproductive system consists of the testicles, epididymis, vasa deferentia, and penis.

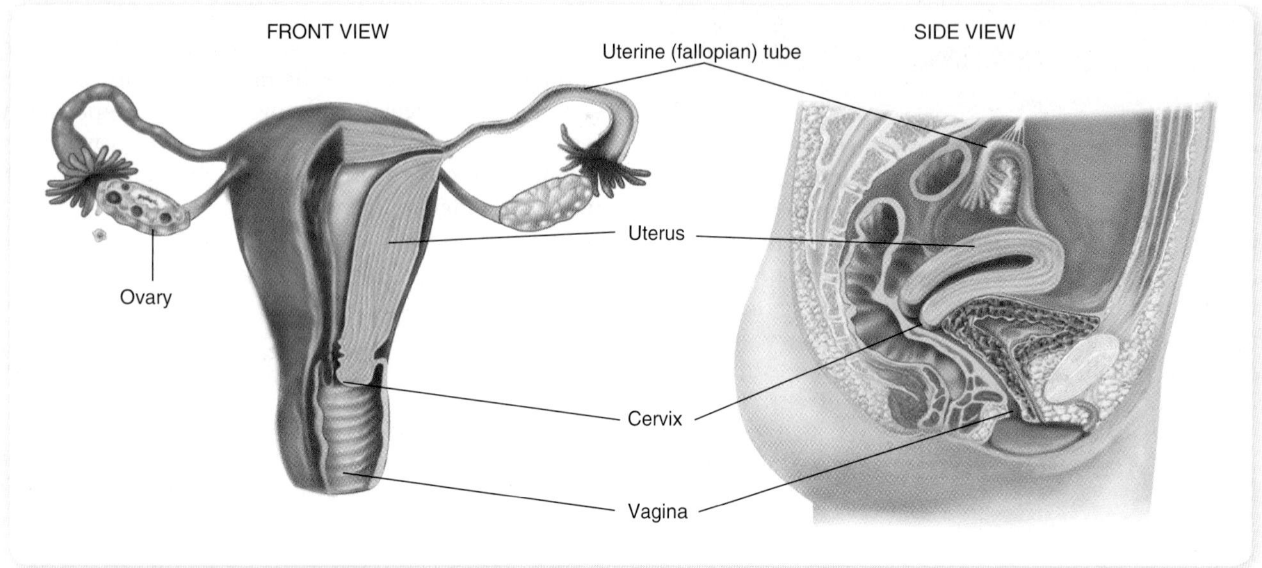

Figure 7-86 The female reproductive system consists of the ovaries, fallopian tubes, uterus, cervix, and vagina.

The fallopian tubes are hollow tubes or ducts that extend from the region of each ovary and carry the ovum into the uterus. Once an ovum is inside the fallopian tube, movement of cilia (hairlike projections) on the cell surfaces results in passage of the ovum toward the uterus. The **uterus** is pear-shaped and hollow, with muscular walls. The innermost layer of the uterus, the **endometrium**, is divided into two layers. The deep basal layer is connected directly to the **myometrium**. The functional layer lines the cavity itself and undergoes menstrual changes and sloughing during the female menstrual cycle. The narrow opening from the uterus to the vagina is the **cervix**. The **vagina** (birth canal) is a muscular distensible tube that connects the uterus with the vulva (the external female genitalia).

The area between the urethral opening and the anus is the **perineum**. It includes skin, the external genitalia, and underlying tissues. Two anatomic triangles make up this area.

The female external genitalia are referred to as the **vulva**. A pair of skin folds, the **labia minora**, borders the vestibule, which is a space into which the vagina and the urethra open. The **clitoris** is located in the anterior margin of the vestibule. It contains erectile tissue which becomes engorged with blood as a result of sexual excitement. The labia minora unite over the clitoris, forming the **prepuce**. Lateral to the labia minora are two prominent, rounded folds of skin, the **labia majora**. These structures unite anteriorly over the pubic symphysis at the **mons pubis**.

During the **menstrual cycle**, an ovum matures, forming a developed ovum. At ovulation, this ovum ruptures through the surface of the ovary. If fertilization occurs, the fertilized egg proceeds through the fallopian tube to implant in the uterus. If fertilization does not occur, a series of hormonal changes causes the remnants of the ovum, called the **corpus luteum**, to be sloughed, along with the uterine lining. The vagina channels the menstrual flow from the uterus out of the body.

The menstrual cycle is a recurring cycle, beginning at **menarche**, which is the time of the first menstrual cycle, and ending at **menopause**. During each cycle, the lining of the uterus thickens in preparation for pregnancy. If pregnancy does not occur, this functional layer is shed during **menstruation**. The average menstrual cycle is 28 days, with day one being the first day of menstrual flow.

The length of menstruation varies somewhat among women. Various hormones, including gonadotropin-releasing hormone (GnRH), FSH, LH, estrogen and progesterone stimulate the uterine lining at different stages during the menstrual cycle. As mentioned earlier, another hormone involved in reproduction is hCG. It stimulates the corpus luteum to produce progresterone.

The vagina receives the penis during sexual intercourse, when **semen** is deposited in it. Mucous membranes on the surface of the vagina secrete a protective fluid and produce lubricating secretions during sexual intercourse. The sperm in the semen may pass into the uterus and fertilize an egg, causing pregnancy. Should the pregnancy come to completion at approximately 40 weeks, the neonate will pass through the vagina and be born.

Breasts contain the organs of milk production (lactation), the **mammary glands**. Mammary glands are actually modified sweat glands. In both male and female breasts, there is an external raised nipple that is surrounded by the pigmented areola. In the female breast, the **areolar glands** produce secretions that protect the nipple and areola during nursing.

The female mammary glands contain 15 to 20 glandular lobes covered by a variable amount of fatty tissue. This superficial fat gives the breast its form. The lobes produce milk, which is stored in and expressed from the nipple.

The functions of the female reproductive system are similar to those of the male reproductive system: reproduction and hormone balance. Urination occurs through the urethra, which in females is not interconnected to the reproductive tract. In males, the urethra is interconnected.

Life Support Chain

The body's cells, tissues, and organs, regardless of their function, all require oxygen, nutrients, and the removal of wastes to perform their job. Oxygen is brought to the cells through the respiratory and circulatory systems. Nutrients are made available to the body after we eat. The digestive system takes the food we eat and breaks it down into glucose, among other things. Glucose is the primary fuel of the body. The circulatory system is the carrier of these supplies and wastes through the process of perfusion. If interference occurs in this delivery system, cells will become damaged or die.

Oxygen is critical for cells; as mentioned earlier, some cells are unable to survive without a constant supply. Most cells in the body are able to continue to function, even without oxygen, in an anaerobic state for a limited period of time. When illness or injury occurs, the body needs to shift available resources to areas in need while ensuring that critical areas, such as the brain and heart, have an uninterrupted supply of resources. Anaerobic metabolism occurs anytime you exercise vigorously and begin to feel a burning sensation. In this state, very limited amounts of energy are able to be released so the body must quickly correct the oxygen deficiency or risk cellular death. An important by-product of anaerobic metabolism is lactic acid, which is the material that causes muscle burning during anaerobic exercise. Lactic acid is converted back to a useful energy source after oxygen is available. Anaerobic metabolism can be supported in most cells for only 1 to 3 minutes.

Words of Wisdom

When cells function with oxygen, they use aerobic metabolism. They generate large amounts of ATP (cellular energy) and produce wastes of carbon dioxide and water.

When cells function without oxygen, they use anaerobic metabolism. They generate small amounts of ATP (cellular energy) and produce waste of lactic acid.

YOU are the Provider SUMMARY

1. **How can knowledge of anatomy and physiology help you care for patients?**

   Familiarity with the structures and function of the body's systems will allow you to better assess a patient as well as predict potential complications resulting from occult injuries (those not visible to the eye).

2. **How can knowledge of medical terminology help you care for patients?**

   AEMTs must be familiar with the language of topographic anatomy. By using proper medical terms, you will be able to communicate correct information with the least possible confusion to other members of the health care team.

3. **What are the components of the respiratory system?**

   The respiratory system consists of all the structures of the body that contribute to respiration, or the process of breathing. It includes the nose, mouth, throat, larynx, trachea, bronchi, and bronchioles, which are all air passages or airways. The system also includes the lungs, where oxygen is passed into the blood and carbon dioxide is removed. Finally, the respiratory system includes the diaphragm, the muscles of the chest wall, and accessory muscles of breathing, which permit normal respiratory movement.

4. **On the basis of your knowledge of anatomy, what possible organs may be damaged as a result of the gunshot wound to the abdomen?**

   In the LUQ, the principal organs are the stomach, the spleen, and a portion of the colon and small intestine. The spleen is almost entirely under the protection of the left rib cage, whereas the stomach may sag well down into the LLQ when full. The spleen lies in the lateral and posterior portion of this quadrant, under the diaphragm and immediately in front of the 9th to 11th ribs. Knowing the anatomic locations of organs and structure will allow you to "picture" possible internal injuries.

5. **What are the possible results of respiratory compromise in this patient?**

   Some possible results of respiratory compromise in this patient include the inability to exhale effectively, resulting in an increase of carbon dioxide in the blood, and the inability to inhale effectively, which causes oxygen levels in the blood to fall. In both situations, the diffusion of respiratory gases will be affected.

6. **What type of shock is this patient most likely experiencing?**

   This patient is most likely experiencing hypovolemic shock, which is a result of loss of circulating volume. Shock is a condition in which organs and tissues are not receiving an adequate flow of blood and oxygen, or perfusion. A patient in shock has difficulty transporting oxygen in the blood, which allows the buildup of wastes. There are several ways a disease can have an effect on tissue perfusion. Essentially, the patient can have insufficient blood volume or a heart that does not pump effectively, or the patient's body can no longer control the blood vessels.

YOU are the Provider SUMMARY (continued)

7. What could be causing the difference in left and right radial pulses in this patient?

The differences in left and right radial pulses are most likely explained by his gunshot wound to the arm. If the projectile severed a major artery, the patient may have diminished circulation to that arm, creating the difference in pulses.

8. Body fluid is divided into two main compartments. What are they and where are they found?

Body fluid is divided into two main compartments: intracellular and extracellular fluid. ICF is found within individual cells and makes up approximately 75% of all body fluid. ECF is the fluid found outside of cell membranes and makes up approximately 25% of all body fluid. ECF is further divided into intravascular fluid and interstitial fluid. Intravascular fluid (plasma), the fluid portion of blood, is noncellular and is found within the blood vessels. Interstitial fluid is the fluid located outside of the blood vessels, in the spaces between the body's cells. There is a delicate balance among the various fluid compartments of the body that is essential in maintenance of homeostasis.

EMS Patient Care Report (PCR)

Date: 10-8-18	**Incident No.:** 54474	**Nature of Call:** Gunshot wound	**Location:** 523 3rd St SW

Dispatched: 0235	**En Route:** 0237	**At Scene:** 0242	**Transport:** 0251	**At Hospital:** 0317	**In Service:** 0350

Patient Information

Age: 18 **Sex:** M **Weight (in kg [lb]):** 79.6 kg (175 lb)	**Allergies:** No known drug allergies **Medications:** None **Past Medical History:** None **Chief Complaint:** Multiple gunshot wounds

Vital Signs

Time: 0243	**BP:** Not obtained	**Pulse:** Not obtained	**Respirations:** 12	**Spo_2:** Not obtained
Time: 0247	**BP:** 86/54	**Pulse:** 126	**Respirations:** 12	**Spo_2:** 95%
Time: 0257	**BP:** 98/58	**Pulse:** 126	**Respirations:** 14	**Spo_2:** 97%

EMS Treatment (circle all that apply)

Oxygen @ 15 **L/min via (circle one):** **NC** **(NRM)** **Bag-mask device**		**Assisted Ventilation**	**Airway Adjunct**	**CPR**
Defibrillation	**(Bleeding Control:** Yes)	**(Bandaging:** Yes)	**Splinting**	**Other:**

Narrative

EMS dispatched to above location for reported shooting. En route, dispatch advised law enforcement on scene with one patient, multiple gunshot wounds. Patient present AO×4, ABCs intact, lying left lateral on ground, covered in blood. States he heard 5–6 shots, but unsure of how many times he was hit. Manual stabilization provided. Rapid exam reveals GSW to left chest, left upper arm, and left upper abdominal quadrant. Chief complaint difficulty breathing. Bleeding controlled via direct pressure and dressings. Chest wound covered with occlusive dressing. 15 L/min via nonrebreathing mask applied. Secured patient to stretcher, loaded into ambulance. 18-gauge IV line established to right arm, with NS TKO due to patient's blood pressure. Clothing removed, no other injuries found. On arrival at Charity hospital, care and report given to ED staff without incident.**End of report**

Prep Kit

▶ Ready for Review

- To properly care for your patients, you must have a thorough understanding of human anatomy and physiology so you can assess the patient's condition and communicate with hospital personnel and other health care providers.
- Cells are the basic functional unit of the body. The cells of the body are extremely varied in their shape and function. Cells with a common job are grouped closely together and are called tissues. Groups of tissues that all perform interrelated jobs form organs. A series of organs working together make up the body systems.
- Cells have a cell membrane, a nucleus, and cytoplasm. Specialized structures within the cell, called organelles, perform specific functions.
- The life cycle of a cell includes interphase, cell division, cytoplasmic division, and differentiation.
- Cellular respiration is the process by which cells use glucose and oxygen to release energy. This process requires three reactions: glycolysis, the Krebs cycle, and the electron transport chain.
- Cell transport mechanisms relate to fluid administration, an AEMT skill. The cell membrane allows some substances to pass through it, but not others. Selective permeability allows normal differences in concentrations between intracellular and extracellular environments to be maintained.
- Several mechanisms, such as diffusion, osmosis, facilitated diffusion, active transport, endocytosis, and exocytosis, allow material to pass through the cell wall.
- Fluid balance in the body must be maintained (homeostasis). Fluid balance is the process of maintaining homeostasis through equal intake and output of fluids. The major mechanisms for maintaining homeostasis include antidiuretic hormone, thirst, kidneys, and water shifts.
- You must be able to identify superficial landmarks of the body and know what lies underneath the skin so that you can perform an accurate patient assessment.
- The skeleton gives the body its recognizable human form through a collection of bones, ligaments, tendons, and cartilage.
- The skeletal system provides protection for fragile organs, allows for movement, and gives the body its shape.
- The contraction and relaxation of the musculoskeletal system gives the body its ability to move.
- Smooth muscle, also called involuntary muscle, is found within blood vessels and intestines and controls involuntary functions. Skeletal muscle, so named because it attaches to the bones of the skeleton, forms the major muscle mass of the body. It is also called voluntary muscle, because all skeletal muscle is under direct voluntary control.
- Cardiac muscle is different from skeletal and smooth muscle because it has the property of "automaticity"; it can generate and conduct electricity, and therefore muscular contraction, without influence from the brain.
- The respiratory system consists of all the structures of the body that contribute to the process of breathing. It includes the nose, mouth, throat, larynx, trachea, bronchi, and bronchioles.
- The primary function of the respiratory system is to conduct respiration. Oxygen is essential for the body to function. Gas exchange of oxygen into the blood and carbon dioxide out of the blood occurs at the lungs' alveoli via diffusion.
- Ventilation is the process of moving air in and out of the lungs.
- The respiratory center in the brainstem controls breathing. Nerves in this area sense the level of carbon dioxide in the blood and spinal fluid. The brain adjusts breathing as needed if the level of carbon dioxide or oxygen in the arterial blood is too high or too low.
- Increases in the level of carbon dioxide in the blood ($Paco_2$) cause decreased pH levels in the respiratory center, which triggers an increase in ventilation. Decreases in the $Paco_2$ result in increased pH levels in the respiratory center and a decrease in ventilation.
- Hypoxic drive is a backup system the body uses to control respiration. Areas in the brain, walls of the aorta, and carotid arteries act as oxygen sensors and stimulate breathing if the oxygen level falls.
- The concentration of hydrogen ions (H^+) determines the level of acidity in the blood. Normal homeostatic functions keep the concentration of H^+ within a fairly narrow range. pH is the most common expression of acidity. pH ranges from 0 (most acidic) to 14 (most basic), with 7.0 being neutral. When pH is higher than this, the blood is too basic, or alkalotic. When pH is lower, the blood is too acidic, or acidotic.
- The circulatory system is a complex arrangement of connected tubes, including the arteries, arterioles, capillaries, venules, and veins. The cardiac cycle begins with myocardial contraction and concludes at the beginning of the next contraction. The heart's contraction results in pressure changes within the cardiac chambers, resulting in the movement of blood from areas of high pressure to areas of low pressure.
- Blood pressure is noted as a fraction, with the systolic reading placed above the diastolic reading (for example, 140/70 mm Hg).

Prep Kit *(continued)*

- The pressure in the aorta against which the left ventricle must pump blood is called the afterload. The greater the afterload, the harder it is for the ventricle to eject blood into the aorta. This reduces the stroke volume—the amount of blood ejected per contraction.
- Cardiac output is the amount of blood pumped through the circulatory system in 1 minute. Cardiac output is expressed in liters per minute (L/min). The cardiac output equals the heart rate multiplied by the stroke volume.
- Increased venous return to the heart stretches the ventricles, resulting in increased cardiac contractility. This relationship is known as the Starling law.
- The nervous system is perhaps the most complex organ system within the human body. It consists of the brain, spinal cord, and nerves.
- The skin is divided into two parts: the superficial epidermis, which is composed of several layers of cells, and the deeper dermis, which contains the specialized skin structures.
- The skin, the largest single organ in the body, serves three major functions: to protect the body in the environment, to regulate the temperature of the body, and to transmit information from the environment to the brain.
- The digestive system is composed of the gastrointestinal tract (stomach and intestines), mouth, salivary glands, pharynx, esophagus, liver, gallbladder, pancreas, rectum, and anus.
- Digestion of food, from the time it is taken into the mouth until essential compounds are extracted and delivered by the circulatory system to nourish all cells in the body, is a complicated chemical process.
- The endocrine system is a complex message and control system that integrates many body functions.
- The urinary system controls the discharge of certain waste materials filtered from the blood by the kidneys.
- The genital system controls the reproductive processes by which life is created.

▶ Vital Vocabulary

abdomen The body cavity that contains the major organs of digestion and excretion. It is located below the diaphragm and above the pelvis.

acetabulum The depression on the lateral pelvis where its three component bones join, in which the femoral head fits snugly.

acid A substance that increases the concentration of hydrogen ions in a solution.

acidosis A pathologic condition that results from the accumulation of acids in the body.

acromioclavicular (AC) separation One or more torn ligaments in the acromioclavicular joint, resulting in a separated shoulder.

acromion process The tip of the shoulder and the site of attachment for the clavicle and various shoulder muscles.

active transport A method used to move compounds across a cell membrane to create or maintain an imbalance of charges.

adenosine triphosphate (ATP) The nucleotide involved in energy metabolism; used to store energy.

adrenal cortex The outer layer of the adrenal gland; it produces hormones that are important in regulating the water and salt balance of the body.

adrenal glands Endocrine glands located on top of the kidneys that release adrenaline when stimulated by the sympathetic nervous system.

adrenaline Hormone produced by the adrenal glands that mediates the "fight-or-flight" response of the sympathetic nervous system; also called epinephrine.

adrenocorticotropic hormone (ACTH) Hormone that targets the adrenal cortex to secrete cortisol (a glucocorticoid).

aerobic Referring to a process that can occur only in the presence of oxygen.

afterload The pressure in the aorta against which the left ventricle must pump blood.

agonist A substance that mimics the actions of a specific neurotransmitter or hormone by binding to the specific receptor of the naturally occurring substance.

agranulocytes Leukocytes that lack granules.

alkalosis The buildup of excess base (lack of acids) in the body.

alpha cells Cells located in the islets of Langerhans that secrete glucagon.

alpha effects Stimulation of alpha receptors that results in vasoconstriction.

alveolar ducts Ducts formed from division of the respiratory bronchioles in the lower airway; each duct ends in clusters known as alveoli.

alveoli The air sacs of the lungs in which the exchange of oxygen and carbon dioxide takes place.

alveolocapillary membrane The very thin membrane, consisting of only one cell layer, that lies between the alveolus and capillary, through which respiratory exchange between the alveolus and the blood vessels occurs.

anaerobic Referring to a process that can occur in the absence of oxygen; the principal product is lactic acid.

Prep Kit (continued)

anatomy The study of the structure of an organism and its parts.

antagonist A molecule that blocks the ability of a given chemical to bind to its receptor, preventing a biologic response.

antibodies Proteins within plasma that react with antigens.

antigens Substances on the surface of erythrocytes that are recognized by the immune system.

aorta The principal artery leaving the left side of the heart and carrying freshly oxygenated blood to the body.

aortic arch One of the three described portions of the aorta; the section of the aorta between the ascending and descending portions that gives rise to the right brachiocephalic (innominate), left common carotid, and left subclavian arteries.

aortic valve The semilunar valve that regulates blood flow from the left ventricle to the aorta.

appendicular skeleton The portion of the skeletal system that comprises the arms, legs, pelvis, and shoulder girdle.

appendix A small tubular structure that is attached to the lower border of the cecum in the lower right quadrant of the abdomen.

arachnoid The middle membrane of the three meninges that enclose the brain and spinal cord.

areolar glands The glands that produce secretions that protect the nipple and areola during nursing.

arteries The blood vessels that carry blood away from the heart.

arterioles The smallest branches of arteries leading to the vast network of capillaries.

ascending aorta The first of three portions of the aorta; originates from the left ventricle and gives rise to two branches, the right and left main coronary arteries.

atlanto-occipital joint The location where the atlas articulates with the occipital condyles.

atlas The first cervical vertebra (C1), which provides support for the head.

atrioventricular (AV) node The site located in the right atrium adjacent to the septum that is responsible for transiently slowing electrical conduction.

atrioventricular valves The two valves through which blood flows from the atria to the ventricles.

atrium One of the two upper chambers of the heart.

atrophy A decrease in cell size as a result of a loss of subcellular components.

auditory ossicles The bones that function in hearing and are located deep within cavities of the temporal bone.

autonomic nervous system The part of the nervous system that regulates functions, such as digestion and sweating, that are not controlled voluntarily.

axial skeleton The part of the skeleton comprising the skull, spinal column, and rib cage.

axillary vein The vein that is formed from the combination of the basilic and cephalic veins; it drains into the subclavian vein.

axis The second cervical vertebra (C2); the point that allows the head to turn.

ball-and-socket joint A joint that allows internal and external rotation, as well as bending.

baroreceptors Receptors in the blood vessels, kidneys, brain, and heart that respond to changes in pressure in the heart or main arteries to help maintain homeostasis.

base A substance that decreases the concentration of hydrogen ions.

basilic vein One of the two major veins of the arm; it combines with the cephalic vein to form the axillary vein.

basophils White blood cells that work to produce chemical mediators during an immune response.

beta cells Cells located in the islets of Langerhans that secrete insulin.

beta effects Stimulation of beta receptors that results in inotropic, dromotropic, and chronotropic states.

biceps The large muscle that covers the front of the humerus.

bile ducts The ducts that convey bile between the liver and the intestine.

bilirubin A waste product of red blood cell destruction that undergoes further metabolism in the liver.

blood The fluid that is pumped by the heart through the arteries, veins, and capillaries and consists of plasma and formed elements or cells, such as red blood cells, white blood cells, and platelets.

blood pressure The pressure that the blood exerts against the walls of the arteries as it passes through them.

bone marrow A substance that manufactures most red blood cells.

brachial artery The major vessel in the upper extremity that supplies blood to the arm.

brain The controlling organ of the body and center of consciousness; functions include perception, control of reactions to the environment, emotional responses, and judgment.

brainstem The area of the brain between the spinal cord and cerebrum, surrounded by the cerebellum; controls functions that are necessary for life, such as respiration.

Prep Kit *(continued)*

bronchioles Fine subdivisions of the bronchi that give rise to the alveolar ducts.

bronchospasm Constriction of the airway passages of the lungs that accompanies muscle spasms.

bruit An abnormal "whooshinglike" sound indicating turbulent blood flow within a blood vessel.

buffer Any substance that can reversibly bind H^+.

buffer system Fast-acting defenses for acid-base changes, providing almost immediate protection against changes in the hydrogen ion concentration of extracellular fluid.

bundle of His Part of the conduction system of the heart; a continuation of the atrioventricular node.

bursa A small fluid-filled sac located between a tendon and a bone that cushions and protects the joint.

calcitonin A hormone produced by the parafollicular cells of the thyroid gland that is important in the regulation of calcium levels in the body.

cancellous bone A type of bone that consists of a lacy network of bony rods called trabeculae.

capillaries The tiny blood vessels between the arterioles and venules that permit transfer of oxygen, carbon dioxide, nutrients, and waste between body tissues and the blood.

cardiac cycle The repetitive pumping process that begins with the onset of cardiac muscle contraction and ends just prior to the beginning of the next contraction.

cardiac muscle The heart muscle.

cardiac output The amount of blood pumped through the circulatory system in 1 minute.

carotid artery The major artery that supplies blood to the head and brain.

carpometacarpal joint The joint between the wrist and the metacarpal bones; the thumb joint.

cartilage The support structure of the skeletal system that provides cushioning between bones; also forms the nasal septum and portions of the outer ear.

catecholamines Hormones produced by the adrenal medulla (epinephrine and norepinephrine) that assist the body in coping with physical and emotional stress by increasing the heart and respiratory rates and the blood pressure.

cecum The first part of the large intestine, into which the ileum opens.

cell membrane The cell wall; the cell membrane is selectively permeable.

cellular respiration A biochemical process resulting in the production of energy in the form of ATP.

central nervous system (CNS) The brain and spinal cord.

central vision The visualization of objects directly in front of you.

cerebellum One of the three major subdivisions of the brain, sometimes called the little brain; coordinates the various activities of the brain, particularly fine body movements.

cerebrospinal fluid (CSF) Fluid produced in the ventricles of the brain that flows in the subarachnoid space and bathes the meninges.

cerebrum The largest part of the three subdivisions of the brain, sometimes called the gray matter; made up of several lobes that control movement, hearing, balance, speech, visual perception, emotions, and personality.

cervical spine The portion of the spinal column consisting of the first seven vertebrae that lie in the neck.

cervix The lower one third, or neck, of the uterus.

chemoreceptors Receptors in the blood vessels, kidneys, brain, and heart that respond to changes in chemical composition of the blood to help maintain homeostasis.

chordae tendineae Thin bands of fibrous tissue that attach to the valves in the heart and prevent them from inverting.

choroid plexus Specialized cells within hollow areas in the ventricles of the brain that produce cerebrospinal fluid.

chromosomes Structures formed from condensed fibers and protein of deoxyribonucleic acid; they are threadlike and are contained within the nucleus of the cells.

chronic obstructive pulmonary disease (COPD) A progressive and irreversible disease of the airway marked by decreased inspiratory and expiratory capacity of the lungs.

chronotropic state Related to the control of the heart's rate of contraction.

chyme The name of the substance that leaves the stomach; a combination of eaten foods with added stomach acids.

circulatory system The complex arrangement of connected tubes, including the arteries, arterioles, capillaries, venules, and veins, that moves blood, oxygen, nutrients, carbon dioxide, and cellular waste throughout the body.

circumflex coronary arteries The two branches of the left main coronary artery.

clavicle The collarbone; it is lateral to the sternum and anterior to the scapula.

clitoris Located in the anterior margin of the vestibule, it contains erectile tissue that becomes engorged with blood as a result of sexual excitement.

Prep Kit (continued)

coccyx The last three to five vertebrae of the spine; the tailbone.

concentration gradient The difference in concentrations of a substance on either side of a selectively permeable membrane.

conduction system A group of complex electrical tissues within the heart that initiate and transmit stimuli that result in contractions of myocardial tissue.

conjunctiva The membranous covering on the anterior surface of the eye that also lines the eyelids.

contractility The strength of heart muscle contraction.

cornea The transparent tissue layer in front of the pupil and iris of the eye.

coronary arteries Arteries that arise from the aorta shortly after it leaves the left ventricle and supply the heart with oxygen and nutrients.

coronary sinus Veins that collect blood that is returning from the walls of the heart.

corpus luteum The remnants of an unfertilized ovum that are sloughed during menstruation.

corticosteroids Any of several steroids secreted by the adrenal gland.

cortisol The most important corticosteroid secreted by the zona fasciculata.

cranial nerves The 12 pairs of nerves that arise from the base of the brain.

cranial vault The bones that encase and protect the brain, including the parietal, temporal, frontal, occipital, sphenoid, and ethmoid bones.

cranium The area of the head above the ears and eyes; the skull. The cranium contains the brain.

crenation Shrinkage of a cell that results when too much water leaves the cell through osmosis.

cribriform plate A horizontal bone perforated with numerous foramina for the passage of the olfactory nerve filaments from the nasal cavity.

cricoid cartilage A firm ridge of cartilage that forms the lower part of the larynx.

cricothyroid membrane A thin sheet of fascia that connects the thyroid and cricoid cartilages that make up the larynx.

crista galli A prominent bony ridge in the center of the anterior fossa to which the meninges are attached.

dead space Any portion of the airway that does contain air and cannot participate in gas exchange, such as the trachea and bronchi.

deep fascia A dense layer of fibrous tissue below the subcutaneous tissue; composed of tough bands of tissue that surround muscles and other internal structures.

dermatome An area of the skin supplied by a specific sensory spinal nerve.

dermis The inner layer of the skin, containing hair follicles, sweat glands, nerve endings, and blood vessels.

descending aorta One of the three portions of the aorta, it is the longest portion and extends through the thorax and abdomen into the pelvis.

diapedesis A process whereby leukocytes leave blood vessels to move toward tissue where they are needed most.

diaphragm A muscular dome that forms the undersurface of the thorax, separating the chest from the abdominal cavity. Contraction of the diaphragm (and the chest wall muscles) brings air into the lungs. Relaxation allows air to be expelled from the lungs.

diastole The relaxation, or period of relaxation, of the heart, especially of the ventricles.

diencephalon Portion of the brain between the brainstem and cerebrum; contains the epithalamus, the thalamus, the hypothalamus, and the subthalamus.

diffusion Movement of a gas from an area of higher concentration to an area of lower concentration.

digestion The processing of food that nourishes the individual cells of the body.

dorsal respiratory group (DRG) A portion of the medulla oblongata where the primary respiratory pacemaker is found.

dorsalis pedis artery The artery on the anterior surface of the foot between the first and second metatarsals.

dromotropic state Related to the control of the heart's conduction rate.

dura mater The outermost of the three meninges that enclose the brain and spinal cord; it is the toughest membrane.

ejection fraction The portion of the blood ejected from the ventricle during systole.

electrolytes Salt or acid substances that become ionic conductors when dissolved in a solvent (ie, water); chemicals dissolved in the blood.

endocardium The thin membrane lining the inside of the heart.

endocrine glands Glands that secrete or release chemicals that are used inside the body.

endocrine system The complex message and control system that integrates many body functions, including the release of hormones.

endometrium The innermost layer of the uterine wall.

endosteum A layer that lines the inner surfaces of bone.

enzymes Substances designed to speed up the rate of specific biochemical reactions.

eosinophils Leukocytes that may play a role following infection in various areas in the body.

Prep Kit *(continued)*

epicardium The layer of the serous pericardium that lies closely against the heart. Also called the visceral pericardium.

epidermis The outer layer of skin, which is made up of cells that are sealed together to form a watertight protective covering for the body.

epiglottis A thin, leaf-shaped valve that allows air to pass into the trachea but prevents food and liquid from entering.

epinephrine A hormone produced by the adrenal medulla that has a vital role in the function of the sympathetic nervous system.

epiphyses The growth plates of a long bone; also called the epiphyseal plates.

erythropoiesis The process by which red blood cells are made.

esophagus A collapsible tube that extends from the pharynx to the stomach; contractions of the muscle in the wall of the esophagus propel food and liquids through it to the stomach.

estrogen A hormone released from the ovaries that stimulates the uterine lining during the menstrual cycle.

exocrine glands Glands that excrete chemicals for elimination.

expiratory reserve volume The amount of air that can be exhaled following a normal exhalation.

extracellular fluid (ECF) Fluid outside of the cell, in which most of the body's supply of sodium is contained.

facilitated diffusion Process whereby a carrier molecule moves substances in or out of cells from areas of higher to lower concentration.

fascia A sheet or band of tough, fibrous connective tissue that covers, supports, and separates muscles.

femoral arteries The principal arteries of the thigh; continuation of the external iliac arteries. These supply blood to the lower abdominal wall, external genitalia, and legs; can be palpated in the groin area.

femoral head The proximal end of the femur, articulating with the acetabulum to form the hip joint.

femoral vein A continuation of the saphenous vein that drains into the external iliac vein.

femur The thighbone; the longest and one of the strongest bones in the body.

fibrin A white insoluble protein formed in the clotting process.

fibula The long bone on the posterior surface of the lower leg.

filtration The movement of fluid from intravascular fluid under high pressure to interstitial fluid, which is generally under lower pressure, through a semipermeable membrane.

fluid balance The process of maintaining homeostasis through equal intake and output of fluids.

follicle-stimulating hormone A hormone released from the pituitary gland at roughly monthly intervals that helps to stimulate one oocyte to undergo cell division.

fontanelles The soft spots in the skull of a newborn and infant where the sutures of the skull have not yet grown together.

foramen magnum A large opening at the base of the skull through which the brain connects to the spinal cord.

foramen ovale An opening between the two atria that is present in the fetus but closes shortly after birth.

foramina Small openings, perforations, or orifices in the bones of the cranial vault.

fossa ovalis A depression between the right and left atria that indicates where the foramen ovale had been located in the fetus.

gallbladder A sac on the undersurface of the liver that collects bile from the liver and discharges it into the duodenum through the common bile duct.

genital system The reproductive system in males and females.

germinal layer The deepest layer of the epidermis where new skin cells are formed.

glands Cells or organs that selectively remove, concentrate, or alter materials in the blood and then secrete them back into the body.

glenoid fossa The part of the scapula that forms the socket in the ball-and-socket joint of the shoulder.

gluconeogenesis A process that stimulates both the liver and the kidneys to produce glucose from noncarbohydrate molecules.

glycogen A long polymer from which glucose is converted in the liver (animal starch).

glycogenolysis The breakdown of glycogen to glucose.

gonads The reproductive glands.

granulocytes Leukocytes that have large cytoplasmic granules that are easily seen with a simple light microscope.

greater trochanter A bony prominence on the proximal lateral side of the thigh, just below the hip joint.

heart A hollow muscular organ that pumps blood throughout the body.

Prep Kit *(continued)*

hemoglobin An iron-containing pigment found in red blood cells; carries 97% of oxygen.

hemostasis Control of bleeding by formation of a blood clot.

heparin A substance found in large amounts in basophils that inhibits blood clotting.

hepatic portal system A specialized part of the venous system that drains blood from the stomach, intestines, and spleen.

hepatic veins The veins into which blood empties after liver cells in the sinusoids of the liver extract nutrients, filter the blood, and metabolize various drugs.

Hering-Breuer reflex A protective mechanism that terminates inhalation, thus preventing overexpansion of the lungs.

hilum The point of entry for the bronchi, vessels, and nerves into each lung.

hinge joints Joints that can bend and straighten but cannot rotate; they restrict motion to one plane.

histamine A substance found in large amounts in basophils that increases tissue inflammation.

hormones Substances formed in specialized organs or glands and carried to another organ or group of cells in the same organism. Hormones regulate many body functions, including metabolism, growth, and body temperature.

human chorionic gonadotropin (hCG) A hormone that stimulates the corpus luteum to produce progesterone during the first eight weeks of gestation.

humerus The supporting bone of the upper arm.

hydrostatic pressure The pressure of water against the walls of its container.

hyoid bone A bone at the base of the tongue that supports the tongue and its muscles.

hyperextension When a body part is extended to the maximum level or beyond the normal range of motion.

hypertonic Concentration of solute is higher compared with another solution.

hypertrophy An increase in the size of the cells as a result of synthesis of more subcellular components, resulting in an increase in tissue and organ size.

hypothalamus The basal part of the diencephalons; it regulates the function of the pituitary gland.

hypotonic A lower concentration of sodium in a solution than exists in the cell; the increased intracellular osmotic pressure lets water flow into the cell, causing it to swell and possibly burst.

hypoxic drive A "backup system" to control respiration; senses drops in the oxygen level in the blood.

ilium One of three bones that fuse to form the pelvic ring.

inferior vena cava One of the two largest veins in the body; carries blood from the lower extremities and the pelvic and the abdominal organs to the heart.

inotropic state Related to the strength of the heart's contraction.

inspiratory reserve volume The amount of air that can be inhaled after a normal inhalation; the amount of air that can be inhaled in addition to the normal tidal volume.

integumentary system The largest organ system in the body, consisting of the skin and accessory structures (eg, hair, nails, glands).

interatrial septum A membrane that separates the right and left atria.

interstitial fluid The fluid located outside of the blood vessels in the spaces between the body's cells.

interstitial space The space in between the cells.

interventricular septum A thick wall that separates the right and left ventricles.

intracellular fluid (ICF) Fluid within cells in which most of the body's supply of potassium is contained.

intravascular fluid (plasma) The noncellular portion of blood found within the blood vessels; also called plasma.

involuntary muscle A muscle over which a person has no conscious control. It is found in many automatic regulating systems of the body.

iris The muscle and surrounding tissue behind the cornea that dilate and constrict the pupil, regulating the amount of light that enters the eye; pigment in this tissue gives the eye its color.

ischium One of three bones that fuse to form the pelvic ring.

isotonic The same concentration of sodium in a solution as in the cell. In this case, water does not shift, and no change in cell shape occurs.

joint (articulation) The place where two bones come into contact.

joint capsule The fibrous sac that encloses a joint.

jugular veins The two main veins that drain the head and neck.

kidneys Two retroperitoneal organs that excrete the end products of metabolism as urine and regulate the body's salt and water content.

labia majora Two prominent, rounded folds of skin lateral to the labia minora of the female external genitalia.

labia minora A pair of skin folds in the female external genitalia that border the vestibule.

Prep Kit (continued)

labored breathing The use of muscles of the chest, back, and abdomen to assist in expanding the chest; occurs when air movement is impaired.

lacrimal glands The glands that produce fluids to keep the eye moist; also called tear glands.

lactic acid A metabolic end product of the breakdown of glucose that accumulates when metabolism proceeds in the absence of oxygen.

large intestine The portion of the digestive tube that encircles the abdomen around the small bowel, consisting of the cecum, the colon, and the rectum. It helps regulate water balance and eliminate solid waste.

lateral malleolus An enlargement of the distal end of the fibula, which forms the lateral wall of the ankle joint.

left anterior descending (LAD) artery One of the two branches of the left main coronary artery that is the largest and shortest of the myocardial blood vessels; this vessel and the circumflex coronary arteries supply blood to the left ventricle and other areas.

lens The transparent part of the eye through which images are focused on the retina.

ligament A band of fibrous tissue that connects bones to bones; supports and strengthens a joint.

limbic system Structures within the cerebrum and diencephalon that influence emotions, motivation, mood, and sensations of pain and pleasure.

liver A large solid organ that lies in the right upper quadrant immediately below the diaphragm; it produces bile, stores glucose for immediate use by the body, and produces many substances that help regulate immune responses.

lumbar spine The lower part of the back, formed by the lowest five nonfused vertebrae; also called the dorsal spine.

lungs The two primary organs of breathing.

luteinizing hormone A hormone released from the pituitary gland at roughly monthly intervals that helps to stimulate one oocyte to undergo cell division.

lymph A thin, plasmalike liquid formed from interstitial or extracellular fluid that bathes the tissues of the body.

lymph nodes Round or bean-shaped structures interspersed along the course of the lymph vessels, which filter the lymph and serve as a source of lymphocytes.

lymph vessels Thin-walled vessels through which lymph circulates through the body; they travel close to the major veins.

lymphatic system A passive circulatory system that transports a plasmalike liquid called lymph, a thin fluid that bathes the tissues of the body.

lymphocytes The smallest of the agranulocytes, they originate in the bone marrow but migrate through the blood to the lymphatic tissues.

lysis The process of disintegration or breakdown of cells that occurs when excess water enters the cell through osmosis.

macrophages Cells that are responsible for protecting the body against infection.

mainstem bronchi The part of the lower airway below the larynx through which air enters the lungs.

mammary glands The organs of milk production in the breasts.

mandible The bone of the lower jaw.

manubrium The upper quarter of the sternum.

mastoid process A prominent bony mass at the base of the skull behind the ear.

maxillae The upper jawbones that assist in the formation of the orbit, the nasal cavity, and the palate and hold the upper teeth.

medial malleolus The distal end of the tibia, which forms the medial side of the ankle joint.

mediastinum The space between the lungs, in the center of the chest, that contains the heart, trachea, mainstem bronchi, part of the esophagus, and large blood vessels.

medulla oblongata Nerve tissue that is continuous inferiorly with the spinal cord; serves as a conduction pathway for ascending and descending nerve tracts; coordinates heart rate, blood vessel diameter, breathing, swallowing, vomiting, coughing, and sneezing.

medullary cavity An internal cavity that contains bone marrow.

meiosis A type of cell division that occurs in the production of eggs and sperm.

menarche The first menstrual cycle; the onset of menses.

meninges A set of three tough membranes, the dura mater, arachnoid, and pia mater, that enclose the entire brain and spinal cord.

menopause The ending of the menstrual cycle (menses).

menstrual cycle A cycle lasting approximately 28 days in which physiologic changes occur in the uterus and associated reproductive organs.

menstruation The period in the menstrual cycle of sloughing and discharge of the functional layer of the endometrium.

metabolic acidosis A pathologic condition characterized by a blood pH of less than 7.35 and caused by accumulation of acids in the body from a metabolic cause.

metabolic alkalosis A pathologic condition characterized by a blood pH of greater than 7.45 and resulting

Prep Kit (continued)

from the accumulation of bases in the body from a metabolic cause.

metacarpal bones The bones that form the hand.

midbrain The part of the brain that is responsible for helping to regulate the level of consciousness.

minute volume The amount of air that moves in and out of the lungs per minute minus the dead space. Also called minute ventilation.

mitral valve The valve in the heart that separates the left atrium from the left ventricle.

monocytes Agranulocytes that migrate out of the blood and into the tissues in response to an infection.

mons pubis A rounded flat pad over the female pubic symphysis.

motor nerves Nerves that carry information from the central nervous system to the muscles of the body.

mucous membranes The lining of body cavities and passages that communicate directly or indirectly with the environment outside the body.

mucus The opaque, sticky secretion of the mucous membranes that lubricates the body openings.

murmur An abnormal heart sound, heard as a "whooshinglike" sound, indicating turbulent blood flow within the heart.

musculoskeletal system The bones and voluntary muscles of the body.

myocardial infarction Blockage of the arteries that supply oxygen to the heart, resulting in death to a portion of the myocardium.

myocardium The heart muscle.

myoglobin A pigment synthesized in the muscles to give skeletal muscles their red-brown color.

myometrium A thick smooth muscle that forms the middle layer of the uterine wall.

nasal cavity The chamber inside the nose that lies between the floor of the cranium and the roof of the mouth.

nasal septum The separation between the right and left nostrils.

nasopharynx The part of the pharynx that lies above the level of the roof of the mouth, or palate.

neoplasm A mass of tissue produced by abnormal cell growth and division that may be malignant (cancerous) or benign; a tumor.

nervous system The system that controls virtually all activities of the body, both voluntary and involuntary.

neutrophils One of the three types of granulocytes; they have multilobed nuclei that resemble a string of baseballs held together by a thin strand of thread; they destroy bacteria, antigen-antibody complexes, and foreign matter.

norepinephrine A neurotransmitter and drug sometimes used in the treatment of shock; produces vasoconstriction through its alpha-stimulator properties.

oculomotor nerve The cranial nerve (III) that innervates the muscles that cause motion of the eyeballs and upper lid.

olfactory nerve The cranial nerve (I) for smell.

oncotic pressure The pressure of water to move, typically into the capillary, as the result of the presence of plasma proteins.

oocytes The precursors to a mature egg.

oogenesis The maturation process that results in production of an ovum, or egg.

optic nerve Either of the second cranial nerves that enter the eyeball posteriorly, through the optic foramen.

orbit The eye socket, made up of the maxilla and zygoma.

oropharynx A tubular structure that extends vertically from the back of the mouth to the esophagus and trachea.

osmosis The movement of a solvent, such as water, from an area of low solute concentration to one of high concentration through a selectively permeable membrane to equalize concentrations of a solute on both sides of the membrane.

osmotic pressure The tendency of water to move by osmosis across a membrane.

ovaries Female glands that produce sex hormones and ova (eggs).

ovulation The release of a mature egg (ovum) into the fallopian tube from the ovary.

ovum A mature egg released by the ovary during ovulation.

pancreas A flat, solid organ that lies below the liver and the stomach; it is a major source of digestive enzymes and produces the hormone insulin.

papillary muscles Specialized muscles that attach the ventricles to the cusps of the valves by muscular strands called chordae tendineae.

paranasal sinuses The sinuses, or hollowed sections of bone in the front of the head, which are lined with mucous membrane and drain into the nasal cavity.

parasympathetic nervous system A subdivision of the autonomic nervous system, involved in control of involuntary, vegetative functions, mediated largely by the vagus nerve through the chemical acetylcholine.

parathyroid glands Four glands that are embedded in the posterior portion of each lobe of the thyroid; they produce and secrete parathyroid hormone.

Prep Kit *(continued)*

parathyroid hormone Hormone produced and secreted by the parathyroid glands; it maintains normal levels of calcium in the blood and normal neuromuscular function.

parietal pleura The pleural membrane that lines the pleural cavity.

partial pressure of carbon dioxide ($Paco_2$) A measurement of the amount of carbon dioxide in the blood.

partial pressure of oxygen (Pao_2) A measurement of the amount of oxygen in the blood.

patella The kneecap; a specialized bone that lies within the tendon of the quadriceps muscle.

pelvis The attachment of the lower extremities to the body, consisting of the sacrum and two pelvic bones.

perfusion The circulation of oxygenated blood within an organ or tissue in adequate amounts to meet the cells' current needs.

pericardial fluid A serous fluid that fills the space between the visceral pericardium and the parietal pericardium and helps to reduce friction.

pericardium The serous membranes that surround the heart.

perineum The area of skin between the scrotum and the anus in males, and the vagina and the anus in females.

periosteum A double layer of connective tissue that lines the outer surface of the bone.

peripheral nervous system (PNS) The part of the nervous system that consists of 31 pairs of spinal nerves and 12 pairs of cranial nerves. These peripheral nerves may be sensory nerves, motor nerves, or connecting nerves.

peripheral vision Visualization of lateral objects while looking forward.

peristalsis The wavelike contraction of smooth muscle by which the ureters or other tubular organs propel their contents.

pH The measure of acidity or alkalinity of a solution.

phalanges The small bones of the digits of the fingers and toes.

physiology The study of the body functions of the living organism.

pia mater The innermost of the three meninges that enclose the brain and spinal cord; it rests directly on the brain and spinal cord.

pituitary gland An endocrine gland, located in the sella turcica of the brain, responsible for directly or indirectly affecting all body functions.

plasma A sticky, yellow fluid that carries the blood cells and nutrients and transports cellular waste material to the organs of excretion.

plasmin An enzyme that dissolves the fibrin in blood clots.

platelets Tiny, disk-shaped elements that are much smaller than the cells; they are essential in the initial formation of a blood clot, the mechanism that stops bleeding.

pleura The serous membrane covering the lungs and lining the thoracic cavity, completely enclosing a potential space known as the pleural space.

pleural cavity The potential space between the visceral and parietal pleura.

pleural space The potential space between the parietal pleura and the visceral pleura. It is described as "potential" because under normal conditions, the space does not exist.

pneumotaxic (pontine) center A portion of the pons that assists in creating shorter, faster respirations.

pons An organ that lies below the midbrain and above the medulla and contains numerous important nerve fibers, including those for sleep, respiration, and the medullary respiratory center.

popliteal artery A continuation of the femoral artery at the knee.

posterior tibial artery The artery just behind the medial malleolus; supplies blood to the foot.

preload The volume of blood returned to the heart.

prepuce A structure in the female external genitalia that is formed where the labia minora unite over the clitoris.

progesterone A hormone released from the ovaries that stimulates the uterine lining during the menstrual cycle in preparation for implantation of a fertilized egg.

prostate gland A small gland that surrounds the male urethra where it emerges from the urinary bladder; it secretes a fluid that is part of the ejaculatory fluid.

pubic symphysis A hard bony and cartilaginous prominence found at the midline in the lowermost portion of the abdomen where the two halves of the pelvic ring are joined by cartilage at a joint with minimal motion.

pubis One of three bones that fuse to form the pelvic ring.

pulmonary artery The major artery leading from the right ventricle of the heart to the lungs; it carries oxygen-poor blood.

pulmonary circulation The flow of blood from the right ventricle through the pulmonary arteries and all of their branches and capillaries in the

Prep Kit (continued)

lungs and back to the left atrium through the venules and pulmonary veins; also called the lesser circulation.

pulmonary veins The four veins that return oxygenated blood from the lungs to the left atrium of the heart.

pulmonic valve The semilunar valve that regulates blood flow between the right ventricle and the pulmonary artery.

pulse The wave of pressure created as the heart contracts and forces blood out the left ventricle and into the major arteries.

pulse pressure The difference between the systolic and diastolic pressures.

quadrants The way to describe the sections of the abdominal cavity. Imagine two lines intersecting at the umbilicus dividing the abdomen into four equal areas.

radius The bone on the thumb side of the forearm.

rectum The lowermost end of the colon.

red blood cells (RBCs) Cells that carry oxygen to the body's tissues; also called erythrocytes.

renal pelvis A cone-shaped collecting area that connects the ureter and the kidney.

renin-angiotensin system System located in the kidney that helps to regulate fluid balance and blood pressure.

residual volume The air that remains in the lungs after maximal expiration.

respiration The inhaling and exhaling of air; the physiologic process that exchanges carbon dioxide from fresh air.

respiratory acidosis A pathologic condition characterized by a blood pH of less than 7.35 and caused by accumulation of acids in the body from a respiratory cause.

respiratory alkalosis A pathologic condition characterized by a blood pH of greater than 7.45 and resulting from the accumulation of bases in the body from a respiratory cause.

respiratory system All the structures of the body that contribute to the process of breathing, consisting of the upper and lower airways and their component parts.

reticular activating system Located in the upper brainstem; responsible for maintenance of consciousness, specifically one's level of arousal.

retina The light-sensitive area of the eye where images are projected; a layer of cells at the back of the eye that changes the light image into electrical impulses, which are carried by the optic nerve to the brain.

retroperitoneum The space behind the peritoneum.

Rh factor An antigen found on the red blood cells of most people; in pregnancy, a woman's body can create antibodies against this, which can be problematic to future pregnancies.

sacroiliac joints The connection points between the pelvis and the vertebral column.

sacrum One of three bones that make up the pelvic ring; consists of five fused sacral vertebrae.

saddle joint Two saddle-shaped articulating surfaces oriented at right angles to each other so that complementary surfaces articulate with each other, such as in the thumb.

salivary glands The glands that produce saliva to keep the mouth and pharynx moist.

saphenous vein The longest vein in the body, it drains the leg, thigh, and dorsum of the foot.

scalp The thick skin covering the cranium, which usually bears hair.

scapula The shoulder blade.

sebaceous glands Glands that produce an oily substance called sebum, which discharges along the shafts of the hairs.

secondary bronchi Airway passages in the lungs that are formed from the division of the right and left mainstem bronchi.

semen Seminal fluid ejaculated from the penis and containing sperm.

semilunar valves The two valves, the aortic and pulmonic valves, that divide the heart from the aorta and pulmonary arteries.

seminal vesicles Storage sacs for sperm and seminal fluid, which empty into the urethra at the prostate.

semipermeable Property of the cell membrane that describes the ability to allow certain elements to pass through while not allowing others to do so.

sensory nerves The nerves that carry sensations of touch, taste, heat, cold, pain, and other modalities from the body to the central nervous system.

shock An abnormal state associated with inadequate oxygen and nutrient delivery to the metabolic apparatus of the cell.

shoulder girdle The proximal portion of the upper extremity, made up of the clavicle, the scapula, and the humerus.

sinoatrial (SA) node The normal site of the origin of electrical impulses; located high in the right atrium, it is the heart's natural pacemaker.

sinusitis An inflammation of the paranasal sinuses.

Prep Kit *(continued)*

skeletal muscle Muscle that is attached to bones and usually crosses at least one joint; striated, or voluntary, muscle.

skeleton The framework that gives the body its recognizable form; also designed to allow motion of the body and protection of vital organs.

skull The structure at the top of the axial skeleton that houses the brain and consists of the 28 bones that comprise the auditory ossicles, the cranium, and the face.

small intestine The portion of the digestive tube between the stomach and the cecum, consisting of the duodenum, jejunum, and ileum.

smooth muscle Involuntary muscle; it constitutes the bulk of the gastrointestinal tract and is present in nearly every organ to regulate automatic activity.

solute A particle, such as salt, that is dissolved in a solvent.

somatic nervous system The part of the nervous system that regulates activities over which there is voluntary control.

sphincters Muscles arranged in circles that are able to decrease the diameter of tubes. Examples are found within the rectum, bladder, and blood vessels.

sphygmomanometer A device used to measure blood pressure.

spinal cord An extension of the brain, composed of virtually all nerves carrying messages between the brain and the rest of the body. It lies inside of and is protected by the spinal canal.

Starling law The force of the heartbeat is determined primarily by the length of the fibers constituting its muscular wall. An increase in diastolic filling equals an increase in the force of the heartbeat.

stem cell A type of cell that can develop into other types of cell in the body; this type of cell retains the ability to divide repeatedly without specializing, and allows for continual growth and renewal.

sternocleidomastoid muscles The muscles on either side of the neck that allow movement of the head.

sternum The breastbone.

stratum corneal layer The outermost or dead layer of the skin.

striated muscle Muscle that is attached to bones and usually crosses at least one joint; also called skeletal or voluntary muscle.

stroke volume (SV) The volume of blood pumped forward with each ventricular contraction.

subarachnoid hemorrhage A hemorrhage between the arachnoid membrane and the pia mater.

subarachnoid space The space located between the pia mater and the arachnoid membrane.

subclavian artery The proximal part of the main artery of the arm, which supplies the brain, neck, anterior chest wall, and shoulder.

subclavian veins The proximal part of the main veins of the arm, which unite with the internal jugular veins.

subcutaneous tissue Tissue, largely fat, that lies directly under the dermis and serves as an insulator of the body.

superior vena cava One of the two largest veins in the body; carries blood from the upper extremities, head, neck, and chest into the heart.

surfactant A liquid protein substance that coats the alveoli in the lungs, decreases alveolar surface tension, and keeps the alveoli expanded; a low level in a premature baby contributes to respiratory distress syndrome.

sutures Attachment points in the skull where the cranial bones join together.

sweat glands The glands that secrete sweat, located in the dermal layer of the skin.

sympathetic nervous system Subdivision of the autonomic nervous system that governs the body's fight-or-flight reactions by inducing smooth muscle contraction or relaxation of the blood vessels and bronchioles.

symphysis A type of joint that has grown together forming a very stable connection.

synovial fluid The small amount of liquid within a joint used as lubrication.

synovial membrane The lining of a joint that secretes synovial fluid into the joint space.

systemic circulation The portion of the circulatory system outside of the heart and lungs.

systemic vascular resistance (SVR) The resistance that blood must overcome to be able to move within the blood vessels. SVR is related to the amount of dilation or constriction in the blood vessel.

systole The contraction, or period of contraction, of the heart, especially that of the ventricles.

temporomandibular joint (TMJ) The joint where the mandible meets with the temporal bone of the cranium just in front of each ear.

tendon The fibrous connective tissue that attaches muscle to bone.

tertiary bronchi Airway passages in the lungs that are formed from branching of the secondary bronchi.

testes The male reproductive organs that produce sperm and secrete male hormones; also called testicles.

Prep Kit (continued)

thalamus Structure of the diencephalon that is the sensory switchboard of the brain, through which almost all signals travel on their way in or out of the brain.

thoracic duct One of two great lymph vessels; it empties into the superior vena cava.

thoracic spine The 12 vertebrae that lie between the cervical vertebrae and the lumbar vertebrae. One pair of ribs is attached to each of the thoracic vertebrae.

thorax The chest cavity that contains the heart, lungs, esophagus, and great vessels.

thrombin An enzyme that causes the conversion of fibrinogen to fibrin, which binds to the platelet plug, forming the final mature clot.

thyroid cartilage A firm prominence of cartilage that forms the upper part of the larynx; the Adam's apple.

thyroid gland A large endocrine gland that is located at the base of the neck and produces and excretes hormones that influence growth, development, and metabolism.

tibia The shin bone, the larger of the two bones of the lower leg.

tidal volume The amount of air moved in and out of the lungs in one relaxed breath; approximately 500 mL for an adult.

tissue plasminogen activator (t-PA) A major component in the fibrinolytic system, in which clots that have already formed are lysed or disrupted, converting plasminogen to plasmin.

trabeculae Bony rods that form the lacy network in cancellous bones and are oriented to increase weight-bearing capacity of long bones.

trachea The windpipe; the main trunk for air passing to and from the lungs.

triceps The muscle in the back of the upper arm.

tricuspid valve The heart valve that separates the right atrium from the right ventricle.

tunica adventitia The outer layer of tissue of a blood vessel wall, composed of elastic and fibrous connective tissue.

tunica intima The smooth, thin, inner lining of a blood vessel.

tunica media The middle and thickest layer of tissue of a blood vessel wall, composed of elastic tissue and smooth muscle cells that allow the vessel to expand or contract in response to changes in blood pressure and tissue demand.

ulna The inner bone of the forearm, on the side opposite the thumb.

ureter A small, hollow tube that carries urine from the kidneys to the bladder.

urethra The canal that conveys urine from the bladder to outside the body.

urinary bladder A sac behind the pubic symphysis made of smooth muscle that collects and stores urine.

urinary system The organs that control the discharge of certain waste materials filtered from the blood and excreted as urine.

uterus A muscular inverted pear–shaped organ that lies situated between the urinary bladder and the rectum.

vagina A muscular distensible tube that connects the uterus with the vulva (the external female genitalia); also called the birth canal.

vagus nerve The cranial nerve (X) that provides motor functions to the soft palate, pharynx, and larynx and carries taste bud fibers from the posterior tongue, sensory fibers from the inferior pharynx, larynx, thoracic, and abdominal organs, and parasympathetic fibers to thoracic and abdominal organs.

vasa deferentia The spermatic duct of the testicles; also called vas deferens.

veins The blood vessels that transport blood back to the heart.

venous sinuses Spaces between the membranes surrounding the brain that are the primary means of venous drainage from the brain.

ventilation The movement of air between the lungs and the environment.

ventral respiratory group (VRG) A portion of the medulla oblongata that is responsible for modulating breathing during speech.

ventricle In the context of the circulatory system, one of two lower chambers of the heart; in the context of the neurologic system, hollow storage areas in the brain.

vertebrae The 33 bones that make up the spinal column.

vertebral column The spine or primary support structure of the body that houses the spinal cord and the peripheral nerves.

visceral pleura The pleural membrane that covers the lungs.

vital capacity The amount of air moved in and out of the lungs with maximum inspiration and exhalation.

voluntary muscle Muscle that is under direct voluntary control of the brain and can be contracted or relaxed at will; skeletal, or striated, muscle.

Prep Kit *(continued)*

vulva The female external genitalia; also called the pudendum.

white blood cells (WBCs) Blood cells that have a role in the body's immune defense mechanisms against infection; also called leukocytes.

xiphoid process The narrow, cartilaginous lower tip of the sternum.

zygoma The quadrangular bone of the cheek, articulating with the frontal bone, the maxillae, the zygomatic processes of the temporal bone, and the great wings of the sphenoid bone.

▶ References

1. Causes of COPD Page. National Heart, Lung, and Blood Institute. https://www.nhlbi.nih.gov/health/health-topics/topics/co/causes. Accessed November 9, 2017.
2. Richerson GB, Boron WF. Control of ventilation. In: Boron WF, Boulpaep EL, eds. *Medical Physiology: A Cellular and Molecular Approach*. 2nd ed. Philadelphia, PA: Saunders; 2012:725-745.
3. Lohr NL, Benjamin IJ. Structure and function of the normal heart and blood vessels. In: Benjamin IJ, Griggs RC, Wing EJ, Fitz JG, eds. *Andreoli and Carpenter's Cecil Essentials of Medicine*. 9th ed. Philadelphia, PA: Saunders; 2016:16-21.
4. Blood cell formation. Encyclopaedia Brittanica website. https://www.britannica.com/science/blood-cell-formation . Accessed December 17, 2017.
5. Haase VH. Regulation of erythropoiesis by hypoxia-inducible factors. *Blood Rev*. 2013;27(1):41-53.
6. Sargis RM. An overview of the pineal gland: maintaining circadian rhythm. endocrineweb website. https://www.endocrineweb.com/endocrinology/overview-pineal-gland. Updated June 10, 2014. Accessed December 17, 2017.

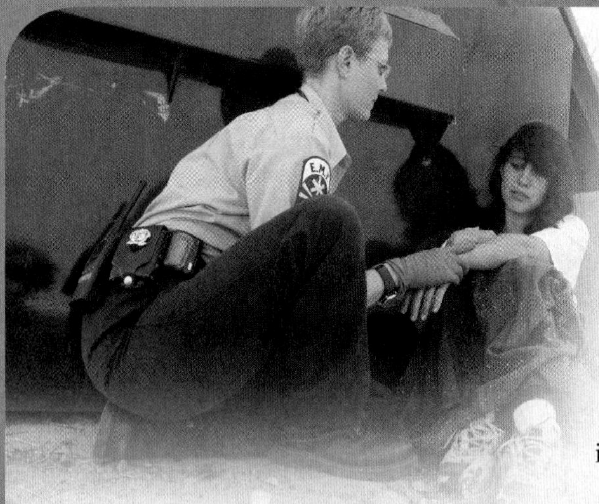

Assessment *in Action*

Your ambulance is dispatched to a local nursing home for an elderly woman who is reporting nonspecific chest pain and bradycardia with some shortness of breath. As you arrive, the nurse hands you the patient's chart, which shows that the patient has a past medical history of three myocardial infarctions, heart failure, and mitral valve prolapse.

1. The mitral valve is also known as the _____ and separates the _____ atrium and ventricle.

- **A.** tricuspid valve, left
- **B.** tricuspid valve, right
- **C.** bicuspid valve, left
- **D.** bicuspid valve, right

2. As you listen to the patient's heart sounds, you note what sounds like a "lub-DUB-da" sound. You know this to be an S_3 sound, and is an abnormal finding. The S_3 sound represents:

- **A.** abnormally increased filling pressures in the atria.
- **B.** decreased compliance of the left ventricle.
- **C.** sudden closure of the pulmonic valve.
- **D.** sudden closure of the tricuspid valve.

Assessment *in Action* *(continued)*

3. The nurse states that the patient has been experiencing bradycardia. The normal electrical impulse of the heart begins in the:

A. AV node.
B. SA node.
C. bundle of His.
D. Purkinje fibers.

4. While listening to breath sounds you note that the patient has pulmonary edema. This is a result of blood backing up that is normally returned to the left atrium via the:

A. circumflex coronary artery.
B. LAD artery.
C. pulmonary artery.
D. pulmonary vein.

5. The result of the fluid backup is a decrease in the amount of blood returned to the heart to be pumped out. The pressure under which the ventricles fill is known as:

A. preload.
B. afterload.
C. stroke volume.
D. ejection fraction.

6. Due to her extensive cardiac history, her cardiac output has been diminished. Cardiac output is measured by:

A. Heart rate × Respiratory rate
B. Blood pressure × Heart rate
C. Stroke volume × Respiratory rate
D. Stroke volume × Heart rate

7. During your assessment, the patient reports she is unable to take a deep breath due to the pain in her chest; this is causing a reduction in her _____, which is the amount of air moved into or out of the lungs in a single breath.

A. minute volume
B. tidal volume
C. residual volume
D. inspiratory reserve volume

8. The pulmonary edema decreases the diffusion of oxygen resulting in dyspnea. RBCs contain ______, which give(s) them their reddish color and transport oxygen throughout the body.

A. bilirubin
B. macrophages
C. hemoglobin
D. erythropoiesis

9. Which blood type is known as the *universal donor*?

10. Explain the *Starling law*.

CHAPTER 8

Pathophysiology

National EMS Education Standard Competencies

Pathophysiology

Integrates comprehensive knowledge of pathophysiology of major human systems.

Knowledge Objectives

1. Define pathophysiology, including its role in diagnosing and treating disease. (p 317)
2. Compare atrophy, hypertrophy, hyperplasia, dysplasia, and metaplasia as means of cellular adaptation. (p 317)
3. List factors that can affect or upset homeostasis. (p 317)
4. Explain the causes, clinical manifestations, assessment, and management of edema. (pp 318-319)
5. Discuss types of fluid deficits and potential resulting complications. (p 319)
6. Explain the physiologic consequences of electrolyte imbalances in sodium, potassium, calcium, phosphate, and magnesium. (pp 319-322)
7. Compare respiratory acidosis, respiratory alkalosis, metabolic acidosis, and metabolic alkalosis. (pp 323-325)
8. Outline how cellular injury occurs in patients with hypoxia, chemical exposures, infection (sepsis), immunologic exposures (hypersensitivity reactions), inflammatory conditions, genetic disorders, nutritional imbalances, physical damage (mechanical injury), and other harmful exposures, such as extremes of hot and cold. (pp 325-329)
9. Examine the concept of apoptosis. (p 329)
10. Define perfusion, including the physiologic consequences of hypoperfusion. (p 330)
11. Analyze the mechanisms by which the body compensates for hypoperfusion. (pp 330-331)
12. Discuss the causes of central and peripheral shock, including cardiogenic, obstructive, hypovolemic, and distributive shock. (pp 331-333)
13. Explain how to treat a patient in shock. (pp 333-334)
14. Describe multiple organ dysfunction syndrome. (pp 334-335)
15. Examine the body's three defense mechanisms against pathogens: anatomic barriers, the immune response, and the inflammatory response. (pp 335-345)
16. Explain how plasma protein systems—the complement system, the coagulation (clotting) system, and the kinin system—modulate the inflammatory response. (pp 342-343)
17. Compare wound healing by primary intention with wound healing by secondary intention. (p 343)
18. Outline each of the four types of hypersensitivity reactions and mechanisms for immunologic injury. (pp 345-347)
19. List several autoimmune reactions. (pp 347-348)
20. Compare inherited and acquired immunodeficiencies. (pp 348-349)
21. Analyze the controllable and uncontrollable risk factors that intersect in order to cause disease. (pp 349-350)
22. Outline how incidence, prevalence, morbidity, and mortality data are used to analyze disease risk. (p 350)
23. Analyze risk factors for cancer and cardiovascular disease. (pp 351-352, 354-355)
24. Describe how hematologic disorders occur. (pp 353-354)
25. Name common renal, gastrointestinal, and neuromuscular disorders. (pp 355-357)
26. List the stages of the general adaptation syndrome, and explore the relationship between stress and disease. (pp 358-360)

Skills Objectives

There are no skills objectives in this chapter.

Introduction

The human body is made up of cells, tissues, and organs. These structures function in a constantly changing microenvironment. The study of the origin, growth, structure, behavior, and reproduction of living organisms is known as *biology*. **Pathophysiology** is the study of the physiology of altered functioning in the presence of disease. The word is derived from the Greek words *pathos*, meaning "suffering," and *physis*, meaning "form." In Chapter 7, *The Human Body*, you learned about the major classes of cells, and cellular structure and function. When the structure and function in cells, tissues, and organs break down in response to stressors and the body can no longer maintain homeostasis, disease may result. Determining the origin of a disease process often helps advanced emergency medical technicians (AEMTs) choose the best approach to patient evaluation and initial treatment.

To understand disease processes, you must understand the ways disease alters the structure and function in cells. We begin this chapter by reviewing how the changes that affect cells disrupt the body's ability to maintain homeostasis and lead to disease. Next, we consider the influence inflammation and shock have on disease development. We also discuss the role of immunity and defense mechanisms in protecting the organism from disease. We conclude with a discussion on the effects genetics and stress have in disease development.

Adaptations in Cells and Tissues

When exposed to adverse conditions, cells undergo a process of adaptation in an attempt to guard against injury. In some situations, the cells change permanently; in others, the structure or function of the cells change only temporarily.

Atrophy is a decrease in cell size due to a loss of subcellular components, which leads to a decrease in the size of the tissue and organ. The actual number of cells remains unchanged. The decreased size represents an attempt to cope with a new steady state in less-than-favorable conditions or a lack of use. For example, a casted, immobilized limb shrinks in muscle mass as a result of disuse atrophy.

Hypertrophy is an increase in the size of the cells due to synthesis of more subcellular components, which leads to an increase in tissue and organ size. For example, the left ventricle in the heart may undergo hypertrophy as a result of chronic high resistance pressures from hypertension (elevated blood pressure).

Hyperplasia is an increase in the actual number of cells in an organ or tissue, usually resulting in an increase in the size of the organ or tissue. For example, a callus represents hyperplasia of the keratinized layer of the epidermis of the foot in response to increased friction or trauma.

Dysplasia is an alteration of the size, shape, and organization of cells. It is most often found in epithelial cells that have undergone irregular, atypical changes in response to chronic irritation or inflammation. For example, the development of cervical dysplasia in women is strongly associated with exposure to certain human papillomaviruses.

Metaplasia refers to the reversible cellular adaptation in which one adult cell type is replaced by another adult cell type. For example, in squamous metaplasia, the ciliated epithelium in the airways of smokers may be replaced by metaplastic epithelium.

Disturbances in Fluid Balance

The human body is composed primarily of water. Therefore, all biochemical reactions taking place within the body are occurring in an aqueous environment. As a result, changes in fluid and electrolyte balance that disrupt homeostasis can either cause or exacerbate various disease processes. The result may be an emergent condition.

Homeostasis can be upset in a number of ways such as excessive output or input of fluids. Profuse sweating can cause dehydration, while excessive salt intake can contribute to hypertension.[1] Not drinking enough water can also alter homeostasis. In fact, a person deprived of water for 3 days or longer may die.

YOU are the Provider — PART 1

You and your partner are dispatched to a single-family residence to assist a 72-year-old man who is having difficulty breathing. On arrival, a neighbor greets you at the door. She tells you the resident of the home—your patient—lives alone, has had numerous heart attacks, and is not doing well. As you approach him, you assess his surroundings. You observe a large number of used facial tissues on the side table, along with an array of prescription medication bottles. The patient is sitting upright in a chair. He is wearing a nasal cannula attached to a home oxygen unit. He is able to speak only a few words at a time. He says he can't breathe, and you note that he looks pale.

1. What is your general impression of the patient?
2. What can you learn about the patient from his surroundings?

The degree of fluid imbalance required to compromise homeostasis and cause illness depends on the patient's size, age, and any underlying medical conditions. In healthy adults, loss of more than 30% of total body fluid is required, but in a small child, a loss of only 10% to 15% of total body fluid could easily produce symptoms of dehydration. Consequently, fluid therapy is a fundamental step in resuscitation.

Special Populations

The total volume of water in the body varies by age and body composition throughout the life span. At birth, a healthy, full-term neonate has approximately 80% total body water; however, this percentage decreases with age Figure 8-1. After several weeks, an infant's total body water drops to approximately 70%.[2] In childhood, the percentage of total body water falls to around 60%. Adults have 50% to 60% total body water, but water may constitute only 45% of body weight in older adults. Dehydration, therefore, can be a serious concern in older adults. Dehydration also remains a concern in the pediatric population. Despite infants having higher total body water content than adults, infants are at higher risk of dehydration due to increased rate of fluid loss during disease and pathologic states.

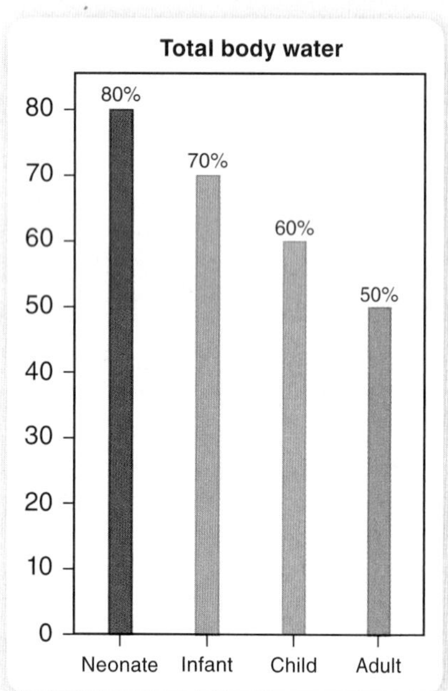

Figure 8-1 Average total water volume in the body by age.

Words of Wisdom

A hypertonic solution has a relatively higher osmotic pressure—that is, it contains more solute—than does the interstitial fluid or the fluid within and surrounding the brain. Administering a hypertonic solution such as mannitol, sodium bicarbonate, or hypertonic saline can cause excess fluid to drain from the tissues and into the blood and can decrease swelling in the brain.

▶ Edema

Edema is swelling caused by excessive fluid trapped in the body tissues Figure 8-2. Edema may have any of several causes. One possible cause is increased capillary hydrostatic pressure, which may be associated with any of the following:

- Arteriolar dilation (for example, from allergic reactions or inflammation)
- Venous obstruction (for example, hepatic obstruction, heart failure, or thrombophlebitis)
- Increased vascular volume, as occurs in patients with heart failure
- An increased level of adrenocortical hormones
- Premenstrual sodium retention
- Pregnancy
- Environmental heat stress
- The effects of gravity from prolonged standing

Decreased colloidal osmotic pressure in the capillaries, another possible cause of edema, can be associated with various processes:

- Decreased production of plasma proteins, such as occurs in starvation and in patients with liver disease or severe protein deficiency
- Increased loss of plasma proteins attributable to protein-losing kidney diseases, extensive burns, or other causes

Obstruction of lymphatic vessels also can cause edema. Such obstruction can be associated with infection, lymphatic disease, or removal of lymphatic structures (for example, removal of lymph nodes during mastectomy can cause upper extremity edema). When lymph vessels are blocked,

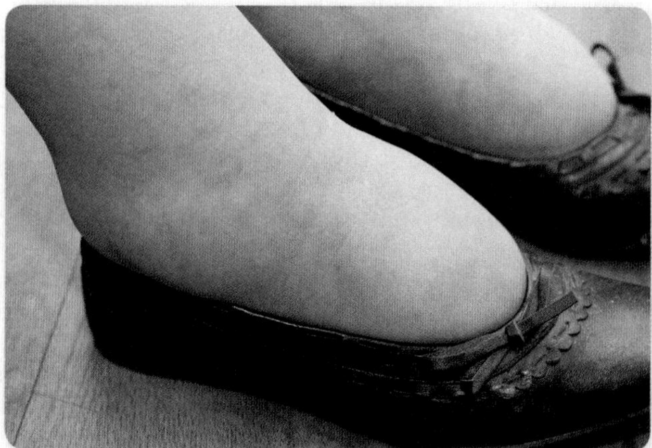

Figure 8-2 Edema is an excessive amount of fluid in the interstitial space.

the amount of fluid exiting through the arterial end of the capillaries is not equal to the amount of fluid being returned to the venous side. Consequently, more fluid leaves the arterial side, where the mean forces favoring outward movement are slightly higher. This additional fluid is picked up by the lymphatic system.

Severe edema, then, may be caused by long-standing lymphatic obstruction. Peripheral edema (as in the ankles and feet) is the most common form. If a person is unable to get out of bed for an extended period, then edema may occur in the sacral area (sacral edema). *Ascites,* the abnormal accumulation of fluid in the peritoneal cavity, is also a type of edema.

The clinical manifestations of edema may be local or generalized. Patients with cardiac disease may have pulmonary edema, or edema may occur due to blast injuries, narcotic overdose, or altitude changes (ie, high altitude pulmonary edema). Patients with acute pulmonary edema have an excessive amount of fluid in their lungs, which impairs the diffusion of oxygen into pulmonary capillaries, making the patient hypoxic and severely short of breath.

AEMTs must perform an in-depth physical assessment that includes auscultation of breath sounds, evaluation for pedal and sacral edema and jugular venous distention, and vital signs. Along with a thorough exam, it is important to determine a patient's medical history and his or her current and past medications. Often, treatment is determined by the patient's chief complaint and presenting problem. The definitive treatment of edema depends on the underlying medical condition that caused it. Possible interventions may include the use of continuous positive airway pressure, supplemental oxygen, positional therapy, nitrates, and diuretics.

Words of Wisdom

When you eat a bag of potato chips, you ingest a large quantity of salt. Acutely, the body responds by holding on to water. Hence, urine output temporarily declines. In healthy people, however, the kidneys and other regulatory mechanisms return both sodium and water levels to normal homeostatic balance.

▶ Isotonic Fluid Deficit

An isotonic fluid deficit is a decrease in extracellular fluid with proportionate losses of sodium and water Table 8-1. This is the most common form of fluid loss, and is often the result of sweating. Excessive sweating or combining increased physical exertion with other comorbidities may complicate the fluid loss and cause additional problems. An isotonic fluid excess is a proportionate increase of sodium and water in extracellular fluid; common causes include kidney and heart failure. The manifestations of these conditions depend on the serum sodium level. When the body becomes dehydrated,

Table 8-1 Isotonic Fluid Deficit/Excess (Hypovolemia/Hypervolemia)

Imbalance	Common Causes
Fluid deficit (proportionate loss in both water and sodium; decreased total body sodium)	Vomiting, diarrhea, loss of plasma or whole blood (eg, burns, hemorrhage), loop diuretic use, excessive sweating, fever, decreased oral fluid intake
Fluid excess (Proportionate gain in both water and sodium; increased total body sodium)	Heart failure, cirrhosis, renal failure, steroid use, excessive sodium intake

Data from: Monahan FD. *Phipps' Medical-Surgical Nursing: Health and Illness Perspectives.* 8th ed. St. Louis, MO: Mosby; 2007:359; and Potter P, PerryA, Stockert P, Hall A. *Basic Nursing.* 7th ed. St. Louis, MO: Mosby; 2011:466.

orthostatic hypotension and decreased urine output (**oliguria**) often occur. When the sodium level is very high (>160 mEq/L), the patient is at risk of delirium and coma. Tonicity and related concepts are covered in detail in Chapter 14, *Vascular Access and Medication Administration*.

Electrolyte Imbalances

▶ Sodium

Sodium, an element essential to the human body, is found primarily in the blood and fluid outside the cells. It regulates fluid balance, total fluid volume, and blood pressure by controlling the movement of water across cellular membranes. It also facilitates muscle contraction and nerve impulse transmission. Abnormal sodium levels may result in nausea, seizures, and cardiac dysrhythmias. A blood test can determine the level of serum sodium (Na); the normal range is 136 to 142 mEq/L.[3] A *hypertonic fluid deficit* occurs when there is water loss in the body without a proportionate loss of sodium—in other words, there is a relative water loss. This condition, called **hypernatremia**, is clinically defined as a serum sodium level of 143 mEq/L or higher. A hypotonic fluid deficit occurs when there is sodium loss in the body without a proportionate loss of water (there is a relative water excess). This deficit causes **hyponatremia**, characterized by a serum sodium level of 135 mEq/L or less.

Causes of hypernatremia and hyponatremia include excessive sweating in the heat or during exercise, gastrointestinal losses through vomiting or diarrhea, and inappropriate use of intravenous (IV) fluids or diuretics. Some patients have nausea and headaches. In others, seizures and coma develop. Clinical findings typically depend not only on the absolute sodium level, but also on when the abnormality developed. People who become hyponatremic over a period of days tend to have fewer symptoms than people in whom the abnormality develops acutely.

▶ Potassium

Potassium (K^+), the major intracellular cation, is crucial to many cellular functions, including neuromuscular control; regulating skeletal, smooth, and cardiac muscles; regulating acid-base balance; facilitating intracellular enzyme reactions; and maintaining intracellular osmolarity. The normal serum level of potassium ranges from 3.5 to 5.0 mEq/L.[3]

Hypokalemia is a decreased serum potassium level. Common causes include the following:

- Decreased dietary potassium intake and absorption
- Decreased shift of potassium into the cells as a result of insulin administration, alkalosis, or beta-adrenergic stimulation, such as with epinephrine
- Renal potassium loss, such as with increased aldosterone activity or diuretic use
- Extrarenal potassium loss, such as with vomiting, diarrhea, or laxative use

Muscular weakness, fatigue, and muscle cramps are the most frequent symptoms associated with mild to moderate hypokalemia.

Hyperkalemia is an elevated serum potassium level. Here are some common causes you may see in the prehospital setting:

- Decreased excretion (from renal failure or from medications that inhibit potassium excretion [spironolactone, angiotensin-converting enzyme inhibitors, nonsteroidal anti-inflammatory drugs])
- Shifts of potassium from within the cell (as with burns, crush injuries, metabolic acidosis, and insulin deficiency)
- Excessive dietary potassium intake

An elevated potassium level interferes with normal neuromuscular function, leading to muscle weakness and, rarely, flaccid paralysis.

▶ Calcium

Nearly all (98%) of the body's calcium (Ca^{+2}) is found in the bones and teeth. This element lends strength and stability to the collagen and ground substance that form the matrix of the skeletal system. Calcium enters the body through the gastrointestinal tract. Its absorption from the intestine is aided by vitamin D **Figure 8-3**, which is manufactured largely by the body in a complex process that begins with exposure of the skin to sunlight. Calcium is then stored in bone tissue and ultimately excreted by the kidney. A normal serum calcium level ranges from 8.2 to 10.2 mg/dL.[3]

Hypocalcemia, a decreased serum calcium level, can be caused by the following:

- Decreased calcium intake or absorption (as in malabsorption and vitamin D deficit)
- Increased calcium loss (as in alcoholism and diuretic therapy)
- Endocrine disease (such as hypoparathyroidism)
- Sepsis

Signs and symptoms of hypocalcemia stem from the increased excitation of the neuromuscular and cardiovascular systems. Skeletal muscle spasm can cause cramps or sustained muscle contraction (tetany). Laryngospasm with stridor can obstruct the airway. Seizures can occur, as can abnormal sensations (paresthesias) affecting the lips and extremities.

Hypercalcemia is an increased serum calcium level. Selected causes are listed below:

- Increased calcium intake or absorption (such as with excessive antacid ingestion)
- Endocrine disorders (such as primary hyperparathyroidism and adrenal insufficiency)
- Neoplasms (cancers)
- Miscellaneous causes (such as diuretics and sarcoidosis)

The signs and symptoms associated with hypercalcemia are sometimes vague and can include fatigue, weakness, nausea, constipation, and frequent urination (**polyuria**). In severe cases, stupor, coma, or renal failure may develop. Treatment of hypercalcemia depends on treating the underlying cause.

▶ Phosphate

Phosphate (PO_4^{-3}), primarily an intracellular anion, is essential to many body functions.

Hypophosphatemia is a decrease in the level of serum phosphate. Causes include the following:

- Decreased supply or absorption, as can occur in starvation, malabsorption, or blocked absorption (such as with aluminum-containing antacids)
- Excessive loss of phosphate associated with use of diuretics, or in patients with hyperparathyroidism, hyperthyroidism, or alcoholism
- Intracellular shift of phosphorus (for example, after administering glucose, anabolic steroids, or oral contraceptives, or in patients with respiratory alkalosis or salicylate poisoning)
- Electrolyte abnormalities, such as hypercalcemia and hypomagnesemia
- Abnormal loss of nutrients followed by inadequate replenishment, as can occur in patients with diabetic ketoacidosis or chronic alcoholism

Respiratory Acidosis

The following equation demonstrates how a diminished rate of respiration can precipitate acidosis:

$$\downarrow \text{Respiration} \rightarrow \uparrow CO_2 \rightarrow \uparrow H_2CO_3 \rightarrow \text{Acidosis}$$

Respiratory acidosis is always related to hypoventilation. Decreased lung tidal volume reduces the amount of carbon dioxide (CO_2) that is exhaled, causing hypercapnia (increased CO_2). Because the acidosis is linked to inadequate breathing, the renal buffer system is initiated as a compensatory mechanism. Some causes of respiratory acidosis include the following:

- Airway obstruction
- Cardiac arrest
- Overdose of a CNS depressant drug, such as heroin
- Submersion
- Respiratory arrest
- Pulmonary edema
- Closed head injury
- Chest trauma

Hypoventilation associated with any of these conditions can devolve quickly into an overwhelming, life-threatening acidosis, making it impossible for the renal system to compensate in time to accomplish a pH shift. The decrease in pH increases permeability of cell membranes, causing a leakage of potassium into the blood. The release of potassium ions into the extracellular fluid can cause a potentially fatal cardiac dysrhythmia. The discharge of calcium into extracellular spaces causes hypercalcemia, characterized by lethargy, a diminished level of consciousness, and a generalized slowing of the nervous system. This nervous system inhibition may also be evidenced by a delayed pupillary response or a weakened or delayed response to painful stimuli.

Signs and symptoms of respiratory acidosis include the following:

- Systemic or cerebral vasodilation (or both)
- Headache, light-headedness
- Warm, flushed skin[7]
- CNS depression
- **Bradypnea** (slow respiratory rate)
- Nausea and vomiting

Chronic obstructive pulmonary disease (COPD) gradually destroys lung tissue and inhibits oxygen and carbon dioxide exchange, eventually resulting in respiratory acidosis **Figure 8-4**. In patients with COPD, the normal stimulus for gas exchange is absent. Carbon dioxide retention leads to an increasing level of carbonic acid. Chemoreceptors eventually become unable to detect the presence of metabolic acids. As a result, the only remaining breathing stimulus is the hypoxic drive, which stimulates breathing by sensing a decreased oxygen level in the blood.

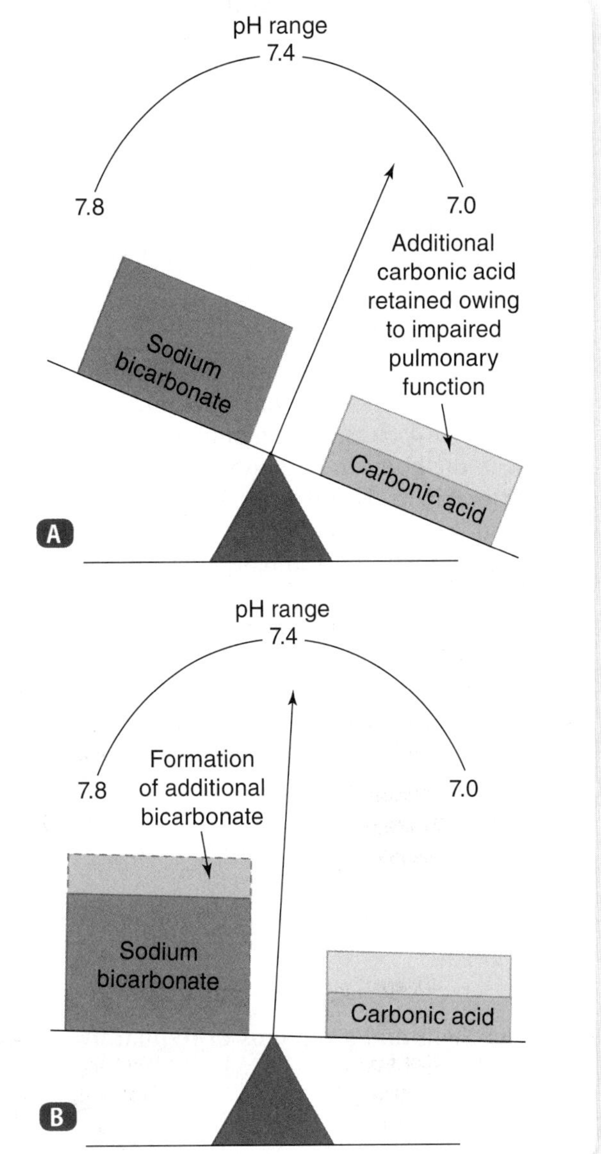

Figure 8-4 A. Derangement of acid-base balance in respiratory acidosis. **B.** Compensation by formation of additional bicarbonate.

The slow onset of this form of respiratory acidosis in patients with COPD makes it survivable. The renal system slowly moderates the acidosis, preventing the

Words of Wisdom

Compensatory mechanisms for pH imbalances bring the pH level closer to normal. Respiratory compensation (acidosis or alkalosis) occurs rapidly and relatively predictably. Metabolic compensation, if it occurs at all, takes hours or days. Acute compensation is never complete. Chronic compensation, such as that which occurs in patients with COPD, often returns the pH level to normal.

life-threatening cardiac dysrhythmias often associated with acute acidosis.

Respiratory Alkalosis

The following equation demonstrates how an increased respiratory rate can produce alkalosis:

$$\uparrow \text{Rate of respiration} \rightarrow \downarrow CO_2 \rightarrow \downarrow H_2CO_3 \rightarrow \text{Alkalosis}$$

Respiratory alkalosis is associated with conditions that result in hyperventilation. Over time, an increased respiratory rate decreases the amount of circulating carbon dioxide in the body. In respiratory alkalosis, the carbon dioxide level in the blood drops, which reduces the level of circulating carbonic acid (H_2CO_3). The renal system then begins to retain H^+ ions to rebalance the depleted acid level. As the same time, H^+ ions begin to shift from the intracellular fluid compartment to the extracellular fluid. Calcium moves into the intracellular fluid to rebalance the depleted hydrogen level. The resulting extracellular hypocalcemia causes muscle contractions. In fact, hyperventilation accompanied by **carpopedal spasm** (a contorted position in which the fingers or toes flex in a clawlike manner) is the classic sign of respiratory alkalosis.

Some causes of hyperventilation and respiratory alkalosis include the following:

- Drug overdose, especially an overdose of aspirin
- Fever
- Overzealous bag-mask ventilation

Some signs and symptoms of respiratory alkalosis are listed below:

- Diminished level of consciousness
- Light-headedness
- Carpopedal spasm
- Paresthesias of the lips and face
- Chest tightness
- Confusion
- Vertigo
- Blurred vision
- Nausea and vomiting

Metabolic Acidosis

The following equation demonstrates how an increased carbonic acid level can produce **metabolic acidosis**:

$$\uparrow H_2CO_3 \rightarrow \uparrow H^+ + HCO_3^- \rightarrow \text{Acidosis}$$

Carbonic acid is broken down into hydrogen and bicarbonate (HCO_3^-). The increased carbonic acid equates to increasing hydrogen, which equates to acidosis.

Any acidosis unrelated to the respiratory system is considered metabolic. An increased rate of breathing (tachypnea) represents the body's attempt to restore acid-base balance, by eliminating excess carbon dioxide through the respiratory system. For example, patients with diabetic ketoacidosis often experience Kussmaul respirations (deep, closely spaced, sighing breaths), in which the body hyperventilates in an attempt to blow off carbon dioxide and correct the acidosis.

As with any acidosis, the extracellular hydrogen ion level increases and extracellular buffers attempt to neutralize the excess acid. Ion shifts occur, hydrogen ions leak into the cells, and potassium shifts into the extracellular spaces, raising the serum potassium level and putting the patient at risk of a life-threatening dysrhythmia. Calcium also shifts into the extracellular spaces. The resulting hypercalcemia obstructs impulse transmission to neurons in muscle and other tissues. Consequently, the patient becomes lethargic and has a decreased level of consciousness.

Causes of metabolic acidosis include the following:

- **Lactic acidosis. Lactic acidosis** is the product of anaerobic cellular respiration, which occurs when tissues and organs are inadequately perfused, as in shock and cardiac arrest.
- **Ketoacidosis. Ketoacidosis** is associated with insulin deficiency or desensitization of cells to insulin. Unable to use glucose for energy, cells must instead begin metabolizing fatty acids. Extremely acidic compounds called **ketones** are the by-products of such metabolism.
- **Aspirin (acetylsalicylic acid) overdose.** A dose of 10 to 30 g aspirin in an adult constitutes an overdose. Aspirin directly stimulates the respiratory centers of the brain, producing tachypnea. Rapid breathing leads to respiratory alkalosis, and initiation of renal compensatory mechanisms leads to metabolic acidosis.
- **Alcohol ingestion.** Ingesting an excessive amount of ethyl alcohol can induce **alcoholic ketoacidosis**. Ingesting as little as 30 mL of either methanol (wood alcohol) or ethylene glycol (antifreeze) can also induce fatal forms of acidosis.
- **Gastrointestinal losses.** Gastrointestinal losses can precipitate metabolic acidosis. Diarrhea, for example, removes bases from the lower intestinal tract.
- Carbon monoxide poisoning.

The clinical presentation of metabolic acidosis is similar to that of respiratory acidosis:[7,8]

- Vasodilation
- CNS depression
- Headaches
- Warm, flushed skin
- Tachypnea
- Nausea and vomiting
- Cardiac dysrhythmias

Metabolic Alkalosis

The following equation demonstrates how a decreased H^+ ion concentration can produce alkalosis:

$$\downarrow H^+ \rightarrow \downarrow H_2CO_3 \rightarrow \text{Alkalosis}$$

Metabolic alkalosis occurs when increased urine output or a decreased gastric acid level leads to an excessive loss of acid. This is rarely an acute condition, but it is common among chronically ill patients, especially those who require nasogastric suctioning.

Several factors associated with upper gastrointestinal losses can lead to metabolic alkalosis:

- **Excessive vomiting.** Illness or an eating disorder, such as anorexia nervosa or bulimia, can be responsible for upper gastrointestinal acid loss. Expelling a great deal of acid from the stomach can trigger a complex metabolic pathway that leads to metabolic alkalosis.
- **Excessive water intake.** Drinking large amounts of water during vigorous exercise not only dilutes the stomach acid, but also stimulates the small intestine to prepare for incoming food from the stomach. An outpouring of strongly alkaline digestive enzymes into the lower gastrointestinal tract exacerbates any existing acid-base imbalance.
- **Nasogastric suctioning.** Removal of contents directly from the gastrointestinal tract eliminates acids from the body, resulting in alkalosis.
- **Excessive intake of alkaline substances.** Metabolic alkalosis can stem from excessive reliance on antacids or similar alkaline substances. This possibility is important to remember when assessing a patient with cardiac disease who reports having self-medicated for hours or days with over-the-counter antacids.

The respiratory system serves as the compensatory mechanism for metabolic alkalosis. Bradypnea develops to correct the diminished H^+ ion level by retaining carbon dioxide, thereby driving up levels of circulating acids.

Signs and symptoms of metabolic alkalosis include the following:

- Confusion
- Muscle tremors and cramps
- Bradypnea
- Hypotension

Cellular Injury

The manifestations of cellular injury or death depend on how many and which types of cells are damaged. Various processes may cause cellular injury:

- Hypoxia (lack of oxygen)
- Ischemia (lack of blood supply)
- Chemical injury
- Infectious injury
- Immunologic (hypersensitivity) injury
- Physical damage (mechanical injury)
- Inflammatory injury

YOU are the Provider — PART 2

You ask your partner to obtain a baseline oxygen saturation level and obtain measurements for baseline vital signs, and to include waveform capnography. While she is setting up her equipment, you ask the patient about his past medical history. With great difficulty, he replies, "Heart failure."

Recording Time: 1 Minute	
Appearance	Awake, in distress, anxious
Level of consciousness	Alert (oriented to person, place, and time)
Airway	Open
Breathing	Accelerated rate; accessory muscle use; productive cough
Circulation	Weak radial pulses; moist, pale, cool skin

3. How does the recruitment of accessory muscles facilitate breathing?
4. How might the productive cough help you identify the source of the patient's breathing difficulty?

Manifestations of cellular injury occur at the microscopic (structural) and functional levels. Common microscopic abnormalities (such as cardiac cell **necrosis** [a process in which the cell breaks down] as a result of long-standing hypoxemia) include cell swelling, rupture of cell membranes or nuclear membranes, and breakdown of nuclear material such as chromosomes **Figure 8-5**. This kind of damage often distorts the shape of a cell and disrupts its function. Functional disturbances may include inefficient oxygen utilization, intracellular acidosis, toxic waste accumulation, and derangement of nutrient metabolization.

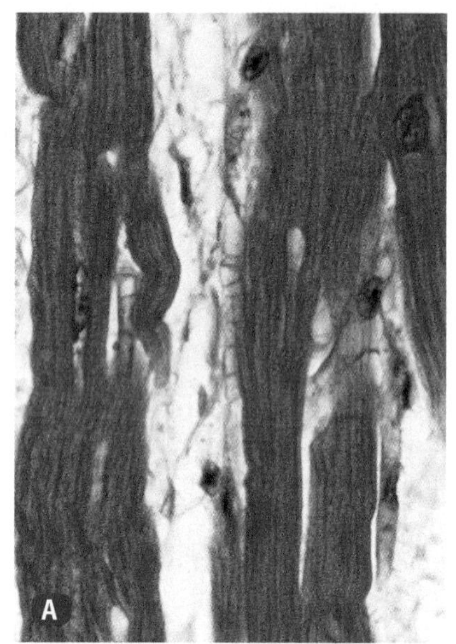

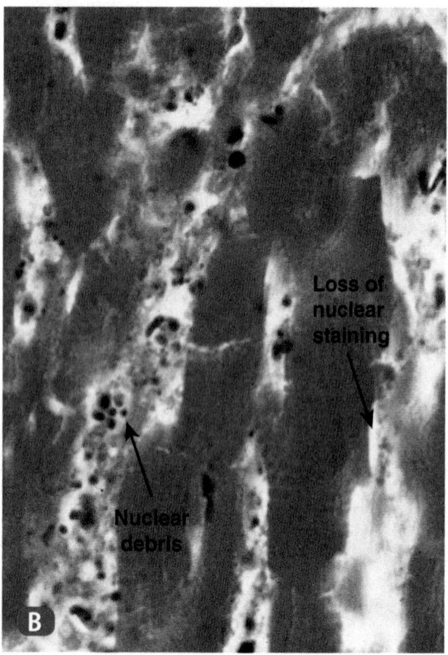

Figure 8-5 Comparison of cardiac muscle fibers **(A)** with necrotic fibers **(B)**. Note fragmentation of fibers, loss of nuclear staining, and fragmented bits of nuclear debris. Cellular injury causes swelling, resulting in nuclear membrane rupture and breakdown of the nuclear material (magnification ×400).

From *An Introduction to Human Disease*, 7th edition. Photo courtesy of Leonard V. Crowley, MD, Century College.

Changes in individual cells often affect the entire organism. In some cases, the changes are associated with only minor systemic abnormalities, such as fever. At other times, such as when renal failure occurs, entire organ systems collapse and the patient's condition becomes critical. Because all body systems are connected, dysfunction in one system inevitably affects the function of other systems, upsetting the homeostatic balance on which the body depends to sustain life.

With proper treatment, cellular injury can be repaired, up to a point; however, when irreversible injury occurs, treatment is futile. Cell death is followed by necrosis. The cell membrane becomes abnormally permeable, allowing an influx of electrolytes and fluids. Then the cell and its organelles swell, and lysosomes release enzymes that destroy intracellular components. These processes occur during and after cell death.

▶ Hypoxic Injury

Hypoxic injury is a common—and often deadly—cause of cellular injury. It may result from decreased amounts of oxygen in the air or loss of hemoglobin function (such as in carbon monoxide poisoning), a decreased number of red blood cells (as from bleeding), disease of the respiratory or cardiovascular system (such as COPD), or loss of cytochromes (mitochondrial proteins that convert oxygen to adenosine triphosphate [ATP], like that seen in cyanide poisoning).

Although hypoxia has deleterious effects on cells, the damage does not stop there. Cells that are hypoxic for more than a few seconds produce mediators (substances) that may damage areas near or far from the initial area of damage in the body. The result is a positive feedback cycle in which mediators lead to more cell damage, which leads to more hypoxia, which leads to further mediator production, and so forth.

The earliest and most dangerous mediators produced by cells in response to hypoxia are **free radicals**. A free radical molecule is missing one electron in its outer shell. The presence of an odd, unpaired electron causes chemical instability as free radicals randomly attack cells and membranes in an attempt to steal back the missing electron. The result is widespread and potentially deadly tissue damage.

▶ Chemical Injury

A variety of chemicals, including poisons, lead, carbon monoxide, ethanol, and pharmacologic agents, may injure and ultimately destroy cells. Common poisons include cyanide and pesticides. Cyanide induces cell hypoxia by blocking oxidative phosphorylation in the mitochondria and preventing the metabolism of oxygen. Pesticides block an enzyme, acetylcholinesterase, thereby preventing proper transmission of nerve impulses.

Long-term ingestion of lead, such as that caused by chewing on windowsills painted with lead-based paint, leads to brain injury and neurologic dysfunction. The ability of lead to substitute for calcium (molecules of lead and calcium are a similar size) is a common factor in many of its toxic actions. Most likely, lead occupies the space normally held for calcium in vital biochemical reactions, leading to abnormal results and dysfunction.

Carbon monoxide binds to hemoglobin more easily than does oxygen, preventing adequate oxygenation of the tissues. A low-level exposure of carbon monoxide causes nausea, vomiting, and headache. A higher level can be rapidly fatal.[9]

At lower doses, ethanol, as found in drinking alcohol, causes the well-known effects of inebriation. Higher doses produce severe CNS depression and hypoventilation, sometimes precipitating cardiovascular collapse.

Some pharmacologic agents produce toxic substances when the agents are metabolized in the body, especially in overdose conditions. For example, acute overdose occurs when an excessive dose of acetaminophen (Tylenol) is ingested. If an adult takes more than 7.5 g in a single dose, the toxins that accumulate can poison the liver and can be fatal.

▶ Infectious Injury

Infectious injury to cells occurs as a result of an invasion of bacteria, fungi, or viruses. Bacteria may cause injury by direct action on cells or by the production of toxins. Viruses often initiate an inflammatory response that leads to cell damage and patient symptoms.

Virulence measures the disease-causing ability of a microorganism. The pathogenicity of any particular microorganism is a function of its ability to reproduce and cause disease within the human body. In particular, the growth and survival of bacteria in the body depend on the effectiveness of the body's own defense mechanisms and on the bacteria's ability to resist the mechanisms. A depressed immune system is less capable of fighting off microorganisms that the body perceives as harmful; populations with weaker immune systems include newborn infants, older adults, people with diabetes, and people with cancer or other chronic diseases.

Bacteria

Many bacteria have a capsule that protects them from ingestion and destruction by **phagocytes**—cells (that is, white blood cells) that engulf and consume foreign material such as microorganisms and cellular debris **Figure 8-6**. However, not all bacteria are encapsulated. *Mycobacterium tuberculosis*, for example, lacks a capsule, yet stubbornly resists destruction; it can be transported by phagocytes throughout the body.

When cells are injured, circulating white blood cells are attracted to the site of injury. White blood cells release endogenous **pyrogens**, which then cause a fever to develop. Indeed, the body's most common reaction to the presence of bacteria is inflammation. Some bacteria have the ability to produce hypersensitivity reactions. The presence of bacteria in the blood is called bacteremia; septicemia (sepsis) is a systemic disease, which may be life threatening, and is caused by the proliferation of microorganisms (or related toxins) in the blood.

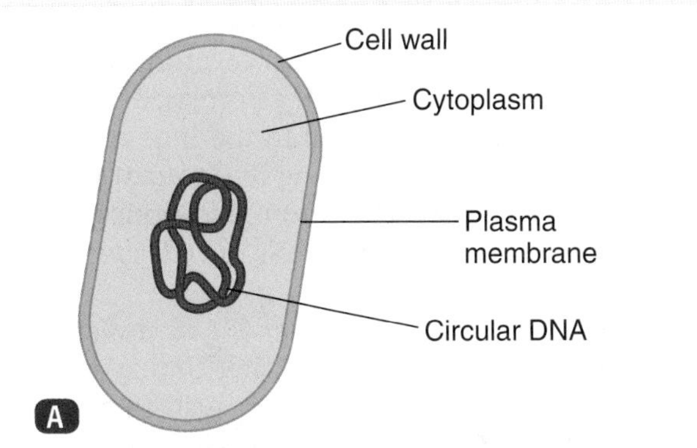

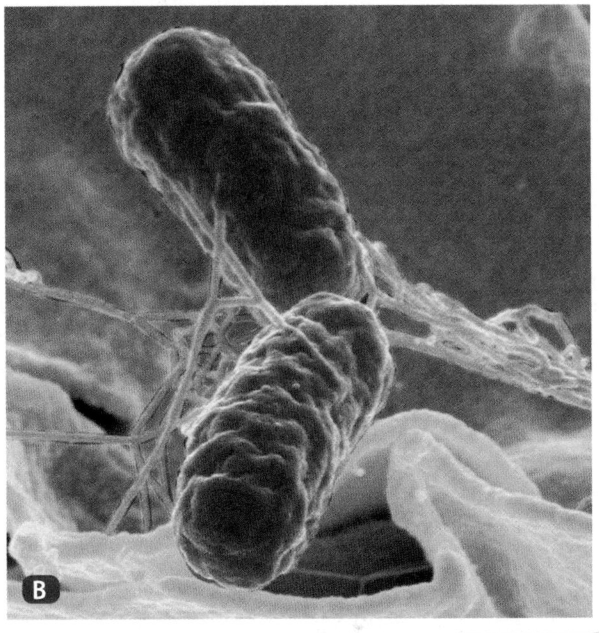

Figure 8-6 General structure of a bacterium. **A.** Bacteria come in many shapes and sizes, but all have a circular strand of deoxyribonucleic acid (DNA), cytoplasm, and a plasma membrane. A cell wall surrounds the membrane in many bacteria. **B.** An electron micrograph of *Salmonella* bacteria. Many bacteria have a capsule that protects them from ingestion and destruction by phagocytes.

A: © Jones & Bartlett Learning; B: Courtesy of Rocky Mountain Laboratory, NIAID, NIH.

Viruses

Viruses are among the most common causes of afflictions. Viruses are intracellular parasites that take over the metabolic processes of the host cell and use the cell to help them replicate. A virus consists of a nucleic acid core of ribonucleic acid (RNA) or deoxyribonucleic acid (DNA). Surrounding the viral core is a protein coat known as the capsid, which protects the virus from phagocytosis. Some viruses have an additional protective coat known as the envelope.

The replication of a virus occurs inside the host cell because viruses do not have their own organelles. Viral infection of a host cell leads to a decreased synthesis of macromolecules that are vital to the host cell. Viruses induce pathology by disrupting the normal metabolic processes, but are protected from antibiotics by living and replicating inside the host cell and effectively hiding from the medication.

A symbiotic relationship may exist between a virus and normal cells that allows the virus to persist without causing an active infection. Viruses such as the human immunodeficiency virus (HIV) can elicit a strong immune response, rapidly producing an irreversible, lethal injury in susceptible cells.

▶ Immunologic and Inflammatory Injury

Inflammation is a protective response occurring in the presence of cellular injury, including trauma, infection, and hypoxia. Infection is characterized by an invasion of microorganisms that causes cell or tissue injury, which leads to the **inflammatory response**. The inflammatory response can be triggered by an agent that is physical (heat or cold), chemical (such as concentrated acid or alkali or another caustic chemical), or microbiologic (such as a bacterium or virus). The inflammatory response is characterized by both local and systemic effects, as shown in **Figure 8-7** and discussed in detail later in this chapter.

Local effects consist of dilation (expansion) of blood vessels and increased vascular permeability. Leukocytes (white blood cells) are attracted to the site of injury. The leukocytes adhere to the endothelium of the small blood vessels, exert force to break through the cell walls, and migrate to the area of tissue damage. The characteristic signs of inflammation are heat, redness, tenderness, swelling, and pain. The increased warmth and redness of the inflamed tissues are caused by dilation of capillaries and slowing of blood flow through the vessels. Swelling occurs because the extravasation (leakage) of plasma from the dilated and more permeable vessels causes the volume of fluid in the inflamed tissue to increase. The tenderness and pain are secondary to irritation of sensory nerve endings at the site of the inflammatory process.

If the inflammatory process is severe, then systemic effects become evident. The person feels ill, and the body temperature is elevated. The bone marrow accelerates its production of leukocytes so the number of leukocytes circulating in the bloodstream increases; this increase in the number of leukocytes in the blood is called **leukocytosis**. The liver produces several proteins called acute phase proteins that are released into the bloodstream in response to tissue injury or inflammation, which help protect the body from the tissue injury caused by the inflammation. The best known of these proteins is called C-reactive protein, which is often measured to monitor the activity of diseases characterized by tissue inflammation.

The outcome of an inflammation response depends on the amount of tissue damage. If the inflammation is mild,

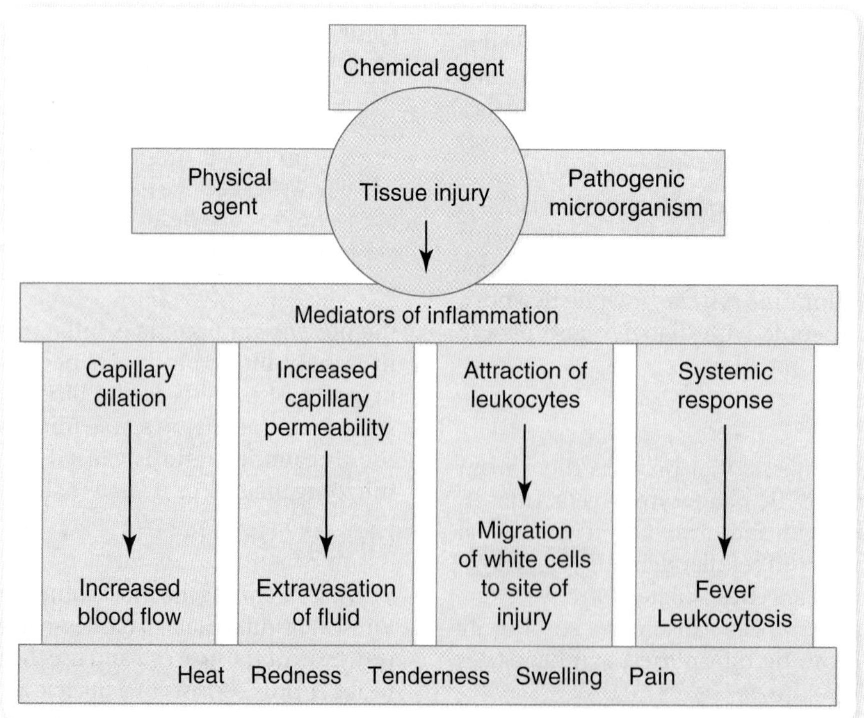

Figure 8-7 Local and systemic effects of tissue injury caused by various agents.

then it soon subsides, and the tissues return to normal. If the inflammatory process is more severe, then tissue is destroyed to some extent and must be repaired. During healing, damaged cells are replaced, and the framework of the injured tissue is repaired as an ingrowth of cells produces connective tissue fibers and new blood vessels. Scar tissue replaces large areas of tissue destruction. Sometimes, the scarring subsequent to a severe inflammation is so severe that function is seriously disturbed.

Cellular membranes may be injured when they come in direct contact with the cellular and chemical components of the immune or inflammatory process, such as phagocytes (neutrophils and macrophages), histamine, antibodies, and lymphokines. In such a case, potassium leaks out of the damaged cell and water flows inward, causing the cell to swell. The nuclear envelope, organelle membranes, and cell membrane may rupture, leading to cell death. The degree of swelling and chance of membrane rupture depend on the severity of the immune and inflammatory responses.

▶ Injurious Genetic Factors

Genetic factors that may damage cells include chromosomal disorders, premature development of atherosclerosis, and, sometimes, obesity. An abnormal gene may develop in a person in one of three ways: by mutation of the gene during meiosis, which affects the newly formed fetus; by heredity; or as a result of other causes later in life. In trisomy 21 (Down syndrome), the child is born with an extra chromosome 21. Rheumatoid arthritis has a genetic link as well.

▶ Injurious Nutritional Imbalances

Good nutrition is required to maintain good health and assist the cells in fighting disease. Injurious nutritional imbalances that can injure cells and the organism as a whole include obesity, malnutrition, vitamin excess or deficiency, and mineral excess or deficiency. These conditions can lead to alterations in physical growth, mental and intellectual retardation, and even death.

▶ Injurious Physical Agents or Conditions

Physical agents, such as heat, cold, and radiation, may also cause cell injury—for example, burns, frostbite, radiation sickness, and tumors. The degree of cell injury that results is determined by the strength of the agent and the length of exposure.

▶ Apoptosis

Apoptosis is normal cell death. It is unique in that it is genetically programmed into the cell as a part of normal development, organogenesis, immune function, and tissue growth. It has a normal role in aging, early development, menses, lactating breast tissue, thymus involution, and red blood cell turnover.

During apoptosis, cells exhibit characteristic nuclear changes, and they typically die in well-defined clusters rather than in a random manner. The molecular mechanism underlying apoptosis involves the activation of genes that encode for proteins known as caspases (*c*ysteine-*asp*artic prote*ases*). The production of these proteins essentially leads to cell suicide. Unlike in the case of cell death from disease processes, proteins and DNA undergo controlled degradation that allows their remnants to be taken up and reused by neighboring cells. In this way, apoptosis allows the body to eliminate a cell but recycle many of its components. Pathologically, areas that have undergone apoptotic death do not show any evidence of inflammation. In contrast, an inflammatory response is typically observed when cells undergo necrosis from hypoxia or cellular toxins.

Apoptosis can be activated prematurely by pathologic factors such as cell injury. This sort of premature stimulation, which occurs in some forms of heart failure, causes early cell death. Another example of pathologic apoptosis is the death of hepatocytes (liver cells) in patients with viral hepatitis. The dying cells form lumps of chromatin known as Councilman bodies. Inhibition of the normal course of apoptosis allows destructive cellular proliferation, such as in cancer and rheumatoid arthritis (uncontrolled synovial tissue proliferation). **Figure 8-8** illustrates the process by which cancerous cells develop from normal cells.

▶ Abnormal Cell Death

If the injury leading to cellular degeneration is of sufficient intensity and duration, then irreversible cell injury leads to cell death. *Necrosis* is the term for tissue death. Necrosis is the result of the morphologic changes that occur following cell death in living tissues. It may be simple necrosis or derived necrosis.

Simple necrosis refers to areas of necrosis where the gross and microscopic tissue and some of the cells are recognizable. It may be caused by acute ischemia, acute toxicity (such as from heavy metals), or direct physical injury (such as from caustic chemicals and burns).

Derived necrosis includes caseation necrosis, dry gangrene, fat necrosis, and liquefaction necrosis. Caseation necrosis is manifested by the loss of all features of the tissue and cells, so they come to resemble cheese when viewed through a microscope. Dry gangrene results from invasion and putrefaction of necrotic tissue, after the blood supply is compromised and the tissue undergoes coagulation necrosis. Fat necrosis results from the destruction of fat cells, usually by enzymes (such as pancreatic proteases and lipases). Liquefaction necrosis results from coagulation necrosis followed by conversion of tissues into a liquid form and invasion by putrefying bacteria that grow rapidly in a warm, moist environment; the bacteria produce lytic enzymes and gas.

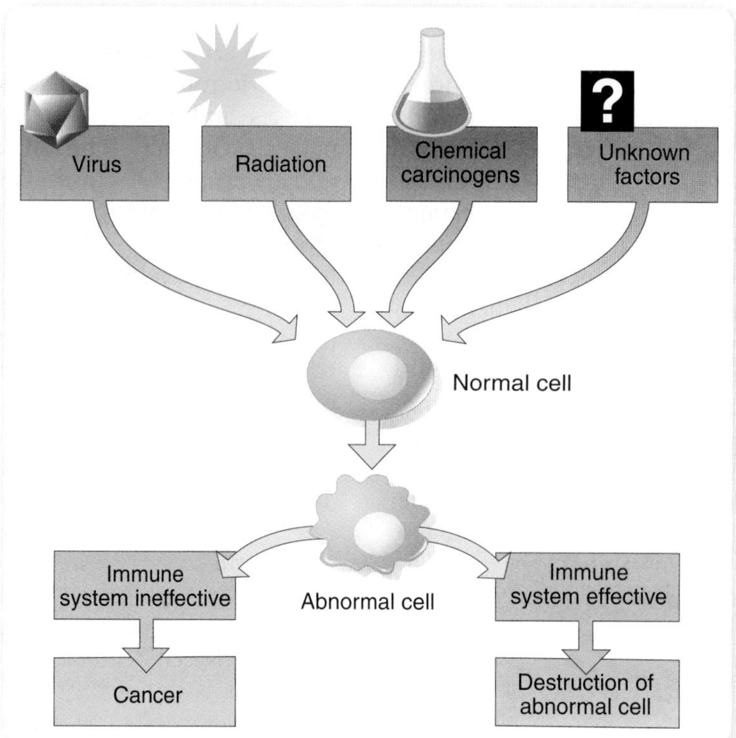

Figure 8-8 The onset of cancer. Viruses and other factors induce a normal cell to become abnormal. When the immune system is working effectively, it destroys the abnormal cells, so no cancer develops. When abnormal cells evade the immune system, they form a tumor and may become a spreading cancer.

Hypoperfusion

Perfusion is defined as the delivery of oxygen and nutrients and removal of wastes from the cells, organs, and tissues by the circulatory system. Adequate circulation depends on a pumping heart, intact vascular system, and an appropriate amount of oxygen-carrying blood. A deficiency in any of these areas will cause problems with perfusion. **Hypoperfusion** occurs when the level of tissue perfusion decreases below normal. It is important to evaluate a patient's level of organ perfusion during emergency medical care, especially in diagnosing shock.

When the body senses tissue hypoperfusion, it sets compensatory mechanisms into motion. In some cases, this action is sufficient to stabilize the patient's condition. At this point, the shock is called compensated shock. In other cases, the hypoperfusion overwhelms the normal compensatory mechanisms and the patient's condition progressively deteriorates; this is called decompensated (hypotensive) shock Table 8-3.

In response to hypoperfusion, the body releases catecholamines (epinephrine and norepinephrine), which produce increased strength of cardiac contraction (positive inotropy), increased pulse rate, vasoconstriction, and, consequently, increased systemic vascular resistance. In addition, the renin-angiotensin-aldosterone system is activated and antidiuretic hormone is released from the pituitary gland. Together, these actions trigger salt and water retention and peripheral vasoconstriction, thereby increasing the amount of fluid in the vascular space and improving blood pressure and cardiac output. Depending on the severity of the insult, variable amounts of fluid will shift from the interstitial tissues into the vascular compartment. The spleen also releases some red blood cells that are normally sequestered there to augment the oxygen-carrying capacity of the blood. The overall response of the initial compensatory mechanisms is to increase the preload (venous return), stroke volume, and heart rate to ensure adequate cardiac output. The result is usually an increase in cardiac output and myocardial oxygen demand.

As hypoperfusion persists, myocardial stress increases. Eventually, the above-normal compensatory mechanisms

Documentation & Communication

The terms *shock* and *hypoperfusion* are often used interchangeably; however, the terms are not synonymous. Localized hypoperfusion, such as from arterial occlusion, is not shock.

Table 8-3 Signs and Symptoms of Compensated and Decompensated Hypoperfusion (Shock)

Compensated	Decompensated
Agitation, anxiety, restlessness	Altered mental status (verbal to unresponsive)
Sense of impending doom	Hypotension
Weak, rapid (thready) pulse	Labored or irregular breathing
Clammy (cool, moist) skin	Thready or absent peripheral pulses
Pallor with cyanotic lips	Ashen, mottled, or cyanotic skin
Shortness of breath	Dilated pupils
Nausea, vomiting	Diminished urine output (oliguria)
Delayed capillary refill time in infants and children	Impending cardiac arrest
Thirst	
Normal blood pressure	

can no longer keep up with the increased oxygen demand. Myocardial function worsens, with decreased cardiac output and ejection fraction. Tissue perfusion decreases, leading to impaired cell metabolism. Often, the blood pressure decreases, especially in progressive hypoperfusion. Fluid may leak from the blood vessels, causing systemic and pulmonary edema. At this point, other signs of hypoperfusion may be present, such as dyspnea, dusky skin, low blood pressure, oliguria, and impaired mentation.

Shock is an abnormal state associated with inadequate oxygen and nutrient delivery to the metabolic apparatus of the cell, resulting in impairment of cellular metabolism and, ultimately, inadequate perfusion of vital organs. After a certain level of tissue hypoperfusion has been reached, cell damage proceeds in a similar manner regardless of the type of initial insult. Impairment of cellular metabolism prevents the body from properly using oxygen and glucose at the cellular level. Cells revert to anaerobic metabolism, which causes increased lactic acid production and metabolic acidosis, decreased oxygen affinity for hemoglobin, decreased ATP production, changes in cellular electrolyte levels, cellular edema, and release of lysosomal enzymes. Glucose impairment raises the level of blood glucose as catecholamines and cortisol are released. In addition, fat breakdown (lipolysis) with ketone formation may occur.

Types of Shock

Shock can occur as a result of inadequacy of the central circulation (the heart and the great vessels) or of the peripheral circulation (the remaining vessels, including the microscopic circulation—that is, arterioles, venules, and capillaries, as illustrated in Chapter 7, *The Human Body*). From a mechanistic approach, two types of shock are distinguished: central and peripheral. **Central shock** consists of cardiogenic shock and obstructive shock. **Peripheral shock** includes hypovolemic shock and distributive shock.

The following sections provide an overview of types of shock. These topics are also discussed in later chapters.

Central Shock

Cardiogenic Shock

Cardiogenic shock occurs when the heart cannot circulate enough blood to maintain adequate peripheral oxygen delivery. In the case of ischemic heart disease, this condition occurs when there is a loss of 40% or more of functioning myocardium. The most common cause of cardiogenic shock is myocardial infarction, as a single event or by cumulative damage. Other forms of cardiac dysfunction may also precipitate cardiogenic shock (such as a large ventricular septal defect or dysrhythmias; see Chapter 18, *Cardiovascular Emergencies*).

Obstructive Shock

Obstructive shock occurs when blood flow becomes blocked in the heart or great vessels. In **pericardial tamponade** Figure 8-9, diastolic filling of the right and left ventricles of the heart is impaired because of relatively large amounts of fluid in the pericardial sac surrounding the heart. Decreased ventricular filling associated with pericardial tamponade leads to a decrease in the cardiac output. Aortic dissection leads to a false lumen (aortic opening), with loss of normal blood flow Figure 8-10. A left atrial tumor may obstruct flow between the atrium

Words of Wisdom

Neurogenic shock can involve bradycardia if the injury is in the high thoracic region because of disruption in the sympathetic autonomic pathway. Cardiogenic shock can involve bradycardia when myocardial infarction is the cause and there is a disruption in the electrophysiologic pathway.

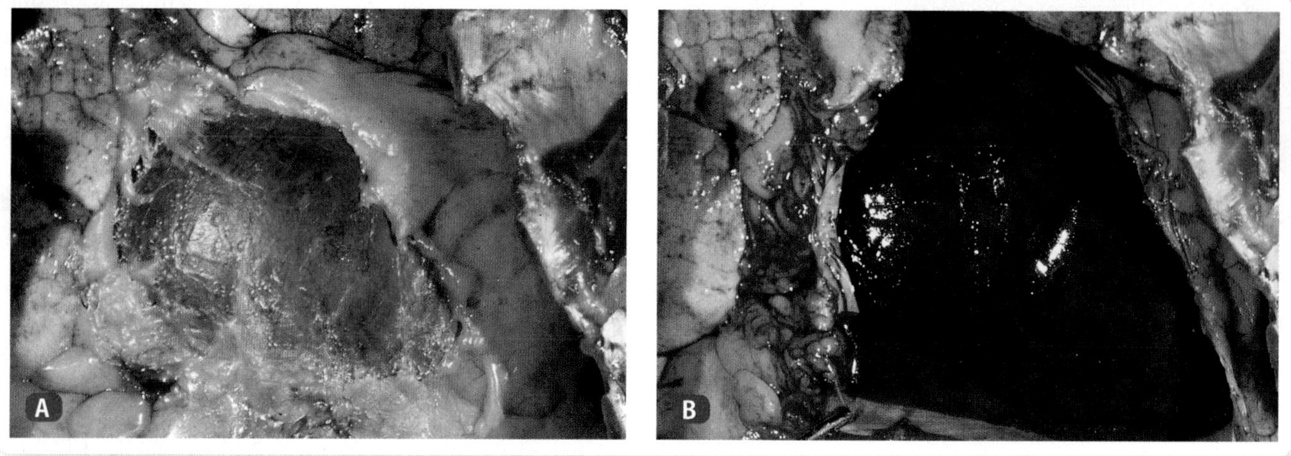

Figure 8-9 Cardiac tamponade following myocardial rupture. **A.** Distended pericardial sac. **B.** Pericardial sac opened, showing clotted blood surrounding the heart, which compressed the heart and prevented filling of the right ventricle in diastole.

Courtesy of Leonard V. Crowley, MD, Century College.

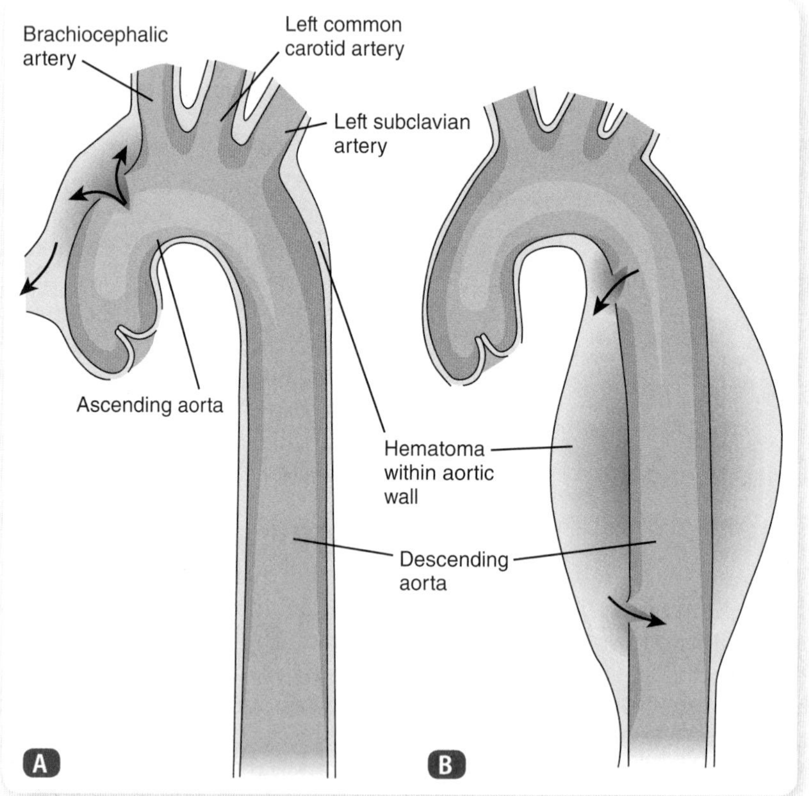

Figure 8-10 Sites of thoracic aortic dissection. **A.** A tear in the ascending aorta causes proximal and distal dissection. **B.** A tear in the descending aorta may cause extensive distal dissection.

and ventricle and decrease cardiac output. Obstruction of the superior or inferior vena cava (vena cava syndrome) decreases cardiac output by decreasing venous return. A large pulmonary embolus (blood clot in the lung) or a tension pneumothorax (lung collapse) may prevent adequate blood flow to the lungs, resulting in inadequate venous return to the left side of the heart.

▶ Peripheral Shock

Hypovolemic Shock

In **hypovolemic shock**, the circulating blood volume is insufficient to deliver adequate oxygen and nutrients to the body. Two types of hypovolemic shock—exogenous and endogenous—are possible, depending on where the fluid loss occurs. The most common type of exogenous hypovolemic shock is external bleeding (such as from an open wound); it may also result from loss of plasma volume caused by diarrhea or vomiting. Endogenous hypovolemic shock occurs when the fluid loss is contained within the body.

Distributive Shock

Distributive shock occurs when there is widespread dilation of the resistance vessels (small arterioles), the capacitance vessels (small venules), or both. The circulating blood volume then pools in the expanded vascular beds, and tissue perfusion decreases. The three most common types of distributive shock are anaphylactic shock, septic shock, and neurogenic shock.

Anaphylactic shock (also called anaphylaxis) occurs when histamine and other vasodilator proteins are released on exposure to an **allergen** (any substance that causes a hypersensitivity reaction). Anaphylactic shock is also accompanied by wheezing and **urticaria** (hives). The result is widespread vasodilation that causes distributive shock and blood vessels that continue to leak. Fluid leaks out of the blood vessels into the interstitial spaces, resulting in intravascular hypovolemia.

Septic shock occurs as a result of widespread infection, usually bacterial. Complex interactions occur between the bacterial invader and the body's defense systems. Initially, the body's own defense mechanisms may keep the infection at bay. If the normal immune mechanisms become overwhelmed, then the body produces a multitude of substances that cause vasodilation and decreased cardiac output. If left untreated, then the result is multiple organ dysfunction syndrome (discussed later) and often death.

> **Words of Wisdom**
>
> In anaphylaxis, interstitial fluid may cause substantial swelling. In some cases, this swelling may occlude the upper airway, resulting in a life-threatening condition manifesting as the adventitious sound of stridor. Recurrent large areas of subcutaneous edema of sudden onset, usually disappearing within 24 hours, are called angioedema. This condition is seen frequently as a result of allergy to food or drugs, such as angiotensin-converting enzyme inhibitors.

> **Words of Wisdom**
>
> Typically, the earliest signs of shock are restlessness and anxiety. The patient looks scared!

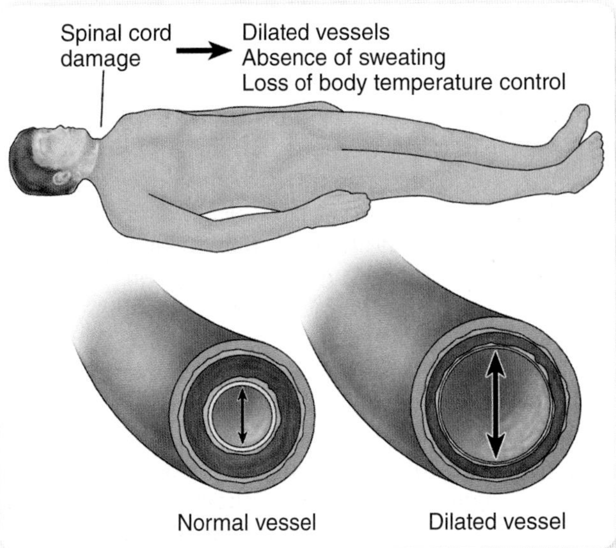

Figure 8-11 Damage to the spinal cord can cause substantial injury to the part of the nervous system that controls the size and muscle tone of blood vessels. If the smooth muscle in the blood vessels is cut off from its impulses to contract, then the vessels dilate widely, increasing the size and capacity of the vascular system. The blood in the body can no longer fill the enlarged vessels, which results in inadequate perfusion and neurogenic shock.

Neurogenic shock usually results from spinal cord injury. The effect is loss of normal sympathetic nervous system tone and vasodilation (Figure 8-11). Patients often have fluid-refractory hypotension as a result of the degree of vasodilation.

▶ Management of Shock

Most types of shock are characterized by reduced cardiac output, circulatory insufficiency, and rapid heartbeat. Although low blood pressure is classically associated with shock, it is a late sign, especially in children.

> **Words of Wisdom**
>
> A possible exception to the standard use of IV fluid therapy to treat shock is hypovolemic shock caused by ongoing bleeding. Permissive hypotension, in which the provider attempts to achieve an appropriate mental status and the presence of peripheral pulses, may be safer than attempting restoration of normotension, which may aggravate ongoing bleeding. As always, follow your local protocols.

Clinically, determining the presence or absence of shock requires you to evaluate the presence and volume of the peripheral pulses and assess end-organ perfusion and function. Strength of the peripheral pulses is related to stroke volume of the heart and pulse pressures. Peripheral pulses should be readily palpable if the person is not in shock, although cold environments or obesity may compromise the presence or strength of these pulses. Normal skin perfusion is indicated by warm, dry, pink extremities, fingers, and toes, whereas a slow, delayed, or prolonged **capillary refill time** indicates shock (although this technique is more reliable in children). To test the capillary refill time, briefly squeeze the toenail or fingernail, and then observe the time it takes for color to return. A normal capillary refill time is less than 2 seconds after blanching of the toe or finger, whereas a person in shock may have a capillary refill time of more than 2 seconds. Mottling, pallor, peripheral or central cyanosis, and delayed capillary refill may signal the presence of shock, whereas altered mental status indicates inadequate brain tissue perfusion. The accuracy of a capillary refill measurement decreases in patients older than 6 years; it is most useful in young children but not as useful in the adult population.

Measuring $ETCO_2$ may also be useful to the astute clinician. Although $ETCO_2$ provides valuable information regarding the respiratory and ventilatory status of the patient, you can also interpret the effectiveness of perfusion in your patient based on changes in capnography and capnometry. Carbon dioxide is one of the by-products of cellular metabolism, so decreasing levels of $ETCO_2$ are an early indicator of shock. Low levels of $ETCO_2$ combined with other signs and symptoms of shock such as hypotension and altered mental status are ominous clinical findings.

Treatment primarily addresses the underlying condition (see Chapter 27, *Bleeding*).

Multiple Organ Dysfunction Syndrome

Multiple organ dysfunction syndrome (MODS), first described in 1975, is a progressive condition that occurs in some critically ill patients. It is characterized by the concurrent failure of two or more organs or organ systems that were initially unharmed by the acute disorder or injury that caused the patient's initial illness. Six organ systems are surveyed in diagnosing MODS: respiratory, hepatic, renal, hematologic, neurologic, and cardiovascular. Each system is assigned a score to determine the patient's overall risk. For example, the Glasgow Coma Scale score is used to score the patient's neurologic system function. Although MODS may begin in one physiologic system, the disease process often progresses in a cyclical method, including multiple organ systems and complicating factors throughout its course.

In MODS, the overall mortality rate varies widely depending on the underlying etiology and ensuing diagnosis and treatment. Despite the inevitability its name suggests, the condition is often reversible, particularly in patients who were healthy before the physiologic insult occurred.[10] MODS is the major cause of death following sepsis, trauma, and burn injuries, with mortality rates of up to 70%.[10]

Primary MODS is a direct result of an insult, such as a pulmonary contusion from striking the chest on the steering wheel during a motor vehicle crash. Secondary MODS is a slower, more progressive organ dysfunction.

MODS occurs when injury or infection (septic shock) triggers a massive systemic immune, inflammatory, and coagulation response accompanied by the release of toxins that are present inside bacterial cells. Overactivating the complement system further increases inflammation and cellular damage. Vascular endothelial damage triggers overactivation of the coagulation system, which leads to uncontrolled coagulation in the venules and arterioles. This coagulation, in turn, causes microvascular thrombus formation and tissue ischemia. In addition, MODS activates the kallikrein-kinin system, stimulating the release of bradykinin, a potent vasodilator. Kallikrein is an inactive enzyme of the pancreas. When activated, kallikrein can dilate blood vessels, influence blood pressure, modulate salt and water excretion by the kidneys, and influence cardiac remodeling after acute myocardial infarction (AMI). Bradykinin increases vascular permeability, dilates blood vessels, contracts smooth muscle, and causes pain when injected into the skin. Vasodilation leads to tissue hypoperfusion and may also contribute to hypotension.

The net outcome of the activation of these systems is maldistribution of systemic and organ blood flow. Often, the body attempts to compensate for this problem by accelerating tissue metabolism. The result is an imbalance in oxygen supply and demand that causes tissue hypoxia, initiating a cascade of ill effects including tissue hypoperfusion, exhaustion of the cells' fuel supply (ATP), metabolic failure, lysosome breakdown, anaerobic metabolism, and acidosis and impaired cellular function.

Typically, MODS develops hours or days following resuscitation. The signs and symptoms include hypotension, insufficient tissue perfusion, uncontrollable bleeding (coagulopathy), and multisystem organ failure. A low-grade fever may develop from the inflammatory response, tachycardia, and dyspnea. Patients may also be difficult to oxygenate because of acute lung injury and acute respiratory distress syndrome.

During a 14- to 21-day period, renal and liver failure can develop in patients with MODS, along with collapse of the gastrointestinal and immune systems. The kidneys depend on adequate perfusion pressure. After the mean arterial pressure drops, kidney function decreases. Oliguria occurs early in shock. Renal studies show elevated blood urea nitrogen and creatinine levels. Many patients require continuous bedside dialysis.

The liver is a complex organ with a key role in excreting wastes and toxins. Adequate liver function is also essential for the synthesis of blood proteins and coagulation proteins, as well as the storage of glycogen, iron, and vitamins. Patients with MODS have elevated levels of total bilirubin and of the liver enzymes aspartate aminotransferase and alanine aminotransferase. Unfortunately, there are no definitive treatments for liver failure. Treatment focuses on minimizing the effects of liver damage.

The brain, adrenal glands, and heart are also affected early in MODS. The level of consciousness deteriorates quickly in hypoxic states, but it declines precipitously in patients with MODS. Cerebral hypoxia and subsequent ischemia can cause permanent deficits as a result of anoxic brain injury.

As the heart struggles to maintain arterial perfusion pressure, it too becomes hypoxic. Hypotension cannot be controlled despite the administration of fluids and vasopressors. Compensatory tachycardia consumes even more oxygen, and dysrhythmias such as bradycardia, ventricular tachycardia, and ventricular fibrillation develop. Cardiovascular collapse and death typically occur within days to weeks of the initial insult.

The Body's Self-Defense Mechanisms

The **immune system** includes all structures and processes associated with the body's defense against foreign substances and disease-causing agents. The body has three lines of defense: anatomic barriers, the inflammatory response, and the immune response.

▶ Anatomic Barriers

Several anatomic barriers decrease the chances of foreign substances invading the body. The skin serves as a major deterrent. Hairs in the upper respiratory tract (the nose) and the lining of the lower respiratory tract (cilia-covered epithelial cells) help repel foreign matter, especially small particles and some bacteria. Acid in the stomach prevents many infectious agents from entering the body via the gastrointestinal tract.

▶ Immune Response

The **immune response** is the body's defense reaction to any substance it recognizes as foreign. This response is often directed toward invading microbes, such as bacteria or viruses. It is also triggered by foreign bodies, such as a splinter, and even abnormal cell growths, such as tumors. The immune response involves only one type of white blood cells, called lymphocytes.

Not all invaders can be destroyed by the body's immune system. In some cases, the best compromise the body can reach is to control the damage and keep the invader from spreading. Often, the immune system succeeds in preventing severe disease following infection. When the normal systems become overwhelmed or fail, serious disease occurs.

The body responds to different kinds of immune challenges in remarkably similar ways. Although the details depend on the particular challenge, the basic pattern is the same—the innate response starts first and is then reinforced by the more specific acquired response. These two pathways are interconnected.

Consider what happens when bacteria enter the body. If the bacteria are not encapsulated, then macrophages

YOU are the Provider PART 3

Your partner is administering high-flow oxygen, attaching the $ETCO_2$, assessing vital signs, and setting up an IV line. You auscultate lung sounds and hear little air movement. You hear coarse crackles (rales) bilaterally in all fields. The patient coughs, and you notice pink, frothy sputum. You ask your partner to assess the medications on the side table while you establish the IV line.

Recording Time: 2 Minutes	
Respirations	22 breaths/min; shallow
Pulse	110 beats/min
Skin	Cool, moist, and pale
Blood pressure	140/90 mm Hg
Oxygen saturation (Spo_2)	89% before high-flow oxygen administration
Pupils	Pupils Equal, Round, and Reactive to Light and Accommodation (PERRLA)

5. On the basis of what you know about physiology, what is causing the pink, frothy sputum?
6. How do you account for the decreased Spo_2 level?

begin immediately to ingest the bacteria. If the bacteria are encapsulated, then antibodies (opsonins) must coat the capsule before it can be ingested by phagocytes.

Components of the cell wall then activate the complement system. Some components of the activated complement system, termed **chemotaxins**, attract leukocytes from the circulation to help fight the infection. The complement cascade ends with the formation of a set of proteins called the **membrane attack complex**. These molecules insert themselves into the bacterial membrane, weakening those areas in the membrane. Ions and water enter the cell through the weakened areas, leading to lysis of the bacterium (a chemical process that does not involve immune cells).

If antibodies to the bacteria are already present in the body, then these antibodies will assist the innate response by acting as opsonins and neutralizing bacterial toxins. Although it often takes several days, memory B cells attracted to the infection site will be activated if a recognized antigen is encountered. If the infection is new to the body—that is, preexisting antibodies are not present—then B cells will be activated. Combined with **helper T cells** and cytokine release, antibodies are produced and memory B and T cells are formed.

Table 8-4 describes the types of immune system cells.

Characteristics of the Immune Response

The native and acquired immune responses protect the body from infectious agents such as viruses and bacteria and from foreign substances that have gained access to the body through the skin or the lining of internal organs.

Natural immunity, also called native immunity, is a nonspecific cellular and humoral (antibody) response that operates as the first line of defense against pathogens. Most natural immunity is associated with the initial inflammatory response.

Table 8-4 Immune System Cells

Type of Cell	Description
Basophil	A type of white blood cell that releases histamine during inflammation.
Eosinophil	A type of white blood cell that phagocytizes the antigen-antibody complex; attacks parasites.
Neutrophil	A type of white blood cell that phagocytizes bacteria.
Monocyte	A type of white blood cell that phagocytizes bacteria, dead cells, and cellular debris.
Lymphocyte	A type of white blood cell involved in immune protection; attacks cells directly or produces antibodies.
Macrophage	White blood cells within tissues; produced by differentiation of monocytes. Functions include phagocytosis and stimulating lymphocytes and other immune cells to respond to pathogens; one of the first lines of defense in the inflammatory process.
Mast cells	Cells that are found in the connective tissues, beneath the skin, in the gastrointestinal mucosa, and in the mucosal membranes of the respiratory system. Functions relate to allergic reactions, immunity, and wound healing.
Plasma cells	White blood cells that develop from B cells and produce large volumes of specific antibodies.
B cells (B lymphocytes)	Cells that mature in the bone marrow, where they differentiate into memory cells or immunoglobulin-secreting (antibody) cells. Functions include eliminating bacteria, neutralizing bacterial toxins, preventing viral reinfection, and producing immediate inflammatory response.
Helper B cell	A type of regulator cell that activates B cells to produce antibodies.
Memory B cell	A type of B cell that aids in the quick response to subsequent exposures to an antigen because memory cells recall the antigen as foreign. These cells rapidly produce antibodies.
T cells (T lymphocytes)	Cells that are produced in the bone marrow and mature in the thymus. Two major types work to destroy antigens—regulator cells and effector cells.
Killer T cell	A type of T cell that destroys cells infected with viruses by releasing lymphokines that destroy cell walls; also called cytotoxic or effector cells.

Acquired immunity (also called adaptive immunity) is a highly specific, inducible, discriminatory method by which armies of cells respond to an immune stimulant, such that the immune system will never fail to recognize the same stimulant when it is subsequently encountered, even years later. It arises when the body is exposed to a foreign substance or disease and produces antibodies to the invader. Passively acquired immunity is the receipt of preformed antibodies to fight or prevent infection. Examples of passively acquired immunity include the transplacental passage of antibodies and the passage of antibodies in colostrum (the mother's initial breast milk to her infant), which protects the infant until his or her immune system matures sufficiently to take over. The injection of immunoglobulin (a concentrated form of antibodies obtained from donors) is also a form of passively acquired immunity.

The primary (initial) immune response takes place during the first exposure to an **antigen** (a foreign substance; a neoantigen is an antigen associated with cancerous cells). Clinical symptoms may not be apparent. Sometimes, the body's initial response is to produce an antibody that triggers symptoms on subsequent exposures. The secondary (amnestic) immune response occurs with reexposure to a foreign substance. The body has already developed a sort of memory for that substance, so a reaction occurs on reexposure to the substance.

An **antibody** binds a specific antigen so the complex can attach itself to specialized immune cells that ingest the complex to destroy it or release biologic mediators such as histamine to induce an allergic or inflammatory response. The specific features of the antigen-antibody interaction depend on the foreign substance involved **Figure 8-12**.

An **immunogen** is an antigen capable of generating an immune response. Thus, an immunogen is an antigen, but an antigen is not necessarily an immunogen. Antigens and immunogens can be categorized by size. Proteins, polysaccharides, and nucleic acids are larger, whereas amino acids, monosaccharides, and fatty acids are smaller.

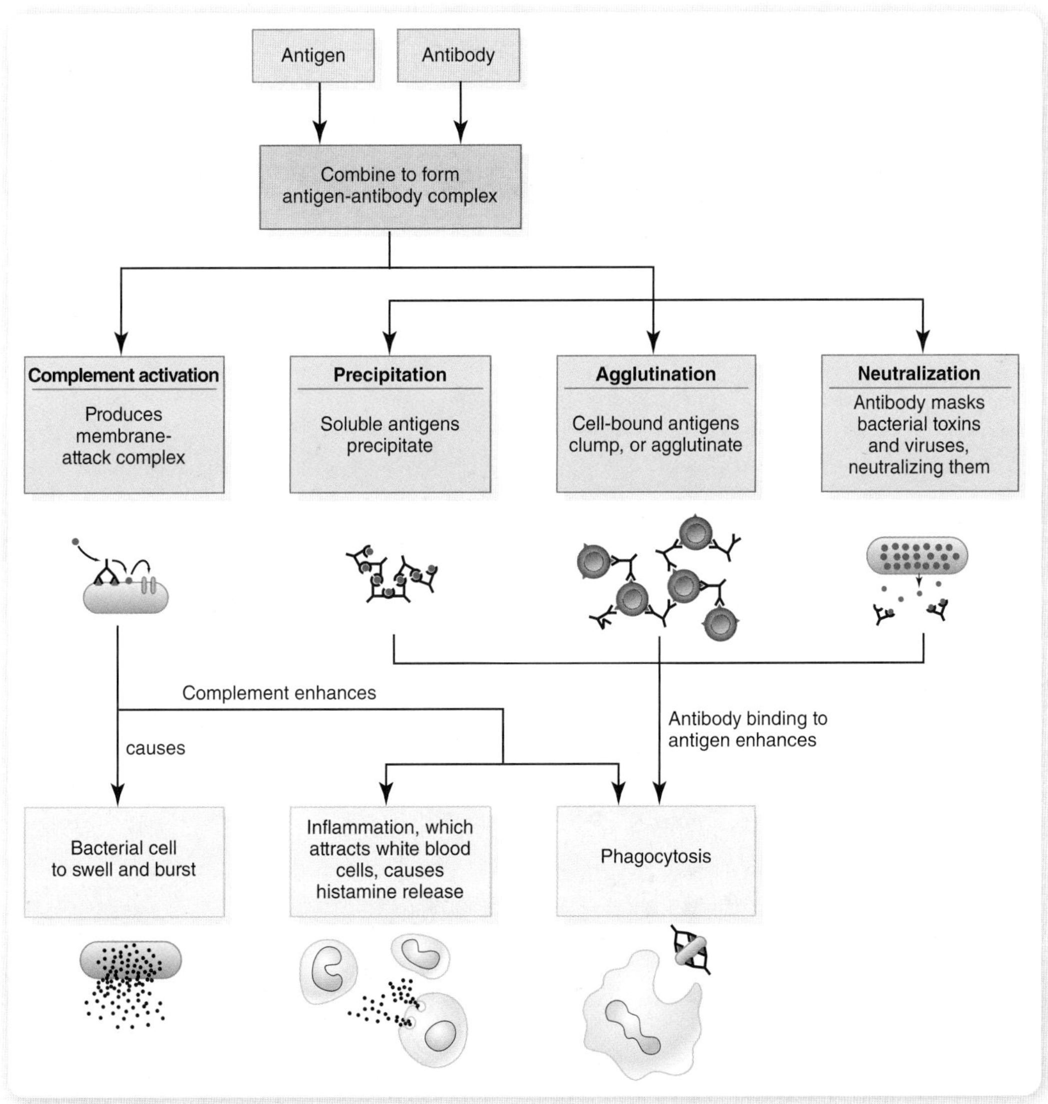

Figure 8-12 How antibodies work.

A **hapten** is a substance that normally does not stimulate an immune response but that can be combined with an antigen and, at a later time, initiate a specific antibody response on its own.

Humoral Immune Response

In **humoral immunity**, B-cell lymphocytes produce antibodies called immunoglobulins, which recognize a specific antigen and then react with it, as shown in **Figure 8-13**.

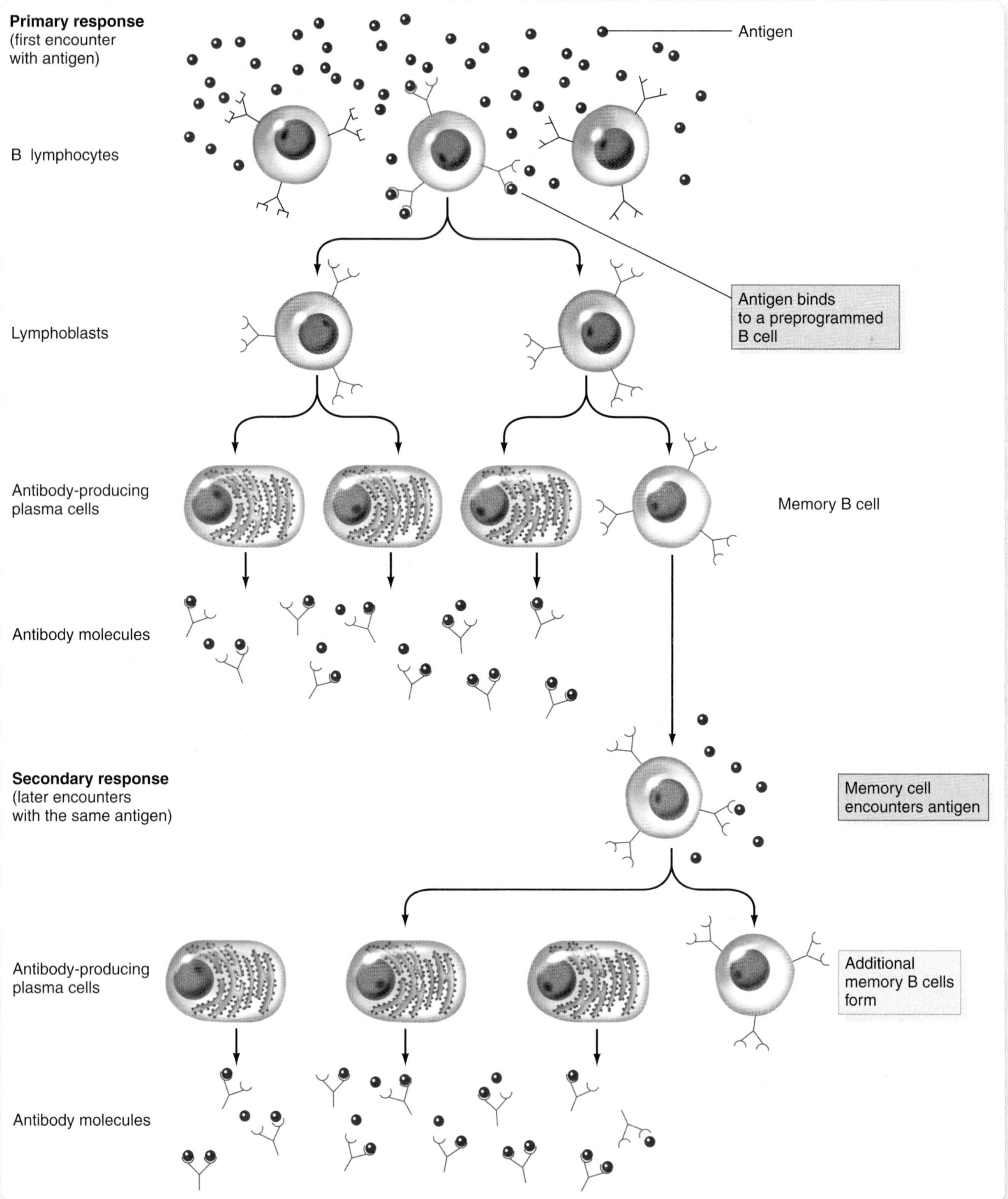

Figure 8-13 B-cell activation. Immunocompetent B cells are stimulated by the presence of an antigen, producing an intermediate cell, the lymphoblast. The lymphoblasts divide, producing plasma cells and some memory B cells. Memory B cells respond to subsequent antigen encroachment, yielding a rapid secondary response.

This differs from cell-mediated immunity, discussed later, in which macrophages and T cells attack and destroy pathogens or foreign substances.

B Lymphocytes. Like all blood cells, B cells are born in the bone marrow, where they are descended from stem cells. The clonal selection theory holds that each B cell makes antibodies that have only one type of antigen-binding region and, therefore, are specific for a particular antigen, known as the cognate antigen. Antibodies are found on the surface of B cells, where they are able to recognize the presence of their cognate antigens. When a B cell recognizes the cognate antigen, it proliferates to make more identical B cells in an exponential manner, each of which can make antibodies that recognize the same antigen.

For B cells to produce antibodies, B cells must first be activated. The most common way this occurs is via helper T cells **Figure 8-14**:

1. A macrophage engulfs the antigen via phagocytosis. It digests the antigen, pushing the discarded particles to the cell surface. These remnants interact with the B cell and a helper T cell.
2. The antigen binds to the B cell and the helper T cell, activating both.
3. The activated helper T cell secretes a lymphokine, a substance that stimulates the B cells to produce a clone. A clone is a group of identical cells formed from the same parent cell. The clone comprises two types of identical cells that have different functions: plasma cells, which make the antibodies, and memory cells, which "remember" the initial encounter with the antigen.

The human body distinguishes between foreign substances and its own cells and tissues by means of the major histocompatibility complex, a group of genes located on a single chromosome that permits a person who is capable of generating an immune response to distinguish *self* from *nonself* (namely, what is foreign). The human leukocyte antigen gene complex is the human

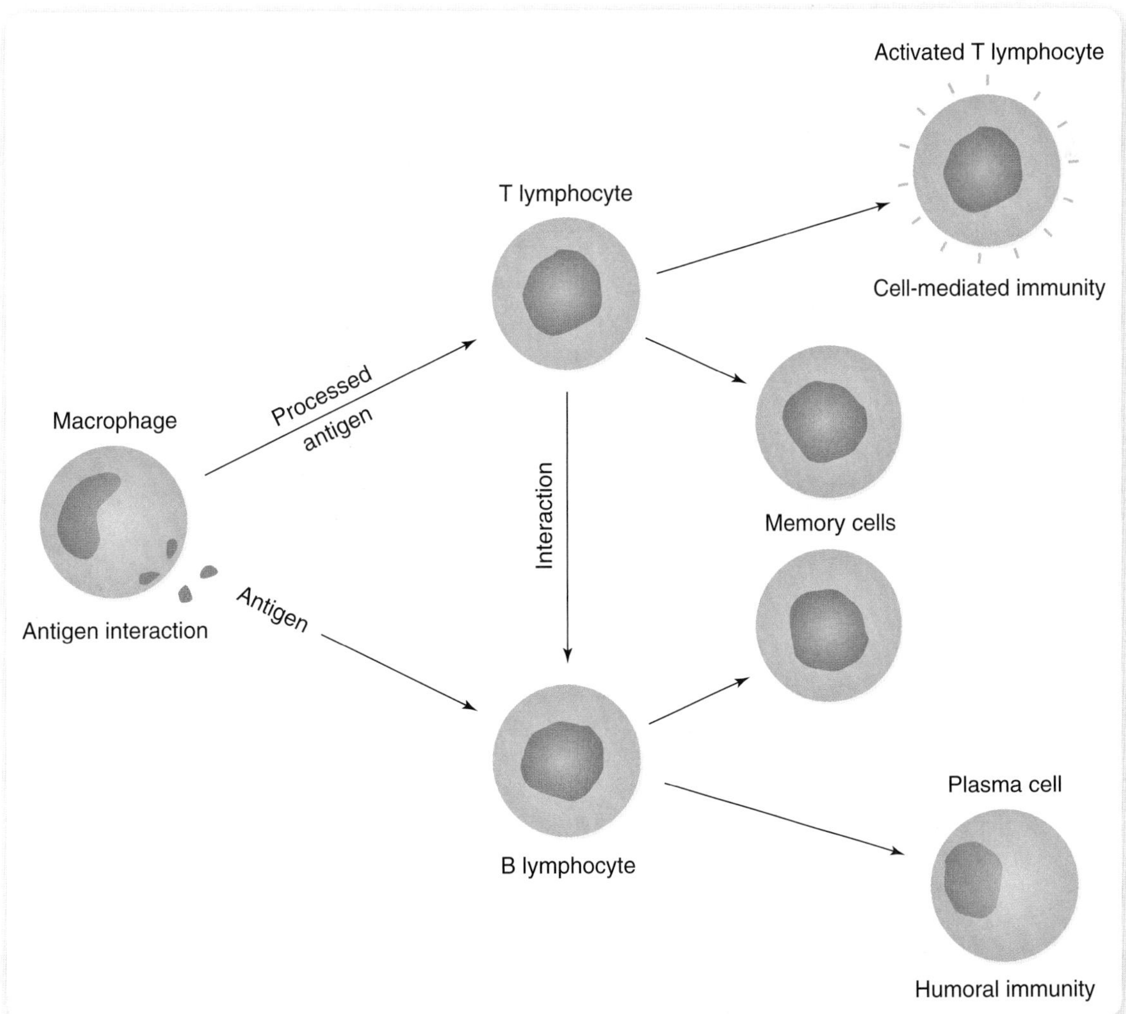

Figure 8-14 Interaction of cell-mediated and humoral immunity. A macrophage presents processed antigen fragments to the T lymphocyte. The B lymphocyte processes the intact antigen and displays fragments of the same antigen on its cell membrane. The T lymphocyte, which has responded to the same antigen, stimulates the B lymphocyte to proliferate, mature into plasma cells, and make antibodies.

major histocompatibility complex and is present in all nucleated human cells. It encodes for numerous antigens that are unique to a person. When the immune system encounters these particular antigens, it recognizes them as self, and no immune response occurs.

Immunoglobulins. The antibodies secreted by B cells are called **immunoglobulins** (this text uses the terms *immunoglobulins* and *antibodies* interchangeably, unless otherwise stated). These Y-shaped proteins consist of a crystallizable fragment (Fc) portion and two antigen-binding fragment (Fab) regions that bind only a specific antigen. The basic antibody molecule has four chains linked into a Y shape. Each side of the Y is identical, with one light chain attached to one heavy chain **Figure 8-15**. The two arms, or Fab regions, contain antigen-binding sites. The stem, or Fc region, determines which of the five immunoglobulin classes an antibody belongs to **Figure 8-16**.

Most antibodies are found in the plasma. Antibodies make up about 20% of the plasma proteins in a healthy person. Antibodies make antigens more visible to the immune system in three ways:

- Antibodies act as opsonins. In **opsonization**, an antibody coats an antigen to facilitate its recognition by immune cells. Antibodies are not toxic, but they label antigens so other immune cells will attack them.

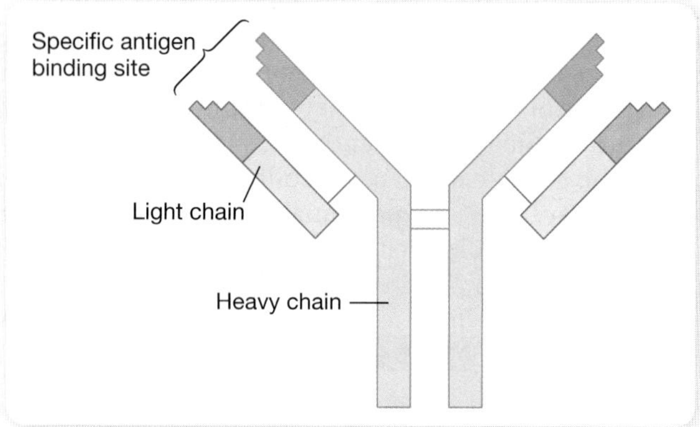

Figure 8-15 Structure of an immunoglobulin molecule.

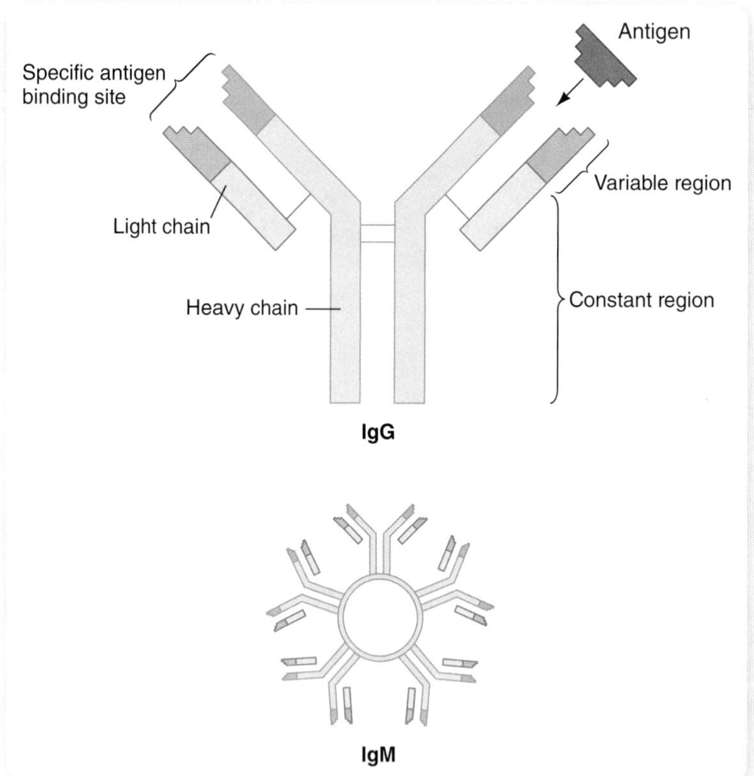

Figure 8-16 General structure of an antibody. Note that immunoglobulin G (IgG) is a monomer; it is one molecule. Immunoglobulin M (IgM) is a pentamer; it is a cluster of five antibodies and is effective in combining with foreign antigens. Also note that the antigen fits exactly into the antigen binding site (if it did not, it would not be able to bind). Antigen binding sites therefore have different structures, depending on the antigen to which they are designed to bind.

Table 8-5 General Classes of Immunoglobulins

Class	Description
IgG	The most common immunoglobulin. Accounts for 75% of the antibodies in the blood. Found in lymph, synovial fluid, peritoneal fluid, cerebrospinal fluid, and breast milk. IgG is the only immunoglobulin that crosses the placenta, giving infants immunity during the first few months of life.
IgA	Accounts for 15% of the antibodies in the blood. Also found in tears, saliva, respiratory tract secretions, and the stomach. IgA combines with a protein in the mucosa and defends body surfaces against invading microorganisms.
IgM	Accounts for 5% to 10% of the antibodies in the blood and is the dominant antibody in ABO (blood type) incompatibilities. IgM is the initial antibody formed in most infections.
IgE	Accounts for less than 1% of the antibodies in the blood and is associated with allergic reactions. When mast cell receptors combine with IgE and antigen, the mast cells degranulate and release chemical mediators such as histamine.
IgD	Accounts for less than 1% of the antibodies in the blood. The physiologic role of IgD is unclear.

- Antibodies cause antigens to clump for easier phagocytosis.
- Antibodies bind to and inactivate some toxins produced by bacteria. Macrophages can then ingest and destroy the inactivated toxins.

Antibodies are divided into five general classes of immunoglobulins Table 8-5.

Cell-Mediated Immune Response

Cell-mediated immunity is characterized by the formation of a population of lymphocytes that can attack and destroy foreign material. It is the main defense against viruses, fungi, parasites, and some bacteria. Cell-mediated immunity is the mechanism by which the body rejects transplanted organs and eliminates the abnormal cells that sometimes arise spontaneously in cell division.

In cell-mediated immunity, T-cell lymphocytes recognize antigens and contribute to the immune response in two major ways: (1) by secreting cytokines that attract other cells or (2) by becoming cytotoxic and killing infected or abnormal cells. There are five subgroups of T cells:

1. **Killer T cells.** Killer T cells (also called cytotoxic T cells) destroy the antigen. Killer T cells help rid the body of cells that have been infected by viruses and cells that have been transformed into cancer cells. Killer T cells are also responsible for the rejection of tissue and organ grafts.
2. **Helper T cells.** Helper T cells activate many immune cells, including B cells and other T cells (also called T4 or $CD4^+$ cells).
3. **Suppressor T cells.** Suppressor T cells (also called T8 or $CD8^+$ cells) suppress the activity of other lymphocytes so they do not destroy normal tissue.
4. **Memory T cells.** Memory T cells remember the reaction for the next time it is needed.
5. **Lymphokine-producing cells.** Secreted by lymphocytes, these cells work to damage cells; for example, lymphokines destroy cells that have been infected with a virus.

During the cell-mediated response, macrophages ingest pathogens. When a macrophage digests a pathogen, it releases small particles of antigen. This antigen pushes its way to the macrophage surface, where it is recognized by specific T cells. Other T cells, such as helper T cells and killer T cells, bind to the antigen and macrophage, destroying the invader.

Special Populations

T-cell and B-cell function is often deficient in older adults. Depressed lymphocyte function is accompanied by a decrease in macrophage activity. Therefore, older adults are more susceptible to infections and recover more slowly. In addition, older adults have an increased level of **autoantibodies** (antibodies directed against the self), which partly explains why older adults are susceptible to autoimmune disease.

▶ Inflammatory Response

The inflammatory response is a response of the tissues of the body to irritation or injury. It is characterized by pain, swelling, redness, and heat. White blood cells of various types are a major component of this response.

The inflammatory reaction and the immune response are independent processes, although the processes often occur simultaneously. Inflammation can be present without activation of the immune response, and vice versa. Inflammation is a dynamic process that, when initiated, triggers a complex cascade involving local and systemic events. The two most common causes of inflammation are infection (such as bacterial or viral) and injury.

Acute Inflammation

The acute inflammatory response involves vascular and cellular components. Initially, the arterioles constrict in an attempt to limit blood loss, but then dilate, allowing an influx of blood under increased pressure. This leads to increased intravascular pressure and causes the blood vessel to expand; as in a balloon that is being inflated, the vessel walls become thinner. The higher pressure combined with increased vessel wall permeability causes fluid to leak into the interstitial spaces (edema). When enough fluid has escaped into the surrounding area and the intravascular pressure has been released, the vessel wall contracts and the flow slows, leading to pooling of blood in the capillaries.

A variety of blood cells participate in tissue inflammatory reactions: white blood cells (leukocytes), platelets, mast cells, and plasma cells (B lymphocytes that create antibodies). Specific cell types include neutrophils, monocytes, lymphocytes, eosinophils, basophils, and activated platelets. Chemical mediators, primarily produced by the mast cells, account for the vascular and cellular events that occur during the acute inflammatory response. Cell-derived mediators include histamine, arachidonic acid derivatives, and cytokines such as interleukins and tumor necrosis factor.

> **Words of Wisdom**
>
> Since corticosteroids can decrease the initial inflammatory response, which is a necessary part of wound healing, this can increase the risk of wound infection. This is an important consideration when obtaining the history of patients with diabetes because of their propensity to develop infections in inadequately healing wounds.

Mast Cells. Mast cells have a major role in inflammation. During inflammation, mast cells degranulate and release a variety of substances. The primary stimuli for the degranulation of mast cells during the inflammatory response are physical injury (trauma), chemical agents (for example, bacterial toxins), and immunologic substances (for example, interaction of an antigen and an immunoglobulin E (IgE) antibody).

After degranulation, mast cells release **vasoactive amines**. The most important of these substances, **histamine** and **serotonin**, increase vascular permeability, cause vasodilation, and can cause bronchoconstriction, nausea, and vomiting. Because histamine is a preformed vasodepressor amine stored in mast cells, it can be released quickly, so its actions are seen early in the inflammatory response. Mast cells also synthesize chemotactic factors that attract neutrophils (neutrophil chemotactic factor) and eosinophils (eosinophilic chemotactic factor).

Mast cells also synthesize leukotrienes. **Leukotrienes**—also known as slow-reacting substances of anaphylaxis—are a family of biologically active compounds derived from arachidonic acid. The clinically important leukotrienes participate in host defense reactions and pathophysiologic conditions that AEMTs commonly see in the field, such as immediate hypersensitivity and inflammation. Leukotrienes have potent actions on many parts of the body, including the cardiovascular, pulmonary, immune, and central nervous systems and the gastrointestinal tract.

Leukotrienes are primarily endogenous mediators of inflammation. They contribute to the signs and symptoms seen in acute inflammatory responses, including responses resulting from the interaction of allergens with IgE antibodies on mast cells. Certain leukotrienes are bronchoconstrictors, stimulate airway mucus secretion, and are very effective at increasing the permeability of postcapillary venules (including those in the bronchial circulation), thereby causing plasma protein exudation (oozing out of the tissue) and edema. Certain leukotrienes may also promote eosinophil migration into the airways of animals and people with asthma, and they may also increase bronchial hyperresponsiveness through an action on sensory nerves.

Finally, mast cells synthesize **prostaglandins**. These substances, which are derived from arachidonic acid, comprise a group of about 20 lipids that are composed of modified fatty acids attached to a five-member ring. Prostaglandins are found in many vertebrate tissues, where they act as messengers in reproduction, the inflammatory response to infection, and pain perception. Aspirin and nonsteroidal anti-inflammatory drugs inhibit prostaglandin synthesis, reducing inflammation and pain.

Plasma Protein Systems. There are plasma-derived mediators that modulate the inflammatory process; these are called plasma protein systems. They include the complement system, the coagulation (clotting) system, and the kinin system. The interaction of these systems is vital to a normal inflammatory response. Each system consists of a cascade of biochemical reactions such that as one compound is produced, it catalyzes the formation of the next compound—similar to knocking over a line of dominoes.

- **Complement system.** The **complement system** is a group of plasma proteins that attract white blood cells to sites of inflammation, activate white blood cells, and directly destroy cells. The central compound in this complement cascade is called C3.
- **Coagulation system.** The **coagulation system** serves a vital role in the formation of blood clots in blood vessels. Inflammation triggers the coagulation cascade, initiating a complex series of reactions that encourage fibrin formation. **Fibrin** is the protein that polymerizes (bonds) to form the fibrous component of a blood clot. The various coagulation factors are counterbalanced by a variety of inhibitors, so the coagulation

is restricted to one area. Simultaneously, the **fibrinolysis cascade** is activated to dissolve the fibrin and create fibrin split products (namely, fragments of the dissolving clot).

- **Kinin system.** The **kinin system** leads to the formation of the vasoactive protein bradykinin from kallikrein. Kallikrein is an enzyme that is normally found in blood plasma, urine, and body tissue in an inactive state. When kallikrein becomes activated, it can dilate blood vessels, influence blood pressure, modulate salt and water excretion by the kidneys, and influence cardiac remodeling after AMI. Bradykinin increases vascular permeability, dilates blood vessels, contracts smooth muscle, and causes pain when injected into the skin.

Cellular Components of Inflammation. The goal of the cellular components of the acute inflammatory response is for inflammatory cells—namely, **polymorphonuclear neutrophils (PMNs)**—to arrive at the sites in the tissue where they are needed. This process involves two major stages: an intravascular phase and an extravascular phase. During the intravascular phase, leukocytes move to the sides of blood vessels and attach to the endothelial cells. During the extravascular phase, leukocytes travel outside of the blood vessels to the site of inflammation and kill organisms. The cellular event sequence is as follows:

1. **Margination.** Loss of fluid from the blood vessels into the inflamed or infected tissue gives the blood that remains in the vessels increased viscosity, which slows the flow of blood and produces stasis. PMNs, which usually travel toward the center of the vessel, settle toward the sides as the blood flow slows. As stasis develops, leukocytes also move (marginate) toward the sides of the vessels, where they bump into the endothelial cells and bind to them. Stress can lead to demargination of some white blood cells, which stimulates the bone marrow to produce more, in turn increasing the white blood cell count.
2. **Activation.** Mediators of inflammation trigger the appearance of selectins and integrins on the surfaces of endothelial cells and PMNs, respectively.
3. **Adhesion.** PMNs attach to endothelial cells, as mediated by selectins and integrins.
4. **Transmigration (diapedesis).** The PMNs permeate the vessel wall, passing into the interstitial space.
5. **Chemotaxis.** The PMNs move toward the site of inflammation in response to chemotactic factors released by bacteria or formed from activated complement, chemokines, or arachidonic acid derivatives (such as leukotrienes) in response to cell injury. **Figure 8-17** illustrates the inflammatory response.

Cellular Products of Inflammation. **Cytokines** are products of cells that affect the function of other cells. Monocytes release monokines, and lymphocytes release lymphokines.

Interleukins include IL-1 (interleukin-1) and IL-2 (interleukin-2), which attract white blood cells to the sites of injury and bacterial invasion. **Interferon** is a protein produced by cells when they are invaded by viruses. This cytokine is released into the bloodstream or intercellular fluid to induce healthy cells to manufacture an enzyme that counters the infection.

Lymphokines stimulate leukocytes. Macrophage-activating factor stimulates macrophages to help engulf and destroy foreign substances. Migration inhibitory factor keeps white blood cells at the site of infection or injury until they can perform their designated task.

Injury Resolution and Repair. Normal wound healing involves four steps—repair of damaged tissue, removal of inflammatory debris, restoration of tissues to a normal state, and regeneration of cells. Healing after tissue injury or loss caused by inflammation depends on the type of cells that make up the affected organ. Labile cells divide continuously, so organs derived from these cells (such as skin, bone, and intestinal mucosa) heal completely. Stable cells are replaced by regeneration of remaining cells, which are stimulated to enter mitosis. These cells are found in the liver and kidney. Permanent cells, such as nerve cells and cardiac myocytes, cannot be replaced; scar tissue is formed instead.

Wounds may heal by primary or secondary intention. Healing by primary intention occurs in clean wounds with opposed margins (such as clean surgical wounds or surgically débrided wounds). First, blood fills the defect and coagulates, forming a scab—a mesh-like structure composed of fibrin and fibronectin. If the inflammatory process was severe, then tissue may be destroyed and may require repair. Next, macrophages remove cellular debris and secrete growth factors. These growth factors stimulate angiogenesis and growth of fibroblasts, encouraging the formation of granulation tissue. The epithelium then regenerates, covering the surface defect. Deposition of collagen produces fibrous union. By the end of the first week, 10% of the preinjury strength is regained. Scar maturation occurs as collagen cross-linking takes place. By the end of 3 months, 80% of the normal tensile strength of the tissue has been restored.

Healing by secondary intention occurs in large, gaping or infected wounds. Wounds that heal by secondary intention have a more pronounced and prolonged inflammatory phase, causing the neutrophils to persist for days. They also have more abundant granulation tissue. Wound contraction is mediated by myofibroblasts, which help to draw the margins of the wound closer to each other as time passes.

Dysfunctional Wound Healing. Factors that can lead to dysfunctional wound healing may be local or systemic. Local factors include infection (when the body's healing

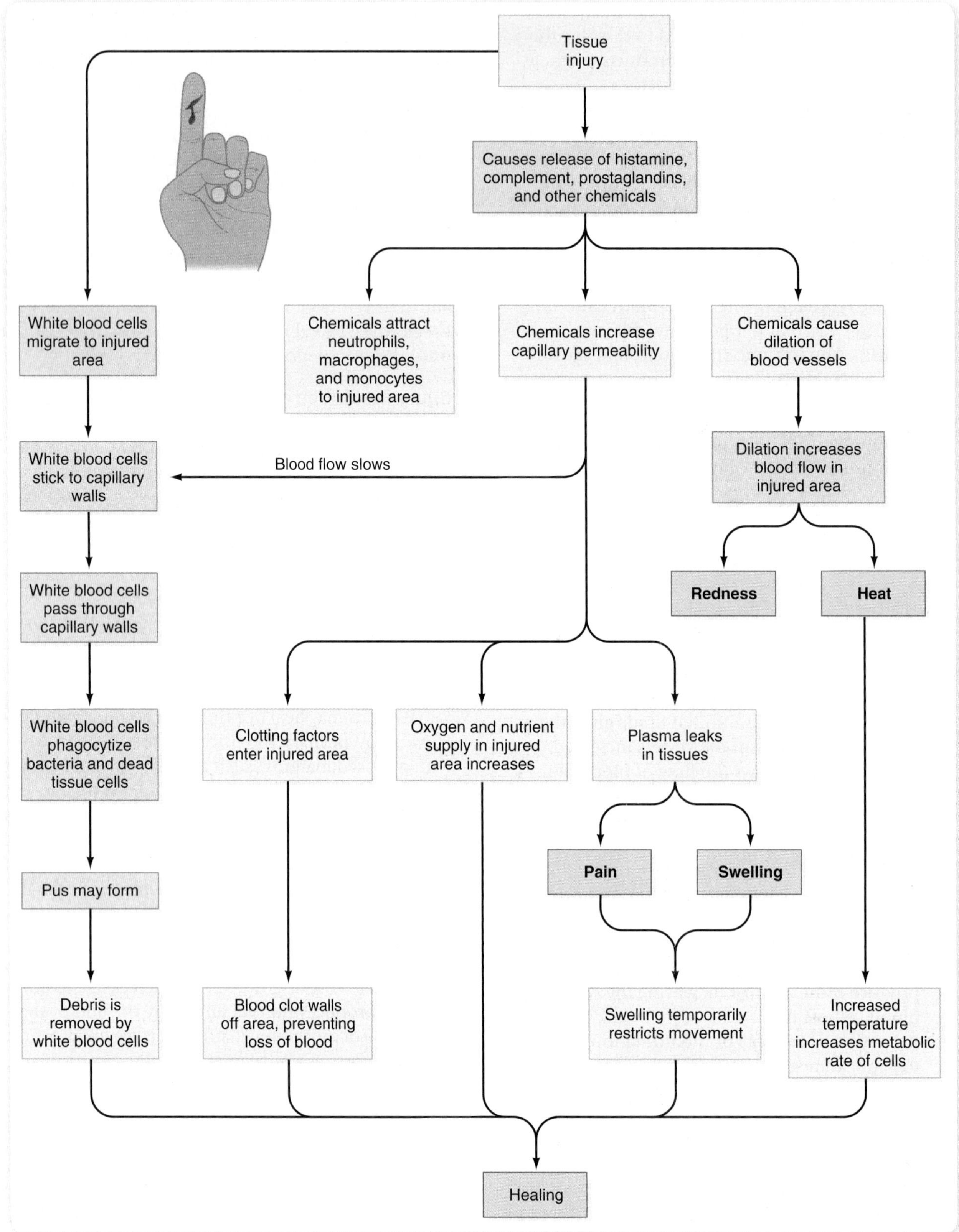

Figure 8-17 The inflammatory response.

efforts are diverted to fight off the cause of the infection); an inadequate blood supply (as in diabetes) that produces tissue hypoxia, which slows wound healing and may promote infection; and foreign bodies (when present in a wound, they stimulate acute and chronic inflammation, both of which interfere with wound healing).

There are several systemic factors that influence wound healing. Collagen is necessary for wound healing, but inadequate nutritional intake can lead to insufficient levels of collagen, which can result in inadequate scar formation and suppression of the immune system. Anything that interferes with epithelialization (the process during which epithelial cells begin to form a scab that protects the wound from the outside world) will prevent proper wound healing. *Wound contraction* is the process during which the size of the wound becomes smaller, as part of healing. Anything that interferes with wound contraction can also prevent healing.

Additional systemic factors that disrupt wound healing include hematologic abnormalities (proper wound healing requires the presence of adequate numbers of white blood cells). Patients who have impaired bone marrow stores of white blood cells are susceptible to infection and their wounds often heal more slowly. Diabetes and acquired immunodeficiency syndrome (AIDS) affect the cells of the immune system, which has a direct role in wound healing, and increase the likelihood of wound infection. Corticosteroids suppress the initial inflammatory response required for the proper formation of scar tissue and increase the risk of wound infection by slowing the immune system response.

Finally, if a wound separates (for example, from physical strain), this will slow down the healing process because healing needs to start over, at least to some extent.

Special Populations

Neonates and older adults often have relative impairment of their immune systems, potentially slowing their inflammatory responses. As a consequence, signs of inflammation may be more subtle in these populations. In addition, wound healing often takes longer, especially in older patients. The immune system is not fully developed until a child is between 2 and 3 years old; therefore, when you treat fever in younger children, you must be aggressive and thorough. Many experts recommend hospital admission for a temperature greater than 100.4°F (38°C) in a child younger than 3 months.

Chronic Inflammatory Responses

Chronic inflammatory responses are usually caused by an unsuccessful acute inflammatory response to a foreign body, a persistent infection, or the presence of an antigen. They are associated with an infiltrate (pus) containing monocytes and lymphocytes and usually involve tissue destruction and repair (or scar formation). The vascular events are similar to those that take place in acute inflammation but also include the growth of new blood vessels (a process known as **angiogenesis**).

Variances in Immunity and Inflammation

Hypersensitivity

Hypersensitivity is any response of the body to any substance to which a patient has increased sensitivity. It is a generic term for a variety of reactions. **Allergy** is a hypersensitivity reaction to the presence of an agent (allergen). **Autoimmunity** is the production of antibodies or T cells that work against the tissues of one's own body, producing hypersensitivity reactions or autoimmune disease (as in systemic lupus erythematosus [SLE]). **Isoimmunity** is the formation of T cells or antibodies directed against the antigens on another person's cells (typically after the transplantation of an organ or tissues). A blood transfusion reaction is an example of an isoimmune reaction to another person's red blood cells. The destruction of cells by antibodies or T cells may be an autoimmune or an isoimmune reaction.

Types of Hypersensitivity Reactions

A hypersensitivity reaction may be immediate, occurring within seconds to minutes, or delayed, occurring hours to days after exposure to an antigen. The speed of symptom evolution depends on the antigen and the type of response the body mounts against it. Hypersensitivity reactions are typically classified based on how the immune system caused the injury. Table 8-6 describes the four types of injuries.

Type I: Immediate Hypersensitivity Reactions. A type I hypersensitivity reaction is an acute reaction that occurs in response to a stimulus (such as a bee sting, penicillin, or shellfish). The mechanism involves interaction between the stimulus (antigen) and a preformed antibody of the IgE type. At first exposure to a specific antigen, specific IgE antibodies bind to mast cells via the nonspecific region (Fc) portion. On secondary exposure to the same antigen, these bound antibodies are cross-linked by the antigen, resulting in degranulation of the mast cell and release of histamine and other mediators Figure 8-18. The released histamine feeds back on mast cells and eosinophils, leading to the release of additional histamine and other mediators. The severity of the symptoms that develop in a particular patient depends on the extent of mediator release.

The degree of severity of hypersensitivity reactions varies from severe, life-threatening reactions, such as anaphylaxis, to milder reactions, such as allergic rhinitis (edema and irritation of the nasal mucosa), bronchial

Table 8-6 Mechanisms of Immunologic Injury

Type	Mechanism	Examples
I: Immediate hypersensitivity	IgE antibodies fix to mast cells and basophils. Later contact with a sensitizing antigen triggers mediator release and clinical manifestations.	Localized response: hay fever, food allergy Systemic response: bee sting, penicillin, anaphylaxis
II: Cytotoxic hypersensitivity reactions	Antibody binds to cell or tissue antigen, and complement is activated, which damages cell, causes inflammation, and promotes destruction of antibody-coated cell by phagocytosis.	Autoimmune hemolytic anemia Blood transfusion reactions Rh hemolytic disease Some types of glomerulonephritis
III: Immune complex disease	Circulating antigen-antibody complexes form, which activate complement and cause inflammatory reaction.	Some types of glomerulonephritis Systemic lupus erythematosus Rheumatoid arthritis
IV: Delayed (cell-mediated) hypersensitivity	Sensitized (delayed hypersensitivity) T cells release lymphokines that attract macrophages and other inflammatory cells.	Tuberculosis Fungus and parasitic infections Contact dermatitis

asthma (bronchial constriction, mucus production, and airway inflammation), wheal and flare (such as an insect bite leading to vasodilation and swelling), and mild food allergy (leading to diarrhea, gastrointestinal distress, and vomiting). A propensity to type I reactions may be diagnosed through skin tests (such as the patch test and scratch test) and other laboratory procedures (measurement of specific IgE antibody levels). Treatment is avoidance of the antigen, but desensitizing injections may be helpful in severe cases.

It is impossible to predict the severity of any given reaction. If a person has had a severe reaction in the past, then he or she is at an increased risk for another one with subsequent antigen exposures. Always assume an IgE-mediated reaction could rapidly become a life-threatening event. These reactions need to be treated quickly in the field, and most prehospital providers are trained to administer epinephrine by using an EpiPen auto-injector or by giving a subcutaneous injection.

Type II: Cytotoxic Hypersensitivity. Type II hypersensitivity reactions are cytotoxic (cell destructive) and classically involve the combination of immunoglobulin G (IgG) or immunoglobulin M (IgM) antibodies with antigens on the cell membrane. Cells are lysed (destroyed) by complement fixation or by other antibodies. This process also destroys many of the body's healthy cells. Histamine release from mast cells is not involved, and IgG-mediated allergic responses occur within a few hours of antigen exposure. Examples of IgG-mediated responses include transfusion reactions and newborn hemolytic disease.

Type III: Tissue Injury Caused by Immune Complexes. Type III hypersensitivity responses involve primarily IgG antibodies that form immune complexes with antigen to recruit phagocytic cells, such as neutrophils, to a site where they can release inflammatory cytokines. Because histamine release from mast cells is not involved, IgG-mediated allergic responses occur within a few hours of antigen exposure. Reactions may be systemic or localized.

The systemic form is called **serum sickness** and results from a large, single exposure to an antigen, such as horse antibody serum. Antigen-antibody complexes formed in the bloodstream are then deposited in sites around the body, most notably in the kidney, with resultant inflammatory reactions (such as serum sickness from penicillin). Signs and symptoms of serum sickness may include fever, malaise, rashes, joint aches, lymphadenopathy, and splenomegaly.

The localized form of a type III response is called an Arthus reaction. Arthus reactions consist of a circumscribed area of vascular inflammation (**vasculitis**). An example of an Arthus reaction is farmer's lung (a type of hypersensitivity pneumonitis reaction in the lung caused by inhalation of moldy hay dust).

Type IV: Delayed (Cell-Mediated) Hypersensitivity. Type IV allergic responses, also known as cell-mediated hypersensitivity, are primarily mediated by soluble molecules that are released by specifically activated T cells. These reactions are classified into two subtypes: delayed hypersensitivity and cell-mediated cytotoxicity.

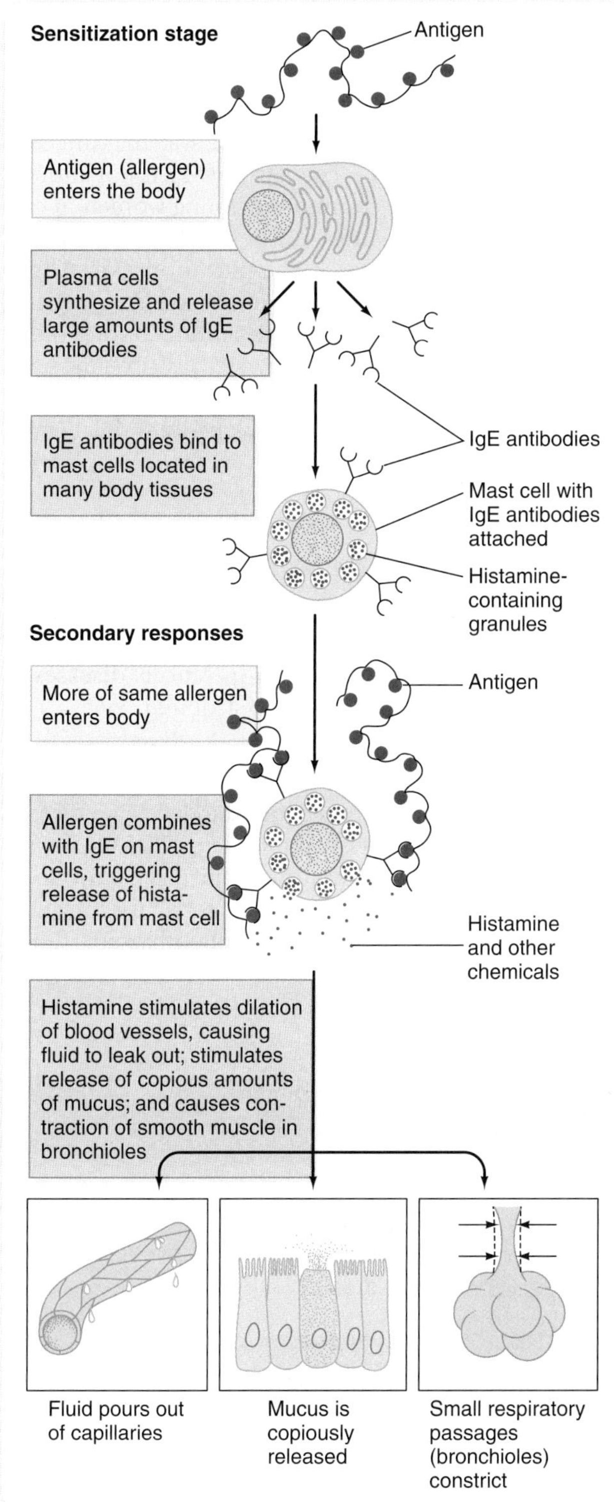

Figure 8-18 Type I allergic reaction. The antigen stimulates the production of massive amounts of immunoglobulin E (IgE), a type of antibody produced by plasma cells; the IgE, in turn, attaches to mast cells. This is a sensitization stage. When the antigen enters again, it binds to the IgE antibodies on the mast cells, triggering a massive release of histamine and other chemicals. Histamine causes blood vessels to dilate and become leaky, and it promotes increased production of mucus in the respiratory tract. Mast cell degranulation may also cause bronchospasm in some people.

Delayed hypersensitivity involves lymphocytes and macrophages. T cells respond to an antigen and activate CD4 (a helper T cell) lymphocytes. These lymphocytes release mediators that are designed to destroy the foreign substance. An example is contact hypersensitivity to poison ivy.

Cell-mediated cytotoxicity involves only sensitized T cells (CD8 lymphocytes or **killer T cells**). These cells kill the antigen-bearing target cells rather than activating the CD4 lymphocyte to do so. Examples include the body's response to viral infections, tumor immune surveillance, and the mechanism by which transplant rejection occurs.

Targets of Hypersensitivity Reactions

The immune system targets different molecules, depending on the type of hypersensitivity reaction. In allergic reactions, the target is an antigen or allergen. Allergens are substances that cause a hypersensitivity reaction, such as those listed in Table 8-7.

Autoimmune Reactions. In autoimmune reactions, the target is a person's own tissues. For reasons that are unclear, normal tolerance of "self" tissues breaks down and the immune system treats the body's own tissues as foreign.

Graves disease is an autoimmune disease caused by thyroid-stimulating or thyroid-growth immunoglobulins. These antibodies activate receptors for thyroid-stimulating hormone, causing increased activity by the thyroid gland. In addition to hyperthyroidism, Graves disease is associated with characteristic eye changes—lid retraction, stare, and exophthalmos (protrusion of the eyes)—and skin

Table 8-7 Allergens That Can Cause Hypersensitivity Reactions

Type	Examples
Inhalants	Pollen, dust, smoke, fungi, plastic, odors
Food	Eggs, dairy, wheat, chocolate, strawberries
Drugs	Aspirin, antibiotics, serums, codeine
Infectious agents	Bacteria, viruses, fungi, animal parasites
Contactants	Animals, plants, metals, chemicals
Physical agents	Light, pressure, radiation, heat and cold

changes (pretibial myxedema—localized edematous skin in the pretibial area).

Type 1 diabetes mellitus is also considered an autoimmune disease. Although the exact insult is unknown (but is suspected to be a viral infection), some agent stimulates the body to produce autoantibodies against beta cells in the pancreas that produce insulin. The results are a deficiency of insulin and, therefore, diabetes.

Rheumatoid arthritis is a chronic systemic disease that affects the entire body. One of the most common forms of arthritis, it is characterized by inflammation of the synovium (the connective tissue membrane lining the joint) with resulting pain, stiffness, warmth, redness, and swelling. Inflammatory cells release enzymes that cause damage to bone and cartilage. The involved joint can lose its shape and alignment, resulting in pain and loss of movement. Rheumatoid arthritis is associated with the formation of rheumatoid factor—that is, IgM antibodies to tissue IgG. In the joints, the synovial membrane is thickened due to infiltration of inflammatory cells (lymphocytes).

Myasthenia gravis is an acquired autoimmune disease that is characterized by autoimmune attack on the nerve-muscle junction. The circulating autoantibodies cause abnormal muscle fatigability and typically involve the smallest motor units first, such as the extraocular muscles. This produces ptosis (droopy eyelid) and diplopia (double vision). Other muscles may be involved, causing problems with swallowing (dysphagia). Characteristically, repeated contraction of the affected muscles makes the symptoms worse. Two-thirds of people with myasthenia gravis have thymic abnormalities, with the most common being thymic hyperplasia. A few of those affected have a tumor of the thymus, called a thymoma.

SLE is a chronic autoimmune disease with many manifestations. In SLE, the body's immune system is directed against the body's tissues. The cause of SLE is not known. Although SLE is more common in young women, it can occur in either sex at any age. The production of autoantibodies leads to immune complex formation. These immune complexes can then be deposited in glomeruli, skin, lungs, synovium, and mesothelium, among other places. Symptoms include arthritis, a red rash over the nose and cheeks, fatigue, weakness, fever, and photosensitivity. Glomerulonephritis (kidney disease), pericarditis, anemia, and neuritis may develop. In addition, many people with SLE have renal complications.

▶ Immune Deficiencies

Immunodeficiency is an abnormal condition in which some part of the body's immune system is inadequate, and, consequently, resistance to infectious diseases is decreased. It may be congenital or acquired.

Congenital Immunodeficiencies

Patients with severe combined immunodeficiency disease have defects that involve lymphoid stem cells. As a consequence, T cells (cellular immunity) and B cells (humoral immunity) are affected. Patients are at risk for infection with all types of organisms (bacteria, mycobacteria, fungi,

YOU are the Provider PART 4

Your partner reports all of the medication bottles are out of date and empty. You ask the patient about this and he states he does not have the means necessary to buy the medications. When you look at the list of medications, you find one for a diuretic. You note that the patient is tachycardic. The $ETCO_2$ waveform appears appropriate in shape and reads 36 mm Hg.

Recording Time: 7 Minutes	
Respirations	24 breaths/min; shallow
Pulse	114 beats/min
Skin	Cool, pale, and moist
Blood pressure	138/88 mm Hg
Oxygen saturation (Spo_2)	92% with high-flow oxygen administration
Pupils	PERRLA

7. Why would a diuretic be prescribed for a patient with heart failure?
8. Why would this patient have a normal or slightly high blood pressure?

viruses, parasites, and prions). There are two forms of this disease, both of which are inherited.

Acquired Immunodeficiencies

Any nutritional deficiency can hamper normal immune function and the inflammatory response. Nutritional deficiencies may depress bone marrow function and diminish white blood cell development. A lack of protein in the diet, for example, decreases the liver's ability to manufacture inflammatory mediators and plasma proteins.

The stress of trauma can also cause immunodeficiency. Other contributors to this condition may include hypoperfusion or shock, mediator production, damage to vital organs, and the decreased nutrition occurring during trauma states.

Iatrogenic (treatment-induced) immunodeficiency is most often caused by medications. For example, corticosteroids, whether taken orally or inhaled, suppress the immune system. This immune system suppression often has therapeutic benefits. However, in a small number of patients, the immunosuppression in the context of exposure to a pathogen leads to other diseases, such as tuberculosis. Because of its potential for adverse effects, physicians are usually cautious about prescribing this therapy for a prolonged period. In addition, idiosyncratic reactions to antibiotics may cause bone marrow suppression. Bone marrow suppression in cancer is often a direct side effect of chemotherapy and not a true idiosyncratic reaction.

Physical or mental stress has been shown to decrease white blood cell and lymphocyte function. It may also lead to decreased production of various antibodies.

AIDS is an immunodeficiency disease that is caused by the RNA retrovirus HIV. HIV binds to the CD4 surface protein of helper T cells, infects these cells, and kills them. The destruction of the cells causes decreased humoral and cell-mediated reactions.

Treatment of Immunodeficiencies

Replacement therapy is available for immunodeficiencies such as common variable immunodeficiency. Intravenous gamma globulin has been used in the treatment of a number of immunologic disorders of the nervous system, especially myasthenia gravis and inflammatory neuropathies, with considerable success. Bone marrow transplantation may restore immune competence in patients with acquired causes of immunodeficiency, such as following chemotherapy to treat cancer. Transfusion is another form of replacement therapy for immunodeficiencies. In the future, gene therapy may be useful to treat congenital and acquired causes of immunodeficiency.

Factors That Cause Disease

Genetic, environmental, age-related, and sex-associated factors can cause or contribute to disease. Genetic factors are present at birth and are passed on through a person's genes to future generations. Environmental factors include microorganisms, immunologic vulnerabilities, personal habits and lifestyle, exposure to chemicals and other toxins, the physical environment, and the psychosocial environment. Family violence, for example, might be a key factor in causing depression or substance abuse, perhaps even years later. A sedentary lifestyle and a high-fat diet can cause or contribute to obesity, diabetes, heart disease, stroke, and other diseases.

Disease also can have anatomic causes. For example, malrotation of the colon is a disease in which the colon does not form properly, resulting in partial blockage. Another example is degenerative diseases of the spine; as intervertebral disks age, they may degenerate to the extent that the patient experiences pain due to nerve compression. *Aortic stenosis* is a condition in which the aortic valve becomes very tight and narrowed, resulting in chest pain from decreased perfusion of the coronary arteries or heart failure.

Finally, an immunologic reaction may result in disease. An example is exposure to an agent that triggers an abnormal immune response against myelin, leading to the development of multiple sclerosis.

▶ Controllable Versus Uncontrollable Risk Factors

Some uncontrollable factors, such as genetics and race, influence the development of disease, but many other factors can be controlled. For example, behaviors such as smoking, drinking alcohol, inadequate nutrition (excessive fat, salt, and sugar intake or insufficient intake of protein, fruits, vegetables, and fiber), lack of physical activity, and stress can be modified.

Age-Related Risk

The risk of a particular disease often depends on a person's age. For example, newborns are at greater risk of certain diseases because their immune systems are not fully developed. Teenagers are at high risk of injury resulting from trauma and illicit drug and alcohol use. As people get older, the risk of having cancer, heart disease, stroke, and Alzheimer disease increases (see Chapter 37, *Geriatric Emergencies*).

Sex-Associated Factors

In some cases, sex is related to the risk of having a certain disease. Note: A person's physical sex and gender are not necessarily the same. In this discussion, we are referring to a person's genetic sex; for example, a person born with an XY sex chromosome is genetically and physically male, even if the person's gender is female.

Some diseases present differently in women compared with men (such as in the presentation of AMI). For example, the hormones found in a premenopausal woman have been shown to have protective benefits in major head trauma and certain cardiac conditions.

Finally, genetic disorders are related to a person's sex when a defective gene is located on a sex chromosome.

Most sex-linked disorders are X linked. X-linked disorders may be either recessive or dominant. Because females have two X chromosomes, those with a defective X gene may not have the disorder; if the disorder is recessive, the X chromosome without the defect will mask the defective X chromosome. Men with a defective X gene will always be affected because they only have one X chromosome; the defect cannot be masked.

▶ Analysis of Disease Risk

Analyzing disease risk involves consideration of disease rates and disease risk factors (causal and noncausal). Risk factors that can directly cause a disease to develop are called causal risk factors. For example, *Mycobacterium tuberculosis* is a causal risk factor for a person becoming infected with tuberculosis. Risk factors that are associated with risk for a disease but not a direct cause are called noncausal risk factors. Poverty is a noncausal risk factor for tuberculosis.

All studies of a disease should consider the incidence, prevalence, and mortality of the disease. The **incidence** is the number of new cases of a disease in a population in a given time period (for example, six new cases of West Nile virus infection developed in the county last year). **Prevalence** refers to the total number of cases of a disease or condition in a particular population within a particular period (for example, last year, more than 100,000 patients in the country had this disease). **Morbidity** refers to the damage or suffering caused by the disease either in an individual patient or in the population as a whole. **Mortality** is most often discussed as the mortality rate, which is the number of deaths from a disease in a given population, expressed as a proportion (for example, 1 in 50 affected people in the United States will die from the disease). Table 8-8 illustrates how the concepts of incidence, prevalence, morbidity, and mortality might be expressed, using statistics on diabetes as an example.

Table 8-8 Incidence, Prevalence, Morbidity, and Mortality Rate of Diabetes in the United States

Term	Example
Incidence	In 2012, 1.7 million people 20 years or older were newly diagnosed with type 1 or type 2 diabetes. An additional 86 million people aged 20 years and older were newly categorized as prediabetic.
Prevalence	9.3% of the total US population (adults and children) had diabetes in 2012.
Morbidity	In 2012, 29.1 million adults and children in the United States had symptoms or complications of diabetes (21.0 million diagnosed and an estimated 8.1 million undiagnosed).
Mortality rate	In 2010, diabetes was responsible for or a key contributor to the deaths of 234,051 people.

Data from: Centers for Disease Control and Prevention. *National Diabetes Statistics Report: Estimates of Diabetes and Its Burden in the United States, 2014.* Atlanta, GA: U.S. Department of Health and Human Services; 2014. http://www.cdc.gov/diabetes/pubs/statsreport14/national-diabetes-report-web.pdf. Accessed January 6, 2017; and American Diabetes Association. Statistics About Diabetes. http://www.diabetes.org/diabetes-basics/statistics/. Accessed January 6, 2017.

Interaction of Risk Factors

Risk factors, age, and sex differences often interact. For example, suppose a person has a genetic tendency toward coronary artery disease; the risk of myocardial infarction or sudden death is higher in this person even if he or she exercises regularly and has no other risk factors. A person who smokes heavily but has no other risk factors may have a similarly elevated risk. Table 8-9 shows the interplay of various risk factors in causing respiratory disease.

▶ Common Familial Diseases and Associated Risk Factors

The terms *genetic risk* and *familial tendency* are often used interchangeably. A true genetic risk is one that is passed through generations by inheritance of a gene. In contrast, diseases with a familial tendency seem to cluster in family groups despite lack of evidence for heritable gene-associated abnormalities.

Immunologic Disorders

Immunologic diseases are caused by hyperactivity or hypoactivity of the immune system. Most immunologic diseases that exhibit familial tendencies involve an overactive immune system—for example, allergies, asthma, and rheumatic fever. Substantial overlap exists often among causative factors, including the person's environment.

Allergies are acquired following initial exposure to an allergen. Repeated exposures cause the immune system to react to the allergen Figure 8-19. Although the clinical presentation varies, it usually includes swelling and itching, runny nose, coughing, sneezing, wheezing, and nasal congestion. A person who has an allergic tendency is said to be **atopic**. Environmental conditions may also increase a person's susceptibility to an allergic reaction.

Asthma is a chronic inflammatory condition of the lower airway resulting in intermittent wheezing and excess mucus production. Nearly 60% of attacks are precipitated

Table 8-9 Common Respiratory Diseases

Disease	Pathology and/or Symptoms	Causes and Possible Contributing Causes
Emphysema	Breakdown of alveoli, shortness of breath	Smoking Air pollution Possible genetic susceptibility Exacerbated by obesity
Chronic bronchitis	Cough, shortness of breath	Smoking Air pollution Possible genetic susceptibility Exacerbated by obesity
Acute bronchitis	Inflammation of the bronchi; coughing up yellow mucus; shortness of breath	Many viruses and bacteria Possible genetic susceptibility Smoking Exacerbated by obesity
Sinusitis	Inflammation of the sinuses; characterized by mucus discharge, blocked nasal passages, and headache	Many viruses and bacteria Poor general health
Laryngitis	Inflammation of larynx and vocal cords, sore throat, hoarseness, mucus buildup, and cough	Many viruses and bacteria Poor general health
Pneumonia	Inflammation of the lungs, ranging from mild to severe; cough and fever, shortness of breath at rest, chills, sweating, chest pain, blood-tinged mucus	Bacteria, viruses, fungi, or inhalation of irritating gases Lack of physical activity
Asthma	Constriction of bronchioles, mucus buildup in bronchioles, periodic wheezing, difficulty breathing	Allergy to pollen, certain foods, food additives; dander (dead skin cells and other debris shed by dogs, cats, or birds) Physical activity (exercise-induced asthma) Probable genetic link

Special Populations

Rheumatic fever is an inflammatory disease that occurs primarily in children. This disease results from a delayed reaction to an untreated streptococcal infection of the upper respiratory tract (such as strep throat). Symptoms, which appear several weeks after the acute infection, may include fever, abdominal pain, vomiting, arthritis, palpitations, and chest pain. Recurrent episodes of rheumatic fever may cause permanent myocardial damage, especially to the cardiac valves. A family history of acute rheumatic fever may predispose a person to the disease.

by viral infections. Allergies account for another 20% of asthma attacks, with stress and emotions causing the remainder. In addition to the familial component, chromosomal differences in certain patients may enhance their susceptibility to asthma.

Cancer

Cancer describes the pathology associated with malignant growths (neoplasms) in various anatomic areas of the human body. The prognosis often depends on the extent of its spread (metastasis) and the effectiveness of treatment.

A major risk factor associated with lung cancer is cigarette smoking. Research has identified eight alterations in the genetic material of lung cancers that suggest a genetic tendency to develop the disease. Other predisposing factors include exposure to asbestos, coal products, and other industrial and chemical products. Symptoms include cough, difficulty breathing, blood-tinged sputum, and repeated infections. Treatment depends on the type, site, and extent of the cancer and may include surgery, chemotherapy, and/or radiotherapy.

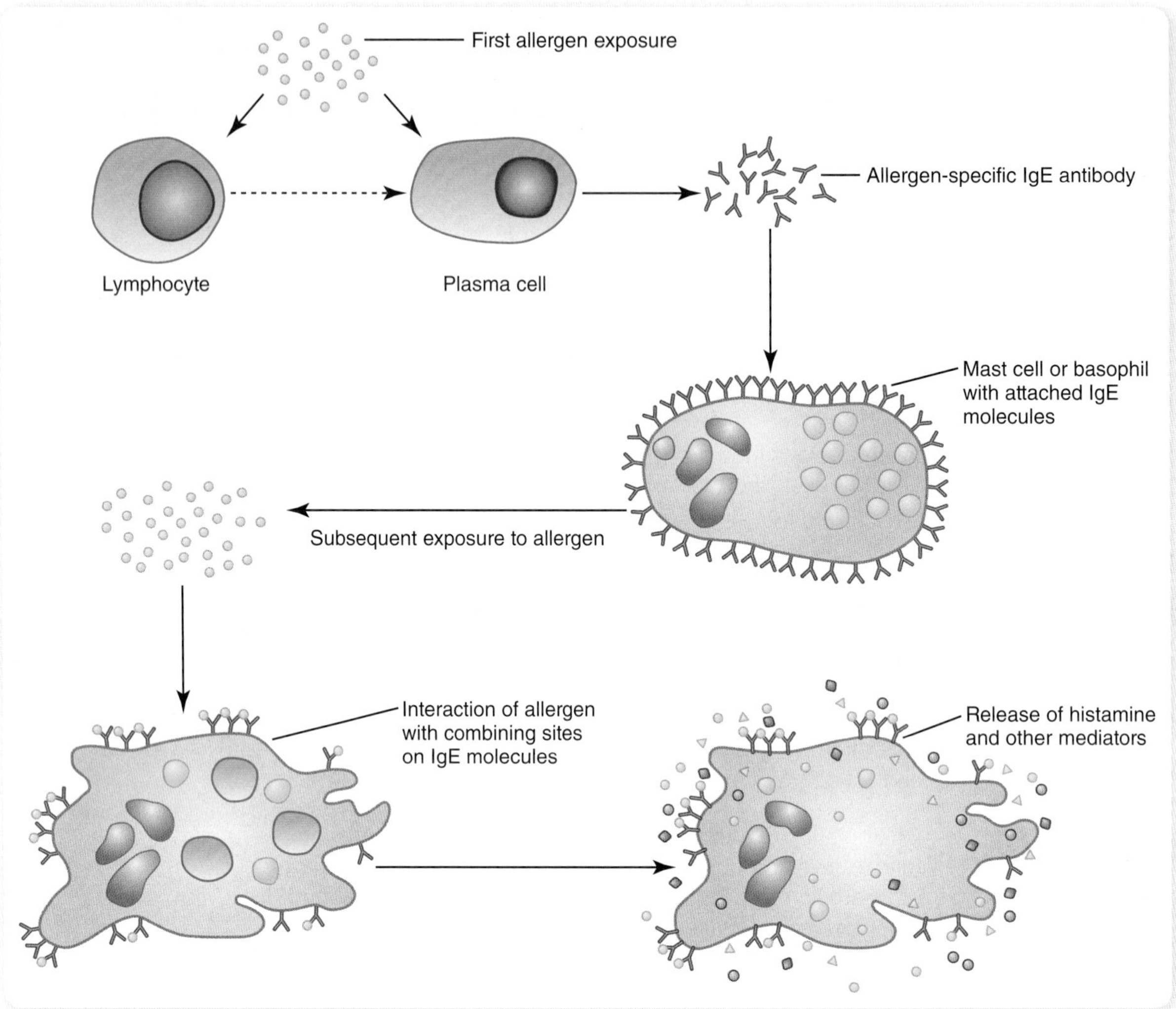

Figure 8-19 Pathogenesis of allergy. First, exposure to an allergen induces formation of specific immunoglobulin E (IgE) antibodies in susceptible patients, which then bind to mast cells and basophils. Subsequent exposure to the same allergen leads to antigen-antibody interaction through activation of memory cells, liberating histamine and other mediators from mast cells and basophils. These mediators induce allergic manifestations.

Breast cancer is the most common type of cancer occurring among women and accounts for as many as 231,840 newly diagnosed cases and 40,290 deaths each year in the United States.[11] Women whose first-degree relatives (such as a parent, sister, or daughter) have breast cancer are 2.1 times more likely to have the disease. Risk varies with the age at which the affected relative was diagnosed; the younger the age at occurrence, the greater the risk posed to relatives. The susceptibility may be inherited through the mother's or the father's side of the family.

Early symptoms of breast cancer are usually detected by the woman during breast self-examination and include a small, painless lump, thick or dimpled skin, or a change in the nipple **Figure 8-20**. Later symptoms include nipple discharge, pain, and swollen lymph glands in the axilla. Treatment depends on the location, size, and metastasis of the tumor.

Colorectal cancer is the third most common type of cancer in men and women. In 2016, the American Cancer Society expected 95,270 new cases and an estimated 49,190 deaths from colorectal cancer in the United States.[11] Relatives of people diagnosed with colorectal cancer are more likely to have the disease themselves, and parents can pass on to their children changes in certain genes that can lead to colorectal cancer. Symptoms may be minimal, consisting only of small amounts of blood in the stool. Treatment involves surgery and sometimes chemotherapy. Periodic rectal examinations and colonoscopy are recommended for adults age 50 years and older to detect the disease at an early stage.

Endocrine Disorders

Diabetes mellitus is one of the most significant endocrine diseases. This chronic disorder of metabolism is associated with partial insulin secretion or total lack of insulin secretion by the pancreas, which in turn affects the body's ability to use glucose. Symptoms include excessive thirst

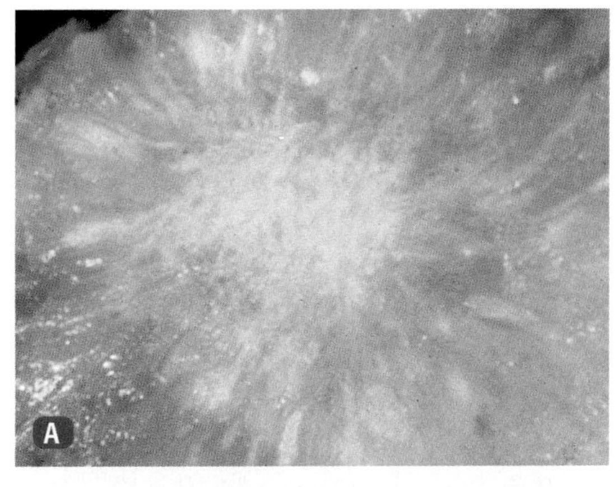

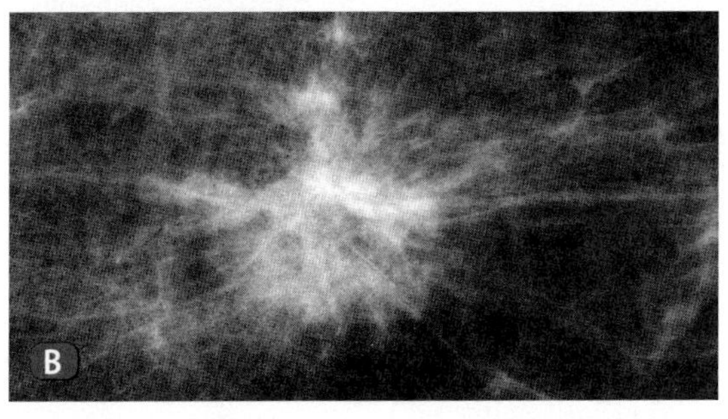

Figure 8-20 Breast carcinoma. **A.** Cross section of breast biopsy specimen. The tumor appears as a firm mass with poorly defined edges that infiltrate the surrounding fatty breast tissue. **B.** Appearance of breast carcinoma in a mammogram. The tumor appears as a white area with infiltrating margins.

and urination, weight abnormalities, and the presence of excessive glucose in the urine and the blood.

Ketoacidosis-prone (type 1) diabetes is also known as insulin-dependent diabetes mellitus because patients need exogenous insulin to survive. Non–ketoacidosis-prone (type 2) diabetes is called non–insulin-dependent diabetes, even though many people with type 2 diabetes require exogenous insulin injections. Both forms have a hereditary predisposition. Type 1 diabetes has no known cure (other than pancreas transplantation) at the present time; type 2 diabetes can occasionally be brought under control with weight loss, regular physical activity, and medications.

Hematologic Disorders

Hemolytic anemia is characterized by increased destruction of red blood cells. This disorder has a number of causes, such as an Rh factor blood transfusion reaction (which would most likely occur in the neonate population), a disorder of the immune system, and exposure to bacterial toxins or chemicals such as benzene. **Figure 8-21** depicts how the body handles iron. Hemolytic anemia following an aspirin overdose or penicillin administration is rare; it is much more common, albeit still rare, with sulfa drugs used to treat urinary tract infections, such as the trimethoprim-sulfamethoxazole combination (known as Septra and Bactrim). An inherited enzyme deficiency (glucose-6-phosphatase dehydrogenase deficiency) markedly increases a person's susceptibility to sulfa drug–induced hemolytic anemia.

Hemophilia is an inherited disorder characterized by excessive bleeding. It is a sex-linked condition, occurring

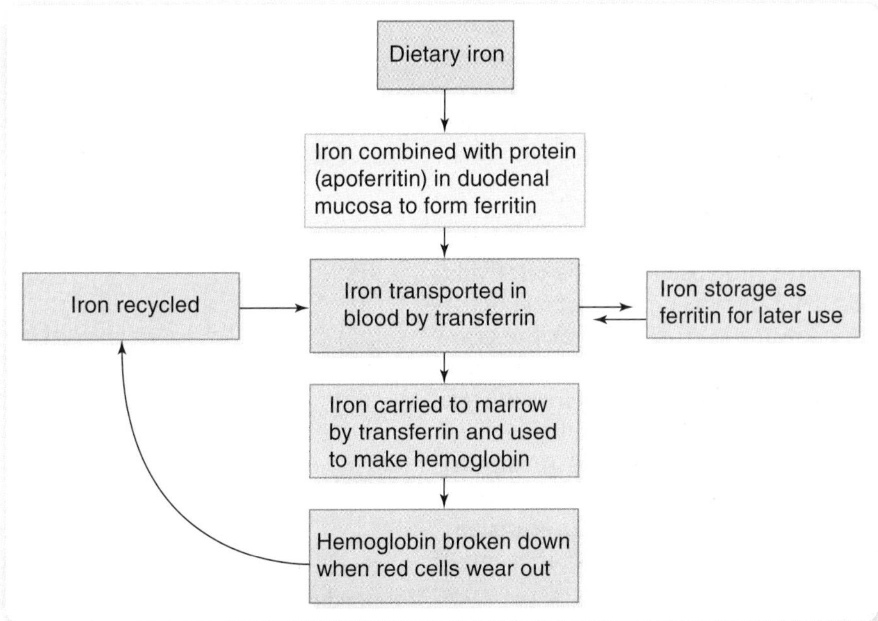

Figure 8-21 Iron uptake, transport, storage, and utilization for hemoglobin synthesis. Most of the iron used for hemoglobin synthesis is recycled from worn-out red blood cells. Chronic blood loss removes iron-containing cells from the circulation, and the iron contained in the red blood cells can no longer be recycled to make hemoglobin, leading to iron deficiency anemia.

predominantly in males, and is passed from asymptomatic mothers to sons.[12] In this disorder, one of the blood-clotting proteins (usually factor VIII) necessary for normal blood coagulation is missing or is present in abnormally low amounts. Patients experience greater-than-usual blood loss in dental extractions and following simple injuries. They may also have bleeding into joints and, rarely, into the brain. Treatment consists of administration of the missing blood-clotting factors.

Hemochromatosis is an inherited disease in which the body absorbs more iron than it needs. The excess iron is stored in various organs, including the liver, kidneys, and pancreas. Hemochromatosis can lead to diabetes, heart disease, liver disease, arthritis, impotence, and a bronzed skin color. These symptoms can be avoided by regularly drawing blood (phlebotomy).

Cardiovascular Disorders

Several cardiovascular disorders are known to follow specific patterns of inheritance. Still others have strong familial tendencies (such as coronary heart disease).

Cardiomyopathy. *Cardiomyopathy* is a general term for diseases of the myocardium (heart muscle) that ultimately progress to heart failure, AMI, or death. These diseases cause the heart muscle to become thin, flabby, dilated, or enlarged. One variant, hypertrophic cardiomyopathy, is genetically predisposed for inheritance in each generation. The main feature of hypertrophic cardiomyopathy is an excessive thickening of the heart muscle (hypertrophy means to thicken or grow excessively) **Figure 8-22**. In addition, microscopic examination of the heart muscle shows that it is abnormal. Patients may have shortness of breath, chest pains, palpitations, or syncope; sudden cardiac death is also possible. Beta-blockers are effective treatment in some patients. Others require surgery or an automatic implantable cardiac defibrillator designed to deliver a shock to the heart.

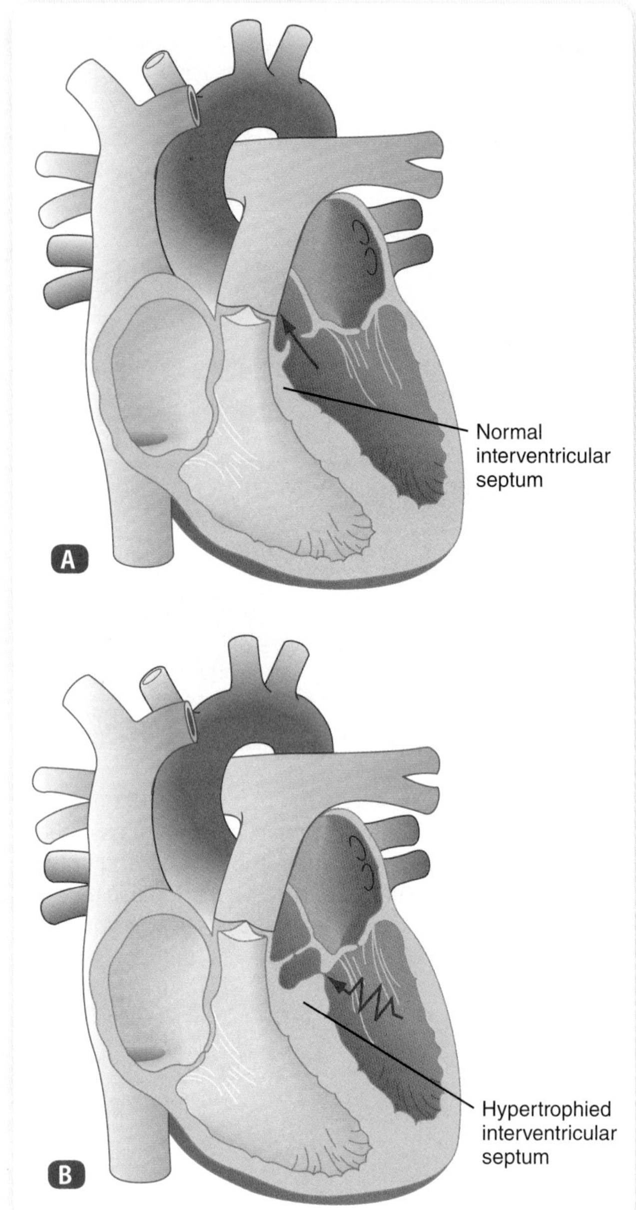

Figure 8-22 Comparison of normal cardiac function with malfunction characteristic of hypertrophic cardiomyopathy. **A.** Normal heart, illustrating unobstructed flow of blood from left ventricle into aorta during ventricular systole. **B.** Hypertrophic cardiomyopathy, illustrating obstruction to outflow of blood from left ventricle by hypertrophied septum, which impinges on the anterior leaflet of mitral valve.

Mitral Valve Prolapse. Also referred to as a floppy mitral valve, mitral valve prolapse (MVP) is relatively common, affecting 2.5% of males and 7.6% of females.[13] A familial tendency toward MVP exists, but the condition is usually associated with other cardiovascular conditions. The mitral valve leaflets balloon into the left atrium during systole. Although MVP is often benign and asymptomatic, some patients have chest pain, fatigue, dizziness, dyspnea, or palpitations. Generally, the only physical finding is a clicking sound heard during cardiac auscultation. Cardiac dysrhythmias develop in a small number of patients.

Sometimes MVP leads to mitral regurgitation (also called mitral insufficiency), in which a large amount of blood leaks backward through the defective valve. Mitral regurgitation can lead to thickening or enlargement of the heart wall, caused by the extra pumping of the heart to make up for the backflow of blood. It sometimes causes people to feel tired or short of breath. Mitral regurgitation usually can be treated with medication, but some people need surgery to repair or replace the defective valve.

Coronary Heart Disease. *Coronary heart disease,* often called coronary artery disease, is caused by impaired circulation to the heart. Typically, patients have occluded coronary arteries from atherosclerotic plaque buildup. The effects can range from ischemia to infarction and necrosis (death) of the myocardium. Almost one-half of all cardiovascular deaths are caused by coronary heart disease.[14] This condition has a familial tendency; significant risk factors for coronary artery disease development include having a father who experienced an AMI or died suddenly younger than 55 years of age or having a mother who experienced an AMI or died suddenly younger than 65 years of age. Other risk factors include hypercholesterolemia, cigarette smoking, hypertension (high blood pressure), age (as age increases, the risk for coronary heart disease increases), and diabetes.

Hypercholesterolemia is an elevation of the blood cholesterol level. The blood cholesterol level is divided into high-density lipoprotein ("good cholesterol") and low-density lipoprotein ("bad cholesterol"). Despite having a normal total cholesterol level, having an abnormally low level of high-density lipoprotein and/or an elevation of low-density lipoprotein increases the risk of coronary heart disease.

Hypertension and Stroke. Hypertension (high blood pressure) is associated with an increased risk of coronary artery disease and is also strongly associated with an increased risk of stroke. Risk factors for developing hypertension can be categorized as genetic or lifestyle-related and include age (as age increases, the risk increases), race (more common in African Americans), sex (men are more likely to experience hypertension), family history, obesity or being overweight, sedentary lifestyle, tobacco use, diet (too much salt, too little potassium, too little vitamin D, too much alcohol), and stress.

Stroke risk factors are also either genetic or lifestyle-related and include age (adults 55 years or older are at increased risk), race (more common in African Americans, Hispanics, and American Indian/Alaska Natives), sex (men are more likely to have a stroke), family history, obesity or being overweight, sedentary lifestyle, hypertension, hypercholesterolemia, tobacco use, diabetes, cardiovascular disease, using birth control pills or hormone therapies, and excessive alcohol consumption.

Renal Disorders

Gout. *Gout* is an abnormal accumulation of uric acid due to a defect in metabolism. As a result of this defect, uric acid accumulates in the blood and joints, causing pain and swelling of the joints, especially the big toe. Often, the patient has fever and chills. Gout is more common among men than women and usually has a genetic basis. If left untreated, gout causes destructive tissue changes in the joints and kidneys. Treatment includes diet and medications to reduce inflammation and to increase the excretion of uric acid or decrease its formation.

Kidney Stones. *Kidney stones* are small masses of uric acid or calcium salts that form in any part of the urinary system (kidney, ureter, or urinary bladder). Kidney stones may cause severe pain, nausea, and vomiting when the body attempts to pass them. Although most stones are small, occasionally they become large enough to adopt the internal contours of the kidney Figure 8-23. Researchers have found a gene that causes the intestines to absorb too much calcium, which can lead to the formation of kidney stones. Uric acid stones also often have a genetic basis. Some are small enough to pass in the urine, with or without pain; others must be removed surgically.

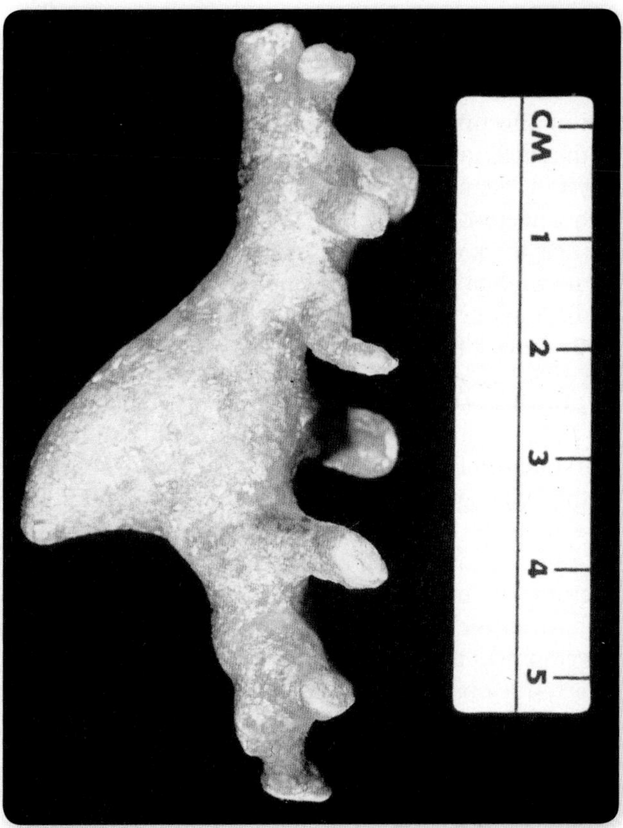

Figure 8-23 Large staghorn-shaped kidney stone.
Courtesy of Leonard V. Crowley, MD, Century College.

Gastrointestinal Disorders

Malabsorption Disorders. *Malabsorption disorders* are caused by defects in the function of the bowel wall that prevent adequate nutrient absorption. The result is a complex of symptoms, including loss of appetite, bloating, weight loss, muscle pain, and stools with high fat content. Diarrhea, which may be bloody, may also be a prominent symptom.

Lactose intolerance is caused by a defect or deficiency of the enzyme lactase, resulting in an inability to digest lactose (milk sugar). Symptoms include bloating, flatulence, abdominal discomfort, nausea, and diarrhea after ingesting dairy or dairy products.

Ulcerative colitis is a serious chronic inflammatory disease of the large intestine and rectum. This disease, which shows a familial tendency, is characterized by recurrent episodes of abdominal pain, fever, chills, and profuse diarrhea, with stools containing pus, blood, and mucus. Treatment consists of anti-inflammatory agents, including corticosteroids. Patients with severe cases may require surgery to remove parts of the intestinal tract.

Patients are at increased risk for the development of colorectal cancer.

Crohn disease is a serious chronic inflammatory condition affecting the colon and/or the terminal portion of the small intestine. It is believed to be associated with as-yet-undetermined gene abnormalities. Symptoms include frequent episodes of diarrhea, melena, abdominal pain, nausea, fever, weakness, and weight loss. Management is by anti-inflammatory agents, antibiotics, proper nutrition, and sometimes surgery to remove the damaged portion of the bowel, fistulas, or scar tissue.

Peptic Ulcer Disease. *Peptic ulcer disease* is characterized by circumscribed erosions (ulcerations) of the mucous membrane lining of the gastrointestinal tract—specifically, in the esophagus, stomach, duodenum, or jejunum. Peptic ulcers may be associated with excess acid production or a breakdown in the normal mechanisms protecting the mucous membranes. Although this disease seems to have a genetic component, a major contributor to its development is infection with the bacterium *Helicobacter pylori*—the observed familial patterns seem to be due to shared infections with *H pylori*. Symptoms include gnawing pain, which is often worse when the stomach is empty, after the person eats certain foods, or when the person is under stress. Treatment includes avoiding irritants such as tobacco, alcohol, and certain foods, antibiotics, and medications to decrease acidity. In refractory cases, surgery may be necessary.

Gallstones. *Gallstones* (choleliths) are stonelike masses in the gallbladder or its ducts caused by precipitation of substances contained in bile (such as cholesterol and bilirubin). Factors that contribute to the formation of gallstones include abnormalities in the composition of bile, or stasis of bile. Gallstones may be asymptomatic, but they cause symptoms when they obstruct the flow of bile. They may cause inflammation of the gallbladder. Small stones that are able to pass into the common duct produce indigestion and biliary colic. Biliary colic pain has a sudden onset and increases steadily to its maximum in approximately 1 hour. The pain is located in the upper right quadrant or the epigastric area and may be referred to the back. Larger stones may cause jaundice (yellow skin and sclerae).

Obesity. **Obesity** is an unhealthy accumulation of body fat and is defined as a body mass index of greater than or equal to 30 kg/m^2. For example, an adult who is 5 feet 9 inches tall (2 m) is considered obese if he or she weighs more than 203 pounds (92 kg). Body mass index, and therefore the definition of obesity, is different for children and adolescents.

Morbid obesity is defined as a body mass index of 40 kg/m^2 or greater. Using the example again of an adult who is 5 feet 9 inches tall (2 m), he or she is considered morbidly obese if he or she weighs more than 270 pounds (122 kg). Morbid obesity includes all of the health risks associated with obesity, but it also makes basic functions such as walking or breathing difficult.

People who are overweight are also at increased risk for disease, although the risk is not as high as for those who are obese. Being **overweight** is defined as a body mass index of 25 to 29.9 kg/m^2. Using the previous example of an adult who is 5 feet 9 inches tall (2 m), he or she would be overweight if he or she weighed between 169 and 202 pounds (77 and 92 kg).

Obesity has a substantial negative impact on a person's health and life span; simply put, it has been statistically proven that the life span of a person with obesity is decreased by an average of 8 to 13 years.[15,16] Obesity has become an epidemic among adults and children in the United States. Approximately two-thirds of adults in the United States are obese or are overweight. Approximately 30% of children and adolescents in the United States are obese.[15,16]

Obesity has many deleterious effects, both medical and social. Health risks associated with obesity include hypertension, hyperlipidemia, cardiovascular disease, glucose intolerance, insulin resistance, diabetes, gallbladder disease, infertility, and cancer of the endometrium, breast, prostate, and colon. Social and psychological effects of obesity include depression, anxiety, shame, rejection, and discrimination in various environments including school and the workplace.

Although some people likely have a genetic predisposition to obesity, the roles of specific genes in its development have yet to be determined. Behavioral and environmental factors are better known. Behavioral factors that contribute to obesity include choosing a sedentary lifestyle, overeating, or eating foods high in calories and low in nutritional value, such as fast food and soda. A person's community or work environment may make it difficult to choose to be physically active or to eat properly. For example, a lack of sidewalks in a community would contribute to the risk of members of that community becoming obese. Large portion sizes offered by restaurants contribute to a lack of understanding of what is a proper portion size. Finally, interest in television and technological media may take time away from physical activity and encourage unhealthy product consumption. Because people tend to snack while watching TV or using a computer, they consume unnecessary additional calories.

Neuromuscular Disorders

Although environmental contributions are highly likely, certain neuromuscular disorders have a familial and genetic basis. The next few sections present several of the better known and more worrisome disorders in this category.

Huntington Disease. *Huntington disease* (also called Huntington chorea), for example, is a hereditary condition characterized by progressive chorea (involuntary rapid, jerky motions) and mental deterioration, leading to dementia. Symptoms usually first appear in the third or fourth decade of life and progress to death, often within 15 years.

Muscular Dystrophy. Muscular dystrophy is a generic term for a group of hereditary diseases of the muscular system characterized by weakness and wasting of groups of skeletal muscles, leading to increasing disability. The various forms differ in age of onset, rate of progression, and mode of genetic transmission. Duchenne muscular dystrophy is a sex-linked recessive disease (affecting only males); symptoms first appear around 4 years of age. Progressive wasting of leg and pelvic muscles produces a waddling gait and abnormal curvature of the spine. Usually, by age 12, the person becomes unable to walk and begins to use a wheelchair. No known treatment exists, and the person often dies, most typically of a heart disorder, by age 20 years.

Multiple Sclerosis. *Multiple sclerosis* is a progressive disease in which the myelin sheath surrounding the nerve fibers of the brain and spinal cord become damaged.[17] Although the disease is not directly inherited, some patients have a familial predisposition, suggesting a genetic influence on susceptibility. The disease usually begins in early adulthood and progresses slowly, with periods of remission and exacerbation. Early symptoms include abnormal sensations in the face or extremities, weakness, and visual disturbances (such as double vision), which progress to ataxia (lack of coordination), abnormal reflexes, tremors, difficulty in urination, and difficulty in walking. Depression is also common. No specific treatment or cure has been developed, but corticosteroids and other drugs are used to treat symptoms.

Special Populations

Never assume that new or worsening confusion in an older adult is due solely to Alzheimer disease, without first considering potentially correctable causes such as new medications, infections, or myocardial infarction. An apparent emotional, psychological, or behavioral disorder may have an organic cause, especially in the older adult population.

Alzheimer Disease. *Alzheimer disease* is characterized by cortical atrophy and loss of neurons in the frontal and temporal lobes of the brain; in addition, as the brain ventricles become enlarged, a loss of brain tissue occurs. Alzheimer disease affects over 5 million Americans.[18] Histologic changes in the brain of a person with Alzheimer disease include neurofibrillary tangles and senile plaques **Figure 8-24**. Studies of the genetics of inherited early-onset Alzheimer disease have been linked to mutations on three genes.

Alzheimer disease is progressive. Early in its progression, it is characterized by memory loss, lack of spontaneity, subtle personality changes, and disorientation to time and date. It may then progress to including impaired cognition and abstract thinking, restlessness and agitation, wandering, inability to perform activities of daily living, impaired judgment, and inappropriate social behavior. Advanced Alzheimer disease involves indifference to food, inability to communicate, urinary and fecal incontinence, and seizures.

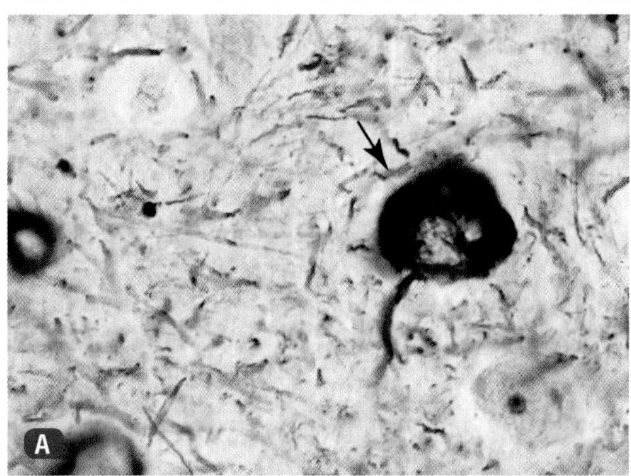

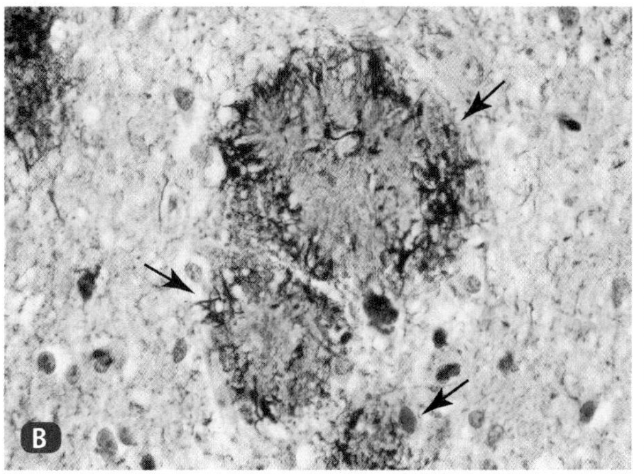

Figure 8-24 Alzheimer disease. **A.** Thickened neurofilaments encircle and obscure the nuclei of nerve cells (arrow), forming a neurofibrillary tangle (magnification, ×400). **B.** Three senile plaques (arrows) composed of broken masses of thickened neurofilaments (magnification, ×100).

Courtesy of Leonard V. Crowley, MD, Century College.

Psychiatric Disorders

Some common psychiatric disorders seem to have a familial and perhaps even genetic component. Two of the most important are schizophrenia and bipolar disorder.

Schizophrenia. *Schizophrenia* comprises a group of mental disorders characterized by gross distortions of reality (psychoses), withdrawal from social contacts, and disturbances of thought, language, perception, and emotional response. Its symptoms are highly varied but may include apathy, catatonia or excessive activity, bizarre actions, hallucinations, delusions, and rambling speech. Although the cause of schizophrenia has not been identified, a combination of hereditary or genetic predisposing factors is likely in most cases.

Bipolar Disorder. *Bipolar disorder* (formerly known as manic-depressive disorder or manic-depressive psychosis) is a mental disorder characterized by episodes of mania and depression. One or the other phase may be dominant at any given time, the phases may alternate, or aspects of both phases may be present at once. The higher rates of bipolar disorder among relatives, identical twins, and biologic parents versus adoptive parents have been cited as evidence of the role of genetics in this disorder; the risk within the general population as a whole is approximately 2.6%.[19] Treatment consists of psychotherapy plus certain atypical antipsychotics.

Stress and Disease

Stress is the medical term for a wide range of strong external stimuli, physiologic and psychological, that can cause a physiologic response. Physiologic stress is defined as a change that makes it necessary for the cells of the body to adapt. Figure 8-25 shows the series of events that occur when the body responds to a stimulus or stressor. Three concepts related to physiologic stress include the stressor itself, its effect in the body, and the body's response to the stress.

The brain and CNS constantly interact with a person's consciousness. Research has shown a strong connection between the human psyche and brain physiology. When a person experiences stress, the body's defense mechanisms are activated. Usually, the response to stress is appropriate and beneficial. However, an unchecked stress response can have deleterious outcomes, including chemical dependency, heart attack, stroke, depression, headache, and abdominal pain.

General Adaptation Syndrome

The **general adaptation syndrome**, a term introduced in the 1920s by Hans Selye, an Austrian endocrinologist, characterizes a three-stage reaction to stressors, physical (such as injury) and emotional (such as loss of a loved one).

Stage 1: Alarm

The body reacts to stress first by releasing catecholamines, chemical compounds derived from the amino acid tyrosine that act as hormones or neurotransmitters. They are produced mainly from the adrenal medulla and the postganglionic fibers of the sympathetic nervous system. Catecholamines are soluble, so they circulate dissolved in blood. The most abundant catecholamines are epinephrine (adrenaline), norepinephrine (noradrenaline), and dopamine. Adrenaline acts as a neurotransmitter in the CNS and as a hormone in the blood. Noradrenaline is primarily a neurotransmitter of the peripheral sympathetic nervous system but is also present in the blood (mostly through spillover from the synapses of the sympathetic system).

As shown in Figure 8-25, stress causes the sympathetic nervous system to be stimulated. When the body

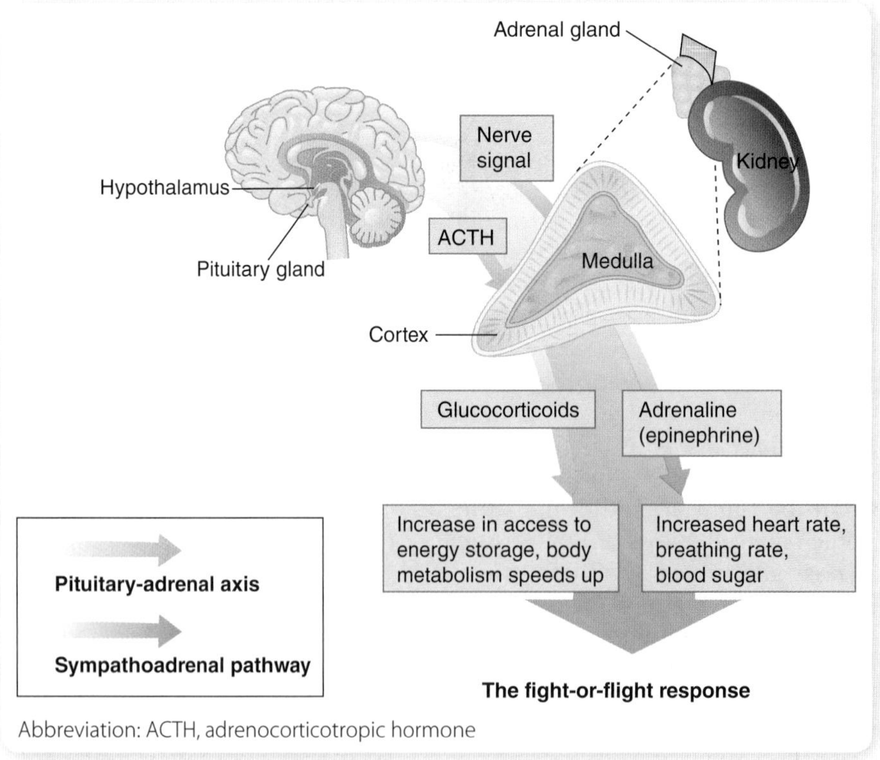

Abbreviation: ACTH, adrenocorticotropic hormone

Figure 8-25 Physiologic response to stress.

senses stress, the brain causes the adrenal medulla of the endocrine system to send catecholamines (the hormones epinephrine and norepinephrine) that activate the sympathetic nervous system by binding to **receptor** sites. In the sympathetic nervous system, the receptors that allow certain responses to be activated are called alpha and beta receptors. When one of these receptors is activated, a predictable sequence of responses occurs. Activation of alpha receptors results in vasoconstriction, while activation of beta receptors results in increased heart rate, increased force of contraction, and increased conduction velocity. Beyond those cardiac effects of catecholamines, other physiologic effects include an increase in respiratory rate, decreased blood flow to the skin, smooth muscle constriction, and various effects on the liver that increase the body's use of glucose.

Normally, the fight-or-flight response that occurs in the alarm reaction prepares the body to deal with stress, but it can also weaken the immune system, leading to infection.

Stage 2: Resistance or Adaptation

During stage 2, the resistance or adaptation stage, the body adapts to stressors primarily by stimulating the adrenal gland to secrete two types of corticosteroid hormones that increase the blood glucose level and maintain blood pressure: glucocorticoids and mineralocorticoids. The most significant glucocorticoid in the body is cortisol, which controls carbohydrate, fat, and protein metabolism. Cortisol also has potent anti-inflammatory actions. Mineralocorticoids (predominantly aldosterone) control electrolyte and water levels in the body, mainly by promoting sodium retention by the kidneys.

During times of stress, the hypothalamus secretes a hormone that stimulates the anterior pituitary to release adrenocorticotropic hormone (ACTH) **Figure 8-26**. ACTH targets the adrenal cortex, resulting in cortisol secretion. Cortisol stimulates body cells to increase their energy production in response to increased stressors; cortisol increases serum glucose levels and impairs the use of glucose by peripheral tissues. It also decreases protein reserves and permits mobilization of fatty acids by epinephrine and growth hormone. It reduces inflammation when inflammation has served its purpose; therefore, it has a role in wound healing. Cortisol also increases red blood cell production and affects electrolyte levels. However, it also decreases the size of lymphoid tissue. Since the lymphatic system has an important role in immunity, this may explain why stress and disease are linked.

Other hormones related to stress include endorphins, which are neurotransmitters released during times of stress. Endorphins help reduce pain and stress by activating opiate receptor sites. They essentially produce a type of analgesia.

Additional hormones include growth hormone, prolactin, and testosterone. Growth factor is a hormone that promotes cell and tissue growth and repair. In the context of stress, growth factor is reduced. Because

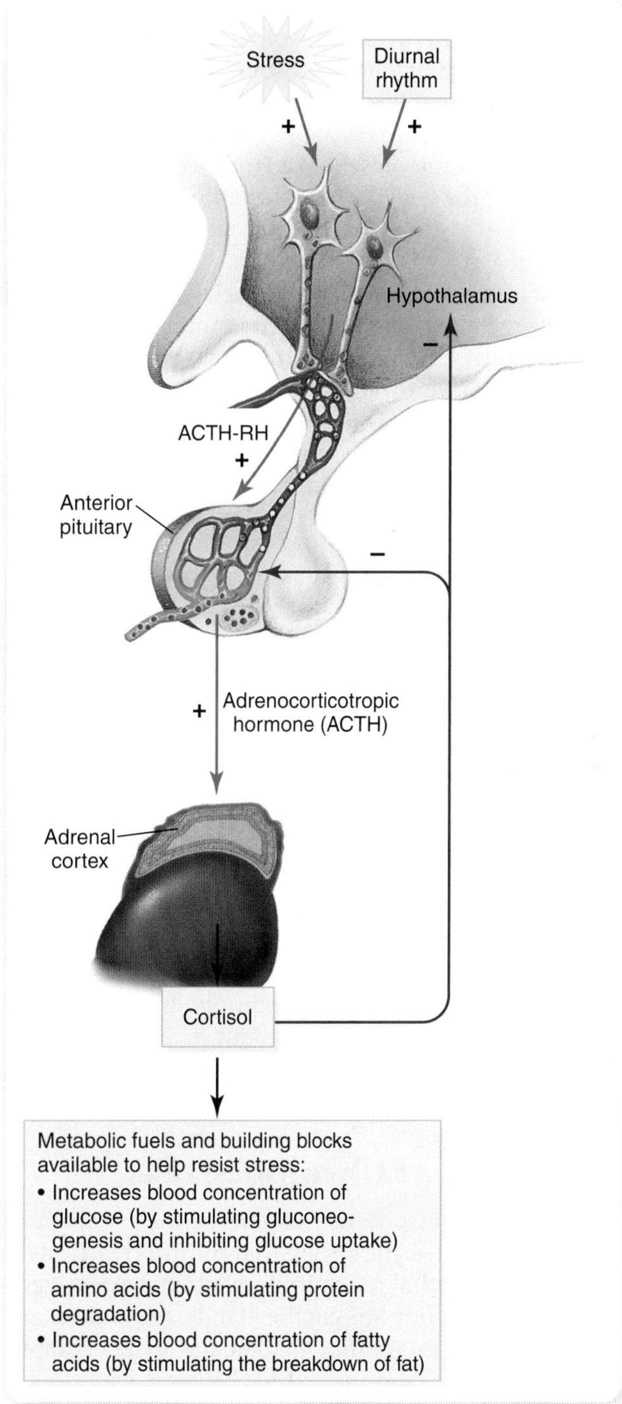

Figure 8-26 Stress triggers secretion of adrenocorticotropic hormone, which results in cortisol secretion.

growth factor correlates to the body's ability to heal, the body's ability to heal is reduced when it is under chronic stress.

Prolactin is a hormone that stimulates breast milk production. It is also believed to play a role in the immune system. In times of stress, prolactin levels increase. Research suggests that prolactin levels increase more in people with ineffective coping mechanisms.

The hormone testosterone is affected by stress. There is a direct link between cortisol levels and testosterone levels; namely, that when cortisol levels are high, testosterone levels are reduced. When the body is not under stress, testosterone levels are protected from cortisol by an enzyme. In the presence of stress, cortisol levels are too high for the enzyme to sufficiently handle them. As a result, the excess cortisol causes testosterone levels to decrease.

It was previously believed that elevated testosterone levels were linked to a suppressed immune system. Now, research suggests that testosterone may be related to the distribution of white blood cells in the body. It is thought that in times of stress, white blood cells are sent to the skin to protect against wound infection. But in the context of chronic stress, this would mean fewer white blood cells in other parts of the body on a regular basis, making those parts more susceptible to infection.

Cortisol levels and the sympathetic nervous system return to normal during this resistance or adaptation stage, causing fight-or-flight symptoms to disappear. Continuation of stress and accompanying corticosteroid release eventually lead to fatigue, lapses in concentration, irritability, lethargy, depression, and a depressed immune system.

Stage 3: Exhaustion

After a long period of stress, the person enters the exhaustion stage. The adrenal glands become depleted, decreasing the blood glucose level, which results in decreased stress tolerance, progressive mental and physical exhaustion, illness, and collapse. At this point, the body's immune system is compromised, substantially reducing a person's ability to resist disease. Heart attack, high blood pressure, or severe infection may result.

▶ Effects of Chronic Stress

The **hypothalamic-pituitary-adrenal axis** is a major part of the neuroendocrine system that controls reactions to stress. The hypothalamic-pituitary-adrenal axis triggers a set of interactions among the glands, hormones, and parts of the midbrain that mediate the general adaptation syndrome. Continued stress, however, leads to loss of these normal control mechanisms. As a result, the adrenals continue to produce cortisol, which exhausts the stress mechanism and leads to fatigue and depression. Cortisol also interferes with serotonin activity, furthering the depressive effect.

A consistently high cortisol level suppresses the immune system by increasing production of interleukin-6, an immune system messenger. Not surprisingly, then, research indicates that stress and depression have a negative effect on the immune system. Reduced immunity makes the body more susceptible to everything from colds and flu to cancer. For example, the incidence of serious illness, including cancer, is substantially higher among people whose spouse has died during the past year.

Although severe, prolonged stress does not cause death directly, it does cause the body to lose its ability to fight disease in its effort to manage the stress. Stress also encourages the body to release fat and cholesterol into the bloodstream, which then block the arteries and can eventually cause a heart attack or stroke. Many people start drinking alcohol to excess to combat their stress. Other diseases and conditions related to chronic stress include depression, headaches, insomnia, ulcers, diuresis, acne, diabetes mellitus, rheumatoid arthritis, and asthma. The variety in this list shows that stress affects most every organ system in the body.

However, it is important to note that a person's reaction to stressful events correlates to elevation or reduction in hormone levels. Therefore, coping mechanisms play a role in the physiologic response to stress. When a healthy person experiences stress, he or she may be able to manage the stress with minimal negative effects to the immune system if he or she has effective coping mechanisms. But in any patient, ineffective coping mechanisms will have deleterious effects on immune status. Effects will be worst in those whose immune systems are already compromised and who do not have effective coping mechanisms to combat the stress. Conversely, effective coping mechanisms can go a long way in helping a patient improve his or her immune system's response. Finally, a person's outlook has been shown to relate to the effectiveness of his or her medical treatment; much like a placebo effect, if a patient believes that the treatment will be effective, it is more likely to be effective.

YOU are the Provider SUMMARY

1. What is your general impression of the patient?

The patient is in obvious respiratory distress because he is not able to speak complete sentences without taking a breath. This finding is very important in the assessment of your patient because it indicates there is not enough oxygen available to the patient to speak effectively.

2. What can you learn about the patient from his surroundings?

The scene assessment gives numerous indications that the patient has a substantial medical history. The first significant finding is you were met at the door by a neighbor. The neighbor tells you the patient has had medical issues and lives alone. After you enter the residence, you observe multiple medication containers and an abundance of used facial tissues adjacent to the patient. These items need to be investigated further. The patient is also wearing a nasal cannula attached to a home oxygen unit, which indicates a preexisting respiratory condition.

3. How does the recruitment of accessory muscles facilitate breathing?

As you have learned, the act of breathing relies on positive and negative pressures. The chest and other related muscles expand and contract to create the pressure. When the act of breathing becomes difficult, accessory muscles assist with the mechanical aspect of breathing. The nasal passages will flare in an attempt to gain as much space as possible to increase airflow into the airways. Musculature in the chest will work visibly harder to move the chest wall and diaphragm to help create the pressure gradient necessary for breathing. Sitting upright aligns the airway to decrease the amount of pressure needed within the chest.

4. How might the productive cough help you identify the source of the patient's breathing difficulty?

The productive cough could indicate many disease processes. The color of the sputum is of particular interest in your assessment. Thick green, brown, or yellow sputum may indicate infection. Pink, frothy sputum indicates pulmonary edema. Hemoptysis may indicate trauma or carcinoma. After you assess the color, determine how much of it is present. In this case, the numerous used facial tissues can help indicate an amount.

5. On the basis of what you know about physiology, what is causing the pink, frothy sputum?

Pink, frothy sputum is an indication of pulmonary edema that, in this case, may be a sign of exacerbation of heart failure. If the left ventricle of the heart is not pumping effectively, then blood backs up in the system. The result of the backup causes an increase in pressure within the pulmonary vasculature. The increased pressure forces fluid through the alveolar membrane and into the alveoli. Blood will enter the alveoli through the alveolar membrane in small amounts, producing a pink rather than red appearance. The froth comes from the additional fluid being exposed to the air in the patient's lungs and airways.

6. How do you account for the decreased Spo_2 level?

In this case, the patient would have a decreased amount of surface area for oxygen exchange due to pulmonary edema. Less surface area means less oxygen will "saturate" the cells, which in turn will be read by the pulse oximeter as a decrease in saturation. It is important to note that the saturation amount shown on the electronic device represents any gas that is saturating the cells. Oxygen is one of many gases that can affect the reading. In addition, saturation levels may be compromised by the patient's own lack of circulation.

7. Why would a diuretic be prescribed for a patient with heart failure?

If a patient has heart failure, then the heart is not pumping blood effectively. This causes a backup within the circulatory system, which in turn causes fluid to back up into the pulmonary vasculature. A diuretic helps to eliminate some of the fluid from the system to lessen the workload on the heart. Most diuretics work on the kidneys to eliminate water and electrolytes. The elimination moves fluid from the extracellular to the intravascular space, which will transport it out of the body. The goal is to reduce the cardiac preload, which will reduce the amount of work the cardiac system has to do and reduce the fluid backup.

8. Why would this patient have a normal or slightly high blood pressure?

In patients with heart failure, the heart is working harder to pump fluid volume. Increased venous return to the heart increases cardiac preload. The heart muscle stretches in response to the increased amount of fluid. According to the Starling law, the heart muscle will then contract with greater force—up to a point—to expel the fluid. This accounts for a normal or higher blood pressure because the body is trying to compensate for the lack of the heart's muscular ability.

YOU are the Provider SUMMARY *(continued)*

EMS Patient Care Report (PCR)					
Date: 08-01-18	**Incident No.:** 1234		**Nature of Call:** Difficulty breathing		**Location:** 420 Beach Street
Dispatched: 2041	**En Route:** 2041	**At Scene:** 2045	**Transport:** 2052	**At Hospital:** 2107	**In Service:** 2122

Patient Information	
Age: 72 **Sex:** M **Weight (in kg [lb]):** 80.2 kg (177 lb)	**Allergies:** No known drug allergies **Medications:** Numerous **Past Medical History:** Heart failure **Chief Complaint:** Difficulty breathing

Vital Signs				
Time: 2047	**BP:** 140/90	**Pulse:** 110	**Respirations:** 22	**Spo_2:** 89%
Time: 2052	**BP:** 138/88	**Pulse:** 114	**Respirations:** 24	**Spo_2:** 92%
Time:	**BP:**	**Pulse:**	**Respirations:**	**Spo_2:**

EMS Treatment (circle all that apply)				
Oxygen @ 15 **L/min via (circle one):** **NC** **(NRM)** **Bag-mask device**		**Assisted Ventilation**	**Airway Adjunct**	**CPR**
Defibrillation	**Bleeding Control**	**Bandaging**	**Splinting**	**Other:**

Narrative
Arrived to find this 72-year-old man being attended by his neighbor. Pt lives alone in this residence. Pt alert (oriented to person, place, and time). Pt unable to speak in complete sentences due to respiratory effort. Pt states he has not been compliant with his medications for a time. Pt states he has a history of "heart failure" and is using 2 L/min O_2 via cannula. Assessment shows vital signs as above; breath sound assessment shows coarse crackles in all fields. Pt has productive cough with pink, frothy sputum. O_2 via NRM applied at 15 L/min on scene and throughout transport. IV line of NS established TKO. $ETCO_2$ waveform appears appropriate in shape and reads 36 mm Hg. Treatment per local protocol, radio report during transport, and verbal report to Halifax Health on arrival. Pt transferred to room A-20.**End of report**

Prep Kit

▶ Ready for Review

- Pathophysiology is the study of the physiology of altered functioning in the presence of disease.
- Pathophysiology in the cellular environment includes disturbances in fluid balance and electrolyte imbalances. These various imbalances can upset homeostasis and may result in or contribute to emergency conditions.
- Cellular injury is caused by factors such as hypoxia, chemical exposure, infectious agents, inappropriate immunologic responses, inflammatory responses, genetic factors, nutritional imbalances, physical agents such as radiation, and adverse conditions such as extreme cold.
- When cells are exposed to adverse conditions, cells undergo a process of temporary or permanent adaptation to protect themselves from injury. Examples of adaptation include atrophy, hypertrophy, hyperplasia, dysplasia, and metaplasia.
- Inflammatory response is characterized by both local and systemic effects. Local effects consist of dilation (expansion) of blood vessels and increased vascular permeability. If the inflammatory process is severe, then systemic effects such as fever become evident. The outcome of an inflammation depends on how much tissue damage has resulted from the inflammation.
- Immunologic diseases occur because of hyperactivity or hypoactivity of the immune system. Allergies are acquired following initial exposure to a stimulant known as an allergen. Repeated exposures generate an immune system reaction to the allergen.
- Perfusion is the delivery of oxygen and nutrients to cells, organs, and tissues through the circulatory system. Hypoperfusion occurs when the level of tissue perfusion falls below normal.
- Shock is an abnormal state associated with inadequate oxygen and nutrient delivery to the metabolic apparatus of the cell, resulting in an impairment of cellular metabolism.
- Central shock consists of cardiogenic shock and obstructive shock. Cardiogenic shock occurs when the heart cannot circulate enough blood to maintain adequate peripheral oxygen delivery. Obstructive shock occurs when blood flow within the heart or great vessels (aorta and pulmonary vein) becomes blocked.
- Peripheral shock includes hypovolemic shock and distributive shock. In hypovolemic shock, the circulating blood volume is insufficient to deliver adequate oxygen and nutrients to the body. Distributive shock occurs when there is widespread dilation of the resistance vessels (small arterioles), the capacitance vessels (small venules), or both.
- Multiple organ dysfunction syndrome (MODS) occurs in acutely ill patients and is characterized by the dysfunction of two or more organs that were not affected by the physiologic insult for which the patient was initially being treated. Six organ systems are surveyed to determine whether a patient has MODS and, if so, how high is the risk of mortality: respiratory, hepatic, renal, hematologic, neurologic, and cardiovascular.
- The immune system includes all of the structures and processes that mount a defense against foreign substances and disease-causing agents.
- The body has three lines of defense: anatomic barriers, the inflammatory response, and the immune response.
- There are two general types of immune response: native and acquired.
- Immunity may be humoral or cell-mediated.
- Important white blood cells in the immune system include neutrophils, eosinophils, basophils, monocytes, and lymphocytes. Other important cells of the immune system include macrophages, mast cells, plasma cells, B cells, and T cells.
- The antibodies secreted by B cells are called immunoglobulins. Antibodies make antigens more visible to the immune system in three ways: by acting as opsonins, by making antigens clump, and by inactivating bacterial toxins.
- The inflammatory response is the reaction of the body's tissues to cellular injury. It is characterized by pain, swelling, redness, and heat.
- The two most common causes of inflammation are infection and injury.
- The plasma protein systems that modulate the inflammatory process include the complement system, the coagulation (clotting) system, and the kinin system.
- Cytokines are products of cells that affect the functioning of other cells; they include interleukins, lymphokines, and interferon.
- Chronic inflammatory responses are usually caused by an unsuccessful acute inflammatory response after the invasion of a foreign body, a persistent infection, or an antigen.
- Normal wound healing involves four steps: repairing damaged tissue, removing inflammatory debris, restoring tissues to a normal state, and regenerating cells.
- Wounds may heal by primary or secondary intention. Healing by primary intention occurs in clean

Prep Kit *(continued)*

wounds with opposed margins. Wounds that heal by secondary intention have a prolonged inflammatory phase and more abundant granulation tissue.

- Hypersensitivity is an increased response of the body to any substance to which the person is abnormally sensitive. A hypersensitivity reaction may be immediate, occurring within seconds to minutes, or delayed, occurring hours to days after exposure to the antigen.
- Hypersensitivity reactions may be classified as autoimmune, idiopathic, or blood incompatibility reactions.
- Immunodeficiency may be congenital or acquired.
- Age- and sex-associated factors interact with a combination of genetic and environmental factors, lifestyle, and anatomic or hormonal differences to cause disease.
- Analyzing disease risk involves consideration of disease rates (incidence, prevalence, morbidity, and mortality) and controllable and uncontrollable disease risk factors (causal and noncausal). These risk factors, age, and sex differences interact to influence a person's level of risk.
- A true genetic risk is passed through generations on a gene. In contrast, a familial tendency may cluster in family groups despite lack of evidence for heritable gene-associated abnormalities.
- Stress does not cause death directly, but it can permit diseases to flourish, ultimately leading to death.
- The general adaptation syndrome describes the body's short- and long-term reactions to stress.
- Stress causes the sympathetic nervous system to be stimulated. This occurs through the release of catecholamines that activate the sympathetic nervous system by binding to alpha and beta receptor sites, resulting in effects categorized as fight-or-flight response.
- Stress also causes secretion of cortisol, which has many useful effects such as increasing serum glucose levels, decreasing protein reserves, and permitting mobilization of fatty acids. However, continuous secretion of cortisol has deleterious effects.

▶ Vital Vocabulary

acidosis An increase in extracellular H^+ ions; a blood pH of less than 7.35.

acquired immunity The immunity that occurs when the body is exposed to a foreign substance or disease and produces antibodies to the invader.

activation Mediators of inflammation trigger the appearance of molecules known as selectins and integrins on the surfaces of endothelial cells and polymorphonuclear neutrophils, respectively.

adhesion The attachment of polymorphonuclear neutrophils to endothelial cells, mediated by selectins and integrins.

alcoholic ketoacidosis The metabolic acidotic state that manifests because of the inadequate nutritional habits associated with chronic alcohol abuse. The liver and body experience inadequate fuel reserves of glycogen and, thus, have to switch to fatty acid metabolism.

alkalosis A decrease in extracellular H^+ ions; a blood pH greater than 7.45.

allergen Any substance that causes a hypersensitivity reaction.

allergy A hypersensitivity reaction to the presence of an agent (allergen) that is intrinsically harmless.

anaphylactic shock A severe hypersensitivity reaction that involves bronchoconstriction and cardiovascular collapse.

angiogenesis The growth of new blood vessels.

antibody A protein secreted by certain immune cells that bind antigens to make them more visible to the immune system.

antigen A foreign substance recognized by the immune system.

apoptosis Normal, genetically programmed cell death.

asthma A chronic inflammatory lower airway condition resulting in intermittent wheezing and excess mucus production.

atopic An allergic tendency.

atrophy A decrease in cell size due to a loss of subcellular components.

autoantibodies Antibodies directed against the person's own proteins.

autoimmunity The production of antibodies or T cells that work against the tissues of a person's body, producing autoimmune disease or a hypersensitivity reaction.

bradypnea A slow respiratory rate.

capillary refill time A test performed on the fingernails or toenails that involves briefly squeezing the toenail or fingernail and evaluating the time it takes for the color to return.

cardiogenic shock A condition caused by loss of 40% or more of the functioning myocardium; the heart is no longer able to circulate sufficient blood to maintain adequate oxygen delivery.

carpopedal spasm A contorted position of the hand or foot in which the fingers or toes flex in a clawlike

Prep Kit (continued)

manner; may result from hyperventilation or hypocalcemia.

cell-mediated immunity The immune process by which T-cell lymphocytes recognize antigens and then secrete cytokines (specifically lymphokines) that attract other cells or stimulate the production of cytotoxic cells that kill the infected cells.

central shock A type of shock caused by central pump failure, including cardiogenic shock and obstructive shock.

chemotaxins Components of the activated complement system that attract leukocytes from the circulation to help fight infections.

chemotaxis The movement of additional white blood cells to an area of inflammation in response to the release of chemical mediators, such as neutrophils, injured tissue, and monocytes.

coagulation system The system that forms blood clots in the body and facilitates repairs to the vascular tree.

complement system A group of plasma proteins whose function is to do one of three things: attract leukocytes to sites of inflammation, activate leukocytes, and directly destroy cells.

cytokines The products of cells that affect the function of other cells.

distributive shock The type of shock caused by widespread dilation of the resistance vessels (small arterioles), the capacitance vessels (small venules), or both.

dysplasia An alteration in the size, shape, and organization of cells.

edema Swelling caused by excessive fluid trapped in the body tissues

fibrin A whitish, filamentous protein formed by the action of thrombin on fibrinogen; the protein that polymerizes (bonds) to form the fibrous component of a blood clot.

fibrinolysis cascade The breakdown of fibrin in blood clots and the prevention of the polymerization of fibrin into new clots.

free radicals A molecule that is missing one electron in its outer shell.

general adaptation syndrome A three-stage description of the body's short- and long-term reactions to stress.

hapten A substance that normally does not stimulate an immune response but can be combined with an antigen and at a later point initiate an antibody response.

helper T cells A type of T lymphocyte that is involved in cell-mediated and antibody-mediated immune responses. It secretes cytokines that stimulate the B cells and other T cells.

hemochromatosis An inherited disease in which the body absorbs more iron than it needs and stores it in the liver, kidneys, and pancreas.

hemolytic anemia A disease characterized by increased destruction of the red blood cells. It can occur from an Rh factor reaction (primarily in Rh-positive neonates born to sensitized Rh-negative mothers), exposure to chemicals, or a disorder of the immune system.

hemophilia An inherited sex-linked disorder characterized by excessive bleeding.

histamine A vasoactive amine that increases vascular permeability and causes vasodilation.

humoral immunity A type of immunity in which B-cell lymphocytes produce antibodies called immunoglobulins, which recognize a specific antigen and then react with it.

hypercalcemia An elevated blood calcium level.

hypercholesterolemia An elevated blood cholesterol level.

hyperkalemia An elevated serum potassium level.

hypermagnesemia An increased serum magnesium level.

hypernatremia A serum sodium level greater than or equal to 143 mEq/L.

hyperphosphatemia An elevated serum phosphate level.

hyperplasia An increase in the actual number of cells in an organ or tissue, usually resulting in an increase in the size of the organ or tissue.

hypersensitivity A generic term for responses of the body to a substance to which a patient has increased sensitivity.

hypertrophy An increase in the size of the cells due to synthesis of more subcellular components, leading to an increase in tissue and organ size.

hypocalcemia A decreased serum calcium level.

hypokalemia A decreased serum potassium level.

hypomagnesemia A decreased serum magnesium level.

hyponatremia A serum sodium level that is less than or equal to 135 mEq/L.

hypoperfusion A condition that occurs when the level of tissue perfusion decreases below that needed to maintain normal cellular functions.

hypophosphatemia A decreased serum phosphate level.

hypothalamic-pituitary-adrenal axis A major part of the neuroendocrine system that controls reactions to stress. It is the mechanism for a set of interactions

Prep Kit *(continued)*

among glands, hormones, and parts of the midbrain that mediate the general adaptation syndrome.

hypovolemic shock A condition that occurs when the circulating blood volume is inadequate to deliver adequate oxygen and nutrients to the body.

immune response The body's defense reaction to any substance that is recognized as foreign.

immune system The body system that includes all of the structures and processes designed to mount a defense against foreign substances and disease-causing agents.

immunodeficiency An abnormal condition in which some part of the body's immune system is inadequate, and, consequently, resistance to infectious disease is decreased.

immunogen An antigen that is capable of generating an immune response.

immunoglobulins Antibodies secreted by the B cells.

incidence The number of new cases of a disease in a population.

inflammatory response A reaction by tissues of the body to irritation or injury, characterized by pain, swelling, redness, and heat.

interferon A protein produced by cells in response to viral invasion that is released into the bloodstream or intercellular fluid to induce healthy cells to manufacture an enzyme that counters the infection.

interleukins Chemical substances that attract white blood cells to the sites of injury and bacterial invasions.

isoimmunity The formation of antibodies or T cells that are directed against antigens or another person's cells.

ketoacidosis An acidotic state created by the production of ketones via fat metabolism.

ketones Acidic by-products of fat metabolism.

killer T cells The cells released during a type IV allergic reaction that kill antigen-bearing target cells.

kinin system A group of polypeptides that mediate inflammatory responses by stimulating visceral smooth muscle and relaxing vascular smooth muscle to produce vasodilation.

lactic acidosis Anaerobic cellular respiration due to hypoperfusion of tissues and organs.

leukocytosis An elevated white blood cell count, often due to inflammation.

leukotrienes Arachidonic acid metabolites that function as chemical mediators of inflammation; also known as slow-reacting substances of anaphylaxis.

lymphokines Cytokines released by lymphocytes, including many of the interleukins, gamma interferon, tumor necrosis factor beta, and chemokines.

margination The loss of fluid from the blood vessels into the tissue, causing the blood left in the vessels to have increased viscosity, which in turn slows the flow of blood and produces stasis.

membrane attack complex Molecules that insert themselves into the bacterial membrane, leading to weakened areas in the membrane.

metabolic acidosis A pathologic condition characterized by a blood pH of less than 7.35 and caused by an accumulation of acids in the body from a metabolic cause.

metabolic alkalosis A pathologic condition characterized by a blood pH of greater than 7.45 and caused by an accumulation of bases in the body from a metabolic cause.

metaplasia A reversible, cellular adaptation in which one adult cell type is replaced by another adult cell type.

morbidity Number of nonfatally injured or disabled people; usually expressed as a rate, meaning the number of nonfatal injuries in a certain population in a given time period divided by the size of the population.

morbid obesity An excessively unhealthy accumulation of body fat, defined as a body mass index of greater than or equal to 40 kg/m^2.

mortality The quality of being mortal; number of deaths from a disease in a given population.

multiple organ dysfunction syndrome (MODS) A grave but sometimes reversible condition in an acutely ill patient characterized by the progressive dysfunction of two or more organs or organ systems not affected by the patient's initial illness or injury.

natural immunity A nonspecific cellular and humoral response that operates as the body's first line of defense against pathogens; also called native immunity.

necrosis The death of tissue, usually caused by a cessation of the blood supply.

neurogenic shock A type of shock that usually results from spinal cord injury; loss of normal sympathetic nervous system tone and vasodilation occur.

obesity An unhealthy accumulation of body fat, defined as a body mass index of greater than or equal to 30 kg/m^2.

obstructive shock The type of shock that occurs when blood flow to the heart or great vessels is obstructed.

oliguria Decreased urine output.

Prep Kit *(continued)*

opsonization The process by which an antibody coats an antigen to facilitate its recognition by immune cells.

overweight An unhealthy accumulation of body fat, defined as a body mass index of 25 to 29.9 kg/m^2.

pathophysiology The study of the physiology of altered functioning in the presence of disease.

perfusion The delivery of oxygen and nutrients to the cells, organs, and tissues of the body; also involves the removal of wastes.

pericardial tamponade The impairment of diastolic filling of the right ventricle due to significant amounts of fluid in the pericardial sac surrounding the heart, leading to a decrease in the cardiac output.

peripheral shock Shock caused by peripheral circulatory abnormalities; includes hypovolemic shock and distributive shock.

phagocytes The cells that engulf and consume foreign material such as microorganisms and debris.

polymorphonuclear neutrophils (PMNs) The type of white blood cells formed by bone marrow tissue that have a nucleus consisting of several parts or lobes connected by fine strands.

polyuria Frequent and plentiful urination.

prevalence The number of cases of a disease in a specific population within a given period.

prostaglandins A group of lipids that act as chemical messengers.

pyrogens Chemicals or proteins that travel to the brain and affect the hypothalamus and stimulate a rise in the body's core temperature.

receptor A specialized area in tissue that initiates certain actions after specific stimulation.

respiratory acidosis A pathologic condition characterized by a blood pH of less than 7.35 and caused by an accumulation of acids in the body from a respiratory cause.

respiratory alkalosis A pathologic condition characterized by a blood pH of greater than 7.45 and caused by an accumulation of bases in the body from a respiratory cause.

septic shock The type of shock that occurs as a result of widespread infection, usually bacterial; untreated, the result is multiple organ dysfunction syndrome and often death.

serotonin A vasoactive amine that increases vascular permeability to cause vasodilation.

serum sickness A condition in which antigen-antibody complexes formed in the bloodstream deposit in sites around the body, most notably the kidneys, with resultant inflammatory reactions.

transmigration (diapedesis) The polymorphonuclear neutrophils permeate through the vessel wall, moving into the interstitial space.

urticaria Multiple small, raised areas on the skin that may be one of the warning signs of impending anaphylaxis; also known as hives.

vasculitis An inflammation of the blood vessels.

vasoactive amines Substances such as histamine and serotonin that increase vascular permeability.

virulence A measure of the disease-causing ability of a microorganism.

▶ References

1. He F, Li J, MacGregor GA. Effect of longer term modest salt reduction on blood pressure: Cochrane systematic review and meta-analysis of randomised trials. *BMJ*. 2013;346:f1325.
2. Friis-Hansen BJ, Holiday M, Stapleton T, Wallace WM. Total body water in children. *Pediatrics*. 1951; 7(3): 321-327.
3. Fontanarosa PB, Christiansen S. Units of measure. Table 2: selected laboratory tests, with reference ranges and conversion factors. In: American Medical Association, ed. *AMA Manual of Style: A Guide for Authors and Editors*. 10th ed. New York, NY: Oxford University Press; 2007:798-815.
4. Paz J, West M. *Acute Care Handbook for Physical Therapists*. 4th ed. St. Louis, MO: Elsevier/Saunders; 2014.
5. Speakman E. *Body Fluids & Electrolytes: A Programmed Presentation*. 8th ed. St. Louis, MO: Elsevier/Mosby; 2002.
6. Stipanuk MH, Caudill M. *Biochemical, Physiological, and Molecular Aspects of Human Nutrition*. 3rd ed. St. Louis, MO: Elsevier/Saunders; 2013.
7. Brown AFT, Cadogan M. *Emergency Medicine: Diagnosis and Management*. 6th ed. Boca Raton, FL: CRC Press; 2011.
8. Goldman L, Schaffer A. *Goldman-Cecil Medicine*, 25th ed. St. Louis, MO: Elsevier/Saunders; 2016.
9. Rose JJ, Wang L, Xu Q, McTiernan CF, Shiva S, Tejero J, Gladwin MT. Carbon monoxide poisoning: pathogenesis, management and future directions of therapy. *Am J Resp Crit Care*. 2016, Oct 18. [Epub ahead of print]
10. Schmidt H, Müller-Werdan U, Hoffmann T, Francis DP, Piepoli MF, Rauchhaus M, Werdan K. Autonomic dysfunction predicts mortality in patients with multiple organ dysfunction syndrome of different age groups. *Crit Care Med*. 2005;33(9), 1994-2002.

Prep Kit (continued)

11. American Cancer Society. *Cancer Facts & Figures 2015*. Atlanta: American Cancer Society; 2015. http://www.cancer.org/acs/groups/content/@editorial/documents/document/acspc-044552.pdf. Accessed October 31, 2016.
12. National Hemophilia Foundation. Hemophilia A. https://www.hemophilia.org/Bleeding-Disorders/Types-of-Bleeding-Disorders/Hemophilia-A. Accessed October 31, 2016.
13. Savage DD, Garrison RJ, Devereaux RB, et al. Mitral valve prolapse in the general population: 1. Epidemiological features: the Framingham study. *Am Heart J*. 1983;106(3):571-576.
14. CDC, NCHS. Underlying Cause of Death 1999-2013 on CDC WONDER Online Database, released 2015. Data are from the Multiple Cause of Death Files, 1999-2013, as compiled from data provided by the 57 vital statistics jurisdictions through the Vital Statistics Cooperative Program. Accessed January 3, 2017.
15. Flegal KM, Carroll MD, Kit BK, Ogden CL. Prevalence of obesity and trends in the distribution of body mass index among US adults, 1999–2010. http://jama.jamanetwork.com/article.aspx?articleid=1104933External Link Disclaimer. *JAMA*. 2012; 307(5):491–97.
16. Ogden CL, Carroll MD, Kit BK, Flegal KM. Prevalence of obesity and trends in body mass index among US children and adolescents, 1999–2010. http://jama.jamanetwork.com/Mobile/article.aspx?articleid=1104932External Link Disclaimer. *JAMA*. 2012; 307(5):483–90.
17. National Multiple Sclerosis Society. What Is MS? http://www.nationalmssociety.org/What-is-MS/What-Causes-MS. Accessed October 31, 2016.
18. Alzheimer's Foundation of America. (Jan 28, 2016). About Alzheimer's Disease. https://www.alzfdn.org/AboutAlzheimers/statistics.html. Retrieved January 3, 2017.
19. Depression and Bipolar Support Alliance. (2016). Bipolar Disorder Statistics. http://www.dbsalliance.org/site/PageServer?pagename=education_statistics_bipolar_disorder. Retrieved January 3, 2017.

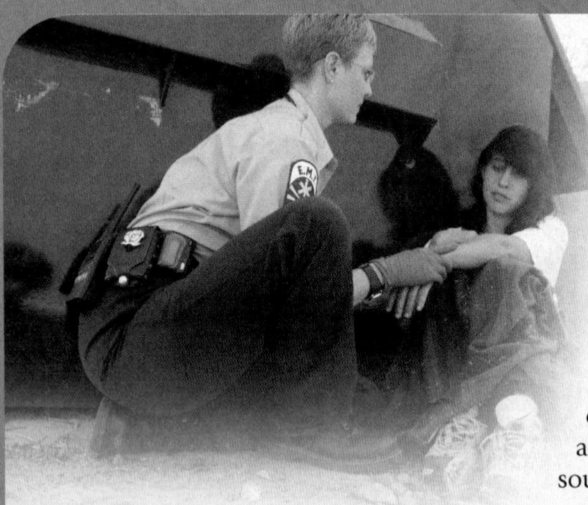

Assessment in Action

You are dispatched to a senior center for an 82-year-old man who was stung by a bee. On arrival, you are met by an aide who directs you to the patient. The patient is sitting upright in a wheelchair in obvious distress. You can see urticaria covering his arms, legs, and face. His tongue is swollen, and you can hear wheezing in all fields when assessing lung sounds. His radial pulses are weak and thready.

1. A(n) _____ is the body's defense reaction to any substance it recognizes as foreign.

- **A.** immunogen
- **B.** cell-mediated immunity
- **C.** immune response
- **D.** humoral immunity

2. Anaphylactic shock is characterized by:

- **A.** hypertension and vasoconstriction.
- **B.** wheezing and widespread vasodilation.
- **C.** hypotension and hives.
- **D.** crackles (rales) and stridor.

Assessment *in Action* *(continued)*

3. When oxygen does not reach the cell, the cell reverts to:

A. anaerobic metabolism.
B. aerobic metabolism.
C. production of ketones.
D. production of bicarbonate.

4. Distributive shock occurs when:

A. blood moves from the core of the body.
B. blood pools in expanded vascular structures.
C. microorganisms attack the body.
D. a significant decrease in stroke volume occurs.

5. An immunogen is a(n) _____ capable of generating an immune response.

A. lymphocyte
B. T cell
C. antibody
D. antigen

6. The worst respiratory sign in this patient with anaphylactic shock is:

A. diminished lung sounds.
B. diffuse expiratory wheezing.
C. diffuse coarse crackles.
D. labored breathing.

7. Based on your knowledge of the pathophysiology of anaphylaxis, what do you anticipate the patient's vital signs to be?

A. Bradycardic and hypertensive with elevated $ETCO_2$
B. Tachycardic and hypotensive with elevated $ETCO_2$
C. Tachycardic and hypotensive with decreased $ETCO_2$
D. Bradycardic and normotensive with a normal $ETCO_2$

8. All of the following are primary stimuli for the degranulation of mast cells during the inflammatory response EXCEPT:

A. physical injury.
B. chemical agents.
C. therapeutic medications.
D. immunologic substances.

9. In arterial blood gas analysis, a patient has a low pH and a high partial pressure of carbon dioxide in arterial blood ($PaCO_2$). What type of acidosis or alkalosis does the patient have?

10. Will a patient who has been hyperventilating have signs and symptoms of respiratory acidosis or respiratory alkalosis?

CHAPTER 9

Life Span Development

National EMS Education Standard Competencies

Life Span Development

Applies fundamental knowledge of life span development to patient assessment and management.

Knowledge Objectives

1. Know the terms used to designate the following developmental stages: infants, toddlers, preschoolers, school-age children, adolescents (teenagers), early adults, middle adults, and older adults. (pp 370, 374, 376, 378, 379)
2. Describe the major physical and psychosocial characteristics of an infant's life. (pp 371-374)
3. Describe the major physical and psychosocial characteristics of a toddler's life. (pp 374-376)
4. Describe the major physical and psychosocial characteristics of a preschooler's life. (pp 374-376)
5. Describe the major physical and psychosocial characteristics of a school-age child's life. (p 376)
6. Describe the major physical and psychosocial characteristics of an adolescent's life. (pp 376-378)
7. Describe the major physical and psychosocial characteristics of an early adult's life. (pp 378-379)
8. Describe the major physical and psychosocial characteristics of a middle adult's life. (p 379)
9. Describe the major physical and psychosocial characteristics of an older adult's life. (pp 379-384)

Skills Objectives

There are no skills objectives for this chapter.

Introduction

One of the most interesting things about humans is that we evolve throughout our life spans—not just as a species, but also as people. Advanced emergency medical technicians (AEMTs) must be aware of the obvious *and* the subtle changes a person undergoes physically and mentally at various stages of life and understand how these changes might alter the approach to patient care.

Neonates (Birth to 1 Month) and Infants (1 Month to 1 Year)

As any parent can attest, infants develop at a startling rate Figure 9-1. **Infants** are defined as children from age 1 month to 1 year. **Neonates** are defined as children from birth to 1 month of age. Neonatal issues and

YOU are the Provider — PART 1

You and your partner are dispatched to a local residence for a 3-month-old girl who has a runny nose. On arrival, you are met at the door by the mother who is holding the infant in her arms. The scene is safe and the house appears to be neat and clean. The patient's mother introduces her older adult mother, whom she also cares for, as well as a 12-year-old sibling.

1. How does the patient's age affect your treatment?
2. What are some physical differences between pediatric and adult patients?

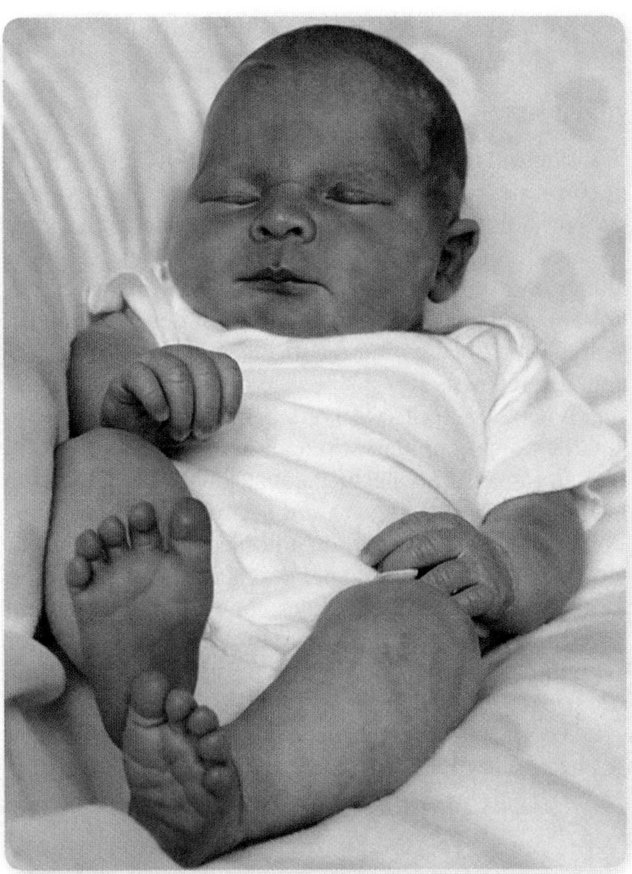

Figure 9-1 An infant.

care are covered in detail in Chapter 35, *Obstetrics and Neonatal Care*.

▶ Physical Changes

Vital Signs

Normal ranges for vital signs for various age groups are outlined in Chapter 10, *Patient Assessment*, and Chapter 36, *Pediatric Emergencies*. The general rule is the younger the person, the faster the pulse rate and respirations. At birth, a pulse rate of 90 to 205 beats/min and a respiratory rate of 30 to 60 breaths/min are considered normal. Within the first half hour after birth, a neonate's pulse rate usually drops to 120 beats/min and the respiratory rate falls to between 30 to 40 breaths/min. By age 1 year, the respiratory rate slows to 20 to 30 breaths/min. The tidal volume in neonates starts at 6 to 8 mL/kg. By the end of the first year, the volume increases to 10 to 15 mL/kg.

Blood pressure directly corresponds to the patient's weight, so it typically increases with age. At birth, the average systolic blood pressure of a neonate is 67 to 84 mm Hg. By 1 year of age, it ranges between 85 and 104 mm Hg. A neonate's normal body temperature ranges from 98°F (37°C) to 100°F (38°C). An infant's normal temperature ranges between 96.8°F (36°C) to 99.6°F (37.5°C).

> **Words of Wisdom**
>
> Infants often land head first when they fall because their heads account for 25% of their total body weight. Also, most infants cannot stretch out their arms in time to cushion or slow their fall. Keep this in mind when considering spinal immobilization of an infant.

Weight

A neonate usually weighs 6 to 8 pounds (3 to 3.5 kg) at birth. Remarkably, the head accounts for 25% of an infant's total body weight. In the first week after birth, neonates will usually have a 5% to 10% birth weight loss due to the loss of fluids. By week 2, the neonate begins to gain weight. From here on, infants grow at a rate of about 1 ounce (30 g) per day, doubling their weight within 4 to 6 months and tripling it by the end of the first year.

Cardiovascular System

Before birth, fetal circulation occurs through the placenta. During the birthing process, hormones and pressure changes help the neonate make the transition from fetal circulation to independent circulation. Chapter 35, *Obstetrics and Neonatal Care*, covers the transition from fetal circulation.

Pulmonary System

Before a neonate's first breath, the lungs have never been inflated. For this reason, a neonate's first breath must be forceful.

Neonates are primarily "nose breathers." Infants younger than 6 months are particularly prone to nasal congestion, which can cause viral upper respiratory infections. If you receive a call for a baby choking, ensure the nasal passages are clear and unobstructed by mucus.

The rib cage of an infant is less rigid than an adult's, and the ribs sit horizontally. This explains the

> **Special Populations**
>
> When you are counting respirations in an infant, count the number of times the abdomen rises instead of concentrating solely on the chest rise.

> **Words of Wisdom**
>
> Fluid and heat loss occur through exhalation. The rapid respiratory rate of infants can lead to significant heat and fluid loss. Keep infants warm, and monitor them for signs of dehydration.

diaphragmatic breathing ("belly breathing") in infants. Owing to the immaturity of the accessory muscles, fatigue sets in quickly.

Two other important anatomic points related to an infant's airway, compared with an adult's, are the proportionally large size of the tongue and the proportionally shorter, narrower, and less stable airway. As a result, the airway in infants can be obstructed much more easily than in older children and adults. There are also fewer alveoli in the lungs, which decreases the surface area for gas exchange.

When providing bag-mask ventilations to an infant, be aware that an infant's lungs are fragile. Ventilations that are too forceful can result in trauma from pressure, or barotrauma **Figure 9-2**. Barotrauma is trauma resulting from increased pressure, for example, from too much pressure in the lungs.

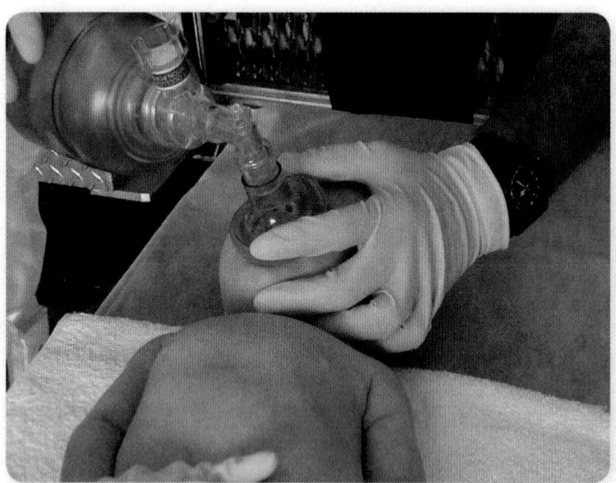

Figure 9-2 An infant's lungs are fragile. Use caution when providing bag-mask ventilations to avoid barotrauma.

Nervous System

Although an infant's nervous system is developed at birth, it continues to evolve after birth. For example, neonates lack the ability to localize and isolate a particular response to sensation. When neonates are born, they tend to move their extremities together in response to stimulation. Motor and sensory development are most developed in the cranial nerves, allowing for strong, coordinated sucking and gag reflexes.

A neonate is born with certain reflexes. The **Moro reflex** (startle reflex) happens when an neonate is surprised by something or someone; the neonate opens his or her arms wide, spreads the fingers, and seems to grab at things. A **palmar grasp** occurs when an object is placed into the neonate's palm. The **rooting reflex** takes place when something touches a neonate's cheek; the neonate will instinctively turn his or her head toward the touch. In conjunction with the **sucking reflex**, which occurs when an infant's lips are stroked, these reflexes are often evident when feeding.

A neonate's **fontanelles** allow the head to be molded—for example, when the neonate passes through the birth canal **Figure 9-3**. The fontanelles are the area or space

> **Special Populations**
>
> Use the fontanelles of infants as an assessment tool: bulging fontanelles may indicate increased intracranial pressure and sunken fontanelles are indicative of dehydration.

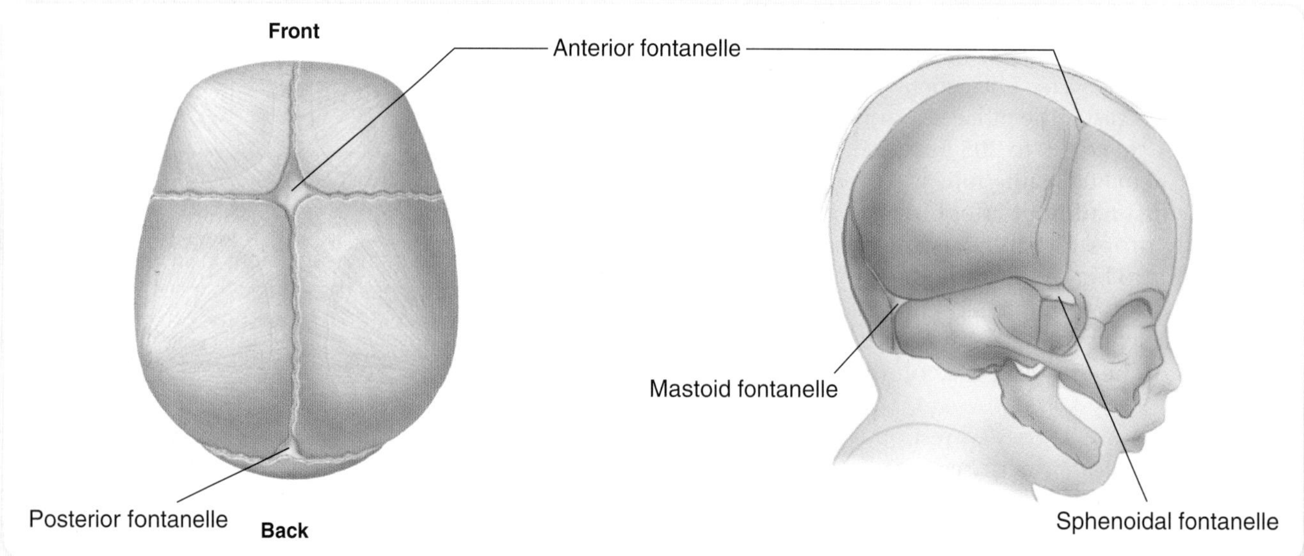

Figure 9-3 Fontanelles.

between the bones that eventually fuse to form the skull. The three or four bones of the skull eventually bind together and form suture joints. The posterior fontanelle normally fuses by 3 months of age. The anterior fontanelle fuses between 9 and 18 months of age. If either of the fontanelles is depressed when you assess the head, the infant is most likely dehydrated. A bulging fontanelle is indicative of increased intracranial pressure.

Perhaps the neurologic development that is of most interest to parents is the development of a sleep pattern. Some physicians suggest parents wake neonates and infants every few hours for feeding and safety (for example, to guard against sudden infant death syndrome, commonly known as SIDS). Others suggest neonates and infants should be left to sleep so they can adjust to family life and develop a circadian rhythm, ideally within 4 months after birth. SIDS is described in more detail in Chapter 36, *Pediatric Emergencies*.

Musculoskeletal System

Growth plates (also known as epiphyseal plates), located on either end of an infant's long bones, aid in lengthening a child's bones.[1] Bones grow in thickness by building on themselves.

Renal System

Infants can become dehydrated easily because their kidneys usually cannot produce concentrated urine. An infant's urine consists mainly of water, which can cause the development of electrolyte imbalances.

Immune System

While in the womb, fetuses collect antibodies from the maternal blood. For the first 6 months of life, the infant maintains some of the mother's immunities, so he or she has naturally acquired passive immunities. Infants can also receive antibodies via breastfeeding, further bolstering their immune system.

▶ Psychosocial Changes

An infant's psychosocial development begins at birth and continues to evolve as the infant interacts with and reacts to the environment. Rapid changes occur during the first year of life. Parents are often very concerned with whether their children are developing within the socially accepted norms. Table 9-1 outlines the typical ages when major psychosocial changes are noticed.

Table 9-1 Noticeable Characteristics at Various Ages

Age	Characteristic
2 months	Recognizes familiar faces; tracks objects with eyes
3 months	Brings objects to the mouth; smiles and frowns
4 months	Reaches out to people; drools
5 months	Sleeps throughout the night; recognizes family members from strangers
6 months	Teething begins; sits upright; speaks one-syllable words
7 months	Afraid of strangers; mood swings
8 months	Responds to "no"; can sit alone; plays peek-a-boo
9 months	Pulls up to a stand; places objects in mouth to explore them
10 months	Responds to own name; crawls efficiently
11 months	Tries to walk without help; frustrated with restrictions
12 months	Knows own name; walks

For most infants, the primary method of communicating distress is through crying. Parents can often tell what is upsetting their children simply by listening to the tone of their cries—that is, they know the difference between a basic cry expressing frustration, fear, hunger, discomfort, and sleepiness and the tears that indicate anger or pain. Infants occasionally make another distinct cry—an alarming distressed cry. This cry may be heard when an unexpected event occurs, causing a situational crisis for the infant.

One key to having a happy, healthy infant is spending time with the infant. Nevertheless, infants often have their own timetable as to when they will become attached to their parents and other family members. **Bonding,** or the formation of a close, personal relationship, is usually based on a secure attachment. A **secure attachment** occurs when an infant understands that parents or caregivers will be responsive to his or her needs. This realization encourages infants to reach out and explore, knowing their parents will provide a "safety net."

Another type of attachment, referred to as **anxious-avoidant attachment,** is observed in infants who are repeatedly rejected. In this attachment style, infants show little emotional response to their parents or caregivers and treat them as they would strangers. These children often develop an isolated lifestyle where they do not have to depend on the support and care of others.

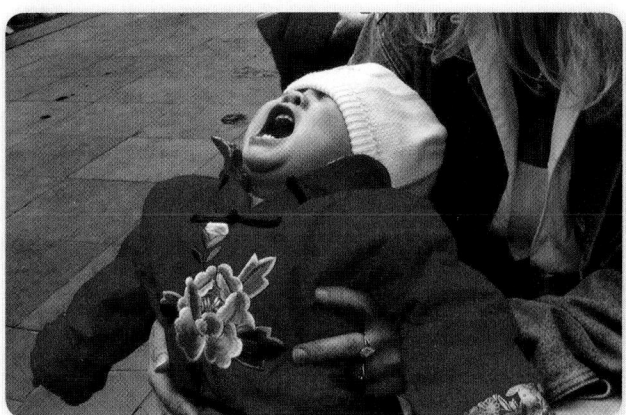

Figure 9-4 Protesting and crying in reaction to unfamiliar places and people is a normal reaction in older infants.

Words of Wisdom

When assessing infants and toddlers, remember that these age groups can experience falls and injuries as a result of their developmental stage (for example, learning to walk or climb). Also remember that they can be victims of abuse and neglect. Look for injuries that are not consistent with the developmental stage, for example, a 15 month old may climb out of a crib and sustain injuries as a result of a fall, but a 4 month old cannot climb out of a crib.

Separation anxiety is common in older infants (10–18 months). The infant may exhibit clingy behavior and fear of unfamiliar places and people. Protesting by crying is another normal reaction in older infants Figure 9-4. As infants become accustomed to their homes and families, they begin to need the security of a predictable environment. If an infant's environment is too unpredictable, the infant may despair and become withdrawn, which leads to trust issues.

Trust and mistrust refers to a stage of development from birth to about 18 months of age. Most infants desire that their world be planned, organized, and routine. When their caregivers and parents provide this environment for them, infants gain trust in those people. If the infant does not perceive the environment as secure, a sense of mistrust will develop.

Toddlers (1 to 3 Years) and Preschoolers (3 to 6 Years)

▶ Physical Changes

In **toddlers** (1 to 3 years), the pulse rate is 80 to 140 beats/min and the respiratory rate is 22 to 37 breaths/min, slower than the corresponding vital signs in infants, whereas the systolic blood pressure is higher (86 to 106 mm Hg). The average temperature of children this age is 96.8°F (36°C) to 99.6°F (38°C), usually leveling off at 98.6°F (37°C) by preschool age Figure 9-5.

In **preschoolers** (3 to 6 years), the pulse rate is 65 to 120 beats/min and the respiratory rate is 20 to 28 breaths/min. The systolic blood pressure is 89 to 112 mm Hg. At the same time, weight gain should level off Figure 9-6.

A toddler's cardiovascular system is not dramatically different from an adult's. A toddler's lungs continue to develop more terminal bronchioles and alveoli. Although

YOU are the Provider — PART 2

The infant appears listless and will only awaken with stimulation. As you are gathering additional information from the mother, the 12-year-old brother comes over and seems very interested in what is going on.

Recording Time: 0 Minute	
Appearance	Lethargic
Level of consciousness	Awakens with tactile stimulation
Airway	Thick yellow secretions from both nares
Breathing	Labored
Circulation	Rapid brachial pulses, cyanosis around the lips

3. Why are the secretions around the infant's nares significant?
4. What are some common psychosocial concerns experienced by pediatric patients?

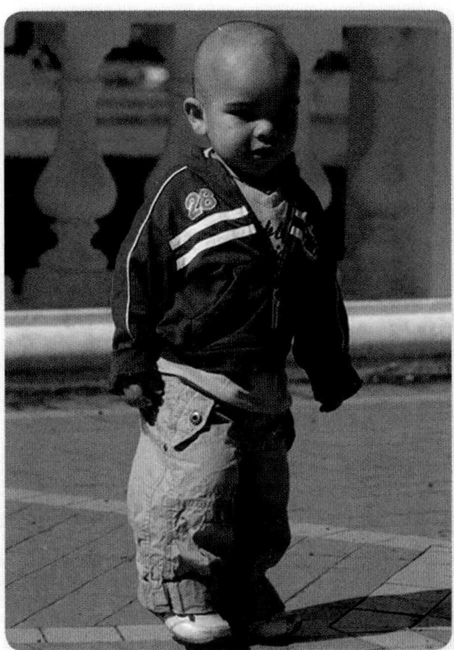

Figure 9-5 A toddler.

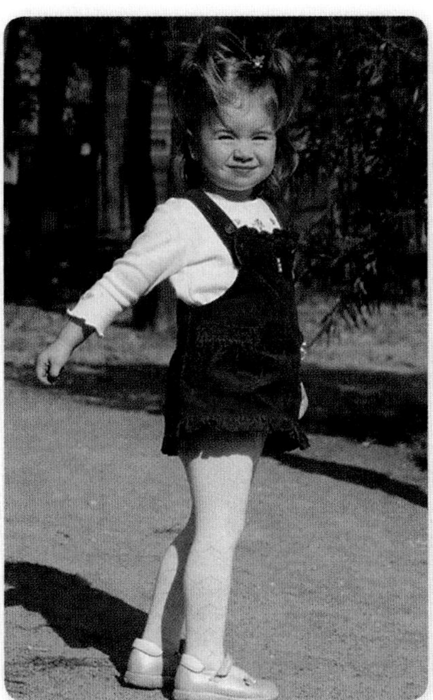

Figure 9-6 A preschooler.

Words of Wisdom

Allow children to remain near family members to decrease anxiety. Invite them to hold or examine medical equipment to reduce their fears of the unknown. In a nonemergency situation, give the child the opportunity to listen to your heartbeat before listening to his or hers. You may also "perform" an examination on a favorite doll or stuffed animal to demonstrate for the child and lessen mistrust.

toddlers and preschoolers have more lung tissue, they do not have well-developed lung musculature. This characteristic prevents them from sustaining deep or rapid respirations for an extended period.

The loss of passive immunity in the immune system is possibly the most obvious development at this stage of human life. Viral infections (colds) often develop that may manifest as gastrointestinal distress or upper respiratory tract infections. As toddlers spend more time around playmates and classmates, they acquire immunities as their bodies are exposed to various viruses and germs.

Neuromuscular growth also makes considerable progress at this age. Toddlers and preschoolers spend a great deal of time finding out exactly how to use their expansive nervous system and the muscles it controls by walking, running, jumping, and playing catch Figure 9-7. Watching the changes in how children play as they age from 1 to 6 years demonstrates how they move from gross motor activities (grabbing an object with the full palm) to fine motor activities (picking up a crayon). By the end of this stage, preschoolers will have a brain that weighs 90% of its final adult weight. In addition, all of this playing places stress on the muscles and bones. Consequently, muscle mass increases, as does bone density.

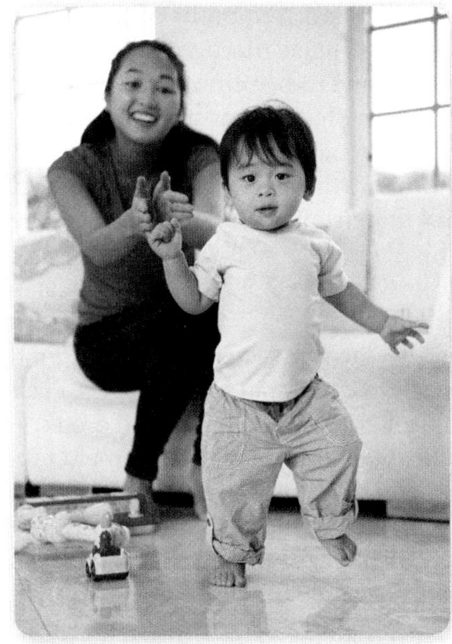

Figure 9-7 A toddler learns to walk, one of the major milestones in life.

This stage also includes the continued development of the renal system and of elimination patterns (ie, toilet training). Physiologically, toddlers have the neuromuscular control needed for bladder control by 12 to 15 months of age. However, the child may not be psychologically ready until 18 to 30 months of age. The average age for completion of toilet training is 28 months of age, but it depends on the individual child.

Other developments that occur during this time frame include the emergence of primary ("baby") teeth. Teething (that is, teeth breaking through the gums) can be painful and accompanied by fever. In addition, parents and toddlers are enthralled with sensory development—for example, as shown by tickling. According to the Centers for Disease Control and Prevention (CDC), the leading cause of death for this age group is unintentional injuries (accidents).[2]

Safety Tips

Do not discount the possibility of an infectious disease in children. Use standard precautions when treating all patients to protect yourself and others.

▶ Psychosocial Changes

This period of development is often exciting for parents. Toddlers or preschoolers are continuing to learn to speak and express themselves, thereby taking a major step toward independence. At the same time, toddlers are very attached to their parents and feel safe with them. Separation anxiety peaks between 10 and 18 months of age. It is fascinating to watch a child struggle through the conflict of wanting to play, yet wanting to be protected.

At 36 months of age, in most toddlers, basic language is mastered. Refinement of this skill is continued throughout childhood. By the age of 3 or 4 years, most children can use and understand full sentences. As they progress through this stage, they will go from using language to communicate what they want to using language creatively and playfully.

This is also the time when toddlers begin to interact with other children and start to play games. Playing games teaches control, following of rules, and even competitiveness. Significant learning and development take place by the child watching his or her peers during group outings, such as "play dates" with other children. By 18 to 24 months, toddlers begin to understand cause and effect. They learn the negative and positive consequences of their actions. For example, "If I move this lever, the water turns on" or "If I take my bath nicely, I will get to listen to a story." Of course, behavior observed on television and computers can also be learned, which is why some parents limit their children's viewing choices or the amount of time they devote to these activities. During this phase of development, children also learn to recognize sexual differences by observing their role models.

School-Age Children (6 to 12 Years)

▶ Physical Changes

During **school age**, from age 6 to 12 years, a child's vital signs and body gradually approach those observed in adulthood **Figure 9-8**. The pulse rate is approximately 58 to 118 beats/min, the respiratory rate is 18 to 25 breaths/min, and the systolic blood pressure is 97 to 120 mm Hg. Obvious physical traits and body function changes become apparent as most children gain about 4 pounds (2 kilograms) and grow 2.5 inches (6 centimeters) each year. Brain function develops further in both hemispheres, and permanent teeth begin to replace children's primary teeth during this period. The CDC sites unintentional injuries as the leading cause of death in this age group.[2]

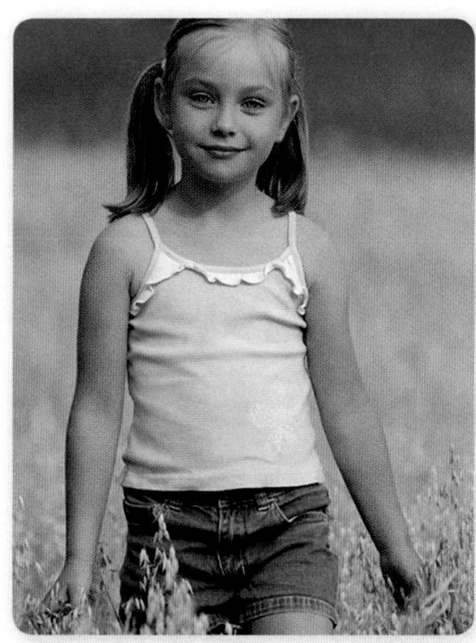

Figure 9-8 A school-age child.

▶ Psychosocial Changes

School-age children are engaged in a lot of psychosocial growth. Parents generally do not devote as much time to their children during this phase as they did in earlier phases. Nevertheless, it is at this crucial time in human de-velopment that children learn various types of reasoning. In **preconventional reasoning**, children act almost purely to avoid punishment and to get what they want. In **conventional reasoning**, they look for approval from their peers and society. In **postconventional reasoning**, children make decisions guided by their conscience.

During school age, children compare themselves with the adults and other children they interact with daily. Through these comparisons, they begin to develop their self-concept and self-esteem. *Self-concept* is our perception of ourselves; *self-esteem* is how we feel about ourselves and how we "fit in" with our peers.

Adolescents (12 to 18 Years)

▶ Physical Changes

In **adolescents** (ages 12 to 18 years), vital signs begin to level off within the adult ranges, with a pulse rate between

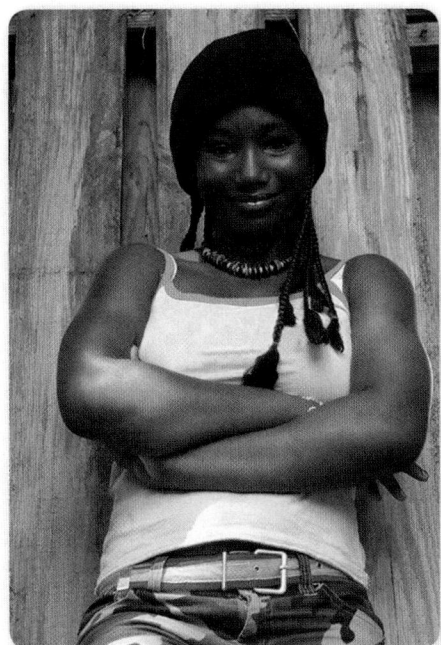

Figure 9-9 An adolescent.

50 to 100 beats/min, respirations in the range of 12 to 20 breaths/min, and a systolic blood pressure generally between 110 and 131 mm Hg **Figure 9-9**.

Adolescence is also the time of life when humans experience a rapid, 2- to 3-year growth spurt (ie, an increase in muscle and bone growth) and body changes. Growth begins with hands and feet, then moves to the long bones of the extremities, and finishes with growth of the torso. Boys typically experience this growth spurt later in life than girls. Girls usually finish their growth spurt by 16 years of age and boys by 18 years of age. When this period of growth has finished, however, boys are generally taller than girls. Muscle mass and bone density are nearly at adult levels.

One change during adolescence is the maturation of the human reproductive system. Secondary sexual development begins, including the enlargement of the external reproductive organs. Pubic hair and axillary hair begin to appear. Voices start to change in range and depth. In girls, the breasts and thighs increase in size as adipose (fat) tissue is deposited there. Menstruation begins during this time. Menarche, the first menstrual bleeding, occurs during this time; however, it is not uncommon for menstruation to begin before a girl becomes a teenager.

These changes in the endocrine and reproductive systems provide the platform for reproduction. By the middle of adolescence, boys are able to produce sperm and a girl's ovaries start releasing eggs for fertilization. Acne can also occur due to hormonal changes. The CDC reports unintentional injuries are also the leading cause of death for adolescents.[2]

▶ Psychosocial Changes

Adolescents and their families often deal with conflict as adolescents try to gain control of their lives and independence from their parents. Privacy becomes an important issue among adolescents, their siblings, and their parents. Self-consciousness also increases. Adolescents may

YOU are the Provider PART 3

After completing your assessment using the Pediatric Assessment Triangle (appearance, work of breathing, circulation), you determine the patient's level of consciousness is altered, her breathing is labored, and she is cyanotic. The mother states the infant has had a runny nose for the past couple of days and she has not had time to take her to the doctor. She states she was just overwhelmed caring for her sick daughter, a school-aged child, and for her older adult mother who has dementia.

Recording Time: 4 Minutes	
Respirations	32 breaths/min; labored
Pulse	Strong and regular; 130 beats/min
Skin	Warm, dry, and pink extremities, cyanosis around the lips and nose
Blood pressure	76/40 mm Hg
Oxygen saturation (Spo_2)	92% while breathing room air
Pupils	Pupils Equal, Round, and Reactive to Light and Accommodation (PERRLA)

5. Are the patient's vital signs consistent with her age?
6. Should you transport the patient to the hospital?

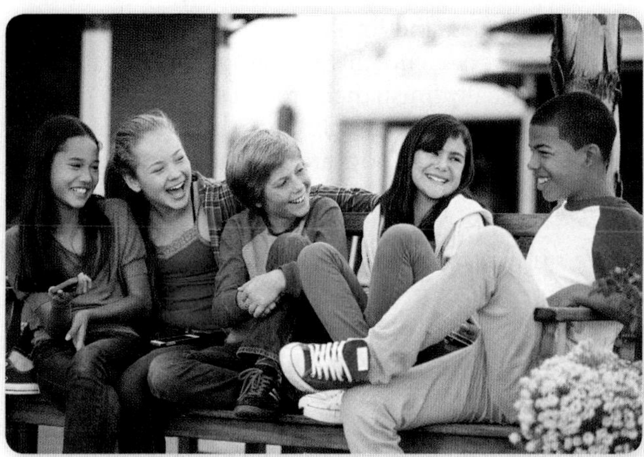

Figure 9-10 Adolescents want to fit in and may struggle to create their identities.

struggle to create their identities—to define themselves Figure 9-10, for example, by dressing in a certain style of clothing to fit their personalities. Adolescents use the feedback from their families and peers to help create their adult image. Adolescents are often caught between two worlds. They want to be treated like adults yet want to be cared for like younger children.

Rebellious behavior can be part of an adolescent trying to find his or her own identity. Adolescents continually compare themselves with their peers, which makes peer pressure a major factor in adolescents' psychological growth. Antisocial behavior peaks during the eighth or ninth grade. Adolescence is also a time when eating disorders may develop as teenagers exhibit self-control through what they eat or become obsessed with body image. Self-destructive behaviors such as smoking, drinking, sex, and other high-risk behaviors may begin. Although these behaviors can be very troubling to parents, the adolescent is trying to determine if he or she is ready to take control of his or her own life. An adolescent's struggle toward independence may include setbacks that can be devastating. Patience and support from family and friends are essential in assisting an adolescent's transition into adulthood.

Adolescents may also show greater interest in sexual relations. Many adolescents are fixated on their public image and are terrified of being embarrassed. At this age, a code of personal ethics is developed, based partly on parents' ethics and values and partly on the influence of the adolescent's environment. At this tumultuous time, teenagers are at a higher risk than other populations for suicide and depression.

Special Populations

When you interview adolescents, treat them as adults to gain better cooperation and honesty. Allow them to express their opinions about the care they will receive, and permit them to voice any disapproval. However, it is important to remember, you are ultimately still dealing with a child.

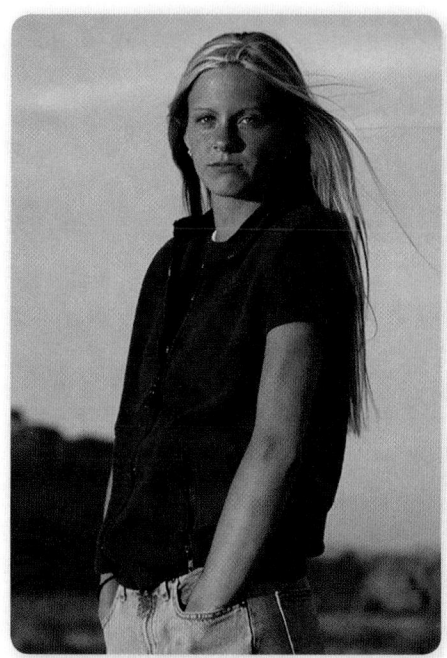

Figure 9-11 An early adult.

Early Adults (19 to 40 Years)

Physical Changes

Early adults range in age from 19 to 40 years Figure 9-11. Their vital signs do not vary greatly from those seen throughout adulthood. Ideally, the human pulse rate will stay around 70 beats/min, the respiratory rate will stay in the range of 12 to 20 breaths/min, and the systolic blood pressure will be approximately between 90 and 140 mm Hg.

From age 19 years to shortly after 25 years, the human body should be functioning at its optimal level. Lifelong habits and routines develop at this age, including eating preferences, exercise, and tobacco use.

At the beginning of the early adult period, the body is working at peak efficiency, but as early adulthood continues, subtle wear and tear on bones and changes in body tissues and muscles begin. The disks in the spine begin to settle, and height can sometimes be affected, causing "shrinking." Being able to eat anything without gaining weight becomes a thing of the past. Fatty tissue increases, which leads to weight gain. Muscle strength decreases, and the reflexes slow. The leading cause of death in this age group is also unintentional injury, according to the CDC.[2]

Psychosocial Changes

Three words best describe a human's world during this stage of life: work, family, and stress. During this period, humans strive to create a place for themselves in the world, and many do everything they can to settle down.

As early adults struggle to find stability in their careers, stress on the job becomes high. Along with this natural tendency to settle down often comes marriage and family. Childbirth is most common in this age group. Despite all of this stress and change, this age group enjoys one of the more stable periods of life. People in early adulthood generally experience fewer psychological problems related to well-being.

Middle Adults (41 to 60 Years)

Physical Changes

Middle adults are age 41 to 60 years Figure 9-12. The average pulse rate for this age remains at 70 beats/min, the respiratory rate continues at 12 to 20 breaths/min, and the systolic blood pressure also remains between 90 and 140 mm Hg. Even though the body is still functioning at a high level, this age group is vulnerable to vision and hearing loss along with other varying degrees of degradation. Cardiovascular health becomes an issue in many people in this age group, as does the greater incidence of cancer. Middle adults may begin having medical symptoms or be unaware of conditions such as diabetes and hypertension. Medications or underlying conditions may affect a patient's response to treatments. In women, menopause—the cessation of menstruation—begins in the late 40s or early 50s. However, it is possible for an unexpected pregnancy after experiencing menopause. Other concerns include an increase in cholesterol levels, a decrease in the efficiency of the heart, and weight control maintenance. However, many of the effects of aging can be diminished with exercise and a healthy diet. The CDC cites unintentional injuries as the leading cause of death of people ages 41 to 44 years. For ages 45 to 60, the leading cause of death is cancer.[2]

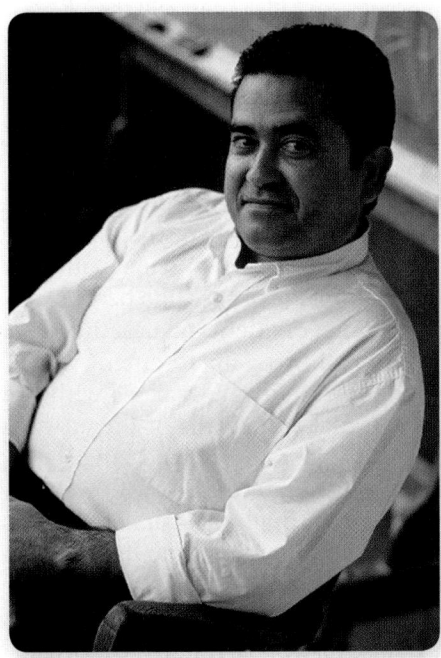

Figure 9-12 A middle adult.

Psychosocial Changes

Middle adults tend to focus on achieving their life's goals, as they approach the halfway point in human life expectancy. After years of nurturing and living with children, parents must readjust their lifestyles as their children leave the home, commonly called the empty nest syndrome. Finances may become a worrisome issue as people prepare for retirement while still managing everyday financial demands. During this time, people often view crisis as a challenge to be overcome and not a threat to be avoided. Generally, their health is stable and they have the physical, emotional, and spiritual reserves to handle life's issues.

The parents of adults in this age group are getting older and now need care. Most of the older adults in the United States are cared for by family members inside the home. Therefore, a person in middle adulthood may need to manage children who are leaving for college while at the same time care for parents who require greater assistance.

Older Adults (61 Years and Older)

Physical Changes

Older adults include people age 61 years or older Figure 9-13. **Life expectancy** is constantly changing. In the early 1900s, life expectancy was 47 years. It is now approximately 78 years, with maximum life expectancy estimated at 120 years.[3] The age to which a person will live is based on many factors. Perhaps surprisingly, the year you were born and the country you live in can have an effect on your life expectancy. These two facts are based on public health advances, changes within diets, attitudes

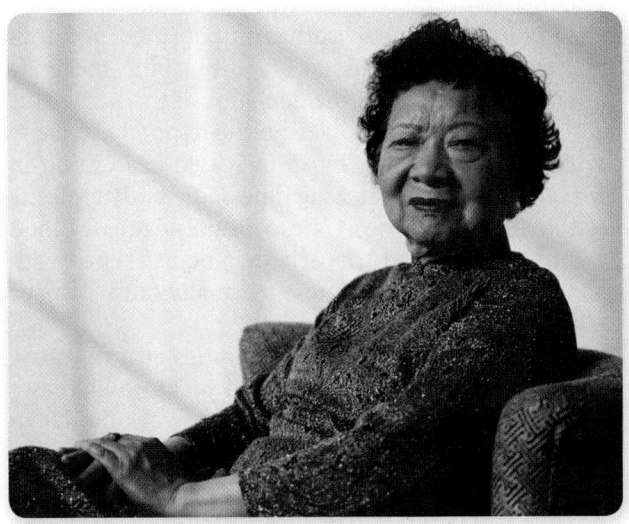

Figure 9-13 An older adult.

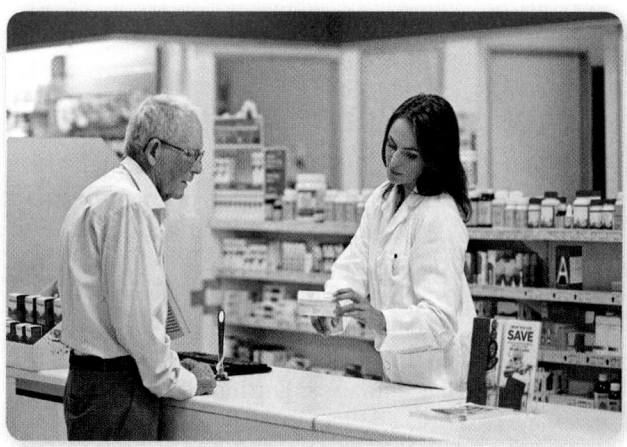

Figure 9-14 Older people are often prescribed multiple medications to help them stay active.

regarding exercise, advances in medical care, access to that medical care, and personal behaviors. According to the CDC, heart disease and cancer are the leading causes of death in ages 65 and older.[2]

Later in life, the vital signs depend on the patient's overall health, medical conditions, and medications taken. Today's older adults are staying active longer than their ancestors did. Thanks to medical advances, they are often able to overcome numerous medical conditions but may need multiple medications to do so Figure 9-14.

Cardiovascular System

Cardiac function declines with age due to anatomic and physiologic changes that are largely related to atherosclerosis. Atherosclerosis most commonly affects coronary vessels. Cholesterol and calcium build up inside the walls of blood vessels, forming plaque. The accumulation of plaque eventually leads to partial or complete blockage of blood flow. The majority of people older than 65 years have some degree of atherosclerotic disease.[4]

Other age-related changes typically include a decrease in heart rate, a decline in cardiac output (the amount of blood circulated each minute), and the inability to elevate cardiac output to match the demands of the body. This translates into a heart that is less able to respond to exercise or disease (for example, by an increased heart rate). In the event of a life-threatening illness, the body typically needs to increase the heart rate to ensure adequate blood pressure. Because heart muscle may be weakened with age, the increase in heart rate can actually cause damage to the heart itself.

The vascular system also becomes stiff. Because of this change, the diastolic blood pressure increases with age. The left ventricle must then work harder to move blood effectively, so it becomes thicker, losing its elasticity in this process. There is increased workload of the heart and reduced blood flow to organs. Decreases in the amount of elastin and collagen in blood vessel walls reduce the elasticity of the peripheral vessels by as much as 70%. Compensation for blood pressure changes is hampered because the vessels are less able to dilate and contract.

Aging also affects blood cells. Blood cells originate from within the bone marrow. As a person ages, more of the bone marrow is replaced with fatty tissue. This decrease in bone marrow causes a decrease in the ability of the bones to manufacture more blood cells when needed. While this change alone typically does not pose a problem, if an older adult sustains trauma, the ability of the body to produce blood cells to replace those lost decreases. Finally, functional blood volume gradually declines over time.

Respiratory System

In older adults, the size of the upper and lower airway increases as the smooth muscle weakens. The surface area of the alveoli decreases. These metabolic changes cause the natural elasticity of the lungs to decrease, forcing people to increasingly rely more on the muscle between their ribs, called intercostal muscle, to breathe. In addition, the chest becomes more rigid because of calcification of the ribs to the sternum, which adds to the difficulty of breathing. As the elasticity of the lungs decreases, the overall strength of the intercostal muscles and diaphragm also decreases. These factors together cause more labor-intensive breathing for older adults. You might think a rigid chest would be more protecting, but this rigidity actually makes the chest more fragile. Overall, the bone structure of older adults is weakened. Instead of the chest being able to bend and give if struck, the calcified bony structure of the chest can fracture. As with all of the physical changes related to aging, however, the changes in the respiratory system are often gradual and go unnoticed until a severe, life-threatening condition occurs. An older adult will then have less respiratory reserve to maintain adequate breathing.

Within the mouth and nose, there is a gradual loss of the mechanisms that protect the upper airway. This loss leads to decreased ability to clear secretions and decreased cough and gag reflexes. The number of cilia that line the airways diminishes with age, resulting in less sensation (and less responsiveness) when structures of the airway are irritated. With a lesser ability to maintain upper airway function, aspiration and obstruction become more likely.

When a younger patient inhales, the airway maintains its shape, allowing air to enter. As the smooth muscle of the lower airway weakens with age, strong inhalation can make the walls of the airway collapse inward and cause inspiratory wheezing Figure 9-15. The collapsing airways result in low flow rates, because less air can move through the smaller airways, and air trapping, because air does not completely exit the alveoli (incomplete expiration).

Also within the airways, the cells of the immune system are less functional. As a result of the overall decrease in the metabolic activity of the older body, the white blood cells found within the airways are less aggressive

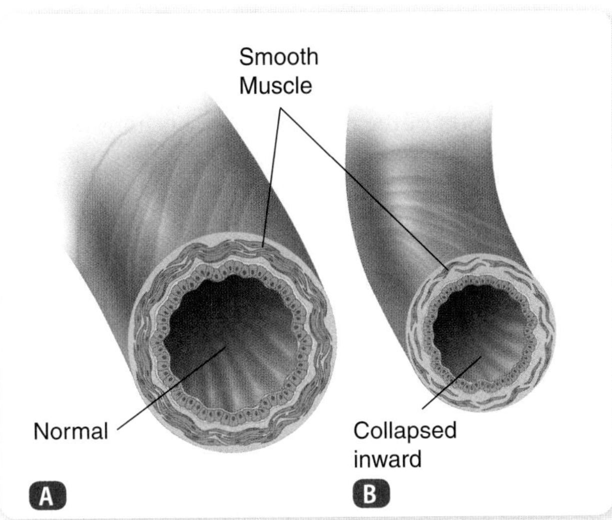

Figure 9-15 A. Healthy muscle in a younger patient's airway helps maintain the open airway during the pressures of inhalation. **B.** Muscle weakening with age can lead to airway collapse that may produce wheezing.

at fighting invading organisms. This leads to an increased risk of lung infections.

By age 75 years, the vital capacity (the volume of air moved during the deepest inspiration and expiration) may amount to only 50% of the vital capacity noted in early adulthood. Factors that contribute to this decline include loss of respiratory muscle mass, increased stiffness of the thoracic cage, and decreased surface area available for the exchange of air.

Physiologically, vital capacity decreases and residual volume (the amount of air left in the lungs after expiration of the maximum possible amount of air) increases with age. As a consequence, stagnant air remains in the alveoli and hampers gas exchange. This effect can produce hypercarbia (increased level of carbon dioxide in the bloodstream) and acidosis, even when the person is at rest.

Endocrine System

As with other systems of the body, the function of the endocrine system gradually declines with age. As people get older, they tend to slow their physical activity. Unfortunately, many do not decrease their food intake. When a person gains weight, more insulin is needed to control the body's metabolism and blood glucose (sugar) level. However, insulin production and glucose metabolism decrease with age, so older adults are more prone to diabetes mellitus. Changes in an older adult's mental status may also be the result of changes in his or her blood glucose level.

The male and female reproductive systems also change with age. Men are able to produce sperm long into their 80s but the rigidity of the penis tends to decrease over time. It is unclear whether this decrease is solely due to aging or other factors such as cardiovascular disease. During menopause, decreased production of regulating hormones results in atrophy of the woman's reproductive organs. The uterus and vagina both decrease in size. Hormone production for both sexes gradually decreases as people age. Sexual desire may diminish with age but does not cease.

YOU are the Provider — PART 4

You suction the infant's nose with a bulb syringe and your partner administers blow-by oxygen. You explain your findings to the mother and inform her the infant needs to be transported to the hospital for further treatment. The mother calls a neighbor to stay with her older child and her mother. While your partner secures the infant in a child safety seat, you take a moment to speak with the woman about the options available to help her care for her aging mother.

Recording Time: 8 Minutes	
Respirations	28 breaths/min; not as labored
Pulse	Strong and regular; 120 beats/min
Skin	Warm, dry, and pink extremities, decreased cyanosis around lips and nose
Blood pressure	76/60 mm Hg
Oxygen saturation (Spo_2)	95% on blow-by oxygen
Pupils	PERRLA

7. What other options could you offer the mother?

Special Populations

Always monitor blood glucose levels in older adult patients presenting with altered mental status. Remember, the symptoms of hypoglycemia can mimic those observed in stroke (for example, facial drooping and hemiparesis).

Renal and Gastrointestinal Systems

In the kidneys, both structural and functional changes occur in older adults. The filtration function of these organs, for example, declines by 50% from age 20 to 90 years. Kidney size decreases by 20% over the same span. This is due in part to the decreased effectiveness of the blood vessels that supply blood to the nephrons. **Nephrons** are sophisticated capillaries that perform filtering in the kidney. They are the structural and functional units of the kidney that form urine. One of the portions of the nephron is the *glomerulus*. The decreased blood supply causes more abnormal glomeruli to be present as a person ages. The number of nephrons also declines between the ages of 30 and 80 years. The loss of renal function means a decrease in the ability to clear wastes from the body. It also means decreased ability to conserve fluids when needed.

Changes in gastrointestinal function may inhibit nutritional intake and utilization in older adults, resulting in vitamin and mineral deficiencies. In the mouth, for example, taste bud sensitivity to salty and sweet sensations decreases. The sense of smell can also be diminished and, along with the decreased taste response, can diminish the flavor of food. Teeth become weaker during this phase of life, making it more difficult for older adults to chew certain foods. The secretion of saliva decreases, which reduces the body's ability to process complex carbohydrates. Gastric motility slows with age because of the loss of intestinal tract neurons, which can lead older adults to feel constipated or not hungry. Likewise, the secretion of gastric acid diminishes. Blood flow in the mesenteric vessels (supplying membranes that connect organs to the abdominal wall) may drop by as much as 50%, decreasing the ability of the intestines to extract nutrients from digested food. Gallstones become increasingly common with age, and anal sphincter changes reduce elasticity and can produce fecal incontinence.

Nervous System

Nervous system changes can result in the most debilitating of age-related ailments. In the central nervous system, the brain weight may decrease 10% to 20% by age 80. Motor and sensory neural networks become slower and less responsive. The metabolic rate in the older brain does not change, however, and oxygen consumption remains constant throughout life. Generally, you have fewer brain cells (neurons) today than you did yesterday. If measured strictly by numbers of brain cells, infants are far more intelligent than any of us. However, this is not how the brain works. Although it is true that older adults have a diminished number of brain cells, there is great flexibility in the operation of the brain. Interconnections between brain cells continue as people age. These new connections provide redundancy within the brain, allowing for loss of neurons without loss of knowledge or skill.

One of the consequences of the loss of neurons is a change in the sleep patterns of older adults. Instead of sleeping through the night, they may take a nap during the day and be up late at night. Their sleep cycle may move into a biphasic (two-phased) sleep cycle—for example, sleep from 0100 hours to 0600 hours and nap from 1200 hours to 1500 hours.

The brain, which is surrounded by the meninges, takes up almost all of the space in the skull. Cerebrospinal fluid protects the brain inside these membranes. Unfortunately, in older adults, age-related shrinkage creates a void between the brain and the outermost layer of the meninges, which provides room for the brain to move when stressed **Figure 9-16**. If trauma moves the brain

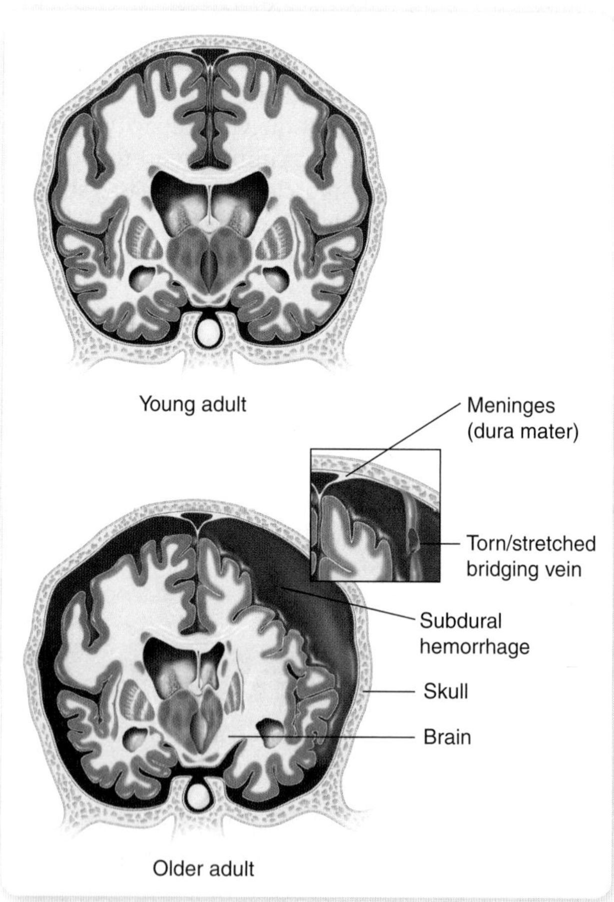

Figure 9-16 Age-related atrophy or shrinkage of the brain results in a space between the brain and its cover, the dura mater. Bleeding into this area can occur more easily from trauma because veins are stretched. Because of the additional space, bleeding in an older brain does not always produce immediate signs of increased intracranial pressure.

forcibly, the bridging veins can tear and bleed. Bleeding can empty into this void and may go unnoticed for some time in this age group.

Functioning of the peripheral nervous system also slows with age. Sensation becomes diminished and misinterpreted. The ability to know where the body is in space (proprioception) can be diminished. Slower reaction times cause longer delays between stimulation and motion. The slowdown in reflexes and decreased kinesthetic sense may contribute to the incidence of falls and trauma. Nerve endings deteriorate, and the ability of the skin to sense the surroundings becomes hindered. Hot, cold, sharp, and wet items can all create dangerous situations because reaction time and pain perception are both diminished in older adults.

Sensory Changes

In addition to a diminished sensation of touch, the other senses are also affected by aging. It is often assumed older adults are hard of hearing and have difficulty seeing. While it is true that there are changes that diminish the effectiveness of the eyes and ears, most older adults hear well and have good vision. They may need eyeglasses or hearing aids, but do not assume your older patient is deaf and nearly blind. Pupillary reaction and ocular movements become more restricted with age. The pupils are generally smaller in older patients, and the opacity of the eye's lens diminishes visual acuity and makes the pupils sluggish when responding to light. Visual distortions are also common in older people. Thickening of the lens makes it more difficult for the eye to focus, especially at close range. Peripheral fields of vision become narrower, and a greater sensitivity to glare constricts the visual field.

Hearing loss is about four times more common than loss of vision in older adults. Changes in several hearing-related structures may lead to a loss of high-frequency hearing or even deafness.

▶ Psychosocial Changes

You should treasure the opportunities to spend time with and communicate with older adults. Many older adults have amazing stories and experiences to share, yet we often take them for granted. They share a great amount of wisdom with us, and we need to remind them of their self-worth. Until about 5 years before death, most late-stage adults retain high brain function. In the 5 years preceding death, however, mental function is presumed to decline, a theory referred to as the **terminal drop hypothesis.**

As the older adult population continues to grow, we have the responsibility to seek unique ways to accommodate their needs during their last 20 to 40 years of life. The increasing number of older adults in the United States as a result of the baby boom of the 1940s through the 1960s has produced a need for more assisted-living facilities. These facilities allow older adults to live in campus-based communities with people in their own age group, while enjoying the privacy of their own apartments and the security of nursing care, maintenance, and food preparation, if desired **Figure 9-17**. Unfortunately, these facilities can be expensive.

Most people need to deal with financial issues throughout their lives. Few things in life produce more worry and

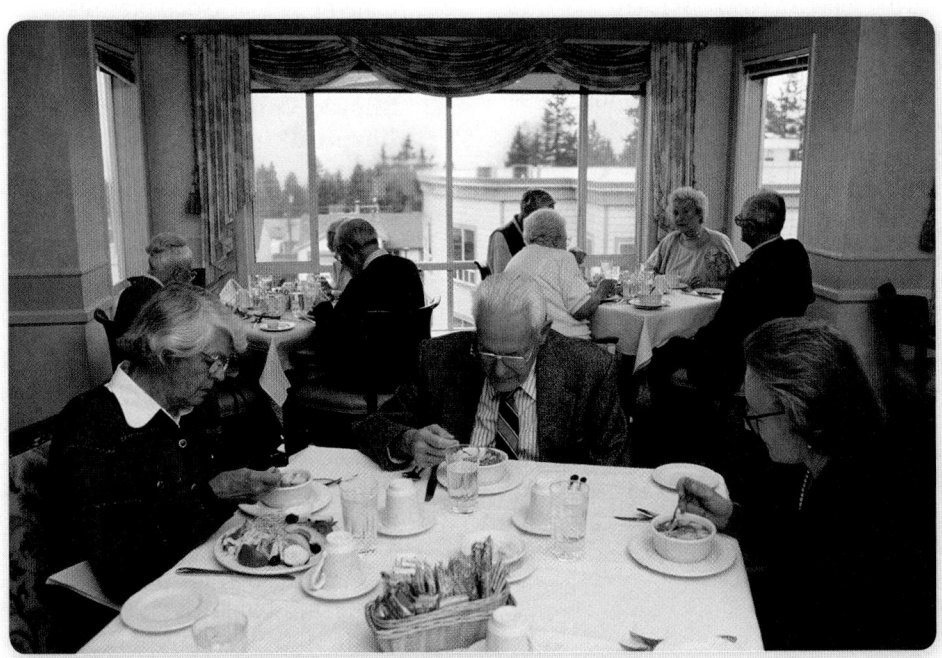

Figure 9-17 An increasing number of older adults live in assisted-living facilities.

stress than money problems. Older adults, in particular, may constantly worry about the rising costs of health care and are often forced to make decisions such as whether to pay for groceries or their medication. Compared with earlier generations, families often take less responsibility for their older adult family members. According to the US government, 10% of people age 65 and older (4.5 million) were below the poverty level in 2014. This problem continues.[5]

One of the important issues that older adults face is mortality. However, the fact is, everyone dies. Yet, for most of us, this concept is an intellectual exercise with a distant connection to reality. It is difficult for older adults to watch as their friends, relatives, and companions grow older and die, leaving them seemingly alone. Older adults may feel useless or worry about being a burden to their families as their health declines and they are no longer able to take care of themselves. Isolation and depression are challenges for older adults.

Fortunately, many older adults are happy and actively participating in life. With good financial resources and a good support system of family and friends, older adults in their 80s and beyond can enjoy life and continue to feel productive.

YOU are the Provider SUMMARY

1. How does the patient's age affect your treatment?

The caregiver will be your primary resource for determining the patient's normal mental status and activity level. The 3-month-old infant should be able to track objects with her eyes and should recognize familiar faces. The development of stranger anxiety does not occur until age 1 year or older.

2. What are some physical differences between pediatric and adult patients?

Compared with an adult, the infant has a proportionately larger tongue and proportionately shorter, narrower, and less stable airway. As a result, the airway in infants can be occluded easily. Infants have fewer alveoli in their lungs, which decreases the surface area for gas exchange. They also continue to be "nose breathers" and have not mastered the ability to breathe through their mouths. The rib cage of an infant is less rigid than an adult's, and the ribs sit horizontally. This explains the diaphragmatic breathing in infants. Owing to the immaturity of the accessory muscles, fatigue sets in quickly.

3. Why are the secretions around the infant's nares significant?

Neonates are primarily "nose breathers" for the first 4 weeks of their lives, but even older infants rely heavily on nose breathing for ease during feeding. Something as simple as nasal congestion can lead to hypoxia in the infant. Infants younger than 6 months are particularly prone to nasal congestion, which can cause viral upper respiratory infections. If you receive a call for an infant choking, ensure the nasal passages are clear and unobstructed by mucus.

4. What are some common psychosocial concerns experienced by pediatric patients?

Infants communicate primarily by crying. Parents can often tell what is upsetting the infant by listening to the tone of the child's crying. Infants occasionally make another distinct cry—an alarming distressed cry. This cry may be heard when an unexpected event occurs, causing a situational crisis for the infant. Because this infant is lethargic and responds only when stimulated, she may be more difficult to evaluate.

5. Are the patient's vital signs consistent with her age?

In infants (1 month to 1 year), the pulse rate is 90 to 180 beats/min and the respiratory rate is 30 to 53 breaths/min. The systolic blood pressure is 72 to 104 mm Hg, so these findings are consistent for the age of the patient.

6. Should you transport the patient to the hospital?

In this scenario, transport is recommended due to the respiratory distress and change in level of consciousness.

7. What other options could you offer the mother?

The mother is feeling overwhelmed because she is caring for three different age groups all needing individual attention. You could suggest possible options for the older child such as an after school program or other adult-led activities. You may also inform the mother of potential resources available in the community to assist in caring for her mother. If she is unable to continue to care for all of them, she may need to evaluate moving her mother into an assisted-living facility or personal care home.

YOU are the Provider SUMMARY (continued)

EMS Patient Care Report (PCR)					
Date: 6-27-18	**Incident No.:** 20102291036	**Nature of Call:** Runny nose		**Location:** 26445 NE Dresser Rd	
Dispatched: 1504	**En Route:** 1505	**At Scene:** 1512	**Transport:** 1517	**At Hospital:** 1523	**In Service:** 1530
Patient Information					
Age: 3 months **Sex:** F **Weight (in kg [lb]):** 7 kg (16 lb)			**Allergies:** No known drug allergies **Medications:** None **Past Medical History:** None **Chief Complaint:** Runny, sore nose		
Vital Signs					
Time: 1516	**BP:** 76/40		**Pulse:** 130	**Respirations:** 32	**Spo_2:** 92%
Time: 1520	**BP:** 76/60		**Pulse:** 120	**Respirations:** 28	**Spo_2:** 95%
EMS Treatment (circle all that apply)					
Oxygen @ 6 **L/min via (circle one):** **NC** **NRM** **Bag-mask device** (Blow-By)			**Assisted Ventilation**	**Airway Adjunct**	**CPR**
Defibrillation	**Bleeding Control**		**Bandaging**	**Splinting**	**Other:**
Narrative					
EMS dispatched to above location for a runny nose. On arrival, met by mother who is holding a 3-month-old infant in her arms. Mother states the patient has had a runny nose for a couple of days and is now less responsive. Physical exam reveals a lethargic infant who responds sluggishly to tactile stimulation. The infant presents with cyanosis around her nose and lips and has yellow drainage from both nares. Nares are suctioned with a bulb syringe and infant is placed on blow-by oxygen at 6 L/min. Advised mother of our findings, and she agreed to transport. The patient was secured in child safety seat and seat was secured in the ambulance. After suctioning and the administration of oxygen, infant is more alert. Patient and mother transported to hospital without incident. Older child and patient's grandmother left in care of neighbor. Mother advised of outreach resources available to assist in caring for her mother. EMS back in service at 1530.**End of report**					

Prep Kit

▶ Ready for Review

- Developmental stages of life include the following: neonate, infant, toddler, preschool age, school age, adolescence, early adulthood, middle adulthood, and older adulthood.
- Each developmental stage is marked by different physical and psychosocial changes and characteristics.
- The pulse rate is fastest during infancy, ranging from 90 to 205 beats/min. This rate slows and levels off during adolescence, reaching the adult range of 60 to 100 beats/min.
- The typical respiratory rate is highest in neonates, at 30 to 60 breaths/min. The respiratory rate levels off during adolescence, reaching the adult range of 12 to 20 breaths/min.
- Blood pressure directly corresponds to the patient's weight, so it typically increases with age. In a neonate, the systolic blood pressure ranges from 67 to 84 mm Hg, while in adults (early, middle, and older) it ranges from 90 to 140 mm Hg.
- By 2 weeks, neonates and infants grow at a rate of about 1 ounce (30 g) per day, doubling their weight within 4 to 6 months and tripling it by the end of the first year.
- Two important points regarding an infant's airway are that an infant's tongue can more easily occlude the airway, and the lungs are fragile. Ventilations that are too forceful can result in barotrauma.
- Toddlers (1 to 3 years) and preschoolers (3 to 6 years) continue to learn to speak and express themselves. Toilet training is usually accomplished around age 28 months.
- School-age children (6 to 12 years) develop self-esteem and reasoning abilities and receive their permanent teeth.
- Adolescents (12 to 18 years) undergo significant reproductive development. They also focus on creating their self-image and are self-conscious. They may also engage in self-destructive behavior such as smoking, drinking alcohol, or taking drugs.
- Early adults (19 to 40 years) focus on work and family. The body should function at an optimal level, and lifelong habits are developed.
- Middle adults (41 to 60 years) focus on achieving life goals. During this stage, medical conditions such as diabetes, hypertension, and cancer become more common.
- While many older adults (61 years and older) are happy and actively participating in life, some focus on their mortality and the mortality of friends and loved ones.
- The vital signs of older adults depend on their health.
- There are significant physical changes in older adults. Cardiac function declines as atherosclerosis develops. Cardiac output decreases, and the vascular system becomes stiff.
- Respiratory changes in older adults include decreased elasticity of the lungs, decreased vital capacity and residual volume, and decreased ability to clear secretions.
- Bones become more rigid in late adulthood, making them more prone to fracture.
- Endocrine changes in older adults include decreases in insulin production and glucose metabolism.
- Renal changes in older adults include decreases in filtration function.
- Gastrointestinal changes in older adults include decreased saliva, slowed gastric motility, and potentially incontinence.
- Nervous system changes affect sleep patterns in older adults and increase the likelihood of falls.
- Age-related shrinkage creates a void that forms between the brain and the outermost layer of meninges. As a result, bleeding may go unnoticed for some time.
- Sensory changes associated with aging include hearing loss and vision problems; however, many older adults hear and see relatively well.

▶ Vital Vocabulary

adolescent A young person age 12 to18 years.

anxious-avoidant attachment An insecure attachment observed in infants who are repeatedly rejected. Children develop an isolated lifestyle that does not depend on the support and care of others.

bonding The formation of a close, personal relationship.

conventional reasoning A type of reasoning in which a child looks for approval from peers and society.

early adult A young adult age 19 to 40 years.

fontanelles Areas where the neonate's or infant's skull bones have not fused together; usually disappear at approximately 18 months of age.

Prep Kit *(continued)*

growth plates Structures located on either end of an infant's long bone, which aid in lengthening bones as the child grows; also known as epiphyseal plates.

infant A young child age 1 month to 1 year.

life expectancy The average number of years a person can be expected to live.

middle adult An adult age 41 to 60 years.

Moro reflex An infant reflex in which, when an infant is caught off guard, the infant opens his or her arms wide, spreads the fingers, and seems to grab at things.

neonate A newborn age birth to 1 month.

nephrons The structural and functional unit of the kidney.

older adult An adult age 61 years or older.

palmar grasp An infant reflex that occurs when something is placed in the infant's palm; the infant grasps the object.

postconventional reasoning A type of reasoning in which a child bases decisions on his or her conscience.

preconventional reasoning A type of reasoning in which a child acts almost purely to avoid punishment or to get what he or she wants.

preschooler A child age 3 to 6 years.

rooting reflex An infant reflex that occurs when something touches an infant's cheek; the infant instinctively turns his or her head toward the touch.

school age A child age 6 to 12 years.

secure attachment A bond between an infant and his or her parent or caregiver in which the infant understands that his or her parents or caregivers will be responsive to his or her needs and take care of him or her when he or she needs help.

separation anxiety An infant behavior that peaks between 10 to 18 months. The child may exhibit clingy behavior and fear of unfamiliar places and people.

sucking reflex An infant reflex in which the infant starts sucking when his or her lips are stroked.

terminal drop hypothesis A theory that a person's mental function declines in the last 5 years preceding death.

toddler A young child age 1 to 3 years.

trust and mistrust Refers to a stage of development from birth to approximately 18 months of age, when infants gain trust of their parents or caregivers if their world is planned, organized, and routine.

▶ References

1. American Academy of Orthopaedic Surgeons. *Growth Plate Fractures.* http://orthoinfo.aaos.org/topic.cfm?topic=A00040. Accessed October 12, 2016.
2. Centers for Disease Control and Prevention. *10 Leading Causes of Death by Age Group, 2014.* http://www.cdc.gov/injury/wisqars/pdf/leading_causes_of_death_by_age_group_2014-a.pdf. Accessed June 28, 2016.
3. Centers for Disease Control and Prevention. *Health, United States, 2015.* http://www.cdc.gov/nchs/fastats/older-american-health.htm. Accessed October 12, 2016.
4. US National Library of Medicine. National Institutes of Health. *The Burden of Cardiovascular Disease in the Elderly: Morbidity, Mortality, and Costs.* https://www.ncbi.nlm.nih.gov/pmc/articles/PMC2797320/. Accessed October 12, 2016.
5. US Department of Health and Human Services, Administration for Community Living. *Profile of Older Americans: 2015.* http://www.aoa.acl.gov/Aging_Statistics/Profile/2015/10.aspx. Accessed October 11, 2016.

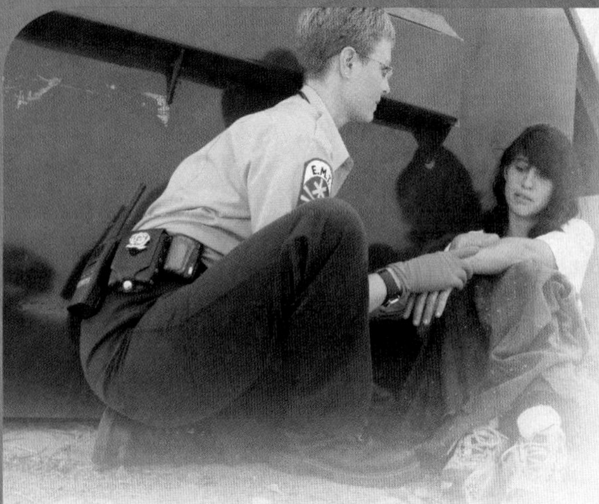

Assessment *in Action*

You were dispatched to a low-income housing apartment for a 1-month-old girl who is "not acting right." On arrival, you are met by the mother who states her daughter has been acting "funny" today. As you approach the infant, she appears to startle.

1. Neonates are born with certain reflexes. What is the medical name for the startle reflex?

A. Moro reflex
B. Rooting reflex
C. Sucking reflex
D. Anxiety reflex

2. Neonates are born with fontanelles. At what age do the posterior fontanelles close?

A. 1 to 2 months
B. 3 to 4 months
C. 4 to 6 months
D. 6 to 8 months

3. In most infants, the primary method of communicating distress is through:

A. speaking.
B. crying.
C. pointing.
D. eye movements.

4. Why is a child's airway more likely to occlude than the airway of an adult?

A. A child's tongue is proportionally smaller and more flexible.
B. A child's airway musculature is less well-developed.
C. A child's airway is proportionally larger in relation to other airway structures.
D. A child's tongue is proportionally larger and the airway is proportionally shorter, narrower, and less stable.

5. School-age children gain approximately how much body weight each year?

A. 1 pounds
B. 2 pounds
C. 3 pounds
D. 4 pounds

6. In older adults, the size of the airway increases and the surface area of the alveoli:

A. increases.
B. decreases.
C. stays the same.
D. depends on the patient.

7. By age 75 years, the vital capacity may amount to only _________ of the vital capacity noted in early adulthood.

A. 25%
B. 50%
C. 75%
D. 100%

8. The brain weight may shrink _________ by age 80 years.

A. 10% to 20%
B. 20% to 30%
C. 30% to 40%
D. 40% to 50%

9. An older patient who presents with an altered mental status after a traumatic incident may have an epidural hematoma or a subdural hematoma. What physiologic changes associated with aging make this injury more likely?

10. School-age children learn various types of reasoning. Explain *preconventional reasoning*.

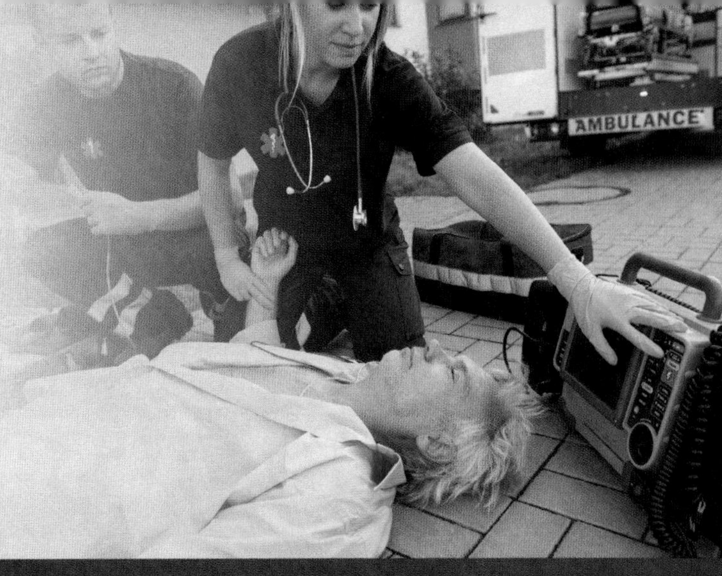

SECTION 3

Patient Assessment

CHAPTER 10

Patient Assessment

National EMS Education Standard Competencies

Assessment

Applies scene information and patient assessment findings (scene size-up, primary and secondary assessment, patient history, reassessment) to guide emergency management.

Scene Size-up

- Scene safety (pp 397-398)
- Scene management (pp 397-398)
  - Impact of the environment on patient care (pp 397-398)
  - Addressing hazards (pp 397-398)
  - Violence (p 398)
  - Need for additional or specialized resources (p 402)
  - Standard precautions (pp 400-401)
  - Multiple patient situations (p 401)

Primary Assessment

- Primary assessment for all patient situations
  - Level of consciousness (pp 403-404)
  - ABCs (pp 405-412)
  - Identifying life threats (pp 415-417)
  - Assessment of vital functions (pp 405-417)
  - Initial general impression (pp 403-405)
- Begin interventions needed to preserve life (pp 405-412)
- Integration of treatment/procedures needed to preserve life (pp 405-412)

History Taking

- Determining the chief complaint (pp 420-422)
- Mechanism of injury/nature of illness (pp 399-400, 419)
- Associated signs and symptoms (pp 421-424)
- Investigation of the chief complaint (pp 420-422)
- Past medical history (pp 424-426)
- Pertinent negatives (p 424)

Secondary Assessment

- Performing a rapid full-body scan (pp 414-416)
- Focused assessment of pain (pp 422-424, 438-439)
- Assessment of vital signs (pp 439-440, 443-448)
- Techniques of physical examination
  - Respiratory system (pp 438-443)
  - Presence of breath sounds (p 441)
  - Cardiovascular system (pp 442-447)
  - Neurologic system (pp 447-449)
  - Musculoskeletal system (pp 449-453)
  - All anatomic regions (pp 449-453)
- Assessment of
  - Lung sounds (pp 441-442)

Monitoring Devices

- Obtaining and using information from patient monitoring devices including (but not limited to)
  - Pulse oximetry (p 431)
  - Noninvasive blood pressure (pp 432, 443-447)
  - Blood glucose determination (pp 433-434)

Reassessment

- How and when to reassess patients (pp 454-455)
- How and when to perform a reassessment for all patient situations (pp 454-455)

Knowledge Objectives

1. Identify the components of the patient assessment process. (p 392)
2. Explain how the different causes and presentations of emergencies will affect how you perform each step of the patient assessment process. (p 392)
3. Describe the key elements of the critical thinking process and how you can apply them in the field. (pp 395-396)
4. Discuss some of the possible environmental, chemical, and biologic hazards that may be present at an emergency scene, ways to recognize them, and precautions to protect personal safety. (p 398)
5. Discuss how to survey a scene for signs of violence and protect yourself and bystanders from real or potential danger. (p 398)
6. Describe how to determine the mechanism of injury or nature of the illness at an emergency and the importance of differentiating trauma patients from medical patients. (pp 399-400)
7. List the minimum standard precautions that should be followed and personal protective

equipment that should be worn at an emergency scene, including examples of when additional precautions would be appropriate. (pp 400-401)

8. Explain why it is important to identify the total number of patients at an emergency scene and how this evaluation relates to determining the need for additional or specialized resources, implementation of the incident command system, and triage. (pp 401-402)

9. Describe the principal goals of the primary survey process. (p 403)

10. Explain the process of forming a general impression of a patient as part of the primary survey and the reasons why this step is critical to patient management. (pp 403-405)

11. Describe the assessment of airway status in patients who are responsive and unresponsive. (pp 405-406)

12. Give examples of possible signs and causes of airway obstruction in patients who are responsive and unresponsive, as well as the appropriate response. (pp 405-406)

13. Describe the assessment of a patient's breathing status, including the key information you must obtain during this process and the emergency medical care required for patients who have both adequate and inadequate breathing. (pp 406-408)

14. List the signs of respiratory distress and respiratory failure. (p 408)

15. Describe the assessment of a patient's circulatory status, including the different methods for obtaining a pulse and appropriate management depending on the patient's status. (pp 408-412)

16. Explain the variations required to obtain a pulse in infant and child patients compared with adult patients. (pp 408-409)

17. Describe the assessment of a patient's skin color, temperature, and condition, including examples of both normal and abnormal findings and the information this provides related to the patient's status. (pp 410-411)

18. Discuss the process of assessing for and methods for controlling external bleeding. (p 411)

19. Explain the importance of assessing a patient's level of consciousness to determine altered mental status. (pp 412-414)

20. Give examples of different methods used to assess alertness, responsiveness, and orientation. (pp 412-414)

21. List the steps to follow during the primary survey of a trauma patient, including examples of abnormal signs and appropriate related actions. (pp 414-416)

22. Discuss the steps used to identify and subsequently treat life-threatening conditions that endanger a patient during an emergency. (pp 415-417)

23. Explain the process for determining the priority of patient care and transport at an emergency scene, including examples of conditions that necessitate rapid transport. (pp 417-418)

24. Discuss the importance of protecting a trauma patient's spine and identifying fractured extremities during patient packaging for transport. (pp 417-418)

25. Discuss the process of taking a patient history, its key components, and its relationship to the primary survey process. (pp 420-425)

26. Describe examples of different techniques you may use to obtain information from patients during the history-taking process. (pp 422-425)

27. Discuss different challenges you may face when taking a patient history on sensitive topics and strategies that can be used to facilitate each situation. (pp 425-429)

28. Describe the purpose of performing a physical exam during secondary assessment, its components, special patient considerations, and methods for determining which aspects of the physical exam will be used. (p 430)

29. Name the devices used to monitor a patient's medical condition during the secondary assessment and reassessment. (pp 431-433)

30. Describe the purpose of a full-body exam, and list the steps used during this process. (pp 433, 435-437)

31. Explain situations in which patients may receive a focused assessment, including examples, by body system, of what each focused assessment should include based on a patient's chief complaint. (pp 438-439)

32. List normal respiratory rate, pulse rate, and blood pressure ranges for adults, children, and infants. (p 440)

33. Explain the importance of performing a reassessment of the patient and the steps in this process. (pp 454-455)

Skills Objectives

1. Demonstrate the techniques for assessing a patient's airway, and correctly obtain information related to respiratory rate, rhythm, quality/character of breathing, and depth of breathing. (pp 405-408, 439-442)

2. Demonstrate how to obtain a pulse rate in a patient. (pp 408-409)

3. Demonstrate how to assess a radial pulse in a responsive patient and an unresponsive patient. (pp 408-409)

4. Demonstrate how to assess a carotid pulse in an unresponsive patient. (pp 408-409)

5. Demonstrate how to palpate a brachial pulse in a child who is younger than 1 year (or a manikin). (p 409)
6. Demonstrate how to assess capillary refill in an adult or child older than 6 years. (p 411)
7. Demonstrate how to assess capillary refill in an infant or child younger than 6 years. (p 411)
8. Demonstrate how to use the AVPU scale to test for patient responsiveness. (pp 412-413)
9. Demonstrate how to evaluate a patient's orientation and document his or her status correctly. (pp 413-414)
10. Demonstrate how to perform a rapid full-body scan during the primary survey of a patient. (pp 414-416, Skill Drill 10-1)
11. Demonstrate the use of a pulse oximetry device to evaluate the effectiveness of oxygenation in the patient. (p 431)
12. Demonstrate the use of electronic and manual devices to assist in determining the patient's blood pressure in the field. (pp 432, 443-447)
13. Demonstrate the use of an end-tidal carbon dioxide monitoring device to assist in determining the patient's concentration of expired carbon dioxide in the field. (pp 432-433)
14. Demonstrate how to assess a patient's blood glucose level. (pp 433-434, Skill Drill 10-2)
15. Demonstrate how to perform a full-body exam. (pp 433, 435-437, Skill Drill 10-3)
16. Demonstrate how to perform a focused assessment. (pp 438-453)
17. Demonstrate how to measure blood pressure by auscultation. (pp 443-445, Skill Drill 10-4)
18. Demonstrate how to measure blood pressure by palpation. (pp 445-446, Skill Drill 10-5)
19. Demonstrate how to test pupil reaction in response to light in a patient and document his or her status correctly. (pp 447-448)

Introduction

The importance of patient assessment cannot be overemphasized. As an emergency medical services (EMS) provider, you must master and be comfortable with the patient assessment process. Patient assessment is used, to some degree, in every patient encounter. You will develop and perfect your own assessment techniques as you complete your education and gain field experience. It is also important to understand the processes of thinking and decision making. By having a better understanding of how your thoughts are formed and processed, you can learn to think more effectively.

The assessment process is divided into five main parts:

1. Scene size-up
2. Primary survey
3. History taking
4. Secondary assessment
5. Reassessment

The five steps of the patient assessment process represent a logical approach to the evaluation of a patient, but the order in which you perform them is dictated by the patient's condition and the environment in which you find him or her. The same components of patient assessment used to evaluate a medical patient are used to assess a trauma patient; the differences lie in your findings and how you effectively care for your patient. Whether you are assessing a medical patient or a trauma patient, the key in both situations is to remain organized.

A **sign** is an objective condition that you can observe (see, hear, feel, smell, or measure) about the patient. A **symptom** is a subjective condition that the patient feels and tells you about. Rarely does one sign or symptom reveal to you the patient's status or underlying problem **Figure 10-1**. Rather, it is the combination of

YOU are the Provider — PART 1

Your EMS crew is dispatched to a motor vehicle crash (MVC). As you are responding, dispatch advises you that law enforcement personnel are already on scene with a one-vehicle crash, sedan versus tree, at an estimated 35 mph. Dispatch also advises you that the patient is unresponsive.

1. What are the components of a scene size-up?
2. What can you do to ensure scene safety?

Patient Assessment

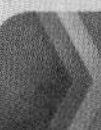

Scene Size-up

Ensure scene safety
Determine mechanism of injury/nature of illness
Take standard precautions
Determine number of patients
Consider additional/specialized resources

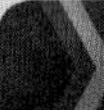

Primary Survey*

Form a general impression

Assess
- Responsiveness/level of consciousness

Assess and Treat
- Exsanguinating hemorrhage
- Airway
- Breathing
- Circulation

Also Assess
- Disability
- Exposure

Identify
- Chief complaint/life threats (treat)
- Priority of patient care
- Transport decision

History Taking

Investigate
- Chief complaint
- History of present illness (OPQRST)
- Past medical history (SAMPLE)

Secondary Assessment

Is the patient medical or trauma?

Assess
- Baseline vital signs
- Monitoring devices (as appropriate)

Systematic physical exam
- Full-body exam or rapid full-body scan
- Focused on injury
- Based on body system (respiratory, cardiovascular, neurologic, reproductive, etc)

Reassessment

- Repeat the primary survey
- Reassess vital signs
- Reassess the chief complaint
- Recheck interventions
- Identify and treat changes in the patient's condition

Reassess patient:
- Unstable patients: every 5 minutes
- Stable patients: every 15 minutes

***Note:** The primary survey usually follows an ABCDE sequence (Airway, Breathing, Circulation, Disability, Exposure) or XABCDE in trauma patients (where X stands for exsanguinating hemorrhage), but if the patient appears lifeless or has severe external bleeding, use a CABDE sequence (Circulation, Airway, Breathing, Disability, Exposure).

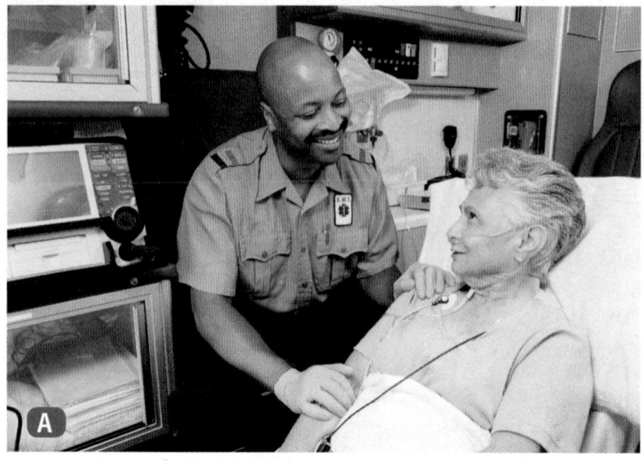

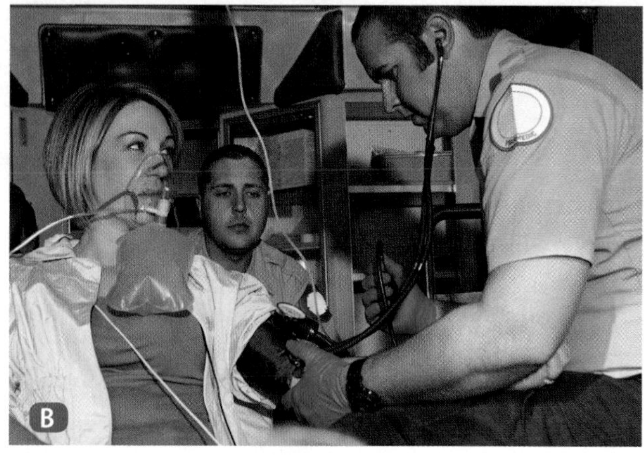

Figure 10-1 A. A symptom is a subjective condition that the patient feels and tells you about. **B.** A sign is an objective condition that you can observe about the patient.

Word of Wisdom

People call 9-1-1 during some of the most difficult times of their lives. In some cases, they call because of a serious illness or injury. In others, they call because the patient or family is frightened, overwhelmed, or unable to cope with a problem any longer. The patient is often fatigued, sick, frightened, angry, or sad, and the family often shares some or all of these feelings. Regardless of the exact nature of the call, the patient, family, and bystanders expect you to bring comfort, control, and resolution of these problems—emotional and physical.

In many ways, good communication skills are as important as technical proficiency, if not more so. As discussed in Chapter 4, *Communications and Documentation*, each step in the assessment process can be impeded by inadequate communication, and each can be enhanced by a good connection between you and the patient and family. Here are five tips that can vastly improve your communication skills during the assessment process:

1. Quickly do whatever you can to make yourself and the patient comfortable. When time permits, sit down and/or position yourself near the patient, introduce yourself, and ask the patient's name. These simple actions signal to the patient that you have time to talk; they open the channels of communication as nothing else will.
2. Actively listen to the patient. In many cases, patients will be able to tell you what is wrong if you are paying attention and truly listening. You can use several skills to actively listen, including leaning in toward the patient, taking selective notes, and periodically repeating back important points to the patient to ensure you understood correctly. Active listening also involves asking follow-up questions related to the information the patient gives you.
3. Make eye contact with the patient. Eye contact signals that you are listening, so the patient is more likely to open up. An added benefit is that you will see facial expressions that, in some cases, communicate information more clearly than the patient's words.
4. Base your initial questions on the patient's complaints. No one likes to think that he or she is "just another patient," but that idea is what you communicate if you always ask the same questions of every patient, regardless of his or complaints. Talk about the patient's problem first; obtain demographic information after tending to the patient's needs.
5. Before you start treatment, stop for a moment and mentally summarize what you have learned and what you are going to do; then tell the patient. By providing necessary information to the patient and family, you help to relieve their anxiety and fear. This practice will also give them an opportunity to give you additional information if you have missed something.

Make it a point to spend your entire EMS career fine-tuning your patient assessment skills, because they are the cornerstone of high-quality prehospital care. An inadequate assessment almost always results in substandard patient care. Therefore, approach each patient with the same thorough assessment. Unless you take a systematic approach to patient assessment, you will systematically fail to find and treat life threats.

Be sure to focus some of your energy on improving the communication process. You will make it easier for patients to feel comfortable around you, which will help them to give honest, direct answers to your questions. As a result, you will get better assessment information in less time.

many signs and symptoms that reveals the underlying problem or condition of your patient. Therefore, it is essential to have a basic understanding of the causes and presentations of emergencies so that you know what to look for.

For example, consider a patient who has crushing chest pain radiating down the left arm and jaw (a symptom) and is diaphoretic and pale (signs). If the onset of his symptoms occurred while he was shoveling snow and his past medical history includes coronary bypass surgery, then you are more likely to suspect and treat myocardial infarction (MI) than other conditions with the same **chief complaint** (the reason EMS was called). In this example, you can see how it is essential to collect all pertinent information and be able to interpret how the pieces of information fit together.

This chapter provides the framework and information necessary for you to understand the fundamental elements that contribute to the critical thinking and decision-making processes, as well as how to conduct the patient assessment process. The patient assessment process is the ground on which all levels of EMS education are built and is the foundation of all emergency medical care. As an advanced emergency medical technician (AEMT), you cannot effectively treat your patients if you cannot correctly assess them. Strong critical thinking and assessment skills will assist you in the process of saving lives.

Clinical Decision Making and Critical Thinking

Effective clinical decision making is dependent on your ability to gather, evaluate, and synthesize patient information; develop an idea of the patient's problem based on gathered information and the patient's presentation; and formulate a field impression on which an appropriate patient treatment plan will be based. This process is called critical thinking.

Gathering, evaluating, and correctly synthesizing patient information will culminate in an appropriate treatment plan. This process requires an understanding of the patient's injury or illness and the impact that your emergency medical care will have on it. You will develop needed critical thinking skills through field experience in dealing with multiple patients with varying problems. In every assessment you perform, practice the following critical thinking skills:

- **Gathering information.** Ensure you have an adequate fund of knowledge and facts. The prehospital setting may be one of controlled chaos; your sources of information may be overwhelming or severely limited. Observe the scene and question the patient and bystanders. Use your knowledge and understanding of anatomy, physiology, pathophysiology, and how injuries and illnesses might or will affect the patient. Knowledge is acquired from initial training, continuing education, and experiences.
- **Evaluating information.** Consider the meaning of the gathered information. Multiple amounts of specific, crucial data, often from multiple sources, must be obtained to direct your assessment and subsequent treatment. You must be able to prioritize this information in a short time, separate relevant from irrelevant data, and provide the most appropriate emergency medical care for the patient. Irrelevant or extraneous data can skew your interpretation of the overall situation, potentially leading to inappropriate patient care. Analyze and compare similar situations from your own experiences.
- **Synthesizing information.** Put together the data you have gathered and evaluated, and then form a plan to manage the scene and/or patient. Your overall understanding of the situation and the treatment that you provide to the patient are only as good as the quality and quantity of data that you obtain.

Although no two patients present in the exact same manner, you must be able to integrate the information you obtain regarding the current incident with similar situations and experiences. This integration will enhance your overall understanding of the current situation and will prepare you to deal with future situations. Recall difficult situations. Recalling and learning from bad experiences enhances your ability to manage the current situation. Articulate assessment-based decisions and construct arguments. You must be able to defend your actions and justify the decisions on which you based your treatment.

Words of Wisdom

Sometimes you will need to think outside the box and do something in a manner inconsistent with guidelines. For example, you may need to use a Kendrick Extrication Device (KED) to remove an unstable patient from entrapment due to space constraints. Under normal circumstances, a KED should only be used on stable patients complaining of neck or back pain. If you do not follow proper procedure because you are acting in the best interest of the patient, then clearly document what you did and the reason for doing it.

The performance of your duties will constantly be challenged by the environment in which you function. Time is perhaps your biggest challenge, especially when managing a critically ill or injured patient. Factors that can hamper your ability to perform emergency medical care—crowds of people, volatile scenes, poor lighting, weather extremes, bumpy ambulances—usually do not exist in other medical settings. Your ability to improvise, adapt, and overcome these unique obstacles—and still provide appropriate emergency medical care—will make you an effective clinical decision maker and a true prehospital professional. Always base your treatment or transport decisions on your assessment of the patient, discussed next.

Words of Wisdom

The fundamental elements that contribute to the critical thinking and clinical decision-making processes are listed below. As you look over each item on the following list, ask yourself, "Do I have this quality already, or do I need to develop it?"

- Adequate knowledge of anatomy, physiology, and pathophysiology
- Ability to gather and organize data and form concepts
- Ability to focus on specific and multiple elements of data
- Ability to identify and deal with **medical ambiguity**—uncertainty regarding the specific cause of the patient's condition. Few 9-1-1 calls follow the scripts in your protocols to the letter.
- Skill in differentiating between relevant and irrelevant data
- Ability to analyze and compare similar and contrary situations
- Ability to articulate your reasoning and construct arguments

Patient Assessment

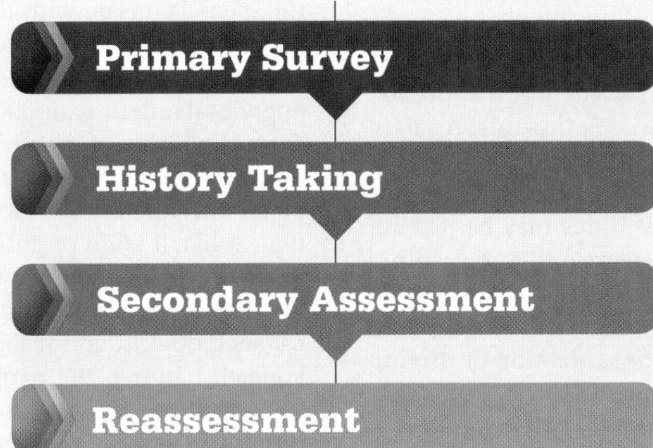

Scene Size-up

The **scene size-up** refers to your evaluation of the conditions in which you will be operating; it is the information gathering stage of the patient assessment process. Although the scene size-up should be the focus of your attention when you first arrive on scene, a continuous **situational awareness** is necessary throughout the entire call to ensure safety. Situational awareness is paying attention to the conditions and people around you at all times, and understanding the potential safety risks those conditions or people pose.

For example, before you know the exact location of an incident, consider the environmental conditions. Is it cold, snowing, raining, dark, hot, or humid? Consider how the weather may affect the physical terrain you may encounter. Even relatively minor weather conditions may present a significant hazard if responders and patients are exposed for a significant amount of time.

You must begin to prepare for a specific situation based on the initial dispatch information. From the moment you are called into action until you reach your patient, you must consider a variety of factors that will have an impact on how you operate on the scene and provide patient care. These factors include road and traffic hazards (which may affect where you park your emergency vehicle) and incident hazards such as fire, hazardous materials (hazmat), or scenes of violence (which may affect if and how you approach the scene). To help ensure safe and effective operations, your scene size-up must combine an understanding of the situation based on the information the dispatcher provides with your observation of the scene itself. Your observation of the scene will help you to identify hazards, safety concerns, the number of patients, and the need for additional resources required to safely and effectively care for the patient.

Safety Tips

Assessing the safety of a scene before entering is the single most important way in which you can attend to your own well-being. Subtle signs of danger that are not recognized and neutralized—or avoided—at this point can quickly become more threatening after you shift your attention to patient assessment and emergency medical care. Remember that scenes are dynamic (constantly changing), so maintain your situational awareness.

Ensure Scene Safety

The prehospital setting is not a controlled and isolated scene; it is unpredictable, dangerous, and unforgiving. What seems relatively safe and secure can change without notice. Every prehospital scene has a potential for injury, and, if you or your partner becomes injured or incapacitated so that you cannot function at the emergency, you have taken away the initial resource to care for the patient. You need to ensure safety for you and your partner first, other responders and bystanders second, and your patient last.

As mentioned previously, dispatch information helps you to anticipate potential hazards prior to arriving on scene. For example, an MVC on a busy roadway indicates, at a minimum, that you must wear a high-visibility Class 2 or Class 3 safety vest approved by the American National Standards Institute. A safety vest helps make you visible to others on the roadway while minimizing interference with other clothing and equipment. It is also likely that fluids may be leaking from the wrecked vehicle. Antifreeze, oil, and gasoline are common chemicals found at the scene of an MVC. These chemicals on the roadway can result in a slippery surface, creating a hazard for those walking or driving past. Consider traffic safety issues. A variety of traffic incident management techniques may be appropriate. These techniques may include the use of personnel and traffic markers such as cones, flares, and signs to divert traffic around the area, and the strategic positioning of emergency vehicles to protect the area. Your ambulance can be a safe haven when caring for patients. Park your vehicle in an area that is a safe distance away, but in a place that allows you rapid access to equipment and your patient. Be aware of the dangers that may not be so apparent.

Look for possible dangers as you approach the scene and before you step out of the vehicle. Hazards found at the scene vary and may include traffic, chemical and biologic agents, electricity from downed power lines or lightning, secondary collapse of structures or terrain, fires, explosions, and carbon monoxide. Observe for unstable surfaces, slopes, ice, water, and wet grass. When gaining access to a patient, it is important to remember that you will typically leave via the same route you entered. When you leave, you will be moving up to a 100-pound (45-kg) stretcher, if it is motorized, and possibly a person weighing 200 pounds (90 kg) or more. If your footing was compromised going in, then you are going to have an even more difficult time coming out.

Working in unfavorable conditions and on unstable surfaces is a large part of prehospital care. Without knowing the infinite number of situations you may become involved in, a good rule to use is that any actions you may take to protect yourself (eg, wearing heavy coats, rain gear, or life jackets; using air conditioned or heated vehicles) should also be considered for the patient. If you are putting on equipment to address environmental hazards, then provide the patient with the same or similar equipment. If you move away from the scene to take cover from an environmental hazard, then move the patient with you if possible. Taking your time to stay focused on what you are doing will go a long way in preventing injuries to yourself and your patients.

Protect bystanders from becoming patients. Many bystanders attempt to help during an emergency; always remember that most are not trained to handle complicated EMS equipment, illnesses, or injuries.

Be aware of scenes that have the potential for violence. Request the assistance of law enforcement personnel if the scene is unsafe with the potential for violence, and do not enter until the scene is declared safe. You will encounter violent patients, distraught family members, angry bystanders, gangs, and unruly crowds. When you enter the home of a patient, look around the immediate area. Are any weapons visible in the area to which a patient or others may have access? Weapons need not be typical like a knife or gun; they can also be items such as a screwdriver, hammer, or simple things sitting on the kitchen table or nightstand by the bed. Always observe for such objects, and if they are not secured, then place yourself between the patient and the potential danger to prevent possible access to the object. If the scene is a potential crime scene, then follow local protocols before entering. Ask for law enforcement personnel to accompany you when needed.

If the scene is unsafe and it is not possible to make it safe, then do not enter. Move to a safe location, and call for additional resources (eg, firefighters, utility workers, or hazmat technicians) **Figure 10-2**. Chapter 40, *Vehicle Extrication, Special Rescue, and Hazardous Materials*, discusses patient rescue and extrication, and the hazards associated with responding to a hazmat incident, in more detail.

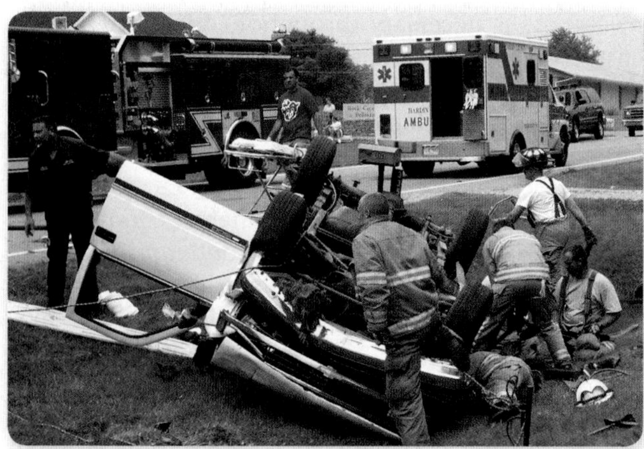

Figure 10-2 If the scene is unsafe, then do not enter until measures have been taken to remedy the problem. An overturned vehicle may be unstable and should be shored up before trying to access the patient.

Words of Wisdom

When you enter a potential crime scene, take care not to disturb possible evidence. If you must move an item (such as a gun laying on a patient's chest), then handle it carefully with a gloved hand and thoroughly document the position in which it was found and to where it was moved. However, patient care takes precedence over evidence preservation. Never delay patient care to preserve a scene.

Determine Mechanism of Injury/Nature of Illness

When you perform the prehospital assessment, do not immediately categorize your patient as either a trauma (injured) patient or a medical (ill) patient. Some patients will have a problem that is not related to trauma, and they are typically referred to as medical patients (for example, patients with chest pain or difficulty breathing). Other patients will have sustained injuries in an incident such as a fall, an MVC, or a shooting, and they are usually considered trauma patients. Some patients fall into both categories. Consider the patient who is involved in an MVC because he or she had a heart attack and lost control of the vehicle. This patient is a trauma patient who also has a medical condition.

Consider an unresponsive man found at the bottom of a ladder. Did he fall off the ladder, strike his head, and become unresponsive? Or did he experience a medical condition (such as hypoglycemia) that caused him to fall off the ladder and then become unresponsive? Early in the assessment, it can be difficult to identify with absolute certainty whether the emergency is of traumatic or medical origin. Remember, the fundamentals of good patient assessment do not change, despite the unique aspects of trauma and medical care.

Considering the mechanism of injury or nature of the illness early will help you prepare for the rest of your assessment. For example, when you begin to gather equipment from the unit to treat your patient, you might collect different equipment for a patient who is reporting chest pain than you would for a pedestrian struck by a vehicle. As an AEMT, you need to be able to identify all of the aspects of the emergency to which you were called to respond.

Mechanism of Injury

Traumatic injuries are the result of physical forces applied to the outside of the body, usually from an object striking the body or a body striking an object **Figure 10-3**. These injuries are generally classified according to the type or amount of force applied to the body, the length of time the force was applied, and where it was applied on the body. The **mechanism of injury (MOI)** describes how the patient became injured. Examples of MOIs may include falls, MVCs, assaults, and industrial accidents.

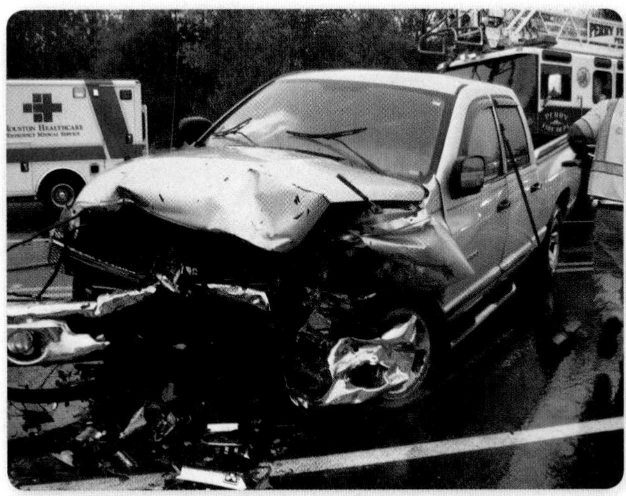

Figure 10-3 With traumatic injuries, the patient has been exposed to some force or energy that has resulted in injury or possibly death. You can learn a great deal about that force by evaluating the mechanism of injury.

Determining the MOI will provide many clues to help you focus your assessment.

As you might expect, certain parts of the body are more easily injured than others. The brain and the spinal cord are fragile and easy to injure. Fortunately, they are protected by the skull, the vertebrae, and several layers of soft tissues. The eyes are also easily injured. Even small forces to the eyes may result in serious injury. The bones and certain organs are stronger and can absorb small forces without sustaining serious injury. A good understanding of anatomy and physiology will help you to identify times when an MOI may lead to injury to parts of the body not directly impacted. For example, consider a patient who has fallen off a roof, landing feetfirst. This patient's MOI would direct attention to possible injury to the feet. But significant energy likely transferred to other body areas and may have caused further injury in the patient's legs, pelvis, and spine.

You will commonly encounter the terms *blunt trauma* and *penetrating trauma*. With blunt trauma, the force of the injury occurs over a broad area, and the skin is not broken **Figure 10-4**. However, the tissues and organs underneath the area of impact may be damaged. With penetrating trauma, the force of the injury occurs at the specific point of contact between the skin and the object. The object pierces the skin and creates an open wound that carries a high potential for infection **Figure 10-5**. The severity of injury depends on the characteristics of the penetrating object, the amount and length of time the force or energy was applied, and the part of the body affected. For more information about blunt and penetrating trauma, see Chapter 26, *Trauma Overview*.

Nature of the Illness

As an AEMT, you are likely to care for more medical patients than trauma patients. For trauma patients, you examine the MOI as part of your scene size-up. For medical patients,

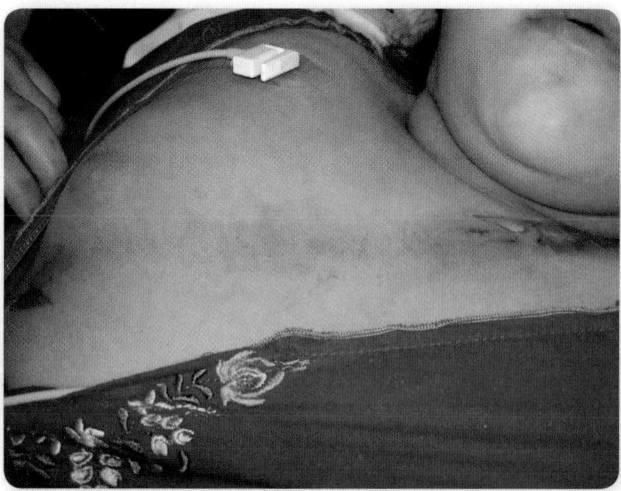

Figure 10-4 With blunt trauma, the force of the injury occurs over a broad area and the skin is not broken. However, the tissues and organs underneath the area of impact may be damaged.

Courtesy of ED, Royal North Shore Hospital/NSW Institute of Trauma & Injury.

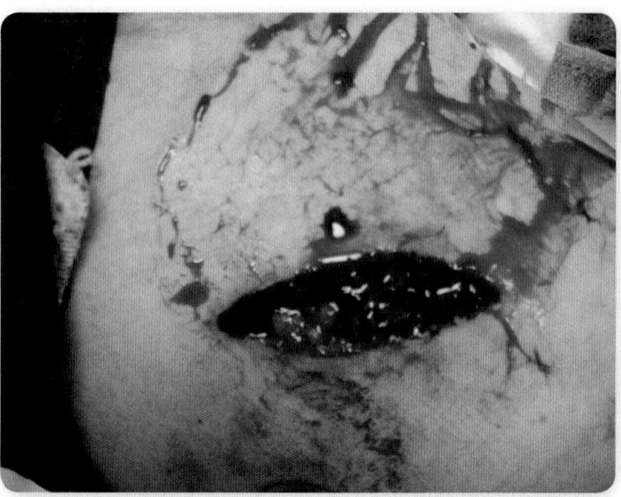

Figure 10-5 With penetrating trauma, an object pierces the skin and creates an open wound that carries a high potential for infection.

Courtesy of Rhonda Hunt.

make an effort to determine the general type of illness, or **nature of the illness (NOI)**. NOIs include seizures, heart attacks, diabetic conditions, and poisonings. The NOI is often best described by the patient's chief complaint and medical history.

To quickly determine the NOI, talk with the patient, family, and/or bystanders about the emergency. At the same time, use your senses to check the scene for clues to the possible cause of the illness. You may see open or spilled medicine containers, poisonous substances, unsanitary living conditions, open food on the counter, oxygen tanks, or home nebulizers. You may smell an unusual or strong odor, such as the odor of fresh paint in a closed room or the nauseating odor associated with gastrointestinal bleeding. You may hear abnormal sounds such as wheezes when the patient attempts to breathe. Keep these observations of the scene in mind as you begin to assess the patient.

Safety Tips

When everyone in the home is sick, consider an environmental cause—and be aware that the scene may be unsafe for you and your partner to enter. For example, when a stomach virus spreads through a family, one person generally gets better as another is affected; they do not all show signs and symptoms at the same time. However, exposure to carbon monoxide from a space heater would cause everyone in the enclosed area to develop signs and symptoms almost simultaneously.

Take Standard Precautions

Standard precautions and **personal protective equipment (PPE)** need to be considered and adapted to the prehospital task at hand. PPE includes clothing and specialized equipment that provides protection to the wearer. The type of PPE used depends on the specific job duties required during a patient care interaction. For example, firefighters may wear PPE such as steel boots, helmets, turnout gear, gloves, heat-resistant outerwear, and self-contained breathing apparatus designed to protect them from injury when performing a forced entry. Hazmat technicians may don a protective suit designed to prevent contamination by potentially lethal materials.

Standard precautions are protective measures that have traditionally been recommended by the Centers for Disease Control and Prevention (CDC) for use in dealing with objects, blood, body fluids, and other potential exposure risks of communicable disease. If you have a primary responsibility for patient care, then you need to take standard precautions when assessing and treating each and every patient. These measures may not provide absolute protection from exposure to infectious diseases or bloodborne pathogens, but they are the most effective way to reduce your risk of exposure. The concept of standard precautions assumes that all blood, body fluids (except sweat), nonintact skin, and mucous membranes may pose a substantial risk of infection. This concept includes potentially infectious materials that are dried, because some viruses (such as hepatitis) can live for days outside the body.

Take standard precautions before you step out of the EMS vehicle and before you make contact with the patient **Figure 10-6**. After you have made contact with a patient, it is too late. The use of standard precautions in EMS may be dictated by local standards or protocols, and include (but are not limited to) consistent handwashing

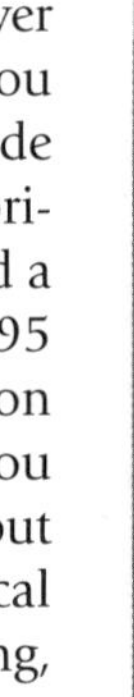

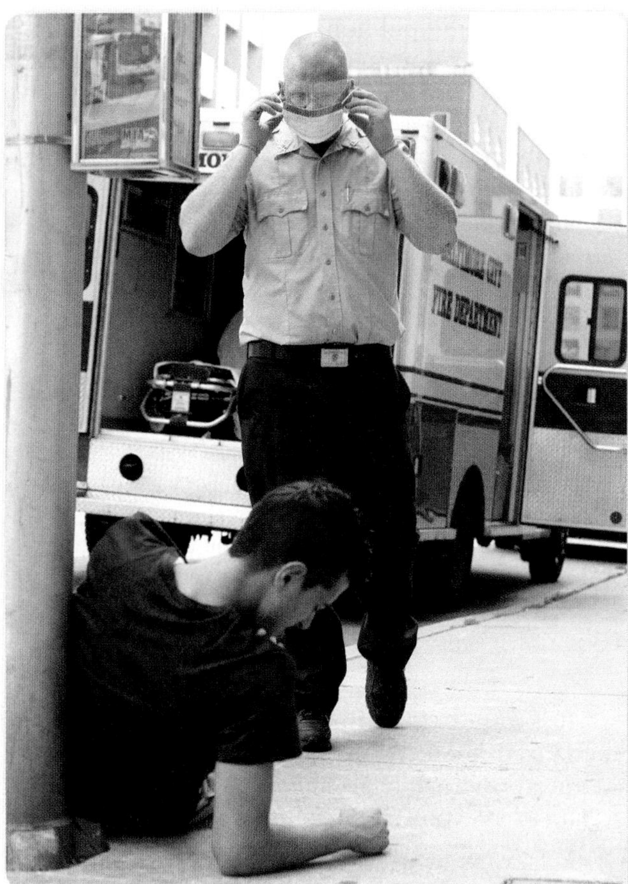

Figure 10-6 Proper protective equipment is vital when you are called to a scene in which you may be exposed to blood or other body fluids.

(with soap and water or alcohol-based hand cleansers) before and after care, gloves, eye protection, a mask, and a gown. At a minimum, gloves must be in place before any patient contact. Remember that after contact with a patient, gloves may be contaminated by infectious materials. Avoid handling EMS equipment with the same gloves used during patient contact, and remember to change gloves before touching another patient. The use of eye protection may be necessary during patient interactions. Standard eyeglasses may not offer enough protection because most are not designed with side splash guards. Eyewear should protect you from potential exposures from all directions. Blood and body fluids that contain potentially infectious materials may become airborne; consider wearing a face mask to reduce the risk of splash or spray. A mask will provide protection from some airborne diseases, but its level of protection will depend on the type of mask, a proper fit, and your ability to apply and wear it properly.

You must be appropriately educated in the use of standard precautions, which should include training in the many types of PPE used in different situations. If you are not trained in the application of PPE that is appropriate for the situation, then do not approach the scene or make patient contact. Instead, call for additional help. If you make contact with the patient and discover a condition that warrants a higher level of PPE than you are using, then do not hesitate to regroup and upgrade your protection. For example, if you discover in your primary survey that a patient has a productive cough and a history of tuberculosis, and you are not wearing an N95 mask, then you and your crew should immediately don appropriate respiratory protection. If you suspect you have been exposed to a communicable disease without the protection of proper PPE, then follow your local agency's protocols for postexposure reporting, testing, and prophylaxis.

Words of Wisdom

Standard precautions are the infection prevention practices intended to reduce the risk of transmission of bloodborne and other pathogens. These precautions include hand hygiene; use of personal protective equipment such as gloves, gowns, and masks; safe injection practices; safe handling of potentially contaminated equipment and surfaces; and respiratory hygiene/cough etiquette. The term *standard precautions* has replaced terms for similar concepts, such as *body substance isolation*, and is promoted by both the CDC and the World Health Organization.

Determine the Number of Patients

As part of the scene size-up, accurately identify the total number of patients. This evaluation is critical in determining your need for additional resources, such as additional ambulances. When multiple patients are present or more patients are present than the responding unit can effectively handle, put your mass-casualty plan into action based on your local protocols. This plan will most likely include establishing the **incident command system (ICS)**, calling for additional units, and then beginning triage Figure 10-7. The ICS is a flexible system implemented to manage disasters and mass-casualty incidents in which section chiefs, including finance, logistics, operations, and planning, report to the person in charge of the incident, the incident commander. **Triage** is the process of sorting patients based on the severity of their conditions; usually, the most experienced EMS provider on scene is assigned to this role. After all patients have been triaged, you can begin to establish treatment and transport priorities. This process helps allocate personnel, equipment, and resources to provide the most effective care to everyone. Be familiar with the ICS and understand your local protocols. Incident command is discussed in more detail in Chapter 41, *Incident Management*.

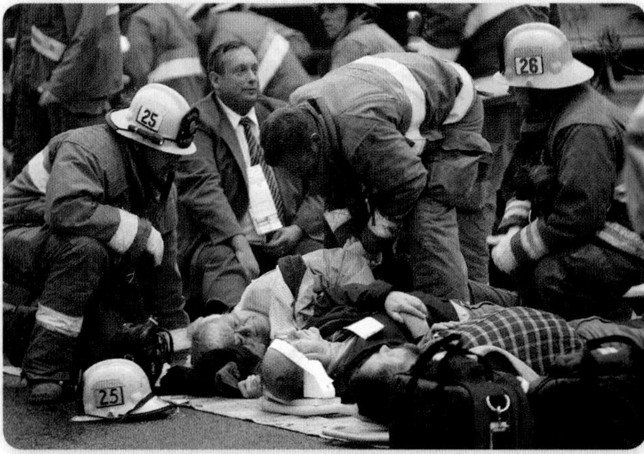

Figure 10-7 When multiple patients are present or more patients are present than the responding unit can effectively handle, use the incident command system, call for additional units, and begin triage.

Consider Additional or Specialized Resources

Some trauma or medical situations may require more ambulances, whereas others may have a need for specialized resources. Basic life support (BLS) units may be all that are needed for some patients; however, you should request paramedic backup for patients with severe injuries or complex medical conditions depending on available resources and local protocols. Air medical support may be another good resource for advanced life support (ALS) in your area.

Fire departments usually provide services beyond fire suppression, including technical rescue, vehicle extrication, high-angle rope rescue, hazmat management, and swift water rescue. Specialized equipment and gear will also be needed for each of these specialized situations.

Words of Wisdom

You are less likely to call for additional assistance after you initiate patient care. Call as soon as you anticipate the need!

Search and rescue teams can help find, package, and transport patients over long distances and across uneven terrain. Law enforcement personnel may also be needed to control traffic or intervene in potentially violent situations. Many police departments throughout the country have officers trained as first responders; they know cardiopulmonary resuscitation (CPR) and may carry an automated external defibrillator (AED). As mentioned previously, law enforcement personnel should be the first to enter crime scenes and hostile environments. Stage yourself and your vehicle at a safe distance until the scene has been secured.

Words of Wisdom

Some law enforcement personnel now carry tourniquets as part of the *Stop the Bleed* campaign, a federal initiative designed to teach bystanders how keep an injured person alive until the arrival of professional emergency responders.[1] This initiative was created to address life-threatening bleeding in situations such as active shooters, bombings, and any violent circumstances where immediate bleeding control may be instrumental in saving lives.

It is important to understand when additional or specialized resources are required and how your EMS system is organized. To determine if you require additional resources, ask yourself the following questions:

- How many patients are present?
- Are enough resources available to respond to their conditions?
- Does the scene pose a threat to you, your patient, or others?

Always call for additional resources as soon as possible, before making contact with patients or beginning triage. It is never wrong to call for backup, even if the extra units are instructed to turn back. Remember, you are less likely to ask for help after you begin patient care because at that point, you are part of the scene, particularly at an MVC in which patients require spinal immobilization or bleeding control.

Words of Wisdom

Based on the MOI or the situation in which the patient is found (such as a patient found on the ground with no witness to verify whether a fall occurred), you should consider cervical spinal immobilization. Assign a partner or another responder to place the head in a neutral inline position and to maintain stabilization until completely immobilized or it is determined that cervical spinal immobilization is not needed.

Patient Assessment

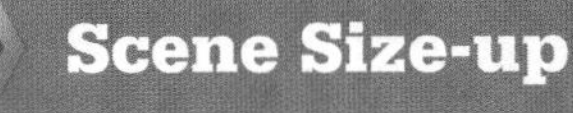

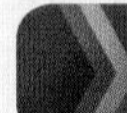

Form a general impression

Assess

- Responsiveness/level of consciousness

Assess and Treat

- Exsanguinating hemorrhage
- Airway
- Breathing
- Circulation

Also Assess

- Disability
- Exposure

Identify

- Chief complaint/life threats (treat)
- Priority of patient care
- Transport decision

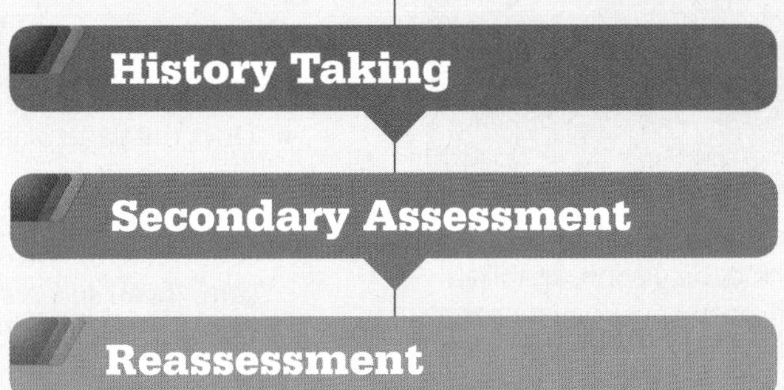

***Note:** The primary survey usually follows an ABCDE sequence (Airway, Breathing, Circulation, Disability, Exposure) or XABCDE in trauma patients (where X stands for exsanguinating hemorrhage), but if the patient appears lifeless or has severe external bleeding, use a CABDE sequence (Circulation, Airway, Breathing, Disability, Exposure).

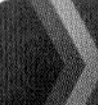

Primary Survey

During the scene size-up, you use dispatch information and your own evaluation of the scene to identify potential hazards and determine if additional resources are needed. These steps are critical prior to the initiation of patient care. The essence of patient assessment, however, begins when you greet your patient and begin the primary survey.

The **primary survey** has a single, all-important goal: to identify and initiate treatment of immediate or imminent life threats. To do this, physically examine the patient to assess the level of consciousness (LOC) and airway, breathing, circulation, disability, and exposure (ABCDEs). **Vital signs** are used to evaluate the patient's condition, but the primary survey is neither an in-depth physical exam nor an assessment of vital signs. Vital signs will be addressed later in the secondary assessment. During the primary survey, always give priority to life threats by assessing the patient's LOC and ABCDEs to ensure life-saving treatment, regardless of what other injuries may exist Figure 10-8.

Form a General Impression

Any time you meet someone new, you form a first impression about that person. Forming the **general impression** of your patient is a similar process that focuses on the rapid identification of potentially life-threatening problems. The formation of a general impression is the first part of the primary survey; it determines the priority of emergency medical care. This step includes noting things such as the person's age, sex, weight, level of distress, overall appearance, and the presence of any obvious bleeding. This information may lead you to anticipate different problems. A woman reporting abdominal pain, for example, may have more serious implications than a man with the same complaint because of the complexity of the female reproductive system.

Think of your general impression as an overall visual assessment that helps you gather information as you approach the patient Figure 10-9. You can feel for pulses, pain, and deformities when you reach the patient. Ensure that you approach the patient from the front to avoid causing the patient to turn to see you, possibly making any injuries worse. Note the patient's position and whether the patient is moving or still.

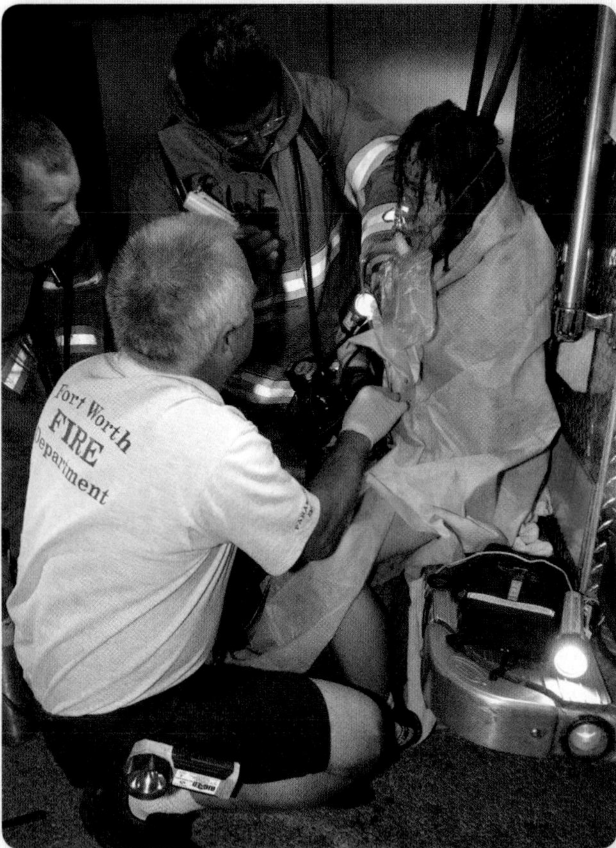

Figure 10-8 An assessment of the patient's level of consciousness and airway, breathing, circulation, disability, and exposure is used to establish whether the patient has a life-threatening condition and what you should do about it.

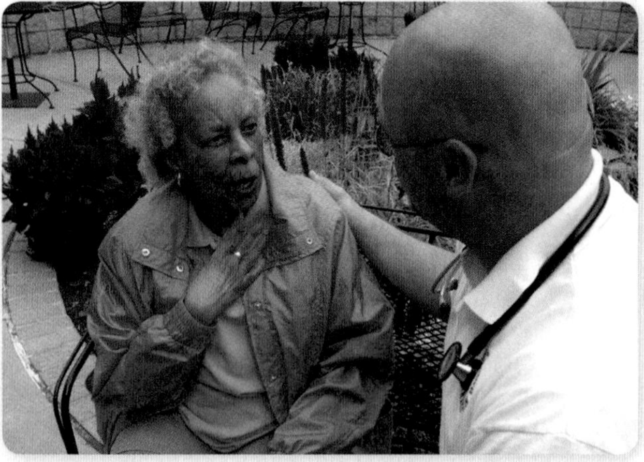

Figure 10-9 As you approach the patient, form a general impression of his or her overall condition.

When you reach the patient, avoid standing over him or her, if possible, especially if he or she is either seated or lying down. Instead, ensure you are at eye level with the patient. This practice shows respect for the patient and helps the patient feel more comfortable as you begin your assessment. Ensure the patient is breathing and assess the patient's skin color and condition as you begin. For example, is the patient's chest moving? Is the patient's skin pink, pale, gray, or cyanotic (blue)? Is it dry, clammy, or diaphoretic? Make note of odors that suggest chemical hazards, smoke, or alcohol on the patient's breath. If the patient is responsive, then introduce yourself and try to learn as much as possible about the chief complaint before you begin your exam. The patient's response can give you insight into the LOC, airway patency, respiratory status, and overall circulatory status before you begin your exam. Sometimes life-threatening conditions are obvious even during the general impression. Treat these conditions as soon as they are found.

> **Words of Wisdom**
>
> Any significant MOI, alteration in mental status, or abnormal finding with the ABCDEs is an indication that this patient is in critical condition!

You must answer the following questions to begin to form your general impression:

- Does the patient appear to have a life-threatening condition? Clues might include unresponsiveness, airway obstructions, obvious difficulty breathing, severe external bleeding, and cyanotic or very pale skin. If you suspect a life-threatening condition, then provide immediate care and transport.
- Was the patient injured? If so, then what was the MOI? On the basis of the MOI, would you expect the patient to be severely injured? If so, then assume the worst and begin treatment, including spinal immobilization.
- Does the patient seem coherent and able to answer questions? If not, then you need to rely more heavily on your physical assessment skills and/or the information that you can obtain from others at the scene.

Determine whether your patient's condition is stable, stable but potentially unstable, or unstable. This determination will direct further treatment and allows prehospital care providers to work together with an appropriate and consistent sense of urgency. However, you must constantly be aware of changes in the patient's condition.

Remember that as an AEMT, you will be called to treat an almost infinite number of different patient problems. If the primary problem appears to be traumatic, then maintain a high index of suspicion and begin treatment, including spinal immobilization. It is important not to have tunnel vision, but to be alert to the possibility that the traumatic event may have a medical origin. As mentioned previously, it is not usually easy or prudent to label patients as either medical or trauma patients until you have finished your assessment. In many cases, medical emergencies and trauma go hand in hand.

Forming your general impression is your opportunity to evaluate "the big picture" before you focus on the patient's specific needs, so use all of your senses in observing the scene and the patient.

Words of Wisdom

Whether the patient is a medical or trauma patient has nothing to do with the severity of the patient's condition. Not every trauma patient is in critical condition, and not every medical patient is in stable condition. A patient who falls over a tree root and breaks two toes is a trauma patient, and a patient experiencing an MI is a medical patient. Categorize patients by the severity of their conditions, not whether their injuries or illnesses are traumatic or medical.

Assess the Airway

As you move through the steps of the primary survey, always be alert for signs of airway obstruction. Regardless of the cause, a mild or severe airway obstruction will result in inadequate or absent airflow into and out of the lungs, and therefore inadequate **perfusion** (the circulation of blood within an organ or tissue to provide necessary oxygen and nutrients and to remove waste) of the entire body. To prevent permanent damage to the brain, heart, and lungs and even death, you must determine if the airway is open (patent) and adequate. Also, you must continually reassess the airway during the rest of patient assessment, care, and transport.

Responsive Patients

Patients of any age who are talking or crying are moving air, regardless of the quality. However, watching and listening to how patients speak, particularly patients with respiratory conditions, may provide important clues about the adequacy of their airways and the status of their breathing. A responsive patient who cannot speak or cry most likely has a severe airway obstruction.

If you identify an airway problem, then stop the assessment process and work to clear the patient's airway. This action may be as simple as positioning the patient so the air moves in and out, suctioning liquids from the airway, or removing an obvious foreign body from the patient's mouth. It may be as complex as providing abdominal thrusts or chest compressions to remove a foreign body from the airway. Do not continue the assessment until the airway is clear. Although airway and breathing problems are not the same, the signs and symptoms often overlap. If your patient has signs of difficulty breathing or is not breathing, then immediately take corrective actions using appropriate airway management techniques.

Words of Wisdom

If the patient has a history of trauma or a potential history of trauma, then use the jaw-thrust maneuver to open the airway. If no risk of trauma exists, then use the head tilt–chin lift maneuver.

YOU are the Provider — PART 2

As you arrive on scene, you note a single vehicle that has driven off the road and collided with a large tree. The grill of the vehicle is crushed in, almost to the firewall, but there is no intrusion into the passenger compartment. As soon as the driver positions your ambulance in a safe location that shields the scene, you grab your jump bag and proceed to the wrecked vehicle. You find the driver of the vehicle restrained in the seat by a lap and shoulder belt, and note that the windshield is cracked in multiple places. Liquid is pooling under the vehicle. You speak to the patient as you open the door. She is now alert and reporting neck pain.

Recording Time: 0 Minutes	
Appearance	Alert
Level of consciousness	Alert, but confused
Airway	Patent
Breathing	Nonlabored
Circulation	Warm, dry, and pink

3. Does this patient present more like a medical patient or a trauma patient?
4. What type of PPE should you wear for this type of call?

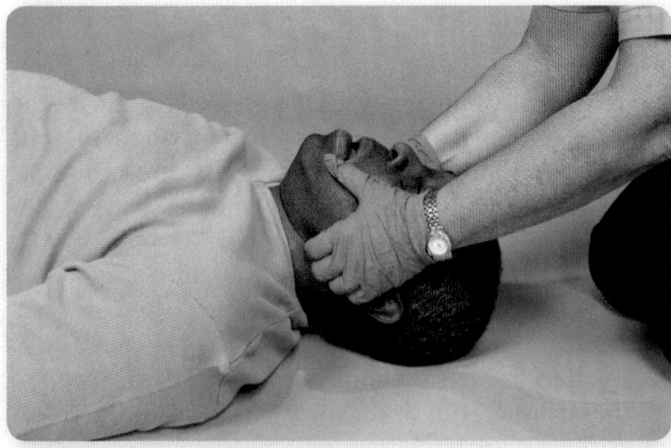

Figure 10-10 The jaw-thrust maneuver.

Unresponsive Patients

With an unresponsive patient or a patient with a decreased LOC, immediately assess the patency of the airway. Unresponsive patients should be considered to have experienced a traumatic event. If the potential for trauma exists, then use the jaw-thrust maneuver to open the airway **Figure 10-10**. If you cannot obtain a patent airway using the jaw-thrust maneuver, or if you can confirm that the patient did not experience a traumatic event, then use the head tilt–chin lift maneuver to open and maintain a patent airway. Both of these techniques are described in Chapter 11, *Airway Management*. Another cause of airway obstruction in an unresponsive patient could be relaxation of the tongue muscles, allowing the tongue to fall to the back of the throat. Address this obstruction by first positioning the airway, followed by placing an oral or nasal airway. Dentures, blood clots, vomitus, mucus, food, and other foreign objects may also create an airway obstruction. These can be cleared with manual techniques and suctioning. These techniques are also described in Chapter 11, *Airway Management*. After you confirm the airway is clear, you can continue your assessment.

Signs of airway obstruction in an unresponsive patient include the following:

- Obvious trauma, blood, or other obstruction
- Noisy breathing, such as snoring, bubbling, gurgling, crowing, stridor, or other abnormal **breath sounds** (Normal or eupneic breathing is quiet.)
- Extremely shallow or absent breathing (Airway obstructions may impair breathing.)

If any of the aforementioned conditions exist, then the airway is considered inadequate. Open the airway using the appropriate method (either the head tilt–chin lift or jaw-thrust maneuver), suction as necessary, and use an airway adjunct as necessary. The body will not be supplied the oxygen needed to survive if the airway is not managed quickly and efficiently. Remember that airway positioning depends on the age and size of your patient. For trauma patients or patients with an unknown illness, manually stabilize the cervical spine while using the jaw-thrust maneuver to open the airway.

Assess Breathing

A patient's breathing status is directly related to the adequacy of his or her airway. After you have made sure the patient's airway is open, ensure the patient's breathing is present and adequate. A patient who is breathing without assistance is said to have **spontaneous respirations** or spontaneous breathing.

As you assess the patient's breathing, ask yourself the following questions:

- Does the patient appear to be choking?
- Is the respiratory rate too fast or too slow?
- Are the patient's respirations shallow or deep?
- Is the patient cyanotic?
- Do you hear abnormal breath sounds when listening to the lungs?
- Is the patient moving air into and out of the lungs on both sides?

Each complete breath includes two distinct phases: inspiration and expiration. During inspiration (inhalation), the diaphragm and intercostal muscles contract and the chest rises up and out, drawing oxygenated air into the lungs. During expiration (exhalation), the muscles relax and the chest returns to its original position, releasing air with an increased carbon dioxide level out of the lungs. Inhalation and exhalation times occur in a 1:3 ratio; the active inhalation phase lasts one-third the amount of time of the passive exhalation phase.

Breathing is a continuous process in which each breath regularly follows the last with no notable interruption. Breathing is normally a spontaneous, automatic process that occurs without conscious thought, visible effort, marked sounds, or pain. Rapidly assess respirations to determine if the:

- Rate is normal, fast, or slow
- Depth is normal or shallow
- Chest rise is equal or unequal

Assess the patient's breathing and listen to breath sounds with a stethoscope over each lung. Chest rise and breath sounds should be equal on both sides of the chest. When you assess breathing, you must obtain the following information:

- Respiratory rate (The normal rate is 12 to 20 breaths/min in adults.)
- Quality and character of breathing
- Degree of distress
- Use of **accessory muscles** in the chest or neck

Never withhold oxygen from any patient who is having difficulty breathing. Oxygen may also be appropriate for patients who are breathing adequately in some situations. Provide positive pressure ventilations for patients who are apneic or whose breathing is too slow, too fast, or too shallow. If the patient is breathing adequately but remains hypoxic, then administer oxygen. The goal for oxygenation for most patients is an oxygen saturation level of approximately 94% to 99%.

If a patient develops difficulty breathing after your primary survey, then immediately reevaluate the airway. If the airway is open and breathing is present and adequate, then consider administering supplemental oxygen. If breathing is present and inadequate because respirations are too fast (generally more than 20 breaths/min), too shallow, or too slow (generally fewer than 12 breaths/min), then administer supplemental oxygen. When respirations exceed 28 breaths/min or are fewer than 8 breaths/min with signs of inadequate tidal volume, then consider providing positive pressure ventilation and using an airway adjunct if the patient will tolerate one. Tidal volume is discussed in more detail later in this chapter. Remember that air exchange is the critical issue, not simply the number of breaths.

Words of Wisdom

When you assess respirations, always pay attention to the events leading up to the assessment. A patient who just completed a marathon will have rapid and deep respirations, whereas a patient who is sleeping will have slow and shallow respirations. These patients do not require positive pressure ventilation. The rate and depth of respirations change with metabolic need.

Observe how much effort is required for the patient to breathe. Normal respirations are not usually shallow or excessively deep. **Shallow respirations** can be identified by little movement of the chest wall (reduced tidal volume) or poor chest excursion. Deep respirations cause a significant rise and fall of the chest. Document when the patient's respirations are shallow or deep.

Normal breathing is an effortless process that does not affect a patient's speech, posture, or positioning. Breathing that becomes progressively more difficult requires progressively more effort. When you can see that effort, the patient's breathing is described as **labored breathing**. Initially, labored breathing is characterized by the patient's position, concentration on breathing, and the increased effort and depth of each breath. As breathing becomes more labored, accessory muscles are used, which include the neck muscles (sternocleidomastoid), the chest pectoralis major muscles, and the abdominal muscles. The presence of **retractions** (indentations above or below the clavicles [supraclavicular and subclavicular] and in the spaces between the ribs [intercostal]) is also a sign of inadequate breathing. The patient may make grunting sounds with each breath. Sometimes the patient may be gasping. In pediatric patients, **nasal flaring**, seesaw breathing, and supraclavicular and intercostal retractions indicate inadequate breathing. Speech

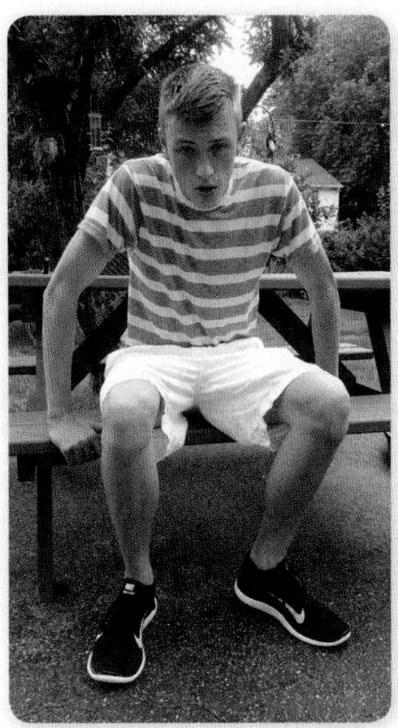

Figure 10-11 A patient in the tripod position will sit leaning forward on outstretched arms with the head and chin thrust slightly forward.

is a good indicator of whether a responsive patient is having difficulty breathing. A patient who can speak smoothly without unusual extra pauses is breathing normally. A patient who can speak only two or three words without pausing to take a breath, a condition known as **two- to three-word dyspnea**, has a serious breathing problem.

Patients who are having marked difficulty breathing will instinctively assume a posture in which it is easier for them to breathe, or will be on their feet pacing around. Two common postures indicate that the patient is trying to increase airflow. The first position is called the **tripod position** Figure 10-11. In this position, a patient is sitting and leaning forward on outstretched arms with the head and chin thrust slightly forward; significant conscious effort is required for breathing. The second position is most commonly seen in children—the **sniffing position**. The patient sits upright with the head and chin thrust slightly forward, and the patient appears to be sniffing Figure 10-12. Those patients who are unable to change position to assist with breathing are often in the most distress.

Infants (age 1 month to 1 year) and small children may have labored breathing for a sustained period, but will then become exhausted, and will no longer have the strength to maintain the necessary energy to breathe. In infants and small children, cardiac arrest is generally caused by respiratory arrest.

Respiratory distress occurs when a patient has difficulty breathing; therefore, the work of breathing is increased. Typically, a person in respiratory distress presents with an increase in respiratory effort and rate. **Respiratory failure** occurs when the blood is inadequately oxygenated or

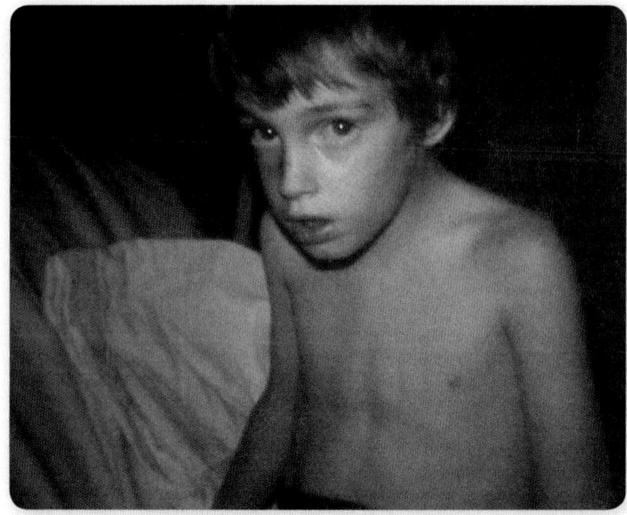

Figure 10-12 A patient in the sniffing position sits upright with the head and chin thrust slightly forward.

Courtesy of Health Resources and Services Administration, Maternal and Child Health Bureau, Emergency Medical Service for Children Program.

Table 10-1 Signs of Respiratory Distress and Failure

Respiratory Distress	Respiratory Failure
Agitation, anxiety, restlessness	Lethargy, difficult to rouse
Stridor, wheezing	Tachypnea (increased respirations) with periods of bradypnea (decreased respirations) or agonal respirations
Accessory muscle use (sternocleidomastoid), intercostal retractions	Inadequate chest rise/ poor excursion
Tachypnea	Inadequate respiratory rate or effort
Mild tachycardia	Bradycardia (decreased heart rate)
Nasal flaring, seesaw breathing, head bobbing	Diminished muscle tone

ventilation is inadequate to meet the oxygen demands of the body and is often caused by a combination of inadequate tidal volume, respiratory rate, and/or airway obstruction. Respiratory arrest is the ultimate result of respiratory failure if the failure is not corrected Table 10-1.

Words of Wisdom

Normal breathing should be quiet and not grossly evident to you. If you see or hear the patient breathe, then he or she may have a problem.

Assess Circulation

Assessing circulation helps you to evaluate how well blood is circulating to the major organs, including the brain, lungs, heart, and kidneys, and the rest of the body. A variety of emergencies can impair circulation, including blood loss, shock, and conditions that affect the heart and major blood vessels. Circulation is evaluated by assessing the patient's mental status, pulse, and skin condition. You will also need to identify and control severe external bleeding.

Special Populations

You can feel the pulse of a child at the carotid artery, as in an adult. However, palpating the carotid pulse in an infant may present a problem. An infant's neck is often short and fat and the pulse is often fast, so it may be difficult to find the carotid pulse. Because of the infant's soft, immature trachea, palpating the carotid artery may cause injury. Therefore, in children younger than 1 year, palpate the brachial artery to assess the pulse (discussed later in this chapter).

Assess Pulse

With each beat of the heart, the ventricles contract, forcefully ejecting blood from the heart and propelling it into the arteries. Often referred to as the heartbeat, the **pulse** is the pressure wave that occurs as each ventricular contraction causes a surge in the blood circulating through the arteries. The pulse is most easily felt at a pulse point where a major artery lies near the surface and can be pressed gently against a bone or solid organ.

Your first consideration when assessing for circulation is to determine whether the patient has a pulse. To do so, hold together your index and long fingers and place the tips over a pulse point, pressing gently against the artery until you feel intermittent pulsations. In responsive patients who are older than 1 year, **palpate** (feel) the radial pulse at the wrist Figure 10-13A. In unresponsive patients older than 1 year, palpate the carotid pulse in the neck Figure 10-13B. When you palpate the carotid pulse, place the tips of your index and long fingers in the center of the throat on the trachea. Next, slide your fingers toward you into the groove between the trachea and the neck muscle to position your fingers directly over the carotid artery. Palpate the carotid pulse on the same side

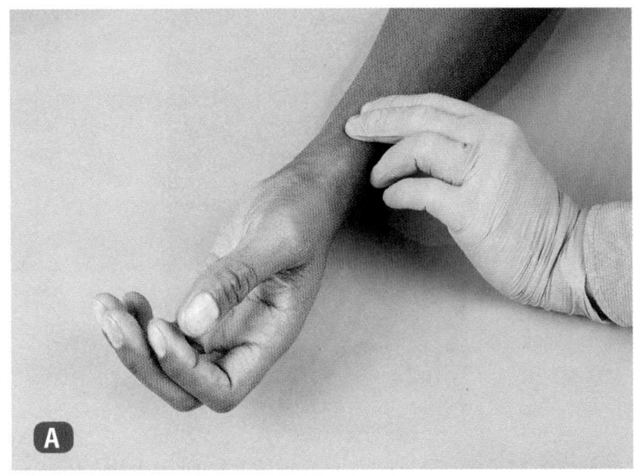

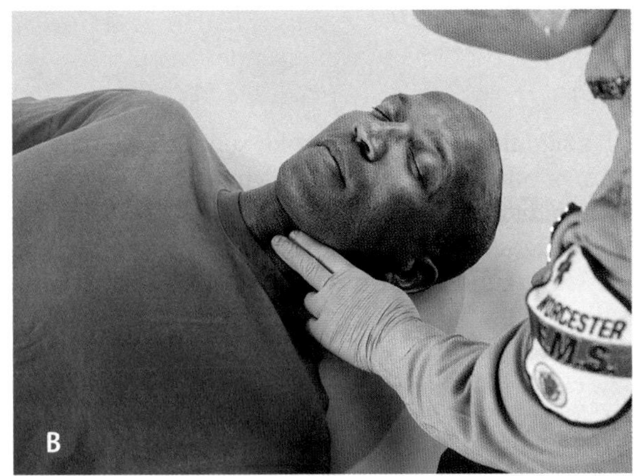

Figure 10-13 A. To palpate the radial pulse, place the tips of your index and long fingers over the radial artery, pressing gently until you feel intermittent pulsations. **B.** To palpate the carotid pulse, place the tips of your index and long fingers over the carotid artery, pressing gently until you feel intermittent pulsations.

of the patient that you are on; palpating on the opposite side of the patient may lead to undue pressure on the neck that may compromise respirations. Use caution when palpating the carotid pulse in a responsive patient, especially an older patient. Only use gentle pressure on one side of the neck. Never press on the carotid arteries on both sides of the neck at the same time. Doing so can reduce circulation to the brain.

Sometimes, you may have to slide your fingertips a little to either side and press again until you feel a pulse. When you palpate a pulse, do not use your thumb because you may mistake the strong pulsing circulation in your thumb for the patient's pulse. The normal pulse rate for an adult is 60 to 100 beats/min.

Palpate the brachial pulse, located at the medial area (inside) of the upper arm, in children younger than 1 year **Figure 10-14**. With the infant lying supine, you can access the brachial pulse by elevating the arm over the infant's head. Because most infants have chubby arms, you need to press your adjacent fingertips firmly along the brachial artery, which lies parallel to the long axis of the upper arm, to be able to palpate the pulse.

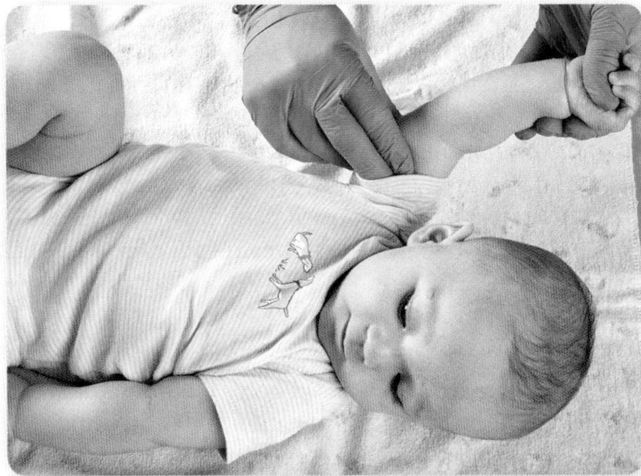

Figure 10-14 To palpate the brachial pulse in an infant, press firmly along the brachial artery on the inside of the upper arm.

During the primary survey, assess the pulse to determine if it is:

- Present or absent
- Normal, fast, or slow
- Weak and thready or strong and bounding

You also need to determine the adequacy of the pulse during the secondary assessment. This step is done by assessing the pulse rate, pulse rhythm, and pulse character, discussed later.

If you cannot palpate a pulse in an unresponsive patient, then begin CPR. If an AED is available, then attach it and follow the voice prompts, following your local protocol. An AED is indicated for use on patients who are unresponsive, apneic, and pulseless. An AED with special pediatric pads and a dose-attenuating system is indicated for use on pediatric patients younger than 8 years; if this equipment is unavailable, then use an adult AED.[2] In infants, it is preferable to perform manual defibrillation or use a dose-attenuating system; if these methods are unavailable, then use an adult AED. More information about CPR and AEDs is available in Chapter 15, *BLS Resuscitation*.

Words of Wisdom

Manual defibrillation is an ALS skill that is not within your scope of practice as an AEMT. If both paramedic backup and pediatric-sized pads are unavailable, then use adult-sized pads with the AED for children and infants. Ensure the pads do not touch on children; for infants, place one pad on the chest and one pad on the back.

If the patient has a pulse but is not breathing, then provide ventilations at a rate of 10 to 12 breaths/min for adults and 12 to 20 breaths/min for an infant or a child. Continue to monitor the pulse to evaluate the effectiveness of your ventilations. If at any time the pulse is lost, then start CPR and apply the AED. The apparent absence of a palpable pulse in a responsive patient is not caused by cardiac arrest. Therefore, never begin CPR or use an AED on a responsive patient.

Assess Skin

The skin has many functions. It helps maintain the water content of the body, acts as insulation and protection from infection, and has a role in regulating body temperature by changing the amount of blood circulating through the surface of skin.

Assessing the skin is one of the most important and most readily accessible ways of evaluating circulation and perfusion, blood oxygen level, and body temperature. A normally functioning circulatory system perfuses the skin with oxygenated blood. A lack of perfusion or hypoperfusion will result in hypoxia of the brain, lungs, heart, and kidneys. The degree of hypoperfusion and how long it lasts will determine if a patient will sustain permanent damage related to the hypoxia. Perfusion is assessed by evaluating a patient's skin color, temperature, moisture, and capillary refill.

Skin Color. Many blood vessels lie near the surface of the skin. The color of the skin is determined by the blood circulating through these vessels and the amount and type of pigment present in the skin. Blood is red when it is adequately saturated with oxygen. As a result, the skin in lightly pigmented people is pink. The pigmentation in most people will not hide changes in the underlying color of the skin, regardless of the person's race. In patients with deeply pigmented skin, changes in color may be apparent only in certain areas, such as the fingernail beds, the mucous membranes in the mouth, the lips, the underside of the arm, and palm (which are usually less pigmented), and the conjunctiva of the eyes. The **conjunctiva** is the delicate membrane lining the eyelids, and it covers the exposed surface of the eye. In addition, you should assess the palms of the hands and soles of the feet in infants and children.

Inadequate peripheral circulation will cause the skin to appear pale, white, ashen, or gray, possibly with a waxy, translucent appearance like a white candle. Abnormally cold or frozen skin may also appear this way. When the blood is not properly saturated with oxygen, it appears blue. Therefore, in a patient with insufficient air exchange and a low level of oxygen in the blood, the blood and vessels become blue, and the lips, mucous membranes, nail beds, and skin over the blood vessels appear blue or gray. This condition is called **cyanosis** Figure 10-15.

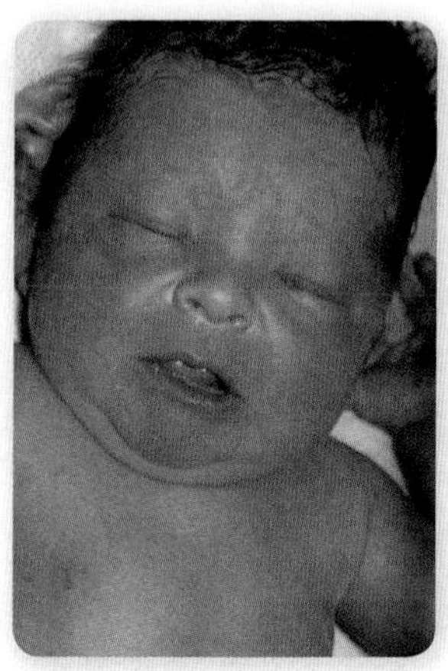

Figure 10-15 Cyanosis occurs when a patient has a low level of oxygen in the blood.

High blood pressure may cause the skin to be abnormally flushed and red. In some patients with extremely high blood pressure, all of the visible blood vessels will be so full that the skin will appear to be a dark red-purple. A patient with a significant fever, heatstroke, sunburn, mild thermal burns, or other conditions in which the body is unable to properly dissipate heat will also appear to have red skin.

Changes in skin color may also result from chronic illness. Liver disease or dysfunction may cause **jaundice**, resulting in the patient's skin and sclera turning yellow. The **sclera** is the normally white portion of the eye and may show color changes even before skin color change is visible.

Skin Temperature. Normal skin temperature will be warm to the touch; normal body temperature is 98.6°F (37°C). Abnormal skin temperatures are hot, cool, cold, and clammy. Clammy is considered cool and moist. When a patient has a significant fever, sunburn, or hyperthermia, the skin feels hot to the touch. The skin will feel cool when the patient is in early shock, has mild hypothermia, or has inadequate perfusion. With poor perfusion, the body pulls blood away from the surface of the skin and diverts it to the core of the body. The result is cool, pale, clammy skin; in your primary survey, this finding is a good indication of hypoperfusion and inadequacy of circulatory system function (shock). The skin will feel cold when the patient is in profound shock, has hypothermia, or has frostbite (frozen tissue).

Body temperature is normally measured with a thermometer in the hospital. However, in the field, feeling the patient's torso, underneath clothing with the back of your hand, is usually adequate to determine whether the patient's temperature is either elevated or decreased.

Skin Moisture. Dry skin is normal. Skin that is wet or moist from sweat, or excessively dry and hot, suggests a problem. In the early stages of shock, the skin will become slightly moist. Skin that is only slightly moist but not covered excessively with sweat is described as clammy, damp, or moist. When the skin is bathed in sweat, such as after strenuous exercise or when the patient is in shock, the skin is described as wet or **diaphoretic**.

Because the color, temperature, and moisture of the skin are often related signs, consider them together.

When you record or report your assessment of the skin, first describe the color, then the temperature, and last, whether the skin is dry, moist, or wet. For example, you could say or write, "Skin: pale, cool, and clammy."

Again, these characteristics are important findings in your primary survey because hypoperfusion can lead to serious consequences if treatment is delayed or ignored.

Capillary Refill. **Capillary refill** is often evaluated in pediatric patients to assess the ability of the circulatory system to restore blood to or perfuse the capillary system in the fingers and toes. When evaluated in an uninjured limb, capillary refill time (CRT) may provide an indication of the pediatric patient's level of perfusion. However, especially in adult patients, capillary refill can be affected by the patient's body temperature, position, preexisting medical conditions, history as a smoker, and medications. Therefore, capillary refill is useful in children and infants, but is not considered an accurate indication of perfusion in adults. Other conditions that are unrelated to the body's circulation may also slow capillary refill. These conditions include exposure to a cold environment, hypothermia, frostbite, and **vasoconstriction** (narrowing of a blood vessel, such as with hypoperfusion or cold extremities). Injuries to bones and muscles of the extremities may cause local circulatory compromise, resulting in hypoperfusion of an extremity rather than hypoperfusion of the body in general.

To test capillary refill, place your thumb on the patient's fingernail with your fingers on the underside of the patient's finger and gently compress Figure 10-16A. The blood will be forced from the capillaries in the nail bed. Remove the pressure applied against the tip of the patient's finger. The nail bed will remain blanched (white) for a brief period. As the underlying capillaries refill with blood, the nail bed will be restored to its normal pink color.

Capillary refill should be prompt, and the nail bed color should be pink. With adequate perfusion, the color in the nail bed should be restored to its normal pink color within 2 seconds, or about the time it takes to say "capillary refill" at a normal rate of speech Figure 10-16B. For a CRT of 2 seconds or less, report and document it as normal. Suspect poor peripheral circulation when capillary refill takes more than 2 seconds or the nail bed remains blanched. In this case, report and document the CRT as delayed, or CRT more than 2 seconds.

A blue color may indicate that the capillaries are refilling with blood drawn from the veins rather than with oxygenated blood from the arteries, making the test invalid. Consider the capillary refill test invalid if the patient is in or has been exposed to a cold environment or if the patient is older. In both situations, delayed capillary refill may be normal.

To assess capillary refill in older infants and children younger than 6 years, press on the skin or nail bed and determine how long it takes for the pink color to return. In newborns and young infants, press on the forehead, chin, or sternum to determine CRT. As with adults, capillary refill should be restored within 2 seconds. Suspect poor peripheral circulation when capillary refill takes more than 2 seconds or the nail bed remains blanched. In this case, report and document the CRT as delayed, or CRT more than 2 seconds. Again, delayed capillary refill is not considered an accurate indication of poor perfusion in adult patients.

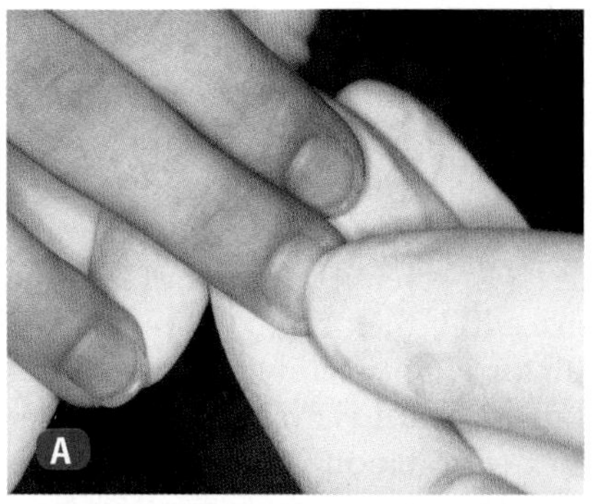

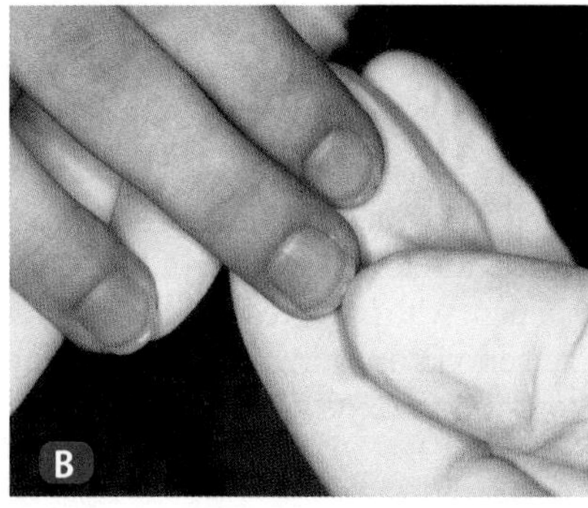

Figure 10-16 A. To test capillary refill, gently compress the fingertip until it blanches. **B.** Release the fingertip, and count until it returns to its normal pink color.

Assess and Control External Bleeding

Identify and immediately control any major external bleeding. In some patients, rapid blood loss can quickly result in shock or even death. Therefore, this step demands your immediate attention and should be performed before addressing airway or breathing concerns. Signs of blood loss include active bleeding from wounds and/or evidence of bleeding such as blood on the clothes or near the patient. Serious bleeding from a large vein may be characterized by steady blood flow. Bleeding from an artery is characterized by a spurting flow of blood. When you evaluate an unresponsive patient, do a sweep for blood quickly and lightly by running your gloved hands from head to toe, pausing periodically to see if your gloves are bloody.

Initially, direct pressure with a gloved hand and followed by a sterile bandage over the wound will control bleeding in most cases. Direct pressure stops the bleeding and helps the blood to coagulate (clot) naturally. Most minor bleeding can be adequately controlled by using direct pressure. When direct pressure is not quickly successful or whenever you encounter obvious arterial hemorrhage of an extremity, apply a tourniquet. More information about controlling bleeding and applying a tourniquet is found in Chapter 27, *Bleeding*.

Restoring Circulation

If a patient has inadequate circulation, then take immediate action to restore or improve circulation, control severe bleeding, and improve oxygen delivery to the tissues. The apparent absence of a palpable pulse in a responsive patient is indicative of a low cardiac output state—not cardiac arrest. However, if you cannot feel a pulse in an unresponsive adult, then begin CPR if an AED or manual defibrillator is not readily available. Once an AED or manual defibrillator is available, immediately assess the need for defibrillation. Remember to take standard precautions, which may include use of a barrier device for ventilation, gloves, and protective eyewear.

Continued impaired circulation is devastating to the body's cells because it deprives the cells of vital oxygen, which is necessary for cell function. CPR and bleeding control are intended to maintain circulation. Oxygen delivery is improved through the administration of 100% supplemental oxygen. Any patient with impaired circulation should receive high-flow oxygen via a nonrebreathing mask or assisted ventilation to improve oxygen delivery at the cellular level.

Assess the Patient for Disability

After you have examined the patient's ABCs and addressed any life-threatening conditions, perform a brief neurologic evaluation of the patient. The patient's LOC can tell you a great deal about the patient's neurologic and physiologic status. The brain requires a constant supply of oxygen and glucose to function properly. In the primary survey, you need to ascertain only the gross LOC by determining which of the following three categories best fits your patient:

- Unresponsive
- Responsive with an altered LOC
- Responsive with an unaltered LOC

Sustained unresponsiveness in a patient indicates that a critical respiratory, circulatory, or central nervous system (CNS) problem may exist. Presume the patient has a critical injury or life-threatening condition until proven otherwise. Therefore, after rapidly assessing the patient and providing emergency treatment, package the patient and provide rapid transport to the hospital.

An altered LOC in a responsive patient may indicate that inadequate perfusion and oxygenation are adversely affecting the brain and its ability to function. An altered LOC in a responsive patient can also be caused by medications, drugs, alcohol, poisoning, hypoglycemia, chemical imbalances, and/or neurologic conditions. Further assessment will be required for any patient with an altered LOC.

It is important to determine, if possible, the patient's normal mental status. A number of circumstances—including ongoing illness and/or history of stroke, traumatic brain injury, developmental delay, Alzheimer disease, and more—may cause a patient to have a baseline mental status that is not fully alert and oriented. Any deviation from alert and oriented to person, place, time, and event, or from a patient's normal baseline, is considered an **altered mental status**.

When you assess a patient, determine the appropriateness of the patient's response by how well it demonstrates the patient's understanding and mental activity, not by how well it reflects your definition of socially acceptable behavior. You can evaluate mental status and LOC in just a few seconds by testing for **responsiveness** (the way in which a patient responds to external stimuli, including verbal stimuli [sound], tactile stimuli [touch], and painful stimuli) and orientation.

If you determine the patient has any of the indicators for spinal immobilization, then ensure the patient's cervical spine is manually stabilized by either you or another provider. If it is impossible to both manually stabilize the patient's cervical spine and continue your assessment to identify and correct life threats, then do your best to ensure the patient's spine remains in a stable position while you continue your primary survey. The indicators for spinal immobilization include the following:[3]

- Either blunt or penetrating trauma with any of the following findings:
  - An MOI that indicates the potential for spinal injury
  - Pain or tenderness on palpation of the neck or spine
  - Patient reports pain in the neck or back
  - Paralysis or neurologic complaint (numbness, tingling, partial paralysis of the legs or arms)
  - **Priapism** (male patients)
- Blunt trauma with any of the following:
  - Altered mental status
  - Intoxication (alcohol or drugs)
  - Difficulty or inability to communicate

Words of Wisdom

The Glasgow Coma Scale (GCS) is the most common method of assessing mental status and neurologic function. Although it may take slightly longer to calculate the patient's GCS score compared with the AVPU scale, it provides much greater insight into the patient's overall neurologic function. The GCS is covered in more detail in the secondary assessment section of this chapter.

Use the mnemonic AVPU to assess a patient's LOC, depending on how well he or she responds to external stimuli. The **AVPU scale** tests the patient's responsiveness based on the following criteria:

- **Awake and alert.** The patient's eyes open spontaneously as you approach. The patient appears to be awake and aware of you. He or she is responsive to the environment, seems to follow commands, and his or her eyes track (follow) people and objects.
- **Responsive to Verbal stimuli.** The patient is not awake and alert. The patient's eyes do not open spontaneously as you approach. However, the patient's eyes open to verbal stimuli, and the patient is able to respond in some meaningful way when spoken to.

- **Responsive to Pain.** The patient does not respond to your questions, but moves or cries out in response to a painful stimulus. Appropriate methods of applying a painful stimulus include pinching the patient's earlobe Figure 10-17. Be aware that some methods may not give an accurate result if a spinal cord injury is present.
- **Unresponsive.** The patient does not respond to a verbal or painful stimulus. Unresponsive patients usually have no cough or gag reflexes and lack the ability to protect their airways. If you are in doubt about whether a patient is truly unresponsive, then assume the worst and treat appropriately.

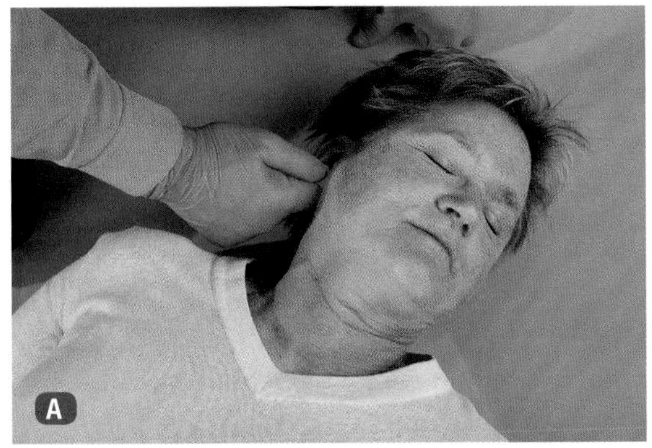

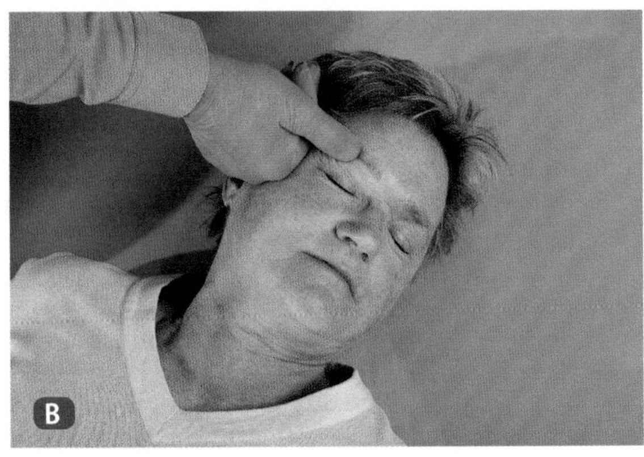

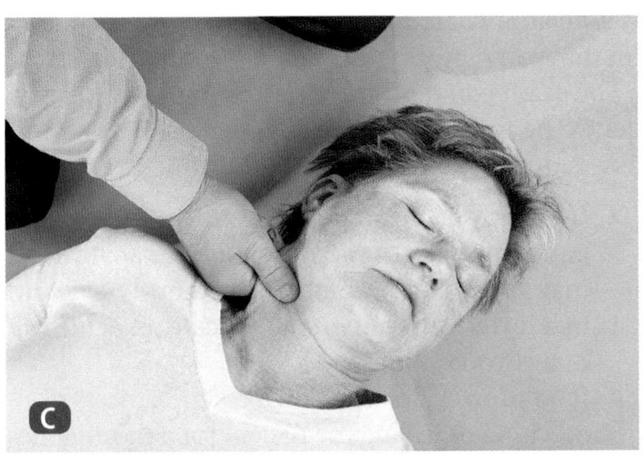

Figure 10-17 Appropriate methods of gauging a patient's responsiveness to painful stimuli. **A.** Gently but firmly pinch the patient's earlobe. **B.** Press on the bone above the eye. **C.** Gently but firmly pinch the muscles of the neck.

A patient who does not respond to your normal speaking voice, but who responds when you speak loudly, is responding to loud verbal stimuli. For a patient who is deaf or hard of hearing, repeatedly tap the patient with your fingers. If the patient responds, then note the patient has a hearing impairment but responds to being tapped.

To determine whether a patient who does not respond to verbal stimuli will respond to a painful stimulus, gently but firmly pinch the patient's skin. Areas where this technique works best are on the patient's earlobe, back of the upper arm (triceps), or the trapezius area (the muscle above the collarbone). A sternal rub is also effective for determining response to pain. Firmly rub your knuckles against the patient's sternum in an up-and-down motion Figure 10-18. Another effective technique is to provide upward pressure along the ridge of the orbital rim along the underside of the eyebrow. A patient who moans or withdraws is responding to the painful stimulus. Be sure to note the type and location of the stimulus and how the patient responded.

If the patient does not respond to a painful stimulus on one side, then try to elicit a response on the other side. A patient who remains flaccid and does not move or make a sound is considered unresponsive.

For a patient who is alert and responsive to verbal stimuli, next evaluate his or her orientation. **Orientation** tests a patient's mental status by checking his or her memory and thinking ability. The most common test evaluates a patient's ability to remember four things:

- **Person.** The patient is able to give his or her name.
- **Place.** The patient is able to identify his or her current location.
- **Time.** The patient is able to tell you the current year, month, and approximate date.
- **Event.** The patient is able to describe what happened (the MOI or NOI).

These questions were not selected at random. They evaluate long-term memory (person and place), intermediate memory (place and time), and short-term memory

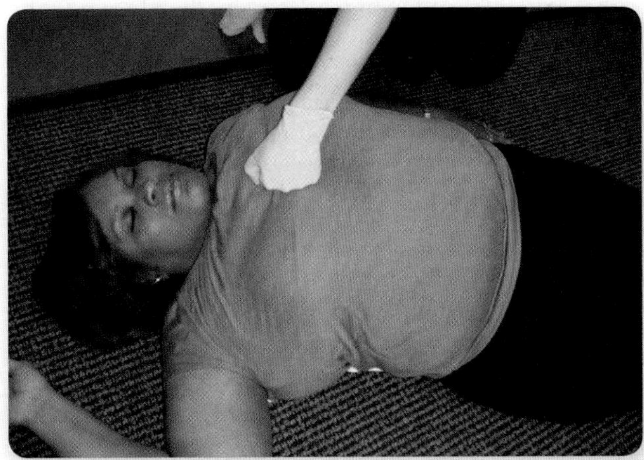

Figure 10-18 Another method for gauging a patient's responsiveness to painful stimuli is to perform a sternal rub.

Table 10-2 Glasgow Coma Scale

Eye Opening		Best Verbal Response		Best Motor Response	
Spontaneous	4	Oriented conversation	5	Obeys commands	6
In response to sound	3	Confused conversation	4	Localizes pain or pressure	5
In response to pressure	2	Words	3	Normal flexion	4
None	1	Sounds	2	Abnormal flexion	3
		None	1	Extension	2
				None	1

Score: 13–15 may indicate mild dysfunction, although 15 is the score a person without neurologic impairment would receive.
Score: 9–12 may indicate moderate dysfunction.
Score: 8 or less is indicative of severe dysfunction.

(time and event). If the patient knows these facts, then the patient is said to be "alert and fully oriented," "alert and oriented to person, place, time, and event," or "alert and oriented × 4."

As mentioned previously, the **Glasgow Coma Scale (GCS)** is the most commonly employed, reliable, and consistent method of assessing mental status and neurologic function. It assigns a point value (score) for eye opening, verbal response, and motor response; these values are added for a total score **Table 10-2**. When you report and record your findings, be sure to include the score for each GCS category, not just a cumulative score.

To illustrate how the GCS works, consider the following scenario. You encounter an older man who tracks you with his eyes as you enter his room. As you speak with the man, you note that his verbal response is disoriented, even though he follows your commands. His GCS values would be 4, 4, and 6, for a total score of 14. By comparison, if the patient opened his eyes only to pain, moaned as the only verbal response, and withdrew to pain, then he would be assigned GCS values of 2, 2, and 4, for a total score of 8.

Special Populations

Mental status may be difficult to evaluate in children. First, determine whether the child is alert. Even infants should be alert to your presence and track you with their eyes. Ask the parent or caregiver whether the child is behaving normally, particularly in regard to alertness. Most children older than 2 years know their own names and the names of their parents and siblings. Evaluate mental status in school-age children by asking about recent holidays, school activities, or the names of teachers.

Expose Then Cover

As you physically examine the patient, visually inspect each area to ensure an accurate and thorough assessment. Although not every patient needs to be completely exposed for appropriate assessment to occur, keep in mind that you cannot assess what you cannot see. Therefore, adequate exposure of each area being examined is essential to the physical exam process. When you are finished, cover up the patient to respect his or her privacy and to maintain body heat. The steps for performing a rapid physical exam are discussed next.

Performing a Rapid Full-Body Scan

It takes about 60 to 90 seconds to perform a **rapid full-body scan** of the patient's body to identify other injuries that must be managed and/or protected before the patient is transported. This scan should be thorough yet quick. This is an abbreviated exam as opposed to the systematic exam that you perform during the secondary assessment.

The exam you perform is based on the needs of your patient. The following are guidelines on how and what to assess during the rapid full-body scan:

- **Inspection.** Inspection is simply looking at your patient for abnormalities. Look for anything that may indicate a problem. For example, swelling in a lower extremity may indicate an acute injury or a chronic illness.
- **Palpation.** Palpation describes the process of touching or feeling the patient for abnormalities. At times palpation is gentle, and at other times it is firmer and will help you to identify where the patient has pain. Your fingertips are best suited for detecting texture and consistency, whereas the back of your hand is best suited for noting temperature.

- **Auscultation.** Auscultation is the process of listening to sounds the body makes by using a stethoscope. For example, when measuring a patient's blood pressure, you listen to the flow of blood against the brachial artery with the head of the stethoscope. This process is auscultation of a blood pressure.

DCAP-BTLS is a mnemonic to remind you what to look for when you are inspecting and palpating various body regions. Each area of the body is evaluated for the following:

- **D**eformities
- **C**ontusions
- **A**brasions
- **P**unctures/penetrations
- **B**urns
- **T**enderness
- **L**acerations
- **S**welling

To perform a rapid full-body scan of the patient to identify and treat life threats, follow the steps in Skill Drill 10-1. Remember, this exam should take no longer than 60 to 90 seconds!

Words of Wisdom

If you are placing the patient on a long backboard, then it is particularly important that you check the back before log rolling the patient onto a backboard. Do not log roll the patient if any instability in the pelvis is present. Instead, use a scoop stretcher to lift the patient onto the backboard.

Identify and Treat Life Threats

Many conditions present an immediate threat to life. The key to your role as an AEMT is to determine if a life threat is present and, if so, to quickly address it. The human body responds quickly and adapts to maintain perfusion when a catastrophic situation occurs. Your role is to recognize the signs and symptoms associated with that response and determine the cause of the patient's presentation.

The first observation that you will most likely make is that the patient is extremely anxious, followed by a loss of meaningful communication between you and the patient. A severely sick or injured person becomes less aware of his or her surroundings and stops making attempts to communicate. After a variable period, loss of consciousness occurs. The patient becomes totally unresponsive to external stimuli. The muscles become slack, among them the muscles of the jaw, thus permitting the tongue to sag against the posterior part of the throat. This in turn leads quickly to airway obstruction. Air can no longer enter the lungs, and within a few minutes the patient stops breathing, cutting off the intake of oxygen and the release of carbon dioxide. The heart cannot continue to function without oxygen, and it stops beating. Within a few minutes, a number of brain cells begin to die, leading to irreversible brain damage. Only a few general conditions can cause sudden death: airway obstruction, respiratory arrest, respiratory failure, primary cardiac arrest, shock, and severe bleeding. Often, these conditions are manageable or even reversible, but you have to be able to recognize them quickly and take immediate steps to correct them. This is the purpose of the primary survey.

Life-saving interventions begin with you opening the airway and assessing its patency. Airway patency is your

Skill Drill 10-1 Performing a Rapid Full-Body Scan

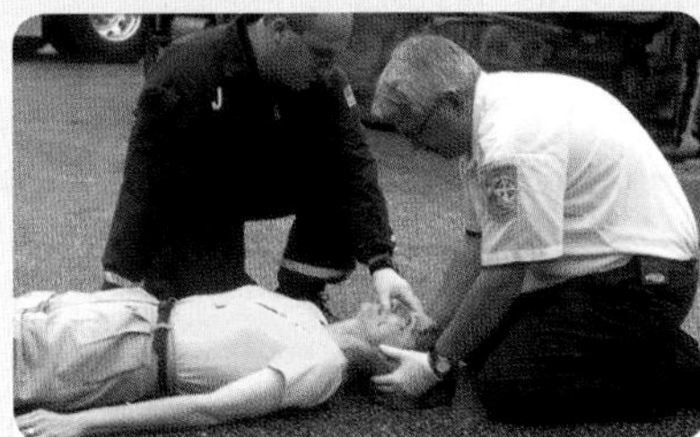

Step 1 Assess the head, looking and feeling for DCAP-BTLS and crepitus (a grating or grinding sensation or sound made when two pieces of broken bone are rubbed together). Have your partner maintain in-line stabilization if trauma is suspected.

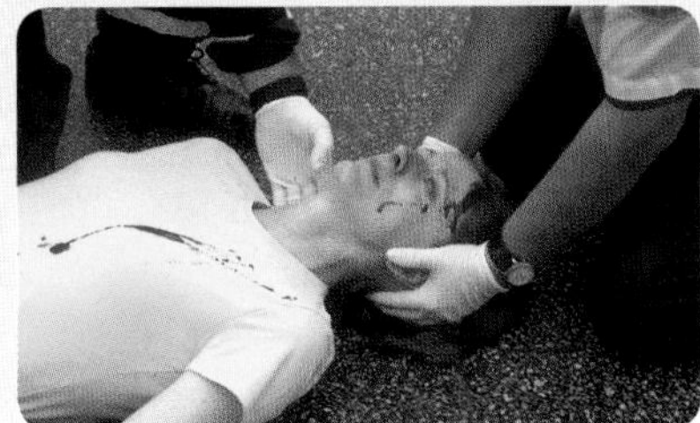

Step 2 Assess the neck, looking and feeling for DCAP-BTLS, step-offs where the cervical vertebrae are not aligned properly, jugular venous distention, tracheal deviation from midline in the neck, and crepitus.

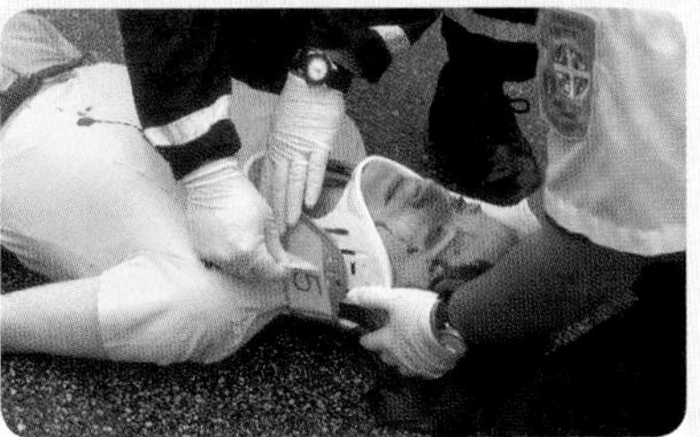

Step 3 In trauma patients, apply a cervical collar.

(continued)

Skill Drill 10-1 Performing a Rapid Full-Body Scan *(continued)*

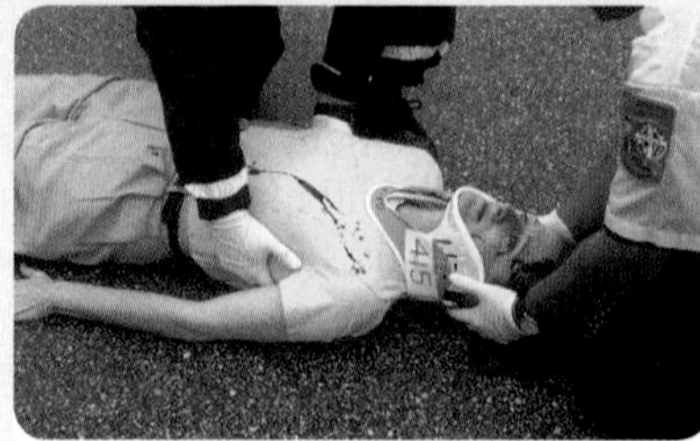

Step 4 Assess the chest, looking and feeling for DCAP-BTLS, paradoxical motion, subcutaneous emphysema, and crepitus. Listen to breath sounds on both sides of the patient's chest.

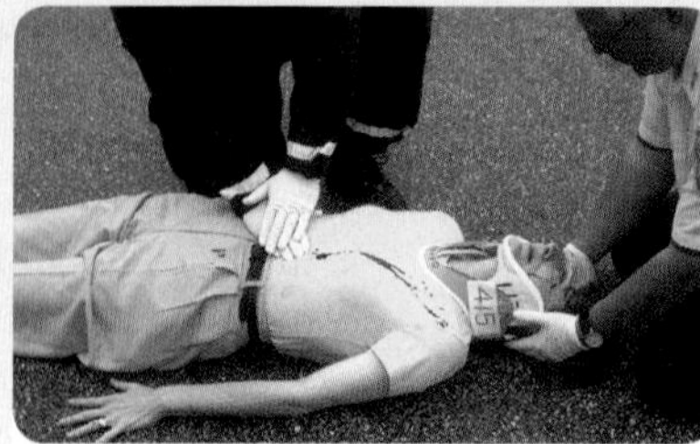

Step 5 Assess the abdomen, looking and feeling for DCAP-BTLS, rigidity (firm or soft), guarding, rebound tenderness, and distention.

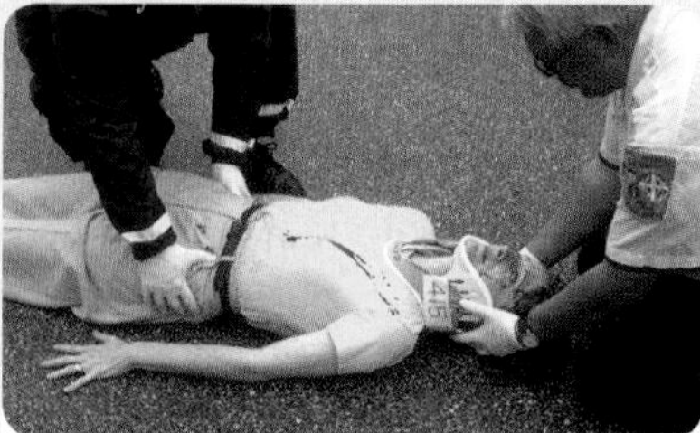

Step 6 Assess the pelvis, looking for DCAP-BTLS. If no pain is present, then gently compress the pelvis downward and inward to look for tenderness and instability.

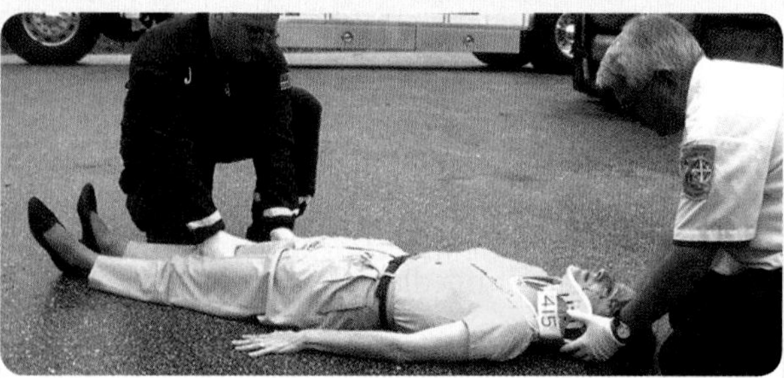

Step 7 Assess all four extremities, looking and feeling for DCAP-BTLS. Also assess bilaterally for distal pulses and motor and sensory function.

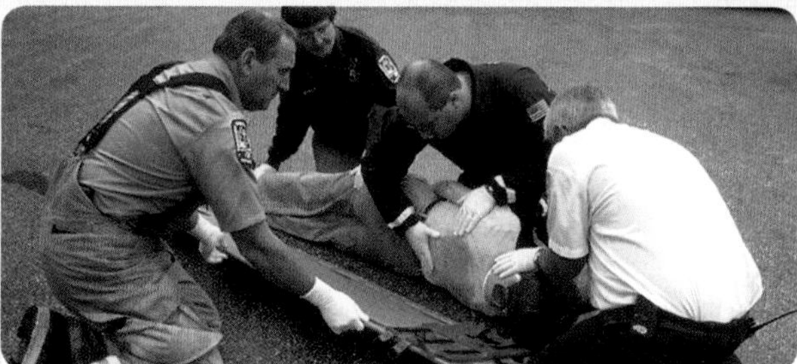

Step 8 Assess the back and buttocks, looking and feeling for DCAP-BTLS. In all trauma patients, maintain in-line stabilization of the spine while log rolling the patient on his or her side in one motion. Do not log roll the patient if any instability in the pelvis is present. Instead, gently run your hands under each side of the patient as far as possible to note any obvious injuries or bleeding.

number one priority. Assess the patient's breathing, and initiate ventilations in patients who have either inadequate respirations or no respirations at all. Although a range of "normal" respiratory rates exist, always assess your patient's overall condition to decide on appropriate treatment. It is important to assess the quality of respirations, mental status, skin color, appearance, and chest rise. Respirations that are shallow may not be ventilating and oxygenating the patient adequately. Next assess the patient's pulse. If the patient is pulseless, then initiate chest compressions. (Chapter 15, *BLS Resuscitation*, covers chest compressions in detail.) Assess the skin for color, moisture, and temperature. If any of these signs are inadequate, then initiate treatment for shock. (Chapter 14, *Shock*, covers the treatment for shock in detail.) If the cause of shock is identifiable, then attempt to correct the problem. A common example of a life-threatening cause of shock is severe bleeding. The detection of severe bleeding is the last life-saving intervention. Severe external bleeding must be controlled using direct pressure and/or a tourniquet.

In most cases, identifying and correcting life-threatening issues begins with the assessment of the ABCDEs. However, when a patient is in cardiac arrest, you should assess the ABCDEs simultaneously in the interest of minimizing the time to first compression. Also, when a patient has life-threatening bleeding, it is more appropriate to first address life threats to circulation, following a sequence of circulation, airway, breathing, disability, and exposure

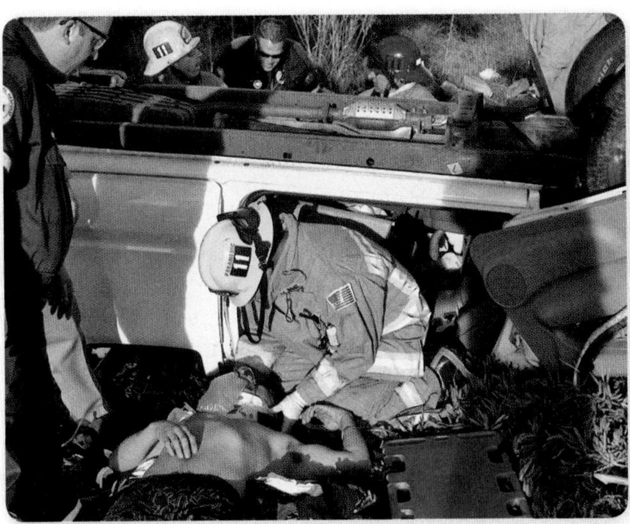

Figure 10-19 Identifying priority patients.

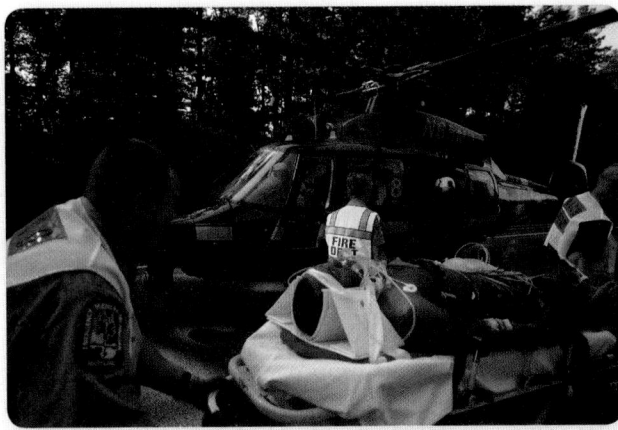

Figure 10-20 If you suspect a spinal injury has occurred, then provide spinal immobilization.

(CABDE). In these cases, controlling life-threatening bleeding takes priority over airway and breathing concerns.

Determine Priority of Patient Care and Transport

As you complete your primary survey, you will need to make some decisions about patient care and transport. If you do not identify any injuries that require treatment or rapid transport when completing your assessment of the ABCDEs, then you may find indications for rapid transport during your rapid full-body scan of the patient's body Figure 10-19. The rapid full-body scan will assist you in determining transport priority. For example, you may identify an internal hemorrhage by the presence of a distended or firm abdomen or bilateral femoral fractures. These types of conditions would be indications for rapid transport.

Would you consider your patient a high, medium, or low priority for transport? Priority designation is used to determine if your patient needs rapid transport or will tolerate a few more minutes on scene. Patients with any of the following conditions are examples of high-priority patients and should be transported immediately:

- Difficulty breathing
- Serious MOI
- Poor general impression
- Any alteration in mental status
- Severe chest pain
- Pale skin or other signs of poor perfusion
- Complicated childbirth
- Uncontrolled bleeding
- Responsive but unable to follow commands
- Severe pain in any area of the body
- Inability to move any part of the body

Protecting the patient's spine and identifying fractured extremities are integral parts of packaging for transport

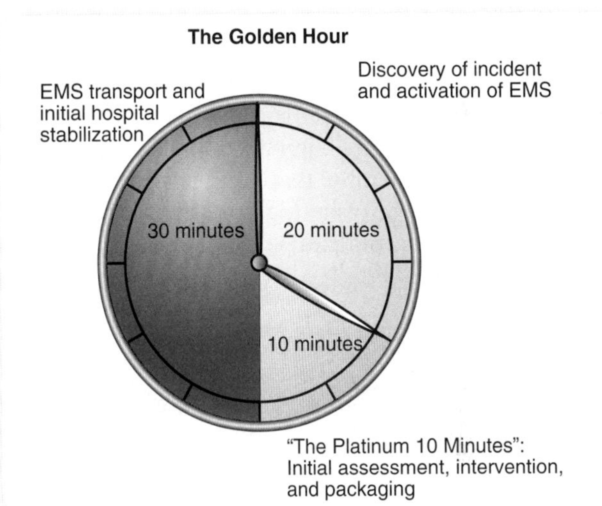

Figure 10-21 The Golden Hour, also called the Golden Period, is the time during which treatment of shock or traumatic injuries is most critical and the potential for survival is best.

Figure 10-20. If you suspect a spinal injury or the MOI is significant enough to cause a possible injury, then consider spinal immobilization early. Be certain to understand your local protocols with regard to which patients warrant immobilization. These injuries can be made worse if you neglect to assess and treat them before moving the patient.

Recognizing the need to transport serious trauma patients is of such importance that you may hear colleagues refer to the **Golden Hour** (sometimes called the Golden Period), which refers to the time from injury to definitive care, during which treatment of shock and traumatic injuries should occur because the potential for survival is best Figure 10-21 Over time, it is increasingly difficult for the body to compensate for shock and traumatic injuries. For this reason, spend as little time as possible on scene with

Primary Survey

patients who have sustained significant or severe trauma. Aim to assess, stabilize, package, and begin transport to the appropriate facility within 10 minutes (often referred to as the "Platinum 10") after arrival on scene whenever possible. However, a difficult or complex extrication may obviously limit possibilities.

Some patients may benefit from remaining on scene and receiving continuing emergency medical care. For example, an older patient with chest pain may be better served on scene by receiving nitroglycerin and aspirin and waiting for paramedic backup than by rapid transport. Call for support from paramedics if a unit is not already en route to the scene. Depending on the travel distance, a paramedic unit can be met while transporting a patient in critical condition. If paramedic assistance is delayed or farther away, then coordinating a rendezvous may be a better decision for a high-priority patient. Your decision to stay on scene or transport immediately will be based on your patient's condition, the availability of more advanced help, the distance you must transport, and your local protocols.

Correct identification of high-priority patients is an essential aspect of the primary survey and helps to improve patient outcome. Although initial treatment is important, it is essential to remember that rapid transport is one of the keys to the survival of any high-priority patient. Initiate transport as soon as practical and possible.

Remember, the goal of your primary survey is to identify and treat life threats, including management of the ABCs, as quickly as possible. Measuring vital signs more exactly is accomplished during the secondary assessment (discussed later), after time and life threats are less of an issue.

If the patient's condition is stable, then reassess vital signs every 15 minutes until you reach the emergency department (ED). If the patient's condition is unstable, then reassess vital signs every 5 minutes (or as often as the situation permits), while looking for trends in the patient's condition, and treat for shock.

Do not be falsely reassured by apparently normal vital signs. The body has amazing abilities to compensate for severe injury or illness, especially in children and young adults. Even patients who have experienced severe medical or traumatic conditions may initially present with fairly normal vital signs. However, the patient's body eventually loses its ability to compensate (decompensated shock), and the vital signs may deteriorate rapidly, especially in children. In fact, this tendency for the vital signs to fall rapidly as the patient decompensates is the reason that it is important to frequently recheck and record vital signs. Treating a patient for shock before obvious signs of shock helps to reduce the overall effects of decompensated shock and, therefore, to potentially increase your patient's chance of survival.

YOU are the Provider — PART 3

You are able to gain access to the patient without difficulty, and you inform your partner to maintain manual stabilization of the spine while you begin your initial assessment. You perform a quick primary survey and find no immediate life threats. She is alert, but confused about the crash. You notice she has a large hematoma on her forehead. Her airway is patent, she is breathing adequately, and she has no bleeding that you can see. Her radial pulses are strong and regular, and her skin is warm and dry. You calculate her GCS score as 14. Her breath sounds are clear and equal bilaterally. Although she has no signs of respiratory distress, you place her on oxygen via nonrebreathing mask due to the MOI. She has good pulses, motor function, and sensation in all extremities, but reports a tingling sensation. No other injuries are found during your rapid exam, but you do find a medic alert bracelet that says "Diabetic."

Recording Time: 10 Minutes	
Respirations	18 breaths/min; clear
Pulse	90 beats/min; regular
Skin	Warm, dry, and pink
Blood pressure	118/76 mm Hg
Oxygen saturation (Spo_2)	99% on oxygen at 15 L/min
Pupils	Pupils Equal, Round, and Reactive to Light and Accommodation (PERRLA)

5. What are the components of the GCS score?
6. How can you rule in or rule out diabetes as the cause of her altered mental status?

> **Words of Wisdom**
>
> Reassess vital signs often, watching for trends such as decreasing mental status that may indicate a patient is unable to compensate for illness or injury. Suspect shock in any patient with tachycardia and pale, cool, clammy skin, and transport immediately.

Reconsider the MOI

As part of the scene size-up, you evaluated the MOI before you began treatment. At this point in the assessment process, look at the MOI again to ensure you have not missed important information. Understanding the MOI helps you to understand the potential severity of the patient's problem and provides valuable information to hospital staff as well. Some patients have experienced a significant MOI; others clearly have not. The MOI will also serve as a guide during the secondary assessment phase, discussed later. Significant MOIs are listed in Table 10-3.

Seat belts and airbags have significantly reduced the death and disability associated with MVCs. However, be aware that seat belts and airbags can also cause injuries. When you evaluate a patient who was involved in an MVC, look for and ask questions to determine whether seat belts and/or an airbag were involved. During your handoff report at the hospital, ensure that you tell hospital personnel whether seat belts were worn, whether the airbag deployed, and the extent of damage to the vehicle.

> **Words of Wisdom**
>
> When you assess a patient, always consider occult injuries. Occult injuries are those that are not visible to the eye. Occult injuries include damage to internal organs such as a lacerated liver from impact with a steering wheel.

Table 10-3 Significant MOIs

Age Group	MOI
Adults	▪ Ejection from a vehicle ▪ Death of another person in the same vehicle ▪ Fall of an adult from a height greater than 20 feet (6m) ▪ Fall of a child from a height greater than 10 feet (3 m), or a height two or three times the child's height ▪ Vehicle rollover ▪ High-speed (>40 mph) vehicle crash ▪ Vehicle-pedestrian collision ▪ Motorcycle crash ▪ Unresponsiveness or altered mental status following trauma ▪ Penetrating trauma to the head, chest, or abdomen
Children	▪ All MOIs in the preceding list for adults, with the following additions or modifications: • Fall greater than 10 feet (3 m) or two to three times the child's height • Fall of less than 10 feet (3) with loss of consciousness • Medium- to high-speed vehicle crash (≥25 mph) • Bicycle crash

Abbreviation: MOI, mechanism of injury

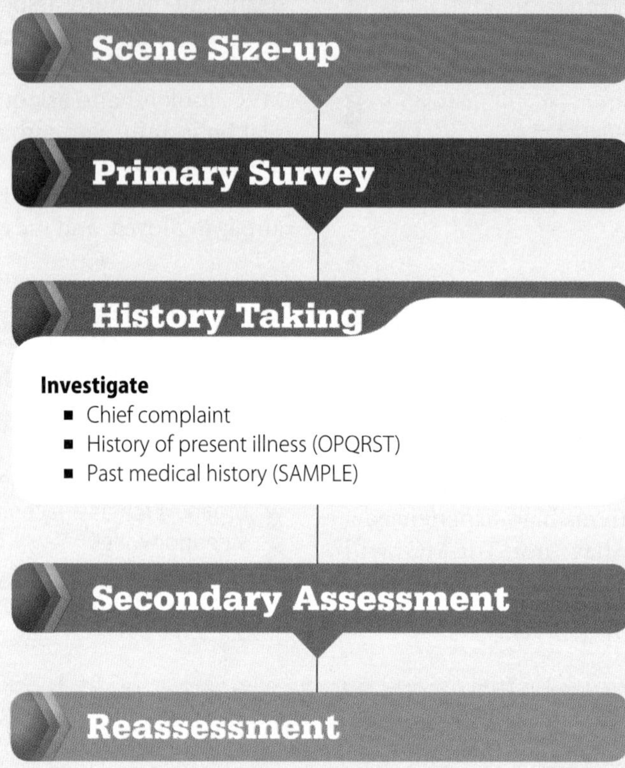

History Taking

History taking provides details about the patient's chief complaint and an account of the patient's signs and symptoms. Although history taking is listed after the primary survey, it is an integral part of the assessment and should be initiated on scene simultaneously with other tasks. You or your partner may ask questions of people in the vicinity while the other initiates patient assessment. It is important to gather as much history as possible on scene from family, friends, and bystanders because this information may be lost forever if not retrieved at this time. Also check for medical identification tags and paperwork to gain essential information concerning events leading up to the incident. If the patient is able to answer questions or a family member is transported in the ambulance with the patient, then history taking can be expanded en route. Sometimes history may be essential to determine the underlying illness or injury. Do not delay transport for patients who are in unstable condition.

It is important to document all of the information gathered during this phase of the assessment process, including demographic information (age, race, sex), past medical history, and current health status of the patient, along with any pertinent family history and recent travel history when relevant.

Investigate the Chief Complaint

The patient's chief complaint is the most serious thing that the patient is concerned about. This is the reason the patient or someone else called 9-1-1 **Figure 10-22**. To investigate the chief complaint, begin by making introductions, make the patient feel comfortable, and obtain permission to treat. Then you can then start your investigation by asking

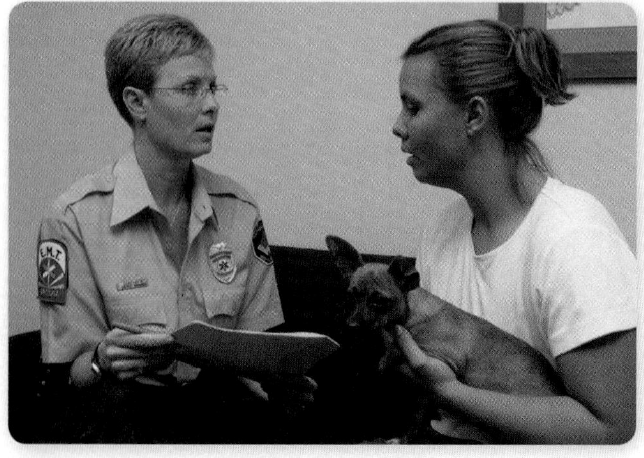

Figure 10-22 The patient's initial response to the question "What's wrong?" is the chief complaint.

a few simple, open-ended questions. Refer to the patient as "Mr.," "Ms.," or "Mrs.," using the patient's last name. Avoid using terms such as "honey" and "sweetie." If you cannot obtain the patient's name, then "ma'am" or "sir" is appropriate. Questions such as, "What seems to be the matter?" or "What's wrong today?" should produce a response that will help determine a chief complaint. These questions and others can help to elicit a response that may determine the patient's highest concern. The response is usually expressed in the patient's own words with simple answers such as, "My chest hurts" or "I have been feeling weak." Use eye contact to encourage the patient to continue speaking, and repeat statements back to the patient to show that you understand the situation. Use eye contact, body position, and language to show you are concerned and to encourage the patient to continue speaking. Do not interrupt, and be empathetic of the patient's situation. As discussed previously, the problems or feelings the patient reports to you are the symptoms. Symptoms cannot be felt or observed by others. Signs are objective conditions that can be seen, heard, felt, smelled, or measured by you or others.

You must consider the wide range of age groups that you will interact with as an AEMT. Information from infants and children may come from a parent or caregiver. Older patients might be slow to respond or have multiple complaints. Over time, you will develop your own particular technique or style for communicating with patients of various ages.

You will also gather information about the chief complaint from observable clues and information received from the original dispatch. If the patient is unresponsive, then you may obtain information about the patient, pertinent past medical history, and clues about the immediate incident from family members, a person who may have witnessed the situation, medical alert jewelry, or other forms of patient medical history documentation **Figure 10-23**. Observable clues may include conditions such as two- to three-word dyspnea (when the patient can only speak two to three words before pausing to take a breath). These clues may indicate the patient's chief complaint is "difficulty breathing," or the clues may be part of a bigger problem that has to do with a lengthy history of cardiac conditions.

Consider the following scenario: you respond to a call to the home of an older man who fell. This information was provided by the dispatcher, and you can use it to help process all of the clues that may be presented in what appears to be a simple fall. You find the patient lying at the bottom of the stairs. How many stairs are there, are they carpeted, and is the floor concrete, wood, or tile? Do you see a throw rug that may have caused the patient to trip and fall? You note that the patient has an obvious deformity of his right arm, and you suspect a possible fracture. Is this deformity the patient's chief complaint, or is the deformity the result of another problem? The patient states he fell, which is how the injury occurred, and he is reporting pain in the right

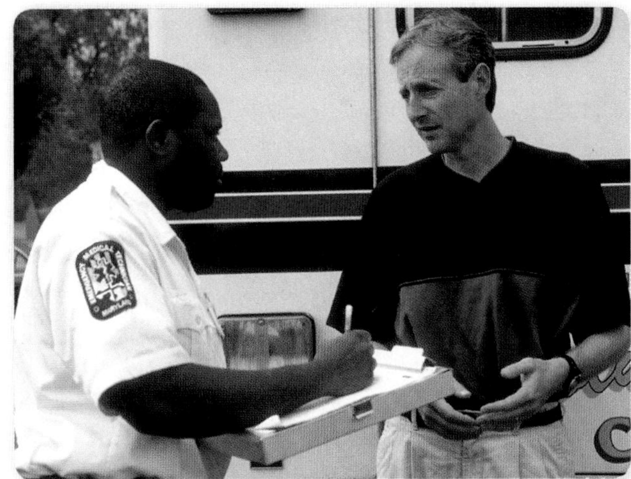

Figure 10-23 If the patient is unresponsive, then try to obtain a pertinent history or patient information from family or bystanders.

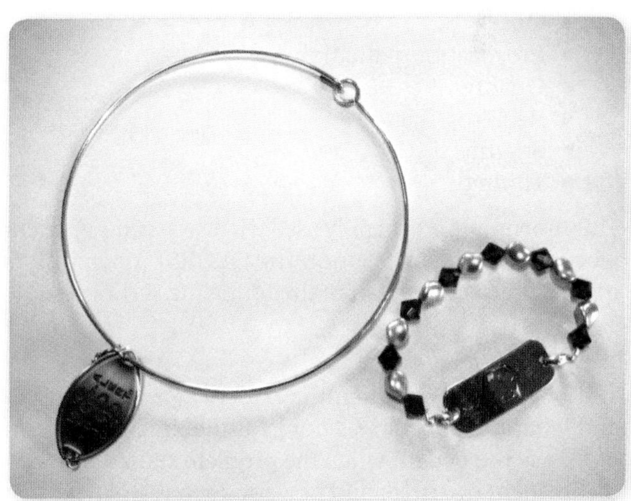

Figure 10-24 Medical identification tags.

arm. However, was the fall the result of tripping on a step, or was it associated with a medical condition such as dizziness, vertigo, or a syncopal episode? It is your responsibility to look at all the possibilities and ask the appropriate questions to determine the patient's chief complaint.

Sorting through the clues from the emergency scene itself, from the patient's complaints, and from the patient's signs and symptoms and past medical history will assist you in understanding the cause of your patient's problem and enable you to make appropriate, timely decisions about your patient's care. Remember to use family members, friends, bystanders, other public safety personnel, and medical identification tags to gain essential information concerning events leading up to the incident **Figure 10-24**. The patient's history will help to tie together your findings from the primary survey.

Words of Wisdom

The chief complaint is what you are actually called for. The primary problem is what is actually wrong with the patient. For example, you may be called out for a patient with difficulty breathing. On assessment, you find that the patient has pulmonary edema and chest pain because of heart failure. The chief complaint is "dyspnea," and the primary problem is "heart failure."

Investigate History of Present Illness (OPQRST)

As you learn about the chief complaint, broaden your knowledge to include the circumstances surrounding the complaint, or the history of the present illness. You can remember the six most important circumstances by using the mnemonic **OPQRST**, which stands for the following:

- **O**nset
- **P**rovocation/palliation
- **Q**uality
- **R**egion/radiation
- **S**everity
- **T**iming

This mnemonic is generally used when assessing a patient who reports pain or dyspnea. The OPQRST mnemonic is discussed in more detail in the following sections.

Onset

The onset refers to when the patient's problem began and what the patient was doing at the time of the incident. Ask the patient when the problem started or when the incident occurred, and how long ago the patient first noticed the problem. Chest pain that started while the patient was sleeping may be more significant than chest pain that started while the patient was pushing a lawn mower in extreme heat. If the patient reports that the problem started a long time ago (days or weeks), then also ask, "What prompted you to call now?" In most cases, the patient will note a sudden worsening of the problem or an additional problem that compounded the first one. For example, a patient who has experienced shortness of breath for the past 3 days may have called because of an onset of chest pain an hour ago. You often will not learn about this second problem unless you ask.

For patients with traumatic problems, there may be a delay between when they were hurt and when they called. Again, ask them why they delayed and what prompted them to call today. The information they give may be valuable to you and the ED staff.

Provocation/Palliation

Learning about provoking and palliating factors (also known as aggravating or alleviating factors) can be extremely helpful in determining the cause and severity of the patient's problem. Provoking factors include anything that seems to bring on the problem or that seems to makes the problem worse, such as increased shortness of breath during exertion. Palliating factors include anything that brings the patient relief from the problem, such as sitting down to rest. Note the position in which the patient is found upon arrival.

The answers to these questions often help you to identify the potential cause. For example, shortness of breath that started when the patient climbed a set of stairs may be respiratory or cardiac in origin. These questions are often the clues to hidden medical conditions from traumatic incidents. When you ask if anything makes the pain better or worse, the patient may report that the pain has been worse "since I fell last week," uncovering a traumatic event that was not previously reported.

Quality

The patient's description of the pain may be useful when trying to determine the cause of the problem. For example, patients who are having a heart attack classically describe their chest pain as "squeezing" or "pressure," although they may also say things such as, "My chest feels heavy." To learn about the quality of the pain, ask the patient to describe how he or she feels. Avoid asking the patient leading questions when possible, such as those that can be simply answered yes or no; this approach may not give you an accurate description of what the patient actually feels. Remember that not all patients experience pain in the same way, and an older patient may deny the presence of chest pain but may state, "My chest just feels heavy."

Patients often initially say, "I don't know," or "It's hard to describe." Once again, the key is for you to have patience. If you wait, then most patients will ultimately describe the quality of their pain. Carefully document in the patient's own words; this information may be significant to other health care providers who become involved in the patient's care. Some patients have limited vocabulary when it comes to their bodies; it may be best to let them simply point to their pain, rather than describe it. Ask patients to point to the area of pain, describe the area of pain, or describe pain anywhere else associated with the problem. If the patient still cannot describe the pain or if the patient cannot speak, then you might consider offering several descriptions of pain and letting the patient choose. For example, you might ask, "Which of these words best describes your pain: Sharp or dull? Burning? Stabbing? Crushing? Throbbing?"

You can learn a great deal about the patient's problem through these questions. For example, a patient who points to a single place for his or her pain has what is known as **focal pain** Figure 10-25A. Many problems, such as fractures and areas of inflammation, commonly cause focal pain. However, some patients cannot point to a single location. Instead, they often rub their hands across their chests or abdomens as they are asked to point to their pain. These patients are experiencing **diffuse pain** Figure 10-25B. A number of conditions, including heart attack and internal bleeding, typically cause diffuse pain.

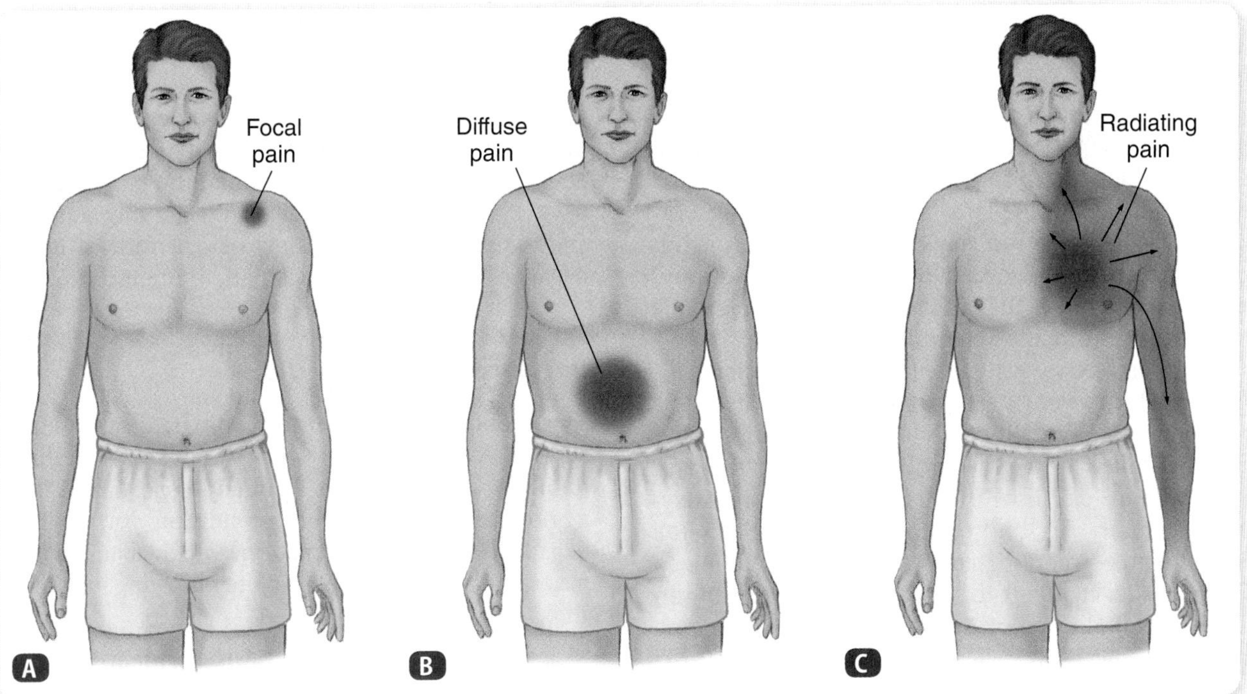

Figure 10-25 A. Focal pain. **B.** Diffuse pain. **C.** Radiating pain.

Words of Wisdom

Your documentation of any pain complaint should include a description in the patient's words and your findings from the other OPQRST questions. Record all pain complaints in detail. Not all pain symptoms are "classic"; the exact description may help hospital personnel make the correct diagnosis in a case that is not typical.

Region/Radiation

Patients can often provide clues about the cause of their problems by describing the region or location of any pain or discomfort. **Radiating pain** refers to an area of the body from which the origin of pain or discomfort may travel **Figure 10-25C**. The presence of radiating pain will not alter your treatment much; however, physicians and nurses caring for the patient in the hospital may be interested in hearing about areas of radiation. For example, a patient who is having a heart attack may report chest pain that radiates to the left arm and jaw. Carefully document what you learn.

Be careful how you ask about radiation of pain. Most patients will not understand if you ask, "Does your pain radiate anywhere else?" The best way to ask patients about radiation is to ask, "Do you have pain or discomfort anywhere else?" or, "Does it feel like the pain moves around?"

Referred pain is pain that exists in more than one place, without a "trail" of pain in between. For example, it is common for a patient with gallbladder disease to report pain in the right upper quadrant of the abdomen and in the right shoulder. However, there is no pain between the right upper quadrant and right shoulder. There may also be pain only in an area that is not the source of the pain.

Severity

Severity refers to the patient's perception of "how bad" the current incident is in comparison with others. In some cases, particularly when the patient has experienced the problem before, his or her perception provides extremely useful information. For example, a patient with asthma may provide helpful information by comparing this episode with previous asthma attacks. However, if the problem has never occurred, the patient's perception of severity may not be useful except as a guide to whether the problem is getting worse or better during transport.

To assess severity, you may ask the following questions:

- "How bad is this episode in comparison with previous ones?" (if the problem is chronic or recurring)
- "What happened the last time you had an episode this bad?" (if the problem is chronic or recurring)
- "How would you rate this problem in numbers, if 0 is normal (that is, pain-free) and 10 is the worst pain or discomfort you can imagine?"

For patients with chronic problems, obtaining the answer to the question, "What happened the last time you had an episode this bad?" is invaluable. In most cases, patients are accurate in their self-assessments of severity. For example, a patient with asthma might tell you that the last time he had an episode this bad, he was intubated and spent 2 weeks in the intensive care unit. The patient's comments tell you that this episode is extremely serious. Complete your assessment and provide rapid transport. At the other extreme, the patient might tell you that he was kept in the ED for about an hour and then discharged. Obviously, these two episodes are very different in urgency, and you can adjust your plans for treatment and transport accordingly. Bear in mind, however, that no relationship may exist between the severity of previous incidents and the current one; treat the patient as he or she presents, keeping past information in mind.

Another way to evaluate changes in the patient's condition during your treatment and transport is to use a numeric rating system. For example, a patient with an apparent broken leg might initially tell you that the pain is an 8 on a scale of 1 to 10. After you have applied oxygen, splinted the leg, and begun transport, recheck the patient's pain perception. If the pain is now a 9, then you might consider changing the position of the leg, using an ice pack, or, if allowed by local protocol, administering analgesic medications such as nitrous oxide. However, if the pain level is now reportedly a 5, then you know that the treatment is effective (at least for now). Remember, patients perceive pain in different ways, so it is inappropriate to compare one patient's numeric rating with another patient's rating.

Time

The questions related to time provide information about when the problem began. You might want to find out whether the problem has been constant or intermittent. If the patient states that the problem is intermittent, then ask what seemed to make it better or worse.

The answers to these questions will further help you and other health care providers involved with the patient's care to understand the nature of the problem. Some conditions, such as those involving abdominal organs, have classically intermittent pain. Other problems, such as fractures, typically have constant pain.

Interventions

You may hear the mnemonic *OPQRST-I* used. The letter *I* refers to interventions. Some patients may self-treat or self-medicate before calling 9-1-1. For example, a patient reporting chest pain may have taken nitroglycerin or aspirin before your arrival. It is pertinent to ask about any treatment prior to EMS arrival to avoid overdosing a patient on any medication he or she may have already taken, and to note the possible interactions between medications. People may try a variety of home remedies for whatever is ailing them. Be sure to ask; this information may affect your treatment of the patient.

Identify Pertinent Negatives

During the process of achieving a thorough history, you must also document pertinent negatives. **Pertinent negatives** are findings you would expect based on the patient's complaint, but that are not present. For example, you would expect a patient reporting severe abdominal pain to have a tender abdomen and possible nausea and/or vomiting. An abdomen that is soft and nontender on palpation or the lack of nausea or vomiting are all pertinent negatives. These are signs and symptoms that the patient does not have. Pertinent negatives also indicate that a thorough and complete exam and history were performed. Pertinent negatives will vary with each patient interaction.

Investigate Past Medical History (SAMPLE History)

As you obtain a patient history from medical and trauma patients, you need to know some of the standard techniques for interviewing patients. By obtaining a **SAMPLE history**, a brief history of the patient's condition, you will be able to gather important information from the patient. Use the mnemonic SAMPLE to obtain the following information:

- **S** *Signs and symptoms*. What signs and symptoms occurred at the onset of the incident? Does the patient report pain?
- **A** *Allergies*. Is the patient allergic to any medication, food, or other pertinent substance? What reactions did the patient have to any of them? If the patient has no known drug allergies, note this on the run report as "no known drug allergies" or "NKDA."
- **M** *Medications*. What medication(s) is the patient prescribed? What dosage is prescribed? How often does the patient take the medication? What prescription, over-the-counter (OTC), and herbal medications has the patient taken in the last 12 hours? Many people do not consider herbal or OTC medications to be medications. They may leave out this information unless specifically questioned. How much was taken and when? Does the patient take recreational drugs or drink alcohol?
- **P** *Pertinent past medical history*. Does the patient have any history of medical, surgical, or trauma occurrences? Has the patient had a recent illness or injury, fall, or blow to the head? Is there important family history that should be known? Has the patient ever had this problem before? If so, then how was it treated previously?
- **L** *Last oral intake*. When did the patient last eat or drink? What did the patient eat or drink, and how much was consumed? Did the patient take any drugs or drink alcohol? Has there been any other oral intake in the last 4 hours?
- **E** *Events leading up to the illness or injury*. What are the key events that led up to this incident? What occurred between the onset of the incident and your arrival? What was the patient doing when this illness started? What was the patient doing when this injury happened?

Words of Wisdom

When you interview a patient about medical history, it is helpful to ask, "What medications do you take?" Otherwise, you may find that the patient denies any history but has multiple prescriptions (polypharmacy). For example, when asked about having seizures, a patient may deny having them even though prescriptions exist in the patient's name for antiseizure medications. The typical answer when asked about the medication is, "No, I don't have seizures as long as I take my medicine."

Obtaining the History on Sensitive Topics

Alcohol and Drugs. The signs and symptoms a patient may present with while under the influence of alcohol or drugs may be confusing, hidden, or disguised. Many patients who abuse alcohol and/or drugs may deny the abuse. Families, friends, and coworkers may be unaware that a patient has any drug or alcohol dependencies. The reasons patients deny using alcohol or drugs can vary greatly. It may be out of fear of losing their employment or driver's license, worry about what friends and others such as health care providers may think about them, and embarrassment or insecurity about their dependency.

The history that you gather from a patient with a chemical dependency may be unreliable **Figure 10-26**. If patients are not telling the people closest to them that they have a problem, then you, as an outsider, may have even less success in obtaining information about a patient's current dependency. The signs and symptoms of alcohol or drug use may be masked by the patient's presentation. Use all of your senses when providing patient care.

Establish a strong rapport with your patients. Do not judge a patient who may have a chemical dependency, and be professional in your approach. Be honest and open. Foremost, impress on the patient that information received will be kept in confidence. Then and only then, a patient may open up to you and provide information that can be valuable in his or her assessment and treatment.

Physical Abuse or Violence. You must report all cases of suspected physical abuse or domestic violence to the appropriate authorities. Follow your state laws and local protocols when dealing with such cases. If you suspect a patient is a survivor of physical abuse or domestic violence, then do not accuse any person of being responsible for the situation. Instead, immediately involve law enforcement.

Because abuse and physical violence are sensitive situations, look for hidden clues that such a situation exists. Information gathered at the scene, during the assessment process, and while transporting a patient may indicate violence or abuse.

What should you look for? When obtaining a history, note whether the information provided by the patient and others present at the scene is inconsistent. Do you observe multiple injuries in various stages of healing? Are some bruises red, black, brown, or even green? In some cases, a survivor of abuse or violence will not tell you what happened because of fear of further violence when EMS is not present. The patients may not answer your questions because the physical aggressor is present and is answering questions for him or her. In these cases, separate the people present and interview both parties about the situation.

In cases of domestic violence, involvement can be extremely dangerous. If you determine that the emergency response is part of a domestic abuse situation, then call law enforcement personnel immediately **Figure 10-27**.

When involved with cases of physical abuse, be observant and open-minded, have a high index of suspicion, and be nonjudgmental. Accurate and thorough documentation is very important in cases of abuse and domestic violence. Your documentation should be an objective report of the facts. Avoid subjective, judgmental

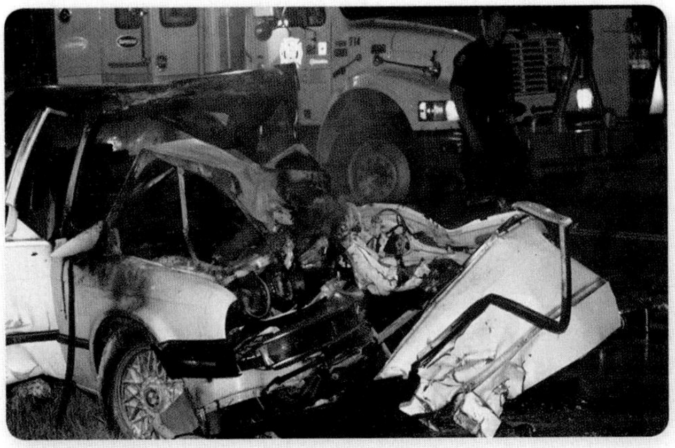

Figure 10-26 Many vehicle crashes involve alcohol. In these cases, the patient history may be unreliable.

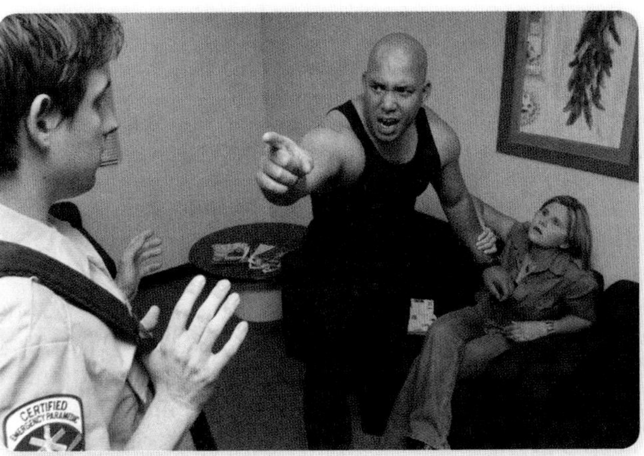

Figure 10-27 Do not handle potentially violent calls alone. Summon law enforcement personnel immediately.

statements, and include any pertinent statements made by the patient or others present using quotation marks. Remember, these prehospital situations will most likely involve some type of legal process later on. You may be summoned at a later date to provide testimony regarding what may have happened.

Sexual History. Your ability to obtain information about a patient's sexual history may be limited. Religious beliefs, cultural stereotypes, and societal expectations may have a major role in a patient choosing not to reveal a personal side of his or her life, including practices considered by some people to be bizarre or exotic. In addition, some patients find sharing information regarding their sexual histories with others to be uncomfortable.

When would information about a patient's sexual history become important? As an AEMT, you will be involved in the care of female patients reporting lower abdominal pain. Consider all female patients of childbearing age who report lower abdominal pain to be pregnant unless ruled out by history or other information. Questions to ask when faced with this prehospital scenario include the following:

- When was your last menstrual period?
- Are your periods normal? (Is any vaginal discharge or bleeding present that is not associated with a menstrual period?)
- Do you have urinary frequency or burning?
- What is the severity of cramping?
- Are any unpleasant odors present?
- Is it possible you may be pregnant?
- Are you taking birth control pills or using other types of birth control?
- How many sexual partners do you have?
- Have you had recent sexual encounters?

When dealing with a male patient, you must inquire about urinary symptoms:

- Do you have any pain associated with urination?
- Do you have any discharge, sores, or an increase in urination?
- Do you have burning or difficulty voiding?
- Has any trauma occurred?
- How many sexual partners do you have?
- Have you had recent sexual encounters?

In obtaining a history in all patients, ask about the potential for sexually transmitted diseases. Providing this information may be difficult and uncomfortable for the patient. Never be judgmental about the response to your questions. All patients should be and expect to be treated with compassion and respect. All information obtained from a patient for the purpose of determining a treatment plan is confidential; do not share it with others unless necessary in the process of treating the patient's medical or traumatic condition.

Special Challenges in Obtaining the Patient History

Each patient presents a unique assessment challenge. Those with physical limitations or unusual behavioral tendencies may prove particularly difficult to understand and therefore assess. As a result, you may miss critical information or become discouraged by the patient's inability to communicate clearly. Therefore, it is important that you develop strategies that assist in gathering pertinent information while at the same time avoiding potential frustration that can come from difficult communications.

Silence. Dealing with patients who say very little or nothing at all can be difficult and frustrating. Patience is extremely important when dealing with patients and their emergency crises. Patients may be thinking about how to answer you, getting the facts straight, or assessing your crew to determine if they feel comfortable answering you. Using a close-ended question that requires a simple yes or no answer may work best. Consider whether the silence is a clue to the patient's chief complaint. Also consider whether something about your communication style could be making the patient uncomfortable, and try to alter your technique to be as sensitive, empathetic, and professional as possible.

Always look for visual signs in the patient's environment that may indicate why a patient is not communicating. In addition, look for nonverbal clues, including facial expressions that may show pain or fear. Is the patient distressed or intimidated by your presence? How is the patient sitting or standing? Is there a communication problem? Is there a language problem? The number of reasons a patient may be silent during the prehospital encounter is endless. A good AEMT will continue to assess the situation and determine a way to communicate with the patient.

Overly Talkative. On the other end of the spectrum is the patient or bystander who is extremely talkative. Some people just talk a lot, and gathering details about their medical conditions may be difficult if they talk around your question or you have a difficult time refocusing the patient's conversation. Some possible causes as to why a patient may be overly talkative could include excessive caffeine consumption, nervousness, and ingestion of cocaine or methamphetamines.

After you have allowed a talkative patient a chance to express himself or herself, you must keep the patient focused on the questions asked. Direct the patient to stick to the facts by summarizing his or her statements frequently, and clarify statements for the purpose of making sure the information you are gathering is correct. Remember, there is no such thing as too much information.

Multiple Symptoms. Some patients present with multiple symptoms, particularly older patients. Be prepared to spend extra time assessing the patient owing to possible challenges with communication. Prioritize the patient's complaints as you would during triage; start with the most serious and end with the least serious. Always ask for additional information to determine why EMS was called.

Keep an open mind, and do not focus on one complaint or detail to determine a treatment plan. Always remember there may be a number of possible medical or traumatic causes for a patient's chief complaint.

Anxiety. When a person is involved in an emergency situation, it is natural for that person to appear excited or anxious. Many people have not been faced with a true emergency during their lifetime, and their reactions may be unpredictable. As an AEMT, you are trained to handle stressful situations. Your patient or bystander may be nervous, pacing, vocal, panicked, or, in some extreme cases, experiencing complete hysteria. It is your responsibility to deal not only with the emergency crisis at hand, but also with the people present who are having difficulties coping with the situation. Frequently, anxious patients can be observed in emergency scenes that involve a large number of patients, such as during a disaster. Anxiety also can be observed or encountered during a routine EMS call when family members or patients cannot cope.

You can expect anxious patients to exhibit signs of psychological shock, such as pallor, diaphoresis, shortness of breath, numbness in the hands and feet, dizziness or light-headedness, and even loss of consciousness. Some anxious people may have no real medical complaint but may be hiding or concealing information, such as trying to keep a family member, friend, or employer from discovering their dependency on alcohol or drugs. Or, the patient may have been involved in a physical abuse or domestic situation that he or she wants to keep quiet. In any situation involving an anxious patient, you must be aware of verbal and nonverbal clues. Is the patient making sense during a verbal conversation? Anxiety can also be an early indicator of low blood glucose level, shock, or hypoxia. Perform the appropriate exam to rule out these potentially life-threatening causes early in your assessment.

During a crisis situation, reassure the patient that any nervous or anxious response is normal and can be overcome. It may be possible for you to control an anxious patient by simply smiling or using a delicate and therapeutic touch, if the patient seems receptive to touch. Be confident in your approach, and have a positive demeanor. In many patient care interactions, your presence may be all that is required to calm the patient.

As in every response, safety is a paramount concern. Be aware that emergency responses involving anxious and possibly hysterical patients can turn violent. A confident but cautious AEMT can prevent a bad situation from getting worse and professionally calm and control anxious patients, friends, and family members.

Special Populations

When you deal with pediatric patients, be sure to involve them in their own care. Give choices, but avoid questions with "yes" or "no" answers. For example, do not ask "Can I touch your tummy?" Rather, give the child a choice, such as the following: "I need to listen to your breathing and also touch your tummy. Which would you like for me to do first?" This practice allows participation without limiting your emergency medical care.

Anger and Hostility. Every patient encounter has the potential for violence and hostility, from a situation involving a 9-year-old boy who was hit by a vehicle to a 90-year-old grandmother experiencing chest pain. Some emergency calls have a high potential for unexpected violence because people in an emergency situation might be afraid and react with anger. Patients, friends, family, or bystanders may direct their anger and rage toward you. Do not take this anger and frustration personally. More important, do not become angry yourself because "anger feeds anger."

When handling potentially violent situations, remain calm, reassuring, and gentle. Always be observant. Be aware of nonverbal clues, such as posture, position, and facial expressions. Look at the patient, and be aware of how the patient is positioned. Is the patient stiff, with the hands clenched and feet wide apart?

If the scene is not safe or secured, then contact law enforcement to secure it. Never let a potentially violent or hostile patient leave the room alone. Understand that everything in reach of a patient has the potential to be used as a weapon.

Intoxication. The number of EMS calls dealing with a patient who is intoxicated has increased over the years. When you attempt to obtain a history for a patient who is intoxicated, be aware the information may not only be difficult to get, but also could be unreliable. A patient who is intoxicated may become impatient with you when he or she is trying to provide you with information. As the patient's impatience increases, so does his or her anger level. Do not put the patient in a position where he or she feels threatened and has no way out. As in other emergency cases, the potential for violence and a physical confrontation is high when a patient is intoxicated.

During the assessment and treatment of a patient who is under the influence, be accepting, diplomatic, objective, and nonjudgmental. Because of the intoxication, the patient may not be telling you everything about how he or she feels. Alcohol dulls a patient's senses, which will make it difficult for a patient who is intoxicated to inform you that something feels painful. Treat the patient with dignity and respect. Never assume the patient's condition is the result of alcohol consumption when an underlying medical condition or trauma may be the cause of the patient's presentation.

Crying. A crying patient is a breathing patient. But why do some patients cry? In the context of an emergency, a patient who cries may be sad, in pain, or emotionally overwhelmed. No matter the reason for crying, you need to remain calm, patient, reassuring and confident and maintain a soft voice.

Your presence may make a crying patient feel more secure. In some extreme cases, additional diplomacy and verbal intervention will help the patient. No matter how you address a crying patient, as with all patients, be sympathetic and treat them with respect and dignity.

Depression. Depression is a common reason patients call EMS. In fact, according to the World Health Organization, depression is the leading cause of disability worldwide, with an estimated 350 million people of all ages suffering from this condition.[4] Some of the symptoms of depression include sadness, a feeling of hopelessness, restlessness, and irritability. The patient may also have sleeping and eating disorders and a decreased energy level. Depression is a normal human response, but it can lead to harmful behavior. When you encounter a patient with depression, be nonjudgmental and compassionate toward the patient's feelings. The most effective prehospital approach to a patient's depression is being a good listener. Often, the patient needs someone to talk to and someone to listen.

Confusing Behavior or History. Patients sometimes provide more history information to hospital personnel than they do to AEMTs because they are embarrassed or frightened and may feel more comfortable talking with hospital staff. Whatever the situation, you must be aware of medical causes that can lead a patient to report a confusing history. Hypoxia, stroke, diabetes, trauma, and drug/medication use could alter a patient's explanation of events. One of the most common causes of confusion is hypoxia. It is not uncommon to encounter an older patient who has dementia, delirium, or Alzheimer disease. (These conditions are discussed in more detail in Chapter 37, *Geriatric Emergencies*.) It is important to verify the baseline mental status of each patient. Do not assume that because a patient is older and confused, he or she has one of these conditions.

> **Words of Wisdom**
>
> An altered mental status in any patient should be considered abnormal until proven otherwise. Immediately consider hypoxia, hypoglycemia, or shock as potential culprits. Even patients with a history of dementia may have hypoxia or hypoglycemia. Do a thorough assessment on every patient, and do not assume that an altered mental status is normal for anyone.

Confused behavior is not a normal response. After you have properly assessed and treated any life threats, attempt to ask the patient again about the chief complaint or ask someone close to the patient, such as family members or friends, to provide additional details.

Limited Cognitive Abilities. Cognitive disabilities can range from those that are barely recognizable to those that are severe. Develop a habitual method for dealing with a patient who has limited cognitive abilities. First, assume you can get an adequate history. Keep your questions simple, and limit the use of medical terms. Be alert for partial answers, and keep asking questions. In cases in which patients have severely limited cognitive function, rely on family, caregivers, and friends to supply answers to your questions. See Chapter 4, *Communications and Documentation*, for more information about communication challenges and techniques.

Language Barriers. We live in a country that is a melting pot of people with diverse nationalities. Not everyone speaks English. For example, imagine that you respond to a call for an older woman who fell at a nursing home. The emergency response seems pretty straightforward until you ask the patient what happened and she answers in French. If you don't speak the language, then how will you ask the patient to describe what happened and what hurts? Keep in mind that some patients may have disabilities that make it difficult to understand them in any language.

To overcome language barriers, consider using interpreters, translation resources, and related mobile device apps. The best answer is to find an interpreter, but it is not always that simple. First, determine whether the patient speaks or understands any English by asking the patient or others who may be present. Start by introducing yourself by using your name. Determine whether the patient understands who you are. If the patient is able to respond by giving you his or her name, then the patient has the ability to understand some English, but more important, the patient has cognitive ability (the ability to understand). Remember that increasing the volume of your questions or of your voice will not increase the patient's understanding of what you are asking him or her. Keep questions straightforward and brief. Simple is best. Use of hand gestures may be helpful.

Be aware of the language diversity in your community. Some dispatch centers and most hospitals have set up programs within the institution that identify various employees who can speak different languages. Provide the hospital with advanced notice that a non–English-speaking patient will be arriving. This practice will allow the hospital the opportunity to make arrangements for an interpreter.

Hearing Impairments. Hearing disabilities in patients range from slight to total deafness. Hearing impairment can make the process of obtaining an in-depth history

Special Populations

Many mobile device apps are available to assist in communication with patients who are hard of hearing or who speak another language.

difficult. When you are treating a patient who has a hearing deficit, ask questions slowly and clearly. You may want to use a stethoscope to function like a hearing aid; have the patient place the stethoscope in his or her ears while you speak softly into the stethoscope bell, which will amplify the sound. Changing the pitch of your voice may also help the patient to hear you.

Oftentimes, a patient who has had a hearing disability for some time will have mastered the technique of reading lips. If the patient has a hearing aid, then ask the patient to use it. Speak slowly and face-to-face with the patient. Some patients will attempt to use sign language for communication, which can be difficult for others to understand. Learning simple sign language during your career will help in the communication process. Probably the simplest way to communicate with a patient who has a hearing deficit is to use a pencil and paper. Write down uncomplicated questions that require simple yes or no answers.

Visual Impairments. Identify yourself verbally when entering the home of a visually impaired patient who has called for help. By announcing yourself when entering a residence, you are letting a patient know that help has arrived and any response from the patient may help you locate the patient's whereabouts. If the patient cannot see clearly and has eyeglasses, then ask the patient to put them on.

During the assessment and subsequent treatment of a patient who is visually impaired, it is important that you put any items that have been moved back into their previous position. Many visually impaired patients can move freely about their homes because they know exactly where everything is placed. If you move something, then put it back.

During the assessment and history-taking process, explain to the patient what is happening and stay in contact with the patient by keeping a hand on the patient's arm or shoulder. Explain that you will be checking vital signs by feeling for the pulse, listening to breath sounds, and applying a blood pressure cuff to the patient's arm. Notify the patient when you prepare to lift and move him or her on the stretcher. Remember, you are a stranger to the patient, and an EMS vehicle is a foreign environment. A little communication can go a long way in easing uncertainty in a visually impaired patient. If the patient is unable to provide you with all of the necessary information, then try to find someone else who can.

Words of Wisdom

Throughout your assessment process, take note of the patient's mental status. Changes in mental status will be your best indicator for improvement or deterioration in your patient's condition. If at any time deterioration in mental status or function occurs, then your immediate attention is required and the severity of your patient's condition should be upgraded.

Patient Assessment

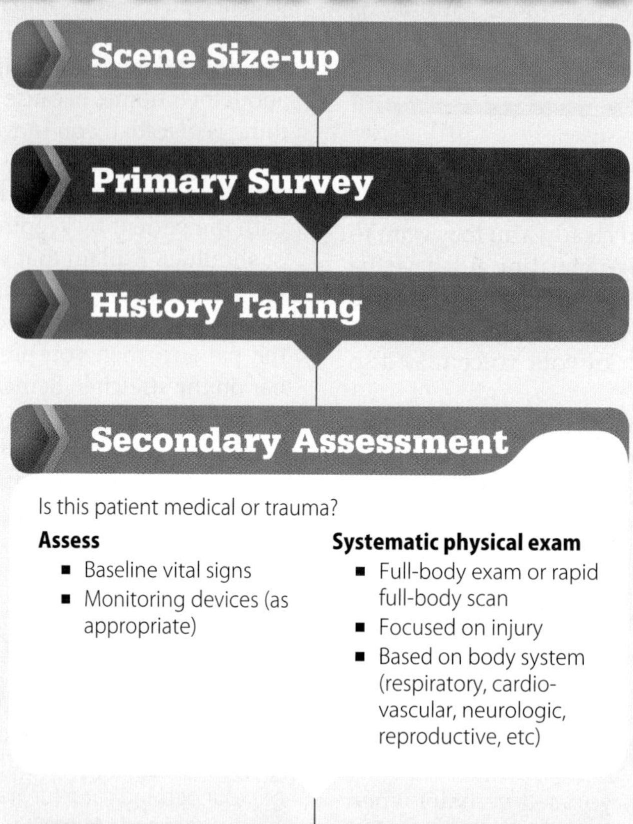

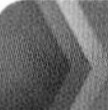

Secondary Assessment

If the patient is in stable condition and has an isolated complaint, then the secondary assessment may occur at the scene. If the secondary assessment is not performed at the scene, then it is performed in the back of the ambulance en route to the hospital. However, in some situations, you may not have time to perform a secondary assessment, such as if you have to continually manage life threats that were identified during the primary survey.

The purpose of the **secondary assessment** is to obtain vital signs and perform a systematic physical exam of the patient. As part of the secondary assessment, you will take a complete set of vital signs. At a minimum, assess and document the following:

- Respirations
- Pulse
- Blood pressure
- Level of consciousness
- Skin condition
- Blood glucose
- Pulse oximetry

The physical exam may be a head-to-toe, **full-body exam** or an exam that focuses on a certain area or region of the body, often determined through the chief complaint. Circumstances will dictate which aspects of the physical exam will be used.

Words of Wisdom

Patients may feel vulnerable and exposed during a physical exam. Display compassion during this difficult time, and clearly explain to your patient what you are doing. It is important to protect the patient's modesty and maintain body temperature by keeping areas covered that you are not currently assessing.

As discussed previously, the physical exam you perform is based on the needs of your patient. Also recall that the exam should include inspection, palpation, and auscultation. The mnemonic DCAP-BTLS, discussed earlier, will help remind you what to look for when inspecting and palpating various body regions.

An integral part of your physical exam is to compare findings on one side of the body with the other side when possible. If one ankle appears swollen, then look at the other. If one shoulder feels "out of joint," then feel the other one to compare. When listening to breath sounds, listen to both sides of the chest. Find out which conditions are new and which ones the patient has been experiencing for some time.

On some occasions, it may even be helpful to note odors during an exam. Odors can indicate anything from infections, to certain medical conditions, to scene safety threats.

Words of Wisdom

Recall that DCAP-BTLS is a mnemonic for assessment in which each area of the body is evaluated for Deformities, Contusions, Abrasions, Punctures/penetrations, Burns, Tenderness, Lacerations, and Swelling.

Assess Vital Signs Using the Appropriate Monitoring Devices

The use of monitoring equipment in the prehospital setting has continued to expand. AEMTs at all levels use a wide variety of devices in the continuous monitoring of patients. It is important to remember that these devices are manufactured and subject to limitations and mechanical failures. Always follow the manufacturer's instructions for operating any device. These devices should never be used to replace your comprehensive assessment of your patient; think of these devices as simply adjuncts to the assessment and treatment of your patient. Obtaining and using information from patient monitoring devices includes, but is not limited to, data from pulse oximetry, noninvasive blood pressure monitoring, end-tidal carbon dioxide measurements, and blood glucose monitoring.

Pulse Oximetry

Pulse oximetry is an assessment tool that is used to evaluate the effectiveness of oxygenation. The pulse oximeter is a photoelectric device that monitors the oxygen saturation of hemoglobin (the iron-containing portion of the red blood cell to which oxygen attaches) in the capillary beds Figure 10-28. The parts that make up the pulse oximeter include a monitor and a sensing probe. The sensing probe clips onto a finger or earlobe.

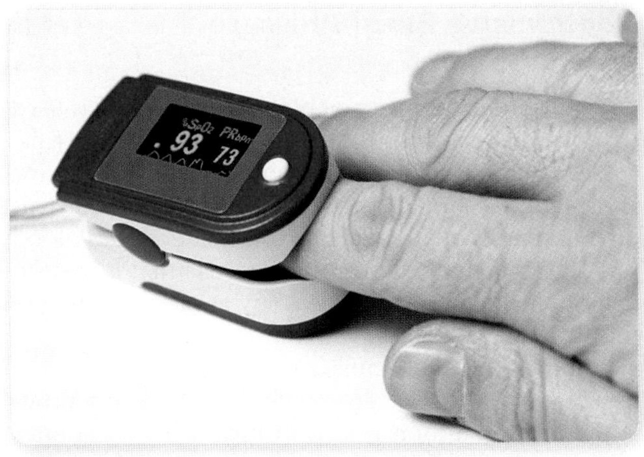

Figure 10-28 The pulse oximeter is a device that measures the saturation of oxygen in the blood as a percentage.

The light source must have unobstructed access to a capillary bed, so dark fingernail polish might need to be removed. Results appear as a percentage on the display screen. Normally, pulse oximetry values in ambient air will vary depending on the altitude, with the majority of values falling between 95% and 99%.

The goal of applying oxygen therapy is to increase oxygen saturation to a normal level. This device is a useful assessment tool to determine the effectiveness of oxygen therapy, bronchodilator therapy, and artificial ventilations. However, the pulse oximeter does not take the place of good assessment skills and should not prevent the application of oxygen to any patient who reports difficulty breathing, regardless of the pulse oximetry value seen on the monitor.

Because the device presumes adequate perfusion and numbers of red blood cells, any situation that causes vasoconstriction (such as hypothermia or shock) or loss of red blood cells (such as bleeding or anemia) will result in inaccurate or misleading values. The device also presumes that oxygen is saturating the hemoglobin. Therefore, any chemical that displaces oxygen (such as carbon monoxide) will also cause misleading values.

The pulse oximeter is a useful tool as long as you remember that the device is only a tool, not a substitute for a good assessment. Do not use the device when hypoperfusion or known anemia is present, carbon monoxide or exposure to other toxic inhalants has occurred, or the patient's extremities are cold.

Words of Wisdom

Always treat your patient, not the diagnostic tools! A patient with dyspnea needs oxygen regardless of the pulse oximeter readings.

Noninvasive Blood Pressure Measurement

The sphygmomanometer, or blood pressure cuff, is used in the measurement of the patient's blood pressure (discussed later in this chapter). Blood pressure is a routine vital sign that should be continuously monitored. This device consists of an inflatable cuff that occludes blood flow and a manometer (pressure meter) that is used to determine the pressure in the artery at various points in the physical exam. These two components are connected via tubing. In manual cuffs, a separate tube connects to an inflation bulb. The auscultatory method (listening) is the most common means of measuring a patient's blood pressure using a sphygmomanometer. In contrast, blood pressure measured by palpation is accomplished by palpating the radial pulse as the cuff is deflated. Only a systolic measurement can be obtained by palpation.

Oscillometric measurement, or electronic measurement, is another method of obtaining blood pressure readings of patients. An electronic device measures changes in pressure oscillations that occur during cuff deflation and are related to systolic, mean, and diastolic pressures. Two types of electronic devices are used in the prehospital setting; the blood pressure cuff deflates differently in each device. The first device measures readings using linear deflation, and the second type measures readings by using stepped deflation. An electronic blood pressure cuff that uses linear deflation allows a uniform decline in pressure in the cuff during deflation. Conversely, stepped deflation allows the cuff to deflate in small steps or intervals. Although both devices are accurate in the prehospital setting, stepped deflation tends to be more accurate in patients who are moving and in patients who may be hypotensive. Stepped deflation can release the pressure in the cuff in intervals at variable lengths, allowing the system to better detect oscillations. Always take the first set of vital signs manually, regardless of the availability of electronic devices.

Electronic devices are prone to inaccurate readings in moving vehicles, noisy environments, or if the cuff is not correctly sized or properly placed on the patient. If you are faced with readings that do not match the clinical presentation of the patient, then obtain manual readings to confirm.

End-Tidal Carbon Dioxide

Although pulse oximetry can evaluate the effectiveness of oxygenation, it cannot measure the amount of oxygen being consumed by a patient's cells during cellular metabolism. To determine oxygen consumption, you will need to measure **carbon dioxide (CO_2)** levels. CO_2 is the by-product of aerobic cellular metabolism and reflects the amount of oxygen being consumed during the process. Metabolism refers to the chemical reactions that occur in the body or cells to maintain life. The two noninvasive methods in which CO_2 is monitored in the field are capnometry and capnography. **Capnometry** typically consists of a disposable or electronic device that provides you with a means of measuring CO_2 output. **Capnography** includes not only a measurement of CO_2 output, but also provides a waveform based on serial measurements **Figure 10-29**.

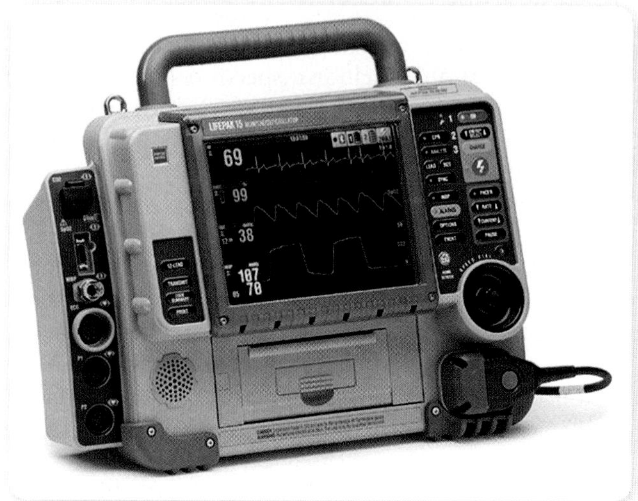

Figure 10-29 This device is capable of monitoring multiple functions simultaneously, including continuous capnography (bottom tracing).

Capnography can quickly and efficiently provide information on a patient's ventilatory status, circulation, and metabolism. Capnography also serves as an indicator of chest compression effectiveness and can detect return of spontaneous circulation. The provision of this information is possible because blood must circulate through the lungs for CO_2 to be exhaled and measured. These devices are typically used in the prehospital setting as a secondary means to determine endotracheal placement, to maximize a patient's ventilatory status, and to avoid inadvertent hyperventilation of patients with head injuries, which has been linked to poor outcomes.

End-tidal carbon dioxide ($ETCO_2$) is the partial pressure or maximal concentration of CO_2 at the end of an exhaled breath, which is expressed as a percentage of CO_2, or in millimeters of mercury (mm Hg). The digital display of $ETCO_2$ is expressed in millimeters of mercury or as a percentage of exhaled gas. The normal range is 35 to 45 mm Hg, or 5% to 6% CO_2. Because CO_2 is not present in the esophagus, use of an $ETCO_2$ detector is a reliable (and essential) method for confirming and monitoring advanced airway placement. When capnography shows an absence of CO_2, it may indicate the endotracheal tube is in the wrong position or there is an absence or decrease in the level of CO_2 in the lungs—possibly from cardiac arrest, ineffective CPR, or shock. When cardiac output increases, the $ETCO_2$ measurement provides information on the adequacy of ventilation and circulation.

$ETCO_2$ is measured or detected by colorimetry, capnometry, and capnography devices. **Colorimetric devices** come in different shapes and sizes but provide continuous end-tidal monitoring by displaying one of three colors **Figure 10-30**. A colorimetric capnographer provides qualitative (that is, it does not assign a numeric value) information regarding the presence of CO_2 in the patient's exhaled breath. It does not measure the exact

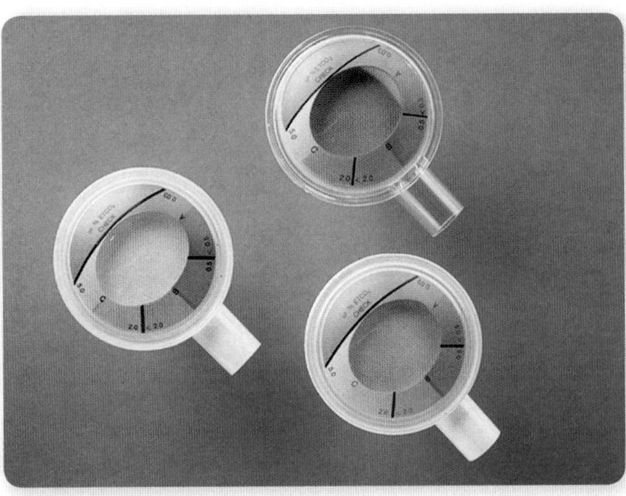

Figure 10-30 Colorimetric capnographers.

Courtesy of Marianne Gausche-Hill, MD, FACEP, FAAP.

amount of CO_2 exhaled, but it indicates whether CO_2 is present in reasonable amounts in the exhaled breath of a patient. The device is attached between the advanced airway and bag-mask device. After six to eight positive pressure ventilations—the amount of time it takes for CO_2 to accumulate in the device—the specially treated paper inside the detector should turn from purple to yellow during exhalation, indicating the presence of exhaled CO_2. Purple indicates a CO_2 level of less than 0.5%, tan indicates a range of 0.5% to 2%, and yellow indicates a level of greater than 2%. A yellow reading indicates adequate circulation. Remember to check these devices regularly for damage, cracks, and blockages caused by gastric secretions because this damage will affect the accuracy of the readings. Colorimetric devices are also sensitive to temperature extremes and humidity.

> **Words of Wisdom**
>
> A colorimetric capnographer is a "spot-check" device that should be used during initial confirmation of advanced airway placement and then replaced as soon as possible with a quantitative device. The monitor may be incorrect (or fooled) if the patient has CO_2 trapped in the stomach from the ingestion of carbonated beverages, so confirm the reading over at least six breaths to be certain it is not a false-positive reading.

Blood Glucometry

The glucometer is used to measure the level of glucose in a patient's bloodstream. If the blood glucose level is low, then this finding can help you identify the reason a patient has a decreased LOC or is unresponsive. If the blood glucose level is high in a patient with nausea, vomiting, abdominal pain, and a change in mental status, then it may signal dangerous complications of high blood glucose.

While determining glucose levels is largely a routine part of the patient assessment process, indications include known diabetes in patients with a decreased LOC, a decreased LOC of unknown origin in any patient, general malaise, weakness, or a poor general impression. In addition, you can assess the blood glucose level of any patient whom you feel has a poor general impression or any alteration in mental status.

Most glucometers operate in much the same manner; however, refer to the manufacturer's instructions for the specific device being used. To obtain a measurement, you will need to use a lancet needle to obtain a drop of blood. Follow the steps in **Skill Drill 10-2** to assess blood glucose level.

There is only a small difference in the blood glucose results when samples are taken from capillary or venous sources. Samples may be obtained from the intravenous (IV) catheter when inserting an IV catheter rather than sticking the patient's finger. A normal glucose level is 80 to 120 mg/dL. Refer to Chapter 21, *Endocrine and Hematologic Emergencies*, for further information and treatment of endocrine conditions.

Like most mechanical devices, the glucometer may fail. Lack of calibration is a common problem for incorrect readings or failure of the device to work. Glucometers also have a set limit and will just read "Hi" above certain levels. Verify that the test strips match the glucometer you are using and are not expired. Most have a shelf life after opening as well, so write the date on the bottle label when it is initially opened. Be familiar with the user manual for the device you are using, and refer to it as needed.

> **Words of Wisdom**
>
> **Medical Assessment Versus Trauma Assessment**
>
> Any patient with a significant MOI or an altered mental status who cannot identify a specific complaint should receive a full head-to-toe assessment or full-body exam. The assessment of a patient without a traumatic injury who has a specific complaint should focus on the body system specific to the complaint.

Systematically Assess the Patient: Full-Body Exam

The goal of the full-body exam is to identify hidden injuries or identify causes that may not have been found during the 60- to 90-second rapid exam that took place during the primary survey. Any patient who has sustained a significant MOI, is unresponsive, or is in critical condition should receive this type of exam after life threats have been managed. An unresponsive patient is unable to tell you what is wrong; therefore, this type of exam may give you clues to identify the problem.

To perform a full-body exam of a patient with no suspected spinal injuries, follow the steps in **Skill Drill 10-3**. To perform a full-body exam in which the patient has sustained significant trauma, ensure manual stabilization is still in place and follow the steps in Skill Drill 10-3.

Skill Drill 10-2 Assessing Blood Glucose Level

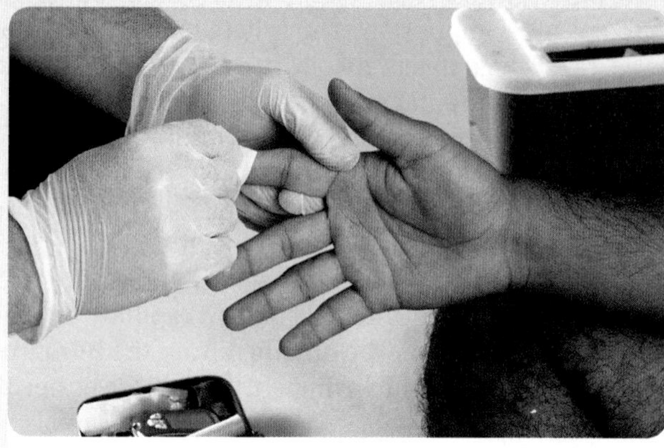

Step 1 Take standard precautions. Select, check, and assemble the equipment (glucometer, test strip, needle or spring-loaded puncture device, alcohol prep pads). Turn on the glucometer and insert a test strip. Cleanse the fingertip with an alcohol prep pad.

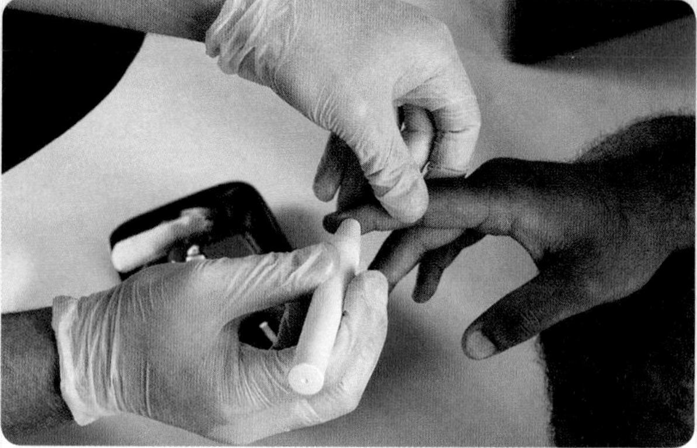

Step 2 Puncture the prepped site with lancet needle or puncture device, drawing capillary blood.

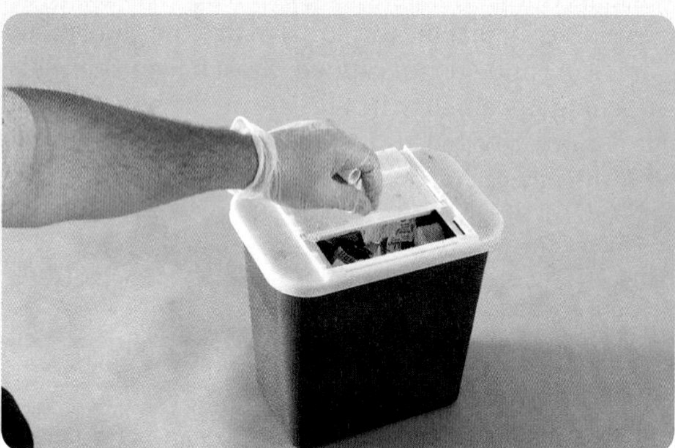

Step 3 Dispose of the lancet needle in a sharps container.

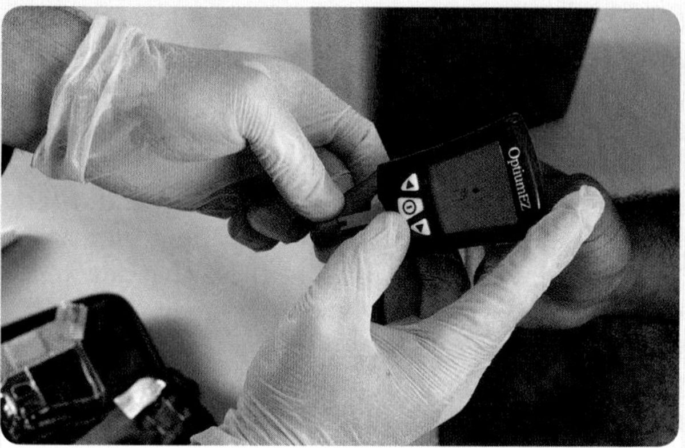

Step 4 Obtain a blood sample and transfer it to the test strip. Insert the test strip into the glucometer and activate the device per the manufacturer's instructions.

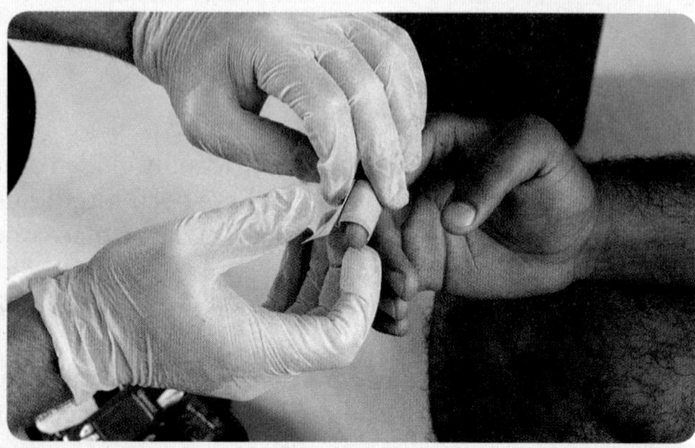

Step 5 Dress the fingertip wound with pressure and an alcohol prep pad, then place a bandage over the puncture site. Record the reading from the glucometer and document appropriately.

Skill Drill 10-3 Performing the Full-Body Exam

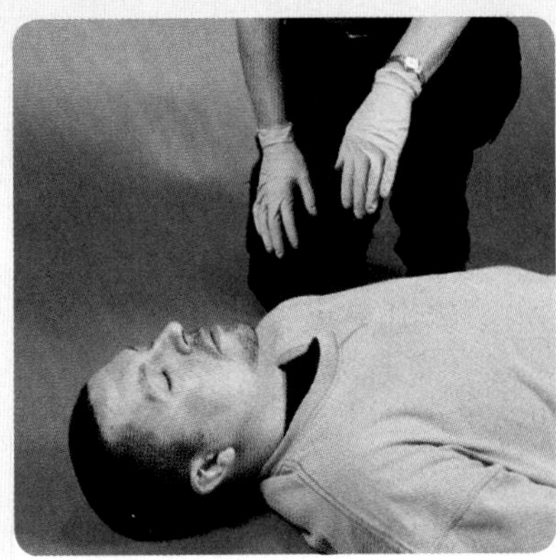

Step 1 Examine the face for obvious lacerations, bruises, and deformities. Maintain manual stabilization if spinal injury is suspected.

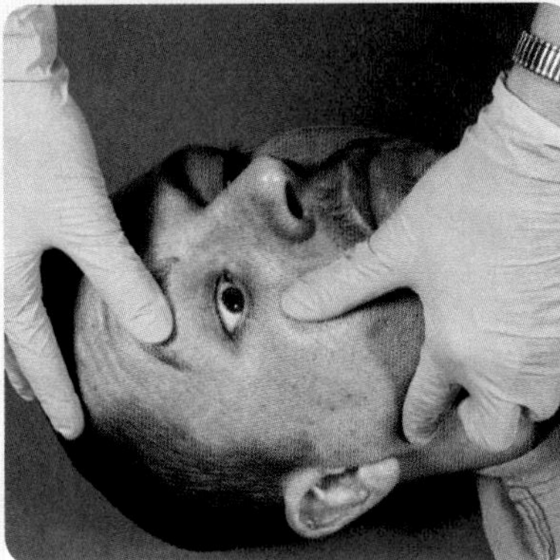

Step 2 Inspect the area around the eyes and eyelids.

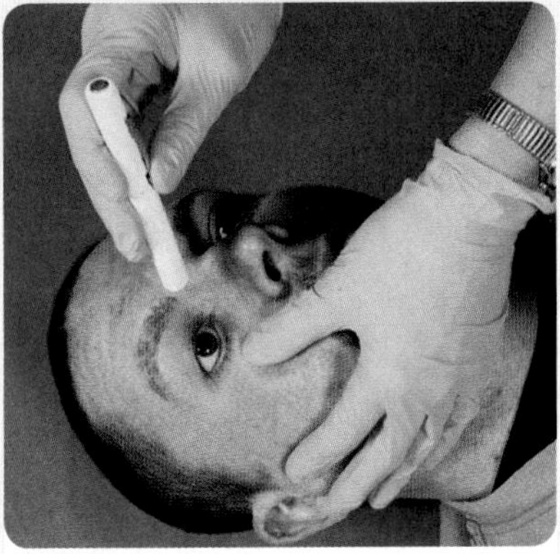

Step 3 Examine the eyes for redness and for contact lenses. Assess pupils using a penlight.

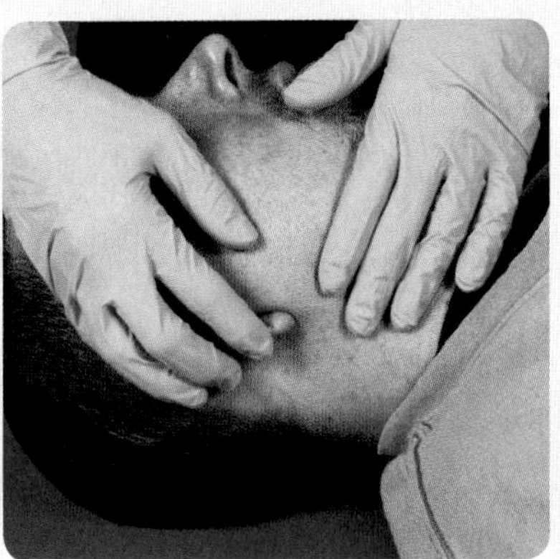

Step 4 Look behind the ears to assess for bruising (Battle sign).

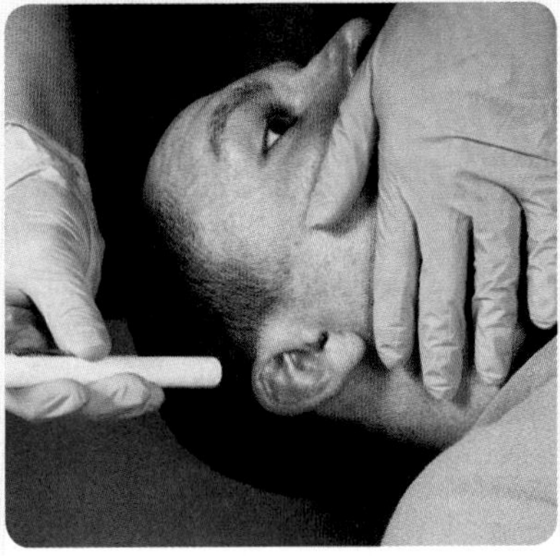

Step 5 Use the penlight to look for drainage of spinal fluid or blood in the ears.

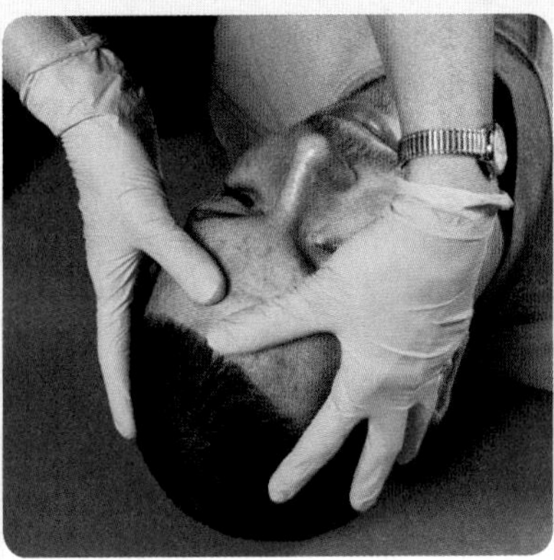

Step 6 Examine the head for bruising and lacerations. Palpate for tenderness, depressions of the skull, and deformities.

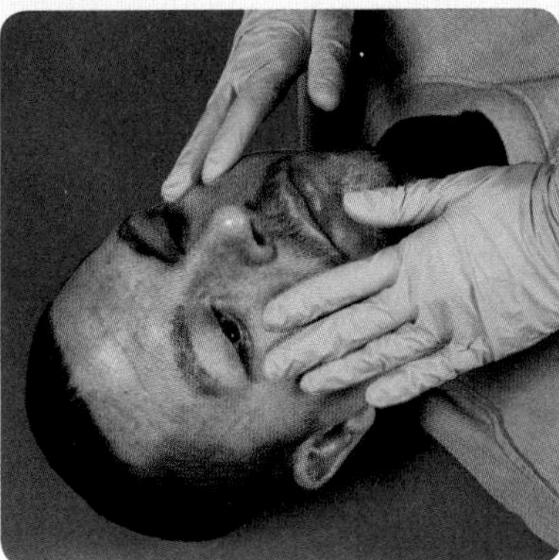

Step 7 Palpate the zygomas (cheekbones) for tenderness or instability.

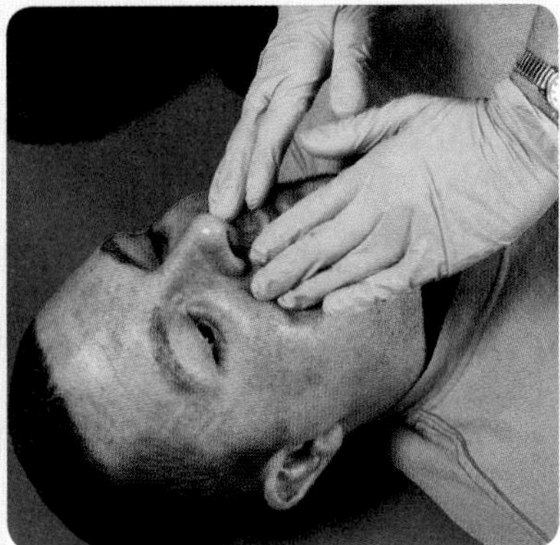

Step 8 Palpate the maxillae.

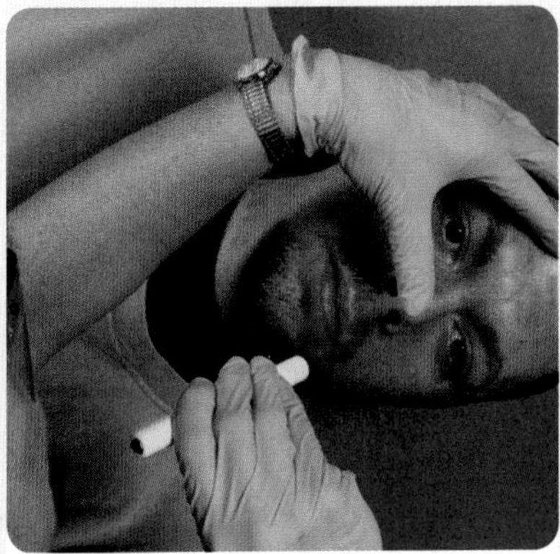

Step 9 Check the nose for blood and drainage.

(continued)

Skill Drill 10-3 Performing the Full-Body Exam *(continued)*

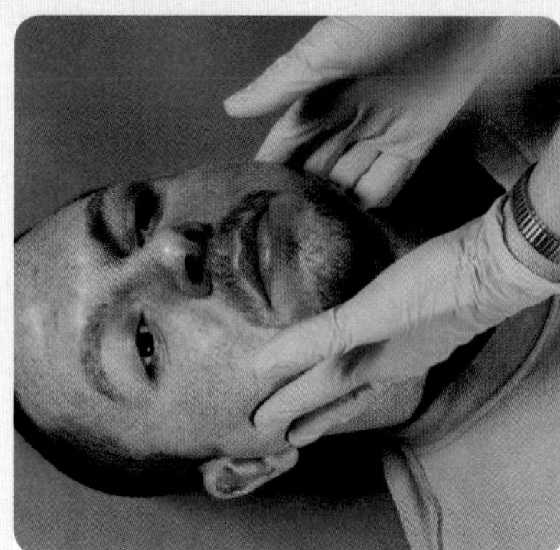

Step 10 Palpate the mandible.

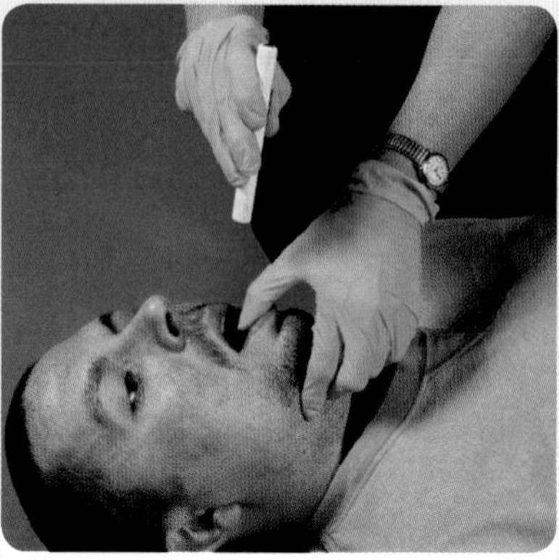

Step 11 Assess the mouth and nose for cyanosis, foreign bodies (including loose teeth or dentures), bleeding, lacerations, and deformities.

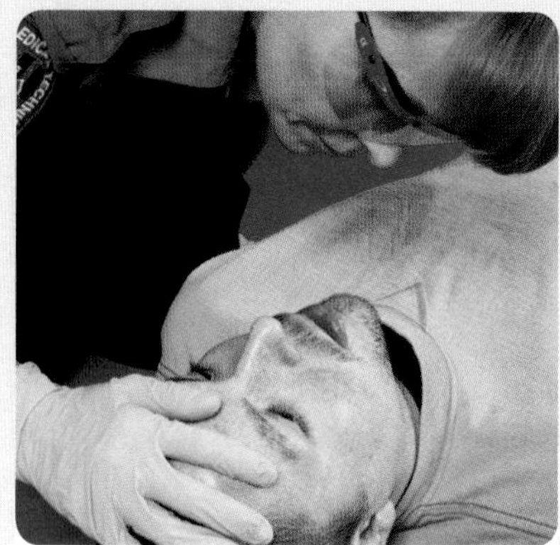

Step 12 Check for unusual odors on the patient's breath.

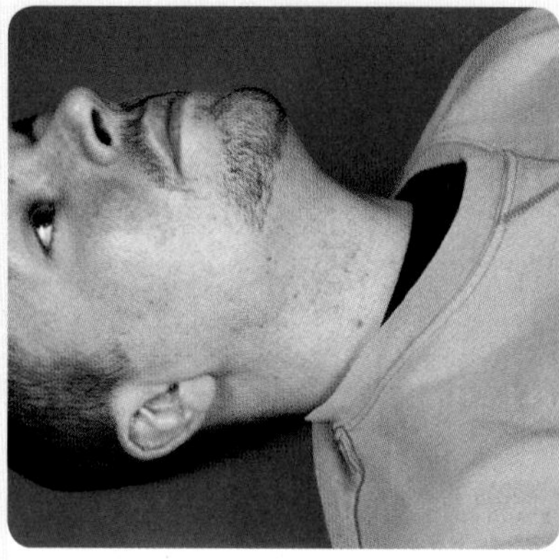

Step 13 Inspect the neck for obvious lacerations, bruises, and deformities. Observe for jugular vein distention and/or tracheal deviation. Apply a cervical collar if spinal injury is suspected.

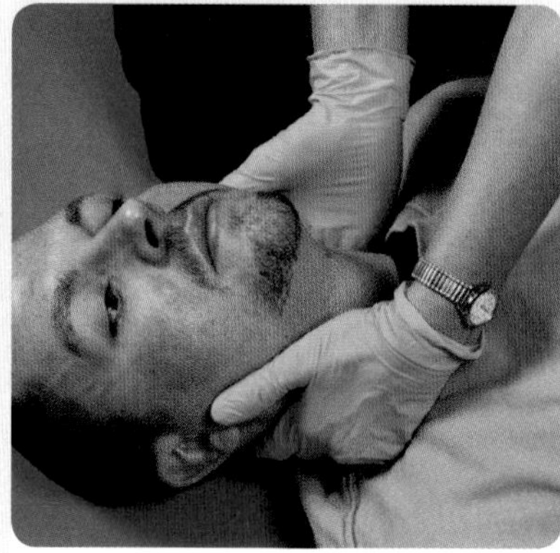

Step 14 Palpate the front and the back of the neck for tenderness and deformity.

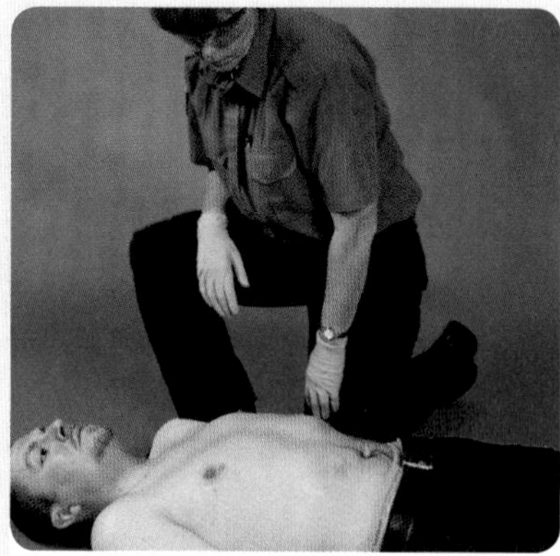

Step 15 Inspect the chest for obvious signs of injury before you begin palpation. Watch for movement of the chest with respirations. Assess the work of breathing.

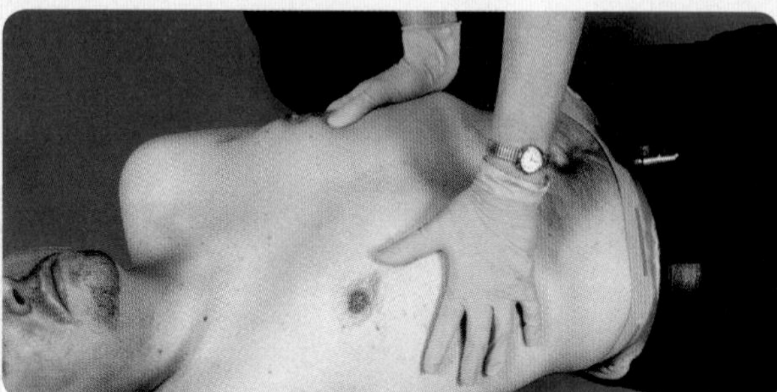

Step 16 Gently palpate over the ribs to elicit tenderness. Avoid pressing over obvious bruises and fractures.

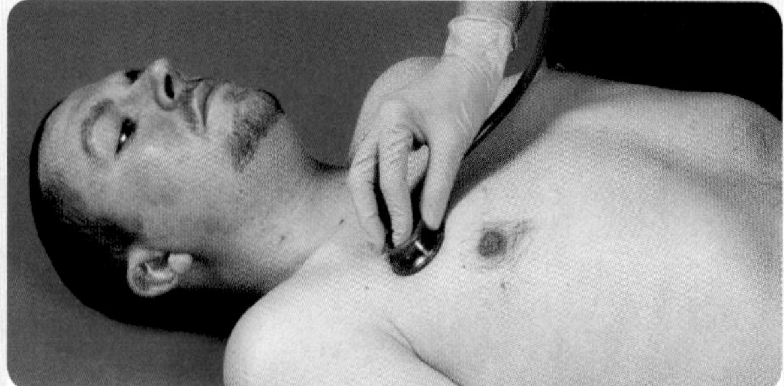

Step 17 Listen for anterior breath sounds over the major airways (midaxillary and midclavicular lines).

Skill Drill 10-3 Performing the Full-Body Exam *(continued)*

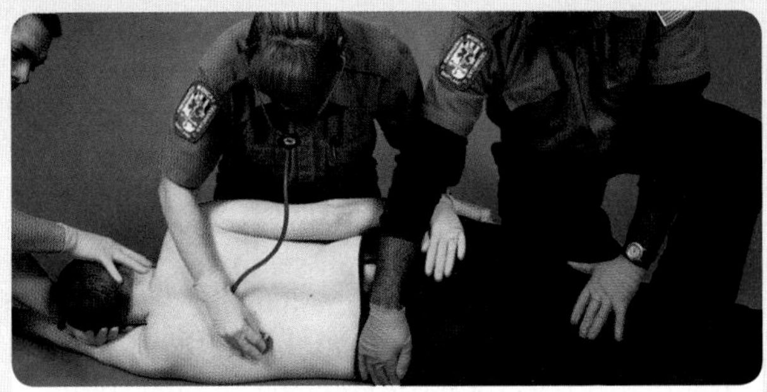

Step 18 Listen also to posterior breath sounds over the lower lungs (bases) and upper lungs (apices). Assess the lungs including the bases and apexes of the lungs. At this point, also assess the back for tenderness and deformities, so you log roll the patient only once. Remember, if you suspect a spinal cord injury, then use spinal precautions as you log roll the patient.

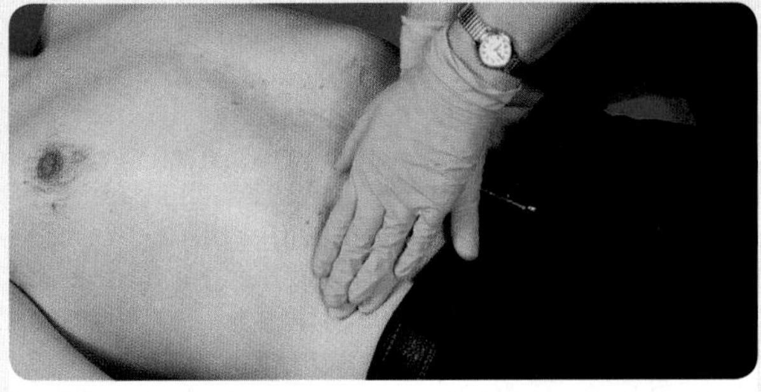

Step 19 Look at the abdomen and pelvis for obvious lacerations, bruises, and deformities. Gently palpate the abdomen for tenderness. If the abdomen is unusually tense, then describe the abdomen as rigid.

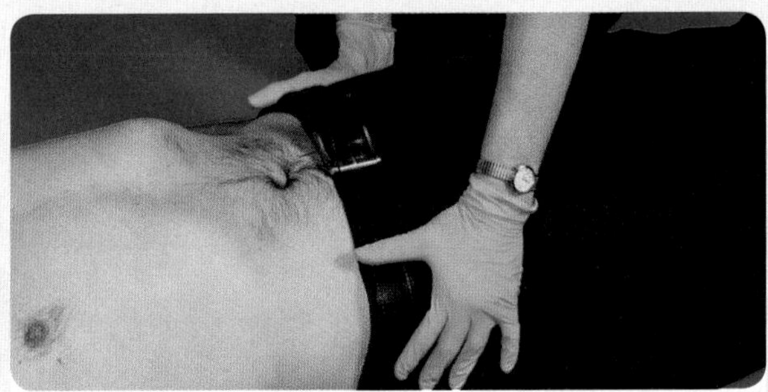

Step 20 Gently compress the pelvis from the sides to assess for tenderness.

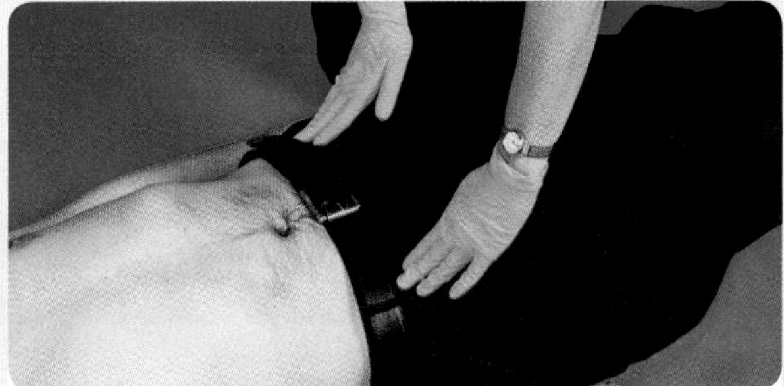

Step 21 Gently press the iliac crests to elicit instability, tenderness, and/or crepitus.

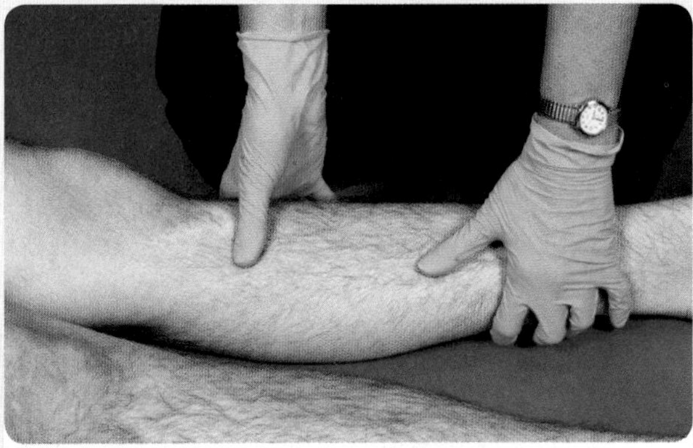

Step 22 Inspect all extremities for lacerations, bruises, swelling, deformities, and medical alert anklets or bracelets. Also assess distal pulses and motor and sensory function in all extremities.

Systematically Assess the Patient: Focused Assessment

A **focused assessment** is generally performed on patients who have sustained nonsignificant MOIs and on responsive medical patients with a specific complaint. This type of exam is based on the chief complaint. Your assessment can focus on a particular body part or system that has been affected. For example, in a person reporting a headache, carefully and systematically assess the head and/or the neurologic system. A person with a laceration on the arm may need to only have that arm evaluated. The goal of a focused assessment is to focus your attention on the immediate problem. Table 10-4 gives examples of common chief complaints and the corresponding focused assessment.

Words of Wisdom

Not all patients present with pedal edema. When you assess for dependent edema, remember that edema collects in the dependent or lowest areas of the body. For a patient who is bedridden, this area is typically in the sacral region of the back.

Respiratory System

You identified and managed life threats during the primary survey. During the secondary assessment, you will perform an exam to help determine which treatment to perform and protocols to follow when the patient's chief complaint is focused on the respiratory system.

Look again for signs of airway obstruction and trauma to the neck and/or chest. Expose the patient's chest, and inspect for overall symmetry. Does the right side of the chest look like the left side? Listen carefully to breath sounds, noting abnormalities. Measure the respiratory rate, chest rise and fall (for tidal volume), and effort. Look for retractions. Is the patient using accessory muscles to help with breathing, and is increased work of breathing present?

Because the location of this complaint is the chest, carefully reevaluate the pulse rate and skin and blood pressure (described in the next section). Inspect and palpate from the clavicles to the shoulder to the abdomen, and reassess breath sounds. Note the presence of subcutaneous emphysema and any abnormalities found, and document those findings on the patient care report. With this information, you can develop a treatment plan and prioritize transport procedures.

YOU are the Provider PART 4

A cervical collar is applied and the decision is made to remove the patient with a vest-type extrication device. Firefighters who have arrived on scene prepare the stretcher and backboard. With the assistance of your partner and a firefighter, you are able to rotate the patient onto the backboard and properly secure her. Pulse, motor, and sensation are reassessed with no change. A quick reassessment determines that the patient is alert and oriented, but does not remember the crash. Respirations and radial pulses are normal and skin is still warm and dry. A quick check of her blood glucose shows 98 mg/dL. The patient is placed in the ambulance and transported to the local trauma center. Reassessment continues and an IV line is started en route. Radiographs show that the patient has a fracture of her sixth cervical vertebra, and the trauma surgeon commends you on a job well done protecting the spine during extrication and transport.

Recording Time: 15 Minutes	
Respirations	16 breaths/min; clear
Pulse	88 beats/min
Skin	Warm, dry, and pink
Blood pressure	116/84 mm Hg
Oxygen saturation (Spo_2)	99% on oxygen at 15 L/min
Pupils	PERRLA

7. How often should you reassess your patients?
8. Why is critical thinking important as an AEMT?

Table 10-4 Common Chief Complaints and Focused Assessments

Chief Complaint	Focused Assessment
Chest pain	Evaluate skin, pulse, and blood pressure. Look for trauma to the chest, assess the external jugular veins, and listen to breath sounds. Assess for peripheral/dependent edema.
Abdominal pain	Evaluate skin, pulse, and blood pressure. Look for trauma to the abdomen, and palpate the abdomen for tenderness or rigidity.
Shortness of breath	Evaluate skin, pulse, blood pressure, and rate and depth of respirations. Assess for airway obstruction. Listen carefully to breath sounds, and assess for hypoxemia (that is, use pulse oximetry). Assess for peripheral/dependent edema.
Dizziness	Evaluate skin, pulse, blood pressure, and adequacy of respirations. Monitor the LOC and orientation carefully. Check the head for signs of trauma. Evaluate for signs of stroke, including facial droop, slurred speech, and one-sided weakness. Use a glucometer to assess blood glucose levels.
Pain associated with bones or joints	Evaluate skin, pulse, movement, and sensation adjacent and distal to the affected area.

Abbreviation: LOC, level of consciousness

Respiratory Rate. As mentioned previously, normal resting respiratory rate varies widely in adults, ranging from approximately 12 to 20 breaths/min. Children breathe at even faster rates. With practice, you will be able to estimate the rate and note whether it is too fast or too slow. Count the number of respirations during your primary survey if you do not feel comfortable with your estimation.

Respirations are determined by counting the number of breaths in a 30-second period and multiplying by two, counting the number of breaths in a 15-second period and multiplying by four, or counting the number of breaths for a full 60 seconds. The result equals the number of breaths per minute. For accuracy, count each breath at the same point in its cycle. This is most easily done by counting each peak chest rise. Although you can see peak chest rise, it is easier to place your hand on the patient's chest and feel it. However, be aware that a responsive patient who knows that you are evaluating his or her breathing will often override the automatic rate and depth by breathing more slowly and deeply. To prevent this from happening, check respirations in a responsive, alert patient without making the patient aware of what you are evaluating. This can be easily done by first taking a radial pulse and then, without releasing the wrist or otherwise suggesting a change, counting the chest rise that you see or feel as the patient's forearm rises and falls with the movement of the chest Figure 10-31. If the patient coughs, yawns, sighs, or talks during the 30-second period, then wait a few seconds and start again. Table 10-5 shows the normal range of respiratory rates of patients who are at rest, as well as normal ranges for other vital signs at various ages.

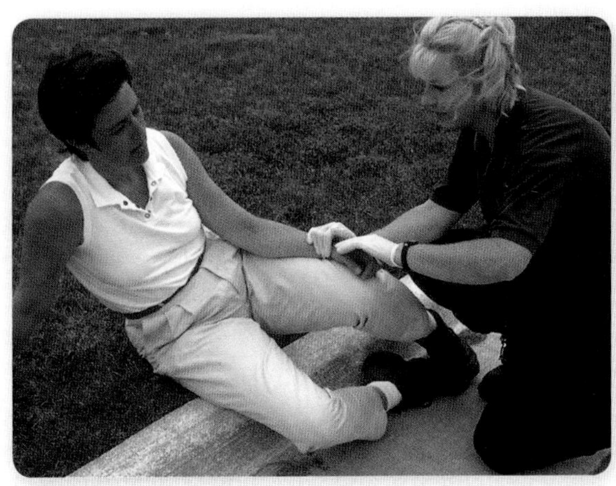

Figure 10-31 Assess respirations in a responsive patient by first taking a radial pulse and then, without releasing the patient's wrist, counting the chest rise and fall for 30 seconds.

Respiratory Rhythm. While counting the patient's respirations, also note the rhythm. If the time from one peak chest rise to the next is fairly consistent, then respirations are considered regular. If respirations vary or change frequently, then they are considered irregular. When you document the vital signs, be sure to note whether the patient's respirations were regular or irregular.

Quality of Breathing. It is helpful to quickly listen to breath sounds on each side of your patient's chest early in the primary survey. This step can help identify the quality

Table 10-5 Normal Vital Signs at Various Ages

Age	Pulse Rate (beats/min)	Respirations (breaths/min)	Blood Pressure (mm Hg)	Temperature (°F)
Neonate (0 to 1 month)	Awake: 100 to 205 Asleep: 90 to 160	30 to 60	Systolic: 67 to 84 Diastolic: 35 to 53 Mean arterial pressure: 45 to 60	98 to 100 (37 to 38°C)
Infant (1 month to 1 year)	Awake: 100 to 180 Asleep: 90 to 160	30 to 53	Systolic: 72 to 104 Diastolic: 37 to 56 Mean arterial pressure: 50 to 62	96.8 to 99.6 (36 to 37.5°C)
Toddler (1 to 2 years)	Awake: 98 to 140 Asleep: 80 to 120	22 to 37	Systolic: 86 to 106 Diastolic: 42 to 63 Mean arterial pressure: 49 to 62	96.8 to 99.6 (36 to 37.5°C)
Preschooler (3 to 5 years)	Awake: 80 to 120 Asleep: 65 to 100	20 to 28	Systolic: 89 to 112 Diastolic: 46 to 72 Mean arterial pressure: 58 to 69	98.6 (37°C)
School-aged child (6 to 12 years)	Awake: 75 to 118 Asleep: 58 to 90	18 to 25	Systolic: 97 to 120 Diastolic: 57 to 80 Mean arterial pressure: 66 to 79	98.6 (37°C)
Adolescent (12 to 15 years)	Awake: 60 to 100 Asleep: 50 to 90	12 to 20	Systolic: 110 to 131 Diastolic: 64 to 83 Mean arterial pressure: 73 to 84	98.6 (37°C)
Early adult (18 to 40 years)	60 to 100	12 to 20	Systolic: 90 to 140	98.6 (37°C)
Middle adult (41 to 60 years)	60 to 100	12 to 20	Systolic: 90 to 140	98.6 (37°C)
Older adult (61 years and older)	60 to 100	12 to 20	Systolic: 90 to 140	98.6 (37°C)

Pediatric data from: American Heart Association (AHA). Vital signs in children. Pediatric Advanced Life Support; Dallas, TX:AHA;2015.

of air movement in both lungs. Decreased or absent breath sounds on one side of the chest and decreased movement in the rise and fall on one side indicate inadequate breathing.

Table 10-6 shows four ways in which the quality or character of respirations can be described. You can determine the quality or character of respirations while you are counting the number of respirations. Use your sense of hearing to listen for breath sounds or use the preferred method of auscultation, listening with a stethoscope.

Normal breathing is silent or, in a quiet environment, accompanied only by the sounds of air movement at the mouth and nose. Through a stethoscope, normal breath sounds include only the sound of air movement through the bronchi accompanied by a soft, low-pitched murmur. Breathing accompanied by other sounds may indicate a significant respiratory condition. If the upper airway has a mild obstruction caused by a foreign body or swelling, then you may hear stridor. If you can hear bubbling or gurgling in the upper airway, then the patient probably has fluid in

Table 10-6 Characteristics of Respirations

Normal (eupneic)	Breathing is neither shallow nor deep Equal chest rise and fall No use of accessory muscles
Shallow	Decreased chest or abdominal wall motion
Labored	Increased breathing effort Use of accessory muscles Possible gasping Nasal flaring, supraclavicular and intercostal retractions in infants and children
Noisy	Increase in sound of breathing, including snoring, wheezing, gurgling, crowing, grunting, and stridor

those passages, potentially impeding the exchange of gases. Suction the patient to avoid **aspiration** of fluid into the lungs. A mild upper airway obstruction is usually a result of the tongue blocking the airway in unresponsive patients. You may hear other sounds, like wheezes or snoring, or a musical sound indicative of a mild lower airway obstruction. The presence of any of these abnormal sounds indicates that an airway or breathing problem exists. With a severe airway obstruction, the patient will not be able to move any air and will no longer be able to cough or talk. Sounds are caused by air moving through small spaces or fluid. If you hear no sounds, then the patient may be moving no air and requires treatment to clear the obstruction.

The following describes how and where to listen to assess breathing:

- First, remember that you can almost always hear a patient's breath sounds better from the patient's back; therefore, if the patient's back is accessible, auscultate (listen) there. If you have stabilized the patient on a backboard or if the patient is in a supine position, then listen from the front and sides Figure 10-32.
- Auscultate over the upper lungs (apices) at approximately 1 inch (2.5 cm) below the clavicle at the midclavicular line, the midlung fields at the third or fourth intercostal space from the patient's posterior, and the lower lungs (bases) at the sixth intercostal space, midaxillary line.
- Lift the clothing or slide the stethoscope under the clothing. When you listen over clothing, you will primarily hear the sound of the stethoscope sliding over the fabric because breath sounds are muted by clothing.
- Place the diaphragm of the stethoscope firmly against the skin to hear the breath sounds.

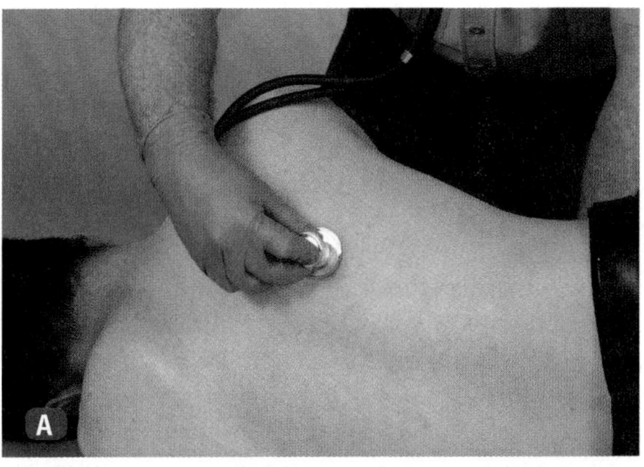

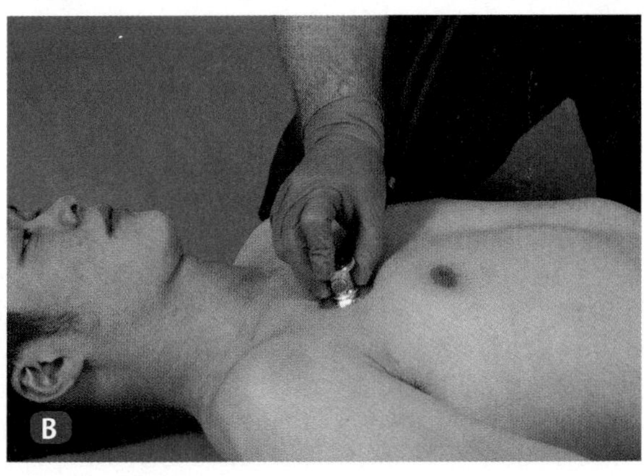

Figure 10-32 A. Listen to breath sounds from the patient's back (if possible), over the apices, the midlung fields, and the bases. **B.** If the patient is immobilized on a backboard or in a supine position, then listen from the front and sides.

During your assessment, you may be able to identify normal breath sounds or **adventitious sounds** (abnormal sounds). Adventitious sounds include crackles, rhonchi, stridor, wheezing, and pleural friction rubs. Breath sounds are described as follows:

- **Normal breath sounds.** These sounds are clear and relatively quiet during inspiration and expiration. Tracheal sounds (noted over the trachea) are loud and harsh. The loud, high-pitched, and hollow sounds noted over the manubrium (over the main stem bronchus) are known as bronchial sounds. The soft, breezy, lower pitched sounds found at the midclavicular line are known as **bronchovesicular sounds**. The finer and somewhat fainter breath sounds noted in the lateral wall of the chest are from the smaller bronchioles and alveoli and are known as **vesicular sounds**.
- **Wheezing breath sounds.** These sounds suggest an obstruction or narrowing of the lower airways. **Wheezing** is a high-pitched whistling sound that is most prominent on expiration, but can also be heard on inspiration in sicker patients. If wheezing is unilateral, then suspect an aspirated foreign body or infection. If wheezing is bilateral, then an inhaled irritant such as chlorine or disease states such as reactive airway disease, asthma, or other less common lung diseases (such as asbestosis) may be the problem.
- **Crackles.** Wet breath sounds may indicate cardiac failure or infection, especially in a young child. Such sounds are often difficult to hear, especially in the back of a moving ambulance. A moist crackling, usually on inspiration and expiration, is called crackles (formerly called rales). Crackles are produced by oxygen passing through moisture in the bronchoalveolar system or by closed alveoli opening abruptly.
- **Rhonchi.** Rhonchi, or congested breath sounds, are continuous sounds with a lower pitch and a rattling quality and are indicative of fluid in the larger airways in the lungs. Rhonchi may indicate the presence of mucus in the lungs, for example, as a result of an infection (such

as pneumonia) or inflammation (such as bronchitis). Expect to hear low-pitched, noisy sounds that are most prominent on expiration. The patient often reports a productive cough associated with these sounds. Aspiration of fluid may also result in rhonchi.

- **Stridor.** **Stridor** is a brassy, crowing sound often heard without a stethoscope. It is caused by the narrowing, swelling, or obstruction of the upper airway and may indicate that the patient has an airway obstruction in the neck or upper part of the chest. It is most prominent on inspiration. Stridor may be caused by bacterial epiglottitis, viral croup, swelling from upper airway burns, anaphylaxis, or a partial foreign body airway obstruction. Onset of crowing or stridor in the presence of fever or upper respiratory infection should be recognized as a potential threat to life.
- **Pleural friction rubs.** These squeaking or grating sounds occur when the pleural linings rub together. If this sound occurs, then the pleural layers have lost their lubrication, most commonly caused by inflammation of the pleura. This condition is usually associated with pain on inspiration. The sounds may be heard any time the chest wall moves; therefore, they can be heard on inspiration, expiration, or both.

A patient who coughs up thick, yellow or green sputum (matter from the lungs) most likely has an advanced respiratory infection. A patient with a chest injury may cough up blood or frothy white or pink sputum caused by blood and fluid mixing with air in the lungs. A patient with congestive heart failure may also cough up frothy sputum. The presence of either substance, regardless of its cause, indicates that an urgent, potentially critical cardiovascular and respiratory problem may exist, possibly requiring oxygenation, ventilation, and other treatments. Without these treatments, the patient's condition may deteriorate rapidly to a point where the patient can no longer breathe.

Depth of Breathing. The amount of air that the patient is exchanging depends on the rate and the tidal volume. **Tidal volume** is a measure of the depth of breathing and is the amount of air in milliliters that is moved into or out of the lungs during one breath. The depth of the breath determines whether the tidal volume is normal, less than normal, or more than normal. Normal tidal volume for an adult is approximately 500 mL or 7 mL/kg per breath. Shallow respirations indicate a decreased tidal volume, and deep respirations indicate an increased tidal volume.

Cardiovascular System. When the patient's chief complaint is associated with chest pain or other discomfort, a physical exam should include looking, listening, and feeling for abnormalities in the patient's thoracic region. Listen for breath sounds and look for trauma to the chest. Consider the pulse and respiratory rate and the blood pressure. Pay particular attention to rate, quality, and rhythm of the pulse. Reevaluate the skin. Check and compare distal pulses to determine any differences in the right and left sides. Consider auscultation for abnormal heart tones, such as those that are muffled; however, keep in mind that obtaining these sounds may be difficult in a noisy prehospital setting.

Pulse Rate. For an adult, the normal resting pulse rate should be between 60 and 100 beats/min and may remain on the higher end of normal in older patients. Generally, in pediatric patients, the younger the patient, the faster the pulse rate. In well-conditioned athletes or in people taking heart medications such as beta blockers, the pulse rate may be considerably lower. See Table 10-5 for the normal ranges of pulse rates for adults and children.

To obtain the pulse rate in most patients, count the number of pulses felt in a 30-second period and then multiply by two, count the number of pulses felt in a 15-second period and multiply by four, or count the number of pulses for a full 60 seconds. A pulse that is weak and difficult to palpate, irregular, or extremely slow should be palpated and counted for a full minute. A pulse rate is counted as beats per minute; however, in reporting the pulse rate, it is not necessary to state or write "beats per minute" after the number.

In an adult patient, a pulse rate that is greater than 100 beats/min is described as **tachycardia**, and a rate of less than 60 beats/min is described as **bradycardia**.

Pulse Quality. Always report the quality, or character, of the pulse whenever reporting or recording the pulse. The pulse is generally palpated at the radial or carotid artery in adults and at the brachial artery in infants, because it is normally strong and easily palpable at these locations. Therefore, if the pulse feels of normal strength, describe it as being strong. Describe a stronger than normal pulse as "bounding" and a pulse that is weak and difficult to feel as "weak" or "thready." With a little experience, you will be able to easily make the necessary distinctions.

Pulse Rhythm. When you are assessing the pulse, you must also determine whether the rhythm is regular or irregular. When the interval between each ventricular contraction of the heart is short, the pulse is rapid. When the interval is longer, the pulse is slower. Regardless of the rate, the interval between each contraction should be the same, and the pulse should occur at a constant, regular rhythm. Document this rhythm as regular.

The rhythm is considered irregular if the heart periodically has an early or late beat or if a pulse beat is missed. Some people have a chronically irregular pulse; however, if an irregular pulse is found in a patient with signs and symptoms that suggest a cardiovascular condition, the patient likely needs advanced cardiac assessment and life support. Therefore, depending on your protocols, call for paramedic backup or initiate rapid transport to definitive care.

With practice, you will be able to assess whether the pulse is too slow, too fast, or irregular without actually counting the pulsations. This will help to speed your assessment of the ABCDEs and allow you to focus on finding other potentially life-threatening problems. A pulse rate that is too slow or too fast may change decisions related to transporting your patient.

Blood Pressure. Adequate blood pressure is necessary to maintain proper circulation and perfusion of the vital organs. **Blood pressure** is the pressure of circulating blood against the walls of the arteries. A decrease in the blood pressure may indicate one of the following:

- Loss of blood or its fluid components
- Loss of vascular tone and sufficient arterial constriction to maintain the necessary pressure even without any actual fluid or blood loss
- A cardiac pumping problem
- An overdose of a beta blocker or other antihypertensive medication

When any of these conditions occurs and results in a decrease in circulation, the body's compensatory mechanisms are activated, resulting in an increased heart rate and constriction of the arteries. Normal blood pressure is maintained, and by decreasing the blood flow to the skin and extremities, available blood volume is temporarily redirected to the vital organs so that they remain adequately perfused. However, as shock progresses, and the body's defense mechanisms can no longer keep up, the blood pressure will fall. Decreased blood pressure is a late sign of shock and indicates that the patient is in the critical phase of decompensated shock unless the patient is experiencing neurogenic (or spinal) shock. Any patient with a markedly low blood pressure has inadequate pressure to maintain proper perfusion of all of the vital organs and needs to have his or her blood pressure and perfusion restored immediately to a normal level.

When the blood pressure becomes elevated, the body's defenses act to reduce it. Some people have chronically high blood pressure from progressive narrowing of the arteries that occurs with age, and during an acute episode, their blood pressure may increase to even higher levels. Head injury or a number of other conditions may also cause blood pressure to rise to high levels. Abnormally high blood pressure may result in a rupture or other critical damage in the arterial system.

Blood pressure contains two key separate components: systolic pressure and diastolic pressure. **Systolic pressure** is the increased pressure that is caused along the artery with each contraction (systole) of the ventricles and the pulse wave that it produces. This is the pumping, or working, phase of the heart. **Diastolic pressure** is the residual pressure that remains in the arteries during the relaxing phase of the cycle of the heart (diastole), when the left ventricle is at rest. This is the resting phase, and it should be significantly lower than the systolic pressure. Systolic pressure represents the maximum pressure to which the arteries are subjected, and the diastolic pressure represents the minimum amount of pressure that is always present in the arteries.

Early blood pressure gauges contained a column of mercury and a linear scale that was graduated in millimeters. Even though different gauges are used today, the blood pressure is still measured in millimeters of mercury (mm Hg). Blood pressure is reported as a fraction in the form of systolic pressure over diastolic pressure. Therefore, if the patient's systolic pressure is 120 and the diastolic pressure is 78, then you would record it as "BP 120/78 mm Hg." You would report the patient's blood pressure verbally as "BP is 120 over 78."

Avoid taking a blood pressure on an arm if the patient has an IV site, a central line catheter, or a port; has a dialysis fistula or shunt; has had a mastectomy on that side; or has an injury to that arm. You can ask the patient if any of these exist if they are not visible; for example, a mastectomy. If a patient has chronic renal failure and is undergoing dialysis, then you may ask if the patient has a fistula or any other reason that you should not take a blood pressure using that arm.

A blood pressure cuff with gauge (sphygmomanometer) contains the following components **Figure 10-33**:

- A wide outer cuff designed to be fastened snugly around the entire arm or leg
- An inflatable wide bladder sewn into a portion of the cuff
- A ball-pump with a one-way valve that allows air to enter and a turn-valve that can be closed or, when opened, will allow air to be released at a controlled speed from the cuff
- A pressure gauge calibrated in millimeters of mercury, which indicates the pressure that exists in the cuff that is being applied against the underlying artery

Most EMS agencies carry at least four sizes of blood pressure cuffs: obese, adult, pediatric, and infant **Figure 10-34**. A thigh cuff is also available. Be sure to

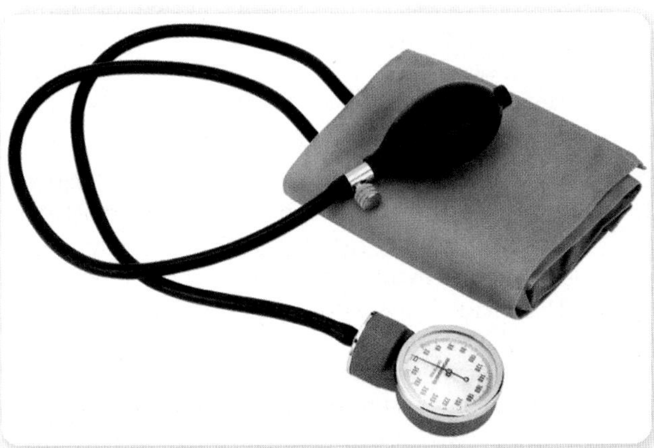

Figure 10-33 A sphygmomanometer.

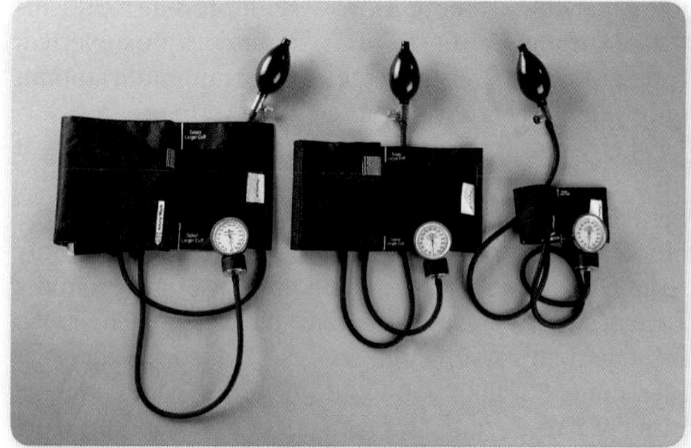

Figure 10-34 Blood pressure cuffs: thigh, adult, and pediatric.

select the appropriately sized cuff. A cuff that is too small may result in falsely high readings; a cuff that is too large may result in falsely low readings. The normal size cuff is designed to wrap around the arm 1 to 1.5 times and take up two-thirds the length from the armpit to the crease in the elbow of most adults. Use an obese or thigh cuff with patients who are obese or have exceptionally well-developed arm muscles, and to take the blood pressure in the thigh in patients who have injuries in both arms. Use a small pediatric cuff with children and exceptionally small adults. Measure the blood pressure in all patients older than 3 years.

The auscultatory method (listening) is the most common means of measuring a patient's blood pressure. A blood pressure cuff is applied to a patient's upper arm, allowing for the compression of the brachial artery when inflated. This compression creates turbulence and arterial vibrations that make sounds that can be heard using a stethoscope. These sounds are known as Korotkoff sounds. As the cuff is released, the blood flow returns to the artery, and Korotkoff sounds will be heard, denoting the systolic pressure. The disappearance of Korotkoff sounds indicates the diastolic pressure reading.

Follow the steps in Skill Drill 10-4 to measure blood pressure by auscultation.

Words of Wisdom

Blood pressure is most often measured by auscultation with the patient in a sitting or semisitting position. Be sure to note whether a different method or position was used. Occasionally when a patient's blood pressure is very low, you will continue to hear pulse sounds from the reading at which they started all the way until the gauge has reached 0. When this occurs, record the diastolic pressure as "0" or "all the way down" to indicate that pulse sounds were heard until the gauge read "0."

Skill Drill 10-4 Obtaining Blood Pressure by Auscultation

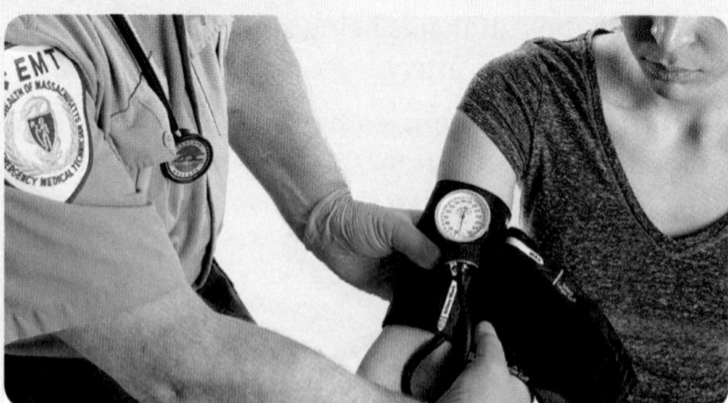

Step 1 Take standard precautions. Check for ports, central lines, mastectomy, dialysis fistula, and injury to the arm. If any are present, then use the brachial artery on the other arm. Apply the cuff snugly. The lower border of the cuff should be about 1 inch (2.5 cm) above the antecubital space (the crease at the inside of the patient's elbow). Ensure the center of the inflatable bladder, which is usually marked by an arrow on the cuff, lies over the brachial artery.

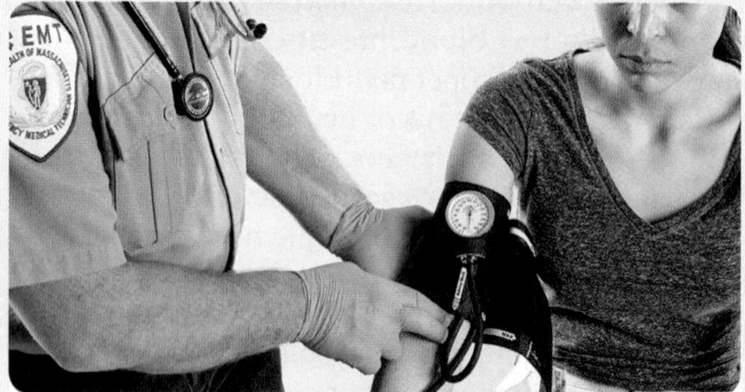

Step 2 Support the exposed arm at the level of the heart. With your nondominant hand, palpate the brachial artery (in the antecubital fossa, the anterior aspect of the elbow) to determine where to place the stethoscope.

Skill Drill 10-4 Obtaining Blood Pressure by Auscultation *(continued)*

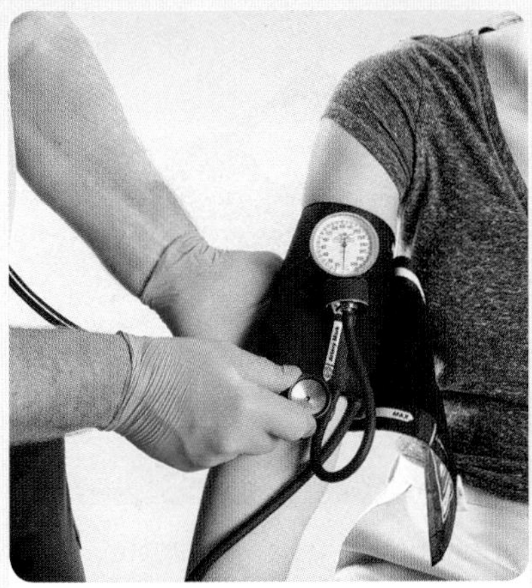

Step 3 Place the bell (if one is present) of the stethoscope over the brachial artery, and hold it firmly against the artery with the fingers of your nondominant hand. Hold the rubber ball-pump in the palm of your other hand and the turn-valve between your thumb and first finger.

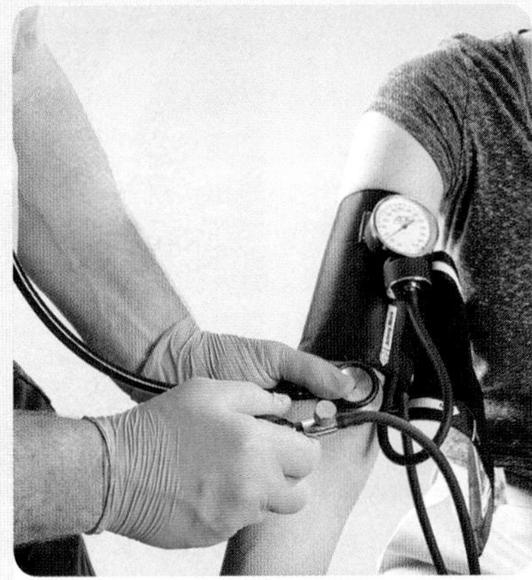

Step 4 Close the valve tightly, and pump to 30 mm Hg above the point at which you stop hearing pulse sounds. Next, slowly turn the valve, opening it until air is steadily escaping from the cuff and you see the needle of the gauge slowly drop. The systolic pressure is the first time you hear the Korotkoff sound. The diastolic pressure is the last time it is heard.

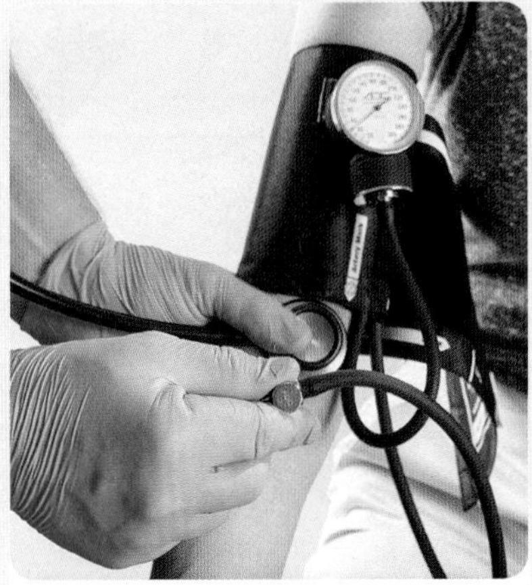

Step 5 As soon as the pulse sounds stop, open the valve, and quickly release remaining air. After you have finished measuring the blood pressure, document your findings and the time at which the blood pressure was taken.

Obtaining a patient's blood pressure accurately by auscultation may be difficult at times. Noisy environments, patient movement from tremors or seizures, external vibrations from the EMS vehicle, and excessive noises may produce sounds that mimic Korotkoff sounds and provide inaccurate readings. Other variables that may make obtaining an accurate blood pressure reading nearly impossible are uncooperative adults, infants and children, and patients who are hypotensive with poor perfusion. In these cases, measure blood pressure by palpation.

The palpation (touch) method does not depend on your ability to hear sounds and should be used in these cases to obtain a patient's blood pressure. If possible, then it is preferable that you first obtain a baseline auscultated blood pressure. Follow the steps in Skill Drill 10-5 to measure blood pressure by palpation.

Normal Blood Pressure. Blood pressure levels vary with age and sex. Refer to Table 10-5 for normal blood pressure ranges.

A patient has **hypotension** when the blood pressure is lower than the normal range and **hypertension** when the blood pressure is higher than the normal range.

Typically, you will assess fewer children than adults; therefore, you might not remember the normal ranges for the various age groups. It is a good idea to carry a chart with you that lists normal blood pressure ranges and other vital signs.

Words of Wisdom

Often, the most important information associated with the blood pressure is not the absolute value at any one point, but the trend in the pressure over the course of time you are caring for a patient.

When assessing a patient's general circulation, the blood pressure, pulse, skin temperature, and capillary refill should not be assessed in an injured limb. However,

Secondary Assessment

Skill Drill 10-5 Obtaining Blood Pressure by Palpation

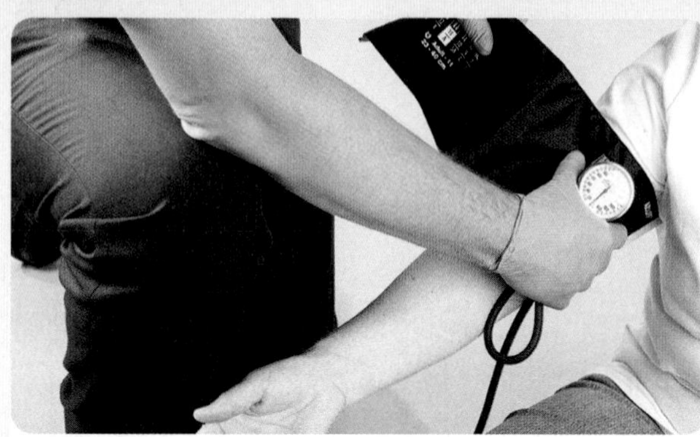

Step 1 Secure the appropriately sized cuff around the patient's upper arm in the manner previously described.

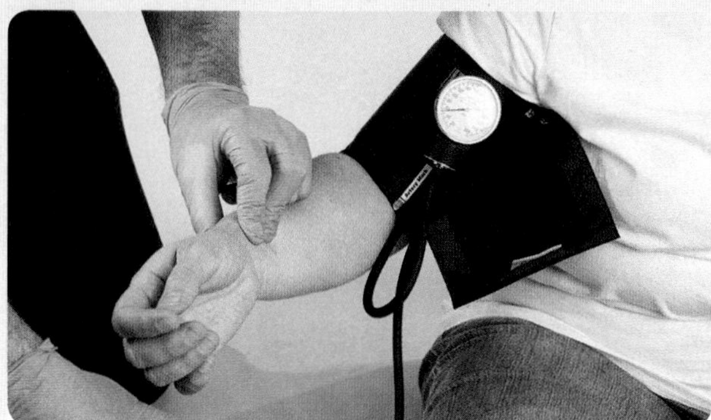

Step 2 With your nondominant hand, palpate the patient's radial pulse on the same arm as the cuff. After you have located it, do not move your fingertips until you have completed taking the blood pressure.

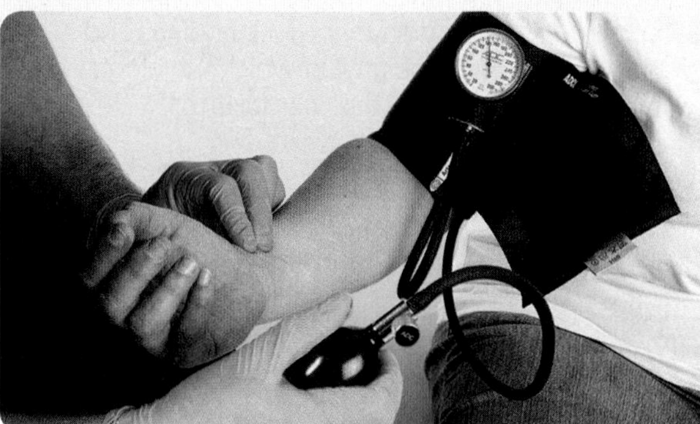

Step 3 While holding the ball-pump in your other hand, close the turn-valve and slowly inflate the cuff until the pulse disappears and then continue to inflate another 30 mm Hg. As the cuff inflates, you will no longer feel the pulse under your fingertips.

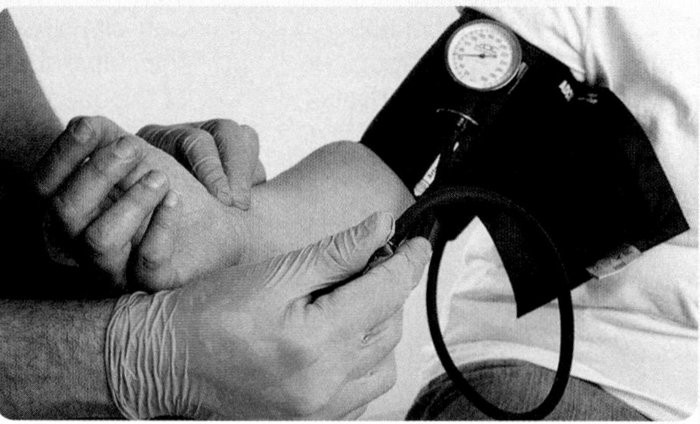

Step 4 Open the turn-valve so that air slowly escapes from the cuff, and carefully observe the gauge. When you can again feel the radial pulse under your fingertips, note the reading on the gauge as the patient's systolic blood pressure.

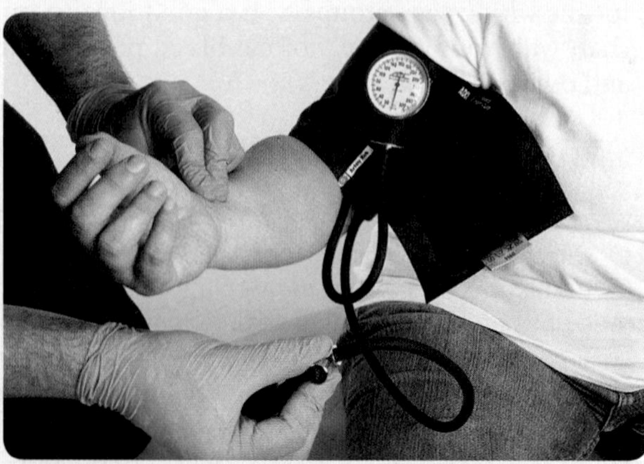

Step 5 Next, open the turn-valve further, and completely deflate the cuff. Document your findings, including the time, and note that the pressure was taken by palpation.

after you have obtained these vital signs from an uninjured limb, you might want to compare the distal skin temperature, quality of the distal pulse, and/or CRT in the injured limb with those found on the uninjured side. This information is useful in evaluating whether the injury may have compromised the circulation in the injured limb.

Neurologic System

A neurologic assessment should be performed any time you are confronted with a patient who has changes in mental status, a possible head injury, stupor, dizziness, drowsiness, or syncope. A neurologic assessment begins without even touching the patient. It can be as simple as talking with the patient, asking questions, and evaluating the reply from the patient. This step may be performed during the primary survey.

Evaluate the LOC and orientation to determine the patient's ability to think. Use the AVPU scale to determine the patient's mental status. Is the person alert, oriented to person, place, time, and event? Is the patient responsive or unresponsive? Does the patient respond to verbal and painful stimuli? If the patient is responsive, then evaluate speech for clarity, speed, organization, and logic. When evaluating speech, assess the patient's thought process and determine if he or she may be delusional or has unusual reasoning. Consider the following questions to help assess the neurologic system:

- What is the patient's activity level?
- What are the patient's mood and thought content?
- What do the patient's facial expressions tell you? Is the patient angry, fearful, depressed, anxious, or restless?
- Does the patient appear uncomfortable?
- Does the patient make incomprehensible or understandable statements?
- Is the patient's memory affected?
- Does the patient remember who family members are?
- What is the patient's perception or view of what is happening?

Inspect the head for trauma. Pulse, blood pressure, and skin changes may indicate hypoperfusion of the brain.

You can further assess mental status by considering whether the patient is alert and oriented (A × O) in four areas: person, place, time, and the event itself, and determining the GCS score, as discussed in the Primary Survey section of this chapter.

Finally, as part of your brief neurologic evaluation, assess for any gross neurologic deficits by having the patient carefully move all extremities to pinpoint any motor deficits. Assess bilaterally for motor strength or weakness by asking the patient to move each extremity against the resistance of your hands. Assess grip strength by having the patient squeeze two of your fingers bilaterally and simultaneously, so that any unilateral neurologic deficits will be obvious. Quickly assess for any loss of sensation by touching the distal portions of the extremities with a blunt or sharp object to assess for any gross sensory defects.

Table 10-7 Pupillary Reactions

Appearance	Possible Causes
Round and equal size	Normal condition
Fixed with no reaction to light	Depressed brain function (head injury or stroke)
Fully dilated and fixed (blown pupil)	Increased intracranial pressure
Dilate with bright light, constrict with low light	Depressed brain function
Constricted	Drugs (opiates) or bright light
Dilated	Drugs (barbiturates) or dim lighting
Sluggish reaction	Severe increase in intracranial pressure
Unequal size	Depressed brain function Medication placed in eye Injury or condition of the eye Congenital **anisocoria** (normally unequal pupils)[a]

[a] Approximately 20% of the population has anisocoria. In such cases, the pupils usually differ in size by less than 1 mm. (Anisocoria and Horner's syndrome. American Association for Pediatric Ophthalmology and Strabismus website. https://www.aapos.org/terms/conditions/27. Updated August 2016. Accessed October 20, 2016.)

Pupils. Assessing the pupils is an important consideration when assessing the neurologic system Table 10-7. The pupil is the black center of the pigmented iris of the eye. The diameter and reactivity to light of the patient's pupils reflect the status of the brain's perfusion, oxygenation, and condition. The pupils are normally round and of approximately equal size and adjust in size depending on the available light. Normally, pupil size changes instantly to any change in light level. In normal room light, the pupil should appear to be midsize. When a bright light is suddenly introduced, the pupils instantly constrict, allowing less light to enter, protecting the sensitive receptors in the inner eye from damage

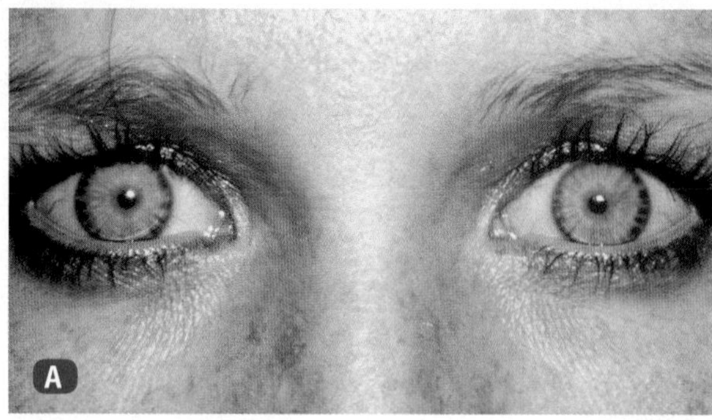

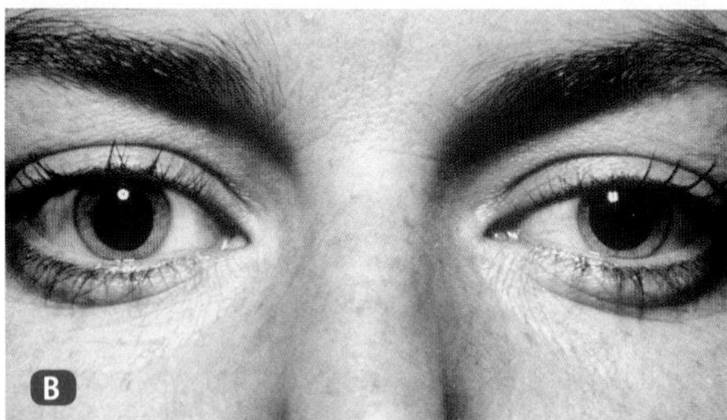

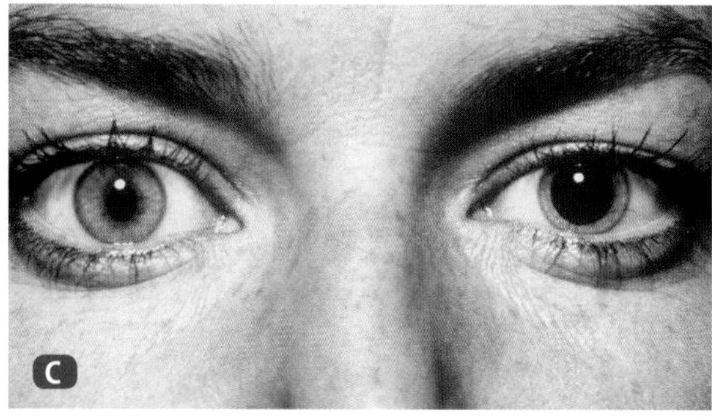

Figure 10-35 **A.** Constricted pupils. **B.** Dilated pupils. **C.** Unequal pupils (anisocoria).

Figure 10-35A. When a bright light is introduced into one eye (or higher levels of light enter one eye only), both pupils should constrict equally to the appropriate size for the pupil receiving the most light.

With less light, the pupils dilate, allowing more light to enter the eye, making it possible to see even in dim light. In the absence of any light, the pupils will become fully relaxed and dilated Figure 10-35B. When light is introduced, each eye sends sensory signals to the brain, indicating the level of light it is receiving. Pupil size is regulated by a series of continuous motor commands that the brain automatically sends through the oculomotor nerves (third cranial nerve) to each eye, causing both pupils to constrict to the same appropriate size. In the presence of light, a single pupil that remains fully dilated is generally caused by pressure on the oculomotor nerve on that side of the head due to increasing intracranial pressure. Bilateral dilated pupils that do not respond to light are usually due to death.

A small number of people have normally unequal pupils (anisocoria), which is usually congenital Figure 10-35C. If the patient or family member cannot confirm the presence of this condition, then you must assume the patient has depressed brain function as a result of CNS depression or injury if the pupils react in any of the following ways:

- Become fixed (either dilated or constricted) with no reaction to changes in light
- Dilate with introduction of a bright light and constrict when the light is removed
- React sluggishly instead of briskly
- Become unequal in size
- Become unequal in size when a bright light is introduced into or removed from one eye

Some of the causes of depressed brain function include the following situations:

- Injury of the brain or brainstem
- Trauma
- Stroke
- Brain tumor
- Inadequate oxygenation or perfusion
- Drugs or toxins (CNS depressants)

Words of Wisdom

Opiates, which are one category of CNS depressants, cause the pupils to constrict significantly, regardless of light. They become so small as to be described as pinpoint. Intracranial pressure from intracranial bleeding may cause sufficient pressure against the oculomotor nerve on one side so that the motor commands can no longer pass from the brain to that eye. When this occurs, the eye no longer receives commands to constrict, and its pupil becomes fully dilated and fixed. This finding is described as a "blown" pupil.

The mnemonic PERRLA is a useful guide in assessing the pupils. The letters stand for the following:

P Pupils
E Equal
R Round and
R Reactive to
L Light and
A Accommodation

For patients with normal pupils, you can report "pupils are equal, round, and reactive to light and accommodation (react properly)" or "Pupils PERRLA." Describe any abnormal findings using the longer form, such as "Pupils are equal and round, the left pupil is fixed and dilated, and the right pupil is regular in size and reacts to light."

Assessing Neurovascular Status. Now perform a hands-on assessment to determine motor and sensory response. How does the patient move? Check for bilateral muscle strength and weaknesses. Complete a thorough sensory assessment. Test for pain, sensations, and position, and compare distal and proximal motor and sensory responses and one side with the other. Remember that a physical exam that deals with a specific chief complaint can be streamlined to assess a specific area of concern.

Anatomic Regions

Head, Neck, and Cervical Spine. Inspect for abnormalities of the head, neck, and cervical spine. Gently palpate the scalp and skull for any pain, deformity, tenderness, **crepitus**, and bleeding **Figure 10-36**. Ask a responsive patient if he or she feels any pain or tenderness. Look at the patient's face. Is it symmetrical? Is any evidence of trauma present, such as ecchymosis or hematomas? Does the patient have any facial expressions such as a smile or grimace? Check the patient's face for the presence of a rash and petechiae (tiny red, purple, or brown spots on the skin caused by bleeding that may look like a rash), which suggest an infectious process and should alert you to the necessity for a mask and goggles. Check the patient's eyes, and assess pupillary function, shape, and response. Are the pupils equal in size and reactive to light, or are they constricted, dilated, or unequal? Check the color of the sclera. Check for foreign objects or blood in the eye and for bruising or discoloration around the eyes and behind the ears; these signs may be associated with head trauma. Assess the patient's zygomas for possible injury. Check the patient's ears and nose for fluid. Next, before opening the patient's mouth, check the upper (maxilla) and lower (mandible) jaws. After the patient's jaws have been assessed and it has been determined that movement will not create additional pain or injury, open the patient's mouth, looking for any broken or missing teeth. Blood and secretions impairing the airway should have been corrected during the primary survey. Before moving on to the neck, note any unusual odors that may be present in the patient's mouth. Odors such as a strong alcohol odor or fruity odor suggest the need to check the blood glucose level.

Words of Wisdom

Because many steps require patient cooperation, you will not be able to assess motor and sensory function in an unresponsive patient. A Babinski test may be used to check for sensation in an unresponsive patient. This test is accomplished by rubbing a pen or other object along the sole of the patient's foot. A normal reaction in young children and infants is for the great toe to flex toward the top of the foot and the other toes to fan out. However, this is an abnormal reaction in older children and adults. Do not perform a Babinski test on a patient who has injuries to the lower extremities. This test could cause the patient to pull the leg back, causing further injury.

Next, check the neck for signs of swelling or bleeding. Palpate the neck for signs of trauma, such as deformities, bumps, swelling, bruising, and bleeding, and for a crackling sound produced by air bubbles under the skin, also known as **subcutaneous emphysema** **Figure 10-37**. Also, in patients in whom spinal injury is not suspected, inspect for pronounced or distended jugular veins with the patient sitting at a 45° angle. This is a normal finding in a person who is lying down; however, jugular venous distention in a patient who is sitting up suggests a problem with blood returning to the heart. Carefully report and record your findings.

Chest. Next, expose the patient's chest. Inspect, visualize, and palpate over the chest area for injury or signs of

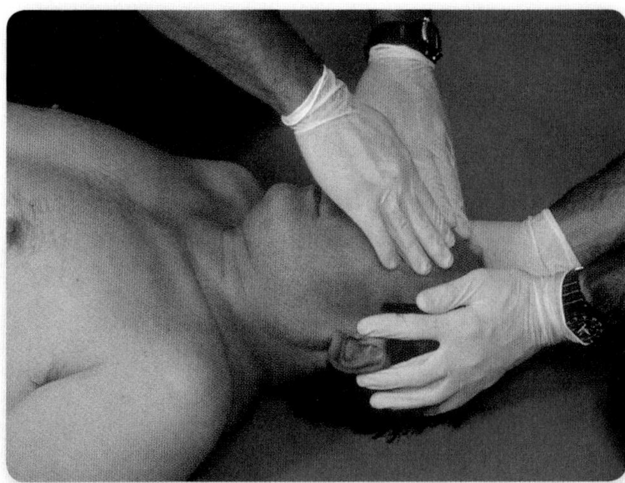

Figure 10-36 Gently palpate the head for any pain, deformity, tenderness, crepitus, and bleeding.

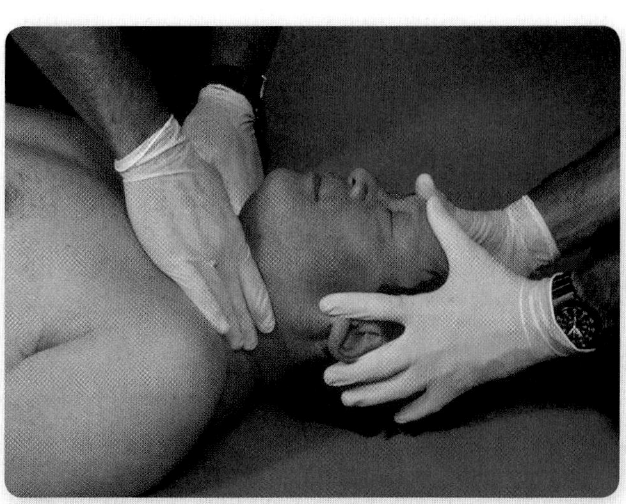

Figure 10-37 Gently palpate the neck.

trauma, including bruising, tenderness, and swelling. Watch the chest rise and fall with breathing. Normal breathing should be symmetric, in which both sides of the chest rise and fall together. Look for signs of abnormal breathing, including retractions (when the skin pulls in around the ribs during inspiration) and **paradoxical motion** (when one section rises on inspiration while the remainder of the chest falls).

Intercostal retractions indicate that the patient has some condition that is impairing the flow of air into and out of the lungs. Paradoxical motion is associated with a fracture of several ribs (flail chest), causing a section of the chest to move independently from the rest of the chest wall. When palpating the chest, note if there is any crepitus, which is indicative of fractured ribs. Do not purposely elicit for crepitus because this action may cause further injury to the patient. Palpate the chest for subcutaneous emphysema, especially in cases of severe blunt chest trauma. This finding could indicate a pneumothorax.

Auscultate breath sounds as described previously. Evaluate air movement in and out of the lungs and to determine the presence of unilaterally diminished or absent breath sounds. You may hear normal breath sounds or adventitious breath sounds (crackles, wheezes, rhonchi, stridor, or pleural friction rub). Remember that breath sounds are easier to hear from the patient's back; place the stethoscope under the patient's clothing, and be sure to compare side to side, listening over the upper part of the lungs (apices), the lower part of the lungs (bases), and the major airways (midclavicular and midaxillary lines). If the patient's breathing is abnormal, then reassess breathing and, if appropriate, assist with ventilations.

Abdomen. Look for trauma to the abdomen and for distention. Palpate the abdomen for tenderness, rigidity, and patient **guarding.** If the patient is alert, then ask about pain as you perform the exam. Expose the site, and visually inspect the abdomen for bruising or other discoloration, bleeding, swelling, masses, and/or a pulsating mass (pulsations of the aorta caused by an abdominal aortic aneurysm). Bruising over the flank area suggests blood collecting in the retroperitoneal space and may occur from trauma or from a ruptured or "leaking" organ such as the aorta or a kidney. Asymmetry may suggest a swollen organ immediately under that area. The most frequently noted asymmetry is the result of an inflamed liver in patients with cirrhosis or hepatitis. Gentle pressure in that area often results in jugular venous distention. Distention may not be readily apparent. Also note changes if the patient is pregnant.

How rapidly the distention has occurred is important for the receiving hospital to know. Severe distention may be caused by fluid in the peritoneal space, as in **ascites**; blood, as in a slow leak from a rupture; obstruction, as in a bowel blockage; or infection, as in some cases of **sepsis**. Reassess frequently to determine if distention is increasing.

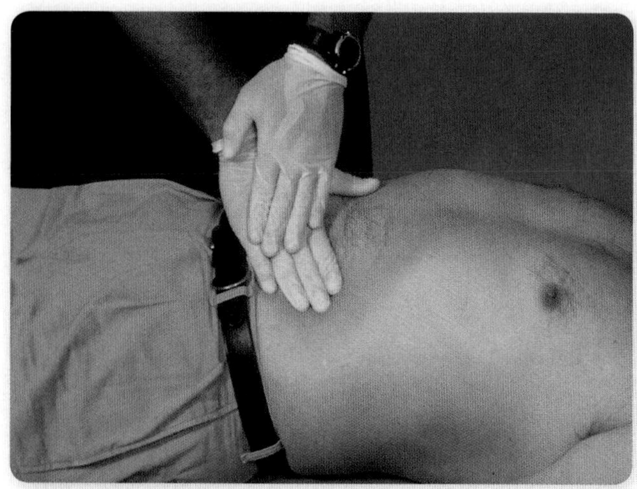

Figure 10-38 Palpate the abdomen, evaluating for symmetry, masses, tenderness, and bleeding.

Be sure to palpate the abdomen, evaluating for symmetry, masses, tenderness, and bleeding **Figure 10-38**. As you palpate the abdomen, use the terms *firm*, *soft*, *tender*, or *distended* (swollen) to report your findings. The abdomen is divided into four quadrants: left upper quadrant (LUQ), left lower quadrant (LLQ), right upper quadrant (RUQ), and right lower quadrant (RLQ). Always start the palpation of the abdomen in the quadrant that is farthest from the patient's pain or obvious injury. Do not palpate obvious soft-tissue injuries, and be careful not to palpate too firmly.

Assess for the presence of **rebound tenderness**. Rebound tenderness is pain that the patient feels when pressure is released as opposed to when pressure is applied and is characteristic of the pain associated with appendicitis. Assessing for rebound tenderness can be done by applying gentle, steady pressure on the abdomen and then releasing quickly. Explain to the patient ahead of time what you intend to do so that you gain valuable information. For example, tell the patient, "I am going to press on your abdomen and hold it for a couple of seconds and then let go. I need you to tell me if the pain is worse when I press down or when I let go." The same assessment can be accomplished by determining whether abdominal pain is produced by having the patient cough or tapping the heel of the

Words of Wisdom

Assess the abdomen for the following:

- Tenderness
- Rigidity
- Swelling
- Guarding
- Distention
- Rebound tenderness

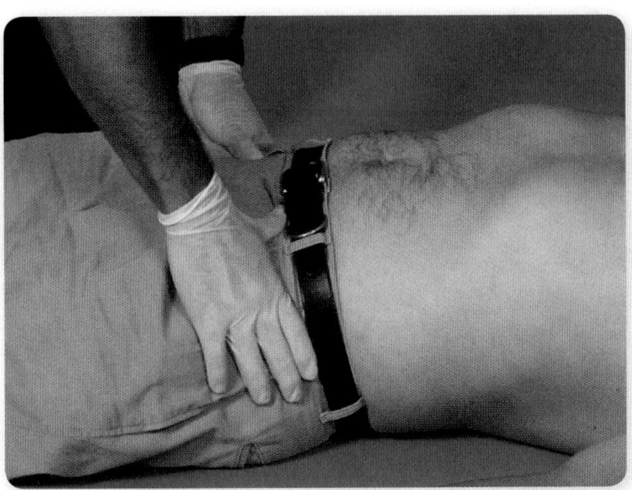

Figure 10-39 Inspect the pelvis for any obvious signs of injury, bleeding, and deformity.

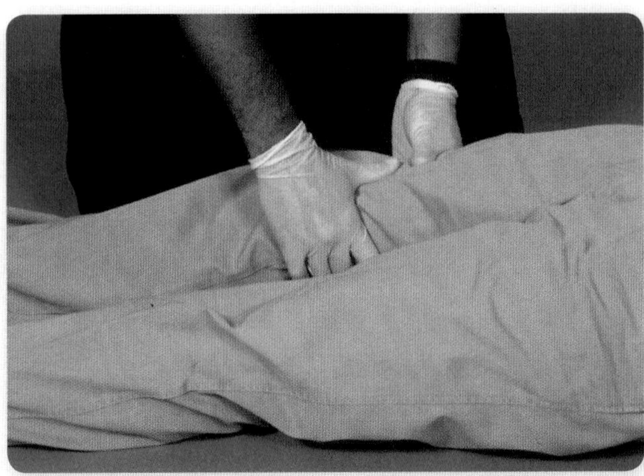

Figure 10-40 Inspect each extremity for DCAP-BTLS (Deformities, Contusions, Abrasions, Punctures/penetrations, Burns, Tenderness, Lacerations, Swelling).

patient's foot on the affected side. Note the position in which the patient is most comfortable.

Pelvis. Inspect the pelvis for symmetry, instability, pain, tenderness, crepitus, bleeding, deformity, and any obvious signs of injury; all findings may indicate a fractured pelvis and the potential for severe internal hemorrhage and shock. If the patient reports no pain, then gently press downward and inward on the iliac crests of the pelvic bones Figure 10-39. Do not rock the pelvis; this action may result in torqueing the spine and creating further injury. If you feel any movement or crepitus or the patient reports pain or tenderness, then severe injury may be present. Injuries to the pelvis and surrounding abdomen may bleed profusely without any obvious external signs, so continue to monitor the patient's mental status, skin condition, and vital signs. Provide supplemental oxygen as needed to minimize the effects of shock.

Inspection of the pelvic area, including the genitalia, is not often done in patients with medical emergencies, except when pain and bleeding is present. In female patients, it is important to determine whether the bleeding is coming from the vaginal opening, the urethra, female external genitalia, or the rectum. In male patients, it is important to determine whether bleeding is coming from the urethra or the rectum.

Extremities. An assessment of the patient's musculoskeletal system typically is done because of a chief complaint associated with some type of trauma or due to the MOI. Do all extremities appear to be properly positioned, and do all extremities appear to be functioning normally? Assess for posture if standing, and look at joints, checking for range of motion. Ask the patient how much he or she can move the extremity or joint. Never force a painful joint to move. Always compare the right side with the left side, looking for weakness or atrophy, and assess equality of grip strength.

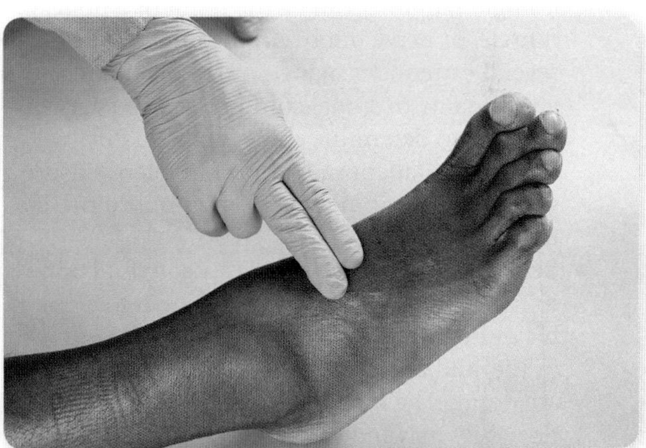

Figure 10-41 Palpation of the dorsalis pedis pulse.

Inspect each extremity for DCAP-BTLS Figure 10-40. Ask the patient about any tenderness or pain. As you evaluate the extremities, check for pulses, motor function, and sensory function:

- **Pulse.** Check the distal pulses on the foot (dorsalis pedis or posterior tibial) Figure 10-41 Figure 10-42 and wrist. Assess the pulses in the lower extremities for rate, quality, and rhythm. Is the pulse fast, slow, or irregular? Is the pulse weak, thready, or bounding? Compare pulses with one another (compare radial, femoral, and pedal pulses). A difference from one side to the other suggests unilateral impairment of arterial blood flow. Also check circulation. Evaluate the skin color and temperature in the hands and feet. Is it normal? How does it compare with the skin color and temperature of the other extremities? Pale or cyanotic skin may indicate poor circulation in that extremity.

Secondary Assessment

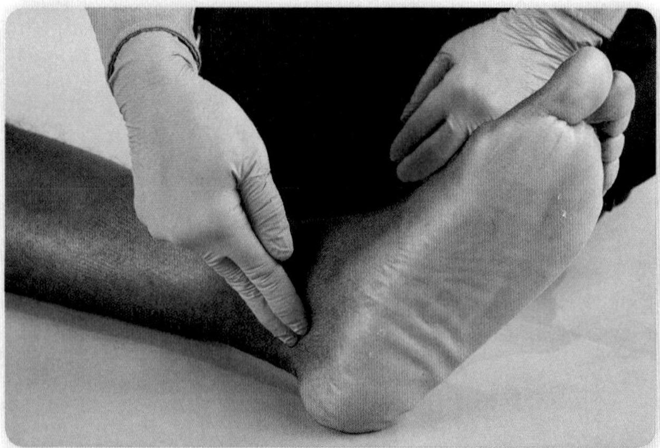

Figure 10-42 Palpation of the posterior tibial pulse.

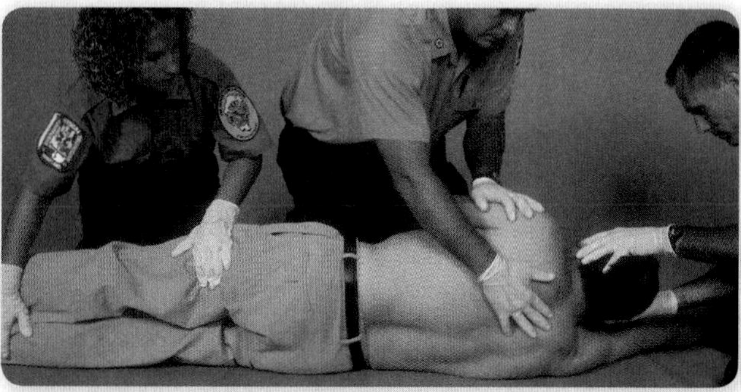

Figure 10-43 Feel the back for tenderness, deformity, and open wounds. Carefully palpate the spine from the neck to the pelvis for tenderness and deformity. Look under the clothing for obvious injuries, including bruising and bleeding.

- **Motor function.** Ask the patient to wiggle his or her fingers and toes. An inability to move a single extremity can be the result of a bone, muscle, or nerve injury. An inability to move several extremities may be a sign of a brain abnormality or spinal cord injury. Assess grip strength to determine ability and equality by having the patient squeeze your fingers. Ensure you are maintaining spinal immobilization, if indicated.
- **Sensory function.** Evaluate sensory function in the extremity by asking the patient to close his or her eyes. Gently squeeze or pinch a finger or toe, and ask the patient to identify what you are doing. The inability to feel sensation in the extremity may indicate a local nerve injury. The inability to feel in several extremities may be a sign of a spinal cord injury. Ensure you are maintaining spinal immobilization, if indicated.

Palpate each extremity individually. Note the temperature of the feet and legs, and attempt to palpate edema in the legs. To do so, press your thumb over the dorsum of the foot and anteriorly over the tibia, holding the thumb with firm, gentle pressure for at least 5 seconds. Pitting edema occurs when depression of the skin causes an indentation that persists for some time after the pressure is released. Bilateral pitting edema is indicative of conditions such as right-sided heart failure, whereas unilateral edema occurs with local conditions such as occlusion of a deep vein.

Pay close attention to the color of the hands and arms in comparison with one another. A ruddy color in one arm suggests obstruction of venous return, whereas edema suggests blockage of the lymphatic system.

Assessment of the hands and feet, particularly the nail beds, can give you clues to adequacy of perfusion and oxygenation. Note the color of the fingers and nail beds. Cyanosis may be noted; an early onset of cyanosis may cause the nail beds to darken and appear gray.

Words of Wisdom

Pitting edema is graded on a scale of 1 to 4, based on the depth of the indentation that occurs when the skin is depressed.

+1 = 0 inch to 0.25 inch (<6.5 mm)
+2 = 0.25 inch to 0.5 inch (6.5 mm to 12.5 mm)
+3 = 0.5 inch to 1 inch (12.5 mm to 2.5 cm)
+4 = >1 inch (>2.5 cm)

Posterior Body. Inspect the back for DCAP-BTLS, symmetry, bleeding, and open wounds **Figure 10-43**. When placing the patient onto a backboard, it is particularly important that you check the back as you log roll the patient. Ensure you keep the spine in line at all times as you log roll the patient onto his or her side. Do not remove the hand that is supporting the shoulder because this could cause the spine to torque and create further injury. Carefully palpate the spine from the neck to the pelvis with the other hand, examining for tenderness or deformity, and look for obvious injuries, including bruising and bleeding. In addition, assess for the presence of rectal bleeding.

Additional Physical Exams. After you have performed the secondary assessment, if time permits during transport, you may decide to perform a focused assessment of each body system (including areas that you did not initially assess). In many cases, you will not have time for this detailed exam, but when time permits, you may learn additional information about the patient's complaint by performing this exam.

When you have time to perform a focused assessment of each body system, begin by asking yourself two questions: "What additional problems can be identified through this exam?" and "How will these findings change my treatment choices?" These exams will provide you with additional information that will enable you to recognize patterns of response, particularly compensatory mechanisms, and help you understand more about the nature of the patient's problem. Actions you may need to take as a result of findings include the following:

- Addressing any potentially life-threatening conditions (this is unlikely this late in the exam but is possible). Certain conditions, such as a pneumothorax or bleeding in the peritoneal cavity, may not be readily apparent during your initial assessment, but may be obvious at this point.
- Performing spinal immobilization if neck or back pain or abnormality in sensation or movement is identified in relationship to trauma (This is unlikely but could occur, especially in the case of a spinal cord contusion in a pediatric or geriatric patient.)
- Modifying any treatment that is underway on the basis of any new information
- Initiating treatment for additional problems identified during the focused exams
- Modifying transport decisions to a more appropriate facility, if the patient's condition deteriorates or potential life threats are found

Patient Assessment

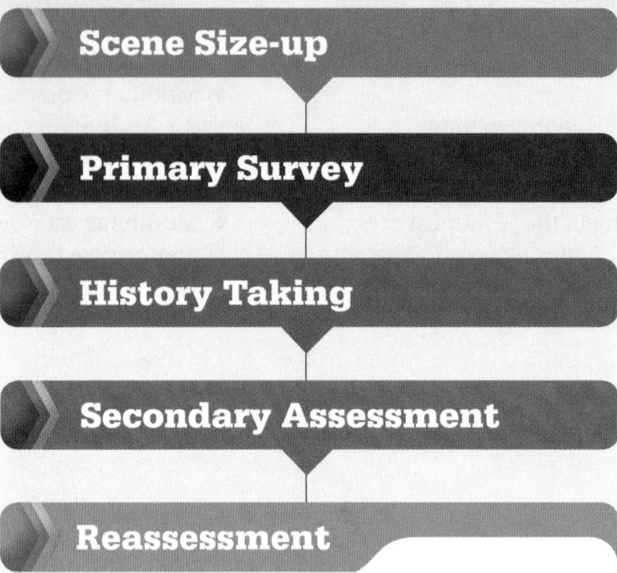

Repeat the primary survey
Reassess vital signs
Reassess the chief complaint
Recheck interventions
Identify and treat changes in the patient's condition
Reassess patient:

- Unstable patients: every 5 minutes
- Stable patients: every 15 minutes

Reassessment

A **reassessment** is performed at regular intervals during the assessment process, and its purpose is to identify and treat changes in a patient's condition. When you perform reassessment, reassess the ABCDEs to ensure you adequately addressed the chief complaint, obtained another set of vital signs, and completed any other tasks related to patient care (such as dressing small wounds or placing ice packs). Reassessment represents a continuous, cyclical process you perform throughout transport, right up to the time you turn over patient care to the ED staff. For patients in stable condition, do a reassessment every 15 minutes or so. For patients in unstable condition, make a concerted effort to repeat the reassessment every 5 minutes.

Words of Wisdom

Reassess stable patients every 15 minutes and unstable patients every 5 minutes.

Repeat the Primary Survey

Reassessment combines repetition of the primary survey, reassessment of vital signs and breath sounds, and repetition of the secondary assessment. First, compare the patient's LOC with your baseline assessment. Is the LOC changing? If so, then how?

Reassess Vital Signs

Reassess and record the vital signs. Compare the baseline vital signs obtained during the primary survey with any and all subsequent vital signs. Look for trends. Have the vital signs changed, improved, declined, or stayed the same? Reassess the mental status and the ABCs. Monitor skin color and temperature. Reassess the blood pressure and pulse.

Reassess the Chief Complaint

Reassess the patient's chief complaint in the light of treatments provided thus far. Ask and answer the following questions about the patient's chief complaint:

- Is the current treatment improving the patient's condition?

- Has an already identified problem gotten better?
- Has an already identified problem gotten worse?
- What is the nature of any newly identified problems?

Recheck Interventions

In the reassessment process, reevaluate everything that has been done to this point in the patient assessment process. Check all interventions. Management of the patient's ABCs is most important. In addition, are the bandages, spinal immobilization devices, extrication equipment, and patient-securing instruments in place and appropriate for transport? Are IV lines flowing properly, or does the rate need to be changed based on patient presentation? Ensure management of bleeding. Ensure adequacy of other interventions, and consider the need for new interventions.

Identify and Treat Changes in the Patient's Condition

No matter what the patient's condition was before your arrival, which interventions were used, or which decisions on treatment and transport priorities were made, a reassessment is necessary to help monitor changes in the patient's condition. If the patient's condition improves, then simply continue whatever treatments you are providing. If the patient's condition deteriorates, then prepare to modify treatments as appropriate. Document any changes, whether negative or positive.

Reassess the Patient

How and when to perform a reassessment depends on the patient's condition. A patient in unstable condition should be reassessed every 5 minutes, whereas a patient in stable condition should be reassessed every 15 minutes.

YOU are the Provider SUMMARY

1. What are the components of a scene size-up?

The components of a scene size-up include information that you receive from your dispatcher and other agencies already on scene, combined with a visual inspection of the scene in an attempt to identify any potential safety hazards to your crew, the patient, and bystanders. Another component is confirming the number of patients to ensure you have adequate resources to care for the patients.

2. What can you do to ensure scene safety?

You must recognize that hazards come in many different forms, shapes, and sizes. Initial information obtained by your dispatcher can alert you to possible scene hazards. Hazards exist at every MVC scene. Strategically position your emergency vehicle in a manner that will minimize risk to responders. Also, fluids leaking from a wrecked vehicle can be extremely slippery when they come into contact with a road surface. Look for possible dangers as you approach the scene and before you step out of the vehicle. Observe unstable surfaces, slopes, ice, water, and wet grass. Consider the location of your patient and the conditions. You are obliged to provide protection for the patient.

Occasionally, you and your partner will not be able to enter a scene safely. If the scene is unsafe, then make it safe. If this is not possible, then do not enter. If the hazard presents a substantial risk to your health and safety, then request the appropriate assistance. If the scene is a potential crime scene, then follow local protocols before entering. Ask for law enforcement personnel to accompany you when needed.

3. Does this patient present more like a medical patient or a trauma patient?

One of the great dangers in performing the prehospital assessment is categorizing your patient immediately as either a trauma (injured) patient or a medical (ill) patient. Early in the assessment, it can be difficult to identify with absolute certainty whether the problem is of traumatic or medical origin. Consider the patient in this scenario. Did she strike the tree and become unresponsive? Or did she experience a medical problem that caused her to strike the tree? Remember, the fundamentals of good patient assessment do not change, despite the unique aspects of trauma and medical care.

4. What type of PPE should you wear for this type of call?

Standard precautions and PPE need to be considered and adapted to the prehospital task at hand. Included in PPE is the clothing or specialized equipment that provides protection to the wearer. The type of PPE required depends on the specific job duties required during a patient care interaction. For an MVC, gloves are usually sufficient for those providing patient care. If there is risk for blood splatter, a gown and goggles should be worn in addition to gloves. These measures may not provide absolute protection from exposure to infectious diseases or bloodborne pathogens, but they are the most effective way to reduce your risk of exposure.

5. What are the components of the GCS score?

The GCS uses parameters that test a patient's eye opening, best verbal response, and best motor response, which provide a numeric score that defines the severity of a patient's brain dysfunction. This information provides baseline data on the patient's overall neurologic status and can be a reliable predictor of the outcome of a patient with a brain injury. When you are reporting the GCS score, document or report each section (eg, Eye opening, 3; Verbal response, 2; Motor response, 4; GCS score, 9) to document baseline function in each area.

6. How can you rule in or rule out diabetes as the cause of her altered mental status?

The glucometer is used to assess blood glucose levels, which can assist you in determining if the glucose level is the cause of the patient's altered mental status. While determining glucose levels is largely a routine part of the patient assessment, indications include known diabetes in patients with a decreased LOC, a decreased LOC of unknown origin in any patient, general malaise, weakness, or a poor general impression. A normal glucose reading is 80 to 120 mg/dL.

7. How often should you reassess your patients?

Reassess patients in critical or unstable condition every 5 minutes and patients in stable or noncritical condition every 15 minutes. Performing reassessments at these intervals provides a method for you to recognize any improvement or deterioration in the patient's status.

8. Why is critical thinking important as an AEMT?

The prehospital setting may be one of controlled chaos; your sources of information can be overwhelming or severely limited. You must be able to prioritize this information in a short time, separate relevant from irrelevant data, and provide the most appropriate care for the patient. These abilities are the cornerstones of being an effective EMS provider.

YOU are the Provider SUMMARY *(continued)*

Gathering, analyzing, and correctly synthesizing patient information will culminate in an appropriate treatment plan. This process requires an understanding of the patient's injury or illness and the impact that your emergency medical care will have on it. You will develop needed critical thinking skills through field experience in dealing with multiple patients with varying problems.

Patient Care Report (PCR)					
Date: 7-12-18	**Incident No.:** 10-85-9		**Nature of Call:** MVC		**Location:** Hwy 81 & Frontage Road
Dispatched: 1142	**En Route:** 1143	**At Scene:** 1150	**Transport:** 1210	**At Hospital:** 1215	**In Service:** 1220

Patient Information	
Age: Mid 30s **Sex:** F **Weight (in kg [lb]):** 50 kg (111 lb)	**Allergies:** Unknown **Medications:** Unknown **Past Medical History:** Diabetes **Chief Complaint:** Neck pain and confusion

Vital Signs				
Time: 1152	**BP:** Not obtained	**Pulse:** Not obtained	**Respirations:** Nonlabored	**Spo_2:** Not obtained
Time: 1202	**BP:** 118/76	**Pulse:** 90	**Respirations:** 18	**Spo_2:** 99%
Time: 1207	**BP:** 116/84	**Pulse:** 88	**Respirations:** 16	**Spo_2:** 99%

Prehospital Treatment (circle all that apply)				
Oxygen @ 15 **L/min via (circle one):** **NC** **(NRM)** **Bag-mask device**		**Assisted Ventilation**	**Airway Adjunct**	**CPR**
Defibrillation	**Bleeding Control**	**Bandaging**	**Splinting**	(**Other:** Spinal immobilization IV line established)

Narrative
EMS requested to a vehicle vs. tree. On arrival, EMS finds an adult female patient sitting in the driver's seat with lap and shoulder belt still in place. There is severe damage to the front of the vehicle and the windshield is cracked in multiple places. Access is gained by opening the driver's door and manual spinal immobilization is maintained. The patient is alert but confused, and she reports neck pain. Respirations are adequate, breath sounds are clear and equal bilaterally, radial pulses are strong and regular, and skin is warm and dry. Blood glucose level is 98 mg/dL. Patient presents with a large hematoma on her forehead and her pupils are equal and reactive to light and accommodation. She has good pulses, motor function, and sensation in all extremities, but reports a "tingling" sensation. Patient is placed on O_2 via NRB mask at 15 L/min. A cervical collar is applied and the patient is removed from the vehicle onto a long backboard using a vest-style extrication device. She is secured to the backboard and placed in the ambulance for transport. En route to the trauma center, patient is reassessed with no changes found and an 18-gauge IV line is established with NS at a TKO rate. Patient left in care of ED staff for further evaluation.**End of report**

Prep Kit

▶ Ready for Review

- Critical thinking includes gathering, evaluating, and synthesizing patient information, developing an idea of the patient's problem based on gathered information and the patient's presentation, and formulating a field impression on which an appropriate patient treatment plan will be based. Learn and practice the key elements of critical thinking so you can apply them when in the field.
- Always base your treatment or transport decisions on your assessment of the patient.
- The assessment process begins with the scene size-up, which identifies real and potential hazards. The patient should not be approached until these hazards have been dealt with in a way that eliminates or minimizes risk to you and the patient(s).
- The primary survey is performed on all patients. It includes forming an initial general impression of the patient, including the level of consciousness, and identifying any life-threatening conditions by assessing the ABCDEs. A primary survey is performed to assist in prioritizing time and mode of transport. Any life threats identified must be treated before moving on to the next step of the assessment.
- History taking includes an exploration of the patient's chief complaint or history of present illness. A SAMPLE history is generally taken during this step of the assessment process. This information may be obtained from the patient, family, friends, bystanders, caregivers, or medical alert devices or documentation.
- The secondary assessment includes physical exam of the patient. The physical exam may be a systematic head-to-toe, full-body exam or a systematic assessment that focuses on a certain area or region of the body, often determined through the chief complaint. Circumstances will dictate which aspects of the physical exam will be used. The secondary assessment is performed on scene or in the back of the ambulance en route to the hospital. If the patient has serious life threats, then you may not have time to perform a secondary assessment.
- The reassessment is performed on all patients. It gives you an opportunity to reevaluate the chief complaint and to reassess interventions to ensure they are still effective. Information from the reassessment may be used to identify and treat changes in the patient's condition.
- A patient in stable condition should be reassessed every 15 minutes, whereas a patient in unstable condition should be reassessed every 5 minutes.
- The assessment process is systematic and dynamic. Each assessment you perform will be slightly different, depending on the needs of the patient. The result will be a process that will enable you to quickly identify and treat the needs of all patients, both medical and trauma related, in a way that meets their unique needs.

▶ Vital Vocabulary

accessory muscles The secondary muscles of respiration that include the neck muscles (sternocleidomastoids), the chest pectoralis major muscles, and the abdominal muscles.

adventitious sounds Abnormal breath sounds that include crackles, rhonchi, wheezes, stridor, and pleural friction rubs.

altered mental status Any deviation from alert and oriented to person, place, time, and event, or any deviation from a patient's normal baseline mental status.

anisocoria A medical condition characterized by normally unequal pupils.

ascites The accumulation of serous fluid in the peritoneal cavity.

aspiration Drawing in or out by suction; may occur in the lungs when the patient is unable to maintain his or her own airway and blood or fluid is present in the mouth.

auscultation A method of listening to sounds within an organ with a stethoscope.

AVPU scale A mnemonic to describe the method of assessing the level of consciousness by determining whether the patient is Awake and alert, responsive to Verbal stimuli or Pain, or Unresponsive; used principally early in the assessment process.

blood pressure The pressure that the blood exerts against the walls of the arteries as it passes through them.

bradycardia A slow heart rate of less than 60 beats per minute.

breath sounds An indication of air movement in the lungs, usually assessed with a stethoscope.

bronchovesicular sounds Soft, breezy, and low-pitched normal breath sounds found at the midclavicular line.

capillary refill A test that evaluates distal circulatory system function by squeezing (blanching) blood from an area such as a nail bed and watching the speed of its return after releasing the pressure.

capnography A noninvasive method that can quickly and efficiently provide information on a patient's ventilatory status, circulation, and metabolism; effectively measures the concentration of carbon dioxide in expired air over time.

Prep Kit *(continued)*

capnometry The use of a capnometer, a device that measures the amount of expired carbon dioxide.

carbon dioxide (CO_2) A component that typically makes up 0.3% of air at sea level; also a waste product exhaled during expiration by the respiratory system.

chief complaint The reason a patient called for emergency medical services; also, the patient's response to questions such as "What's wrong?" or "What happened?"

colorimetric devices End-tidal carbon dioxide detectors that use a chemical reaction to detect the amount of carbon dioxide present in expired gases.

conjunctiva The delicate membrane that lines the eyelids and covers the exposed surface of the eye.

crackles A crackling, rattling breath sound that signals fluid in the air spaces of the lungs; formerly called rales.

crepitus A grating or grinding sensation caused by fractured bone ends or joints rubbing together; also, air bubbles under the skin that produce a crackling sound or crinkly feeling.

cyanosis A blue-gray skin color that is caused by a reduced level of oxygen in the blood.

DCAP-BTLS A mnemonic for assessment in which each area of the body is evaluated for Deformities, Contusions, Abrasions, Punctures/penetrations, Burns, Tenderness, Lacerations, and Swelling.

diaphoretic Characterized by light or profuse sweating.

diastolic pressure The pressure that remains in the arteries during the relaxing phase of the cycle of the heart (diastole) when the left ventricle is at rest.

diffuse pain Pain that is not identified as being specific to a single location but is spread out over an area of the body or felt all over the body.

end-tidal carbon dioxide ($ETCO_2$) The partial pressure or maximal concentration of carbon dioxide at the end of an exhaled breath.

focal pain Pain that is easily identified as being specific to a single location of the body.

focused assessment A type of physical assessment typically performed on patients who have sustained nonsignificant mechanisms of injury or on responsive medical patients. This type of exam is based on the chief complaint and focuses on one body system or part.

full-body exam A systematic head-to-toe exam that is performed during the secondary assessment of a patient who has sustained a significant mechanism of injury, is unresponsive, or is in critical condition.

general impression The overall initial impression that determines the priority for patient care; based on the patient's surroundings, the mechanism of injury, nature of the illness, signs and symptoms, and the chief complaint.

Glasgow Coma Scale (GCS) The most commonly employed, reliable, and consistent method of assessing mental status and neurologic function.

Golden Hour The time from injury to definitive care, during which treatment of shock and traumatic injuries should occur because survival potential is best; sometimes called the Golden Period.

guarding Involuntary muscle contractions of the abdominal wall to minimize the pain of abdominal movement; a sign of peritonitis.

history taking A step within the patient assessment process that provides detail about the patient's chief complaint and an account of the patient's signs and symptoms.

hypertension Blood pressure that is higher than the normal range.

hypotension Blood pressure that is lower than the normal range.

incident command system (ICS) A system implemented to manage disasters and mass-casualty incidents in which section chiefs, including finance, logistics, operations, and planning, report to the incident commander. Also referred to as the incident management system.

jaundice Yellow skin or sclera caused by liver disease or dysfunction.

labored breathing Breathing that requires greater than normal effort; may be slower or faster than normal and characterized by grunting, stridor, and use of accessory muscles.

mechanism of injury (MOI) The forces, or energy transmission, applied to the body that cause injury.

medical ambiguity Uncertainty regarding the specific cause of the patient's condition.

nasal flaring Widening of the nostrils, indicating that an airway obstruction is present.

nature of the illness (NOI) The general type of illness a patient is experiencing.

OPQRST A mnemonic used in evaluating a patient's pain: Onset, Provocation/palliation, Quality, Region/radiation, Severity, and Timing of pain.

orientation The mental status of a patient as measured by memory of person (name), place (current location), time (current year, month, and approximate date), and event (what happened).

Prep Kit *(continued)*

palpate To examine by touch.

paradoxical motion A condition in which one section of the chest wall rises on inspiration while the remainder of the chest falls.

perfusion The flow of blood through body tissues and vessels.

personal protective equipment (PPE) Equipment that blocks exposure to a pathogen or a hazardous material.

pertinent negatives Expected signs or symptoms with negative findings that warrant no care or intervention.

pleural friction rubs Squeaking or grating sounds that occur when the pleural linings rub together, which may be heard on inspiration, expiration, or both; commonly caused by inflammation of the pleura.

priapism A painful, tender, and persistent erection of the penis; can result from spinal cord injury, use of erectile dysfunction drugs, or sickle cell disease.

primary survey A step within the patient assessment process that identifies and initiates treatment of immediate and potential life threats.

pulse The pressure wave that occurs as each heartbeat causes a surge in the blood circulating through the arteries.

pulse oximetry An assessment tool that measures oxygen saturation of hemoglobin in the capillary beds.

radiating pain An area of the body from which the origin of pain or discomfort may travel.

rapid full-body scan A thorough, 60- to 90-second review of the patient's body to identify injuries that must be managed or protected immediately; conducted during the primary survey.

reassessment A step within the patient assessment process that is performed at regular intervals during the assessment process to identify and treat changes in a patient's condition. A patient in unstable condition should be reassessed every 5 minutes, whereas a patient in stable condition should be reassessed every 15 minutes.

rebound tenderness Pain that the patient feels when pressure is released as opposed to when pressure is applied; characteristic of appendicitis.

referred pain Pain in two separate locations of the body, without a "trail" of pain between the two locations, or pain in an area of the body that is not the source of the pain.

respiratory distress A clinical state characterized by increased respiratory rate, effort, and/or work of breathing.

respiratory failure A clinical state of inadequate oxygenation, ventilation, or both.

responsiveness The way in which a patient responds to external stimuli, including verbal stimuli (sound), tactile stimuli (touch), and painful stimuli.

retractions Movements in which the skin pulls in around the ribs during inspiration.

rhonchi Coarse, low-pitched breath sounds heard in patients with chronic mucus in the upper airways.

SAMPLE history A brief history of a patient's condition to determine signs and symptoms, allergies, medications, pertinent past history, last oral intake, and events leading up to the illness or injury.

scene size-up A step within the patient assessment process that involves a quick assessment of the scene and the surroundings to provide information about scene safety and the mechanism of injury or nature of the illness before you enter and begin patient care.

sclera The tough, fibrous, white portion of the eye that protects the more delicate inner structures.

secondary assessment A step within the patient assessment process in which a systematic physical exam of the patient is performed. The exam may be a full-body exam or an assessment that focuses on a certain area or region of the body, often determined through the chief complaint.

sepsis The spread of an infection from its initial site into the bloodstream.

shallow respirations Respirations characterized by little movement of the chest wall (reduced tidal volume) or poor chest excursion.

sign Objective findings that can be seen, heard, felt, smelled, or measured.

situational awareness Knowledge and understanding of one's surroundings and the ability to recognize potential risks to the safety of the patient or the emergency medical services team.

sniffing position An upright position in which the patient's head and chin are thrust slightly forward to keep the airway open.

spontaneous respirations Breathing that occurs without assistance.

standard precautions Protective measures that have traditionally been recommended by the Centers for Disease Control and Prevention for use in dealing with objects, blood, body fluids, and other potential exposure risks of communicable disease.

stridor A harsh, high-pitched breath sound, generally heard during inspiration, that is caused by partial

Prep Kit *(continued)*

blockage or narrowing of the upper airway; may be audible without a stethoscope.

subcutaneous emphysema The presence of air in soft tissues, causing a characteristic crackling sensation on palpation.

symptom Subjective findings that the patient feels but that can be identified only by the patient.

systolic pressure The increased pressure in an artery with each contraction of the ventricles (systole).

tachycardia A rapid heart rate of more than 100 beats per minute.

tidal volume The amount of air (in milliliters) that is moved into or out of the lungs during one breath.

triage The process of establishing treatment and transportation priorities according to severity of injury and medical need.

tripod position An upright position in which the patient leans forward onto two arms stretched forward and thrusts the head and chin forward.

two- to three-word dyspnea A severe breathing condition in which a patient can speak only two to three words at a time without pausing to take a breath.

vasoconstriction The narrowing of a blood vessel.

vesicular sounds Fine and faint normal breath sounds noted in the lateral wall of the chest from the smaller bronchioles and alveoli.

vital signs Clinical measurements that indicate the current state of the body and how well it is functioning.

wheezing A high-pitched, whistling breath sound that is most prominent on expiration, and which suggests an obstruction or narrowing of the lower airways; occurs in asthma and bronchiolitis.

▶ References

1. Stop the Bleed. Department of Homeland Security website. https://www.dhs.gov/stopthebleed. Published October 11, 2016. Accessed November 7, 2016.
2. Berg MD, Schexnayder SM, Chameides L, Terry M, Donoghue A, Hickey RW, Berg RA, Sutton RM, Hazinski MF. Part 13: pediatric basic life support: 2010 American Heart Association Guidelines for Cardiopulmonary Resuscitation and Emergency Cardiovascular Care. *Circulation*. 2010;122(suppl 3): S862–S875.
3. National Association of Emergency Medical Technicians. *PHTLS: Prehospital Trauma Life Support*. 8th ed. Burlington, MA: Jones & Bartlett Learning; 2014: 298–301.
4. Depression. World Health Organization website. http://www.who.int/mediacentre/factsheets /fs369/en/. Updated February 2017. Accessed October 20, 2016.

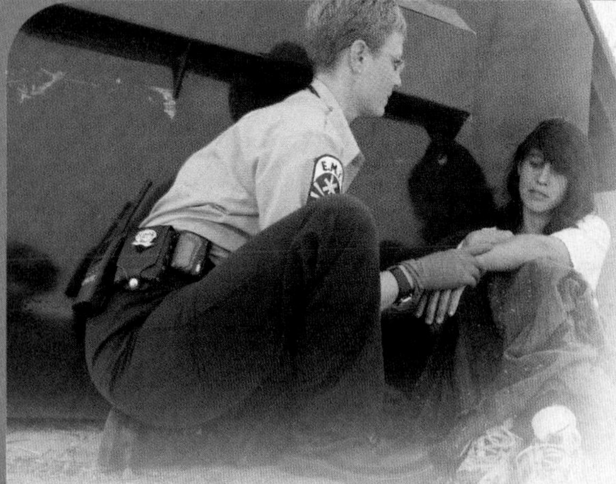

Assessment *in Action*

Your ambulance is dispatched for a reported asthma attack. On arrival, you immediately perform your primary survey and obtain a patient history. The patient states that he has a past medical history of asthma, which is almost always resolved at home with his rescue inhaler. He further states that his inhaler is now empty, and that is why he called 9-1-1.

1. Which step of the primary survey includes noting things such as the person's age, sex, and weight?

A. Form a general impression.
B. Assess LOC.
C. Identify the chief complaint.
D. Identify priority of patient care and transport.

2. At which step in the assessment process do you initially obtain vital signs?

A. Primary survey
B. History taking
C. Secondary assessment
D. Reassessment

3. Which breath sounds would you expect to hear in a patient reporting an asthma attack?

A. Crackles
B. Rhonchi
C. Wheezing
D. Stridor

4. Wheezing in a patient with asthma is:

A. a sign.
B. a symptom.
C. a sign and a symptom.
D. neither a sign nor a symptom.

5. The normal range for exhaled carbon dioxide is:

A. 15 to 25 mm Hg.
B. 25 to 35 mm Hg.
C. 35 to 45 mm Hg.
D. 45 to 55 mm Hg.

6. Which of the following questions would be the MOST appropriate for the *P* portion of the OPQRST mnemonic?

A. "Does the pain move anywhere?"
B. "How long has this pain been going on?"
C. "What were you doing when this pain started?"
D. "Does anything make the pain worse?"

7. Which of the following findings is a pertinent negative for this patient?

A. Breath sounds are clear and equal.
B. Heart tones are crisp.
C. Patient has no motor or sensory deficit.
D. Pain does not radiate.

8. At which step in the assessment process do you obtain vital signs using monitoring devices?

A. Primary survey
B. History taking
C. Secondary assessment
D. Reassessment

9. How should you obtain a history on a patient who has limited cognitive abilities?

10. What is the purpose of measuring $ETCO_2$?

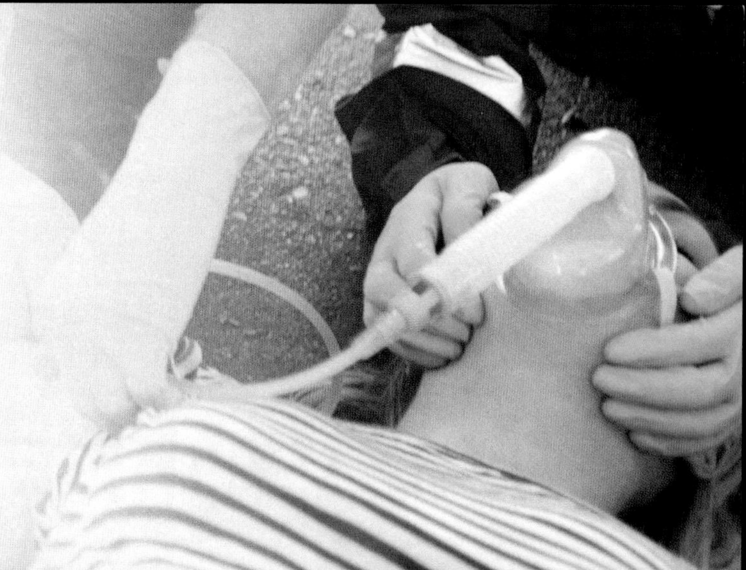

SECTION 4

Airway

CHAPTER 11

Airway Management

National EMS Education Standard Competencies

Airway Management, Respiration, and Artificial Ventilation

Applies knowledge (fundamental depth, foundational breadth) of upper airway anatomy and physiology to patient assessment and management in order to assure a patent airway, adequate mechanical ventilation, and respiration for patients of all ages.

Airway Management

Airway anatomy (pp 466-469)
Airway assessment (pp 483-487)
Techniques of assuring a patent airway (pp 487-497)

Respiration

Anatomy of the respiratory system (pp 466-469)
Physiology and pathophysiology of respiration

- Pulmonary ventilation (pp 471-473, 476-477)
- Oxygenation (pp 473, 477-478)
- Respiration
  - External (p 474)
  - Internal (pp 474-475)
  - Cellular (pp 473-474)

Assessment and management of adequate and inadequate respiration (pp 483-530)
Supplemental oxygen therapy (pp 498-503)

Artificial Ventilation

Assessment and management of adequate and inadequate ventilation

- Artificial ventilation (pp 506-513)
- Minute ventilation (pp 472-473)
- Alveolar ventilation (pp 472, 476-477)
- Effect of artificial ventilation on cardiac output (p 478)

Pathophysiology

Applies comprehensive knowledge of the pathophysiology of respiration and perfusion to patient assessment and management.

Knowledge Objectives

1. Review the major structures of the respiratory system. (pp 466-469)
2. Discuss the physiology of breathing. (pp 469-475)
3. Describe factors related to ventilation, including partial pressure and volumes. (pp 471-473)
4. Describe factors related to the pathophysiology of respiration, including ventilation-perfusion ratio mismatch, hypoventilation, hyperventilation, and circulatory compromise. (pp 475-479)
5. Review the concept of acid-base imbalance. (pp 479-480)
6. Explain how to assess for adequate and inadequate respiration, including the use of pulse oximetry. (pp 480-485)
7. List the signs of adequate breathing. (p 480)
8. List the signs of inadequate breathing. (p 481)
9. Explain how to assess for a patent airway. (pp 481-482)
10. Describe abnormal breathing patterns to recognize when assessing a patient's breathing. (pp 482-483)
11. Discuss the methods for end-tidal carbon dioxide assessment, including its importance. (pp 485-487)
12. Describe the assessment and care of a patient with apnea. (pp 487-513)
13. Describe how to perform the head tilt–chin lift maneuver. (pp 487, 489)
14. Describe how to perform the jaw-thrust maneuver. (pp 489-490)
15. Explain the use of the recovery position to maintain a clear airway. (pp 490-491)
16. Discuss the importance and techniques of suctioning. (pp 491-493)
17. Explain the AEMT's role in performing tracheobronchial suctioning. (p 493)
18. Explain how to measure and insert an oropharyngeal (oral) airway. (pp 494-495)
19. Explain how to measure and insert a nasopharyngeal (nasal) airway. (pp 496-497)
20. Describe the importance of giving supplemental oxygen to patients who are hypoxic. (p 498)

21. Describe the basics of how oxygen is stored and the various hazards associated with its use. (pp 498-501)
22. Explain how to use a nonrebreathing mask, and state the oxygen flow requirements for its use. (pp 503-504)
23. Describe the indications for using a nasal cannula rather than a nonrebreathing face mask. (p 504)
24. Describe the indications for use of a humidifier during supplemental oxygen therapy. (p 505)
25. Describe the use of a one-, two-, or three-person bag-mask device and a manually triggered ventilation (MTV) device. (pp 505-512)
26. Explain how to perform mouth-to-mouth or mouth-to-mask ventilation. (pp 507-508)
27. Describe the signs associated with adequate and inadequate artificial ventilation. (pp 511-512)
28. Describe the indications, contraindications, and complications of use of continuous positive airway pressure (CPAP). (pp 513-516)
29. Explain the considerations surrounding gastric distention. (p 516)
30. Discuss airway management considerations for patients with a laryngectomy, tracheostomy, or stoma. (pp 516-519)
31. Discuss supraglottic and multilumen airway devices, including how they work, their indications, contraindications, and complications, and the procedure for inserting them. (pp 520-529)
32. Describe how to recognize and care for a foreign body airway obstruction. (pp 529-530)

Skills Objectives

1. Demonstrate use of pulse oximetry. (pp 483-485)
2. Demonstrate how to position the unresponsive patient. (pp 487-488, Skill Drill 11-1)
3. Demonstrate the steps in performing the head tilt–chin lift maneuver. (p 489)
4. Demonstrate the steps in performing the jaw-thrust maneuver. (pp 489-490)
5. Demonstrate the steps in performing the tongue–jaw lift maneuver. (p 490)
6. Demonstrate how to place a patient in the recovery position. (pp 490-491)
7. Demonstrate how to operate a suction unit. (pp 491-492)
8. Demonstrate how to suction a patient's airway. (pp 492-493, Skill Drill 11-2)
9. Demonstrate how to perform tracheobronchial suctioning. (p 493)
10. Demonstrate the insertion of an oral airway. (pp 494-495, Skill Drill 11-3)
11. Demonstrate the insertion of an oral airway with a 90° rotation. (pp 494-495, Skill Drill 11-4)
12. Demonstrate the insertion of a nasal airway. (p 497, Skill Drill 11-5)
13. Demonstrate how to place an oxygen cylinder into service. (pp 501-502, Skill Drill 11-6)
14. Demonstrate the use of a partial rebreathing mask in providing supplemental oxygen therapy to patients. (p 504)
15. Demonstrate the use of a Venturi mask in providing supplemental oxygen therapy to patients. (p 504)
16. Demonstrate the use of a humidifier in providing supplemental oxygen therapy to patients. (p 505)
17. Demonstrate how to assist a patient with ventilations using the bag-mask device for one and two rescuers. (pp 505-506, 510-511)
18. Demonstrate mouth-to-mask ventilation. (pp 507-508, Skill Drill 11-7)
19. Demonstrate the use of a MTV device to assist in delivering artificial ventilation to the patient. (pp 511-512)
20. Demonstrate the use of an automatic transport ventilator to assist in delivering artificial ventilation to the patient. (pp 512-513)
21. Demonstrate the use of CPAP. (pp 513-516, Skill Drill 11-8)
22. Demonstrate how to suction a stoma. (pp 516-517, Skill Drill 11-9)
23. Demonstrate mouth-to-stoma ventilation with a resuscitation mask. (pp 516, 518, Skill Drill 11-10)
24. Demonstrate bag-mask device-to-stoma ventilation. (pp 516, 519, Skill Drill 11-11)
25. Demonstrate insertion of the King LT airway. (pp 521-522, Skill Drill 11-12)
26. Demonstrate insertion of the laryngeal mask airway. (pp 523-524, Skill Drill 11-13)
27. Demonstrate insertion of an i-gel supraglottic airway. (pp 525-526, Skill Drill 11-14)
28. Demonstrate insertion of the Cobra perilaryngeal airway. (p 527)
29. Demonstrate insertion of the Combitube. (p 529)

Introduction

The single most important steps in caring for any patient are to obtain and maintain a patent airway and to ensure that the patient is breathing adequately. Within a few minutes of being deprived of oxygen, vital organs such as the heart and brain may not function normally. Brain cell death occurs within 4 to 6 minutes without oxygen.

Oxygen reaches body tissues and cells through two separate but related processes: breathing and circulation. During inhalation, oxygen moves from the atmosphere into our lungs and then passes from the alveoli in the lungs into the capillaries to oxygenate the blood. The blood, enriched with oxygen, travels through the body by the pumping action of the heart. At the same time, carbon dioxide, produced by cells in the body tissues, moves from the capillaries into the alveoli. The carbon dioxide then leaves the body during exhalation. The primary objective of emergency care is to ensure optimal ventilation—movement of air into and out of the lungs—to facilitate the delivery of oxygen and elimination of carbon dioxide.

Basic airway management skills tend to be taken for granted as more advanced skills are learned, yet they are among the most crucial skills any emergency medical services (EMS) provider learns. This chapter reviews the anatomy and physiology of the respiratory system. It then describes how to assess patients quickly and carefully to determine their airway and ventilation status. The equipment, procedures, and guidelines that you will need to manage a patient's airway and breathing are described in detail. You will learn several ways to open a patient's airway and manage situations that place the airway in jeopardy. Because artificial airway equipment can cause harm to the patient if used improperly, the chapter will thoroughly discuss airway adjuncts, oxygen therapy devices, definitive airway equipment, and artificial ventilation methods.

Anatomy Review

The respiratory system consists of all the structures in the body that make up the **airway** and help us breathe, or ventilate Figure 11-1. The airway is divided into the upper and lower airways. Structures that help us breathe include the diaphragm, the muscles of the chest wall, accessory muscles of breathing, and the nerves from the brain and spinal cord to those muscles. Ventilation is the exchange of air between the lungs and environment. The diaphragm and muscles of the chest wall are responsible for the regular rise and fall of the chest that accompany normal breathing.

▶ The Upper Airway

The airway is divided into upper and lower airways. The larynx is considered the dividing line between the upper and lower airways.

The major functions of the upper airway are to warm, filter, and humidify air brought into the body. Air enters the body through the mouth and nose. Warming protects the patient from becoming hypothermic. Humidification is accomplished as the air picks up moisture from the tissues of the airway. The pharynx—the muscular tube that extends from the nose and mouth to the level of the esophagus and trachea—is composed of the nasopharynx, oropharynx, and the laryngopharynx (also called the hypopharynx) Figure 11-2. The laryngopharynx is the lowest portion of the pharynx. At the base, it splits into two lumens (a lumen is a channel within a tube), the larynx anteriorly and the esophagus posteriorly.

Nasopharynx

The union of the facial bones forms the nasopharynx. The nasopharynx is divided by the septum. The nasopharynx is lined with a ciliated mucosal membrane that keeps dust and small particles from entering the respiratory system. Cilia help move contaminants out of the body. During an illness, the body produces more mucus to trap potentially infectious agents.

From the lateral walls of the nose, three bony shelves called **turbinates** extend into the nasal passageway. They are parallel to the nasal floor. The turbinates serve to increase the surface area of the nasal mucosa, thereby improving filtration, warming, and humidification of inhaled air. The sinuses are cavities formed by the cranial bones. They further trap bacteria and viruses and act as tributaries for fluid to and from the eustachian tubes and tear ducts, and they commonly become infected. Because the cranial

YOU are the Provider — PART 1

Your station is dispatched to a local assisted living center for a man in respiratory distress. As you call in, dispatch advises you that an ambulance is responding and is approximately 15 minutes away. As your engine arrives on scene, you are met by a frantic patient care attendant who states that the patient was just admitted to the facility earlier this morning, but now he does not seem to be breathing normally; however, she is unsure if this is normal for him or not. As you approach the patient's room, you ask if he is a full code, to which the patient care attendant replies "Yes."

1. How does the body regulate ventilation?
2. What are some of the factors that affect pulmonary ventilation?

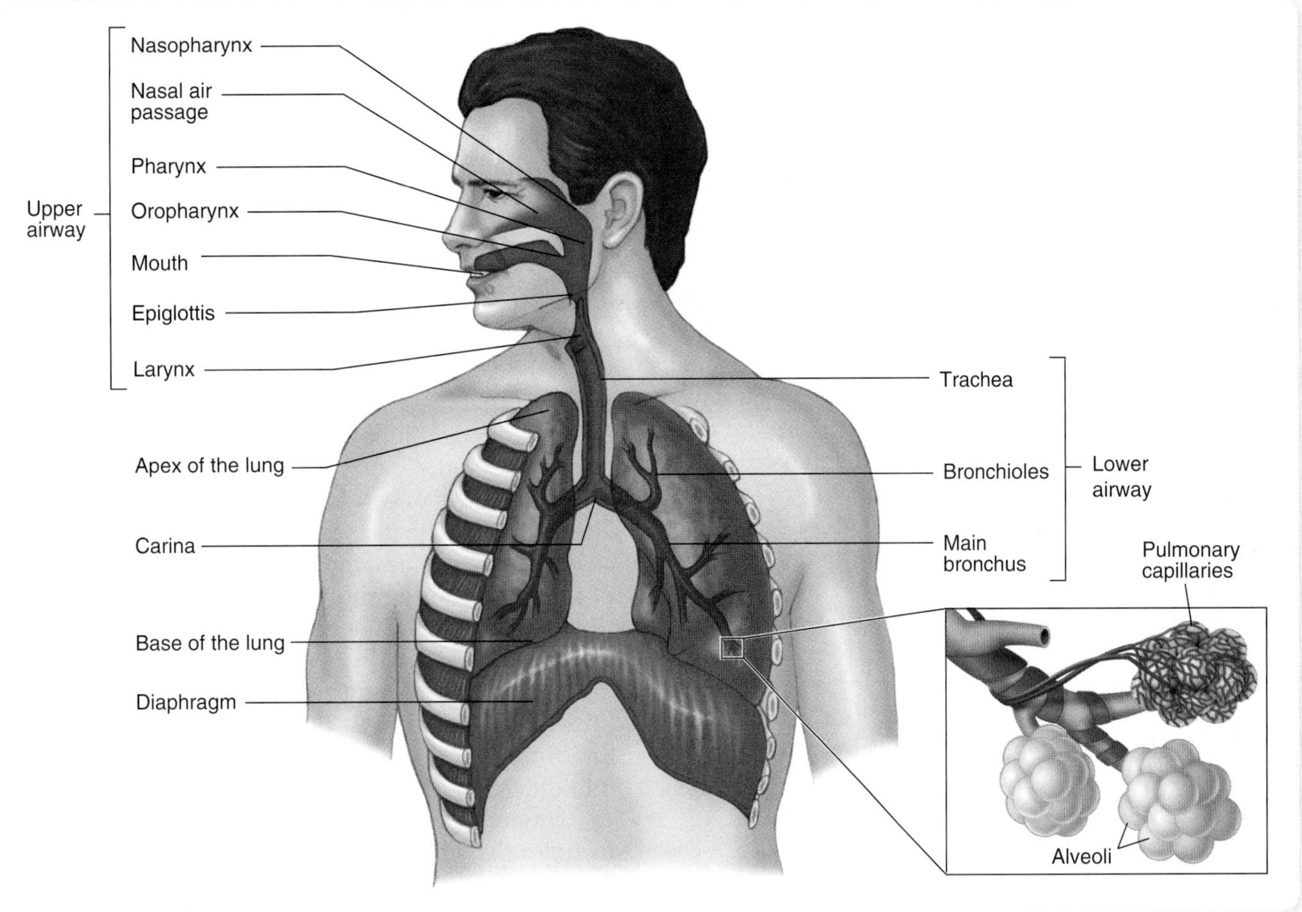

Figure 11-1 The upper and lower airways contain the structures in the body that help us breathe.

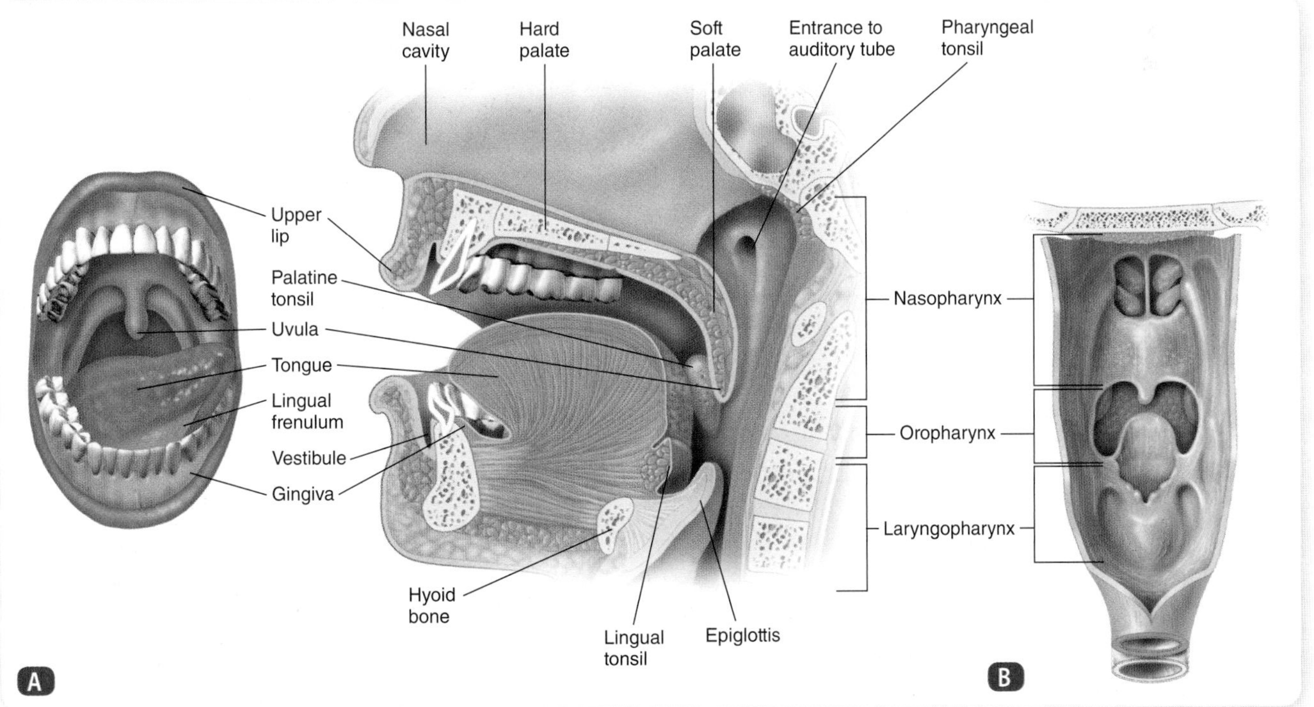

Figure 11-2 A. The oral cavity. **B.** The pharynx.

bones form the sinus cavities, fractures of certain sinus bones may cause a leakage of cerebrospinal fluid (CSF) into the nasal passageways and auditory canal.

The tissues of the nasopharynx are extremely delicate and highly vascular. Improper or overly aggressive placement of airway devices may cause substantial bleeding that cannot be controlled by direct pressure.

Oropharynx

The oral cavity begins with the mouth and teeth. The oral cavity is an alternate airway to the nose and is the entrance to the digestive system. The oropharynx is the part of the throat found at the posterior of the oral cavity. Recall from Chapter 7, *The Human Body*, that it contains the back third of the tongue, hyoid bone, soft palate, and the tonsils and adenoids.

The epiglottis is a leaf-shaped cartilaginous flap located at the base of the tongue and above the larynx at the superior border of the oropharynx that prevents food and liquid from entering the larynx during swallowing. When swallowing begins, laryngeal muscles contract to cause downward movement of the epiglottis and upward movement of the glottis. Combined with closure of the vocal cords, these actions protect the airway from **aspiration** (introduction of foreign material into the lungs) during eating and drinking.

Larynx

The **larynx** is a complex structure formed by many independent cartilaginous structures that all work together Figure 11-3. The main laryngeal structure is the thyroid cartilage, which is suspended from the hyoid bone by the thyroid ligament. The inferior aspect of the thyroid cartilage articulates with the cricoid cartilage or cricoid ring.

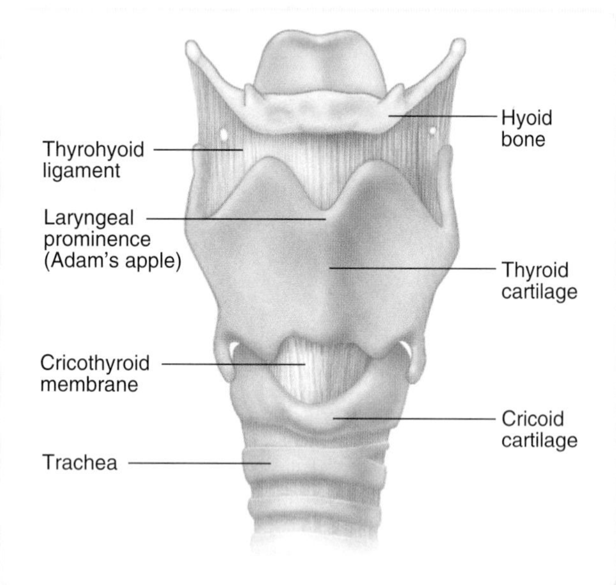

Figure 11-3 The larynx.

The **glottic opening** is the narrowest portion of the adult trachea. Airway patency in this area depends heavily on muscle tone. Airway devices are occasionally inadvertently inserted into the piriform fossae (hollow pockets along the lateral borders of the larynx), resulting in "tenting" of the skin under the jaw. The jugular notch, or suprasternal notch, is the large, visible dip located at the top of the manubrium between the neck and the two clavicles.

▶ The Lower Airway

The function of the lower airway is to exchange oxygen and carbon dioxide. Its external boundaries are the fourth cervical vertebra and the xiphoid process, which is the narrow cartilaginous lower tip of the sternum. Internally, it spans the glottis to the pulmonary capillary membrane.

The **trachea**, or windpipe, is the conduit for air entry into the lungs. The trachea begins directly below the cricoid cartilage and descends anteriorly down the midline of the neck into the thoracic cavity. When the trachea reaches the thoracic cavity, it divides at the level of the **carina**, which externally is approximately at the level of the jugular (sternal) notch at the top of the manubrium, into the two mainstem bronchi (right and left). The hollow bronchi are supported by cartilage and distribute air into the right and left lungs.

The lungs consist of the entire mass of tissue that includes the smaller bronchi, bronchioles, and alveoli Figure 11-4. The lungs are surrounded by a serous membrane called the pleura. All lung tissue is covered with a thin, slippery outer membrane called the **visceral pleura**. The **parietal pleura** lines the inside of the thoracic cavity. A small amount of fluid is found between these two layers and serves as a lubricant to prevent friction during breathing.

On entering the lungs, each bronchus divides into increasingly smaller bronchi, which subdivide into bronchioles. The **bronchioles** are thin, hollow tubes made of smooth muscle. The tone of these smooth muscles allows the bronchioles to dilate or constrict in response to various stimuli. The smaller bronchioles branch into alveolar ducts that end at the alveolar sacs.

The alveoli, located at the end of the airway, are millions of thin-walled, balloonlike sacs that serve as the functional site for the exchange of oxygen and carbon dioxide. Surrounding each of these sacs is an intricate bed of blood vessels, known as pulmonary capillaries. Oxygen diffuses through the lining of the alveoli into the pulmonary capillaries where, depending on adequate blood volume and pressure, it is carried back to the heart for distribution to the rest of the body. At the same time, carbon dioxide (waste) diffuses from the pulmonary capillaries into the alveoli where it is exhaled and removed from the body. A substance called **surfactant** lines the alveoli; surfactant decreases surface tension and helps keep the alveoli expanded. If the amount of surfactant is inadequate or the alveoli

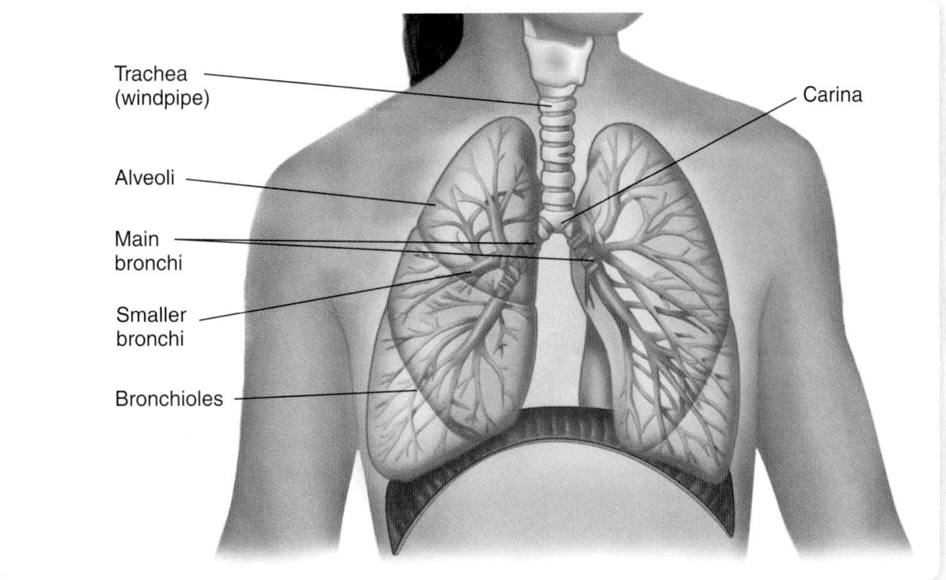

Figure 11-4 The trachea and the lungs are lower airway structures.

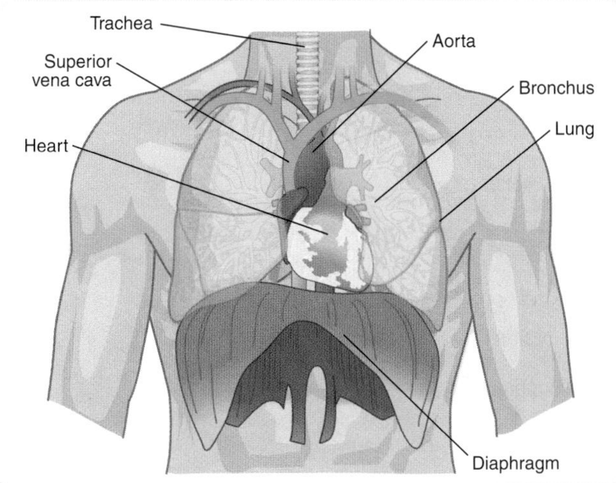

Figure 11-5 The thoracic cavity contains important anatomic structures for respiration, including the lungs and bronchi, heart, great vessels (the vena cava and aorta), and trachea.

are not inflated, the alveoli collapse, which results in a condition known as **atelectasis**.

The chest cage (thoracic cavity) contains the lungs, one on each side **Figure 11-5**. The ribs protect the thorax. Between each rib are intercostal muscles that can assist with breathing; however, they generally are not used unless the patient is in respiratory distress. Between the lungs is a space called the **mediastinum**, which is surrounded by tough connective tissue. This space contains the heart, the great vessels, the esophagus, the trachea, the major bronchi, and many nerves. The mediastinum effectively separates the right lung space from the left lung space.

In addition to the respiratory and circulatory structures found in the chest cage, the **phrenic nerves** travel through the chest to the diaphragm. The phrenic nerve innervates the diaphragmatic muscle, allowing it to contract. Contraction of the diaphragm occurs in a downward direction and is necessary for adequate inspiration to occur. When the phrenic nerves stop stimulation of the diaphragms, the diaphragm muscle relaxes and rises upward, allowing exhalation to occur.

Physiology of Breathing

The respiratory and cardiovascular systems work together to ensure that a constant supply of oxygen and nutrients are delivered to every cell in the body and that carbon dioxide and waste products are removed from every cell. The following sections describe the processes of **ventilation**, **oxygenation**, and **respiration**; however, you first need to understand how the processes of breathing and circulation are connected.

As air enters the body, it passes through the vocal cords, into the glottis, and down the trachea, where it is distributed through the mainstem bronchi into the bronchioles of the lungs. This occurs because negative pressure is created in the chest. Eventually the air reaches the alveolar sacs where the oxygen is diffused across the alveolar membrane into the pulmonary capillaries. At the same time, carbon dioxide is diffused across this membrane and is exhaled from the body. The oxygen in the pulmonary capillaries is transported back to the heart, where it is distributed to the rest of the body.

The heart pumps blood to the tissues of the body through a series of arteries and veins. Arteries carry

Special Populations

Although the maneuvers, techniques, and indications for airway management are essentially the same in children as they are in adults, several anatomic differences in children make mastery of these techniques difficult.

Infants and small children have a proportionately larger occiput (posterior portion of the cranium), which causes the head to flex when the child lies supine; this position itself can cause an airway obstruction. When positioning the airway of an infant or a child, you should place a folded towel under his or her shoulders to maintain a neutral position of the head.

Compared with adults, children have a proportionately smaller mandible and a proportionately larger tongue **Figure 11-6**. Both factors increase the incidence of airway obstruction in children.

The child's epiglottis is more floppy and omega-shaped (Ω) than an adult's **Figure 11-7**.

In general, the airway in infants and children is smaller and narrower at all levels. The larynx lies more superior and anterior than an adult's. The larynx is also funnel-shaped due to the narrow, underdeveloped cricoid cartilage. In children younger than 8 years, the *narrowest* portion of the airway is at the cricoid ring. Further narrowing of the child's inherently narrow airway, such as that caused by soft-tissue swelling or foreign body aspiration, can result in a major decrease in airway resistance and breathing inadequacy.

Children do not have well-developed chest musculature, and their ribs and cartilage are softer and more pliable than an adult's. As a result, the thoracic cavity cannot optimally contribute to lung expansion. Children rely heavily on their diaphragm for breathing, which moves their abdomen in and out. For this reason, infants and children are commonly referred to as belly breathers. When infants and children need to use the accessory muscles for breathing, they quickly tire and progress into respiratory distress, followed by respiratory arrest.

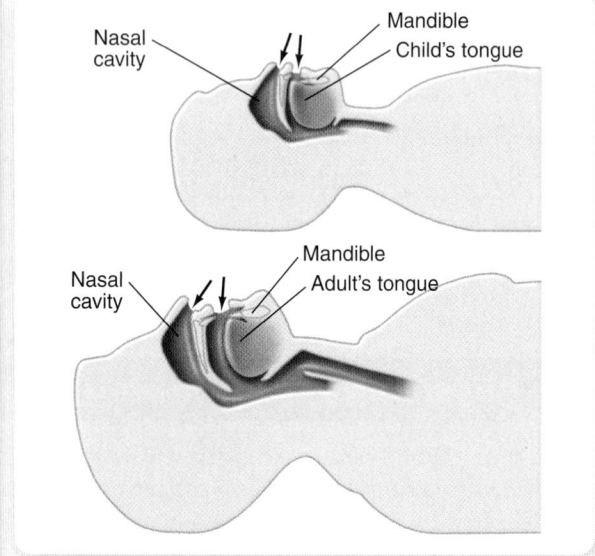

Figure 11-6 In children, the mandible is proportionately smaller and the tongue is proportionately larger than in an adult.

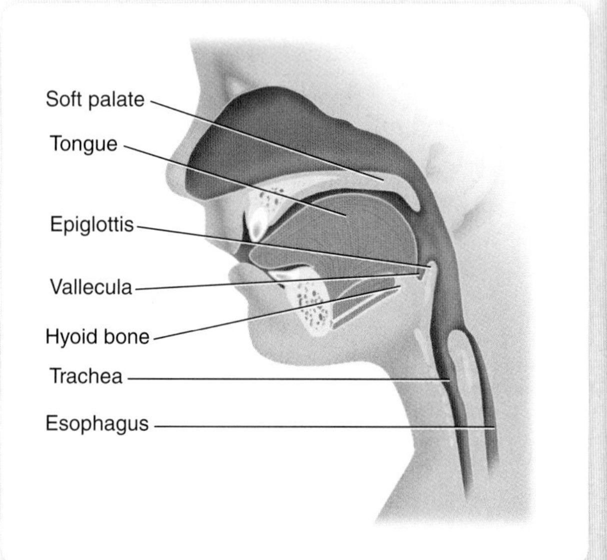

Figure 11-7 The child's epiglottis and surrounding structures.

oxygenated blood away from the heart and branch into arterioles and capillaries. When in the capillaries, the exchange of nutrients and waste products takes place. Oxygen and nutrients leave the capillaries and enter the cells. At the same time, waste products, such as carbon dioxide, diffuse from the cells back into the blood of the capillaries. From here, the blood travels through a series of venules that connect to larger veins. All veins (except the pulmonary vein) carry deoxygenated blood to the heart. The deoxygenated blood enters the right side of the heart through the right atrium, where it is pumped through the tricuspid valve, right ventricle, and pulmonary artery before being pumped to the lungs for oxygenation and removal of carbon dioxide. The oxygenated blood then travels through the pulmonary vein to the left atrium through the bicuspid valve and into the left ventricle, where it is again pumped to the rest of the body. Refer to Chapter 7, *The Human Body*, for an illustration of this process.

It is important to understand that the respiratory and circulatory systems work together to facilitate oxygen delivery to the tissues of the body **Table 11-1**. When one of these systems is compromised, oxygen delivery is not effective and cellular death could result.

Table 11-1	Ventilation, Oxygenation, and Respiration
Function	**Definition**
Ventilation	The physical act of moving air into and out of the lungs
Oxygenation	The process of loading oxygen molecules onto hemoglobin molecules in the bloodstream
Respiration	The actual exchange of oxygen and carbon dioxide in the alveoli and the tissues of the body

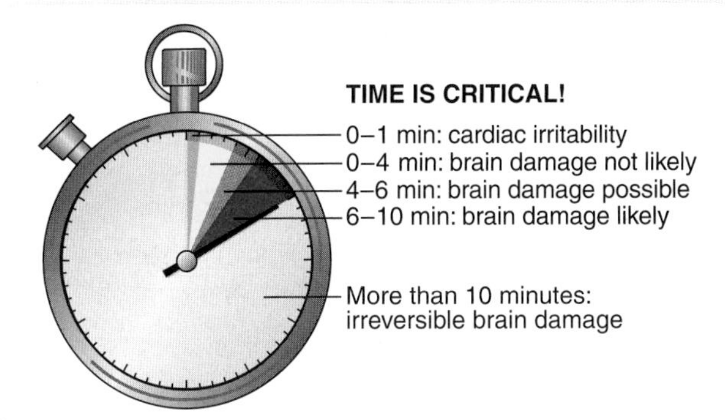

Figure 11-8 Cells need a constant supply of oxygen to survive. Some cells may be severely or permanently damaged after 4 to 6 minutes without oxygen.

Every cell in the body needs a constant supply of oxygen to survive. Whereas some tissues are more resilient than others, eventually all cells will die if deprived of oxygen **Figure 11-8**. To deliver adequate amounts of oxygen to the tissues of the body, sufficient levels of external ventilation and perfusion—circulation of blood within an organ or tissue in adequate amounts to meet the cells' current needs—must take place.

▶ Ventilation

Pulmonary ventilation, the process of moving air into and out of the lungs, is necessary for oxygenation and respiration to occur. Adequate, continuous ventilation is essential for life and, therefore, is one of the highest priorities in treating any patient. If a patient is not breathing or is breathing inadequately, you must immediately intervene to ensure adequate ventilation.

Inhalation

The active, muscular part of breathing is called **inhalation**. When a person inhales, air enters the body through the mouth and nose and moves to the trachea. This air travels to and from the lungs, filling and emptying the alveoli. During inhalation, the diaphragm and intercostal muscles contract. When the diaphragm contracts, it moves down slightly and enlarges the thoracic cage from top to bottom, and when the intercostal muscles contract, they lift the ribs up and out. The combined actions of these structures enlarge the thorax in all directions. Maximum inspiration occurs when the diaphragm and intercostal muscles are contracted and the lungs fill with air.

The lungs have no muscle tissue; therefore, they cannot move on their own. They need the help of other structures to be able to expand and contract during inhalation and exhalation. Therefore, the ability of the lungs to function properly is dependent on the movement of the chest and supporting structures. These structures include the thorax, the thoracic cage (chest), the diaphragm, the intercostal muscles, and the accessory muscles of breathing. Accessory muscles are secondary muscles of respiration.

The diaphragm is a specialized skeletal muscle. Innervated by the phrenic nerve, the diaphragm is attached to the costal arch and the vertebrae and functions as both a voluntary and involuntary muscle. It acts as a voluntary muscle when you are taking a deep breath, coughing, or holding your breath—all actions that are under voluntary control. However, unlike other skeletal or voluntary muscles, the diaphragm also performs an automatic function. Breathing continues during sleep and at all other times. Although you can hold your breath or temporarily breathe more quickly or slowly, you cannot continue these variations in breathing indefinitely. When the concentration of carbon dioxide rises within the blood, the autonomic regulation of breathing resumes under the control of the brainstem.

Words of Wisdom

Ventilation is the physical act of moving air in and out of the lungs. Ventilation is required for adequate respiration. If ventilation is adequate, other problems may hinder respiration. Examples of conditions that produce interruptions of ventilation include trauma such as a flail chest, foreign body airway obstruction, and an injury to the spinal cord that disrupts the function of the phrenic nerve that innervates the diaphragm.

Partial pressure is the term used to describe the amount of gas in air or dissolved in fluid, such as blood. Partial pressure is measured in millimeters of mercury (mm Hg). The partial pressure of oxygen in air residing in the alveoli is 104 mm Hg. Carbon dioxide enters the alveoli from the blood and causes a partial pressure of carbon dioxide of 40 mm Hg.

Deoxygenated arterial blood from the right side of the heart has a partial pressure of oxygen (called the PaO_2) that is lower than the partial pressure of oxygen in the alveoli.

The body attempts to equalize the partial pressure, which results in oxygen diffusion across the membrane into the blood; carbon dioxide diffuses into the alveoli and is eliminated as waste during exhalation. Oxygen and carbon dioxide both diffuse until partial pressures in the alveoli and blood are equal. This process occurs in reverse when the arterial blood reaches the tissues. Oxygen diffuses into the tissue fluid and then into the cells, and carbon dioxide diffuses out of the cells into the tissue fluid and blood.

The air pressure outside the body, called the atmospheric pressure, is normally higher than the air pressure within the thorax. During inhalation, the thoracic cage expands and the air pressure within the thorax decreases, creating a slight vacuum. This pulls air in through the trachea, causing the lungs to fill. When the air pressure outside equals the air pressure inside, air stops moving. Gases, such as oxygen, will move from an area of higher pressure to an area of lower pressure until the pressures are equal. At this point, the air stops moving, and inhalation stops.

It may help you to understand this if you think of the thoracic cage as a bell jar in which balloons are suspended. In this example, the balloons are the lungs. The base of the jar is the diaphragm, which moves up and down slightly with each breath. The ribs, which are the sides of the jar, maintain the shape of the chest. The only opening into the jar is a small tube at the top, similar to the trachea. During inhalation, the bottom of the jar moves down slightly, causing a decrease in pressure in the jar and creating a slight vacuum. As a result, the balloons fill with air **Figure 11-9**.

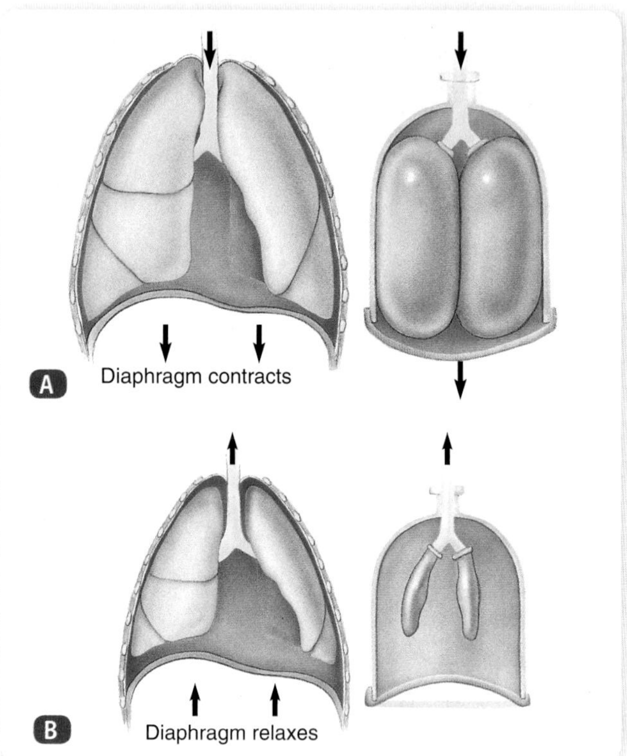

Figure 11-9 The mechanism of ventilation can be illustrated by a bell jar. **A.** Inhalation and chest expansion, anatomic (left) and bell jar (right). **B.** Exhalation and chest contraction, anatomic (left) and bell jar (right).

The entire process of **inspiration** is focused on delivering oxygen to the alveoli. However, not all of the air you breathe actually reaches the alveoli. **Table 11-2** reviews terminology discussed in Chapter 7, *The Human Body*, as it relates to the process of inspiration and ventilation.

It is important to note that variations in tidal volume, **respiratory rate** (the number of times a person breathes

Table 11-2 Ventilation Terminology

Term	Definition
Tidal volume	The amount of air (in milliliters) that is moved in or out of the lungs during one breath.
Residual volume	The air that remains in the lungs after maximal expiration.
Alveolar ventilation	The volume of air that reaches the alveoli; calculated by subtracting the amount of dead space air from the tidal volume.
Minute volume	The volume of air moved through the lungs in 1 minute; calculated by multiplying tidal volume and respiratory rate.
Alveolar minute volume	The volume of air moved through the lungs in 1 minute minus the dead space; calculated by multiplying tidal volume (minus dead space) and respiratory rate.
Vital capacity	The amount of air that can be forcibly expelled from the lungs after breathing in as deeply as possible.
Dead space	The portion of the tidal volume that does not reach alveoli and thus does not participate in gas exchange.

in 1 minute), or both will affect the minute volume. For example, if a patient is breathing at a rate of 12 breaths/min, but the tidal volume is reduced (shallow breathing), minute volume will decrease. Likewise, if a patient is breathing at a rate of 12 breaths/min and the tidal volume increases (deep breathing), minute volume will increase.

Exhalation

Unlike inhalation, **exhalation** does not normally require muscular effort; therefore, it is a passive process. As the chest expands, mechanical receptors, known as stretch receptors, in the chest wall and bronchioles send a signal to the apneustic center via the vagus nerve to inhibit the inspiratory center, and exhalation occurs. This feedback loop, a combination of mechanical and neural control, is known as the **Hering-Breuer reflex** and terminates inhalation to prevent overexpansion of the lungs. The diaphragm and intercostal muscles relax, which increases intrapulmonary pressure. The natural elasticity, or recoil, of the lungs passively removes the air. When the size of the thoracic cage decreases, air in the lungs is compressed into a smaller space. The air pressure within the thorax then becomes higher than the outside pressure, and the air is pushed out through the trachea. Maximum **expiration** occurs when the diaphragm and intercostal muscles relax and air is exhaled forcefully as opposed to the normal passive process.

Remember that air will reach the lungs only if it travels through the trachea. This is why clearing and maintaining an open airway is so important. Clearing the airway means removing obstructing material, tissue, or fluids from the nose, mouth, and throat. Maintaining the airway means keeping the airway **patent** so that air can enter and leave the lungs freely Figure 11-10.

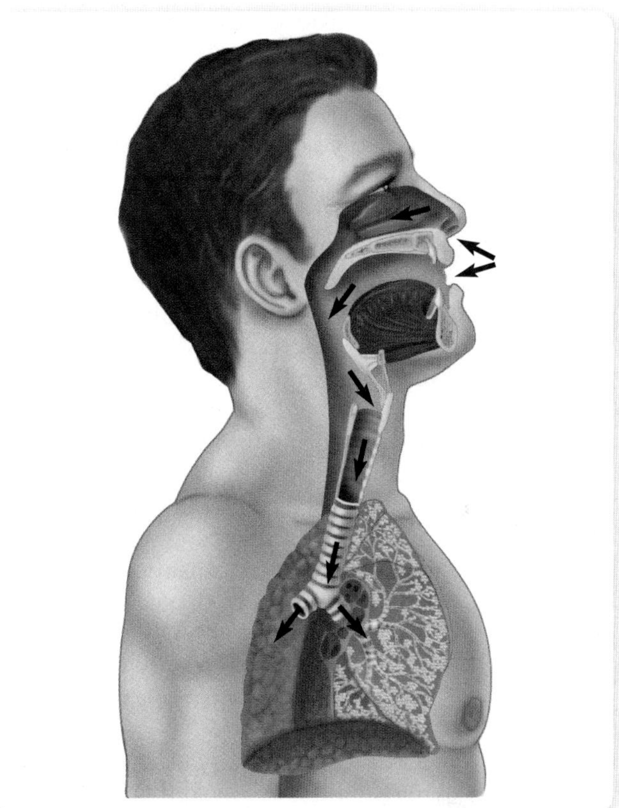

Figure 11-10 Air reaches the lungs only if it travels through the trachea. Maintaining the airway means keeping the airway patent so that air can enter and leave the lungs freely.

Air may also pass into the chest cavity through an abnormal opening in the throat or chest wall as a result of trauma, remaining outside the bronchi and never reaching the alveoli. In later chapters, you will learn how to recognize and manage these potentially life-threatening conditions.

Regulation of Ventilation

The body's need for oxygen is dynamic. The respiratory system must be able to accommodate the changes in oxygen demand by altering the rate and depth of ventilation. The regulation of ventilation involves a complex series of receptors and feedback loops that sense gas concentrations in the body fluids and send messages to the respiratory center in the brain to adjust the rate and depth of ventilation accordingly. For most people, the drive to breathe is based on pH changes (related to the carbon dioxide level) in the blood and CSF. In healthy people, when the oxygen level rises, the respiratory center suspends respiration until a rising carbon dioxide level stimulates the respiratory center to begin breathing again.

▶ Oxygenation

Oxygenation is the process of loading oxygen molecules onto hemoglobin molecules in the bloodstream. Adequate oxygenation is required for internal respiration to take place; however, it does not guarantee internal respiration is taking place. Oxygenation requires that the air used for ventilation contains an adequate percentage of oxygen. Although a person generally cannot oxygenate without ventilation, it is possible to ventilate without oxygenation. This situation occurs in places where the oxygen level in the breathing air has been depleted, such as in mines and confined spaces. Ventilation without adequate oxygenation also occurs in climbers who ascend too quickly to an altitude with inadequate atmospheric pressure. At high altitudes, the percentage of oxygen remains the same, but the atmospheric pressure makes it difficult to adequately bring sufficient amounts of oxygen into the body.

▶ Respiration

All living cells perform a specific function and need energy to survive. Cells take energy from nutrients through a series of chemical processes. The name given to these processes as a whole is **metabolism (cellular respiration)**. During metabolism, each cell combines nutrients (such as sugar) and oxygen and produces energy and waste products, primarily water and carbon dioxide. Each cell in the body requires a continuous supply of oxygen and a regular means of disposing of waste (carbon dioxide). The body provides for these requirements through respiration.

Respiration is the process of exchanging oxygen and carbon dioxide. This exchange occurs by diffusion, a process in which a gas moves from an area of greater concentration to an area of lower concentration. In the body, gases diffuse rapidly across a short distance of only micrometers.

External Respiration

External respiration (pulmonary respiration) is the process of breathing fresh air into the respiratory system and exchanging oxygen and carbon dioxide between the alveoli and the blood in the pulmonary capillaries Figure 11-11.

Fresh air that is inspired into the lungs contains about 21% oxygen, 78% nitrogen, and 0.3% carbon dioxide. As this air reaches the alveoli, it comes into contact with surfactant. As discussed, surfactant reduces surface tension within the alveoli and keeps them expanded, making it easier for the gas exchange between oxygen and carbon dioxide to take place. It is important to remember that although adequate ventilation is necessary for external respiration to take place, it does not guarantee that external respiration is being achieved.

After the oxygen crosses the alveolar-capillary membrane, it is bound to hemoglobin, an iron-containing protein molecule that has a great affinity for oxygen molecules, and is found in red blood cells. Hemoglobin molecules low in oxygen concentration are pumped from the right side of the heart into the capillaries of the pulmonary circulation. The capillaries surround alveoli containing high concentrations of oxygen (from inspired air). The hemoglobin molecules pick up fresh oxygen as it crosses the alveolar membrane and transport it back to the left side of the heart, where it is pumped out to the rest of the body. Under normal conditions, 96% to 100% of the hemoglobin receptor sites contain oxygen.

Words of Wisdom

The blood does not use all the inhaled oxygen as it passes through the body. The air that we exhale contains approximately 16% oxygen and 3% to 5% carbon dioxide; the rest is nitrogen. Therefore, when you provide mouth-to-mouth (or mask) ventilation to a patient who is not breathing, the patient is receiving a 16% concentration of oxygen with each of your exhaled breaths.

Internal Respiration

The exchange of oxygen and carbon dioxide between the systemic circulatory system and the cells of the body is called **internal respiration**. As blood travels through the body, it supplies oxygen and nutrients to various tissues and cells. As the oxygenated blood travels through the arteries and capillaries, the oxygen passes from the blood in the capillaries to tissue cells, while carbon dioxide and cell waste pass in the opposite direction: from tissue cells through capillaries and into the veins Figure 11-12.

In the presence of oxygen, the mitochondria of the cells convert glucose into energy using a process known as **aerobic metabolism**. Energy in the form of adenosine triphosphate (ATP) is produced through a series of processes known as the Krebs cycle and oxidative phosphorylation. Together, these chemical processes yield nearly 40 molecules of energy-rich ATP for each molecule of glucose metabolized. Without adequate oxygen, the cells do not completely convert glucose into energy, and lactic acid and other toxins accumulate in the cell. This process, **anaerobic metabolism**, cannot meet the metabolic demands of the cell. Although another intracellular process, glycolysis, also contributes to ATP production and does not require oxygen, this process results in less ATP production, and lactic acid waste products and toxins are produced. If this process is not

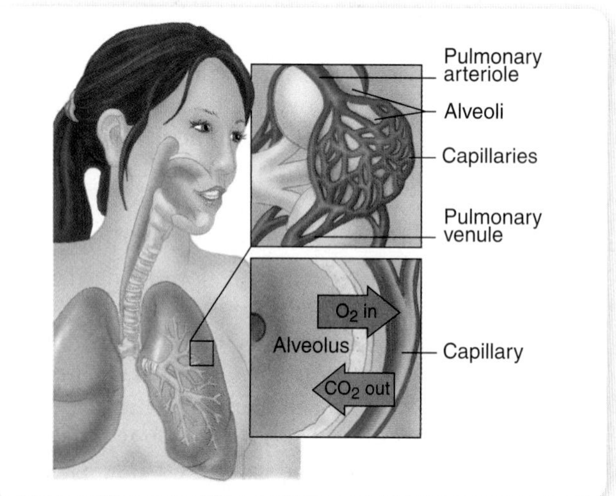

Figure 11-11 External respiration.

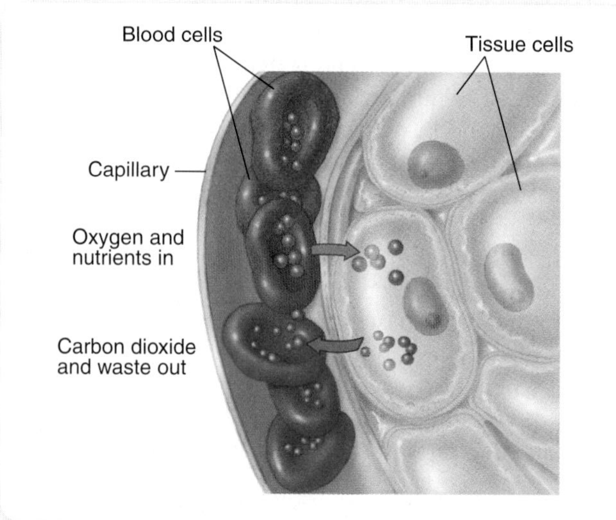

Figure 11-12 Internal respiration.

corrected, the cells will eventually die. Therefore, adequate levels of perfusion (circulation of blood within an organ or tissue) and external ventilation must be present for aerobic internal respiration to take place. However, although these elements are necessary for internal respiration, they do not guarantee that aerobic internal respiration will take place.

When the mitochondria within each cell use oxygen to convert glucose to energy, carbon dioxide (the main waste product) accumulates in the cell. Carbon dioxide is then transported through the circulatory system and back to the lungs for exhalation.

When oxygen is not present, anaerobic metabolism occurs. It creates a series of events that will eventually result in cellular death. Initially, cells become hypoxic, and as stores of glucose are used up, lactic acid, which is the by-product of glycolysis, remains. The increasing acidic environment destroys the cellular proteins, which in turn results in cellular death and infarction of tissue as more cells become ischemic and then necrotic.

Understanding the process of ventilation, oxygenation, and respiration is an important concept for AEMTs. The overall goal of these mechanisms is to deliver an adequate supply of oxygen to the cells of the body. When one of these processes fails or becomes disrupted, cells will die. By recognizing the signs and symptoms of inadequate tissue perfusion and oxygenation, you can immediately intervene and correct a potentially life-threatening condition.

▶ Neural Control

The neural control of breathing originates in the brain and brainstem. Primary control comes from the medulla and pons. The medulla is the primary involuntary respiratory center. It is connected to the respiratory muscles by the vagus nerve. The medullary respiratory centers control the rate, depth, and rhythm of breathing in a negative feedback interaction with centers in the pons.

The apneustic center of the pons is the secondary control center if the medulla fails to initiate respiration. The apneustic center influences the respiratory rate by increasing the number of inspirations per minute. This is balanced by the pneumotaxic center, which has an inhibitory influence on inspiration. The respiratory rate, therefore, results from the interaction between these two centers. In times of increased demand, the pneumotaxic center decreases its influence, thereby increasing the respiratory rate.

▶ Chemical Stimuli

The goal of the respiratory system is to keep the blood's concentrations of oxygen and carbon dioxide and its acid-base balance within very narrow normal ranges. The body has many receptors that monitor variables and provide feedback to the respiratory centers to modify the respiratory rate and depth based on the body's needs. These **chemoreceptors** have important effects on respiratory rate and depth.

Chemoreceptors that constantly monitor the chemical composition of body fluids are located throughout the body to provide feedback on many metabolic processes. Three sets of chemoreceptors affect respiratory function. The first two, which monitor the carbon dioxide level in the blood and the pH of the CSF, have a much greater effect on ventilatory depth and rate than does the third.

The chemoreceptors that measure the amount of carbon dioxide in arterial blood are located in the carotid bodies and the aortic arch. These receptors sense minute changes in the carbon dioxide level and send signals to the respiratory center via the glossopharyngeal nerve (9th cranial nerve) and the vagus nerve (10th cranial nerve).

Central chemoreceptors, which constantly monitor the pH of the CSF, are located adjacent to the respiratory centers in the medulla. The acidity of the CSF is an indirect measure of the amount of carbon dioxide in arterial blood because the carbon dioxide in the blood readily diffuses across the blood-brain barrier and combines with water to form carbonic acid (H_2CO_3). The carbonic acid dissociates, and the pH decreases as the hydrogen ion (H^+) concentration increases. An increase in the acidity of CSF triggers the central chemoreceptors to increase the rate and depth of respiration. These central chemoreceptors are sensitive to small changes in pH and provide for "fine-tuning" of the body's acid-base balance.

Although the primary control of ventilation is the pH of the CSF, the amount of oxygen dissolved in the plasma (PaO_2) has a secondary and protective role. The chemoreceptors located in the aortic arch and carotid bodies also respond to decreases in PaO_2 by sending messages to the respiratory control center to increase respiration. Under normal conditions, these chemoreceptors serve as a backup to the primary control of ventilation, which is based on the level of carbon dioxide in the blood and the pH of the CSF.

When serum carbon dioxide or hydrogen ion levels increase because of medical or traumatic conditions involving the respiratory system, chemoreceptors stimulate the dorsal and ventral respiratory groups in the medulla to increase the respiratory rate, thus removing more carbon dioxide or acid from the body. The **dorsal respiratory group** is responsible for initiating inspiration based on the information received from the chemoreceptors. The **ventral respiratory group** is primarily responsible for motor control of the inspiratory and expiratory muscles.

Pathophysiology of Respiration

Multiple conditions inhibit the body's ability to effectively deliver oxygen to the cells. Disruption of pulmonary ventilation, oxygenation, and respiration will cause immediate effects on the body. As an AEMT, you need to recognize these conditions and correct them immediately.

Hypoxia

Failure to meet the body's needs for oxygen may result in **hypoxia**. Hypoxia is an extremely dangerous condition in which the tissues and cells of the body do not get enough oxygen. If this process is not corrected, patients may die quickly.

Patients with chronic obstructive pulmonary disease (COPD) have difficulty eliminating carbon dioxide through exhalation; thus, they always have higher levels of carbon dioxide. This potentially can alter their drive for breathing. The theory is that respiratory centers in the brain gradually accommodate to a high level of carbon dioxide. In patients with COPD in the end-stage of their disease, the body uses a "backup system" to control breathing. This theory of secondary control of breathing, called **hypoxic drive**, stimulates breathing when the arterial oxygen level falls. However, the nerves in the brain, the walls of the aorta, and the carotid arteries that act as oxygen sensors are easily satisfied with a minimal level of oxygen. Therefore, the hypoxic drive is much less sensitive and less powerful than the carbon dioxide sensors in the brainstem.

Hypoxic drive is typically found in end-stage COPD and not in the patient with a recent diagnosis. Providing high concentrations of oxygen could potentially negatively affect the body's drive to breathe in patients dependent on hypoxic drive. This effect is rare, however, and easily addressed with coaching or ventilator assistance. A high concentration of oxygen should never be withheld from any patient who needs it.

Patients who are breathing inadequately will show varying signs and symptoms of hypoxia. The onset and degree of tissue damage caused by hypoxia often depend on the quality of ventilations. Early signs of hypoxia include restlessness, irritability, apprehension, fast heart rate (tachycardia), and anxiety. Late signs of hypoxia include mental status changes, a weak (thready) pulse, and cyanosis. Responsive patients will report shortness of breath (**dyspnea**) and may not be able to talk in complete sentences. You should administer supplemental oxygen to a patient with respiratory distress before signs and symptoms of hypoxia appear.

Words of Wisdom

A patient who is breathing inadequately (hypoventilating) requires oxygen regardless of history. Withholding oxygen from a patient with COPD in an attempt to preserve the hypoxic drive may be detrimental to the patient. If vital organs are not perfused, cells and tissue may die, resulting in irreversible damage. Even after the cause of the problem is addressed, if substantial damage has occurred, the patient may not recover. By ventilating the hypoxic patient, vital organs are perfused. If the hypoxic drive is eliminated, organs are still oxygenated. After the cause of the original problem has been corrected, the patient can be weaned off the ventilator and may return to a normal, productive life.

Ventilation-Perfusion Ratio and Mismatch

The lungs have a functional role of placing ambient (room) air in proximity to circulating blood to permit gas exchange by simple diffusion. To accomplish this action, air and blood flow must be directed to the same place at the same time. In other words, ventilation and perfusion must be matched. A failure to match ventilation and perfusion, or **$\dot{V}/\dot{Q}$ mismatch**, contributes to most abnormalities in oxygen and carbon dioxide exchange.

In most people, the normal resting minute ventilation is approximately 6 L/min. Approximately one-third of this volume fills dead space; therefore, resting alveolar ventilation is approximately 4 L/min. However, pulmonary artery blood flow is approximately 5 L/min. This yields an overall ratio of ventilation to perfusion of four-fifths L/min, or 0.8 L/min. Because neither ventilation nor perfusion is distributed equally, both are distributed to dependent regions of the lungs at rest. However, the increase in gravity-dependent flow is more marked with perfusion (blood) than with ventilation (air). Hence, the ratio of ventilation to perfusion is highest at the apex (top) of the lung and lowest at the base (bottom).

When ventilation is compromised but perfusion continues, blood passes over some alveolar membranes without gas exchange taking place; therefore, not all alveoli are enriched with oxygen. This results in a lack of oxygen diffusing across the membrane and into the circulatory system. Along the same lines, carbon dioxide is also unable to diffuse across the membrane and is recirculated in the bloodstream. The $\dot{V}/\dot{Q}$ mismatch that results limits the ability of the lungs to oxygenate the blood and to filter carbon dioxide from the blood. When this affects a large portion of the lung, the result can be fatal.

Similar problems can occur when perfusion across the alveolar membrane is disrupted. Even though the alveoli are filled with fresh oxygen, disruption in blood flow does not allow for exchange of gases across the membrane in affected areas of the lung. The result of inadequate perfusion is less oxygen absorption in the bloodstream and less carbon dioxide removal. This $\dot{V}/\dot{Q}$ ratio mismatch can also result in hypoxia, and when severe, the patient needs immediate intervention to prevent further damage or death.

Factors Affecting Ventilation

Maintaining a patent airway is critical to the delivery of oxygen to the tissues of the body. Many intrinsic and extrinsic factors cause airway obstruction. Intrinsic conditions such as infections, allergic reactions, and unresponsiveness (possibly resulting in airway obstruction by the tongue) can cause substantial restrictions on the ability to maintain an open airway. Swelling from infections and allergic reactions can be fatal if not aggressively managed with medications and, possibly, advanced airway management techniques. The tongue is the most common airway obstruction in an unresponsive patient. This airway obstruction, although easily corrected, can result in hypoxia and hinder adequate tissue perfusion. Snoring respirations and an improper position of the head and/or neck are good indicators that the tongue may be obstructing the airway. Prompt correction of this obstruction is necessary for adequate ventilation and oxygenation.

Some factors affecting pulmonary ventilation are not necessarily directly part of the respiratory system. The central and peripheral nervous systems have key roles in the regulation of breathing. Interruptions to these systems can have a drastic effect on the ability to breathe efficiently. Medications that depress the central nervous system lower the respiratory rate and tidal volume. This lower rate and volume will decrease the overall minute volume and alveolar ventilation. As a result, the amount of carbon dioxide in the respiratory and circulatory systems is increased, resulting in an overall increase of the carbon dioxide level in the bloodstream, known as **hypercapnia**. Trauma to the head and spinal cord can also interrupt nervous control of ventilation, resulting in decreased respiratory function and even failure. Neuromuscular disorders, such as muscular dystrophy, can also affect the ability of the nervous system to control breathing. Muscular dystrophy causes degeneration of muscle fibers, slowing motor development, and loss of muscle contractility. Curvature of the spine is also likely in patients with muscular dystrophy and can impair pulmonary function.

Patients with allergic reactions might have not only a potential airway obstruction from swelling (angioedema), but also a decrease in pulmonary ventilation from bronchoconstriction. As the bronchioles constrict, air is forced through smaller lumens resulting in decreased ventilation. Bronchoconstriction is also associated with conditions such as COPD and asthma.

Extrinsic factors affecting pulmonary ventilation can include trauma and foreign body airway obstruction. Trauma to the airway or chest requires immediate evaluation and intervention. Blunt or penetrating trauma and burns can disrupt airflow through the trachea and into the lungs, quickly resulting in oxygenation deficiencies. In addition, trauma to the chest wall can result in structural damage to the thorax, resulting in inadequate pulmonary ventilation. For example, a patient with numerous rib fractures or a flail chest may purposely breathe shallowly in an attempt to alleviate the pain caused by the injury. This practice is called respiratory splinting and can result in decreased pulmonary ventilation. Swelling, punctures, and lung tissue bruising can all have a tremendous effect on the ability to deliver oxygen to the alveoli and into the bloodstream. Proper airway management and ventilatory support are crucial to the outcome in these situations.

If carbon dioxide production exceeds the body's ability to eliminate it by ventilation, then the partial pressure of carbon dioxide ($Pa{CO_2}$) rises, resulting in hypoventilation (slow and/or shallow breathing). Theoretically, hypoventilation can occur in two ways: either carbon dioxide production can exceed the body's ability to eliminate it, or carbon dioxide elimination can be depressed to the extent that it no longer keeps up with normal metabolism.

At the other extreme is **hyperventilation** (rapid and/or deep breathing), which occurs when carbon dioxide elimination exceeds carbon dioxide production. For example, a patient experiencing an anxiety attack tends to breathe very deeply and rapidly, so he or she eliminates carbon dioxide at a rate faster than the body produces it. The level of carbon dioxide in his or her blood then falls below normal, and the patient experiences symptoms such as dizziness and numbness or tingling in the face and extremities.

Hypoventilation and hyperventilation could represent the body's attempt to compensate for various abnormal conditions. For example, if the pH of the blood is too high (**alkalosis**), the patient's breathing may become slow and/or shallow in an attempt to retain carbon dioxide (and therefore, hydrogen ions [H^+]) in an attempt to decrease the pH. Conversely, hyperventilation could be a compensatory response of the body to a decrease in the pH of the blood (**acidosis**), such as what occurs with hyperglycemic ketoacidosis or aspirin overdose.

In addition to factors discussed thus far, decreases or increases in minute volume can result in problems with carbon dioxide levels in the blood **Table 11-3**. A decrease in the minute volume decreases carbon dioxide elimination, resulting in a buildup of carbon dioxide in the blood (hypercapnia). An increase in the minute volume increases carbon dioxide elimination, which lowers the carbon dioxide content of the blood (hypocapnia).

Factors Affecting Oxygenation and Respiration

External elements in the environment can affect the overall process of respiration. For proper respiration to take place at the cellular level, both oxygenation and perfusion need to function efficiently.

Table 11-3 Carbon Dioxide Balance

	Hypoventilation	Hyperventilation
Minute volume	↓	↑
CO_2 elimination	↓	↑
$Pa{CO_2}$	↑ (hypercapnia)	↓ (hypocapnia)

Abbreviations: CO_2, carbon dioxide; $Pa{CO_2}$, partial pressure of carbon dioxide

External Factors

Adequate respiration requires proper ventilation and oxygenation. External factors such as atmospheric pressure and the partial pressure of oxygen (Pa_{O_2}) in the ambient air have a key role in the overall process of respiration. At high altitudes, the percentage of oxygen remains the same, but the partial pressure decreases because the total atmospheric pressure decreases. The low Pa_{O_2} can make it difficult (or impossible) to adequately oxygenate tissue, thus interrupting internal respiration. In addition, closed environments, such as mines and trenches, may also have decreases in ambient oxygen, resulting in poor oxygenation and respiration.

Carbon monoxide, along with other toxic gases, displaces oxygen in the environment and makes proper oxygenation and respiration difficult. Particularly, carbon monoxide has a much greater affinity for hemoglobin than does oxygen (200 to 250 times greater). The attachment of carbon monoxide molecules to the hemoglobin molecules, which forms carboxyhemoglobin (COHb), inhibits the proper transport of oxygen to tissues and can cause false pulse oximeter readings.

Internal Factors

Conditions that reduce the surface area for gas exchange also decrease the body's oxygen supply, resulting in inadequate tissue perfusion. Medical conditions such as pneumonia, **pulmonary edema**, and COPD may also result in a disturbance of cellular metabolism. These conditions decrease the surface area of the alveoli by damaging the alveoli or by resulting in an accumulation of fluid in the lungs.

Nonfunctional alveoli inhibit the diffusion of oxygen and carbon dioxide. As a result, blood entering the lungs from the right side of the heart bypasses the alveoli and returns to the left side of the heart in an unoxygenated state, a condition called **intrapulmonary shunting**.

Patients who are submerged in water and patients with pulmonary edema have fluid in the alveoli. This accumulation of fluid inhibits adequate gas exchange at the alveolar membrane and results in decreased oxygenation and respiration. In addition, exposure to certain environmental conditions (such as high altitudes) or occupational hazards (such as epoxy resins) can result in fluid accumulation in the alveoli over time, resulting in an overall decrease in respiration. Respirations increase or decrease based on the body's need at any given time. As body temperature rises, the number of respirations increase in response to the increased metabolic activity. Certain medications cause the respiratory rate to increase or decrease, depending on their physiologic action. Pain and strong emotions can also increase respirations. Hypoxia, which is a powerful stimulus to breathe, increases respirations in an effort to bring in more oxygen. Conversely, to eliminate carbon dioxide from the body, respirations increase when carbon dioxide production is increased. Respirations decrease as metabolism slows, such as during sleep.

Other conditions that affect the cells of the body include hypoxia, hypoglycemia (low blood glucose level), and infection. As oxygen and glucose levels decrease, the body is unable to maintain a homeostatic balance regarding energy production. At this point, the energy production cannot meet the needs of the body, and cellular death is likely if the condition is not corrected. Infection also increases the metabolic needs of the body and disrupts homeostasis. If not corrected, the cells will die as well. If the levels of the hormone insulin decrease in the body, then the cellular uptake of glucose will decrease. Without sufficient glucose, the cells will metabolize fatty acids, resulting in ketoacidosis—a form of metabolic acidosis.

Words of Wisdom

During normal breathing, the negative pressure created by each breath increases venous return of blood to the heart. Just as negative intrathoracic pressure draws air into the chest cavity through the airway (**negative pressure ventilation**), the same pressure also draws venous blood back to the heart from the head (via the superior vena cava) and abdomen (via the inferior vena cava).

When patients transition from negative pressure ventilation to positive pressure ventilation (the forcing of air into the lungs [ie, bag-mask ventilation]), they lose this stimulus for venous return, and some patients may experience decreased cardiac output and hypotension as a result. The increased intrathoracic pressure caused by positive pressure ventilation creates a pressure gradient against which the heart must pump. This process also increases the afterload (the amount of resistance against which the ventricle must contract), which can further decrease cardiac output. The greater the pressure used to ventilate an apneic or a hypoventilating patient, the greater the decrease in **preload** (the volume of blood that returns to the heart), which occurs when the heart is literally squeezed by increased intrathoracic pressure.

Patients who are hypotensive, in shock, or are otherwise hemodynamically unstable may experience profound changes in blood pressure as a result of the hemodynamic effects of positive pressure ventilation. The best way to minimize this complication is to ventilate the patient for a period of 1 second—just enough to cause visible chest rise—and avoid ventilating the patient too fast.

Circulatory Compromise

For respiration to take place, the circulatory system must function efficiently to deliver oxygen to the tissues of the body. When this system becomes compromised, perfusion becomes inadequate and the body's oxygen demands will not be met.

Obstruction of blood flow to individual cells and tissue is typically related to trauma emergencies. Conditions you may encounter include pulmonary embolism, a simple or tension **pneumothorax**, open pneumothorax (sucking chest wound), hemothorax, and hemopneumothorax. All of these conditions inhibit gas exchange at the tissue level as a result of their effects on the respiratory and circulatory systems. In addition, conditions such as heart failure and cardiac tamponade inhibit the ability of the heart to effectively pump oxygenated blood to the tissues.

Blood loss and anemia—a deficiency of red blood cells—reduce the oxygen-carrying capacity of the blood. Without sufficient circulating red blood cells, not enough hemoglobin molecules are available to bind with oxygen.

When the body is in a state of shock, oxygen is not delivered to the cells efficiently. Hemorrhagic shock (a form of **hypovolemic shock**) is an abnormal decrease in blood volume that causes inadequate oxygen delivery to the body. In contrast, **vasodilatory shock** is not determined by the amount of circulating blood, but by the size of the blood vessels. As the diameter of the blood vessels increases, the blood pressure in the circulatory system decreases; oxygen is not delivered to the tissues in an effective manner. Both forms of shock result in poor tissue perfusion that results in anaerobic metabolism. You should aggressively treat any patient suspected of being in shock to prevent further interruptions in tissue perfusion.

Acid-Base Balance

Both hypoventilation and hyperventilation, along with hypoxia, cause disruptions in the acid-base balance in the body that may result in rapid deterioration and death. The respiratory system and the renal system have roles in maintaining homeostasis in the body. Homeostasis is a tendency toward stability in the body's internal environment and requires a balance between the acids and bases in the body. When there is an excess of acid in the body, the fastest way to eliminate it is through the respiratory system. Excess acid can be expelled as carbon dioxide from the lungs. Conversely, slowing respirations will increase the level of carbon dioxide. The renal system regulates pH by filtering out more hydrogen and retaining bicarbonate when needed, or doing the reverse. The fastest way the body can eliminate excess H^+ ions is to create water and carbon dioxide, which can be expelled from the lungs.

Anything that inhibits respiratory function can result in acid retention and acidosis. Any time a patient is in respiratory distress or is unable to breathe, acidosis quickly develops. Acidosis can develop as a result of abnormal respiratory function (such as with **bradypnea**, labored breathing, or shallow breathing [reduced tidal volume]). Alkalosis can develop if the respiratory rate is too high (**tachypnea**) or the volume too great.

Recall that the four main clinical presentations of acid-base disorders are:

- **Respiratory acidosis**
- **Respiratory alkalosis**
- **Metabolic acidosis**
- **Metabolic alkalosis**

Fluctuations in pH due to the available bicarbonate level result in metabolic acidosis or alkalosis. Fluctuations in pH due to respiratory disorders result in respiratory acidosis or alkalosis. The focus here is on respiratory acidosis and respiratory alkalosis.

YOU are the Provider — PART 2

As you approach the patient, you note snoring respirations approximately every 10 to 12 seconds, with cyanosis around the patient's lips and nail beds. You attempt to speak to the patient, but he responds with only a low moaning sound when you do a sternal rub. You direct your partner to immediately establish bag-mask ventilations at a rate of 10 breaths/min, with supplemental oxygen. As you perform your primary survey of the patient, you note no abnormal findings beyond his cyanosis, and no readily identifiable cause for his hypoxia and bradypnea. You apply your pulse oximeter and obtain a reading of 78%.

Recording Time: 1 Minute	
Appearance	Poor
Level of consciousness	Moans to pressure stimulation
Airway	Patent
Breathing	Shallow, slow
Circulation	Cool, clammy, cyanotic

3. Which acid-base disorder do you suspect this patient is experiencing?
4. How does the pulse oximeter guide your treatment of this patient?

Acid-base disorders that are not immediately correctable by the body's buffering systems initiate compensatory mechanisms to help return levels to normal. For example, metabolic acidosis may create respiratory alkalosis as a compensatory response. Often, patient treatment involves treating more than one form of acid-base imbalance.

Treatment for the classic hyperventilation syndrome focuses on restoring the normal respiratory rate to increase the carbon dioxide level. However, increasing the carbon dioxide level can aggravate other more serious medical conditions that cause hyperventilation. Therefore, you must carefully evaluate the patient to determine the underlying cause of the hyperventilation before you attempt to correct it.

Patient Assessment: Airway Evaluation

Recognizing Adequate Breathing

You can think of a normal breathing pattern as a bellows system. Breathing should appear easy, not labored. As with a bellows used to move air to start a fire, breathing should be a smooth flow of air into and out of the lungs. A patient with adequate breathing should be able to speak in full sentences and in a normal voice. Generally, if you can see or hear a patient breathe, there is a problem.

Normal respirations in an adult are characterized by a rate of between 12 and 20 breaths/min with adequate depth (tidal volume), a regular pattern of inhalation and exhalation, and clear and equal **bilateral** breath sounds (on both sides of the chest) Table 11-4. Breathing at rest should be effortless; changes may be subtle in rate or regularity.

> **Words of Wisdom**
>
> Recognition of an extremely rapid rate, an incredibly slow rate, any unusual respiratory pattern, or poor tidal volume should immediately result in consideration of bag-mask ventilations if the patient will tolerate it.

Table 11-4 Normal Respiratory Rate Ranges

Age	Range (breaths/min)
Adults	12 to 20
Children (ages 1 to 18 years)	12 to 37
Infants (ages 1 month to 1 year)	30 to 53

Pediatric data from: American Heart Association (AHA). Vital signs in children. In: *Pediatric Advanced Life Support.* Dallas, TX: AHA; 2015.

Recognizing Inadequate Breathing

An adult patient who is breathing at a rate of fewer than 12 breaths/min or more than 20 breaths/min should be evaluated for other signs of inadequate breathing, such as shallow breathing (reduced tidal volume), an irregular pattern of breathing, altered mentation, or abnormal breath sounds. Irregular respiratory patterns are clinically important until proven otherwise.

Patients with respiratory distress often compensate with preferential positioning, such as an upright sniffing position (in which the patient is sitting up, with the head moved forward until the earlobes are on the same vertical plane as the manubrium of the sternum), or a tripod position (in which the patient is sitting up and leaning forward with elbows bent). A patient experiencing breathing difficulty will avoid a supine position because this position typically increases respiratory distress.

Respiratory distress may be the result of upper and/or lower airway obstruction, inadequate ventilation, impairment of the respiratory muscles, or impairment of the nervous system. Any difficulty in respiratory rate, regularity, or effort is defined as dyspnea. Dyspnea may be the result of or result in **hypoxemia**—a deficiency of oxygen in the arterial blood. If left untreated, hypoxemia will progress to hypoxia (lack of oxygen to the body's cells and tissues). Untreated hypoxia will result in anoxia and death of the body's cells and tissues.

> **Words of Wisdom**
>
> *Hypoxemia* is defined as a low level of oxygen in arterial blood. *Hypoxia*, as discussed earlier, is a deficiency of oxygen at the tissue and cellular levels. Although these terms are often used interchangeably, they are different processes. Hypoxemia can often be reversed by administering supplemental oxygen, whereas hypoxia may require more aggressive oxygenation and, in some cases, metabolic correction. Left untreated, hypoxia will result in **anoxia**—a lack of oxygen that results in tissue and cellular death.

Recognition and treatment of dyspnea are crucial to patient survival. Careful assessment and treatment of a patient with dyspnea are essential. The brain can survive only a few minutes of anoxia. After 4 to 6 minutes without oxygen, brain cells may be severely and permanently damaged and may even die. Dead brain cells can never be replaced. Treatment of the patient will be ineffective if the airway is not patent and the patient is not breathing adequately.

Evaluation of the patient in respiratory distress includes observations, palpation, and auscultation. Use visual techniques at first sight of the patient—literally from the door as you are entering the room. Determine answers to the following questions when you assess a patient with respiratory distress:

- How is the patient positioned? Is he or she in a tripod position (elbows out)?
- Is the patient experiencing **orthopnea** (positional dyspnea)?
- Is there adequate rise and fall of the chest?
- Is the patient gasping?
- What is the color of the skin? Is the skin moist or clammy?
- Is there flaring of the nares present?
- Is the patient breathing through pursed lips?
- Do you note any **retractions** (skin pulling in around the ribs during inspiration):
  - Intercostal?
  - At the suprasternal notch?
  - At the supraclavicular fossa?
  - Subcostal?
- Is the patient using accessory muscles to breathe?
- Is the patient's chest wall moving symmetrically? (**Asymmetric chest wall movement**, when one side of the chest moves less than the other, indicates that airflow into one lung may be decreased.)
- Is the patient taking a series of quick breaths, followed by a prolonged exhalation phase?

A patient with inadequate breathing may appear to be working hard to breathe. This type of breathing pattern is called **labored breathing**. It requires effort and, especially among children, may involve the use of accessory muscles. Accessory muscles include the neck muscles (sternocleidomastoid), the chest pectoralis major muscles, and the abdominal muscles **Figure 11-13**.

Accessory muscles are not used during normal breathing. More information about recognizing labored breathing and respiratory distress in children is found in later chapters. Signs of inadequate breathing in adults are as follows:

- Respiratory rate of fewer than 12 breaths/min or more than 20 breaths/min in the presence of shortness of breath (dyspnea)
- Irregular rhythm, such as a patient taking a series of deep breaths followed by periods of **apnea** (absence of breathing)
- Diminished, absent, or noisy auscultated breath sounds
- Abdominal breathing
- Reduced flow of expired air at the nose and mouth
- Unequal or inadequate chest expansion, resulting in reduced tidal volume

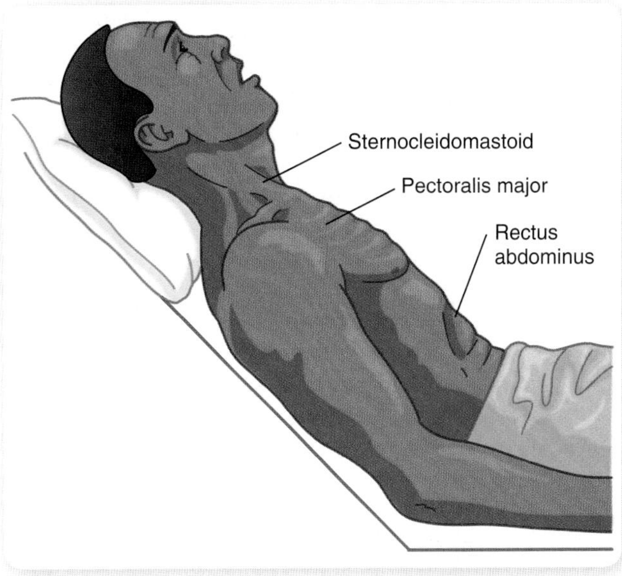

Figure 11-13 The accessory muscles of breathing are used when a patient is having difficulty breathing, but not during normal breathing. The accessory muscles include the sternocleidomastoid, pectoralis major, and abdominal muscles.

- Increased effort of breathing—use of accessory muscles
- Shallow depth (reduced tidal volume)
- Skin that is pale, cyanotic (blue), cool, mottled or moist (clammy)
- Retractions
- Staccato speech patterns (one- to two-word dyspnea)

When you are assessing a patient with a potential airway compromise, pay particular attention to the external environment, such as high altitude, enclosed spaces, or potential poisonous gases. Remember personal safety if the environment is unsafe.

Next, auscultate breathing with and without a stethoscope. Is air movement noted at the mouth and nose? Can clear, equal, and bilateral breath sounds be heard over all lung fields?

Feel for air movement at the mouth and nose. Observe the chest for symmetry, and note any **paradoxical motion**—the inward movement of the chest during inhalation and outward movement of the chest during exhalation, which is the opposite of normal chest wall movement during breathing and occurs on the side of injury (flail segment).

Evaluate for pulsus paradoxus, a condition in which the systolic blood pressure drops more than 10 mm Hg with inspiration. A change in pulse quality, or even the disappearance of a pulse, may also be detected. Pulsus paradoxus is generally seen in patients with decompensating COPD or severe pericardial tamponade. It may also indicate an increase in intrathoracic pressure (such as tension pneumothorax or a severe asthma attack).

A history of the present illness is a vital part of your assessment. Determine the evolution of this particular event:

- Was its onset sudden or gradual?
- Is there any known cause or "trigger" of the event?
- What was the duration (is the problem constant or recurrent)?
- Does anything alleviate or exacerbate the problem?
- Are there any other associated symptoms, such as a productive cough (if yes, what does the sputum look like?), chest pain or pressure, or fever?
- Were any interventions attempted before EMS arrival?
- Is the patient currently taking any medications, and is he or she compliant with the prescribed regimens?
- Is this a constant (chronic) or recurrent (episodic) problem?
- Has the patient been evaluated by a physician or admitted to the hospital for this condition in the past?
- Has the patient ever been intubated for this problem? If so, how does today's episode compare to that experience? This is one of the most important questions to ask; a condition bad enough to warrant intubation needs urgent attention to prevent a repeated occurrence.

Note protective reflexes of the airway, including coughing, sneezing, and gagging. A cough is a forceful, spastic exhalation that aids in clearing the bronchi and bronchioles. Sneezing clears the nasopharynx and is often caused by an irritant, such as dust. The gag reflex is a spastic pharyngeal and esophageal reflex as a result of a stimulus of the posterior pharynx to prevent foreign objects from entering the trachea.

Sighing and hiccuping are other modified forms of respiration. Sighing is an involuntary deep breath that increases opening of the alveoli, preventing atelectasis. The average person sighs approximately once per minute. Hiccuping is a sudden inhalation, caused by spastic contraction of the diaphragm cut short by closure of the glottis. Persistent hiccuping may be clinically important.

Respiratory pattern changes indicate serious injury or illness. Table 11-5 shows various respiratory patterns and causes. Irregular respiratory breathing patterns may be related to a specific condition. For example, Cheyne-Stokes respirations are often seen in patients with stroke and patients with serious head injuries Figure 11-14.

Serious head injuries may also cause changes in the normal respiratory rate and pattern of breathing. The result may be irregular, ineffective respirations that may or may not have an identifiable pattern (**ataxic respirations**). Patients experiencing a metabolic or toxic disorder may display other irregular respiratory patterns such as Kussmaul respirations.

Table 11-5 Respiratory Pattern Changes

Pattern	Characteristics
Cheyne-Stokes respirations	Rhythmic, gradually increasing rate and depth of respirations followed by gradual decrease of respirations with intermittent periods of apnea; associated with brainstem injury
Kussmaul respirations	Deep, rapid respirations; common in patients with diabetic **ketoacidosis**
Biot (ataxic) respirations	Irregular pattern, rate, and depth of breathing with intermittent periods of apnea; results from increased intracranial pressure
Central neurogenic hyperventilation	Deep, rapid respirations similar to Kussmaul; also results from increased intracranial pressure
Apneustic respirations	Prolonged, gasping inhalation followed by extremely short, ineffective exhalation; associated with brainstem insult
Agonal gasps	Slow, shallow, irregular or occasional gasping breaths; results from brain anoxia. Agonal gasps may be seen when the heart has stopped but the brain continues to send signals to the muscles of respiration. This is not considered a form of respiration.

Data from: Fontanarosa PB, Christiansen S. Units of measure. Table 2: Selected laboratory tests, with reference ranges and conversion factors. In: American Medical Association, ed. *AMA Manual of Style: A Guide for Authors and Editors.* 10th ed. New York, NY: Oxford University Press; 2007:798-815.

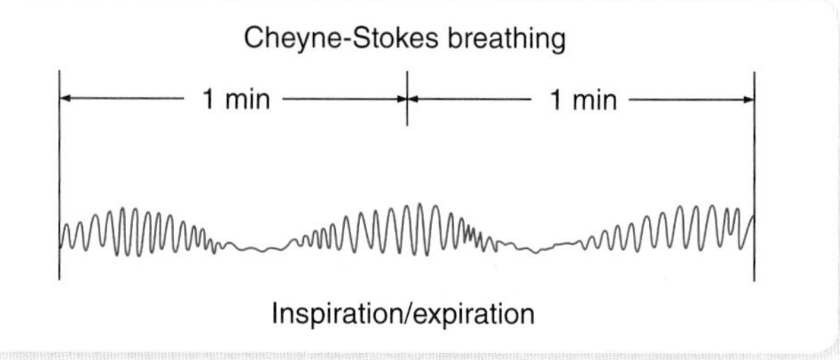

Figure 11-14 Cheyne-Stokes breathing shows irregular respirations followed by a period of apnea.

You should be aware that a patient may appear to take a breath after his or her heart has stopped. During these occasional, **agonal gasps**, the patient is not breathing. In patients with agonal gasps, you will need to provide artificial ventilations and, very likely, chest compressions.

Whereas rapid breathing is a compensatory mechanism to help patients in respiratory distress, some patients are so ill that their body is not able to compensate for their respiratory distress. The patients may look like they are compensating; however, no clinical improvement will be noticeable. You need to be vigilant when monitoring patients in respiratory distress because their condition may decline rapidly.

Patients with inadequate breathing have inadequate minute volume and need to be treated immediately. This condition is most easily recognized in patients who are unable to speak in complete sentences when at rest or who have a fast or slow respiratory rate, either of which may result in a reduction in tidal volume. Emergency medical care includes airway management, supplemental oxygen, and ventilatory support.

Words of Wisdom

If more than one patient with similar symptoms requires treatment, consider the presence of toxic gases. For example, carbon monoxide may be present in a residence with improperly vented heating systems and may be poisoning the occupants. Fire departments generally carry carbon monoxide detectors, and even some EMS services carry handheld carbon monoxide detectors to aid in the process of assessing ambient air.

▶ Assessment of Respiration

A patient's level of consciousness (LOC) and skin color are excellent indicators of respiration. During normal respiration, oxygen and carbon dioxide diffuse in and out of tissues and allow aerobic metabolism to take place. When you are assessing the brain and skin tissues, it will be apparent if the patient has adequate oxygen reaching these areas. A patient presenting with an altered LOC may not have adequate oxygen reaching the brain. This lack of oxygen can cause rapid changes in the patient's mental status. Therefore, when treating patients with an altered mental status, always consider the possibility that the patients may not be getting adequate oxygen to the brain and that you need to consider the possible underlying causes. However, remember to determine a baseline mental status on the patient. Some patients naturally have an abnormal mental status because of a previous medical condition. Ask family members what the patient's normal mental status is.

Just as an altered LOC indicates inadequate respiration, the same is true for patients with poor skin color. As oxygen fails to reach the skin from a lack of perfusion or poor oxygenation, the color of the skin changes to reflect the inadequate oxygen. Pale skin and mucous membranes are typically associated with poor perfusion caused by illness or shock. As this condition worsens, cyanosis becomes noticeable first peripherally, in the fingertips, and then centrally, in the mucous membranes and around the lips. Eventually, if the poor perfusion or oxygenation is not corrected, anaerobic metabolism will take place. This could cause the skin to become marked with blotches of different colors, commonly referred to as mottling.

Whereas assessment of a patient's baseline mental status and color of the skin and mucous membranes provides good indicators of respiration, you should also consider proper oxygenation when assessing patients. Several methods can be used to assess proper oxygenation, including assessing skin color, mental status, and **pulse oximetry**.

Pulse Oximetry

Pulse oximetry is a simple, rapid, safe, and noninvasive method of measuring—minute by minute—how well a person's hemoglobin is saturated. Pulse oximetry is considered a routine vital sign and can be used as part of any patient assessment.

A pulse oximeter measures the percentage of hemoglobin in the arterial blood that is saturated with oxygen **Figure 11-15**. Under normal circumstances, hemoglobin is saturated with oxygen. A sensor probe, clipped to the patient's finger or earlobe, uses a light-emitting diode to transmit light through the vascular bed to a light-sensing detector. The amount of light transmitted across the vascular bed depends on the proportion of hemoglobin that is saturated with oxygen. To ensure that the instrument is measuring arterial and not venous **oxygen saturation (Spo_2)**, pulse oximeters are designed to assess only pulsating blood vessels. Subsequently, pulse oximeters also measure the patient's pulse. One way to check the

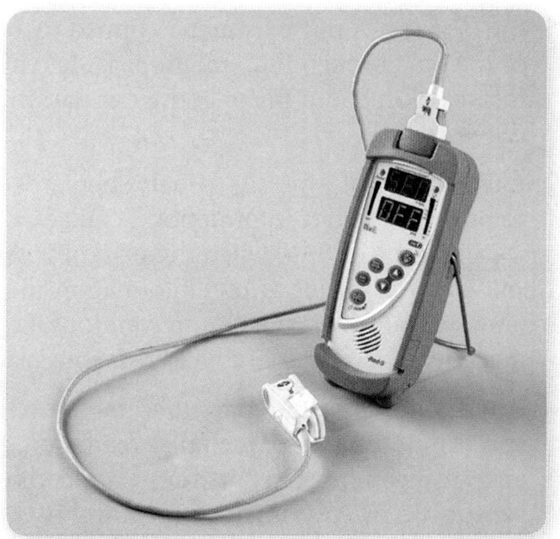

Figure 11-15 Pulse oximetry is a noninvasive method of assessing arterial oxygen saturation.

functioning of a pulse oximeter is to compare the pulse reading it provides with your own measurement of the patient's pulse by palpation.

A person with normal oxygenation and normal perfusion should have an Spo_2 level of greater than 95% while breathing room air. A reading of less than 95% in a nonsmoker suggests hypoxemia and a need for supplemental oxygen therapy.

Situations in which pulse oximeters may be useful in prehospital emergency medical care include the following:

- **Monitoring the oxygenation status of a patient during an attempt to insert an advanced airway or during suctioning.** The low-saturation alarm on the pulse oximeter can signal that you should abort the attempt and ventilate the patient.
- **Identifying deterioration in the condition of a trauma patient.** In a patient with multiple trauma, the signs of a developing tension pneumothorax may not be evident until the condition is advanced. A declining Spo_2 level can alert you to a problem and prompt a search for the cause of the problem.
- **Identifying deterioration in the condition of a patient with cardiac disease.** Pulse oximetry may enable early identification of patients who are experiencing heart failure in the wake of acute myocardial infarction.
- **Identifying high-risk patients with respiratory conditions.** For example, pulse oximetry may identify patients with asthma who are having serious attacks or patients with emphysema who are in severe decompensation.
- **Assessing vascular status in orthopaedic trauma.** Pulse oximetry is routine practice in assessing a fractured extremity to evaluate circulation distal to the fracture. Loss of a pulse means that the limb is in jeopardy and may require urgent action in the field if transport time is long. A pulse oximeter clipped to a finger or toe on a broken limb might provide critical information about the ongoing circulation to the limb.

The usefulness of a pulse oximeter depends on its ability to provide accurate information. A pulse oximeter that gives a reading of 99% when the patient is severely hypoxemic will not provide helpful information and could result in inadequate or erroneous interventions. Be aware of circumstances that might produce erroneous readings:

- **Bright ambient light** may enter the spectrophotometer of the pulse oximeter and create an incorrect reading. Protect the sensor clip by covering it with a towel or aluminum foil.
- **Patient motion** can confuse the pulse oximeter because it may mistake motion for arterial pulsation and read the oxygen saturation level from a vein rather than an artery.
- **Poor perfusion** makes it difficult for the pulse oximeter to sense a pulse and therefore to generate a reading. Poor perfusion occurs in states such as shock, cardiac arrest, and cold exposure. If the vessels in a patient's limbs are constricted and the limbs are cold, then it may be necessary to place the pulse oximeter clip on the earlobe or nose.
- **Nail polish** will prevent the sensor from working properly. Carry disposable acetone (nail polish remover) swabs to quickly remove nail polish.
- **Venous pulsations** may occur in some patients with right-side heart failure as a result of the systemic backup of blood. If a vein is pulsating, then the pulse oximeter may regard it as an artery and measure venous oxygen saturation.
- **Abnormal hemoglobin** may produce a falsely normal Spo_2 level. Examples include situations such as anemia where there is a deficiency of hemoglobin, so even if the hemoglobin is fully saturated, there is still a lack of oxygen, and carbon monoxide poisoning where the hemoglobin is fully saturated, but with carbon monoxide instead of oxygen.

Remember, do not make treatment decisions based solely on pulse oximetry, and be aware of its limitations.

Words of Wisdom

Remember that a pulse oximeter can detect only the saturation of hemoglobin. It cannot identify the gas that is saturating the hemoglobin. When carbon monoxide is present in the inspired gas, it displaces oxygen from the hemoglobin. Carbon monoxide, which has an affinity for hemoglobin that is 200 to 250 times greater than that of oxygen for hemoglobin, has similar characteristics to arterial blood. Therefore, the dual wavelengths of infrared light used by the pulse oximeter may not be able to distinguish between carbon monoxide and oxygen, producing a falsely high reading. Therefore, in cases of carbon monoxide poisoning, the Spo_2 reading can be normal in the context of hypoxia.

It is essential to pay close attention to the scene size-up and to treat the patient instead of the diagnostic equipment. The pulse oximeter is designed to detect gross abnormalities, not subtle changes.

- In patients with substantial vasoconstriction or low perfusion states (including cardiac arrest), there may not be enough peripheral perfusion to be detected by the sensor. In these cases, move the sensor to a more central location (bridge of the nose or ear lobe). Always consult the manufacturer's guidelines for proper placement and troubleshooting of these devices.

The pulse oximeter is a valuable adjunct to aid in decision making, but it is not a replacement for a complete assessment. Because of many factors, the pulse oximeter may give falsely high or low readings. When you are conducting a complete patient assessment, consider using pulse oximetry readings as one additional measure to use while obtaining all other comprehensive information you need. Assess the patient for signs and symptoms of adequate oxygenation. If a patient has signs, such as cyanosis or pale or clammy skin, or symptoms, such as shortness of breath, and a normal Spo_2 reading, treat the patient's condition, not the diagnostic device.

Peak Expiratory Flow Measurement

In patients with certain reactive airway diseases (such as asthma), you can evaluate bronchoconstriction by measuring the peak rate of a forceful exhalation with a peak expiratory flowmeter Figure 11-16. An increasing peak expiratory flow suggests that the patient is responding to treatment (such as inhaled bronchodilators). A decreasing peak expiratory flow may be an early indication that the patient's condition is deteriorating.

Peak expiratory flow varies based on sex, height, and age. Healthy adults have a peak expiratory flow rate of 350 to 750 mL. To assess peak expiratory flow, place the patient in a seated position with legs dangling. Assemble the flowmeter, and ensure that it reads zero. Ask the patient to take a deep breath, place the mouthpiece in his or her mouth, and exhale as forcefully as possible (ensure no air leaks around the device or comes from the patient's nose). Perform the test three times, and take the best peak flow rate of the three readings.

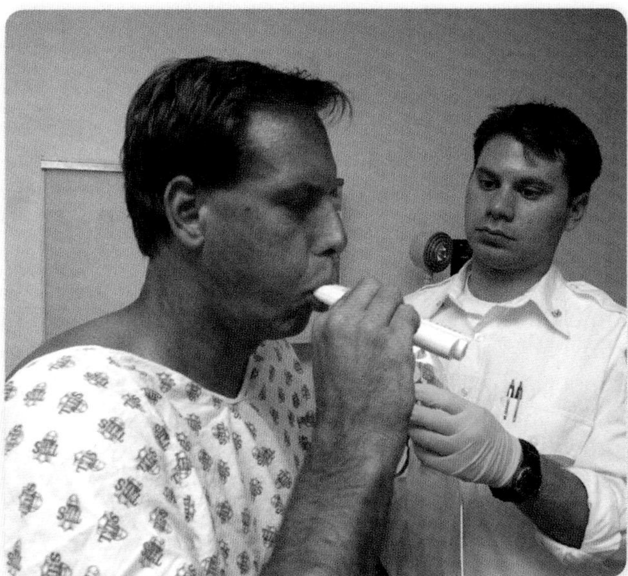

Figure 11-16 Peak expiratory flowmeters are used to quantify the degree of bronchoconstriction.

Arterial Blood Gas Analysis

AEMTs are not typically trained to obtain arterial blood specimens and do not carry the equipment needed to analyze the patient's blood. As a result, you will rely on noninvasive methods of assessing ventilation and oxygenation (such as pulse oximetry and capnography/capnometry).

Analysis of arterial blood gases (ABGs) provides the most comprehensive quantitative information about the respiratory system. In this procedure, blood is obtained from a superficial artery, such as the radial or femoral artery. The blood is then analyzed for pH, $Paco_2$, Pao_2, Hco_3- (concentration of bicarbonate ions), base excess (indicating acidosis or alkalosis), and Spo_2 levels. Normal ABG values are summarized in Table 11-6.

With ABG measurements, the values of pH and Hco_3- are used to evaluate the acid-base status of the patient. The $Paco_2$ value is an indicator of the effectiveness of ventilation. The values of Pao_2 and Spo_2 are indicators of oxygenation. To maintain normal ABG values, a balance between alveolar volume and perfusion of the alveolar capillaries must be maintained.

End-Tidal Carbon Dioxide Assessment

Carbon dioxide can be described as the "smoke of metabolism." The body uses oxygen as its fuel and makes carbon dioxide as its by-product. As long as oxygen is delivered to the cells and tissues, the production of carbon dioxide continues. A helpful analogy is a motor vehicle engine. As long as gasoline continues to burn, exhaust is produced. In the human body, carbon dioxide is the exhaust.

An **end-tidal carbon dioxide ($ETCO_2$) monitor** detects the presence of carbon dioxide in exhaled air. These

Table 11-6	Normal Arterial Blood Gas Values
pH	7.35 to 7.45
Pao_2	80 to 100 mm Hg
$Paco_2$	35 to 45 mm Hg
Hco_3-	21 to 28 mEq/L
Base (excess or deficit)	−2 to 3 mEq/L
Sao_2	>95%

Abbreviations: Hco_3-, concentration of bicarbonate ions; $Paco_2$, partial pressure of carbon dioxide; Pao_2, partial pressure of oxygen; Sao_2, oxygen saturation

Data from: Fontanarosa PB, Christiansen S. Units of measure. Table 2: selected laboratory tests, with reference ranges and conversion factors. In: American Medical Association, ed. *AMA Manual of Style: A Guide for Authors and Editors*. 10th ed. New York, NY: Oxford University Press; 2007:798-815.

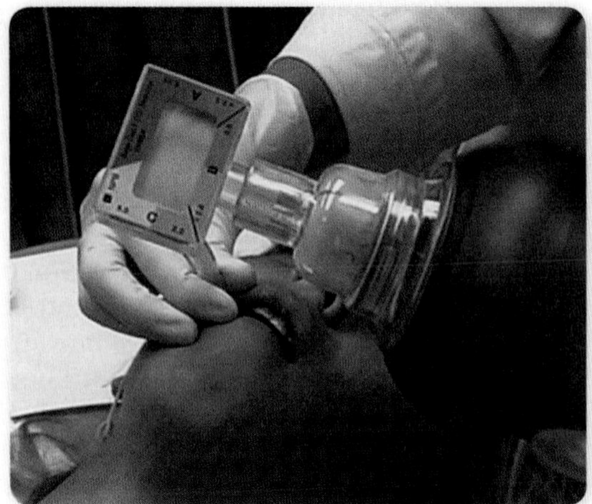

Figure 11-17 The paper inside the colorimetric carbon dioxide detector should turn from purple to yellow during exhalation, indicating the presence of exhaled carbon dioxide.

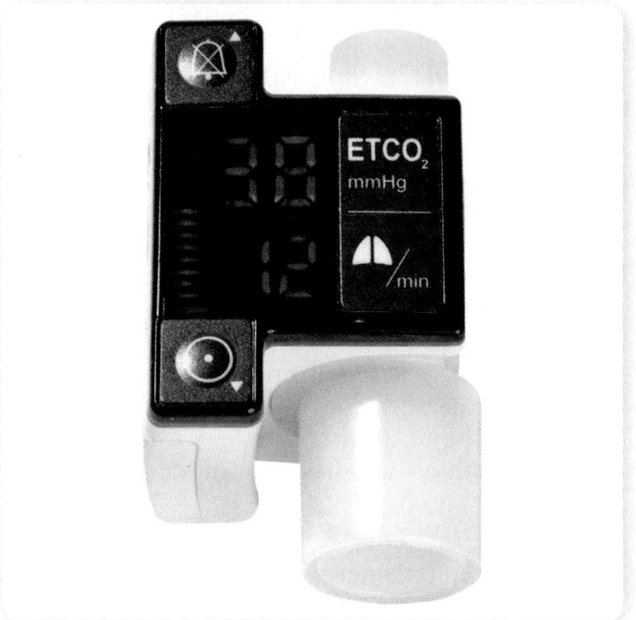

Figure 11-18 A capnometer.

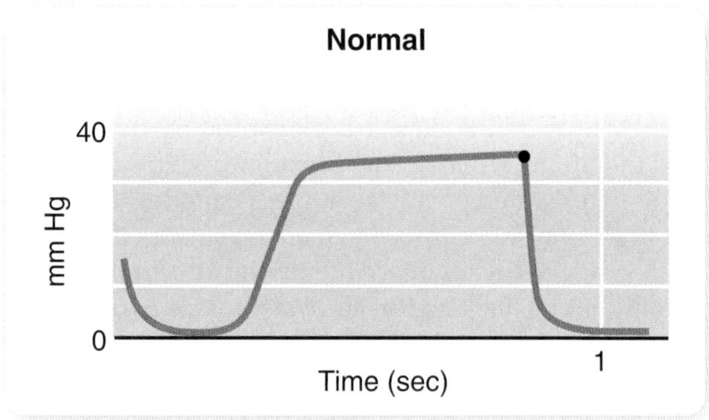

Figure 11-19 A normal capnographic waveform.

monitoring tools are important adjuncts for determining the adequacy of ventilations and proper placement of advanced airways. The types of $ETCO_2$ monitors include colorimetric, digital, and digital/waveform.

A **colorimetric carbon dioxide detector** provides qualitative information regarding the presence of carbon dioxide in the patient's exhaled breath; that is, it does not assign a numeric value. The colorimetric CO_2 detector is attached between any tube inserted into the trachea and the ventilation device. After six to eight positive pressure breaths—the amount of time it takes for carbon dioxide to accumulate in the device—the specifically treated paper inside the detector should turn from purple to yellow during exhalation **Figure 11-17**. Air exhaled through a tube that has been properly placed in the trachea of a patient with adequate perfusion should contain 4% to 5% carbon dioxide, which will cause the paper to turn yellow during exhalation. If the tube is in the esophagus, a negligible amount (less than 0.5%) of carbon dioxide will be present in the exhaled gas; this amount will cause the paper to remain purple during exhalation.

Several limitations exist with the colorimetric CO_2 detector. The device might give a false-positive reading if the patient has carbon dioxide trapped in the stomach from the ingestion of carbonated beverages. Furthermore, the device is sensitive to extremes of temperature and humidity; it may be less reliable if vomitus or other secretions get inside it; and the paper inside the device degrades over time, resulting in a less reliable reading.

A **capnometer** provides quantitative information, in real time, by displaying a numeric reading of exhaled carbon dioxide levels. It uses a special adapter, which attaches between the advanced airway device and ventilation device **Figure 11-18**. Because it provides quantitative data, the capnometer is more reliable than the colorimetric CO_2 detector.

A **capnographer** is a device that provides a graphic representation of exhaled carbon dioxide levels. It performs the same function and attaches in the same way as the capnometer. The two types of capnographers are waveform and digital/waveform.

Waveform capnography provides quantitative, real-time information regarding the patient's exhaled carbon dioxide level. Unlike capnometry, however, waveform capnography displays a graphic waveform **Figure 11-19**. In most cases, portable cardiac monitors/defibrillators provide a numeric reading and a waveform (also called digital/waveform capnography and quantitative waveform capnography).

Quantitative waveform capnography has many applications in emergency medicine, including the detection of bronchospasm, hypoventilation, and hyperventilation. Quantitative waveform capnography is the recommended method of monitoring initial and ongoing placement of an advanced airway device. Capnography can also serve as

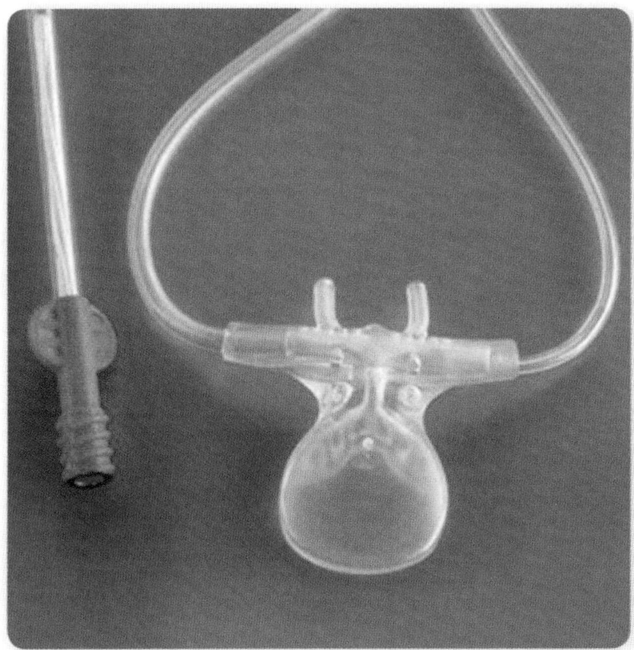

Figure 11-20 FilterLine® nasal cannula device for monitoring end-tidal carbon dioxide in a spontaneously breathing patient.

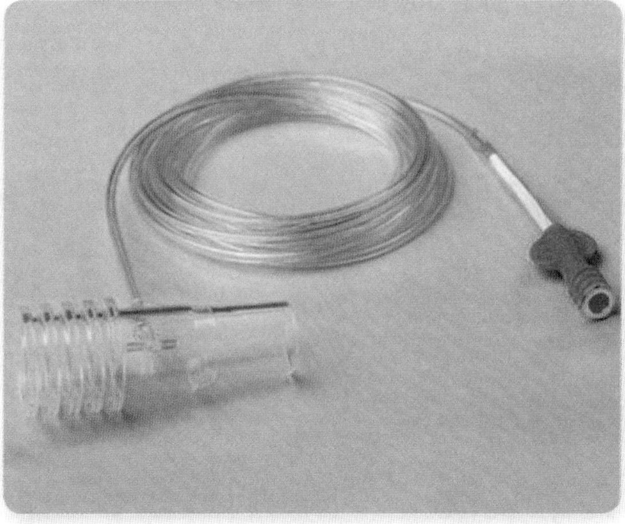

Figure 11-21 FilterLine® in-line end-tidal carbon dioxide device for use in the patient with an advanced airway.

an indicator of the effectiveness of chest compressions and to detect return of spontaneous circulation (ROSC). The provision of this information is possible because blood must circulate through the lungs for carbon dioxide to be exhaled and measured. When ROSC occurs, you would expect a large amount of carbon dioxide to be returned to the lungs. Waveform capnography can be monitored in spontaneously breathing patients with an adequate airway by applying a special nasal cannula device to the patient and connecting the sampling line to the cardiac monitor/defibrillator Figure 11-20. If the patient has an advanced airway, then place an in-line adapter between the advanced airway device and ventilation device and connect the sampling line to the cardiac monitor/defibrillator Figure 11-21.

Because carbon dioxide rapidly equilibrates in the alveolar gases, the carbon dioxide concentration in exhaled gases—particularly the gases present near the end of exhalation—can be used to grossly approximate arterial $Paco_2$ levels, which normally range between 35 and 45 mm Hg. Typically, $ETCO_2$ level is approximately 2 to 5 mm Hg lower than the arterial $Paco_2$ level, but this amount varies depending on the volume of alveolar dead space and any $\dot{V}/\dot{Q}$ mismatch present. Because carbon dioxide is present only in negligible (0.5% or less) concentrations in the esophagus, use of an $ETCO_2$ detector—specifically, quantitative waveform capnography—is a reliable (and essential) method for confirming and monitoring advanced airway placement.

Use of $ETCO_2$ monitoring is limited with patients in cardiac arrest. In a patient with a short arrest interval, exhaled carbon dioxide may be detected despite a lack of perfusion. Patients with prolonged cardiac arrest, however, will have minimal levels of exhaled carbon dioxide because of severe acidosis and minimal carbon dioxide return to the lungs.

Opening the Airway

Emergency medical care begins with ensuring an open airway. If you cannot immediately open and maintain an airway, you cannot provide effective patient care.

When you respond to a call and find an unresponsive patient, you need to assess and determine immediately whether the patient has an open airway and breathing is adequate and if he or she has a pulse. The patient needs to be in the supine position to adequately open the airway and assess breathing. If your patient is found in the prone position, he or she must be properly positioned to allow for assessment of airway and breathing and to begin cardiopulmonary resuscitation (CPR) should it be necessary. Currently, health care workers are taught to begin CPR with high-quality compressions if cardiac arrest is suspected. The patient should be log rolled as a unit so the head, neck, and spine all move together without twisting. To position an unresponsive patient to open the airway, follow the steps in Skill Drill 11-1.

In an unresponsive patient, the most common airway obstruction is the patient's tongue, which falls back into the throat when the muscles of the throat and tongue relax Figure 11-22. Dentures (false teeth), blood, vomitus, mucus, food, and other foreign objects may also create a blockage. Therefore, you should always be prepared to help clear and maintain a patent airway.

▶ Head Tilt–Chin Lift Maneuver

Opening the airway to relieve an obstruction can often be done quickly and easily by simply tilting the patient's

Skill Drill 11-1 Positioning an Unresponsive Patient

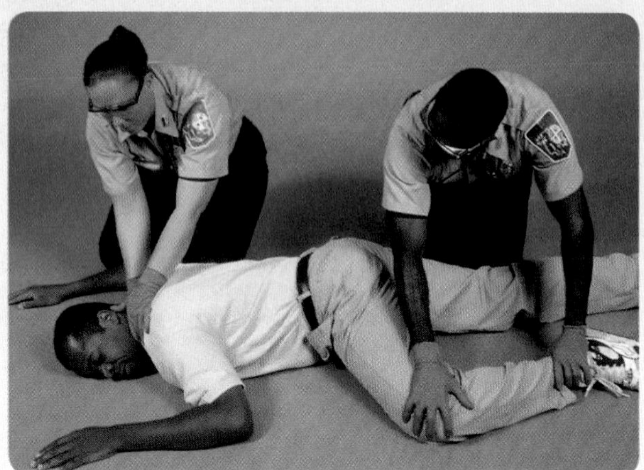

Step 1 Kneel beside the patient. Kneel far enough away so that the patient, when rolled toward you, does not come to rest in your lap. Place your hands behind the back of the patient's head and neck to provide in-line stabilization of the cervical spine as your partner straightens the patient's legs.

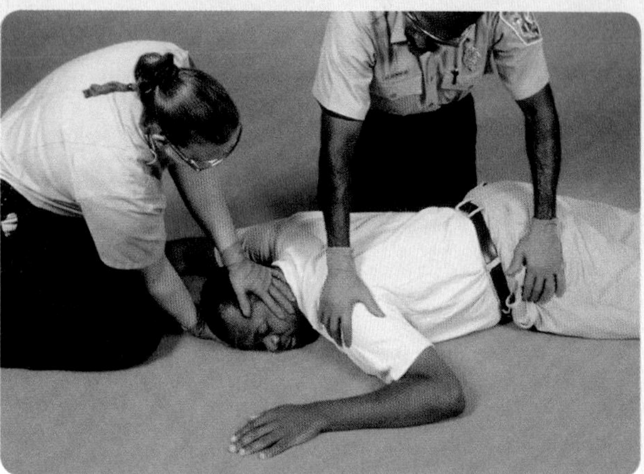

Step 2 Have your partner place his or her hands on the patient's far shoulder and hip.

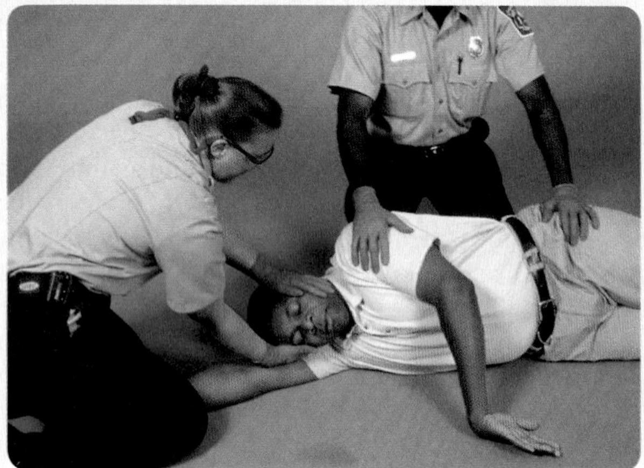

Step 3 As you call the count to control movement, have your partner turn the patient toward you by pulling on the far shoulder and hip. Control the head and neck so that they move as a unit with the rest of the torso. In this way, the head and neck stay in the same vertical plane as the back. This single motion will minimize aggravation of any spinal injury. Replace the patient's farther arm back at his or her side.

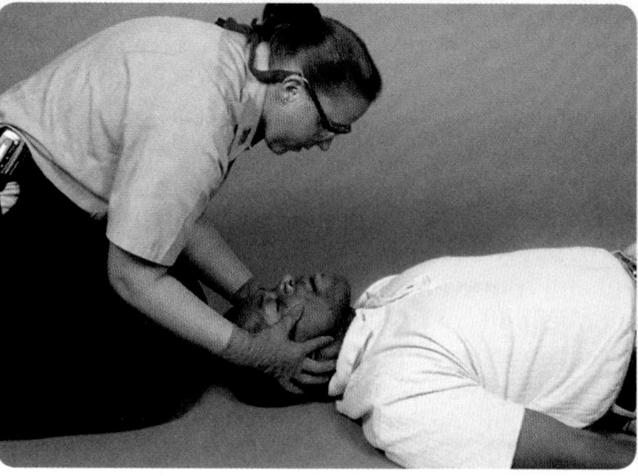

Step 4 After the patient is positioned, maintain an open airway and assess the patient's airway and breathing status.

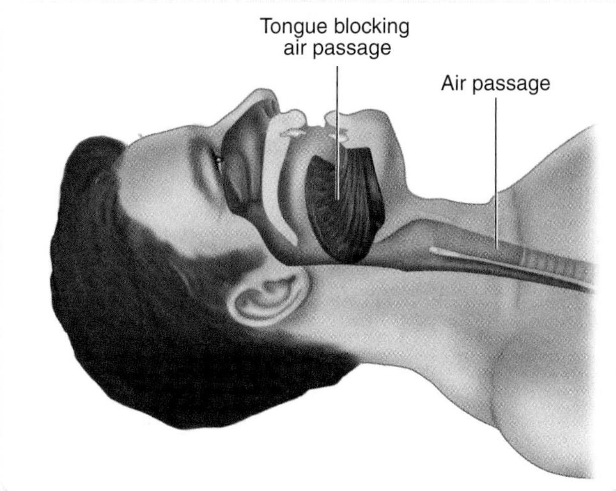

Figure 11-22 The most common airway obstruction is the patient's tongue, which falls back into the throat when the muscles of the throat and tongue relax.

head back and lifting the chin in what is known as the **head tilt–chin lift maneuver**. For patients who have not sustained trauma, this simple maneuver is sometimes all that is needed for the patient to resume breathing.

To perform the head tilt–chin lift maneuver, follow these steps Figure 11-23:

1. With the patient in a supine position, position yourself beside of the patient's head.
2. Place the heel of one hand on the patient's forehead, and apply firm backward pressure with your palm to tilt the patient's head back. This extension of the neck will move the tongue forward, away from the back of the throat, and clear the airway if the tongue is blocking it.
3. Place the fingertips of your other hand under the patient's chin. Do not compress the soft tissue under the chin because this may block the airway.
4. Lift the chin upward, bringing the entire lower jaw with it, helping to tilt the head back. Do not compress the soft tissue under the chin. Lift so that the teeth are nearly brought together, but avoid closing the mouth completely. Continue to hold the forehead to maintain the backward tilt of the head.

▶ Jaw-Thrust Maneuver

The head tilt–chin lift maneuver will open the airway in most patients; however, if you suspect a cervical spine injury, use the jaw-thrust maneuver. The **jaw-thrust maneuver** is a technique to open the airway by placing the fingers behind the angle of the jaw and lifting the jaw upward. The jaw is displaced forward at the mandibular angle. You can easily seal a mask around the mouth while performing the jaw-thrust maneuver. This is the method of choice for patients with suspected cervical spine injury. Perform the jaw-thrust maneuver on an adult in the following manner Figure 11-24:

1. Kneel above the patient's head. Place your fingers behind the angles of the lower jaw, and move the jaw upward. Use your thumbs to help position the lower jaw to allow breathing through the mouth and nose.

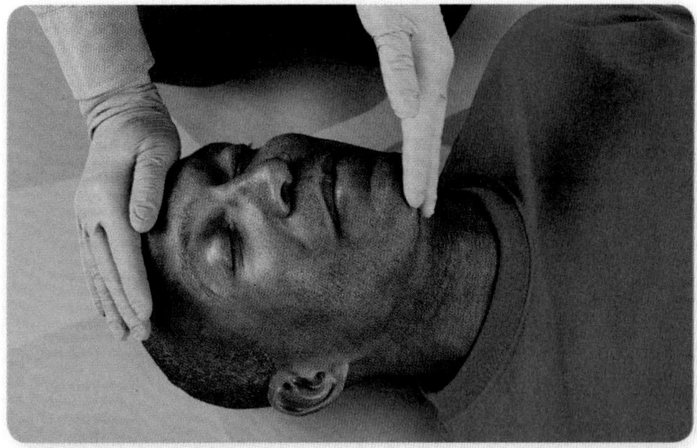

Figure 11-23 The head tilt–chin lift maneuver is a simple technique for opening the airway in a patient without a suspected cervical spine injury.

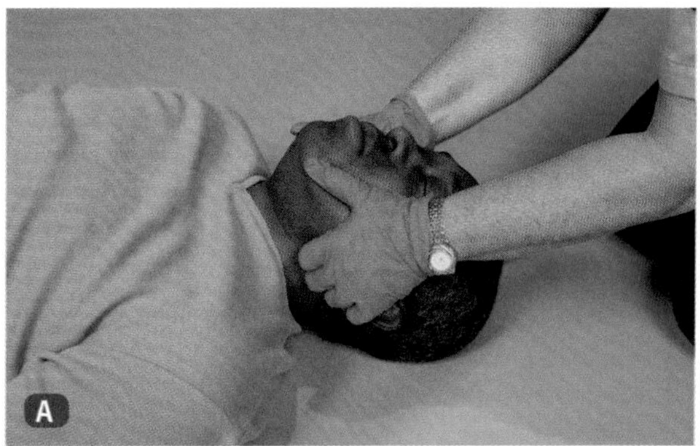

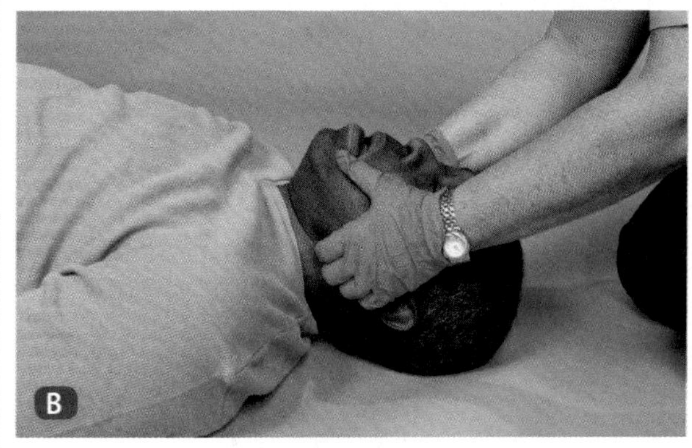

Figure 11-24 Performing the jaw-thrust maneuver. **A.** Kneeling above the patient's head, place your fingers behind the angles of the lower jaw, and move the jaw upward. Use your thumbs to help position the lower jaw. **B.** The completed maneuver should look like this.

2. The completed maneuver should open the airway with the mouth slightly open and the jaw jutting forward.

After the airway has been opened, the patient may start to breathe on his or her own. Assess whether breathing has returned.

With complete airway obstruction, there will be no movement of air. However, you may see the chest and abdomen rise and fall considerably with the patient's frantic attempts to breathe. This is why the presence of chest wall movement alone does not indicate breathing is present. Regular chest wall movement indicates that respiratory effort is present. Observing chest and abdominal movement is often difficult with a fully clothed patient. You may see little, if any, chest movement, even with normal breathing. This is particularly true in some patients with chronic lung disease. If you are not sure if the patient is moving enough air, begin ventilations.

▶ Tongue-Jaw Lift Maneuver

The **tongue-jaw lift maneuver** is used more frequently to open a patient's airway to facilitate oropharyngeal suctioning. It cannot be used to ventilate a patient because it will not allow for an adequate mask seal on the patient's face. To perform the tongue-jaw lift maneuver, follow these steps Figure 11-25:

1. Position yourself at the patient's side.
2. Place the hand closest to the patient's head on the forehead.
3. With your other hand, reach into the patient's mouth and hook your first knuckle under the incisors or gumline. While holding the patient's head and maintaining the hand on the forehead, lift the jaw straight up.

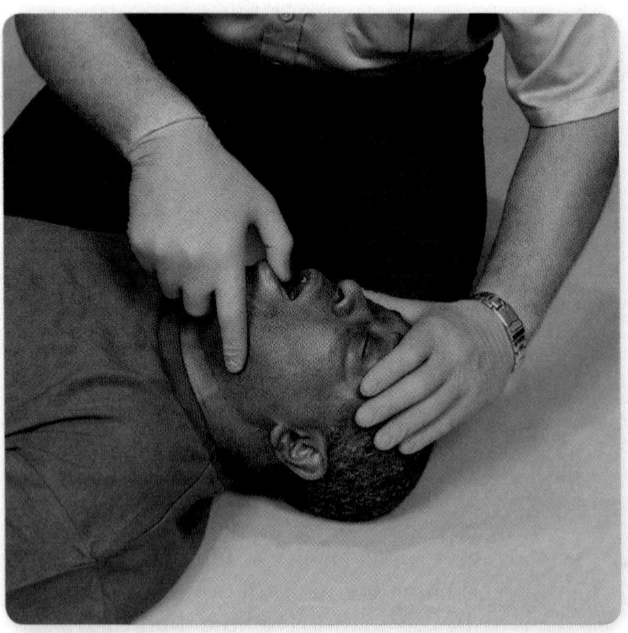

Figure 11-25 The tongue-jaw lift maneuver.

Special Populations

Routine procedures for patients with obesity can become extremely complicated. Airway procedures are made more difficult by a larger tongue, larger patient head size, and limited neck mobility associated with obesity. Bag-mask ventilation may be ineffective with patients in a supine position. Multiple studies have demonstrated that ramped positioning of the patient with obesity has a positive effect on the chances of successful airway management.[1-6]

Ramping of the patient with obesity may be accomplished by utilizing pillows and/or blankets to achieve the desired position or with commercially manufactured ramping devices Figure 11-26. Both methods carry equivalent rates of success and complication.[1-6]

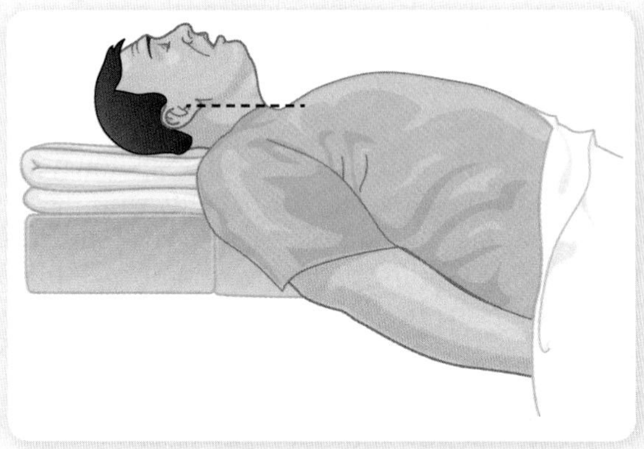

Figure 11-26 The ramped position with the head and shoulders elevated approximately 25° to 30° increases the chance of successful airway management. It is important to confirm that the external auditory meatus is in line with the sternal notch.

Data from: Miller RD, Cohen NH, Erikkson LI, et al. Chapter 55: Airway management in the adult. In: *Miller's Anesthesia*. 8th ed. Philadelphia, PA: Elsevier; 2015:1666.

Maintaining the Airway

After you have evaluated the airway, if the patient is breathing on his or her own with a normal rate and adequate tidal volume (depth of breathing) and does not have a traumatic injury, place him or her in the **recovery position** to help maintain a clear airway Figure 11-27. Take the following steps to put the patient in the recovery position:

1. Roll the patient onto the side so that the head, shoulders, and torso move at the same time without twisting.
2. Place the patient's lower arm and upper hand under his or her cheek.

After patients have resumed spontaneous breathing after being resuscitated, the recovery position will prevent the aspiration of vomitus. However, this position is not appropriate for patients with suspected spinal, hip, or pelvic injuries; nor is it adequate for patients who are

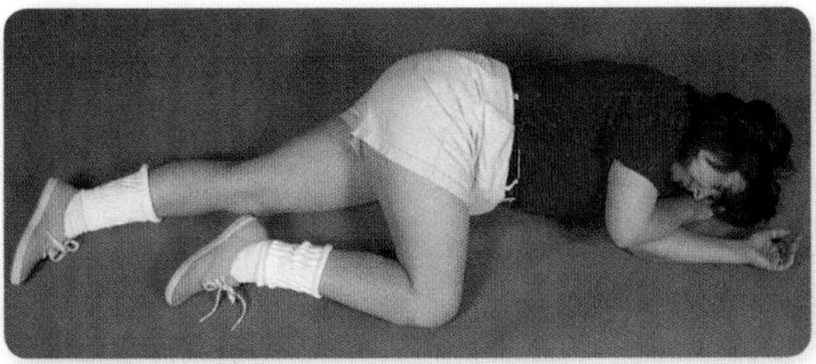

Figure 11-27 In the recovery position, the patient is rolled onto his or her left or right side.

unresponsive and require ventilatory assistance. Reposition such patients to provide access to the airway.

Suctioning

You must keep the airway clear so that you can ventilate the patient properly. If the airway is not clear, you will force material into the lungs and possibly cause a complete airway obstruction. Therefore, suctioning is your first priority. If you have any doubt about the situation, remember this rule: If you hear gurgling, the patient needs suctioning!

▶ Suctioning Equipment

Portable, hand-operated, battery-operated, and fixed (mounted) types of suctioning equipment are essential for resuscitation Figure 11-28. A portable suctioning unit must provide enough vacuum pressure and flow to allow you to suction the mouth and oropharynx effectively. Hand-operated suctioning units with disposable chambers are reliable, effective, and relatively inexpensive. A fixed suctioning unit should generate an airflow of more than 40 L/min and a vacuum of more than 300 mm Hg when the tubing is clamped.

A portable and fixed suctioning unit should be fitted with the following:

- Wide-bore, thick-walled, nonkinking tubing
- Soft and rigid suction catheters
- A nonbreakable, disposable collection bottle
- A supply of water for rinsing the tips

A **suction catheter** is a hollow, cylindrical device that is used to remove fluids and secretions from the airway. A **tonsil-tip catheter** is the best kind of catheter for suctioning the pharynx in adults and the preferred method for infants and children. These plastic tips have a large diameter and are rigid, so they do not collapse Figure 11-29.

Tips with a curved contour allow easy, rapid placement in the oropharynx. Soft plastic, nonrigid catheters, sometimes called French or whistle-tip catheters, are used to suction the nose and liquid secretions in the back of the mouth and in situations in which you cannot use a rigid catheter, such as for a patient with a **stoma** Figure 11-30. A stoma is an opening through the skin

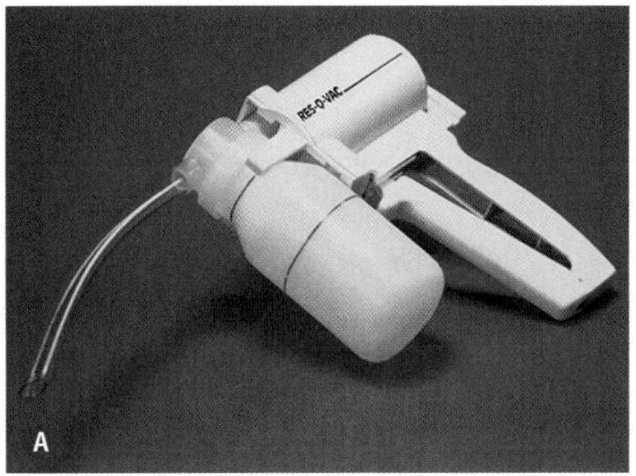

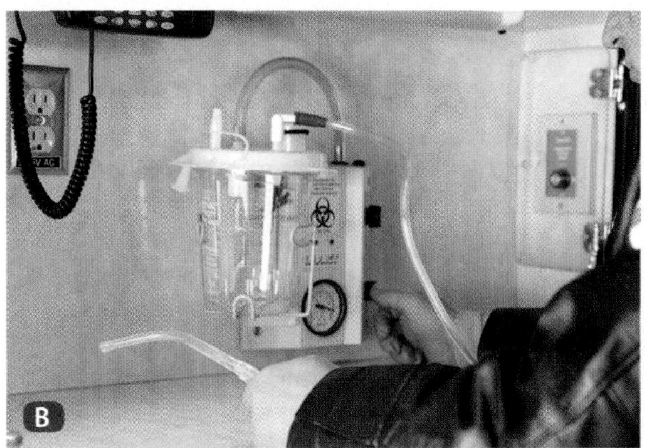

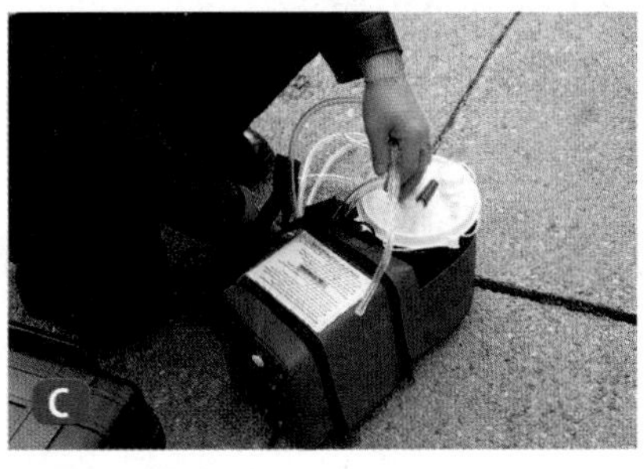

Figure 11-28 Suctioning equipment is essential for resuscitation. **A.** Hand-operated device. **B.** Fixed unit. **C.** Portable unit.

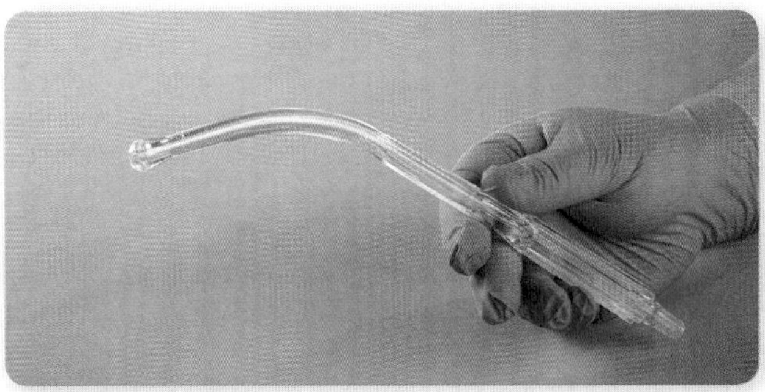

Figure 11-29 Tonsil-tip catheters are the best for suctioning the oropharynx because they have wide-diameter tips and are rigid.

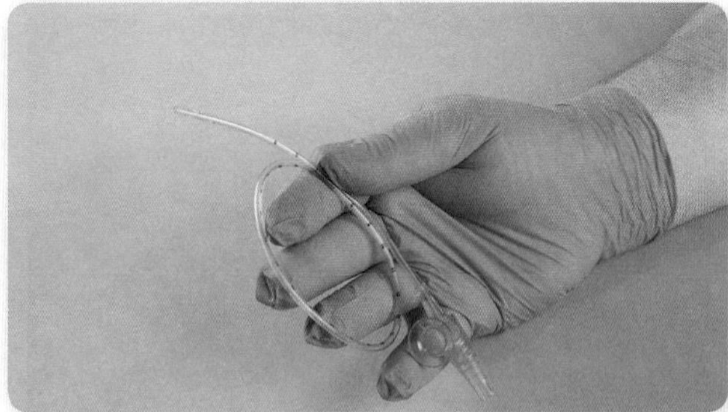

Figure 11-30 French, or whistle-tip, catheters are used in situations in which rigid catheters cannot be used, such as with a patient who has a stoma, patients whose teeth are clenched, or if suctioning the nose is necessary.

that goes into an organ or other structure. For example, a rigid catheter could break off a patient's tooth, whereas a flexible catheter may be inserted along the cheeks without injury.

Before you insert any catheter, make sure to measure for the proper size. Use the same technique as you would use when measuring for an oropharyngeal airway. You should use extreme caution when suctioning a responsive patient. Put the tip in only as far as you can visualize. Never insert a catheter past the base of the tongue because this action may result in gagging and vomiting and increases the possibility of aspiration.

▶ Techniques of Suctioning

Inspect your suctioning equipment regularly to make sure it is in proper working condition. Turn on the suction, clamp the tubing, and make sure that the unit generates a vacuum of more than 300 mm Hg. Check that a battery-charged unit has charged batteries. Ensure that your suctioning equipment is at the patient's head and is easily accessible. Follow these steps to operate the suction unit:

1. Check the unit for proper assembly of all its parts.
2. Turn on the suctioning unit, and test it to ensure a vacuum pressure of more than 300 mm Hg.
3. Select and attach the appropriate catheter to the tubing.

Limit suctioning time to no more than 15 seconds at one time for adult patients, 10 seconds for children, and 5 seconds for infants. Suctioning removes oxygen from the airway along with obstructive material. Rinse the catheter and tubing with water to prevent clogging of the tube with dried vomitus or other secretions. Repeat suctioning only after the patient has been ventilated and reoxygenated.

To properly suction a patient's airway, follow the steps in Skill Drill 11-2.

At times, a patient may have secretions or vomitus that cannot be suctioned quickly and easily. Some suction units cannot effectively remove solid objects such as teeth, foreign bodies, and food. In these situations, remove the catheter from the patient's mouth, log roll

NR Skill

Skill Drill 11-2 Suctioning a Patient's Airway

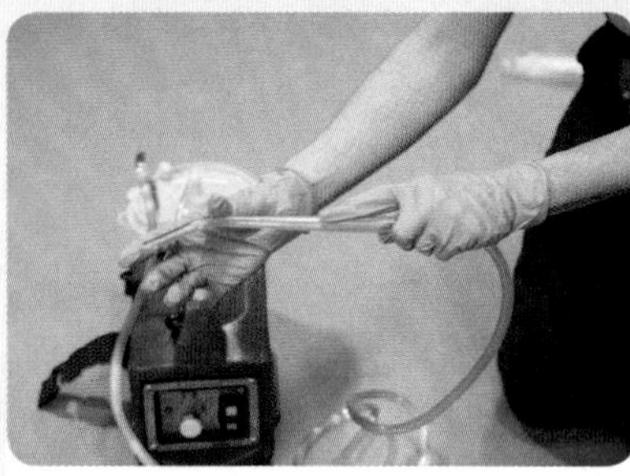

Step 1 Make sure the suctioning unit is properly assembled, and turn on the suction unit. Test the suction by clamping the tubing and making sure the unit generates a vacuum of more than 300 mm Hg.

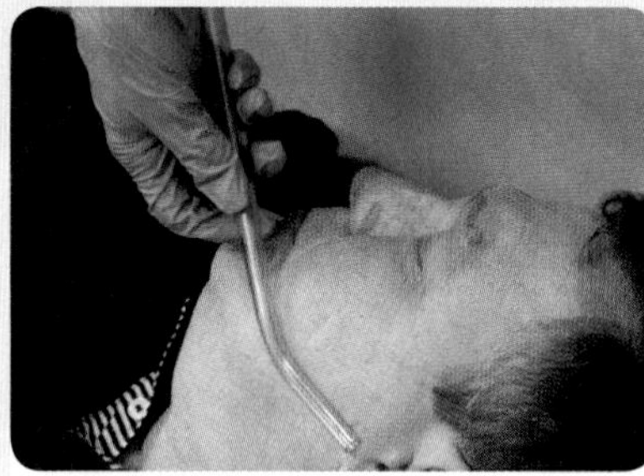

Step 2 Measure the catheter from the corner of the patient's mouth to the tip of the earlobe or angle of the jaw.

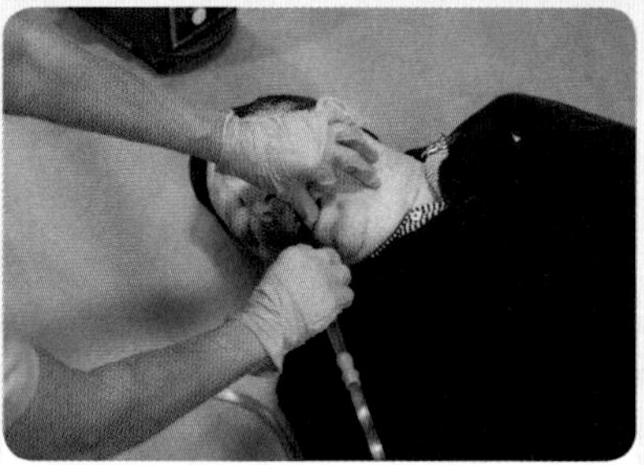

Step 3 Before applying suction, turn the patient's head to the side (unless you suspect cervical spine injury). Open the patient's mouth by using the cross-finger technique or tongue-jaw lift, and insert the catheter to the depth measured, without using force. Do not suction while inserting the catheter.

Skill Drill 11-2 Suctioning a Patient's Airway *(continued)*

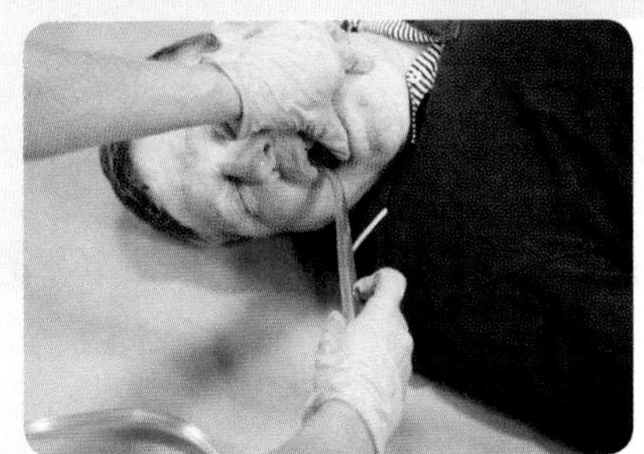

© Jones & Bartlett Learning. Courtesy of MIEMSS.

Step 4 Insert the catheter to the premeasured depth, and apply suction in a circular motion as you withdraw the catheter. Remember that you are removing oxygen while suctioning, so limit suctioning time to no more than 15 seconds in an adult, 10 seconds in a child, and 5 seconds in an infant.

the patient onto his or her side, and then clear the mouth carefully with your gloved finger. Only attempt to remove an object if it is visible during examination of the open mouth; blind sweeps of the back of the oropharynx may push an object farther down in the airway, making the obstruction worse. Copious frothy secretions may be produced as quickly as you can suction them from the airway. In this situation, you should suction the patient's airway for 15 seconds (less time in infants and children), then ventilate the patient for 2 minutes. This alternating pattern of suctioning and ventilating should continue until all secretions have been cleared from the patient's airway. Continuous ventilation is not appropriate if vomitus or other particles are present in the airway.

Clean and decontaminate your suctioning equipment after each use according to the manufacturer's guidelines. Place all disposable suctioning equipment (such as catheter, suction tubing) in a biohazard bag.

Words of Wisdom

Suctioning time limits:

Adult: 15 seconds
Child: 10 seconds
Infant: 5 seconds

Pediatric patients are very susceptible to vagal stimuli and their heart rate will decrease if suctioning or stimulating the back of the throat occurs for too long.

Safety

A mask, protective eyewear, and gloves should be worn whenever airway management involves suctioning. Body fluids can become aerosolized, and can come into contact with the mucous membranes of your mouth, nose, eyes, and hands.

Tracheobronchial Suctioning of an Intubated Patient

Endotracheal (ET) intubation is a paramedic skill in which an ET tube is passed through the glottic opening to manage the airway when other less invasive methods are not sufficient. Following ET intubation, thick pulmonary secretions or other fluids may occlude the ET tube, preventing effective ventilation. You may at times assist with tracheobronchial suctioning of an intubated patient.

In such cases, you must pass a suction catheter into the ET tube to remove the secretions. Use sterile technique if possible; do not reinsert a catheter that is not sterile. Monitor the patient's oxygen saturation level during the procedure. Preoxygenation is essential before tracheobronchial suctioning. Lubricate a soft-tip (whistle-tip) catheter, and hyperoxygenate for 30 seconds to 1 minute. It may be necessary to inject 3 to 5 mL of sterile water down the ET tube to loosen secretions. Gently insert the catheter until you feel resistance **Figure 11-31**. Apply suction as the catheter is extracted, taking care not to exceed 15 seconds in an adult patient. Continue to ventilate and oxygenate the patient.

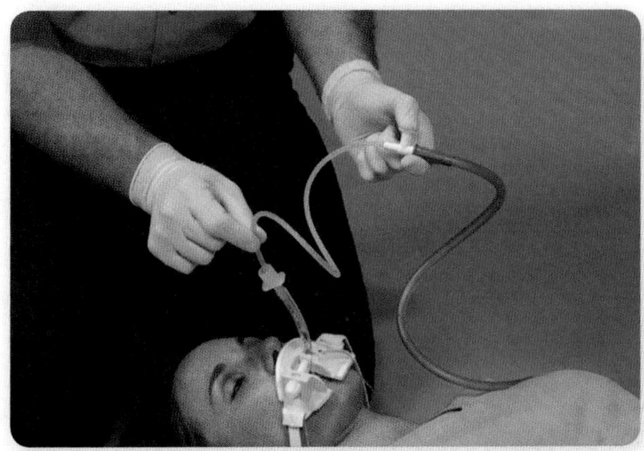

Figure 11-31 Tracheobronchial suctioning involves passing a suction catheter into an endotracheal tube to remove secretions.

© Jones & Bartlett Learning.

Basic Airway Adjuncts

The primary function of an airway adjunct is to prevent obstruction of the upper airway by the tongue and allow the passage of air and oxygen to the lungs.

▶ Oropharyngeal Airway

An **oropharyngeal (oral) airway** is a hard, plastic airway designed to prevent the tongue from obstructing the glottis **Figure 11-32**. This type of airway device is often used in conjunction with bag-mask ventilation.

Indications for the oral airway include the following:

- Unresponsive patients without a gag reflex (breathing or apneic)
- Any patient being ventilated with a bag-mask device who does not have a gag reflex

Contraindications for the oral airway include the following:

- Responsive patients
- Any patient (responsive or unresponsive) who has an intact gag reflex

An oropharyngeal airway should be inserted promptly in unresponsive patients who have no gag reflex. The patients may or may not be breathing on their own. The **gag reflex** is a protective reflex mechanism that prevents food and other particles from entering the airway. Inserting an oral airway in a patient with a gag reflex may result in vomiting or a spasm of the vocal cords. An oral airway is a safe, effective way to help maintain the airway of a patient with a possible spinal injury.

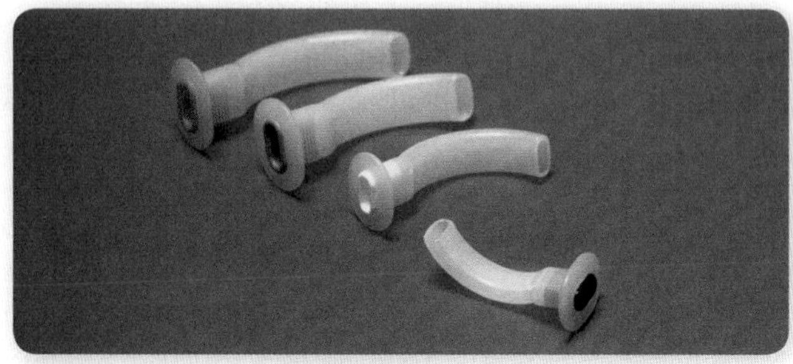

Figure 11-32 An oral airway is used for unresponsive patients who have no gag reflex. It works to keep the tongue from blocking the airway.

You must clearly understand when and how this device is used. If the oropharyngeal airway is not the proper size or is inserted incorrectly, it could actually push the tongue back into the pharynx, blocking the airway. Conversely, an oral airway that is too small could block the airway directly, just like any foreign body obstruction. Follow the steps in **Skill Drill 11-3** to insert an oropharyngeal airway.

Take care to avoid injuring the hard palate as you insert the airway. Roughness in your technique can cause bleeding that may aggravate airway problems or even cause vomiting.

If you encounter difficulty while inserting the oral airway, an alternative method may be used—inserting the oral airway with a 90° rotation. To do so, follow the steps in **Skill Drill 11-4**.

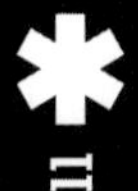

NR Skill

Skill Drill 11-3 Inserting an Oral Airway Into an Adult

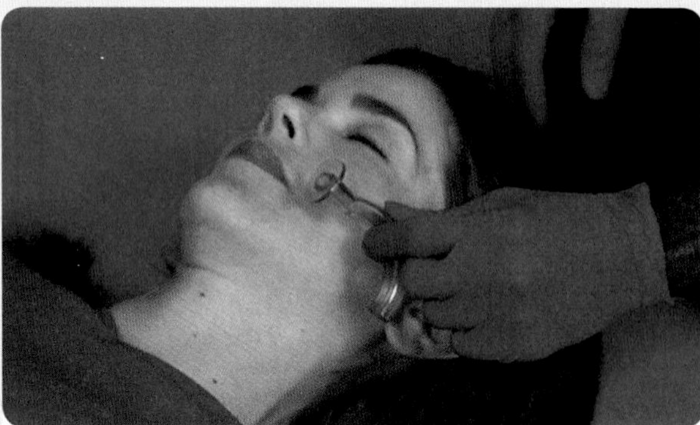

Step 1 To select the proper size, measure the distance from the patient's earlobe to the corner of the mouth. Another acceptable method is to measure from the center of the mouth to the angle of the jaw.

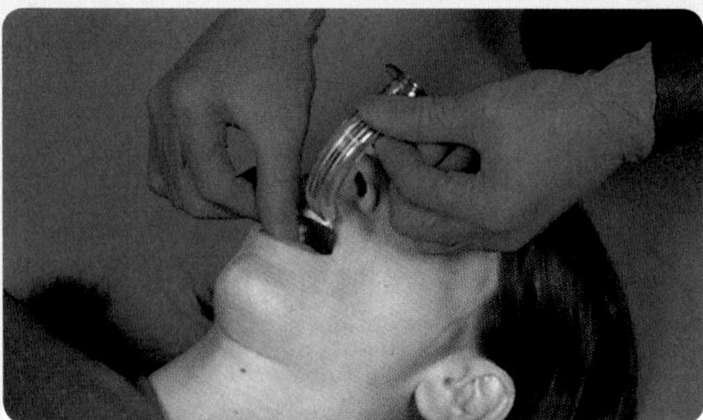

Step 2 Open the patient's mouth with the cross-finger technique. Hold the airway upside down with your other hand. Insert the airway with the tip facing the roof of the mouth and slide it in until it touches the roof of the mouth.

Skill Drill 11-3 Inserting an Oral Airway Into an Adult *(continued)*

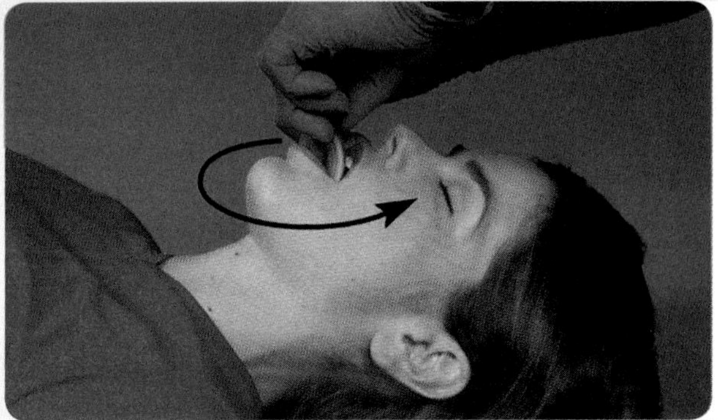

Step 3 Rotate the airway 180° after it passes the soft palate. When inserted properly, the airway device will rest in the mouth with the curvature of the airway device following the contour of the anatomy. The flange should rest against the patient's lips or teeth. In this position, the airway will hold the tongue forward.

Skill Drill 11-4 Inserting an Oral Airway With a 90° Rotation

NR Skill

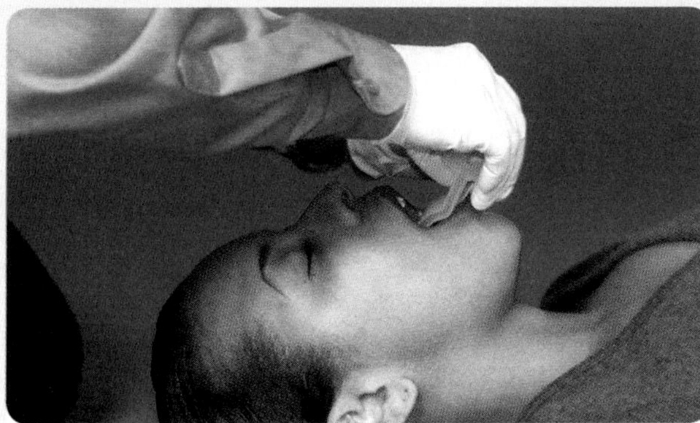

Step 1 Use a tongue depressor or bite stick to depress the tongue, ensuring the tongue remains forward.

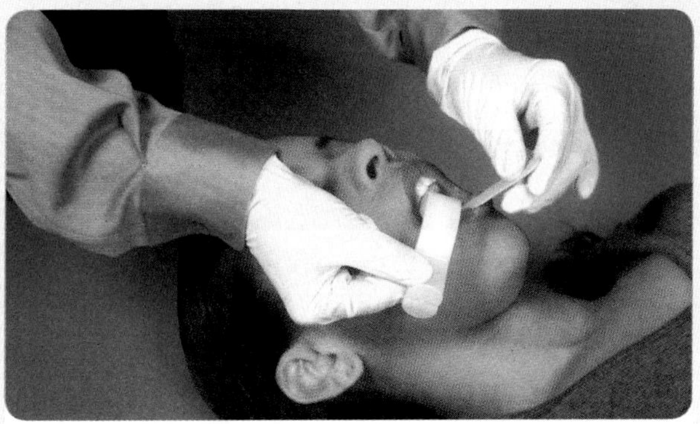

Step 2 Insert the oral airway sideways from the corner of the mouth, until the flange reaches the teeth.

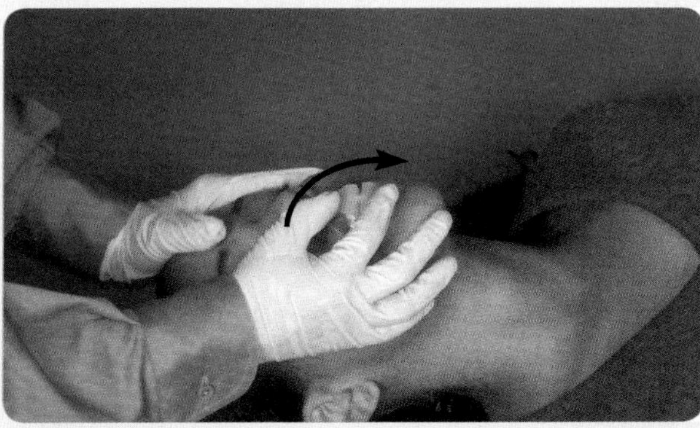

Step 3 Rotate the oral airway 90°, removing the depressor or bite stick as you exert gentle backward pressure on the oral airway until it rests securely in place against the lips and teeth.

In some cases, a patient may become responsive and regain a gag reflex after you have inserted an oral airway. If this occurs, gently remove the airway by pulling it out, following the normal curvature of the mouth and throat. Be prepared for the patient to vomit. Have suction available, and log roll the patient onto his or her side to allow any fluids to drain out.

▶ Nasopharyngeal Airway

A **nasopharyngeal (nasal) airway** is soft rubber with a beveled tip and usually is used in a patient who has an intact gag reflex and is not able to maintain an airway Figure 11-33. Patients with altered mental status or patients who have just had a seizure may also benefit from this type of airway. If a patient has sustained severe trauma to the head or face, consult medical control before inserting a nasopharyngeal airway. Use extreme care with such trauma patients. Although rare, if the airway is accidentally pushed through the hole caused by a basilar skull fracture, it may penetrate through the cranium and into the brain.

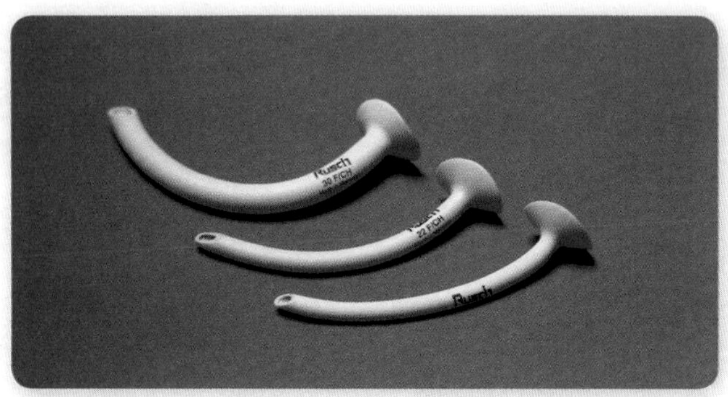

Figure 11-33 A nasal airway is better tolerated by patients who have an intact gag reflex.

Special Populations

In children, the only acceptable method of inserting an oral airway is to use a tongue blade to hold the tongue down while inserting the airway straight in. Because the airways of children are undeveloped, rotating an oropharyngeal airway in the posterior pharynx may cause damage to the uvula and soft palate.

This type of airway is usually better tolerated by patients who have an intact gag reflex. It is not as likely as the oropharyngeal airway to cause vomiting. The distal tip of the nasopharyngeal airway rests in the hypopharynx behind the tongue. You should coat the airway well with a water-soluble lubricant (ie, KY®, Lubifax®, Surgilube®, etc) before

YOU are the Provider PART 3

Your partner indicates that he is having difficulty maintaining an effective mask seal because of the patient's dentition, and you notice that the pulse oximetry reading is not increasing. On the basis of these findings and the seriousness of the patient's condition, you decide that he is a candidate for insertion of the King LT airway. You quickly remove the King LT (size 5) from your airway bag and check the patency of the balloons by inflating them with the recommended 80 mL of air. Finding no leakage, you position the patient's head and gently insert the airway until the base of the connector is aligned with the gums. After the King LT airway has been inserted, you quickly fill the balloon with 80 mL of air and direct your partner to resume ventilations while you assess for breath sounds.

Recording Time: 8 Minutes	
Respirations	12 breaths/min; clear
Pulse	120 beats/min; regular
Skin	Clammy, cyanotic
Blood pressure	90/42 mm Hg
Oxygen saturation (Spo_2)	82% and increasing with 15 L/min
Pupils	Pupils Equal, Round, and Reactive to Light and Accommodation (PERRLA)

5. What are the indications for insertion of an advanced airway?
6. What are the contraindications for insertion of a King LT airway?

it is inserted. Be aware that slight bleeding may occur even when the airway is inserted properly. However, you should never force the airway into place. If you meet resistance, then try to pass the airway device down the other nostril.

Indications for the nasopharyngeal airway include the following:

- Patients with an altered mental status who still have an intact gag reflex
- Patients who otherwise will not tolerate an oropharyngeal airway

Contraindications for the nasopharyngeal airway include the following:

- Severe head injury with blood draining from the nose (epistaxis)
- Potential for basilar skull fracture
- History of fractured nasal bone
- Meeting with resistance during insertion (ie, deviated septum; try other nare)

Follow the steps in Skill Drill 11-5 to ensure correct placement of the nasopharyngeal airway.

Skill Drill 11-5 Inserting a Nasal Airway

NR Skill

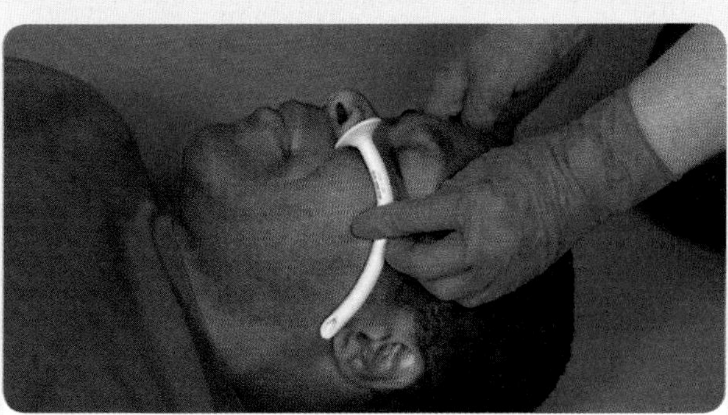

Step 1 Before inserting the airway device, be sure you have selected the proper size. Measure the distance from the tip of the patient's nose to the earlobe or the angle of the jaw. The diameter should be roughly equal to the diameter of the patient's little finger. If the nasopharyngeal airway is too long, it will obstruct the patient's airway. Coat the tip with a water-soluble lubricant.

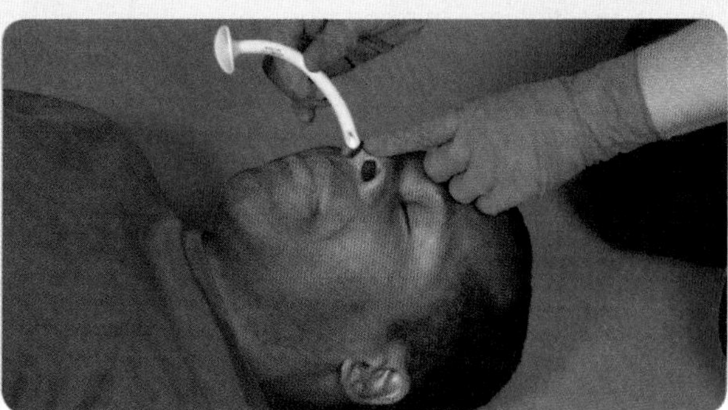

Step 2 In almost all patients, one nostril is slightly larger than the other. Insert the lubricated airway device into the larger nostril with the curvature following the floor of the nose. If using the right nare, the bevel should face the septum. If using the left nare, insert the airway device with the tip of the airway pointing upward, which will allow the bevel to face the septum.

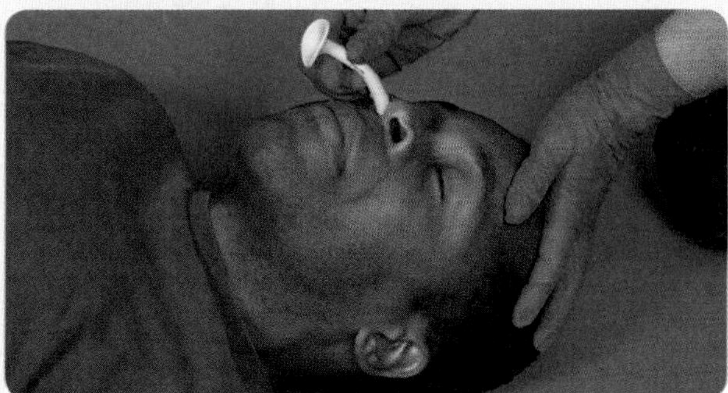

Step 3 Gently advance the airway. If using the left nare, insert the nasopharyngeal airway until you feel resistance. Then rotate the nasopharyngeal airway 180° into position. This rotation is not required if using the right nare.

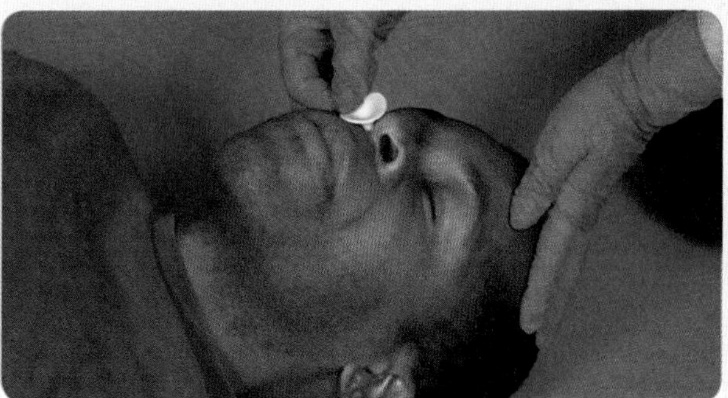

Step 4 Continue until the flange rests against the skin. If you feel any resistance or obstruction, remove the nasal airway and insert it into the other nostril. When completely inserted, the flange rests against the nostril. The other end of the airway opens into the posterior pharynx. If the patient becomes intolerant of the nasal airway, you may have to remove it. Precautions similar to those used when removing an oral airway should be followed.

Supplemental Oxygen

You should administer supplemental oxygen to any patient with potential hypoxia, even if the patient's clinical appearance is otherwise normal. By enriching atmospheric air with supplemental oxygen, you subsequently increase oxygen to the cells, thereby reducing pain and further damage; for example, to myocardial tissue. Increasing the available oxygen also enhances the body's compensatory mechanisms during shock and other distressed states. The oxygen delivery method must be reassessed frequently and adjusted accordingly based on the patient's clinical condition and breathing adequacy.

Historically, oxygen was administered to patients whose clinical condition did not otherwise indicate its use (that is, no evidence of respiratory compromise, with an oxygen saturation level greater than 94%). Limited evidence suggests that supplemental oxygen in a well-oxygenated patient may not be in his or her best interest, because issues such as oxidative stress and hyperoxic injury are of concern. However, the evidence that oxygen is helpful to a patient with hypoxia is profound, so if you are in doubt as to the patient's oxygenation status, then administer supplemental oxygen.[7,8]

Current guidelines from the American Heart Association for patients with chest pain or evidence of acute coronary syndromes state that if the patient is not experiencing respiratory distress and has an oxygen saturation level that is greater than or equal to 94%, then supplemental oxygen is not indicated.[9] Follow your local protocols regarding supplemental oxygen administration.

Some tissues and organs need a constant supply of oxygen to function normally. *Never withhold oxygen from any patient who might benefit from it, especially if you must assist ventilations.*

▶ Supplemental Oxygen Equipment

In addition to knowing when and how to give supplemental oxygen, you must understand how oxygen is stored and the various hazards associated with its use.

Oxygen Cylinders

The oxygen that you will give to patients is usually supplied as a compressed gas in green, seamless steel or aluminum cylinders. Some cylinders may be silver or chrome with a green area around the valve stem on top. Newer cylinders are often made of lightweight aluminum or spun steel; older cylinders are much heavier.

Check to make sure that the cylinder is labeled for medical oxygen. You should look for letters and numbers stamped into the metal on the collar of the cylinder **Figure 11-34**. Of particular importance are the month and year stamps, which indicate when the cylinder was last tested. Generally, aluminum cylinders are tested every 5 years; composite cylinders are tested every 3 years.

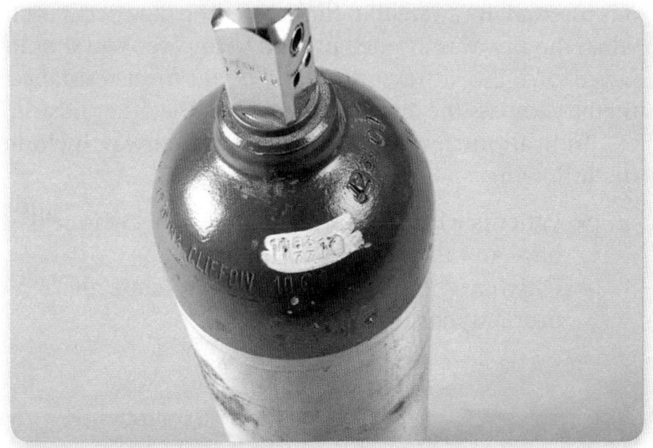

Figure 11-34 Oxygen tanks for medical use have a series of letters and numbers stamped into the metal on the collar of the cylinder.

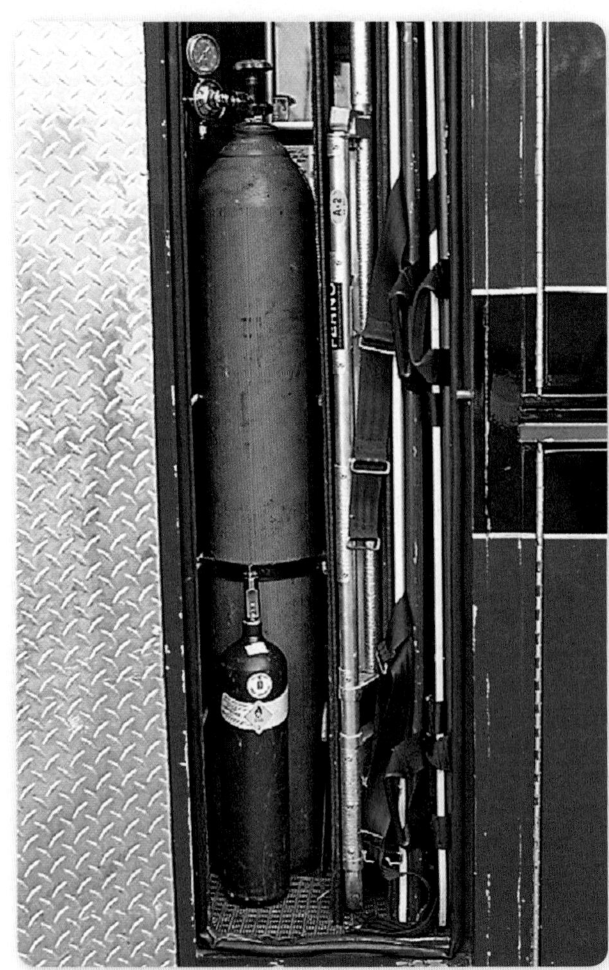

Figure 11-35 The cylinders most commonly found on an ambulance are the D (or jumbo D) and M size cylinders.

Oxygen cylinders are available in several sizes. The two sizes that you will most often use are the D (or jumbo D) cylinder, which contains 350 L, and the M cylinder, which contains 3,000 L **Figure 11-35**. The D (or jumbo D) cylinder can be carried from your unit to the patient.

The M tank remains on board your unit as a main supply tank. Other sizes that you will see are A, E, G, H, and K Table 11-7. Another naming system for identifying the size of the oxygen cylinder has been introduced. Per this naming convention, cylinders are labeled with M (for medical), followed by a number.

The length of time you can use an oxygen cylinder depends on the pressure in the cylinder and the flow rate. A method of calculating cylinder duration, or tank life, is shown in Table 11-8.

Table 11-7 Oxygen Cylinder Sizes Carried on the Ambulance

Size	Volume, Liters
D	350
Jumbo D	500
E	625
M	3,000
G	5,300
H, A, K	6,900

Table 11-8 Oxygen Cylinders: Duration of Flow

Formula:

(Tank pressure in psi − 200 psi [the safe residual pressure]) × Cylinder constant/Flow rate in L/min = Duration of flow in minutes

Cylinder constant for a given cylinder size:

A = 3.14	G = 2.41
D = 0.16	H = 3.14
E = 0.28	K = 3.14
M = 1.56	

Steps:

Determine the life of an M cylinder that has a pressure of 2,000 psi and a flow rate of 10 L/min.

$$\frac{(2{,}000 - 200) \times 1.56}{10} = \frac{2{,}808}{10} = 281 \text{ min, or } 4 \text{ h } 41 \text{ min}$$

Abbreviation: psi, pounds per square inch

Liquid Oxygen

Liquid oxygen is oxygen that is cooled to its aqueous state. It converts to the gaseous state when warmed. Liquid oxygen is becoming more commonly used as an alternative to compressed gas oxygen. There are advantages and disadvantages of liquid oxygen. A much larger volume of gaseous oxygen can be stored in the liquid state, and containers do not need to be filled as often. Liquid oxygen units also weigh less than aluminum or steel tanks. For these reasons, many people who receive long-term oxygen therapy use liquid oxygen units. Unfortunately, units for liquid oxygen generally require upright storage and have special requirements for filling, large-volume storage, and cylinder transfer.

Safety Considerations

Compressed gas cylinders must be handled very carefully because their contents are under pressure. Cylinders are fitted with pressure regulators to make sure that patients receive the right amount and type of gas. Make sure that the correct pressure regulator is firmly attached before you transport the cylinders. A puncture or hole in the tank can cause the cylinder to become a deadly missile. Do not handle a cylinder by the neck assembly alone. Cylinders should be secured with mounting brackets when they are stored on the ambulance. Oxygen cylinders that are in use during transport should be positioned and secured to prevent the tank from falling and to protect the valve-gauge assembly from damage. Contact with the liquid oxygen should be prevented at all costs. Severe tissue damage, including frostbite and tissue necrosis from frostbite, can occur.

Pin-Indexing System

The compressed gas industry has established a **pin-indexing system** for portable cylinders to prevent an oxygen regulator from being connected to a carbon dioxide cylinder, and so on. When preparing to administer oxygen, always check to be sure that the pinholes on the cylinder exactly match the corresponding pins on the regulator.

The pin-indexing system features a series of pins on a yoke that must be matched with the holes on the valve stem of the gas cylinder. The arrangement of the pins and holes varies for different gases according to accepted national standards Figure 11-36. Other gases that are supplied in portable cylinders, such as acetylene, carbon dioxide, and nitrogen, use regulators and flowmeters that are similar to those used with oxygen cylinders. Each cylinder of a specific gas has a given pattern and a given number of pins. These safety measures make it impossible for you to attach a cylinder of nitrous oxide to an oxygen regulator. The oxygen regulator will not fit.

The outlet valves on E size or smaller cylinders are designed to accept yoke-type pressure-reducing gauges, which conform to the pin-indexing system Figure 11-37.

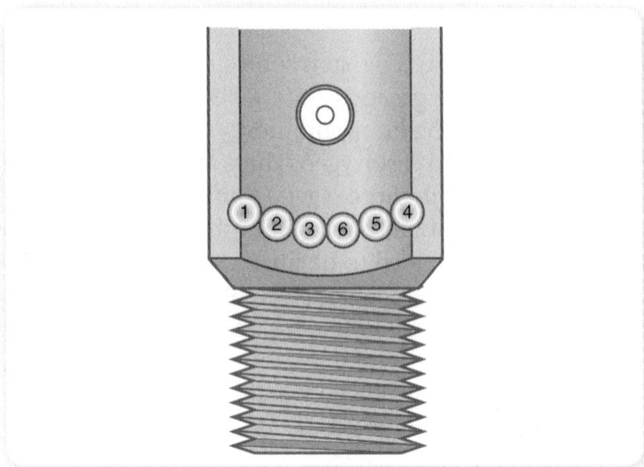

Figure 11-36 The locations of the pin-indexing safety system holes in a cylinder valve face. Each cylinder of a specific gas has a given pattern and a given number of pins.

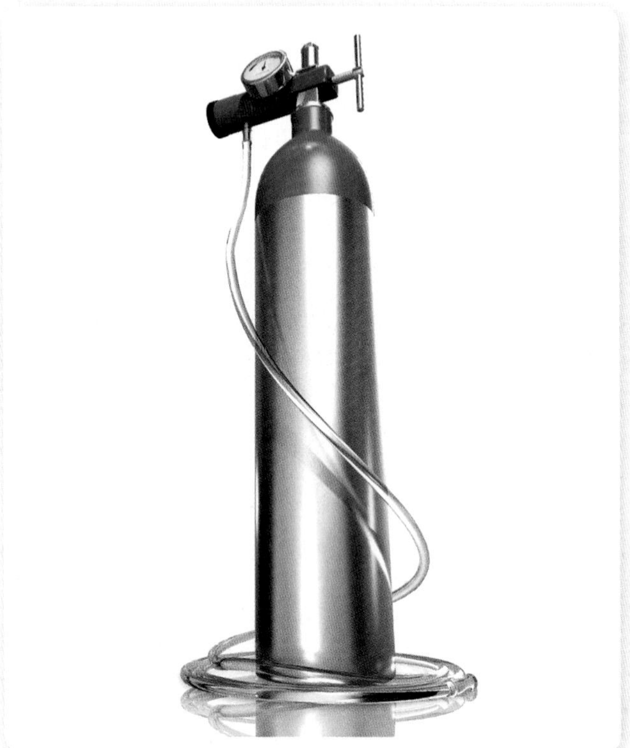

Figure 11-37 A yoke-type pressure-reducing gauge is used with a portable oxygen cylinder.

The safety system for large cylinders is known as the **American Standard System**. In this system, cylinders larger than E size are equipped with threaded gas outlet valves. The inside and outside thread sizes of these outlets vary depending on the gas in the cylinder. The cylinder will not accept a regulator valve unless it is properly threaded to fit that regulator. The purpose of these safety devices is the same as in the pin-indexing system: to prevent the accidental attachment of a regulator to a wrong cylinder.

Pressure Regulators

The pressure of gas in a full oxygen cylinder is approximately 2,000 psi. This is far too much pressure to be safe or useful for your purposes. Regulators reduce the pressure to a more useful range, usually 40 to 70 psi. Most pressure regulators that are currently in use reduce the pressure in a single stage, although multistage regulators exist. A two-stage regulator will reduce the pressure first to 700 psi and then to 40 to 70 psi.

After the pressure is reduced to a workable level, the final attachment for delivering the gas to the patient is usually one of the following:

- A quick-connect female fitting that will accept a quick-connect male plug from a pressure hose or ventilator or resuscitator
- A flowmeter that will permit the regulated release of gas measured in liters per minute

Flowmeters

Flowmeters are usually permanently attached to pressure regulators on emergency medical equipment. The two types of flowmeters that are commonly used are pressure-compensated flowmeters and Bourdon-gauge flowmeters.

A pressure-compensated flowmeter incorporates a float ball within a tapered calibrated tube. The float rises or falls according to the gas flow within the tube. The flow of gas is controlled by a needle valve located downstream from the float ball. This type of flowmeter is affected by gravity and must always be maintained in an upright position for an accurate flow reading Figure 11-38.

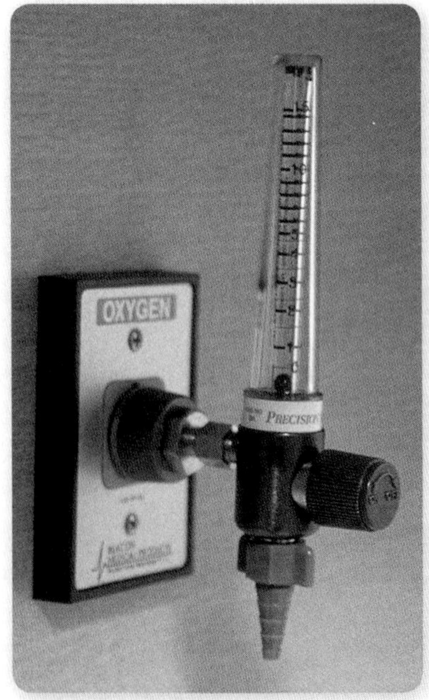

Figure 11-38 Pressure-compensated flowmeters contain a float ball that rises or falls according to the gas flow within the tube. It must be maintained in an upright position for an accurate reading.

By contrast, the **Bourdon-gauge flowmeter** is not affected by gravity and can be placed in any position. This pressure gauge is calibrated to record the flow rate Figure 11-39. The major disadvantage of this type of flowmeter is that it does not compensate for backpressure.

As a result, it will usually record a higher flow rate when there is any obstruction to gas flow downstream.

▶ Operating Procedures

To place an oxygen cylinder into service, follow the steps in Skill Drill 11-6.

Open the flowmeter to the desired flow rate. Flow rates will vary based on the oxygen-delivery device being used. Remember that you must be completely familiar with the equipment before attempting to use it on a patient. After the oxygen is flowing at the desired rate, confirm

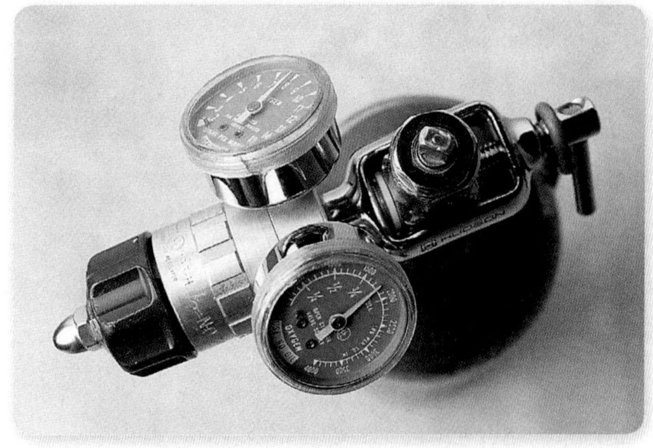

Figure 11-39 The Bourdon-gauge flowmeter is not affected by gravity and can be placed in any position.

Skill Drill 11-6 Placing an Oxygen Cylinder Into Service

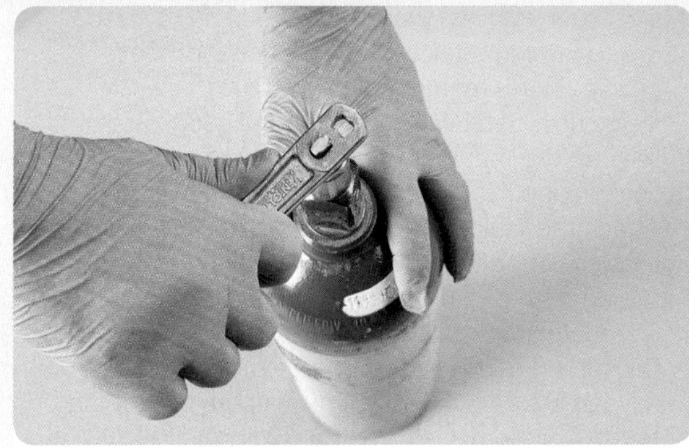

Step 1 Inspect the cylinder and its markings. If the cylinder was commercially filled, it will have a plastic seal around the valve stem covering the opening in the stem. Remove the seal, and inspect the opening to make sure that it is free of dirt and other debris. The valve stem should not be sealed or covered with adhesive tape or any petroleum-based substances. These can contaminate the oxygen and can contribute to combustion when mixed with pressurized oxygen.

"Crack" the cylinder by slowly opening and then reclosing the valve to help make sure that the dirt particles and other possible contaminants do not enter the oxygen flow. Never face the tank toward yourself or others when cracking the cylinder. Open the tank by attaching a tank key (wrench) to the valve and rotating the valve counterclockwise. You should be able to hear clearly the rush of oxygen coming from the tank. Close the tank by rotating the valve clockwise.

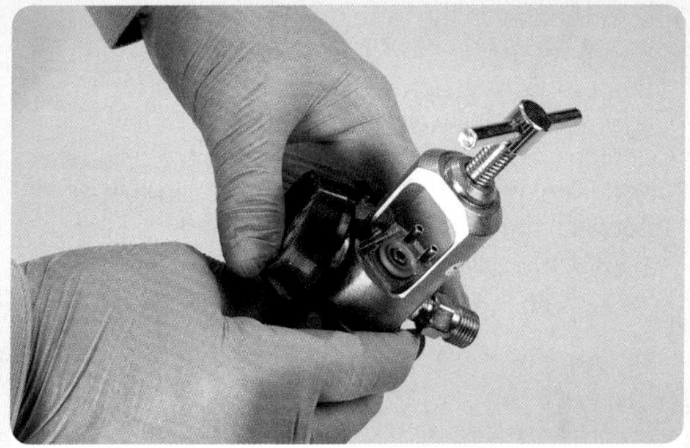

Step 2 Attach the regulator/flowmeter to the valve stem after clearing the opening. On one side of the valve stem, you will find three holes. The larger one, on top, is a true opening through which the oxygen flows. The two smaller holes below it do not extend to the inside of the tank. They provide stability to the regulator. Following the design of the pin-indexing system, these two holes are very precisely located in positions that are unique to the oxygen cylinders.

Above the pins on the inside of the collar is the actual port through which oxygen flows from the cylinder to the regulator. A metal-bound elastomeric sealing washer (also called a gasket) is placed around the oxygen port to optimize the airtight seal between the collar of the regulator and the valve stem. In the past, crush gaskets made of plastic and nylon were used, but are no longer recommended. If used, crush gaskets can be used only once and then they must be replaced.

(continued)

Skill Drill 11-6 Placing an Oxygen Cylinder Into Service *(continued)*

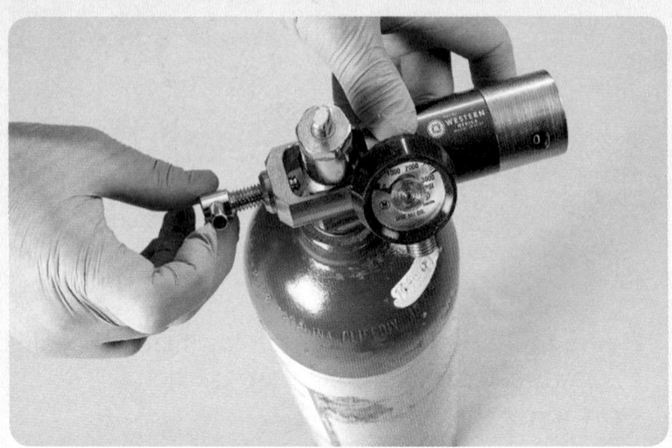

Step 3 Place the regulator collar over the cylinder valve, with the oxygen port and pin-indexing pins on the side of the valve stem that has the three holes. Open the screw bolt just enough to allow the collar to fit freely over the valve stem. Move the regulator so that the oxygen port and the pins fit into the correct holes on the valve stem. The screw bolt on the opposite side should be aligned with the dimple depression. As you hold the regulator securely against the valve stem, hand tighten the screw bolt until the regulator is firmly attached to the cylinder. At this point, you should not see any open spaces between the sides of the valve stem and the interior walls of the collar.

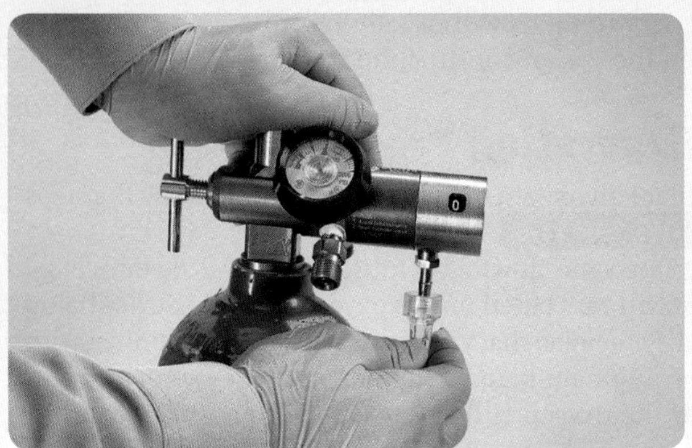

Step 4 With the regulator firmly attached, open the cylinder completely, check for air leaking from the regulator–oxygen cylinder connection, and read the pressure level on the regulator gauge. Most portable cylinders have a maximum pressure of approximately 2,000 psi. Most EMS systems consider a cylinder with less than 500 to 1,000 psi to be too low to keep in service. Learn your department's policies in this regard and follow them.

The flowmeter will have a second gauge or a selector dial that indicates the oxygen flow rate. Several popular types of devices are widely used. Attach the selected oxygen device to the flowmeter by connecting the universal oxygen connecting tubing to the "Christmas tree" nipple on the flowmeter. Most oxygen-delivery devices come with this tubing permanently attached; however, some oxygen masks do not. You must attach this tubing to the oxygen-delivery device if it is not already attached.

flow from the device, then apply the oxygen device to the patient and make any necessary adjustments. Monitor the patient's reaction to the oxygen and to the oxygen device, and periodically recheck the regulator gauge to make sure there is sufficient oxygen in the cylinder. Disconnect the tubing from the flowmeter nipple and turn off the cylinder valve when oxygen therapy is complete or when the patient has been transferred to the hospital and is using the hospital's oxygen system. In a few seconds, the sound of oxygen flowing from the nipple will cease. This indicates that all the pressurized oxygen has been removed from the flowmeter. Turn off the flowmeter. The gauge on the regulator should read zero with the tank valve closed. This confirms that there is no pressure left above the valve stem. As long as there is a pressure reading on the regulator gauge, it is not safe to remove the regulator from the valve stem.

Safety

Slowly open the oxygen tank after attaching the regulator, and check for leaks. Remember that although oxygen itself is not combustible, it supports combustion, and any ignition source may cause a fire or an explosion in an oxygen-rich environment—especially if oxygen is being released too quickly from the cylinder at the time or if the seal between the regulator and oxygen cylinder is not secure.

Hazards of Supplemental Oxygen

Oxygen does not burn or explode. However, it supports combustion. The more oxygen that is around, the faster the combustion process. A small spark, even a glowing cigarette, can become a flame in an oxygen-rich atmosphere. Therefore, you must keep any possible source of fire away from the area while oxygen is in use. Make sure the area is adequately ventilated, especially in industrial settings where hazardous materials may be present and where sparks are easily generated. Be extremely cautious in any enclosed environment in which oxygen is being administered because an oxygen-rich environment increases the chance of fire if a spark or flame is introduced. A smoking bystander or a vehicle extrication that generates sparks are possible ignition sources. Never leave an oxygen cylinder standing unattended. The cylinder could be knocked over, injuring the patient or damaging the regulator.

Oxygen Toxicity

The administration of oxygen to patients is a common practice. Although many patients in the prehospital environment require high concentrations of oxygen, not all patients do. Excessive supplemental oxygen can have a detrimental effect on patients with certain illnesses (ie, COPD, bronchopulmonary dysplasia).

Recent research has shown that although the administration of oxygen benefits many patients and is rarely problematic, high concentrations of oxygen are potentially harmful for a select population. **Oxygen toxicity** refers to damage to cellular tissue as a result of excessive oxygen levels in the blood. Previously, high concentrations of oxygen were thought to benefit all patients in the prehospital environment. However, current evidence suggests that increased cellular oxygen levels contribute to the production of oxygen free radicals. These radicals may result in tissue damage and cellular death in some patients.

Tailor oxygen therapy to patient needs and use caution with administration. Understand that hypoxemia is much worse than oxygen toxicity; when in doubt, or if unable to measure oxygen saturation reliably, supplemental oxygen should be administered.

Oxygen-Delivery Devices

In general, the oxygen-delivery equipment that is used in the field should be limited to nonrebreathing masks, bag-mask devices, and nasal cannulas, depending on local protocol. However, you may encounter other devices during transports between medical facilities. Flow rates for various oxygen-delivery devices are shown in Table 11-9.

Table 11-9 Oxygen-Delivery Devices

Device	Flow Rate	Oxygen Delivered
Nasal cannula	1 to 6 L/min	24% to 44%
Nonrebreathing mask	10 to 15 L/min	Up to 90%
Bag-mask device with reservoir	15 L/min	Nearly 100%
Mouth-to-mask device	15 L/min	Nearly 55%

Nonrebreathing Mask

The **nonrebreathing mask** is the preferred device to use when giving oxygen in the prehospital setting to patients who have adequate tidal volume but are suspected of having or are showing signs of hypoxia. Contraindications include apnea and poor respiratory effort. The nonrebreathing mask delivers oxygen passively and requires adequate tidal volume for the oxygen to be effectively drawn into the lungs. With a good mask-to-face seal and a flow rate of 15 L/min, it is capable of providing up to 90% inspired oxygen.

The nonrebreathing mask is a combination mask and reservoir bag system. Oxygen fills a reservoir bag that is attached to the mask by a one-way valve Figure 11-40. The system is called a nonrebreathing mask because the exhaled gas escapes through flapper valve side ports covered by a one-way disk at the cheek areas of the mask. The valve between the mask and reservoir prevents the patient from rebreathing exhaled gases. The patient inhales enriched oxygen from the reservoir bag rather than residual air.

In this system, you must be sure that the reservoir bag is full before the mask is placed on the patient. Adjust

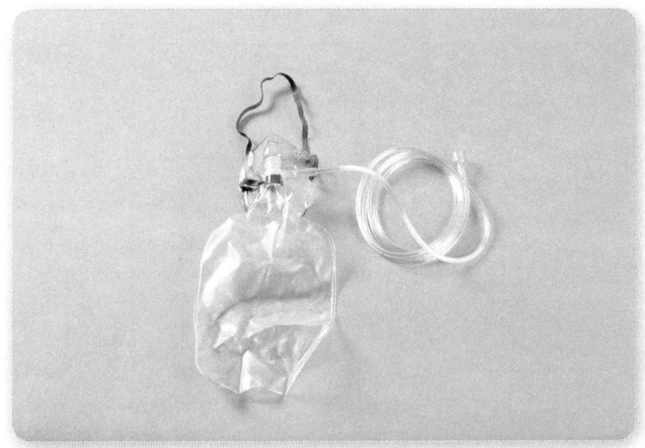

Figure 11-40 The nonrebreathing mask contains flapper valve ports at the cheek areas of the mask to prevent the patient from rebreathing exhaled air.

the flow rate so that the bag does not fully collapse when the patient inhales, to approximately two-thirds of the bag volume, or 12 to 15 L/min. Make sure the bag stays inflated. Should the bag collapse when the patient inhales, increase the flow rate of oxygen. In addition, if oxygen therapy is discontinued, remove the mask from the patient's face. Leaving the mask in place, while oxygen is not flowing, allows the patient to rebreathe exhaled carbon dioxide. Use a pediatric mask, which has a smaller reservoir bag, for infants and children because they inhale a smaller volume.

▶ Nasal Cannulas

A **nasal cannula** delivers oxygen through two small, tubelike prongs that fit into the patient's nostrils Figure 11-41. This device can provide 24% to 44% inspired oxygen when the flowmeter is set at 1 to 6 L/min. For the comfort of your patient, flow rates above 6 L/min are not recommended with the nasal cannula.

A nasal cannula has limited use in the prehospital setting. It is ineffective for patients with poor respiratory effort, severe hypoxia, apnea, or mouth breathing. The primary use of a nasal cannula in the prehospital setting is for a patient who will not tolerate a nonrebreathing mask. In addition, a nasal cannula would be appropriate for patients requiring long-term oxygen therapy for certain diseases (such as COPD) whose current complaint is unrelated to their respiratory disease.

The advantage of a nasal cannula is that it is well tolerated. Even patients who are claustrophobic can tolerate the nasal cannula. Unfortunately, it does not deliver high volumes or high concentrations of oxygen.

The nasal cannula delivers dry oxygen directly into the nostrils. Therefore, when you anticipate a long transport time, you should consider the use of humidification.

▶ Partial Rebreathing Mask

The **partial rebreathing mask** is similar to a nonrebreathing mask except that there is no one-way valve between the mask and the reservoir. Consequently, patients rebreathe a small amount of their exhaled air. This has some benefit when you want to increase the patient's partial pressure of carbon dioxide, which makes this the ideal mask for patients whom you think are experiencing hyperventilation syndrome. The oxygen enriches the air mixture and delivers a gas mix of approximately 80% to 90% oxygen. You can easily convert a nonrebreathing mask to a partial rebreathing mask by removing the one-way valve between the mask and the reservoir bag.

▶ Venturi Mask

A Venturi mask has a number of attachments that enable you to vary the percentage of oxygen delivered to the patient while a constant flow is maintained from the regulator Figure 11-42. The patient receives a highly specific concentration of oxygen because of the Venturi principle, which causes air to be drawn into the flow of oxygen as it passes a hole in the line. The Venturi mask is a medium-flow device that delivers 24% to 40% oxygen, depending on the manufacturer.

The main advantage of the Venturi mask is the use of its fine adjustment capabilities in the long-term treatment of patients in physiologically stable condition. However, in the emergency setting, such fine adjustments are not necessary or even generally desirable. When you need to adjust the oxygen concentration in an emergency, it is typically done by adjusting the flow rate or changing the delivery device.

▶ Tracheostomy Masks

A patient with a **tracheostomy** does not breathe through the mouth and nose. A face mask or nasal cannula therefore cannot be used to treat these patients. Masks designed specifically for patients with tracheostomies cover the tracheostomy hole and have a strap that goes around the neck. These masks are usually available in intensive care units, where many patients have tracheostomies, and may not be available in an emergency setting. If you do not

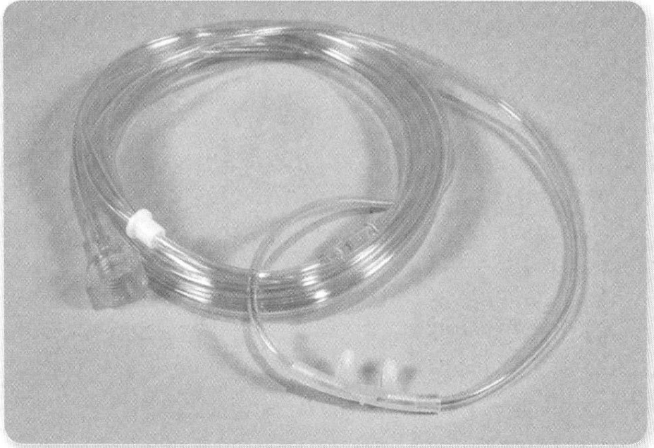

Figure 11-41 The nasal cannula delivers oxygen directly through the nostrils.

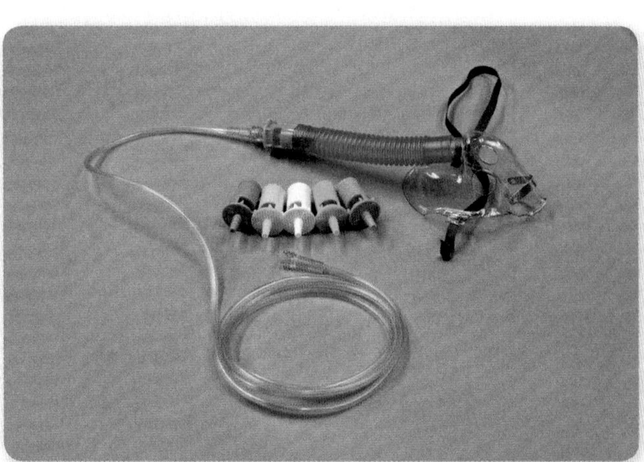

Figure 11-42 A Venturi mask.

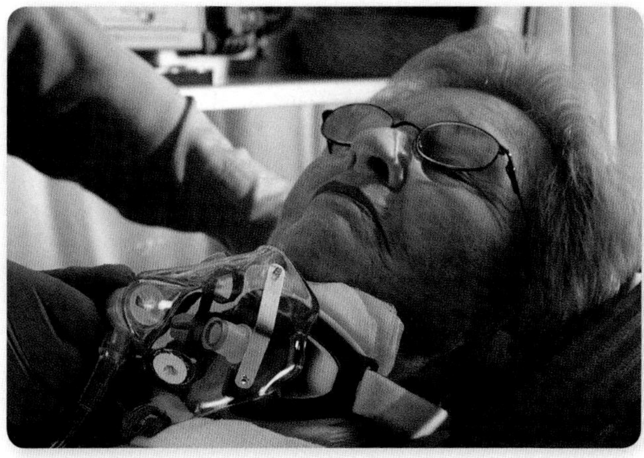

Figure 11-43 If you do not have a tracheostomy mask, use a face mask instead.

have a tracheostomy mask, you can improvise by placing a face mask over the stoma. Even though the mask is shaped to fit the face, you can usually get an adequate fit over the patient's neck by adjusting the strap Figure 11-43.

> **Words of Wisdom**
>
> A nebulizer with saline or sterile water placed in the medication chamber may be used in place of humidified oxygen. Simply attach an oxygen mask to the aerosol chamber and set the flowmeter at 6 L/min.

▶ Oxygen Humidifiers

Some EMS systems provide humidified oxygen to patients during transport Figure 11-44, especially patients receiving long-term oxygen therapy. A sterile water reservoir is needed for humidifying the oxygen. However, humidified oxygen is usually indicated only for long-term oxygen therapy, prolonged transport time, and conditions such as croup, epiglottitis, and bronchiolitis. Many EMS systems do not use humidified oxygen in the prehospital setting, especially if their transport times to the hospital are short. Always refer to local protocols for guidance involving patient treatment issues.

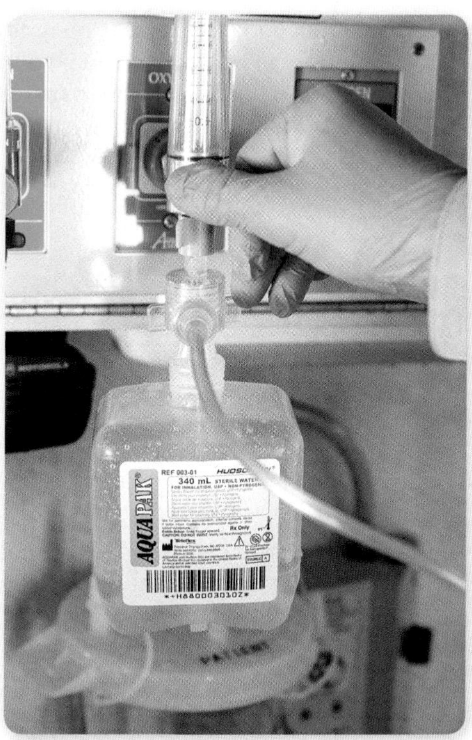

Figure 11-44 Administering humidified oxygen may be preferred with long transport times. However, this type of oxygen-delivery system is not used in all EMS systems.

Assisted and Artificial Ventilation

A patient who is not breathing needs artificial ventilation and 100% supplemental oxygen. Assisted and artificial ventilation are probably the most important skills in EMS—at any level. Basic airway and ventilation techniques are extremely effective when administered appropriately. Mastery of these techniques is imperative.

Patients who are breathing inadequately, such as patients who are breathing too fast or too slowly with reduced tidal volume, are typically unable to speak in complete sentences. An irregular breathing pattern will also require artificial ventilation to assist patients in maintaining adequate minute volume. Keep in mind that fast, shallow breathing can be just as dangerous as extremely slow breathing. Fast, shallow breathing moves air primarily in the larger airway passages (dead air space) and does not allow for adequate exchange of air and carbon dioxide in the alveoli. Signs of altered mental status and inadequate minute volume are indications for assisted ventilation. In addition, excessive accessory muscle use and fatigue from labored breathing are signs of potential respiratory failure. Patients exhibiting these signs need immediate treatment. Two treatment options are available for patients in severe respiratory distress or respiratory failure: assisted ventilation and **continuous positive airway pressure (CPAP)**. The purpose of assisted ventilation is to improve the overall oxygenation and ventilatory status of the patient. CPAP is discussed later in this chapter; the focus of this section will be on assisted ventilation.

Follow these steps to assist a patient with ventilation using a bag-mask device. Remember to follow standard precautions as needed when managing the patient's airway.

1. Explain the procedure to the patient.
2. Place the mask over the patient's nose and mouth.
3. Squeeze the bag each time the patient breathes, maintaining the same rate as the patient, and coaching the patient as needed.

4. After the initial 5 to 10 breaths, slowly adjust the rate and deliver an appropriate tidal volume.
5. Adjust the rate and tidal volume to maintain an adequate minute volume.

Words of Wisdom

Methods of ventilation (listed in order of preference):

- Mouth-to-mask with one-way valve
- Two-person bag-mask device with reservoir and supplemental oxygen
- Manually triggered ventilation (MTV) device (flow-restricted, oxygen-powered ventilation device)
- One-person bag-mask device with oxygen reservoir and supplemental oxygen

Note: This order of preference has been stated because research has demonstrated that personnel who infrequently ventilate patients have great difficulty maintaining an adequate seal between the mask and the patient's face.

Words of Wisdom

Ventilation rates for an apneic patient with a pulse:

Adult: 1 breath every 5 to 6 seconds
Child: 1 breath per 3 to 5 seconds
Infant: 1 breath per 3 to 5 seconds

▶ Artificial Ventilation

Without immediate treatment, patients who are in respiratory arrest will die. However, the act of breathing for a patient, or artificial ventilation, is not a skill you should take lightly. After you determine that a patient is not breathing, you should begin artificial ventilation immediately. The methods that you may use to provide artificial ventilation include the mouth-to-mask technique; a one-, two-, or three-person bag-mask device; and the **manually triggered ventilation (MTV) device**.

Normal Ventilation Versus Positive Pressure Ventilation

It is important to understand that although artificial ventilations are necessary to sustain life, they are not the same as normal breathing. As discussed earlier, the act of air moving in and out of the lungs is based on pressure changes within the thoracic cavity. During normal ventilation, the diaphragm contracts and negative pressure is generated in the chest cavity. This essentially sucks air into the chest through the trachea in an attempt to equalize the pressure in the chest with the atmospheric pressure. However, positive pressure ventilation generated by a device, such as a bag-mask device, forces air into the chest cavity from the external environment, rather than based on pressure changes. This difference between normal ventilation and positive pressure ventilation can create some challenges Table 11-10.

The physical act of the chest wall expanding and retracting during breathing serves to aid the circulatory system in returning blood to the heart. During normal

Table 11-10 Normal Ventilation Versus Positive Pressure Ventilation

	Normal Ventilation	Positive Pressure Ventilation
Air movement	Air is drawn into the lungs due to the negative intrathoracic pressure created when the diaphragm contracts.	Air is forced into the lungs by means of mechanical ventilation.
Blood movement	Normal breathing allows blood to naturally be pulled back to the heart.	Intrathoracic pressure is increased, not allowing blood to be drawn back to the heart as efficiently. This causes the amount of blood pumped by the heart to be reduced.
Airway wall pressure	Not affected during normal breathing	More volume is required to have the same effects as normal breathing. As a result, the walls are pushed out of their normal anatomic shape.
Esophageal opening pressure	Not affected during normal breathing	Air is forced into the stomach, causing gastric distention that could result in vomiting and aspiration.
Overventilation	Overventilation is not typical of normal breathing.	Forcing volume and rate results in increased intrathoracic pressure, gastric distention, and a decrease in cardiac output (hypotension).

ventilation, the chest wall movement works similar to a pump. The pressure changes in the thoracic cavity help draw venous return back to the heart. However, positive pressure ventilation causes the walls of the chest cavity to push out of their normal anatomic shape. As a result, there is an increase in the overall intrathoracic pressure within the chest cavity. This pressure increase affects the venous return of blood to the heart. The blood flow is decreased due to the increased pressure in the chest. This causes decreased venous return to the heart, and the amount of blood pumped out of the heart is reduced. Therefore, it is imperative that AEMTs regulate the rate and volume of artificial ventilations to avoid overdistention of the chest wall and thus help prevent this decrease in cardiac output.

Another difference between normal ventilation and positive pressure ventilation is the control of airflow. When a person breathes, air enters the trachea and, generally, not the esophagus. However, the force generated from positive pressure ventilation allows air to enter not only the trachea, but also the esophagus. Ventilations that are too forceful can result in excessive air in the stomach. This potential complication, called gastric distention, will be discussed later in this chapter.

▶ Mouth-to-Mouth and Mouth-to-Mask Ventilation

As you learned in your CPR course, mouth-to-mouth ventilation is routinely performed with a barrier device, such as a mask or face shield. A **barrier device** is a protective item that features a plastic barrier placed on a patient's face with a one-way valve to prevent the backflow of secretions, vomitus, and gases. Barrier devices provide adequate protection **Figure 11-45**.

Mouth-to-mouth is the most basic form of ventilation. Indications for this type of ventilation include apnea when other ventilation devices are not available.

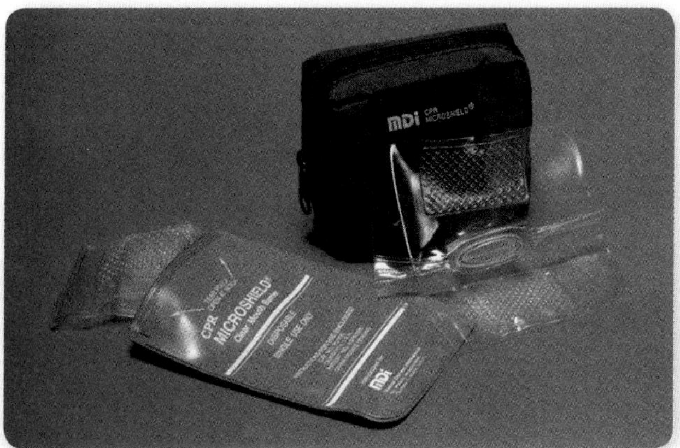

Figure 11-45 Barrier devices, such as a plastic shield or pocket mask with a one-way valve, provide adequate protection.

Although mouth-to-mouth ventilation requires no special equipment and can deliver effective tidal volume, there are other methods of providing artificial ventilation that are safer for the rescuer. The disadvantages of the mouth-to-mouth technique include the risk of unknown communicable diseases and psychological barriers associated with this method.

Mouth-to-mask ventilation (or ventilation using another barrier device) is preferred over the mouth-to-mouth technique. Advantages of using a mask include placing a physical barrier between the rescuer's mouth and the patient's mouth. Most masks offer a one-way valve to prevent the rescuer's exposure to blood and body fluids. It is also easier to secure an effective seal with a mask because the rescuer can use both hands, which enables the provision of adequate tidal volume to the patient.

A mask with an oxygen inlet provides oxygen during mouth-to-mask ventilation to supplement the air from your own lungs. Remember that the gas you exhale contains 16% oxygen, which is adequate to sustain the patient's life. With the mouth-to-mask system, however, the patient gets the additional benefit of substantial oxygen enrichment with inspired air.

The mask may be shaped like a triangle or a doughnut, with the apex (top) placed across the bridge of the nose. The base (bottom) of the mask is placed in the groove between the lower lip and the chin. In the center of the mask is a chimney with a 15-mm connector.

Follow the steps in **Skill Drill 11-7** to use mouth-to-mask ventilation.

You know that you are providing adequate ventilation if you see the patient's color improving and chest rise adequately and you do not meet resistance when ventilating. Feel for resistance of the patient's lungs as they expand. You should also hear and feel air escape as the patient exhales. Make sure that you are providing the correct number of breaths per minute for the patient's age. Color improvement may not be instantaneous.

To increase the oxygen concentration, administer high-flow oxygen at 15 L/min through the oxygen inlet valve of the mask. This, when combined with your exhaled breath, will deliver approximately 55% oxygen to the patient. Ventilate over 1 second to produce visible chest rise.

▶ The Bag-Mask Device

With an oxygen flow rate of 15 L/min and an adequate seal, a **bag-mask device** with an oxygen reservoir can deliver nearly 100% oxygen **Figure 11-46**. Most bag-mask devices on the market include modifications or accessories (reservoirs) that permit the delivery of oxygen concentrations approaching 100%. However, the device can deliver only as much volume as you can squeeze out of the bag by hand. The bag-mask device provides less tidal volume than mouth-to-mask ventilation; however, it delivers a much higher oxygen concentration.

The bag-mask device is the most common method used to ventilate patients in the field. An experienced

Skill Drill 11-7 Mouth-to-Mask Ventilation

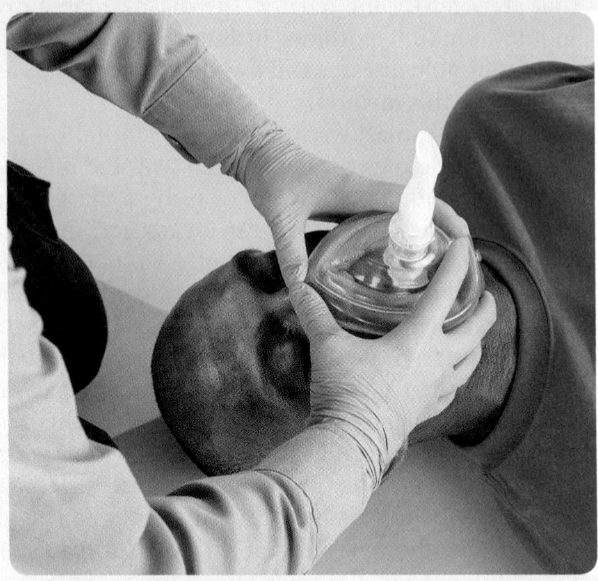

Step 1 Kneel at the patient's head. Open the airway using the head tilt–chin lift maneuver or the jaw-thrust maneuver if trauma is suspected. Insert an oral or nasal airway, if possible, to help maintain airway patency. Connect the one-way valve to the face mask and place the mask on the patient's face. Make sure the top is over the bridge of the nose and the bottom is in the groove between the lower lip and the chin. Hold the mask in position by placing your thumbs over the top part of the mask and your index fingers over the bottom half. Grasp the lower jaw with the remaining three fingers on each hand, making an airtight seal by pulling the lower jaw into the mask. Maintain an upward and forward pull on the lower jaw with your fingers to keep the airway open. This method of securing the mask to the patient's face is known as the EC-clamp method.

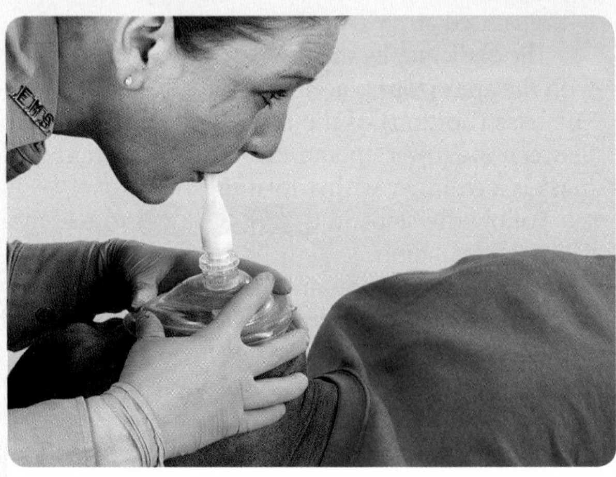

Step 2 Take a deep breath and exhale through the open port of the one-way valve. Breathe slowly into the patient's mask until you observe adequate chest rise.

Step 3 Remove your mouth from the valve, and watch the patient's chest fall during passive exhalation.

AEMT will be able to supply adequate tidal volumes with a bag-mask device. Use of the device, however, is a difficult skill to master. Mask seal on a medical patient may be difficult to obtain and maintain with only one rescuer. Because it takes two hands to perform a jaw-thrust maneuver, it takes two rescuers to use a bag-mask device on a trauma patient unless an advanced airway has been inserted already. The amount of tidal volume and the concentration of oxygen delivered to the patient are dependent on mask seal integrity. Be sure to practice on ventilation manikins several times before using a bag-mask device on a patient.

A bag-mask device should be used when you need to deliver high concentrations of oxygen to patients who are not ventilating adequately. The bag-mask device may be used with or without oxygen. However, it is most effective when used with supplemental oxygen and a reservoir. Depending on the patient's LOC, you should use an oral or a nasal airway adjunct in conjunction with the bag-mask device to maintain patency of the patient's airway. Generally, a bag-mask device should not be used on any patient who is intolerant of its use; however, if the patient is responsive and breathing inadequately (that is, reduced tidal volume), ventilatory assistance with a bag-mask device

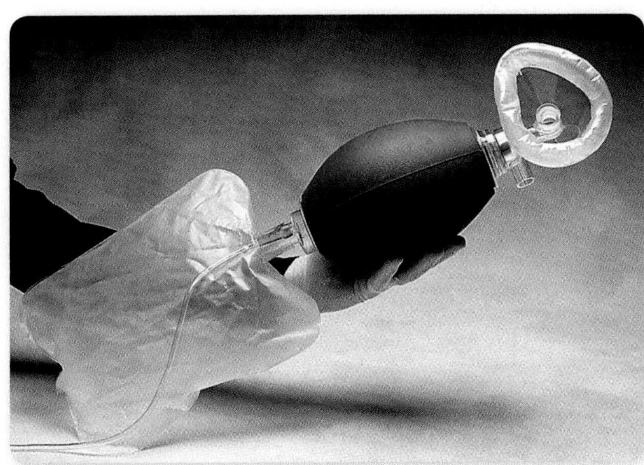

Figure 11-46 A bag-mask device with an oxygen reservoir can deliver nearly 100% oxygen if a good seal between the mouth and mask is achieved and if supplemental oxygen is used.

will be required to maintain adequate minute volume. In such cases, you must explain the procedure to the patient, advising that each time he or she takes a breath, you will squeeze the bag-mask to assist breathing efforts.

Bag-Mask Device Components

All adult bag-mask devices should have the following components and characteristics:

- A disposable self-refilling bag
- No pop-off valve or, if one is present, the capability of disabling the pop-off valve
- An outlet valve that is a true valve for nonrebreathing
- An oxygen reservoir that permits delivery of a high concentration of oxygen
- A one-way, no-jam inlet valve system that provides an oxygen inlet flow at a maximum of 15 L/min with standard 15/22-mm fittings for face mask and/or advanced airway (ie, ET tube, LMA, King LT, i-gel)
- A transparent face mask
- Ability to perform under extreme environmental conditions, including extreme heat and cold

The total amount of gas in the reservoir bag of an adult bag-mask device is usually 1,200 to 1,600 mL. The pediatric bag contains 500 to 700 mL, and the infant bag holds 150 to 240 mL.

The volume of air (oxygen) to deliver to the patient is based on one key observation—visible chest rise. A delivered tidal volume of 500 to 600 mL (6 to 7 mL/kg) per breath will produce visible chest rise in most adults. When using a bag-mask device, whether supplemental oxygen is attached to it or not, you should deliver each breath during a period of 1 to 2 seconds—just enough to produce visible chest rise—at the appropriate rate. Breaths

YOU are the Provider PART 4

Your partner states that he is now able to ventilate the patient with ease, and you note adequate chest rise and fall and an increase in the patient's pulse oximetry level. You contact dispatch and are advised that the transporting ambulance is approximately 4 minutes away and requests that you switch to the fireground channel and provide a quick update to the ambulance. You change channels on your radio, and, after making contact, you provide a quick update to the responding paramedics. They ask whether the patient had any abnormal respiratory patterns before insertion of the airway, to which you reply "negative." They then advise that they are pulling into the parking lot now. As the paramedics arrive, you give a more detailed report and assist in loading the patient onto their stretcher. They thank you for your prompt treatment and release you back in service.

Recording Time: 14 Minutes	
Respirations	12 breaths/min; assisted
Pulse	112 beats/min
Skin	Cool, dry, and pink
Blood pressure	100/54 mm Hg
Oxygen saturation (Spo_2)	88% on 15 L/min
Pupils	PERRLA

7. What are some possible respiratory patterns you may encounter?
8. If the patient's respiratory rate increases to an acceptable level, should the King LT airway be removed?

that are delivered too forcefully or too fast can result in two negative effects: gastric distention (and the associated risks of vomiting and aspiration) and decreased blood return to the heart because of increased intrathoracic pressure.

Improper technique, an ineffective mask-to-face seal, or the presence of gastric distention may cause you to deliver inadequate tidal volume and oxygen. Training and practice are key to the proper use of a bag-mask device.

Bag-Mask Device Technique

Whenever possible, you and your partner should work together to provide ventilation with the bag-mask device. One AEMT can maintain a good mask seal by securing the mask to the patient's face with two hands while the other AEMT squeezes the bag. Ventilation using a bag-mask device is a challenging skill: it may be very difficult for one EMS provider to maintain a proper seal between the mask and the face with one hand while squeezing the bag well enough to deliver an adequate volume to the patient. Also, performance of this skill depends on having enough personnel to carry out other actions that need to be done at the same time, such as chest compressions, putting the stretcher in place, or helping to lift the patient onto the stretcher.

There are three major considerations when using a bag-mask device to ventilate a patient. First, the typical adult bag-mask device holds a much larger volume of air than is needed. Not only can excessive volume cause barotrauma, it can also result in an increase in intrathoracic pressure that decreases venous return to the heart. You should squeeze the bag slowly, over 2 seconds, and just until you have adequate chest rise. Second, quick, forceful delivery of breaths may result in gastric distention as it only takes a small amount of pressure to override the lower esophageal sphincter. This may trigger regurgitation of stomach contents or may expand the stomach, causing it to compress the diaphragm and impede ventilation by inhibiting lung expansion. And last, be conscientious of the rate of delivery of breaths. Hyperventilation is only helpful in very few specific incidences. If possible, monitor $ETCO_2$ and maintain at 35 to 45 mm Hg. If the $ETCO_2$ drops below 35 mm Hg, you are ventilating too fast; if it rises above 45 mm Hg, you are ventilating too slowly.

Follow these steps to use the two-person bag-mask device technique:

1. Kneel above the patient's head. If possible, your partner should be at the side of the head to squeeze the bag while you hold a seal between the mask and the patient's face with two hands. Select the proper size mask.
2. Maintain the patient's neck in a hyperextended position unless you suspect a cervical spine injury. In that case, you should immobilize the patient's head and neck in a neutral position and use the jaw-thrust maneuver. Have your partner squeeze the bag.
3. Connect the bag-mask device to supplemental oxygen.
4. Open the patient's mouth, and suction as needed. Insert an oral or nasal airway to maintain airway patency.
5. Place the mask on the patient's face. Ensure the top is over the bridge of the nose and the bottom is in the groove between the lower lip and the chin. If the mask has a large, round cuff around the ventilation port, center the port over the patient's mouth. Inflate the collar to obtain a better fit and seal to the face if necessary.
6. Bring the lower jaw up to the mask with your last three fingers. Pull the face up to the mask instead of pushing the mask onto the face. This will help to maintain an open airway. Make sure you do not grab the fleshy part of the neck because you may compress structures and create an airway obstruction. If you think the patient may have a spinal injury, make sure your partner immobilizes the cervical spine as you move the lower jaw.
7. Hold the mask in place while your partner squeezes the bag with two hands until the patient's chest visibly rises **Figure 11-47**. If a

Special Populations

The flat nasal bridge of pediatric patients makes achieving an effective mask-to-face seal more difficult. Compressing the mask against the face to improve mask seal may result in obstruction. The best mask seal is achieved by the two-person ventilation method with jaw displacement.

For full-term neonates and infants, use a pediatric bag-mask device with a minimum tidal volume of 450 mL. In children (ages 1 year to the onset of puberty [ages 12 to 14 years]), consider the size of the child when determining bag size. You may use an adult bag-mask device with a 1,500-mL tidal volume, but a pediatric bag-mask device is preferred. Children older than 12 to 14 years require the adult-sized bag-mask device for adequate ventilation. Choose a size to ensure a proper mask fit. The mask should reach from the bridge of the nose to the cleft of the chin. A length-based resuscitation tape may also be used to determine the proper size of the bag-mask device for pediatric patients who weigh up to 75 pounds (34 kg).

When you are ventilating a pediatric patient, ensure a proper mask seal by using the EC clamp technique (as discussed previously in this chapter). Avoid placing pressure on the soft area under the chin. Deliver each ventilation over 1 second—just enough to produce visible chest rise. *Do not overinflate.* Deliver one breath every 3 to 5 seconds, and allow adequate time for exhalation. While ventilating, look for adequate chest rise. Listen for breath sounds at the third intercostal space on the midaxillary line bilaterally. Also assess for improvement in skin color and pulse rate.

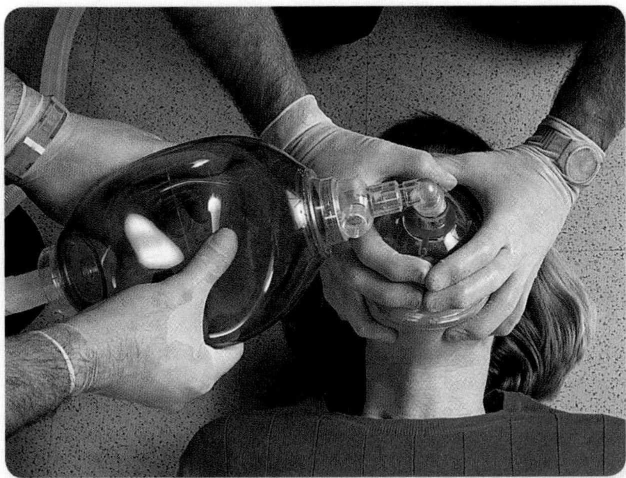

Figure 11-47 With two-person bag-mask device ventilation, you should hold the mask in place while your partner squeezes the bag with two hands until the patient's chest rises.

spinal injury is suspected, stabilize the patient's head and neck with your forearms while maintaining an adequate mask-to-face seal with your hands. Continue squeezing the bag once every 5 to 6 seconds for adults and once every 3 to 5 seconds for infants and children.

8. If you are alone, then place your thumb and index finger as high up on the mask as you can to form a C. Maintain the airway by lifting the bony prominence of the chin with your remaining fingers to form an E. Do not push the mask to the face; pull the lower jaw into the mask. This is known as the EC-clamp method and can be used to maintain an effective face-to-mask seal Figure 11-48. Use the head tilt–chin lift maneuver to make sure the neck is extended. Squeeze the bag with your other hand in a rhythmic manner once every 5 to 6 seconds for adults and once every 3 to 5 seconds for infants and children.
9. Observe for gastric distention, changes in compliance of the bag with ventilation, and improvement or deterioration of the patient's condition.

When using the bag-mask device to assist ventilation, you should squeeze the bag as the patient breathes in. Then, for the next 5 to 10 breaths, slowly adjust the rate and delivered tidal volume until an adequate minute volume is achieved.

To assist respirations of a patient who is breathing too fast (hyperventilation) with reduced tidal volume, you must first explain the procedure to the patient if the patient is coherent. Initially assist respirations at the rate at which the patient has been breathing, squeezing the bag each time the patient inhales. Then, for the next 5 to 10 breaths, slowly adjust the rate and the delivered tidal volume until an adequate minute volume is achieved.

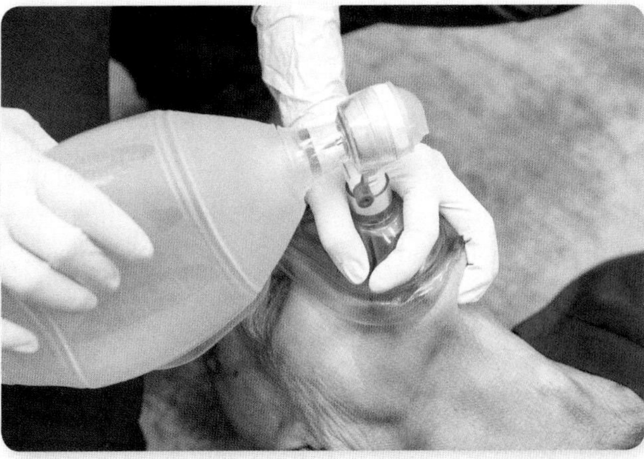

Figure 11-48 Maintain the seal of the mask to the face using the EC-clamp technique if you must ventilate alone.

As you are assisting ventilation with a bag-mask device, evaluate the effectiveness of your ventilations Table 11-11. Artificial ventilation is not adequate if the patient's chest does not rise and fall with each ventilation or the rate of ventilation is too slow or too fast for the patient's age, or the heart rate does not return to normal. If the patient's chest does not rise and fall, you may need to reposition the head or insert an airway adjunct.

If the patient's stomach, rather than the chest, seems to be rising and falling, you should reposition the head. In a patient with a possible spinal injury, you should reposition the jaw rather than the head. If too much air is escaping from under the mask, reposition the mask for a better seal. If the patient's chest still does not rise and fall after you have made these corrections, check for an airway obstruction. If an obstruction is not present, you should attempt ventilation with another airway device.

Advanced airway techniques are beneficial when ventilation with basic means is not effective, the patient has a cervical spine injury, or the patient's condition warrants.

▶ Manually Triggered Ventilation Devices

Another method of providing artificial ventilation is with the MTV device, also known as flow-restricted, oxygen-powered ventilation devices. They are mainly used to ventilate apneic or hypoventilating patients, although these devices can also be used to provide supplemental oxygen to breathing patients. MTV devices have a "demand valve" that is triggered by the negative pressure generated by inhalation Figure 11-49. This valve automatically delivers 100% oxygen as the patient begins to inhale and stops the flow of gas at the end of the inspiratory phase of the respiratory cycle. Because the MTV device makes an airtight seal with the patient's face, the gas that the patient inspires is almost 100% oxygen.

The major advantage to this device is that it allows a single rescuer to use both hands to maintain a mask-to-face

Table 11-11	Evaluating Effectiveness of Artificial Ventilations
Adequate artificial ventilation:[a]	▪ Visible and equal chest rise and fall with ventilation ▪ Breath sounds can be heard during auscultation of the chest ▪ Ventilations delivered at the appropriate rate • 10 to 12 breaths/min for adults • 12 to 20 breaths/min for infants and children • In patients with ongoing CPR and an advanced airway in place, 1 breath every 6 seconds ▪ Pulse rate returns to normal range ▪ Patient's color is improving ▪ Oxygen saturation level improves
Inadequate artificial ventilation:	▪ Minimal or no chest rise and fall ▪ Breath sounds cannot be heard during auscultation of the chest ▪ Ventilations delivered too fast or too slowly for patient's age ▪ Pulse rate does not return to normal range ▪ Patient's color remains cyanotic or mottled or deteriorates ▪ Oxygen saturation level does not improve

Abbreviation: CPR, cardiopulmonary resuscitation
[a]In patients who are apneic with a pulse.

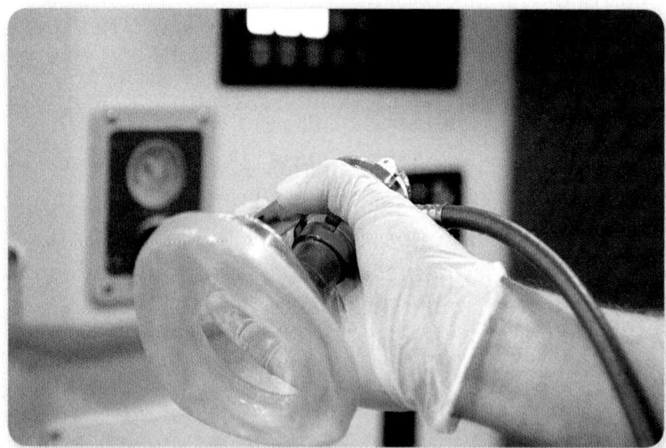

Figure 11-49 A manually triggered ventilation device can provide up to 100% oxygen.

seal while providing positive pressure ventilation to a spontaneously breathing patient. It also reduces rescuer fatigue associated with using a bag-mask device on extended transports. However, findings suggest that MTV devices are associated with difficulty in maintaining adequate ventilation without assistance and should not be used routinely because of the high incidence of gastric distention and possible damage to structures within the chest cavity. Another disadvantage is that a special unit and additional training are required when using the MTV device on infants and children. Because the rescuer is not actively squeezing a bag, it is virtually impossible to assess for lung compliance. As a result, the rescuer should take extra care when ventilating; the high ventilatory pressures generated by the device may damage lung tissue if not carefully monitored.

Learning how to use these devices correctly requires proper training and considerable practice. As with bag-mask devices, you must make sure there is an airtight fit between the patient's face and the mask. The amount of pressure that is necessary to ventilate a patient adequately will vary according to the size of the patient, the patient's lung volume, and the condition of the lungs. Pressures that are too great can cause a pneumothorax. Always follow local medical protocols carefully when you use these devices.

▶ Automatic Transport Ventilators/Resuscitators

The **automatic transport ventilator (ATV)** allows the variables of ventilation—ventilator rate, tidal volume, and peak inspiratory time—to be precisely set; these features allow for consistent ventilation Figure 11-50. Many types of ATVs are available, some with basic settings and others with more advanced settings and features. The steps for using the ATV are as follows:

1. Attach the ATV to the wall-mounted oxygen source.
2. Set the ventilator rate, tidal volume, and peak inspiratory time on the ATV as appropriate for the patient's condition.
3. Connect the ATV to the 15/22-mm fitting on the ET tube or other advanced airway device.
4. Auscultate the patient's breath sounds, and observe for equal chest rise to ensure adequate ventilation.

Although the ATV lacks the sophisticated control of a hospital ventilator, it frees your hands to perform other tasks, such as maintaining a mask seal or ensuring continued patency of the airway. You can even perform other, non–airway-related tasks if the patient is intubated and being ventilated with the ATV. However, even though an ATV is

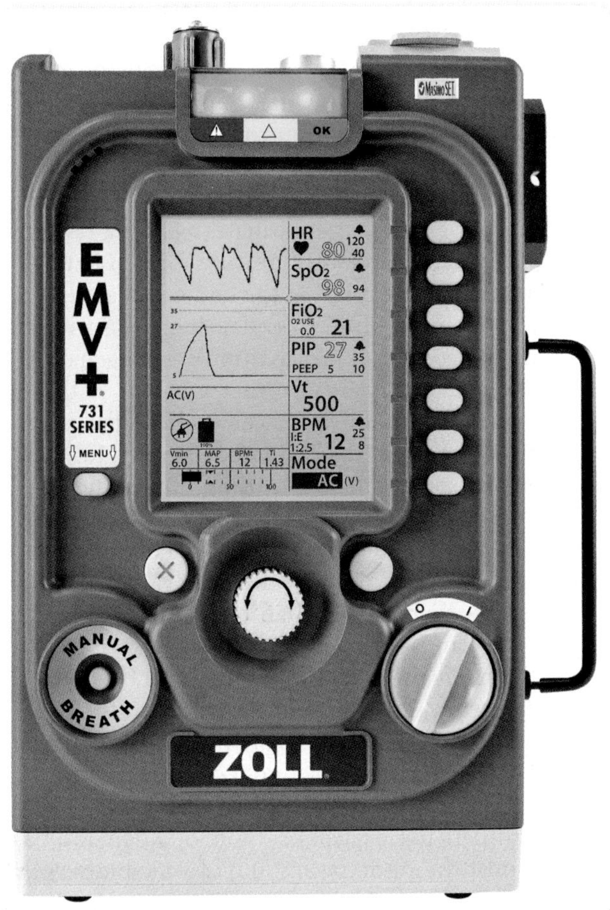

Figure 11-50 An automatic transport ventilator.

Provided with permission by ZOLL Medical.

helpful, you must always have a bag-mask device and mask prepared and ready for use should the ATV malfunction.

Most models have adjustments for respiratory rate and tidal volume. In most cases, the respiratory rate is set at the midpoint or average for the patient's age. The machine or respiratory therapist estimates tidal volume using a formula based on 6 to 7 mL/kg because ATVs are oxygenpowered and provide oxygen-enriched breathing gas. The tidal volume can be adjusted based on the patient's chest rise and physiologic response. The ATVs are considered volume-cycled–rate-controlled ventilators. This means that they deliver a preset volume at a preset ventilatory rate, although this does not guarantee that all of the volume is being delivered to the lungs. In the event of cardiac arrest, you may need to revert to ventilations with a bag-mask device. The ATV is set at a fixed rate and will not cycle in conjunction with the timing of chest compressions.

The ATV is oxygenpowered, although some models may require an external power source. Whereas this device requires oxygen, it generally consumes 5 L/min of oxygen, unlike a bag-mask device that uses 15 to 25 L/min. In addition, the ATV has a pressure-relief valve, which can result in hypoventilation in patients with poor lung compliance, increased airway resistance, or airway obstruction. **Lung compliance** is the ability of the alveoli to expand when air is drawn in during inhalation; poor lung compliance is the inability of the alveoli to fully expand during inhalation. Remember that there is the possibility of barotrauma (trauma resulting from excessive pressure) if the relief valve fails or if ventilation is overzealous.

Continuous Positive Airway Pressure

CPAP is a noninvasive means of providing ventilatory support for patients experiencing respiratory distress. Many people with obstructive sleep apnea wear a CPAP unit at night to maintain their airway while they sleep. The use of CPAP in the prehospital environment has proven to be an excellent adjunct in the treatment of respiratory distress associated with obstructive pulmonary disease, acute bronchospasm, and acute pulmonary edema. Typically, many of the patients would be treated with advanced airway devices, such as ET intubation. Early intervention with CPAP is an alternative means for providing ventilatory assistance and can prevent the need for ET intubation, thereby improving the patient's chance of survival. Because of the simplicity of the device and its great benefit to patients, CPAP is becoming widely used in EMS.

CPAP increases pressure in the lungs, opens collapsed alveoli, pushes more oxygen across the alveolar membrane, and forces interstitial fluid back into the pulmonary circulation. The desired effect of CPAP is to improve pulmonary compliance and make spontaneous ventilation easier. The therapy is typically delivered through a face mask that is held to the head with a strapping system. A good seal with minimal leakage between the face and mask is essential.

The face mask is fitted with a pressure-relief valve that determines the amount of pressure delivered to the patient (such as 5 cm water [cm H_2O]). This pressure results in a high inspiratory flow and the need to push a pressure valve open with exhalation. Although this may appear to require a great deal of effort from the patient, especially while in respiratory distress, many patients make a dramatic turnaround when CPAP is applied.

▶ Indications for CPAP

CPAP is indicated for patients experiencing respiratory distress in which their own compensatory mechanisms cannot keep up with their oxygen demand. Although the condition of most patients improves after the application of CPAP, it is important to remember that CPAP is merely treating the symptoms and not necessarily the underlying pathology.

The following are some general guidelines for CPAP candidates:

- Patient is alert and able to follow commands
- Obvious signs of moderate to severe respiratory distress (such as accessory muscle use, retractions, or tripod position) from an underlying

disease such as heart failure with pulmonary edema, obstructive pulmonary disease (such as COPD), acute bronchospasm (such as in acute asthma), and suspected pneumonia
- Respiratory distress after a submersion incident
- Rapid breathing (more than 26 breaths/min), such that it affects overall minute volume
- Pulse oximetry reading of less than 90%

Whereas these guidelines should be considered when assessing the need for CPAP, it is important that you follow your local guidelines and protocols.

▶ Contraindications to CPAP

CPAP has proven to be immensely beneficial to patients experiencing respiratory distress from acute pulmonary edema, acute bronchospasm, and obstructive pulmonary disease; however, there are some times that CPAP is not appropriate.

The following are general contraindications for CPAP use:

- Patient is unresponsive or otherwise unable to follow verbal commands
- Respiratory arrest or agonal respirations
- Patient is unable to speak
- Patient is unable to protect his or her own airway
- Hypoventilation (slow respiratory rate and/or reduced tidal volume)
- Hypotension (systolic blood pressure is less than 90 mm Hg)
- Signs and symptoms of a pneumothorax or chest trauma (either blunt or penetrating)
- Closed head injury
- Facial trauma
- Cardiogenic shock
- Tracheostomy
- Active gastrointestinal bleeding, nausea, or vomiting
- History of recent gastrointestinal surgical procedure
- Patient is unable to sit up
- Inability to properly fit the CPAP system mask and strap
- Excessive facial hair or dysmorphic facial features that can impede your ability to ensure a proper-fitting mask
- Patient cannot tolerate the mask

In addition, always reassess the patient for signs of deterioration and/or respiratory failure. CPAP is an excellent tool to assist with ventilation; however, not all patients will experience an improvement in condition with this device. After signs of respiratory failure become apparent or the patient is no longer able to follow commands, remove the CPAP device and initiate positive pressure ventilation with a bag-mask device attached to high-flow oxygen.

▶ Application of CPAP

Several varieties of CPAP units are available to EMS services; however, most follow the same general guidelines for use and setup. CPAP units are generally composed of a generator, a mask, a circuit that contains corrugated tubing, a bacteria filter, and a one-way valve. During the expiratory phase, the patient exhales against a resistance called **positive end-expiratory pressure (PEEP)**. PEEP maintains pressure in the lungs at the end of exhalation and keeps the open alveoli from collapsing. It also recruits, or opens, closed alveoli, which improves oxygenation by increasing the surface area for gas exchange. Within the CPAP generator is a valve that determines the amount of PEEP; however, some CPAP models have PEEP valves that connect separately. Depending on the device, the PEEP is controlled by manually adjusting the PEEP using a manometer or predetermined by a fixed setting on the PEEP valve. A PEEP of 5.0 to 10.0 cm H_2O is generally an acceptable therapeutic range for a patient using CPAP, although it can be adjusted higher or lower if needed. Always consult the operations manual of a particular CPAP device for proper assembly instructions.

Because most CPAP units are powered by oxygen, it is important to have a full cylinder of oxygen when using CPAP. Some CPAP units use a continuous flow of oxygen, whereas others use oxygen on more of a demand basis. Continuously monitor the amount of available oxygen in your cylinder. Some CPAP units will empty a D cylinder in as little as 5 to 10 minutes. Therefore, proper planning for oxygen consumption is necessary when considering the application of CPAP. In addition, some newer CPAP devices allow the provider to adjust the fraction of inspired oxygen (FIO_2). Most CPAP devices are set to deliver a fixed FIO_2 of 30% to 35%; however, some can deliver as high as 80%.

Follow the steps in Skill Drill 11-8 to use a CPAP.

▶ Complications of CPAP

The application and administration of CPAP is a relatively easy process. However, some patients may find CPAP claustrophobic and will resist the application. As patients become more hypoxic, the application of a mask to their face is sometimes perceived as suffocation, rather than helping them breathe. In any event, it is important to explain the application to patients and coach them through the process. Do not force the mask on patients. Forceful application will create a higher level of anxiety and increase oxygen demand. Coach patients through the application of CPAP, allowing them to adjust to the situation. Coaching patients is not always an easy task; it takes practice and a willingness to work closely with your patient during a rather difficult time.

Because of the high volume of pressure generated by CPAP, it is possible to cause a pneumothorax as a result of barotrauma. You should be aware of this risk and continually assess your patients for signs and symptoms of a pneumothorax.

Skill Drill 11-8 Using CPAP

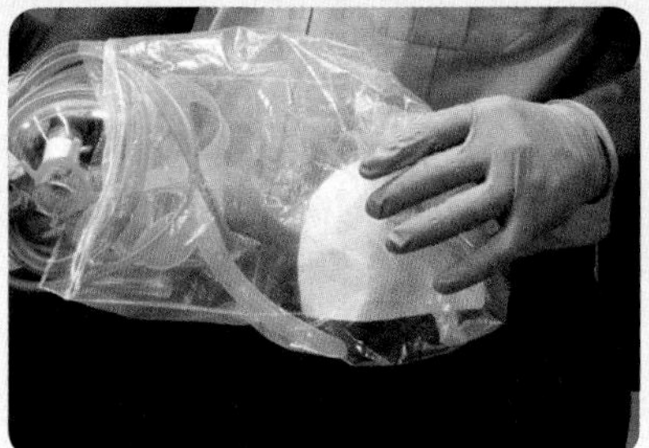

Step 1 Take standard precautions. Assess the patient for indications and contraindications for CPAP. Confirm the patient's blood pressure, and explain the procedure to him or her. Check your equipment, then connect the circuit to the CPAP device.

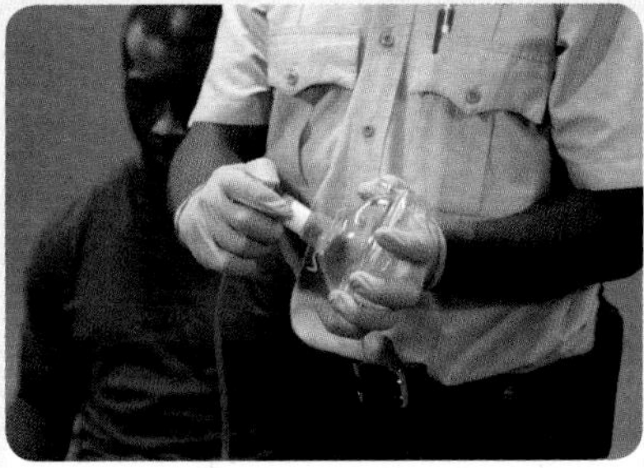

Step 2 Connect the face mask to the circuit tubing. After the system is connected, look for an on/off button or switch. Some models have this feature. Confirm the device is powered on and working before you apply CPAP to the patient.

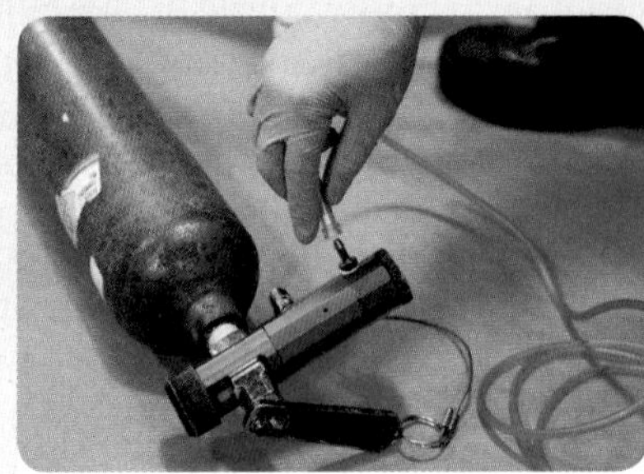

Step 3 Connect the tubing to the oxygen tank.

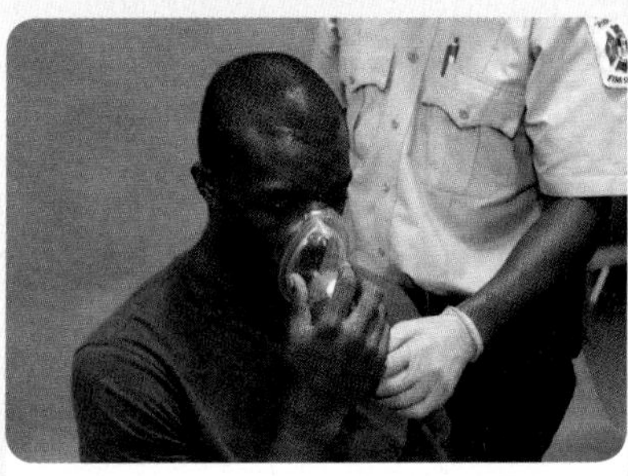

Step 4 Place the mask over the patient's mouth and nose, creating as much of an airtight seal as possible. Place the patient in a high Fowler position to facilitate breathing, and coach him or her through the initial application of the mask. To reduce some of the stress and anxiety associated with the application of CPAP, it may be beneficial to initially allow the patient to hold the mask to his or her face. Allow the patient to get used to the mask.

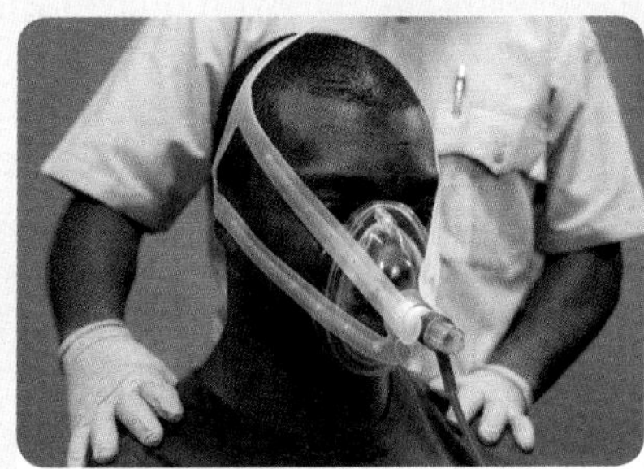

Step 5 After the mask is placed on the face and the patient adjusts to it, use the strapping mechanism to secure it to the patient's head. Ensure the seal between the mask and face remains intact. Consult the manufacturer's guidelines for specific strapping instructions.

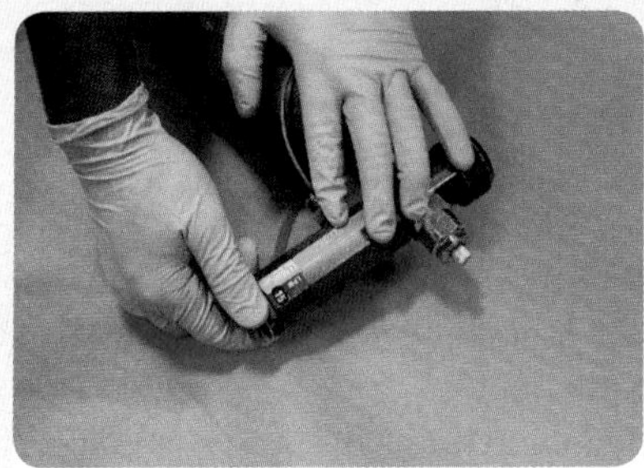

Step 6 Adjust the PEEP valve and the F_{IO_2} level according to the manufacturer's recommendations to maintain adequate oxygenation and ventilation. With CPAP in place, the patient's oxygenation saturation level should improve, the work of breathing should decrease, the ease of speaking should increase, and breath sounds should improve. Constantly reassess the patient for signs of clinical deterioration and/or complications (ie, pneumothorax).

In addition to pneumothoraces, increased pressure in the chest cavity can result in hypotension. As the intrathoracic pressure increases, venous blood returning to the heart (preload) meets resistance from the increased pressure in the chest, which can cause hypotension. Although this is not common with lower levels of CPAP, continuous monitoring of blood pressure is necessary.

As with any form of positive pressure ventilation in the unprotected airway, air may enter the stomach, which increases the risk of vomiting and therefore the potential for aspiration.

Words of Wisdom

Bilevel positive airway pressure (BPAP), another form of noninvasive positive pressure ventilation, is also used to treat patients with obstructive lung disease, acute bronchospasm, and acute pulmonary edema. Whereas CPAP delivers a single pressure (which is most beneficial to the patient during exhalation), BPAP delivers two pressures: a higher inspiratory positive airway pressure (IPAP), which opens the lower airways, and a lower expiratory positive airway pressure (EPAP), which helps keep the lower airways open. Common BPAP settings deliver 10 cm H_2O during inhalation and 5 cm H_2O during exhalation; the difference between the IPAP and EPAP is called pressure support. The indications, contraindications, and precautions for BPAP are the same as they are for CPAP. Follow your EMS system protocols regarding the use of BPAP and the desired IPAP and EPAP settings.

Special Considerations

Gastric Distention

Any form of artificial ventilation that blows air into the patient's mouth—as opposed to blowing air directly into the trachea via an ET tube—may result in inflation of the patient's stomach with air. Gastric distention—inflation of the patient's stomach with air—is especially likely to occur if excessive pressure is used to inflate the lungs, if ventilations are performed too fast or too forcefully, or if the airway is partially obstructed during ventilation attempts. The pressure in the airway forces open the esophagus, and air flows into the stomach. Gastric distention occurs most often in children but is common in adults as well.

A distended stomach is harmful for at least two reasons. First, it promotes regurgitation of stomach contents, which creates the potential for aspiration. Second, a distended stomach pushes the diaphragm upward into the chest, reducing the amount of space in which the lungs can expand.

Signs of gastric distention include an increase in the diameter of the stomach, an increasingly distended abdomen, and increased resistance to bag-mask ventilations. If you observe these signs, reassess and reposition the airway as needed and observe the chest for adequate rise and fall as you continue ventilating. In addition, limit ventilation times to 1 second or the time needed to produce adequate chest rise.

Laryngectomy, Tracheostomy, Stoma, and Tracheostomy Tubes

A **laryngectomy** is a surgical procedure in which the larynx is removed. This procedure is performed by making a tracheostomy, thus creating a stoma. The tracheal stoma is located in the midline of the anterior part of the neck. Surgical removal of the entire larynx is called **total laryngectomy**. A person who has undergone this procedure breathes through the stoma in his or her neck. Because a connection no longer exists between the patient's pharynx and lower airway, you cannot ventilate the patient through the nose and mouth with a bag-mask device or other face mask. The air blown into the mouth or nose can only go down the esophagus into the stomach; it will not reach the lower airway.

A **partial laryngectomy** entails surgical removal of a portion of the larynx. In practice, you may be unable to tell whether a person has had a total or partial laryngectomy until you attempt artificial ventilation. As opposed to a total laryngectomy, artificial ventilation through the nose and mouth may still be effective after a partial laryngectomy.

Suctioning of a Stoma

You may encounter patients who require suctioning of thick secretions from the stoma. Failure to recognize and identify this need could result in hypoxia. It is not uncommon for a patient's stoma to become occluded with mucous plugs. Patients with a laryngectomy have a less efficient cough and, therefore, have difficulty spontaneously clearing the stoma.

You must perform suctioning of the patient's stoma with extreme care, especially if you suspect laryngeal swelling. Even the slightest irritation of the tracheal wall can result in a violent **laryngospasm** and complete airway closure. Limit suctioning of the stoma to 10 seconds at a time.

The steps for suctioning a stoma are shown in Skill Drill 11-9.

Ventilation of Stoma Patients

Neither the head tilt–chin lift nor the jaw-thrust maneuver is required for ventilating a patient with a stoma. If the patient has a stoma and no tracheostomy tube (discussed next) in place, then you can perform ventilation using the mouth-to-stoma (with a resuscitation mask) technique or with a bag-mask device. Regardless of the technique used, you should use an infant- or child-size mask to make an adequate seal over the stoma. Seal the patient's nose and mouth with one hand to prevent the leakage of air up the trachea. Release the seal of the patient's mouth and nose following each ventilation, allowing exhalation to occur through the upper airway. Two rescuers are needed to perform bag-mask device-to-stoma ventilation: one to seal the nose and mouth and the other to squeeze the bag-mask device. If you are unable to ventilate a patient who has a stoma, then try suctioning the stoma and mouth with a soft-tip (French) catheter before providing artificial ventilation through the nose and mouth. Note that this technique would only work if the patient had a partial laryngectomy, not if he or she had a total laryngectomy. If you seal the stoma during ventilation, then the ability to artificially ventilate the patient in this way may be improved, or it may help to clear any obstructions.

Skill Drill 11-9 Suctioning of a Stoma

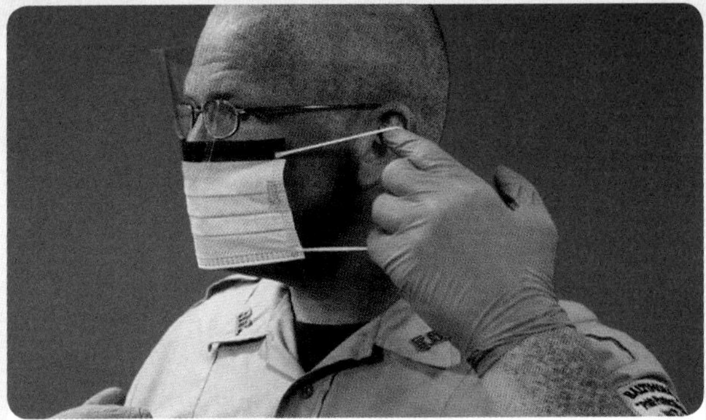

Step 1 Take standard precautions.

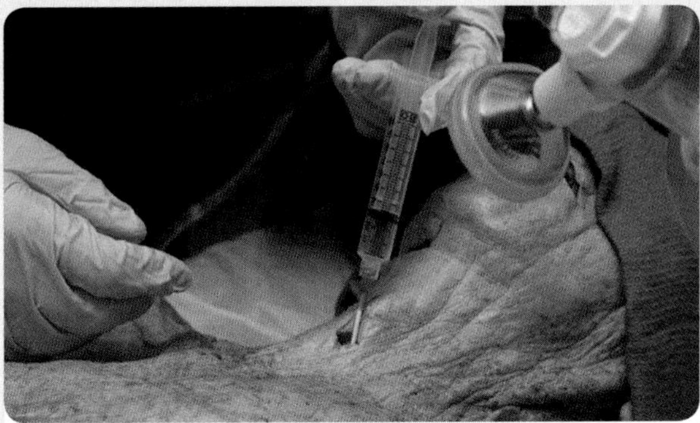

Step 2 Inject 3 mL of sterile saline through the stoma and into the trachea.

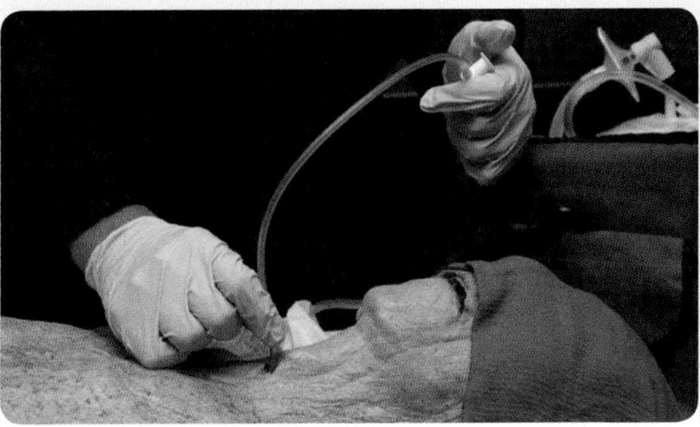

Step 3 Instruct the patient to exhale (if he or she is responsive), and insert the catheter without providing suction until resistance is felt (no more than 12 cm).

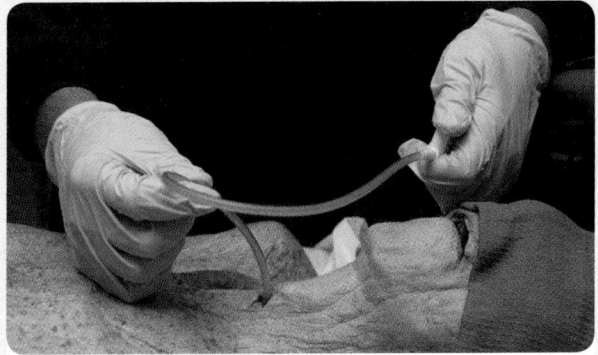

Step 4 Suction while withdrawing the catheter.

The steps for performing mouth-to-stoma ventilation with a resuscitation mask are shown in Skill Drill 11-10.

The steps for performing bag-mask device-to-stoma ventilation are shown in Skill Drill 11-11.

▶ Tracheostomy Tubes

A **tracheostomy tube** is a plastic tube placed within the tracheostomy site (stoma) Figure 11-51. It requires a 15/22-mm adapter to be compatible with ventilatory devices, such as a mechanical ventilator or bag-mask device. Patients with a tracheostomy tube may receive supplemental oxygen via tubing designed to fit over the tube or by placing an oxygen mask over the tube. Ventilation is accomplished by simply attaching the bag-mask device to the 15-mm adapter on the tracheostomy tube.

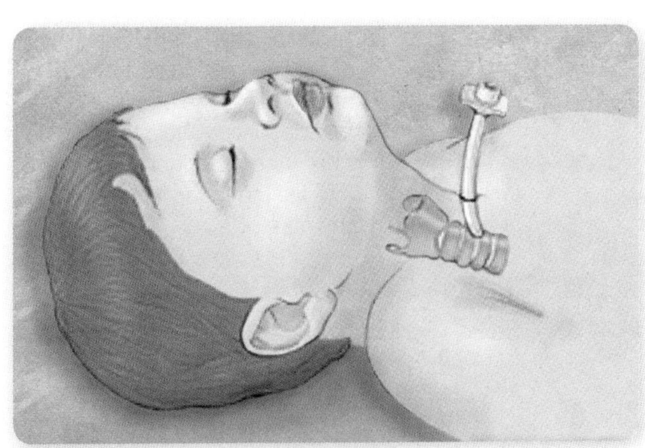

Figure 11-51 A tracheostomy tube.

Skill Drill 11-10 Ventilating Through a Stoma Using a Resuscitation Mask

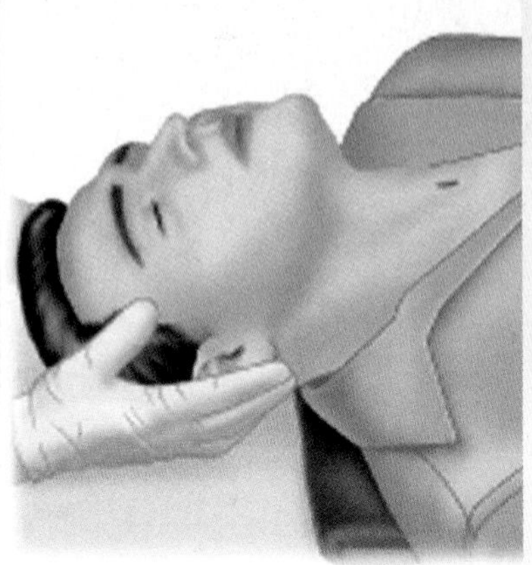

Step 1 Position the patient's head in a neutral position with the shoulders slightly elevated.

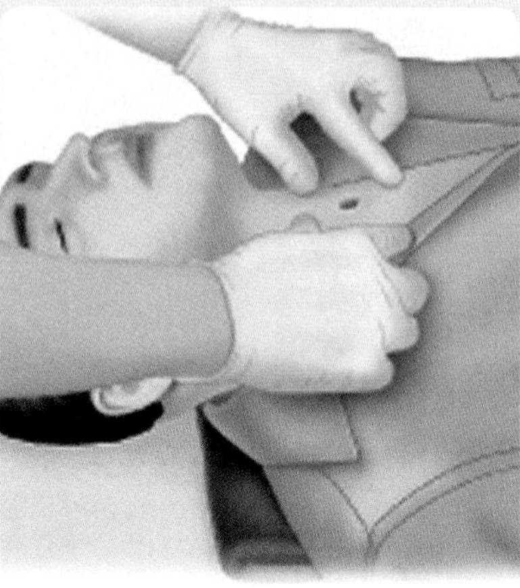

Step 2 Locate and expose the stoma site.

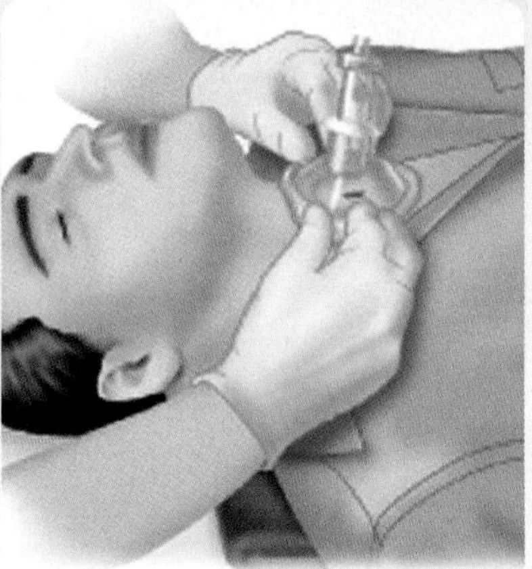

Step 3 Place the resuscitation mask over the stoma, and ensure an adequate seal. For best results, use a pediatric mask.

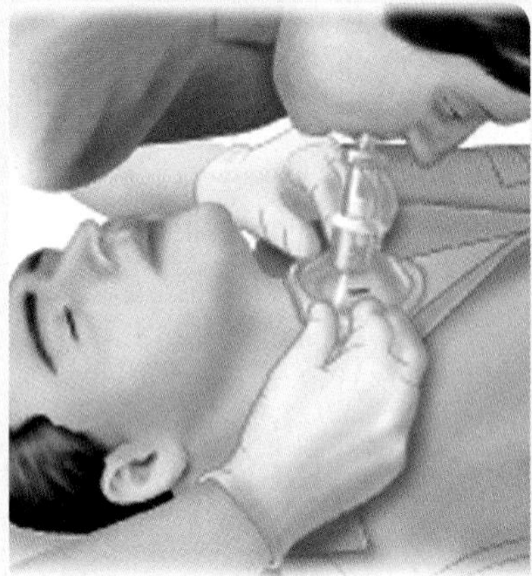

Step 4 Maintain the patient's neutral head position, and ventilate the patient by exhaling directly into the resuscitation mask. Assess the patient for adequate ventilation by observing his or her chest rise and feeling for air leaks around the mask.

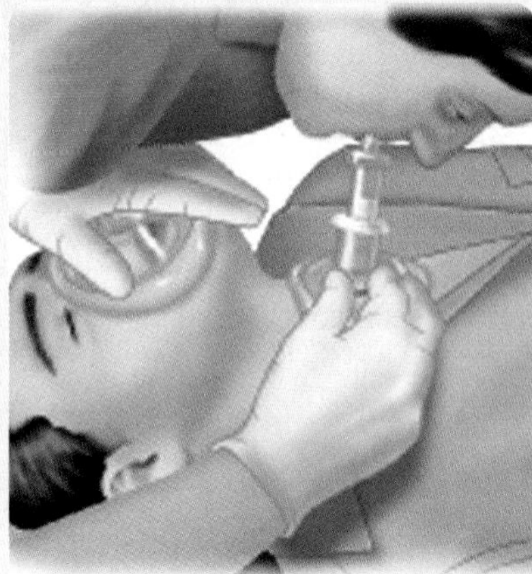

Step 5 If air leakage is evident, then seal the patient's mouth and nose and ventilate.

Skill Drill 11-11 Ventilating a Stoma With a Bag-Mask Device

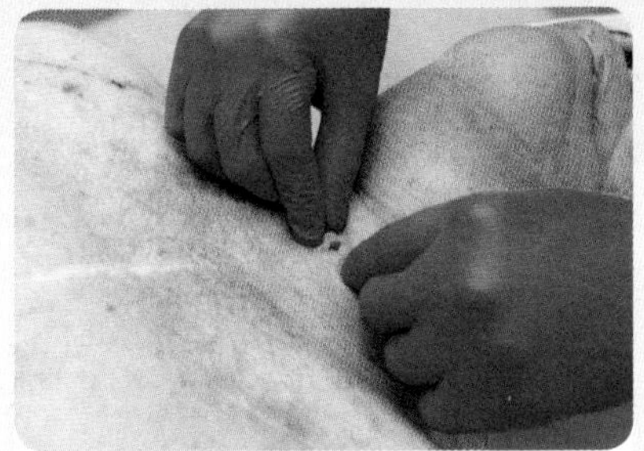

Step 1 With the patient's head in a neutral position, locate and expose the stoma.

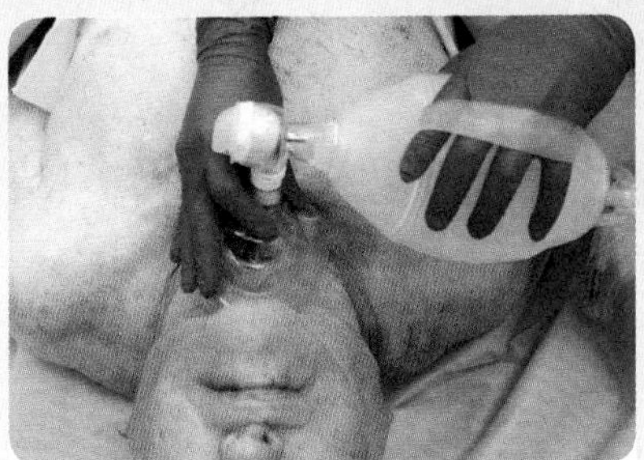

Step 2 Place the bag-mask device (with a pediatric mask) over the stoma, and ensure an adequate seal. Ventilate the patient by squeezing the bag-mask device, and assess for adequate ventilation by observing chest rise and feeling for air leaks when using a mask. Seal the mouth and nose if an air leak is evident from the upper airway.

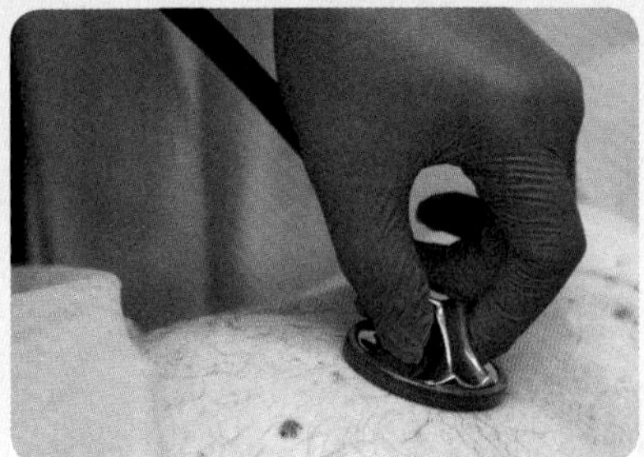

Step 3 Auscultate over the lungs to confirm adequate ventilation.

Patients with a tracheostomy tube who experience sudden dyspnea often have thick secretions in the tube. In this case, perform suctioning through the tracheostomy tube as you would through a stoma.

When a tracheostomy tube becomes dislodged, stenosis (narrowing) of the stoma may occur. Stenosis is potentially life threatening because soft-tissue swelling decreases the diameter of the stoma and impairs the patient's ventilatory ability. Call early for paramedic backup if needed. Because a patient with a stoma already has a substantial medical injury or illness (such as brain injury or chronic respiratory insufficiency), he or she may be less tolerant of even brief periods of hypoxia.

▶ Dental Appliances

Many dental appliances can cause an airway obstruction. If a dental appliance, such as a crown or bridge, dentures, or even a piece or section of braces, has become loose, you should manually remove it before providing ventilation. Simple manual removal may relieve the obstruction and allow the patient to breathe on his or her own.

Providing bag-mask device or mouth-to-mask ventilation is usually much easier when dentures can be left in place. Leaving the dentures in place provides more "structure" to the face and will generally assist you to provide a good face-to-mask seal. Dentures and appliances may become loose or be completely out of place following an accident or as you are providing care. Periodically reassess the patient's airway to make sure the devices are firmly in place.

Special Populations

When managing the airway of an older patient, you must be aware of the presence of dentures or other dental appliances. If dentures are tightfitting and allow for effective airway management, they should be left in place. However, if the dentures are loose, they must be removed to avoid potential airway obstruction.

▶ Facial Bleeding

Airway problems can be especially challenging in patients with serious facial injuries **Figure 11-52**. Because the blood supply in the face is so rich, injuries to the face can result in severe tissue swelling and bleeding into the airway. Control bleeding with direct pressure and suction as necessary.

Facial injuries are also associated with a high suspicion for cervical spine injury. When inserting any type of airway device, it is imperative to maintain in-line stabilization of the cervical spine.

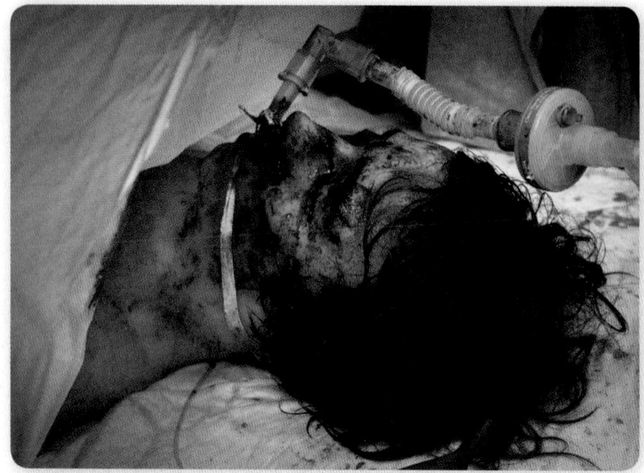

Figure 11-52 Airway problems can be especially challenging in patients with serious facial injuries.

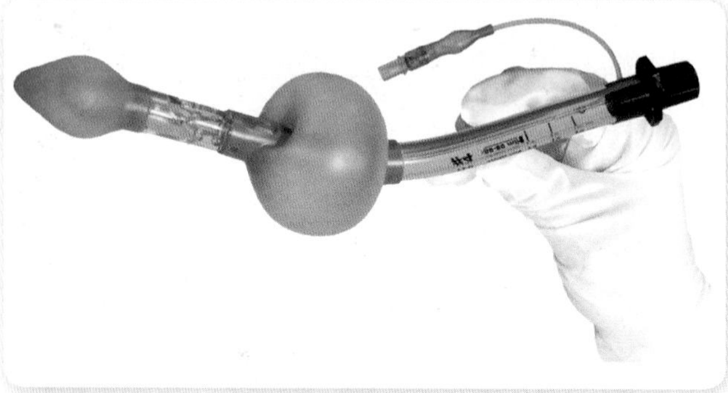

Figure 11-53 The King LT is a single-lumen airway that is blindly inserted into the esophagus. The King LT-D model is shown here.

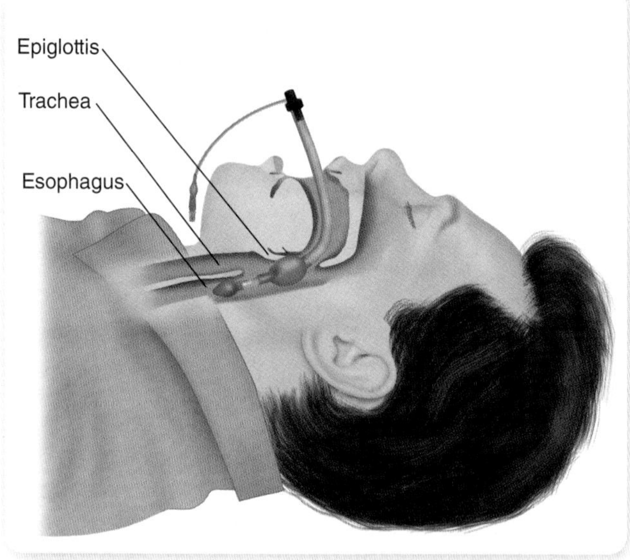

Figure 11-54 Placement of the King LT airway. When properly placed, the distal cuff seals the esophagus, and the proximal cuff seals the oropharynx.

Supraglottic Airway Devices

▶ King LT Airway

The **King LT airway** is a latex-free, single-use, single-lumen airway that is blindly inserted into the esophagus **Figure 11-53**. You can use the King LT to provide positive pressure ventilation to apneic patients and maintain a patent airway in unresponsive patients who are breathing spontaneously, but who require advanced airway management. The King LT is available in both adult and pediatric sizes.

The device consists of a curved tube with ventilation ports located between two inflatable cuffs. Both cuffs are inflated simultaneously using a single valve/pilot balloon. When the airway is properly placed in the esophagus, the distal cuff seals the esophagus, and the proximal cuff seals the oropharynx **Figure 11-54**. Openings located between these two cuffs provide ventilation of the lungs after positioning is confirmed. You can use the King LT as a rescue airway device.

Two types of King LT airway are available: the King LT-D and the King LTS-D. The King LTS-D is the more commonly used device; it is available in seven sizes that are based on the patient's height and/or weight. Each size has a different color of proximal connector and requires different cuff inflation pressures. **Table 11-12** lists sizes and patient criteria for the King LTS-D. Each kit contains a single King LT, a syringe for cuff inflation, water-soluble gel, and instructions for use.

The King LT-D (see Figure 11-53) and the King LTS-D share most of the same features. Both have a proximal pharyngeal cuff and a distal cuff and several ventilation outlets at the distal part of the tube. The distal end of the King LT-D is closed, whereas the distal end of the King LTS-D is open. This opening permits insertion of a suction catheter (up to size 18F) through a gastric access lumen on the proximal end of the King LTS-D for gastric decompression **Figure 11-55**.

Indications and Contraindications for the King LT Airway

The King LT airway should be considered an alternative to bag-mask ventilation when a rescue device is required for a failed intubation attempt. The King LT airway is intended for airway management in patients who are taller than 4 feet. It has the same disadvantages, complications, and special considerations as the Combitube (discussed later in this chapter).

Regarding contraindications, the King LT airway does not protect the airway from the effects of vomiting and aspiration. High airway pressures may cause air to leak into the stomach or out of the mouth. The King LT airway should not be used in patients with an intact gag reflex, patients with known esophageal disease, or patients who

Table 11-12 Sizes and Patient Criteria for the King LTS-D

Size	Connector Color	Patient Criteria: Height and Weight[a]	Cuff Volume
0	Transparent	11 lb (5 kg)	10 mL
1	White	11-26 lb (5-12 kg)	20 mL
2	Green	35-45 in. (90-115 cm) or 26-55 lb (12-25 kg)	35 mL
2.5	Orange	41-51 in. (105-130 cm) or 55-77 lb (25-35 kg)	40-45 mL
3	Yellow	4-5 ft (122-155 cm)	50-60 mL
4	Red	5-6 ft (155-180 cm)	70-80 mL
5	Purple	>6 ft (180 cm)	80-90 mL

[a]Sizes 0 and 1 are weight based. Sizes 2 and 2.5 are weight and/or height based. Adult sizes (sizes 3-5) are height based.

Data from: Ambu King LTS-D Disposable Laryngeal Tube. Ambu USA website. December 2015 version. http://www.ambuusa.com/usa/products/anesthesia/product/king_lts-d%E2%84%A2_disposable_laryngeal_tube-prod17813.aspx. Accessed February 21, 2017.

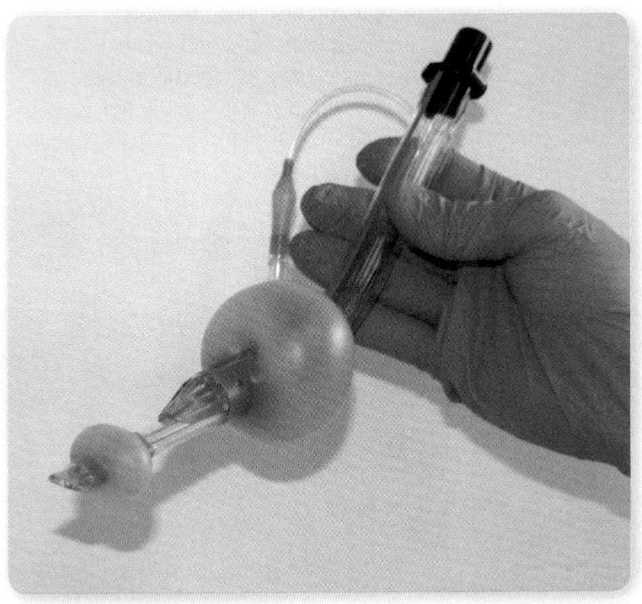

Figure 11-55 The King LTS-D.

Courtesy of Candice M. Thompson, NREMT-P.

have ingested caustic substances. As with other advanced airway devices, confirm proper placement by observing chest rise, auscultating the epigastrium and lungs, and using a secondary confirmation device.

Complications of the King LT Airway

It is reasonable to assume that laryngospasm, vomiting, and possible hypoventilation may occur. Trauma may also result from improper insertion technique. Ventilation may be difficult if the pharyngeal balloon pushes the epiglottis over the glottic opening. If this occurs, withdraw the device while gently bagging the patient to assess ventilation—without deflating the cuffs—until ventilation becomes easier.

Insertion Technique

As previously discussed, the King LT airway comes in five sizes; the patient's height and weight will determine the size that you should use. The steps for inserting the King LT airway are shown in Skill Drill 11-12.

▶ The Laryngeal Mask Airway

The **laryngeal mask airway (LMA)** Figure 11-56 was originally developed for use in the operating room. It provides a viable option for cases that require more airway support than mask ventilation but do not require intubation.

The LMA is designed to provide a conduit from the glottic opening to the ventilation device. This is achieved by surrounding the opening of the larynx with an inflatable silicone cuff positioned in the hypopharynx. When properly inserted, the opening of the LMA is positioned right at the glottic opening. The tip is inserted into the proximal esophagus, the lateral portions in the piriform fossae, and the upper border at the base of the tongue. The inflatable cuff conforms to the contours of the airway and makes a relatively airtight seal Figure 11-57.

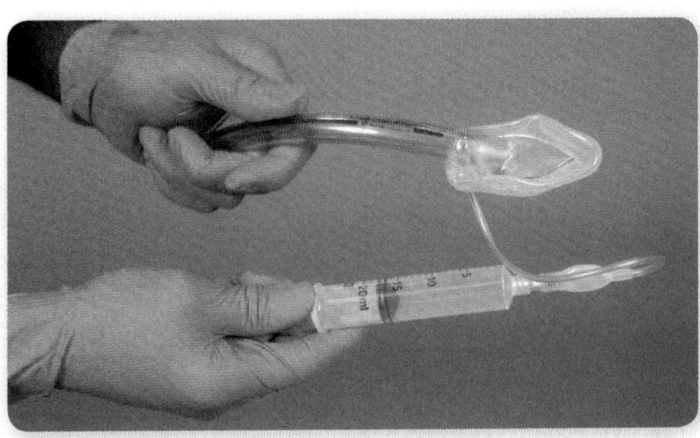

Figure 11-56 The laryngeal mask airway.

© Jones & Bartlett Learning.

NR Skill

Skill Drill 11-12 Inserting a King LT Airway

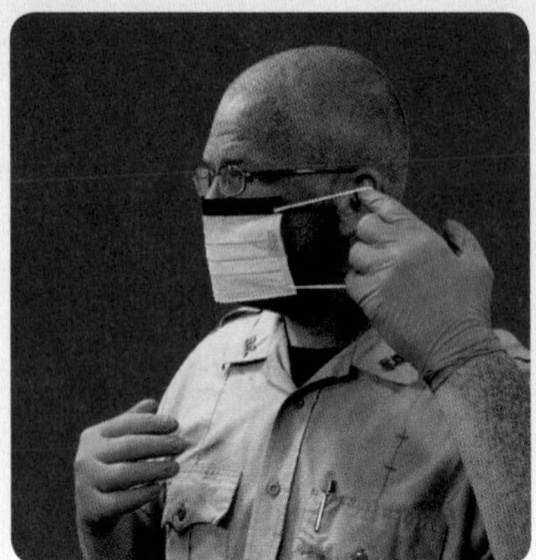

Step 1 Take standard precautions.

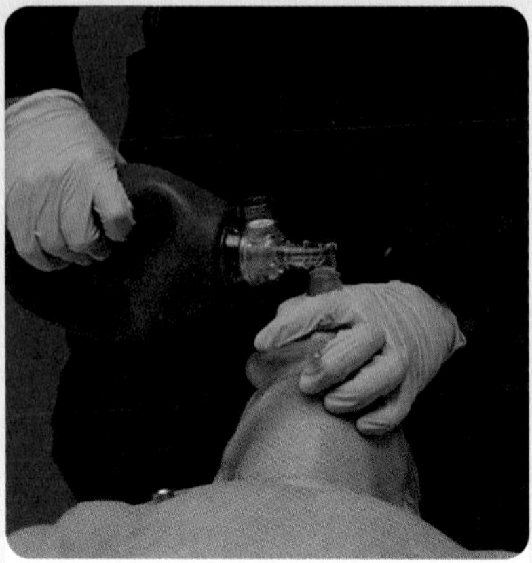

Step 2 Preoxygenate the patient with a bag-mask device and 100% oxygen.

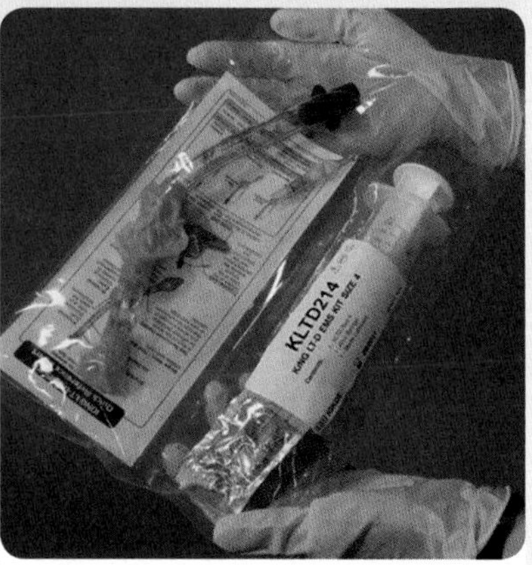

Step 3 Gather your equipment. Choose the proper size of King LT airway for the patient. Test the cuff for proper inflation. Ensure all air is removed from the cuff before insertion. Lubricate the tip of the device with a water-soluble gel for easy insertion and minimal airway damage.

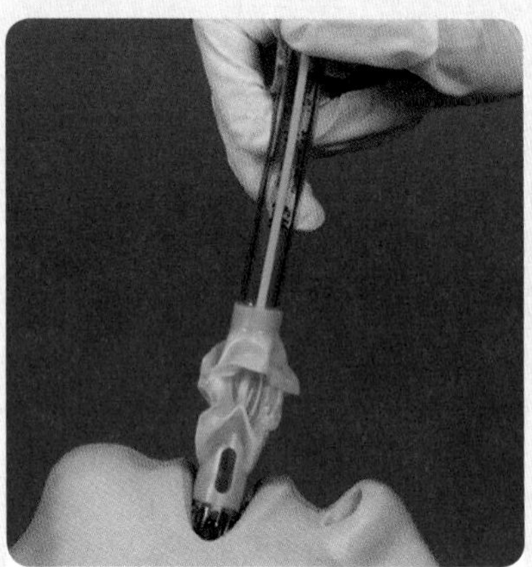

Step 4 Place the patient's head in a neutral position, unless contraindicated (use the jaw-thrust maneuver if you suspect trauma). In your dominant hand, hold the King LT at the connector. With your other hand, hold the patient's mouth open while positioning the head. Insert the tip of the King LT airway into the midline of the mouth.

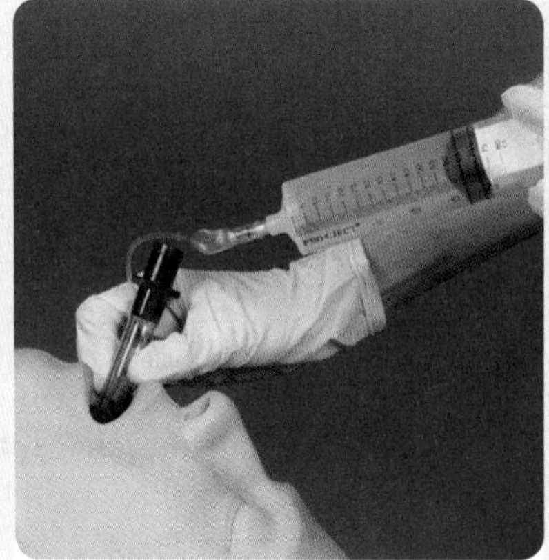

Step 5 Advance the tip beyond the base of the tongue. If you meet resistance, then rotate the device slightly, change your angle, and advance it again. Continue to gently advance the device until the base of the connector is aligned with the patient's teeth or gums. Do not use excessive force. Inflate the cuff with the recommended amount of air or just enough to seal the device.

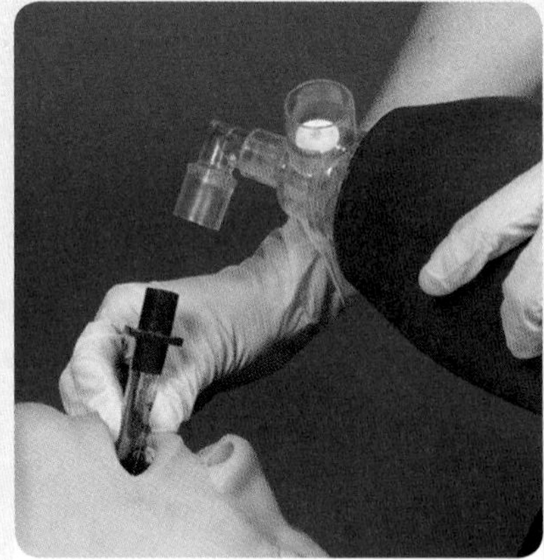

Step 6 Attach the tube to the ventilation device, and confirm tube placement by auscultating the lungs and epigastrium and attaching waveform capnography. Add additional air to the cuff to maximize airway seal, if needed; however, avoid exceeding the manufacturer's recommended maximum amount of air. After placement is confirmed, continue to ventilate the patient.

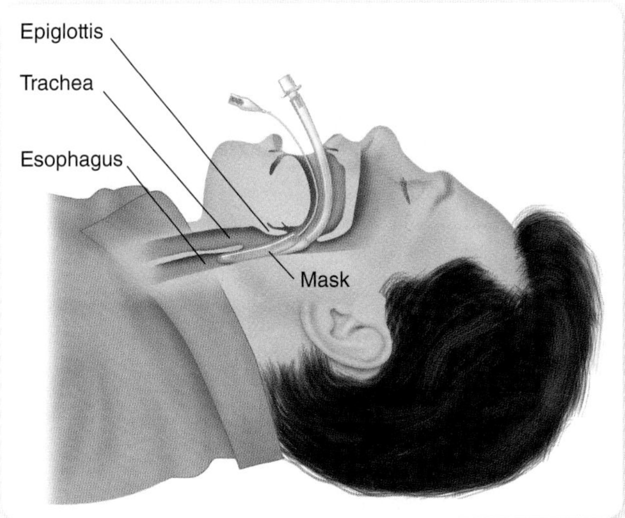

Figure 11-57 When properly positioned, the opening of the laryngeal mask airway is at the glottic opening, the tip is at the entrance of the esophagus, the lateral portion is in the piriform fossae, and the upper border is at the base of the tongue.

The LMA has many advantages compared with ventilating the unprotected airway with a mask. The LMA has been shown to provide better oxygenation than mask ventilation with an oral airway, and ventilation with an LMA does not require the continual maintenance of a mask seal. Compared with an ET tube, LMA insertion is easier. There is substantially less risk of soft-tissue, vocal cord, tracheal wall, and dental trauma than with ET intubation and other forms of intubation that rely on blocking the esophagus. The LMA provides protection from upper airway secretions, and the tip of the LMA wedged into the proximal esophagus most likely provides some obturation.

The main disadvantage of the LMA, especially in emergencies, is that it does not provide as much protection against aspiration as does endotracheal intubation. The LMA may actually increase the risk of aspiration if the patient regurgitates because the patient's stomach contents would most likely be directed into the trachea.

During prolonged LMA ventilation, some air may be insufflated into the stomach because the seal made in the airway is not airtight. Because of the risk of aspiration, it is unlikely that the LMA will ever replace ET intubation in prehospital emergency care. The LMA should not be considered a primary airway for emergency patients, but it may have a role. For a patient who cannot be intubated, the LMA should be considered superior to mask ventilation.

Indications and Contraindications for the LMA

The LMA should be considered as one possible alternative to mask ventilation only when the patient cannot be intubated. Do not consider the LMA as a primary airway in emergency situations.

The LMA is less effective in obese patients and should not be used in patients with morbid obesity. Patients who are pregnant or have a hiatal hernia are at an increased risk for regurgitation and must be evaluated carefully if LMA use is considered. The LMA is ineffective for the ventilation of patients requiring high pulmonary pressures (such as patients with COPD or heart failure).

Complications of Using the LMA

The most substantial complications associated with use of the LMA involve regurgitation and subsequent aspiration. The product literature states that the LMA should be used only in patients who are fasting. Unfortunately, this would eliminate all patients in emergency situations. You must weigh the risk of aspiration against the risk of hypoventilation with bag-mask ventilation in the context of a given clinical scenario.

Observe the patient for clinical indications of adequate ventilation (chest rise, breath sounds) during LMA ventilation. Hypoventilation of patients who require high ventilatory pressures can also occur, and the patient should be monitored for evidence of upper airway swelling.

Equipment for the LMA

The LMA comes in seven sizes and is sized based on the patient's weight. The device consists of a tube and the mask or inflatable cuff. The cuff provides a collar that is designed to position the opening of the tube at the glottic opening when inflated. Two vertical bars are present at the opening of the tube to prevent occlusion. The proximal end of the tube is fitted with a standard 15/22-mm adapter that is compatible with any ventilation device. The cuff has a one-way valve assembly and should be inflated with a predetermined volume of air (based on the size of the airway) **Figure 11-58**.

Insertion Technique

Before insertion, check and prepare all equipment. The steps for using an LMA are summarized in **Skill Drill 11-13**.

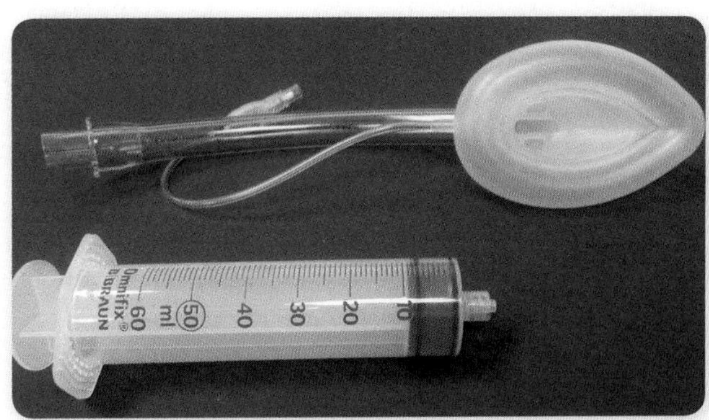

Figure 11-58 The laryngeal mask airway with the cuff inflated.

NR Skill

Skill Drill 11-13 LMA Insertion

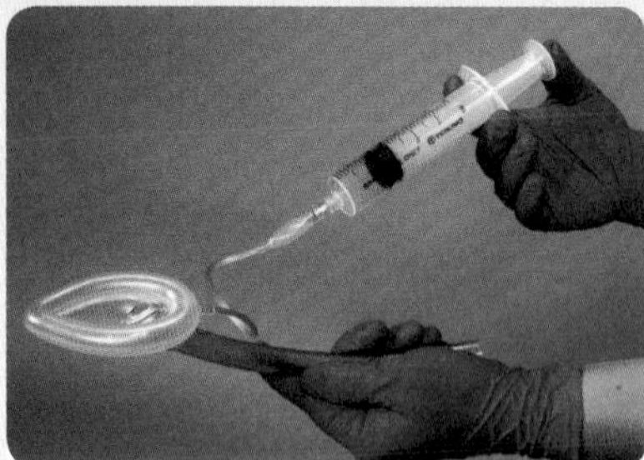

Step 1 Take standard precautions. Check the cuff of the LMA by inflating it with 50% more air than is required for the size of airway to be used.

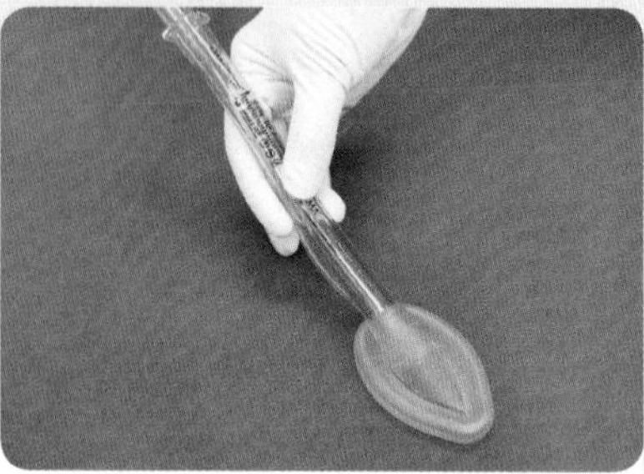

Step 2 Deflate the cuff completely so that no folds appear near the tip. Deflation is best accomplished by pressing the device, cuff down, on a flat surface to remove all wrinkles from the cuff.

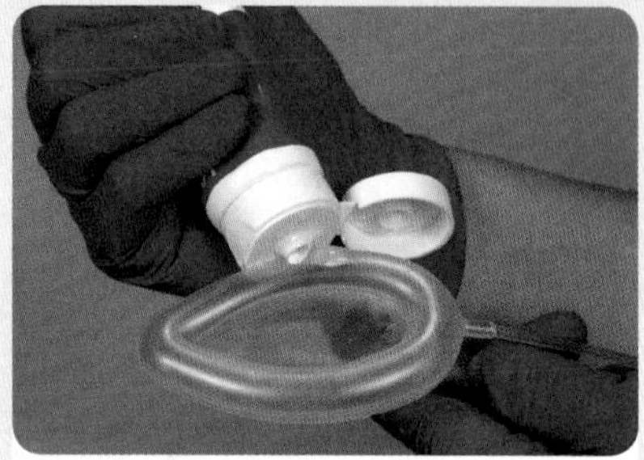

Step 3 Lubricate the outer rim of the device.

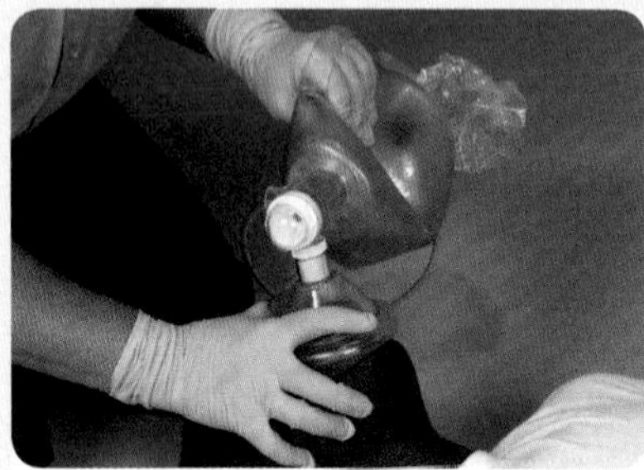

Step 4 Preoxygenate the patient before insertion. Do not interrupt ventilation for more than 30 seconds to accomplish airway placement. Place the patient in the sniffing position.

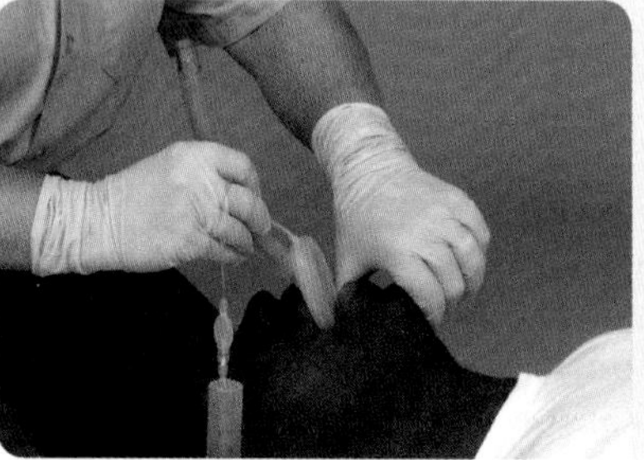

Step 5 Insert your finger between the cuff and the tube. Place the index finger of your dominant hand in the notch between the tube and the cuff. Open the patient's mouth. Lift the jaw with one hand, and begin to insert the device with the other hand.

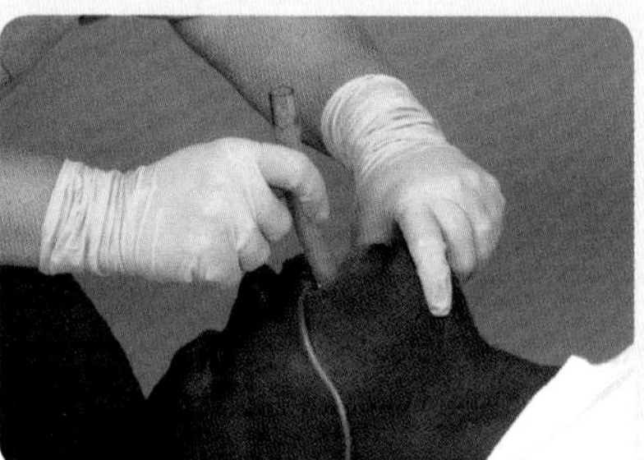

Step 6 Insert the LMA along the roof of the mouth. The key to proper insertion is to slide the convex surface of the airway along the roof of the mouth. Use your finger to push the airway against the hard palate. After it slides past the tongue, the LMA will move easily into position.

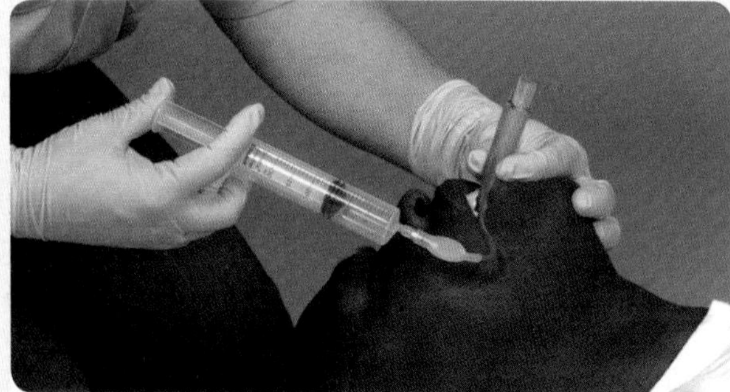

Step 7 Inflate the cuff with the amount of air indicated for the airway being used. If the LMA is properly positioned, then it will move out of the airway slightly (0.5 to 0.75 inch [1 to 2 cm]) as it moves into position (a good indication that the LMA is in the correct position).

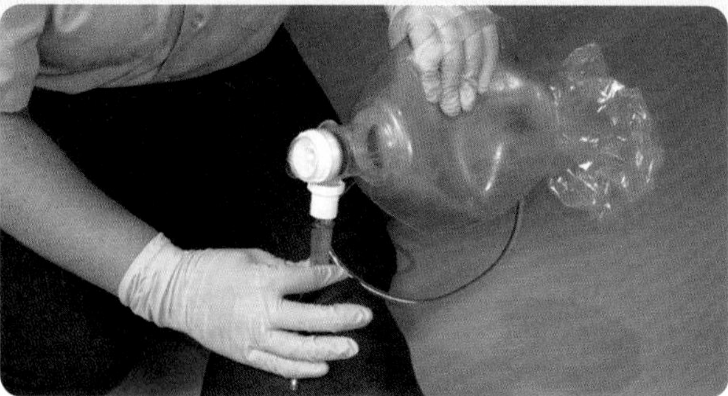

Step 8 Begin to ventilate the patient. Confirm chest rise and the presence of breath sounds. Continuously and carefully monitor the patient. Monitor $ETCO_2$ if available.

Continuously and carefully monitor for regurgitation in the tube. The LMA can be easily dislodged because it was not designed for patients who are being transported. Carefully attend to the airway during any patient movement, and be prepared to mask ventilate if the LMA becomes dislodged.

Documentation & Communication

If adverse events, such as bleeding or trauma, occur with the use of advanced airway devices, then be sure to document these occurrences on the PCR.

▶ i-gel

The **i-gel** supraglottic airway is inserted in a manner similar to the LMA. This particular airway device was designed to create a noninflatable, anatomic seal of the pharyngeal, laryngeal, and perilaryngeal structures, while avoiding compression trauma that may occur from devices with an inflatable cuff **Figure 11-59**. The i-gel is a common rescue airway device and is a reasonable alternative when intubation is unsuccessful.

The i-gel features an integral bite block, a gastric access channel that allows for passage of a 12F gastric tube, a supplemental oxygen inlet port to facilitate passive oxygenation, and a support strap to secure the i-gel in position. A color-coded, proximal hook ring indicates the size of the i-gel and serves as an anchor for the support strap. Furthermore, the size and weight range for the i-gel is printed on the device.

Similar to the LMA, the tip of the i-gel is designed to fit into the proximal esophagus, and the sides and proximal parts of the device form a seal around the hypopharynx. This position facilitates air entry into the trachea **Figure 11-60**. **Table 11-13** lists three adult-sized i-gel supraglottic airways and patient weight criteria.

The steps for inserting an i-gel supraglottic airway are shown in **Skill Drill 11-14**.

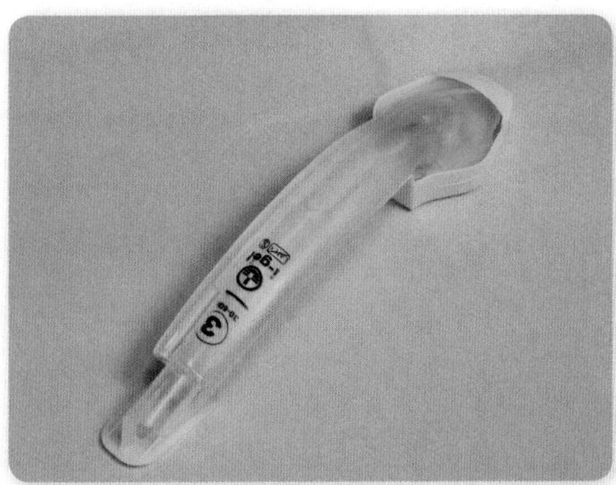

Figure 11-59 The i-gel supraglottic airway.

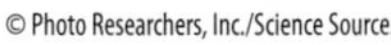

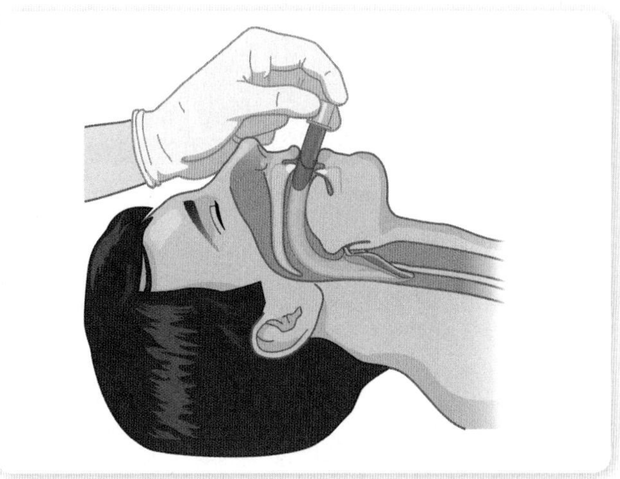

Figure 11-60 Correct position of the i-gel in the airway.

Table 11-13 Sizes and Patient Criteria for Adult i-gel Supraglottic Airway

Size	Connector Color	Weight Criteria
3	Yellow	66-132 lb (30-60 kg)
4	Green	110-198 lb (50-90 kg)
5	Orange	>198 lb (>90 kg)

Data from: i-gel user guide. 9989 issue 1 01.10. Intersurgical Ltd website. http://docsinnovent.com/downloads/igel_User_Guide_English.pdf. Accessed February 21, 2017.

▶ The Cobra Perilaryngeal Airway

The **Cobra perilaryngeal airway (CobraPLA)** was first introduced as a device to ventilate patients with difficult airways. It is so named because of the "cobra" shape of the distal part of the airway **Figure 11-61**. The shape allows the device to slide easily along the hard palate and to hold the soft tissue away from the laryngeal inlet (hence, *perilaryngeal*) when in place. It is a supraglottic device with a tube for ventilation and a circumferential cuff (that sits in the hypopharynx at the base of the tongue) proximal to the distal end, which is the ventilation outlet. It also has a 15-mm standard adapter, and the distal widened end that holds soft tissue apart and allows ventilation of the trachea. The distal tip is proximal to the esophagus and seals the hypopharynx. When the cuff is inflated, it raises the tongue and creates an airway seal allowing for ventilation. Because the insertion technique is simple, it is possible to successfully place the device with minimal or no experience.

The CobraPLA is available in eight sizes. Proper size is determined by the one that comfortably fits through the patient's mouth.

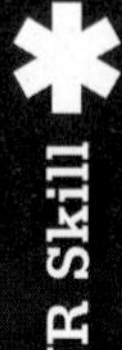

Skill Drill 11-14 Inserting an i-gel Supraglottic Airway

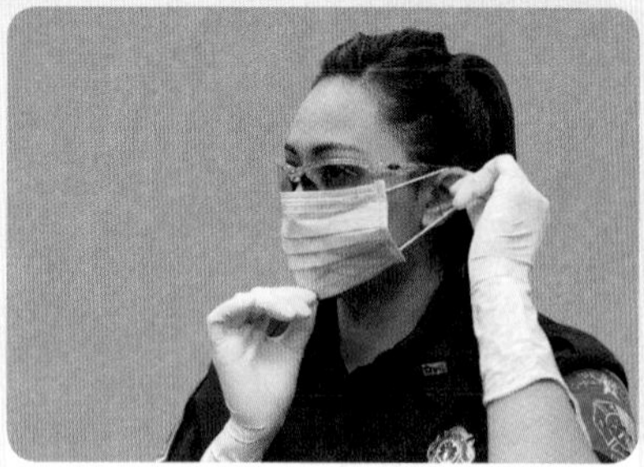

Step 1 Take standard precautions.

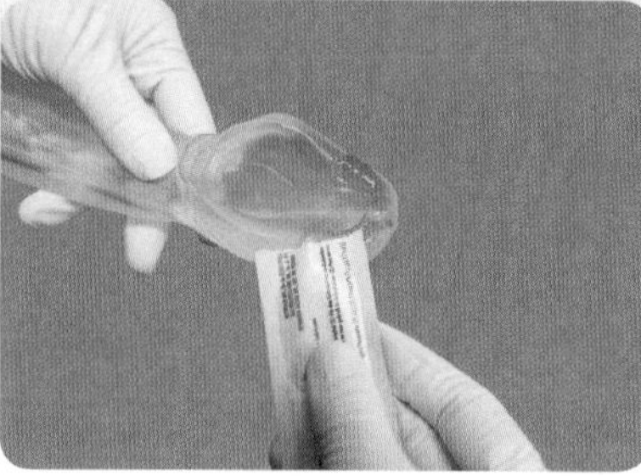

Step 2 Lubricate the back, sides, and front of the cuff with a thin layer of water-soluble gel.

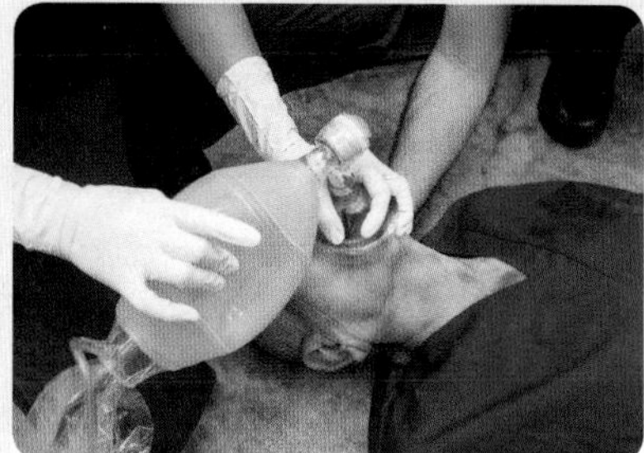

Step 3 Preoxygenate the patient before insertion. Do not interrupt ventilation for more than 30 seconds to accomplish airway placement. Place the patient in the sniffing position.

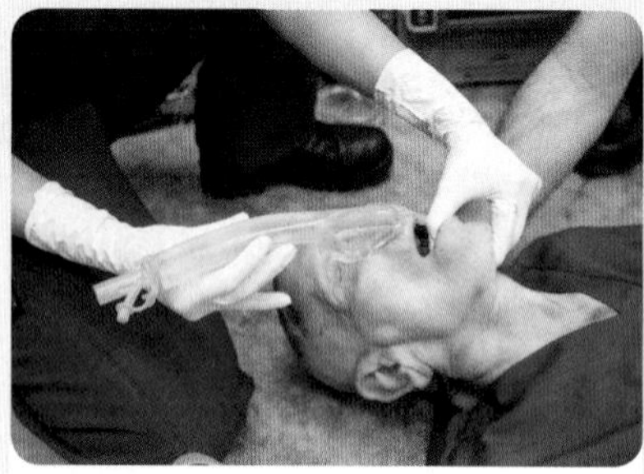

Step 4 Open the airway with the tongue-jaw lift maneuver and position the i-gel so that the cuff outlet is facing toward the patient's chin.

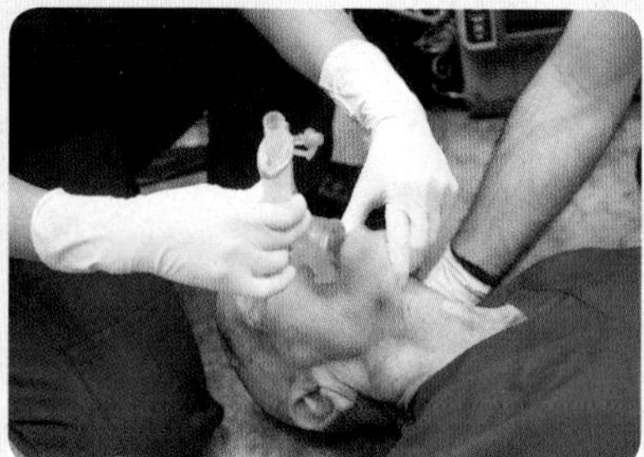

Step 5 Introduce the leading soft tip of the i-gel into the patient's mouth, directing it toward the hard palate.

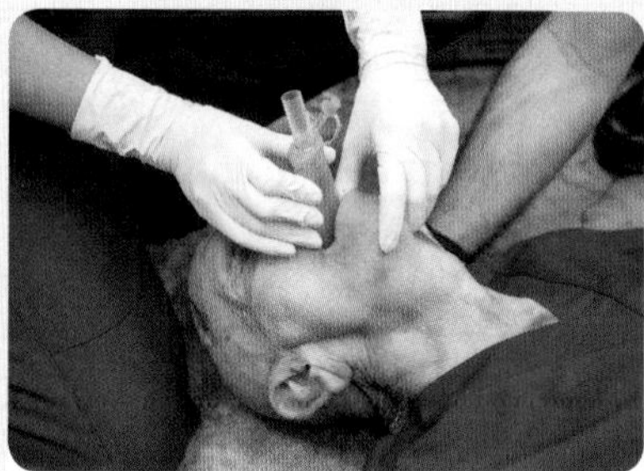

Step 6 Glide the i-gel downward and backward along the hard palate with a continuous but gentle push until a definitive resistance is felt.

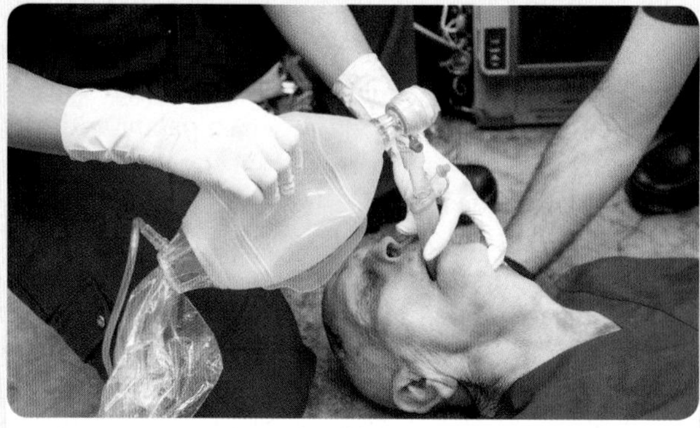

Step 7 Begin to ventilate the patient. Confirm chest rise and the presence of breath sounds. Ensure proper tube placement with waveform capnography. Continuously and carefully monitor the patient's condition.

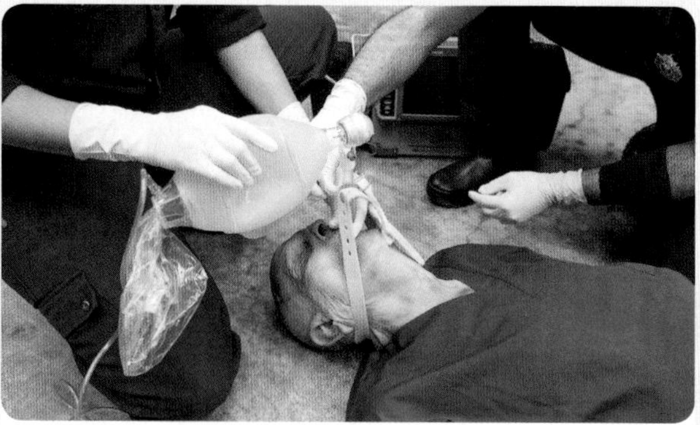

Step 8 Secure the i-gel in place with the provided strap.

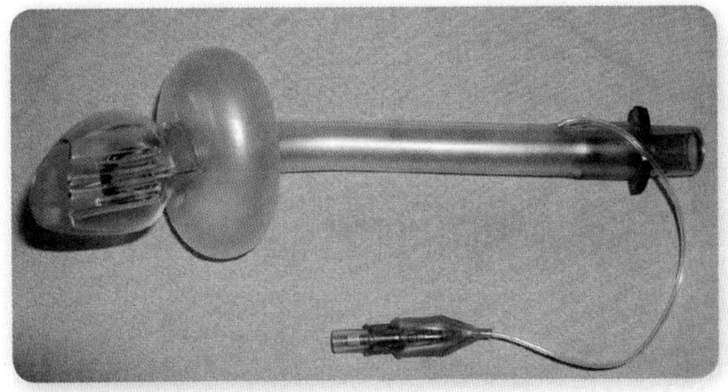

Figure 11-61 The Cobra perilaryngeal airway.

Reproduced from: Sunder RA, Sinha R, Agarwal A, Perumal BCS, Paneerselvam SR. Comparison of Cobra perilaryngeal airway (CobraPLATM) with flexible laryngeal mask airway in terms of device stability and ventilation characteristics in pediatric ophthalmic surgery. *J Anaesthesiol Clin Pharmacol*. 2012;28(3):322-325.

Indications and Contraindications for the CobraPLA

The CobraPLA is used in a manner similar to other supraglottic airways and can be used on pediatric patients. Because the device does not provide protection against aspiration, it is recommended for use only in patients who are not at risk of vomiting.

Contraindications include risk for aspiration and massive trauma to the oral cavity.

Complications of the CobraPLA

If the patient has an intact gag reflex, laryngospasm may occur. If the Cobra is not inserted far enough, inflation of the cuff may cause the tongue to protrude from the mouth, disrupting an adequate seal. Using the proper size is vital because the patient cannot be ventilated if the device is too small and passes into the laryngeal inlet. However, in such an instance, it can be removed and another size inserted with minimal trauma to the oropharynx.

Insertion Technique

To insert the CobraPLA, fully deflate the cuff and apply a water-soluble gel to the front and back of the device and to the cuff. With the patient's head in the sniffing position, open the airway with the tongue-jaw lift maneuver and direct the distal end of the CobraPLA straight back between the tongue and hard palate. Continue advancing the CobraPLA until modest resistance is felt Figure 11-62A. Inflate the cuff with only enough air to achieve a good seal; do not overinflate the cuff. Ventilate the patient while observing for chest rise and auscultating over the neck, chest, and epigastrium. Use a detection device for further confirmation and secure the device in place Figure 11-62B.

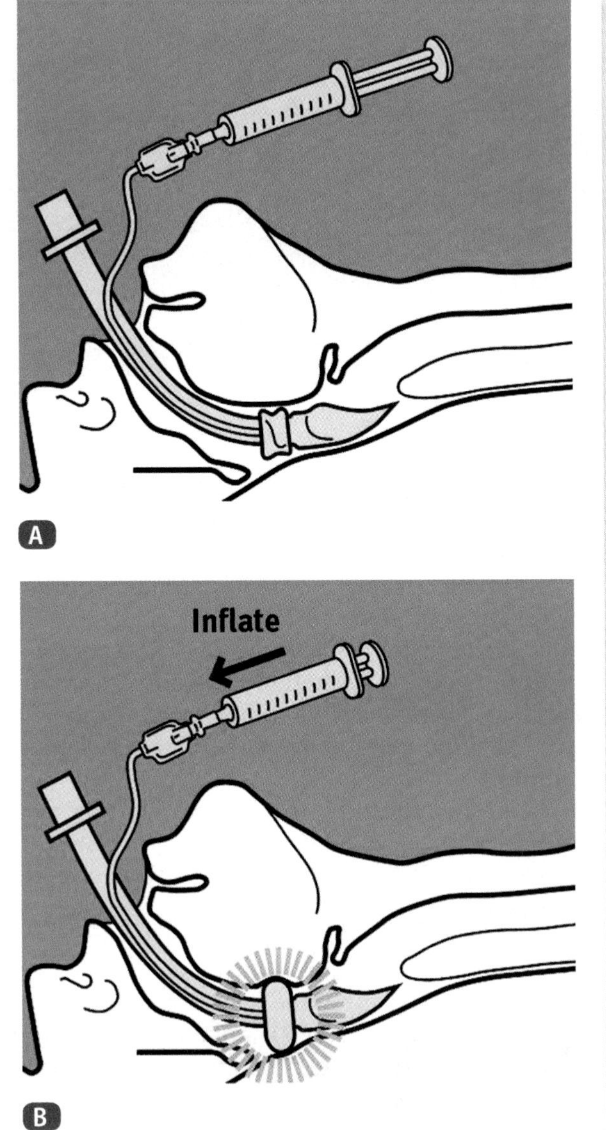

Figure 11-62 A. Open the airway with the tongue-jaw lift maneuver and advance the Cobra perilaryngeal airway until modest resistance is felt. **B.** Inflate the cuff with only enough air to achieve a good seal. Ventilate the patient, confirm proper placement, and secure the device in place.

Multilumen Airway Devices

▶ Combitube

The **Combitube** is a **multilumen airway device** with a long tube that is inserted blindly into the airway Figure 11-63. It is a reasonable alternative to ET intubation and has been clinically proven to secure the airway and allow for better ventilation than a bag-mask device and simple airway adjunct in most cases.

In contrast with single-lumen airways, the tube can be used for ventilation whether it is inserted into the esophagus or trachea. Although this device almost always comes to rest in the esophagus, it can function as an ET tube if inserted into the trachea Figure 11-64. The Combitube contains two lumens, which function appropriately based on tube position and ventilating through the correct lumen. Each lumen has a standard 15/22-mm ventilation adapter, which accommodates any ventilation device (such as a bag-mask device or mechanical ventilator). The

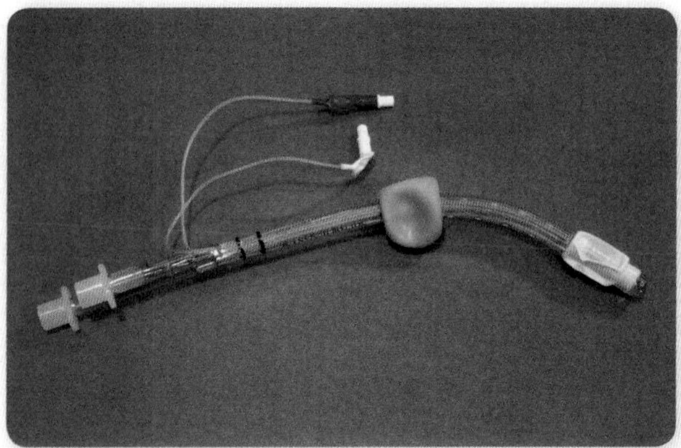

Figure 11-63 A Combitube.

proper port for ventilation depends on where the tube is located. It also contains an oropharyngeal balloon, which eliminates the need for a mask seal.

The major advantage of the multilumen airway is that, in effect, it cannot be improperly placed; effective ventilation is possible whether the tube enters the esophagus or the trachea. Furthermore, because insertion of the airway is performed with the patient's head in the neutral position, cervical spine movement is kept to a minimum.

The Combitube also provides some patency to the airway. If the tube is placed in the trachea, it allows the airway to be maintained, and no upper airway positioning is required. If the tube is placed into the esophagus (as most commonly occurs), the pharyngeal balloon creates an airtight seal in the oropharynx, making the tongue position less of a factor in the maintenance of a patent airway. A jaw-thrust maneuver should easily alleviate any ventilatory difficulty that occurs if the epiglottis partially obstructs the airway.

Use of the Combitube requires strict attention and good assessment skills because ventilation in the wrong port results in no pulmonary ventilation. Multilumen airways are usually considered temporary airways and should be replaced as soon as possible. The pharyngeal balloon reduces—but does not completely eliminate—the risk of aspiration.

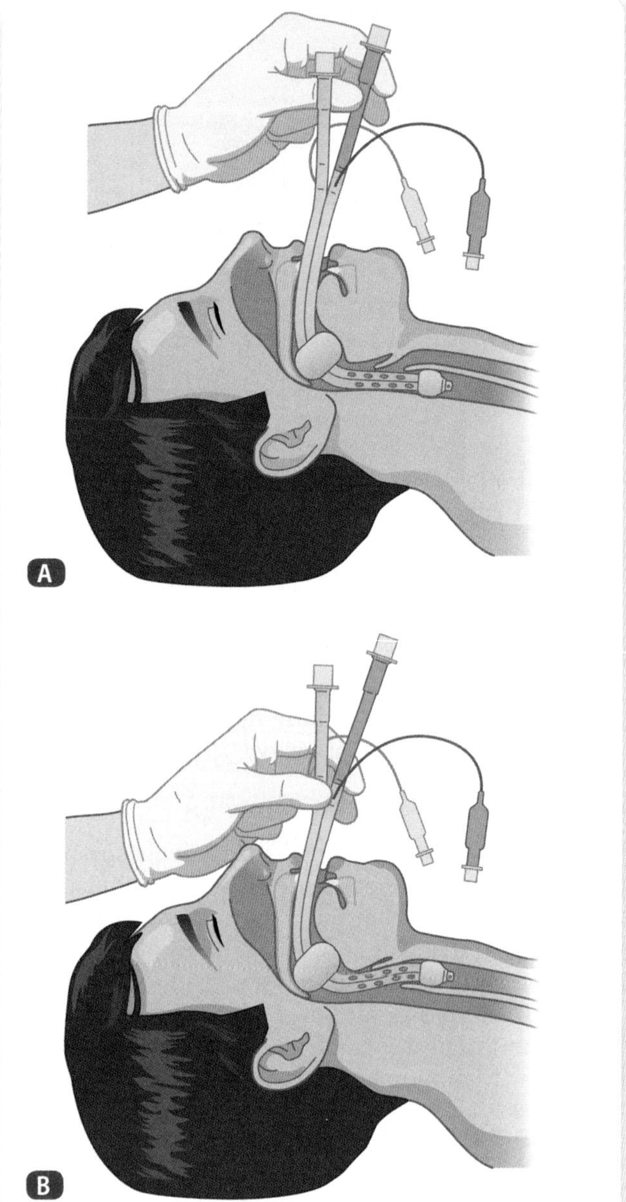

Figure 11-64 A. If the Combitube is inserted into the esophagus, then ventilations can still be provided to the patient. **B.** If the Combitube is inserted into the trachea, then it functions as an endotracheal tube, with ventilations provided directly into the trachea.

Indications and Contraindications for the Combitube

The Combitube is indicated for the airway management of deeply unresponsive, apneic patients with no gag reflex in whom ET intubation is not possible or has failed.

The Combitube cannot be used in pediatric patients younger than 16 years, and it should be used only for patients between 5 and 7 feet (1.5 to 2 m) tall. (A smaller version of the Combitube, called the Combitube SA [small adult], can be used for patients between 4 and 5.5 feet [approximately 1 to 2 m] tall.) Because most of the time the tube is inserted into the esophagus, the Combitube should not be used in patients with a known pathologic condition of the esophagus (such as esophageal varices), patients with esophageal trauma, patients who have ingested a caustic substance, or patients who have a history of alcoholism.

Complications of the Combitube

The most significant complication associated with the use of a Combitube is unrecognized displacement of the tube into the esophagus. (It is acceptable if the tube is placed in the esophagus, but you must realize this to effectively ventilate.) Therefore, good assessment skills are essential to properly confirm tube placement, and use rigorous confirmation protocol following insertion of the device.

Laryngospasm, vomiting, and possible hypoventilation may occur during insertion of a Combitube. Trauma to the pharynx or esophagus may also result from improper insertion technique.

Ventilation may be difficult if the pharyngeal balloon pushes the epiglottis over the glottic opening. In such cases, ventilation should become easier if the device is withdrawn 1 to 1.5 inches (2 to 4 cm).

Insertion Techniques

The Combitube consists of a single tube with two lumens, two balloons, and two ventilation ports. One of the lumens is open at its distal end, and the other is closed. The closed lumen has side holes distal to the pharyngeal balloon. The proximal balloon is designed to be inflated with 100 mL of air and provide a pharyngeal seal. The distal balloon is inflated with 15 mL of air and makes an airtight seal with the walls of the trachea (in case of tracheal placement) or provides esophageal obturation (in case of esophageal placement).

Before inserting the Combitube, check and prepare all equipment. Check both cuffs, and ensure that they hold air. The patient should be preoxygenated before insertion. Ventilation should not be interrupted for longer than 30 seconds to accomplish airway placement. For insertion, the patient's head should be placed in the neutral position.

- **Forwardly displace the jaw.** With the patient's head in the neutral position, insert the thumb of your gloved nondominant hand into the patient's mouth and lift the jaw. This action lifts the hyoid bone and pulls the base of the tongue off the posterior pharyngeal wall.
- **Insert the device.** Following the curvature of the tube, insert the device blindly into the posterior pharynx. The Combitube is inserted until the incisors are between the two black lines printed on the tube. Be gentle, and stop advancing the tube if you meet resistance.
- **Inflate the cuffs.** The Combitube has two independent inflation valves that must be inflated sequentially. The first inflation valve goes to the pharyngeal balloon (on the blue No. 1 tube) and is inflated with 100 mL of air (this is printed on the pilot balloon). The second inflation valve inflates the distal balloon (on the clear No. 2 tube) and is filled with 15 mL of air.

Remember that when inserting a multilumen airway, confirmation of ventilation is very critical. If you used the wrong port, the patient would receive no pulmonary ventilation and you could be instilling air directly into the stomach.

Following inflation of the balloons, begin to ventilate the patient. With the Combitube, ventilate the longer (blue) tube. Confirm the patient's chest rise and the presence of breath sounds. If there are no breath sounds, the chest does not rise and fall with ventilation, or epigastric sounds are present, switch immediately to the other inflation port. Be sure to continuously monitor ventilation. The Combitube is generally secure in the airway because of the large pharyngeal balloon; however, it is still important to secure the device in place after ventilations are confirmed.

Foreign Body Airway Obstruction

A foreign body that *completely* blocks the airway in a patient is a true emergency that will result in death if not treated immediately. In an adult, sudden foreign body airway obstruction usually occurs during a meal. In a child, it occurs while eating, playing with small toys, or crawling around the house. An otherwise healthy child who has sudden difficulty breathing has probably aspirated a foreign object.

By far, the most common airway obstruction in an unresponsive patient is the tongue, which relaxes and falls back into the throat, occluding the posterior pharynx. There are other causes of airway obstruction that do not involve foreign bodies in the airway. These include laryngeal edema (from infection or acute allergic reactions), laryngeal spasm, and trauma (tissue damage from injury). With airway obstruction from medical conditions such as infection and acute allergic reactions, repeated attempts to clear the airway as if there were a foreign body will be unsuccessful and potentially dangerous. These patients require specific emergency medical care and rapid transport to the hospital.

▶ Recognition

Early recognition of airway obstruction is crucial for you to be able to provide emergency medical care effectively.

Words of Wisdom

Possible causes of airway obstruction:

- Relaxation of the tongue in an unresponsive patient
- Foreign objects—food, small toys, dentures
- Blood clots, bone fragments, broken teeth, or damaged oral tissue following trauma
- Airway tissue swelling—infection, allergic reaction
- Aspirated vomitus (stomach contents)

Obstruction by a foreign body can result in a **mild airway obstruction** or a **severe airway obstruction**.

Patients with a mild airway obstruction (partially obstructed airway) are still able to exchange air but will have varying degrees of respiratory distress. Great care must be taken to prevent a mild airway obstruction from becoming a severe airway obstruction.

With a mild airway obstruction, the patient can cough forcefully, although you may hear **wheezing** between the coughs. As long as the patient can breathe, cough forcefully, or talk, you should not interfere with the patient's efforts to expel the foreign object on his or her own. Continue to monitor the patient closely, and encourage the patient to continue coughing. Abdominal thrusts are usually not effective for dislodging a mild airway obstruction. Attempts to remove the object manually could force the object farther down into the airway and cause a severe obstruction. Continually reassess the patient's condition, and be prepared to provide immediate treatment if the mild obstruction becomes a severe obstruction.

With poor air exchange, the patient has a weak, ineffective (not forceful) cough and may have increased difficulty breathing, **stridor** (a high-pitched noise heard primarily on inspiration), and cyanosis. Stridor is an indication of a mild upper airway obstruction. You must quickly recognize this situation and provide immediate care.

For patients with mild airway obstruction with poor air exchange, treat immediately as if there is a severe airway obstruction.

Patients with a severe airway obstruction (completely obstructed airway) cannot breathe, talk, or cough. One sure sign of a severe obstruction is the sudden inability to speak or cough immediately after eating. The person may clutch or grasp his or her throat (universal distress signal), begin to turn cyanotic, and make frantic attempts to breathe. There is little or no air movement. Ask the responsive patient, "Are you choking?" If the patient nods "yes," provide immediate treatment. If the obstruction is not cleared quickly, the amount of oxygen in the patient's blood will decrease dramatically. If not treated, the patient will become unresponsive and die.

Some patients with a severe airway obstruction will be unresponsive. You may not know that an airway obstruction is the cause of their condition. There are many other causes of unresponsiveness and respiratory distress, including stroke, heart attack, trauma, seizures, and drug overdose. A complete and thorough patient assessment by you, therefore, is key in providing appropriate emergency medical care.

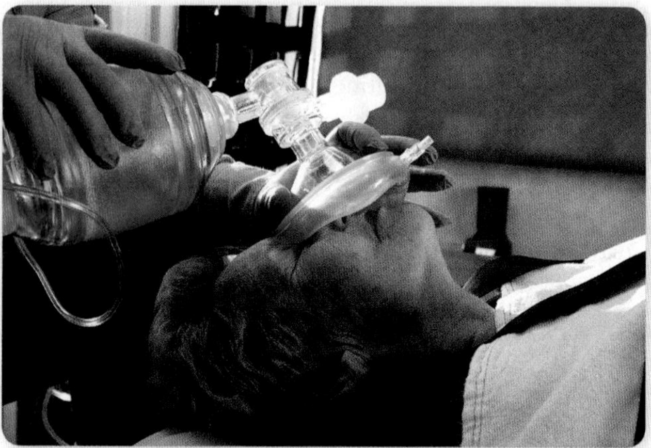

Figure 11-65 When you open the airway and attempt ventilations, it will be obvious to you if the airway is still blocked.

If a patient is found unresponsive and does not appear to be breathing, you should begin CPR with high-quality chest compressions. After 30 compressions, when you open the airway and attempt two ventilations, it will become clear that the airway is blocked **Figure 11-65**. Often the compressions may have been enough to clear the airway; however, if this has not cleared the obstruction and you are unable to ventilate the patient after two attempts (the chest does not visibly rise), or you feel resistance when ventilating, consider the possibility of an airway obstruction. Resistance to ventilation can also be a result of poor lung compliance.

Chapter 15, *BLS Resuscitation*, discusses steps for emergency medical care of a foreign body airway obstruction in detail. Recall that aspiration of blood or other fluid is dangerous for the patient. In addition to potentially obstructing the airway, aspiration destroys delicate bronchiolar tissue, introduces pathogens into the lungs, and decreases the patient's ability to ventilate (or be ventilated). Suction should be readily available for any patient who is unable to maintain his or her own airway. Always assume that patients who require emergency medical care have a full stomach.

YOU are the Provider SUMMARY

1. How does the body regulate ventilation?

The respiratory system must be able to accommodate the changes in oxygen demand by altering the rate and depth of ventilation. For most people, the drive to breathe is based on pH changes (related to the carbon dioxide level) in the blood and CSF. In healthy people, when the oxygen level rises, the respiratory center suspends respiration until a rising carbon dioxide level stimulates the respiratory center to begin breathing again.

2. What are some of the factors that affect pulmonary ventilation?

There are many factors that affect pulmonary ventilation, both intrinsic and extrinsic. Intrinsic causes include infections, allergic reactions, and airway obstructions (primarily due to tongue occlusion). Extrinsic factors include trauma or foreign body airway obstructions. The most common cause of obstruction in an unresponsive patient is the tongue obstructing the airway.

3. Which acid-base disorder do you suspect this patient is experiencing?

This patient is most likely experiencing respiratory acidosis as a result of his ineffective ventilation. The acidosis that results is quick and overwhelming, making it impossible for the slower-reacting renal system to compensate in time for the pH shift; this results in potentially fatal cardiac dysrhythmia and is usually fatal. Signs and symptoms of respiratory acidosis include vasodilation, headaches, central nervous system depression, bradypnea, nausea, and vomiting.

4. How does the pulse oximeter guide your treatment of this patient?

A pulse oximeter measures the percentage of hemoglobin saturation. Under normal conditions, the Spo_2 should be 98% to 100% while breathing room air. An Spo_2 of 94% or lower generally requires treatment unless the patient has a chronic condition causing a perpetually low oxygen saturation. Although the pulse oximeter should not directly guide your treatment, it can be used as a confirmatory adjunct that will confirm the patient's hypoxic state and give a numeric display as to the effectiveness of your interventions.

5. What are the indications for insertion of an advanced airway?

Indications for insertion of an advanced airway include deeply unresponsive, apneic patients without an intact gag reflex and patients in whom ET intubation is not possible or has been unsuccessful.

6. What are the contraindications for insertion of a King LT airway?

As with other advanced airway devices, contraindications for insertion of a King LT airway include responsive patients with an intact gag reflex, patients with known esophageal disease, and patients who have ingested caustic substances.

7. What are some possible respiratory patterns you may encounter?

Some of the possible respiratory pattern changes that you may encounter include Cheyne-Stokes respirations, Biot respirations, Kussmaul respirations, central neurologic hyperventilation, and agonal gasps. Any changes in respiratory pattern indicate a seriously ill patient and warrant aggressive airway management.

8. If the patient's respiratory rate increases to an acceptable level, should the King LT airway be removed?

The decision of whether to remove an advanced airway after it is inserted should be made in accordance with local protocols and consultation with medical direction. Typically, if a patient regains consciousness and is able to maintain his or her own airway adequately, the advanced airway can be removed, provided that a suction device is readily available at the patient's bedside.

YOU are the Provider SUMMARY *(continued)*

EMS Patient Care Report (PCR)

Date: 7-22-18	**Incident No.:** 56712	**Nature of Call:** Respiratory distress	**Location:** 421 Golden Acres Lane

Dispatched: 1720	**En Route:** 1723	**At Scene:** 1726	**Transport:** N/A	**At Hospital:** N/A	**In Service:** 1750

Patient Information

Age: 102 **Sex:** M **Weight (in kg [lb]):** 43 kg (95 lb)	**Allergies:** Unknown **Medications:** Unknown **Past Medical History:** Unknown **Chief Complaint:** Respiratory distress; decreased LOC

Vital Signs

Time: 1728	**BP:** Not obtained	**Pulse:** Not obtained	**Respirations:** 6-8	**Spo$_2$:** 78% on room air
Time: 1734	**BP:** 90/42	**Pulse:** 120	**Respirations:** 12 assisted	**Spo$_2$:** 82% on 15 L/min
Time: 1740	**BP:** 100/54	**Pulse:** 112	**Respirations:** 12 assisted	**Spo$_2$:** 88% on 15 L/min

EMS Treatment (circle all that apply)

Oxygen @ 15 **L/min via (circle one):** **NC** **(NRM)** **Bag-mask device**	(**Assisted Ventilation:** Yes)	(**Airway Adjunct:** King LT)	**CPR**

Defibrillation	**Bleeding Control**	**Bandaging**	**Splinting**	**Other:**

Narrative

Engine 9938 dispatched to above location, room 107, for man with respiratory distress. On arrival, met by patient care attendant, Stephanie, who states patient was admitted to facility earlier this AM and is breathing "funny." Patient presents with initial GCS of 7 (E-1, V-2, M-4), respirations of 6-8 breaths/min, cyanosis present around lips and nail beds. Bag-mask ventilations established at a rate of 10/min, O_2 administered at 15 L/min. Initial Spo$_2$ of 78%. Unable to get history from PCA; only information she is able to provide is that the patient is a "full code." Firefighter Hollister states she is having poor compliance with bag-mask ventilations due to patient's dentition. Prepared patient for insertion of King LT. After establishing patency, head aligned, size 5 King LT inserted without difficulty. Balloon inflated with 80 mL. Placement confirmed with clear bilateral breath sounds, equal/adequate chest rise, and increasing Spo$_2$. Dispatch contacted for transporting ambulance ETA. Made contact with paramedics, who advise quick ETA. On arrival of paramedics, report given, care released.**End of report**

Prep Kit

▶ Ready for Review

- The respiratory system includes the diaphragm, the muscles of the chest wall, and the accessory muscles of breathing.
- The upper airway includes the nose, mouth, jaw, oral cavity, pharynx, and larynx. Its function is to warm, filter, and humidify air as it enters the nose and mouth.
- The lower airway includes the trachea and lungs, and its function is to exchange oxygen and carbon dioxide.
- The respiratory system and the renal system have roles in maintaining a balance between acids and bases in the body. The respiratory system works to quickly remove excess acid as carbon dioxide from the lungs. Conversely, slowing respirations will increase carbon dioxide. The renal system regulates pH by filtering out more hydrogen and retaining bicarbonate when needed, or doing the reverse.
- Adequate breathing features a normal rate of 12 to 20 breaths/min, a regular pattern of inhalation and exhalation, bilateral clear and equal lung sounds, regular and equal chest rise and fall, and adequate tidal volume.
- Inadequate breathing for an adult features a respiratory rate of fewer than 12 breaths/min or more than 20 breaths/min, shallow depth (reduced tidal volume), an irregular pattern of inhalation and exhalation, and breath sounds that are diminished, absent, or noisy.
- Patients who are breathing inadequately show signs of hypoxia, a dangerous condition in which the body's tissues and cells do not have enough oxygen.
- Patients with inadequate breathing need to be treated immediately. Emergency medical care includes airway management, supplemental oxygen, and ventilatory support.
- Clearing the airway means removing obstructing material; maintaining the airway means keeping it open.
- Basic techniques for opening the airway include the head tilt–chin lift maneuver and the jaw-thrust maneuver.
- Suctioning is the next priority after opening the airway. Rigid tonsil-tip catheters are the best to use when suctioning the pharynx; soft, plastic catheters are used to suction the nose and liquid secretions in the back of the mouth. AEMTs may also need to perform tracheobronchial suctioning in patients who have been intubated by paramedics.
- One basic airway adjunct is the oropharyngeal or oral airway, which keeps the tongue from blocking the airway in unresponsive patients with no gag reflex. If the oral airway is not the proper size or is inserted incorrectly, it can push the tongue back into the pharynx, causing an obstruction.
- Another basic airway adjunct is the nasopharyngeal or nasal airway, which is usually used with patients who have a gag reflex and is better tolerated than the oral airway.
- The recovery position is used to help maintain the airway in patients without traumatic injuries who are breathing adequately on their own.
- You must provide immediate artificial ventilations with supplemental oxygen to patients who are not breathing on their own. Patients with inadequate breathing may also require artificial ventilations to maintain effective tidal volume.
- Handle compressed gas cylinders very carefully; their contents are under pressure. Always make sure the correct pressure regulator is firmly attached before transporting a cylinder. The pin-indexing safety system features a series of pins on a yoke that must be matched with the holes on the valve stem of the gas cylinder. Pressure regulators reduce the pressure of gas in an oxygen cylinder to between 40 and 70 psi. Pressure-compensated flowmeters and Bourdon-gauge flowmeters permit the regulated release of gas measured in liters per minute.
- When oxygen therapy is complete, disconnect the tubing from the flowmeter nipple, and turn off the cylinder valve; then turn off the flowmeter. As long as there is a pressure reading on the regulator gauge, it is not safe to remove the regulator from the valve stem. Keep any possible source of fire away from the area while oxygen is in use.
- Nasal cannulas and nonrebreathing masks are used most often to deliver oxygen in the field. The nonrebreathing mask is the delivery device of choice for providing supplemental oxygen to patients who are breathing adequately but are suspected of having or are showing signs of hypoxia. With a flow rate set at 15 L/min and the reservoir bag preinflated, the nonrebreathing mask can provide more than

Prep Kit (continued)

90% inspired oxygen. If the patient will not tolerate a nonrebreathing mask, apply a nasal cannula.

- Pulse oximetry, an assessment tool to evaluate the effectiveness of oxygenation, does not take the place of a good assessment. This measurement depends on adequate perfusion to the capillary beds and is inaccurate when the patient is cold or in shock or has been exposed to carbon monoxide.
- The methods of providing artificial ventilation include mouth-to-mask ventilation, one-person bag-mask device ventilation, two-person bag-mask ventilation, and the manually triggered ventilation (MTV) device. The MTV device is not a recommended ventilation device by most standards. Your own exhaled breath combined with high-flow oxygen at 15 L/min through the oxygen inlet valve will give your patient up to 55% oxygen; a bag-mask device with an oxygen reservoir and supplemental oxygen can deliver nearly 100% oxygen.
- Continuous positive airway pressure is a noninvasive method of providing ventilatory support for patients in respiratory distress or suffering from sleep apnea.
- It is imperative to be familiar with indications, contraindications, advantages, disadvantages, and special considerations when choosing the appropriate device. This is especially important when dealing with pediatric patients. Regardless of the method, aggressive airway management is essential to a positive patient outcome.
- When you are providing artificial ventilation, remember that ventilating too forcefully can cause gastric distention. Slow, gentle breaths during artificial ventilation can help to prevent gastric distention. Patients who have a tracheal stoma or a tracheostomy tube need to be ventilated through the tube or the stoma.
- Advanced devices that can be used by AEMTs to provide definitive airway management to patients unable to maintain their own airway include esophageal airways and multilumen airways.
- The King LT is a single-lumen airway that is blindly inserted into the esophagus. When it is properly placed in the esophagus, the distal cuff seals the esophagus while the proximal cuff seals the oropharynx. Openings located between these two cuffs provide for ventilation of the lungs.
- The laryngeal mask airway (LMA) is designed to provide a conduit from the glottic opening to the ventilation device. When properly inserted, the opening of the LMA is positioned right at the glottic opening. The inflatable cuff conforms to the contours of the airway and makes a relatively airtight seal.
- The Cobra perilaryngeal airway is designed to slide easily along the hard palate and to hold the soft tissue away from the laryngeal inlet when in place. The distal tip is proximal to the esophagus and seals the hypopharnyx. When the cuff is inflated, it raises the tongue and creates an airway seal allowing for ventilation.
- Multilumen airways have two tubes and can be inserted blindly. The Combitube is an example of such a device. A multilumen airway can be used to ventilate via the esophagus or the trachea based on placement.
- Foreign body airway obstruction usually occurs during a meal in an adult or while a child is eating, playing with small objects, or crawling about the house. The earlier you recognize any airway obstruction, the better. You must learn to recognize the difference between airway obstruction caused by a foreign object and that caused by a medical condition.
- Foreign body airway obstructions are classified as being mild or severe. Patients with a mild airway obstruction are able to move adequate amounts of air and should be left alone. Patients with a severe airway obstruction cannot move any air at all and require immediate treatment. Perform abdominal thrusts on a responsive adult or child with a severe airway obstruction. If the patient becomes unresponsive, begin CPR with high-quality chest compressions, and attempt to ventilate the patient.
- Check for loose dental appliances in a patient before assisting ventilation. Loose appliances should be removed to prevent them from obstructing the airway. Tight-fitting appliances should be left in place.
- Airway problems can be especially challenging in patients with serious facial injuries. Control bleeding with direct pressure and suction as necessary.

Prep Kit *(continued)*

▶ Vital Vocabulary

acidosis A pathologic condition that results from the accumulation of acids in the body.

aerobic metabolism Metabolism that can proceed only in the presence of oxygen.

agonal gasps Occasional gasps that are ineffective attempts at breathing, occurring after the heart has stopped.

airway The upper airway tract or the passage above the larynx, which includes the nose, mouth, and throat, and the lower airway, which includes the trachea and lungs. Also used to refer to devices used to open and maintain a patient's airway.

alkalosis The buildup of excess base (lack of acids) in the body.

alveolar minute volume The volume of air moved through the lungs in 1 minute minus the dead space; calculated by multiplying tidal volume (minus dead space) and respiratory rate.

alveolar ventilation The volume of air that reaches the alveoli. It is determined by subtracting the amount of dead space air from the tidal volume.

American Standard System A safety system for oxygen cylinders larger than size E, designed to prevent the accidental attachment of a regulator to a cylinder containing the wrong type of gas.

anaerobic metabolism The metabolism that takes place in the absence of oxygen; the principal product is lactic acid.

anoxia An absence of oxygen.

apnea Absence of breathing; periods of not breathing.

aspiration The introduction of vomit or other foreign material into the lungs.

asymmetric chest wall movement Unequal movement of the two sides of the chest; indicates decreased airflow into one lung.

ataxic respirations Irregular, ineffective respirations that may or may not have an identifiable pattern.

atelectasis A condition of airless or collapsed alveoli that causes pulmonary shunting, ventilation-perfusion mismatching, and possibly hypoxemia.

automatic transport ventilator (ATV) A mechanical ventilator that is used to ventilate intubated patients during transport; has settings for the tidal volume and ventilatory rate.

bag-mask device A device with a face mask attached to a ventilation bag containing a reservoir and connected to oxygen; delivers more than 90% supplemental oxygen.

barrier device A protective item, such as a pocket mask with a valve, that limits exposure to a patient's body fluids.

bilateral A body part or condition that appears on both sides of the midline.

bilevel positive airway pressure (BPAP) A form of noninvasive positive pressure ventilation that delivers two pressures (a higher inspiratory positive airway pressure and a lower expiratory positive airway pressure).

Bourdon-gauge flowmeter An oxygen flowmeter that is commonly used because it is not affected by gravity and can be placed in any position.

bradypnea Slow respiratory rate.

bronchioles Small airways made of smooth muscle that lead to the alveoli.

capnographer A device that attaches between the endotracheal tube and ventilation device; provides graphic information about the presence of exhaled carbon dioxide.

capnometer A device that performs the same function and attaches in the same way as a capnographer but provides a digital reading of the exhaled carbon dioxide.

carina Point at which the trachea bifurcates (divides) into the left and right mainstem bronchi.

cellular respiration A biochemical process resulting in the production of energy in the form of adenosine triphosphate.

chemoreceptors Peripheral and central receptors that monitor the levels of chemicals in the blood.

Cobra perilaryngeal airway (CobraPLA) A supraglottic airway device with a shape that allows the device to slide easily along the hard palate and to hold the soft tissue away from the laryngeal inlet.

colorimetric carbon dioxide detector A device that attaches between the endotracheal tube and

Prep Kit *(continued)*

ventilation device; uses special paper that should turn from purple to yellow during exhalation, indicating the presence of exhaled carbon dioxide.

Combitube A dual-lumen airway device that is inserted blindly; permits ventilation of the patient whether the tube is placed in the esophagus or the trachea.

continuous positive airway pressure (CPAP) A method of ventilation used primarily in the treatment of critically ill patients with respiratory distress; can prevent the need for endotracheal intubation.

dead space The amount of inhaled air that does not participate in respiration.

dorsal respiratory group A portion of the medulla oblongata where the primary respiratory pacemaker is found.

dyspnea Shortness of breath or difficulty breathing.

end-tidal carbon dioxide ($ETCO_2$) monitor A detection device for monitoring the amount of carbon dioxide in exhaled air that can be used to adjust oxygen administration or ventilations.

exhalation The part of the breathing process in which the diaphragm and the intercostal muscles relax, forcing air out of the lungs.

expiration The process of moving air out of the lungs.

external respiration The exchange of gases between the lungs and the blood cells in the pulmonary capillaries; also called pulmonary respiration.

gag reflex A normal reflex mechanism that causes retching; activated by touching the soft palate or the back of the throat.

glottic opening The narrowest portion of the adult's airway; space between the vocal cords.

head tilt–chin lift maneuver A combination of two movements to open the airway by tilting the forehead back and lifting the chin; used for nontrauma patients.

Hering-Breuer reflex The nervous system mechanism that terminates inhalation and prevents lung overexpansion.

hypercapnia Increased carbon dioxide level in the bloodstream.

hyperventilation An increased amount of air entering the alveoli, which lowers the blood carbon dioxide level and usually is a result of rapid or deep breathing.

hypovolemic shock A condition in which low blood volume, due to massive internal or external bleeding or extensive loss of body water, results in inadequate perfusion.

hypoxemia A deficiency of oxygen in arterial blood.

hypoxia A dangerous condition in which the body's tissues and cells do not have enough oxygen.

hypoxic drive A backup system to control respirations when the oxygen level falls.

i-gel A supraglottic airway device that uses a noninflatable, gel-like mask to isolate the larynx and facilitate ventilation.

inhalation The active, muscular part of breathing that draws air into the airway and lungs.

inspiration The process of moving air into the lungs.

internal respiration The exchange of gases between the blood cells and the tissues.

intrapulmonary shunting Bypassing of oxygen-poor blood past nonfunctional alveoli to the left side of the heart.

jaw-thrust maneuver Technique to open the airway by placing the fingers behind the angle of the jaw and bringing the jaw forward; used when a patient may have a cervical spine injury.

ketoacidosis An acidotic state created by the production of ketones via fat metabolism.

King LT airway A single-lumen airway that is blindly inserted into the esophagus; when properly placed in the esophagus, one cuff seals the esophagus, and the other seals the oropharynx.

labored breathing Breathing that requires greater than normal effort; may be slower or faster than normal and usually requires the use of accessory muscles.

laryngeal mask airway (LMA) An airway device that is inserted into the mouth blindly and comes to rest at the glottic opening. A flexible cuff is inflated, creating an almost airtight seal.

laryngectomy A surgical procedure in which the larynx is removed.

laryngospasm The spasmodic contraction of the vocal cords, accompanied by an enfolding of the arytenoid and aryepiglottic folds.

larynx A complex structure formed by the epiglottis, thyroid cartilage, cricoid cartilage, arytenoid cartilage,

Prep Kit (continued)

corniculate cartilage, and cuneiform cartilage; the voice box.

lung compliance The ability of the alveoli to fully expand when air is drawn in during inhalation.

manually triggered ventilation (MTV) device A fixed flow rate ventilation device that delivers a breath every time its button is pushed; also referred to as a flow-restricted, oxygen-powered ventilation device.

mediastinum Space within the chest that contains the heart, major blood vessels, vagus nerve, trachea, major bronchi, and esophagus; located between the lungs.

metabolic acidosis A pathologic condition characterized by a blood pH of less than 7.35 and caused by accumulation of acids in the body from a metabolic cause.

metabolic alkalosis A pathologic condition characterized by a blood pH of greater than 7.45 and resulting from the accumulation of bases in the body from a metabolic cause.

metabolism The chemical processes that provide the cells with energy from nutrients.

mild airway obstruction A condition in which an obstruction leaves the patient able to exchange some air, but also causes some degree of respiratory distress.

minute volume The amount of air moved in and out of the respiratory tract per minute, which is determined by the tidal volume multiplied by the respiratory rate.

multilumen airway device A type of airway device with a single long tube that can be used for esophageal obturation or endotracheal tube ventilation, depending on where it comes to rest following blind positioning.

nasal cannula An oxygen-delivery device in which oxygen flows through two small, tubelike prongs that fit into the patient's nostrils.

nasopharyngeal (nasal) airway An airway adjunct inserted into the nostril of a responsive patient who is not able to maintain a natural airway.

negative pressure ventilation Drawing of air into the lungs; airflow from a region of higher pressure (outside the body) to a region of lower pressure (the lungs); occurs during normal (unassisted) breathing.

nonrebreathing mask A combination mask and reservoir bag system that is the preferred way to give oxygen in the prehospital setting; delivers up to 90% inspired oxygen.

oropharyngeal (oral) airway An airway adjunct inserted into the mouth to keep the tongue from blocking the upper airway and to make suctioning the airway easier.

orthopnea Positional dyspnea.

oxygenation The process of delivering oxygen to the blood by diffusion from the alveoli following inhalation into the lungs.

oxygen saturation (Spo_2) The measure of the percentage of oxygen molecules that are bound to hemoglobin in arterial blood.

oxygen toxicity A condition of excessive oxygen consumption resulting in cellular and tissue damage.

paradoxical motion The inward movement of the chest during inhalation and outward movement during exhalation; the opposite of normal chest wall movement during breathing.

parietal pleura Thin membrane that lines the chest cavity.

partial laryngectomy Surgical removal of a portion of the larynx.

partial pressure The term used to describe the amount of gas in air or dissolved in fluid, such as blood.

partial rebreathing mask A mask that is similar to a nonrebreathing mask except there is no one-way valve between the mask and the reservoir; therefore, patients rebreathe a small amount of their exhaled air.

patent Open, clear of obstruction.

phrenic nerves The nerves that innervate the diaphragm; necessary for adequate breathing.

pin-indexing system A system established for portable cylinders to ensure that a regulator is not connected to a cylinder containing the wrong type of gas.

pneumothorax A partial or complete accumulation of air in the pleural space.

positive end-expiratory pressure (PEEP) Mechanical maintenance of pressure in the airway at the end of expiration to increase the volume of gas remaining in the lungs.

Prep Kit *(continued)*

preload The pressure of blood that is returned to the heart (venous return).

pulmonary edema A buildup of fluid in the lungs, usually as a result of congestive heart failure.

pulse oximetry An assessment method that measures the oxygen saturation of hemoglobin in the capillary beds.

recovery position A side-lying position used to maintain a clear airway in patients without injuries.

residual volume The air that remains in the lungs after a maximal expiration.

respiration The process of exchanging oxygen and carbon dioxide.

respiratory acidosis A pathologic condition characterized by a blood pH of less than 7.35 and caused by accumulation of acids in the body from a respiratory cause.

respiratory alkalosis A pathologic condition characterized by a blood pH of greater than 7.45 and resulting from the accumulation of bases in the body from a respiratory cause.

respiratory rate The number of ventilatory cycles in a unit of time, usually 1 minute; also known as the ventilation rate.

retractions Movements in which the skin pulls in around the ribs during inspiration.

severe airway obstruction Occurs when a foreign body completely obstructs the patient's airway. Patients cannot breathe, talk, or cough.

stoma A surgical opening in the body that connects an internal structure to the skin, such as a stoma in the neck that connects the trachea directly to the skin.

stridor A harsh, high-pitched respiratory sound, generally heard during inspiration, that is caused by partial blockage or narrowing of the upper airway; may be audible without a stethoscope.

suction catheter A hollow, cylindrical device used to remove fluids and secretions from the airway.

surfactant The proteinaceous substance that lines the inside of the alveoli and allows for easy expansion and recoil of the alveoli.

tachypnea Rapid respiratory rate.

tidal volume The amount of air moved during one breath.

tongue-jaw lift maneuver A method of opening the airway for suctioning or inserting an oral airway; involves grasping the incisors or gums and lifting the jaw.

tonsil-tip catheter A suction catheter with a large, semirigid suction tip, recommended for suctioning the pharynx; also called Yankauer tip.

total laryngectomy Surgical removal of the entire larynx.

trachea The windpipe; the main conduit for air passing to and from the lungs.

tracheostomy Surgical creation of a hole in the trachea.

tracheostomy tube A tube inserted through the hole created by a tracheostomy.

turbinates Bony shelves that extend from the lateral walls of the nose into the nasal passageway; increase the surface area of the nasal mucosa, improving filtration, warming, and humidification of inhaled air.

vasodilatory shock A type of shock related to relaxation of the blood vessels, allowing blood to pool and impairing circulation.

ventilation The exchange of air between the lungs and the air of the environment, spontaneously by the patient or with assistance.

ventral respiratory group A portion of the medulla oblongata that is responsible for modulating breathing during speech.

visceral pleura Thin membrane that covers the lungs.

vital capacity The amount of air that can be forcibly expelled from the lungs after breathing in as deeply as possible.

$\dot{V}/\dot{Q}$ mismatch A measurement that examines how much gas is being moved effectively and how much blood is gaining access to the alveoli.

wheezing A high-pitched, whistling breath sound that is most prominent on expiration, and which suggests an obstruction or narrowing of the lower airways; occurs in asthma and bronchiolitis.

▶ References

1. Collins JS, Lemmens HJ, Brodsky JB, et al. Laryngoscopy and morbid obesity: a comparison of the "sniff" and "ramped" positions. *Obes Surg.* 2004;14(9):1171-1175.
2. Frappier J, Guenoun T, Journois D, et al. Airway management using the intubating laryngeal mask airway for the morbidly obese patient. *Anesth Analg.* 2003;96(5):1510-1515, table of contents.

Prep Kit (continued)

3. Lee BJ, Kang JM, Kim DO. Laryngeal exposure during laryngoscopy is better in the 25 degrees back-up position than in the supine position. *Br J Anaesth*. 2007;99(4):581-586.
4. Navarro Martínez MJ, Pindado Martínez ML, Paz Martín D, et al. [Perioperative anesthetic management of 300 morbidly obese patients undergoing laparoscopic bariatric surgery and a brief review of relevant pathophysiology]. *Rev Esp Anestesiol Reanim*. 2011;58(4):211-217.
5. Neligan PJ, Porter S, Max B, et al. Obstructive sleep apnea is not a risk factor for difficult intubation in morbidly obese patients. *Anesth Analg*. 2009;109(4):1182-1186.
6. Rao SL, Kunselman AR, Schuler HG, DesHarnais S. Laryngoscopy and tracheal intubation in the head-elevated position in obese patients: a randomized, controlled, equivalence trial. *Anesth Analg*. 2008;107(6):1912-1918.
7. O'Connor RE, Al Ali AS, Brady WJ, et al. Part 9: acute coronary syndromes: 2015 American Heart Association Guidelines Update for Cardiopulmonary Resuscitation and Emergency Cardiovascular Care. *Circulation*. 2015;132(suppl 2):S487.
8. O'Gara PT, Kushner FG, Ascheim DD, et al. 2013 ACCF/AHA guideline for the management of ST-elevation myocardial infarction: executive summary: a report of the American College of Cardiology Foundation/American Heart Association Task Force on Practice Guidelines. *J Am Coll Cardiol*. 2013;61:485-510.
9. O'Connor RE, Al Ali AS, Brady WJ, et al. Part 9: acute coronary syndromes: 2015 American Heart Association Guidelines Update for Cardiopulmonary Resuscitation and Emergency Cardiovascular Care. *Circulation*. 2015;132(suppl 2): S483-S500.

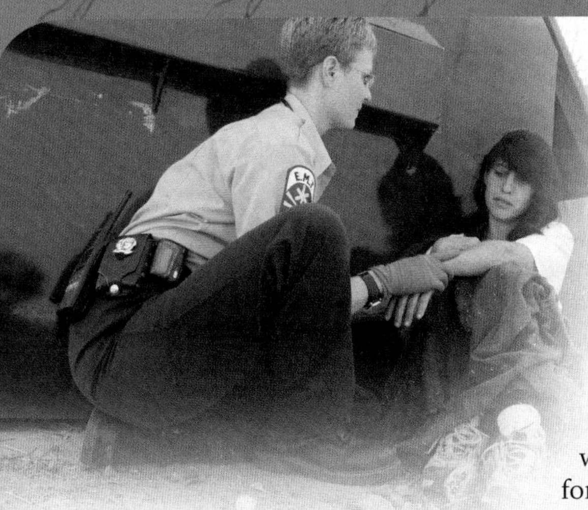

Assessment *in Action*

Your ambulance is dispatched to the local homeless shelter to assist a volunteer with a 60-year-old woman with a history of "heart problems." On arrival, you find a woman in obvious respiratory distress who states that she "feels like I'm drowning." As you are discussing the patient's recent history with the volunteer, he tells you that she has been at the shelter for 3 days and has taken no medication during this time.

1. The immediate treatment for this patient should include:

A. opening the airway.
B. suctioning the airway.
C. oxygen via the appropriate delivery device.
D. starting chest compressions.

2. When listening to her breath sounds, what would you expect to hear based on her description and presentation?

A. Crackles
B. Rhonchi
C. Stridor
D. Wheezing

Assessment *in Action* (continued)

3. The patient states that she has "heart failure." After listening to breath sounds and noting the presence of pulmonary edema, which airway therapy would you feel is most appropriate for this patient?

A. Bag-mask ventilation
B. CPAP
C. Nonrebreathing mask
D. Venturi mask

4. You assist the patient with the placement of CPAP and monitor for signs of improvement. Which of the following indicates the therapy is working?

A. An increase in Spo_2
B. An increase in $ETCO_2$
C. An increase in anxiety
D. An increase in heart rate

5. You notice the patient's blood pressure dropping and her mental status is now altered. What should you do next?

A. Stimulate the patient and coach her breathing.
B. Gain intravenous access and give a fluid bolus.
C. Remove the CPAP device and initiate positive pressure ventilations.
D. Switch her to an NRM and monitor her $ETCO_2$.

6. Which of the following is a contraindication for the use of CPAP?

A. Ability to follow commands
B. Lack of facial trauma
C. Hypertension
D. Hypotension

7. In this scenario, the primary indication for the use of CPAP is:

A. inability to ventilate.
B. history of "heart failure."
C. pulmonary edema.
D. lack of medication.

8. CPAP __________ pressure in the lungs.

A. increases
B. decreases
C. initially decreases, then increases
D. initially increases, then decreases

9. List the contraindications for insertion of a Combitube.

10. List five possible causes of airway obstruction.

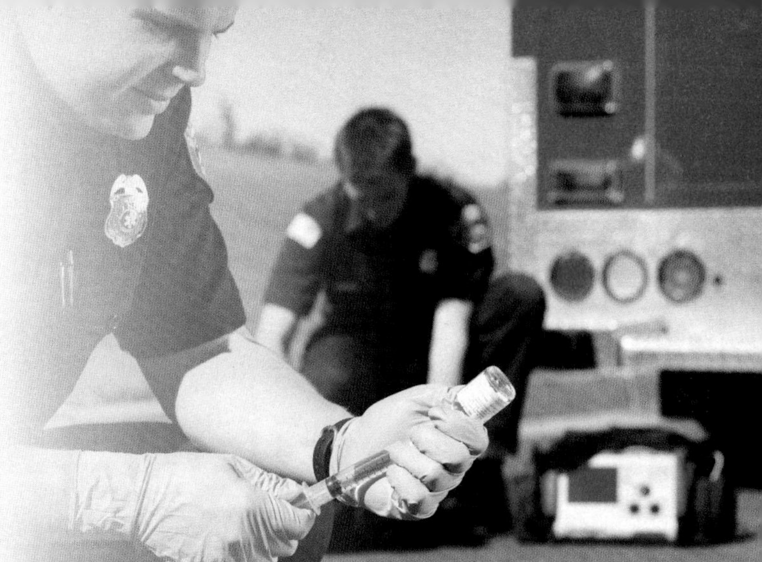

SECTION 5

Pharmacology

CHAPTER 12

Principles of Pharmacology

National EMS Education Standard Competencies

Pharmacology

Applies to patient assessment and management fundamental knowledge of the medications carried by AEMTs that may be administered to a patient during an emergency.

Principles of Pharmacology

- Medication safety (p 548)
- Kinds of medications used during an emergency (pp 569-577)
- Medication legislation (pp 546-547)
- Naming (pp 544-545)
- Classifications (pp 550-556)
- Storage and security (p 548)
- Autonomic pharmacology (pp 551-552)
- Metabolism and excretion (pp 561-562)
- Mechanism of action (pp 551, 563-564)
- Medication response relationships (p 564)
- Medication interactions (pp 564-566)
- Toxicity (p 544)

Knowledge Objectives

1. Discuss important drug terminology, including intended effects, unintended effects, untoward effects, indications, and contraindications. (p 544)
2. Discuss the differences between generic, trade, chemical, and official medication names, and provide an example of each. (pp 544-545)
3. Discuss the US laws and regulations that relate to medication manufacturing and distribution. (pp 546-547)
4. List the five schedules of drugs with the highest abuse potential per the Controlled Substances Act. (p 546)
5. Discuss the US Food and Drug Administration (FDA) approval process. (p 547)
6. Describe the proper storage for drugs and security concerns. (p 548)
7. Describe the medication administration considerations that must be applied to special populations, including pediatric, geriatric, and pregnant patients. (pp 548-550)
8. Discuss legal, moral, and ethical considerations related to drug administration. (p 550)
9. Explain the term mechanism of action. (pp 551, 563-564)
10. Describe the roles and functions of the sympathetic and parasympathetic nervous systems. (pp 551-552)
11. Discuss the concept of receptor sites, including adrenergic receptors, and how medications may take advantage of these. (pp 551-552)
12. Discuss the concepts of agonists and antagonists as they relate to medications. (pp 551-552)
13. List the types of drugs that affect the sympathetic nervous system, including sympathomimetics and sympatholytics, and describe how they create their effects. (pp 551-552)
14. List the types of drugs that affect the parasympathetic nervous system, including parasympathomimetics and parasympatholytics, and describe how they create their effects. (p 552)
15. Discuss the effects of opioid agonists, opioid antagonists, and opioid agonist-antagonists. (pp 552-553)
16. Discuss types of sedative-hypnotics, including benzodiazepines, barbiturates, and nonbarbiturate hypnotics. (p 553)
17. Discuss central nervous system stimulants and depressants. (p 553)
18. Discuss drugs that affect the cardiac system, including cardiac glycosides, antidysrhythmics, and antihypertensive medications, and describe how they exert their effects. (pp 554-555)
19. Describe drugs that affect the respiratory system, including oxygen, over-the-counter medications, bronchodilators, and xanthines. (pp 555-556)
20. Explain the solid, liquid, and gas forms of medication, provide examples of each, and discuss how the form of a medication dictates its route of administration. (pp 556-558)
21. Describe the enteral and parenteral routes of medication administration and explain how they differ. (p 559)

22. Describe the following routes of medication administration and discuss their individual rates of absorption: oral, intravenous, intraosseous, subcutaneous, intramuscular, sublingual, intranasal, and inhalation. (pp 559-560)
23. Define the term pharmacokinetics and describe the stages a medication goes through while being processed in the body. (pp 560-562)
24. Define the term pharmacodynamics, and describe the types of predictable and unpredictable responses a drug may create. (pp 563-566)
25. Discuss the concepts of serum sickness, idiosyncratic reaction, cumulative effect, summation, potentiation, drug dependence, and medication interaction. (pp 564-566)
26. Give the generic and trade names, actions, indications, contraindications, routes of administration, side effects, interactions, and doses of 10 medications and 3 intravenous fluids that may be administered by an AEMT in an emergency as directed by state protocols and local medical direction. (pp 569-577)

Skills Objectives

There are no skills objectives for this chapter.

Introduction

Administering medications is a serious business. Used appropriately, medication may alleviate pain, ease suffering, and improve a patient's well-being. However, used inappropriately, medication may cause harm and even death. *All medications are poisons if they are given to the wrong patient or in toxic quantities*. As an advanced emergency medical technician (AEMT), you will be responsible for administering certain medications to patients and helping them to self-administer others. You will ask patients about their medication allergies, and you will report this information to hospital personnel. To act without understanding how medications work will place both patients and you in danger.

This chapter describes the various forms of medications, the different ways in which they can be administered, and their mechanisms of action. It then takes a close look at each of the forms of medications you may be called on to administer or help patients to self-administer.

Table 12-1 lists components of a drug profile and serves as an introduction to the type of information covered in this chapter. A drug profile gives all specifics about the drug. This is the information included on the package insert and listed in various pharmaceutical publications. As an AEMT, you should familiarize yourself with the drug profiles of the medications you may be expected to administer.

Drug Terminology

Pharmacology is the study of the properties (characteristics) and effects of drugs and medications on the body. **Drugs** are substances that produce a physiologic effect, whether therapeutic or not; clinically, they are chemical agents used in the diagnosis, treatment, and prevention of disease. Although the terms *drugs* and *medications* are often used interchangeably, the word *drugs* may make some people think of narcotics or illegal substances. For this reason, you should try to use the word *medications*, especially when interviewing patients and families. In general terms, a **medication** is a chemical substance that is used to treat or prevent disease or relieve pain.

YOU are the Provider — PART 1

Your ambulance is dispatched to a man lying unresponsive in an alley. On arrival, you find a law enforcement officer leaning over a man who is in his mid 30s. The patient is unresponsive and not breathing. The officer has opened the airway, is providing ventilations with a pocket mask, and states that the patient is well known to him and has an extensive history of intravenous (IV) drug use, with his drug of choice being heroin.

1. Are there any potential hazards with this scene?
2. What medication might the AEMT carry that would be appropriate to administer in this situation?

Table 12-1 Components of a Drug Profile

Drug names—This includes the generic name, trade name, and chemical name.
Classification—What type of drug is this? What is it used for?
Mechanisms of action—How does the drug work? What is its intended purpose?
Indications—What are the reasons for taking this drug?
Contraindications—When should the drug not be given? Does it affect certain medical conditions or react with other medications adversely?
Pharmacokinetics—How is the drug absorbed, metabolized, and so forth? What is its **half-life**?
Side and adverse effects—Are there any side effects? What are the adverse effects?
Routes of administration—How is the drug given?
How supplied—What is the total quantity of the medication? What form?
Dosages—This generally includes proper dosages for adult, pediatric, and special considerations, such as when to modify the dosage based on the patient's history.
Special considerations—These are considerations for certain groups such as pediatric, geriatric, and pregnant patients and other special patient groups.
Other—The drug profile may include any other information that is vital to the user.

The **dose** of the medication is the amount that is given. The dose depends on the patient's size and age; adults and children may receive different amounts of the same medication. The dose also depends on the desired action of the medication. The **action** is the therapeutic effect or **intended effect** that a medication is expected to have on the body. For example, nitroglycerin relaxes the walls of the blood vessels and may dilate the arteries. This effect increases the blood flow and, thus, the supply of oxygen to the heart muscle. In this way, nitroglycerin relieves the squeezing or crushing pain that occurs with angina. Nitroglycerin is therefore indicated for chest pain associated with angina. **Unintended effects** are the effects that are undesirable but pose little risk to the patient. **Untoward effects** are the effects that can be harmful to the patient. **Toxicity** is the risk that a substance will pose a health hazard to an individual or organism.

Words of Wisdom

An *indication* is a reason for giving a drug. A *contraindication* is a reason not to give a drug. The number one contraindication for any medication is hypersensitivity (allergy) to that drug.

Indications are the therapeutic uses for a particular medication. There are times when you should not give a patient medication, even if it usually is indicated for that person's condition. Such situations are called **contraindications**. A medication is contraindicated when it would harm the patient or have no positive effect on the patient's condition. For example, administration of oral glucose is indicated when a patient has a low blood glucose level. Because of the high sugar content, it rapidly raises blood glucose levels. However, oral glucose would be contraindicated if the patient were unresponsive and could not swallow or had an altered mental status and could not maintain his or her airway.

Medication Names

The medications we use are derived from four principal sources: animal, vegetable, mineral, and synthetic compounds. Plant sources of medications include a variety of roots, leaves, flowers, and seeds. For example, digitalis, which is used in the treatment of heart failure, is prepared from the dried leaves of a wildflower called purple foxglove. In contrast, insulin, a medication taken by diabetics, is usually prepared from the pancreas of animals (primarily pigs). Minerals used in the treatment of medical problems include calcium, iron, and magnesium. Drugs that are manufactured synthetically include synthetic forms of vitamins, steroids, narcotics, and many others.

Medications have different types of names. A **trade name** is the brand name that a manufacturer gives to a medication, such as Tylenol and Lasix. As a proper noun, a trade name begins with a capital letter. Trade names are used in every aspect of our daily lives, not just in medications. Well-known examples include Jell-O gelatin, Band-Aid adhesive bandages, and Hershey's chocolate candy. A medication may have many different trade names, depending on how many companies manufacture it. Advil, Nuprin, and Motrin all are trade names for the same generic medication, ibuprofen.

The **generic name** of a medication (such as ibuprofen) is usually its original chemical name, which is not capitalized, and is usually suggested by the first manufacturer and approved by the US Food and Drug Administration (FDA). Sometimes a medication is called by its generic name more often than by any of its trade names. For example, you may hear the term *nitroglycerin* used more often than the trade names Isordil and

Nitrostat. All medications that are licensed for use in the United States are listed by their generic names in the *United States Pharmacopeia (USP)*.

The **chemical name** of a medication is a precise description of the drug's chemical composition and molecular structure. The **official name** is the name assigned by the *USP*. In most cases, the official name is generally the generic name followed by "USP."

Examples of the four names for a drug are as follows:

- **Chemical name:** 9-chloro-11β,17,21-trihydroxy-16β-methylpregna-1,4-diene-3,20-dione 17,21-dipropionate
- **Generic name:** beclomethasone dipropionate
- **Trade name:** Vanceril
- **Official name:** beclomethasone dipropionate, USP

Medications may be **prescription medications** or **over-the-counter (OTC) medications**. Only pharmacists, according to a physician's order, can legally distribute prescription medications to patients. However, OTC medications may be purchased directly from a wholesale or retail source, such as a discount store or supermarket, without a prescription. In recent years, the number of prescription medications that have become available OTC has increased dramatically. Therefore, many of the problems attributable to prescription medications may become more common. You may also come into contact with patients who have taken "street" drugs such as heroin or cocaine. Although street drugs lack the pharmaceutical purity of OTC or prescribed medications, they are still pharmacologically active and will cause an effect.

Sources of Drug Information

There are numerous references to learn more about a particular drug. Publications include the *American Medical Association (AMA) Drug Evaluations* and the *Physicians' Desk Reference (PDR)*. Information regarding drugs can also be obtained through the use of a hospital formulary—a local publication that delineates which drugs are used in a particular facility. Medications come packaged with drug inserts that give information specific to preparation, dosage, effects, possible **side effects**, and other information. There are also numerous other texts and sources, including the Internet. AEMTs should be familiar with these resources and other field references, particularly regarding medications commonly encountered in the prehospital setting. Table 12-2 lists some of the most up-to-date and reliable sources.

Table 12-2 Sources of Drug Information

Source	Description
US FDA Center for Drug Evaluation and Research	Mission is to ensure that safe and effective drugs are available in the United States
Physicians' Desk Reference	Compiles data on most medications available in the United States; uses the information on file with the FDA; includes all of the necessary information on indications, dosages, contraindications, and adverse reactions. The size of the book makes it difficult for use on an ambulance, but a CD-ROM version makes it more accessible in the field.
Hospital formulary	A list of drugs, dosage forms, package sizes, and drug strengths stocked by hospitals and pharmacies; published as a quick reference to assist the physician and nursing staffs; divided into four general sections: introduction, therapeutic index, drug monographs, and general reference
Drug inserts	Printed document included in the packaging provided by the drug's manufacturer; generally the same information submitted and approved by the FDA; when available, serves as a valuable reference; should not be confused with the information provided by a pharmacy when a patient receives a prescription, which is useful in obtaining information pertaining to a drug but is not necessarily all inclusive
AMA Drug Evaluations	A nonofficial compendium that provides another source of useful and miscellaneous drug information for pharmacists and medical practitioners; includes generic and trade names; information may not be limited to drugs approved for use by the FDA

Abbreviations: AMA, American Medical Association; FDA, Food and Drug Administration

US Regulation of Pharmaceuticals

The manufacture of pharmaceuticals in the United States and most other countries is subject to a variety of laws and regulations. The goal of these laws and regulations is to protect consumers. In particular, they prohibit manufacturers from making false claims about the benefits of their drugs and prohibit advising patients on the administration of the drugs, which may be incorrect. These laws also seek to protect patients from drugs that might cause harm and require drug manufacturers to publish information about side effects and known potential harmful effects of their products.

Laws and regulations also outline standards for drug manufacture to ensure that drugs produced by different manufacturers are uniform in strength and purity. In the United States, these drug standards are published in the *USP* and the *National Formulary*. In addition, several federal laws have been enacted to protect consumers (patients) from unsafe substances and unscrupulous manufacturers and distributors.

▶ Drug-Related Legislation

The Pure Food and Drug Act (1906) was the first federal legislation in the United States aimed at protecting the public from mislabeled, poisonous, or otherwise harmful foods, medications, and alcoholic beverages. It required little more than the labeling of drugs, and it was replaced by more comprehensive legislation in 1938.

The Food, Drug, and Cosmetic Act (1938, amended in 1952 and 1962) added several new provisions:

- Required drug makers to label their products, indicating whether they contain potentially habit-forming substances and to include warnings about possible side effects
- Authorized the creation of the FDA, discussed later in this chapter
- Mandated that dangerous drugs could be dispensed only with a prescription from a physician, dentist, or veterinarian

The Harrison Narcotic Act (1914) regulated the import, manufacture, prescription, and sale of several nonnarcotic drugs and cocaine, opium, and their derivatives. Precise record keeping about the dispensing of controlled drugs and registration of distributors, such as pharmacists, are required. Penalties—namely, fines and imprisonment—are specified for illegal possession or distribution of controlled drugs.

The Narcotic Control Act (1956) increased the penalties for violation of the Harrison Act, made the possession of heroin illegal, and outlawed the acquisition and transportation of marijuana.

In 1970, Congress enacted the Controlled Substances Act, comprehensive legislation dealing with narcotic and nonnarcotic drugs that have potential for abuse. This act specifies requirements for registration, procurement, storage, distribution, and record keeping for these drugs and penalties for failure to comply with these requirements. The drugs covered by the Controlled Substances Act are classified into five categories, or *schedules*, according to their abuse potential. Schedule I includes drugs with the highest abuse potential, and Schedule V includes drugs with the lowest abuse potential. Table 12-3 lists these schedules, including descriptions and examples.

Schedule I drugs have the highest abuse potential and a propensity for severe **drug dependence**; none of them have any accepted medical application. In general, Schedule I drugs are completely outlawed. On rare occasions, and under the strictest control by the FDA and Drug Enforcement Agency (DEA), these drugs may be used for research, analysis, and instruction only.

Some states have enacted their own laws or regulations related to the use, storage, and handling of controlled

Table 12-3 Classification of Medications Considered Controlled Substances

Schedule	Description	Examples
I	High abuse potential; no recognized medical purpose	Heroin, marijuana, LSD
II	High abuse potential; legitimate medical purpose	Fentanyl (Sublimaze), methylphenidate (Ritalin), cocaine
III	Less potential for abuse than Schedule II medications	Hydrocodone (Vicodin), acetaminophen with codeine (Tylenol #3 with codeine), ketamine
IV	Less potential for abuse than Schedule III drugs	Diazepam (Valium), lorazepam (Ativan)
V	Less potential for abuse than Schedule IV drugs	Narcotic cough medicines

Abbreviation: LSD, lysergic acid diethylamide

substances. If the state law is more stringent than the federal law, the state law takes precedence.

While marijuana is still a Schedule I narcotic, as of September, 2017, 29 states along with the District of Columbia have enacted laws that legalize marijuana in some form. Included in this number are seven states and the District of Columbia who also have approved marijuana for recreational use. Some states who have not adopted laws broadly legalizing medical marijuana still provide limited access under certain circumstances such as Alabama and Mississippi, which have very limited laws permitting the use of medical marijuana for severe epileptic conditions.[1] The laws regarding the use of medical marijuana and the types of medical conditions for which its use is allowed vary from state to state. As an AEMT, you should be aware of the laws in your state and always follow local protocols.

▶ Manufacturing-Related Regulations

Federal legislation also focuses on guaranteeing standardization of doses. Standardization assures patients that when they take a medication with a stated amount of the active ingredient, they will, in fact, receive that amount of the drug. Clearly, no one would want to be prescribed a certain dose of a drug and find that the actual medication contained twice (or one-half) the amount of active ingredient stated on the drug's label. For a drug to have the USP label, the amount of active ingredients must be within 95% to 105% of that stated on the label. For example, if the label says "300 mg of amiodarone," the medication must contain between 285 and 315 mg of the drug.

▶ Government Agencies That Regulate Drugs

Today, regulation of drugs in the United States falls under the jurisdiction of several agencies:

- The FDA enforces the Food, Drug, and Cosmetic Act. As part of its responsibilities, the FDA is charged with determining the safety and efficacy of drugs before they are allowed to enter the US market.
- The DEA, formerly the Bureau of Narcotics and Dangerous Drugs, was created by the Federal Controlled Substances Act of 1970. The DEA, which is a division of the Justice Department, is responsible for executing the provisions of the Controlled Substances Act, including the registration of physicians who are permitted to dispense controlled substances.
- The Public Health Service regulates biologic products—that is, medications made from living organisms such as antitoxins and vaccines.
- The Federal Trade Commission (FTC) monitors drug advertising and ensures that it is not misleading or inappropriate. The FTC has become involved in making recommendations to the FDA regarding direct-to-consumer (DTC) advertisements. The FTC found that DTC advertisements "generally benefit consumers" but stated that DTC ads should contain a "major statement of drug risks along with adequate provision for more complete risk information."

The Drug-Approval Process

New drugs are constantly being developed. The commercialization process, however, takes years—the average time for a drug to be developed, tested, and approved is approximately 9 years. In some cases, manufacturers spend most of those 9 years developing a drug only to find out that the drug does not work as envisioned or is too dangerous for human consumption.

All new drugs must go through animal studies and clinical trials in humans before they are approved for distribution.

▶ Animal Studies

Animal studies are designed to learn more about the properties of a drug and to identify tissues and organs that are sensitive to the actions of the drug. Testing in at least two animal species is required by law. After successful completion of animal studies, an investigational new drug may enter clinical trials in humans.

▶ Clinical Trials

Clinical trials proceed in four phases:

- **Phase I.** The new drug is tested in healthy volunteers to compare human data with those in animals to determine safe doses of the drug and to assess its safety.
- **Phase II.** These trials are performed in homogeneous populations of patients (50 to 300 patients). In double-blind studies, one group receives the drug and the other group receives a placebo. These studies are designed to evaluate the efficacy and safety of the drug and to establish which form is the most effective dose.
- **Phase III.** In these clinical trials, the drug is made available to a larger group of patients (several thousand). These studies, which usually last several years, evaluate the efficacy of the drug and monitor the nature and incidence of side effects.
- **Phase IV.** After successful completion of Phase III clinical trials, the drug company can apply to the FDA for approval to market the drug. Phase IV trials compare the new drug with others on the market and examine the drug's long-term efficacy and cost-effectiveness.

Drug Storage and Security of Controlled Substances

All drug containers or "boxes" should be carefully guarded against possible theft. This requires that the boxes not only be locked, but also secured within the ambulance. Certain precepts should guide the manner in which drugs are secured, stored, distributed, and accounted for. Your local protocols will determine the manner in which the drugs are maintained.

If controlled substances, such as narcotics, are administered, the records must be kept separate from other paperwork. As mentioned earlier, the DEA strictly regulates these substances. If drugs are lost or stolen, the supervisor and law enforcement personnel must be notified immediately.

All medications should be stored in an environment with a constant temperature if possible. Temperature, light, moisture, shelf life, and exposure to air all affect the potency of medications. If controlled medications are not used before their expiration dates, they must be destroyed. The destruction must be witnessed by two employees and documented on the proper forms.

Special Considerations in Drug Therapy

▶ Pregnant Patients

Before you administer any medications to a female of childbearing age, the patient should be asked whether she could possibly be pregnant. In an emergency situation, the health of the woman is the priority. However, before using any drug during pregnancy, the expected benefits should be considered against the possible risk to the fetus. Drugs, whether prescription or OTC, have the potential to harm the fetus by crossing the placental barrier, as well as through lactation. A **teratogenic** drug is one that poses a risk to the normal development or health of the unborn fetus.

Changes in a pregnant woman's body also affect the way drugs are processed and may increase the chance of harm to the fetus. Metabolism of drugs in the liver is decreased during pregnancy, along with an increased rate of excretion owing to increased cardiac output.

The FDA has established the following scale with the categories A, B, C, D, and X to indicate drugs that have documented problems in animals and/or humans during pregnancy. Category A drugs pose the least risk to the fetus, while Category X drugs pose the greatest risk. This five-category system is being replaced by a more detailed system that uses narrative summaries to convey prescribing information related to pregnancy (including labor and delivery), lactation, and the risks of a medication to male and female users with reproductive potential. Medications approved after June 2015 have only the narrative summary. Medications approved before June 2015 have a 3-year period to transition to this new format.[2,3] This change was driven by concerns that the five-category system oversimplified risks related to pregnancy and lactation, resulting in poor prescribing decisions.[2] Table 12-4 outlines the pregnancy categories for both classification systems.

There are still many drugs used with unknown effects during pregnancy. For this reason, it is better to

YOU are the Provider — PART 2

You quickly assess the scene for hazards. Finding none, you begin your assessment. You find no obvious trauma, but note fresh needle track marks on the patient's left arm. Assessment of the eyes reveals slightly reactive pupils that are constricted bilaterally. You believe that your patient is experiencing an acute narcotic overdose and prepare a dose of naloxone. You direct your partner to insert an oropharyngeal airway and begin assisting ventilations with a bag-mask device.

Recording Time: 1 Minute	
Appearance	Unresponsive
Level of consciousness	Unresponsive
Airway	Patent
Breathing	Assisted at 10 breaths/min
Circulation	Strong radial pulse, skin is warm, dry, and pink

3. By which route or routes may naloxone be administered?
4. What class of medication is naloxone?

Table 12-4 FDA Drug Category Classification in Pregnant Women

Drug Categories by Letter	Implications
A	Controlled studies in women fail to demonstrate a risk to the fetus in the first trimester (and there is no evidence of a risk in later trimesters), and the possibility of fetal harm appears remote.
B	Either animal reproduction studies have not demonstrated a fetal risk but there are no controlled studies in pregnant women, or animal reproduction studies have shown an adverse effect (other than a decrease in fertility) that was not confirmed in controlled studies in women in the first trimester (and there is no evidence of a risk in later trimesters).
C	Either studies in animals have revealed adverse effects on the fetus (teratogenic or embryocidal or other) and there are no controlled studies in women, or studies in women and animals are not available. Drugs should be given only if the potential benefit justifies the potential risk to the fetus.
D	There is positive evidence of human fetal risk, but the benefits from use in pregnant women may be acceptable despite the risk (eg, if the drug is needed in a life-threatening situation or for a serious disease for which safer drugs cannot be used or are ineffective).
X	Studies in animals or humans have demonstrated fetal abnormalities, there is evidence of fetal risk based on human experience, or both, and the risk of the use of the drug in pregnant women clearly outweighs any possible benefit. The drug is contraindicated in women who are or may become pregnant.
Drug Categories (Pregnancy, Lactation, and Reproductive Potential)[a]	**Type of Information in Narrative Summary[b]**
Pregnancy (includes labor and delivery)	Pregnancy exposure registry Risk summary Clinical considerations Data
Lactation (includes nursing mothers)	Risk summary Clinical considerations Data
Female and male users with reproductive potential	Pregnancy testing Contraception Infertility

[a] Effective June 30, 2015.

[b] Medications approved after June 2015 will have only the narrative summary. Medications approved before June 2015 have a 3-year period to transition to this new format.

Data from: US National Archives and Records Administration. *Code of Federal Regulations*. Title 21, Volume 4, Parts 200 to 299. Revised as of April 1, 1997; FDA pregnancy categories. Drugs.com website. https://www.drugs.com/pregnancy-categories.html. Accessed March 9, 2017; and Pregnancy and lactation labeling (drugs) final rule. US Food and Drug Administration website. http://www.fda.gov/Drugs/DevelopmentApprovalProcess/DevelopmentResources/Labeling/ucm093307.htm. Updated November 18, 2016. Accessed March 9, 2017.

delay pharmacologic treatments for pregnant patients until they reach the hospital, except in life-threatening situations.

In the field, you must be able to quickly evaluate the risks versus the benefits of drug administration. Does the potential benefit to the pregnant woman outweigh the risk to the fetus? If the drug is the only option for saving the woman's life, then that consideration would be paramount. When in doubt, contact medical control to discuss the situation.

▶ Pediatric Patients

Medications have much different effects in adults than they do in children—whether the pediatric patient is a newborn, a neonate, an infant, or a toddler. Young infants have a sharply reduced metabolic capacity. The incomplete development of the gastrointestinal tract in young infants slows **absorption** of oral medications and delays elimination, so the same medication may be more potent in an infant than in an adult.

However, children can metabolize some medications much more quickly than adults do, so they may require relatively higher doses or more frequent administration of some medications. Also, the products of metabolism in children can vary from those seen in adults, which may sometimes result in unexpected responses.

Special Populations

When you are treating pediatric patients, it is imperative to remember that they are not just little adults. Medication dosage is usually based on a child's weight or body surface area as opposed to age because size varies greatly from child to child. If possible, determine the exact weight of the child by asking the parent or guardian. With infants and toddlers, a length-based resuscitation tape works well for estimating and also gives accurate dosage information for most emergency drugs and sizes for endotracheal tubes and IV catheters.

When you are treating neonates, it is important to remember that they have immature body systems and are unable to metabolize drugs as quickly as an older child or adult can. Medications tend to remain in the system for longer periods, resulting in lengthened times of drug effect. Dosages may need to be altered to prevent inadvertent overdose.

Geriatric Patients

The changes in pharmacokinetics in geriatric patients are comparable to those observed in young children. In elderly people, hepatic functions and gastrointestinal activity slow, which delays absorption and elimination. In addition, geriatric patients are often taking several medications; these concomitant therapies may interact and modify the effects of each medication. Furthermore, because geriatric patients may take a large number of medications and may have alterations in their normal mental status, geriatric patients may unintentionally overdose on a particular drug or forget to take it.

Scope of Practice

As an AEMT, you are legally, morally, and ethically responsible for each drug you administer. You must have a good foundation of knowledge of OTC and prescription medications that may interact with drugs you may give, and you must have enough knowledge to obtain a medical history for patients who are unable to communicate.

Drug administration must be safe and therapeutically effective. You should always keep a field guide or other medication reference handy to look up medications that are unfamiliar to you. Follow the standardized national guidelines listed in Table 12-5 when providing drug therapy.

Table 12-5 Guidelines for Providing Drug Therapy
Understand pharmacology.
Use correct precautions and techniques.
Observe and document the effects of drugs, good or bad.
Obtain a drug history from patients, including prescribed medications (name, strength, and daily dosage), over-the-counter medications, vitamins, herbal preparations, and drug reactions. If possible, gather all medications to take along to the hospital with the patient.
Perform an evaluation to identify drug indications and contraindications.
Establish and maintain professional relationships.
Keep your knowledge base current for changes and trends in pharmacology.
Seek drug reference literature.
Consult with medical direction.

Methods of Drug Classification

Classifications of drugs are based on the effect the drugs will have on a particular part of the body or on a specific condition. Antiemetic medications, for example, suppress the sensation of nausea. Many medications fall into more than one classification. For example, promethazine (Phenergan) is an antiemetic and an antihistamine. This section discusses a few of the classifications of drugs and their subcategories.

Drugs or medications can be classified into the following three categories:

- **By body system.** Classification by body system is simply categorizing by the system affected by that drug. Nitroglycerin is a vasodilator that is used predominantly for cardiac ischemia; therefore, it is classified as a cardiac drug. Understanding which systems are affected by which drugs will help you make the appropriate decisions for patient care.

- **Class of agent.** The class of a medication tells how it affects the system. For example, an antipyretic is given to reduce fever, and an antiemetic is used to control vomiting.
- **Mechanism of action.** The mechanism of action is the particular action by which the drug creates its desired effect on an organism. Again, using the example of nitroglycerin, it is a potent vasodilator given for cardiac ischemia because it opens the vessels to allow oxygenated blood to pass through.

Nervous System Classifications

As discussed in Chapter 7, *The Human Body*, the nervous system is the body's principal control system. It is composed of the central nervous system (CNS), made up of the brain and spinal cord, and the peripheral nervous system, which includes all nervous tissue outside the CNS.

Recall that the peripheral nervous system contains the **autonomic nervous system (ANS)**, which controls all of the automatic, or involuntary, functions. The ANS is divided into the sympathetic nervous system and the parasympathetic nervous system. The **sympathetic nervous system** is responsible for the body's response to shock and stress and is known as the "fight-or-flight" division. This response is associated with the release of adrenaline from the adrenal glands. The sympathetic nervous system response is called **adrenergic** because special adrenergic nerve fibers ultimately cause the release of the hormones epinephrine (adrenaline) and norepinephrine (noradrenaline). Sympathetic responses include shunting of blood from the extremities to the vital core organs, increasing the heart rate and respirations, increasing blood pressure, dilation of the pupils, and reduction of digestive system activity.

The **parasympathetic nervous system** relaxes the body. It controls automatic functions during nonstressful times and is referred to as the "rest and relax" division. Stimulation of the parasympathetic nervous system results in effects opposite from those of the sympathetic nervous system. Heart and respiratory rates decrease, lowering the blood pressure, constricting the pupils, and increasing digestive system activity.

The sympathetic and parasympathetic divisions work in constant opposition to each other to maintain basic harmony in the body, with each division taking more precedence in the proper circumstances.

The hormones released by sympathetic system stimulation are carried throughout the body where they cause their intended effects by acting directly on hormone receptors. This stimulates tissues that are not innervated by sympathetic nerves and also prolongs the effects of direct sympathetic stimulation. Adrenergic receptors are located throughout the body and, after stimulation by the appropriate hormone, they cause a response in the target organ. Adrenergic receptors are generally divided into four types Table 12-6.

Table 12-6 Alpha and Beta Responses

Type of Receptor	Response
Alpha-1 (α_1)	Peripheral vasoconstriction
Alpha-2 (α_2)	Peripheral vasodilation Little or no bronchoconstriction
Beta-1 (β_1)	Increased heart rate Increased automaticity Increased contractility Increased conductivity
Beta-2 (β_2)	Bronchodilation Vasodilation

Drugs Affecting the Sympathetic Nervous System

To give the best patient care, it is imperative for you to recognize how certain medications affect the body. Drugs can be given that produce the same effects on a body system as the hormones of the sympathetic nervous system that are released naturally in the body. These drugs are known as **sympathomimetics** because they mimic the effects of the sympathetic nervous system. Medications that have the opposite effect, or inhibit the sympathetic nervous system, are known as **sympatholytics** (also known as antiadrenergics), which antagonize, or fight against the effects of the sympathetic nervous system. Drugs that counteract the action of something else are called **antagonists**, while drugs that bind to a receptor and cause a response are called **agonists**.

Words of Wisdom

Think of the hormones of the sympathetic nervous system as a key that starts a car. When the key is placed in the ignition (or the hormone is placed in the receptor site) and the key is turned, a certain sequence of events occurs to start the car. If you have a duplicate key made and use it to start the car, the same sequence of events takes place. This is exactly what happens when a sympathomimetic drug (the duplicate key) is introduced into the body. The same sequence of events takes place when the duplicate is joined with the receptor site.

Some medications stimulate alpha and beta receptors, whereas others are selective to specific receptors. A medication that is an agonist of an alpha-1 receptor stimulates the receptor, causing vasoconstriction of the vessels, thereby increasing blood pressure, cardiac preload, and afterload. When these receptors are antagonized (suppressed), the blood pressure is lowered by preventing vasoconstriction.

Many patients take medications that belong to the **beta blocker** class. These are used to control blood pressure in some patients and heart rhythm disturbances in others. Beta blockers work by filling a portion of the beta receptor sites—the portion to which beta stimulators would normally bind. In this way, beta effects are prevented.

> **Words of Wisdom**
>
> Imagine beta blockers as the plastic plugs that are placed in electric sockets to prevent children from sticking things into the sockets. The plugs do not do anything; they only plug up the holes. Beta blockers work the same way. They have no effect on the body; they only plug up the receptor sites, preventing beta agonists from binding.

In the prehospital setting, you will often administer drugs that agonize the beta-1 receptors to treat cardiac arrest and hypotension. Stimulation of these receptors increases myocardial contractility. In contrast, antagonizing the beta-1 receptors lowers the blood pressure by limiting the myocardial contractility and the heart rate. It also decreases impulse generation in the heart and slows the conduction at the atrioventricular node, thereby treating tachycardia.

Beta-2-selective drugs cause bronchodilation with little effect on the heart, which only has beta-1 receptor sites. Stimulation of the beta-2 receptors allows you to treat asthma and other diseases that cause excessive narrowing of the bronchioles.

Drugs Affecting the Parasympathetic Nervous System

Like the sympathetic division, agonists to the parasympathetic nervous system are known as **parasympathomimetics** and antagonists are known as **parasympatholytics**. One of the most commonly used parasympatholytics is the drug atropine, which is used for symptomatic bradycardia and exposure to organophosphates and certain chemical nerve agents.

Parasympathomimetics are also called **cholinergic** medications because they stimulate the cholinergic receptors, to which acetylcholine (ACh) normally binds. ACh is an important neurotransmitter in the parasympathetic nervous system. Cholinergic medications may act directly or indirectly on cholinergic receptors. A drug that has direct action binds with cholinergic receptors, thereby blocking ACh. If it acts to prevent activation of the receptor by binding, its function is described as **anticholinergic**. A drug that has indirect action interacts with acetylcholinesterase (AChE), which normally deactivates ACh. When a drug

> **Words of Wisdom**
>
> Atropine is a potent *parasympatholytic* that is used to increase the heart rate in symptomatic bradycardia. Because increasing the heart rate is an effect of the sympathetic nervous system, you might think that atropine is classified as a sympathomimetic. However, atropine has no effect on the heart itself. Instead, it acts as a roadblock to the vagus nerve and prevents innervation by ACh. It does not directly affect the target organ, in this case the heart, but prevents anything from passing through. Because it decreases the effects of the parasympathetic nervous system (which slows the heart rate), it is an antagonist to the parasympathetic division, or a parasympatholytic.

interacts with AChE, deactivation of ACh does not occur. If excessive cholinergics are present, the patient may exhibit the SLUDGEM symptoms: increased Salivation, sweating; Lacrimation (excessive tearing of the eyes); Urination; Defecation, drooling, diarrhea; Gastrointestinal upset and cramps; Emesis (vomiting); Muscle twitching/miosis (pinpoint pupils). Patients exposed to certain fertilizers, insecticides, VX (a nerve agent), and sarin gas exhibit SLUDGEM symptoms because all of these substances have cholinergic properties.

Parasympatholytics are also called anticholinergic medications; they block the two types of cholinergic receptors (muscarinic and nicotinic). **Muscarinic cholinergic antagonists** block ACh exclusively at the muscarinic receptors. Atropine, for example, is a muscarinic cholinergic antagonist; it decreases secretions, increases the heart rate, dilates the pupils, and decreases gastrointestinal system activity. On the other hand, nicotinic cholinergic antagonists block ACh exclusively at the nicotinic receptors. This inhibition effectively disables the ANS, so it is virtually never used.

▶ Analgesics and Antagonists

Analgesics include medications that relieve pain—that is, induce analgesia (the absence of the sensation of pain). Sometimes the analgesic itself is not sufficient to relieve pain, in which case an adjunct medication may be given to enhance the effects of the analgesic.

The most common class of medications used for analgesia in the prehospital setting is opioid agonists. **Opioid agonists**, which are similar to or derived from the opium plant, bind to opiate receptors. By blocking these receptors, they prevent the neurons from sending pain signals.[4] These medications are also CNS depressants. Fentanyl (Sublimaze) is a popular opioid agonist because it is rapid-acting, is very potent, and has a relatively short **duration of action**. The patient will experience analgesia within approximately 90 seconds, and the drug's effective duration is approximately 30 minutes. Morphine is a popular option for prehospital analgesia. In addition to analgesia, morphine has a tendency to cause a euphoric feeling.

Several **nonopioid analgesics** exist, many of which are available as OTC drugs. Many of these nonopioid analgesics have antipyretic properties as well, meaning they can reduce the patient's fever. All of these medications alter the production of prostaglandins and cyclooxygenase (COX) to produce their effects. Three forms of nonopioid analgesics are particularly popular: salicylates (such as aspirin); **nonsteroidal anti-inflammatory drugs (NSAIDs)** (such as ibuprofen); and para-aminophenol derivatives (such as acetaminophen [Tylenol]).

The NSAIDs are designed to reduce pain, inflammation, and fever. They work by inhibiting the COX enzymes, which produce the chemical prostaglandin; prostaglandin promotes pain, inflammation, and fever. Aspirin differs slightly from other NSAIDs in that it targets the COX-1 enzymes to reduce platelet aggregation, which provides great benefit in patients who are suspected of experiencing a myocardial infarction by helping to keep clots from forming and propagating. This also explains why you cannot substitute another NSAID such as ibuprofen, which is a nonselective COX inhibitor, for aspirin in this situation.

Opioid antagonists reverse the effects of opioid drugs. They bind with the opiate receptors in an antagonistic manner; as a result of this binding, the opioid molecules cannot get to the receptor, and the receptor cannot initiate its action. The most common opioid antagonist used in the prehospital setting is naloxone (Narcan).

Finally, **opioid agonist-antagonists** have agonistic and antagonistic properties. They are often preferred because they can decrease pain but do not diminish the function of the respiratory system or result in dependence or addiction, unlike some other analgesics.

▶ Antianxiety, Sedative, and Hypnotic Drugs

Drugs that produce sedation are used to help a patient sleep through a medical procedure. To ensure that the patient sleeps through the event, he or she also receives drugs that produce hypnosis. Drugs that create sedation and hypnosis include benzodiazepines, barbiturates, opioid agonists, and nonbarbiturate hypnotics. There are currently no drugs in these categories that are within the scope of practice of the AEMT.

Benzodiazepines are the sedatives most commonly used to prepare patients for invasive procedures. Although their exact mechanism of action is not fully understood, these drugs are believed to affect the neurotransmitter gamma-aminobutyric acid (GABA) in the brain. Benzodiazepine molecules bind to a receptor near GABA binding sites, which is thought to enhance their affinity for GABA. This increased affinity causes brain activity to slow. **Barbiturates** are believed to work similarly to benzodiazepines by increasing the affinity between receptor sites and the neurotransmitter GABA.

The **nonbarbiturate hypnotics** have almost identical properties to benzodiazepines and barbiturates in how they affect GABA receptors. The difference is that nonbarbiturate hypnotics tend to have comparatively fewer side effects, particularly regarding cardiovascular compromise.

▶ Anticonvulsants

A seizure is a state of neurologic hyperactivity. Active seizures generally require treatment in the prehospital setting because of the complications associated with them. Although the exact mechanism behind **anticonvulsant medications** is not completely clear, these drugs are believed to work by inhibiting the influx of sodium into cells. This halt of sodium transport decreases the cells' ability to depolarize and propagate the seizures. Several other types of drugs are used as anticonvulsants, including benzodiazepines, barbiturates, hydantoins, and valproic acids.

▶ Stimulants

A common group of CNS agents is **stimulants**, which exert their action by excitation of the CNS. The CNS can be stimulated in one of two ways: by increasing excitatory neurotransmitters or by decreasing inhibitory neurotransmitters. Caffeine, cocaine, and amphetamines (prescription and illicit) are examples of CNS stimulants. They increase the release of dopamine and norepinephrine to increase wakefulness and awareness and reduce drowsiness and fatigue. They also increase tachycardia and hypertension and can cause seizures and psychosis. High doses of these agents can cause increased nervousness, irritability, tremors, and headache. Some people may also experience withdrawal symptoms when they stop taking stimulants.

▶ Depressants

In other cases, patients may be prescribed CNS **depressants**. These agents are used to slow brain activity. They may be prescribed to treat anxiety, muscle tension, pain, insomnia, stress, panic attacks, and, in some cases, seizures. Some other CNS depressants are used as anesthetics. Examples of CNS depressants include lorazepam (Ativan), triazolam (Halcion), chlordiazepoxide (Librium), diazepam (Valium), alprazolam (Xanax), and zolpidem tartrate (Ambien).

▶ Psychotherapeutic Drugs

Most psychotherapeutic drugs work by blocking dopamine receptors in the brain. Schizophrenia is often treated with medications that fit into the phenothiazine and butyrophenone classifications. These medications are associated with a host of side effects, which may include extrapyramidal symptoms, orthostatic hypotension, and sedation. They also tend to cause sexual dysfunction. **Extrapyramidal symptoms** include a wide array of symptoms such as involuntary movements, tremors, rigidity, muscle contractions, restlessness, and changes in breathing and heart rate.

Depression is a common disorder for which many treatments are available. In particular, depression is often treated with selective serotonin reuptake inhibitors and monoamine oxidase inhibitors, which block the metabolism of monoamines in the brain. Although their popularity is waning, tricyclic antidepressants are still occasionally used as antidepressants.

▶ Drugs Affecting the Cardiovascular System

The walls of the heart are composed of many interconnected cells. These cells are specialized to perform particular functions: some conduct electrical impulses; others cause the heart to contract. Medications targeting the cardiovascular system are classified according to their effects on these specialized cells.

The various effects on the heart are categorized as follows. A **chronotropic** effect is one that affects the heart rate. An **inotropic** effect changes the force of contraction. A **dromotropic** effect is when a drug alters the velocity of the conduction of electricity through the heart. All three types of effects can be positive or negative. For example, if there is a positive chronotropic effect, the heart rate has increased. If there is a negative inotropic effect, the heart is not squeezing as forcefully.

Cardiac Glycosides

Cardiac glycosides are a class of medications that are derived from plants. These drugs block certain ionic pumps in the heart cell membranes, which indirectly increases calcium concentrations. However, cardiac glycosides generally have a small therapeutic index (margin of safety) and are associated with numerous side effects.

Antidysrhythmic Medications

Antidysrhythmic medications have long been used in the prehospital setting to treat and prevent cardiac rhythm disorders. These medications can have direct and indirect effects on cardiac tissue. Antidysrhythmics are further classified into the following four groups according to their fundamental mode of action on the heart:

- **Sodium channel blockers** slow the conduction through the heart; in other words, they have a negative dromotropic effect.
- Beta blockers reduce the adrenergic stimulation of the beta receptors.
- **Potassium channel blockers** increase the heart's contractility (positive inotropy) and work against the reentry of blocked impulses.
- **Calcium channel blockers** block the inflow of calcium into the cardiac cells, thereby decreasing the force of contraction and automaticity. They may also decrease the conduction velocity (negative dromotropic effect).

Antihypertensive Medications

Approximately 75 million people in the United States have hypertension.[5] Medications administered to treat

YOU are the Provider PART 3

Because you note numerous track marks on the patient's arms and extensive scar tissue, you opt to administer naloxone via the intranasal route. You proceed to draw 0.4 mg of naloxone in a 1-mL syringe, attach your mucosal atomizer device (MAD) to the syringe, and, while instructing your partner to temporarily stop ventilations, inject the medication into the patient's left nares. As soon as you have administered the medication, you instruct your partner to continue ventilations. Knowing that narcotic overdose patients often become combative after the naloxone begins to work, you advise your partner and the law enforcement officer to stay alert for the possibility of a combative patient.

Recording Time: 8 Minutes	
Respirations	Assisted at 12 breaths/min
Pulse	Strong and regular, 82 beats/min
Skin	Warm, dry, and pink
Blood pressure	124/66 mm Hg
Oxygen saturation (Spo_2)	100% on 15 L/min via bag-mask device
Pupils	Constricted

5. What is the mechanism of action of naloxone?

hypertension, known as **antihypertensives**, have the following treatment goals: keep blood pressure within normal limits, maintain or improve blood flow, and reduce the stress placed on the heart.

Diuretic medications cause the kidneys to remove excess amounts of salt and water in the body. By lowering the total fluid volume, they reduce the level of stress placed on the cardiovascular system. In particular, diuretics lower the preload on the heart and decrease the stroke volume. **Vasodilator medications** act on the smooth muscles of the arterioles and veins. This property explains why nitroglycerin, a vasodilator, is so beneficial in treating myocardial ischemia. Unfortunately, the dilation of these vessels prompts a response from the sympathetic nervous system. Consequently, when vasodilators are used to lower blood pressure, the patient must also take medications that inhibit the sympathetic nervous system.

Sympathetic blocking agents include beta blockers and adrenergic inhibitors. Beta blockers, mentioned earlier, compete with epinephrine to bind with available receptor sites, thereby diminishing the effects of beta stimulation.

Angiotensin-converting enzyme (ACE) inhibitors target the renin-angiotensin-aldosterone system, which partially controls blood pressure. ACE inhibitors suppress the conversion of angiotensin I to angiotensin II, thereby decreasing blood pressure. Angiotensin II is a potent vasoconstrictor that promotes smooth muscle contraction in the arterioles throughout the body. This constriction raises the blood pressure by increasing peripheral resistance.

Calcium channel blockers, mentioned earlier, have antidysrhythmic and antihypertensive properties. By causing the dilation of coronary arteries, calcium channel blockers enable more oxygen to reach the heart via coronary artery dilation. In addition, they prevent the contraction of smooth vascular muscle, which reduces resistance in the peripheral vascular system.

Anticoagulants, Fibrinolytics, and Blood Components

Platelets repair damage in the blood vessels. This function is critical because defects in blood vessels can cause blood flow to slow, sometimes enough to result in the formation of a blood clot (also known as a thrombus). Abnormal thrombi may cause a life-threatening crisis such as acute coronary syndrome or stroke. A variety of medications are used to prevent or minimize the detrimental effects of thrombi.

Antiplatelet agents interfere with the aggregation, or collection, of platelets. They do not break down aggregated platelets but simply prevent further buildup of these blood cells. Notably, salicylic acid (aspirin) has substantial antiplatelet properties and has proved important in the prehospital setting because of its ability to minimize the damage to the myocardium in acute coronary syndrome.

Anticoagulant drugs, as their name suggests, work against coagulation, thereby preventing thrombi from forming. Some patients can be prescribed anticoagulants on a long-term basis as a preventive measure, thereby avoiding the formation of thrombi associated with surgeries and certain cardiovascular conditions. You need to be aware of anticoagulant use, particularly when patients have sustained a traumatic injury. Just as anticoagulants prevent blood coagulation in the vascular system, they can also prevent the life-saving coagulation needed to prevent blood loss.

After a blood clot has formed, a **fibrinolytic agent** may be administered to dissolve the thrombus and prevent it from breaking off and entering the bloodstream, where it might do further damage. Fibrinolytic agents promote the digestion of fibrin (the protein involved in forming a blood clot). The use of fibrinolytic medications in the prehospital setting remains controversial, and, in some circumstances, other forms of reperfusion therapy may be indicated.

▶ Drugs Affecting the Respiratory System

Oxygen is the most commonly used medication in the prehospital setting. And it is, in fact, a medication—which means it has appropriate and inappropriate uses and some side effects. Supplementary oxygen therapy is covered in depth in Chapter 11, *Airway Management*.

Patients may be taking a gamut of medications to treat respiratory problems, depending on their symptoms. Especially during the cold and influenza seasons, use of OTC decongestant medications is common. Patients may also take antihistamines during allergy season. Try to find out which medications your patient is taking, and know the effects that these drugs may have on other medications and the signs and symptoms they can produce. Although each decongestant varies slightly in its mechanism of action, all such medications seek to reduce tissue edema, facilitate drainage, and maintain the patency of the sinuses.

Unfortunately, the fact that these and other medications are readily available sometimes results in their illicit use. People looking to get high have been known to overdose on pseudoephedrine (a decongestant), dextromethorphan (an antitussive), or diphenhydramine (an antihistamine).

Serious respiratory emergencies often arise from severe narrowing of any portion of the respiratory tract. The respiratory tract is lined by smooth muscle fibers that influence the diameter of the airway. Control of the smooth muscles is maintained by the ANS.

Many respiratory emergency treatments attempt to expand the respiratory tract by using sympathomimetic medications. Complications arise when patients with respiratory emergencies eventually experience decreased amounts of oxygen to the vital organs, including the heart. Increased heart rate and greater force of contraction result in a higher demand for oxygen—but oxygen is already in short supply in a respiratory emergency. Therefore, stimulation of the beta-2 receptors, which produces bronchodilation and vasodilation, is the most beneficial to patients with respiratory emergencies. These drugs produce smaller increases in heart rate and force of contraction, which in turn decreases the amount of oxygen needed for the myocardium to function.

A second-line treatment in a respiratory emergency is from **xanthines**. This class of drugs relieves airway constriction by relaxing the smooth muscles of the bronchioles and stimulating cardiac muscles to work harder, thereby increasing blood flow. These drugs also stimulate the CNS—one notable xanthine is caffeine, the well-known CNS stimulant.

Other respiratory medications suppress the inflammatory response that typically causes acute distress for patients with restrictive airway diseases. In the acute care setting, corticosteroids—including methylprednisolone (Solu-Medrol) and dexamethasone (Decadron)—can be administered for this purpose.

Drugs Affecting the Pancreas

A variety of hypoglycemic medications are available to affect the pancreas. Still others may not act on the pancreas directly, but instead alter the way insulin (produced by the pancreas) is used by the body. In the absence of pancreatic function, patients may take insulin injections.

To directly affect the pancreas, sulfonylureas increase insulin secretion from the pancreatic beta cells. This medication is effective only if patients have residual beta cell function. Insulin sensitivity is increased by thiazolidinediones and biguanides, which are oral hypoglycemic agents.

Drugs Affecting the Immunologic System

Patients who undergo organ transplantation or have an autoimmune disease are often prescribed **immunosuppressant medications**. Immunosuppressants are intended to inhibit the body's ability to attack the "foreign" organ, or, in the case of autoimmune diseases, the medications inhibit the body's attack on itself. These drugs are generally derived from fungi or bacteria and tend to have a complicated mechanism of action. Put succinctly, they inhibit lymphocytes and T cells from carrying out their immune functions.

Vitamins and Minerals

Vitamins and minerals are necessary substances that allow for normal metabolism, growth and development, and cellular function. Patients may be taking vitamin and mineral supplements to replace deficient items or as a preventive measure. Vitamins affect a wide variety of functions, but one particular vitamin used in the prehospital setting is thiamine (vitamin B_1). Thiamine aids in converting carbohydrates into energy. People with alcoholism, among others, tend to be deficient in this vitamin.

Fluids and Electrolytes

Several types of IV fluids may be administered to patients. Crystalloid solutions are typically used in the prehospital setting and can be isotonic, hypotonic, or hypertonic. Isotonic solutions provide a stable medium for the administration of medication and provide effective fluid and electrolyte replacement. Hypertonic solutions help provide nutrition. Hypotonic solutions are beneficial in dehydration situations but not in hypovolemic cases. In addition to crystalloids, you may administer colloid solutions to your patients. IV fluids are discussed in detail in Chapter 13, *Vascular Access and Medication Administration*.

> **Words of Wisdom**
>
> When you are questioning a patient about medications, be sure to mention the pertinence of any herbal or OTC preparations. Patients may use herbal alternatives as a substitute for more expensive prescription medications. Most patients do not consider these agents to be "medications" because they do not require a prescription. Any of these may interact with prescribed pharmaceuticals and may produce allergic or idiosyncratic reactions. There are generally no FDA requirements for the manufacture and distribution of herbal preparations. With no regulation, they may be incorrectly prepared or labeled, resulting in serious complications.

Drug Forms

The form that a medication comes in usually determines its route of administration. For example, a tablet or a spray cannot be administered through a needle. The manufacturer chooses the form to ensure the proper route for the medication, the timing of its release into the bloodstream, and its effects on the target organs or body systems. As an AEMT, you should be familiar with the following seven medication forms.

Solid Drugs

Most medications that are given by mouth to adult patients are in tablet or capsule form **Figure 12-1**. Capsules are gelatin shells filled with powdered or liquid medication. If the capsule contains liquid, the shell is sealed and usually soft. If the capsule contains powder, the shell can usually be pulled apart. Tablets often contain other materials that are mixed with the medication and compressed under high pressure.

Some tablets are designed to dissolve very quickly in small amounts of liquid so that they can be given sublingually (SL) and absorbed rapidly. An example is the SL nitroglycerin tablet used for chest pain by patients with cardiac conditions. These medications are especially useful in emergency situations. Tablets may also be ground into a powder, allowing them to be absorbed more quickly. Generally, a medication that must be swallowed is less useful in an emergency because the digestive tract provides a slower route of delivery. For example, an oral pain

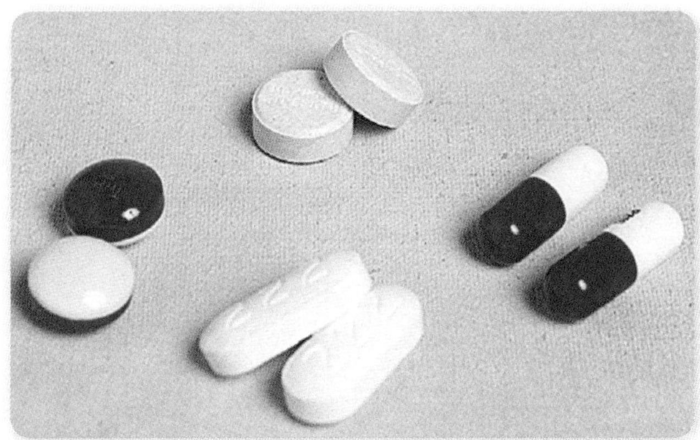

Figure 12-1 Tablets and capsules are typically taken by mouth and enter the bloodstream through the digestive system.

medication is less useful than an IV pain medication when pain relief is needed within minutes.

Pills are solid drugs that are shaped into a ball or oval to be swallowed. They are often coated to disguise an unpleasant taste.

Suppositories are another form of solid drugs that are administered by inserting them into the rectum. These medications are more rapidly absorbed through the rectal mucosa than those that must travel through the upper portion of the digestive tract. Suppositories are not administered by AEMTs.

Liquid Drugs

A **solution** is a liquid mixture of one or more substances that cannot be separated by filtering or allowing the mixture to stand. Solutions can be given by almost any route. When given by mouth, solutions may be absorbed from the stomach rather quickly because the medication is already dissolved. Solutions that irritate the stomach may be applied topically to the skin, sprayed SL, or inhaled. For example, you may need to assist in the SL delivery of a nitroglycerin spray Figure 12-2. Many solutions can be given as an IV, intramuscular (IM), or subcutaneous injection. If a patient has a severe allergic reaction, you may help administer a solution of epinephrine IM using an auto-injector.

Many substances do not dissolve well in liquids. Some of these can be ground into fine particles and evenly distributed throughout a liquid by shaking or stirring. This type of mixture is called a **suspension**. An example of a suspension is activated charcoal, which you may give to patients who have taken overdoses of certain medications or ingested certain poisons.

There are several other types of liquid drugs that you may encounter occasionally that include alcohol in their preparation. Tinctures are liquid preparations that are alcohol based. The name of the material contained in the tincture other than alcohol is added to the name of the tincture, such as tincture of iodine. Spirits are also

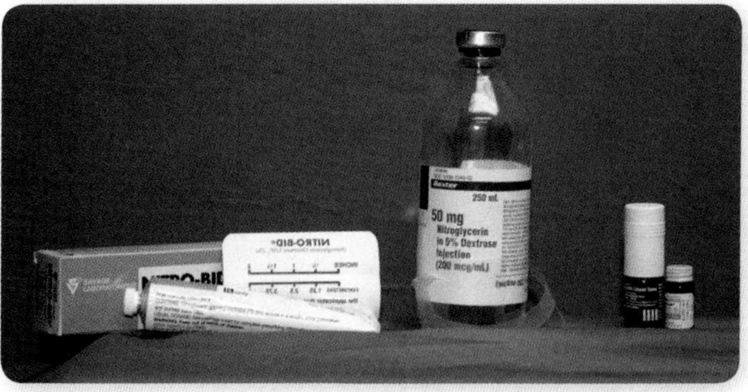

Figure 12-2 Nitroglycerin, which is prescribed for chest pain, is often given sublingually as a spray or as a tablet.

alcohol solutions that are volatile. Elixirs constitute one of the most common types of medicinal preparations taken orally in liquid form and are made up of a sweetened, aromatic, hydroalcoholic liquid.

> **Words of Wisdom**
>
> Suspensions separate if they stand or are filtered. It is important that you shake a suspension well before administering it to ensure that the patient receives the right amount of medication.

Syrups are mixtures with a high sugar content that are designed to disguise the taste of the medication. These are most commonly used for children's medications. An emulsion is a mixture of two liquids that are not mutually soluble. Emulsions are generally a mixture of water and oil that must be thoroughly shaken to mix.

Metered-Dose Inhalers

If liquids or solids are broken into small enough droplets or particles, they can be inhaled. A **metered-dose inhaler (MDI)** is a miniature spray canister used to direct such substances through the mouth and into the lungs Figure 12-3. An MDI delivers the same amount of medication each time it is used. Because an inhaled medication usually is a suspension, the MDI must be shaken vigorously before the medication is administered. Patients with respiratory illnesses such as asthma and emphysema often use MDIs.

Topical Medications

Lotions, creams, and ointments all are **topical medications**, that is, they are applied to the surface of the skin and affect only that area. Of these three, lotions contain the largest amount of water and are absorbed the quickest. Calamine lotion is an example of a medical lotion. Creams, in turn, are absorbed more slowly than lotions but faster than ointments. Hydrocortisone cream, used to diminish skin itching, is an example of a medical cream. Ointments contain the smallest amount of water, resulting in a slower

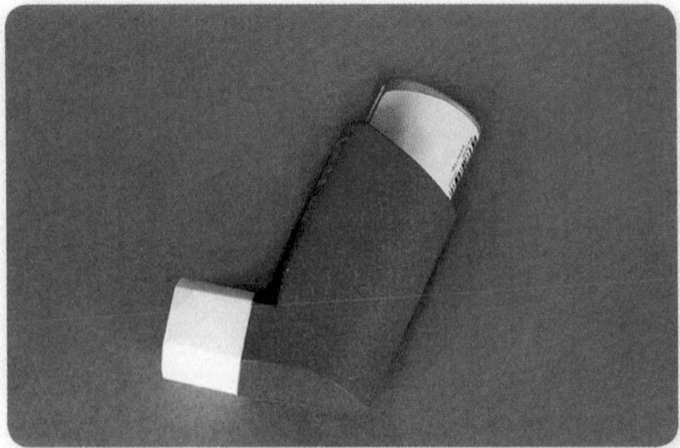

Figure 12-3 Some medications are inhaled into the lungs with a metered-dose inhaler so that they can be absorbed into the bloodstream more quickly.

rate of absorption of the medication. Neosporin first aid ointment is an example of a medical ointment.

▶ Transcutaneous Medications

Transcutaneous or transdermal medications are designed to be absorbed through the skin, or transcutaneously. These medications can affect other areas of the body. Nitroglycerin for patients with chest pain and fentanyl for pain management, for example, are commonly encountered medications that are administered transdermally through a paste or a patch **Figure 12-4**. Nitroglycerin paste usually has properties or delivery systems that help to dilate the blood vessels in the skin, thus speeding absorption into the bloodstream. In contrast to most topical medicines, which work directly on the application site, transcutaneous medications are usually intended for systemic effects.

Safety

If a medication that can be absorbed transdermally comes in contact with your skin while administering it, you can absorb it just as readily as the patient can. When you are removing a medication patch from a patient's skin, be sure not to touch the medication even with your gloves on. Grasp the edge of the dressing or patch with your fingers and gently pull it away from the skin. Use a 4- x 4-inch gauze to wipe the excess medication off the patient.

▶ Gels

A **gel** is a semiliquid substance that is administered orally through capsules or plastic tubes. Gels usually have the consistency of pastes or creams but are transparent. Depending on your local protocol, as an AEMT you may give **oral glucose** in gel form to a conscious patient with a low blood glucose level **Figure 12-5**.

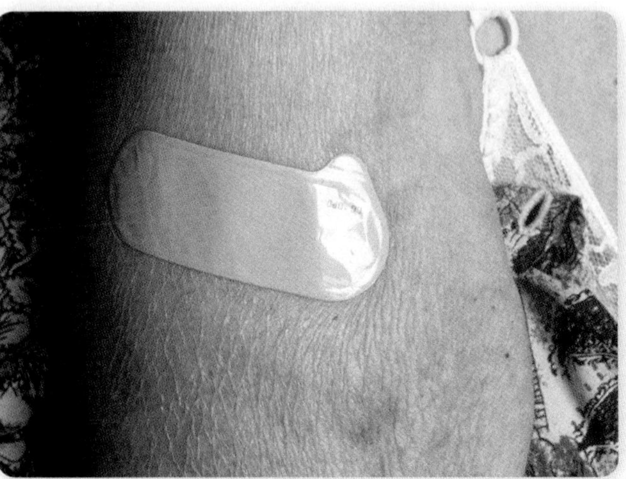

Figure 12-4 Some medications are transcutaneous, or administered through the skin, such as the nitroglycerin patch shown.

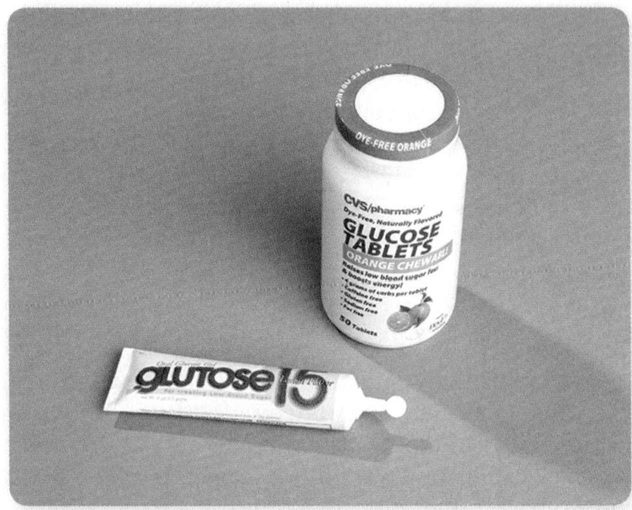

Figure 12-5 Oral glucose, used in diabetic emergencies, is available in gel and tablet form.

▶ Gases

Gaseous medications are neither solid nor liquid and often are delivered in an operating room. The medication that is most commonly used in gas form in the prehospital setting is oxygen. You might not think of oxygen as a medication because it is all around us and we all use it. However, in its concentrated form, it is a potent medication that has systemic effects. You will usually administer oxygen through a nasal cannula, a nonrebreathing mask, or bag-mask device when ventilating a patient.

Nitrous oxide is another medication that comes in gaseous form and has been used in the prehospital environment. It is an analgesic that may be administered by AEMTs to reduce pain. Nitrous oxide is administered simply by inhalation through a mask and has both analgesic and euphoric effects.

Routes of Drug Administration

The route of drug administration affects the rate at which the onset of action occurs and may affect the therapeutic response that results. The choice of the route of administration is crucial in determining the suitability of a drug. Drugs are given for their local or systemic effects. Absorption is the process by which medications travel through body tissues until they reach the bloodstream.

Enteral drugs are those that are administered along any portion of the gastrointestinal tract. They include the following:

- **Oral**. Many medications are taken by mouth, per os (PO), and enter the bloodstream through the digestive system. This process can take as long as 1 hour.
- **Rectal**. Per rectum (PR) means "by rectum." There are no AEMT medications that are administered rectally, with the possible exception of 50% dextrose (D_{50}) if allowed by local protocols, and if allowed, rectal administration of D_{50} would be done only as a last resort.

Parenteral drugs are those that are administered through any route other than the gastrointestinal tract. There are many parenteral routes. Ones with which the AEMT may need to be familiar include the following:

- **Intravenous (IV) injection**. Intravenous means "into the vein." Medications that need to enter the bloodstream immediately may be injected directly into a vein. This is the fastest way to deliver a medication, but the IV route cannot be used for all medications. For example, aspirin, oxygen, and charcoal cannot be given by the IV route.
- **Intraosseous (IO)**. Intraosseous means "into the bone." Medications that are delivered via this route reach the bloodstream through the bone marrow. To administer medication into the marrow requires drilling a needle through the bone cortex. Because this is painful, the IO route of delivery is used most often in patients who are unresponsive as a result of cardiac arrest or extreme shock. Most commonly, the IO route is reserved for children who have fewer available (or difficult to access) IV sites.
- **Subcutaneous injection**. Subcutaneous means "beneath the skin." A subcutaneous injection is given into the tissue between the skin and the muscle. Because there is less blood here than in the muscles, medications that are delivered via this route are generally absorbed

YOU are the Provider — PART 4

Approximately 2 minutes after administration of the naloxone, the patient begins to stir. You inform your partner to stop assisting ventilations and place the patient on a nonrebreathing mask at 15 L/min. He is groggy at first, but quickly regains a more normal mental status, asking what happened. You explain to the patient that you believe that he overdosed on narcotics, to which he states, "Not again." You inform the patient that the medication that you gave him to reverse his overdose might not last as long as the substances are in his system and that he should be transported to the emergency department. He reluctantly agrees to transport. You assist the patient onto the stretcher and initiate nonemergent transport to the hospital. During this time, you are monitoring his airway and mental status to ensure that the naloxone continues to work. On arrival at the emergency department, you turn over care to the awaiting staff.

Recording Time: 16 Minutes	
Respirations	16 breaths/min
Pulse	Strong and regular, 68 beats/min
Skin	Warm, dry, and pink
Blood pressure	122/74 mm Hg
Oxygen saturation (Spo_2)	100% on 15 L/min via nonrebreathing mask
Pupils	Pupils Equal, Round, and Reactive to Light and Accommodation (PERRLA)

6. What is the half-life of naloxone?

more slowly, and their effects last longer. A subcutaneous injection is a useful way to deliver medications that cannot be taken by mouth, as long as they do not irritate or damage the tissue. Commonly, a daily insulin shot is given this way to a patient with diabetes. Also, epinephrine can be given by this route. Like the IM route, subcutaneous-administered medications are less effective in patients with decreased peripheral perfusion.

- **Intramuscular (IM) injection**. Intramuscular means "into the muscle." Usually, medications that are administered via IM injection are absorbed quickly because muscles are highly vascular. Some types of medications, though, are designed for a slower, sustained release from the muscle. Many such medications have the prefix "depo" in their names, meaning that they form a deposit in the muscle after being injected. Not all medications can be administered IM. IM injections can cause damage to muscle tissue and result in uneven, unreliable absorption. This is especially true in people who are experiencing decreased peripheral perfusion (as in shock).
- **Sublingual (SL)**. Sublingual means "under the tongue." Medications that take the SL route, such as nitroglycerin tablets, are absorbed by the venous plexus under the tongue and enter the bloodstream through the oral mucous membranes within minutes. This route not only is faster, it also protects medications from chemicals in the digestive system such as acids that can weaken or inactivate them.
- **Buccal**. The buccal route is similar to the SL route. The medication is placed between the cheek and gums, where it is absorbed into the bloodstream. This is a common route for glucose gel.
- Transcutaneous or transdermal. Both these terms refer to the route of absorbing medication through the layers of the skin and into the bloodstream. Some medications can be absorbed transcutaneously, such as the nicotine in nicotine patches used by people who are trying to quit smoking. On occasion, a medication that comes in another form is administered transcutaneously to achieve a slower, longer-lasting effect. An example is an adhesive patch containing nitroglycerin.
- **Intranasal (IN)**. Intranasal is a relatively new format for the delivery of medication. In this route, a medication is pushed through a specialized atomizer device called a **mucosal atomizer device (MAD)**. The liquid medication is turned into a spray and is administered into a nostril. Blood flow to the head and face is very high; therefore, absorption is rather quick with this route. Naloxone can be administered via this route to some patients who are experiencing an overdose.
- **Inhalation**. Drugs administered by the inhalation route are aerosolized and drawn into the lungs through the mouth or nose as the patient breathes. These include nebulized medications and MDIs. Some medications are inhaled into the lungs so that they can be absorbed into the blood more quickly. Others are inhaled because they actually work in the lungs. Generally, inhalation helps to minimize the effects of the medication in other body tissues. Inhaled medications come in the form of aerosols, fine powders, and sprays.

Table 12-7 Routes of Administration and Rates of Absorption

Route	Rate
Enteral	
Sublingual (SL)	Rapid
Per rectum (PR)	Rapid
Ingestion (oral)	Slow
Parenteral	
Intravenous (IV)	Immediate
Intraosseous (IO)	Immediate
Inhalation	Rapid
Intranasal (IN)	Rapid
Intramuscular (IM)	Moderate
Subcutaneous	Slow
Transcutaneous	Slow

Table 12-7 lists common routes of medication administration and rates of absorption.

Pharmacokinetics: Movement of Drugs Through the Body

The effectiveness of a drug relates to its pharmaceutical properties, pharmacokinetics, and pharmacodynamics. Pharmaceutical properties determine a drug's concentration at its site of action.

Drugs modify the existing functions of tissues and organs; they do not give new functions to tissues or organs. Also, drugs generally cause multiple actions rather than a single effect. A drug action, as previously discussed, is the result of a physiochemical interaction between the drug and a molecule in the body, such as a receptor.

Once administered, drugs go through four stages: absorption, distribution, metabolism, and excretion. The study of these four stages and the actions of drugs is **pharmacokinetics**.

Principles of Pharmacokinetics

You must carefully consider the pharmacokinetic properties of any medication you are thinking of administering to a patient. As a medication is administered, the body begins a complex process of moving the medication, possibly altering the structure of the medication, and ultimately removing the medication from the body. The medication dose, route of administration, and clinical status of a patient will largely determine the duration and effectiveness of the medication (called pharmacodynamics, and discussed later in this chapter). The actions of absorption, distribution, biotransformation, and elimination are discussed in detail in the following text.

The pharmacokinetics section of medication profiles typically states the **onset of action**, **peak**, and duration of action for most medications. These values vary by route of administration and may have a broad range, depending on characteristics of individual patients. The onset and peak of a medication are generally related to absorption and distribution. A minimum dose or concentration of medication must be present at certain sites in the body for clinical effects to occur.

The duration of action is generally related to medication metabolism and elimination. As the amount of a medication near cell receptors (or other site of action) decreases, the clinical effects caused by the medication begin to decrease and normal function resumes.

If a medication permanently binds with a receptor site or irreversibly alters the function of a cell, the duration of the medication is determined by the body's ability to regenerate cells. In these cases, the duration of action of a medication may be almost entirely unrelated to the dose or concentration present in the body. A single dose of aspirin, for example, is rapidly eliminated by the body, usually within several hours, but can cause an inhibition of platelet activity lasting for 3 to 10 days.

Drug Absorption

The passage of a substance through some surface of the body into body fluids and tissues is known as absorption. Numerous variables affect drug absorption, including the nature of the absorbing surface, blood flow to the site of administration, solubility of the drug, pH, drug concentration, dosage form, route of administration, bioavailability, diffusion, osmosis, and filtration. Table 12-8 describes these primary factors.

Table 12-8 Primary Factors of Drug Absorption

Factor	Discussion
Nature of the absorbing surface	Some surfaces are highly permeable. It is much easier for a drug to travel through a single layer of cells than through multiple layers. The greater the surface area exposed to the substance, the greater the absorption.
Blood flow to the site of administration	Blood flow to a particular area regulates how fast the medication is absorbed into the central circulation. This is why administering medications intramuscularly to a patient having a seizure produces a minimal effect. Because of the seizure activity, blood flow to the extremities is diminished. Medications introduced intramuscularly tend to stay in the tissues until the seizure activity stops. When blood flow resumes, the patient may experience the effects of an overdose if multiple doses were given.
Solubility of the drug	The more soluble (dissolvable) the drug, the faster it enters the circulatory system.
pH	The pH of the body and that of the drug can affect the rate of absorption. Some medications are coated to keep them from being absorbed before they reach the small intestine because the acid environment of the stomach can destroy the drug.
Drug concentration	The more of a drug available for absorption, the more that will be absorbed and the more that will remain in the system. Often, a loading dose (bolus) of a medication is given, followed by a continuous infusion to maintain a constant therapeutic level.

(continued)

Table 12-8 Primary Factors of Drug Absorption *(continued)*

Factor	Discussion
Dosage form	Form has a lot to do with the speed of absorption. A liquid will be absorbed much more quickly than a pill, which must be dissolved before it is absorbed.
Routes of administration	IV administration is the most rapid route for delivering drugs in the prehospital environment. The medication bypasses the gastrointestinal absorption process because it is introduced directly into the vascular system. Intramuscular and subcutaneous routes are much slower because they depend on blood flow to the area in which the medication is administered.
Bioavailability	Bioavailability is the rate and extent to which an active drug enters the general circulation, permitting access to the site of action. It is determined by measurement of the concentration of the drug in body fluids.
Diffusion	Diffusion is the movement of solutes (molecules) from an area of higher concentration to an area of lower concentration.
Osmosis	Osmosis is the movement of a solvent (fluid) from an area of lower solute concentration to an area of higher solute concentration.
Filtration	Filtration is the removal of particles from a solution by allowing the liquid portion to pass through a membrane or other partial barrier. The semipermeability of the membrane allows fluid to pass through, but the openings are too small for solid particles.

Abbreviations: IV, intravenous; pH, potential of hydrogen

▶ Drug Distribution

Drugs pass freely and quickly out of the vascular space and into the interstitial fluid. Therefore, blood flow to the area determines the amount of a drug reaching a particular part of the body. Most drugs tend to pass fairly easily from the intravascular compartment, through the interstitial spaces, and on to their target tissue. These drugs tend to have a rapid onset and a short duration of action. Other drugs become bound to serum proteins in the blood and are not immediately available to act on receptor sites. With the drug bound to the protein, it cannot produce an effect in a receptor site or diffuse through the tissues.

Some areas of the body, such as the brain and placenta, are less accessible to certain drugs than others. Drugs that are protein-bound or in an ionized form are weak penetrators of the blood-brain barrier. The blood-brain barrier and the placental barrier are both less permeable to provide protection to the brain and fetus, respectively.

▶ Biotransformation

Many drugs are inactive when administered and only become active once they have been absorbed and converted into an active form in the blood or by the target tissue. The chemical alteration that a substance undergoes in the body is known as **biotransformation**. The primary organ for biotransformation is the liver. If the liver is diseased, inactivation (detoxification) of drugs may be impaired. This will also increase elimination time of the drug from the body, possibly resulting in toxic blood levels. The liver performs synthetic reactions that yield inactive products (metabolites) that can be secreted by the kidneys, and nonsynthetic reactions, which may result in products that are more active, charged in activity, or less active. The drugs that are biotransformed to an inactive metabolite very quickly have limited effects on the body and must be administered frequently to continue the effect. Epinephrine (administered by paramedics) during a cardiac arrest is an example of a drug that is rendered inactive very quickly and must be administered every 3 to 5 minutes as needed or alternatively as a continuous infusion.

▶ Drug Elimination

Excretion is the elimination of waste products from the body. Drugs are eliminated in their original forms or as metabolites. Organs of excretion include the kidneys via the urine, the intestines through the feces, the lungs via respiration, sweat through the salivary glands, and the mammary glands through breast milk. The rate of elimination varies with the amount of drug in the body and the underlying condition of the excretion organs. During shock, when the kidneys are poorly perfused, drugs may remain in the circulation for longer periods. This also holds true for geriatric patients whose kidneys may not function as well owing to the normal deterioration associated with aging and for patients with chronic kidney disease. A patient's poor ability to eliminate a drug may result in an accumulation of the drug if subsequent doses are given, resulting in toxic effects.

Special Populations

Geriatric patients often take many medications. They might also save medications left over from previous medical conditions to use if they need them in the future. Make every effort to identify which medications are current and what conditions they are being used to treat. Ask family members to help distinguish current from outdated medications, or look at the expiration dates on the medication labels. Take a list of the current medications or the drugs themselves with you to the emergency department.

Elderly patients can become confused about their medication regimen. Uncertainty about whether they missed a dose may cause them to repeat the medication, possibly resulting in an overdose. If you think an overdose has occurred, contact medical control.

Along with the potential for overdosing, the physiologic effects of aging can result in altered pharmacodynamics and pharmacokinetics. As the body ages and organs (such as the liver and kidneys) function less effectively, medications are not processed and filtered out of the system as quickly as in a younger person. Each time a dose of a particular drug is taken, it results in overaccumulation of that drug in the body. Decreased gastric motility can result in greater absorption time, and a decrease in total body water along with an increase in fat can result in a greater concentration of drugs with weight-based dosages.

Medications can interact with each other, creating potentially harmful conditions for the patient. Even though a medication may be indicated for a certain condition, it might be contraindicated in the presence of another medication. For example, if the patient is taking the heart medication propranolol (Inderal), which is a beta blocker, and has an acute episode of shortness of breath, any asthma remedy might be rendered ineffective. Bronchodilation is a beta effect of most emergency asthma medications.

Medications such as sildenafil (Viagra), tadalafil (Cialis), and vardenafil (Levitra)—all of which are used to treat erectile dysfunction—can have potentially fatal interactions with common heart medications, specifically nitroglycerin. If used in combination with any of these medications, nitroglycerin can cause life-threatening hypotension due to severe vasodilation. Ask a patient who has been prescribed nitroglycerin if he has used Viagra in the past 24 hours, or Cialis or Levitra within the past 48 hours. Report this to medical control.

Although medications help people to recover from acute conditions and adjust to chronic diseases, they can pose serious problems for geriatric patients. You should distinguish current from previous medications, suspect accidental or intentional overdoses, and be prepared for potentially lethal medication interactions. Document all findings, and inform medical control.

Pharmacodynamics

Pharmacodynamics is the way in which a medication produces the response we intended, also known as the mechanism of action. A medication's pharmacodynamics also includes factors that may alter the intended response and any side effects or unexpected effects.

▶ Mechanism of Action

To produce optimal desired or therapeutic effects, a drug must reach appropriate concentrations at its site of action. Molecules of the chemical compound must proceed from the point of entry into the body to the tissues with which they react. The magnitude of the response depends on the dose and the time that it takes the drug to travel in the body.

Drugs may produce their effects locally, systemically, or both. Local effects are those that result from the direct application of a drug to a tissue. An example of a local effect would be when cortisone cream is applied to the skin to relieve itching. Systemic effects occur after the drug is absorbed by any route and distributed by the bloodstream. Systemic effects almost always involve more than one organ, although the response of one or another organ may predominate.

Medications cause their action on the body by the following four mechanisms:

- They may bind to a receptor site.
- They may change the physical properties of cells—typically, by changing the osmotic balance.
- They may chemically combine with other chemicals (such as with the goal of turning the substance into a nonproblematic chemical).
- They may alter a normal metabolic pathway (such as by interrupting the normal growth process of cells).

Medications that bind to a receptor site are the most prevalent, particularly in the prehospital setting. Cellular responses can be wide ranging depending on the chemical mediator and the cells being stimulated. The medication molecule must compete with the naturally occurring chemical mediator. To win this battle, the medication molecule must have a higher affinity for the receptor than the naturally occurring chemical mediator does, or it must be present in a higher concentration. In addition, more than one medication may vie for the same receptor.

After the medication binds to the receptor site, it initiates a chemical change that produces the expected

Table 12-9 Factors Altering Drug Responses

Factor	Description
Age	As the body ages, metabolism slows and the organs of excretion do not always function as well as those in younger patients. This can cause a toxic level of drugs in the system if not considered when administering multiple doses. Likewise, infants and small children have immature organs and systems and cannot metabolize the same amount of drug as an adult.
Body mass	Many medications are given based on the patient's weight. This is especially true of children. To have a therapeutic dose, concentrations within the tissues must meet the desired level.
Sex	Owing to different body compositions of fat, water, and hormones, certain medications affect males and females differently and must be adjusted accordingly.
Environmental conditions and time of administration	Factors such as time of day, temperature, altitude, and even noise may alter the body's response to a drug.
Genetic factors	Patients who may already have some compromise in function as a result of an existing condition may not be adversely affected by certain medications because of changes in absorption, distribution, metabolism, and excretion.
Psychological factors	Mental stresses can have negative effects on the entire system, resulting in an inability to properly metabolize medications.

effect. In some cases, this chemical change *is* the intended effect. In other cases, the initial chemical change releases a second compound (known as a second messenger) that causes the intended effect.

▶ Drug-Response Relationship

After the medication finds the target tissue, it needs to accumulate to a sufficient concentration to produce its desired effect. The drug-response relationship correlates the amount of medication given and the response it causes.

When administering a medication, you need to know the onset of action and duration of action. The **termination of action** is the amount of time after the concentration level falls below the minimum level to the time it is eliminated from the body. All of these factors affect the **therapeutic index**—the ratio of a drug's lethal dose for 50% of the population (LD_{50}) to its effective dose for 50% of the population (ED_{50}). In other words, the therapeutic index gives an indication of a medication's margin of safety. Each medication also has a biologic half-life—that is, the time it takes the body to eliminate one-half of the drug. For example, the half-life of naloxone is typically 45 minutes.

The minimum concentration required to produce the desired response is referred to as the **therapeutic threshold** or the minimum effective concentration. A concentration lower than the therapeutic threshold will not induce a clinical response. A concentration higher than the therapeutic threshold may actually be detrimental and possibly fatal. The goal of drug therapy is to give the minimum concentration of a drug that will produce the desired effects.

Table 12-9 lists factors that alter drug responses.

Factors Influencing Medication Interactions

There are many variables that influence **medication interaction**. When you are administering medications, it is important to know not only how they affect the patient, but also how they may affect other medications that were previously administered. An interaction between medications occurs whenever the actions of one drug on the body are in some way modified by another chemical substance. This chemical substance may be another prescription medication, herbal or OTC, or something like nicotine from cigarette smoking, something in the patient's diet, or anything to which the person is exposed. One example is the use of bronchodilators that may be exacerbated by ingesting caffeine. The caffeine stimulates the CNS and may produce adverse effects.

It is important to be aware of the potential interactions of medications that are prescribed and those that the patient may be self-administering. Many patients, especially elderly patients, may take several medications each day (**polypharmacy**). The chance of developing an undesired medication interaction increases rapidly with the number of medications used. This also is true when patients take medications that may interact with other substances such as particular foods and alcohol. Warning labels on prescription bottles warn against the substances that may cause interactions. Unfortunately, however, many people do not read the warning labels.

▶ Predictable Responses

Because of the extensive research that goes into developing and testing a medication before it is approved, there is common knowledge about what effect a particular medication will have on the patient. Obviously, an AEMT expects to see the desired response after administering the medication. At the same time, you should anticipate responses beyond the desired effect. *Side effects* are any actions of a medication other than the desired ones. Side effects may occur even when a medication is administered properly and under the appropriate circumstances. For example, giving epinephrine to a patient who is having an allergic reaction should dilate the bronchioles and decrease wheezing. However, two side effects of epinephrine are cardiac stimulation and constriction of the arteries, which may elevate the patient's heart rate and blood pressure. These side effects are predictable.

▶ Iatrogenic Responses

An **iatrogenic response** is an adverse condition inadvertently induced in a patient by the treatment given. One example is a urinary tract infection that develops in a patient after insertion of an indwelling catheter (such as a Foley catheter). When the administration of medications results in symptoms that mimic naturally occurring disease states, it is known as an iatrogenic medication response.

▶ Unpredictable Responses

Some patients may have adverse effects that are not anticipated. The most common unpredictable response encountered in the prehospital setting is an allergic reaction. An allergy develops when a person has previously been exposed to a particular antigen and develops antibodies against that substance (sensitization). After a person has become sensitized, subsequent exposure to that same substance results in **hypersensitivity**. Because the patient is hypersensitive, the medication activates the immune system. Allergic reactions are unpredictable—unless the patient has had an allergic reaction to the same medication in the past—and may result in life-threatening anaphylaxis. Anaphylaxis is an acute systemic reaction that is usually life threatening. An allergic reaction may be immediate or delayed. Before administering any medication, if possible, question the patient carefully about any known medication allergies. The AEMT should remain alert for an allergic reaction after administering *any* medication.

A delayed reaction is known as **serum sickness**. This type of reaction is a hypersensitivity similar to an allergy and occurs a considerable time after a stimulus, such as a skin inflammation occurring hours or days after exposure to the allergen. Unlike other allergic reactions to medications that occur soon after administration, serum sickness can develop 7 to 14 days after the first exposure to a medication.

In rare cases, the patient may experience a completely unique response that is specific to that person; it is not seen in other patients. This situation is known as an **idiosyncrasy**. An **idiosyncratic reaction** is a peculiar or individual reaction to a drug. For example, if a patient were administered nitroglycerin and then experienced a seizure, this would be an idiosyncratic reaction because seizure is not an expected reaction when administering nitroglycerin.

Patients who take a particular medication for an extended period can build up **tolerance** to it. In these cases, the patient will have a decreased response to the same amount of medication, often requiring higher doses than normal. Also, a patient can develop a tolerance to other drugs in a certain class as a result of prolonged administration of another medication in that same class. Known as **cross-tolerance**, this phenomenon is often seen in patients who take many pain medications. When patients are taking a medication such as oxycodone, they become tolerant to opiate-based medications. If morphine is administered for pain, the patient may not have the same response as other patients because of cross-tolerance. A disease or condition that does not respond to treatment is known as **refractory**.

Any medication needs to reach a minimum concentration in the target tissue before it becomes effective; that concentration is reached by providing a specific dose. If several doses are given in a relatively short time, the patient may experience a cumulative effect. A **cumulative effect** is the increased effect when a medication is given in several successive doses, which might result in therapeutic or nontherapeutic effects.

With prolonged administration of a medication, a patient can become drug-dependent. *Drug dependence* is a psychological and sometimes physical state resulting from continued use of a substance. Characteristic behavioral response includes a compulsion to take the drug on a continuous or periodic basis to experience its effects or to avoid the discomfort of its absence. A person will have significant symptoms if he or she stops using the medication. **Habituation** is the term for physical tolerance of and psychological dependence on a drug or drugs.

Many patients take multiple medications at one time. It is possible for the effects of one medication to alter the response of another medication, a phenomenon known as a drug interaction. A drug interaction can be fatal. The interaction may not always be anticipated. Even if two medications are sympathomimetics, for example, it does not necessarily mean the patient will experience a more dramatic sympathetic response. It is possible to see the opposite response or a completely unrelated response. When a patient is taking multiple medications, one medication could block the body's response to another medication (**drug antagonism**). You can use this fact as an advantage. For example, if the patient has taken an opiate-based drug such as morphine, you have the ability to administer another medication, naloxone, to block the response to the morphine.

A **summation effect** is an additive effect—that is, two drugs that have the same or similar effect increase the patient's response when both are administered to the patient. When the patient receives two drugs that have the same effect but produce a response greater than the sum of their individual responses, the result is known as **synergism**. At times, the interaction between two medications can cause one drug to enhance the effect of another, known as **potentiation**. For example, acetaminophen (Tylenol) and alcohol interact. In this case, it is well known that high doses of acetaminophen are damaging to the liver. When alcohol is ingested along with acetaminophen, more of the medication is taken up into the liver and may result in acute liver failure. Some potentiation effects are known and can be exploited to achieve a desired effect; in other cases, potentiation may occur unexpectedly. A direct biochemical interaction that takes place between two drugs is referred to as **interference**.

Reducing Medication Errors

As an AEMT, you will have the difficult task of assessing patients, performing invasive procedures, and administering medications in the uncontrolled prehospital setting. In this environment, patient history is often limited, inaccurate, or nonexistent. AEMTs do not always have the time or resources for a careful evaluation of the risks and benefits associated with medications that they are considering administering to a patient. Medication decisions are often based on memory and frequently occur in the context of a stressful, life-threatening patient situation. AEMTs are constantly at risk for a cognitive error such as choosing the wrong medication or dose, or a technical error such as administering more volume of medication than was intended. Table 12-10 lists the ten rights of medication administration.

Table 12-10 The Ten Rights of Medication Administration

1. Right Patient

Although you will typically treat one patient at a time, sometimes you may have to treat multiple patients. It is essential to confirm the identity of a patient before administering any medication—especially when patients are unconscious or are unable to communicate (because of extremes of age, altered consciousness, or other factors). Always attempt to have the patient confirm his or her identity verbally, or confirm the identity of the patient yourself through identification devices (such as bracelets or identification cards), to the extent possible. A critical issue, as identified in the SAMPLE history, is to ensure that the patient does not have allergies to the medication(s) you intend to give Figure 12-6.

2. Right Medication

Administration of the wrong medication is the most common pharmacology-related error. Several factors may lead to "wrong medication" errors, including similar packaging and labeling, similar names and storage practices, and ineffective communication. Always repeat (echo) the medication order (out loud and in the presence of your partner), and confirm that the packaging matches the intended order. While checking the packaging, confirm that the medication is not expired by reading the expiration date out loud to your partner. Avoid using abbreviations, and always recheck the order before administration.

3. Right Dose

Doses of nearly every medication depend on patient-specific factors (such as condition, weight, and age). The actual dose needed is often not equal to the amount supplied in an ampule or a prefilled syringe in the prehospital setting. Therefore, you will have to calculate the patient-specific dose. When calculating the correct dose, always recheck your math, and if possible, have your partner recheck and verify the final dose.

4. Right Route

Many medications can be administered by a variety of routes; the optimal route depends on the patient's condition and the speed with which the medication needs to take effect. Errors can occur when medication doses and routes are confused. For example, IV drip doses can be different from doses for the same medication injected into an IV as a bolus. Another important route-related issue is the patient's condition. If a patient is in profound shock, you must consider how well the medication will be absorbed and distributed to target tissues. Choosing the right route helps enable the medication to have the correct effect. Always verify the route of administration.

5. Right Time
Because all medications take a certain amount of time to take effect and may have the potential to interfere with other medications, you must always follow the recommended guidelines for the proper frequency of medication administration. Evaluate the patient's condition before and after you administer any medication, and document any noted response or change in the patient's condition. Also remember that some medications require a specific administration frequency to maintain a therapeutic level.
6. Right Documentation and Reporting
Because AEMTs frequently transfer care of a patient to other health care providers, it is critical to document in writing the medications administered, the dose, when they were administered, and the effects the patient experienced. Whenever possible, communicate this information in writing (on the patient care report), and in a verbal report to the next level of care.
7. Right Assessment
Confirm indications and contraindications. Ensure that the medication is appropriate for the patient's medical condition and medical history.
8. Right to Refuse
Respect patient autonomy. Patients with decision-making capacity or a surrogate decision maker may refuse medications and other interventions, even if refusing a medication may result in harm. Consult online medical control in any high-risk situation. Make sure the patient is aware of the potential consequences of refusing a medication or treatment.
9. Right Evaluation
Continually monitor your patient. Observe for desired effects and any possible adverse reactions for any medication administered. Certain medications may require careful monitoring; other medications may require multiple doses to achieve the desired effect.
10. Right Patient Education
Patient education should begin as soon as possible. Responsive patients should be informed of any pertinent risks and benefits prior to medication administration. Involve responsive patients in ongoing evaluation and monitoring by informing them of any important symptoms they may experience or that should be reported.

Abbreviations: AEMT, advanced emergency medical technician; IV, intravenous; SAMPLE, Signs and symptoms, Allergies, Medications, Pertinent past medical history, Last oral intake, Events leading up to the illness or injury

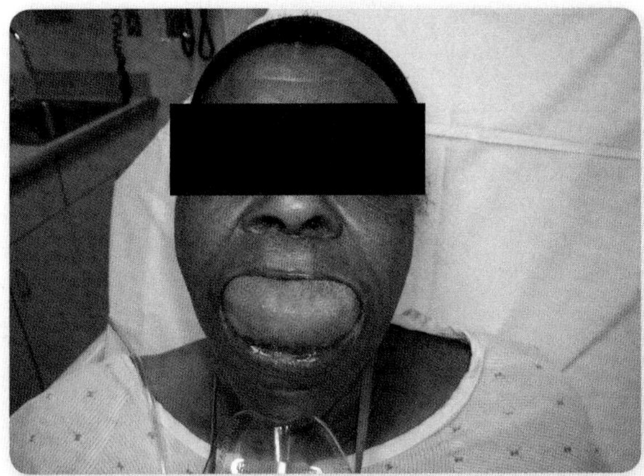

Figure 12-6 Angioedema is acute swelling, sometimes of the lips and tongue, that may be caused by an allergic reaction. Some medications cause angioedema after the first or second dose.

Use a current, reliable medication reference source whenever administering potentially unfamiliar medications or whenever an unusual dose or route of administration is being considered. Technical errors can be avoided by having a partner confirm the volume in a syringe or a weight-based medication calculation. Many health care settings require that two providers check pediatric and high-risk medication calculations. AEMTs should also evaluate for a patient medication allergy or hypersensitivity before each medication administration.

The Institute for Safe Medication Practices has developed a list of medication abbreviations prone to causing errors. When these symbols and abbreviations are used by physicians, AEMTs, and other health care providers, there is an increased likelihood of a medication error as a result of miscommunication. The full list is exhaustive. Table 12-11 lists several important sources of error relevant to the prehospital setting.

Words of Wisdom

Wichita-Sedgwick County EMS System in Kansas developed a tool known as Medication Administration Cross-Check© (MACC) Figure 12-7.[6] This tool uses principles of crew resource management by requiring a process for verification for every medication, every time. The tool employs job aids to help reduce cognitive load and ensure the process is completed each time a medication is administered.

Because EMS systems vary in configuration—for example, an AEMT working with an EMT—the tool is designed to work with all provider levels. Although BLS providers may lack familiarity with all medications, they can verify quantities, medication names, expiration dates, etc.

More important, the second provider, regardless of certification level, acts as a sounding board for the first provider. This forces the first provider to validate the medication administration. Some providers may catch the error as they read it back to themselves. Others may catch it when the second provider asks them to repeat something that did not sound right. Sometimes the second provider can catch the error and bring it to the first provider's attention. The tool will not eliminate all medication errors. However, with proper use of this tool, medication errors can be significantly reduced.

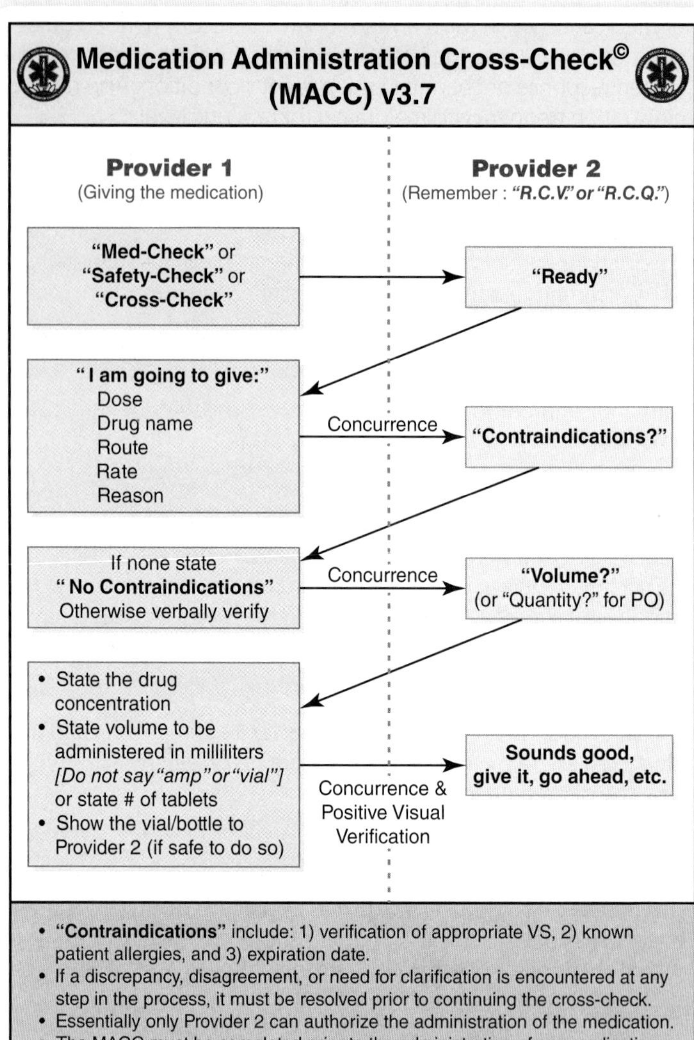

Abbreviations: PO, per os (orally); R.C.Q, Ready, Contraindications, Quantity; R.C.V, Ready, Contraindications, Volume; VS, vital signs

Figure 12-7 Medication Administration Cross-Check© job aid.

Reproduced from: Misasi P, Braithwaite S. The Medication Administration Cross-Check© (MACC) User's Manual. Wichita-Sedgwick County EMS System. March 2012.

Table 12-11 Examples of Errors and Misinterpretations in Reporting

Error Source	Intended Meaning	Possible Misinterpretation	Correction
Trailing zero after the decimal point (eg, 4.0 mg)	4 mg	40 mg	Avoid trailing zeros when decimal place is not needed.
No leading zero before decimal point (eg, .8 mg)	0.8 mg	8 mg	Use a zero before the decimal point when the dose is less than 1 unit.
SC	Subcutaneous	SL (sublingual)	Write out "subcutaneous."
IN	Intranasal	IV (intravenous) or IM (intramuscular)	Write out "intranasal."

Documentation & Communication

Documenting medication administration is extremely important. You must list the dose administered, name of the medication, route, rate, time of administration, who administered the drug, who helped perform the medication check, and the patient's response.

Specific Medications

A certified AEMT is allowed to administer or help patients self-administer numerous medications. Details about each of these are provided in Table 12-12. As an AEMT, you may administer the following:

- Oxygen
- Oral glucose
- Glucagon
- IV dextrose (eg, D_{50}, D_{25}, or D_{10})
- IV fluids—D_5W (5% dextrose), normal saline, lactated Ringer solution
- Epinephrine (IM or subcutaneous)
- MDI medications—albuterol
- Nebulized medications—albuterol
- Nitroglycerin—spray, tablets, paste
- Nitrous oxide
- Naloxone
- Aspirin
- Others based on local protocols

The table uses "tall man" lettering. This is sometimes used to avoid confusion of medications with similar spellings.[7] With tall man lettering, capitalized letters highlight the area that differentiates the medication from others with similar names. Use of tall man lettering is intended to help reduce medication-related errors.

However, you may administer or help to administer these medications only under the following conditions:

- A licensed physician gives you a direct order to administer a medication, and/or the local medical protocols under which you are working permit you to administer that medication. Some local protocols exclude one or more of the medications listed in Table 12-12.
- The local medical protocols under which you are working include standing orders for the use of a medication in defined situations.
  It is imperative that you do not give or help patients take any other medications under any circumstances.

Table 12-12 Medications, Fluids, and Routes Used at the AEMT Level[a]	
Albuterol (Proventil, Ventolin)	
Class	Sympathomimetic, bronchodilator
Mechanism of action	Selective beta-2 agonist that stimulates adrenergic receptors of the sympathomimetic nervous system. Causes smooth muscle relaxation in the bronchial tree and peripheral vasculature.
Indications	Treatment of bronchospasm in patients with reversible obstructive airway disease (COPD/asthma). Prevention of exercise-induced bronchospasm.
Contraindications	Known prior hypersensitivity reactions to albuterol. Tachycardia dysrhythmias, especially those caused by digitalis. Synergistic with other sympathomimetics.
Adverse reactions/side effects	Often dose-related and include headache, fatigue, light-headedness, irritability, restlessness, aggressive behavior, pulmonary edema, hoarseness, nasal congestion, increased sputum, hypertension, tachycardia, dysrhythmias, chest pain, palpitations, nausea/vomiting, dry mouth, epigastric pain, and tremors.
Drug interactions	Tricyclic antidepressants may potentiate vasculature effects. Beta blockers are antagonistic and may block pulmonary effects. May potentiate hypokalemia caused by diuretics.
Route	Inhalation (nebulizer or MDI)
Dosage and administration	*Adult*: Administer 2.5 mg. Dilute in 0.5 mL of 0.5% solution for inhalation with 2.5 mL normal saline in nebulizer and administer over 10–15 minutes. MDI: 1–2 inhalations (90–180 mcg); wait 5 minutes between inhalations. *Pediatric*: <20 kg: 1.25 mg/dose via handheld nebulizer or mask over 20 minutes; >20 kg: 2.5 mg/dose via handheld nebulizer or mask over 20 minutes. Repeat once in 20 minutes.
Duration of action	*Onset*: 5–15 minutes. *Peak effect*: 30 minutes to 2 hours. *Duration*: 3–4 hours.
Special considerations	Pregnancy safety: Category C. May precipitate angina pectoris and dysrhythmias. In prehospital emergency care, albuterol should be administered only via inhalation. Patients may need to be coached on proper use of MDI, particularly with spacer.
Aspirin (Acetylsalicylic Acid)	
Class	Platelet inhibitor, anti-inflammatory agent
Mechanism of action	Prevents the formation of thromboxane A_2, which causes platelets to clump together (aggregate) and form plugs that cause obstruction or constriction; has antipyretic and analgesic properties.
Indications	New onset chest discomfort that suggests ACS.
Contraindications	Hypersensitivity. Relatively contraindicated in patients with active ulcer disease or asthma.
Adverse reactions/side effects	Bronchospasm, anaphylaxis, wheezing in allergic patients, prolonged bleeding, GI bleeding, epigastric distress, nausea/vomiting, heartburn, Reye syndrome.
Drug interactions	Use with caution in patients allergic to NSAIDs.
Route	Oral (chewable tablet[s])
Dosage and administration	*Adult*: 160 to 325 mg PO. Chewing is preferred to swallowing. *Pediatric*: Not recommended.
Duration of action	*Onset*: 5–30 minutes. *Peak effect*: 1–3 hours. *Duration*: 3–6 hours.

Special considerations	Pregnancy safety: Category D. Use cautiously during pregnancy, weighing risks and benefits. If there are no contraindications, non–enteric-coated, chewable aspirin should be given as soon as possible to all patients with a suspected ACS as soon as possible after symptom onset. Not recommended in pediatric population.
Dextrose	
Class	Carbohydrate, antihypoglycemic, hypertonic solution
Mechanism of action	Rapidly increases serum glucose levels. Short-term osmotic diuresis.
Indications	Hypoglycemia, altered level of consciousness, coma of unknown origin, seizure of unknown origin, status epilepticus.
Contraindications	Intracranial hemorrhage with normal blood glucose level
Adverse reactions/side effects	Extravasation leads to tissue necrosis. Cerebral hemorrhage; cerebral ischemia; pulmonary edema; warmth, pain, burning from IV infusion, hyperglycemia.
Drug interactions	Sodium bicarbonate, warfarin (Coumadin)
Route	IV, IO
Dosage and administration	*Adult*: D_{50} 25 g slow IV push. May be repeated as necessary. 10% dextrose (D_{10}) may be an option. D_{10} can be as effective as D_{50} and D_{25}, with fewer potential side effects. Consult your local protocols regarding the concentrations used in your system. *Pediatric*: 1 year and older; dextrose 25% 0.5–1 g/kg/dose slow IV push. May be repeated as necessary. As with adults, in pediatric patients other concentrations of dextrose, such as D_{10}, may be used depending on local protocol. *Neonates and infants*: D_{10} 200–500 mg/kg slow IV push (see below). May be repeated as necessary. Maximum concentration of 12.5% (vasculature extremely sensitive to high concentrations).
Duration of action	*Onset*: Less than 1 minute. *Peak effect*: Variable. *Duration*: Variable.
Special considerations	Pregnancy safety: Category C. Draw blood to determine glucose level before administering. Do not administer to patients with known CVA unless hypoglycemia documented. Due to potential medication shortages, this may not be available in bolus form.
Epinephrine (Adrenalin) 1 mg/mL (1:1,000)	
Class	Sympathomimetic
Mechanism of action	Direct-acting alpha and beta agonist. Alpha: vasoconstriction. Beta-1: positive inotropic, chronotropic, and dromotropic effects. Beta-2: bronchial smooth muscle relaxation and dilation of skeletal vasculature. Blocks histamine receptors.
Indications	Allergic reaction, anaphylaxis, asthma
Contraindications	None in the emergency setting. Relative contraindications include hypertension, hypothermia, pulmonary edema, myocardial ischemia, hypovolemic shock.
Adverse reactions/side effects	Nervousness, restlessness, headache, tremor, pulmonary edema, dysrhythmias, chest pain, hypertension, tachycardia, nausea/vomiting
Drug interactions	Potentiates other sympathomimetics; MAOIs may potentiate effect. Beta blockers may blunt effect.
Route	IM, subcutaneous
Dosage and administration	*Adult*: Allergic reactions and asthma: 0.3–0.5 mg (0.3–0.5 mL of 1 mg/mL [1:1,000]) IM. *Pediatric*: Anaphylaxis/severe status asthmaticus: 0.01 mg/kg (0.01 mL/kg) IM of a 1 mg/mL (1:1,000) solution (maximum single dose: 0.3 mg).

(continued)

Table 12-12	Medications, Fluids, and Routes Used at the AEMT Level[a] (continued)
	Epinephrine (Adrenalin) 1 mg/mL (1:1,000)
Duration of action	*Onset*: Immediate. *Peak effect*: Minutes. *Duration*: Several minutes.
Special considerations	Pregnancy safety: Category C. May cause syncope in asthmatic children. May increase myocardial oxygen demand.
	Glucagon (GlucaGen)
Class	Hyperglycemic agent, pancreatic hormone, insulin antagonist.
Mechanism of action	Increases blood glucose level by stimulating glycogenesis. Unknown mechanism of stabilizing cardiac rhythm in beta blocker overdose. Minimal positive inotropic and chronotropic response. Decreases GI motility and secretions.
Indications	Altered level of consciousness when hypoglycemia is suspected. May be used as a reversal agent in beta blocker overdose.
Contraindications	Hyperglycemia, hypersensitivity
Adverse reactions/side effects	Dizziness, headache, hypertension, tachycardia, nausea/vomiting, rebound hypoglycemia.
Drug interactions	Incompatible in solution with most other substances. No significant drug interactions with other emergency medications.
Route	IM
Dosage and administration	*Adult*: Hypoglycemia: 1 mg IM/IN; may repeat in 7–10 minutes. *Pediatric*: Hypoglycemia: 1 mg IM/IN if 20 kg or greater (or 5 years or more); 0.5 mg IM/IN if less than 20 kg or younger than 5 years.
Duration of action	*Onset*: 1 minute. *Peak effect*: 5–20 minutes. *Duration*: 60–90 minutes.
Special considerations	Pregnancy safety: Category B. Use in pregnancy only if clearly indicated. Not recommended for use in lactating women. Ineffective if glycogen stores depleted. Should always be used in conjunction with D_{50} whenever possible. If patient does not respond to a second dose of glucagon, D_{50} must be administered. Requires reconstitution with the supplied solution.
	Naloxone Hydrochloride (Narcan)
Class	Opioid antagonist, antidote
Mechanism of action	Competitive inhibition at narcotic receptor sites. Reverses respiratory depression secondary to opiate drugs. Completely inhibits the effect of morphine.
Indications	Opiate overdose, complete or partial reversal of CNS and respiratory depression induced by opioids, decreased level of consciousness, coma of unknown origin. Narcotic agonist for the following: morphine sulfate, heroin, HYDROmorphone (Dilaudid), methadone, meperidine (Demerol), paregoric, fentaNYL (Sublimaze), oxycodone (Percodan), codeine, propoxyphene (Darvon). Narcotic agonist and antagonist for the following: butorphanol (Stadol), pentazocine (Talwin), nalbuphine (Nubain).
Contraindications	Use with caution in narcotic-dependent patients. Use with caution in neonates of narcotic-addicted mothers.
Adverse reactions/side effects	Restlessness, seizures, dyspnea, pulmonary edema, tachycardia, hypertension, dysrhythmias, nausea/vomiting, withdrawal symptoms in opioid-addicted patients, diaphoresis.
Drug interactions	Incompatible with bisulfite and alkaline solutions

Route	IV, IN, IO, IM (auto-injector)
Dosage and administration	*Adult*: 0.4–2.0 mg IM/IV/IO; minimum single dose recommended, 2 mg. Repeat at 5-minute intervals to a maximum total dose of 10 mg (medical control may request higher amounts). For IN route, administer one-half of the dose in each nostril; maximum dose is 1 mL per nostril. *Pediatric*: 0.1 mg/kg per dose IV/IO/IM every 2 minutes as needed. Maximum total dose of 2 mg. If no response in 10 minutes, administer an additional 0.1 mg/kg per dose.
Duration of action	*Onset*: Less than 2 minutes. *Peak effect*: Variable. *Duration*: 30–60 minutes.
Special considerations	Pregnancy safety: Category C. Any use during pregnancy. Use in breastfeeding women should be clearly indicated. Assist ventilations prior to administration to avoid sympathetic stimulation. Seizures without causal relationship have been reported. May not reverse hypotension. Use caution when administering to narcotic addicts (potential violent behavior). Half-life of naloxone is often shorter than the half-life of narcotics; repeat dosing may be required. In cardiac arrest, naloxone is generally not beneficial.

Nitroglycerin (Nitrostat, Nitro-Bid, Tridil)	
Class	Vasodilator
Mechanism of action	Smooth muscle relaxant acting on vasculature, bronchial, uterine, intestinal smooth muscle. Dilation of arterioles and veins in the periphery. Reduces preload and afterload, decreasing workload of the heart and thereby myocardial oxygen demand.
Indications	Acute angina pectoris, ischemic chest pain, hypertension, heart failure, pulmonary edema
Contraindications	Hypotension, hypovolemia, intracranial bleeding or head injury, pericardial tamponade, severe bradycardia or tachycardia, previous administration in the last 24 hours: sildenafil (Viagra) or 48 hours: vardenafil (Levitra) or tadalafil (Cialis).
Adverse reactions/side effects	Headache, dizziness, weakness, reflex tachycardia, syncope, hypotension, nausea/vomiting, dry mouth, diaphoresis, muscle twitching
Drug interactions	Additive effects with other vasodilators. Incompatible with other IV drugs.
Route	SL (rapid absorption)
Dosage and administration	*Adult*: 0.4 mg SL; may repeat in 3–5 minutes to maximum of 3 doses. Nitroglycerin spray: 0.4 mg under the tongue; 1–2 sprays. Nitroglycerin IV infusion: begin at 10 to 20 mcg/min; increase by 5–10 mcg/min every 5 minutes until desired effect. *Pediatric*: Not recommended.
Duration of action	*Onset*: 1–3 minutes. *Peak effect*: 5–10 minutes. *Duration*: SL: 20–30 minutes; IV: 1–10 minutes after discontinuation of infusion.
Special considerations	Pregnancy safety: Category C. Has been used safely during pregnancy. Use caution with breastfeeding women and monitor infants for adverse effects. Hypotension more common in older patients. Nitroglycerin decomposes when exposed to light or heat; must be kept in airtight containers. Active ingredient may have a stinging effect when administered.

Nitropaste (Nitro-Bid Ointment)	
Class	Vasodilator
Mechanism of action	Smooth muscle relaxant acting on vasculature, bronchial, uterine, intestinal smooth muscle. Dilation of arterioles and veins in the periphery. Reduces preload and afterload, decreasing workload of the heart and thereby myocardial oxygen demand.

(continued)

Table 12-12	Medications, Fluids, and Routes Used at the AEMT Level[a] *(continued)*
Nitropaste (Nitro-Bid Ointment)	
Indications	Angina pectoris, chest pain associated with AMI, hypertension, heart failure, pulmonary edema.
Contraindications	Hypotension, hypovolemia, intracranial bleeding or head injury, previous administration in the last 24 hours of sildenafil (Viagra) or in the last 48 hours of vardenafil (Levitra) or tadalafil (Cialis).
Adverse reactions/side effects	Headache, dizziness, weakness, reflex tachycardia, syncope, hypotension, nausea, vomiting, dry mouth, muscle twitching, diaphoresis.
Drug interactions	Additive effects with other vasodilators
Route	Transdermal
Dosage and administration	*Adult*: Paste: Apply 1/2- to 3/4-inch (1- to 2-cm) line (15–30 mg), cover with wrap, and secure with tape. Maximum: 5-inch (12.5-cm) line (75 mg) per application. Transdermal: Apply unit to intact skin (usually chest wall) in varying doses. *Pediatric*: Not recommended.
Duration of action	*Onset*: 30 minutes. *Peak effect*: variable. *Duration*: 18–24 hours.
Special considerations	Pregnancy safety: Category C. Has been used safely during pregnancy. Use caution with breastfeeding women and monitor infants for adverse effects. Not a great value in prehospital arena. Wear gloves when applying paste. Store paste in cool place with tube tightly capped. Erratic absorption rates quite common.
Nitrous Oxide 50:50 (Nitronox)	
Class	Gaseous analgesic and anesthetic
Mechanism of action	Exact mechanism unknown; affects CNS phospholipids.
Indications	Moderate to severe pain, anxiety, apprehension
Contraindications	Impaired level of consciousness, head injury, inability to follow or comply with instructions, decompression sickness (nitrogen narcosis, air embolism, air transport), undiagnosed abdominal pain or marked distention, bowel obstruction, hypotension, shock, COPD, cyanosis, chest trauma with pneumothorax.
Adverse reactions/side effects	Light-headedness, drowsiness, respiratory depression, apnea, nausea/vomiting, malignant hyperthermia.
Drug interactions	None of significance
Route	Inhalation
Dosage and administration	*Adult*: Instruct the patient to inhale deeply through demand valve and mask or mouthpiece. *Pediatric*: Same as adult.
Duration of action	*Onset*: 2–5 minutes. *Peak effect*: Variable. *Duration*: 2–5 minutes.
Special considerations	Pregnancy safety: Category C. Nitrous oxide increases the incidence of spontaneous abortion. Ventilate patient care area during use. Nitrous oxide is nonflammable and nonexplosive. Nitrous oxide is ineffective in 20% of the population.

Oral Glucose (Insta-Glucose)	
Class	Hyperglycemic, carbohydrate
Mechanism of action	After absorption in the GI tract, glucose is distributed to the tissues providing an increase in circulating blood glucose levels.
Indications	Alert patients with suspected hypoglycemia
Contraindications	Decreased level of consciousness, nausea, vomiting
Adverse reactions/side effects	Nausea, vomiting
Drug interactions	None
Route	Oral, buccal
Dosage and administration	*Adult*: 25 g PO in patients with intact gag reflex and ability to manage their own secretions. Pastes or gels should be placed between the cheek and gum for absorption. *Pediatric*: 0.5–1 g PO in patients with intact gag reflex and ability to manage their own secretions.
Duration of action	*Onset*: 10 minutes. *Peak effect*: Variable. *Duration*: Variable.
Special considerations	Must be swallowed. Glucose is not absorbed sublingually or buccally. Check a glucometer reading before administering oral glucose and repeat at least 10 minutes after.

Oxygen	
Class	Naturally occurring atmospheric gas
Mechanism of action	Reverses hypoxemia
Indications	Confirmed or expected hypoxemia, ischemic chest pain, respiratory insufficiency, prophylactically during air transport, confirmed or suspected carbon monoxide poisoning, all other causes of decreased tissue oxygenation, decreased level of consciousness.
Contraindications	Certain patients with COPD or emphysema who will not tolerate oxygen concentrations over 35%, hyperventilation.
Adverse reactions/side effects	Decreased level of consciousness (COPD patients), decreased respiratory drive in COPD patients, dry mucous membranes.
Drug interactions	None
Route	Inhalation
Dosage and administration	*Adult*: Cardiac arrest and carbon monoxide poisoning: 100%. Hypoxemia: 10–15 L/min via nonrebreathing mask. COPD: 0–2 L/min via nasal cannula or 28%–35% Venturi mask. Be prepared to provide ventilatory support if higher concentrations of oxygen needed. *Pediatric*: Same as for adult with exception of premature infant.
Duration of action	*Onset*: Immediate. *Peak effect*: Not applicable. *Duration*: Less than 2 minutes.
Special considerations	Be familiar with liter flow rates and each type of delivery device used. Supports combustion.

(continued)

Table 12-12	Medications, Fluids, and Routes Used at the AEMT Level[a] *(continued)*
IV Solutions **Lactated Ringer (Hartmann) Solution**	
Class	Isotonic crystalloid solution
Mechanism of action	Lactated Ringer solution replaces water and electrolytes.
Indications	Hypovolemic shock; keep open IV line, hypoperfusion.
Contraindications	Lactated Ringer solution should not be used in patients with heart failure or renal failure.
Adverse reactions/side effects	Rare in therapeutic dosages
Drug interactions	Few in the emergency setting
Route	IV
Dosage and administration	Hypovolemic shock; titrate according to patient's physiologic response.
Duration of action	Short-term therapy
Special considerations	None
5% Dextrose in Water	
Class	Hypotonic dextrose-containing solution
Mechanism of action	D_5W provides nutrients in the form of dextrose as well as free water.
Indications	IV access for emergency medications; for dilution of concentrated medications for IV infusion.
Contraindications	D_5W should not be used as a fluid replacement for hypovolemic states.
Adverse reactions/side effects	Rare in therapeutic dosages
Drug interactions	D_5W should not be used with phenytoin (Dilantin) or amrinone (Inocor).
Route	IV
Dosage and administration	D_5W is usually administered through a minidrip (60 drops/mL) set at a rate of "to keep open."
Duration of action	Short-term therapy
Special considerations	None
0.9% Sodium Chloride (Normal Saline)	
Class	Isotonic crystalloid solution
Mechanism of action	Normal saline replaces water and electrolytes.
Indications	Heat-related problems (heat exhaustion, heat stroke), freshwater drowning, hypovolemia, diabetic ketoacidosis, keep open IV.

Contraindications	The use of 0.9% sodium chloride should not be considered in patients with heart failure because circulatory overload can be easily induced.
Adverse reactions/side effects	Rare in therapeutic dosages
Drug interactions	Few in the emergency setting
Route	IV
Dosage and administration	The specific situation being treated will dictate the rate at which normal saline will be administered. In severe heatstroke, diabetic ketoacidosis, and freshwater drowning, it is likely that you will be called on to administer the fluid quite rapidly. In other cases, it is advisable to administer the fluid at a moderate rate (for example, 100 mL/h). *Neonates*: Fluid bolus: 10-mL/kg IV given over 5–10 minutes; multiple boluses may be administered if the patient remains clinically hypovolemic. In a neonate, a 10-mL/kg normal saline bolus may aid in improved perfusion and clearance of acid.
Duration of action	Short-term therapy
Special considerations	None

[a] Local protocols vary and may not include all of these medications, or may include some of the above routes but not others, and medication concentrations may vary. Always follow local protocols regarding medications to administer, forms, routes, and dosages.

Abbreviations: ACS, acute coronary syndrome; AMI, acute myocardial infarction; CNS, central nervous system; COPD, chronic obstructive pulmonary disease: CVA, cerebrovascular accident; D_5W, 5% dextrose in water; D_{50}, dextrose 50%; GI, gastrointestinal; IM, intramuscular; IN, intranasal; IO, intraosseous; IV, intravenous; MAOIs, monoamine oxidase inhibitors; MDI, metered-dose inhaler; NS, normal saline; NSAID, nonsteroidal anti-inflammatory drug; PO, per os (orally); SL, sublingual

Data sources: Hazard Vallerand A, Sanoski CA. *Davis' Drug Guide for Nurses*. 14th ed. Philadelphia, PA: FA Davis Company; 2016; Truven Health Analytics. Micromedex database. http://www.micromedexsolutions.com/. Accessed February 29, 2017; Lexi-Comp website. online.lexi.com. Accessed April 2017; American Heart Association. 2015 American Heart Association Guidelines for CPR and ECC. https://eccguidelines.heart.org/index.php/circulation/cpr-ecc-guidelines-2/. Accessed February 29, 2017; National Model EMS Clinical Guidelines. National Association of State EMS Officials. V.08-16. https://www.nasemso.org/Projects/ModelEMSClinicalGuidelines/index.asp. Accessed April 7, 2017; Society of Critical Care Medicine. Surviving Sepsis Campaign. http://www.survivingsepsis.org/Pages/default.aspx. Accessed February 29, 2017; National Association of Emergency Medical Technicians (NAEMT). Tactical Combat Casualty Care Guidelines for Medical Personnel. http://www.naemt.org/education/TCCC/guidelines_curriculum. Published June 3, 2016. Accessed February 29, 2017; Hypoglycemia/Hyperglycemia. In: *National Model EMS Clinical Guidelines*. National Association of State EMS Officials. V.08-16:58. https://www.nasemso.org/Projects/ModelEMSClinicalGuidelines/index.asp. Accessed April 7, 2017; Bronchospasm (due to Asthma and Obstructive Lung Disease). In: *National Model EMS Clinical Guidelines*. National Association of State EMS Officials. V.08-16:135. https://www.nasemso.org/Projects/ModelEMSClinicalGuidelines/index.asp. Accessed April 7, 2017; Glucagon for injection. Lilly USA, LLC website. http://pi.lilly.com/us/rglucagon-pi.pdf. Revised September 19, 2012. Accessed March 29, 2017; Naloxone hydrochloride. Hospira, Inc. website. http://labeling.pfizer.com/ShowLabeling.aspx?id=4542. Revised January 2007. Accessed March 29, 2017; Pulmonary Edema. In: *National Model EMS Clinical Guidelines*. National Association of State EMS Officials. V.08-16:143. https://www.nasemso.org/Projects/ModelEMSClinicalGuidelines/index.asp. Accessed April 7, 2017; Pulmonary Edema. In: *National Model EMS Clinical Guidelines*. National Association of State EMS Officials. V.08-16:141. https://www.nasemso.org/Projects/ModelEMSClinicalGuidelines/index.asp. Accessed April 7, 2017; Hypoglycemia/Hyperglycemia. In: *National Model EMS Clinical Guidelines*. National Association of State EMS Officials. V.08-16:57. https://www.nasemso.org/Projects/ModelEMSClinicalGuidelines/index.asp. Accessed April 7, 2017.

YOU are the Provider SUMMARY

1. Are there any potential hazards with this scene?

As with any call that you respond to, scene safety is paramount. This patient has a known history of IV drug abuse; therefore, contaminated uncapped needles may be present. Also, when the patient regains consciousness, he may become hostile and combative.

2. What medication might the AEMT carry that would be appropriate to administer in this situation?

An AEMT may be approved by the medical director to carry and administer the medication naloxone (Narcan), which is given to patients with an acute narcotic overdose.

3. By which route(s) may naloxone be administered?

Naloxone may be administered IV, IM, subcutaneously, intranasally, and IO. Each route of administration has its own risks and benefits and should be carefully evaluated to ensure that you are administering the medication by the best route for that patient.

The standard adult dose of naloxone is 0.4 to 2 mg by slow IV push. Naloxone administration may be repeated at 5-minute intervals if needed. If no response is seen after a total of 10 mg has been administered, you need to consider another cause of the patient's unresponsiveness.

YOU are the Provider SUMMARY (continued)

Precautions to naloxone administration include using caution when administering to patients with supraventricular dysrhythmias, head injuries, and increased intracranial pressure. Naloxone may also cause seizures, so you should use caution in administering the drug to patients with convulsive disorders. Because the duration of action of naloxone is shorter than that of narcotics, repeated doses of naloxone may be necessary when treating a patient who is not an addict but has overdosed on narcotics.

4. What class of medication is naloxone?

Naloxone is classified as an opioid antagonist. An opioid antagonist competitively binds with the opiate receptors. As a result of this binding, the opioid molecules cannot get to the receptor.

5. What is the mechanism of action of naloxone?

Naloxone works by competitively inhibiting at narcotic receptor sites. This competitive action displaces narcotic analgesics from their receptor sites, blocking their effects, which include CNS depression and respiratory depression.

6. What is the half-life of naloxone?

Naloxone generally begins acting within 2 minutes, and its effects typically last for 30 to 60 minutes.

EMS Patient Care Report (PCR)

Date: 4-20-18	**Incident No.:** 20183724	**Nature of Call:** Unresponsive	**Location:** Main & Central		
Dispatched: 0112	**En Route:** 0116	**At Scene:** 0120	**Transport:** 0131	**At Hospital:** 0140	**In Service:** 0200

Patient Information

Age: 39 **Sex:** M **Weight (in kg [lb]):** 55 kg (122 lb)	**Allergies:** None **Medications:** None **Past Medical History:** IV drug abuser per PD **Chief Complaint:** Unresponsive

Vital Signs

Time: 0121	**BP:** Not obtained	**Pulse:** Not obtained	**Respirations:** 10, assisted	**Spo_2:** Not obtained
Time: 0128	**BP:** 124/66	**Pulse:** 82	**Respirations:** 12, assisted	**Spo_2:** 100% on 15 L/min via bag-mask device
Time: 0136	**BP:** 122/74	**Pulse:** 68	**Respirations:** 20	**Spo_2:** 100% on 15 L/min via NRM

EMS Treatment (circle all that apply)

Oxygen @ 15 **L/min via (circle one):** **NC** **(NRM)** **(Bag-mask device)**		**(Assisted Ventilation)**	**Airway Adjunct**	**CPR**
Defibrillation	**Bleeding Control**	**Bandaging**	**Splinting**	**(Other:** 0.4 mg naloxone IN)

Narrative

EMS dispatched to above location for unresponsive male. On arrival find Denville Police Department officer with patient. Patient is unresponsive and apneic. Police officer assisting ventilations with pocket mask. Officer states patient is well known to him, known history of IV heroin use. Ventilations assisted with bag-mask device. Rapid assessment reveals fresh track marks found on arms, no obvious trauma. Pupils constricted and sluggish. 0.4 mg naloxone given intranasally (left naris). After approximately 2 minutes, patient begins to arouse, but groggy. Ventilations stopped, patient placed on nonrebreathing mask at 15 L/min. Informed patient that he overdosed on narcotics, to which he replied, "Not again." Advised of need to be evaluated at ED, to which patient reluctantly agreed. Assisted patient to stretcher, secured, transported nonemergent. En route: Patient maintains patent airway, AO×4, calm and cooperative throughout transport. On arrival at ED, care and report given to ED staff without incident.**End of report**

Prep Kit

▶ Ready for Review

- Pharmacology is the study of the properties (characteristics) and effects of drugs and medications on the body. Drugs are substances that produce a physiologic effect, whether therapeutic or not. Medications are chemical agents used to treat or prevent disease or relieve pain. They have intended effects, unintended effects, and may have untoward effects (those that can be harmful to the patient).
- There are indications and contraindications for each medication. Indications are the therapeutic uses for a particular medication. Contraindications are cases in which you should not give a patient medication.
- As an AEMT you must be familiar with the various names of medications (trade, generic, chemical, official), the sources of medications, their classification, and sources where information on medications may be obtained.
- The manufacture of pharmaceuticals in most countries is regulated to protect consumers. For example, standardized manufacturing is required for uniform strength and purity.
- The Controlled Substances Act of 1970 is comprehensive legislation dealing with narcotic and non-narcotic drugs that have a potential for abuse and consists of five categories or schedules according to abuse potential. Schedule I represents the highest abuse potential and Schedule V is the lowest.
- Medications must go through an approval process that includes animal studies and clinical trials in humans before being approved for distribution.
- There are special considerations for certain groups of patients when administering medications: geriatric, pediatric, and pregnant patients. With pregnant patients, the health of the mother is the priority in emergency situations. US Food and Drug Administration Categories A, B, C, D, and X rate risk to the fetus, with Category X representing the greatest risk. This system is being replaced by a more detailed system that uses narrative summaries regarding pregnancy, lactation, and reproductive effects.
- There are several medication concerns related to geriatric patients. Effects of a medication may be delayed. Geriatric patients often take several medications, making drug interaction possible. Alterations in mental status can result in overdosing or underdosing.
- As an AEMT, you are held responsible for safe and therapeutically effective medication administration. This includes legal, moral, and ethical considerations.
- Drugs are grouped into classifications based on their effect on a body system, or their mechanism of action (how they create the effect).
- To understand the effects drugs have on the body, you must have an understanding of the nervous system. The sympathetic nervous system is responsible for the body's response to shock and stress ("fight or flight"). The parasympathetic nervous system relaxes the body, controlling automatic functions during nonstressful times ("rest and relax").
- Adrenergic receptors cause a response in the target organ and are grouped as alpha-1, alpha-2, beta-1, and beta-2. Some medications stimulate alpha and beta receptors, whereas others may block specific receptors.
- Drugs that produce the same effects as sympathetic nervous system hormones are sympathomimetics. Drugs that have the opposite effect are sympatholytics.
- Agonists aid or increase effects. Antagonists antagonize or fight the effects of another substance.
- Beta blockers are used to control blood pressure in some patients and heart rhythm disturbances in others. Beta blockers work by filling a portion of the beta receptor sites to prevent binding by beta stimulators that occur naturally in the body and can be introduced as a medication.
- Agonists to the parasympathetic nervous system are known as parasympathomimetics, and antagonists are known as parasympatholytics. One of the most commonly used parasympatholytics is the drug atropine that is used for symptomatic bradycardia and exposure to organophosphates and certain chemical nerve agents.
- Analgesics include medications that relieve pain. The most common class of medications used for analgesia in the prehospital setting comprises the opioid agonists. Opioid antagonists reverse the effects of opioid drugs. Opioid agonist-antagonists have agonistic and antagonistic properties. They are often preferred because they can decrease pain but do not diminish the function of the respiratory system or result in dependence or addiction.
- Sedative-hypnotics do what their name suggests: sedate and produce hypnosis. They are preferred for invasive procedures. Drugs that create sedation and hypnosis include benzodiazepines, barbiturates, opioid agonists, and nonbarbiturate hypnotics.
- Stimulants excite the central nervous system, while depressants slow brain activity.
- Drugs that affect the cardiac system may affect heart rate, force of contraction, or velocity of conduction through the heart. Cardiac glycosides,

Prep Kit *(continued)*

antidysrhythmics, and antihypertensive medications are included in this group.

- Antihypertensive medications include diuretics, vasodilator medications, angiotensin-converting enzyme inhibitors, and calcium channel blockers.
- Certain medications prevent or minimize the effects of thrombi. These include antiplatelet agents, anticoagulants, and fibrinolytics.
- Drugs that affect the respiratory system include oxygen, over-the-counter decongestants, bronchodilators, and xanthines.
- Drugs come in many different forms, including solid, liquid, inhaled, topical, transcutaneous, gels, and gases. Liquid intravenous (IV) medications are some of the most common medications in the prehospital setting.
- You should also know the various routes of medication administration and which routes are used for the drugs you may administer in the prehospital setting. Routes include enteral and parenteral.
- Enteral drugs are those that are administered along any portion of the gastrointestinal tract, including the oral and rectal routes.
- Parenteral drugs are those that are administered through any route other than the gastrointestinal tract and include IV, intraosseous (IO), subcutaneous, intramuscular (IM), sublingual (SL), buccal, transcutaneous, intranasal, and inhalation.
- After drugs are administered, they go through four stages: absorption, distribution, metabolism, and excretion.
- Pharmacokinetics is the study of the metabolism and action of drugs with particular emphasis on the time required for absorption, duration of action, distribution in the body, and method of excretion. The onset of action, peak, and duration of action are important concepts in pharmacokinetics.
- Pharmacodynamics is the way in which a medication produces the response we intended, also known as the mechanism of action. It also encompasses the factors that may alter the intended response and any side effects or unexpected effects.
- Factors that alter drug response include age, body mass, sex, environmental conditions, time of administration, genetic factors, and psychological factors.
- Responses beyond the desired effect are side effects and may occur even when a medication is administered properly.
- Unpredictable responses may occur when a medication is administered. These include allergic reaction, serum sickness, and idiosyncratic reaction. Other effects that may occur include cumulative effect, summation, potentiation, drug dependence, and drug interaction.
- Administering medication includes the risk of making an error. To minimize errors, follow the ten rights of medication administration. Follow a procedure such as a medication administration cross-check to ensure safe administration.
- Certain medication abbreviations are prone to causing errors. Become familiar with these so you can decrease the chance of misinterpretation.
- Overall, it is important to learn as much as you can about the medications you may be allowed to administer in your area. Carry a pharmacologic reference to look up medications that may be unfamiliar.
- You should also be aware of proper medication storage and security. Follow local protocols for medication administration, and review pharmacology often.

▶ Vital Vocabulary

absorption The process by which medications travel through body tissues until they reach the bloodstream.

action The expected therapeutic effect of a medication on the body.

adrenergic Pertaining to nerves that release the neurotransmitter norepinephrine or noradrenaline; also pertains to the receptors acted on by norepinephrine.

agonists Drugs that bind to a receptor and cause a response.

analgesics A classification for medications that relieve pain or induce analgesia.

angiotensin-converting enzyme (ACE) inhibitors Medications that suppress the conversion of angiotensin I to angiotensin II.

antagonists In the pharmacologic sense, drugs that counteract the action of something else, such as a muscle or drug.

anticholinergic Of or pertaining to blockage of acetylcholine receptors, resulting in inhibition of transmission of parasympathetic nerve impulses.

Prep Kit *(continued)*

anticoagulant drugs The medications used to prevent intravascular thrombosis by preventing blood coagulation in the vascular system.

anticonvulsant medications The medications used to treat seizures, which are believed to work by inhibiting the influx of sodium into cells.

antidysrhythmic medications The medications used to treat and prevent cardiac rhythm disorders.

antihypertensives The medications used to control blood pressure.

antiplatelet agents The medications that interfere with the collection of platelets.

autonomic nervous system (ANS) The part of the nervous system that regulates functions, such as digestion and sweating, that are not controlled voluntarily.

barbiturates Any medications of a group of barbituric acid derivatives that act as central nervous system depressants and are used as sedatives or hypnotics.

benzodiazepines Sedative-hypnotic drugs that provide muscle relaxation and mild sedation; includes drugs such as diazepam (Valium) and midazolam (Versed).

beta blocker A common class of cardiac drugs that blocks beta effects, causing a decrease in the workload of the heart by reducing the speed of contraction, as well as reducing blood pressure.

bioavailability The rate at and extent to which an active drug enters the general circulation, permitting access to the site of action.

biotransformation The chemical alteration that a substance undergoes in the body.

buccal A medication route in which the medication is placed between the cheek and gums, where it is absorbed into the bloodstream.

calcium channel blockers The medications that suppress dysrhythmias, provide more oxygen to the heart via coronary artery dilation, and reduce peripheral vascular resistance.

cardiac glycosides A classification of medications that naturally occur in plant substances and that block certain ionic pumps in the membranes of heart cells, which indirectly increases calcium concentrations; an example is digoxin.

chemical name Precise description of a drug's chemical composition and molecular structure.

cholinergic Fibers in the parasympathetic nervous system that release a chemical called acetylcholine.

chronotropic Affecting the rate of contraction of the heart.

contraindications Situations in which a medication should not be given because it would not help or may actually harm a patient.

cross-tolerance A tolerance to a particular drug that crosses over to other drugs in the same class.

cumulative effect Action of increased intensity after administration of several doses of a drug.

depressants Agents used to slow brain activity.

diffusion The movement of solutes (molecules) from an area of higher concentration to an area of lower concentration.

diuretic medications The medications designed to promote elimination of excess salt and water by the kidneys.

dose The amount of medication given on the basis of the patient's size and age.

dromotropic Affecting the velocity of conduction in the heart.

drug antagonism A decrease in the action of a drug by the administration of another drug.

drug dependence A psychological and sometimes physical state resulting from continued use of a substance, characterized by a compulsion to take the drug on a continuous or periodic basis to experience its effects or to avoid the discomfort of its absence.

drugs Chemical agents used in the diagnosis, treatment, and prevention of disease.

duration of action The amount of time a medication concentration can be expected to remain above the minimum level needed to provide the intended action.

enteral Drugs that are administered along any portion of the gastrointestinal tract, including the oral and rectal routes.

excretion The elimination of waste products from the body.

extrapyramidal symptoms A wide array of symptoms such as involuntary movements, tremors, rigidity, muscle contractions, restlessness, and changes in breathing and heart rate, usually as a result of taking antipsychotic drugs.

Prep Kit *(continued)*

fibrinolytic agent Medication that dissolves blood clots after they have already formed; promotes the digestion of fibrin.

filtration The removing of particles from a solution by allowing the liquid portion to pass through a membrane or other partial barrier.

gel A semiliquid substance that is administered orally through capsules or plastic tubes.

generic name The original chemical name of a medication (in contrast with one of its trade names); not capitalized.

habituation The situation in which there is a physical tolerance and psychological dependence on a drug or drugs.

half-life The time required by the body, tissue, or organ to metabolize or inactivate one-half of the amount of a substance taken in; an important consideration in determining the proper dose of drug and frequency of administration.

hypersensitivity Occurs when a patient reacts with exaggerated or inappropriate allergic symptoms after coming in contact with a substance the body perceives as harmful.

iatrogenic response An adverse condition induced in a patient by the treatment given.

idiosyncrasy An abnormal sensitivity or reaction to a drug or other substance that is peculiar to an individual.

idiosyncratic reaction A peculiar or individual response to a drug or medication through unusual susceptibility.

immunosuppressant medications The medications intended to inhibit the body's ability to attack the "foreign" transplanted organ or in the case of autoimmune diseases, the medications that inhibit the body's attack on itself.

indications Therapeutic uses for a specific medication.

inhalation Breathing into the lungs; a medication delivery route.

inotropic Affecting the contractility of muscle tissue, especially cardiac muscle.

intended effect The effect that a medication is expected to have on the body.

interference A direct biochemical interaction between two drugs.

intramuscular (IM) injection Injection into a muscle; a medication delivery route.

intranasal (IN) Into the nasal mucosa; a medication delivery route.

intraosseous (IO) Into the bone; a medication delivery route.

intravenous (IV) injection Injection directly into a vein; a medication delivery route.

mechanism of action The way in which a medication produces the intended response.

medication A chemical substance that is used to treat or prevent disease or relieve pain.

medication interaction A situation in which the effects of one medication alter the response of another medication.

metered-dose inhaler (MDI) A miniature spray canister through which droplets or particles of medication may be inhaled.

mucosal atomizer device (MAD) A device that attaches to the end of a syringe that is used to spray (atomize) certain medications via the intranasal route.

muscarinic cholinergic antagonists Medications that block acetylcholine exclusively at the muscarinic receptors; an example is atropine.

nonbarbiturate hypnotics Medications designed to sedate without the side effects of a barbiturate.

nonopioid analgesics Medications designed to relieve pain without the side effects of opioids.

nonsteroidal anti-inflammatory drugs (NSAIDs) Medications with analgesic and fever-reducing properties.

official name Drug name assigned by the *United States Pharmacopeia* (*USP*), generally the generic name followed by "USP."

onset of action The time needed for the concentration of the medication at the target tissue to reach the minimum effective level.

opioid agonist-antagonists Medications designed to relieve pain without the side effects of opioids.

opioid agonists Chemicals that are similar to or derived from the opium plant.

opioid antagonists A classification of medications that reverses the effects of opioid drugs.

oral By mouth; a medication delivery route.

oral glucose A simple sugar that is readily absorbed by the bloodstream; it is carried on the EMS unit.

osmosis The movement of a solvent (fluid) from an area of lower solute concentration to an area of higher solute concentration.

over-the-counter (OTC) medications Medications that may be purchased directly by a patient without a prescription.

parasympathetic nervous system The part of the autonomic nervous system that relaxes the body.

Prep Kit *(continued)*

parasympatholytics Drugs that block the actions of the parasympathetic nervous system; also known as anticholinergics.

parasympathomimetics Drugs that produce the same effects as those of the parasympathetic nervous system; also known as cholinergics.

parenteral Drug administration through any route other than through the gastrointestinal tract; includes intravenous, intraosseous, subcutaneous, intramuscular, sublingual, buccal, transcutaneous, intranasal, and inhalation.

peak In a pharmacologic context, the point of maximum effect of a drug.

pH The measure of acidity and alkalinity of a solution.

pharmacodynamics The study of drugs and their actions on living organisms.

pharmacokinetics The study of the metabolism and action of drugs with a particular emphasis on the time required for absorption, duration of action, distribution in the body, and method of excretion.

pharmacology The study of the properties and effects of medications.

polypharmacy The use of many drugs by the same patient.

potassium channel blockers Medications that increase the contractility of the heart and work against the reentry of blocked impulses.

potentiation Enhancement of the action of a drug by the administration of another drug.

prescription medications Medications that are distributed to patients only by pharmacists according to a physician's order.

rectal Through the rectum; a medication delivery route.

refractory Describes a disease or condition that does not respond to treatment.

serum sickness A condition in which antigen-antibody complexes formed in the bloodstream deposit in sites around the body, most notably in the kidney, with resultant inflammatory reactions.

side effects Any effects of a medication other than the desired ones.

sodium channel blockers Antidysrhythmic medications that slow conduction through the heart.

solution A liquid mixture that cannot be separated by filtering or allowing the mixture to stand.

stimulants An agent that increases the level of body activity.

subcutaneous injection Injection into the tissue between the skin and muscle; a medication delivery route.

sublingual (SL) Under the tongue; a medication delivery route.

summation effect Increased effect that may occur when two drugs that have the same or similar action are given together.

suspension A mixture of ground particles that are distributed evenly throughout a liquid but do not dissolve.

sympathetic blocking agents An antihypertensive medication that decreases cardiac output and renin secretions.

sympathetic nervous system Part of the autonomic nervous system that is responsible for the body's response to shock and stress.

sympatholytics Drugs that block the actions of the sympathetic nervous system.

sympathomimetics Drugs that produce the same effects as the hormones of the sympathetic nervous system.

synergism Combined effect of two drugs that is greater than the sum of their individual effects.

teratogenic Poses a risk to the normal development or health of the unborn fetus.

termination of action The amount of time after the concentration of a medication falls below the minimum effective level until it is eliminated from the body.

therapeutic index The difference between the minimum effective concentration and the toxic level of a drug.

therapeutic threshold The minimum concentration of a drug necessary to cause the desired response.

tolerance The capacity for enduring a large amount of a substance without an adverse effect and showing decreased sensitivity to subsequent doses of the same substance.

topical medications Lotions, creams, and ointments that are applied to the surface of the skin and affect only that area; a medication delivery route.

toxicity The risk that a substance will pose a health hazard to an individual or organism.

trade name The brand name that a manufacturer gives a medication; capitalized.

transcutaneous Through the skin; a medication delivery route; also called transdermal.

unintended effects Actions that are undesirable but pose little risk to the patient.

Prep Kit (continued)

untoward effects Actions that can be harmful to the patient.

vasodilator medications The medications that work on the smooth muscles of the arterioles and/or the veins.

xanthines A classification of medications that affect the respiratory smooth muscle and that relax bronchiole smooth muscles, stimulate cardiac muscle, and stimulate the central nervous system.

▶ References

1. State Marijuana Laws in 2017 Map. Governing website. http://www.governing.com/gov-data/state-marijuana-laws-map-medical-recreational.html. Accessed October 30, 2017.
2. FDA pregnancy categories. Drugs.com website. https://www.drugs.com/pregnancy-categories.html. Accessed March 9, 2017.
3. Pregnancy and lactation labeling (drugs) final rule. U.S. Food and Drug Administration website. http://www.fda.gov/Drugs/DevelopmentApprovalProcess/DevelopmentResources/Labeling/ucm093307.htm. Page last updated November 18, 2016. Accessed March 9, 2017.
4. Opioid (narcotic) pain medications. WebMD website. http://www.webmd.com/pain-management/guide/narcotic-pain-medications#1. Accessed September 20, 2017.
5. Nwankwo T, Yoon SS, Burt V, Gu Q. Hypertension among adults in the US: National Health and Nutrition Examination Survey, 2011-2012. NCHS Data Brief, No. 133. Hyattsville, MD: National Center for Health Statistics, Centers for Disease Control and Prevention, US Dept of Health and Human Services; 2013.
6. Misasi P, Braithwaite S. The Medication Administration Cross-Check© (MACC) User's Manual. Wichita-Sedgwick County EMS System. https://kansasemstransition.files.wordpress.com/2012/08/macc-user-manual-v2-0.pdf. Published 2012. Accessed May 26, 2016.
7. FDA and ISMP Lists of Look-Alike Drug Names and Recommended Tall Man Letters. Horsham, PA: Institute for Safe Medication Practices; 2016:1-6. Table 12-10

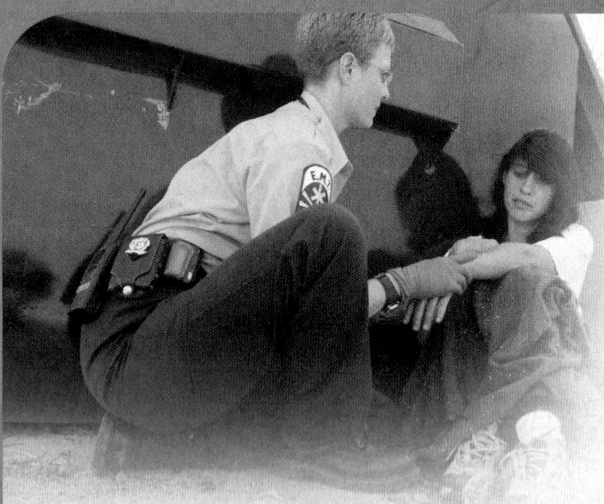

Assessment in Action

You arrive on scene to find an elderly man complaining of chest pain, which he describes as a constant pressure radiating to his left arm and jaw. You believe that the patient may be experiencing an acute myocardial infarction and prepare your treatment.

1. Which of the following is NOT an indication for the use of nitroglycerin?

A. Angina pectoris
B. Pulmonary edema
C. Hypertension
D. Commotio cordis

2. Nitroglycerin does NOT come in which of the following forms?

A. Gel
B. Transcutaneous
C. Tablet
D. Intravenous

Assessment *in Action* *(continued)*

3. Nitroglycerin can be administered by which of the following routes?

A. Inhalation
B. Intramuscular
C. Sublingual
D. Intradermal

4. Medications such as sildenafil (Viagra), tadalafil (Cialis), and vardenafil (Levitra) can have potentially fatal interactions with nitroglycerin due to their _____ effects.

A. vasodilatory
B. vasoconstriction
C. beta-1 agonist
D. beta-1 antagonist

5. After you administer the appropriate dose of nitroglycerin to your patient, he begins to have a seizure. This would be an example of a(n):

A. contraindication.
B. side effect.
C. idiosyncratic reaction.
D. allergic reaction.

6. Which term describes the interaction between two medications that causes one drug to enhance the effect of another?

A. Summation
B. Synergism
C. Potentiation
D. Interference

7. Valium (Diazepam) is categorized by the Controlled Substances Act of 1970 as a __________ medication.

A. Schedule I
B. Schedule II
C. Schedule III
D. Schedule IV

8. This category of medications is defined as "Risk of adverse effects has clearly been demonstrated in humans; therefore, these drugs should not be administered to pregnant or potentially pregnant women."

A. Category A
B. Category B
C. Category C
D. Category X

9. List the ten rights of medication administration.

10. Explain the difference between *enteral* and *parenteral* drugs.

CHAPTER 13

Vascular Access and Medication Administration

National EMS Education Standard Competencies

Pharmacology

Applies (to patient assessment and management) fundamental knowledge of the medications carried by advanced emergency medical technicians (AEMTs) that may be administered to a patient during an emergency.

Medication Administration

- Routes of administration (pp 627-644)
- Self-administer medication (pp 627-628)
- Peer-administer medication (pp 628-644)
- Assist/administer medications to a patient (pp 627-644)

Emergency Medications

- Names (Chapter 12, *Principles of Pharmacology*)
- Effects (Chapter 12, *Principles of Pharmacology*)
- Indications (Chapter 12, *Principles of Pharmacology*)
- Routes of administration (pp 627-644)
- Dosages for the medications administered (pp 588-589, and Chapter 12, *Principles of Pharmacology*)
- Actions (Chapter 12, *Principles of Pharmacology*)
- Contraindications (Chapter 12, *Principles of Pharmacology*)
- Complications (Chapter 12, *Principles of Pharmacology*)
- Side effects (p 590, and Chapter 12, *Principles of Pharmacology*)
- Interactions (Chapter 12, *Principles of Pharmacology*)

Knowledge Objectives

1. Describe the role of medical direction in medication administration, and explain the difference between direct orders (online) and standing orders (offline). (p 588)
2. Explain the 10 rights of medication administration and describe how each one relates to emergency medical services. (pp 588-590)
3. Explain why determining a patient's prescription and over-the-counter (OTC) medications is a critical aspect of patient assessment. (p 589)
4. Discuss basic cell physiology and how it relates to intravenous (IV) therapy. (pp 590-597)
5. List commonly used IV fluid compositions and types of IV solutions. (pp 595-597)
6. Discuss the techniques for performing IV therapy. (pp 597-610)
7. Discuss the factors to consider when choosing an IV solution. (p 598)
8. Discuss the factors to consider when choosing an administration set. (pp 598-600)
9. Discuss the factors to consider when choosing an IV site. (pp 601-603)
10. List types of IV catheters. (pp 603-604)
11. Discuss alternative IV sites and techniques. (pp 609-610)
12. Describe complications that can occur as a result of IV therapy. (pp 610-613)
13. Describe special considerations when performing IV therapy on a pediatric or geriatric patient. (pp 613-614)
14. Discuss the techniques for establishing an intraosseous (IO) line. (pp 615-616, 618-620)
15. List the types of IO devices available. (pp 616-618)
16. Discuss the possible complications of IO infusion. (pp 620-621)
17. Discuss the systems of weights and measures used when administering medication. (pp 622-623)
18. Explain principles of drug dose calculations, including desired dose, concentration on hand, volume on hand, volume to administer, and IV drip rate. (pp 624-626)
19. Discuss the advantages, disadvantages, and techniques for administering the following routes:
    - Oral administration (pp 627-628)
    - Rectal administration (p 628)
    - Subcutaneous administration (pp 632-634)
    - Intramuscular administration (pp 633-636)
    - Sublingual administration (pp 636-637)
    - Intranasal administration (pp 636-638)
    - Administration by inhalation (pp 637, 639-642)
    - IV administration (pp 641-643)
    - IO administration (pp 643-644)

Skills Objectives

1. Demonstrate the process an AEMT should follow when following the 10 rights of medication administration. (pp 588-590)

2. Demonstrate how to spike an IV bag. (pp 600-601, Skill Drill 13-1)
3. Demonstrate how to obtain vascular access. (pp 606-608, Skill Drill 13-2)
4. Demonstrate how to gain IO access. (pp 618-620, Skill Drill 13-3)
5. Demonstrate how to administer oral medication to a patient. (pp 627-628)
6. Demonstrate how to draw medication from an ampule. (pp 629-630, Skill Drill 13-4)
7. Demonstrate how to draw medication from a vial. (pp 629, 631-632, Skill Drill 13-5)
8. Demonstrate how to administer a subcutaneous medication to a patient. (pp 632-634, Skill Drill 13-6)
9. Demonstrate how to administer an intramuscular medication to a patient. (pp 633-636, Skill Drill 13-7)
10. Demonstrate how to administer a sublingual medication to a patient. (pp 636-637, Skill Drill 13-8)
11. Demonstrate how to administer an intranasal medication to a patient. (pp 636-638, Skill Drill 13-9)
12. Demonstrate how to administer a medication via inhalation to a patient. (pp 637, 639-642)
13. Demonstrate how to assist a patient with a metered-dose inhaler (MDI). (pp 639-640, Skill Drill 13-10)
14. Demonstrate how to assist a patient with a small-volume nebulizer. (pp 639, 641-642, Skill Drill 13-11)
15. Demonstrate how to administer a medication via the IV bolus route. (pp 641-643, Skill Drill 13-12)
16. Demonstrate how to administer a medication via the IO route. (pp 643-644, Skill Drill 13-13)

Introduction

Before you administer any medication to a patient, you must have a thorough understanding of how the medication will affect the body—both negatively and positively. This includes familiarity with the medication's mechanism of action, indications, contraindications, routes of administration, dose, adverse reactions, and what to do in the event of an adverse reaction; this information was discussed in Chapter 12, *Principles of Pharmacology*. This also is true of medications belonging to the patient that you may assist the patient in taking.

The first rule of medicine is "First, do no harm." For example, administering the medication glucagon to a patient who is not hypoglycemic could result in hyperglycemia and potential compromise and cause harm to the patient. It is therefore paramount to ensure that a particular medication is clearly indicated to treat the patient's condition. A careful assessment of the patient will help ensure that only beneficial medications are administered **Figure 13-1**.

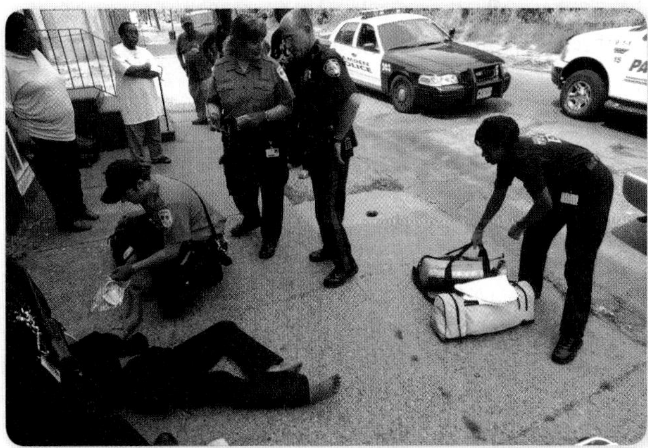

Figure 13-1 Carefully assess the patient before administering a medication.

Intravenous (IV) therapy is one of the most invasive procedures an advanced emergency medical technician (AEMT) learns. During your career in emergency medical

YOU are the Provider — PART 1

Your ambulance is dispatched to a local intersection for a motor vehicle crash. On arrival, you find a single vehicle that hit a telephone pole at approximately 45 miles per hour. Your patient is a 35-year-old woman seated in the driver's seat. She is responsive, alert, oriented, and complaining of severe abdominal pain. You instruct your partner to hold manual spinal immobilization as you apply an appropriate-size cervical collar. With the assistance of the fire department responders, you extricate the patient onto a long backboard and begin your assessment.

1. On the basis of the information given, do you think this patient will require intravenous (IV) access?
2. What is the appropriate-size IV catheter for this patient?

services (EMS), few procedures will require more training or practice. Proficiency in IV therapy and technique is required for most advanced life support procedures.

A medical problem of any type alters a person's established balance among the systems (internal environment) of the body. This balance, called **homeostasis**, produces optimal physical performance. It is the job of health care providers to fully assess a patient's condition and to identify and treat life-threatening injuries and illnesses that alter homeostasis. AEMTs are often first on the scene and provide the first care for persons who need their homeostatic balance restored.

In addition to knowledge of the medications you may administer as an AEMT, you must also understand basic math for pharmacology to calculate the appropriate medication dose.

Drug doses and flow rate calculations are common areas of confusion for many prehospital personnel, yet they are skills you will need to perform frequently in the field. As an AEMT, you must learn to quickly and accurately calculate doses to maximize the chance for a positive patient outcome. Disastrous results, including death, may occur if you administer an inappropriate medication or dose, give a medication by the wrong route, or give the medication too rapidly or too slowly.

Medication Administration

Medical Direction

Medication administration is governed by your local protocols and/or online medical direction. The medical director for your service may allow the administration of certain medications as long as the patient meets certain criteria. Most EMS services carry drug boxes with a variety of cardiac medications, pain medications, anticonvulsants, antiemetics, and other medications specific to their service.

For example, for an unresponsive diabetic patient with a confirmed blood glucose reading of 40 mg/dL, the AEMT may be allowed by written protocols (standing orders) to administer 50% dextrose (D_{50}). As discussed in Chapter 1, *EMS Systems*, standing orders are a form of offline or indirect medical control, in which the AEMT performs certain predefined procedures before contacting the physician.

Some EMS system medical directors require AEMTs to contact them before performing certain procedures (for example, administering medications), referred to as online (direct) medical control.

Local policies and procedures are designed to guide you in specific situations. When questions or unusual situations arise—even if you function primarily by standing orders—contact medical control for direction. *If you have any doubt as to the correct action, consult with medical control!*

AEMT's Responsibility Associated With Drug Orders

The danger of something going wrong when administering a medication—for example, administering the wrong medication or the wrong dose of a medication—can be minimized by confirming the 10 rights of medication administration discussed in Chapter 12, *Principles of Pharmacology*:

- Right patient
- Right medication
- Right dose
- Right route
- Right time
- Right documentation and reporting
- Right assessment
- Right to refuse
- Right evaluation
- Right patient education

These principles are included in the following set procedure for administering any medication. These steps also incorporate several safety precautions:

1. **Obtain an order from medical control.** This order may be given to you directly, through online medical control via telephone or radio. Or it may be indirect, through protocols that contain standing orders for the administration of certain medications. For example, your system may use a protocol that describes how the medical director wants you to deal with a patient who is having respiratory difficulties. Part of this protocol may direct you to use a nonrebreathing mask to deliver oxygen to such a patient at 15 L/min. You may do this without calling online medical control if the patient meets the criteria of the protocol.

   When you are communicating with medical control about administering a particular medication, make sure that the medication is indicated for the patient's condition. Knowledge of the indications, contraindications, therapeutic effects, side effects, and appropriate doses for each of the medications that you carry on your ambulance is critical to safe patient care. Given the patient's clinical presentation, you must know the *right time* to administer a medication (that is, when the medication is indicated). Of equal if not greater importance is knowing when *not* to administer a medication (that is, when the medication is contraindicated). Furthermore, some of the medications you carry on the ambulance have specific intervals for repeated doses; you must be aware of these medications and the appropriate intervals at which they are administered.

Make sure medical control understands the situation. The decision to order the administration of any given medication is complex, involving such considerations as the patient's age, weight, clinical status, allergy history, concomitant medical problems, and other drugs he or she may be taking, including prescription medications, over-the-counter (OTC) medications, and recreational drugs. Thus, it is critical that you obtain and communicate complete, accurate information about the patient to enable the physician to make prudent, correct decisions about medication administration.

Verify that your patient is indeed the *right patient.* In situations in which there are multiple patients, reconfirm the patient's name and compare it with the wrist band or triage tag. If you are assisting a patient with his or her medication, be sure it is prescribed to that patient.

2. **Make sure you understand the physician's orders.** If the orders are unclear or seem inappropriate for the patient's condition (for example, the dosage is more than the usual range or an unusual route of administration is requested), *ask the physician to repeat the order.* Do not assume that the physician is infallible.
3. **Repeat any orders, word for word, for verification.** This will help ensure that you understand the order and that the physician did not inadvertently give you an incorrect dosage order. In the repetition, state the *name of the medication,* the *dose,* and the *route* by which it is to be given. As an AEMT, you are just as responsible for the administration of the medication and its possible consequences as the physician giving the order, so be absolutely certain which medication is to be administered, in what dose, and by which route. If your partner does not hear the exchange of information, you should repeat the order to him or her as an additional safety measure.
4. **Inquire about any medication allergies the patient may have.** If the patient is unresponsive, try to obtain this information from another reliable source of information. Check for medic alert jewelry or tags as well.
5. **Verify the proper medication and prescription.** You have received and confirmed the medication order and determined that the patient is still a candidate for the medication. You must now make sure that the medication you are about to give is the correct medication. Carefully read the label. If it is the patient's own prescription, the bottle may show the trade name or the generic name. If you have any questions at all, contact online medical control. Examine the label to confirm that the medication is prescribed to the patient and not to a family member or friend. You should never give a medication to a patient that has been prescribed for someone else. Note the **concentration** printed on the label.

   Note that you should read the medication label at least three times before administration to ensure that you have the *right medication:*
   - When it is still in the drug box it came in
   - When you prepare the medication for administration
   - Before actually administering the medication to the patient
6. **Verify the form, dose, and route of the medication.** At this point, you have confirmed your order and verified that the medication is correct. Now you must make sure that the form of the medication, the dose, and the route are all consistent with the order you received. For example, suppose that you are told to administer a sublingual nitroglycerin tablet. The patient's nitroglycerin bottle is empty, but he has another bottle of nitroglycerin capsules. These are to be swallowed four times per day. The medication is the same, but the form, dose, and route of delivery are different from the order given. You may not substitute the capsules for the tablets without specific orders from medical control.

   You are responsible for knowing the appropriate doses for the medications you carry on your ambulance. You are also responsible for accurately calculating the appropriate dose of the medication. Always recheck your medication calculations before administration to ensure that you are administering the *right dose.*

   It is imperative that you know the *right route* for the medication(s) you are about to administer. A medication given by an inappropriate route—even if it is the right medication—could have disastrous and possibly fatal consequences.
7. **Check the expiration date and condition of the medication.** The last step before administering a medication is to make sure the expiration date has not passed. Prescription and OTC medications should have an expiration date on their labels. Check the date. If no date can be found, you should examine the medication with suspicion. Check for defects in the vial, preloaded syringe, or ampule, noting whether the container appears to be cracked or damaged. If the medication looks suspicious in any way, do *not* use it. In addition, if you find discoloration, cloudiness, or particles in a liquid medication, you should

not administer it. If a patient with asthma gives you a metered-dose inhaler (MDI) and the expiration date on it is smudged, you should not administer it.

8. **Confirm medication compatibility.** If you have orders to administer more than one medication, make sure that the medications are compatible. Some medications will not mix with others, which could cause a precipitate to form in the solution. Should any cloudiness occur after a medication has been injected into IV tubing, *clamp the tubing immediately* and replace it with a new **administration set**.
9. **Dispose of any syringes and needles safely.** Do *not* try to recap a needle, for the likelihood of sticking yourself in the process is quite high; rather, immediately dispose of the needle and syringe in a sharps container.
10. **Monitor the patient for possible adverse side effects.** Reassess the vital signs, especially heart rate and blood pressure, at least every 5 minutes or as the patient's condition warrants.
11. **Document.** Always document your actions and the patient's response on the patient care report after administering a medication. Include the:
    - Name of the medication
    - Dose of the medication
    - Time you administered the medication
    - Route of administration
    - Your name or the name of the person who administered the medication
    - Patient's response to the medication, whether positive or negative

    Did the patient's condition improve, get worse, or not change at all? Were there any side effects? If your performance should ever be questioned, documentation is your best defense.

Specific Medications

Chapter 12, *Principles of Pharmacology*, listed the specific medications that a certified AEMT is allowed to administer or help patients self-administer. Recall that as an AEMT, you may administer the following:

- Oxygen
- Oral glucose
- Glucagon
- 50% dextrose in water ($D_{50}W$)
- IV fluids—**D_5W** (5% dextrose in water), **normal saline**, **lactated Ringer solution**
- Epinephrine (intramuscular [IM] or subcutaneous)
- MDI medications—albuterol
- Nebulized medications—albuterol
- Nitroglycerin—spray, paste, tablets
- Nitrous oxide
- Naloxone
- Aspirin
- Others based on local protocols

Recall that you may only administer or help to administer these medications when allowed by local protocols or ordered by a licensed physician.

Basic Cell Physiology

Basic cell physiology provides an understanding of how administering fluids to a patient, for example via IV access, can be beneficial depending on the patient's condition. A human cell can exist only in a special balanced environment. Understanding how this environment is created and maintained will give you the foundation you need to determine how IV therapy will affect the patient and what is needed to protect that delicate homeostasis.

Because cells are completely enclosed by a cell membrane, compounds must move through the membrane to enter a cell. Small compounds such as water (H_2O), carbon dioxide (CO_2), hydrogen ions (H^+), and oxygen (O_2) can easily pass through the membrane. Larger charged compounds need assistance to cross a cell membrane and enter the cell.

The composition of the cell membrane allows it to have **selective permeability**. The cell membrane is a **phospholipid bilayer**, which is an important barrier to fluid movement and the acid-base balance. Everything discussed in this section will in some way be related to the cell membrane barrier and movement across that barrier.

Electrolytes

Atoms carry charges—some positive, some negative. Two or more atoms that bond together form a molecule. When atoms bond together, they share and disperse their charges throughout the molecule. Molecules containing carbon atoms—for example, table sugar ($C_6H_{12}O_6$)—are called organic molecules. Molecules created without carbon—for example, table salt (NaCl)—are called inorganic molecules. Inorganic molecules give rise to **electrolytes** when they disassociate in water into their charged components. For example, table salt disassociates into sodium (Na^+) and chloride (Cl^-).

Charged atoms and charged compounds are called electrolytes because of their ability to conduct electricity. Electrolytes, also called **ions**, are reactive and dangerous if left to circulate in the body, but the body uses the energy stored in these charged particles. Electrolytes help to regulate everything from water levels to cardiac function and muscle contractions. Water in the body helps to stabilize the electrolyte charges so that the electrolytes can be used to perform the **metabolic** functions that are necessary to life.

Each electrolyte has a unique property or value to the body and is used in a different way. If the electrolyte has an overall positive charge, it is called a **cation**; an electrolyte with an overall negative charge is called an **anion**. The major cations of the body include sodium, potassium, and calcium; conversely, bicarbonate, chloride, and phosphorus are the major anions.

Sodium (Na^+) is the principal extracellular cation needed to regulate the distribution of water throughout the body in the **intravascular** and **interstitial** fluid compartments, making it a major factor in adequate **cellular perfusion**. This gives rise to the saying, "Where sodium goes, water follows." Sodium is also a major component of the circulating **buffer**, sodium bicarbonate ($NaHCO_3$).

Potassium is the principal intracellular cation. Approximately 98% of all the body's potassium (K^+) is found inside the cells of the body. Potassium plays a major role in neuromuscular function as well as in the conversion of glucose into glycogen. Cellular potassium levels are regulated by insulin. The **sodium/potassium (Na^+/K^+) pump** is helped by the presence of insulin and epinephrine. Low potassium levels—**hypokalemia**—in the serum (blood plasma) can result in decreased skeletal muscle function, gastrointestinal (GI) disturbances, and alterations in cardiac function. High potassium levels in the serum—**hyperkalemia**—can result in hyperstimulation of neural cell transmission, resulting in cardiac arrest.

Calcium (Ca^{+2}) is the principal cation needed for bone growth. It plays an important part in the functioning of heart muscle, nerves, and cell membranes and is necessary for proper blood clotting.

Low serum calcium levels—**hypocalcemia**—can result in overstimulation of nerve cells, resulting in the following signs and symptoms:

- Skeletal muscle cramps
- Abdominal cramps
- Carpopedal spasms (hand/foot spasms)
- Hypotension
- Vasoconstriction

High serum calcium levels—**hypercalcemia**—can result in decreased stimulation of nerve cells, resulting in the following signs and symptoms:

- Skeletal muscle weakness
- Lethargy
- **Ataxia**
- Vasodilation
- Hot, flushed skin

Bicarbonate (HCO_3^-) levels are related to the conditions of **acidosis** and **alkalosis** in the body. Sodium bicarbonate is the primary buffer used in all circulating body fluids.

Chloride (Cl^-) primarily regulates the **pH** of the stomach. It also regulates extracellular fluid (ECF) levels.

Finally, phosphorus (P) is an important component in the formation of adenosine triphosphate (ATP), the powerful energy supplier of the body.

Body Fluid Composition

The fluids found in the body are composed of dissolved elements and water, a combination known as a solution. A solution is a mixture of two things:

- **Solvent.** The fluid that does the dissolving, or the solution that contains the dissolved components (in the body, the solvent is water)
- **Solute.** The dissolved particles contained in the solvent

YOU are the Provider — PART 2

You quickly remove the patient's clothing and find bruising around the lower abdominal area, presumably from the seat belt, with abdominal distention. The patient describes significant pain when the abdomen is palpated. Finding no other injuries, you quickly place the patient into the ambulance and initiate rapid transport to the closest Level 1 trauma center. A rolled-up blanket is placed under the patient's knees to help relieve some of the pressure on her abdomen.

Recording Time: 5 Minutes	
Appearance	Poor
Level of consciousness	Alert and oriented
Airway	Patent
Breathing	20 breaths/min
Circulation	Strong radial pulse; skin is cool, pale, and clammy

3. Does this patient require any medications, and, if so, by what route should they be administered?
4. What are the 10 rights of medication administration?

A good example of making a solution is the process of brewing a cup of coffee. Passing hot water (solvent) over the coffee grounds leaches out the oils (the solute) to create the solution known as coffee. Remember, as the solute concentration increases, the solvent concentration decreases. Is a strong cup of coffee created by using less water (solvent) or by adding more coffee (solute)? Either one could be true, as they both end up creating stronger coffee.

Understanding the composition of body fluids will help you understand the concepts of fluid and electrolyte movement, discussed next.

▶ Fluid and Electrolyte Movement

Water and electrolytes move among the body's fluid compartments according to some basic chemical and biologic rules. One such rule is that unequal concentrations on different sides of a cell membrane will move to balance themselves equally on both sides of the membrane. Balance across a cell membrane has two components:

- Balance of compounds (such as water or electrolytes) on either side of the cell membrane
- Balance of charges (the one or two charges carried on the atoms) on either side of the cell membrane

When concentrations of charges or compounds are greater on one side of the cell membrane than on the other, a gradient is created. The natural tendency for materials is to flow from an area of higher concentration to one of lower concentration. This movement establishes a **concentration gradient**. The process of flowing down a gradient depends on whether the cell membrane will allow the material to pass through it. Certain compounds can travel freely across the cell membrane, whereas others require more effort to move across the membrane, either because of the size of the compound or because of an incompatible charge.

Diffusion

Compounds or charges concentrated on one side of a cell membrane will move across it to an area of lower concentration to balance themselves across the membrane, a process called **diffusion** Figure 13-2. To visualize this, imagine that too many people show up for a theater performance. The management decides to open another seating area to accommodate the crowd. Patrons (charges or compounds) are concentrated in the small seating area (the cell) outside the door (the cell membrane) leading to the new seating area. When the theater manager opens the door, patrons can move through (selective cell membrane permeability) from the congested seating area (down a concentration gradient). The patrons spread themselves out evenly (diffuse) throughout the total area, some choosing to stay behind in the original seating area as others move into the new area, so that they all have an equal amount of room.

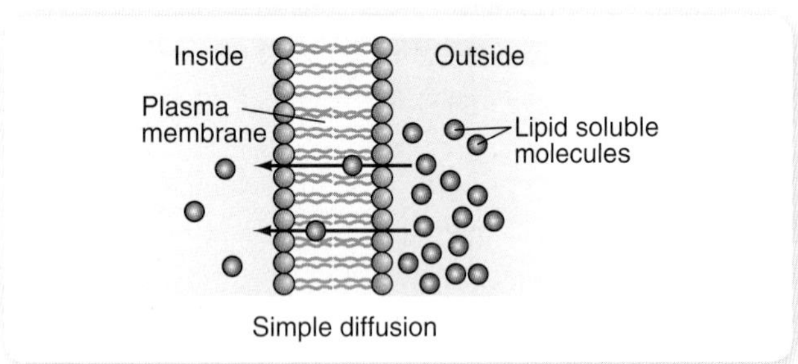

Figure 13-2 Diffusion.

Filtration

Filtration is another type of diffusion, commonly used by the kidneys to clean blood. Water carries dissolved compounds across the cell membranes of the tubules of the kidney. The tubule membrane traps these dissolved compounds but lets the water pass through in much the same way that a coffee filter traps the grounds as water passes through it. This cleans the blood of wastes and removes the trapped compounds from circulation so they can be flushed out of the body.

Active Transport

Often, the cell must maintain an imbalance of compounds across its membrane to achieve some metabolic purpose. **Active transport** is a method used to move compounds to create or maintain an imbalance of charges Figure 13-3. An example is the sodium/potassium pump. The cell uses sodium outside the cell and potassium inside the cell for an important cellular function called **depolarization**. To maintain this imbalance, the cell must use energy in the form of ATP and actively transport compounds across its membrane. Even though active transport demands a high-energy expenditure, the benefits outweigh the initial utilization of ATP. Pumping sodium out of the cell and potassium into the cell has the added benefit of moving glucose into the cell at the same time.

Osmosis

Osmosis is movement of water across a cell membrane Figure 13-4. Osmosis occurs when there are different concentrations on each side of a membrane, and equal numbers of molecules on either side are displaced to the other side. For example, if 10 sodium ions are added to the fluid surrounding a cell, this causes 10 molecules of water to be displaced from that fluid. As a result, the fluid surrounding the cell contains 10 fewer water molecules relative to the fluid within the cell, and a concentration gradient has been created. Water will then move down the concentration gradient to balance itself across the cell membrane. Essentially, osmosis is diluting a solution by

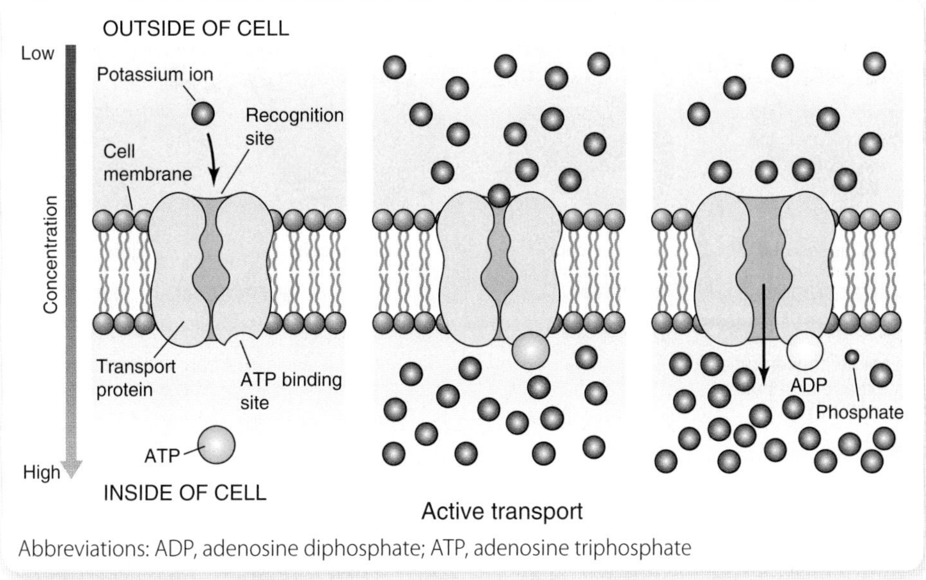

Abbreviations: ADP, adenosine diphosphate; ATP, adenosine triphosphate

Figure 13-3 Active transport uses energy from adenosine triphosphate to open a pathway for compounds to move against a concentration gradient.

adding water, whereas diffusion is moving solid particles to accomplish the same thing.

An important point to take away here is that increasing the concentration of sodium in the surrounding (extracellular) fluid decreases the water in that fluid. Water moves out of the cell to create a balance of water molecules and to dilute the increased concentrations of sodium. Remember, where sodium goes, water follows.

The movement of water adds additional molecules to the extracellular compartment to create a balanced solution. This increased, yet balanced, volume puts pressure against the cell wall, called **osmotic pressure**. Osmotic pressure drives several important metabolic functions in the body, including cellular perfusion.

The effects of osmotic pressure on a cell are referred to as the **tonicity** of the solution Figure 13-5. Tonicity is the concentration of sodium in a solution and the movement of water in relation to the sodium levels inside and outside the cell:

- An **isotonic solution** has the same concentration of sodium as does the cell. In this case, water does not shift and no change in cell shape occurs.
- A **hypertonic solution** has a greater concentration of sodium than does the cell. Water is drawn out of the cell, and the cell may collapse from the increased extracellular osmotic pressure.
- A **hypotonic solution** has a lower concentration of sodium than does the cell. Water flows into the cell, causing it to swell and possibly burst from the increased intracellular osmotic pressure.

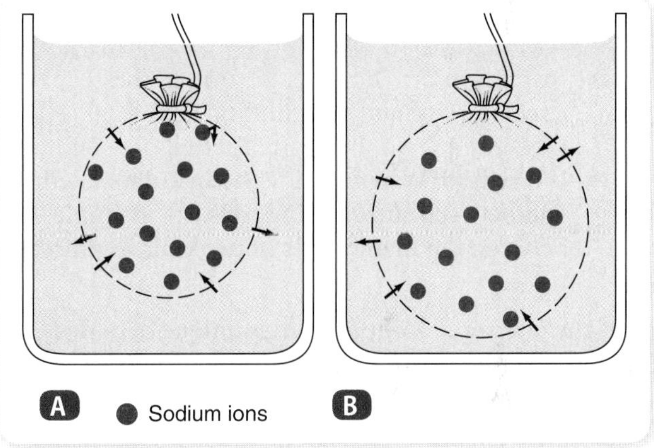

Figure 13-4 A. An example of osmosis occurs when a semipermeable bag of salt water is immersed in a solution of pure water. **B.** Water moves into the bag (toward the area with lower water concentration) and sodium moves out into the water until there is an equal amount of sodium and water on each side.

IV fluids introduced into the circulatory system can affect the tonicity of the ECF, resulting in dire consequences unless care is used.

▶ Fluid Compartments

The body stores water in various locations called fluid compartments. The fluid compartments are defined by their relationship to cells—the water is either inside the cell (intracellular) or outside the cell (extracellular). Although water levels in these compartments constantly

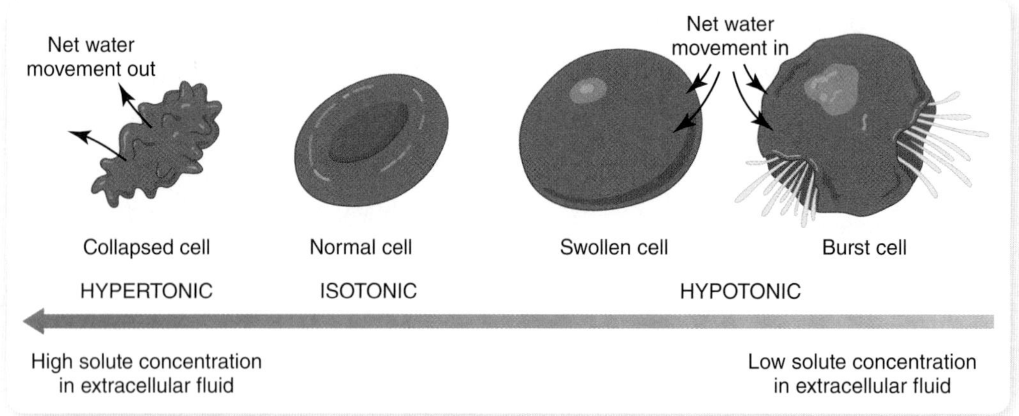

Figure 13-5 Tonicity.

shift, homeostatic control mechanisms ensure that balance is restored whenever water is lost.

The body's circulatory (vascular) system functions as a fluid highway, but it also contains cells. Thus, it can be thought of as another fluid compartment.

The extracellular compartment is broken down into two subareas:

- **Intravascular:** The water portion of the circulatory system surrounding the blood cells (for example, in the heart, arteries, or veins)
- **Interstitial:** Water outside the vascular system and between surrounding cells (for example, between the membranes of two cells in muscle tissue)

The interstitial compartment is unique because it acts as the buffer between the other compartments. As fluid levels fluctuate between the intravascular and intracellular compartments, the interstitial compartment first responds by shifting fluid reserves between the two compartments **Figure 13-6**.

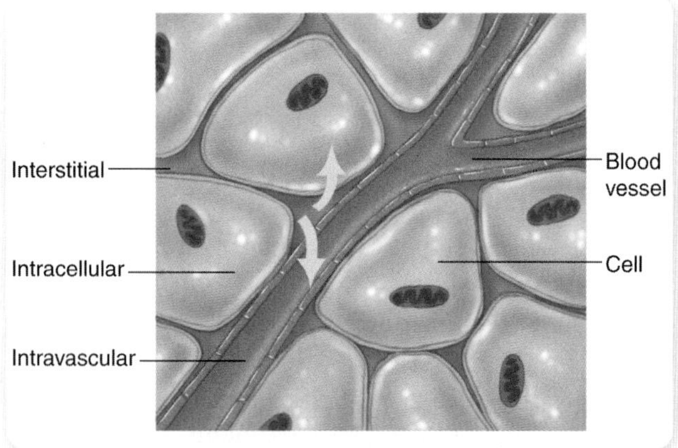

Figure 13-6 Fluid shifts from the intravascular compartment to and from the intracellular compartment via the interstitial compartment.

Therefore, there are three fluid compartments in the human body: intravascular (extracellular), interstitial (extracellular), and intracellular. The fluids within these compartments account for 60% of total body weight.

ECF occupies any area that is not inside the cells. ECF compartments act as conduits for transferring gases and nutrients between the vascular and intracellular fluid (ICF) compartments. ECF is found in the interstitial and intravascular compartments. ECF levels in the intravascular and interstitial compartments are regulated by the presence of sodium. Interstitial fluid accounts for 16% of total body weight and occupies the microscopic spaces between the cells. Interstitial fluid consists of a gel-type protein that helps disperse water evenly throughout the interstitial compartment. This protein gel helps move water freely between the cells and vasculature. Perfusion occurs in the capillaries as a result of high hydrostatic pressures and osmosis in the **capillary beds**. The high arterial capillary pressures placed on the capillary beds push fluids from the vascular compartment into the interstitial compartment.

ICF is within all the cells of the body. Large proteins within the cell can draw fluid into the cell because their overall negative charge attracts positively charged atoms such as potassium, sodium, and the positive end of the water molecule (H_2O). The cell membrane prevents too many positively charged compounds, including water, from entering the cell and causing it to rupture. The sodium ions drawn into the cell are quickly removed via the sodium/potassium pump to prevent cellular **lysis** (rupture of the cell).

▶ Fluid Balance

Some form of water surrounds all cells. Cells survive as long as this environment remains stable and is compatible for the life of the cell; any alteration in the supply of water, nutrients, oxygen, or food can result in cellular death. Water exists both inside and outside the cell.

The role of water in the body is diverse; it plays a part both in cellular metabolism and in the maintenance of homeostasis. Without the presence of water in the body, people would quickly succumb to illness and disease, cellular function would cease, and body systems would shut down.

The role water plays in helping to maintain homeostasis is related to the size of the water molecule itself. Composed of only three atoms (two hydrogen and one oxygen), water has some unique properties. Water is a polar molecule; that is, it has two positive poles (hydrogen) and a negative pole (oxygen). This property means that water can surround charged particles and stabilize their charges, allowing the particles to remain in solution. Water can also move across cell membranes easily, because it is a relatively small molecule.

The body adjusts to changes in the balance between ICF and ECF by retaining or eliminating water. Fluid levels in the body are balanced when intakes equal outputs. Daily intakes of water include fluid from liquid, food, and cellular metabolism; daily outputs occur from respiration and excretion of urine, feces, and perspiration.

Maintenance of the internal environment of the cell is regulated by elaborate systems of checks and balances. As systems in the body become imbalanced and begin to shift, feedback systems create an appropriate response to return the internal environment to normal. This normally balanced condition is referred to as homeostasis, or the resistance to change. When disturbances in homeostasis occur as a result of water shifting within the body, certain conditions may develop related to the type of shifting that occurs.

Dehydration

Dehydration is defined as depletion of the body's total systemic fluid volume. Dehydration is more common in older adults and young children. It may take days to manifest and may be a result of a medical condition. As fluid is lost from the vascular compartment, the body reacts by shifting interstitial fluid into the vascular area. This then forces a shift of fluid from the intracellular to the extracellular compartments. A total systemic fluid deficit occurs.

Signs and symptoms of dehydration include:

- Decreased level of consciousness (LOC)
- **Orthostatic hypotension**
- Dry mucous membranes
- **Tachycardia**
- Poor skin turgor
- Flushed, dry skin
- Decreased urine output

Causes of dehydration include:

- Diarrhea
- Vomiting
- GI drainage
- Hemorrhage
- Insufficient fluid/food intake
- Infection

Overhydration

When the body's total systemic fluid volume increases, overhydration occurs. Fluid fills the vascular compartment, filters into the interstitial compartment, and finally is forced from the engorged interstitial compartment into the intracellular compartment. This fluid backup can result in death **Figure 13-7**.

Signs and symptoms of overhydration include:

- Shortness of breath
- Puffy eyelids
- Edema
- **Polyuria** (excessive urination)
- Moist crackles (rales)
- Acute weight gain

Causes of overhydration include:

- Unmonitored IV lines
- Kidney failure
- Prolonged hypoventilation

▶ IV Fluid Composition

IV solutions are tools designed to facilitate patient treatment. Considering the cell physiology discussed thus far, the use of IV fluids can substantially alter the patient's condition. Compounds and ions dissolved in the solution are identical to the ones found in the body. Each solution is a concentration of solute and solvent.

Sodium is used as the benchmark to calculate a solution's tonicity. The concentration of sodium in the cells of the body is approximately 0.9%. A common IV fluid

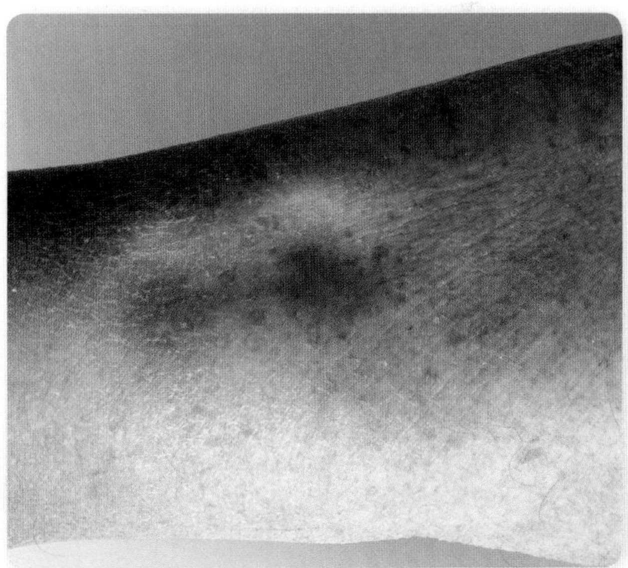

Figure 13-7 One sign of fluid backup is pitting edema, shown in this patient. Pitting edema occurs when the skin is pressed with a finger and an indentation remains after removal of the finger, as seen here.

that AEMTs administer is normal saline, which is 0.9% sodium chloride. Other percentages of sodium chloride may also be used. Altering the concentration of sodium in the IV solution can move the water into or out of any fluid compartment in the body. (Where sodium goes, water follows.)

▶ Types of IV Solutions

IV solutions are categorized in two different ways. They are categorized as crystalloid or colloid based on their dissolved components, or makeup. They are also categorized as isotonic, hypotonic, or hypertonic based on their tonicity. For example, 5% dextrose in water (D_5W) is a hypotonic crystalloid solution because of its tonicity and makeup.

Crystalloid Solutions

A **crystalloid solution** contains dissolved crystals (for example, salts or sugars) in water. These solutions contain compounds that quickly disassociate in solution. The ability of these fluids to cross membranes and alter the various fluid levels makes them the best choice for the prehospital care of injured patients who need fluid replacement for body fluid loss. When you are using an isotonic crystalloid for fluid replacement to support blood pressure from blood loss, remember the 3-to-1 replacement rule: *3 mL of isotonic crystalloid solution is needed to replace 1 mL of patient blood.* This amount is needed because approximately two-thirds of the infused isotonic crystalloid solution will leave the vascular spaces in about 1 hour.

When you replace lost volume, it is imperative to remember that crystalloid solutions do not have the capability to carry oxygen. Boluses of 250 mL should be given to maintain perfusion (radial pulses), but not to restore blood pressure to the patient's normal level. (A **bolus** is a single dose given via the IV route.) Increasing blood pressure with IV solutions not only dilutes remaining blood volume, thereby decreasing the proportion of hemoglobin, but also may increase internal bleeding by interfering with hemostasis—the body's internal blood-clotting mechanism. Blood pressure should be titrated to 90 mm Hg systolic in adults, unless otherwise noted by local protocol.[1]

> **Words of Wisdom**
>
> Standard IV solutions replace volume, but do not have the capacity to carry oxygen. Replace lost volume to maintain perfusion, and recognize the need for rapid transport.

Colloid Solutions

A **colloid solution** contains molecules (usually proteins) that are too large to pass out of the capillary membranes and therefore remain in the vascular compartment. These large protein molecules give colloid solutions a high osmolarity. As a result, they draw fluid from the interstitial and intracellular compartments into the vascular compartments. Colloid solutions work well in reducing edema (as in pulmonary or cerebral edema) while expanding the vascular compartment. They could cause dramatic fluid shifts and place the patient in considerable danger if they are not administered in a controlled setting. Examples of colloids are albumin and hetastarch. Whole blood and blood products are also colloid solutions.

Isotonic Solutions

As mentioned, IV solutions are also categorized by their tonicity. The three categories related to tonicity are:

- **Isotonic:** 0.9% sodium chloride (normal saline), lactated Ringer
- **Hypotonic:** D_5W
- **Hypertonic:** 3.0% saline, blood products, and albumin

Isotonic solutions such as normal saline (0.9% sodium chloride) possess nearly the same **osmolarity** as serum and other body fluids. Osmolarity is technically the concentration of certain particles in a solution—the particles that influence the movement of water across a semipermeable membrane. Therefore, a solution's osmolarity indicates how easily (or not easily) water will move.

Because normal saline has similar osmolarity as serum and other body fluids, it stays inside the intravascular compartment. Isotonic solutions expand the contents of the intravascular compartment without shifting fluid to or from other compartments. Awareness of this fact is useful when dealing with hypotensive or hypovolemic patients. Although isotonic fluid does a good job of hydrating, this fluid remains in the vascular compartment, so you must be careful to avoid fluid overloading. Patients with hypertension and heart failure are at greatest risk of fluid overload. The extra fluid increases the workload of the heart, creating fluid backup in the lungs.

Lactated Ringer solution is generally used in the field for patients who have lost large amounts of blood. It contains the buffering compound lactate, which is metabolized in the liver to form bicarbonate—the key buffer that combats the intracellular acidosis associated with severe blood loss. Lactated Ringer solution should not be given to patients with liver problems because they cannot metabolize the lactate.

D_5W is a special type of isotonic solution. As long as it remains in the bag, it is considered an isotonic solution. After administration, the dextrose is quickly metabolized, and the solution becomes hypotonic.

Hypotonic Solutions

As mentioned, hypotonic fluid has a lower concentration of sodium than the cell. When this fluid is placed in the vascular compartment, it begins diluting the serum by introducing more solvent. Soon the serum osmolarity is less than the interstitial fluid; water is pulled from the vascular compartment into the interstitial fluid compartment and, eventually, the same process is repeated, pulling water from the interstitial compartment into the cells.

Hypotonic solutions hydrate the cells while depleting the vascular compartment. These solutions may be needed for a patient on dialysis when diuretic therapy dehydrates the cells. They may also be used for hyperglycemic conditions such as diabetic ketoacidosis, in which high serum glucose levels draw fluid out of the cells and into the vascular and interstitial compartments. Hypotonic solutions can be dangerous to use because they can cause a sudden fluid shift from the intravascular space to the cells, causing cardiovascular collapse and increased intracranial pressure from shifting fluid into the brain cells. For example, giving D_5W for an extended period can cause increased intracranial pressure. Therefore, hypotonic solutions are dangerous to use with patients experiencing a stroke or any head trauma. Using hypotonic solutions on patients with burns, trauma, malnutrition, or liver disease is also hazardous, because these patients are at risk for **third spacing**, an abnormal fluid shift into the serous linings of the body (the thick membranes that cover the organs).

Hypertonic Solutions

A hypertonic solution has an osmolarity higher than serum, which means the solution has more **ionic concentration** than serum and pulls fluid and electrolytes from the intracellular and interstitial compartments into the intravascular compartment. Hypertonic solutions shift body fluids into the vascular spaces and help stabilize blood pressure, increase urine output, and reduce edema. These fluids are rarely, if ever, used in the prehospital setting. Often, the term hypertonic refers to solutions that contain high concentrations of proteins. They have the same effect on fluid as sodium. Careful monitoring is needed to guard against fluid overloading when hypertonic fluids are used, especially in patients with impaired heart or kidney function. Also, hypertonic solutions should not be given to patients with diabetic ketoacidosis or others at risk of cellular dehydration. Hypertonic solutions have been studied in the treatment of patients experiencing hemorrhaging to help restore blood pressure while minimizing fluid overloading.

> **Words of Wisdom**
>
> When deciding on a type of IV fluid, use the prefixes to help make the decision:
>
> - *iso* means equal
> - *hypo* means low
> - *hyper* means high
>
> We are comparing the osmolarity of the fluid to the patient's blood. An *isotonic* solution will remain in the vascular space, a *hypotonic* solution will quickly leave the vascular space, and a *hypertonic* solution will draw fluid into the vascular space.

IV Techniques and Administration

The most important point to remember about IV techniques and fluid administration is to keep the IV equipment sterile. Forethought will help prevent mental and procedural errors while starting the IV line.

One way to ensure proper technique is to develop a routine to follow as you assemble the appropriate equipment. A routine will help you keep track of your equipment and the steps necessary to complete a successful IV line.

Assembling Your Equipment

To avoid delays or the possibility of IV site contamination, gather and prepare all your equipment before you attempt to start an IV line. Sometimes the condition and presentation of the patient make full preparation difficult. This is where working as a team becomes critical. It is often the members of your own crew who, by anticipating your needs, help make the IV equipment assembly possible. Equipment includes **Figure 13-8**:

- Elastic constricting band (preferably nonlatex) (these are sometimes called tourniquets; not to be confused with tourniquets used for bleeding control)
- Antiseptic wipe or solution
- Gauze
- Tape or adhesive bandage

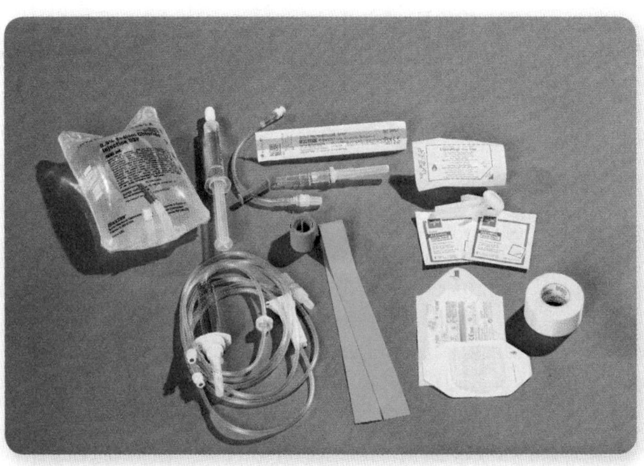

Figure 13-8 Intravenous equipment.

- Appropriate-size IV **catheter** (a hollow, laser-sharpened needle inside a hollow plastic tube inserted into a vein to keep the vein open)
- IV extension set
- A saline flush
- IV administration set

Table 13-1 shows a logical sequence of steps in assembling your equipment and performing IV therapy; each will be described later.

Words of Wisdom

Helpful IV therapy hints:

- Allow the hand or arm to hang off the stretcher.
- Pat or rub the area, without being too firm.
- Apply chemical hot packs for approximately 60 seconds.
- If you meet resistance from a valve, elevate the extremity.
- After two misses, let your partner try.
- Try sticking without the constricting band if the vein keeps infiltrating.
- Never pull the catheter back over or through the needle.
- The more you set up IV sites for medication or fluid administration, the more proficient you will become.

Choosing an IV Solution

Prehospital patient care and IV therapy center on identifying the type of situation and the needs of the patient. Ask yourself:

- Is the patient's condition critical?
- Is the patient's condition stable?
- Does the patient need fluid replacement?

Each IV solution bag is wrapped in a protective sterile plastic bag and is guaranteed to remain sterile until the posted expiration date. After the protective wrap is torn and removed, the IV solution has a shelf life of 24 hours. The bottom of each IV bag has an **access port** for connecting the administration set. A removable pigtail that represents a point-of-no-return line protects the sterile access port. After this pigtail is removed, the bag must be used immediately or discarded.

Words of Wisdom

Whether the patient is a trauma patient or medical patient has nothing to do with the amount of fluid that needs to be administered. Instead, consider how much fluid the patient has lost and consider the patient's clinical presentation. Any patient who has lost a substantial amount of fluid needs rapid replacement with large-bore IV catheters. This applies to a medical patient with GI bleeding as well as a trauma patient with an unstable pelvis and bilateral femur fractures.

Table 13-1 Steps in Assembling IV Equipment and Performing IV Therapy

Assembling IV Equipment

1. Always wear gloves! Standard precautions cannot be emphasized strongly enough.
2. Choose a solution. Check the solution for clarity and the expiration date and to ensure it is the correct one. Explain the procedure to the patient.
3. Choose an administration set appropriate for the needs of the patient.
4. Choose an appropriate IV site.
5. Choose an appropriately sized catheter.
6. Recheck your work before you go any further.
7. Tear tape for securing the IV site.
8. Have blood tubes close by.
9. Set up the Luer adapter and the Vacutainer barrel, or have a syringe close by for drawing blood, if indicated.
10. Have a couple of catheters ready for insertion.
11. Open an alcohol wipe.
12. Have 4- × 4-inch pieces of gauze ready for catching blood.
13. Have a constricting band ready.

Steps in Performing IV Therapy

1. Spike the bag.
2. Apply a constricting band (the last thing done before inserting the IV line).
3. Insert the catheter and draw blood, if indicated.
4. Adequately dispose of sharps.
5. Hook up the IV tubing and adjust the flow.
6. Secure the site and the blood tubes.
7. Administer medication if necessary.
8. Document every procedure.

Abbreviation: IV, intravenous

IV solution bags come in different fluid volumes Figure 13-9. Volumes commonly used in hospitals are 1,000 mL, 500 mL, 250 mL, and 100 mL; the more common prehospital volumes are 1,000 mL and 500 mL.

Choosing an Administration Set

An administration set moves fluid from the IV bag into the patient's vascular system. As with IV solution bags, IV administration sets are sterile as long as they remain in their protective packaging. Each IV administration set has

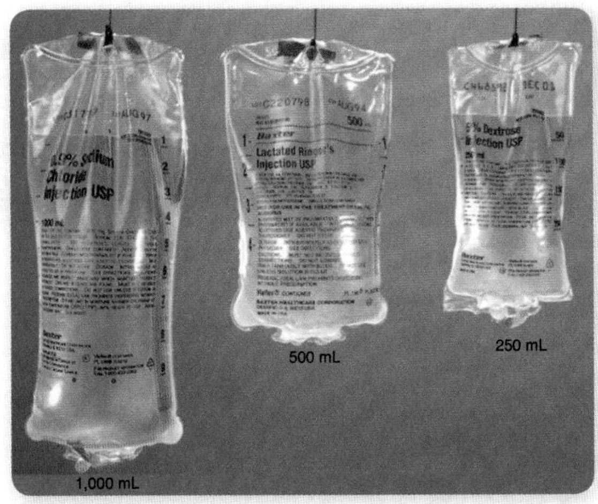

Figure 13-9 Intravenous solution bags come in different fluid volumes.

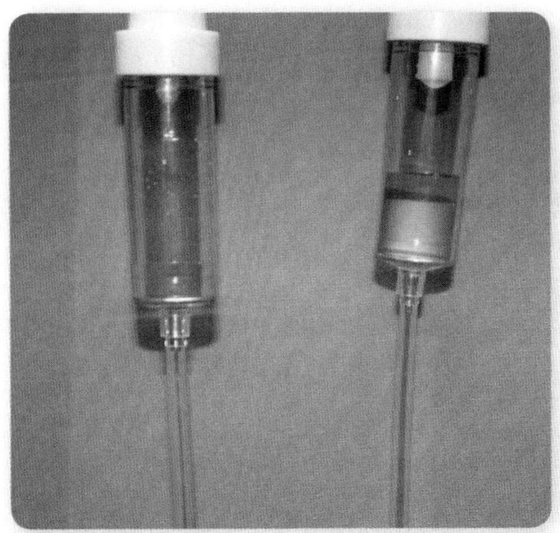

Figure 13-10 Drip chambers from two different-size drip sets are shown here.

a **piercing spike** protected by a plastic cover. Again, after the piercing spike is exposed and the seal surrounding the cap is broken, the set must be used immediately or discarded.

There are different sizes of administration sets for different situations and patients. A **drip set** is another term for an administration set. Most drip sets have a number visible on the package, which indicates the number of drops it takes for 1 milliliter of fluid to pass through the orifice and into the **drip chamber** Figure 13-10 . Drip sets come in two primary sizes: microdrip and macrodrip. A **microdrip set** allows 60 **gtt** (drops)/mL through the small, needlelike orifice inside the drip chamber. Microdrips are ideal for medication administration or pediatric fluid delivery because it is easy to control their fluid flow. A **macrodrip set** allows 10 to 15 gtt/mL through a large opening between the piercing spike and the drip chamber. Macrodrip sets are best used for rapid fluid replacement.

A blood set is a special type of macrodrip set designed to facilitate rapid fluid replacement by manual infusion of either multiple IV bags or IV/blood replacement

YOU are the Provider PART 3

You administer oxygen to the patient by placing her on a nonrebreathing mask at 15 L/min, and after obtaining a SAMPLE history (Signs and symptoms, Allergies, Medications, Pertinent past medical history, Last oral intake, Events leading up to the illness or injury), you place an 18-gauge IV catheter in each antecubital fossa vein. The patient continues to complain of severe abdominal pain, and you notice her skin is becoming pale.

Recording Time: 11 Minutes	
Respirations	20 breaths/min
Pulse	Strong and regular, 121 beats/min
Skin	Cool, pale, and clammy
Blood pressure	76/40 mm Hg
Oxygen saturation (Spo_2)	100% on 15 L/min via nonrebreathing mask
Pupils	Pupils Equal, Round, and Reactive to Light and Accommodation (PERRLA)

5. What type of fluid should you administer to this patient?
6. How much fluid should be administered to this patient?

combinations. Most blood sets have dual piercing spikes that allow two bags of fluid to be hung simultaneously for the same patient Figure 13-11.

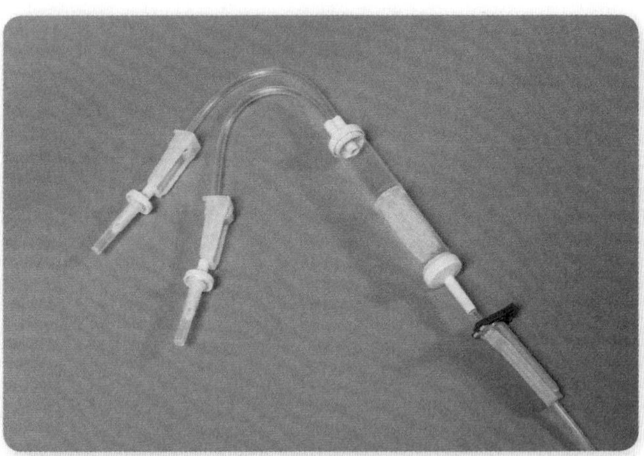

Figure 13-11 Most blood sets have dual piercing spikes that allow two bags of fluid to be hung simultaneously for the same patient.

Words of Wisdom

To differentiate between macrodrip and microdrip sets, remember that the prefixes refer to the size of the drops, not the size of the tubing.

Macro means *large*. A 10-gtt set, which is a macrodrip set, has 10 drops that equal 1 mL of fluid. *Micro* means *small*. A 60-gtt set, which is a microdrip set, has 60 drops that equal 1 mL of fluid.

Preparing an Administration Set

To prepare to spike the bag with the administration set, follow the steps in Skill Drill 13-1.

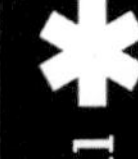

NR Skill

Skill Drill 13-1 Spiking the Bag

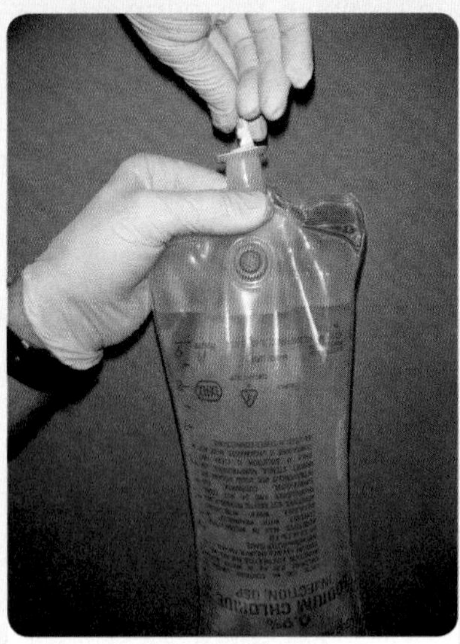

Step 1 Take standard precautions. Ensure you've chosen the correct administration set, tubing is not tangled, and protective covers are in place. Ensure you have the proper solution, that it is clear and has not expired, and that the protective tail port covers are in place. Move the roller clamp to the off (or open) position.

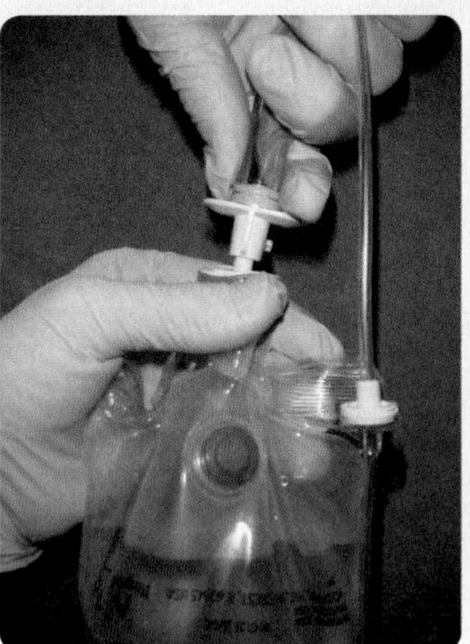

Step 2 Remove the protective covering found on the end of the IV bag. The bag is still sealed and will not leak until the piercing spike punctures this port. Remove the protective cover from the piercing spike (remember, this spike is sterile and sharp!) and slide the spike into the IV bag port until it is seated against the bag.

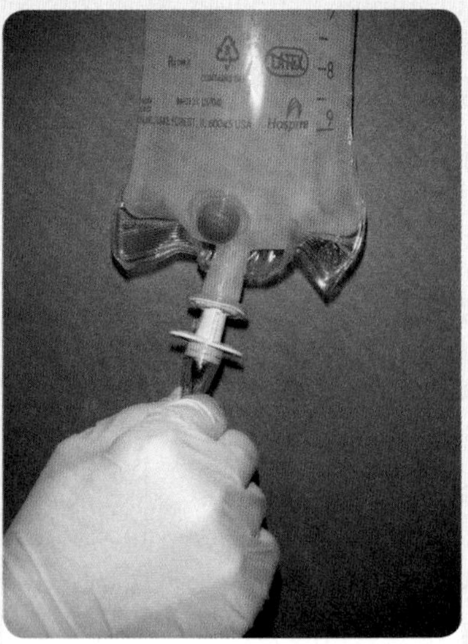

Step 3 Squeeze the drip chamber to fill to the line marking the chamber (half full) and then run fluid into the line to flush the air out of the tubing.

Skill Drill 13-1 Spiking the Bag *(continued)*

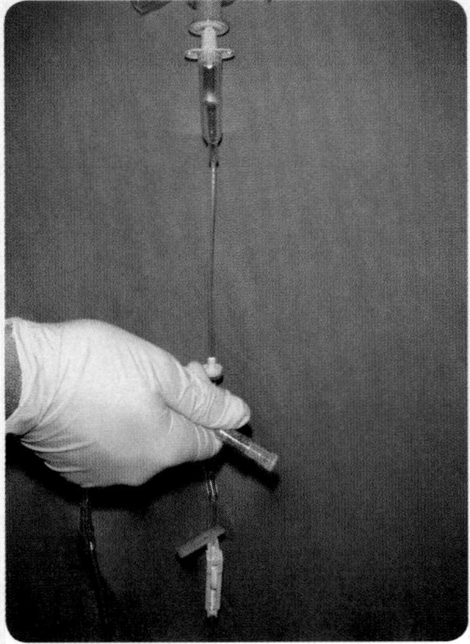

Step 4 Twist the protective cover on the opposite end of the IV tubing to allow air to escape. Do not remove this cover yet because the cover keeps the tubing end sterile until it is needed. Let the fluid flow until air bubbles are removed from the line before turning the roller clamp wheel to stop the flow.

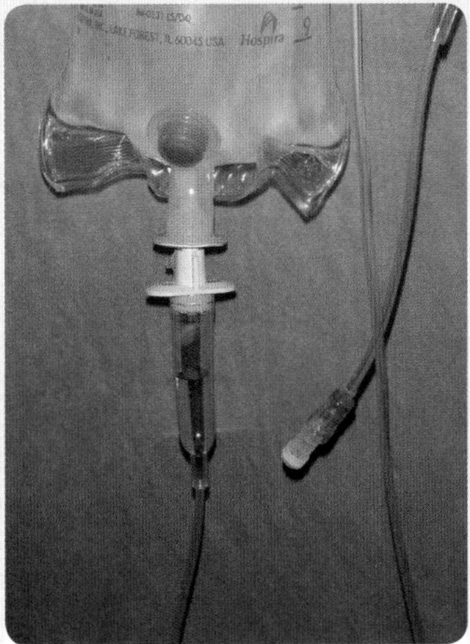

Step 5 Next, go back and check the drip chamber; it should be only half filled. The fluid level must be visible to calculate drip rates. If the fluid level is too low, squeeze the chamber until it fills properly; if the chamber is too full, with the roller clamp in the off (open) position, invert the bag and the chamber and squeeze the chamber to empty the fluid back into the bag. Hang the bag in an appropriate location with the end of the IV tubing easily accessible.

▶ Choosing an IV Site

It is important to select the most appropriate vein for IV catheter insertion. Common sites for IV catheter insertion are shown in Figure 13-12. Avoid areas of the vein that contain valves because a catheter will not pass through these areas easily and the needle may cause damage. Valves can be recognized as small bumps located in the vein. Use the following criteria to select a vein:

- Locate the vein section with the straightest appearance Figure 13-13.
- Choose a vein that has a firm, round appearance or is springy when palpated.
- Avoid areas where the vein crosses over joints.
- Avoid any extremity that shows signs of trauma, injury, or infection.
- Avoid any extremity that shows signs of edema.
- Avoid any extremity with a dialysis fistula.
- Avoid any extremity on the same side as a prior mastectomy or lymph node dissection surgery.

Words of Wisdom

When starting an IV on a pregnant woman who may be in labor, try to avoid using the antecubital vein. Most women will need to prop on their elbows or bend their arms to pull on the bed rails while pushing, which will cut off the flow of the IV line. Choose an area on the dorsal hand or forearm for these patients.

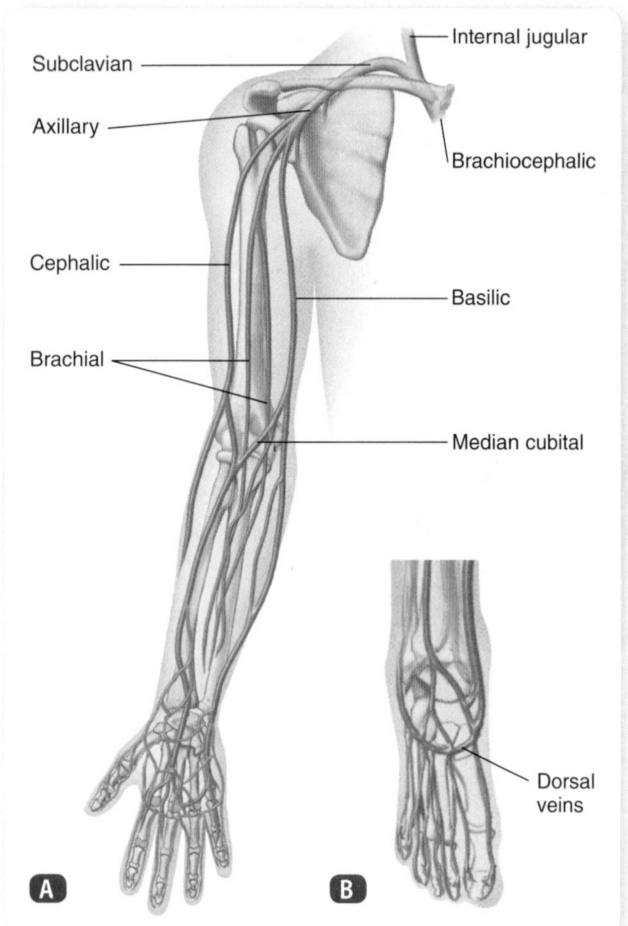

Figure 13-12 A. Common intravenous (IV) sites in the upper extremity include the brachial and cephalic veins in the arm, the radial and ulnar veins in the forearm, the antecubital veins that lie anterior to the elbow, and the dorsal veins of the hands. **B.** Common IV sites in the lower extremity include the dorsal veins of the feet.

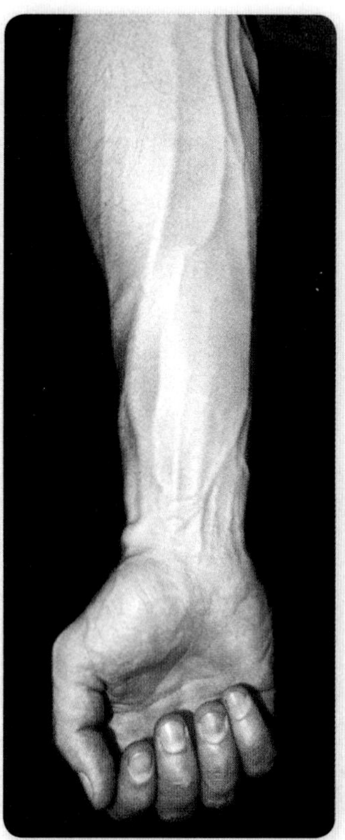

Figure 13-13 Look for veins that are relatively straight and spring back when palpated.

Courtesy of Rhonda Hunt.

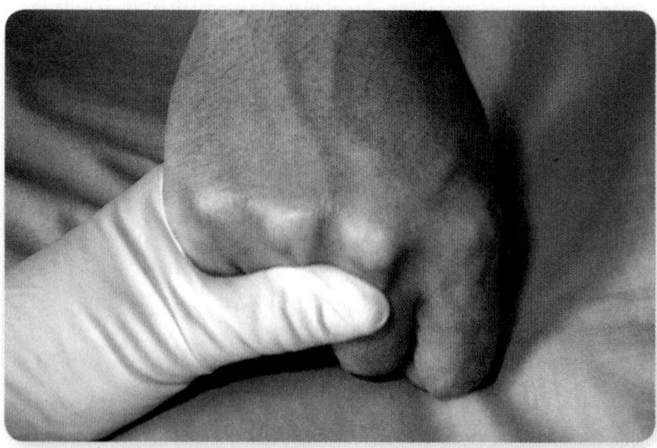

Figure 13-14 Hold hand veins in place by pulling the skin over the vein taut with the thumb of your free hand as you flex the patient's hand.

Courtesy of Rhonda Hunt.

Also pay careful attention to areas of the vein that have tract marks, because this is usually a sign of **sclerosis** (hardening of a vein from scar tissue) caused by frequent puncture or **cannulation** (insertion of a hollow tube into a vein).

If IV therapy is being given for a life-threatening illness or injury, choice is often limited to the areas that remain open during hypoperfusion. For patients who are in critical condition, always start at the antecubital fossa or higher. Otherwise, limit IV access to the more distal areas of the extremities. An important concept to remember is "Start distally, work proximally." First, select areas that are as distal as possible, for example, the hand. If the distal site ruptures, or infiltrates, you can move up the extremity to the next appropriate site (for example, the forearm). Because the failed cannulation creates a possibility of leakage into the surrounding tissues, any fluid introduced immediately below an open wound has the potential to enter the tissue and possibly cause damage.

Large, protruding arm veins can be deceiving in their ease of cannulation. Often these bulging veins can move side to side during cannulation, causing you to miss the vein and resulting in possible **infiltration** (escape of fluid into the surrounding tissue). A remedy is to apply manual traction to the vein to lock it into position. Traction techniques differ depending on the location chosen for cannulation. Hold hand veins in place by pulling the skin over the vein taut with the thumb of your free hand as you flex the patient's hand **Figure 13-14**. Stabilize wrist veins by flexing the wrist and pulling the skin taut over the vein. Applying lateral traction to the vein with your free hand can stabilize veins in the forearm and **antecubital** areas.

The patient's opinion should also be considered when selecting an IV site because he or she may know an IV location that has worked in the past.

Some protocols allow IV cannulation of leg veins. Caution must be used when cannulating these areas, because there is some thought that these might potentially place the patient at greater risk of infection or of **venous thrombosis** and subsequent **pulmonary embolus**.

▶ Choosing a Catheter

The most common types of catheter found in the prehospital setting are **over-the-needle catheters** Figure 13-15 (also called Angiocaths, Insytes) and **butterfly catheters** Figure 13-16. Catheter selection should reflect the need for IV administration, the age of the patient, and the location site.

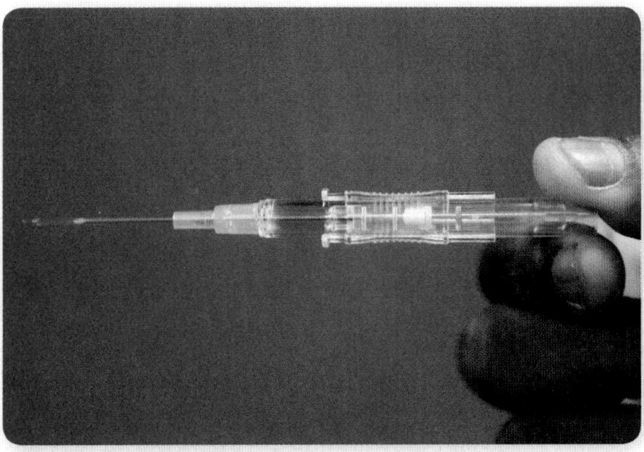

Figure 13-15 A catheter is a hollow tube that is inserted into a vein to keep the vein open, allowing a passageway into the vein. This photo shows an over-the-needle catheter (needle plus catheter).

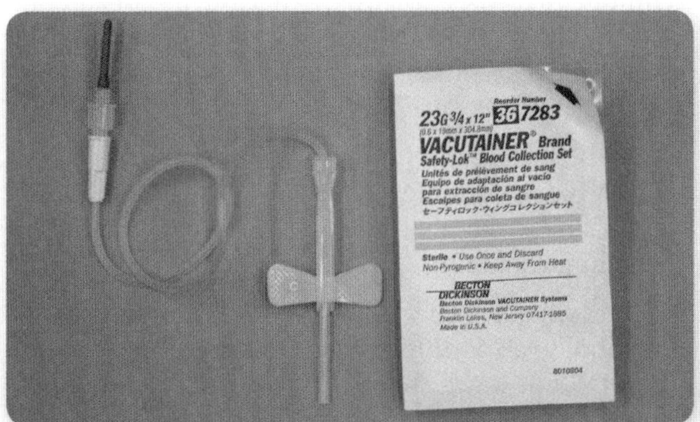

Figure 13-16 A butterfly catheter is a hollow, stainless steel needle with two plastic wings to facilitate handling.

Over-the-needle catheters are sized by their diameter, which is referred to as the **gauge**. The larger the diameter of the catheter, the smaller the gauge. Thus, a 14-gauge catheter has a greater diameter than a 22-gauge catheter. The larger the diameter, the more fluid can be delivered through the catheter.

Select the largest-diameter catheter that will fit the vein you have chosen or that will be the most appropriate and comfortable for the patient. A good rule of thumb to follow is: the more distal the IV site, the smaller the catheter. An 18-gauge catheter is usually a good size for adult patients. Metacarpal veins of the hand accommodate 18- to 20-gauge catheters; antecubital veins of the upper arm can often accommodate larger gauge catheters.

Words of Wisdom

New ATLS and PHTLS recommendations include revised fluid resuscitation guidelines.[2] Instead of 20 mL/kg boluses of crystalloid solutions for resuscitation, they recommend 250-mL boluses with reassessment after each bolus. These boluses may be repeated up to four times prior to medical consultation. In that context, 18-gauge catheters are generally sufficient to support flow rates necessary for rapid administration of the boluses. If unsuccessful with establishment of an 18-gauge IV line in the context of hemodynamic or physiologic instability, rapid transition to intraosseous access is recommended. Establishment of a second line with an 18-gauge catheter is recommended soon after establishment of the first but without delaying transport of the patient. The purpose of the second line is redundancy of intravenous access and medication administration. Use of larger catheters results in increased pain for the patient, decreased likelihood of successful venous cannulation on the first attempt, and therefore likely increased scene time for patients in physiologic or hemodynamic extremis. Routine use of catheters with diameters larger than 18 gauge is therefore not recommended.

Over-the-needle catheters can be used for all adults and most children for long-term IV therapy Figure 13-17. The plastic catheter allows for greater patient movement and often does not require immobilizing the entire limb. Over-the-needle catheters come in different gauges as well as in different lengths. The most common lengths are 1 inch and 1¼ inches. The shorter the catheter, the faster fluid can flow through it.

Butterfly catheters derive their name from the plastic tabs attached to the sides of the needle. These allow for a stable anchoring platform.

In recent years, an attempt has been made to create over-the-needle catheters that minimize the risk of a contaminated stick. A **contaminated stick** occurs when an AEMT punctures his or her skin with the same catheter

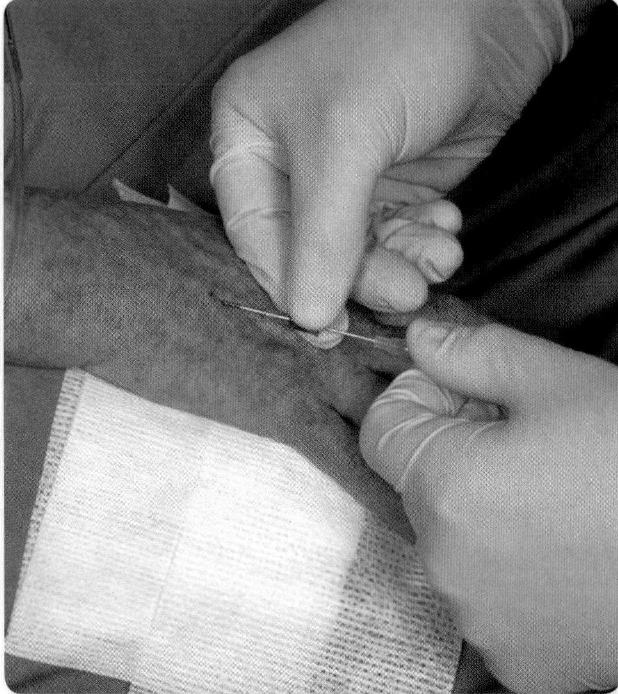

Figure 13-17 The over-the-needle sheath slides off the needle during cannulation and remains inside the vein to keep the vein open.

that was used to cannulate the vein of a patient. Newer over-the-needle catheters use several different methods to protect an AEMT from the possibility of a contaminated stick. One of the more common methods is automatic needle retraction after insertion, usually accomplished with a locking slide mechanism or a spring-loaded slide mechanism.

Words of Wisdom

Always start low and work your way up. For patients who need rapid fluid replacement or who are in cardiac arrest, the antecubital vein or one more proximal should be used.

Words of Wisdom

If you have trouble getting a catheter to feed completely, it may be against a valve. Remove the needle and attach the flush syringe or IV line to the hub of the catheter. Gently "float" the catheter into the vein as the fluid pushes the valve open. Watch carefully for infiltration around the site and if swelling is present, discontinue IV administration immediately, remove the catheter, and document the event.

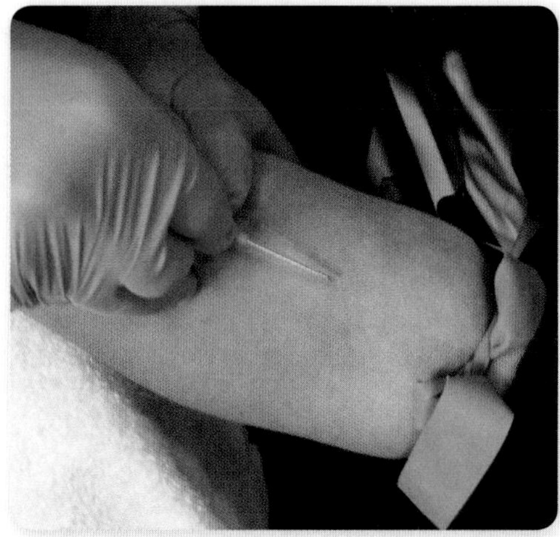

Figure 13-18 Keep the beveled side of the catheter up when inserting the needle in a vein.

▶ Inserting the IV Catheter

Each AEMT has a unique technique for inserting an IV line, and it is important for you to observe many different techniques to determine what works best for you. The following considerations, however, apply to any technique:

- Keep the beveled side of the catheter up when inserting the needle in a vein Figure 13-18.
- Maintain adequate traction on the vein during cannulation.

Apply a constricting band above the site you have chosen for the insertion to allow blood to fill the veins. A constricting band is used to help create additional vascular pressure to engorge the veins with blood below the constricting band. Constricting bands should be snug enough to substantially diminish venous flow but should not hamper arterial flow. The constricting band should be left in place only long enough to complete the IV insertion, blood draws, and line attachment. *Do not leave the constricting band applied while you assemble IV equipment.*

Constricting bands can be difficult to manage, especially if you are wearing gloves. You should develop a technique that will allow you to release the constricting band with a small tug on one end. If a commercial device is not available, constricting bands can be made of any available material, such as:

- A **Penrose drain** (a type of surgical drain)
- A blood pressure cuff Figure 13-19
- Gloves
- Surgical tubing

After you have selected an insertion site, prep it with an alcohol swab, iodine swab, or chlorhexidine (ChloraPrep). Do not touch the site after it has been prepped. Apply gentle downward or lateral traction on the vein with your free hand while holding the catheter, bevel side up, in your dominant hand. Use caution as you apply

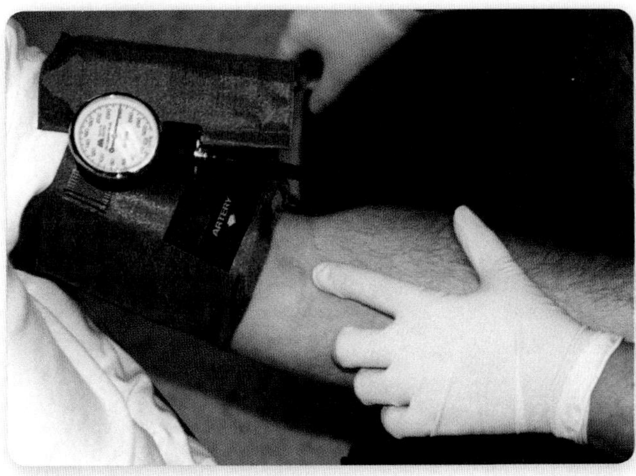

Figure 13-19 A blood pressure cuff may be used in the absence of a constricting band.

traction to avoid collapsing the vein. Begin by establishing an insertion angle of approximately 45°. Advance the catheter through the skin until the vein is pierced (there may or may not be a flash of blood in the catheter **flash chamber**); then immediately drop the angle down to approximately 15° and advance the catheter a few more millimeters to ensure the catheter sheath is in the vein. Slide the sheath off the needle and into the vein; do not advance the needle too far because it can lacerate the back wall of the vein. After the catheter is fully advanced, apply pressure to the vein just proximal to the end of the indwelling catheter, remove the needle, and dispose of it in a sharps container.

Words of Wisdom

Use an **aseptic technique** when cleansing the site Figure 13-20. With an alcohol prep or iodine swab, start from the center of the area you intend to stick and wipe in a circular motion from the inside out. Take a second swab and wipe straight down the center over the area you intend to stick.

Words of Wisdom

Using iodine to prep an IV site helps to make veins more visible in dark-skinned individuals.[3,4]

▶ Drawing Blood

AEMTs may need to draw blood when establishing IV access, depending on the patient's condition and local protocols. If blood is drawn, it must be drawn first, before fluids or medications are administered. Drawing blood,

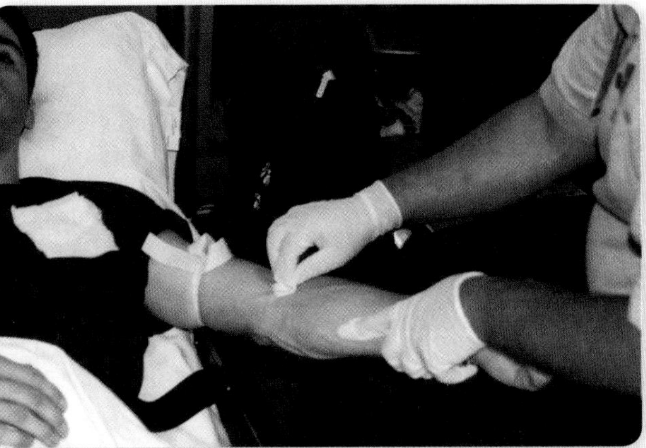

Figure 13-20 Always use an aseptic technique when cleansing the site for intravenous cannulation. Use the first alcohol pad to clean in a circular motion from the inside out, and then use the second to wipe straight down the center.

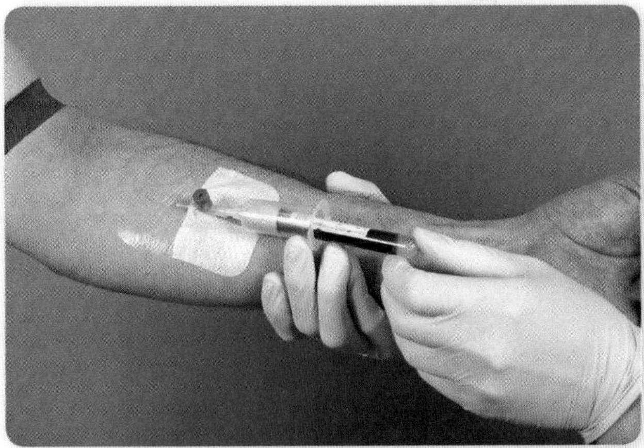

Figure 13-21 A Vacutainer.

while preferable, is not always possible. Often a patient is so compromised that it is impossible to draw blood. If you are having difficulty drawing blood, stop and finish establishing the IV line. Do not allow the constricting band to remain tied too long around the patient's arm because this will allow waste products to build up in the blood and will skew lab results.

A blood collection tube with a vacuum, called a Vacutainer, connects to a catheter to assist with blood collection Figure 13-21. Attach the Vacutainer to the hub of the catheter sheath and release the hand holding pressure because you now have a sealed system. Grasp the Vacutainer in one hand to stabilize it while you insert the tubes for the blood draws. If you do not have a Vacutainer setup, you can draw blood from the IV site using a 15- to 20-mL syringe. Follow local protocols for the types of blood tubes to draw.

Label all the tubes with the patient's name, the date, the time, and your name as soon as possible to avoid mixing tubes with those of another patient.

Safety

Assume that any needle withdrawn from a patient's skin after giving an injection is contaminated with potentially infectious fluids. Handle contaminated "sharps" accordingly, and dispose of them immediately according to your service's procedures for preventing infectious exposures.

▶ Securing the Line

After the catheter is in position, the IV line has been attached, and the contents of the IV bag are flowing properly, the site must be secured. Tape the area so that the catheter and tubing are securely anchored in case of a sudden pull on the line Figure 13-22. You should tear the tape before you start IV administration because you will need one hand to stabilize the site while you tape the site. Double back the tubing to create a loop that will act as a shock absorber if the line gets pulled accidentally. Commercial coverings may be used in place of tape. Avoid any circumferential taping around any extremity, because circumferential taping can act like a constricting band and may impair circulation.

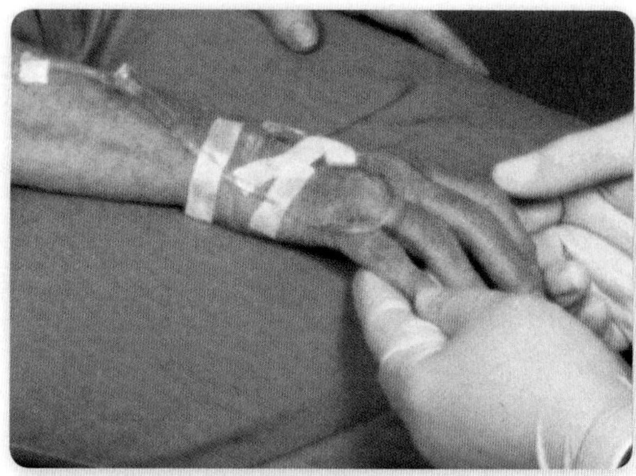

Figure 13-22 Tape the area so that the catheter and tubing are securely anchored.

The steps in performing IV therapy are summarized in Skill Drill 13-2.

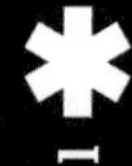

NR Skill

Skill Drill 13-2 Obtaining Vascular Access

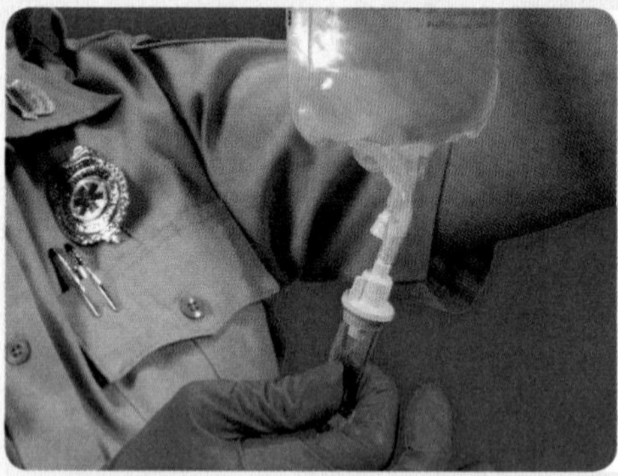

Step 1 Choose the appropriate fluid and examine for clarity and expiration date. Ensure that no particles are floating in the fluid and that the fluid is appropriate for the patient's condition.

Choose the appropriate drip set and attach it to the fluid. A macrodrip set (eg, 10 gtt/mL) should be used for a patient who needs volume replacement, and a microdrip set (eg, 60 gtt/mL) should be used for a patient who mainly needs a route for medication. If an IV extension set is available, attach it to the end of the tubing to assist the hospital staff in manipulating the IV tubing at the hospital.

Fill the drip chamber by squeezing it together.

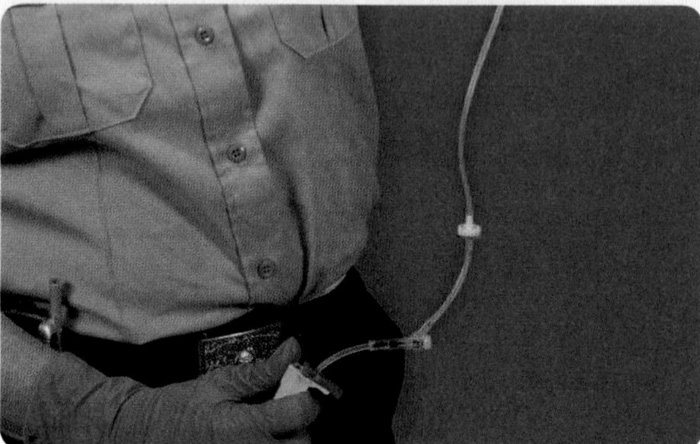

Step 2 Flush or "bleed" the tubing to remove any air bubbles by opening the roller clamp. Make sure no errant bubbles are floating in the tubing.

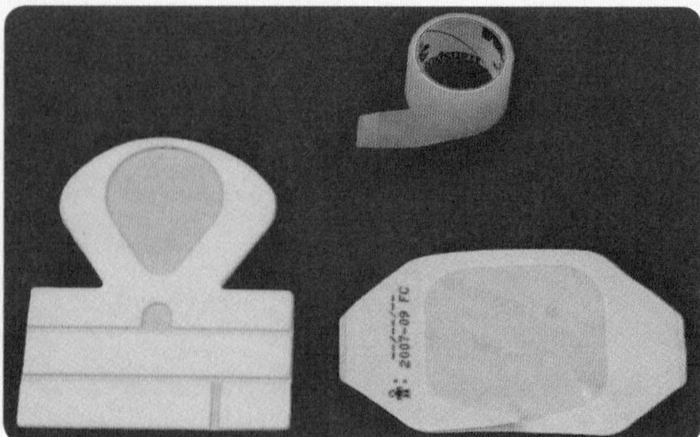

Step 3 Tear tape prior to venipuncture or have a commercial device available. Collect and open antiseptic swabs, gauze pads, and anything else needed for vascular access per local practice.

Skill Drill 13-2 Obtaining Vascular Access *(continued)*

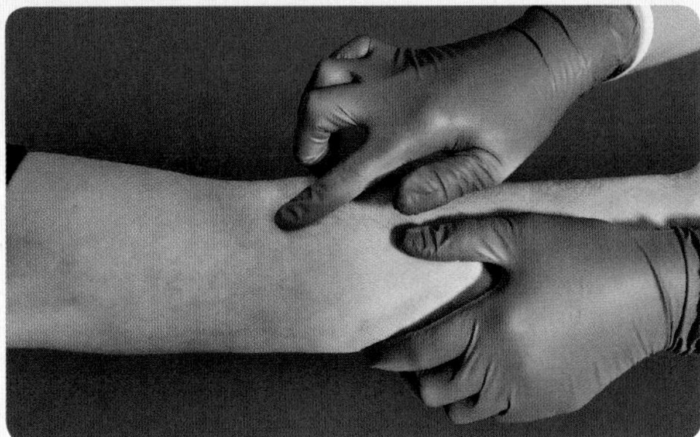

Step 4 Take standard precautions before making contact with the patient. Palpate a suitable vein. Veins should be "springy" when palpated. Stay away from areas that are hard when palpated.

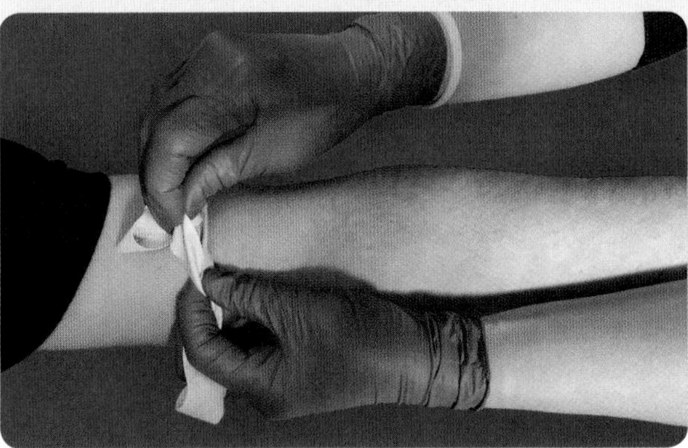

Step 5 Apply the constricting band above the intended IV site. It should be placed approximately 4 to 8 inches above the intended site.

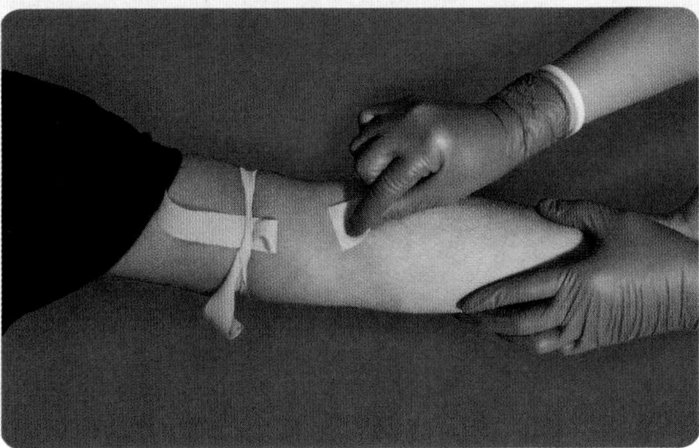

Step 6 Clean the area using an aseptic technique. Use an alcohol pad to cleanse in a circular motion from the inside out. Use a second alcohol pad to wipe straight down the center.

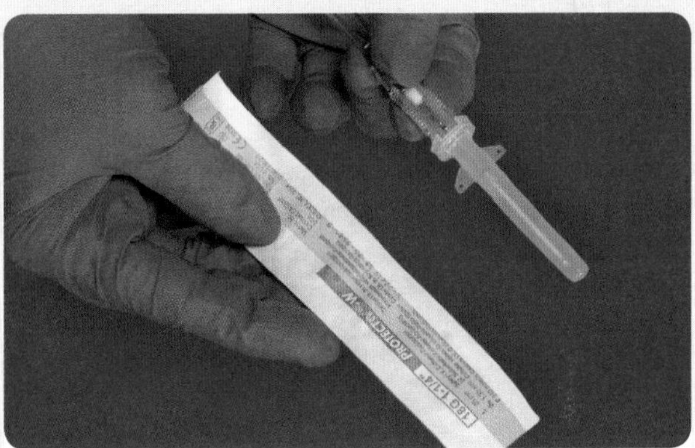

Step 7 Choose the appropriate-size catheter, and twist the catheter to break the seal. Do not advance the catheter upward as this may cause the needle to shear the catheter. Examine the catheter and discard it if you discover any imperfections, such as "burrs" on the edge of the catheter. Loosen the catheter hub.

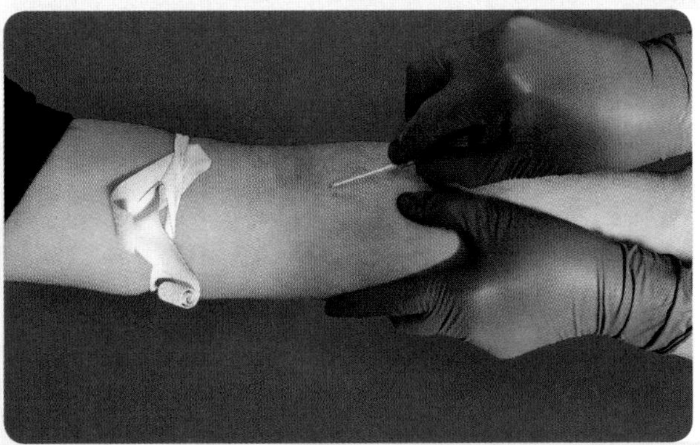

Step 8 Advise the patient to expect a needlestick. While applying distal traction at the site with one hand, insert the catheter at approximately 45° with the bevel up. This traction will stabilize the vein and help to keep it from "rolling" as you stick.

(continued)

Skill Drill 13-2 Obtaining Vascular Access *(continued)*

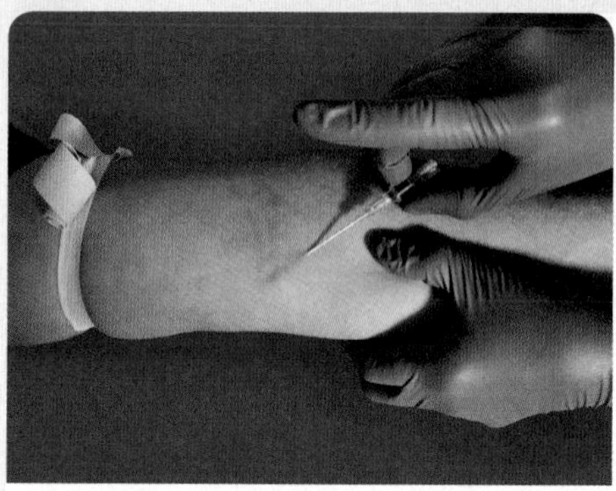

Step 9 Feel for a "pop" as the stylet enters the vein, and observe for "flashback" as blood enters the catheter. The clear chamber at the top of the catheter should fill with blood when the catheter enters the vein. If you note only a drop or two, you should gently advance the catheter farther into the vein, approximately ⅛ to ¼ inch (0.3 to 0.6 cm).

Apply pressure to occlude the catheter to prevent blood leaking while removing the stylet. Place the thumb of the hand not holding the catheter over the end of the catheter that is currently situated inside the vein, so as not to pull the catheter and to prevent blood running out when you remove the needle. With practice, you will be able to feel the catheter.

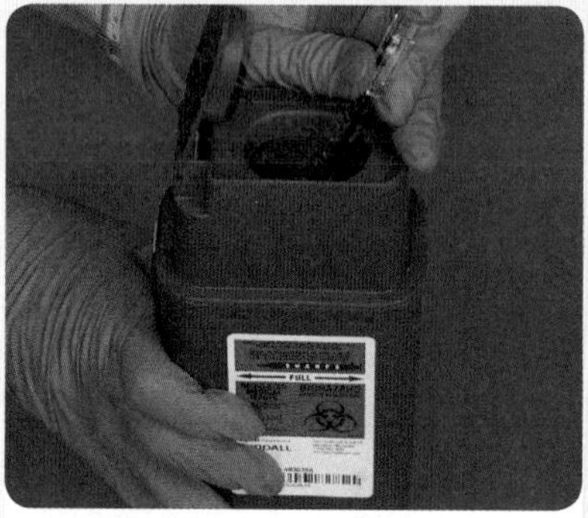

Step 10 Immediately dispose of all sharps in the proper container.

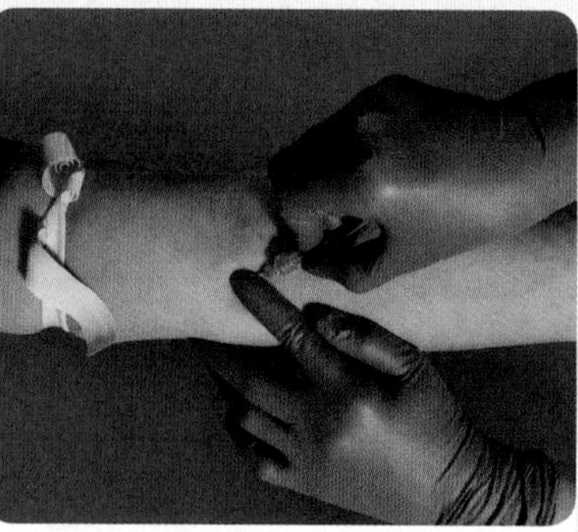

Step 11 Attach the prepared IV line. Hold the hub of the catheter while connecting the IV line.

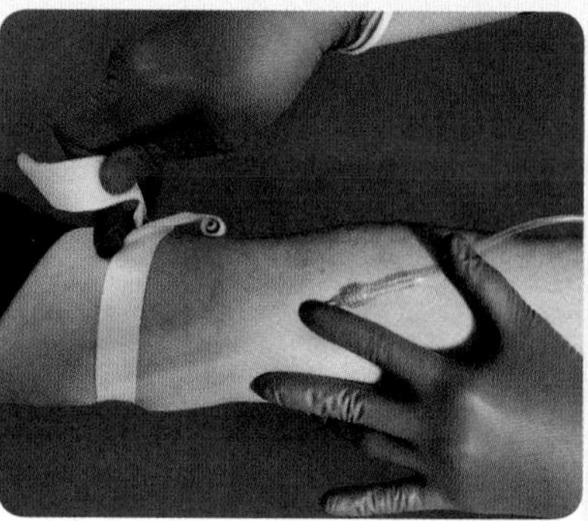

Step 12 Remove the constricting band.

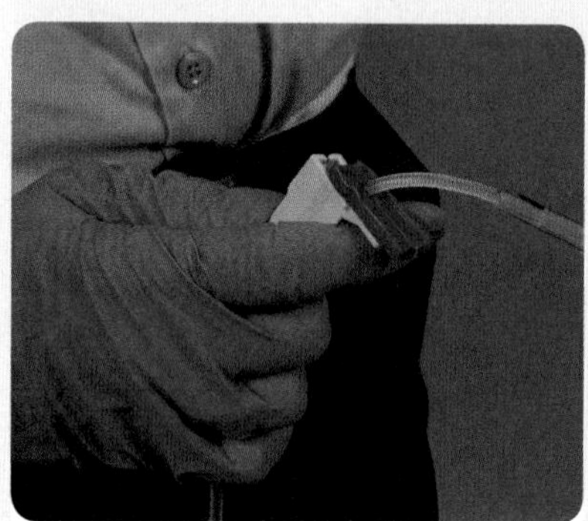

Step 13 Open the IV line to ensure fluid is flowing and the line is patent. Observe for any swelling or infiltration around the IV site. If the fluid does not flow, check to see if the constriction band has been released. If infiltration is noted, immediately stop the infusion and remove the catheter while holding pressure over the site with a piece of gauze to prevent bleeding.

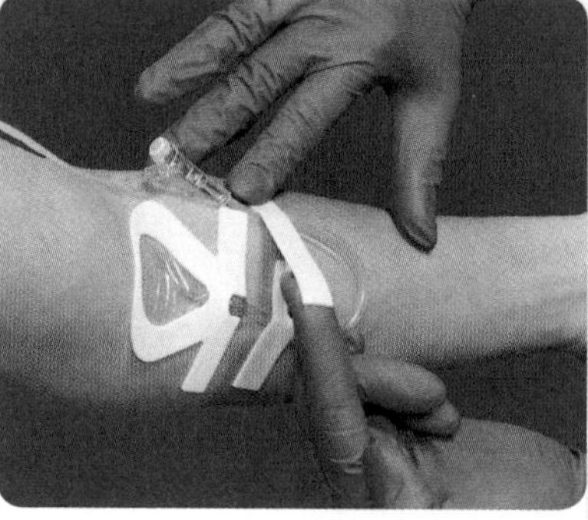

Step 14 Secure the catheter with tape or a commercial device.

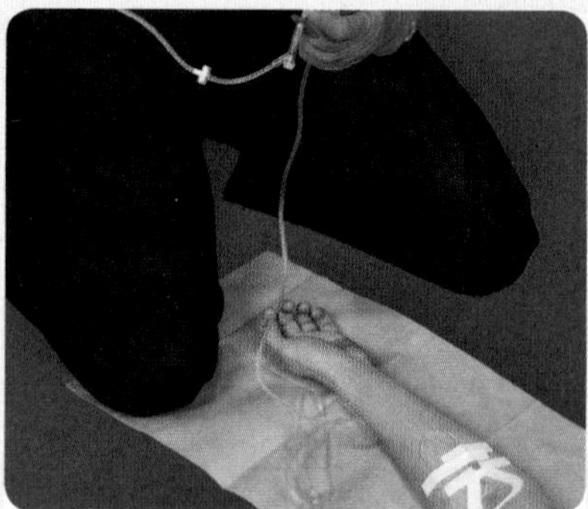

Step 15 Secure IV tubing and adjust the flow rate while monitoring the patient.

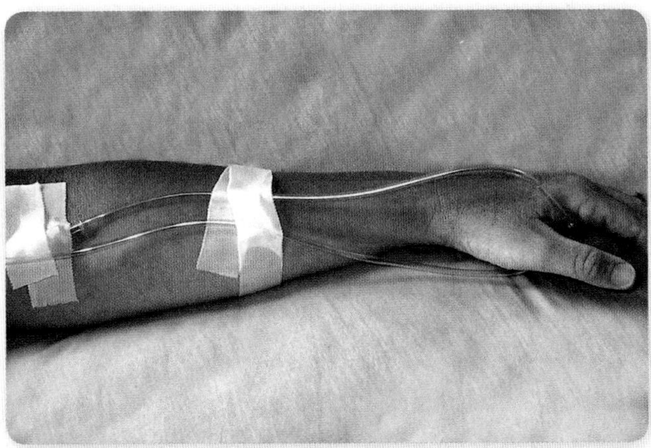

Figure 13-23 Loosely wrap the intravenous line around the patient's thumb and secure it to the forearm.

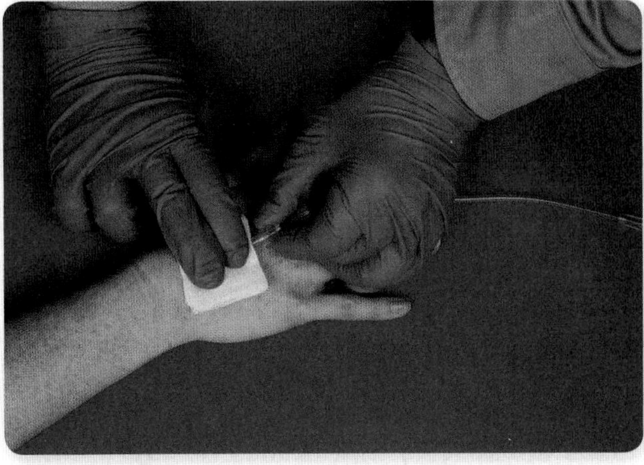

Figure 13-24 When removing a catheter and intravenous line, pull gently and apply pressure to control bleeding.

Words of Wisdom

To further stabilize the IV line, loosely wrap it around the patient's thumb and secure it to the forearm. This will prevent disruption of the administration if the line is pulled **Figure 13-23**.

▶ Changing an IV Bag

You may have to change the IV bag for some patients, particularly those who require larger volumes of IV fluid (ie, for hypovolemic shock). Do not allow an IV fluid bag to become *completely* empty. Change the bag when approximately 25 mL of fluid is left. This will reduce the risk of air embolus.

As with the initial setup of the IV bag and administration set, replacing the IV bag is a sterile process. If the equipment becomes contaminated, then replace it and use new equipment. Always ensure some fluid remains in the drip chamber and tubing of the set. This will prevent air from entering the patient's vein.

The steps for changing an IV fluid bag are as follows:

1. Stop the flow of fluid from the depleted bag by closing the roller clamp.
2. Prepare the new IV bag by removing the pigtail from the piercing spike port. Inspect the new bag of IV fluid for clarity and discoloration, as well as the expiration date.
3. Remove the piercing spike from the depleted bag and insert it into the port on the new bag. *Do not touch the piercing spike of the administration set.*
4. Ensure the drip chamber is appropriately filled, and then open the roller clamp and adjust the fluid rate accordingly.

▶ Discontinuing the IV Line

To discontinue the IV line, shut off the flow from the line with the roller clamp. Gently peel the tape back toward the IV site. As you get closer to the site and the catheter, stabilize the catheter while you loosen all the remaining tape holding the catheter in place. Do not remove the IV tubing from the hub of the catheter. Fold a 4- × 4-inch piece of gauze and place it over the site, holding it down while you pull back on the hub of the catheter. Gently pull the catheter and the IV line from the patient's vein while applying pressure to control bleeding **Figure 13-24**.

▶ Alternative IV Sites and Techniques

Some additional IV sites and techniques available to prehospital providers require training beyond the scope of this chapter. However, because you may need to assist in these types of IV administration, you can benefit from understanding how they work.

Saline Locks

A **saline lock** is a way to maintain an active IV site without having to run fluid through the vein. These access devices are used primarily for patients who do not need additional fluids but may need rapid medication delivery. Saline locks are access ports commonly used with patients who have disorders such as heart failure or pulmonary edema. A saline lock is attached to the end of an IV catheter and filled with approximately 2 mL of normal saline to keep blood from clotting at the end of the catheter **Figure 13-25**. Because this is a sealed-access site, the saline remains in the port without entering the vein, thus preventing clotting. These are also known as intermittent, or INT, sites because they eliminate the need to reestablish an IV line each time the patient needs medication or fluid.

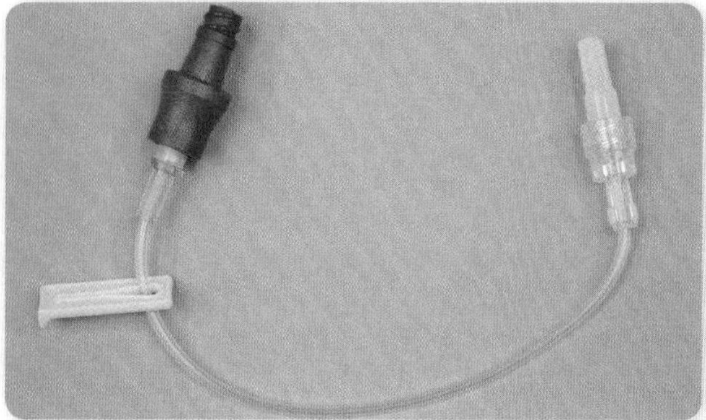

Figure 13-25 A saline lock is attached to the end of an intravenous catheter and filled with approximately 2 mL of normal saline to keep blood from clotting at the end of the catheter.

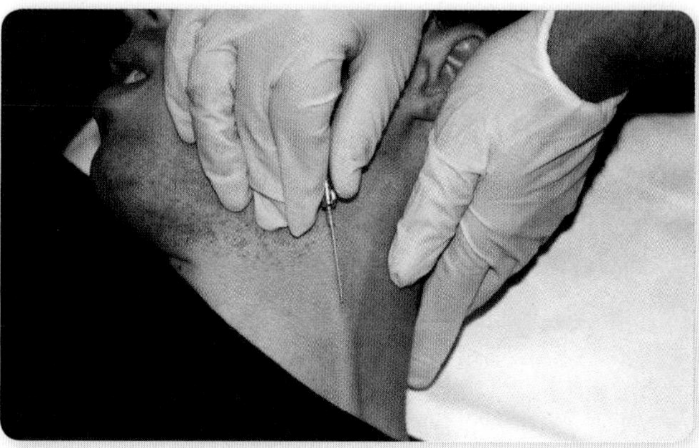

Figure 13-26 External jugular vein catheterization requires a specific insertion site midway between the angle of the jaw and the midclavicular line with the catheter pointed toward the shoulder on the same side as the puncture.

External Jugular IV Lines

External jugular IV lines provide venous access through the external jugular veins of the neck. These are the same veins used to assess jugular vein distention. The vein is tamponaded by placing a finger or the edge of a tongue depressor on the vein just above the clavicle, causing the vein to fill. If the vein is difficult to find, place the patient supine to facilitate venous return. The catheter is inserted into the vein in the same manner as a normal IV line, except the insertion point is very specific. The catheter is inserted midway between the angle of the jaw and the midclavicular line, with the catheter pointed toward the shoulder on the same side as the puncture site **Figure 13-26**. These punctures are difficult because a tough fibrous sheath that makes access difficult surrounds these veins.

These techniques require more advanced education and training than this chapter will provide. Understanding their application and use is important because you may need to perform these procedures depending on local protocols or assist with the performance of these procedures.

Words of Wisdom

Always feel very carefully for a pulse prior to cannulating an external jugular vein. It is imperative not to pierce the carotid artery.

▶ Troubleshooting IV Therapy

Several factors can influence the flow rate of an IV line. For example, if the IV bag is not hung high enough, the flow rate will not be sufficient. It is always helpful to perform the following checks after completing IV administration. Also, if there is a flow problem, rechecking these items will help determine the cause of the problem.

- **Check your IV fluid.** Thick, viscous fluids such as blood products and colloid solutions infuse slowly and may be diluted, if needed, to help speed delivery. Cold fluids run slower than warm fluids. If you can, warm IV fluids before administering them in cold weather.
- **Check your administration set.** Macrodrips are used for rapid fluid delivery, whereas microdrips are designed to deliver a more controlled flow.
- **Check the height of your IV bag.** The IV bag must be hung high enough to overcome the patient's own blood pressure. Hang the bag as high as possible.
- **Check the type of catheter used.** The wider the catheter (the smaller the gauge), the more fluid can be delivered—14 gauge is the widest, 27 gauge the narrowest. Catheter length also affects flow—the shorter the catheter, the more rapid the flow.
- **Check your constricting band.** One of the most overlooked factors is leaving the constricting band on the patient's arm after completing the IV line setup.

Words of Wisdom

To document IV administration, you need to include four things:

- The gauge of the needle
- The site
- The type of fluid you are administering
- The rate the fluid is running

▶ Possible Complications of IV Therapy

Problems associated with IV therapy can be categorized as either local or systemic reactions. **Local reactions** include problems such as infiltration; phlebitis; occlusion; vein irritation; hematoma; nerve, tendon, or ligament damage; and arterial puncture. **Systemic complications** include allergic reactions, circulatory overload, air embolus, vasovagal reactions, and catheter shear.

Local IV Site Reactions

Most local reactions require that you discontinue the administration, reestablish the IV line in the opposite extremity, and document the event.

Infiltration. Infiltration is the escape of fluid into the surrounding tissue. This escape of fluid causes a localized area of edema. Some of the more common reasons for infiltration include the following:

- The IV line has passed completely through the vein and out the other side.
- The patient is moving excessively, causing the catheter to become dislodged from the vein.
- The tape used to secure the area has become loose or dislodged (again causing the catheter to become dislodged from the vein).
- The catheter was started at an angle that is too shallow and has only entered the **fascia** surrounding the vein (this is more common with IV lines in larger veins, such as those in the upper arm and neck).

Some of the associated signs and symptoms of infiltration include the following:

- Edema at the catheter site
- Continued IV flow after occlusion of the vein above the insertion point
- Patient complaints of tightness and pain around the IV site

To correct the infiltration, discontinue administration and reestablish the IV line in the opposite extremity or at a more proximal location on the same extremity. Apply direct pressure over the swollen area to reduce further swelling or bleeding into the tissue. Avoid wrapping tape around the extremity for direct pressure because this could create a constricting band.

Thrombophlebitis. Thrombophlebitis is inflammation of the vein. Thrombophlebitis is not usually seen with the emergency prehospital patient. You may encounter it in patients who abuse drugs, as well as in patients who are receiving long-term IV therapy in a hospital, home care, or hospice setting.

Often, thrombophlebitis is associated with fever, tenderness, and red streaking up the associated vein. Hardening of the vein can occur if a vein has been repeatedly punctured, as seen with drug abuse. Some of the more common causes for thrombophlebitis include localized irritation and infection from nonsterile equipment, prolonged IV therapy, or irritating IV solutions.

Vein irritation is usually caused by an infusion that is too rapid. If redness develops at the IV site with rapidly developing thrombophlebitis, discontinue the infusion and save the equipment for later analysis. Reestablish the IV line in the other extremity with all new equipment in case there were unseen contaminants in the old equipment. Be sure to document the event and the patient's response.

Occlusion. Occlusion is the physical blockage of a vein or catheter. If the flow rate is not sufficient to keep fluid moving out of the catheter tip and if blood enters the catheter, a clot may form and occlude the flow. The first sign of a possible occlusion is a decreasing **drip rate** or the presence of blood in the IV tubing. A positional IV site can cause occlusion, which means that fluid flows at different rates depending on the position of the catheter within the vein. Proximity to a valve is often the reason for occlusion. Other causes can be related to patient movement that allows the line to become physically blocked from either resting on the line or crossing the arms. Occlusion may also develop if the IV bag nears empty and the blood pressure overcomes the flow and backs up in the line.

To determine whether an IV line should be reestablished, you may use a syringe prefilled with saline, or you may draw the saline from an IV bag. After you have a full syringe of clean IV fluid, you will use it to add pressure to the line. Gently apply pressure to the plunger to disrupt the occlusion and reestablish flow **Figure 13-27**. If flow is reestablished, ensure that the line is free and the rate is sufficient. If the occlusion does not dislodge, discontinue the administration and reestablish an IV line in the opposite extremity or at a proximal location on the same extremity.

Hematoma. A **hematoma** is an accumulation of blood in the tissues surrounding an IV site. Hematomas result from vein perforation or improper catheter removal that allows blood to accumulate in the surrounding tissues. Blood can be seen rapidly pooling around the IV site, resulting

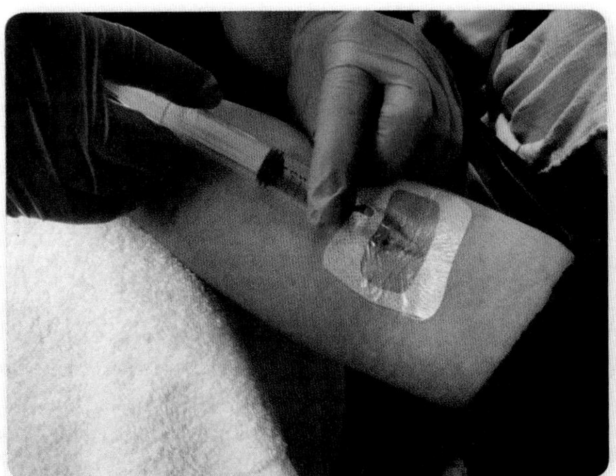

Figure 13-27 To check if an intravenous line is viable, gently flush the catheter to disrupt the occlusion and reestablish flow. This photo shows a syringe prefilled with saline.

Courtesy of Rhonda Hunt.

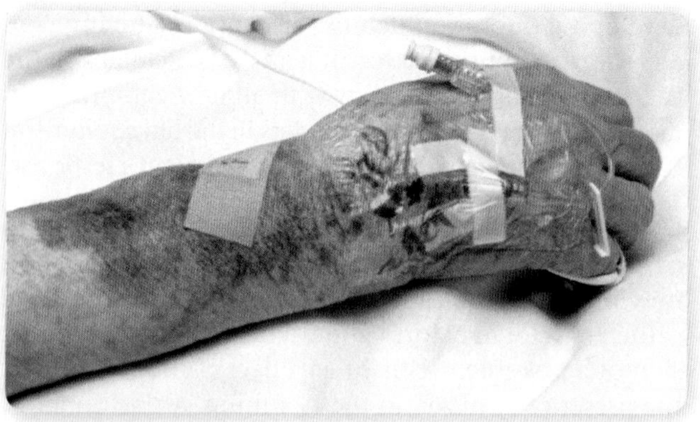

Figure 13-28 Hematomas can be caused by the improper removal of a catheter, resulting in the pooling of blood around the intravenous site, causing tenderness and pain and in extreme cases, skin necrosis and slough.

Courtesy of Rhonda Hunt.

in tenderness and pain and in extreme cases, skin necrosis and slough Figure 13-28. Patients with a history of vascular diseases (including diabetes) or patients receiving certain medications (such as corticosteroids) can have a predisposition to vein rupture or have tendencies for hematomas to develop rapidly on IV insertion.

If a hematoma develops while you are attempting to insert a catheter, stop and apply direct pressure to help minimize bleeding. If a hematoma develops after a successful catheter insertion, evaluate the IV flow and the hematoma. If the hematoma appears to be controlled and the flow is not affected, monitor the IV site and leave the line in place. If the hematoma develops as a result of removing the IV line, apply direct pressure with a 4- × 4-inch gauze pad to the site.

Nerve, Tendon, or Ligament Damage. Improper identification of anatomic structures around the IV site can result in perforation of tendons, ligaments, or nerves. An IV site choice around joints increases the risk for perforation of these structures. Patients will experience sudden, severe shooting pain when a nerve, tendon, or ligament is perforated. Numbness in the extremity after the incident can be common. Immediately remove the catheter and select another IV site. Be sure to document the event.

Arterial Puncture. Occasionally, cannulation of an artery may occur. Cannulation of an artery is easily recognized because bright red blood is quickly seen either spurting from the catheter after the needle is withdrawn, or backing up into the IV tubing and the IV bag because of the high pressure that exists in the arteries. If cannulation of an artery occurs, you must stop IV administration, remove the catheter, and apply direct pressure to the site with gauze for at least 15 minutes and certainly until any bleeding is controlled.

Systemic Complications

Systemic complications can develop from reactions or complications associated with IV insertion. Systemic complications usually involve other body systems and can be life threatening. If the IV line is established and patent, do not remove it, because it may be needed for treatment of the patient.

Allergic Reactions. Often, allergic reactions are minor, but anaphylaxis is possible and therefore any allergic reaction must be treated aggressively. Allergic reactions can be related to an individual's unexpected sensitivity to medication being infused with the intravenous fluid or to a prep solution such as iodine used to prepare the site for intravenous administration. Such sensitivity could be an unknown condition to the patient; thus, vigilance must be maintained with any IV line for a possible reaction.

Patient presentation depends on the extent of the reaction. Common signs and symptoms of an allergic reaction include:

- Itching
- Shortness of breath
- Edema of face and hands
- Urticaria
- Bronchospasm
- Anaphylaxis
- Wheezing

If an allergic reaction occurs, discontinue IV administration of the medication and remove the solution. Leave the catheter in place as an emergency medication route. Notify medical control immediately and maintain an open airway. Monitor the patient's airway, breathing, and circulation and vital signs. Document the event and keep the IV bag or medication for evaluation by the hospital. Further treatment for anaphylaxis is covered in Chapter 22, *Immunologic Emergencies*.

Air Embolus. The amount of air a healthy adult can tolerate entering the circulatory system varies, but patients who are already ill or injured can be affected if any air is introduced into the IV line. Properly flushing an IV line will help eliminate any potential of introducing air into a patient. IV bags are designed to collapse as they empty to help prevent this problem, but collapse does not always occur. Be sure to replace empty IV bags with full ones. Entrapment of air may also occur if IV catheters in large vessels, such as external jugular veins, are left open to the air. Be sure to quickly attach the IV line to prevent such an occurrence.

If your patient begins to experience respiratory distress with unequal breath sounds, consider the possibility of an **air embolus**, an air bubble that blocks blood flow. Other associated signs and symptoms include the following:

- Cyanosis (even in the presence of high-flow oxygen)
- Signs and symptoms of shock
- Loss of consciousness
- Respiratory arrest

Treat a patient with a suspected air embolus by placing the patient on his or her left side with the head down to trap any air inside the right atrium or right ventricle, and rapidly transport to the closest most appropriate facility. Be prepared to assist ventilations if the patient experiences increasing shortness of breath or inadequate tidal volume. Document the event.

Catheter Shear. **Catheter shear** occurs when part of the catheter is pinched against the needle, and the needle slices through the catheter, creating a free-floating segment. The catheter segment can travel through the circulatory system and possibly end up in the pulmonary circulation, causing a pulmonary embolus. Blockage of other vessels may result in a myocardial infarction, stroke, or other problems. If you suspect a catheter shear, then place the patient in a left lateral recumbent position with the legs down and the head elevated to try to keep the catheter remnant out of the pulmonary circulation.

Treatment involves surgical removal of the sheared tip. Catheter hubs are radiopaque (that is, they will appear white on a radiograph) to aid in diagnosing this type of problem. Never rethread a catheter. Dispose of the used one and use a new one.

Patients who have experienced catheter shear with pulmonary artery occlusion may present with sudden dyspnea, shortness of breath, and possibly diminished breath sounds. They will mimic the presentation of a patient with an air embolus and can be treated the same way. These patients will need continued IV access, and you must try to obtain an IV line in the other extremity.

Circulatory Overload. An unmonitored IV bag can result in circulatory overload. Healthy adults can handle as much as 2 to 3 extra liters of fluid without compromise. Problems occur when the patient has cardiac, pulmonary, or renal dysfunction; these types of dysfunction do not tolerate any additional demands from increased circulatory volume. In trauma patients, increased circulatory volume from overaggressive resuscitation can disrupt clot formation and actually increase ongoing hemorrhage. The most common cause of circulatory overload in the prehospital setting is failure to readjust the drip rate after flushing an IV line immediately after insertion. Always monitor IV bags to ensure the proper drip rate.

Patient presentation includes dyspnea, jugular vein distention, and increased blood pressure. Crackles are often heard when evaluating breath sounds. Acute peripheral edema can also be an indication of circulatory overload.

To treat a patient with circulatory overload, slow the IV rate to keep the vein open and raise the patient's head to ease respiratory distress. Administer high-flow oxygen and monitor vital signs and breathing adequacy. Contact medical control immediately and inform personnel of the developing problem because medications can be administered to reduce the circulatory volume. Document the event.

Vasovagal Reactions. Some patients have anxiety concerning needles or the sight of blood. Such anxiety may cause vasculature dilation, resulting in a decrease in blood pressure and patient collapse. A patient can present with anxiety, diaphoresis, nausea, and a **syncopal episode**.

Treatment for a patient with a **vasovagal reaction** (also known as vagaling down) centers on treatment for shock:

1. Place patient in the position dictated by protocol for shock management.
2. Apply high-flow oxygen.
3. Monitor vital signs.
4. Establish an IV line in case fluid resuscitation is needed.

▶ Pediatric IV Therapy Considerations

The same IV solutions and equipment can be used on pediatric patients as on adults, with a few exceptions.

Catheters

Catheters come in various sizes Figure 13-29. If you are using over-the-needle catheters to start a pediatric IV line, the 20-, 22-, 24-, or 26-gauge catheters are best for insertion depending on the size of the patient and the size of available veins. Butterfly catheters are ideal for pediatric patients and can be placed in the same locations as over-the-needle catheters and in visible scalp veins. Scalp veins are best used in young infants.

IV Locations

When you are starting an IV line, explain what you are doing to both the child and the parent. A parent can become as stressed as a child, so take time to thoroughly explain the procedure.

The younger the pediatric patient, the fewer choices you have for IV sites. Hand veins are painful and difficult to manage in younger pediatric patients but remain the location of choice for starting peripheral IV lines. Protecting the IV site after it has been established is critical and is sometimes best accomplished by immobilizing the site before cannulation with an arm board.

One of the better techniques for starting pediatric IV lines is to use a penlight to illuminate the veins on the

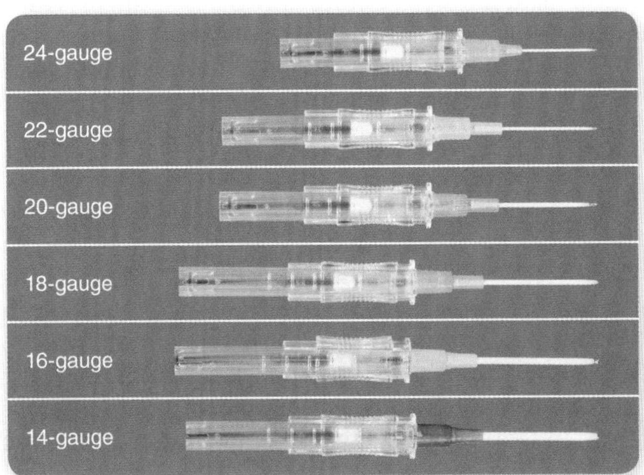

Figure 13-29 Note the difference in sizes of the catheters.

back of the hand. Shine the light through the palm side of the hand to illuminate the veins on the back side of the hand. Be sure not to burn the patient with the penlight, even though this is unlikely. After a suitable site is located, slightly graze the surface of the hand with your fingernail so you can find the location after you turn off the penlight. Proceed with the IV insertion, using the mark you created as a guide. Sometimes the best choice is an antecubital vein line with full arm immobilization to avoid dislodging the IV line.

Scalp vein cannulation is often aesthetically unpleasant for both the child and the parents and can produce apprehension in both simply because of the location. In addition, scalp veins can be difficult to cannulate and do not allow for rapid fluid resuscitation. When you are securing a scalp vein, tape a paper cup over the site to avoid applying any direct pressure to the butterfly catheter. Pressure may cause the needle to puncture the other side of the vein and let fluids escape into the tissues (extravasation).

Geriatric IV Therapy Considerations

Smaller catheters may be preferable with older adult patients unless rapid fluid replacement is needed. Some medications commonly used by older adults have the tendency to create fragile skin and veins. Often, simply puncturing the vein will cause a massive hematoma. The use of tape can result in skin damage, so be careful when establishing IV lines in older adults. Consider using alternative options such as paper tape or commercial devices that reduce the risk of skin damage.

Catheters

Try using smaller catheters (such as 20-, 22-, or 24-gauge) because they may be more comfortable for the patient and can reduce the risk of extravasation.

IV Sets

Be careful when you are using macrodrips because they can allow rapid infusion of fluids, which may result in edema if they are not monitored closely. With both geriatric and pediatric patients, fluid overloading is potentially serious. Always monitor fluid administration carefully.

Locations

In choosing an IV site, you should consider the possibility of poor vein elasticity. One of the consequences of aging is the loss of elasticity in the body tissues. Veins become sclerosed, making them brittle. Certain medications, such as prednisone, can also affect the structure of the vein, making the veins of geriatric patients even more fragile and easily ruptured. Avoid small, spidery veins that weave back and forth Figure 13-30 because they may rupture easily. Do not use **varicose veins**; although they often appear to be ideal choices for IV starts, they are almost completely closed off and allow very little circulation.

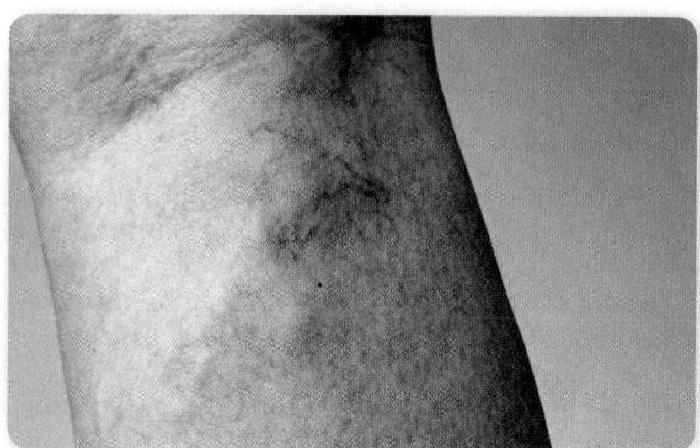

Figure 13-30 When you are looking for an intravenous site, avoid small, spidery veins and varicose veins.

Intraosseous Infusion

Intraosseous (IO) means "within the bone." **Intraosseous infusion** is a technique of administering fluids, blood and blood products, and medications into the **intraosseous space** of the proximal tibia, humeral head, or sternum. Long bones, such as the tibia, consist of a shaft (**diaphysis**), the ends (**epiphyses**), and the growth plate (**epiphyseal plate**) Figure 13-31.

The IO space collectively comprises the spongy cancellous bone of the epiphyses and the medullary cavity of the diaphysis. Its vasculature drains into the central circulation by a network of venous sinuses and canals.

When a patient is in shock, cardiac arrest, or an otherwise hemodynamically compromised condition, peripheral veins often collapse, making IV access extremely difficult, if not impossible. However, the IO space remains patent unless trauma has been sustained to its bony structure (eg, a fracture). For this reason, the IO space is commonly referred to as a "noncollapsible vein." It quickly absorbs IV fluids and medications and rapidly gets them to the central circulation—as rapidly as is possible with the IV route. Anything that can be given via the IV route—crystalloids, medications, and blood and blood products—can be given via the IO route.

IO infusion is indicated when you are unable to rapidly obtain IV access in a critically ill or injured patient (eg, in profound shock, cardiac arrest, or status epilepticus). Depending on local protocol, you will typically attempt one or two IV lines within 90 seconds prior to an IO infusion attempt. Some situations, such as cardiac arrest, may warrant going immediately to an IO infusion due to the time savings, likelihood of success, and ease of use. Vascular access times and flow rates for various IO sites are presented in Table 13-2.

IO Sites

Common sites you will use for IO insertion are the sternum, humerus, proximal tibia, and distal tibia. The technique for performing IO infusion requires proper anatomic landmark identification. To locate the humeral IO site,

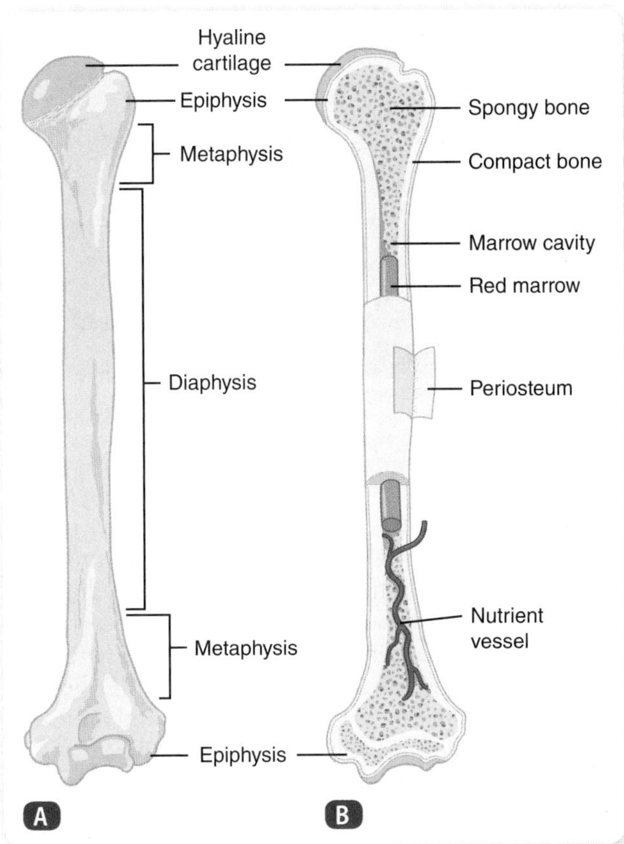

Figure 13-31 The components of a long bone. **A.** The humerus. Note the long shaft and dilated ends. **B.** Longitudinal section of the humerus showing compact bone, cancellous (spongy) bone, and marrow.

Table 13-2 Vascular Access Time and Flow Rate for Various IO Sites

IO Site	Reported Flow Rate (mL/min)
Sternal	469
Humeral	148.1-286
Proximal tibial	154-204.6

Abbreviation: IO, intraosseous

Data from: Pasley J, Miller CHT, DuBose JJ, et al. Intraosseous infusion rates under high pressure: a cadaveric comparison of anatomic sites. *J Trauma Acute Care Surg*. 2015;78(2):295-299; Ngo ASY, Oh JJ, Chen Y, et al. Intraosseous vascular access in adults using the EZ-IO in an emergency department. *Int J Emerg Med*. 2009;2(3):155-160; and Ong MEH, Chan YH, Oh JJ, Ngo AS-Y. An observational, prospective study comparing tibial and humeral intraosseous access using the EZ-IO. *Amer J Emerg Med*. 2009;27:8-15.

you will need to manipulate the patient's arm and palpate the humeral head **Figure 13-32**. Begin by placing the patient's hand over his or her abdomen, which causes an internal rotation of the humeral head. Place the ulnar aspect of one of your hands vertically over the axilla near the humeral head that will be used for insertion. Place

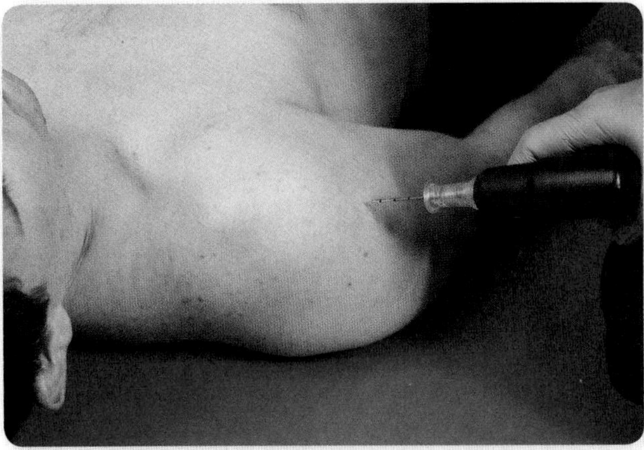

Figure 13-32 The humeral site for intraosseous insertion.

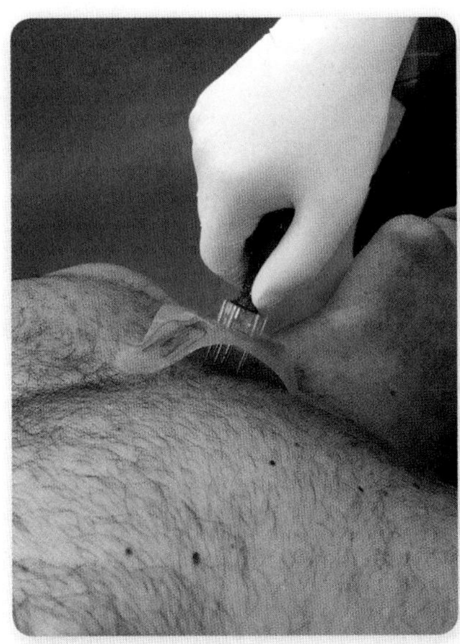

Figure 13-33 The sternal site for intraosseous insertion.

the ulnar aspect of your other hand laterally along the midline of the upper portion of the patient's humerus. Place your thumbs together, palpating up the surgical neck to the humeral head. When this site is used, medications can reach the right atrium within 3 seconds of rapid IV push. Appropriate needle selection and stabilization are crucial to use this site successfully.

Identify the sternal IO site by palpating the sternal notch and using the IO device's adhesive target **Figure 13-33**. The sternal site has an extremely rapid flow rate. The device location is near the chest compression landmarks; however, the device does not impede chest compressions.

The flat bone of the proximal tibia is located medial to the tibial tuberosity, the bony protuberance just below the knee. It is necessary to feel the leg to know the difference between the first and second landmarks (these cannot be seen; they must be felt). To locate the proximal tibia IO site, palpate the tibial tuberosity, then palpate 2 cm

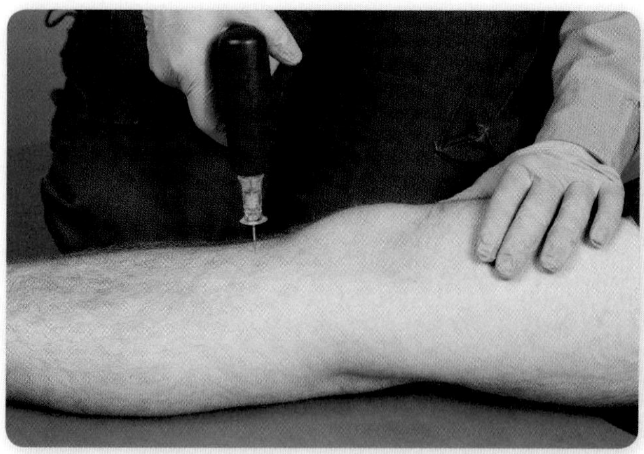

Figure 13-34 The proximal tibia site for intraosseous insertion in adults.

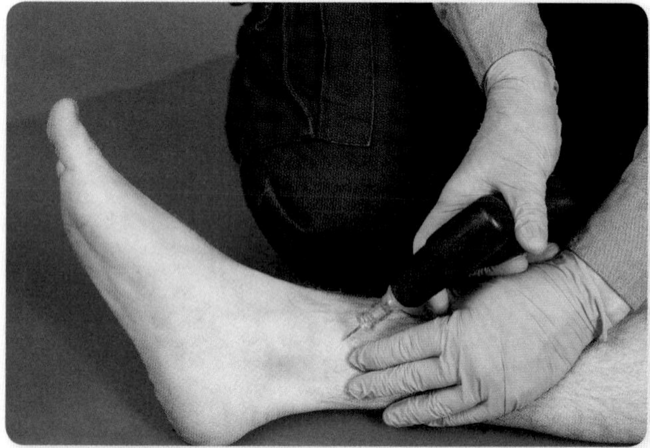

Figure 13-35 The distal tibia site for intraosseous insertion in adults.

medially. This is the site for adult patients Figure 13-34. For pediatric patients, palpate 1 to 2 cm distally to avoid the epiphyseal plate.

For the distal tibia IO site, use palpation as well. First, identify the medial malleolus. Then palpate 2 to 3 cm above that site Figure 13-35. For pediatric patients, you should palpate 1 to 2 cm above the medial malleolus.

▶ Equipment for IO Infusion

Several products are used for placing an IO needle into the IO space: manually inserted IO needles, the FAST1, the EZ-IO, the Bone Injection Gun (BIG), and the New Intraosseous (NIO) device. Use of these devices requires specialized training and thorough familiarity with each device's features, functionality, and clinical application.

If your EMS system uses any of these devices, then follow local protocols regarding their application. Manually inserted IO needles (ie, Jamshedi needle, Cook catheter) were the original devices used for establishing IO access in children and are still widely used in the prehospital setting. They consist of a solid boring needle (**trocar**) inserted through a sharpened hollow needle Figure 13-36. The IO needle is pushed into the bone with a screwing, twisting action. After the needle pops through the bone, the solid needle is removed, leaving the hollow steel catheter in place. The IV tubing is attached to this catheter. Because manually inserted IO needles are long, rest at a 90° angle to the bone, and are easily dislodged, they require full, careful immobilization. Stabilization is critical for these lines to maintain adequate flow. Stabilize the IO needle in the same manner that you would any impaled object.

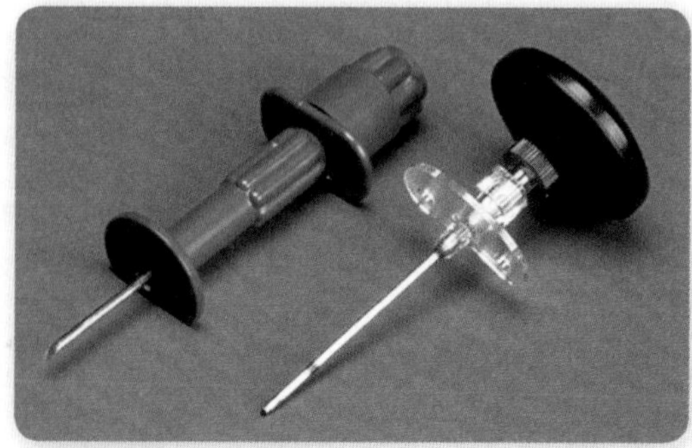

Figure 13-36 Manually inserted intraosseous needles.

FAST Devices

The **FAST devices** (First Access for Shock and Trauma) were the first IO devices approved for use in patients age 12 years and older. Four design elements allow IO placement in the sternum using FAST devices: an infusion tube and subcutaneous portal, an introducer, a target/strain relief patch, and a protective dome. FAST devices can be used during cardiac arrest. Although chest compressions can coincide with FAST IO use, mechanical cardiopulmonary resuscitation (CPR) devices must be paused during the insertion phase. Mechanical CPR can continue after the FAST device is stabilized.

The company that developed the FAST devices chose sternum placement based on the ease of locating the manubrium and because it is easier to penetrate than other bones. The landmarks can be felt on most adults even in low-light situations. The target device is shaped so that it lines up with the sternal notch, minimizing the margin of error.

The FAST1 is the original sternal IO device Figure 13-37. It consists of a 14-gauge infusion tube and 10 stabilization needles. It has been field tested in the military and used in civilian EMS for over a decade. The device is completely manual (no batteries required).

The FAST Responder (FASTR) is an updated device that has some advantages. Many of the components are already assembled, expediting the insertion process. For example, the adhesive target comes attached to the device. The device also has a safety lock that must be removed

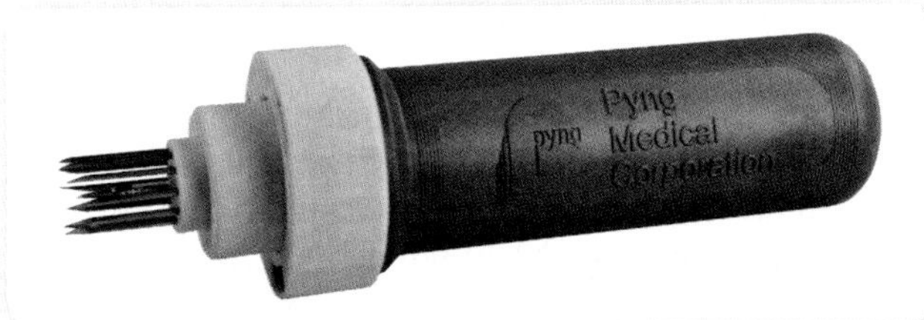

Figure 13-37 The FAST1 intraosseous insertion device.

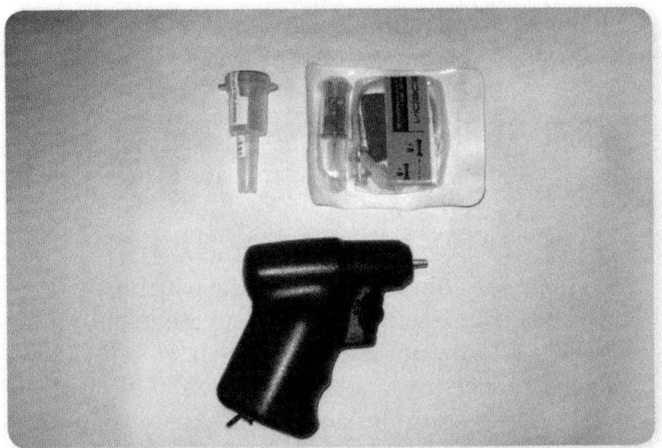

Figure 13-38 The EZ-IO insertion device features a handheld battery-powered driver, to which a special intraosseous needle is attached. The battery-powered driver of the EZ-IO is universal, but different sizes of needles are available.

Courtesy of VidaCare Corporation.

before insertion. The FASTR only requires 32 pounds (15 kg) of pressure for insertion. If sternal IOs are the preference for your EMS system, then familiarize yourself with both devices.

Both devices are designed to remain in place for a maximum of 24 hours. To remove either FAST device, firmly grasp the insertion tube and pull steadily until the device is dislodged. Use one continuous motion for removal; avoid starting and stopping.

EZ-IO Device

The **EZ-IO** features a handheld battery-powered driver, to which a special IO needle is attached Figure 13-38. This device is used to insert an IO needle into the proximal or distal tibia of adults and children and the humeral head in adults when IV access is difficult or impossible to obtain. The battery-powered driver of the EZ-IO is universal, but different sizes of needles are available depending on the patient. The needle size is estimated based on the insertion site and patient's weight; however, the ultimate determining factor in needle size selection is the amount of subcutaneous tissue present over the insertion site Table 13-3. When sizing the needle, you should ensure at least one hash mark (5 mm) can be seen after insertion.

Table 13-3 EZ-IO Needle Sizes and Determination Criteria

EZ-IO Needle[a]	EZ-IO Needle Size (mm)	Needle Determination Criteria[b]
	15	3-39 kg
	25	> 40 kg
	45	Excessive subcutaneous tissue and humeral IO insertion

[a]All needles are 15 gauge.
[b]Determination criteria may vary based on the amount of subcutaneous tissue present.
Abbreviation: IO, intraosseous

Data from: Arrow EZ IO Intraosseous Vascular Access. EZ-IO Intraosseous Vascular Access Needles: Instructions for Use. 8082 Rev A. July 2014. http://www.teleflex.com/en/usa/ezioeducation/documents/8082_Rev_A_US_FDA_Intraosseous_Infusion_System_IFU.pdf. Accessed February 15, 2017.

Courtesy of VidaCare Corporation (www.vidacare.com).

Use a 10-mL syringe to remove an EZ-IO. Attach the syringe to the IO's Luer lock, twist the syringe clockwise, and pull the device out in one swift motion.

Bone Injection Gun Device

The **Bone Injection Gun (BIG)** is a spring-loaded device that is used to insert an IO needle into the proximal tibia of adult and pediatric patients and the humeral head in adults Figure 13-39. It comes in an adult size and a pediatric size. Although both versions offer the same operational

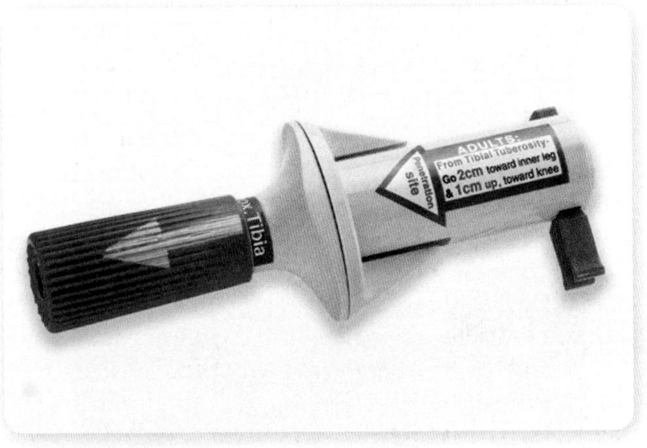

Figure 13-39 The Bone Injection Gun (BIG).

Courtesy of PerSys Medical.

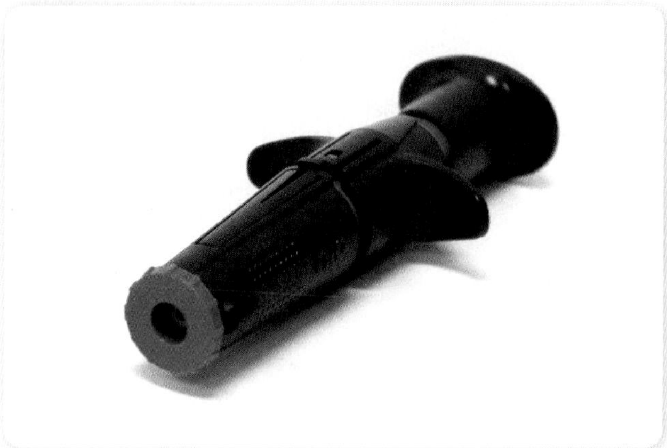

Figure 13-40 The New Intraosseous (NIO) device.
Courtesy of PerSys Medical.

features, the depth of insertion is different for the adult and pediatric devices.

The BIG uses the safety lock as the stabilization device after the device has been inserted. When you are ready to remove the device, use the stabilization device as the removal tool. Place the wider side of the removal tool over the connection port. Pull the device out in one swift motion while grasping onto the removal tool.

New Intraosseous Device

The **New Intraosseous (NIO) device** is a device that is placed in the proximal tibia of an adult patient Figure 13-40. The humeral head is an alternative site for this device. The spring-loaded device contains neither drill nor battery. It is inserted by unlocking a safety cap. Then, while applying downward pressure with the dominant hand, the fingers of the other hand are used to pull trigger wings up to deploy the device. The device is then pulled up in a rotating motion while the needle stabilizer is held against the skin. After the introducing trocar is removed, any Luer-lock tubing can be attached.

A pediatric version, NIO Pediatric (NIO-P), is also available. This device has an adjustable dial, allowing the provider to adjust by age or depth (if excessive girth for the age is anticipated). At the time of this writing, the NIO-P is approved for placement in the proximal tibia only.

▶ Performing IO Infusion

Follow these steps to perform IO infusion using an EZ-IO device Skill Drill 13-3.

To attach a FAST1 device, follow these steps:

1. Align the adhesive target on the patient and prepare to insert the device into the manubrium. The manubrium is approximately 15 mm below the sternal notch, and at 13.3 mm, it is the thickest part of the sternum. The stabilization needles prevent you from pushing the insertion tube to an inappropriate depth.
2. Prepare the insertion site on the patient's manubrium.
3. Position yourself behind the patient's head, place two hands on the FAST1 device, align the stabilization needles with the target, and apply

Skill Drill 13-3 Gaining Intraosseous Access With an EZ-IO Device

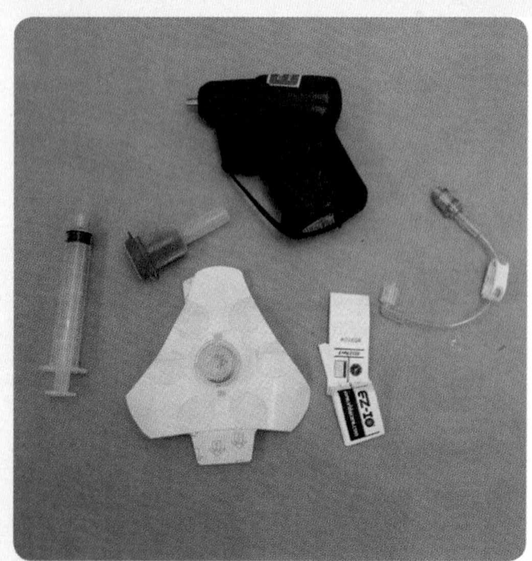

Step 1 Check the selected IV fluid for proper fluid, clarity, and expiration date. Look for discoloration and for particles floating in the fluid. If particles are found in the fluid, discard the bag and choose another bag of fluid.

Select the appropriate equipment, including an IO needle, syringe, saline, extension set, antiseptic swabs, and gauze pads.

A three-way stopcock may also be used to facilitate easier fluid administration.

Select the proper administration set. Connect the administration set to the bag. Prepare the administration set. Fill the drip chamber and flush the tubing. Ensure all air bubbles are removed from the tubing.

Prepare the syringe and extension tubing. Ensure the tubing is not tangled.

Cut or tear the tape and prepare bulky dressings. This can be done at any time before IO puncture.

Skill Drill 13-3 Gaining Intraosseous Access With an EZ-IO Device *(continued)*

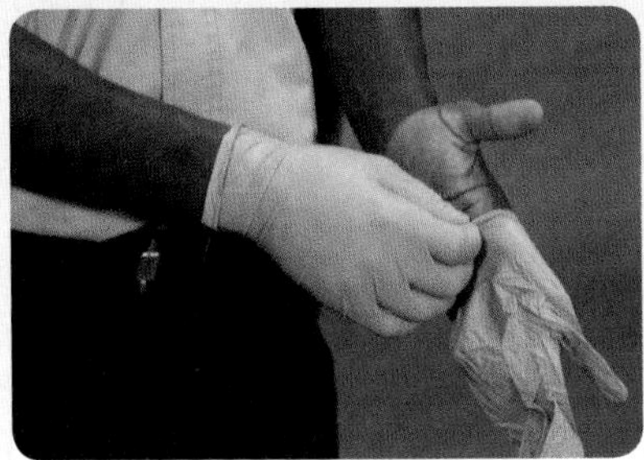

Step 2 Take standard precautions.

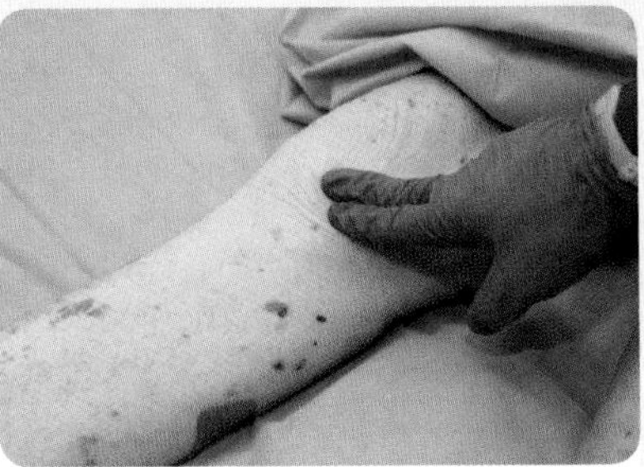

Step 3 Identify the proper anatomic site for IO puncture. Palpate the landmarks and then prepare the site.

- **Tibia placement.** This site is reserved for the EZ-IO and the BIG.
- **Humerus placement.** Humeral placement is typically reserved for adults when using the EZ-IO or the BIG.

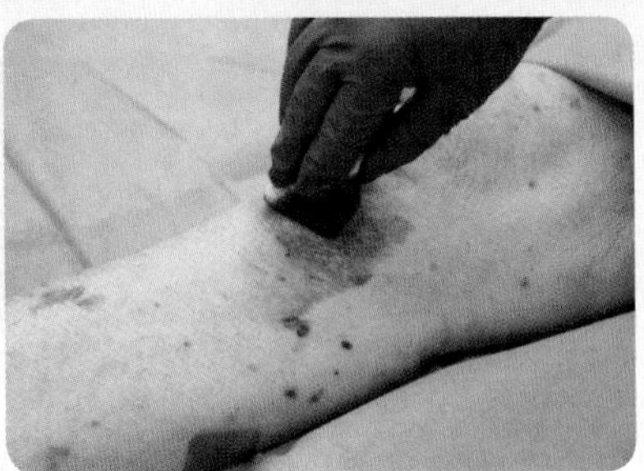

Step 4 Cleanse the site appropriately. Follow aseptic technique by cleansing in a circular manner from the inside out.

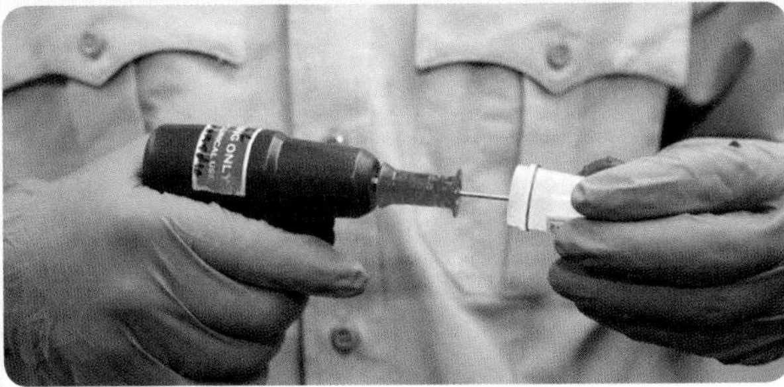

Step 5 Attach the needle to the EZ-IO gun and remove the protective cover. Examine the needle. If you find any imperfections, discard the needle and select another one.

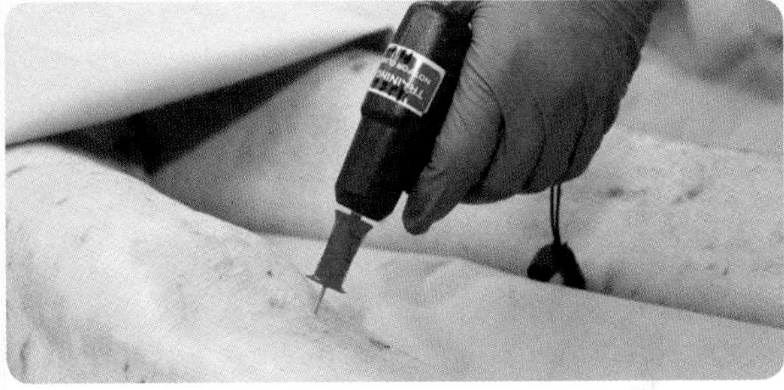

Step 6 Perform the IO puncture by first stabilizing the tibia, then placing a folded towel under the knee, and finally holding the extremity in a manner to keep your fingers away from the site of puncture. For humeral placement, continue to apply pressure on the anterior and inferior aspects of the humerus. Insert the needle at a 90° angle to the insertion site. Advance the needle with a twisting motion until a "pop" is felt. Unscrew the cap, and remove the stylet from the needle.

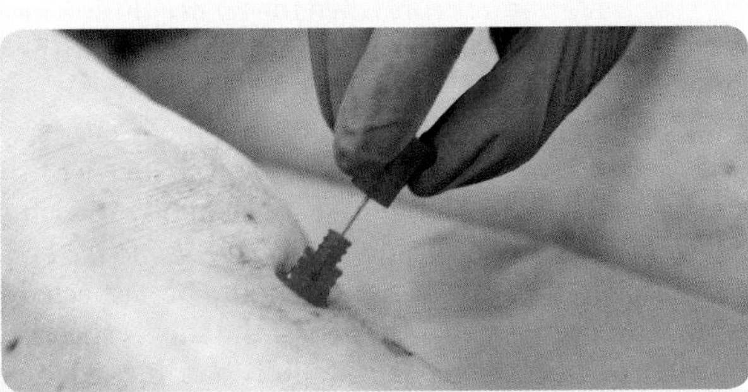

Step 7 Remove the stylet from the catheter.

(continued)

Skill Drill 13-3 Gaining Intraosseous Access With an EZ-IO Device *(continued)*

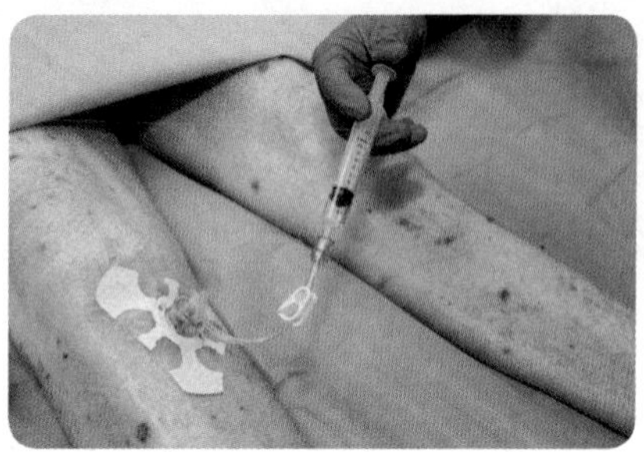

Step 8 Attach the syringe and extension set to the IO needle. Pull back on the syringe to aspirate blood and particles of bone marrow to ensure proper placement. The absence of marrow does not mean the access failed. Check the site for other signs of extravasation. Slowly inject saline to ensure proper placement of the needle. Responsive patients should receive 1% lidocaine prior to infusion of fluids. Watch for extravasation, and stop the infusion immediately if any evidence of extravasation is noted. It is possible to fracture the bone during insertion of the IO needle. If this happens, then remove the IO needle and switch to the other insertion site.

Connect the administration set and adjust the flow rate as appropriate. Fluid does not flow as rapidly through an IO catheter as through an IV line; therefore, crystalloid boluses should be given with a syringe in children and a **pressure infuser device** (a sleeve placed around the IV bag and inflated to force fluid from the IV bag) in adults.

Secure the needle with tape, and support it with a bulky dressing. Stabilize in place in the same manner that an impaled object is stabilized. Use bulky dressings around the catheter, and tape securely in place. Be careful not to tape around the entire circumference of the leg because this could impair circulation and potentially result in compartment syndrome.

Dispose of the needle in the proper container.

approximately 45 pounds (20 kg) of pressure until you feel the infusion tube separate from the FAST1 introducer Figure 13-41.

4. Discard the stabilization needle in a sharps container and attach the IV tubing to the insertion tube's Luerlock. Aspirate blood and particles of bone marrow to ensure proper placement. Slowly inject the IV solution to ensure proper placement of the needle. Adjust the flow rate as appropriate. Place the protective dome, and begin using the device.

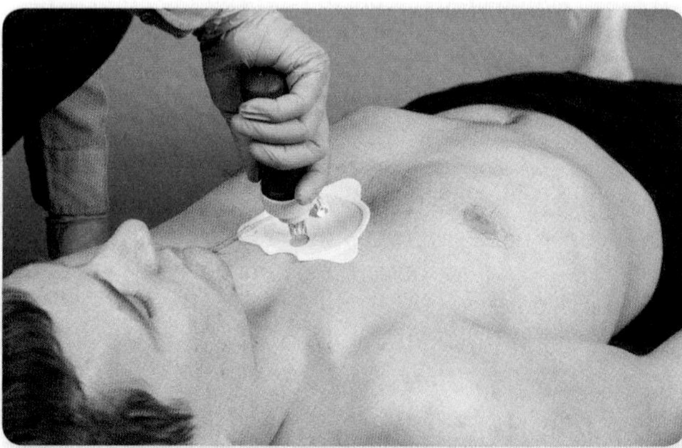

Figure 13-41 To use the FAST1 device, first align the adhesive target along the patient's sternal notch, and match the insertion site with the patient's manubrium. Position yourself behind the patient's head, place your hand on the FAST1 device, align the stabilization needles with the target, and apply pressure until you feel the infusion tube separate from the FAST1 introducer.

▶ Potential Complications of IO Infusion

If the proper technique is used (ie, proper anatomic landmark identification, aseptic technique), then IO infusion is associated with a relatively low complication rate. The same potential complications associated with IV therapy—thrombophlebitis, local irritation, allergic reaction, circulatory overload, and air embolism—can occur with IO infusion, as well as several others unique to this method of infusion.

Extravasation occurs when the IO needle does not rest in the IO space, but rather rests outside the bone (because the bone was missed completely or is fractured or because the needle becomes dislodged from the bone). In such a case, IV fluid will collect in the soft tissues. The risk of extravasation can be reduced substantially by using the proper insertion technique: *insert the IO needle at a 90° angle to the bone*. Extravasation should be suspected if the infusion does not run freely or if the site—especially the posterior aspect of the leg—rapidly becomes edematous. If this occurs, discontinue the infusion immediately and reattempt insertion in the opposite leg. Undetected extravasation could result in compartment syndrome.

Osteomyelitis is inflammation of the bone and muscle caused by an infection. Osteomyelitis can occur from IO insertion, but is rare.

Failure to identify the proper anatomic landmark can damage the growth plate, potentially resulting in long-term bone growth abnormalities in children. If your insertion technique is too forceful, or if you use an IO needle that is too large for the patient's age or size, then fractures can occur. Through-and-through insertion occurs when the IO needle passes through *both* sides of the bone. To avoid this, stop inserting the needle when you feel a pop. If you feel a "pop, pop," then you have likely passed the needle through both sides of the bone. If either occurs, then remove the needle and attempt insertion on the opposite extremity.

Words of Wisdom

With the exception of the FAST1 sternal IO device, all IO devices—manual, spring-loaded, and battery-powered—are primarily used to insert an IO needle into the IO space of the proximal tibia, distal tibia, or humeral head. However, other anatomic locations, such as the distal femur, may also be acceptable locations for IO needle insertion.

A pulmonary embolism can occur if particles of bone, fat, or marrow enter into the systemic circulation and lodge in a pulmonary artery. You should suspect a pulmonary embolism if the patient experiences acute shortness of breath, pleuritic chest pain, and cyanosis.

Words of Wisdom

When you start an IV line for the purpose of administering a medication, you should set the flow rate just slow enough to keep the vein patent. This slow flow rate can be documented using the acronym TKO, which stands for To Keep Open.

▶ Contraindications to IO Infusion

Cannulation of a peripheral vein remains the preferred route for administering IV fluids and medications. If a functional IV line is available—in a pediatric patient or an adult—IO cannulation is *not* indicated. Other contraindications to IO cannulation and infusion include fracture of the bone intended for IO cannulation, osteoporosis, **osteogenesis imperfecta** (a congenital disease resulting in fragile bones), bilateral knee replacements (humeral and sternal sites remain an option), and a prosthetic limb at the IO site.

Mathematical Principles Used in Pharmacology

As mentioned, you will need an understanding of some basic mathematical principles to calculate accurate medication dosages. This section reviews some basic principles and discusses formulas for medication calculations.

▶ Mathematical Principles Used in Pharmacology

Mathematics Review

This section discusses the use of fractions, percentages, and decimals. Having basic math skills is imperative for paramedics to appropriately administer medications.

Understanding fractions is important in formula calculation. Fractions represent a portion of a whole number expressed. Fractions are expressed as a numerator (the top number representing the portion available) over the denominator (representing the total quantity). For example, if you have four EMS units available and one of them is dispatched to an emergency, then one-fourth ($\frac{1}{4}$) of your units are occupied. Think of fractions as the numerator divided by the denominator. For example, $\frac{1}{4}$ is the same as $1 \div 4$.

Decimals distinguish numbers that are greater than zero from numbers that are smaller than zero. Whole numbers appear to the left side of the decimal point, and fractions of numbers on the right. Fractions can be easily converted to decimals by dividing the numerator by the denominator. For example, when you are administering atropine to bradycardic adult patients, you administer $\frac{1}{2}$ of 1 milligram. By dividing 1 by 2, you get 0.5 ($1 \div 2 = 0.5$).

Dividing or multiplying by 10 is simple when you remember the following method. If you are dividing a number by 10, then simply move the decimal point to the left. If you are multiplying a number by 10, then simply move the decimal point to the right. In other words, if you are dividing the number 20 by 10, moving the decimal point one space to the left results in 2, which is the correct answer. The following examples show this method.

Multiplication problem: 20×10

Step 1: Place the decimal point:

20.0

Step 2: To multiply by 10, move the decimal point one space to the right:

200.0 →

The answer is 200.

Division problem: 20 ÷ 10

Step 1: Place the decimal point:

20.0

Step 2: To divide by 10, move the decimal point one space to the left:

2.00
←

The answer is 2.

Percentages are a part of 100 and are denoted by the % symbol. Percentages can be represented as a fraction with the denominator being 100; for example, 21% = 21/100. Decimals can also be turned into percentages easily by moving the decimal point over two places (0.21 is equal to 21%).

The Metric System

The **metric system** is a decimal system based on multiples of 10. It is used to measure length, volume, and weight, which are represented as follows:

- Meter (m): The basic unit of length
- Liter (L): The basic unit of volume
- Gram (g): The basic unit of weight

In the metric system, prefixes demonstrate the fraction of the base being used. Commonly used prefixes, from smallest to largest, include the following:

- micro- = 0.000001
- milli- = 0.001
- centi- = 0.01
- kilo- = 1,000.0

Table 13-4 illustrates the symbols of weight and volume used in the metric system. It is important to be able to recognize these symbols because medications will be supplied in a variety of weights and volumes and

Table 13-4 Symbols Used in the Metric System

Unit	Symbol
Weight (smallest to largest)	
Microgram	mcg
Milligram	mg
Gram	g (or gm)
Kilogram	kg
Volume (smallest to largest)	
Milliliter	mL
Deciliter	dL
Liter	L

YOU are the Provider PART 4

You administer an initial 250-mL bolus of 0.9% normal saline. After the initial fluid bolus is infused, you recheck her blood pressure and breath sounds. You find no increase in her blood pressure, and breath sounds remain clear, so you administer another 250-mL bolus of 0.9% normal saline. On arrival at the trauma center, you turn over care to the awaiting trauma team without incident.

Recording Time: 21 Minutes	
Respirations	20 breaths/min
Pulse	Strong and regular, 130 beats/min
Skin	Cool, pale, and clammy
Blood pressure	86/48 mm Hg
Oxygen saturation (Spo_2)	100% on 15 L/min
Pupils	PERRLA

7. Why is it important to constantly reassess breath sounds when you are administering fluid to a patient?
8. What are some possible complications of vein cannulation?

Table 13-5 Metric Units

Unit	Equivalent
Weight (smallest to largest)	
1 mcg	0.001 mg
1 mg	1,000 mcg
1 g	1,000 mg
1 kg	1,000 g
Volume (smallest to largest)	
1 mL	1 cc[a]
100 mL	1 dL
1,000 mL	1 L

[a] Cubic centimeters (cc) is a unit also used to represent milliliters (mL); therefore, 1 cc is the same as 1 mL (1 cc = 1 mL).

you will be required to convert these weights to volume to administer the appropriate dose of a medication to your patient.

Table 13-5 illustrates the metric units of weight and volume and their equivalents. Again, you must be able to understand these metric unit equivalents for proper drug conversion and subsequent administration.

To administer the appropriate dose of a medication to a patient, you must be able to convert larger units of volume to smaller ones (for example, liters to milliliters) and larger units of weight to smaller ones (for example, grams to milligrams). Conversely, you must also be able to convert smaller units of volume to larger ones (for example, milliliters to liters) and smaller units of weight to larger ones (for example, milligrams to grams).

Medications are packaged in different units of volume and weight; however, the volume (for example, milliliters) and weight (for example, micrograms, milligrams, grams) of the medication to be administered is usually only a fraction of the total amount of its packaged form. For example, a physician may order 50 mg of a medication for a patient, but the medication is packaged in grams. Therefore, you must be able to convert grams to milligrams and then determine how much volume is required to achieve the desired dose. (**Desired dose** refers to the amount of a medication that the physician orders, or protocol dictates, you to give to a patient.)

Volume Conversion. In the prehospital setting, you will usually be dealing with only two measurements of volume: milliliters and liters. Because 1 L equals 1,000 mL, simply divide or multiply by 1,000 or move the decimal point three places to the left or right.

When you are converting milliliters to liters, divide the smaller unit of volume by 1,000 *or* simply move the decimal point three places to the left, as demonstrated in the following examples:

Example 1:
Converting 100 mL to L (100 mL = X L)

100 mL ÷ 1,000 = 0.1 L *or* 100. = 0.1 L
←

Example 2:
Converting 250 mL to L (250 mL = X L)

250 mL ÷ 1,000 = 0.25 L *or* 250. = 0.25 L
←

Conversely, when you are converting liters to milliliters, multiply the amount in liters by 1,000 *or* simply move the decimal point three places to the right, as demonstrated in the following examples:

Example 1:
Converting 1.5 L to mL (1.5 L = X mL)

1.5 L × 1,000 = 1,500 mL *or* 1.500 = 1,500 mL
→

Example 2:
Converting 25 L to mL (25 L = X mL)

25 L × 1,000 = 25,000 mL *or* 25.000 = 25,000 mL
→

Weight Conversion. You will likely only need to convert weight when assisting a paramedic with administering a medication to a pediatric patient. Converting weight from g to mg is simply a matter of multiplying or dividing by 1,000 or moving the decimal point three places to the right or left. To convert g to mg, multiply the larger unit of weight by 1,000 *or* simply move the decimal point three places to the right, as demonstrated in the following examples:

Example 1:
Converting 2 g to mg (2 g = X mg)

2 g × 1,000 = 2,000 mg *or* 2.000 = 2,000 mg
→

Example 2:
Converting 5 mg to mcg (5 mg = X mcg)

5 mg × 1,000 = 5,000 mcg *or* 5.000 = 5,000 mcg
→

Conversely, to convert a smaller unit to a larger unit when the difference is 1,000 (such as milligrams to grams or micrograms to milligrams), divide the mg by 1,000 *or* simply move the decimal point three places

Words of Wisdom

When you are converting units of volume, remember these basic rules:

Volume conversion

Smaller to larger (for example, mL to L): Divide the smaller unit by 1,000 or move the decimal point three places to the left.
Larger to smaller (for example, L to mL): Multiply the larger unit by 1,000 or move the decimal point three places to the right.

to the left, as demonstrated in the following examples. Remember that 1 g equals 1,000 mg and 1 mg equals 1,000 mcg.

Example 1:
Converting 200 mcg to mg (200 mcg = X mg)

200 mcg ÷ 1,000 = 0.2 mg *or* 200. = 0.2 mg

Example 2:
Converting 250 mg to g (250 mg = X g)

250 mg ÷ 1,000 = 0.25 g *or* 250. = 0.25 g

Converting Pounds to Kilograms. It would be a luxury if your patients were able to tell you how much they weighed in kilograms (kg); however, the chances of this happening are slim to none. For patients who do not know their weight in pounds or who are unresponsive and unable to provide you with this information, you must do the following:

1. Estimate the patient's weight in pounds (lb)
2. Convert pounds to kilograms (kg)

Although many of the medications given in emergency medicine are administered in a standard dose (for example, 1 mg of epinephrine), other paramedic-level medications are administered based on the patient's weight in kilograms (for example, 1 to 1.5 mg/kg of lidocaine). In addition, most medications administered to pediatric patients are based on their weight in kilograms.

There are two formulas that can be used to convert pounds to kilograms; use the one that is easiest for you to remember.

Formula 1:

Divide the patient's weight in pounds by 2.2
(1 kg = 2.2 lb)

For example, when converting a 170-lb man's weight to kilograms, the formula would be as follows:

170 lb ÷ 2.2 = 77.27 kg

Because the value following the decimal point in the preceding example is less than 0.5, you may round the patient's weight in kg to 77.0. If the value after the decimal point had been greater than 0.5, you would round the weight in kg to 78.0. Although this may seem negligible, it is important to administer the most appropriate amount of the medication to the patient; it's good practice.

Formula 2:

Divide the patient's weight in pounds by 2
and subtract 10%

For example, when converting a 120-lb woman's weight to kg, the formula would be as follows:

Step 1: 120 lb ÷ 2 = 60 lb

Step 2: 60 lb × 10% = 6

Step 3: 60 − 6 = 54 kg

Calculating Drip Rates

As an AEMT, you will sometimes administer IV fluid, such as normal saline, lactated Ringer, or D_5W. IV fluid hydrates the patient and may treat shock, but it does not include medication. When you administer IV fluid, you will need to calculate the drip rate.

One of the easiest ways to calculate drip rates is to use dimensional analysis. Dimensional analysis uses the same simple conversions as equations, and you will not need to memorize the equation! Dimensional analysis allows you to compare seemingly unrelated items by setting up a relationship (that is, a comparison between two items).

An example of a relationship could be a car and the wheels on a car. Every car rides on four wheels, so there are four wheels for every car.

$$\frac{\text{1 car}}{\text{4 wheels}} = \frac{\text{4 wheels}}{\text{1 car}}$$

Another way to look at these comparisons is as a ratio, which is by nature a relationship. Dimensional analysis uses ratios as conversion factors.

To calculate a drip rate, you need to know:

- Which administration set to use
- Length of time for the infusion
- Amount to flow

You may need the conversion factor of 1 hour equals 60 minutes.

Example:

- Order given is for 250 mL normal saline over 90 minutes.
- Administration set 5 macrodrip (10 gtt/mL).

Determine how many drops per minute should be given.

Set up the equation:

$$\frac{?\text{ gtt}}{\text{min}} = \frac{10\text{ gtt}}{1\text{ mL}} \times \frac{250\text{ mL}}{90\text{ min}}$$

Cancel out what you can and reduce the fractions:

$$\frac{?\text{ gtt}}{\text{min}} = \frac{1\cancel{0}\text{ gtt}}{1\ \cancel{\text{mL}}} \times \frac{250\ \cancel{\text{mL}}}{9\cancel{0}\text{ min}}$$

Multiply and divide:

$$= \frac{250\text{ gtt}}{9\text{ min}} = \frac{27.77\text{ gtt}}{\text{mL}} = 28\text{ gtt}$$

You will need to set the drip rate at 28 gtt/min normal saline to achieve the desired order.

> **Words of Wisdom**
>
> The volume in milliliters (mL) is the "doctor's order." The drip set is always drops per mL, and the time is always in minutes. Multiply the doctor's order (in mL) times the drip set (in drops/mL) and divide by the time (in minutes). This yields the number of drops per minute.

Another useful formula to remember is a simple drip rate calculation that gives you the number of drops per minute:

$$\frac{(\text{volume in mL}) \times (\text{drip set})}{(\text{time in minutes})} = \frac{\text{gtt}}{\text{min}}$$

> **Words of Wisdom**
>
> TKO means "to keep open." This is an abbreviation for a rate equal to about 8 to 15 drops/min that is used to allow just enough fluid through the IV line to keep blood from clotting at the end of the catheter.

Calculating Medication Doses

When you administer a medication, you will need to calculate the dose. There are multiple formulas for calculating medication doses. It is beyond the scope of this chapter to demonstrate every one of these calculation formulas. Therefore, the discussion in this chapter is limited to formulas that most students find easy to understand. For other calculation formulas, consult with your instructor. The method of drug dose calculation demonstrated in this chapter is based on the following three factors:

1. Desired dose
2. Concentration of the medication available (dose on hand)
3. Volume to be administered

Desired Dose

The desired dose (that is, the drug order) is the amount of a medication that the physician orders you to administer to a patient. It may be expressed as a standard dose (for example, 25 g of dextrose), or it may be expressed as a specific number of grams or milligrams per kilogram of body weight (for example, 0.1 mg/kg is the pediatric dose for naloxone).

Medication Concentration

After receiving a drug order (that is, the desired dose), you must determine how much of the medication that you have available. In other words, you must know its *concentration*—the total weight (micrograms, milligrams, or grams) of the medication contained in a specific volume (mL or L). An example of a common prepackaged drug concentration is 50% dextrose, 25 g/50 mL.

Note that medications are contained in different volumes of solution. This is your **volume on hand**. *To administer a medication, you must know the weight of the medication that is present in 1 mL.* This will tell you the concentration of the medication that you have on hand. The formula for calculating this is as follows:

$$\text{Total weight of the medication} \div \text{Total volume in milliliters} = \text{Weight per milliliter}$$

By using this formula and the examples of common prepackaged medications, you will calculate how much of the medication is contained in each milliliter (dose on hand). For example, if the drug order is for dextrose, 25 g/50 mL, you would calculate the concentration as follows:

$$25\text{ g (total weight)} \div 50\text{ mL (total volume)} = 0.5\text{ g/mL}$$

Volume to Be Administered

After you have determined the concentration of the medication present in each milliliter (dose on hand), you must calculate how much volume is needed to give the amount of the medication ordered (desired dose). Use the following formula to calculate the volume to be administered:

Desired dose (mg) ÷ Concentration on hand (mg/mL) = Volume to be administered (mL)

Notice that the desired dose is in milligrams and the concentration on hand is in milligrams per milliliter. There may be instances where the desired dose is in a different unit, such as grams or micrograms. Before using the above formula, the units in the desired dose must match the units in the top of the concentration-on-hand fraction. If they do not, you will need to do a quick calculation to convert the desired dose units to match the units in the top half of the concentration on hand.

On the basis of the preceding formula, you will be able to determine how much volume to give to achieve the required dose. Here is an example:

Example 1:
You are ordered to administer 12.5 g of dextrose to a hypoglycemic patient. You have a prefilled syringe containing 25 g of D_{50} in 50 mL. How many milliliters of dextrose will you give?

Step 1: Determine the concentration/dose on hand (in g/mL).

25 g ÷ 50 mL = 0.5 g/mL (dose on hand)

Step 2: Determine how much volume to administer.

12.5 g (desired dose) ÷ 0.5 g/mL (dose on hand) = 25 mL

You will need to administer 25 mL, or half of the 50-mL syringe.

Example 2:
You are ordered to administer 70 mg of medication "Y" to a patient. The medication is prepared as follows: 100 mg in 5 mL of saline. How many milliliters must you give to achieve the ordered dose?

Step 1: Determine the concentration/dose on hand (in mg/mL).

100 mg ÷ 5 mL = 20 mg/mL (dose on hand)

Step 2: Determine how much volume to administer.

70 mg (desired dose) ÷ 20 mg/mL (dose on hand) = 3.5 mL

You will need to administer 3.5 mL of the medication.

Weight-Based Medication Doses

As previously discussed, some medication doses are based on the patient's weight in kilograms. Determining the appropriate dose for the patient requires simply converting the patient's weight in pounds to kilograms and then proceeding with the formula that was just discussed. Remember, 1 kg equals 2.2 lb. As an AEMT, medications that you may administer and whose orders may be weight-based include pediatric dosages for dextrose, epinephrine, and naloxone.

The following are some examples of how to calculate the appropriate medication dose based on the patient's weight:

Example 1:
You are ordered to give 0.1 mg/kg of naloxone (Narcan) to your 40-lb pediatric patient. You have a prefilled syringe of the medication containing 100 mg in 10 mL. How many milligrams will you give to this patient? How much volume will you give to achieve the required dose?

Step 1: Convert the patient's weight in pounds to kilograms.

Formula 1: 40 lb ÷ 2.2 = 18.18 kg (round to 18 kg)

Formula 2: 40 lb ÷ 2 = 20 − 10% = 18 kg

Step 2: Determine the desired dose.

0.1 mg/kg × 18 kg = 1.8 mg (desired dose)

Step 3: Determine the concentration/dose on hand (in mg/mL).

100 mg ÷ 10 mL = 10 mg/mL (dose on hand)

Step 4: Determine how much volume to administer.

1.8 mg (desired dose) ÷ 10 mg/mL (dose on hand) = 0.18 mL (round to 0.2 mL)

Example 2:
A 4-year-old boy in asystole requires 0.01 mg/kg of epinephrine. You have a prefilled syringe of epinephrine containing 1 mg in 10 mL. The child's mother tells you that he weighs 35 lb. How many milligrams will you give to this patient (that is, what is the desired dose)? How much volume will you give to achieve the required dose?

Step 1: Convert the patient's weight in pounds to kilograms.

Formula 1: 35 lb ÷ 2.2 = 15.9 kg (round to 16 kg)

Formula 2: 35 lb ÷ 2 = 17.5 − 10% = 15.75 kg (round to 16 kg)

Step 2: Determine the desired dose.

0.01 mg × 16 kg = 0.16 mg/kg (desired dose)

Step 3: Determine the concentration/dose on hand (in mg/mL).

1 mg ÷ 10 mL = 0.1 mg/mL (dose on hand)

Step 4: Determine how much volume to administer.

0.16 mg (desired dose) ÷ 0.1 mg/mL (dose on hand) = 1.6 mL (round to 2 mL)

Special Populations

It is important to administer the most appropriate dose of a medication to a child. Many parents or caregivers know how much their children weigh in pounds, which you can easily convert to kilograms (1 kg = 2.2 lb). If a parent or caregiver is available, simply ask the child's weight; do not attempt to estimate the child's weight if it is not necessary.

▶ Pediatric Doses

There are several methods for determining the appropriate dose of medication for a pediatric patient. Many rescuers use length-based resuscitation tapes; others may carry a field guide with tables or charts for reference. Most medications used in pediatric emergency medicine are based on the child's weight in kilograms. The calculations for pediatric drug dosing and medication infusions are the same as they are for adults, but the doses and volumes will be obviously smaller.

Steps for Administering by Specific Routes

Up to this point, this chapter has covered principles of medication administration, basic cell physiology, IV therapy, and mathematical principles. This last section will discuss steps for administering medications by the specific routes. Steps for administering medications for system-specific emergencies are given in later chapters; such instances are noted.

▶ Administering Enteral Medications

Enteral medications are those that are given through some portion of the digestive or intestinal tract. This includes medications that are administered orally, through a feeding tube, or rectally.

Oral Administration

Forms of solid and liquid oral medications include capsules, timed-release capsules, lozenges, pills, tablets, elixirs, emulsions, suspensions, and syrups. Oral medications are used when the desired effect is systemic and the medications are taken up by the intestines. To give oral medications, you may use a small medicine cup, a medicine dropper, a teaspoon, an oral syringe, or a nipple. Gather the appropriate equipment for the form of medication you are administering. As with any medication, check for indications, contraindications, precautions, and the 10 rights before administering an oral medication. Medications administered by AEMTs using the oral route include aspirin and oral glucose.

Follow these steps when administering an oral medication Figure 13-42:

1. Take standard precautions.
2. Determine the need for the medication based on patient presentation.

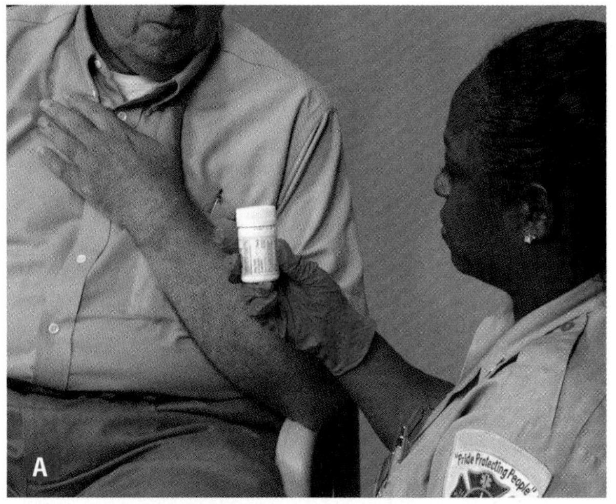

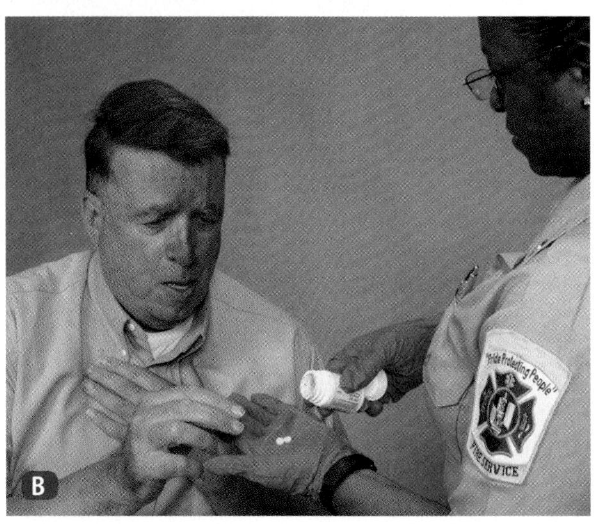

Figure 13-42 Administering an oral medication. **A.** Check the 10 rights of medication administration. **B.** Have the patient take the medication. Administer a cup of water if necessary.

3. Obtain a history, including any medication allergies.
4. Follow standing orders, or contact medical control for permission.
5. Check the medication to be sure it is the right medication and not cloudy or discolored and that its expiration date has not passed. Check the 10 rights of medication administration.
6. Determine the appropriate dose. If the medication is liquid, pour the desired amount into a calibrated cup.
7. Instruct the patient to swallow the medication with water, if administering a pill or tablet.
8. Monitor the patient's condition, and document the medication given, route, time of administration, and patient response.

Safety

Standard precautions should be used any time you are administering a medication.

Rectal Administration

Some AEMTs may be allowed to administer D_{50}, but whether rectal administration is allowed depends on local protocols. If it is allowed, administering D_{50} by this route is a last resort, when a patient is hypoglycemic and no other route is an option (IV access cannot be established). Check for indications, contraindications, and precautions before giving D_{50} rectally **Figure 13-43**.

Follow these steps to administer a medication rectally:

1. Take standard precautions.
2. Determine the need for the medication based on patient presentation.
3. Obtain a history, including any medication allergies.
4. Follow standing orders, or contact medical control for permission.
5. Determine the appropriate dose, and check that the medication is the right medication, there is no cloudiness or discoloration, and the expiration date has not passed.
6. When inserting a suppository, use a water-soluble gel for lubrication. Insert the suppository into the rectum approximately 1 to 1½ inches while instructing the patient to relax and not to bear down.
7. For medications that are in liquid form, some modifications are needed. You may use a nasopharyngeal airway, a small endotracheal (ET) tube, an 18-gauge IV catheter without a needle, or a commercial device as your delivery device.
   a. Lubricate the end of the nasal airway or ET tube with a water-soluble gel, and gently insert it approximately 1 to 1½ inches into the rectum. Instruct the patient to relax and not to bear down.
   b. With a *needleless* syringe, gently push the medication through the tube.
   c. After the medication has been delivered, remove and dispose of the tube or syringe in an appropriate container.
8. Monitor the patient's condition, and document the medication given, route, time of administration, and patient response.

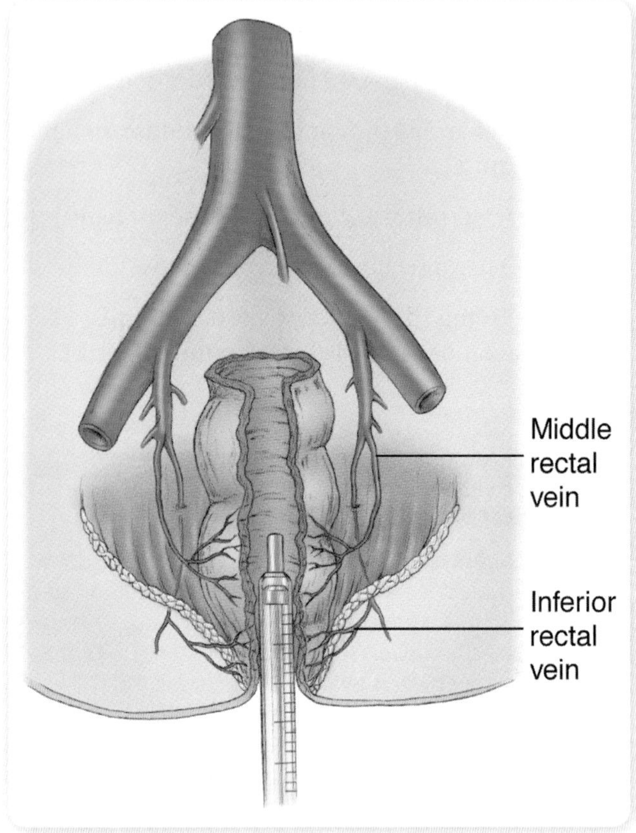

Figure 13-43 The rectal mucosa is highly vascular and rapidly absorbs medications.

▶ Administering Parenteral Medications

Parenteral medications are those that are given through any route other than the GI tract. Parenteral routes used by the AEMT include subcutaneous, IM, IV bolus, IO, sublingual, transcutaneous, transdermal, and inhalation. Of the parenteral medication routes, IV administration is the most common route used in the prehospital setting and generally is the quickest route for getting medication into the central circulation.

Equipment

A variety of needles and syringes are used for administering parenteral medications. Most syringes come prepackaged in color-coded packs with a needle already

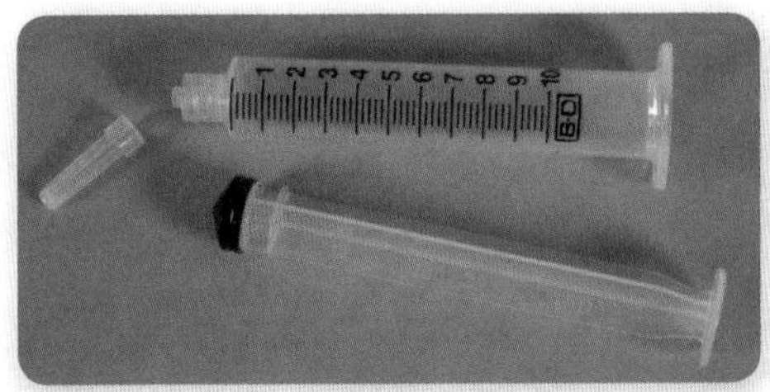

Figure 13-44 A syringe consists of a plunger, body or barrel, flange, and tip.

attached. The needles and syringes may also be packaged separately. You must choose the appropriate-size syringe and appropriate needle length for the desired route. Syringes consist of a plunger, body or barrel, flange, and tip **Figure 13-44**. Most syringes are marked with 10 calibrations per milliliter on one side of the barrel, where each small line represents 0.1 mL. The 3-mL syringe is the most commonly used for injections, but others are available as needed. Needle lengths vary from 3/8 inch to 2 inches for standard injections.

Packaging

Parenteral medications are most commonly packaged in ampules, vials, and prefilled syringes. **Ampules** are breakable sterile glass containers that are designed to carry a single dose of medication **Figure 13-45**. **Vials** may contain single or multiple doses **Figure 13-46**. Vials have a rubber-stopper top and are made of glass or plastic. Many medications used in prehospital care are carried in vials.

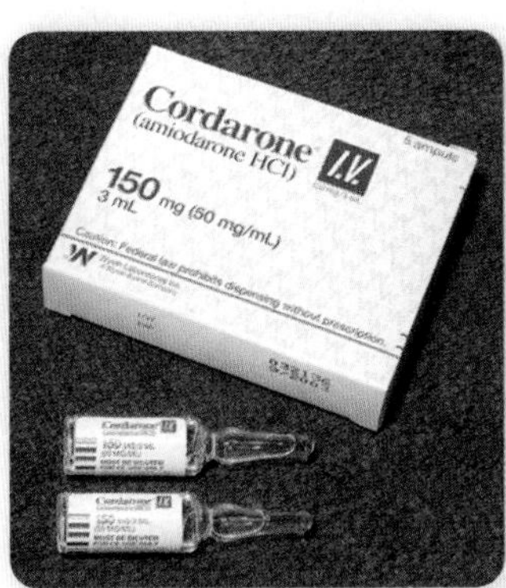

Figure 13-45 Medication stored in ampules.

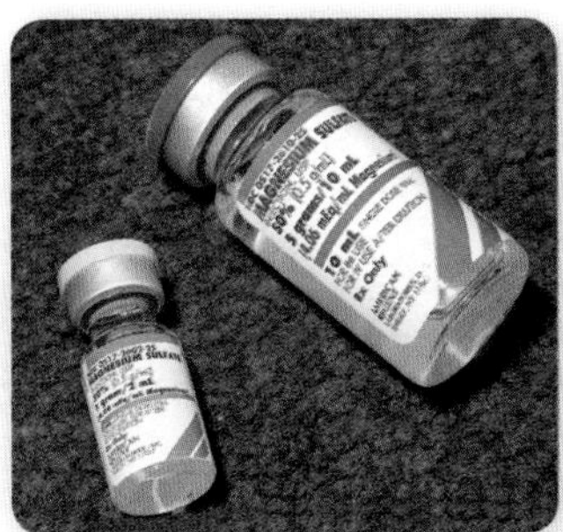

Figure 13-46 Vials (single-dose and multidose).

Prefilled syringes are designed for ease of use. It is much easier and quicker to use a prefilled syringe when you are treating a patient in cardiac arrest than it is to draw up each individual dose. There are also single-dose disposable cartridges that use a reusable syringe such as a Tubex or Abboject **Figure 13-47**. Some medications may need to be reconstituted, such as methylprednisolone sodium succinate (Solu-Medrol) and glucagon. These come with two vials, one with a powdered form of the medication and one with sterile water. **Drug reconstitution** involves injecting the sterile water from one vial into the vial that contains the powder, making a solution for injection. Glucagon is an example of a medication that must be reconstituted before administration.

Ampules. Naloxone (Narcan) is an example of a medication that comes in the form of an ampule. When drawing a medication from an ampule, follow the steps in **Skill Drill 13-4**.

> **Safety**
>
> Anytime you are using a needle to draw up medication or to inject blood into blood tubes, always hold the syringe against your palm with the needle pointing up and draw the vial or blood tube down onto the needle using the thumb and forefinger of the palm the syringe is braced against to avoid sticking yourself. This especially applies if you are in a moving ambulance.

Vials. Epinephrine and naloxone (Narcan) are two examples of medications that may come in vials. When you are administering a vial of medication, you must first determine how much of the medication you will need and how many doses are in the vial.

When drawing medication from a vial, follow the steps in **Skill Drill 13-5**.

For a single-dose vial, you will draw up the entire amount in the vial. For multiple-dose vials, you should draw out only the amount needed. Remember that after you remove the cover from a vial, it is no longer sterile. If you need a second dose, the top of the vial should be cleaned with alcohol before withdrawing the medication.

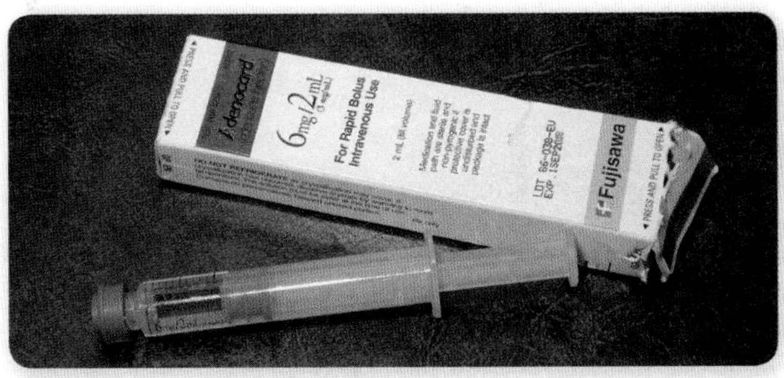

Figure 13-47 A preassembled prefilled syringe.

Skill Drill 13-4 Drawing Medication From an Ampule

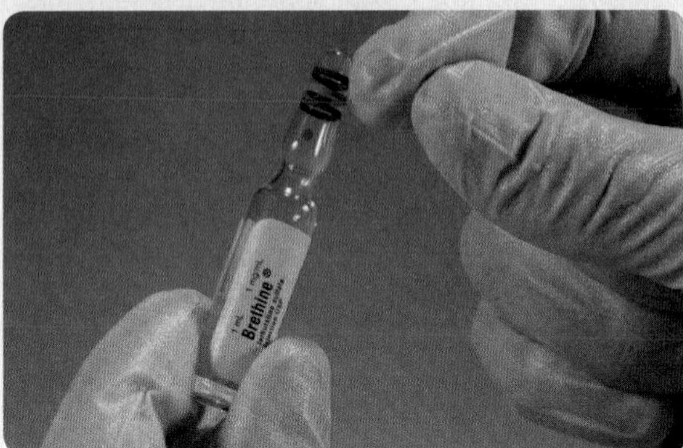

Step 1 Check the medication to be sure that the expiration date has not passed and that it is the correct medication and concentration.

Shake the medication down into the base of the ampule. If some of the medication appears to be stuck in the neck, gently thump or tap the stem.

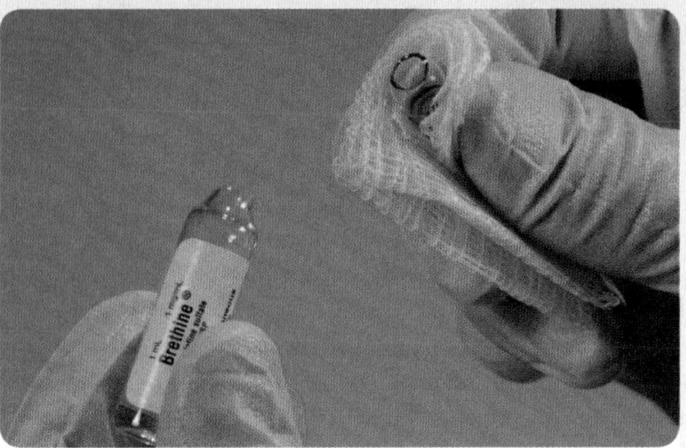

Step 2 Using a 4- × 4-inch (10- × 10-cm) gauze pad or an alcohol prep, grip the neck of the ampule and snap it off where the ampule is scored. If the ampule is not scored and an attempt is made to break it, some sharp edges may be present. Drop the stem in the sharps container.

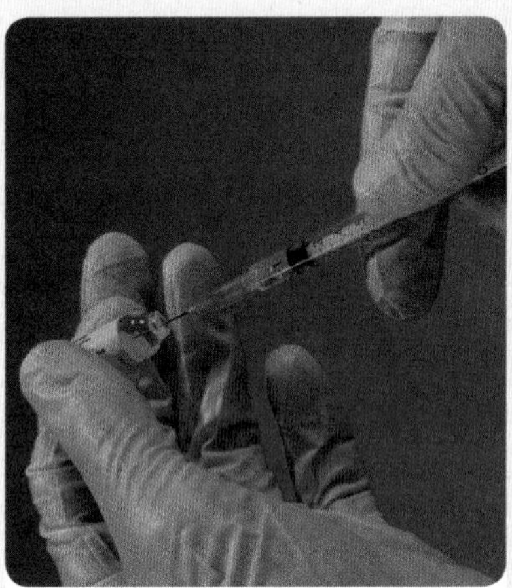

Step 3 Insert a filtered needle into the ampule without touching the outer sides of the ampule. Draw the solution into the syringe, and dispose of the ampule in the sharps container.

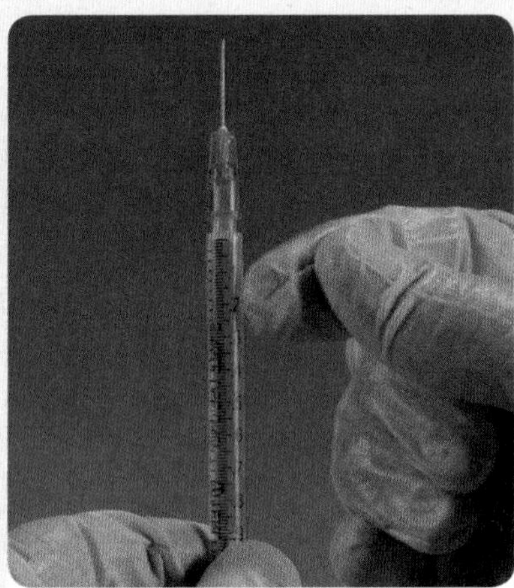

Step 4 Hold the syringe with the needle pointing up, and gently tap the barrel to loosen air trapped inside and cause it to rise.

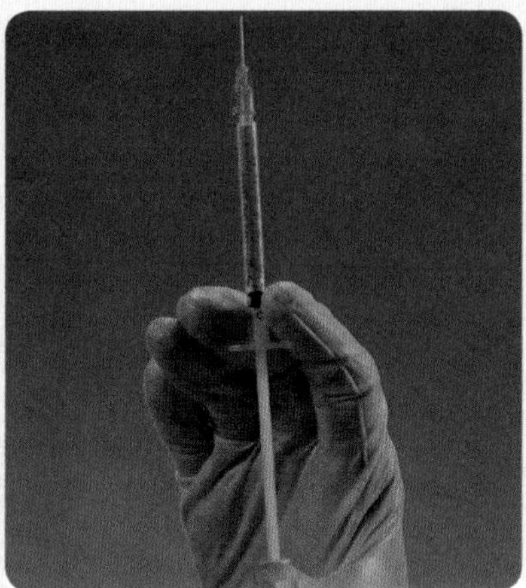

Step 5 Press gently on the plunger to dispel any air bubbles. Recap the needle using the one-handed method to avoid contamination. Dispose of the needle in the sharps container and attach a standard hypodermic needle to the syringe if necessary to administer the medication.

Skill Drill 13-5 Drawing Medication From a Vial

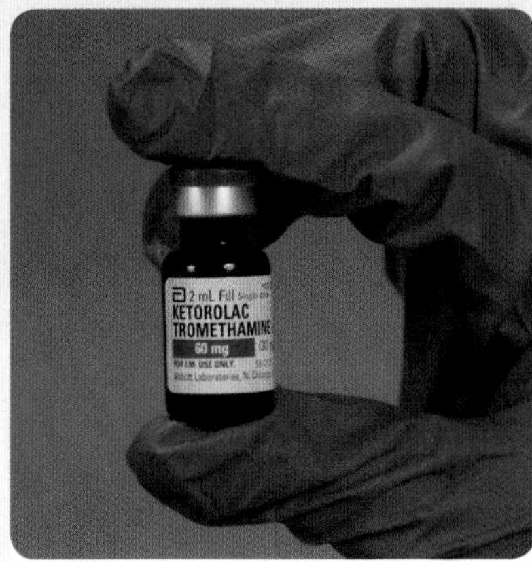

Step 1 Check the medication to be sure that the expiration date has not passed, and that it is the correct medication and concentration. Check that it is not discolored.

Remove the sterile cover, or clean the top with alcohol if it was previously opened.

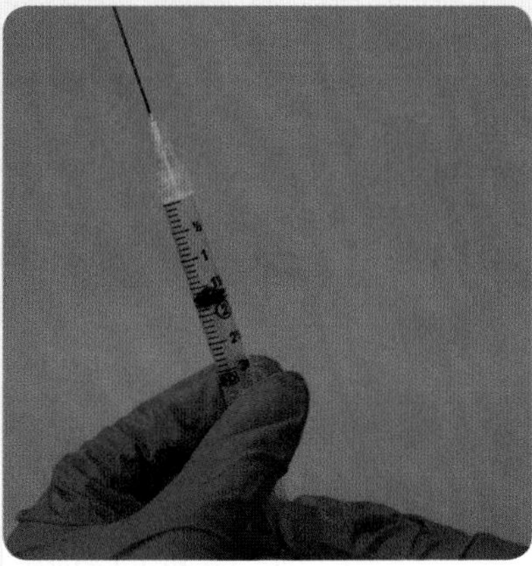

Step 2 Determine the amount of medication that you will need, and draw that amount of air into the syringe. Allow a little extra room to expel some air while removing air bubbles.

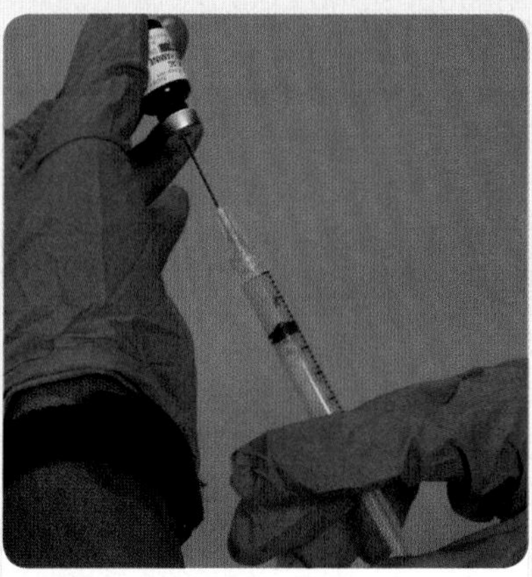

Step 3 Invert the vial, clean the rubber stopper with an alcohol prep, and insert the needle through the rubber stopper into the medication. Expel the air in the syringe into the vial and then withdraw the amount of medication needed.

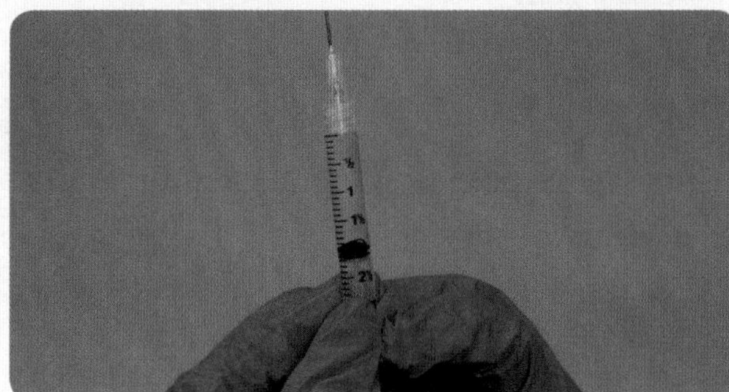

Step 4 After you have the correct amount of medication in the syringe, withdraw the needle and expel any air in the syringe.

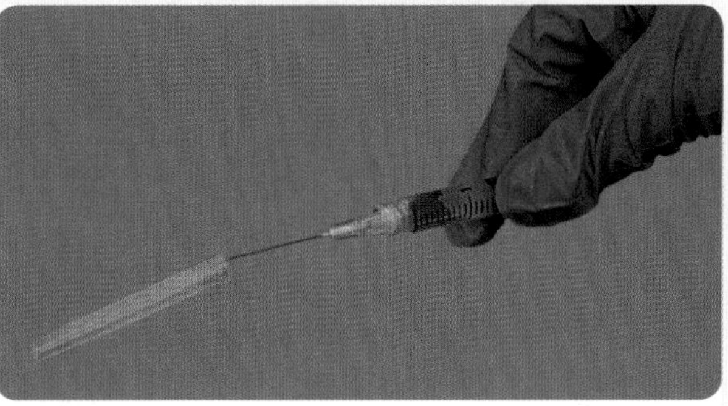

Step 5 Recap the needle using the one-handed method and avoiding contamination. Label the syringe if it is not immediately given to the patient.

Some medications that are stored in vials need to be reconstituted; these may come in two separate vials or in a single vial divided into two compartments by a rubber stopper. An example of the latter is an Act-o-Vial Figure 13-48. To reconstitute a medication contained in an Act-o-Vial, squeeze the two vials together, which releases the center stopper and allows the contents to mix. Shake vigorously to mix the contents before drawing out the medication.

To mix the contents of two separate vials, draw the fluid out of the first vial as described. Insert the syringe into the top of the second vial, and expel all fluid into it. Shake vigorously to mix. After the medication is reconstituted, regardless of the manner, draw up the medication as described for single- and multiple-dose vials.

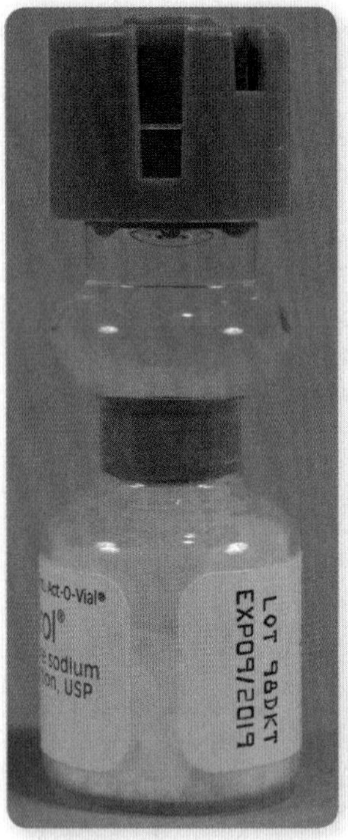

Figure 13-48 An Act-o-Vial.

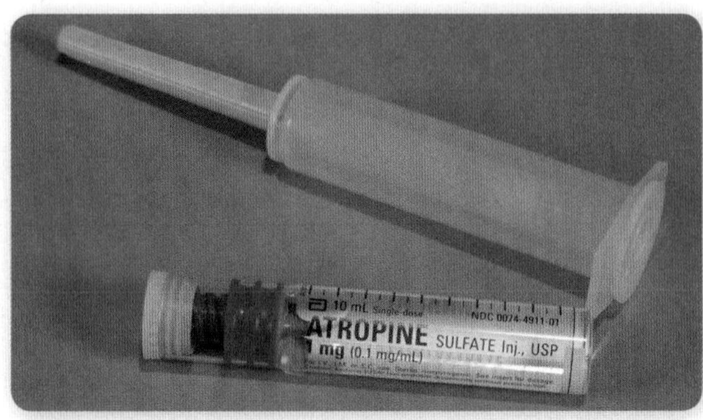

Figure 13-49 Prefilled syringes come in two parts, the glass medication cartridge and a syringe.

Prefilled Syringe. Prefilled syringes come in tamper-proof boxes and are separated into the glass medication cartridge and a syringe Figure 13-49. $D_{50}W$ is an example of a medication that comes as a prefilled syringe.

To assemble the two-part prefilled syringe, pop the yellow caps off of the syringe and the medication cartridge, insert the drug cartridge into the barrel of the syringe, and screw them together. Remove the needle cover, and expel air in the manner previously described. Follow the steps for the route the medication is to be given.

Subcutaneous Administration

Subcutaneous injections are given into the loose connective tissue between the dermis and the muscle layer Figure 13-50. Volumes of a medication administered subcutaneously are usually 1 mL or less. The injection is performed using a 24- to 26-gauge ½-inch to 1-inch needle. Common sites include the upper part of the arms, anterior part of the thighs, and the abdomen Figure 13-51. Patients who take insulin injections usually vary the sites owing to the multiple number of injections they require (usually daily). An example of an AEMT medication that is administered subcutaneously is epinephrine.

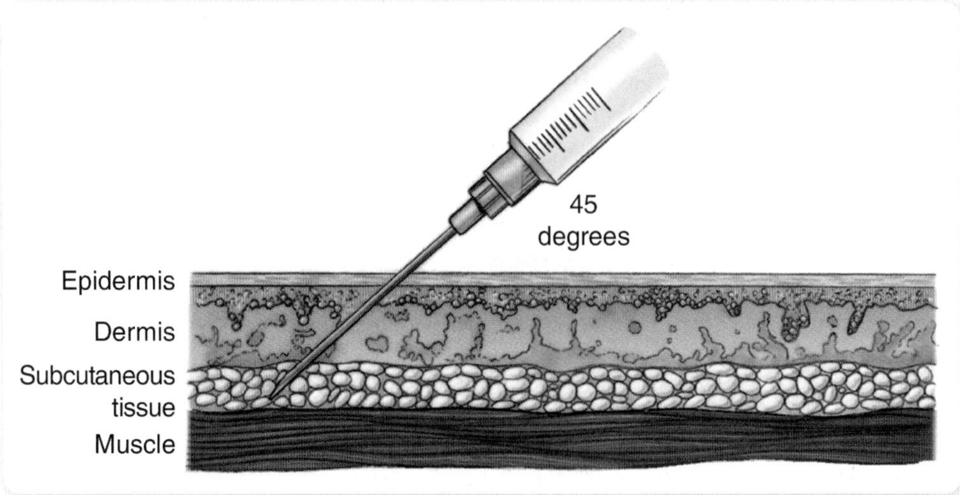

Figure 13-50 A subcutaneous injection is below the dermis and above the muscle.

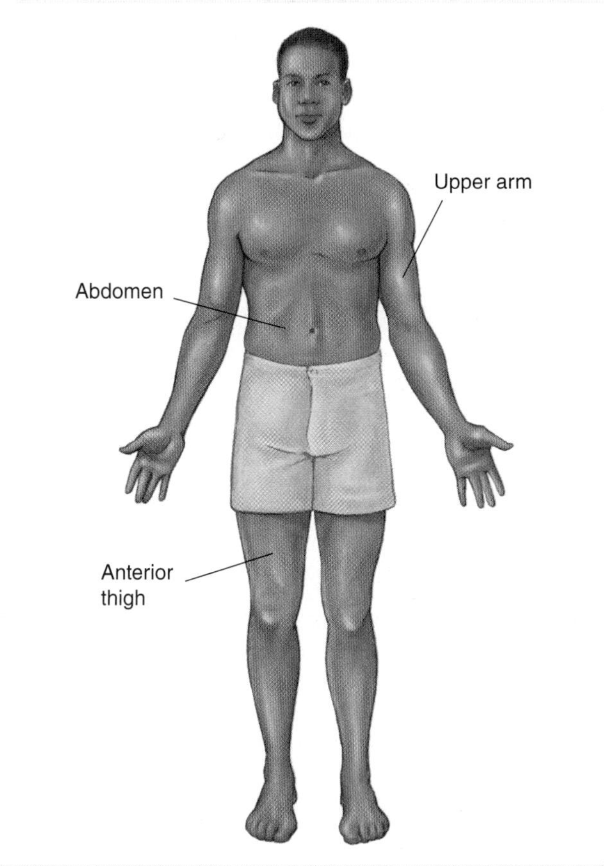

Figure 13-51 Common sites for subcutaneous injections.

When you are preparing to administer fluid or medication, you will need to use aseptic technique, also called medical asepsis. This is a method of cleansing used to prevent contamination of a site when performing an invasive procedure such as starting an IV line or administering a medication. Aseptic technique may be accomplished via the sterilization of equipment used, antiseptics, or disinfectants.

Follow the steps in Skill Drill 13-6 to administer a medication via the subcutaneous route.

Intramuscular Administration

Intramuscular (IM) injections are made by penetrating a needle through the dermis and subcutaneous tissue into the muscle layer Figure 13-52. This allows administration of a larger volume of medication (up to 5 mL) than the subcutaneous route. Because there is also the potential for damage to nerves because of the depth of the injection, it is important to choose the appropriate site. Common anatomic sites for IM injections for adults and children include the following:

- **Deltoid muscle**—the muscle of the upper part of the arm that covers the prominence of the shoulder. The site for injection is approximately 1½ to 2 inches below the acromion process on the lateral side Figure 13-53.
- **Vastus lateralis muscle**—the large muscle on the lateral side of the thigh

Skill Drill 13-6 Administering Medication via the Subcutaneous Route

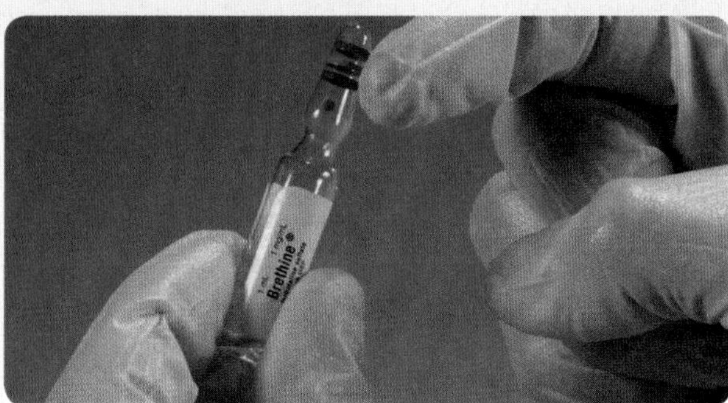

Step 1 Take standard precautions. Determine the need for the medication based on patient presentation. Obtain a history, including any medication allergies and vital signs. Follow standing orders, or contact medical control for permission. Check the medication to be sure that it is not cloudy, that the expiration date has not passed, and that it is the correct medication and concentration, and determine the appropriate dose.

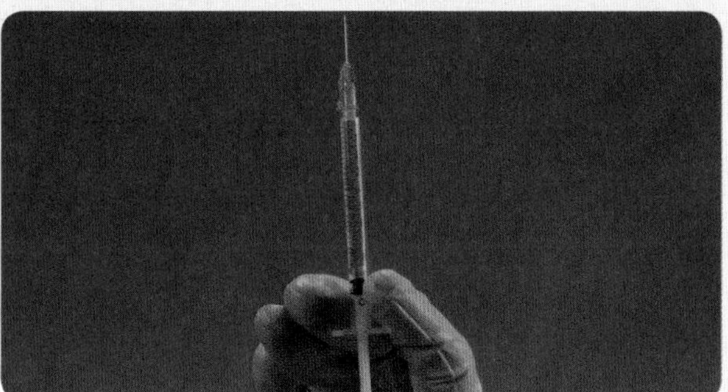

Step 2 Advise the patient of potential discomfort while explaining the procedure.

Assemble and check the equipment needed: alcohol preps and a 3-mL syringe with a 24- to 26-gauge needle. Draw up the correct dose of medication.

(continued)

Skill Drill 13-6 Administering Medication via the Subcutaneous Route *(continued)*

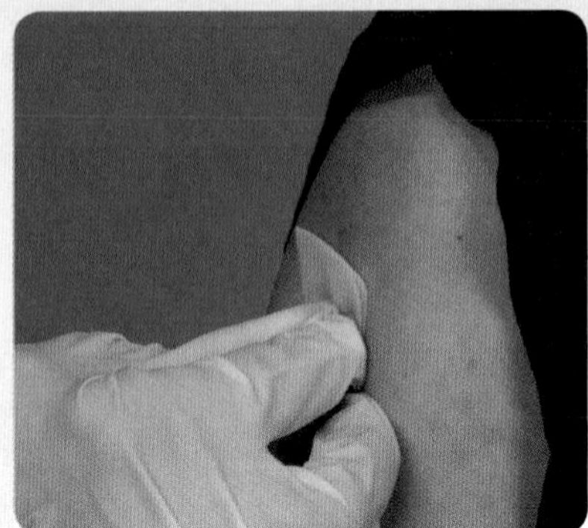

Step 3 Cleanse the area for the administration (usually the upper part of the arm or thigh) using aseptic technique.

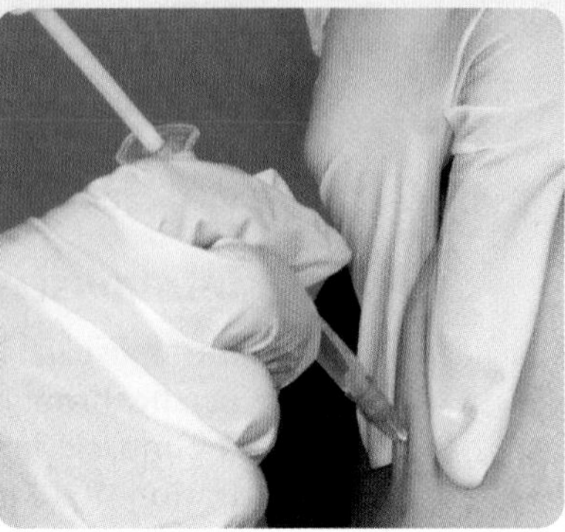

Step 4 Pinch the skin surrounding the area, advise the patient of a stick, and insert the needle at a 45° angle.

Pull back on the plunger to aspirate for blood. The presence of blood in the syringe indicates you may have entered a vein. Remove the needle, and hold pressure over the site. Discard the syringe and needle in the sharps container. Prepare a new syringe and needle and select another site.

If there is no blood in the syringe, inject the medication and remove the needle. Immediately place it in the sharps container.

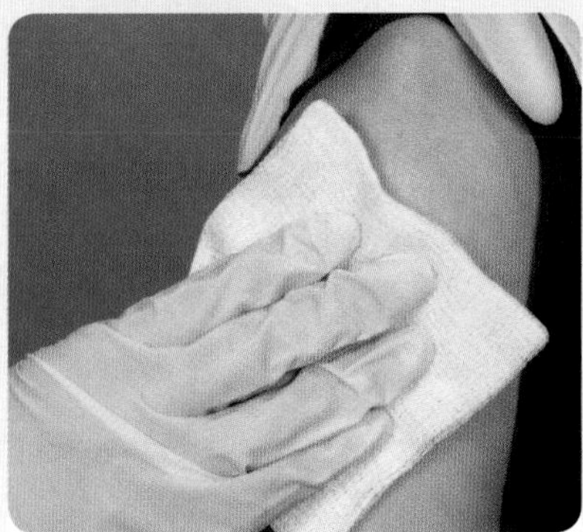

Step 5 To disperse the medication through the tissue, rub the area in a circular motion with your gloved hand. Properly store any unused medication. Monitor the patient's condition, and document the medication given, route, administration time, and patient response.

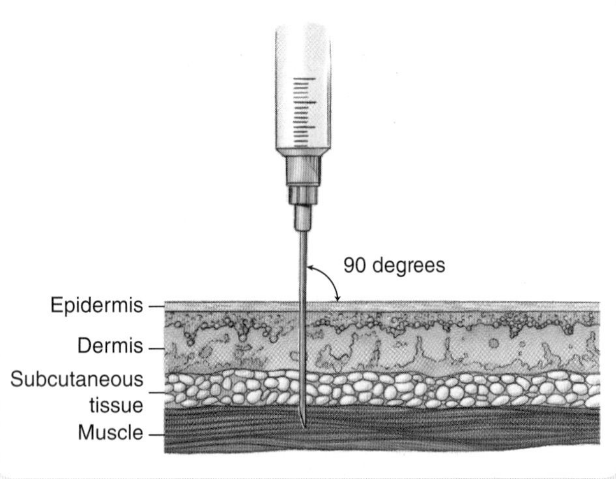

Figure 13-52 An intramuscular injection is below the dermis and subcutaneous layer and into the muscle.

- **Rectus femoris muscle**—the large muscle on the anterior side of the thigh
- **Gluteal area**—the buttocks, specifically the upper lateral aspect of either side

AEMT medications that may be administered intramuscularly include epinephrine and glucagon. Follow the steps in Skill Drill 13-7 to administer an IM injection.

Words of Wisdom

When administering an IM medication, rub the area in a circular motion with your gloved hand to disperse the medication through the tissue.

Patients may also have their own auto-injector for certain medications such as epinephrine for anaphylactic

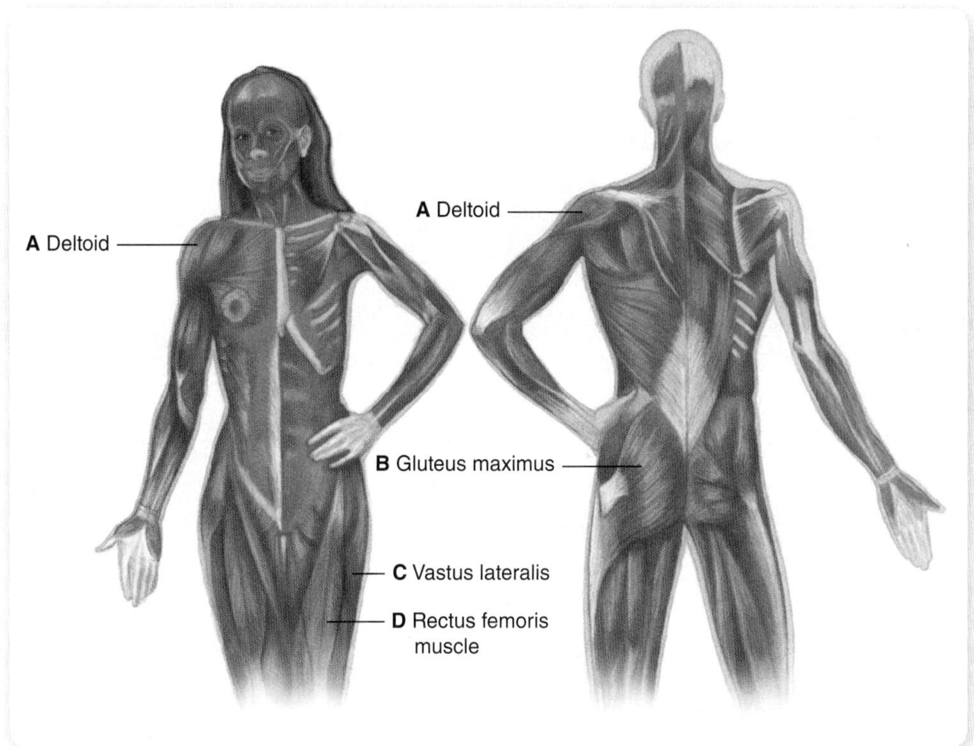

Figure 13-53 Common sites for intramuscular injections. **A.** Deltoid muscles. **B.** Gluteal area. **C.** Vastus lateralis muscle. **D.** Rectus femoris muscle.

Skill Drill 13-7 Administering Medication via the Intramuscular Route

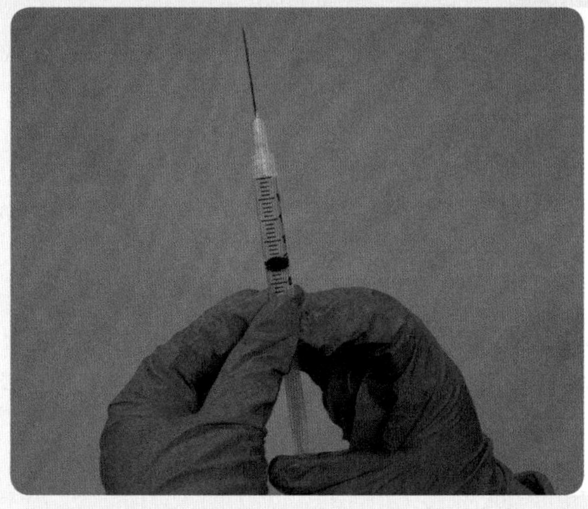

Step 1 Take standard precautions. Determine the need for the medication based on patient presentation. Obtain a history, including any medication allergies and vital signs. Follow standing orders, or contact medical control for permission.

Check the medication to be sure it is the correct one, that it is not discolored, and that the expiration date has not passed, and determine the appropriate dose.

Advise the patient of potential discomfort while explaining the procedure.

Assemble and check equipment needed: alcohol preps and a 3- to 5-mL syringe with a 21-gauge, 1-inch or 2-inch (4-cm or 5-cm) needle. Draw up the correct dose of medication and dispel air while maintaining sterility.

(continued)

Skill Drill 13-7 Administering Medication via the Intramuscular Route *(continued)*

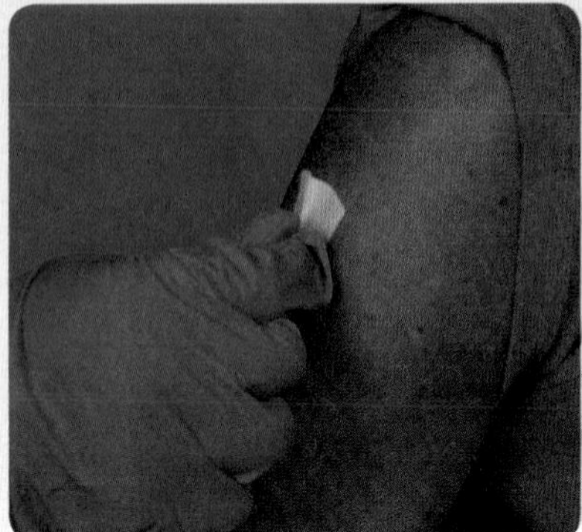

Step 2 Cleanse the area for the administration (usually the upper arm or the hip) using aseptic technique.

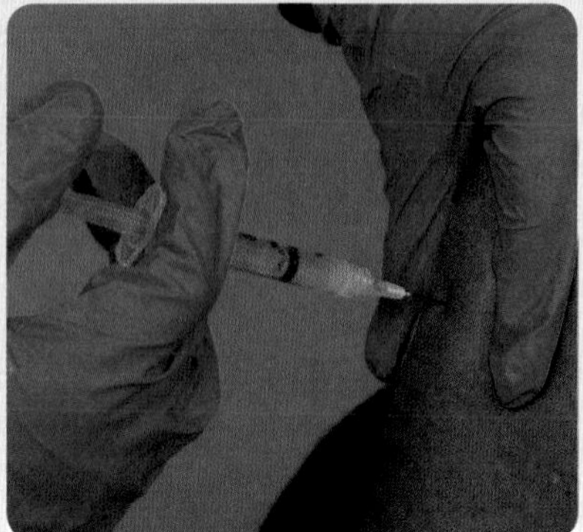

Step 3 Stretch the skin over the cleansed area, advise the patient of a stick, and insert the needle at a 90° angle.
Pull back on the plunger to aspirate for blood. The presence of blood in the syringe indicates you may have entered a blood vessel. Remove the needle, and hold pressure over the site. Discard the syringe and needle in the sharps container. Prepare a new syringe and needle, and select another site.

If there is no blood in the syringe, inject the medication and remove the needle.

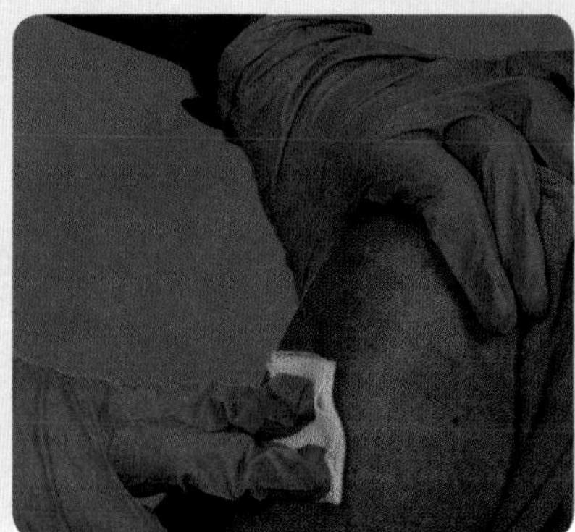

Step 4 Cover the puncture site. Immediately dispose of the needle and syringe in the sharps container. Store any unused medication properly. Monitor the patient's condition, and document the medication given, route, administration time, and patient response.

reactions. Steps for administering specific injector devices are detailed in Chapter 22, *Immunologic Emergencies*.

Sublingual Administration

Sublingual and **buccal** medications enter the circulatory system much faster than those that travel through the enteral route. There is a vast network of vessels under the tongue (sublingual) and in the cheek (buccal). For a sublingual or buccal medication to work effectively, mucous membranes must be moist to allow the medication to dissolve. Medications given via the sublingual or buccal route may also be taken up in the proximal part of the GI tract without reaching the intestines.

Medications given by the sublingual route come in tablet, liquid, and spray forms. Nitroglycerin is a medication that is commonly given via the sublingual route, and it comes in tablet and spray forms. To administer a sublingual medication, follow the steps in Skill Drill 13-8.

Oral glucose is an example of an AEMT medication administered via the buccal route. The technique for administering oral glucose is shown in Chapter 21, *Endocrine and Hematologic Emergencies*.

Words of Wisdom

When you are administering or assisting with sublingual medications, have the patient rinse his or her mouth with a little water to help the medication dissolve if the mucous membranes are dry.

Intranasal Administration

Intranasal (within the nose) medications include nasal spray for congestion or solutions to moisten the nasal mucosa. In recent years, this route of medication administration has become increasingly more popular in the prehospital

Skill Drill 13-8 Administering Medication via the Sublingual Route

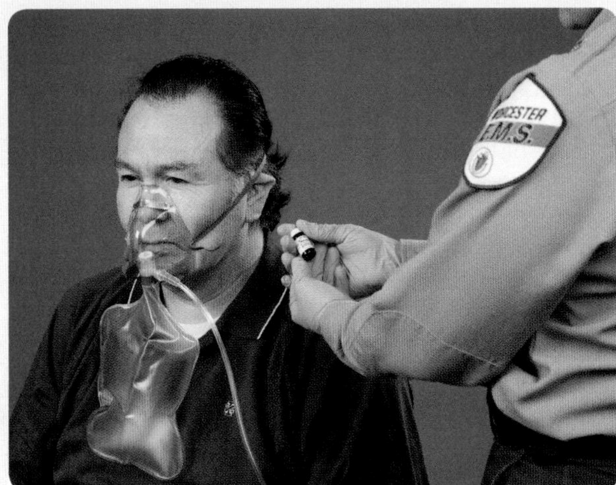

Step 1 Take standard precautions. Determine the need for the medication based on patient presentation. Obtain a history, including any medication allergies and vital signs. Follow standing orders, or contact medical control for permission. Check the medication to make sure that it is the correct one and that its expiration date has not passed, and determine the appropriate dose.

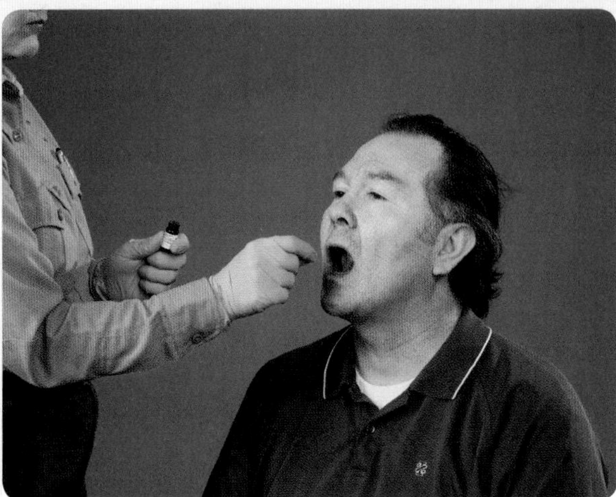

Step 2 Ask the patient to rinse his or her mouth with a little water if the mucous membranes are dry. Explain the procedure, and ask the patient to lift his or her tongue.

Place the tablet or spray the dose under the tongue, or ask the patient to do so. Advise the patient not to chew or swallow the tablet, but to let it dissolve slowly.

Monitor the patient's condition, and document the medication given, route, administration time, and patient response.

setting. Intranasally administered medications are rapidly absorbed, providing a more rapid onset of action than IM injections. Administration of emergency medications via the intranasal route is performed with a **mucosal atomizer device** Figure 13-54. The device attaches to a syringe and allows you to spray (atomize) select medications into the nasal mucosa.

Only a few emergency medications can be given intranasally, including naloxone (Narcan). Follow local protocol, or consult with medical control about the appropriate doses of these medications and any other medications that may be administered intranasally.

To administer a medication via the intranasal route, follow the steps in Skill Drill 13-9.

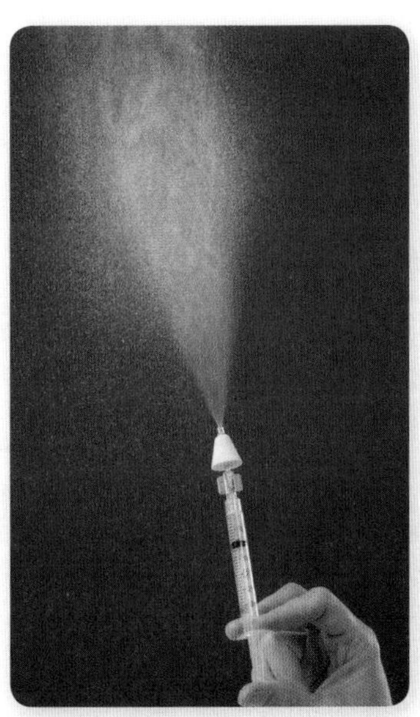

Figure 13-54 Mucosal atomizer device.

Courtesy of LMA North America.

Medications Administered by the Inhalation Route

Many medications used in the treatment of respiratory emergencies are administered via the **inhalation** route. The most common inhaled medication is oxygen. Beta-2

Skill Drill 13-9 Administering Medication via the Intranasal Route

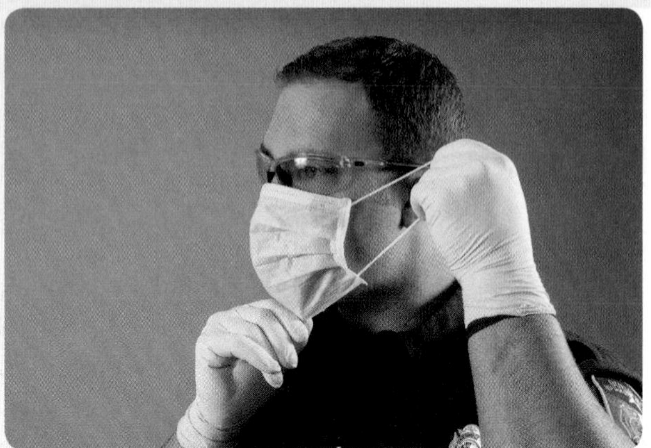

Step 1 Take standard precautions. Determine the need for the medication based on patient presentation. Obtain a history, including any medication allergies and vital signs. Assemble and collect the needed equipment, including the mucosal atomizer device. Follow standing orders, or contact medical control for permission. Check the 10 rights of medication administration out loud with your partner.

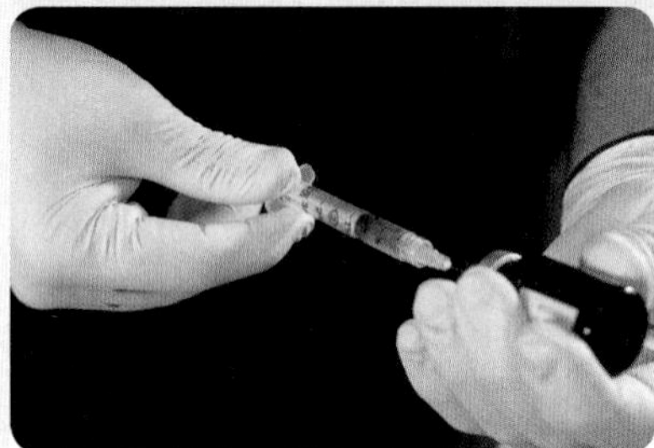

Step 2 Draw up the appropriate dose of medication in the syringe, dispel air, and reconfirm medication. Dispose of the needle properly.

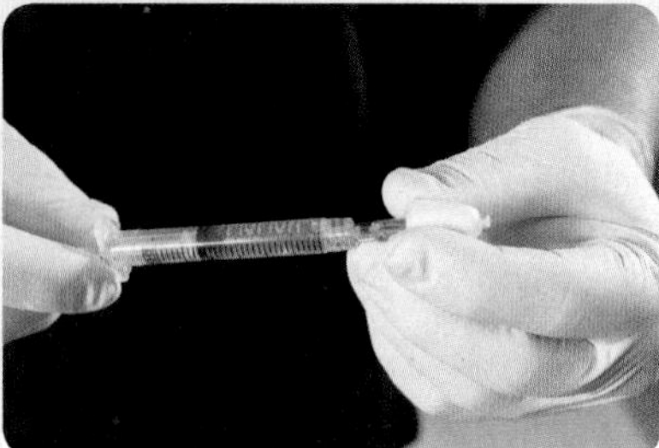

Step 3 Attach the mucosal atomizer device to the syringe, maintaining sterility.

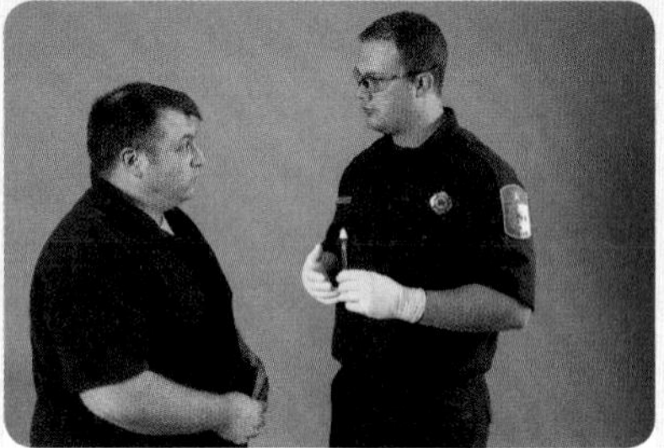

Step 4 Explain the procedure to the patient (or to a relative if the patient is unresponsive) and the need for the medication. Stop ventilation of the patient if necessary; remove any masks. Insert the mucosal atomizer device into the larger and less deviated or less obstructed nostril while pinching off the opposite nostril.

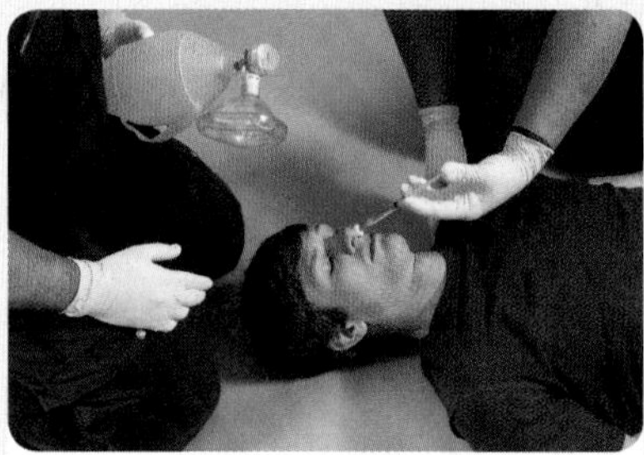

Step 5 Quickly spray the medication dose into a nostril.

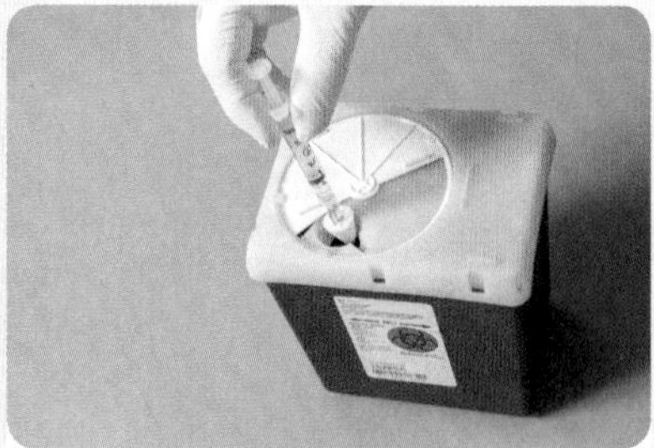

Step 6 Dispose of the atomizer device and syringe in the appropriate container.

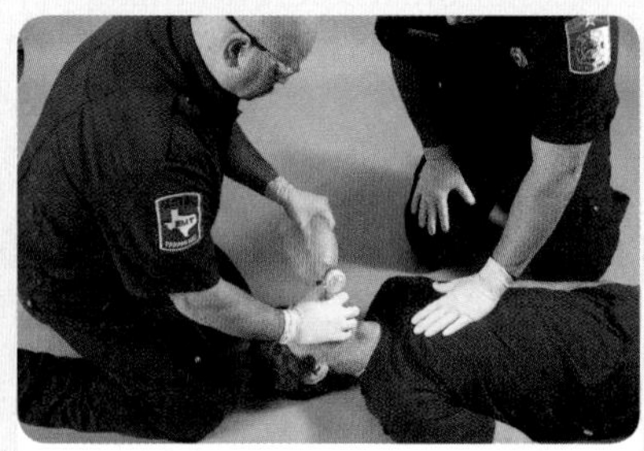

Step 7 Monitor the patient's condition, and document the medication given, route, time of administration, and patient response.

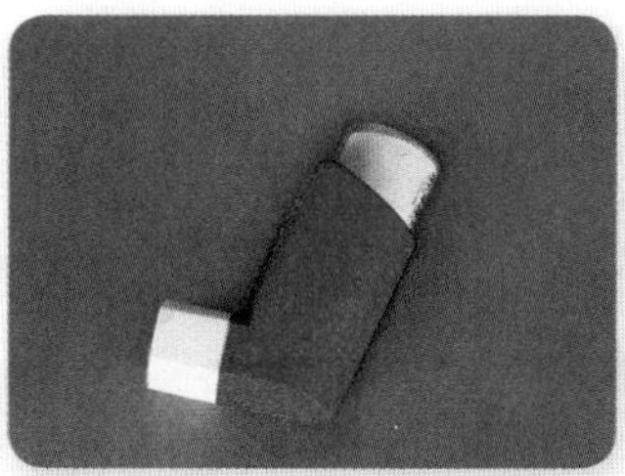

Figure 13-55 Some medications are inhaled into the lungs with a metered-dose inhaler so that they can be absorbed quickly into the bloodstream.

agonist bronchodilators (eg, albuterol [Ventolin, Proventil], isoetharine [Bronkosol], metaproterenol [Alupent]) are often administered in the prehospital setting for patients experiencing respiratory distress caused by certain obstructive airway diseases, such as asthma, bronchitis, and emphysema. Other medications, such as ipratropium bromide (Atrovent)—an anticholinergic bronchodilator—are also administered via the inhalation route. Check your drug reference guide or the package insert for the indications, contraindications, and precautions before giving any of these medications.

A patient with a history of respiratory problems will usually have a **metered-dose inhaler (MDI)** to use on a regular basis or as needed Figure 13-55. MDIs are usually administered by the patient using the patient's own prescribed medications, but AEMTs must know how to administer via this route because they may assist the patient with administration. Medications administered by the MDI can be delivered through a mouthpiece held by the patient or by a mask—with or without a spacer device—for young children and patients who are unable to hold the mouthpiece Figure 13-56.

Follow the steps in Skill Drill 13-10 to help a patient self-administer medication from an inhaler.

Words of Wisdom

MDIs are also called HFAs, after the propellant hydrofluoroalkane that is now used instead of chlorofluorocarbons.

For more severe problems, liquid bronchodilators may be aerosolized in a **nebulizer** for inhalation. Small-volume nebulizers (also called updraft or handheld nebulizers) are the most commonly used method of administration of inhaled medications in the prehospital setting Figure 13-57. Oxygen or a compressed air source is connected to the nebulizer to produce the aerosolized mist.

Some nebulizers have been adapted with child-friendly shapes and images to ease the use with pediatric patients. They may allow for blow-by administration to help the patient tolerate the medication. Other methods used on patients include a nebulized mask that does not require the patient to hold the device. Some adapters have been designed to allow providers to administer nebulized medications to intubated patients with each ventilation Figure 13-58. These devices may also be adapted for use with continuous positive airway pressure (CPAP) masks Figure 13-59.

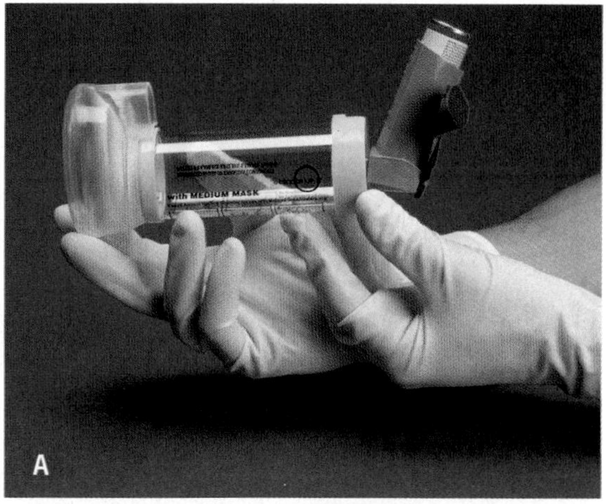

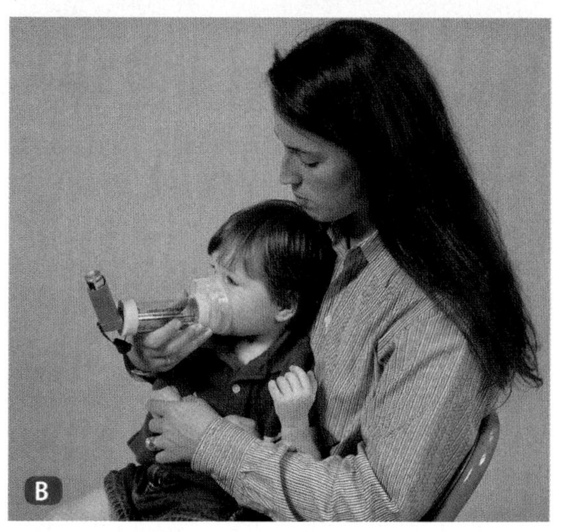

Figure 13-56 A. In children, a metered-dose inhaler and spacer can be used with or without a mask. **B.** Children as young as 6 months can use a mask and spacer device.

Follow the steps in Skill Drill 13-11 to administer a medication via a small-volume nebulizer.

Some patients with respiratory emergencies may be breathing inadequately (ie, inadequate tidal volume, fast or slow respiratory rate) and will not be able to effectively inhale beta agonist medications into the lungs via a nebulizer or an MDI. In this case, use a small-volume nebulizer in-line with the assistive device. If the patient is intubated, then assist with bag-mask ventilation or a ventilator by placing a short piece of corrugated tubing, separated by a T piece, to connect the nebulizer. When utilizing CPAP, most manufacturers have a nebulizer that is designed to work with their device. The nebulizer should be placed between the assistive device and mask, or ET tube if the patient is intubated, with a separate oxygen line connected to the nebulizer.

Skill Drill 13-10 Assisting a Patient With a Metered-Dose Inhaler

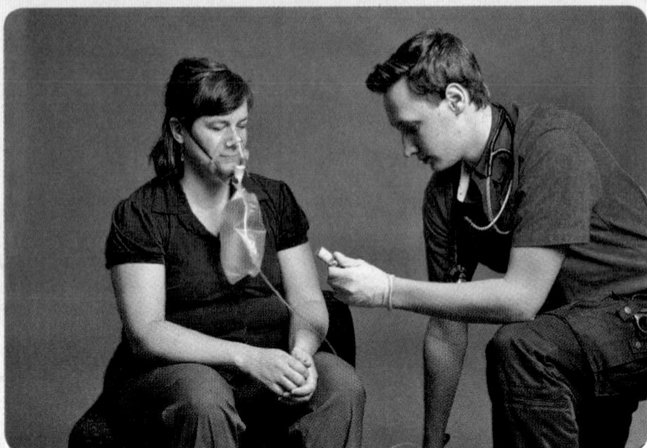

Step 1 Take standard precautions. Obtain an order from medical control or follow local protocol. Assemble the needed equipment.

Ensure you have the right medication, right patient, right dose, right route, and that the medication is not expired.

Ensure the patient is alert enough to use the inhaler. Check to see whether the patient has already taken any doses. Obtain baseline breath sounds for comparison after a few minutes of inhaler use. Ensure the inhaler is at room temperature or warmer.

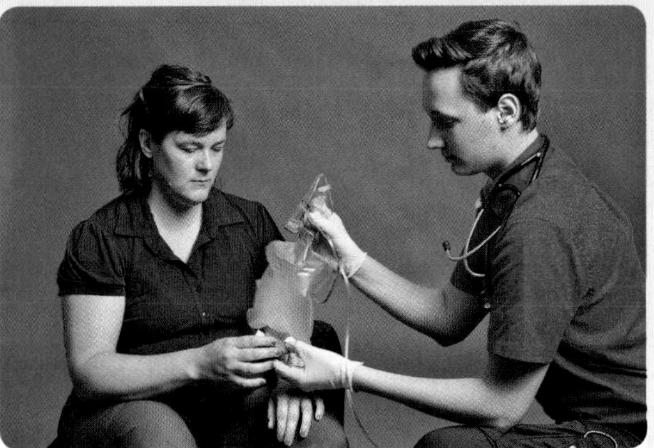

Step 2 Shake the inhaler vigorously several times. Stop administering supplemental oxygen and remove any mask from the patient's face. Ask the patient to exhale deeply and, before inhaling, to put his or her lips around the opening of the inhaler.

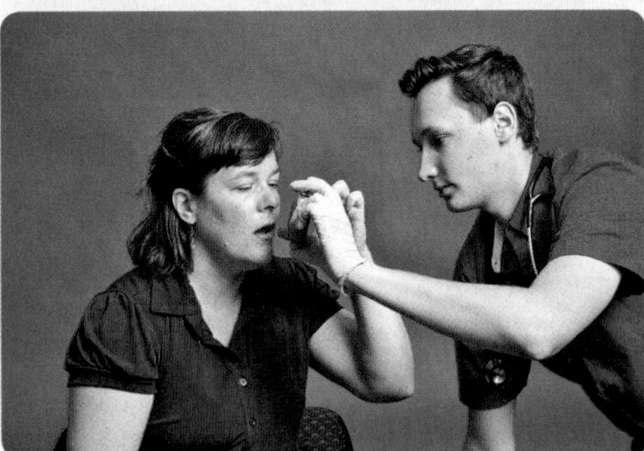

Step 3 If the patient has a spacer, then attach it to allow more effective use of the medication. Have the patient depress the handheld inhaler as he or she begins to inhale deeply.

Instruct the patient to hold his or her breath for as long as he or she comfortably can to help the lungs absorb the medication.

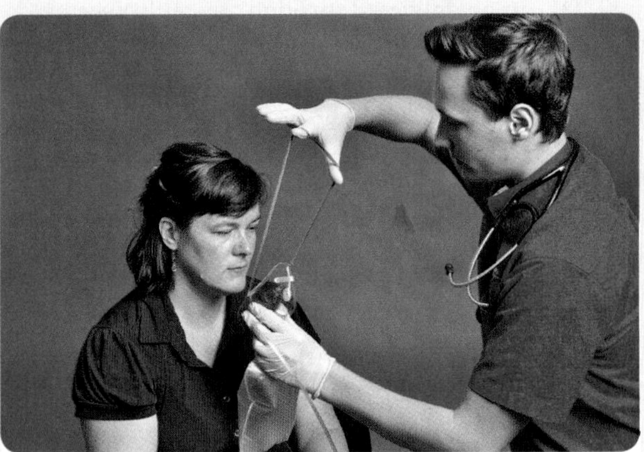

Step 4 Continue administering supplemental oxygen.

Allow the patient to breathe a few times, then give the second dose per direction from medical control or according to local protocol. Monitor the patient's condition, and document the medication given, route, administration time, and response of the patient.

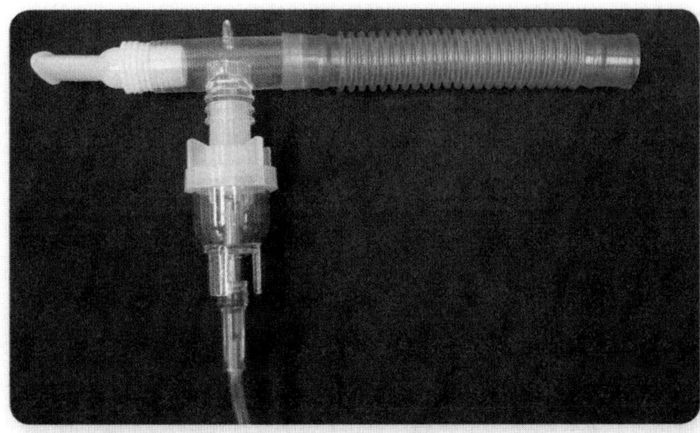

Figure 13-57 A small-volume nebulizer is used to deliver medications via aerosolized mist.

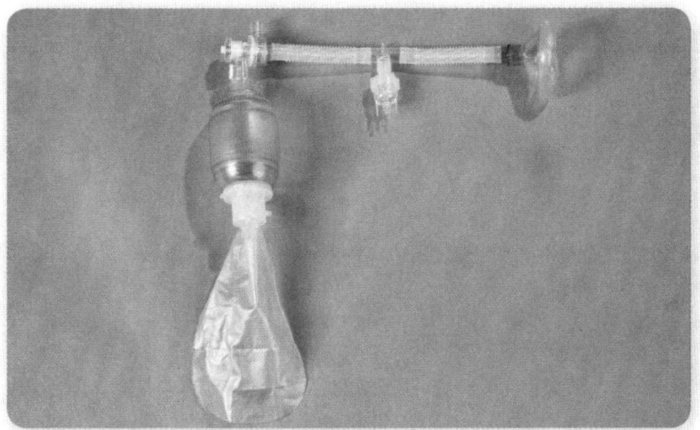

Figure 13-58 A nebulizer can be attached to a bag-mask device and administered through the mask.

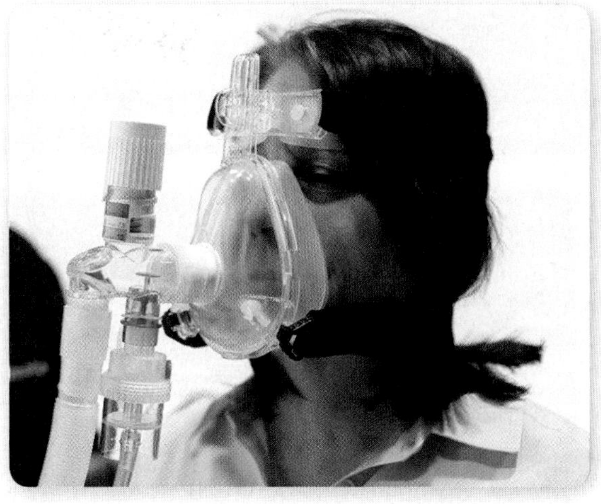

Figure 13-59 A nebulized medication being administered through a continuous positive airway pressure mask.

Intravenous Medication Administration

The IV route places the medication directly into the circulatory system. This is the fastest route of medication administration for AEMTs to administer because it bypasses most barriers to drug absorption. This also means that there is no room for error. Medications are administered by direct injection with a needle and syringe into an established peripheral IV line. Many services now use needleless systems to provide protection against needlesticks. In a needleless system, the syringe simply screws into the injection port.

As mentioned earlier, a bolus is a single dose given by the IV route. A bolus (in one mass) can be a small

Skill Drill 13-11 Administering a Medication via a Small-Volume Nebulizer

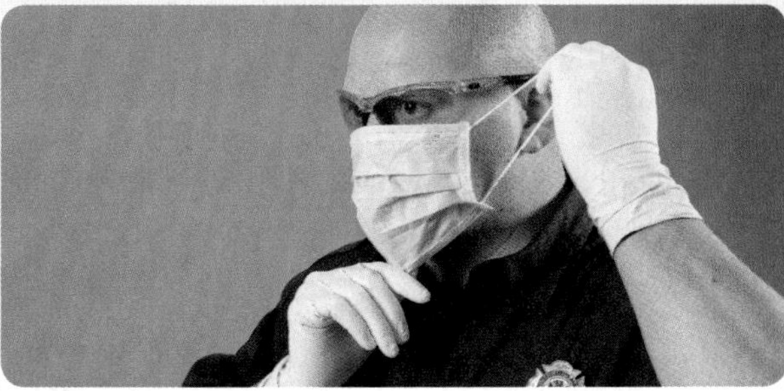

Step 1 Take standard precautions. Determine the need for an inhaled bronchodilator based on patient presentation. Obtain a history, including any medication allergies and vital signs.

Follow standing orders, or contact medical control for permission. Check the 10 rights of medication administration. Assemble and check needed equipment.

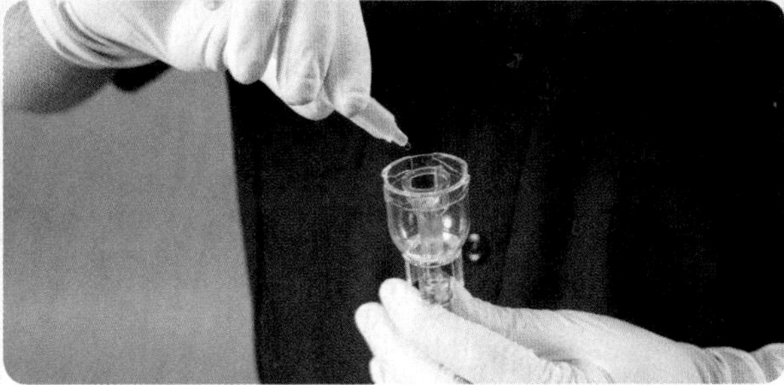

Step 2 If the medication is in a premixed package, then add it to the bowl of the nebulizer. If it is not premixed, then add the medication to the bowl and mix it with the specified amount of normal saline, usually 2.5 to 3 mL.

(continued)

Skill Drill 13-11 Administering a Medication via a Small-Volume Nebulizer *(continued)*

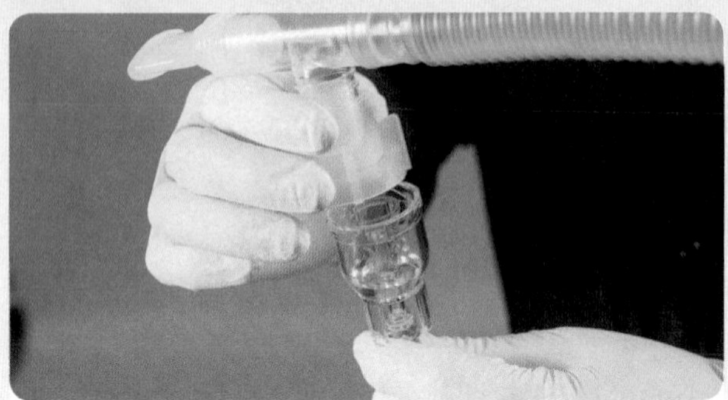

Step 3 Connect the T piece with the mouthpiece to the top of the bowl, or the mask to the bowl, and connect it to the oxygen tubing.

Set the flowmeter at 6 L/min to produce a steady mist. Remove the oxygen mask from the patient if oxygen is being administered.

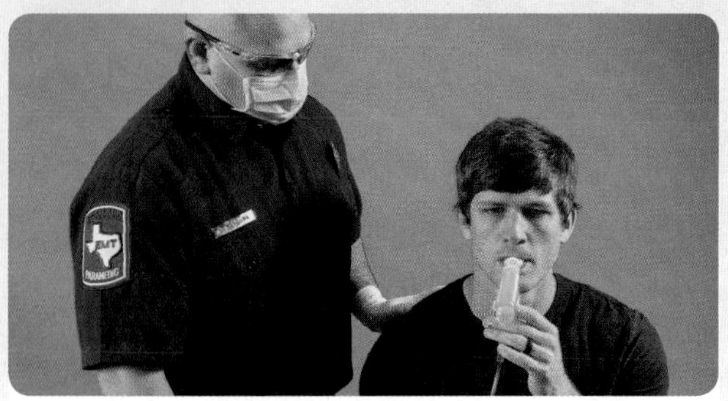

Step 4 With the MDI or handheld nebulizer in position, instruct the patient on the proper way to breathe. Have the patient breathe as deeply as possible and hold his or her breath for 3 to 5 seconds before exhaling. Continue to coach the patient as needed.

Monitor the patient's condition, and document the medication given, route, time of administration, and response of the patient to the medication.

or large quantity of a drug. Some medications require an initial bolus and then a continuous IV infusion to maintain a therapeutic level of the medication. Recall that complications may arise from using the IV route, including the local and systemic complications discussed earlier in this chapter.

Follow the steps in Skill Drill 13-12 when administering a medication via the IV bolus route.

Follow these steps to administer a medication through a saline lock, or intermittent site:

1. Take standard precautions.
2. Determine the need for the medication based on patient presentation.
3. Obtain a history, including any medication allergies and vital signs.
4. Follow standing orders, or contact medical control for permission.
5. Check the 10 rights of medication administration including ensuring that it is not cloudy or discolored and that its expiration date has not passed.
6. Explain the procedure to the patient and the need for the medication.
7. Assemble needed equipment, and draw up the medication. Draw up 20 mL of normal saline to use as a flush for the medication.
8. Cleanse the injection port with alcohol, or remove the protective cap if using the needleless system.
9. Insert the needle into the port while holding it carefully, or screw the syringe onto the port.
10. Pull back slightly on the syringe plunger, and observe for blood return. If blood appears, slowly inject the medication, watching for infiltration. If resistance is felt, or if the patient complains of any discomfort, discontinue administration immediately. A new site will need to be established.
11. Place the needle and syringe into the sharps container.
12. Clean the port, and insert the needle with the syringe containing the flush.
13. Flush the saline lock, and place the needle in the sharps container.
14. Store any unused medication properly.
15. Monitor the patient's condition, and document the medication given, route, time of administration, and patient response.

Skill Drill 13-12 Administering Medication via the IV Bolus Route

NR Skill

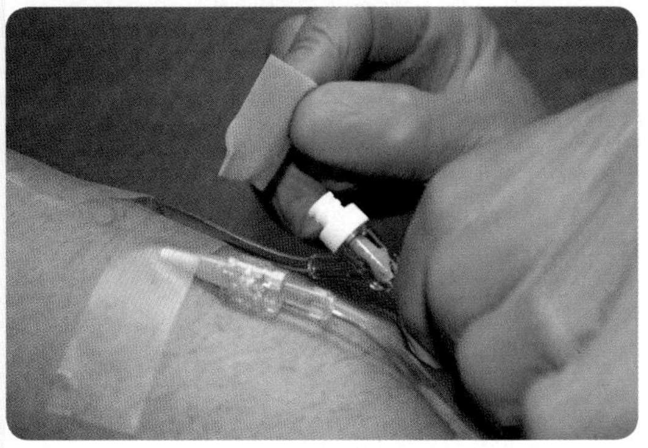

Step 1 Take standard precautions. Determine the need for the medication based on patient presentation. Obtain a history, including any medication allergies and vital signs. Follow standing orders, or contact medical control for permission.

Check the medication to be sure that it is the correct one, that it is not cloudy or discolored, and that its expiration date has not passed, and determine the appropriate dose.

Explain the procedure to the patient and the need for the medication. Assemble needed equipment, and draw up the medication. Expel any air in the syringe. Draw up 20 mL of normal saline to use as a flush for the medication.

Cleanse the injection port with alcohol, or remove the protective cap if using the needleless system.

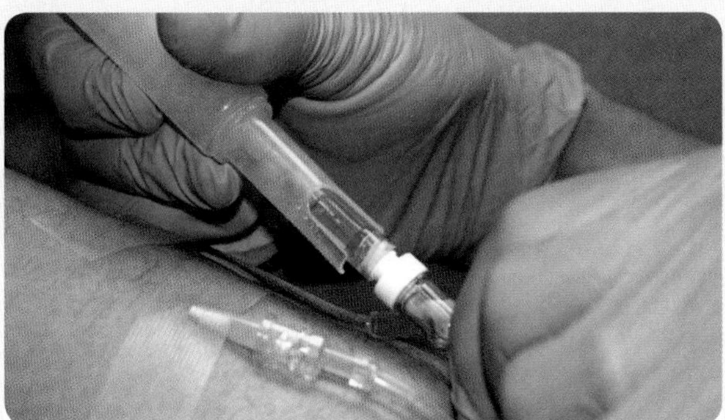

Step 2 Insert the needle into the port (or screw the syringe into the needless hub), and pinch off the IV tubing proximal to the administration port. Failure to shut off the line will result in the medication taking the pathway of least resistance and flowing into the bag instead of into the patient.

Administer the correct dose of the medication at the appropriate rate. Some medications must be administered very quickly, whereas others must be pushed slowly to prevent adverse effects.

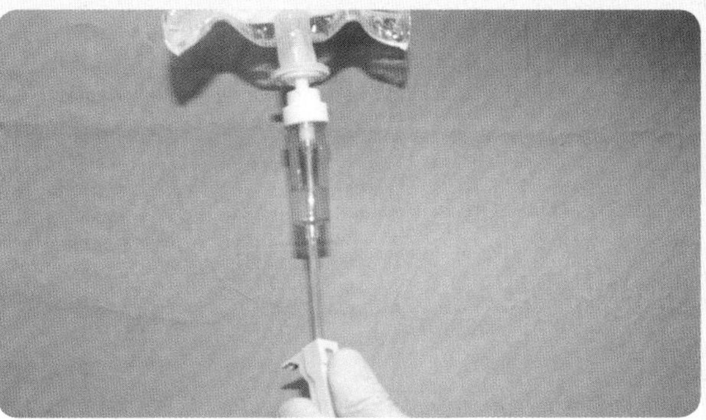

Step 3 Place the needle and syringe into the sharps container.

Unclamp the IV line to flush the medication into the vein. Allow it to run briefly wide open, or flush with a 20-mL bolus of normal saline.

Readjust the IV flow rate to the original setting.

Properly store any unused medication.

Monitor the patient's condition, and document the medication given, route, time of administration, and patient response.

Intraosseous Medication Administration

The IO route is used for critically ill or injured children and adults when IV access is difficult or impossible to obtain. Any fluid or medication that may be given through an IV line—bolus or maintenance infusion—can be given by the IO route. Shock, status epilepticus, and cardiac arrest are a few of the reasons for establishing IO access.

Unlike with an IV line, fluid does not flow well into the bone because of resistance; therefore, it is necessary to use a large syringe to infuse the fluid. A pressure infuser device—a sleeve placed around the IV bag and inflated to force fluid from the IV bag—should be used when infusing fluids in adults.

Complications of using the IO route are similar to those of the IV route. Along with the complications discussed earlier in this chapter, there is also the potential for compartment syndrome if fluid leaks outside the bone and into the osteofascial compartment.

Follow the steps in Skill Drill 13-13 to administer a medication via the IO route.

Skill Drill 13-13 Administering Medication via the Intraosseous Route

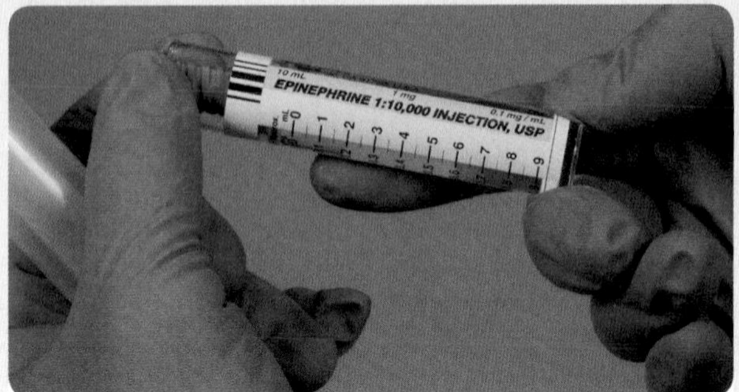

Step 1 Take standard precautions. Determine the need for the medication based on patient presentation. Obtain a history, including any medication allergies and vital signs. Follow standing orders, or contact medical control for permission. Check the medication to ensure that it is the correct one, that it is not cloudy or discolored, and that the expiration date has not passed, and determine the appropriate amount and concentration for the correct dose.

Explain the procedure to the patient and/or parent and the need for the medication. Assemble needed equipment and draw up the medication. Also draw up 20 mL of normal saline for a flush.

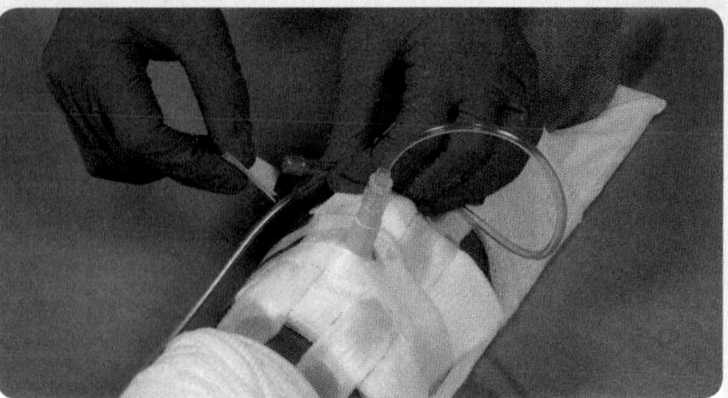

Step 2 Cleanse the injection port of the extension tubing with alcohol, or remove the protective cap if using the needleless system.

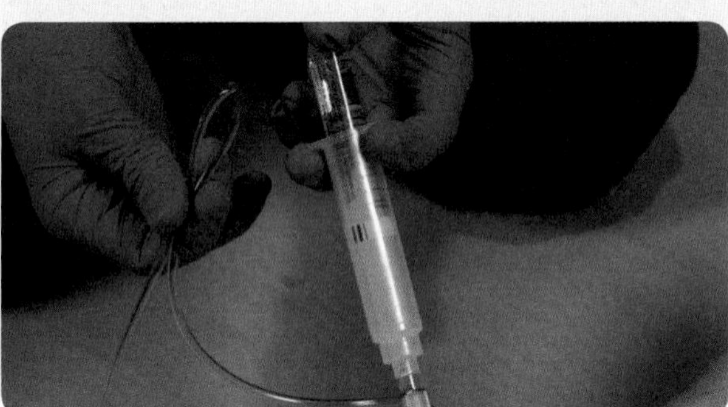

Step 3 Insert the needle into the port, and clamp off the IV tubing proximal to the administration port. This is usually managed with a three-way stopcock. Failure to shut off the line will result in the medication taking the pathway of least resistance and flowing into the bag instead of into the patient. Administer the correct dose of the medication at the proper push rate. Some medications must be administered quickly, whereas others must be pushed slowly to prevent adverse effects.

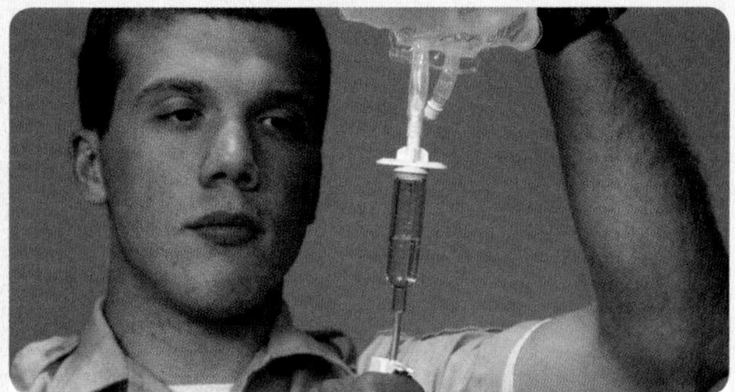

Step 4 Place the needle and syringe into the sharps container. Unclamp the IV line to flush the medication into the site. Flush with at least a 20-mL bolus of normal saline. Readjust the IV flow rate to the original setting. Store any unused medication properly.

Monitor the patient's condition, and document the medication given, route, time of administration, and response of the patient.

YOU are the Provider SUMMARY

1. On the basis of the information given, do you think this patient will require IV access?

The patient's mechanism of injury and complaint of abdominal pain indicate that a minimum of one IV line should be initiated, with preferably two IV lines. Because this patient is reporting abdominal pain, it is important to have IV access in case she becomes hypotensive and requires fluid administration.

2. What is the appropriate-size IV catheter for this patient?

This patient requires fluid resuscitation. Previously, the largest IV catheter that you could successfully place would have been the correct answer. Because the goals of fluid resuscitation are to administer up to four boluses of 250 mL each followed by a reassessment of the blood pressure after each bolus, the catheter should be large enough to allow for rapid administration of the 250-mL bolus. Current recommendations in hemorrhagic shock are to use at least one 18-gauge angiocatheter. This decreases the risk of an unsuccessful cannulation attempt relative to use of a larger catheter. A second IV catheter of similar diameter or larger should be established during transportation. Remember that the more distal the IV site, the smaller the catheter. Metacarpal veins of the hand accommodate 18- to 20-gauge catheters with more difficulty than do more proximal veins. Antecubital veins of the upper part of the arm can accommodate larger catheters.

3. Does this patient require any medications, and, if so, by what route should they be administered?

Given the mechanism of action and your physical exam findings, this patient requires oxygen administration. It is important to remember that medical-grade oxygen is a medication and, as such, requires you to ascertain a thorough medical history prior to administration. Oxygen is given via the inhalation route, either through a mask, nasal cannula, or a nebulizer. In trauma patients, oxygen should always be given via a nonrebreathing mask.

4. What are the 10 rights of medication administration?

Prior to administering any medication, you must ensure the 10 rights of medication administration. These are the right patient, right medication, right dose, right route, right time, right documentation and reporting, right assessment, right to refuse, right evaluation, and right patient education.

5. What type of fluid should you administer to this patient?

This patient should be given an isotonic solution such as 0.9% sodium chloride or lactated Ringer solution. Because normal saline has almost the same osmolarity as serum and other body fluids, it stays inside the intravascular compartment. Isotonic solutions expand the contents of the intravascular compartment without shifting fluid to or from other compartments. Awareness of this fact is useful when dealing with hypotensive or hypovolemic patients. Although isotonic fluid does a good job of hydrating, this fluid remains in the vascular compartment, so you must be careful to avoid fluid overloading.

6. How much fluid should be administered to this patient?

In trauma patients, AEMTs should administer up to four boluses of 250 mL each titrated to achieve a systolic blood pressure greater than 80 mm Hg with reassessment of the blood pressure and heart rate after each bolus. Check with medical control before administering more medication.

7. Why is it important to constantly reassess breath sounds when you are administering fluid to a patient?

An unmonitored IV bag can result in circulatory overload. Healthy adults can handle as much as 2 to 3 extra liters of fluid without compromise. Problems occur when the patient has cardiac, pulmonary, or renal dysfunction or has recently been experiencing active bleeding. These types of dysfunction do not tolerate any additional demands from increased circulatory volume. The most common cause of circulatory overload in the prehospital setting is failure to readjust the drip rate after flushing an IV line immediately after insertion. Always monitor IV bags to ensure the proper drip rate. Patient presentation of circulatory overload includes dyspnea, jugular vein distention, and increased blood pressure. Crackles are often heard when evaluating breath sounds. Acute peripheral edema can also be an indication of circulatory overload. In the case of recent active bleeding, driving the blood pressure to or even above normal levels risks disrupting clots that may have formed and which have helped control hemorrhage. This clot disruption can actually exacerbate underlying bleeding.

8. What are some possible complications of vein cannulation?

Peripheral IV insertion carries associated risks. The problems associated with IV lines can be categorized as either local or systemic reactions. Local reactions include problems such as infiltration; thrombophlebitis; occlusion; vein irritation; hematoma; nerve, tendon, or ligament damage; and arterial puncture. Systemic complications include circulatory overload, air embolus, vasovagal reactions, and catheter shear.

YOU are the Provider SUMMARY *(continued)*

EMS Patient Care Report (PCR)			
Date: 10-1-18	**Incident No.:** 20100152	**Nature of Call:** MVC	**Location:** Main & 1st Street

Dispatched:	**En Route:**	**At Scene:**	**Transport:**	**At Hospital:**	**In Service:**
1218	1220	1225	1234	1256	1324

Patient Information

Age: 35 **Sex:** F **Weight (in kg [lb]):** 75 kg (165 lb)	**Allergies:** None **Medications:** None **Past Medical History:** None **Chief Complaint:** Severe abdominal pain

Vital Signs

Time: 1230	**BP:** Not obtained	**Pulse:** Not obtained	**Respirations:** 20	**Spo_2:** Not obtained
Time: 1236	**BP:** 76/40	**Pulse:** 121	**Respirations:** 20	**Spo_2:** 100% on 15 L/min
Time: 1246	**BP:** 86/48	**Pulse:** 130	**Respirations:** 20	**Spo_2:** 100% on 15 L/min

EMS Treatment (circle all that apply)

Oxygen @ 15 **L/min via (circle one):** **NC** **(NRM)** **Bag-mask device**	**Assisted Ventilation**	**Airway Adjunct**	**CPR**
Defibrillation / **Bleeding Control**	**Bandaging**	**Splinting**	**Other:**

Narrative

EMS dispatched to above location for reported MVC. On arrival find single-vehicle MVC, where sedan impacted telephone pole at approximately 45 miles per hour. Patient found seated in driver's seat, AO×4, ABCs intact. Immediate manual stabilization performed, cervical collar applied, patient extricated to long backboard. Rapid assessment reveals severe pain and bruising to lower abdominal area, coupled with distention. Secured to stretcher, transport emergent to Charity hospital. En route – Vitals as above. Nonrebreathing mask at 15 L/min applied. Bilateral 18-gauge IVs established to AC, with initial 250-mL normal saline bolus administered because of patient's hypotension. Report called to online medical control with condition and ETA. At conclusion of fluid bolus, breath sounds clear bilaterally, patient remains hypotensive. 2nd 250-mL bolus given, with slight increase in blood pressure. On arrival, care and report given to ED staff without incident.**End of report**

Prep Kit

▶ Ready for Review

- As an AEMT, it is your responsibility to thoroughly understand how medications affect the body.
- The danger of something going wrong when administering a medication—for example, administering the wrong medication or the wrong dose of a medication—can be minimized by confirming the "10 rights" of medication administration: right patient, right medication, right dose, right route, right time, right documentation and reporting, right assessment, right to refuse, right evaluation, and right patient education.
- Follow a set procedure when you administer any medication. A safe procedure begins with obtaining an order from medical control and making sure you understand the physician's orders. Repeat any orders word for word for verification.
- You must inquire about any medication allergies that the patient may have. Verify the proper medication and prescription. Verify the form, dose, and route of the medication.
- You must also check the expiration date and condition of the medication before its administration and confirm medication compatibility.
- The final steps of medication administration are to notify the physician when the medication has been administered, monitor the patient for effects, and advise medical control of any changes in the patient's condition. Document your actions and the patient's responses.
- Dispose of any syringes and needles safely in a sharps container, and do not recap needles.
- A certified AEMT is allowed to administer or help patients self-administer numerous medications: oxygen, oral glucose, glucagon, dextrose, epinephrine, metered-dose inhaler medications, nebulized medications, nitroglycerin, nitrous oxide, naloxone, aspirin, and possibly others based on local protocol.
- AEMTs may administer intravenous (IV) fluids, including 5% dextrose in water, normal saline, and lactated Ringer solution.
- AEMTs may only administer medications and fluids when either directly ordered by medical control or allowed by local protocols or standing orders.
- An understanding of basic cell physiology can help an AEMT understand why different types of IV fluids are administered for different conditions. The cellular environment contains ions, or electrolytes, that are used by the cell for different purposes, depending on its needs. These ions include sodium, potassium, calcium, bicarbonate, chloride, and phosphorus. Their electrical charges must remain in balance on either side of the cell membrane.
- There must be a balance of compounds on either side of the cell membrane. If an imbalance occurs, the cell can move chemicals or charges across its membrane by various methods, including diffusion, filtration, active transport, and osmosis.
- Becoming familiar with the various types of IV solutions will give you an understanding of their use in relation to patient conditions. IV solutions are categorized by dissolved components (crystalloid and colloid) and by tonicity (isotonic, hypotonic, hypertonic).
- Crystalloid solutions are dissolved crystals in water and contain compounds that quickly disassociate in solution. These solutions are the best choice for the patients who need fluid replacement.
- Colloid solutions contain molecules that are too large to pass out of the capillary membranes and therefore remain in the vascular compartment. These are not generally used in the prehospital setting. Examples of colloids are albumin and corticosteroids.
- Isotonic solutions have nearly the same osmolarity as serum and other body fluids; therefore, these solutions stay inside the intravascular compartment. Hypotonic solutions have a lower concentration of sodium than the cell; these solutions pull fluid from the vascular compartment into the interstitial fluid compartment. Hypertonic solutions have a higher osmolarity than serum and shift fluids into the intravascular compartment.
- Successful IV administration technique takes practice. Several factors, from the patient's condition to the available IV equipment, influence every IV start. Mastery of IV therapy skills comes when you understand and can overcome all the variables. Take your time when you practice inserting an IV line and gain a solid understanding of what you are doing. This understanding will be useful when you need to start a quick and flawless IV line in less than optimum conditions.
- During IV therapy, it is critical to always keep equipment sterile.
- You will need to choose an IV solution and administration set. There are different sizes of administration sets for different situations and patients. Administration sets come in two primary sizes: microdrip and macrodrip. Microdrip sets are ideal for medication administration; macrodrip sets are best for fluid replacement.
- Before administering IV fluid, you will need to choose an IV site, spike the bag, and choose a catheter. Catheters are sized by their diameter

Prep Kit *(continued)*

and referred to by the gauge of the catheter. The larger the diameter of the catheter, the smaller the gauge. The larger the diameter, the more fluid can be delivered through the catheter.

- After you have gained vascular access, you will need to secure the line and remove the constricting band.
- Possible complications of IV therapy include local reactions and systemic reactions.
- Infiltration is the escape of fluid into the surrounding tissue. This escape of fluid causes a localized area of edema. To correct the infiltration, discontinue administration and reestablish an IV line in the opposite extremity or at a more proximal location on the same extremity. Apply direct pressure over the swollen area to reduce further swelling or bleeding into the tissue.
- Occlusion is the physical blockage of a vein or catheter. If the flow rate is not sufficient to keep fluid moving out of the catheter tip and if blood enters the catheter, a clot may form and occlude the flow.
- A hematoma is an accumulation of blood in the tissues surrounding an IV site. Blood can be seen rapidly pooling around the IV site, resulting in tenderness and pain. If a hematoma develops while you are attempting to insert a catheter, stop and apply direct pressure to help minimize bleeding. If a hematoma develops after a successful catheter insertion, evaluate the IV flow and the hematoma.
- Any allergic reaction must be treated aggressively. Patient presentation depends on the extent of the reaction. If an allergic reaction occurs while administering medication through an IV, discontinue administration and remove the solution. Notify medical control immediately and maintain an open airway.
- Treat a patient with a suspected air embolus by placing the patient on his or her left side with the head down to trap any air inside the right atrium or right ventricle and rapidly transport to the closest most appropriate facility. Be prepared to assist ventilations if the patient experiences increasing shortness of breath or inadequate tidal volume. Document the event.
- Catheter shear occurs when part of the catheter is pinched against the needle, and the needle slices through the catheter, creating a free-floating segment. Treatment involves surgical removal of the sheared tip.
- An unmonitored IV bag can result in circulatory overload. Always monitor IV bags to ensure the proper drip rate. To treat a patient with circulatory overload, slow the IV rate to keep the vein open and raise the patient's head to ease respiratory distress. Administer high-flow oxygen and monitor vital signs and breathing adequacy. Contact medical control immediately and document the event.
- Administering IV therapy to pediatric and geriatric patients requires special care. Both populations are at a higher risk for certain medical conditions that can affect both the patient's need for IV therapy and the effectiveness of the therapy. By understanding the risks and concerns of these populations, you will be better equipped to properly administer IV therapy. Finally, in any medical situation involving pediatric or geriatric patients, remember to be sensitive to the patient's personal issues.
- Intraosseous administration (administration of fluids or medications into the bone) is an alternative if IV access is difficult or impossible. Any fluid or medication that can be administered via the IV route can be administered via the intraosseous route and can travel to the central circulation just as rapidly.
- Good math skills, along with an understanding of the metric system, are imperative to providing the correct dose for the patient. Practice your math skills frequently to stay proficient.
- As an AEMT, you should be familiar with the various routes of medication administration. This includes an understanding of the proper use of equipment and proper anatomic locations for administration. Enteral administration includes the administration of all medications that may be given through any portion of the digestive tract. The parenteral route includes any method of medication administration that does not go through the digestive tract.
- When in doubt, always follow local protocols or contact medical control for direction.

▶ Vital Vocabulary

access port A sealed hub on an administration set designed for sterile access to the intravenous fluid.

acidosis A pathologic condition resulting from the accumulation of acids in the body.

active transport A method used to move compounds across a cell membrane to create or maintain an imbalance of charges.

administration set Tubing that connects to the intravenous bag access port and the catheter to deliver the intravenous fluid.

air embolus The presence of air in the veins, which can result in cardiac arrest if it enters the heart.

Prep Kit *(continued)*

alkalosis A pathologic condition resulting from the accumulation of bases in the body.

ampules Small glass containers that are sealed and the contents sterilized.

anion An ion that contains an overall negative charge.

antecubital The anterior aspect of the elbow.

aseptic technique A method of cleansing used to prevent contamination of a site when performing an invasive procedure, such as inserting an intravenous line.

ataxia A staggered walk or gait caused by injury to the brain or spinal cord.

bolus A term used to describe "in one mass"; in medication administration, a single dose given by the intravenous route; may be a small or large quantity of the drug.

Bone Injection Gun (BIG) A spring-loaded device that is used for inserting an intraosseous needle into the proximal tibia in adult and pediatric patients.

buccal Relating to the cheek or mouth.

buffer A substance or group of substances that controls the hydrogen levels in a solution.

butterfly catheters Rigid, hollow, venous cannulation devices identified by plastic "wings" that act as anchoring points for securing the catheter.

cannulation The insertion of a hollow tube into a vein to allow for fluid flow.

capillary beds The terminal ends of the vascular system where fluids, food, and wastes are exchanged between the vascular system and the cells of the body.

catheter A flexible, hollow structure that delivers fluid.

catheter shear A free-floating segment of a catheter in the circulatory system, created if the needle slices through the catheter while it is being inserted.

cation An ion that contains an overall positive charge.

cellular perfusion The ability of a cell to take in oxygen and remove carbon dioxide.

colloid solution A type of intravenous solution that contains compounds that are too large to pass out of the capillary membranes and therefore remain in the vascular compartment; for example, used to help reduce edema.

concentration The total weight of a drug contained in a specific volume of liquid.

concentration gradient The natural tendency for substances to flow from an area of higher concentration to an area of lower concentration, either within the cell or outside the cell.

contaminated stick The puncturing of an emergency care provider's skin with a catheter that was used on a patient.

crystalloid solution A type of intravenous solution that contains compounds that quickly disassociate in solution and can cross membranes; considered the best choice for prehospital care of injured patients who need fluids to replace lost body fluid.

D_5W An intravenous solution made up of 5% dextrose in water.

depolarization The rapid movement of electrolytes across a cell membrane that changes the cell's overall charge. This rapid shifting of electrolytes and cellular charges is the main catalyst for muscle contractions and neural transmissions.

desired dose The amount of a drug that the physician orders for a patient; the drug order.

diaphysis The shaft of a long bone.

diffusion A process in which molecules move from an area of higher concentration to an area of lower concentration.

drip chamber The area of the administration set where fluid accumulates so that the tubing remains filled with fluid.

drip rate Number of drops per minute.

drip set Another name for an administration set.

drug reconstitution Injecting sterile water (or saline) from one vial into another vial containing a powdered form of the drug.

electrolytes Charged atoms or compounds that result from the loss or gain of an electron. These are ions that the body uses to perform certain critical metabolic processes.

enteral medications Medications that are given through a portion of the gastrointestinal tract.

epiphyseal plate The growth plate of a bone; a major site of bone development during childhood.

epiphyses The ends of a long bone.

external jugular IV lines Intravenous catheters established in the jugular veins of the neck.

EZ-IO A handheld, battery-powered driver to which a special intraosseous needle is attached; used for insertion of the intraosseous needle into the proximal tibia of children and adults.

fascia The fiberlike connective tissue that covers arteries, veins, tendons, and ligaments.

FAST devices (First Access for Shock Trauma) Manual sternal intraosseous devices used in patients age 12 years and older; include an infusion tube,

Prep Kit *(continued)*

subcutaneous portal, an introducer, a target/strain relief patch, and a protective dome.

filtration A type of diffusion in which water carries dissolved compounds across the cell membrane; commonly used by the kidneys to clean blood.

flash chamber The area of a catheter that fills with blood to help indicate when a vein is cannulated.

gauge In the medication administration sense, the interior diameter of a catheter or needle.

gtt A measurement that indicates drops.

hematoma An accumulation of blood in the tissues surrounding an intravenous site.

homeostasis The balance of all systems of the body.

hypercalcemia High serum calcium levels.

hyperkalemia High serum levels of potassium.

hypertonic solution A solution that has a greater concentration of sodium than does the cell; the increased extracellular osmotic pressure can draw water out of the cell and cause it to collapse.

hypocalcemia Low serum calcium levels.

hypokalemia Low levels of potassium.

hypotonic solution A solution that has a lower concentration of sodium than the cell does; the increased intracellular osmotic pressure lets water flow into the cell, causing it to swell and possibly burst.

infiltration The escape of fluid into the surrounding tissue.

inhalation Breathing into the lungs; a medication delivery route.

interstitial Water between the vascular system and the surrounding cells (for example, between the membranes of two cells located outside the vascular compartment in the body).

intramuscular (IM) Into a muscle; a medication delivery route.

intranasal A delivery route in which a medication is pushed through a specialized atomizer device, called a mucosal atomizer device, into the naris.

intraosseous (IO) Into the bone; a medication delivery route.

intraosseous infusion A technique of administering fluids, blood and blood products, and medications into the intraosseous space of a long bone, usually the proximal tibia.

intraosseous space The spongy cancellous bone of the epiphyses and the medullary cavity of the diaphysis, collectively.

intravascular The water portion of the circulatory system surrounding the blood cells (for example, in the heart, arteries, or veins).

intravenous (IV) Into a vein; a medication delivery route.

ions Charged atoms or compounds that result from the loss or gain of an electron.

ionic concentration The amount of charged particles found in a particular area.

isotonic solution A solution that has the same concentration of sodium as does the cell. In this case, water does not shift, and no change in cell shape occurs.

lactated Ringer solution A sterile crystalloid isotonic intravenous solution of specified amounts of calcium chloride, potassium chloride, sodium chloride, and sodium lactate in water.

local reactions Mild to moderate allergic reactions occurring in a localized area.

lysis The rupturing of a cell caused by either the presence of certain enzymes or the uncontrolled influx of material into the cell.

macrodrip set An administration set named for the large orifice between the piercing spike and the drip chamber; allows for rapid fluid flow into the vascular system.

metabolic Relating to the breakdown of ingested foodstuffs into smaller and smaller molecules and atoms that are used as energy sources for cellular function.

metered-dose inhaler (MDI) A miniature spray canister used to direct medications through the mouth and into the lungs.

metric system A decimal system based on tens for the measurement of length, weight, and volume.

microdrip set An administration set named for the small orifice between the piercing spike and the drip chamber; allows for carefully controlled fluid flow and is ideally suited for medication administration.

mucosal atomizer device A device that attaches to the end of a syringe that is used to spray (atomize) certain medications via the intranasal route.

nebulizer A device for producing a fine spray or mist that is used to deliver inhaled medications.

New Intraosseous (NIO) device A spring-loaded device that contains neither drill nor battery, used for inserting an intraosseous needle into the proximal tibia of an adult patient.

normal saline 0.9% sodium chloride; an isotonic crystalloid.

occlusion Blockage, usually of a tubular structure such as a blood vessel.

orthostatic hypotension Symptomatic drop in blood pressure related to the patient's body position,

Prep Kit *(continued)*

detected by measuring pulse and blood pressure while the patient is lying supine, sitting up, and standing. An increase in pulse rate and a decrease in blood pressure in any one of these positions is considered a positive sign for this condition.

osmolarity The ability to influence the movement of water across a semipermeable membrane.

osmosis The movement of water across a cell membrane from an area of lower to higher solute molecules.

osmotic pressure Pressure created against the cell wall by the presence of water.

osteogenesis imperfecta A congenital bone disease that results in fragile bones.

osteomyelitis Inflammation of the bone and muscle caused by infection.

over-the-needle catheters The prehospital standard for intravenous cannulation, these consist of a hollow tube over a laser-sharpened steel needle; also referred to as an angiocath.

parenteral medications Medications that are given through any route other than through the gastrointestinal tract.

Penrose drain A type of surgical drain; can be used as a constricting band.

pH A measure of the acidity of a solution.

phospholipid bilayer The cell membrane's double layer, consisting of a hydrophilic outer layer composed of phosphate groups, and a hydrophobic inner layer made up of lipids, or fatty acids. It is this structure and composition that allows the cell membrane to have selective permeability.

piercing spike The hard, sharpened plastic spike on the end of the administration set designed to pierce the sterile membrane of the intravenous bag.

polyuria The passage of an unusually large volume of urine in a given period. In diabetes, this can result from excreting excess glucose in the urine.

pressure infuser device A sleeve that is placed around the IV bag and inflated to force fluid to flow from the IV bag and into the tubing.

pulmonary embolus A blood clot trapped within the pulmonary circulation.

saline lock A type of intravenous (IV) access device that allows an active IV site to be maintained without having to run fluids through the vein, also called a buff cap or intermittent site.

sclerosis The hardening of a vein from scar tissue after repeated cannulation.

selective permeability The ability of the cell membrane to selectively allow compounds into the cell based on the cell's current needs.

sodium/potassium (Na^+/K^+) pump The mechanism by which the cell brings in two potassium (K^+) ions and releases three sodium (Na^+) ions.

subcutaneous Into the tissue between the skin and muscle; a medication delivery route.

sublingual Under the tongue; a medication delivery route.

syncopal episode Fainting; brief loss of consciousness caused by transiently inadequate blood flow to the brain.

systemic complications Moderate to severe allergic reaction affecting the systems of the body.

tachycardia Rapid heart rhythm, more than 100 beats/min.

third spacing The shifting of fluid into the tissues, creating edema.

thrombophlebitis Inflammation of a vein.

tonicity The osmotic pressure of a solution, based on the relationship between sodium and water inside and outside the cell, that takes advantage of chemical and osmotic properties to move water to areas of higher sodium concentration.

trocar A solid boring needle.

varicose veins Veins on the leg that are large, twisted, and ropelike and can cause pain, swelling, or itching.

vasovagal reaction A reaction consisting of precordial distress, anxiety, nausea, and sometimes syncope.

venous thrombosis The development of a stationary blood clot in the venous circulation.

vials Small glass bottles for medications; may contain single or multiple doses.

volume on hand The amount of fluid you have on hand, such as the amount of fluid in an intravenous bag or the amount of fluid in a vial of medication.

▶ References

1. National Association of Emergency Medical Technicians (NAEMT). *Advanced Medical Life Support*. 2nd ed. Burlington, MA: Jones and Bartlett Learning; 2017:159.
2. The Committee on Trauma. *Advanced Trauma Life Support® Student Course Manual*. 10th ed. Chicago, IL: American College of Surgeons; 2018.
3. Cantor-Peled G, Halak M, Ovadia-Blechman Z. Peripheral vein locating techniques. Open Access Journals. http://www.openaccessjournals.com/articles/peripheral-vein-locating-techniques.html. Accessed February 17, 2017.
4. Mbamalu D, Banerjee A. Methods of obtaining peripheral venous access in difficult situations. *Postgrad Med J*. 1999;75(886):459-462.

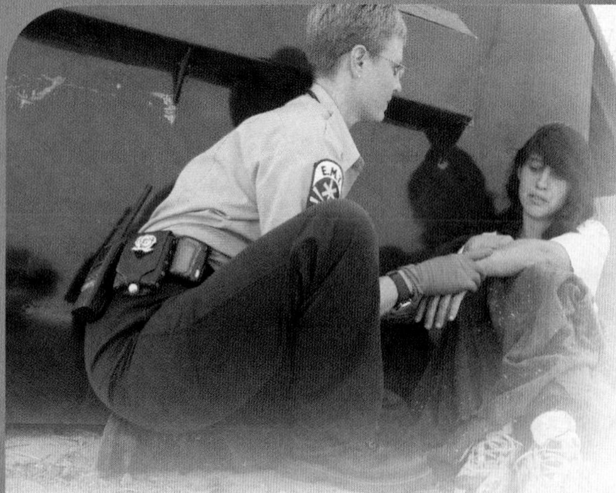

Assessment *in Action*

You arrive to a local halfway house to find a middle-aged man seated on the sofa complaining of nausea, a rash, and shortness of breath. He states that he was just prescribed atenolol by his physician yesterday, and he took his first dose approximately 90 minutes ago.

1. What type of medication name is atenolol?

A. Trade name
B. Generic name
C. Chemical name
D. Official name

2. The patient was prescribed atenolol to slow his heart rate. This therapeutic use is referred to as the medication's:

A. indication.
B. contraindication.
C. intended effect.
D. side effect.

3. The symptoms that occurred following the patient's dose of atenolol are considered:

A. indications.
B. contraindications.
C. intended effects.
D. side effects.

4. What medication does the AEMT carry that may be useful in treating the patient's problem?

A. Aspirin
B. Nitroglycerin
C. Albuterol
D. Diphenhydramine

5. While you are obtaining the SAMPLE history from the patient, he states that he uses an albuterol "puffer" twice a day for asthma. Albuterol is administered by which route?

A. Intravenous
B. Rectal
C. Inhalation
D. Subcutaneous

6. Albuterol is a(n) __________ medication that causes bronchial dilation.

A. alpha-1
B. alpha-2
C. beta-1
D. beta-2

7. Macrodrips are ideal for medication administration or pediatric fluid delivery because it is easy to control their fluid flow.

A. True
B. False

8. At what point should intraosseous lines typically be used if you are unable to gain IV access?

A. After 2 tries or 60 seconds
B. After 2 tries or 90 seconds
C. After 3 tries or 60 seconds
D. After 3 tries or 90 seconds

9. To calculate a drip rate, which of the following information is NOT necessary to know?

A. The type of administration set
B. The length of time for infusion
C. The amount to flow
D. The patient's weight

10. What is the formula used to calculate the drip rate for IV fluids?

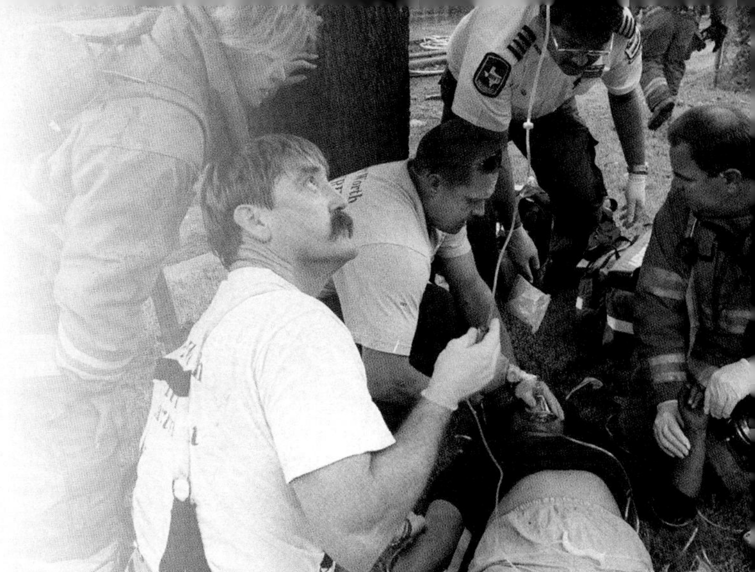

SECTION 6

Shock and Resuscitation

CHAPTER 14

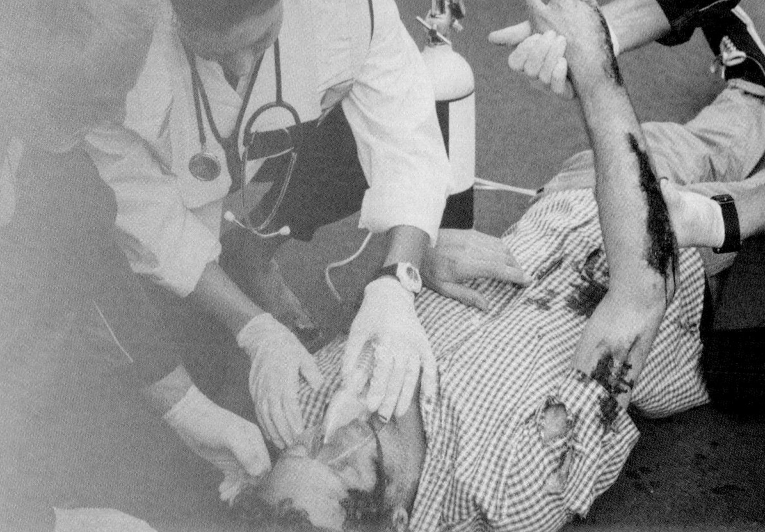

Shock

National EMS Education Standard Competencies

Shock and Resuscitation

Applies fundamental knowledge to provide basic and selected advanced emergency care and transportation based on assessment findings for a patient in shock, respiratory failure or arrest, cardiac failure or arrest, and post resuscitation management.

Pathophysiology

Applies comprehensive knowledge of the pathophysiology of respiration and perfusion to patient assessment and management.

Knowledge Objectives

1. Describe the physiology of perfusion, including the role of the autonomic nervous system in controlling blood pressure. (pp 655-657)
2. Discuss cardiac output, heart rate, stroke volume, and systemic vascular resistance. (p 655)
3. Discuss myocardial contractility, afterload, and preload, and how they relate to shock. (p 655)
4. Discuss the pathophysiology of shock (hypoperfusion). (pp 657-662)
5. Describe how the body compensates for decreased perfusion. (pp 659-660)
6. Explain how the body progresses to multiple-organ dysfunction syndrome (MODS). (p 662)
7. Recognize the causes of shock. (p 663)
8. Describe the various types of shock, including hypovolemic shock, cardiogenic shock, obstructive shock, and distributive shock. (pp 663-669)
9. Describe the signs and symptoms of shock. (pp 664-665, 668-669)
10. Describe the three stages of shock. (pp 670-672)
11. Explain the progression of shock, including the three distinct phases. (pp 670-672)
12. Discuss the assessment of a patient who could be in shock. (pp 672-674)
13. Describe the steps to follow in the emergency care of the patient with signs and symptoms of shock. (pp 674-680)
14. Discuss the role of fluid administration in treating a patient in potential shock. (pp 675-677)
15. Discuss special considerations in fluid resuscitation. (p 677)

Skills Objectives

1. Demonstrate how to complete an emergency medical services patient care report for a patient with bleeding and/or shock. (pp 673-674)
2. Demonstrate how to treat a patient in potential shock. (pp 674-680)

YOU are the Provider PART 1

Your ambulance is dispatched to a local residence to evaluate an elderly male patient reporting weakness and nausea. You find the patient lying supine in bed holding his hand over his abdomen. He states that he has not felt well over the past couple of days and feels as if he could pass out. He is pale, cool, and clammy.

1. What is shock and how does it relate to perfusion?
2. What factors does perfusion depend on?

Introduction

Shock has several meanings. In this chapter, shock (hypoperfusion) describes a state of collapse and failure of the cardiovascular system. When the circulation of blood in the body becomes inadequate, the oxygen and nutrient needs of the cells cannot be met. In the early stages of shock, the body will attempt to maintain **homeostasis** (a balance of all systems of the body); however, as shock progresses, blood circulation slows and eventually ceases. This abnormal state of inadequate oxygen and nutrient delivery to the cells of the body causes organs and then organ systems to fail. If not treated promptly, shock can be fatal.

Shock can occur because of medical or traumatic events such as a heart attack, severe allergic reaction, internal or external bleeding from injuries sustained as a result of an automobile crash, or as a result of a gunshot wound. As an advanced emergency medical technician (AEMT), you will respond to these different types of emergencies to provide care and transportation for these patients. Therefore, you must be constantly alert to the signs and symptoms of shock. Maintain a high index of suspicion. The goal is to recognize shock in its early stages and provide appropriate treatment.

This chapter begins with a close-up look at **perfusion**, the function that fails in shock. Next, it looks at the physiologic causes of shock and describes each of its major forms. Finally, it discusses the assessment and emergency treatment of shock in general and of each kind of shock in particular. See Chapter 15, *BLS Resuscitation*, for resuscitation techniques.

Physiology of Perfusion

Perfusion is the circulation of blood within an organ or tissue in adequate amounts to meet the cells' current needs for oxygen, nutrients, and waste removal. Perfusion requires having a working cardiovascular system. It also requires adequate gas exchange in the lungs, adequate nutrients in the form of glucose in the blood, and adequate waste removal, primarily through the lungs.

The body is perfused via the circulatory system. The circulatory system is a complex arrangement of connected tubes, including the arteries, arterioles, capillaries, venules, and veins. There are two circuits in the body: the systemic circulation in the body and the pulmonary circulation in the lungs. The systemic circulation, the circuit in the body, carries oxygen-rich blood from the left ventricle through the body and back to the right atrium. In the systemic circulation, as blood passes through the tissues and organs, it gives up oxygen and nutrients and absorbs cellular wastes and carbon dioxide. Carbon dioxide is one of the primary waste products of cellular work (metabolism) in the body and is removed from the body by the lungs. This is the reason why one of your primary concerns for your patient should be ensuring adequate ventilation and oxygenation.

Words of Wisdom

The following elements are collectively known as the **Fick principle**, which states that the movement and use of oxygen in the body is dependent on:

1. Adequate concentration of inspired oxygen (FIO_2 [fraction of inspired oxygen])
2. Appropriate movement of oxygen across the alveolar-capillary membrane into the arterial bloodstream
3. Adequate number of red blood cells (RBCs) to carry the oxygen
4. Proper tissue perfusion
5. Efficient off-loading of oxygen at the tissue level

Cardiac Output

Cardiac output (CO) is the volume of blood that the heart can pump per minute, and it depends on several factors. First, the heart must have adequate strength, which is largely determined by the ability of the heart muscle to contract. This ability to contract is referred to as **myocardial contractility**. Second, the heart must receive adequate blood to pump. As the volume of blood coming to the heart increases, the precontraction pressure in the heart builds up. This precontraction pressure is known as **preload**. As preload increases, the volume of blood within the ventricles increases, which causes the heart muscle to stretch. When the heart muscle is stretched, the strength of its contractions increases, resulting in increased cardiac output. Last, the resistance to flow in the peripheral circulation must be appropriate. The force or resistance against which the heart pumps is known as **afterload**.

Blood pressure, the pressure that is generated by the contractions of the heart and the dilation and constriction of the blood vessels, is usually carefully controlled by the body so that there is always sufficient circulation in the various tissues and organs, and it is a rough measure of perfusion. Because the heart cannot pump out what is not in its holding chambers, blood pressure varies directly with cardiac output, **systemic vascular resistance (SVR)**, and blood volume. (SVR is the resistance to blood flow within all blood vessels except the pulmonary vessels.) Remember that blood pressure is the pressure of blood within the vessels at any one time. The systolic pressure is the peak arterial pressure, or pressure generated every time the heart contracts; the diastolic pressure is the pressure maintained within the arteries while the heart rests between heartbeats.

Perfusion depends on cardiac output, SVR, and transport of oxygen.

$$\text{CO} = \text{HR} \times \text{SV}$$
$$\text{Cardiac Output} = \text{Heart Rate} \times \text{Stroke Volume}$$
$$\text{BP} = \text{CO} \times \text{SVR}$$
$$\text{Blood Pressure} = \text{Cardiac Output} \times \text{Systemic Vascular Resistance}$$

Mean arterial pressure (MAP) is generally considered to be the patient's blood pressure. However, MAP is ultimately the blood pressure required to sustain organ perfusion and is roughly 60 mm Hg in the typical resting adult. If the MAP falls substantially below 60 mm Hg for an appreciable amount of time, the result will be ischemia of the organs from lack of perfusion. MAP is approximated using this formula:

$$\text{MAP} \approx \text{Diastolic blood pressure} + \tfrac{1}{3}\text{ Pulse pressure (Systolic blood pressure} - \text{Diastolic blood pressure)}$$

Note this equation approximates MAP, as designated by the ≈ symbol.

▶ The Role of the Nervous System

Control of the cardiovascular system is a function of the **autonomic nervous system**, which is composed of competing subsystems **Table 14-1**. One of the subsystems, the sympathetic nervous system, which is sometimes known as the fight-or-flight system, prepares the body for physical activity during a stressful situation. This preparation includes increasing the pulse rate, blood pressure, and respiratory rate while dilating blood vessels in areas required for physical activity and constricting those in areas primarily involved with reproduction and restoration.

The autonomic nervous system is primarily regulated from the upper part of the medulla oblongata of the brain. Nerve signals caused by stimulation of the sympathetic nervous system travel between the brain and the body via nerves through the spinal cord. These nerves leave the spinal cord between each pair of vertebrae and spread out to affect the tissues in those areas **Figure 14-1**. Another mechanism used by the sympathetic nervous system is the chemical release of epinephrine and norepinephrine from the adrenal glands into the bloodstream. These chemicals travel through the bloodstream to all parts of the body to activate a sympathetic response in those areas.

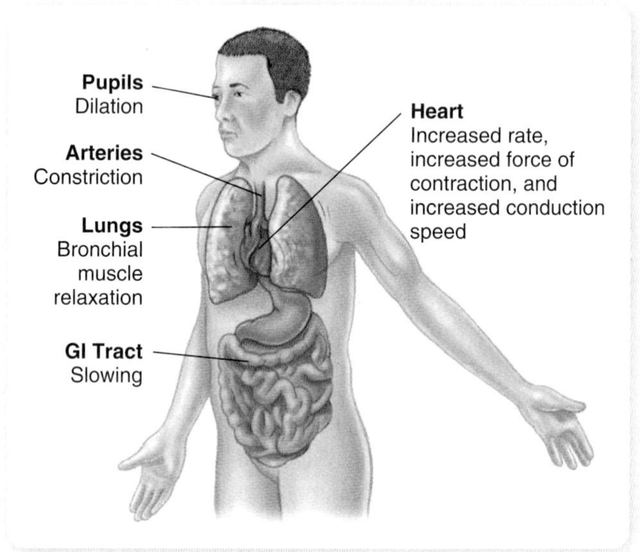

Figure 14-1 The sympathetic nervous system.

Table 14-1 Comparison of Sympathetic and Parasympathetic Nervous Systems

Features	Parasympathetic	Sympathetic
Other name for system	Cholinergic, "rest and digest"	Adrenergic, "fight or flight"
Natural chemical mediator	Acetylcholine	Norepinephrine, epinephrine
Primary nerve(s)	Vagus	Nerves from the thoracic and lumbar ganglia of the spinal cord
Effect of stimulation	Decreases cardiac contractility (negative **inotropic effect**) Slows conduction velocity (negative **dromotropic effect**) Slows the heart[a] (negative **chronotropic effect**) Constricts pupils Increases gut motility Increases salivation	Increases cardiac contractility (positive inotropic effect) Speeds conduction velocity (positive dromotropic effect) Speeds the heart[a] (positive chronotropic effect) Dilates pupils Slows the gut Dilates the bronchi

[a]Slowing or speeding occurs mostly in the atria.

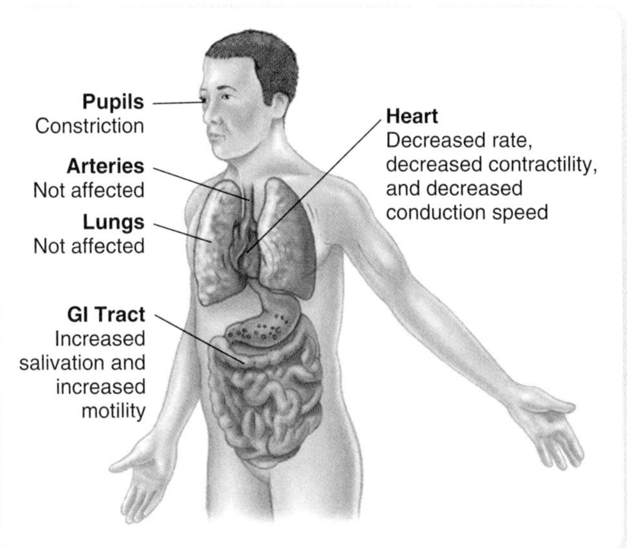

Figure 14-2 The parasympathetic nervous system.

The other subsystem of the autonomic nervous system is the parasympathetic nervous system, which is primarily responsible for rest and regeneration Figure 14-2. The parasympathetic nervous system opposes every action of the sympathetic nervous system. Where the sympathetic system increases the pulse rate, blood pressure, and respiratory rate, the parasympathetic system decreases these. The parasympathetic system also constricts blood vessels in muscular tissue and dilates those in the digestive system.

Regulation of Blood Flow

Blood flow through the capillary beds is regulated by the capillary **sphincters**, circular muscular walls that constrict and dilate, acting as a gate to increase or decrease flow. These sphincters are under the control of the autonomic nervous system. Capillary sphincters also respond to other stimuli such as heat, cold, the need for oxygen, and the need for waste removal. Under normal circumstances, not all cells have the same needs at the same time. For example, the stomach and intestines have a high need for blood flow during and shortly after eating, when digestion is at a peak. Between meals, blood flow is lessened, and blood is diverted to other areas. The brain, by contrast, needs a constant and consistent supply of blood to function.

Regulation of blood flow is determined by cellular need and is accomplished by vessel constriction or dilation, together with sphincter constriction or dilation. Maintenance of blood flow, or perfusion, is accomplished by the heart, blood vessels, and blood working together.

Respiration and Oxygenation

Each time you take a breath, the alveoli (microscopic, thin-walled air sacs) receive a supply of oxygen-rich air. The oxygen then dissolves in the blood plasma and attaches to the blood's hemoglobin. The oxygenated blood passes through the alveolar wall into the walls of a fine network of pulmonary capillaries that are in close contact with the alveoli. If the oxygenated blood is not properly circulated, some of the cells and organs will not receive proper nutrients, possibly resulting in cellular death.

Oxygen and carbon dioxide pass rapidly across these thin tissue layers through diffusion. Diffusion, as discussed in Chapter 13, *Vascular Access and Medication Administration*, is a passive process in which molecules move from an area with a higher concentration of molecules to an area of lower concentration. There are more oxygen molecules in the alveoli than in the blood; therefore, the oxygen molecules move from the alveoli into the blood. Because there are more carbon dioxide molecules in the blood than in the inhaled air, carbon dioxide moves from the blood into the alveoli.

Just like oxygen, a large portion of carbon dioxide is bound to the hemoglobin while the remainder is dissolved in the plasma, some of which combines with water to form carbonic acid. Carbonic acid concentrations become high just as the blood is moving toward the lungs. After it reaches the lungs, the carbonic acid breaks down and the carbon dioxide is exhaled. This action takes place to maintain the delicate balance between the gases and maintain the pH of the body.

Pathophysiology

Shock can result from inadequate cardiac output, decreased SVR, or the inability of RBCs to deliver oxygen to tissues. If there is a disturbance in the transportation of oxygen and removal of carbon dioxide, dangerous waste products will build up, resulting in cellular death and eventually death of the entire organ. If the shock state persists, it will ultimately result in death of the entire organism (the body). As mentioned, shock, or hypoperfusion, is a state of collapse and failure of the cardiovascular system that results in inadequate circulation. To protect vital organs, the body attempts to compensate by shunting (directing) blood flow from organs that are more tolerant of low flow (such as the skin and intestines) to vital organs that cannot tolerate hypoperfusion (such as the heart, brain, and lungs). If the cause of shock is not promptly addressed, the patient will soon die.

The cardiovascular system consists of three parts: a pump (the heart), a set of pipes (the blood vessels or arteries that act as the container), and the contents of the container (the fluid or blood) Figure 14-3. These three parts can be referred to as the perfusion triangle Figure 14-4. When a patient is in shock, one or more of the three parts is not working properly.

Blood is the vehicle for carrying oxygen and nutrients through the vessels to the capillary beds to tissue cells, where these supplies are exchanged for waste products created during metabolism. For this process to happen, the vessels (container) must be intact. Blood contains

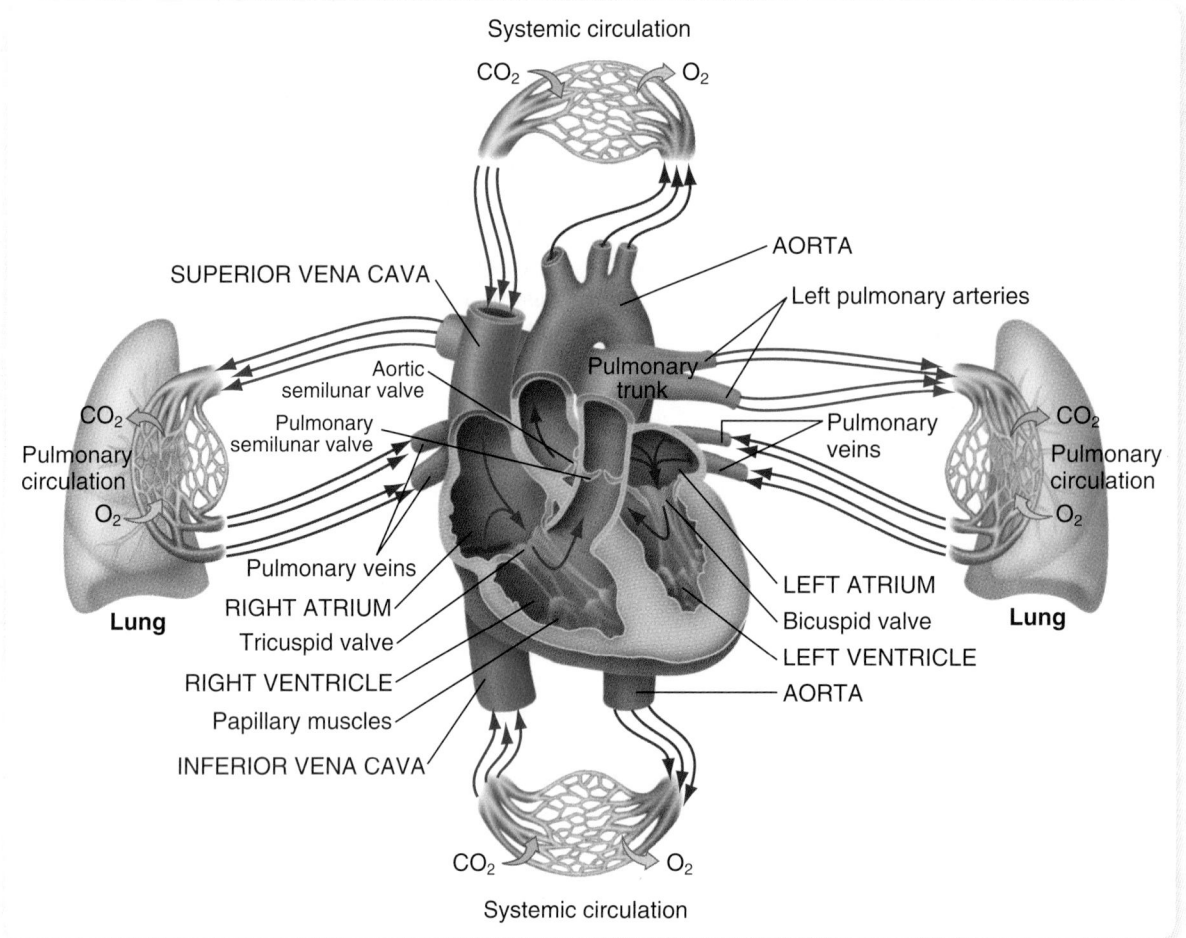

Figure 14-3 The cardiovascular system consists of three parts: the pump (heart), the container (vessels), and the contents (blood). The blood carries oxygen (O_2) and nutrients through the vessels to the capillary beds, where they are exchanged for waste products (such as carbon dioxide [CO_2]).

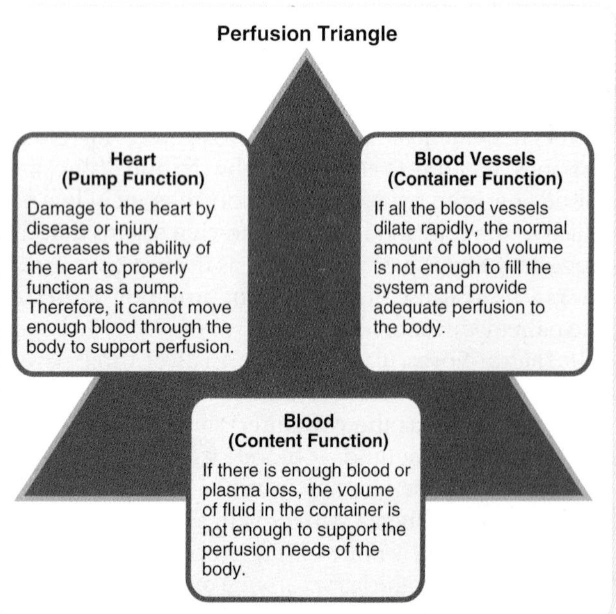

Figure 14-4 The heart, the blood vessels, and the blood represent the three legs of the perfusion triangle.

RBCs, white blood cells, platelets, and plasma (the liquid portion of the blood). As discussed in Chapter 7, *The Human Body*, hemoglobin (the protein inside RBCs) is responsible for the transportation of oxygen to the cells and for transporting carbon dioxide (a waste product of cellular metabolism) away from the cells to the lungs, where it is exhaled and removed from the body. White blood cells help the body to fight infection. Platelets are responsible for forming blood clots.

Blood clots are an important response from the body to control blood loss. In the body, a blood clot forms depending on one of the following principles: retention of blood because of blockage in blood circulation (blood stasis), changes in the vessel wall (such as a wound), and the blood's ability to clot (as the result of a disease process or medication). When injury occurs to tissues in the body, platelets begin to aggregate at the site of injury; this causes the RBCs to become sticky and clump together. As the RBCs begin to clump, another substance in the body called fibrinogen reinforces the RBCs. This is the final step in the formation of a blood clot. Clots can become unstable and susceptible to rupture because blood is continually moving as a result of the blood pressure.

The result may be an embolus at a distant site if the clot is venous or rebleeding if the clot is arterial.

The body's neural and hormonal mechanisms, including the autonomic nervous system and hormones, are triggered when the body senses that the pressure in the system is falling and the need for perfusion of vital organs is increased. The sympathetic side of the autonomic nervous system, which is responsible for the fight-or-flight response, will assume more control of the body's functions during a state of shock. The parasympathetic nervous system is a division of the autonomic nervous system that controls involuntary functions by sending signals to the cardiac, smooth, and glandular muscles and takes over during nonstressful situations. The sympathetic division of the autonomic nervous system causes the release of hormones such as epinephrine and norepinephrine. These hormones cause changes in certain body functions such as an increase in the heart rate and in the strength of cardiac contractions and vasoconstriction in nonessential areas, primarily in the skin, muscles, and gastrointestinal tract (peripheral vasoconstriction). Together, these actions are designed to maintain pressure in the system and, as a result, sustain perfusion of the vital organs (ie, brain, heart, lungs, kidneys, and liver).

Eventually, there is also a shifting of body fluids to help maintain pressure within the system. However, the response of the autonomic nervous system and hormones comes within seconds. It is this response that causes all the signs and symptoms of shock in a patient.

Words of Wisdom

The Frank-Starling mechanism states that the length of the muscle fibers of the heart's wall determines the force of the contraction.[1] In other words, an increase in diastolic filling increases the force of the contraction, and a decrease in diastolic filling decreases the force of the contraction. Decreased perfusion in shock is the result of a decrease in cardiac contraction, which may be the result of loss of fluid, increased container size, or a damaged pump.

▶ Compensation for Decreased Perfusion

Central among the homeostatic mechanisms that regulate cardiovascular dynamics are those that maintain blood pressure. When any event results in decreased perfusion (such as in blood loss, myocardial infarction, loss of vasomotor tone, or **tension pneumothorax**), the body must respond immediately to preserve the vital organs. **Baroreceptors** located in the aortic arch and carotid sinuses (as well as in most of the large arteries of the neck and thorax) sense the decreased blood pressure and flow and activate the vasomotor center in the medulla oblongata, which oversees changes in the diameter of blood vessels, to begin constriction of the vessels, therefore increasing blood pressure. Along with baroreceptors are **chemoreceptors**, which measure subtle shifts in the amounts of carbon dioxide in the arterial blood. In Chapter 7, *The Human Body*, you learned that these shifts have an effect on the regulation of the respiratory rate as well as control of the acid/base balance in the body.

Normally, stimulation occurs when the systolic pressure is between 60 and 80 mm Hg in adults or even lower in children. A decrease in the systolic pressure to less than 80 mm Hg stimulates the vasomotor center to increase the arterial pressure by constricting vessels. As the arterial pressure decreases, the walls of the arteries are not stretched as much, thereby decreasing baroreceptor stimulation. Normally, baroreceptor stimulation prevents the vasoconstrictor center of the medulla from constricting the vessels, resulting in vasodilation in the peripheral circulatory system and a decrease in pulse rate and contractility, causing a concomitant decrease in arterial pressure. With decreasing pressure, the baroreceptors are not stimulated to allow for vasodilation, so the vessels constrict to raise the blood pressure. The sympathetic nervous system is also stimulated as the body recognizes a potential catastrophic event. This message is sent to the adrenal glands to release epinephrine and norepinephrine into the bloodstream. These two naturally occurring "medications" will cause tachycardia and increase the contractility of the heart. Additionally, they will cause venous and arteriolar constriction, resulting in a decrease in blood flow to the skin, muscles, the gastrointestinal tract, and often the kidneys. This allows for a relative redistribution of blood to the brain and heart. Capillary hydrostatic pressure decreases in the compensated phase of shock, allowing fluid from the interstitial compartment to flow into the vessels.

Also, in response to hypoperfusion, the renin-angiotensin-aldosterone system in the kidneys is activated and antidiuretic hormone is released from the pituitary gland. Together, these mechanisms trigger salt and water retention and peripheral vasoconstriction. The result is an increase in the patient's blood pressure and maintenance of cardiac output. Depending on the severity of the insult, variable amounts of fluid will shift from the interstitial tissues into the vascular compartment. The spleen also releases some RBCs that are normally sequestered there to augment the blood's oxygen-carrying capacity. The overall response of the initial compensatory mechanisms is to increase the preload, stroke volume, and pulse rate, which usually results in an increase in cardiac output. This "autotransfusion" effect, along with the subtle effects in other response systems of the body (ie, osmosis, insulin and glucagon production in the pancreas, as well as the effects of the hormones arginine vasopressin (also known as antidiuretic hormone [ADH]), the adrenocorticotropic hormone cortisol system, and somatotropin), allows the body to compensate adequately for a volume loss of up to 25%. Remember that shock is a *normal compensatory response* of the body, and disease can occur or become exacerbated when normal response systems are activated under abnormal conditions.

As hypoperfusion persists, the myocardial oxygen demand exceeds its supply. Eventually, the accelerated compensatory mechanisms are no longer able to keep up with the body's demand. Myocardial function then worsens, with decreased cardiac output and ejection fraction. Tissue perfusion decreases, resulting in impaired cell metabolism. Often, the systolic blood pressure decreases, especially in progressive hypoperfusion or "decompensated" shock. Fluid may leak from the blood vessels, as in the case of a severe allergic reaction, causing systemic and pulmonary edema.

As the patient decompensates, perfusion to the brain and coronary arteries decreases. Cells switch from aerobic to anaerobic metabolism. In **anaerobic metabolism**, cellular processes occur in the absence of oxygen; in contrast, in **aerobic metabolism** all cell processes occur with an adequate oxygen supply. This switch is a critical point, and lactic acidosis begins to develop from this inefficient form of metabolism. This also decreases cardiac function and makes the heart more susceptible to the effect of the circulating catecholamines (causing dysrhythmias). Other signs of hypoperfusion may also be present, such as dusky skin color, oliguria, and impaired mentation.

The body produces its own "medicines," epinephrine and norepinephrine, in the adrenal glands in response to hypoperfusion. These substances are released by the body as part of the global compensatory state. Release of epinephrine improves cardiac output by increasing the pulse rate and strength of contractions. The alpha-1 response to its release includes vasoconstriction, increased peripheral vascular resistance, and increased afterload from the arteriolar constriction. Alpha-2 effects ensure a regulated release of alpha-1. Beta responses from the release of epinephrine primarily affect the heart and lungs. Increases in pulse rate, contractility, conductivity, and automaticity occur in tandem with bronchodilation.

Effects of norepinephrine are primarily alpha-1 and alpha-2 in nature and center on vasoconstriction and increasing peripheral vascular resistance. Table 14-2 lists the alpha and beta effects of epinephrine and norepinephrine. This vasoconstriction allows the body to shunt blood from areas of lesser need to areas of greater need, keeping the brain and other vital organs perfused in the early phases of shock. To maintain circulation to the brain, the body will shunt blood away from the following tissues in the following order: placenta, skin, muscles, gut, kidneys, liver, heart, lungs. This planned shunting of blood is often referred to as the pecking order. The skin and muscles can survive with minimal blood flow from vasoconstriction for a much longer period than can major organs such as the kidneys, liver, heart, and lungs. If the blood supply is inadequate to the major organs for more than 60 minutes, they often develop complications that will result in death, such as renal failure and shock lung. This concept has been traditionally referred to as the Golden Hour or the Golden Period in recognition of the fact that the time frame actually varies with the severity of the disruption in the blood supply and the resilience

Table 14-2 Effects of Epinephrine and Norepinephrine

Receptor	Effects
Epinephrine	
Alpha-1	Vasoconstriction Increase in peripheral vascular resistance Increased afterload from arteriolar constriction
Alpha-2	Inhibit insulin release Relax gastrointestinal smooth muscle
Beta-1	Positive chronotropic effects (increase in the heart's rate of contraction) Positive inotropic effects (increase in the contractility of the heart muscle) Positive dromotropic effects (increase in the heart's velocity of conduction)
Beta-2	Bronchodilation Gastrointestinal smooth muscle dilation
Norepinephrine	
Alpha-1 and alpha-2	Vasoconstriction Increase in peripheral vascular resistance Increased afterload from arteriolar constriction

of the tissues, yet it describes why it is so important for you to treat the cause of the shock immediately.

Failure of compensatory mechanisms to preserve perfusion results in decreases in preload and cardiac output. Myocardial blood supply and oxygenation decrease, reducing myocardial perfusion. As cardiac output further decreases, coronary artery perfusion also decreases, resulting in myocardial ischemia. While all of these changes are occurring, other organ systems are affected too. The normal functions of the liver and pancreas are affected by the low perfusion state inhibiting insulin release, which is why patients in shock have been described as being in a diabetic-like state. Gastrointestinal motility is decreased, causing stress ulcers to develop. When kidney perfusion is diminished, so is urine production; this results in kidney failure if reperfusion does not occur within a sufficient time frame.

Shock-Related Events at the Capillary and Microcirculatory Levels

As perfusion decreases, cellular ischemia occurs. Minimal blood flow passes through the capillaries, causing the cells to switch from aerobic metabolism to anaerobic metabolism (all cell processes occurring in the absence of oxygen), which can quickly result in metabolic acidosis. With reduced circulation, the blood stagnates in the capillaries. The precapillary sphincter relaxes in response to the buildup of lactic acid, vasomotor center failure, and increased amounts of carbon dioxide. The postcapillary sphincters remain constricted, causing the capillaries to become engorged with fluid.

The capillary sphincters—circular muscular walls that constrict and dilate—regulate blood flow through the capillary beds. These sphincters are under the control of the autonomic nervous system, which regulates involuntary functions such as sweating and digestion. Capillary sphincters also respond to other stimuli such as heat, cold, increased demand for oxygen, and the need for waste removal. Thus, the regulation of blood flow is determined by cellular need and is accomplished by vessel constriction or dilation, working in tandem with sphincter constriction or dilation.

The body can tolerate anaerobic metabolism for only a limited time. Anaerobic metabolism is much less efficient than aerobic metabolism and results in systemic acidosis and depletion of the body's normally high energy reserves (adenosine triphosphate [ATP]). Although hypoxia decreases the rate of ATP synthesis in cells, it will not damage the mitochondria unless it is sustained and severe. During anaerobic metabolism, incomplete glucose breakdown results in an accumulation of pyruvic acid. However, pyruvic acid cannot be converted to acetyl coenzyme A without oxygen, so it is transformed in greater amounts to lactate and other acid by-products, resulting in acidosis.

At the same time, ischemia stimulates increased carbon dioxide production by the tissues. The higher the body's metabolic rate, the higher the carbon dioxide level in hypoperfused states. The excess carbon dioxide combines with intracellular water to produce carbonic acid. Increased tissue acid levels will react with other buffers to form more intracellular acidic substances. Thus, acidosis serves as an indirect measure of tissue perfusion. The acidic condition of the blood inhibits hemoglobin in the RBCs from binding with and carrying oxygen.

Meanwhile, sodium, which is usually more abundant outside the cells than inside them, is naturally inclined to diffuse into the cells. Normally the sodium/potassium pump acts like a "bouncer" at the cell membrane, sending the sodium back out against the concentration gradient. This mechanism involves active transport and requires an ample supply of ATP to fuel the bouncer. Reduced levels of ATP, however, result in a dysfunctional sodium/potassium pump and alter the cell membrane function. Excessive sodium begins to diffuse into the cells, along with water, which ultimately depletes the interstitial compartment.

The intracellular enzymes that usually help digest and neutralize bacteria introduced into a cell are bound in a relatively impermeable membrane inside cells in structures known as lysosomes. Cellular flooding explodes the lysosomal membrane and releases these lysosomal enzymes, which then autodigest the cell. If enough cells are destroyed in this way, organ failure will become evident. The release of the lysosomes opens the floodgates for the progression of shock to the point where it may quickly be fatal and the damage irreversible.

To compound these problems, accumulating acids and waste products act as potent vasodilators, further decreasing venous return and diminishing blood flow to the vital organs and tissues. The arterial pressure falls to the point at which even the "protected organs" such as the brain and heart are no longer adequately perfused. When aortic pressures fall below an MAP of 60 mm Hg, the coronary arteries no longer fill as effectively, the heart is underperfused, and the cardiac output falls.

Eventually, the reduced blood supply to the vasomotor center in the brain results in slowing and then stopping of sympathetic nervous system activity. The metabolic wastes are released into the slower-flowing blood. The blood's sluggish flow, coupled with its acidity, results in platelet agglutination and formation of microthrombi. Because the capillary walls are stretched, they lose their ability to retain large molecules, allowing them to leak into the surrounding interstitial spaces. Hydrostatic pressure forces plasma into the interstitial spaces, further increasing the distance from the capillaries to the cells. In turn, oxygen transport decreases, further increasing cellular hypoxia.

The continuing buildup of lactic acid and carbon dioxide acts as a potent vasodilator, resulting in relaxation of the postcapillary sphincters. The accumulated hydrogen, potassium, carbon dioxide, and thrombosed (clotted) RBCs wash out into the venous circulation, increasing the metabolic acidosis. This has been referred to as the capillary washout phase. The result is an even greater decrease in cardiac output. This process ultimately results in multiple-organ dysfunction syndrome (MODS), in which various organ systems fail in succession.

In conjunction with all this injury occurring, the white blood cells and blood clotting system are impaired. There is a decreased resistance to infection, and disseminated intravascular coagulation (DIC) may occur. DIC is a serious

Words of Wisdom

Capillary hydrostatic pressure tends to force fluids through capillary walls, whereas interstitial fluid hydrostatic pressure pushes fluid back into the cells.

Oncotic pressure pulls fluids from the surrounding tissue into the capillaries as a result of a difference in the concentration of solutes in the fluid inside the capillaries. Fluid leaves the capillaries as a result of hydrostatic pressure, while albumin and other large proteins remain inside, resulting in a greater concentration of solutes inside the capillaries. The oncotic pressure increases, pulling more water into the capillaries to balance the solute concentration. If capillary hydrostatic pressure is greater, fluid will leave the capillaries. If capillary oncotic pressure is greater, fluid will be pulled into the capillaries.

disorder whereby the circulating proteins that normally control clotting become depleted and ineffective, resulting in paradoxical spontaneous uncontrolled bleeding while also causing small vessel thrombosis throughout the body, further compromising perfusion to those sites and leading to ischemic injury. Yet again, a normal function becomes activated under abnormal circumstances. DIC has also been found to complicate **septic shock**.

Words of Wisdom

Recall from Chapter 8, *Pathophysiology*, that ion concentration is altered during acidosis and alkalosis. Table 14-3 shows a reminder of increases and decreases during those states.

Buffer systems respond in the following order:

- Chemical (bicarbonate) buffer
- Respiratory system
- Renal system

Table 14-3 Acid/Base Balance

Acidosis	Alkalosis
↓ pH	↑ pH
↑ H^+	↓ H^+
↑ CO_2	↓ CO_2
↓ HCO_3^-	↑ HCO_3^-
↑ H_2CO_3	↓ H_2CO_3

Metabolic = H^+ and HCO_3^-

Respiratory = CO_2 and O_2

Abbreviations: CO_2, carbon dioxide; H^+, hydrogen ion; HCO_3^-, bicarbonate; H_2CO_3, carbonic acid; O_2, oxygen; pH, potential of hydrogen

Multiple-Organ Dysfunction Syndrome

Multiple-organ dysfunction syndrome (MODS) is a progressive condition characterized by combined failure of several organs, such as the lungs, liver, and kidney, along with some clotting mechanisms, which occurs after severe illness or injury. It is a major cause of death following septic, traumatic, and burn injuries.

MODS occurs when injury or infection (as in septic shock) triggers a massive systemic immune, inflammatory, and coagulation response, resulting in the release of numerous inflammatory mediators and activation of the following systems:

- **The complement system.** Normally, this group of plasma proteins functions to eliminate invading bacteria. In MODS, an overactive complement system induces further inflammation and damage to cells.
- **The coagulation system.** Endothelial damage and coagulation, especially in the microscopic venules and arterioles, become uncontrolled in MODS, which results in microvascular thrombus formation and tissue ischemia.
- **The kallikrein-kinin system.** The release of bradykinin, a potent vasodilator, results in tissue hypoperfusion and may contribute to hypotension.

The net outcome of overactivity in these systems is maldistribution of systemic and organ blood flow. Often, tissues attempt to compensate by accelerating their metabolism. The result is an oxygen supply-demand imbalance that leads to tissue hypoxia, tissue hypoperfusion, exhaustion of the cells' fuel supply (ATP), metabolic failure, lysosome breakdown, anaerobic metabolism, acidosis, and impaired cellular function. As MODS progresses, various organs begin to malfunction as a result of cell and tissue hypoxia.

MODS typically develops within hours to days following resuscitation. In a 14- to 21-day period, renal and liver failure can develop, along with collapse of the gastrointestinal and immune systems. If the patient does not respond to treatment of the underlying condition, cardiovascular collapse and death typically occur within days to weeks of the initial injury.

Signs and symptoms of MODS include hypotension, insufficient tissue perfusion, uncontrollable bleeding, and multisystem organ failure caused mainly by hypoxia, tissue acidosis, and severe local alterations of metabolism. Patients can have a low-grade fever from the inflammatory response and are tachycardic and dyspneic. They may prove difficult to oxygenate owing to the presence of adult respiratory distress syndrome, which is discussed in Chapter 17, *Respiratory Emergencies*.

Respiratory Insufficiency

A patient with a severe chest injury, such as flail chest, or obstruction of the airway, may be unable to breathe in an adequate amount of oxygen. This affects the ventilation process of respiration; enough oxygen cannot be inspired to meet the metabolic demand.

An insufficient concentration of oxygen in the blood can produce shock as rapidly as vascular causes, even if the volume of blood, the volume of the vessels, and the action of the heart are all normal. Without oxygen, the organs in the body cannot survive, and their cells promptly start to deteriorate.

Certain types of poisoning may affect the ability of cells to metabolize or carry oxygen. Carbon monoxide has a 200- to 250-fold greater affinity for hemoglobin than does oxygen. If a patient is in an environment where he or she inhales carbon monoxide, it will bind to the hemoglobin, forming carboxyhemoglobin, rather than allowing oxygen to bind. This results in a hypoxic state if not corrected. Cyanide impairs the ability of cells to metabolize oxygen within the cell, and cellular asphyxia may occur.

Anemia is defined as an abnormally low number of RBCs. RBCs contain hemoglobin, an iron-containing protein. Hemoglobin transports oxygen from the lungs to the tissues. Each hemoglobin molecule can carry four oxygen molecules. Anemia may be the result of either chronic or acute bleeding, a deficiency in certain vitamins or minerals, or an underlying disease process. If severe anemia is present, tissues may be hypoxic because the blood may not be able to carry adequate oxygen, even though the hemoglobin is fully saturated. In this situation, a pulse oximeter may indicate that there is adequate saturation, even though the tissues are hypoxic. This type of hypoxia is known as hypoxemic hypoxia.

Causes of Shock

Shock can result from many conditions, including bleeding, respiratory failure, acute allergic reactions, and overwhelming infection. In all cases, however, the damage occurs because of insufficient perfusion of organs and tissues. As soon as perfusion stops or becomes impaired, tissues start to die, affecting all local body processes. If the conditions causing shock are not promptly arrested and reversed, death soon follows.

You should have a high index of suspicion for shock in many emergency medical situations. For example, you would expect **hemorrhagic shock** to accompany massive external or internal bleeding. You should also expect shock if a patient has any one of the following conditions:

- Multiple severe fractures
- Abdominal or chest injury
- Spinal injury
- A severe infection
- A major heart attack (acute myocardial infarction)
- **Anaphylaxis**

Understanding the basic physiologic causes of shock will better prepare you to treat it. There are three basic causes of shock Figure 14-5.

Words of Wisdom

Shock is a complex physiologic process that gives subtle signs to its presence before it becomes severe. These early signs relate very closely to the events that result in more severe shock, so it is important for you to know the underlying processes thoroughly. If you understand what causes shock, you will be able to recognize it in many patients before it becomes out of control.

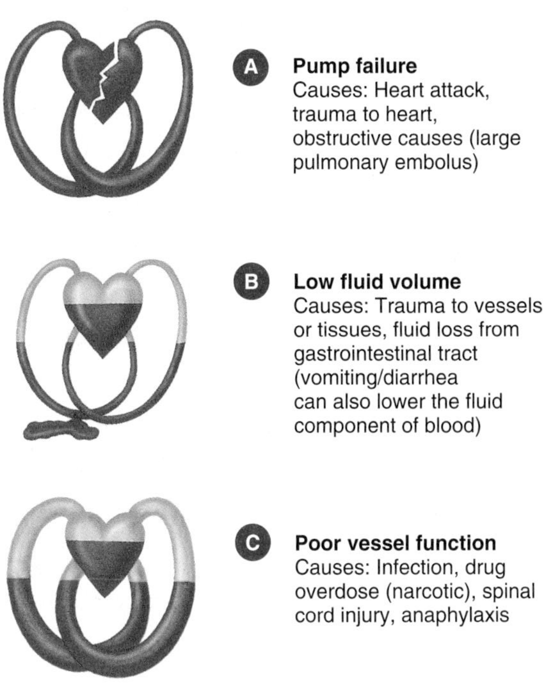

A
Pump failure
Causes: Heart attack, trauma to heart, obstructive causes (large pulmonary embolus)
B
Low fluid volume
Causes: Trauma to vessels or tissues, fluid loss from gastrointestinal tract (vomiting/diarrhea can also lower the fluid component of blood)
C
Poor vessel function
Causes: Infection, drug overdose (narcotic), spinal cord injury, anaphylaxis

Figure 14-5 There are three basic causes of shock and impaired tissue perfusion. **A.** Pump failure occurs when the heart is damaged by disease, injury, or obstructive causes. The heart may not generate enough energy to move the blood through the system. **B.** Low fluid volume, often a result of bleeding, leads to inadequate perfusion. **C.** Poor vessel function—if blood vessels dilate excessively, the blood within them, even though it is of normal volume, is inadequate to fill the system and provide efficient perfusion.

Types of Shock

Shock may be the result of a variety of causes, but hypovolemia from blood or fluid loss is a common culprit. Table 14-4 explains the differences between the types of nonhypovolemic shock and how to differentiate them from **hypovolemic shock** (shock that arises from inadequate blood volume). Specific types of shock are discussed next.

Hypovolemic Shock

When shock comes about because of inadequate blood volume, it is termed *hypovolemic shock* (*hypo* = deficient + *vol* = volume + *emia* = in the blood). There are hemorrhagic and nonhemorrhagic causes of hypovolemic shock. Volume can be lost as blood (internal or external hemorrhagic shock), plasma (burns), or electrolyte solution (vomiting, diarrhea, sweating) (nonhemorrhagic shock).

Nonhemorrhagic hypovolemic shock will be discussed in this chapter. See Chapter 27, *Bleeding*, for information on treatment of hemorrhagic shock.

Nonhemorrhagic shock occurs when the fluid loss is contained within the body, as in dehydration, burn injury, crush injury, and anaphylaxis. With severe thermal burns,

Table 14-4 Differentiating Nonhypovolemic Causes of Shock

Type	How to Differentiate
Cardiogenic shock	Differentiated from hypovolemic shock by the presence of one or more of the following: ▪ Chief complaint: chest pain, dyspnea, tachycardia ▪ Heart rate: bradycardia or excessive tachycardia ▪ Signs of heart failure: jugular vein distention, rales ▪ Dysrhythmias
Distributive shock	Differentiated from hypovolemic shock by the presence of one or more of the following: ▪ Mechanism that suggests vasodilation: spinal cord injury, drug overdose, sepsis, anaphylaxis ▪ Warm, flushed skin, especially in dependent areas ▪ Lack of tachycardic response: this is not reliable because a substantial number of hypovolemic patients never experience tachycardia.
Obstructive shock	Differentiated from hypovolemic shock by the presence of signs and symptoms suggestive of: ▪ **Cardiac tamponade** ▪ Tension pneumothorax ▪ Pulmonary embolism

for example, intravascular plasma leaks from the circulatory system into the burned tissues that are adjacent to the injury. By comparison, crushing injuries may result in the loss of blood and plasma from damaged (crushed) vessels into injured tissues.

Abnormal losses of fluids and electrolytes (dehydration) may occur through a variety of mechanisms listed as follows:

- Gastrointestinal losses, especially through vomiting and diarrhea
- Increased loss as a result of fever, hyperventilation, or high environmental temperatures (through the lungs)
- Increased and excessive sweating
- Internal losses ("third-space" losses), as in peritonitis, pancreatitis, and ileus
- Plasma losses from burns, drains, and granulating wounds

Other causes of body fluid deficits include ascites (buildup of free fluid in the abdomen), diabetes insipidus (inappropriate excretion of excess fluid from the kidneys), and osmotic diuresis secondary to hyperosmolar states (ie, diabetic ketoacidosis).

Most of the typical symptoms and signs of shock result from inadequate tissue oxygenation and the body's attempts to compensate for volume loss. The earliest signs of shock are restlessness and anxiety: the patient looks scared! The decline in tissue perfusion may not be enough to produce obvious asphyxia, but it *is* setting off alarms all over the body, to which the patient responds with a feeling of apprehension—a "gut" feeling that something is not right. If conscious, the patient may report being thirsty, reflecting the deficit of fluids in the body; at the same time, the patient may feel nauseated and even vomit. The diversion of blood flow away from low-priority peripheral tissues causes the skin to become pale, cold, and clammy; sometimes it has a mottled appearance. Meanwhile, the heart speeds up to circulate the remaining RBCs more rapidly, producing a rapid, weak pulse—rapid because the heart is beating faster, weak because the blood vessels are now narrow and the volume moving through them is decreased.

In each case, the fluid lost has a unique electrolyte composition, and long-term therapy aims to restore the deficient body chemicals. For treatment in the field, however, all excessive fluid losses can be considered to result in dehydration.

Symptoms of dehydration include loss of appetite (anorexia), nausea, vomiting, and sometimes fainting when standing up (postural syncope). Physical examination of a dehydrated patient reveals poor skin turgor (the skin over the forehead or sternum will "tent" when pinched); a shrunken, furrowed tongue; and sunken eyes. The pulse will be weak and rapid, rising more than 15 beats/min when the patient is raised from a recumbent to a sitting position (a maneuver that may cause the patient to feel faint). When fluid and electrolyte depletion are severe, shock and coma may be present.

As bleeding or fluid loss continues, the blood pressure finally falls in the shock patient. Do not wait until the blood pressure falls before you suspect shock and begin treatment! Falling blood pressure is a *late* sign in shock (decompensated shock, discussed later), signaling the collapse of all compensatory mechanisms and the fact that the patient may have already lost 30% or more fluid volume. Furthermore, the blood pressure measured at the arm provides you with little information about perfusion of vital organs; it tells only about perfusion of the arms.

Table 14-5 summarizes the signs and symptoms of hypovolemic shock.

Table 14-5	Signs and Symptoms of Hypovolemic Shock

- Mental status changes
- Rapid, weak pulse
- Thirst
- Low blood pressure (late sign)
- Cool, clammy, pale skin

The goal in treating shock is to save the brain, lungs, and kidneys; these organs must remain perfused if the patient is to survive and return to a healthy life. The best indication of brain perfusion is the patient's level of consciousness (LOC). If the patient is alert and oriented, the brain is being perfused adequately despite what the blood pressure findings show. If the patient has an altered mental status, perfusion of the brain is inadequate.

▶ Cardiogenic Shock

Cardiogenic shock is caused by inadequate function of the heart, or pump failure. Circulation of blood throughout the vascular system requires the constant pumping action of a normal and vigorous heart muscle. Many diseases or injuries can cause destruction or inflammation of this muscle. Within certain limits, the heart can adapt to these problems. However, if too much muscular damage occurs, as sometimes happens after a massive heart attack, the heart no longer functions well. A major effect is the backup of blood into the lungs. The resulting buildup of fluid within the pulmonary tissue is called pulmonary edema. **Edema** is the presence of abnormally large amounts of fluid between cells in body tissues, causing swelling of the affected area **Figure 14-6**. Pulmonary edema results in impaired ventilation, which may be manifested by an increased respiratory rate and abnormal breath sounds secondary to fluid buildup within the alveoli.

The muscular contraction of the heart moves blood through the vessels at distinct pressures. For blood to circulate efficiently throughout the entire system, there must be the right amount of pressure and an adequate number of heartbeats. For this reason, the heart has its own electrical system that initiates and regulates its beating. Disease or injury can damage or destroy this system, causing irregular and uncoordinated beats, a heart rate that is too slow (fewer than 60 beats/min), or a heart rate that is too fast (more than 100 beats/min).

Cardiogenic shock develops when the heart cannot maintain sufficient output (cardiac output) to meet the demands of the body. In general, as afterload increases, cardiac output decreases. Increased afterload may also cause the heart to overwork while trying to maintain adequate cardiac output. High afterload is often the reason that heart failure develops in patients with hypertension.

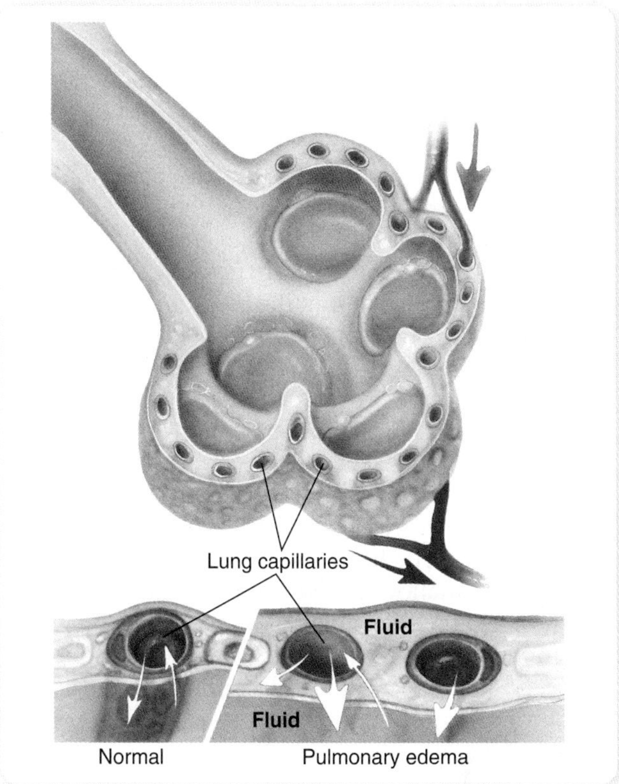

Figure 14-6 Pulmonary edema develops as a result of fluid buildup within the pulmonary tissue. The edema causes swelling and results in impaired ventilation.

Cardiogenic shock may result from low cardiac output due to high afterload, low preload, poor contractility, or any combination of the three.

▶ Obstructive Shock

Obstructive shock results when conditions that cause mechanical obstruction of the cardiac muscle also affect pump function. Three of the most common examples of obstructive shock are cardiac tamponade, tension pneumothorax, and pulmonary embolism.

Cardiac tamponade, or pericardial tamponade, occurs when blood leaks into the tough fibrous membrane known as the pericardium, causing an accumulation of blood within the pericardial sac. It is caused by blunt or penetrating trauma and can progress rapidly. This accumulation results in compression of the heart. Because the pericardium has a limited ability to stretch, each contraction of the heart allows more blood accumulation between the heart and the sac. The accumulated blood prevents the heart from opening up to allow complete refilling. Continued pressure within the pericardial sac obstructs the flow of blood into the heart, resulting in decreased outflow from the heart. Signs and symptoms of cardiac tamponade are referred to as the Beck triad, and include the presence of jugular vein distention, muffled heart sounds, and a narrowing **pulse pressure** (the difference between the systolic and diastolic pressures).

Another obstructive condition occurs with a tension pneumothorax. A tension pneumothorax is caused by damage to the lung tissue. This damage allows air normally held within the lung to escape into the chest cavity. If a pneumothorax progresses, a sufficient amount of air will accumulate within the chest cavity and begin applying pressure to the structures in the mediastinum. The primary organs in this area are the heart and great vessels (aorta, venae cavae, and pulmonary arteries and veins). When the trapped air begins to shift the chest organs toward the uninjured side, a pneumothorax becomes known as a tension pneumothorax, which is a serious and life-threatening condition. As pressure from one side of the chest begins to push the mediastinum toward the other side, the vena cava loses its ability to stay fully expanded. This mechanical compression of the vessel results in reduced return of blood to the heart. The patient becomes anxious and short of breath. The heart and respiratory rates increase and become shallower. Blood pressure decreases. You may notice difficulty when attempting to ventilate the patient with a bag-mask device. The affected side will have decreased or absent breath sounds and the patient will become cyanotic. Tracheal deviation is a late sign of tension pneumothorax.

A massive, centrally located pulmonary embolism can also result in obstructive shock. A pulmonary embolism is a blood clot that occurs in the pulmonary circulation and blocks the flow of blood through the pulmonary vessels. When a massive pulmonary embolism occurs, it can prevent blood from being pumped from the right side of the heart to the left, resulting in complete backup of blood in the right ventricle and leading to catastrophic obstructive shock and complete pump failure.

▶ Distributive Shock

Distributive shock results when there is widespread dilation of the small arterioles, small venules, or both. As a result, the circulating blood volume pools in the expanded vascular beds and tissue perfusion decreases. The four most common types of distributive shock are septic shock, **neurogenic shock**, **anaphylactic shock**, and **psychogenic shock**.

Septic Shock

Septic shock occurs as a result of severe infections, usually bacterial, in which toxins (poisons) are generated by the bacteria or by infected body tissues. In this condition, the toxins damage the vessel walls, causing increased cellular permeability. The vessel walls leak and are unable to contract well. Widespread dilation of vessels, in combination with plasma loss through the injured vessel walls, results in shock.

Septic shock is a complex problem. First, there is an insufficient volume of fluid in the container, because much of the plasma has leaked out of the vascular system (hypovolemia). Second, the fluid that has leaked out often collects in the respiratory system, interfering with ventilation. Third, the vasodilation results in a larger-than-normal vascular bed to contain the smaller-than-normal volume of intravascular fluid.

YOU are the Provider PART 2

You identify that the patient is exhibiting signs and symptoms of hypoperfusion. You partner places a nonrebreathing mask on the patient and administers oxygen at 15 L/min. You continue your primary survey and find no other life threats. While performing your secondary assessment, you note a distended abdomen that is tender to palpation. Your SAMPLE history (Signs and symptoms, Allergies, Medications, Pertinent past medical history, Last oral intake, Events leading up to the illness or injury) reveals that the patient has no allergies and has a history of hypertension and peptic ulcers. He has been unable to eat since last night and reports a "burning" pain in his epigastric region. There is no incidence of trauma or physical activity. You send your partner to retrieve the stretcher.

Recording Time: 1 Minute	
Appearance	Poor
Level of consciousness	Alert and oriented
Airway	Patent
Breathing	25 breaths/min, labored and irregular
Circulation	Cool, clammy, pale

3. Which type of shock do you suspect this patient is experiencing?
4. Which stage of shock is this patient experiencing?

Septic shock presents similarly to hemorrhagic shock in that the patient will have a weak, thready pulse; shallow, rapid respirations; and altered mental status. One major difference is that patients with septic shock often present with warm or hot skin as a result of the elevated core body temperature associated with the infection. Septic shock is almost always a complication of a serious illness, injury, or surgery.

Neurogenic Shock

Damage to the spinal cord, particularly at the upper cervical levels, may cause substantial injury to the part of the nervous system that controls the size and muscular tone of the blood vessels. Neurogenic shock is usually the result. Although not as common, there are medical causes as well. These include brain conditions, tumors, pressure on the spinal cord, and spina bifida. In neurogenic shock, the muscles in the walls of the blood vessels are cut off from the sympathetic nervous system and nerve impulses that cause them to contract. This prevents the natural catecholamine release that is seen with other types of shock resulting in the classic symptoms. As a result of the lack of sympathetic innervation, all vessels below the level of the spinal injury dilate widely, increasing the size and capacity of the vascular system and causing blood to pool **Figure 14-7**. The available 6 L of blood in the body can no longer fill the enlarged vascular system. Even though no blood or fluid has been lost, perfusion of organs and tissues becomes inadequate, and shock occurs. In this condition, a radical change in the size of the vascular system has caused shock. Characteristic signs of this type of shock are the absence of sweating below the level of injury, normal warm skin, and the lack of an elevated pulse.

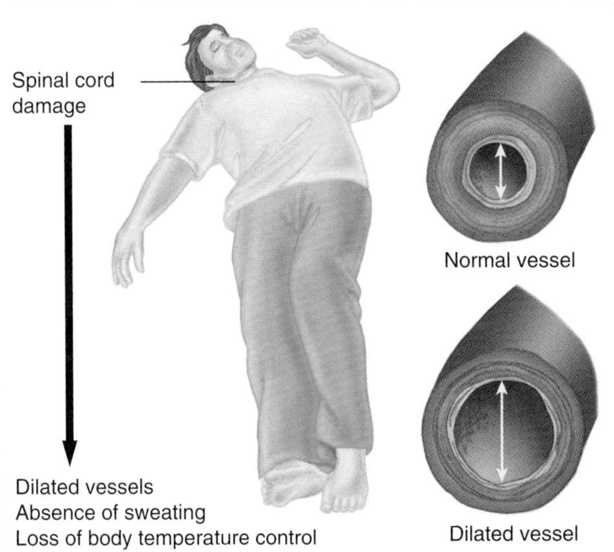

Figure 14-7 Damage to the spinal cord can result in nerves no longer being able to make the vessels contract. Instead, vessels dilate widely. The blood in the body can no longer fill the enlarged vessels; inadequate perfusion results.

Words of Wisdom

With neurogenic shock, many other functions that are under the control of the same part of the nervous system are also lost. The most important of them, in an acute injury setting, is the ability to control body temperature. Body temperature in a patient with neurogenic shock can rapidly fall to match that of the environment. In many situations, substantial hypothermia occurs, severely complicating the situation. **Hypothermia** is a condition in which the internal body temperature falls below 95°F (35°C), usually after prolonged exposure to cool or freezing temperatures. Maintenance of body temperature is always an important element of treatment for a patient in shock.

Words of Wisdom

Microcirculation is a term used to describe the small vessels in the vasculature that are embedded within organs and responsible for the distribution of blood within tissues. Capillaries are part of microcirculation. They branch off the arterioles and allow for exchange between cells and circulation. The arteriole-venule shunts are short vessels that connect the arteriole and venule at opposite sides, bypassing the capillary beds. The main functions of microcirculation include the regulation of blood flow and tissue perfusion, blood pressure, tissue fluid, delivery of oxygen, removal of carbon dioxide, and the regulation of body temperature and inflammation.

Anaphylactic Shock

Anaphylaxis, or anaphylactic shock, occurs when a person reacts violently to a substance to which he or she has been sensitized. **Sensitization** means becoming sensitive to a substance that did not initially cause a reaction. Do not be misled by a patient who reports no history of allergic reaction to a substance on first or second exposure. Each subsequent exposure after sensitization tends to produce a more severe reaction.

In anaphylactic shock, there is no loss of blood, no mechanical vascular damage, and only a slight possibility of direct cardiac muscular injury. Instead, there is widespread vascular dilation, increased permeability, and bronchoconstriction. The combination of poor oxygenation and poor perfusion in anaphylactic shock may easily prove fatal.

In anaphylaxis, immune system chemicals, such as histamine and other vasodilator proteins, are released when exposed to an allergen. Their release causes the severe bronchoconstriction that accounts for wheezing if the patient is actually moving enough air. Anaphylaxis is also accompanied by urticaria (hives). The results are widespread vasodilation, which causes distributive shock, and blood vessels that continue to leak. Fluid leaks out of the blood vessels and into the interstitial space, resulting in hypovolemia and potentially causing substantial swelling. In some cases, this swelling may occlude the upper airway, resulting in a life-threatening condition.

Instances that cause severe allergic reactions commonly fall into the following four categories of exposure:

- Injections (tetanus antitoxin, penicillin)
- Stings (honeybee, wasp, yellow jacket, hornet)
- Ingestion (shellfish, nuts, fruit, medication)
- Inhalation (dust, pollen)

Anaphylactic reactions can develop within minutes or even seconds after contact with the substance to which the patient is allergic. The signs of such allergic reactions are very distinct and not seen with other forms of shock. Signs of anaphylactic shock are summarized later in this chapter and discussed in Chapter 22, *Immunologic Emergencies*. Note that **cyanosis** (bluish color of the skin) is a late sign of anaphylactic shock.

Recurrent large areas of subcutaneous edema of sudden onset, usually disappearing within 24 hours and mainly seen in young women (frequently as a result of allergy to food or drugs), are called **angioedema**.

Psychogenic Shock

A patient in psychogenic shock has had a sudden reaction of the nervous system that produces a temporary, generalized vascular dilation, resulting in fainting, or **syncope**. Blood pools in the dilated vessels, reducing the blood supply to the brain; as a result, the brain ceases to function normally, and the patient faints. Whereas there are many causes of syncope, it is important to realize that some are of a serious nature but others are not. Causes of syncope that are potentially life-threatening result from events such as an irregular heartbeat or a brain **aneurysm**. Other non–life-threatening events that cause syncope may be the receipt of bad news or experiencing fear or unpleasant sights (such as the sight of blood).

Table 14-6 summarizes potential causes and signs and symptoms of the various types of shock.

Table 14-6 Potential Causes and Signs and Symptoms of Various Types of Shock

Type of Shock	Examples of Potential Causes	Signs and Symptoms
Cardiogenic	Inadequate heart function Disease of muscle tissue Impaired electrical system Disease or injury	Chest pain Irregular pulse Weak pulse Low blood pressure Cyanosis (lips, under nails) Cool, clammy skin Anxiety Crackles (rales) Pulmonary edema
Obstructive	Mechanical obstruction of the cardiac muscle causing a decrease in cardiac output 1. Tension pneumothorax 2. Cardiac tamponade 3. Pulmonary embolism	Dependent on cause: ▪ Dyspnea ▪ Rapid, weak pulse ▪ Rapid, shallow breaths ▪ Decreased lung compliance ▪ Unilateral, decreased, or absent breath sounds ▪ Decreased blood pressure ▪ Jugular vein distention ▪ Subcutaneous emphysema ▪ Cyanosis ▪ Tracheal deviation toward affected side ▪ Beck triad (cardiac tamponade): • Jugular vein distention • Narrowing pulse pressure • Muffled heart tones
Septic	Severe bacterial infection	Warm skin or fever Tachycardia Low blood pressure

Type of Shock	Examples of Potential Causes	Signs and Symptoms
Neurogenic	Damaged cervical spine, which causes widespread blood vessel dilation	Bradycardia (slow pulse) or normal pulse Low blood pressure Signs of neck injury
Anaphylactic	Extreme life-threatening allergic reaction	Can develop within seconds Mild itching or rash Burning skin Vascular dilation Generalized edema Coma Rapid death
Psychogenic (fainting)	Temporary, generalized vascular dilation Anxiety, bad news, sight of injury or blood, prospect of medical treatment, severe pain, illness, tiredness	Rapid pulse Normal or low blood pressure
Hypovolemic	Loss of blood or fluid	Rapid, weak pulse Low blood pressure Change in mental status Cyanosis (lips, under nails) Cool, clammy skin Increased respiratory rate
Respiratory insufficiency	Severe chest injury, airway obstruction	Rapid, weak pulse Low blood pressure Change in mental status Cyanosis (lips, under nails) Cool, clammy skin Increased respiratory rate

Words of Wisdom

Mental status is the best determinant of how well the brain and likely the other vital organs are being perfused.

Words of Wisdom

You should consider any patient exhibiting signs and symptoms of shock without obvious external injury to have probable internal bleeding, usually in the abdominal cavity.

Special Populations

When you are treating pediatric patients, remember that their bodies can compensate well until they have lost about 30% to 35% of their blood volume; then their condition declines rapidly. Their ability to compensate relies on an increasing pulse rate and SVR. These measures cause the body to rapidly burn glucose. Unfortunately, children have little stored glucose.

Pediatric patients compensate through vasoconstriction and increased peripheral vascular resistance, but this is not enough to perfuse the brain, heart, and lungs to stay alive. Blood pressure may be the last measurable factor to change in shock. By the time you detect a decrease in blood pressure, shock is well developed. This is particularly true in infants and children, who can maintain their blood pressure until they have lost more than one-half of their blood volume. By the time blood pressure decreases in infants and children who are in shock, they are close to death. *Never* wait to see a decrease in the systolic blood pressure to aggressively manage a child you suspect may be in the early phase of shock.

Treat pediatric patients aggressively and early if there is any indication of developing shock. Provide oxygen, manage the body temperature, place the patient in the appropriate position, and initiate intravenous (IV) access en route to the appropriate facility. See Chapter 36, *Pediatric Emergencies*, for more information on shock in pediatric patients.

The Progression of Shock

Shock occurs in two successive stages—compensated and decompensated. Although you cannot see shock, you can see its signs and symptoms Table 14-7. The early stage of shock, while the body can still compensate for blood loss, is called **compensated shock** (nonprogressive shock). The late stage, when blood pressure is falling, is called **decompensated shock** (progressive shock).

Words of Wisdom

Your goal as an AEMT is to recognize the signs of the early stages of shock and begin immediate treatment before permanent damage occurs. To accomplish this, you must be aware of the subtle signs exhibited in compensated shock and treat the patient aggressively. Anticipate the potential for shock from the scene size-up. Recognize the signs of poor perfusion that precede hypotension, and do not rely on any one sign or symptom to determine the degree of shock. Always err on the side of caution when treating a potential shock patient. Rapid assessment and immediate transportation are essential to minimize organ damage and to preserve any chance of patient survival.

Sometimes the term **irreversible shock** is used to describe shock that has progressed to a terminal stage.[2] In this case, even if the cause of shock is treated and reversed, vital organ damage may be permanent, and the patient may eventually die.

Compensated Shock

Compensated shock is the earliest stage of shock. At this stage, the level of responsiveness is a better indicator of tissue perfusion than most other vital signs. Release of chemical mediators by the autonomic nervous system as it recognizes a potential catastrophic event causes the arterial blood pressure to remain normal or slightly elevated. There is an increase in the rate and depth of respirations to bring in more oxygen and remove more carbon dioxide. This helps to maintain the acid-base balance by creating respiratory alkalosis to offset the metabolic acidosis.

At this stage, the blood pressure is maintained. There is a narrowing of the pulse pressure, which is the difference between the systolic and diastolic pressures.

$$\text{Pulse pressure} = \text{Systolic pressure} - \text{Diastolic pressure}$$

The pulse pressure reflects the tone of the arterial system and is more sensitive to changes in perfusion than the systolic or diastolic blood pressure alone. Patients in the compensated stage may have positive **orthostatic vital signs**

YOU are the Provider — PART 3

You assess the patient's vital signs. He has absent radial pulses and you note that his carotid pulse is rapid. A decision is made to establish an IV line and initiate fluid resuscitation based on his blood pressure, skin condition, and the absence of radial pulses. You insert an 18-gauge catheter in the patient's right antecubital fossa and initiate a bolus of normal saline, monitoring carefully for a return of radial pulses. While you are transferring the patient to the stretcher, he reports severe dizziness and has a brief syncopal episode. You and your partner quickly place the patient in the ambulance and begin rapid transport to the closest emergency department (ED).

Recording Time: 8 Minutes	
Respirations	26 breaths/min, irregular
Pulse	160 beats/min, regular
Skin	Clammy, cool, pale
Blood pressure	72/40 mm Hg
Oxygen saturation (Spo_2)	98% on 15 L/min
Pupils	Pupils Equal, Round, and Reactive to Light and Accommodation (PERRLA)

5. How much IV fluid should this patient receive?
6. How should the patient be positioned on the stretcher for transport?

Table 14-7 Progression of Shock	
Stage	**Signs and Symptoms**
Compensated shock	▪ Agitation, anxiety, restlessness ▪ Sense of impending doom ▪ Weak, rapid (thready) pulse ▪ Clammy (cool, moist) skin ▪ Pallor, with cyanotic lips ▪ Shortness of breath ▪ Nausea, vomiting ▪ Delayed capillary refill in infants and children ▪ Thirst ▪ Narrowing pulse pressure
Decompensated (progressive) shock	▪ Altered mental status (verbal to unresponsive)[a] ▪ Hypotension (systolic blood pressure of 90 mm Hg or lower in an adult) ▪ Narrowing of the pulse pressure, indicating impairment of circulation ▪ Labored or irregular breathing ▪ Thready or absent peripheral pulses ▪ Additional increase in pulse and respirations ▪ Ashen, mottled, or cyanotic skin ▪ Dull eyes, dilated pupils ▪ Diminished urine output ▪ Diaphoresis ▪ Thirst (the body's call for increased volume) ▪ Decreased capillary refill time ▪ Dry mucosa ▪ Nausea and vomiting (caused by shunting of blood from abdominal organs)
Irreversible shock	▪ Marked decrease in level of responsiveness (Glasgow Coma Scale score <7) ▪ Decreased respiratory rate and effort ▪ Inability to palpate a pulse ▪ Decrease in pulse rate ▪ Profound hypotension ▪ Impending cardiac arrest ▪ Appears moribund or dead

[a]Mental status changes are late indicators.

(an increase in pulse rate and decrease in systolic blood pressure when changing from a supine position to a sitting or standing position, which is commonly seen with dehydration). Treatment at this stage will typically result in recovery.

▶ Decompensated Shock

The next stage, decompensated shock, is when blood pressure is falling; blood volume decreases more than 30%. The compensatory mechanisms are beginning to fail, and signs and symptoms are much more obvious. Cardiac output falls dramatically, resulting in further reductions in blood pressure and cardiac function. The signs and symptoms become more obvious as blood is shunted to the brain, heart, lungs, and kidneys. At this point, vasoconstriction can have a disastrous effect if allowed to continue. Cells in the nonperfused tissues become hypoxic, resulting in anaerobic metabolism. Treatment at this stage will sometimes result in recovery.

Special Populations

You must use caution when caring for geriatric patients. As a result of the aging process, older patients generally have more serious complications than younger patients. Although illness is a common problem among the geriatric population, you must understand that it is not just part of aging. When treating these patients, keep in mind the following physiologic changes that accompany the aging process:

- The central nervous system often has a delayed response.
- The cardiovascular system has a variety of changes that result in a decrease in the efficiency of the system. On assessment, be alert for higher resting heart rates and irregular pulse rates.
- The respiratory system undergoes substantial changes as the elasticity of the lungs and their size and strength decrease. On assessment, be alert for higher respiratory rates, lower tidal volume, and a decreased gag reflex. In addition, you must remember that cervical arthritis may be present and that dentures may cause an airway obstruction.
- The skin becomes thinner, drier, less elastic, and more fragile, thus providing less protection and thermal regulation (cold and hot).
- The renal system decreases in function and may not respond well to unusual demands such as illness.
- The gastrointestinal system sustains changes in gastric motility that may result in slower gastric emptying.

Along with the normal physiologic changes associated with aging, it is important to remember that medications may interfere with normal coping mechanisms and the patient may not exhibit the same signs and symptoms of shock as another patient. Beta blockers and calcium channel blockers are common medications used for hypertension and cardiac conditions that may prevent compensation.

Irreversible Shock

In what is sometimes called the irreversible stage, arterial blood pressure is abnormally low. A rapid deterioration of the cardiovascular system occurs that cannot be reversed by compensatory mechanisms or medical interventions. There are life-threatening reductions in cardiac output, blood pressure, and tissue perfusion. Blood is shunted away from the liver, kidneys, and lungs to keep the heart and brain perfused. Cells begin to die, and, even if the cause of shock is treated and reversed, vital organ damage cannot be repaired, and the patient may eventually die. The distinction between decompensated shock and irreversible shock is made based on the failure of the shock state to reverse with appropriate treatment including surgical intervention if appropriate and intensive care management. It is not possible to distinguish irreversible shock from severe decompensated shock in the prehospital environment.

Patient Assessment

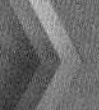

Scene Size-up

As you approach the scene, be alert to potential hazards to your safety. Once on scene, look for and address hazards and threats to the safety of the crew, bystanders, and the patient. If this is a trauma scene or bleeding is suspected, put on gloves and eye protection, at a minimum. Put several pairs of gloves in your pocket for easy access in case your gloves tear or there are multiple patients with bleeding.

Safety

When you are caring for a bleeding patient or a patient with severe vomiting or diarrhea, be sure to take necessary precautions to protect yourself from splashing or splattering. Wear appropriate protective equipment including gloves, gown, mask, and eye protection. This is especially essential when arterial bleeding is present. Also remember that frequent, thorough handwashing between patients and after every call is a simple yet important protective measure.

Words of Wisdom

When you first visualize your patient, quickly form an initial general impression. This includes age, sex, signs of distress, obvious life-threatening injuries, abnormal positioning, and skin color. These observations will help you develop an early sense of urgency for care of a patient who appears "sick."

When you first see the patient, observe the scene and patient for clues to determine the nature of the illness or the mechanism of injury. This could help you anticipate the potential for development of shock. Remember that the more traumatic injuries a patient has sustained, the less likely the patient will be able to compensate.

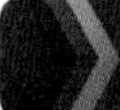

Primary Survey

The primary survey for a patient with suspected shock should include a rapid full-body scan of the patient to determine LOC, identify and manage life-threatening concerns, and determine priority of the patient and transport. Threats to circulation, airway, or breathing are considered life threatening and must be treated *immediately* to prevent mortality.

Life-threatening bleeding should be treated first. A patient with massive hemorrhage may require a tourniquet (or direct pressure dressings when tourniquets are not feasible or available) prior to opening the airway. When possible, direct another rescuer to control bleeding and continue your assessment of the airway and breathing, Treatment of shock should begin as quickly as possible once initial life threats are addressed. Such treatment includes administering high-flow oxygen to assist in perfusion of damaged tissues. Also, early in your assessment, determine the need for manual spinal immobilization.

After addressing life-threatening bleeding, quickly assess the airway to ensure it is patent. If the patient is awake and answering questions, the airway is patent. Be alert to abnormal airway sounds such as gurgling (suction the airway) or stridor, indicating partial airway obstruction. Consider an adjunct such as an oropharyngeal or nasopharyngeal airway combined with assisted ventilations for a patient with airway impairment and inadequate ventilations.

Quickly assess the patient's breathing. Observe the patient for signs of accessory muscle use such as the muscles of the neck, intercostal retractions, or abnormal use of the abdominal muscles. An increased respiratory rate is often an early sign of impending shock. Assess the patient's breath sounds with a stethoscope, listening for wheezes or other abnormal breath sounds.

Assessing the patient's circulatory status can reveal important clues regarding the presence of shock. Check for the presence of a distal pulse. If you cannot obtain a distal pulse, assess for a central pulse. If the patient has no pulse and is not breathing, immediately begin cardiopulmonary resuscitation (CPR). Quickly determine if the pulse is fast, slow, weak, strong, or altogether absent. A rapid pulse suggests compensated shock. In shock or compensated shock, the skin may be cool, clammy, or ashen. Assess skin temperature, condition, and color; also check for capillary refill time. Maintain a high index of suspicion for occult injuries, especially when the patient is exhibiting signs of shock with no obvious cause.

If the patient shows signs of hypoperfusion, gain IV access, treat aggressively, and provide rapid transport to the closest, most appropriate facility. Request paramedic backup as necessary to assist with more aggressive shock management.

Sometimes, local protocols dictate that a patient should be transported to the nearest hospital for stabilization prior to transfer to a definitive treatment center. If travel time is lengthy, air medical transportation may be the best option. Rapid transport to an appropriate facility without unnecessary scene delays is imperative. Administer fluid en route. Do not delay transport to complete non–life-saving treatments such as splinting extremity fractures; instead, perform these treatments en route.

Also provide psychological support en route. Even unresponsive patients can sometimes hear and understand. Remember to speak calmly and reassuringly to the patient throughout assessment, care, and transport.

Words of Wisdom

For the patient exhibiting signs of a tension pneumothorax, needle chest decompression (performed in-hospital or by paramedics) is necessary to improve cardiac output. In cases of suspected cardiac tamponade, you must recognize the need for expeditious transport for pericardiocentesis at the ED. Either of these conditions further impairs circulation by compression of the heart and decreasing cardiac output.

History Taking

After the life threats have been managed during the primary survey, determine the chief complaint. You should obtain a medical history and be alert for injury-specific signs and symptoms that might cause you to look for evidence of trauma as an etiology for the patient's complaints as well as any pertinent negatives such as loss of sensation.

Quickly obtain a SAMPLE history from the patient. Remember, if the patient experiences a substantial change in LOC before arrival at the hospital, you should provide the hospital personnel with this important information. Note that patients taking beta blockers or calcium channel blockers are less able to compensate for hypoperfusion or early shock because their vessels do not vasoconstrict as well as a result of the medication they are taking. Also, blood thinners can make bleeding injuries considerably worse.

Secondary Assessment

Begin the secondary assessment by repeating the primary survey to identify injuries not yet found, then follow with a focused assessment. In some instances, such as a critically injured or ill patient or short transport time, you may not have time to conduct a secondary assessment.

If substantial trauma has likely affected multiple systems, start with a full-body exam to be sure that you have identified all injuries.

If your patient is one who gives you a poor general impression, is not responsive, or if you found problems in the primary survey, perform a rapid full-body scan. These scans should be performed quickly but thoroughly to ensure that you do not miss any substantial or life-threatening problems or delay needed care.

Whether your examination is rapid or focused, if a life-threatening problem is found, treat it immediately.

When time permits and the patient's condition is stable, perform a thorough examination of the patient. This includes a complete neurologic assessment.

Obtain a complete set of baseline vital signs. If the patient's condition is unstable or could become unstable, reassess vital signs every 5 minutes. If the patient is in stable condition, reassess vital signs every 10 to 15 minutes. Baseline vital signs will help you track changes in your patient that correlate to the progression of shock.

In addition to hands-on assessment, you should use monitoring devices to quantify the patient's oxygenation and circulatory status. Use a pulse oximeter to evaluate the effectiveness of oxygenation. Use a manual technique to monitor blood pressure first (a sphygmomanometer and stethoscope), before using a noninvasive blood pressure monitor. Use a glucometer to monitor blood glucose levels.

Words of Wisdom

Just as they make for thorough written reporting, taking and recording frequent vital signs—and observing perfusion indicators such as skin condition and mental status—will give you a window into the progression of shock in your patient. Use your documentation to remind you to suspect shock early and treat it aggressively.

Reassessment

Reassessment is extremely important in patient care. The rule of thumb is assess—intervene—reassess. This portion of the assessment revisits the primary survey, the vital signs, the chief complaint, and any treatment performed on the patient, including oxygen administration. You must assess the patient to determine whether the interventions you performed are having any effect on the patient. This step prepares you to present the patient at the hospital with a complete, concise account of the patient encounter and care.

You must determine what interventions are needed for your patient at this point based on the findings of your assessment. Focus on supporting the cardiovascular system. Treating for shock early and aggressively will help to prevent inadequate perfusion from harming your patient. Specific interventions are discussed in the emergency medical care section later in this chapter.

Special Populations

In older patients, dizziness, syncope, or weakness may be the first sign of nontraumatic internal hemorrhage or cardiac dysrhythmias.

Patients who are in decompensated shock will need rapid interventions to restore adequate perfusion. The hospital may or may not have suggestions on how best to support a patient's failing cardiovascular system. Most of the interventions used to treat shock do not require a specific physician's order; however, some do. Determine, based on the signs and symptoms found in your assessment, whether your patient is in compensated or decompensated shock. Document these findings after you have treated for shock.

Emergency Medical Care for Shock

As mentioned, much of your treatment for shock will begin during the assessment process as soon as you discover life threats and realize shock may be present. Key interventions are addressing life-threatening bleeding, and airway and breathing concerns.

Control all obvious external bleeding by the methods discussed in Chapter 27, *Bleeding*. These include placing dry, sterile dressings over the bleeding sites, securing with bandages, and applying a tourniquet if direct pressure does not rapidly control bleeding from an extremity.

Another key intervention is placing the patient in the position dictated by local protocol for shock patients. This will usually be a supine position. Some patients may find it easier to breathe in a sitting or semisitting position. If spinal immobilization is indicated, splint the patient on a backboard.

Further key interventions are to provide warmth, gain IV access, and administer fluid as needed based on patient presentation. To prevent the loss of body heat, place blankets under and over the patient. Be careful not to overload the patient with covers or attempt to warm the body too much; it is best for the patient to maintain a normal body temperature. Do not use external heat

YOU are the Provider — PART 4

En route, you reassess the patient's vital signs and note that the radial pulse is barely palpable and the carotid pulse has increased slightly. His skin continues to be pale and diaphoretic. You elect to give a second bolus and to establish a second peripheral IV line in the left arm and administer normal saline at a to-keep-open (TKO) rate. You also note that the patient's abdomen is becoming more distended and rigid during the transport. His Glasgow Coma Scale score is evaluated at a 10. In anticipation of further deterioration, you prepare the bag-mask device. You notify the receiving hospital of the patient's condition and your arrival of 10 minutes. While preparing additional equipment that you may need, you arrive at the ED. No further changes are noted on arrival at the hospital.

Recording Time: 16 Minutes	
Respirations	26 breaths/min
Pulse	164 beats/min
Skin	Cool, pale, and clammy
Blood pressure	68/P
Oxygen saturation (Spo_2)	99% on 15 L/min
Pupils	PERRLA

7. Did this patient require a second IV line?

Words of Wisdom

Take care when placing all potential shock patients in a completely supine position. Although this may help temporarily increase perfusion in some shock patients, it may have detrimental effects in others. In patients with chest injuries or difficulty breathing due to heart failure with cardiogenic shock (pump failure), this position may worsen symptoms. In patients with head injury, it may cause a detrimental increase in intracranial pressure. In these instances, consider elevating the head of the long backboard for patients who are fully immobilized to reduce pressure in the head and chest. As always, follow your local protocols or consult medical control.

sources, such as hot water bottles or heating pads. They may harm a patient in shock by causing vasodilation and decreasing blood pressure even more.

Transport the patient and treat additional problems en route. Consider rendezvousing with paramedics if possible, and consider aeromedical transport. The Golden Hour refers to the first 60 minutes after injury, which is thought to be a critically important period. Since this time frame varies (more than an hour in some patients, less in others), the concept is often referred to as the Golden Period for the early resuscitation and treatment of severely injured trauma patients. This concept underscores the importance of rapid evaluation, stabilization, and transport. The goal of emergency medical services (EMS) is to limit on-scene time (time on scene until transport to hospital is started) to 10 minutes or less (the platinum 10).

If time allows, splint individual extremity fractures during transport. This minimizes pain, bleeding, and discomfort, all of which can aggravate shock. It also prevents the broken bone ends from further damaging adjacent soft tissue.

Do not give the patient anything by mouth, no matter how urgently you are asked. To relieve the intense thirst that often accompanies shock, give the patient a moistened piece of gauze to chew or suck. Never give a patient in shock an alcoholic drink or other depressant. A stimulant, such as coffee, also has no role in treating shock.

Finally, comfort, calm, and reassure the patient; speak calmly and reassuringly to a responsive patient throughout assessment, care, and transport.

The following list summarizes initial management for shock:

1. Manage the airway.
2. Administer supplemental oxygen to all patients with trauma, and to patients who are in respiratory distress or who have an Spo_2 of less than 94%.
3. Place the patient in a position of comfort.
4. Obtain vital signs, including Spo_2 and glucose level.
5. Obtain IV/intraosseous access for medication or fluid bolus.
6. Maintain body heat.

Words of Wisdom

You are never wrong to treat for shock, and many patients will experience some degree of shock even if signs and symptoms are minimal. Consider whether or not you need to treat for shock for each patient you encounter.

Table 14-8 lists the general supportive measures for the major types of shock. Not every measure is used for every type of shock.

Special Populations

Treatment for a pediatric or geriatric patient in shock is no different than treatment of any other shock patient. However, remember that the very young and the very old compensate differently, so you must maintain a high index of suspicion and treat aggressively.

▶ IV Therapy

IV lines are inserted for one of three purposes: (1) to provide a route for *immediate replacement* of fluid in patients who have already lost substantial volumes of fluid or blood, (2) to provide a route for *potential replacement* in patients who are at risk of losing substantial volumes of fluid or blood, and (3) to provide a route for the administration of medication. The IV fluid of choice is an isotonic crystalloid such as normal saline or lactated Ringer solution.

Specifically, all patients in hypovolemic shock need IV fluid replacement. In addition, IV access should be obtained in patients who are likely to develop hypovolemic shock due to loss of blood (internal or external), fluid (vomiting, diarrhea, burns), or because of widespread vasodilation.

In case of need for emergency administration of medications, IV lines should also be inserted TKO. When a patient has poor cardiac output (as in shock), blood is shunted away from the skin and skeletal muscles. Therefore, medications administered subcutaneously or intramuscularly are absorbed at a low and unpredictable rate. Administering a medication directly into the vein ensures that the desired dose of the drug reaches the circulation. Patients who need a vein TKO include those at risk of cardiac arrest (it is easier to start the IV line before the arrest) and patients who may need parenteral

Table 14-8 Shock Treatment

Type of Shock	Treatment
Hypovolemic	Manage the airway Administer oxygen or assist ventilations as needed Control external bleeding Place supine Keep warm Transport promptly Gain IV access; provide fluid resuscitation en route
Cardiogenic	Place patient in a position of comfort Administer oxygen or assist ventilations as needed Transport promptly Gain IV access; administer fluid at a TKO rate
Obstructive	Dependent on cause: ▪ Paramedic assist and/or rapid transport ▪ Administer oxygen or assist ventilations as needed ▪ Gain IV access as a medication route; administer fluid at a TKO rate
Septic	Transport promptly Administer high-flow oxygen or assist ventilations as needed Keep patient warm Gain IV access en route; administer fluid boluses to maintain radial pulses
Neurogenic	Manage the airway Spinal immobilization Administer oxygen or assist ventilations as needed Preserve body heat Transport promptly Gain IV access; administer warmed IV fluids to maintain radial pulses
Anaphylactic	Manage the airway Administer oxygen or assist ventilations as needed Determine cause Assist with administration of epinephrine Gain IV access as a medication route; administer fluid at a TKO rate Transport promptly
Psychogenic (fainting)	Determine duration of unresponsiveness Position patient supine Record initial vital signs and mental status Suspect head injury if patient is confused or slow to respond Transport promptly
Respiratory insufficiency	Manage the airway Administer high-flow oxygen or assist ventilations as needed Seal hole in chest Stabilize impaled objects Transport promptly Gain IV access en route; administer fluid at a TKO rate

Abbreviations: IV, intravenous; TKO, to keep open

medication (such as patients with seizures, diabetes, heart failure, or coma).

Techniques for vascular access were discussed in Chapter 13, *Vascular Access and Medication Administration*. Establish IV access with at least one 18-gauge catheter or larger, and administer an isotonic crystalloid solution to replace fluid loss. The goal of volume replacement is to maintain perfusion without increasing hemorrhage or overloading a strained heart. Therefore, most protocols advise administration of IV fluid in boluses of 20 mL/kg up to 30 mL/kg in 250- to 500-mL increments until radial pulses return. The presence of radial pulses is thought to equate to a systolic blood pressure of approximately 80 to 90 mm Hg, which, in most people, is sufficient to perfuse the brain and other vital organs. This belief has been contested in recent studies.[3] Raising blood pressure further may result in worsening cardiac failure or internal hemorrhage. Monitor the patient's response to IV therapy carefully and document any changes.

If vital signs return to within normal limits, or reach the desired status, slow IV fluid administration to a TKO rate and reassess frequently, adjusting the flow as needed. If the patient's response to initial treatment shows no improvement or slow deterioration, there may be ongoing bleeding or fluid loss. Maintain the patient's blood pressure around 90 mm Hg systolic (maintain radial pulses), depending on local protocol.

Call early for paramedic intervention to administer vasopressors if needed. The vasodilation that accompanies distributive shock creates relative hypovolemia. Regardless of the cause, the problem is still a lack of fluid for the size of the container.

Words of Wisdom

Using larger-diameter and shorter-length catheters results in greater fluid flow. Choose a catheter that is size 18-gauge or larger and which is no longer than 1 to 1.5 inches. For maximum volume infusion, use a blood set or macrodrip set (10 to 15 drops/min) without a saline lock that restricts flow. Administer a bolus of 250 mL of an isotonic crystalloid solution. A second 18-gauge IV line may be established when it is safe to do so and time allows, but this is not necessary to initiate effective resuscitation.

▶ Special Considerations in Fluid Resuscitation

For instances where increasing blood pressure may be detrimental to the patient, such as cardiogenic shock or massive internal bleeding, it may be necessary to administer only enough fluid to maintain radial pulses. Aggressive fluid therapy increases the workload on the heart, worsening cardiogenic shock and increasing internal bleeding by breaking up clots that are forming or increasing the pressure in the vessels.

Temperature control is vital to maintaining perfusion in children and infants. If fluid replacement is required and IV access cannot be obtained, consider using intraosseous infusion. Use a Broselow tape or other reference to remember normal vital signs by age. Infuse a 20-mL/kg bolus of a warmed isotonic crystalloid solution, considering a second infusion if there is no response to the first. While administering fluids, it is imperative to remember that a patient who has lost blood needs to replace RBCs. Carefully monitor patient status and treat conservatively in instances of uncontrolled hemorrhage. Use a continuous infusion to maintain adequate perfusion levels of critical organs en route to the hospital. A third infusion of 20 mL/kg may be considered after medical consultation.

Geriatric patients can present a challenge when providing IV therapy in instances of shock. Patients who have chronic hypertension may require a higher blood pressure to achieve the same level of end-organ perfusion than those who maintain a normal blood pressure. The geriatric patient may be in shock and his or her systolic blood pressure may be above 100 mm Hg. Even modest amounts of fluid loss can be detrimental and result in shock in these patients because of a reduced circulating blood volume. Geriatric patients may also be less able to tolerate excessive fluids that may cause harmful electrolyte alterations. Anemia may be yet another complication because aggressive fluid resuscitation may further reduce the relative concentrations of RBCs. For these patients, rapid transport is essential.

When you are treating obstetric patients, it is imperative to remember that there are two patients involved: the pregnant woman and the fetus. Because states of shock result in shunting of blood away from the fetus, the only way to maintain fetal perfusion is to aggressively treat the woman. Remember to place pregnant patients in a left lateral recumbent position, or tilt the backboard if the patient is immobilized, to increase perfusion. Provide fluid resuscitation to maintain radial pulses of the mother. The closer the maternal blood pressure is to normal, the better the perfusion of the fetus.

Assessment and Management of Specific Types of Shock

▶ Treating Hypovolemic Shock

The emergency treatment of hypovolemic shock or hemorrhagic shock includes control of all obvious external bleeding. If bleeding is not controlled with direct pressure, consider use of a tourniquet, as discussed in Chapter 27, *Bleeding*.

En route to the ED, establish at least one 18-gauge or larger peripheral IV line using an over-the-needle catheter. Unless local medical policy favors a different resuscitation fluid, administer normal saline or lactated Ringer solution in an initial bolus of 250 mL. For guidance, refer to your local protocol. Then reassess the patient to see the effect of the intervention. Use warmed fluids when available.

Although you cannot control internal bleeding in the field, you must recognize its existence and provide aggressive general support. Secure and maintain an airway and provide respiratory support, including supplemental oxygen and, if needed, assisted ventilations. Administer oxygen as soon as you suspect shock, and continue providing it during transport; with too little circulating blood, additional oxygen may be lifesaving. Be sure the patient does not aspirate blood or vomitus; keep suction at hand to clear the mouth and pharynx

Words of Wisdom

Introducing large quantities of IV fluid may exacerbate internal bleeding. Give fluid judiciously and only enough to maintain palpable radial pulses. This equates to a systolic blood pressure of 80 to 90 mm Hg.

Do not give the patient anything by mouth because he or she is likely to vomit. Keep the patient at normal temperature, covering the patient with a blanket and warming the patient compartment of the ambulance—patients in hypovolemic shock are often unable to conserve body heat effectively and are easily chilled.

Monitor the patient's mental status, pulse rate, blood pressure, Spo_2, and if required by your system, end-tidal carbon dioxide ($ETCO_2$). (However, $ETCO_2$ does not provide additional actionable information on hypovolemic shock.) In a patient with substantial vasoconstriction, the blood pressure sounds may be difficult to hear, especially under field conditions. If you can feel a pulse over the femoral artery, but not over the radial artery, the systolic blood pressure is most likely between 70 and 80 mm Hg. The pulse oximetry and $ETCO_2$ findings will help you assess adequacy of oxygenation efforts. Monitoring $ETCO_2$, if available, can help you assess adequacy of ventilation and the potential need for ventilatory assistance.

Provide rapid transport to the closest, most appropriate facility. Consider calling for paramedic backup for advanced treatment or air transport when time is of the essence and the distance to definitive care is substantial.

▶ Treating Cardiogenic Shock

The patient who is in cardiogenic shock as a result of a heart attack does not need excess fluid. This can actually be detrimental to the patient. The damaged heart muscle simply cannot generate the necessary power to pump blood throughout the circulatory system.

Keep in mind that chronic lung disease will aggravate cardiogenic shock. If the patient has chronic obstructive pulmonary disease and heart disease, oxygenation of the blood passing through the lungs is impaired. Because fluid is collecting in the lungs, this patient is often able to breathe better in a sitting or slightly reclining upright position. Usually, patients with cardiogenic shock do not have any injury, but they may be having chest pain as a result of ischemia from lack of perfusion. Before administering nitroglycerin to any patient with the potential for cardiogenic shock, be sure systolic blood pressure is greater than 90 mm Hg and consult with medical control for instructions. Assess the patient's blood pressure, and gain IV access prior to nitroglycerin administration. Patients in cardiogenic shock are often already hypotensive. Administration of nitroglycerin will only exacerbate the problem and most likely have detrimental effects. Other signs of cardiogenic shock include a weak, irregular pulse, cyanosis about the lips and underneath the fingernails, anxiety, and nausea.

Treatment of cardiogenic shock should begin by placing the patient in a position of comfort and administering high-flow oxygen. Be ready to assist ventilations as necessary, and have suction nearby in case the patient vomits. Provide prompt transport to the ED. Gain IV access and administer fluid at a TKO rate. Remember also to approach a patient who has had a suspected heart attack with calm reassurance. Frequently checking for a pulse in an unresponsive patient is important to identify early whether an automated external defibrillator is needed.

▶ Treating Obstructive Shock

As discussed previously, three of the most common examples of obstructive shock are pulmonary embolus, cardiac tamponade and tension pneumothorax.

Increasing cardiac output should be the priority in treating cardiac tamponade. As the heart is being squeezed by the increasing pressure in the pericardium, the preload must be increased. Apply high-flow oxygen. Oxygen should never be withheld from a patient who needs it; however, you must weigh the need for positive pressure ventilations against the possibility of hypoventilation. The only definitive treatment for cardiac tamponade is surgery or pericardiocentesis (inserting a needle into the pericardium and withdrawing the accumulated blood from the pericardial sac). Because neither of these is performed in the field, the only treatment available to prehospital providers is early recognition and rapid transport for definitive care.

In treating tension pneumothorax, high-flow oxygen via a nonrebreathing mask should be applied early to prevent hypoxia. Be cautious about providing positive pressure ventilation to a patient with a tension pneumothorax because the increase of air will increase the pressure in the chest. Usually, the only action that can prevent eventual death from a tension pneumothorax is decompression of the injured side of the chest, relieving the pressure in the chest and allowing the heart to expand fully again. Needle chest decompression (needle thoracostomy) is a skill that paramedics are trained to perform. Rapid transport or paramedic backup, if available, is the key treatment available to AEMT providers. In patients with tension pneumothorax, gain IV access as a medication route and administer fluid at a TKO rate.

In treating pulmonary embolus in the prehospital setting, assess blood pressure; provide a fluid bolus of 250 mL of crystalloid solution; and recheck blood pressure. Multiple boluses may be indicated if you are unable to restore blood pressure to greater than 90 mm Hg systolic.

The patient may breathe more comfortably in an upright or partially upright position. Definitive treatment involves anticoagulation to prevent progression, ventilatory and circulatory support, and occasionally thrombolytic therapy or clot retrieval. None of these is possible in the prehospital setting, so rapid transport to an appropriate facility is indicated.

▶ Treating Septic Shock

The proper treatment of septic shock requires complex hospital management, including antibiotics. If you suspect that a patient has septic shock, you must use appropriate standard precautions and transport as promptly as possible. Use high-flow oxygen during transport. Ventilatory support may be necessary to maintain adequate tidal volume. Use blankets to conserve body heat. Gain IV access en route and administer fluid boluses to maintain radial pulses.

▶ Treating Neurogenic Shock

Shock that accompanies spinal cord injury is best treated by a combination of all known supportive measures. The patient who has sustained this kind of injury usually will require hospitalization for a long time. Emergency treatment must be directed at obtaining and maintaining a proper airway, providing spinal immobilization, assisting inadequate breathing as needed, conserving body heat, and providing the most effective circulation possible.

This patient usually is not losing blood. However, the capacity of his or her blood vessels has become substantially greater than the volume of blood these vessels contain. Supplemental oxygen will boost the concentration of oxygen in the blood. If respirations are weak or inadequate, provide assisted ventilations. Keep the patient as warm as possible with blankets, because the injury may have disabled the body's normal temperature controls. Gain IV access and administer warmed IV fluids to maintain radial pulses. Transport promptly.

▶ Treating Anaphylactic Shock

The only truly effective prehospital treatment for a severe, acute allergic reaction is to administer epinephrine by way of subcutaneous or intramuscular injection. For more information on the emergency care for allergic reactions, see Chapter 22, *Immunologic Emergencies*. A patient who is aware of having a specific sensitivity may carry a bee-sting kit containing epinephrine **Figure 14-8**. If he or she is unable to inject the medication, you may have to do so if you are allowed by local protocol. If the patient's signs and symptoms recur or the patient's condition deteriorates, you should repeat the injection after consulting with medical control.

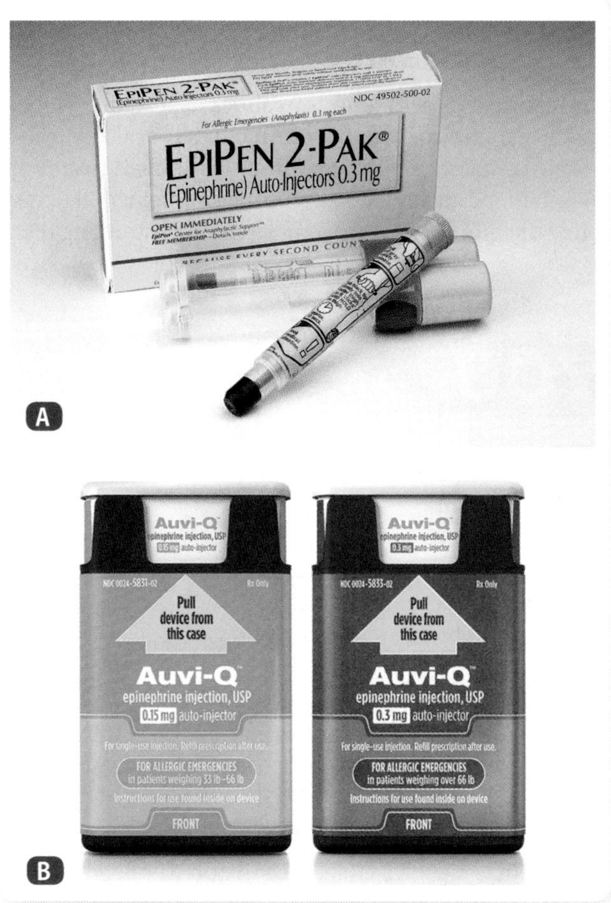

Figure 14-8 Patients who are known to have anaphylaxis often carry kits with an intramuscular injector or auto-injector, containing epinephrine. **A.** An EpiPen. **B.** Auvi-Q epinephrine auto-injectors.

Promptly transport the patient to the ED while providing all possible support, primarily supplemental oxygen and ventilatory assistance. Try to determine what agent caused the reaction (for example, a drug, an insect bite or sting, a food item) and how it was received (for example, by mouth, by inhalation, or by injection). The severity of allergic reactions can vary greatly, with symptoms ranging from mild itching to profound coma and rapid death. Keep in mind that a mild reaction may worsen suddenly or over time. Gain IV access as a medication route and administer fluid at a TKO rate. Consider requesting paramedic backup, if available.

▶ Treating Psychogenic Shock

In an uncomplicated case of fainting, after the patient collapses and becomes supine, circulation to the brain is usually restored and, with it, a normal state of functioning. Remember that psychogenic shock can substantially worsen other types of shock. If the attack has caused the patient to fall, you must check for injuries, especially in older patients. If, after regaining consciousness, the patient is unable to walk without weakness, dizziness, or pain, you should suspect another problem, such as head injury. Transport the patient promptly.

Be sure to record your initial observations of vital signs and LOC. In addition, try to learn from bystanders whether the patient reported any problems before fainting and how long he or she was unresponsive.

▶ Treating Respiratory Insufficiency

In treating a patient who is in shock as a result of inadequate respiration, you must immediately seal any hole in the chest, stabilize impaled objects in the chest, secure and maintain the airway, and administer supplemental oxygen. Clear the mouth and throat of anything obstructing the air passages, including mucus, vomitus, and foreign material. Assess the Spo_2 as well as vital signs, and determine the need to assist ventilations with a bag-mask device and supplemental oxygen. If available based on local protocol, monitoring $ETCO_2$ can provide additional information about adequacy of ventilatory efforts. Determine the most appropriate transportation destination based on the patient's condition and local protocols.

YOU are the Provider SUMMARY

1. What is shock and how does it relate to perfusion?

Shock (hypoperfusion) describes a state of collapse and failure of the cardiovascular system. When the circulation of blood in the body becomes inadequate, the oxygen and nutrient needs in the cells cannot be met. In the early stages of shock, the body will attempt to maintain homeostasis (a balance of all systems of the body); however, as shock progresses, blood circulation slows and eventually ceases. This abnormal state of inadequate oxygen and nutrient delivery to the cells of the body causes organs, and then organ systems, to fail. If not treated promptly, shock can be fatal.

Perfusion is the circulation of blood within an organ or tissue in adequate amounts to meet the cells' current needs for oxygen, nutrients, and waste removal. Perfusion requires a working cardiovascular system. It also requires adequate oxygen exchange in the lungs, adequate nutrients in the form of glucose in the blood, and adequate waste removal, primarily through the lungs.

2. What factors does perfusion depend on?

Perfusion depends on cardiac output, SVR, and transport of oxygen. SVR is the resistance to blood flow within all blood vessels except the pulmonary vessels.

3. Which type of shock do you suspect this patient is experiencing?

This patient is most likely experiencing hypovolemic shock based on the lack of other findings. He does not have any signs or symptoms that would indicate cardiogenic shock, and has no history of spinal cord injury, infections, or anaphylaxis. Therefore, you must consider any patient presenting with signs and symptoms of shock without external injury to have probable internal bleeding or fluid loss, usually in the abdominal cavity.

4. Which stage of shock is this patient experiencing?

This patient is in decompensated shock, in which the circulating blood volume has decreased more than 25%. The compensatory mechanisms are beginning to fail, and signs and symptoms are much more obvious. In this stage, cardiac output falls dramatically, resulting in further reductions in the blood pressure and cardiac function. The signs and symptoms become more obvious as blood is shunted to the brain, heart, and kidneys. At this point, vasoconstriction can have a disastrous effect if allowed to continue. Cells in the nonperfused tissues become hypoxic, resulting in anaerobic metabolism. Treatment at this stage sometimes results in recovery.

5. How much IV fluid should this patient receive?

This patient should receive fluid boluses of 20 mL/kg in 250- to 500-mL increments until systolic blood pressure exceeds 80 mm Hg. The presence of radial pulses equates roughly to a systolic blood pressure of 80 to 90 mm Hg, but this is variable and only a rough guide. Use actual cuff pressure measurements whenever possible. Raising the blood pressure further may result in worsening internal hemorrhage. You should monitor the patient's response to IV therapy carefully and document any changes.

6. How should the patient be positioned on the stretcher for transport?

The patient should be placed supine on the stretcher. Placing the patient in this position will assist in increasing perfusion to the vital organs, thus increasing the patient's overall perfusion.

7. Did this patient require a second IV line?

This patient could benefit from a second IV line, if time allows. With the suspicion of a bleeding or perforated ulcer and the patient's presentation of decompensated shock, it is likely that this patient will further decompensate and need larger fluid boluses and, potentially, surgical intervention. You should always remember that it is easier to establish IV access while the patient is still relatively perfused, as opposed to profoundly hypotensive.

YOU are the Provider SUMMARY *(continued)*

EMS Patient Care Report (PCR)					
Date: 09-8-18		**Incident No.:** 0247	**Nature of Call:** Weakness and nausea	**Location:** 521 4th Street	
Dispatched: 1542	**En Route:** 1550	**At Scene:** 1555	**Transport:** 1607	**At Hospital:** 1618	**In Service:** 1632

Patient Information	
Age: 67 **Sex:** M **Weight (in kg [lb]):** 79 kg (174 lb)	**Allergies:** None **Medications:** Lisinopril, Zantac **Past Medical History:** HTN, peptic ulcers **Chief Complaint:** Weakness, nausea, epigastric pain

Vital Signs				
Time: 1556	**BP:** Not obtained	**Pulse:** Not obtained	**Respirations:** 25	**Spo_2:** Not obtained
Time: 1603	**BP:** 72/40	**Pulse:** 160	**Respirations:** 26	**Spo_2:** 98% on 15 L/min
Time: 1611	**BP:** 68/P	**Pulse:** 164	**Respirations:** 26	**Spo_2:** 99% on 15 L/min
Time: 1616	**BP:** 70/P	**Pulse:** 160	**Respirations:** 24	**Spo_2:** 99% on 15 L/min

EMS Treatment (circle all that apply)				
Oxygen @ 15 L/min via (circle one): **NC** (**NRM**) **Bag-mask device**		**Assisted Ventilation**	**Airway Adjunct**	**CPR**
Defibrillation	**Bleeding Control**	**Bandaging**	**Splinting**	**Other:**

Narrative

EMS requested to respond to a patient reporting weakness and nausea with a "burning" epigastric pain. Patient states that he has not felt well over the past couple of days and his weakness and nausea became much worse this morning. He has a history of peptic ulcers and HTN. He has no drug allergies and medications are listed above. EMS found the patient lying supine in bed. He is alert and oriented but slow to respond. He is tachypneic with a respiratory rate of 25. Patient placed on a nonrebreathing mask at 15 L/min. His lungs are clear and he has a pulse oximetry reading of 98% on 15 L/min O_2 via NRM. His skin is cool and clammy with absent radial pulses. Carotid is rapid. He denies any trauma or physical activity. His abdomen is distended and tender to palpation. An 18-gauge IV catheter was established in the patient's right AC and a 250-mL bolus of NS was given. Patient placed supine and loaded into ambulance for rapid transport to the ED. A second bolus of 250-mL NS was delivered and an additional IV established with NS wide open while en route to the hospital. While en route the patient's LOC decreased and abdomen appears more distended. Airway continues to be open and clear. Respirations continue to be rapid. Weak radial pulses regained with fluid bolus, but rate continuing to increase. Patient rapidly transported to the ED without further incident.**End of report**

Prep Kit

▶ Ready to Review

- Perfusion is the circulation of blood within an organ or tissue in adequate amounts to meet the cells' current needs for oxygen, nutrients, and waste removal. Perfusion requires an intact cardiovascular system and a functioning respiratory system.
- Blood is the vehicle for carrying oxygen and nutrients through the vessels to the capillary beds to tissue cells, where these supplies are exchanged for waste products.
- Blood flow through the capillary beds is regulated by the capillary sphincters that are under the control of the autonomic nervous system. Regulation of blood flow occurs by vessel constriction or dilation, along with sphincter constriction or dilation.
- The *systolic* pressure is the peak arterial pressure, or pressure generated every time the heart contracts; the *diastolic* pressure is the pressure maintained within the arteries while the heart rests between heartbeats.
- Perfusion depends on cardiac output, systemic vascular resistance, and transport of oxygen. Cardiac output is the volume of blood that the heart can pump per minute. Systemic vascular resistance is the resistance to blood flow within all blood vessels except the pulmonary vessels.
- Most types of shock (hypoperfusion) are caused by dysfunction in one or more parts of the perfusion triangle:
  - The pump (the heart)
  - The pipes, or container (blood vessels)
  - The content, or volume (blood)
- Shock (hypoperfusion) is the collapse and failure of the cardiovascular system, when blood circulation slows and eventually stops.
- The autnonomic nervous system has a role in regulation of pulse rate, blood pressure, and respiratory rate. Activation of the sympathetic nervous system increases these; activation of the parasympathetic nervous system decreases these.
- The body has neural and hormonal mechanisms for regulating blood pressure, which is important to maintaining homeostasis. If perfusion decreases, baroreceptors sense the decreased flow and activate the vasomotor center, which oversees changes in the diameter of blood vessels, to begin constriction of the vessels and increase blood pressure. Chemoreceptors measure subtle shifts in the amounts of carbon dioxide in arterial blood and are important in regulating respiration.
- Failure of compensatory mechanisms to preserve perfusion results in decreases in preload and cardiac output. Myocardial blood supply and oxygenation decrease, reducing myocardial perfusion. As cardiac output further decreases, coronary artery perfusion also decreases, resulting in myocardial ischemia.
- Multiple-organ dysfunction syndrome is a progressive condition in which several organ systems fail. This occurs when injury or infection triggers a massive systemic immune, inflammatory, and coagulation response.
- Suspect shock if the patient has substantial external or internal bleeding, multiple severe fractures, abdominal or chest injury, spinal injury, severe infection, major heart attack, or anaphylaxis.
- The various types of shock are hypovolemic, cardiogenic, septic, neurogenic, anaphylactic, and psychogenic.
- Signs of compensated shock include agitation, anxiety, or restlessness; a sense of impending doom; weak, rapid pulse; pale, cool, moist skin; shortness of breath; nausea and vomiting; and increased thirst. If there is any question on your part, treat for shock. It is never wrong to treat for shock.
- Notable signs of decompensated shock include altered mental status; hypotension; labored or irregular breathing; thready or absent pulses; ashen, mottled, or cyanotic skin; dilated pupils; diminished urine output; dry mucosa; and nausea and vomiting.
- Remember, by the time a decrease in blood pressure is detected, shock is usually in an advanced stage. Early recognition and treatment are crucial.
- Treating a pediatric or geriatric patient in shock is no different than treating any other shock patient.
- Treat all patients suspected to be in shock from any cause as follows:
  - Address life threats; control obvious external bleeding, then airway and breathing concerns.
  - If cardiac arrest is suspected, focus on high-quality chest compressions prior to airway and breathing.
  - Provide high-flow oxygen and, as needed, provide bag-mask-assisted ventilations.
  - Place the patient supine.
  - Maintain normal body temperature with blankets.
  - Provide prompt transport to the appropriate hospital.
  - Gain intravenous (IV) access.

Prep Kit (continued)

- Starting an IV line and administering fluids is part of treating a patient who is in shock. Administer IV volume expanders (warmed if possible) to replace fluid loss. Isotonic crystalloids, such as normal saline or lactated Ringer solution, should be used (synthetic solutions may also be used). Call early for paramedic intervention to administer vasopressors if needed.

▶ Vital Vocabulary

aerobic metabolism Metabolism that can proceed only in the presence of oxygen.

afterload The force or resistance against which the heart pumps.

anaerobic metabolism The metabolism that takes place in the absence of oxygen; the principal product is lactic acid.

anaphylactic shock Severe shock caused by an allergic reaction.

anaphylaxis An unusual or exaggerated allergic reaction to foreign protein or other substances.

aneurysm A swelling or enlargement of part of an artery, resulting from weakening of the arterial wall.

angioedema Recurrent large areas of subcutaneous edema of sudden onset, usually disappearing within 24 hours, which is seen mainly in young women, frequently as a result of allergy to food or drugs.

autonomic nervous system The part of the nervous system that regulates involuntary functions, such as heart rate, blood pressure, digestion, and sweating.

baroreceptors Receptors in the blood vessels, kidneys, brain, and heart that respond to changes in pressure in the heart or main arteries to help maintain homeostasis.

cardiac output (CO) The amount of blood pumped through the circulatory system in 1 minute.

cardiac tamponade Compression of the heart caused by a buildup of blood or other fluid in the pericardial sac.

cardiogenic shock Shock caused by inadequate function of the heart, or pump failure.

chemoreceptors Receptors in the blood vessels, kidneys, brain, and heart that respond to changes in chemical composition of the blood to help maintain homeostasis.

chronotropic effect Affecting the heart's rate of contraction.

compensated shock The early stage of shock, in which the body can still compensate for blood loss; also called nonprogressive shock.

cyanosis Bluish color of the skin resulting from poor oxygenation of the circulating blood.

decompensated shock The late stage of shock when blood pressure is falling; also called progressive shock.

distributive shock A condition that occurs when there is widespread dilation of the small arterioles, small venules, or both.

dromotropic effect Affecting the heart's velocity of conduction.

edema The presence of abnormally large amounts of fluid between cells in body tissues, causing swelling of the affected area.

Fick principle States that the movement and use of oxygen in the body is dependent on adequate concentration of inspired oxygen (FIO_2 [fraction of inspired oxygen]), appropriate movement of oxygen across the alveolar-capillary membrane into the arterial bloodstream, adequate number of red blood cells to carry the oxygen, proper tissue perfusion, and efficient off-loading of oxygen at the tissue level.

hemorrhagic shock A condition in which low blood volume due to massive internal or external bleeding results in inadequate perfusion.

homeostasis A balance of all systems of the body.

hypothermia A condition in which the internal body temperature falls below 95°F (35°C), usually as a result of prolonged exposure to cool or freezing temperatures.

hypovolemic shock Shock caused by fluid or blood loss.

inotropic effect Affecting the contractility of the heart muscle.

irreversible shock The final stage of shock, resulting in death.

mean arterial pressure (MAP) The average pressure against the arterial wall during a cardiac cycle; generally considered to be the same as blood pressure.

multiple-organ dysfunction syndrome (MODS) A progressive condition usually characterized by combined failure of several organs, such as the lungs, liver, and kidney, along with some clotting mechanisms, which occurs after severe illness or injury.

Prep Kit (continued)

myocardial contractility The ability of the heart muscle to contract.

neurogenic shock Circulatory failure caused by paralysis of the nerves that control the size of the blood vessels, resulting in widespread dilation; seen in patients with spinal cord injuries.

nonhemorrhagic shock Shock that occurs as a result of fluid loss contained within the body, such as in dehydration, burn injury, crush injury, and anaphylaxis.

obstructive shock Shock that occurs when there is a block to blood flow in the heart or great vessels, causing an insufficient blood supply to the body's tissues.

orthostatic vital signs Multiple sets of vital signs taken from the patient in different positions (for example, in the supine and sitting or standing positions) to determine the degree of hypovolemia.

perfusion Circulation of blood within an organ or tissue in adequate amounts to meet the cells' current needs.

preload The precontraction pressure in the heart as the volume of blood builds up.

psychogenic shock Shock caused by a sudden, temporary reduction in blood supply to the brain that causes fainting (syncope).

pulse pressure Difference between the systolic and diastolic pressures.

sensitization Developing a sensitivity to a substance that initially caused no allergic reaction.

septic shock Shock caused by severe infection, usually a bacterial infection.

shock A condition in which the circulatory system fails to provide sufficient circulation to enable every body part to perform its function; also called hypoperfusion.

sphincters Circular muscles that surround and, by contracting, constrict a duct, tube, or opening.

syncope Fainting.

systemic vascular resistance (SVR) The resistance that blood must overcome to be able to move within the blood vessels; related to the amount of dilation or constriction in the blood vessel.

tension pneumothorax An accumulation of air or gas in the pleural space that progressively collapses the lung with potentially fatal results.

▶ References

1. Frank O. Zur dynamik des herzmuskels. *J Biol.* 1895;32:370-447. Translation from German: Chapman CP, Wasserman EB. On the dynamics of cardiac muscle. *Am Heart J* . 1959;58:282-317.
2. Healey MA, Samphire J, Hoyt DB, et al. Irreversible shock is not irreversible; a new model of massive hemorrhage and resuscitation. *J Trauma.* 2001;50(5):826-834.
3. Rezaie S. Is ATLS wrong about palpable blood pressure estimates? ALiEM: Academic Life in Emergency Medicine website. https://www.aliem.com/2013/is-atls-wrong-about-palpable-blood-pressure/. Published March 31, 2013. Accessed January 23, 2017.

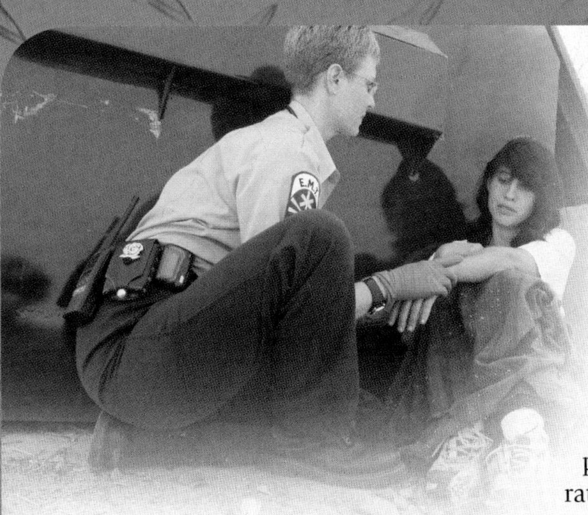

Assessment *in Action*

Your ambulance is dispatched to a local residence for a 55-year-old man reporting chest pain. On arrival, you find the patient seated in a recliner in the tripod position. He states that he has chest pain and shortness of breath. He is pale and diaphoretic and his vital signs are as follows: blood pressure, 74/48 mm Hg; pulse rate, 49 beats/min; and respirations, 22 breaths/min and labored.

1. On the basis of the vital signs, which type of shock is this patient most likely experiencing?

- **A.** Neurogenic
- **B.** Cardiogenic
- **C.** Septic
- **D.** Hypovolemic

2. Cardiogenic shock develops when the heart cannot maintain sufficient:

- **A.** cardiac output.
- **B.** automaticity.
- **C.** oxygenation.
- **D.** excitability.

3. Causes of cardiogenic shock may include all of the following EXCEPT:

- **A.** inadequate heart function.
- **B.** disease of muscle tissue.
- **C.** impaired electrical system.
- **D.** inadequate respirations.

4. Initial treatment for this patient should include:

- **A.** administration of nitroglycerin for the patient's chest pain.
- **B.** placing the patient in a position of comfort.
- **C.** administration of a 250-mL fluid bolus.
- **D.** administration of one 325-mg aspirin tablet.

5. What differentiates septic shock from hemorrhagic shock?

- **A.** Altered mental status
- **B.** Warm or hot skin
- **C.** Weak, thready pulse
- **D.** Shallow, rapid respirations

6. A collection of fluid within the pericardial sac that is causing compression on the heart is called:

- **A.** myocardial contusion.
- **B.** myocardial dysrhythmia.
- **C.** pericardial tamponade.
- **D.** cardiac compromise.

7. The only effective prehospital treatment for anaphylactic shock is:

- **A.** epinephrine.
- **B.** oxygen.
- **C.** rapid transport.
- **D.** diphenhydramine.

8. A patient in decompensated shock presents with a narrowing pulse pressure indicating:

- **A.** profound hypotension.
- **B.** impairment of circulation.
- **C.** weakness.
- **D.** impairment of respirations.

9. Give the three purposes for IV lines.

10. List the signs and symptoms of compensated shock.

CHAPTER 15

BLS Resuscitation

National EMS Education Standard Competencies

Shock and Resuscitation

Applies fundamental knowledge to provide basic and selected advanced emergency care and transportation based on assessment findings for a patient in shock, respiratory failure or arrest, cardiac failure or arrest, and post resuscitation management.

Knowledge Objectives

1. Explain the elements of basic life support (BLS), how it differs from advanced life support (ALS), and why BLS must be applied rapidly. (pp 688-689)
2. Explain the goals of cardiopulmonary resuscitation (CPR) and when it should be performed on a patient. (p 689)
3. Explain the components of CPR, the five links in the American Heart Association (AHA) chain of survival, and how each one relates to maximizing patient survival. (pp 689-690)
4. Discuss guidelines for circumstances that require the use of an automated external defibrillator (AED) on both adult and pediatric patients experiencing cardiac arrest. (pp 692-693)
5. Explain four special situations related to the use of an AED. (pp 693-694)
6. Describe the proper way to position an adult patient to receive BLS care. (p 694)
7. Describe the purpose of external chest compressions. (pp 694-695)
8. Describe the two techniques advanced emergency medical technicians (AEMTs) may use to open an adult patient's airway and the circumstances that would determine when to use each technique. (pp 697-698)
9. Describe the recovery position and circumstances that would warrant its use as well as situations in which it would be contraindicated. (p 699)
10. Describe the process of providing artificial ventilations to an adult patient, ways to avoid gastric distention, and modifications required for a patient with a stoma. (pp 699-701)
11. Explain the steps in providing one-rescuer adult CPR. (pp 701-702)
12. Explain the steps in providing two-rescuer adult CPR, including the method for switching positions during the process. (pp 701-704)
13. Explain crew resource management and the roles of the team member and the team leader. (pp 704-705)
14. Summarize the steps of postcardiac arrest care. (p 705)
15. Describe the different mechanical devices that are available to assist emergency medical care providers in delivering improved circulatory efforts during CPR. (pp 705-709)
16. Describe the different possible causes of cardiopulmonary arrest in children. (pp 709-710)
17. Explain pediatric BLS procedures and how they differ from BLS procedures used in an adult patient. (pp 709-713)
18. Describe the ethical issues related to patient resuscitation, including examples of when not to start CPR on a patient. (pp 714-716)
19. Explain the various factors involved in the decision to stop CPR after it has been started on a patient. (pp 716-717)
20. Explain common causes of foreign body airway obstruction in both children and adults and how to distinguish mild or partial airway obstruction from complete airway obstruction. (p 717)
21. Describe the different methods for removing a foreign body airway obstruction in an infant, child, and adult, including the procedure for a patient with an obstruction who becomes unresponsive. (pp 717-722)
22. Describe special resuscitation circumstances, such as opioid overdose or cardiac arrest in pregnancy. (pp 722-723)
23. Discuss how to provide grief support for a patient's family members and loved ones after resuscitation has ended. (pp 723-724)
24. Discuss the importance of frequent CPR training for AEMTs, as well as public education programs that teach compression-only CPR. (p 724)

Skills Objectives

1. Demonstrate how to position an unresponsive adult for CPR. (p 694)
2. Demonstrate how to check for a pulse at the carotid artery in an unresponsive child or adult. (p 694)
3. Demonstrate how to perform external chest compressions on an adult. (pp 694-697, Skill Drill 15-1)
4. Demonstrate how to perform a head tilt–chin lift maneuver on an adult. (pp 697-698)
5. Demonstrate how to perform a jaw-thrust maneuver on an adult. (pp 697-698)
6. Demonstrate how to place a patient in the recovery position. (p 699)
7. Demonstrate how to perform artificial ventilations in an adult. (pp 699-701)
8. Demonstrate how to perform one-rescuer adult CPR. (pp 701-702, Skill Drill 15-2)
9. Demonstrate how to perform two-rescuer adult CPR. (pp 701-704, Skill Drill 15-3)
10. Demonstrate the use of mechanical devices that assist emergency responders in delivering improved circulatory efforts during CPR. (pp 706-709)
11. Demonstrate how to check for a pulse at the brachial artery in an unresponsive infant. (p 710)
12. Demonstrate how to perform external chest compressions on an infant. (pp 710-711, Skill Drill 15-4)
13. Demonstrate how to perform CPR on a child who is between 1 year of age and the onset of puberty. (pp 710-712, Skill Drill 15-5)
14. Demonstrate how to perform a head tilt–chin lift maneuver on a pediatric patient. (p 712)
15. Demonstrate how to perform a jaw-thrust maneuver on a pediatric patient. (pp 712-713)
16. Demonstrate how to perform rescue breathing on a child. (p 713)
17. Demonstrate how to perform rescue breathing on an infant. (p 713)
18. Demonstrate how to remove a foreign body airway obstruction in a responsive adult patient using abdominal thrusts (Heimlich maneuver). (pp 717-718)
19. Demonstrate how to remove a foreign body airway obstruction in a responsive pregnant patient or patient with obesity using chest thrusts. (p 718)
20. Demonstrate how to remove a foreign body airway obstruction in a responsive child older than 1 year using abdominal thrusts (Heimlich maneuver). (p 720)
21. Demonstrate how to remove a foreign body airway obstruction in an unresponsive child. (p 721, Skill Drill 15-6)
22. Demonstrate how to remove a foreign body airway obstruction in an infant. (pp 721-722)

Introduction

The principles of basic life support (BLS), or cardiopulmonary resuscitation (CPR), were introduced in 1960. Since then, the specific techniques for the management of cardiac arrest and the *Guidelines for Cardiopulmonary Resuscitation and Emergency Cardiac Care* have been reviewed and revised every 5 years by the American Heart Association (AHA), in concert with the International Liaison Committee on Resuscitation (ILCOR). However, in 2015, it was determined a 5-year cycle is insufficient to keep pace with the rapidly evolving research in resuscitation science, so it is planned for the guidelines to be updated on a more regular basis. The goal is to produce the best recommendations possible given the available scientific evidence. The updated guidelines are published in peer-reviewed journals: *Circulation* in the United States and *Resuscitation* in Europe. The most recent review conducted by ILCOR occurred as a result of a rigorous and systematic review of the newest scientific evidence surrounding the treatment of cardiac arrest and the provision of emergency and cardiac care, using validated, transparent, and scientifically rigorous methodology to

YOU are the Provider — PART 1

It is a very hot summer day. At 1445 hours, you and your partner respond to the local farmer's market for an unresponsive patient sitting in a pickup truck. While you are en route to the scene, dispatch informs you that bystander CPR is in progress. Your response time is less than 5 minutes.

1. What should you immediately do on receiving this update from dispatch?
2. What should be your initial actions on arriving at this scene?

produce the best recommendations possible given the available evidence.

This chapter begins with a definition and general discussion of BLS. It then reviews methods for opening and maintaining a patent (open) airway, providing artificial ventilation to a person who is not breathing, providing artificial circulation to a person with no pulse, removing a foreign body airway obstruction, and post-resuscitation care for those with a return of spontaneous circulation. Each of these topics is followed by a review of the changes in technique that are necessary to treat infants and children. Chapter 2, *Workforce Safety and Wellness,* discusses the methods of preventing the transmission of infectious diseases during CPR. Chapter 7, *The Human Body,* discusses the anatomy and physiology of the respiratory and cardiovascular systems. Working as a team during an emergency is crucial to give the patient the best chance for a successful outcome. Uninterrupted chest compressions offers the best chance of survival for victims of cardiac arrest while awaiting **advanced life support (ALS)** intervention. Effective teamwork with good communication increases the potential for a positive outcome.

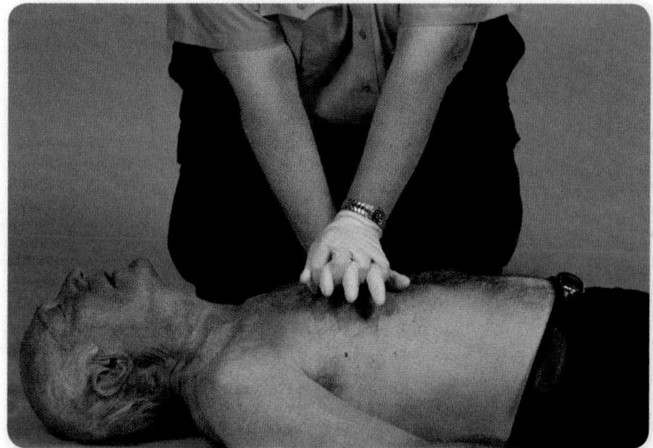

Figure 15-1 Chest compressions are essential and must be started as quickly as possible.

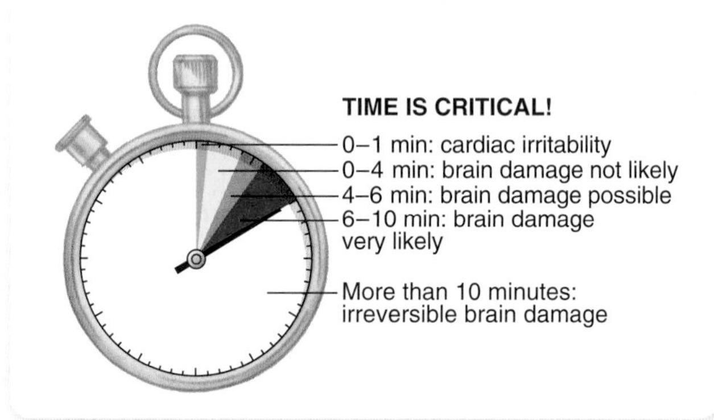

Figure 15-2 Time is critical for patients who are not breathing. If the brain is deprived of oxygen for 4 to 6 minutes, brain damage is possible.

Words of Wisdom

Although your chances of contracting a disease during CPR training or actual CPR on a patient are very low, both common sense and Occupational Safety and Health Administration (OSHA) guidelines demand you take reasonable precautions to prevent unnecessary exposure to an infectious disease. By taking standard precautions, you can significantly reduce your risk of being exposed to an infectious disease.

Elements of BLS

Basic life support (BLS) is noninvasive emergency life-saving care that is used to treat medical conditions, including airway obstruction, respiratory arrest, and cardiac arrest. BLS follows a specific sequence for adults and for infants and children. This care focuses on the ABCDEs: Airway (obstruction), Breathing (respiratory arrest), Circulation (cardiac arrest or severe bleeding), Disability (brief neurologic evaluation), and Exposure (adequate exposure of each area being examined). If the patient is in cardiac arrest, then a CABDE sequence (Compressions, Airway, Breathing, Disability, and Exposure) is used because chest compressions are essential and must be started as quickly as possible **Figure 15-1**. Ideally, only seconds should pass between the time you recognize that a patient needs BLS and the start of treatment. Remember, brain cells die every second that they are deprived of oxygen. Permanent brain damage is possible after only 4 to 6 minutes without oxygen **Figure 15-2**.

If a patient is not breathing adequately or at all, then you may be able to restore normal breathing simply by opening the airway. However, if the patient has no pulse, then you must combine artificial ventilation with artificial circulation (chest compressions). If breathing stops before the heart stops, then the patient may have enough oxygen in the lungs to stay alive for several minutes. But when cardiac arrest occurs first, the heart and brain stop receiving oxygen immediately.

Cardiopulmonary resuscitation (CPR) is used to establish circulation and artificial ventilation in a patient who is not breathing and has no pulse. The steps for CPR include the following:

1. First, open the airway with the jaw-thrust or head tilt–chin lift maneuver.
2. Next, perform 30 high-quality compressions to a depth of 2 inches to 2.4 inches (5 cm to 6 cm) in an adult at the rate of 100 to 120 per minute to circulate blood to the vital organs.
3. Last, provide rescue breaths (via mouth-to-mask ventilation or bag-mask ventilation). Administer 2 breaths, each over 1 second, while visualizing for chest rise.

The goal of CPR is to help restore spontaneous breathing and circulation; however, defibrillation and advanced interventions (ie, medication therapy) are often necessary to achieve this outcome. For CPR to be effective, you must be able to quickly identify a patient who is in respiratory and/or cardiac arrest and immediately begin BLS measures **Figure 15-3**.

BLS differs from ALS, which involves advanced life-saving procedures, such as cardiac monitoring, administration of intravenous (IV) or intraosseous (IO) fluids and medications, and the use of advanced airway adjuncts. However, when done correctly, BLS care can maintain life for a short time until ALS measures can be started. In some cases, such as choking, near drowning, or lightning injuries, early BLS measures may be all that is needed to restore a patient's pulse and breathing. Of course, these patients still require transport to the emergency department (ED) for evaluation.

The BLS measures are only as effective as the person who is performing them. Your skills may be good immediately after training, but as time goes on, skills will deteriorate unless you practice them regularly.

To survive cardiac arrest, effective CPR at an adequate rate and depth with minimal interruptions is essential until defibrillation can be administered. Therefore, the BLS care you provide as an advanced emergency medical technician (AEMT) is an extremely critical factor in the patient's chance for survival and, in many ways, is as important as the ALS care you will provide.

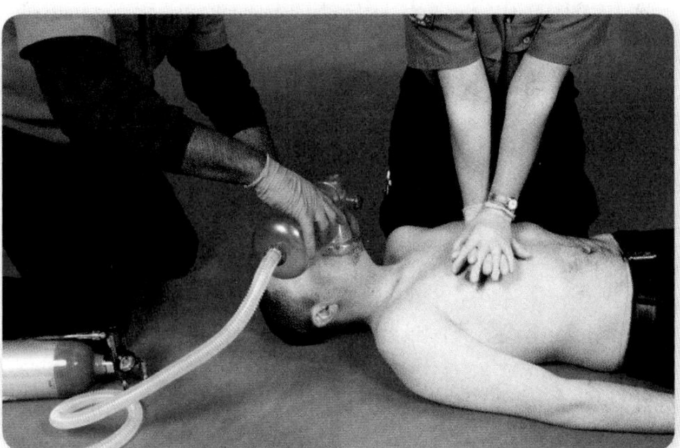

Figure 15-3 You must quickly identify patients in respiratory and/or cardiac arrest so basic life support measures can begin immediately.

Words of Wisdom

Remember to push hard and push fast! Some BLS classes use music to set the beat while teaching CPR. Songs such as the 1970s disco classic "Staying Alive" offer an enjoyable learning experience and just may serve as a reminder for a provider who is actually performing chest compressions.

The Components of CPR

According to the AHA, 70% of prehospital cardiac arrests occur in the home.[1] Few patients who experience cardiac arrest in the prehospital environment survive unless a rapid sequence of events takes place. The AHA has determined an ideal sequence of events, termed the chain of survival, that if taken can improve the chance of successful resuscitation of a patient who experiences sudden cardiac arrest **Figure 15-4**. A successful resuscitation is defined not only by the **return of spontaneous circulation (ROSC)**, but also the survival of the patient to

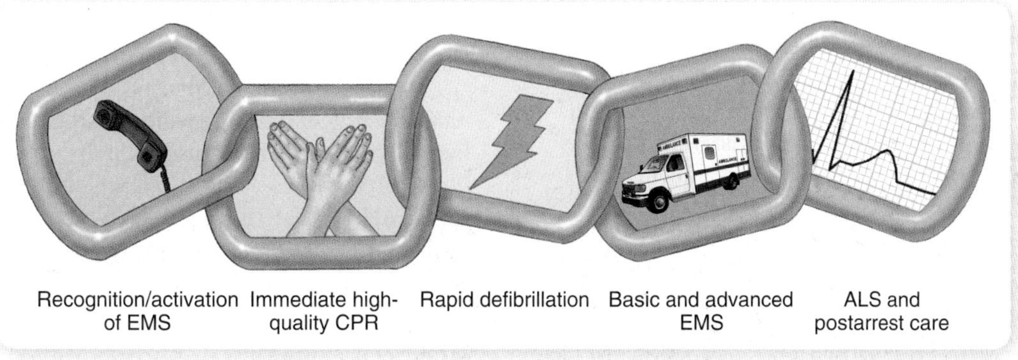

Figure 15-4 The five links of the chain of survival.

hospital discharge. The five links in the chain of survival are as follows:[2]

1. **Recognition and activation of the emergency response system.** The first step in the chain of survival requires public education and awareness. Laypeople must learn to recognize the early warning signs of a cardiac emergency and immediately activate emergency medical services (EMS) by calling 9-1-1. This step ensures emergency responders are dispatched to the scene quickly, thus allowing the other links of the chain to be more effective. In modern EMS systems, the 9-1-1 dispatcher can provide prearrival instructions and direct the caller to provide CPR if needed.
2. **Immediate, high-quality CPR.** The initiation of immediate CPR by a bystander is essential for successful resuscitation of a person in cardiac arrest. CPR will keep blood, and, therefore, oxygen, flowing to the vital organs to keep the patient alive until the other components of the chain are available. The more people trained in CPR in the community, the better the chances of CPR being administered quickly to a person in cardiac arrest. Immediate, high-quality CPR markedly increases the patient's chance of survival, whereas a delay in CPR leads to poor patient outcomes. The lay public as well as emergency responders should all be trained in CPR. Unfortunately, many bystanders are hesitant to perform CPR on a stranger for fear of contracting a disease from mouth-to-mouth breathing, or out of fear of liability. A perception that bystander CPR involves both mouth-to-mouth breathing and chest compressions persists. Laypeople should be educated in performing compression-only (hands-only) CPR.

   For chest compressions to be most effective, they must be given hard and fast. The AHA recommends compressions be started as quickly as possible after onset of cardiac arrest. Compressions should be between 2 inches and 2.4 inches in depth (5 to 6 cm) and given at a rate of 100 to 120 per minute. The chest should completely recoil between each compression to maximize blood return to the heart. The rescuer should never lean on the chest between compressions. Interruptions between compressions for any reason should be minimized.
3. **Rapid defibrillation.** Provided that immediate, high-quality CPR with minimal interruption is performed, early defibrillation offers the best opportunity to achieve a successful patient outcome. Automated external defibrillators (AEDs) have become readily available in many schools, fitness clubs, concert venues, sports arenas, government buildings, and other mass gathering places. The simple design of the AED makes it easy for emergency medical providers and laypeople to use with very little training.
4. **Basic and advanced emergency medical services.** This link in the chain describes care provided by AEMTs and other ALS providers before the patient arrives at the ED. Such care includes continuing high-quality CPR; basic airway management (ie, oral airway insertion, bag-mask ventilation); advanced airway management (ie, endotracheal [ET] intubation or use of supraglottic airway devices); manual defibrillation; vascular access; transcutaneous pacing; and medication administration.

   In addition to the care you provide in the prehospital setting, be familiar with the cardiac resuscitation centers in your service area.

   Your agency should implement a process to ensure early notification and transport to the appropriate receiving facility.
5. **Advanced life support and postarrest care.** After your team delivers the patient to the ED, further cardiopulmonary and neurologic support is provided to improve the patient's recovery when indicated. This support can include additional medication therapy to support blood pressure; targeted temperature management (ie, therapeutic hypothermia); maintenance of blood glucose levels; cardiac catheterization; an electroencephalogram to detect seizure activity; and admission to the intensive care unit for critical care management.

If any one of the links in the chain is absent or not maintained, the patient is more likely to die. For example, few patients survive cardiac arrest if CPR is not administered within the first few minutes. Likewise, if the time from cardiac arrest to defibrillation is more than 10 minutes, the chance of survival is minimal. The patient's best chance of survival occurs when all links in the chain are continuously maintained.

Figure 15-5 shows an algorithm with the components of providing advanced cardiac life support to a patient in cardiac arrest, including defibrillation, CPR, IV/IO access, and postcardiac care. The rest of this chapter will discuss these components in depth.

As soon as resources permit, IV or IO access should be established as a fluid and medication route. A patient may be hypoglycemic, and administration of dextrose ($D_{50}W$) may help with the ROSC. Use the Hs & Ts mnemonic described by the AHA to determine possible reversible causes of the cardiac arrest, many of which are treatable on an AEMT level.[3]

- Hypovolemia
- Hypoxia
- Hydrogen ion (acidosis)
- Hypo-/hyperkalemia
- Hypothermia
- Tension pneumothorax

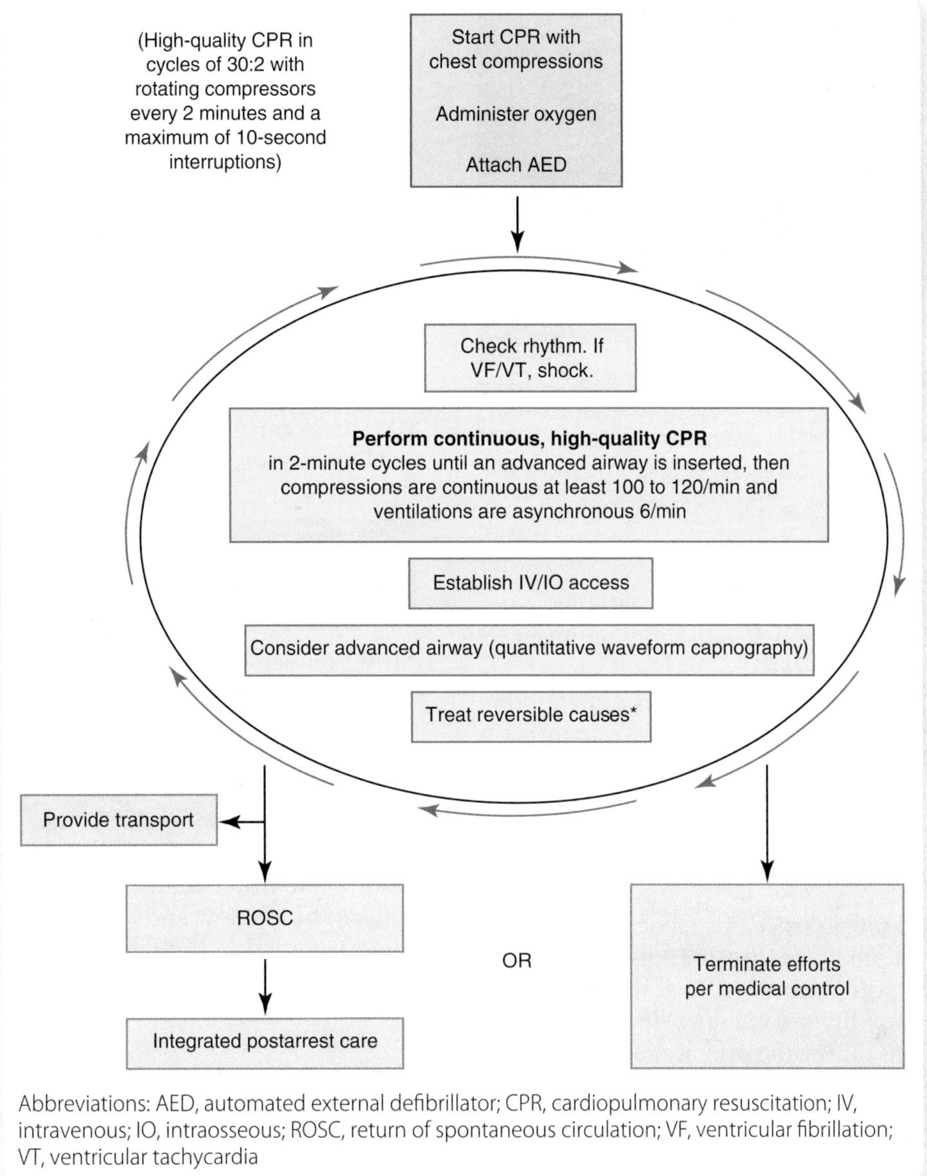
(High-quality CPR in cycles of 30:2 with rotating compressors every 2 minutes and a maximum of 10-second interruptions)
Start CPR with chest compressions
Administer oxygen
Attach AED
Check rhythm. If VF/VT, shock.
Perform continuous, high-quality CPR
in 2-minute cycles until an advanced airway is inserted, then compressions are continuous at least 100 to 120/min and ventilations are asynchronous 6/min
Establish IV/IO access
Consider advanced airway (quantitative waveform capnography)
Treat reversible causes*
Provide transport
ROSC
Integrated postarrest care
OR
Terminate efforts per medical control

Abbreviations: AED, automated external defibrillator; CPR, cardiopulmonary resuscitation; IV, intravenous; IO, intraosseous; ROSC, return of spontaneous circulation; VF, ventricular fibrillation; VT, ventricular tachycardia

Figure 15-5 Algorithm for providing advanced cardiac life support. *Reversible causes in adults that can be treated by AEMTs include Hs and Ts: hypovolemia, hypoxia, hydrogen ion (acidosis), hypothermia, tension pneumothorax, toxins (Narcan can be administered), and pulmonary and coronary thrombosis. In pediatric patients, hypoglycemia is also a reversible cause.

- Tamponade, cardiac
- Toxins
- Thrombosis, pulmonary
- Thrombosis, coronary

Assessing the Need for BLS

As always, begin by surveying the scene. Is the scene safe? How many patients are present? What is your general impression of the patient? Are bystanders present who may have additional information? What is the mechanism of injury or nature of illness? Do you suspect trauma? Do you need additional assistance? If you were dispatched to the scene, then does the dispatch information match what you see?

Because of the urgent need to start CPR in a pulseless, apneic patient, you must complete a primary survey as

Words of Wisdom

If you anticipate the need for additional assistance, alert dispatch *immediately!* Do not wait until you are actually performing CPR and have to stop to use the radio.

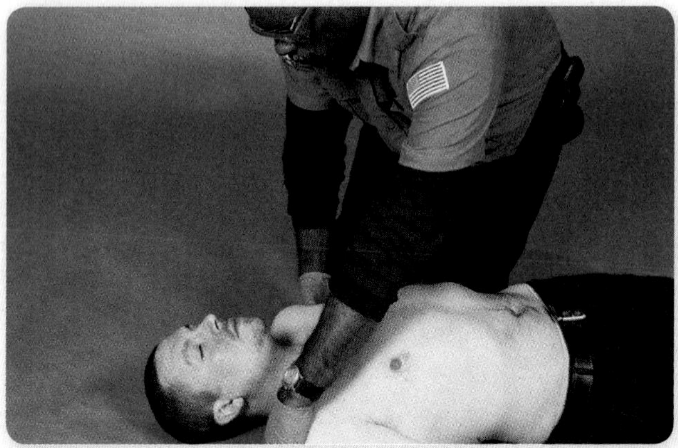

Figure 15-6 Assess an unresponsive patient by first attempting to rouse him or her by tapping on the shoulder.

soon as possible and begin CPR, starting with chest compressions. The first step is to determine unresponsiveness. Gently tap the patient on the shoulder and shout, "Are you okay?" **Figure 15-6**. If the patient does not respond to verbal or physical stimuli, he or she is unresponsive. A patient who is responsive does not need CPR. Continue your assessment by simultaneously checking for breathing and a pulse; this step should take no more than 10 seconds. If the patient is in cardiac arrest, then begin CPR immediately.

If you suspect the presence of a cervical spine injury then take precautions to protect the spinal cord from further injury as you perform CPR. If there is even a remote possibility of this type of injury, then begin taking appropriate actions during the primary survey.

You may encounter a cardiac arrest patient while off duty. If you are alone and off duty, use your mobile phone to call 9-1-1. Recall from Chapter 3, *Medical, Legal, and Ethical Issues,* that you must be familiar with the laws and policies that apply in your service area regarding your duty to act. If you are alone and do not have a mobile phone, then leave the patient to call 9-1-1 and then return to begin CPR. If you choose to intervene while off duty, you must continue to provide competent care until an equal or higher medical authority assumes care of the patient.

▶ Basic Principles of BLS

The basic principles of BLS are the same for infants, children, and adults. For the purposes of BLS, anyone younger than 1 year is considered an infant. A child is between 1 year of age and the onset of puberty (approximately 12 to 14 years of age), as signified by breast development in girls and underarm, chest, and facial hair in boys. Adulthood is from the onset of puberty and older. Children vary in size. Some small children may best be treated as infants, some larger children as adults. There are two basic differences in providing CPR for infants, children, and adults. The first is that the emergencies in which infants and children require CPR usually have different underlying causes. The second is that there are anatomic differences in adults, children, and infants, such as smaller airways in infants and children than in adults.

Although cardiac arrest in adults usually occurs before respiratory arrest, the reverse is true in infants and children. In most cases, cardiac arrest in children results from respiratory arrest. If untreated, respiratory arrest will quickly lead to cardiac arrest and death. Respiratory arrest in infants and children has a variety of causes, including aspiration of foreign bodies into the airway, such as parts of hot dogs, peanuts, candy, or small toys; airway infections, such as croup and epiglottitis; near-drowning incidents or electrocution; and sudden unexpected infant death.[4]

Automated External Defibrillation

Most prehospital cardiac arrests occur as the result of a sudden cardiac rhythm disturbance (dysrhythmia), such as ventricular fibrillation (VF) or pulseless ventricular tachycardia (VT). The normal heart rhythm is known as a sinus rhythm and originates in the sinoatrial (SA) node. VF is the disorganized quivering of the ventricles generated by ectopic foci (electrical activity originating from a site other than the SA node) resulting in no forward blood flow and a state of cardiac arrest. VT is a rapid contraction of the ventricles that does not allow for normal filling of the heart. As mentioned previously, according to the AHA, early defibrillation is the link in the chain of survival that is most likely to improve survival rates. The likelihood of survival decreases rapidly over time as long as VF or pulseless VT persists.

Words of Wisdom

The heart is the only muscle that has the property of automaticity—the ability to generate its own electrical impulses. Ectopic means outside of the normal area (think of an ectopic pregnancy—the embryo is implanted somewhere other than inside the uterus). Ectopic electrical activity in the heart is generated from cells other than the sinoatrial node (the normal area for initiation of electrical impulses) and causes cardiac dysrhythmias.

When a patient is in cardiac arrest, begin CPR, starting with high-quality chest compressions, and apply an AED as soon as it is available. If indicated, defibrillate immediately. Chapter 18, *Cardiovascular Emergencies,* covers AED use in detail.

Words of Wisdom

If you witness a cardiac arrest and an AED is available, immediately apply and activate it. Next, begin CPR. However, if you did not witness the patient's cardiac arrest or if an AED is unavailable, then perform CPR and apply the AED as soon as it is available. If two or more rescuers are present, one rescuer should begin chest compressions while the other prepares to defibrillate using the AED.

▶ AED Use in Children

AEDs can safely be used in children using the pediatric-sized pads and a dose-attenuating system (energy reducer). However, if these items are unavailable, use adult-sized AED pads. Apply the AED to infants or children after the first five cycles of CPR have been completed. Recall, cardiac arrest in children is usually the result of respiratory failure; therefore, oxygenation and ventilation are vitally important. After the first five cycles of CPR, use the AED to deliver shocks in the same manner as with an adult patient.

If the patient is an infant (between 1 month and 1 year of age) and paramedics are available, then a manual defibrillator is preferred. As with any cardiac arrest situation, immediately call for paramedic backup. If paramedic backup with a manual defibrillator is unavailable, then an AED equipped with pediatric-sized pads and a dose attenuator is preferred over using adult-sized pads. If neither is available, then use an AED with adult-sized pads.

If you use adult-sized AED pads on an infant or small child, never cut the pads to adjust the size. Instead, use the anterior-posterior placement, following the manufacturer's recommendation.

Words of Wisdom

Never apply an AED to a patient with a pulse. The AED is designed to detect ventricular fibrillation and ventricular tachycardia, but cannot detect the presence of a pulse. Some patients with ventricular tachycardia actually have a pulse and are treated differently from those in cardiac arrest. Defibrillating a patient with a pulse will most likely result in cardiac arrest.

▶ Special AED Situations

It is essential to ensure your safety, the safety of others at the scene, and the patient. As such, keep the following factors in mind when using an AED.

Pacemakers and Implanted Defibrillators

You may encounter a patient who has an automated implanted cardioverter-defibrillator (AICD) or pacemaker. These devices are used in patients who are at a high risk for certain cardiac dysrhythmias and cardiac arrest. It is easy to recognize AICDs or pacemakers because they create a hard lump beneath the skin, usually on the upper left side of the chest (just below the clavicle). If the AED pads are placed directly over the device, then the effectiveness of the shock delivered by the AED may be blocked, and the shock could potentially damage the implanted device. Therefore, if you identify an AICD or pacemaker, then place the AED pads at least 1 inch (2.5 cm) away from the device.

Occasionally, the implanted device will deliver shocks to the patient. If you observe the patient's muscles twitching as if he or she was just shocked, then continue CPR and wait 30 to 60 seconds before delivering a shock from the AED.

Special Populations

If you encounter an infant or small child in cardiac arrest who has an existing cardiac condition, then assess the chest and abdomen carefully for the presence of an implanted device. Small infants and children do not have sufficient musculature in the chest to support the device, so it is typically implanted in the abdomen. By the time the child reaches school age, it has generally been moved to the upper left chest under the clavicle.

Water

Water conducts electricity. Therefore, the AED should not be used in water. If the patient's chest is wet, the electrical current may move across the skin rather than between the pads to the patient's heart. If the patient is submerged in water, pull him or her out of the water and quickly dry the skin before attaching the AED pads. Do not delay CPR to dry the patient thoroughly; instead, quickly wipe off as much moisture as possible from the chest. If the patient is lying in a small puddle of water or in the snow, the AED can be used, but again, the patient's chest should be quickly dried as much as possible.

Hair

Occasionally, you will encounter a patient with enough chest hair to prevent the AED pads from adhering properly. The pads must be in direct contact with the chest to effectively defibrillate the patient. You may receive a "check electrodes" or "check pads" error message from the AED when you attempt to analyze if the pads are not adhering to the chest or if the cable is not properly connected to the AED. EMS providers generally carry small razors for removing hair; however, this will not be available if you are responding as a layperson. The quickest way to remove hair is to press the AED pads firmly against the chest in the appropriate area and then quickly pull them off, taking the hair with the pad. Take a new set of pads and place over the areas where the hair has been removed. Ensure you have at least two sets of AED pads before using the first set of pads to remove hair.

Transdermal Medication Patches

You may encounter a patient who is receiving medication through a transdermal medication patch, such as nitroglycerin, nicotine, hormones, or various pain medications. The patch could reduce the flow of the electrical current from the AED to the heart and may burn the skin. If the medication patch interferes with AED pad placement, remove the patch with your gloved hands and wipe the skin with gauze to remove any residue prior to attaching the AED pad. Since the medication is absorbed through the skin, it will be absorbed through your skin if you are exposed to it. Patches should be removed as soon as possible, but should not take precedence over chest compressions. The medication delivered through the patch may be instrumental in the cause of the cardiac arrest. For example, nitroglycerin is a potent vasodilator that may cause hypotension and narcotic patches are a common source of overdoses.

Positioning the Patient

For CPR to be effective, the patient must be lying supine on a firm, flat surface, with enough clear space around the patient for at least two rescuers to perform CPR and use the AED. If the patient is crumpled up or lying face down (prone), you need to move him or her to a supine position with attention to cervical spine control if a potential injury is suspected **Figure 15-7**. If the patient is found in a bed, then move him or her to the floor. You cannot effectively perform chest compressions on a soft or pliable surface.

If possible, log roll the patient onto a long backboard as you position him or her for CPR. A backboard will provide support for CPR and offer an easy medium for moving the patient as a unit.

Check for Breathing and a Pulse

After you determine a patient is unresponsive, quickly check for breathing and a pulse. These assessments can occur simultaneously and should take no longer than 10 seconds in total.

Visualize the chest for signs of breathing while palpating for a carotid pulse. Feel for the carotid artery by locating the larynx at the front of the neck and then sliding two fingers toward one side (the side closest to you). The pulse is felt in the groove between the larynx and sternocleidomastoid muscle, with the pads of the index and middle fingers held side by side **Figure 15-8**. Light pressure is sufficient to palpate the pulse.

Provide External Chest Compressions

If the patient is not breathing (or is breathing only slowly or occasionally, known as agonal gasps) and does not have a pulse, then begin CPR, starting with chest compressions. It is critical to perform compressions properly. Chest compressions are administered by applying rhythmic pressure and relaxation to the lower half of the sternum. The heart is located slightly to the left of the middle of the chest between the sternum and the spine **Figure 15-9**. Compressions squeeze the heart, thereby acting as a pump to circulate blood. Allow the chest to completely recoil between compressions, which enhances blood return to the heart. Do not lean on the

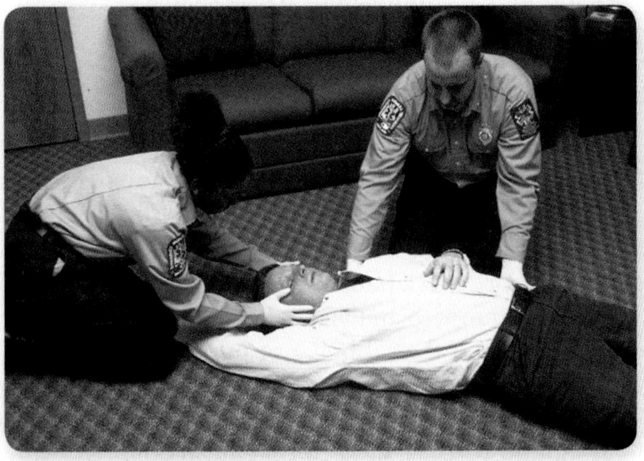

Figure 15-7 Ensure the patient is in a supine position. Protect the patient's neck in case a spinal injury is present, and move him or her as a unit, without twisting.

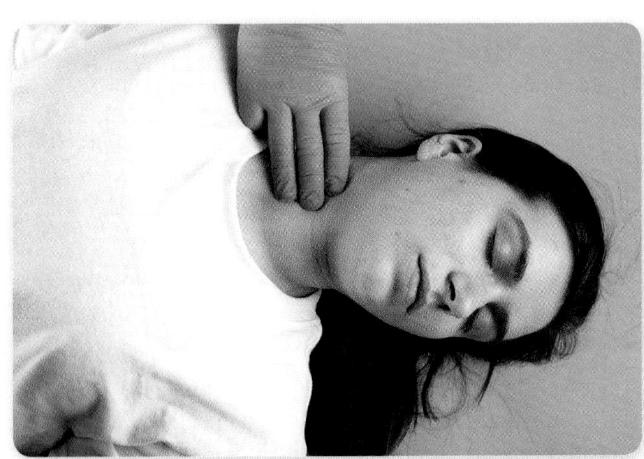

Figure 15-8 Feel for the carotid artery by locating the larynx, then slide your index and middle fingers toward one side. You can feel the pulse in the groove between the larynx and sternocleidomastoid muscle.

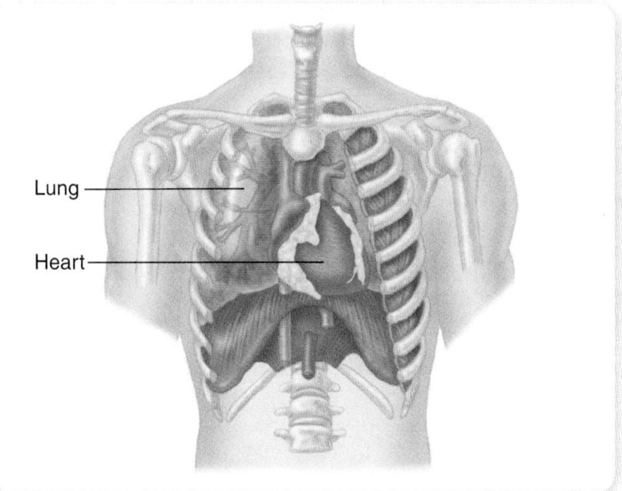

Figure 15-9 The heart lies slightly to the left of the middle of the chest between the sternum and spine.

chest between compressions. When artificial ventilation is provided, the blood that is circulated through the lungs during chest compressions is likely to receive adequate oxygen to maintain tissue perfusion. However, even when external chest compressions are performed properly, they circulate only one-third of the blood that is normally pumped by the heart.

Proper Hand Position and Compression Technique

With the adult patient, correct hand position is established by placing the heel of one hand on the sternum in the center of the chest (lower half of the sternum). Your technique may be improved or made more comfortable if you interlock the fingers of your lower hand with the fingers of your upper hand.

To perform chest compressions, follow the steps in Skill Drill 15-1.

Skill Drill 15-1 Performing Chest Compressions

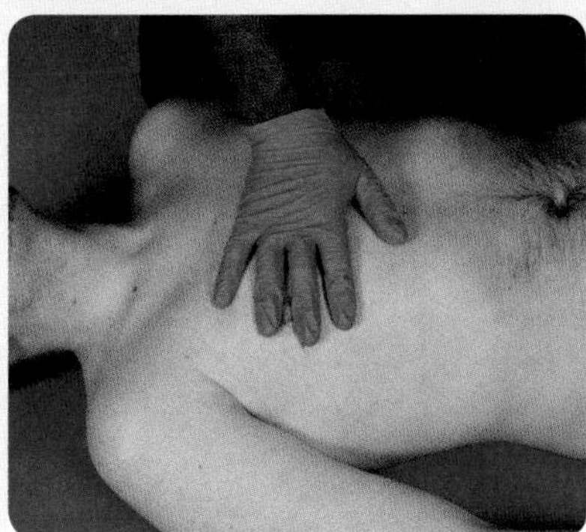

Step 1 Take standard precautions. Place the heel of one hand on the center of the chest over the lower half of the sternum.

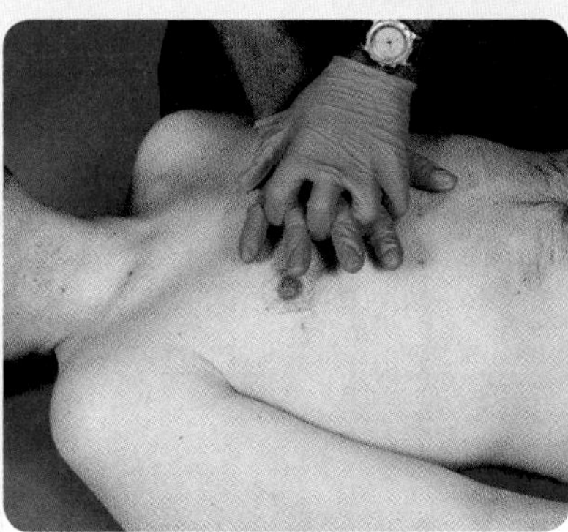

Step 2 Place the heel of your other hand over the first hand.

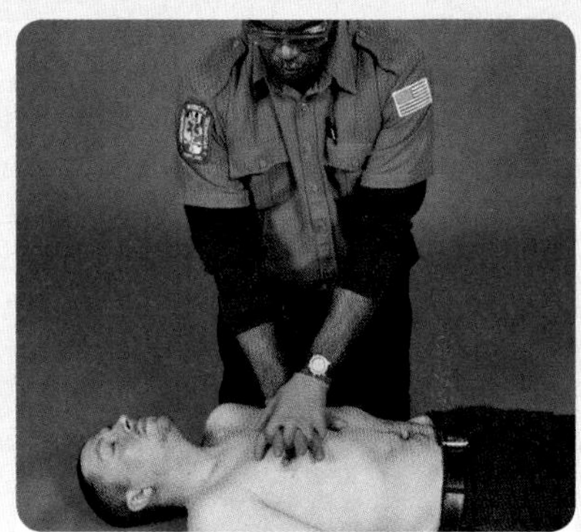

Step 3 With your arms straight, lock your elbows and position your shoulders directly over your hands, so the thrust of each compression is straight down on the sternum. Do not rock forward on the ribs during compressions. Depress the sternum at a rate of 100 to 120 compressions per minute and to a depth of 2 inches to 2.4 inches (5 cm to 6 cm) using a downward movement. Allow the chest to return to its normal position; do not lean on the patient's chest between compressions. Compression and relaxation should be of equal duration.

Words of Wisdom

An alternate technique for chest compressions may be helpful for those with arthritis or other joint conditions. Place the first hand in the proper position on the sternum and use the second hand to grasp the wrist of the first hand to provide support during the compressions.

Complications from chest compressions are rare but can include fractured ribs, a lacerated liver, and a fractured sternum. Although these injuries cannot be entirely avoided, you can minimize the chance that they will occur if you use good technique and proper hand placement.

Words of Wisdom

If you hear a popping or crunching noise, or if you feel crepitus during chest compressions, then stop long enough to reassess your hand position. You may fracture the patient's ribs if your hands are to the left or right of the sternum. If your hand placement is correct, then continue with compressions.

Your motions must be smooth, rhythmic, and uninterrupted **Figure 15-10A**. Short, jabbing compressions are not effective in producing artificial blood flow. Do not remove the heel of your hand from the patient's chest during relaxation, but ensure you completely release pressure on the sternum so it can return to its normal resting position between compressions **Figure 15-10B**.

Special Populations

Proper hand position and depth of compression, which are always important, take on added priority in geriatric patients who are likely to have brittle bones and chest cartilage. There is no guarantee against causing injury to these tissues, and you must compress adequately to provide adequate perfusion of vital organs. Pay particular attention to your compression technique and hand placement, to help reduce avoidable injuries.

Words of Wisdom

When performing chest compressions on an adult, compress the chest to a depth of at least 2 inches (5 cm), but not more than 2.4 inches (6 cm). It is difficult to achieve such a precise depth without the use of a monitoring device that provides immediate feedback **Figure 15-11**. If such a device is available to you, then use it.

It is more dangerous to compress the chest too lightly than it is to compress too forcefully. Compressing hard can lead to fatigue, and as you become tired, your compressions will become shallower. Therefore, it is critical to push hard and push fast and switch compressors (the person providing chest compressions) every 2 minutes—even if the compressor does not feel tired.

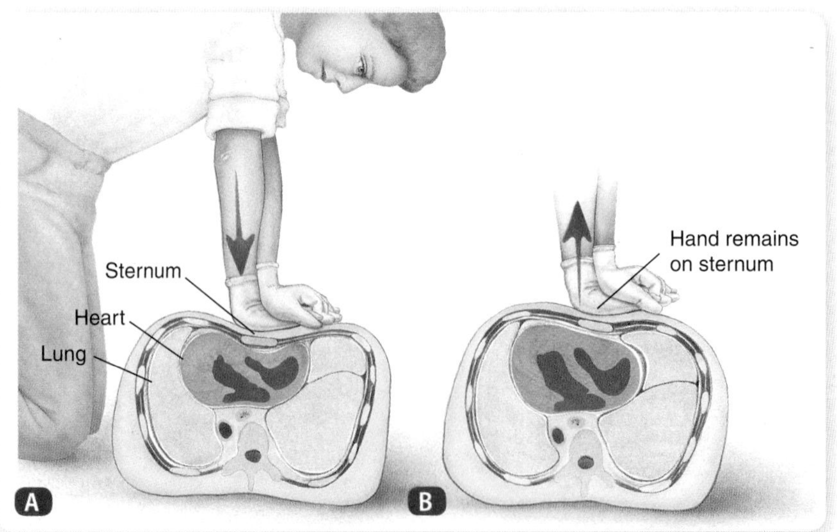

Figure 15-10 A. Compression and relaxation should be rhythmic and of equal duration (a 1:1 ratio). **B.** Pressure on the sternum must be released so the sternum can return to its normal resting position between compressions.

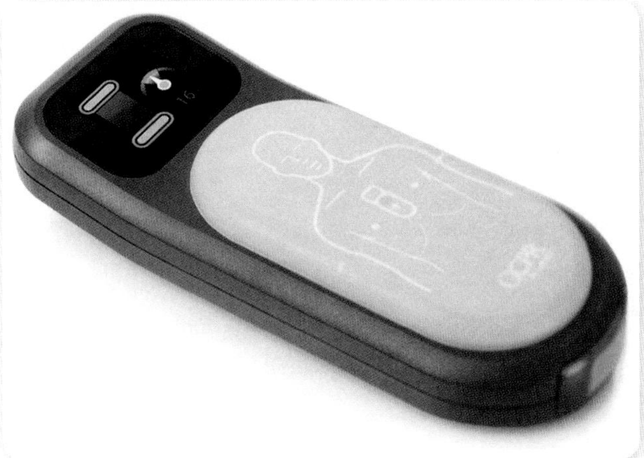

Figure 15-11 Cardiopulmonary resuscitation feedback devices help ensure a consistent rate and depth of compressions.

Words of Wisdom

Chest compressions create blood flow to the heart through filling of the coronary arteries. Every time compressions are stopped, blood flow—and, thus, perfusion—to the heart (and brain) drops to zero. It takes 5 to 10 compressions to reestablish effective blood flow to the heart after chest compressions are resumed. Avoid frequent or prolonged interruptions in chest compressions, which lead to poor patient outcomes.

Opening the Airway and Providing Artificial Ventilation

Opening the Airway in Adults

Without an open airway, rescue breathing will not be effective. As discussed in Chapter 11, *Airway Management*, the two techniques for opening the airway in adults are the head tilt–chin lift maneuver and the jaw-thrust maneuver. These manual maneuvers are designed to bring the tongue forward and off the back of the throat. The **head tilt–chin lift maneuver** is effective for opening the airway in most patients when there is no indication of a spinal injury Figure 15-12.

In patients who have not sustained trauma, this simple maneuver is sometimes all that is required for the patient to resume breathing. If the patient has any foreign material or vomitus in the mouth, then quickly remove it. Liquids may be removed with a suction device, and solid materials may be removed by using your hooked index finger. If suction is not readily available, roll the patient to the side to remove foreign materials. Figure 15-13 reviews how to perform the head tilt–chin lift maneuver in an adult.

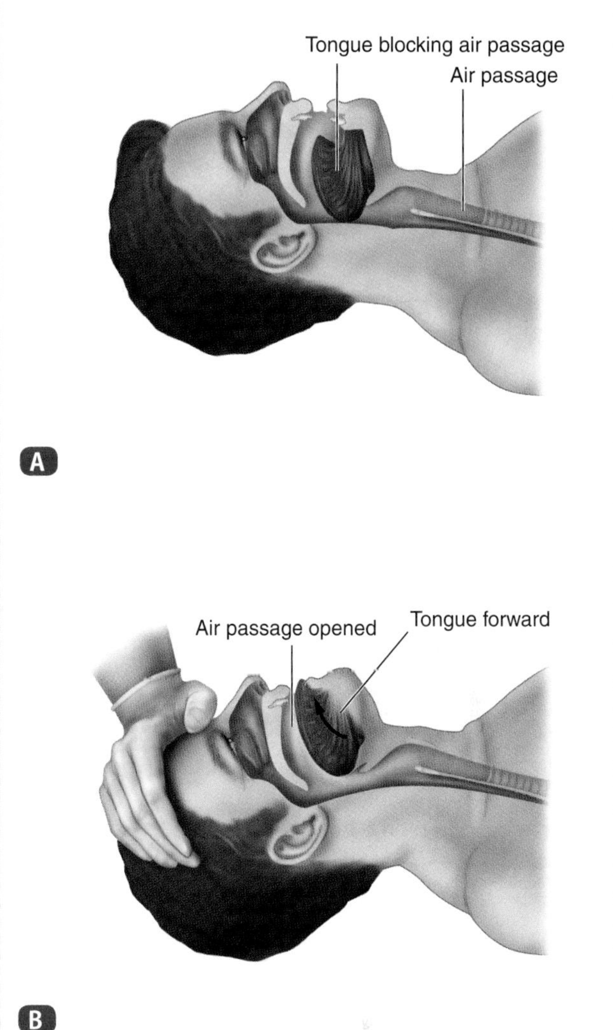

Figure 15-12 A. Relaxation of the tongue back into the throat causes airway obstruction. **B.** The head tilt–chin lift maneuver combines two movements of opening the airway; head tilt is shown here.

Special Populations

When caring for older patients who wear dentures, the head tilt–chin lift maneuver has the added advantage of holding loose dentures in place, which makes obstruction by the lips less likely. Performing ventilation is much easier when dentures are in place. However, remove dentures that do not stay in place. Partial dentures (plates) may become loose as a result of an injury or as you are providing care, so check these periodically.

If spinal injury is suspected, then use the **jaw-thrust maneuver**. To perform a jaw-thrust maneuver, place your fingers behind the angles of the patient's lower

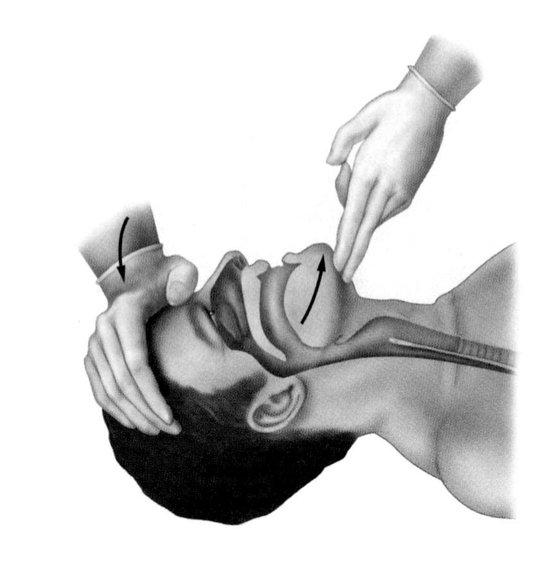

Figure 15-13 To perform the head tilt–chin lift maneuver, place one hand on the patient's forehead and apply firm backward pressure with your palm to tilt the head back. Next, place the tips of the index and middle fingers of your other hand under the lower jaw near the bony part of the chin. Lift the chin upward, bringing the entire lower jaw with it, helping to tilt the head back.

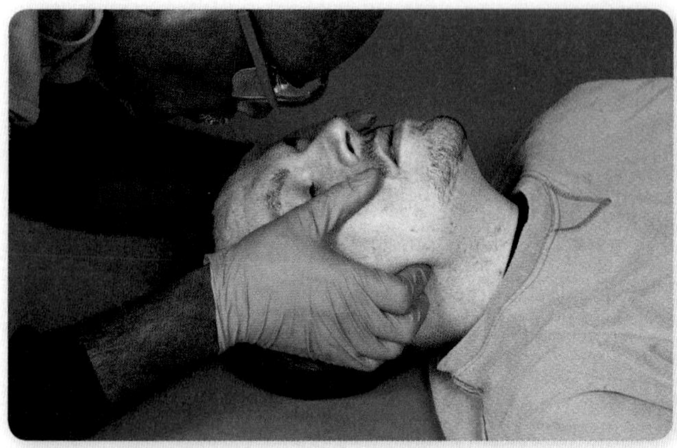

Figure 15-14 To perform the jaw-thrust maneuver, maintain the head in neutral alignment and place your fingers behind the angles of the lower jaw, and move the jaw upward. The completed maneuver should look like this.

jaw and then move the jaw upward. Keep the head in a neutral position as you move the jaw upward and open the mouth. If the patient's mouth remains closed, then use your thumbs to pull down the patient's lower lip to allow breathing. **Figure 15-14** reviews how to perform the jaw-thrust maneuver in an adult.

YOU are the Provider PART 2

You arrive at the scene and find two bystanders performing CPR on the patient, who appears to be in his late 40s. A second BLS ambulance is en route to the scene and will arrive in about 5 minutes. You perform a primary survey as your partner opens the AED.

Recording Time: 1 Minute	
Appearance	Motionless; cyanosis of the face
Level of consciousness	Unresponsive
Airway	Open; clear of secretions or foreign bodies
Breathing	Absent
Circulation	No carotid pulse; skin, cool and pale; no gross bleeding

Your partner takes over performing compressions while one of the bystanders delivers mouth-to-mask ventilations. The other bystander tells you the patient had just dropped off a load of produce and sat down in his truck, and then he slumped over the steering wheel. By the time the bystander reached him, he was unresponsive and not breathing. The bystander further tells you he immediately called 9-1-1 and then began CPR.

3. What links in the chain of survival have been maintained at this point?
4. Why is it so crucial to minimize interruptions in CPR?

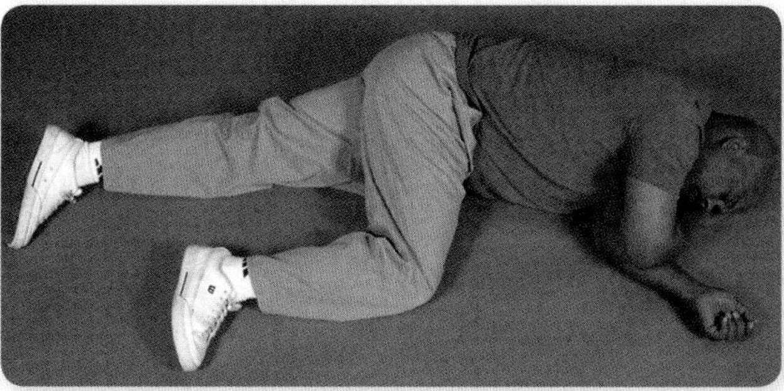

Figure 15-15 The recovery position is used to maintain an open airway in an adequately breathing patient with a decreased level of consciousness who has no spine, hip, or pelvic injuries. It allows vomitus, blood, and any other secretions to drain from the mouth.

▶ Recovery Position

If the patient is breathing adequately on his or her own and has no signs of injury to the spine, hip, or pelvis, then place him or her in the **recovery position**. This position helps to maintain a clear airway in a patient with a decreased level of consciousness who has not sustained traumatic injuries and is breathing adequately on his or her own Figure 15-15. It also allows vomitus or secretions to drain from the mouth. Roll the patient onto his or her side so the head, shoulders, and torso move as a unit, without twisting. Then place the top hand under his or her cheek. Never place a patient who has a suspected head or spinal injury in the recovery position because in this position, the spine is not aligned, spinal stabilization is not possible, and further spinal injury could result. Likewise, if the patient has a hip or pelvic injury, then positioning the patient on his or her side could cause fractured bone ends to compress or sever large arteries and veins, resulting in severe internal bleeding. You should suspect an associated spinal injury in any unresponsive patient with a hip or pelvic injury until proven otherwise.

▶ Breathing

A lack of oxygen (hypoxia), combined with too much carbon dioxide in the blood (hypercapnia), is lethal. Ventilations should be delivered over 1 second. This gentle, slow method of ventilating the patient prevents air from being forced into the stomach resulting in gastric distention.

▶ Provide Artificial Ventilations

Ventilations, the exchange of air between the lungs and the environment, can be given by one or two EMS providers. Use a barrier device when you administer ventilations in the prehospital environment, such as a pocket mask with a one-way valve or a bag-mask device Figure 15-16. Use devices that supply supplemental oxygen when possible. Devices with an oxygen reservoir will provide higher percentages of oxygen to the patient. Regardless of whether you ventilate the patient with or without supplemental oxygen, you should observe the chest for visible rise to assess the effectiveness of your ventilations.

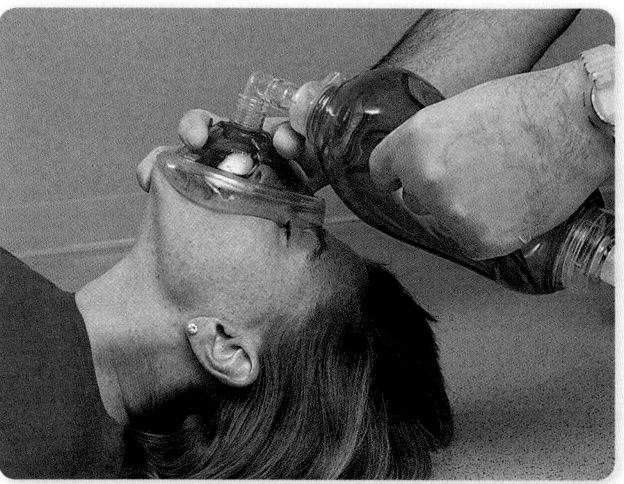

Figure 15-16 When you provide ventilations, use a bag-mask device (shown here) or a pocket mask with one-way valve.

The specific steps of CPR are discussed later in this chapter. Adult BLS procedures are summarized in Table 15-1. Pediatric BLS procedures are summarized in Table 15-2 later in this chapter. Resuscitation of a neonate is discussed in Chapter 35, *Obstetrics and Neonatal Care*.

Hyperventilation, ventilating too fast or with too much force, may cause increased intrathoracic pressure (pressure inside the chest cavity). Increased intrathoracic pressure reduces the amount of blood that returns to the heart, thus decreasing the effectiveness of chest compressions and resulting in the heart and brain receiving decreased amounts of oxygen. Rapid, forceful ventilations also increase the risk of gastric distention and may result in expulsion of gastric contents and aspiration of fluid or vomitus into the lungs.

Words of Wisdom

Atmospheric air is 21% oxygen. We exhale approximately 16% oxygen, which means we only use about 5%. This is why mouth-to-mask or mouth-to-mouth ventilations are still effective until we can ventilate the patient with 100% oxygen. When providing ventilations via mouth-to-mask without an oxygen inlet, you can increase the percentage of expired oxygen by placing a nasal cannula on yourself.

Stoma Ventilation

Patients who have undergone a laryngectomy (surgical removal of the larynx) often have a permanent tracheal stoma at the midline in the neck. In this case, a stoma is an opening that connects the trachea directly to the skin Figure 15-17. Because it is at the midline, the stoma is the only opening that will move air into the patient's lungs. Patients with a stoma should be ventilated with a bag-mask device or pocket mask device placed directly over the stoma.

Table 15-1 Review of Adult BLS Procedures

Procedure	
Circulation	
Pulse check	Carotid artery
Compression area	Center of the chest, in between the nipples
Compression depth	2 in. to 2.4 in. (5 cm to 6 cm)
Compression rate	100 to 120/min
Compression-to-ventilation ratio (until advanced airway is inserted)	30:2
Foreign body obstruction	Responsive: abdominal thrusts (Heimlich maneuver); chest thrusts if patient is pregnant or has obesity Unresponsive: CPR
Airway	
Airway positioning	Head tilt–chin lift maneuver; jaw-thrust maneuver if spinal injury is suspected
Breathing	
Ventilations	1 breath every 5 to 6 seconds (10 to 12 breaths/min); about 1 second per breath; visible chest rise
Ventilations with advanced airway placed	1 breath every 6 seconds (a rate of 10 breaths/min)

Abbreviations: BLS, basic life support; CPR, cardiopulmonary resuscitation

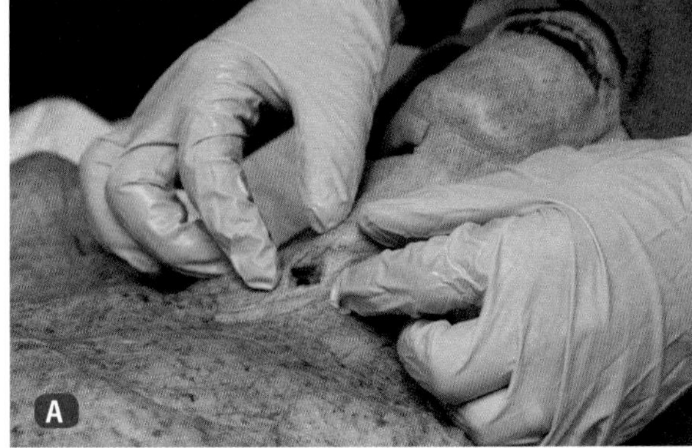

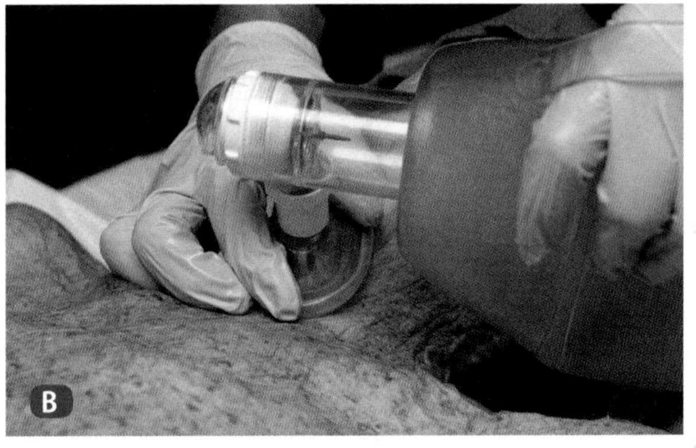

Figure 15-17 A. This stoma connects the trachea directly to the skin. **B.** Use a bag-mask device or pocket mask device to ventilate a patient with a stoma.

Not all stomas are disconnected from the nose and mouth. If air leakage through the nose and mouth interferes with ventilation through the stoma, then cover the nose and mouth with your hand to make a seal. Use a pediatric or infant mask to ventilate through the stoma.

Gastric Distention

Artificial ventilation may result in the stomach becoming filled with air, a condition called **gastric distention.** Although it occurs more easily in children, this condition also happens frequently in adults. Gastric distention is likely to occur if you hyperventilate the patient. If you ventilate too forcefully, or if the patient's airway is not opened adequately, then the excess pressure opens the esophagus and allows air to enter the stomach. Therefore, it is important for you to give slow, gentle breaths. Such breaths are also more effective in ventilating the lungs. Excessive inflation of the stomach is dangerous because it can cause the patient to vomit during CPR. It can also reduce lung volume by exerting pressure on the diaphragm.

If massive gastric distention interferes with adequate ventilation, then contact medical control. Check the airway again and reposition the patient, watch for rise and fall of the chest, and avoid giving forceful breaths. Have a suction unit available in case the patient vomits. Remember, mortality increases significantly if aspiration occurs. Advanced airway adjuncts can also eliminate gastric distention because the air goes directly into the lungs. Chapter 11, *Airway Management,* lists adjuncts appropriate at the AEMT level. If a paramedic is available he or she can insert an orogastric or nasogastric tube to decompress the stomach or may intubate the patient to ensure ventilation without the possibility of gastric distention or aspiration.

One-Rescuer Adult CPR

When you provide CPR alone, you must provide a continuous cycle of 30 chest compressions followed by two artificial ventilations (a ratio of 30:2). To perform one-rescuer adult CPR, follow the steps in Skill Drill 15-2.

Two-Rescuer Adult CPR

You and your team should be able to perform one-rescuer and two-rescuer CPR with ease. Two-rescuer CPR is preferred because it is less tiring and it facilitates effective chest compressions. In fact, a team approach to CPR and AED use is far superior to the one-rescuer approach. Once one-rescuer CPR is in progress, additional rescuers can be easily added to the procedure. Before assisting with CPR, a second rescuer should apply the AED and then set up airway adjuncts, including a bag-mask device and suction, and insert an oropharyngeal (oral) airway. When the first rescuer completes a cycle of 30 compressions, the first rescuer should move to the head and give two ventilations while the second rescuer moves into position to provide chest compressions. To perform two-rescuer adult CPR, follow the steps in Skill Drill 15-3.

Skill Drill 15-2 Performing One-Rescuer Adult CPR

NR Skill

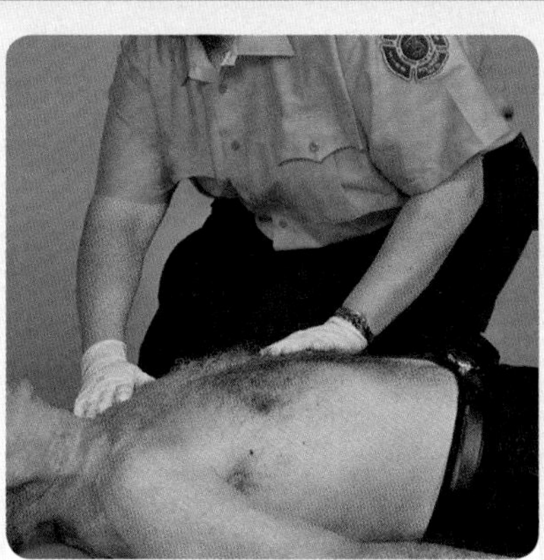

Step 1 Take standard precautions. Establish unresponsiveness and call for additional help.

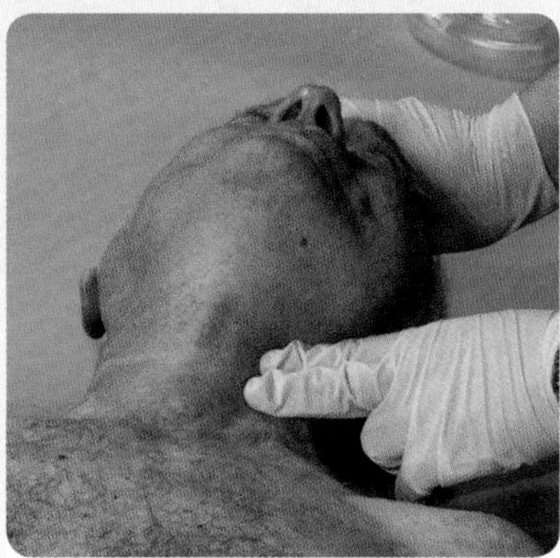

Step 2 Position the patient properly (supine) on a flat surface. Check for breathing and a carotid pulse for no more than 10 seconds.

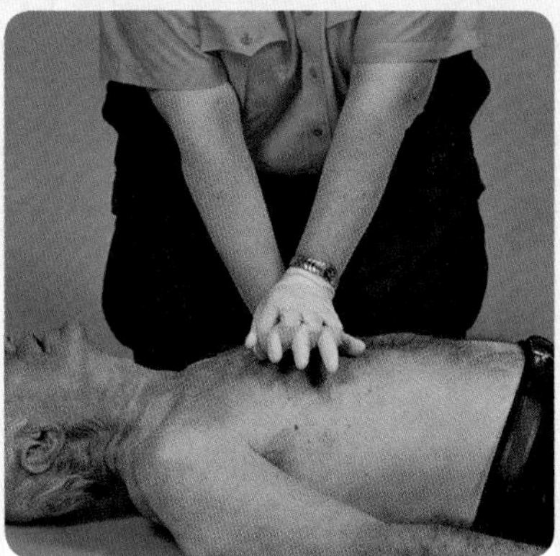

Step 3 If pulse and breathing are absent, then perform CPR until an AED is available. Kneel at the patient's side. Place your hands in the proper position for delivering external chest compressions, as described previously. Give 30 chest compressions at a rate of 100 to 120 per minute for an adult. Each set of 30 compressions should take about 17 seconds.

(continued)

Skill Drill 15-2 Performing One-Rescuer Adult CPR *(continued)*

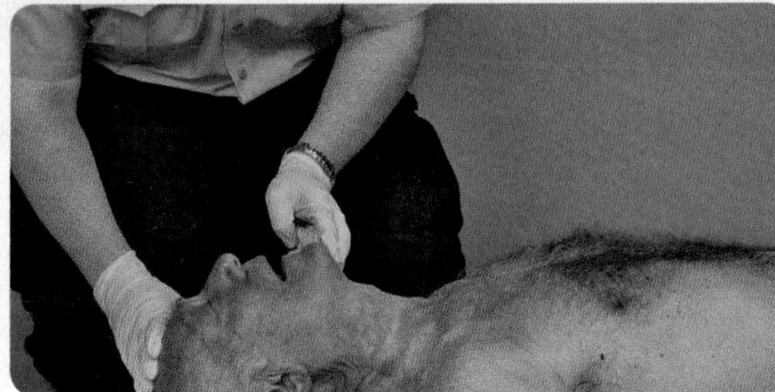

Step 4 Open the airway according to your suspicion of spinal injury.

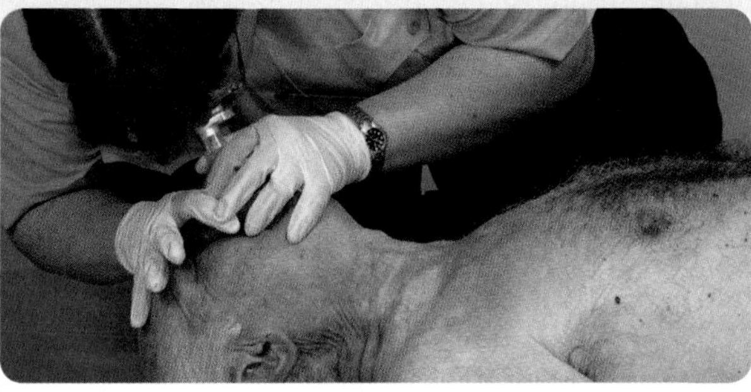

Step 5 Give two ventilations of 1 second each and observe for visible chest rise. Continue cycles of 30 chest compressions and two ventilations until additional personnel arrive or the patient starts to move.

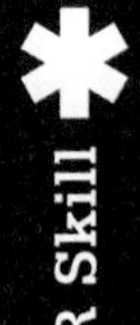

NR Skill

Skill Drill 15-3 Performing Two-Rescuer Adult CPR

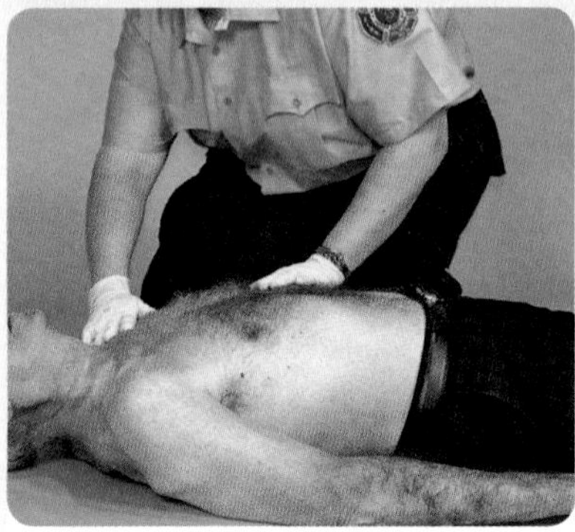

Step 1 Take standard precautions. Establish unresponsiveness while your partner moves to the patient's side to be ready to deliver chest compressions.

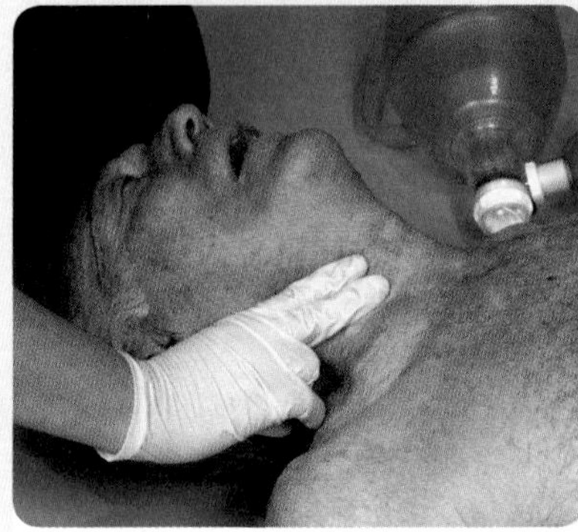

Step 2 If the patient is unresponsive, then simultaneously check for breathing and palpate for a carotid pulse; take no more than 10 seconds to do this.

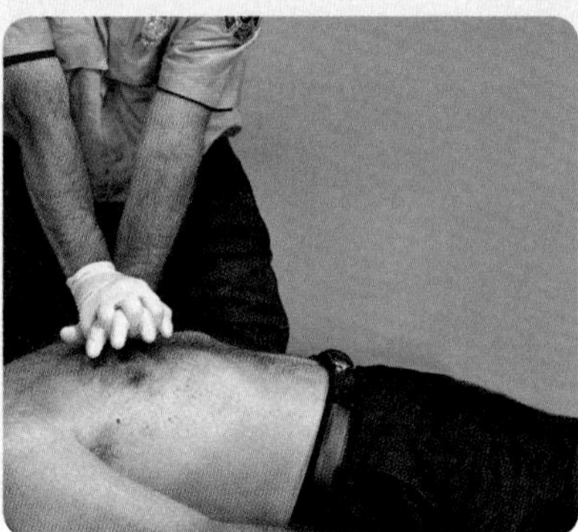

Step 3 If the patient is not breathing and has no pulse, then begin CPR, starting with chest compressions. Give 30 chest compressions at a rate of 100 to 120 per minute. If an AED is available, then apply it and follow its voice prompts. Do not interrupt chest compressions to apply the AED pads.

Skill Drill 15-3 Performing Two-Rescuer Adult CPR *(continued)*

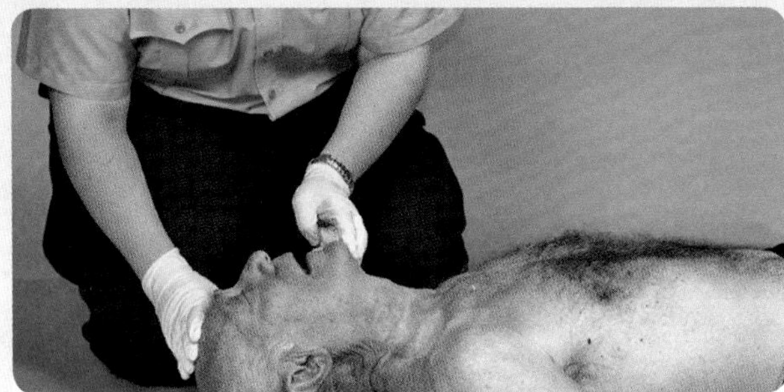

Step 4 Open the airway according to your suspicion of spinal injury.

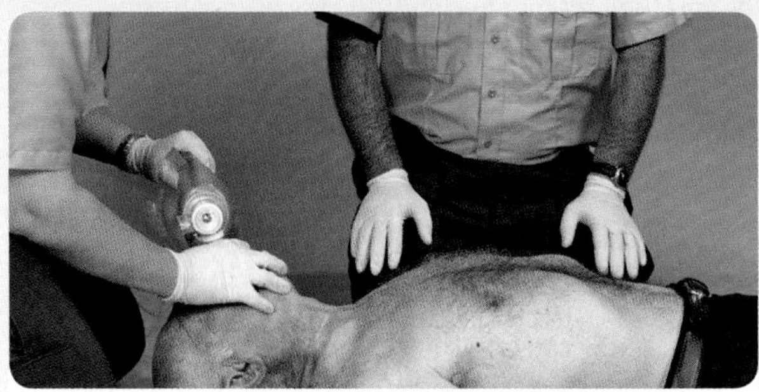

Step 5 Give two ventilations of 1 second each and observe for visible chest rise. Perform five cycles of 30 compressions and two ventilations (this should take about 2 minutes). After 2 minutes of CPR, the compressor and ventilator should switch positions. It should not take longer than 5 seconds to switch positions. Reanalyze the patient's cardiac rhythm with the AED every 2 minutes and deliver a shock if indicated. Continue cycles of 30 chest compressions and two ventilations until other providers take over or the patient starts to move. Perform five cycles of 30 compressions and two ventilations (this should take about 2 minutes). After 2 minutes of CPR, the compressor and ventilator should switch positions. It should not take longer than 5 seconds to switch positions. Reanalyze the patient's cardiac rhythm with the AED every 2 minutes and deliver a shock if indicated. Continue cycles of 30 chest compressions and two ventilations until additional providers arrive allowing you to initiate ALS care, or until the patient starts to move.

Words of Wisdom

When CPR is in progress on a patient who has an advanced airway device in place (eg, ET tube, King LT supraglottic airway, i-gel supraglottic airway), cycles of CPR are not indicated. Compressions should be continuous at a rate of 100 to 120 per minute and ventilations should occur at a rate of one breath every 6 seconds (10 breaths/min). While there is no synchronization of compressions and ventilations, it is more effective to deliver ventilations during the recoil of the chest than during the actual compression.

▶ Switching Positions

It is critical to switch rescuers during CPR to maintain high-quality compressions. After five cycles of CPR (about 2 minutes), the rescuer providing compressions to the patient (the compressor) will begin to tire, and compression quality will decrease. Therefore, compressors should switch positions every 2 minutes. If there are only two rescuers on scene, the two rescuers will alternate positions. If additional rescuers are available, the compressor should rotate every 2 minutes. During switches, every effort should be made to minimize the time that no compressions are being administered. It should take less than 5 seconds to switch compressors.

The switch between the two rescuers can be easily accomplished. Rescuer one (the first compressor) should finish the cycle of 30 compressions while the second rescuer moves to the opposite side of the chest and moves into position to begin compressions. Rescuer one should deliver two rescue breaths and then rescuer two should take over compressions by administering 30 chest compressions. Rescuer one will then deliver two ventilations and the CPR cycles will continue as needed until the next 2-minute mark (five cycles) is reached, at which time the process will be repeated.

Crew Resource Management

In the past, EMS training focused on mastering individual skills and did not always include the benefits of an effective team-based approach. Specifically, there was a lack of focus on the behavioral and communication skills that were necessary when in a team environment. Also known as the "pit crew" approach, this approach can be particularly effective in cardiac arrest resuscitation. Each member is assigned a particular role prior to treating an actual patient in cardiopulmonary arrest. This helps to prevent the potential confusion and lack of direction that may occur on a chaotic scene.

Crew resource management (CRM) is a way for team members to work together with the team leader to develop and maintain a shared understanding of the emergency situation. CRM allows team members with different skill sets to collaborate and communicate, fulfill their roles and responsibilities, and achieve the shared goal of the best possible patient outcome **Figure 15-18**. Under the CRM model, each team member is responsible for maintaining situational awareness of the patient's current condition and sharing any crucial information with the team leader. Likewise, the team leader is responsible for listening to any crucial information you or other team members provide and incorporating that information into his or her decision-making process.

Even in the often loud and hectic environment in which EMS providers work, when you believe there is an immediate or potential problem you must bring it to the team leader's attention. CRM recommends using the PACE mnemonic:

- P *Probe.* Look or ask to confirm the problem.
- A *Alert.* Communicate the problem to the team leader.
- C *Challenge.* If the issue is not corrected, challenge the team's present course of action that is leading to the problem. For example, "Lieutenant, I think this additional action should be taken. Do you agree?"
- E *Emergency.* If the problem is clear and critical (such as an immediate safety issue), then immediately communicate the emergency to the entire team.

The CRM model does not mean you are free to ignore the chain of command within the incident command system. It means you are empowered to provide the team leader and other team members with immediate feedback in the event of a potential threat to the patient's or crew's safety. It means the team, as a whole, recognizes the importance of getting input from each individual and that the team is committed to fostering open communication. CRM empowers people to speak up clearly and concisely when they detect a problem or potential problem.

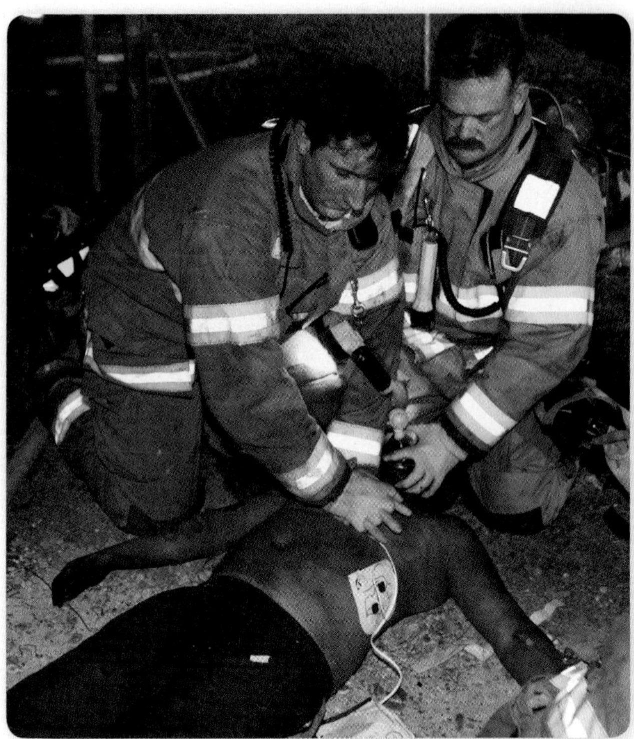

Figure 15-18 Collaboration and communication are crucial aspects of crew resource management.

Whether you are a code team member or a code team leader, know your role and the roles of the other team members during the resuscitation attempt. This helps you anticipate and understand what steps are coming next and how essential your role is as part of the resuscitation attempt. Regardless of the skills you are trained and appropriately authorized to perform, it is essential to the success of the resuscitation that you are prepared, have practiced regularly, have mastered the algorithms, and are committed to success.

Code Team Member Roles

A code team member may be called on to perform all of the following roles (and more):

- **Ventilator**—manages the airway. This team member's duties include suctioning the patient, ventilating the patient with a bag-mask device, inserting an advanced airway device (eg, LMA, Combitube, or King LT), and maintaining manual in-line stabilization of the head and neck.

- **Active compressor**—provides high-quality chest compressions. The responsibility of this team member is to compress for 2 minutes and be the on-deck compressor for 2 minutes.
- **On-deck compressor**—At the 2-minute point, this team member needs to be ready to relieve the compressor without any interruption in compressions. Other functions include assisting with application of a mechanical CPR adjunct device (if available), assessing vital signs, and preparing the patient for transport.
- **Other support personnel**—responsible for operating the AED, gaining venous (IV or IO) access, providing documentation for the patient care report, and supporting family members.

▶ Code Team Leader Roles

Every resuscitation team needs a leader to organize the efforts of the group. Clearly, the code team leader must know all of the specific skills and be able to expertly perform each skill—occasionally the code team leader will serve as the backup for a team member who may be having difficulty inserting a tube or gaining IV/IO access. The code team leader is often responsible for ensuring everything gets done at the right time in the right way.

The roles of the code team leader may include all of the following:

- Obtaining the patient's history and performing the physical exam
- Keeping track of the time
- Making a medication decision following the algorithm
- Clearly delegating tasks to code team members
- Completing documentation after the resuscitation attempt
- Talking with medical control
- Controlling the resuscitation scene

Code team leaders must also model excellent behavior and leadership skills for their team and all others who may be involved in the resuscitation. The code team leader helps train future team leaders, seeks to improve the effectiveness of the entire team through continuous quality improvement, and evaluates processes after the resuscitation to help prepare for the next code.

Postresuscitation Support

Postresuscitative care is an important component of caring for cardiac arrest patients. If an effective cardiac rhythm is restored in the field, you should provide immediate transport because the patient needs careful monitoring and titrated therapy that can most effectively be provided in an intensive care unit. During transport it is imperative that you monitor the patient's blood glucose level and ensure effective ventilation with the proper rate and tidal volume. Always leave AED pads in place. In the event the patient goes into cardiopulmonary arrest again, you will save valuable time if you can immediately analyze the rhythm without replacing the AED pads.

The following is a summary of postcardiac arrest care:[5]

1. Optimize ventilation and oxygenation
   a. Maintain oxygen saturation ≥94%
   b. Consider advanced airway and waveform capnography
   c. Do not hyperventilate
2. Treat hypotension (SBP <90 mm Hg)
   a. IV/IO bolus
   b. Consider treatable causes (H's & T's)
   c. Paramedic backup for administration of a vasopressor infusion
3. Advanced critical care in the ED including:
   a. 12-Lead ECG to rule out STEMI (ST-elevation myocardial infarction) or AMI (acute myocardial infarction)
   b. Coronary reperfusion
   c. Targeted temperature management for comatose patients

Devices and Techniques to Assist Circulation

The effectiveness of CPR depends on the amount of blood circulated throughout the body as a result of chest

Words of Wisdom

Many EMS systems have implemented a *pit crew approach* to the management of cardiac arrest. The term originated in motor racing, in which teams of technicians rapidly assess and repair vehicles in a matter of seconds. Following this model, each resuscitation team member is assigned a specific role before beginning care of the cardiac arrest patient. For example:

- AEMT 1 will be the team leader.
- AEMT 2 and AEMT 3 will perform CPR.
- AEMT 4 will operate the AED.

This model clarifies each team member's role and responsibilities and minimizes confusion on the scene. If there are only two AEMTs on scene initially—as is the situation in many cases—then a plan should be developed to integrate additional rescuers into the resuscitation effort as they arrive. This preplanned approach allows rescuers to accomplish multiple steps and assessments simultaneously, rather than the slower, sequential manner used by individual rescuers. Therefore, the pit crew model minimizes the time to first compression. The success of this team approach depends on preplanning, practice, and thorough familiarity with the cardiac arrest algorithm.

Special Populations

On occasion, you may encounter a patient who has a left ventricular assist device (LVAD). The LVAD is a mechanical pump that is implanted in the chest and helps pump blood from the left ventricle to the aorta. A tube from the device passes through the skin and is attached to an external power source that patients wear on their belts or on over-the-shoulder harnesses. The LVAD is commonly implanted in patients with severe heart failure or in those who are awaiting a heart transplant. If the LVAD is working, then you will hear a humming sound when listening to the chest with a stethoscope. Blood flows continuously through the LVAD, and the more assistance the LVAD is providing to the heart, the weaker the patient's pulse will be. In some LVAD patients, you may not feel a pulse at all, even though they are responsive and alert. When transporting a patient who has an LVAD, be sure to bring all of the LVAD equipment with you and ensure the receiving facility is capable of caring for the patient's specific needs.

Know the location of LVAD patients in your service area. If possible, visit with the patient prior to any emergency to determine his or her specific device and to obtain instructions. Family members are usually knowledgeable about the device; use them as a source of information.

LVAD coordinators are usually available for consult 24 hours a day. These medical professionals typically work at the same facility that placed the device, so they should also be familiar with the patient. Follow your local protocols or contact medical control regarding the treatment of a patient with an LVAD. For more information on the LVAD, see Chapter 38, *Patients With Special Challenges.*

compressions. However, even under ideal conditions, manual chest compressions cannot equate to normal cardiac output. In addition, factors such as rescuer fatigue or inaccurate depth or rate of compressions can further impede the resuscitation process. Before you consider using mechanical devices to assist circulation, ensure your manual chest compressions are of consistently high quality.

Several mechanical devices are available to assist emergency responders in maximizing blood flow during CPR. Although improved patient outcomes have not yet been documented, these devices may be considered for use as an adjunct to CPR in select settings when used by properly trained personnel for patients in cardiac arrest in the prehospital or in-hospital setting. These specific settings include instances when limited rescuers are available, when CPR is prolonged, or when CPR is required in a moving ambulance.

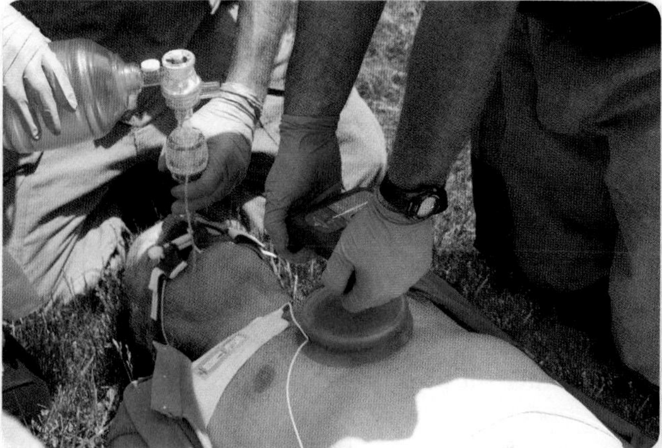

Figure 15-19 An active compression-decompression cardiopulmonary resuscitation device.

▶ Active Compression-Decompression CPR

Active compression-decompression CPR is a technique that involves compressing the chest and then actively pulling it back up to its neutral position or beyond (decompression). This technique may increase the amount of blood that returns to the heart and, thus, the amount of blood ejected from the heart during the compression phase. **Figure 15-19** shows an active compression-decompression CPR device. It features a suction cup that is placed in the center of the chest. After compressing the chest to the proper depth, the rescuer pulls up on the handle of the device to provide active decompression of the chest, thus ensuring the chest returns to at least its neutral position or even beyond neutral.

▶ Impedance Threshold Device

An **impedance threshold device (ITD)** is a valve device placed between the ET tube and a bag-mask device; it

Words of Wisdom

Another alternative to conventional CPR is *interposed abdominal compression.* The same standard sequence of CPR steps is followed with the addition of abdominal compressions in counterpoint to chest compressions. Always follow local protocols and current American Heart Association guidelines.[6]

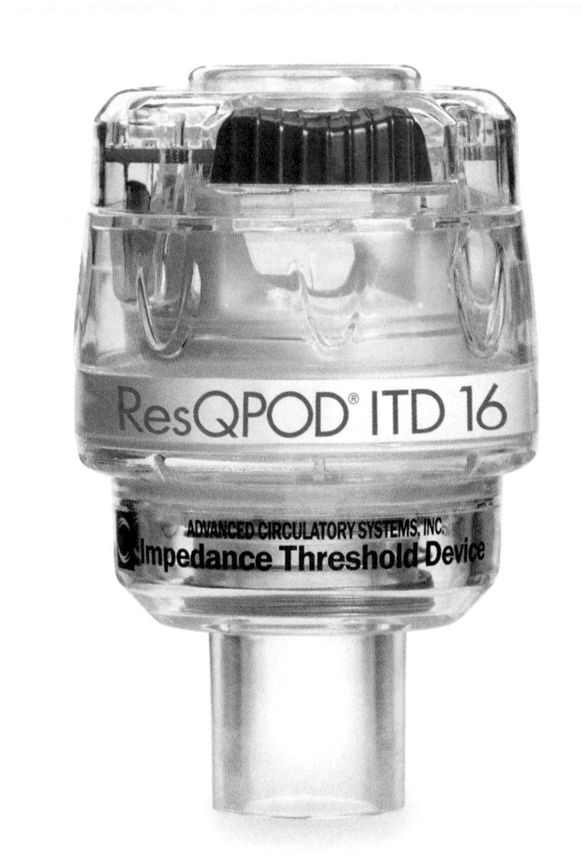

Figure 15-20 An impedance threshold device.

Courtesy of Advanced Circulatory Systems, Inc.

may also be placed between the bag and mask if an ET tube is not in place. The ITD is designed to limit the air entering the lungs during the recoil phase between chest compressions **Figure 15-20**. This results in negative intrathoracic pressure that may draw more blood toward the heart, ultimately resulting in improved cardiac filling and circulation during each chest compression. An ITD selectively prevents unnecessary air from rushing into the chest, maximizing the vacuum during the recoil phase of the compression. This results in enhanced return of blood that increases cardiac output, blood pressure, and perfusion to vital organs, and ultimately improves survival rates. Use an ITD to help improve circulation during CPR and increase the ROSC in cardiac arrest patients. The ITD may be considered when used together with devices that provide active compression-decompression CPR. It is *not* currently recommended for use with conventional CPR. If the patient's pulse returns, then the ITD should be removed from the ventilation system because it is designed to be used in conjunction with compressions. Ensure you understand research trends regarding the effectiveness of the ITD.

▶ Mechanical Piston Device

A **mechanical piston device** is a device that depresses the sternum via a compressed gas-powered or electric-powered plunger mounted on a backboard **Figure 15-21**. The patient is positioned supine on the backboard, with the piston positioned on top of the patient with the plunger centered over the patient's thorax in the same manner as with manual chest compressions. The device is then secured to the backboard.

The mechanical piston device allows rescuers to configure the depth and rate of compressions, resulting in consistent delivery. This frees the rescuer to complete

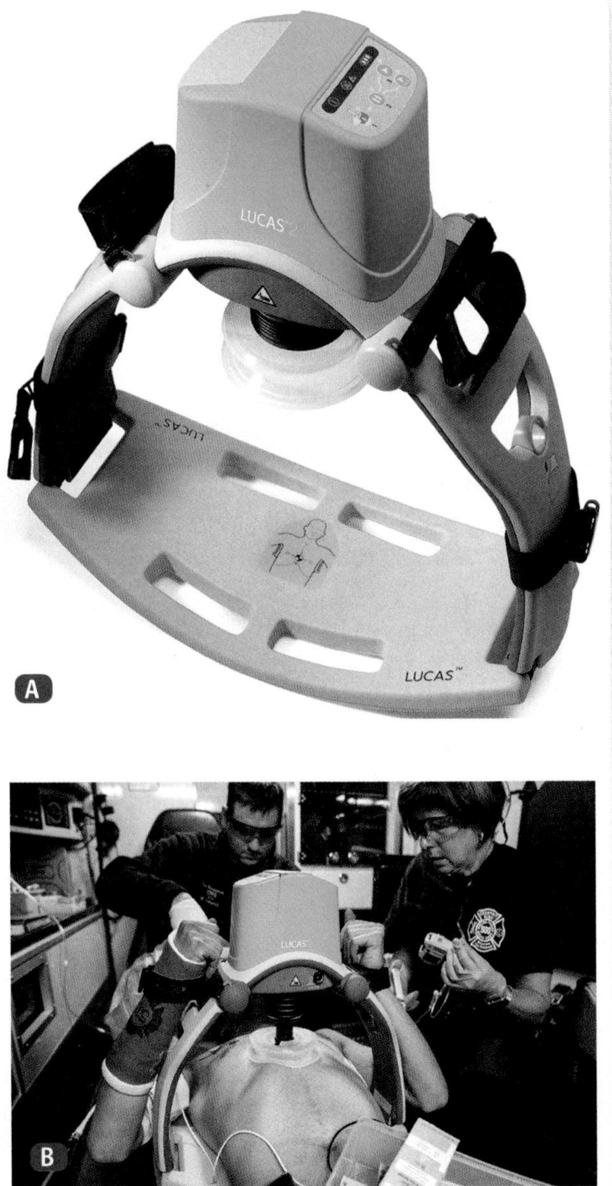

Figure 15-21 A. A mechanical piston device. **B.** The device in use.

A: Courtesy of LUCAS CPR (Physio Control Inc.); **B:** © Jones & Bartlett Learning.

other tasks and eliminates rescuer fatigue that results from continuous delivery of manual chest compressions. These devices have been available for many years. The latest versions of these devices offer you the option of providing compressions using a battery instead of an oxygen tank or a compressed air system, thus eliminating the tanks and hoses.

▶ Load-Distributing Band CPR or Vest CPR

The **load-distributing band (LDB)** is a circumferential chest compression device composed of a constricting band and backboard Figure 15-22. The device is either electrically or pneumatically driven to compress the heart by putting inward pressure on the thorax.

As with the mechanical piston device, use of the LDB frees up the rescuer to complete other tasks. The device weighs less than the early-version mechanical piston devices and can be easier to apply.

Although a mechanical CPR device may be a reasonable alternative to conventional CPR in specific settings, manual chest compressions remain the standard of care. If your EMS system uses a mechanical CPR device, then it is crucial to practice using it frequently to

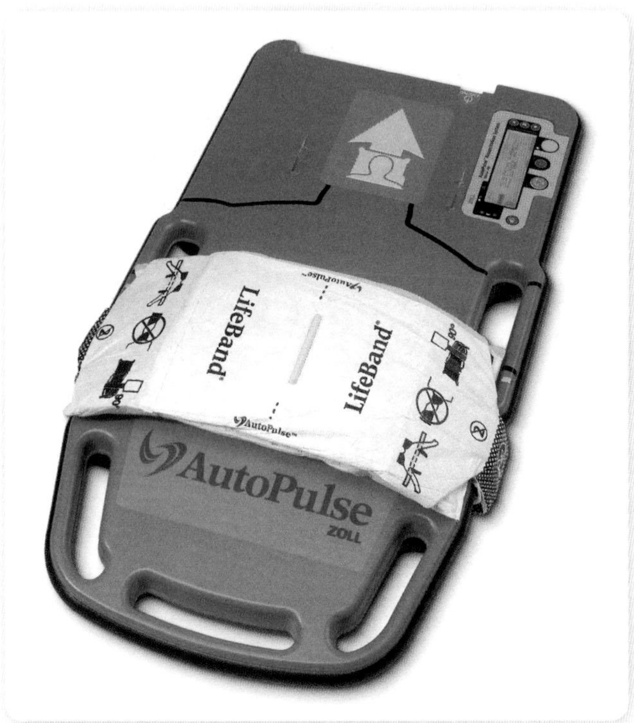

Figure 15-22 A load-distributing band.
Provided with permission by ZOLL Medical.

YOU are the Provider — PART 3

With CPR ongoing, you open the AED pads and prepare to apply them to the patient's chest. You note the patient has a medication patch on the right upper part of his chest. You also see a bulge with a scar on the left upper part of his chest. You apply the AED pads, analyze the patient's cardiac rhythm, and receive a "shock advised" message. After delivering the shock, you and your partner resume CPR. The second ambulance arrives, and one EMT moves into position to take over compressions at the end of the cycle and a second EMT prepares to take over ventilations.

Recording Time: 4 Minutes	
Level of consciousness	Unresponsive
Respirations	Absent (baseline); 2 breaths are being given after every 30 chest compressions; chest rise is visible with each breath
Pulse	Absent (baseline); femoral pulse is palpable with chest compressions
Skin	Pale
Blood pressure	Not measurable
Oxygen saturation (Spo_2)	Not measurable

5. Should you remove the medication patch or leave it in place? Why or why not?
6. What does the bulge and scar over the patient's left chest indicate? How will this affect the way you treat the patient?
7. Which rhythms will the AED defibrillate?

ensure you can rapidly apply it. Remember to minimize interruptions to chest compressions while the device is being applied.

Infant and Child CPR

In most cases, cardiac arrest in infants and children follows respiratory arrest, which triggers hypoxia and **ischemia** (decreased oxygen supply) of the heart. Children consume oxygen two to three times as rapidly as adults, so you must first focus on opening the airway and providing artificial ventilation. Often, this will be enough to allow the child to resume spontaneous breathing and, thus, prevent cardiac arrest. Therefore, airway and breathing are the focus of pediatric BLS Table 15-2.

Respiratory issues leading to cardiopulmonary arrest in children can have a number of different causes, including:

- Injury, both blunt and penetrating
- Infections of the respiratory tract or another organ system (croup, epiglottitis)

Table 15-2 Review of Pediatric BLS Procedures

Procedure	Infants (between age 1 month and 1 year[a])	Children (1 year to onset of puberty[b])
Circulation		
Pulse check	Brachial artery	Carotid or femoral artery
Compression area	Just below the nipple line	In the center of the chest, in between the nipples
Compression width	Two-finger technique or two-thumb-encircling-hands technique	Heel of one or both hands
Compression depth	At least one-third anterior-posterior diameter (about 1.5 in. [4 cm])	At least one-third anterior-posterior diameter (about 2 in. [5 cm])
Compression rate	100 to 120/min	100 to 120/min
Compression-to-ventilation ratio (until advanced airway is inserted)	30:2 (one rescuer); 15:2 (two rescuers)[c]	30:2 (one rescuer); 15:2 (two rescuers)[c]
Foreign body obstruction	Responsive: Back slaps and chest thrusts Unresponsive: CPR	Responsive: Abdominal thrusts (Heimlich maneuver) Unresponsive: CPR
Airway		
	Head tilt–chin lift maneuver; jaw-thrust maneuver if spinal injury is suspected	Head tilt–chin lift maneuver; jaw-thrust maneuver if spinal injury is suspected
Breathing		
Ventilations	1 breath every 3 to 5 seconds (12 to 20 breaths/min); about 1 second per breath; visible chest rise	1 breath every 3 to 5 seconds (12 to 20 breaths/min); about 1 second per breath; visible chest rise
Ventilations with advanced airway placed	1 breath every 6 seconds (a rate of 10 breaths/min)	1 breath every 6 seconds (a rate of 10 breaths/min)

Abbreviations: BLS, basic life support; CPR, cardiopulmonary resuscitation

[a]The American Heart Association defines neonatal patients as birth to age 1 month, and infants as age 1 month to 1 year. Neonatal resuscitation is covered in Chapter 35, *Obstetrics and Neonatal Care.*

[b]Onset of puberty is approximately 12 to 14 years of age, as defined by secondary characteristics (eg, breast development in girls and armpit hair in boys).

[c]Pause compressions to deliver ventilations.

- A foreign body in the airway
- Submersion (drowning)
- Electrocution
- Poisoning or drug overdose
- Sudden infant death syndrome (SIDS)

▶ Determining Responsiveness

Never shake a child to determine whether he or she is responsive, especially if the possibility of a neck or back injury exists. Instead, gently tap the child on the shoulder, and say loudly, "Are you okay?" Figure 15-23. With an infant, gently tap the soles of the feet. If a child is responsive but struggling to breathe, allow the child to remain in whatever position is most comfortable.

If you find an unresponsive, apneic, and pulseless child while you are alone and off duty, and you did not witness the child's collapse, perform CPR beginning with chest compressions for approximately five cycles (about 2 minutes), and then stop to call 9-1-1 and retrieve an AED. Do not call 9-1-1 right away, as you would with an adult. Remember, cardiopulmonary arrest in children is most often the result of respiratory failure, not a primary cardiac event. Therefore, children will require immediate restoration of oxygenation, ventilation, and circulation, which can be accomplished by immediately performing five cycles (about 2 minutes) of CPR before activating the EMS system.

▶ Check for Breathing and a Pulse

After you establish responsiveness, assess breathing and circulation. As with an adult, this assessment can occur simultaneously and should take no longer than 10 seconds. Visualize the chest for signs of breathing and palpate for a pulse in a large central artery. You can usually palpate the carotid or femoral pulse in children older than 1 year, but it is difficult in infants. Therefore, in infants, palpate the brachial artery, which is located on the inner side of the arm, midway between the elbow and shoulder. Place the tips of your index and middle fingers on the inside of the biceps, and press lightly toward the bone. CPR is required if the infant or child is not breathing or is not breathing normally (agonal gasps), and a pulse is absent (or less than 60 beats/min).

As with an adult, an infant or child must be lying on a hard, flat surface for effective chest compressions. If you need to carry an infant while providing CPR, your forearm and hand can serve as the flat surface. Use your palm to support the infant's head. In this way, the infant's shoulders are elevated, and the head is slightly tilted back in a position that will keep the airway open. Ensure the infant's head is not higher than the rest of the body.

The technique for chest compressions in infants and children differs from adults because of a number of anatomic differences, including the position of the heart, the size of the chest, and the fragile organs of a child. The liver (immediately under the right side of the diaphragm) is relatively large and fragile, especially in infants. The spleen, on the left, is smaller and more fragile in children than in adults. These organs are easily injured if you are not careful in performing chest compressions, so be sure your hand position is correct before you begin. The chest of an infant is smaller and more pliable than that of an older child or adult; therefore, use only two fingers to compress the chest. If two rescuers are performing CPR on an infant, use the two-thumb-encircling-hands technique to deliver chest compressions Figure 15-24. In children, especially those older than 8 years, you can use the heel of one or both hands to compress the chest.

Follow the steps in Skill Drill 15-4 to perform infant chest compressions.

Coordinate compressions and ventilations in a 30:2 ratio if you are working alone, and 15:2 if you are working with a trained bystander or another health care provider. Ensure the infant's chest fully recoils in between compressions and that the chest visibly rises with each ventilation. You will find this easier to do if you use your

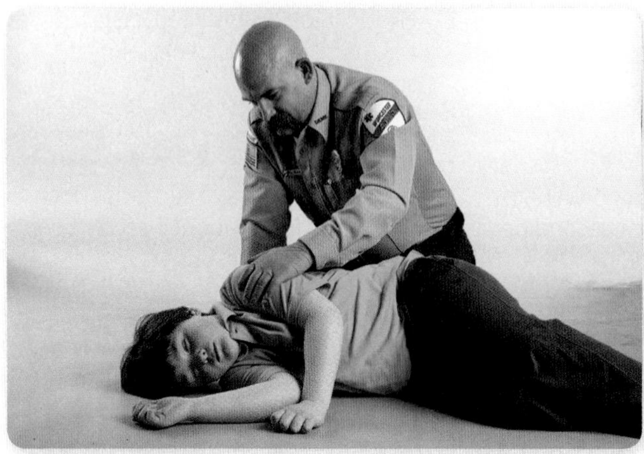

Figure 15-23 Never shake a child to determine responsiveness. Instead, gently tap on the shoulder (child) or tap the soles of the feet (infant), and speak loudly.

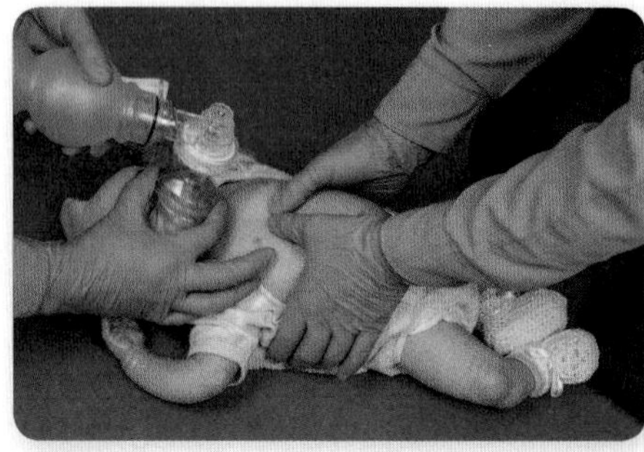

Figure 15-24 Chest compressions should be given with the hands encircling the infant and thumbs side by side.

Skill Drill 15-4 Performing Infant Chest Compressions

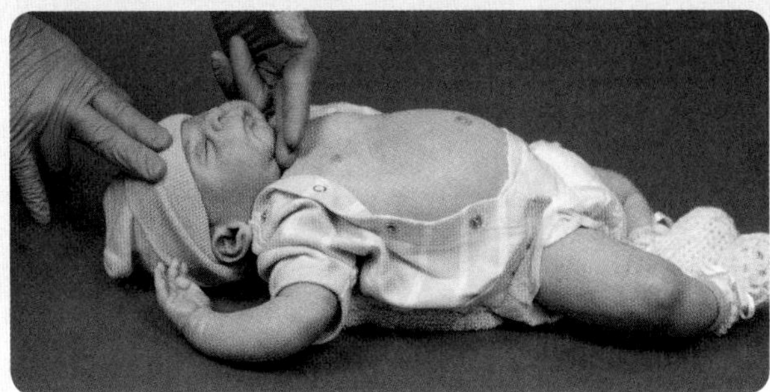

Step 1 Take standard precautions. Place the infant on a firm, flat surface, and keep the head in an open airway position. You can also use a pad or wedge under the shoulders and upper body to keep the head from tilting forward.

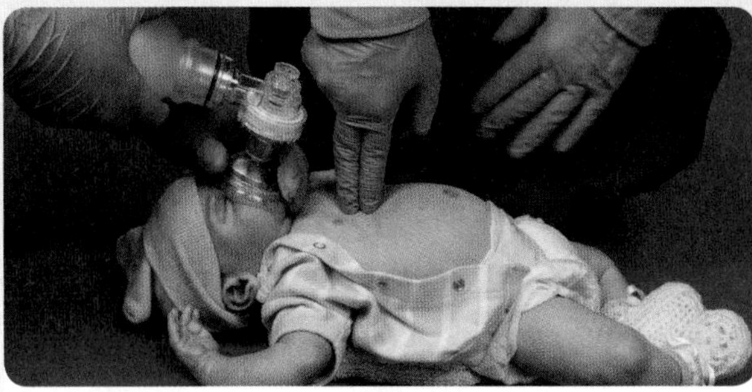

Step 2 Imagine a horizontal line drawn between the nipples. Place two fingers in the middle of the sternum, just below the nipple line. Use two fingers to compress the sternum at least one-third the anterior-posterior diameter of the chest (approximately 1.5 inches [4 cm] in most infants). Compress the chest at a rate of 100 to 120 per minute. After each compression, allow the sternum to return briefly to its normal position. Allow equal time for compression and relaxation of the chest. Do not remove your fingers from the sternum, and avoid jerky movements.

free hand to keep the head in the open airway position. If the chest does not rise, or rises only a little, then use a head tilt–chin lift to open the airway. Reassess the infant for signs of spontaneous breathing or a pulse after five cycles (about 2 minutes) of CPR.

Skill Drill 15-5 shows the steps for performing CPR in children between 1 year of age and the onset of puberty.

Switching rescuer positions is the same for children as it is for adults: every five cycles (2 minutes) of CPR. Remember, if the child is past the onset of puberty, use the adult CPR sequence, including the use of the AED.

▶ Airway

Infants and toddlers often put toys and other objects in their mouths; therefore, foreign body obstruction of the upper airway is common. Make sure the upper airway is patent when managing pediatric respiratory emergencies or cardiopulmonary arrest. If the child is unresponsive and lying in a supine position, the airway may become obstructed when the tongue and throat muscles relax and the tongue falls backward.

If the child is unresponsive but breathing adequately, place the child in the recovery position to maintain an open airway and allow drainage of saliva, vomitus, or other secretions from the mouth Figure 15-25. Do not use this position if you suspect injury to the spine, hips, or pelvis unless you can secure the child to a backboard that can be tilted to the side. If the child is responsive, but breathing is labored, provide prompt transport to the closest appropriate hospital.

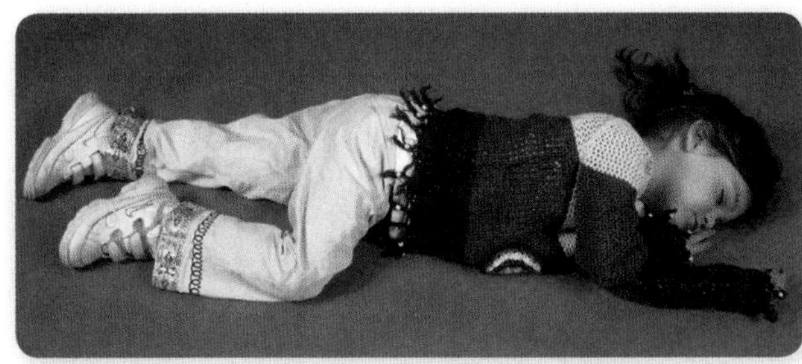

Figure 15-25 A child who is unresponsive but breathing adequately should be placed in the recovery position to allow saliva or vomitus to drain from the mouth.

Opening the airway in an infant or child is done by using the same techniques as used for an adult. However, because a child's neck is so flexible, the techniques should be slightly modified. The jaw-thrust maneuver is the best method to use if you suspect a spinal injury in a child. If a second rescuer is present, he or she should immobilize the child's cervical spine. If you do not suspect spinal injury,

Skill Drill 15-5 Performing CPR on a Child

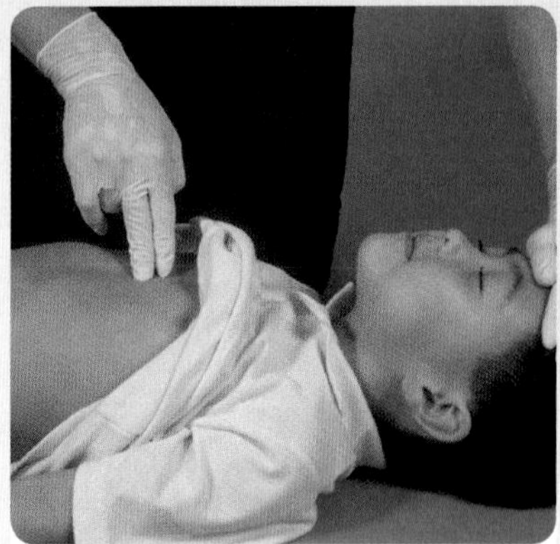

Step 1 Take standard precautions. Place the child on a firm, flat surface. Place the heel of one or two hands (if treating a larger child) in the center of the chest, in between the nipples. Avoid compression over the lower tip of the sternum, which is called the xiphoid process.

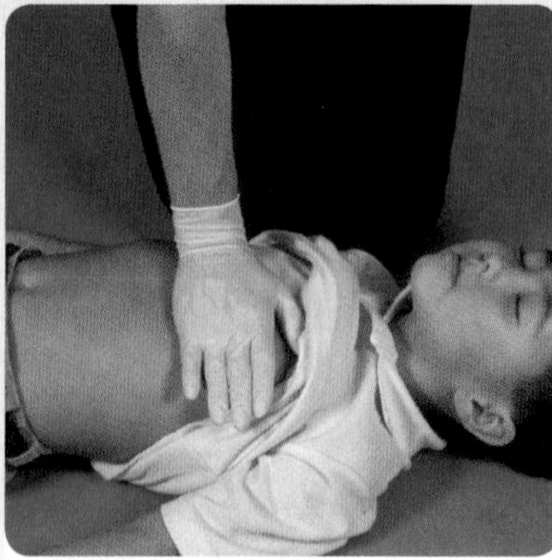

Step 2 Compress the chest at least one-third the anterior-posterior diameter of the chest (approximately 2 inches [5 cm] in most children) at a rate of 100 to 120 times/min. Coordinate compressions with ventilations in a 30:2 ratio for one rescuer or 15:2 ratio for two rescuers, making sure the chest rises with each ventilation. At the end of each cycle, pause for two ventilations. Reassess for a pulse after 2 minutes. If there is no pulse and an AED is available, resume CPR and apply the AED pads.

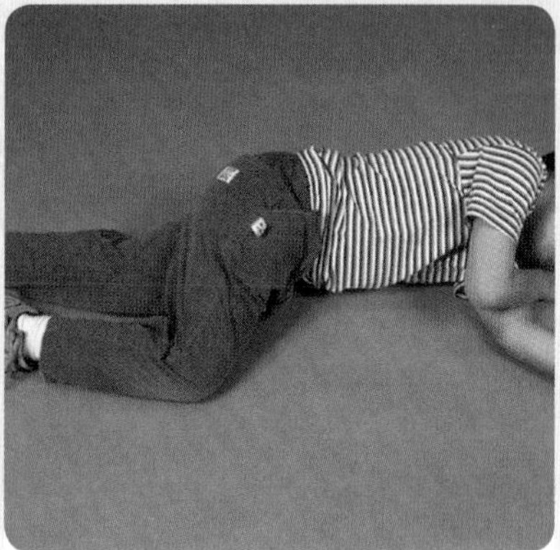

Step 3 If the child regains a pulse of greater than 60 beats/min and resumes effective breathing, then place him or her in a position that allows for frequent reassessment of the airway and vital signs during transport.

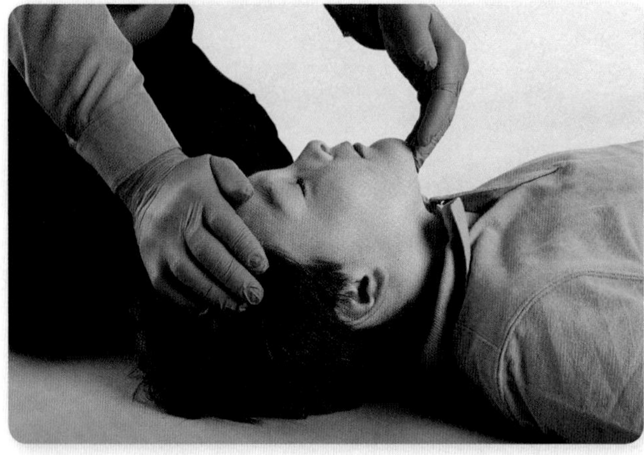

Figure 15-26 Use the head tilt–chin lift maneuver to open the airway in a child who has not sustained a traumatic injury. Do not overextend the neck.

then use the head tilt–chin lift maneuver but modified so that, as you tilt the head back, you are moving it only into the neutral position or a slightly extended position **Figure 15-26**.

Head Tilt–Chin Lift Maneuver

Perform the head tilt–chin lift maneuver in a child in the following manner:

1. Place one hand on the child's forehead, and gently tilt the head back, with the neck slightly extended.
2. Place two or three fingers (not the thumb) of your other hand under the child's chin, and lift the jaw upward and outward. Do not close the mouth or push under the chin; either move may obstruct rather than open the airway.
3. Remove any visible foreign body or vomitus.

Jaw-Thrust Maneuver

Perform the jaw-thrust maneuver in a child in the following manner:

1. Place two or three fingers under each side of the angle of the lower jaw; lift the jaw upward and outward.

2. If the jaw thrust alone does not open the airway and cervical spine injury is not a consideration, tilt the head slightly. If cervical spine injury is suspected, use a second rescuer to immobilize the cervical spine.

Remember, the head of an infant or young child is disproportionately large in comparison with the chest and shoulders. As a result, when a child is lying flat on his or her back, especially on a backboard, the head will bend forward (hyperflexion) onto the upper chest. This position can partially or completely obstruct the upper airway. To avoid this possibility, place a wedge of padding under the child's upper chest and shoulders (torso).

▶ Provide Rescue Breathing

If the child is not breathing but has a pulse, open the airway and deliver one breath every 3 to 5 seconds (12 to 20 breaths/min) Figure 15-27. If the child is not breathing and does not have a pulse, deliver 2 rescue breaths after every 30 chest compressions (15 chest compressions if two rescuers are present). Each ventilation should last about 1 second and should produce visible chest rise. Use the proper-sized mask and ensure an adequate mask-to-face seal.

If an infant or small child is breathing, provide prompt transport. Again, a child who is in respiratory distress should be allowed to stay in whatever position is most comfortable. Children who are unresponsive but breathing with difficulty should be kept in a position that allows you to manage the airway and provide ventilatory support, if needed.

In a child with a tracheostomy tube in the neck, remove the mask from the bag-mask device and connect it directly to the tracheostomy tube to ventilate the child. If a bag-mask device is unavailable, a face mask with one-way valve or other barrier device over the tracheostomy site can be used. Place your hand firmly over the child's mouth and nose to prevent the artificial breaths from leaking out of the upper airway.

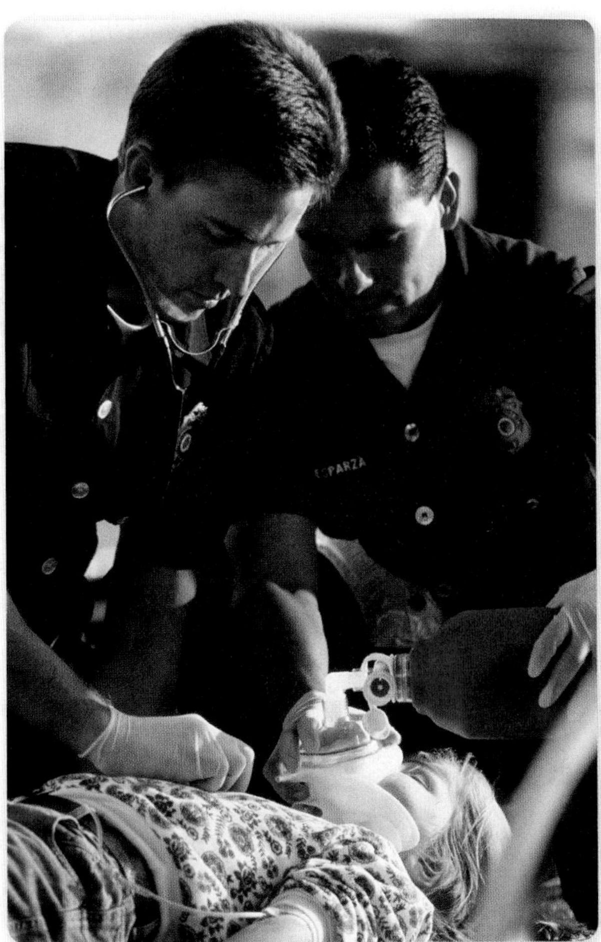

Figure 15-27 Open the child's airway and provide rescue breathing.

Words of Wisdom

An injured child with a serious airway or breathing problem is likely to need full-time attention from two providers. Therefore, it is important for you to arrange for backup from another unit as soon as possible—perhaps even before you arrive at the scene. Paramedic backup is preferable to provide support as needed.

Special Populations

Neonatal resuscitation is quite different from that of infant CPR. Follow the steps listed for any newborn requiring resuscitation:

1. Perform the initial steps in stabilization (provide warmth, clear airway if necessary, dry, stimulate).
2. Provide positive-pressure ventilation with SpO_2 (oxygen saturation) monitoring.
3. Administer chest compressions if the heart rate is below 60 beats/min.
4. Consider laryngeal mask airway, or paramedic backup for intubation, continue chest compressions, and coordinate with positive pressure ventilation.
5. If the heart rate remains below 60 beats/min, gain IV/IO access, and call paramedic backup for administration of IV epinephrine, and consider hypovolemia or pneumothorax.

Following the initial steps of resuscitation, the need for and extent of further resuscitation is based on the assessment of three key parameters: respiratory effort, heart rate, and color. See Chapter 35, *Obstetrics and Neonatal Care*, for more information on neonatal resuscitation.

Interrupting CPR

CPR is a crucial, life-saving procedure that provides minimal circulation and ventilation until the patient can receive defibrillation, ALS treatment, and definitive care at the ED. No matter how well CPR is performed, however, it is rarely enough to save a patient's life. If paramedic backup is unavailable at the scene, you must provide transport based on your local protocols and continue CPR en route. Keep in mind, movement from a vehicle can interfere with analyzation by an AED. Contact the manufacturer to confirm whether the model you have can be used in a moving vehicle. Otherwise, the ambulance must be stopped each time you utilize the AED. En route to the ED, consider requesting a paramedic rendezvous if available. This will provide further ALS care to the patient sooner, thereby improving the patient's chance for survival. However, not all EMS systems have paramedic backup support available to them, especially in rural settings. For those areas where it is available, consider calling early for air transport. Their goal is to provide service to rural areas where advanced care may not be readily available or transport times are long.

Special Populations

Children in respiratory distress are often struggling to breathe. As a result, they usually position themselves in a way that keeps the airway open enough for air to move. Let the child stay in that position as long as his or her breathing remains adequate. If you and your partner arrive at the scene and find that the infant or child is not breathing or has cyanosis, immediate management (including rescue breathing and supplemental oxygen) is essential. Consider requesting paramedic assistance, if available.

Remember, too, a child's airway is smaller than an adult's. Therefore, there is greater resistance to air flow. As a result, you will need to use *slightly* more ventilatory pressure to inflate the lungs. You will know you are giving the correct tidal volume when you see the chest rise. Infants and children should be ventilated once every 3 to 5 seconds (at a rate of 12 to 20 breaths/min). Do not ventilate too fast or use too much force.

If air enters freely with your initial breaths and the chest rises, then the airway is clear. If air does not enter freely, then check the airway for obstruction. Reposition the patient to open the airway, and attempt to give another breath. If air still does not enter freely, you must take steps to relieve the obstruction.

Try not to interrupt CPR for more than a few seconds, except when it is absolutely necessary. For example, if you have to move a patient up or down stairs, then continue CPR until you arrive at the head or foot of the stairs, interrupt CPR at a mutually agreed-on signal, and move quickly to the next level where you can resume CPR. Do not move the patient until all transport arrangements are made so that interruptions to CPR can be kept to a minimum. See Chapter 6, *Lifting and Moving Patients*, to review patient lifting and moving techniques.

Chest compression fraction is the total percentage of time during a resuscitation attempt in which chest compressions are being performed. Make every effort to maintain a chest compression fraction of at least 60% (the higher the better). The more frequent the interruptions in chest compressions, the lower the compression fraction will be. Low compression fractions lead to worse patient outcomes. Most modern cardiac monitors will provide information about chest compression fraction that you can review after a cardiac arrest. If possible, routinely review this information after every arrest so you can learn ways to improve the chest compression fraction and improve on other key performance indicators.

When Not to Start CPR

As an AEMT, it is your responsibility to start CPR on virtually all patients who are in cardiac arrest. There are only three general exceptions to the rule.

First, do not start CPR if the scene is unsafe. Ensure scene safety in cardiac arrest situations, just as you would on any other call.

Second, do not start CPR if the patient has obvious signs of death. Obvious signs of death include an absence of a pulse and breathing, along with any one of the following findings:

- **Rigor mortis**, or stiffening of the body after death
- **Dependent lividity** (livor mortis), a discoloration of the skin caused by pooling of blood Figure 15-28
- Putrefaction (decomposition of the body tissues)
- Mortal injury, such as decapitation, dismemberment, or burned beyond recognition.

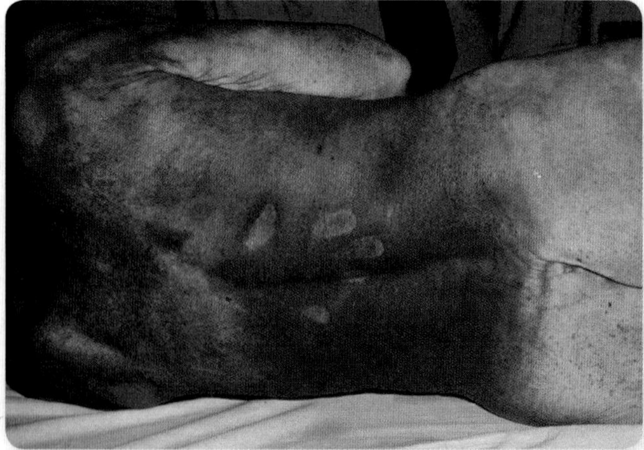

Figure 15-28 Dependent lividity is an obvious sign of death, caused by blood settling to the areas of the body not in firm contact with the ground. The lividity in this figure is seen as purple discoloration of the back, except in areas that are in firm contact with the ground (scapula and buttock).

Figure: 25 TAC §157.25 (h)(2)

OUT-OF-HOSPITAL DO-NOT-RESUSCITATE (OOH-DNR) ORDER

TEXAS DEPARTMENT OF STATE HEALTH SERVICES

STOP DO NOT RESUSCITATE

This document becomes effective immediately on the date of execution for health care professionals acting in out-of-hospital settings. It remains in effect until the person is pronounced dead by authorized medical or legal authority or the document is revoked. Comfort care will be given as needed.

Person's full legal name ______ Date of birth ______ ☐ Male ☐ Female

A. Declaration of the adult person: I am competent and at least 18 years of age. **I direct that none of the following resuscitation measures be initiated or continued for me: cardiopulmonary resuscitation (CPR), transcutaneous cardiac pacing, defibrillation, advanced airway management, artificial ventilation.**

Person's signature ______ Date ______ Printed name ______

B. Declaration by legal guardian, agent or proxy on behalf of the adult person who is incompetent or otherwise incapable of communication:

I am the: ☐ legal guardian; ☐ agent in a Medical Power of Attorney; OR ☐ proxy in a directive to physicians of the above-noted person who is incompetent or otherwise mentally or physically incapable of communication.

Based upon the known desires of the person, or a determination of the best interest of the person, **I direct that none of the following resuscitation measures be initiated or continued for the person: cardiopulmonary resuscitation (CPR), transcutaneous cardiac pacing, defibrillation, advanced airway management, artificial ventilation.**

Signature ______ Date ______ Printed name ______

C. Declaration by a qualified relative of the adult person who is incompetent or otherwise incapable of communication: I am the above-noted person's:

☐ spouse, ☐ adult child, ☐ parent, OR ☐ nearest living relative, and I am qualified to make this treatment decision under Health and Safety Code §166.088.

To my knowledge the adult person is incompetent or otherwise mentally or physically incapable of communication and is without a legal guardian, agent or proxy. Based upon the known desires of the person or a determination of the best interests of the person, **I direct that none of the following resuscitation measures be initiated or continued for the person: cardiopulmonary resuscitation (CPR), transcutaneous cardiac pacing, defibrillation, advanced airway management, artificial ventilation.**

Signature ______ Date ______ Printed name ______

D. Declaration by physician based on directive to physicians by a person now incompetent or nonwritten communication to the physician by a competent person: I am the above-noted person's attending physician and have:

☐ seen evidence of his/her previously issued directive to physicians by the adult, now incompetent; OR ☐ observed his/her issuance before two witnesses of an OOH-DNR in a nonwritten manner.

I direct that none of the following resuscitation measures be initiated or continued for the person: cardiopulmonary resuscitation (CPR), transcutaneous cardiac pacing, defibrillation, advanced airway management, artificial ventilation.

Attending physician's signature ______ Date ______ Printed name ______ Lic# ______

E. Declaration on behalf of the minor person: I am the minor's: ☐ parent; ☐ legal guardian; OR ☐ managing conservator.

A physician has diagnosed the minor as suffering from a terminal or irreversible condition. **I direct that none of the following resuscitation measures be initiated or continued for the person: cardiopulmonary resuscitation (CPR), transcutaneous cardiac pacing, defibrillation, advanced airway management, artificial ventilation.**

Signature ______ Date ______

Printed name ______

TWO WITNESSES: (See qualifications on backside.) We have witnessed the above-noted competent adult person or authorized declarant making his/her signature above and, if applicable, the above-noted adult person making an OOH-DNR by nonwritten communication to the attending physician.

Witness 1 signature ______ Date ______ Printed name ______

Witness 2 signature ______ Date ______ Printed name ______

Notary in the State of Texas and County of______. The above noted person personally appeared before me and signed the above noted declaration on this date:______.

Figure 15-29 Do not start cardiopulmonary resuscitation (CPR) if the patient and his or her physician have previously agreed on do not resuscitate or no-CPR orders. Learn your local protocols for treating terminally ill patients.

Rigor mortis and dependent lividity develop after a patient has been dead for a long period.

Third, do not start CPR if the patient and his or her physician have previously agreed on a do not resuscitate (DNR) order or no-CPR order **Figure 15-29**. DNR orders give you permission not to attempt resuscitation. This may apply only in situations in which the patient is known to be in the terminal stage of an incurable disease. In this situation, CPR would only prolong the patient's death. However, end-of-life issues can be complicated. Advance directives, such as living wills, may express the patient's wishes; however, these documents may not be readily producible by the patient's family or caregiver. In such cases, the safest course is to begin CPR under the rule of implied consent and then contact medical control for further guidance. However, if a valid DNR document or living will is produced, resuscitative efforts may be withheld. Learn your local protocols and the standards in your EMS system for treating terminally ill patients. Some EMS systems have electronic notes on patients who are preregistered with the system. These notes usually specify the amount and extent of treatment that is desired. Other states have specific DNR forms that allow EMS providers to withhold care when the patient, family, and physician have agreed in advance that such a course is most appropriate. It is essential that you understand your local protocols and are aware of the specific restrictions these advance directives imply.

You may also encounter Physician Orders for Life-Sustaining Treatment (POLST) or Medical Orders for

Life-Sustaining Treatment (MOLST) forms. These legal documents describe acceptable interventions for the patient in the form of medical orders and must be signed by an authorized medical provider to be valid. Be familiar with POLST or MOLST forms, and learn your local protocols and state laws with regard to withholding end-of-life medical interventions. If you are presented with a POLST or MOLST form, then contact medical control for guidance.

In all other cases, begin CPR on anyone who is in cardiac arrest. It is usually impossible to know how long the patient's brain and vital organs have gone without oxygen. Factors such as air temperature and the basic health of the patient's tissues and organs can affect survivability. Most legal advisers recommend that, when in doubt, always give too much care rather than too little care. Always start CPR if any doubt exists.

Words of Wisdom

When you choose not to start CPR on a patient in cardiac arrest, you must ensure you are in compliance with local protocols and you have detailed and accurate documentation. Specifically, record signs from the physical exam that led to your decision and make reference to the local protocol that states these signs as a reason not to start CPR. If extenuating circumstances such as entrapment physically prevent resuscitation attempts, then record the conditions thoroughly. These decisions occasionally give rise to questions that can often be put to rest immediately by reference to a well-written report.

When to Stop CPR

As an AEMT, you are generally not responsible for making the decision to stop CPR. After you begin CPR in the field, you must continue until one of the following events occurs (the STOP mnemonic):

S The patient *Starts* breathing and has a pulse.
T The patient's care is *Transferred* to another provider of equal or higher-level training.
O You are *Out* of strength or too tired to continue CPR.
P A *Physician* who is present or providing online medical direction assumes responsibility for the patient and directs you to discontinue CPR.

Out of strength does not merely mean weary; rather, it means you are no longer physically able to perform CPR. In short, always continue CPR until the patient's care is transferred to a physician or higher medical authority in the field. In some cases, your medical director or a designated medical control physician may order you to stop CPR on the basis of the patient's condition.

Words of Wisdom

Patients who do not achieve ROSC may be potential kidney or liver donors in select situations (eg, short transport times, rapid access to an organ recovery program). High-quality CPR maintains end organ perfusion. Follow your local protocols regarding the care of potential organ donors.

YOU are the Provider — PART 4

After 2 minutes of CPR, you reanalyze the patient's cardiac rhythm and receive a "no shock advised" message. The two EMTs immediately resume CPR. During CPR, your partner ventilates the patient with a bag-mask device and administers high-flow oxygen and considers insertion of an advanced airway. As the EMT who is ventilating the patient attempts to insert an oral airway, the patient starts to gag. You quickly reassess him.

Recording Time: 7 Minutes	
Level of consciousness	Unresponsive
Respirations	Occasional agonal gasps; 4 breaths/min
Pulse	100 beats/min; strong carotid pulse; absent radial pulses
Skin	Skin color is improving
Blood pressure	70/40 mm Hg
Oxygen saturation (Spo_2)	82% (on oxygen)

8. How should you continue to treat this patient?
9. Because the patient is no longer in cardiac arrest, should you remove the AED pads? Why or why not?

Every EMS system should have clear standing orders or protocols that provide guidelines for starting and stopping CPR. Your medical director and your system's legal adviser should agree on these protocols, which should be closely administered and reviewed by your medical director.

Foreign Body Airway Obstruction in Adults

Occasionally, a foreign body will be aspirated and block the upper airway. An airway obstruction may be caused by various factors, including relaxation of the throat muscles in an unresponsive patient, vomited or regurgitated stomach contents, blood, damaged tissue after an injury, dentures, or foreign bodies such as food or small objects.

Large objects that are visible but cannot be removed from the airway with suction, such as loose dentures, large pieces of food, or blood clots, should be swept forward and out with your gloved index finger. Suctioning can then be used as needed to keep the airway clear of thinner secretions such as blood, vomitus, and mucus.

Recognizing Foreign Body Airway Obstruction

An airway obstruction by a foreign body in an adult usually occurs during a meal. In children, it usually occurs during mealtime or at play. If the foreign body is not removed quickly, then the lungs will use up their oxygen supply, and unresponsiveness and death will follow. Management is based on the severity of the airway obstruction.

Mild Airway Obstruction

Patients with a mild (partial) airway obstruction are able to exchange adequate amounts of air, but still have signs of respiratory distress. Breathing may be noisy; however, the patient usually has a strong, effective cough. Leave these patients alone! Your main concern is to prevent a mild airway obstruction from becoming a severe (complete) airway obstruction. Abdominal thrusts are *not* indicated for patients with a mild airway obstruction.

For the patient with a mild airway obstruction, first encourage him or her to cough or to continue coughing if they are already doing so. Do not interfere with the patient's own attempts to expel the foreign body. Instead, administer supplemental oxygen if needed and provide prompt transport to the ED. Closely monitor the patient and observe for signs of a severe airway obstruction (weak or absent cough, decreasing level of consciousness, cyanosis).

Responsive Patients

A sudden, severe airway obstruction is usually easy to recognize in someone who is eating or has just finished eating. The person is suddenly unable to speak or cough, grasps his or her throat, turns cyanotic, and makes exaggerated efforts to breathe. Either air is not moving into and out of the airway, or the air movement is so slight that it is not detectable. At first, the patient will be responsive and able to clearly indicate the problem. Ask the patient, "Are you choking?" The patient will usually respond by nodding yes. Alternatively, he or she may use the universal sign to indicate airway blockage Figure 15-30.

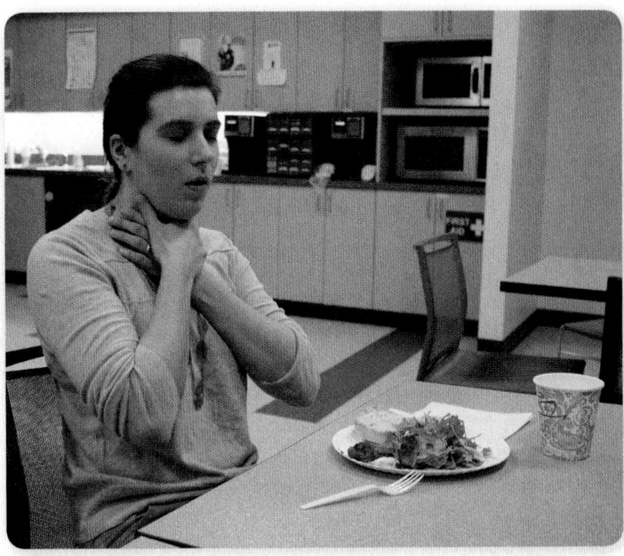

Figure 15-30 Placing the hands at the throat is the universal sign to indicate choking.

If there is a minimal amount of air movement, then you may hear a high-pitched sound called **stridor**. This occurs when the object is not fully blocking the airway, but the small amount of air entering the lungs is not enough to sustain life and the patient will eventually become unresponsive if the obstruction is not relieved.

Unresponsive Patients

When you discover an unresponsive patient, your first step is to determine whether he or she is breathing and has a pulse. The unresponsiveness may be caused by airway obstruction, cardiac arrest, or a number of other conditions. If the patient has a pulse, but is not breathing, then you must make sure the airway is open and unobstructed.

You should suspect an airway obstruction if the standard maneuvers to open the airway and ventilate the lungs are ineffective. If you feel resistance when attempting to ventilate, then the patient probably has some type of obstruction. Reposition the airway and attempt to ventilate. If you still meet resistance, then follow the steps for removing a foreign body airway obstruction.

Removing a Foreign Body Airway Obstruction in an Adult

The manual maneuver recommended for removing severe airway obstructions in responsive adults and children older than 1 year is the **abdominal-thrust maneuver** (also called the Heimlich maneuver). This maneuver creates an artificial cough by causing a sudden increase in intrathoracic pressure when thrusts are applied to the subdiaphragmatic region; it is a very effective method for removing a foreign body obstruction from the airway. If the patient with a severe airway obstruction is unresponsive, then perform chest compressions.

Responsive Patients

Abdominal-Thrust Maneuver. The goal of the abdominal-thrust maneuver is to compress the lungs upward and force residual air from the lungs to flow upward and expel the object. In responsive patients with a severe airway obstruction, repeat abdominal thrusts until the foreign body is expelled or the patient becomes unresponsive. Each thrust should be deliberate, with the intent of relieving the obstruction.

To perform abdominal thrusts on a responsive adult **Figure 15-31**, do the following:

1. Stand behind the patient, and wrap your arms around his or her abdomen. Straddle your legs outside the patient's legs. This will allow you to easily slide the patient to the ground if he or she becomes unresponsive.
2. Make a fist with one hand; grasp the fist with the other hand. Place the thumb side of the fist against the patient's abdomen just above the umbilicus and well below the xiphoid process.
3. Press your fist into the patient's abdomen with a quick inward and upward thrust.
4. Continue abdominal thrusts until the object is expelled from the airway or the patient becomes unresponsive.

Chest Thrusts. You can safely perform the abdominal-thrust maneuver on all adults and children. However, for women in advanced stages of pregnancy and patients with obesity, use chest thrusts instead.

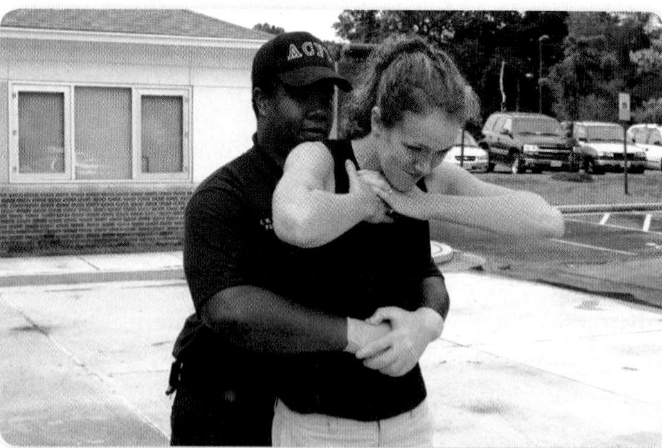

Figure 15-31 The abdominal-thrust maneuver in a responsive adult. Stand behind the patient and wrap your arms around the patient's abdomen. Place the thumb side of one fist against the patient's abdomen while holding your fist with your other hand. Press your fist into the patient's abdomen, using inward and upward thrusts.

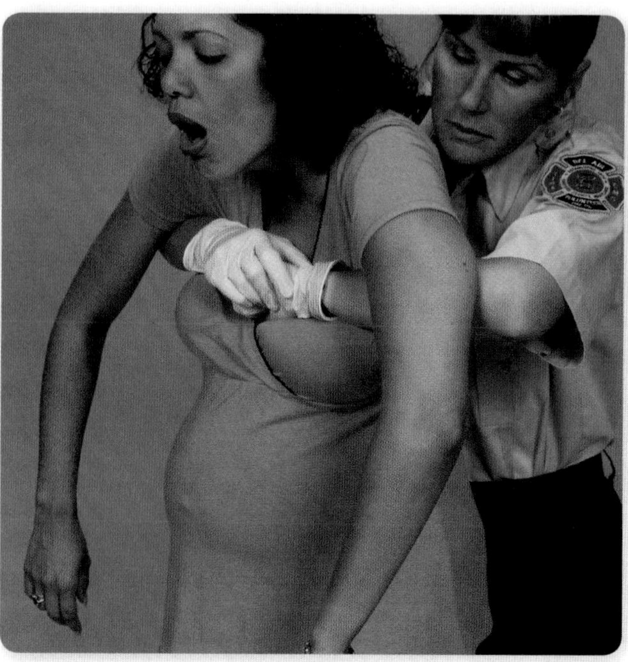

Figure 15-32 Remove a foreign body airway obstruction in a responsive pregnant adult using chest thrusts. Stand behind the patient and wrap your arms around the patient's chest. Place the thumb side of one fist against the chest while holding your fist with your other hand. Press your fist into the patient's chest with backward thrusts.

To perform chest thrusts on responsive pregnant adults and adults with obesity do the following **Figure 15-32**:

1. Stand behind the patient with your arms directly under the patient's armpits, and wrap your arms around the patient's chest.
2. Make a fist with one hand; grasp the fist with the other hand. Place the thumb side of the fist against the patient's sternum, avoiding the xiphoid process and the edges of the rib cage.
3. Press your fist into the patient's chest with backward thrusts until the object is expelled or the patient becomes unresponsive.
4. If the patient becomes unresponsive, then begin CPR, starting with chest compressions **Figure 15-33**.

Words of Wisdom

If a responsive choking patient is found lying on the floor, then administer abdominal thrusts by straddling the patient's legs, place your hands just above the umbilicus, and give rapid thrusts inward and upward under the rib cage, using the heel of your hand with your other hand on top of it.

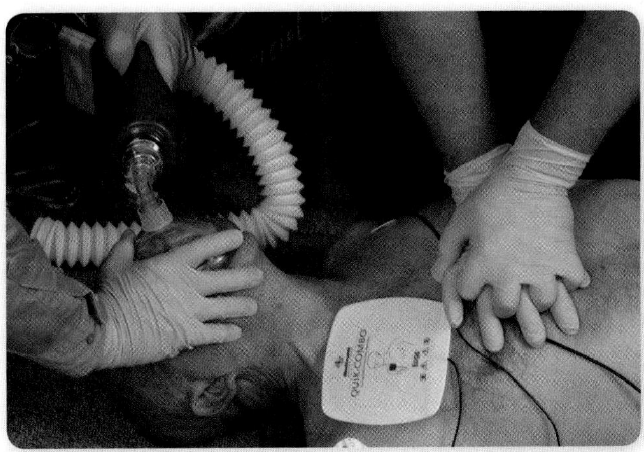

Figure 15-33 An unresponsive patient with a foreign body airway obstruction requires cardiopulmonary resuscitation.

Responsive Patients Who Become Unresponsive

A patient with a foreign body airway obstruction may become unresponsive while you are attempting to remove the obstruction. In this case, begin CPR, starting with chest compressions. Follow these steps to manage the patient's foreign body airway obstruction:

1. Carefully support the patient to the ground and immediately call for help (or send someone to call for help).
2. Perform 30 chest compressions, using the same landmark as you would for CPR (center of the chest, between the nipples). Do not check for a pulse before performing chest compressions.
3. Open the airway and look in the mouth. If you see an object that can easily be removed, then remove it with your fingers and attempt to ventilate. If you do not see an object, then resume chest compressions.
4. Repeat steps 2 and 3 until the obstruction is relieved or paramedics take over.

If you are able to remove an object from the mouth, then attempt to ventilate. If ventilation produces chest rise, then continue to ventilate and check for a pulse. If a pulse is present but the patient is not breathing, then continue rescue breathing and monitor the pulse. If a pulse is absent, then continue CPR (compressions and ventilations) and apply the AED as soon as it is available.

Unresponsive Patients

When a patient is found unresponsive, it is unlikely you will know what caused the problem. Begin CPR by determining unresponsiveness and checking for breathing and a pulse. If a pulse is present but breathing is absent, open the airway and attempt to ventilate. If the first ventilation does not produce visible chest rise, reposition the airway and reattempt to ventilate. If both ventilation attempts do not produce visible chest rise, perform 30 chest

YOU are the Provider PART 5

You package the patient, load him into the ambulance, and begin transport to a hospital located 5 miles away. An EMT from the backup ambulance accompanies you in the back and continues rescue breathing. En route, you reassess the patient and establish an 18-gauge IV line in his left antecubital fossa with normal saline running wide open. Next, you call in your radio report to the receiving hospital.

Recording Time: 12 Minutes	
Level of consciousness	Unresponsive
Respirations	8 breaths/min; shallow depth
Pulse	94 beats/min; strong carotid pulse, weak radial pulses
Skin	Pink, cool, and dry
Blood pressure	86/66 mm Hg
Oxygen saturation (Spo_2)	95% (on oxygen)

10. Would an ITD benefit your patient at this point?
11. What further treatment, if any, is indicated for this patient?
12. What options do you have if you are unable to obtain IV access?

compressions, and then open the airway and look in the mouth. If an object is visible and can easily be removed, remove it with your fingers and attempt to ventilate. Never perform blind finger sweeps on any patient; doing so may push the obstruction farther into the airway. If an object is not visible or cannot easily be removed, then resume chest compressions. Continue the sequence of chest compressions, open the airway, and look inside the mouth until the airway is clear or paramedics arrive.

Foreign Body Airway Obstruction in Infants and Children

As mentioned previously, airway obstruction is common in infants and children, usually caused by a foreign body (such as food or a toy) or by an infection, resulting in swelling and narrowing of the airway. Try to identify the cause of the obstruction as soon as possible. In patients who have signs and symptoms of an airway infection, do not waste time trying to dislodge a foreign body. Administer supplemental oxygen if needed and immediately transport the child to the ED.

A previously healthy child who is eating or playing with small toys or an infant who is crawling about the house and who suddenly has difficulty breathing has probably aspirated a foreign body. As in adults, foreign bodies may cause a mild or a severe airway obstruction.

With a mild airway obstruction, the child can cough forcefully, although he or she may wheeze between coughs. As long as the patient can breathe, cough, or talk, do not interfere with his or her attempts to expel the foreign body. As with the adult, encourage the child to continue coughing. Administer supplemental oxygen if needed (and tolerated), and provide transport to the ED.

Intervene only if signs of a severe airway obstruction develop, such as a weak, ineffective cough; cyanosis; stridor; absent air movement; or a decreasing level of consciousness.

Removing a Foreign Body Airway Obstruction in a Child

Responsive Child

If you determine a child older than 1 year has an airway obstruction, stand or kneel behind the child and provide abdominal thrusts in the same manner as an adult, but use less force, until the object is expelled or the child becomes unresponsive. If the child becomes unresponsive, follow the same steps as for the unresponsive adult.

To perform the abdominal-thrust maneuver in a responsive child who is in a standing or sitting position, follow these steps Figure 15-34:

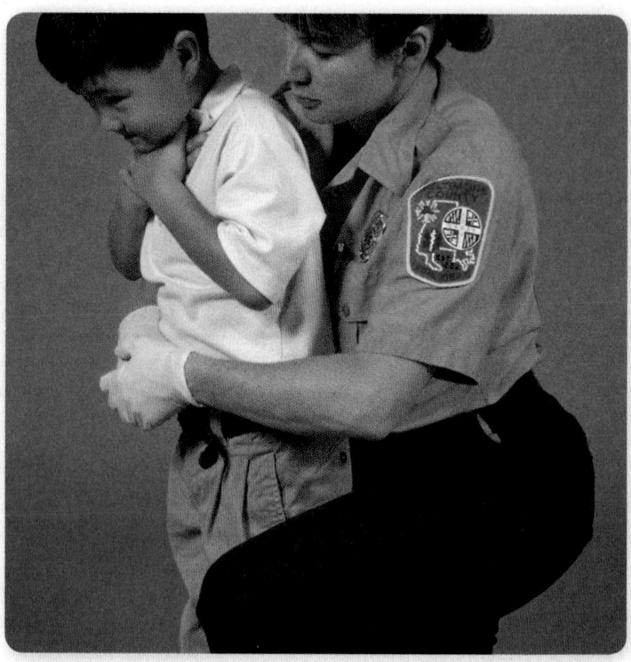

Figure 15-34 To perform the abdominal-thrust maneuver on a child, kneel on one knee behind the child, wrap your arms around his or her body, and place your fist just above the umbilicus and well below the lower tip of the sternum.

1. Kneel on one knee behind the child, and circle both of your arms around the child's body. Prepare to give abdominal thrusts by placing your fist just above the patient's umbilicus and well below the xiphoid process. Place your other hand over that fist.
2. Give the child abdominal thrusts in an upward direction. Avoid applying force to the lower rib cage or sternum.
3. Repeat this technique until the child expels the foreign body or becomes unresponsive.
4. If the child becomes unresponsive, position the child on a firm, flat surface and immediately call for help (or send someone to call for help).
5. Give 30 chest compressions (one cycle of 15 compressions if two rescuers are present), using the same landmark as you would for CPR. Do not check for a pulse before performing chest compressions.
6. Open the airway and look inside the mouth. If you see an object that can easily be removed, then remove it with your fingers and attempt to ventilate. If you do not see an object, then resume chest compressions.
7. Repeat steps 5 and 6 until the obstruction is relieved or paramedics take over.

If you manage to clear the airway obstruction in an unresponsive child but he or she still has no spontaneous breathing or circulation, then perform CPR (compressions and ventilations) and apply the AED as soon as it is available.

Unresponsive Child

If a child older than one year with an airway obstruction becomes unresponsive, he or she is managed in the same manner as an adult. Skill Drill 15-6 demonstrates the steps for removing a foreign body airway obstruction in an unresponsive child.

▶ Removing a Foreign Body Airway Obstruction in Infants

Responsive Infants

Do not use abdominal thrusts on a responsive infant with a foreign body airway obstruction because of the

Skill Drill 15-6 Removing a Foreign Body Airway Obstruction in an Unresponsive Child

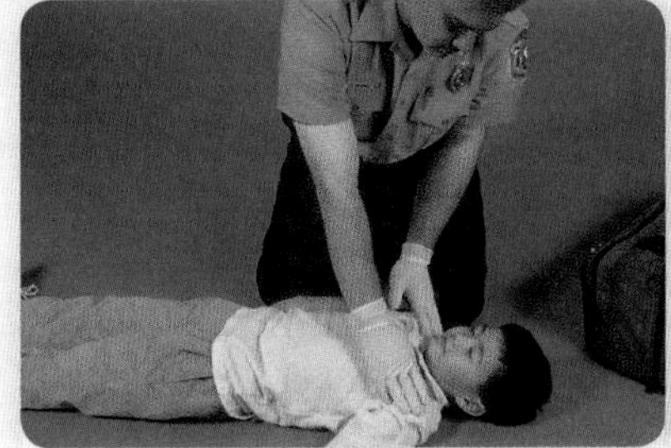

Step 1 Take standard precautions. Carefully place the child in a supine position on a firm, flat surface.

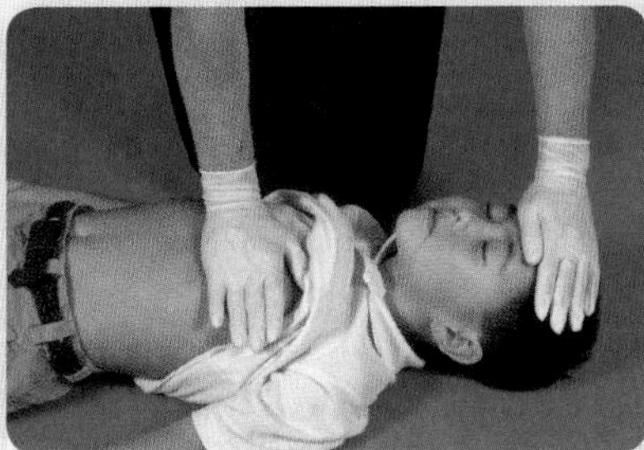

Step 2 Perform 30 chest compressions (15 compressions if two rescuers are present) using the same landmark as you would for CPR (lower half of the sternum). Do not check for a pulse before performing chest compressions.

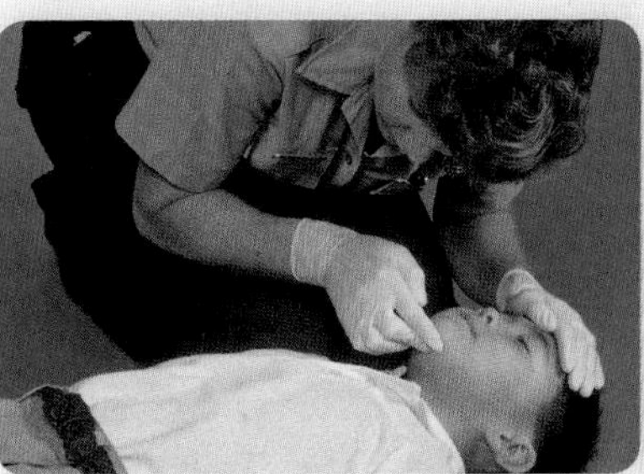

Step 3 Open the airway and look inside the mouth.

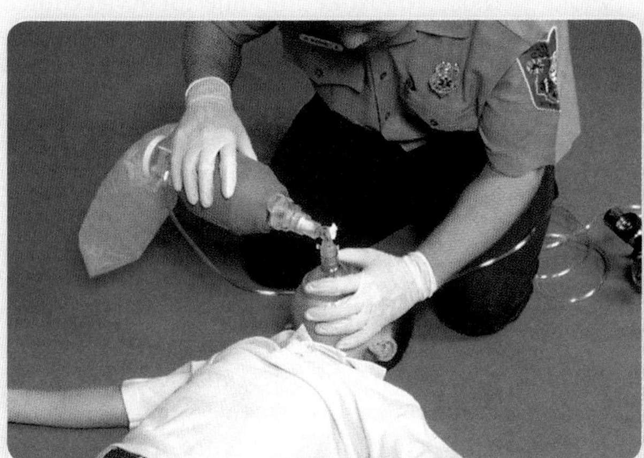

Step 4 If an object is visible and can easily be removed, then remove it with your fingers and attempt to ventilate.

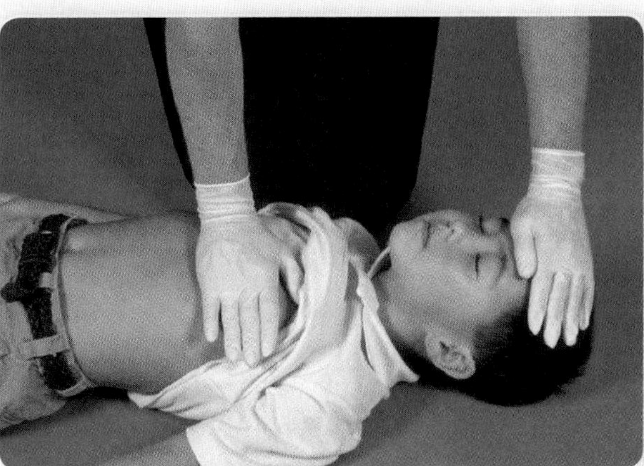

Step 5 If you do not see an object in the mouth, then resume chest compressions. Continue the sequence of chest compressions, opening the airway, and looking inside the mouth until the obstruction is relieved or the patient is transferred to a higher level of care.

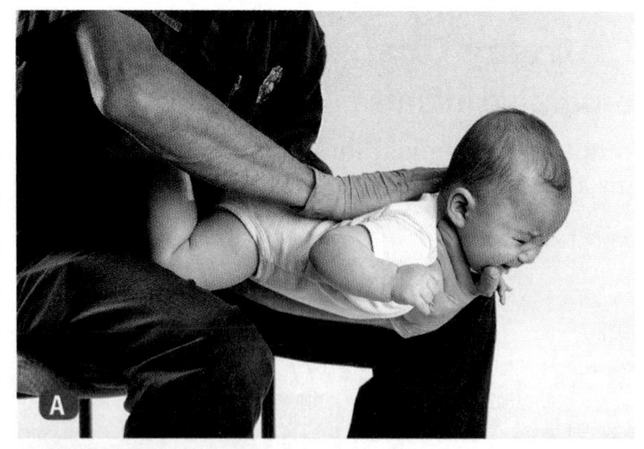

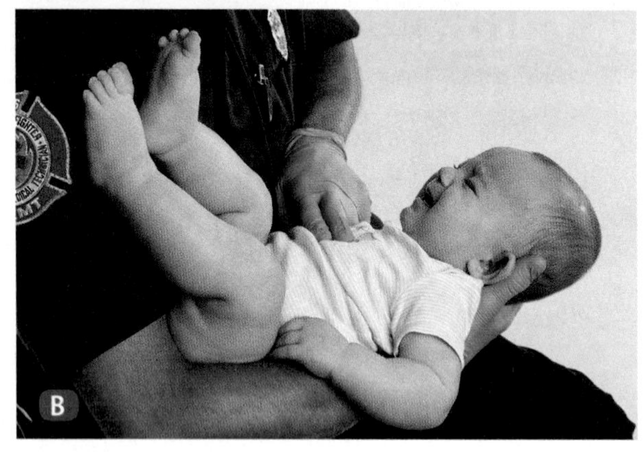

Figure 15-35 A. Hold the infant facedown with the body resting on your forearm. Support the jaw and face with your hand, and keep the head lower than the rest of the body. Give the infant five back slaps between the shoulder blades, using the heel of your hand. **B.** Give the infant five quick chest thrusts, using two fingers placed on the lower half of the sternum.

risk of injury to the immature organs of the abdomen. Instead, perform back slaps and chest thrusts to try to clear a severe airway obstruction in a responsive infant, as follows Figure 15-35:

1. Hold the infant facedown, with the body resting on your forearm. Support the infant's jaw and face with your hand, and keep the head lower than the rest of the body.
2. Deliver five back slaps between the shoulder blades, using the heel of your hand.
3. Place your free hand behind the infant's head and back, and turn the infant faceup on your other forearm and thigh, sandwiching the infant's body between your two hands and arms. The infant's head should remain below the level of the body.
4. Give five quick chest thrusts in the same location and manner as chest compressions, using two fingers placed on the lower half of the sternum. For larger infants, or if you have small hands, you can perform this step by placing the infant in your lap and turning the infant's whole body as a unit between back slaps and chest thrusts.
5. Check the airway. If you can see the foreign body, then remove it. If you do not see a foreign body, repeat the cycle as often as necessary.
6. If the infant becomes unresponsive, then begin CPR and follow the same sequence as for a child and adult.

Unresponsive Infants

If the infant becomes unresponsive during your attempts to relieve an airway obstruction, then perform CPR starting with chest compressions. Do not check for a pulse before starting compressions. Open the airway and look in the mouth. If you see an object that can easily be removed, then remove it with your finger and attempt to ventilate. If you do not see an object, then resume chest compressions. Continue the sequence of chest compressions, open the airway, and look inside the mouth until the obstruction is relieved or paramedics take over.

Special Resuscitation Circumstances

▶ Opioid Overdose

An opioid is a narcotic drug that, when taken in excess, depresses the central nervous system and causes respiratory arrest followed by cardiac arrest. Examples of opioids include heroin and oxycodone. In situations where opioid overdose is the suspected cause of a patient's cardiac arrest, bystanders may have administered the antidote naloxone (Narcan) to the patient prior to EMS arrival. Naloxone blocks opiate receptors in the body and reverses the effect of opioid overdose. Naloxone auto-injector devices, intended for use by laypeople (as well as health care providers), are now available in the United States. If you respond to a patient who has possibly overdosed on an opioid and naloxone was administered by a bystander prior to your arrival, then determine how much of the medication was given and the route by which it was given.

As an AEMT, naloxone is one of the medications that you can administer through local protocols written by your EMS medical director in cases of suspected opioid overdose. The recommended algorithm for implementing naloxone into the cardiac arrest management sequence is discussed in Chapter 23, *Toxicology*.

Standard resuscitative measures (ie, high-quality chest compressions, ventilation, defibrillation) take priority over naloxone administration; do not delay other interventions while awaiting the patient's response to naloxone therapy. Many patients who have overdosed on an opioid have a pulse (although slow) but are not breathing. In these patients, bag-mask ventilation is the most critical treatment, followed by administration of naloxone if it is available.

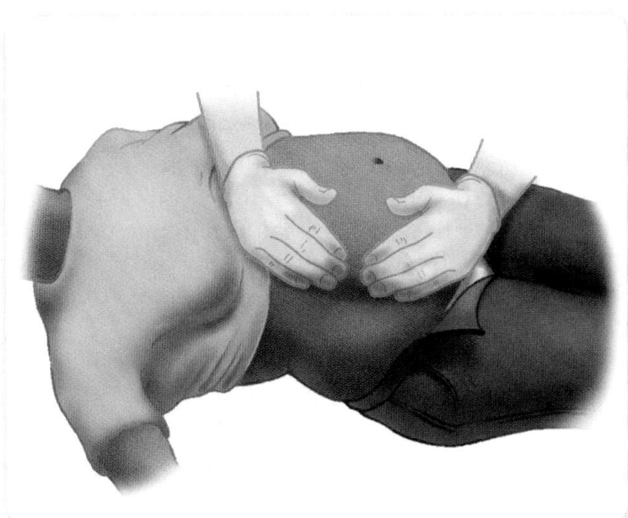

Figure 15-36 Manual left displacement of the uterus. The two-handed technique is shown. Alternatively, one hand can be used.

▶ Cardiac Arrest in Pregnancy

If you encounter a pregnant patient who is in cardiac arrest, your priorities are to provide high-quality CPR and relieve pressure off the aorta and vena cava. When the patient lies supine, the pregnant uterus can compress the aorta and vena cava (aortocaval compression). Compression of the vena cava causes a significant decrease in blood return to the heart and, secondarily, in the forward flow of blood to the vital organs.

If the pregnant patient is not in cardiac arrest, then position the patient on the left side to relieve pressure on the great vessels. However, if the patient is in cardiac arrest, this approach is impractical, because the patient must remain in a supine position to maximize the effectiveness of compressions. Therefore, if the top of the patient's uterus (fundus) can be felt at or above the level of the umbilicus, perform manual displacement of the uterus to the patient's left to relieve aortocaval compression while CPR is being performed. This step will improve the effectiveness of compressions Figure 15-36.

Grief Support for Family Members and Loved Ones

Whenever you assist a patient, remember his or her loved ones may also be affected by the emergency. Serious illness, injury, and pediatric patients create an especially high level of anxiety for family members. A health emergency is often hard for family members to understand. In some cases, family members may experience a psychological crisis that turns into a medical crisis and may become patients themselves.

Consider the scenario of a cardiac arrest in an otherwise healthy 57-year-old man. The family is watching your team perform CPR. Family members may assume you will bring him back or, at the very least, will expect you to transport. After 30 minutes or so, you stop resuscitation and start packing up your gear, then turn the scene over to the police. The patient is lying dead on the floor.

A trend in cardiac arrest care is to stay on the scene and perform the entire resuscitation in the location where the patient was found, particularly when ALS care is provided at the scene. Many EMS systems advocate this practice because continuous compressions are an important part of an effective resuscitation effort. CPR in the back of an ambulance is generally not as effective. If the patient has not responded to treatment after 20 to 30 minutes (or longer), many protocols suggest discontinuing resuscitative efforts and not transporting. However, this may create an uncomfortable situation at the scene.

For EMS crews, wanting to help but not knowing what to do can be very stressful. Is it the responsibility of EMS to explain the death to the family? Would you consider the bereaved widow the legal or moral responsibility of EMS? How is good patient care defined here? If you consider a spouse and perhaps other family members to be your patients as well, then it is appropriate to interact with them. Using the above scenario as an example, consider the following things that may make grief support in the field a little easier.

Whereas this cardiac arrest may be one of many similar calls in your career, family members and loved ones will remember this event in detail for the rest of their lives. Your reaction to them will form a lasting impression. Conversely, a mismanaged death notification or poor interaction could leave the family feeling disrespected or ignored. A compassionate and sensitive approach will leave a positive impression of you and your agency. Most important, appropriate and supportive care at the onset of grief may positively affect the family's grieving process.

Families do not typically expect EMS providers to stop resuscitation and leave their loved one on scene. When death appears imminent and resuscitative efforts are unsuccessful, make the family members aware the patient is not responding to treatment. Discuss with them what is happening so they may be better prepared for the inevitable. Keep family members informed throughout the resuscitation process because it may also help them feel more in control.

Sequential notification starts during resuscitative efforts; family members should be updated as the resuscitation progresses, if possible. Designate one provider to communicate the patient's status to family members, so information is streamlined from one source rather than from multiple providers. Be concise and clear. For example, say, "Your husband is not breathing and his heart has stopped. We are attempting to restart his heart." After resuscitation efforts have stopped, it is appropriate to tell them, "As you know, when we arrived, your husband wasn't breathing and did not have a pulse. He has not responded to any of our treatments. I'm sorry, but he has died." Avoid euphemisms such as "passed away" or "passed on," because these expressions may be confusing or misinterpreted. Law enforcement personnel may be involved in the official death declaration and will likely be responsible for what happens next, such as determining whether the medical examiner should be notified.

In a situation where ROSC occurs prior to transport, family members may wish to interact with the patient. This can give them comfort, especially if the patient ultimately does not survive.

After resuscitation has stopped, these other measures can be helpful:

- Take the family to a quiet, private place.
- Introduce yourself and anyone with you.
- Use clear language and speak in a warm, sensitive, and caring manner.
- Try to exhibit calm, reassuring authority.
- Use the patient's name.
- Use eye contact and appropriate touch.
- Expect family members to show emotion as they begin the grieving process. Be prepared for different reactions, including anger.
- While you are still on scene, be supportive but do not hover.
- Ask if a friend or family member can be called to come and help support them.
- When you need to leave, turn over the family to someone else, for example, a police officer.

Some family members will want to see the deceased. Being able to touch or talk to their loved ones may be helpful to them. This may not be advisable in a medical examiner's case. Law enforcement personnel will make that determination. It is appropriate to make the body presentable, but follow local protocols regarding movement of the patient or removal of resuscitation equipment.

Another consideration is to ensure children are not ignored. They may not understand death. Preschool-aged children may be less affected, whereas older children understand death but do not expect it to happen to someone they know. Younger children tend to blame themselves. Teenagers may be highly affected but may mask their feelings.

It is never easy to be the bearer of bad news, but it can help to know you did your best for the family during a difficult situation. Lastly, consider your own feelings in this stressful situation and make sure you seek assistance if needed. See Chapter 2, *Workforce Safety and Wellness*, for a discussion of the emotional aspects of emergency care and stress management.

Education and Training for the AEMT

You may go weeks or months without performing CPR on a human, depending on how busy your EMS system is. Like any skill, CPR skills can deteriorate over time. Practice this skill often using manikin-based training—ideally, more frequently than the standard recertification that occurs every 2 years.

You are encouraged to use high-fidelity manikins for CPR training, if your system's budget allows. If this is not an option, then CPR devices that provide corrective feedback are preferred over devices that provide only voice prompts (ie, a metronome).

CPR self-instruction through videos and/or computer-based modules with hands-on practice may be a reasonable alternative to instructor-led courses, because it may facilitate frequent retraining.

Education and Training for the Public

As an AEMT, you are a patient advocate. You are not only responsible for providing the best possible care for your patient, but you must also do your part to facilitate the training of laypeople in the critical skills of CPR and AED operation. Training in CPR and AED usage should not be limited to health care providers. Not enough laypeople are trained to perform these life-saving skills. Ask yourself, "Who is the *real* first responder?" Obviously, the layperson is likely to be at the scene before you and your team arrive.

As discussed previously, many laypeople assume CPR requires both mouth-to-mouth rescue breathing and chest compressions. As long as this misconception remains, fewer people will be willing to help during an emergency, which means fewer lives will be saved. If you are asked to train members of your community how to perform compression-only CPR, then you should consider it your professional responsibility and be willing to assist.

It is likely that some citizens in your service area are at increased risk for cardiac arrest. Your agency should make an effort to identify these potential patients and educate their families to recognize cardiac arrest and to train them to perform compression-only CPR.

YOU are the Provider SUMMARY

1. What should you immediately do on receiving this update from dispatch?

After you are informed that CPR is in progress, you should immediately request additional assistance. Effective treatment of a patient in cardiac arrest requires adequate personnel at the scene and during transport. As an AEMT, familiarize yourself with the resources that are available to you and know when it is appropriate to request them.

The type of backup you receive (ie, BLS versus paramedic) will depend on your EMS system and the resources that are available to you. High-quality CPR and defibrillation, combined with early advanced care, increase the patient's chance for survival.

If you do not have access to other AEMTs or to paramedics, then request assistance from the fire department. Fire departments are often staffed with at least one or two emergency medical responders who are able to perform CPR and assist with certain BLS interventions.

Regardless of the resources available to you, request them as soon as possible—in this case, as soon as you are advised CPR is in progress. One AEMT cannot effectively treat a cardiac arrest patient during transport; you would have to perform continuous CPR while your partner drives the ambulance (or vice versa), which could result in rescuer fatigue and decreased effectiveness of chest compressions.

2. What should be your initial actions on arriving at this scene?

After you ensure your safety, approach this patient as you would any other patient, by performing a primary survey. Although the dispatcher has advised you that bystander CPR is in progress, you must still assess the patient to confirm he is indeed apneic and pulseless and requires CPR.

Your primary survey should take only a few seconds, just long enough to confirm the patient is in cardiac arrest. If he is in cardiac arrest, then begin CPR immediately, apply the AED as soon as it is available, and analyze the patient's cardiac rhythm. To avoid interrupting CPR, you should apply the AED pads around your partner's hands as he or she is performing chest compressions (do not stop compressions to do this).

If the AED advises you to shock, then deliver the shock and immediately resume CPR, starting with chest compressions. If the AED does not advise you to shock, then immediately resume CPR, starting with chest compressions. During CPR, ask the two bystanders if they witnessed the event and determine whether they know anything about the patient (ie, past medical history, events leading up to the arrest).

Regardless of how a call is dispatched and whether or not you assume patient care from bystanders or other health care providers, it is important for you to always perform a primary survey of the patient.

3. What links in the chain of survival have been maintained at this point?

The following links in the chain of survival have been maintained:

- Recognition and activation of the emergency response system, because the bystanders quickly recognized the patient was experiencing a cardiac emergency and immediately called 9-1-1.
- Immediate, high-quality CPR, because the bystanders began CPR directly after calling 9-1-1.
- Basic and advanced emergency medical services, because EMS providers are at the scene providing specialized care to the patient.

The following links in the chain of survival have not been maintained:

- Rapid defibrillation, because it has not yet occurred. Of all the links in the chain of survival, early defibrillation has the most profound impact on patient survival. With early access and early CPR, defibrillation may successfully terminate lethal cardiac dysrhythmias in a significant number of patients. For each minute that defibrillation is delayed, the patient's chance for survival decreases by 7% to 10%.
- Advanced life support and postarrest care, because ROSC has not been established and the patient has not arrived at the hospital.

4. Why is it so crucial to minimize interruptions in CPR?

Even when CPR is performed correctly (that is, at a rate of 100 to 120 compressions per minute and a depth of 2 inches to 2.4 inches [5 cm to 6 cm] in the adult), chest compressions deliver only about one-third of a person's normal cardiac output. When CPR is performed properly and with minimal interruption, it is often enough to keep the patient's vital organs viable until defibrillation and more advanced care can be provided at the ED. Of course, this assumes that defibrillation and advanced care are provided within a short period of time.

Within a few seconds of stopping chest compressions, the pressure generated in the arteries drops to near zero; therefore, frequent or prolonged interruptions in chest compressions will not even provide the minimum perfusion needed to keep the vital organs viable. This has been clearly linked to low survival rates from cardiac arrest. Remember to maintain a chest compression fraction of at least 60%.

As soon as cardiac arrest has been confirmed, it is crucial to begin CPR immediately and apply the AED as soon as it is available. Even when the AED pads are being applied, your partner should continue chest compressions; you should apply the pads around your partner's hands.

YOU are the Provider SUMMARY *(continued)*

5. Should you remove the medication patch or leave it in place? Why or why not?

The patch is located on the patient's right upper chest, which is where you will place one of the AED pads. Because of its location, the patch could interfere with the electrical current to the heart and may cause burns to the patient's skin. To prevent this complication, remove the patch, wipe any residue from the skin, and then apply the AED pads. Remember to take standard precautions!

6. What does the bulge and scar over the patient's left chest indicate? How will this affect the way you treat the patient?

A hard lump or bulge on the patient's chest, usually with a corresponding scar, indicates an AICD or pacemaker. These devices are used in patients who are at high risk for certain cardiac dysrhythmias and cardiac arrest. The AICD will deliver shocks directly to the heart if it detects a lethal cardiac dysrhythmia. Implanted pacemakers are used to increase the patient's heart rate if it falls below a given value.

If the AED pads are placed directly over the device, then shocks delivered by the AED may be less effective. Therefore, if you identify an AICD or pacemaker, place the AED pad at least 1 inch (2.5 cm) away from the device. Because most of these devices are implanted in the upper left chest, this should not be an issue. The pads are placed to the right of the upper sternum and to the lower left chest, just below the nipple, so they should be well beyond 1 inch (2.5 cm) from the device. Follow your local protocols regarding patients with AICDs or implanted pacemakers.

7. Which rhythms will the AED defibrillate?

AEDs are designed to shock VF and pulseless VT. It is important to remember AEDs will not shock all cardiac rhythms, just lethal ventricular rhythms. However, remember an AED cannot detect the presence of a pulse and may shock a patient in VT who has a pulse. This is why you should not apply the AED to a patient with a pulse.

8. How should you continue to treat this patient?

You have restored a pulse in your patient; however, his breathing is not adequate. Agonal gasps are ineffective and do not produce adequate minute volume.

Some patients may have an intact gag reflex, despite being unresponsive; in these cases, an oropharyngeal airway is contraindicated. Insert a nasopharyngeal (nasal) airway and continue to provide rescue breathing. Deliver one breath every 5 to 6 seconds (10 to 12 breaths/min); each breath should be delivered over 1 second (just enough to produce visible chest rise). Closely and carefully monitor the patient's pulse and be prepared to resume CPR if necessary.

Assume the patient has a full stomach and have a suction unit ready in case he regurgitates. Remember, mortality increases significantly if aspiration occurs. It is also important to avoid hyperventilating the patient.

9. Because the patient is no longer in cardiac arrest, should you remove the AED pads? Why or why not?

Although the patient is not in cardiac arrest, he is still at high risk for redeveloping cardiac arrest. Therefore, do not remove the AED pads; simply continue rescue breathing, and prepare the patient for prompt transport.

10. Would an ITD benefit your patient at this point?

An ITD is a valve device that is placed between the ET tube and resuscitation bag; it can also be placed in between the resuscitation bag and mask if the patient is not intubated. It is used only for patients who are apneic and pulseless. At this point, your patient has a pulse and is breathing (albeit slowly and shallowly); therefore, the ITD is not indicated. Furthermore, the ITD *may* be of benefit when used during active compression-decompression CPR, but it is not recommended for use during conventional CPR. If ROSC occurs, the ITD must be removed.

11. What further treatment, if any, is indicated for this patient?

Further treatment of your patient should consist of careful monitoring because he remains at high risk for recurrence of cardiac arrest. In patients who are responsive and alert, the presence of a pulse is obvious; however, when a patient is unresponsive, you must frequently reassess for a pulse.

Unresponsive patients are at an increased risk for regurgitation, which could lead to aspiration and increased mortality. Vigilantly monitor the patient's airway status and be prepared to turn his head to the side if he regurgitates. Maintain his airway with manual positioning and a basic airway adjunct, in this case, a nasal airway.

Although the patient is breathing, his breaths are slow and shallow. Slow, shallow (reduced tidal volume) respirations will not produce adequate minute volume; therefore, continue to assist the patient's ventilations with a bag-mask device, but *do not hyperventilate him.* Deliver each breath over 1 second while observing for visible chest rise. Monitor his oxygen saturation (Spo_2) level and heart rate to help you determine if your assisted ventilations are adequate.

YOU are the Provider SUMMARY *(continued)*

As mentioned earlier, do not remove the AED pads. Turn off the AED, but be prepared to stop the ambulance if cardiac arrest redevelops.

The patient's blood pressure (86/66 mm Hg) is still low. Follow your local protocols regarding positioning of the patient to improve his blood pressure.

12. What options do you have if you are unable to obtain IV access?

You have limited options if you are unsuccessful at obtaining intravenous (IV) access. In the setting of a cardiac arrest, you should limit yourself to two attempts to gain IV access, prior to obtaining intraosseous (IO) access.

EMS Patient Care Report (PCR)					
Date: 8-20-18	**Incident No.:** 011122		**Nature of Call:** Cardiac arrest	**Location:** 483 Farmer's Market Road	
Dispatched: 1445	**En Route:** 1447	**At Scene:** 1454	**Transport:** 1508	**At Hospital:** 1518	**In Service:** 1528
Patient Information					
Age: 48 **Sex:** M **Weight (in kg [lb]):** 77 kg (170 lb)			**Allergies:** Unknown **Medications:** Unknown **Past Medical History:** Unknown **Chief Complaint:** Cardiac arrest		

Vital Signs				
Time: 1455	**BP:** N/A	**Pulse:** 0	**Respirations:** 0	**Spo_2:** N/A
Time: 1458	**BP:** N/A	**Pulse:** 0	**Respirations:** 0	**Spo_2:** N/A
Time: 1501	**BP:** 70/40	**Pulse:** 100	**Respirations:** 4	**Spo_2:** 82% on O_2
Time: 1506	**BP:** 86/66	**Pulse:** 94	**Respirations:** 8	**Spo_2:** 95% on O_2
EMS Treatment (circle all that apply)				
Oxygen @ 15 **L/min via (circle one):** **NC** **NRM** **Bag-mask device** (circled)		**Assisted Ventilation** (circled)	**Airway Adjunct** (circled)	**CPR** (circled)
Defibrillation (circled)	**Bleeding Control**	**Bandaging**	**Splinting**	**Other:**

Narrative

EMS dispatched to local farmer's market for "CPR in progress." On arrival at the scene, found two bystanders performing CPR on the patient, a 48-year-old male. Medic 22 (BLS) was dispatched to the scene to assist. Primary survey revealed that the patient was apneic and pulseless. Continued two-rescuer CPR for 2 minutes while the AED was being prepared. Per one of the bystanders, the patient delivered a load of produce then sat down in his truck and slumped over the steering wheel. There was no trauma involved. The bystander further stated that by the time he got to the patient, he was unresponsive, apneic, and pulseless. After 2 minutes of CPR, EMS analyzed patient's cardiac rhythm with the AED and received a shock advised message. Delivered single shock and immediately resumed CPR. Medic 22 arrived at scene and assisted with CPR and airway management. The patient's past medical history was unknown, although he had an AICD and was wearing a medication patch, which was removed. Continued CPR for 2 minutes, reanalyzed the patient's cardiac rhythm, and received a no shock advised message. Continued CPR and attempted to insert an oral airway; however, the patient began to gag. Immediate reassessment revealed that he had a strong carotid pulse, but was not breathing adequately. Inserted a nasal airway, continued ventilations at 12 breaths/min, packaged the patient, and loaded him into the ambulance. EMT Smith from Medic 22 assisted with patient care en route to the hospital. En route, reassessed patient and found that he remained unresponsive; his respiratory rate increased, but the depth of his breathing remained shallow. Established an 18-gauge IV left AC with NS wide open to give a 20 mL/kg bolus. Continued assisted ventilation and called in radio report to the receiving facility. Monitored the patient's pulse, provided additional supportive care, and delivered him to the ED without incident. Gave verbal report to attending physician. Cleared the hospital and returned to service at 1528.**End of report**

Prep Kit

▶ Ready for Review

- BLS is noninvasive emergency life-saving care that is used to treat medical conditions, including airway obstruction, respiratory arrest, and cardiac arrest.
- BLS care focuses on the ABCs: airway (obstruction), breathing (respiratory arrest), and circulation (cardiac arrest or severe bleeding). If the patient is in cardiac arrest, then use a CAB sequence (compressions, airway, breathing).
- CPR is used to establish artificial ventilation and circulation in a patient who is not breathing and has no pulse.
- The goal of CPR is to help restore spontaneous breathing and circulation; however, advanced procedures such as medications and defibrillation are often necessary for this to occur.
- ALS involves advanced life-saving procedures, such as cardiac monitoring, administering intravenous fluids and medications, and using advanced airway adjuncts.
- The five links in the chain of survival are (1) recognition and activation of the emergency response system; (2) immediate, high-quality CPR; (3) rapid defibrillation; (4) basic and advanced emergency medical services; and (5) ALS and postarrest care.
- Apply an AED to any nontrauma cardiac arrest patient as soon as it is available.
- When using an AED on a child between ages 1 and 8 years, use pediatric-sized pads and a dose-attenuating system (energy reducer). If these items are unavailable, then use adult-sized AED pads. In infants (age 1 month to 1 year), manual defibrillation is preferred. If a manual defibrillator is unavailable, then use an AED equipped with pediatric-sized pads and a dose attenuator. If neither option is available, then use adult-sized AED pads.
- As an AEMT, it is your responsibility to start CPR in virtually all patients who are in cardiac arrest. The three general exceptions to the rule are as follows: (1) do not start CPR if the scene is unsafe; (2) do not start CPR if the patient has obvious signs of death; and (3) do not start CPR if the patient and his or her physician have a previously agreed-on DNR or no-CPR order.
- As an AEMT, you are generally not responsible for making the decision to stop CPR. After you begin CPR in the field, you must continue until one of the following events occurs (the STOP mnemonic):
  - **S**, the patient *Starts* breathing and has a pulse.
  - **T**, the patient's care is *Transferred* to another provider of equal or higher-level training.
  - **O**, you are *Out* of strength or too tired to continue.
  - **P**, a *Physician* who is present or providing online medical direction assumes responsibility for the patient and gives direction to discontinue CPR.
- An airway obstruction may have various causes, including relaxation of the throat muscles in an unresponsive patient; vomited or regurgitated stomach contents; blood; damaged tissue after an injury; dentures; or foreign bodies such as food or small objects.
- The manual maneuver recommended for removing severe airway obstructions in the responsive adult and child is the abdominal-thrust maneuver (the Heimlich maneuver). Use back slaps and chest thrusts to treat a responsive infant with a severe airway obstruction.
- If the adult, child, or infant with a severe airway obstruction is unresponsive, then perform CPR, starting with chest compressions.
- As an AEMT, you will encounter situations in which grief support for family and loved ones will be part of your role. After resuscitation has stopped, turn your attention to the family and loved ones, and provide clear communication and emotional support.

▶ Vital Vocabulary

abdominal-thrust maneuver The preferred method to dislodge a severe airway obstruction in adults and children; also called the Heimlich maneuver.

active compression-decompression CPR A technique that involves compressing the chest and then actively pulling it back up to its neutral position or beyond (decompression); may increase the amount of blood that returns to the heart and, thus, the amount of blood ejected from the heart during the compression phase.

advanced life support (ALS) Advanced life-saving procedures used to treat medical conditions, such as cardiac monitoring, administration of intravenous fluids and medications, and the use of advanced airway adjuncts. EMTs and AEMTs may be trained in some of these areas.

basic life support (BLS) Noninvasive emergency life-saving care used to treat medical conditions, including airway obstruction, respiratory arrest, and cardiac arrest.

cardiopulmonary resuscitation (CPR) The combination of chest compressions and rescue breathing used to establish adequate ventilation and circulation in a patient who is not breathing and has no pulse.

chest compression fraction The total percentage of time during a resuscitation attempt in which active chest compressions are being performed.

Prep Kit *(continued)*

crew resource management (CRM) A way for team members to work together with the team leader to develop and maintain a shared understanding of the emergency situation; to collaborate and communicate, fulfill their roles and responsibilities, and achieve the shared goal of the best possible patient outcome.

dependent lividity Blood settling to the lowest point of the body, causing discoloration of the skin; a definitive sign of death.

gastric distention A condition in which air fills the stomach, often as a result of high volume and pressure during artificial ventilation.

head tilt–chin lift maneuver A combination of two movements to open the airway by tilting the forehead back and lifting the chin; not used for trauma patients.

hyperventilation Rapid or deep breathing that lowers the blood carbon dioxide level below normal; may lead to increased intrathoracic pressure, decreased venous return, and hypotension when associated with bag-mask device use.

impedance threshold device (ITD) A valve device placed between the endotracheal tube and a bag-mask device that limits the amount of air entering the lungs during the recoil phase between chest compressions.

ischemia A lack of oxygen that deprives tissues of necessary nutrients, resulting from partial or complete blockage of blood flow; potentially reversible because permanent injury has not yet occurred.

jaw-thrust maneuver Technique to open the airway by placing the fingers behind the angle of the jaw and bringing the jaw forward; used for patients who may have a cervical spine injury.

load-distributing band (LDB) A circumferential chest compression device composed of a constricting band and backboard that is either electrically or pneumatically driven to compress the heart by putting inward pressure on the thorax.

mechanical piston device A device that depresses the sternum via a compressed gas-powered or electric-powered plunger mounted on a backboard.

recovery position A side-lying position used to maintain a clear airway in unresponsive patients who are breathing adequately and do not have suspected injuries to the spine, hips, or pelvis.

return of spontaneous circulation (ROSC) The return of a pulse and effective blood flow to the body in a patient who previously was in cardiac arrest.

rigor mortis Stiffening of the body muscles; a definitive sign of death.

stridor A harsh, high-pitched respiratory sound, generally heard during inspiration, that is caused by partial blockage or narrowing of the upper airway; may be audible without a stethoscope.

ventilation Exchange of air between the lungs and the environment, spontaneously by the patient or with assistance from another person, such as an EMT.

▶ References

1. American Heart Association. CPR Facts and Stats. http://cpr.heart.org/AHAECC/CPRAndECC/AboutCPRFirstAid/CPRFactsAndStats/UCM_475748_CPR-Facts-and-Stats.jsp. Accessed July 26, 2016.
2. Out-of-hospital Chain of Survival. © 2016 American Heart Association, Inc. All rights reserved. http://cpr.heart.org/AHAECC/CPRAndECC/AboutCPRFirstAid/CPRFactsAndStats/UCM_475731_CPR-Chain-of-Survival.jsp. Accessed October 27, 2016.
3. Link MS, Berkow LC, Kudenchuk PJ, Halperin HR, Hess EP, Moitra VK, Neumar RW, O'Neil BJ, Paxton JH, Silvers SM, White RD, Yannopoulos D, Donnino MW. Part 7: adult advanced cardiovascular life support: 2015 American Heart Association Guidelines Update for Cardiopulmonary Resuscitation and Emergency Cardiovascular Care. Circulation. 2015;132(suppl 2):S452.
4. Sudden Unexpected Infant Death Syndrome and Sudden Infant Death Syndrome – about SUID and SIDS. Centers for Disease Control and Prevention website. https://www.cdc.gov/sids/aboutsuidandsids.htm. Updated February 1, 2017. Accessed September 7, 2017.
5. American Heart Association. Web-based Integrated Guidelines for Cardiopulmonary Resuscitation and Emergency Cardiovascular Care – Part 8: Post-Cardiac Arrest Care. ECCguidelines.heart.org. Accessed September 7, 2017.
6. Babbs, CF. Interposed abdominal compression CPR: a comprehensive evidence-based review. *Resuscitation.* 2003;59(1):71-82.

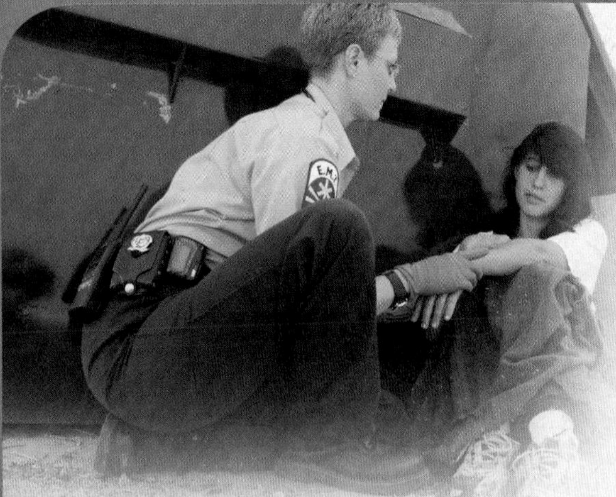

Assessment in Action

Your EMS supervisor is conducting a so-called tabletop exercise with your crew in preparation for the next cardiac arrest call and wants to assess your crew's knowledge of cardiac arrest management. She presents your crew with the following scenario questions.

1. Which intervention(s) would have the MOST positive impact on the cardiac arrest patient's outcome?

- **A.** Advanced airway management
- **B.** Early CPR and defibrillation
- **C.** IV fluid administration
- **D.** Cardiac medications

2. The AED gives a "no shock advised" message to a patient who is in cardiac arrest. You should:

- **A.** resume chest compressions.
- **B.** check for a carotid pulse.
- **C.** reanalyze the cardiac rhythm.
- **D.** deliver two rescue breaths.

3. What is the maximum amount of time you should spend checking for spontaneous breathing in an unresponsive child?

- **A.** 5 seconds
- **B.** 10 seconds
- **C.** 15 seconds
- **D.** 20 seconds

4. When performing CPR on an adult, you should compress the chest to a depth of ___ at a rate of ___ compressions per minute.

- **A.** 1 inch to 1.4 inches (2.5 cm to 3.5 cm); 80 to 100
- **B.** 2 inches to 2.4 inches (5 cm to 6 cm); 80 to 100
- **C.** 1 inch to 1.4 inches (2.5 cm to 3.5 cm); 100 to 120
- **D.** 2 inches to 2.4 inches (5 cm to 6 cm); 100 to 120

5. What is the proper compression-to-ventilation ratio for two-rescuer adult CPR?

- **A.** 15:2
- **B.** 30:2
- **C.** 50:2
- **D.** 75:2

6. When checking for a pulse in an infant, you should palpate which of the following arteries?

- **A.** Carotid
- **B.** Femoral
- **C.** Brachial
- **D.** Dorsalis pedis

7. When you are performing CPR on an adult or child, you should reassess the patient for return of respirations and/or circulation approximately every __________ minutes.

- **A.** 5
- **B.** 3
- **C.** 2
- **D.** 1

8. What is the preferred method of removing a foreign body in an unresponsive child?

- **A.** Back slaps
- **B.** Abdominal thrusts
- **C.** Chest compressions
- **D.** Manual removal

9. After you have started CPR in the field, under what circumstances can you stop?

10. Explain why the presence of gastric distention is dangerous to the patient.

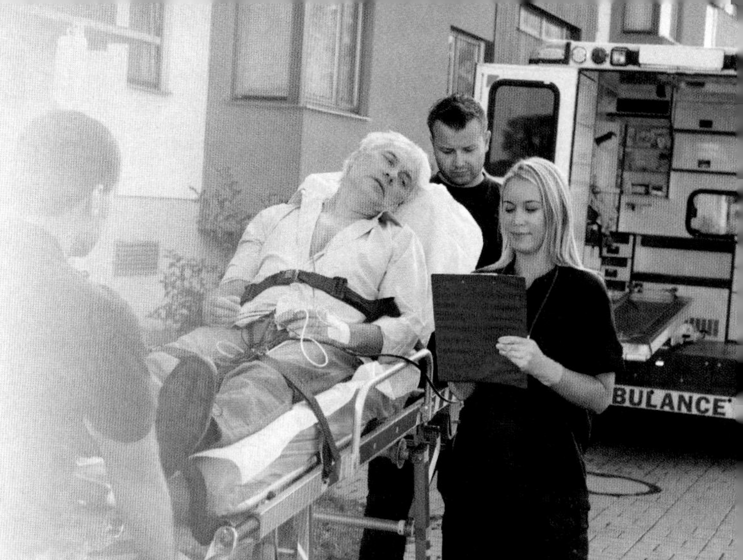

SECTION 7

Medical

CHAPTER 16

Medical Overview

National EMS Education Standard Competencies

Medicine

Applies fundamental knowledge to provide basic and selected advanced emergency care and transportation based on assessment findings for an acutely ill patient.

Medical Overview

Assessment and management of a

- Medical complaint (pp 733-737)

Pathophysiology, assessment, and management of medical complaints to include

- Transport mode (pp 737-738)
- Destination decisions (p 738)

Infectious Diseases

Awareness of

- A patient who may have an infectious disease (p 739)

Assessment and management of

- A patient who may have an infectious disease (p 739)
- A patient who may be infected with a bloodborne pathogen (pp 740-743)
  - Human immunodeficiency virus (HIV) (pp 740-741)
  - Hepatitis B (pp 741-743)
- Antibiotic-resistant infections (p 745)
- Current infectious diseases prevalent in the community (pp 741, 744-747)

Knowledge Objectives

1. Differentiate between medical emergencies and trauma emergencies, remembering that some patients may have both. (p 733)
2. Name the various categories of common medical emergencies and give examples. (p 733)
3. Describe the evaluation of the nature of illness. (p 734)
4. Identify elements and steps in the assessment of a patient with a medical emergency. (pp 734-736)
5. Explain the importance of transport time and destination selection for a medical patient. (pp 737-738)
6. Describe the general assessment and management principles when working with a patient who may have an infectious or communicable disease. (p 739)
7. Define *epidemic* and *pandemic*. (pp 739-740)
8. Discuss the pathophysiology, signs and symptoms, and management of a patient with HIV or acquired immunodeficiency syndrome. (p 740)
9. Discuss precautions to protect against exposure to HIV. (pp 740-741)
10. Discuss the pathophysiology, signs and symptoms, and management of a patient with influenza, and describe ways to protect against its transmission. (p 741)
11. Discuss the pathophysiology, signs and symptoms, and management of a patient with hepatitis. (pp 741-743)
12. Discuss precautions to protect oneself against exposure to hepatitis. (pp 742-743)
13. Discuss other infectious diseases of special concern and their routes of transmission, including herpes simplex, syphilis, meningitis, tuberculosis, pertussis, and methicillin-resistant *Staphylococcus aureus*. (pp 744-745)
14. Identify other new and emerging diseases, including West Nile virus, severe acute respiratory syndrome, and avian flu. (pp 745-746)
15. Discuss infections that are global health issues, including Middle East respiratory syndrome coronavirus and Ebola. (pp 746-747)
16. Understand the procedure for taking a travel history, and apply its findings to the patient's present condition. (p 747)

Skills Objectives

There are no skills objectives for this chapter.

Introduction

Patients who need emergency medical services (EMS) assistance generally have experienced either a medical emergency or trauma emergency; in some cases, both have occurred. **Trauma emergencies** involve injuries resulting from physical forces applied to the body. **Medical emergencies** involve illnesses or conditions caused by disease. Although it is important for you to be able to make the distinction between medical and trauma patients, it is equally important for you to remember that patients may have a combination of medical and trauma conditions affecting their health. For example, a person who has a heart attack while driving may be involved in a crash, or a diabetic patient whose blood glucose level is too low may fall and be injured. This chapter discusses medical emergencies. Chapter 26, *Trauma Overview*, discusses trauma emergencies.

Words of Wisdom

Patients are classified as critical or stable based on their presentation—not based on whether they have a medical illness or a traumatic injury. A myocardial infarction is a critical medical condition, whereas an isolated broken toe is a stable traumatic injury.

Types of Medical Emergencies

There are many types of medical emergencies Table 16-1. Respiratory emergencies occur when patients have trouble breathing or when the amount of oxygen supplied to the tissues is inadequate. Diseases that can lead to respiratory emergencies include asthma, emphysema, and chronic bronchitis. Cardiovascular emergencies are caused by conditions affecting the circulatory system. The most common examples that require EMS intervention include myocardial infarction and heart failure. Neurologic emergencies involve the brain and may be caused by a seizure, stroke, or fainting (syncope). Many gastrointestinal conditions are true emergencies and can result in a call to EMS for help. The most well-known of these gastrointestinal emergencies is appendicitis, although there are many others, including diverticulitis and pancreatitis. A urologic emergency can involve kidney stones. The most common endocrine emergencies are caused by complications of

Table 16-1 Common Medical Emergencies

Type of Medical Emergency	Examples of Conditions
Respiratory	Asthma, emphysema, chronic bronchitis
Cardiovascular	Myocardial infarction, heart failure
Neurologic	Seizure, stroke, syncope
Gastrointestinal	Appendicitis, diverticulitis, pancreatitis
Urologic	Kidney stones, pyelonephritis
Endocrine	Diabetes mellitus
Hematologic	Sickle cell disease, hemophilia
Immunologic	Anaphylactic reaction (severe allergy to beestings, food, or other substances)
Toxicologic	Substance abuse, food, plant, or chemical poisoning
Psychiatric	Alzheimer disease, schizophrenia, depression
Gynecologic	Vaginal bleeding, sexually transmitted disease, pelvic inflammatory disease, ectopic pregnancy

YOU are the Provider PART 1

At 1422 hours, your ambulance is dispatched for a call involving a 47-year-old woman with back pain and difficulty urinating. You and your partner proceed to the scene, with a response time of about 6 minutes. On arrival, you are met by the patient's husband, who directs you to the patient. She is lying on the bed in the fetal position. A quick glance around the room reveals no visible hazards to you or your partner. The patient states that she has sharp pain in her right side towards the back, which increases in intensity when she tries to urinate. She further states that she has had this pain for 3 days and has not been eating or drinking as much as normal.

1. Which systems of the body may be causing the patient's signs and symptoms?
2. Does this patient require immediate transport?

diabetes mellitus. Hematologic (blood-related) emergencies may be the result of sickle cell disease or various types of blood clotting disorders such as hemophilia. Immunologic emergencies involve the body's response to foreign substances. When the body overreacts to a foreign substance, the condition is commonly referred to as an allergic reaction. Allergic reactions are a type of immunologic medical emergency that can range from fairly minor conditions to life-threatening anaphylaxis. Toxicologic emergencies, including poisoning and substance abuse, result in other types of medical emergencies. Some medical emergencies are caused by psychological or behavioral problems. Behavioral emergencies may be especially difficult to manage because patients often do not present with typical signs and symptoms. Some conditions, such as gynecologic conditions, will most likely be challenging for you because there is little that you can do to treat patients with these conditions in the prehospital setting. The chapters in this section discuss each of these medical emergencies.

Patient Assessment

Assessment of a medical patient is similar to the assessment of a trauma patient but with a different focus. Whereas trauma assessments focus on the mechanism of injury or physical injuries, most of which are visible through a physical examination, medical patient assessment focuses on the **nature of illness (NOI)**, symptoms, and the patient's chief complaint. Information received from dispatch can be helpful in anticipating what you might find when you arrive on scene, but it is conceivable that what appears to be a traumatic emergency may in fact be a medical emergency or vice versa. For example, a patient may have a medical condition that resulted in a motor vehicle crash, or the patient may have sustained a large laceration and you fail to recognize that the patient has experienced a hypoglycemic event. Tunnel vision occurs when you become focused on one aspect of the patient's condition and exclude all others, which may cause you to miss an important injury or illness.

As discussed in Chapter 10, *Patient Assessment*, the major components of patient assessment include the following:

- Scene size-up
- Primary survey
- History taking
- Secondary assessment
- Reassessment

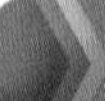

Scene Size-up

You must complete a scene size-up. The most important aspect of this step is to make sure the scene is safe. Although hazards are not as obvious with medical emergencies as with trauma situations, they still exist and must be considered. For example, patients who are substance abusers may need help in potentially dangerous locations, and some patients may have guard dogs or weapons that could pose a threat to you.

It is also important that you follow standard precautions when you respond to an emergency, including wearing gloves and other protective equipment. After determining the number of patients who need assistance and considering whether you need additional help, your next task is to determine the NOI. What signs and symptoms is the patient experiencing? Evaluation of the NOI for a medical patient will provide you with an index of suspicion for different types of serious or life-threatening underlying illnesses. The **index of suspicion** is your awareness and concern for potentially serious underlying and unseen injuries or illness.

Words of Wisdom

Use the patient's chief complaint to guide your assessment, but do not get tunnel vision. A patient initially reporting dyspnea may present with difficulty breathing, rales, and coughing up pink, frothy sputum. While the chief complaint may be shortness of breath, the underlying problem in such a case is heart failure. An inability to recognize the patient's actual condition may result in a delay in providing definitive treatment or inappropriate care.

Primary Survey

As you approach a medical patient, you should form a general impression of his or her condition. Do not let a relatively normal impression lull you into complacency; the conditions of many medical patients may not appear serious at first. Quickly determine the patient's level of consciousness using the AVPU (*Alert*—is awake, follows commands, visually tracks people or objects—and oriented to person, place, and time; responsive to *Verbal* stimuli; responsive to *Pain*; *Unresponsive*) scale.

Identify life threats by quickly assessing the patient's Airway, Breathing, Circulation, Disability, and Exposure (ABCDEs). In responsive patients, ensure the airway is open and breathing is adequate. Consider applying oxygen at this time if there is any indication that breathing has been affected. For unresponsive patients, make sure to open the airway using the proper technique for their condition and take several seconds to evaluate their breathing. Apply oxygen to patients in shock, with difficulty breathing, and when low oxygen saturations are measured (SpO_2 less than 94%). Unresponsive patients may need airway adjuncts and ventilatory assistance with a bag-mask device. Quickly assess the circulation by checking the radial pulse in a responsive patient and the carotid pulse in the unresponsive patient, and by observing the patient's skin color, temperature, and condition **Figure 16-1**.

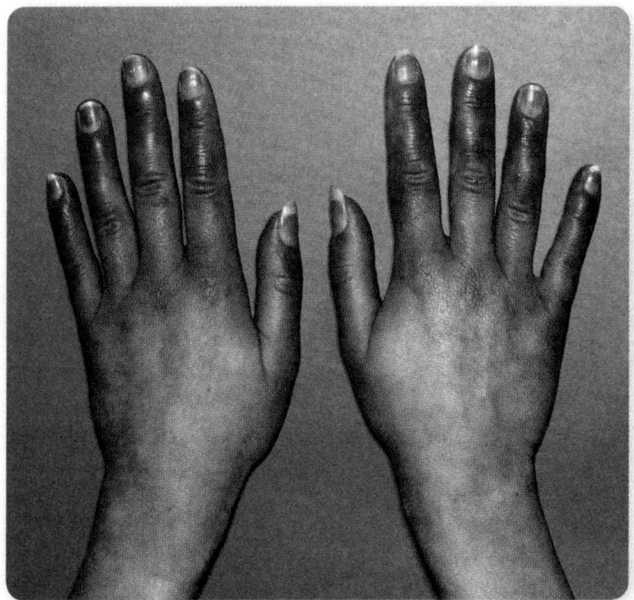

Figure 16-1 Skin color can provide an early and fast indication of several disease processes. Cyanosis presents as blue skin.

Also quickly glance around the patient to identify any life threats such as severe bleeding or injury to the chest that affects the breathing. If any life threats are found, address them immediately.

Once you have completed the primary survey, you should have enough information to make a preliminary transport decision. The following patients should be considered in serious condition and in need of rapid transport: patients who are unresponsive or who have an altered mental status, patients with airway or breathing problems, and patients with obvious circulation problems such as severe bleeding or signs of shock.

Words of Wisdom

A **sign** is something you can see or measure (a laceration or the patient's blood pressure). A **symptom** is what the patient tells you ("My head hurts").

History Taking

With a medical patient, history taking may be the only way to determine what the problem is or what may be causing the problem **Figure 16-2**. This information may include both a history of present illness (why the patient called EMS today) and a medical history (previously experienced conditions that may or may not be influencing the present illness). Investigate the NOI by asking questions about the chief complaint—for example, about signs and symptoms associated with the chief complaint and the history of the present illness. Obtain a SAMPLE (Signs and symptoms, Allergies, Medications, Pertinent past medical history, Last oral intake, Events leading up to the illness or injury) history and ask questions about the history of the present illness using the OPQRST (Onset, Provocation/palliation, Quality, Region/radiation, Severity, and Timing) mnemonic and ask follow-up questions such as, "Has

YOU are the Provider — PART 2

The patient says that her symptoms began spontaneously 3 days ago. Urination is painful, but even when she is not urinating she is still in pain. The pain is described as stabbing in the right flank area that seems to radiate to her groin. In tears, the patient says this is the worst pain she has ever felt in her life. She rates the severity a 10 out of 10. She tells you that she has no known allergies and takes no medications. Her medical history includes kidney stones approximately 13 years ago, but she does not remember them hurting this much.

Recording Time: 1 Minute	
Appearance	Anxious
Level of consciousness	Alert and oriented to person, place, time, and event
Airway	Patent
Breathing	Nonlabored
Circulation	Strong, rapid radial pulses; skin warm, dry, and pink

3. What are some other pertinent questions that you may want to ask the patient?
4. On the basis of the patient's presentation, what do you suspect is the most likely cause of her discomfort?

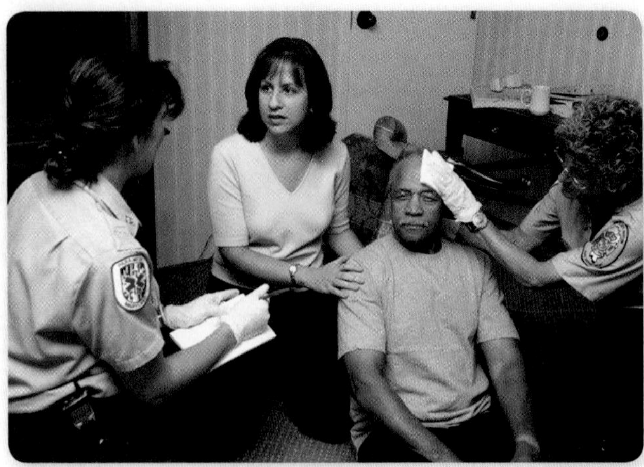

Figure 16-2 History taking is an important part of the assessment process.

anything like this ever happened before?" and if the patient answers yes, then ask, "What was done at that time?" and "How does this episode compare with previous episodes?"

Record any allergies, medical conditions, and any medications that the patient takes. If the patient has a current list of medications, bring that along; if not, it may be necessary to collect the medications and take them to the hospital with the patient. Inquire about any over-the-counter medications and any herbal remedies the patient may have taken. Ask patients who are taking medications whether they are compliant with their drug regimen—that is, whether they are taking their medications in the dosages and at the times prescribed.

While you are obtaining the history from the patient, look around the scene for evidence that may also help you determine the history of the patient—for example, evidence of medication containers or medical devices that the patient may have been using. Look for medic alert tags, which can offer a wealth of information.

If the patient is unresponsive, try to obtain as much of the patient's medical history as possible from family members, friends, or bystanders, or from the scene itself. (If the advanced emergency medical technician [AEMT] does not obtain and document this information, it may be lost forever.) Family members or friends may know the patient's allergies, medications, or medical conditions. Ask whether the patient was complaining of any symptoms before he or she became unresponsive.

Secondary Assessment

The secondary assessment is designed to identify any signs or symptoms of illness or injury that were not found during the primary survey. If the patient is critically ill or injured or the transport time is short, you may not have time to conduct a secondary assessment. In other cases, the secondary assessment may occur on scene or en route to the emergency department (ED).

Unresponsive patients are unable to tell you what is wrong, so you should always perform a full-body exam of these individuals. In contrast, responsive medical patients may not need a full-body exam, but you should perform a limited or focused assessment based on their chief complaint. For example, if you suspect a neurologic problem, you should check for a pulse and motion and sensation in all of the patient's extremities and check the patient's pupillary reactions.

Obtain a baseline set of vital signs. Often your partner can begin this process while you are asking about the medical history. Consider using the automatic blood pressure cuff for future assessments at regular intervals after first obtaining a manual reading. Depending on your local protocol, other important information to consider obtaining includes a blood glucose level and a pulse oximetry reading. End-tidal carbon dioxide monitoring should be considered if the patient complains of respiratory problems or if you suspect a stroke. Additionally, any patient who has a cardiac-related symptom should be placed on a cardiac monitor. Consider calling for paramedic backup if this is the case. The cardiac monitor enables the AEMT or the paramedic to monitor and record 3-lead electrocardiogram (ECG) tracings, and record 12-lead ECGs in the field. It also enables him or her to quickly identify a suspected acute myocardial infarction, transmit the findings electronically to the receiving facility, and make sound transport decisions regarding patient destination based on the ECG findings.

Reassessment

Once the assessment and treatment have been completed, reassessment should begin and continue throughout transport. During the reassessment, you should repeat the primary survey and reassess the chief complaint. Look for any changes in the level of consciousness; reassess the patient's vital signs; and reexamine the transport decision. Reconsider the need for paramedic backup. The reassessment also includes reviewing all treatments that have been performed and ensuring they are still effective. Document any changes that have developed as a result of the treatments and, if needed, adjust any of the treatments accordingly. Alert the ED before the arrival of potentially critical patients.

Management: Transport and Destination

Most medical emergencies require a level of treatment beyond that available in the prehospital setting. Also, the treatments depend on an accurate diagnosis of the exact medical condition, which may require advanced testing in a hospital. The primary prehospital treatments for medical emergencies address the symptoms more than the actual disease process.

The ability to administer medications that are stored in the ambulance is limited for AEMTs and depends on the scope of practice, along with state and local protocols. A few of these protocols include administering oral glucose or glucagon to a patient with diabetes and a low blood glucose level, administering naloxone to a patient with a narcotic overdose, and administering albuterol to a patient with respiratory difficulty. The administration of activated charcoal to a patient who has ingested a poison is also allowed when it may be beneficial.

Each of these situations and any other administration of medications by an AEMT require that direct permission be obtained from medical control. Written protocols may allow the administration of certain medications without calling for online medical control, so it is important to be familiar with the guidelines for your EMS agency. The process of obtaining permission includes completing a thorough assessment of the patient before calling medical control. After you give a report to the physician and obtain permission, the medication may be administered. Never administer any medication without first obtaining permission from medical control (either online or off-line), and always follow your state and local protocols.

You may also use an automated external defibrillator (AED) on a patient who is pulseless and apneic. In some cases of cardiac arrest, immediate treatment with an AED may provide the best option to resuscitate the patient. The AED is discussed in more detail in Chapter 18, *Cardiovascular Emergencies*. Familiarize yourself with the equipment and medications carried on your ambulance and use them appropriately under a medical director's instruction.

▶ Scene Time

In many cases, the time on scene may be longer for medical patients than for trauma patients. If the patient is not in critical condition, gather as much information as possible from the scene so that you can transmit that information to the physician at the ED. Critical patients include those with altered mental status, airway or breathing difficulties, or any sign of circulatory compromise. In addition, a patient who is very old or very young may be considered critical even if they appear to be relatively stable. Critical patients always need rapid transport. The time on scene should be limited to 10 minutes or less for these patients.

▶ Type of Transport

Serious consideration should be given to how to best transport a medical patient. If a life-threatening condition exists, the transportation should include lights and sirens, but if the patient is not critical, consider nonemergency transport. Many patients experiencing a medical emergency do not have immediate life-threatening conditions; therefore, they can be transported without the use of lights and sirens. This is a much safer method of transport and will often result in arrival only a few minutes later than an emergency transport using lights and sirens.

Differentiating a high-priority transport from a low-priority transport is a skill developed with experience, but it is a skill that can be learned. A good rule of thumb for determining the priority of transport is to consider the results of the patient's primary survey. Patients with an altered mental status, especially if it is still present at the completion of your assessment and treatment, should be considered a high-priority transport. Patients with circulatory compromise, including signs and symptoms of shock, should also be considered a high-priority transport. Most patients with circulatory conditions cannot be stabilized in the prehospital setting and need to receive treatment at a hospital quickly but safely. Patients with difficulty breathing generally require high-priority transport. However, if the patient has responded well to your initial treatment, such as oxygen and albuterol administration, lights and sirens may not be necessary.

Words of Wisdom

When transporting a patient who has had a seizure, do not use lights and sirens unless the patient is in status epilepticus and actively seizing. The additional stimulus may precipitate a new onset of seizures.

Modes of transport ultimately come in one of two categories: ground **Figure 16-3** or air **Figure 16-4**. Ground transportation EMS units are generally staffed by emergency medical technicians (EMTs) and advanced life support providers (AEMTs or paramedics). Air transportation EMS units or critical care transport units are generally staffed by critical care transport professionals such as critical care nurses and paramedics. While it is not as common to summon an air ambulance for a medical patient, there are instances where it is advisable. In rural areas with long ground transport times, patients who have possibly experienced a heart attack, a stroke, or a complication of pregnancy could benefit from air

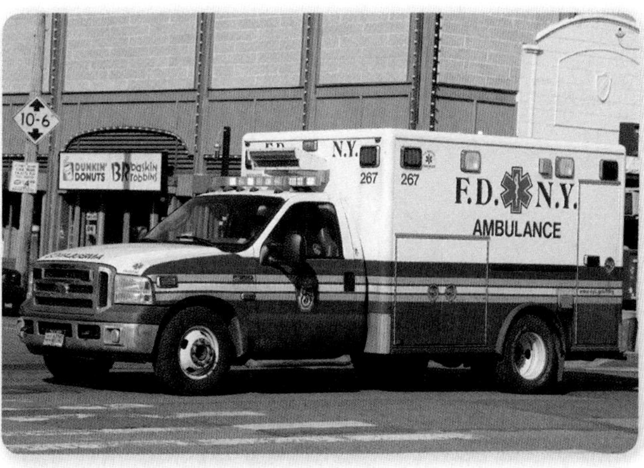

Figure 16-3 Ground transport.

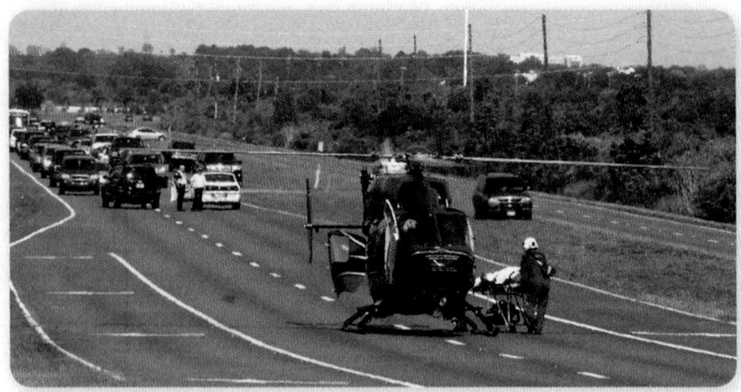

Figure 16-4 Air transport.

transport to the most appropriate facility. Children with serious medical conditions can also benefit from air transport. When you are considering additional paramedic support for a patient, compare the total time for a ground unit to respond and transport to the time required for a helicopter to respond and transport as well as the urgent resources needed by the patient. Follow local protocols and medical direction.

For more information on air ambulances, see Chapter 39, *Transport Operations*.

▶ Destination Selection

It is generally appropriate to select the closest ED as your destination. However, there are times when the closest hospital is not necessarily the most appropriate choice. Patients with chest pain as the result of a myocardial infarction may need a facility that is capable of performing heart catheterization, which may not necessarily be available at the closest hospital. If the patient is in cardiac arrest or experiences cardiac arrest during transport, immediately reroute to the closest hospital with emergency facilities. Patients with stroke can also benefit from specialized hospital selection. Although most hospitals now have designated stroke teams, taking a patient with a possible stroke to a hospital without a stroke team may result in a delay in definitive treatment and may lead to a worse outcome for the patient. Your local protocols should provide guidance on the appropriate facility, but contact medical control when unsure.

Some medical patients may benefit from on-scene treatment provided by paramedics. It is important to recognize early when paramedics can provide added value on a scene so that, if they are readily available, they can be called to respond in a timely manner or intercept the transport en route to the hospital.

Words of Wisdom

An *infectious* disease is a medical condition caused by the growth and spread of harmful organisms within the body. A *communicable* disease is a disease that can be spread from one person or species to another. Most of these diseases are much harder to transmit than is commonly believed. In addition, there are many immunizations, protective techniques, and devices that can be used to minimize your risk of infection. When these protective measures are used, the risk of your contracting a serious infectious disease is reduced.

YOU are the Provider — PART 3

After explaining to the patient that you believe she is experiencing her pain as the result of a new kidney stone, you obtain consent for treatment and transport and assist her to the stretcher. As you are securing her, she requests to be placed on her left side because it helps to slightly reduce the pain.

Recording Time: 6 Minutes	
Respirations	22 breaths/min, normal
Pulse	Strong and rapid, 114 beats/min
Skin	Warm, dry, and pink
Blood pressure	164/92 mm Hg
Oxygen saturation (Spo_2)	100% on room air
Pupils	Pupils Equal, Round, and Reactive to Light and Accommodation (PERRLA)

5. Does this patient require an intravenous (IV) line?
6. Does this patient require treatment at a specific hospital, or should you transport her to the closest community hospital?

Infectious Diseases

As discussed in Chapter 2, *Workforce Safety and Wellness,* you will be called on to treat and transport patients with a variety of infectious or communicable diseases. Chapter 2 discussed the routes of transmission and standard precautions that responders need to take to reduce risk and increase prevention. This chapter discusses the management, awareness, and assessment of a patient who may have a communicable or infectious disease. Chapter 39, *Transport Operations,* discusses decontamination techniques for transport.

▶ General Assessment Principles

The assessment of a patient suspected to have an infectious disease should be approached much like any other medical patient. First, the scene must be sized up and standard precautions taken with consideration for the potential infectious agent. Once you can be assured that the scene is safe, proceed with the primary survey by assessing the patient's ABCDEs. Prioritize the treatment of the patient. With most patients who have a potentially infectious disease in the prehospital setting, the next step is to gather patient history, using OPQRST to elaborate on the patient's chief complaint. Typical chief complaints include fever, nausea, rash, pleuritic chest pain, and difficulty breathing. Obtain a SAMPLE history and a set of baseline vital signs, paying particular attention to medications the patient is currently taking and the events leading up to today's problem. Also ask whether the patient has recently traveled. Always show respect for the feelings of the patient, family members, and others at the scene.

▶ General Management Principles

The general management of the patient with a suspected infectious disease first focuses on any life-threatening conditions that were identified in the primary survey (airway maintenance, oxygen and ventilatory assistance, bleeding control, and circulatory support). Remember to be empathetic. Because most of these patients will have a fever of unexplained origin or mild breathing problems, place the patient in the position of comfort on the stretcher to keep warm. Remember to use standard precautions for your own safety. Always follow your agency's exposure control plan in cleaning equipment and properly discard any disposable supplies as well as linens.

Words of Wisdom

The ability of your EMS service to support you in the event of exposure to a communicable disease depends on your understanding of how an exposure can occur and your immediate reporting of exposure to potentially infectious materials. Make notes right away to ensure that you remember all pertinent information, and report the possible exposure immediately after the response, following your local protocol.

▶ Epidemic and Pandemic Considerations

An **epidemic** occurs when new cases of a disease in a human population substantially exceed the number

Words of Wisdom

Causes of Infectious Disease

Type of Organism	Description	Example
Bacteria	Grow and reproduce outside the human cell in the appropriate temperature and with the appropriate nutrients	*Salmonella*
Viruses	Smaller than bacteria; multiply only inside a host and die when exposed to the environment	Human immunodeficiency virus
Fungi	Similar to bacteria in that they require the appropriate nutrients and organic material to grow	Mold
Protozoa (parasites)	Single-celled microscopic organisms, some of which cause disease	Amoebas
Helminths (parasites)	Invertebrates with long, flexible, rounded, or flattened bodies	Worms

expected based on recent experience. A **pandemic** is an outbreak that occurs on a global scale. For example, a flu pandemic occurs when a new influenza virus for which people have little or no immunity emerges. The disease can then spread easily from person to person, cause serious illness, and be found in multiple countries in a short time. Obviously, there would be no specific vaccine immediately available.

Common or Serious Communicable Diseases

Human Immunodeficiency Virus Infection

Human immunodeficiency virus (HIV) type 1 was first identified in the late 1970s. According to the US Centers for Disease Control and Prevention (CDC), more than 1.2 million people in the United States are infected with this virus and 1 in 8 do not know they are infected.[1] Nevertheless, a 19% decline in the annual number of new HIV diagnoses occurred from 2005 to 2014 that may be attributed to targeted prevention efforts.[1] Gay and bisexual men—and particularly young African American gay and bisexual men—account for the majority of new diagnoses.[1]

HIV infection is a potential hazard only when deposited on a mucous membrane or directly into the bloodstream. It is primarily a sexually transmitted disease, but it is also a bloodborne disease. It can also be transmitted from a pregnant woman to her infant in the birthing process. HIV is also transmitted through blood transfusions, although such transmission is not common because donated blood is now tested for a protein indicating the presence of HIV.

In a person with HIV infection, the entire immune system begins to fail, allowing life-threatening opportunistic infections to flourish. The HIV pathogen envelops infected cells and attacks the immune system and other body organs. The immune system is then unable to assist in protecting the infected person from other diseases. It takes approximately 7 days for the virus to envelop a cell, and this process may occur 4 to 6 weeks after the exposure event. The communicable period is unknown, but is believed to span from the onset of infection possibly throughout life.

Many patients who are infected with HIV do not show any symptoms. For those who are symptomatic, signs and symptoms may include acute febrile illness, malaise, fatigue, sore throat, swollen spleen and lymph glands, headache, weight loss, and possibly rash. Following initial infection, most patients present with enlargement of the lymph nodes and appear healthy. However, the immune system ultimately becomes weakened.

Acquired immunodeficiency syndrome (AIDS) is the end-stage disease process caused by HIV infection. A patient with AIDS is extremely vulnerable to numerous bacterial, viral, and fungal infections that would be easily brushed aside in a person with an intact immune system. These opportunistic infections include pneumonia in infants or people with compromised immune systems, loss of vision due to cytomegalovirus, reddish/purple skin lesions, atypical tuberculosis, and cryptococcal meningitis.

The incubation period of AIDS spans the time between documented infection (ie, becoming HIV positive) and development of the end-stage disease. The communicable period for HIV infection begins before clinically apparent AIDS develops.

Prehospital management of HIV/AIDS is supportive. Support the airway and respiratory status, assisting ventilations as needed. Establish IV access and give a fluid bolus of an isotonic crystalloid solution if the patient is hypovolemic. Use a nonrebreathing mask or other mask for respiratory isolation if the patient is coughing.

Exposure to HIV is a risk that AEMTs face on a regular basis. It is this prospect that led to the development of standard precautions. There is no vaccine to protect against HIV infection, and despite great progress in drug treatments, AIDS can still be fatal. Fortunately, HIV is not easily transmitted in your work setting. For example, it is far less contagious than hepatitis B. Because HIV infection can only occur via sexual contact or exposure to blood or body fluids, your risk of infection is limited to exposure to an infected patient's blood and body fluids. Exposure can take place in the following ways:

- The patient's blood is splashed or sprayed into your eyes, nose, or mouth or into an open sore or cut, however tiny; even a microscopic opening in the skin is an invitation for infection with a virus. The risk of HIV transmission after exposure of the eye, nose, or mouth to HIV-infected blood is estimated at only 1 in 1,000; the risk after cut exposure is approximately 1 in 300.[2]
- You have blood from the infected patient on your hands and then touch your own eyes, nose, mouth, or an open sore or cut.
- A needle used to inject the patient breaks your skin. The risk to you from a single injection, even with a hollow-bore needle, is small, probably less than 1 in 300.[2] However, this is by far the most dangerous form of exposure.
- Broken glass at a motor vehicle crash or other incident penetrates your glove (and skin), which may have already been covered with blood from an infected patient.

Because many patients who are infected with HIV do not show any symptoms, health care workers should wear gloves any time they are likely to come into contact with secretions or blood from any patient. Always put on gloves before leaving the ambulance to care for a patient. Also, take great care in handling and properly disposing of needles and other sharp objects in a sharps container so that you and others are not inadvertently exposed to them. Finally, cover any open wounds that you have whenever you are on the job.

If you have any reason to think that a patient's blood or secretions may have entered your system, especially through contact with a patient's blood, seek medical advice as soon as possible and notify your infectious disease officer. If you know that the patient is infected with HIV, current recommendations from the CDC include immediate prophylactic treatment as soon as possible after exposure to prevent you from becoming infected. Treatment should continue for a 4-week duration and expert consultation should be sought. If testing proves negative, treatment may be discontinued.[3]

As scientists learn more about HIV infection, testing and treatment recommendations change. It is important that you immediately see your physician (or your program's designated physician) anytime you have a significant exposure to a communicable or infectious disease. Know the policy for your system, and take time now to consider what you would do in the event of exposure.

Words of Wisdom

An AEMT with a cold or the flu can be extremely hazardous to a patient who is immunocompromised.

▶ Influenza

Influenza, commonly known as flu, is primarily an animal respiratory disease that has mutated to infect humans. It can affect all people, but those with chronic medical conditions, compromised immune systems, the very young, and the very old are particularly susceptible to complications of the disease. All strains of influenza are transmitted by direct contact with nasal secretions and aerosolized droplets from coughing and sneezing by infected people.

The H1N1 virus, which was initially identified as the swine flu in 2009, is a specific form of influenza.[4] This virus has been present for years in animals. Many deaths have been caused by the H1N1 virus, although deaths caused by other influenza viruses have also occurred. The most positive effect of the outbreak of the H1N1 virus has been the general public's greater awareness of the routes of transmission of contagious diseases. This increased awareness could result in a reduction of all communicable diseases, not only H1N1.

General treatment for a patient with influenza includes supportive treatment. Place the patient in a position of comfort and be alert for potential vomiting. Oxygen is generally not needed for patients with influenza, but potential comorbid conditions may warrant the application. Gain IV access and consider the administration of a 20-mL/kg bolus of an isotonic crystalloid solution. Patients with influenza may quickly dehydrate from vomiting or lack of fluid intake. Keep the patient warm during transport.

In addition to influenza, many potentially serious diseases can be passed by the respiratory route; therefore, you need to wear personal protective equipment (PPE), such as gloves, eye protection, and a high-efficiency particulate air (HEPA) respirator, at a minimum. Viruses can live for several days on surfaces, so frequent handwashing is also important. Maintain your vaccinations and stay up-to-date on the latest CDC recommendations. Place a surgical mask on patients with suspected or confirmed respiratory disease. Wear a HEPA respirator during any aerosol-generating procedures such as suctioning of airway secretions, performing cardiopulmonary resuscitation, or assisting with endotracheal intubation.

An annual influenza immunization is important, especially for EMS personnel, to protect both providers and patients. The influenza virus is constantly changing. Experts adjust vaccines from year to year to provide protection against the strains most likely to affect the population. Vaccination effectively decreases transmission rates and limits (though does not eliminate) the disease incidence. Complications of the vaccine are far less common and severe than complications of the flu, which causes approximately 36,000 deaths each year in the United States.[5] The theory that immunizations cause autism has been proven through research to be untrue. Remember, people die each year from influenza virus, which is often transmitted by people who have failed to be immunized. Health care workers should not become the source of such transmission. Make sure you are immunized annually, and if you are sick, do not come to work and expose your patients to a disease that could prove fatal to them.

▶ Hepatitis

The term **hepatitis** refers to an inflammation (and often infection) of the liver. Hepatitis can be caused by a number of different viruses and toxins. Complications of hepatitis include scarring of the liver, liver cancer, and liver failure. According to the CDC, of the three types of viral hepatitis (designated as A, B, and C), hepatitis C accounted for the greatest number of deaths and the highest mortality rate in the United States, estimated at 5.0 deaths per 100,000 population in 2014.[6]

Depending on the severity of the infection, patients with hepatitis may be asymptomatic or may have a variety of signs and symptoms. Early signs of viral hepatitis include loss of appetite, vomiting, fever, fatigue, sore throat, cough, and muscle and joint pain. Several weeks later, jaundice (yellow eyes and skin) and right upper quadrant abdominal pain develop Figure 16-5. Acute liver failure, also known as fulminant hepatitis, is a rare but potentially fatal disease that may occur after infection with viral hepatitis. The severity of toxin-induced hepatitis depends on the amount of agent absorbed and the duration of exposure. Toxin-induced hepatitis is not contagious.

Management of patients with any type of hepatitis is strictly supportive. Maintain a patent airway, give 100%

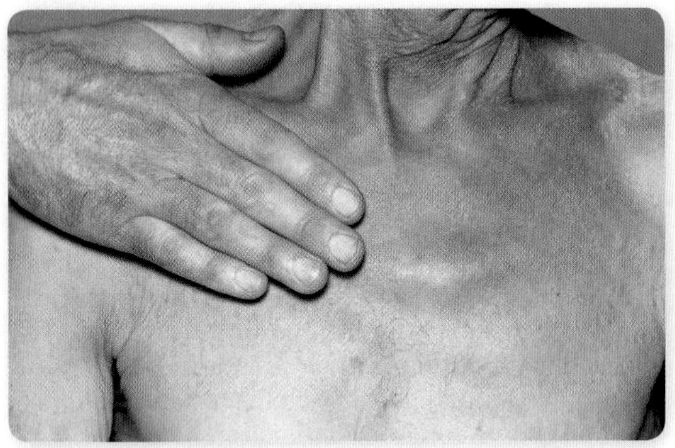

Figure 16-5 Jaundice is a sign of a hepatitis infection.

oxygen, and assist ventilations as needed. Establish IV access, and if fluid resuscitation is needed, give a 20-mL/kg bolus of an isotonic crystalloid solution. If no trauma is suspected, transport in a position of comfort to the closest, most appropriate facility.

There is no sure way to tell which patients with hepatitis have a contagious form of the disease and which do not. Table 16-2 lists the characteristics of different types of hepatitis, from which you can assess your risk of exposure. Hepatitis A can be transmitted only from a patient who has an acute infection, whereas hepatitis B and hepatitis C can be transmitted from long-term carriers who have no signs of illness. A carrier is a person (or animal) in whom an infectious organism has taken up permanent residence and may or may not cause any active disease. Carriers may never know that they harbor the organism; however, they can infect other people.

Hepatitis A is transmitted orally through oral or fecal contamination. This means that, generally, you must eat or drink something that is contaminated with the virus. The organisms that cause hepatitis B, C, and G are transmitted through vehicles other than food or water. For example, these organisms may enter the body through a transfusion or needlestick with infected blood, which puts health care workers at high risk for contracting hepatitis B, the more contagious and virulent form. **Virulence** is the strength or ability of a pathogen to produce disease. Hepatitis B is far

Table 16-2 Characteristics of Hepatitis

Type	Route of Infection	Incubation Period	Chronic Infection	Vaccine and Treatment	Comments
Viral Hepatitis					
Hepatitis A (infectious)	Fecal–oral, infected food or drink	2–6 weeks	Chronic condition does not exist	Vaccine is available; no specific treatment is available; body will clear the infection on its own	Mild illness; mortality is approximately 0.02 patients per 100,000 population; after acute infection, the patient has lifelong immunity
Hepatitis B	Blood, sexual contact, saliva, urine, breast milk	4–12 weeks	Chronic infection affects 2% to 6% of adult patients and up to 90% of newborns who have the disease	Vaccine is available; treatment is minimally effective	Chronic carriers are asymptomatic and without signs of liver disease, but they may infect others; mortality is approximately 0.5 deaths per 100,000 population
Hepatitis C	Blood, sexual contact	2–10 weeks	Chronic infection affects 75% to 85% of patients	No vaccine is available; treatment is costly but effective for many strains of hepatitis C	Cirrhosis of the liver develops in 5% to 20% of patients with hepatitis C; chronic infection increases the risk of cancer of the liver; mortality is approximately 5.0 deaths per 100,000 population

Type	Route of Infection	Incubation Period	Chronic Infection	Vaccine and Treatment	Comments
Viral Hepatitis					
Hepatitis D	Blood, sexual contact	4–12 weeks	Chronic infection develops in only 5% of patients with acute infection	No vaccine is available; no treatment is available	Occurs only in patients with active hepatitis B infection; superinfection of hepatitis D in the presence of chronic hepatitis B leads to more severe disease in 70% to 90% of cases
Hepatitis E (epidemic non-A, non-B hepatitis)	Fecal–oral, contaminated water or food	15–60 days	Usually resolves on its own over several weeks to months	No vaccine is available; no treatment is available	Mild illness; fatal in approximately 1% of all cases; fulminant disease may develop, especially in pregnant patients; mortality is as high as 20% to 25% in pregnant women in the third trimester who develop fulminant hepatitis E
Hepatitis G (hepatitis GB)	Blood, sexual contact, breast milk	Possibly 15–50 days	Mild and usually short-lived	No vaccine is available; no treatment is available	Can cause severe liver damage resulting in liver failure; often seen in conjunction with hepatitis B, hepatitis C, or both
Toxin-Induced Hepatitis					
Medications, drugs, and alcohol	Inhalation, skin or mucous membrane exposure, oral ingestion, or intravenous administration	Within hours to days following exposure	Some chemicals may initiate an inflammatory response that continues to cause liver damage long after the chemical is out of the body	No vaccine is available; treatment is to stop exposure; in patients with an overdose of acetaminophen, certain drugs may minimize liver injury if given early enough	Not contagious; patients with toxin-induced hepatitis may have liver damage and jaundice; not every exposure to a toxin will cause liver damage

Data from: Surveillance for viral hepatitis—United States, 2014. Centers for Disease Control and Prevention website. June 22, 2016. https://www.cdc.gov/hepatitis/statistics/2014surveillance/commentary.htm#summary. Accessed January 20, 2017; Viral hepatitis: hepatitis B information. Centers for Disease Control and Prevention website. May 31, 2015. https://www.cdc.gov/hepatitis/hbv/index.htm. Accessed January 20, 2017; Hepatitis C FAQs for health professionals. Centers for Disease Control and Prevention website. July 21, 2016. https://www.cdc.gov/hepatitis/hcv/hcvfaq.htm. Accessed January 20, 2017; World Health Organization. Hepatitis D. July 2016. http://www.who.int/mediacentre/factsheets/hepatitis-d/en/. Accessed January 20, 2017; Hepatitis E FAQs for health professionals. Centers for Disease Control and Prevention website. December 18, 2015. https://www.cdc.gov/hepatitis/hev/hevfaq.htm. Accessed January 20, 2017; and World Health Organization. Hepatitis E. July 2016. http://www.who.int/mediacentre/factsheets/fs280/en/. Accessed January 20, 2017.

more contagious than HIV. For this reason, vaccination with hepatitis B vaccine is highly recommended for AEMTs. Unfortunately, immediate immunity to the virus does not develop in everyone who is vaccinated. Sometimes, but not always, an additional dose will provide immunity. You should be tested after vaccination to determine your immune status.

If you are stuck with a needle or injured in some other way while caring for a patient who might have hepatitis, see your physician immediately.

Herpes Simplex

Herpes simplex is a common virus strain carried by humans. More than 85% of people carrying the virus are asymptomatic,[7] but symptomatic infections cause eruptions of tiny fluid-filled blisters called vesicles that often appear on the lips or genitals. Herpes simplex can also cause more serious illnesses like pneumonia and meningitis in the very young, very old, and immunocompromised patients. The primary mode of infection is through close personal contact, so standard precautions are generally sufficient to prevent spread to or from health care workers.

Syphilis

Although syphilis is commonly thought of as a sexually transmitted disease, it is also a bloodborne disease. There is a small risk for transmission through a contaminated needlestick injury or direct blood-to-blood contact.

The initial infection with syphilis produces a lesion called a chancre. Chancres are most commonly located in the genital region. For more information on syphilis, see Chapter 25, *Gynecologic Emergencies*.

Meningitis

Meningitis is an inflammation of the meningeal coverings of the brain and spinal cord. Patients with meningitis develop signs and symptoms such as fever, headache, stiff neck, and altered mental status. This uncommon but very frightening infectious disease can be caused by viruses or bacteria, most of which are not contagious. However, one form, **meningococcal meningitis**, is highly contagious. The meningococcal bacterium colonizes the human nose and throat and only rarely causes an acute infection. When it does, it can be lethal. Patients with this kind of infection often have red blotches on their skin, fever, and nuchal rigidity; however, many patients with forms of meningitis that are not contagious also have red blotches.

Only laboratory tests can sort out the different forms of meningitis; therefore, you should take standard precautions with any patient who is suspected of having meningitis. Wearing gloves and a mask will go a long way toward preventing the patient's secretions from getting into your nose and mouth. Be aware that the risk of infection is low, even if the organism is transmitted. For this reason, vaccines, which are available for most types of meningococcus, are rarely used. Meningitis can be treated at the ED with antibiotics.

After treating a patient with meningitis, contact your employer health representative. Many states consider meningitis "reportable" and will notify you that one of your patients was diagnosed with meningitis. Prophylactic treatment may be recommended for you.

Safety

Place a surgical mask on any patient suspected of having tuberculosis and a HEPA mask on yourself.

Tuberculosis

Most patients who are infected with *Mycobacterium tuberculosis* (the tubercle bacillus) are well most of the time. If the disease involves the brain or kidneys, the patient is only slightly contagious. In the United States, however, **tuberculosis** is a chronic mycobacterial disease that usually strikes the lungs. Disease that occurs shortly after infection is called primary tuberculosis. Except in infants, this infection is not usually serious. After the primary infection, the tubercle bacillus is rendered dormant by the patient's immune system. However, even after decades of lying dormant, this germ can reactivate. Reactive tuberculosis is common and can be much more difficult to treat, especially because an increasing number of tuberculosis strains have grown resistant to most antibiotics.

Although tuberculosis is often difficult to distinguish from other diseases, patients who pose the highest risk almost invariably have a cough. Therefore, for your own safety, you should consider respiratory tuberculosis to be the only contagious form because it is the only one that is spread by airborne transmission. The droplets produced by coughing are not the real problem, but rather the droplet nuclei—that is, the remnants of the droplets after the excess water has evaporated. These particles are tiny enough to be invisible and can remain suspended in the air for a long time. In fact, as long as these particles are shielded from ultraviolet light, they can remain alive for decades. Particles that are the size of droplet nuclei are not stopped by routine surgical masks. When inhaled, they are carried directly to the alveoli of the lungs, where the bacteria may begin to grow. N95 or HEPA masks are required to prevent the inhalation of droplet nuclei. For a patient with dyspnea, wearing a nonrebreathing mask has two benefits: it oxygenates the patient while providing a barrier to prevent the droplets from spreading to the AEMT. If the patient is not having difficulty breathing, place a surgical mask on the patient and a HEPA mask on yourself.

Why is tuberculosis not more common than it is? After all, absolute protection from infection with the tubercle bacillus does not exist: everyone who breathes is at risk. According to the CDC, one-third of the world's population is infected with tuberculosis.[8] The vaccine for tuberculosis, called bacillus Calmette-Guérin, is only rarely used in the United States because of the low risk of infection.[9] It is only recommended in specific situations. Under normal circumstances, however, the mechanism of transmission used by *M tuberculosis* is not very efficient. Infected air is easily diluted with uninfected air. *M tuberculosis* is one of those germs that typically cause no illness in a new host. In fact, many patients with tuberculosis do not even transmit the infection to family members. However, in crowded environments with poor ventilation, the disease spreads more easily.

If you are exposed to a patient who is found to have pulmonary tuberculosis, you will be given a tuberculin skin test. This simple skin test determines whether a person has been infected with *M tuberculosis*. A positive result means that exposure has occurred; it does not mean that the person has active tuberculosis. It takes at least 6 weeks for the bacteria to show up in the laboratory test. So if you are tested for the disease within a few weeks of the exposure and your results are positive, this outcome means that you were exposed to tuberculosis at an earlier time from somebody else. You will probably never identify the source. Most transmissions occur silently, so it is necessary that you have tuberculin skin tests regularly. If the infection is found before you become ill, preventive therapy is almost 100% effective. Usually, a daily dose of the medication isoniazid will prevent the development of active infection.

Special Populations

Everyone has body defenses that help protect against illness, but the aging process can pose a threat to the body's natural defense mechanisms against invading microorganisms. As a person ages, his or her physical defenses weaken or are eliminated. Thinning and loss of supportive collagen in the skin and a reduction in the number of blood vessels, for example, can allow bacteria or viruses to enter the body with less resistance. The respiratory system cannot trap and eliminate bacteria and viruses in the airways as efficiently as it once did. Moreover, the gastrointestinal system allows easier entry for bacteria or viruses through the intestines. As the body ages, physical barriers to entry weaken, the immune system deteriorates, and invading organisms are not as easily identified as abnormal. Infectious agents can take hold in elderly patients much more easily because of reduced defenses.

When transporting an elderly patient, protect the patient from the environment because extremes in heat or cold can further reduce the body's defenses. If the patient has a cold or the flu, protect yourself. However, remember that your defense system is probably much stronger than that of the patient.

▶ Pertussis

Pertussis, also called whooping cough, is an airborne disease caused by bacteria that previously affected primarily children younger than 6 years, but is becoming more common in adults whose vaccination was years prior and whose immunity has decreased. Signs and symptoms include fever and a "whoop" sound that occurs when the patient tries to inhale after a coughing attack.

The best way to prevent infection from pertussis is to be vaccinated with a diphtheria, tetanus, and acellular pertussis (DTaP) vaccine. Providers who have previously received this vaccine should make sure they are up-to-date with a booster. For added protection, place a mask on the patient and on yourself.

▶ Methicillin-Resistant *Staphylococcus aureus*

Methicillin-resistant *Staphylococcus aureus* (MRSA) is a bacterium that causes infections and is resistant to many antibiotics. **Nosocomial** infections with MRSA are believed to be transmitted from patient to patient via the unwashed hands of health care providers. Studies have shown that 1% to 5% of health care providers carry MRSA in their nares.[10] The pathogen can subsequently be transferred to skin and other areas of the body through a break in the skin. Surfaces contaminated with MRSA do not seem to be important in transmission. Factors that increase the risk for developing MRSA include antibiotic therapy, prolonged hospital stays, a stay in an intensive care or burn unit, and exposure to an infected patient.

The incubation period for MRSA appears to be between 5 and 45 days. The communicable period varies, as patients who have active infection may carry MRSA for months. MRSA results in soft-tissue infections. Its signs and symptoms may involve localized skin abscesses, and sepsis may be found in older patients with the infection.

To prevent MRSA transmission, use standard precautions (gloves and good handwashing technique) when in contact with patient wounds and nonintact skin. If you are in direct contact with wound drainage but your skin is intact, no exposure will occur. If you have a true exposure, no postexposure treatment is recommended. The incident must still be documented, however.

▶ New and Emerging Diseases

Newly recognized diseases, such as those caused by Hantavirus (a rare but deadly virus transmitted through rodent urine and droppings) and enteropathogenic *Escherichia coli* (a common cause of pediatric diarrhea in developing countries), are being reported. These diseases are not transmitted from person to person directly; rather, they are carried by a vehicle, such as food, or a vector, such as rodents.

West Nile Virus

Although not a newly discovered illness, West Nile virus has caused some concern in the past. The virus' vector, the mosquito, affects humans and birds. The virus is tracked by tests done on birds suspected of being killed by the virus. These diseases are not communicable and do not pose a risk to you during patient care.

Severe Acute Respiratory Syndrome

A virus that has caused significant concern in the recent past is **severe acute respiratory syndrome (SARS)**. SARS is a serious, potentially life-threatening viral infection caused by a recently discovered family of viruses. SARS usually starts with flulike symptoms, which may progress to pneumonia, respiratory failure, and, in some cases, death. The SARS virus strain probably spread from Guangdong province in southern China to Hong Kong, Singapore, and Taiwan.[11] Canada experienced a significant outbreak in the Toronto area in 2003.[11] SARS is thought to be primarily transmitted by close person-to-person contact. Most cases have involved people who lived with or cared for a person with SARS or who had exposure to contaminated secretions from a patient with SARS.

Avian Flu

Avian (bird) flu is caused by a virus (designated as H5N1) that occurs naturally in the bird population. This virus is carried in the intestinal tract of wild birds and does not usually cause illness. However, in domestic bird populations (eg, chickens, ducks, and turkeys), it is very contagious. Birds acquire the illness from contact with contaminated excretions or surfaces that are contaminated with excretions. If an infected bird is used for food and is cooked, it does not pose a risk to those who eat it.

The first case of this flu was reported in Hong Kong in 1997; 18 people became infected and 6 died in the outbreak. Since then, the incidence has been decreasing, but influenza can still be fatal.[12] No cases of rapid human-to-human transmission of this disease have been reported. Instead, the cases occurring in humans have involved close contact with infected birds. The transmission risk for humans is low.

Global Health Issues

▶ Middle East Respiratory Syndrome Coronavirus

Middle East respiratory syndrome coronavirus (MERS-CoV) is a virus most commonly found in bats and camels living in the Middle East. The first human case of MERS-CoV was discovered in 2012 in Saudi Arabia. While most clusters of human infections are found in the Middle East, cases of MERS-CoV have also been reported in Europe and the United States. Common patient symptoms include high fever, cough, muscle aches, vomiting, and diarrhea. In some cases, renal failure, respiratory failure, and death have been reported. There is presently no cure or vaccine for this virus. If you suspect your patient might have MERS-CoV, place a surgical mask on him or her and notify the receiving facility.

▶ Ebola

In 2014, an outbreak of the Ebola virus in West Africa caused international concern. Several infected people with the virus traveled to other countries, including the United States, motivating EMS and health care facilities to prepare for further outbreaks. The incubation period is approximately 6 to 12 days after exposure; however, symptoms may not begin to appear for as long as 21 days after infection. Symptoms include watery diarrhea, vomiting, fever, body aches, and bleeding. The fatality rate can be as high as 70% if effective supportive treatment in an intensive care unit is not initiated promptly.[13]

YOU are the Provider — PART 4

On the basis of the patient's vital signs and physical examination, you elect to establish an IV line and administer a 250-mL bolus of normal saline. After you administer the bolus, you note that the patient's skin turgor is poor and that her skin is tenting. Because of this finding, you elect to administer a second 250-mL bolus of normal saline. On arrival at the ED, you give a report to the receiving nurse and prepare your unit for another call.

Recording Time: 12 Minutes	
Respirations	20 breaths/min, normal
Pulse	Strong and regular, 100 beats/min
Skin	Warm, dry, and pink
Blood pressure	158/88 mm Hg
Oxygen saturation (Spo_2)	100% on room air
Pupils	PERRLA

7. What is the likely cause of the patient's hypertension?
8. With the administration of the second fluid bolus, which sounds should you listen for?

If you suspect the patient may have this condition, place a surgical mask on him or her and follow PPE precautions as outlined by local protocols and the CDC. Immediately notify the receiving facility that the patient may have or may have been exposed to the Ebola virus.

Words of Wisdom

Travel history should be a routine part of patient assessment.

Zika Virus

Zika virus is a vector-borne infection first noted in the United States in mid-2015. Cases are typically related to travel to areas where the Zika virus is prevalent. The virus is transmitted by the bite of the *Aedes aegypti* mosquito. There are multiple countries in the Caribbean and South America where the virus is prevalent, and certain areas in the continental United States and Puerto Rico. South Florida and Brownsville, Texas are two areas in the United States where travel precautions are advised.[14] There is no vaccine for the virus, and prevention is aimed at protecting against mosquito bites.[15]

According to the CDC, most people infected with Zika virus present with few or no symptoms.[16] The most common symptoms of Zika include fever, rash, joint pain, and conjunctivitis. Other symptoms may include muscle pain and/or headache. Symptoms are usually mild and last from several days to a week. Zika virus can be diagnosed with a urine or blood test.[17]

The most significant complication of Zika virus affects pregnant women.[18] The fetus is at risk for serious birth defects including microcephaly in which the baby's head is small because the brain has not properly developed or stops growing after birth.[19] Other than mother to fetus, the most common route of human-to-human transmission is through sexual contact.[15]

There have been no documented cases of blood transfusion transmission of Zika virus in the United States, but there have been cases of transmission through platelet transfusions in Brazil.[20] All blood donations in the United States are screened for Zika virus, and potential donors are questioned about travel to areas where the virus is prevalent.

Care is supportive. Place the patient in a position of comfort, and provide oxygen and IV fluids as needed. Question travel history for any patient suspected of Zika virus. Use routine standard precautions for patient care. There are currently no recommendations for special protective equipment for medical personnel, except to prevent person-to-person transmission through blood or body fluids.

Travel Medicine

Every day, thousands of people travel to various countries. While humans share many common germs, some are confined to certain areas of the world. As an EMS provider, you must be aware of this when assessing a patient who recently traveled outside the United States.

Patients who acquire an illness from another country can present with a variety of symptoms, depending on the illness. They may have a fever, cough, vomiting, bloody diarrhea, body aches, or rashes. In many cases, the patient experiences mild symptoms and does not require EMS care. However, some patients become extremely ill, requiring urgent evaluation and treatment. When you encounter an ill patient with a recent travel history, place a mask on the patient and gather as much information as possible. Important questions to ask the patient include the following:

- Where did you recently travel?
- Did you receive any vaccinations before your trip?
- Were you exposed to any infectious diseases?
- Is there anyone else in your travel party who is sick?
- Which types of food did you eat?
- What was your source of drinking water?

If you suspect the patient has a communicable illness, follow appropriate PPE precautions and notify the receiving facility. While treatment for many travel-related illnesses is primarily supportive in the prehospital environment, always be prepared to manage life-threatening conditions should the patient become unstable.

Conclusion

Although trauma patients often present with dramatic signs and symptoms, the assessment and treatment you provide for them are fairly straightforward. The assessment and treatment of medical patients, by comparison, can be very challenging, and the medical patient's condition may not be as readily apparent as in a trauma patient. Therefore, treatment may not be as straightforward. You must remember that delays of any kind in an attempt to diagnose a condition can be harmful to the patient and thus are not recommended. Your best approach is to keep calm, use your patient assessment skills, treat the patient's symptoms while maintaining a high index of suspicion for underlying problems, report to medical control, and transport the patient safely to the closest most appropriate facility. Finally, keep in mind that patients sometimes have more than one isolated problem, so you must be prepared to handle any combination of conditions, including conditions of medical patients who have been involved in traumatic situations.

YOU are the Provider SUMMARY

1. Which systems of the body may be causing the patient's signs and symptoms?

This patient's symptoms could be the result of a gastrointestinal problem such as appendicitis or diverticulitis. They could also be a result of reproductive problems such as pelvic inflammatory disease or another sexually transmitted disease. A urinary problem such as a kidney stone is another possibility. On the basis of the patient's history and physical examination, a kidney stone should be high on your list of probabilities.

2. Does this patient require immediate transport?

This patient does not require immediate transport. You do not note any immediate life threats, so you should spend time on scene continuing your assessment and performing any treatment you may elect to initiate.

3. What are some other pertinent questions that you may want to ask the patient?

You may want to ask questions about the patient's sexual history. Is she still sexually active? Is she in a monogamous relationship? If so, is her partner also monogamous? Does she still have her menstrual cycle? If so, when was her last cycle and was it normal for her? Does she have a medical history of sexually transmitted diseases? You may also want to further question the patient regarding her urinary output—specifically, the frequency, color, and any associated odors. All of these questions will assist you in narrowing down the specific medical cause(s).

4. On the basis of the patient's presentation, what do you suspect is the most likely cause of her discomfort?

This patient presents with typical signs and symptoms of a kidney stone. The flank pain is a result of the stone traveling in the kidney, and the pain on urination is from the stone attempting to pass through the ureter. Based on the length of transport, you may want to consider a paramedic intercept for the administration of pain medications.

5. Does this patient require an IV line?

On the basis of the patient's statement that she has not had adequate fluid intake for 3 days, the patient is most likely dehydrated and would benefit from IV fluid administration. Fluid may also help to flush out the stone. Because of the patient's age and lack of a cardiac history, you recognize that the risk of pulmonary edema with a 250-mL fluid bolus is very small. Nonetheless, it is prudent to listen to lung sounds to exclude fluid overload after administration of the second 250-mL bolus.

6. Does this patient require treatment at a specific hospital, or should you transport her to the closest community hospital?

This patient should be transported to the closest hospital. There is no increased benefit in transporting her to a specialty hospital. The local community hospital should have the appropriate resources to treat a common problem such as a kidney stone.

7. What is the likely cause of the patient's hypertension?

The cause of this patient's hypertension can likely be attributed to one of two causes. The first potential cause is the severe pain that the patient is experiencing; pain and anxiety are common causes of elevated blood pressure. The second cause might be chronic, undiagnosed hypertension. In other words, this may be the patient's normal blood pressure.

8. With the administration of the second fluid bolus, which sounds should you listen for?

With the administration of IV fluid, the AEMT would want to pay careful attention to the patient's lung sounds. In a patient with a history of pulmonary edema (either diagnosed or undiagnosed), the administration of two fluid boluses may exacerbate the condition, causing an increase in the work of breathing.

YOU are the Provider SUMMARY *(continued)*

EMS Patient Care Report (PCR)					
Date: 5-2-18	**Incident No.:** 20100086-M		**Nature of Call:** Urinary difficulty	**Location:** 474 Big Mountain Rd	
Dispatched: 1422	**En Route:** 1423	**At Scene:** 1428	**Transport:** 1442	**At Hospital:** 1510	**In Service:** 1524
Patient Information					
Age: 47 **Sex:** F **Weight (in kg [lb]):** 84 kg (186 lb)			**Allergies:** None **Medications:** None **Past Medical History:** Kidney stones **Chief Complaint:** Flank pain/urinary difficulty		
Vital Signs					
Time: 1434	**BP:** 164/92	**Pulse:** 114	**Respirations:** 22	$\mathbf{Spo_2}$**:** 100% R/A	
Time: 1440	**BP:** 158/88	**Pulse:** 100	**Respirations:** 20	$\mathbf{Spo_2}$**:** 100% R/A	
Time: 1455	**BP:** 152/84	**Pulse:** 96	**Respirations:** 18	$\mathbf{Spo_2}$**:** 100% R/A	
EMS Treatment (circle all that apply)					
Oxygen @ ______ L/min via (circle one): **NC NRM Bag-mask device**		**Assisted Ventilation**	**Airway Adjunct**	**CPR**	
Defibrillation	**Bleeding Control**	**Bandaging**	**Splinting**	**Other:**	
Narrative					
EMS dispatched to 474 Big Mountain Road for a 47-year-old woman with flank pain and difficulty with urination. On arrival, met by husband who directs us to the patient, who is found lying in bed in the fetal position. Patient is AO×4, ABCs intact, complains of sharp, stabbing pain in right-side flank area for 3 days. Further states pain on urination that radiates to her groin in "waves," which has decreased her fluid intake. Complains of 10/10 pain. No past medications or known allergies. Past medical history of kidney stones 13 years ago, but states this pain is worse. Remainder of physical exam is unremarkable, with the exception of poor skin turgor and tenting. Consent obtained for treatment and transport. Assisted patient to cot, secured on left side per patient request. Transported to Pembina County Memorial Hospital (PCMH), nonemergent. En route: Vitals as above. 18-ga IV established to right hand with 250-mL NS bolus. After bolus, patient still shows signs of dehydration. Additional 250-mL bolus administered. On arrival at PCMH, care and report given to ED staff without incident.**End of report**					

Prep Kit

▶ Ready for Review

- Trauma emergencies are injuries that are the result of physical forces applied to the body. Medical emergencies require emergency medical services (EMS) attention because of illnesses or conditions not caused by an outside force.
- The assessment of a medical patient is similar to the assessment of a trauma patient but with a different focus. Whereas a trauma assessment focuses on physical injuries, most of which are visible through a physical examination, medical patient assessment is usually more focused on symptoms and depends more on establishing an accurate medical history.
- Evaluation of the nature of illness (NOI) for a medical patient can provide an index of suspicion for different types of serious or life-threatening underlying illnesses.
- For responsive medical patients, obtaining a thorough patient history can be one of the most beneficial aspects of the patient assessment. Try to determine the NOI by asking questions about the patient's chief complaint.
- Responsive medical patients seldom need a full-body exam, but all should get a focused examination based on their chief complaint. On the other hand, you should always perform a full-body exam on unresponsive patients; this head-to-toe assessment may give you clues to help identify the problem. Your secondary assessment of an unresponsive or unstable patient should never delay transport.
- Most medical emergencies require a level of treatment beyond what is available in the prehospital setting. Also, the treatments depend on an accurate diagnosis of the exact medical condition; therefore, advanced testing in the hospital may be required.
- If the patient is not in critical condition, you should gather as much important information as possible from the scene so that you can transmit that information to the physician at the emergency department.
- Written protocols may allow the advanced emergency medical technician (AEMT) to administer certain medications without calling for online medical control, so it is important to be familiar with the guidelines for your EMS agency.
- Many medical patients will benefit from being transported to a specific hospital capable of handling their particular condition—for example, a patient with myocardial infarction may need a facility that is capable of performing heart catheterization, and a patient with stroke may need a facility with a designated stroke team.
- Because it is often impossible to tell which patients have infectious diseases, you should avoid direct contact with the blood and body fluids of all patients. Always wear gloves, cover any open wounds you may have, wash hands properly and frequently, routinely clean your vehicle after transport, and take great care in handling and disposing of needles. Be sure to follow the proper steps when dealing with potential exposure situations.
- If you think you may have been exposed to an infectious disease, or you are stuck with a needle or injured in some other way while caring for a patient who might have a disease of concern, see your physician (or your employer's designated physician) immediately.
- AEMTs are especially likely to encounter certain infectious diseases, including human immunodeficiency virus (HIV), influenza, hepatitis, herpes simplex, syphilis, meningitis, tuberculosis, pertussis, and methicillin-resistant *Staphylococcus aureus*.
- Patients with HIV infection or hepatitis may be asymptomatic or have a variety of signs and symptoms. Prehospital treatment is supportive.
- Acquired immunodeficiency syndrome (AIDS) is the end-stage disease process caused by HIV. A patient with AIDS is extremely vulnerable to infection, so it is important to protect him or her from contracting additional infections.
- There is no vaccine to protect against HIV infection, but it is only a potential hazard when deposited on a mucous membrane or directly into the bloodstream.
- There is no sure way to tell which patients have a contagious form of hepatitis. Vaccination with hepatitis B vaccine is highly recommended for AEMTs.
- Newly recognized or emerging diseases include Hantavirus, enteropathogenic *Escherichia coli*, West Nile virus, severe acute respiratory syndrome, and avian flu. Some of these diseases were first noted outside the United States, but have since become established in US vectors.
- Global health issues include Middle East respiratory syndrome coronavirus and Ebola. When these diseases are suspected, travel history may provide valuable insights into the patient's condition.

▶ Vital Vocabulary

acquired immunodeficiency syndrome (AIDS) The end-stage disease process caused by the human immunodeficiency virus (HIV). A person with AIDS is extremely vulnerable to numerous infections.

Prep Kit (continued)

epidemic A situation in which new cases of a disease in a human population substantially exceed the number expected based on recent experience.

hepatitis Inflammation of the liver, usually caused by a viral infection, that causes fever, loss of appetite, jaundice, fatigue, and altered liver function.

herpes simplex A common virus caused by human herpes viruses 1 and 2, characterized by small blisters whose location depends on the type of virus. Type 2 results in blisters on the genital area, while type 1 results in blisters on nongenital areas.

human immunodeficiency virus (HIV) The virus that causes infection and ultimately causes acquired immunodeficiency syndrome (AIDS), which damages the cells in the body's immune system so that the body is unable to fight infection or certain cancers.

index of suspicion Awareness that unseen life-threatening injuries or illness may exist.

influenza A virus that has crossed the animal/human barrier and infected humans and that kills thousands of people every year.

medical emergencies Emergencies caused by illnesses or conditions, not by an outside force.

meningitis An inflammation of the meningeal coverings of the brain and spinal cord; it is usually caused by a virus or a bacterium.

meningococcal meningitis An inflammation of the meningeal coverings of the brain and spinal cord; can be highly contagious.

methicillin-resistant *Staphylococcus aureus* (MRSA) A bacterium that can cause infections in different parts of the body and is often resistant to commonly used antibiotics; it is transmitted by different routes, including the respiratory route, and can be found on the skin, in surgical wounds, and in the bloodstream, lungs, and urinary tract.

nature of illness (NOI) The general type of illness a patient is experiencing.

nosocomial Hospital acquired.

pandemic An outbreak of a disease that occurs on a global scale.

pertussis An airborne disease caused by bacteria that mostly affects children younger than 6 years; it presents with fever and a "whoop" sound that occurs when the patient tries to inhale after a coughing attack; also called whooping cough.

severe acute respiratory syndrome (SARS) Potentially life-threatening viral infection that usually starts with flulike symptoms.

sign Something you can see or measure (eg, a laceration or the patient's blood pressure) when assessing a patient to establish illness or injury.

symptom Something the patient tells you ("My head hurts") when assessing a patient to establish illness or injury.

trauma emergencies Emergencies that are the result of physical forces applied to the body; injuries.

tuberculosis A chronic bacterial disease, caused by *Mycobacterium tuberculosis*, that usually affects the lungs but can also affect other organs such as the brain and kidneys; it is spread by cough and can lie dormant in a person's lungs for decades and then reactivate.

virulence The strength or ability of a pathogen to produce disease.

Zika A type of virus that is transmitted by the *Aedes aegypti* mosquito in which the majority of infected persons are asymptomatic; transmission can occur from an infected mother to her fetus, and from an infected male to his sexual partners.

▶ References

1. HIV in the United States: at a glance. Centers for Disease Control and Prevention website. December 2, 2016. https://www.cdc.gov/hiv/statistics/overview/ataglance.html. Accessed January 20, 2017.
2. Frequently asked questions: bloodborne pathogens—occupational exposure. Centers for Disease Control and Prevention website. October 25, 2013. https://www.cdc.gov/OralHealth/infectioncontrol/faq/bloodborne_exposures.htm. Accessed January 20, 2017.
3. Kuhar DT, Henderson DK, Struble KA, et al. Updated U.S. Public Health Service Guidelines for the Management of Occupational Exposures to HIV and Recommendations for Postexposure Prophylaxis. Centers for Disease Control and Prevention website. https://stacks.cdc.gov/view/cdc/20711. Accessed September 10, 2017.
4. Mayo Clinic. Swine flu (H1N1 flu). August 13, 2015. http://www.mayoclinic.org/diseases-conditions/swine-flu/basics/definition/CON-20034916. Accessed January 20, 2017.
5. Influenza (flu): prevention strategies for seasonal influenza in healthcare settings. Centers for Disease Control and Prevention website. http://www.cdc.gov/flu/professionals/infectioncontrol/healthcaresettings.htm. Accessed March 29, 2017.
6. Surveillance for viral hepatitis—United States, 2014. Centers for Disease Control and Prevention website.

Prep Kit *(continued)*

June 22, 2016. https://www.cdc.gov/hepatitis/statistics/2014surveillance/commentary.htm#summary. Accessed January 20, 2017.

7. *Disease Surveillance 2014*. Atlanta, GA: U.S. Department of Health and Human Services, Centers for Disease Control and Prevention, National Center for HIV/AIDS, Viral Hepatitis, STD, and TB Prevention, Division of STD Prevention; November 2015. https://www.cdc.gov/std/stats14/surv-2014-print.pdf. Accessed January 20, 2017.
8. Tuberculosis: data and statistics. Centers for Disease Control and Prevention website. December 9, 2016. https://www.cdc.gov/tb/statistics/. Accessed January 20, 2017.
9. Tuberculosis (TB)—Fact Sheets—BCG Vaccine. Centers for Disease Control and Prevention website. https://www.cdc.gov/tb/publications/factsheets/prevention/bcg.htm. Updated September 12, 1016. Accessed September 10, 2017.
10. Dulon M, Peters C, Schablon A, Nienhaus A. MRSA carriage among healthcare workers in non-outbreak settings in Europe and the United States: a systematic review. *BMC Infect Dis.* 2014;14:363. http://bmcinfectdis.biomedcentral.com/articles/10.1186/1471-2334-14-363. Accessed January 20, 2017.
11. CDC SARS response timeline. Centers for Disease Control and Prevention website. April 26, 2013. https://www.cdc.gov/about/history/sars/timeline.htm. Accessed January 20, 2017.
12. World Health Organization. Cumulative number of confirmed human cases for avian influenza A(H5N1) reported to WHO, 2003–2016. December 29, 2016. http://www.who.int/influenza/human_animal_interface/2016_12_19_tableH5N1.pdf?ua=1. Accessed January 20, 2017.
13. WHO Ebola Response Team. Ebola virus disease in West Africa: the first 9 months of the epidemic and forward projections. *N Engl J Med.* 2014;371:1481-1492. http://www.nejm.org/doi/full/10.1056/NEJMoa1411100. Accessed January 20, 2017.
14. Areas with Zika, Key Facts. Centers for Disease Control and Prevention website. January 13, 2017. https://www.cdc.gov/zika/geo/index.html. Accessed February 13, 2017.
15. Zika Virus, About Zika. Centers for Disease Control and Prevention website. September 29, 2016. https://www.cdc.gov/zika/about/index.html. Accessed February 13, 2017.
16. Zika Virus, Symptoms, Testing, and Treatment. Centers for Disease Control and Prevention website. June 21, 2016. https://www.cdc.gov/zika/symptoms/index.html. Accessed February 13, 2017.
17. Zika Virus, Symptoms. Centers for Disease Control and Prevention website. January 24, 2017. https://www.cdc.gov/zika/symptoms/symptoms.html. Accessed February 13, 2017.
18. Zika Virus, Pregnancy. Centers for Disease Control and Prevention website. January 23, 2017. https://www.cdc.gov/zika/pregnancy/index.html. Accessed February 13, 2017.
19. Zika Virus, Microcephaly and Other Birth Defects. Centers for Disease Control and Prevention website. January 17, 2017. https://www.cdc.gov/zika/healtheffects/birth_defects.html. Accessed February 13, 2017.
20. Zika Virus, Zika and Blood Transfusion. Centers for Disease Control and Prevention website. November 18, 2016. https://www.cdc.gov/zika/transmission/blood-transfusion.html. Accessed February 13, 2017.

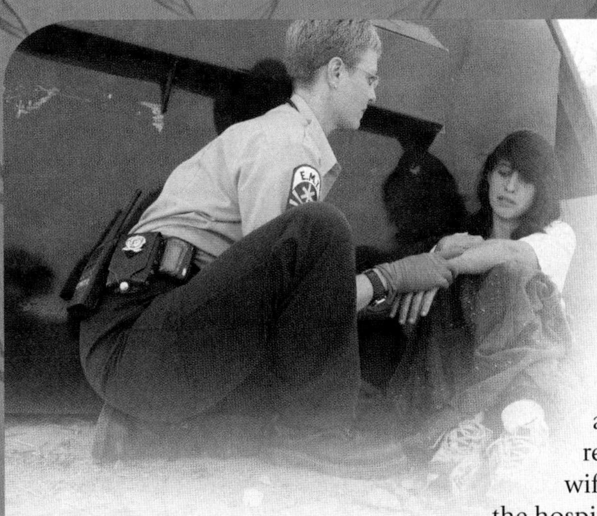

Assessment in Action

You are dispatched to a "general medical" complaint. On arrival, you find a 35-year-old man complaining of feeling "ill" with a severe headache and a stiff neck. On further questioning of the patient, you are able to detect a slightly altered mental status. Your physical examination reveals patchy red blotches throughout the patient's upper body. The patient's wife states, "This happened one time before and he was put in the hospital for meningitis."

1. Based on the patient's presentation, which standard precautions would be appropriate?

A. Gloves and mask
B. Gown and gloves
C. Mask and goggles
D. Gloves and goggles

2. Meningitis is an inflammation of the meningeal coverings of the:

A. brain and spinal cord.
B. spinal cord.
C. nerve fibers.
D. cerebellum.

3. Which of the following is a cause of meningitis?

A. Bacteria
B. Fungi
C. Protozoa
D. Parasite

4. Which of the following is NOT a sign or symptom of meningitis?

A. Fever
B. Back pain
C. Headache
D. Stiff neck

5. In health care settings, which type of infection is believed to be transmitted from patient to patient via the unwashed hands of health care providers?

A. Methicillin-resistant *Staphylococcus aureus* (MRSA)
B. Tuberculosis
C. Hantavirus
D. Severe acute respiratory syndrome (SARS)

6. When questioning a patient with potential meningitis, it is important to ask about the "T" part of the history. The "T" in OPQRST stands for:

A. temperature.
B. tenderness.
C. timing.
D. tympany.

7. Which of the following is NOT a sign or symptom of Ebola?

A. Watery diarrhea
B. Dilated pupils
C. Body aches
D. Bleeding

8. In rural settings with long transport times, patients with which of the following conditions would NOT benefit from aeromedical transport?

A. Stroke
B. Heart attack
C. Complication of pregnancy
D. Fracture of the radius with good perfusion

9. How should you treat a patient suspected of having tuberculosis to prevent the spread of the infection?

10. What is the appropriate way to assess for level of consciousness?

CHAPTER 17

Respiratory Emergencies

National EMS Education Standard Competencies

Medicine

Applies fundamental knowledge to provide basic and selected advanced emergency care and transportation based on assessment findings for an acutely ill patient.

Respiratory

Anatomy, signs, symptoms, and management of respiratory emergencies including those that affect the

- Upper airway (pp 755-756, 759, 761, 764, 768-773, 777-778, 781, 783-795)
- Lower airway (pp 755-756, 759, 761, 764, 772-773, 777-795)

Anatomy, physiology, pathophysiology, assessment, and management of

- Epiglottitis (pp 761, 764-765, 773, 778, 794)
- Spontaneous pneumothorax (pp 761, 769-770, 789, 792-793)
- Pulmonary edema (pp 764, 766-767, 790-791)
- Asthma (pp 761, 768-769, 774-775, 778, 780-781, 786, 791-792)
- Chronic obstructive pulmonary disease (pp 767-769, 774-775, 778, 780, 782, 785-786, 791)
- Environmental/industrial exposure (pp 771-772, 776, 793-794)
- Toxic gas (pp 766, 771-772, 776, 793-794)
- Pertussis (pp 761, 773, 794)
- Cystic fibrosis (p 772)
- Pulmonary embolism (pp 770-771, 793)
- Pneumonia (pp 761, 764, 773, 778, 794)
- Viral respiratory infections (pp 764, 772-773, 794)
- Obstructive/restrictive disease (pp 767-769, 774-775, 780-781, 786, 791)

Knowledge Objectives

1. Review the structures and functions of the upper and lower airways, lungs, and accessory structures of the respiratory system. (pp 755-758)
2. Explain the physiology of respiration and list the signs of normal breathing. (pp 756-759)
3. Explain the special patient assessment and care considerations that are required for pediatric patients who are experiencing respiratory distress. (pp 757, 766, 776, 786-787, 792, 794)
4. Discuss the pathophysiology of respiration and provide examples of the common signs and symptoms a patient with inadequate breathing may present with in an emergency situation. (pp 759-760)
5. Explain the concept of hypoxic drive. (p 760)
6. Describe the various respiratory conditions that cause dyspnea, including their causes, assessment findings and symptoms, complications, and specific prehospital management and transport decisions. (pp 763-795)
7. List and review the characteristics of infectious diseases that are frequently associated with dyspnea. (pp 764, 772-773)
8. Explain the special patient assessment and care considerations that are required for geriatric patients who are experiencing respiratory distress. (pp 773, 776, 794-795)
9. Describe the assessment of a patient who is in respiratory distress and the relationship of the assessment findings to patient management and transport decisions. (pp 776-783)
10. Describe the primary emergency medical care of a person who is in respiratory distress. (pp 777, 783-790)
11. List and define five different types of adventitious breath sounds, their signs and symptoms, and the disease process associated with each one. (p 778)
12. Summarize the steps in emergency medical care of a patient with dyspnea. (pp 783-790)
13. State the generic name, medication forms, dose, administration, indications, actions, and contraindications for medications that are administered via metered-dose inhalers and small-volume nebulizers. (pp 785-786)
14. Discuss the application of a continuous positive airway pressure/bilevel positive airway pressure unit. (pp 789-790)
15. Discuss some epidemic and pandemic considerations related to the spread of influenza type A and strategies advanced emergency

medical technicians should use to protect themselves from infection during a possible crisis situation. (p 795)

Skills Objectives

1. Demonstrate the process of history taking to obtain more information related to a patient's chief complaint based on a case scenario. (pp 779-780)
2. Demonstrate how to use the OPQRST assessment to obtain more specific information about a patient's breathing problem. (pp 779-780)
3. Demonstrate how to assist a patient with the administration of a small-volume nebulizer. (p 785)
4. Demonstrate how to assist a patient with the administration of a metered-dose inhaler. (pp 787-788)

Introduction

Dyspnea, or difficulty breathing, is a complaint that you will encounter often. It is a symptom of many different conditions, from the **common cold** and **asthma** to heart failure and **pulmonary embolism**. Several different problems occurring at the same time may contribute to a patient's dyspnea, including some that are serious or life threatening. You may or may not be able to determine the cause of dyspnea in a particular patient. Regardless, you may still be able to save a life.

This chapter begins with a basic explanation of how the lungs function. It then looks at common medical problems that can impede normal functioning and cause dyspnea, including acute pulmonary edema, chronic obstructive pulmonary disease (COPD), and asthma. You will learn the signs and symptoms of each condition. You should keep all of these possible medical problems in mind as you obtain the patient's medical history and perform a physical assessment. The information that you obtain will help you determine the best treatment, which may differ based on the underlying cause of the dyspnea.

Remember, the sensation of not getting enough air can be terrifying, regardless of its cause. As an advanced emergency medical technician (AEMT), you must be prepared to treat not only the patient's symptoms and underlying problem, but the anxiety produced as well.

Anatomy and Physiology Review

Anatomy Review

The anatomy and physiology of the respiratory system was discussed in Chapter 11, *Airway Management*, and is reviewed here. The respiratory system consists of all the structures of the body that contribute to the breathing process. The upper airway includes all anatomic airway structures above the level of the vocal cords. Air flows through the structures shown in Figure 17-1.

Gas exchange is the process by which deoxygenated blood from the pulmonary circulation releases carbon dioxide and is resupplied with oxygen before it enters the cardiac circulation. This process occurs at the level of the alveoli, the tiny air sacs clustered around the terminal bronchioles in the lungs Figure 17-2. These terminal bronchioles are very thin and have little structure. This is helpful for gas exchange, but it also means that these bronchioles lack cilia, a mucous blanket, smooth muscle, or rigid structures.

The pulmonary circulation begins at the right ventricle, where the pulmonary artery (the only artery that primarily carries deoxygenated blood) branches into increasingly smaller vessels until the pulmonary capillary bed surrounds the alveoli and terminal bronchioles

YOU are the Provider — PART 1

Medic One is requested to respond to an assisted living center for a patient with difficulty breathing. You and your partner are greeted by the staff who state that the 86-year-old patient has been getting progressively worse over the past couple of days. They suggested she go to the hospital at the onset of symptoms, but the patient kept insisting that it would "get better" after her oxygen was increased and she used her "puffer." The patient has a history of hypertension, emphysema, and asthma. She is currently on oxygen at 4 L/min via nasal cannula.

1. What are some potential causes of shortness of breath in older adults?
2. What equipment would you need immediately after you arrive on scene?

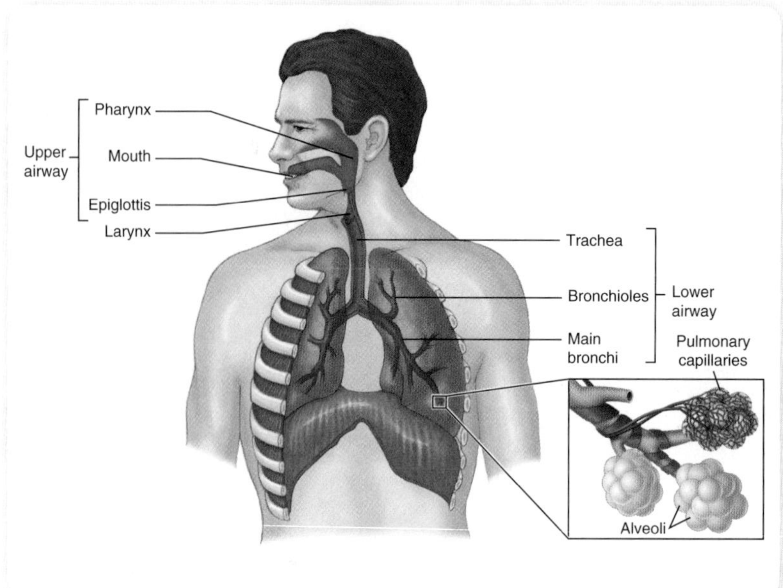

Figure 17-1 The upper airway includes the nasopharynx, nasal air passages, pharynx, mouth, oropharynx, and epiglottis. The larynx is considered the dividing line between the upper and lower airways. The lower airway includes the trachea, alveoli, bronchioles, and main bronchi.

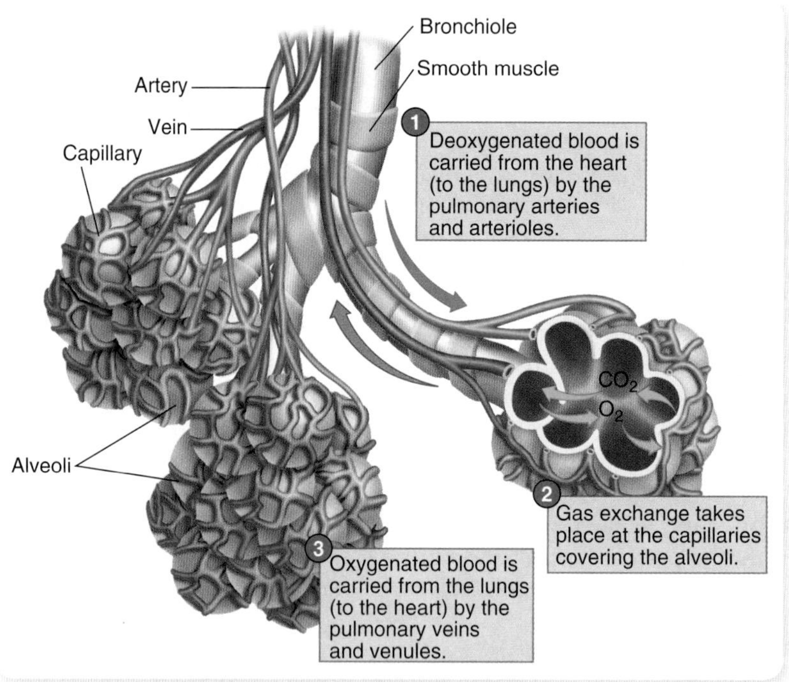

Figure 17-2 An enlarged view of a single alveolus (air sac) showing where the exchange of oxygen and carbon dioxide between air in the sac and blood in the pulmonary capillaries takes place.

Figure 17-3. There is substantially more circulation to the lung bases than there is to the lung apices. Because humans are upright, gravity-dependent creatures, most infections and pathologic conditions occur at the base of the lung.[1]

▶ Physiology Review

Respiration

The principal function of the lungs is **respiration**, which is the exchange of oxygen and carbon dioxide. The two

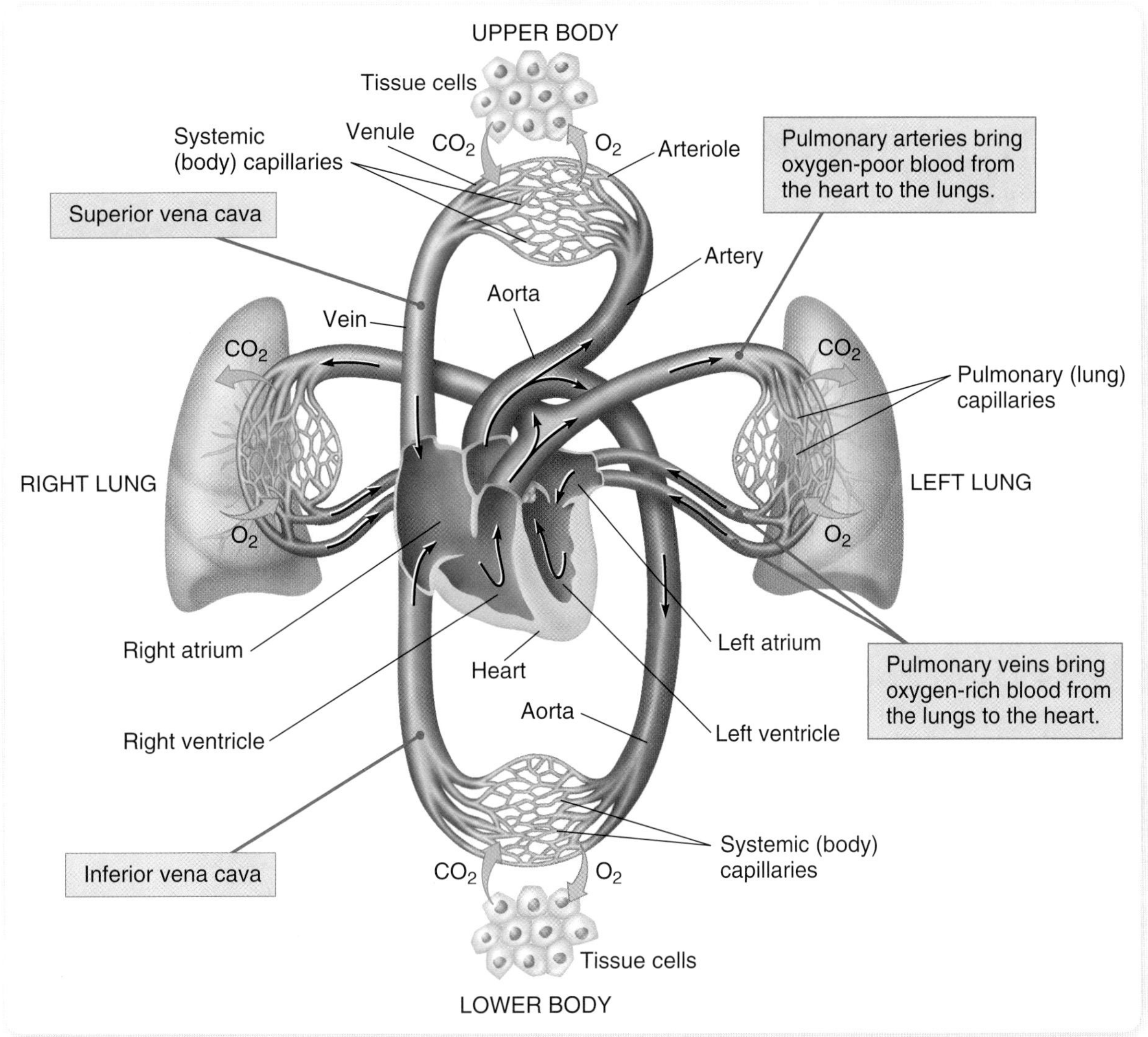

Figure 17-3 Pulmonary circulation begins as blood leaves the right ventricle via the pulmonary artery. The pulmonary capillary bed brings red blood cells close to the terminal bronchioles. After picking up oxygen, the blood returns to the left atrium via the pulmonary veins.

Special Populations

The anatomy of the respiratory system in children is proportionately smaller and less rigid than that in an adult **Figure 17-4**. A child's nose and mouth are much smaller than those of an adult. The larynx, cricoid cartilage, and trachea are smaller, softer, and more flexible as well. This makes the mechanics of breathing much more delicate. A child's pharynx is also smaller and less deeply curved. The tongue takes up proportionately more space in a child's mouth than in an adult's mouth.

These anatomic differences are important for your assessment. For example, the smaller larynx of a child becomes obstructed more easily. The chest wall in children is softer. Therefore, children depend more heavily on the diaphragm for breathing. You will notice that the abdomen moves in and out considerably with each breath, especially in an infant. Young infants do not know how to breathe through the mouth. Therefore, as you assess an infant or a child, you must carefully consider these differences.

processes that occur during respiration are inspiration (inhaling) and expiration (exhaling). **Ventilation** is the mechanical process of moving air into and out of the lungs for gas exchange. During pulmonary respiration, oxygen is provided to the blood, and carbon dioxide is removed from it. Oxygen entering the alveoli from inhalation passes through tiny passages in the alveolar wall into the capillaries, which carry the oxygen to the heart. The heart, in turn, pumps oxygenated blood throughout the body. Carbon dioxide produced by the body's cells

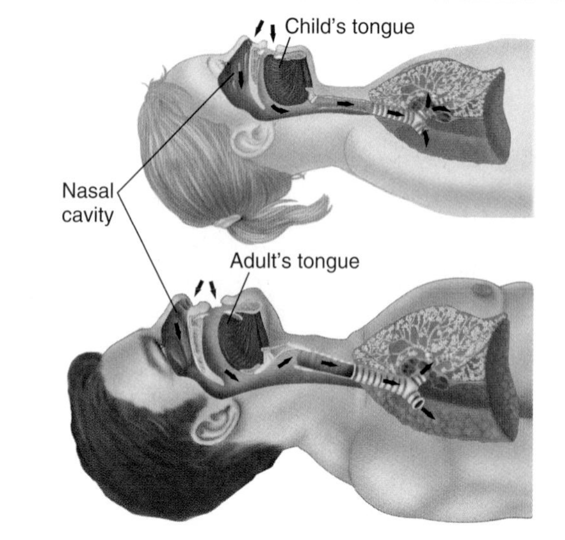

Figure 17-4 The respiratory system of a child is proportionally smaller and less rigid than that of an adult.

Figure 17-5A returns to the lungs in the blood that circulates through and around the alveolar air spaces. The carbon dioxide diffuses back into the alveoli and travels back up the bronchial tree and out the upper airways during exhalation Figure 17-5B. Again, carbon dioxide is "exchanged" for oxygen, which travels in exactly the opposite direction (during inhalation).

Words of Wisdom

Ventilation is the act of air going into and out of the lungs. *Respiration* is the exchange of gases at the pulmonary or cellular level.

Inspiration

The stimulus to breathe comes from the respiratory center located in the medulla. The involuntary control of breathing originates in the brainstem, specifically in the pons and medulla. The impulses for automatic breathing descend through the spinal cord and can be overridden (to a point) by voluntary control. The motor nerves of respiration are the phrenic nerves, which innervate the diaphragm, and the intercostal nerves, which innervate the external intercostal muscles (muscles between the ribs).

During inspiration, the diaphragm and intercostal muscles contract, causing the diaphragm to flatten and the ribs to move up and out. The combined actions of these structures enlarge the thorax in all directions, causing intrapulmonary pressure to fall slightly below atmospheric pressure (the air pressure outside the body). As the diaphragm and intercostal muscles contract and the thoracic cage expands, air pressure within the thorax decreases, creating a slight vacuum. This pulls air in through the trachea and fills the lungs, inflating the alveoli. When the air

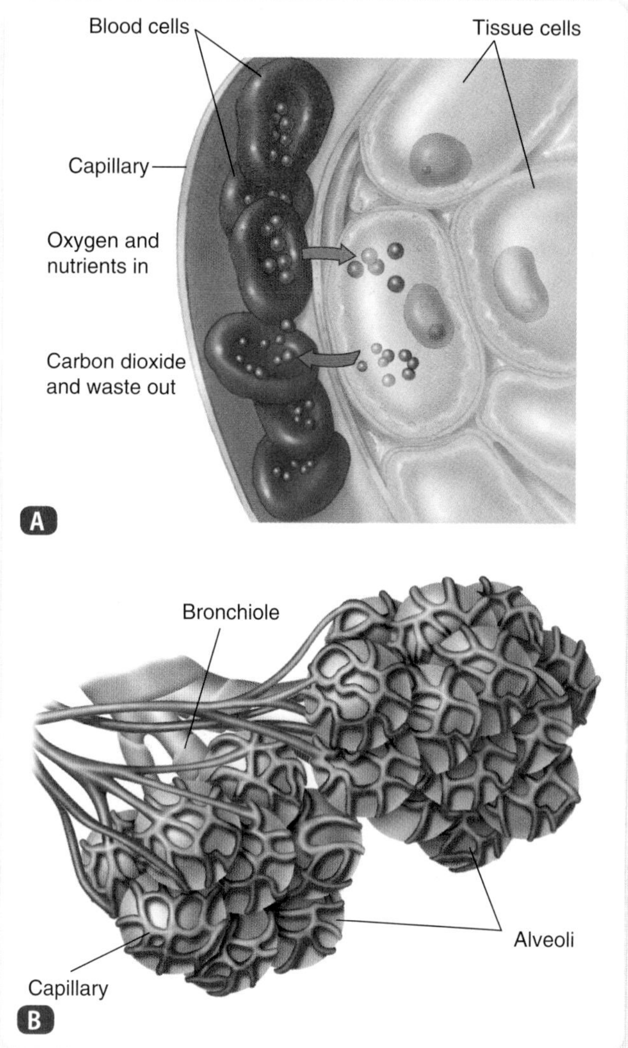

Figure 17-5 The exchange of oxygen and carbon dioxide during respiration. **A.** Oxygen passes from the blood through capillaries to tissue cells. Carbon dioxide passes from tissue cells through capillaries to the blood. **B.** In the lungs, oxygen is picked up by the blood and carbon dioxide is given off.

pressure outside the thorax equals the air pressure inside the thorax, air stops moving, and a person stops inhaling. Oxygen and carbon dioxide are then able to diffuse across the alveolar membrane from an area of higher pressure to an area of lower pressure until the pressures are equal. Normal inspiratory reserve volume, the amount of air that can be inhaled in addition to normal tidal volume (about 500 mL), is about 3,000 mL in a typical adult male and 2,300 mL in a typical adult female.

Expiration

As the chest expands, mechanical receptors, known as stretch receptors, in the chest wall and bronchioles send a signal to the apneustic center via the vagus nerve to inhibit the inspiratory center, and expiration occurs. This feedback loop, a combination of mechanical and neural control, is

Table 17-1 Signs of Normal Breathing

- A normal rate (adult: 12 to 20 breaths/min; child: 15 to 30 breaths/min; infant: 25 to 50 breaths/min)
- A regular pattern of inhalation and exhalation
- Clear and equal breath sounds on both sides of the chest
- Regular and equal chest rise (chest expansion) and fall
- Adequate depth (tidal volume)
- Unlabored; without **adventitious breath sounds** (abnormal breath sounds) (**wheezing**, **stridor**)

Note: Respiratory ranges are per the NHTSA 2009 EMT National EMS Education Standards. Ranges presented in other sources may vary.

Pediatric data from: American Heart Association (AHA). Vital signs in children. In: *Pediatric Advanced Life Support*. Dallas, TX: AHA; 2015.

known as the **Hering-Breuer reflex** and terminates inhalation to prevent overexpansion of the lungs. The diaphragm and intercostal muscles relax, moving the ribs down and in and the diaphragm back into its dome shape, which increases intrapulmonary pressure. The natural elasticity, or recoil, of the lungs passively removes the air. Normal expiratory reserve volume, the amount of air that can be exhaled following normal exhalation, is about 1,200 mL.

Normally, expiration lasts twice as long as inspiration. This relationship is expressed by the **inspiratory/expiratory (I/E) ratio**; a normal I/E ratio is 1:2. When a patient's lower airway is obstructed and he or she has difficulty getting air out (such as in asthma), the expiratory phase is prolonged and may be four to five times as long as inspiration. In the case of a patient with asthma, the I/E ratio would be 1:4 or 1:5. In a patient with **tachypnea** (rapid respiratory rate), the expiratory phase is short and approaches that of inspiration; the I/E ratio may be 1:1.

Table 17-1 lists the characteristics of adequate breathing, and Table 17-2 lists characteristics of inadequate breathing.

Table 17-2 Signs and Symptoms of Inadequate Breathing

Signs and Symptoms of Inadequate Breathing
Dyspnea or shortness of breath.
An altered mental status associated with shallow or slow breathing.
The adult patient appears anxious or restless; the pediatric patient appears sleepy or listless.
The respiratory rate is too fast or too slow.
The breathing rhythm is irregular.
The skin is pale, cool, clammy, or cyanotic.
Adventitious breath sounds are heard, including wheezing, gurgling, snoring, crowing, or stridor (harsh, high-pitched, barking sounds).
Decreased or noisy breath sounds are heard on one or both sides of the chest.
An inability to speak more than a few words between breaths (two- to three-word dyspnea). Ask the patient "How are you doing?" If the patient cannot speak at all, he or she most likely has a respiratory emergency.
Accessory muscle use, **retractions**, or labored breathing.
Unequal or inadequate chest expansion.
Coughing excessively.
The patient is sitting up, leaning forward with his or her palms flat on the bed or the arms of the chair. This is called the tripod position because the patient's back and both arms are working together to support the upper body.
Pursed lips (pursed lip breathing) or nasal flaring.

Pathophysiology

For the body to receive the required nutrients and oxygen and to dispose of waste products, adequate ventilation, **diffusion**, and **perfusion** must occur. There are multiple complications that interfere with an ample intake of oxygen. These can be separated into four areas:

1. Upper airway obstruction may be from a foreign body obstruction, trauma, or an inflammation such as tonsillitis or **epiglottitis**.
2. Lower airway obstruction may be caused by trauma. Obstructive lung disease and other complications, such as mucus accumulation, smooth-muscle spasm, and airway edema, can also create narrowing and blockage of the lower airways.
3. Chest wall impairment is another cause of impaired ventilation. Trauma, hemothorax, **pneumothorax**, empyema (**pleural effusion**), pleural inflammation, and neuromuscular diseases such as multiple sclerosis or muscular dystrophy prevent adequate chest wall excursion.
4. Problems in neurologic control can impair ventilation. These include brainstem malfunction from central nervous system depressant drugs, stroke or other medical neurologic condition, or trauma. Trauma and neuromuscular diseases can also cause

phrenic or spinal nerve dysfunction, preventing normal neurologic control. By rapidly assessing the patient and providing the necessary interventions, problems associated with oxygenation and ventilation can be minimized or avoided altogether.

Regardless of the reason for breathing difficulty, the critical issue is that you must be able to immediately recognize the signs and symptoms of inadequate breathing and know what to do. Table 17-3 provides key signs and symptoms to help you recognize and differentiate between different respiratory complaints.

Gas Exchange Interface

It is often helpful to think of alveoli as small balloons at the end of a straw. Alveoli are made up of two types of cells:

1. Type I alveolar cells (pneumocytes) are almost empty, allowing for better gas exchange. They lack cellular components that would permit them to reproduce.
2. Each alveolus has several type II pneumocytes, which can make new type I cells and produce a substance known as surfactant, which reduces surface tension and helps keep the alveoli expanded. When alveoli are damaged by infection, cigarette smoking, or other trauma, their ability to repair themselves correlates directly to the number of type II cells that remain. After all type II cells in an alveolus have been destroyed, the alveolus cannot make new cells or surfactant and is essentially dead.

Alveoli function best when they are kept partially inflated. Blowing up a balloon takes a lot of pressure. After the balloon is partially inflated, however, it is much easier to inflate it the rest of the way. The same is true of alveoli. By reducing the surface tension of the alveoli, surfactant makes it easier for them to expand. When surfactant is washed out of the alveoli, as may occur in pulmonary edema, submersion incidents, or severe shock, they are much more likely to collapse.

After foreign material gets into the terminal bronchioles and alveoli, it typically never comes out. Emphysema may affect this area of the lung, damaging or destroying the few structural components that are present. When that happens, the terminal branches of the tracheobronchial tree become so weak that they collapse during exhalation and trap air in the alveoli.

Collapsed, fluid-filled, or pus-filled alveoli do not participate in gas exchange. Instead, these alveoli contribute to a shunt, in which blood from the right side of the heart bypasses the alveoli and returns to the left side of the heart in an unoxygenated state, perhaps resulting in hypoxemia. Conditions related to ventilation, perfusion, or both can prevent oxygen from reaching the bloodstream.

Like all capillaries in the body, the pulmonary capillaries are narrow and normally allow red blood cells to pass through only in single file. People with chronic lung disease and chronic **hypoxia** often generate a surplus of red blood cells over time, which makes their blood thick (polycythemia). Viscous blood that is pushed through the tiny pulmonary capillaries can place a substantial strain on the right side of the heart. When the alveoli are distended by COPD, they push against the capillary bed, further narrowing the capillaries and straining the right side of the heart. Right-side heart failure because of chronic lung disease is known as cor pulmonale.

Words of Wisdom

The body's immediate response to mild hypoxemia is to increase the heart rate (possibly to a rate of more than 130 beats/min, or tachycardia). Severe hypoxia often causes bradycardia. Any uncorrected hypoxic insult may trigger a lethal cardiac dysrhythmia, such as ventricular fibrillation or ventricular tachycardia.

Carbon Dioxide Retention and Hypoxic Drive

You will sometimes encounter patients who have an elevated level of carbon dioxide in their arterial blood. The level can rise for several reasons. Various types of lung disease may impair the exhalation process. The body may also produce too much carbon dioxide, either temporarily or chronically, depending on the disease or abnormality. If, over a period of years, arterial carbon dioxide levels rise slowly to an abnormally high level and remain there (as in late COPD), the respiratory centers in the brain, which sense carbon dioxide levels and control breathing, may work less efficiently.

The failure of those centers to respond normally to a rise in arterial levels of carbon dioxide is a result of chronic **carbon dioxide retention**. Recall that normally, chemoreceptors sense the levels of carbon dioxide (based on the pH) in the blood and cerebrospinal fluid. When carbon dioxide levels become elevated, the respiratory centers in the brain increase the rate and depth of ventilation accordingly. However, patients with chronic lung diseases have difficulty eliminating carbon dioxide through exhalation; thus, they always have higher levels of carbon dioxide. The theory is that the brain gradually accommodates high levels of carbon dioxide and then uses a "backup system" to control breathing based on low levels of oxygen, rather than high levels of carbon dioxide. This condition is called **hypoxic drive**.

In these patients, the stimulus to breathe is the detection of low blood oxygen levels. If the arterial level of oxygen is raised, as happens when the patient is given additional oxygen, there is less stimulus to breathe; both the high carbon dioxide and low oxygen drives are decreased. Therefore, giving too much oxygen to these patients may actually depress, or completely stop, the respirations. However, as will be discussed later in this chapter, you should never withhold oxygen from a patient who needs it.

Table 17-3 Signs and Symptoms Seen in Various Respiratory Conditions

Condition	Signs and Symptoms	Condition	Signs and Symptoms
Asthma	▪ Wheezing on inspiration/expiration ▪ Bronchospasm	Epiglottitis	▪ Dyspnea ▪ High fever ▪ Stridor ▪ Drooling ▪ Difficulty swallowing ▪ Severe sore throat ▪ Tripod or sniffing position
Anaphylaxis	▪ Flushed skin or hives (urticaria) ▪ Generalized edema ▪ Decreased blood pressure (hypotension) ▪ Laryngeal edema with dyspnea ▪ Wheezing or stridor	**Influenza type A (flu)**	▪ Cough ▪ Fever ▪ Sore throat ▪ Fatigue
Bronchiolitis	▪ Shortness of breath ▪ Wheezing ▪ Coughing ▪ Fever ▪ Dehydration ▪ Tachypnea ▪ Tachycardia	**Pertussis (whooping cough)**	▪ Coughing spells ▪ "Whooping" sound ▪ Fever
Bronchitis	▪ Chronic cough (with sputum production) ▪ Wheezing ▪ Cyanosis ▪ Tachypnea (increased breathing rate)	**Pneumonia**	▪ Dyspnea ▪ Chills, fever ▪ Cough ▪ Green, red, or rust-colored sputum ▪ Localized wheezing or crackles
Heart failure	▪ Dependent edema ▪ Crackles (pulmonary edema) ▪ Orthopnea ▪ Paroxysmal nocturnal dyspnea	Pneumothorax	▪ Sudden chest pain with dyspnea ▪ Decreased breath sounds (affected side) ▪ **Subcutaneous emphysema**
Common cold	▪ Cough ▪ Runny or stuffy nose ▪ Sore throat	Pulmonary embolus	▪ Sharp chest pain ▪ Sudden onset ▪ Dyspnea ▪ Tachycardia ▪ Clear breath sounds initially
Croup	▪ Fever ▪ Barking cough ▪ Stridor ▪ Mostly seen in pediatric patients	Tension pneumothorax	▪ Severe shortness of breath ▪ Decreased/altered level of consciousness ▪ Neck vein distention ▪ Tracheal deviation (late sign) ▪ Hypotension; signs of shock (late sign)
Diphtheria	▪ Difficulty breathing and swallowing ▪ Sore throat ▪ Thick, gray buildup in throat or nose ▪ Fever	**Respiratory syncytial virus (RSV)**	▪ Cough ▪ Wheezing ▪ Fever ▪ Dehydration
Emphysema	▪ Barrel chest ▪ Pursed lip breathing ▪ Dyspnea on exertion ▪ Cyanosis ▪ Wheezing/decreased breath sounds	**Tuberculosis**	▪ Cough ▪ Fever ▪ Fatigue ▪ Productive/bloody sputum

Special Populations

People older than 65 years are especially susceptible to problems with respiration, from occult (not obvious) stroke, lung disease, cardiovascular disease, liver disease, or certain medications.[2]

▶ Hypoventilation

When the lungs fail to work properly, the body cannot efficiently dispose of carbon dioxide, and it accumulates in the blood. The excess carbon dioxide combines with water to form bicarbonate ions and hydrogen (H^+) ions, also known as carbonic acid (H_2CO_3). The result is **respiratory acidosis**.

Acidosis can occur if **hypoventilation** is not recognized. Impaired ventilation can be attributed to a variety of factors, as shown in Table 17-4.

Recall that pH is an inverse expression of how many free hydrogen ions (H^+) are in a solution. Thus, the carbon dioxide level in the blood is also directly related to pH (acid-base balance). Patients who are hyperventilating usually have respiratory alkalosis with a high pH. As their carbon dioxide level decreases, their pH level rises. Patients who are hypoventilating usually have respiratory acidosis. As their carbon dioxide level increases, their pH level decreases.

Table 17-4 Selected Causes of Impaired Ventilation

Category	Conditions
Upper airway obstruction	Foreign body obstruction Infection Trauma
Lower airway obstruction	Trauma Obstructive disease Increased mucus production Airway swelling (edema)
Chest wall impairment	Pneumothorax Flail chest Pleural effusion Restrictive disease (scoliosis, kyphosis)
Neuromuscular impairment	Overdose Lou Gehrig disease (amyotrophic lateral sclerosis) Carbon dioxide narcosis

Many types of problems can cause patients to hypoventilate:

- **Conditions that impair lung function.** When a patient is breathing but gas exchange is impaired, the carbon dioxide level in the blood rises. This situation can occur in patients with severe atelectasis, pneumonia, pulmonary edema, asthma, and COPD.
- **Conditions that impair the mechanics of breathing.** Gas flow can be suppressed by a high cervical fracture with chest wall paralysis, flail chest, diaphragmatic rupture, severe retractions, an abdomen full of air or blood, abdominal or chest binding (using a pneumatic antishock garment or immobilization straps), and anything else that restricts the pressure changes that facilitate respiration.

  Obesity hypoventilation syndrome (also known as pickwickian syndrome) is respiratory compromise related to morbid obesity. One of the earliest descriptions of the combination of obesity, respiratory compromise, and sleep apnea is found in the character of Joe the "fat boy" in Charles Dickens's *Pickwick Papers*. Joe would fall asleep in midsentence, snore loudly, and generally have signs of hypercapnia. This syndrome is becoming more common, given the nationwide increase in the occurrence of obesity.
- **Conditions that impair the neuromuscular apparatus.** A patient who has experienced head trauma, an intracranial infection, or a brain tumor may have sustained damage to the respiratory centers of the brain, which may then compromise ventilation. Other conditions also may impair the neuromuscular apparatus:
  - Serious injury to the spinal cord (above the level of the fourth cervical vertebra [C4]) may block the nerve impulses that stimulate breathing.
  - **Guillain-Barré syndrome**, characterized by progressive muscle weakness and paralysis advancing up the body from the feet, can result in ineffective breathing if the paralysis reaches the diaphragm.
  - Amyotrophic lateral sclerosis (ALS; also known as Lou Gehrig disease) also causes progressive muscle weakness. This disease is progressive, with death usually attributable to respiratory failure as the muscles of respiration become unable to maintain adequate ventilation.
  - **Botulism** is caused by the bacterium *Clostridium botulinum*. This somewhat rare disease is usually caused by food poisoning or by giving infants raw (unpasteurized) honey,

which may be contaminated with spores of the bacterium. Botulism can cause muscle paralysis and is usually fatal when it reaches the muscles of respiration.

- **Conditions that reduce respiratory drive.** The stimulus to breathe is often called respiratory drive. Anything that interrupts or decreases the involuntary stimulus to breathe can result in hypoventilation or even apnea. Perhaps the most common hypoventilation crisis emergency medical services (EMS) providers see is acute opioid narcotic overdose (heroin, for example). Intoxication with alcohol, narcotics, and a host of other drugs and toxins can reduce the respiratory drive. Head injury, hypoxic drive, and asphyxia are all associated with grossly low respiratory rate and volume. The ultimate expression of hypoventilation is respiratory arrest followed by cardiac arrest.

In these circumstances, aggressive treatment must be initiated to assist the patient's respiratory efforts.

Hyperventilation

Hyperventilation is defined as overbreathing to the point that the level of arterial carbon dioxide falls below normal. This may be an indicator of a major, life-threatening illness. For example, a patient with diabetes who has an extremely high blood glucose level, a patient who has taken an overdose of aspirin, or a patient with a severe infection is likely to hyperventilate. In these cases, rapid, deep breathing is the body's attempt to compensate for acidosis, the buildup of excess acid in the blood or body tissues, resulting from the primary illness. Because carbon dioxide, mixed with water in the bloodstream, can add to the blood's acidity, lowering the level of carbon dioxide helps to compensate for the other acids.

Similarly, in an otherwise healthy person, tachypnea without physiologic demand for increased oxygen causes **respiratory alkalosis**, or a buildup of excess base (lack of acids) in the body fluids. The shift in the acid-base balance moves toward the base end of the scale.

Alkalosis is the cause of many of the symptoms associated with **hyperventilation syndrome (panic attack)**, including anxiety, dizziness, numbness, tingling of the hands and feet (which can progress to actual spasms of the phalanges known as **carpopedal spasm**, in which the hands and feet become clenched into a clawlike position), and even a sense of dyspnea despite the rapid breathing. Although hyperventilation can be the body's response to illness and a buildup of acids, hyperventilation syndrome is not the same thing. Instead, this syndrome occurs in the absence of other physical problems. It commonly occurs when a person is experiencing psychological stress. The respirations of a person who is experiencing hyperventilation syndrome may be as high as 40 shallow breaths/min or as low as only 20 very deep breaths/min.

Causes of Dyspnea

Dyspnea is shortness of breath or difficulty breathing. Many different medical problems may cause dyspnea. Be aware that if the problem is severe and the brain is deprived of oxygen, the patient may not be alert enough to report shortness of breath. More commonly, altered mental status is a sign of hypoxia of the brain.

In addition to the conditions listed in Table 17-3, patients with the following medical conditions often experience breathing difficulty or hypoxia:

- Pulmonary edema
- Hay fever
- Pleural effusion
- Obstruction of the airway
- Rib fractures (flail segment)
- **Cystic fibrosis**
- Hyperventilation syndrome
- Prolonged seizures
- Neuromuscular disease (such as multiple sclerosis or muscular dystrophy)
- Environmental or industrial exposure to toxic gases
- Carbon monoxide poisoning
- Drug overdose

As you treat patients with disorders of the lung, you should be aware that one or more of the following situations most likely exists:

- Gas exchange between the alveoli and pulmonary circulation is obstructed by fluid in the lung, infection, or collapsed alveoli (**atelectasis**).
- The alveoli are damaged and cannot transport gases properly across their own walls.
- The air passages are obstructed by muscle spasm, mucus, or weakened airway walls.
- Blood flow to the lungs is obstructed by blood clots.
- The pleural space is filled with air or excess fluid, so the lungs cannot properly expand.

All of these conditions prevent the proper exchange of oxygen and carbon dioxide. In addition, the pulmonary blood vessels themselves may have abnormalities that interfere with blood flow and thus with the transfer of gases.

Besides shortness of breath, a patient with dyspnea may also report the sensation of chest tightness and air hunger. Air hunger is when a person reports the feeling of "not getting enough air" and has a strong need to breathe. Chest tightness is described as an uncomfortable feeling in the chest, and it is commonly reported by patients with asthma.

Dyspnea is also a common complaint in patients with cardiopulmonary diseases. In some cases, it may be caused by physical exertion that has been made difficult because the patient's heart is damaged. Heart failure is a troublesome cause of breathlessness because the heart is not pumping efficiently and, therefore, the body does not have adequate oxygen. Another condition commonly associated with heart failure is pulmonary edema, in which the alveoli are filled with fluid.

Severe pain can cause a patient to experience rapid, shallow breathing without the presence of a primary pulmonary dysfunction. In some patients, breathing deeply causes pain because it causes expansion of the chest wall.

When you assess your patient for complaints of dyspnea, ask about chest pain; conversely, when you are evaluating your patient for chest pain, ask about dyspnea.

Words of Wisdom

Never withhold oxygen from any patient exhibiting signs of distress. If a patient with COPD stops breathing spontaneously (rare) as a result of increased levels of oxygen, it is a simple matter to coach breathing or to ventilate the patient and continue oxygenating organs and tissues. Withholding oxygen may result in an insufficient amount of inspired oxygen, and because of the decreased rate, depth, or other obstructive problem, vital organ damage may occur.

Upper or Lower Airway Infection

Infectious diseases causing dyspnea may affect all parts of the airway. Some cause mild discomfort; others require aggressive respiratory support. Infections that impair airflow through the airways are problems of respiration. Inadequate oxygen delivery to the tissues is a problem of oxygenation. Infections may cause dyspnea by obstructing airflow in the larger airways as a result of the production of mucus and secretions (colds, diphtheria) or by causing swelling of soft tissues located in the larger, upper airways (epiglottitis, croup). Infections may also impair exchange of gases between the alveoli and the capillaries (pneumonia). Table 17-5 shows infectious diseases that are associated with some degree of dyspnea.

Acute Pulmonary Edema

Pulmonary edema is an accumulation of fluid in the lungs and has various causes. The fluid accumulation causes a decrease in gas exchange and results in severe dyspnea. Severe myocardial damage caused by an acute problem (such as acute myocardial infarction) or a chronic problem (such as cardiomyopathy) results in reduced contractile force of the myocardium. In these cases, the left side of the heart cannot remove blood from the lungs as fast as the right side delivers it. As a result, fluid backs up

Table 17-5 Infectious Diseases Associated With Dyspnea

Disease	Characteristics
Bronchitis	• An acute or chronic inflammation of the lung that may damage lung tissue, usually associated with cough, production of sputum, and, depending on its cause, sometimes fever • Fluid also accumulates in the surrounding normal lung tissue, separating the alveoli from their capillaries. (Sometimes, fluid can also accumulate in the pleural space.) • The lung's ability to exchange oxygen and carbon dioxide is impaired. • The breathing pattern in bronchitis does not indicate major airway obstruction, but the patient may experience tachypnea, an increase in the breathing rate, which is an attempt to compensate for the reduced amount of normal lung tissue and for the buildup of fluid.
Common cold	• A viral infection usually associated with swollen nasal mucous membranes and the production of fluid from the sinuses and nose • Dyspnea is not severe; patients complain of "stuffiness" or difficulty breathing through the nose.
Croup	• Inflammation and swelling of the whole airway (pharynx, larynx, and trachea) typically seen in children between ages 6 months and 3 years Figure 17-6 • The common signs of croup are stridor and a seal-bark cough, which signal a substantial narrowing of the air passage of the larynx that may progress to marked obstruction. • Croup often responds well to the administration of humidified oxygen. • Croup is rarely seen in adults because the airways are larger.
Diphtheria	• Although well controlled during the past decade, it is still highly contagious and serious when it occurs. • The disease causes the formation of a diphtheritic membrane lining the pharynx that is composed of debris, inflammatory cells, and mucus. This membrane can rapidly and severely obstruct the passage of air into the larynx.

Disease	Characteristics
Epiglottitis	▪ Inflammation of the epiglottis due to a bacterial infection that can produce severe swelling of the flap over the larynx. Severe, rapidly progressive infection of the epiglottis and surrounding tissue that may be fatal because of sudden respiratory obstruction. ▪ In preschool and school-aged children (ages 4 to 7 years) especially, the epiglottis can swell to two or three times its normal size. ▪ The airway may become almost completely obstructed, sometimes quite suddenly **Figure 17-7**. ▪ Stridor (harsh, high-pitched, continued, rough, barking inspiratory sounds) may be heard late in the development of airway obstruction. ▪ Acute epiglottitis in the adult is characterized by a severe sore throat. ▪ Less common in children than it was 20 years ago because of a vaccine that can help to prevent most cases
Influenza type A	▪ A virus that has crossed the animal/human barrier and has infected humans ▪ Flu that has the potential to spread at a **pandemic** level
Meningococcal meningitis	▪ An inflammation of the meningeal coverings of the brain and spinal cord that can be highly contagious ▪ The bacteria can be spread through the exchange of respiratory and throat secretions through coughing and sneezing. ▪ The effects are lethal in some cases. Patients who survive can be left with brain damage, hearing loss, or learning disabilities. ▪ Patients may present with flulike symptoms, but unique to meningitis are high fever, severe headache, photophobia (light sensitivity), and a stiff neck in adults. Patients sometimes have an altered level of consciousness and can have red blotches on the skin. ▪ Use respiratory protection and report any potential cases.
Methicillin-resistant *Staphylococcus aureus* (MRSA)	▪ A bacterium that can cause infections in different parts of the body ▪ Transmitted by different routes, including the respiratory route; can enter the body through nonintact skin or respiratory droplets when patients cough ▪ Difficult to treat because it is resistant to many commonly used antibiotics, especially methicillin ▪ Most common in people with weakened immune systems, including those in hospitals and nursing homes
Pertussis (whooping cough)	▪ An airborne bacterial infection that affects mostly children younger than 6 years ▪ Patient will be feverish and exhibit a "whoop" sound on inspiration after a coughing attack. ▪ Highly contagious through droplet infection ▪ Coughing spells can last for more than a minute; child may turn red or purple. ▪ Does not cause the typical whooping illness in adults; causes severe upper respiratory infection that could be an entry pathway to pneumonia in older persons
Pneumonia	▪ An acute bacterial or viral infection of the lung that damages lung tissue, usually associated with fever, cough, and production of sputum ▪ Fluid also accumulates in the surrounding normal lung tissue, separating the alveoli from their capillaries. (Sometimes fluid can also accumulate in the pleural space.) ▪ The lung's ability to exchange oxygen and carbon dioxide is impaired. ▪ The breathing pattern does not indicate major airway obstruction, but the patient may experience tachypnea, an increase in the breathing rate, which is an attempt to compensate for the reduced amount of normal lung tissue and for the buildup of fluid.
Respiratory syncytial virus	▪ A major cause of illness in young children ▪ Causes an infection of the lungs and breathing passages ▪ Can result in other serious illnesses that affect the lungs or heart, such as bronchiolitis and pneumonia ▪ Highly contagious and spread through droplets ▪ Survives on surfaces, including hands and clothing ▪ Look for signs of dehydration. ▪ Humidified oxygen is helpful, if available.

(continued)

Table 17-5 Infectious Diseases Associated With Dyspnea *(continued)*

Disease	Characteristics
Severe acute respiratory syndrome (SARS)	▪ A virus that has caused substantial concern ▪ A serious, potentially life-threatening viral infection caused by a recently discovered family of viruses best known as the second most common cause of the common cold ▪ Usually starts with flulike symptoms, which may progress to pneumonia, respiratory failure, and, in some cases, death ▪ Thought to be transmitted primarily by close person-to-person contact
Tuberculosis	▪ A disease that can lay dormant in a person's lungs for decades, then reactivate ▪ Dangerous because many tuberculosis strains are resistant to many antibiotics ▪ Spread by cough; droplet nuclei can remain intact for decades. ▪ Use a high-efficiency particulate air (HEPA) respirator.

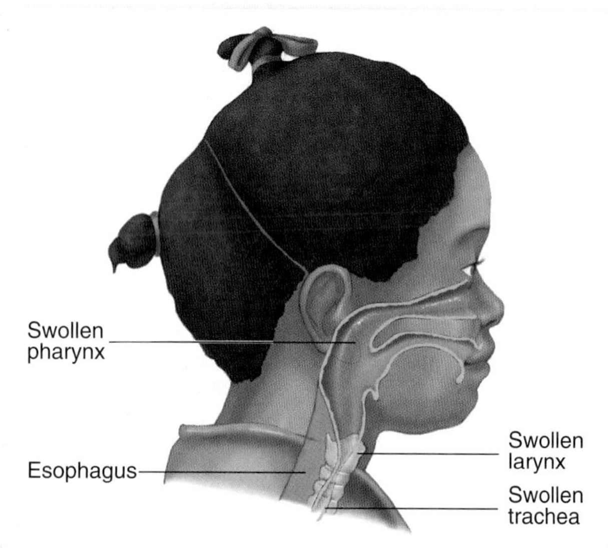

Figure 17-6 Croup swells the lining of the larynx, which is the narrowest point in the child's airway.

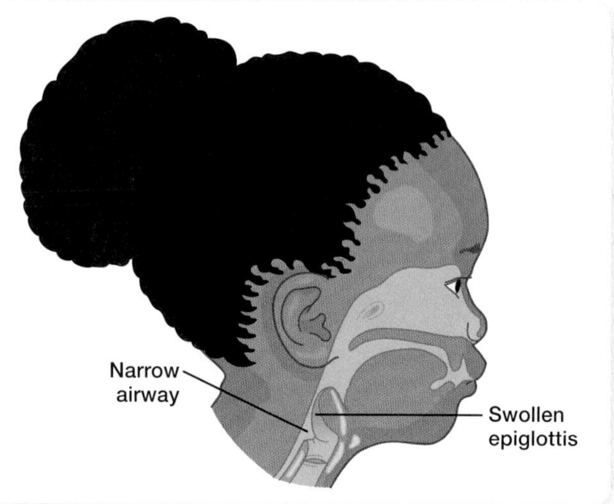

Figure 17-7 Epiglottitis is caused by a bacterial infection resulting in severe swelling of the epiglottis.

into the alveoli and in the lung tissue between the alveoli and the pulmonary capillaries. By physically separating the alveoli from the pulmonary capillary vessels, the edema interferes with the exchange of carbon dioxide and oxygen **Figure 17-8**. There is not enough room left in the lung for slow, deep breaths.

Pulmonary edema can develop quickly, especially following a major cardiovascular insult. The patient usually experiences dyspnea with rapid, shallow respirations. In the most severe instances, you will see frothy pink sputum at the nose and mouth.

Not all patients with pulmonary edema have heart disease. Poisonings from inhaling large amounts of smoke or toxic chemical fumes can produce pulmonary edema, as can traumatic injuries of the chest and exposure to high altitudes. In these cases, fluid collects in the alveoli and lung tissue in response to damage of the tissues of the lung or the bronchi.

Regardless of the initial cause, the resulting assessment findings are similar. Patients with pulmonary edema that is cardiogenic in origin may present with signs and symptoms of a cardiac emergency. Patients with non-cardiogenic pulmonary edema tend to have a history of associated factors such as a hypoxic episode, shock, chest trauma, recent acute inhalation of toxic gases or particles, or recent ascent to a high altitude without acclimatizing. In both cases, patients may also present with dyspnea, **orthopnea** (severe dyspnea experienced when lying down or in a position that is not upright, and relieved by sitting or standing up), fatigue, reduced exercise capacity, and pulmonary **crackles** (formerly known as rales).

Words of Wisdom

Any nontrauma patient experiencing difficulty breathing should immediately be placed in a position of comfort.

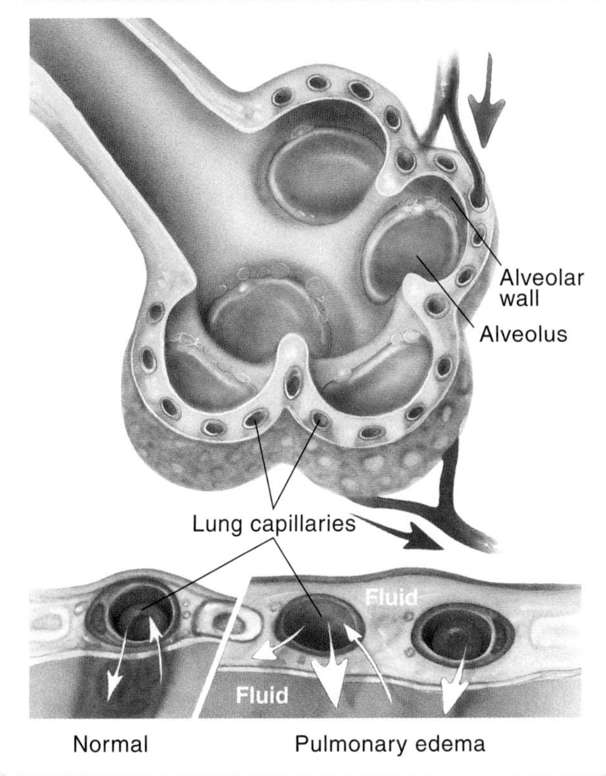

Figure 17-8 In pulmonary edema, fluid fills the alveoli and separates the capillaries from the alveolar wall, interfering with the exchange of oxygen and carbon dioxide.

Chronic Obstructive Pulmonary Disease

Chronic obstructive pulmonary disease (COPD) is a common lung condition that is a slow process of dilation and disruption of the airways and alveoli caused by chronic bronchial obstruction. COPD is an umbrella term used to describe a few lung diseases including emphysema and **chronic bronchitis**.

COPD may be a result of direct lung and airway damage from repeated infections or inhalation of toxic gases and particles, but most often it results from cigarette smoking. Obstruction occurs in the bronchioles. The cilia are unable to remove excess mucus, creating a buildup. The bronchioles dilate naturally on inspiration, enabling air to enter the alveoli despite the presence of obstruction. The bronchioles naturally constrict on expiration, and air becomes trapped distal to the obstruction on exhalation.

Tobacco smoke is a bronchial irritant and can create chronic bronchitis, an ongoing irritation of the trachea and bronchi. Chronic bronchitis results from overgrowth of the airway mucous glands and excess secretion of mucus, which blocks the airway. Patients have a chronic productive cough. The clinical definition of chronic bronchitis is a productive cough for at least 3 months per year for 2 or more consecutive years.[3]

Pneumonia develops easily when the passages are persistently obstructed. Ultimately, repeated episodes of irritation and pneumonia cause scarring in the lung

YOU are the Provider — PART 2

You find the patient sitting on the bed in a tripod position. She has cyanosis around her lips and is in obvious respiratory distress. She is slow to respond to questions and is unable to answer in complete sentences. Her pulse oximetry (Spo_2) is 91%. On auscultation of her chest you note wheezing in the upper lobes and diminished breath sounds in the lower lobes. Her skin is warm and dry to touch and she has strong, rapid radial pulses. Your partner places her on a nonrebreathing mask at 15 L/min and begins to take vital signs while you complete your assessment. A quick check shows no signs of peripheral edema. The patient states she has not felt well for a couple of days and she was discharged from the hospital about a month ago for exacerbation of her emphysema. Your partner relays her vital signs and you note that she is tachycardic and tachypneic. You advise the patient of your findings and recommendations and she consents to treatment and transport.

Recording Time: 1 Minute	
Appearance	Pale, cyanotic, and anxious
Level of consciousness	Alert, lethargic, but slow to respond to questions due to dyspnea
Airway	Patent
Breathing	30 breaths/min
Circulation	Bounding radial pulses; skin is warm, pale, and cyanotic

3. What would your next course of action be?
4. Should this patient be loaded on the stretcher and treated in the ambulance, or should you treat her at the scene?

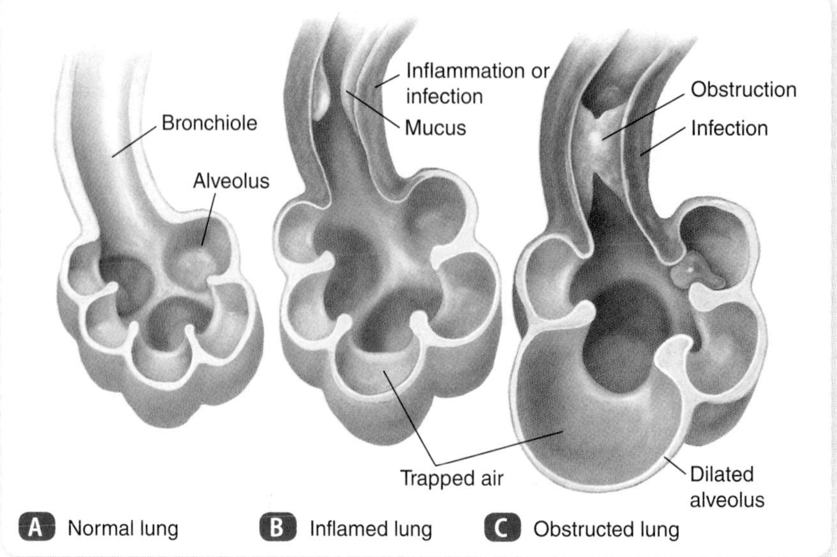

Figure 17-9 Repeated episodes of irritation and inflammation in the alveoli result in the obstruction, scarring, and some dilation of the alveolar sac characteristic of chronic obstructive pulmonary disease. **A.** Normal alveolus. **B.** Infection produces mucus and swelling. **C.** A mucous plug creates an obstruction and further dilation of the alveolus.

and some dilation of the obstructed alveoli, resulting in COPD **Figure 17-9**.

The most common form of COPD is emphysema. Emphysema is a degenerative condition characterized by destruction of the alveolar walls related to the destruction of pulmonary surfactant. Surfactant is a substance that lines and lubricates the alveolar walls, allowing them to easily expand and recoil. After the amount of surfactant is reduced, elasticity is diminished. With emphysema, elastic material in the lungs is lost when the alveolar air spaces are chronically stretched as a result of inflamed airways and obstruction of airflow out of the lungs. Normally, the lungs act like spongy balloons that are inflated; after they are inflated, they will naturally recoil because of their elastic nature, expelling gas rapidly. However, when they are constantly obstructed or when the elasticity is diminished, air is no longer expelled rapidly, and the walls of the alveoli eventually fall apart, leaving large "holes" in the lung that resemble large air pockets or cavities.

Emphysema is an irreversible condition; however, with proper treatment, its progression can be slowed. Emphysema also makes the alveoli susceptible to collapse (atelectasis). Chronically low oxygen levels associated with emphysema stimulate the production of red blood cells, sometimes in excessive quantity (polycythemia). As a result, the patient's skin tends to remain pink.

Most patients with COPD have elements of both chronic bronchitis and emphysema. They have a history of recurring lung problems and are almost always long-term cigarette smokers. Some patients will have more elements of one condition than the other; few patients will have only emphysema or bronchitis. Therefore, most patients with COPD will produce sputum, have a chronic cough, and have difficulty expelling air from their lungs, with long expiration phases and wheezing.

Words of Wisdom

Normal breathing should be quiet and not grossly evident to you. If you can see or hear the patient breathe, there is a problem.

The patient in an acute COPD episode will complain of shortness of breath with gradually increasing symptoms over a period of days and often exhales through pursed lips. Patients with COPD may complain of tightness in the chest and constant fatigue. Because air has been gradually and continuously trapped in their lungs in increasing amounts, their chests often have a barrel-like appearance **Figure 17-10**. If you listen to the chest with a stethoscope, you will hear abnormal breath sounds, discussed in detail later in this chapter.

Asthma

Asthma is an acute spasm of the smaller air passages called bronchioles that is associated with excessive mucus production and spasm of the bronchiolar muscles **Figure 17-11**.[4] It is a common but serious disease. Asthma is a reversible obstruction that is caused by a combination of smooth-muscle spasm (bronchospasm), mucus production, and edema. **Status asthmaticus** is

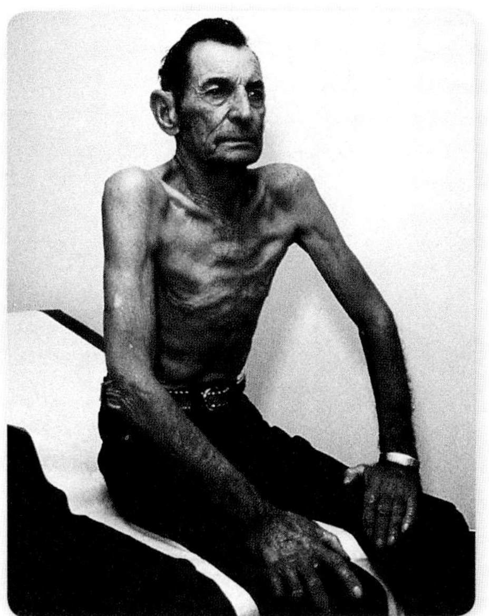

Figure 17-10 Typically, a patient with chronic obstructive pulmonary disease has a barrel-shaped chest and uses accessory muscles and pursed lips for breathing. Notice also that the patient is sitting in the tripod position.

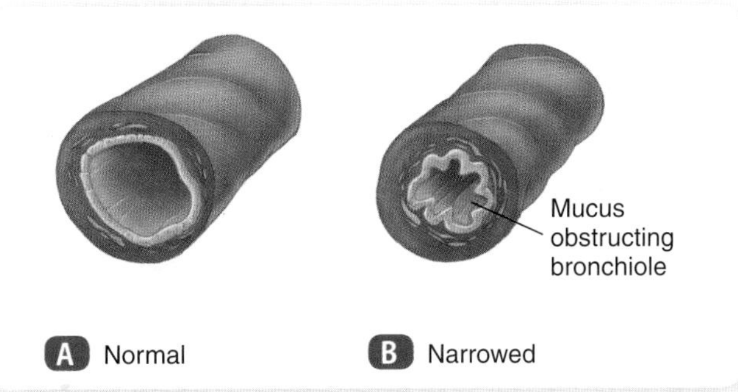

Figure 17-11 Asthma is an acute spasm of the bronchioles. **A.** Cross section of a normal bronchiole. **B.** The bronchiole in spasm; a mucous plug has formed and partially obstructed the bronchiole.

a severe, prolonged asthmatic attack that cannot be resolved with conventional treatment. It is a dire medical emergency.

Asthma produces a characteristic wheezing as the patient attempts to exhale through partially obstructed air passages; wheezing is indicative of a narrowed lower airway. These same air passages open easily during inspiration so that breathing appears relatively normal; the wheezing is heard only when they exhale. This wheezing may be so loud that you can hear it without a stethoscope, which is known as audible wheezing.[5] Continuous wheezing occurs during inspiration and expiration and is generally diffuse, or heard throughout the lungs, not just over one particular lobe. In other cases, the airways are so blocked that no air movement is heard (a silent chest). In severe cases, the actual work of exhaling is very tiring, and cyanosis, respiratory arrest, or both may develop.

Asthma affects people of all ages and is usually the result of an allergic reaction to an inhaled, ingested, or injected substance. It may also be induced by exercise, severe emotional stress, or respiratory infections.

Most patients with asthma are familiar with their symptoms and know when an attack is imminent. Typically, they will have appropriate medication with them or at home. Listen carefully to what patients tell you; they often know exactly what they need.

▶ Anaphylactic Reactions

Patients who do not have asthma may still have severe allergic reactions. Anaphylaxis is a severe allergic reaction characterized by airway swelling and dilation of blood vessels all over the body, which may substantially lower blood pressure. The pathophysiology of anaphylaxis is covered in detail in Chapter 22, *Immunologic Emergencies*. This condition is sometimes referred to as anaphylactic shock. Anaphylactic shock may cause respiratory distress that is severe enough to result in coma and death.

Anaphylaxis may be associated with widespread hives (urticaria), itching, signs of shock, and signs and symptoms similar to those of asthma. The airway may swell so much that breathing problems can progress from extreme difficulty in breathing to total airway obstruction in a matter of a few minutes. Most anaphylactic reactions occur within 30 minutes of exposure to the **allergen**, which can be anything from certain nuts or other foods to a penicillin injection. Because this may be the first time such a reaction to the substance has occurred, some patients may not know what caused the swelling and allergic reaction. In other cases, the patient may know of the allergen but not be aware of exposure. This is a true emergency.

Words of Wisdom

To determine the degree of nocturnal dyspnea, ask the patient how many pillows he or she sleeps on at night. If a patient cannot breathe well while lying flat and needs to adjust his or her sleep position to breathe, there is a problem. The greater the number of pillows needed, the greater the degree of respiratory difficulty.

▶ Spontaneous Pneumothorax

Normally, the "vacuum" pressure in the pleural space keeps the lung inflated. When the surface of the lung is disrupted, however, air escapes into the pleural cavity, and the negative vacuum pressure is lost; the natural elasticity of the lung tissue causes the lung to collapse. The accumulation of air in the pleural space, which may be partial or complete, is called a pneumothorax **Figure 17-12**. Pneumothorax is most often caused by trauma, but it also can be caused by some medical conditions without any

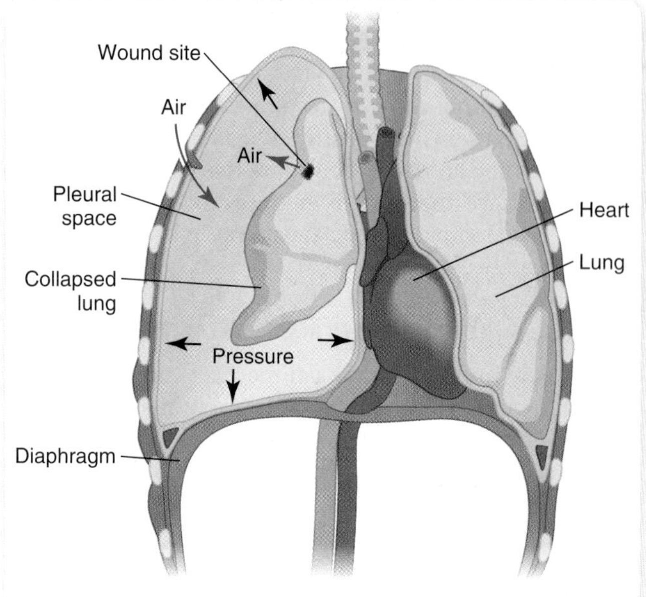

Figure 17-12 A pneumothorax occurs when air leaks into the pleural space from an opening in the chest wall or the surface of the lung. The lung collapses as air fills the pleural space and the two pleural surfaces are no longer in contact.

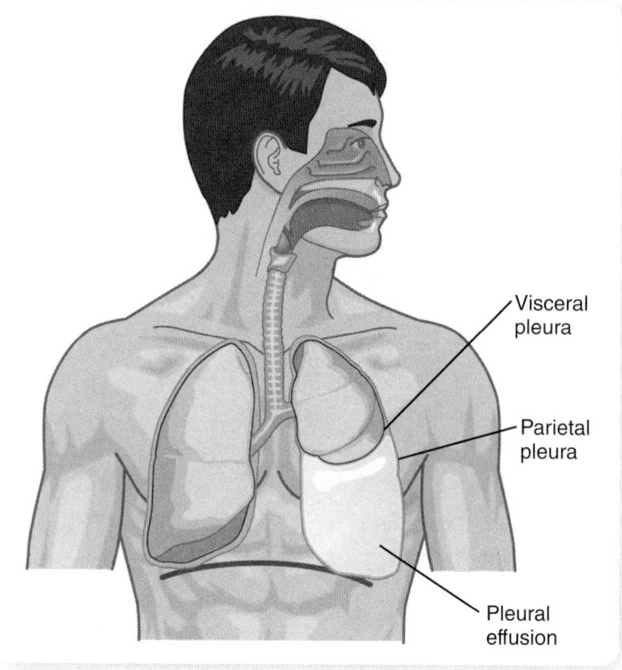

Figure 17-13 With a pleural effusion, fluid may accumulate in large volumes on one or both sides, compressing the lungs and causing dyspnea.

injury. In these cases, the condition is called spontaneous pneumothorax.

Spontaneous pneumothorax may occur in patients with certain chronic lung infections or in young people born with weak areas of the lung. Patients with emphysema and asthma are at high risk for spontaneous pneumothorax when a weakened portion of lung ruptures, often during severe coughing. Tall, thin, athletic males are also at higher risk for spontaneous pneumothorax, particularly while performing strenuous activities, such as heavy lifting.

A patient with a spontaneous pneumothorax becomes acutely dyspneic (short of breath) and typically complains of **pleuritic chest pain**, a sharp, stabbing pain on one side that is worse during breathing or with certain movement of the chest wall. Patients may also present with subcutaneous emphysema, or air bubbles trapped under the skin in the subcutaneous tissue, that may be found while palpating the chest. By listening to the chest with a stethoscope, you may note that breath sounds are absent or decreased on the affected side. However, altered breath sounds are difficult to detect in patients with severe emphysema. Spontaneous pneumothorax may be the cause of a sudden worsening of dyspnea in a patient with underlying emphysema. Patients experiencing minor problems may be pale, diaphoretic, and tachypneic. Severe findings include altered mental status, cyanosis, tachycardia, unilaterally decreased breath sounds, local hyperresonance to percussion, and subcutaneous emphysema. Tracheal deviation may be seen as a late sign. These patients require immediate care to survive.

▶ Pleural Effusion

A pleural effusion is a collection of fluid outside the lung on one or both sides of the chest. By compressing one or both lungs, it causes dyspnea **Figure 17-13**. This fluid may collect in large volumes in response to any irritation, infection, heart failure, or cancer. Although it can build up gradually over days or even weeks, patients often report that their dyspnea began suddenly. Pleural effusions should be considered a possibility in any patient with lung cancer and shortness of breath.

When you listen with a stethoscope to the chest of a patient with dyspnea resulting from pleural effusion, you will hear decreased breath sounds over the region of the chest where fluid has moved the lung away from the chest wall. These patients frequently feel better if they are sitting upright. Definitive care for the patient with a pleural effusion includes removing the fluid, a procedure that must be performed by a physician.

▶ Pulmonary Embolism

An **embolus** is anything in the circulatory system that moves from its point of origin and travels to a distant site where it lodges, creating a perfusion disorder by obstructing subsequent blood flow in that area. Beyond the point of obstruction, circulation can be markedly decreased or completely cut off, causing deep vein stasis or stagnation of blood, which can result in a serious life-threatening condition. Emboli can be fragments of blood clots in an artery or vein that break off and travel through the bloodstream. They also can be foreign bodies

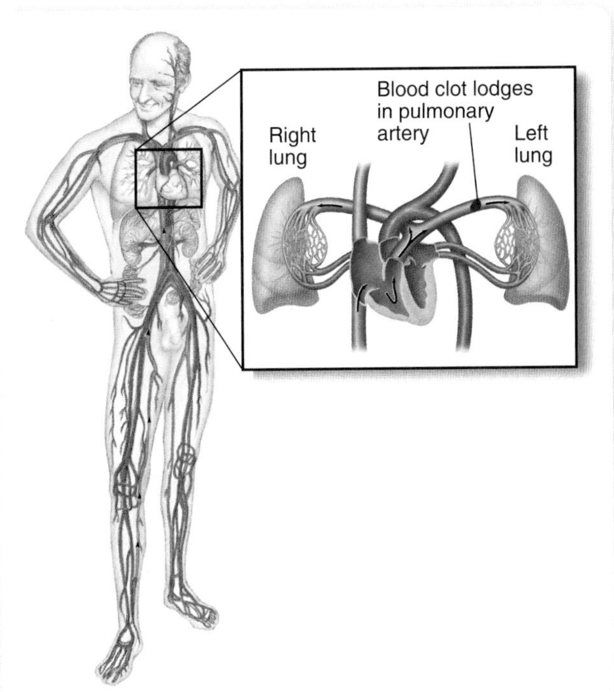

Figure 17-14 A pulmonary embolism is a blood clot from the vein that breaks off, circulates through the venous system, and moves through the right side of the heart into a pulmonary artery. Here, it can become lodged and substantially obstruct blood flow.

that enter the circulation, such as a piece of the material from a catheter shear or a bubble of air.

A pulmonary embolism is a blood clot (thrombus) formed in a vein, usually in the legs or pelvis, that breaks off and circulates through the venous system. The large clot moves through the right side of the heart and into a pulmonary artery, where it becomes lodged, substantially decreasing or blocking blood flow Figure 17-14. Even though the lung is actively involved in inhalation and exhalation of air, no exchange of oxygen or carbon dioxide takes place in the areas of blocked blood flow because there is no effective circulation. As a result of the ventilation-perfusion mismatch, the level of arterial carbon dioxide rises, and the oxygen level may drop substantially, perhaps to a point at which cyanosis develops.

Pulmonary emboli may occur as a result of damage to the lining of vessels, causing platelet aggregation, a tendency for blood to clot unusually fast (hypercoagulability), or, most often, slow blood flow in a lower extremity. Slow blood flow in the legs can occur when patients are bedridden, which can result in the collapse of veins. Patients whose legs are immobilized following a fracture or recent surgery are at risk for pulmonary emboli for days or weeks after the incident. Pregnancy and active cancer are other risk factors. Additional risk factors include recent surgery, pregnancy, oral contraceptives, smoking, infection, cancer, sickle cell anemia, and prolonged inactivity; patients who are bedridden also are at risk. Pulmonary emboli occur less commonly in active, healthy people without other risk factors.

Estimates suggest that 300,000 to 900,000 people in the United States are affected each year by pulmonary emboli, and 10% to 30% will die within 1 month of diagnosis.[6] Signs and symptoms, when they occur, include the following:

- Dyspnea
- Tachycardia
- Tachypnea
- Varying degrees of hypoxia
- Cyanosis
- Acute chest pain
- Hemoptysis (coughing up blood)

When a patient has a possible pulmonary embolus, the chief complaint is usually a sudden onset of inspiratory chest pain, dyspnea, and nonproductive cough. Identifying possible risk factors may help to narrow the causes for the chief complaint. With a large enough embolus, complete, sudden obstruction of the output of blood flow from the right side of the heart can result in sudden death.

▶ Obstruction of the Airway

As an AEMT, you should always be aware of the possibility that a patient with dyspnea may have a mechanical obstruction of the airway and be prepared to treat it quickly. In an unresponsive patient, the obstruction may be the result of vomitus or a foreign object Figure 17-15A or improper positioning of the head so that the tongue is blocking the airway Figure 17-15B.

Always consider upper airway obstruction from a foreign body first in patients who were eating just before becoming short of breath.

▶ Environmental/Industrial Exposure

Many accidental exposures that cause inhalation injury and dyspnea occur at industrial sites. Pesticides, cleaning solutions, chemicals, chlorine, and other gases can be accidentally released and inhaled by employees. Sometimes chemicals such as ammonia and chlorine bleach are mixed and create a hazardous by-product. Carbon monoxide is another toxic, odorless, highly poisonous gas that is produced in industrial settings by vehicles, gasoline-powered tools, and heaters.

The type of damage from the substance depends in large part on the water solubility of the toxic gas. Highly water-soluble gases such as ammonia will react with the moist mucous membranes of the upper airway and cause swelling and irritation. If the substance gets in the patient's eyes, they will also burn and feel inflamed and irritated. Less water-soluble gases such as phosgene and nitrogen dioxide may get deep into the lower airway, where they may cause pulmonary edema up to 24 hours later.

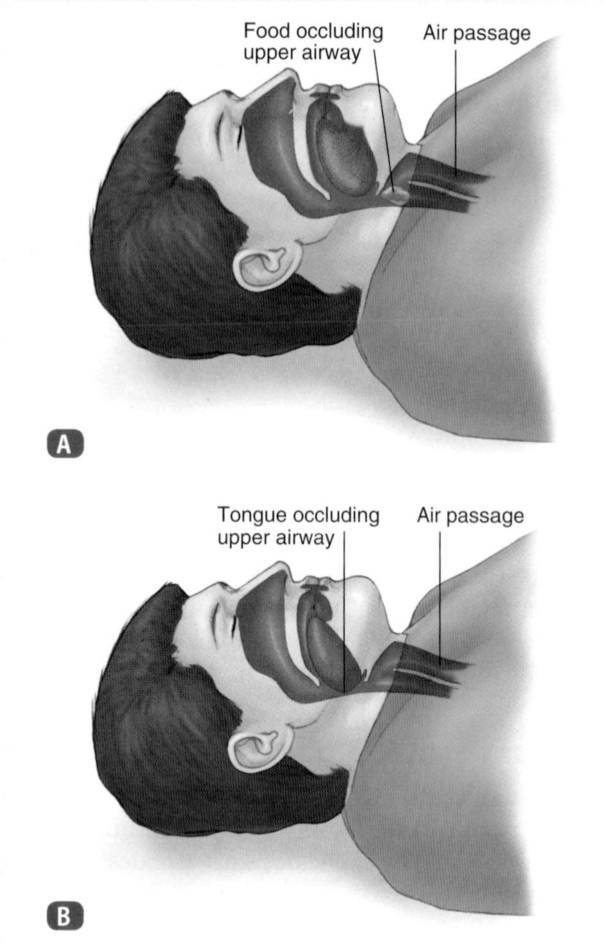

Figure 17-15 A. Foreign body obstruction occurs when an object, such as food, is lodged in the airway. **B.** Mechanical obstruction also occurs when the head is not properly positioned, causing the tongue to fall back into the throat.

Safety

If you suspect that a patient has an airborne disease, place a surgical mask (or a nonrebreathing mask if needed) on the patient. When you have specific reason to suspect tuberculosis, do this and also place a high-efficiency particulate air (HEPA) respirator on yourself.

▶ Cystic Fibrosis

Cystic fibrosis (CF) is a genetic disorder that affects the lungs and digestive system. The disease is usually fatal, with most children not living past their teens; however, because of advances in treatment, the life expectancy for patients with CF becomes better each year. With aggressive management and careful monitoring, some patients may live well into their 30s.

CF is caused by a defective gene, which makes it difficult for chloride to move through cells. This causes unusually high sodium loss and abnormally thick mucus secretions. The secretions in the lungs cause breathing difficulties and provide an ideal growing medium for bacteria, leaving the patient highly susceptible to infection. Ultimately, the lung damage from the condition results in lung disease, the primary cause of death in affected persons.

In CF, the child's symptoms range from sinus congestion to wheezing and asthma-like complaints. The child may have a chronic cough that produces thick, heavy, discolored mucus. He or she may also present with tachypnea, shortness of breath, barrel chest, clubbed fingers, and cyanosis. The thick mucus may also collect in the intestines. The child often has dyspnea; this generally results in the parents calling EMS. Treat the child with suction and oxygen using age-appropriate adjuncts. Keep a keen eye out for respiratory insufficiency, signs of a respiratory infection, and intestinal blockage.

CF often causes death in childhood because of chronic pneumonia secondary to the thick pathologic mucus in the airway. Adults with CF are predisposed to other medical conditions, including arthritis, osteoporosis, diabetes, and liver problems.

▶ Age-Related Conditions

Bronchiolitis

Bronchiolitis is an inflammation of the small airways (bronchioles) in the lower respiratory tract as a result of viral infection. The most common source of this disease is respiratory syncytial virus (RSV), although a new virus, *Metapneumovirus*, has also been found to cause this illness. These viruses occur with highest frequency during the late fall and winter months,[7] and they primarily affect infants and children younger than 2 years. Severity ranges from mild to moderate respiratory distress with hypoxia and respiratory failure.

The signs and symptoms of bronchiolitis can be difficult to distinguish from those of asthma, but note the child's age. Asthma is rare in children younger than 1 year; an infant with a first-time wheezing episode occurring in late fall or winter likely has bronchiolitis. Mild to moderate retractions, tachypnea, diffuse wheezing, diffuse crackles, and mild hypoxia are characteristic findings. As with asthma, a sleepy or obtunded patient or one with severe retractions, diminished breath sounds, or moderate to severe hypoxia (oxygen saturation $<90\%$) is in danger of respiratory failure and requires immediate ventilatory support and transport.

Respiratory Syncytial Virus

As mentioned, RSV is a common cause of illness in young children. It causes an infection in the lungs and breathing passages and can result in other serious illnesses such as bronchiolitis and pneumonia, as well as serious heart and lung problems in premature infants and children who have depressed immune systems.

RSV is highly contagious and can be spread through droplets when the patient coughs or sneezes. The virus can also survive on surfaces, including hands and clothing. Therefore, the infection tends to spread rapidly through schools and in child care centers.

RSV can also cause severe upper respiratory infections and typical asthma symptoms in adults and geriatric patients.

Croup

Croup is caused by inflammation and swelling of the pharynx, larynx, and trachea. This disease is often secondary to an acute viral infection of the upper respiratory tract and is typically seen in children between ages 6 months and 3 years. It is easily passed between children.

The disease starts with a cold, cough, and a low-grade fever that develop over 2 days. The hallmark signs of croup are stridor and a seal-bark cough, which signal a substantial narrowing of the air passage of the trachea that may progress to marked obstruction. Peak seasonal outbreaks of this disease occur in the late fall and during the winter.

Croup is rarely seen in adults because their breathing passages are larger and can accommodate the inflammation and mucus production without producing symptoms. The airways of adults are wider, and the supporting tissue is firmer than in children.

Croup often responds well to the administration of humidified oxygen.

Epiglottitis

Epiglottitis is a life-threatening inflammatory disease of the epiglottis, the small flap of tissue at the back of the throat that protects the larynx and trachea during swallowing. It is usually caused by a bacterial infection that produces severe swelling of the flap over the larynx. Although epiglottitis may be seen at any age, it is much more predominant in children. The development of a childhood vaccine against *Haemophilus influenzae* has dramatically decreased the incidence of this disease.

In preschool and school-aged children especially, the epiglottis can swell to two to three times its normal size. This puts the airway at risk of complete obstruction. Patients with epiglottitis will look very sick. Epiglottitis usually has a sudden onset in an otherwise healthy child; children with this infection look ill, complain of a very sore throat, and have a high fever. They will usually be in the tripod position and drooling. Patients may also have stridor, high-pitched inspiratory sounds indicating partial airway obstruction.

Occasionally, the constellation of symptoms of epiglottitis can also appear in an adult or a geriatric patient, especially if the patient has other issues such as diabetes, which affect his or her ability to fight off disease. In adults, epiglottitis, or supraglottitis, can be caused by different bacterial or viral organisms. Acute epiglottitis in an adult or geriatric patient can be potentially life threatening and not recognized because it more commonly occurs in pediatric patients. Deterioration can occur quickly in adults with acute epiglottitis. You should be concerned if your patient is an adult presenting with stridor or any other sign of anatomic airway obstruction.

Pneumonia

Pneumonia is a ventilation disorder caused by an infection of the lung parenchyma, which is the tissue of the lung itself. It is the eighth leading cause of death in the United States and is not a single disease, but a group of specific infections.[8] Young children are at risk for pneumonia because of their immature immune systems. Older adults are also at risk because of age-related weakening of the immune system.

Pneumonia presents as a localized infection in the lungs that may cause atelectasis, or alveolar collapse. If not treated promptly, the infection may become systemic, resulting in sepsis and septic shock. Typical findings with pneumonia include an acute onset of fever and chills, productive cough with purulent (thick) sputum, pleuritic chest pain, and excessive mucus causing pulmonary consolidation that may be detected by auscultation in the form of rales or rhonchi.

Pertussis

Pertussis (whooping cough) is an airborne bacterial infection that primarily affects children younger than 6 years. It is highly contagious and is passed through droplet infection. In infants younger than 6 months, pertussis can be life threatening.

A patient with pertussis will be feverish and exhibit a "whoop" sound on inspiration after a coughing attack. Symptoms of pertussis are generally similar to those of colds, and you should look for signs of dehydration. The coughing spells can last for more than 1 minute, during which the child may turn red or purple. This may frighten the parents into calling 9-1-1.

Pertussis in adults does not cause the typical whooping illness that it does in infants and toddlers, but can cause severe coughing spells that can actually result in fracture of the ribs, and if the patient is already weak, pertussis can result in hospitalization.

Airway Obstruction

Always consider upper airway obstruction from a foreign body first when a young child becomes short of breath. This is especially true of crawling babies, who might have swallowed and choked on a small object. Inflammation of the tonsils may also partially occlude the airway, creating an obstruction. Dysfunction of a tracheostomy may also create an upper airway obstruction, especially if plugged with mucus or other secretions.

The obstruction may be in the lower airway, below the vocal cords. Trauma to the trachea may result in a crushing injury, fractured larynx, or edema that obstructs the lower airway. Obstruction may also be in the form of obstructive lung disease, mucus accumulation, or smooth muscle spasm. Edema also may be present when a patient has been exposed to toxic chemicals or superheated air, as in a structural fire.

Heart Failure

Sometimes, the heart muscle is so injured after a heart attack or other illness that it cannot circulate blood properly. The heart is not able to maintain cardiac output that meets the needs of the body; thus the heart is failing as a pump. In these cases, the left side of the heart cannot remove blood from the lung as fast as the right side delivers it. As a result, fluid builds up within the alveoli and in the lung tissue between the alveoli and the pulmonary capillaries. This accumulation of fluid is referred to as pulmonary edema, and it is usually a result of heart failure.

Patient risk factors for heart failure include hypertension and a history of coronary artery disease and/or atrial fibrillation, a condition in which the atria no longer contract, but instead quiver.

In most cases, patients have a long-standing history of chronic heart failure that can be controlled with medication. However, an acute onset may occur if the patient stops taking the medication, eats food that is too salty, or has a stressful illness, a new heart attack, or an abnormal heart rhythm.

Signs and symptoms of heart failure include difficulty breathing with exertion because the heart cannot keep up with the body's need for oxygen. Patients may also report a sudden attack of respiratory distress that wakes them at night when they are in a reclining position. This is caused by fluid accumulation in the lungs. Patients also report coughing, feeling suffocated, cold sweats, and tachycardia.

Wet Lungs Versus Dry Lungs and "Cardiac Asthma"

Confusion sometimes exists between the concepts *wet lungs* in pulmonary edema, caused most often by heart failure, and *dry lungs* in COPD. Table 17-6 compares the differences between COPD and heart failure.

Suppose you are called to assist an 80-year-old man who has had shortness of breath for 45 minutes. Physical examination reveals that his pulse and respirations are elevated and you can see that he has pedal edema and jugular vein distention. His lung sound check reveals wheezing. He has a history of hypertension, heart failure, and myocardial infarction; however, he has no history of smoking.

Are patients with heart failure supposed to have crackles rather than wheezing? Breath sounds are extremely helpful but can also be confusing. In a case in which the alveoli are so full of fluid, bubbles (the condition that gives the sound of crackles) cannot form. The bronchi also become constricted, which produces wheezing. This

Table 17-6 Comparison of Chronic Obstructive Pulmonary Disease and Heart Failure

	Chronic Obstructive Pulmonary Disease	Heart Failure
Description	▪ A slow process of dilation and disruption of the airways and alveoli caused by chronic bronchial obstruction ▪ Usually in long-term smokers	▪ A disease of the heart characterized by shortness of breath, edema, and weakness ▪ Patient may or may not smoke
Pathophysiology	Emphysema: ▪ Destruction of the airways distal to the bronchiole ▪ Destruction of the pulmonary capillary bed ▪ Decreased ability to oxygenate the blood ▪ Lower cardiac output and hyperventilation ▪ Development of muscle wasting and weight loss Chronic bronchitis: ▪ Excessive mucus production with airway obstruction ▪ Pulmonary capillary bed undamaged ▪ Compensation by decreasing ventilation and increasing cardiac output ▪ Poorly ventilated lungs, resulting in hypoxemia ▪ Increased carbon dioxide retention	▪ Damaged ventricles and failure of heart as a pump ▪ Attempt by heart to compensate with increased rate ▪ Enlarged left ventricle ▪ Backup of fluid into the body as the heart fails to pump adequately

	Chronic Obstructive Pulmonary Disease	Heart Failure
Appearance	▪ Use of accessory muscles Emphysema: ▪ Thin appearance with barrel chest ▪ "Puffing" (pursed-lip) style of breathing ▪ Tripod position Chronic bronchitis: ▪ May be obese ▪ Difficulty with expiration	▪ Abdominal distention ▪ Dependent edema (sacral or pedal) ▪ Tachycardia ▪ Increased respiratory rate ▪ Anxiety ▪ Inability to lie flat ▪ Ashen or cyanotic
Level of consciousness	Normal or altered	Confusion
Neck veins	▪ Flat ▪ Distended when heart failure also present	Distended
Skin color	▪ In emphysema, pink ▪ In chronic bronchitis, blue, often cyanotic	Blue
Lung condition	▪ In emphysema, dry ▪ In chronic bronchitis, wet when heart failure also present	Wet
Breathing	▪ Shortness of breath (mostly on exertion) ▪ Breathing worsens over time (progressive)	▪ Shortness of breath all the time ▪ Sudden onset of shortness of breath
Breath sounds	Rhonchi, wheezing	Crackles, wheezing
Circulation	No dependent edema	Dependent edema
Cough	▪ In emphysema, little or none ▪ In chronic bronchitis, frequent or chronic cough	Coughing may be present; increases when supine
Sputum	▪ In emphysema, no mucus ▪ In chronic bronchitis, excessive, thick mucus	Pink, frothy sputum
Medications	Home oxygen, bronchodilators, and steroids help open the airways	Diuretics and antihypertensives help promote cardiac function and reduce fluid loads on the heart

patient is experiencing cardiac asthma, which is even more confusing because the patient has no history of asthma.

Patients with COPD wheeze because of bronchial constriction and present with shortness of breath. Their breathing becomes progressively worse, and they have the most trouble breathing on exertion. Patients with COPD have chronic coughing and thick sputum. They do not have jugular vein distention or dependent edema and are usually long-term smokers with a thin, barrel chest appearance. Their medications would include home oxygen, bronchodilators, and corticosteroids.

You should suspect heart failure in this patient because of the patient's elevated blood pressure, pedal edema, and history of heart failure. Unlike a typical patient with COPD, he has no history of smoking and takes diuretics and medications to reduce preload.

Patients with COPD have a slower onset of symptoms because their disease is worsened by infection and other stressors. Patients with heart failure experience a fluid overload in the lung, which develops quickly from a failing pump.

As you try to discern between COPD and heart failure, do not assume that *all* COPD patients have wheezing and *all* heart failure patients have crackles; keep an open mind so that you do not miss important differences. The best advice is to treat the patient, not the breath sounds. In some cases, a patient with COPD may have air passages that are so constricted that you do not hear anything.

Special Populations

Normal aging processes alter the respiratory system and the ability to exchange oxygen and carbon dioxide. Geriatric patients are at an increased risk of pneumonia or a worsening of asthma or COPD if the airways have lost muscle mass or tone. Secretions might not be expelled from the airways, allowing pneumonia to develop. Provide adequate ventilation and oxygenation according to the patient's needs. Geriatric patients may need ventilatory support for conditions that, in younger adults, are easily accommodated by the respiratory system.

Geriatric patients may also have a decreased ability to generate heat during a fever. Even a low-grade fever in a geriatric patient may have a serious underlying cause. Fever may also result in confusion or an altered mental status.

Patient Assessment

Assessment of patients in respiratory distress should be conducted as a calm, systematic process. Patients in respiratory distress are usually quite anxious, and they may be some of the most ill and challenging patients you will encounter.

Safety

Scene safety is crucial in a toxic environment, but you will not always be told that you are entering a toxic environment. Stay alert for clues. If you enter a house for a patient who is not feeling well and you notice others with the same symptoms, suspect a toxic emergency. Remain alert for clues throughout the call; clues may not always be apparent when you first arrive.

Scene Size-up

As always, first consider standard precautions and use of personal protective equipment (PPE). Follow local protocols.

Pulmonary complaints may be associated with exposure to a wide variety of toxins, including carbon monoxide, toxic products of combustion, or environments that have deficient ambient oxygen (such as silos and enclosed storage spaces). It is critical to ensure a safe environment for all EMS personnel before making patient contact. If necessary, personnel with specialized training and equipment should remove the patient from a hazardous environment.

After you have determined that the scene is safe, determine how many patients there are and whether you need additional or specialized resources. If there are multiple people with dyspnea, consider the possibility of an airborne hazardous material release.

If the nature of the illness is in question, ask why 9-1-1 was activated. By questioning the patient and family and/or bystanders, you should be able to determine the nature of the illness.

Primary Survey

The major focus of the primary survey is to recognize and treat life threats or potential life threats. A variety of pulmonary conditions pose a high risk for death. Recognition of life threats and the initiation of resuscitation take priority over performing a detailed assessment. Signs of life-threatening respiratory distress in adults, listed from most ominous to least severe, include the following:

- Altered mental status
- Severe cyanosis
- Absent or abnormal breath sounds
- Audible stridor
- Two- to three-word dyspnea
- Coughing
- Tachycardia of more than 130 beats/min
- Abdominal breathing
- Change in respiratory rate or rhythm
- Pallor and diaphoresis
- The presence of retractions and/or the use of the accessory muscles
- Tripod positioning

Special Populations

In children, foreign bodies such as pencil erasers, candy, and beans frequently obstruct a nostril. These items often sit in the nose for a day or two before the child presents with pain and a foul-smelling nasal discharge. Do not try to remove the obstruction yourself.

Note your general impression of the patient. A patient in substantial respiratory distress will want to sit up. In a worst-case scenario, you will arrive to see the patient in the tripod position.

Does the patient appear calm? Is he or she anxious or restless? Is he or she listless and tired? How severe is his or her breathing complaint? This initial impression will help you decide whether the patient's condition is stable or unstable. Use the AVPU (Awake and alert, responsive to Verbal stimuli, responsive to Pain, Unresponsive) scale to check for responsiveness. If the patient is alert or responding to verbal stimuli, you know that the brain is still receiving oxygen. Ask the patient about his or her chief complaint. If the patient is responsive only to painful stimuli or unresponsive, the brain may not be oxygenating well and the potential for an airway or breathing problem is more likely. If there is no gag or cough reflex, you need to immediately assess the patient's airway status. Within seconds, you will be able to determine if there are any immediate threats to life.

To evaluate airway and breathing, begin with these questions: Is the airway open and clear? Is the patient breathing? Provide the appropriate oxygen therapy for a patient with spontaneous breathing, or immediately provide positive pressure ventilations for one who is apneic. If ventilating, determine if ventilations are effective. Is there equal rise and fall of the chest, and is the heart rate decreasing appropriately?

If not, try to reposition the airway and insert an airway adjunct to keep the tongue from blocking the airway. Refer to Chapter 11, *Airway Management*, for a review of airway management and ventilation techniques. Continue to monitor the airway for fluid, secretions, and other problems as you move on to assess the adequacy of your patient's breathing.

The next step in assessing breathing in a patient with a respiratory emergency is to assess breath sounds. Techniques for this assessment are described at the end of this section.

After assessing breath sounds, evaluate circulation. Assess the pulse rate, rhythm, and character. Tachycardia or bradycardia indicates the patient may not be getting enough oxygen. An increased pulse rate is the body's way of responding to respiratory distress and can be an indicator of shock. Tachycardia is also a normal response to pain, fear, excitement, and exertion.

Assess for the presence of shock and bleeding. Respiratory distress in a patient could be caused by an insufficient number of red blood cells to transport the oxygen. Assess capillary refill in infants and children. Capillary refill is not considered a reliable assessment tool in the adult patient. Also assess perfusion by evaluating skin color, temperature, and condition.

You should now to be able to identify any life threats in your patient by the following signs or symptoms:

- Problems with airway, breathing, and circulation (ABCs)
- Poor initial general impression
- An altered mental status
- Potential hypoperfusion or shock
- Chest pain associated with low blood pressure
- Severe pain anywhere
- Excessive bleeding

If the patient's condition is unstable and there is a possible life threat, address the life threat and proceed with rapid transport. This means you will keep your scene time short, providing only life-saving interventions. Perform a secondary assessment en route to the hospital. If the patient's condition is stable and there are no life threats, you may decide to perform a thorough secondary assessment on scene, after obtaining the patient history.

YOU are the Provider — PART 3

You and your partner assist the patient onto the stretcher in a position of comfort while continuing the oxygen via nonrebreathing mask. The patient is placed in the ambulance, and per your protocols, you elect to administer a nebulized breathing treatment consisting of 2.5 mg of albuterol sulfate mixed in 3 mL of normal saline. After completion of the treatment, the patient continues to report shortness of breath and you note that she is still tachycardic. You notify the receiving facility of the treatments administered and patient response as well as current status. Medical control denies orders for a second nebulized treatment of albuterol because of the patient's tachycardia.

Recording Time: 7 Minutes	
Respirations	28 breaths/min, wheezes bilaterally
Pulse	Strong and regular, 148 beats/min
Skin	Warm, pale, and cyanotic
Blood pressure	148/92 mm Hg
Oxygen saturation (Spo_2)	91% on 100% oxygen
Pupils	Pupils Equal, Round, and Reactive to Light and Accommodation (PERRLA)

5. How can you explain the patient's elevated heart rate?
6. With this patient's history of COPD, should you be concerned about the hypoxic drive?

Assessing Breath Sounds

Auscultating breath sounds, or lung sounds, is one of the most important vital signs for your patient in respiratory distress. Listen over the bare chest. Trying to listen through clothing may give you inaccurate information. The diaphragm of the stethoscope must be in firm contact with the skin. If your patient is lying down, bring him or her to a sitting position when possible based on the patient's overall condition, which is a better position for assessing breath sounds.

You need to determine whether your patient's breath sounds are normal (**vesicular breath sounds** represent air moving in and out of the alveoli, and **bronchial breath sounds** represent air moving through the bronchi) or decreased, absent, or abnormal (adventitious breath sounds). With your stethoscope, check breath sounds on the right and left sides of the chest, and compare each side Figure 17-16. When you are listening on the patient's back, place the stethoscope head between and below the scapulae, not over them, or your assessment will not be accurate.

Make sure that you listen for a full respiratory cycle so you can detect the adventitious sounds that may be heard at the end of the inspiratory or expiratory phase. When you are assessing for fluid collection, pay special attention to the lower lung fields. Start from the bottom up and determine at which level you start hearing clear breath sounds.

You want to hear clear flow of air in both lungs. Not hearing the flow of air is considered an absent lung sound. The lack of air movement in the lung is a substantial finding. Listen carefully and do not confuse absent breath sounds with clear breath sounds. Table 17-7 provides examples of breath sounds, the diseases that may be associated with them, and important signs and symptoms.

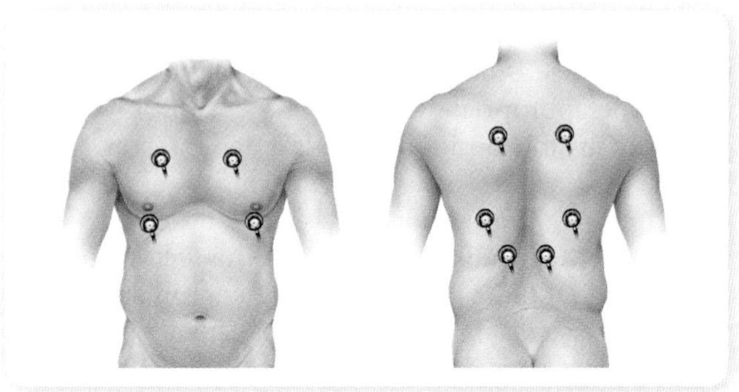

Figure 17-16 Stethoscope placement for auscultation of breath sounds.

Table 17-7 Signs, Symptoms, and Adventitious Breath Sounds Associated With Specific Respiratory Diseases

Breath Sounds	Disease	Signs and Symptoms
Wheezes	Asthma COPD Heart failure/pulmonary edema Pneumonia Bronchitis Anaphylaxis	Dyspnea Productive or nonproductive cough Dependent edema, pink frothy sputum Fever, pleuritic chest pain Clear or white sputum Hives, facial swelling, stridor, nonproductive cough
Rhonchi	COPD Pneumonia Bronchitis	Productive cough Fever, pleuritic chest pain Clear or white sputum
Crackles	Heart failure/pulmonary edema Pneumonia	Dependent edema, pink frothy sputum Fever, pleuritic chest pain
Stridor	Croup Epiglottitis	Fever, barking cough Fever, sore throat, drooling
Decreased or absent breath sounds	Asthma COPD Pneumonia Hemothorax Pneumothorax Atelectasis	Nonproductive cough, dyspnea Productive cough Fever, pleuritic chest pain Shock, respiratory distress Dyspnea, pleuritic chest pain Fever, decreased oxygen saturation

Abbreviation: COPD, chronic obstructive pulmonary disease

Abnormal breath sounds may include crackles (rales), which are sounds of air trying to pass through fluid in the alveoli. They are usually related to chronic scarring of small airways. It is a crackling or bubbling sound typically heard on inspiration. There are high-pitched sounds called fine crackles and low-pitched sounds called coarse crackles. These sounds are often a result of heart failure, pulmonary edema, or fluid in the lungs caused by heart failure.

Rhonchi are lower pitched sounds caused by secretions or mucus in the larger airway. The sound resembles rattling. This can be heard with infections such as pneumonia, bronchitis, or in cases of aspiration.

Stridor is a high-pitched sound heard on inspiration as air tries to pass through an obstruction in the upper airway. This sound indicates a partial obstruction of the trachea and is seen in patients with anatomic or foreign body airway obstruction.

Wheezing is a high-pitched whistling sound typically heard on expiration. It indicates constriction and/or inflammation in the bronchus. Wheezing is common in patients with asthma and sometimes in patients with COPD. Because of large emphysematous air pockets and diminished airflow, sounds of breathing are frequently difficult to hear and may be detected only high up on the posterior portion of the chest.

A **pleural friction rub** is a squeaking or grating sound that occurs when the pleural linings rub together. If this occurs, the pleural layers have lost their lubrication, most commonly because of pleural inflammation. This condition is usually associated with pain on inspiration. The sounds may be heard anytime the chest wall moves; therefore, they can be heard on inspiration, expiration, or both.

Finally, snoring sounds are indicative of a partial upper airway obstruction, usually in the oropharynx.

History Taking

After you form your general impression and have completed the primary survey, ask the patient to describe the problem to determine the chief complaint.

Questioning a Patient With Difficulty Breathing

With patients in respiratory distress, the SAMPLE history (Signs and symptoms, Allergies, Medications, Pertinent past medical history, Last oral intake, Events leading up to the illness or injury) can be obtained from the family or bystanders if they are present. Limit the number of questions to pertinent ones—a patient who is in respiratory distress does not need to be using any additional air to answer questions.

Be sure to ask the following questions about a patient in respiratory distress:

- What is the patient's general state of health?
- Has the patient had any childhood or adult diseases?
- Have there been any recent surgeries or hospitalizations?
- Have there been any traumatic injuries?
- Is there any dyspnea or chest pain?

If time allows, also ask about the patient's immunization history.

Because chronically ill patients live with their condition every day, when they call EMS, something has changed for the worse. Ask about previous episodes, medication allergies, and current medications. The patient's subjective description of the problem is an accurate indicator of the acuity of this episode if the disease is chronic. Start by asking the patient "What happened the last time you had an attack this bad?" or "What did the doctor do then?" The answer provides an extremely useful predictor of the current episode's course. If you do not know the diagnosis, try to learn whether the problem is related primarily to ventilation, diffusion, perfusion, or a combination. Any history of intubation is an accurate indicator of severe pulmonary disease and suggests that intubation by paramedics may be required again.

Find out what the patient has already done for the breathing problem. Pay close attention to the medications the patient is currently taking. Does the patient use a prescribed inhaler or a small-volume nebulizer? If so, when was it used last? How many doses have been taken? Are there any pulmonary medications, and if so, are they inhaled, oral, or parenteral? Consult medical control. Remember to report the name of the medication, when the patient last took a puff, how many puffs were used at that time, and what the label states regarding dosage. If medical control permits, you may administer a bronchodilator via nebulizer, which is discussed later.

Words of Wisdom

The presence of corticosteroids or other steroids in the patient's daily medication regimen strongly suggests severe chronic disease.

If the patient does not have a prescribed inhaler, continue with the history taking and secondary assessment. Despite use of the inhaler, the patient's condition may continue to worsen. You need to reassess breathing frequently and be prepared to assist ventilation in severe cases.

Also, find out whether the patient has any allergies or history of medication reactions.

Use the OPQRST-I mnemonic to determine the specifics of pain and obtain specific information about the breathing problem:

- When did the breathing problem begin (Onset)?
- What makes the breathing difficulty worse or better (Provocation or palliation)?
- How does the breathing feel (Quality)?
- Does the discomfort move (Radiation/region)?

- How much of a problem is the patient having (Severity)? On a scale of 1 to 10, with 10 being the worst pain the patient has ever had, how bad is it?
- Is the problem continuous or intermittent? If it is intermittent, how frequently does it occur and long does it last (Timing)?
- What has been done to alleviate the problem prior to EMS arrival (Interventions)? Any medications taken?

Other questions to ask include:

- Does the patient have a cough? Is it productive or nonproductive? If it is productive, what color is the sputum?
- Is there any hemoptysis? Wheezing? Fever? Chills?
- Any increased sputum production?
- Has there been any exposure to smoke or does the patient have a history of smoking?

Chronic Respiratory Conditions

Different respiratory complaints offer different clues and different challenges. Patients with chronic conditions may have long periods in which they are able to live relatively normal lives but then sometimes experience acute worsening of their conditions. That is when you are called, and it is important for you to be able to determine your patient's baseline status, in other words, his or her normal condition, and what is different this time that made the patient call you. For example, patients with COPD (emphysema and chronic bronchitis) do not cope well with pulmonary infections because the existing airway damage makes them unable to cough up the mucus or sputum produced by the infection. The chronic lower airway obstruction makes it difficult for the patient to breathe deeply enough to clear the lungs. Gradually, the arterial oxygen level falls, and the carbon dioxide level rises. If a new infection of the lung occurs in a patient with COPD, the arterial oxygen level may fall rapidly. In a few patients, the carbon dioxide level may become high enough to cause sleepiness. In these cases, patients require respiratory support and administration of supplemental oxygen.

Patients with COPD usually have a long history of dyspnea with a sudden increase in shortness of breath. There is rarely a history of chest pain. More often, they will remember having had a recent "chest cold" with fever and either an inability to cough up mucus or a sudden increase in sputum. If the patient is able to cough up sputum, it will be thick and is often green or yellow. The blood pressure of patients with COPD is normal; however, the pulse is rapid and occasionally irregular. Pay particular attention to the respirations. They may be rapid, or they may be slow.

Patients with asthma may have different "triggers," including allergens, cold, exercise, stress, infection, and noncompliance with medication prescriptions. It is important to try to determine what may have triggered the attack so that it can be treated appropriately. For example, an

Words of Wisdom

Dyspneic patients might resort to using—and sometimes misusing—over-the-counter medications in addition to their prescribed medications. The following is a list of over-the-counter medications that a patient may be using in conjunction with his or her prescribed medications:

- *Antihistamines* dry secretions and should not be taken by people who have asthma. Antihistamines are a common ingredient in many over-the-counter cough and cold medications.
- *Antitussives* are used to suppress coughs. Because coughing helps clear secretions from the airways, suppressing a cough might not be helpful. Coughs can be annoying, particularly if they interrupt sleep. However, the need for comfort must be weighed against the need to rid the airway of excess secretions. Overuse of antitussives can cause sedation, reduce respiratory drive, and cause excessive plugging of the airway with secretions. Many over-the-counter cough syrups also contain antihistamines that can cause problems if not used appropriately.
- *Bronchodilators* are available in some over-the-counter preparations. They often produce a nonspecific response, meaning that the medication may also have a substantial effect on the heart and blood vessels, particularly when taken in addition to prescription bronchodilators. The most common over-the-counter bronchodilators are simply attenuated (diluted) forms of epinephrine.
- *Diuretics* can be found in diet pills and caffeine-containing products, including many beverages. People are often told to drink plenty of fluids to maintain hydration, but overindulging in beverages that contain alcohol or caffeine has the opposite effect.
- *Expectorants* thin out pulmonary secretions so that they can be coughed up. Most common expectorants can be purchased over the counter. Many products combine expectorants with antitussives or antihistamines. These combinations are often at odds with each other. People with increased mucus production should avoid antihistamine products, taking only products that contain the expectorant guaifenesin.

asthma attack that occurred while your patient was jogging in the cold will probably not respond to antihistamines, whereas one brought on by a reaction to pollen might.

Patients with heart failure often walk a fine line between compensating for their diminished cardiac capacity and decompensating. Many take several medications, most often including diuretics (also known as water pills) and blood pressure medications. Your history taking should include obtaining a list of all their medications and paying special attention to the events leading up to the current problem.

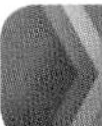

Words of Wisdom

Always treat your patient, not diagnostic test results!

Secondary Assessment

The secondary assessment is a more in-depth assessment of body systems, and it addresses the specific chief complaint, for example, difficult breathing (dyspnea) or shortness of breath. The secondary assessment includes a physical examination and taking vital signs.

As always, you should only proceed to history taking and the secondary assessment after all life threats have been identified and treated during the primary survey. If you are busy treating airway or breathing problems, you may not have the opportunity to proceed to a physical examination prior to arriving at the emergency department. Never compromise the assessment and treatment of airway and breathing problems to conduct a physical examination.

Sometimes it is not possible to quickly and definitively determine what is causing your patient's respiratory distress. For example, a 20 year old at a picnic who experiences rapid onset of difficult breathing and hives after being stung by a bee will likely have a different problem than an older woman in a nursing home who is on multiple medications and has a cough and increasing shortness of breath that developed over the past week. Keep an open mind, gather as complete a history as possible, and perform a secondary assessment.

Additional pieces to the assessment and treatment puzzle may be revealed during the physical examination. For example, you are treating a patient in acute respiratory distress who is breathing at a rate of 40 breaths/min and has audible wheezing. Given this information, you may be unsure as to whether the patient is in heart failure or is having an asthma attack. The secondary assessment may provide you with some clues, such as a consistently elevated blood pressure and swollen legs and feet (pedal edema) that would lead you in the direction of heart failure.

Conduct an in-depth assessment when a patient reports shortness of breath. In addition to the signs of air hunger present in all patients with respiratory distress, such as tripod positioning, rapid breathing, and use of accessory muscles, restriction of the small lower airways in patients with asthma often causes wheezing. Patients may have a prolonged expiratory phase of breathing as they attempt to exhale trapped air from the lungs. In severe cases, you may not actually hear wheezing because of insufficient airflow. As your patient tires from the effort of breathing and his or her oxygen levels decrease, the respiratory and heart rates may decrease, and your patient may seem to relax or fall asleep. A change in mental status is one of the early warning signs of respiratory inadequacy and indicates a lack of perfusion to the brain. This may manifest itself as confusion, lack of coordination, bizarre behavior, or even combativeness.

When you are performing a secondary assessment on the respiratory system, look for overall symmetry of the chest, adequate rise and fall of the chest, and evidence of retractions or accessory muscle use. Does the patient have increased work of breathing? Assess breath sounds, and do a physical assessment, if warranted.

What is the patient's respiratory status? The respiratory rate is not an accurate indicator of respiratory status unless it is extremely slow. However, respiratory trends are essential for evaluating chronically ill patients. A slowing respiratory rate in the face of an unimproved condition suggests physical exhaustion and impending respiratory failure. The patient's respiratory pattern should be noted; respiratory patterns are listed in Table 17-8.

As you perform your physical examination, look for signs of increased work of breathing. Are the patient's lips pursed? Do you see any accessory muscle use in the neck? Many smokers and people with chronic respiratory diseases cough up sputum every day (especially first thing in the morning), so determine if the color or amount of

Table 17-8 Respiratory Patterns

- Eupnea (normal breathing pattern)
- Tachypnea (rapid respiratory rate)
- Cheyne-Stokes respirations (a rhythmic breathing pattern characterized by periods of rapid and slow respirations alternating with periods of apnea; commonly seen in patients with head injury)
- Central neurogenic hyperventilation (deep, rapid respirations commonly seen in patients with head injury)
- Kussmaul respirations (deep, rapid respirations accompanied by an acetone or fruity odor on the patient's breath; seen in patients with diabetic ketoacidosis)
- Ataxic (Biot) respirations (rapid, irregular respirations with periods of apnea)
- Apneustic respirations (impaired respirations with sustained inspiratory effort)
- Apnea (cessation of breathing)

Table 17-9 Classic Sputum Types

Type of Sputum	Causes
Frothy, sometimes with a pink tinge	Heart failure
Thick	Dehydration or antihistamine use
Purulent	Infectious process (because the pus contains dead white blood cells)
Yellow, green, brown	Older secretions in various stages of decomposition
Clear or white	Bronchitis
Blood-streaked	Tumor, tuberculosis, pulmonary edema, or trauma from coughing

this sputum has changed Table 17-9. Jugular venous distention may accompany right-side heart failure, which may be caused by severe pulmonary arterial obstruction. It is important to note whether the mucus is **purulent** (puslike).

A secondary assessment of the cardiovascular system, especially when there is associated chest pain, should include checking and comparing distal pulses, reassessing the skin condition, and being alert for bradycardia and tachycardia.

When you are examining the chest, are there any obvious signs of trauma? Any retractions? Is the chest symmetric? A barrel chest indicates the presence of long-standing COPD. Listen to breath sounds if not previously done. Examine the extremities for skin color, condition, and temperature. Numbness, tingling, and carpopedal spasm may be associated with hypocapnia resulting from periods of rapid, deep respiration.

Blood pressure should be auscultated (by listening) when possible to obtain the systolic and diastolic measurements. If you are in an environment where you cannot hear well enough to auscultate the blood pressure, then palpation (by feeling) is an alternative. It is preferable to auscultate when you can because palpation does not provide a diastolic value that may be pertinent when a patient has a condition such as hypertension.

Words of Wisdom

What is the patient's pulse rate? Tachycardia is a sign of hypoxemia or might be a result of sympathomimetic medications taken for respiratory difficulty. Bradycardia in a patient experiencing dyspnea is an ominous sign of severe hypoxemia and imminent cardiac arrest. What is the patient's blood pressure? Hypertension may be associated with the use of sympathomimetic medication.

When there is inadequate oxygen in the blood, the body will attempt to divert blood from the extremities to the core to help keep the vital organs, including the brain, perfused. This action will result in pale skin and delayed capillary refill in the hands and feet. Feel for the skin temperature, and look for color changes in the extremities and in the core of the body. Cyanosis is an ominous sign that requires immediate, aggressive intervention.

It is important to assess the neurologic system frequently because the level of consciousness can change. Check the patient's mental status, and determine if the patient's activity can be described as anxious or restless. If so, that would be an indicator of hypoxia. Does the patient have clear thought processes? Disorientation may be another indicator of hypoxia.

Use monitoring devices if you have them available, including, but not limited to, a pulse oximeter. Under normal circumstances, a pulse oximeter is a noninvasive device that measures the percentage of a patient's hemoglobin that has oxygen attached to it. Oxygen saturation greater than 94% is considered normal, and most healthy people would feel short of breath at a saturation rate of less than 88%. Diagnostic testing will provide baseline information and indicate the severity of respiratory difficulty. Pulse oximetry is used to evaluate or confirm the adequacy of oxygen saturation.

Words of Wisdom

Most pulse oximeters also display the patient's pulse rate; this reading should match the patient's palpated heart rate. Always palpate the patient's pulse and compare it to the reading on the pulse oximeter.

Pulse oximetry readings may be inaccurate in the presence of conditions that abnormally bind hemoglobin, including carbon monoxide poisoning as well as any condition that causes a decrease in perfusion. For example, if the patient's hemoglobin level is low (as a result of trauma or hemorrhage, for example), the pulse oximetry result will be correspondingly high. If the reading shows only 6 g/dL of hemoglobin (normal level, 12 to 14 g/dL), ideally all hemoglobin will have oxygen attached and the oxygen saturation will be 100%. Such a patient needs more hemoglobin in the form of whole blood or packed red cells. A patient with an abnormally high hemoglobin level, as is common in chronic hypoxia such as in cases of COPD, or a patient who lives at a high altitude will have a correspondingly low oxygen saturation.

Another more accurate tool available to AEMTs in some EMS systems is end-tidal carbon dioxide ($ETCO_2$) monitoring, which is a method for measuring the amount of exhaled carbon dioxide. $ETCO_2$ monitoring is accomplished with a device that measures the amount of carbon dioxide exhaled during a specific time (minutes or hours) and plots the resulting values graphically as a waveform as well as giving numeric readouts. $ETCO_2$ monitoring can be extremely valuable in assessing patients, but rarely results in different prehospital care for AEMTs.

The exact percentage of carbon dioxide contained in the last few milliliters of the patient's exhaled air can be measured using a special sensor. For example, some electronic $ETCO_2$ detectors use a photoelectric sensor that relies on absorption of infrared light by carbon dioxide to provide this measurement. The sensor can evaluate $ETCO_2$ in a spontaneously breathing patient via a specialized nasal cannula–type device, or it can be attached to the end of an endotracheal tube. These devices typically display a waveform that can provide additional data about the patient's respiratory status. In addition, such monitors serve as alarms that can alert providers to changes in respiratory rate or depth. This kind of monitoring is called waveform capnography.

The recent realization that the amount of $ETCO_2$ in the exhaled breath of a patient in cardiac arrest is an important indicator of the effectiveness of cardiopulmonary resuscitation (CPR) has resulted in a substantially increased awareness of this important value. In cardiac arrest, an $ETCO_2$ of less than 10 torr (torr = mm Hg) may indicate suboptimal CPR compressions. A sudden increase in $ETCO_2$ (for example, from 10 to 35 mm Hg) may be the earliest indicator of the return of spontaneous circulation. Keep in mind that the $ETCO_2$ value can be dramatically affected by the rate and depth of ventilation. The ultimate value of this parameter depends on a provider's ability to maintain ventilation at recommended levels (8 to 10 breaths/min at 6 to 7 mL/kg in an adult in a state of cardiac arrest).

Another tool is the peak flow meter. This device provides a baseline assessment of expiratory airflow for patients with obstructive lung disease. The peak flow is the maximum flow rate at which a patient can expel air from the lungs. Normal peak flow values vary by age, sex, and height, but generally range from approximately 350 to 700 L/min; a peak flow less than 150 L/min is considered inadequate and signals substantial distress. Some people with chronic asthma have a peak flow that never exceeds 100 L/min. Many patients with chronic pulmonary diseases may already use a peak flow meter at home. Encourage these patients to take their records and medications with them to the hospital for evaluation of the progression of their illness.

Reassessment

After the assessment and treatment have been completed, you need to reassess the patient and closely watch patients with shortness of breath. Repeat the primary survey, and maintain an open airway. Monitor the patient's breathing, and reassess circulation.

Determine if there have been changes in the patient's condition. Confirm the adequacy of interventions and patient status. If the changes you find are improvements, simply continue the treatments; however, if your patient's condition deteriorates, prepare to modify treatments. Be prepared to assist ventilations with a bag-mask device. Monitor the skin color and temperature. Reassess and record vital signs at least every 5 minutes for a patient in unstable condition and/or after the patient uses an inhaler. If the patient's condition is stable and no life threat exists, vital signs should be obtained at least every 15 minutes.

Contact medical control with any change in level of consciousness or difficulty breathing. Depending on local protocols, contact medical control prior to assisting with any prescribed medications. Be sure to document any changes (and at what time) and any orders given by medical control.

Emergency Medical Care

This section will discuss how to manage a patient with dyspnea. Later in the chapter, the management of specific diseases and conditions will be discussed.

Perform Standard Interventions

In treating a patient with dyspnea, a variety of standard interventions should be implemented before administering medication. Oxygen to keep the saturation above 94% and an intravenous line are typical interventions for any patient who needs advanced life support.[9]

Psychological support is also an important consideration for a patient with dyspnea. Always speak with assurance and assume a calm, professional, and caring demeanor to reassure the patient, who, no doubt, will be very frightened. Your efforts to reduce that patient's anxiety can help lower the patient's heart rate and blood pressure and allow the patient to maximize breathing effectiveness.

Decrease the Work of Breathing

Even under normal circumstances, muscles must work to allow breathing, and they must work much harder during respiratory distress. People with asthma, for example, can often compensate for respiratory distress by devoting substantial energy to breathing. They can maintain their oxygen and carbon dioxide levels in an acceptable range as long as they continue to recruit their muscles for this effort. The tremendous workload uses large amounts of energy, which requires even more oxygen and ventilation. A patient in such a condition typically is not able to eat and drink normally, so he or she becomes progressively more dehydrated, malnourished, and fatigued. At some point, the patient will tire and be unable to continue the necessary work of breathing; he or she will look sleepy, the rate and depth of respirations will slowly decrease, and he or she will experience decompensation (respiratory failure). Some patients with asthma may compensate for days, hoping that their steroids and bronchodilators will resolve an attack. By the time they realize that those approaches aren't working, they may be in too much distress to seek care except by calling 9-1-1.

The supine position with or without the legs raised, especially for an overweight patient, causes the abdominal organs to compress the diaphragm. With each breath, the patient must move the abdominal contents out of the way to expand the thorax and breathe. Abdominal distention with air or blood compounds the situation. Shortness of breath induced by lying flat is called orthopnea. It explains why most people maintain a sitting position when they are short of breath. To decrease the work of breathing, help the patient sit up if he or she is more comfortable in that position. Remove constricting clothing, such as belts and tight collars. *Do not make the person walk.*

▶ Provide Supplemental Oxygen

It is essential to provide supplemental oxygen to any patient who needs it. As with any other medication, you must administer oxygen in the concentrations necessary to be effective. Patients who are not breathing adequately should receive bag-mask ventilation with supplemental oxygen, or more advanced airway management techniques. Closely reassess the patient's breathing status, and adjust treatment accordingly. Pulse oximetry is a useful guide to oxygenation if it is accurate (the pulse rate on the oximeter matches the palpated pulse) and if the patient's hemoglobin level is relatively normal.

It is safe to administer oxygen in concentrations less than 50% to almost anyone, and it is appropriate to do so when there is a reasonable chance the patient would benefit from it. Oxygen concentrations higher than 50% should be reserved for patients with hypoxia that does not respond to lower concentrations. The use of 100% oxygen should be limited to the shortest period necessary.

Of the oxygen in the body, 97% is bound to hemoglobin. The other 3% is dissolved in the plasma. After all hemoglobin in the blood has been saturated with oxygen, further exposure to high concentrations of oxygen begins to damage the lung tissue.

As an AEMT, you will treat many patients who require high-concentration oxygen to maintain acceptable oxygen saturation. You should never hesitate to administer oxygen aggressively to those patients who need it. At the same time, however, most patients with good oxygen saturation (at least 94%) do not benefit from supplemental oxygen.[9-11] Even patients with trauma, stroke, and acute coronary syndrome derive no benefit from supplemental oxygen therapy if oxygen saturation is already at or above 94%.[12] It remains common practice to administer low-flow oxygen to such patients, but **hyperoxia** (an excess of oxygen) should be avoided. In general, the American Heart Association recommends maintaining oxygen saturation between 94% and 99%.[12] Oxygen saturation of 100% should be avoided, because it's impossible to predict how high the blood oxygen level may rise when the hemoglobin is completely saturated.

Also, remember to consider the possibility that the pulse oximeter may provide falsely elevated assessment of the patient's overall level of oxygenation, such as in cases of carbon monoxide poisoning or anemia due to acute blood loss or chronic anemia. In such cases, providing supplemental oxygen sufficient to achieve an oxygen saturation of 100% may be extremely valuable. There is no evidence that short-term hyperoxia is detrimental to any group of patients. There is some evidence that long-term hyperoxia (several hours) may be associated with worse outcomes (acute coronary syndrome and traumatic brain injury). In the context of very prolonged transport times, these factors and conditions should be considered. In the context of very short transport times (less than an hour) there is essentially no danger to hyperoxia, and oxygen therapy should be employed liberally.

Always consider insertion of an advanced airway in unresponsive patients to protect the airway. Call for paramedic backup if needed.

Special Populations

In the 1950s, scientists began to understand that administering high concentrations of oxygen could cause blindness in premature neonates. Thus began the medical community's recognition that oxygen can have toxic effects. Current protocols now discourage the use of 100% oxygen in neonatal care, even during initial resuscitation (100% oxygen is still given, however, in neonatal cardiac arrest).[13] Further research is being done on the effects of free radicals and the impact of high-concentration oxygen on all patients.

▶ Administer a Bronchodilator

Many patients with respiratory distress receive some benefit from bronchodilation, and some patients benefit substantially. Today's aerosol bronchodilators rarely harm patients, so AEMTs tend to use them aggressively in the field. However, patients who do not have bronchospasm usually benefit only slightly from aerosol bronchodilators, and the oxygen concentration delivered is often reduced during a typical aerosol treatment. Under these circumstances, application of a nonrebreathing mask is a better choice than the aerosol treatment. Follow local protocol, but remember bronchodilators are of little value in treating conditions such as pneumonia, pulmonary edema, and heart disease.

Respiratory Medications

Some of the most common medications used for dyspnea are called inhaled beta agonists, which, through stimulation of selective beta-2 receptors in the lungs, dilate the bronchioles. Typical trade names are Proventil, Ventolin, Alupent, Metaprel, and Brethine. The generic name for Proventil and Ventolin is albuterol; for Alupent and Metaprel, it is metaproterenol; and for Brethine, it is terbutaline. The action of most of these medications is to relax the smooth muscles within the bronchioles in the lungs, resulting in enlargement (dilation) of the airways and easier passage of air.

Bronchodilators relax the smooth muscle around the larger bronchi and are an important therapy for bronchoconstriction. Administered via so-called rescue inhalers, fast-acting bronchodilators provide almost instant relief, a property that sometimes results in their misuse. Strictly speaking, bronchodilators do not reduce swelling, kill bacteria, push fluid out of the lungs, or open closed alveoli. However, patients with pneumonia, heart failure, or atelectasis may have a small amount of secondary bronchoconstriction that could be reversed with a bronchodilator.

In the past, the strategy was to disperse atropine (the most common parasympathetic blocker) through an aerosol. Currently, a medication specifically designed for aerosol use, ipratropium, is available. It is also available in a **metered-dose inhaler (MDI)**. The combination of albuterol (a beta-2 agonist) and ipratropium (an anticholinergic) is also available as a so-called premixed cocktail, as an aerosol, or as an MDI.

Anticholinergics have emerged as a central component in the management of COPD. Tiotropium (Spiriva), a once-per-day anticholinergic for this indication, is taken via a type of dry-powder inhaler. Patients taking tiotropium would not typically also use aerosol ipratropium.

Table 17-10 lists medications used for acute and chronic respiratory symptoms. Those used for acute symptoms are designed to give the patient rapid relief from symptoms if the condition is reversible. Medications used for chronic symptoms are administered for preventive measures or as maintenance doses. The medications for chronic use will provide little relief of acute symptoms. Common side effects of inhalers used for acute shortness of breath include increased pulse rate, nervousness, and muscle tremors.

Some of these medications are administered in the home by using an aerosol nebulizer, an MDI, or a dry-powder inhaler.

Aerosol Therapy

An aerosol treatment is a simple method of delivering medications, such as bronchodilators. Aerosol nebulizers deliver liquid medications in the form of a fine mist Figure 17-17. To generate the optimal particle size, most nebulizers need to have gas (oxygen) flow of at least 6 L/min. Running the gas more slowly generates particles that are too large and cannot make it into the lower airways; running it substantially faster makes the treatment go faster, with the potential of less medication delivery.

In the home, most people run their aerosol treatments off of a small air compressor. In the ambulance, this therapy usually runs off of tanked oxygen or a wall unit attached to the main oxygen supply. As a result, the patient might receive only 30% to 40% oxygen via an aerosol treatment, which is still more than the 21% oxygen contained in room air but may be less than needed by a patient with substantial hypoxia.

A nebulizer can be attached to a mouthpiece (pipe), a face mask, or a tracheostomy collar, or it can simply be held in front of the patient's face (called the blow-by technique). The smaller the amount of mist the patient inhales, however, the less medication he or she receives. Blow-by and mouthpiece treatments are ineffective if patients continually turn their heads or remove the mouthpiece to answer questions. As such, after the decision has been made to deliver a breathing treatment, try to stop the conversation and let the patient focus on inhaling the medication.

Controversies

In some systems, aerosol treatments are given to anyone who is dyspneic under the belief that they might help and are usually harmless; in other systems, the use of aerosol bronchodilators is restricted to situations in which they are clearly indicated. Be sure to consult medical direction and your local protocols to keep abreast of how this class of medications is used in your region.

Nebulizers also deliver substantial humidity to the airway. A quick way to provide a cooling mist to the swollen upper airway of a patient with burns or a child with croup is to give an aerosol treatment of saline solution or sterile water.

The newer aerosol bronchodilators cause far less tachycardia than those that are older and less beta-2–specific. As a result, it has become possible to give repeated treatments to patients with bronchospasm. Continuous nebulizers are available that hold up to 10 times the usual medication dosages and run for 1 hour or longer. However, the potential for some beta-1 stimulation (causing tachycardia) remains, and some physicians are concerned that aerosol bronchodilators could worsen tachycardia in a patient with underlying cardiac disease. Tachycardia is almost always already present in patients with dyspnea, so be sure to consult medical control or local protocols for guidance. The steps for administering medications via **small-volume nebulizer** are shown in Chapter 13, *Vascular Access and Medication Administration*.

Table 17-10 Respiratory Inhalation Medications

Medication			Indications			Use	
Generic Drug Name	Trade Names	Action	Asthma	Bronchitis	COPD	Acute	Chronic
Albuterol	Proventil, Ventolin, Volmax	Dilates bronchioles	Yes	Yes	Yes	Yes	No
Beclomethasone	Beclovent Beconase, Qvar, Vanceril	Anti-inflammatory, reduces swelling	Yes	No	No	No	Yes
Cromolyn	Intal	Decreases release of histamines	Yes	No	No	No	Yes
Fluticasone	Flovent Diskus	Anti-inflammatory, reduces swelling	Yes	No	No	No	Yes
Fluticasone, salmeterol	Advair Diskus	Decreases secretions	Yes	No	No	No	Yes
Ipratropium bromide	Atrovent	Dilates bronchioles	Yes	Yes	Yes	Yes	No
Levalbuterol	Xopenex	Dilates bronchioles	Yes	Yes	Yes	Yes	No
Metaproterenol sulfate	Alupent, Metaprel	Dilates bronchioles	Yes	Yes	Yes	Yes	No
Montelukast	Singulair	Anti-inflammatory, reduces swelling	Yes	No	Yes	No	Yes
Salmeterol	Serevent Diskus	Dilates bronchioles	Yes	Yes	Yes	No	Yes

Abbreviation: COPD, chronic obstructive pulmonary disease

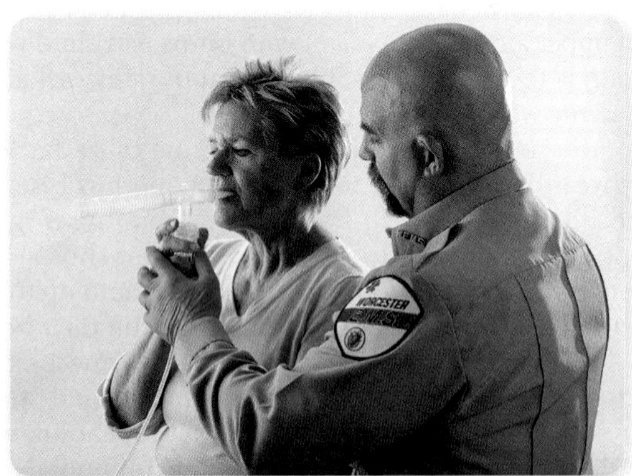

Figure 17-17 Aerosol nebulizers are often used to deliver medications directly to the respiratory tract. Unfortunately, they may supply only 30% to 40% oxygen during a treatment. Flow rate is an important factor in how much medication reaches the lungs.

Words of Wisdom

Albuterol is one of the most commonly administered bronchodilators given via nebulizer and can be administered by AEMTs. Dosages are as follows:

- **Adult:** Administer 2.5 mg diluted with 2.5 mL of normal saline.
- **Pediatric:** Administer as follows:
  - *Patients who weigh less than 20 kg*: 1.25 mg/dose via handheld nebulizer or mask over 20 minutes.
  - *Patients who weigh more than 20 kg*: 2.5 mg/dose via handheld nebulizer or mask over 20 minutes.
  - Repeat once in 20 minutes; consult medical control regarding the second dose, depending on local protocols.

Metered-Dose Inhalers

An MDI is a miniature spray canister used to direct medication through the mouth and into the lungs. When properly used, an MDI should deliver the same amount of medication as an aerosol treatment. This device is small, easy for patients to carry and use, and convenient. Because it does not require additional equipment (such as a nebulizer or air compressor), it is usually the delivery method of choice for bronchodilators and corticosteroids in the home setting **Figure 17-18**. Because patients use (and may misuse) their own inhalers in the home, be sure to document how often the patient has been taking an extra puff. Do not forget to consult medical control before administering additional doses if this is required in your system.

Each MDI on the ambulance should ideally be equipped with a **spacer**. A spacer is a device that collects the medication as it is released from the canister, allowing more to be delivered to the lungs and less to be lost to the environment. When a spacer is used, the patient does not have to worry about timing the inhalation to coincide with the discharge of the inhaler. Spacers also reduce deposition of the drug into the mouth and oropharynx, which is a problem with inexperienced users.

Achieving the proper technique when using an MDI is not difficult, but it requires constant reinforcement. The steps for administering medication with an MDI are shown in Chapter 13, *Vascular Access and Medication Administration*.

The following are some tips on how to avoid common errors when using or administering an MDI:

- **The mist from an MDI must enter the lungs.** Patients must inhale deeply as they discharge the inhaler to draw the medication deep into their lungs. Placing the inhaler directly into the mouth (without a spacer) often causes much of the medication to fall on the posterior pharynx, where it is swallowed and digested, thus negating its intended effect.
- **Some patients mistakenly blow into the spacer.** Tell them to think of the spacer as a big straw from which they should try to suck the medication out of the bottom.
- **Many spacers make a harmonica-like sound if the patient sucks too hard.** The best particle deposition comes from smooth, low-pressure, laminar flow. Inhaling too forcefully causes turbulent flow, which makes many of the particles stick to the trachea and large bronchi, where they are not as effective.
- **Patients should try to inhale the medication deeply and then hold their breath for a few seconds.** This is a lot to ask of someone who is dyspneic, and it is not always possible. Sometimes the inhalation causes the patient to cough immediately after inhaling the medication, which precludes delivery of a full dose but may be unavoidable.
- **Make sure the inhaler contains medication.** The labels of most inhalers list the number of puffs of medication in the canister. Patients should be encouraged to keep track of how many times they have used the inhaler and to discard it when they reach the recommended number of uses. The sound of fluid sloshing around when the canister is shaken doesn't indicate that there is medication left in it.
- **Keep the spacer and canister holder clean.** The spacer and canister holder should occasionally be rinsed off to avoid inhaling dust and other particles. In addition, respiratory devices should be dried after they are cleaned to avoid the growth of microorganisms.
- **After using a corticosteroid inhaler, patients should rinse out the mouth with water or mouthwash.** Residual corticosteroid in the pharynx can predispose patients to thrush, an annoying fungal infection in the pharynx or mouth.

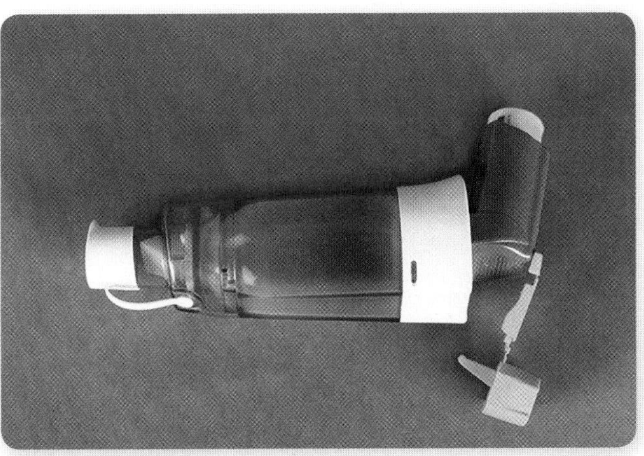

Figure 17-18 Metered-dose inhalers are a common delivery platform for respiratory medications. Their effectiveness is greatly increased by using a spacer device (shown here), which regulates the release of medication into the inhaler.

Special Populations

In asthma education programs children learn to take a puff from a bronchodilator inhaler, turn over an hourglass egg timer, and wait 1 or 2 minutes before taking the next puff. This strategy lets the medication delivered in the first puff open up the airways a little so the second puff can go deeper into the airways.

If a patient with shortness of breath has a prescribed MDI, read the label carefully to make sure that the medication has been prescribed to the patient and that it is not expired. The patient should take repeated doses of the medication if the maximum dose has not been exceeded and he or she is still experiencing shortness of breath. Contraindications for the use of an MDI include the following:

- The patient is unable to help coordinate inhalation with depression of the trigger on an MDI or is too confused to effectively administer medication through a small-volume nebulizer. These devices will be only minimally effective when patients are in respiratory failure and have only minimal air movement.
- The MDI or small-volume nebulizer is not prescribed for this patient.
- You did not obtain permission from medical control and/or it is not permissible by local protocol.
- The patient had already met the maximum prescribed dose before your arrival.
- The medication is expired.
- There are other contraindications specific to the medication.

Words of Wisdom

Positioning the patient in an upright position to loosen mucus and relieve buildup can be effective in treating a patient with a respiratory emergency.

You must carefully monitor patients with dyspnea. About 5 minutes after the patient uses an inhaler, repeat the vital signs and the primary survey. Ask the patient whether the treatment was effective. Look at the patient's chest to see whether the patient is still using accessory muscles to breathe. Listen to the patient's speech pattern. Be prepared to assist ventilations with a bag-mask device if the patient's condition deteriorates.

After helping the patient with the inhaler treatment or administering a bronchodilator via nebulizer, transport the patient to the closest, most appropriate emergency department. While en route, continue to assess the patient's breathing. Provide reassurance and continue to give supplemental oxygen. In cases of severe distress, do not delay transport. Using MDIs as well as administering nebulized treatments may be done en route.

Dry-Powder Inhalers

Some respiratory medications are most stable in the form of a fine powder. Several common corticosteroids and slow-acting bronchodilators are often dispensed by this means. Each time the device is opened, the small plastic blister that holds a dose is rotated into position. The patient then pushes a small lever to puncture the blister, presses the disk to his or her lips over the opening, and

Documentation & Communication

Teach patients to use their rescue inhalers before taking corticosteroids, slow-acting bronchodilators, and other medications. A rescue inhaler dilates the bronchi so that subsequent medications are more effective.

YOU are the Provider — PART 4

You auscultate the patient's lungs again, and while you still note wheezing, you also are able to note increased air movement, and the patient's cyanosis is resolving slightly. You place the patient back on a nonbreathing mask at 15 L/min and establish an intravenous (IV) line with a 20-gauge catheter in her left antecubital fossa with normal saline at a to-keep-open rate. The patient states that her breathing is much easier en route, but you note that she is still experiencing a degree of dyspnea. On arrival, you turn over care to the awaiting triage nurse without incident.

Recording Time: 15 Minutes	
Respirations	26 breaths/min, clear bilaterally
Pulse	Strong and regular, 142 beats/min
Skin	Warm, dry, and pink
Blood pressure	134/82 mm Hg
Oxygen saturation (Spo_2)	95% on 100% oxygen

7. Should paramedic backup have been requested for this patient?
8. Should this patient have received an IV line?

inhales deeply to suck the powder out of the device. These devices are reasonably convenient and easy to use, but they are rarely used during emergency care.

Other dry-powder devices require the patient to insert a capsule of powdered medication, which is then pierced when the patient compresses a button or lever on the device. The patient sucks the powder out using a technique similar to that previously described.

▶ Consider Fluid Balance

Rehydration is supplemental therapy for patients with respiratory problems who are dehydrated (for example, some patients who have pneumonia or asthma). It is common practice to give a fluid bolus to younger patients with these conditions. In any older adult or other patient with cardiac dysfunction, administering too much fluid could cause pulmonary edema. Always assess breath sounds *before* and *after* giving a fluid bolus to make certain the patient does not become overhydrated. Of course, patients who have respiratory problems can quickly become extremely ill, and you will almost always want to have an IV line in place as a medication route.

▶ Support or Assist Ventilation

If the patient becomes fatigued, breathing might need to be supported more aggressively. Therapy using continuous positive airway pressure (CPAP) and bilevel positive airway pressure (BPAP) is becoming increasingly common and can preclude the need for intubation in many patients. Some patients may simply require bag-mask ventilation for a short period to reoxygenate, improve hemoglobin saturation, and reduce the partial pressure of arterial carbon dioxide ($PaCO_2$).

Trying to assist breathing for a patient who is *already breathing on his or her own* is one of the most difficult interventions. To avoid worsening a patient's condition, it is important to be confident in your bag-mask ventilation technique. Gastric distention and vomiting from overaggressive ventilation can complicate an already worsening situation. As always, *do no harm*.

Continuous Positive Airway Pressure

CPAP is used in two distinctly different ways: to treat obstructive sleep apnea and to treat respiratory failure. Many people with obstructive sleep apnea wear a CPAP unit at night to maintain their airways during sleep. This type of CPAP may be applied via nasal pillows, a nasal mask, a face mask that resembles a typical mask used for bag-mask ventilation, or a mask that covers the entire face. This is *not* the type of CPAP used for critically ill patients. In people who are not critically ill, the positive pressure delivered maintains the stability of the posterior pharynx, thereby preventing obstruction of the upper airway when the person sleeps. This pressure limits hypoxic episodes and snoring.

The CPAP used as therapy for respiratory failure is almost always delivered through a mask that is secured

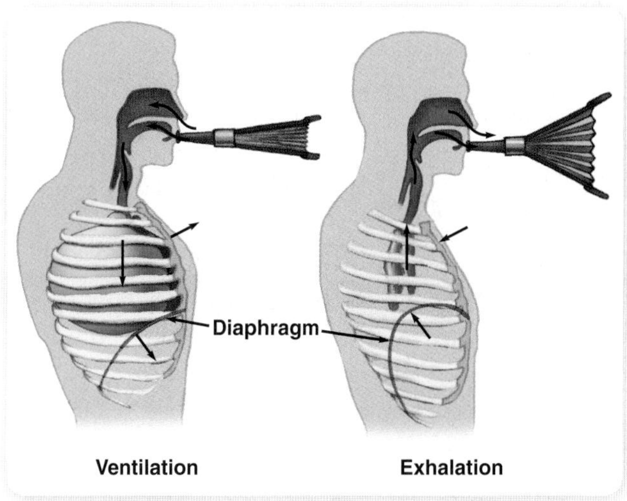

Figure 17-19 Positive pressure ventilation is physiologically the opposite of normal ventilation. Air is pushed into the respiratory tract with bag-mask ventilation and can enter the esophagus and stomach unless careful technique is used.

to the face by some type of strap. When positive pressure ventilation (that is, with a pocket mask or bag-mask ventilation) is given, air is forced into the upper airway and flows into the trachea and esophagus unless steps are taken to help direct it into the trachea **Figure 17-19**. Indeed, positive pressure ventilation with bag-mask ventilation or a pocket mask is physiologically the opposite of normal (negative pressure) ventilation.

Using a bag-mask device for ventilation produces positive pressure in the chest. The more forcefully the bag is squeezed, the higher the pressure. Pressure that is too high can cause several problems. Simple pneumothorax can evolve into tension pneumothorax, air leaks can produce huge amounts of subcutaneous air, and high intrathoracic pressure can retard, or even completely block, venous return. In recent years, prehospital providers have begun to understand the ramifications of positive pressure ventilation during low-flow states such as shock and cardiac arrest. This understanding has resulted in CPR guidelines that stress lower ventilation rates, smaller volumes, and lower pressures. CPR is based on principles of hemodynamics, and the rate, volume, and pressure of delivered breaths can quickly do more harm than good during resuscitation.

Similarly, administering CPAP increases pressure in the chest. If the patient's blood pressure is already low, too much CPAP can stop venous return to the heart and cause a sudden decrease in blood pressure. This problem is uncommon with lower levels of CPAP, but blood pressure should be carefully monitored whenever CPAP is used (especially at levels greater than 10 cm H_2O). Keep in mind that CPAP can turn a simple pneumothorax into a tension pneumothorax in only a few breaths.

Ensure a good seal with minimal leakage **Figure 17-20**. In the field, 100% supplemental oxygen is the most

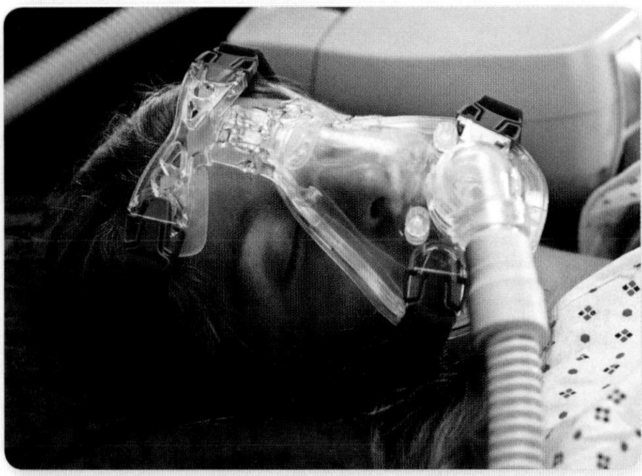

Figure 17-20 The continuous positive airway pressure used in the acute setting is usually administered via face mask, which must make a tight seal to function properly.

common driving gas for the positive pressure. Be vigilant about monitoring the gas supply—depending on the flow and the patient's respiratory rate, some CPAP units may empty a D cylinder in as little as 5 or 10 minutes. The mask is fitted with a pressure-relief valve that determines the amount of pressure delivered (such as 5 cm H_2O). The effect is similar to being in a gale-force wind (high inspiratory flow) and having to push a pressure valve open with exhalation. This would seem to require a great deal of effort and tire out a patient in decompensating respiratory failure, but many patients in critical condition make a dramatic turnaround when CPAP is applied.

Sometimes patients find the CPAP mask claustrophobic and fight its application. Some patients can be talked through the mask application with good results, but other patients simply cannot tolerate the mask. Don't struggle with a patient who is unwilling to use the mask; doing so will increase the patient's anxiety, cardiac workload, and cardiac oxygen consumption. When CPAP works as intended, it can provide dramatic relief and avoid intubation. When it fails, it is critical to recognize a deteriorating condition and be prepared to move to the next step. Within several minutes of application, the patient's oxygen saturation should increase and the respiratory rate should decrease. The success of CPAP is inversely related to the patient's respiratory rate soon after its application. If this rate *increases*, the therapy is likely to fail; if this rate *decreases*, the therapy is likely to succeed.

Bilevel Positive Airway Pressure

In BPAP, one pressure can be delivered during inspiration (inspiratory positive airway pressure) and a different pressure can be delivered during exhalation (expiratory positive airway pressure). Instead of delivering 20 cm H_2O as in CPAP, BPAP set at 20/8 gives 20 cm H_2O pressure during inhalation and 8 cm H_2O pressure during exhalation. Because this type of positive airway pressure is more like normal breathing, it is often more comfortable for patients. It causes a pressure variation in the chest, which allows for more normal blood flow. The BPAP device is also more complex and expensive, and it is not commonly used in the field.

Assessment and Management of Specific Conditions

Upper or Lower Airway Diseases

Patients with obstructive airway disease typically present with signs of severe respiratory impairment. These may include one- to two-word dyspnea (able to say only one or two words between breaths), diminished or absent breath sounds, and altered mental status. The chief complaint is typically that of dyspnea, cough, or nocturnal dyspnea (awakens the person from sleep).

Obtain a thorough history, including any personal or family history of asthma and allergies. Determine whether the patient has had an acute exposure to any pulmonary irritant or any previous similar episodes. Ask the patient if he or she has ever been intubated.

Wheezing may be present in all types of obstructive lung disease. Look for retractions and the use of accessory muscles. Use a peak flow meter to establish the baseline expiratory airflow and a pulse oximeter to document the degree of hypoxemia and response to therapy. Remember that the pulse oximeter is designed to detect gross abnormalities, not subtle changes.

Begin management of obstructive airway disease by placing the patient in a position of comfort. Consider calling early for paramedic backup if the patient is in severe distress. Monitor the airway, apply high-flow oxygen, and assist ventilation if needed. Use humidified oxygen if available. Establish IV access and provide circulatory support. IV therapy may be necessary to improve hydration and to thin and loosen mucus. Assist patients with their MDIs as needed. Continue monitoring, and transport the patient to the closest appropriate facility. Contact medical control for further orders. Airway problems can be very frightening. Provide psychological support en route to the hospital.

Acute Pulmonary Edema

Dyspnea caused by acute pulmonary edema may be associated with cardiac disease or direct lung damage. In either case, administer 100% oxygen and, if necessary, carefully suction any secretions from the airway. Place the patient in a position of comfort. Provide assisted ventilation as needed. CPAP has proven to be immensely beneficial to patients experiencing respiratory distress from obstructive pulmonary disease and acute pulmonary edema. Establish IV access. Monitor flow rates carefully to avoid fluid excess, which will exacerbate the patient's pulmonary edema.

Consider calling for paramedic backup for intubation, and provide prompt transport.

▶ Aspiration

The inhalation of anything other than gases is called **aspiration**. Patients can aspirate fresh or salt water, blood, vomitus, or food. Patients who receive tube feedings are at particular risk for aspiration if they are placed supine immediately after receiving a large feeding. Aspiration is associated with a high mortality rate. It is a common but profoundly dangerous complication in patients who have had cardiac arrest and in patients who are unresponsive as a result of trauma or overdose. Such patients are at risk for aspirating vomitus. The aspiration of stomach contents carries the additional risk of aspiration **pneumonitis**, in which the gastric acid irritates lung tissue. This risk is in addition to the risk of pneumonia from any bacteria in the aspirated material.

Aspiration of foreign bodies, such as nuts or broken teeth, may also occur. Most adults choke only when they are intoxicated or traumatized or have a reduced gag reflex from a stroke or aging. Chronic aspiration of food is also a common cause of pneumonia in older patients.

Follow these guidelines when treating patients at risk for aspiration or who have aspirated:

1. Aggressively reduce the risk of aspiration by avoiding gastric distention when ventilating.
2. Aggressively monitor the patient's ability to protect his or her own airway, and protect the patient's airway with an advanced airway when needed.
3. Aggressively treat aspiration with suction and airway control if steps 1 and 2 fail.

Patients at risk for aspiration should not eat when they are having difficulty breathing.

▶ Chronic Obstructive Pulmonary Disease

Patients with COPD may have an altered level of consciousness or be unresponsive from hypoxia or from carbon dioxide retention. Patients with COPD often find breathing difficult when lying down. Assist with the patient's prescribed inhaler if there is one. Often, a patient with COPD will overuse an inhaler, so watch for side effects. Transport patients with COPD as promptly as possible to the emergency department, allowing them to sit upright if this is most comfortable.

Words of Wisdom

While one AEMT is getting oxygen ready, the second AEMT should try to coach the patient with asthma or COPD to use pursed-lip breathing. This further opens the bronchioles to help air to escape.

Auto-PEEP

Not everyone should be ventilated the same way. When ventilating a patient who has severe obstructive disease, such as patients with decompensated asthma or COPD, remember the difficulty exhaling. Complete exhalation must be allowed before the next breath is delivered or pressure in the thorax will continue to rise. This phenomenon, which is called auto-PEEP (positive end-expiratory pressure), can eventually cause a pneumothorax or cardiac arrest. If the pressure in the chest exceeds the pressure of blood returning to the heart, limiting venous return, cardiac arrest may occur.

Patients in whom auto-PEEP is a concern should be ventilated at a rate of as little as 4 to 6 breaths/min. Such restraint is difficult, but it is an absolute necessity to avoid the dire consequences of raising the thoracic pressure with each breath. Remember that the standard ventilation rate for adults in cardiac arrest is only 10 breaths/min in patients without COPD.

▶ Asthma

Many lung problems are incorrectly labeled "asthma"; therefore, your assessment of the patient is critical. Asthma is often a recurring pathologic condition. Confirm whether the patient is able to breathe normally at other times. If possible, ask family members to describe the patient's asthma. Even if they only identify wheezing as a problem, be aware that some forms of heart failure, foreign body aspiration, toxic fumes inhalation, or allergic reactions may cause wheezing.

Bronchial asthma is characterized by an increased reactivity of the trachea and bronchi to a variety of stimuli. The hyperreactivity results in widespread, reversible narrowing of the airways, or bronchospasm. Three components of asthma are bronchospasm, airway edema, and increased mucus production Figure 17-21. Asthma makes it difficult to exhale. Air is trapped in the distal portions of the lung and does not allow air from the next inhalation to enter the alveoli.

As you assess the patient's vital signs, note that the pulse rate will be normal or elevated, the blood pressure may be slightly elevated, and respirations will be increased. Ask questions about how and when the symptoms began.

Asthma is a common childhood illness. When you are assessing a pediatric patient, look for retraction of the skin above the sternum and between the ribs. Retractions are typically easier to see in children than in adults. Cyanosis is a late finding in children. Keep in mind that a cough may not be a symptom of a cold; it could signal pneumonia or asthma. Even if you do not hear much wheezing, the presence of a cough can indicate some degree of reactive airway disease (for example, asthma or bronchiolitis).

As you care for the patient, be prepared to suction and to administer oxygen. Allow some time for oxygenation between suction attempts. If the patient is unresponsive, you may have to provide airway management.

If the patient has medication, such as an inhaler for an asthma attack, you may help with its administration

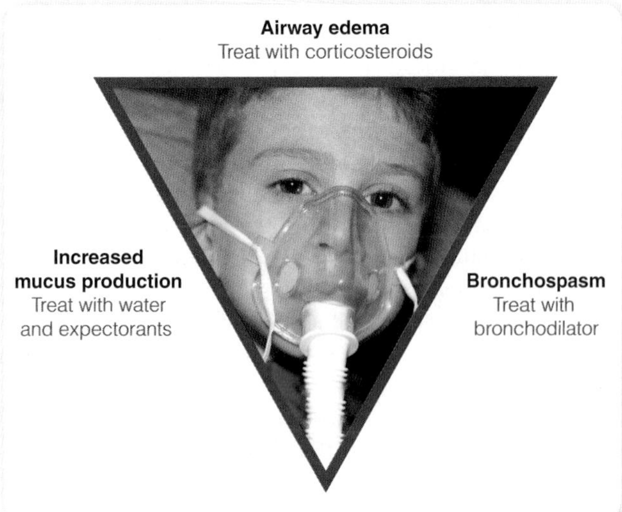

Figure 17-21 The asthma triad demonstrates the three primary components of asthma and the corresponding treatments for each component. Asthma presents differently in different people, so individual treatments need to vary as well.

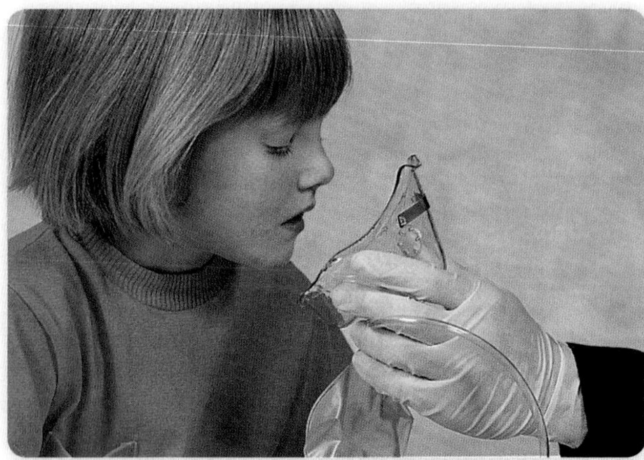

Figure 17-22 Because children may refuse to wear an oxygen mask, you may have to hold the mask in front of the child's face. If the child still refuses, enlist the parent's help.

or administer nebulized medication, as directed by local protocol. Even patients who use their inhaler may continue to get worse. Reassess breathing frequently and be prepared to assist ventilations with a bag-mask device in severe cases. If you must assist ventilations in a patient who is having an asthma attack, use slow, gentle breaths. Remember, the problem in asthma is getting the air out of the lungs, not into them. Resist the temptation to squeeze the bag hard and fast. Always assist with ventilations as a last resort, and then provide only about 10 to 12 shallow breaths/min.

The emergency care of a child with shortness of breath is the same as it is for an adult, including the use of supplemental oxygen. However, many small children will not tolerate (or may refuse to wear) a face mask. Rather than fighting with the child, hold the oxygen mask in front of the child's face or ask the parent to hold the mask Figure 17-22. Many children with asthma have home nebulizers and are familiar with them. Administering a treatment with a bronchodilator may stabilize the event.

Status asthmaticus is a severe, prolonged asthmatic attack that cannot be stopped with conventional treatment. *It is a dire medical emergency.* Just as a person with COPD ordinarily does not call for an ambulance unless his or her condition has markedly changed, a person with asthma does not usually dial 9-1-1 unless the attack is much worse than usual. It is reasonable to assume that *any person with asthma who feels sick enough to call an ambulance may be in status asthmaticus until proved otherwise*.

On examination, a patient in status asthmaticus will be desperately struggling to move air through obstructed airways, with prominent use of the accessory muscles of breathing. The chest will be maximally hyperinflated. Breath sounds and wheezes may be entirely inaudible because air movement is negligible, and the patient will usually be exhausted, severely acidotic, and dehydrated.

The effort to breathe during an asthma attack is very tiring, and the patient may be exhausted by the time you arrive at the hospital. An exhausted patient may have stopped feeling anxious or even struggling to breathe. This patient is not recovering; he or she is at a very critical stage and is likely to stop breathing. Aggressive airway management, oxygen administration, and prompt transport are essential in this situation. Paramedic backup should be considered. Follow local protocol.

Anaphylactic Reactions

In severe anaphylactic reactions, first remove the offending agent. Maintain the airway—the airway is always a priority regardless of the situation. If the patient is still awake, allow him or her to assume a position that does not compromise breathing. Use an appropriate oxygen device for supplemental oxygen administration, and consider early transport. Be prepared to assist breathing as needed. Epinephrine is the treatment of choice. Rapid transport and the early administration of epinephrine, if allowed by protocol, should be a priority. Because epinephrine has immediate action, it can rapidly reverse the effects of anaphylaxis. Management of anaphylaxis is covered in detail in Chapter 22, *Immunologic Emergencies*.

Spontaneous Pneumothorax

Management of a spontaneous pneumothorax begins with the ABCs. Provide airway and ventilatory support, including high-flow oxygen and assisting ventilation as needed. Be alert for the signs of the development of a tension pneumothorax.

Consider IV initiation if severe symptoms are present. Pharmacologic interventions are not typically necessary, because the patient is generally treated symptomatically. Place the patient in a position of comfort and transport to the closest appropriate facility. The patient's condition should determine the transport mode. Provide reassurance en route. Consider calling for a paramedic unit if the patient shows signs of developing a tension pneumothorax.

▶ Pleural Effusion

Treatment of pleural effusion consists of removal of fluid collected outside the lung, which must be done by a physician in a hospital setting. However, you should provide oxygen and other routine support measures to these patients.

▶ Pulmonary Embolism

Manage the airway and provide high-flow oxygen, assisting ventilation as needed. Initiate CPR if the patient is pulseless and apneic. Establish an IV line with a bolus of an isotonic crystalloid solution, and give fluid for hydration based on clinical symptoms. Other interventions are supportive, and the most severe cases will be managed as a cardiac arrest of unknown origin. Transport the patient in the appropriate mode to the most appropriate facility. Offer reassurance and psychological support en route. Call for paramedic backup if needed.

▶ Hyperventilation

The decision whether hyperventilation is caused by a life-threatening illness or a panic attack should not be made outside the hospital. All patients who are hyperventilating should be given supplemental oxygen and transported to the hospital.

Management of hyperventilation syndrome depends on the cause of the syndrome. Oxygen should never be withheld from any patient complaining of dyspnea. The rate of oxygen administration is based on symptoms and pulse oximetry readings. Remember that factors such as carbon monoxide toxicity, which could also result in hyperventilation, may produce a falsely high oxygen saturation reading. If, through the patient's history, anxiety-related hyperventilation is confirmed, coached ventilation should be considered. When in doubt, always provide 100% oxygen.

Interventions for circulatory support and pharmacologic interventions are rarely required. Provide psychological support for the patient with anxiety-related hyperventilation. Have the patient mimic your respiratory rate and volume. Never place a paper bag over a hyperventilating patient's mouth and nose; if the hyperventilation is the result of hypoxia or other life-threatening condition, rebreathing carbon dioxide could be lethal. Provide transport to the closest appropriate facility; the patient's condition determines the transport mode.

▶ Obstruction of the Airway

If the patient is a small child or someone who was eating just before dyspnea developed, you may assume that the problem is an inhaled or aspirated foreign body. If the patient is old enough to talk but cannot make any noise, upper airway obstruction is the likely cause.

Upper airway obstruction may be either partial or complete. If your patient is able to talk and breathe, the wisest course may be to provide supplemental oxygen and transport carefully in a position of comfort to the hospital. As long as the patient is able to obtain sufficient oxygen, avoid doing anything that might turn a partial airway obstruction into a complete airway obstruction.

No condition is more immediately life threatening than a complete airway obstruction. The obstructing body must be removed before any other actions will be effective. Clear the patient's upper airway according to basic life support guidelines. Opening the airway with the head tilt–chin lift maneuver (or the jaw-thrust maneuver for patients with suspected spinal trauma) may solve the problem. You should perform this maneuver only after you have ruled out a head or neck injury. If simply opening the airway does not correct the breathing problem, you will have to assess the upper airway for the obstruction. Then, whether or not you are successful in clearing the airway, administer supplemental oxygen and transport the patient promptly to the emergency department.

▶ Environmental/Industrial Exposure

In many cases, industrial sites have their own medical/fire/hazardous materials teams that are familiar with all the chemicals used at their site and know what to do in case of exposure. They will begin immediate decontamination and medical care. In these cases, the patient needs to undergo decontamination by trained responders prior to you taking responsibility.

After the patient is decontaminated, gather information from the first responders about the substance and the cause of dyspnea. Assess the patient, paying special attention to lung sounds. Inhalation injuries can cause aspiration pneumonia that can result in eventual pulmonary edema. The inhaled substance can also cause lung damage. Blood coming from the airway is a particularly ominous sign.

Provide 100% supplemental oxygen or assisted ventilation if breathing is impaired (there is reduced tidal volume). If the upper airway is compromised, aggressive airway management (such as intubation or a cricothyrotomy by a paramedic) may be required.

Safety

The most important aspect of treatment in toxic inhalations is to remove the patient from the toxic environment, but do not enter a known toxic environment without protective breathing apparatus.

▶ Age-Related Assessment and Management

Bronchiolitis

The treatment of infants and young children with bronchiolitis is entirely supportive. Leave the patient in a position of comfort (eg, in the caregiver's arms, if the child does not seem to be in respiratory failure), and provide supplemental oxygen. Be prepared to assist ventilation with a bag-mask device or call for paramedic backup for endotracheal intubation if needed.

Respiratory Syncytial Virus

When you are assessing a child, look for signs of dehydration. Infants with RSV often refuse liquids and become dehydrated. Treat airway and breathing problems as appropriate. Humidified oxygen is helpful, if available.

Words of Wisdom

Immunizations have substantially reduced the incidence of many infectious diseases, such as diphtheria; however, an increasing number of people in the United States do not receive immunizations (because of poverty, lack of access to health care, geographic isolation) or refuse to be immunized (because of fears that immunizations cause other diseases or beliefs that immunizations are unnecessary), causing the resurgence of some diseases. In addition, because the effects of immunizations do not last forever, conditions such as epiglottitis may be seen (albeit rarely) in adults in their 20s and 30s.

Croup

As mentioned earlier, croup often responds well to the administration of humidified oxygen. Allow the patient to assume a position of comfort, and avoid agitating him or her. Administer nebulized epinephrine if dictated by local protocol. Transport rapidly to an appropriate facility.

Epiglottitis

Treat children with epiglottitis gently and try not to do anything that will make them cry. Keep them in a position of comfort, and give them high-flow oxygen. *Do not* put anything in their mouths because this could create a complete airway obstruction. Treatment of an adult patient with potential epiglottitis should be focused on maintaining a patent airway.

Pneumonia

Management of pneumonia includes monitoring the ABCs and providing high-flow oxygen and ventilatory support as needed. Administration of IV fluids may improve hydration and thin and mobilize mucus. If a high fever is present, cool the patient. Transport to the closest appropriate facility while providing psychological support.

Pertussis

Some infants and younger children with pertussis should be treated in a hospital because they are at greater risk for complications such as pneumonia, which occurs mostly in children younger than 1 year. In infants younger than 6 months, pertussis can sometimes be life threatening.[14]

Children with pertussis may vomit or not want to eat or drink. Watch for signs of dehydration. You may have to suction thick secretions to clear the airway. Give oxygen by the most appropriate means.

Pertussis in adults or geriatric patients does not cause the typical whooping illness that it does in infants and toddlers. However, it can cause a very severe upper respiratory infection, which in older people can result in pneumonia. The infection can cause coughing spells that last for weeks and can be so severe that patients find it hard to breathe, eat, or sleep. In the worst cases, coughing can result in cracked ribs. For patients who are already weak from other chronic conditions, pertussis can result in hospitalization. The disease has become a serious enough issue that physicians are becoming more aggressive about immunizing adults with the pertussis vaccine.

Pertussis is easily prevented with a vaccine. All AEMTs should check their immunization status and/or get a booster.

Airway Obstruction

If there is evidence of a partial or complete airway obstruction in a young child, especially a crawling baby, consider that the child may have swallowed and choked on a small object. One sign of aspiration may be an abnormality in the voice. Perform the appropriate airway clearing technique; if the patient is a child, use techniques specific to the child's age. Provide oxygen, and transport any patient with a suspected aspiration. A radiograph will be needed to confirm the aspiration, its location, and the treatment.

Heart Failure

When patients with heart failure decompensate, they will often experience pulmonary edema, as fluid backs up in their circulatory system and into the lungs. High blood pressure and low cardiac output often trigger this flash (sudden) pulmonary edema. These patients are among the most sick, frightened, and worrisome patients you will encounter. They are literally drowning in their own fluid. In addition to the classic signs of respiratory distress, they may have pink, frothy sputum coming from the mouth. They will have adventitious breath sounds, most often wet (crackles, rhonchi) but sometimes dry sounding (wheezes). Their legs and feet may be swollen (pedal edema) from the backup of fluid. You might find the patient has cool, diaphoretic, cyanotic skin. The patient's pulse will be tachycardic. The patient may have hypertension early, followed by deterioration to hypotension as a late finding.

Treatment should consist of airway, ventilatory, and circulatory support. Provide oxygen with adjuncts appropriate to the patient's condition, and prepare for the next level of deterioration. CPAP is often indicated for patients who have moderate to severe respiratory distress from an underlying disease, such as pulmonary edema from heart failure or obstructive pulmonary disease, and are alert and able to follow commands.

Tracheostomy Dysfunction

Children with chronic pulmonary medical conditions may use a home ventilator that is connected by a tracheostomy tube. This tube is placed in an opening in the neck (stoma) and can sometimes become obstructed by secretions, mucus, or foreign bodies. Other tracheostomy tube complications include bleeding, leaking, dislodgement, and infection. Your main goal is to establish a patent airway. Place the patient in a position of comfort and provide suctioning to clear the obstruction. If you are unable to clear the airway, consider paramedic intervention. After the obstruction is clear, oxygenate the patient and treat based on the patient's presentation.

Geriatric patients may have a tracheostomy tube in place because of airway obstruction, laryngeal cancer, severe infection, trauma, or the inability to manage secretions. As with children, in geriatric patients, the tube can become obstructed by secretions, foreign bodies, or airway swelling. The stoma itself can become infected. Establishing airway patency is the immediate goal.

Epidemic and Pandemic Considerations

An **epidemic** occurs when new cases of a disease occur in a human population and substantially exceed what is "expected," based on recent experience. A pandemic is an outbreak that occurs on a global scale. A flu pandemic occurs when a new influenza virus emerges for which people have little or no immunity. The disease can spread easily from person to person, cause serious illness, and be found in multiple countries in a short time. Obviously, there would be no specific vaccine immediately available.

Influenza type A is primarily an animal respiratory disease that has mutated to infect humans. Human infections have occurred and are spreading. In 2009, the H1N1 strain of influenza type A became pandemic.[15] Like seasonal flu, it may make chronic medical conditions worse. All strains of influenza type A are transmitted by direct contact with nasal secretions and aerosolized droplets from coughing and sneezing by infected people.

Many potentially serious diseases can be passed by the respiratory route; therefore, you need to be especially compliant with wearing of PPE (gloves, eye protection, and HEPA respirator at a minimum). Viruses can live for several days on surfaces, so frequent handwashing is also important. Maintain your vaccinations and stay up to date on the latest Centers for Disease Control and Prevention recommendations. Place a surgical mask on patients with suspected or confirmed respiratory disease. Wear a HEPA respirator during any aerosol-generating procedures such as suctioning of airway secretions, CPR, and when assisting with endotracheal intubation.

YOU are the Provider — SUMMARY

1. What are some potential causes of shortness of breath in older adults?

Some possible causes of shortness of breath in geriatric patients are the possibility of a foreign body airway obstruction, an acute disease process such as asthma, anaphylaxis, chronic conditions such as COPD and chronic bronchitis, and myocardial infarction. Because myocardial infarction is a possible cause, you must request paramedic intercept for the purpose of cardiac monitoring to ensure that no substantial dysrhythmias are present. Also, never rule out the possibility of a toxic exposure; however, in this case, that possibility is unlikely because no other patients are experiencing breathing difficulty.

2. What equipment would you need immediately after you arrive on scene?

Because you can never be sure of what you may encounter, you should take in all of the equipment that you believe that you will need based on dispatch information and your company's policy. In a situation such as shortness of breath, you should take in supplemental oxygen, masks such as nasal cannulas and nonrebreathing masks, nebulized medications, and an appropriate-size bag-mask device.

3. What would your next course of action be?

The next course of action for this patient will depend on local protocols. If allowed per protocols, the administration

YOU are the Provider SUMMARY (continued)

of an inhaled beta agonist such as albuterol should be considered based on the patient's presentation and wheezing.

4. **Should this patient be loaded on the stretcher and treated in the ambulance, or should you treat her at the scene?**

   This patient needs immediate treatment. She has an acute respiratory problem associated with cyanosis. Initiate treatment and then consider moving the patient while she is receiving the medication. Make every effort to treat an acute respiratory problem immediately and then provide transport.

5. **How can you explain the patient's elevated heart rate?**

   This patient's elevated heart rate can be attributed to two causes. The first cause is a compensatory mechanism, which is a result of the dyspnea. To increase oxygenation, the body has increased the heart rate to circulate the available oxygen faster. The second likely cause is the administration of albuterol. Tachycardia is a common side effect of inhaled beta agonists.

6. **With this patient's history of COPD, should you be concerned about the hypoxic drive?**

   You should never withhold oxygen from a patient who needs it for fear of depressing or stopping breathing, even in patients with COPD. Even though this patient has a history of COPD, she is experiencing a hypoxic episode and needs supplemental oxygen.

7. **Should paramedic backup have been requested for this patient?**

   Paramedic backup should always be considered for patients reporting shortness of breath. Paramedics may be able to provide different medications for the patient's condition and provide endotracheal intubation, if needed. Also, paramedic backup should be requested to address any underlying cardiac condition that may have triggered this episode of dyspnea.

8. **Should this patient have received an IV line?**

   Rehydration is supplemental therapy for patients with respiratory problems who are dehydrated, such as for some patients who have pneumonia or asthma. It is also useful to thin mucus secretions in those with reactive airway diseases. It is common practice to give a fluid bolus to younger patients with these conditions. However, any geriatric patient or patient who has a cardiac dysfunction could be pushed into pulmonary edema by too much fluid. Always assess breath sounds *before* and *after* giving a fluid bolus to make certain you have not overhydrated the patient. Of course, patients who have respiratory problems can quickly become ill, and you will almost always want to have an IV line in place.

EMS Patient Care Report (PCR)

Date: 9-12-18	**Incident No.:** 9587	**Nature of Call:** Dyspnea	**Location:** 330 S Central Ave		
Dispatched: 1724	**En Route:** 1730	**At Scene:** 1737	**Transport:** 1754	**At Hospital:** 1804	**In Service:** 1822

Patient Information

Age: 86 **Sex:** F **Weight (in kg [lb]):** 61 kg (135 lb)	**Allergies:** Sulfa **Medications:** Lisinopril, albuterol **Past Medical History:** Asthma, COPD, hypertension **Chief Complaint:** Dyspnea

Vital Signs

Time: 1738	**BP:** Not yet obtained	**Pulse:** Bounding	**Respirations:** 30	**Spo_2:** Not yet obtained
Time: 1744	**BP:** 148/92	**Pulse:** 148	**Respirations:** 28	**Spo_2:** 91% on 100% oxygen
Time: 1752	**BP:** 134/82	**Pulse:** 142	**Respirations:** 26	**Spo_2:** 95% on 100% oxygen

YOU are the Provider SUMMARY *(continued)*

EMS Treatment (circle all that apply)				
Oxygen @ 15 L/min via (circle one): **NC** **(NRM)** **Bag-mask device**		**Assisted Ventilation**	**Airway Adjunct**	**CPR**
Defibrillation	**Bleeding Control**	**Bandaging**	**Splinting**	(**Other:** 2.5 mg albuterol sulfate)

Narrative
Medic One responded to an assisted living center for a patient with dyspnea. Caregiver advised EMS that the patient has been short of breath x 2 days but refused to go to the hospital. She has a prior Hx of HTN, emphysema, and asthma. EMS found pt sitting in tripod position on the edge of her bed in obvious respiratory distress. Pt AO×3, but lethargic and slow to respond to questions. Pt presents with wheezes in upper lobes and diminished breath sounds in both lower lobes. On arrival pt on O_2 @ 4 L/min via NC with an Spo_2 of 91%. Placed pt on O_2 via NRM @ 15 L/min. Skin warm and dry with bounding radial pulses at 148 bpm. Pt has good ROM in all extremities and no peripheral edema noted. Placed pt on stretcher in position of comfort and initiated nebulized treatment of albuterol per protocol. Established 20 g IV left AC with NS TKO. Pt stated breathing was "better" after nebulized tx, but still dyspneic and wheezes still present in upper lobes. Requested orders for second nebulized albuterol treatment but denied due to pt's persistent tachycardia. Provided rapid transport to the ED for evaluation. Gave report to triage nurse and returned to service.**End of report**

Prep Kit

▶ Ready for Review

- Dyspnea is a common complaint that may be caused by numerous medical problems, including infections of the upper or lower airways, acute pulmonary edema, chronic obstructive pulmonary disease, spontaneous pneumothorax, asthma or allergic reactions, pleural effusions, mechanical obstruction of the airway, pulmonary embolism, and hyperventilation.
- Lung disorders interfere with the exchange of oxygen and carbon dioxide that takes place during respiration through problems with ventilation, diffusion, perfusion, or a combination of these.
- Signs and symptoms of breathing difficulty include adventitious breath sounds, nasal flaring, pursed-lip breathing, cyanosis, inability to talk, use of accessory muscles to breathe, and sitting in the tripod position.
- Respiratory conditions that occur more commonly in children include bronchiolitis, epiglottitis, croup, and pertussis.
- Assessment of patients in respiratory distress should be conducted as a calm, systematic process. The patients are usually quite anxious.
- Remember to use standard precautions. A patient with a respiratory emergency may have an infection that could be passed to you through sputum and/or air droplets.
- Pulmonary complaints may be associated with exposure to a wide variety of toxins. Suspect toxic inhalation if more than one patient has dyspnea, and immediately remove yourself from the scene until it is safe.
- In treating dyspnea, it is important to reassure the patient and provide supplemental oxygen. Remember to maintain the patient in a position that is comfortable for breathing, usually sitting upright.
- If the patient is not breathing or is breathing inadequately, administer 100% oxygen. You may need to provide positive pressure ventilations with a bag-mask device. Establish IV access and administer fluids as needed.
- You will need to listen to the patient's breath sounds. Listen for a full respiratory cycle. You want to hear clear flow of air in both lungs. Not hearing the flow

Prep Kit (continued)

of air is considered an absent lung sound. The lack of air movement in the lung is an important finding.
- Rales are fine, crackling sounds of air trying to pass through fluid in the alveoli, typically heard on inspiration. These are often a result of pulmonary edema, or fluid in the lungs caused by heart failure.
- Rhonchi are lower pitched sounds caused by secretions or mucus in the larger airway. These can be heard with infections such as pneumonia and bronchitis, or in cases of aspiration.
- Stridor is a high-pitched sound heard on inspiration as air tries to pass through an obstruction in the upper airway. This sound indicates a partial obstruction of the trachea and is seen in patients with anatomic or foreign body airway obstruction.
- Wheezing is a high-pitched whistling sound typically heard on expiration. It indicates constriction and/or inflammation in the bronchus and may be heard in patients with asthma or chronic obstructive pulmonary disease.
- If there are life-threatening conditions, there may not be time to take a history or perform a secondary assessment. If you can, obtain a thorough history, asking the patient to describe the problem to determine the chief complaint.
- If the patient has a prescribed inhaler or other respiratory medication, consult medical control to assist with appropriate use.
- Transport the patient to the hospital, monitoring his or her condition en route.
- Reassess and record vital signs at least every 5 minutes for a patient in unstable condition and/or after the patient uses an inhaler.
- Consider rehydration; it is supplemental therapy for patients with respiratory problems who are dehydrated. It is common practice to give a fluid bolus to younger patients with respiratory problems, but a patient with cardiac dysfunction could experience pulmonary edema by having too much fluid.
- Breathing may need to be supported more aggressively with continuous positive airway pressure or bilevel positive airway pressure.
- Remember that pulse oximetry readings may be inaccurate in the presence of conditions that abnormally bind hemoglobin, including carbon monoxide poisoning.
- Remember, a patient who is breathing rapidly may not be getting a sufficient amount of oxygen as a result of respiratory distress from a variety of problems. In every case, prompt recognition of the problem, giving oxygen or providing ventilatory support, and prompt transport are essential.

▶ Vital Vocabulary

adventitious breath sounds Abnormal breath sounds such as wheezes, rhonchi, and rales.

allergen A substance that causes an allergic reaction.

aspiration The inhalation of liquid or solid matter into the lungs through the trachea, typically as a result of an incompetent gag reflex or overaggressive resuscitation technique.

asthma A disease of the lungs in which muscle spasm in the small air passageways and the production of large amounts of mucus result in airway obstruction.

atelectasis Collapse of the alveoli.

botulism Poisoning characterized by severe muscle paralysis and usually caused by eating food containing botulinum toxin.

bronchial breath sounds Normal breath sounds made by air moving through the bronchi.

bronchiolitis Inflammation of the bronchioles that usually occurs in children younger than 2 years and is often caused by the respiratory syncytial virus.

carbon dioxide retention A condition characterized by a chronically high level of carbon dioxide in blood as the result of a respiratory disease.

carpopedal spasm Tingling and spasms of the phalanges resulting from hyperventilation.

chronic bronchitis Irritation and inflammation of the major lung passageways, from either infectious disease or irritants such as smoke.

chronic obstructive pulmonary disease (COPD) A slow, degenerative process that causes destructive changes in the alveoli and bronchioles in the lungs.

common cold A viral infection usually associated with swollen nasal mucous membranes and the production of fluid from the sinuses.

crackles Crackling, moist breath sounds signaling fluid in the smaller air passages of the lungs; formerly called rales.

croup An infectious disease of the upper respiratory system that may cause partial airway obstruction and is characterized by a barking cough; usually seen in children; also referred to as laryngotracheobronchitis.

cystic fibrosis A genetic disorder of the endocrine system that makes it difficult for chloride to move through cells; primarily targets the respiratory and digestive systems.

diffusion The movement of gases from a higher concentration to a lower concentration.

diphtheria An infectious disease in which a membrane lining the pharynx is formed that can severely obstruct passage of air into the larynx.

Prep Kit *(continued)*

dyspnea A feeling of shortness of breath or difficulty breathing.

embolus A blood clot or other substance in the circulatory system that breaks free from its site of origin and obstructs blood flow in a distant blood vessel.

emphysema A disease of the lungs in which there is extreme dilation and eventual destruction of pulmonary alveoli with poor exchange of oxygen and carbon dioxide; it is one form of chronic obstructive pulmonary disease.

epidemic Occurs when new cases of a disease occur in a human population and substantially exceed what is "expected," based on recent experience.

epiglottitis An infectious disease in which the epiglottis becomes inflamed and enlarged and may cause upper airway obstruction; also referred to as acute supraglottic laryngitis.

Guillain-Barré syndrome A disease of unknown cause characterized by progressive paralysis moving from the feet to the head (ascending paralysis); if paralysis reaches the diaphragm, the patient may require respiratory support.

Hering-Breuer reflex The nervous system mechanism that terminates inhalation and prevents lung overexpansion.

hyperoxia An excess of oxygen.

hyperventilation Rapid or deep breathing.

hyperventilation syndrome (panic attack) A syndrome that occurs in the absence of other physical problems and whose symptoms include anxiety, dizziness, numbness, tingling of the hands and feet, and dyspnea despite rapid breathing.

hypoventilation The movement of inadequate volumes of air into the lungs.

hypoxia A condition in which the body's cells and tissues do not have enough oxygen.

hypoxic drive Backup system to control respirations when oxygen levels fall dangerously low.

influenza type A (flu) A virus that has crossed the animal/human barrier and has infected humans, recently reaching a pandemic level with the H1N1 strain.

inspiratory/expiratory (I/E) ratio An expression for comparing the length of inspiration with that of expiration, normally 1:2, meaning that expiration is twice as long as inspiration (not measured in seconds).

meningococcal meningitis An inflammation of the meningeal coverings of the brain and spinal cord; can be highly contagious.

metered-dose inhaler (MDI) A miniature spray canister used to direct medications through the mouth and into the lungs.

methicillin-resistant *Staphylococcus aureus* (MRSA) A bacterium that can cause infections in different parts of the body.

orthopnea Severe dyspnea experienced when lying down and relieved by sitting up.

pandemic An outbreak that occurs on a global scale.

perfusion Supplying an organ or tissue with required nutrients and oxygen.

pertussis (whooping cough) An airborne bacterial infection that causes fever and a "whoop" sound on inspiration after a coughing attack; affects mostly children younger than 6 years; highly contagious through droplet infection.

pleural effusion A collection of fluid between the lung and chest wall that may compress the lung.

pleural friction rub A squeaking or grating sound that occurs when the pleural linings rub together, which may be heard on inspiration, expiration, or both; commonly caused by inflammation of the pleura.

pleuritic chest pain Sharp, stabbing pain in the chest that is worsened by a deep breath or other chest wall movement; often caused by inflammation or irritation of the pleura.

pneumonia An infectious disease of the lung that damages lung tissue.

pneumonitis Lung inflammation from an irritant, such as a chemical, dust, or radiation, or from aspiration, such as aspiration of gastric contents.

pneumothorax A partial or complete accumulation of air in the pleural space.

pulmonary edema A buildup of fluid in the lungs, usually as a result of left-side heart failure.

pulmonary embolism A blood clot that breaks off from a large vein and travels to the blood vessels of the lung, causing obstruction of blood flow.

purulent Full of pus; having the character of pus.

respiration The exchange of gases that occurs at the pulmonary and cellular levels.

respiratory acidosis A pathologic condition characterized by a blood pH of less than 7.35 and caused by an accumulation of acids in the body from inadequate ventilation.

respiratory alkalosis A pathologic condition characterized by a blood pH of greater than 7.45 and resulting from the accumulation of bases in the body from overaggressive ventilation.

respiratory syncytial virus (RSV) A virus that causes an infection of the lungs and breathing passages; can result in other serious illnesses that affect the lungs or heart, such as bronchiolitis and pneumonia; highly contagious and spread through droplets.

Prep Kit (continued)

retractions The drawing in of the intercostal muscles and the muscles above the clavicles that can occur in respiratory distress.

rhonchi Coarse, rattling breath sounds heard in patients with chronic mucus in the larger lower airways.

severe acute respiratory syndrome (SARS) A potentially life-threatening viral infection that usually starts with flulike symptoms.

small-volume nebulizer A respiratory device that holds liquid medicine that is turned into a fine mist. The patient inhales the medication into the airways and lungs as a treatment for conditions like asthma.

spacer A device that collects medication as it is released from the canister of a metered-dose inhaler, allowing more medication to be delivered to the lungs and less to be lost to the environment.

status asthmaticus A prolonged exacerbation of asthma that does not respond to conventional therapy.

stridor A harsh, high-pitched respiratory sound, generally heard during inspiration, that is caused by partial blockage or narrowing of the upper airway; may be audible without a stethoscope.

subcutaneous emphysema Air bubbles trapped underneath the skin in the subcutaneous tissue.

tachypnea Rapid respiratory rate.

tuberculosis A disease that can lay dormant in a person's lungs for decades, then reactivate; many strains are resistant to many antibiotics; spread by cough.

ventilation The movement of air into and out of the lungs.

vesicular breath sounds Normal breath sounds made by air moving in and out of the alveoli.

wheezing A high-pitched, whistling breath sound that is most prominent on expiration, and which suggests an obstruction or narrowing of the lower airways; occurs in asthma and bronchiolitis.

▶ References

1. Khan AN, Al-Jahdali H, AL-Ghanem S, Gouda A. Reading chest radiographs in the critically ill (Part II): radiography of lung pathologies common in the ICU patient. *Ann Thorac Med.* 2009; 4(3):149-157. https://www.ncbi.nlm.nih.gov/pmc/articles/PMC2714572/. Accessed September 26, 2017.
2. Sharma G, Goodwin J. Effect of aging on respiratory system physiology and immunology. *Clin Interv Aging.* 2006; Sep; 1(3):253-260. https://www.ncbi.nlm.nih.gov/pmc/articles/PMC2695176/. Accessed September 26, 2017.
3. Kim V, Criner GJ. Chronic bronchitis and chronic obstructive pulmonary disease. *Am J Respir Crit Care Med.* 2013;187. http://www.atsjournals.org/doi/full/10.1164/rccm.201210-1843CI. Accessed September 26, 2017.
4. What Is Asthma? National Heart, Lung, and Blood Institute. https://www.nhlbi.nih.gov/health/health-topics/topics/asthma/. Updated August 4, 2014. Accessed November 20, 2017.
5. Health Guide: breath sounds. *The New York Times* website. Review date: 11/2/2009. http://www.nytimes.com/health/guides/symptoms/breath-sounds/overview.html?mcubz=0. Accessed September 26, 2017.
6. What is pulmonary embolism? Health After 50 website; School of Public Health at the University of California. March 31, 2017. https://www.healthafter50.com/respiratory-health/article/what-is-a-pulmonary-embolism. Accessed September 27, 2017.
7. Bronchiolitis. MedlinePlus website. https://medlineplus.gov/ency/article/000975.htm. Updated November 6, 2017. Accessed November 20, 2017.
8. Centers for Disease Control and Prevention. Leading causes of death. https://www.cdc.gov/nchs/fastats/leading-causes-of-death.htm. Accessed September 27, 2017.
9. Kane B, Decalmer S, O'Driscoll BR. Emergency oxygen therapy: from guideline to implementation. *Breathe.* 2013 9:246-253. http://breathe.ersjournals.com/content/9/4/246. Accessed October 18, 2017.
10. Hale KE, Gavin C, O'Driscoll BR. Audit of oxygen use in emergency ambulances and in a hospital emergency department. *Emerg Med J.* 2008;25:773-776.
11. O'Driscoll BR, Howard LS, Bucknall C, Welham SA, Davison AG. British Thoracic Society emergency oxygen audits. *Thorax.* 2011;66:734-735.
12. Berg RA, Hemphill R, Abella BS, et al. Part 5: adult basic life support: 2010 American Heart Association Guidelines for Cardiopulmonary Resuscitation and Emergency Cardiovascular Care. *Circulation.* 2010;122(suppl 3):S685-S705.
13. Perrone S, Bracciali C, Nicola Di Virgilio N, Buonocore G. Oxygen use in neonatal care: a two-edged sword. *Front Pediatr.* 2016; 4:143. https://www.ncbi.nlm.nih.gov/pmc/articles/PMC5220090/. Accessed October 19, 2017.
14. Centers for Disease Control and Prevention. Whooping cough is deadly for babies. https://www.cdc.gov/pertussis/pregnant/mom/deadly-disease-for-baby.html. Accessed October 19, 2017.
15. Centers for Disease Control and Prevention. The 2009 H1N1 pandemic: summary highlights, April 2009-April 2010. https://www.cdc.gov/h1n1flu/cdcresponse.htm. Accessed September 27, 2017.

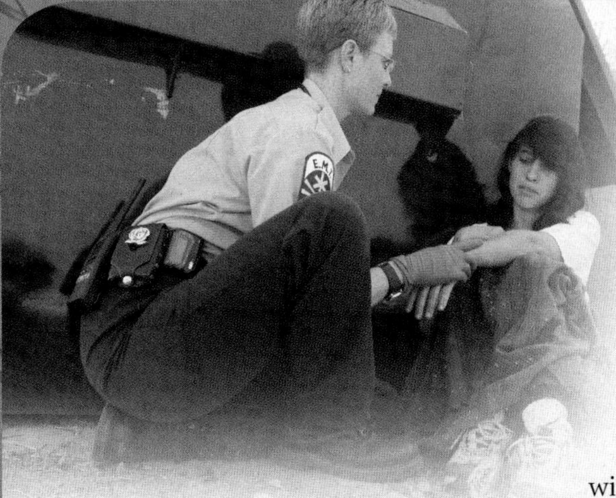

Assessment *in Action*

You are dispatched to a local motel for a 53-year-old man who is reporting severe shortness of breath. On arrival, you are met by a woman who states the patient started coughing uncontrollably and became short of breath. You see the obese patient seated in the tripod position on the bed.

The patient states that his severe shortness of breath started with exertion when he lifted two suitcases. He further states that he has a history of chronic bronchitis and chronic obstructive pulmonary disease (COPD) and smokes 1.5 packs of unfiltered cigarettes per day.

1. What is COPD?

A. The end of a slow process that results in disruption of the airways
B. An infectious disease of the lung that damages lung tissue
C. A potentially life-threatening viral infection that usually starts with flulike symptoms
D. A disease of the lungs in which there is extreme dilation of the alveoli

2. Which one of the following is NOT a common cause for exacerbation of COPD?

A. Smoking
B. H1N1 vaccine
C. Air pollution
D. Tuberculosis

3. The clinical definition of chronic bronchitis is a productive cough for at least ___ months per year for ___ or more consecutive years.

A. 2, 2
B. 3, 3
C. 2, 3
D. 3, 2

4. Which term indicates coarse rattling sounds caused by mucus in the larger lower airways?

A. Stridor
B. Wheezing
C. Rhonchi
D. Rales

5. The patient is in a tripod position. _____ is severe difficulty breathing experienced when lying down or in a position that is not upright.

A. Apnea
B. Orthopnea
C. Dyspnea
D. Eupnea

6. What is the most common source of bronchiolitis?

A. Prolonged exposure to tobacco smoke
B. Foreign body airway obstruction
C. Respiratory syncytial virus
D. A bacterial upper respiratory infection

7. How does a pleural effusion cause shortness of breath?

A. By compressing one or both lungs
B. By obstructing the airway
C. By causing damage to the alveoli
D. By causing the lungs to fill with fluid

8. _____ is an irreversible condition that makes the alveoli susceptible to atelectasis.

A. Emphysema
B. Asthma
C. Pertussis
D. Bronchiolitis

9. What is the purpose of using *a spacer* with a metered dose inhaler?

10. List three possible complications that may occur when a bag-mask device is used too forcefully for ventilation.

CHAPTER 18

Cardiovascular Emergencies

National EMS Education Standard Competencies

Pathophysiology

Applies comprehensive knowledge of the pathophysiology of respiration and perfusion to patient assessment and management.

Medicine

Applies fundamental knowledge to provide basic and selected advanced emergency care and transportation based on assessment findings for an acutely ill patient.

Cardiovascular

Anatomy, signs, symptoms, and management of

- Chest pain (pp 809-813, 822-824)
- Cardiac arrest (pp 811-813, 826-835)

Anatomy, physiology, pathophysiology, assessment, and management of

- Acute coronary syndrome (pp 810-811, 817-824)
  - Angina pectoris (pp 810-811, 817-824)
  - Myocardial infarction (pp 811-813, 817-822, 826-835)
- Aortic aneurysm/dissection (pp 816-824)
- Thromboembolism (pp 809-810, 817-824)
- Heart failure (pp 815-816, 817-824)
- Hypertensive emergencies (pp 816-824)

Knowledge Objectives

1. Review the basic anatomy and physiology of the cardiovascular system. (pp 803-808)
2. Discuss the regulation of heart function. (p 807)
3. Describe the cardiac cycle, including the concepts of afterload, stroke volume, and cardiac output. (pp 807-808)
4. Describe the pathophysiology of angina pectoris, thromboembolism, and myocardial infarction. (pp 809-812)
5. List the dangerous dysrhythmias that may follow a myocardial infarction. (pp 812-814)
6. Discuss the pathophysiology of cardiogenic shock and its signs, symptoms, and treatment. (pp 813, 815)
7. Discuss the pathophysiology of heart failure and its signs, symptoms, and treatment. (pp 815-816)
8. Discuss the pathophysiology of pulmonary edema. (p 816)
9. Describe the pathophysiology, signs and symptoms, and management of hypertensive emergencies. (pp 816-817)
10. Describe the pathophysiology, assessment, and management of aortic aneurysm/dissection. (pp 816-817)
11. Explain patient assessment procedures for cardiovascular problems. (pp 817-822)
12. Explain the relationship between airway management and the patient with cardiac compromise. (p 818)
13. Discuss emergency medical care for cardiovascular emergencies, including angina pectoris, thromboembolism, and myocardial infarction. (pp 822-824, 829-835)
14. List the indications and contraindications for the use of nitroglycerin. (p 823)
15. Explain that many patients will have had cardiac surgery and may have implanted pacemakers. (pp 823, 825)
16. Define cardiac arrest. (p 826)
17. Discuss the different types of AEDs. (pp 826-827)
18. Describe the difference between the fully automated and the semiautomated defibrillator. (p 827)
19. List the advantages of using AEDs. (p 828)
20. List the indications and contraindications for use of an automated external defibrillator (AED). (p 828)
21. Explain the use of remote, adhesive defibrillator pads. (pp 828, 831)
22. Explain why not all patients in cardiac arrest need to be attached to an AED. (pp 828, 831)
23. List the reasons for early defibrillation. (p 828)
24. Describe AED maintenance procedures. (pp 828-829)
25. Explain the circumstances that may result in inappropriate shocks from an AED. (p 829)
26. Explain the role played by medical direction in the use of AEDs. (p 829)
27. Explain the need for a case review of each incident in which an AED is used. (p 829)

28. Discuss the importance of practice and continuing education with the AED. (p 829)
29. Explain the reason not to touch the patient, such as by delivering cardiopulmonary resuscitation, while the AED is analyzing the heart rhythm and delivering shocks. (pp 829, 831)
30. Describe the emergency medical care for the patient with cardiac arrest. (pp 829-833)
31. Explain the relationship of age to defibrillation. (p 831)
32. Discuss the procedures to follow for standard operation of the various types of AEDs. (pp 831-833)
33. Describe the components of care following AED shocks. (pp 833-834)
34. Explain criteria for transport of the patient following CPR and defibrillation. (pp 834-835)
35. Discuss the role of cardiac monitoring. (p 835)

Skills Objectives

1. Demonstrate how to assess and provide emergency medical care for a patient with chest pain or discomfort. (pp 822-824)
2. Demonstrate the administration of aspirin to a patient with chest pain. (p 823)
3. Demonstrate the administration of nitroglycerin. (pp 823-824, Skill Drill 18-1)
4. Demonstrate how to perform maintenance of an AED. (pp 828-829)
5. Demonstrate how to use an AED and perform CPR. (pp 831-833, Skill Drill 18-2)
6. Demonstrate how to place electrodes for cardiac monitoring. (pp 835-837, Skill Drill 18-3)

Introduction

The American Heart Association estimates that one person has an acute myocardial infarction (AMI) in the United States approximately every 40 seconds.[1] In the United States, emergency medical services (EMS) personnel treat approximately 60% of out-of-hospital cardiac arrests each year.[1] Heart disease has been the leading cause of death of Americans since the early 1900s.[2,3]

It is important for EMS providers to understand that many deaths caused by cardiovascular disease occur from problems that may have been avoided by people living healthier lifestyles and by access to improved medical technology. We can help to reduce these numbers of deaths with better public awareness, early access to EMS, increased numbers of laypeople trained in and willing to perform cardiopulmonary resuscitation (CPR), increased use of evolving technology in dispatch and cardiac arrest response, public access to defibrillation devices, the recognition of the need for advanced life support (ALS) services, and transportation to hospitals that can provide coronary catheterization and postarrest care.

This chapter begins with a brief description of the heart and how it works. It then discusses the relationship between chest pain and ischemic heart disease. It explains how to recognize and treat AMI (classic heart attack) and its complications—sudden death, cardiogenic shock, and heart failure. The use of nitroglycerin and aspirin are described. The last part of the chapter is devoted to the use and maintenance of the automated external defibrillator (AED) and placement of electrodes for cardiac monitoring.

Anatomy and Physiology Review

Anatomy Review

The cardiovascular system consists of the heart (the pump), the blood vessels (the container), and the blood

YOU are the Provider — PART 1

Your ambulance is dispatched to a local residence for a woman who reports chest pain. As you arrive on scene, the patient's husband greets you at the front door and states that his wife is on the sofa, complaining of "really bad" chest pain. On walking into the residence, you find the wife in the fetal position on the sofa, rocking back and forth, moaning in pain. She states that she is 56 years old and has had multiple heart attacks in the past.

1. How does the heart become oxygenated?
2. What is the most common cause of chest pain?

(the fluid). All components must interact effectively to maintain life.

Structures of the Heart

As you know from Chapter 7, *The Human Body*, the **heart** is a muscular, cone-shaped organ whose function is to pump blood throughout the body **Figure 18-1**.

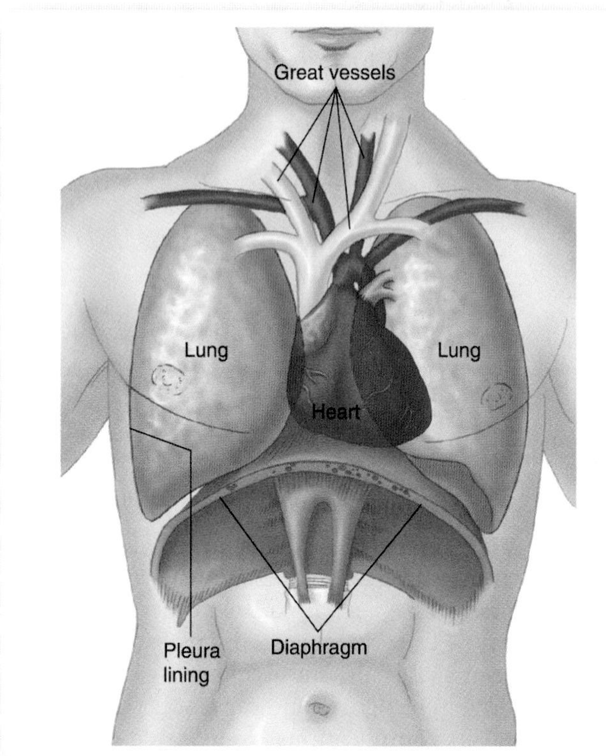

Figure 18-1 The anterior aspect of the thorax shows the relative position of the heart beneath the surface.

The heart muscle is referred to as the **myocardium**. The **pericardium**, or **pericardial sac**, is a thick, fibrous membrane that surrounds the heart. The inner membrane of the pericardium contains the visceral layer and the parietal layer. The visceral layer of the pericardium lies against the heart and is also called the **epicardium**. The second layer of the pericardium, the parietal layer, is separated from the visceral layer by a small amount of **pericardial fluid** that reduces friction within the pericardial sac. The **endocardium** is the smooth inner lining of the chambers of the heart and the surface of the valves.

Two atria and two ventricles make up the upper and lower chambers of the heart, respectively. Each **atrium** receives blood that is returned to the heart from other parts of the body; each **ventricle** pumps blood out of the heart. The left ventricle is the strongest and largest of the four cardiac chambers because it is responsible for pumping blood through blood vessels throughout the body.

Valves of the Heart

The valves of the heart include the **atrioventricular valves** (these are the **tricuspid valve** and the **mitral valve** [also known as the bicuspid valve]) and the **semilunar valves** (these are the **aortic valve** and the **pulmonic valve**) **Figure 18-2**. **Papillary muscles** in the ventricles contract to tighten the **chordae tendineae**, preventing blood from flowing backward into the atria.

Coronary Circulation

The heart, like any other muscle, requires oxygen and nutrients. These are supplied via the **coronary arteries**, which arise from the **aorta** shortly after it leaves the left ventricle. The coronary circulation emanates from the left and right coronary arteries **Figure 18-3**.

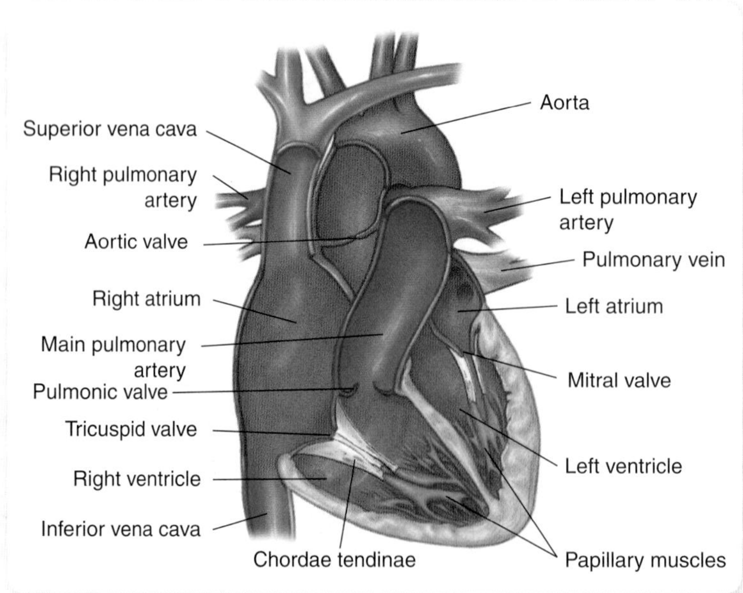

Figure 18-2 Anatomy of the heart, including its valves.

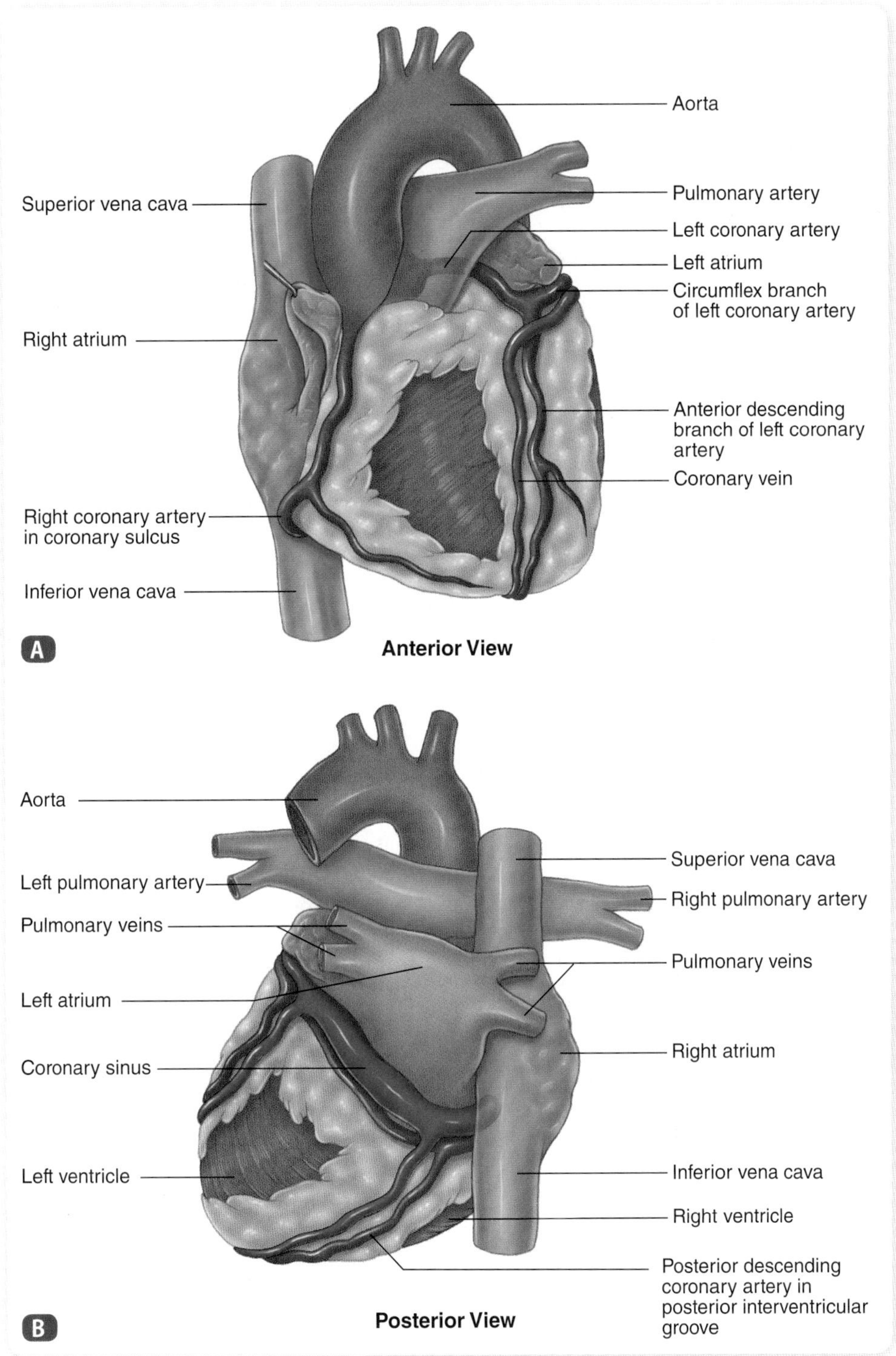

Figure 18-3 The coronary arteries supply oxygen and nutrients to the heart. **A.** Anterior view. **B.** Posterior view.

The left main coronary artery is the largest and shortest of the myocardial blood vessels. It rapidly divides into two branches, the **left anterior descending (LAD) artery** and the **circumflex coronary artery**. These arteries subdivide further, supplying blood to most of the left ventricle, the interventricular septum (the thick walls between the ventricles), and, at times, the **atrioventricular (AV) node**.

Blood Vessels

Blood is transported through the body via the **arteries**, which carry blood away from the heart, and **veins**, which carry blood back to the heart. The aorta is the body's largest artery. Arteries become smaller as they get farther from the heart. Eventually, they branch into many small

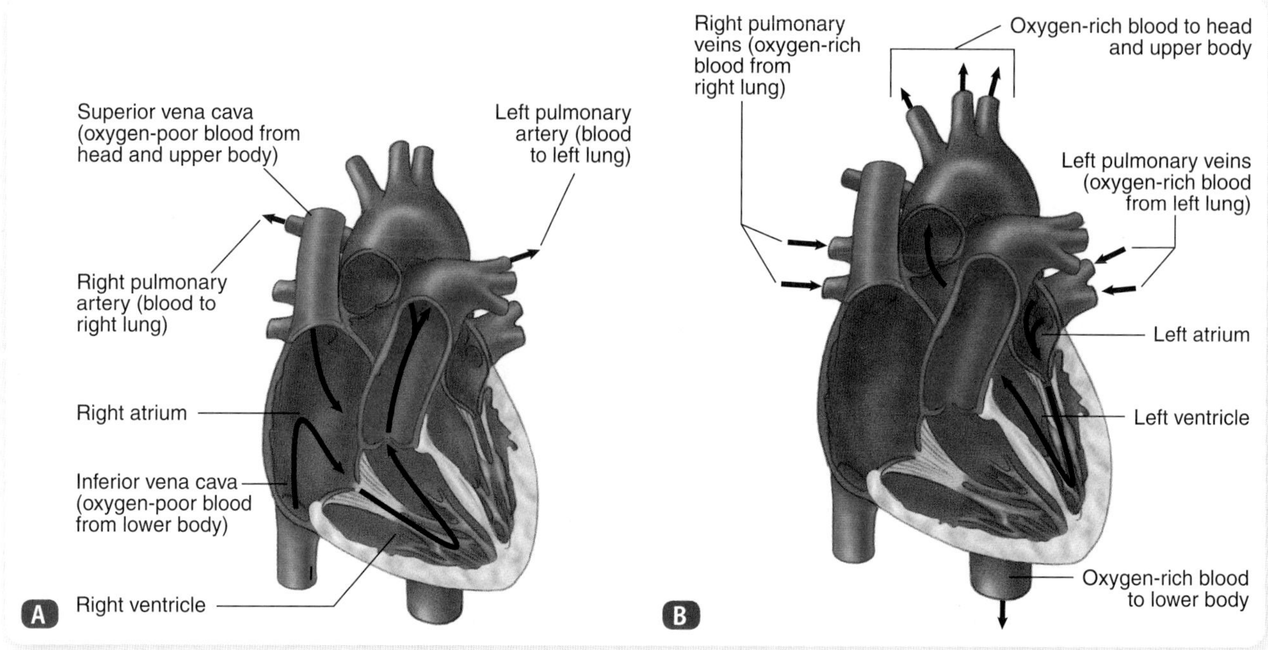

Figure 18-4 Blood flow through the heart. **A.** Flow of oxygen-poor blood from the venous circulation. **B.** Flow of oxygen-rich blood from the pulmonary veins, through the left side of the heart and into the aorta.

arterioles that divide even further into **capillaries**, which are microscopic, thin-walled blood vessels. The capillaries eventually enlarge to form **venules**, which merge and form veins.

Two large veins, the **superior vena cava** and the **inferior vena cava**, return deoxygenated blood from the body to the right atrium. The inferior vena cava is the larger of the two veins.

In the heart, blood enters the right atrium via the superior and inferior venae cavae and the **coronary sinus** (the end of the great cardiac vein) collects blood returning from the walls of the heart. Blood from four pulmonary veins enters the left atrium Figure 18-4.

Blood and Its Components

Blood consists of **plasma** and formed elements or cells (**red blood cells (RBCs)**, **white blood cells (WBCs)**, and platelets). Plasma accounts for more than one-half of total blood volume. RBCs (erythrocytes) carry oxygen to the tissues. These disk-shaped cells flow in the plasma, which moves them along through the circulatory system. RBCs contain the protein **hemoglobin**, which binds to oxygen and carries it to the tissues. WBCs (leukocytes) fight infection either via antibodies or direct attack on bacteria. Finally, **platelets** play an important role in the blood clotting process (coagulation); they begin the process by clumping together, after which clotting proteins solidify the remainder of the clot.

The Electrical Conduction System

The brain partially controls the heart's rate and strength of contraction via the autonomic nervous system. However, pumping of the heart occurs in response to an electrical stimulus initiated by a group of complex electrical tissues that are part of a **conduction system**. The cardiac conduction system consists of six parts, as shown in Figure 18-5.

The **sinoatrial (SA) node,** located high in the right atrium, is the normal site of origin of the electrical impulse. It is the heart's natural pacemaker and has an intrinsic rate of 60 to 100 beats/min. If the SA node is not functioning properly, the AV node may take over as the heart's pacemaker. The intrinsic rate of the AV node is 40 to 60 beats/min. Rhythms originating below the AV node have an intrinsic rate of 20 to 40 beats/min. Impulses originating in the SA node travel through the right and left atria, resulting in atrial contraction. The impulse then travels to the AV node, located in the right atrium adjacent to the septum, where it transiently slows. Electrical stimulation of the heart muscle then continues toward the bundle of His, which is a continuation of the AV node. From here, it proceeds rapidly to the right and left bundle branches, stimulating the interventricular septum. The impulse then spreads out through the rest of the conduction system, resulting in ventricular contraction, or systole.

Electrical Properties of Cardiac Cells

The ability of cells to respond to electrical impulses is referred to as the property of **excitability**. The ability of the cells to conduct electrical impulses is referred to as the property of **conductivity**.

Cardiac muscle cells have a special characteristic called **automaticity** that is not found in any other type of muscle cells. Automaticity allows a cardiac muscle cell to contract

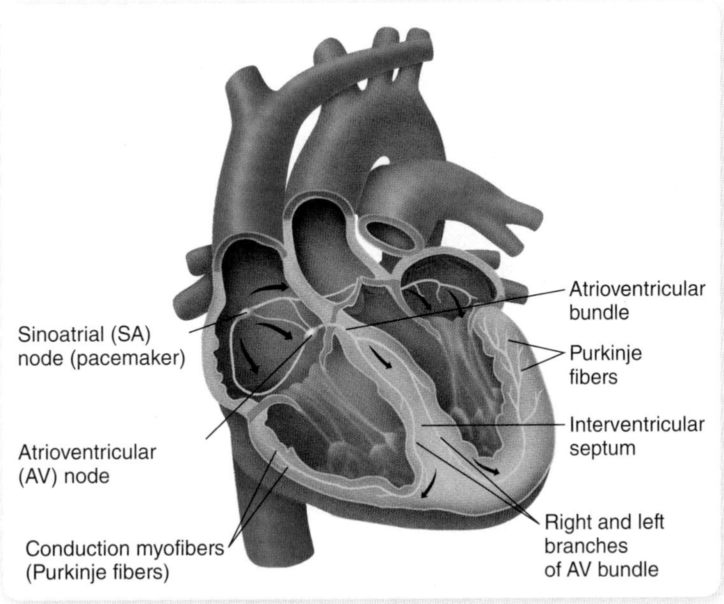

Figure 18-5 The electrical conduction system of the heart initiates an electrical impulse throughout the heart. The impulse travels through the six parts of the cardiac conduction system.

spontaneously without a stimulus from a nerve source. Normal impulses in the heart start at the SA node. As long as impulses come from the SA node, the other myocardial cells will contract when the impulse reaches them. If no impulse arrives, however, the other myocardial cells are capable of creating their own impulses and stimulating a contraction of the heart, although at a generally slower rate.

▶ Physiology Review

Regulation of Heart Function

Recall from Chapter 7, *The Human Body*, that the electrical stimulus that causes the heart to contract originates from impulses from the brain via the **autonomic nervous system**. The heart's **chronotropic state** (control of the rate of contraction), **dromotropic state** (control of electrical conduction), and **inotropic state** (control of the strength of contraction) are controlled by the autonomic nervous system, the hormones of the endocrine system, and the heart tissue.

Receptors in the blood vessels, kidneys, brain, and heart constantly monitor body functions to help maintain homeostasis. **Baroreceptors** respond to changes in pressure, usually within the heart or the main arteries. **Chemoreceptors** sense changes in the chemical composition of the blood. If abnormalities are sensed, nerve signals are transmitted to the appropriate target organs, and hormones or neurotransmitters are released to correct the situation. After conditions normalize, the receptors stop firing and the signals cease.

The Cardiac Cycle

The process that creates the pumping of the heart is known as the **cardiac cycle**. This cycle begins with myocardial contraction and concludes at the beginning of the next contraction. The heart's contraction results in pressure changes within the cardiac chambers, causing blood to move from areas of high pressure to areas of low pressure.

Systole refers to the contraction of the ventricles and the pumping of blood into the systemic circulation; during this phase, systolic blood pressure is measured. **Diastole** refers to relaxation of the heart; during this phase, diastolic blood pressure is measured.

Preload is the amount of blood returned to the heart to be pumped out and directly affects **afterload**. Afterload is the pressure in the aorta or the peripheral vascular resistance, against which the left ventricle must pump blood. The greater the afterload, the harder it is for the ventricle to eject blood into the aorta, reducing the **stroke volume**, or the amount of blood ejected per contraction. To a large degree, afterload is governed by arterial blood pressure. Afterload is greater with vasoconstriction and less with vasodilation.

Cardiac output (the amount of blood pumped through the circulatory system in 1 minute) is expressed in liters per minute (L/min) and is expressed with this equation:

$$\text{Cardiac output} = \text{Stroke volume} \times \text{Heart rate}$$

Factors that influence the heart rate, the stroke volume, or both will affect cardiac output and, thus, **perfusion** (flow of blood) to the body's tissues. The presence of pulses is a good indicator of blood pressure. Weak or absent peripheral pulses indicate decreased perfusion. Weak central pulses indicate substantial hypotension and decompensated shock.

Increased venous return to the heart stretches the ventricles to some extent, resulting in increased cardiac **contractility**. This relationship is called the **Starling law** of the heart.

The heart has several ways of increasing stroke volume. According to the Starling law, the more cardiac muscle is stretched, the greater the force with which it contracts. If an increased volume of blood is returned to the right or left side of the heart, the muscle surrounding the cardiac chambers will have to stretch to accommodate the larger volume. The more the cardiac muscle stretches, the greater will be the force of its contraction, the more completely it will empty, and, therefore, the greater will be the stroke volume. The amount of blood returning to the right atrium may vary somewhat from minute to minute, but the normal heart continues to pump out the same percentage of blood returned. This is called the **ejection fraction**. This system allows the heart to function at the same capacity regardless of changes in the body's position or what the person is doing, whether sitting, moving, sneezing, or other activity.

Words of Wisdom

Three components are required to have adequate tissue perfusion: pump (heart), container (vessels), and fluid (blood).

Blood Flow Within the Heart

Blood from the upper part of the body returns to the heart through the superior vena cava, and blood from the lower part of the body returns through the inferior vena cava. From the right atrium, blood passes through the tricuspid valve into the right ventricle. Blood is then pumped by the right ventricle through the pulmonic valve into the pulmonary artery and to the lungs. In the lungs, blood is oxygenated and, at the same time, carbon dioxide and other waste products are removed.

Freshly oxygenated blood is returned to the left atrium through the pulmonary veins. Blood then flows through the mitral valve into the left ventricle, which pumps the oxygenated blood through the aortic valve, into the aorta, and then to the entire body. In the body, oxygen and nutrients pass out of the capillaries into the cells, and carbon dioxide and waste products pass from the cells into the capillaries in a process called diffusion.

After oxygenated blood has been delivered by the capillaries, deoxygenated blood is returned to the heart, starting from the capillaries, to the venules, and to the veins. Eventually the veins empty into the heart, then the blood is sent to the lungs to be reoxygenated and returned to the heart where the process begins again.

Pulmonary Circulation

Within the body, the **pulmonary circulation** carries blood from the right side of the heart to the lungs and back to the left side of the heart, and the **systemic circulation** is responsible for blood flow to the rest of the body. Deoxygenated blood from the right ventricle is pumped through the pulmonic valve into the pulmonary artery. This artery rapidly divides into the right and left pulmonary arteries. These arteries transport the blood to the lungs. Inside the lungs, the arteries branch, becoming smaller and smaller. At the level of the capillary, waste products are exchanged and the blood is reoxygenated. The reoxygenated blood travels through venules into the pulmonary veins. The four pulmonary veins empty into the left atrium, two from each lung.

Systemic Arterial Circulation

Oxygenated blood leaves the heart through the aortic valve and passes into the aorta. From the aorta, blood is distributed to all parts of the body. All arteries of the body are derived from the aorta.

Special Populations

The cardiovascular system is affected by aging. You should be aware of the changes, seeking to distinguish what is normal from what is chronic for the patient and from what is an acute condition. Sometimes the weakening of the heart muscle, the deterioration of its electrical conduction system, and the hardening of the arteries make the task of assessing and caring for geriatric patients more difficult.

As the heart's muscle mass and tone decrease, the amount of blood pumped out of the heart per beat is decreased. The residual (reserve) capacity of the heart is also reduced; therefore, when the vital organs of the body need additional blood flow, the heart cannot meet the increased need. If blood flow to the brain is inadequate, the patient may report weakness, fatigue, or dizziness and syncope may develop.

Under normal conditions, electrical impulses travel throughout the heart, resulting in the contraction of the heart muscle and the pumping of blood from the heart's chambers. With aging, the electrical conduction system can deteriorate, causing the heart's contraction to weaken or, if blood flow to the heart muscle is affected, extra beats to form. With decreased strength of contraction, the heartbeat is weaker and blood flow to the tissues is reduced. If extra beats are produced, the patient's heart rhythm will be irregular. Although some irregular heart rhythms are benign, others can be potentially lethal.

The arteries are also affected by aging. Arteriosclerosis (hardening of the arteries) can develop, affecting perfusion of the tissues. There is an increased chance of heart attack or stroke from decreased blood flow or plaque formation (atherosclerosis) in the narrowed arteries.

In some older patients, particularly those with diabetes, chest pain is absent, and the clinical picture can be confused with other, noncardiac conditions.

Pathophysiology

Chest pain or discomfort that is related to the heart usually stems from cardiac cell **ischemia**, which is decreased blood flow to the heart muscle. Because of a partial or complete blockage of blood flow through the coronary arteries, heart tissue fails to get enough oxygen and nutrients. The tissue soon begins to starve and eventually dies if blood flow is not restored. Therefore, ischemic heart disease is disease involving a decrease in blood flow to one or more portions of the heart muscle.

▶ Atherosclerosis

Most often, diminished blood flow to the myocardium is caused by coronary artery **atherosclerosis**. Atherosclerosis is a disorder in which a fatty material called cholesterol and other fatty substances build up and form plaque inside the walls of blood vessels, obstructing flow and interfering with their ability to dilate or contract **Figure 18-6**. Eventually, atherosclerosis can cause complete **occlusion**, or blockage, of a coronary artery. Atherosclerosis usually involves other arteries of the body, as well.

The problem begins when the first deposit of cholesterol is laid down on the inside of an artery. This may happen during the teenage years. As a person ages, more of this fatty material is deposited; the **lumen**, or the inside diameter of the artery, narrows. As the cholesterol deposits grow, calcium deposits can form as well. The inner wall of the artery, which is normally smooth and elastic, becomes rough and brittle with these atherosclerotic plaques. Damage to the coronary arteries may become so extensive that they cannot accommodate increased blood flow at times of increased need, resulting in an inappropriate circulating volume.

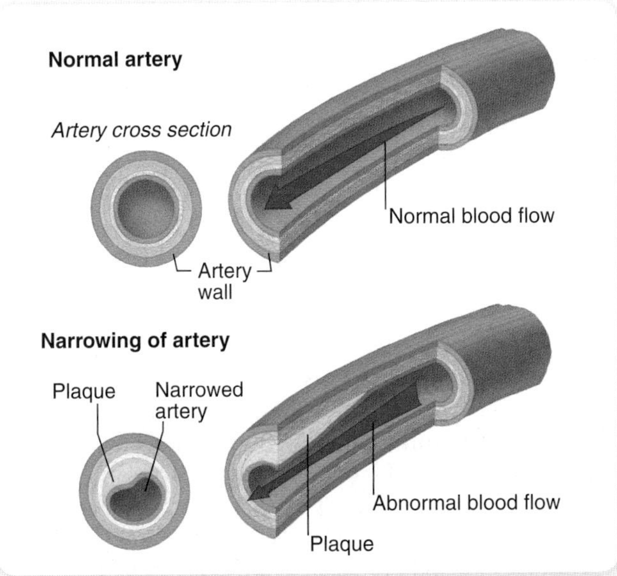

Figure 18-6 In atherosclerosis, cholesterol and other fatty substances build up inside the walls of the blood vessels, causing an obstruction in blood flow to the heart.

Arteriosclerosis can also cause a reduction in blood flow. Arteriosclerosis is a thickening of the arterial walls, which causes a loss of elasticity (hardening of the arteries).

Words of Wisdom

Various changes in the walls of coronary arteries can result in certain disease states. Atherosclerosis is a disorder characterized by the formation of plaques of material, mostly lipids and cholesterol, on the intima of the artery. This process gradually narrows the lumen (opening or hollow part of the artery), resulting in a reduction in arterial blood flow. Arteriosclerosis is hardening of the arteries so they cannot compensate for atherosclerosis by dilating.

For reasons that are still not completely understood, brittle plaque will sometimes develop a crack, exposing the inside of the atherosclerotic wall. Acting like a torn blood vessel, the jagged edge of the crack activates the blood-clotting system, just as it does when an injury has caused bleeding. In this situation, however, the resulting blood clot will partially or completely block the lumen of the artery. If it does not occlude the artery at that location, the blood clot may break loose and begin floating in the blood, becoming what is known as a thromboembolism. A **thromboembolism** is a blood clot that is floating through blood vessels until it reaches an area too narrow for it to pass, causing it to stop and block the blood flow at that point. Tissues downstream from the blood clot will experience a lack of oxygen (hypoxia). If blood flow is resumed in a short time, the hypoxic tissues will recover. However, if too much time goes by before blood flow is resumed, the tissues become necrotic (die). If a blockage occurs in a coronary artery, the condition is known as an **acute myocardial infarction (AMI)**, a classic heart attack **Figure 18-7**. Infarction means the death of tissue. The same sequence may also cause the death of cells in other organs, such as the brain. The death of heart muscle can result in severe diminishment of the heart's ability to pump or cause it to stop completely (cardiac arrest).

In the United States, coronary artery disease is the number one cause of death for men and women[3] and can strike at any age. You must be alert to the possibility that, although less likely than in an older person, a 26-year-old person with chest pain could actually be having a heart attack, especially if he or she has a higher than usual risk.

Factors that place a person at higher risk for a myocardial infarction are called risk factors. The major controllable factors are cigarette smoking, high blood pressure, elevated cholesterol levels, an elevated blood glucose level (diabetes), lack of exercise, and stress. The major risk factors that cannot be controlled are older age,

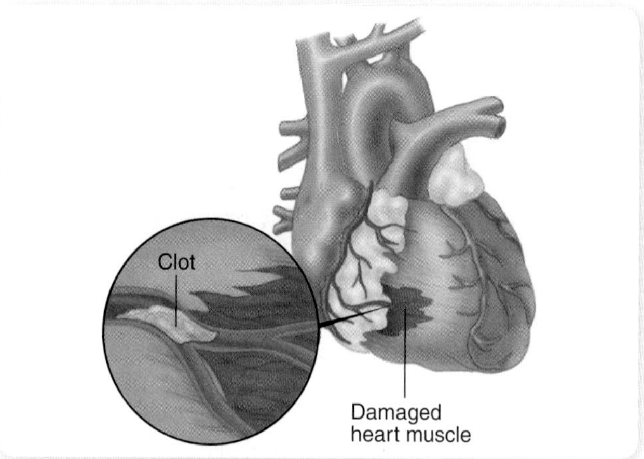

Figure 18-7 An acute myocardial infarction occurs when a blood clot prevents blood flow to an area of the heart muscle. If left untreated, this results in death of heart tissue.

family history of atherosclerotic **coronary artery disease**, race, ethnicity, and male sex.

▶ Acute Coronary Syndrome

Many patients who call for EMS assistance because of chest pain have acute coronary syndrome. **Acute coronary syndrome (ACS)** is the term used to describe any group of symptoms consistent with acute myocardial ischemia. Myocardial ischemia is a decrease in blood flow to the heart, which results in chest pain through reduction of oxygen and nutrients to the tissues of the heart. This can be a temporary situation known as angina pectoris, or a more serious condition, an AMI. Because the signs and symptoms of these two conditions are very similar, they are treated basically the same under the designation of ACS. To understand them better, we will discuss each one separately.

Angina Pectoris

Chest pain does not always mean that a person is having an AMI. When, for a brief period, heart tissues are not getting enough oxygen (ischemia), the pain is called **angina pectoris**, or angina. It is defined as a brief discomfort that has predictable characteristics and is relieved promptly. There is no change in the heart rhythm pattern with angina. Although it can result from a spasm of the artery (also known as vasospastic angina or Prinzmetal angina), angina is most often a symptom of atherosclerotic coronary artery disease. Angina occurs when the heart's need for oxygen exceeds its supply, usually during periods of physical or emotional stress when the heart is working hard. A large meal or sudden fear may also trigger an attack. When the increased oxygen demand goes away (for example, the person stops exercising), the pain typically goes away.

Angina pain is typically described as crushing, squeezing, or "like somebody standing on my chest." It is usually felt in the midchest, under the sternum (substernal). However, it can radiate to the jaw, the arms (frequently the left arm), the midback, or the epigastrium (the upper-middle region of the abdomen). The pain usually lasts from 3 to 8 minutes, rarely longer than 15 minutes. It may be associated with shortness of breath, nausea, or sweating. It disappears promptly with rest, supplemental oxygen, or nitroglycerin (NTG), all of which increase the supply of oxygen to the heart. Although angina pectoris is frightening, it does not mean that heart cells are dying; nor does it usually result in death or permanent heart damage. It is, however, a warning that you and the patient should both take seriously. A single episode may be a precursor to a myocardial infarction. Even with angina, because oxygen supply to the heart is diminished, the electrical system can be compromised and the person is at risk for substantial cardiac rhythm problems. Even though chest pain may dissipate, myocardial ischemia and injury can continue.

The first episode of angina is called initial angina. Angina is generally classified as stable or unstable. Stable angina occurs at a relatively fixed frequency and is usually relieved by rest and/or medication. Unstable angina occurs without a fixed frequency and may or may not be relieved by rest and/or medication. Progressive angina is stable or unstable angina that is accelerating in frequency and duration. Preinfarction angina presents with pain that occurs at rest when the patient is sitting or lying down.

EMS usually becomes involved when stable angina becomes unstable, such as when a patient whose pain is normally relieved by sitting down and taking one NTG tablet has taken three tablets with no relief. Keep in mind that it can be very difficult even for physicians in hospitals to distinguish between the pain of angina and the pain of a myocardial infarction. For this reason, any complaint of chest pain should be treated as a myocardial infarction until proven otherwise.

Of course, not all chest pain is caused by cardiac ischemia or injury. Many other conditions—such as pulmonary embolism, pneumothorax, pneumonia,

Words of Wisdom

Prinzmetal angina is a rare chronic condition that almost always occurs when a person is at rest and usually in younger patients than those who have other types of angina. Attacks can be extremely painful and typically occur between midnight and early morning.

The pain from Prinzmetal angina is caused by a spasm in the coronary arteries (which supply blood to the heart muscle). The spasm may be the result of stress, smoking, cocaine use, exposure to cold weather, or medications that cause vasoconstriction. Symptoms can generally be relieved by taking medications that include calcium antagonists and nitrates. Other names for Prinzmetal angina include *variant angina*, *Prinzmetal variant angina*, and *angina inversa*.[4]

pericarditis, aortic dissection, indigestion, and peptic ulcer—may cause chest pain that can be mistaken for angina or a myocardial infarction.

Acute Myocardial Infarction

Heart disease is the leading cause of death in the United States.[3] Most deaths from AMI are caused by **dysrhythmia** (an irregular or abnormal heart rhythm), usually ventricular fibrillation, which typically occurs during the early hours of the infarct. Dysrhythmias can often be prevented or treated, so *most deaths from AMI are preventable.*

The pain of AMI signals the actual death of cells in the area of the heart where blood flow is obstructed. Once dead, the cells cannot be revived. Instead, they will eventually turn to scar tissue and become a burden to the beating heart. This is why fast action is critical in treating a heart attack. The sooner the blockage can be cleared, the fewer the cells that may die. Approximately 30 minutes after blood flow is cut off, some heart muscle cells begin to die. After approximately 2 hours, as many as one-half of the cells in the area can be dead. In many cases, opening the coronary artery with "clot-busting" medications, two classes of medications called thrombolytics and fibrinolytics, can prevent or minimize damage to the heart muscle if administered within the first few hours after the onset of symptoms. Angioplasty or percutaneous coronary intervention (PCI), which is the mechanical clearing of the artery, has been shown to be the most effective treatment for a patient experiencing an AMI if performed promptly. Therefore, immediate treatment and transport to an emergency department with cardiac capabilities is essential.

An AMI is more apt to occur in the larger, thick-walled left ventricle, which needs more blood and oxygen, than in the right ventricle.

As with angina, precipitating causes may include atherosclerosis, occlusions, and traumatic or nontraumatic injury. Persistent angina may also be a factor.

Signs and Symptoms of Acute Myocardial Infarction.

A patient with an AMI may show any of the following signs and symptoms:

- Sudden onset of weakness, nausea, and sweating without an obvious cause
- Chest pain, discomfort, or pressure that is often crushing or squeezing and that does not change with each breath
- Pain, discomfort, or pressure in the lower jaw, arms, back, abdomen, or neck
- Irregular heartbeat and syncope (fainting)
- Shortness of breath, or dyspnea
- Pink, frothy sputum (indicating possible pulmonary edema)
- Sudden death

YOU are the Provider PART 2

You perform a primary survey of the patient while your partner obtains a set of baseline vital signs; findings show a pulse rate of 74 beats/min, respirations of 24 breaths/min, a blood pressure of 146/88 mm Hg, and Spo_2 of 92% on room air. Your partner places the patient on a nonrebreathing mask at 15 L/min. On completion of your assessment you find no signs of trauma. The patient states that she was taking her normal afternoon nap, and she woke up with a pain in her chest, which radiates to her left arm. When you ask her to describe the pain, she describes it as "an elephant sitting on my chest." You further question the patient and ascertain that these symptoms started approximately 20 minutes ago, nothing makes the pain better or worse, and the patient describes the pain as 9/10, not quite as bad as her previous heart attacks, but almost. After confirming that the patient has no allergies and takes no medications, per your protocols you administer 324 mg of aspirin orally and 0.4 mg of nitroglycerin sublingually.

Recording Time: 1 Minute	
Respirations	24 breaths/min
Pulse	74 beats/min
Skin	Warm, dry, and pink
Blood pressure	146/88 mm Hg
Oxygen saturation (Spo_2)	92% on room air

3. In which medication class is aspirin, and what are the indications and contraindications for administration?
4. What is the mechanism of action of nitroglycerin, and what are the indications and contraindications?
5. What are the various routes available to administer nitroglycerin?

The Pain of Acute Myocardial Infarction. The most common symptom of AMI is chest pain. A patient with chronic angina will be aware that something different from previous anginal attacks is happening. The pain of an AMI differs from the pain of angina in three ways:

- It may or may not be caused by exertion but can occur at any time, sometimes when a person is sitting quietly or even sleeping.
- It does not resolve in a few minutes; rather, it can last between 30 minutes and several hours. It also increases in frequency and/or duration.
- It may or may not be relieved by rest or NTG.

The pain of AMI is typically felt just beneath the sternum and is variously described as heavy, squeezing, crushing, or tight. The pain may radiate to the arms (most often the left arm) and into the fingers; it may also radiate to the neck, jaw, upper back, or epigastrium. The pain of AMI is not influenced by coughing, deep breathing, or other body movements.

Not all patients who are having an AMI experience pain or recognize it when it occurs. In fact, approximately one-third of patients never seek medical attention. This can be attributed, in part, to the fact that people are afraid of dying and do not wish to face the possibility that their symptoms may be serious. Middle-aged men are particularly likely to minimize or deny their symptoms. However, a few patients, particularly older people, women, and people with diabetes, do not experience any pain during an AMI but have other common complaints associated with ischemia. This is often referred to as a silent MI because of the lack of pain. These patients may present with symptoms related to a decrease in cardiac output. It is not unusual for sudden dyspnea to develop, progressing rapidly to pulmonary edema, a sudden loss of consciousness, an unexplained drop in blood pressure, an apparent stroke, or simply confusion. Others may feel only mild discomfort and call it indigestion. It is not uncommon for the only complaint, especially in older women, to be fatigue. Heart disease is the number one cause of death of women in the United States;[5] you should consider AMI even when the classic symptom of chest pain is not present. This is also true for older people and people with diabetes.

Words of Wisdom

More men have heart disease, but more women die of heart disease, in part because their symptoms are less clear cut.

Physical Findings of Acute Myocardial Infarction and Cardiac Compromise. The physical findings of AMI vary, depending on the extent and severity of heart muscle damage. The following are common:

- **General appearance.** The patient often appears frightened. There may be nausea, vomiting, and a cold sweat. The skin is often pale or ashen gray because of poor cardiac output and the loss of perfusion, or blood flow through the tissue. Occasionally, the skin will have a bluish tint, called cyanosis; this is the result of poor oxygenation of the circulating blood.
- **Pulse.** Generally, the pulse rate increases as a normal response to pain, stress, fear, or actual injury to the myocardium. Because dysrhythmias are common in an AMI, you may feel an irregularity or even a slowing of the pulse. The pulse may also depend on the area of the heart that has been affected by the AMI. Damage to the inferior area of the heart often presents with bradycardia.
- **Blood pressure.** Blood pressure may fall as a result of diminished cardiac output and diminished capability of the left ventricle to pump. However, most patients with an AMI will have a normal or, most likely, elevated blood pressure.
- **Respiration.** A complaint of difficulty breathing is common with cardiac compromise, so even if the rate seems normal, look at the work of breathing and treat the patient as if respiratory compromise were present, especially in patients with a history of heart failure.
- **Mental status.** Patients with AMIs sometimes experience an almost overwhelming feeling of impending doom. If a patient tells you, "I think I am going to die," pay attention.

Consequences of Acute Myocardial Infarction. An AMI can have three serious consequences:

- Sudden death
- Cardiogenic shock
- Heart failure

Sudden Death

Many patients with AMI never reach the hospital. Sudden death is usually the result of **cardiac arrest**, in which the heart fails to generate an effective blood flow. Although you cannot feel a pulse in someone experiencing cardiac arrest, there may still be electrical activity, though chaotic. The heart is using up energy without pumping. Such an abnormality of heart rhythm is a ventricular dysrhythmia, known as ventricular fibrillation.

A variety of other lethal and nonlethal dysrhythmias may follow AMI, usually within the first hour. In most cases, it is premature ventricular contractions (PVCs), or extra beats from the damaged ventricle. PVCs by themselves are harmless and are common among healthy people, as well as in sick people. Other dysrhythmias are much more dangerous **Figure 18-8**. These include the following:

- **Tachycardia**. Rapid beating of the heart, greater than 100 beats/min.
- **Bradycardia**. Unusually slow beating of the heart, less than 60 beats/min.
- **Ventricular tachycardia (VT)**. Rapid heart rhythm, usually at a rate of 150 to 200 beats/min. The electrical activity starts in the ventricle instead of the atrium. This rhythm usually does not allow adequate time between beats for the left ventricle to fill with blood. Therefore, the patient's blood pressure may fall. He or she may also feel weak or lightheaded or may even become unresponsive. In some cases, existing chest pain may worsen or chest pain that was not there before onset of the dysrhythmia may develop. The appearance of three or more PVCs in a row is called a "run of VT." Most cases of ventricular tachycardia will be more sustained and may deteriorate into ventricular fibrillation.
- **Ventricular fibrillation (VF)**. Disorganized, ineffective quivering of the ventricles caused by unorganized electrical activity. No blood is pumped through the body, and the patient usually becomes unresponsive within seconds. The only way to treat this dysrhythmia is to electrically defibrillate the heart. To **defibrillate** means to shock the heart with a specialized electrical current to stop all electrical activity in an attempt to restore a normal, rhythmic beat. By stopping the dysrhythmia, it gives the conduction system the chance to resume its normal activity. Defibrillation is highly successful in saving a life if delivered within 1 to 2 minutes after the onset of ventricular fibrillation. If a defibrillator is not immediately available, CPR with high-quality chest compressions must be initiated to buy a few more minutes for arrival of an AED or manual defibrillator. Even if CPR is begun right at the time of collapse, chances of survival diminish each minute until defibrillation is accomplished.

If uncorrected, unstable ventricular tachycardia or ventricular fibrillation will eventually result in **asystole**, the absence of all cardiac electrical and mechanical activity. Without CPR, this may occur within minutes. Because it reflects a long period of ischemia, nearly all patients you find in asystole will die.

▶ Cardiogenic Shock

Shock is a simple concept but one that few people without medical training really understand. For that reason, Chapter 14, *Shock*, provides a more in-depth discussion of shock. The discussion of shock in this chapter is limited to that associated with cardiac problems.

For an AEMT, shock is a critical concept. Shock is present when body tissues do not get enough oxygen and nutrients to function normally, causing body organs to malfunction. In **cardiogenic shock**, often caused by a myocardial infarction, the problem is that the heart lacks enough power to force the proper volume of blood through the circulatory system. Cardiogenic shock can occur immediately or as late as 24 hours after the onset of an AMI. The various signs and symptoms of cardiogenic shock are produced by the improper functioning of the body's organs. The challenge for you is to recognize shock in its early stages, when treatment is likely to be more successful.

Cardiogenic shock may be differentiated from hypovolemic shock by one or more of the following:

- Chief complaint (chest pain, dyspnea, tachycardia)
- Heart rate (bradycardia or excessive tachycardia)
- Peripheral edema
- Dysrhythmias
- Jugular venous distention
- Crackles (rales) on auscultation of breath sounds

A patient with suspected cardiogenic shock should receive the same initial evaluation and treatment as any patient who is reporting chest pain. Pay particular attention to respiratory effort and the presence of peripheral or pulmonary edema. It is imperative to recognize the urgency of transport and to make sure the patient is taken to the closest, most appropriate facility.

Signs and Symptoms of Cardiogenic Shock

One of the first signs of shock is anxiety or restlessness as the brain becomes relatively starved for oxygen. The patient may report "air hunger." Think of the possibility of shock when the patient is yelling, "I can't breathe." Obviously, the patient can breathe because he or she can talk. However, the patient's brain is sensing that it is not getting enough oxygen.

As the shock continues, the body shunts blood to the most important organs, such as the brain and heart, and away from less important organs, such as the skin. Therefore, you may see pale, clammy skin in patients with shock.

As the shock gets worse, the body will attempt to compensate by increasing the amount of blood pumped through the heart. Therefore, the pulse rate will be higher than normal. In severe shock, the heart rate will usually, but not always, be more than 120 beats/min.

Shock can also be characterized by rapid and shallow breathing, nausea and vomiting, and a decrease in body temperature.

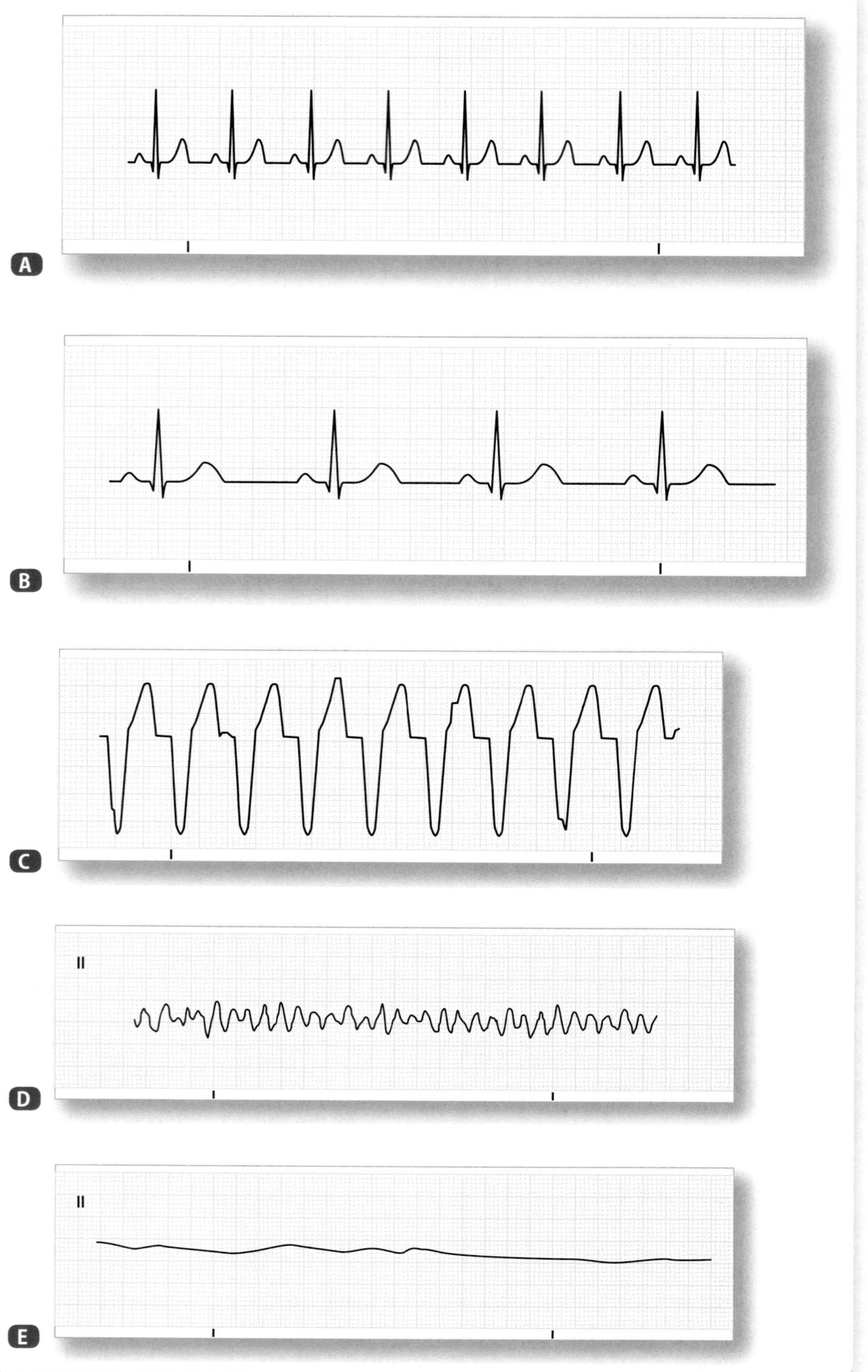

Figure 18-8 Common cardiac dysrhythmias. **A.** Sinus tachycardia. **B.** Sinus bradycardia. **C.** Ventricular tachycardia. **D.** Ventricular fibrillation. **E.** Asystole.

A-C: From 12-Lead ECG: The Art of Interpretation, Second Edition, courtesy of Tomas B. Garcia, MD; **D** and **E:** From Arrhythmia Recognition: The Art of Interpretation, courtesy of Tomas B. Garcia, MD.

Finally, as the heart and other organs begin to malfunction, the blood pressure will fall below normal. A systolic blood pressure of less than 90 mm Hg is easy to recognize, but it is a late finding that indicates decompensated shock. Do not assume that shock is not present just because the blood pressure is normal (compensated shock).

Treatment of Patients With Cardiogenic Shock

Take the following steps when treating patients with signs and symptoms of cardiogenic shock:

1. Position the patient comfortably. Most patients with heart failure will be more comfortable in the semi-Fowler position; however, those with low blood pressure may not tolerate this position. These patients may be more comfortable and more alert in a supine position.
2. Administer oxygen as needed to maintain an Spo_2 of greater than 94%.
3. Assist ventilation as necessary.
4. Cover the patient with sheets or blankets as indicated to preserve body heat. Be sure to cover the patient's head in cold weather; this is where the most heat is lost.
5. Gain intravenous (IV) access, and give fluid boluses of 250 mL up to a total of 1,000 mL if necessary of an isotonic crystalloid solution to achieve a systolic blood pressure of at least 80 mm Hg. Monitor breath sounds for the development of pulmonary edema.
6. Provide prompt transport to the closest, most appropriate emergency department.
7. Call for paramedic backup if available and timely for the administration of vasopressors.

▶ Heart Failure

Failure of the heart occurs when the ventricular myocardium is so damaged that it can no longer keep up with the return flow of blood from the atria. **Heart failure** can occur any time after a myocardial infarction, heart valve damage, or long-standing high blood pressure, but it usually happens between the first few hours and the first few days after an AMI.

Left-Side Heart Failure

Just as the pumping function of the left ventricle can be damaged by coronary artery disease, it can also be damaged by diseased heart valves or chronic hypertension. In any of these cases, when the myocardium can no longer contract effectively, the heart tries other ways to maintain an adequate cardiac output. Two specific changes in heart function occur: the heart rate increases, and the left ventricle enlarges to increase the amount of blood pumped each minute.

When these adaptations can no longer make up for the decreased heart function, heart failure eventually develops. It is called congestive heart failure because the lungs become congested with fluid when the heart fails to pump the blood effectively. Blood tends to back up in the pulmonary veins, increasing the pressure in the capillaries of the lungs. When the pressure in the capillaries exceeds a certain level, fluid (mostly water) passes through the walls of the capillary vessels and into the alveoli. This condition is called pulmonary edema. It may occur suddenly, as in an AMI, or slowly over months, as in chronic heart failure. Sometimes, in patients with an acute onset of heart failure, severe pulmonary edema will develop, in which the patient has pink, frothy sputum and severe dyspnea.

Right-Side Heart Failure

If the right side of the heart is damaged, fluid collects in the body, often showing up as swelling in the feet and legs. The collection of fluid in the part of the body that is closest to the ground is called **dependent edema** (which may be in the sacral area of the back in a bedridden patient). **Pedal edema** is swelling specifically in the feet and lower legs. The swelling causes relatively few symptoms other than discomfort. However, chronic pedal edema may indicate underlying heart disease (right-side heart failure) even in the absence of pain or other symptoms.

Words of Wisdom

When assessing the patient for peripheral edema, remember that fluid collects in dependent areas. Check the sacral area in patients who are bedridden and the lower extremities in those who are sitting upright.

Signs and Symptoms of Heart Failure

Watch for the following signs and symptoms in a patient you suspect has heart failure:

- **Orthopnea**. The patient finds it easier to breathe when sitting up. When the patient is lying down, more blood is returned to the right ventricle and lungs, causing further pulmonary congestion and shortness of breath.
- Often, the patient is mildly or severely agitated.
- Chest pain may or may not be present.
- The patient often has distended neck veins that do not collapse even when the patient is sitting.
- The patient may have swollen ankles from pedal edema. If the patient is bedridden, the edema may be seen in the sacral area.
- The patient generally will have hypertension, tachycardia, and tachypnea.
- The patient will usually be using accessory breathing muscles of the neck and ribs, reflecting the additional hard work of breathing.

- The fluid surrounding small airways may produce crackles (also called rales), best heard by listening to either side of the patient's chest, about midway down the back. In severe heart failure, these soft sounds can be heard even at the top (apex) of the lung.
- The patient may have a productive cough, or you may note the presence of pink, frothy sputum.
- The patient may have delayed capillary refill time. With damage to the myocardium, the pumping mechanism is effectively reduced; therefore, there is a lack of perfusion in the extremities, causing delayed capillary refill time.

After heart failure develops, it can be treated but not cured. Regular use of medications may alleviate the symptoms. However, these patients often become ill again and are frequently hospitalized.

Treatment of Heart Failure

Treat a patient with heart failure the same way as a patient with chest pain:

1. Obtain vital signs, monitor heart rhythm, and administer oxygen as needed, ventilating if needed. Continuous positive airway pressure (CPAP) may also be beneficial for patients who meet the requirements; see Chapter 11, *Airway Management*, for information on CPAP.
2. Allow the patient to remain sitting in an upright position with the legs down.
3. Gain IV access. You may also give fluid if the patient becomes hypotensive. Frequently assess breath sounds for the development of pulmonary edema.
4. Be reassuring; many patients with heart failure are quite anxious because they cannot breathe.
5. Patients who have had problems with heart failure before will usually have specific medications for its treatment. Gather these medications and take them along to the hospital.
6. NTG may be of value if the patient's systolic blood pressure is above 100 mm Hg. If the patient has been prescribed NTG, and medical control advises you to do so, you can administer it sublingually.

Provide prompt transport to the closest, most appropriate emergency department.

▶ Pulmonary Edema

Pulmonary edema is a common complication of myocardial ischemia that may or may not be the result of an AMI. Without treatment, pulmonary edema can result in acute respiratory failure and death. Precipitating causes include heart failure (left-side and/or right-side), myocardial infarction, pulmonary embolism, hypertension, and cardiomegaly (enlarged heart).

Preload and afterload can greatly influence the buildup of pulmonary edema. As the left ventricle loses its ability to pump effectively, blood backs up into the pulmonary veins and, subsequently, into the lungs. This increased pressure causes fluid to leak from the capillaries into the interstitial tissue and the alveoli. This is common in heart failure as the loss of contractile ability results in fluid overload. Pulmonary edema may be acute as the result of an AMI, or may be chronic as a result of multiple events or chronic heart failure.

Treatment is focused on maintaining the airway, breathing, and circulation and transporting the patient for definitive care. Obtain a thorough history from the patient, and provide psychological support en route.

▶ Hypertensive Emergencies

Hypertension is defined as any systolic blood pressure of greater than 140 mm Hg or a diastolic blood pressure of greater than 90 mm Hg. Another cardiac-related condition is a hypertensive emergency. A **hypertensive emergency** usually occurs only with a systolic pressure of greater than 180 mm Hg, a rapid increase in the systolic pressure, or a diastolic pressure of 120 mm Hg.[6] Because blood pressure cannot be directly felt by the patient, the signs and symptoms of a hypertensive emergency are related to the effects of the hypertension. Some patients with chronic hypertension may not experience signs or symptoms until their systolic pressure is substantially higher than this value. One of the most common signs is a sudden severe headache. Often described as "the worst headache I have ever felt," this may also be a sign of cerebral hemorrhage. Other signs and symptoms include a strong bounding pulse, ringing in the ears, nausea and vomiting, dizziness, warm skin (dry or moist), nosebleed, altered mental status, and even the sudden development of pulmonary edema. Untreated hypertensive emergencies can result in a stroke or a dissecting aortic aneurysm.

If you suspect your patient is experiencing a hypertensive emergency, attempt to make him or her comfortable and monitor the blood pressure regularly. Position the patient with the head elevated, transport rapidly to the emergency department, and establish IV access. Call early for paramedic backup if needed for medication administration.

Aortic/Dissecting Aneurysm

An **aortic aneurysm** is a weakness in the wall of the aorta. The aorta dilates at the weakened area, which makes it susceptible to rupture. A **dissecting aneurysm** occurs when the inner layers of the aorta become separated, allowing blood (at high pressures) to flow between the layers. Uncontrolled hypertension is the primary cause of dissecting aortic aneurysms. This separation of layers weakens the wall of the aorta substantially, making it more likely to rupture under conditions of continued high blood pressure. If the aorta ruptures completely, the amount of internal blood loss will be so large that the patient will die almost immediately.

The signs and symptoms of a dissecting thoracic aortic aneurysm include very sudden chest pain located in the anterior part of the chest or in the back between the shoulder blades. It may be difficult to differentiate the chest pain of a dissecting thoracic aortic aneurysm from that of an AMI, but several distinctive features may help. The pain from an AMI is often preceded by other symptoms—nausea, indigestion, weakness, and sweating—and tends to come on gradually, becoming more severe with time and often described as "pressure" rather than "stabbing." By contrast, the pain of a dissecting aortic aneurysm usually comes on full force from one minute to the next with a description more consistent of "a tearing, burning sensation" originating in the back or scapular area and radiating anteriorly; in some cases patients describe pain that originates in the anterior chest and radiates posteriorly **Table 18-1**. A patient with a dissecting aortic aneurysm also may exhibit a difference in blood pressure between the arms or diminished pulses in the lower extremities.

Thoracic aortic aneurysms are almost impossible to diagnose in the prehospital setting, but you must consider them a possibility in any patient with substantial hypertension. Transport the patient without delay.

Table 18-1 Acute Myocardial Infarction Versus Dissecting Thoracic Aortic Aneurysm

	Acute Myocardial Infarction	Dissecting Thoracic Aortic Aneurysm
Onset of pain	Gradual, with additional symptoms	Abrupt, without additional symptoms
Quality of pain	Tightness or pressure	Sharp or tearing
Severity of pain	Increases with time	Maximal from onset
Timing of pain	May wax and wane	Does not abate after it has started
Region/ radiation	Substernal; back is rarely involved	Back possibly involved, between the shoulder blades
Clinical signs	Peripheral pulses equal	Blood pressure discrepancy between arms or decrease in a femoral or carotid pulse

Patient Assessment

When you are called to a scene where a patient's chief complaint is chest pain, perform a thorough assessment, no matter what the patient says. Any complaint of chest pain or discomfort or other symptoms suggestive of a cardiac etiology is a serious matter.

It is imperative that you recognize a sense of urgency for reperfusion when the patient receives no relief with medications or presents with hypotension or signs of hypoperfusion. Throughout the call, provide emotional support for the patient and an explanation for the family or significant others.

Scene Size-up

While en route to the scene, consider the minimum and maximum standard precautions that will be needed.

Always ensure that the scene is safe for you, your partner, your patient, and bystanders. As you approach the scene, look for and address any hazards, and assess the scene for the potential of violence. Determine how many patients there are. From the nature of the call and first glance at your patient, consider whether you will need additional resources to assist in moving the patient or patients.

It is important to identify the nature of illness to start your patient assessment on the right track. Use the dispatch information, clues at the scene, and comments of bystanders or family members to begin to develop an idea about the type of problem your patient might be experiencing. For patients with cardiac problems, the clues often include a report of chest pain, difficulty breathing, or sudden loss of consciousness. After you establish a preliminary nature of illness, you will be able to guide your assessment to find the important information much more effectively. Remember not to become fixated on a specific condition at this early point in the assessment; sometimes the situation turns out to be extremely different from how it initially appeared.

Primary Survey

As you approach the patient, form a general impression of his or her condition to recognize and address life threats. You will likely begin by determining whether the patient is responsive. A decreased level of consciousness may be an indication of decreased perfusion to the brain. If the patient is responsive, determine if he or she is experiencing dizziness and if any loss of consciousness occurred before EMS arrival.

Perform a rapid full-body scan of the patient. If the patient is not responsive and is not breathing, begin

CPR, starting with chest compressions, and call for an AED. An AED should be applied as soon as it is available if the patient is pulseless, not breathing (apneic), and unresponsive. Use of the AED is discussed in the section on cardiac arrest later in this chapter. Consider calling for paramedic backup if needed and available.

Quickly assess for any major bleeding that needs to be controlled or any substantial edema in dependent areas.

Unless the patient is unresponsive, the airway will most likely be patent. Is there any evidence of debris, blood, or frothy sputum in the airway? Responsive patients should be able to maintain their own airway. Some episodes of cardiac compromise may produce dizziness or even syncopal episodes. If dizziness or fainting has occurred, consider the possibility of injuries from a fall, including potential spinal injuries.

Determine the rate, quality, and degree of distress of respirations. If the rate is too fast or too slow, the depth of respiration seems to be too shallow, or the patient is struggling to breathe, respirations are inadequate. Auscultate breath sounds at this time because these can also be important indicators of patient condition. With cardiac patients, breath sounds may be affected by the presence of fluid buildup. Auscultate for crackles or congestion that indicates pulmonary edema. Some patients feel short of breath even though there are no obvious signs of respiratory distress. Apply oxygen as needed, or if the patient is not breathing or has inadequate breathing, ensure adequate ventilation with a bag-mask device and 100% oxygen to maintain an Spo_2 of greater than 94%.

If available, consider the use of CPAP when needed. For example, patients experiencing pulmonary edema may require positive pressure ventilation with a bag-mask device or CPAP. CPAP is the most effective way to assist a person with heart failure to breathe effectively and avert the need to use an invasive airway management technique. Be aware of the indications and contraindications of CPAP and be competent in using this equipment.

After assessing airway and breathing, assess the patient's circulation. Determine the rate, rhythm, and quality of the patient's pulse. Is the pulse rhythm regular or irregular? Is the pulse too fast or too slow? Abnormalities in the pulse may indicate substantial problems. It is also important to question patients with an irregular pulse about any past history of dysrhythmias. Assess the patient's skin condition, color, moisture, and temperature, as well as capillary refill time and skin turgor. The patient may present with pallor during the episode, and diaphoresis is usually present. Assess blood pressure; it may be elevated during the episode and normalize afterward. Also, the patient's temperature may vary. Changes in perfusion may indicate more serious cardiac compromise. Begin treatment for cardiogenic shock early to reduce the workload of the heart. Place the patient in a position of comfort, usually sitting up and well supported.

Make a transport decision based on whether you were able to stabilize life threats during the primary survey. The remainder of the assessment can be performed en route, if time allows. In general, most patients with chest pain should be transported immediately. Whether to use the lights and sirens during transport is determined for each patient individually and may be partially based on the estimated transport time. Use lights and sirens sparingly when transporting patients with cardiac problems to alleviate some of the stress associated with emergency transport. Little time is saved by using the lights and sirens, but you can do a lot to calm your patient and reduce the release of heart-damaging adrenaline through your reassurance and by creating a ride to the hospital that is as nonstressful as possible. Try not to allow the patient to exert himself or herself, strain, or walk.

Transport patients to the closest appropriate facility. If your service is served by one hospital, follow local protocols, and consider alternative destinations when available if the patient would be better served by transport to another facility. This requires that you understand local protocols and any differences in treatment capabilities of various institutions in your area.

History Taking

After you have stabilized life threats, you will want to determine and investigate the chief complaint and the history of the present illness. If the patient is responsive, begin by taking a brief past pertinent history, identifying associated signs and symptoms, and identifying pertinent negatives. If the patient has an altered mental status, friends or family members who are present may have helpful information.

Remember that not all patients experiencing an AMI have the same signs and symptoms. A chief complaint of chest pain or discomfort, shortness of breath, or dizziness should be taken seriously. Many patients who suspect that something is wrong experience restlessness, appear anxious, and perhaps have a sense of impending doom. Answer questions in a professional manner and provide emotional support. Your professional attitude may be the single most important factor in winning the patient's cooperation and helping the patient through this event. Patients often have a good idea about what is happening, so do not lie and offer false reassurance.

Begin by asking questions about the current situation. Determine whether the patient is experiencing chest pain or discomfort and whether there are any other signs and symptoms. Ask the patient about recurring events along

Special Populations

It is important to ask the patient, "How do you feel? Describe it to me." Remember that older patients may not experience pain, only weakness or syncope. Listen for descriptive terms such as pressure, crushing, squeezing, tightness, shortness of breath, dizziness, etc.

with any increase in frequency and/or duration of an event. Remember that typical angina has a sudden onset of discomfort that is generally of brief duration, lasting only 3 to 5 minutes, not 30 minutes to 2 hours, and is usually relieved by rest and/or medication.

Determine whether the patient is having respiratory difficulty; this is common among patients with chest pain. If the patient is experiencing dyspnea, find out whether it is related to exertion and whether it is related to the patient's position. Also determine whether the dyspnea is continuous or if it changes, especially with deep breathing. Note whether the patient has a productive cough. Ask about other signs and symptoms that are commonly found such as nausea and vomiting, fatigue, headache, and palpitations (a feeling of the heart "skipping a beat" or racing). Make sure to ask about any trauma the patient might have experienced during the past few days. Be sure to record your findings, including those that are negative (known as pertinent negatives).

Words of Wisdom

When you are assessing a patient with a complaint of chest pain or dyspnea, it is common to ask, "How many pillows do you sleep on at night?" Many patients with a history of heart failure will tell you that they sleep on multiple pillows to keep their head up or are unable to sleep lying down and spend their nights in a recliner or similar position. The more upright the patient must sit, the more severe the condition.

Words of Wisdom

Paroxysmal means sudden onset. An episode of paroxysmal nocturnal dyspnea is a sudden onset of shortness of breath at night—usually when a person lies down. This is often the result of heart failure or pulmonary edema.

If the patient is responsive, obtain the SAMPLE history (Signs and symptoms, Allergies, Medications, Pertinent past medical history, Last oral intake, Events leading up to the illness or injury) and ask the following questions specific to a cardiovascular emergency:

- Have you ever had a heart attack?
- Have you been told that you have heart problems?
  - Have you ever been diagnosed with angina, heart failure, or heart valve disease?
  - Have you ever had high blood pressure?
  - Have you ever been diagnosed with an aneurysm?
  - Do you have any respiratory diseases such as emphysema or chronic bronchitis?
- Do you have diabetes or have you ever had any problems with your blood sugar?
- Have you ever had kidney disease?
- Do you have any risk factors for coronary artery disease, such as smoking, high blood pressure, or high-stress lifestyle?
  - Is there a family history of heart disease?
  - Do you currently take any medications?

The SAMPLE history provides basic information on the patient's overall medical history. The more signs and symptoms a patient has, the easier it is to identify a particular problem. In addition, ask whether the patient has had the same pain before. If so, ask "Do you take any medications for the pain?" and "Do you have any of the medication with you?" Determine whether the patient has taken NTG, aspirin, or any other medications before your arrival. If the patient has had a heart attack or angina before, ask whether the pain is similar.

Make sure to ask about medication allergies. If the patient is taking medications, determine whether they are prescribed, over-the-counter, herbal medications, and/or if there is any recreational drug use, as well as for what condition they are taken. Even when a patient may not be able to articulate his or her exact medical condition, knowing the patient's medications may give you important clues. For example, a patient may say he has "heart problems." You see that he is taking furosemide (Lasix), digoxin, and amiodarone (Cordarone). Furosemide is a diuretic, digoxin increases the strength of heart contractions, and amiodarone controls certain types of dysrhythmias. These drugs are often prescribed together for patients with heart failure and may alert you to carefully evaluate the lungs for the presence of crackles (rales), which indicate fluid in the lungs and a need to increase the amount of oxygen being delivered. Ask about any other medical conditions the patient may have. Asking about the last oral intake may seem unnecessary, but this information can be very important; it is always better to have too much information rather than not enough. Also remember to ask about any home remedies the patient might have used.

Words of Wisdom

When questioning a patient about medications, remember to ask about the use of herbal remedies or home remedies. Most patients do not consider these substances to be medications or realize that they can interact with prescribed medications.

Be sure to include the OPQRST-I questions (Onset, Provocation/palliation, Quality, Region/radiation, Severity, Timing–Interventions) when you are obtaining the symptoms as part of the SAMPLE history. Using OPQRST-I

Table 18-2 OPQRST-I Mnemonic for Assessing Pain

Onset	When did the problem begin, and what does the patient think may have caused it?
Provocation/palliation	Ask what makes the pain or discomfort better or worse. Is it positional? Does a deep breath or palpation of the chest make it worse? Did the patient take anything for it (including anything nonprescribed)?
Quality	Ask the patient to describe his or her pain. Let the patient use his or her own words to describe what is happening. If the patient is unable to describe the pain, try to avoid supplying the patient with only one option. Do not ask, "Does it feel like an elephant is sitting on your chest?" Instead, say, "Tell me what the pain feels like." If the patient cannot answer an open-ended question, then provide a list of alternatives: "There are lots of different kinds of pain. Is your pain more like a heaviness, pressure, burning, tearing, dull ache, stabbing, crampy, or needlelike?"
Region/radiation	Ask where the pain or discomfort is located and whether it has spread to another part of the body.
Severity	Ask the patient to rate the pain on a simple scale. Often, a scale ranging from 0 to 10 is used, in which 0 represents no pain at all and 10 represents the worst pain imaginable. Do not use the patient's answer to determine whether the pain has a serious cause. Instead, use this scale to determine whether the pain is getting better or worse. After a few minutes of oxygen or administration of NTG, ask the patient to rate the pain again.
Time	Find out how long the pain has been going on, how long it lasts when it is present, and whether it has been intermittent or continuous. Ask whether it is worsening or improving and if it is associated with rest or activity.
Intervention	Ask what has been done prior to EMS arrival. Has the patient taken prescribed NTG or other medication? If so, when? How many? Has there been any change?

Abbreviations: EMS, emergency medical services; NTG, nitroglycerin

helps you to understand the details of specific complaints, such as chest pain Table 18-2. Ask whether the patient has taken anything for the pain and, if so, whether it helped. If the patient reports having taken NTG without relief, it is important to establish *why* the patient did not obtain relief.

At least two reasons might explain this failure. One possibility is that the patient is, indeed, having an AMI, for which NTG would not provide complete pain relief. The other possibility is that the NTG has simply gone stale. To retain its potency, NTG must be stored in a dark, airtight container; if it is left out in the open for any period (for example, if the patient stores the medicine on the windowsill above the kitchen sink), it loses its therapeutic effectiveness. To distinguish between the two explanations, ask the patient whether he or she noticed the usual effects of the NTG. NTG tablets that are therapeutically active may cause a slight burning under the tongue, may make the patient feel flushed, or may give the patient a transient throbbing headache. If the patient confirms that he or she felt one of those effects but the chest pain still would not go away, then you know there was most likely nothing wrong with the NTG but there may be something very wrong with the patient. A third possibility is that the patient's symptoms are not related to a cardiac problem.

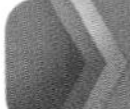

Secondary Assessment

Circumstances will determine which aspects of the physical examination will be used. A physical examination of a patient with chest pain would typically focus primarily on the cardiovascular system. Evaluate the patient's circulation by assessing pulses at various locations, and assess skin color, temperature, and condition. Is the skin cool or moist? How do the mucous membranes look? Are they pink, ashen, or cyanotic? Are the pulses of equal strength bilaterally? Does the patient have any edema in the extremities, especially the lower extremities? All of these physical findings can help identify poor circulation, which may be caused by a failure of the cardiovascular system.

In addition to the cardiovascular system, examine the respiratory system for signs of inadequate ventilation.

These two systems are closely related, and some problems with the respiratory system can be caused by cardiovascular issues. Auscultate breath sounds for depth, equality, and any adventitious sounds such as crackles or wheezing. Listen for gurgling, and look for blood-tinged or foamy froth from the mouth and/or nose. Wet-sounding lungs indicate fluid is being moved into the lungs from the circulatory system, possibly because of a problem with the heart. Are the breath sounds equal? Are the neck veins distended? Is the trachea deviated, or is it midline? The answers to these questions can help determine whether a problem exists with the lungs or with the heart. Although the physical examination is not usually as important as the history in a patient with a possible cardiac problem, it may produce important clues to the patient's condition.

Reassess the level of consciousness. Is the patient diaphoretic? Is there nausea or vomiting, fatigue, or palpitations? Note the presence of edema in the extremities or sacral area. Has the patient had a headache or a syncopal episode? Has the patient's behavior changed? Note any anguished facial expressions or activity limitations. Inspect the neck, looking at the position of the trachea and the appearance of the neck veins. Palpate for any areas of crepitus or tenderness in the thorax and any pulsation or distention in the epigastrium.

Measure and record the patient's vital signs, including pulse, respirations, and blood pressure. You must obtain readings for systolic and diastolic blood pressures. If available, use pulse oximetry. Pulse oximetry may not give an accurate measurement if the patient has poor circulation, has been exposed to a toxic chemical, or is in cardiac arrest, but it should be used and the readings noted for all patients with possible cardiac problems. Assess blood glucose levels.

If you suspect stroke or aortic aneurysm, obtain blood pressure readings in both arms and compare the measurements. Conditions such as these may cause the blood pressure to vary from the left to the right. Markedly elevated pressures may also contribute to stroke, aortic dissection, or heart failure. A normal pulse pressure is 30 to 40 mm Hg. If the pulse pressure is narrowed (below 30 mm Hg), the patient may be tachycardic or experiencing a cardiac tamponade. If the pulse pressure is widened (above 40 mm Hg), the patient may be in late shock.

Repeatedly obtain the vital signs at appropriate intervals. Be sure to note the time that each set of vital signs is obtained.

Reassessment

Repeat the primary survey by checking to see whether the patient's chief complaint and condition have improved or are deteriorating. Vital signs should be reassessed at least every 5 minutes or any time substantial changes in the patient's condition occur. It is essential to monitor the patient with a suspected AMI closely because sudden cardiac arrest is always a risk. If cardiac arrest occurs, you must be ready to begin automated defibrillation or chest compressions immediately. If an AED is immediately

YOU are the Provider PART 3

As soon as the medications have been administered, you assist the patient onto the stretcher, secure her, and place her in the back of the ambulance. She states that her pain now rates about 2 out of 10, and the pressure has greatly diminished. You direct your partner to repeat the patient's vital signs while you prepare to obtain IV access. The patient states that even though she has an extensive cardiac history, she really does not like needles, and asks if it is necessary for you to stick her.

Recording Time: 10 Minutes	
Respirations	20 breaths/min
Pulse	68 beats/min, regular
Skin	Warm, dry, and pink
Blood pressure	122/84 mm Hg
Oxygen saturation (Spo_2)	96% on 15 L/min
Pupils	Pupils Equal, Round, and Reactive to Light and Accommodation (PERRLA)

6. Does this patient require IV access?
7. Should paramedic backup be requested for this patient?

available, use it; if not, perform CPR until the AED is available, as discussed in the later section on cardiac arrest. Reassess your interventions to see whether they are helping and whether the patient's condition is improving. Reassessment will also determine whether further interventions are indicated or contraindicated.

Provide prompt transport to the closest appropriate facility so that treatments such as clot-busting medications or angioplasty can be initiated. To be most effective, these treatments must be started as soon as possible after the onset of the attack. Alert the emergency department about the status of your patient and your estimated time of arrival. Do not delay transport to assist with administration of NTG. The medication can be given en route.

Report to the hospital by radio or cellular telephone while en route. Include information about the patient's history, vital signs, the reassessment of vital signs, medications taken, and any treatment you are giving. Follow the instructions of medical control. Describe the patient's condition to the emergency department staff on arrival.

It is important to document your assessment of the patient. You must record the interventions performed. All interventions should be initiated according to protocol. If the intervention required an order from medical control, document the intervention and/or medication requested and whether approval was granted. It must be clear in your documentation that the patient was reassessed appropriately following any intervention. The patient's response to the intervention and the time of each intervention must also be recorded.

Emergency Medical Care for Chest Pain or Discomfort

Your treatment of the patient begins with proper positioning. As mentioned before, some patients will not tolerate being positioned supine, so they should be allowed to sit up (leaning back on the stretcher). Also, loosen tight clothing, to make the patient as comfortable as possible.

Provide oxygen as needed and maintain Spo_2 at 94% or higher. For patients with mild dyspnea, a nasal

Special Populations

Cardiovascular emergencies are relatively rare in children. When such problems arise, they are often related to volume or infection rather than a primary cardiac cause, unless the child has congenital heart disease. Through the primary survey, you can quickly identify a cardiovascular emergency, understand the likely cause, and institute potentially lifesaving treatment. Call early for paramedic backup if a need is suspected.

The child's appearance gives an overview of perfusion, oxygenation, ventilation, and neurologic status. For a suspected cardiovascular problem, an abnormal appearance may indicate inadequate brain perfusion and the need for rapid intervention.

Tachypnea, without retractions or abnormal airway sounds, is common in an infant or child with a primary cardiac problem; it is a mechanism for blowing off carbon dioxide to compensate for metabolic acidosis related to poor perfusion. In contrast, when cardiac compromise progresses to heart failure, pulmonary edema results in increased work of breathing and a fast respiratory rate. The presence of pallor, cyanosis, or mottling may tip you off to this problem.

Bradycardia in children is most often a result of hypoxia, rather than of a primary cardiac problem (such as heart block). Airway management, supplemental oxygen, and assisted ventilation as needed are always first-line treatment. Also, treat any underlying respiratory problem. Less common causes of bradycardia include congenital or acquired heart block and toxic ingestion of beta blockers, calcium channel blockers, or digoxin. Elevated intracranial pressure can also cause bradycardia and should be considered in children with ventricular shunts, a history of head injury, or suspected child abuse without a consistent injury history.

Tachycardia, a pulse rate higher than normal for the patient's age, is common in children. Although it may be a sign of serious underlying illness or injury, it may also be caused by fever, pain, or anxiety. Interpret the presence of tachycardia in the context of the remainder of the primary survey. For example, if a child appears well but has a fever, tachycardia is likely and treatment with antipyretics is all that is necessary. If a tachycardic child has a history of copious vomiting or diarrhea, fluid resuscitation is the appropriate treatment.

For suspected cardiovascular compromise, start with airway and breathing, and provide supportive care as needed. Ensure adequate oxygenation and ventilation, and then assess the circulation by checking heart rate; pulse quality; skin condition, color, moisture, and temperature; and blood pressure when possible. Use information from the primary survey to make an initial decision about the likely underlying cause, the patient's priority, and the need for immediate treatment or transport.

If you determine that the patient's condition is stable enough for you to continue the assessment on site, continue with the SAMPLE history and the secondary assessment. Repeat the primary survey after each intervention, and monitor trends over time.

cannula may be all that is needed, whereas patients with more serious respiratory difficulty will respond better to a nonrebreathing mask. A patient who is unresponsive or in obvious respiratory distress may need assistance with breathing. Use a bag-mask device or a positive pressure ventilation device such as positive end-expiratory pressure, CPAP, bilevel positive airway pressure, or, if an advanced airway is in place, a manual or automatic transport ventilator if available and you have been approved to use one of these methods in your service.

Gain IV access as long as it doesn't cause a delay in transport. A saline lock is sufficient unless the patient is hypotensive. If so, consider a 250-mL bolus of an isotonic crystalloid solution such as normal saline.

Depending on local protocol, prepare to administer aspirin and assist with prescribed NTG. Aspirin (acetylsalicylic acid) prevents clots from forming or getting bigger. Administer aspirin according to local protocol. Low-dose aspirin comes in 81-mg chewable tablets. The recommended dose is 162 mg (two tablets) to 324 mg (four tablets). Be sure you have verified that the patient is not allergic to aspirin before you give it, because many people are. Also, ask the patient if he or she has any history of internal bleeding such as stomach ulcers, and, if so, contact medical control before giving the patient aspirin.

NTG relieves the pain of angina by increasing the size of the vessels to increase oxygenation to the hypoxic tissue. NTG comes in several forms—as a small white pill, placed sublingually (under the tongue); as a spray, also taken sublingually; and as a skin patch applied to the chest. In any form, the effect is the same. NTG relaxes the muscle of blood vessel walls, dilates coronary arteries, increases blood flow and the supply of oxygen to the heart muscle, and decreases the workload of the heart. NTG also dilates blood vessels in other parts of the body and can sometimes cause low blood pressure and/or a severe headache. Other side effects include changes in the patient's pulse rate, including tachycardia or bradycardia. For this reason, you should take the patient's blood pressure within 5 minutes after each dose. If the systolic blood pressure is less than 100 mm Hg, do not give more NTG. Other contraindications include the presence of a head injury, use of erectile dysfunction drugs within the previous 24 to 72 hours, and the maximum prescribed dose has already been given (usually three doses). Nitrous oxide may also provide a measure of pain relief. Follow local protocols for administration.

▶ Administering Nitroglycerin

Check the condition of the medication and its expiration date. Be sure to wear gloves when handling NTG tablets or spray because it is easily absorbed through the skin. If the patient has an NTG patch on when you arrive, be sure to carefully remove it if the patient is hypotensive or in cardiac arrest (before use of an AED).

After you obtain permission from medical control, administer prescribed NTG to the patient. NTG works in most patients within 5 minutes. Most patients who have been prescribed NTG carry a supply with them. Patients take one dose of NTG under the tongue whenever they have an episode of angina that does not immediately go away with rest. If the pain is still present after 5 minutes, patients are typically instructed by their physicians to take two subsequent doses as needed, up to a total of three doses. Follow local protocols for administration of additional doses of NTG.

Be aware that NTG will lose its potency over time, especially if exposed to light. Patients who take it only rarely may keep a bottle in their pocket for months. It may lose its potency even before its expiration date.

To safely assist the patient with NTG, follow the steps listed in Skill Drill 18-1.

Words of Wisdom

Allowing a patient with a dry mouth to rinse his or her mouth with water prior to administration of NTG will help the tablet dissolve faster. Make sure he or she does not swallow the water. This is not necessary when using the spray form of NTG.

Heart Surgeries and Cardiac Assistive Devices

During the past 30 years, hundreds of thousands of open-heart procedures have been performed to bypass damaged segments of coronary arteries in the heart. In a coronary artery bypass graft, a blood vessel from the chest or leg is sewn directly from the aorta to a coronary artery beyond the point of the obstruction. Another procedure is percutaneous transluminal coronary angioplasty, which aims to dilate, rather than bypass, the coronary artery. In this procedure, usually called an angioplasty or balloon angioplasty, a tiny balloon is attached to the end of a long, thin tube. The tube is introduced through the skin into a large vein, usually in the groin, and then threaded into the narrowed coronary artery, with radiographs serving as a guide. After the balloon is in position inside the coronary artery, it is inflated. The balloon is then deflated, and the tube is removed from the body. Sometimes, a metal mesh called a stent is placed inside the artery instead of or after the balloon. The stent is left in place permanently to help keep the artery from narrowing again.

A patient who has had an AMI or angina will almost certainly have undergone one of these procedures. Patients

Skill Drill 18-1 Administering Nitroglycerin

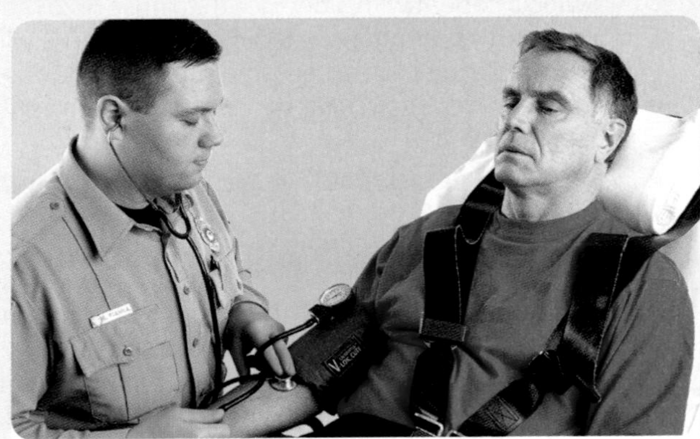

Step 1 Obtain an order from medical control—online or off-line protocol. Take the patient's blood pressure. Administer NTG only if the systolic blood pressure is greater than 100 mm Hg.

Attempt IV access prior to administration of NTG in patients who have not received it previously or who are known to respond to NTG with hypotension. If the patient has a prescription for NTG and you are assisting with his own medication, an IV line should not be necessary first.

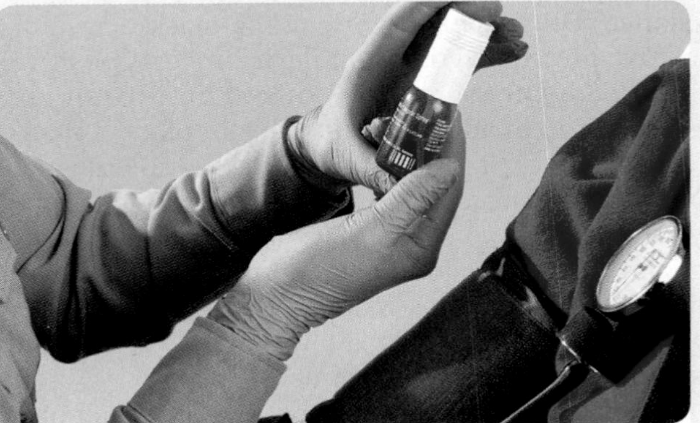

Step 2 Check that you have the right medication, the right patient, and the right delivery route. Check the expiration date. Make sure the patient has no contraindications, such as having taken a medication for erectile dysfunction in the past 24 to 72 hours.

Ask the patient about the last dose he or she took and its effects. Make sure that the patient understands the route of administration. Be prepared to have the patient lie down to prevent fainting if the NTG substantially lowers the patient's blood pressure (the patient gets dizzy or feels faint).

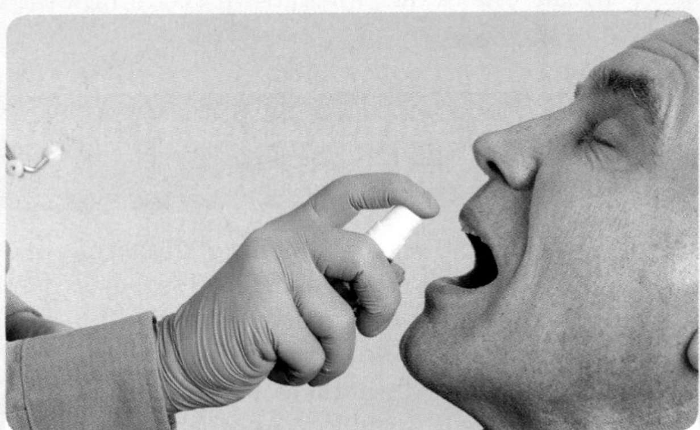

Step 3 Ask the patient to lift his or her tongue. Place the tablet or spray the dose under the tongue (while wearing gloves), or have the patient do so. Have the patient keep his or her mouth closed with the tablet or spray under the tongue until it is dissolved and absorbed. Caution the patient against chewing or swallowing the tablet.

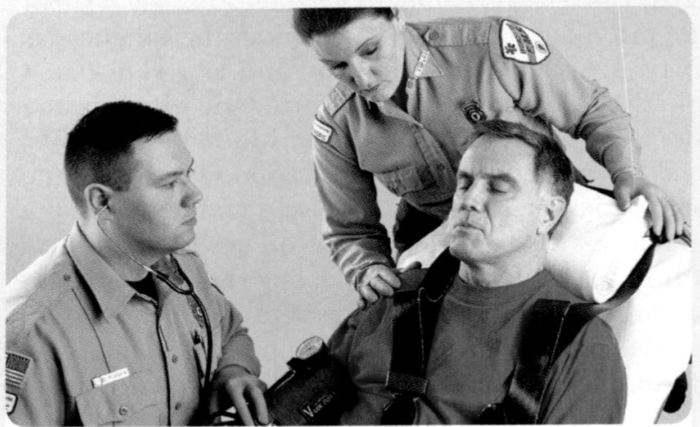

Step 4 Recheck the blood pressure within 5 minutes. Record the medication and the time of administration. Reevaluate the chest pain and blood pressure, and note the response to the medication. If the chest pain persists and the patient still has a systolic blood pressure of greater than 100 mm Hg, repeat the dose every 5 minutes as authorized by medical control. In general, a maximum of three doses of NTG is given for any one episode of chest pain. If protocols allow, consider administering 160 to 325 mg of aspirin.

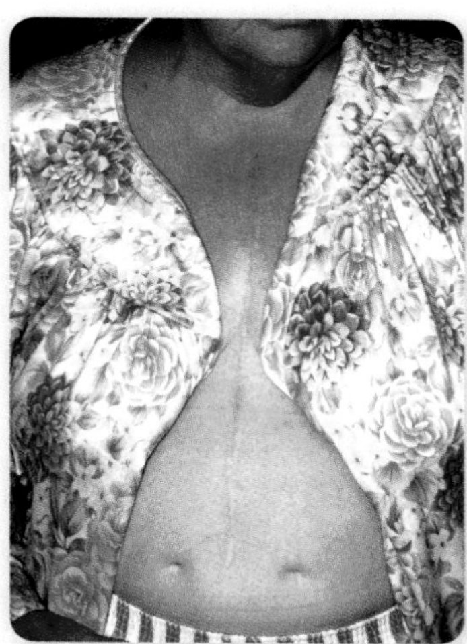

Figure 18-9 A long vertical surgical scar on a patient's chest suggests previous coronary artery bypass graft surgery.
Courtesy of Rhonda Hunt.

who have undergone a bypass graft will have a long surgical scar on their chest from the procedure Figure 18-9. Patients who have undergone an angioplasty or coronary artery stent usually will not. However, newer "keyhole" surgical techniques may not produce a large scar. You should not assume that a patient who has a small scar has not had bypass surgery. Chest pain in a patient who has undergone any of these procedures should be treated the same as chest pain in patients who have not undergone any heart surgery. Perform all the described tasks, and transport the patient promptly to the emergency department of the closest, most appropriate hospital. If CPR is required, begin with compressions and perform the procedure in the usual way, regardless of the scar on the patient's chest. Similarly, if indicated, an AED should be used as soon as possible.

Many people with heart disease in the United States have cardiac pacemakers to maintain a regular cardiac rhythm and rate Figure 18-10. Pacemakers are inserted when the electrical conduction system of the heart is so damaged that it cannot function properly. These battery-powered devices deliver an electrical impulse through wires that are in direct contact with the myocardium. The generating unit is generally placed under a heavy muscle or a fold of skin; it typically resembles a small silver dollar under the skin in the left upper part of the chest.

Normally, you do not need to be concerned about problems with pacemakers. Thanks to modern technology, an implanted unit will not require replacement for years. Wires are well protected and rarely broken. Previously, pacemakers sometimes malfunctioned when a patient got too close to an electrical radiation source, such as a microwave oven, but this is no longer the case. Every patient with a pacemaker still should be aware of the precautions, if any, which must be taken to maintain its proper functioning.

If a pacemaker does not function properly, as when the battery wears out, the patient may experience syncope,

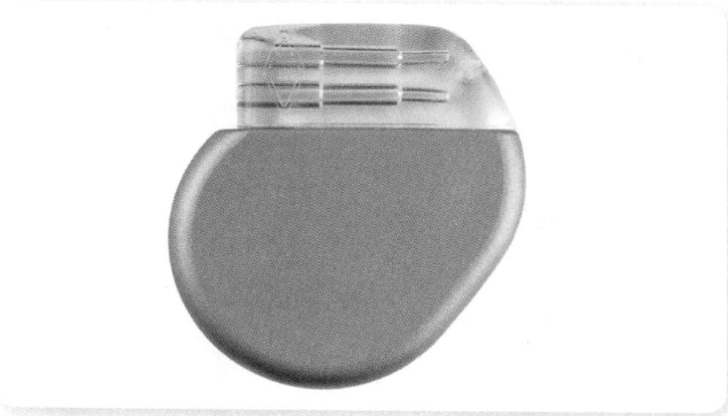

Figure 18-10 A pacemaker, which is typically inserted under the skin in the left upper part of the chest, delivers an electrical impulse to regulate heartbeat.
© Carolina K. Smith, MD/Shutterstock.

dizziness, or weakness because of an excessively slow heart rate. The pulse ordinarily will be less than 60 beats/min because the heart is beating without the stimulus of the pacemaker and without the regulation of its own electrical conduction system, which may be damaged. In these circumstances, the heart tends to assume a fixed slow rate that is not fast enough to allow the patient to function normally. A patient with a malfunctioning pacemaker should be promptly transported to the emergency department for evaluation and possible repair of the pacemaker. When an AED is used, the patches should not be placed directly over the pacemaker. This will ensure a better flow of electricity through the patient's body.

▶ Automatic Implantable Cardiac Defibrillators

More and more patients who survive cardiac arrest due to ventricular fibrillation have a small automatic implantable cardiac defibrillator (AICD) implanted Figure 18-11. Some patients who are at particularly high risk for a cardiac arrest have them as well. These devices are attached directly to the heart and can prolong lives. They continuously monitor the heart rhythm, delivering shocks as needed. Regardless of whether a patient having an AMI has an AICD, he or she should be treated like all other AMI patients. Treatment should include performing CPR, beginning with compressions, and using an AED if the patient goes into cardiac arrest. Generally, the electricity from an AICD is so low that it will have no effect on rescuers and, therefore, should not be of concern to you.

▶ External Defibrillator Vest

An alternative to the AICD is the external defibrillator vest. This device is a vest with built-in monitoring electrodes and defibrillation pads, which is worn by the patient under his or her clothing. The vest is attached to a monitor worn on a belt or hung from a shoulder strap. The monitor provides alerts and voice prompts when it recognizes a

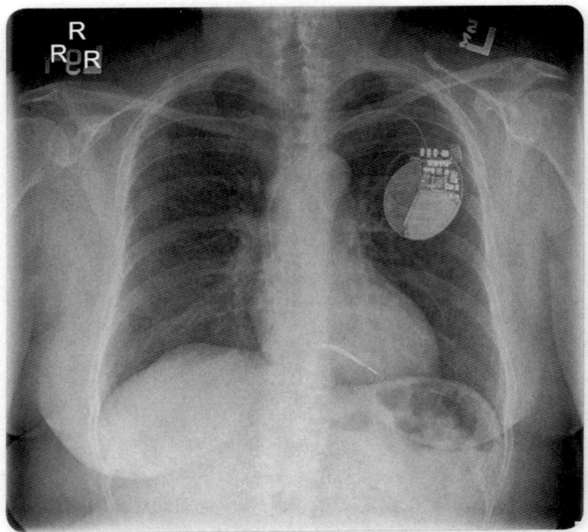

Figure 18-11 An automatic implantable cardiac defibrillator (AICD) is attached directly to the heart and continuously monitors heart rhythm, delivering shocks as needed. The electricity from the AICD is so low that it has no effect on rescuers.

dangerous rhythm and before a shock is delivered. Unlike the implantable defibrillator, this device uses high-energy shocks similar to an AED, so you should avoid contact with the patient if the device warns that it is about to deliver a shock. Blue gel under the large defibrillation pads indicates that the device has already delivered at least one shock.

If the patient is in cardiac arrest, the vest should remain in place while CPR is being performed unless it interferes with compressions. If it is necessary to remove the vest, simply remove the battery from the monitor and then remove the vest. You can then use your own AED on the patient. Any patient who is wearing a device that has already delivered a shock should be transported to the hospital for further evaluation.

▶ Left Ventricular Assist Devices

Left ventricular assist devices (LVADs) are used to enhance the pumping of the left ventricle in patients with severe heart failure or in patients who need a temporary boost due to a myocardial infarction. There are several types of LVADs; the most common ones have an internal pump unit and an external battery pack. These pumps may be pulsatile, meaning they pump the blood in pulsations just like the natural heart, or they may be continuous, in which case, the patient will not have any palpable pulses. If you encounter a patient with a LVAD, he or she (or his or her family members) may be able to tell you about the unit. Unless it malfunctions, you should not need to deal with it. If you are unsure of what to do, contact medical control for assistance. Also, LVADs provide a number to call for assistance. Transport all LVAD supplies and battery packs to the hospital with the patient.

Cardiac Arrest

Cardiac arrest is the complete cessation of functional cardiac activity—either electrical, mechanical, or both. It is indicated in the field by the absence of a carotid pulse. Cardiac arrest may be the result of trauma or numerous medical conditions, such as end-stage renal disease, hyperkalemia with renal disease, or hypothermia, to name a few.

▶ Automated External Defibrillation

In the late 1970s and early 1980s, scientists developed a small computer that could analyze electrical signals from the heart and determine when ventricular fibrillation was taking place. This development, along with improved battery technology, made possible the portable automated defibrillator, which can automatically administer an electrical shock to the heart when needed.

The AED machines come in models with different features Figure 18-12. All of them require a certain degree of operator interaction, beginning with applying the pads

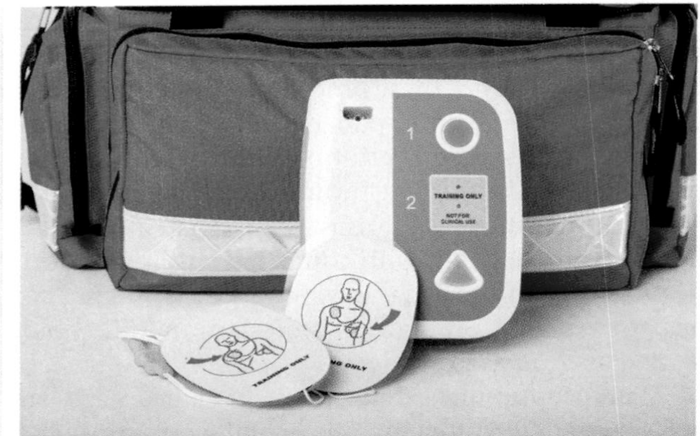

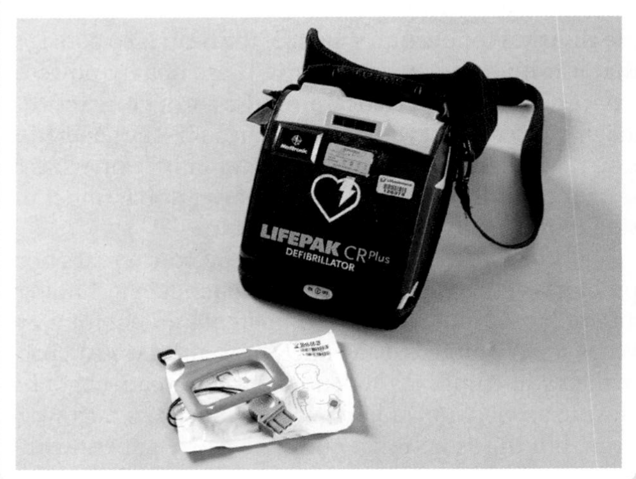

Figure 18-12 Automated external defibrillators vary in their design, features, and operation. Two devices are shown here.

and turning the machine on. The operator also has to push a button to deliver an electrical shock, depending on the model. Many AEDs use a computer voice synthesizer to advise the operator what steps to take on the basis of the AED's analysis. Some have a button that tells the computer to analyze the heart's electrical rhythm; other models start doing this as soon as they are turned on. Even though most defibrillators are now semiautomated, the acronym AED is used as the general term to describe all of these machines. Fully automated AEDs were among the first AEDs made; however, unlike the semiautomated AED, they delivered the shock automatically (the operator had no control over when the shock was delivered). Because of the safety concerns, there are few, if any, fully automated AEDs left; all manufacturers now produce only semiautomated external defibrillators.

AEDs also come equipped to give a monophasic shock or a biphasic shock. Monophasic means to send the energy in one direction, from negative to positive, and biphasic means to send the energy in two directions simultaneously. The advantage of biphasic shock is that it produces a more efficient defibrillation and may require a lower energy setting. The initial and subsequent energy setting for ventricular fibrillation and pulseless ventricular tachycardia on a monophasic machine is 360 joules. With the biphasic technology, the energy can be 120 joules for the first and all subsequent shocks or can start at 120 joules and then escalate to 200 joules for subsequent shocks. The optimum energy setting for biphasic AEDs is still being studied, and no recommendation is currently supported in the literature. Most AEDs currently in use are biphasic.

The computer inside the AED is specifically programmed to recognize rhythms that require defibrillation to correct, most commonly ventricular fibrillation and pulseless ventricular tachycardia. The current programs are extremely accurate. It would be rare for an AED to recommend a shock when a shock would not be indicated, and an AED rarely fails to recommend one when it would be indicated. Therefore, if the AED recommends a shock, you can believe it is indicated.

YOU are the Provider — PART 4

After you establish IV access, you contact your dispatch on the radio to request a paramedic intercept. You are advised that there are no paramedic units available and you will have to transport this patient on your own. You inform your partner to transport emergent to First Care Hospital, which is approximately 22 minutes away. Your partner asks why you are bypassing Unity Hospital, which is only 10 minutes away, to which you reply that Unity does not have a cardiac catheterization laboratory, and First Care does, and according to local protocols, any patient suspected of having an AMI is to be diverted to the closest facility with a catheterization lab. You contact First Care, and inform them that you are coming in with a "Heart alert" and you relay your findings. You continue to monitor your patient, and when asked, she states that her pain is increasing back up to a 7 out of 10. Per your protocols, you administer a second 0.4-mg dose of nitroglycerin sublingually. After approximately 90 seconds, the patient appears to become unresponsive. You quickly palpate a carotid pulse, and finding none, begin chest compressions while attaching the AED electrodes to the patient. Your partner stops the ambulance to allow the AED to analyze. On receiving the message "Shock advised," you defibrillate the patient after and begin CPR. You inform your partner of the need to divert to Unity Hospital and ask him to contact both facilities and advise them of the change in the patient's status. Your partner advises that you are approximately 2 minutes from Unity Hospital. With the relatively short ETA, you elect to withhold insertion of an advanced airway and continue ventilations with a bag-mask device. On arrival at Unity Hospital, you continue CPR while the patient is wheeled into the resuscitation bay, at which point you turn over care to the awaiting physician while hospital staff take over CPR.

Recording Time: 20 Minutes	
Respirations	0 breaths/min
Pulse	0 beats/min
Skin	Warm, dry, and pink
Blood pressure	Not obtained
Oxygen saturation (Spo_2)	Not obtained
Pupils	Not assessed

8. What is the most common error with AED operation?
9. What are the five links in the chain of survival?

The AED provides several advantages. First, the machine is fast, and delivers the most important treatment for the patient in ventricular fibrillation or pulseless ventricular tachycardia: an electrical shock. It can be delivered within 1 minute of your arrival at the patient's side. Second, you will find AEDs are easy to operate. Paramedics do not have to be on the scene to provide this critical intervention.

Current AEDs offer two other advantages. The shock can be given through remote, adhesive defibrillator pads, which are safe to use. Also, the pad area is larger than manual paddles, which means that the transmission of electricity is more efficient. Usually, there are pictures on the pads to remind you where they are placed on the patient's chest. As a safety measure, make sure the patient is not lying on wet ground or touching metal objects when he or she is being shocked.

Not all patients in cardiac arrest require an electrical shock. Although all patients in cardiac arrest should be analyzed with an AED, some do not have shockable rhythms (eg, pulseless electrical activity and asystole). Asystole (flatline) indicates that no electrical or mechanical activity is present, whereas pulseless electrical activity usually refers to a state of cardiac arrest despite an organized cardiac rhythm. In both cases, CPR should be initiated as soon as possible, beginning with chest compressions.

Rationale for Early Defibrillation

Few patients who experience sudden cardiac arrest outside of a hospital survive unless a rapid sequence of events takes place. The chain of survival is a way of describing the ideal sequence of events that should take place when such an arrest occurs.

The five links in the chain of survival are as follows **Figure 18-13**:

- Recognition of early warning signs and immediate activation of EMS
- Immediate CPR with emphasis on high-quality chest compressions
- Rapid defibrillation
- Basic and advanced EMS care
- ALS and postarrest care

If any one of the links in the chain is absent or delayed, the patient's chances for survival diminish. For example, few patients benefit from defibrillation when more than 10 minutes elapse before administration of the first shock or if CPR is not performed in the first 2 to 3 minutes. If all links in the chain are strong, the patient has the best possible chance of survival. The link that is the greatest determinant for survival is the third link—rapid defibrillation.

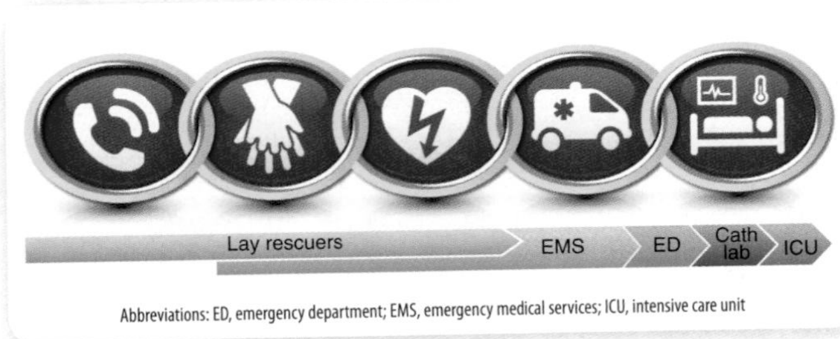

Figure 18-13 The five links in the out-of-hospital chain of survival.

Reprinted with permission Web-based Integrated 2010 & 2015 AHA Guidelines for CPR & ECC-Part 4: Systems of Care & Continuous Quality Improvement ©2015 American Heart Association, Inc.

CPR helps patients in cardiac arrest because it maintains myocardial and cerebral perfusion, thus prolonging the period during which defibrillation can be effective. Rapid defibrillation has successfully resuscitated many patients with cardiac arrest from ventricular fibrillation. However, defibrillation works best if it takes place within 2 minutes of the onset of the cardiac arrest. To try to achieve better survival rates among cardiac arrest victims, many communities are exploring the idea that nontraditional first responders should be trained to administer early defibrillation. These responders would include police officers, security personnel, lifeguards, maintenance workers, and flight attendants. As an AEMT, you should support these efforts to shorten the time until defibrillation. Remember, seconds really matter when the patient is in cardiac arrest.

The final step in the chain of survival is ALS and postarrest care. This refers to controlling temperature to optimize neurologic recovery in the field and maintaining glucose levels in the patient who is hypoglycemic. Ventilations should be delivered at less than 12 breaths/min or as needed to achieve an end-tidal carbon dioxide of 35 to 40 mm Hg; maintain oxygen saturation between 94% and 99%; and ensure blood pressure is above 90 mm Hg. It also includes cardiopulmonary and neurologic support at the hospital, PCIs when indicated, and an electroencephalogram to detect seizure activity.

Integrating the Automated External Defibrillator and Cardiopulmonary Resuscitation

Because most cardiac arrests occur in the home, a bystander at the scene may already have started CPR before you arrive. For this reason, you must know how to work the AED into the CPR sequence. Remember that the AED is not very complex; it may not be able to distinguish other movements from ventricular fibrillation. Therefore, do not touch the patient while the AED is analyzing the heart rhythm and delivering shocks. Stop CPR, and let the AED do its job.

Automated External Defibrillator Maintenance

It is crucial at the beginning of your shift to ensure that you have a functioning AED. You must become familiar with the maintenance procedures required for the brand of AED your service uses. Read the operator's manual. If your defibrillator does not work on the scene, someone will want to know what went wrong. That person may be your system's administrator, your medical director, the local newspaper reporter, or the family's attorney.

You will be asked to show proof that you maintained the defibrillator properly and attended any mandatory in-service sessions.

When an error occurs, it is usually because of one of the following:

- **Failure to charge or maintain the AED.** The most common error is not having a charged battery. To avoid this problem, many defibrillator companies have built smarter machines that will warn the operator that the battery is unlikely to work. However, some of the older models do not have this feature.
- **Failure to use the AED correctly.** Another form of operator error is failing to push the *Analyze* or *Shock* buttons when the machine advises you to do so or failing to apply the AED to a patient in cardiac arrest.
- **Application of an AED to a patient who has a pulse.** The computer may be unable to tell the difference between electrical signals from the heart and electrical signals from the arms and chest muscles that are moving. Additionally, most AEDs identify a regular rhythm of faster than 150 or 180 beats/min as ventricular tachycardia, which, if pulseless, should be defibrillated. However, a patient in ventricular tachycardia with a pulse should be cardioverted (a paramedic skill); defibrillating this patient will most likely result in cardiac arrest. Avoid these errors by using the AED only for pulseless patients.

The main legal risk in using the AED is failing to deliver a shock when one was needed. Of course, the AED is like any other manufactured item. It can fail, although this is rare. Ideally, you will encounter any such failure while performing routine maintenance, not while caring for a patient in cardiac arrest. Check your equipment, including your AED, at the beginning of each shift and exercise the battery as often as the manufacturer recommends. Ask the manufacturer for a checklist of items that should be checked daily, weekly, or less often Figure 18-14.

If the AED fails while you are caring for a patient, you must report the problem to the manufacturer and the US Food and Drug Administration. Be sure to follow the appropriate EMS procedures for notifying these organizations.

Medical Direction

Defibrillation of the heart is a medical procedure. Although AEDs have made the process of delivering electricity much simpler, there is still a benefit in having a physician's involvement. The medical director of your service should help to teach you how to use the AED. At the least, he or she should approve the written protocol that you will follow in caring for patients in cardiac arrest. In most states, AED training in an AEMT course is not permitted without approval by state laws, rules, and local medical direction authority.

There should be a review of each incident in which the AED is used. After returning from the hospital or the scene, discuss with the rest of the team what happened. This discussion will help all members of the team learn from the incident. Review such events by using the written report, any voice-electrocardiogram (ECG) tape recorder, and the device's solid-state memory modules and magnetic tape recordings, if applicable.

There should also be a review of the incident by your service's medical director or quality improvement officer. Quality improvement involves people using AEDs and the responsible EMS system managers. This review should focus on speed of defibrillation, that is, the time from the call to the time of the shock. Few systems will achieve the ultimate goal: shocking 100% of patients within 1 minute of the call. However, all systems should continuously work on improving patient care. Mandatory continuing education with skill competency review is generally required for EMS providers, with a continuing competency skill review every 3 to 6 months for the AEMT.

Safety

When operating an AED, make sure that no one is injured, including yourself. Be sure no one is touching the patient. Do not defibrillate a patient who is in pooled water. Do not defibrillate someone who is touching metal that others are touching. Finally, carefully remove any medication patches from a patient's chest with your gloved hands, and wipe the area with a dry towel before defibrillation to prevent ignition of the patch.

Emergency Medical Care for Cardiac Arrest

Cardiopulmonary Resuscitation

Recall the five links of the chain of survival from Chapter 15, *BLS Resuscitation*. The second and third links in this chain are immediate high-quality CPR and rapid defibrillation, respectively. The importance of high-quality chest compressions during CPR cannot be overstated. This is perhaps the most important intervention you will offer, even more important than defibrillation. Immediate, high-quality CPR markedly increases the patient's chance of survival; a delay leads to poor patient outcomes. Remember to push hard and fast, and ensure the chest completely recoils between each compression; this maximizes blood return to the heart. Finally, do not interrupt compressions unless absolutely necessary.

Preparation for Defibrillation

When dispatch reports an unresponsive patient with CPR in progress, the AED should be one of the first pieces

AUTOMATED EXTERNAL DEFIBRILLATOR

Inspection Checklist

Serial # ____________ **Date** ____________ **Time** ____________

Model # ____________ **Inspected by** ____________

Item	**Pass**	**Fail**
Exterior/Cables		
Nothing stored on top of unit		
Carry case intact and clean		
Exterior/LCD/cables/connectors clean and undamaged		
Cables securely attached to unit		
Batteries		
All chargers plugged in and operational (if applicable)		
All batteries fully charged (battery in unit, spare battery)		
Valid expiration date on both batteries		
Supplies		
Two sets of electrodes in sealed packages with valid expiration dates		
Razor		
Hand towel		
Alcohol wipes		
Memory/voice recording device—module, card, microcassette		
Manual override—module, key (if applicable)		
Printer paper (if applicable)		
Operation		
Unit self-test per manufacturer's recommendation/instructions		
Display (if applicable)		
Visual indicators		
Verbal prompts		
Printer (if applicable)		
Attach AED to simulator/tester		
Recognizes shockable rhythm		
Charges to correct energy level within manufacturer's specifications		
Delivers charge		
Recognizes nonshockable rhythm		
Manual override system in working order (if applicable)		

Signature:

Figure 18-14 A sample daily checklist for the automated external defibrillator.

of equipment you obtain from the ambulance. As the operator of the AED, you are responsible for ensuring its safe operation. Remote defibrillation using pads allows you to distance yourself safely from the patient. Do not defibrillate a patient who is in pooled water. Electricity follows the path of least resistance; instead of traveling between the pads and through the patient's heart, it will diffuse into the water. You can defibrillate a wet patient, but first wipe the water from the patient's chest. Prior to defibrillation, ensure that no one is touching any metal that the patient may be in contact with. Carefully remove any NTG or other medication patch from the patient's chest and wipe the area with dry gauze before defibrillation to prevent ignition of the patch. The medication may also be contributing to the cause of the arrest. It is also helpful to shave a hairy patient's chest before pad placement to increase conductivity. Be sure to consult local protocols for issues such as pad placement and preparation of the pad site.

Words of Wisdom

If the AED pads will not stick well due to the amount of hair on the patient's chest, a quick and easy way to remove it is to place the pads firmly in the proper position and then rip them off, pulling the hair out with them. Then place a second set of pads over the area where the hair has been removed. Always make sure you have two sets of pads before using one set for hair removal!

Special Populations

In general, your approach to pediatric patients with a cardiac emergency should be the same as that for an adult. You should attempt to reassure the patient. If possible, administer oxygen. If the patient will not wear a face mask, have the parent hold the oxygen in front of the child's face.

Cardiac arrest in infants and children is usually the result of respiratory failure, not a primary cardiac event. However, the American Heart Association has determined that AEDs are safe to use on infants and children. If the patient is 8 years old or younger, pediatric-sized pads and a dose-attenuating system (energy reducer) are preferred. However, if these are unavailable, a regular adult AED can be used. If the child is between 1 month and 1 year of age (an infant), a manual defibrillator is preferred to an AED. If a manual defibrillator is not available, an AED equipped with a pediatric dose attenuator is preferred. If neither is available, an AED without a pediatric dose attenuator may be used. Chapter 35, *Obstetrics and Neonatal Care*, discusses neonatal resuscitation for infants younger than 1 month.

Determine the nature of illness and/or mechanism of injury. If the incident involves trauma, perform spinal immobilization as you begin the primary survey. Is there only one patient? If you are in a tiered system and the patient is in cardiac arrest, call for paramedic assistance.

Indications for not initiating resuscitative techniques include rigor mortis, dependent lividity, and decapitation. Local protocols may also dictate other circumstances, such as advance directives (that is, living wills) and do not resuscitate orders.

▶ Performing Defibrillation

Prepare with standard precautions en route to the scene. On arrival at the scene, make sure that the scene is safe. Ask any bystanders or first responders who are performing CPR to stop so that you can check for a pulse and apply the AED. Make sure to minimize the time that you are not performing chest compressions; research has shown the best survival rates for patients in whom compressions were interrupted for the least amount of time.[7] Immediately after each defibrillation, resume high-quality CPR with compressions first. Take the steps shown in Skill Drill 18-2 to use an AED.

Safety

When you are "clearing" the patient before an AED shock, ensure that no one is touching the patient and that no one is in contact with any object that is touching the patient, such as the stretcher or a bag-mask device.

If the AED advises no shock and the patient has a pulse, check the patient's breathing. If the patient is breathing adequately, administer oxygen via a nonrebreathing mask and transport. If the patient is not breathing adequately, provide ventilations with a bag-mask device or pocket mask device attached to 100% oxygen and transport. Ensure that proper airway techniques are used at all times.

Words of Wisdom

Optimally, while performing CPR and using the AED, your patient will regain a pulse. Although you should never use an AED on a patient with a pulse, in this situation, you would leave it in place. However, DO NOT press the *Analyze* button or the *Shock* button as long as the patient maintains a pulse. The AED cannot detect the presence of a pulse, only electrical activity. Defibrillating a patient with a pulse will most likely result in cardiac arrest. In most cases, the AED will not allow you to do this.

NR Skill

Skill Drill 18-2 AED and CPR

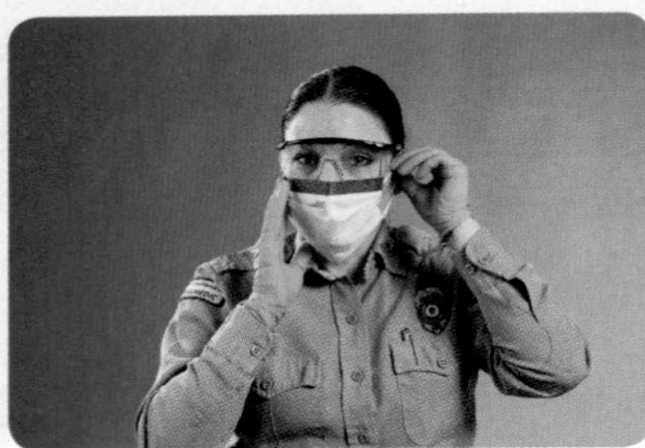

Step 1 Assemble equipment, including AED, AED pads, oxygen, and oxygen administration device. Take standard precautions. Ensure scene safety.

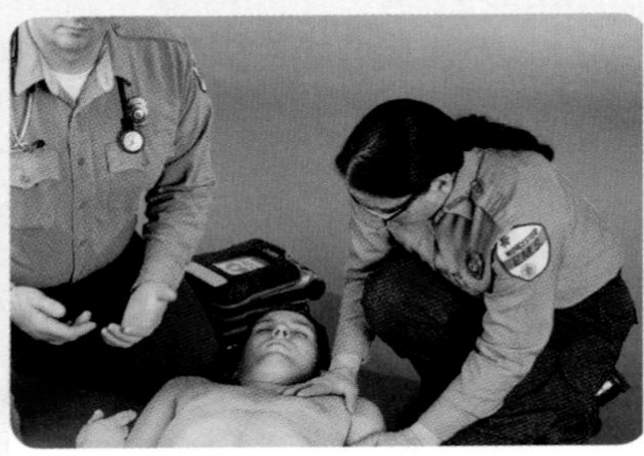

Step 2 Assess responsiveness. If the patient is responsive, do not apply the AED. Gather additional information about the arrest event.

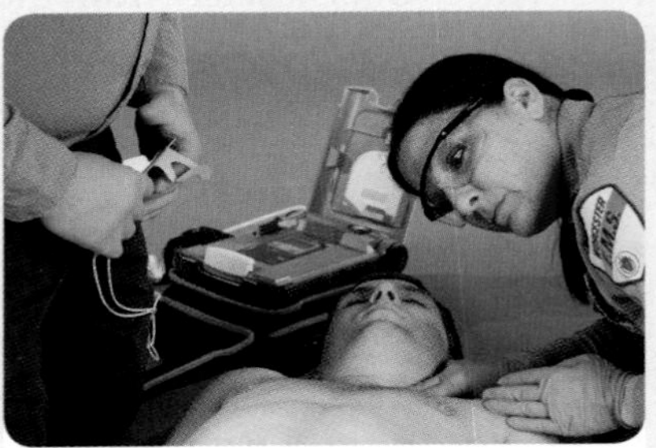

Step 3 Check for a carotid pulse while assessing the patient's breathing.

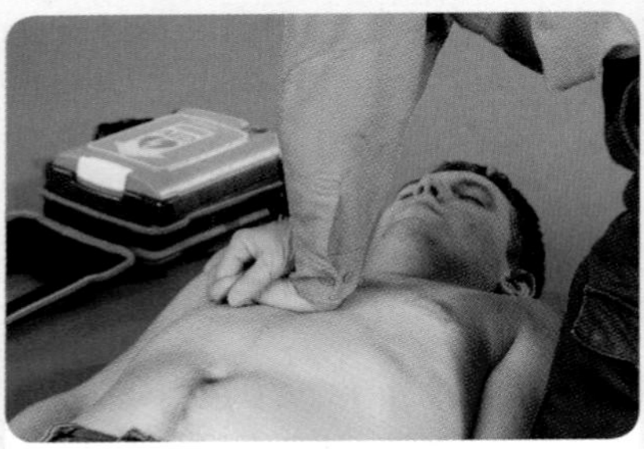

Step 4 If CPR is in progress, assess the effectiveness of chest compressions. If the patient is pulseless and CPR has not been started yet, begin providing chest compressions and rescue breaths at a ratio of 30 compressions to 2 breaths, continuing until an AED arrives and is ready for use. It is important to start chest compressions and use the AED as soon as possible. Compressions provide vital blood flow to the heart and brain, improving the patient's chance of survival.

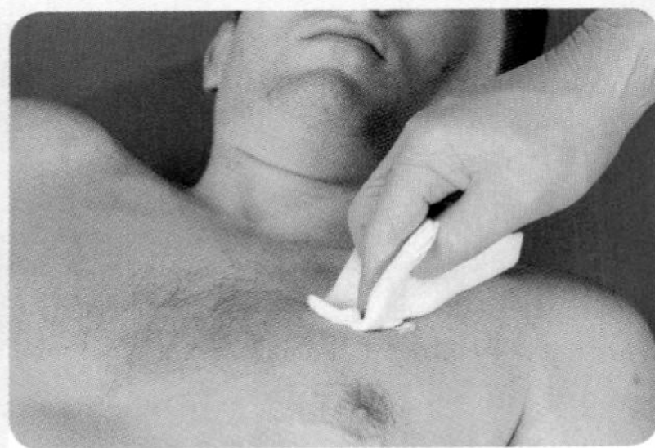

Step 5 Turn on the AED. Remove clothing from the patient's chest area. With gloves, remove medication paste or patches from the patient's chest, if present, and wipe away any residue.

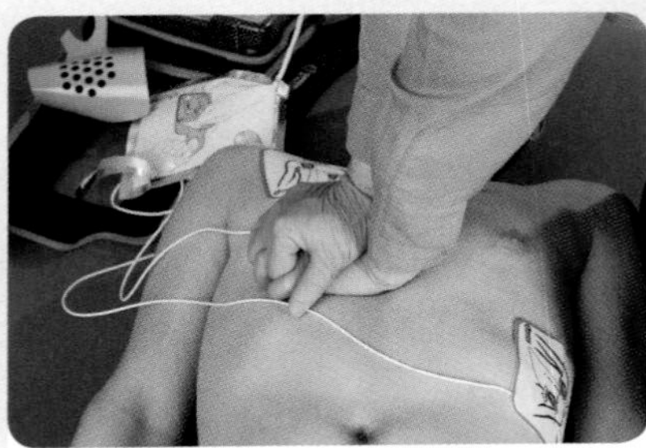

Step 6 Apply the AED pads to the chest and attach the pads to the AED: one just to the right of the breastbone (sternum) just below the collarbone (clavicle), the other on the left lower chest area with the top of the pad 2 to 3 inches below the armpit. Do not place the pads on top of breast tissue. If necessary, lift the breast out of the way and place the pad underneath. Ensure that the pads are attached to the patient cables (and that they are attached to the AED in some models). Plug in the pads' connector to the AED.

Skill Drill 18-2 AED and CPR *(continued)*

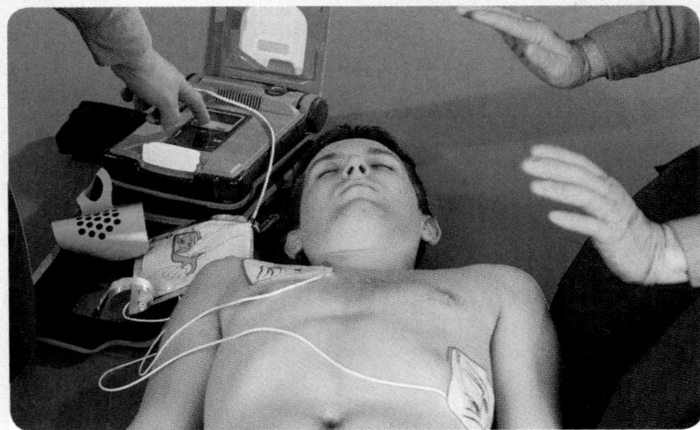

Step 7 Stop CPR. Verbally and visually clear the patient by stating aloud, "Clear the patient," and ensure that no one is touching the patient. Push the *Analyze* button, if there is one. Wait for the AED to determine whether a shockable rhythm is present. If no shock is advised, perform five cycles (2 minutes) of CPR beginning with chest compressions, then reanalyze the cardiac rhythm. If a shock is advised, restart compressions until the AED is charged, reconfirm that no one is touching the patient, and push the *Shock* button.

Step 8 After the shock is delivered, immediately resume CPR beginning with chest compressions. After five cycles (2 minutes) of CPR, reanalyze the cardiac rhythm. Do not interrupt chest compressions for more than 10 seconds. After five cycles (2 minutes) of CPR, reanalyze the cardiac rhythm. Repeat the cycle of 2 minutes of CPR, one shock (if indicated), and 2 minutes of CPR. Transport, and contact medical control as needed.

Gain IV access, and initiate fluid therapy based on patient status. Give a 250-mL bolus of an isotonic crystalloid solution if hypovolemia is suspected. Determine blood glucose level and give IV dextrose or glucagon if the patient is hypoglycemic.

Provide psychological support for the family and significant others. On arrival at the emergency department, give a full report to the attending staff, including length of time since resuscitation efforts were initiated, how long the patient was "down" before EMS arrival, and any treatment given.

▶ Patient Care After Automated External Defibrillator Shocks

The care of the patient after the AED delivers its shock depends on your location and the EMS system; therefore, you should follow your local protocols. After the AED protocol is completed, the patient will have had one of the following occur:

- Pulse is regained
- No pulse, and the AED indicates that no shock is advised
- No pulse, and the AED indicates that a shock is advised

Commonly, in patients who are successfully defibrillated by an AED a normal heart rhythm will develop. However, if the heart still is not receiving optimal amounts of oxygen, ventricular fibrillation will often recur.

Patients who do not regain a pulse on the scene of the cardiac arrest usually do not survive. What you do with these patients, again, depends on your EMS system's protocols. Whether you should transport the patient or wait for a paramedic unit to arrive should be in the local protocols established by medical control. If paramedics are responding to the scene, the best option usually is to stay where you are and continue the sequence of shocks and CPR. Administering CPR while patients are being moved or transported is usually not effective. The best chance for patient survival occurs when the patient is resuscitated where found, unless the scene is unsafe. See Chapter 15, *BLS Resuscitation*, for a review of BLS for adults, children, and infants.

If paramedics are not responding to the scene and your local protocols agree, you should begin transport when one of the following occurs:

- The patient regains a pulse.
- Six to nine shocks have been delivered (or as directed by local protocol).

- The machine gives three consecutive messages (separated by 2 minutes of CPR) that no shock is advised (or as directed by local protocol).

If you transport a patient while performing CPR, you need a plan for treating the patient in the ambulance. Ideally, you should have two EMS providers in the patient compartment while a third provider drives. You may deliver additional shocks at the scene or en route with the approval of medical control. *Keep in mind that some AEDs cannot analyze rhythm while the vehicle is in motion;* therefore, it is pertinent to be familiar with your equipment and stop if needed. Be sure to memorize the protocol of your EMS service **Figure 18-15**.

▶ Cardiac Arrest During Transport

If you are traveling to the hospital with an unresponsive patient, check the pulse at least every 30 seconds. If a pulse is not present, take the following steps:

1. Stop the vehicle.
2. If the AED is not immediately ready, perform CPR, beginning with chest compressions, until it is available.
3. Analyze the rhythm.
4. Deliver one shock, if indicated, and immediately resume CPR.

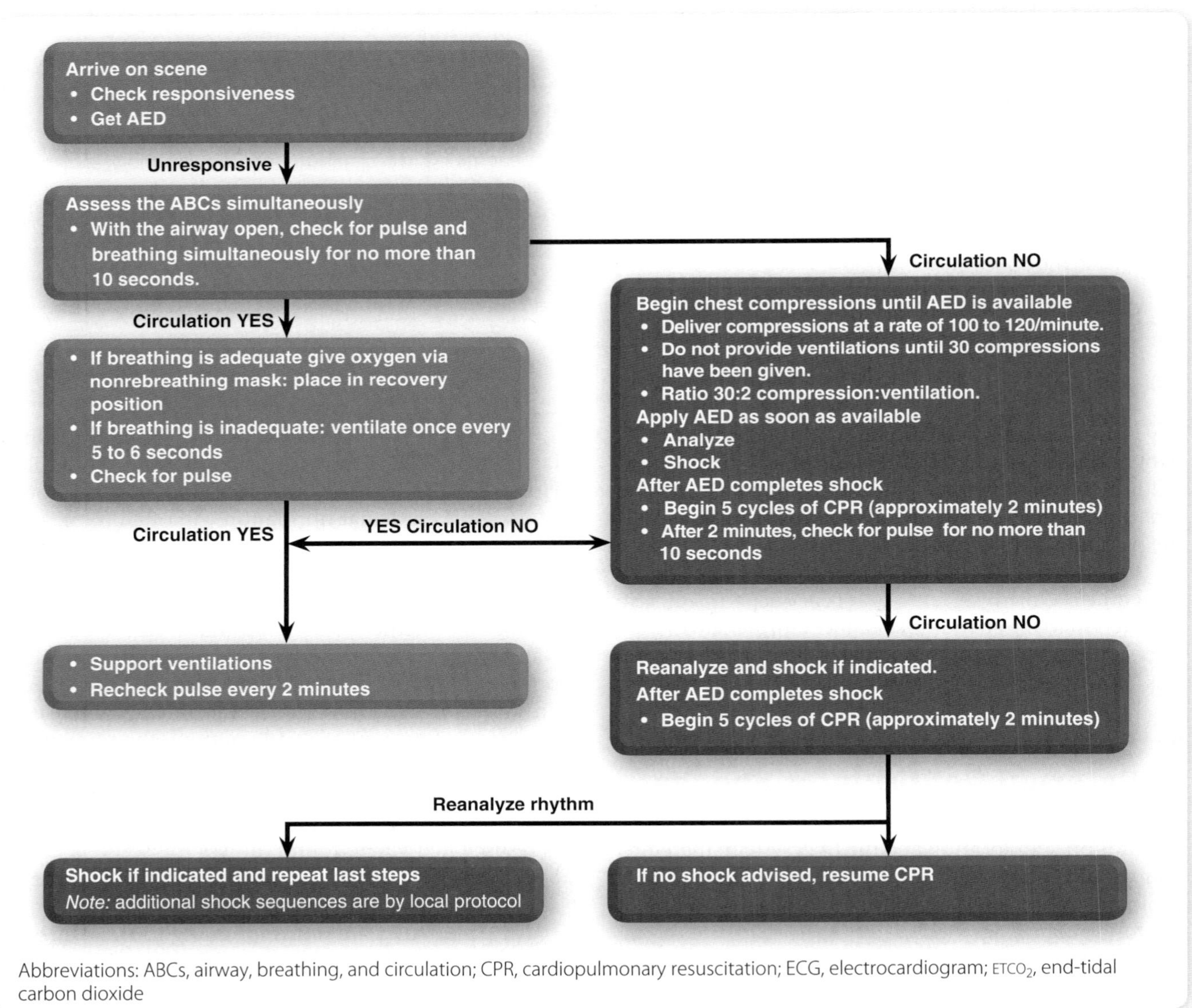

Figure 18-15 Automated external defibrillator (AED) algorithm. Follow procedures for return of spontaneous circulation for your region (ie, transport to the appropriate facility; monitor $ETCO_2$ and vital signs; consider hypothermia; consider obtaining a 12-lead ECG; etc).

5. Continue resuscitation according to your local protocol.

If you are en route with an alert adult patient who is having chest pain and becomes unresponsive, take the following steps:

1. Check for a pulse.
2. Stop the vehicle if no pulse is present.
3. If the AED is not immediately ready, perform CPR, beginning with chest compressions, until it is ready.
4. Analyze the rhythm.
5. Deliver one shock, if indicated, and immediately begin CPR.
6. Begin compressions, and continue resuscitation according to your local protocol, including transporting the patient.

▶ Management of Return of Spontaneous Circulation

Restoration of a pulse after cardiac arrest is called return of spontaneous circulation. If you are able to restore a pulse through the use of CPR and/or an AED, the next steps can be crucial for patient survival. Monitor for spontaneous respirations, provide oxygen via bag-mask device at 10 to 12 breaths/min to maintain $ETCO_2$ between 35 and 45 mm Hg, and maintain an oxygen saturation between 95% and 99%. Assess blood pressure, and determine if the patient can follow commands such as "Squeeze my fingers." Transport patient to the closest appropriate facility depending on local protocol.

Cardiac Monitoring

Some EMS systems will allow AEMTs to place electrodes, attach the leads, and obtain an ECG tracing prior to transport. If your service allows you to perform this skill, the following information will guide you.

For an ECG to be reliable and useful, the electrodes must be placed in consistent positions on each patient. **Figure 18-16** shows placement of limb lead electrodes, which are used to obtain a 3-lead ECG. **Figure 18-17** shows placement of limb lead electrodes and 12-lead ECG electrodes, both of which are used when obtaining a 12-lead ECG. To maintain consistency in monitoring and obtaining a useful ECG, there are predetermined locations for each electrode. Electrodes used in the prehospital setting are generally adhesive and have a gel center to aid in skin contact. Whichever type is used, certain basic principles should be followed to achieve the best skin contact and minimize **artifact** in the signal. Artifact refers to an ECG tracing that is the result of interference, such as patient movement, rather than the heart's electrical activity. Guiding principles are as follows:

- To maintain the correct lead placement, it may occasionally be necessary to shave body hair from the electrode site. A hairy chest may initially appear to have good skin contact, but the electrode will rise off the skin and stick to the hair. If you must shave the site, be very careful to avoid nicking the skin. If one is

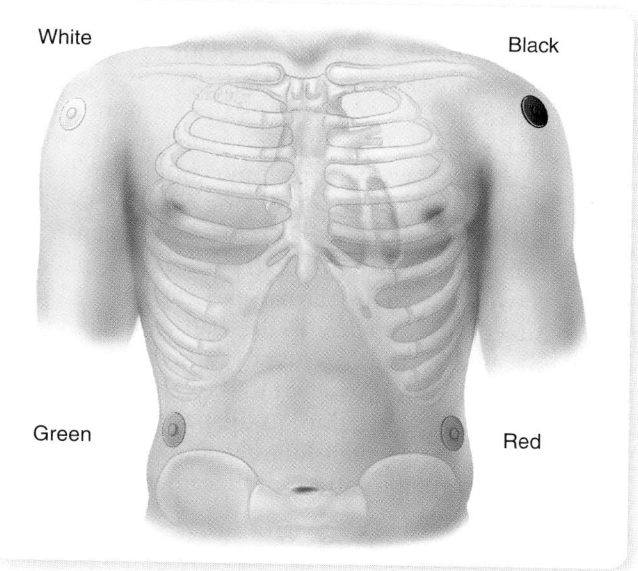

Figure 18-16 Limb electrode placement for acquisition of a 3-lead electrocardiogram and cardiac monitoring.

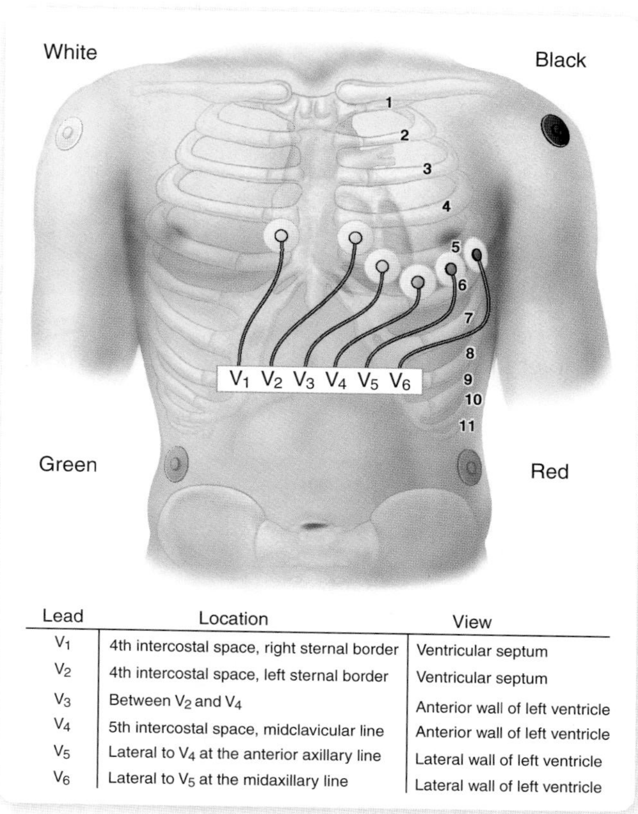

Lead	Location	View
V_1	4th intercostal space, right sternal border	Ventricular septum
V_2	4th intercostal space, left sternal border	Ventricular septum
V_3	Between V_2 and V_4	Anterior wall of left ventricle
V_4	5th intercostal space, midclavicular line	Anterior wall of left ventricle
V_5	Lateral to V_4 at the anterior axillary line	Lateral wall of left ventricle
V_6	Lateral to V_5 at the midaxillary line	Lateral wall of left ventricle

Figure 18-17 12-lead ECG electrode placement.

available, it is best to use an electric razor to remove hair, because single-blade manual razors irritate the skin and can easily cut a patient.
- To remove oils and dead tissues from the surface of the skin, rub the electrode site briskly with an alcohol swab before application. Wait for the alcohol to dry before applying electrodes or dry it with a quick wipe of a 4- × 4-inch gauze pad. This step may have to be repeated if the patient is sweaty, as many cardiac patients are.
- Attach the electrodes to the ECG cables before placement. Confirm that the appropriate electrode (now attached to the cable) is placed at the correct location on the patient's chest or limbs. (Each cable is marked and color coded as to the correct location for placement.)
- When all electrodes are in place, switch on the monitor and print a sample rhythm strip. If the strip shows any interference (artifact), verify that the electrodes are firmly applied to the skin and the monitor cable is plugged in correctly.

Artifact on the monitor can be tricky. Patient movement, including deep breathing or muscle tremor, may cause a wavy baseline or small up-and-down squiggles on the baseline. These will prevent the ECG from being usable. Make sure that the patient is supine if possible or in the semi-Fowler position if he or she is having difficulty breathing. Also make sure that the patient's arms are relaxed by his or her side and his or her feet are uncrossed.

Skill Drill 18-3 shows the steps for performing cardiac monitoring.

Skill Drill 18-3 Performing Cardiac Monitoring

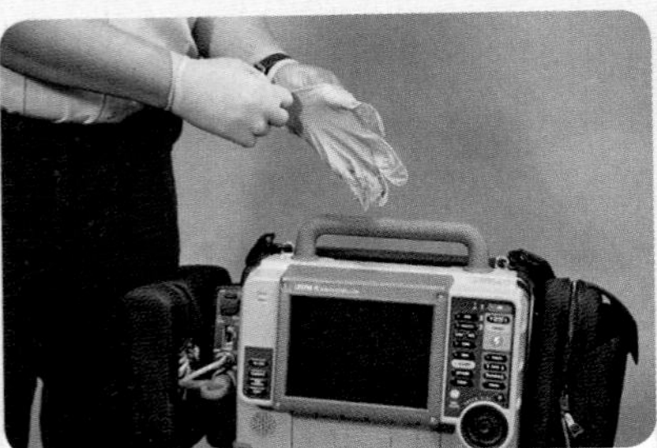

Step 1 Take standard precautions.

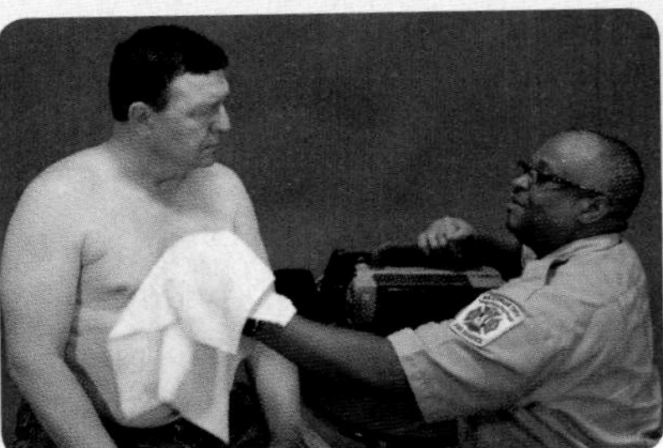

Step 2 Explain the procedure to the patient. Prepare the skin for electrode placement.

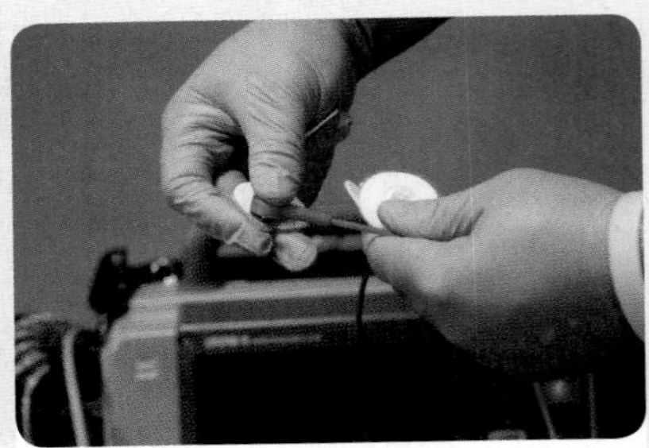

Step 3 Attach the electrodes to the leads before placing them on the patient.

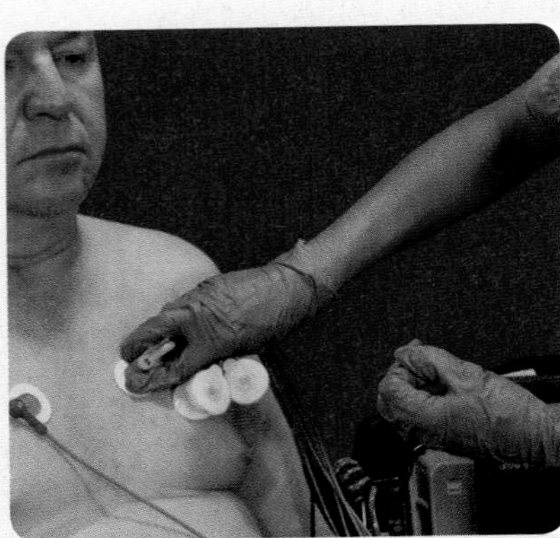

Step 4 Position the limb electrodes on the patient, on the torso if performing continuous monitoring, on the limbs if you will be acquiring a 12-lead ECG. The RA (right arm) electrode goes on the right arm distal to the shoulder or on the wrist (avoid placing it directly over a bone). The LA (left arm) electrode goes on the left arm at the same location as you placed the RA electrode on the right arm. The LL (left leg) electrode is placed on the left leg on the thigh or ankle, although if you do not plan to obtain a 12-lead ECG tracing, this electrode is often placed on the lower left side of the abdomen (slightly lower than an AED pad would be placed). Place the RL (right leg) electrode at the same location on the right side of the body as the LL electrode on the left.

Skill Drill 18-3 Performing Cardiac Monitoring (continued)

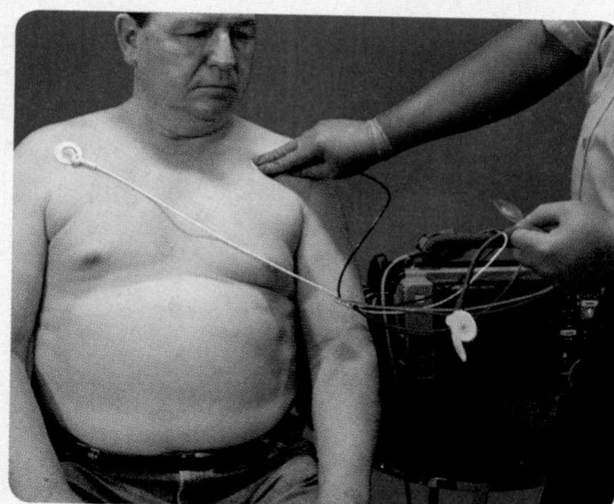

Step 5 If you plan to obtain a 12-lead ECG tracing, place the chest leads on the chest as shown.

- The V_1 electrode is placed on the right side of the sternum between the fourth and fifth ribs.
- The V_2 electrode is placed on the left side of the sternum directly across from V_1.
- The V_4 is placed next, between the fifth and sixth ribs in a straight line down from the middle of the clavicle.
- The V_3 is then placed halfway between V_2 and V_4.
- The V_6 is placed next and is located horizontally even with V_4 in a straight line down from the middle of the armpit.
- Finally, V_5 is placed halfway between V_4 and V_6.

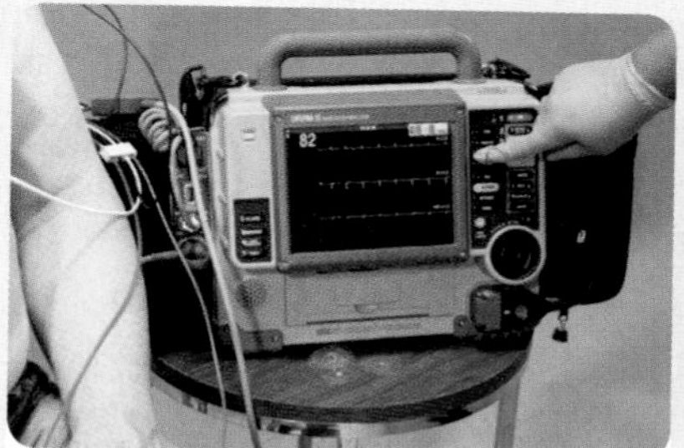

Step 6 Turn on the monitor.

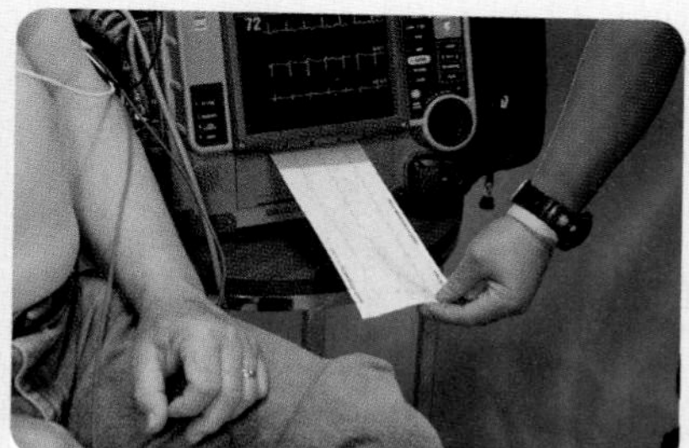

Step 7 Record tracings. As soon as a rhythm is visible on the screen, press the print button on the monitor and print a strip while counting slowly to six or seven. Then press the print button again to stop the printout. If the time is not printed correctly on the strip, write it on the edge of the strip. If you are obtaining a 12-lead ECG tracing, ask the patient to hold his or her breath or to take very shallow breaths. Press the 12-lead button and wait for the machine to acquire, analyze, and print or transmit the 12-lead ECG tracing. Gently tear off the tracing when the printer automatically stops.

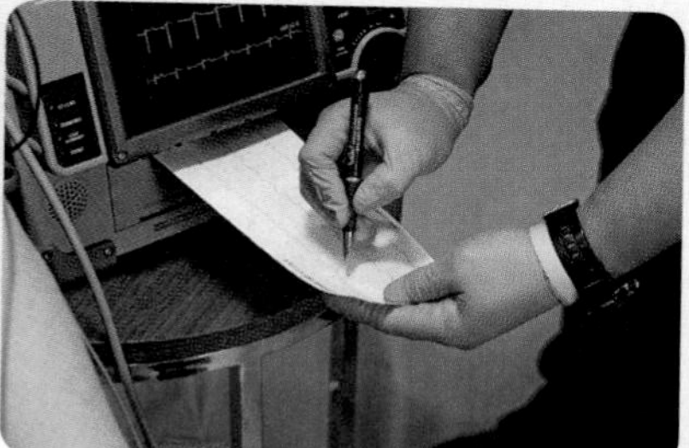

Step 8 Label each strip.

YOU are the Provider SUMMARY

1. How does the heart become oxygenated?

The heart, like any other muscle, requires oxygen and nutrients. These substances are supplied via the coronary arteries, which arise from the aorta shortly after it leaves the left ventricle. The coronary circulation emanates from the left and right coronary arteries.

The right coronary artery generally divides into nine branches. These branches supply blood to the walls of the right atrium and ventricle, a portion of the inferior part of the left ventricle, and portions of the conduction system.

The left main coronary artery is the widest and shortest of the myocardial blood vessels. It rapidly divides into two branches: the left anterior descending artery and the circumflex coronary artery. These arteries subdivide further, supplying blood to most of the left ventricle, the interventricular septum, and, at times, the AV node.

2. What is the most common cause of chest pain?

Chest pain or discomfort that is related to the heart usually stems from a condition called ischemia, which is decreased blood flow, in this case, to the heart. Because of a partial or complete blockage of blood flow through the coronary arteries, heart tissue fails to get enough oxygen and nutrients. The tissue soon begins to starve and, if blood flow is not restored, eventually dies.

3. In which medication class is aspirin, and what are the indications and contraindications for administration?

Aspirin, acetylsalicylic acid, is classified as a platelet inhibitor and a nonsteroidal anti-inflammatory agent. Indications for administration of aspirin include new-onset chest pain, suggesting AMI. Contraindications for administration include hypersensitivity to aspirin; also, aspirin is relatively contraindicated in patients with active ulcer disease or asthma. Adverse reactions you may encounter include heartburn, gastrointestinal bleeding, nausea, and vomiting.

4. What is the mechanism of action of nitroglycerin, and what are the indications and contraindications?

NTG is a vasodilator. It relaxes smooth muscles in the body, including those in the vasculature. This causes dilation of the arterioles and veins in the periphery, which reduces preload and afterload. In doing this, NTG reduces the workload of the heart which also reduces myocardial oxygen demand. NTG is indicated in patients with acute angina pectoris, ischemic chest pain, hypertension, heart failure, and pulmonary edema. NTG should not be given to patients experiencing hypotension, hypovolemia, intracranial bleeding, or head injuries. NTG should also not be given to patients who have taken Viagra, Revatio, Levitra, Cialis, or similar agents within the past 24 to 36 hours.

5. What are the various routes available to administer nitroglycerin?

NTG comes in several forms and may be administered several ways. Forms include a small white pill given sublingually, a spray administered sublingually, or a topical paste applied to the skin. NTG can also be administered as a liquid continuous infusion by paramedics or in the hospital. Regardless of the form or route that it is administered, the effects are the same.

6. Does this patient require IV access?

It might be beneficial to establish IV access (a saline lock) in this patient. However, establishing IV access should not take precedence over transport. Whereas this patient is not currently hypovolemic, she may require the administration of IV fluid en route to the hospital, should hypovolemia develop as a result of the administration of NTG or deterioration of the cardiovascular system (the pump). Patients who are experiencing a possible AMI are also potential candidates for cardiac arrest. It is much easier to obtain IV access while the patient actually has a pulse.

7. Should paramedic backup be requested for this patient?

Again, if you suspect that this patient is experiencing an AMI, paramedic backup should be requested. This patient has the potential to go into cardiac arrest from potential dysrhythmias, as well as potentially benefiting from narcotic administration if the chest pain persists. Having paramedics treat this patient may increase her chance of survival. Do not delay transport while waiting; instead, have the paramedic unit rendezvous at a point on the way to the hospital.

8. What is the most common error with AED operation?

The most common error with AED operation is failure to have a charged and operable battery. To avoid this problem, many defibrillator companies have built smarter machines that will warn the operator that the battery is unlikely to work. However, some of the older models do not have this feature. You should check the AED daily, and exercise the battery as often as the manufacturer recommends.

YOU are the Provider SUMMARY *(continued)*

9. What are the five links in the chain of survival?

The five links in the chain of survival are immediate recognition of warning signs and activation of EMS, immediate CPR with emphasis on high-quality chest compressions, rapid defibrillation, effective basic and advanced EMS care, and ALS postarrest care.

If any one of the links in the chain is absent or delayed, the patient's chances for survival diminish. For example, few patients benefit from defibrillation when more than 10 minutes elapse before administration of the first shock or if CPR is not performed in the first 2 to 3 minutes. If all links in the chain are strong, the patient has the best possible chance of survival.

EMS Patient Care Report (PCR)

Date: 11-27-18	**Incident No.:** 6284	**Nature of Call:** Chest pain	**Location:** 1894 Port Sulphur Avenue

Dispatched: 1532	**En Route:** 1534	**At Scene:** 1538	**Transport:** 1548	**At Hospital:** 1600	**In Service:** 1649

Patient Information

Age: 56 **Sex:** F **Weight (in kg [lb]):** 111 kg (245 lb)	**Allergies:** None **Medications:** None **Past Medical History:** MI x 4, last 2016 **Chief Complaint:** Chest pain

Vital Signs

Time: 1539	**BP:** 146/88	**Pulse:** 74	**Respirations:** 24	**Spo_2:** 92% on room air
Time: 1549	**BP:** 122/84	**Pulse:** 68	**Respirations:** 20	**Spo_2:** 96% on 15 L/min
Time: 1558	**BP:** None	**Pulse:** 0	**Respirations:** 0	**Spo_2:** Not obtained

EMS Treatment (circle all that apply)

Oxygen @ 15 **L/min via (circle one):** **NC** **NRM** **Bag-mask device** (circled)		**Assisted Ventilation:** Yes (circled)	**Airway Adjunct:** OPA (circled)	**CPR:** Yes (circled)
Defibrillation: Yes x 1 (circled)	**Bleeding Control**	**Bandaging**	**Splinting**	**Other:** Medication administration (circled)

Narrative

EMS dispatched to above location for a 56 y/o female complaining of chest pain. On arrival, patient found in fetal position on sofa, rocking back and forth, moaning in pain. Patient presents AO×4, ABCs intact, states she has an extensive cardiac history, with last MI in 2016. Placed patient on 15 L/min, primary survey reveals no signs of trauma. States pain woke her up from a nap, described as an "elephant sitting on her chest," which radiates to left arm. Pain 9/10. Vitals obtained as above. In accordance with protocols, patient administered 324 mg aspirin orally, and 0.4 mg of NTG via sublingual route, which brought pain to 2/10. Placed patient on stretcher and secured, loaded into ambulance. Vital signs reassessed, 22-gauge saline lock established to right wrist. Contacted Central Medical dispatch for paramedic intercept, advised no units available. Transport emergent to First Care ED due to Unity not having cardiac services available. At 1555, patient reports increasing chest pain, per protocols, 0.4 mg NTG given via SL route. Approximately 90 seconds after administration, patient becomes pulseless and apneic. Ambulance stopped, AED applied, and patient analyzed. Patient defibrillated once per AED. One-person CPR initiated and diverted to Unity Hospital. On arrival, care and report given to ED staff without further incident.**End of report**

Prep Kit

▶ Ready for Review

- Cardiovascular diseases are the number one cause of death in men and women. Although older people are at a higher risk, such a sweeping generalization overlooks a large number of younger people. For these reasons, early recognition and early treatment are the keys to survival.
- The heart is divided down the middle into two sides, right and left, each with an upper chamber called the atrium and a lower chamber called the ventricle.
- The largest of the four heart valves that keep blood moving through the circulatory system in the proper direction is the aortic valve, which lies between the left ventricle and the aorta, the body's main artery.
- The heart's electrical conduction system controls heart rate and helps to keep the atria and ventricles working together. The mechanical pumping action of the heart can occur only in response to an electrical stimulus.
- Cardiac muscle cells have a special characteristic called automaticity. Automaticity allows a cardiac muscle cell to contract spontaneously without a stimulus from a nerve source. Impulses from the sinoatrial node cause the other myocardial cells to contract.
- Regulation of heart function is provided by the brain via the autonomic nervous system, the hormones of the endocrine system, and the heart tissue. Baroreceptors and chemoreceptors sense abnormalities in pressure and chemical composition.
- The two phases of the cardiac cycle are systole, the pumping phase, and diastole, the resting phase.
- During periods of exertion or stress, the myocardium requires more oxygen. This is supplied by dilation of the coronary arteries, which increases blood flow.
- Chest pain or discomfort that is related to the heart usually stems from ischemia (decreased blood flow) to the heart. The tissue soon begins to starve and, if blood flow is not restored, eventually dies.
- Diminished blood flow to the myocardium is usually caused by atherosclerosis, a disorder in which cholesterol and other fatty substances build up and form plaque inside the walls of blood vessels.
- Occasionally, brittle plaque will crack, causing a blood clot to form. A blood clot may break loose and begin floating in the blood, becoming what is known as a thromboembolism. A thromboembolism is a blood clot that is floating through blood vessels until it reaches an area too narrow for it to pass, causing it to stop and block the blood flow at that point.
- Heart tissue downstream suffers from a lack of oxygen and, within 30 minutes, will begin to die. This is called an acute myocardial infarction (AMI), or heart attack.
- Chest pain may be caused by a brief period when heart tissues do not get enough oxygen. The discomfort associated with this is called angina. Angina pain is similar to the pain of an AMI, but responds to nitroglycerin (NTG) administration. However, angina can be a sign that an AMI will occur in the future.
- Myocardial tissues that are ischemic but are not yet dying can cause pain called angina. The pain of AMI is different from that of angina in that it can come at any time, not just with exertion; it lasts up to several hours, rather than just a few moments; and it is not relieved by rest or NTG.
- In addition to chest pain or pressure, signs of AMI include sudden onset of weakness, nausea, and sweating; sudden dysrhythmia; pulmonary edema; and even sudden death.
- Heart attacks can have three serious consequences. One is sudden death, usually the result of cardiac arrest caused by abnormal heart rhythms called dysrhythmias. These include tachycardia, bradycardia, ventricular tachycardia (VT), and, most commonly, ventricular fibrillation (VF).
- The second consequence is cardiogenic shock. Symptoms include restlessness; anxiety; pale, clammy skin; pulse rate higher than normal; and blood pressure lower than normal. Patients with these symptoms should receive oxygen, assisted ventilation as needed, and immediate transport.
- The third consequence of AMI is heart failure, in which the damaged myocardium can no longer contract effectively enough to pump blood through the system. The lungs become congested with fluid, breathing becomes difficult, the heart rate increases, and the left ventricle enlarges.
- Signs of heart failure include swollen ankles from pedal edema, high blood pressure, rapid heart rate and respirations, rales, and sometimes the pink sputum and dyspnea of pulmonary edema.
- Treat a patient with heart failure as you would a patient with chest pain. Monitor the patient's vital signs. Give the patient oxygen via a nonrebreathing mask. Allow the patient to remain sitting up.
- In treating patients with chest pain, obtain a SAMPLE history, following the OPQRST-I mnemonic to assess the pain; measure and record vital signs; ensure that the patient is in a comfortable position, usually semireclining or half sitting up; administer

Prep Kit *(continued)*

prescribed NTG and oxygen; and transport the patient, reporting to medical control as you do.

- Follow local protocols to treat a patient in cardiac arrest. Ensure a patent airway, and obtain an advanced airway as soon as possible. Establish intravenous access.
- Termination of efforts should be based on local protocol and direct communication with online medical control.
- The automated external defibrillator (AED) requires the operator to apply the pads, power on the unit, follow the AED prompts, and press the *Shock* button if indicated. The computer inside the AED recognizes rhythms that require shock.
- The most common errors in using certain AEDs are operator failure (such as failure to keep a charged battery), failure to use the AED correctly, and applying the AED to a patient with a pulse.
- Do not touch the patient while the AED is analyzing the heart rhythm or delivering shocks.
- Approach to pediatric patients with a cardiac emergency should be the same as that for an adult. If the patient is 8 years old or younger, pediatric-sized pads and a dose-attenuating system (energy reducer) are preferred. If these are not available, an adult AED can be used. For a child between age 1 month and 1 year (an infant), a manual defibrillator is preferred to an AED.
- Effective cardiopulmonary resuscitation (CPR) and rapid defibrillation with an AED are critical interventions to the survival of a patient in cardiac arrest. If the patient is in cardiac arrest, start CPR, beginning with high-quality chest compressions, and apply the AED as soon as it is available.
- If paramedics are responding to the scene, stay where you are and continue CPR and defibrillation as needed. Do not wait for the paramedics to arrive to begin defibrillation. If paramedics are not responding, begin transport if the patient regains a pulse, if you have delivered six to nine shocks, or if the AED gives three consecutive messages (separated by 2 minutes of CPR) that no shock is advised. Follow your local protocols regarding when it is appropriate to transport the patient.
- If an unresponsive patient has a pulse but loses it during transport, you must stop the vehicle, reanalyze the rhythm, and defibrillate again or begin CPR, as appropriate.
- The chain of survival, which is the sequence of events that must happen for a patient in cardiac arrest to have the best chance of survival, includes recognition of early warning signs and immediate activation of EMS, immediate CPR with emphasis on high-quality chest compressions, rapid defibrillation, basic and advanced EMS care, and ALS and postarrest care. Seconds count at every stage.
- Your role as the advanced emergency medical technician may include obtaining an electrocardiogram. For example, you may place electrodes, attach leads, and obtain the tracing. Whether for 3-lead or 12-lead monitoring, it is important for electrode placement to be consistent.

▶ Vital Vocabulary

acute coronary syndrome (ACS) A term used to describe a group of symptoms caused by myocardial ischemia; includes angina and myocardial infarction.

acute myocardial infarction (AMI) Heart attack; death of heart muscle following obstruction of blood flow to it. Acute in this context means new or happening right now.

afterload The resistance the heart must pump against, or the systemic vascular resistance.

angina pectoris Transient (short-lived) chest discomfort caused by partial or temporary blockage of blood flow to the heart muscle.

aorta The main artery that receives blood from the left ventricle and delivers it to all the other arteries that carry blood to the tissues of the body.

aortic aneurysm A weakness in the wall of the aorta that makes it susceptible to rupture.

aortic valve The one-way valve that lies between the left ventricle and the aorta; keeps blood from flowing back into the left ventricle after the left ventricle ejects its blood into the aorta and is one of four heart valves.

arteries Vessels of the circulatory system that carry oxygenated blood away from the heart.

arterioles The smallest branches of arteries leading to the vast network of capillaries.

arteriosclerosis The thickening of the arterial walls that results in a loss of elasticity and concomitant reduction in blood flow.

artifact A tracing on an electrocardiogram that is the result of interference, such as patient movement, rather than the heart's electrical activity.

asystole Complete absence of heart electrical activity.

Prep Kit (continued)

atherosclerosis A disorder in which cholesterol and possibly calcium build up inside the walls of blood vessels, eventually leading to partial or complete blockage of blood flow.

atrioventricular (AV) node The site located in the right atrium adjacent to the septum that is responsible for transiently slowing electrical conduction.

atrioventricular valves The two valves through which blood flows from the atria to the ventricles.

atrium One of two (right and left) upper chambers of the heart.

automaticity The ability of cardiac cells to generate an impulse to contract even when there is no external nervous stimulus.

autonomic nervous system The part of the nervous system that regulates involuntary functions, such as heart rate, blood pressure, digestion, and sweating.

baroreceptors Receptors in the blood vessels, kidneys, brain, and heart that respond to changes in pressure in the heart or main arteries to help maintain homeostasis.

bradycardia Slow heart rate, less than 60 beats/min.

capillaries Microscopic, thin-walled blood vessels through which oxygen and nutrients and carbon dioxide and waste products are exchanged.

cardiac arrest A state in which the heart fails to generate an effective and detectable blood flow; pulses are not palpable in cardiac arrest, even if muscular and electrical activity continues in the heart.

cardiac cycle The repetitive pumping process that begins with the onset of cardiac muscle contraction and ends just before the beginning of the next contraction.

cardiac output The amount of blood pumped through the circulatory system in 1 minute.

cardiogenic shock A state in which not enough oxygen is delivered to the tissues of the body, caused by low output of blood from the heart; can be a severe complication of a large acute myocardial infarction, as well as other conditions.

chemoreceptors Receptors in the blood vessels, kidneys, brain, and heart that respond to changes in chemical composition of the blood to help maintain homeostasis.

chordae tendineae Small muscular strands that attach the ventricles and the valves, preventing regurgitation of blood through the valves from the ventricles to the atria.

chronotropic state Related to the control of the heart's rate of contraction.

circumflex coronary artery One of the two branches of the left main coronary artery.

conduction system A group of complex electrical tissues within the heart that initiate and transmit stimuli that result in contractions of myocardial tissue.

conductivity The ability of the cardiac cells to conduct electrical impulses.

contractility The strength of heart muscle contraction.

coronary arteries Blood vessels that carry blood and nutrients to the heart muscle.

coronary artery disease The condition that results when atherosclerosis or arteriosclerosis is present in the arterial walls.

coronary sinus The end of the great cardiac vein that collects blood returning from the walls of the heart.

defibrillate To shock a fibrillating (chaotically beating) heart with specialized electrical current in an attempt to restore a normal rhythmic beat.

dependent edema Swelling in the part of the body closest to the ground, caused by collection of fluid in the tissues; a possible sign of congestive heart failure.

diastole The relaxation phase of the heart, when the ventricles are filling with blood.

dissecting aneurysm A condition in which the inner layers of an artery, such as the aorta, become separated, allowing blood (at high pressures) to flow between the layers.

dromotropic state Related to the control of the heart's electrical conduction.

dysrhythmia An irregular or abnormal heart rhythm.

ejection fraction The portion of the blood ejected from the ventricle during systole.

endocardium The thin membrane lining the inside of the heart.

epicardium The layer of the serous pericardium that lies closely against the heart; also called the visceral pericardium.

excitability A property of cardiac cells that provides the cells with the ability to respond to electrical impulses.

heart A muscular, cone-shaped organ whose function is to pump blood throughout the body.

heart failure A disorder in which the heart loses part of its ability to effectively pump blood, usually as a result of damage to the heart muscle and usually resulting in a backup of fluid into the lungs.

hemoglobin An iron-containing protein within red blood cells that has the ability to combine with oxygen.

Prep Kit *(continued)*

hypertensive emergency An emergency situation created by excessively high blood pressure, which can lead to serious complications such as stroke or aneurysm.

inferior vena cava The principal vein draining blood from the lower portion of the body.

inotropic state Related to the strength of the heart's contraction.

ischemia A lack of oxygen that deprives tissues of necessary nutrients, resulting from partial or complete blockage of blood flow; potentially reversible because permanent injury has not yet occurred.

left anterior descending (LAD) artery One of the two branches of the left main coronary artery, which is the largest and shortest of the myocardial blood vessels; this and the circumflex coronary arteries supply blood to the left ventricle and other areas.

lumen The inside diameter of an artery or other hollow structure.

mitral valve The valve in the heart that separates the left atrium from the left ventricle.

myocardium Heart muscle.

occlusion Blockage, usually of a tubular structure such as a blood vessel.

orthopnea Severe dyspnea experienced when lying down that is relieved by a change in position, such as sitting up or standing.

papillary muscles Specialized muscles that attach the ventricles to the cusps of the valves by muscular strands called chordae tendineae cordis.

pedal edema Swelling of the feet and ankles caused by collection of fluid in the tissues; a possible sign of congestive heart failure.

perfusion The flow of blood through body tissues and vessels.

pericardial fluid A serous fluid that fills the space between the visceral pericardium and the parietal pericardium and helps to reduce friction.

pericardial sac A thick, fibrous membrane that surrounds the heart. Also called the pericardium.

pericardium A thick, fibrous membrane that surrounds the heart. Also called the pericardial sac.

plasma A sticky, yellow fluid that carries the blood cells and nutrients and transports cellular waste material to the organs of excretion.

platelets Tiny, disk-shaped elements that are much smaller than the blood cells; they are essential in the initial formation of a blood clot, the mechanism that stops bleeding.

preload The amount of blood returned to the heart to be pumped out; directly affects afterload.

pulmonary circulation The circulatory system in the body that carries blood from the right side of the heart to the lungs and back to the left side of the heart.

pulmonic valve The semilunar valve that regulates blood flow between the right ventricle and the pulmonary artery.

red blood cells (RBCs) Cells that carry oxygen to the body's tissues; also called erythrocytes.

semilunar valves The two valves, the aortic and pulmonic valves, that divide the heart from the aorta and pulmonary arteries.

sinoatrial (SA) node The normal site of the origin of electrical impulses; located high in the right atrium, it is the heart's natural pacemaker.

Starling law A principle that states that if a muscle is stretched slightly before stimulation to contract, the muscle will contract harder; describes how increased venous return to the heart stretches the ventricles and allows for increased cardiac contractility.

stroke volume The amount of blood that the left ventricle ejects into the aorta in each contraction.

superior vena cava The principal vein draining blood from the upper portion of the body.

systemic circulation The circulatory system in the body that is responsible for blood flow in all areas of the body, except for areas covered by the pulmonary circulation (blood flow from the right side of the heart to the lungs and back to the left side of the heart).

systole Contraction of the ventricular mass with its concomitant pumping of blood into the systemic circulation.

tachycardia Rapid heart rhythm, more than 100 beats/min.

thromboembolism A blood clot that has formed within a blood vessel and is floating within the bloodstream.

tricuspid valve The heart valve that separates the right atrium from the right ventricle.

veins The blood vessels that transport unoxygenated blood back to the heart.

ventricle One of two (right and left) lower chambers of the heart. The left ventricle receives blood from the left atrium (upper chamber) and delivers blood to the aorta. The right ventricle receives blood from the right atrium and pumps it into the pulmonary artery.

Prep Kit *(continued)*

ventricular fibrillation (VF) Disorganized, ineffective twitching of the ventricles, resulting in no blood flow and a state of cardiac arrest.

ventricular tachycardia (VT) Rapid heart rhythm in which the electrical impulse begins in the ventricle (instead of the atrium), which may result in inadequate blood flow and eventually deteriorate into cardiac arrest.

venules Very small, thin-walled vessels.

white blood cells (WBCs) Blood cells that have a role in the body's immune defense mechanisms against infection; also called leukocytes.

▶ References

1. Mozaffarian D, Benjamin EJ, Go AS, et al. Heart disease and stroke statistics—2016 update: a report from the American Heart Association. *Circulation*. 2016;133(4):e38-e360.
2. Leading Causes of Death, 1900-1998. Centers for Disease Control and Prevention/National Center for Health Statistics website. https://www.cdc.gov/nchs/data/dvs/lead1900_98.pdf. Accessed December 26, 2017.
3. 10 leading causes of death by age group, United States – 2015. National Vital Statistics System, National Center for Health Statistics, Centers for Disease Control and Prevention. https://www.cdc.gov/injury/wisqars/LeadingCauses.html. Accessed September 22, 2017.
4. Prinzmetal's or Prinzmetal Angina, Variant Angina, and Angina Inversa. American Heart Association website. http://www.heart.org/HEARTORG/Conditions/HeartAttack/DiagnosingaHeartAttack/Prinzmetals-or-Prinzmetal-Angina-Variant-Angina-and-Angina-Inversa_UCM_435674_Article.jsp#.WhGcPkqnGUk. Updated August 21, 2017. Accessed December 15, 2017.
5. Women and Heart Disease Fact Sheet. Centers for Disease Control and Prevention website. https://www.cdc.gov/dhdsp/data_statistics/fact_sheets/fs_women_heart.htm. Updated August 23, 2017. Accessed December 26, 2017.
6. Sheps SG. Hypertensive crisis: What are the symptoms? Mayo Clinic website. https://www.mayoclinic.org/diseases-conditions/high-blood-pressure/expert-answers/hypertensive-crisis/faq-20058491. July 21, 2017. Accessed December 26, 2017.
7. Yu T, Weil MH, Tang W, et al. Adverse outcomes of interrupted precordial compression during automated defibrillation. *Circulation*. 2002;106:368-372.

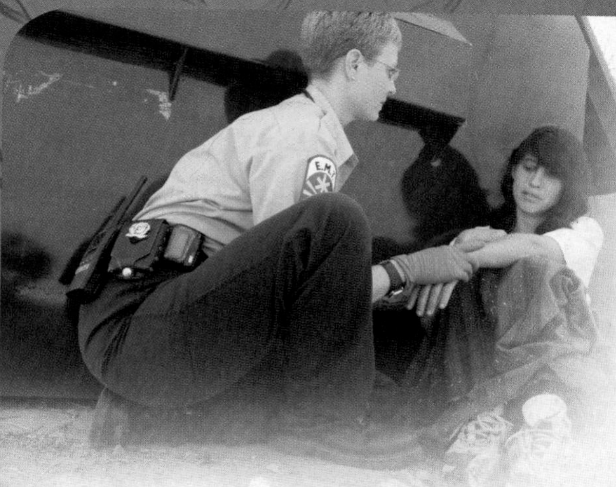

Assessment *in Action*

Your ambulance is dispatched to a local residence for a man reporting chest pain and shortness of breath. On your arrival, you find an elderly, obese man seated in the tripod position at the kitchen table. He states he has had these symptoms for a few days, and they are getting progressively worse.

1. As you look at the patient, you note substantial swelling in his feet. This swelling is called:

A. dependent edema.
B. angioedema.
C. sacral edema.
D. pulmonary edema.

2. Patients with heart failure have difficulty breathing in the supine position that resolves with sitting partially upright. This is known as:

A. dyspnea.
B. orthopnea.
C. hypoxia.
D. apnea.

3. Your assessment of the patient reveals frothy pulmonary edema, as well as rales bilaterally. If available, you should consider the use of:

A. an oropharyngeal airway.
B. a nasopharyngeal airway.
C. continuous positive airway pressure (CPAP).
D. a supraglottic airway.

4. As you review the patient's medications, you note that he takes furosemide. You know that furosemide is what type of medication?

A. Antacid
B. Diuretic
C. Antihypertensive
D. Bronchodilator

5. Peripheral edema is a sign of:

A. right-side heart failure.
B. left-side heart failure
C. renal failure.
D. hepatic failure.

6. A special characteristic of cardiac muscle cells, not found in any other type of muscle cells, is called:

A. excitability.
B. conductivity.
C. automaticity.
D. contractility.

7. You decide to give nitroglycerin for the chest pain. Nitroglycerin is contraindicated if the systolic blood pressure is less than:

A. 90 mm Hg.
B. 100 mm Hg.
C. 110 mm Hg.
D. 120 mm Hg.

8. Nitroglycerin is administered through the _____ route.

A. oral
B. intranasal
C. intramuscular
D. sublingual

9. List five possible causes of an episode of Prinzmetal angina.

10. List the possible signs and symptoms of a hypertensive emergency.

CHAPTER 19

Neurologic Emergencies

National EMS Education Standard Competencies

Medicine

Applies fundamental knowledge to provide basic and selected advanced emergency care and transportation based on assessment findings for an acutely ill patient.

Neurology

Anatomy, presentations, and management of

- Decreased level of responsiveness (pp 860-861, 869-870)

Anatomy, physiology, pathophysiology, assessment, and management of

- Seizure (pp 856-859, 861-869, 871, 873)
- Stroke/transient ischemic attack (pp 852-856, 861-869, 870-872)
- Status epilepticus (pp 858, 861-869, 871, 873)
- Headache (pp 861-869, 873)

Knowledge Objectives

1. Review the anatomy and physiology of the brain and spinal cord. (pp 848-851)
2. List the various ways blood flow to the brain may be interrupted and cause a stroke. (pp 852-853)
3. Discuss the causes of ischemic strokes, hemorrhagic strokes, and transient ischemic attacks (TIAs) and their similarities and differences. (pp 852-855)
4. Discuss the different types of headaches, the possible causes of each, and how to distinguish a harmless headache from a potentially lifethreatening condition. (pp 853, 855, 857, 861)
5. Describe the dangers associated with increased intracranial pressure (ICP) and the processes that occur in the brain with increased ICP. (p 854)
6. List the general signs and symptoms of stroke, and identify those symptoms that manifest if the left hemisphere of the brain is affected, if the right hemisphere of the brain is affected, and if there is bleeding in the brain. (p 855)
7. Discuss three conditions with symptoms that mimic stroke and the assessment techniques the advanced emergency medical technician (AEMT) may use to identify them. (pp 855-856)
8. Define a generalized seizure, partial seizure, and status epilepticus, including their effects on a patient and how they differ from each other. (pp 856-858)
9. Describe the different phases of a seizure. (pp 856-857)
10. List the different types of seizures and their possible causes. (pp 856-858)
11. Explain why it is important for the AEMT to recognize when a seizure is occurring or whether one has already occurred in a patient and to identify other problems that may be associated with the seizure. (p 859)
12. Describe the postictal state and the specific patient care interventions that may be necessary to assist the patient. (p 859)
13. Define altered mental status, its various possible causes, and the patient assessment considerations that apply to each. (pp 859-861)
14. Discuss scene safety considerations when responding to a patient with a neurologic emergency. (p 861)
15. Describe the steps involved in performing a primary survey of a patient who is experiencing a neurologic emergency and the necessary interventions that may be required to address all life threats. (p 864)
16. Discuss the special considerations required for pediatric patients who exhibit altered mental status. (pp 864, 865, 873)
17. Discuss special considerations for geriatric patients who are experiencing a neurologic emergency. (p 865)
18. Describe the process of history taking for a patient who is experiencing a neurologic emergency, and explain how this process varies depending on the nature of the patient's illness. (pp 865-866)
19. Discuss how to use a stroke assessment tool to identify a stroke patient rapidly, giving examples of two commonly used tools. (pp 866-867)
20. List the key information an AEMT must obtain and document for a stroke patient during assessment and reassessment. (pp 866-869)

21. Explain why a patient who is suspected of experiencing a stroke is placed on stroke alert and requires treatment within the first 3 to 6 hours after the stroke begins. (pp 869-871)
22. Describe the patient management, treatment, and transport of patients who are experiencing headaches, stroke, seizure, or altered mental status. (pp 869-873)

Skills Objectives

1. Demonstrate how to use a stroke assessment tool such as the Cincinnati Prehospital Stroke Scale to test a patient for aphasia, facial weakness, and motor weakness. (p 866)

Introduction

The National Center for Health Statistics lists two of the top 10 causes of death in the United States in 2015 as neurologic in nature.[1] **Stroke**, a serious medical condition in which blood supply to areas of the brain is interrupted, is the fifth leading cause of death in the United States, after heart disease and cancer.[1] In the United States, someone experiences a stroke every 45 seconds.[1] The sixth leading cause of death is Alzheimer disease.[1] As you consider these statistics, it is important to place them in context. Clearly, advanced emergency medical technicians (AEMTs) will encounter many neurologic emergencies.

Over the past 20 years, there has been a revolution in the treatment of stroke.[2] Treatments are based on the type of stroke—ischemic or hemorrhagic—and range from more traditional medications for breaking up clots to new, innovative surgical procedures such as mechanical clot removal in cerebral ischemia (MERCI) and arteriovenous malformation repair.[3] Emergency physicians, neurologists, and neurosurgeons can help some patients with acute stroke avoid the most devastating consequences of this disease, providing that signs and symptoms are recognized early on and that they receive prompt care.

Seizures and altered mental status also occur when there is a disorder in the brain. Seizures may occur as a result of a recent or an old head injury, a brain tumor, a metabolic problem, a genetic predisposition, scar tissue from a stroke, or an unknown cause. Your ability to recognize when a seizure has occurred or is occurring is critical for the patient because this information helps direct the most appropriate treatment.

Altered mental status is a common presentation in patients with a wide variety of medical problems. You should not make assumptions about the cause of altered mental status, which can range from alcohol intoxication to head injury to diabetic emergency to stroke. Treatment varies widely, depending on the underlying cause. The care for patients with altered mental status presents a particular challenge because the patients may be difficult to handle and frustrating to treat at times. Your professionalism is paramount in these situations.

Neurologic patients can be extremely vulnerable or even helpless. Many of the reflexes that protect an awake person may not function when the nervous system is depressed. The eyelids do not blink away dust and irritants. The pharynx does not produce the gag reflex and the cough reflex is not stimulated in reaction to secretions draining down or foreign matter in the airway. The body does not seek a more comfortable position in response to compression of a limb in an awkward position. The tongue becomes flaccid. The airway is at risk.

In this chapter, you will learn how to approach and assess a patient with a brain disorder and the indications for prompt transport to an appropriate medical facility.

YOU are the Provider — PART 1

At 0354 hours, just as you are leaving the emergency department from your last call, dispatch advises you to respond to a local homeless shelter for a severely intoxicated person with slurred speech. You and your partner give each other a knowing look and respond to the scene. On your arrival, you encounter a 62-year-old man who is a patient you frequently see because of intoxication. He is sitting on the ground, leaning against the wall for support. As you begin your assessment, you notice slurred speech, which is common for him when he is intoxicated. However, you also notice some right-side facial droop and possible left-side weakness.

1. What mnemonic is useful for assessing adult patients with altered mental status?
2. What are the two types of abnormal posturing, and what do they indicate?

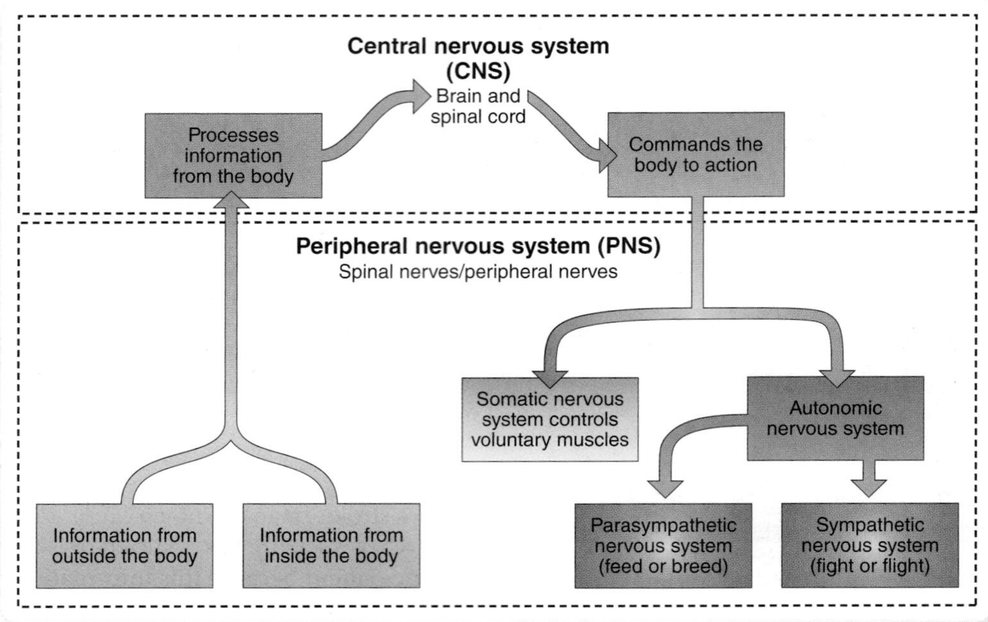

Figure 19-1 Basic organization of the nervous system.

Anatomy and Physiology Review

The nervous system is the most complex organ system within the human body. It consists of two major structures, the brain and spinal cord, plus thousands of nerves allowing communication among all parts of the body. This system is responsible for fundamental functions such as controlling breathing, heart rate, blood pressure, and temperature and higherlevel activities such as memory, understanding, communication, and thought.

The basic organization of the nervous system is shown in **Figure 19-1**. Recall from Chapter 7, *The Human Body*, that the major structures of the nervous system are divided into two main categories: the central nervous system (CNS), which is responsible for thought, perception, feeling, and autonomic body functions; and the peripheral nervous system (PNS), which transmits commands from the brain to the body and receives feedback from the body.

The brain controls breathing, speech, and all other body functions. Different parts of the brain perform different functions. For example, some parts of the brain receive input from the senses, including sight, hearing, taste, smell, and touch; some control the muscles and movement, whereas others control the formation of speech.

The brain is divided into three major parts: the brainstem, the cerebellum, and the largest part, the cerebrum **Figure 19-2**. The brainstem controls the most basic functions of the body, such as breathing, blood pressure, swallowing, and pupil constriction. Located just behind the brainstem, the cerebellum controls muscle and body coordination. It is responsible for coordinating complex tasks that involve voluntary movement of muscles, such as walking, writing, and playing the piano.

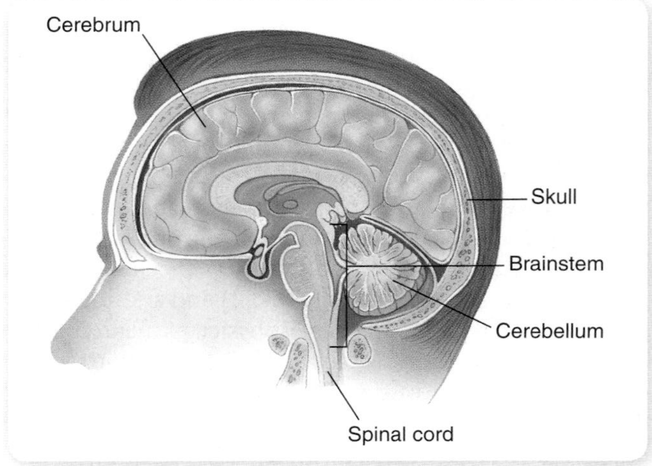

Figure 19-2 The brain is well protected within the skull. The brain's major parts are the cerebrum, the cerebellum, and the brainstem.

The cerebrum, located above the cerebellum, is divided down the middle into the right and left cerebral hemispheres. Each hemisphere controls activities on the opposite side of the body. The front part of the cerebrum controls emotion and thought, and the middle part controls touch and movement. The back part of the cerebrum processes sight. In most people, speech is controlled on the left side of the brain near the middle of the cerebrum.

Messages sent to and from the brain travel through nerves. Twelve cranial nerves run directly from the brain to various parts of the head, such as the eyes, ears, nose,

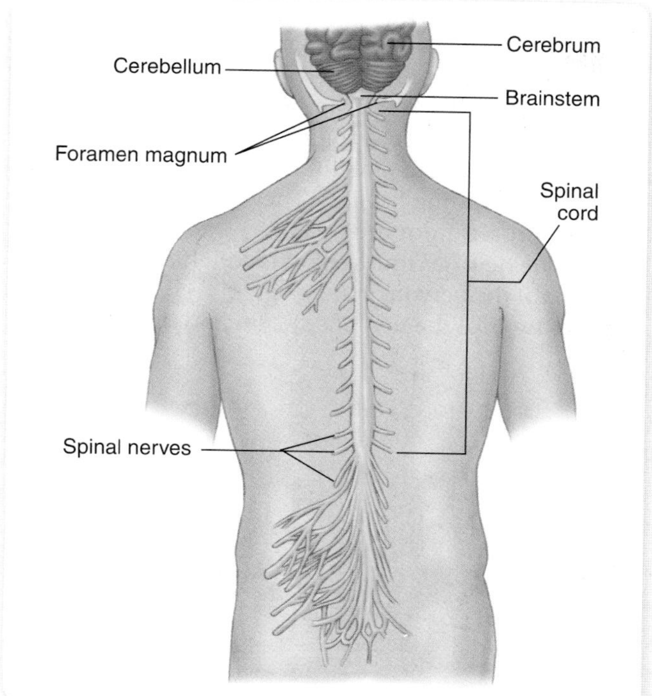

Figure 19-3 The spinal cord is the continuation of the brainstem. It exits the skull at the foramen magnum and extends down to the level of the second lumbar vertebra.

and face. All the rest of the nerves join in the spinal cord and exit the brain through a large opening in the base of the skull called the foramen magnum Figure 19-3. At each vertebra in the neck and back, two nerves, called spinal nerves, branch out from the spinal cord and carry signals to and from the body; the areas of skin sensation corresponding to specific spinal nerves are called dermatomes Figure 19-4.

▶ Neurons and Impulse Transmission

A neuron is a nerve cell and is the fundamental element of the nervous system. Neurons are composed of three basic parts: the cell body, the axon, and dendrites. The cell body contains the nucleus. The **axon** is a projection from the cell body that extends toward another cell carrying signals away from the neuron. The axon may or may not be wrapped in a sheath of **myelin**, an insulating substance that allows the cell to transmit its signal efficiently and consistently, without "shorting out" or losing electricity to surrounding fluids and tissues. Myelin also increases the speed of conduction. Most of the neurons within the body have a myelin sheath.

Synapses

Interaction between two neurons occurs at a junction known as a **synapse**. Nerve cells do not actually come in direct contact with each other. There is a slight gap between each cell. This allows for a far greater level of

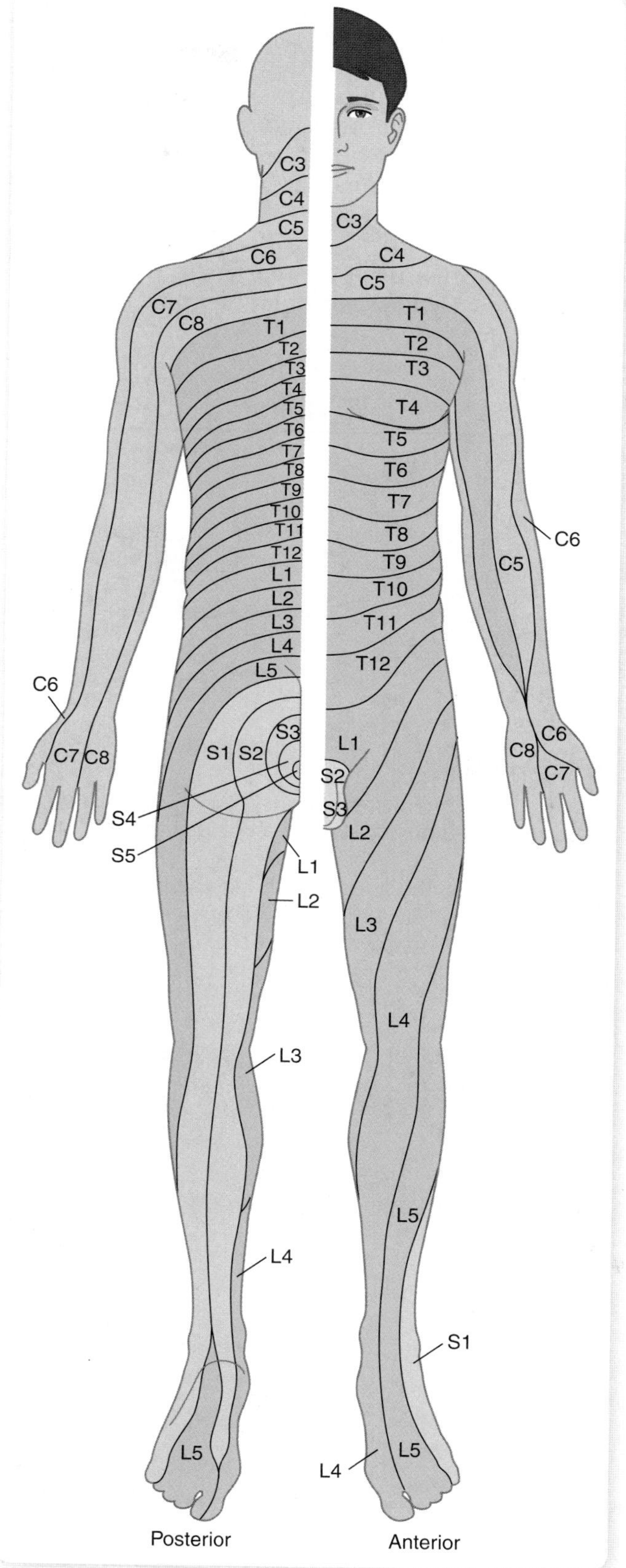

Figure 19-4 Dermatome map showing the association of the spinal nerves and the skin sensation throughout areas of the body.

fine control than if each cell were in direct contact with the next. The synapse, which is present wherever a nerve cell terminates, "connects" one nerve cell to the next cell. This communication occurs through the release of chemicals called neurotransmitters from the first cell. These chemicals cross the synapse and interact with the second cell triggering a message.

Neurotransmitters

Most neurons use **neurotransmitters** to transmit their signal across a synapse to other neurons. Dopamine, acetylcholine, epinephrine, and serotonin are examples of neurotransmitters. These chemicals take the electrically conducted signal from one nerve cell (a neuron) and relay it to the next cell (either another neuron or a target cell such as a muscle fiber) Figure 19-5.

It is important to remember that nerve cells respond in an all-or-nothing fashion. They either fire or they do not; a neuron cannot fire weakly.

This review has touched on highlights of the various portions of the nervous system. Table 19-1 summarizes the structures of the nervous system and their functions.

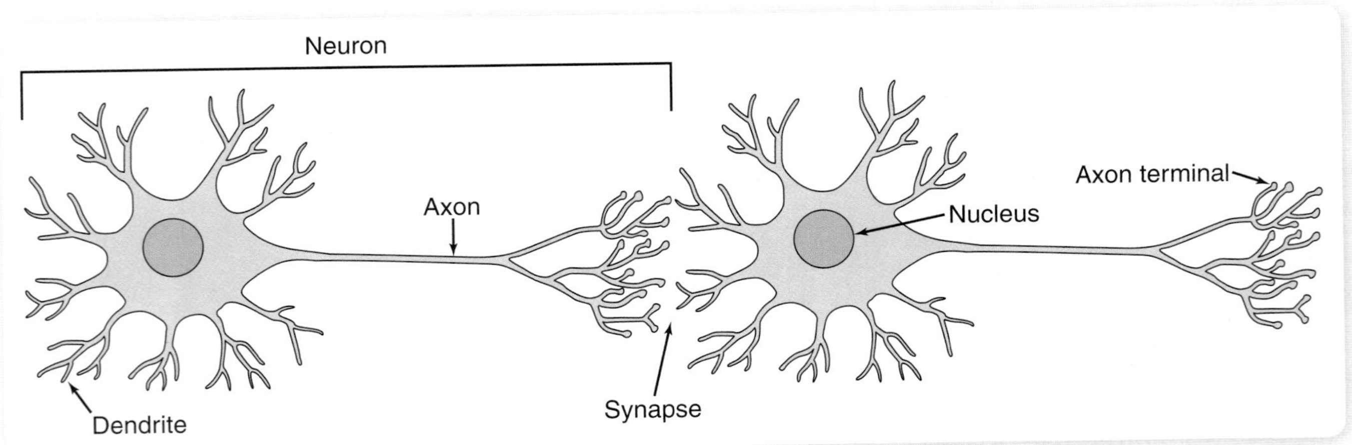

Figure 19-5 Neuron and synapse. The signal travels from the left to the right in this diagram: First, the neuron fires and sends a signal along its axon to the axon terminal. Next, the impulse reaches the axon terminal, where neurotransmitters are released and trickle across the synapse. Although neurons have only one axon, they have many dendrites. When the neuron's dendrites detect these chemicals, the sum total of excitation determines if a signal is sent to the next cell via its axon. Dendrites also release neurotransmitter deactivators, so that a single impulse from the first neuron generates a single response from the second.

Table 19-1 Structures and General Functions of the Nervous System

Major Structure	Subdivision	General Function
		Central Nervous System
Brain	Occipital	▪ Vision and storage of visual memories
	Parietal	▪ Sense of touch and texture and storage of tactile memories
	Temporal	▪ Hearing and smell ▪ Language ▪ Storage of sound and odor memories
	Frontal	▪ Motor cortex: Voluntary muscle control and storage of spatial memories ▪ Prefrontal cortex: Judgment and prediction of consequences of a person's actions; abstract intellectual functions
	Limbic system	▪ Basic emotions ▪ Basic reflexes (such as chewing and swallowing)
	Diencephalon (thalamus)	▪ Relay center that prioritizes signals to hone in on important messages

Brainstem	Diencephalon (hypothalamus)	▪ Emotions ▪ Temperature control ▪ Interface with the endocrine system
	Midbrain	▪ Level of consciousness ▪ Location of the reticular activating system, which controls arousal and consciousness ▪ Muscle tone and posture
	Pons	▪ Respiratory pattern and depth
	Medulla oblongata	▪ Pulse rate; blood pressure; respiratory rate
Spinal cord	Not applicable	▪ Reflexes ▪ Relays information to and from body
Peripheral Nervous System		
Cranial nerves	Not applicable	▪ Special peripheral nerves that connect directly from the brain to body parts to relay information from the brain
Peripheral nerves	Not applicable	▪ Brain to spinal cord to body part ▪ Receive stimulus from body; send commands to body
Central Nervous System and Peripheral Nervous System		
Neuron	Cell body	▪ Portion of the neuron where the nucleus resides; site of protein synthesis
	Axon	▪ Projection from the cell body that reaches out to connect with other neurons or target organs; signals are sent away from the cell body ▪ Some axons are covered with insulation called myelin; myelin increases speed of nerve conduction
	Dendrite	▪ Projections from cell body that receives signals from axons of other neurons; most neurons have multiple dendrites
	Synapse	▪ The gap between an axon and a dendrite
	Neurotransmitter	▪ A chemical released into a synapse that helps make the connection between one neuron and another (eg, serotonin, dopamine, and epinephrine)

Data from: Bailey R. Neurons. About.com website. http://biology.about.com/od/humananatomybiology/ss/neurons.htm. Updated December 15, 2016. Accessed January 8, 2017.

Pathophysiology

Many different disorders may cause brain dysfunction or other neurologic symptoms and may affect the patient's level of consciousness (LOC), speech, and voluntary muscle control. The brain is most sensitive to changes in oxygen, glucose, and temperature levels. A substantial change in any one of these three levels will result in a neurologic change. In general, if the problem is caused primarily by disorders in the heart and lungs, the entire brain will be affected. For example, when blood flow is stopped (cardiac arrest), the patient will go into a **coma**, a state of profound unresponsiveness, and permanent brain damage can result within minutes. However, if the primary problem is in the brain, such as a poor blood supply to one side of the brain, the patient may have signs and symptoms affecting only one side of the body. A low oxygen level in the bloodstream will affect the entire brain, often causing anxiety, restlessness, and confusion. Extremely low blood glucose levels (hypoglycemia) can cause a wide spectrum of symptoms ranging from mild confusion to symptoms that mimic stroke.

Other brain disorders include conditions such as infection and tumor. Although not all specific problems are addressed, the seizures or altered mental status that often accompanies them is discussed. The information in this section will help you better understand, communicate with, and care for patients who have experienced some type of brain disorder.

▶ Stroke

A stroke, or **cerebrovascular accident (CVA)**, is an interruption of blood flow to the brain that often is sudden and results in the loss of function in the affected part of the brain. People older than 65 years represent almost 75% of all patients who have experienced stroke.[4] The American Heart Association (AHA) reports that a substantial number of patients who experience strokes either deny their symptoms or do not understand what their symptoms mean.[5] Many patients fail to activate emergency medical services (EMS) and subsequently delay care. The goal of treatment, as recommended by the AHA, is early recognition and rapid, appropriate intervention. The longer the stroke continues, the less likely the patient will have a promising outcome because "time is brain." Early recognition begins with an EMS system that can effectively identify potential strokes at dispatch and rapidly request the appropriate resources. As an EMS provider, do not delay your response to a patient with a potential stroke. According to the AHA, one-fifth of patients with an intracranial hemorrhage will have a substantial decrease in their LOC between emergency medical care provided by EMS and care on transfer to the emergency department.

Without oxygen, brain cells cease to function and begin to die. These dead cells are called **infarcted cells**. After the cells are infarcted, medical science has little to offer. However, because cell death is not immediate and may take several hours or more to occur, infarction may be prevented with prompt care that leads to restoration of blood flow to the affected cells. Alternately, if a small amount of blood is still able to reach the affected area of the brain, it may supply enough oxygen to keep a larger group of brain cells, called **ischemic cells**, alive, but not enough to let the cells function properly and may result in temporary or permanent disability. If normal blood flow is restored to an ischemic area of the brain in a timely manner, the patient may have less residual damage.

Words of Wisdom

A stroke is also called a "brain attack." This phrase is used with the general public to emphasize that rapid recognition of the signs and symptoms and prompt transport to an appropriate facility can mean the difference between the patient regaining function and suffering lifelong disability.

Interruption of cerebral blood flow may result from a **thrombus**, a clot that has developed locally, in this case, in a cerebral artery; an **arterial rupture**, a rupture of a cerebral artery; or a **cerebral embolism**, an obstruction of a cerebral artery caused by a clot that was formed elsewhere, detached, and traveled to the brain.

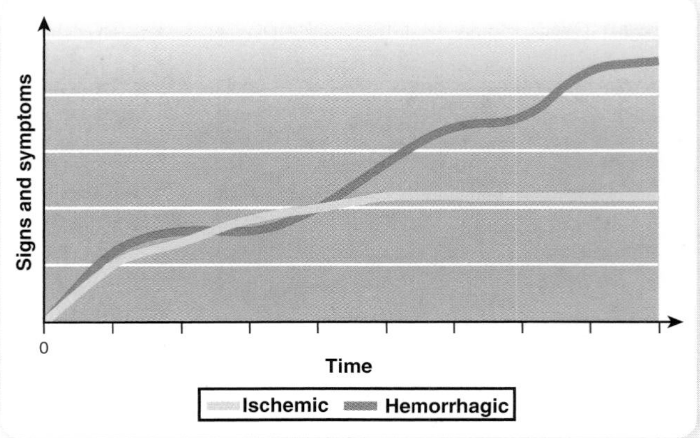

Figure 19-6 Symptom patterns for hemorrhagic compared with ischemic stroke.

The two basic types of stroke are **hemorrhagic stroke** (from arterial rupture) which account for 13% of all strokes according to the AHA, and **ischemic stroke** (from an embolism or thrombus), which account for 87%.[6] These two causes of strokes have differing presentation patterns, but ultimately, advanced radiographic imaging such as computed tomography (CT) scanning in a hospital is necessary to differentiate them. The graph shown in **Figure 19-6** provides some insight into the evolution of a stroke.

Ischemic Stroke

In an ischemic stroke, a blood vessel is blocked so the tissue distal to the blockage becomes ischemic. Eventually, that tissue will die if blood flow is not restored. But this pathology is self-limiting. Only the tissue beyond the blockage is affected, so the area or areas of the brain involved are limited. This blockage can be from a thrombus or an embolism that obstructs blood flow.

As with coronary artery disease, atherosclerosis in the blood vessels is usually the cause of stroke. **Atherosclerosis** is a disorder in which calcium and cholesterol build up, forming a plaque inside the walls of blood vessels. This plaque obstructs blood flow, interfering with the vessels' ability to dilate. Eventually, atherosclerosis can cause complete occlusion (blockage) of an artery **Figure 19-7**. In other cases, an atherosclerotic plaque in a carotid artery will rupture or crack. A blood clot will form over the disruption in the plaque, sometimes growing big enough to completely block all blood flow through that artery.

Deprived of oxygen, the parts of the brain supplied by the artery will become ischemic. As oxygen and glucose levels drop, brain cells turn to anaerobic metabolism to stay alive. This mechanism, however, is only a stopgap measure. Anaerobic metabolism creates only miniscule amounts of energy for the cell and produces acidic by-products. If circulation is not returned quickly, the cell will not have enough fuel to survive and will die.

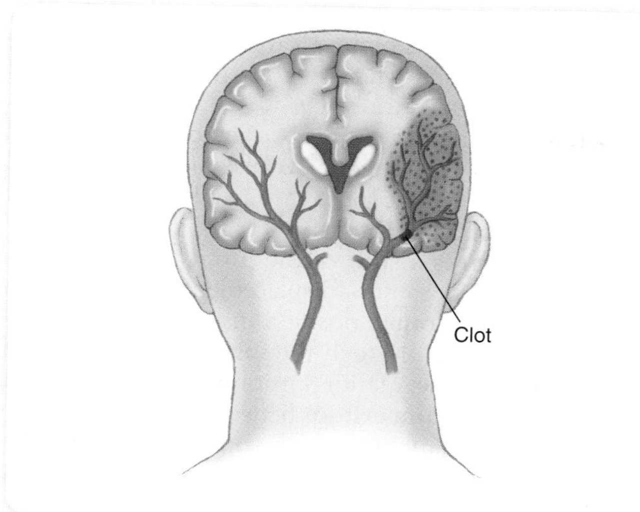

Figure 19-7 Atherosclerosis can damage the wall of a cerebral artery, producing narrowing or a clot. When the vessel is narrowed or completely blocked, blood flow to that part of the brain may be blocked, and the cells begin to die.

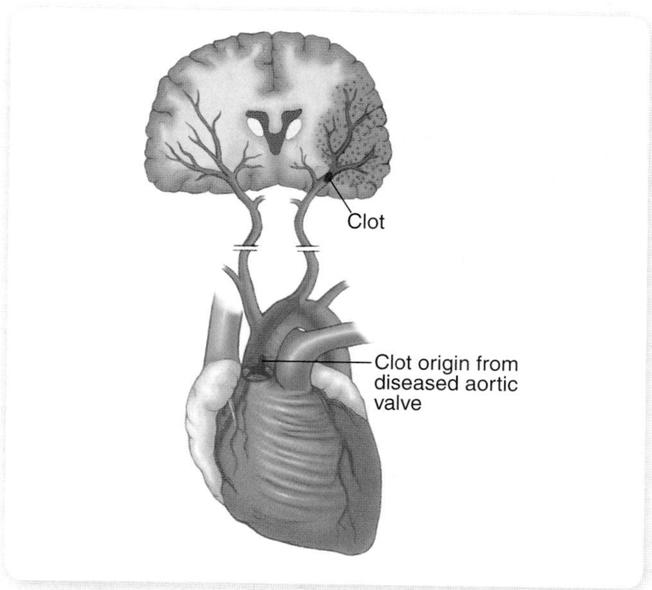

Figure 19-8 An embolus, a blood clot usually formed on a diseased heart valve, can travel through the body's vascular system, lodge in a cerebral artery, and cause a stroke.

If the blockage in the carotid artery is incomplete, smaller pieces of the clot may embolize (break off and be carried by the normal flow of blood) deep into the brain. There, a piece of clot may become lodged in a branch of a smaller branch of a blood vessel. This cerebral embolism then obstructs blood flow **Figure 19-8**. Depending on the location of the obstruction, the patient's symptoms can vary widely, from nothing at all to an inability to move one side of the body or complete paralysis.

Patients with ischemic strokes will have dramatic symptoms, including, among others, loss of movement on the opposite side of the body, confusion, and the inability to speak.

Hemorrhagic Stroke

A hemorrhagic stroke occurs as a result of bleeding within the brain, typically when a blood vessel ruptures and the accumulated blood then forms a blood clot. The severity of the hemorrhagic stroke depends on the location and size of the ruptured cerebral vessel. As bleeding continues within the brain, **intracranial pressure (ICP)** increases and compresses brain tissue. When brain tissue is compressed, oxygenated blood cannot get into the area, and the surrounding cells begin to die.

Certain patients are at higher risk for hemorrhagic stroke. The patients at highest risk are those who have chronic, poorly controlled hypertension. Many years of high blood pressure weaken the blood vessels in the brain, making them prone to rupture. Cerebral hemorrhages are often fatal, although proper treatment of high blood pressure can help to prevent this long-term damage to the blood vessels, reducing morbidity and mortality.

Arterial walls consist of three layers of tissue. People who are born with a weakness in one or more of those layers are also at increased risk for hemorrhagic stroke. Aneurysms occur in the following way:

1. A small tear or defect occurs within the wall of an artery.
2. Blood penetrates between the layers of the artery.
3. Pressure builds up, and the initial small tear increases in size.

If this process continues, the arterial wall will become so damaged that it can no longer withstand the normal pressure of blood flowing through the artery. The weakened wall will begin to bulge. If the damage is severe, the bulging artery can leak or fail catastrophically, causing an intracranial hemorrhage.

Many people with a hemorrhagic stroke due to a ruptured aneurysm have a sudden onset of a severe headache, frequently described as "the worst headache of my life," which signals the rupture of the aneurysm. Shortly after experiencing the severe headache, it is common for the patient's LOC to decrease rapidly, indicating increased ICP. When a hemorrhagic stroke occurs in an otherwise healthy young person, it is often the result of a berry aneurysm. This type of aneurysm resembles a tiny balloon (or berry) that protrudes from a cerebral artery. When the aneurysm is overstretched and ruptures, bleeding occurs in the subarachnoid space—the area between the coverings (meninges) of the brain. These types of strokes are therefore called subarachnoid hemorrhages. With prompt care, surgical repair of the aneurysm is sometimes possible. Continued bleeding within the brain will cause the ICP to increase further, thus decreasing cerebral perfusion pressure. Eventually, the brain, which is substantially compressed, may be forced out of the cranial vault through the foramen magnum in a process called **herniation** (the movement of a structure from its normal location into another space). With herniation, pressure on the medulla oblongata (located directly above the spinal cord) can result in rather bizarre vital signs and other findings, including slowed heart and erratic respiratory rates, eventually leading to death.

Intracranial Pressure

Hemorrhagic strokes that cause bleeding into the brain place patients at risk for increased ICP. Treatment is directed at providing some degree of control over this potentially deadly effect.

The skull (cranial vault) is filled with three substances: brain, blood, and cerebrospinal fluid. These three substances exert a pressure against the skull and the skull exerts a reflected pressure. This balanced exchange allows the brain to fit snugly within the skull without permitting any voids. If the skull contained empty spaces, with head movement, the brain would slam into the skull and cause damage.

When the pressure within the cranial vault begins to increase and remains high (increased ICP), the amount of blood available to the brain decreases. Cerebral perfusion pressure (CPP), the pressure of blood within the cranial vault, then begins to fall.

As with most readings within the body, ICP changes constantly. For example, coughing, vomiting, or bearing down tends to increase the ICP. These momentary spikes in ICP are not harmful. By contrast, if there is blood, swelling, pus, or a tumor within the cranial vault, the ICP will increase and remain high. Because the volume of the cranial vault is limited and inflexible, pressure increases as more substances squeeze into this space. As long as there is no substantial decrease in blood pressure **Figure 19-9** or significant increase in ICP, the heart will still be able to get blood into the brain. However, patients can have life-threatening issues when ICP rises sharply and/or blood pressure becomes critically low.

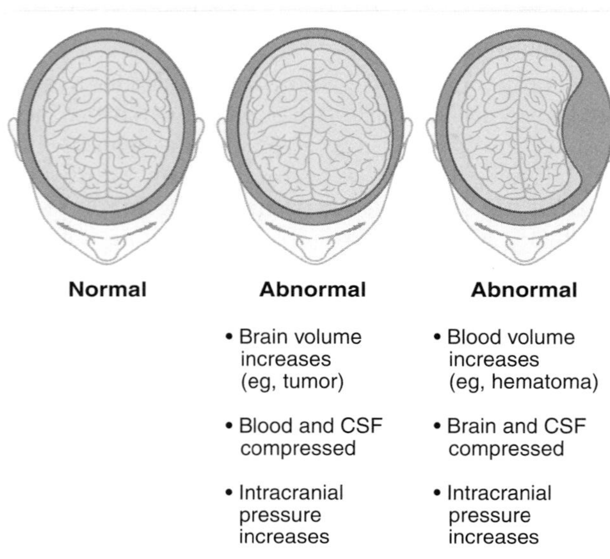
Normal
Abnormal
• Brain volume increases (eg, tumor)
• Blood and CSF compressed
• Intracranial pressure increases
Abnormal
• Blood volume increases (eg, hematoma)
• Brain and CSF compressed
• Intracranial pressure increases

Figure 19-9 Normal and abnormal intracranial pressure.

As the ICP rises, it creates two major problems. The brain may become ischemic because of a lack of blood supply and/or herniate (push through the ligaments that compartmentalize the brain).

Herniation is a shift of the intracranial contents within the cranial vault or displacement of the contents away from their normal position inside the skull.[7] Herniation may occur through the foramen magnum, the large opening at the inferior portion of the skull through which the spinal cord exits or between spaces inside the skull such as the tentorium (a horizontal projection of the dura that separates the cerebellum from the cerebrum). A herniation will eventually compress and strangulate the brainstem, at which point the patient will lose control of his or her vegetative functions. Prehospital treatment is not very effective at decreasing ICP and preventing or reversing herniation.

Documentation & Communication

Patients with strokes can present with a wide range of communication difficulties.

- Patients who are multilingual may lose understanding of one language but not another.
- Patients may be able to understand the written word but not the spoken word.
- Patients may not be able to understand any form of communication.

Be open to trying various ways to communicate. Remember, communication problems do not indicate that the patient is not thinking. The problem is that the patient cannot get you to understand what he or she is thinking.

Transient Ischemic Attack

In some patients, normal processes in the body will destroy a blood clot in the brain. When that happens quickly, blood flow is restored to the affected area, and the patient will regain use of the affected region of the body. When stroke symptoms subside within 24 hours, the event is called a **transient ischemic attack (TIA)**, also referred to as a "small stroke" or a "ministroke."

No residual damage to brain tissue occurs, and no signs and symptoms appear after the episode ends. However, these ministrokes are often signs of a serious vascular condition that requires medical evaluation. The National Institute of Neurological Disorders and Stroke reports that approximately one-third of patients with TIAs will have an acute stroke sometime in the future.[8] Think of the relationship between TIA and stroke as the equivalent of the relationship between angina and myocardial infarction.

Although most patients with TIAs do well, it is still a neurologic emergency. For this reason, all patients with a TIA should be evaluated by a physician to determine whether preventive action can be taken to prevent a stroke in the future.

Signs and Symptoms of Stroke

The general signs and symptoms of stroke include the following:

- Facial drooping
- Sudden weakness or numbness in the face, arm, leg, or one side of the body
- Decreased or absent movement and sensation on one side of the body
- **Ataxia** (lack of muscle coordination) or loss of balance
- Sudden vision loss in one eye; blurred or double vision (diplopia)
- **Dysphagia** (difficulty swallowing)
- Decreased level of responsiveness
- Aphasia; difficulty expressing thoughts or inability to use the right words (expressive aphasia) or difficulty understanding spoken words (receptive aphasia)
- Slurred speech (dysarthria)
- Sudden and severe headache
- Confusion
- Dizziness
- Weakness
- Combativeness
- Restlessness
- Tongue deviation
- Coma

Left Hemisphere Problems. If the left cerebral hemisphere has been affected by a stroke, the patient may exhibit a speech disorder called **aphasia**, the inability to produce or understand speech. Speech problems vary widely. Patients may have trouble understanding speech but can speak clearly. This condition is called receptive aphasia. You can detect aphasia by asking the patient a question such as "What day is today?" In response, a patient with aphasia may say, "Green." The speech is clear, but the answer does not make sense. Other patients will be able to understand the question but cannot produce the right sounds to provide an answer. Only grunts or other incomprehensible sounds emerge. This type of aphasia is expressive. Strokes that affect the left side of the brain also can cause paralysis on the right side of the body and vice versa.

Right Hemisphere Problems. If the right cerebral hemisphere of the brain is not getting enough blood, patients will have trouble moving the muscles on the left side of the body. Usually, they will understand language and be able to speak, but their words may be slurred and difficult to understand. Slurred speech is one characteristic of **dysarthria**.

It is interesting that patients with right hemisphere strokes may be completely oblivious to their problem. If you ask the patients to lift the left arm and they cannot, they will lift the right arm instead. They seem to have forgotten that the left arm even exists. This symptom is called neglect. Patients with a problem affecting the posterior aspect of the cerebrum (occiput) may neglect certain parts of their vision. Generally, this is difficult to detect in the field, but you should be aware of the possibility. Try to sit or stand on the patient's unaffected side, because he or she may be unable to see things on the affected side.

Neglect and lack of pain cause many patients who have had large strokes to delay seeking help. Unless caused by a ruptured cerebral artery, in which case the patient will complain of a severe headache, strokes are typically not painful. Therefore, a patient may be unaware that there is a problem until a family member or friend points out that some part of the patient's body is not working correctly.

Bleeding in the Brain. Patients who have bleeding in the brain (intracerebral hemorrhage) may present with hypertension. Sometimes hypertension is the cause of the bleeding but, many times, it is a response to the bleeding; hypertension may be a response of the body to shunt more oxygenated blood to the injured portion of the brain. Remember, the brain is located inside a box (skull) with only a few openings. When bleeding occurs inside the brain, the pressure inside the skull increases. The body must increase the blood pressure to get blood to the brain's tissues, increasing the pressure even further.

High blood pressure in stroke patients should not be treated in the field. Monitoring the blood pressure and watching for a trend of increasing blood pressure is important. Blood pressure may return to normal or decrease substantially on its own. Substantial decreases in blood pressure may also occur as the patient's condition worsens.

▶ Conditions That May Mimic Stroke

The following three conditions may present similarly to stroke:

- **Hypoglycemia** (a condition characterized by a low blood glucose level)
- A **postictal state** (the reset period of the brain after a seizure, lasting between 5 and 30 minutes and characterized by labored respirations and some degree of altered mental status)
- Subdural or epidural bleeding (a collection of blood near the skull that presses on the brain)

Because oxygen and glucose are needed for brain metabolism, a patient with hypoglycemia may look like a patient who is experiencing a stroke. You should check the patient's blood glucose level and find out whether

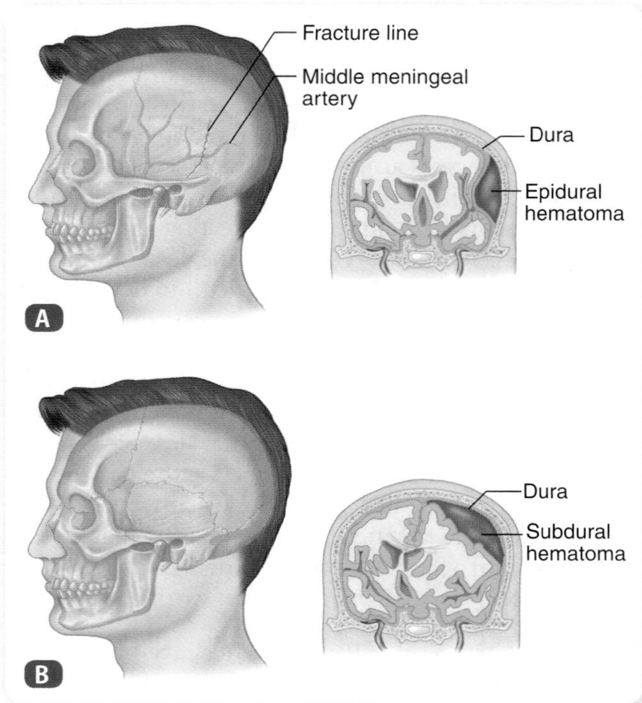

Figure 19-10 Trauma to the head can result in intracranial bleeding. **A.** Bleeding outside the dura but under the skull is epidural. **B.** Bleeding beneath the dura but outside the brain is subdural.

the patient has diabetes and takes insulin or a glucose-lowering medication.

A patient in the postictal state may appear to be experiencing a stroke; however, in most cases, a patient in a postictal state will recover without assistance, whereas a patient experiencing a stroke will not.

Subdural bleeding and epidural bleeding usually occur as results of trauma. These conditions are thoroughly discussed in Chapter 30, *Head and Spine Injuries*. The dura is a leathery covering over the brain, next to the skull. A fracture near the temporal region of the skull may cause an artery (usually the middle meningeal artery) to bleed on top of the dura, resulting in pressure on the brain Figure 19-10A. Because the source of bleeding is from an artery, the onset of symptoms from epidural bleeding is usually very rapid after the injury. In other cases, the veins just below the dura may be torn and bleed, which is known as subdural bleeding Figure 19-10B. Because veins tend to bleed slowly, the onset of symptoms occurs more slowly, sometimes over several days.

With subdural and epidural bleeding, the onset of strokelike signs and symptoms may be subtle. The patient or family may not even remember the original injury that is causing the bleeding.

▶ Seizures

Seizures are sudden, erratic firings of neurons. Patients who have epilepsy commonly have seizures, for example.

Table 19-2 Classification of Seizures

Grouping	Type	Presentation
Generalized	▪ Tonic-clonic (formerly grand mal) ▪ Absence (formerly petit mal) ▪ Pseudoseizures	▪ Full-body, violent jerking movements ▪ Freezing or staring ▪ Tonic-clonic but caused by a psychiatric mechanism (the patient is not faking the seizure)
Partial	▪ Simple partial ▪ Complex partial	▪ Shaking of one area of the body ▪ Sensation in one area of the body ▪ Subtle alterations in LOC

Abbreviation: LOC, level of consciousness

Patients can experience a wide array of signs and symptoms when having seizures, such as muscle spasms, increased secretions, diaphoresis, and cyanosis. A seizure can be limited to one hand shaking or a metallic taste in the mouth, or it can involve the movement of every limb or the complete loss of consciousness. Patients may be aware of the seizure or wake up afterward not knowing what happened.

Types of Seizures

Seizures can be classified as generalized (affecting large portions of the brain) or partial (affecting a limited area of the brain). The classification of seizures is outlined in Table 19-2.

Tonic-Clonic Seizures. **Tonic-clonic seizures**, formerly called grand mal seizures, present you with the greatest assessment challenges.[9] Most tonic-clonic seizures follow a pattern, traveling through each of the following steps in order, although some patients may not experience every step:

1. **Aura.** A sensation the patient experiences before the seizure occurs (for example, muscle twitch, odd taste, seeing lights, hearing a high-pitched noise)
2. **Loss of consciousness**

3. **Tonic phase.** Body-wide rigidity
4. **Hypertonic phase.** Arched back and rigidity
5. **Clonic phase.** Rhythmic contractions of major muscle groups; arms, legs, head movement; lip smacking; biting; teeth clenching. Contractions are chaotic, disorganized, and of small amplitude. Imagine ventricular fibrillation of the brain—that is what a seizure is electrically.
6. **Postseizure.** Major muscles relax; nystagmus (involuntary, rhythmic eye movement) may still occur; eyes possibly "rolled back."
7. **Postictal phase.** Reset period of the brain. The reset can take several minutes to hours before the patient gradually returns to the preseizure LOC. During this time, patients are often initially aphasic (unable to speak), confused or unable to follow commands, emotional, or tired and may be incontinent of urine and/or feces. They may present with a headache. Gradually the brain will begin to function normally.

Tonic-clonic seizures are disconcerting for both family and health care providers to watch. During the seizure process, respiration may become erratic, loud, and obviously abnormal. Alternatively, the patient may stop breathing and become cyanotic. These periods of apnea are usually short lived and do not require intervention. If the patient is apneic for more than 30 seconds, immediately begin ventilatory assistance. Another disconcerting aspect of seizures, particularly for the patient, is incontinence.

Pseudoseizures. Pseudoseizures, or psychogenic nonepileptic seizures, are a generalized neurologic event. Symptomatically, you may not notice any difference from a tonic-clonic seizure. Tonic-clonic motion, loss of consciousness, and a postictal phase are all present during these events. The difference is that in pseudoseizures, the root cause is of psychiatric origin. It is important to understand that in most cases of pseudoseizure, the patient is not intentionally causing this behavior.

Patients with pseudoseizures present with loss of consciousness, which is usually triggered by some emotional event, stress, lights, or pain. Pseudoseizures conspicuously occur with witnesses. This fact may lead health care providers to believe pseudoseizures are contrived. Motion that occurs during the seizure is relatively organized—side-to-side movement of the head, pedaling movements of the legs (such as riding a bicycle), weeping, or stuttering. These patients often have a psychiatric history and/or other medical history, such as fibromyalgia, chronic pain, or chronic fatigue.

Absence Seizures. In contrast with tonic-clonic seizures, **absence seizures** present with little or no movement. The typical patient with absence seizures is a child. Classically, the child will simply stop moving; he or she may be walking and just stop, may be speaking and stop midsentence, or may be playing and freeze with a toy in the hand. The child will rarely fall. These seizures usually last no more than several seconds. There is no postictal period and no confusion. These may be brought on by flashing lights or hyperventilation.

YOU are the Provider — PART 2

Realizing that this call is not just a "normal" intoxication, you conduct a Cincinnati Prehospital Stroke Scale screening. The patient fails all tests. Per your protocols, you ask your partner to call the local hospital which has a stroke team to advise them that you have a "stroke alert" patient. You and a shelter worker assist the patient onto a stretcher, and you quickly obtain a set of vital signs. The worker states that he saw the patient maybe 20 or 30 minutes ago and he was acting normal at that time.

Recording Time: 1 Minute	
Appearance	Slurred speech, right-side facial droop, and possible left-side weakness
Level of consciousness	Alert and confused
Airway	Patent
Breathing	12 breaths/min
Circulation	Strong radial pulse; skin is warm, dry, and pink

3. What are the two types of strokes that this patient may be experiencing?
4. Should you move the patient into the back of the ambulance for evaluation?

Partial Seizures. **Partial seizures** may be classified as simple partial or complex partial. Such seizures involve only a limited portion of the brain. They may be localized to just one spot within the brain, or they may begin in one spot and move in a wavelike manner to other locations.

Simple partial seizures involve movement of one part of the body (when originating in the frontal lobe) or altered sensations in one part of the body (when originating in the parietal lobe). This movement may stay in one body part or spread from one part to another in a wave. An example of such a wave in a simple partial seizure is shaking of the left hand, which moves to the left arm, then shoulder, then head, then right arm, then right hand, and finally moves out of the body. **Complex partial seizures** involve subtle changes in the LOC. The patient may become confused or less alert, experience hallucinations, or be unable to speak. The head or eyes may make small movements. Patients typically do not become unresponsive.

Words of Wisdom

Always assess glucose levels for any patient with an altered mental status and especially those who have had seizures. Although hypoglycemia may result in seizure activity, it is also important to remember that the muscular activity involved in a tonic-clonic seizure may rapidly decrease glucose stores. A patient who was not hypoglycemic at the onset may become hypoglycemic as a result of the seizure activity.

Status Epilepticus

Status epilepticus is a seizure that lasts for longer than 4 or 5 minutes or consecutive seizures that occur without the return of consciousness between seizure episodes. This time frame is arbitrary, however, and some authors suggest that status epilepticus does not occur until 30 minutes of uninterrupted seizure activity. Refer to your local protocols for guidelines on how long a seizure can continue before you should intervene. Status epilepticus is a life-threatening neurologic disorder and it should not be taken lightly. The authors of a 2015 study report that the mortality rate for patients in refractory status epilepticus was 70%.[10]

During a seizure, neurons are in a hypermetabolic state (using large amounts of glucose and producing lactic acid). For a short period, this state does not produce long-term damage. If the seizure continues then the body becomes unable to remove waste products effectively or ensure adequate glucose supplies. Such a hypermetabolic state can result in neurons being damaged or killed. The goals of prehospital care are to stop the seizure and ensure adequate ABCs (airway, breathing, and circulation), including adequate glucose levels.

Table 19-3 Common Causes of Seizures

- Abscess
- Alcohol
- Birth anomaly
- Brain infections (meningitis, encephalitis)
- Brain trauma
- Diabetes mellitus
- Fever (rapid rate of rise)
- Hypertension during pregnancy (eclampsia)
- **Idiopathic** (of no known cause)
- Inappropriate medication dosage
- Organic brain syndromes
- Recreational drug use (cocaine)
- Stroke or TIA
- Systemic infection
- Tumor
- **Uremia** (kidney failure)

Abbreviation: TIA, transient ischemic attack

Causes of Seizures

There are various reasons why a patient may have a seizure, ranging from a congenital disorder, to a diabetic emergency, to fever (a possible cause if the patient is an infant). Knowing the cause will help direct management.

Some seizure disorders, such as epilepsy, are congenital, which means that the patient was born with the condition. Other types of seizures may be a result of a high fever, structural problems in the brain, or metabolic or chemical problems in the body Table 19-3. Epileptic seizures can usually be controlled with medications such as phenytoin (Dilantin), phenobarbital (for example, Solfoton), carbamazepine (for example, Tegretol), levetiracetam (Keppra), gabapentin (Gabarone, Neurontin), or lamotrigine (Lamictal). Patients with epilepsy often have seizures if they stop taking their medications or if they do not take the prescribed dose on a regular basis. In fact, most seizures are the result of medication noncompliance. In the emergency department, blood analysis will frequently show a subtherapeutic level of the antiepileptic drug.

Seizures can also result from sudden high fevers, particularly in infants and small children. Such seizures, known as **febrile seizures**, are usually unnerving for parents to observe but are generally well tolerated by the child. Nevertheless, you must transport a child who has had a febrile seizure because this condition needs to be evaluated in the hospital. It is possible a second seizure may occur. If it does, the patient requires rapid evaluation in a hospital to identify possible causes, such as serious inflammation in the brain or tissues covering the brain (conditions known as encephalitis and meningitis, respectively; an abscess may also be present). Febrile seizures result from a rapid increase in body temperature. In other

Words of Wisdom

Use the mnemonic **FACTS** to obtain pertinent history for patients having a seizure:

Focus (Generalized or focal?)
Activity (Type of movements?)
Color or **C**ocaine (Cyanosis? Indications of cocaine use?)
Time (How long did the seizure last?)
Secondary information (Medications? Events leading up to the seizure? Incontinence? Tongue biting?)

words, it is not necessarily how high the fever gets, but how quickly it gets there.

The Importance of Recognizing Seizures

Regardless of the type or cause of a seizure, it is extremely important for you to recognize when a seizure is occurring or whether one has already occurred. You must also determine whether this episode differs from any previous ones. For example, if a previous seizure occurred on only one side of the body and this seizure occurred over the entire body, some additional or new problem may be involved. In addition to recognizing that seizure activity has occurred and/or that something different may now be occurring, you must also recognize the postictal state and the complications of seizures.

Because most seizures involve vigorous twitching of the muscles, the muscles use a lot of oxygen. This excessive demand consumes oxygen that was being delivered by the circulation to support the vital functions of the body. A seizure is similar to a situation in which you exercise vigorously without giving your body a chance to rest. As a result, there is a buildup of acids in the bloodstream, and the patient may turn cyanotic (bluish lips, mucous membranes, and skin) from the lack of oxygen. Often the seizures themselves prevent the patient from breathing normally, making the problem worse. In a patient with diabetes, the blood glucose level may decrease because of the excessive muscular contraction of a seizure. If your local protocol allows, closely monitor the blood glucose level after a patient with diabetes has a seizure.

Recognizing seizure activity also means looking at other problems associated with the seizure. For example, the patient may have fallen during the seizure episode and injured some part of the body; head injury is the most serious possibility. Patients having a generalized seizure may experience **incontinence**, meaning that they may lose bowel and bladder control. Therefore, one clue that unresponsive or confused patients may have had a seizure is to find that they were incontinent. Although incontinence is possible with other medical conditions, sudden incontinence is likely a sign that a seizure has occurred.

Safety

Be aware that a patient may behave violently during the postictal phase. The patient might not know what has happened and might be frightened by "strangers" providing care or trying to move him or her into the ambulance. Alcohol and/or drugs are not always associated with violent behavior during the postictal phase, but signs of their use or abuse should heighten your awareness of the potential for dangerous behavior.

The Postictal State

After a seizure has stopped, the patient's muscles relax, becoming almost flaccid, or floppy, and breathing becomes labored (fast and deep) in an attempt to compensate for the buildup of acids in the bloodstream. By breathing faster and more deeply, the body can balance the pH in the bloodstream. With normal circulation and liver function, the acids clear away within minutes, and the patient will begin to breathe normally. The longer and more intense the seizure was, the longer it will take for this imbalance to correct itself. Similarly, longer and more severe seizures will result in a longer postictal phase.

In some situations, the postictal state may be characterized by **hemiparesis**, or weakness on one side of the body, resembling a stroke. Unlike the typical stroke, hypoxic hemiparesis spontaneously resolves within a short period. Most commonly, the postictal state is characterized by lethargy and confusion to the point that the patient may be combative and appear angry. You must be prepared for these circumstances in your approach to scene control and in your treatment of the patient's symptoms. If the patient's condition does not improve, you should consider other possible underlying problems, including hypoglycemia and infection.

Words of Wisdom

Physician evaluation of a patient who has had a seizure depends heavily on reports of the seizure pattern and changes in that pattern. For example, was this seizure different from previous ones? If so, how? Record all pertinent information about the seizure in terms of duration, areas of body movement, and possible precipitating factors (such as recent trauma, fever, and medication noncompliance). Effective interviewing of available witnesses, family members, or caregivers is needed to obtain the required information.

▶ Altered Mental Status

Aside from stroke and seizures, the most common type of neurologic emergency that you will encounter is a patient with altered mental status. Simply put, altered mental

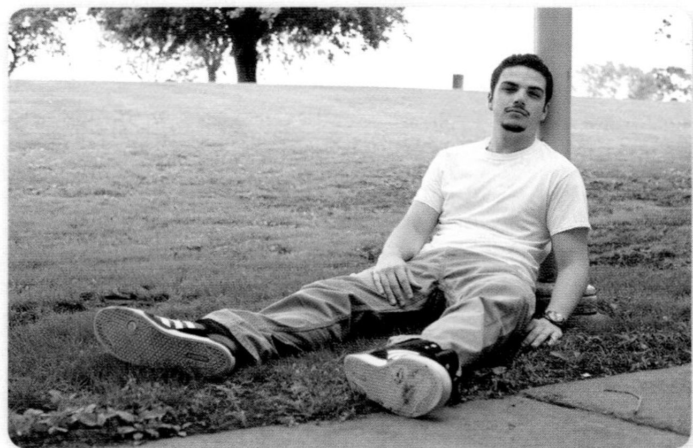

Figure 19-11 A patient with altered mental status can be unresponsive in some cases; in others, the patient may be responsive but confused.

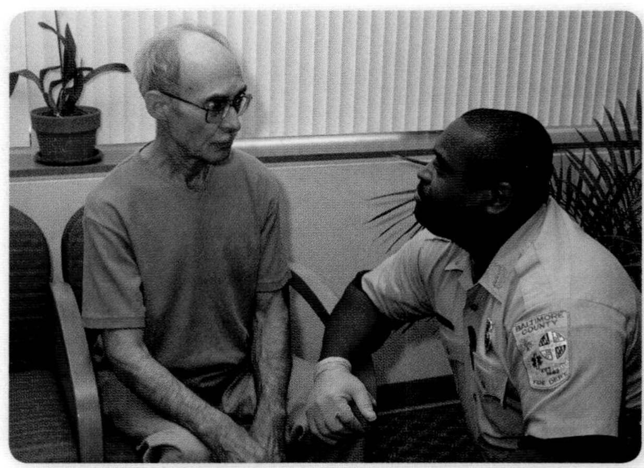

Figure 19-12 During your assessment of a patient with an altered or decreased level of consciousness, consider the possibility of hypoglycemia and check the patient's blood glucose level.

status means that the patient is not thinking clearly or is incapable of being aroused. In some cases, patients will be unresponsive **Figure 19-11**; in others, they may be responsive but confused. The range of problems is wide, and the causes are many, including common problems such as hypoglycemia, hypoxemia, intoxication, drug overdose, unrecognized head injury, brain infection, body temperature abnormalities, and uncommon conditions such as brain tumors, glandular abnormalities, and overdoses and/or poisonings.

Hypoglycemia

The clinical picture of patients with altered mental status caused by hypoglycemia is complex. Because oxygen and glucose are needed for brain function, hypoglycemia can mimic the signs and symptoms of stroke and seizures. Patients may have hemiparesis, similar to what occurs as a result of a stroke. However, the principal difference is that a patient who has experienced a stroke may be alert and attempting to communicate normally, whereas a patient with hypoglycemia almost always has an altered mental status **Figure 19-12**.

Patients with hypoglycemia commonly, but not always, take medications that lower the blood glucose level. Therefore, if the patient appears to have signs and symptoms of stroke and an altered mental status, you should report your findings to medical control and treat the patient accordingly. Check for and report medications, but remember that not all patients who have diabetes take insulin or other medications to lower the blood glucose level. Remember, also, that patients with a decreased LOC may not be able to adequately protect their airways in which case they should not be given anything by mouth. Local protocols should guide your actions.

Patients with hypoglycemia can also experience seizures, and you may arrive at the scene to find a patient in a postictal state: confused and disoriented or unresponsive. The mental status of a patient who has had a typical seizure is likely to improve soon after the seizure stops; however, in a patient with hypoglycemia, the mental status is not likely to improve, even after several minutes. Therefore, you should consider the possibility of hypoglycemia in a patient who has had a seizure, especially if the blood glucose reading is low.

Likewise, you should consider hypoglycemia in a patient who has altered mental status after an injury such as a motor vehicle crash, even when there is the possibility of an accompanying head injury. As with any other patient, you should look for medical identification bracelets or medications that might confirm your suspicions.

Other Causes of Altered Mental Status

In addition to hypoglycemia, three other possible causes of altered mental status include hypoxia (regardless of the cause), unrecognized head injury, and severe alcohol or drug intoxication. Your consideration of these and other possibilities becomes important because a patient with altered mental status may be combative and refuse treatment and transport. You should be prepared for difficult patient encounters and follow local protocols for dealing with these situations, recognizing the potential for serious underlying problems.

In most cases, a patient who appears intoxicated is just that; however, the patient might have other problems as well. People with alcoholism can have abnormalities in liver function, blood clotting, and immune system abnormalities, which can predispose them to intracranial bleeding, brain and bloodstream infections, and hypoglycemia.

Psychological problems and adverse effects of medications are also possible causes of altered mental status. In addition, a person who appears to have a psychological problem may also have an underlying medical condition.

Infections are another possible cause, particularly those involving the brain or bloodstream. Infections in these areas are life threatening and need immediate attention.

Patients may not demonstrate typical signs of infection, such as fever, particularly if they are very young or very old or have an impaired immune system.

Altered mental status can also be caused by drug overdose and poisonings; therefore, you should monitor patients closely for accompanying cardiac and respiratory problems.

The presentation of altered mental status varies widely from simple confusion to coma. Regardless of the cause, you should consider altered mental status to be an emergency that requires immediate attention, even when it appears that the culprit may be alcohol intoxication or a minor car crash or fall.

▶ Syncope

Syncope (fainting) is the sudden and temporary loss of consciousness with accompanying loss of postural tone. Syncope can be a sign of life-threatening cardiac dysrhythmia, stroke, or other serious medical condition. It affects mainly adults and accounts for 1% to 3% of all emergency department visits.[11] The brain uses glucose at a high rate and has no ability to store glucose, so even a 3- to 5-second interruption in blood flow can cause loss of consciousness. The question then becomes: "What caused the sudden decrease in cerebral perfusion?" Potential causes include problems with cardiac rhythm or conduction, problems with cardiac muscle, myocardial infarction, dehydration, hypoglycemia, and a vasovagal episode.

▶ Headache

One of the most common complaints of pain you will hear from your patients is headache. Because a headache is subjective, it may be a symptom of another condition or it may be considered a neurologic condition on its own. Millions of people experience a headache every year, but only a small percentage of these are caused by a serious medical condition. The brain and skull do not actually sense pain because neither contains pain receptors. The pain associated with a headache is felt from the surrounding areas of the face; scalp, meninges (membranes that cover the brain and spinal cord); larger blood vessels; and the muscles of the head, neck, and face.

Tension headaches, migraines, and sinus headaches are the most common types of headaches and are not considered life threatening, although they may be debilitating for the patient. Tension headaches may be caused by stress, altered cortisol levels, and/or depression, which causes residual muscle contractions (tension) within the face and head. The jaw, neck, or shoulders may be stiff or sore. Patients usually describe the pain as squeezing or dull or as an ache. This type of headache does not have any associated symptoms and usually does not require medical attention.

A migraine headache is a complex condition thought to be caused by minor instability within certain clusters of neurons and also by changes in blood vessel size at the base of the brain. The patient may experience an aura (for example, seeing bright lights) and unilateral, focused pain that then spreads over time. The patient often describes the pain as throbbing, pounding, or pulsating and may have nausea or vomiting. During a migraine headache, patients prefer dark, quiet environments. Migraines can last several days.

Two other types of headaches are cluster headaches and sinus headaches. Cluster headaches are rare vascular headaches that occur in groups, or clusters, and last 30 to 45 minutes. However, a person may have several cluster headaches per day. The headaches can recur for days and then stop entirely. They may return at the same time the following month or the same time the next day. The pattern consists of minor pain around one eye. The pain—described as sharp and excruciating, or as if someone is pushing the eyeball out—quickly intensifies and spreads to one side of the face and causes a feeling of anxiety. Sinus headaches are caused by inflammation or infection within the sinus cavities of the face. The pain is located in the superior portions of the face and increases with bending the head forward.

Patient Assessment

The brain is the organ that is most sensitive to fluctuating levels of oxygen, glucose, and temperature; it responds to alterations in these levels with changes in its function. The brain is relatively resilient to internal environmental changes: it does not simply shut down when the oxygen level falls. The key to identifying a neurologic problem is to look for obvious changes and subtle changes.

Scene Size-up

Remember to take standard precautions. A patient having a tonic-clonic seizure, for example, may be incontinent.

Patients with altered levels of consciousness or who are combative may require additional assistance with lifting and moving. Request additional resources early in the call, and ensure you have a way to remove yourself from the scene if needed.

Look for clues at the scene as to what may have happened: for example, an overturned table with blood on the corner indicating where a patient fell. Information from the scene size-up is key to the hospital staff who will be caring for the patient.

As always, consider the need for spinal precautions based on dispatch information and your assessment of the scene as you approach the patient.

Consider the mechanism of injury (MOI) or history of present illness. Look for signs of potential trauma (MOI), indications of a previous medical condition such as diabetic supplies or medical alert tags, and evidence of a seizure. Did anyone witness what happened? When was the last time anyone saw the patient appearing healthy? Most patients with a neurologic emergency have a change in their LOC and their ability to interact with their environment and others.

The AEIOU-TIPS mnemonic is helpful for remembering causes of a decreased LOC. When assessing a patient with an altered mental status, consider these causes Table 19-4.

Examine the scene to ascertain the number of patients. One patient with a headache does not stand out. If an entire family in the same house complains of headache, consider the possibility of carbon monoxide exposure. In such a case, the scene may be unsafe.

Table 19-4 AEIOU-TIPS: Altered Mental Status Causes

Letter	Name	Signs and Symptoms
A	Alcohol	Intoxication; slurred speech; ataxia; odor of alcohol on breath; tremors; hallucinations
	Acidosis	Multiple causes; tachypnea and hyperpnea are common
E	Epilepsy (seizure)	Aura; hypertonic, tonic-clonic activity; postictal state
	Endocrine	For thyroid conditions, increased metabolism (hyperthermia, hypertension, tachypnea, tachycardia) OR decreased metabolism (hypothermia, bradycardia, bradypnea, and hypotension)
	Electrolytes	Dehydration; renal failure; liver failure; ECG changes, etc.
I	Insulin	Diaphoresis; tachycardia; tremors; ataxia
O	Opiates	Constricted pupils; decreased LOC; bradypnea; cyanosis
	Other drugs	Varies depending on agent involved; track marks; drug paraphernalia
U	Uremia (kidney failure)	Nausea/vomiting; uremic frost; muscle cramping; dysrhythmias; pulmonary edema
T	Trauma	Generally, hypotension causes altered LOC or direct head injury.
	Temperature	Hyperthermia (exertional, environmental, or endocrine); hypothermia (environmental, endocrine, situational [eg, immobile person lying on floor for days])
I	Infection	Fever; rash; malaise; tachycardia; tachypnea; skin may be cold or warm depending on degree of infection
P	Poisoning	Varies depending on agent involved; empty pill bottles; chemical odors within a child's mouth; broken leaves of plants, open containers of pesticide
	Psychogenic causes	Delusions; hallucinations; disorganization; bizarre behavior or posture
S	Shock	Decreased blood pressure and other signs of poor perfusion
	Stroke	Facial droop; slurred speech; ataxia; abnormal/irregular respiratory pattern; potential bradycardia
	Syncope	Prodrome of weakness or loss of peripheral vision, then LOC which resolves quickly.
	Space-occupying lesion	Headache; new onset seizures; strokelike symptoms
	Subarachnoid hemorrhage	Thunderclap headache; worst headache of life; signs and symptoms of stroke; seizures

Abbreviations: ECG, electrocardiogram; LOC, level of consciousness

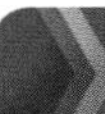

Finally, if the time it takes to get to the nearest stroke center is greater than 1 hour, then request air medical transport early if available.

Primary Survey

As you approach the patient, note the patient's body position and LOC. Observe for seizure activity. Most seizures will be over by the time you arrive. If the seizure is still occurring, the potentially life-threatening condition of status epilepticus may be present. If the patient is in a postictal state, he or she may be unresponsive or starting to regain awareness of the surroundings. Determining the patient's LOC should be first course of action.

If the patient does not respond to verbal stimuli, consider whether he or she may be displaying abnormal posturing; this may indicate severe brain dysfunction. There are two main abnormal postures that the patient may demonstrate with painful stimulation—decorticate and decerebrate. If you see either posture, you should immediately consider the patient to be in critical condition, because these postures represent substantial ICP.

In **decorticate posturing** (abnormal flexion), the patient contracts the arms and curls them toward the chest. At the same time, he or she points the toes. Finally, the wrists are flexed. This posture may indicate damage to the area directly below the cerebral hemispheres **Figure 19-13**. You can easily remember the meaning because with decorticate posturing, the patient's hands are flexed toward his or her core. In **decerebrate posturing** (extension), the patient again points the toes, but now extends the arms outward and rotates the lower arms in a palms-down manner (**pronation**). The wrists and hands are again flexed **Figure 19-14**. This posture is

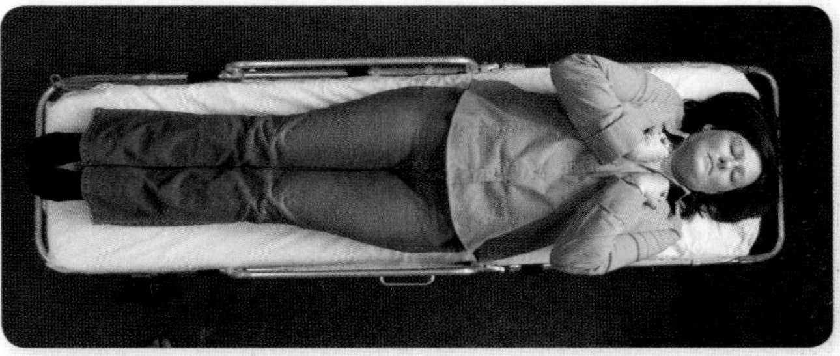

Figure 19-13 Decorticate posturing (abnormal flexion).
Courtesy of Chuck Sowerbrower, MED, NREMT-P.

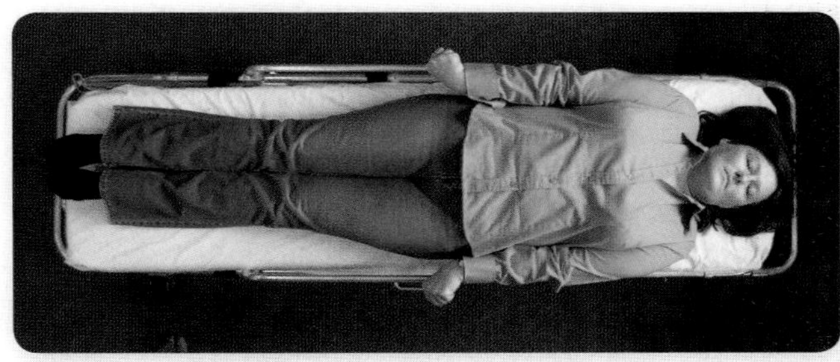

Figure 19-14 Decerebrate posturing (extension).
Courtesy of Chuck Sowerbrower, MED, NREMT-P.

YOU are the Provider — PART 3

After calling the hospital, your partner advises you that medical control has directed you to transport the patient to Miami General Hospital (MGH), approximately 25 minutes away. There is no neurologist on duty at the local hospital today. You inform your partner of the patient's serious condition and proceed to load him into the ambulance. Your partner applies a nonrebreathing mask with oxygen at 15 L/min, while you insert an 18-gauge IV line. After the IV line is secured, you instruct your partner to initiate emergency transport to MGH.

Recording Time: 12 Minutes	
Respirations	12 breaths/min
Pulse	Strong and regular; 74 beats/min
Skin	Warm, dry, and pink
Blood pressure	246/168 mm Hg
Oxygen saturation (Spo_2)	100% at 15 L/min via nonrebreathing mask
Pupils	Left pupil nonreactive

5. What conditions mimicking stroke should AEMTs consider?
6. Should this patient receive a bolus of IV fluid?

a more severe finding than decorticate posturing. In decerebrate posturing, the level of damage is within or near the brainstem (diencephalon/pons/midbrain).

Focus on the patient's airway and breathing on arrival. If the patient is unresponsive and apneic, immediately assess for a pulse and begin chest compressions if pulseless. Evaluate the airway of an unresponsive patient to make sure it is patent and will remain that way. Patients who have experienced a stroke may have difficulty swallowing and are at risk for choking on their own saliva. Continually reassess the airway for patency and respiratory rate and quality. If the patient requires assistance maintaining an airway, consider an oropharyngeal or nasopharyngeal airway. Provide suction and position the patient to prevent aspiration. If you determine that the patient cannot protect his or her airway, place the patient in the recovery position to help prevent secretions from entering the airway.

A patient who has had or is having a seizure may have been eating or chewing gum at the time of the seizure, and there may be a foreign body obstruction. Bystanders may have tried to put objects in the patient's mouth to keep the person from "swallowing the tongue," even though this practice is not advised. A seizure patient may clench his or her teeth (**trismus**) and require sedation. Call early for paramedic backup if dealing with a difficult airway.

Assess the patient's breathing. Be sure to check the rate and rhythm of breathing. Rhythms can have subtle changes or be dramatically different from normal. Generally, the greater the deviation from normal, the more severely the nervous system is affected.

Standard stroke care includes titrating oxygen therapy to the patient's need. Evaluate the patient's pulse oximetry to maintain an Spo_2 of greater than 94%.[5] Ensure that your Spo_2 reading is accurate. Use other assessment techniques, such as end-tidal carbon dioxide ($ETCO_2$) if available and necessary, to ensure your patient is breathing adequately. From a respiratory point of view, if the patient is in stable condition, the nasal cannula is probably sufficient.

Unless you are concerned about possible spine fracture, elevate the head 30°. Provide ventilatory support at 10 to 12 breaths/min unless the patient presents with signs of cerebral herniation. Do not increase the rate any higher than 20 breaths/min because hyperventilation will cause vasoconstriction and decrease perfusion to the brain. Do not suction vigorously. Stimulating the cough and gag reflexes will increase ICP.

Assess circulation beginning with the pulse. As mentioned, if no pulse is found, immediately begin cardiopulmonary resuscitation beginning with chest compressions, and attach an automated external defibrillator. If the pulse is present, determine whether it is fast or slow, weak or strong, or if it is bounding. Evaluate the peripheral and central pulse pressures. Are they the same? The absence of a peripheral pulse with a central pulse present should cause you to suspect shock. What are the characteristics of the skin? Do you see evidence of gross bleeding?

Assess vital signs for evidence of increased ICP. With increased ICP, the blood pressure rises, the heart rates decrease, respiratory rates become irregular, and the pulse pressure widens (systolic hypertension). This set of conditions—known as the Cushing reflex—is the opposite of what is expected in shock.

> **Special Populations**
>
> When you are assessing an infant for increased ICP, consider the quality of the cry. As the ICP increases, the pitch of the cry will increase until a shriek similar to that of a cat can be heard. At the same time, the shape of the pupils can change from round to more oval. These two findings lead to the saying related to infants and increased ICP: "cat's eyes and cat's cries."

At this point in the examination, you should make a transport decision. Unstable patients—those with inadequate or deteriorating ABCs or a substantial MOI or nature of illness—should be transported rapidly to the closest most appropriate facility. Defer gathering detailed information about patients in critical condition; instead, focus on stabilizing and maintaining ABCs. With stable patients—those with normal primary survey findings and a minor MOI or nature of illness—you have more time to gather detailed information at the scene.

If you suspect the patient is experiencing a stroke, you should rapidly transport the patient to an appropriate facility, preferably a stroke center, to ensure that every chance is available to reduce the disability caused by an ischemic stroke. Fibrinolytic medications, commonly referred to as "clot busters," have been shown to reverse symptoms, thus aborting the stroke, if administered within 3 to 4.5 hours after the onset of symptoms for strokes caused by thrombotic or embolic events. Interview family members or bystanders to determine when the patient was last seen "normal" and document the time. Rapid recognition and transport to an appropriate facility may prevent permanent damage and decrease mortality.

Some facilities will need to contact technicians to operate the CT scanners during night hours or weekends; early notification to the emergency department can decrease the time to begin obtaining the scan. If the patient's condition is rapidly decompensating or you suspect a potential stroke, consider transport to a designated stroke center.

If you suspect the patient may have experienced a stroke, place him or her in a comfortable position, usually on one side, with the paralyzed side down and well protected with padding **Figure 19-15**. The patient's head should be elevated approximately 6 inches.

After you begin transport, you should relay the information you have obtained to the receiving hospital, including the time that the patient was last seen to be normal, the findings of your neurologic examination, and the time you anticipate arriving at the hospital.

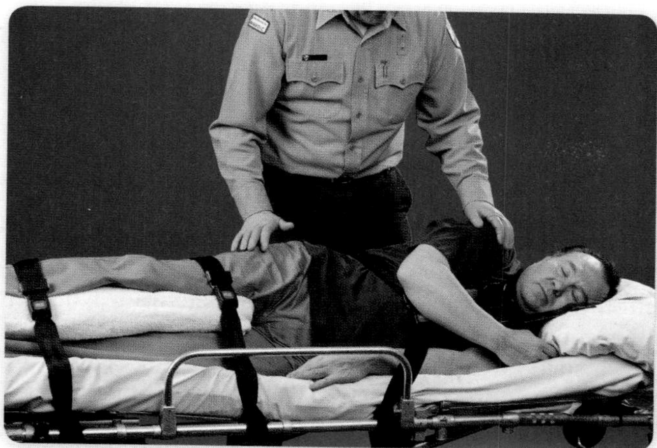

Figure 19-15 A patient who has experienced a stroke should be positioned with the paralyzed side down and well protected with padding. Elevate the head approximately 6 inches.

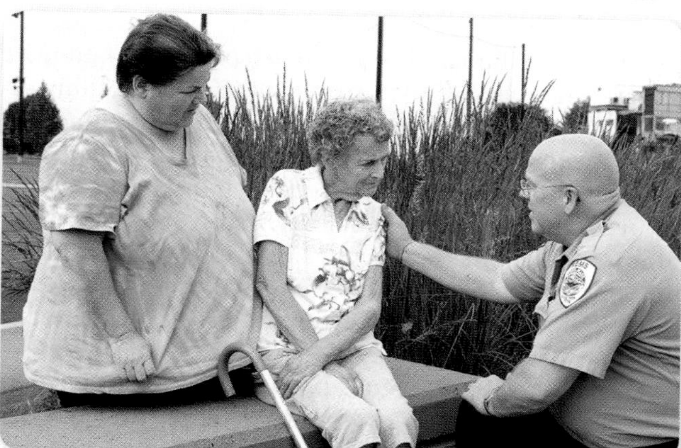

Figure 19-16 Try to speak with family members or bystanders who may have seen what happened. They may also be able to tell you when the patient last appeared "normal."

Special Populations

When you are working with geriatric patients, take their past medical history into account. Patients with a history of dementia could be complicated to manage. The primary question is: "How much change has occurred in the patient's LOC?" Do not assume that the patient's baseline LOC is what you would consider "normal"; speak to the family, friends, or other caregivers to determine the patient's baseline LOC and document that level clearly. It is also important to remember that stroke is common in this age group.

History Taking

Obtain a history from patients who are in stable condition and have minor complaints.

If the patient is unresponsive, you will need to gather any history of the present illness from family or bystanders **Figure 19-16**. If no one is around, quickly look for explanations for the altered mental status (for example, signs of trauma, medical alert tags, track marks, and environmental clues such as empty alcohol or medication containers).

Question the responsive patient about the chief complaint. If the mental status is altered, look for signs and symptoms that may indicate a cause, such as a stroke (eg, hemiparalysis or single-side weakness), and determine whether there is any evidence of a seizure (eg, incontinence or a bitten tongue). Evaluate the patient's speech. Is the patient making any sense? Is speech slurred?

Look for any obvious trauma or explanations if you suspect the patient may have had a seizure.

Special Populations

Meningitis is a consideration when dealing with pediatric patients exhibiting signs of increased ICP. A patient with bacterial meningitis can progress rapidly from appearing mildly ill to coma and even death.

The symptoms of meningitis vary depending on the age of the child and the infectious agent. In general, the younger the child, the vaguer the symptoms. A newborn with early bacterial meningitis may have a fever as the only symptom. Young infants will often have fever and perhaps localized signs such as lethargy, irritability, poor feeding, and a bulging fontanelle. They rarely show typical signs such as nuchal rigidity until they are older. Verbal children will often complain of headaches and neck pain. An altered LOC and seizures are ominous symptoms at any age.

Children with meningococcal sepsis and meningitis get sick extremely fast, so move quickly through your assessment. Form a general impression and perform a primary survey as usual, keeping in mind that symptoms may be quite varied. Look for fever, altered mental status, bulging fontanelle, photophobia, nuchal rigidity, irritability, petechiae (small, pinpoint red spots), purpura (larger purple or black spots), and signs of shock. Assess glucose levels because hypoglycemia may result from the hypermetabolic state. Treat symptomatically and provide prompt transport to the closest, most appropriate facility.

If the patient has a headache, try to determine the patient's level of stress, possible infections, and history of headaches. Stroke patients can also experience headaches. If you suspect a more complicated problem, perform a rapid scan to ensure that you give the patient the best possible care.

Obtain a SAMPLE history (Signs and symptoms, Allergies, Medications, Pertinent past medical history, Last oral intake,

Events leading up to the illness or injury) from the patient or bystanders if possible. Also try to speak with family or friends who may be able to explain the events leading up to the altered mental status, remembering that time can be critical in a neurologic emergency. Many times, you will find out only that the patient seemed normal when he or she went to sleep the night before. In such an instance, the time the patient was last seen to be normal was at bedtime, not when the patient awoke with symptoms. In some cases, pinning down the exact time the stroke began can be difficult, such as with patients who live alone.

Obtain or list all medications the patient has taken, and record the patient's general health before this episode. When possible, determine allergies and the patient's last oral intake.

Although a patient who has experienced a stroke may appear to be unresponsive and unable to speak, the patient may still be able to hear and understand what is taking place. Therefore, you should treat the patient as if he or she is able to hear. Try to communicate with the patient by looking for indications that the patient can understand you, such as a glance, gaze, motion or pressure of the hand, effort to speak, or head nod. Allow the patient to write responses if he or she is able. Reassure the patient often. Establishing effective communication can help you to calm the patient and lessen the fear that accompanies an inability to communicate.

For patients who have had a seizure, your SAMPLE history should reveal whether the patient has a history of seizures. If so, it is important to find out how the patient's seizures typically occur and whether this episode differs in some way from previous episodes. You should also ask what medications the patient has been taking and if he or she is compliant. If the patient takes phenytoin (Dilantin) and phenobarbital (for example, Solfoton), he or she most likely has a seizure disorder. You might find that the patient ran out of medication or stopped taking the medication for a time. Patients who have a history of seizures *and* diabetes may use up all the glucose in the body to fuel the seizure resulting in hypoglycemia and an altered mental status that does not resolve spontaneously after the patient's seizure stops.

If the patient does not have a history of seizures and now suddenly has a seizure, a serious condition, such as a brain tumor, intracranial bleeding, or serious infection should be suspected. You should also determine whether the patient takes medications that lower the blood glucose level, such as insulin and oral hypoglycemic agents. In other situations, you may want to inquire about drug use or exposure to poisons.

Secondary Assessment

As soon as possible, perform a secondary assessment. Look for potential causes of neurologic signs and symptoms, such as trauma not previously noticed. Does the patient have any complaints related to the abdomen? Signs of nausea and vomiting are common with some neurologic conditions, such as headaches and increased ICP. Note whether the patient is incontinent; urinary and fecal incontinence are common findings with seizures or syncope. The patient should also be assessed for injuries, including head lacerations, shoulder dislocation, bitten tongue, and long bone fractures.

Rapid identification of a stroke is imperative. You should perform at least three key physical tests on patients you suspect of having experienced a stroke: tests of speech, facial movement, and arm movement. If any one of the three is positive (abnormal), you should assume that the patient is experiencing (or has had) a stroke.

Common stroke assessment tools include the Cincinnati Prehospital Stroke Scale **Table 19-5** and the

Table 19-5 Cincinnati Prehospital Stroke Scale

Assessment	Normal	Abnormal
Facial Droop		
Ask the patient to smile and show his or her teeth.	Both sides of face move equally well.	One side of face does not move as well as the other side.
Arm Drift		
Ask the patient to close the eyes and hold both arms out with palms up for 10 seconds.	Both arms move the same or neither arm moves. (If neither arm moves, then this may indicate the patient did not understand the instructions. Perform the test again.)	One arm does not move, or one arm drifts down compared with the other.
Speech		
Ask the patient to say, "The sky is blue in Cincinnati."	Patient uses correct words with no slurring.	Patient slurs words, uses inappropriate words, or is unable to speak.

Interpretation: If any one item is abnormal, then the probability of a stroke is 72%.

Table 19-6 Los Angeles Prehospital Stroke Screen

Criteria	Yes	Unknown	No
1. Age > 45 years	☐	☐	☐
2. History of seizures or epilepsy absent	☐	☐	☐
3. Symptoms < 24 hours	☐	☐	☐
4. At baseline, patient does not use a wheelchair or is not bedridden.	☐	☐	☐
5. Blood glucose between 60 and 400 mg/dL	☐	☐	☐
6. Obvious asymmetry (right vs left) in any of the following three exam categories (must be unilateral):	☐	☐	☐
	Equal	**Right Weak**	**Left Weak**
Facial smile/grimace	☐	☐ Droop	☐ Droop
Grip	☐	☐ Weak grip ☐ No grip	☐ Weak grip ☐ No grip
Arm strength	☐	☐ Drifts down ☐ Falls rapidly	☐ Drifts down ☐ Falls rapidly

Interpretation: If criteria 1–6 are marked yes, the probability of a stroke is 97%.

Los Angeles Prehospital Stroke Screen Table 19-6. Also, the checklist presented in Table 19-7 will help you focus on gathering the information that the emergency department physician will need before administration of fibrinolytic medications can be considered.

All patients with altered mental status (stroke, TIA, seizure, of unknown cause) should also have a Glasgow Coma Scale (GCS) score calculated Table 19-8.

Given how critical normal perfusion of the brain is, blood pressure must be closely monitored in any patient with a potential ICP problem. Frequent assessment becomes even more essential when a decrease in blood pressure is also present. For any patient at risk for increased ICP, ensure a systolic blood pressure of at least 110 to 120 mm Hg is maintained.

Changes in pupil size and reactivity may indicate herniation typically associated with substantial bleeding and/or pressure on the brain. As pressure is increased, the pupil on the injured side of the brain will become larger or fully dilated (blown) as the oculomotor nerve is compressed by the swelling. If the patient has an altered mental status (regardless of the cause), you should check the blood glucose level. During most active seizures, it is impossible to evaluate vital signs. Unless the situation is unusual, vital signs in a postictal state will approximate normal. Obtain pulse rate, rhythm, and character; respiratory rate, quality, and degree of distress; blood pressure; skin color, temperature, and condition; blood glucose level; and pupil size and reactivity.

Glucose levels of less than 10 mg/dL are incompatible with brain functioning and typically lethal. Chapter 10, *Patient Assessment*, discusses the use of a glucometer in detail.

Determine the pulse oximeter reading, remembering that normal readings are greater than 94% and that this number is affected by the amount of hemoglobin within the body, perfusion status, cold environments, and the presence of carbon monoxide. If possible, monitor $ETCO_2$ levels. Normal readings are 35 to 45 mm Hg. Higher levels suggest inadequate ventilation.

Reassessment

Reassessment is intended to reassess ABCDEs (Airway, Breathing, Circulation, Disability, and Exposure), vital signs, and interventions and to monitor patients for changes. Casual conversation will allow you to closely monitor brain functions. If the patient is nonverbal, keep a close eye on respiratory patterns and eye and body movements, and monitor for seizure activity.

Routine monitoring should include heart rate, blood pressure, respiratory rate and pattern, pulse oximetry and/or $ETCO_2$, repeated glucose level (if the level was

Table 19-7 Sample Prehospital Fibrinolytic Checklist for Stroke

Use this checklist for all patients suspected of experiencing a stroke.

DATE: __________ TIME: __________		Time signs and symptoms began (record time). If unknown, answer the next question.
DATE: __________ TIME: __________		Time patient was last seen to be normal (record time)
__________ mg/dL		Blood glucose level (record number)
_______/_______ Manual Automatic Right arm Left arm		Blood pressure (record readings, circle method and location)
Yes	No	(Check Yes or No for each item.)
☐	☐	Facial droop?
☐	☐	Slurred speech?
☐	☐	Arm drift (eyes closed and held for 10 seconds)?
☐	☐	In the past 7 days, has the patient undergone a procedure in which an artery was punctured?
☐	☐	In the past 14 days, has the patient undergone a major operation or serious trauma?
☐	☐	In the past 21 days, has the patient had any bleeding from the gastrointestinal or urinary tract?
☐	☐	In the past 3 months, has the patient experienced a myocardial infarction, stroke, or head trauma?
☐	☐	When the signs and symptoms began, did the patient experience a seizure?
☐	☐	Are current bleeding or clotting problems evident?
☐	☐	Is the patient taking anticoagulant medication?
☐	☐	Does the patient have intracranial bleeding either now or in the past?
☐	☐	Are the patient's signs and symptoms of stroke rapidly improving?

Table 19-8 Glasgow Coma Scale

Eye Opening		Best Verbal Response		Best Motor Response	
Spontaneous	4	Oriented conversation	5	Obeys commands	6
In response to sound	3	Confused conversation	4	Localizes pain or pressure	5
In response to pressure	2	Words	3	Normal flexion	4
No response	1	Sounds	2	Abnormal flexion	3
		No response	1	Extension	2
				No response	1

Score: 13–15 may indicate mild dysfunction, although 15 is the score a person without neurologic impairment would receive.
Score: 9–12 may indicate moderate dysfunction.
Score: 8 or less is indicative of severe dysfunction.

low and glucose was given to the patient), and GCS scores. Provide oxygenation and ventilation as needed. Monitor the IV fluids closely to ensure that accidental fluid overload does not occur. Modify treatment based on patient changes.

Observe for recurrent seizures. If another seizure occurs, note whether it starts at a focal part of the body (for example, one arm or one leg) and then progresses to the rest of the body. Most important, evaluate the patient's mental status and monitor it frequently to verify progressive improvement.

Always provide emotional support. Many patients who experience seizures are frustrated with their condition and may refuse transport. Kindness and professional behavior are required to help convince a reluctant patient that transport is necessary for definitive care.

Notify the receiving facility of your patient's chief complaint and your assessment findings. Most designated stroke centers will want you to call a stroke alert for patients you have assessed and found to be experiencing a stroke (check local protocol). This will alert the stroke team members at the hospital and give them time to assemble their resources to treat the patient without delay. Be sure to communicate the time that the patient was last seen to be healthy, the findings of your neurologic examination, and estimated time of arrival.

Document your findings from your stroke scale and the score results of the GCS, along with any changes you found in your reassessment. Document all interventions, including the position in which the patient was placed.

For patients who have experienced a seizure, give a description of the seizure activity, if known. Include bystanders' comments if they witnessed the seizure. Document the onset and duration of the seizure, and whether the patient noticed an aura. Record any evidence of trauma and interventions performed. Document whether the patient has a history of seizures and, if so, the frequency of the seizures and whether there is a history of status epilepticus. Record interventions performed and the patient's response along with the findings of continued reassessments.

Words of Wisdom

You may be the only provider to witness some patient activity, so accurate and complete documentation is critical to ensure continuity of care.

Emergency Medical Care

A patient with stroke, seizure, hypoglycemia, or hypoxia typically shows identifiable signs or symptoms, and treatment options are readily available. With other neurologic emergencies, the cause of the patient's symptoms will not always be obvious and more diagnostic testing may be needed to determine the cause. Most of your interventions will be based on your assessment findings. Your best treatment is determined by performing a thorough assessment and maintaining the ABCs.

Two medications are available for prehospital treatment of hypoglycemia: dextrose and glucagon. In patients suspected of experiencing a stroke, and *ONLY* if the patient's blood glucose level is low, give dextrose. Consider the administration of glucagon for hypoglycemia as an alternative. Use an isotonic crystalloid solution at a to-keep-open (TKO) rate unless the patient is hypovolemic. If hypotensive, give a fluid bolus of 20 mL/kg to maintain adequate perfusion (for example, to maintain the radial pulses), reducing the flow to a TKO rate after radial pulses have returned. Excessive fluids will increase bleeding in patients with hemorrhagic strokes as well as increase ICP.

If you cannot check the patient's blood glucose level because of equipment failure, you need to be more cautious in administering dextrose. In a situation in which the patient is unresponsive or has a decreased LOC and no blood glucose monitor is available, administer 12.5 g (one-half of a syringe) and then reassess the response. Proceed with additional dextrose cautiously, based on responses to previous doses. Hyperglycemia can increase the morbidity rate among stroke patients. Remember, however, that hypoglycemia is *more lethal* than hyperglycemia. If in doubt, err on the side of administering glucose.

When administering intravenous dextrose in the form of D_{50}, you must establish IV access with a large-bore catheter (preferrably 18 gauge) within a large vessel because D_{50} is quite viscous. Ensure that the IV line is patent before you attempt to give the D_{50}. Extravasation of D_{50} into the interstitial space can cause severe damage to muscles, nerves, and skin or even death of these tissues. The usual dose is 25 g of D_{50} or one full syringe. The effects from dextrose typically begin in 30 seconds to 2 minutes. If no effect is apparent or the patient's blood glucose level remains low, ensure adequate IV access and administer additional dextrose.

Words of Wisdom

Many jurisdictions and agencies do not use D_{50} because of the risk to local tissues associated with the high viscosity and the need for a relatively large-gauge catheter to facilitate administration. Hypoglycemia can be treated as effectively and with fewer risks using the same total dose of glucose in a lower concentration (D_{25} or D_{10}). Although administration of the same dose of glucose requires more fluid, the solution is less viscous, less toxic to local tissues, and generally more comfortable to the patient.

Dextrose is commonly supplied in these formats. Note that these all contain the same total dose of dextrose, but the volume of fluid that must be administered increases as the concentration decreases.

- D_{50}: 25 g in 50 mL
- D_{25}: 25 g in 100 mL
- D_{10}: 25 g in 250 mL

If you cannot obtain vascular access, administer 0.5 to 1 mg of glucagon subcutaneously or intramuscularly or consider intraosseous access for glucose administration. The LOC and blood glucose level should increase within 20 minutes after administration of glucagon. If the blood glucose level remains low, repeat the glucagon for a maximum of three doses.

Oral glucose administration is another option for patients with a decreased LOC who can protect their own airways (generally determined by their ability to speak clearly) and therefore swallow safely. Assess the patients carefully, confirming that they are awake enough to follow commands. First give them a small amount of water to drink—maybe 10 mL. If they can swallow that amount, consider administering oral glucose, 25 g (one tube). Alternatives to oral glucose include cake icing, a plain chocolate bar, or orange juice with sugar added. Administration of sugar by mouth will take longer to raise the blood glucose level. Constantly supervise patients as they consume the sugar. To the extent possible, make sure they do not aspirate.

Currently, there is no safe way to lower a high blood glucose level in the field. For patients with hyperglycemia, provide standard care and ensure adequate blood pressure. Hyperglycemic patients are often dehydrated and usually need volume support. Note that rehydration alone in a severely dehydrated patient with hyperglycemia can dramatically lower the patient's blood glucose level.

Finally, provide emotional support for the patient and family. Neurologic emergencies can produce confusion, fear, anger, and helplessness. Consider a therapeutic gentle touch on the shoulder. Touch can communicate compassion. Use a calm, reassuring voice to show that you are there to help. Try to reorient the patient often because confusion is often present in neurologic emergencies.

▶ Stroke

Because it is often impossible to differentiate the symptoms of a TIA from a stroke, assume that a patient with TIA or stroke symptoms is experiencing a stroke. Administer supplemental oxygen to maintain Spo_2 at greater than 94% or, if needed, assist ventilations.[12,13] Establish IV access, and obtain blood samples for analysis. Transport the patient to the closest appropriate facility for evaluation.

In most patients with a suspected stroke, CT is needed for a physician to determine whether there is bleeding in the brain. If there is no bleeding, the patient may be a candidate for clot-dissolving medication that may help brain cells survive.

Most treatments for stroke must be started as soon as possible after the onset of the event Table 19-9. Current treatments are often effective if they are started within 3 hours after the stroke begins. However, for certain patients, treatment may be effective if started up to 4.5 hours after onset.[14-16] Therefore, even if 3 hours have passed since the onset of symptoms, prompt action on your part is essential.

In patients who are unresponsive and demonstrate other signs of increased ICP, administer fluids as needed. Unless you are concerned about possible spinal injury, elevate the patient's head 30°.[5] This change will cause a slight decrease in ICP. Ensure that the airway is clear, but do not vigorously suction because stimulating the cough and gag reflexes will increase ICP. Watch for seizures and call early for paramedic backup. The patient may also be bradycardic because of the ICP. Notify the hospital and provide rapid transport.

YOU are the Provider — PART 4

As you are transporting the patient, you perform a rapid full-body scan to rule out the possibility of trauma as a cause of his symptoms. Finding no trauma and having ruled out the possible conditions mimicking stroke, you are confident in your initial suspicion that this patient has experienced a stroke. You attempt to ask the patient about onset, symptoms, and other pertinent findings. However, you are unable to obtain useful information because of the patient's slurred speech.

Recording Time: 23 Minutes	
Respirations	12 breaths/min
Pulse	Strong and regular; 71 beats/min
Skin	Warm, dry, and pink
Blood pressure	266/174 mm Hg
Oxygen saturation (Spo_2)	100% at 15 L/min via nonrebreathing mask
Pupils	Left pupil nonreactive

7. What is the most important piece of information to give to the receiving physician regarding this patient's stroke?

Table 19-9 Tips on Patient Care for a Possible Stroke Patient
Patients who experience a TIA typically have the same signs and symptoms as patients who experience a stroke. These signs and symptoms can last from minutes up to 24 hours. Therefore, the signs of stroke that you note on arrival may gradually resolve. Patients who appear to have had a TIA should be transported for further evaluation.
Place the patient's affected or paralyzed extremity in a secure, safe position during patient movement and transport. Consider elevating the head 30° (6 inches) to assist with intracranial pressure if there is no concern for spinal injury.
Some patients who have experienced a stroke may be unable to communicate, but they can often understand what is being said around them. Be aware of this possibility.
New therapies for stroke must be used shortly after the onset of symptoms. Minimize time on the scene, and notify the receiving hospital as soon as possible.

Abbreviation: TIA, transient ischemic attack

It is important for you to monitor blood pressure closely in any patient with a potential problem with ICP. Frequent assessment becomes even more critical when a decrease in blood pressure is also present. For any patient at risk for ICP, ensure that the systolic blood pressure remains at least 110 to 120 mm Hg.

Carbon dioxide and oxygen levels are important in patients with increased ICP. A low carbon dioxide level causes constriction of the cerebral arteries. This vasoconstriction further impairs perfusion to the brain. Low oxygen levels markedly increase mortality in patients with brain injury. Never allow a patient with brain injury or stroke to become hypoxic. Restoration of normal levels of ventilation is critically important. In general, do not hyperventilate patients, as this may decrease cerebral perfusion pressure.

In select situations associated with evidence of markedly increased intracranial pressure and impending herniation, slight increase in the ventilatory rate to approximately 20 breaths/min with a goal of decreasing the $ETCO_2$ levels to 30 to 35 mm Hg may be valuable.[5,17] These circumstances include patients with an acute deterioration in their GCS score by 2 or more points and resultant GCS that is below 9. In addition, patients with a GCS score below 9 in whom a unilateral pupillary constriction develops that is unresponsive to light (blown pupil) are at risk for acute herniation and might benefit from limited hyperventilation.

Consider the AHA algorithm that shows goals for the treatment of patients with suspected stroke Figure 19-17. Treatment at the hospital takes different paths of care for each type of stroke. One feature, however, is common to both: time is essential. For ischemic strokes, fibrinolytics need to be administered within 3 to 4.5 hours of onset. In hemorrhagic strokes, the more the patient bleeds into the cranium, the greater the potential for increased ICP and brainstem damage.

Regarding hypertension, currently, there is no AHA/American Stroke Association guideline for its control in the prehospital setting. Do not administer aspirin in the field; it is helpful in patients with ischemic stroke but is harmful in patients with hemorrhagic stroke. Aspirin should be administered only after CT or magnetic resonance imaging has been completed in the hospital.

Finally, because patients may not be able to feel or move their arms or legs, make sure to protect them from injury.

Transient Ischemic Attack

As with strokes, management of TIAs begins with standard care. Follow the same management guidelines as for stroke. Close neurologic assessment is needed. Patients may experience multiple TIAs in a short time frame.

Strongly encourage the patient to be transported. If the patient refuses transportation, appeal to the patient's family for assistance. Encourage the patient to seek medical care very soon. Offer to return, and tell the patient to call 9-1-1 again if he or she wants. It is important to reinforce the message that the TIA is a warning sign of a serious and potentially deadly problem with the blood vessels in the brain.

Seizures

In most situations, patients who have had a seizure require definitive evaluation and treatment in the hospital. Even a patient who has a history of chronic epilepsy that is controlled with medications may have an occasional seizure, commonly referred to as a breakthrough seizure, and should also be taken to the hospital for evaluation. At the hospital, blood levels of seizure medications are checked to ensure that patients are receiving the correct dose. Clearly, patients who have just had their first seizure and patients with chronic seizures who have had an episode that is "different" require immediate evaluation to rule out life-threatening conditions.

For patients who are having a seizure, protect them from harm, maintain a clear airway by suctioning as necessary, and provide oxygen as quickly as possible. If trauma is suspected, provide spinal immobilization. With recurrent seizures, protect the patient from further injury, and manage the airway after the seizure ceases.

For patients who continue to have a seizure, as in status epilepticus, suction the airway, provide positive-pressure ventilations (bag-mask ventilations), and transport quickly to the hospital. If you have the option to rendezvous with paramedics, you should do so. Paramedics can administer medications that can stop a prolonged seizure.

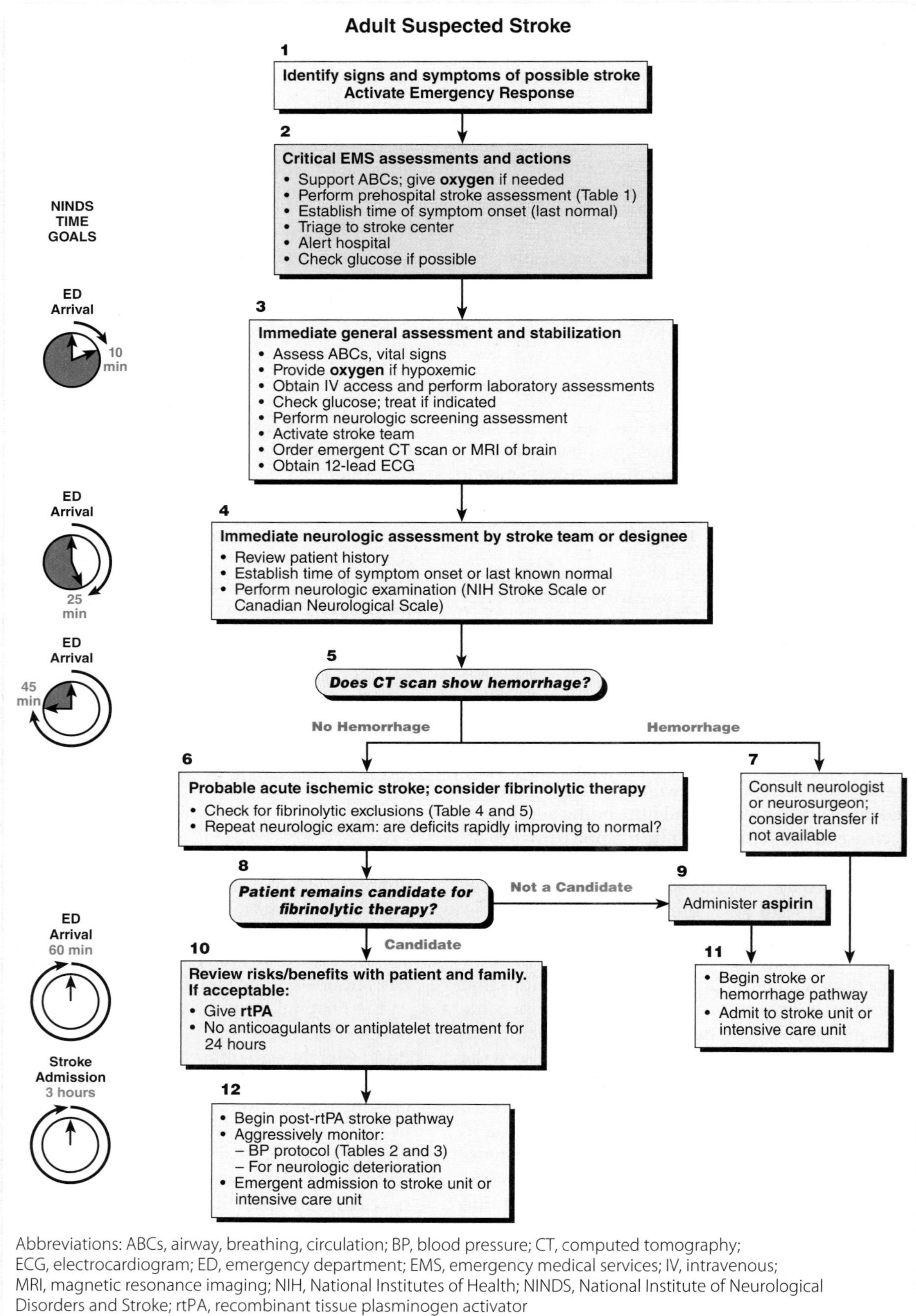

Adult Suspected Stroke
1
Identify signs and symptoms of possible stroke
Activate Emergency Response
2
Critical EMS assessments and actions
• Support ABCs; give oxygen if needed
• Perform prehospital stroke assessment (Table 1)
• Establish time of symptom onset (last normal)
• Triage to stroke center
• Alert hospital
• Check glucose if possible
NINDS TIME GOALS
ED Arrival
10 min
3
Immediate general assessment and stabilization
• Assess ABCs, vital signs
• Provide oxygen if hypoxemic
• Obtain IV access and perform laboratory assessments
• Check glucose; treat if indicated
• Perform neurologic screening assessment
• Activate stroke team
• Order emergent CT scan or MRI of brain
• Obtain 12-lead ECG
ED Arrival
25 min
4
Immediate neurologic assessment by stroke team or designee
• Review patient history
• Establish time of symptom onset or last known normal
• Perform neurologic examination (NIH Stroke Scale or Canadian Neurological Scale)
ED Arrival
45 min
5
Does CT scan show hemorrhage?
No Hemorrhage
Hemorrhage
6
Probable acute ischemic stroke; consider fibrinolytic therapy
• Check for fibrinolytic exclusions (Table 4 and 5)
• Repeat neurologic exam: are deficits rapidly improving to normal?
7
Consult neurologist or neurosurgeon; consider transfer if not available
8
Patient remains candidate for fibrinolytic therapy?
Not a Candidate
9
Administer aspirin
ED Arrival
60 min
Candidate
10
Review risks/benefits with patient and family.
If acceptable:
• Give rtPA
• No anticoagulants or antiplatelet treatment for 24 hours
11
• Begin stroke or hemorrhage pathway
• Admit to stroke unit or intensive care unit
Stroke Admission
3 hours
12
• Begin post-rtPA stroke pathway
• Aggressively monitor:
– BP protocol (Tables 2 and 3)
– For neurologic deterioration
• Emergent admission to stroke unit or intensive care unit
Abbreviations: ABCs, airway, breathing, circulation; BP, blood pressure; CT, computed tomography; ECG, electrocardiogram; ED, emergency department; EMS, emergency medical services; IV, intravenous; MRI, magnetic resonance imaging; NIH, National Institutes of Health; NINDS, National Institute of Neurological Disorders and Stroke; rtPA, recombinant tissue plasminogen activator

Figure 19-17 The Adult Suspected Stroke Algorithm from the American Heart Association.

Administer oxygen as necessary to maintain an Spo_2 greater than 94% to any patient who has experienced a seizure, whether it is the first or whether the patient has chronic seizures. This intervention will help ameliorate any associated hypoxia. Gain IV access as a medication route even if fluid resuscitation is not needed. Note any medications the patient is currently taking and any previous seizures, the time of onset, the duration of the seizure activity, the number of seizures, and whether the patient was responsive between seizures. Provide spinal immobilization if trauma was involved or cannot be ruled out.

Depending on local protocols, you should assess and treat the patient for possible hypoglycemia (for example, a person with diabetes who has altered mental status and takes insulin or oral agents that lower the blood glucose level). Look for tongue lacerations and bleeding that may create an obstruction or lead to aspiration. With recurrent seizures, protect the patient from further injury and manage the airway as needed.

If you are treating a child whom you suspect is having a febrile seizure, you should attempt to lower the body temperature by removing the child's clothing and cooling the child with tepid water, particularly around the head and neck, and then fanning the moistened areas. Be careful not to make the patient shiver, which will further increase temperature and precipitate another seizure.

In all cases, you exhibit patience and tolerance because many of the patients are likely to be confused and, occasionally, frightened. Many patients who experience seizures are frustrated with their condition and may refuse transport. Compassion and professional behavior are required to help convince the patient that transport is necessary for definitive care.

▶ Syncope

Begin with standard care. Determine whether the patient may have experienced trauma during the fall, and take cervical spine precautions as needed. Focus on the blood glucose level and likely cardiac causes. Obtain orthostatic vital signs, if possible. Provide supplemental oxygen and gain IV access. Evaluate the blood glucose level and oxygen saturation level, and obtain orthostatic vital signs. If the patient's blood pressure remains low, then provide fluids as appropriate, based on the cause of the hypotension. It is important to transport any patient who has a syncopal episode to the hospital to determine the cause.

Provide emotional support; a syncopal episode can be embarrassing. Syncope can be a sign of life-threatening cardiac dysrhythmias, stroke, and other serious medical conditions. Call early for paramedic backup if needed.

▶ Headache

Be cautious because headaches can indicate a more serious problem. Give standard care. Ask which medications the patient has taken. Many patients will appreciate a darkened, quiet environment, so do not use lights and sirens if transporting.

Special Populations

Children can have altered mental status caused by strokes, seizures, and other brain emergencies. However, children who have subarachnoid hemorrhages may not have a berry aneurysm; instead, they may have a congenital problem with the blood vessels in the brain known as an arteriovenous malformation. Children who have sickle cell anemia are at particularly high risk for ischemic stroke. Treat stroke in children the same way that you do in adults.

As mentioned, seizures can result from sudden high fever, particularly in children. Remember that although febrile seizures are generally well tolerated by children, you must transport them to the hospital. The possibility of a second seizure makes transport mandatory so that if other problems develop, the child is in the hospital and can receive immediate, definitive care.

Always assess glucose levels in any patient with an altered mental status. The alteration may be entirely a result of hypoglycemia, or there may be another cause. Either way, hypoglycemia is easy to rule out and can be corrected if present. Also, patients with hypoglycemia require close monitoring, particularly of the airway, en route to the hospital.

YOU are the Provider SUMMARY

1. What mnemonic is useful for assessing adult patients with altered mental status?

When assessing adult patients with altered mental status, consider the mnemonic AEIOU-TIPS. This mnemonic will assist in ruling in or out possible causes of altered mental status.

2. What are the two types of abnormal posturing, and what do they indicate?

There are two main abnormal postures that the patient may demonstrate with painful stimulation: decorticate and decerebrate. If you see either posture, you should immediately consider the patient to be in critical condition, because these postures represent substantial impairment in brain function. In decorticate posturing, the patient demonstrates abnormal flexion by flexing the arms and curling them toward the chest. At the same time, he or she points his or her toes. Finally, the wrists are flexed. You can easily remember the meaning of de*cor*ticate posturing because the patient's hands are flexed toward his or her *core*. In decerebrate posturing (also known as extension posturing), the patient again points the toes, but now extends the arms outward and rotates the lower arms in a palms-down manner (called pronation). The wrists are

YOU are the Provider SUMMARY (continued)

again flexed. This posture is a more severe finding than decorticate posturing.

3. What are the two types of strokes that this patient may be experiencing?

There are two main types of stroke: hemorrhagic and ischemic. An ischemic stroke is caused when blood flow to a particular part of the brain is cut off by a blockage (clot) inside a blood vessel. This can be from a thrombosis or an embolism that blocks blood flow. A hemorrhagic stroke occurs as a result of bleeding inside the brain, typically when a cerebral artery ruptures. The severity of the hemorrhagic stroke depends on the location and size of the ruptured cerebral vessel. As bleeding continues within the brain, ICP increases and compresses brain tissue. When brain tissue is compressed, oxygenated blood cannot get into the area, and the surrounding cells begin to die.

4. Should you move the patient into the back of the ambulance for evaluation?

Further assessments should be deferred until the patient is in the back of the ambulance. If you believe that the patient is experiencing a stroke, "time is brain," and the sooner you are able to transfer the patient to definitive care, the better the patient outcome will be. You should also have a suction unit ready as these patients are likely to vomit.

5. What conditions mimicking stroke should AEMTs consider?

The following three conditions may present similarly to stroke:

- Hypoglycemia (a condition characterized by a low blood glucose level)
- A postictal state (a period following a seizure that lasts between 5 and 30 minutes, characterized by labored respirations and some degree of altered mental status)
- Subdural or epidural bleeding (a collection of blood near the skull that presses on the brain)

Because oxygen and glucose are needed for brain metabolism, a patient with hypoglycemia may present like a patient who is experiencing a stroke. Find out whether the patient's medical history includes diabetes.

A patient in the postictal state may appear to be experiencing a stroke. However, in most cases, a patient having a seizure will recover rapidly (within several minutes), whereas a patient experiencing a stroke will not.

Subdural and epidural bleeding usually occur as a result of trauma. With subdural and epidural bleeding, the onset of strokelike signs and symptoms may be subtle. The patient or family may not even remember the original injury that is causing the bleeding.

6. Should this patient receive a bolus of IV fluid?

A bolus of IV fluid for this patient is absolutely contraindicated because of his current hypertension. By administering fluid, you could potentially increase the patient's blood pressure, which could increase the patient's ICP, causing his condition to worsen.

7. What is the most important piece of information to give to the receiving physician regarding this patient's stroke?

The most important piece of information you can give the receiving physician is the onset of symptoms, or the time the patient was last seen as normal. This information will help physicians in the emergency department decide whether it is safe to begin certain treatments (such as thrombolytic therapy) that must be given within a narrow time frame after the onset of symptoms. You may be the only person with the opportunity to speak with bystanders to obtain this critical information. Many times, you will be able to find out only that the patient seemed normal when he or she went to sleep the night before. In such cases, the time the patient was last seen to be normal was at bedtime, not when the patient awoke with symptoms.

EMS Patient Care Report (PCR)					
Date: 10-07-18	**Incident No.:** 20107184		**Nature of Call:** Intoxicated subject		**Location:** Bearpaw Medicine Shelter
Dispatched: 0354	**En Route:** 0357	**At Scene:** 0408	**Transport:** 0417	**At Hospital:** 0447	**In Service:** 0513
Patient Information					
Age: 62 **Sex:** M **Weight (in kg [lb]):** 85 kg (189 lb)			**Allergies:** Unknown **Medications:** Unknown **Past Medical History:** Ethanol abuse **Chief Complaint:** Altered mental status		

YOU are the Provider SUMMARY *(continued)*

Vital Signs				
Time: 0409	**BP:** Not obtained	**Pulse:** Not obtained	**Respirations:** 12	**Spo_2:** Not obtained
Time: 0420	**BP:** 246/168	**Pulse:** 74	**Respirations:** 12	**Spo_2:** 100% on 15 L/min
Time: 0431	**BP:** 266/174	**Pulse:** 71	**Respirations:** 12	**Spo_2:** 100% on 15 L/min

EMS Treatment (circle all that apply)				
Oxygen @ 15 **L/min via (circle one):** **NC** **(NRM)** **Bag-mask device**		**Assisted Ventilation**	**Airway Adjunct**	**CPR**
Defibrillation	**Bleeding Control**	**Bandaging**	**Splinting**	**Other:**

Narrative

EMS dispatched to above location for possible intoxicated patient. On arrival, met by shelter staff who direct us to patient, well known to EMS, who is found seated on floor, leaning against wall. Patient is alert but has very slurred speech and is unable to answer any questions appropriately. Right-side facial droop noted, along with possible left-side weakness. Cincinnati Prehospital Stroke Scale screening performed; patient "failed" all portions of test. Online medical control (OLMC) contacted with "stroke alert," but OLMC informed us to transport patient to MGH due to lack of neurologist services available. Center staff states patient has alcoholism, but he does not believe that he had a drink yet today. He further states that he last saw the patient as normal about 20 or 30 minutes before calling EMS. Placed patient on cot, secured × 3, initiated emergency transport to MGH. En route: Vitals as above. 18-gauge IV established in left antecubital vein, TKO. Patient is able to maintain a patent airway and handle his own secretions. Rapid scan performed; no obvious trauma noted. Blood glucose noted to be 112 mg/dL. Report called to MGH with condition and ETA. On arrival, care and report given to awaiting stroke team without incident.**End of report**

Prep Kit

▶ Ready for Review

- The nervous system is the most complex organ system within the human body and consists of the brain and spinal cord and thousands of nerves. This system is responsible for fundamental functions such as controlling breathing, heart rate, and blood pressure and higher-level activities. Many disorders can cause neurologic symptoms.
- The central nervous system is responsible for thought, perception, feeling, and autonomic body functions. The peripheral nervous system transmits commands from the brain to the body and receives feedback from the body.
- The cerebrum, the largest part of the brain, is divided into right and left hemispheres, each controlling the opposite side of the body.
- A cerebrovascular accident or stroke is an interruption of blood flow to the brain that often is sudden and results in the loss of function in the affected part of the brain. Loss of brain function occurs within minutes, and brain cells begin to die. Signs and symptoms of stroke include receptive or expressive aphasia, dysarthria, muscle weakness or numbness on one side, facial droop, and, sometimes, hypertension.
- After cells are infarcted, they are dead and cannot be restored; however, cell death may take several hours to occur. Ischemic cells are those that are alive but do not have enough oxygen to function properly; however, function can be restored if normal blood flow is restored to that area of the brain in a timely manner.
- The two types of stroke are hemorrhagic and ischemic. Ischemic stroke occurs when blood flow to part of the brain is cut off by a blockage inside a

Prep Kit (continued)

cerebral artery. Hemorrhagic stroke occurs as a result of bleeding within the brain, typically when a cerebral artery ruptures.

- Hemorrhagic strokes place patients at risk for increased intracranial pressure. Increased pressure within the cranial vault may cause the brain to become ischemic or to herniate.
- In a transient ischemic attack, normal body processes break up the blood clot, restoring blood flow and ending symptoms in less than 24 hours. However, patients with transient ischemic shock are at high risk for a full stroke.
- Because current treatments must be administered within 3 to 4.5 hours of the onset of symptoms to be most effective, you should provide prompt transport.
- Seizures are characterized by unresponsiveness and generalized twitching of all or part of the body. There are types of seizures that you should learn to recognize: generalized, partial, and febrile.
- Seizures may be caused by a congenital disorder, a diabetic emergency, or a fever (if the patient is an infant or child).
- Most seizures last between 3 and 5 minutes and are followed by a postictal state in which the patient may be unresponsive, have labored breathing and hemiparesis, and may have been incontinent. It is important for you to recognize the signs and symptoms of seizures so that you can provide emergency department staff with information during transport.
- Altered mental status is also a common neurologic problem that you will encounter. Signs, symptoms, and causes vary widely. Common causes include hypoglycemia, alcohol intoxication, drug overdose, and poisoning.
- Patients with hypoglycemia can have signs and symptoms that mimic stroke and seizures. The principal difference is that a patient who has experienced a stroke may be alert and attempting to communicate normally, whereas a patient with hypoglycemia almost always has an altered mental status.
- Types of headaches include tension headaches, migraines, and sinus headaches; these are not life threatening, but patients have real pain and need emergency medical services assistance.
- Look for scene clues such as overturned furniture or medical alert tags. Note the patient's position and level of consciousness and, as always, immediately address the airway, breathing, and circulation. Do not suction vigorously. Stimulating the cough and gag reflexes will increase the intracranial pressure.
- Be alert for the Cushing reflex, a combination of three conditions: rising blood pressure, falling heart and respiratory rates, and widened pulse pressure (systolic hypertension). These findings indicate increased intracranial pressure.
- Rapidly transport patients in critical condition and patients in whom you suspect stroke. If possible, stroke patients should be taken to a facility that has the ability to administer fibrinolytic drugs.
- Always notify the hospital as soon as possible that you are bringing in a patient with a possible stroke so that staff can prepare to test and treat the patient without delay.
- When obtaining the patient's history, ask what happened, evaluate the patient's speech, find out when the patient's symptoms began, and find out if the patient has a history of stroke, transient ischemic attack, seizure, or diabetic conditions.
- You should always perform at least three neurologic tests on patients you suspect of experiencing a stroke: speech, facial movement, and arm movement. You may use a stroke assessment tool such as the Cincinnati Prehospital Stroke Scale or the Los Angeles Prehospital Stroke Screen.
- All patients with altered mental status should also have a Glasgow Coma Scale score calculated.
- Interventions will be based on assessment findings and may include providing 100% oxygen, assisting ventilations, providing spinal immobilization, administering oral glucose, establishing intravenous access, obtaining blood samples, administering intravenous dextrose, administering glucagon, and administering fluid.

▶ Vital Vocabulary

absence seizures The seizures that may be characterized by a brief lapse of attention in which the patient may stare and does not respond; formerly known as a petit mal seizure.

aphasia The inability to understand or produce speech.

arterial rupture The rupture of an artery. Involvement of a cerebral artery may contribute to interruption of cerebral blood flow.

ataxia The inability to perform coordinated motions such as walking.

atherosclerosis A disorder in which cholesterol and calcium build up inside the walls of blood vessels, forming plaque, which eventually leads to partial or complete blockage of blood flow; a plaque can become a site where blood clots can form, detach, and travel elsewhere in the circulatory system (embolize).

aura Sensations experienced before an attack occurs; common in seizures and migraine headaches.

Prep Kit *(continued)*

axon A projection from a neuron that makes connections with adjacent cells.

cerebral embolism Obstruction of a cerebral artery caused by a clot that was formed elsewhere in the body and traveled to the brain.

cerebrovascular accident (CVA) interruption of blood flow to the brain that results in the loss of brain function; also referred to as a stroke or brain attack.

clonic phase Seizure movement marked by repetitive muscle contractions and relaxations in rapid succession.

coma A state in which a person does not respond to either verbal or painful stimuli.

complex partial seizures The seizures that involve subtle changes in the level of consciousness that may include confusion, reduced alertness, hallucinations, and inability to speak.

decerebrate posturing A body position in which the patient extends the arms outward and rotates the lower arms in a palms-down manner and points the toes; indicates severe brain dysfunction.

decorticate posturing A body position in which the patient flexes the arms and curls them toward the chest, flexes the wrists, and points his or her toes; indicates severe brain dysfunction.

dysarthria The inability to pronounce speech clearly, often due to loss of the nerves or brain cells that control the small muscles in the larynx.

dysphagia Pain, discomfort, or difficulty in swallowing.

febrile seizures The seizures that result from sudden high fever, particularly in children.

hemiparesis Weakness on one side of the body.

hemorrhagic stroke One of the two main types of stroke; occurs as a result of bleeding inside the brain.

herniation A process in which tissue is forced out of its normal position, such as when the brain is forced from the cranial vault, either through the foramen magnum or over the tentorium.

hypoglycemia A condition characterized by a low blood glucose level.

idiopathic Of no known cause.

incontinence Loss of bowel and bladder control; can be due to a generalized seizure and to other conditions.

infarcted cells The cells that die as a result of loss of blood flow.

intracranial pressure (ICP) The pressure within the cranial vault; normally 0 to 15 mm Hg in adults.

ischemic cells cells that receive enough blood after an event, such as a cerebrovascular accident, to stay alive but not enough to function properly.

ischemic stroke One of the two main types of stroke; occurs when blood flow to a particular part of the brain is cut off by a blockage (for example, a clot) inside a blood vessel.

myelin An insulating layer, or sheath, made up of fatty substances and protein that form around the nerves.

neurotransmitters The chemicals produced by the body that stimulate electrical reactions in adjacent neurons.

partial seizures The seizures affecting a limited portion of the brain.

postictal state The period following a seizure that lasts between 5 and 30 minutes, characterized by labored respirations and some degree of altered mental status.

pronation The act of rotating the forearms in a palms-down manner.

seizures Episodes often characterized by generalized, uncoordinated muscular activity associated with loss of consciousness; a convulsion.

simple partial seizures The seizures involving movement of one part of the body or altered sensations in one part of the body; the movement may stay in one body part or spread from one part to another in a wave.

status epilepticus A condition in which seizures recur every few minutes without a lucid interval or last more than 4 or 5 minutes.

stroke A loss of brain function in certain brain cells that do not get enough oxygen during a cerebrovascular accident. Usually caused by obstruction of the blood vessels in the brain that feed oxygen to the brain cells.

synapse The gap between nerve cells across which nervous stimuli are transmitted.

syncope The temporary loss of consciousness and postural tone caused by diminished cerebral blood flow.

thrombus In neurologic emergencies, the local clotting of blood in the cerebral arteries that may result in the interruption of cerebral blood flow and subsequent stroke.

tonic-clonic seizures The seizures characterized by severe twitching of all of the body's muscles that may last several minutes or more; formerly known as a grand mal seizure.

tonic phase In a seizure, the steady, rigid muscle contractions with no relaxation.

transient ischemic attack (TIA) A disorder of the brain in which brain cells temporarily stop working because

Prep Kit (continued)

of insufficient oxygen, causing strokelike symptoms that resolve completely within 24 hours of onset.

trismus The involuntary contraction of the mouth resulting in clenched teeth; occurs during seizures and head injuries.

uremia Severe renal failure resulting in the buildup of waste products within the blood; eventually impairs brain function.

References

1. Deaths and mortality. Centers for Disease Control and Prevention website. http://www.cdc.gov/nchs/fastats/deaths.htm. Published October 7, 2016. Accessed January 2, 2017.
2. Stroke: A Life-Saving Revolution. Heart and Stroke Foundation of Canada website. http://www.heartandstroke.ca/stroke/stroke-news/a-life-saving-revolution. Accessed November 1, 2017.
3. How Is a Stroke Treated? National Heart, Lung, and Blood Institute website. https://www.nhlbi.nih.gov/health/health-topics/topics/stroke/treatment. Updated January 27, 2017. Accessed November 1, 2017.
4. Jauch EC. Ischemic stroke. Medscape website. http://emedicine.medscape.com/article/1916852-overview. Updated November 23, 2015. Accessed March 31, 2016.
5. Jauch EC, Saver JL, Adams HP Jr, Bruno A, Connors JJ, Demaerschalk BM, Khatri P, McMullan PW Jr, Qureshi AI, Rosenfield K, Scott PA, Summers DR, Wang DZ, Wintermark M, Yonas H; on behalf of the American Heart Association Stroke Council, Council on Cardiovascular Nursing, Council on Peripheral Vascular Disease, and Council on Clinical Cardiology. Guidelines for the early management of patients with acute ischemic stroke: a guideline for healthcare professionals from the American Heart Association/American Stroke Association. *Stroke*. 2013;44:870–947.
6. Mozaffarian D, Benjamin EJ, Go AS, Arnett DK, Blaha MJ, Cushman M, Das SR, de Ferranti S, Després J-P, Fullerton HJ, Howard VJ, Huffman MD, Isasi CR, Jiménez MC, Judd SE, Kissela BM, Lichtman JH, Lisabeth LD, Liu S, Mackey RH, Magid DJ, McGuire DK, Mohler ER III, Moy CS, Muntner P, Mussolino ME, Nasir K, Neumar RW, Nichol G, Palaniappan L, Pandey DK, Reeves MJ, Rodriguez CJ, Rosamond W, Sorlie PD, Stein J, Towfighi A, Turan TN, Virani SS, Woo D, Yeh RW, Turner MB; on behalf of the American Heart Association Statistics Committee and Stroke Statistics Subcommittee. Heart disease and stroke statistics—2016 update: a report from the American Heart Association. *Circulation*. 2016;133(4):e38-360.
7. Brain herniation. MedlinePlus website. https://medlineplus.gov/ency/article/001421.htm. Updated October 3, 2017. Accessed November 3, 2017.
8. Transient Ischemic Attack Information Page: National Institute of Neurological Disorders and Stroke (NINDS). https://www.ninds.nih.gov/Disorders/All-Disorders/Transient-Ischemic-Attack-Information-Page. Accessed January 18, 2017.
9. Ko DY. Epilepsy and seizures. Medscape website. http://emedicine.medscape.com/article/1184846-overview. Updated July 12, 2016. Accessed April 8, 2016.
10. Moghaddasi M, Joodat R, Ataei E. Evaluation of short-term mortality of status epilepticus and its risk factors. *J Epilepsy Res*. 2015;5(1):13-16. https://www.ncbi.nlm.nih.gov/pmc/articles/PMC4494989/. Accessed January 7, 2017.
11. Morag R. Syncope. Medscape website. http://emedicine.medscape.com/article/811669-overview. Updated December 7, 2015. Accessed April 8, 2016.
12. Powers WJ, Derdeyn CP, Biller J, Coffey CS, Hoh BL, Jauch EC, Johnston KC, Johnston SC, Khalessi AA, Kidwell CS, Meschia JF, Ovbiagele B; Yavagal DR; on behalf of the American Heart Association Stroke Council. 2015 AHA/ASA focused update of the 2013 guidelines for the early management of patients with acute ischemic stroke regarding endovascular treatment: a guideline for healthcare professionals from the American Heart Association/American Stroke Association. *Stroke.* 2015;46.
13. Early Management of Acute Ischemic Stroke Quick Sheet. American Heart Association/American Stroke Association. http://www.strokeassociation.org/idc/groups/stroke-public/@wcm/@hcm/@sta/documents/downloadable/ucm_491890.pdf. Accessed November 3, 2017.
14. Leggett H. Time window for stroke treatment should be extended. Stanford News website. https://news.stanford.edu/news/2009/june3/med-tpa-060309.html. June 20, 2009. Accessed November 1, 2017.
15. DeNoon DJ. Stroke treatment window widens. WebMD website. https://www.webmd.com/stroke/news/20090528/stoke-treatment-window-widens. May 28, 2009. Accessed November 1, 2017.
16. About Stroke. American Heart Association/American Stroke Association website. http://www.strokeassociation.org/STROKEORG/AboutStroke/Treatment/Stroke-Treatment_UCM_492017_SubHomePage.jsp. Accessed November 1, 2017.
17. Badjatia N, Carney N, Crocco T, et al. Guidelines for prehospital management of traumatic brain injury, 2nd edition. *Prehosp Emerg Care*. 2008;12 Suppl 1:S1-S52.

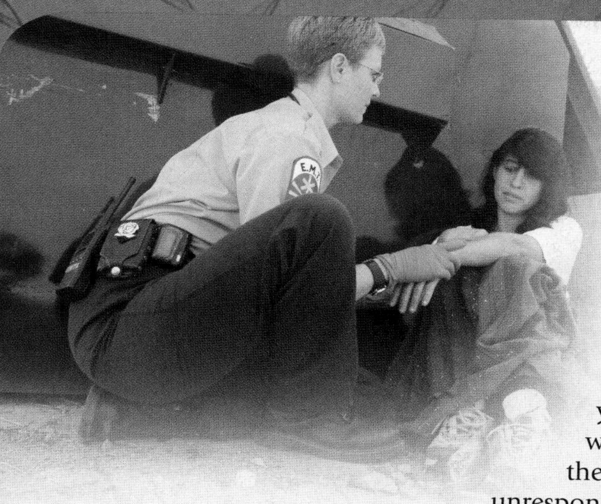

Assessment *in Action*

You are dispatched to a local apartment complex for a person having a seizure. On arrival, you are greeted by a visibly upset middle-aged woman, who states her teenaged son had a seizure that lasted approximately 5 minutes. When you interview the woman, she describes the seizure as "his whole body was shaking" and states that he was "rolling on the ground, foaming at the mouth." Currently the patient is unresponsive but breathing.

1. Which type of seizure is characterized by a loss of consciousness, followed by generalized muscle contractions alternating with rhythmic "jerking" movements?

A. Absence
B. Tonic-clonic
C. Simple partial
D. Complex partial

2. The __________ state is a common finding after someone has had a seizure.

A. preictal
B. bi-ictal
C. postictal
D. semi-ictal

3. What is the first step in caring for a patient who is actively having a seizure?

A. Maintain a clear airway.
B. Protect the patient from harm.
C. Apply oxygen.
D. Initiate chest compressions.

4. Increased ICP will have what effect on the blood pressure?

A. Raises
B. Lowers
C. No change
D. Rhythmically raises and lowers

5. During a seizure, the patient's respirations may become sporadic or stop. You should initiate assisted ventilations after __________ seconds of apnea.

A. 15
B. 30
C. 45
D. 60

6. What cause of seizures is more common in infants and children than in adults?

A. Elevated body temperature
B. Infection
C. Virus
D. Hypoglycemia

7. Emergency treatment of a child having a febrile seizure includes removing the child's clothing and cooling with __________ water.

A. tepid
B. cool
C. cold
D. warm

8. Trismus in an unresponsive patient may indicate all but which of the following?

A. Head injury
B. Seizure
C. Diabetes
D. Hypoxia

9. Assessment of a patient with an altered mental status should be performed with consideration of the mnemonic AEIOU-TIPS. What does AEIOU-TIPS stand for?

10. Explain the difference between a TIA and a stroke.

CHAPTER 20

Gastrointestinal and Urologic Emergencies

National EMS Education Standard Competencies

Medicine

Applies fundamental knowledge to provide basic and selected advanced emergency care and transportation based on assessment findings for an acutely ill patient.

Abdominal and Gastrointestinal Disorders

Anatomy, presentations, and management of shock associated with abdominal emergencies

- Gastrointestinal bleeding (pp 881-882, 886-888, 894-900)

Anatomy, physiology, pathophysiology, assessment, and management of

- Acute and chronic gastrointestinal hemorrhage (pp 881-882, 886-888, 894-900)
- Peritonitis (pp 881-885, 894-900)
- Ulcerative diseases (pp 881-883, 887, 889-890, 894-900)

Genitourinary/Renal

- Blood pressure assessment in hemodialysis patients (p 895)

Anatomy, physiology, pathophysiology, assessment, and management of

- Complications related to:
  - Renal dialysis (pp 900-901)
  - Urinary catheter management (not insertion) (p 901)
- Kidney stones (pp 883, 891, 894-900)

Knowledge Objectives

1. Review the anatomy and physiology of the gastrointestinal and renal systems. (pp 881-883)
2. Define the term *acute abdomen*. (p 884)
3. Define peritonitis and list its potential signs and symptoms. (pp 884-885)
4. Explain the concept of referred pain. (p 884)
5. Recognize that abdominal pain can arise from other body systems. (p 885)
6. Discuss the various potential causes of acute abdomen, including gastrointestinal hemorrhage (eg, from esophagitis, gastroesophageal reflux disease, peptic ulcer disease, Mallory-Weiss tear, esophageal varices, or hemorrhoids) and nonhemorrhagic conditions (eg, gallstones, pancreatitis, appendicitis, gastroenteritis, diverticulitis). (pp 886-889)
7. Discuss the pathophysiology of chronic inflammatory abdominal conditions, including ulcerative colitis, irritable bowel syndrome, and Crohn disease. (pp 889-890)
8. Discuss the various types of urologic pathophysiology, including urinary tract infections. (p 891)
9. Discuss the various types of renal pathophysiology, including kidney stones, acute kidney injury, chronic kidney disease, and end-stage renal disease. (pp 891-892)
10. Identify gynecologic conditions that can cause abdominal pain, including pelvic inflammatory disease and ectopic pregnancy. (p 892)
11. Identify male genital tract conditions that can cause abdominal pain, including epididymitis, priapism, benign prostate hypertrophy, testicular masses, and testicular torsion. (pp 892-893)
12. Identify pathophysiologies of other organ systems that can lead to gastrointestinal and urologic conditions, including aneurysm and hernia. (p 893)
13. Describe the assessment process for patients with an acute abdomen or urologic emergency. (pp 894-899)
14. Describe the procedures to follow in managing the patient with shock associated with abdominal emergencies. (pp 895, 899)
15. Discuss general management of a patient with an acute abdomen or urologic emergency. (pp 899-900)
16. Explain the purpose of renal dialysis. (p 900)
17. Describe potential complications of dialysis or a missed dialysis treatment. (p 901)

Skills Objective

1. Demonstrate the assessment of a patient's abdomen. (pp 897-898)

Introduction

Abdominal pain is a common complaint among patients, but the cause is often difficult to identify, even for a physician. As an advanced emergency medical technician (AEMT), you do not need to determine the exact cause of acute abdominal pain: you simply need to be able to recognize a life-threatening problem and act swiftly in response. Remember, the patient is in pain and is probably anxious, requiring all your skills of rapid assessment and emotional support.

This chapter begins by explaining the anatomy and physiology of the gastrointestinal (GI) and genitourinary systems. It then discusses the pathophysiology of an acute abdomen, including signs and symptoms of the acute abdomen and the procedure for examining the abdomen. Next, it discusses the different causes of an acute abdomen and appropriate emergency medical care.

Anatomy and Physiology Review

The abdominal cavity contains solid and hollow organs that make up the GI, genital, and urinary systems Figure 20-1. Solid organs include the liver, spleen, pancreas, kidneys, and ovaries (in women). Technically, organs such as the kidneys, ovaries, and the majority of the pancreas are retroperitoneal (behind the peritoneum). However, because they are located next to the peritoneum, they can cause abdominal pain. An injury to a solid organ can cause shock and bleeding because of the amount of blood vessels that the organ contains.

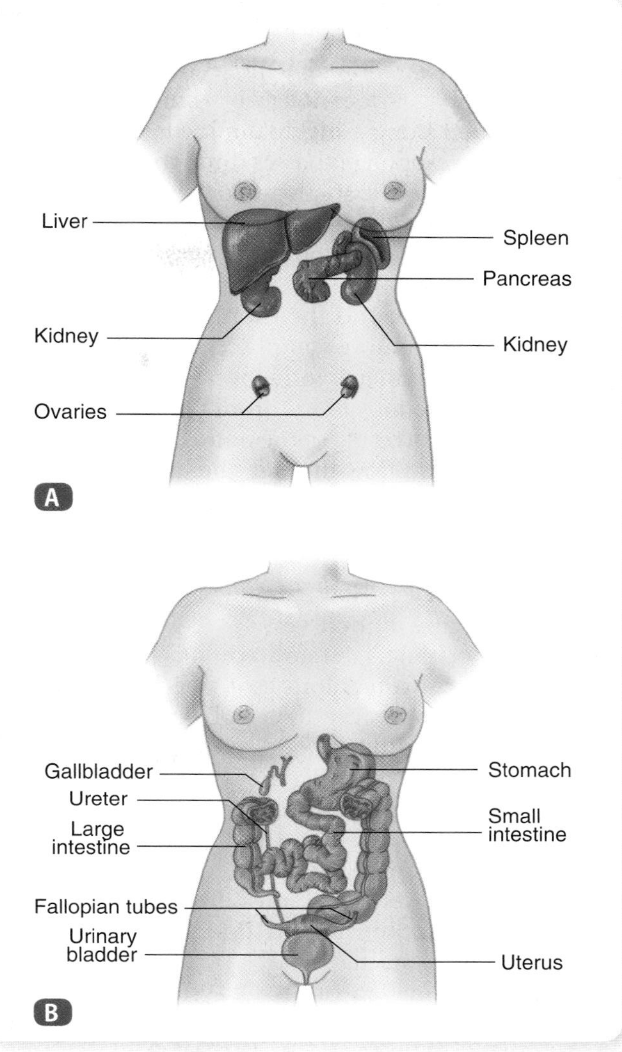

Figure 20-1 The solid and hollow organs of the abdomen. **A.** Solid organs include the liver, spleen, pancreas, kidneys, and ovaries (in women). **B.** Hollow organs include the gallbladder, stomach, small intestine, large intestine, and bladder.

The Gastrointestinal System

The main function of the GI system, which is also known as the digestive tract, is to absorb the products of digestion to fuel the cells within the body. This system consists of the mouth, intestines, salivary glands, pharynx, esophagus, liver, gallbladder, pancreas, rectum, and anus; it is covered in detail in Chapter 7, *The Human Body*.

The entire digestion process takes 8 to 72 hours. It begins when food is put into the mouth and chewed. The salivary glands secrete saliva to help lubricate the food, allowing it to be more easily swallowed. Saliva also contains enzymes that begin the chemical breakdown of foods—starches in particular (and some initial breakdown of triglycerides). These complex carbohydrates can

YOU are the Provider — PART 1

You are dispatched to a local dialysis clinic for a patient who "needs transport to the emergency department." On arrival, you are greeted by clinic staff, who state that the patient undergoes dialysis every Monday, Wednesday, and Friday because of anuria, and today (Monday) when he came in he "wasn't acting right" and seemed a little short of breath. The clinic staff tells you that they are unable to perform dialysis on this patient until his mental status improves.

1. What are some potential causes of altered mental status in a patient receiving dialysis?
2. On the basis of the information provided, which type of dialysis does this patient receive?
3. What is anuria?

be disassembled into simple sugars that are more easily absorbed.

Once food is swallowed, it moves through the esophagus. The esophagus does not absorb nutrients but rather pushes the food along using rhythmic contractions called **peristalsis**. The esophagus passes through the diaphragm and food comes to the sphincter located at the junction of the esophagus and the stomach. The cardiac sphincter is designed to prevent food from backing up into the esophagus.

Intertwined around the esophagus are veins that drain into an even more complex series of veins, which ultimately join together to form the **portal vein**. The portal vein transports venous blood from the GI tract directly to the liver for processing of the nutrients that have been absorbed. If blood flow through the liver slows for any reason, the blood may back up throughout the entire GI system because this series of veins lacks any valves. The veins surrounding the stomach and esophagus then become dilated. Even a low amount of pressure may cause leaking or rupture of these vessels.

As the food enters the stomach, this muscular organ begins to secrete hydrochloric acid, which helps to break down the food to a form that can be used by the body. To mix the acid with the food more evenly, the stomach also contracts, churning the acid and food mixture together until a relatively smooth consistency is achieved. The stomach absorbs some substances, such as water, alcohol, caffeine, and some medications. Once the food is thoroughly converted, a semisolid mass called chyme exits the pyloric sphincter, the doorway at the inferior portion of the stomach.

The main function of the GI system is revealed in the next portion of the GI system, the duodenum, where the GI system begins to absorb resources for use by other cells in the body.

The duodenum is the first part of the small intestine. It is where the pancreas, liver, and gallbladder connect to the digestive system. The stomach is designed to release only small amounts of the food into the duodenum, thereby enabling the small intestine to better manage digestion. The exocrine portion of the pancreas secretes several enzymes into the duodenum that assist with digestion of fats, proteins, and carbohydrates. Amylase, which breaks down starches into sugar, is one enzyme the pancreas secretes. The pancreas also produces bicarbonate and insulin. Bicarbonate neutralizes the stomach acid in the duodenum, and insulin helps regulate the levels of glucose in the bloodstream.

The liver assists in digestion by secreting bile. Bile is an enzyme used by the body to help break down fats. The liver also filters toxic substances produced by digestion, creates glucose stores, and produces substances necessary for blood clotting and immune function. The gallbladder is a hollow pouch located beneath the liver that acts as a reservoir for bile.

The small intestine, where 90% of absorption occurs, produces enzymes that work with the pancreatic enzymes to turn chyme into substances that can be directly absorbed by the capillaries of the small intestine and thereby move into the bloodstream. Blood filled with these nutrients exits the intestinal circulation and heads to the liver, where additional metabolism of fats and proteins takes place. The blood then leaves the liver and enters the subclavian vessels. Water-soluble vitamins are absorbed into the bloodstream for use by cells.

Words of Wisdom

The liver affects the GI system indirectly, through carbohydrate metabolism. Brain cells can burn only one fuel source—glucose. If the blood glucose level falls, the liver can convert glycogen into glucose. Dramatic drops in blood glucose level will cause the liver to convert fats and proteins into sugar. As blood flows through the liver, fat and protein metabolism continues. Without a functioning liver, a person would soon die because he or she would not be able to use any of the proteins that were absorbed from the GI system. In addition, the liver detoxifies drugs, completes the breakdown of dead red and white blood cells, and stores vitamins and minerals.

The jejunum, the next part of the small intestine, comprises a large amount of the surface area of the small intestine and does much of the work. The final part of the small intestine is the ileum. The ileum absorbs nutrients that were not absorbed earlier. It also absorbs bile acids so they can be returned to the liver for future use and vitamin B_{12} for making nerve cells and red blood cells.

The large intestine, or colon, is the next destination. Substances not broken down and used as nutrients enter the colon as waste products, or feces. The primary role of the large intestine is to complete the reabsorption of water. Water is absorbed, which helps to solidify the digested material, and stool is formed. Although most water is reabsorbed in the small intestine, the osmotic function within the colon helps to solidify the digested material into a formed stool. The colon is also the site of bacterial digestion. Bacteria normally found within the colon help to finish the breakdown of the chyme. This breakdown produces gas as a by-product. Flatulence may be considered impolite, but it is certainly normal.

Attached to the last portion of the colon is the rectum. The colon terminates at a sphincter called the anus, where the feces are expelled from the body.

▶ Additional Abdominal Organs

The spleen is also located in the abdomen but has no digestive system function. The spleen is part of the lymphatic system and plays a significant role in relation to red blood cells and the immune system. It assists in the filtration of blood, aids in the development of red blood cells, and serves as a blood reservoir. The spleen also produces antibodies to help the body fight off disease and infection.

▶ The Genital System

The abdominal space also holds the male and female reproductive organs. The male reproductive system consists of the testicles, epididymis, vasa deferentia, seminal vesicles, prostate gland, and penis. The female reproductive system includes the ovaries, fallopian tubes, uterus, cervix, and vagina.

▶ The Urinary System

The urinary system consists of the kidneys, which filter the blood and produce urine; the urinary bladder, which stores the urine until it is released from the body; the ureters, which transport the urine from the kidneys to the bladder; and the urethra, which transports the urine from the bladder out of the body **Figure 20-2**. Overall, the urinary system performs two main functions for the body: (1) it regulates electrolytes, water content, and acids in the blood; and (2) it removes metabolic wastes, drug metabolites, and excess fluids. The kidneys perform these functions continuously, filtering 200 L of blood each day. In addition, the kidneys produce hormones that generate new red blood cells and help the liver convert glycogen to glucose. Nephrons, found in the cortex, are the structural and functional units of the kidney that form urine. Each kidney contains approximately 900,000 to 1 million nephrons, though these numbers can vary dramatically.[1]

The kidneys play a major role in maintaining homeostasis, including calcium, magnesium, and phosphate balance. They preserve this balance by eliminating metabolic waste products such as urea from the blood. When the kidneys fail, the patient loses the ability to excrete urea from the body, leading to a condition called **uremia**. Urea that is normally excreted through the kidneys then builds up in the blood.

Once the urine enters the collecting ducts, it passes through the minor calyx, into the major calyx, and then into the renal pelvis. From there, the urine moves through the ureter (one ureter from each kidney) and is stored in the urinary bladder. Normally, the brain exerts control over the urge to void, keeping the external urinary sphincter contracted until conditions are favorable for urination. At this point, the inhibition of the external urinary sphincter is reduced and the urine passes from the urinary bladder into the urethra.

The beginning of the urethra, through which urine is expelled, sits at the inferior aspect of the bladder. In females, the urethra exits at the site of the external genitalia. The female urethra is shorter than the male urethra (1.5 versus 8 inches [4 versus 20 cm]).

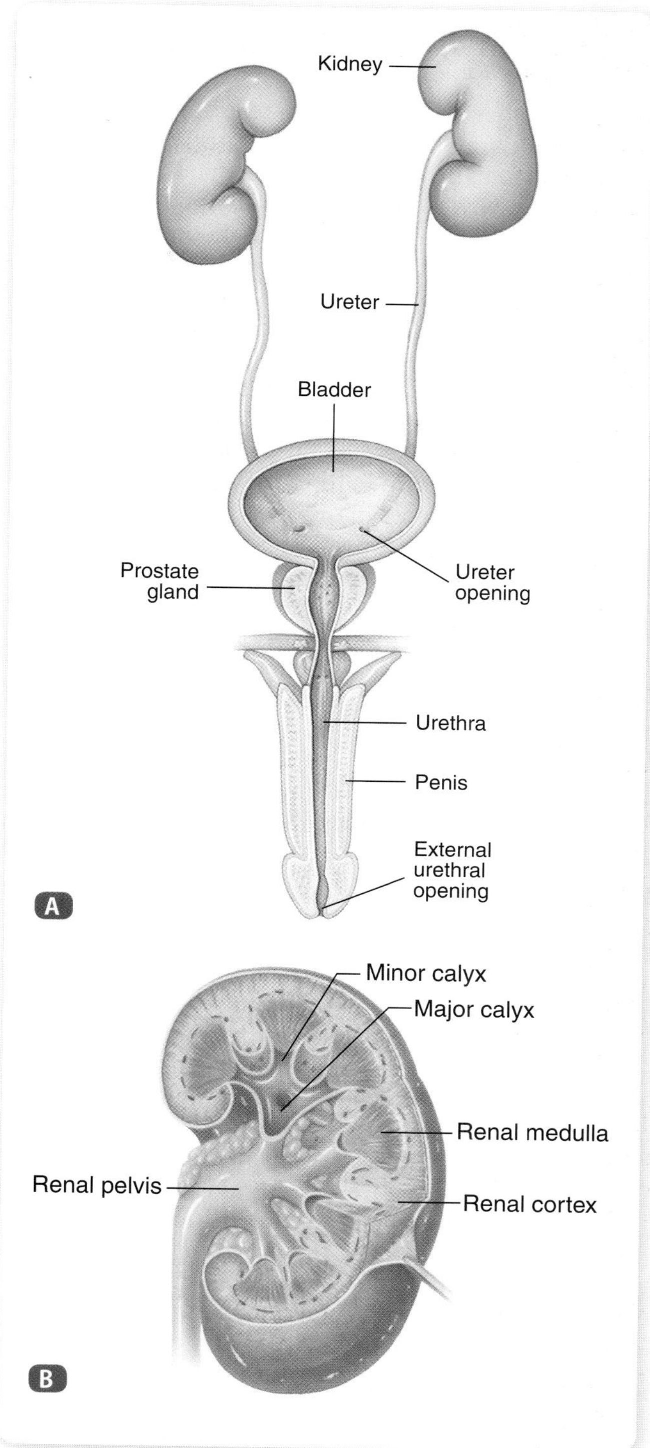

Figure 20-2 The urinary system. **A.** Anterior view showing the relationship of the kidneys, ureters, urinary bladder, and urethra. **B.** Cross section of the human kidney showing the renal cortex, renal medulla, and renal pelvis.

Words of Wisdom

The normal adult forms 1.5 to 2 L of urine per day.

Pathophysiology

Acute abdomen is a medical term referring to the sudden onset of abdominal pain that indicates an irritation of the **peritoneum**, the thin membrane that lines the entire abdominal cavity. This condition, called **peritonitis**, can be caused by an infection, a penetrating abdominal wound, a blunt injury severe enough to damage abdominal organs, and many diseases. In all cases, the major symptom is the same: severe pain. The major clinical signs are abdominal tenderness and distention.

Anatomically, the peritoneum is not one membrane, but two. The parietal peritoneum lines the walls of the abdominal cavity; the visceral peritoneum covers the surface of each of the organs in the abdominal cavity.

Two different types of nerves supply these two areas of the peritoneum. The parietal peritoneum is supplied by the same nerves from the spinal cord that supply the skin overlying the abdomen; it can therefore perceive many of the same sensations—pain, touch, pressure, heat, and cold. These sensory nerves can easily identify and localize a point of irritation. In contrast, the visceral peritoneum is supplied by the autonomic nervous system. These nerves are far less able to localize sensation. The visceral peritoneum is stimulated when distention or contraction of the hollow abdominal organs activates the stretch receptors. This sensation is usually interpreted as **colic**, a severe, intermittent cramping pain.

When receptors at the affected organs are stimulated, they send impulses along the nerves to the brain, where the impulses are evaluated and interpreted as pain. **Visceral pain**— the type of pain most commonly associated with urologic problems—usually occurs when receptors in the hollow structures, such as the ureters, urinary bladder, and urethra, are stimulated. Pinpointing the source of such pain is challenging because only a few nerve fibers may be involved in the pain transmission. Because many different nerve fibers travel to the brain through the spinal cord, pain that originates in one area of the body (eg, the urinary bladder) may be perceived by the brain as coming from a different area of the body (eg, the neck or shoulder). Other painful sensations that occur because of an irritated visceral peritoneum may be perceived at a distant point on the surface of the body, such as the back or shoulder. This phenomenon is called **referred pain**.

Referred pain is the result of connections between the body's two separate nervous systems. The spinal cord supplies sensory nerves to the skin and muscles; these nerves are a part of the somatic (voluntary) nervous system. The autonomic nervous system controls the function of the abdominal organs and the caliber of the blood vessels. The nerves connecting these two systems cause the stimulation of the autonomic nerves to be perceived as stimulation of the spinal sensory nerves. For example, acute cholecystitis (inflammation of the gallbladder) may cause referred pain to the right shoulder because the autonomic nerves serving the gallbladder lie near the spinal cord at the same anatomic level as the spinal sensory nerves that supply the skin of the shoulder[2] **Figure 20-3**.

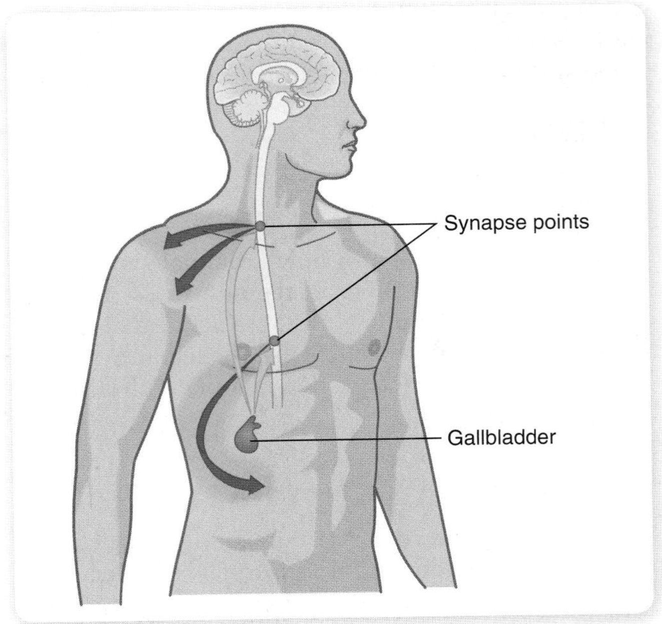

Figure 20-3 Acute cholecystitis can cause referred pain to the shoulder, as well as abdominal pain.

Peritonitis typically causes **ileus**, or paralysis of the muscular contractions that normally propel material through the intestine (peristalsis). The retained gas and feces, in turn, cause abdominal distention. In the presence of such paralysis, nothing that is eaten can pass normally out of the stomach or through the bowel. The only way the stomach can empty itself, then, is by **emesis**, or vomiting. For this reason, peritonitis is almost always associated with nausea and vomiting. These complaints do not point to a particular cause because they can accompany almost every type of GI disease or injury.

Peritonitis is associated with a loss of body fluid into the abdominal cavity. Abnormal shifts of fluid from the bloodstream into body tissues decrease the volume of circulating blood and may eventually cause hypovolemic shock. This problem can be compounded by massive internal or external bleeding, resulting in severe inadequate perfusion (shock). The patient may have normal vital signs or, if the peritonitis has progressed further, signs of shock (such as restlessness, tachycardia, and hypotension). When peritonitis is accompanied by hemorrhage, the signs of shock are much more apparent.

Fever may or may not be present, depending on the cause of the peritonitis. Patients with **diverticulitis** (an inflammation of small pockets in the colon) or **cholecystitis** (inflammation of the gallbladder) may have a substantial elevation in temperature, which may be due to the inflammatory process itself or an underlying

Table 20-1 Common Abdominal Conditions

Condition	Localization of Pain
Appendicitis	Around navel (referred); right lower quadrant (direct); rebound tenderness (pain felt on the rebound after palpation)
Cholecystitis	Right shoulder (referred); right upper quadrant (direct)
Ulcer	Upper midabdomen or upper back area
Diverticulitis	Left lower quadrant
Abdominal aortic aneurysm (ruptured or dissecting)	Low part of back and lower quadrants
Cystitis (inflammation of the bladder)	Lower midabdomen (retropubic)
Kidney infection (pyelonephritis)	Costovertebral angle
Kidney stone	Right or left flank, radiating to genitalia (referred)
Pelvic inflammation (in women)	Both lower quadrants
Pancreatitis	Upper abdomen (both quadrants); back
Pneumonia	Referred pain to the upper abdomen
Hernia	Anywhere in the abdominal area
Peritonitis	Anywhere in the abdominal area

infection. However, patients with acute **appendicitis** may have a normal temperature until the appendix ruptures and an abscess starts to form.

Diseases and conditions of the renal and urologic systems range from mild (urinary tract infections) to true emergencies (acute kidney injury). Although the prehospital care for many urologic diseases is supportive, your ability to recognize the signs and symptoms of these conditions, especially when they are genuine emergencies, is critical to providing your patients with the best chance of a positive outcome. The most common abdominal emergencies, with the most common locations of direct and referred pain, are listed in Table 20-1.

Many conditions discussed in this section can cause **urinary retention**—that is, incomplete emptying of the bladder or a complete lack of ability to empty the bladder. Some of these conditions are listed in Table 20-2.

Table 20-2 Conditions That May Cause or Lead to Urinary Retention

Kidney stones
Benign prostate hypertrophy
Urethral obstructions
Urinary tract infections
Nerve damage

Data from: Urinary Retention. National Institute of Diabetes and Digestive and Kidney Diseases website. https://www.niddk.nih.gov/health-information/urologic-diseases/urinary-retention. Accessed September 15, 2017; and Urinary Retention. Baylor College of Medicine website. https://www.bcm.edu/healthcare/care-centers/obstetrics-gynecology/conditions/urinary-retention. Accessed September 15, 2017.

Causes of Acute Abdomen

The entire abdominal cavity normally contains a very small amount of peritoneal fluid that bathes and lubricates the organs. Any condition that allows pus, blood, feces, urine, gastric juice, intestinal contents, bile, pancreatic juice, amniotic fluid, or other foreign material to accumulate within or adjacent to this cavity can cause peritonitis and, therefore, an acute abdomen. Technically, organs such as kidneys, ovaries, and other genitourinary structures are retroperitoneal (behind the peritoneum). However, because they lie next to the peritoneum, problems in these organs can lead to an acute abdomen. Ultimately, nearly every kind of abdominal problem can cause an acute abdomen.

▶ Gastrointestinal Hemorrhage

Bleeding within the GI tract is a symptom of a disease, not a disease itself. GI hemorrhage can be acute, which may be shorter in duration and more severe, or chronic, which may be longer in duration and less severe. All complaints of bleeding from the GI tract should be considered serious. Causes of GI bleeding are shown in Table 20-3.

A GI hemorrhage can occur in the upper or lower GI tract. The upper GI tract spans from the esophagus to the upper part of the small intestine. In the esophagus, bleeding conditions might stem from esophagitis, esophageal varices, or a Mallory-Weiss tear, which results from excessive retching or vomiting. **Hematemesis** (vomiting blood) is frequently seen in patients with upper GI bleeding. The blood is either bright red or has the appearance of coffee grounds, depending on where in the GI tract it originated and how briskly it is occurring.

The lower GI tract spans the upper part of the small intestine to the anus. Bowel inflammation, diverticulosis, diverticulitis, cancer, and hemorrhoids are common causes of bleeding in the lower GI tract. In lower GI tract bleeding, the bleeding often manifests as **melena** (dark tarry stools), as a result of partial digestion of the blood.

Esophagitis

As its name suggests, **esophagitis** is an inflammation of the esophagus. This can be caused by an infectious process or by reflux of gastric secretions into the esophagus. Additionally, some medications can be irritating, as can chemotherapy or radiation therapy. Esophagitis also is associated with eosinophils, a type of white blood cell.

Regardless of the underlying cause, the effects are irritation and swelling. Generally speaking, patients will present with either heartburn or choking as their primary complaint. Esophagitis most commonly occurs in patients with gastroesophageal reflux disease, discussed next.

Gastroesophageal Reflux Disease

Gastroesophageal reflux disease (GERD) is a condition in which the sphincter between the esophagus and the stomach opens, allowing stomach acid to move superiorly. This condition, which is also referred to as acid reflux disease, can cause a burning sensation within the chest (heartburn). Various factors can make some people more susceptible to this condition. Smoking, obesity, and pregnancy all increase the chances of GERD. Eating fatty fried foods, drinking alcohol, and eating citrus fruits are also factors that are associated with GERD. If the reflux continues over a long period, damage can occur to the esophageal wall. This damage could result in weakened portions that are more susceptible to bleeding.

Heartburn is the predominant clinical finding for this condition. This pain may be increased with positional changes—sitting upright is preferred, whereas lying flat makes the condition worse. Some patients may not have pain, but experience coughing or have difficulty swallowing. Bleeding can occur if the damage is long term, resulting in hematemesis and melena.

YOU are the Provider — PART 2

As you begin to interview the patient, you find that he is able to answer all questions appropriately; however, he is very slow to formulate his answers. According to the patient and staff, the patient is normally as "sharp as a tack," and this delay in responding is abnormal for him. The patient denies engaging in any abnormal activities over the weekend but states that he went to his granddaughter's birthday party on Saturday and may have overexerted himself.

Recording Time: 1 Minute	
Appearance	Pale; "sick" looking
Level of consciousness	Alert; oriented to person, place, time, and event; however, slow to respond to questions
Airway	Patent
Breathing	36 breaths/min; normal rhythm
Circulation	Bounding radial pulses; skin warm, dry, and pink

4. The patient seems to be answering all questions appropriately, but more slowly than what is reported to be normal. Should you approach the dialysis staff and request that he undergo dialysis in an attempt to help improve his mental status?
5. You note a "lump" in the patient's left forearm. What is this lump, and why is it important for you to note?

Table 20-3 GI Bleeding by Organ and Cause

Organ	Causes	Location	Substances
Esophagus	Inflammation (esophagitis) Varices Mallory-Weiss tear Cancer Dilated veins (cirrhosis, liver disease) Gastroesophageal reflux disease	Upper GI	Melena, hematemesis, vomitus with gross blood
Stomach	Ulcers Cancer Inflammation (gastritis)	Upper GI	Melena, hematemesis, vomitus with gross blood
Small intestine	Ulcer (duodenal) Cancer Inflammation (irritable bowel disease)	Upper or lower GI	Melena, hematemesis, vomitus with gross blood
Large intestine	Infections Inflammation (ulcerative colitis) Colorectal polyps Colorectal cancer Diverticular disease	Lower GI bleed	Hematochezia
Rectum	Hemorrhoids	Lower GI bleed	Hematochezia, gross bleeding

Abbreviation: GI, gastrointestinal

Peptic Ulcer Disease and Gastritis

Both the stomach and the duodenum are subjected to high levels of acidity. High levels of acidity can result in **ulcers**, which are abrasions of the stomach or small intestine. To prevent damage to these organs, protective layers of mucus line both organs. In peptic ulcer disease (PUD), this protective layer is eroded, allowing the acid to eat into the organ itself over the course of weeks, months, or even years. **Gastritis** is caused by the same imbalance between stomach acid and the protective layers. Gastritis is a preulcerative state in which the stomach is inflamed, but erosions have not yet occurred.

Most peptic ulcers are the result of infection of the stomach with *Helicobacter pylori*. Another major cause is erosive gastritis, often resulting from chronic use of nonsteroidal anti-inflammatory drugs (NSAIDs). In erosive gastritis, the mucosal lining of the stomach slowly erodes and ulcerates. Alcohol and smoking can also affect the severity of these conditions by increasing gastric acidity.

PUD affects men and women equally, but tends to occur more often in older age groups. As people age, the immune system's ability to fight infection decreases, making infection more likely. The geriatric population, in general, also uses NSAIDs more frequently for arthritis and other age-related musculoskeletal conditions.

All of the cited factors for PUD can also cause gastritis. Foodborne infections and food allergies also can cause inflammation of the stomach.

Patients with peptic ulcers and gastritis experience a classic sequence of burning or gnawing pain in the stomach that subsides or diminishes immediately after eating and then reemerges 2 to 3 hours later. The pain usually presents in the upper abdomen, but sometimes may be found below the sternum. With some patients, the pain occurs immediately after eating. Nausea, vomiting, belching, and heartburn are common symptoms. If the erosion is severe, gastric bleeding can occur, resulting in hematemesis and melena.

Some ulcers heal without medical intervention, but complications often can occur from bleeding or perforation (a hole through the wall of the stomach). More serious ulcerative conditions can cause severe peritonitis and an acute abdomen.

Mallory-Weiss Tear

A **Mallory-Weiss tear** is a tear in the junction between the esophagus and the stomach, causing severe bleeding and potentially death. Primary risk factors include alcoholism and eating disorders. Mallory-Weiss tears have a sudden onset and affect people of any age.

Vomiting is the principal symptom of a Mallory-Weiss tear. In women, this syndrome may be associated with severe vomiting related to pregnancy. The extent of the bleeding can range from very minor bleeding, resulting in very little blood loss, to severe bleeding and extreme fluid loss. In extreme cases, patients may experience signs and symptoms of shock, upper abdominal pain, hematemesis, and melena.

Similar to a Mallory-Weiss tear, **Boerhaave syndrome** also occurs during vomiting. In this case, the esophagus tears longitudinally and the tear travels entirely through the wall of the esophagus. This creates a passage for blood, air, and food out of the esophagus into the mediastinum. Occurring more often in men, Boerhaave syndrome typically presents after a large meal that included alcohol consumption.

Esophageal Varices

Esophageal varices occur when the amount of pressure within the blood vessels surrounding the esophagus increases. The esophageal blood vessels eventually drain their blood into the liver. If the liver becomes damaged and blood cannot flow through it easily, blood begins to back up into these portal vessels, dilating the vessels and causing the capillary network of the esophagus to begin leaking. If pressure continues to build, the vessel walls may fail, causing massive upper GI bleeding and, quickly afterward, hematemesis.

In industrialized countries, alcohol is the main cause of portal hypertension. Long-term alcohol consumption damages the interior of the liver (cirrhosis), leading to slower blood flow. In developing countries, viral hepatitis is the main cause of liver damage.

Presentation of esophageal varices takes two forms. Initially, the patient shows signs of liver disease—fatigue, weight loss, jaundice, anorexia, edema in the abdomen, abdominal pain, nausea, and vomiting. This very gradual disease process takes months to years before the patient reaches a state of extreme discomfort.

By contrast, rupture of the varices occurs far more suddenly. The patient may report sudden-onset discomfort in the epigastric region or sternum. He or she may have severe difficulty swallowing, vomiting of bright red blood, hypotension, and signs of shock. If the bleeding is less dramatic, hematemesis and melena are likely. Regardless of the rate of bleeding, damage to these vessels can be life threatening. Spontaneous rupture is often life threatening, and significant blood loss at the scene may be evident. Major ruptures can lead to death in a matter of minutes.

Hemorrhoids

Hemorrhoids are created by swelling and inflammation of the blood vessels surrounding the rectum. They are a common problem, with almost one-half the population having at least one hemorrhoid by age 50 years.[3] Hemorrhoids may result from conditions that increase pressure on the rectum or from irritation of the rectum. Pregnancy, straining at stool, and chronic constipation cause increased pressure. Diarrhea can cause irritation.

Hemorrhoids present as bright red blood during defecation. This bleeding, which is called **hematochezia**, tends to be minimal and is easily controlled. Additionally, patients may experience itching and a small mass on the rectum. Typically, this mass is a clot formed in response to the mild bleeding.

▶ Nonhemorrhagic Conditions

Gallstones

The gallbladder is a storage pouch for digestive juices and waste from the liver. Gallstones can form and block the outlet from the gallbladder, causing pain. Sometimes the blockage will pass. If it does not, it can lead to inflammation of the wall of the gallbladder, called cholecystitis. In severe cases, the gallbladder may rupture, causing inflammation to spread and irritate surrounding structures such as the diaphragm and bowel. This condition presents as a constant, severe pain in the right upper or midabdominal region that may refer to the right upper back, shoulder area, or flank. The pain may steadily increase for hours, or it may come and go. Cholecystitis commonly produces symptoms about 30 minutes after consumption of a particularly fatty meal and usually at night. Other symptoms include general GI distress such as nausea and vomiting, indigestion, bloating, gas, and belching.

Pancreatitis

The pancreas forms digestive juices and is also the source of insulin. Inflammation of the pancreas, called **pancreatitis**, can be caused by an obstructing gallstone, alcohol abuse, and other diseases. Severe pain may present in the upper left and right quadrants and often radiates to the back. Other signs and symptoms may include nausea and vomiting, abdominal distention, and tenderness. Complications such as sepsis or hemorrhage can occur, in which case assessment may also reveal fever or tachycardia.

Appendicitis

The appendix is a small recess in the large intestine. Inflammation or infection in the appendix is called appendicitis and is a frequent cause of acute abdomen. This inflammation can eventually cause the tissues to die and/or rupture, causing an abscess, peritonitis, or shock. Initially, the pain caused by appendicitis is generalized, dull, and diffuse and may center in the umbilical area. The pain later localizes to the right lower quadrant of the abdomen. Appendicitis can also cause referred pain. In addition, the patient may report nausea and vomiting, anorexia (lack of appetite for food), fever, and chills.

A classic symptom of appendicitis is **rebound tenderness**. Rebound tenderness is a result of peritoneal irritation. This can be assessed by pressing down gently and firmly on the abdomen—the patient will feel pain when the pressure is released. Women who are pregnant may not exhibit this symptom.

Gastroenteritis

Acute **gastroenteritis** comprises a family of conditions revolving around a central theme of infection combined with diarrhea, nausea, and vomiting. Bacterial and viral organisms can cause this condition. These organisms typically enter the body through contaminated food or water. Patients may begin to experience an upset stomach

Special Populations

Appendicitis can be difficult to diagnosis. Consider that appendicitis occurs most often in young people, even young women who are pregnant. As the uterus expands to accommodate the growing fetus, it moves the appendix out of its normal position. A woman in her third trimester of pregnancy will more likely present with upper right quadrant or right flank pain instead of lower right pain if she has appendicitis. Even the most attentive paramedic will have difficulty determining if this pain is appendicitis, cholecystitis, or kidney stones (renal calculi).

and diarrhea as soon as several hours or several days after contact with the contaminated matter. The disease can then run its course in 2 to 3 days or continue for several weeks.

Gastroenteritis may also be caused by noninfectious conditions such as adverse reactions to medications, exposure to certain toxins, or chemotherapy. The symptoms are similar regardless of the underlying cause.

Diarrhea is the principal symptom in both infectious and noninfectious gastroenteritis. Patients may experience large dumping-type diarrhea or frequent small liquid stools. The diarrhea may contain blood and/or pus, and it may have a foul odor or be odorless. Abdominal cramping is frequently reported. Nausea, vomiting, fever, and anorexia are also present. If the diarrhea continues, dehydration will result. As the volume of fluid loss increases, the likelihood of shock increases.

Diverticulitis

Diverticulitis was first recognized around 1900, when the types of foods people ate began to change dramatically. In particular, the amount of fiber within the US diet plummeted as the amount of processed foods eaten increased.

As the amount of fiber consumed as part of the diet decreases, the consistency of the normal stool becomes more solid. This hard stool requires more intestinal contractions to expel, subsequently increasing pressure within the colon. In this environment, small defects within the colonic wall that would otherwise never pose a problem now fail, resulting in bulges in the wall. These small outcroppings eventually turn into pouches, called diverticula. As feces travel through the colon, some may become trapped within these pouches. When bacteria grow there, they cause localized inflammation and infection.

The main symptom of diverticulitis is abdominal pain, which tends to be localized to the left side of the lower abdomen. Classic signs of infection include fever, malaise, body aches, chills, nausea, and vomiting. Bleeding is rare with this condition. Because of the local infections of these pouches, adhesions may develop, narrowing the diameter of the colon and resulting in constipation and bowel obstruction. In severe cases, these infected outcroppings may burst, causing perforation of the affected segment of colon. This event may lead to peritonitis, severe infection, and, if left untreated, septic shock.

Special Populations

Many of the conditions discussed in this chapter are more prevalent in older patients. Older patients can have diminished abilities to detect pain and tend to have a higher pain threshold. As a result, they may not display rigidity or guarding. This presentation can hamper diagnosis and—more importantly—delay access to health care. Because an older patient has decreased body temperature regulation and response, conditions such as an acute abdomen, including peritonitis, may not present with fever. Even if fever is present, it can be minimal. If an older patient does not feel pain, he or she may not know why a fever has occurred. The patient may try to treat it at home. Thus, by the time emergency medical services (EMS) is activated, the patient is already septic and seriously ill.

Abdominal pain can also be a symptom of a cardiac condition. Imagine how difficult it would be to initially distinguish the source of abdominal pain in a 75-year-old man with a history of gastric ulcers, diverticulitis, and heart disease. Additionally, vascular pathology such as an abdominal aortic aneurysm can cause abdominal pain.

Comorbidity creates great difficulties for health care providers, but success can be achieved by obtaining a complete history and performing a thorough physical examination. You should ask about the patient's medical history, especially the history of recent illness, to identify a potential illness. Ask about abdominal discomfort, when the patient last had a bowel movement, whether she or he was constipated or had diarrhea, when the patient last ate, and whether he or she vomited. Asking these questions can help to rule out appendicitis, bowel obstruction, and ruptured bowel. Remember, however, that history taking should not delay transport.

Consider establishing intravenous (IV) access in most patients with abdominal pain who have comorbid factors. Finally, monitor vital signs, provide rapid transport, and be ready for any changes in the patient's status.

Chronic Inflammatory Conditions

▶ Ulcerative Colitis

Ulcerative colitis is caused by inflammation of the colon. This inflammation is generalized, affecting the inner lining of the intestine, and does not occur in patches, as in Crohn disease. It is unclear what causes the chronic inflammation, though genetics, stress, and autoimmunity have been speculated to be responsible. In ulcerative colitis, the inflammation causes a thinning of the wall of the intestine, resulting in a weakened, dilated rectum.

The damaged lining of the colon is highly susceptible to infections by bacteria and bleeding. These two states establish the foundation on which the signs and symptoms develop.

In the United States, approximately 238 per 100,000 people have ulcerative colitis.[4] In the past, ulcerative colitis was thought to peak between age 15 and 25 years and then again between 55 and 65 years, although recent studies contradict this supposition.[5,6] It occurs more often in men than in women.[7] There is a strong family history component for this disease. For example, having a sibling with ulcerative colitis increases the risk of developing the disease more than fourfold.[8] This fact supports the hypothesis that genetics plays some role in this disease. Ulcerative colitis is more prevalent in Caucasians and people of Jewish descent.[7]

The presentation of this condition is characterized by gradual onset of bloody diarrhea, hematochezia, and mild to severe abdominal pain. Other signs and symptoms can be joint pain and skin lesions. These effects lend credence to the idea of an autoimmune component to the disease. Finally, the patient can experience fever, fatigue, and loss of appetite from the infection.

▶ Irritable Bowel Syndrome

Irritable bowel syndrome (IBS) is a condition in which patients have abdominal pain and changes in their bowel habits. One diagnostic criterion is that patients have pain at least 3 days per month for at least 3 months. The pathology of the disease is unclear. The following three main factors are typically observed in patients with IBS:

- Hypersensitivity of bowel pain receptors. Normal stretching of the bowel can cause pain in these patients.
- Hyperresponsiveness of the smooth muscles in the bowel, which produces the cramping sensations and diarrhea.
- Psychiatric disorder connection and IBS. It is unclear if the bowel disorder causes the psychiatric disorder, or vice versa.

Hyperresponsiveness of the bowel in IBS can cause areas of spasm. These spasms can stop fecal movement, creating constipation and bloating. Conversely, if the spasms are more wavelike than localized, the patient can experience diarrhea as the feces are moved quickly through the bowel.

Patients typically begin to have problems with bowel habits during childhood, with 50% of IBS cases developing in patients younger than age 35 years.[9] In Western countries, women are more susceptible to this disease; in contrast, in South Asia, South America, and Africa, the typical patient is a man.[10]

IBS can be triggered by various stimuli. Stress, large meals, and certain foods such as wheat, rye, chocolate, alcohol, milk products, and caffeinated drinks can trigger an attack.

IBS is a chronic condition. Prehospital presentations will typically involve a flare-up of the condition. Patients may present with abdominal pain or discomfort. This pain is relieved by a bowel movement. When the pain starts, there is usually a change in the frequency and consistency of bowel movements. Patients may experience diarrhea, **steatorrhea**, or constipation. They may also feel bloated.

▶ Crohn Disease

Crohn disease is similar to ulcerative colitis, but can involve the entire GI tract from mouth to anus. The main part of the GI tract that tends to be affected is the ileum—the last portion of the small intestine before it joins the large intestine. There are several theories as to the cause of Crohn disease, though no definitive cause has been identified.

Crohn disease affects 201 adults per 100,000 population.[4] Most patients are between age 15 and 35 years,[11] although a second peak in incidence among older adults (age 60 to 70 years) has also been identified.[12] Men are diagnosed as often as women.[11] This condition generally affects more whites than African Americans, and people of Jewish descent have a notably increased incidence of the disease.[13]

Of interest with Crohn disease and colitis is the presence of signs and symptoms outside the GI system. This evidence helps to support the theory that an autoimmune component is functioning within this disease. It is unclear what causes this immune reaction: Does the presence of antigens in the GI tract trigger an immune response? Is the immune system itself not working correctly? Another theory is that the immune system creates antibodies for an antigen that does not exist, thereby triggering a cascade of reactions to a nonexistent invader.

Family history and genetics play a role with this disease. Medical researchers are discovering that how the body is made and how it is able to function are important characteristics in whether a person gets a disease and how that disease progresses. The fact that many people with Crohn disease have family members who have some type of bowel disease suggests a familial/genetic component.[14]

Regardless of the underlying reason for the development of Crohn disease, the result is a series of attacks by the immune system on the GI tract. This activity of white blood cells damages all layers of the portion of GI tract involved. The result is most often a scarred, narrowed, stiff, and weakened portion of the small intestine. This patch of damage is found among areas of intestine that are normal, and narrowing of this segment can cause bowel obstruction.

Patients with Crohn disease present with a chronic complaint of abdominal pain, often in the lower right area. This pain corresponds to the location of the ileum. Rectal bleeding, weight loss, diarrhea, arthritis, skin problems, and fever may also be present. Bleeding tends to involve small blood losses over a long period of time. Acute severe hemorrhage is rare, but chronic bleeding resulting in anemia and hypotension does occur. Patients can have episodes of mild to severe signs and symptoms.

Pathophysiology of the Urinary System

Diseases and conditions of the urinary system can cause acute abdominal pain. These conditions range from mild (urinary tract infections) to true emergencies (acute kidney injury). Although the prehospital care for many urologic diseases is supportive, your ability to recognize the signs and symptoms of the true emergencies is critical to providing your patients with the best chance of a positive outcome.

Urinary tract infections (UTIs), also known as bladder inflammation or **cystitis**, usually develop in the lower urinary tract (urethra and bladder) when either normal bacteria flora, which exist naturally on the skin, or other bacteria enter the urethra and grow. These infections are common, especially in women, owing to the relatively short urethra and the proximity of the urethra to the vagina and rectum. A UTI in the upper urinary tract (ureters and kidneys) occurs most often when a UTI in the lower urinary tract remains untreated. Upper UTIs can lead to **pyelonephritis** (inflammation of the kidney and renal pelvis) and abscesses, which eventually reduce kidney function. In severe cases, and more commonly in the elderly, untreated UTIs can lead to sepsis.

Common symptoms in patients with a lower UTI include painful urination, frequent urges to urinate, and difficulty in urination. The pain usually begins as a visceral discomfort but then converts to an extreme burning pain, especially during urination. The pain, which remains localized in the pelvis, is often perceived as bladder pain in women and as prostate pain in men. Sometimes the pain may be referred to the shoulder or neck. In addition, the urine may have a foul odor or may appear cloudy.

Pathophysiology of the Renal System

Kidney stones (renal calculi) originate in the renal pelvis and arise when an excess of insoluble salts or uric acid crystallizes in the urine **Figure 20-4**. This excess of salts is typically due to water intake that is insufficient to dissolve the salts. The stones consist of different types of chemicals, depending on the precise imbalance in the urine.

The most common stones—calcium stones—occur more frequently in men than in women and may have a hereditary component. These stones also occur in patients with metabolic disorders such as gout or with hormonal disorders.

Patients who have kidney stones will almost always be in pain. (Many rate kidney stone pain as 11 on a scale of 1 to 10.) The pain usually starts as a vague discomfort in the flank but becomes very intense within 30 to 60 minutes. It may migrate forward and toward the groin as the stone passes through the system.

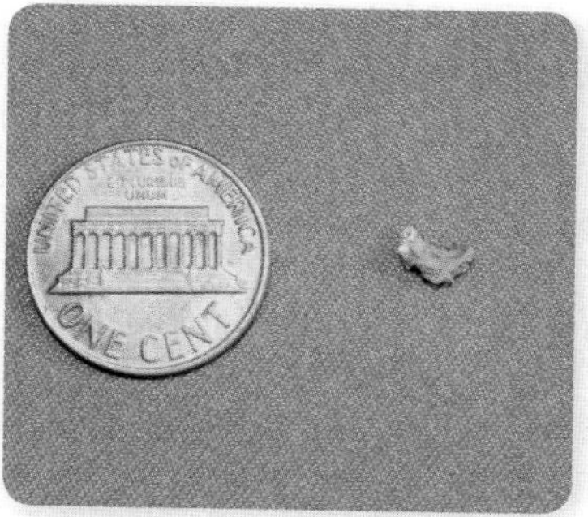

Figure 20-4 A kidney stone.

Some patients will be agitated and restless as they walk and move in an attempt to relieve the pain. Others will attempt to remain motionless and guard the abdomen. Either behavior makes palpation of the abdomen difficult. Vital signs will vary, depending on the severity of pain. The greater the pain, the higher the blood pressure and pulse will be.

If a stone has become lodged in the lower part of the ureter, signs and symptoms of a UTI (frequency and urgency of urination, painful urination, and/or **hematuria**) may be present, but the patient will not have a fever. If a kidney stone is suspected, be sure to obtain a patient history and a family history; both can supply important information.

Kidney disease may be categorized as either acute or chronic. In the United States, the prevalence of chronic kidney disease is approximately 14%.[15] The two leading causes of kidney disease are high blood pressure and uncontrolled diabetes.[15]

Acute kidney injury (AKI) is a sudden (possibly over a period of days) decrease in kidney function. It is accompanied by an increase of toxins in the blood. In 2008, according to the National Kidney and Urologic Diseases Information Clearinghouse, AKI accounted for more than 23,000 hospitalizations in the United States.[16] However, hospitalization rates declined significantly from 2012 to 2013, and by 10% for patients with acute kidney disease.[15] More than 48,000 people with kidney disease died in 2014,[17] but AKI is often reversible if promptly diagnosed and treated.

If the urine output drops to less than 500 mL per day, the condition is called **oliguria**. If urine production stops completely, the condition is called **anuria**. Whenever AKI occurs, the patient may experience generalized edema, acid buildup, and high levels of waste products in the blood. If left untreated, AKI can lead to heart failure, hypertension, and metabolic acidosis.

Chronic kidney disease is progressive and irreversible inadequate kidney function that is the result of permanent loss of nephrons. This disease develops over months or years. It is often caused by systemic diseases, such as diabetes or hypertension. In addition, chronic kidney disease can be caused by congenital disorders or prolonged pyelonephritis or can be a secondary effect of some infections, such as strep throat.

As the **nephrons** of the kidney become damaged and cease to function, scarring occurs. The tissue begins to shrink and waste away as the scarring progresses, leading to a loss of nephrons and renal mass. As kidney function diminishes, waste products and fluid build up in the blood. Systemic complications can develop, such as hypertension, congestive heart failure, anemia, and electrolyte imbalances.

Patients with chronic kidney disease may exhibit a wide variety of signs and symptoms, beginning with an altered level of consciousness. In later stages, seizures and coma are possible. Additional signs and symptoms include lethargy, nausea, headaches, cramps, and signs of anemia. The patient's skin will be pale, cool, and moist, and the patient may appear jaundiced because of the buildup of wastes. A powdery accumulation of uric acid, called **uremic frost**, may also be present, especially on the face. The skin may appear bruised, and muscle twitching may be present. Patients with chronic kidney disease exhibit edema in the extremities and face because of fluid imbalances; they will also be hypotensive and have tachycardia. Pericarditis and pulmonary edema are common as well, and should be considered during auscultation of the chest.

Health expenditures for patients with chronic kidney disease are notoriously high. In 2013, Medicare spending for patients with chronic kidney disease age 65 years and older exceeded $50 billion, representing 20% of all Medicare spending in this age group.[18]

▶ End-Stage Renal Disease

If left untreated, AKI or chronic kidney disease will progress to **end-stage renal disease (ESRD)**. In a patient with ESRD, the kidneys have lost most of their ability to function, and toxic waste materials build up in the patient's blood. ESRD is fatal unless treated by dialysis or renal transplantation. In 2013, nearly 120,000 new cases of ESRD were reported in the United States.[18] The prevalence of ESRD exceeded 670,000 patients in the first quarter of 2014, and it continues to rise as mortality rates decline among this population.[18] Of more than 120,000 people waiting for life-saving organ transplants in the United States, nearly 100,000 are awaiting kidney transplants (as of December 2016).[19] Fewer than 18,000 people receive a transplant each year.[19]

Confusion, shortness of breath, peripheral edema, bruising, chest pain, and bone pain are initial signs of ESRD. As toxins continue to accumulate, pruritus, nausea and vomiting, muscle twitching and tremors, and hallucinations may occur. Patients may also present with lethargy, headaches, cramps, and signs of anemia. The skin is pale, cool, and moist and may appear jaundiced or bruised. Uremic frost may be present around the face. Edema of the extremities and face is apparent, and patients are hypotensive and tachycardic. Pericarditis and pulmonary edema are also common and should be evaluated during auscultation of the chest. In the late stages, seizures and coma are possible and the patient may ultimately die.

Pathophysiology of Female Reproductive Organs

Gynecologic conditions are a common cause of acute abdominal pain. Always consider that a woman with lower quadrant abdominal pain and tenderness may have a problem related to her ovaries, fallopian tubes, or uterus. While pain may be related to the normal menstrual cycle or the release of an egg from an ovary, a common cause of an acute abdomen in women is **pelvic inflammatory disease (PID)** (infection of the fallopian tubes and the surrounding tissues of the pelvis). With PID, acute pain and tenderness in the lower part of the abdomen may be intense and accompanied by a high fever.

Between 1% and 2% of all pregnancies are ectopic.[20] The term **ectopic pregnancy** means that a fertilized egg has come to lie in an area outside the uterus, usually in a fallopian tube. A fallopian tube is simply not large enough to support the growth of a fetus and placenta for more than about 6 to 8 weeks. When the tube ruptures, it produces massive internal hemorrhage and acute abdominal pain, generally on one side. In this situation, the acute abdomen may be associated with the onset of hypovolemic shock. Chapter 25, *Gynecologic Emergencies*, covers gynecologic emergencies in depth.

Pathophysiology of the Male Genital Tract

▶ Epididymitis and Orchitis

One possible complication of male UTI is **epididymitis**, an infection that causes inflammation of the epididymis along the posterior border of the testis. When one or both testes become infected, this condition is called **orchitis**. With orchitis, the infection causes one or both testes to become enlarged and tender, leading to pain and swelling in the scrotum. Swelling may occur in the groin on the affected side. The pain may increase during bowel movements. The patient will have a fever, and the urine will have a foul odor. Prehospital management of these conditions is supportive.

▶ Priapism

Priapism, a painful, tender, persistent erection, can result from diseases such as leukemia and tumors, as well as from blunt perineal trauma, spinal cord injury, and use of cocaine, certain prescription medications, or drugs for erectile dysfunction. When this condition is present, be sure to maintain the patient's privacy and do not make assumptions about the cause of the condition. Whatever the cause, treat all patients with respect. If a spinal cord injury is suspected, ensure proper immobilization techniques.

▶ Benign Prostate Hypertrophy

Benign prostate hypertrophy (BPH) is an age-related nonmalignant (noncancerous) enlargement of the prostate gland. It occurs in approximately 50% of men older than 60 years.[21] BPH may be asymptomatic, or it may lead to difficulty starting urine flow, a slow weak urine flow once started, incomplete emptying of the bladder, increased urination at night, and urinary retention.

▶ Testicular Masses

Testicular masses rarely require prehospital treatment. They may be painful or painless, and if painful, the pain may radiate up the spermatic cord or be localized to a specific scrotal point. Most are benign cystic masses or a varicocele—a painless mass of dilated veins posterior to the testicle. Testicular cancer usually presents as a painless solid lump on the testicle. Incidence of testicular cancer is on the rise, with rates rising from 3.7 cases per 100,000 population from 1969 to 1971, to 5.4 cases per 100,000 population from 1995 to 1999.[22] In 2014, more than 8,800 new cases of this cancer were reported in the United States, with 380 deaths from this cause.[22]

▶ Testicular Torsion

Testicular torsion is a twisting of the testicle on the spermatic cord, from which it is suspended. This condition is associated with the sudden onset of scrotal pain and swelling. It is a medical emergency if the twisting of the vessels reduces blood flow to the testis. The torsion is usually unilateral, occurring in only one testis at a time. Torsions may occur with or without blunt trauma, a testicular lump, or blood in the semen. Patients should be carefully and promptly transported and allowed to assume the position of greatest comfort.

Pathophysiology of Other Organ Systems

The aorta lies immediately behind the peritoneum. In older people, the wall of the aorta sometimes develops weak areas that swell to form an **aneurysm** (a swelling or enlargement of a part of an artery, resulting from weakening of the arterial wall). The development of an aneurysm, unless acutely dissecting, is rarely associated with symptoms because it occurs slowly. If the aneurysm tears and ruptures, however, massive hemorrhage may occur, and the patient will present with signs of acute peritoneal irritation and hemorrhagic shock. The patient may also report radiation of severe pain to the back because the peritoneum can be stripped away from the wall of the main abdominal cavity by the hemorrhage. Pain can also be associated with the pressure of blood on the back itself. In such cases, bleeding usually leads to profound shock.

A **hernia** is a protrusion of an organ or tissue through a hole or opening into a body cavity where it does not belong. Hernias can occur as a result of the following:

- A congenital defect, as around the umbilicus
- A surgical wound that has failed to heal properly
- A natural weakness in an area, such as in the groin

Hernias do not always produce a mass or lump that the patient will notice. Extreme obesity may interfere with the ability to identify the mass. At times, the mass will disappear back into the body cavity in which it belongs. In this case, the hernia is said to be reducible. If the mass cannot be pushed back within the body, it is said to be incarcerated.

Reducible hernias pose little risk to the patient; some people live with them for years. When a hernia is incarcerated, however, its contents may become seriously compressed by the surrounding tissue, eventually compromising the blood supply. This situation, called **strangulation**, is a serious medical emergency. Immediate surgery is required to remove any dead tissue and repair the hernia. In the abdomen, there are several common locations for hernias Figure 20-5.

The following signs and symptoms indicate a serious hernia problem:

- A formerly reducible mass is no longer reducible
- Pain at the hernia site
- Tenderness when the hernia is palpated
- Red or blue skin discoloration over the hernia

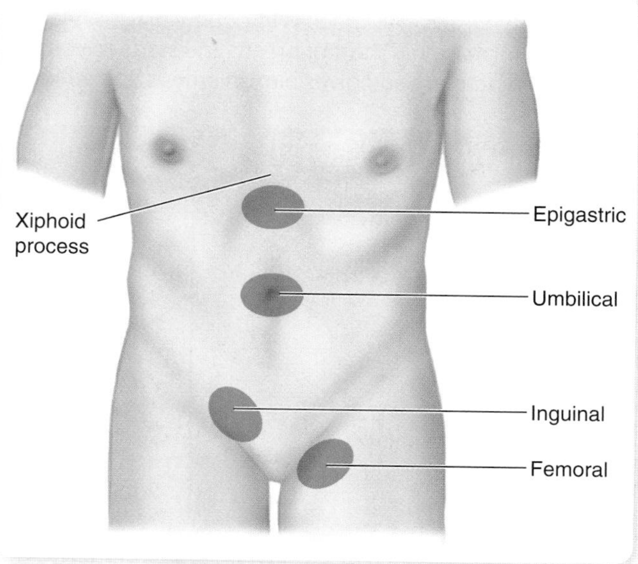

Figure 20-5 Common locations of abdominal hernias.

Patient Assessment

Scene Size-up

As always, ensure that the scene is safe and be alert for clues to help you determine the nature of illness (NOI) or the mechanism of injury. Acute abdomen can be the result of violence, such as blunt or penetrating trauma, so always be vigilant. Chapter 32, *Abdominal and Genitourinary Injuries*, discusses traumatic injuries in detail.

Take standard precautions, using a minimum of gloves and eye protection. Consider donning a gown and covering your shoes with disposable, protective covers because there may be feces and urine on the floor and some patients may have active projectile vomiting. Examples of additional resources for a GI patient include extra gloves, mask, gowns, change of uniform, suction equipment, extra linens, blankets, washcloths, towels, and adult and child diapers.

Determine the number of patients at the scene. Note that most calls for GI problems will not involve multiple patients. However, a call for assistance at an office building where several people are complaining about GI symptoms should lead you to suspect release of an agent. Biologic or chemical agents, for example, can cause people to have abdominal pain, nausea, vomiting, diarrhea, and other GI signs and symptoms.

Primary Survey

The first step of the primary survey is to form your general impression and determine whether a patient has an acute abdomen. The following is a checklist of common signs and symptoms of irritation or inflammation of the peritoneum.

- Local or diffuse abdominal pain or tenderness
- A quiet patient who is guarding the abdomen
- Rapid and shallow breathing
- Referred (distant) pain
- Anorexia, nausea, and vomiting
- Hematemesis (bright red or "coffee-ground" emesis)
- Tense, often distended, abdomen
- Sudden constipation or bloody diarrhea
- Dark, tarry stool (melena)
- Painful or frequent urination
- Discolored urine accompanied by a strong odor
- Tachycardia
- Hypotension
- Fever

Patients who are experiencing renal or genital problems may exhibit many of the same symptoms as a patient with other abdominal problems—nausea and vomiting, constipation or diarrhea, flank pain, and abdominal pain.

YOU are the Provider — PART 3

You explain your concerns to the patient, and he agrees to allow you to transport him to the emergency department (ED), even though he says, "All I need is to get my dialysis." As you place the patient on the stretcher and secure him, he begins to become increasingly short of breath and starts to vomit. Your partner provides the patient with 100% oxygen via a nonrebreathing mask and gives him an emesis bag while you attempt to insert an IV line.

Recording Time: 10 Minutes	
Respirations	36 breaths/min, rales bilaterally
Pulse	Strong and regular, 140 beats/min
Skin	Warm, dry, and pink
Blood pressure	226/108 mm Hg
Oxygen saturation (Spo_2)	94% on 100% oxygen
Pupils	Pupils Equal, Round, and Reactive to Light and Accommodation (PERRLA)

6. Does this patient need IV access?
7. What are your treatment options for this patient?
8. What could be a cause of this patient's shortness of breath?

In forming your general impression, closely examine the location where the patient is found, because it can provide hints about what happened. Was the patient walking to the bathroom when he or she passed out? Has the patient been sick for several days and camped out on the couch? Was the patient at work when a sudden bout of pain doubled him or her over?

A patient with urologic or renal problems may exhibit extremes of activity. Is the patient constantly changing positions in an attempt to find a comfortable position (the kidney stone dance)? Or is the patient sitting very still, with the knees drawn to the chest? Is the abdomen distended or rigid?

In some situations, patients are comfortable only when lying in one particular position, which tends to relax muscles adjacent to the inflamed organ and thus lessen the pain. Therefore, the position of the patient may provide you with an important clue. For example, a patient with appendicitis may draw up the right knee, whereas a patient with pancreatitis may lie curled up on one side.

One aspect of the general impression that is different for GI patients is odor. What is the smell of the room or location of the patient? There are few EMS calls that rise to the level of noxious odor as those that involve upper GI bleeding. The foul-smelling stool that accompanies these calls can make even an experienced AEMT nauseous. When dealing with these strong odors, the key is to hold your ground. The sense of smell is the most acute for approximately 1 minute, but then the intensity of an odor is lost due to the olfactory nerve becoming tired of sending the same signal. If you are faced with a strong odor on a call, stay in the environment. After 2 to 5 minutes, the smell may be barely noticeable.

It is not critical for you to determine the cause of acute abdomen; rather, your priority is to recognize potential causes and provide the correct supportive care.

Special Populations

Use a hands-off assessment to establish a general impression when dealing with pediatric patients. Until a rapport is established, touching a child may cause anxiety and distress, which can alter assessment findings.

Evaluate the patient's airway, breathing, circulation, disability, and exposure (ABCDEs), and immediately care for any life threats. Airway patency becomes a pertinent concern with a GI patient. A patient who is vomiting has a greater chance to aspirate. In patients who are awake and responsive, positioning is key to maintaining a patent airway. In patients who have an altered mental status, open the airway using the appropriate maneuvers. Inspect the airway closely for foreign bodies. Remove or suction any obstructions that are found. While evaluating the airway, notice any unusual odors emanating from the mouth. Patients who have extremely advanced bowel obstructions can have feculent breath, smelling of stool.

GI problems rarely affect breathing directly. If a breathing problem is encountered, it typically stems from a severe complication. Ensure that the airway is clear. In particular, if the patient has aspirated a substance, it can affect his or her ability to oxygenate and ventilate. Also, as a result of the abdominal pain, the patient may show shallow or inadequate respirations because deep breaths often intensify the pain.

The assessment of the circulatory system is essential in understanding how the GI issue is affecting the body. The patient's pulse rate and quality, as well as skin condition, may indicate shock. Check the pulses in both arms because a difference in pulse strength may indicate an aortic dissection. Expose the patient and assess for major bleeding.

Words of Wisdom

When measuring the blood pressure in a dialysis patient, always use the arm that does not have the shunt.

Many GI diseases involve pain and/or hemorrhage. Shock may be caused by hypovolemia or may be the result of a severe infection (sepsis). If evidence of shock (inadequate perfusion) is present, interventions should include high-flow oxygen, keeping the patient warm, and placing the patient in the position dictated by local protocol for shock patients. Ensure that you provide prompt treatment for life threats, and do not delay in providing transport.

Orthostatic vital signs, assessing vital signs in two different patient positions, will help you determine the extent of bleeding that has occurred, if any. First, have the patient assume a position of comfort, usually seated or lying down. Take an accurate blood pressure and heart rate. Next, have the patient change positions (that is, have the patient stand or sit up). Use caution, because the patient may lose consciousness with a positional change. Wait a minute or two, and then repeat the blood pressure and heart rate measurements. Normally, there should be little change in the blood pressure or heart rate with such a positional change. When a patient has a significant loss of fluid within the vascular space, however, there may be a 10-beat increase in the heart rate and/or a 10-mm Hg drop in blood pressure. A decrease in a patient's blood pressure while sitting up from a lying position or when standing up from a sitting position is called **orthostatic hypotension**.

When you examine a patient with a GI problem for gross bleeding, it is not unusual to find large amounts of blood. Take note of the amount of blood lost, focusing on being accurate. The emotional effects of seeing large amounts of blood could lead people to overestimate the volume lost. The amount of blood in a toilet is particularly difficult to estimate owing to dilution. To practice volume estimation, measure the amount of water in a glass, and then spill it on a carpet; note the size of the puddle. Spill another volume of water on a hard surface such as a tile floor; again note the size of the puddle.

When making your transport decision, integrate the information obtained in the primary survey. If the patient has positive orthostatic vital signs (that is, serial vital signs change with a change in position), thoughtfully consider how the patient will be moved. Can the patient sit up in a stair chair, or will he or she pass out? Is the patient in critical condition so that he or she needs to be moved urgently?

Patients who have airway, breathing, or circulation problems, including problems with pulse and perfusion, and those with suspected internal bleeding require rapid transport. Included in the group to package quickly and transport rapidly are patients who have a poor general impression, especially pediatric and geriatric patients. Pale, cool, diaphoretic skin; tachycardia; hypotension; and altered level of consciousness are all signs of significant illness.

Ensure that the ride during transport is as gentle as possible for the patient. Drive smoothly and steadily. Rapid driving can result in increased vehicle movement, potentially aggravating and possibly worsening the patient's abdominal pain.

Words of Wisdom

An acute abdomen is characterized by abdominal pain and tenderness.

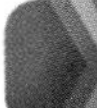

History Taking

Pain is often a finding of importance in patients with GI problems because it can indicate trauma, hemorrhage, infection, or obstruction. As with the primary survey, use OPQRST (**O**nset, **P**rovocation/palliation, **Q**uality, **R**egion/radiation, **S**everity, and **T**iming) to elaborate on the chief complaint. Table 20-4 describes the types of pain that may be experienced with an abdominal problem.

In patients with a urologic problem, the patient history and physical examination will provide the information needed to successfully manage the patient. Determining that the pain actually started in the flank and not in its present location of the lower right quadrant could mean the difference between a correct field diagnosis of a kidney stone and an incorrect field diagnosis of appendicitis. Similarly, determining that the patient has a history of diabetes and hypertension along with signs of uremia can help confirm your impression of chronic kidney disease.

The SAMPLE (Signs and symptoms, Allergies, Medications, Pertinent past medical history, Last oral intake, Events leading up to the illness or injury) history will help elicit the relevant current and past medical history. It may not affect the interventions you perform, but it will help provide needed information for the physician in the ED to aid in determining the cause of the acute abdomen.

When asking patients about their complaints, you often need to discuss subjects that are not commonly described with everyday language. It is important that you and your patient have a common frame of reference. For example, one person's "diarrhea" may be another person's "soft stool."

Table 20-4 Types of Abdominal Pain

Abdominal Pain Type	Origin	Description	Cause
Visceral discomfort	Hollow organs	Difficult to localize Described as burning, cramping, gnawing, or aching Usually felt superficially	Organ contracts too forcefully or is distended (stretched)
Parietal pain/rebound pain	Peritoneum	Steady, achy pain Easier to localize than visceral Increases with movement	Inflammation of the peritoneum (caused by bleeding or infection)
Somatic pain	Peripheral nerve tracts	Localized pain, usually felt deeply	Irritation of or injury to tissue, causing activation of peripheral nerve tracts
Referred pain	Peripheral nerve tracts	Pain originating in the abdomen and causing the perception of pain in distant locations Usually occurs after initial visceral, parietal, or somatic pain	Similar paths for the peripheral nerves of the abdomen and the distant location

Ask the following questions specific to the signs and symptoms of a GI or urologic emergency:

- **Nausea and vomiting.** Do you feel nauseous? Have you vomited? How many times? In which period of time? Was there red blood? Did it look like coffee grounds?
- **Changes in bowel habits.** Has there been any change in your bowel habits? Have you been constipated? Did the stool look dark and tarry? Have you had diarrhea? How many bowel movements have occurred, and over what period of time? Was there any red blood in it?
- **Urination.** Have you been urinating more or less often than usual? Is there pain when you urinate? Is the color of the urine dark or unusual? Is there an unusual odor?
- **Weight loss.** Have you lost weight recently? How many pounds?
- **Belching or flatulence.** Have you experienced belching or flatulence? For how long?
- **Pain.** What does the pain feel like? How long have you had this pain? Is the pain constant or intermittent?
- **Other.** Ask about any other signs or symptoms related to this complaint, such as "Are there any changes you have noted recently that may be contributing to your pain?"
- **Concurrent chest pain.** If the patient reports chest pain, use OPQRST.

Continue with the SAMPLE history. Has the patient experienced this kind of abdominal pain before? If the patient is female and of childbearing age, identify the date of her last menstrual period. This will help determine if the patient could possibly be pregnant or raise the suspicion of an ectopic pregnancy. Has the patient had any surgery or recent hospitalizations?

It is important to determine whether the patient has ingested any substance that could be causing the acute abdomen. If eating causes pain, discomfort, vomiting, or diarrhea, the patient will eat less often or stop eating. Do not give the patient anything by mouth, as food or fluid may aggravate many of the symptoms. Also, the presence of food in the stomach increases the risk of aspiration, especially if the patient needs emergency surgery.

Finally, determine the events that led up to the patient's present illness. It is important to determine whether this is a medical emergency or related to trauma.

Secondary Assessment

Information gathered in the history-taking portion of the patient assessment may be used to focus your physical examination of the abdomen. A normal abdomen is soft and not tender. In contrast, an acute abdomen is characterized by pain and tenderness. The pain may be sharply localized or diffuse and will vary in its severity. Localized pain gives a clue to the problem organ or area causing it. Tenderness may be minimal or so great that the patient will not allow you to touch the abdomen. In some instances, the muscles of the abdominal wall become rigid in an involuntary effort to protect the abdomen from further irritation. This boardlike muscle spasm, called **guarding**, can be seen with major problems such as a perforated ulcer or pancreatitis. You may also note the presence of **ascites**, a collection of edema in the abdomen typically caused by liver failure.

Words of Wisdom

When you are palpating the abdomen, always begin on the side opposite from the site of pain.

Words of Wisdom

An acute abdomen may indicate peritonitis, in which generalized signs can make it challenging to determine exactly where the problem lies, even for physicians. Knowing the abdominal assessment steps well and recording your findings in detail are important early components of the process that leads to diagnosis.

A patient with peritonitis usually has abdominal pain, even when lying quietly. The patient may have difficulty breathing and may take rapid, shallow breaths because of the pain. Usually, you will find tenderness on palpation of the abdomen or when the patient moves. The degree of pain and tenderness is usually related directly to the severity of peritoneal inflammation.

Use the following steps to assess the abdomen:

1. Explain to the patient what you are going to do in terms of assessing the abdomen.
2. Place the patient in a supine position with the legs drawn up and flexed at the knees to relax the abdominal muscles. If trauma is involved, the patient should remain supine and stabilized. Determine whether the patient is restless or quiet and whether motion causes pain.
3. Expose the abdomen and visually assess it. Does the abdomen appear distended (enlarged)? Do you see any pulsating masses (indicates an aortic aneurysm)? Is there bruising to the abdominal wall? Are there any surgical scars?
4. Ask the patient where the pain is most intense. Palpate in a clockwise direction beginning with the quadrant *after* the one the patient indicates is tender or painful; end with the quadrant the patient indicates is tender or painful. If the most

painful area is palpated first, the patient may guard against further examination, making your assessment more difficult and less reliable.

5. Be very gentle when palpating the abdomen. Occasionally, an organ within the abdomen will be enlarged and very fragile, such that rough palpation could cause further damage. If you see a pulsating mass, do not touch it; doing so could cause the aorta to rupture.
6. Palpate the four quadrants of the abdomen gently to determine whether each quadrant is tense (guarded) or soft when palpated **Figure 20-6**.
7. Note whether the pain is localized to a particular quadrant or diffuse (widespread).
8. Palpate and wait for the patient to respond, looking for a facial grimace or a verbal "ouch." Do not ask the patient, "Does it hurt here?" as you palpate.
9. Determine whether the patient exhibits rebound tenderness (may be tender when direct pressure is applied, but very painful when pressure is released). This is an indicator of peritonitis.
10. Determine whether the patient can relax the abdominal wall on command. Guarding or rigidity may be present, which can indicate peritoneal irritation.

Words of Wisdom

When assessing for rebound tenderness, it is important to describe to the patient what you are going to do prior to touching. Explain by stating, "I am going to press down on your abdomen and then hold it for a few seconds before I release it. I need you to tell me whether it hurts more when I press down or when I let go."

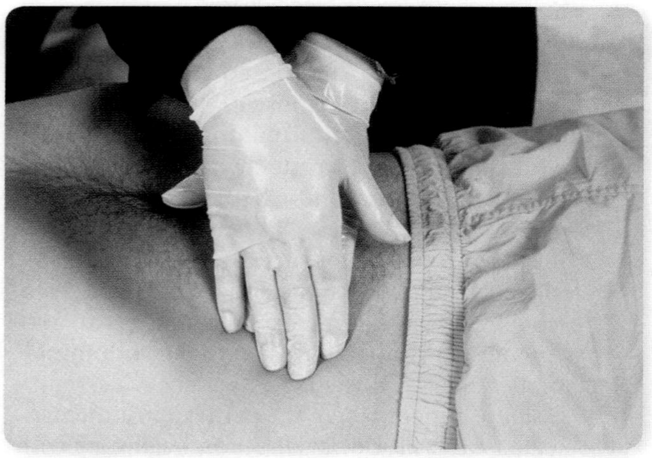

Figure 20-6 Check for tenderness or rigidity by gently palpating the abdomen.

Findings of a high respiratory rate with a normal pulse rate and blood pressure may indicate the patient is unable to ventilate properly because deep breathing causes pain. A high respiratory rate and pulse rate with signs of shock, such as pallor and diaphoresis (profuse sweating), may indicate septic or hypovolemic shock.

Use pulse oximetry and noninvasive blood pressure devices when these monitoring devices are available. It is recommended that you always obtain the patient's first blood pressure reading manually with a sphygmomanometer (blood pressure cuff) and stethoscope.

Special Populations

Abdominal injuries are the third leading cause of trauma-related deaths in children (after head and chest injuries).[23] In pediatric patients, the intra-abdominal organs are relatively large, making them vulnerable to blunt trauma. For example, the abdomen in an infant or toddler often seems protuberant because of the large liver. The liver and spleen extend below the rib cage in young children and, therefore, do not have as much bony protection as they do in an adult. These organs have a rich blood supply, so injuries to them can result in large blood losses. The kidneys are also more vulnerable to injury in children because they are more mobile and less well supported than in adults. Finally, the duodenum and pancreas are likely to be damaged in handlebar injuries.

Owing to their smaller fluid volume, children dehydrate quickly from vomiting. Abdominal pain in children often is the result of constipation; however, appendicitis is also another frequent cause of abdominal pain. Remember to assess for GI bleeding as well. Management of pediatric patients with abdominal complaints is the same as that for adults. Use a hands-off approach to get a general impression of the patient before touching to adequately assess any signs of distress.

Reassessment

Because it is often difficult to determine the cause of an acute abdominal emergency, it is extremely important to reassess the patient frequently to determine whether the patient's condition has changed. Remember, the condition of a patient with an acute abdomen can change rapidly from stable to unstable.

Vital signs must be reassessed and compared with the patient's baseline vital signs. If anything changes en route to the hospital, manage the problem and document any changes or additional treatment.

Reassess the patient and then ask and answer the following questions (where appropriate):

- Has the patient's level of consciousness changed?
- Has the patient become more anxious?

- Has the appearance of the skin changed?
- Has the pain gotten better or worse?
- Has bleeding become increased or decreased?
- Is the current treatment improving the patient's condition?
- Has an already identified problem gotten better or worse?
- What is the nature of any newly identified problems?

If the patient has GI bleeding, continue to assess for signs of shock. Before giving additional fluid boluses, listen to the patient's lung sounds to determine whether acute pulmonary edema is developing. If the patient wants to lie on his or her side, try to make that possible. Be sure that you can observe and maintain the patient's airway because vomiting is common in patients with GI conditions.

If the patient's condition is unstable, call for paramedic backup. If transport time is extended and rapid transport is needed, consider air medical transport if available.

Patients with urologic emergencies, especially patients with signs and symptoms of renal failure, also need reassessment. The electrolyte imbalances caused by the buildup of toxins can cause major, rapid changes in the functioning of the body's organs. Serial vital signs should be obtained and documented on the prehospital care report—at least every 5 minutes in cases of possible renal failure. Note any trends in the vital signs and level of consciousness, because they can be indicators of disease progression. Patients with possible urologic disease should not be given anything by mouth because this may induce vomiting or complicate surgical procedures.

Emergency Medical Care

The signs and symptoms of an acute abdomen signal a serious medical or surgical emergency. Ensure that you provide prompt, gentle transport for the patient; do not delay transport. Carry out the following steps as quickly as possible before transport:

1. Do not attempt to diagnose the cause of the acute abdomen.
2. Clear and maintain the airway.
3. Anticipate vomiting. Place the patient in the recovery position or position of comfort. Most patients feel better in a lateral recumbent position with the knees pulled in toward the chest.
4. Administer 100% supplemental oxygen, and be prepared to assist ventilation if the patient has a reduced tidal volume (shallow breathing).
5. Do not give the patient anything by mouth. Food or fluid will merely aggravate many of the symptoms, because intestinal paralysis will prevent it from passing out of the stomach. In addition, the stomach will have to be emptied before surgery if it is required.
6. Document all pertinent information. Use the OPQRST mnemonic. Note the presence of abdominal tenderness, distention, or guarding.
7. Anticipate the development of hypovolemic shock. Monitor blood pressure. Treat the patient for shock when it is evident. Place the patient in the position dictated by local protocol for shock patients.
8. Establish IV access, and give a 20-mL/kg bolus of an isotonic crystalloid if the patient presents with signs of hypovolemia. Otherwise, administer fluids at a to-keep-open rate. If kidney function is present, administer a bolus of fluid to the patient with a UTI and to the patient with a kidney stone. The fluid will rehydrate the patient, and an increased volume of urine will help flush any infection from the system. For a patient with kidney stones, the increased urine formation will help move the stone through the system.
9. Make the patient as comfortable as possible for transport. Patients are usually more comfortable with their legs pulled up toward the abdomen, because this position takes the pressure off the abdominal wall and diminishes pain. Conserve body heat with blankets, as needed. Provide gentle but rapid transport and constant psychological support.
10. Monitor vital signs; these may change quickly.
11. Consider calling for additional paramedic backup if the patient's condition shows any signs of instability.

Remember that in female patients with PID, acute pain and tenderness in the lower part of the abdomen may be intense and accompanied by a high fever. If you suspect PID, promptly transport the patient to the ED for treatment.

The combination of acute abdominal pain and hypovolemic shock mandates immediate transport to the hospital. Consider an ectopic pregnancy in any female of childbearing age who presents with acute abdominal distress, especially in the presence of hypotension.

Pneumonia, especially in the lower parts of the lung, may cause both ileal and abdominal pain. In this case, the problem lies in an adjacent body cavity, but the intense inflammatory response can affect the abdomen. Treat and transport this patient as you would any patient with abdominal pain.

The association of acute abdominal signs and symptoms with shock could also signify an aneurysm and requires prompt transportation. Because this is a fragile situation with a large, leaking artery, avoid unnecessary and vigorous palpation of the abdomen. Handle the patient gently during transport. Administer fluid only if the patient is hypotensive *and* symptomatic. Increasing blood pressure could cause rupture of an aneurysm.

Any signs and symptoms of a hernia in a patient with acute abdominal pain are cause for prompt transport to the ED as the pain could be caused by an incarceration or strangulation of the hernia.

Finally, AKI and chronic kidney disease can lead to life-threatening emergencies. Support of the ABCs is imperative. Be alert for the possibility of hypotension or pulmonary edema. Because of possible toxic buildup and electrolyte problems, medications to regulate acidosis and electrolyte imbalance and fluids for volume regulation may be required. Emergency transport and supportive care are often preferred over aggressive management in these patients.

Renal Dialysis

The only definitive treatment other than transplantation in cases of ESRD is **renal dialysis**. More than 468,000 patients are currently on dialysis in the United States.[24] In this process, the patient's blood is filtered and cleansed of the toxins and then returned to the body. The treatment eliminates waste, normalizes the blood chemistry, and reduces excess fluid. Renal dialysis and problems associated with it may prompt calls for prehospital care.

Two types of dialysis may be performed—peritoneal dialysis and hemodialysis. In peritoneal dialysis, large amounts of specially formulated dialysis fluid are infused into (and back out of) the abdominal cavity. This fluid stays in the cavity for 1 to 2 hours, allowing equilibrium to occur. Peritoneal dialysis is very effective but carries a high risk of peritonitis; consequently, aseptic technique is essential. With proper training, however, peritoneal dialysis can be performed in the home.

In hemodialysis, the patient's blood circulates through a dialysis machine that functions in much the same way as the normal kidneys. Most patients undergoing long-term hemodialysis have some sort of **shunt**; that is, a surgically created connection between a vein and an artery that is usually located in the forearm or upper arm. The patient is connected to the dialysis machine through this shunt, which allows blood to flow from the body into the dialysis machine and back to the body. Other patients have a small, button-shaped device called a HemaSite, which has a rubber septum that can be punctured with dialysis needles during treatment. HemaSites are usually placed in the upper arm or proximal anterior thigh. Finally, some patients have an **internal shunt** (an arteriovenous [AV] fistula), which is an artificial connection between a vein and an artery that is usually located in the forearm or upper arm **Figure 20-7**.

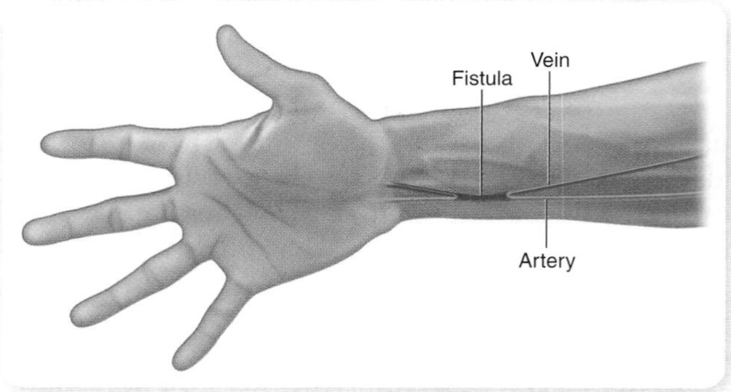

Figure 20-7 With an arteriovenous fistula, a bulge is created beneath the skin by arterial pressure at the site where the artery and the vein have been directly connected.

YOU are the Provider — PART 4

Venous access is difficult in this patient, but you are able to place a 22-gauge saline lock in the patient's right hand to be used as a medication route. You radio medical control, advising of the patient's condition, and are informed to withhold any IV fluid in this patient. You advise medical control that you have an approximately 7-minute estimated time of arrival.

Recording Time: 15 Minutes	
Respirations	36 breaths/min; rales bilaterally
Pulse	Strong and regular; 142 beats/min
Skin	Warm, dry, and pink
Blood pressure	210/102 mm Hg
Oxygen saturation (Spo_2)	95% on 100% oxygen

You continue monitoring the patient en route to the hospital. On arrival, you give your report to the ED nurse and complete your patient care report while your partner readies the ambulance for your next call.

9. Why did the medical control physician order that no IV fluid be administered to this patient?

In patients with a life-threatening emergency, the internal shunt may be used for IV access. In all other instances, an alternative IV site should be selected. AV shunts should not be used for routine blood draws.

You will most likely see a dialysis machine only if your service transports patients to and from dialysis centers. If there is a dialysis machine in a private residence, treatments will most likely be performed by a trained dialysis technician and only rarely by the patient or family members.

Patients requiring long-term dialysis usually undergo this process every 2 or 3 days for a period of 3 to 5 hours. Many receive dialysis in the hospital or in community dialysis facilities, but a significant number have home dialysis units. Patients undergoing dialysis at home usually have extensive training in the procedures, and often someone else in the home has also been trained. If a problem with the machine occurs, the patient may know a lot more about it than you do, so always ask what the patient has done before your arrival!

Although patients undergoing chronic dialysis can experience the same spectrum of illnesses and injuries as other patients, they are particularly vulnerable to certain conditions, either because of the dialysis itself or because of the underlying renal failure. Conditions associated with dialysis may result from accidental disconnection from the machine, malfunction of the machine, or rapid shifts in fluids and electrolytes. In addition, many adverse effects and complications can occur with dialysis; these are listed in Table 20-5.

A sudden drop in blood pressure is not uncommon during or immediately after dialysis, but it can lead to cardiac arrest if not promptly detected and treated. The patient may feel lightheaded or become confused, and often he or she yawns more than usual. Because dialysis alters the blood's chemistry, an electrolyte imbalance may develop. For this reason, you should consider the possibility of cardiac dysrhythmias and the need for advanced life support backup. Shock secondary to bleeding is also possible from any number of causes. Patients with chronic kidney disease, for example, are highly susceptible to duodenal ulcers; bleeding from those ulcers is not unusual. Bleeding may also occur from the dialysis cannula.

Also, if a patient misses a dialysis treatment, he or she may experience weakness, pulmonary edema, or excesses of electrolytes. If your call involves a patient on dialysis, start with the ABCDEs and manage them as necessary. Provide high-flow oxygen if indicated and manage any bleeding from the access site. Position the patient sitting up in cases of pulmonary edema or supine if the patient is in shock, and transport promptly.

When you find a shunt leaking during the dialysis cycle, see if you can tighten the connection. If it has become disconnected at the vein, clamp the cannula and disconnect the patient from the machine. In a suicide attempt, the patient may open up the cannula and allow himself or herself to exsanguinate. Keep in mind that patients receiving dialysis have often endured numerous medical interventions to simply survive. If you encounter this situation, immediately clamp off the cannula and apply direct pressure.

Some dialysis patients also have urinary catheters. The catheter is placed in the bladder so the urine can run into a bag. These catheters can often be a source of infection. The patient may report fever and general malaise (illness) in addition to any symptoms specific to kidney failure. Leave the device in place. Treat any signs and symptoms and transport the patient for further evaluation.

During transport, unless there is a life-threatening event, make all attempts to deliver the patient to a hospital with dialysis capability.

Table 20-5 Complications and Adverse Effects of Dialysis
Hypotension
Muscle cramps
Nausea/vomiting
Hemorrhage, especially from the access site
Infection at the access site
Altered mentation, loss of consciousness
Air embolism
Electrolyte imbalance
Myocardial ischemia

▶ Disequilibrium Syndrome

Dialysis rapidly lowers the concentration of urea in the blood, whereas the concentration of solutes in the cerebrospinal fluid (CSF) remains high. Water moves by osmosis from a solution of lower concentration into a solution of higher concentration. Thus, as a consequence of dialysis, water initially shifts from the bloodstream into the CSF, thereby mildly increasing intracranial pressure. In such a circumstance, the patient may experience **disequilibrium syndrome**, a condition characterized by

Words of Wisdom

In the field, it may be impossible to distinguish between disequilibrium syndrome and subdural hematoma, to which dialysis patients are particularly vulnerable. In such a case, transport the patient to the hospital immediately for a full neurologic evaluation.

nausea, vomiting, headache, and confusion. After a few hours, the fluid will re-equilibrate between the blood and CSF, and the patient's symptoms will improve on their own.

▶ Air Embolism

If any of the fittings and connections in the dialysis system are loose, air may enter the system, producing an **air embolism** in the patient. Symptoms of an air embolism include sudden dyspnea, hypotension, and cyanosis. If you suspect an air embolism, disconnect the patient from the dialysis machine. Per the Advanced Renal Education program, flat supine position for such a patient may be better than the traditionally advocated left lateral (Duran) and Trendelenburg position (position in which the body is supine with the head lower than the feet).[25] Transport the patient immediately.

YOU are the Provider SUMMARY

1. What are some potential causes of altered mental status in a patient receiving dialysis?

Common causes of altered mental status in a patient receiving dialysis are the same causes of altered mental status in patients who do not receive dialysis. However, when the dialysis patient has missed a dialysis appointment or has gone longer than normal in between treatments, he or she is particularly vulnerable to an electrolyte imbalance that is the result of the buildup of toxins in the bloodstream.

2. On the basis of the information provided, which type of dialysis does this patient receive?

The two types of dialysis are peritoneal dialysis and hemodialysis. In peritoneal dialysis, large amounts of specially formulated dialysis fluid are infused into (and back out of) the abdominal cavity. In hemodialysis, the patient's blood circulates through a dialysis machine that functions in much the same way as the normal kidneys. The patient is connected to the dialysis machine through a shunt, which allows blood to flow from the body into the dialysis machine and back to the body. Because of the large machines required for hemodialysis, this type of dialysis is almost exclusively found in dialysis centers. Hemodialysis is the type of dialysis this patient is receiving.

3. What is anuria?

Anuria is the complete cessation of urine production. If the urine output drops to less than 500 mL per day, the condition is called oliguria.

4. The patient seems to be answering all questions appropriately, but more slowly than what is reported to be normal. Should you approach the dialysis staff and request that he undergo dialysis in an attempt to help improve his mental status?

This treatment would be a possibility, but it would probably not be recommended. Dialysis needs to be performed on a routine basis, and missing or delaying a treatment may have a major impact on the patient's well-being. The patient's slowness to respond to questions, coupled with the patient's statement that this condition is not normal for him, warrants a trip to the ED.

5. You note a "lump" in the patient's left forearm. What is this lump, and why is it important for you to note?

Some patients receiving dialysis have a shunt, which is a surgically created access port usually located in the forearm or upper arm. It is important for AEMTs to recognize the presence and location of this shunt because the arm without the shunt should be used, if at all possible, for blood pressure measurements and IV lines.

6. Does this patient need IV access?

This patient could benefit from IV access for multiple reasons. First, he has an altered mental status and shortness of breath. Those two conditions alone are reason enough to insert an IV line, not only for possible fluid administration, but also as a medication route. Because this patient has a chronic medical condition, he may have poor venous access. In such a case, it would be prudent to establish IV access in this patient while he is still in somewhat stable condition, before he starts to decompensate, when it will be more difficult to establish access.

7. What are your treatment options for this patient?

There are multiple options for treatment in this patient, and some are better than others. This patient presents with rales bilaterally. Call for paramedic backup to administer medications or to administer continuous positive airway pressure, which may also be beneficial in clearing up the rales. Regardless of the treatment path you decide to take, 100% oxygen is indicated, but careful attention must be given to the patient in case of more emesis.

YOU are the Provider SUMMARY *(continued)*

8. What could be a cause of this patient's shortness of breath?

Because there is a longer time frame between dialysis treatments over the weekend (2 days) as opposed to the more frequent treatments during the week, this patient's shortness of breath is probably caused by an accumulation of fluid inside of the body, exacerbated by the possibility of increased salt, sugar, and fluid intake during the birthday party.

9. Why did the medical control physician order that no IV fluid be administered to this patient?

Owing to this patient's anuric state, hypertension, presence of rales, and unknown time until his next dialysis treatment, the medical control physician most likely thought that the patient was already fluid overloaded.

EMS Patient Care Report (PCR)

Date: 4-20-18	**Incident No.:** 20090154657	**Nature of Call:** Unknown medical	**Location:** 512 E Main St

Dispatched: 0800	**En Route:** 0801	**At Scene:** 0809	**Transport:** 0832	**At Hospital:** 0839	**In Service:** 0903

Patient Information

Age: 52 **Sex:** M **Weight (in kg [lb]):** 82 kg (182.2 lb)	**Allergies:** Penicillin **Medications:** Insulin **Past Medical History:** End-stage renal failure, diabetes mellitus **Chief Complaint:** Altered mental status, dyspnea

Vital Signs

Time: 0810	**BP:** Not yet obtained	**Pulse:** Not yet obtained	**Respirations:** 36	**Spo_2:** Not yet obtained
Time: 0819	**BP:** 226/108	**Pulse:** 140	**Respirations:** 36, rales	**Spo_2:** 94% on 15 L/min NRM
Time: 0824	**BP:** 210/102	**Pulse:** 142	**Respirations:** 36, rales	**Spo_2:** 95% on 15 L/min NRM

EMS Treatment (circle all that apply)

Oxygen @ 15 **L/min via (circle one):** **NC** **(NRM)** **Bag-mask device**		**Assisted Ventilation**	**Airway Adjunct**	**CPR**
Defibrillation	**Bleeding Control**	**Bandaging**	**Splinting**	**Other:**

Narrative

EMS called to above location for a male patient to be transported to the ED. On arrival, met by dialysis clinic staff, who stated patient regularly receives dialysis on M, W, and F. Today patient came in for regularly scheduled treatment, but staff found him slow to answer questions and mildly short of breath. Patient is AO×3 but is slow to answer questions. Both patient and staff state this is abnormal for him. Patient has mild dyspnea, with rales bilaterally. Patient was assisted onto stretcher and secured. While preparing patient for transport, patient vomited × 1. Administered oxygen @ 15 L/min, via nonrebreathing mask. Transported nonemergency to Upson Regional Hospital. 22-gauge saline lock established in right hand. No fluid administered per medical control. Patient remains moderately short of breath. Report called to ED with condition and ETA. On arrival at ED, report given to nurse without incident.**End of report**

Prep Kit

▶ Ready for Review

- The gastrointestinal (GI) system is also known as the digestive tract. Its main function is to absorb the products of digestion to fuel the cells within the body.
- The digestive process begins with saliva to lubricate food. Once food is swallowed, it moves through the esophagus via rhythmic contractions called peristalsis.
- Veins intertwine around the esophagus and join together to form the portal vein, which transports blood from the GI tract to the liver. If blood flow through the liver slows, blood may back up throughout the entire GI system.
- The stomach secretes hydrochloric acid to help break down food. The material then moves into the small intestine.
- The small intestine is divided into the duodenum, the jejunum, and the ileum. The small intestine produces enzymes that turn digested food into substances that can be moved into the bloodstream.
- The duodenum is where the active stage of absorption begins. The pancreas and liver secrete enzymes and bile, respectively, which ultimately assist digestion in the small intestine.
- The liver also converts glycogen into glucose, the essential and only fuel source for brain cells. The liver also detoxifies drugs, completes the breakdown of dead red and white blood cells, and stores vitamins and minerals.
- The large intestine, or colon, is the next step in the digestive process. The primary role of the large intestine is to complete the reabsorption of water. This process helps solidify the digested material into a formed stool. The colon is also the site of digestion by bacteria, which helps to finish the breakdown of chyme.
- The genitourinary system includes the kidneys, urinary bladder, ureters, urethra, male and female reproductive organs, and specific structures within the kidneys.
- Any condition that allows pus, blood, feces, urine, gastric juice, intestinal contents, bile, pancreatic juice, amniotic fluid, or other foreign material to lie within or adjacent to the peritoneum in the abdominal cavity can cause peritonitis and, therefore, an acute abdomen.
- Acute abdomen can be caused by GI or renal sources, diverticulitis, cholecystitis, appendicitis, perforated gastric ulcer, aortic aneurysm, hernia, cystitis, kidney infection, kidney stone, pancreatitis, urinary tract infection, and, in women, ectopic pregnancy and pelvic inflammation.
- Peritonitis typically causes ileus—paralysis of peristalsis—and ultimately abdominal distention. It is almost always associated with nausea and vomiting and can lead to hypovolemic shock.
- GI hemorrhage can be acute, which may be shorter term in duration and more severe, or chronic, which may be of longer duration and less severe. All complaints of bleeding should be considered serious. Sources of GI hemorrhage may include esophagitis, peptic ulcer disease, Mallory-Weiss tears, esophageal varices, gastroesophageal reflux disease, and hemorrhoids.
- Nonhemorrhagic conditions affecting the GI system include gallstones, pancreatitis, appendicitis, gastroenteritis, and diverticulitis. All of these conditions are characterized by abdominal pain, which is often localized to a particular quadrant depending on the source.
- Chronic inflammatory conditions of the colon include ulcerative colitis, irritable bowel syndrome, and Crohn disease. These conditions are all characterized by changes in bowel habits and can range from mild to severe in their signs and symptoms.
- Symptoms of urinary tract infection include painful urination, frequent urges to urinate, difficulty urinating, and possibly referred pain to the shoulder or neck. The urine may have a foul odor and be cloudy.
- Kidney stones result from crystallization of an excess of insoluble salts or uric acid in the urine. Symptoms include severe pain in the flank that may migrate forward to the groin.
- Acute kidney injury is a sudden decrease in kidney filtration, resulting in a release of toxins into the blood. Chronic kidney disease is progressive and irreversible inadequate kidney function. In end-stage renal disease, the kidneys have lost all ability to function, and toxic waste materials build up in the patient's blood; this condition is fatal unless treated by dialysis or renal transplant.
- Gynecologic problems are a common cause of acute abdominal pain. Always consider that a woman with lower abdominal pain and tenderness may have a problem related to her ovaries, fallopian tubes, or uterus.
- Conditions related to the male genital tract include epididymitis and orchitis (which stem from infection of the epididymis and testes, respectively), priapism (painful tender, persistent erection), benign prostate hypertrophy, testicular masses, and testicular torsion.

Prep Kit *(continued)*

- Abdominal pain may stem from other organ systems. If an abdominal aortic aneurysm ruptures, massive hemorrhage may occur and signs of acute peritoneal irritation will present. A hernia (protrusion of an organ or tissue through a hole in the body) may eventually compromise blood supply to the tissue or organ protruding through, causing a serious emergency.
- GI complaints often involve body substances. Take extra gloves, masks, gowns, and other protective equipment and supplies with you to the scene.
- In a patient with an acute abdomen, the first priorities are to assess airway, breathing, and circulation and then apply oxygen. Assist ventilation if the patient is breathing inadequately.
- When taking the patient's history, ask when the symptoms began, how they have changed, where the pain is located (be precise), and how it feels. Also ask if there has been vomiting or diarrhea.
- Airway concerns may arise with a patient who is vomiting. Open the airway using the appropriate maneuvers, and closely inspect it for foreign bodies. Remove or suction any obstructions that are found.
- Abnormal abdominal assessment findings include excessive nausea/vomiting or hematemesis, changes in bowel habits/stool, painful or frequent urination that is discolored or has a strong odor, weight loss, belching/flatulence, concurrent chest pain, and abdominal pain, tenderness, guarding, or distention.
- Pain is commonly located directly over the inflamed area of the peritoneum, or it may be referred to another part of the body.
- A healthy or normal abdomen should be soft and not tender. The pain in an acute abdomen may be sharply localized or diffuse, and will vary in severity. Localized pain gives a clue to the problem organ or area causing it. The abdominal muscles may have become rigid, called guarding.
- In a patient with a GI condition, take vital signs, and gently palpate the abdomen. If the abdomen is tender, the patient needs to be transported urgently.
- Note the degree of abdominal distention; it can provide clues to the severity of the patient's condition.
- Patients with acute abdomen may be comfortable only when lying in one particular position—for example, curled up on one side or with the right knee drawn up. Note the patient's position.
- Do not give the patient with an acute abdomen anything by mouth; establish intravenous access; consult with medical control to administer pain medication, and transport the patient promptly but gently.
- Renal dialysis is a procedure for removing toxic wastes and excess fluids from the blood. Patients receiving dialysis usually have a shunt through which they are connected to the dialysis machine. They are vulnerable to problems such as hypotension, potassium imbalance, disequilibrium syndrome, and air embolism.

▶ Vital Vocabulary

acute abdomen A condition of sudden onset of pain within the abdomen, usually indicating peritonitis; demands immediate medical or surgical treatment.

acute kidney injury A sudden decrease in filtration through the glomeruli of the kidneys.

air embolism The presence of air in the venous circulation, which forms a gas bubble that can block the outflow of blood from the right ventricle to the lung; can lead to cardiac arrest, shock, or other life-threatening complications.

aneurysm A swelling or enlargement of a part of an artery, resulting from weakening of the arterial wall.

anuria A complete halt in the production of urine.

appendicitis Inflammation of the appendix.

ascites Abdominal edema typically signaling liver failure.

benign prostate hypertrophy (BPH) Age-related nonmalignant (noncancerous) enlargement of the prostate gland.

Boerhaave syndrome Forceful vomiting that results in a tear in the esophagus that extends entirely through the esophageal wall, creating a hole.

cholecystitis Inflammation of the gallbladder.

chronic kidney disease Progressive and irreversible inadequate kidney function as a result of permanent loss of nephrons.

colic Acute, intermittent, cramping abdominal pain.

Crohn disease Inflammation of the ileum and possibly other portions of the gastrointestinal tract, in which the immune system attacks portions of the intestinal walls, causing them to become scarred, narrowed, stiff, and weakened.

cystitis Another name for urinary tract infection.

disequilibrium syndrome A condition characterized by nausea, vomiting, headache, and confusion, which results when, as a consequence of dialysis, water initially shifts from the bloodstream into the cerebrospinal fluid, mildly increasing intracranial pressure.

diverticulitis Inflammation of a diverticulum, usually in the colon, creating abdominal discomfort; a *diverticulum* is an abnormal pouch or sac.

Prep Kit (continued)

ectopic pregnancy A pregnancy in which the ovum implants somewhere other than the uterine endometrium.

emesis Vomiting.

end-stage renal disease (ESRD) A condition in which the kidneys have lost all ability to function, and toxic waste materials build up in the patient's blood; occurs after acute or chronic kidney disease.

epididymitis An infection that causes inflammation of the epididymis along the posterior border of the testis; a possible complication of male urinary tract infection.

esophageal varices A condition in which the amount of pressure within the blood vessels surrounding the esophagus increases, causing blood to back up into the portal vessels and ultimately causing the capillary network of the esophagus to leak.

esophagitis Inflammation of the lining of the esophagus.

gastritis Inflammation of the stomach.

gastroenteritis A family of conditions resulting in diarrhea, nausea, and vomiting; some have infectious causes.

gastroesophageal reflux disease (GERD) A condition in which the sphincter between the esophagus and the stomach opens, allowing stomach acid to move superiorly; can cause a burning sensation within the chest (heartburn); also called acid reflux disease.

guarding Involuntary muscle contractions (spasm) of the abdominal wall; an effort to protect the inflamed abdomen.

hematemesis Vomit with blood; can either look like coffee grounds, indicating the presence of partially digested blood, or contain bright-red blood, indicating active bleeding.

hematochezia The passage of stool in which bright red blood can be distinguished; caused by lower gastrointestinal bleeding.

hematuria The presence of blood in the urine.

hernia The protrusion of a loop of an organ or tissue through an abnormal body opening.

ileus Paralysis of the bowel, arising from any one of several causes; it stops the contractions that normally move material through the intestine.

internal shunt Also called an arteriovenous fistula, this device is an artificial connection between a vein and an artery, usually in the forearm or upper arm.

irritable bowel syndrome (IBS) A condition in which patients have abdominal pain and changes in their bowel habits; generally the pain must be present for at least 3 days a month for at least 3 months to be considered this disease.

kidney stones Solid crystalline masses formed in the kidney, resulting from an excess of insoluble salts or uric acid crystallizing in the urine; these masses may become trapped anywhere along the urinary tract.

Mallory-Weiss tear A tear in the mucous membrane, or inner lining, where the esophagus and the stomach meet, causing severe bleeding and potentially death.

melena Dark, tarry, malodorous stools caused by upper gastrointestinal bleeding.

nephrons The structural and functional units of the kidney that form urine; composed of the glomerulus, the glomerular (Bowman) capsule, the proximal convoluted tubule, loop of Henle, and the distal convoluted tubule.

oliguria A decrease in urine output to the extent that total urine output drops to less than 500 mL per day.

orchitis A complication of a male urinary tract infection in which one or both testes become infected, enlarged, and tender, causing pain and swelling in the scrotum.

orthostatic hypotension A drop in systolic blood pressure when moving from a lying or sitting to a standing position.

orthostatic vital signs Assessing vital signs in two different patient positions to determine the degree of hypotension; also known as the tilt test.

pancreatitis Inflammation of the pancreas.

pelvic inflammatory disease (PID) An infection of the female upper organs of reproduction, specifically the uterus, ovaries, and fallopian tubes.

peristalsis Waves of alternate circular contraction and relaxation of the intestines or other tubular structure to propel the contents forward.

peritoneum The membrane lining the abdominal cavity (parietal peritoneum) and covering the abdominal organs (visceral peritoneum).

peritonitis Inflammation of the peritoneum.

portal vein The blood vessel that transports blood from the gastrointestinal tract to the liver.

priapism A painful, tender, persistent erection of the penis; can result from spinal cord injury, erectile dysfunction drugs, or sickle cell disease.

pyelonephritis Inflammation of the kidney and renal pelvis.

rebound tenderness Parietal pain that occurs when pressure is removed rather than applied; suggestive of a serious and potentially life-threatening condition.

Prep Kit *(continued)*

referred pain The pain felt in an area of the body other than the area where the cause of pain is located.

renal dialysis A technique for "filtering" the blood of its toxic wastes, removing excess fluids, and restoring the normal balance of electrolytes.

shunt A passageway that allows fluid to move from one part of the body to another or to a dialysis machine.

steatorrhea Foamy, fatty stools associated with liver failure or gallbladder problems.

strangulation Complete obstruction of blood circulation in a given organ as a result of compression or entrapment; an emergency situation causing death of tissue.

testicular torsion Twisting of the testicle on the spermatic cord, from which it is suspended; associated with scrotal pain and swelling, and is a medical emergency.

ulcerative colitis Generalized inflammation of the inner lining of the colon that results in a weakened, dilated rectum, making it susceptible to infection and bleeding.

ulcers Abrasions of the stomach or small intestine.

uremia The presence of excessive amounts of urea and other waste products in the blood.

uremic frost A powdery buildup of uric acid, especially on the face.

urinary retention Incomplete emptying of the bladder or a complete lack of ability to empty the bladder.

urinary tract infections (UTIs) Infections, usually of the lower urinary tract (urethra and bladder), which occur when normal flora bacteria or other bacteria enter the urethra and grow.

visceral pain Crampy, aching pain deep within the body, the source of which is usually difficult to pinpoint; common with urologic problems.

▶ References

1. Bertram JF, Douglas-Denton RN, Diouf B, Hughson MD, Hoy WE. Human nephron number: implications for health and disease. *Pediatr Nephrol.* 2011;26(9):1529-1533. https://www.ncbi.nlm.nih.gov/pubmed/21604189. Accessed December 29, 2016.
2. Markman J, Narasimhan SK. Overview of pain. Merck Manual website. http://www.merckmanuals.com/home/brain,-spinal-cord,-and-nerve-disorders/pain/overview-of-pain. Accessed September 15, 2017.
3. Baker H. Hemorrhoids. In: Longe JL ed. *Gale Encyclopedia of Medicine*. 3rd ed. Detroit: Gale; 2006:1766-1769. http://www.medscape.com/viewarticle/805040_2. Accessed January 25, 2017.
4. Kappelman MD, Rifas-Shiman SL, Kleinman K, et al. The prevalence and geographic distribution of Crohn's disease and ulcerative colitis in the United States. *Clin Gastroenterol Hepatol.* 2007;5:1424-1429. http://www.medscape.com/medline/abstract/17904915. Accessed December 27, 2016.
5. Herrinton LJ, Liu L, Lewis JD, Griffin PM, Allison J. Incidence and prevalence of inflammatory bowel disease in a Northern California managed care organization, 1996–2002. *Am J Gastroenterol.* 2008;103(8):1998-2006. https://www.ncbi.nlm.nih.gov/pubmed/18796097. Accessed December 27, 2016.
6. Loftus EV Jr. Clinical epidemiology of inflammatory bowel disease: incidence, prevalence, and environmental influences. *Gastroenterology.* 2004;126(6):1504-1517. http://www.sciencedirect.com/science/article/pii/S0016508504004627. Accessed December 27, 2016.
7. Centers for Disease Control and Prevention. Epidemiology of the IBD. https://www.cdc.gov/ibd/ibd-epidemiology.htm. Accessed December 27, 2016.
8. Bengtson MB, Aamodt G, Vatn MH, Harris JR. Concordance for IBD among twins compared to ordinary siblings: a Norwegian population-based study. *J Crohns Colitis.* 2010;4(3):312-318. https://www.ncbi.nlm.nih.gov/pubmed/21122520. Accessed December 27, 2016.
9. Maxwell PR, Mendall MA, Kumar D. Irritable bowel syndrome. *Lancet.* 1997;350(9092):1691-1695. http://www.thelancet.com/journals/lancet/article/PIIS0140-6736(97)05276-8/abstract. Accessed December 27, 2016.
10. Canavan C, West J, Card T. The epidemiology of irritable bowel syndrome. *Clin Epidemiol.* 2014;2014(6):71-80. https://www.dovepress.com/the-epidemiology-of-irritable-bowel-syndrome-peer-reviewed-fulltext-article-CLEP. Accessed December 27, 2016.
11. Crohn's and Colitis Foundation of America. About the epidemiology of IBD. June 1, 2012. http://www.ccfa.org/resources/epidemiology.html. Accessed December 27, 2016.
12. Rendi M. Crohn disease pathology: epidemiology. September 17, 2015. http://emedicine.medscape.com/article/1986158-overview#a2. Accessed December 27, 2016.
13. Sandler RS, Golden AL. Epidemiology of Crohn's disease. *J Clin Gastroenterol.* 1986;8(2):160-165. https://www.ncbi.nlm.nih.gov/pubmed/3745850. Accessed December 27, 2016.
14. Crohn's and Colitis Foundation of America. IBD Genetics Initiative: unraveling the genetic

Prep Kit (continued)

components to the development of Crohn's and colitis. http://www.ccfa.org/science-and-professionals/research/current-research-studies/genetics-initiative.html. Accessed December 27, 2016.

15. National Institutes of Health, National Institute of Diabetes and Digestive and Kidney Diseases. Kidney disease statistics for the United States. December 2016. https://www.niddk.nih.gov/health-information/health-statistics/Pages/kidney-disease-statistics-united-states.aspx. Accessed December 28, 2016.
16. National Kidney and Urologic Diseases Information Clearinghouse. Kidney disease statistics for the United States. July 17, 2013. http://ww1.prweb.com/prfiles/2013/07/17/10940519/Kidney%20Diseases%20Statistics%20for%20the%20United%20States%20-%205-year%20survival%20rate.pdf. Accessed December 28, 2016.
17. Kochanek KD, Murphy SL, Xu J, Tejada-Vera B. Deaths: final data for 2014. *Natl Vital Stat Rep.* 2016;65(4). https://www.cdc.gov/nchs/data/nvsr/nvsr65/nvsr65_04.pdf. Accessed December 28, 2016.
18. Saran R, Li Y, Robinson B, et al. US Renal Data System 2015 annual data report: epidemiology of kidney disease in the United States. *Am J Kidney Dis.* 2016;67(3)(suppl 1):S1-S434. http://www.ajkd.org/article/S0272-6386(15)01490-0/fulltext. Accessed December 28, 2016.
19. United Network for Organ Sharing. Transplant trends. December 23, 2016. https://www.unos.org/data/transplant-trends/#waitlists_by_organ. Accessed December 28, 2016.
20. Jurkovic D, Wilkinson H. Diagnosis and management of ectopic pregnancy. *BMJ.* 2011;342:d3397. http://www.bmj.com/content/342/bmj.d3397. Accessed December 28, 2016.
21. Cunningham GR, Kadmon D. Epidemiology and pathogenesis of benign prostatic hyperplasia. *UpToDate.* August 11, 2015. http://www.uptodate.com/contents/epidemiology-and-pathogenesis-of-benign-prostatic-hyperplasia. Accessed December 28, 2016.
22. Hanna NH, Albany C, Loehrer PJ, et al. Testicular cancer. Cancer Network. November 1, 2015. http://www.cancernetwork.com/cancer-management/testicular. Accessed December 28, 2016.
23. Avarello JT, Cantor RM. Pediatric major trauma: an approach to evaluation and management. *Emerg Med Clin North Am.* 2007;25:803-836. http://anes-som.ucsd.edu/intranet/Peds_Resources/Trauma/Pediatric%20major%20trauma.pdf. Accessed December 28, 2016.
24. National Kidney Foundation. Fast facts: kidneys. https://www.kidney.org/news/newsroom/factsheets/FastFacts. Accessed December 29, 2016.
25. Advanced Renal Education Program. Air embolism. http://advancedrenaleducation.com/content/air-embolism. Accessed December 29, 2016.

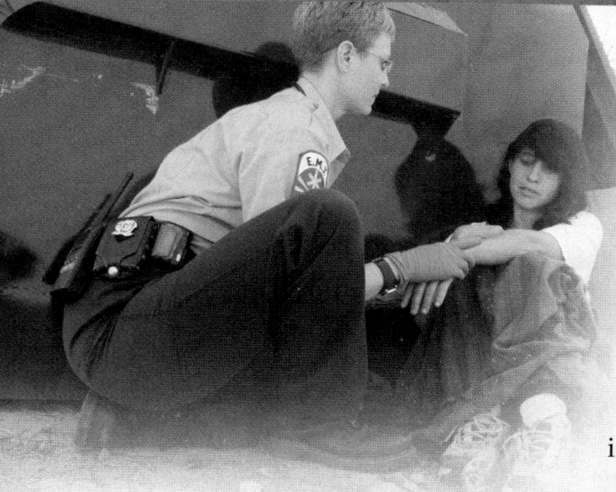

Assessment *in Action*

You are dispatched to a well-kept, upscale residential home for a 46-year-old woman who is complaining of severe abdominal pain. On arrival, you are met by the patient's husband, who directs you to the back bedroom. There, you find the patient lying in bed, in the fetal position, moaning in pain.

The patient states that she has severe abdominal pain that she rates as a "10" on a 1 to 10 scale. The pain started approximately 30 minutes ago, after she ate fried chicken and a baked potato with "a lot of butter." Nothing she does makes the pain any better or worse.

1. What is the most likely cause of the patient's discomfort?

A. Diverticulitis
B. Cholecystitis
C. Appendicitis
D. Gastritis

2. What is the medical term for inflammation of the gallbladder?

A. Acute cholecystitis
B. Acute appendicitis
C. Acute pyelonephritis
D. Acute bronchiolitis

3. Where is referred pain from acute cholecystitis typically found?

A. Jaw
B. Groin
C. Left shoulder
D. Right shoulder

4. Which of the following types of pain is described as difficult to localize and as burning, cramping, gnawing, or aching and is usually felt superficially?

A. Visceral
B. Parietal
C. Somatic
D. Referred

5. The gallbladder is a storage pouch for digestive juices and waste from the:

A. stomach.
B. liver.
C. pancreas.
D. spleen.

6. Eating any of the following might precede the symptoms of cholecystitis EXCEPT:

A. fried chicken.
B. bacon.
C. boiled eggs.
D. french fries.

7. Which membrane lines the walls of the abdominal cavity?

A. Visceral peritoneum
B. Parietal peritoneum
C. Potential peritoneum
D. Somatic peritoneum

8. Where is pain commonly felt by a patient experiencing acute cholecystitis?

A. Right upper quadrant
B. Right lower quadrant
C. Left upper quadrant
D. Left lower quadrant

9. List the signs and symptoms associated with gastroesophageal reflux disease.

10. What are the signs and symptoms associated with ulcerative colitis?

CHAPTER 21

Endocrine and Hematologic Emergencies

National EMS Education Standard Competencies

Medicine

Applies fundamental knowledge to provide basic and selected advanced emergency care and transportation based on assessment findings for an acutely ill patient.

Endocrine Disorders

Awareness that

- Diabetic emergencies cause altered mental status (pp 914, 918, 921, 923, 925-926)

Anatomy, physiology, pathophysiology, assessment, and management of

- Acute diabetic emergencies (pp 914-932)

Hematology

Anatomy, physiology, pathophysiology, assessment, and management of

- Sickle cell crisis (pp 934-935, 937-939)
- Clotting disorders (pp 936-940)

Knowledge Objectives

1. Review the anatomy and physiology of the endocrine system and its main function in the body. (pp 911-913)
2. Discuss the role of glucose as a major source of energy for the body and its relationship to insulin. (pp 913-914)
3. Compare hypothyroidism with hyperthyroidism. (p 914)
4. Define the term diabetes. (p 914)
5. Discuss complications of diabetes. (pp 915-916)
6. Distinguish between the two types of diabetes and how their onset patterns differ. (pp 917-919)
7. Explain some age-related considerations when managing a geriatric patient who has undiagnosed diabetes. (p 917)
8. Identify risk factors associated with prediabetes, including the role of hemoglobin A1c blood tests, in distinguishing prediabetes from diabetes. (pp 919-920)
9. Discuss diagnosis and management of gestational diabetes. (p 920)
10. Explain some age-related considerations when managing a pediatric patient who is experiencing a hyperglycemic or hypoglycemic crisis. (pp 918, 926)
11. Describe the differences and similarities between hyperglycemic and hypoglycemic diabetic emergencies, including their onset, signs and symptoms, and management considerations. (pp 920-924)
12. Discuss the steps to follow when conducting a primary survey and secondary assessment of a patient with an altered mental status who is a suspected diabetic patient. (pp 927-928)
13. Explain the process for assessing and managing the airway of a patient with an altered mental status, including ways to differentiate a hyperglycemic patient from a hypoglycemic patient. (p 927)
14. Describe the interventions for providing emergency medical care during a hypoglycemic crisis to responsive and unresponsive patients who have a history of diabetes. (pp 929-931)
15. Describe the interventions for providing emergency medical care during a hyperglycemic crisis to responsive and unresponsive patients with a history of diabetes. (pp 929, 931-932)
16. Provide the generic and trade names, form, dose, administration, indications, and contraindications for giving oral glucose to a patient with a decreased level of consciousness who has a history of diabetes. (pp 929-930 and Chapter 12, *Principles of Pharmacology*)
17. Explain when it is appropriate to obtain medical direction when providing emergency medical care to a patient with diabetes. (p 930)
18. Provide the generic and trade names, form, dose, administration, indications, and contraindications for administering dextrose to a patient with hypoglycemia. (pp 930-931 and Chapter 12, *Principles of Pharmacology*)
19. Provide the generic and trade names, form, dose, administration, indications, and contraindications

for administering glucagon to a patient with hypoglycemia. (p 931 and Chapter 12, *Principles of Pharmacology*)

20. Discuss the composition and functions of blood. (pp 932-934)
21. Describe the pathophysiology of sickle cell disease and the four main types of sickle cell crises. (pp 934-935)
22. Describe blood clotting disorders and the risk factors, characteristics, and management of each. (pp 936-940)
23. Describe the assessment and management of a patient with suspected sickle cell disease. (pp 937-939)

Skills Objectives

1. Demonstrate the assessment and care of a patient with hypoglycemia and a decreased level of consciousness. (pp 929-931)
2. Demonstrate how to administer glucose to a patient with an altered mental status. (pp 929-930)
3. Demonstrate how to administer dextrose to a patient with hypoglycemia. (pp 930-931)
4. Demonstrate how to administer glucagon to a patient with hypoglycemia. (p 931)
5. Demonstrate the assessment and care of a patient with sickle cell crisis. (pp 937-939)
6. Demonstrate the assessment and care of a patient with a blood clotting disorder. (pp 937-940)

Introduction

The endocrine system directly or indirectly influences almost every cell, organ, and function of the body. Consequently, patients with an endocrine disorder often are seen with a multitude of signs and symptoms that require a thorough assessment and immediate treatment. This chapter also discusses hematologic emergencies, which rarely occur in most emergency medical services (EMS) systems. Although hematologic disorders can be difficult to assess and treat in a prehospital setting, your actions may not only offer support, but you may save the patient's life.

Anatomy and Physiology Review: The Endocrine System

The major components of the **endocrine system** include the hypothalamus; the pineal gland, pituitary gland, thyroid gland, thymus gland, parathyroid gland, and adrenal glands; the pancreas; and the gonads, including the ovaries and testes.

The endocrine system comprises a network of glands that produce and secrete chemical messengers called hormones. A **hormone** is a chemical substance produced by a gland that has special regulatory effects on other organs and tissues. Hormones travel in the bloodstream to target tissues Figure 21-1. Hormones are involved in regulation of mood, growth and development, metabolism, tissue function, and sexual development and function. **Endocrine glands** secrete or release chemicals, such as hormones, inside the body.

The main function of the endocrine system and its hormone messengers is to maintain homeostasis and promote permanent structural changes. Maintaining homeostasis requires a response to any change in the body, such as low glucose or calcium levels in the blood.

Pituitary Gland

Located at the base of the brain, the pituitary gland is divided into anterior and posterior regions.

YOU are the Provider — PART 1

At 1130 hours, your ambulance is dispatched to an unresponsive 41-year-old man. On arrival, you are greeted by the patient's wife, who states that the patient has a medical history of diabetes. She tells you that as she was fixing lunch, he became confused and then unresponsive. Your primary survey of the patient reveals that he is responsive to deep painful stimuli, with adequate respirations. The patient's wife states that the patient has an insulin pump, but she didn't know if she should turn it off or not.

1. What are the two types of diabetes, and how do they differ?
2. What is the function of an insulin pump?
3. Should you instruct the patient's wife to turn off the insulin pump?

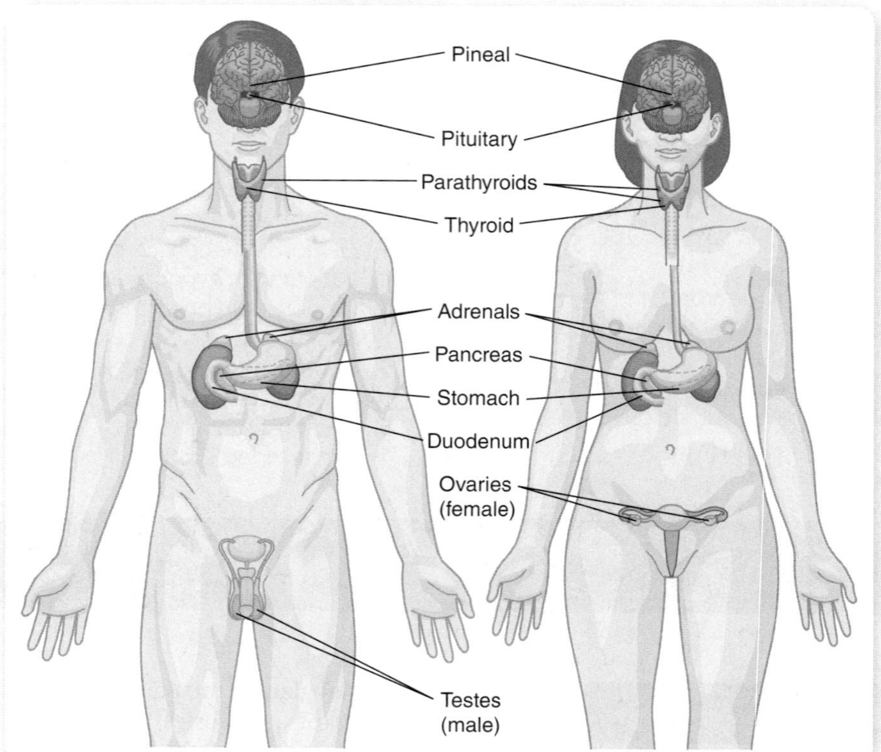

Figure 21-1 The endocrine system uses the various glands within the system to deliver chemical messages to organ systems throughout the body.

Six of the hormones secreted by the pituitary gland stimulate other endocrine glands and are referred to as tropic (from the Greek *tropos*, meaning "to turn" or "change") hormones. These include adrenocorticotropic hormone (ACTH), follicle-stimulating hormone, growth hormone, luteinizing hormone, prolactin, and **thyroid-stimulating hormone**. The other two hormones, antidiuretic hormone and oxytocin, control other body functions.

During times of stress, the hypothalamus secretes a hormone that stimulates the anterior pituitary to release ACTH. ACTH targets the adrenal cortex and causes it to secrete **cortisol**. Cortisol stimulates most body cells to increase their energy production.

▶ Thyroid Gland

Thyroid hormones, which affect metabolism, are secreted in response to stimulation of the thyroid gland by the anterior pituitary gland. The anterior pituitary gland secretes thyroid-stimulating hormone in response to the hypothalamus's secretion of thyrotropin-releasing hormone.

The thyroid gland secretes thyroxine (T_4) when the body's metabolic rate decreases. Thyroxine, the body's major metabolic hormone, stimulates energy production in cells, which increases the rate at which cells consume oxygen and use carbohydrates, fats, and proteins. Without the proper intake level of dietary iodine, thyroxine cannot be produced, and the patient's physical and mental growth are diminished.

The thyroid gland also secretes **calcitonin**, which helps maintain normal calcium levels in the blood. This hormone is secreted when the thyroid detects high levels of calcium. Calcitonin travels to the bones, where it stimulates the bone-building cells to absorb the excess calcium. It also stimulates the kidneys to absorb and excrete excess calcium.

▶ Pancreas

The **pancreas** is considered both an endocrine gland and an **exocrine gland**. It has a role in hormone production as well as in digestion. The exocrine component secretes digestive enzymes into the duodenum via the pancreatic duct. The endocrine component secretes hormones from cell groups called the **islets of Langerhans**. These cell groups within the pancreas act like "an organ within an organ," secreting the polypeptide hormones **glucagon** (from alpha cells, and which raises blood glucose levels), **insulin** (from beta cells, and which lowers blood glucose levels), and somatostatin (from delta cells, and which is responsible

Words of Wisdom

The brain is the only organ that can utilize glucose without insulin.

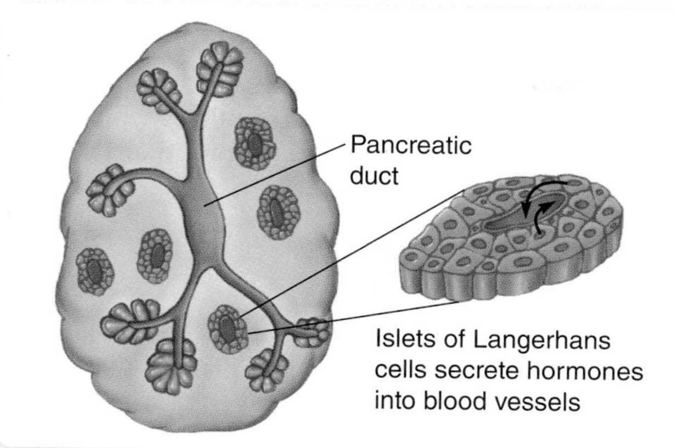

Figure 21-2 The islets of Langerhans secrete hormones into blood vessels that modulate serum glucose levels.

for the inhibition of insulin and glucagon secretion) **Figure 21-2**. In a healthy patient, the body regulates blood glucose levels using both insulin and glucagon.

▶ The Role of Glucose and Insulin

Glucose, or dextrose, is one of the basic sugars in the body and, along with oxygen, is the primary fuel for cellular metabolism. Glucose is the major source of energy for the body, and all cells need it to function properly. Some cells will not function at all without glucose. The brain needs a constant supply of glucose, just as it does oxygen. Without glucose, or with an extremely low glucose level, brain cells rapidly suffer permanent damage. A normal blood glucose level in nonfasting adults and children is approximately 70 to 120 mg/dL.

Special Populations

The normal range for glucose levels in blood in nonfasting children is the same as adults: 70 to 120 mg/dL. The blood glucose level in neonates should be above 70 mg/dL.

Insulin is a hormone produced by the pancreas that facilitates the uptake of glucose from the bloodstream into the cell. With the exception of the brain, insulin is needed to allow glucose to enter individual body cells to fuel their functioning. For this reason, insulin is said to be a cellular key.

Regulation of glucose levels in the body is a complex and dynamic process that begins when absorbed carbohydrates stimulate the release of insulin from the beta cells of the islets of Langerhans in the pancreas **Figure 21-3**. Insulin is responsible for the removal of glucose from the blood for storage as glycogen, fats, and protein.

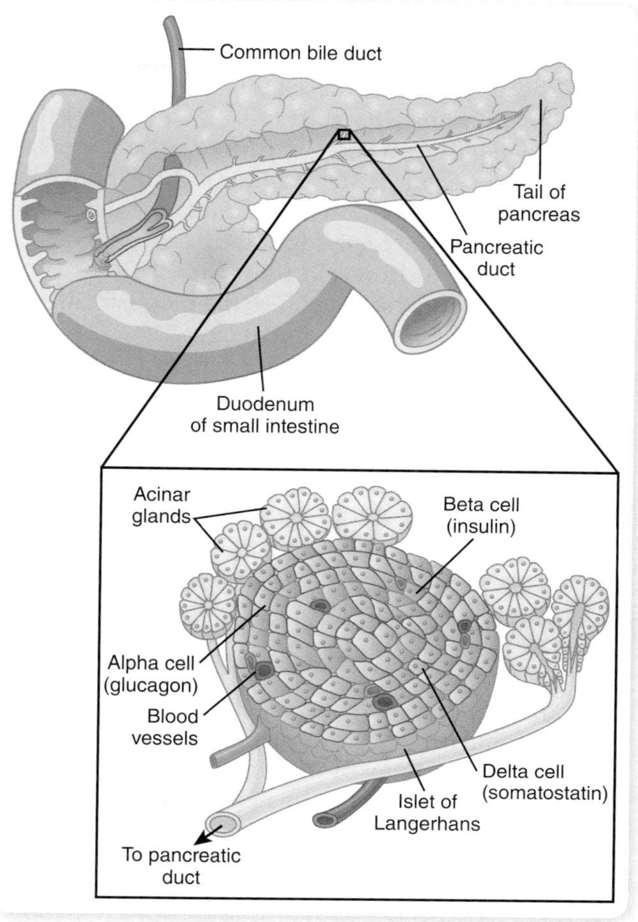

Figure 21-3 The alpha, beta, and delta cells are in the islets of Langerhans, which are in the pancreas.

When blood glucose levels are elevated, the following process occurs:

- The islets of Langerhans secrete insulin, which is carried by the bloodstream to the cells.
- Insulin increases cell membrane permeability and mediates the transport of glucose across the cell membrane into the cells, where it is used to produce energy.
- The cells use glucose to produce energy through processes that include **glycolysis**, the conversion of glucose into energy via metabolic pathways, and the Krebs cycle. (Recall from Chapter 7, *The Human Body*, that when oxygen is present during this process, **aerobic metabolism** occurs, the by-products of which are carbon dioxide and water.)

Insulin also stimulates the liver to store excess glucose, and the skeletal muscles store glycogen for later use by the body. Insulin is the only hormone that decreases blood glucose levels. After blood glucose levels have returned to normal, the islets of Langerhans discontinue the secretion of insulin.

When the blood glucose level decreases, such as between meals, the following process occurs:

- The alpha cells of the islets of Langerhans release the hormone glucagon.
- When glucagon enters the bloodstream, it raises the blood glucose level and brings the body's energy back to normal by stimulating the liver to convert stored glycogen back into glucose through a process called **glycogenolysis**.
- The glucose is secreted into the bloodstream, where cells can use it for energy.
- If stored glycogen levels are depleted, the cells begin to metabolize fats, proteins, and other noncarbonate sources, thus producing new glucose—a process called **gluconeogenesis**.

In healthy endocrine systems, these shifts in metabolism are tolerated and never allowed to proceed to extremes.

Pathophysiology of the Endocrine System

Endocrine disorders can be caused by either hypersecretion or insufficient secretion of a gland. Hypersecretion presents as overactivity of the target organ regulated by the gland. Insufficient secretion results in underactivity of the organ controlled by the gland. Hyperthyroidism and hypothyroidism are two serious illnesses of the endocrine system. However, most of the endocrine emergencies you will encounter will be related to diabetic emergencies secondary to abnormal insulin secretion.

Hypothyroidism and Hyperthyroidism

Hyperthyroidism increases metabolism, while hypothyroidism decreases metabolism. Table 21-1 summarizes the major effects of hypothyroidism and hyperthyroidism. Although approximately 20 million Americans have some type of thyroid disorder,[1] many are unaware of their condition. Treatment of these patients should be symptomatic with transport to the closest most appropriate facility.

Words of Wisdom

Thyroid storm is a rare, life-threatening condition that may occur in patients with thyrotoxicosis (a toxic condition caused by excessive levels of circulating thyroid hormone). The condition is usually triggered by a stressful event or increased volume of thyroid hormones in the circulation. In addition to the normal signs and symptoms of hyperthyroidism, patients may present with fever, severe tachycardia, nausea, vomiting, altered mental status, and possibly heart failure.

Diabetes Mellitus

Diabetes is a metabolic disorder that is now thought to be associated with a group of complex diseases with many causes (ie, **diabetes mellitus** [a disease characterized by the body's inability to sufficiently metabolize glucose], **gestational diabetes** [diabetes that develops during pregnancy in women who did not have diabetes before pregnancy], hypoglycemia/hyperglycemia, diabetic ketoacidosis [DKA], hyperosmolar hyperglycemic syndrome [HHS]). These pathologic conditions reflect a flaw in the production or function of insulin, or both. Insulin assists in the metabolism of carbohydrates and the transport of glucose into the cells. The end result of diabetes is hyperglycemia, also known as high blood glucose. Medically, the term *diabetes* refers to a metabolic disorder in which the body's ability to metabolize simple

Table 21-1 Comparison of Major Effects of Hypothyroidism and Hyperthyroidism

	Hypothyroidism	Hyperthyroidism
Cardiovascular effects	Slow pulse, reduced cardiac output	Rapid pulse, increased cardiac output
Metabolic effects	Decreased metabolism, cold skin, weight gain	Increased metabolism, skin hot and flushed, weight loss
Neuromuscular effects	Weakness, sluggish reflexes	Tremor, hyperactive reflexes
Mental, emotional effects	Mental processes sluggish, personality placid	Restlessness, irritability, emotional lability
Gastrointestinal effects	Constipated	Diarrhea
General somatic effects	Cold, dry skin	Warm, moist skin

carbohydrates (glucose) is impaired. It is characterized by the following symptoms:

- **Polyphagia**, an increased appetite caused by the inability of glucose to be transported across the cell membrane.
- **Polydipsia**, a substantial thirst caused by dehydration brought about by an increase in diuresis (the production of large amounts of urine by the kidney).
- **Polyuria**, the passage of large quantities of urine. In diabetes, excess glucose is excreted in the urine (glycosuria) and attracts water, resulting in excessive diuresis.

Diabetes mellitus is characterized by the body's inability to sufficiently metabolize glucose. *Mellitus*, from the Greek word for honeybee, means "sweet"—a reference to the presence of glucose in the urine. In people with this disease, the pancreas does not produce enough insulin or the body's cells do not respond to the effects of the insulin that is produced. In either case, the result is the same: an elevated level of glucose in both the blood and the urine. Glucose builds up in the blood, overflows into the urine, and flows out of the body. Because the lack of effective insulin prevents the sugar from moving inside the cells where it can be metabolized, cells can actually "starve," or be deprived of glucose, even when the blood contains large amounts of glucose **Figure 21-4**.

According to the 2014 National Diabetes Statistics Report, more than 29 million people in the United States (approximately 9.3% of the population) have diabetes;[2] of these, 8.1 million remain undiagnosed. Thus, one in four people with diabetes is unaware of his or her disease status.[2,3] In 2013, diabetes was the seventh leading cause of death in United States, although the US Centers for Disease Control and Prevention (CDC) suggest diabetes may be underreported as a source of mortality.[2]

Diabetes mellitus is responsible for myriad life-altering complications, some of which are listed here:

- **Kidneys.** Diabetes is the principal cause of kidney failure, accounting for 44% of new cases in 2011.[3] The glomeruli of the kidney become sclerotic, causing necrosis of the papillary tissue and resulting in nephropathy (end-stage renal disease) and renal failure. High levels of glucose in the blood cause the kidneys to work harder than normal and can result in decreased kidney function over time.
- **Heart.** Adults with diabetes are approximately two times more likely to die of heart disease or to experience a stroke than those who do not have diabetes.[3] When diabetes is poorly controlled, the process of **lipolysis** (from *lipo-*, meaning "fat," and *-lysis*, meaning "breakdown") raises the level of fat in the blood. As a result of the raised fat level, the risk of atherosclerosis and coronary artery disease increases. The fat circulating through the bloodstream adheres to the vessel walls, eventually causing them to be stiff and brittle. In addition, glucose crystals are sharp and can damage the blood vessels. The microscopic deterioration of the vessel walls, called **microangiopathy**, results in swelling of basement membrane cells, which then restricts the flow of blood to organs and tissues. Inadequate blood flow (ischemia) causes necrosis, or tissue death. Chronic heart failure develops over a period of several years and is twice as prevalent among people with diabetes than among those without the disease.[3] Central nervous system damage can cause cardiac dysrhythmias, which can result in cardiac arrest

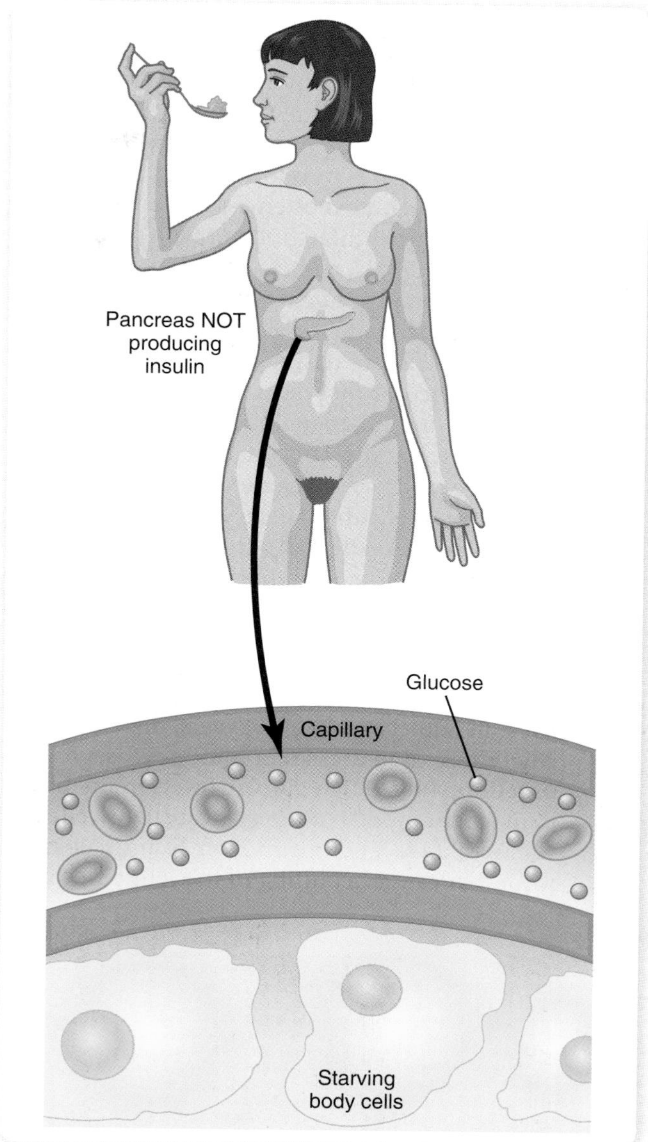

Figure 21-4 Diabetes is defined as a lack of or ineffective action of insulin. Without insulin, cells begin to "starve" because insulin is needed to allow glucose to enter and nourish the cells.

and sudden death. Microangiopathy and nerve damage contribute to an increased risk for a *silent* myocardial infarction to be experienced by a patient with diabetes. These pathologies combine and result in the patient with diabetes not perceiving the common signs of chest pain, pressure, or tightness often associated with an acute myocardial infarction (AMI). Therefore, an AMI should always be assumed until proved otherwise for any patient with diabetes who reports a syncopal episode, fainting, weakness, fatigue, malaise, or dyspnea on exertion.

- **Cerebrovascular disease, stroke, and hypertension.** Microangiopathy results in cerebrovascular disease and an increased incidence of stroke. Hypertension is present in 71% of people with diabetes.[3] Hypertension further increases the risk of heart disease, stroke, kidney disease, and blindness.

Peripheral artery disease is also common in people with diabetes and impairs circulation to the lower extremities **Figure 21-5**.

- **Eyes.** In adults age 20 to 74 years, diabetes is the chief cause of new cases of blindness as a result of retinopathy.[4] High glucose levels in the blood damage the vessels of the eye, causing swelling, wall weakness, and obstruction. Scar tissue can form that causes a pulling of the retina from the eye, or retinal detachment. Cataracts are a cloudy film that forms when fructose and sorbitol are deposited in the lens of the eye.
- **Neuropathy.** Neuropathy is nerve damage that results in a loss of sensation and function in the area innervated by the affected nerves. Such damage can cause sexual impotence, neurogenic bladder, constipation, or diarrhea. Neuropathy associated with diabetes often affects peripheral nerves, causing diminished sensation and function in the extremities. Patients with peripheral neuropathy often have paresthesia, a pinprick sensation in the hands, feet, arms, or legs. Paresthesia and dysesthesia—the absence of sensation—can blunt pain perception, making it possible for foot ulcers to go unnoticed until they become seriously infected. Because many of these patients also have poor circulation in the extremities, gangrene can develop in adjacent tissues and infection may spread to the bone. In fact, more than 60% of nontraumatic lower limb amputations can be attributed to diabetes.[3]

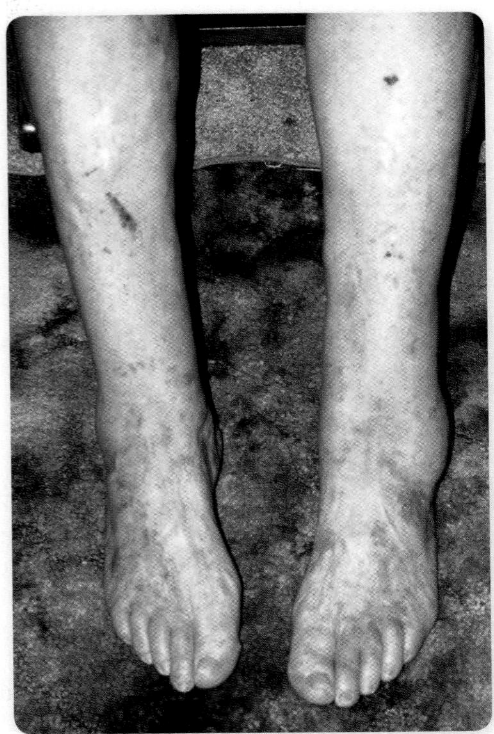

Figure 21-5 Peripheral edema and poor circulation are complications associated with long-term diabetes.

Courtesy of Rhonda Hunt.

Because of the widespread effect of diabetes on all systems of the body, any preexisting condition will be more difficult to manage after diabetes develops in the patient. The more closely patients adhere to the recommended management of their diabetes, the better the outcome of their other conditions will be. Conditions that develop subsequent to the onset of diabetes will respond more effectively when diabetes is managed appropriately. Many conditions associated with the presence of diabetes can be delayed or prevented with appropriate lifestyle changes and continued management of diabetes. Conversely, any kind of distress can have a negative effect on the patient and result in a 9-1-1 call because blood glucose levels are more difficult to control in the setting of increased physical activity or emotional stress.

Both chronic and acute complications are associated with diabetes mellitus. Although these complications are present in both forms of the disease (type 1 and type 2), they tend to be more severe in people with diabetes who require insulin. Left untreated, diabetes results in organ system dysfunction, wasting of body tissues, and death. Even with excellent medical care, some patients with particularly aggressive forms of diabetes will die at a relatively young age from complications of the disease. The severity of diabetic complications correlates with the average blood glucose level and the age of onset. Although some patients with well-controlled diabetes have a normal life span, they must be willing to adjust their lives to the demands of the disease, especially their eating habits and physical activity levels. There is no cure for the disease, so treatment focuses on maintaining the level of blood glucose within the patient's normal range.

Two forms of diabetes mellitus exist: type 1 (formerly known as juvenile-onset diabetes) and type 2 (formerly known as adult-onset diabetes). The age of onset of the patient's symptoms is less important than whether the patient requires insulin to survive. Both types of diabetes mellitus are serious conditions that affect many tissues and functions other than the glucose-regulating mechanism, and both require lifelong medical management. In addition, the condition known as **prediabetes** is now recognized as a warning sign that may precede the development of type 2 diabetes, and is discussed later in this chapter.

Special Populations

You might encounter an older adult patient who has undiagnosed diabetes. These patients report that they have not been feeling well for a while but have not seen a physician. A patient with undiagnosed diabetes or one who is in denial or ignores the advice of his or her physician may call 9-1-1 when the signs and symptoms get worse. Nonhealing wounds, blindness, renal failure, and other complications are associated with poorly controlled or uncontrolled diabetes. It is important that you recognize the signs and symptoms of diabetes because you might be the first health care provider to suggest medical treatment to an older adult patient who might otherwise ignore the condition.

Older adult patients and those with diabetes commonly present atypically with an AMI. They often do not present with classic crushing substernal chest pain or pressure because of the neuropathy associated with increasing age and diabetes. Older adults also generally have a higher pain tolerance than do younger patients. Other causes of an altered perception of pain can include impaired cognition or slowed nerve conduction. You should maintain a high index of suspicion when these populations experience a syncopal episode, fatigue, shortness of breath, or nausea and diaphoresis.

Older adult patients are also more susceptible to dehydration and infections. As we age, our bodies tend to lose approximately 10% of the total body fluid.[5] Older adult patients may not become thirsty or react to thirst until they are extremely dehydrated. Medications can also cause an increase in diuresis, compounding the problem.

▶ Type I Diabetes Mellitus

As mentioned, **type 1 diabetes** has historically been referred to as insulin-dependent diabetes mellitus or juvenile-onset diabetes because it generally affects children. Although type 1 diabetes has a hereditary predisposition, it is believed that environmental factors may play a role—for example, with an infection that triggers an autoimmune disorder. With type I diabetes, the body develops autoantibodies that incorrectly identify the body's own tissues or substances as foreign invaders to be destroyed. Contributing to pancreatic destruction are autoantibodies to the insulin-secreting beta cells in the islets of Langerhans, to insulin, and to other pancreatic substances. The rate of beta-cell destruction is variable, occurring rapidly in some patients (mainly children) and slowly in others (mainly adults).[6] Eventually, the pancreatic beta cells become incapable of secreting insulin and regulating intracellular glucose. Because beta cells are the only source of insulin, it must then be administered by injection or with a pump when the cells are destroyed.

Latent autoimmune diabetes in adults is a variant of type 1 diabetes that occurs in adults older than 30 years. The pathophysiology is the same as that of young-onset diabetes, with the body's immune system destroying the beta cells. Thus, adult patients with latent autoimmune diabetes will ultimately require insulin therapy.

When the endocrine system (or pancreas) fails to produce insulin (as is the case in most patients with type 1 diabetes), people require daily injections of supplementary, synthetic insulin throughout their lives to control their blood glucose levels. In addition to daily insulin injections, strict dietary control must be observed, which can be difficult to achieve with young children. Increased activity and alcohol consumption can result in low blood glucose levels (alcohol depletes glycogen stores in the liver). Therefore, in adults with type 1 diabetes, alcohol consumption also must be controlled.

In terms of management, type 1 diabetes always requires the use of insulin that is administered by injection or an insulin pump, also called continuous subcutaneous insulin infusion therapy. Insulin cannot be ingested orally because the digestive process will render it inactive.

You will likely encounter patients with diabetes who use insulin pumps to treat their disease. An alternative to multiple daily injections of insulin, insulin pumps provide improved control of blood glucose levels and better quality of life for many patients. These small devices consist of an infusion set, a reservoir for insulin, and the pump itself. The pump is approximately the size of a deck of cards, weighs approximately 3 ounces, and can be worn on a belt or carried in a pocket **Figure 21-6**.

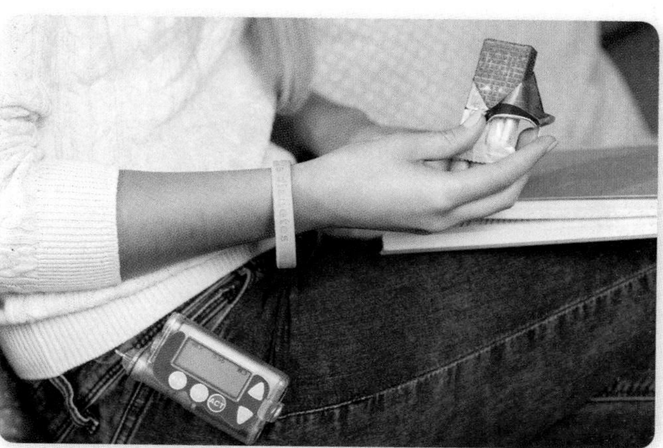

Figure 21-6 An insulin pump is a small electronic device that automatically delivers insulin to maintain the desired blood glucose level.

Insulin is administered through a catheter under the skin. The pump is often set to deliver a basal amount of insulin continuously throughout the day. Alternatively, the pump can be set to deliver a bolus of insulin at specific times such as mealtimes, when blood glucose levels are high.

Special Populations

Pediatric patients with type 1 diabetes are susceptible to seizures and dehydration in hyperglycemia. In late stages of hyperglycemia, cerebral edema may also develop. Treat pediatric patients with an altered mental status aggressively and provide rapid transport.

Type 2 Diabetes Mellitus

The most common form of diabetes is **type 2 diabetes** (sometimes called adult-onset diabetes), in which blood glucose levels are elevated because the body becomes resistant to the insulin produced and cannot produce enough insulin to overcome that resistance effectively. Type 2 diabetes can also be caused by a deficiency in insulin production. Type 2 diabetes typically develops when a person is middle aged, although the disease is becoming more common in younger people.

In some cases, an abnormal increase in the production of glucose by the liver causes an increase in blood glucose levels. Normally, when blood glucose and insulin levels are low, the pancreas releases glucagon and stimulates the liver to produce and release glucose into the blood. In some people, however, the levels of glucagon stay high. When glucagon levels remain high, excess amounts of glucose are produced, resulting in high blood glucose levels.

According to the World Health Organization, approximately 8.5% of the world's population is affected by diabetes, mostly type 2, making it a global health concern.[7] Approximately 90% of all people with diabetes in the United States have type 2 diabetes.[8] The development of type 2 diabetes has been associated with obesity and physical inactivity, two characteristics becoming more common in today's populations.

Symptoms of untreated type 2 diabetes may include the following:

- Fatigue
- Nausea
- Frequent urination
- Thirst
- Unexplained weight loss
- Blurred vision
- Frequent infections and slow healing of wounds
- Being cranky, confused, or shaky
- Unresponsiveness
- Seizure

These symptoms tend to develop gradually and usually become noticeable in middle age. In fact, the onset

YOU are the Provider PART 2

Recognizing that this patient is probably hypoglycemic, you instruct the patient's wife to turn off the insulin pump. After the pump is turned off, you proceed to check the patient's blood glucose level, to which your glucometer displays "Lo." The reading from the glucometer confirms your suspicion that the patient is experiencing an acute hypoglycemic episode. Because the patient has a decreased level of consciousness, the administration of oral glucose is contraindicated. You ask your partner to place the patient on a nonrebreathing mask and administer oxygen at 15 L/min. Finding a large vein in the patient's arm, you establish an 18-gauge intravenous (IV) line and ensure that the line is patent as you prepare a 50% dextrose (D_{50}) solution.

Recording Time: 1 Minute	
Appearance	Poor
Level of consciousness	Responsive to deep painful stimuli
Airway	Patent
Breathing	12 breaths/min
Circulation	Strong radial pulse; skin is warm, dry, and pink

4. By which route or routes may D_{50} be administered?
5. What are the indications and contraindications for dextrose?
6. What is the usual adult dosage of dextrose?

of type 2 diabetes may be so insidious that patients may not realize they have the disease. In some instances, the symptoms can develop over several years in overweight adults older than 40 years. A small percentage of patients do not display any symptoms.

Weight loss is an important factor in helping to control type 2 diabetes. Exercise and a well-balanced, nutritious diet are key components in combating the complications of diabetes. To maintain glucose levels within the normal range, food intake must be spread throughout the day in coordination with daily oral medications and/or insulin injections and monitoring of glucose levels with a glucometer **Figure 21-7**. Metformin, the medication most commonly prescribed for the management of type 2 diabetes, causes a decrease in glucose production. You can help patients by reinforcing this message to the patient and by helping the family understand how to reduce the patient's risk of diabetic complications.

▶ Prediabetes

As mentioned, *prediabetes* is a condition identified in people who have certain risk factors associated with type 2 diabetes and exists when blood glucose levels or hemoglobin A1c levels are above normal levels, yet not high enough to be diagnosed as diabetes. The A1c blood test reveals information about the patient's blood glucose levels over the prior 3 months. A normal A1c level is less than 5.7%, prediabetes is diagnosed with an A1c level between 5.7% and 6.4%, and type 2 diabetes is diagnosed with an A1c level greater than 6.4%. A patient with uncontrolled diabetes over a long period may have a level higher than 8%.[9] The goal for a diabetic patient is an A1c level of 7% or less.

Words of Wisdom

A portion of the glucose in the blood attaches to the hemoglobin and is called hemoglobin A1c (or HbA1c). The higher the glucose level in the bloodstream, the higher the amount that binds to the hemoglobin. Because the red blood cells (RBCs) live and circulate in the bloodstream for several months, a measurement can be obtained that determines the average level of blood glucose over a couple of months.

The hemoglobin A1c test does not require fasting and can be performed at any time of the day. Factors that affect hemoglobin may alter accurate A1c test results, and include:

- Heavy or chronic bleeding may deplete hemoglobin stores and result in falsely low A1c results.
- Iron-deficiency **anemia** may cause A1c results to be falsely high.
- Recent blood transfusions or hemolytic anemia may result in falsely low results.
- People with an uncommon form of hemoglobin, known as a hemoglobin variant, may have test results that are falsely low or falsely high. This is most often found in people of African, Mediterranean, or Southeast Asian descent. In such cases, tests should be performed at specialized labs for the most accurate results.
- People with kidney or liver failure, or who have a family history of sickle cell anemia, may also have inaccurate A1c results.

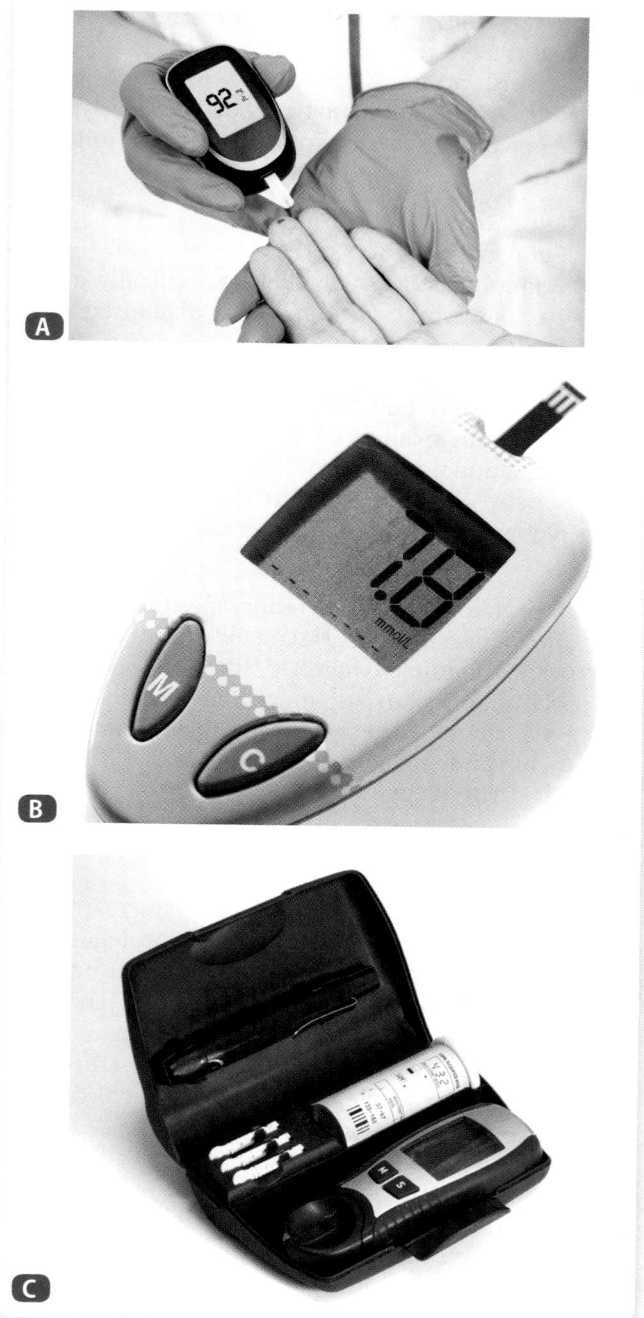

Figure 21-7 The blood glucose self-monitoring kit with digital meter is a device used by patients at home and by EMS providers in the field. Three types are shown.

According to the CDC, prediabetes affects 1 out of 3 adults in the United States, or approximately 86 million people, and 90% are unaware of their status. Within 5 years and with no intervention, 15% to 30% of people with prediabetes will develop type 2 diabetes. Risk factors for experiencing this disease course include the following characteristics:[10]

- Older than 45 years
- Being overweight
- A family history of diabetes—specifically, a parent or sibling who has been diagnosed as having type 2 diabetes
- Being of African American, Hispanic/Latino, American Indian, Pacific Islander, and some Asian American racial or ethnic backgrounds
- Gestational diabetes or having given birth to a baby who weighed more than 9 pounds (4 kg)
- Being physically active fewer than 3 times per week

Although some of the risk factors affecting the pathway from prediabetes to type 2 diabetes cannot be altered, others can. According to the CDC, interventions affecting two specific factors can help prevent or delay the onset of type 2 diabetes by 58%, specifically, losing 5% to 7% of the patient's body weight and getting at least 150 minutes of physical activity per week.[11]

Gestational Diabetes

Gestational diabetes does not have a pancreatic component, but rather is a form of glucose intolerance that can occur during pregnancy. This condition has been identified more often in African American, Hispanic/Latino, and Native American populations, as well as in women with obesity or who have a family history of diabetes. Women who experience gestational diabetes during pregnancy have a 40% to 60% increased risk of developing type 2 diabetes within one decade.[12,13] For most women, gestational diabetes will resolve before delivery. In a few women, however, diabetes will not resolve or type 2 diabetes will develop.

Blood glucose crosses the placental barrier. When a pregnant woman is hyperglycemic, high levels of glucose enter the fetus, causing increased production of insulin by the fetus in an attempt to normalize blood glucose levels. The extra glucose is converted into fat in the fetus, such that women experiencing gestational diabetes often deliver large babies (macrosomia) and may encounter difficult deliveries. Often, cesarean sections are required.

Gestational diabetes is usually diagnosed at 28 weeks' gestation and peaks in the third trimester of pregnancy. It is thought that two hormones produced by the placenta, progesterone and estrogen, result in *insulin resistance*. Because this condition does not occur until later in pregnancy, it does not produce birth defects. Infants of mothers in whom gestational diabetes developed are at higher risk for obesity and diabetes in their lifetime.

Words of Wisdom

The oral glucose tolerance test is used to diagnose gestational diabetes. This test should be used until the pregnant woman is within 12 weeks of delivery. The hemoglobin A1c test can be used during the first pregnancy visit to identify the presence of preexisting diabetes or prediabetes.

Management of gestational diabetes should be initiated as soon as possible to stabilize blood glucose levels and minimize potential complications to both mother and baby. Management includes diet modification, exercise, and blood glucose testing. Oral medications are not prescribed for this form of diabetes, and insulin injections may be required.

Hypoglycemia

Hypoglycemia in a person with type 1 diabetes is often the result of having taken too much insulin, too little food, or both. The tissues of the central nervous system (including the brain), unlike other tissues that can usually metabolize fat or protein in addition to sugar, depend entirely on glucose as their source of energy. If the level of glucose in the blood decreases dramatically, the brain is literally starved. **Hypoglycemic crisis**, also known as *insulin shock*, is the result of hypoglycemia, or insufficient glucose in the blood.

Counterregulation is the body's natural defensive ability to maintain blood glucose at an appropriate level. An understanding of this concept is critical because it will help you treat (and ideally prevent) severe hypoglycemia.

The body's first line of defense against low blood glucose is to reduce insulin production by the pancreas and to increase glucagon production by the alpha cells. When cells are deprived of glucose, a distress signal goes out over the sympathetic nervous system, causing the release of various stress hormones. The body's second line of defense is the secretion of catecholamines—including epinephrine and norepinephrine—by the adrenal gland. The effects of this catecholamine release can be seen as tachycardia and diaphoresis in the hypoglycemic patient. This second line of defense also includes cortisol, an adrenocorticoid (a steroid produced in the adrenal gland). Cortisol release results in an increase in blood glucose levels, which counteracts insulin's actions. Other hormones produced by the intestine and growth hormone produced by the pituitary gland also increase blood glucose levels.

Last, stimulation of the autonomic nervous system generates signals that allow production of counterregulatory hormones to increase. The same stimulation also triggers symptoms telling the body that the blood glucose level is low; ideally, the affected patient will recognize these symptoms and consume a source of sugar to remedy the imbalance. In response to the action of these hormones, the body mobilizes fatty acids and amino acids from adipose and muscle, respectively. The liver uses these products to make new glucose for the body in a process called gluconeogenesis.

In patients with type 1 diabetes, the islets of Langerhans do not make insulin. As a result, the body's first line of defense against hypoglycemia is lost because the ability to decrease insulin levels via this mechanism is not possible. Often, a low blood glucose level in a patient with diabetes is caused by an elevated level of exogenous insulin (insulin prescribed to the patient for injection) from inaccurate dosing, intentional overdose, or perhaps a mismatch with carbohydrate intake and exogenous insulin intake. In addition, increased use of glucose, such as what occurs during exercise, causes the blood glucose level to drop sharply, resulting in hypoglycemia.

In patients with type 2 diabetes, the pancreas can generate insulin, so these patients can suppress insulin production from within their own bodies. However, their bodies may be resistant to the effects of insulin, or they may not make enough insulin over time to lower the blood glucose level adequately. Medications given to treat type 2 diabetes act by either stimulating the body's ability to secrete insulin or by improving insulin's actions. These medications also tend to contribute to hypoglycemia, especially in certain groups of patients such as older adults and those who are not metabolizing these medications properly because of liver or kidney disease. Often, if the hypoglycemia is caused by excessive insulin dosing by the patient or by the prolonged or exaggerated effects of oral diabetes medications, the low blood glucose level will have a prolonged effect and more long-term treatment may be needed.

Some patients who have had type 1 diabetes for many years, and to a lesser degree, patients who have had type 2 diabetes for many years, may not experience a glucagon release from the pancreas in response to hypoglycemia.[14] Lack of glucagon response makes the body more dependent on epinephrine to overcome the effects of hypoglycemia, yet there may be some lack of responsiveness to epinephrine in diabetes as well.[15,16] Prolonged disease can also decrease a patient's ability to recognize having a low blood glucose level (a state called hypoglycemic unawareness), preventing him or her from taking the necessary measures of self treatment.

The patient with hypoglycemia will experience trembling; a rapid heart rate; rapid, shallow respirations; sweating; and a feeling of hunger. The brain is highly sensitive to glucose levels, and so these symptoms reflect both the disordered function of hungry brain cells and the alarm reaction (sympathetic nervous system discharge) set off by the brain's distress signals. If hypoglycemia persists, cerebral dysfunction progresses quickly to permanent brain damage.

Some of the most common signs and symptoms of hypoglycemia include:

- Blood glucose level less than 70 mg/dL
- Hunger
- Agitation, irritability, or combative behavior that cannot be explained
- Altered mentation or confusion
- Nausea
- Weakness, dizziness, or fainting
- Tachycardia (poor cardiac output)
- Cool, clammy skin

Additional signs and symptoms associated with hypoglycemia include headache, mental confusion, memory loss, incoordination, slurred speech, irritability, dilated pupils, and seizures and coma in severe cases.

Hypoglycemia is a common problem experienced by patients with either type 1 or type 2 diabetes. It develops *rapidly*, over a period ranging from minutes to a few hours, and should be suspected in any patient with diabetes who presents with bizarre behavior, neurologic signs such as altered mental status or weakness or facial drooping similar to a stroke, or coma. Often, a hypoglycemic patient appears intoxicated because of slurred speech and lack of coordination, and may be paranoid, hostile, and aggressive.

Although it is not completely preventable, hypoglycemia can be treated easily. This condition can be detected with regular blood glucose monitoring and rarely results in complications for the patient if identified and treated promptly.

In contrast, severe hypoglycemia, resulting in loss of consciousness or altered mental status, is a more common reason for a call to 9-1-1 and requires intervention and treatment. As an EMS professional, you will need to promptly provide treatment to these patients. If untreated or not detected, serious hypoglycemia can result in coma or death.

Words of Wisdom

The longer a patient remains unresponsive from hypoglycemia, the more likely there will be permanent brain damage! If more than 20 to 30 minutes go by, toxic compounds (free radicals) in the brain are produced that can cause permanent damage.

Of course, people with diabetes are not the only ones who are likely to have episodes of hypoglycemia. Patients with alcoholism, patients who have ingested certain poisons or overdosed with certain drugs (notably aspirin), and patients with certain cancers, liver disease, kidney disease, and some other conditions may also experience hypoglycemic episodes. Do not discount the possibility of hypoglycemia in a comatose patient just because the patient is not known to have diabetes. Conversely, do not let a known diagnosis of diabetes prevent you from considering other causes of coma. People with diabetes can also experience head injury, stroke, seizures, meningitis, and other traumatic injuries or conditions; the presentation of these conditions may appear similar to diabetic emergencies. Keep an open mind and assess the patient thoroughly.

Words of Wisdom

A patient experiencing a hypoglycemic event may be confused with a patient having a cerebrovascular accident (CVA). D_{50} is *contraindicated* in CVA in the presence of normal blood glucose levels. Thus, the blood glucose level should be assessed and verified carefully in patients with signs associated with CVA prior to administering D_{50}. The hypertonic properties of D_{50} may result in increased cerebral edema in the event of a cerebrovascular event.

▶ Hyperglycemia and Diabetic Ketoacidosis

Without insulin, glucose from food remains in the blood and gradually rises to extremely high levels. Normally, high carbohydrate levels are tolerated and return to normal by means of metabolic pathways. Problems arise when the blood glucose level remains elevated and the mechanisms that normally correct this have failed. This condition is called **hyperglycemia**. Hyperglycemia can be caused by excessive food intake, insufficient insulin dosages, infection or illness, injury, surgery, and emotional stress. **Hyperglycemic crisis**, also known as diabetic coma, is a state of unresponsiveness resulting from several problems, including ketoacidosis, hyperglycemia, and dehydration because of excessive urination.

Common early signs include frequent and excessive thirst accompanied by frequent and excessive urination. Hyperglycemia occurs when blood glucose levels exceed the normal range (70 to 120 mg/dL).

Onset of hyperglycemia may be rapid (within minutes) or gradual (hours to days), depending on the cause. For example, excessive food intake may cause blood glucose levels to increase quickly, whereas an infection or illness will result in hyperglycemia over the course of several days.

Some patients with type 2 diabetes can go undiagnosed for several years. Over time, however, repeated episodes of hyperglycemia will cause several physiologic changes that have detrimental long-term effects. Largely because of the increased hyperosmolarity it causes, hyperglycemia puts undue strain on the cardiovascular system, kidneys, and other end organs that are sensitive to increased serum viscosity and the subsequent pressures exerted by the thicker serum. The eventual result is an increased incidence of disorders such as renal failure, heart failure, retinopathy, coronary artery disease, and neuropathy.

When serum glucose levels rise above tolerable levels, physiologic changes occur. These changes represent actual pathologic conditions called **diabetic ketoacidosis (DKA)** (blood glucose level greater than approximately 350 mg/dL) and **hyperosmolar hyperglycemic syndrome (HHS)** (blood glucose level greater than approximately 600 mg/dL). DKA is associated predominately with people with type 1 diabetes. A life-threatening condition, DKA occurs when certain acids accumulate in the body because insulin is not available **Figure 21-8**. Common causes of DKA include infection, injury, alcohol use, emotional distress, and illness such as stroke or myocardial infarction. In patients with DKA, hyperglycemia continues—that is, glucose continues to accumulate in the blood. Eventually, the patient undergoes massive osmotic diuresis (passing large amounts of urine because of the high solute concentration of the blood).

The process of excreting so much glucose in the urine requires a large amount of water. The loss of water in such large amounts causes the classic symptoms of uncontrolled diabetes, the "3 Ps": polyuria, polydipsia, and polyphagia. This, together with vomiting, causes dehydration and even shock. Along with water, the body also loses electrolytes

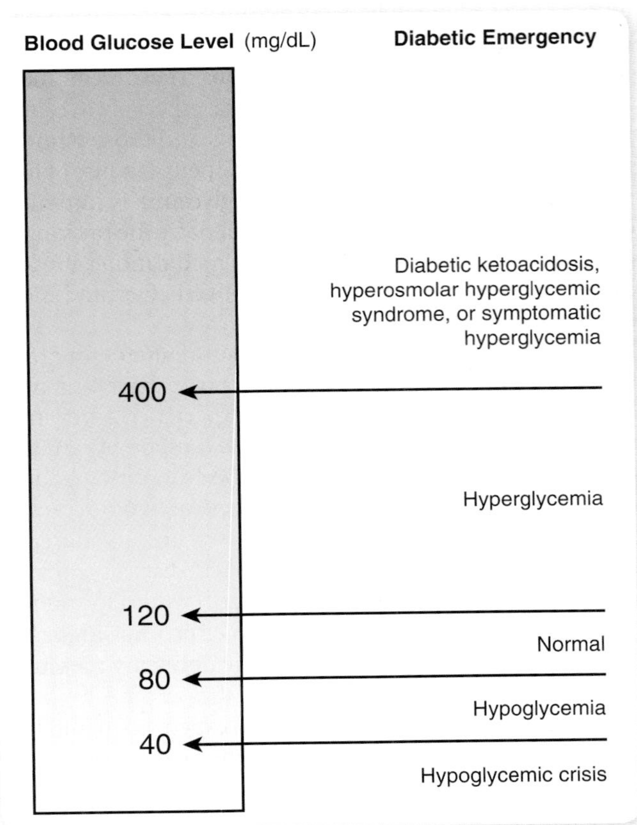

Figure 21-8 The two most common diabetic emergencies, diabetic ketoacidosis and hypoglycemic crisis, occur when the patient has too much or too little glucose in the blood, respectively. The left column illustrates blood glucose levels; the right column illustrates the conditions associated with that particular level of blood glucose. Notice that the normal range is rather small in comparison to the other ranges.

Words of Wisdom

In DKA, the body does not have sufficient insulin to transport glucose into the cells. Therefore, it uses stored fat as an energy source, producing ketones and acids as waste products. This increase in acids causes a decrease in the body's pH level, resulting in metabolic acidosis. The body must then rely on its buffer systems to attempt to return the pH balance to normal.

$$\uparrow H^+ + HCO_3^- = \uparrow H_2CO_3 = H_2O + \uparrow CO_2$$

(↑ Hydrogen + Bicarbonate = ↑ Carbonic acid = Water + ↑ Carbon dioxide)

The chemical buffer system initially breaks down the acid into a form that can be readily expelled from the body. Remember that with metabolic acidosis, the compensatory mechanism is the respiratory system. Because carbon dioxide is an acid, an increase in the rate and depth of respirations (Kussmaul respirations) will attempt to decrease the amount of acid in the body.

(sodium and potassium), which may result in disturbances in water balance and acid-base balance.

Without glucose to supply energy for cells, the body must turn to other fuel sources, the most abundant of which is fat. Unfortunately, when fat is used as an immediate energy source, chemicals called ketones and fatty acids are formed as waste products and are difficult for the body to excrete.

Fatty acids are broken down primarily by the mitochondria in liver cells. As part of this process, ketone bodies are released into the bloodstream. Large quantities of ketone bodies in the bloodstream cause a decrease in the blood's pH and result in metabolic **acidosis**. This acidosis triggers the body's attempts to buffer the acidity with bicarbonate (HCO_3^-), and the blood pH decreases because of the inability to keep up with the ongoing acidity. In addition to fat tissue breaking down its stores of energy, muscle tissue mobilizes its stores in an effort to create more glucose for the body. This process creates amino acids that may be used by the liver to make glucose (gluconeogenesis). In addition, lactate increases in the bloodstream and contributes to lowering the body's pH. This form of acidosis is known as DKA.

The ketones are responsible for the sweet, fruity breath odor associated with DKA. When the acid levels in the body become too high, individual cells will cease to function. If the patient is not given proper fluid rehydration and insulin to reverse fat metabolism and restore the use of glucose as a source of energy, ketoacidosis will progress to unresponsiveness, diabetic coma, and, eventually, death. However, patients in DKA are seldom deeply comatose; therefore, a totally unresponsive patient likely has another problem, such as head injury, stroke, or drug overdose.

Signs and Symptoms of Hypoglycemia Versus Hyperglycemia

The signs and symptoms of hypoglycemia and hyperglycemia can be similar Table 21-2. The signs and symptoms of simple hyperglycemia are usually mild, if present at all. They can include blurred vision, polyuria, polydipsia, polyphagia, orthostatic syncope, frequent infections, and skin ulcerations. If you encounter a patient with simple hyperglycemia who has not progressed to a more serious syndrome, treatment should include supportive care and transport.

Hyperglycemia usually progresses slowly, over a period of 12 to 48 hours, with the patient's level of consciousness deteriorating only gradually. The load of glucose present within the kidneys during hyperglycemia results in glucose spilling into the urine, causing the body to become hyperosmotic. As the kidneys remove excess glucose, water is removed via increased urination, resulting in dehydration. The kidneys also help clear ketone bodies from the blood. As part of the substantial amount of water lost through diuresis, patients lose excessive amounts of sodium, potassium, and phosphates in the urine. As mentioned, this combination of effects results in both dehydration and metabolic acidosis with associated electrolyte imbalances.

The resulting signs and symptoms manifest these etiologic factors:

- Polyuria (excessive urine output), because of osmotic diuresis
- Polydipsia (excessive thirst), because of dehydration
- Polyphagia (excessive eating), probably related to inefficient use of nutrients
- Nausea and vomiting, the latter worsening the patient's dehydration
- Tachycardia as a consequence of dehydration
- Deep, rapid respirations (**Kussmaul respirations**)—the body's attempt to compensate for acidosis by blowing off carbon dioxide (CO_2)
- Warm, dry skin and dry mucous membranes, also reflecting dehydration
- Fruity odor of ketones (acetone smell) on the breath
- Abdominal pain
- Sometimes fever

Patients usually appear thin or dehydrated and have warm, dry skin. Patients also may exhibit orthostatic hypotension, supine hypotension, fatigue, altered mental status, and, with time, weight loss from the hypermetabolic state.

The respiratory rate is usually elevated and the tidal volume is increased (Kussmaul respirations) because of **ketonemia** (excess amounts of ketone bodies in the blood), acidosis, and the body's attempt to relieve itself of the excessive burden of CO_2. These respiratory changes result in hypocapnia, which is recognized by lower-than-normal

Table 21-2 Comparison of Hypoglycemia and Hyperglycemia

	Hypoglycemia	Hyperglycemia: Diabetic Ketoacidosis[a]	Hyperglycemia: HHS[b]
Food intake	Insufficient	Excessive	Excessive
Insulin dosage	Excessive	Insufficient	Insufficient
Onset	Rapid, within minutes	Gradual—hours to days	Gradual—days to weeks
Skin	Pale to moist	Warm and dry	Warm and dry
Infection	Uncommon	Common	Usual
Thirst	Absent	Intense	Very intense
Hunger	Intense	Excessive	Excessive
Vomiting	Uncommon	Common	Uncommon
Breathing	Normal or rapid	Rapid, deep (Kussmaul respirations)	Tachycardia
Odor of breath	Normal	Sweet, fruity (nail polish remover/acetone smell)	No ketone body produced; therefore there is no fruity odor
Blood pressure	Low	Normal to low	Hypotension
Pulse	Rapid, weak	Normal or rapid and full	Rapid, weak
Level of consciousness	Irritability, confusion, seizure, or coma	Restless merging to coma	Restless merging to coma
Urine: Sugar	Absent	Present	Present
Urine: Acetone	Absent	Present	Absent
Blood glucose level (mg/dL)	<60	>250	>600
Response to treatment	Immediately after administration of glucose	Gradual, within 6 to 12 hours following medical treatment	

Abbreviation: HHS, hyperosmolar hyperglycemic syndrome

[a] Usually associated with type 1 diabetes
[b] Usually associated with type 2 diabetes

end-tidal CO_2 ($ETCO_2$) levels. Because $ETCO_2$ levels are affected, capnography is another tool you can use to confirm your diagnosis. DKA results in both Kussmaul respirations and metabolic acidosis; an $ETCO_2$ value less than 25 mm Hg corroborates your suspicions.[17]

In patients with type 2 diabetes, DKA is rare because insulin is still present, at least early in the course of the disease. Despite the elevated blood glucose levels, the level of insulin is sufficient to prevent uncontrolled breakdown of glycogen, adipose tissue, and muscle. In all patients with type 2 diabetes, regardless of the duration of the disease, ketone bodies can be found in the urine when the patient experiences hyperglycemia. With increased duration of type 2 diabetes, a loss of pancreatic insulin production may occur. In fact, patients can develop elevated serum ketone levels, reduced blood pH levels, and DKA similar to those patients with type 1 diabetes.

▶ Hyperosmolar Hyperglycemic Syndrome

HHS is also called **hyperosmolar nonketotic coma (HONK)**, a metabolic derangement that occurs principally in patients with type 2 diabetes.[18-21] This condition is characterized by hyperglycemia, hyperosmolarity, and an absence of substantial ketosis. The term *hyperosmolarity* describes highly concentrated blood as a result of relative dehydration. Key signs and symptoms of HHS include:

- Hyperglycemia
- Altered mental status, drowsiness, and lethargy
- Severe dehydration, thirst, and dark urine
- Visual or sensory deficits
- Partial paralysis or muscle weakness
- Seizures

Oddly enough, less than 20% of patients present in a comatose state.[22] Instead, most patients have severe dehydration and focal or global neurologic deficits. In addition, AMI is frequently associated with HHS/HONK. The clinical features of HHS/HONK and DKA tend to overlap and are often observed simultaneously.

HHS/HONK often develops in patients with diabetes who have a secondary illness that results in reduced fluid intake. Although infection (in particular, pneumonia and urinary tract infection) is the most common cause, many other conditions can cause altered mentation or dehydration. In most cases, the secondary illness is not identified.

Words of Wisdom

Certain medications—including diuretic medications, beta blockers, histamine-2 (H_2) blockers, dialysis, total parenteral nutrition, and dextrose-containing fluids—may contribute to the development of HHS/HONK by increasing serum glucose levels, inhibiting insulin, or causing dehydration. Hyperglycemia and hyperosmolarity lead to osmotic diuresis and an osmotic shift of fluid to the intravascular space, resulting in further intracellular dehydration.

Words of Wisdom

There is no predictable correlation between the increase in a patient's blood glucose level and the degree of ketoacidosis in the blood. Not all patients with increased blood glucose levels have DKA or HHS/HONK. Many people have glucose intolerance and hyperglycemia with absolutely no symptoms. Rely on the patient's clinical presentation rather than the "number."

Unlike patients with DKA, patients with HHS/HONK do not experience ketoacidosis. The onset of DKA can occur in as little as a few hours, whereas HHS/HONK can take up to weeks to develop. Blood glucose levels tend to be substantially higher in HHS/HONK as compared with DKA (Table 21-3). Although most patients diagnosed as having HHS/HONK have a known history of diabetes (usually type 2), as many as 20% do not have a prior diagnosis of diabetes.[23] The stress response to any acute illness tends to increase hormones that favor elevated glucose levels: cortisol, catecholamines (epinephrine and norepinephrine), glucagon, and many other hormones have effects that tend to counter those of insulin. Various neurologic changes may be noted, including drowsiness and lethargy, delirium and coma, focal or generalized seizures, visual disturbances, hemiparesis, and sensory deficits.

Table 21-3 Comparison of Hyperglycemic Conditions

	Hyperosmolar Hyperglycemic Syndrome/Hyperosmolar Nonketotic Coma	Diabetic Ketoacidosis
Glucose	>600 mg/dL	>250 mg/dL
Arterial pH	>7.3	<7.3
Ketone bodies	Absent	Present
Type of diabetes mellitus	Type 2	Type 1

Words of Wisdom

Occasionally, patients with hypoglycemia or hyperglycemia are thought to be intoxicated, especially if their condition has caused a motor vehicle crash or other incident. Confined by police in a "drunk tank," a patient with diabetes is at risk. In such situations, an emergency medical identification bracelet, necklace, or card may help to save the patient's life. Often, only a blood glucose test performed at the scene or in the emergency department will identify the actual problem.

Certainly, diabetes and alcoholism can coexist in a patient. But you must be alert to the similarity in symptoms of acute alcohol intoxication and diabetic emergencies. Likewise, hypoglycemia and a head injury can coexist, and you must appreciate the potential even when the head injury is obvious.

Patient Assessment of Endocrine Emergencies

Assessment of a patient with a history of diabetes will be similar to your assessment of any other medical patient. Keep in mind that, in addition to hyperglycemic and hypoglycemic crises, patients with diabetes may have silent, or painless, heart attacks. A patient's only symptom may be "not feeling so well." This is especially true of geriatric patients. It is imperative to maintain a high index of suspicion and treat patients aggressively.

Special Populations

Diabetes in children may pose a particular management problem. First, the high levels of activity of children mean that they can use up circulating glucose more quickly than adults do, even after a normal insulin injection. Second, they do not always eat correctly and on schedule. Third, they have limited stores of liver glycogen that can be rapidly depleted. As a result, hypoglycemic crisis can develop more rapidly and more severely in children than in adults.

Safety

When managing problems related to diabetes and altered mental status, exposure to body fluids is generally extremely limited. Follow standard precautions, as you would with any other patient. Always use gloves, and wash your hands carefully after obtaining and checking a blood sample or if you perform airway techniques.

Also, remain aware that patients with diabetic emergencies can become confused, and possibly aggressive or dangerous.

Scene Size-up

Evaluate scene safety as you arrive on scene and as you approach the patient. Make sure that all hazards are addressed. Remember that diabetic patients often use syringes to administer insulin. It is possible you may be stuck by a used needle that was not disposed of properly. Insulin syringes on the bed stand, insulin bottles in the refrigerator, a plate of food, or a glass of orange juice are important clues that may help you decide what is possibly wrong with your patient. Evaluate each situation quickly and make sure the necessary personal protective equipment

YOU are the Provider — PART 3

After reconfirming that the IV line is patent, you slowly administer 25 g of D_{50} over 4 minutes, per your protocols. As you are completing a bolus of D_{50}, the patient begins to moan and move around. You begin to reassess the patient. Approximately 5 minutes after the dextrose has been infused, the patient is able to communicate appropriately. According to his wife, he is now acting normally. You inform the patient of what you believe has happened, and state that he should be transported to the local emergency department for evaluation. The patient states, "I don't need to go to the hospital, my insulin pump should keep my sugar up."

Recording Time: 8 Minutes	
Respirations	18 breaths/min
Pulse	Strong and regular, at 77 beats/min
Skin	Warm, dry, and pink
Blood pressure	154/88 mm Hg
Oxygen saturation (Spo_2)	100% at 15 L/min via nonrebreathing mask
Pupils	Pupils Equal, Round, and Reactive to Light and Accommodation (PERRLA)

7. Does this patient require transport to the emergency department?

is readily available. Standard precautions should consist of gloves and eye protection at a minimum.

As you approach, question bystanders on events leading up to your arrival. Determine whether this is your only patient and whether trauma was involved. Decide whether you will need any additional resources. Do not let your guard down even on what appears to be a routine call.

Primary Survey

Perform a rapid scan of the patient to form a general impression. How does the patient look? Does he or she appear anxious, restless, or listless? Is the patient apathetic or irritable? Is the patient interacting with his or her environment appropriately? These initial observations may lead you to suspect high or low blood glucose values. In patients with altered mental status, suspect a low blood glucose level. Remember that hypoglycemia is a potentially life-threatening event.

Identify life threats, and provide lifesaving interventions, particularly airway management. Determine the patient's level of consciousness using the AVPU (*Awake* and alert, responsive to *Verbal* stimuli, responsive to *Pain*, *Unresponsive*) scale. An unresponsive patient may have undiagnosed diabetes. Perform cervical spine immobilization, when indicated, and provide rapid transport. At the emergency department, diabetes and its complications can be quickly diagnosed.

As you are forming your general impression, assess the patient's airway and breathing. Patients showing signs of inadequate breathing, an altered mental status, or oxygen saturation (Spo_2) of 94% or less should receive high-flow oxygen at 12 to 15 L/min via nonrebreathing mask or ventilations via bag-mask device. A patient who is hyperglycemic may have rapid, deep respirations (Kussmaul respirations) and a sweet, fruity breath odor. A patient who is hypoglycemic will have normal or shallow to rapid respirations. If the patient is not breathing or is having difficulty breathing, open the airway and insert an airway adjunct, and assist ventilations. Continue to monitor the airway as you provide care. Consider calling for paramedic backup if the patient needs a definitive airway.

If the patient is unresponsive, treat him or her as any other unresponsive patient, with attention to the airway. If dextrose is indicated, use of an advanced airway should be avoided until dextrose has been administered. If the patient remains unresponsive, an advanced airway can be considered.

Patients with altered mental status, particularly those who are difficult to awaken, are at risk for losing their gag reflex. When the gag reflex is absent, patients cannot reject foreign materials in their mouth (including vomit), and their tongue will often relax and obstruct the airway. Therefore, you must carefully monitor the airway in patients with hypoglycemia, hyperglycemic crisis, or other complications such as stroke or seizure. Place the patient in a lateral recumbent position, and have suction readily available.

Words of Wisdom

A patient with Kussmaul respirations may have an oxygen saturation of close to 100% because of their increased rate and depth of respirations. These patients still need high-flow oxygen via nonrebreathing mask. The respirations are in response to the increased acidosis in the body.

After you have assessed airway and breathing and have performed the necessary lifesaving interventions, check the patient's circulatory status. A patient with dry, warm skin indicates hyperglycemia, whereas a patient with moist, pale skin indicates hypoglycemia. The patient in hypoglycemic crisis will have a rapid, weak pulse.

History Taking

Investigate the chief complaint or the history of the present illness. Responsive patients usually are able to provide their own medical history. If the patient has eaten but has not taken insulin, it is more likely that hyperglycemia is developing. If the patient has taken insulin but has not eaten, the problem is more likely to be hypoglycemia. A patient with diabetes will often know what is wrong. If the patient is not thinking or speaking clearly, or is unresponsive, attempt to obtain a medical history from family members or bystanders.

Physical signs such as tremors, diaphoresis, abdominal cramps, vomiting, a fruity breath odor, or a dry mouth may guide you in determining whether the patient is hypoglycemic or hyperglycemic.

You will need to obtain a SAMPLE history (Signs and symptoms, Allergies, Medications, Pertinent past medical history, Last oral intake, Events leading up to the illness or injury) from your patient. In addition, be sure to ask the following questions of any ill patient who has a history of diabetes:

- Do you take insulin or any pills that lower your blood glucose?
- Have you taken your usual dose of insulin (or pills) today?
- Have you eaten normally today?
- Have you had any illnesses, unusual amount of activity, or stress today?

Also ask the patient or family about the following (these questions will help determine whether the patient is compliant with the management of his or her disease):

- The patient's last meal and insulin dose
- Any vision changes, headaches, dizziness, or bleeding
- A recent change in the patient's bowel movements or eating habits

- Tingling, numbness, or swelling of the extremities. Patients with long-standing diabetes may have undergone amputation, and their residual limb may become infected or septic.

When you are assessing a patient who might have diabetes, check to see whether he or she has an emergency medical identification device—a wallet card, necklace, or bracelet—or ask the patient or a family member. Remember that the environment, bystanders, and medical identification devices may provide important clues about your patient's condition.

Special Populations

Be aware of the possibility of diabetes complicating a pregnancy. If you encounter a woman who is pregnant with an altered mental status, be sure to check her blood glucose level. If hypoglycemia is present, administer 25 g of dextrose 50% IV. If hyperglycemia or DKA is present, isotonic crystalloid fluid boluses may be necessary to treat the associated dehydration.

Secondary Assessment

If time allows, conduct a secondary assessment.

Assess unresponsive patients with a full-body exam, looking for clues to their condition. With unresponsive patients or patients with an altered mental status, you must look for problems or injuries that are not obvious because the patient is unable to communicate these to you. Although an altered mental status may be caused by a blood glucose level that is too high or too low, the patient may have sustained trauma resulting from dizziness or from changes in level of consciousness, or may have another metabolic problem. An altered mental status may also be caused by something else, such as intoxication, poisoning, or a head injury. Also, because patients may have an altered perception of pain, particularly in their extremities, it is important to assess for any signs of sores or infections. A systematic examination of the patient may provide you with information essential to proper patient care.

When you suspect a diabetes-related problem, a secondary assessment should focus on the patient's mental status and ability to swallow and protect the airway. Obtain a Glasgow Coma Scale score to track the patient's neurologic status.

Obtain a complete set of vital signs. Pulse and respiratory rates will vary, depending on the diabetic emergency the patient is experiencing; at times the blood pressure may be low as a result of dehydration from polyuria. It should be easier for you to identify abnormal vital signs when you know the blood glucose level is too high or too low. Remember, the patient may have abnormal vital signs and a normal blood glucose value. In this case, something else may be causing the patient's symptoms.

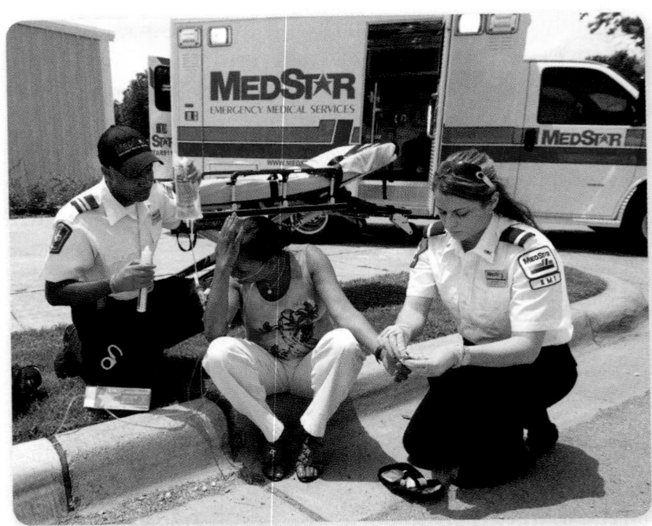

Figure 21-9 Obtain the blood glucose level in any patient with an altered mental status.

It is important to always obtain a blood glucose level in any patient with an altered mental status as described in Chapter 10, *Patient Assessment* **Figure 21-9**. Glucometers measure the glucose level in whole blood using either capillary or venous samples.

It is important to read and understand the operator's manual before use because the specifications of the device may vary depending on the manufacturer. Some glucometers indicate low (Lo) when they detect a glucose reading of less than 20 mg/dL, whereas others display Lo when they detect a reading of less than 30 mg/dL. Conversely, the same is true with a high (Hi) reading; some glucometers read Hi at 550 mg/dL and some at 600 mg/dL; therefore, it is important to know both the upper and lower ranges at which your glucometer functions.

As mentioned earlier, the normal range for glucose levels in blood in nonfasting adults and children is 70 to 120 mg/dL; the blood glucose level in neonates should be higher than 70 mg/dL.

Reassessment

It is important to reassess the diabetic patient frequently to assess changes. Is there an improvement in the patient's mental status? Are the ABCs (airway, breathing, and circulation) still intact? Monitor the airway carefully and be alert for potential vomiting, especially if glucose has been administered orally. When patients who are hypoglycemic are given large quantities of glucose orally, they tend to become nauseated.

How is the patient responding to the interventions performed? How must you adjust or change the interventions? In many patients with diabetes, you will note marked improvement with appropriate treatment. Document each assessment, your findings, the time of the interventions, and any changes in the patient's condition. Base your administration of glucose on serial readings.

The administration of glucose, glucagon, and IV fluids will be based on your service's protocols and standing orders.

Keep hospital personnel informed about the patient's history, the present situation, assessment findings, and your interventions and their results.

Emergency Medical Care of Endocrine Emergencies

▶ General Management

When you are treating the patient, place him or her in a position of comfort. If the patient has an altered mental status, establish an IV line with 0.9% normal saline or a saline lock. Measure the blood glucose level immediately and initiate treatment if the reading is less than 60 mg/dL and the patient is symptomatic. Give 12.5 to 25 g of dextrose in a concentration consistent with your local protocols (eg, D_{50}—25 g of dextrose per every 50 mL, or 50% concentration); this dose will reverse most cases of hypoglycemia. Some EMS systems no longer carry D_{50} and may use D_{25} (25% dextrose concentration), D_{10} (10% dextrose concentration), or glucagon. Glucagon is administered 1 mg intramuscularly (IM), with a greatly increased recovery time as compared with IV D_{50}, D_{25}, or D_{10}. D_{25} and D_{10} are less concentrated and less hypertonic. The decreased osmolarity in these concentrations is less caustic to the veins and tissues. They also cause less fluctuation in blood glucose levels after administration. For these reasons, many agencies are moving to one or more of the dilute solutions rather than using D_{50}.

If the patient's condition does not improve after a dose of dextrose, and if you have reason to suspect a narcotic overdose (based on signs of pinpoint pupils, needle tracks, depressed respirations), consider administering naloxone (Narcan).

Transport the unresponsive patient supine or in the lateral recumbent or recovery position (unless any injuries preclude that position). If there are indications of increasing intracranial pressure such as the Cushing reflex (slowing pulse, rising blood pressure, and an erratic respiratory pattern), posturing, or unequal pupils, transport with the head elevated to a 30° to 45° angle and the head midline to assist in venous return and minimize intracranial pressure. Always keep the mouth and pharynx suctioned free of secretions, vomitus, and blood.

▶ Management of Hypoglycemia

Hypoglycemic patients may experience permanent cerebral damage if blood glucose levels are not restored rapidly. Management of hypoglycemia includes immediately increasing blood glucose levels, with the precise treatment depending on several factors. It is always preferable to provide the least invasive method of treatment possible that will successfully address the condition.

If the hypoglycemic patient is alert and able to swallow without the risk of aspiration, administer sugar by mouth. Provide juice sweetened with sugar, a candy bar, or any item that contains sugar. Do not be afraid to give too much sugar. Do not give sugar-free drinks that are sweetened with saccharin or other synthetic sweetening compounds because they will have little or no effect. Oral glucose may also be given, but most patients prefer the taste of *regular* food or drink as opposed to the taste of oral glucose and will be more cooperative.

The first-line medical treatment for patients with hypoglycemia is to administer oral glucose as discussed in the next section, assuming the patient is responsive and there is no risk of aspiration. If this is not possible, you should administer dextrose via the IV route. Finally, if IV access cannot be obtained, you should administer glucagon via the IM route.

Words of Wisdom

Fluids and dextrose solutions may also be given through an IO (intraosseous) line. However, IO access is usually reserved for critical situations where IV access cannot be obtained.

Words of Wisdom

When you are unable to measure a patient's glucose level and are unsure whether the patient is hypoglycemic or hyperglycemic, always err on the side of caution and give glucose. More glucose in a hyperglycemic patient will not cause harm, but it may save the life of a hypoglycemic patient, especially if the patient is in hypoglycemic crisis.

One exception to this is the potential for a head injury. If the patient has a mechanism of injury that may lead you to suspect a head injury, do not administer glucose. Instead, focus on oxygenation and provide rapid transport.

If you are treating an older adult or a patient whose clinical history suggests that the problem may be stroke, note that it is especially important to measure the patient's blood glucose level *prior* to administration of dextrose. Administration of concentrated glucose solutions in a situation of suspected stroke may exacerbate cerebral damage.

Situations in which you are unable to measure a patient's blood glucose level should be extremely rare, particularly if you are diligent about checking all of your equipment, including your glucometer prior to every shift.

Administering Oral Glucose

Oral glucose is commercially available in tablet and gel forms that dissolve when placed in the mouth Figure 21-10. Trade names for the gel include Glutose and Insta-Glucose. The only contraindications to glucose

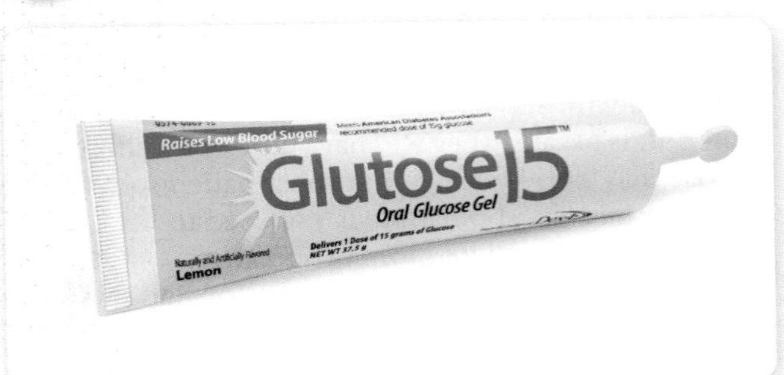

Figure 21-10 Oral glucose is commercially available in gel and tablet form. One tube of gel equals one dose.

are an inability to swallow or unresponsiveness because aspiration (inhalation of the substance) can occur. Oral glucose itself has no side effects if it is administered properly; however, aspiration in a patient who does not have a gag reflex can have lethal results.

If your hypoglycemic patient is unresponsive, or if there is any risk of aspiration, do not give anything by mouth! Although patients with hypoglycemia and altered mental status need glucose, *never give anything by mouth to an unresponsive patient*, even if you suspect hypoglycemic crisis. Instead, administer IV/IO glucose or IM glucagon.

Words of Wisdom

A tube of commercially prepared cake icing is an excellent substitute for oral glucose. You may be able to find some in the patient's kitchen.

A patient who is alert can administer his or her own glucose gel or tablets. For those who need assistance, the gel can be squeezed into the open mouth in small increments to allow time to swallow. Have water available—the gel is extremely sweet and viscous. Another option is to place the gel on a tongue depressor and place it between the patient's cheek and gum for absorption with the gel side turned toward the cheek. The patient will usually become more alert within minutes.

Reassess the patient frequently after administering glucose, even if you see rapid improvement in the patient's condition. Remain alert for airway problems, sudden loss of consciousness, or seizures. Provide prompt transport to the hospital; do not delay transport just to give additional oral glucose if the patient has an altered mental status.

When there is any doubt about whether a responsive patient with diabetes is going into hypoglycemic or hyperglycemic crisis, most protocols will err on the side of giving glucose. The risk of increasing the glucose level of a patient who is already hyperglycemic is minimal compared with the benefit of increasing the glucose level of one who is hypoglycemic. Hypoglycemia is detrimental to the patient's overall health and can quickly result in other systemic problems. The patient with diabetes who is unresponsive and having seizures is more likely to be in a hypoglycemic crisis. When in doubt, consult medical control.

For patients presenting with signs of dehydration, administer a 20-mL/kg bolus of an isotonic crystalloid solution such as normal saline or lactated Ringer solution. Treatment is aimed at rehydrating the patient and providing prompt transport to an appropriate facility. Reassess the patient after the initial bolus and repeat if needed. Reassure the patient en route, and provide general comfort measures.

Administering Intravenous Dextrose

If the hypoglycemic patient has an altered mental status or is unable to swallow, you will need to administer IV dextrose.

Exercise caution when using dextrose; contraindications include the presence of increased intracranial pressure or possible intracranial bleeding. When the unresponsive patient is older than 55 years or the family gives a history of recent transient ischemic attacks or stroke, assess glucose levels to rule out hypoglycemia prior to administering IV dextrose.

Also use caution with patients suspected of having hypokalemia (low potassium levels), such as patients who are taking diuretics. Administering glucose in the presence of hypokalemia worsens the effects of low potassium. However, the potential for worsening the patient's hypokalemia should not be a factor when dealing with a severely hypoglycemic patient.

Dextrose comes packaged in various concentrations. D_{50} is 25 g in 50 mL; D_{25} is 25 g in 100 mL; and D_{10} is 25 g in 250 mL. The total dose of dextrose in these formats is the same, though the concentration and volumes differ.

Doses of dextrose are as follows. D_{50} is usually supplied in a prefilled container called a bristojet containing 25 g of dextrose dissolved in 50 mL of water.

- **Adults:** 12.5 to 25 g (50 mL) of D_{50} (or follow local protocol)
- **Children 1 year and older:** 0.5 to 1 g/kg per dose of D_{25} or D_{10} via slow IV push. (Empty one-half of the bristojet of D_{50} and draw up normal saline to fill the tube; this will give a concentration of 25% if your service does not carry the prefilled syringes of D_{25}.)
- **Neonates and infants:** 200 to 500 mg/kg of D_{10} solution via slow IV push. (Put 2 mL of D_{50} into a syringe and add 8 mL of normal saline.)

Dextrose may cause serious damage to tissue from extravasation outside the vein. Therefore, you must give dextrose by IV push while carefully monitoring for infiltration into local tissue.

The steps for performing IV infusion are covered in Chapter 13, *Vascular Access and Medication Administration*.

The steps for administering dextrose to a patient with an altered level of consciousness are summarized here:

1. Insert an IV line with the largest catheter possible for the patient and in the largest possible vein.
2. Attach an IV bag of an isotonic crystalloid solution such as 0.9% normal saline. Check the IV line carefully to confirm that it is patent and flowing freely. Inject a test bolus of 10 to 20 mL of normal saline, making sure the IV line is not susceptible to infiltration. Recheck the status of the line by lowering the IV bag and looking for backflow of blood into the infusion set.
3. After you are certain the IV line is reliable, open the line wide, crimp the line superior to the administration port, and administer 12.5 to 25 g (25 to 50 mL) of dextrose slowly, over at least 3 minutes. Depress the plunger slowly to avoid rupturing the vein.

   When administering D_{50}, to ensure patency of the line, draw back on the syringe (eg, bristojet) to observe a blood return. Keep in mind that D_{50} can also be given IO or rectally.
4. Recheck after one-half of the dose has been given by pulling back on the plunger again to check for blood return. Flush the IV line by opening the line for a few seconds. If the cause of unresponsiveness is hypoglycemia, the patient will often quickly awaken—although in cases of severe hypoglycemia, another 25 g of D_{50} may be required to restore a normal level of consciousness.

Administering Glucagon

Administering glucagon IM is an option when IV access (for administering dextrose) cannot be obtained in a hypoglycemic patient. However, it is important to remember that glucagon is only effective when there are stores of glycogen to draw from. If glycogen stores are depleted, glucagon will be ineffective.

Glucagon is supplied in 1-mg ampules and requires reconstitution with the provided diluent **Figure 21-11**. The dosage for an adult is 1 mg IM and may be repeated in 7 to 10 minutes. The pediatric dosage is 0.5 mg or 20 to 30 mcg/kg IM for children who weigh less than 20 kg. For children weighing greater than 20 kg, the dose is the same as for adults.[24]

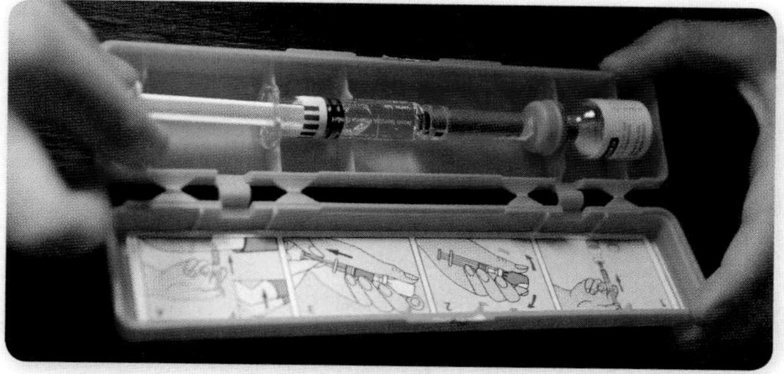

Figure 21-11 Glucagon is supplied in 1-mg ampules and requires reconstitution.

Glucagon should be used in conjunction with dextrose whenever possible. If the patient does not respond to the second dose of glucagon, dextrose must be administered. Review Chapter 13, *Vascular Access and Medication Administration*, for the steps to administer a medication via the IM route.

Management of Hyperglycemia and DKA

Patients with DKA will generally present with a markedly elevated glucose level and signs and symptoms consistent with severe hyperglycemia; if your field measurement of the patient's glucose level is more than 250 mg/dL, the physician will probably order treatment for DKA. The goals of prehospital treatment of DKA are to begin rehydration and to correct the patient's electrolyte and acid-base abnormalities. Specific treatment with insulin will occur on the patient's arrival at the hospital, where therapy can be closely monitored with laboratory determinations of blood glucose levels, ketones, and other values.

Maintain the patient's airway and administer oxygen. Be particularly alert for vomiting, and have suction ready. Consider paramedic backup for definitive airway control if needed. Gain IV access and administer a 20-mL/kg bolus of an isotonic crystalloid solution for signs of dehydration or if the patient is hypotensive. Reassess and provide additional boluses as needed.

Hyperglycemic patients who have not reached the stage of DKA may not need large quantities of fluid. Treat the patient symptomatically, providing oxygen and IV fluid as needed.

Management of HHS/HONK

The treatment of HHS/HONK in the prehospital setting follows the pathway for dehydration and altered mental status. Airway management is the top priority because the unresponsive patient often is unable to maintain and protect his or her airway. For this reason, advanced airway management may be indicated and should be completed as early as possible. Cervical spine immobilization should be considered for all unresponsive patients with a possible mechanism of high-energy injury. Obtain a blood glucose level as soon as possible. Large-bore IV access (18 gauge) should be gained as soon as possible

After you have initiated the IV line, a bolus of 500 mL of 0.9% normal saline is appropriate for almost all adults who are clinically dehydrated. In patients with a history of heart failure and/or renal insufficiency, give fluid sparingly (250 mL may be a more appropriate starting point) while monitoring breath sounds for developing pulmonary edema. Fluid deficits in patients with HHS/HONK may amount to 10 L or more. These patients may receive 1 to 2 L within the first hour. You may also need to treat for hypoglycemia if glucose levels are low and the patient is symptomatic.

Hematologic Emergencies

Hematology is, by definition, simply the study of blood; however, the specialty addresses not only the blood, but also the ways in which its constituent parts are involved in health and disease. These components include **red blood cells (RBCs)**, **white blood cells (WBCs)**, platelets, and individual proteins involved in the bleeding and clotting cascades, as well as the **hematopoietic system**—that is, organs and tissues involved in the production of blood components (primarily bone marrow, spleen, and lymph nodes). Most EMS systems rarely respond to hematologic emergencies.

The blanket term **hematologic disorder** refers to any disorder of the blood. Within this general category, **hemolytic disorders** refer to disease processes that cause the breakdown of RBCs, and **hemostatic disorders** refer to bleeding and clotting abnormalities. These disorders can be complex, difficult to assess, and challenging to treat in the prehospital setting.

As an AEMT, you should have a basic understanding of the hematopoietic system and hematologic disorders, and know how to respond to these kinds of emergencies appropriately. Although you may be able to provide only limited interventions in the field for patients with hematologic disorders, your actions may not just offer support, but actually save the patient's life.

Anatomy and Physiology Review: Hematology

Blood and Plasma

Without blood, we would not be able to live. Blood performs the following functions:

- **Respiratory function.** Transports oxygen from the lungs to the tissues and carbon dioxide from the tissues to the lungs
- **Nutritional function.** Carries nutrients (glucose, proteins, and fats) from the digestive tract to cells throughout the body
- **Excretory function.** Ferries the waste products of metabolism from the cells where they are produced to the excretory organs
- **Regulatory function.** Transports hormones to their target organs and transmits excess internal heat to the surface of the body to be dissipated
- **Defensive function.** Carries defensive cells and antibodies, which protect the body against foreign organisms

Blood is made up of two main components: plasma and formed elements (cells). **Plasma**, a straw-colored

YOU are the Provider PART 4

You inform the patient that you believe that his insulin pump is not functioning correctly and that he should be evaluated in the emergency department. The patient again states that he does not wish to be transported, but you are able to persuade him to speak with your medical control physician. You proceed to contact online medical control and explain the situation to the physician, who readily agrees with you that the patient should be evaluated and asks to speak with the patient. After approximately 2 minutes, the patient agrees to transport, and you thank the medical control physician for his assistance. You assist the patient onto the stretcher and begin transport to the hospital. En route, you continue administering high-flow oxygen, ensure that the IV line is still patent, and recheck the patient's blood glucose level, which is found to be 189 mg/dL. On arrival at the emergency department, you turn over care to the awaiting nurse; the patient thanks you for your prompt treatment.

Recording Time: 16 Minutes	
Respirations	20 breaths/min
Pulse	Strong and regular, at 68 beats/min
Skin	Warm, dry, and pink
Blood pressure	154/78 mm Hg
Oxygen saturation (Spo_2)	100% at 15 L/min via nonrebreathing mask
Pupils	PERRLA

8. Why is it important to reassess the patient's blood glucose level during transport?

fluid, is essentially 92% water and 6% to 7% proteins; the remainder consists of a variety of other elements (including electrolytes, clotting factors, and glucose). Plasma accounts for 55% of the total blood volume. All of the formed element components—RBCs, WBCs, and platelets—are transported through the body in plasma.

Most of the formed elements (99%) are RBCs (erythrocytes). Within the RBCs, iron-rich hemoglobin is responsible for carrying oxygen to the tissues. RBC production occurs within **stem cells** (cells that develop into other types of cells in the body); the production of RBCs is stimulated by a protein secreted by the kidneys in response to circulatory need. RBCs may take as long as 5 days to mature and have an average life of approximately 4 months. Oxygen attached to hemoglobin gives blood its characteristic red color, although many other factors can change the color of blood (such as carbon monoxide poisoning).

WBCs (leukocytes) are larger than RBCs and are also found in the bloodstream. They provide the body with immunity against "foreign invaders," fighting infection and removing dead cells. WBCs are derived from stem cells. Several types of WBCs exist, each of which performs a specific task in relation to maintaining the immune system.

Platelets (thrombocytes) are the smallest of the formed elements and are responsible for clot formation.

Words of Wisdom

Platelets form the initial plug following vascular injury. Clotting proteins then toughen and complete the blood clot.

Approximately two-thirds of the body's platelets circulate throughout the blood; the rest are stored in the spleen. Platelets are also derived from stem cells. They have an average life span of approximately 7 to 10 days. When damage occurs to a blood vessel, platelets are sent to the site of injury to help create a blood clot to stop the bleeding.

Platelets form the initial plug following vascular injury; the clotting proteins then toughen and complete the blood clot. Without platelets, our bodies would not be able to stop bleeding. However, there can be too much of a good thing with platelets: conditions such as **thrombocytosis**, in which the body produces too many platelets, can result in other dangerous medical conditions, such as **thrombosis**, which is coagulation or clotting of blood inside of a blood vessel.

Hemostasis is a highly complex process that allows the body to stop bleeding through vascular spasm, coagulation, and platelet plugging. The opposite of hemostasis is hemorrhage. Clots themselves are made up of fibrin. When injury is detected, thrombin converts fibrinogen to fibrin, and the clotting process begins. Calcium acts as a binding agent, holding fibrin fibers close together to form the meshwork of the clot.

Any process that interferes with the activation or continuation of the clotting cascade or hemostasis is known as a **coagulopathy**. Coagulopathies can result in heavy or prolonged bleeding. One such bleeding disorder is von Willebrand disease, in which the blood's ability to clot is decreased because of the absence of a key protein, von Willebrand factor, that is necessary for platelet adhesion.

Words of Wisdom

In a normal adult, the WBC count initially increases in response to infection. As the infection continues, the WBC count may decrease as the WBCs are exhausted faster than they can regenerate. Thus, a low WBC count does not necessarily indicate absence of infection.

▶ Blood-Forming Organs and Red Blood Cell Production

Although many parts and organs of the human body can alter or affect the hematologic system, the major players are the bone marrow, liver, and spleen **Figure 21-12**.

The bone marrow is the primary site for cell production within the human body. Bone marrow may be found in most of the long bones plus the pelvis, skull, and vertebrae.

The liver produces the **clotting factors** found in the blood. It filters the blood to remove toxins and is essential to normal metabolism and homeostasis. As old RBCs enter the liver, they are broken down into bilirubin, a protein that is excreted by the liver within the bile. The liver is a highly vascular organ that also stores some blood within itself.

The spleen is also quite vascular. It is involved with the filtering and breakdown of RBCs, assists with the

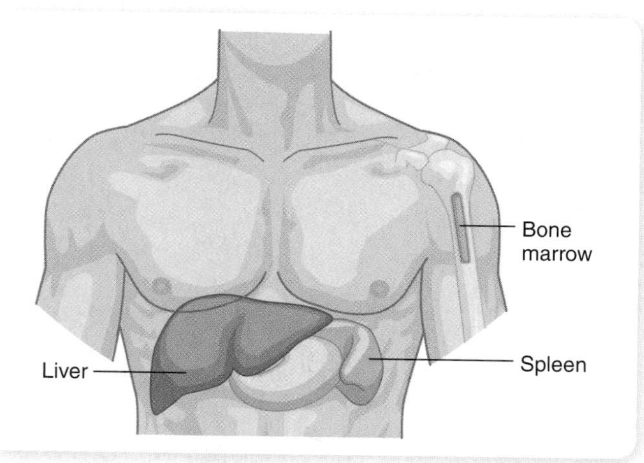

Figure 21-12 The bone marrow, liver, and spleen are the main components of the body related to the blood system.

production of WBCs, and has an important role in providing homeostasis and infection control. The spleen stores approximately one-third of the body's platelets. If the spleen is removed, then the platelets formed after that time remain in the blood throughout their life span.

Blood Classifications

To ensure compatibility and prevent medical problems during blood component replacement, blood type classifications have been developed. As discussed in Chapter 7, *The Human Body*, the **ABO system** uses the RBC classification types O, A, B, and AB to indicate which antigens are found in the plasma membrane Table 21-4.

Blood contains a secondary antigen, known as the Rh antigen (the name signifies that the antigen was first found in the Rhesus monkey). In the United States, approximately 85% of all Americans have this antigen.[25] In blood types that are positive (for example, A+), the blood contains the Rh antigen.

Transfusion Reactions

Some patients may be receiving or may have previously received a blood transfusion. It is important to determine a patient's blood type and the type of blood received. When a patient receives blood or plasma that matches his or her classification (A+ into A+) or the universal donor blood type (O), problems rarely arise. However, if a patient receives a blood type that is different than his or her own—for example, a patient with type A receives type B—a transfusion reaction will occur. Also, if a patient with A− blood receives an A+ transfusion, a transfusion reaction could occur, but this is rare. Blood reactions are similar to an anaphylactic reaction—they occur rapidly and can cause severe circulatory collapse and even death. High-flow oxygen should be administered. When a patient receives a blood transfusion, it is important to monitor the patient very closely for the first 30 to 60 minutes because transfusion reactions typically begin within this time frame.

Table 21-4 Blood Types

Blood Type	ABO Antigens	ABO Antibodies	Acceptable Blood Donor Types
A	A	Anti-B	A, O
B	B	Anti-A	B, O
AB	A, B	None	A, B, AB, O
O	None	Anti-A Anti-B	O

Pathophysiology of Hematologic Emergencies

Sickle Cell Disease

Sickle cell disease is—by far—the most common inherited blood disorder. Although it primarily affects African American, Puerto Rican, and European populations, it can occur in anyone. As of 2016, approximately 100,000 people in the United States had sickle cell disease.[26] Mortality at younger ages is common; the average life expectancy is 42 years for men with sickle cell anemia and 48 years for women with this disorder.[27]

Sickle cell disease starts with a genetic defect of the adult-type hemoglobin (HbA). When the RBCs are first developing their membranes, they may become rigid and deformed. The defective RBCs have an oblong shape instead of a smooth, round shape Figure 21-13. This shape makes the RBC a poor oxygen carrier, which means a patient with this disease is highly susceptible to hypoxia. Since sickle cells also have a much shorter life span than normal erythrocytes, the patient is also more susceptible to develop anemia.

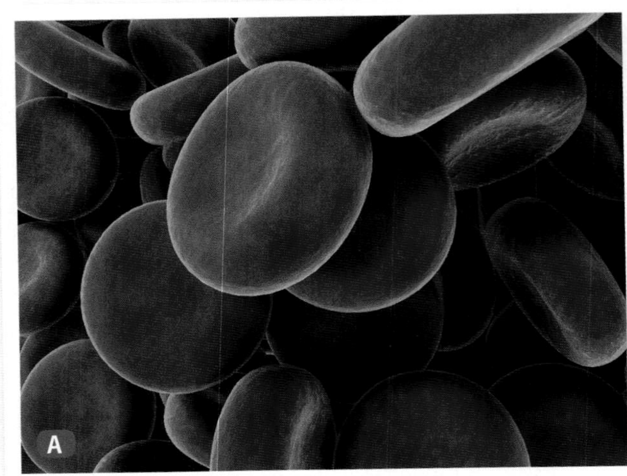

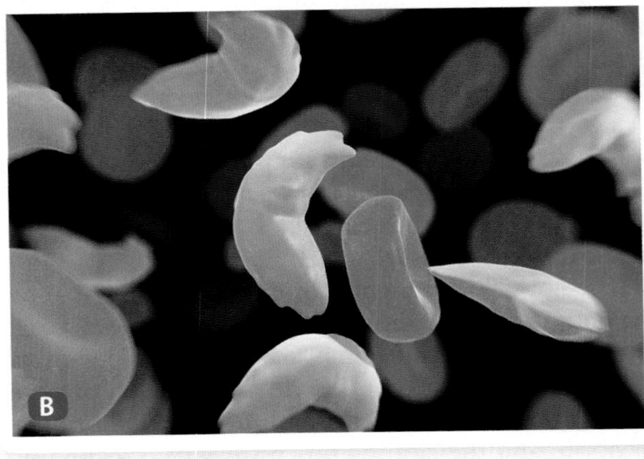

Figure 21-13 A. Normal red blood cells. **B.** Sickle cells.

The odd shape may also cause RBCs to lodge in small blood vessels, resulting in thrombosis. Defective RBCs may migrate to the spleen, causing the organ to swell and rupture, which can result in death.

Sickle cell disease may result in an aplastic crisis, a hemolytic crisis, or thrombosis. In an aplastic crisis, the body temporarily stops RBC production, causing the patient to become easily tired, anemic, pale, and short of breath. In contrast, a hemolytic crisis arises when acute RBC destruction results in jaundice. In both cases, the patient may have rapidly evolving anemia, **leukocytosis**, and fever. The odd shape of the RBCs may also cause these cells to become lodged in small blood vessels, resulting in thrombosis. A sickle cell crisis may manifest in several ways:

- A **vaso-occlusive crisis** results from blood flow to an organ becoming restricted, causing pain, ischemia, and often organ damage. Most vaso-occlusive crises last between 5 and 7 days. Frequently, circulation to the spleen becomes obstructed as a result of its narrow vessels and function of removing damaged RBCs.
- **Acute chest syndrome** is a vaso-occlusive crisis that can be associated with pneumonia. Common signs and symptoms include chest pain, fever, and cough. Vaso-occlusion in the brain may result in a CVA (stroke).
- An **aplastic crisis** is a worsening of the patient's baseline anemia (lack of circulating RBCs in the body), which causes tachycardia, pallor, and fatigue. This may be caused by the parvovirus B19, which affects the production of RBCs, almost stopping new production for 2 to 3 days.
- A **hemolytic crisis** is an acute accelerated drop in the patient's hemoglobin level. Caused by RBCs breaking down at a faster than normal rate, this type of crisis is common in patients with glucose-6-phosphate dehydrogenase deficiency (a common enzyme deficiency).
- A **splenic sequestration crisis** is caused by painful, acute enlargement of the spleen, causing the abdomen to become hard and bloated.

In acute crises, patients may have substantial pain resulting from congested vessels that do not allow for the passage of oxygen and nutrients into tissues and joints. They may experience frequent infections, which can result in sepsis and death. Over time, various organs may be destroyed as circulation is impeded. Patients may often have signs of mild dehydration, splenomegaly, cardiomegaly, and many other complaints.

Special Populations

Acute splenic sequestration syndrome is a life-threatening complication in which RBCs become trapped in the spleen, causing a dramatic decline in the amount of hemoglobin available in the circulation. Patients present not only with a painful, acute abdomen, but also with sudden weakness, pallor, tachypnea, and tachycardia. Acute splenic sequestration syndrome usually occurs in infants or toddlers.

Words of Wisdom

Patients may report multisystem involvement, including chest, abdominal, and arthritic-type pain, although some may report only fatigue or achiness along with fever. Pediatric patients will typically present with initial pain in the hands and feet, whereas adult patients will report back and proximal extremity pain.

Patients with chronic sickle cell attacks are susceptible to severe, life-threatening complications of which you must be aware. Although some of these complications take days to weeks to develop, some complications are acute and life threatening. Some of the potential complications of sickle cell disease are as follows:

- Cerebrovascular attack
- Gallstones
- Jaundice
- Osteonecrosis
- Splenic infections
- Osteomyelitis
- Opiate tolerance
- Leg ulcers
- Retinopathy
- Chronic pain
- Pulmonary hypertension
- Chronic renal failure

Anemia

Anemia is defined as a hemoglobin or RBC level that is lower than normal. Usually, this condition is associated with some type of underlying disease process. Anemia may also result from acute or chronic blood loss, or from a decrease in production or an increase in destruction of erythrocytes. Anemia may be an outcome of a preexisting hemolytic disorder (a disorder related to the breakdown of RBCs).

Iron-deficiency anemia is the most common type of anemia. Other typical causes include gastrointestinal blood loss, menstrual bleeding, and blood loss as a result of frequent donations or diagnostic tests for patients hospitalized for long periods. In children, it is most often related to premature birth or low birth weight.

Anemia may sometimes be caused by an inherited hemolytic disorder, such as sickle cell disease or thalassemia. In these disorders, when the RBCs are first developing their membranes, they become rigid and deformed. The RBCs may then become lodged in small blood vessels, resulting in a thrombosis (blood clot).

Anemia may also be caused by hematologic disorders resulting from a deficiency of an enzyme known as glucose-6-phosphate dehydrogenase. This enzyme helps protect RBCs during infections. When levels of this enzyme are low, cells can become damaged. Although glucose-6-phosphate dehydrogenase deficiency is most commonly seen in African Americans, it can occur in people of any race.

The most common type of acquired anemia develops when the flow of RBCs is disrupted owing to problems with blood vessel linings (such as aneurysms and weaknesses) or blood clots. In autoimmune disorders, RBCs are destroyed by the body's own antibodies, which erroneously perceive the normal blood cells as foreign invaders. RBCs can also be destroyed by microorganisms in the blood.

Anemia can also have serious consequences for people who travel to high-altitude areas. The combination of a smaller number of RBCs and the reduced partial pressure of oxygen in the atmosphere can result in serious conditions that a healthy person would not experience, such as hypoxia, difficulty breathing, and chest pain.

Your basic assessment should be the same for all patients, although you may want to ask some specific questions when anemia is suspected. Most commonly, patients with anemia will report feeling worn down, having no energy, or feeling as if they have overexerted themselves. Patients may also report that they "can't catch their breath." Owing to the reduction in their hemoglobin level, some may have angina-type chest pain related to decreased oxygen availability to the heart muscle. The reduction in functional RBCs can also result in pale skin. Subtle variations may be seen by assessing the conjunctiva of the eyes, the inside of the lips, and the creases of the palms of the hand. These areas can be instrumental in identifying pallor, especially in patients with darker skin. Other conditions that are common in patients with anemia include **leukopenia** (reduction in WBCs) and **thrombocytopenia** (reduction in platelets); both conditions can induce more frequent infections, fevers, cutaneous bleeding, and nosebleeds.

Words of Wisdom

When abnormalities of the blood cells are suspected, note the following:

- Anemia commonly results in complaints of fatigue, lethargy, and dyspnea.
- Low WBC counts (leukopenia) often result in infection and fever.
- Low platelet counts (thrombocytopenia) often cause cutaneous bleeding (including petechiae) and bleeding from mucous membranes (such as nosebleeds and rectal bleeding).

▶ Clotting Disorders

A clotting disorder is a condition in which there is an abnormality in the blood's clotting ability. The development of a blood clot is called thrombosis and can occur in either arterial or venous blood vessels. The patient's symptoms are related to the part of the vascular system in which the clot occurs, the size of the clot, and whether the clot becomes dislodged and travels to another part of the body.

Thrombophilia

Thrombophilia, or the tendency to develop blood clots, affects a large number of people around the world.

Thrombosis is a common medical problem and may manifest itself as the formation of a blood clot in a blood vessel or in one of the chambers of the heart. Pulmonary emboli secondary to deep vein thromboses are a leading cause of death in hospitalized patients.

Many patients with thrombophilia receive anticoagulant medications that thin the blood, which helps decrease the tendency to form a clot. Examples of these medications include aspirin, heparin, and warfarin (Coumadin). Typically, pediatric patients do not experience blood clots.

The following are some risk factors for increased clotting:

- Recent surgery
- Impaired mobility
- Congestive heart failure
- Cancer
- Respiratory failure
- Infectious diseases
- Age older than 40 years
- Being overweight/obesity
- Smoking
- Oral contraceptive use

Hemophilia

Hemophilia is a genetic bleeding disorder in which clotting does not occur or occurs insufficiently (von Willebrand disease). In people with hemophilia, the body is not able to control bleeding by developing spontaneous clots as normal, resulting in an increased bleeding time. This condition occurs predominately in males and the most common—hemophilia A—occurs in approximately 1 in every 5,000 births.[28] The disease is classified into two primary types:

- **Hemophilia A.** The most common type, hemophilia A is a result of low levels of factor VIII.
- **Hemophilia B.** This second most common type is associated with a deficiency of factor IX.

The levels of factors VIII and IX determine the severity of the disease.

Both type A and type B have the same signs and symptoms. Acute and chronic bleeding can occur at any time and may or may not be life threatening. Any injury or illness that can cause bleeding should not be taken lightly in a person with hemophilia. Spontaneous intracranial bleeding is common in hemophilia and is a frequent cause of death in these patients. Patients with substantial acute bleeding episodes require hospitalization for transfusion and often require infusion of factors VIII or IX.

When you are obtaining the patient's history, you may learn that the patient has a history of conditions associated with hemophilia. In addition to managing the ABCs, be alert for signs of acute blood loss (pallor, weak pulse, and hypotension). Note any bleeding of unknown origin, such as nosebleeds, bloody sputum, and blood in the urine or stool (melena). Patients may exhibit signs of hypoxia owing to the reduction in oxygen-carrying capacity as a result of blood loss.

▶ Disseminated Intravascular Coagulation

Disseminated intravascular coagulation (DIC) may result from any number of life-threatening conditions, including massive injury and hypotension resulting from trauma. Sepsis and obstetric complications also may cause DIC.

This condition progresses in two stages. First, free thrombin and fibrin deposits in the blood increase, and platelets begin to aggregate. In this stage, defibrination, or a breakdown of the fibrin clots, occurs owing to excessive bleeding, massive blood loss, or tissue injury. Second, uncontrolled hemorrhage results from the severe reduction in clotting factors.

The mortality rate for patients with DIC is quite high, especially in acute cases; some studies have shown it to be 60% to 65%.[29] The primary causes of death relate to uncontrolled bleeding, hypotension, and shock.

Words of Wisdom

Patients with DIC experience simultaneous multiple organ failure (such as kidneys, lungs, and heart), accompanied by bleeding from IV sites, bleeding into joints, and, possibly, intracranial hemorrhage.

As you assess and care for critically injured or ill patients, keep in mind the issues that may result in DIC. Your goal is to identify signs and symptoms commonly associated with DIC or progression toward this coagulopathy. In cases involving severe trauma, patients may have episodes of respiratory difficulty, signs of shock, and skin changes ranging from cold and clammy to pallor to small black-and-blue marks (purpura) on the chest and abdomen.

Patient Assessment of Hematologic Emergencies

Assessment of a patient suspected of having a hematologic disorder should be no different from assessment of any other patient, albeit with a few additional items to consider and questions to ask. Also, be supportive of the patients and their families—some patients with a blood disorder may not be willing to disclose the condition because they may feel that they will be treated differently.

Scene Size-up

Although your report from dispatch may be for a patient with an unknown medical problem, most patients presenting with a sickle cell crisis have experienced a crisis before and will relay that information to the dispatcher. As always, ensure the scene is safe for entry, consider the mechanism of injury and/or nature of illness, determine the number of patients, and assess for hazards and the need for additional help. Standard precautions should consist of gloves and eye protection at a minimum. Remember to evaluate each situation quickly and make sure the necessary personal protective equipment is readily available.

Patients experiencing a vaso-occlusive crisis are often in extreme pain and would benefit from administration of analgesics. Call for paramedic backup early.

Primary Survey

An African American patient or any patient of Mediterranean descent who reports severe pain may have undiagnosed sickle cell disease.

Remember that even though a person has a history of sickle cell disease, sickle cell disease may not be causing the current problem; trauma or another type of medical emergency may be the cause. For this reason, you must always perform a thorough, careful primary survey, paying attention to the ABCs and immediately correcting any life-threatening issues.

Perform a rapid full-body scan of the patient to form an initial general impression of the patient. How does the patient look? Does the patient appear anxious, restless, or listless? Is the patient apathetic or irritable? Determine the patient's level of consciousness.

As you are forming your general impression, assess the patient's airway and breathing. Patients showing signs of inadequate breathing, an altered mental status, or Spo_2 of 94% or less should receive high-flow oxygen at 12 to 15 L/min via nonrebreathing mask or ventilation via bag-mask as needed. Should you need to provide additional airway support with suctioning and/or basic or advanced airways, be aware that even minor trauma during these procedures can result in bleeding into the airway and increase the risk of airway compromise. A patient who is experiencing a sickle cell crisis may have increased respirations as a result of severe pain or exhibit signs of pneumonia. Continue to monitor the airway as you provide care.

After you have assessed the airway and breathing and have performed the necessary interventions, check the patient's circulatory status. An increased heart rate represents a compensatory mechanism, in an attempt to "force" the sickled cells through smaller vasculature. Look for signs of shock, such as a rapid pulse rate and low blood pressure. If you find any life-threatening conditions, take immediate steps to manage them and provide urgent transport to an appropriately equipped receiving facility.

In patients with suspected hemophilia, be alert for signs of acute blood loss such as pallor, weak pulse, and hypotension. Note any bleeding of unknown origin, such as nosebleeds, bloody sputum, and blood in the urine or stool. Patients with hemophilia may exhibit signs of hypoxia or shock because of blood loss. Fluid resuscitation may be necessary for these patients; however, it must be administered with care so as not to "wash out" the clots that are forming.

Whether you decide to rapidly transport the patient will depend on the severity of the patient's condition and the patient's wishes. Patients with a history of sickle cell disease, but who have not had a crisis in some time, may require emotional support and refuse transport. However, transport to an emergency department should always be recommended to any patient who is experiencing a sickle cell crisis or has a history of hemophilia and is bleeding.

History Taking

It is extremely important to understand the chief complaint; to do so, you may need to be inquisitive about the patient's history and SAMPLE history. When you are obtaining the patient's history, you may discover previous or current sickle cell disease or hemophilia conditions.

Responsive medical patients are usually able to provide their own medical history to help you identify a cause for their severe pain. Do not take a call for a person having a sickle cell crisis lightly. Patients are often in life-threatening situations, characterized by shortness of breath and signs of pneumonia. Their skin will show signs of inadequate perfusion, accompanied by hypotension. Physical signs, such as swelling of the fingers and toes, priapism, and jaundice may also guide you in determining whether the patient is experiencing a sickle cell crisis.

If the patient reports pain, ascertain whether the pain is isolated to a single location or whether it is felt throughout the entire body. Has the patient experienced muscle pain or stiffness for unknown reasons? Be alert for signs of acute blood loss (pallor, weak pulse, and hypotension). Look for changes in level of consciousness and symptoms such as vertigo, feelings of fatigue, or syncopal episodes. Ask if the patient has had skin changes such as color changes, burning, or itching. Is the patient having any visual disturbances? Note any bleeding of unknown origin, such as nosebleeds, bloody sputum, and blood in the urine or stool. Is the patient experiencing any gastrointestinal problems, such as nausea, vomiting, or abdominal cramping? Is the patient reporting any chest pain or shortness of breath?

Words of Wisdom

Many anti-inflammatory drugs (aspirin, ibuprofen) and some herbals (ginkgo, garlic, ginger, ginseng, feverfew) decrease platelet aggregation. Although this effect may be beneficial (such as in myocardial infarction or stroke prevention), these drugs may also increase the tendency to bleed. Always ask patients about medications, including over-the-counter and herbal medications.

In a patient with known sickle cell disease, ask the following questions in addition to obtaining a SAMPLE history:

- Have you had a crisis before?
- When was the last time you had a crisis?
- How did your last crisis resolve?
- Have you had any illness, unusual amount of activity, or stress lately?

Secondary Assessment

The secondary assessment may be performed on scene, en route to the emergency department, or not at all. This will depend on transport time and the patient's condition.

Systematically examine the patient, focusing on major joints at which cells congregate, and obtain your patient's baseline vital signs. Evaluate and document mental status using the AVPU scale. Table 21-5 shows common findings in patients with blood disorders.

Obtain a complete set of vital signs, including a measurement of the patient's oxygen saturation level. In patients experiencing a sickle cell crisis, respirations are normal to rapid, pulse is weak and rapid, and skin is typically pale and clammy with a low blood pressure.

Use pulse oximetry, if available. However, keep in mind that the oxygen saturation reading you obtain may be inaccurate as a result of the patient's anemic state.

Reassessment

It is important to reassess the patient frequently to determine if there have been changes in his or her condition. For example, are there changes in the patient's mental status? Are the ABCs still intact? How is the patient responding to the interventions performed? Should you adjust or change the interventions? In many patients, you will note marked improvement with appropriate treatment. Document each assessment, your findings, the time of the interventions, and any changes in the patient's condition.

Communication with hospital staff is important for continuity of care. Hospital personnel need to be informed about the patient's history, the present situation, your

Table 21-5 Common Findings With Blood Disorders

System	Examples of Common Findings
Level of consciousness	Alterations in level of consciousness, ranging from excitability, agitation, and combativeness, to complete unresponsiveness
Skin	Uncontrolled bleeding, unexplained or chronic bruising, itching, pallor or jaundice (yellow appearance usually indicates liver problems)
Visual disturbances	Visual disturbances, including blurred vision, decreased vision, tunnel vision, and seeing black or gray spots
Gastrointestinal	Epistaxis (bloody nose), bleeding or infected gums, ulcers, melena (blood in the stool), and liver failure (causes jaundice)
Skeletal	Chronic joint or bone pain or rigidity
Cardiovascular	Dyspnea, tachycardia, chest pain, hemoptysis (coughing up blood)
Genitourinary	Hematuria, menorrhagia, chronic or recurring infections

assessment findings, and your interventions and their results.

Your run report is the only legal document that shows appropriate care was provided. Document your assessment findings clearly as the basis for your treatment. Follow your local protocols for patients who refuse treatment or transport.

Emergency Medical Care of Hematologic Emergencies

Emergency medical care for any patient with problems related to a blood disorder should include the following:

- **Oxygen.** The amount needed and how it is given (that is, bag-mask ventilation, nonrebreathing mask) depend on the severity of the patient's condition and respiratory status. High levels of oxygen are recommended for patients with sickle cell disease to maximize oxygen delivery to the tissues and mitigate the crisis.
- **Fluids.** Initiate IV fluid replacement as indicated for the specific disorder or chief complaint. You may need to give IV fluid therapy to counter the patient's dehydration.
- **Transport.** Provide rapid transport to the closest, most appropriate facility.
- **Pharmacology.** Pain management is often necessary, especially in the case of a sickle cell crisis. Follow local protocols.
- **Comfort and rest.** Place the patient in a position of comfort, and cover the patient to maintain his or her body temperature.
- **Psychological support.** Be supportive and communicate with the patient.

Remember that patients may have lived with the disease for a long time and, thus, may have a high pain threshold. As a consequence, they often require a higher level of analgesia. Nitrous oxide may provide a measure of relief. Follow local protocols for pain management.

Management of Specific Conditions

Distinguishing a true sickle cell crisis from other nonspecific causes of pain can be difficult. In these situations, perform a thorough assessment and contact the hospital to help sort out the signs and symptoms. Medical control should be a resource for you to help problem-solve situations and provide guidance on how to treat your patient. After the patient has arrived at the hospital, care for sickle cell disease might include analgesics for pain, antibiotics to prevent infection, and, depending on the severity of the crisis, a blood transfusion.

In cases of anemia, check and monitor the airway and the patient's breathing closely, administering high-flow oxygen when necessary. The patient's oxygen-carrying capacity is limited, so you want to make sure that the RBCs that are present are being maximized. Check vital signs frequently. Monitor patients closely during fluid replacement—IV fluids do not contain RBCs or blood components, so they may induce unwanted or unexpected bleeding. Do not be surprised if you have to control substantial nosebleeds in any patient with anemia. For patients reporting chest pain, call early for paramedic backup.

Although patients with hemophilia may require IV therapy in cases of unstable hypotension, understand that the patient actually needs a transfusion or plasma. The patient may also exhibit worsening signs of hypoxia as IV fluid dilutes the blood, further diminishing oxygen levels. Some patients will have substantial pain, so analgesics may be appropriate. Cover patients to maintain body temperature. Although you may be called to treat someone with bleeding of unknown cause only to find that the bleeding stopped before you arrive on scene, you should suggest that the patient receive immediate transport to the hospital or physician follow-up.

It is important to identify DIC and establish treatment early, while not delaying transport to an appropriate facility. Maintain the patient's airway, administer supplemental oxygen, and treat the patient for shock (keep the patient warm, control bleeding, administer IV fluids for hypotension) per local protocol. Patients who have DIC have a poor survival rate; both patients and their family members need strong support. Be optimistic but honest with patients and family, and do not give false hope regarding survival.

YOU are the Provider SUMMARY

1. **What are the two types of diabetes, and how do they differ?**

   There are two common types of diabetes: type 1 and type 2. Typically, type 1 diabetes develops during childhood. However, type 1 diabetes can, in many cases, develop later in life as well. In type 1 diabetes, no insulin is produced and the patient requires daily injections of supplemental, synthetic insulin to control blood glucose levels.

   The most common form of diabetes is type 2 diabetes. In type 2 diabetes, patients produce insufficient amounts of insulin or insulin that does not function effectively. Type 2 diabetes typically develops when the patient is a middle-age adult, although the disease is becoming more common in younger people. In many people with type 2 diabetes, the pancreas actually produces enough insulin; however, the body cannot effectively utilize it.

2. **What is the function of an insulin pump?**

   An insulin pump is a small device that consists of an infusion set, a reservoir for insulin, and the pump itself. Such pumps provide improved control of blood glucose levels for many diabetic patients.

3. **Should you instruct the patient's wife to turn off the insulin pump?**

   Yes, instruct the patient's wife to turn off the insulin pump, at least until you are able to obtain the patient's blood glucose level. If the patient is hypoglycemic and the pump is allowed to remain on, if it is functioning inappropriately, it may decrease the patient's blood glucose level. If the patient is found to be hyperglycemic then, depending on local protocols, the pump may be turned back on and the patient may be treated for hyperglycemia per protocols.

4. **By which route or routes may D_{50} be administered?**

   D_{50} may be administered via the IV or the IO route. Some local protocols may also allow it to be administered rectally, but this is usually a last resort.

5. **What are the indications and contraindications for dextrose?**

   Dextrose should be administered to patients with symptomatic hypoglycemia, altered level of consciousness for unknown reasons, and unresponsiveness with no obtainable patient history, among other reasons. Contraindications for dextrose administration include the presence of increased intracranial pressure or possible intracranial bleeding. Unless the patient is severely hypoglycemic, dextrose should be used with caution in patients suspected of having hypokalemia (low potassium levels), such as patients who are taking diuretics.

6. **What is the usual adult dosage of dextrose?**

   The usual adult dosage of dextrose is 12.5 to 25 g, in 50 to 250 mL of fluid depending on local protocols. It is therefore important to consult local protocols prior to the administration of any medication.

7. **Does this patient require transport to the emergency department?**

   Yes, this patient requires transport to the emergency department for evaluation. The patient's blood glucose level should not have been low because he has an insulin pump. On the basis of this finding, it is likely that the patient's insulin pump is malfunctioning. If the patient is allowed to refuse transport, he may experience another hypoglycemic episode.

8. **Why is it important to reassess the patient's blood glucose level during transport?**

   It is important to recheck the patient's blood glucose level because of the half-life of dextrose. In the case of a patient with a faulty insulin pump, the insulin may have a longer half-life than that of dextrose, causing rebound hypoglycemia.

YOU are the Provider SUMMARY *(continued)*

EMS Patient Care Report (PCR)					
Date: 03-17-18	**Incident No.:** 201040051	**Nature of Call:** Unresponsive		**Location:** 178 Stutzman Street	
Dispatched: 1130	**En Route:** 1130	**At Scene:** 1133	**Transport:** 1208	**At Hospital:** 1216	**In Service:** 1226

Patient Information

Age: 41 **Sex:** M **Weight (in kg [lb]):** 96 kg (212 lb)	**Allergies:** None **Medications:** Insulin **Past Medical History:** Type 1 DM **Chief Complaint:** Unresponsive

Vital Signs

Time: 1134	**BP:** Not obtained	**Pulse:** Not obtained	**Respirations:** 12	**Spo_2:** Not obtained
Time: 1141	**BP:** 154/88	**Pulse:** 77	**Respirations:** 18	**Spo_2:** 100% on 15 L/min
Time: 1149	**BP:** 154/78	**Pulse:** 68	**Respirations:** 20	**Spo_2:** 100% on 15 L/min

EMS Treatment (circle all that apply)

Oxygen @ 15 **L/min via (circle one):** **NC** (**NRM** circled) **Bag-mask device**	**Assisted Ventilation**	**Airway Adjunct**	**CPR**
Defibrillation	**Bleeding Control**	**Bandaging**	**Splinting**
(circled) **Other:** 25 g D_{50}			

Narrative

EMS dispatched to above location for unresponsive man. On arrival, greeted by patient's wife, who states patient has past medical history of type 1 diabetes and while she was making lunch he became confused and then unresponsive. Patient presents responsive to deep painful stimuli, airway patent. Wife asks if she should turn off patient's insulin pump, advised "yes." Initial blood glucose level reads "Lo" (less than 25 mg/dL). Nonrebreathing mask applied at 15 L/min, 18-gauge IV line established to right arm, infusing well with no signs of infiltration. 25 g of D_{50} administered over 4 minutes, followed by 250-mL bolus of normal saline. Approximately 5 minutes after administration, the patient is AO×4, ABCs intact, refusing all further treatment. Advised the patient of the need to be evaluated at the emergency department because of the possibility of a malfunctioning insulin pump. Patient remains adamant about refusal of services. Contacted Dr. Anderson at Park County Memorial Hospital (PCMH) who spoke to patient. Patient reluctantly agreed to transport. Assisted to ambulance, secured × 3, transport nonemergent to PCMH. En route: vitals, O_2, and IV line as above. Repeat blood glucose level reading of 189 mg/dL. On arrival at PCMH, care and report given to ED staff without incident.**End of report**

Prep Kit

▶ Ready for Review

- The endocrine system comprises a network of glands that produce and secrete hormones—chemical substances produced by a gland that have special regulatory effects on other organs and tissues.
- The major components of the endocrine system are the hypothalamus, pineal gland, pituitary, thyroid gland, thymus gland, parathyroid gland, adrenal glands, and reproductive organs (gonads). The pancreas is also part of this system; it has a role in hormone production as well as in digestion.
- The main function of the endocrine system is to maintain homeostasis. Maintaining homeostasis requires a response to any change in the body, such as low glucose levels in the blood.
- Thyroid disorders include hyperthyroidism and hypothyroidism. Learn the effects of these on the body so you can distinguish these disorders. Ensure you know how to recognize thyroid storm because it can be life threatening.
- Diabetes is a metabolic disorder in which the body does not sufficiently metabolize glucose. Diabetes can be caused by a lack of insulin, or the body's inability to respond to insulin. Insulin is a hormone that enables glucose to enter the cells, where it can be used for energy. Diabetes is typically characterized by polyphagia (increased appetite), polydipsia (substantial thirst), and polyuria (excessive urination), along with deterioration of body tissues.
- There are two types of diabetes. Type 1 diabetes usually starts in childhood and requires daily insulin to control the blood glucose level. Type 2 diabetes usually develops in middle-age patients and can often be controlled with diet and oral medications. Both are serious systemic diseases that affect the kidneys, eyes, small arteries, and peripheral nerves, especially if the disease is uncontrolled or poorly controlled.
- Prediabetes exists when blood glucose levels or hemoglobin A1c levels are above normal levels, yet not high enough to be diagnosed as diabetes.
- Gestational diabetes is diabetes that a woman develops during pregnancy. It should be managed to stabilize blood glucose levels and minimize potential complications to mother and baby.
- Patients with diabetes have chronic complications that place them at risk for other diseases such as myocardial infarction, stroke, and infections. Most often, however, you will be summoned to treat the acute complications of blood glucose imbalance. These include hyperglycemia (excess blood glucose) and hypoglycemia (low blood glucose).
- Symptoms of hypoglycemia classically include confusion; rapid respirations; rapid pulse; cool, pale skin; diaphoresis; trembling; dizziness; fainting; and a feeling of hunger. This condition, called hypoglycemic crisis, is rapidly reversible with the administration of glucose in oral or intravenous (IV) form, or glucagon intramuscularly. Without treatment, permanent brain damage and death can occur.
- Hyperglycemia is usually associated with dehydration and diabetic ketoacidosis. It can result in hyperglycemic crisis, marked by rapid (often deep) respirations; warm, dry skin; a weak, rapid pulse; and a fruity breath odor. Hyperglycemia must be treated in the hospital with insulin and IV fluid rehydration.
- Hyperosmolar hyperglycemic syndrome (HHS), also called hyperosmolar nonketotic coma (HONK), is a metabolic derangement that occurs principally in patients with type 2 diabetes who have a secondary illness. It is characterized by hyperglycemia, hyperosmolarity, and an absence of substantial ketosis.
- Because either too much or too little blood glucose can result in an altered mental status, you must perform a thorough history and patient assessment. Check for an emergency medical identification device—a wallet card, necklace, or bracelet—or ask the patient or a family member.
- A patient in hypoglycemic crisis (rapid onset of altered mental status, hypoglycemia) needs sugar immediately. A patient in hyperglycemic crisis (acidosis, dehydration, hyperglycemia) needs insulin and IV fluid therapy. These patients need prompt transport to the hospital for appropriate medical care.
- When you cannot determine the nature of the problem, it is best to treat the patient for hypoglycemia. The risk of increasing the glucose level of a patient who is already hyperglycemic is minimal compared with the benefit of increasing the glucose level of a patient who is hypoglycemic.
- Be prepared to give oral glucose to a responsive patient who is confused or has a slightly decreased level of consciousness and IV or intraosseous dextrose to an unresponsive patient. Do not give oral glucose to a patient who is unresponsive or otherwise unable to swallow properly or protect his or her own airway.
- Dextrose is available in various concentrations: 50% (D_{50}), 25% (D_{25}), and 10% (D_{10}). The total dose of dextrose in these formats is the same; the concentration and volumes differ.
- You may administer glucagon intramuscularly when you cannot obtain IV access and therefore cannot administer dextrose.

Prep Kit *(continued)*

- Hematology is the study and treatment of blood-related diseases, such as sickle cell disease or hemophilia.
- Blood is made of two main components: plasma and formed elements (cells). The formed elements include red blood cells (RBCs), white blood cells (WBCs), and platelets, which are transported through the body in plasma.
- RBCs carry oxygen to the tissues. WBCs provide the body with immunity, fight infection, and remove dead cells. Platelets are responsible for clot formation. The bone marrow is the primary site for cell production, and the liver and spleen also have important roles.
- During a blood transfusion, if a patient receives a different blood type than his or her own, a transfusion reaction will occur. Such a reaction is similar to an anaphylactic reaction; both occur rapidly and can be fatal. Patients receiving blood transfusions must be monitored closely for 30 to 60 minutes.
- Sickle cell disease is an inherited blood disorder that results in the RBCs having an oblong shape instead of a smooth, round shape. This shape inhibits the ability of RBCs to carry oxygen effectively.
- Symptoms of sickle cell disease are typically characterized by pain in the joints, fever, respiratory distress, and abdominal pain.
- Patients with sickle cell disease have chronic complications that place them at risk for other diseases, such as heart attack, stroke, and infection. Most often, however, you will be called on to treat the acute complications of severe pain.
- Anemia is a hemoglobin or RBC level that is lower than normal. Patients with anemia may report feeling worn down, having no energy, or feeling as if they have overexerted themselves. They may also have angina-like pain and be pale.
- Thrombophilia and hemophilia are clotting disorders. Thrombophilia is a tendency to develop blood clots, which can result in thrombosis and obstruct blood flow. Patients with hemophilia are not able to control bleeding because clots do not develop as they should.
- Disseminated intravascular coagulation is uncontrolled hemorrhage that results from a life-threatening condition, for example, massive injury and hypotension owing to trauma. Remain alert for signs of coagulopathy as you assess and care for critically injured and ill patients.
- Obtain a thorough patient history and SAMPLE history with any patient with a potential blood disorder. The history may reveal that the patient has a known blood disorder, or reveal signs and symptoms that could suggest an undiagnosed blood disorder.
- Do not take a call from a person having a sickle cell crisis lightly. Patients are often in life-threatening situations. They will have signs of inadequate perfusion and of hypotension, and may have muscle pain, swelling of the fingers and toes, priapism, and jaundice.
- Emergency care for patients with sickle cell disease or a clotting disorder includes oxygen administration, IV fluid therapy, pain management, comfort measures, psychological support, and transport.

▶ Vital Vocabulary

ABO system The antigen classification given to blood.

acidosis A pathologic condition resulting from the accumulation of acids in the body.

acute chest syndrome A vaso-occlusive crisis that can be associated with pneumonia; common signs and symptoms include chest pain, fever, and cough.

aerobic metabolism Metabolism that can proceed only in the presence of oxygen.

anemia A lower-than-normal hemoglobin or red blood cell level.

aplastic crisis A condition in which the body stops producing red blood cells; typically caused by infection.

calcitonin The hormone secreted by the thyroid gland that helps maintain normal calcium levels in the blood.

clotting factors Substances in the blood that are necessary for clotting; also called coagulation factors.

coagulopathy Any type of bleeding disorder that interferes with the activation or continuation of the clotting cascade or hemostasis.

cortisol Hormone that stimulates most body cells to increase their energy production.

diabetes mellitus A metabolic disorder in which the ability to metabolize carbohydrates (sugars) is impaired due to a lack of insulin.

diabetic ketoacidosis (DKA) A form of acidosis in uncontrolled diabetes in which certain acids accumulate when insulin is not available.

disseminated intravascular coagulation (DIC) A condition that begins with widespread activation of the clotting cascade, which depletes the clotting factors and platelets, and eventually results in uncontrolled hemorrhage.

endocrine glands Glands that secrete or release chemicals that are used inside the body.

Prep Kit (continued)

endocrine system Regulates metabolism and maintains homeostasis.

exocrine gland A gland that excretes chemicals for elimination.

gestational diabetes Diabetes that develops during pregnancy in women who did not have diabetes before pregnancy.

glucagon The hormone released from the alpha cells in the islets of Langerhans that converts glycogen to glucose when the body's blood glucose level drops.

gluconeogenesis The production of new glucose through the metabolization of noncarbohydrate sources.

glucose One of the basic sugars; it is the primary fuel, along with oxygen, for cellular metabolism.

glycogenolysis The process by which glycogen is converted to glucose; facilitated by glucagon.

glycolysis The conversion of glucose into energy via metabolic pathways.

hematologic disorder Any disorder of the blood.

hematology The study and prevention of blood-related disorders.

hematopoietic system The system that includes all blood components and the organs involved in their development and production.

hemolytic crisis A rapid destruction of red blood cells that occurs faster than the body's ability to create new cells.

hemolytic disorders Disorders relating to the breakdown of red blood cells.

hemophilia A congenital abnormality in which the body is unable to produce clots, which results in uncontrollable bleeding.

hemostasis The body's natural blood-clotting mechanism.

hemostatic disorders Bleeding and clotting abnormalities.

hormone A chemical substance, produced by a gland, that regulates the activity of body organs and tissues.

hyperglycemia Abnormally high glucose level in the blood.

hyperglycemic crisis Unresponsiveness caused by dehydration, a very high blood glucose level, and ketoacidosis.

hyperosmolar hyperglycemic syndrome (HHS) A metabolic derangement that occurs principally in patients with type 2 diabetes; it is characterized by hyperglycemia, hyperosmolarity, and an absence of significant ketosis. Also known as hyperosmolar nonketotic coma.

hyperosmolar nonketotic coma (HONK) Condition characterized by severe hyperglycemia, hyperosmolality, and dehydration but no ketoacidosis; also called hyperosmolar hyperglycemic nonketotic coma (HHNC) or HONK/HHNC.

hypoglycemia Abnormally low glucose level in the blood.

hypoglycemic crisis Unresponsiveness or altered mental status in a patient with diabetes caused by significant hypoglycemia; usually the result of excessive exercise or activity, failure to eat after a routine dose of insulin, or an inadvertent overdose of insulin.

insulin A hormone produced by the islets of Langerhans (an exocrine gland in the pancreas) that enables sugar in the blood to enter the cells of the body; used in synthetic form to treat and control diabetes mellitus.

islets of Langerhans Structures found in the pancreas that are composed of four types of cells; one type, the beta cell, is responsible for the production of insulin.

ketonemia Excess amounts of ketone bodies in the blood.

Kussmaul respirations Deep, rapid breathing; the result of an accumulation of certain acids when insulin is not available in the body.

leukocytosis An increase in the total number of white blood cells.

leukopenia A reduction in the number of white blood cells.

lipolysis The metabolism (breakdown or destruction) of stored fat that has been released into the circulation.

microangiopathy Microscopic deterioration of vessel walls caused primarily by adherence of blood lipids to vessel walls.

pancreas The digestive gland that secretes digestive enzymes into the duodenum through the pancreatic duct; considered both an endocrine gland and an exocrine gland.

plasma A component of blood made mostly of water, but also electrolytes, clotting factors, and glucose; formed elements are transported in this.

platelets Small cells in the blood that are responsible for clot formation; also called thrombocytes.

polydipsia Excessive thirst persisting for long periods despite reasonable fluid intake; often the result of excessive urination.

polyphagia Excessive eating; in diabetes, the inability to use glucose properly can cause a sense of hunger.

Prep Kit *(continued)*

polyuria The passage of an unusually large volume of urine in a given period; in diabetes, this can result from wasting of glucose in the urine.

prediabetes A condition identified in people who have certain risk factors associated with type 2 diabetes and exists when blood glucose levels or hemoglobin A1c levels are above normal levels, yet not high enough to be diagnosed as diabetes.

red blood cells (RBCs) The formed elements in the blood that contain hemoglobin and are responsible for carrying oxygen to the tissues; also called erythrocytes.

sickle cell disease A hereditary disease that causes normal, round red blood cells to become oblong, or sickle shaped.

splenic sequestration crisis An acute, painful enlargement of the spleen caused by sickle cell disease.

stem cells Cells that can develop into other types of cells in the body.

thrombocytopenia A reduction in the number of platelets.

thrombocytosis A condition in which the body produces too many platelets.

thrombophilia A tendency toward the development of blood clots as a result of an abnormality of the system of coagulation.

thrombosis A blood clot, either in the arterial or venous system.

thyroid-stimulating hormone Hormone that stimulates the release of thyroid hormone from the thyroid gland.

thyroid storm A rare, life-threatening condition that may occur in patients with thyrotoxicosis. The condition is usually triggered by a stressful event or increased volume of thyroid hormones in the circulation.

type 1 diabetes The type of diabetic disease that usually starts in childhood and requires insulin for proper treatment and control.

type 2 diabetes The type of diabetic disease that usually starts later in life and often can be controlled through diet and oral medications.

vaso-occlusive crisis Ischemia and pain caused by sickle-shaped red blood cells that obstruct blood flow to a portion of the body.

white blood cells (WBCs) The formed elements in the blood that provide immunity, fight infection, and remove dead cells; also called leukocytes.

References

1. General Information/Press Room. American Thyroid Association website. https://www.thyroid.org/media-main/about-hypothyroidism/. Accessed December 6, 2017.
2. Diabetes. Centers for Disease Control and Prevention website. https://www.cdc.gov/chronicdisease/resources/publications/aag /diabetes.htm. Updated July 25, 2016. Accessed March 6, 2017.
3. Statistics About Diabetes. American Diabetes Association. http://www.diabetes.org/diabetes-basics/statistics/. Last edited December 12, 2016. Accessed March 6, 2017.
4. Lee R, Wong TY, Sabanayagam C. Epidemiology of diabetic retinopathy, diabetic macular edema and related vision loss. *Eye Vis (Lond)*. 2015;2:17.
5. Health Information for Older Adults. Centers for Disease Control and Prevention website. https://www.cdc.gov/aging/aginginfo/index.htm. Updated January 31, 2017. Accessed March 6, 2017.
6. Lough ME. Endocrine disorders and therapeutic management. In: Urden LD, Stacy KM, Lough ME, eds. *Critical Care Nursing: Diagnosis and Management.* 7th ed. St. Louis, MO: Mosby; 2014:809-848.
7. Diabetes Fact Sheet. World Health Organization website. http://www.who.int/mediacentre/factsheets/fs312/en/. Reviewed November 2016. Accessed March 8, 2017.
8. NIH Fact Sheets—Diabetes, Type 2. National Institutes of Health website. https://www.report.nih.gov/nihfactsheets/ViewFactSheet.aspx?csid=121. Updated March 29, 2013. Accessed March 6, 2017.
9. A1C Test. Mayo Clinic Website. https://www.mayoclinic.org/tests-procedures/a1c-test/details/results/rsc-20167939. Accessed November 19, 2017.
10. About Prediabetes & Type 2 Diabetes. Centers for Disease Control and Prevention website. http://www.cdc.gov/diabetes/prevention/prediabetes-type2/index.html. Updated July 19, 2016. Accessed March 8, 2017.
11. National Diabetes Prevention Program. Centers for Disease Control and Prevention website. https://www.cdc.gov/diabetes/prevention/prediabetes-type2/preventing.html. Updated January 14, 2016. Accessed March 8, 2017.
12. Gestational Diabetes and Pregnancy. Centers for Disease Control and Prevention website. https://www.cdc.gov/pregnancy/diabetes-gestational.html. Updated September 16, 2015. Accessed March 6, 2017.
13. Diabetes and Pregnancy: Gestational Diabetes. Centers for Disease Control and Prevention website. https://www.cdc.gov/pregnancy/documents/Diabetes_and_Pregnancy508.pdf. Accessed March 6, 2017.

Prep Kit (continued)

14. Gerich JE, Langlois M, Noacco C, et al. Lack of glucagon response to hypoglycemia in diabetes: evidence for an intrinsic pancreatic alpha cell defect. *Science*. 1973;182(4108):171-173.
15. Sandoval DA, Guy DL, Richardson MA, et al. Effects of low and moderate antecedent exercise on counterregulatory responses to subsequent hypoglycemia in type 1 diabetes. *Diabetes*. 2004;53(7):1798-1806.
16. Cryer P. Hypoglycemia during therapy of diabetes. In: DeGroot LJ, Chrousos G, Dungan K, et al, eds. Endotext [Internet]. South Dartmouth, MA: MDText.com, Inc.; 2000. https://www.ncbi.nlm.nih.gov/books/NBK279100/. Updated May 28, 2015. Accessed March 23, 2017.
17. Soleimanpour H, Taghizadieh A, Niafar M, et al. Predictive value of capnography for suspected diabetic ketoacidosis in the emergency department. *West J Emerg Med*. 2013;14(6):590-594.
18. Diabetic hyperglycemic hyperosmolar syndrome. U.S. National Library of Medicine Medline website. https://medlineplus.gov/ency/article/000304.htm. Updated April 4, 2017. Accessed May 1, 2017.
19. Crandall J, Shamoon H. Diabetes mellitus. In: Goldman L, Schafer AI, eds. *Goldman-Cecil Medicine*. 25th ed. Philadelphia, PA: Saunders; 2016:1527-1548.
20. Cydulka RK, Maloney GE. Diabetes mellitus and disorders of glucose homeostasis. In: Marx JA, Hockberger RS, Walls RM, eds. *Rosen's Emergency Medicine*. 8th ed. Philadelphia, PA: Saunders; 2014:1652-1666.
21. Whitlatch HB. Hyperosmolar hyperglycemic syndrome. In: Ferri FF, ed. *Ferri's Clinical Advisor 2017*. Philadelphia, PA: Elsevier; 2017:632-633.
22. Collopy K, Kivlehan S, Snyder S. Prehospital Treatment of Hyperglycemia. 2013 (September 1). http://www.emsworld.com/article/11112993/prehospital-treatment-of-hyperglycemia. Accessed March 6, 2017.
23. Pasquel FJ, Umpierrez GE. Hyperosmolar hyperglycemic state: a historical review of the clinical presentation, diagnosis, and treatment. *Diabetes Care*. 2014;37(11):3124-3131.
24. Sandoval DA, Guy DL, Richardson MA, et al. Effects of low and moderate antecedent exercise on counterregulatory responses to subsequent hypoglycemia in type 1 diabetes. *Diabetes*. 2004;53(7):1798-1806.
25. Do you have Rh Negative Blood? The Rh-Negative Registry website. http://www.rhnegativeregistry.com/welcome.html. Accessed January 2, 2018.
26. Sickle cell disease (SCD). Centers for Disease Control and Prevention website. https://www.cdc.gov/ncbddd/sicklecell/data.html. Updated August 31, 2016. Accessed March 13, 2017.
27. Platt OS, Brambilla DJ, Rosse WF, et al. Mortality in sickle cell disease: life expectancy and risk factors for early death. *N Engl J Med*. 1994;330:1639-1644. http://www.nejm.org/doi/full/10.1056/NEJM199406093302303#t=article. Accessed March 13, 2017.
28. Fast Facts. National Hemophilia Foundation website. https://www.hemophilia.org/About-Us/Fast-Facts. Accessed January 2, 2018.
29. Lee JH, Song JW, Song KS. Diagnosis of overt disseminated intravascular coagulation: a comparative study using criteria from the International Society versus the Korean Society on Thrombosis and Hemostasis. *Yonsei Med J*. 2007;48(4):595-600. https://www.ncbi.nlm.nih.gov/pmc/articles/PMC2628057/. Accessed March 13, 2017.

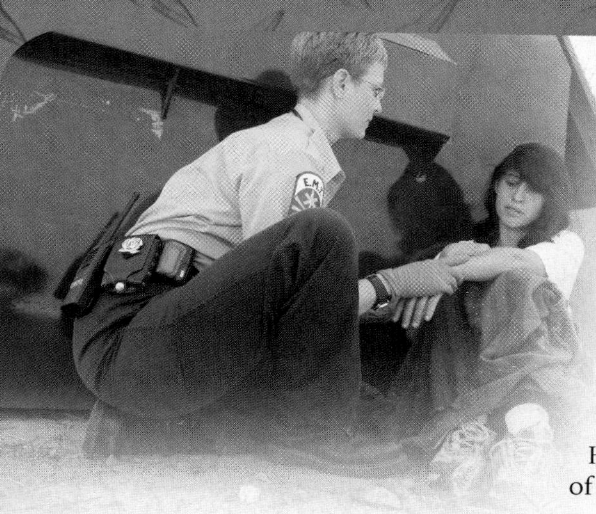

Assessment in Action

EMS is requested at 0300 hours to evaluate a 26-year-old African American man with a history of sickle cell disease reporting back and knee pain and shortness of breath. His pain started midafternoon and has become progressively worse. The shortness of breath started about 20 minutes ago. He states that he takes hydrocodone for pain, but has been out of the medication for 3 days.

1. The first priority when treating this patient is to:

A. gain IV access.
B. administer an analgesic.
C. administer oxygen.
D. place him in a position of comfort.

2. When assessing this patient's vital signs, you expect to find all of the following except:

A. respirations normal to rapid.
B. pulse weak and rapid.
C. skin pale and clammy.
D. high blood pressure.

3. Since sickle cells also have a much shorter life span than normal erythrocytes, the patient is more susceptible to the development of:

A. thrombophilia.
B. anemia.
C. infections.
D. hemophilia.

4. Potential complications of sickle cell disease include all of the following except:

A. osteonecrosis.
B. pulmonary hypertension.
C. opiate intolerance.
D. leg ulcers.

5. Which of the following is not a standard treatment for a patient with a sickle cell crisis?

A. Oxygen
B. Immobilization
C. IV fluid
D. Analgesics

6. High levels of oxygen are recommended for patients with sickle cell disease to prevent further destruction of the RBCs due to:

A. dehydration.
B. thrombosis.
C. hypoperfusion.
D. hypoxia.

7. In a(n) _____ crisis, the body temporarily stops RBC production, causing the patient to become easily tired, anemic, pale, and short of breath.

A. aplastic
B. hemolytic
C. vaso-occlusive
D. splenic sequestration

8. ________ is one of the basic sugars in the body and, along with ______, is the primary fuel for cellular metabolism.

A. Glucose; oxygen
B. Glucose; glucagon
C. Glucose; dextrose
D. Glucose; insulin

9. What is *prediabetes*?

10. In order for glucagon to be effective, what must be present?

CHAPTER 22

Immunologic Emergencies

National EMS Education Standard Competencies

Medicine

Applies fundamental knowledge to provide basic and selected advanced emergency care and transportation based on assessment findings for an acutely ill patient.

Immunology

Recognition and management of shock and difficulty breathing related to

- Anaphylactic reactions (pp 954-956, 960-963)

Anatomy, physiology, pathophysiology, assessment, and management of hypersensitivity disorders and/or emergencies

- Allergic and anaphylactic reactions (pp 949-963)

Knowledge Objectives

1. Understand and define the terms *allergic reaction* and *anaphylaxis*. (p 949)
2. Describe the purpose of the immune system. (p 949)
3. Discuss the process that begins when a foreign substance is detected in the body (primary response). (pp 950-951)
4. Explain the roles of basophils and mast cells in the immune response process. (p 950)
5. Describe the process that occurs when the body undergoes a secondary response. (p 951)
6. Explain the difference between a local response and a systemic response to allergens. (p 952)
7. Explain the roles of two types of chemical mediators, histamines and leukotrienes, in the immune response process. (pp 953-954)
8. List and compare the signs and symptoms of an allergic reaction with those of anaphylaxis. (pp 954-956)
9. Describe the assessment process for a patient with an allergic reaction. (pp 955-959)
10. Explain the importance of managing the airway, breathing, and circulation of a patient who is having an allergic reaction. (p 957)
11. Review the process for providing emergency medical care to a patient who is experiencing an allergic reaction. (pp 960-963)
12. Explain the rationale, including communication and documentation considerations, when determining whether to administer epinephrine to a patient who is having an allergic reaction. (pp 959-960)
13. List the types of insect stings that may cause an allergic reaction, and describe specific treatment of patients with such stings. (pp 963-964)
14. Discuss patient education related to prevention and management of anaphylaxis and allergic reactions. (p 964)

Skills Objectives

1. Demonstrate how to use an EpiPen auto-injector. (p 961, Skill Drill 22-1)
2. Demonstrate how to remove a stinger from a bee sting and proper patient management following its removal. (p 964)

YOU are the Provider — PART 1

You are dispatched to the home of a 46-year-old man with a possible allergic reaction. On arrival, you are greeted by the patient's wife. She directs you to the patient, who is seated on the sofa. The patient states that he just started a new antibiotic for an upper respiratory infection, and now he itches all over and a large rash is developing on his torso.

1. What is the major difference between an allergic reaction and anaphylaxis?
2. How are the treatments for these two conditions the same? How do they differ?

Introduction

Every year, at least 1,500 Americans die of acute allergic reactions.[1] When managing allergy-related emergencies, you must be aware of the possibility of acute airway obstruction and cardiovascular collapse and be prepared to treat these life-threatening complications. You must also be able to distinguish between the body's usual response to an allergen and an **allergic reaction**—an exaggerated immune response to any substance—that may require **epinephrine**, or **anaphylaxis**—an extreme systemic form of an allergic reaction involving two or more body systems. Your ability to recognize and manage the many signs and symptoms of allergic reactions may be the only thing standing between a patient's life and imminent death.

This chapter begins by describing the physiology of the body's immune response and the pathophysiology of an allergic reaction—that is, how an immune response can evolve into a potentially life-threatening event. It discusses the general assessment of patients who may be having an allergic reaction and how to care for them, including the administration of epinephrine. Finally, the chapter describes specific stings and bites from bees, wasps, yellow jackets, hornets, and fire ants.

Anatomy and Physiology Review

Anatomy Review

The **immune system** protects the human body from substances and organisms that are foreign to the body. Without the immune system for protection, life as you know it would not exist. You would be under constant attack from any type of invader, such as a bacterium or virus, that wanted to make your body a home. Fortunately, most people have immune systems that are well equipped to detect unauthorized visits or invading attacks by foreign substances.

The body protects itself via two types of systems: cellular immunity and humoral (ie, related to the body's fluids) immunity. In **cellular immunity**, also called *cell-mediated immunity*, the body produces specialized white blood cells called *T cells* that attack and destroy invaders. In **humoral immunity**, B cell lymphocytes produce antibodies that dissolve in the plasma and lymph to wage war on invading organisms. The cells producing immunity factors are located throughout the body in the lymph nodes, spleen, and gastrointestinal tract. Their goal is to intercept foreign invaders as they enter the body, thereby limiting the spread and damage of these organisms.

Given the right person and the right circumstances, almost any substance can trigger the body's immune system and cause an allergic reaction. For example, animal bites, food, latex gloves, and even semen can all be **allergens**, the antigens or substances that produce allergic symptoms in a patient. The most common allergens, however, fall into one of the following five general categories:

- **Insect bites and stings.** When an insect bites or stings you, the act of injecting its venom is called **envenomation**. Envenomation by a honeybee, wasp, ant, yellow jacket, or hornet may cause a localized reaction, causing swelling and itching at the site, or a severe and systemic reaction (ie, anaphylaxis).
- **Medications.** If the medication is injected, the reaction may be immediate (within 30 minutes) and severe. Reactions to oral medications may take more than 30 minutes to appear, but can also be very severe. The fact that a person has taken a medication once without experiencing an allergic reaction is no guarantee that he or she will not have an allergic reaction to the same medication with subsequent exposure.
- **Plants.** People who inhale dust, pollen, mold, mildew, or other organic materials to which they are sensitive may experience an allergic reaction. Some common plant allergens include ragweed, ryegrass, maple, and oak.
- **Foods.** Eating certain foods such as shellfish and peanuts may result in a relatively slow (more than 30 minutes) reaction; however, the reaction still can be quite severe. It is possible for a patient to be unaware of the exposure; for example, a person allergic to peanuts may eat something without knowing that one of the ingredients is peanuts.
- **Chemicals.** Certain chemicals, makeup, soap, hair dye, latex, and various other substances can cause severe allergic reactions. Latex is of particular concern to health care providers. For some, simply being in the same room as someone wearing powdered latex gloves can cause a reaction. It is a good practice to routinely use latex alternatives such as nitrile gloves. Follow your local protocol.

Most allergens are usually harmless substances that do not pose a threat to other people—for example, milk, eggs, chocolate, and strawberries. An **antibody** is a protein the body produces in response to an **antigen** (the foreign invader). This protein (globulin) is found in the plasma—a characteristic that inspired its other name, *immunoglobulin* (Ig). Table 22-1 lists the common antibodies, their actions, and locations.

Foreign substances can invade the body through the skin, the respiratory tract, or the gastrointestinal tract Table 22-2. Invasion through the skin may come in the form of injection or absorption. In **injection**, the invading substance pierces the skin and deposits foreign material into the skin. Bees and hornets are often the cause of this type of invasion. **Absorption** occurs when foreign material is deposited on the skin and slowly absorbed through the skin. Invasion by allergens does not stop at the skin; they may also enter the respiratory tract as the patient quietly

Table 22-1 Antibodies or Immunoglobulins

Antibody	Action	Location
IgA	Provides localized protection to mucous membranes. Stress can lower the IgA level, making the body more susceptible to infection.	Tears, saliva, mucus, breast milk, gastrointestinal secretions, blood, and lymph
IgD	Thought to stimulate antibody-producing cells to make antibodies.	Blood, lymph, and the surface of B cells
IgE[a]	Responds in allergic reactions.	Located on mast and basophil cells
IgG	Provides protection against bacteria and viruses; enhances phagocytosis; neutralizes toxins; triggers the complement system.	Blood, lymph, and intestines
IgM	One of the first antibodies to appear; causes agglutination and lysis of microbes. ABO agglutinins are IgM antibodies.	Blood, lymph, and the surface of B cells

Abbreviation: Ig, immunoglobulin

[a]The IgE antibody is the primary antibody of concern during allergic and anaphylactic reactions.

Table 22-2 Allergen Routes of Entry Ingestion

- Injection
- Inhalation
- Absorption
- Ingestion

breathes. Following this kind of **inhalation** exposure, the foreign substance may advance through the respiratory system and launch its attack from the lungs. Pet hair and dander, peanuts, and many plants may enter the body through this type of exposure. The final way allergens attack the body is through the gastrointestinal tract via **ingestion**. Many different foods, such as strawberry shortcake, a mushroom and cheese omelet, or peanut butter pie, can cause an allergic reaction; medications also can cause a reaction through this route. Allergens that are injected or inhaled tend to cause the most severe reaction.

▶ Physiology Review

When a foreign substance invades the body, the body goes on alert and initiates a series of responses. The first encounter with the foreign substance begins the **primary response** and mainly involves the white blood cells—the cells that fight infection in the body. Cells (macrophages) immediately greet, confront, and engulf the invaders to determine whether they are allowed in the body. If the body is unable to identify the invader, it uses immune cells to record the salient features of this substance. These cells record one or two of the proteins on the surface of the invading substance and then design antibodies to match each substance. These antibodies are intended to match up with the antigen and inactivate it.

Through the primary response, the body develops **sensitivity**—that is, the ability to recognize the foreigner the next time it is encountered. To determine whether the substance is "one of us," the body records enough details to assist in future identification of the substance and production of antibodies that match up perfectly with the invading antigen. The body then sends out these details to the rest of the body, by placing the specific antibodies on two types of cells: **basophils** and **mast cells**. Basophils are stationed in specific sites within the tissues. Mast cells are on patrol through the connective tissues, bronchi, gastrointestinal mucosa, and other vulnerable border areas that act as barriers to foreign invaders.

The basophils and mast cells produce the body's "chemical weapons," known as **chemical mediators**. These cells contain granules filled with a host of powerful substances that are ready to be released to fight invading forces of antigens. As long as the body is not invaded by one of the previously identified foreign substances, the granules are kept encapsulated in their protective walls and remain inactive. However, if an antigen invades the body and combines with one of the antibodies, the granules are ejected from the mast cells and detonated. Degranulation is the process in which granules burst, releasing their powerful contents. The chemical mediators are then released into the surrounding tissue and the bloodstream.

The chemical mediators launch and maintain the immune response. They summon more white blood cells to the area to battle the invading force. They also increase blood flow to the area under attack by dilating the blood vessels and increasing capillary permeability.

These actions are useful when a small invasion occurs to a limited area but can be extremely dangerous when they spread throughout the body. Chemical mediators cause the local effects of an allergic reaction seen in the body. When they have systemic effects, the chemical mediators cause the signs and symptoms of anaphylactic reactions Figure 22-1.

As a health care provider, you exploit the body's ability to protect itself. For example, vaccines are administered to produce **immunity** against a disease. A vaccine contains a killed or weakened version of a disease-causing organism or one of its proteins. The body develops antibodies in response to the vaccine that enable it to produce an immune response that neutralizes an invading disease (caused by a more potent form of the pathogen found in the vaccine) before it can establish itself and damage the body. Thus, the body develops antibodies in a controlled way through vaccination. When the hepatitis B vaccine is administered, for example, a small amount of the inactivated parts of the hepatitis B virus (HBV) enters the body. The body identifies this virus and produces antibodies to it; these antibodies then become distributed throughout the body. If an immunized person is later exposed to HBV, the virus may invade the body. Once in the body, the virus begins to set up residency and reproduce. At this point, the wandering immune cells identify the HBV as something that does not belong in that area of the body. The alarm sounds, and the body begins aggressive production of the "antihepatitis" antibodies, sending these cells to kill the HBV and clean up residual traces of the invasion. This intense response to the invading virus is called the **secondary response**. Meanwhile, the "contaminated," immunized person remains unaware of the battle raging inside his or her body.

This battle is termed **acquired immunity**. In this type of immunity, the administration of a vaccine allows the body to produce antibodies without having to experience the disease. Vaccinations against measles, mumps, and poliomyelitis are examples of acquired immunity. By contrast, in **natural immunity**, the body encounters the antigen and experiences a full immune response but with all the effects of the disease. Having the measles, for example, causes the body to produce antibodies to this pathogen, but the drawback is that the person has the itching, rash, and high fever associated with the disease.

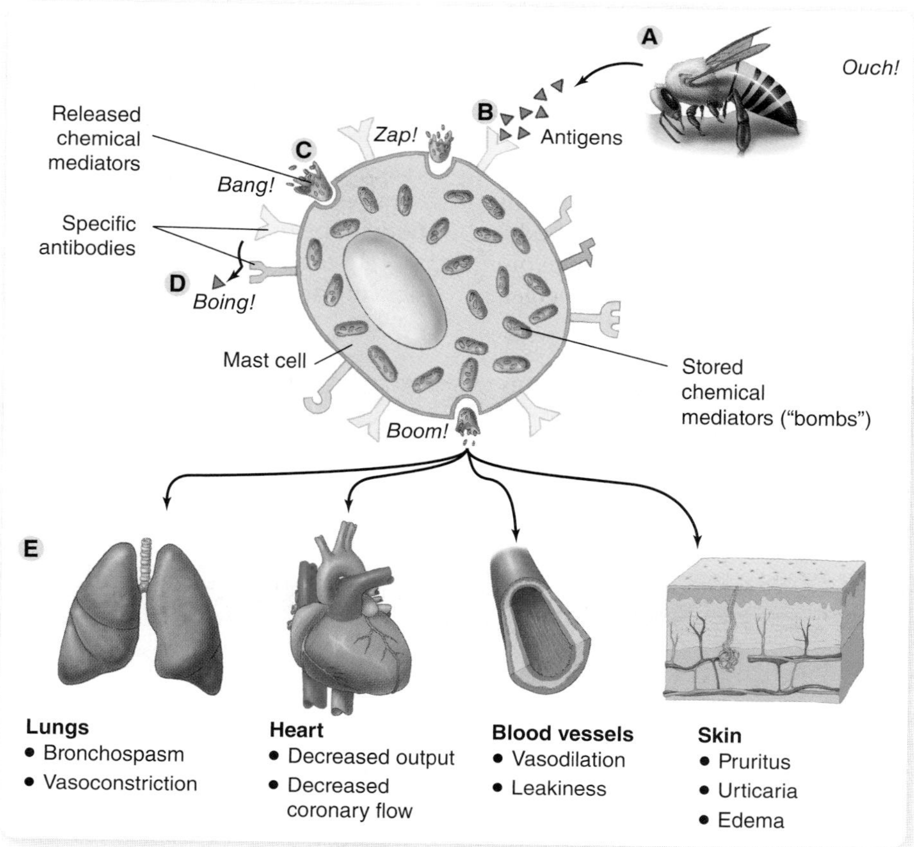

Figure 22-1 The sequence of events in anaphylaxis. **A.** The antigen is introduced into the body. **B.** The antigen-antibody reaction occurs at the surface of a mast cell. **C.** The mast cell chemical mediators release. **D.** The specific antibody reacts with its corresponding antigen. **E.** Chemical mediators exert their effects on end organs.

Words of Wisdom

Use of the poliomyelitis vaccine has resulted in herd immunity, which occurs when a group of people are immunized against a substance. This immunization protects the entire group by decreasing the number of people who are able to contract the disease, thereby protecting all members of the group. Other vaccines that have led to herd immunity include the measles, mumps, and rubella (MMR) vaccine as well as the pertussis vaccine. Herd immunity can be lost when pediatric immunization rates decline, leaving more members of the group vulnerable to developing a disease.

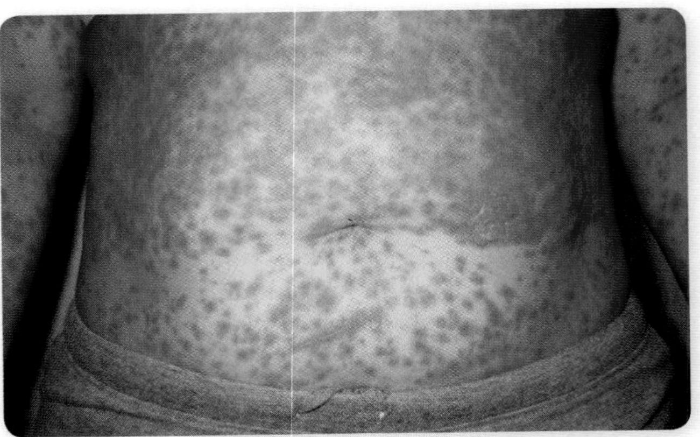

Figure 22-2 A severe allergic reaction to medication.

Courtesy of Carol B. Guerrero.

▶ Pathophysiology

An ever-watchful and responsive immune system is essential to life and health. Unfortunately, sometimes the immune system becomes overzealous in defending the body. The resulting conditions may range in severity from hay fever to anaphylaxis, and exist along the spectrum from a simple annoyance to a life-threatening crisis. During these abnormal reactions, the immune system becomes hypersensitive to one or more substances. The body often has these reactions to substances that should not be identified as harmful by the immune system—substances such as ragweed, strawberries, and penicillin **Figure 22-2**.

Contrary to what many people might think, an allergic reaction is not caused directly by an outside stimulus, such as a bite or sting. Rather, it is a reaction by the body's immune system that occurs when a person has been previously exposed or sensitized to a substance or allergen.

▶ Allergic Reactions Versus Anaphylaxis

An allergic reaction may be mild and localized, or it may be systemic. In a **local reaction**, the body limits its response to a specific area after being exposed to a foreign substance; the swelling around an insect bite is an example. By comparison, a **systemic reaction** occurs throughout the body, possibly affecting multiple body systems. This kind of reaction is seen when a person who is allergic to strawberries, for example, has swelling and hives all over his body after eating strawberries or a food containing strawberries. The patient may also experience **hypersensitivity**, which occurs when a person reacts with exaggerated or inappropriate allergic symptoms after coming into contact with a substance perceived by the body to be harmful.

Up to 15% of the US population is at risk for experiencing an anaphylactic reaction, which can be fatal for

YOU are the Provider — PART 2

As you expose the patient's chest, you observe the following:

Recording Time: 1 Minute	
Appearance	Anxious, flushed
Level of consciousness	Alert and oriented to person, place, time, and event
Airway	Patent; mild audible wheezes; no stridor
Breathing	Rapid at 36 breaths/min
Circulation	Absent distal pulses; skin is mottled

3. What is the significance of stridor not being present during airway assessment?

approximately 1% of the people exposed.[1] Most (possibly as many as 45 million) of these individuals have preexisting allergies that make them more susceptible to anaphylaxis.[1] However, the number of patients who die from anaphylaxis may even be greatly underreported because not all anaphylactic deaths are recognized as such. Anaphylactic events may be mistaken for heart attacks, heat stroke, or many other conditions.[2] In cases of anaphylaxis with known causes, medications produce the most allergy-related deaths.[3]

Words of Wisdom

The term *anaphylaxis* was first used in 1902, when Portier and Richet were vaccinating dogs with sea anemone toxin. After the second dose of the toxin, one of the dogs died. Because this response was against a substance intended to provide protection, it was referred to as *anaphylaxis* (meaning "without protection"). The term is not entirely accurate, however; the fundamental problem in an anaphylactic reaction is not a lack of protection but rather overprotection. That is, anaphylaxis is a form of allergy—an extreme and devastating form—and an allergy represents the body's protective immune system gone overboard.

To anticipate anaphylaxis, of course, it would be useful to be able to identify people who are at greatest risk for this type of reaction. Neither race nor gender seems to affect the incidence of anaphylaxis. Diseases related to allergies, such as allergic rhinitis, asthma, and atopic dermatitis, increase the potential for anaphylactic reactions.

The other major factors associated with anaphylaxis are the route of exposure to the allergen and the time between exposures. While a severe reaction can occur by any route, the longer the time between exposures to a substance, the less likely it is that a severe anaphylactic reaction will occur. This pattern is thought to reflect the decreased production of the specific Ig or antibody cells in the body over time.

Anaphylaxis is classified as a response mediated by IgE antibodies, whereas an **anaphylactoid reaction** is a response that does not involve IgE antibody mediation. The exact mechanism is unknown, but an anaphylactoid event may occur without the patient being previously exposed to the offending agent. Examples of triggers of anaphylactic reactions include nuts, fish, and latex. Anaphylactoid triggers, by comparison, include some contrast materials given before radiography, morphine-derived medications, and aspirin. Although the process that causes the reaction is different, the patient presentation is the same and the reactions should be treated in the same manner because both can be life threatening.

Words of Wisdom

Anaphylaxis and anaphylactoid responses are clinically indistinguishable and should be treated in the same manner because both can be life threatening.

Pathophysiologic Response

The immune cells of the person with allergies are more sensitive than the immune cells of a person without allergies. Although these cells have the capability to recognize and react to dangerous invaders such as bacteria and viruses, they also identify harmless substances as potential threats.

When the invading substance enters the body, the mast cells recognize it as potentially harmful and begin releasing chemical mediators. The two types of chemical mediators are histamine and leukotrienes. **Histamine** causes the blood vessels in the local area to dilate and the capillaries to leak. **Leukotrienes**, which are even more powerful, are released and cause additional dilation and leaking. White blood cells are called to the area to help engulf and destroy the enemy, and platelets begin to collect (aggregate) and clump together. In most cases, this overreaction to harmless invaders is usually restricted to the local area being invaded. The runny, itchy nose and swollen eyes associated with hay fever are examples of a local allergic reaction.

In the case of anaphylaxis, the person is not so lucky. Chemical mediators are released, and the effect involves more than one system throughout the body Table 22-3. An initial effect may be seen from the release of histamine, with secondary effects following a few hours later when the remainder of the chemicals are released.

The release of histamine causes immediate vasodilation, which often presents as flushed (erythematous) skin and sometimes leads to hypotension. It also increases vascular permeability, which results in **angioedema** (swelling of the face and tongue), fluid secretion, and fluid loss. Edema can present as **urticaria** (hives) Figure 22-3, airway constriction, and increased fluids in the airway. Histamine

Words of Wisdom

- Inotropic effect: affecting the strength of the contraction of cardiac muscle
- Chronotropic effect: affecting the heart's rate of contraction
- Dromotropic effect: affecting the conduction speed in the atrioventricular node and, consequently, the rate of electrical impulses through the heart

Table 22-3 Physiologic Effects of Chemical Mediators

Mediator	Physiologic Effects
Histamine	▪ Systemic vasodilation ▪ Increased permeability of blood vessels ▪ Decreased cardiac contractility ▪ Decreased coronary blood flow ▪ Dysrhythmias ▪ Bronchoconstriction ▪ Pulmonary vasoconstriction
Leukotrienes (slow-reacting substance of anaphylaxis)	▪ Vascular permeability ▪ Bronchoconstriction ▪ Decreased force of cardiac contraction ▪ Decreased coronary blood flow ▪ Dysrhythmias • More potent than histamine (thousands of times) • React more slowly than histamine
Platelet-activating factor	▪ Platelet aggregation ▪ Causes histamine release
Serotonin	▪ Pulmonary vasoconstriction ▪ Bronchoconstriction

similarly causes smooth muscle contraction, especially in the respiratory and gastrointestinal systems. This results in laryngospasm or bronchospasm and abdominal cramping. Finally, histamine decreases the contractility (inotropic effects) of the heart. When this effect is coupled with vasodilation, the person may experience profound hypotension. Dysrhythmias resulting from hypoperfusion and hypoxia are also common.

Later responses from the much more powerful leukotrienes compound the effects of histamine. The person's respiratory status will become even more compromised as these highly potent bronchoconstrictors are released. In addition, the release of leukotrienes causes coronary vasoconstriction, which contributes to a worsening cardiac condition and myocardial irritability. Leukotrienes are also associated with increased vascular permeability, further contributing to the state of hypoperfusion.

The remaining chemical mediators continue to worsen the situation as they undertake what they determine as steps to protect the body from this foreign invader. As a result of these activities, when the body undergoes an anaphylactic reaction, the person may not survive without immediate intervention.

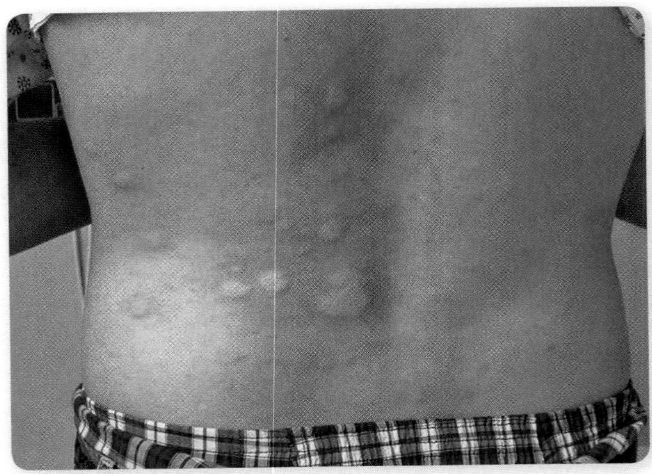

Figure 22-3 Urticaria, or hives, may appear following exposure to an allergen and is characterized by multiple, small, raised areas on the skin. Urticaria may be one of the warning signs of an impending anaphylactic reaction.

▶ Clinical Symptoms of Anaphylaxis

The skin is the body's first line of defense against would-be invaders, so skin symptoms are often the first indications of anaphylaxis. Initially, the person may be aware of feeling warm and flushed. **Pruritus** (itching) is another early sign, which is a result of vasodilation and capillary leaking. The area around the eyes is often susceptible to this effect, which causes swollen, red eyes. Angioedema may contribute to airway compromise. You may also note swelling of the hands and feet. Histamine is responsible for the urticaria experienced by a patient with anaphylaxis.

The most common complaints are usually respiratory symptoms, which often present as dyspnea (shortness of breath) and tightness in the throat and chest. You may also note **stridor** and/or hoarseness. These signs and symptoms are often due to upper airway swelling in the laryngeal and epiglottic areas. Affected patients may complain of a lump in the throat. The lower airway is often involved as well. Bronchoconstriction and increased airway secretions may result in wheezes and crackles. It is not uncommon for the patient to cough or sneeze as the body tries to clear the airway. These symptoms may progress slowly or alarmingly fast. You may have only 1 to 3 minutes to halt this rapid, life-threatening process.

Cardiovascular symptoms are serious complications of anaphylaxis. Histamines and leukotrienes work directly on the heart to decrease its contractility. The resulting decrease in cardiac output is complicated by vasodilation (in which the blood vessels widen) and increased capillary permeability, leading to blood pooling at the capillary beds, further decreasing the amount of fluid returned to the heart, despite constriction of the coronary arteries. As cardiac output declines, perfusion decreases, resulting in ischemia and the potential for cardiac dysrhythmias. As the fluid leaks out of the capillaries, the intravascular system is left short on fluid. (Up to 50% of the vascular volume can be shifted to the extravascular space within 10 minutes of exposure to an antigen.) Instead of responding normally to the fluid loss and constricting, the blood vessels do just the opposite: they dilate. The already low vascular volume becomes totally inadequate, and hypotension reigns. In response to the low blood pressure, the heart rate increases, putting stress on an already compromised heart. In this situation, tachycardia, flushed skin, and hypotension are synonymous with anaphylactic shock.

Remember that the body will not tolerate an acute blood loss of greater than 20% of blood volume. When significant volume moves from the intravascular space to the extravascular space, it has the same effect as external blood loss. The patient will exhibit signs of shock, including substantial changes in vital signs: increased heart rate, increased respiratory rate, and decreased blood pressure. Hypotension is seen sooner in patients with anaphylactic shock, as opposed to hypovolemic shock, owing to vasodilation caused by the release of histamines, preventing the body from compensating.

Gastrointestinal symptoms also may be part of an anaphylactic response, particularly if the offending antigen has been ingested. Abdominal cramping is a common presentation, but nausea, bloating, vomiting, abdominal distention, and profuse, watery diarrhea also may be present.

Patients may present with central nervous system symptoms in response to decreased cerebral perfusion and hypoxia. These symptoms include headache, dizziness, confusion, and anxiety. A sense of "impending doom" aptly represents the patient's sense of being near death. A patient who expresses a sense of impending doom requires rapid assessment and treatment.

Table 22-4 summarizes the signs and symptoms of anaphylaxis compared with those of an allergic reaction. Anaphylaxis may present as affecting any two or more of these body systems, so the picture can be confusing at times. Think of a patient with anaphylaxis as experiencing three types of shock: (1) cardiogenic shock due to decreased cardiac output, (2) hypovolemic shock due to fluids leaking into the tissues, and (3) neurogenic shock due to inability of the blood vessels to constrict.

Patient Assessment

Assessment of a patient who is experiencing an anaphylactic reaction can be highly challenging. You may have to simultaneously assess the patient, identify the problem, and intervene within seconds of arriving on the scene to save the patient's life. Suspicion for anaphylaxis must be high if any of the pertinent symptoms are present. You may not have a second opportunity because the patient's condition may deteriorate before your eyes.

YOU are the Provider — PART 3

The local fire unit arrives on scene and assists your partner in bringing in the stretcher while you continue your assessment. The patient states that he visited his primary physician this morning; the physician prescribed the penicillin for an upper respiratory infection. The patient got the prescription filled after his visit and took the initial dose approximately 1 hour ago, with lunch. Approximately 30 minutes ago, an itching sensation developed, along with the rash. While the patient is talking, you notice an increase in his work of breathing. You place the patient on 100% oxygen via nonrebreathing mask and begin taking vital signs.

Recording Time: 5 Minutes	
Respirations	40 breaths/min; wheezes bilaterally
Pulse	Absent radial pulses; carotid, 138 beats/min
Skin	Red, swollen patches on torso, extending to arms and legs
Blood pressure	76/32 mm Hg
Oxygen saturation (Spo_2)	93% on 100% oxygen
Pupils	Pupils Equal, Round, and Reactive to Light and Accommodation (PERRLA)

4. In which position should this patient be placed?
5. Based on his presentation, what is the definitive treatment for this patient?

Table 22-4 Common Signs and Symptoms of Allergic Reactions and Anaphylaxis

	Allergic Reaction	Anaphylaxis[a]
Respiratory system	▪ Sneezing or an itchy, runny nose (initially) ▪ Tightness in the chest or throat ▪ Irritating, persistent, dry cough ▪ Hoarseness ▪ Rapid, labored, or noisy respirations ▪ Wheezing, stridor, or both	▪ Sneezing ▪ Tightness in the chest or throat ▪ Coughing ▪ Stridor ▪ Hoarseness ▪ Lump in throat ▪ Dyspnea ▪ Wheezes ▪ Crackles
Circulatory/cardiovascular system	▪ Increase in pulse rate (initially) ▪ Decrease in blood pressure ▪ Pale skin and dizziness	▪ Tachycardia ▪ Hypotension (can be profound) ▪ Dysrhythmias
Skin	▪ Flushing, itching, or burning skin ▪ Hives (urticaria) ▪ Swelling, especially of the face, neck, hands, feet, and tongue ▪ Swelling and cyanosis or pallor around the lips ▪ Warm, tingling feeling in the face, mouth, chest, feet, and hands	▪ Warm, flushed skin ▪ Itching (pruritus) ▪ Hives (urticaria) ▪ Swollen, red eyes ▪ Swelling of the face, neck, hands, feet, and tongue
Gastrointestinal system	▪ Abdominal cramping	▪ Abdominal cramping ▪ Nausea ▪ Bloating ▪ Vomiting ▪ Abdominal distention ▪ Profuse, watery diarrhea
Neurologic system	▪ Anxiety; a sense of impending doom ▪ Headache ▪ Decreasing mental status	▪ Anxiety and restlessness ▪ Sense of impending doom ▪ Headache ▪ Altered mental status ▪ Dizziness ▪ Confusion ▪ Loss of consciousness and coma
Other findings	▪ Itchy, watery eyes	▪ Not applicable

[a]Signs and symptoms of anaphylaxis include the signs and symptoms of allergic reactions, plus additional signs and symptoms. Anaphylaxis is a systemic reaction, whereas allergic reactions are usually mild and localized.

The response to antigens may occur in a multistep manner, with the immediate acute response being followed later by a delayed response. Alternatively, the reaction can be either acute or delayed. Acute reactions have a rapid onset and typically result in the most life-threatening situations. Delayed reactions may take hours or longer to manifest, and the response is not usually as exaggerated. A *prolonged, persistent reaction* is one in which anaphylaxis symptoms continue over time from 5 to 72 hours.[4] In a *biphasic response*, the patient experiences an initial reaction, appears to recover, and then experiences a recurrence of symptoms. To help minimize the effects of a delayed reaction that occurs alone or as part of a biphasic response, all patients who experience an allergic reaction should be encouraged to seek medical attention.

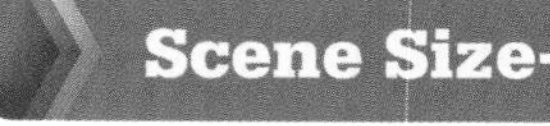

Scene Size-up

First and foremost, ensure the scene is safe. The patient's environment or recent activity may indicate the source of the reaction, such as an insect sting or bite, a food allergy triggered by eating at a restaurant, or a new medication regimen. A respiratory problem reported by dispatch may be an allergic reaction. If many people are affected, however, the scene could involve an inhaled poison or a terrorist event. Never enter a scene where more than one person is experiencing the same symptoms with a similar onset. Consider the need for additional or specialized resources, and call for those resources earlier rather than later.

Do not neglect the possibility that traumatic injury may also be present, secondary to the medical emergency. Determine the mechanism of injury or nature of illness. Look for bee stingers or contact with chemicals and other indications of a reaction. Do not let your guard down, even on what appears to be a routine call.

Words of Wisdom

Evidence of the exact source of an allergic reaction or envenomation may be scarce when you arrive, or bystanders may give you incorrect information. The cause of such an incident is more likely to pose a risk to responders and added risk to the patient if you draw incorrect conclusions about its nature. Keep your eyes and ears open, avoid making unsupported assumptions, and be curious about things that do not quite make sense.

Primary Survey

Perform the primary survey of the patient. The patient's presentation will give you an indication of the severity of the problem. Any change in mental status in an anaphylactic patient should direct you to immediately begin airway evaluation and management.

Quickly assess the patient for respiratory symptoms, such as dyspnea, tightness in the throat and chest, increased work of breathing, use of accessory muscles, head bobbing, tripod positioning, nostril flaring, prolonged expiration, and abnormal breath sounds. A noisy upper airway is a concern in any patient, but even more so in an anaphylactic patient because it may be an early sign of impending airway occlusion. Assess breath sounds for **wheezing**. Exhalation, normally the passive, relaxed part of breathing, becomes harder as the patient tries to cough up the secretions or move air past the constricted airways. As the patient's condition worsens and the lungs become tighter (closed) and less ventilated (hypoventilation), breath sounds may even diminish to the point of being almost silent. Stridor, a harsh, high-pitched sound heard on inspiration, occurs when swelling in the upper airway (near the vocal cords and throat) begins to close off the airway. It can eventually lead to total obstruction.

Position an alert patient in a tripod position, leaning forward; this position will facilitate air entry into the lungs and may help the patient to relax. Do not hesitate to initiate high-flow oxygen therapy. For unresponsive patients or those with an altered mental status who are in severe respiratory distress, you may have to assist ventilations using a bag-mask device, attached to a high concentration of oxygen. The positive pressure ventilations you provide will force air through the swelling in the airway and into the lungs while you await more definitive treatment. Standard airway procedures and positive pressure ventilation are described in detail in Chapter 11, *Airway Management*.

Although respiratory complaints are most common, some patients in anaphylaxis may present primarily with signs and symptoms of circulatory distress, such as hypotension. Palpate for the presence and quality of a radial pulse to quickly identify how the patient's circulatory system is responding to the reaction. If the patient is unresponsive and pulseless, begin basic life support measures and use an automated external defibrillator if necessary. Assess for a rapid pulse rate; pale, cool, cyanotic or red, moist skin; and delayed capillary refill, all of which may indicate hypoperfusion. Treatment for shock includes administering oxygen, placing the patient supine, and preventing the loss of body heat. The definitive treatment for shock resulting from anaphylaxis is epinephrine, discussed later in this chapter.

Words of Wisdom

The definitive treatment for anaphylaxis is epinephrine!

Expose and evaluate the skin for erythema, rashes, edema, moisture, pruritus, and urticaria. Pallor and cyanosis may be present as well. Bite or sting marks may be observed, depending on the cause of the allergic reaction.

If anaphylaxis is suspected, or if a relatively mild allergic reaction appears to be worsening, immediate transport to the closest, most appropriate facility is warranted. Before leaving the scene, be sure to take along the patient's medications (eg, auto-injectors and inhalers). Make your transport decision based on findings in the primary survey. Anaphylaxis may present as affecting two or more body systems, so the picture can be confusing at times. You will need to use your assessment skills to identify the potential for anaphylaxis, take aggressive action to treat the patient, and stop the anaphylactic process as rapidly as possible. If the patient has signs of respiratory distress or shock, treat those conditions and transport. (For information on how to treat shock, see Chapter 14, *Shock*.) In contrast, if the patient is calm and does not exhibit severe signs and symptoms, continue the assessment at the scene.

Words of Wisdom

Think of a patient with anaphylaxis as simultaneously experiencing three types of shock:

- Cardiogenic shock due to decreased cardiac output
- Hypovolemic shock due to fluids leaking into the tissues
- Neurogenic shock due to inability of the blood vessels to constrict

History Taking

Investigate the patient's chief complaint or history of the present illness. Identify associated signs and symptoms such as wheezing or a rash, and pertinent negatives such as lack of nausea or vomiting or no chest pain.

If the patient is responsive, begin by obtaining the SAMPLE (Signs and symptoms, Allergies, Medications, Pertinent past medical history, Last oral intake, Events leading up to the illness or injury) history (including OPQRST [Onset, Provocation/palliation, Quality, Region/radiation, Severity, Timing]) and the following information specific to allergic reactions:

- **Have any interventions already been completed?** Prior to your arrival, the patient or other emergency medical responders may have begun treatment with medication, such as an epinephrine auto-injector, antihistamines such as chlorpheniramine (Chlor-Trimeton) or diphenhydramine (Benadryl), or an inhaler that contains a bronchodilator (such as albuterol or metaproterenol) or aerosolized epinephrine (such as Primatene Mist or racemic epinephrine). If the patient has an EpiPen or used one, be aware that some EpiPens come with two doses. Do not discard the second dose.
- **Has the patient experienced a severe allergic reaction in the past?** If so, what happened? The patient's answers may indicate how severe the present reaction may become.
- **Be alert for any statements regarding previous exposure to common antigens.** For example, if the patient just ate peanuts, asking about previous ingestions may be useful. A severe reaction may occur at the second exposure to an antigen, so the patient might not know about the allergy. Asking about medications, and in particular new medications, may also help identify the antigen.

Secondary Assessment

Next, perform a physical examination. If the patient is exhibiting life-threatening signs and symptoms, perform the examination en route to the hospital.

If you have not already done so, auscultate for abnormal breath sounds such as wheezing or stridor, and carefully inspect the skin for swelling, rashes, hives, and signs of the source of the reaction—for example, bite, sting, or contact marks. A rapidly spreading rash can be concerning because it may indicate a systemic reaction. The skin may appear pale or cyanotic and cool; however, red, hot skin is typical in the early stages, suggesting a systemic reaction as the blood vessels lose their ability to constrict and blood moves outward and closer to the skin. If a systemic reaction continues, the body will have difficulty supplying blood and oxygen to the vital organs. One of the first signs that this has occurred will be altered mental status, as the brain is deprived of oxygen and glucose.

Vital signs help determine whether the body is compensating for the stress imposed upon the body by the reaction. Assess baseline vital signs, including the pulse and respiratory rate, blood pressure, pupillary response, and oxygen saturation. Rapid respiratory and pulse rates may indicate respiratory distress or systemic shock. Tachycardia and hypotension are ominous signs, indicating systemic vascular collapse and shock. Remember that skin signs may be unreliable indicators of hypoperfusion, as they may vary widely or be hidden by rashes and swelling.

You should use a cardiac monitor in your assessment because dysrhythmias may be associated with anaphylaxis. Monitoring through pulse oximetry may alert you to low oxygen saturation, which will assist in identifying the patient's degree of respiratory distress. However, it is important to remember that factors such as decreased circulation and exposure to carbon monoxide can alter pulse oximetry readings. End-tidal carbon dioxide ($ETCO_2$) levels should be monitored because they may be elevated in anaphylaxis and are more reliable than pulse oximetry in low-perfusion states. In nonintubated patients, the waveform is more important than the numeric value obtained during capnography because capnography results are not always reliable in such patients. The partial pressure of carbon dioxide will be elevated, and the $ETCO_2$ value will be normal to low because of poor alveolar gas exchange. The decision to administer oxygen to a patient experiencing an allergic reaction should be based on careful assessment of the patient's airway patency, work of breathing, and abnormal breath sounds upon auscultation, not solely on the pulse oximetry readings.

Reassessment

Reassessment is conducted typically en route to the receiving hospital. A patient experiencing a suspected allergic reaction should be monitored with vigilance. Deterioration of the patient's condition can be rapid and fatal, so special attention should be given to any signs of airway compromise. The patient's anxiety level and mental status should be monitored as well because these may provide additional indications of the course of the reaction. Monitor for signs of shock, and, if present, treat immediately.

To treat allergic reactions, you must first identify the severity of the reaction. Mild reactions may only require supportive care and monitoring. On the other hand, anaphylaxis can produce severe or rapidly progressing signs and symptoms, requiring more aggressive treatment, including epinephrine and ventilatory support. In either situation, the patient should be transported to a medical facility for further evaluation.

Recheck your interventions. If you administered epinephrine, what was the effect? Has the patient's condition improved? Does the patient need a second dose? More than one injection of epinephrine may be appropriate if the patient has decreasing mental status, increased breathing difficulty, or decreasing blood pressure. Remember to consult medical control before administering any subsequent doses for which you have not already obtained authorization. Identify and treat changes in the patient's condition.

The point at which you contact medical control depends on your assessment findings and the urgency of care required. In some allergic reactions, you may use standing orders to administer epinephrine before ever calling medical control. At other times, the reaction may be less severe and you may question whether the patient needs an injection of epinephrine. Medical control will be most helpful when the reaction is less severe. Follow your local protocols, which may guide you in providing life-saving care without needing to contact medical control.

Your documentation should not only include the signs and symptoms found during your assessment, but should also clearly show *why* you chose to administer the care you provided. If anyone should later question your care, your documentation will show the reasoning for your actions. Finally, be certain to record the patient's response to your treatment.

Words of Wisdom

While one advanced emergency medical technician is getting oxygen ready, the other should be assisting the patient into semi-Fowler position. This positioning will improve perfusion to the brain while easing the patient's respiratory effort.

YOU are the Provider — PART 4

As your emergency medical technician (EMT) partner returns with the stretcher, you inform him of the patient's worsening condition and indicate that you plan to treat the patient initially on scene before transporting. Because your service carries adult EpiPens, you are able to rapidly administer the epinephrine in his lateral thigh. You also initiate intravenous (IV) access with a large-bore IV catheter while your partner assembles a handheld nebulizer. Once IV access is established, you establish a line of normal saline at a wide-open rate and administer a 20-mL/kg bolus. After confirming that the patient has no known allergies (other than a possible new penicillin allergy), and following local protocols, you add 2.5 mg of albuterol sulfate to the nebulizer and instruct the patient on its proper use.

Recording Time: 8 Minutes	
Respirations	40 breaths/min; severe wheezes bilaterally; audible stridor
Pulse	Absent radial pulses; carotid, 144 beats/min
Skin	Red, swollen patches on torso, extending to arms and legs; seems to be progressing
Blood pressure	72/34 mm Hg
Oxygen saturation (Spo_2)	93% on 100% oxygen

6. What will administering albuterol sulfate do to the respirations? What will it do to the patient's oxygen saturation level?
7. What is the purpose of the IV fluid bolus?

Emergency Medical Care

You will need to differentiate between anaphylaxis and other conditions with similar symptoms. People who are having allergic reactions are separated into two groups for treatment purposes. The first group includes patients who have signs of an allergic reaction (for example, hives) but no signs of anaphylaxis. The drug of choice in this case is diphenhydramine. Continue to monitor for changes in the patient's condition, but recognize that most patients in this group will recover with no further problems.

The second group includes patients with signs of anaphylaxis. These patients require 100% oxygen, epinephrine, and antihistamines (usually diphenhydramine). Whenever dyspnea and/or signs of shock are present with signs of an allergic reaction, you should administer epinephrine, closely monitor the patient, and provide rapid transport.

Words of Wisdom

Maintain a high index of suspicion if a reaction has occurred previously and the patient has been exposed to the same substance.

If the patient appears to be having a severe allergic or anaphylactic reaction, you should administer basic life support and provide prompt transport to the hospital. When possible, remove the patient from the situation involving the antigen or the antigen from the patient. For example, if the patient is allergic to peanuts and is being exposed to peanuts through inspiration, you may need to remove the patient from the room because you may not be able to eliminate the peanut allergen from the air.

Maintain the airway. If the patient is alert, allow him or her to assume a position of comfort that does not compromise breathing. If the patient cannot sit up, have suction readily available to maintain a clear airway. Use an appropriate oxygen delivery device for supplemental oxygen administration, and consider early transport. Administer high-flow oxygen via a nonrebreathing mask at 15 L/min if the patient is breathing inadequately, and be prepared to assist ventilations. Also, maintain a high index of suspicion for the potential for airway occlusion because of swelling or edema. Consider calling early for advanced life support backup, and be prepared to assist breathing as needed. If necessary, treat the patient for shock by placing him or her in the position dictated by local protocol, maintain body heat with a blanket, and initiate IV therapy as discussed in Chapter 13, *Vascular Access and Medication Administration*.

Special Populations

Because epinephrine can stress the heart, it is important to use this drug only as needed in older patients and patients with a history of cardiovascular disease. Monitor patients closely for cardiac problems or hypertension.

Maintain circulation. Insert at least one large-bore IV catheter, such as a 16- or 18-gauge, to administer an isotonic solution (lactated Ringer solution or normal saline) at a wide-open rate. Ideally, you should initiate two IV lines en route to the emergency department. This step is crucial, especially if the patient is hypotensive and does not respond to epinephrine. Initially, administer 20 mL/kg of isotonic fluid (normal saline or lactated Ringer) rapidly over 15 minutes intravenously or via intraosseous administration, repeating as needed.[5] If there is no response, consider calling for paramedic backup for administration of a vasopressor in conjunction with fluid administration.

Find out which interventions have been completed before your arrival. Determine whether the patient has any prescribed, preloaded medications for allergic reactions (such as an epinephrine auto-injector), and then inform medical control of the patient's condition.

Words of Wisdom

Whether naturally occurring in the body (endogenous) or made by a drug manufacturer, epinephrine works rapidly to raise the blood pressure by constricting the blood vessels and increasing the strength of cardiac contractions. Epinephrine also dilates the bronchioles, thereby improving the patient's breathing.

- **Indications:** Severe allergic reaction or hypersensitivity to exposed substance or anaphylaxis
- **Contraindications:** None in a life-threatening emergency; however, consult medical control when the patient has a history of heart disease or acute coronary syndrome
- **Actions:** Vasoconstriction and increased cardiac contractility, bronchodilation
- **Side effects:** Tachycardia, sweating, pale skin, dizziness, headache, anxiety, cardiac dysrhythmias
- **Dosage:**
  - Adults: 0.3 to 0.5 mg of a 1-mg/mL (1:1,000) epinephrine solution subcutaneously or intramuscularly (IM)
  - Children: 0.01 mg/kg of a 1-mg/mL (1:1,000) epinephrine solution subcutaneously or IM

Early administration of epinephrine should be a priority. It is much easier to obtain IV access before the patient's blood pressure starts to decrease. Use the IM route if the patient shows evidence of airway or respiratory compromise or hypotension. IM administration of epinephrine is preferred for anaphylaxis because it provides more rapid absorption than does subcutaneous administration. Administration in the thigh is preferred over the deltoid site for more rapid absorption. Subcutaneous administration of epinephrine is unpredictable and may have delayed effects in the presence of shock.

Epinephrine is the drug of choice for anaphylactic reactions because its effects are immediate: It can rapidly reverse the histamine-related effects of anaphylaxis. The alpha-adrenergic properties of epinephrine cause the blood vessels to constrict, which reverses vasodilation and hypotension. This elevates the diastolic pressure and improves coronary blood flow. The beta-1 adrenergic effects increase cardiac contractility, reversing the depressing effects on the heart and improving the strength of cardiac contractions. The beta-2 adrenergic effects cause bronchodilation, relieving bronchospasm in the lungs.

Many patients and EMTs carry epinephrine in the form of an EpiPen, so the patient may have administered this medication before your arrival. Patients who receive epinephrine must be monitored closely for adverse effects. Use a cardiac monitor, if available, to watch for dysrhythmias, and reassess the patient's vital signs at least every 5 minutes.

If the patient is able to use the auto-injector on his or her own, your role is limited to helping the patient do so. To use, or help the patient use, the auto-injector, you should first receive a direct order from medical control or follow local protocol. Follow standard precautions, and make sure the medication has been prescribed specifically for that patient. If it is discolored or has expired, do not give the medication.

Follow the steps in **Skill Drill 22-1** to use an EpiPen auto-injector. In a life-threatening situation, do not delay administration of epinephrine to expose the thigh. An EpiPen can be administered directly through clothing. Note that the injection time, which was formerly recommended as 10 seconds, has been reduced to 3 seconds; also, take steps to ensure the patient's leg does not move during administration. These steps may help decrease the chance of patient harm during the administration process.[6] See Chapter 13, *Vascular Access and Medication Administration*, for more information on administering a medication from a vial.

After the medication has been administered, properly dispose of the injector in a biohazard container. Record the time and dose, patient's vital signs, and any response to the medication. If there is no improvement after 5 minutes, consider administration of a second dose. You may also need to give more than one injection of epinephrine if the patient displays decreased mental status, increased breathing difficulty, or decreased blood pressure. Be sure to consult medical control first.

Skill Drill 22-1 Using an EpiPen Auto-injector

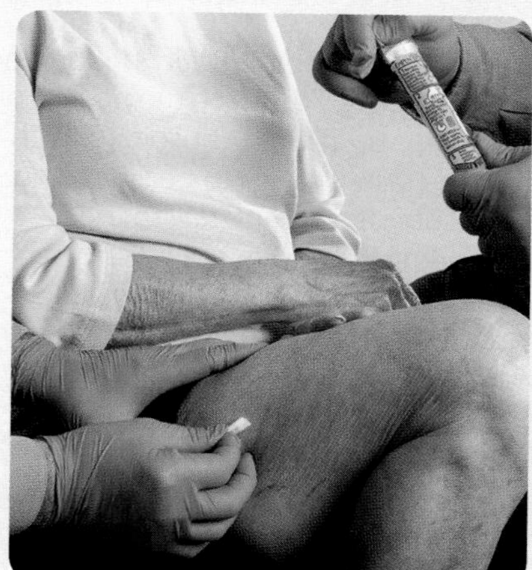

Step 1 Remove the auto-injector's safety cap. Expose and quickly wipe the thigh with antiseptic, if time permits.

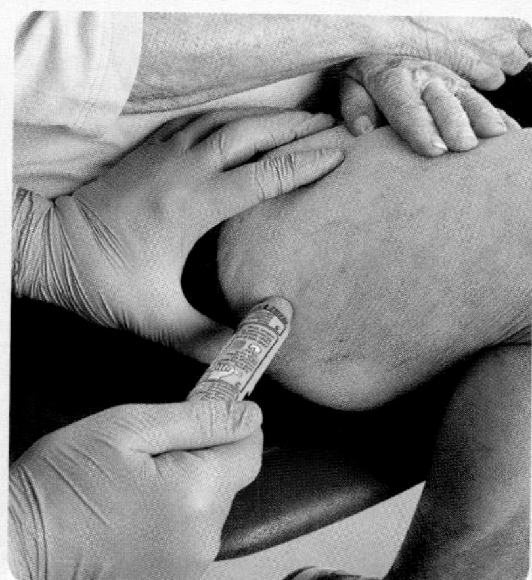

Step 2 Place the tip of the auto-injector against the lateral part of the thigh. Push the auto-injector firmly against the thigh until a click is heard. Hold it in place until all the medication has been injected (3 seconds). Ensure the patient's leg does not move during administration.

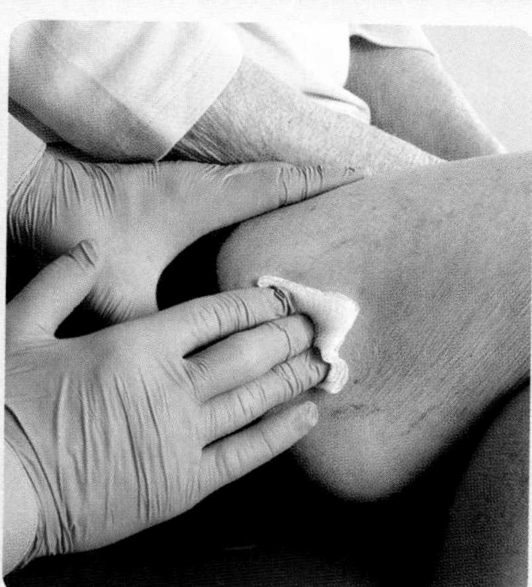

Step 3 Rub the area for 10 seconds.

Words of Wisdom

The adult EpiPen delivers 0.3 mg of a 1-mg/mL (1:1,000) solution of epinephrine IM. The EpiPen Jr, which contains 0.15 mg of a 0.5-mg/mL (1:2,000) solution, is used for children who weigh less than 33 lb (15 kg).

Other allergy kits may contain oral or IM antihistamines, agents that block the effect of histamine. These medications work relatively slowly, within several minutes to 1 hour. Because epinephrine can have an effect within 1 minute, it is the primary way to save the life of someone having a severe anaphylactic reaction. However, epinephrine and antihistamines work synergistically, and both play key roles in reversing and stopping the effects of histamine.

Because epinephrine constricts blood vessels, it may cause the patient's blood pressure to increase significantly. Monitor IV fluid administration carefully to prevent inadvertent fluid overload. Other side effects of epinephrine include tachycardia, anxiety, pallor, dizziness, chest pain, headache, nausea, and vomiting. In a life-threatening situation, the administration of epinephrine outweighs the risk of side effects. However, patients who do not exhibit signs of respiratory compromise or hypotension and do not meet the criteria for a diagnosis of anaphylaxis should not be given epinephrine.

Whether or not your emergency treatment includes epinephrine, you should always provide prompt transport for any patient who is experiencing an allergic reaction or has experienced a poisonous envenomation or bite. Continue to reassess the patient's vital signs en route; remember that signs and symptoms may change rapidly when a patient has an allergic or anaphylactic reaction. If the patient's condition improves, provide supportive care, including continuing oxygen therapy during transport.

Consider early transport or calling for paramedic backup if the patient needs resources beyond your capabilities. Even if you are able to stop the reaction and the patient begins to recover, it is recommended that patients be observed in a medical facility. Up to 20% of patients will experience a recurrence of the symptoms within the next 8 hours, even if they have been symptom-free for a time.[7] After the patient has been symptom-free for 4 hours, he or she can be released from the facility but should be instructed to return or call an ambulance if the symptoms recur.

YOU are the Provider — PART 5

After administering epinephrine and albuterol, you note that the patient's work of breathing has decreased, and stridor is no longer present. Mild angioedema is apparent, however, and the wheezing is still present bilaterally. You place the patient on the stretcher, being sure to continue the administration of 100% oxygen, and initiate rapid transport to the hospital, which is 14 minutes away. You note that the patient's blood pressure has increased slightly, but the rash appears to be spreading. You opt to contact medical control because you are concerned that the patient has not responded completely to the administration of the epinephrine. Online medical control orders administration of a second dose of 0.5 mg of a 1-mg/mL (1:1,000) concentration epinephrine subcutaneously. After confirming the order, you draw up 0.5 mg of epinephrine and administer it to the patient. After several minutes, you note that the rash appears to be decreasing, and the patient states that he does not itch as badly any more. His respirations are regular with equal chest rise and no accessory muscle use.

Recording Time: 18 Minutes	
Respirations	24 breaths/min; clear bilaterally
Pulse	Strong distal pulse; 92 beats/min
Skin	Small area of redness on anterior torso; area appears to be decreasing
Blood pressure	104/72 mm Hg
Oxygen saturation (Spo_2)	98% on 100% oxygen

You continue monitoring the patient en route to the hospital. On arrival, you give your report to the emergency department nurse and complete your patient care report while your partner readies the ambulance for your next call.

8. What are some possible side effects of epinephrine administration?

Table 22-5 Management of Anaphylaxis
▪ Remove the offending agent. ▪ Position the patient as appropriate. ▪ Apply high-flow oxygen, or assist ventilation as needed. ▪ Obtain IV access. ▪ Give fluid resuscitation as needed. ▪ Administer epinephrine and an antihistamine (eg, diphenhydramine) as indicated. ▪ Transport promptly. ▪ Frequently reassess the patient, and provide psychological support.

Abbreviation: IV, intravenous

Words of Wisdom

Allergic reactions and responses to bites and stings can become rapidly life threatening. With prompt care, severe signs and symptoms may subside just as quickly. Thus, performing a multisystem examination and documenting your findings is important before and after treatment. Give particular attention to the patient's skin condition and to the status of respiratory, circulatory, and mental functions.

Table 22-5 summarizes the management of anaphylaxis.

▶ Assessment and Management of Insect Stings

Thousands of people in the United States are stung by insects each year.[8] Deaths resulting from anaphylactic reactions to stinging insects far outnumber deaths due to snake bites: This type of allergy accounts for approximately 90 to 100 deaths each year in the United States.[8]

The stinging organ of most bees, wasps, and hornets is a small, hollow spine projecting from the abdomen. Venom can be injected through this spine directly into the skin. The stinger of the honeybee is barbed, so the bee cannot withdraw it Figure 22-4A. Instead, the bee leaves a part of its abdomen embedded with the stinger and dies shortly after flying away. In contrast, wasps and hornets do not have this handicap; they can sting repeatedly Figure 22-4B. Because these insects usually fly away after stinging, it is often impossible to identify which species was responsible for the injury.

Some ants, especially the fire ant (*Solenopsis*), also strike repeatedly, injecting a particularly irritating **toxin**, or poison, at the bite sites Figure 22-5A. It is not uncommon for a patient to rapidly sustain multiple ant bites, usually on the feet and legs Figure 22-5B.

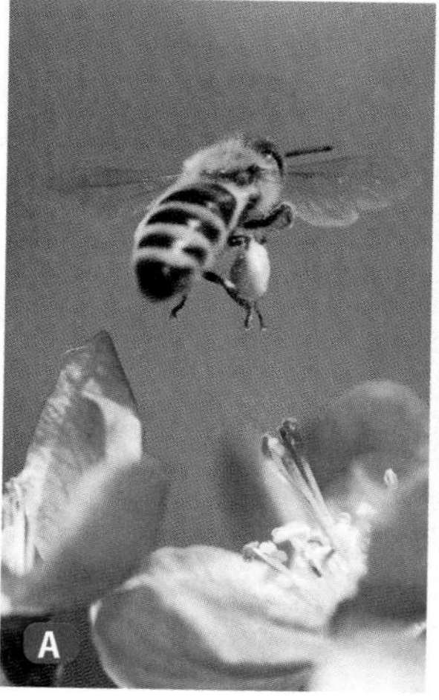

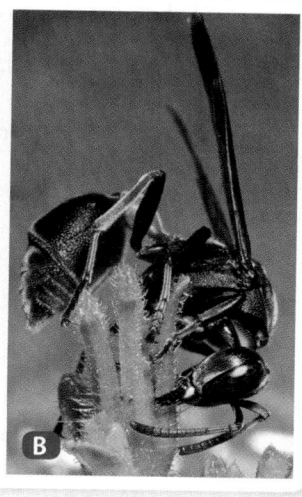

Figure 22-4 Most stinging insects inject venom through a small, hollow spine that projects from the abdomen. **A.** The stinger of the honeybee is barbed; the honeybee cannot withdraw its stinger once it has stung someone. **B.** The wasp's stinger is unbarbed, meaning that it can inflict multiple stings.

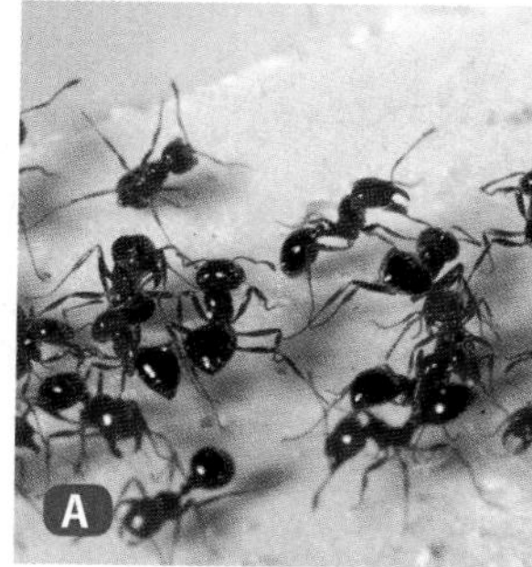

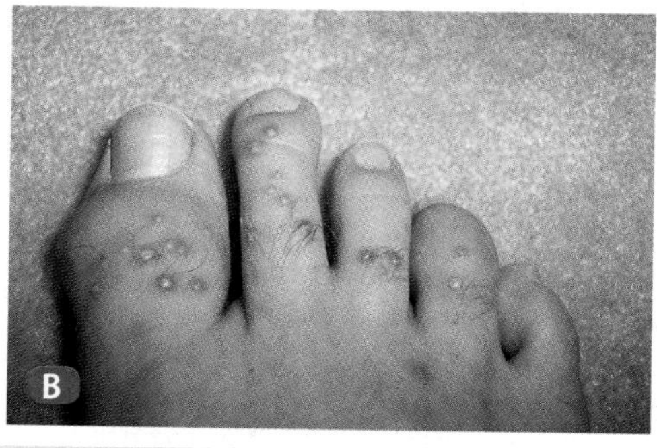

Figure 22-5 A. The fire ant. **B.** Fire ants inject an irritating toxin at multiple sites. Bites are generally found on the feet and the legs and appear as multiple small, raised pustules.

Signs and symptoms of insect stings and bites include sudden pain, swelling, localized heat, widespread urticaria, and redness in light-skinned people, usually at the site of injury. There may be itching and sometimes

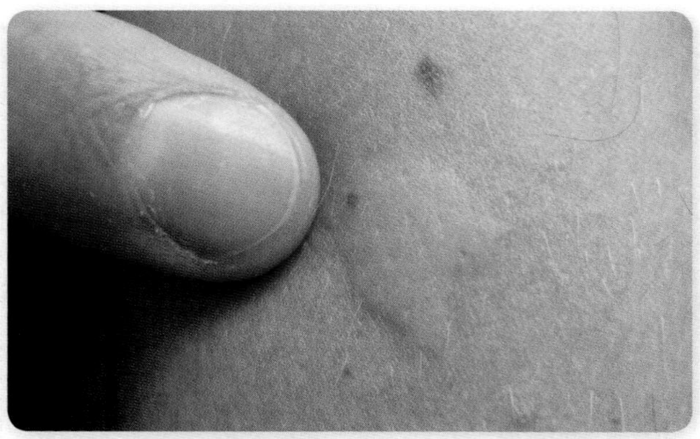

Figure 22-6 A wheal is a whitish, firm elevation of the skin that occurs after an insect sting or bite.

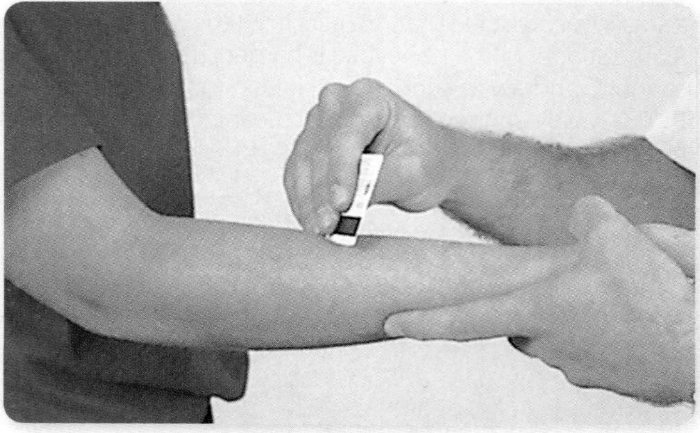

Figure 22-7 To remove the stinger of a honeybee, gently scrape the skin with the edge of a sharp, stiff object such as a credit card.

a **wheal**, which is a raised, swollen, well-defined area on the skin Figure 22-6. Applying ice sometimes makes wheals less irritating. The swelling associated with an insect bite may be dramatic and sometimes frightening to the patient or to you. However, as long as these manifestations remain localized, they are not usually serious.

Because the stinger of a honeybee remains in the wound created by its sting, it can continue to inject venom for up to 20 minutes following the actual sting. Thus, if the stinger is still in place, attempt to remove the stinger by scraping the skin with the edge of a sharp, stiff object such as a credit card Figure 22-7. Do not use tweezers or forceps to remove the stinger because this may squeeze more venom into the wound.

Gently wash the area of the insect sting with soap and water or a mild antiseptic. Try to remove any jewelry from the area before swelling begins. Position the injection site slightly below the level of the heart, and apply ice or cold packs to the area. Placing ice over the injury site may slow absorption of the toxin, diminish swelling, and relieve pain.

Be alert for signs of airway swelling and other signs of anaphylaxis such as nausea, vomiting, and abdominal cramps, and do not give the patient anything by mouth. Place the patient in the supine position if indicated, and give oxygen if needed. Monitor the patient's vital signs, and be prepared to provide further support as needed.

Patient Education

The best management of anaphylaxis and allergic reactions is to educate patients about prevention and self-preservation. At a minimum, discuss the following topics:

- **Avoid the antigen.** Review information on the offending item. For example, if the patient is allergic to penicillin, he or she should be provided with a list of drugs that include penicillin and the alternative names for penicillin. Drugs that may produce a cross-reaction should also be discussed. Food allergies can be even more difficult to avoid. For example, peanuts can be found in many other foods: Peanut oil may be used to prepare foods that do not actually contain peanuts, and peanut butter may be an ingredient in various foods. Some patients are so allergic to peanuts that just using the same devices to process non–peanut-containing foods can cause a reaction. Patients must be educated to avoid the allergen, read labels, and ask about how food is prepared to avoid exposure. Latex allergies are also a concern, so advising patients to notify care providers of latex allergies is essential. Many services are latex-free, but not all of them, so patients must inform providers of their allergies so exposures can be avoided.
- **Notify all health personnel of the allergy.** Review the need to alert health personnel to the allergy. This step is important because patients often think only a physician would need this information, not an emergency medical services (EMS) provider.
- **Wear identification tags or bracelets.** These items notify providers of allergies in case the patient is unable to do so.
- **Carry an anaphylaxis kit or EpiPen.** A reaction may occur rapidly or worsen before help can arrive. Make sure the patient and his or her family knows how to use the kit or EpiPen.
- **Report symptoms early.** Ideally, interventions should begin before the situation becomes life threatening. The patient should recognize that reactions can occur more rapidly and with greater severity with repeated exposures.

YOU are the Provider SUMMARY

1. What is the major difference between an allergic reaction and anaphylaxis?

The major difference between an allergic reaction and anaphylaxis is that an allergic reaction is more of an "annoyance," whereas anaphylaxis is a potentially life-threatening problem. Anaphylaxis typically involves two or more organ systems, whereas an allergic reaction typically involves only one system.

2. How are the treatments for these two conditions the same? How do they differ?

Treatment for an allergic reaction is typically supportive. The signs and symptoms can usually be relieved by supplemental oxygen to decrease anxiety and administration of an antihistamine, such as diphenhydramine, to decrease the size and intensity of the rash. Anaphylaxis typically involves the airway, causing stridor or bronchospasm. These effects can be relieved by administration of medication by an inhaled bronchodilator, such as albuterol sulfate. Epinephrine may need to be administered to attempt to cause vasoconstriction and improve contractility, thereby increasing the blood pressure, and to ensure bronchodilation.

3. What is the significance of stridor not being present during airway assessment?

Stridor indicates an upper airway obstruction due to swelling, which, in this patient, is not present yet. Since stridor is absent, you can assume that the patient currently has a patent airway.

4. In which position should this patient be placed?

This patient should be placed in the position of comfort. Any position that maximizes oxygenation and ventilation, while minimizing anxiety, should be considered.

5. Based on his presentation, what is the definitive treatment for this patient?

The patient is showing signs of respiratory and cardiovascular compromise indicating anaphylaxis. Epinephrine is the definitive treatment for anaphylaxis.

6. What will administering albuterol sulfate do to the respirations? What will it do to the patient's oxygen saturation level?

The administration of albuterol sulfate may initially cause the patient's respirations to increase; this patient already has increased work of breathing and will be attempting to get the medication into his respiratory tract to alleviate the respiratory distress more quickly. However, once the albuterol sulfate begins to work by dilating the bronchioles, the patient's respirations will decrease and his oxygen saturation level will increase.

7. What is the purpose of the IV fluid bolus?

The IV fluid bolus is intended to maintain circulation. Insert at least one large-bore IV catheter to administer an isotonic solution (lactated Ringer solution or normal saline) at a wide-open rate. Ideally, you should place two IV lines en route to the emergency department. This step is crucial, especially if the patient is hypotensive and does not respond to the epinephrine. Initially, a 20-mL/kg bolus should be administered. If there is no response, contact medical control prior to administering more fluid, and consider paramedic rendezvous or backup.

8. What are some possible side effects of epinephrine administration?

Common side effects of epinephrine are tachycardia, palpitations, sweating, pale skin, headache, anxiety, dizziness, and cardiac dysrhythmias.

<table>
<tr><th colspan="6">EMS Patient Care Report (PCR)</th></tr>
<tr><td>Date: 5-7-18</td><td colspan="2">Incident No.: 3472</td><td colspan="2">Nature of Call: Possible allergic reaction</td><td>Location: 209 Branson Street</td></tr>
<tr><td>Dispatched: 1346</td><td>En Route: 1347</td><td>At Scene: 1353</td><td>Transport: 1408</td><td>At Hospital: 1422</td><td>In Service: 1446</td></tr>
<tr><th colspan="6">Patient Information</th></tr>
<tr><td colspan="3">Age: 46
Sex: M
Weight (in kg [lb]): 74 kg (163 lb)</td><td colspan="3">Allergies: No known drug allergies
Medications: Possible allergy to penicillin
Past Medical History: Upper respiratory infection
Chief Complaint: Rash, itch</td></tr>
</table>

YOU are the Provider SUMMARY (continued)

Vital Signs				
Time: 1354	**BP:** Not obtained	**Pulse:** Not obtained	**Respirations:** 36	**Spo_2:** Not obtained
Time: 1358	**BP:** 76/32	**Pulse:** 138	**Respirations:** 40	**Spo_2:** 93% on 100% O_2
Time: 1401	**BP:** 72/34	**Pulse:** 144	**Respirations:** 40	**Spo_2:** 93% on 100% O_2
Time: 1411	**BP:** 104/72	**Pulse:** 92	**Respirations:** 24	**Spo_2:** 98% on 100% O_2
EMS Treatment (circle all that apply)				
Oxygen @ 15 **L/min via (circle one):** **NC** **(NRM)** **Bag-mask device**		**Assisted Ventilation**	**Airway Adjunct**	**CPR**
Defibrillation	**Bleeding Control**	**Bandaging**	**Splinting**	**Other:**
Narrative				

EMS called to above location for a 46 y/o male with a possible allergic reaction. On arrival, patient found seated on sofa, AO×4, but anxious. Patient presents with mild respiratory distress, absent peripheral pulses, and mottled skin. Patient states that he had a doctor's appointment this morning and his physician prescribed a new medication, penicillin. Patient states that he has never taken this medication before, and took it approximately 1 hour ago. Approximately 30 minutes later, a large rash developed on anterior part of torso, with profuse itching. Patient presents with increased work of breathing, progression of rash, and audible stridor. Supplemental oxygen applied via nonrebreathing mask at 15 L/min. 0.3 mg of 1 mg/mL (1:1,000) epinephrine administered IM to right lateral thigh, 2.5 mg albuterol sulfate administered via nebulizer, and 16-gauge IV line established in left AC, with 20-mL/kg bolus of normal saline initiated. After administration of medications, patient presents with decreased work of breathing, no stridor, and diminished areas of rash. Patient assisted to stretcher and secured in position of comfort. Transported nonemergency to North Keen Medical Center. En route, patient has increasing angioedema and wheezing, and rash continues to spread. Per medical control, second dose of 0.5 mg of 1 mg/mL (1:1,000) epinephrine for progressing anaphylaxis given subcutaneously in left forearm. On reassessment, patient began showing marked improvement in signs and symptoms, with wheezing decreased and size of rash shrinking. Report called to emergency department with condition and ETA. On arrival, care transferred and report given to nurse without incident.**End of report**

Prep Kit

▶ Ready for Review

- An allergic reaction is a response to chemicals the body releases to combat certain stimuli, called *allergens*. Almost any substance can trigger the body's immune system and cause an allergic reaction. Allergic reactions occur most often in response to five categories of stimuli: insect bites and stings, medications, foods, plants, and chemicals.
- Anaphylaxis is a life-threatening allergic reaction mounted by multiple organ systems that must be treated with epinephrine. Wheezing and skin wheals can be signs of anaphylaxis.
- The immune system protects the human body from substances and organisms that are considered foreign to the body.
- Allergens enter the body through oral ingestion, injection or envenomation, inhalation, or topical absorption. Injected and inhaled allergens tend to cause the most severe reactions, but a severe reaction can occur by any route.
- When a foreign substance first invades the body, the primary response begins. If the body is unable to identify the substance, immune cells record the features of the outside substance and produce antibodies to inactivate the foreign substance. This process is called *development of sensitivity*.
- Basophils and mast cells contain antibodies and can recognize the foreign substance should it

Prep Kit *(continued)*

enter the body again. Basophils are stationed in specific sites within the tissues. Mast cells are on patrol throughout the body.

- Chemical mediators are essentially the body's weapons against foreign substances. They release substances when an antigen invades the body and combines with one of the antibodies. If this response spreads throughout the body (becoming systemic), it causes the signs and symptoms of an anaphylactic reaction. Allergic reactions are more localized.
- Histamines are some of the primary chemical mediators. They cause the blood vessels in the local area to dilate and the capillaries to leak; this translates into flushed skin, hypotension, tissue swelling, and fluid secretion.
- Other chemical mediators include the leukotrienes, which cause additional dilation and leaking of fluid into the tissues.
- Signs and symptoms of an anaphylactic or allergic reaction vary but can include hives, pruritus (itching), flushed skin, swelling, respiratory symptoms (wheezing, stridor, dyspnea, and angioedema), cardiovascular symptoms, gastrointestinal symptoms, neurologic symptoms, and even shock if the reaction is severe.
- When assessing a person who may be having an allergic reaction, check for flushing, itching, and swelling skin; hives; wheezing and stridor; a persistent cough; a decrease in blood pressure; a weak pulse; dizziness; abdominal cramps; and headache.
- The patient history will help to identify problems specific to the allergic reaction. When assessing a patient with an allergic reaction, ask if the patient has a history of allergies, what the patient was exposed to, when the exposure occurred, and how the patient was exposed. Determine the onset of symptoms, the effects of the exposure, and the progression of those effects.
- The airway is always a priority in every situation, and assessing for the presence of stridor and hoarseness should indicate the severity of the airway compromise in a patient with an anaphylactic or allergic reaction. All patients with suspected anaphylaxis require oxygen.
- People who know that they are allergic to bee, hornet, yellow jacket, or wasp venom often carry a bee sting kit that contains epinephrine in an auto-injector. You may help to administer this medication in this form with authorization from medical control.
- Always provide prompt transport to the hospital for any patient who is having an allergic reaction or has been bitten by a poisonous insect. Remember that the patient's condition can deteriorate rapidly. Carefully monitor the patient's vital signs en route, especially for airway compromise.
- Patients having allergic reactions are separated into two groups for treatment purposes. Those with signs and symptoms of an allergic reaction but no signs of anaphylaxis should be treated with diphenhydramine. Those with signs of anaphylaxis require 100% oxygen, epinephrine, and antihistamines. Early administration of epinephrine should be a priority.
- Management also includes removing the offending agent, providing fluid resuscitation as needed, and transporting promptly.
- Patient education related to anaphylaxis and allergic reactions includes the following points:
  - Avoid the antigen.
  - Notify all health personnel of the allergy.
  - Wear identification tags or bracelets.
  - Carry an anaphylaxis kit or EpiPen.
  - Report symptoms early.

▶ Vital Vocabulary

absorption In allergic reactions, when foreign material is deposited on and moves into the skin.

acquired immunity The immunity the body develops as part of exposure to an antigen.

allergen A substance that causes an allergic reaction.

allergic reaction The body's exaggerated immune response to an internal or a surface antigen.

anaphylactoid reaction An extreme allergic response that does not involve IgE antibody mediation. The exact mechanism is unknown, but an anaphylactoid event may occur without the patient being previously exposed to the offending agent.

anaphylaxis An extreme, life-threatening, systemic allergic reaction that may include shock and respiratory failure.

angioedema Localized areas of swelling beneath the skin, often around the eyes and lips, but can also involve other body areas as well.

antibody A protein the body produces in response to an antigen; an immunoglobulin.

antigen An agent that, when taken into the body, stimulates the formation of specific protective proteins called antibodies.

basophils White blood cells that work to produce chemical mediators during an immune response.

cellular immunity The immunity provided by special white blood cells called T cells that attack and destroy invaders.

Prep Kit *(continued)*

chemical mediators Chemicals that work to cause the immune or allergic response—for example, histamines.

envenomation The act of injecting venom.

epinephrine A substance produced by the body (commonly called adrenaline), and a drug produced by pharmaceutical companies that increases pulse rate and blood pressure; the drug of choice for treating an anaphylactic reaction.

histamine Chemical substance released by the immune system in allergic reactions that is responsible for many of the symptoms of anaphylaxis, such as vasodilation.

humoral immunity The use of antibodies dissolved in the plasma and lymph to destroy foreign substances.

hypersensitivity Abnormal sensitivity; a condition in which the body manifests an exaggerated response to the stimulus of a foreign agent.

immune system The body system that includes all of the structures and processes designed to mount a defense against foreign substances and disease-causing agents.

immunity The body's ability to protect itself from acquiring a disease.

ingestion Eating or drinking materials for absorption through the gastrointestinal tract.

inhalation In allergic reactions, breathing in foreign substances through the respiratory system.

injection In allergic reactions, piercing of the skin, followed by deposition of foreign material into the skin.

leukotrienes Chemical substances that contribute to anaphylaxis; released by the immune system in allergic reactions.

local reaction When the body limits a response to a specific area after being exposed to a foreign substance.

mast cells Cells located in the tissues that release chemical mediators in response to an antigen-antibody reaction.

natural immunity The immunity the body develops as part of being exposed to an antigen and developing antibodies—for example, exposure to measles, having the measles, and developing immunity to the measles.

primary response The first encounter with the foreign substance that initiates the immune response.

pruritus Itching.

secondary response The body's reaction when it is exposed to an antigen for which it already has antibodies, in which it responds by killing the invading substance.

sensitivity The ability of the body to recognize a foreign substance the next time it is encountered.

stridor A harsh, high-pitched respiratory sound, generally heard during inspiration, that is caused by partial blockage or narrowing of the upper airway; may be audible without a stethoscope.

systemic reaction A reaction that occurs throughout the body, possibly affecting multiple body systems.

toxin A poisonous or harmful substance.

urticaria Small areas of generalized itching and/or burning that appear as multiple raised areas on the skin; hives.

wheal A raised, swollen, well-defined area on the skin resulting from an insect bite or allergic reaction.

wheezing A high-pitched, whistling breath sound that is most prominent on expiration, and which suggests an obstruction or narrowing of the lower airways; occurs in asthma and bronchiolitis.

▶ References

1. PIMS Multimedia. Anaphylaxis fact files: II. Anaphylaxis statistics. http://www.pimsmultimedia.com/anaphylaxisfactfiles/docs/download.php?file=II_Statistics_2_29_08.pdf. Accessed February 7, 2017.
2. National Institute for Occupational Safety and Health. Insects and scorpions. July 1, 2016. https://www.cdc.gov/niosh/topics/insects/. Accessed February 7, 2017.
3. Asthma and Allergy Foundation of America. Research: allergy facts and figures. http://www.aafa.org/page/allergy-facts.aspx. Accessed February 7, 2017.
4. Johnson RF, Peebles RS. Anaphylactic shock: pathophysiology, recognition, and treatment. Medscape website. http://www.medscape.com/viewarticle/497498_8. Accessed April 4, 2017.
5. National Model EMS Clinical Guidelines. National Association of State EMS Officials. V.08-16:49-52. https://www.nasemso.org/Projects/ModelEMSClinicalGuidelines/index.asp. Revised September 15, 2014. Accessed April 7, 2017.
6. EPIPEN – epinephrine injection, EPIPENJR – epinephrine injection. DailyMed U.S. National Library of Medicine website. https://dailymed.nlm.nih.gov/dailymed/fda/fdaDrugXsl.cfm?setid=7560c201-9246-487c-a13b-6295db04274a&type=display. Revised May 2016. Accessed April 5, 2017.
7. Campbell RL, Li JT, Nicklas RA, et al. Emergency department diagnosis and treatment of anaphylaxis: a practice parameter. *Ann Allergy Asthma Immunol.* 2014;113:606.
8. National Institute for Occupational Safety and Health. Insects and scorpions. July 1, 2016. https://www.cdc.gov/niosh/topics/insects/. Accessed February 9, 2017.

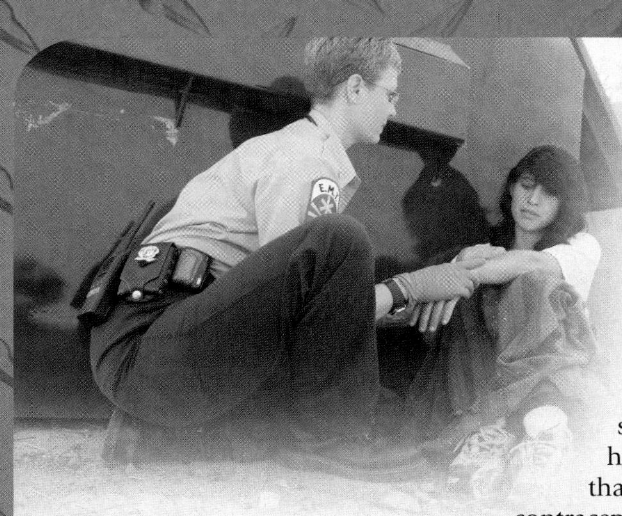

Assessment *in Action*

You are eating lunch at a local seafood restaurant when a young female employee comes up to you and says that another customer may be having an allergic reaction. As you examine the patient, you note that she is anxious with swelling and cyanosis around her mouth, a rash is visible on her chest, and she is itching profusely. The patient tells you that she is 28 years old, has no medical problems, takes an oral contraceptive daily, and has no known allergies.

1. What is the most likely route by which an allergen entered the patient's body?

A. Adsorption
B. Ingestion
C. Inhalation
D. Injection

2. The chemicals that are released during an allergic reaction cause vasodilation and vascular leakage resulting in the rash visible on her chest, known as:

A. angioedema.
B. erythema.
C. leukopenia.
D. urticaria.

3. The rash on her chest is the result of the release of which chemical mediator?

A. Histamine
B. Leukotrienes
C. Platelet-activating factor
D. Serotonin

4. As you assess the patient, you hear a harsh, high-pitched inspiratory sound. The sound that occurs when swelling in the upper airway (near the vocal cords and throat) closes off the airway, and can eventually lead to total obstruction, is called:

A. stridor.
B. rales.
C. rhonchi.
D. wheezing.

5. Which of the following medications might be prescribed for a patient with a history of seafood allergies?

A. Antipyretics
B. Antibiotics
C. Antihistamines
D. Beta-blockers

6. In the setting of anaphylaxis, administration of epinephrine causes:

A. constriction of the blood vessels.
B. dilation of the blood vessels.
C. constriction of the bronchioles.
D. dilation of adrenal glands.

7. What is the adult dose of epinephrine in an EpiPen?

A. 0.15 mg
B. 0.3 mg
C. 0.45 mg
D. 0.5 mg

8. Of the signs and symptoms the patient presents with, which should most concern you?

A. Her anxiety
B. The swelling and cyanosis around her mouth
C. The rash on her chest
D. Her perfuse itching

9. What is the proper way to remove a stinger from a patient?

10. What are the three types of shock that may affect a patient with anaphylaxis?

CHAPTER 23

Toxicology

National EMS Education Standard Competencies

Medicine

Applies fundamental knowledge to provide basic and selected advanced emergency care and transportation based on assessment findings for an acutely ill patient.

Toxicology

Recognition and management of

- Carbon monoxide poisoning (p 993)
- Nerve agent poisoning (p 992)

How and when to contact a poison control center (pp 971-972)

Anatomy, physiology, pathophysiology, assessment, and management of

- Inhaled poisons (pp 973-974)
- Ingested poisons (pp 972-973)
- Injected poisons (p 974)
- Absorbed poisons (pp 974-975)
- Alcohol intoxication and withdrawal (pp 982-983)
- Opiate toxidrome (pp 975, 983-986)

Knowledge Objectives

1. Define the terms toxicology, poison, and overdose. (p 971)
2. Describe the routes by which poisons are absorbed in the body. (pp 972-975)
3. Discuss major toxidromes and their use in assessment and management of toxicologic emergencies. (p 975)
4. Identify the common signs and symptoms of poisoning. (p 976)
5. Discuss substance abuse and concepts associated with it. (p 977)
6. Describe the assessment and treatment of a patient with suspected poisoning. (pp 978-982)
7. Describe the assessment and treatment of a patient with a possible overdose. (pp 978-982)
8. Understand the role of airway management in a patient with poisoning or overdose. (p 979)
9. Explain the use of activated charcoal, including indications, contraindications, and the need to obtain approval from medical control before its administration. (pp 981-982)
10. Discuss emergencies related to severe intoxication, including alcoholism. (pp 982-983)
11. Explain the effects of each of the specific types of poisons: alcohol, narcotics, opiates, opioids, stimulants, marijuana, hallucinogens, sedative-hypnotic drugs, cardiac medications, other medications, organophosphates, inhalants, metals, and caustics. (pp 982-996)
12. Describe the assessment and treatment for the patient with suspected food poisoning. (p 996)
13. Describe the assessment and treatment for the patient with suspected plant poisoning. (pp 997-998)

Skills Objectives

1. Demonstrate the steps in the assessment and treatment of the patient with suspected poisoning. (pp 978-982)
2. Demonstrate the steps in the assessment and treatment of the patient with suspected overdose. (pp 978-982)
3. Demonstrate the steps required to administer activated charcoal. (pp 981-982)

Introduction

In the course of their duties, advanced emergency medical technicians (AEMTs) treat patients who have taken drugs of abuse (including alcohol) on an almost daily basis. Given the nature of drug use and abuse, it is impossible to accurately identify how many users of such substances exist. Sometimes the abused substance is legal (**licit**), as in the case of alcohol and oxycodone (when the patient has a prescription). At other times, the substance is illegal (**illicit**), as in the case of heroin and ecstasy.

Before delving into this challenging area of AEMT practice in depth, it is important to define some key terms. A **poison** is a substance that is toxic by nature, no matter how it gets into the body or in which quantity it is taken. At a minimum, a poison has the potential to make people ill; in the worst-case scenario, it will kill them. By contrast, a **drug** is a substance that has a physiologic effect—for example, reducing inflammation, fighting bacteria, or producing euphoria—when given in the appropriate circumstances and in the appropriate dose. (A medication refers to a substance used to treat an illness or medical condition.) When a drug (licit or illicit) is taken in excess, the person is said to have overdosed; an **overdose** is a toxicologic emergency, because the person has been poisoned. In a nutshell, a poison is always a poison, whereas a licit or illicit substance can poison a person if it is taken to excess.

Types of Toxicologic Emergencies

Toxicology is the study of toxic or poisonous substances. **Toxicologic emergencies** usually fall under one of two general headings: intentional or unintentional. Poisoning in adults is commonly intentional. In particular, suicide is often accomplished with the use of drugs.

An unintentional toxicologic emergency can occur in many ways. For example, medication dosing errors are common problems in clinical practice. In some cases, the event may be idiosyncratic: 2 mg of midazolam (Versed) may relax one patient but cause respiratory arrest in another person.

Childhood poisonings are common, especially in young children. Young children may put anything into their mouths, such as colorful berries found on a house or garden plant that draw their attention. In addition, a parent's prescription medication may be mistaken for candy.

Nature is fraught with toxicologic perils. For example, wild mushrooms, once in the body, can produce a wide spectrum of reactions—from nausea to death.

The workplace also harbors its share of toxic hazards. Unfortunately, some of these hazards are not identified until after an exposure has occurred. For example, countless people who worked with polychlorinated biphenyls (PCBs) on a daily basis in the electric energy field developed cancer later in life; only then was the harmful nature of PCBs recognized. Similarly, thousands of people developed asbestosis after continued exposure to asbestos in the workplace, and their illnesses prompted research that identified the true toxicity of this material.

Sometimes unintentional toxicologic emergencies may occur as a result of simple neglect or oversight. For example, a geriatric person with diabetes and comorbid early-onset dementia or Alzheimer disease may take his or her insulin in the morning, but later be unable to remember whether the dose was taken. If the patient then takes another dose, the result may be a call to 9-1-1 for an unresponsive person in need of assistance.

The risks associated with chemical and biologic warfare have drawn increasing attention in recent years owing to the heightened awareness of bioterrorism, but intentional poisoning or overdose more commonly occurs during much smaller-scale crimes. In recent years, date rape drugs such as flunitrazepam (Rohypnol) have been used to facilitate sexual assault. Chloral hydrate ("knockout drops") has been used to commit assault for decades, and pharmacologic agents are used in homicides as well.

Poison Centers

Given the wide variety of illicit drugs, coupled with the continued growth in the number of licit drugs, even the most well-read veteran AEMT may find it difficult to keep up-to-date on the myriad drugs sold in the streets today. For this reason, the American Association of Poison Control

YOU are the Provider — PART 1

You and your partner are dispatched to assist local law enforcement officers with an unknown medical problem. When you arrive on scene, you note the presence of four police cars in the immediate vicinity, increasing your index of suspicion for violence. A police captain approaches your ambulance and tells you that police were called to the location for a "person acting strange." When the first officer arrived, she found a naked man standing in the front yard of a residence, with both arms bloodied, screaming unintelligible words. Officers have tried to calm the man, but he refuses to comply with their commands, and the captain states that they are trying to decide on the best way to subdue him.

1. What are the potential hazards with this scene?
2. What is a likely explanation for this patient's presentation?

Centers' Poison Help line (1-800-222-1222) may be an indispensable aid in a suspected toxicologic emergency.[1]

Suppose you are called to a home where a frantic mother is hovering over a toddler who sits beside the remains of a planted philodendron, most of which he apparently just ate. Is the plant poisonous? How poisonous? Should you make the child vomit? Is an antidote available? In such a scenario, you can call a poison center and get a fast rundown on the ingestion, its toxic potential, and steps to negate its effects, thereby providing proper patient care.

Poison centers have access to information about almost all commonly used medications, chemicals, and substances that could possibly be poisonous. Never hesitate to use these resources when confronted with a call involving *any* **toxin** (poison) with which you have limited or no familiarity. In addition to assisting with the current incident, your call helps the center collect data on poisonings in your region. These data are analyzed to help detect trends, identify developing public health problems, and evaluate current treatment protocols for different poisonings.

Some mobile medical reference apps, such as Epocrates, will assist with pill identification. You input basic information about the pills (shape, color, or markings), and the software identifies a list of potential medications. Poison Control also offers an online triage tool and mobile device app called webPOISONCONTROL that can be used by laypeople or health care providers.

Pathophysiology: Routes of Absorption

Toxins cannot exert their effects until they enter the human body. The four primary methods of entry are ingestion, inhalation, injection, and absorption. Just as each of these methods of entry is unique, so is the rate at which a given toxin is absorbed into the body by that route. Once a toxin is in the body, the combination of the amount of toxin and the relative speed at which it is metabolized determine its effects and excretion rate.

▶ Poisoning by Ingestion

Medications around the home and household chemicals (such as cleaning agents or laundry detergent capsules) are the most common sources of poisoning by ingestion. Ingested poisons may produce immediate damage to tissues, or their toxic effects may be delayed for several hours. With ingestion of a caustic substance (ie, a strong acid or alkali), these effects occur immediately. By contrast, some poisons must be absorbed into the bloodstream before they will produce toxic effects.

Assessment clues pointing toward ingestion can be as obvious as a plant with partially chewed leaves or a section of a plant with berries missing. Stained fingers, lips, or tongue are other indicators of ingestion. Any patient complaining of a sudden onset of stomach cramps with or without nausea, vomiting, or diarrhea may have an ingestion-related problem. Empty pill bottles are another obvious clue, as is the date on which the prescription was filled. The bottle for a prescription filled 6 months ago is not likely to be full today; an empty bottle for a prescription filled yesterday is far more ominous.

Entry of a toxin into the body by the oral route generally provides a more forgiving time frame for treatment. Little absorption occurs in the stomach; indeed, the ingested substance may stay there for a variable period, with the majority of absorption actually taking place in the small intestine. As a consequence, managing a patient with poisoning by ingestion should focus on removing or neutralizing the poison before it enters the intestines.

In the past, syrup of ipecac was widely used to induce vomiting. Unfortunately, when this treatment is used, people who have ingested substances that may cause diminished alertness over time may potentially vomit and inhale the vomitus into the lungs as they become less responsive. As a result, syrup of ipecac is now recommended in only a few situations in which the risk of losing consciousness is clearly low, and it is usually not carried on ambulances.

In specific ingestion emergencies some emergency medical service (EMS) systems may allow AEMTs to use activated charcoal as an alternative treatment **Figure 23-1**. Activated charcoal, which comes as a suspension, binds to the poison in the stomach and carries it out of the patient's system. Because of this mechanism of action, it is more effective and safer for patients than syrup of ipecac. However, its administration carries the risk of severe pulmonary injury if aspirated. Administration of activated charcoal is discussed later in this chapter.

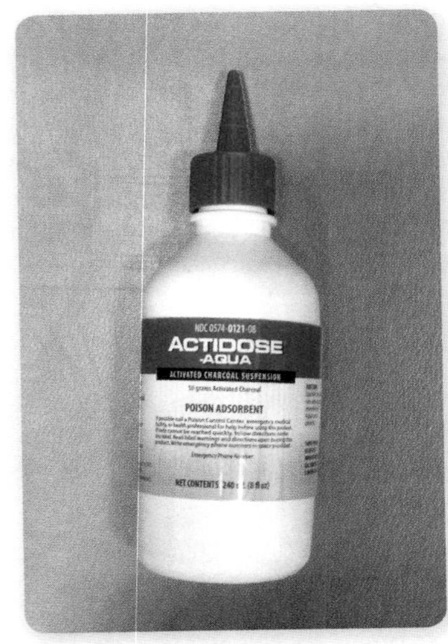

Figure 23-1 Activated charcoal comes as a premixed suspension that you should administer, if local protocol allows, in a covered cup with a straw.

As always, you should immediately assess the airway, breathing, and circulation (ABCs) of a patient with suspected poisoning. Many patients have died as a result of problems with their ABCs that might have been managed easily. Provide aggressive ventilatory support and cardiopulmonary resuscitation (CPR) to a patient who has ingested an opiate, a sedative, or a barbiturate, as all of these types of drugs can cause depression of the central nervous system (CNS) and slow breathing.

Whenever ingestion poisoning is suspected, you should provide prompt transport to the emergency department (ED). The patient may need intravenous (IV) support and may require other treatments that can be given only in the hospital.

Words of Wisdom

Because e-cigarettes are becoming more popular due to their low cost, flavored options, and approved use indoors, they are also becoming a rare but emerging source of poisonings. The liquid nicotine contained in an e-cigarette is often the offending agent. The most common route of exposure is inhalation, but there are reported cases of ingestion and absorption through the eyes.[2] Nausea, vomiting, and eye irritation are common symptoms following an exposure.[3] Pediatric exposures have also increased further, conveying the need to keep e-cigarettes out of the reach of children.[3]

▶ Poisoning by Inhalation

Home medications and household chemical products (such as bleach and cleaning agents) are responsible for the most common types of inhalation emergencies. A person can be poisoned by inhalation only if the poison is present in the surrounding atmosphere. That fact has important implications. First, so long as the patient remains in the toxic environment, he or she will keep inhaling the poison—and so will you. For example, **carbon monoxide (CO)**, an odorless, colorless, tasteless, and highly poisonous gas, is a hazard for rescuers as well as for patients. Therefore, you should not enter the hazardous environment; instead, call for additional responders with specialized protective equipment. Second, when poisoning occurs because of a toxic environment, you are likely to encounter more than one patient at the emergency scene.

Words of Wisdom

An encounter with multiple patients with similar complaints—at the same time and inside the same building or area—equals poisoning until it is proven otherwise! Take necessary precautions for personal safety.

Inhaled toxins quickly reach the alveoli, which then allow the toxins almost instant access to the circulation. Carbon monoxide, for example, binds to hemoglobin on the red blood cells 200 to 250 times more readily than do oxygen molecules, which leads to rapidly diminished oxygen-carrying capacity. In turn, patients experience a rapid onset of signs and symptoms. For this reason, the window of opportunity for treating an inhalation poisoning is limited.

When you are dealing with an inhalation emergency, the first general management consideration is to ensure scene safety. Specialized personnel will likely need to access the patient, and the patient may need to be decontaminated by special rescuers after removal from the toxic environment. Consult with poison control or local hazardous materials team members regarding the need for patient decontamination. Remove the patient's clothing in this process because it may contain trapped gases that can be released later, thereby exposing you or other responders to the toxin. Do not administer emergency care until this step has been completed and there is no danger of the poison contaminating you.

Safety

Never pull a shirt over the head of a patient who may have been exposed to a toxin. Doing so may introduce the toxin into the patient's eyes, nose, or mouth. Instead, unbutton or cut the shirt to remove it. Pulling clothing over a patient's head could also introduce the toxin into the air, causing a hazard to you or other providers.

Inhaled toxins produce a wide range of signs and symptoms, many of which are unique to the toxin involved. For example, a patient with CO poisoning does not exhibit the same signs and symptoms as a person who has sniffed glue, who in turn looks nothing like a patient poisoned by a furniture stripper containing methylene chloride.

As with other types of poisoning, it is helpful to take any suspicious containers, bottles, and labels with you when you transport the patient with inhalation poisoning to the hospital. Often patients use inhaled poisons to commit suicide, such as when a person sits inside a vehicle with the engine running in an enclosed garage. The exhaust fumes from the vehicle contain high levels of CO that will cause the patient to lose consciousness and eventually stop breathing. A recent variation on the use of automobiles for suicide, called **chemical suicide**, involves people using a tightly sealed vehicle as a type of gas chamber. Fairly common household chemicals are mixed inside the vehicle to produce hydrogen sulfide gas, which is quickly fatal. When you approach such a vehicle and open the door, you may be overcome by the gas as well.

Signs of chemical suicide include taped or sealed windows, locked doors, posted warning signs, a suicide note, empty chemical containers, and unusual odor. If you suspect this type of poisoning has taken place, contact hazardous materials responders and have them remove the patient from the vehicle.

Frequently, the emergency scene itself provides clues about the identity of the toxin. That information, coupled with the assistance of the poison center and direction from the medical control physician, will drive your treatment plan. You must treat hypoxia immediately, so administer a high concentration of oxygen. Establish vascular access, and perform pulse oximetry. Call early for paramedic backup.

Words of Wisdom

Always treat the patient, rather than the diagnostic tool. Pulse oximeters, for example, are notorious for giving false readings when patients have been exposed to many chemicals, including carbon monoxide and cyanide. Administer oxygen as appropriate without regard to pulse oximetry readings if the patient has difficulty breathing.

▶ Poisoning by Injection

Poisoning by injection is usually the result of drug abuse, such as with heroin or cocaine.

Depending on the specific toxin injected, signs and symptoms can vary greatly. Frequently, the patient may be able to identify the source, greatly simplifying the assessment process.

In general, injected poisons are impossible to dilute or remove because they are usually absorbed quickly into the body or cause intense local tissue destruction. If you suspect that rapid absorption has occurred, monitor the patient's airway, administer high-flow oxygen, and be alert for nausea and vomiting. Remove rings, watches, and bracelets from areas around the injection site if swelling occurs. Prompt transport to the ED is essential. Take all containers, bottles, and labels with the patient to the hospital.

Bites and stings are also considered to be a form of poisoning by injection. Managing specific bites and stings is covered in Chapter 22, *Immunologic Emergencies*, and Chapter 34, *Environmental Emergencies*.

▶ Poisoning by Absorption

Some poisons gain access to the body by being absorbed through the skin. Of the various poisonings that occur by absorption, those caused by pesticides such as organophosphates and similar substances are often the most serious.

Many corrosive substances will damage the skin, mucous membranes, or eyes, causing chemical burns, telltale rashes, or lesions. For example, acids, alkalis, and some petroleum (hydrocarbon) products have very destructive local effects. Other substances are absorbed into the bloodstream through the skin and have systemic effects. Still other substances, such as poison ivy or poison oak, may just cause an itchy rash without being dangerous to the patient's health. It is important, therefore, to distinguish between contact burns and contact absorption.

Words of Wisdom

Absorption of toxic substances through the skin is a common problem in agriculture and manufacturing. Most solvents and "cides"—insecticides, herbicides, and pesticides—are toxic and can be readily absorbed through the skin.

Signs and symptoms of absorption poisoning include a history of exposure, liquid or powder on a patient's skin, burns, itching, irritation, redness of the skin in light-skinned people, or typical odors of the substance.

As always, emergency medical treatment for a typical contact poisoning begins with avoiding contamination for both yourself and others. Once you accomplish this step and you protect yourself from exposure, remove the irritating or corrosive substance from the patient as rapidly as possible. Cut off all clothing that has been contaminated with poisons or irritating substances. Never pull clothing over a patient's head; doing so could introduce the material into the eyes, nose, and mouth. Note that the order of these steps is important. You should never flush off a dry powder, as that could activate a chemical reaction. Dry off thoroughly first, then flush the skin with running water, and then wash the skin with soap and water. When a large amount of material has been spilled on a patient, flooding the affected part for at least 20 minutes may be the fastest and most effective treatment.

If the patient has a chemical agent in the eyes, irrigate the eyes quickly and thoroughly. To avoid contaminating the other eye as you irrigate the affected eye, ensure the fluid runs from the bridge of the nose outward **Figure 23-2**. This action should be started initially on the scene and continued during transport.

Many chemical burns occur in industrial settings, where showers and specific protocols for handling surface burns are available. If you are called to such a scene, trained people usually will be there to assist you. Do not spend time trying to neutralize substances on the skin with additional chemicals, as this action may actually be more harmful than leaving the original chemical intact. Instead, brush off as much as possible if the material is a solid, and then immediately wash off the substance with plenty of water. Obtain material safety data sheets from industrial sites and transport them with the patient, if available.

The only time you should not irrigate the contact area with water after brushing it off is when a patient has

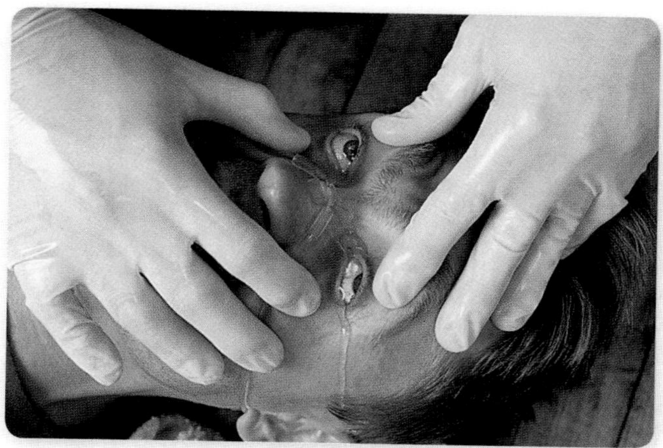

Figure 23-2 If chemical agents are in the patient's eyes, then irrigate the eyes quickly and thoroughly, ensuring that the irrigation fluid runs from the bridge of the nose outward. (Use of a nasal cannula is pictured.)

been contaminated with a poison that reacts violently with water, such as phosphorus or elemental sodium. These substances ignite when they come into contact with water. In such a case, you should brush off the chemical from the patient, remove contaminated clothing, and apply a dry dressing to the burn area. Ensure you wear appropriate protective gloves and the proper protective clothing when performing these steps.

For all patients with absorption poisoning, provide prompt transport to the ED for definitive care. En route, continue irrigation and administer oxygen if possible.

Understanding and Using Toxidromes

Although the sheer number of substances of abuse may seem daunting, the good news is that many drugs, upon entering the body, result in similar signs and symptoms. For example, whether a narcotic substance is a natural product derived from opium (ie, an opiate) or a synthetic, non–opium-derived narcotic (ie, an opioid), all drugs in this group work in a similar manner, so they produce similar signs and symptoms. The syndrome-like symptoms of a poisonous agent are termed a toxic syndrome or **toxidrome**. Toxidromes are useful for remembering the elements in assessing and managing different substances that fall under the same clinical umbrella. The major toxidromes are produced by stimulants, narcotics, sympathomimetics, sedatives and hypnotics, cholinergics, and anticholinergics Table 23-1.

Table 23-2 lists common signs and symptoms of poisoning. If you look at the patient's history and physical examination findings in conjunction with the vital signs, you can often develop a working diagnosis that will allow you to provide appropriate care until the patient reaches the receiving facility.

Table 23-1 Major Toxidromes

Toxidrome	Signs and Symptoms
Stimulant (Examples: amphetamine, methamphetamine, cocaine, diet aids, nasal decongestants)	Restlessness, agitation, incessant talking; insomnia; anorexia; dilated pupils, tachycardia; tachypnea, hypertension or hypotension; paranoia, seizures, cardiac arrest
Narcotic (opiate and opioid) (Examples: heroin, morphine, hydromorphone [Dilaudid], fentanyl, oxycodone)	Pinpoint pupils, marked respiratory depression; drowsiness, stupor, coma
Sympathomimetic (Examples: epinephrine, albuterol, cocaine, methamphetamine)	Hypertension, tachycardia, dilated pupils, agitation and seizures, hyperthermia
Sedative-hypnotic (Examples: diazepam [Valium], secobarbital [Seconal], flunitrazepam [Rohypnol])	Drowsiness, disinhibition, ataxia, slurred speech, mental confusion, respiratory depression, progressive central nervous system depression, hypotension
Cholinergic (Examples: diazinon, orthene, parathion, nerve gas)	Increased salivation, lacrimation (tearing), excess defecation or urination, nausea or vomiting, airway compromise, seizures, coma
Anticholinergic (Examples: atropine, scopolamine, antihistamines, antipsychotics, Jimsonweed)	Tachycardia, hyperthermia, dry skin and mucous membranes, dilated pupils, blurred vision, sedation; agitation, seizures, coma, or delirium

Table 23-2 Common Signs and Symptoms of Poisoning

Sign or Symptom	Type	Possible Causative Agents
Odor	Bitter almonds	Cyanide
	Garlic	Arsenic, organophosphates, phosphorus
	Acetone	Methyl alcohol, isopropyl alcohol, aspirin, acetone
	Wintergreen	Methyl salicylate
	Pears	Chloral hydrate
	Violets	Turpentine
	Camphor	Camphor
	Alcohol	Alcohol
Pupils	Constricted	Narcotics, organophosphates, Jimsonweed, nutmeg, propoxyphene (Darvon)
	Dilated	Barbiturates, atropine, amphetamine, glutethimide (Doriden), LSD, cyanide, CO
Mouth	Salivation	Organophosphates, arsenic, strychnine, mercury, salicylates
	Dry mouth	Atropine (belladonna), amphetamines, diphenhydramine (Benadryl), narcotics
	Burns in mouth	Formaldehyde, iodine, lye, toxic plants, phenols, phosphorus, pine oil, silver nitrate, acids
Skin	Pruritus	Jimsonweed, belladonna, boric acid
	Dry, hot skin	Atropine (in belladonna), botulism, nutmeg
	Sweating	Organophosphates, arsenic, aspirin, amphetamines, barbiturates, mushrooms, naphthalene
Respiratory	Depressed respirations	Narcotics, alcohol, propoxyphene, CO, barbiturates
	Increased respirations	Aspirin, amphetamines, boric acid, cyanide, kerosene, methyl alcohol, nicotine
	Pulmonary edema	Organophosphates, petroleum products, narcotics, CO
Cardiovascular	Tachycardia	Alcohol, amphetamines, arsenic, atropine, aspirin, cocaine, some antiasthma drugs
	Bradycardia	Digitalis, gasoline, nicotine, mushrooms, narcotics, cyanide, mistletoe, rhododendron
	Hypertension	Amphetamines, lead, nicotine, antiasthma drugs
	Hypotension	Barbiturates, narcotics, tranquilizers, house plants, mistletoe, nitroglycerin, antifreeze
Central nervous system	Seizures	Amphetamines, camphor, cocaine, strychnine, arsenic, carbon monoxide, petroleum products, scorpion sting
	Coma	All depressant drugs (such as narcotics, barbiturates, tranquilizers, alcohol), CO, cyanide
	Hallucinations	Atropine, LSD, mushrooms, organic solvents, phencyclidine, nutmeg
	Headache	CO, alcohol, disulfiram (Antabuse)
	Tremors	Organophosphates, CO, amphetamine, tranquilizers, poisonous marine animals
	Weakness or paralysis	Organophosphates, botulism, eel, hemlock, puffer fish, pine oil, rhododendron
Gastrointestinal	Cramps, nausea, vomiting, and/or diarrhea	Many, if not most, ingested poisons

Abbreviations: CO, carbon monoxide; LSD, lysergic acid diethylamide

Overview of Substance Abuse

The area of medicine dealing with drugs of abuse is highly challenging because of uncertainty about the prevalence of the problem and the continual evolution of the substances themselves. Substance abuse can be broadly defined as the self-administration of licit or illicit substances in a manner not in accordance with approved medical or social practice. Part of that definition is cultural—and there is great variation in what is considered substance abuse.

Any given society's definition of abuse may have little relation to the potential harm from the abused substance. For example, US culture places no restrictions on the long-term and compulsive use of tobacco, even though this substance is a major contributor to cardiovascular and respiratory disease. By comparison, use of marijuana may be punishable by fines or imprisonment (although some states have made it legal to use small amounts for personal recreational purposes, and some states allow the use of "medical marijuana" to treat pain, nausea, and some other symptoms).

The following list defines some basic terms and concepts related to substance abuse:

- **Drug abuse.** Any use of drugs that causes physical, psychological, economic, legal, or social harm to the user or to others affected by the drug user's behavior.
- **Habituation.** Psychological dependence on a drug or drugs.
- **Physical dependence.** A physiologic state of adaptation to a drug, usually characterized by tolerance to the drug's effects and a withdrawal syndrome if the drug is stopped, especially if it is stopped abruptly.
- **Psychological dependence.** The emotional state of craving a drug to maintain a feeling of well-being.
- **Tolerance.** Physiologic adaptation to the effects of a drug such that increasingly larger doses of the drug are required to achieve the same effect.
- **Withdrawal syndrome.** A predictable set of signs and symptoms, usually involving altered CNS activity, that occurs after the abrupt cessation of a drug or after rapidly decreasing the usual dosage of a drug.
- **Drug addiction.** A chronic disorder characterized by the compulsive use of a substance resulting in physical, psychological, or social harm to the user, who continues to use the substance despite the harm.
- **Antagonist.** Something that counteracts the action of something else. In relation to drugs, a drug that is an antagonist has an affinity for a cell receptor; by binding to the receptor, the antagonist prevents the cell from responding.
- **Potentiation.** Enhancement of the effect of one drug by another drug.
- **Synergism.** The action of two substances such as drugs, in which the total effect is greater than the sum of the independent effects of the two substances (that is, 2 + 2 = 5).

Drug abuse is not limited to members of the younger generation or to any particular stratum of society. It occurs in all age groups and at all social levels. However, adolescents are susceptible to experimentation with drugs of abuse because of curiosity and peer pressure.

YOU are the Provider — PART 2

The police officers are able to successfully subdue the patient using minimal force and place him in handcuffs. The officers then motion you over. Your initial impression reveals a severely agitated, thin-appearing man who is screaming incoherently and who has what appears to be severe abrasions on each forearm. The patient has a patent airway as evidenced by his screaming, and the bleeding appears to be superficial. You immediately place a blanket over the patient. As you question the patient, he keeps screaming, "Don't let them get me! I'm burning! God help me!" A family member who has arrived at the scene approaches you.

Recording Time: 1 Minute	
Appearance	Anxious, agitated
Level of consciousness	Alert, but does not appear to be oriented to person, place, time, or event
Airway	Patent
Breathing	Rapid, panting
Circulation	Strong radial pulses; skin warm, dry, and pink

3. Does this patient's presentation warrant transport via EMS, or should he be transported via law enforcement?
4. Should you request paramedic backup for this patient?

Patient Assessment

Generally, patients with toxicologic emergencies are considered medical patients, although toxicologic emergencies may also lead to trauma. The general assessment approach is the same for all patients: scene size-up, primary survey, history taking, secondary assessment, and reassessment.

Words of Wisdom

While at the scene, take thorough (and legible) notes about the nature of the poisoning. You can then quickly state the type and amount of substance and the time and route of exposure in your radio, verbal, and written reports. Clear notes that can be handed over on arrival will be appreciated by busy hospital staff.

Scene Size-up

When you have a situation that involves a toxicologic emergency, a well-trained dispatcher is of great value. Dispatchers with an appropriate set of protocols and excellent interrogation skills can obtain important information pertaining to a poisoning call that will help you anticipate the proper protection needed to ensure your safety. If this information is not obtained before your arrival, you must take the time to thoroughly assess the scene to ensure your safety. Determine the nature of the illness and any mechanism of injury, as well as the number of patients involved, the need for additional resources, and the need for spinal immobilization.

Because of the risk of possible cross-contamination by poisons that can be inhaled, absorbed, ingested, and injected, you must take appropriate standard precautions. Wear the appropriate personal protective equipment necessary to avoid being contaminated.

Patients who have taken an overdose may be extremely dangerous. If necessary, call for law enforcement backup.

As you approach the scene, look for clues that might indicate the substance or poison involved:

- Are there medication bottles lying around the patient and the scene? If so, is there medication missing that might indicate an overdose?
- Are there alcoholic beverage containers present?
- Are there syringes or other drug paraphernalia on the scene?
- Is there an unpleasant or odd odor in the room? If so, is the scene safe? An odor could also be a clue to an inhaled poison.
- Is there a suspicious odor or drug paraphernalia present that may indicate the presence of a drug laboratory? Drug laboratories can be very volatile, so ensure scene safety before trying to access the patient Figure 23-3.

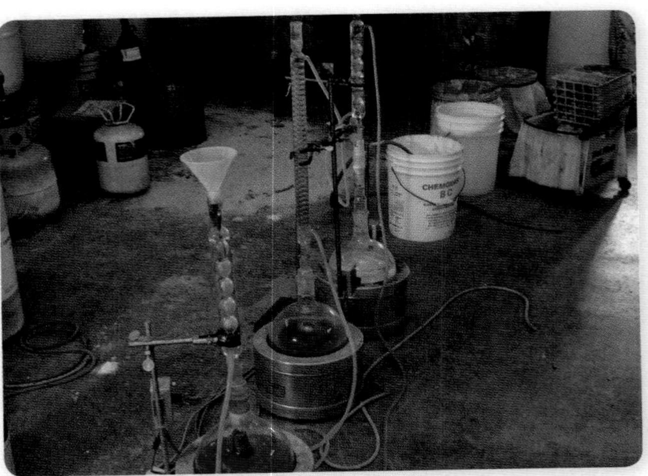

Figure 23-3 A "meth lab"—a laboratory capable of producing large quantities of methamphetamine.

Courtesy of U.S. Drug Enforcement Administration.

Keep a constant observant eye on the surroundings, and keep an open mind when questioning the patient or bystanders to avoid coming to mistaken conclusions.

Safety

Scene safety is your primary concern when you are called to an inhalation incident. Whenever you encounter more than one patient but find no evidence of the mechanism of injury, be suspicious. Toxic fumes may be odorless and colorless, and they can affect you as well as the patients. Be suspicious of toxic fumes when encountering patients with changes in level of consciousness, especially at an industrial site or enclosed space.

Primary Survey

The primary survey of a drug-overdosed or poisoned patient begins with your general impression. That impression can be as simple as "a young adult man snoring in a public bathroom stall." Conversely, do not be fooled into thinking that a patient who is responsive, alert, and oriented is in stable condition and has no apparent life threats. In some cases, the patient may have a harmful or even lethal amount of poison in his or her system that has just not had enough time to produce a systemic reaction.

Begin your assessment by identifying any life threats (assess airway, breathing, circulation, disability, and exposure [ABCDEs]). The primary survey may also identify the mechanism of injury or nature of illness, suggest the need for additional units, and set the priority and "tone" of the call. A primary survey that reveals a patient with signs of distress or altered mental status gives you early confirmation that the poisonous substance is causing a systemic reaction.

Manage life threats quickly. Ensure the patient has an open airway and adequate ventilation. Do not hesitate to begin oxygen therapy for the patient. If the patient is unresponsive to painful stimuli, then consider inserting an airway adjunct to ensure the airway remains open. Have suction available; patients who have been poisoned are susceptible to vomiting. You may also have to assist a patient's ventilations with a bag-mask device, because some substances act as depressants on the body's systems. As you assess and manage the patient's airway and breathing, consider the potential for spinal injury. Spinal precautions in an unresponsive patient must begin when the airway is first opened and be continued if positive pressure ventilations are needed.

Use diagnostic tools such as the pulse oximeter, but remember, if the patient has been exposed to CO, the reading will be inaccurate. CO has a 200 to 250 times greater affinity for hemoglobin than does oxygen, which causes oxygen molecules to be displaced from hemoglobin. Thus, the reading on the pulse oximeter will be at or near 100% in a patient with CO poisoning because the hemoglobin is completely saturated—though it is saturated with CO molecules rather than oxygen. Always treat the patient, not the diagnostic tool; never withhold oxygen based on a pulse oximeter reading if you suspect CO poisoning or if it's even a remote possibility! Treatment for CO poisoning consists of high-flow oxygen and transport of the patient to the closest, most appropriate facility.

Once you have assessed the patient's airway and breathing and performed the appropriate interventions, assess the patient's circulatory status. Patients' circulatory status will vary depending on the substance involved in a poisoning. Assess the pulse and skin condition. Remember that some poisons are stimulants, and others are depressants. Stimulant exposure may result in restlessness, agitation, incessant talking; insomnia; anorexia; dilated pupils, tachycardia; tachypnea, hypertension or hypotension; paranoia, seizures, and/or cardiac arrest, whereas depressant exposure generally presents with respiratory depression, bradycardia, drowsiness, and possible coma. Some poisons cause vasoconstriction, whereas others trigger vasodilation. Although bleeding may not be obvious, alterations in consciousness may have contributed to trauma and bleeding.

Also, assess for disability, and expose the patient to identify any additional conditions.

Patients with obvious alterations in the ABCs and patients whom you assess as having a poor general impression should be considered for immediate transport. A delay on the scene to further assess and treat such patients is rarely indicated.

Some industrial settings may have specific decontamination stations and antidotes for specific toxic substances present at the site. Some of the time, decontamination and antidote administration will have been initiated by the industrial response team before your arrival and should not delay rapid transport. Your own decontamination of the patient may sometimes be needed before transport depending on the poison involved. For example, this action is necessary if a patient continues to off-gas or if your crew has the potential to become exposed in the confined space of the ambulance during transit. Decontamination is especially important when transporting exposed patients in a helicopter.

History Taking

After completing the primary survey, begin obtaining the history. Many poisoning and overdose cases involve patients with medical conditions, so you will need to elaborate on their chief complaint using the OPQRST mnemonic (Onset, Provocation/palliation, Quality, Region/radiation, Severity, Timing). Obtain the patient's medical history. In many situations, this step can be performed in the ambulance en route to the hospital. If the patient is responsive and can answer questions, begin with an evaluation of the exposure and the SAMPLE (Signs and symptoms, Allergies, Medications, Pertinent past medical history, Last oral intake, Events leading up to the illness or injury) history. If the patient is not responsive, attempt to obtain the history from other sources, such as friends or family members. Medical identification jewelry and cards in wallets may also provide information about the patient's medical history.

In toxicologic emergencies, the SAMPLE history guides your focus as you continue to assess the patient's complaints. The physical exam helps to determine the visible signs of a reaction to the toxin. Vital signs may indicate any physiologic response to the exposure as well as give you an indication of the urgency. These three assessments are important in that they give you direction in determining the best interventions for the patient. To choose the appropriate course of action in a toxicologic emergency, obtain at least the following specific information:

- **What is the agent?** If you know the substance involved, you will be better able to access the appropriate resource, such as the poison center, to determine lethal doses, time before harmful effects begin, effects of the substance at toxic levels, and appropriate interventions.
- **When was the poison ingested, injected, absorbed, or inhaled?** This information will let you know if and when the harmful effects will begin. It will also tell the emergency physician which harmful effects can be reversed and which cannot because of the length of time that the patient has been exposed to the substance. The decision to induce vomiting (infrequently done—check local protocols) or to flush out (lavage) the stomach (also rare) is strongly

influenced by the amount of time that has elapsed since the exposure. Also, acute-onset events often indicate a more serious patient scenario—for example, if the patient smoked crack cocaine 15 minutes ago and immediately began to have crushing chest pain.

- **How much was taken, injected, absorbed, or inhaled?** Based on this information, the poison center will be able to determine whether the patient has received a harmful or lethal dose. For example, if the patient says that she took four tabs of Ecstasy, that amount is four times the single dose. In toxicologic emergencies, there is almost always a direct correlation between dose and toxic effects.
- **What else was taken?** The majority of intentional self-poisonings (suicide attempts) or illicit drug overdoses involve polydrug ingestions, with alcohol often being one of the drugs taken.[4,5] The patient may also have tried to take something to counteract the effect of the poison. This information can be invaluable to the ED staff when deciding which tests to order.
- **Over which period did the patient take the substance?** All at once or over minutes or hours?
- **Has the patient or a bystander performed any intervention?** Has the intervention helped? The patient's or bystander's intervention may cause more complications. The emergency physician will also need to know this information to be able to adjust subsequent interventions accordingly.
- **Has the patient vomited or aspirated?** If so, how soon after the ingestion or exposure? How much?
- **How much does the patient weigh?** If activated charcoal is indicated, you will need to determine the dose based on the patient's weight. The antidote or neutralizing agent given by the emergency physician may be based on the patient's weight as well.
- **Why was the substance taken?** Although you may not get a reliable answer from someone abusing illicit drugs, this is still a question worth asking. Do not assume every patient is trying to get high. Drug use could be a coping mechanism for a person who is being abused, or it could be a suicide attempt. Put the reason in "quotation marks" on your patient care report.

If the patient has overdosed on a prescription drug, take the pill bottle and the remaining pills to the ED with the patient **Figure 23-4**. If the substance was a commercial product, take the container and its remaining contents to the ED. If the patient ingested a plant, find out which part (roots, leaves, stem, flower, or fruit) and take a sample of the plant to the ED for identification. If the patient vomits, save a sample of the vomitus in a clean, closed container.

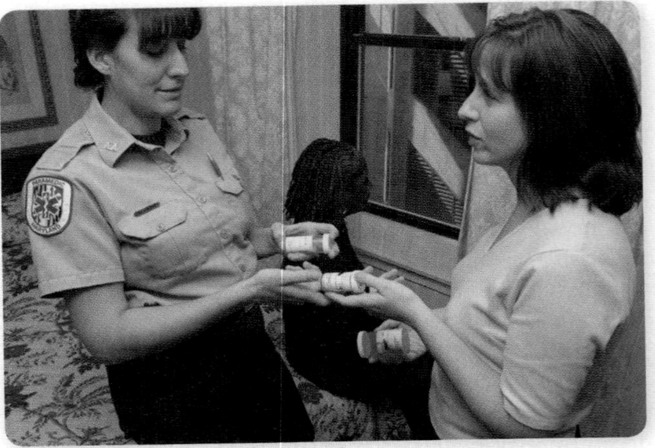

Figure 23-4 Take any bottles, containers, and their remaining contents to the emergency department.

Secondary Assessment

Your physical examination of a patient with a toxicologic emergency should focus on the area of the body involved with the poisoning or the route of exposure. For example, if the patient has ingested a poison, inspect the mouth for indications of poisoning. Are there burns from caustic chemicals? Are there plant or pill fragments? If the person's skin came in contact with a poison, is there a rash or burns? How large is the involved area? If a respiratory exposure occurred, auscultate the lungs. Is there good air movement in and out of the lungs? Do you hear any wheezing or crackles? The specific focus of your physical exam is largely based on the route of exposure and the particular drug or chemical that was involved. Take the time to become knowledgeable about the effects of general classes of drugs and chemicals so you will become familiar with how to assess and treat patients who are exposed to specific and common poisons.

Managing life threats during the primary survey is the priority assessment and treatment goal. Once the life threats have been addressed, conducting a thorough physical exam will often provide additional information on the patient's toxicologic exposure. A general review of all body systems may help to identify systemic problems. This review should be performed, at a minimum, on patients with extensive chemical burns or other significant trauma and on patients who are unresponsive. This should be done en route, so as not to delay transport.

A complete set of baseline vital signs is an important tool for you to use to determine how the patient is doing. Many poisons produce no outward indications of the seriousness of the exposure. Alterations in the level of consciousness, pulse, respirations, blood pressure, and skin are more sensitive indicators that something serious is wrong. Be aware that exposure to CO may produce false pulse oximetry readings.

Special Populations

A geriatric patient may have become confused about his or her drug regimen, resulting in an accidental overdose or poisoning. He or she may have forgotten that a medication was taken earlier, and repeat the dose one or more times. The patient could also have forgotten or misunderstood the doctor's instructions to stop a medication and may have taken both the current and older drugs, resulting in increased effects or unwanted drug interactions. A geriatric patient may also intentionally overdose in a suicide attempt.

Reassessment

The condition of patients exposed to poisons may change suddenly and without warning. You should continually reassess the adequacy of the patient's ABCDEs. Repeat the vital signs, and compare them with the baseline set obtained earlier in your assessment. Evaluate the effectiveness of any interventions you have provided. If your assessment has obtained specific, pertinent information about the poisonous substance, you may be able to anticipate changes in the patient's condition. If the patient has consumed a harmful or lethal dose of a poisonous substance, you must reassess the patient's vital signs every 5 minutes, or more often if necessary. If the patient is in stable condition and there are no life threats, reassess your patient every 15 minutes. If the poison or the level of exposure is unknown, then it is mandatory for you to perform a careful and frequent reassessment.

The treatment you provide for poisoned patients depends a great deal on the substance to which they were exposed, the route of exposure, and other signs and symptoms uncovered in your assessment. Supporting these patients' ABCs is your most important task. Some poisons can be easily diluted or patients decontaminated before transport or en route to the hospital: dilute airborne exposures with oxygen, remove contact exposures with copious amounts of water unless contraindicated, and consider administering activated charcoal for ingested poisons. Remember, these patients may vomit at any time, so continuously monitor the airway. Contact medical control or a poison center to discuss treatment options for particular poisonings.

Once you have completed your primary survey, history taking, and secondary assessment, contact medical control for advice on necessary interventions. Report to the hospital as much information as you have about the poison or chemical to which the patient was exposed. If a safety data sheet is immediately available in a work setting, take it with you to the hospital. If this document is not immediately available, ask the company to send it (eg, via email or fax) to the receiving hospital while you are en route. This information will help hospital providers identify and quickly make available specific interventions and potential antidotes.

Words of Wisdom

Have someone count the medications left in the prescription bottle and compare to the date filled to figure out the maximum quantity the patient might have taken.

Emergency Medical Care

First, ensure scene safety by taking standard precautions and performing external decontamination, if indicated after consulting poison control and/or medical control. Remove tablets or fragments from the patient's mouth, and wash or brush poison from the patient's skin. Treatment focuses on support: assessing and maintaining the patient's ABCs and monitoring the patient's breathing. Administer oxygen to the patient as needed, and assist ventilations if necessary. If the patient has signs and symptoms of shock, provide treatment according to your local protocol.

In some cases, you may administer activated charcoal to patients who have ingested certain poisons, if approved by medical control or local protocol. Activated charcoal is not indicated for patients who have ingested an acid, an alkali, or a petroleum product; who have a decreased level of consciousness and cannot protect their airways; or who are unable to swallow.

Activated charcoal adsorbs, or sticks to, many commonly ingested poisons, preventing the toxin from being absorbed into the body by the stomach or intestines. If your local protocol permits, you will likely carry plastic bottles of premixed suspension, each containing up to 50 g of activated charcoal. Some common trade names for the suspension form are Insta-Char, Actidose, and Liqui-Char. The usual dose is 1 g of activated charcoal per kilogram of body weight, which translates into 25 to 50 g for adults and 12.5 to 25 g for children.

As mentioned earlier, administration of activated charcoal carries with it severe risk of aspiration. Never administer activated charcoal to anyone who is not alert or is unable (or may become unable) to protect his or her own airway. Always check with medical control and/or poison control prior to administering.

Once medical control has given orders to administer activated charcoal, shake the bottle vigorously to mix the suspension. This medication looks like mud, so it is best to cover the outside of the container so the fluid is not visible and ask the patient to drink it with a straw. Activated charcoal is an inky, messy fluid, so you may have to do some coaxing to get the patient to drink it; try to give it in a covered cup with a straw. Remember, you should never force this (or any other) liquid into a patient's mouth. If the patient takes a long time to drink the mixture, you will have to shake the container frequently to keep the medication mixed. Once the patient has finished, discard the container from which the charcoal was administered. Ensure you record the time when you administered the activated charcoal.

A major side effect of ingesting activated charcoal is black stools. If the patient has ingested a poison that causes nausea, he or she may vomit after taking activated charcoal, and the dose will have to be repeated. As you reassess the patient, be prepared for vomiting, nausea, and possible airway problems.

Pathophysiology, Assessment, and Management of Specific Poisons

▶ Alcohol

Alcohol is the most widely abused drug in the United States and around the world. In the 2015 National Survey on Drug Use and Health, 86% of US adults reported drinking alcohol at some point in their lifetime; 15 million people in the United States have alcoholism.[6] **Alcoholism**, a state of physical and psychological addiction, is the fourth leading cause of death in the United States, with an estimated 88,000 alcohol-related deaths annually.[6] Worldwide, nearly 6% of all deaths (more than 3 million deaths in 2012) are attributable to alcohol consumption.[6] In addition, people with alcoholism tend to have chronic malnutrition and fall frequently, increasing the likelihood of head injury or other trauma.

Alcohol is a powerful CNS depressant. It is both a sedative (it decreases activity and excitement) and a hypnotic (it induces sleep). In general, alcohol dulls the sense of awareness, slows reflexes, and reduces reaction time. It may also cause aggressive and inappropriate behavior and lack of coordination. However, a person who appears intoxicated may have other medical conditions as well. When you are treating a patient, look for signs of head trauma, toxic reactions, or uncontrolled diabetes. Severe acute alcohol ingestion may cause hypoglycemia, which may contribute to the symptoms. At the very least, you should assume all intoxicated patients are experiencing a drug overdose and require a thorough exam by a physician.

Severe alcohol intoxication is a form of poisoning and carries the same lethal potential as poisoning with any other CNS depressant. The most immediate danger to an acutely intoxicated person is death from respiratory depression and/or aspiration of vomitus or stomach contents secondary to a suppressed gag reflex.

Physical dependence on alcohol results from the regular consumption of large quantities. This dependence becomes apparent when a person abruptly stops consuming alcohol and withdrawal symptoms result. The severity of the withdrawal can vary according to the length and intensity of the alcoholic habit. Minor withdrawal is characterized by restlessness, anxiousness, sleeping problems, agitation, and tremors. Major withdrawal symptoms include increased blood pressure, vomiting, and hallucinations. **Delirium tremens (DTs)**, or alcohol withdrawal delirium, results in tremors and restlessness, weakness, fever, diaphoresis, disorientation, hallucinations, confusion, hypotension, seizures, and possibly death.

Because of the toxic effects of alcohol, a person with alcoholism is considerably more susecptible than a sober person to a number of serious illnesses and injuries **Table 23-3**. The most common long-term effect is liver damage; up to 35% of heavy drinkers will develop alcoholic hepatitis, and 10% to 20% of alcoholics will develop cirrhosis.[7] Other long-term effects of alcoholism include an increased incidence of pancreatitis, development of erosive gastritis, and an increased risk for breast and colorectal cancer. The long-term abuse of alcohol leads to atrophy of the cerebrum, possibly resulting in permanently reduced mental function.

If an intoxicated patient is unresponsive, treat him or her as you would any unresponsive patient. As always, first establish and maintain the airway. If the patient has an intact gag reflex, place the patient in left lateral recumbent position with suction ready; the patient may vomit forcefully and the vomit may be bloody because large amounts of alcohol irritate the stomach. If there is no gag reflex, place an appropriate airway adjunct and ventilate the patient with a bag-mask device or consider calling for paramedic backup for intubation and cardiac monitoring. In addition, administer high-concentration supplemental oxygen, and assist ventilation as needed. Establish vascular access. Assess the patient's blood glucose level, treating hypoglycemia if it is found. Finally, transport the patient to an appropriate facility.

Suspect internal bleeding if the patient appears to be in shock (hypoperfusion). Blood might not clot effectively in a patient who has a prolonged history of alcohol abuse.

A person who has been drinking heavily for an extended period and suddenly stops drinking may have a variety of withdrawal phenomena. Seizures usually occur within 12 to 48 hours of the last drink. Use the same care plan described for alcohol intoxication, and call for paramedic backup to administer benzodiazepines for seizure control.

The treatment for a patient in DTs is aimed at protecting him or her from injury and supporting the cardiovascular system. The often-terrifying hallucinations associated with DTs typically make for an agitated, often combative patient. Try to keep the patient calm. In addition, administer oxygen by nasal cannula and establish vascular access. Manage hypotension with an infusion of normal saline, and, during the reassessment, reassess breath sounds. Maintain an ongoing dialogue with the patient throughout transport to help orient and reassure the patient.

Table 23-3 Medical Conditions to Which People With Alcoholism Are Particularly Susceptible

Condition	Contributing Factors
Subdural hematoma	Frequent falls; impaired clotting mechanisms; brain atrophy allows for significant movement during impact
Gastrointestinal bleeding	Irritated stomach lining, leading to gastritis; impaired clotting mechanisms; cirrhosis (excess scar tissue) of the liver, leading to engorgement of esophageal veins (esophageal varices)
Pancreatitis	Secretion of enzymes, causing inflammation
Hypoglycemia	Damaged liver; impairs gluconeogenesis
Pneumonia	Aspiration of vomitus occurring during intoxication and coma; suppressed immune system by alcohol
Burns	Risky behaviors during intoxication; decreased pain sensitivity during intoxication
Hypothermia	Insensitivity to extreme temperatures while intoxicated; falling asleep outside in the cold; impaired thermoregulation
Seizures	Effects of alcohol withdrawal; neurotransmitter or electrolyte imbalance
Dysrhythmias (atrial fibrillation or ventricular tachycardia)	Toxic effects of alcohol on the heart; hypertension; electrolyte imbalance
Cancer	Damaged liver from heavy alcohol use; may cause alterations in normal cellular pathways
Esophageal varices	Obstructed blood flow to the liver, causing blood to back up into smaller, more fragile blood vessels in the esophagus

▶ Narcotics, Opiates, and Opioids

A **narcotic** is a drug that produces sleep or altered mental status. Historically, narcotics have been classified into two major divisions: opiates and opioids. The term **opiate** is used to describe natural drugs derived from opium (that is, from poppy juice); the term **opioid** refers to non–opium-derived synthetics. We use the term *opioids* to describe licit therapeutic agents and illicit substances in this group. Abuse of narcotics remains one of the most common causes of overdose deaths reported to poison centers, and the majority of deaths from drug overdoses (more than six out of 10) in the United States involve an opioid.[8] Since 1999, the rate of overdose deaths involving opioids, including prescription opioid pain relievers and heroin, has nearly quadrupled, leading to a veritable opioid epidemic today.[9] In 2015, more than 33,000 deaths from drug overdoses in the United States involved an opioid.[9] The number continues to rise; in 2016, there were over 50,000 deaths from accidental overdose.[9]

Narcotic agents include morphine, codeine, heroin, fentanyl, oxycodone, meperidine, propoxyphene, and dextromethorphan. Although these drugs share certain commonalities, they exhibit highly diverse effects and vary widely in their potency. Opioids are used primarily in clinical medicine for analgesia, whereas the illicit drug heroin is abused for the unique euphoria it produces. Some of these drugs, such as fentanyl and its derivatives, are so potent that they can present a danger to you and other providers if you are exposed while caring for a patient.

Opioids produce their major effects on the CNS by binding with receptor sites in the brain and other tissues. These agents are readily absorbed from the gastrointestinal tract but can also be absorbed from the nasal mucosa (when snorted) or from the lungs (opium smoking). When taken orally, the effects of opioid drugs are lessened compared with their effects when given parenterally. When heroin passes through the liver, it is metabolized into acetyl morphine, which continues to exert narcotic effects that may outlast the effects of naloxone (a narcotic antagonist discussed next). An AEMT who does not understand this concept can be fooled into thinking that a dose of naloxone has permanently reversed the effects of the heroin, only to have the patient lapse into unresponsiveness 15 or 20 minutes later.

Morphine is a commonly used analgesic in the prehospital setting and is a potent vasodilator. When given to young adults, its half-life is roughly 2 to 3 hours, but it typically takes longer to metabolize in older adults.

The classic presentation of opioid use features euphoria, hypotension, respiratory depression, and pinpoint pupils. Depending on the particular agent, nausea, vomiting, and constipation may occur as well. Allergic phenomena may also occur with opioid use, albeit rarely. With increased doses, coma, seizures (usually secondary to hypoxia), and cardiac arrest (usually secondary to respiratory arrest) are common.

Morphine and heroin produce an impressive dreamlike state. Shortly after injecting heroin, a user will appear to pass out. However, the user is typically quite lucid and remains aware of what is being done or said.

Patient Safety

A relatively new safety hazard for responders has surfaced in the form of synthetic opioids that are analogs of fentanyl. They have been associated with an epidemic of opioid-related overdose deaths.[10] One such drug, *carfentanil*, is 10,000 times more powerful than morphine. Fentanyl is similar to heroin and morphine, but is 50 to 100 times more potent than either.[11] These drugs are also being mixed with heroin to make them even more potent.

Carfentanil was designed for use by veterinarians to treat large animals such as horses, elephants, and the like. It acts quickly to depress the respiratory centers and CNS. Very small amounts can be detrimental to humans and possible fatal. While supplied in patches, powder, tablets, and spray, routes of exposure for first responders typically include absorption through the skin and inhalation via the respiratory tract. Law enforcement, firefighters, EMS, and even police dogs are at risk of exposure.[12]

While naloxone will work for overdoses, it may take significant amounts to make a difference. Personal protective equipment should include mask, gloves, and eye protection. Do not touch any substance that looks suspicious. Along with the risk of exposure to the substances, responders also face the potential for violent attacks from the patient when naloxone is used to reverse the effects of the drugs. Be prepared and call early for paramedic or law enforcement assistance.

Naloxone (Narcan) is an antidote that reverses the effects of opiate or opioid overdose. This medication can be administered via IV line, intramuscularly (IM), or intranasally. Ideally, naloxone is administered via IV access. However, in many instances, IV access is difficult to obtain in the chronic user of illicit intravenous drugs such as heroin. These patients have venous scarring, called track marks, from repeated use of needles on peripheral veins. Therefore, the intranasal route is becoming a preferred alternative route for administering naloxone. It is safer than administering an IM injection because a needle is not required to administer the medication. The dosage of naloxone is 0.4 to 2 mg.

Some EMS systems allow AEMTs to administer naloxone by the intranasal route, in which the antidote is atomized through the nares into the nasal mucosa. Be aware that the administration of naloxone may precipitate withdrawal symptoms resulting in violent behavior and/or seizure activity. Also, acute narcotic reversal may lead to vomiting and aspiration.[13] This medication should only be used when the patient has agonal respirations or apnea. Place an oropharyngeal (oral) or nasopharyngeal (nasal) airway and ventilate the patient using a bag-mask device prior to administering naloxone. Provide adequate ventilation while administering naloxone to decrease the risk of permanent brain damage related to hypoxia.

Words of Wisdom

In some areas, laypeople are permitted to administer naloxone. Be aware that it may have been administered prior to your arrival. Find out from bystanders what has occurred and who was given naloxone.

Closely monitor the patient. As the patient's level of consciousness rises, the patient will no longer tolerate the oropharyngeal airway, so you will have to remove it to prevent aspiration.

If a patient goes into cardiac arrest, follow the algorithm shown in **Figure 23-5**, including administering naloxone if it is available. However, providing bag-mask ventilations is a critical treatment for these patients as well. Whether or not naloxone is available, provide ventilations and rapid transport.

If the patient does not respond to naloxone, it is possible that the person has a "mixed-bag overdose"—that is, the patient may have taken multiple drugs, some of which are not opioids and will not respond to naloxone or may need a subsequent dose.[14] Alternatively, the lack of responsiveness may be from another source altogether, such as a head injury. In such a scenario, insert an advanced airway (eg, a Combitube, King airway, or laryngeal mask airway), provide other care as needed, and transport the patient to an appropriate facility. Call early for paramedic backup if needed.

Patient Safety

Remember the importance of performing a rapid full-body scan of patients who have overdosed on opioids. People may use multiple routes of administration when abusing opioids, including transdermal patches. Missing a fentanyl patch that was covered by clothing could lead to the patient lapsing back into respiratory arrest. Look in discreet areas such as between the cheeks of the buttocks, the inner thighs, and other areas that are not readily visible when clothing is removed. If you have not found and removed the patch, then you may not be successful in treating the life-threatening overdose.

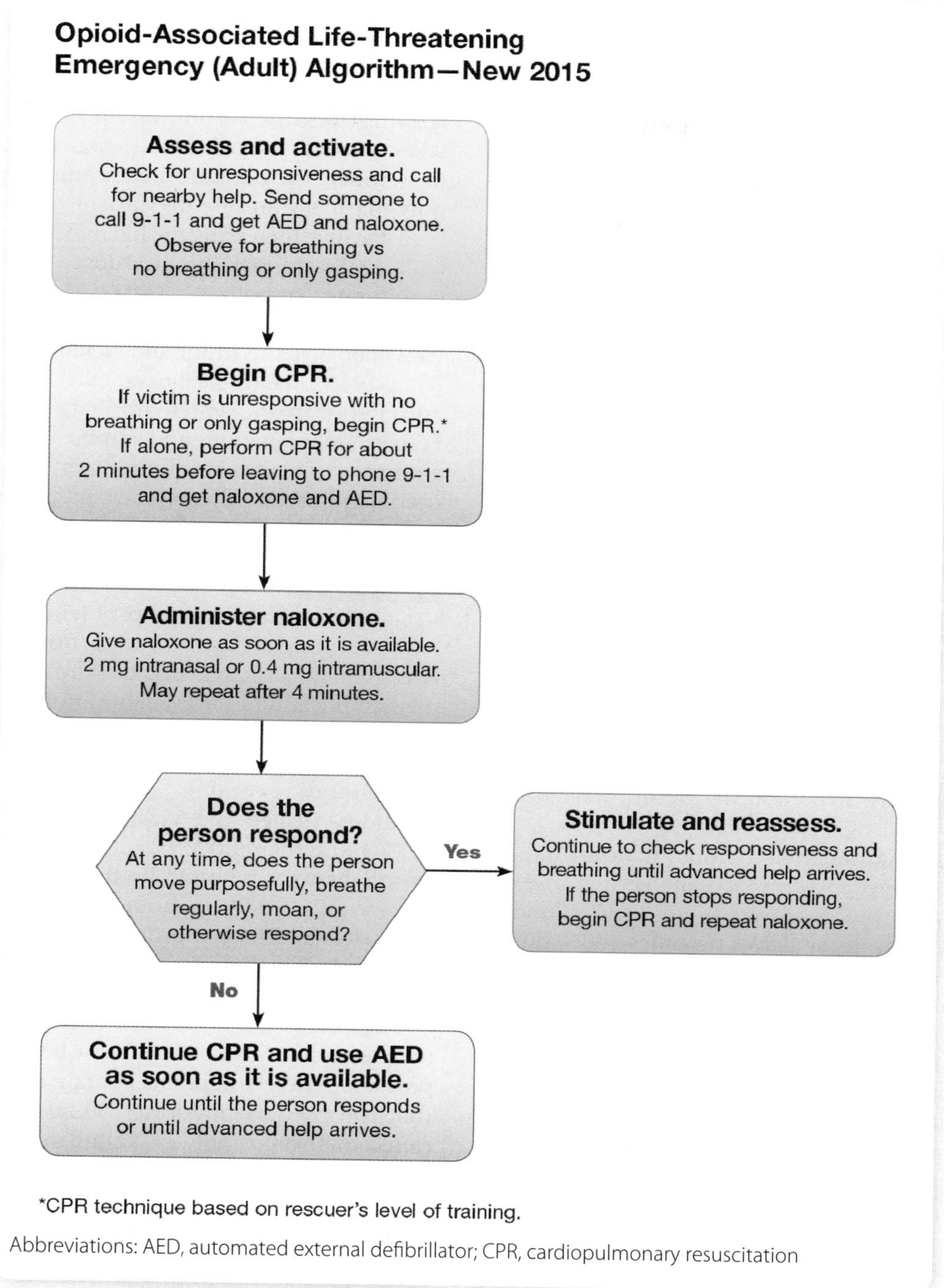

Opioid-Associated Life-Threatening
Emergency (Adult) Algorithm—New 2015
Assess and activate.
Check for unresponsiveness and call for nearby help. Send someone to call 9-1-1 and get AED and naloxone. Observe for breathing vs no breathing or only gasping.
Begin CPR.
If victim is unresponsive with no breathing or only gasping, begin CPR.* If alone, perform CPR for about 2 minutes before leaving to phone 9-1-1 and get naloxone and AED.
Administer naloxone.
Give naloxone as soon as it is available. 2 mg intranasal or 0.4 mg intramuscular. May repeat after 4 minutes.
Does the person respond?
At any time, does the person move purposefully, breathe regularly, moan, or otherwise respond?
Yes
Stimulate and reassess.
Continue to check responsiveness and breathing until advanced help arrives. If the person stops responding, begin CPR and repeat naloxone.
No
Continue CPR and use AED as soon as it is available.
Continue until the person responds or until advanced help arrives.
*CPR technique based on rescuer's level of training.
Abbreviations: AED, automated external defibrillator; CPR, cardiopulmonary resuscitation

Figure 23-5 The American Heart Association's algorithm for life-threatening opioid overdose.

When caring for a patient who has overdosed on opiates, it is important to remember that the patient may have other underlying chronic illnesses or conditions, such as hepatitis, human immunodeficiency virus (HIV)/acquired immunodeficiency syndrome (AIDS), malnutrition, or sepsis. Medications taken for any of these conditions may interact with the opioid, creating a myriad of signs and symptoms.

Older patients often take multiple medications for pain due to arthritis, degenerative diseases, and other conditions. For those patients who have chronic pain and regularly take large doses of narcotics, dependency may become a major problem. Using a narcotic antagonist in such a patient may cause withdrawal and result in seizures or other problems. Closely monitor these patients and provide prompt transport to the closest appropriate facility.

When you prepare your patient care report, ensure you document whether the ingestion was intentional or accidental, how much was taken, and what was taken. Also document whether the patient has vomited since ingestion. Take any pills or bottles to the hospital with the patient. Report all findings to receiving personnel at the ED, and also report any illicit substances to law enforcement.

▶ Stimulants

Few drugs compare with **stimulants** in potential for abuse—particularly cocaine, **amphetamines**, and **methamphetamine**. As with opioids, a first-time user may become an addict to one of these substances within just a few days.[15] If the person decides to quit using the stimulant, it is unlikely that the abstinence will be successful. In 2014, more than 900,000 people in the United States had a stimulant use disorder because of cocaine use, and more than 470,000 people had a stimulant use disorder as a result of using other stimulants besides methamphetamines.[16]

Depending on the formulation, stimulant drugs may be taken orally, smoked, or via IV injection. The clinical presentation of the stimulant abuser includes excitement, delirium, tachycardia, hypertension with a fast pulse rate or hypotension with a fast pulse rate, and dilated pupils. As toxic levels are reached, the patient may experience psychosis, hyperpyrexia, tremors, seizures, and cardiac arrest.

Cocaine is a naturally occurring alkaloid that is extracted from the *Erythroxylon coca* plant leaves found in South America. Once processed into cocaine hydrochloride, the active ingredient in the leaves becomes 100% pure, dramatically increasing its toxic potential. Cocaine is sold under many street names (blow, Coke, stash, nose candy, snow, dust). It is a local anesthetic and a CNS stimulant that can create euphoria that features enhanced alertness and a tremendous sense of well-being. Collectively, these effects make cocaine one of the most—if not the most—psychologically addictive drug available.

Cocaine is quickly absorbed across all mucosal membranes, allowing it to be applied topically, swallowed, snorted, or via IV injection. Also, this drug may be mixed with two inexpensive ingredients, baking soda and water. Once mixed together into a pastelike slurry and cooked or baked, the end result is smokable cocaine (known as crack).

When cocaine is snorted nasally, the effects are felt within 1 to 2 minutes, and peak effects occur in 20 to 30 minutes. When it is smoked, the onset of effects is much more rapid (8 to 10 seconds) and the high is more intense, though the effects do not last as long, leading to binge redosing.

When the effects of cocaine wear off, the user experiences a "crash," characterized by depression, irritability, sleeplessness, and exhaustion. Depending on the amount and length of cocaine use, the person may experience a cascade of adverse effects collectively referred to as *cocaine washout syndrome*. This syndrome presents as a hypoactive state related to a lack of synaptic neurotransmitters. To avoid this crash, the user will often seek more cocaine. Adding to the problem, a person addicted to cocaine, who is trying to escape the unpleasant effects of a crash, often takes a sedative (such as diazepam [Valium], alcohol, or heroin). Thus, a chronic cocaine user may practice polypharmacy and be dependent on more substances than cocaine, increasing the likelihood that he or she will need EMS care, possibly overdosed on amphetamines, barbiturates, or both.

Amphetamines are structurally similar to the derivatives of phenylethylamine and include methamphetamine (crank or ice), methylenedioxyamphetamine (MDA, Adam), and methylenedioxymethamphetamine (MDMA, Eve, Ecstasy). Amphetamine and amphetaminelike drugs have a number of legitimate clinical applications. Most nasal decongestants and diet pills are members of this family, as are the drugs used to treat narcolepsy, attention-deficit disorder, and attention-deficit/hyperactivity disorder **Figure 23-6**.

Methamphetamine is problematic because it is a low-cost, long-acting (up to 12 hours) stimulant that is extremely addictive. Because the ingredients to cook methamphetamine are available locally within the United States and the drug is easily and quickly made, its manufacturer avoids the hassle, risk, and high cost associated with importing cocaine. "Meth labs" are dangerous and should be treated as a hazardous materials incident. In 2014, more than 9,000 incidents involving clandestine meth labs were reported by the US Drug Enforcement Agency;[17] thus, AEMTs should be prepared to encounter these sites and take appropriate precautions when one is suspected, including calling for law enforcement and specialty responder assistance.

Synthetic cathinones, marketed as "bath salts" under unique names such as "Blaze," have become a public health problem. These stimulants contain an active ingredient that is a pseudoephedrine (Sudafed) reduction drug called methcathinone, or a similar methamphetamine

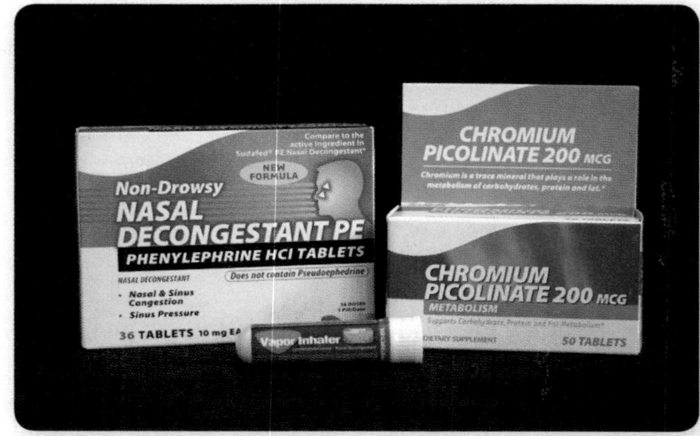

Figure 23-6 Nasal decongestants and diet pills generally fall into the category of amphetamines.

knock-off. Users typically snort, smoke, or ingest these drugs, which couple the intensity and long-acting effects of methamphetamine with the euphoric effects of crack cocaine. The more serious side effects of these designer drugs include agitation, hallucinations, and paranoia. Many states have now made it illegal to manufacture or possess these drugs, which are often sold online. In addition, in 2012, the federal government banned the two main active ingredients of synthetic cathinones, mephedrone and methylenedioxypyrovalerone, although new compounds continue to emerge.[18]

Signs and symptoms of stimulant abuse may appear as a patient with a wild-eyed but thin-as-a-rail appearance, and nervous or jittery movements. For a serious abuser, week-long runs without sleeping are not unusual, and the person often goes days without eating during such a period. As the days pass by, increasing paranoia makes encounters risky. Patients are usually "amped up" when you encounter them, and it often takes very little to set off a violent tirade.

A person who has overdosed on cocaine may exhibit any of these signs and symptoms. Cocaine may also cause a variety of serious, potentially fatal complications: lethal electrocardiograph dysrhythmias, acute myocardial infarction, seizures, stroke, apnea, and hyperthermia. In addition, a crack smoker risks pneumothorax and pneumomediastinum. The clinical presentation of the patient abusing amphetamine or methamphetamine is almost identical to that of a person abusing cocaine, except the effects last many hours longer than those of cocaine. Use of synthetic cathinones is associated with significant paranoia, hallucinations, incredible strength, excited delirium, and other bizarre behaviors. Tachycardia, diaphoresis, nausea, and hyperthermia may also be present. Pay careful attention to your personal safety when assessing and treating patients suspected of using these drugs.

The treatment for patients abusing cocaine, amphetamines, synthetic cathinones, or methamphetamine is fundamentally the same: maintain maximum oxygen saturation levels, prevent seizures with adequate sedation, and monitor serial vital signs. Consider paramedic backup for an advanced airway as needed. Establish vascular access and manage hypotension with a fluid infusion of normal saline. Apply the pulse oximeter. Call for paramedic backup to control anxiety and seizures and to administer benzodiazepines per local protocol. If the patient has a seizure, protect the airway. Finally, transport the patient to the appropriate facility.

In severe cases of stimulant overdose, the patient may present with hyperthermia, which can be lethal. Apply ice packs or mist the patient's skin to help reduce his or her body temperature.

Throughout the resuscitation process, it is essential to maintain peripheral perfusion with aggressive fluid therapy. Regular assessment of breath sounds to avoid inadvertent overhydration is necessary.

Remember the potential for the patient who has abused stimulants to be emotionally or psychologically unstable. With chronic abuse, each passing day without sleep and little or no food intake may make the patient increasingly paranoid and even psychotic. The patient's behavior can suddenly become violent, so consider the situation a potential hazard. Contact law enforcement for support when you first suspect the possibility that violence may occur.

▶ Marijuana and Cannabis Compounds

When the leaves and flower buds of the *Cannabis sativa* plant are harvested and dried, the end product is referred to as **marijuana** (known as weed, pot, dope, smoke, and bud). Over the past decade, some states have legalized the use of marijuana and some of the compounds from the plant for medical use; other states have legalized it for recreational use. According to the 2014 National Survey on Drug Use and Health, marijuana remains the most commonly used illicit drug in the United States, with approximately 32% of people ages 18 to 25 reporting using marijuana within the prior year.[19] For these reasons, it is important to have a thorough understanding of marijuana and cannabis compounds.

Marijuana is usually smoked but can be ingested (such as when baked in cookies or brownies). The onset of effects from smoking marijuana occurs in a matter of minutes; oral ingestion slows the onset time to several hours.

Marijuana users may have a distorted sense of time and space and, occasionally, a feeling of unreality. Smoking marijuana results in bronchodilation and slight tachycardia. Other signs and symptoms of marijuana use include euphoria, drowsiness, decreased short-term memory, diminished motor coordination, increased appetite, and bloodshot eyes.

Management focuses on supportive care, because there is relatively low likelihood of a serious medical complication from marijuana use. A novice user may exhibit some behavioral symptoms such as paranoia and (rarely) psychosis. Reassurance is generally helpful with either issue.

Another illicit drug that is growing in popularity is **spice**, a mixture of dried plant material that is sold as incense in efforts to avoid existing drug laws. This psychoactive drug is a blend of synthetic cannabinoids (knock-offs of the naturally occurring psychoactive elements in marijuana), where the active substance is sprayed onto a plant-like material for smoking or sold as a liquid for vaporizing in e-cigarettes. Unlike marijuana, which typically has relaxing effects, the adverse effects of spice use include psychosis, hallucinations, tachycardia, vomiting, renal problems, and seizures. In some cases, these effects are reported to last as long as 3 months.

It can be challenging to obtain a good assessment and form a treatment plan for someone who has used spice. Remember that various chemicals may have been used in the spice, so you may be faced with patient presentations related more to those chemicals than to the plant-like material the patient is smoking. Supportive care with fluids and airway maintenance is often appropriate. Benzodiazepines are the recommended medication for patients experiencing a seizure. In these cases, call for paramedic backup to administer benzodiazepines or antiemetics.

▶ Hallucinogens

A **hallucinogen** alters a person's sensory perception, causing the individual to see, hear, or feel things that are not actually present. Experiences involving hallucinogens can vary markedly, with people taking the same dose of the same drug from the same batch experiencing totally different effects. In 2014, 1.2 million people in the United States (0.4% of the total population) reported using hallucinogens in the past month; this rate has remained steady for more than 1 decade.[20]

The classic hallucinogen is lysergic acid diethylamide (LSD). LSD primarily affects the senses rather than changing physiologic functions. Synthesthesias (crossing of the senses) often prompt a user to respond to the question "What were you doing?" with a reply such as "I was watching the music play" or "I was listening to that painting." With higher doses, the effects of LSD can last as long as 12 hours, although 3 to 4 hours is more typical. Effects of LSD often consist of tachycardia, mild hypertension, and dilated pupils. In a "bad trip," the user has a frightening experience, resulting in an acute anxiety attack and the physical effects secondary to increased anxiety.

Psilocybin mushrooms are among the most frequently used hallucinogens by teens and young adults in the United States Figure 23-7.[21] The onset of symptoms and hallucinogenic effects (similar to LSD but less intense) is within 30 minutes of ingestion, and effects usually last 4 to 6 hours. Signs and symptoms include nausea and vomiting, mydriasis, mild tachycardia, and mild hypertension. The likelihood of any serious medical side effects is low, though seizures and hyperthermia may occur.

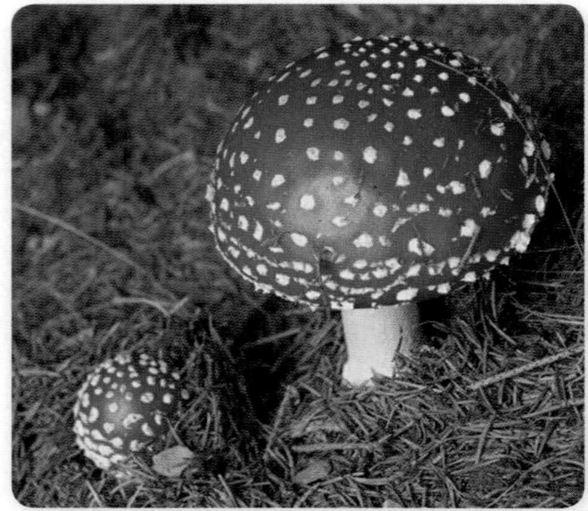

Figure 23-7 Certain mushrooms are hallucinogenic if ingested.

Abuse of phencyclidine (PCP, angel dust), another hallucinogen, is relatively uncommon among young adults. Nevertheless, there were more than 75,000 ED visits related to PCP use in 2011 (up from 14,000 visits in 2005), with more than two-thirds of these visits involving men.[22] PCP is typically smoked or snorted, although it can be injected. Slurred speech, staggering gait, tachycardia, hypertension, staring blankly for extended periods, and horizontal nystagmus (involuntary, rhythmic movement of the eyes) are common with PCP use. Muscle rigidity and especially grinding of the teeth prompt many users to resort to pacifiers in an effort to avoid pronounced jaw aches. More problematic are the hallmarks of PCP use, which include mind–body separation, related hallucinations, and violent outbreaks. Users may make bizarre comments such as "I can fly" and then jump off a balcony to prove it. Users have an almost unfathomable ability to withstand pain with no reaction and exhibit almost superhuman strength.

Ketamine (known as Special K, Vitamin K) is similar in chemical structure to PCP. Most ketamine available on the street is stolen from veterinary clinics, but this drug is increasingly being used in emergency medicine. Although its abuse in the general population is low (prevalence of recreational use in the US population is estimated between 0.1% and 4%), ketamine is a popular "club drug" used in nightclubs, raves, and other party settings. It is frequently used in combination with other club drugs, alcohol, and stimulants.[23] Illicit ketamine is colorless and odorless and is commonly found in powdered form. It is often mixed in a drink, although it can be snorted. It is physically and psychologically addicting.

Ketamine is a dissociative anesthetic. At low doses, a user presents with mild inebriation, lethargy, dreamy or erotic thoughts, and increased sociability. At higher doses, a patient may have pronounced nausea, difficulty moving, and report "entering another reality." In extreme cases, users will enter the "K-hole," which involves out-of-body experiences that may cause hallucinations, delusions, or a near-death experience.[24] Long-term use can result in extensive problems with memory, cognitive impairment, and/or an inability to properly speak or see.[25]

Mescaline, the dried flower "buttons" of the peyote cactus, is also a hallucinogen. Peyote and mescaline are Schedule I substances with a high potential for abuse and no currently accepted medical use in the United States. Few statistics are available on their use. Profound vomiting occurs shortly after ingestion of mescaline. The psychedelic experience then typically begins with feelings of increased sensitivity to sensory stimulation. Users may experience hallucinations, a distortion of time and space, or out-of-body experiences. The physical effects of mescaline are similar to those of LSD, including dilated pupils, increased heart rate, mild hypertension, and increased body temperature.

The treatment for a patient using hallucinogens is primarily supportive. A person having a bad trip is in a vivid dream or nightmare that will not end until the drug wears off. Try to limit sensory stimulation as much as possible—for example, by avoiding the use of emergency lights and siren. Routine transport to the appropriate facility plus psychological support is usually all that is required in the prehospital setting.

For patients who have used PCP or ketamine, secure the patient well, assess the ABCDEs and manage any life threats, administer oxygen therapy, establish vascular access if the patient is receptive, and provide safe transport to the appropriate facility. Keep a close eye on the patient, because violent behavior can suddenly occur. Benzodiazepines may help calm an agitated patient who is experiencing significant delirium; call for paramedic backup in such a case. *Note:* PCP can cause some of the most violent and difficult behavior you will encounter in the field, so protect the patient and the EMS team from attacks involving poor judgment and impaired behavior.

Care for mescaline users and psilocybin mushroom users is primarily supportive. Pay attention to the ABCDEs, administer oxygen therapy, monitor vital signs, provide positive psychological support, and provide safe transport. If time and circumstances allow, establish vascular access to provide a medication route.

▶ Sedatives and Hypnotics

Sedative-hypnotic drugs have a wide range of applications. Drugs with sedative qualities reduce anxiety and calm agitated patients. Drugs with hypnotic qualities help produce drowsiness and sleep. In either case, sedative-hypnotic drugs function primarily as CNS depressants.

Barbiturates have a long history of use as sleep aids, antianxiety drugs, and seizure control medications. In the past, the frequent combination of alcohol and barbiturates used by people to attempt suicide and the high incidence of accidental overdoses pushed researchers to develop sedative-hypnotic drugs that had fewer depressive effects on the respiratory system and were less lethal.

With mild to moderate barbiturate intoxication, patients present similarly to those with alcohol intoxication; their symptoms include drowsiness, decreased inhibitions, ataxia, mental confusion, and staggering gait. As the dose increases, patients become increasingly lethargic and demonstrate an increasingly lower level of responsiveness until they are unresponsive (Glasgow Coma Scale score of 3).

Barbiturate abusers quickly develop tolerance and require ever-larger doses to produce the desired effects. Long-term use results in physical addiction. Abrupt cessation in a long-term barbiturate abuser will produce typical signs and symptoms of withdrawal syndrome in approximately 24 hours. In the case of minor withdrawal, the patient may present with symptoms similar to those observed in a patient with alcohol withdrawal: restlessness, tremulousness, insomnia, diaphoresis, abdominal cramping, and nausea and vomiting. Patients in severe withdrawal may present with delirium, hallucinations,

YOU are the Provider — PART 3

The patient's sister introduces herself and tells you her brother has used meth for about 5 years and has never sought drug treatment. You and your partner agree the patient requires transport to the ED via ambulance, and you also agree that law enforcement must ride in the back of the ambulance with you. When you speak with the police captain about this issue, he agrees to send one of his officers with you in the back, with another officer following the ambulance. Because the patient remains highly agitated and your department's policies prohibit patients from being handcuffed in the ambulance, with police assistance you place each of the patient's extremities in soft restraints.

Recording Time: 4 Minutes	
Respirations	32 breaths/min, rapid
Pulse	Strong and regular, 120 beats/min
Skin	Hot, dry, and pink
Blood pressure	84/52 mm Hg
Oxygen saturation (Spo_2)	95% on room air
Pupils	Dilated, equal, and reactive to light

5. Which treatment does this patient require en route to the hospital?
6. Why should you have a law enforcement officer in the back of the ambulance during this transport?

psychosis, hyperthermia, and cardiovascular collapse. Life-threatening withdrawal, similar to DTs, is possible with abrupt cessation of large doses of barbiturates.

Benzodiazepines are also members of the sedative-hypnotic family. These medications are most commonly used to treat anxiety, seizures, and alcohol withdrawal. Effects of benzodiazepines include sedation, reduced anxiety, and relaxation of striated muscle. Assessing a patient who is abusing benzodiazepines can be complicated, because the person is also likely to use other drugs and alcohol. The most common clinical effects of benzodiazepine overdose include altered mentation, drowsiness, confusion, slurred speech, ataxia, and general uncoordination. Today, the likelihood of death after the ingestion of a single sedative-hypnotic such as diazepam is small.

Withdrawal from benzodiazepines may include tachycardia, tremulousness, confusion, and possibly seizures. Withdrawal is rarely a life-threatening event, but it can be complicated by withdrawal from other substances, such as alcohol.

Airway management is the first priority in caring for a patient who has overdosed on barbiturates or benzodiazepines. Call for paramedic backup to intubate the patient and monitor the electrocardiographic rhythm. Next, administer high-concentration oxygen and establish venous access. If the patient develops shock, then a rapid infusion of a 20-mL/kg bolus of normal saline and possibly repeated doses up to 2 L may be needed. Assess breath sounds before and after each bolus, rather than infusing an entire liter and then assessing breath sounds. A reversal agent is available for managing a benzodiazepine overdose—flumazenil (Romazicon), a benzodiazepine receptor antagonist—although its use in the prehospital setting is rarely warranted, as it can precipitate withdrawal symptoms in susceptible patients. Call for paramedic backup for administration if needed.

Activated charcoal may also be an option for treating patients with sedative-hypnotic overdose. However, do not administer it to patients who are at risk of becoming unresponsive or of losing the ability to protect their airways, as vomiting can occur and aspiration of activated charcoal can be exceedingly dangerous.

▶ Cardiac Medications

The medications used to treat patients with cardiac and cardiac-related problems continue to increase in number and sophistication. The major classes of drugs used as part of these treatment regimens include antidysrhythmics, beta-blockers, calcium-channel blockers, cardiac glycosides, and angiotensin-converting enzyme inhibitors. Many patients take a combination of drugs—sometimes three or more—in attempts to control hypertension, electrocardiographic rhythm disturbances, or other problems. An overdose with these drugs is usually accidental.

Signs and symptoms of overdose with cardiac drugs vary, but may include hypotension, weakness or confusion, nausea and vomiting, rhythm disturbances (most commonly bradycardia or heart block), headache, and difficulty breathing. As with all emergencies, ensure a patent airway, provide adequate ventilation, and administer high-flow supplemental oxygen.

Establish vascular access in case of overdose with these agents. Several therapeutic interventions and antidotes are available if the specific agent is identified. In case of hypotension, sequential fluid boluses of normal saline will often bring the blood pressure into an acceptable range.

Because of the sophistication of cardiac drugs and the likelihood that the patient may be taking multiple cardiac and other medications, making contact with medical control to consult with a physician is prudent.

▶ Other Medications

Erectile dysfunction medications are the most dangerous of the various drugs that increase sexual gratification. These drugs, such as sildenafil (Viagra), tadalafil (Cialis), or vardenafil (Levitra), are contraindicated for patients who take nitrates for cardiac conditions. In these patients, erectile dysfunction medications may result in severe hypotension or total cardiovascular collapse, ultimately leading to death. If patients develop hypotension after taking one of these drugs, then repeated boluses of normal saline can increase the blood pressure to an acceptable level. If cardiac arrest occurs, follow your protocols.

Patients taking a variety of psychiatric medications may experience toxicologic emergencies. **Tricyclic antidepressants (TCAs)** carry a high risk of intentional overdose. Also, minimal dosing errors may produce toxic effects. The most common signs and symptoms of a TCA overdose are altered mental status (drowsy, confused, slurred speech), dysrhythmias (usually sinus tachycardia or supraventricular tachycardia), dry mouth, blurred vision or dilated pupils, urinary retention, constipation, and pulmonary edema. With a more serious toxic exposure, be alert for ventricular tachycardia, hypotension, respiratory depression, and seizures; dysrhythmias may be life threatening. Managing patients with a TCA overdose includes the following measures:

- Maintain the airway. If the patient's mental status suddenly deteriorates (as is often the case), insert an advanced airway.
- Call for paramedic backup as needed for cardiac monitoring, intubation, and medication administration.
- Administer high-flow supplemental oxygen.
- Establish vascular access.
- Administer activated charcoal per medical control orders.
- Manage hypotension with sequential boluses of normal saline. Be alert to the possibility of pulmonary edema, which occurs frequently in cases of TCA overdose.
- Assess blood glucose levels. Administer dextrose 50% in water if the patient is hypoglycemic.

- Rule out head trauma as a possible cause of decreased mental status.
- Monitor for agitation or violence. Provide rapid transport to the closest appropriate facility.

Monoamine oxidase inhibitors (MAOIs) are sometimes used to treat depression, but have a high potential for drug interactions. MAOIs can precipitate a hypertensive crisis if taken in conjunction with tyramine-containing foods (such as beer, wine, aged cheese, chopped liver, pickled herring, sour cream, yogurt, and fava beans). Symptoms of MAOI toxicity are often delayed, occurring 6 to 12 hours after ingestion and, in some cases, as long as 24 hours later. Once signs and symptoms begin to appear, you should prepare to manage a life-threatening event. Early signs and symptoms of MAOI overdose include hyperactivity, dysrhythmias (usually sinus tachycardia), hyperventilation, and nystagmus. With increased levels of toxicity, be alert for chest pain, palpitations, hypertension, diaphoresis, agitated or combative behavior, marked hyperthermia, and hallucinations.

Unfortunately, there is no antidote available for an MAOI overdose. Establish and maintain the airway. Administer high-flow supplemental oxygen or provide positive pressure ventilation if needed. Establish vascular access. Consider administration of activated charcoal if recommended by medical control. Do *not* give syrup of ipecac. With a patient in deteriorating condition, treat hypotension with sequential fluid boluses of normal saline. If seizures occur, call for paramedic backup for medication administration.

Selective serotonin reuptake inhibitors (SSRIs) are among the widely used medications for managing depression. Patients with an SSRI overdose may be asymptomatic. When symptoms are present, they most commonly include nausea, vomiting, dysrhythmias (usually sinus tachycardia), sedation, and tremors, and possibly dilated pupils, agitation, blood pressure changes (hypotension or hypertension), seizures, and hallucinations. Managing a patient with an SSRI overdose follows the general approach for poisoned patients:

- Establish and maintain the airway.
- Administer high-flow supplemental oxygen.
- Establish vascular access.
- Call for paramedic backup as needed.
- Consider a single dose of activated charcoal per medical control.
- Transport the patient to the appropriate facility.

Despite the major advances made in many areas of psychiatric medicine, **lithium** remains the cornerstone drug for treating a bipolar disorder. Lithium is excreted from the body slowly, meaning the threat of toxic levels and overdosing is always present. Signs and symptoms of lithium overdose include nausea, vomiting, hand tremors, excessive thirst, and slurred speech; as toxicity increases, patients may develop ataxia, muscle weakness and incoordination, blurred vision, and hyperreflexia (twitching). Eventually, patients may have seizures and become comatose.

Managing a patient with a suspected lithium overdose is mostly supportive. Establish and maintain the airway, inserting an advanced airway as needed. Administer high-flow supplemental oxygen, and ensure vascular access. If the patient experiences hypotension, administer serial boluses of normal saline. Transport the patient to an appropriate facility.

Medications used for pain management account for a large portion of the over-the-counter (OTC) drug market. Nonsteroidal anti-inflammatory drugs (NSAIDs) are some of the most popular options for pain relief, fever control, and anti-inflammatory action. Most of the problems associated with NSAIDs involve long-term use; patients may experience gastrointestinal bleeding and kidney dysfunction with chronic use. Signs and symptoms of NSAID overdose may include headache, altered mentation, behavioral changes, seizures, bradydysrhythmias, hypotension, abdominal pain, nausea, and vomiting.

For symptomatic patients with NSAID overdose, care in the prehospital setting is usually supportive. Establish and maintain the airway, inserting an advanced airway as needed. Administer high-flow supplemental oxygen, and establish vascular access. If hypotension develops, administer fluid boluses of normal saline. If hypotension persists after sequential fluid boluses, consider calling for paramedic backup for medication administration. Transport the patient to an appropriate facility.

Although aspirin (acetylsalicylic acid, or ASA) can be involved in a toxicologic emergency, more typically other OTC products containing **salicylates** cause toxicity (eg, Pepto-Bismol and hot-air vaporizers). With continued use of these products over a period of days, infants or young toddlers may ingest toxic levels of the salicylate. Chief complaints are usually nausea, vomiting, abdominal pain, diaphoresis, hyperpnea, ringing in the ears, pulmonary edema, and acid–base disturbances. Severe toxicity may produce metabolic acidosis or combined respiratory alkalosis–metabolic acidosis.

No salicylate antidote or antagonist is available, so field management is primarily supportive. Establish and maintain the airway, inserting an advanced airway as needed. Administer high-flow supplemental oxygen, and establish vascular access. If hypotension develops (from volume depletion), administer serial boluses of normal saline. Monitor carbon dioxide levels with capnometry if available. Following consultation with medical control, administer one dose of activated charcoal if appropriate. Call for paramedic backup as needed. Transport the patient to the closest, most appropriate facility.

Acetaminophen is a well-tolerated drug with few side effects that is available OTC. It is important to try to accurately estimate the time of its ingestion, because this information drives the decision-making process for patient care in the field and the hospital following acetaminophen overdose. An antidote for acetaminophen toxicity exists, although not as a prehospital intervention, and should be given less than 8 hours after the ingestion.

Prehospital management of acetaminophen toxicity first focuses on establishing and maintaining the airway, with an advanced airway being inserted as needed. Administer high-flow supplemental oxygen, and establish vascular access. For recent ingestions, consider administration of activated charcoal after consulting with medical control, and only if the patient is alert and able to follow commands. Transport the patient to an appropriate facility.

Drugs used to facilitate sexual assault—commonly known as "date rape" drugs—are often administered unknowingly to an individual, frequently in an alcoholic drink. **Gamma-hydroxybutyrate (GHB)** is a drug that is frequently associated with sexual assaults. GHB is available as an odorless and colorless liquid. It has a salty taste, but this may not be noted when placed in a drink. GHB produces a pronounced hypnotic effect along with disinhibition, severe passivity, and antegrade amnesia. Treatment for GHB intoxication focuses on the CNS depression and the risks associated with the patient being unable to protect the airway. Establish and maintain the airway; insert an advanced airway as needed. Carefully monitor the patient's level of consciousness. Assist breathing as necessary, and administer high-flow supplemental oxygen. Establish vascular access. Apply the pulse oximeter. Finally, provide rapid transport to the ED.

▶ Organophosphates

Organophosphates are a major component in many insecticides (Orthene, diazinon, and malathion) used in agriculture and in the home. Similar-performing compounds are used as "nerve gases" designed for chemical warfare, and like organophosphates, are categorized as cholinergic agents. These agents overstimulate normal body functions that are controlled by the parasympathetic nerves, resulting in salivation, mucus secretion, urination, crying, and an abnormal heart rate. You are unlikely to encounter patients who have been exposed to nerve gases, but you may be called to care for patients who have been exposed to one of the organophosphate insecticides (pesticides) or certain wild mushrooms, which are also cholinergic agents.

Suicide attempts account for a considerable share of organophosphate poisonings. When suicide is the goal, the poison is usually taken by mouth. Accidental agricultural exposure is another common source of AEMT calls for organophosphate poisoning, and persons involved in the manufacture of organophosphates and similar compounds are all at risk for this type of exposure.

The symptoms of organophosphate poisoning are fundamentally the same regardless of the chemical's route of entry—anxiety and restlessness; headache, dizziness, and confusion; tremors or seizures; dyspnea, diffuse wheezing, and respiratory depression; and loss of consciousness. A patient poisoned with organophosphates will usually present with signs and symptoms within the first 8 hours. In addition, the CNS signs and symptoms associated with cholinergic excess are often expressed using the SLUDGEM mnemonic:

S Salivation, sweating
L Lacrimation (excessive tearing of the eyes)
U Urination
D Defecation
G Gastric upset and cramps
E Emesis
M Muscle twitching/miosis (pinpoint pupils)

Alternatively, you can use the mnemonic DUMBELS:

D Diarrhea
U Urination
M Miosis (constriction of the pupils), muscle weakness
B Bradycardia, bronchospasm, bronchorrhea (discharge of mucus from the lungs)
E Emesis
L Lacrimation
S Seizures, salivation, sweating

To assess and treat a patient with organophosphate poisoning, start with decontaminating and removing all contaminated clothing *before* initiating care or loading the patient into the ambulance. Contaminated clothing should be placed in plastic bags and disposed of as hazardous materials. Ideally, the patient should be scrubbed with soap and water. After that, patient care includes the following measures:

- Establish and maintain the airway. Consider an advanced airway as needed.
- Suction as needed.
- Administer high-flow supplemental oxygen.
- Establish vascular access.
- Call for paramedic backup for medication administration and cardiac monitoring.
- Apply the pulse oximeter.
- Transport immediately to the closest appropriate facility.

In the unlikely event of a terrorist attack involving cholinergic agents, be aware that the US military has developed antidotes to nerve gas agents that can be administered if they are available and indicated. The most common of these antidotes are the DuoDote kit, the Antidote Treatment Nerve Agent Auto-Injector (ATNAA), and the Mark 1 kit (which is no longer manufactured but may still be present in stocked supplies). The indications for these antidotes are a known exposure to nerve agents or organophosphates with manifestation of signs and symptoms. Removal of the patient from the source of the exposure is also critical in these cases. If your service carries these antidote kits, ask to receive training on the proper use prior to being cleared to administer them. Nerve agent treatment, and these kits, are covered in Chapter 42, *Terrorism Response and Disaster Management*.

▶ Carbon Monoxide

Carbon monoxide is one of the most common fatal poisonings.[26] This gas is produced during the incomplete combustion of organic fuels, such as in an automobile engine or a home-heating device. CO poisoning may occur when a flue or ventilating system becomes blocked, or it may be a method of suicide (an automobile running in a closed garage). CO is also a major contributor to death in house fires.

Because CO is a colorless, odorless, tasteless gas, people who are exposed to it often have no idea that they are inhaling a toxic substance until it is too late. The toxicity arises primarily from the affinity of CO for hemoglobin in red blood cells; carbon dioxide displaces oxygen, thereby preventing the red blood cells from carrying oxygen to the tissues and leading to suffocation at the cellular level. The atmospheric level of CO does not need to be very high for poisoning to occur.

Because the overall ability of the blood to transport oxygen is drastically reduced when CO reaches toxic levels, anything that increases the body's oxygen requirements, such as physical exertion or a fever, will increase the severity of the poisoning. Children, whose metabolic rate is intrinsically higher than that of adults, tend to have more severe symptoms at any given level of exposure.

CO poisoning can be difficult to diagnose in the field unless it is the direct result of an easily identifiable cause, such as a fire or intentional exposure to exhaust fumes from an automobile. Its signs and symptoms are highly variable and vague, often resembling the early onset of the flu—for example, headache, nausea, and vomiting. With acute poisoning, the patient may be confused and unable to think clearly. Complaints of a sensation of pressure in the head or roaring in the ears are common. The physical exam often reveals bounding pulses, dilated pupils, and pallor or cyanosis. The cherry red color of the skin that is mentioned in many textbooks is a very late sign of CO poisoning. Consider the possibility of CO poisoning whenever you are confronted with several (possibly many) people who have shared the same accommodations for any period, especially if they have been quartered together in a closed area, such as one house in the winter.

Words of Wisdom

Carbon monoxide is a hazard for providers, as well as for patients. When you have multiple patients with medical complaints—at the same time and inside the same building—consider CO poisoning.

Recent developments in technology have given AEMTs the ability to perform noninvasive identification of CO poisoning (% Sp_{CO}, or CO saturation of the blood) in the field, which helps address the problem of delayed diagnosis. *Note:* Pulse oximetry *will not* provide a true assessment of arterial oxygenation because the device cannot determine whether CO or oxygen is bound to the hemoglobin. A reading of 99% on the pulse oximeter would be excellent in a normal environmental setting, but would be a grave finding in the presence of carboxyhemoglobin because the hemoglobin is saturated with the wrong chemical! Special CO monitoring devices are available that use the same probe used to measure oxygen saturation, but specifically measure CO saturation instead. If your service carries a CO monitoring device, ensure you know how to use it.

Treat CO poisoning in the field by administering the highest concentration of oxygen possible in an attempt to displace CO molecules from the hemoglobin. For patients with only mild symptoms, such as headache, nausea, and flulike symptoms, the elimination half-time of carboxyhemoglobin is roughly 4 hours. By comparison, if the patient is breathing 100% oxygen, the half-time can be reduced to approximately 1.5 hours. Hyperbaric oxygen therapy can further reduce the elimination time in some cases of severe exposure with markedly elevated CO levels.

If you suspect CO poisoning:

- Remove the patient from the exposure environment.
- Establish and maintain the airway, inserting an advanced airway as needed.
- Administer high-flow supplemental oxygen by a tight-fitting nonrebreathing mask.
- Establish vascular access.
- Keep the patient quiet and at rest to minimize oxygen demand.
- Monitor the patient's level of consciousness.
- Transport the patient to the appropriate facility. If the patient is unresponsive or has signs of serious CO poisoning, then direct transport to a facility capable of providing hyperbaric medicine is preferred.
- For patients with injuries or illness from a structural or vehicular fire, consider the possibility of combined CO/cyanide poisoning, especially if the patient has signs of shock.

▶ Metals

Despite the bans on lead in gasoline, paint, canning processes, and plumbing, lead poisoning remains the leading cause of chronic metal poisoning.[27] It has long been known that elevated levels of lead exposure may significantly hamper intellectual development in children.

With inorganic lead, absorption usually occurs via the respiratory or gastrointestinal tract. Once inside the body, approximately 90% of the lead is stored in the teeth and bones.[28] From this site, it eventually makes its way into the bloodstream. Inorganic lead can also cross the placental barrier and negatively affect fetal development. Its excretion from the body is incredibly slow, with the half-life of lead in bone estimated at 30 years.

Table 23-4 Body Systems Affected by Lead Poisoning	
Body System	**Signs and Symptoms**
Central nervous	Altered mentation, including irritability, mood changes, memory deficit, sleep disturbances; headache; seizures; ataxia
Gastrointestinal	Abdominal pain (usually occurs with acute poisoning); constipation; diarrhea
Renal	Renal insufficiency; hypertension; gout
Hematologic	Anemia

Most organic lead (tetraethyl lead) exposures occur in occupational settings,[29] although they can also occur from gas sniffing where leaded gasoline is available. Once inside the body, tetraethyl lead is metabolized to inorganic lead and triethyl lead, with triethyl lead being the primary cause of CNS toxicity.

Lead poisoning is associated with a long list of signs and symptoms Table 23-4. In particular, encephalopathy is a major cause of mortality and morbidity from lead poisoning.

In the field, you have few treatment options for lead poisoning. Your most helpful move may be to identify the source of the lead, which can assist the appropriate government agency to prevent more occurrences by removing the toxin. When you are managing the patient, first establish and maintain the airway, inserting an advanced airway as needed. Administer high-flow supplemental oxygen. Establish vascular access with a saline or heparin lock. Unless hypotension is present, do not provide fluid therapy—it may worsen cerebral edema. Transport the patient to an appropriate facility.

Iron is another metal that is commonly ingested. Although only a small amount of iron is required as part of a healthy diet, many adult and pediatric multivitamins contain iron. Children younger than 6 years have frequent iron exposures, usually secondary to ingesting chewable vitamins that are flavored or in cartoon shapes. By comparison, most toxic exposures in adults are intentional.

In the average 154-pound (70-kg) adult, the body's entire iron supply consists of only about 4 g. Of that total, roughly 65% is found in hemoglobin, with the remainder sequestered elsewhere. Because of its toxic potential, iron is stored in the body by several mechanisms, which permit access to the supply as needed. The body of a healthy person does not contain "free" (unbound) iron.

From a practical perspective, the toxic effects of an iron exposure reflect the amount of elemental iron ingested. You should expect mild to moderate toxicity if a patient ingests 20 to 60 mg/kg. With dosing of more than 60 mg/kg, severe and potentially lethal toxicity is a possibility.

Two broad categories of iron poisoning can be distinguished: gastrointestinal and systemic. With gastrointestinal toxicity, the symptoms consist of abdominal pain, vomiting (the most common sign), and diarrhea. With systemic toxicity, patients may be hypotensive or in frank shock from coagulopathy and vomiting blood. These patients are commonly in metabolic acidosis and become tachypneic as the body attempts to adjust its pH by increasing the elimination of carbon dioxide.

Children typically remain asymptomatic when they have a low-level iron exposure. However, children who ingest a large dose of iron are at risk of dying unless aggressive and immediate interventions are taken. Unfortunately, there is little you can do in the field for iron poisoning, other than provide basic attention to the ABCs and transport the patient to the closest, most appropriate facility for further evaluation and laboratory studies.

Special Populations

Children younger than 6 years have frequent iron exposures, usually secondary to ingesting chewable vitamins. Children typically remain asymptomatic when they have a low-level iron exposure. However, children who ingest a large dose of iron are at risk of dying unless aggressive and timely interventions take place. Unfortunately, little can be done in the field for iron poisoning, other than providing basic attention to the ABCs and transporting the patient to the closest, most appropriate facility for further evaluation and laboratory studies.

▶ Miscellaneous Substances

Many other substances may cause toxicologic emergencies. Additional substances are discussed in this section.

Incidents involving chlorine gas are relatively common because of the widespread use of chlorine compounds in the home and occupational settings. Cases of chlorine gas exposure occur both inside (eg, from mixing bleach and other cleaning products) and outside the home. The signs and symptoms of chlorine gas exposure include burning sensations in the eyes, nose, and throat along with a slight cough. With a more intense exposure, patients may develop chest tightness, choking, paroxysmal cough, headache, nausea and vomiting, diffuse wheezing, cyanosis, crackles in the chest, shock, seizures, and loss of consciousness. Remove patients from the area of exposure. Once you are in a safe environment, quickly triage the patients, prioritizing those with breathing problems. Irrigate burning or itching eyes with water, as well as any areas of the skin that have come in contact with the chlorine.

Cyanide poisoning can occur as a result of combustion of certain materials in a fire, through industrial exposure, or after ingestion of products that contain cyanide. Within the body, cyanide blocks the utilization of oxygen at the cellular level. The results are cellular suffocation and death of the patient within seconds if the cyanide was inhaled or within minutes to possibly an hour or two if it was ingested. A patient who has been poisoned with cyanide may have an altered mental state. If the patient is alert enough to answer questions, he or she may report headache, palpitations, or dyspnea. A classic odor of bitter almonds on the patient's breath is highly suggestive of cyanide poisoning. Initially, respirations are usually rapid and labored; however, as the poisoning progresses, respirations can become slow and gasping. The pulse is usually rapid and thready. Vomiting, seizures, and coma are common. Treatment must be instituted as fast as possible. Administer 100% oxygen via nonrebreathing mask or positive pressure ventilations. In the prehospital setting, hydroxocobalamin or sodium thiosulfate may be ordered by medical control to counteract cyanide; if it is given in time, this treatment is usually effective. Call for paramedic backup if needed for advanced airway management or treatment of seizures. Notify the receiving hospital of the probable diagnosis so staff can make preparations. Transport the patient without delay to an appropriate facility.

Caustics include strong acids and strong alkalis. Both types of chemicals are commonly used in industry, agriculture (anhydrous ammonia), and the home (eg, bleach). Most cases of caustic poisoning involve accidental dermal or ocular exposure. If the patient is an adult, oral ingestion of caustics is usually an intentional suicide attempt. Most patients who have swallowed caustic substances present with severe pain in the mouth, throat, or chest. Usually, the airway is not a problem and the patient is not in shock. Respiratory distress, if present, is most likely due to soft-tissue swelling in the larynx, epiglottis, or vocal cords, which means that the patient is in immediate danger of complete airway obstruction. Establish vascular access, usually en route, because immediate transport to the ED is needed. If the patient was exposed to a strong alkali, diluting and flushing away the caustic substance is the main goal. With an eye exposure, continuously irrigate the eyes; if only one eye was exposed, ensure you do not contaminate the other eye while washing.

Some alcohols, including methyl alcohol and ethylene glycol, are even more toxic than ethyl alcohol (drinking alcohol). Methyl alcohol is found in dry gas products and Sterno; ethylene glycol is found in some antifreeze products. Both cause a "drunken" feeling. If patients are not treated for ingestion of these alcohols, both will also cause severe tachypnea, blindness (methyl alcohol), renal failure (ethylene glycol), and eventually death. Even ethyl alcohol (typical drinking alcohol) can stop a patient's breathing if taken too fast or in a dose that is too high,

YOU are the Provider — PART 4

As your partner initiates transport to the local hospital, you administer 100% oxygen to the patient via a nonrebreathing mask and establish IV access with an 18-gauge catheter. You decide to administer a 20-mL/kg bolus of normal saline in an attempt to increase his blood pressure, and you apply ice packs in the axillary regions to cool the patient down. As you are attempting to clean and bandage the abrasions on the patient's arms, he continually tries to pull away and get out of the restraints. The remainder of your transport remains uneventful, and on arrival at the ED, you turn over care to the staff without incident.

Recording Time: 12 Minutes	
Respirations	30 breaths/min, rapid
Pulse	Strong and regular, 118 beats/min
Skin	Hot, dry, and pink
Blood pressure	102/74 mm Hg
Oxygen saturation (Spo_2)	98% on 100% oxygen
Pupils	Dilated, equal, and reactive to light

7. What are the possible complications of use of restraints?
8. Should you be concerned about the possibility of infectious disease in this patient?

Words of Wisdom

There are a number of significant "don'ts" for caustic ingestions: *don't* give any neutralizing substances, *don't* induce vomiting, *don't* perform gastric lavage, and *don't* give activated charcoal.

Patient Safety

Some chemicals react with water. Although small amounts can usually be flushed safely with large quantities of water, larger amounts of such chemicals can give off toxic fumes or explode when wet. Ensure you check the relevant warnings or placards or call poison control for assistance.

Words of Wisdom

Many poisonous items are commonly found in households. For example, many household cleaning agents are toxic if ingested. Laundry pods are especially troubling because small children are often attracted to their small size and bright colors. Household plants may have poisonous leaves or berries. Pesticides and herbicides used in lawn and garden care are potentially poisonous. Paint thinners and solvents can cause permanent neurologic damage or death if inhaled in the right amount; the same is true of glue fumes.

particularly in children. Although they may be used as a substitute by a chronic alcoholic who is unable to obtain ethyl alcohol, these types of alcohols are more often taken by someone attempting suicide. In either case, immediate transport to the ED is essential.

Hydrocarbons are found in a variety of products around the home, including cleaning and polishing agents, glues, spot removers, lighter fluids, paints, paint thinners and paint removers, other fuels, and pesticides. The vast majority of intentional hydrocarbon inhalations are "recreational," but hydrocarbons may also be ingested by young children who mistake them for a beverage. Hydrocarbon inhalation is achieved by pouring the volatile material onto a rag, placing it in a trash bag, and then holding the bag over the face to breathe in the fumes. Breathing fumes directly off a soaked rag or towel is termed *huffing*, whereas the use of a trash bag is called *bagging*. Frequently, people who "bag" or "huff" are young—middle-school age and, occasionally, younger children. A single hydrocarbon substance exposure may cause life-threatening toxicity and, on occasion, sudden death.

Treat a patient who has inhaled hydrocarbons by removing the patient from the noxious environment, administering high-concentration supplemental oxygen, and promptly transporting to the appropriate facility. Patients who have symptoms such as coughing, choking, or vomiting within a few minutes of ingestion are likely to have aspirated and need immediate attention. Signs of respiratory distress—air hunger, intercostal retractions, tachypnea, and cyanosis—must be considered danger signals. Hypoglycemia and cardiac dysrhythmias may occur; call for paramedic backup if needed. The patient may have severe abdominal pain, diarrhea, and belching, sometimes lasting for hours after the incident. Management should include the following measures:

- Remove contaminated clothing and decontaminate the patient, ideally before placing the patient in the ambulance.
- Establish and maintain the airway, and ensure adequate ventilation.
- Administer high-flow supplemental oxygen.
- Establish vascular access.
- Administer sequential bolus infusions of normal saline to treat hypotension.
- Transport the patient to the most appropriate facility.

▶ Food Poisoning

Whenever you encounter two or more people who are sick at the same time and at the same scene, think food poisoning or CO poisoning—your hunch will likely be correct.

Four pathogens—*Salmonella* (28%), *Toxoplasma* (24%), *Listeria* (19%), and *Norovirus* (11%)—are the leading causes of food-related deaths in the United States.[30] Poisoning with *Clostridium botulinum*, an extremely deadly toxin, is usually the result of improper food storage or canning. In addition, the toxins produced by dinoflagellates in "red tides" may contaminate bivalve shellfish such as oysters, clams, and mussels and produce life-threatening or fatal paralytic shellfish poisoning.

Depending on the toxin, onset of signs and symptoms can range from several hours after ingestion to days or weeks. The longer the time until symptom onset, the more difficult it will be to link the patient's problem to the event at which the toxin was ingested. Gastrointestinal complaints are the most common and include abdominal pain and cramping, nausea, vomiting, and diarrhea. With prolonged episodes of vomiting or diarrhea, hypotension secondary to fluid loss and electrolyte imbalance becomes likely. Respiratory distress or arrest can occur with toxins such as *C botulinum* or those found in paralytic shellfish poisoning.

Treatment for patients with food poisoning is usually supportive. Most of the cases you will encounter will not be life threatening, and the signs and symptoms of acute gastroenteritis are typically self-limiting. Establish and maintain the airway, inserting an advanced airway as needed. Administer high-flow supplemental oxygen, and establish vascular access. For hypotension secondary to fluid loss, administer fluid boluses of normal saline. Call for paramedic backup as needed. Finally, transport the patient to an appropriate facility.

Words of Wisdom

Herbal preparations can cause potentially serious interactions with traditional medications and, in some cases, overdose.[31] Ensure you inquire about all medications the patient may have taken, including herbal medications or supplements.

▶ Poisonous Plants

Of the thousands of plant varieties, only a few are poisonous Figure 23-8. Oddly enough, poisonous plants represent some of the most common ornamental garden shrubs and houseplants. Most plant-related exposures involve children younger than 6 years; nearly 28,000 such incidents were reported to US poison control centers in

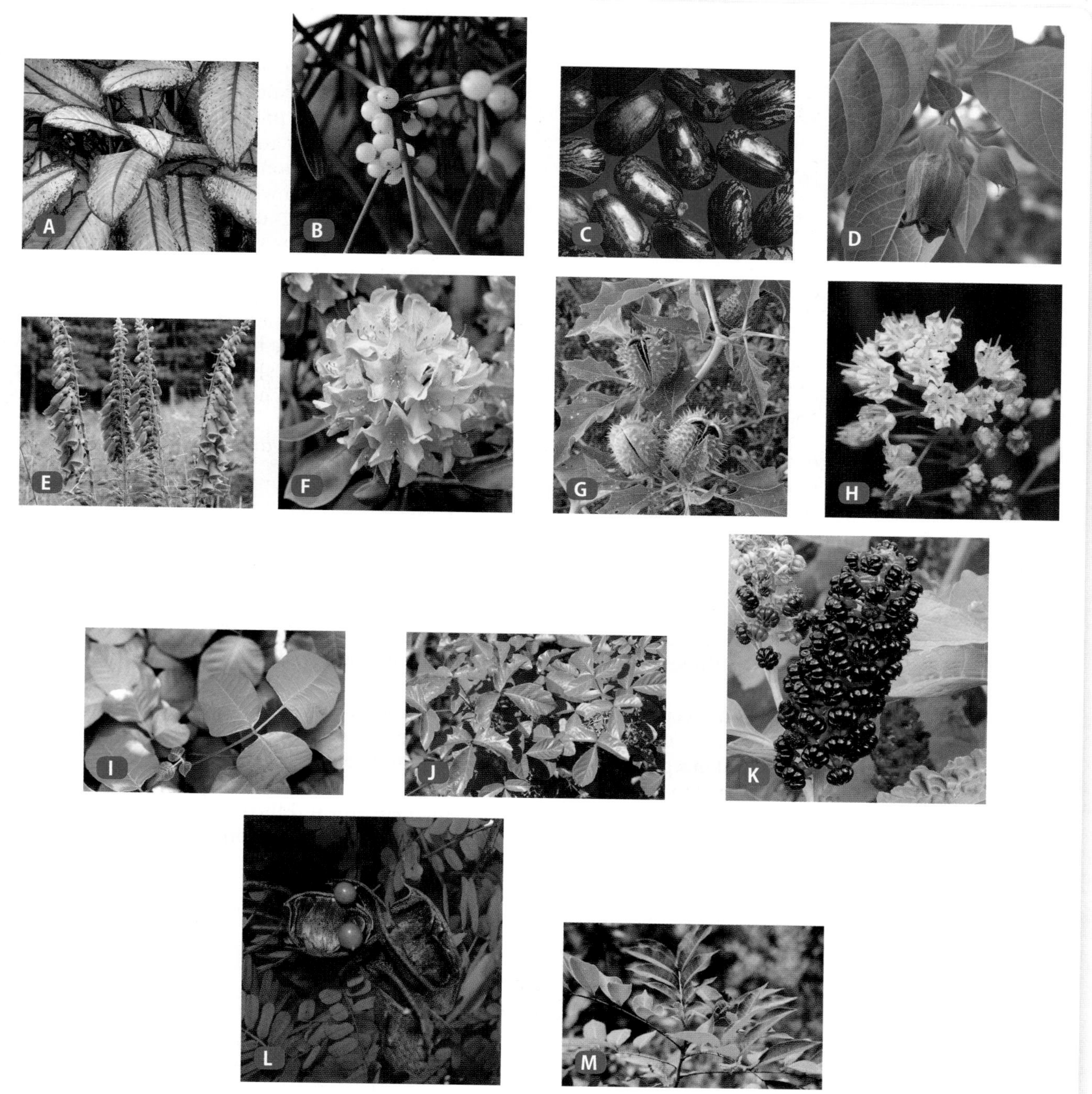

Figure 23-8 The toxins in these common poisonous plants are often ingested or absorbed through the skin. **A.** Dieffenbachia. **B.** Mistletoe. **C.** Castor bean. **D.** Nightshade. **E.** Foxglove. **F.** Rhododendron. **G.** Jimsonweed. **H.** Death camas. **I.** Poison ivy. **J.** Poison oak. **K.** Pokeweed. **L.** Rosary pea. **M.** Poison sumac.

Table 23-5 Common Toxic Plants	
Scientific Name	**Common Name**
Abrus precatorius	Jequirity bean/rosary pea
Cicuta species	Water hemlock/wild carrot
Colchicum autumnale	Autumn crocus
Conium maculatum	Poison hemlock
Convallaria majalis	Lily of the valley
Datura stramonium	Jimsonweed/stinkweed
Dieffenbachia	Dumb cane
Digitalis purpurea	Foxglove
Nerium oleander	Oleander or rose laurel
Nicotiana glauca	Tree tobacco
Phoradendron	Mistletoe
Phytolacca americana	Pokeweed
Rhododendron	Rhododendron or azalea
Ricinus communis	Castor bean/ricin
Solanum nigrum	Deadly nightshade/ atropa belladonna
Zigadenus species	Death camas

Data from: U.S. Food and Drug Administration. FDA Poisonous Plant Database. www.accessdata.fda.gov/scripts/plantox/textResults.cfm. Accessed 10/16/15.

2014.[32] Deaths from plant ingestions are rare, however. Table 23-5 lists common toxic plants.

Some poisonous plants cause local irritation of the skin; others can affect the circulatory system, the gastrointestinal tract, or the CNS. It is impossible for you to memorize every plant and poison, let alone their effects, but there are two worth mentioning.

The ubiquitous **dieffenbachia** is a green plant with broad, variegated leaves. It is nicknamed "dumb cane," because eating dieffenbachia can result in a person being unable to speak. In severe cases, edema of the tongue and larynx may lead to airway compromise. Dieffenbachia ingestion is common in children and cats.

Castor bean seeds originate from an attractive shrub but are highly poisonous—chewing on just a few seeds (and, in some cases, just one) can kill a child. Ricin, the poison in castor beans, causes a variety of toxic effects: burning of the mouth and throat; nausea, vomiting, diarrhea, and severe stomach pains; prostration; failing vision; and kidney failure (the usual cause of death).

When you encounter a case of plant poisoning, get all the information you can from the patient or parent and then consult your regional poison center for advice:

- **When was the plant ingested?** If it was more than 12 hours ago and the patient is still asymptomatic, chances are good that the patient will not experience symptoms. Most plant poisonings produce signs and symptoms of toxicity, if they are going to do so, within 4 hours of ingestion. One notable exception is castor bean, for which symptoms may not appear until 1 to 3 days after ingestion.
- **What, exactly, was eaten?** Try to find out not just which type of plant, but also which parts of the plant (eg, leaves, root, stem, flower, or fruit) were eaten. If possible, estimate how much was ingested (such as a bite or two from a leaf versus three or four leaves). If you transport the patient, take along the offending plant—or whatever is left of it.
- **Which signs or symptoms, if any, does the patient have?**

Most plant-related exposures require no treatment—a decision that can be made after consulting with the poison center and medical control per local protocol. If there is a responsible adult who can keep a close eye on the child for at least 4 to 6 hours after the ingestion, there is no need to transport the child to the hospital. Conversely, a child with any signs and symptoms should be evaluated in the ED.

Emergency medical treatment of dieffenbachia poisoning includes maintaining an open airway, administering oxygen, and promptly transporting the patient to the closest hospital for respiratory support. Continue to assess the patient for airway difficulties throughout transport. If necessary, provide positive pressure ventilation.

YOU are the Provider SUMMARY

1. What are the potential hazards with this scene?

This scene presents numerous hazards for EMS, law enforcement, and the patient, as well as any additional bystanders. This is a highly volatile situation with a patient who is not obeying commands by law enforcement, and could easily escalate. It is imperative that EMS providers remain in a safe staging area away from potentially unsafe areas to minimize the potential for injury.

2. What is a likely explanation for this patient's presentation?

A multitude of reasons might have led to this patient's presentation. The most likely explanation is the patient is experiencing an acute psychotic episode. Other possibilities for his behavior include agitated delirium, drug or alcohol withdrawal, or drug abuse.

3. Does this patient's presentation warrant transport via EMS, or should he be transported via law enforcement?

This patient definitely requires transport via EMS. He is experiencing an altered mental status for an unknown reason. Also, he has abrasions to his arms with active bleeding; this medical problem rules out the option of transport via law enforcement. There is also the possibility that the patient might experience a seizure, which would be better managed by an AEMT.

4. Should you request paramedic backup for this patient?

Whether you request paramedic backup depends on your system's policies and procedures. Presently, this patient does not require any skills that would mandate the presence of a paramedic. However, if the patient's condition deteriorates at any point, paramedic backup should be requested.

5. Which treatment does this patient require en route to the hospital?

This patient requires supportive care. Obviously, the bleeding needs to be controlled and the wounds dressed. An IV line should be established and a fluid bolus administered in an attempt to increase his blood pressure. Administer oxygen to prevent hypoxia, and ice packs should be applied to promote cooling of the core temperature.

6. Why should you have a law enforcement officer in the back of the ambulance during this transport?

Depending on system policies and procedures, law enforcement may be required whenever a patient has been placed in handcuffs. Regardless of policies, having a law enforcement officer in the back of the ambulance lessens the potential for injury for EMS providers should the patient get out of his restraints and become a threat.

7. What are the possible complications of use of restraints?

The potential complications of use of restraints include loss of distal circulation if the restraints are applied too tightly. That is the conundrum: if restraints are applied too tightly, distal circulation is lost; if they are applied too loosely, the patient may be able to become free from the restraints. Also, depending on the degree of compliance of the patient, there is a potential for injury from fractures or strains if the patient continues to struggle.

8. Should you be concerned about the possibility of infectious disease in this patient?

Yes. Whenever blood or body fluids are present on a patient, there is the potential for transmission of infectious disease. In this scenario, the patient's history of drug use exponentially increases the possibility for infectious disease.

YOU are the Provider SUMMARY *(continued)*

EMS Patient Care Report (PCR)

Date: 10-3-18	Incident No.: 20108732711	Nature of Call: Police assist	Location: 1843 Seville Loop		
Dispatched: 0320	**En Route:** 0324	**At Scene:** 0329	**Transport:** 0412	**At Hospital:** 0421	**In Service:** 0455

Patient Information

Age: 24 **Sex:** M **Weight (in kg [lb]):** 69 kg (152 lb)	**Allergies:** Unknown **Medications:** Unknown **Past Medical History:** IV methamphetamine use **Chief Complaint:** AMS, acute psychotic episode

Vital Signs

Time: 0405	**BP:** 84/52	**Pulse:** 120	**Respirations:** 32	**Spo_2:** 95%
Time: 0413	**BP:** 102/74	**Pulse:** 118	**Respirations:** 30	**Spo_2:** 98% on 100% NRM
Time:	**BP:**	**Pulse:**	**Respirations:**	**Spo_2:**

EMS Treatment (circle all that apply)

Oxygen @ 15 **L/min via (circle one):** **NC** (**NRM**) **Bag-mask device**		**Assisted Ventilation**	**Airway Adjunct**	**CPR**
Defibrillation	(**Bleeding Control:** Yes–applied pressure)	(**Bandaging:** Yes)	**Splinting**	**Other:**

Narrative

EMS dispatched to above location for "unknown medical, police request." On arrival, spoke with the Captain of the Police Dept, who states they received multiple reports of a "naked person covered in blood, acting bizarre." The patient can be seen standing in the front yard of a residence, with both arms covered in blood, yelling incoherently. The Captain states they will probably have to physically subdue the patient, and to stand by for further orders. After approximately 20 minutes on scene, law enforcement subdued the patient and subsequently placed him in handcuffs. After we were directed to the patient, the patient's sister arrived on scene.

The patient presents as alert, but unable to give us any additional information. Airway is patent, minimal bleeding noted to each forearm, appears to be abrasions. Patient remains screaming at the top of his lungs, "Don't let them get me. I'm burning. God help me." Patient's sister provides medical history of 5 years of methamphetamine use. With law enforcement assistance, handcuffs were removed and each of patient's extremities placed in soft restraints. Transport initiated to North Regional Medical Center with patrolman Steele accompanying in back of ambulance. 100% oxygen via a nonrebreathing mask administered. 18-gauge IV line with 20-mL/kg bolus of 0.9% normal saline administered. Ice pack applied to axillary regions, and abrasions cleaned and bandaged. Patient remains agitated and hostile throughout transport. Distal circulation checked numerous times, with +PMS to all extremities. On arrival at NRMC, care and report given to ED staff without incident.**End of report**

Prep Kit

▶ Ready for Review

- Toxicologic emergencies usually fall under one of two general headings: intentional or unintentional.
- Even the most well-read veteran AEMT may find it difficult to stay up-to-date with the myriad drugs sold in the streets today. For this reason, poison centers may be an indispensable aid in a suspected toxicologic emergency.
- The four primary methods whereby a toxin commonly enters the body are ingestion, inhalation, injection, and absorption.
- Although the sheer number of substances of abuse may seem daunting, many drugs, on entering the body, result in similar signs and symptoms. The syndromelike symptoms of a poisonous agent are termed a toxic syndrome or toxidrome. The major toxidromes are produced by stimulants, narcotics, sympathomimetics, sedatives and hypnotics, cholinergics, and anticholinergics.
- Substance abuse is self-administration of licit or illicit substances in a manner not in accordance with approved medical or social practice. A person may become physically or psychologically dependent on a substance through this practice and develop a tolerance.
- A person who is addicted to a substance can experience withdrawal syndrome—a predictable set of signs and symptoms—if he or she abruptly stops using a drug or rapidly decreases the usual dosage.
- Toxicologic emergency scenes can present hazards to the AEMT, including potential contamination with the substance or potentially dangerous patients. AEMTs must properly protect themselves and thoroughly assess every scene before entering it.
- Generally, patients with toxicologic emergencies are considered medical patients, although toxicologic emergencies may lead to trauma too.
- At the scene of a potential toxicologic emergency, look for clues that might indicate that a substance or poison is involved, such as medication bottles, alcoholic beverage containers, syringes, drug paraphernalia, or an unusual odor.
- Managing the airway, breathing, and circulation (ABCs) are the top priority with toxicologic patients, as always. Have suction available, as these patients are susceptible to vomiting.
- Consider decontamination of the patient before transport depending on the poison to which the patient was exposed. In some cases, a patient may need to be decontaminated prior to assessment and treatment by specially trained and equipped personnel.
- Ask which agent the patient was exposed to, when the patient was exposed to it, how much of the substance was involved, whether anything else was taken, over what time period the patient was exposed to the substance, whether any interventions were performed, how much the patient weighs, and why the substance was taken. Also find out if the patient has vomited or aspirated and why the substance was taken.
- Transport any containers, the remainder of the substance, and vomit with the patient if possible for identification.
- The condition of patients exposed to poisons may change suddenly and without warning. Continually reassess airway, breathing, circulation, disability, and exposure and repeatedly obtain vital signs. If the poison or the level of exposure is unknown, careful and frequent reassessment is required.
- The treatment for poisoned patients depends a great deal on the toxin, the route of exposure, and other signs and symptoms found in your assessment.
- Emergency medical care for a patient with a toxicologic emergency includes ensuring scene safety, managing the ABCs, administering oxygen, establishing vascular access, and being prepared to manage shock, coma, seizures, and dysrhythmias. In some cases, activated charcoal may need to be administered.
- Alcohol—a powerful central nervous system depressant—is the most widely abused drug in the United States. A patient may be acutely intoxicated with alcohol or may be a chronic alcohol abuser. In either case, manage the ABCs and expect vomiting. A patient with delirium tremens may be agitated or combative and needs reassurance.
- Narcotics (opiates and opioids) produce sleep or altered mental status; some opioids may produce euphoria. In the case of a narcotic overdose, manage the ABCs, establish vascular access, administer naloxone as indicated, and call for paramedic backup for further medication administration and cardiac monitoring. In the case of a cardiac arrest from an opioid overdose, follow the American Heart Association algorithm for assessment and management.
- The main stimulants of concern for AEMTs include cocaine, amphetamines, methamphetamine, and synthetic cathinones. The classic presentation of stimulant overdose includes excitement, delirium, tachycardia, hypertension with a fast pulse rate or hypotension with a fast pulse rate, and dilated pupils. Treatment is managing the ABCs, calling for paramedic backup to control anxiety and seizures, administering benzodiazepines per local protocol

Prep Kit (continued)

(or calling for paramedic backup to do so), and providing reassurance.

- Treatment of the patient who has used marijuana or cannabis compounds focuses on supportive care, because there is little likelihood of a serious medical complication from marijuana use.
- A hallucinogen alters a person's sensory perception, causing the individual to see, hear, or feel things that are not actually present. Hallucinogenic substances include lysergic acid diethylamide, psilocybin mushrooms, phencyclidine, ketamine, and mescaline. Treat patients using hallucinogens by providing transport to the appropriate facility and psychological support.
- Sedative-hypnotic drugs may reduce anxiety and produce drowsiness and sleep. Barbiturates and benzodiazepines are the main drugs of concern in this category. Patients present much like patients with alcohol intoxication. Manage the ABCs, monitor for shock, and administer fluids if needed.
- Signs and symptoms of overdose with cardiac drugs vary, but may include hypotension, weakness or confusion, nausea and vomiting, rhythm disturbances, headache, and difficulty breathing. As with all emergencies, ensure a patent airway, provide adequate ventilation, and administer high-flow supplemental oxygen.
- Other medications that may prompt calls related to overdose include erectile dysfunction medications, psychiatric medications (eg, tricyclic antidepressants, monoamine oxidase inhibitors, selective serotonin reuptake inhibitors, lithium), over-the-counter pain-relief medications (eg, nonsteroidal anti-inflammatory drugs, salicylates, acetaminophen), and drugs used to facilitate sexual assault (eg, gamma-hydroxybutyrate). After administering the appropriate on-scene care (which may sometimes include activated charcoal), these patients should be transported to the appropriate facility.
- Cholinergic agents include organophosphates and nerve gases. These agents overstimulate normal body functions that are controlled by the parasympathetic nerves, resulting in salivation, mucus secretion, urination, crying, and an abnormal heart rate. Patients must be decontaminated before initiating care.
- Carbon monoxide is a common cause of fatal poisoning. Signs and symptoms of carbon monoxide poisoning vary and are vague, often resembling the onset of the flu. Remove the patient from the environment, administer 100% oxygen via nonrebreathing mask or bag-mask–assisted ventilations, and consider performing carbon monoxide monitoring.
- Lead poisoning is associated with a long list of signs and symptoms, with encephalopathy being a major cause of mortality and morbidity in these patients. The toxic effects of an iron exposure reflect the amount of elemental iron ingested. With both of these types of metal poisoning, AEMT should provide supportive care as there is little that can be done for these patients in the field.
- In case of chlorine gas poisoning, first remove patients from the area of exposure, then quickly triage the patients, prioritizing those with breathing problems. Irrigate burning or itching eyes with water, as well as any areas of the skin that have come in contact with the chlorine.
- Immediate treatment is required for cyanide poisoning. Administer 100% oxygen via nonrebreathing mask or bag-mask–assisted ventilations. Most patients who have swallowed caustic substances present with severe pain in the mouth, throat, or chest. Provide immediate transport to the emergency department (ED). Establish vascular access en route. If the patient was exposed to a strong alkali, diluting and flushing away the caustic substance is the first priority.
- Some alcohols, including methyl alcohol and ethylene glycol, are even more toxic than ethyl alcohol (drinking alcohol). Immediate transport to the ED is essential when patients have ingested these substances.
- Treat patients who have inhaled hydrocarbons by removing the patient from the noxious environment, administering high-concentration supplemental oxygen, and providing prompt transport to the appropriate facility.
- Patients with food poisoning develop gastrointestinal complaints. Hypotension secondary to fluid loss and electrolyte imbalance becomes likely, and respiratory distress or arrest can occur. Treatment for patients with food poisoning is usually supportive.
- Most poisonous plant–related exposures involve children younger than 6 years. Plants may irritate the skin, affect the circulatory system, or cause abdominal complaints. Most plant-related exposures require no treatment. Consult a poison center and medical control per local protocol.

▶ Vital Vocabulary

alcoholism A state of physical and psychological addiction to ethanol.

amphetamines A class of drugs that increase alertness and excitation (stimulants); includes methamphetamine

Prep Kit (continued)

(crank or ice), methylenedioxyamphetamine (MDA, Adam), and methylenedioxymethamphetamine (MDMA, Eve, Ecstasy).

antagonist Something that counteracts the action of something else; a drug of this type has an affinity for a cell receptor and, when it binds to that receptor, the cell is prevented from responding.

barbiturates Potent sedative-hypnotics historically used as sleep aids, as antianxiety drugs, and as part of the regimen for seizure control.

benzodiazepines The family of sedative-hypnotics most commonly used to treat anxiety, seizures, and alcohol withdrawal.

carbon monoxide (CO) An odorless, highly poisonous gas that results from the incomplete oxidation of carbon during combustion.

caustics Chemicals that are acids or alkalis; they cause direct chemical injury to the tissues they contact.

chemical suicide A method of suicide that involves mixing certain household chemicals in an enclosed space to create toxic gases, such as hydrogen sulfide and hydrogen cyanide, as the chemicals combine; also called detergent suicide.

delirium tremens (DTs) A severe withdrawal syndrome seen in people with alcoholism who are deprived of ethyl alcohol, which is characterized by restlessness, fever, sweating, disorientation, agitation, and seizures; it can be fatal if untreated.

dieffenbachia A common houseplant that resembles "elephant ears"; its ingestion leads to burns of the mouth and tongue and, possibly, paralysis of the vocal cords and nausea and vomiting. In severe cases, ingestion may cause edema of the tongue and larynx, leading to airway compromise.

drug A substance that has some therapeutic effect (such as reducing inflammation, fighting bacteria, or producing euphoria) when given in the appropriate circumstances and in the appropriate dose.

drug abuse Any use of drugs that causes physical, psychological, economic, legal, or social harm to the user or others affected by the user's behavior.

drug addiction A chronic disorder characterized by the compulsive use of a substance that results in physical, psychological, or social harm to the user who continues to use the substance despite the harm.

gamma-hydroxybutyrate (GHB) A sedative and central nervous system depressant.

habituation The situation in which there is a physical tolerance and psychological dependence on a drug or drugs.

hallucinogen An agent that produces false perceptions in any one of the five senses.

hydrocarbons Compounds made up of hydrogen and carbon atoms; they are frequently obtained from the distillation of petroleum.

illicit In relation to drugs, illegal drugs such as marijuana, cocaine, and lysergic acid diethylamide.

licit In relation to drugs, legalized drugs such as coffee, alcohol, and tobacco.

lithium The cornerstone drug for the treatment of bipolar disorder.

marijuana The dried leaves and flower buds of the *Cannabis sativa* plant, which are smoked to achieve a high.

methamphetamine A highly addictive drug in the amphetamine family.

monoamine oxidase inhibitors (MAOIs) Psychiatric medication used primarily to treat atypical depression by increasing norepinephrine and serotonin levels in the central nervous system.

narcotic A generic term for opiates and opioids; a drug that acts as a central nervous system depressant and produces insensibility or stupor.

opiate Any of the various alkaloids derived from the opium or poppy plant.

opioid A synthetic narcotic not derived from opium.

organophosphates A class of chemicals found in many insecticides used in agriculture and in the home.

overdose Consumption of an excessive quantity of a drug that, when taken or administered, can have toxic or lethal consequences.

physical dependence A physiologic state of adaptation to a drug, usually characterized by tolerance to the drug's effects and a withdrawal syndrome if use of the drug is stopped, especially abruptly.

poison A substance whose chemical action could damage structures or impair function when it is introduced into the body.

potentiation Enhancement of the effect of one drug by another drug.

psychological dependence The emotional state of craving a drug to maintain a feeling of well-being.

salicylates Aspirin-like drugs.

sedative-hypnotic A drug used to reduce anxiety, calm agitated patients, and help produce drowsiness and sleep; a central nervous system depressant.

selective serotonin reuptake inhibitors (SSRIs) A class of antidepressants that inhibit the reuptake of serotonin.

Prep Kit (continued)

spice An illicit drug consisting of a blend of synthetic cannabinoids; it can produce short- and long-term psychotic effects.

stimulants Medications or chemicals that temporarily enhance central nervous system and sympathetic nervous system functioning and produce an excited state.

synergism The action of two substances such as drugs, in which the total effects are greater than the sum of the independent effects of the two substances.

tolerance Physiologic adaptation to the effects of a drug, such that increasingly larger doses of the drug are required to achieve the same effect.

toxicologic emergencies Medical emergencies caused by toxic agents such as poisons.

toxicology The study of toxic or poisonous substances.

toxidrome The syndromelike symptoms of a poisonous agent.

toxin A poison or harmful substance produced by bacteria, animals, or plants.

tricyclic antidepressants (TCAs) A group of drugs used to treat severe depression and manage pain; even minimal dosing errors with these agents can cause toxic results.

withdrawal syndrome A predictable set of signs and symptoms, usually involving altered central nervous system activity, that occurs after the abrupt cessation of a drug or after rapidly decreasing the usual dosage of a drug.

▶ References

1. American Association of Poison Control Centers website. http://www.aapcc.org/. Accessed October 6, 2017.
2. Kamboj A, Spiller HA, Casavant MJ, et al. Pediatric exposure to e-cigarettes, nicotine, and tobacco products in the United States. *Pediatrics*. 2016;137(6).
3. Centers for Disease Control and Prevention. New CDC study finds dramatic increase in e-cigarette-related calls to poison centers. April 3, 2014. https://www.cdc.gov/media/releases/2014/p0403-e-cigarette-poison.html. Accessed March 19, 2017.
4. European Monitoring Centre for Drugs and Drug Addiction. Polydrug use: patterns and responses. 2009. http://www.emcdda.europa.eu/attachements.cfm/att_93217_EN_EMCDDA_SI09_polydrug%20use.pdf. Accessed March 17, 2017.
5. Warner M, Trinidad JP, Bastian BA, Miniño AM, M.P.H., Hedegaard H. Drugs most frequently involved in drug overdose deaths: United States, 2010–2014. *Natl Vital Stat Rep*. 2016;65(10):5-6. https://www.cdc.gov/nchs/data/nvsr/nvsr65/nvsr65_10.pdf. Accessed March 17, 2017.
6. National Institute on Alcohol Abuse and Alcoholism. Alcohol facts and statistics. February 2017. http://niaaa.nih.gov/alcohol-health/overview-alcohol-consumption/alcohol-facts-and-statistics. Accessed March 18, 2017.
7. American Liver Foundation. Alcohol-related liver disease. November 30, 2016. http://www.liverfoundation.org/abouttheliver/info/alcohol/. Accessed March 18, 2017.
8. US Department of Health and Human Services. The opioid epidemic: by the numbers. June 2016. https://www.hhs.gov/sites/default/files/Factsheet-opioids-061516.pdf. Accessed March 18, 2017.
9. Rudd RA, Seth P, David F, Scholl L. Increases in drug and opioid-involved overdose deaths—United States, 2010–2015. *MMWR*. 2016;65(50-51):1445-1452. https://www.cdc.gov/mmwr/volumes/65/wr/mm655051e1.htm. Accessed March 18, 2017.
10. Fentanyl: Preventing Occupational Exposure to Emergency Responders—Illegal Use of Fentanyl. Centers for Disease Control and Prevention website. https://www.cdc.gov/niosh/topics/fentanyl/illegaluse.html. Updated November 28, 2016. Accessed October 6, 2017.
11. Fentanyl: Preventing Occupational Exposure to Emergency Responders—Overview. Centers for Disease Control and Prevention website. https://www.cdc.gov/niosh/topics/fentanyl/default.html. Updated November 28, 2016. Accessed October 6, 2017.
12. Fentanyl: Preventing Occupational Exposure to Emergency Responders—Protecting Workers at Risk. Centers for Disease Control and Prevention website. https://www.cdc.gov/niosh/topics/fentanyl/risk.html. Updated August 30, 2017. Accessed October 6, 2017.
13. van Dorp E, Yassen A, Dahan A. Naloxone treatment in opioid addiction: the risks and benefits. *Expert Opin Drug Saf*. 2007;6(2):125-132.
14. Orciari Herman A. CDC: Multiple Naloxone Doses May Be Needed for Fentanyl Overdoses. NEJM Journal Watch. October 27, 2015. http://www.jwatch.org/fw110784/2015/10/27/cdc-multiple-naloxone-doses-may-be-needed-fentanyl. Accessed October 6, 2017.
15. Badiani A, Belin D, Epstein D, et al. Opiate versus psychostimulant addiction: the differences do matter. *Nat Rev Neurosci*. 2011;12(11)685-700.
16. Substance Abuse and Mental Health Services Administration. Substance use disorders. October 27, 2015. https://www.samhsa.gov/disorders/substance-use. Accessed March 18, 2017.
17. US Drug Enforcement Agency. Methamphetamine lab incidents, 2004–2014. https://www.dea.gov/resource-center/meth-lab-maps.shtml. Accessed March 18, 2017.

Prep Kit *(continued)*

18. Haggin P. Obama signs federal ban on "bath salt" drugs. *Time.* July 10, 2012. http://newsfeed.time.com/2012/07/10/obama-signs-federal-ban-on-bath-salt-drugs/. Accessed March 18, 2017.
19. National Institute on Drug Abuse. National Survey of Drug Use and Health. https://www.drugabuse.gov/national-survey-drug-use-health. Accessed June 4, 2016.
20. Substance Abuse and Mental Health Services Administration. Hallucinogens. October 30, 2015. https://www.samhsa.gov/atod/hallucinogens. Accessed March 18, 2017.
21. US Department of Justice, National Drug Intelligence Center. Psilocybin: fast facts. https://www.justice.gov/archive/ndic/pubs6/6038/index.htm. Accessed March 18, 2017.
22. Substance Abuse and Mental Health Services Administration. Emergency department visits involving phencyclidine (PCP). *DAWN Rep.* November 12, 2013. http://archive.samhsa.gov/data/2k13/DAWN143/sr143-emergency-phencyclidine-2013.pdf. Accessed March 18, 2017.
23. Kalsi SS, Wood DM, Dargan PI. The epidemiology and patterns of acute and chronic toxicity associated with recreational ketamine use. *Emerg Health Threats J.* 2011;4. http://journals.co-action.net/index.php/ehtj/article/view/7107. Accessed March 18, 2017.
24. What is a K-Hole and How is it Dangerous? Ketamine.com website. http://ketamine.com/ketamine-effects/what-is-a-k-hole-and-how-is-it-dangerous/. Accessed October 6, 2017.
25. Morgan CJ, Riccelli M, Maitland CH, et al. Long-term effects of ketamine: evidence for a persisting impairment of source memory in recreational users. *Drug Alcohol Depend.* 2004;75(3):301–308.
26. QuickStats: Average Annual Number of Deaths and Death Rates from Unintentional, Non-Fire-Related Carbon Monoxide Poisoning, *† by Sex and Age Group – United States, 1999-2010. *MMWR*. 2014;63(03):65. https://www.cdc.gov/mmwr/preview/mmwrhtml/mm6303a6.htm. Updated January 24, 2014. Accessed October 6, 2017.
27. Adal A. Heavy metal toxicity. *Medscape.* June 30, 2016. http://emedicine.medscape.com/article/814960-overview#a6. Accessed March 18, 2017.
28. Holstege CP. Pathophysiology and Etiology of Lead Toxicity. Medscape website. http://emedicine.medscape.com/article/2060369-overview. Updated December 9, 2015. Accessed October 6, 2017.
29. Lead. United States Department of Labor website. https://www.osha.gov/SLTC/lead/. Accessed October 6, 2017.
30. Scallan E, Hoekstra RM, Angulo FJ, et al. Foodborne illness acquired in the United States—major pathogens. *Emerg Infect Dis.* 2011;17(1):7-15. https://wwwnc.cdc.gov/eid/article/17/1/p1-1101_article. Accessed March 18, 2017.
31. Barrueto F Jr. Herb poisoning: pathophysiology. *Medscape.* February 11, 2016. http://emedicine.medscape.com/article/817427-overview#a5. Accessed March 18, 2017.
32. National Capital Poison Center. Poison statistics: national data 2014. http://www.poison.org/poison-statistics-national. Accessed March 18, 2017.

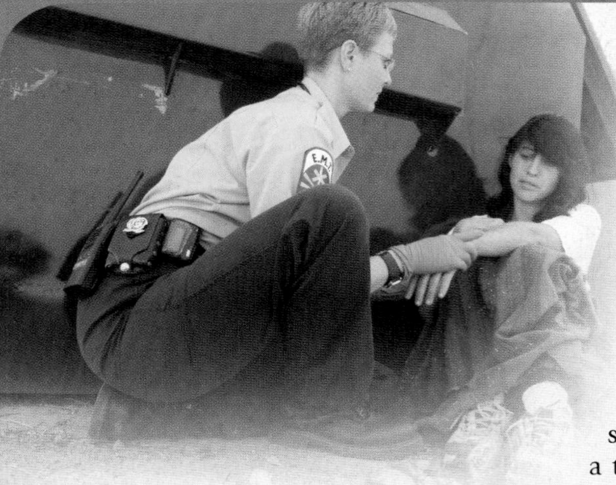

Assessment *in Action*

You are dispatched to a rural farming community for a man who has collapsed. On arrival, you are directed to a barn, where you find the patient lying on the ground. His respirations are shallow and gasping. The patient appears to be unresponsive. As you begin to assist ventilations, you start to feel lightheaded and you begin to cough. Suspecting a toxic environment, you safely extricate the patient to the outside of the barn.

1. Which of the following is the most likely route of exposure in this scenario?

- **A.** Inhalation
- **B.** Absorption
- **C.** Ingestion
- **D.** Intoxication

2. Which of the following is a sign or symptom of organophosphate poisoning?

- **A.** Dry mouth
- **B.** Constipation
- **C.** Dilated pupils
- **D.** Emesis

3. The CNS signs and symptoms associated with cholinergic excess are often expressed using the SLUDGEM mnemonic. What does the D stand for in this mnemonic?

- **A.** Drooling
- **B.** Defecation
- **C.** Dyspnea
- **D.** Diaphoresis

4. What is the first step in the assessment and treatment of a patient with an organophosphate exposure?

- **A.** Airway
- **B.** Breathing
- **C.** Circulation
- **D.** Decontamination

5. The signs and symptoms present in the patient are the result of:

- **A.** overstimulation of normal body functions controlled by the parasympathetic nerves.
- **B.** overstimulation of normal body functions controlled by the sympathetic nerves.
- **C.** understimulation of normal body functions controlled by the parasympathetic nerves.
- **D.** understimulation of normal body functions controlled by the sympathetic nerves.

6. The "U" in the SLUDGEM mnemonic for organophosphate exposure stands for:

- **A.** urination.
- **B.** unique.
- **C.** unremarkable.
- **D.** ubiquitous.

Assessment *in Action* *(continued)*

7. What should be done with this patient's clothing?

- **A.** Clothing should be given to housekeeping at the hospital for cleaning and returned to the patient.
- **B.** Clothing should be placed in a belongings bag and returned to the patient.
- **C.** Clothing should be placed in plastic bags and disposed of as hazardous materials.
- **D.** Nothing, the hospital will dispose of the clothing when the patient is placed in a hospital gown.

8. What is the proper treatment for a patient exposed to carbon monoxide?

9. List the signs and symptoms of a lithium overdose.

10. Explain the differences between the two categories of iron poisoning: gastrointestinal and systemic.

CHAPTER 24

Psychiatric Emergencies

National EMS Education Standard Competencies

Medicine

Applies fundamental knowledge to provide basic and selected advanced emergency care and transportation based on assessment findings for an acutely ill patient.

Psychiatric

Recognition of

- Behaviors that pose a risk to the AEMT, patient, or others (pp 1014, 1016-1017)

Assessment and management of

- Basic principles of the mental health system (pp 1009-1010)
- Acute psychosis (pp 1020-1021)
- Suicidal/risk (pp 1021-1023)
- Agitated delirium (p 1023)

Knowledge Objectives

1. Discuss the potential causes of behavioral emergencies, including organic and functional causes. (pp 1010-1012)
2. Identify psychiatric signs and symptoms. (p 1013)
3. Describe the assessment process for patients with psychiatric emergencies, including safety guidelines and specific questions to ask. (pp 1014-1019)
4. Discuss risk factors that help indicate whether a patient may become violent. (pp 1014, 1016-1017)
5. Discuss the importance of history taking when assessing a patient with a psychiatric emergency. (pp 1017-1018)
6. Discuss general management of a patient with a psychiatric emergency. (p 1020)
7. Explain the safe management of a potentially violent patient. (pp 1020, 1028-1029)
8. Discuss assessment and management of specific psychiatric emergencies. (pp 1020-1027)
9. Describe the care for a patient experiencing a psychotic episode. (p 1021)
10. Explain how to recognize the behavior of a patient at risk of suicide, and discuss the management of such a patient. (pp 1021-1023)
11. Define agitated delirium and describe the care for a patient with agitated delirium. (p 1023)
12. Discuss types of mood disorders and their management, including mania and depression. (pp 1024-1025)
13. Discuss types of neurotic disorders and their management, including generalized anxiety disorder, phobias, and panic disorder. (pp 1025-1027)
14. Discuss medicolegal considerations and their relevance in psychiatric emergencies. (pp 1027-1029)
15. Describe situations where restraint may be justified. (p 1028)
16. Describe methods used to restrain patients. (pp 1028-1029)
17. Explain the causes of posttraumatic stress disorder (PTSD), along with its signs and symptoms. (p 1029)
18. Describe the special needs of combat veterans and their management. (p 1030)

Skills Objective

1. Demonstrate the techniques used to mechanically restrain a patient. (p 1028)

Introduction

As an advanced emergency medical technician (AEMT), you can expect to be called on to care for patients who are experiencing a psychological or behavioral crisis. This kind of crisis may be caused by a medical condition, a mental illness, use of mind-altering substances, stress, and many other reasons. This chapter discusses various kinds of behavioral emergencies, including those involving overdoses, violent behavior, and mental illness. You will learn how to assess a person who exhibits signs and symptoms of a behavioral emergency and how to determine the kind of emergency care that may be required in these situations. The chapter also covers legal concerns when caring for patients who are disturbed. Finally, it describes how to identify and manage the potentially violent patient, including the use of restraints.

Myth and Reality

Everyone experiences an emotional crisis at some point in life, some more severe than others. Even perfectly healthy people may have some of the signs and symptoms of mental illness from time to time. Therefore, you should not assume that you have a mental illness when you behave in certain ways that are discussed in this chapter. With that caveat in mind, you should also avoid making the same assumption about a patient in any given situation.

The most common misconception about mental illness is that if you are feeling "bad" or "depressed," you must be "sick." That is simply untrue. There are many justifiable reasons for feeling depressed, including divorce, loss of a job, and the death of a relative or friend. For a teenager who just broke up with his girlfriend of 12 months, it is quite normal to withdraw from ordinary activities and to feel sad. This is a normal reaction to a crisis situation. However, when a person finds that Monday morning blues start to last until Friday and that this pattern continues week after week, he or she may have a behavioral problem.

Many people believe that all people with mental health disorders are dangerous, violent, or otherwise unmanageable; this is also untrue. Only a small percentage of people with mental health problems fall into these categories. However, as an AEMT, you may be exposed to a higher proportion of violent patients because dealing with them is part of your job. You are seeing people who are, by definition, considered to be having an emergency; otherwise, your assistance would not have been requested. You are there because family members or friends felt unable to manage the patient by themselves. The situation could be a result of the use or abuse of drugs or alcohol. Alternatively, your assistance may have been requested because the patient has a long history of mental illness and is reacting to a particularly stressful event.

Whereas you cannot determine what has caused a person's behavioral problem, you may be able to predict when a person will become violent. The ability to predict violence is an important assessment tool for the AEMT.

Defining Behavioral Emergencies

Behavior is what you can see of a person's response to the environment—that is, his or her actions. Sometimes, it is obvious what a person is responding to. For example, if a person is punched, he or she may run away, burst into tears, or hit back. Sometimes, the source of distress is less clear, such as when someone is depressed for complex reasons.

Most of the time, people respond to the environment in reasonable ways. Over the years, they have learned to adapt to a variety of situations in daily life, including various stressors. This process is called adjustment. At other times, however, the stress is so great that the normal methods of adjusting do not work. When this happens, a person's behavior is likely to change, even if only temporarily. This new behavior may not be appropriate or normal.

Regarding the concept of normal behavior, there exists some disagreement over what is "normal." There is no clear idea or ideal model. The idea of what is normal tends to vary by cultural or ethnic group. Normal behavior is basically classified as whatever behavior society accepts. In contrast, abnormal or maladaptive behavior is anything that deviates from society's norms and expectations. It tends to interfere with the person's well-being and ability to function. It may also be harmful to an individual or group.

The definition of a **behavioral crisis** or emergency is any reaction to events that interferes with **activities of daily living (ADLs)** or has become unacceptable to the patient, family, or community. For example, when a person

YOU are the Provider — PART 1

You are dispatched to a 70-year-old man who is complaining of chest pain. Law enforcement has also been dispatched to the scene. The patient is well-known and has a history of posttraumatic stress disorder (PTSD). He has been violent with responders in the past and has a tendency to hallucinate and have flashbacks after having served in Vietnam.

1. Does this scene need to be treated differently than other scenes just because the patient has a mental illness?
2. Who has overall control of this scene, emergency medical services (EMS) or law enforcement?

experiences an interruption of his or her daily routine, such as washing, dressing, and eating, it is likely that the individual's behavior has become a problem. For that person, at that time, a behavioral emergency may exist. If the interruption of the daily routine tends to recur on a regular basis, the behavior is now also considered a *mental health* problem. It is now a pattern, rather than an isolated incident.

For example, a person who experiences a panic attack after having a heart attack is not necessarily mentally ill. Likewise, you would expect a person who is fired from a job to have some type of reaction, often sadness and depression. These behavioral problems are short-term and isolated events. However, the person who reacts with a fit of rage, attacking people and property or going on a drinking or drug spree for a week, has gone beyond what society considers appropriate or normal behavior. This person is clearly undergoing a behavioral emergency. Usually, if an abnormal or disturbing pattern of behavior lasts for at least a month, it is regarded as a matter of concern from a mental health standpoint. For example, chronic **depression** is a medical diagnosis of a persistent feeling of sadness, despair, and discouragement. This type of long-term problem would be considered a mental health disorder.

A person who is no longer able to respond appropriately to the environment may be having what is called a psychological or psychiatric emergency. When a psychiatric emergency arises, the patient may show agitation or violence or become a threat to him- or herself or to others. This situation is more serious than a more typical behavioral emergency that causes inappropriate behavior such as interference with ADL or intolerable actions. An immediate threat to the person involved or to others in the immediate area, including family, friends, bystanders, and emergency responders (including AEMTs), should be considered a psychiatric emergency. For example, a person might respond to the death of a spouse by attempting suicide. However, not all major life disruptions necessarily involve violent behavior or harm to an individual. Disruption can take many forms; not all include violence, nor are they all psychiatric emergencies.

Words of Wisdom

The medicolegal issues associated with responses to behavioral emergencies put added emphasis on thorough and specific documentation of the call. Record detailed, objective findings that support the conclusion of abnormal behavior (eg, withdrawn, will not talk, crying uncontrollably) and quote the patient's own words when appropriate (eg, "Life isn't worth living anymore" or "The voices are telling me to kill people"). Avoid subjective, judgmental statements, because they create the impression that you based your care on personal bias rather than the patient's needs.

Table 24-1 Common Causes of Behavioral Alterations

Common Causes of Behavioral Alterations
Hypoglycemia
Hypoxia
Hypoperfusion
Head trauma
Mind-altering substances
Psychogenic—resulting in psychotic thinking, depression, or panic
Environmental exposure (excessive cold, excessive heat)
Meningitis
Seizure disorders
Toxic ingestions/overdose
Withdrawal from drugs or alcohol

The Magnitude of Mental Health Problems

According to the National Institute of Mental Health, at one time or another, nearly one in five Americans has some type of **mental disorder**, an illness with psychological or behavioral symptoms that may result in impaired functioning.[1] Such a mental disorder can be caused by a social, psychological, genetic, physical, chemical, or biologic disturbance. Common causes of behavioral alterations are listed in Table 24-1.

Pathophysiology of Abnormal Behavior

Although sudden grief, emotional conflicts, and other psychological problems can cause behavioral emergencies, sudden illness, recent trauma, drug or alcohol intoxication, and diseases of the brain, such as Alzheimer disease, can produce abnormal behavior as well. Likewise, altered mental status can arise from hypoglycemia, hypoxia, and exposure to excessive heat or cold. Behavioral emergencies constitute serious mental health problems and incapacitate more people than all other health problems combined.[2] As an AEMT, you are not responsible for diagnosing the underlying cause of a behavioral or psychiatric emergency. However, you should know the two basic categories of diagnosis a physician will use: organic (physical) and functional (psychological).

Organic Causes of Behavioral Emergencies

Organic brain syndrome is a temporary or permanent dysfunction of the brain caused by a disturbance in the physical or physiologic functioning of brain tissue. Causes of organic brain syndrome include sudden illness; recent trauma to the head; seizure disorders; drug and alcohol intoxication, overdose, or withdrawal; and diseases of the brain, such as Alzheimer disease and meningitis.

Altered mental status can arise from a low blood glucose level, lack of oxygen, inadequate blood flow to the brain, and excessive heat or cold. An altered mental status, or a change in the way a person thinks or behaves, may be one indicator of a psychiatric disease such as bipolar disorder. A patient displaying bizarre behavior may actually have an acute medical illness that is the cause, or a partial cause, of the behavior. Recognizing this possibility may allow you to save a life.

Environmental Causes

A person's environment exerts a tremendous influence on behavior. Typically, that environment includes both psychosocial and sociocultural influences on behavior.

When people are consistently exposed to stressful psychosocial events (eg, childhood trauma) or developmental influences (eg, parents who deprived them of love, care, support, and encouragement), they may develop abnormal reactions. When a person's basic needs are threatened, that individual faces a crisis. A person in crisis has two alternatives for dealing with

Special Populations

As the population ages, you will begin to see more geriatric patients. In responding to an increasing number of patients older than 65 years, you will probably notice some behavioral or mental health problems, including depression, dementia, and delirium. These mental status changes can affect your ability to thoroughly assess and treat the ill or injured geriatric patient. Understanding the causes of altered behavior in an older patient will help you provide better patient care.

Depression is one of the more common mental status problems that you will see in the older population. Whereas much attention has been given to depression in younger adults, the media have not given as much coverage to older adults' mental health challenges. As an AEMT, you can recognize a problem and perhaps suggest resources that may improve the person's day-to-day quality of living or prevent suicide in the depressed older person.

Depression has a number of causes: some organic, some psychological, and some cultural. Organic causes of depression may include an emotional response to a major illness such as cancer or dementia. In addition, some medications can induce a feeling of depression, especially if they interact with other prescription or over-the-counter drugs. Changes in the endocrine system, such as menopause, can elicit depression. Psychological causes of depression include dealing with the effects of getting older—an older adult could have the feeling that life has passed him or her by, leading to depression. Some cultural attitudes may also cause stress for the older person: whereas some cultures revere their elders, others tend to view them as a burden, causing anguish and feelings of uselessness in older adults.

Given the many possible causes of depression, an older adult can feel helpless and hopeless. Some people with depression can be argumentative; others can be placid. Some patients with depression may trivialize complaints, not wanting to be a bother to anyone. Someone who sees no way out of his or her situation may turn to suicide. You should be alert for suicidal gestures and ideation, even though the signs may not be obvious.

Whereas depression can create behavioral problems in older patients, dementia is another cause of abnormal behavior. The most common cause of dementia is primary progressive dementia, also known as Alzheimer dementia. According to the Alzheimer's Association, an estimated 11% of the US population older than 65 years and 32% of the population older than 85 years have Alzheimer dementia, and the patient's life expectancy can range from 4 to 20 years following diagnosis.[4] Currently, there is no cure for Alzheimer disease, but several prescription medications have been introduced that may reduce the symptoms of Alzheimer disease, such as memory loss, or may help slow the progression of the disease.

During the progression of Alzheimer disease, the patient may exhibit openly hostile behavior and may kick, yell at, pinch, and hit you, your partner, or the caregiver. You might need to restrain the violent patient, but do so gently and only to the point at which the violent behavior stops.

Other causes of altered behavior may include diabetic emergencies, heat- and cold-related illnesses, poisoning, overdose, strokes and transient ischemic attacks, and infection. It is interesting to note that a urinary tract infection or constipation can alter an older person's behavior; however, the mechanism by which this behavior change evolves is not fully understood.

When you respond to a call for help, you should accept the possibility of depression and other potential mental health problems in the older patient. Do not discount the patient's feelings or devalue his or her emotions. Be alert for suicide gestures, and pay attention to any statements the patient may make about death. To obtain the patient's cooperation, you can elicit his or her help in providing care for the acute illness or injury. A smile and a touch can go a long way toward alleviating fear in many of your patients, especially older patients.

this threat: (1) cope with it, by finding ways to alter the situation or the individual's perception of it so that the threat is no longer so stressful, or (2) attempt to alleviate the discomfort by escaping from the stress. Escape may take many forms, including use of alcohol and drugs, psychiatric symptoms, and even suicide.

Humans are social beings, preferring to live in groups. Not surprisingly, then, sociocultural factors directly affect biology, behavior, and responses to the stress of emergencies. For example, the effects of assault, rape, racial attacks, or the death of a loved one may produce significant changes in a person's behavior.

Injury and Illness as Causes

Acute illness can overwhelm a person, causing changes in his or her behavior. Medical problems such as severe infections, electrolyte abnormalities, and many types of metabolic disorders result in stress on coping mechanisms and can cause abnormal behaviors.

The number of traumatic events occurring in the general population has increased in both frequency and intensity in recent years. An acute traumatic situation creates a great deal of stress for the person experiencing the trauma as well as those around the individual. As an AEMT, you are not immune to this stress. **Posttraumatic stress disorder (PTSD)** is a severe form of anxiety that stems from a traumatic experience; it is characterized by the individual reliving the stress of the original situation. Causes of PTSD can range from combat military service and terrorist attacks to a car crash or sexual assault.

Words of Wisdom

You should know the two basic types of underlying causes of behavioral emergencies: organic (physical) and functional (psychological).

Substance-Related Causes

Substance-related mental disorders may stem from the use of alcohol, cigarettes, illicit drugs, and other substances that change the way a person feels, behaves, or thinks. These disorders cost thousands of lives and billions of dollars annually. It was not until the late 20th century that substance-related disorders were recognized as a complex biologic and psychological problem rather than a sign of moral weakness. Currently, an estimated 7.9 million adults in the United States have both a substance use disorder and a mental disorder.[3]

▶ Functional Disorders

A **functional disorder** is one in which the etiology cannot be traced to an obvious change in the actual structure or physiology of the brain itself. Something has gone wrong, but the root cause cannot be identified definitively as brain dysfunction. Schizophrenia, anxiety conditions, and depression are good examples of mental disorders. There may be a chemical or physical cause for these disorders, but it is not always obvious or well understood.

YOU are the Provider — PART 2

The patient is sitting in a recliner in the living room and appears to have just finished lunch. There is an empty plate with a fork and knife next to his chair. He is mumbling to himself, but acknowledges your presence and does not appear to be aggressive. The patient reluctantly agrees to allow you to perform a physical examination. He states his chest feels "full," but it doesn't hurt and he hasn't had any difficulty breathing.

Recording Time: 1 Minute	
Appearance	Anxious, agitated
Level of consciousness	Alert and oriented to person, place, time, and event; however, experiencing auditory hallucinations
Airway	Patent
Breathing	Normal rate and rhythm
Circulation	Strong radial pulses; skin warm, dry, and pink

3. This patient has a known history of mental illness. Does he need to be transported to the hospital?
4. Does this patient require an ambulance transport to the emergency department, or should law enforcement transport him?

▶ Psychiatric Signs and Symptoms

When a person's physical health is challenged, the human body mobilizes various defenses to correct the abnormality. The patient experiences the effects of those abnormalities and corrective measures as symptoms, and you observe them as signs. Physical symptoms and signs reflect the body's attempts to maintain its balance in the face of physical stress. When a person's mental health is challenged, similar psychological mechanisms or behaviors are mobilized to help return the person's mental state to homeostasis. These defensive mechanisms present as various types of psychiatric signs and symptoms or behaviors that you may also observe.

Like the symptoms and signs of physical illness, psychiatric symptoms and signs can be grouped according to the "systems" they affect. Here, however, the focus is on systems of psychological (rather than physiologic) functioning. The psychological functions involved are consciousness, motor activity, speech, thought, affect, memory, orientation, and perception. Psychiatric signs and symptoms can affect the following areas: consciousness, motor activity, speech, thinking, mood and affect, memory, orientation, perception, and intelligence. The signs and symptoms of these disorders are listed in Table 24-2.

Table 24-2 Classification of Psychiatric Signs and Symptoms

Function Affected	Psychiatric Signs and Symptoms
Consciousness	Distractibility and inattention Confusion Delirium Stupor and coma
Motor activity	Restlessness **Stereotyped movements** (repetition of movements that do not seem to serve any useful purpose) **Compulsions** (repetitive actions that are carried out to relieve the anxiety of obsessive thoughts) Slow movements
Speech	Slow speech Acceleration or **pressure of speech** (the pouring out of words like water escaping under pressure) **Neologisms** (words the patient invents) **Echolalia** (the patient echoes words he or she hears) **Mutism** (the patient does not speak at all)
Thought progression	**Flight of ideas** (accelerated thinking in which the mind skips very rapidly from one thought to the next) Slowness of thought **Perseveration** (repetition of the same idea over and over again) **Circumstantial thinking** (the inclusion of many irrelevant details)
Thought content	**Delusions** (false beliefs) Obsessions **Phobias** (obsessive, irrational fears of specific things or situations, such as fear of heights, fear of open places, fear of confined spaces, or fear of certain animals)
Mood and **affect**	Anxiety Euphoria Depression **Inappropriate affect** (emotion that is out of synch with the situation—for example, wearing a smile while discussing a parent's death) **Flat affect** (the absence of emotion; appearing to feel no emotion at all)
Memory	Amnesia **Confabulation** (inventing experiences to fill gaps in memory)
Orientation	Disoriented to person, place, and time
Perception	Illusions **Hallucinations**
Intelligence	Difficulty learning

Patient Assessment

Scene Size-up

When evaluating a situation that is considered a behavioral emergency, you should first consider your safety and then determine how the patient is responding to the environment. Is the situation unduly dangerous to you and your partner? Do you need immediate law enforcement backup? Does the patient's behavior seem typical or normal given the circumstances? For example, a patient who has just been assaulted has good reason to be fearful of other people, including you. Conversely, if you ask a person, "Do you know where you are?" and he or she replies, "The planet Venus" (and does not seem to be joking), you may conclude that the person is disoriented, regardless of the cause.

Assessment of the environment can help give clues to the patient's condition or the cause of the emergency. Is the home too hot or too cold? Is the home well kept and secure? Are there hazardous conditions? Look for potential clues from the patient's social history; general living conditions; availability of social and family support; activity level; medications; overall appearance with respect to nutrition, general health, cleanliness, and personal hygiene; and attitude and mental well-being.

All the regular AEMT skills—assessment, providing care, patient approach, history taking, and patient communication—are used in behavioral emergencies. With behavioral emergencies, you should recognize that patient assessment is also part of the treatment. As soon as you speak to the patient, your voice and manner will affect his or her condition, for better or worse.

In addition, some other management techniques may be necessary. It is beyond the scope of this chapter to discuss all of these techniques, but you should follow general guidelines to ensure your safety at the scene of a behavioral emergency Table 24-3.

Table 24-3 Safety Guidelines for Behavioral Emergencies
Assess the scene. If the patient is armed or has potentially harmful objects in his or her possession, ensure that these objects have been removed by law enforcement personnel before you provide care.
Be prepared to spend extra time. It may take longer to assess, listen to, and prepare the patient for transport.
Have a definitive plan of action. Decide who will do what. If restraint is needed, how will it be accomplished?
Identify yourself calmly. Try to gain the patient's confidence. If you begin shouting, the patient is likely to shout louder or become more excited. A low, calm voice is often a quieting influence.
Be direct. State your intentions and what you expect of the patient.
Stay with the patient. *Do not let the patient leave the area, and do not leave the area yourself unless law enforcement personnel can and will stay with the patient.* Otherwise, the patient may go to another room and obtain weapons, lock himself or herself in the bathroom, or take pills.
Encourage purposeful movement. Help the patient get dressed and gather appropriate belongings to take to the hospital.
Express interest in the patient's story. Let the patient tell you what happened or what is going on now in his or her own words. However, do not play along with auditory or visual disturbances.
Keep a safe distance from the patient. Everyone needs personal space. Furthermore, you want to be sure you can move quickly if the patient becomes violent or tries to run away. Do not physically talk down to or directly confront the patient. A squatting, 45° angle approach is usually not confrontational; however, it may hinder your movements. Do not allow the patient to get between you and the exit.
Avoid fighting with the patient. You do not want to get into a power struggle. Remember, the patient is not responding to you in a normal manner; he or she may be wrestling with internal forces over which neither of you has control. You and others may be stimulating these inner forces without knowing it. If you can respond with understanding to the feeling that the patient is expressing, whether this is anger, fear, or desperation, you may be able to gain his or her cooperation. If it is necessary to use force, ensure that you have adequate help and move toward the patient quietly and with assured firmness.
Be honest and reassuring. If the patient asks whether he or she has to go to the hospital, the answer should be, "Yes, that is where you can receive medical help."
Do not judge. You may see behavior that you dislike. Set those feelings aside, and concentrate on providing emergency medical care.

Determine the mechanism of injury and/or nature of illness. For example, a patient with diabetes may have an altered mental status because of a low blood glucose level.

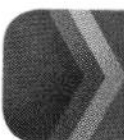

Primary Survey

As you approach the patient, respect the patient's territory and limit physical touching without permission. Approach slowly and purposefully while avoiding threatening actions, statements, and questions. Assess the patient's pupils carefully, because they may indicate other causes of altered mental status. For example, constricted pupils may indicate opiate ingestion, or unequal pupils may indicate cerebral trauma. Form a general impression of your patient Table 24-4.

A behavioral crisis puts tremendous stress on a person's coping mechanisms, including natural abilities and training. The person is actually incapable of responding reasonably to the demands of the environment. This state may be temporary, as in an acute illness, or longer-lived, as in a complex, chronic mental illness. In either situation, the patient's perception of reality may be compromised or distorted.

Table 24-4 Evaluating a Behavioral Crisis

General
How is the patient dressed? Is the dress appropriate for the time of year and occasion? Are the clothes clean or dirty?
Has the patient harmed himself or herself? Is there damage to the surroundings?
Speech
How does the patient respond to you? ▪ How does the patient feel? ▪ Is there trauma involved? ▪ Is there a medical problem?
Does the patient answer your questions appropriately?
Are the patient's vocabulary and expressions what you would expect under the circumstances? Are they in line with the patient's social and educational background?
Is the patient alert and able to speak logically and coherently?
Skin
What is the quality of the patient's skin? ▪ Color? ▪ Temperature? ▪ Condition?
Posture/Gait
Are the patient's movements coordinated or jerky and awkward? Does he or she appear to be agitated?
Are the patient's movements purposeful? Are the movements helping to accomplish a task, such as sitting down and putting on a pair of shoes, or do they appear to be aimless, such as rocking back and forth in the chair?
Does the patient appear relaxed or stiff and guarded?
Mental Status
Does the patient understand why you are there?
Mood
Is the patient withdrawn or detached?
Is the patient hostile or friendly? Too friendly?

(continued)

Table 24-4 Evaluating a Behavioral Crisis *(continued)*

What are the patient's facial expressions? Are they bland and flat or expressive? Does the patient show joy, fear, or anger as appropriate? To what degree?
What is the patient's mood? Does he or she seem agitated, elated, or abnormally depressed?
Does the patient appear fearful or worried?
Thought
Does the patient express disordered thoughts, delusions, or hallucinations? Does he or she appear to be seeing, hearing, or responding to people or situations that are not evident to you?
Perception
Are the patient's responses to what is going on around him or her appropriate?
Judgment
Does the patient exhibit rational judgment?
Memory
Is the patient's memory intact? Check orientation to time, place, and person by asking the patient the following questions: ▪ Do you know what day/month/year it is? ▪ Do you know where you are? ▪ Do you know who I am?
Attention
Is the patient easily distracted? Is the patient able to concentrate?

When performing your assessment, it is important to limit the number of people around the patient. Remember to stay alert to potential danger. A patient in unstable condition may become violent at any time. Watch for signs of agitation or aggression. It is important to separate the patient from bystanders or family members who seem to be exacerbating the patient's condition. You may ask them to step into another room and speak to your partner, or you may take the patient to the ambulance before beginning your primary survey, if appropriate.

Violent patients make up only a small percentage of those experiencing a behavioral or psychiatric crisis. Nevertheless, the potential for violence by such a patient should always be an important consideration for you. Although a patient with a large body size may be intimidating, there is no correlation between the size of the patient and the potential for violence.

Consider the following risk factors when assessing the level of danger:

- **History.** Has the patient previously exhibited hostile, overly aggressive, or violent behavior? Ask people at the scene, or request this information from law enforcement personnel or family.
- **Posture.** How is the patient sitting or standing? Is the patient tense, rigid, or sitting on the edge of his or her seat? Such physical tension is often a warning signal of impending hostility.
- **The scene.** Is the patient holding or near potentially lethal objects such as a knife, gun, glass, scissors, or bat (or near a window or glass door)? Also take note of conventional household objects that the patient could use as weapons, such as lamps, heavy dishes, hand tools, or figurines.
- **Vocal activity.** Which kind of speech is the patient using? Loud, obscene, erratic, and bizarre speech patterns usually indicate emotional distress. Someone using quiet, ordered speech is not as likely to strike out as someone who is yelling and screaming. However, do not discount the possibility of violent behavior in the quiet patient.
- **Physical activity.** The motor activity of a person experiencing a psychiatric crisis may be the most telling factor of all. The patient who has tense muscles, clenched fists, glaring eyes, or is pacing, cannot sit still, or is fiercely protecting personal space requires careful watching. Agitation may predict a quick escalation to violence.

Other factors to consider in assessing a patient's potential for violence include the following:

- Poor impulse control
- A history of truancy, fighting, and uncontrollable temper
- Low socioeconomic status, unstable family structure, or inability to keep a steady job (note, however, that violence occurs among all classes and that socioeconomic class is a relative concept, depending on geographic areas)
- Tattoos, especially those with gang identification or statements such as "Born to Kill" or "Born to Lose," or jail-related tattoos (jail-related tattoos tend to be homemade and on the hands or forearms)
- Substance abuse
- Depression (Depression is associated with a threefold increased risk of violence compared to the general population.[5])
- Functional disorder (If the patient says that voices are telling him or her to kill, believe it.)

As with any patient, determine the presence of any life-threatening medical conditions by performing an assessment of the patient's ABCDEs (Airway, Breathing, Circulation, Disability, and Exposure). Assess the airway to make sure it is patent and adequate. Next, evaluate the patient's breathing. Provide any appropriate interventions on the basis of your assessment findings. You will need to assess the pulse rate, quality, and rhythm. Obtain the systolic and diastolic blood pressures when possible. Assessing a patient's circulation includes an evaluation for the presence of shock and bleeding. Assess the patient's perfusion level by evaluating skin color, temperature, and condition.

While you are assessing the patient's mental status, note any evidence of rage, elation, hostility, depression, fear, anger, anxiety, confusion, or any other abnormal behavior. Observe for any signs of overt behavior and give close attention to body language, such as abnormal posture or threatening gestures. Talk to the patient as you continue your assessment, and explain all procedures that you intend to perform.

Unless the patient's condition is unstable from a medical problem or trauma, prepare to spend time at the scene with the patient. Depending on your local protocol, there may be a specific facility to which patients with mental problems are transported.

Safety

When you are assessing a patient who is experiencing a behavioral emergency, it can be useful to obtain information separately from a relative or caregiver. Obtaining the patient's history in this way often yields valuable information and can help reduce the potential for violence when there is tension between the people involved.

History Taking

Once any life-threatening emergencies have been addressed, remove the patient from the crisis or disturbing situation. You should focus your questions during the history taking on the immediate problem to avoid confusion. Establishing a good rapport with the patient will enable you to provide better care. Use therapeutic interviewing techniques by engaging in active listening, being supportive and empathetic, limiting interruptions, and respecting the patient's personal space. Limit physical contact to minimize patient apprehension. Avoid using any threatening actions, statements, or questions. Approach the patient slowly and purposefully.

When you are talking with the patient, it is important to evaluate the potential for suicide or harm to others. Factors that increase these risks include recent depression, recent loss of a family member or friend, financial setback, drug use, or evidence of a detailed plan. If you are able to determine that the patient has actually established a plan for suicide or violence, there is a great risk of the patient carrying it out. In particular, a patient who has a very detailed plan and access to the means to complete it is all the more likely to carry out the plan. For example, a patient who actually has a bottle of pills is much more likely to overdose than one who does not have ready access to pills.

Reflective listening, also called active listening, is a technique frequently used by mental health professionals to gain insight into a patient's thinking. It involves repeating back to patients what they have said, encouraging them to expand on their thoughts. Although it often requires more time to be effective than is available in an EMS setting, it may be a helpful tool for you to use when other communication techniques are unsuccessful. It is important to actively listen and to be supportive and empathetic. Allow time for the patient to answer and limit interruptions.

Sometimes a patient experiencing a behavioral or psychiatric emergency will not respond to any of your questions. In those situations, you may be able to determine much about the patient's emotional state from facial expressions, pulse rate, and respirations. Take note of the presence of tears, sweating, and blushing—these findings may be significant indicators of the patient's state of mind. Also, make sure that you look at the patient's eyes; a patient who has a blank gaze or rapidly moving eyes may be experiencing central nervous system depression or some type of extra stress **Figure 24-1**.

Family, friends, and observers may also be of great help in answering patient history questions. Together with your observations and interaction with the patient, they should provide enough data for you to assess the situation. This part of the patient assessment has two primary goals: recognizing major threats to life and reducing the stress of the situation as much as possible.

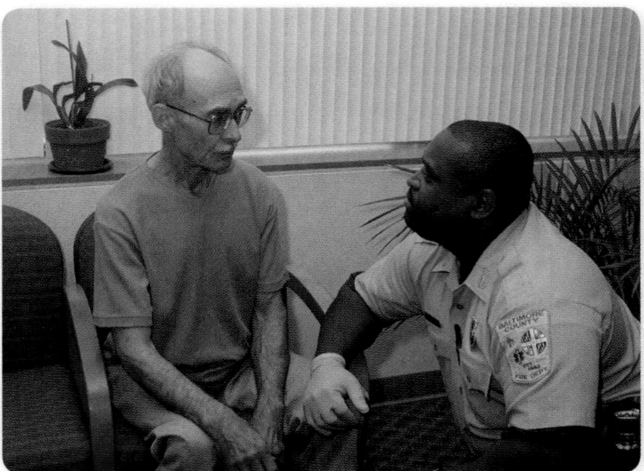

Figure 24-1 Looking at the patient's eyes can provide useful clues about the individual's emotional state.

Special Populations

Although not all elderly patients have Alzheimer disease or dementia, consider these conditions as possible causes of abnormal behavior. In patients with any sort of dementia, it is essential to obtain information from relatives, friends, or extended-care facility staff. Facility staff such as certified nurse's aides may be a particularly useful resource for this information because they spend a significant amount of time interacting directly with their patients. Determining the patient's baseline mental status will be essential in guiding your treatment and transport decisions. However, it is important to remember that any patient with an altered mental status, regardless of history, should receive a complete assessment, including a check for hypoxia and hypoglycemia.

When trying to determine the etiology of the patient's condition, you should consider four major areas as possible contributors:

- Is the patient's central nervous system functioning properly? For example, the patient may be experiencing diabetic problems, particularly hypoglycemia. He or she may have been poisoned or may be responding to physical trauma. Any of these situations could cause the patient to behave in an unusual or irrational manner.
- What is the general condition of the patient's environment? Is the patient dressed appropriately? Clean?
- Is there any evidence of substance abuse? Are hallucinogens or other drugs or alcohol a factor? Does the patient see strange things? Is everything distorted? Do you smell alcohol on the patient's breath?
- Are **psychogenic** circumstances, symptoms, or illness (caused by mental rather than physical factors) involved? These might include the death of a loved one, severe depression, a history of mental illness, threats of suicide, or some other major interruption of ADL.

Be sure to note any physical assessment findings or complaints of physical symptoms. Document the intellectual function: Is the patient oriented? Is the patient's memory intact? Is the patient able to concentrate and use the appropriate judgment? Does the patient have disordered thoughts, delusions, hallucinations, unusual worries or fears, or express suicidal or homicidal threats? Also note the speech pattern and content. Is the speech garbled or unintelligible? What is the patient's mood like? What about appearance and hygiene? Finally, is the patient's motor activity normal? Be sure to accurately document all findings.

Secondary Assessment

Whereas much of your assessment involves interviewing the patient about any psychiatric history, you must also look for signs of an organic cause of the patient's behavior:

- Obtain the vital signs to look for signs of fever or indications of increased intracranial pressure.
- Examine the skin temperature and moisture, and note any prominent tattoos. Certain tattoos may suggest a tendency toward violence. Scars may indicate self-mutilation.
- Inspect the head for evidence of trauma.
- Check the pupils for size, equality, and reaction to light. Pupillary abnormalities may indicate a toxic ingestion or an intracranial process as the source of the patient's behavior.
- Note any unusual odors on the patient's breath such as poisons, alcohol, or ketones from diabetic ketoacidosis.
- Examine the extremities, looking for needle tract marks, tremors, and unilateral weakness or loss of sensation.

Unless a significant traumatic problem exists, a secondary assessment may be conducted to provide helpful information. Alternatively, on the basis of your transport time and the patient's mental status, the secondary assessment may be deferred.

Obtain vital signs when doing so will not exacerbate the patient's emotional distress. Make every effort to assess blood pressure, pulse, respirations, skin, and pupils. Remember that a behavioral crisis can be caused or precipitated by physiologic problems such as a head injury or diabetic disorder and that such a crisis can aggravate preexisting conditions. Do not forget that the physical person and the emotional person are one.

When it will not exacerbate the patient's emotional distress, you may use monitoring devices to measure and assess the patient's oxygenation and circulatory status. It is recommended that you always assess the patient's first blood pressure with a sphygmomanometer (blood pressure cuff) and a stethoscope. A pulse oximeter, if available, can be used to assess the level of the patient's oxygenation, but only if there is no impairment of perfusion or exposure to substances such as carbon monoxide that will interfere with accurate readings.

Reassessment

Reassessment is routinely performed during transport. This is a good time to assess more details of the patient's mental status.

Many times, patients with abnormal behavior may have settled down physically, but their minds may still be in a state of flux—this could lead to very impulsive behavior. Monitor patients vigilantly for sudden changes in thought or behavior, particularly as you near the hospital. If patients do not want help, they may try to jump from the ambulance or hurt themselves. Patients will not hesitate to hurt you while attempting to exit the vehicle. Do not put yourself at risk. Medical and traumatic conditions may cause deterioration in a condition identified earlier in the assessment.

You should try to give the receiving hospital advance warning when a patient experiencing a psychiatric emergency is coming in. Many hospitals require extra preparation to ensure that appropriate staff and room are available to accommodate the patient's needs and to ensure safety for all. Report whether restraints will be required when the patient arrives at the hospital.

Provide thorough and careful documentation in your patient care report. Think about what you are going to write before you write it, so that you can describe what are often confusing scenes as clearly as possible. Because psychiatric emergencies may present with few or no physical signs, your report may be the only documentation of the patient's distress. Psychiatric emergencies are fraught with legal dangers, so it is wise to document everything that occurred on the call, particularly in a situation that required restraints. When restraints are implemented to protect you or the patient from harm, include why and which type of restraints were used. This information is essential if the case is reviewed for medicolegal reasons.

YOU are the Provider PART 3

As your partner is placing the blood pressure cuff on his arm, the patient suddenly jumps to his feet and makes shooting noises while pointing an imaginary gun around the room. He shouts, "Did I get them? Did I get them?" You and your partner quickly move back from the patient. The officer on scene calls for additional law enforcement. The patient paces back and forth and appears very anxious and agitated. Once additional law enforcement arrives, the decision is made to restrain the patient with handcuffs for his own protection as well as that of the EMS crew. Because his chief complaint is chest pain, you recommend that the patient be transported by ambulance.

Recording Time: 10 Minutes	
Respirations	26 breaths/min, clear bilaterally
Pulse	Strong and regular, 120 beats/min
Skin	Warm, dry, and pink
Blood pressure	176/102 mm Hg
Oxygen saturation (Spo_2)	97% on room air
Pupils	Pupils Equal, Round, and Reactive to Light and Accommodation (PERRLA)

5. What is the minimum number of providers who should be present when attempting to physically restrain a patient?
6. In which position should this patient be restrained?
7. Should a law enforcement officer accompany you in the back of the ambulance or should the officer follow behind the ambulance in the patrol car?

Emergency Medical Care

Treatment of the patient with a psychiatric problem follows the approach stressed throughout this text. First, ensure scene safety; then, when safety is confirmed, focus on life-threatening conditions. If the erratic behavior might possibly be caused by a medical disorder (eg, hypoglycemia, overdose, or hypoxia), treat the patient for the medical disorder before presuming that the patient's behavior is due to an emotional or psychiatric cause. These treatment measures may include oxygen therapy, testing of the blood glucose level, and administration of D_{50} (25 grams of dextrose in 50 mL of water), as well as general interventions for hypothermia or shock management.

Throughout your care of the patient, maintain safety for the patient and for yourself. By placing the patient on the stretcher with the straps in place, you will be more in control of the situation if it turns violent. Control violent situations by restraining the patient, if needed. Call immediately for law enforcement assistance if the patient is potentially violent.

Remain with the patient at all times unless an unsafe situation exists. Avoid challenging the patient's personal space. Always ask permission before touching the patient, and explain procedures before you perform them. Attempt to eliminate or decrease any condition that may distress the patient, such as loud sirens or fast movements. Refrain from performing procedures that may not be absolutely pertinent, such as starting an intravenous line, if no medical issue exists. Remember to document only objective findings and avoid being judgmental. The patient did not ask for this problem, and you must view it as any other type of illness. If there is any indication of overdose or reason to suspect the patient may have taken something, bring any medications or drugs found to the medical facility.

Words of Wisdom

Altered mental status may be a sign of hypoxia or hypoglycemia. Never withhold oxygen from any patient or discount its use because the patient has a history of mental problems. Check the patient's blood glucose level to rule out hypoglycemia.

Assessment and Management of Specific Emergencies

Acute Psychosis

Psychosis is a state of delusion in which the person is out of touch with reality. Affected people live in their own reality of ideas and feelings. To the person experiencing a psychotic episode, the line between reality and fantasy is blurred. That reality may make patients belligerent and angry toward others. Patients may become silent and withdrawn as they give all their attention to the voices and feelings within.

Psychoses or psychotic episodes occur for many reasons. The use of mind-altering substances is one of the most common causes, and that experience may be limited to the duration over which the substance is metabolized within the body. Other causes may include intense stress, delusional disorders, and, more commonly, schizophrenia. Some psychotic episodes last for brief periods; others last a lifetime.

Disorganization and **disorientation** are *not* diagnoses, but rather ways in which various conditions such as schizophrenia and organic brain syndromes may present themselves. These presentations account for a large number of EMS calls, particularly those involving older people. Although you do not need to make a specific diagnosis in such cases, you do need to know how to manage these patients in the field.

Schizophrenia

Schizophrenia is a complex disorder that is not easily defined or easily treated, yet has a dramatic effect on society. According to the Centers for Disease Control and Prevention, estimates of the worldwide prevalence of schizophrenia range from 0.5% to 1%.[6] The typical onset occurs during early adulthood, with dysfunctional symptoms becoming more prominent over time. Some people diagnosed with schizophrenia display signs during early childhood; their disease may be associated with brain damage sustained early in life. Other influences thought to contribute to this disorder include genetics, neurobiologic influences, and psychological and social influences.

People with schizophrenia may experience delusions, hallucinations, apathy, mutism, a flat affect, a lack of interest in pleasure, erratic speech, emotional responses, and motor behavior (either a lack of motor behavior or excessive motor behavior). Because the precise cause of schizophrenia remains unknown, treatments focus on eliminating these symptoms.[7]

Assessment of Psychosis

The most characteristic feature of psychosis is a profound thought disorder, often accompanied by disturbances in mood and perception. Patients are usually incoherent or rambling in their speech, although they may be oriented to person and place. Often these patients are found wandering aimlessly down the street, dressed oddly, uttering meaningless words and sentences. A thorough examination of the patient is rarely possible, and the principal objective for the AEMT is to transport the patient to the hospital in an atraumatic fashion.

The COASTMAP mnemonic is one way to remember the signs and symptoms commonly associated with patients experiencing a psychotic episode:

- **Consciousness.** The patient is awake and alert, but may be easily distracted, especially if paying attention to hallucinations. If the patient's level of consciousness fluctuates, suspect an organic brain syndrome.

- **Orientation.** Disturbances in orientation are more common in organic disorders than in psychoses, but the patient experiencing severe psychosis may be disoriented as to time and place.
- **Activity.** Activity is most commonly accelerated, with agitation and hyperactivity, but it may also be diminished. Bizarre, stereotyped movements are common.
- **Speech.** Speech may be pressured or sound strange because of unusual words that the patient has invented (neologisms).
- **Thought.** Thought is disturbed in progression and content and may show any of the following disorders:
  - Flight of ideas, with the patient's mind plunging from one thought to another.
  - **Loosening of associations**, in which the logical connection between one idea and the next becomes obscure, at least to the listener. In extreme cases, the patient's speech may be entirely incomprehensible.
  - Delusions, especially of persecution.
  - **Thought broadcasting** (the patient's belief that his or her thoughts are broadcast aloud and can be heard by others).
  - **Thought insertion** (the patient's belief that thoughts are being thrust into his or her mind by another person) and **thought withdrawal** (the patient's belief that his or her thoughts are being removed).
- **Memory.** Memory can be relatively or entirely intact in psychosis. It may be difficult to obtain the cooperation of the patient for formal memory testing.
- **Affect and mood.** Mood is likely to be disturbed in psychosis. The disturbance may take the form of euphoria, sadness, or wide swings in mood; affect may reflect those inner states or be flat.
- **Perception.** Auditory hallucinations are common in psychosis. Patients hear voices commenting on their behavior or telling them what to do. Suspect that patients are hearing such voices when they seem to be attending a conversation other than yours or talking to themselves.

Management of Psychosis

Dealing with a patient with acute psychosis is difficult. The usual methods of reasoning with a patient are unlikely to be effective because the person experiencing a psychotic episode has his or her own rules of logic that may be quite different from those that govern nonpsychotic thinking. Furthermore, you are likely to feel uncomfortable in the presence of a person experiencing a psychotic episode. Those uncomfortable feelings are one of your built-in diagnostic instruments. They are elicited by the fear, suspicion, and hostility that the patient is broadcasting through body language. Use your uncomfortable feelings to help make a tentative diagnosis that the patient is experiencing a psychotic problem.

The disorganized patient needs structure. You should explain in plain language what is being done and what the patient's role will be. Directions should be simple, consistent, and firm. It may be impossible to obtain a detailed history directly from the patient; a name and address may be all the information that you can gather. Explain to the patient that he or she needs to be seen by a physician and that you will take the individual to the hospital to get help.

In managing the disoriented patient, the key is to *keep orienting the patient* to time, place, and the people in the environment. Tell the patient who you are, and explain what you are doing. You may have to repeat that information several times en route. Reassure the patient, and point out landmarks to help orient the patient.

Nonpharmacologic techniques, such as maintaining an emotional distance, explaining each step of the assessment, and involving people whom the patient trusts, should be the methods you try first. Consider paramedic backup for administration of a sedative or antianxiety drug if the patient is not compliant and possibly represents a danger to him- or herself or to others.

▶ Suicide

The single most significant factor that contributes to suicide is depression.[8] Any time you encounter a patient experiencing depression, you must consider the possibility of suicide. Risk factors for suicide are listed in Table 24-5.

It is a common misconception that people who threaten suicide never commit it. This is not correct. Suicide is a cry for help. Threatening suicide is an indication that someone is in a crisis he or she cannot handle. Immediate intervention is necessary.

Whether or not the patient has any of these risk factors, you must be alert to the following warning signs:

- Does the patient have an air of tearfulness, sadness, deep despair, or hopelessness that suggests depression?
- Does the patient avoid eye contact (although this may sometimes be a culturally based behavior), speak slowly or haltingly, and project a sense of vacancy, as if he or she really is not there?
- Does the patient seem unable to talk about the future? Ask the patient whether he or she has any vacation plans. Suicidal people consider the future so uninteresting that they do not think about it; people who are seriously depressed consider the future so distant that they may not be able to think about it at all.
- Is there any suggestion of suicide? Even vague suggestions should not be taken lightly, even if presented as a joke. If you think that suicide is a possibility, do not hesitate to bring the subject up. You will not "give the patient ideas" if you ask directly, "Are you considering suicide?"

Table 24-5 Risk Factors for Suicide
Ideation or defined lethal plan of action that has been verbalized and/or written
Purposelessness
Feeling trapped, no way out
Anxiety, agitation, unable to sleep, or sleeping all the time
Withdrawal from friends, family, and society
Anger and/or aggressive tendencies
Recklessness or engaging in risky activities
Dramatic mood changes
History of trauma or abuse
Some major physical illness (eg, cancer, heart failure)
Easy access to lethal means
Certain cultural and religious beliefs
Depression, any age
Previous suicide attempt (In one study, when the initial suicide attempt was not successful, 80% of the individuals later went on to have a completed suicide.[9])
Current expression of wanting to commit suicide or sense of hopelessness
Family history of suicide
Age older than 40 years, particularly for single, widowed, or divorced people and people with alcoholism or depression (Men in this category who are older than 55 years have an especially high risk.)
Recent loss of spouse, significant other, family member, or support system and sense of isolation
Chronic debilitating illness or recent diagnosis of serious illness
Holidays (especially Christmas)
Financial setback, loss of job, police arrest, imprisonment, or some sort of social embarrassment
Alcohol and substance abuse, particularly with increasing use
Parent with alcoholism
Severe mental illness
Anniversary of death of loved one, job loss, divorce, or other important event
Unusual gathering or new acquisition of things that can cause death, such as purchase of a gun, a large volume of pills, or increased use of alcohol

- Does the patient have any specific plans relating to death? Has the patient recently prepared a will? Given away significant possessions or advised close friends what he or she would like done with them? Arranged for a funeral service? These are critical warning signs.

Consider also the following risk factors for suicide:

- Are there any unsafe objects in the patient's hands or nearby (eg, a sharp knife, glass, poisons, or a gun)?
- Is the environment unsafe (eg, an open window in a high-rise building, a patient standing on a bridge or precipice)?
- Is there evidence of self-destructive behavior (eg, partial cuts on the body; lacerations in various stages of healing on the thighs, upper arms, or other areas that can be easily covered; large alcohol or drug intake)?
- Is there an imminent threat to the patient or others?
- Is there an underlying medical problem?

Remember, the patient considering suicide may be homicidal as well. Do not jeopardize your life or the lives of your fellow AEMTs. If you have reason to believe that you are in danger, you must enlist the aid of law enforcement personnel. In the meantime, try not to frighten the patient or make him or her suspicious.

When a person has *attempted* suicide, medical treatment takes priority. The patient who has taken an overdose of sedative or depressant drugs must be managed for possible respiratory depression or circulatory collapse. The patient who has slashed his or her wrists must be treated to control bleeding and restore circulating volume. Nonetheless, if the patient is still conscious, try to establish communication and ask the patient to talk about the situation.

Special Populations

Behavioral disorders are estimated to affect as many as 11% to 20% of all children and adolescents, yet only one in eight children with a mental health problem receives proper treatment.[10] When not treated properly, such a problem will most likely persist into adulthood. Given that suicide was the second leading cause of death in US adolescents in 2014,[11] more attention has recently been given to mood disorders, anxiety, and other behavioral problems in this population. Children are also more likely to have coexisting problems (eg, attention deficit/hyperactivity disorder, conduct disorder, and oppositional defiant disorder) along with the more traditional mental health disorders.

Mental health problems in children are difficult to diagnose because the lines between normal and abnormal behavior are less clear in this population. Diagnosis and treatment may be difficult when trying to distinguish between organic, genetic, and environmental causes. Cultural and ethnic factors may also blur the line between normal and abnormal coping mechanisms. The mental status assessment of the child is similar to that of an adult, but it takes the child's developmental level into consideration. Abnormal findings in the developmental and mental status examination are often related to adjustment disorders and stress rather than the more serious disorders. Remember that aggressive behavior may be a symptom of an underlying disorder or disability. Your assessment must include an assessment of suicide risk in any child.

▶ Agitated Delirium

A problem you will sometimes encounter in an EMS response is a patient who is experiencing agitated delirium. **Agitated delirium**, also called excited delirium or exhaustive mania, is a state of global cognitive impairment that is acute in onset and associated with fluctuations in mental status and behavior, inattention, disorganized thinking, and an altered level of consciousness. Delirium is a condition of impairment in cognitive function that can present with disorientation, hallucinations, or delusions. Agitation is a behavior that is characterized by restless and irregular physical activity. By comparison, **dementia** is a more chronic process that produces severe deficits in memory, abstract thinking, and judgment. Although patients experiencing delirium are generally not dangerous, if they exhibit agitated behavior, they may strike out irrationally. One of the most important factors to consider in these situations is your personal safety.

The symptoms of agitated delirium may include hyperactive irrational behavior with inattentiveness and possible vivid hallucinations. Common physical symptoms include hypertension, tachycardia, diaphoresis, and dilated pupils. Because hallucinations are erroneous perceptions of reality, the patient may perceive you as a threat. Agitation is recognized as a biologic attempt to release nervous tension; it can result in sudden, unpredictable physical actions in the patient.

If you think that you can safely approach the patient, be very calm, supportive, and empathetic. Be an active listener by nodding, indicating understanding, and by limiting your interruptions of the patient's comments. It is extremely important to approach the patient slowly and purposefully and to respect the patient's territory. Limit physical contact with the patient as much as possible. It is also imperative that the patient not be left unattended, unless the situation becomes unsafe for you or your partner.

Carefully use interviewing techniques to assess the patient's cognitive functioning. Try to indirectly determine the patient's orientation, memory, concentration, and judgment by asking simple questions such as "When did you first begin to notice these feelings?" Through interviewing, try to determine what the patient is thinking. Are the patient's thoughts disorganized? For example, does the patient begin to answer your question and then drift off, only to begin discussing a childhood friend? Is the patient experiencing delusions or hallucinations? Does the patient have any unusual worries or fears? For example, does the patient express anxiety if you go too close to a pile of old newspapers?

Pay particular attention to the patient's ability to communicate clearly, and make notes on the patient's apparent mood. Is the patient anxious, depressed, elated (extremely happy or joyful) under inappropriate circumstances, or agitated? Pay attention to the patient's appearance, dress, and personal hygiene. If you determine that the patient requires restraint because he or she is a threat to him- or herself or to others, make sure you have adequate, well-trained personnel available to help you before approaching the patient. If the patient appears to be experiencing an overdose, take all medication bottles or illegal substances with you to the medical facility. The patient should be transported to a hospital with psychiatric facilities capable of handling his or her condition. Whenever possible, refrain from using lights and sirens because these sights and sounds may aggravate the patient's condition.

Mood Disorders

Mood disorders, formally known as affective disorders, are among the most prevalent mental disorders. Up to 21% of the US population will experience a mood disorder, such as a **manic–depressive illness** or major depression, at some point in their lives.[12] Although feelings such as depression and joy are universal, mood disorders differ from normal bouts of sadness or happiness. In mood disorders, the changes in affect are accompanied by other symptoms, and the net effect is to cause a major disturbance in the person's ability to function. Patients who experience either depression or mania have a unipolar mood disorder; that is, their mood remains at only one pole of the depression–mania continuum. Patients who alternate between mania and depression (both poles of the continuum) have **bipolar mood disorder**. Most patients with a unipolar mood disorder are depressed. Unipolar mania is relatively rare, with only 5% to 7% of all patients with bipolar disorder having this subtype.[13]

Manic Behavior

Mania is one of the most striking psychiatric conditions. Typically, a bystander or family member calls for an ambulance because the patient is unlikely to believe that anything is wrong. To the contrary, the patient with mania is more apt to report being "on top of the world—never felt better in my life." People experiencing mania typically have abnormally exaggerated happiness, joy, or euphoria with hyperactivity and insomnia.

Patients experiencing mania are typically awake and alert but are easily distracted. They are also often markedly hyperactive and may report being unable to concentrate. Almost all patients experiencing mania report a significantly decreased need for sleep, and they may go for days without sleeping. In conversation, people experiencing mania are talkative, with pressured and rapid speech. Flight of ideas and delusions of grandeur make it difficult for them to focus on one thing. Patients may report that their thoughts are racing; their monologues may skip rapidly from one topic to another (**tangential thinking**). Their ideas are often grandiose, such as unrealistic plans to embark on a large business venture or to run for high public office. Patients may also believe that they have special powers or that they are famous and wealthy. Their memory is usually intact but may be distorted by underlying delusions. Their affect is elated (the hallmark of mania). The patient seems to be on a "high," and is unusually and infectiously cheerful. The good cheer may be quite brittle, however, and the person may quickly become irritable, sarcastic, and hostile with little provocation. A person having an acute manic episode may show psychotic symptoms such as hallucinations.

People experiencing acute manic episodes have a high probability of getting themselves into trouble of one sort or another—for example, going on wild spending sprees, making foolish business investments, driving recklessly, committing sexual indiscretions, or picking fights. Often, it is when the person has gotten into some sort of trouble, or when his or her behavior has become intolerably disruptive, that an ambulance is summoned.

Because patients with mania are unlikely to consider themselves ill, they may not agree that they need treatment. In dealing with the manic individual, be calm, firm, and patient; do not argue or get into a power struggle. Minimize external stimulation. Talk to the patient in a quiet place, away from other people. (Meanwhile, have your partner obtain the history separately from relatives or bystanders.) When it is time to transport the patient, do not use sirens.

If the patient refuses transport, consult medical control. Obtain law enforcement assistance for transport if medical control indicates that hospital evaluation is necessary.

Depression

Depression is the leading cause of disability in people between age 15 and 44 years.[14] It affects women more frequently than men and may occur at any age (the mean age of onset is 32 years).[14] The patient with depression is often readily identified by a sad expression, bouts of crying, and listless or apathetic behavior. He or she expresses feelings of worthlessness, guilt, and pessimism. These patients may want to be left alone, asserting that no one understands or cares and that their problems are hopeless.

Depression may occur in episodes with a sudden onset and limited duration; this is common in major depressive disorder, in which the patient feels substantial suffering and pain that interfere with social or occupational functioning. In other cases, the onset of depression may be insidious and chronic in nature. When a person experiences signs and symptoms of depression for more days than not for a period of at least 2 years, he or she may be experiencing a chronic form of depression known as dysthymic disorder. The signs and symptoms of dysthymic disorder cause social and occupational distress but rarely require hospitalization unless the person becomes suicidal.

The diagnostic features of depression are most easily remembered by the mnemonic GAS PIPES:

- **Guilt.** Guilt and self-reproach are characteristic features of depression. One way to try to get at the patient's guilt feelings is to ask a question such as "Are you down on yourself?" or "Do you ever feel as if you're worthless?"
- **Appetite.** Appetite is abnormal in depression. Usually it is decreased, but a minority of patients with depression may report increased appetite.
- **Sleep.** Sleep disturbance usually takes the form of insomnia. The typical patient with depression will report that he or she awakens at 0300 or 0400 hours and cannot get back to sleep.
- **Paying attention.** The patient with depression has an impaired ability to concentrate; the impairment is sometimes severe. Ask the patient, "When you're reading a book or a newspaper, can you get all the way through what you're

reading, or does your mind start to wander after a couple of minutes?"

- **Interest.** The patient with depression loses interest in things that were once important. He or she can no longer summon enthusiasm for work or hobbies. You might ask the patient, "Are you a [local team name] fan?" If the answer is yes, ask, "How are they doing this season?" The patient with depression will tell you, "Well, I haven't really been following them lately."
- **Psychomotor abnormalities.** In the patient with depression, psychomotor abnormalities can be increased (from agitation) or slowed. Although many patients with depression seem to do everything in slow motion, a significant percentage show agitated behavior such as pacing, wringing their hands, or picking at themselves.
- **Energy.** People with depression have no energy. They are tired all the time and do not feel like doing anything.
- **Suicidal thoughts.** Most worrisome, people with depression tend to have pervasive and recurrent thoughts of suicide.

▶ Neurotic Disorders

Neurotic disorders are a collection of mental disorders without psychotic symptoms and lacking the intense psychopathology of other mood disorders. These disorders cause many problems for patients, their families, and society in general. Treating neurotic disorders comes at a substantial price; however, the cost to society of not treating these disorders (in terms of lost production and lost efficiency) is probably even greater.

This category of conditions includes **anxiety disorders**, which are mental disorders in which the dominant moods are fear and apprehension. Everyone experiences anxiety occasionally, and a certain amount of anxiety helps people adapt constructively to stress. Patients with anxiety disorders, by contrast, experience persistent, incapacitating anxiety in the absence of external threat. An estimated 18% of adults will experience some form of anxiety disorder in any given year, and nearly 30% will develop such a disorder at some point in their lifetime.[15] Several types of anxiety disorders, including generalized anxiety disorder, phobias, and panic disorder, are likely to elicit a call for an ambulance or affect the delivery of prehospital care.

Generalized Anxiety Disorder

Although some anxiety in everyday activity is normal, when a person worries about everything for no particular reason, or if that worrying is unproductive and the person cannot decide what to do about an upcoming situation, the person may be experiencing **generalized anxiety disorder (GAD)**. To make a diagnosis of GAD, symptoms (anxiety and worry) must be present more days than not for a period of at least 6 months and the worry must be difficult to turn off or control. Nearly 6% of all individuals will experience this type of anxiety disorder at some point in their lifetime.[16] Patients experiencing GAD are often treated with both pharmacologic agents and counseling. The acute symptoms of anxiety and worry can become overwhelming in GAD, however, prompting a family member or coworker to call for an ambulance.

When you are dealing with a patient with GAD, identify yourself in a calm, confident manner. Listen attentively to the patient and talk with the person generally about his or her feelings.

Phobias

Phobic disorders involve an unreasonable fear, apprehension, or dread of a specific situation or thing. The patient with a **simple phobia** focuses all his or her anxieties onto one class of objects (eg, mice, spiders, dogs) or situations (eg, high places, darkness, flying). At some point in their lifetime, an estimated 12% of adults have social phobias, or fear of everyday social situations such as fear of going to parties, meeting new people, speaking, or eating in public.[17] When confronted with the feared object or situation, the person with a phobia experiences intolerable anxiety and all of the autonomic symptoms that anxiety brings. The patient usually recognizes that the fear is unreasonable but is unable to do anything about it.

In managing a patient with a phobia, explain each step of treatment in detail before you carry it out: "First we'll give you oxygen to help you breathe. Then we're going to move you onto the stretcher, so that we can carry you downstairs."

Panic Disorder

Panic disorder is characterized by sudden, usually unexpected and overwhelming feelings of fear and dread, accompanied by a variety of other symptoms produced by a massive activation of the autonomic nervous system. Women are more likely to be affected by this condition than are men (the female-to-male ratio is estimated at 72:28[18]), and the disorder tends to run in families. The attacks usually begin when the patient is in his or her 20s. Most affected people can identify a stressful event that preceded their first attack, such as an illness or loss of a loved one. Thereafter, the attacks may come "out of the blue," without any apparent precipitating stress. If allowed to continue, panic attacks may cause severe restrictions in the patient's lifestyle. The person may become afraid to go to work, to go shopping, or to leave the house at all, out of fear that an attack will occur away from home. The fear of going into public places is called **agoraphobia** (literally, "fear of the marketplace").

The classic signs and symptoms of panic disorder are summarized in Table 24-6. A large percentage of these signs and symptoms—such as palpitations and sweating—are a consequence of autonomic nervous system discharge, whereas others (chest discomfort, paresthesias) may reflect hyperventilation. The symptoms usually peak in intensity within about 10 minutes and last around an hour altogether.

Table 24-6 Signs and Symptoms of a Panic Attack	
▪ Shortness of breath or a sensation of being smothered ▪ Palpitations or tachycardia ▪ Sweating ▪ Nausea or abdominal distress ▪ Chills or hot flashes ▪ Fear of dying ▪ Feelings of unreality or of being detached from oneself	▪ Feeling dizzy, unsteady, light-headed, or faint ▪ Trembling or shaking ▪ Feeling of choking ▪ Paresthesias ▪ Chest pain or discomfort ▪ Feeling of losing control or going crazy

Data from: American Psychiatric Association. *Diagnostic and Statistical Manual of Mental Disorders*. 5th ed. Washington, DC: American Psychiatric Association; 2013.

By the time you arrive at the scene, the patient having a panic attack may be surrounded by many anxious and excited people, who will themselves contribute to the problem. Accordingly, you will need to take the following steps to control the situation quickly:

- Separate the patient from panicky bystanders. If you can find a calm friend or member of the patient's family, however, having this person present may be helpful.
- Provide a calm environment. The environment should be as calm as possible while you transport the patient to the hospital.
- Be tolerant of the patient's disability. The patient having an anxiety attack may not be able to cooperate or answer questions at first because of intense fear and distress. Your manner must convey that everything is under control.
- Reassure the patient that he or she is safe. The word *safe* can be a magic pill that will often deescalate symptoms to a more manageable level: "We're going to take you down these stairs on the stretcher. It's going to be okay; we'll go slowly and be careful to keep you safe while we move you."
- Give the patient's symptoms a name. Once you have checked the vital signs and the electrocardiogram monitor, you should be in a position to reassure the patient that he or she is not in immediate danger of dying: "I know that your feeling of panic is distressing, but it is not life threatening."
- Help the patient regain control. Encourage the patient to do things for himself or herself to the extent that he or she is able, to help regain a sense of being in control.

YOU are the Provider — PART 4

Since handcuffing the patient required that he be placed temporarily in police protective custody, the officer rides with you in the back of the ambulance. As you transport the patient nonemergently to the hospital, you attempt to rule out any medical causes of the patient's irrational behavior. You are able to obtain a capillary blood glucose level of 146 mg/dL.

The patient is now calm and appears relaxed. He asks you to take the handcuffs off. He tells you they are uncomfortable and hurting his wrist. You continue monitoring the patient en route to the hospital. You work with the officer to adjust them to decrease the discomfort. On arrival, you give your report to the emergency department nurse and complete your patient care report while your partner readies the ambulance for your next call.

Recording Time: 17 Minutes	
Respirations	20 breaths/min, clear bilaterally
Pulse	Strong and regular, 90 beats/min
Skin	Warm, dry, and pink
Blood pressure	124/82 mm Hg
Oxygen saturation (Spo_2)	97%

8. Is it possible that the patient may be suffering from a traumatic brain injury?
9. If the patient is now cooperating, should you ask the officer to remove the patient's handcuffs?

Panic attacks may mimic a range of physical disorders in their presentation. Conversely, symptoms of anxiety may be the presenting complaint in medical conditions such as cardiac dysrhythmias, withdrawal states, anaphylaxis, hyperthyroidism, and certain tumors. For that reason, any patient experiencing a panic attack—especially a first panic attack—should be fully evaluated in the hospital. Hyperventilating patients should not be treated with "paper bag therapy;" that is, rebreathing their exhaled air from a paper bag. Patients whose anxiety results from an unsuspected pulmonary embolism or cardiac problem may experience serious complications and even die of hypoxemia if a paper bag is used. Hyperventilation is best managed initially by coaching patients to slow their breathing until they regain control.

Medicolegal Considerations

The medical and legal aspects of emergency medical care become more complicated when the patient is undergoing a behavioral or psychiatric emergency. Nevertheless, legal problems are greatly reduced when an emotionally disturbed patient consents to care. Therefore, gaining that patient's confidence is a critical task for the AEMT.

Mental incapacity can take many forms, including unresponsiveness (as a result of hypoxia, drugs, or hypoglycemia), temporary but severe stress, or depression. Once you have determined that a patient has impaired mental capacity, you must decide whether he or she requires immediate emergency medical care. A patient in a mentally unstable condition may resist your attempts to provide care. Nevertheless, you must not leave the patient alone—doing so may expose you to civil action for abandonment or negligence. In such situations, you should request that law enforcement personnel handle the patient. Another reason for seeking law enforcement support is that a patient who resists treatment often threatens AEMTs and others. Violent or dangerous people who do not require medical care must be taken into custody by the police.

Special Populations

Some communities have crisis intervention teams (CIT) staffed by law enforcement officers with specialized training in recognizing and managing people experiencing a mental health crisis. The primary role of the CIT is to keep patients from revolving through the criminal justice system and the hospital. Such programs have been successful in establishing long-term care and solutions for people with chronic and persistent mental health issues who may not otherwise have the resources or support to get the help they need.

▶ Consent

When a patient is not mentally competent to grant consent for emergency medical care, the law assumes that consent is implied. For example, the consent of an unresponsive patient is implied. The law refers to this concept as the emergency doctrine: consent is implied because of the necessity for immediate emergency treatment, and if the patient were conscious, there is an inherent implication that he or she would consent to emergency care. In a situation that is not immediately life threatening, emergency medical care or transportation may be delayed until the proper consent is obtained. Contact medical control or follow local protocols when in doubt.

In situations involving psychiatric emergencies, however, the matter is not always clear-cut. Does a life-threatening emergency exist or not? If you are not sure, you should obtain online medical direction and request the assistance of law enforcement personnel.

▶ Limited Legal Authority

As an AEMT, you have limited legal authority to require or force a patient to undergo emergency medical care when no life-threatening emergency exists. Patients have the right to refuse care. However, most states have legal statutes regarding the emergency care of mentally ill and drug-impaired people. These statutory provisions permit law enforcement personnel to place such a person in protective custody so that emergency care can be provided. Medical direction may also order transport of a patient against his or her will. You should be familiar with your local and state laws regarding these situations.

The typical provision may state that:

> Any police officer who has reasonable cause to believe that a person is mentally ill and dangerous to himself, herself, or others, or gravely disabled, may take such person into custody and take or cause such person to be taken to a general hospital for emergency examination.

Again, because these provisions vary, you should become familiar with those in your state.

The general rule of law is that a competent adult has the right to refuse treatment, even if life-saving care is involved. In psychiatric cases, however, a court of law would consider your actions in providing life-saving care to be appropriate, particularly if you have a reasonable belief that the patient will harm himself or herself or others without your intervention. Additionally, a patient who is in any way impaired—whether by mental illness, medical condition, or intoxication—may not be considered competent to refuse treatment or transportation. These situations are among the most perilous you will encounter from a legal standpoint. When in doubt, consult your supervisor, police, and/or medical control. Always maintain a pessimistic attitude toward your patients' condition: assume the worst and hope for the best. Err on the side of treatment and transport. It is far easier to defend yourself against charges of battery than it is to justify abandonment.

Words of Wisdom

When a patient is not mentally competent to grant consent for emergency medical care, the law assumes that there is implied consent to treat immediately life-threatening conditions.

▶ Restraint

Ordinarily, restraint of a person must be ordered by a physician, a court order, or a law enforcement officer. If you restrain a person without authority in a nonemergency situation, you expose yourself to a possible lawsuit, as well as to personal danger. Legal actions that can be taken against you can involve charges of assault, battery, false imprisonment, and violation of civil rights. You may use restraints only to protect yourself or others from bodily harm or to prevent the patient from causing injury to himself or herself Figure 24-2. In either case, you may use only reasonable force as necessary to control the patient—and different courts may define "reasonable force" differently. For this reason, you should always consult medical control and contact law enforcement for help before restraining a patient.

In fact, you should routinely involve law enforcement personnel if you are called to assist a patient in a severe behavioral or psychiatric crisis. They will provide physical backup in managing the patient, can serve as the necessary witnesses, and will provide legal authority should physical restraint become necessary. A patient who is restrained by law enforcement personnel is in their custody.

Always try to transport a disturbed patient without restraints if possible. However, once the decision has been made to restrain a patient, you should carry it out quickly. Take proper standard precautions. If the patient is spitting, for example, place a surgical mask over his or her mouth and make sure that you and your partner do the same.

Make sure you have adequate help to restrain a patient safely. *At least five trained, able-bodied people should be present to carry out the placement of restraints*, with each person being responsible for one extremity. Before you begin, discuss the plan of action. As you prepare to restrain the patient, stay outside the patient's range of motion.

When subduing a disturbed patient, use the minimum force necessary. Avoid acts of physical force that may cause injury to the patient. The level of force will vary depending on the following factors:

- The degree of force that is necessary to keep the patient from injuring himself or herself, or others.
- A patient's sex, size, strength, and mental status.
- The type of abnormal behavior the patient is exhibiting. You should use only restraint devices that have been approved by the relevant authority in your area (sometimes the state health department). Soft, wide leather or cloth restraints are preferred over police-type handcuffs.

Acting at the same time, the law enforcement personnel should secure the patient's extremities with approved equipment. Someone—preferably you or your partner—should continue to talk to the patient throughout the process. Remember to treat the patient with dignity and respect at all times. Also, monitor the patient for vomiting, airway obstruction, and cardiovascular stability: once the patient is restrained, he or she cannot fend for himself or herself. Drug or alcohol intoxication initially may cause violent behavior but then lead to physical problems such as vomiting or aspiration. Never place a patient facedown, because it is impossible to adequately monitor the patient and this positioning may inhibit the breathing of an impaired or exhausted patient. Be careful not to place restraints in such a way that the patient's respirations are compromised. Reassess the patient's airway and breathing continuously. You should make frequent checks of circulation on all restrained extremities, regardless of patient position Figure 24-3. Document the reason for the restraint and the technique that was used.

Be especially careful if a combative patient suddenly becomes calm and cooperative. This is not the time to relax; rather, you should remain vigilant. The patient may suddenly become combative again and injure someone.

Safety

If you do not have five people to restrain a violent patient, you should call the dispatcher and request additional assistance.

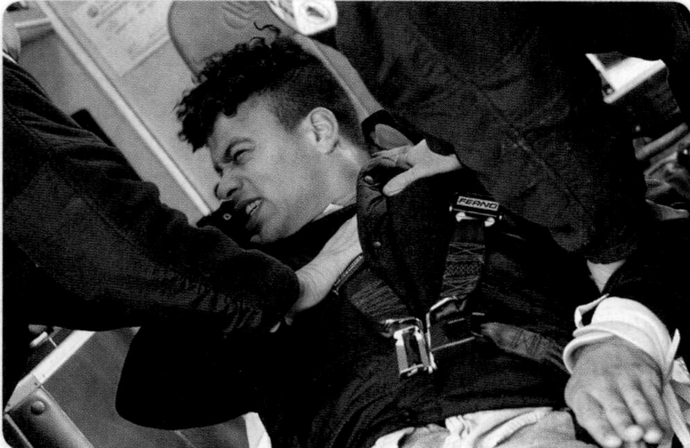

Figure 24-2 You may use restraints only to protect yourself or others or to prevent a patient from causing injury to himself or herself.

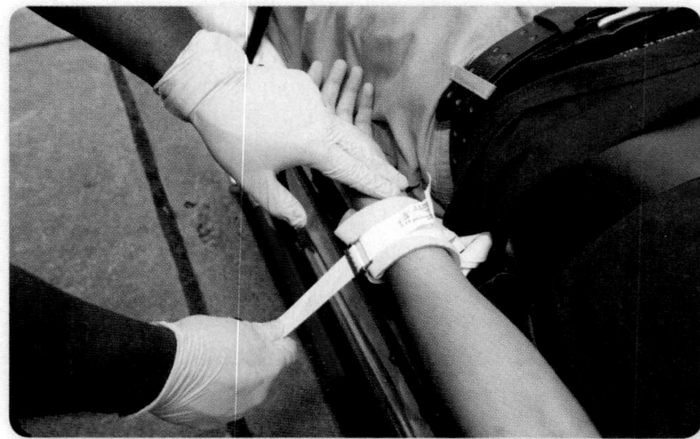

Figure 24-3 Assess the airway and distal circulation frequently while the patient is restrained.

Keep in mind that you may use reasonable force to defend yourself against an attack by an emotionally disturbed patient. It is extremely helpful to have (and document) witnesses in attendance, even during transport, to protect against false accusations. AEMTs may be accused of sexual misconduct and other physical abuse in such circumstances.

Words of Wisdom

After restraining a patient, document the reason for doing so and the method you used. Check the pulse and motor and sensory function in all extremities, make any adjustments needed to ensure adequate function, and record your actions and findings in detail.

Posttraumatic Stress Disorder and Returning Combat Veterans

PTSD can occur after exposure to, or injury from, a traumatic event. Such events may include sexual or physical assault, child abuse, a serious accident, a natural disaster, war, loss of a loved one, or stressful life changes. People may have experienced fear of danger, helplessness, or a severe reaction during the event. The reaction could be to trauma that occurred long ago, or it may be the result of multiple traumatic events over time. It is not necessarily the result of one isolated or recent event.

It is estimated that 7% to 8% of the general population will experience signs of PTSD at some point in their lives.[19] For health care workers returning from a warfare environment, which could include disaster workers, threat of personal harm is considered a predictive factor in determining in whom PTSD will develop.

Military personnel who experienced combat have a high incidence of PTSD. PTSD occurred in 11% to 20% of veterans of the Iraq and Afghanistan wars, 12% of Gulf War veterans, and 30% of Vietnam veterans.[19] Reminders of their experiences in the military such as news coverage or gatherings of veterans can also be triggers.

Signs and Symptoms of PTSD

Symptoms of PTSD include feelings of helplessness, anxiety, anger, and fear. People with PTSD may avoid things that remind them of the trauma, including loud noises or smells, and sometimes they may avoid interactions with other people. This emotional and physical distancing from others can have a negative impact on the individual's quality of life. Memories of the trauma linger and continue to be disruptive. Symptoms of PTSD may be made worse in the context of other mental health challenges.

The sympathetic nervous system provides the fight-or-flight response as a means to help protect us in a perceived dangerous situation. This mechanism is not intended to be activated for any longer than it takes to mitigate the threat. People with PTSD, however, suffer nervous system arousal that continues and is not easily suppressed. Heart rate increases to channel blood into the heart, lungs, and brain; pupils dilate; and systolic blood pressure is increased. Senses are sharpened and mental acuity is heightened. The patient may be hypervigilant or display an exaggerated startle response to perceived danger.

People with PTSD can relive the traumatic event through intrusive thoughts, nightmares, or even flashbacks. Flashbacks are uncontrollable events triggered by a sound, sight, or smell. The patient may experience the same visceral response he or she did during the initial encounter with the stress. These episodes can last seconds or hours and can occur at any time, even years after the exposure. The person fears his or her inability to control a flashback and worries that it will present as irrational behavior. Recent traumatic events may also trigger old memories and create a reflex reaction of preparing for the worst. A person who has experienced flashbacks may become preoccupied with the perception of danger. Hypervigilance and trouble sleeping are not unusual.

Dissociative PTSD occurs when the person attempts to find an escape from constant internal distress or a particularly disturbing event. The individual's altered consciousness allows him or her to continue functioning under negative conditions. Some people may undergo an out-of-body experience; others experience delusions. Other psychological conditions such as personality disorders and increased functional impairment can develop in those individuals with a dissociative subtype of PTSD.

Guilt, shame, paranoia, hostility, and depression are not uncommon in combat veterans. Alcohol and/or drug use often represents an attempt to suppress the sympathetic nervous system activity and slow down the body. This attempt at anesthesia can easily become addictive.

Suicide is sometimes sought to end the pain. Veterans are much more likely to harm themselves or try to harm themselves. The US Department of Veterans Affairs reported that an average of 20 veterans take their lives each day.[20] They also experience a host of physical conditions—some from injuries sustained in combat, and sometimes vague, unfocused pain not associated with any specific part of the body. This perception of physical pain may be a sign of their anguish. Combat veterans, in particular, may develop heart disease earlier than expected given their age, have a higher incidence of type 2 diabetes, and sustain a loss of brain gray matter. High cholesterol and hypertension are not uncommon and are often undiagnosed or misdiagnosed.

Another consideration for the combat veteran is the higher incidence of traumatic brain injury (TBI) sustained from trauma secondary to the explosion of an improvised explosive device (IED). In some cases, the TBI may go undiagnosed because its manifestations are similar to the symptoms of PTSD or because the patient downplays the symptoms. People with TBI can experience sensory dysfunction, confusion headaches, memory loss, and general disorientation. Memory loss can include retrograde and anterograde amnesia (affecting memories formed before and after the event, respectively).

When treating a combat veteran with PTSD, try to eliminate excess noise. Do not touch or do anything to the veteran without an explanation. Interestingly, diesel fumes can be a trigger for combat veterans, so keep your diesel equipment far enough away that its odors are not noticeable by the patient.

▶ Caring for the Combat Veteran

How do you recognize returning veterans? They often continue to adhere to their military identity by having short haircuts and wearing military clothing with combat patches, and many have military-themed tattoos. Their homes may have flags, memorials, commendations, and military photos. They may have a military appearance and use military vocabulary. They tend to show respect for authority but may be reluctant to talk to you about PTSD. They may not be aware that they have this condition, or do not want to be considered "mental." They might have trouble asking for help. Questions such as "How do you want me to help you?" or "What do you need right now?" are good ways to open the conversation.

The returning combat veteran is a patient who will require a unique level of understanding, compassion, and specialized attention. These patients experience pain that is emotional as well as physical. You will need to take time to establish the history of this patient and listen to his or her concerns. Approach this patient with sensitivity and respect. Be careful how you phrase your questions. "Were you in combat?" is an appropriate question, but in some cases, veterans may be in denial or do not believe they were in combat. A better question might be "Were you shot at or under fire?" If you served in combat, you can create trust by letting the patient know. Ask questions about the patient's service (eg, branch, rank). You may get enough information out of that conversation to eliminate probing with specific questions.

YOU are the Provider SUMMARY

1. Does this scene need to be treated differently than other scenes just because the patient has a mental illness?

This scene needs to be treated the same as any other call, with the exception of maintaining an increased situational awareness for the potential of violence. It is necessary to rule out the possibility of a medical cause being the reason for the patient's altered mental status.

2. Who has overall control of this scene, EMS or law enforcement?

This kind of situation requires coordinated management by all agencies involved. A mental illness call is not just a "law enforcement problem" or an "EMS problem," but rather a problem that takes a team approach to achieve the best outcome for all people involved.

3. This patient has a known history of mental illness. Does he need to be transported to the hospital?

This patient is having homicidal ideations and is a threat to others. He also has an extensive documented history of PTSD. This patient definitely needs to be evaluated in an emergency department.

4. Does this patient require an ambulance transport to the emergency department, or should law enforcement transport him?

Whether this patient requires transport via EMS or law enforcement depends on local protocols. Once all possible medical causes have been ruled out as the cause of his behavior, some agencies may defer transport to law enforcement. However, knowing who will transport patients such as this before the time comes is imperative to having a smoothly run scene.

5. What is the minimum number of providers who should be present when attempting to physically restrain a patient?

In an ideal environment, at least five providers should be present to physically restrain the patient: one provider to take each extremity, and a fifth provider to control the head. Using five providers will minimize the potential for any injuries, while still providing positive control over the patient.

6. In which position should this patient be restrained?

This patient should be restrained in the supine position. Under no circumstances should a patient be transported restrained in the prone position because of the possibility of positional asphyxia.

7. Should a law enforcement officer accompany you in the back of the ambulance or should the officer follow behind the ambulance in the patrol car?

When a patient is restrained in handcuffs, it is necessary that the officer accompany EMS personnel in the back of the ambulance with the patient. This will allow for easy removal of the handcuffs should the patient's condition deteriorate. If the officer follows along behind the ambulance and there is an emergency that requires that the handcuffs be removed, an unacceptable delay in getting the officer into the back of the ambulance would result. Furthermore, placing the patient into handcuffs for his own

YOU are the Provider SUMMARY *(continued)*

protection is possible only if the officer effectively takes the patient into protective custody. The patient should therefore not be transported without being escorted by a law enforcement officer.

8. Is it possible that the patient may be suffering from a TBI?

Yes, it is possible the patient may be suffering from TBI. A consideration for the combat veteran is the higher incidence of TBI sustained from trauma secondary to the explosion of an IED. In some cases, the TBI may go undiagnosed because its manifestations are similar to the symptoms of PTSD or because the patient downplays the symptoms. People with TBI can experience sensory dysfunction, confusion headaches, memory loss, and general disorientation. Memory loss can include retrograde and anterograde amnesia (affecting memories formed before and after the event, respectively).

9. If the patient is now cooperating, should you ask the officer to remove the patient's handcuffs?

Under no circumstances should you remove the handcuffs of a psychiatric patient just because the patient states he or she will cooperate or reports "feeling better." The only reason to remove physical restraints after they have been applied would be if the patient's condition deteriorated and the restraints hindered access to the patient. If the patient is complaining of discomfort related to the handcuffs however, it is important to check and to adjust the tightness of the cuffs if necessary to prevent skin breakdown secondary to pressure from the metal.

EMS Patient Care Report (PCR)					
Date: 9-7-18	**Incident No.:** 20090715641	**Nature of Call:** Chest pain		**Location:** 152 Rolette St	
Dispatched: 0345	**En Route:** 0352	**At Scene:** 0401	**Transport:** 0432	**At Hospital:** 0438	**In Service:** 0500

Patient Information	
Age: 70 **Sex:** M **Weight (in kg [lb]):** 103 kg (226.6 lb)	**Allergies:** No known drug allergies **Medications:** Lithium, carbamazepine, metoprolol **Past Medical History:** Bipolar disorder, PTSD, HTN **Chief Complaint:** Chest pain

Vital Signs				
Time: 0411	**BP:** 176/102	**Pulse:** 120	**Respirations:** 26	**Spo_2:** 97%
Time: 0418	**BP:** 124/82	**Pulse:** 90	**Respirations:** 20	**Spo_2:** 97%
Time:	**BP:**	**Pulse:**	**Respirations:**	**Spo_2:**

EMS Treatment (circle all that apply)					
Oxygen @ _______ L/min via (circle one): **NC** **NRM** **Bag-mask device**		**Assisted Ventilation**	**Airway Adjunct**	**CPR**
Defibrillation	**Bleeding Control**	**Bandaging**	**Splinting**	**Other:**

Narrative

On arrival 70-year-old male patient sitting in recliner is AO×3 and slightly agitated. Patient complains of a "fullness" in his chest, but denies any dyspnea. Skin is warm and dry with strong and regular radial pulses. PERRLA, glucose—146 mg/dL. While attempting to take patient's BP, patient became very agitated and jumped to his feet while shooting an imaginary gun. He began shouting repeatedly, "Did I get them?" Law enforcement on scene restrained patient with handcuffs and he was placed on the stretcher in a position of comfort. Patient was loaded into ambulance without incidence and law enforcement accompanied EMS in the ambulance due to patient being restrained. Patient calm en route and patient transport was uneventful. Report given to receiving nurse.**End of report**

Prep Kit

▶ Ready for Review

- Behavioral emergencies can present you with great difficulties in patient management. Your major responsibility in these situations is to defuse potentially life-threatening incidents and reduce the impact of the stressful condition without exposing yourself to unnecessary risks.
- Whereas only a small percentage of people with mental health disorders are dangerous to themselves or others, you may be exposed to a higher proportion of violent situations in your daily activities as an AEMT. Warning signs of violence include a history of hostile behavior, rigidity, loud and erratic speech patterns, agitation, and depression.
- A behavioral emergency or psychiatric emergency is any reaction to events that interferes with activities of daily living. A person who is no longer able to respond appropriately to the environment may be having a more serious psychiatric emergency. Not all behavioral emergencies involve a mental health problem, however: some emergencies are a temporary response to a traumatic event.
- Underlying causes of behavioral emergencies fall into two categories: organic and functional disorders.
- Organic brain syndrome is a temporary or permanent dysfunction of the brain caused by a disturbance in the physical or physiologic functioning of brain tissue.
- Altered mental status is a change in the way a person thinks or behave, and is an indicator of central nervous system disease.
- A person's environment includes both psychosocial and sociocultural influences on behavior; when these influences cause stress, they may precipitate a behavioral crisis. Other organic causes of behavioral emergencies may include injury or illness and substance use.
- A functional disorder is one in which the etiology cannot be traced to an obvious change in the actual structure or physiology of the brain itself.
- Psychiatric signs and symptoms can affect the following areas: consciousness, motor activity, speech, thinking, mood and affect, memory, orientation, perception, and intelligence.
- Violent patients make up only a small percentage of those experiencing behavioral or psychiatric crises, but it is important to assess for risk factors for such a patient. History, posture, the scene, vocal activity, and physical activity can show clues as to the likelihood of the patient becoming violent.
- Assessing a person who may be having a behavioral crisis involves observing the person, talking with the person, and talking with friends, family members, and witnesses to the person's behavior. Look for indications that the person's thoughts, feelings, and reactions are inappropriate for the circumstances. Remember to always assess the ABCDEs (Airway, Breathing, Circulation, Disability, and Exposure).
- Consider contributing factors in four areas: central nervous system dysfunction, environmental factors or clues, drug or alcohol use, and psychogenic circumstances such as the death of a loved one or other major interruption of normal life.
- Look for organic causes of a behavioral emergency. Measure vital signs, examine the patient's skin, inspect for evidence of trauma, check the pupils, note unusual odors, and examine the extremities.
- In providing emergency medical care for a patient experiencing a behavioral emergency, be direct, honest, and calm; have a definitive plan of action; stay with the patient at all times, but do not get too close; and express interest in the patient's story, but do not judge his or her behavior. Always treat patients with respect.
- Psychosis is a state of delusion in which the person is out of touch with reality. Patients with psychosis may be belligerent and angry, or silent and withdrawn. The usual methods of reasoning with a patient are unlikely to be effective with psychotic individuals, so be sure to learn the guidelines in caring for such patients, including being calm, direct, straightforward, and nonconfrontational.
- The threat of suicide requires immediate intervention. Depression is the most significant risk factor for suicide, but other risk factors include personal or family history of suicide attempts, chronic debilitating illness, financial setback, and severe mental illness. Be aware that the patient considering suicide may be homicidal as well.
- You may encounter patients with agitated delirium. This impairment of cognitive function can present with disorientation, hallucinations, or delusions and is characterized by restless and irregular physical activity. One of the most important factors to consider when caring for these patients is your personal safety. Use careful interviewing techniques and refrain from upsetting the patient further.
- In mood disorders, changes in the patient's affect are accompanied by other symptoms, and the net effect is to cause a major disturbance in the person's ability to function. People experiencing mania typically have abnormally exaggerated happiness, joy, or euphoria with hyperactivity and insomnia. In contrast, the patient with depression is often readily

Prep Kit *(continued)*

identified by a sad expression, bouts of crying, and listless or apathetic behavior; he or she expresses feelings of worthlessness, guilt, and pessimism.

- Several types of anxiety disorders, including generalized anxiety disorder, phobias, and panic disorder, are likely to elicit a call for an ambulance or affect the delivery of prehospital care. Panic attacks may mimic a range of physical disorders in their presentation; given the possibility of misdiagnosis, any patient experiencing a panic attack—especially a first panic attack—should be fully evaluated in the hospital.
- As an AEMT, you have limited legal authority to require a patient to undergo emergency medical care in the absence of a life-threatening emergency. Most states have provisions allowing law enforcement personnel to place mentally impaired people in custody so that such care can be provided. You should always involve law enforcement personnel anytime you are called to assist a patient with a severe behavioral or psychiatric crisis.
- Always consult medical control and contact law enforcement for help before restraining a patient. If the patient poses an immediate threat, leave the area until law enforcement secures the scene. If restraints are required, use the minimum force necessary. Assess the airway and circulation frequently while the patient is restrained, and maintain a constant dialogue with the patient throughout the restraining process.
- Symptoms of posttraumatic stress disorder (PTSD) include feelings of helplessness, anxiety, anger, and fear. In addition, people with PTSD can relive the traumatic event through intrusive thoughts, nightmares, or flashbacks.
- The returning combat veteran is a patient who will require a unique level of understanding, compassion, and specialized attention. Take the time to establish the history of this patient and listen to his or her concerns; approach the individual with sensitivity and respect.

▶ Vital Vocabulary

activities of daily living (ADLs) The basic activities a person usually accomplishes during a normal day, such as eating, dressing, and washing.

affect The outward expression of a person's inner feelings (happy, sad, angry, fearful, withdrawn).

agitated delirium An acute confrontational state characterized by global impairment of thinking, perception, judgment, and memory; also called excited delirium or exhaustive mania.

agoraphobia Literally, "fear of the marketplace"; fear of entering a public place from which escape may be impeded.

altered mental status A change in the way a person thinks and behaves, which may signal disease in the central nervous system or other contributing factors.

anxiety disorders Mental disorders in which the dominant mood is fear and apprehension.

behavior How a person functions or acts in response to his or her environment.

behavioral crisis The point at which a person's reactions to events interfere with activities of daily living; a behavioral crisis becomes a psychiatric emergency when it causes a major life interruption, such as attempted suicide.

bipolar mood disorder A disorder in which a person alternates between mania and depression.

circumstantial thinking Situation in which the patient includes many irrelevant details in his or her account of things.

compulsions Repetitive actions carried out to relieve the anxiety of obsessive thoughts.

confabulation The invention of experiences to cover gaps in memory, seen in patients with certain organic brain syndromes.

delusions Fixed beliefs that are not shared by others of a person's culture or background and that cannot be changed by reasonable argument; false beliefs.

dementia The slow onset of progressive disorientation, shortened attention span, and loss of cognitive function.

depression A mental health disorder characterized by a persistent mood of sadness, despair, and discouragement.

disorganization A condition in which a person is characterized by uncontrolled and disconnected thought, is usually incoherent or rambling in speech, and may or may not be oriented to person and place.

disorientation A condition in which a person may be confused about his or her identity, the location, and the time of day; one of the ways in which various conditions such as schizophrenia or organic brain syndrome may present.

echolalia Meaningless echoing of the interviewer's words by the patient.

flat affect The absence of emotion; appearing to feel no emotion at all.

flight of ideas Accelerated thinking in which the mind skips very rapidly from one thought to the next.

Prep Kit (continued)

functional disorder A disorder in which there is no known physiologic reason for the abnormal functioning of an organ or organ system.

generalized anxiety disorder (GAD) A disorder in which a person worries about everything for no particular reason, or the worrying is unproductive and the person cannot decide what to do about an upcoming situation.

hallucinations Sense perceptions not founded on objective reality; false perceptions.

inappropriate affect Emotion that is out of synch with the situation (for example, wearing a waxy smile while discussing a parent's death).

loosening of associations A situation in which the logical connection between one idea and the next becomes obscure, at least to the listener.

mania A mental disorder characterized by abnormally exaggerated happiness, joy, or euphoria with hyperactivity, insomnia, and grandiose ideas.

manic–depressive illness A bipolar disorder in which mood fluctuates between depression and mania. The alterations in mood are usually episodic and recurrent.

mental disorder An illness with psychological or behavioral symptoms and/or impairment in functioning, caused by a social, psychological, genetic, physical, chemical, or biologic disturbance; may also be referred to as a psychiatric disorder.

mood disorders Disorders in which the disturbance of mood is accompanied by full or partial manic or depressive syndrome.

mutism The absence of speech.

neologisms Invented words that have meaning only to their inventor.

neurotic disorders A collection of mental disorders without psychotic symptoms and lacking the intense psychopathology of other mood disorders; includes anxiety disorders, phobias, and panic disorder.

organic brain syndrome Temporary or permanent dysfunction of the brain, caused by a disturbance in the physical or physiologic functioning of brain tissue.

panic disorder A disorder characterized by sudden, usually unexpected, and overwhelming feelings of fear and dread, accompanied by a variety of other symptoms produced by a massive activation of the autonomic nervous system.

perseveration Repeating the same idea over and over again.

phobias Obsessive, irrational fears of specific things or situations, such as fear of heights, fear of open places, fear of confined spaces, or fear of certain animals.

posttraumatic stress disorder (PTSD) A severe form of anxiety that stems from a traumatic experience; characterized by the reliving of the stress and nightmares of the original situation.

pressure of speech Speech in which words seem to tumble out under immense emotional pressure.

psychogenic A symptom or illness that is caused by mental factors as opposed to physical ones.

psychosis A mental disorder characterized by the loss of contact with reality.

schizophrenia A complex, difficult-to-identify mental disorder with typical onset occurring during early adulthood. Dysfunctional symptoms typically become more prominent over time and include delusions, hallucinations, apathy, mutism, flat affect, a lack of interest in pleasure, erratic speech, emotional responses, and motor behavior.

simple phobia A fear that is focused on one class of objects (eg, mice, spiders, dogs) or situations (eg, high places, darkness, flying).

stereotyped movements Repetitive movements that do not appear to serve any purpose.

tangential thinking Leaving the current topic in midconversation to talk about something else, inhibiting interpersonal communication.

thought broadcasting The belief that thoughts are broadcast aloud and can be heard by others.

thought insertion The belief that thoughts are being thrust into one's mind by another person.

thought withdrawal The belief that thoughts are being removed from one's mind.

References

1. National Institute of Mental Health. Any mental illness (AMI) among U.S. adults. https://www.nimh.nih.gov/health/statistics/prevalence/any-mental-illness-ami-among-us-adults.shtml. Accessed January 3, 2017.
2. Reeves WC, Strine TW, Pratt LA, et al. Mental illness surveillance among adults in the United States. *MMWR.* 2011;60(3);1–32. https://www.cdc.gov/mmwr/preview/mmwrhtml/su6003a1.htm. Accessed January 3, 2017.
3. Center for Behavioral Health Statistics and Quality. *Behavioral Health Trends in the United States: Results From the 2014 National Survey on Drug Use and Health* (HHS Publication No. SMA 15-4927, NSDUH Series H-50). Rockville, MD: Center for Behavioral Health Statistics and Quality, Substance Abuse and Mental Health Services Administration; 2015. https://www.samhsa.gov/data/sites/default/files/NSDUH-FRR1-2014/NSDUH-FRR1-2014.pdf. Accessed January 3, 2017.

Prep Kit (continued)

4. Alzheimer's Association. 2014 Alzheimer's disease facts and figures. *Alzheimer's & Dementia.* 2014;10(2). http://www.alz.org/downloads/facts_figures_2014.pdf. Accessed January 3, 2017.
5. Fazel S, Wolf A, Chang Z, Larsson H, Goodwin GM, Lichtenstein P. Depression and violence: a Swedish population study. *Lancet Psychiatry.* 2015;2(3): 224–232. http://www.thelancet.com/journals/lanpsy/article/PIIS2215-0366(14)00128-X/fulltext. Accessed January 3, 2017.
6. Centers for Disease Control and Prevention. Burden of mental illness. October 4, 2013. https://www.cdc.gov/mentalhealth/basics/burden.htm. Accessed January 3, 2017.
7. National Institute of Mental Health. Schizophrenia. February 2016. https://www.nimh.nih.gov/health/topics/schizophrenia/index.shtml. Accessed January 3, 2017.
8. McLean J, Maxwell M, Platt S, Harris F, Jepson R. *Risk and Protective Factors for Suicide and Suicidal Behaviour: A Literature Review.* Edinburgh, UK: Scottish Government Social Research; 2008. http://www.gov.scot/Publications/2008/11/28141444/0. Accessed January 3, 2017.
9. Bostwick JM, Pabbati C, Geske JR, McKean AJ. Suicide attempt as a risk for completed suicide: even more lethal than we knew. *Am J Psychiatry.* 2016;173(11):1094–1100. http://ajp.psychiatryonline.org/doi/abs/10.1176/appi.ajp.2016.15070854?journalCode=ajp. Accessed January 3, 2017.
10. American Academy of Pediatrics. Early interventions for behavioral and emotional disorders: AAP clinical report. January 26, 2015. https://www.aap.org/en-us/about-the-aap/aap-press-room/pages/Early-Interventions-for-Behavioral-and-Emotional-Disorders-AAP-Clinical-Report.aspx. Accessed January 4, 2017.
11. Centers for Disease Control and Prevention, National Center for Health Statistics, National Vital Statistics Programs. 10 leading causes of death by age group, United States—2014. https://www.cdc.gov/injury/images/lc-charts/leading_causes_of_death_age_group_2014_1050w760h.gif. Accessed January 4, 2017.
12. National Institute of Mental Health. Any mood disorder among adults. https://www.nimh.nih.gov/health/statistics/prevalence/any-mood-disorder-among-adults.shtml. Accessed January 4, 2017.
13. Baek JH, Eisner LR, Nierenberg AA. Epidemiology and course of unipolar mania: results from the National Epidemiologic Survey on Alcohol and Related Conditions (NESARC). *Depress Anxiety.* 2014;31(9):746–755. https://www.ncbi.nlm.nih.gov/pubmed/24677651. Accessed January 4, 2017.
14. American Psychological Association. Data on behavioral health in the United States. http://www.apa.org/helpcenter/data-behavioral-health.aspx. Accessed January 4, 2017.
15. National Institute of Mental Health. Any anxiety disorder among adults. https://www.nimh.nih.gov/health/statistics/prevalence/any-anxiety-disorder-among-adults.shtml. Accessed January 4, 2017.
16. National Institute of Mental Health. Generalized anxiety disorder among adults. https://www.nimh.nih.gov/health/statistics/prevalence/generalized-anxiety-disorder-among-adults.shtml. Accessed January 4, 2017.
17. National Institute of Mental Health. Social phobia among adults. https://www.nimh.nih.gov/health/statistics/prevalence/social-phobia-among-adults.shtml. Accessed January 4, 2017.
18. *Psychology Today.* Stats on panic disorder: crunching the numbers on panic disorder. June 9, 2016. https://www.psychologytoday.com/articles/199307/stats-panic-disorder. Accessed January 4, 2017.
19. US Department of Veterans Affairs, National Center for PTSD. How common is PTSD? October 3, 2016. http://www.ptsd.va.gov/public/PTSD-overview/basics/how-common-is-ptsd.asp. Accessed January 5, 2017.
20. Department of Veterans Affairs. VA Suicide Prevention Program. *Facts About Veteran Suicide.* July 2016. https://www.va.gov/opa/publications/factsheets/Suicide_Prevention_FactSheet_New_VA_Stats_070616_1400.pdf. Accessed January 27, 2017.

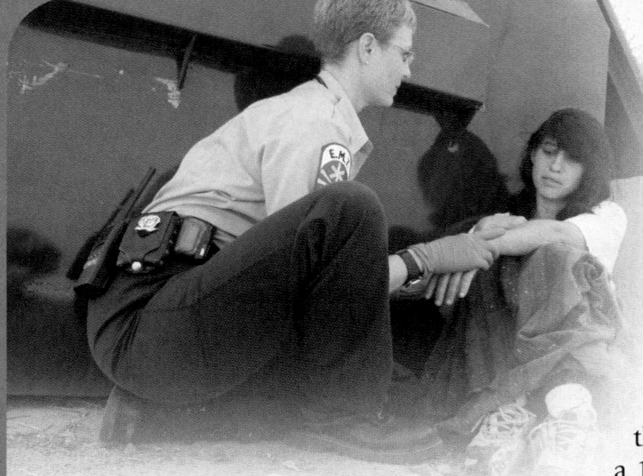

Assessment in Action

You are dispatched to an apartment complex for a woman who is screaming and throwing things. On arrival, you note that there are no law enforcement personnel at the scene, so you advise dispatch that you will be staging until law enforcement arrives and secures the scene. Once law enforcement has secured the scene, you proceed into the apartment and find the patient, a 17-year-old woman, screaming: "Martians put a probe in my brain and they are trying to steal my thoughts to use to invade the Earth!"

Her mother tells you that the young woman has a history of schizophrenia and has refused to take her medication for several days. The patient finally agrees to go to the hospital, but she wants to get a change of clothes from her bedroom first.

1. What is the appropriate way to respond to the patient's altered perceptions?

A. Go along with her delusions, telling her not to resist the voices in her head.
B. Tell her that everything will be alright.
C. Place restraints on the patient to keep her from harming herself.
D. Tell her that while you cannot hear the voices, you do not doubt that she is hearing them and that you feel she needs to go to the hospital and be evaluated.

2. Should this patient be allowed to go to her bedroom to get a change of clothes?

A. Yes, the patient can be allowed to get a change of clothes because she is likely to be hospitalized for a long period of time.
B. Yes, the patient can be allowed to get a change of clothes as long as she is escorted by someone, preferably a law enforcement officer, and her belongings are thoroughly searched prior to her being allowed to have them.
C. No, the patient should not be allowed to get a change of clothes because this call needs to be resolved quickly so that you can get your ambulance back into service.
D. Yes, the patient can be allowed to get a change of clothes but only if restraints are applied to her wrists so that she cannot become physically violent.

3. ________________________ is defined as a state of delusion in which the person is out of touch with reality.

A. Behavioral crisis
B. Psychosis
C. Mental disorder
D. Organic brain syndrome

4. The *M* in the COASTMAP acronym stands for:

A. mood.
B. memory.
C. mental.
D. method.

5. What is the key in managing a disoriented patient?

A. Go along with the patient's hallucinations.
B. Administer an antianxiety medication.
C. Keep orienting the patient.
D. Give complex explanations of medical procedures.

6. The first *A* in the COASTMAP acronym stands for:

A. activity.
B. anxiety.
C. association.
D. agitation.

Assessment *in Action* *(continued)*

7. Causes of psychotic episodes include all of the following EXCEPT:

A. schizophrenia.
B. intense stress.
C. delusional disorders.
D. hypoxia.

8. ________ is basically classified as whatever behavior society accepts.

A. Activities of daily living
B. Maladaptive behavior
C. Normal behavior
D. Abnormal behavior

9. List the signs and symptoms of a panic attack.

10. You are assessing a patient who has been diagnosed with PTSD and is experiencing flashbacks. What are flashbacks and what causes them?

CHAPTER 25

Gynecologic Emergencies

National EMS Education Standard Competencies

Medicine

Applies fundamental knowledge to provide basic and selected advanced emergency care and transportation based on assessment findings for an acutely ill patient.

Gynecology

Recognition and management of shock associated with

› Vaginal bleeding (pp 1045, 1047-1049)

Anatomy, physiology, assessment findings, and management of

› Vaginal bleeding (pp 1043, 1045, 1047-1049)
› Sexual assault (to include appropriate emotional support) (pp 1044-1045, 1048, 1050-1051)
› Infections (pp 1041-1042, 1049)

Knowledge Objectives

1. Review the anatomy and physiology of the female reproductive system. (pp 1039-1041)
2. Describe abnormalities associated with the menstrual cycle, including premenstrual syndrome, mittelschmerz, and amenorrhea. (pp 1040-1041)
3. Discuss the pathophysiology of gynecologic emergencies, including pelvic inflammatory disease, sexually transmitted diseases, vaginal yeast infections, ruptured ovarian cyst, ectopic pregnancy, vaginal bleeding, endometritis, endometriosis, postpartum eclampsia, and sexual assault. (pp 1041-1044)
4. Explain the assessment process for patients with gynecologic emergencies. (pp 1045-1048)
5. Discuss the importance of history taking when assessing a patient with a gynecologic emergency. (pp 1045-1047)
6. Discuss the general management of a patient with a gynecologic emergency. (pp 1048-1049)
7. Discuss assessment and management of specific gynecologic emergencies, including pelvic inflammatory disease, ruptured ovarian cyst, ectopic pregnancy, and vaginal bleeding. (pp 1049-1050)
8. Discuss special considerations in the assessment and management of victims of sexual assault, including those related to maintaining patient confidentiality and preserving evidence of the crime. (pp 1050-1051)

Skills Objectives

There are no skills objectives for this chapter.

YOU are the Provider PART 1

You are requested by law enforcement at a residential dwelling for a 19-year-old woman who reports she was sexually assaulted. On arrival, you find a scared-looking patient who is crying. She states she was sexually assaulted by an unknown assailant who broke into her home, and that she just wants to bathe because she feels "dirty." She is also concerned that the attacker did not use a condom.

1. Should this patient be encouraged to bathe?
2. What are the possible medical impacts of a sexual assault on this patient?

Introduction

Occasionally, girls, women in their childbearing years, and older adult women will have major gynecologic emergencies requiring urgent medical care. These emergencies include excessive bleeding and soft-tissue injuries to the external genitalia. The genitalia have a rich nerve supply; thus, soft-tissue injuries can be very painful. Some gynecologic conditions can be life threatening without prompt intervention. The reproductive system is extremely vascular, and the potential for bleeding is great. You may be called to care for patients with exacerbations or conditions related to sexually transmitted diseases (STDs). Also, vaginal discharge (nonbleeding) is a common problem, though not necessarily a true emergency.

This chapter will help you learn how to determine whether a life-threatening emergency exists, which prehospital interventions are required, and if transport is needed. Finally, the chapter discusses gynecologic emergencies unrelated to childbirth.

Anatomy and Physiology Review

Anatomy Review

The female reproductive organs include the external female genitalia, uterus, vagina, fallopian tubes, ovaries, and the perineum. The **ovaries** are almond-shaped organs that lie on each side of the upper pelvic cavity Figure 25-1. The two functions of the ovaries are to produce ova (mature **oocytes**, or female sex cells; singular, ovum) and the hormones estrogen and progesterone. These hormones are secreted by the corpus luteum, a small yellow endocrine structure that develops within a ruptured ovarian follicle (sac), and are responsible for development and maintenance of secondary sexual characteristics, preparation of the uterus for pregnancy, and development of the mammary glands. The **fallopian tubes**, or uterine tubes, are tubes or ducts that extend from the uterus and terminate near the ovary on each side. Their purpose is to carry an ovum from the ovary to the uterus and spermatozoa from the uterus toward the ovary.

The **uterus**, or womb, is the muscular organ where the fertilized egg implants and grows. It is responsible for contractions during labor and ultimately helps push the infant through the birth canal. The uterus is made up of the **fundus**, the uppermost part of the uterus, farthest from the cervical opening; the body, the principal mass of the uterus; the uterine cavity, the space within the uterus; the **endometrium**, the inner layer of the uterine wall; and the **myometrium**, the muscular wall of the uterus.

The **vagina** is the outermost cavity of a woman's reproductive system and forms the lower part of the birth canal. It is about 8 to 12 centimeters long, begins at the **cervix** (the neck of the uterus), and ends as an external opening of the body. Essentially, the vagina completes the passageway from the uterus to the outside world for the delivering infant. The cervical canal is the passageway from the uterus to the opening into the vagina.

The external female genitalia, or **vulva**, includes the **mons pubis**, the pad of fatty tissue and coarse skin that lies over the symphysis pubis; the **labia majora**, the

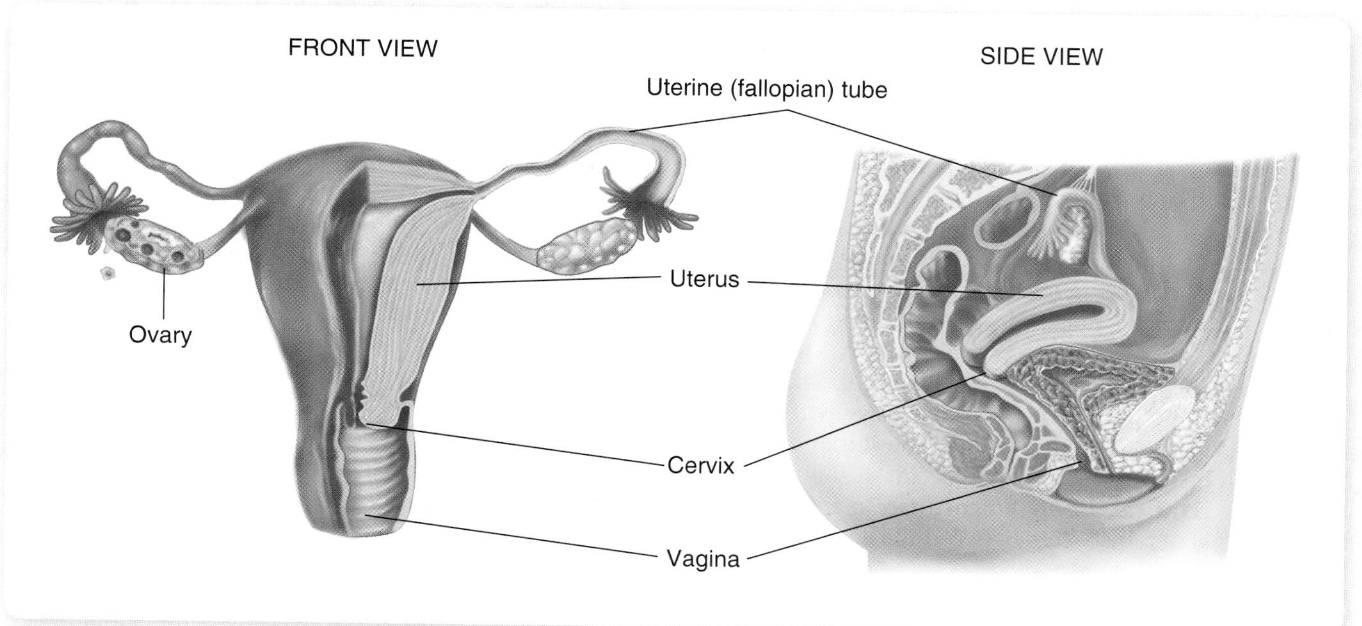

Figure 25-1 Front and side views of the female reproductive system.

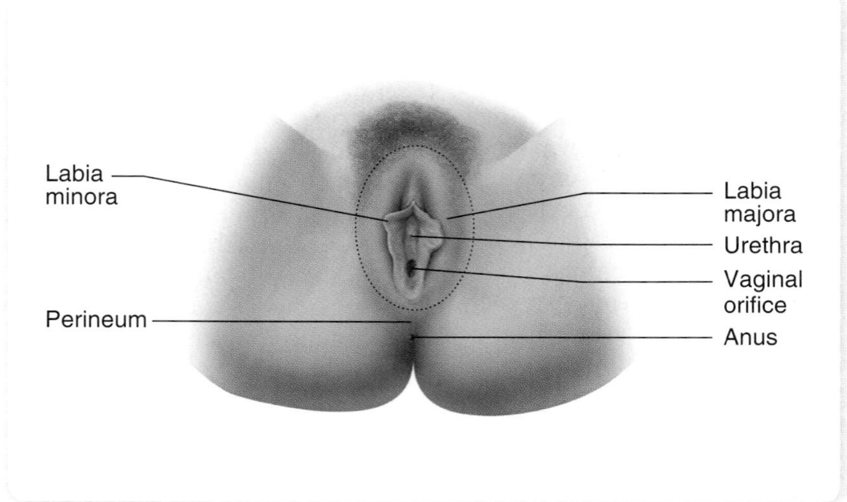

Figure 25-2 The external genitalia of the female reproductive system.

outer lip-shaped structure; the **labia minora**, the inner lip-shaped structure; the **clitoris**, the small erectile body partially hidden by the labia minora and covered by the **prepuce** or foreskin; the **vestibule**, the small space at the beginning of the vagina, and its glands; the opening of the **urethra**, the canal for the discharge of urine extending from the urinary bladder to the outside of the body; and the **vaginal orifice**, the opening of the vagina. The vaginal orifice is protected by the **hymen**. This membrane forms a border around the vaginal orifice, partially enclosing it. Contrary to popular belief, the presence or absence of the hymen does not denote virginity. Pregnancy has occurred with the hymen intact. The **perineum**, or pelvic floor, lies between the vulva and the **anus** (the outlet of the rectum) **Figure 25-2**.

▶ Physiology Review

Each month as the level of hormones rises in the female, certain characteristic changes take place. The hormones stimulate the development of the eggs in the ovaries and cause the endometrium of the uterus to thicken in anticipation of implantation of a fertilized egg. If an egg is fertilized and implants in the uterus, menses is suspended until such time as the pregnancy ends. If no fertilized egg implants, **menstruation** begins; menstruation is the cyclic shedding of the uterine lining that occurs approximately every 28 days. A typical cycle lasts 4 to 6 days, with blood loss of approximately 25 to 60 mL. The initial onset of menstruation, known as **menarche**, occurs during puberty. **Menopause** is the cessation of menstruation and ovarian function. It generally occurs between the ages of 45 and 55 years.

A number of conditions are associated with the menstrual cycle and may be encountered by advanced emergency medical technicians (AEMTs) caring for premenopausal women. Note, however, that these conditions are not necessarily emergencies. **Premenstrual syndrome (PMS)** is a cluster of troubling symptoms that normally occurs 7 to 14 days before the onset of the menstrual flow and then generally subsides once the flow begins. PMS affects approximately 20% to 30% of all premenopausal women, with one meta-analysis showing worldwide prevalence to be more than 45%,[1] and may be significantly debilitating. Stress, diet, alcohol consumption, and prescription or nonprescription drug use may exacerbate PMS symptoms. In addition, some women may experience reactive hypoglycemia, resulting in increased fatigue. This may be a strong clue as to what is troubling the patient, especially if the history elicits a recent intense craving for sweets or decreased alcohol tolerance. Prehospital treatment is predominantly supportive. Supportive field treatment may include administering oral or intravenous (IV) glucose, if blood glucose levels support the need, or administering a small dose of analgesics or anxiolytics to reduce patient anxiety.

Some women may experience abdominal pain and cramping in the 2 weeks before the beginning of menses. This pain and its accompanying symptoms result from the ovulatory process and are collectively called mittelschmerz (pronounced "MITT-ul-shmurz"; German for "middle pain"). Mittelschmerz, which may start at any time during ovulation (midcycle), affects approximately 20% of women.[2] In most cases, the pain is not severe; it may last only a few minutes or as long as 48 hours (average, 6 to 8 hours). Signs and symptoms include sharp, cramping pain in the lower abdomen, often localized to one side, beginning midcycle, with a history of similar pain episodes during previous periods. The pain may also be reported as "switching sides" from month to month. Some women report feeling nauseated or experiencing minor blood spotting. The condition itself is not serious, and the pain can often be relieved by over-the-counter analgesics. Any persistent pain or any abnormal symptoms are cause for concern and should be evaluated by a physician.

Amenorrhea is the absence or cessation of menses. This condition may be caused by a number of factors, but the most common cause is pregnancy. Exercise-induced amenorrhea is common in female athletes, particularly those who participate in physically intense sports. Amenorrhea may occur when a woman's body fat drops below a certain percentage. Amenorrhea can also be caused by emotional problems or extreme stress. In adolescents or young adults, the condition may have its origin in an eating disorder such as anorexia nervosa or bulimia; in this case, it is a symptom of the patient's malnutrition and emotional state.

Pathophysiology

Disorders in the female reproductive system can lead to gynecologic emergencies. These disorders include acute or chronic infection, hemorrhage, rupture of a cyst, and rupture of an ectopic pregnancy. The pathophysiology of these emergencies is discussed in this section. Specific assessment and management are discussed later in this chapter.

Pelvic Inflammatory Disease

Pelvic inflammatory disease (PID) is an acute or chronic infection of the upper female reproductive organs. Disease-causing organisms enter the vagina during sexual activity and migrate through the opening of the cervix and into the uterine cavity. The infection may then expand to the fallopian tubes, eventually involving the ovaries.

The chief symptoms of PID are pelvic pain and fever. Complications may include sepsis, abscess formation, generalized peritonitis, and infertility. Scarring may cause tubal infertility and increase the risk of ectopic pregnancy.

Sexually Transmitted Diseases

STDs can lead to more serious conditions. For example, PID is typically a secondary infection, with the primary infection being an STD—often chlamydia or gonorrhea. STDs are reviewed briefly here, with the exception of infection with human immunodeficiency virus (HIV), which is discussed in Chapter 16, *Medical Overview*. Treatment of a patient with an STD-related emergency typically involves placing the patient in a position of comfort and providing supportive care.

Bacterial vaginosis is the most common vaginal infection in women age 15 to 44.[3] In this infection, normal bacteria in the vagina are replaced by an overgrowth of other bacterial forms. Symptoms may include itching, burning, or pain and may be accompanied by a "fishy," foul-smelling discharge. Pregnant women with bacterial vaginosis may have premature babies or babies born with low birth weight. If it is left untreated, then bacterial vaginosis can lead to more serious infections or result in PID. It is treated with metronidazole, an antibiotic. If the patient consumes alcohol while taking this medication, then severe nausea and vomiting may develop.

Chancroid is caused by the bacterium *Haemophilus ducreyi*. This highly contagious yet curable disease causes painful sores (ulcers), usually of the genitals. Swollen, painful lymph glands or inguinal buboes in the groin area may be present as well. Women may be asymptomatic and, therefore, unaware they have the disease.

Chlamydia is caused by the bacterium *Chlamydia trachomatis*. It is currently the most commonly reported STD in the United States.[4] Although the symptoms of chlamydia are usually mild or absent, some women may report lower abdominal pain, low back pain, nausea, fever, pain during sexual intercourse, and/or bleeding between menstrual periods. Chlamydial infection of the cervix can spread to the rectum, leading to rectal pain, discharge, or bleeding. If it is left untreated, then the disease can progress to PID. In rare cases, chlamydia causes arthritis that may be accompanied by skin lesions and inflammation of the eye and urethra (Reiter syndrome).

Cytomegalovirus (CMV) is a member of the herpesvirus family. This common viral infection has no known cure, and the virus can remain dormant in the body for years. In its active stages, CMV infection may produce symptoms including prolonged high fever, chills, headache, malaise, extreme fatigue, and an enlarged spleen. People with an increased risk for active infection and more serious complications (such as fever, pneumonia, liver infection, and anemia) include people with immune disorders, those receiving chemotherapy, and pregnant women. Newborns who acquire CMV are susceptible to lung conditions, blood conditions, liver conditions, swollen glands, rash, and poor weight gain.

Genital herpes is an infection of the genitals, buttocks, or anal area caused by herpes simplex virus, type 1 or type 2. Type 1, which is the most common form, infects the mouth and lips, causing cold sores or "fever" blisters; it may also produce sores on the genitals. Type 2, the more serious infection, can affect the mouth as well, but is more commonly known as the primary cause of genital herpes. Genital herpes infection is more prevalent in women than in men.[5]

In an active herpes infection (called an outbreak), symptoms generally appear within 2 weeks of primary infection and can last for several weeks. Symptoms may include tingling or sores near the area where the virus has entered the body, such as on the genital or rectal area, on the buttocks or thighs, or on other parts of the body where the virus has entered through broken skin. In women, the sores may occur inside the vagina, on the cervix, or in the urinary passage. Small red bumps appear first, develop into small blisters, and finally become itchy, painful sores that might develop a crust and heal without leaving a scar. Other symptoms that may accompany the first outbreak, and possibly subsequent outbreaks, include fever, muscle aches and pains, headache, dysuria, vaginal discharge, and swollen glands in the groin area.

Gonorrhea is caused by *Neisseria gonorrhoeae*, a bacterium that can grow and multiply rapidly in the warm, moist areas of the reproductive tract, including the cervix, uterus, and fallopian tubes in women and in the urethra in women and men. The bacterium can also grow in the mouth, throat, eyes, and anus. Symptoms, which are generally more severe in men than in women,[6] appear approximately 2 to 10 days after exposure. Women may be infected with gonorrhea for months but not have any symptoms, or only mild ones, until the infection has spread to other parts of the reproductive system. When symptoms do appear in women, they generally present as dysuria (painful urination), with associated burning or itching; a yellow or bloody vaginal discharge, usually with a foul odor; and occult blood associated with vaginal intercourse. More severe infections may present with cramping and abdominal pain, nausea and vomiting, and bleeding between menstrual periods; these symptoms indicate that the infection has progressed to PID. Rectal infections generally present with anal discharge and itching and occasional painful bowel movements with fecal blood spotting. Infection of the throat (for which oral sex is the introducing factor) is called gonococcal pharyngitis. Its symptoms are usually mild, consisting of painful or difficult swallowing, sore throat, swollen lymph glands, and fever. Headache and nasal congestion may also be present. If the infection is not treated, then the bacterium may enter the bloodstream and spread to other parts of the body, including the brain—a condition known as disseminated gonococcemia.

Genital warts (also called condylomata acuminata and venereal warts) are caused by the **human papillomavirus (HPV)**. HPV is the most common STD, with an estimated 79 million people being infected and approximately 14 million new cases occurring every year; one-half of new cases occur in young adults, ages 15 to 24 years.[7] Some infected people have no symptoms. In others, multiple growths develop in the genital areas—that is, the vagina, vulva, cervix, or rectum, or the penis and scrotum in men. HPV has been identified as a causative agent in cervical, vulvar, and anal cancers. In pregnant women, warts may develop that become large enough to impede urination or obstruct the birth canal. If the virus is passed to the fetus, then laryngeal papillomatosis (throat warts that block the airway), a potentially life-threatening condition, may develop.

Syphilis is caused by the bacterium *Treponema pallidum*. Because many of its signs and symptoms mimic those of other diseases, syphilis is sometimes called the "great imitator" by clinicians. The disease manifests in three stages: primary, secondary, and tertiary. Transmission occurs through direct contact with open sores, which may arise anywhere on the body, but tend to appear on the genitals, anus, rectum, lips, or mouth. A person with syphilis may remain asymptomatic for years, not realizing that his or her sores are manifestations of a disease.

The primary stage of syphilis is usually marked by the appearance of a single sore (a chancre), although some people develop multiple sores. The chancre is usually painless and is small, firm, and round. It usually goes away after 3 to 6 weeks, at which point the disease has progressed to the second stage.

The secondary stage of syphilis is characterized by the development of mucous membrane lesions and a rash. The characteristic rash may present on the palms of the hands and the bottoms of the feet as rough, red or red-brown spots. Alternatively, it may be barely discernible or resemble rashes from other diseases. The rash generally does not itch. Symptoms of secondary syphilis may include fever, swollen lymph glands, sore throat, patchy hair loss, headache, weight loss, muscle ache, and fatigue. Like the chancre of the primary stage, these symptoms will resolve without treatment. Left untreated, the secondary stage invariably leads to tertiary syphilis.

In the tertiary stage of syphilis, internal damage is accumulating. Syphilis attacks the brain, nerves, eyes, heart, blood vessels, liver, bones, and joints, although it can take years for syphilis to progress from the primary stage to the tertiary stage; thus, the damage may not become evident for years. Paralysis, numbness, dementia, gradual blindness, and difficulty coordinating muscle movements are possible physical manifestations and may be serious enough to cause death. Pregnant women with syphilis may have stillborn babies, babies who are born blind, developmentally delayed babies, or babies who die shortly after birth.

Trichomoniasis is caused by a single-celled protozoan parasite, *Trichomonas vaginalis*. This parasite is transmitted through sexual contact, with the vagina being the most common site of infection. The infected person may be asymptomatic or may experience signs and symptoms including a frothy, yellow-green vaginal discharge with a strong odor. The infection may also cause irritation and itching of the female genital area, discomfort during intercourse, dysuria, and lower abdominal pain. When present, symptoms usually appear in women within 5 to 28 days of exposure to *T vaginalis*. If it is left untreated, then the infection can lead to low birth weight or premature birth in pregnant women and increase the patient's susceptibility to HIV infection.

▶ Vaginal Yeast Infections

Vaginal yeast infections are typically caused by the *Candida albicans* fungus. Yeasts are tiny organisms that normally live in small numbers inside the vagina and on the skin. The normal acidic environment of the vagina helps keep yeast from growing. If the vagina becomes less acidic, however, the yeast population may increase dramatically and result in infection. Conditions that may alter the acidic balance of the vagina, allowing yeast overgrowth, include the use of oral contraceptives, menstruation, pregnancy, diabetes, and some antibiotics. Moisture and irritation of the vagina also seem to encourage yeast growth. Stress from lack of sleep, illness, and poor diet are other contributing factors. Women with immunosuppressive diseases such as HIV infection or diabetes are also at increased risk. Symptoms include itching, burning, soreness in the vagina and around the vulva, and vulvar swelling. Some women may report a thick, white vaginal discharge ("cottage cheese" appearance), pain during sexual intercourse, and burning on urination.

▶ Ruptured Ovarian Cyst

An ovarian cyst is a fluid-filled sac attached to the inside or outside of the ovary. As the cyst enlarges, it can become filled with an enormous amount of fluid. The cyst may need to be removed surgically to relieve pressure or to treat infection. Complications include possible significant internal bleeding; however, this is rare.

▶ Ectopic Pregnancy

Ectopic pregnancy—a pregnancy that develops outside the uterus, most often in a fallopian tube—occurs in nearly 20 of every 1,000 pregnancies.[8] Vaginal bleeding may be the only sign of an ectopic pregnancy. The leading cause of maternal death during the first trimester is internal hemorrhage into the abdomen following rupture of an ectopic pregnancy.[8] For this reason, you should consider the possibility of an ectopic pregnancy in women who have missed a menstrual cycle and report sudden stabbing and usually unilateral pain in the lower abdomen. A history of PID, tubal ligation, or previous ectopic pregnancy should heighten your suspicions for a possible ectopic pregnancy. Consider the possibility of an ectopic pregnancy in any female of reproductive age who has abdominal pain.

An ectopic pregnancy occurs when the ovum develops outside the uterus. Numerous causes may affect the normal pathway of the ovum, preventing it from implanting in the uterus. Previous surgical adhesions, PID, a tubal ligation (having the fallopian tubes surgically tied to prevent pregnancy), or an intrauterine device (IUD) may interfere with the movement of a fertilized egg. Generally, it is the fallopian tubes that are affected, but on rare occasions, implantation may occur elsewhere in the pelvic cavity. Because the fallopian tubes are extremely narrow, even the slightest growth of the egg will cause symptoms; therefore, ectopic pregnancy is an early first-trimester emergency, typically, occurring within the first 6 to 8 weeks of pregnancy.

In ectopic pregnancy, the cells begin to divide and the zygote grows, even though this process occurs without the aid of oxygen or nutrients. Therefore, there is no viable fetus that can be removed and implanted in the uterus. Eventually, the fallopian tube will rupture if the ectopic pregnancy is not caught in time; this rupture can lead to a life-threatening emergency.

Special Populations

Vaginal bleeding in a young girl may be the result of menarche. There is no set age for the beginning or cessation of menstruation. Likewise, unusual signs and symptoms in an older adult patient going through menopause may be an indication of an unexpected pregnancy.

▶ Vaginal Bleeding

Vaginal bleeding can be as simple as a normal menstrual cycle or as extreme as a ruptured uterus. Never assume an emergency call for vaginal hemorrhage is bleeding from normal menstruation.

Bleeding that occurs during the first or second trimester of a known or possible pregnancy might indicate a spontaneous **abortion** or miscarriage, especially if the last menstrual cycle was more than 60 days ago.

Any vaginal bleeding during the third trimester of pregnancy is a serious emergency. **Placenta previa** presents with bright red bleeding, and **abruptio placenta** presents with dark bleeding. However, these color differences can be difficult to discern in the prehospital setting. It may be more helpful to note that patients who have placenta previa tend to have significant bleeding and mild pain, whereas patients with abruptio placenta tend to have little bleeding and moderate to severe abdominal pain. These topics will be addressed further in Chapter 35, *Obstetrics and Neonatal Care*.

Other causes of vaginal bleeding include the following:

- Onset of labor
- Ruptured ectopic pregnancy
- PID and other infections
- Trauma
- Lesions from previous surgeries or disease processes

Vaginal bleeding may result from the following traumatic causes:

- **Straddle injury.** This type of injury occurs when a female falls onto an object, such as the bar of a boy's bicycle, causing trauma to the external genitalia and perineum.
- **Blows to the perineum.** A blow to the perineum may be associated with falls or assault.
- **Blunt force to the lower abdomen from assault or seat belt injuries.** Any blunt force to the lower abdomen has the potential to rupture organs or cause serious injury, such as a lap belt causing injury in a motor vehicle crash or blows to the abdomen during an assault.
- **Foreign bodies inserted into the vagina.** This injury may be self-inflicted or the result of a sexual assault.
- **Abortion attempt.** Trauma occurs when a female uses an object such as a clothes hanger in an attempt to abort her pregnancy. This can cause massive trauma and extensive bleeding.
- **Soft-tissue injury.** Sexual assault and vigorous sexual activity can cause soft-tissue injury. Any or all of the pelvic organs may be affected.

▶ Endometritis

Endometritis is an inflammation or irritation of the endometrium (uterine lining). Women are more likely to have endometritis after having a baby or after a miscarriage. This condition is most commonly caused by an infection, frequently by an STD (gonorrhea and chlamydia, predominantly).

Symptoms of endometritis may include malaise, fever (high or low grade), constipation or uncomfortable bowel movements, vaginal bleeding or discharge (or both), abdominal distention, and lower abdominal or pelvic pain. Abdominal auscultation may reveal decreased bowel sounds, and pain may be elicited by palpation of the abdomen.

Endometritis is treated with antibiotics. Provide reassurance to the patient and transport in a position of comfort. If necessary, then start an IV line and titrate to the patient's vital signs. Left untreated, endometritis may lead to septic shock or cause spontaneous abortion in a pregnant patient. Most patients fully recover after antibiotic treatment.

▶ Endometriosis

Endometriosis is believed to develop in more than 5 million women in the United States every year.[9] This condition can be extremely painful, yet some women may not have any symptoms. It results when endometrial tissue grows outside the uterus, generally on the surface of abdominal and pelvic organs. Organs of the pelvic cavity are the most common locations for the ectopic growths, but endometrial tissue can occasionally be found in the lungs or other parts of the body. Endometriosis is one of the leading causes of infertility in women, with nearly 50% of infertile women having this condition.[10] Many women do not even realize they have endometriosis until they encounter difficulties trying to get pregnant.

In women who experience symptoms, the most common complaint is pain (sometimes chronic pain), generally localized in the lower back, pelvic, and abdominal regions. Other symptoms include painful intercourse (during and after), gastrointestinal pain, dysuria and painful bowel movements during the menstrual cycle, fatigue (perhaps leading to misdiagnosis as chronic fatigue syndrome), extremely painful and escalating menstrual cramping, and very heavy menstrual periods. Patients may also experience bleeding between periods or report premenstrual spotting.

Prehospital care for endometriosis is based on the patient's signs and symptoms. If the patient reports severe pain, then provide pain relief with analgesics if allowed in your protocol. Let the patient position herself so she is as comfortable as possible. Use dressings or towels as needed to absorb any significant vaginal bleeding.

▶ Postpartum Eclampsia

You may not think of eclampsia when treating patients with gynecologic emergencies, but after a baby is born, the mother is at risk for eclampsia for several weeks. Postpartum eclampsia usually presents within the first 24 hours after delivery, but may occur as late as 4 weeks following the birth. You may receive a call to care for a woman with seizures and hypertension who has delivered a baby a few weeks earlier. A thorough history is important to determine whether the seizure could be caused by postpartum eclampsia. In such a scenario, paramedic backup is required. Eclampsia is covered in more detail in Chapter 35, *Obstetrics and Neonatal Care*.

▶ Sexual Assault

Unfortunately, sexual assault and rape are all too common occurrences in today's society. Although most victims are women, men and children are also victims. Often, there is little you can do beyond providing compassion and transportation to the emergency department (ED). In some cases, the patients will have sustained multiple-system trauma and will also need treatment for shock. This is discussed in more detail later in this chapter.

YOU are the Provider — PART 2

You explain to the patient that if she were to bathe, she would be removing potential evidence from her body. Therefore, she reluctantly agrees to be transported to the ED for a sexual assault examination.

Recording Time: 1 Minute	
Appearance	Visibly upset
Level of consciousness	Alert and oriented to person, place, time, and event
Airway	Patent
Breathing	Normal rate and rhythm
Circulation	Strong radial pulses; skin warm, dry, and pink

3. If available, should a female provider accompany the patient in the rear of the ambulance?
4. What kind of care does this patient require en route to the hospital?

Patient Assessment

Obtaining an accurate and detailed patient assessment is crucial when dealing with gynecologic emergencies. You may not be able to make a specific diagnosis in the field, but a thorough patient assessment will help determine just how sick the patient is and whether you should initiate life-saving measures. This is especially true when caring for patients with abdominal pain.

Women have many of the same conditions that cause abdominal pain in men, for example, ulcers and appendicitis. In addition, there are numerous gynecologic causes of abdominal pain. An old medical axiom states, "Anyone who neglects to consider a gynecologic cause in a woman of childbearing age who reports abdominal pain will miss the diagnosis at least 50% of the time." Missing the diagnosis may be fatal for the patient.

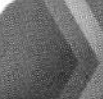

Scene Size-up

Every emergency call—including calls involving gynecologic emergencies—begins with a thorough scene size-up. Gynecologic emergencies can be very messy, sometimes involving significant amounts of blood and body fluids contaminated with organisms that can potentially cause communicable diseases. Take standard precautions.

Where and in what position is the patient found? If she is at home, what is the condition of the residence? Is it clean or dirty? Do you see evidence of a fight? Is alcohol or evidence of drug use present? Are there photos of loved ones or is there a noticeable absence of photos? Does the patient live alone or with other people? All of the information you obtain contributes to your assessment of the patient's overall health and the safety of the scene. In the case of a crime scene, you may also be required to testify in court regarding the conditions on your arrival. Your documentation needs to be accurate and thorough. Involve law enforcement if any type of assault is suspected. In cases of sexual assault, it is valuable to have a female AEMT provide patient care, so consider calling for one early if you and your partner are men.

Often the mechanism of injury (MOI) or nature of illness (NOI) in patients with gynecologic problems will be understood from the dispatch information, such as in cases of sexual assault. In other patients, the exact nature of the condition will not emerge until you gather patient history information. For example, the patient may present with vague symptoms such as abdominal pain, and you may not be able to determine the exact NOI until you gather more information during the patient history.

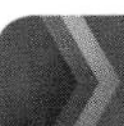

Primary Survey

The general impression is an important aspect of all patient assessments. As you approach the patient, you should quickly determine if her condition is stable or unstable. Use this information to help you as you proceed further with the assessment. Use the AVPU (Alert to person, place, and time; responsive to Verbal stimuli; responsive to Pain; Unresponsive) scale to determine the patient's level of consciousness, and immediately assess airway, breathing, circulation, disability, and exposure (ABCDEs).

If the patient has experienced significant blood loss because of vaginal bleeding, she may not demonstrate obvious signs of shock but may still be hypovolemic. If the patient has a weak or rapid pulse or has pale, cool, or diaphoretic skin, then place the patient in a supine position. Cover the patient to keep her warm, and then transport to the nearest appropriate receiving facility for treatment. Most cases of gynecologic emergencies are not life threatening; however, if signs of shock exist because of bleeding, then rapid transport is necessary. The remainder of the assessment can be performed en route to the hospital.

History Taking

Begin by asking about the patient's chief complaint, but realize that some of the questions you must ask may be considered extremely personal. Be sensitive to the patient's feelings and ensure her privacy and dignity are protected. Gynecologic emergencies can be highly embarrassing for the patient, and many women may be extremely uncomfortable with discussing their sexual history in front of strangers or even close family members. An adolescent girl may want to keep her sexual history from her parents.

When asking patients about sensitive subjects, ensure you do so in a quiet manner away from bystanders. If the patient seems to be emotionally distressed, then assess the cause and degree of distress. This may require moving the patient to the ambulance to remove her from the source of the problem. This is especially true in cases of suspected abuse. Ask only the questions pertinent to your evaluation of her physical status. Your sensitive and caring manner can help you serve as a role model to others.

Gynecologic emergencies often have the same signs and symptoms as emergencies involving other abdominal organs. Assess the patient carefully to determine the nature and extent of the condition. Include the following elements in your assessment:

- SAMPLE (Signs and symptoms, Allergies, Medications, Pertinent past medical history, Last oral intake, Events leading up to the illness or injury)
- Ask about the patient's last menstrual period.
- What, if any, associated symptoms are noted:
  - Fever?
  - Diaphoresis?
  - Syncope?
  - Diarrhea?
  - Constipation?
  - Painful or difficult urination (dysuria)?

The nature and location of pain may also give clues to the origin of the problem. Is the pain localized or diffuse? Is it constant, or does it come and go? Is there any radiation or referred pain? Rebound tenderness? Remember to ask specifically:

- Describe any pain or discomfort.
  - OPQRST (Onset, Provocation/palliation, Quality, Region/radiation, Severity, Timing)?
  - Abdominal pain?
  - **Dysmenorrhea**—does the patient have painful menstruation?
- Are there any aggravating factors?
  - Ambulation—does it hurt the patient to move?
  - Dyspareunia—does the patient have pain during sexual intercourse?
  - Defecation—does it hurt to pass stool?
- Are there any alleviating factors?
  - Positioning—does the patient feel better when in a different position **Figure 25-3**?
  - Ceasing activity—does the pain decrease when the patient stops moving?

Other medical conditions may present as an abdominal condition. Cardiac pain, for example, may be misinterpreted as epigastric pain. Other conditions may also exacerbate gynecologic emergencies. Besides obtaining a SAMPLE history, be sure to ask the patient about previous episodes of this type of condition.

- What is the patient's present health?
  - Any preexisting conditions?
  - Any previous surgeries?

Determine whether the patient has a history of gynecologic conditions and whether she has had any infections. If so, did she seek medical treatment? What was the diagnosis? If she thinks she may be having a repeat episode, has she taken any medication or used any over-the-counter treatment?

Ask the patient if she has had any recent surgeries or procedures (eg, abortion, biopsies, dilation and curettage), because these procedures can cause vaginal bleeding.

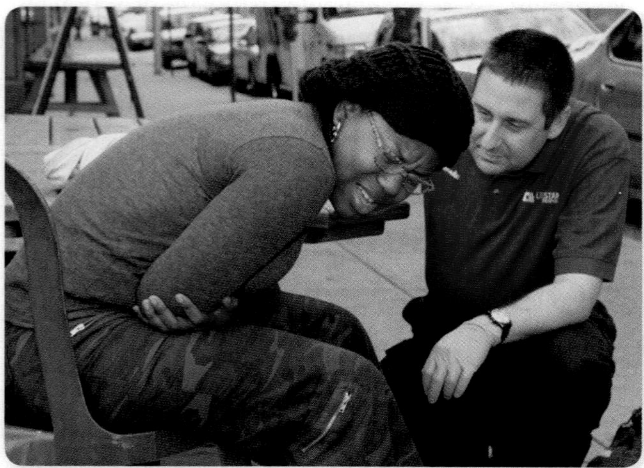

Figure 25-3 Note the position of the patient during your assessment.

Some office-based procedures can cause bleeding but the patient may not think of them as surgeries.

Ask about previous pregnancies. How many times has she been pregnant? How many pregnancies have been carried to full term resulting in live birth? Have there been any miscarriages or clinical abortions, and if so, how many?

Words of Wisdom

Suppose your patient is pregnant and has given birth to two children with no miscarriages. This information can be documented on the patient care report as G3, P2, A0. Gravida [G] is the number of pregnancies including the current pregnancy; para [P] is the number of pregnancies carried to term; and abortus [A] represents the number of miscarriages, stillbirths, or surgical abortions.

Ask whether the patient has ever had an ectopic pregnancy. If so, how far along was the pregnancy? Has she ever had a cesarean section? A patient with a history of an obstetric condition tends to be more susceptible to repetitive problems.

If the patient is currently bleeding, then try to estimate the amount of blood loss. What color is the blood? Is it dark, like the normal menstrual flow, or is it bright red? How many pads are soaked per hour? Take any clots or soaked pads along with the patient to the hospital in a plastic bag. How long has the bleeding been going on? Remember that some women will continue to have menstrual cycles even though they are pregnant. The flow tends to be lighter and may be only "spotting." Therefore, the presence of bleeding does not rule out pregnancy.

Special Populations

Vaginal or urinary bleeding is not common in older adult women who are postmenopausal and is a definite cause for concern. When the patient is an older woman who reports genitourinary bleeding, be sure to take a thorough history, including the use of anticoagulants in her daily medication regimen. Treatment for the most part is strictly supportive unless the bleeding is severe and the patient is exhibiting signs of shock.

If the patient reports any vaginal discharge, then note the color, amount, consistency, and any odor. Is there any irritation or pain associated with the discharge? Is there any burning or irritation with urination?

Inquire about the use of contraceptives. What type is used? Is the patient consistent with its use?

Ask the patient about a missed or late period. When was the patient's last menstrual cycle? How long did it last? Was it normal in duration and amount of flow? Also ask the patient about any bleeding between periods (breakthrough bleeding). A patient who has a regular menstrual cycle is more likely to recognize a problem than one who has an irregular cycle. Determine regularity and how this occurrence differs from the usual pattern.

Consider the possibility of pregnancy in any woman of childbearing age (approximately 12 to 60 years) even if contraception has been used. Also consider the possibility of pregnancy even if the patient denies a history of sexual activity, because this denial may be based on cultural factors or age-related stigma. Is there any breast tenderness? Has the patient noticed a need to urinate frequently without an increased fluid intake? Is there any nausea or vomiting that may be morning sickness? While maintaining the patient's privacy, question the patient to determine whether she is sexually active and whether she has had unprotected sex.

Finally, address any trauma. Determine whether there has been any history of trauma to the reproductive system.

Special Populations

Most teenage girls feel uncomfortable discussing gynecologic emergencies in front of their parents. They may even refuse to seek help to avoid the embarrassment of the situation. Allow them the opportunity to talk privately, and assure them of your discretion **Figure 25-4**. In most cases, a parent will be required to authorize treatment of a minor, but in the case of pregnancy the minor becomes "emancipated" and is legally able to give or refuse consent. STDs are also confidential issues in some areas and do not require parental consent for treatment. Regardless, stress the need for the patient to seek treatment for any gynecologic emergency.

Become familiar with the laws in your area regarding privacy and minors. These laws differ by state, and you should know them before finding yourself in a situation requiring knowledge of them.

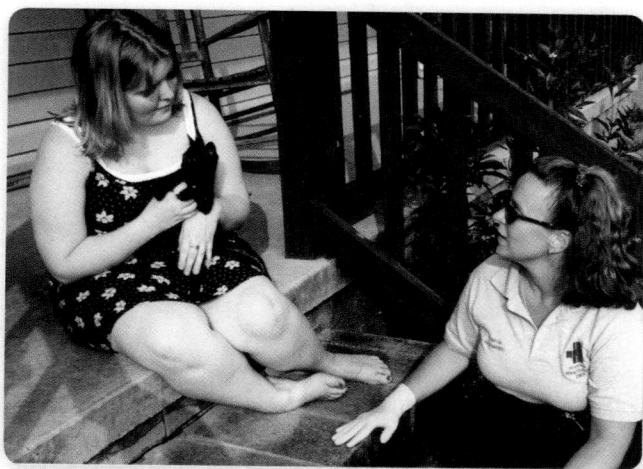

Figure 25-4 Respect the privacy of teenagers by questioning them away from parents or other bystanders.

Courtesy of Rhonda Hunt.

Secondary Assessment

The secondary assessment may be performed on scene, en route to the ED, or, in some instances, not at all. If the patient is critically ill or injured or the transport time is short, then you may not have time to conduct this part of the patient assessment process.

The physical exam is performed in the same manner as the exam for other medical emergencies, with special consideration for the female reproductive system. Approach the patient with a comforting attitude. Protect the patient's modesty by placing a sheet over her and removing only the items of clothing necessary to perform your assessment. Maintain privacy during the exam and while interviewing the patient. Be considerate of the patient's needs and the reason for her discomfort. If the patient has a history of an STD (eg, acquired immunodeficiency syndrome, genital herpes, gonorrhea), then treat her appropriately and without moral judgment.

Focus your physical exam on the NOI and the patient's chief complaint. Assessment of the external genitalia should be done only when necessary and should be a visual inspection only. If vaginal bleeding is the NOI, then you should visualize the bleeding and ask about its quality and quantity. Use external sanitary pads to control the bleeding, and keep the possibility of hypoperfusion or shock in mind. Always ask if there is pain associated with the vaginal bleeding or discharge. Never insert anything into the vagina to control bleeding, including a tampon.

Vaginal discharge is another condition that should be observed if possible. Make observations about the discharge, and ask the patient about any qualities she noticed and the history of the discharge.

Fever, nausea, and vomiting are common with many medical conditions but should be considered especially significant with gynecologic emergencies. Fever should always be considered a sign of an infectious process. Any report of syncope by the patient, especially if she reports vaginal bleeding, is considered significant. Treat the patient reporting this symptom as being in shock until proven otherwise.

Assess the patient's vital signs. Include any orthostatic changes. Hypotension in a patient with abdominal pain may be a sign of internal bleeding in the absence of external hemorrhage. Tachycardia and changes in respiration might also signal shock. Note the color and amount of any bleeding or discharge. If there is any evidence of clots and/or tissue, then transport the patient to the hospital.

Expose and examine the abdomen to look for any discoloration or swelling. Palpate for any masses, tenderness, guarding, distention, or rebound tenderness. If the patient reports discomfort in a particular area, then always begin your assessment in the quadrant farthest away from the area of pain, and palpate the painful area last.

Use the appropriate monitoring devices, such as pulse oximetry, to track the patient's condition. Also consider using noninvasive blood pressure monitoring to continuously track the patient's blood pressure. Assess the patient's first blood pressure manually with a sphygmomanometer (blood pressure cuff) and stethoscope.

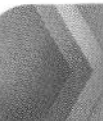

Reassessment

Very few interventions can or should be done for a patient with a gynecologic emergency. If a patient has vaginal bleeding, then treat her for hypoperfusion or shock. Keep her warm, place her in a supine position, and provide her with supplemental oxygen even if she is not experiencing difficulty breathing. Then transport to the nearest appropriate receiving facility.

En route to the receiving hospital, reassess vital signs and watch for trending. Recheck your interventions and note any improvement (or decline) in the patient's condition. Pay specific attention to the needs of the patient, and accommodate her desire for conversation or silence. These patients may be particularly emotionally vulnerable. Do not focus on your paperwork; the paperwork, while important, can wait until the patient has been delivered to the receiving facility.

Notify staff at the receiving hospital of all relevant information, including the possibility of pregnancy, so a proper response can be prepared. Carefully document the patient's condition, her chief complaint, the scene, any findings including vital signs, and all interventions, especially in cases of sexual assault.

Emergency Medical Care

Whenever you care for patients with gynecologic emergencies, you must maintain the patient's privacy and modesty as much as possible. Gain the patient's confidence by communicating appropriately and answering questions honestly. Provide psychological support en route to the hospital. Remain calm, and provide reassuring, gentle care. Call for paramedic backup if needed.

Excessive internal vaginal bleeding can have many causes and can possibly lead to hypoperfusion or shock. Determining the cause of the bleeding should be less important than treating for shock and transporting the patient to an appropriate facility. Use sanitary pads on the external genitalia to absorb the blood, and discourage the use of tampons. Document the number of sanitary pads that were saturated with blood to help the physician estimate blood loss.

If the patient is demonstrating signs of shock or has excessive vaginal bleeding, then place her in a supine position and keep her warm. Establish at least one IV line using a large-bore IV catheter in a large vein. Administer a 20-mL/kg bolus of an isotonic crystalloid solution such as normal saline or lactated Ringer solution if the patient is showing signs of hypovolemia and adjust the flow rate to maintain radial pulses. Consider establishing a second IV line.

If the patient is not demonstrating signs of shock, then place her in a position of comfort based on her presentation. Some patients with abdominal pain find it

YOU are the Provider — PART 3

As you transport the patient to the hospital, the patient states, "I don't know what I did to deserve this." She further states she just wants to be left alone.

Recording Time: 15 Minutes	
Respirations	22 breaths/min, crying
Pulse	Strong and regular, 120 beats/min
Skin	Warm, dry, and pink
Blood pressure	102/68 mm Hg
Oxygen saturation (Spo_2)	99%
Pupils	Pupils Equal, Round, and Reactive to Light and Accommodation (PERRLA)

5. Does this type of call require any special documentation?
6. If you are able to preserve the patient's clothing in a bag for evidence, then in what type of bag should you place the clothing?

more comfortable to lie in a lateral recumbent position. Place the patient on the left side so that she will be facing you instead of the wall of the ambulance. Some patients prefer a knee–chest position, whereas others prefer the hips raised and the knees bent.

Treat any external lacerations, abrasions, and tears with sterile compresses, using local pressure to control bleeding and a diaper-type bandage to hold the dressings in place. Leave any foreign bodies in place after stabilizing them with bandages. Under no circumstances should you pack or place dressings inside the vagina. Continue to assess the patient while transporting her to the receiving facility. Contusions and other blunt trauma will require careful in-hospital evaluation.

Consider the possibility of pregnancy, and be prepared for a possible miscarriage. Anticipate the presence of an ectopic pregnancy on the basis of signs and symptoms. If an ectopic pregnancy is suspected, then be alert for possible hypovolemic shock in the event of rupture. Evaluation by a physician is necessary. Transport the patient to the closest appropriate facility. This may include one with a labor and delivery department or a trauma center with surgical intervention capabilities. Consider emergency transport based on the patient's presentation.

Assessment and Management of Specific Emergencies

The pathophysiology of gynecologic emergencies was discussed earlier in this chapter. This section discusses assessment and management of specific gynecologic emergencies.

Pelvic Inflammatory Disease

Assessment findings of PID include lower abdominal pain, fever, vaginal discharge, and dyspareunia (pain during sexual intercourse). The patient will generally walk doubled-over and guard the abdomen, and she may present with a distinctive gait that appears as a shuffle to avoid excessive movement of the abdominal muscles. The patient will also appear ill.

Care includes placing the patient in a position of comfort and providing transport to an appropriate facility.

Ruptured Ovarian Cyst

When an ovarian cyst ruptures, a sudden onset of severe lower abdominal pain may be noted. Most patients have unilateral pain that may radiate from the abdomen to the back. Rupture of the cyst may result in some vaginal bleeding. Management of vaginal bleeding is discussed later in this section.

Ectopic Pregnancy

A patient with an ectopic pregnancy usually presents with signs of hypovolemic shock. The patient may report severe abdominal pain that radiates to the back. Vaginal bleeding may be absent or minimal. The patient will generally report amenorrhea even if she does not know she is pregnant. If rupture occurs, then bleeding may be excessive. Expect signs and symptoms of shock. Ask the patient about additional relevant history. If the patient has previously undergone abdominal surgery, then surgical adhesions may be present. Ask whether she has experienced PID or a tubal ligation, uses an IUD, or has previously had an ectopic pregnancy.

Monitor the patient for impending shock, including orthostatic vital signs. Note the presence and volume of vaginal blood. A ruptured ectopic pregnancy is a true medical emergency. In addition to the general management, if signs and symptoms of shock are present, establish a second IV line and treat appropriately. Transport the patient rapidly to the closest appropriate facility.

Vaginal Bleeding

A patient may experience menorrhagia, or heavy vaginal bleeding. Carefully ask the patient about the amount of bleeding, and treat her appropriately based on presenting signs and symptoms.

Always assume that any bleeding during the first or second trimester of a known or possible pregnancy might indicate a spontaneous abortion or miscarriage, especially if the last menstrual cycle was more than 60 days ago. Ask the patient about any previous similar events. Are there any large clots or pieces of tissue? If so, then take the patient to the ED for further evaluation. This experience can be a very tragic time for the patient, so emotional support is extremely important.

Any vaginal bleeding during the third trimester of pregnancy is a serious emergency and could be the result of placenta previa or abruptio placenta. A physician should evaluate any vaginal bleeding differing in amount and duration from the normal menstrual cycle. The reproductive organs are very vascular, and any bleeding may be life threatening. Hemorrhage can quickly lead to hypovolemic shock and death. Bleeding related to obstetric emergencies is covered in detail in Chapter 35, *Obstetrics and Neonatal Care*.

When you are assessing a patient who has vaginal bleeding, ensure that you inquire about the onset of symptoms. Does the onset coincide with the normal menstrual cycle? Was there any trauma involved? Is there any chance of pregnancy? Is there a history of bleeding? Check for signs of impending shock, including orthostatic vital signs. Note the presence and volume of bleeding, and remember to take any tissue or clots to the hospital for evaluation.

Patients who have experienced abdominal trauma generally present with a variety of signs and symptoms that can include severe bleeding, pain, and hypovolemic shock **Figure 25-5**. Specific assessment findings are consistent with severe internal injuries. Management should be based on patient presentation.

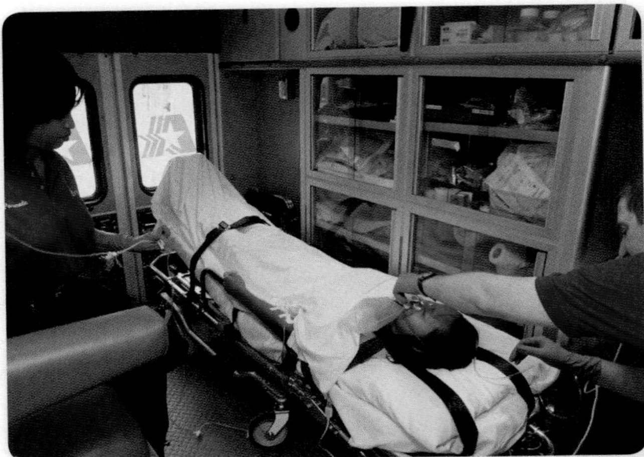

Figure 25-5 A patient with gynecologic trauma should be transported lying down.

▶ Sexual Assault

Sexual assault can take many forms, but the most common is **rape**. In the United States, 12% of women will be raped during their lives (though only 16% to 19% of victims file a crime report),[11] and one of every four will be sexually molested, often before the age of 12 years.[12]

Because rape is a crime, you can generally expect police involvement early in the situation. In many cases, emergency medical services (EMS) may be called by the police. Police officers generally have rudimentary medical training, with many states requiring at least basic training at the first responder level. Nevertheless, primary training for police officers focuses on investigation, not patient care.

A rape victim has just experienced a purposeful "major vehicle crash" of her mind and body. The act was most likely perpetrated by someone she knew and trusted. The last thing she wants to do is give a concise, detailed report of what she has just experienced, and attempting to elicit information in this manner will most likely cause the patient to "shut down." Whenever possible, a female rape victim should be given the option of being treated by a female AEMT because the patient may be experiencing ambivalent feelings toward men in general; these feelings will hinder assessment and the patient's well-being.

It is the job of law enforcement officers to solve the crime, arrest the perpetrator, and ensure justice is served. The job of AEMTs is to manage the medical aspects of the case and to act as the patient's advocate. In this capacity, it is important for you to focus on several key issues Table 25-1.

AEMTs called on to treat a victim of sexual assault, molestation, or actual or alleged rape face many complex issues, ranging from the obvious medical ones to the serious psychological and legal issues. In particular, you may be the first person the victim has contact with after the encounter, and how the situation is managed from the first contact throughout treatment and transport may have lasting effects for the patient and you. Professionalism, tact, kindness, and sensitivity are of paramount importance. First, ask the patient if she would be more comfortable with a female AEMT (or, if it is a male patient, a male AEMT), and make every effort to fulfill this request.

Table 25-1 Treatment Principles for Sexual Assault

In addition to the usual treatment principles that apply to all patients, follow these special steps with patients who have been sexually assaulted:

1. Document the patient's history, assessment, treatment, and response to treatment in detail because you may have to appear in court as long as 2 or 3 years later. Do not speculate. Record only the facts.
2. Complete the SAMPLE history objectively.
3. Follow any crime scene policy established by your system to protect the scene and any potential evidence for police, particularly that for evidence collection. If the patient will tolerate being wrapped in a sterile burn sheet, this may help investigators to find any hair, fluid, or fiber from the alleged offender.
4. Do not examine the genitalia unless there is major bleeding. If an object has been inserted into the vagina or rectum, then do not attempt to remove it.
5. To reduce the patient's anxiety, ensure the AEMT is the same gender as the patient, whenever possible.
6. Discourage the patient from bathing, voiding, or cleaning any wounds until the hospital staff has completed an assessment. Handle the patient's clothes as little as possible, placing articles and any other evidence in paper bags. If the patient insists on urinating, then ask the patient to do so in a sterile urine container (if available). Also, deposit the toilet paper in a paper bag. Seal and mark the bag for the police. This can be critical evidence.

Abbreviations: AEMT, advanced emergency medical technician; SAMPLE, Signs and symptoms, Allergies, Medications, Pertinent past medical history, Last oral intake, Events leading up to the illness or injury

Words of Wisdom

During the assessment, explain to the patient what you are about to do and why. This will help gain her trust and confidence.

Limit any physical exam to a brief survey for life-threatening injuries. Expose and examine the vaginal area only if there is evidence of bleeding that needs to be treated. Do everything possible to protect the patient's privacy and give some sense of control back to the patient.

Examine and interview the patient with a minimum of people present, moving her to the ambulance if necessary to ensure privacy.

The first issue is the medical treatment of the patient. Is she physically injured? Are any life-threatening injuries present? Does the patient complain of any pain?

The second issue is your psychological care of the patient. Do not cross-examine her or attempt to elicit information for the benefit of the police. These issues will be handled later in the ED. Do not pass judgment on the patient, and protect her from the judgment of others on the scene. It does not matter how the patient is dressed, what her local reputation is, where she was, or what she was doing when the assault occurred. The concept of a woman "deserving" to be raped is just as ludicrous as you "deserving" to be assaulted for wearing the colors of a rival sports team. A crime has been committed, and you need to remain cognizant of that fact. Many women report feeling as though they have been "raped again" when subjected to interrogation, criticism, or incredulity.

Remember, you are at a crime scene. Although your job is to treat the *medical* aspects of the incident and not collect evidence, you still have a responsibility to *preserve* evidence. Do not cut through any clothing or throw away anything from the scene. Place bloodstained articles in separate paper (not plastic) bags. Obtain evidentiary bags from the police if necessary. Paper bags allow wet items to dry naturally, whereas plastic allows mold to grow and may destroy biologic evidence.

It may also be necessary to gently persuade the patient to *not* clean up. This will be a natural desire on the part of the patient, stemming from the desire to "wash away" the humiliation and embarrassment of the assault. Valuable evidence can be destroyed in this process. The patient also needs to be discouraged from using hand sanitizer, urinating, changing clothes, moving her bowels, or rinsing out her mouth. She will need to be photographed by law enforcement personnel as well, and the photographic record needs to be as accurate as possible. If the patient cannot be dissuaded from taking these actions, then respect her feelings.

Some patients may refuse transport altogether. For adults who are mentally competent, this is the patient's right. In such cases, you should follow your system's refusal of treatment policy or procedure for sexual assault victims without judging or being condescending to the patient. In no instance should you simply accept the patient's refusal and leave. Offer to call the local rape crisis center for the patient. Many communities have rape crisis centers, with victim advocates on-call. Getting a professional advocate to the scene may help the patient deal with the trauma, and the advocate can better explain the necessities of evidence preservation in more compassionate detail. Many victim advocates are rape-trauma survivors themselves.

Follow your protocol concerning this type of call. Some EMS systems may consider administering a sedative to a patient in this situation.

The patient care report is a legal document and, should the case result in an arrest and subsequent trial, may be subpoenaed. Keep the report concise, and record only what the patient stated in her own words. Use quotation marks to indicate that you are reporting the patient's version of events. Do not insert your own opinion as to whether the patient was raped or offer any conclusions that would validate or invalidate the patient's account of the event. Focus on the facts. Record your observations during the physical examination—the patient's emotional state, the condition of her clothing, and any obvious injuries. Bear in mind that rape is a *legal* diagnosis, not a medical diagnosis. The medical team can establish only whether sexual intercourse occurred; a court must decide whether intercourse was inflicted forcibly on the victim, against her will.

Drugs Used to Facilitate Rape

It is not uncommon for drugs to be involved when a rape or other sexual assault has taken place. Alcohol is a common element to rape scenes. Other drugs used in the commission of the crime of rape include "club drugs" such as Rohypnol (roofies), GHB (liquid E or liquid ecstasy), ketamine (Special K), Klonopin, and Xanax. These drugs can be put into a person's drink and may go undetected because they often do not have a color, smell, or taste. The effects may be immediate. The patient may become weak and confused and may even have a loss of consciousness. If the drugs are still in the patient's system during your assessment, then you may see hypotension, bradycardia, difficulty breathing, seizures, coma, and even death.

▶ Sexual Practices and Vaginal Foreign Bodies

There is a variety of ways in which men and women engage in sexual acts. Your exposure to these practices will most likely occur when these private sexual practices go bad, resulting in an embarrassing call to 9-1-1.

The most common sexual gynecologic emergency you may encounter is simply a foreign object (a beverage or beer bottle, or a sex toy) that has become stuck in the vagina or rectum. For example, a bottle may develop a vacuum inside of the body and stick to an interior structure. Attempts at removal by the patient may result in intense pain or even vaginal bleeding as internal structures tear. Bleeding and pain may cause the patient to panic. With this type of call, keep the patient calm, protect his or her dignity as much as possible, and transport. Do not attempt to remove any foreign objects from the vagina or anus. If at all possible, do not let the patient walk. Overpenetration of any item may lead to internal injury, and should be managed as such.

Some cases of bottle insertion may be associated with rape, so bear in mind that the patient may be an assault victim. Some gangs have been known to insert beer bottles in a woman's vagina after rape, and then take turns punching the woman in the lower abdomen until the bottle breaks. If this is the case, use extreme care and do not move the patient more than necessary to prevent even more internal damage.

Among the more unusual sexual practices you may encounter is the technique known as "fisting," which involves placing the closed fist and wrist into a body orifice (vagina or rectum) for sexual stimulation. Whether the patient is male or female, organ rupture (rectum, vagina) is possible. Life-threatening peritonitis may result. Another sexual practice is the insertion of live animals into the vagina or rectum, including fish, eels, snakes, worms, and hamsters. The patient becomes alarmed when the animal goes in but does not come out.

Assessment in this situation is sensitive. Maintain your patient's privacy. Depending on the circumstances, you may need to inspect the genital area for bleeding, wounds, or objects that may need to be stabilized. Avoid focusing on only one part of your patient; you still need to conduct a thorough patient assessment including vital signs and history.

Treat such a case as you would with any other foreign object, remain nonjudgmental, and transport. Do not attempt to retrieve the object, even if it is an animal, from inside the vagina or rectum. Transport the patient in a knees-flexed, legs-together position.

YOU are the Provider SUMMARY

1. Should this patient be encouraged to bathe?

This patient should be discouraged from bathing, voiding, or cleaning any wounds until hospital personnel have completed a sexual assault assessment. If she insists on urinating, then have her do so in a sterile urine container (if available). Also, have her deposit the toilet paper in a paper bag. Seal and mark the bag for the police. This can be critical evidence.

2. What are the possible medical impacts of a sexual assault on this patient?

Because of the unknown health status of the assailant, the patient could be exposed to any number of STDs, including chlamydia, gonorrhea, HIV, cytomegalovirus, genital herpes, and syphilis. The risk of transmission of several diseases can be mitigated by appropriate postexposure prophylaxis, which can be provided at the hospital.

3. If available, should a female provider accompany the patient in the rear of the ambulance?

Having a same-gender provider accompany the patient in the rear of the ambulance may relieve the patient's anxiety. Because of the vulnerable nature of these types of patients, a provider of the same gender may be better able to provide emotional support for the patient.

4. What kind of care does this patient require en route to the hospital?

This patient requires supportive care, as well as strong emotional support.

5. Does this type of call require any special documentation?

Documentation of a sexual assault call will need to be completed in extreme detail, to include the patient's history, assessment, treatment, and response to treatment. It is important to not speculate or interject opinion, but only to record the facts.

6. If you are able to preserve the patient's clothing in a bag for evidence, then in what type of bag should you place the clothing?

The patient's clothing should be placed in paper—not plastic—bags that are either carried on the ambulance or provided by law enforcement officers on scene. Plastic bags will allow for condensation to form, altering the evidence.

YOU are the Provider SUMMARY *(continued)*

EMS Patient Care Report (PCR)					
Date: 11-9-18	**Incident No.:** 20098256379		**Nature of Call:** Sexual assault	**Location:** 125 W. Bellevue Ln	
Dispatched: 2313	**En Route:** 2315	**At Scene:** 2320	**Transport:** 2341	**At Hospital:** 2349	**In Service:** 0022
Patient Information					
Age: 19 **Sex:** F **Weight (in kg [lb]):** 51 kg (112.2 lb)			**Allergies:** No known drug allergies **Medications:** None **Past Medical History:** None **Chief Complaint:** Sexual assault		
Vital Signs					
Time: 2321	**BP:** Not obtained	**Pulse:** Not obtained	**Respirations:** Not obtained	**Spo_2:** Not obtained	
Time: 2335	**BP:** 102/68	**Pulse:** 120	**Respirations:** 22	**Spo_2:** 99%	
Time:	**BP:**	**Pulse:**	**Respirations:**	**Spo_2:**	
EMS Treatment (circle all that apply)					
Oxygen @ _______ L/min via (circle one): **NC NRM Bag-mask device**		**Assisted Ventilation**	**Airway Adjunct**	**CPR**	
Defibrillation	**Bleeding Control**	**Bandaging**	**Splinting**	**Other:**	
Narrative					
EMS called to above location for a female who was sexually assaulted. On arrival, patient found ambulatory on scene, speaking with Officer Feakes with GCSO (Badge #302). Patient states she was making a late-night snack in her kitchen when an unknown Caucasian male broke into her house and sexually assaulted her with vaginal penetration. Patient is visibly upset, stating that the "Bastard didn't even use a condom" and that she feels dirty and would like to bathe. GCSO 302 and I relay the importance of evidence preservation by not bathing, and the patient states she will wait until she gets to the ED. Patient denies any vaginal bleeding or other associated trauma from the assault. Assisted the patient to the stretcher and secured in a position of comfort. En route to Northern Rockies Medical Center the patient states, "I don't know what I did to deserve this" and that she "just wants to be left alone." Patient reassured that this was not her fault and she did nothing to deserve it. Report called to ED with condition and ETA. On arrival, care and report given to RN without incident.**End of report**					

Prep Kit

▶ Ready for Review

- Occasionally, you will be called for a patient experiencing a gynecologic emergency unrelated to pregnancy. The problem may include excessive bleeding, soft-tissue injuries, or infection.
- The reproductive system is very vascular, and there is a great potential for massive hemorrhage. Familiarity with a woman's anatomy and normal physiology will prepare you to assess and treat most common gynecologic conditions.
- Menstruation is the cyclic shedding of the uterine lining that usually occurs when no fertilized egg implants. Conditions associated with abnormalities of the menstrual cycle include premenstrual syndrome, mittelschmerz, and amenorrhea; prehospital treatment for these conditions is predominantly supportive.
- Disorders in the female reproductive system can lead to gynecologic emergencies. These disorders include acute or chronic infection, hemorrhage, rupture of a cyst, and rupture of an ectopic pregnancy.
- Pelvic inflammatory disease (PID) is caused by an acute or chronic infection in the organs of the female pelvic cavity. The chief symptoms of PID are pelvic pain and fever, which typically occur within 1 week of the menstrual period.
- Sexually transmitted diseases are the primary infection that can lead to PID.
- Bacterial vaginosis is an infection in which normal bacteria in the vagina are replaced by an overgrowth of other bacteria. Symptoms may include itching, burning, or pain and may be accompanied by a "fishy," foul-smelling discharge.
- Chancroid is caused by infection. Signs and symptoms include painful sores (usually of the genitals), and swollen, painful lymph glands or inguinal buboes in the groin area; some women may be asymptomatic.
- Chlamydia is a very common sexually transmitted disease with symptoms that are usually mild or absent, although some women may have lower abdominal pain, low back pain, nausea, fever, pain during intercourse, or bleeding between menstrual periods.
- Cytomegalovirus is a member of the herpesvirus family. In its active stages, this infection may produce prolonged high fever, chills, headache, malaise, extreme fatigue, and an enlarged spleen.
- Genital herpes is an infection of the genitals, buttocks, or anal area caused by herpes simplex virus, type 1 or type 2. An outbreak of herpes first causes small red bumps that develop into small blisters, then become itchy, painful sores. Other symptoms include fever, muscle aches and pains, headache, dysuria, vaginal discharge, and swollen glands in the groin area.
- Gonorrhea is a sexually transmitted disease whose symptoms include dysuria (painful urination), with associated burning or itching, a yellowish or bloody vaginal discharge, usually with a foul odor, and occult blood associated with vaginal intercourse. More severe infections may present with cramping and abdominal pain, nausea and vomiting, and bleeding between periods; these symptoms indicate that the infection has progressed to PID.
- Genital warts are caused by the human papillomavirus. Some infected people have no symptoms. In others, multiple growths develop in the genital areas.
- Syphilis causes signs and symptoms that mimic other diseases. A person with syphilis may remain asymptomatic for years, or have symptoms such as sores, rash, mucous membrane lesions, fever, swollen lymph glands, sore throat, patchy hair loss, headaches, weight loss, muscle aches, and fatigue.
- Trichomoniasis is caused by a single-celled protozoan parasite. The infected person may be asymptomatic or may experience signs and symptoms including a frothy, yellow-green vaginal discharge with a strong odor, as well as irritation and itching of the female genital area, discomfort during intercourse, dysuria, and lower abdominal pain.
- Symptoms of a vaginal yeast infection include itching, burning, soreness in the vagina and around the vulva, and vulvar swelling. Some women may report a thick, white vaginal discharge ("cottage cheese" appearance), pain during sexual intercourse, and burning on urination.
- A ruptured ovarian cyst can cause gynecologic/abdominal pain. An ovarian cyst is a fluid-filled sac attached to the inside or outside of the ovary. Such cysts may need to be removed surgically to relieve pressure or to treat infection.
- Ectopic pregnancy is a pregnancy that develops outside the uterus, most often in a fallopian tube. Symptoms include vaginal bleeding. Consider the possibility of an ectopic pregnancy in any female of reproductive age who has abdominal pain.
- Vaginal bleeding may be caused by normal menstruation, spontaneous abortion (miscarriage), placenta previa, abruptio placenta, or trauma, among other causes.
- Endometritis is an inflammation or irritation of the endometrium; it is treated with antibiotics. Left untreated, it may lead to septic shock or cause spontaneous abortion in a pregnant patient.

Prep Kit *(continued)*

- Endometriosis is a painful condition in which endometrial tissue grows outside the uterus; it often causes infertility. Prehospital care of the patient with endometriosis includes pain relief, placing the patient in a position of comfort, and use of dressings in case of vaginal bleeding.
- Postpartum eclampsia should be suspected when a woman has seizures and hypertension and has delivered a baby a few weeks earlier. Paramedic backup is required in such a case.
- Most patients experiencing a gynecologic emergency will be treated in the same manner regardless of the cause. Bleeding should be controlled, and the patient's ABCDEs should be assessed and monitored closely. Watch for developing signs of shock, and treat appropriately. Provide transport to the closest appropriate facility.
- Patient history has a major role when you are caring for a patient with a gynecologic emergency. Along with a detailed history of the present illness, ask the patient about any previous gynecologic problems and her obstetric history. Consider the possibility of ectopic pregnancy in any patient of childbearing age with abdominal pain.
- Always question the patient in privacy to maintain confidentiality.
- Perform a detailed physical examination, with close attention to preserving the patient's privacy. Expose only the areas that you need to examine, and cover the patient with a sheet. Monitor the patient closely for changes that may indicate shock is developing.
- Excessive bleeding is a serious emergency. Cover the vagina with a sterile pad; change the pad as often as necessary, and take all used pads to the hospital for examination. Pharmacologic interventions are generally not indicated. Contact medical control for further instructions.
- Use local pressure and a diaper-type bandage to hold dressings in place when treating nonobstetric injuries to the external genitalia. Never place dressings in the vagina. Treat patients with these injuries as you would any other victim of blood loss.
- When the patient is potentially in shock, place her in the shock position dictated by local protocol and keep her warm.
- Patients with PID generally walk doubled over guard the abdomen, and appear ill. Care includes placing the patient in a position of comfort and transport to an appropriate facility.
- Patients with a ruptured ovarian cyst usually have unilateral pain that may radiate from the abdomen to the back. Rupture of the cyst may result in some vaginal bleeding.
- Patients with a potential ectopic pregnancy usually present with signs of hypovolemic shock. Monitor the patient and establish a second intravenous line with a large-bore catheter. Place the patient in the shock position dictated by local protocol. Transport the patient rapidly to the closest appropriate facility.
- Treat patients with heavy vaginal bleeding on the basis of presenting signs and symptoms.
- Patients who have experienced abdominal trauma generally present with a variety of signs and symptoms that can include severe bleeding, pain, and hypovolemic shock. Management should be based on patient presentation.
- In the case of sexual assault or rape, treat for shock if necessary, and record all the facts in detail. Follow any crime scene policy established by your system to protect the scene and any potential evidence. Discourage the patient from washing, douching, or voiding until a physician has examined him or her.
- A common sexual gynecologic emergency an AEMT may encounter is a foreign object that has become stuck in the vagina or rectum. Keep the patient calm, protect his or her dignity as much as possible, and transport; do not attempt to remove the foreign object.

▶ Vital Vocabulary

abortion Delivery of the fetus and placenta before 20 weeks' gestation; a spontaneous abortion is called a miscarriage.

abruptio placenta Premature separation of the placenta from the wall of the uterus.

amenorrhea Absence of menstruation.

anus The outlet of the rectum.

bacterial vaginosis An overgrowth of bacteria in the vagina, characterized by itching, burning, or pain, and possibly a "fishy" smelling discharge.

cervix The lower one-third, or neck, of the uterus.

chancroid A highly contagious sexually transmitted disease caused by the bacteria *Haemophilus ducreyi*, which causes painful sores (ulcers), usually of the genitals.

chlamydia A sexually transmitted disease caused by the bacterium *Chlamydia trachomatis*.

clitoris The small erectile body partially hidden by the labia minora. It is covered by the prepuce, or foreskin.

Prep Kit *(continued)*

cytomegalovirus (CMV) A herpesvirus that can produce the symptoms of prolonged high fever, chills, headache, malaise, extreme fatigue, and an enlarged spleen.

dysmenorrhea Painful menstruation.

ectopic pregnancy A pregnancy that develops outside the uterus, typically in a fallopian tube.

endometriosis A condition in which endometrial tissue grows outside the uterus.

endometritis An inflammation of the endometrium that often is associated with a bacterial infection.

endometrium The inner layer of the uterine wall.

fallopian tubes Tubes or ducts that extend from near the ovaries and terminate at the uterus; also called uterine tubes.

fundus The uppermost part of the uterus, farthest from the cervical opening.

genital herpes An infection of the genitals, buttocks, or anal area caused by herpes simplex virus, which may cause sores of the genitals, mouth, or lips.

gonorrhea A sexually transmitted disease caused by *Neisseria gonorrhoeae*.

human papillomavirus (HPV) The most common sexually transmitted disease, caused by a virus, which may cause no symptoms or cause multiple growths in the genital areas.

hymen A fold of mucous membrane that partially covers the entrance to the vagina.

labia majora The outer lip-shaped structure of the vagina.

labia minora The inner lip-shaped structure of the vagina.

menarche The initial onset of menstruation occurring during puberty.

menopause The cessation of the menstrual cycle and ovarian function.

menstruation The cyclic shedding of the uterine lining that occurs approximately every 28 days.

mons pubis The pad of fatty tissue and coarse skin that lies over the pubic symphysis.

myometrium The muscular wall of the uterus.

oocytes Female sex cells.

ovaries Almond-shaped organs that lie on either side of the pelvic cavity. Their functions are to produce ova and certain hormones.

pelvic inflammatory disease (PID) An infection of the female upper organs of reproduction, specifically the uterus, ovaries, and fallopian tubes.

perineum The area of skin between the vagina and the anus.

placenta previa A condition in which the placenta develops over and partially or completely covers the cervix.

premenstrual syndrome (PMS) A cluster of all or some of the troubling symptoms that occur during a woman's menstrual phase that can include fluid retention, breast pain and tenderness, headache, severe cramping, and emotional changes, including agitation, irritability, depression, and anger.

prepuce The foreskin that covers the clitoris.

rape Sexual intercourse inflicted forcibly on another person, against that person's will.

sexual assault An attack against a person that is sexual in nature, the most of common of which is rape.

syphilis A sexually transmitted disease caused by the bacterium *Treponema pallidum*, which manifests in three stages—primary, secondary, and tertiary—and is transmitted through direct contact with open sores.

trichomoniasis A parasitic infection.

urethra Canal for the discharge of urine extending from the urinary bladder to the outside of the body.

uterus The muscular organ where the fetus grows, also called the womb; responsible for contractions during labor.

vagina The outermost cavity of a woman's reproductive system; the lower part of the birth canal.

vaginal orifice Opening of the vagina.

vaginal yeast infection An infection caused by the fungus *Candida albicans*, in which fungi overpopulate the vagina.

vestibule Small space at the beginning of an opening.

vulva The visible external female genitalia.

► References

1. Direkvand-Moghadam A, Sayehmiri K, Delpisheh A, Kaikhavandi S. Epidemiology of premenstrual syndrome (PMS): a systematic review and meta-analysis study. *J Clin Diagn Res.* 2014;8(2):106–109. https://www.ncbi.nlm.nih.gov/pmc/articles/PMC3972521/. Accessed January 25, 2017.
2. Mittelschmerz. *MedlinePlus.* May 9, 2015.https://medlineplus.gov/ency/article/001503.htm. Accessed January 25, 2017.
3. Bacterial vaginosis (BV) statistics. Centers for Disease Control and Prevention website. December 17, 2015. https://www.cdc.gov/std/bv/stats.htm. Accessed February 13, 2017.
4. Chlamydia statistics. Centers for Disease Control and Prevention website. December 9, 2016. https://www.cdc.gov/std/chlamydia/stats.htm. Accessed February 13, 2017.

Prep Kit *(continued)*

5. Genital herpes: CDC fact sheet (detailed). Centers for Disease Control and Prevention website. November 17, 2015. https://www.cdc.gov/std/herpes/stdfact-herpes-detailed.htm. Accessed January 25, 2017.
6. Gonorrhea: CDC fact sheet (detailed version). Centers for Disease Control and Prevention website. October 28, 2016. https://www.cdc.gov/std/gonorrhea/stdfact-gonorrhea-detailed.htm. Accessed January 25, 2017.
7. Human papillomavirus. Centers for Disease Control and Prevention website. November 15, 2016. https://www.cdc.gov/vaccines/pubs/pinkbook/hpv.html. Accessed January 25, 2017.
8. Tulandi T. Ectopic pregnancy: incidence, risk factors, and pathology. *UpToDate*. April 13, 2016. http://www.uptodate.com/contents/ectopic-pregnancy-incidence-risk-factors-and-pathology. Accessed January 25, 2017.
9. U.S. Department of Health and Human Services, National Institutes of Health, National Institute of Child Health and Human Development. How many people are affected by or at risk for endometriosis? https://www.nichd.nih.gov/health/topics/endometri/conditioninfo/Pages/at-risk.aspx. Accessed January 25, 2017.
10. American Society for Reproductive Medicine. Endometriosis: a guide for patients. 2012. http://www.asrm.org/uploadedFiles/ASRM_Content/Resources/Patient_Resources/Fact_Sheets_and_Info_Booklets/endometriosis.pdf. Accessed January 25, 2017.
11. Illinois Coalition Against Sexual Assault. The prevalence of rape in the United States. December 22, 2011. http://www.icasa.org/docs/misc/cq%20rape%20stats%2012-11%20final.pdf. Accessed January 25, 2017.
12. National Sexual Violence Resource Center. Statistics about sexual violence. 2015. http://www.nsvrc.org/sites/default/files/publications_nsvrc_factsheet_media-packet_statistics-about-sexual-violence_0.pdf. Accessed January 25, 2017.

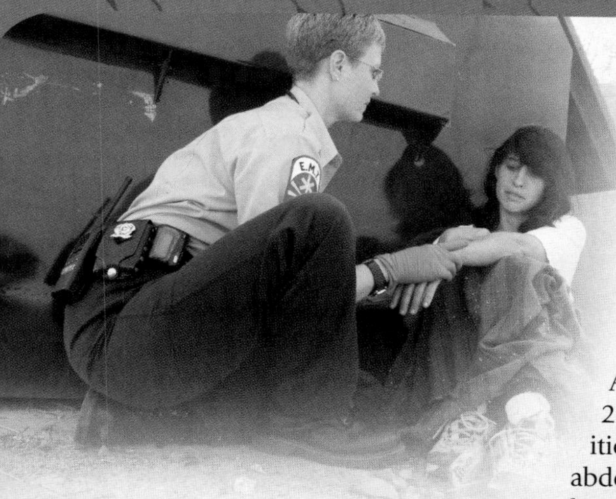

Assessment *in Action*

You are dispatched to a low-rise apartment building for a woman reporting abdominal pain. As you exit the ambulance, you can hear a woman screaming out in pain from the apartment. After you ensure the scene is safe for you to enter, you find a 22-year-old woman in the back bedroom lying in the fetal position on the bed. The patient states she is having severe cramping abdominal pain that has lasted approximately 90 minutes. You note a large amount of blood pooling around the patient's vaginal area.

When questioned about her medical history, the patient states her last menstrual period was 3 months ago. She was seen at her obstetrician's office last week, when he informed her she was approximately 8 weeks pregnant. This is her first pregnancy.

1. On the basis of the history provided, you believe this patient is experiencing:

A. abruptio placenta.
B. placenta previa.
C. a ruptured ectopic pregnancy.
D. a heavy menstrual period.

2. In the case of an ectopic pregnancy, where does the fertilized egg most often become implanted?

A. Fundus
B. Fallopian tube
C. Ovary
D. Vestibule

Assessment in Action (continued)

3. Ectopic pregnancies are usually recognized during the first __________ weeks of pregnancy.

A. 2 to 3
B. 3 to 4
C. 4 to 6
D. 6 to 8

4. How would you document this patient's obstetric history if she has had a miscarriage?

A. G1 P0 A0
B. G1 P1 A0
C. G1 P1 A1
D. G1 P0 A1

5. As part of your physical exam of this patient, you should evaluate the blood for all of the following, EXCEPT:

A. tissue.
B. clots.
C. volume.
D. odor.

6. Yeast infections are typically caused by:

A. *Candida albicans.*
B. *Trichomonas vaginalis.*
C. *Treponema pallidum.*
D. *Haemophilus ducreyi.*

7. All of the following are signs of pelvic inflammatory disease EXCEPT:

A. abdominal pain.
B. vaginal discharge.
C. dyspareunia.
D. dysuria.

8. If your patient is a female teenager who is uncomfortable discussing her gynecologic problems, then what steps can you take to make her comfortable?

A. Postpone taking the patient's history until transport begins, ensuring the patient's parents, if present, travel in a separate vehicle to the hospital.
B. Gently explain to the patient that because she is a minor, her parents must be a part of the conversation, and encourage her to answer your questions in their presence.
C. Find a way to allow the patient to talk with you privately, and assure her of your discretion.
D. Forgo taking the patient's history, since her answers may not be true.

9. What is the proper way to preserve evidence when treating a sexual assault patient?

10. List the signs and symptoms of endometritis.

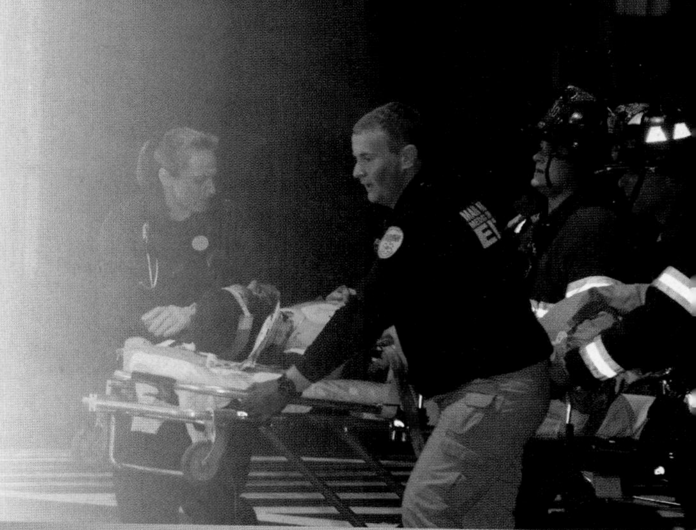

SECTION 8

Trauma

CHAPTER 26

Trauma Overview

National EMS Education Standard Competencies

Trauma

Applies fundamental knowledge to provide basic and selected advanced emergency care and transportation based on assessment findings for an acutely injured patient.

Trauma Overview

Pathophysiology, assessment, and management of the trauma patient

- Trauma scoring (pp 1085, 1087)
- Rapid transport and destination issues (pp 1083-1085)
- Transport mode (pp 1083-1084)

Multisystem Trauma

Recognition and management of

- Multisystem trauma (pp 1080-1081)

Pathophysiology, assessment, and management of

- Multisystem trauma (pp 1080-1081)
- Blast injuries (pp 1077-1080)

Knowledge Objectives

1. Define the term *mechanism of injury* (MOI), and explain its relationship to potential energy, kinetic energy, and work. (pp 1061-1063)
2. Define the term *index of suspicion*, and explain its relationship to the advanced emergency medical technician's (AEMT's) assessment of trauma. (pp 1061, 1063)
3. Define the terms *blunt trauma* and *penetrating trauma*, and provide examples of the MOI that would cause each one to occur. (pp 1063-1077)
4. Describe the five types of motor vehicle collisions, the injury patterns associated with each one, and how each relates to the index of suspicion of life-threatening injuries. (pp 1066-1072)
5. Discuss the three specific factors to consider during assessment of a patient who has been injured in a fall, plus additional considerations for pediatric and geriatric patients. (pp 1074-1076)
6. Discuss the effects of high-, medium-, and low-velocity penetrating trauma on the body and how an understanding of each type helps the AEMT form an index of suspicion about unseen life-threatening injuries. (pp 1076-1077)
7. Discuss primary, secondary, tertiary, and miscellaneous blast injuries, and describe the anticipated damage each one will cause to the body. (pp 1077-1080)
8. Describe multisystem trauma and the special considerations that are required for patients who fit this category, and provide a general overview of multisystem trauma patient management. (pp 1080-1081)
9. Outline the major components of trauma patient assessment, including considerations related to whether the MOI was significant or nonsignificant. (p 1081)
10. Discuss the special assessment considerations related to a trauma patient who has injuries in each of the following areas: head, neck and throat, chest, and abdomen. (pp 1081-1082)
11. Describe trauma patient management in relation to scene time, type of transport, and destination selection and list the Association of Air Medical Services criteria for the appropriate use of emergency air medical services. (pp 1083-1085)
12. Discuss the facilities and transport resources available through emergency medical services (EMS) trauma systems. (pp 1084-1085)
13. Describe the American College of Surgeons' Committee on Trauma classification of trauma centers and how it relates to making an appropriate destination selection for a trauma patient. (pp 1085-1086)

Skills Objectives

There are no skills objectives for this chapter.

Introduction

According to the US Centers for Disease Control and Prevention (CDC), unintentional injury is the primary cause of death and disability in people between ages 1 and 44 years.[1,2] Proper prehospital evaluation and care can do much to minimize suffering, long-term disability, and death from trauma. Understanding the basic physical concepts that determine how injuries occur and affect the human body will allow you to size up a crash scene and use that information as a vital part of patient assessment.

This chapter begins with a basic discussion of energy and trauma. Next, different types of vehicle crashes and their effects on the body are explained. Evaluation of the **mechanism of injury (MOI)** for the trauma patient will provide the advanced emergency medical technician (AEMT) with an **index of suspicion** for different types of serious and/or life-threatening underlying injuries. Certain injury patterns occur with certain types of injury events. The index of suspicion is your awareness and concern for potentially serious underlying and unseen injuries. The amount of energy exchanged also has a major role in the severity of injuries, along with the anatomic structures potentially involved. All of these factors will influence your approach to assessing and treating trauma patients in the field.

Energy and Trauma

Traumatic injury occurs when the body's tissues are exposed to energy levels beyond their tolerance **Figure 26-1**. The MOI is the way in which traumatic injuries occur; it describes the forces (or energy transmission) acting on the body that cause injury. Three concepts of energy are typically associated with injury (not including thermal energy, which causes burns): **potential energy**, **kinetic energy**, and the energy of **work**. When considering the effects of energy on the human body, it is important to remember that energy can be neither created nor destroyed but can only be converted or transformed. It is not the objective of this section to help you to reconstruct the scene of a motor vehicle crash. Rather, you should have a sense of the effects of the event on the human body and understand, in a broad sense, how that work is related to potential and kinetic energy.

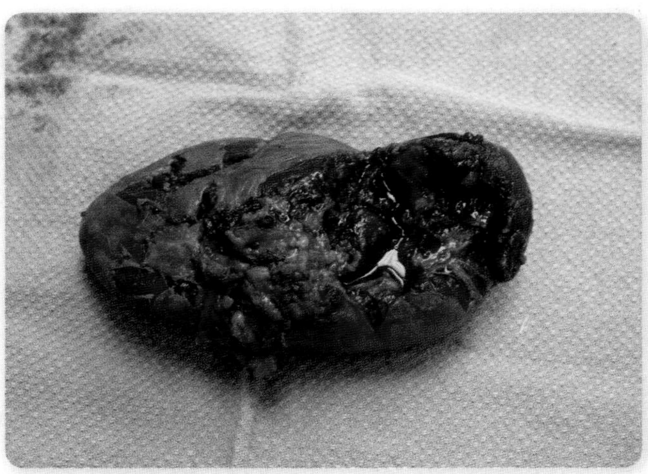

Figure 26-1 Traumatic injury occurs when the body's tissues are exposed to energy levels beyond their tolerance. This photo shows a ruptured spleen.

Work is defined as force acting over a distance. For example, the force needed to bend metal multiplied by the distance over which the metal is bent is the work that crushes the front end of a vehicle that is involved in a frontal impact. Similarly, forces that bend, pull, or compress tissues beyond their inherent limits result in the work that causes injury.

Different forms of energy produce different kinds of trauma. These external energy sources can be mechanical, chemical, thermal, electrical, and barometric.

Mechanical energy is energy from motion. Mechanical energy is subdivided into two types mentioned previously: kinetic energy (such as a moving vehicle) and potential energy (energy stored in an object, such as a brick sitting on a building ledge).

Kinetic energy reflects the relationship between the mass (weight) of the object and the velocity (speed) at which it is traveling and would be found in the force of two moving vehicles colliding. Kinetic energy is expressed as:

$$\text{Kinetic energy} = (\tfrac{1}{2} \times \text{Mass}) \times \text{Velocity}^2,$$
$$\text{or KE} = \tfrac{1}{2}\text{m} \times \text{v}^2$$

YOU are the Provider PART 1

Your ambulance is dispatched to a motor vehicle collision just outside of town. As you advise your dispatch that you are responding, you are told this incident is the result of a high-speed police pursuit and the fleeing car rear-ended a small pickup truck at a stop sign. Officers advise the impact was approximately 85 to 90 mph, and they believe that the driver of the fleeing car is dead.

1. On the basis of the information provided, what are some possible injuries you may encounter?
2. With the understanding that patients at this scene are most likely critical, how long should you remain on scene?

Remember that energy cannot be created or destroyed, only converted. In the case of a motor vehicle crash, the kinetic energy of the speeding vehicle is converted into the work of stopping the vehicle, usually by crushing the vehicle's exterior Figure 26-2. Similarly, the passengers of the vehicle have kinetic energy because they were traveling at the same speed as the vehicle. Their kinetic energy is converted to the work of bringing them to a stop. It is this work on the passengers that results in injury. Notice that, according to the equation for kinetic energy, the energy that is available to cause injury *doubles* when an object's weight doubles but *quadruples* when its speed doubles. When a vehicle's speed increases from 50 to 70 mph, the energy that is available to cause injury

Words of Wisdom

Newton's First Law

Newton's first law states that objects at rest tend to stay at rest and objects in motion tend to stay in motion unless acted on by some outside force. An example of the first part of the law is an empty soda can that will not move spontaneously unless some force, such as a gust of wind, acts on it. An example of the second part might be as follows: in a vehicle going 50 mph that strikes a concrete barrier and comes to a sudden stop, the passengers continue to travel forward at 50 mph. They stay in motion until they are acted on by an external force—most likely the seat belt, windshield, steering wheel, or dashboard. The same thing happens to the driver's internal organs, which are acted on by the sternum, rib cage, or other body structure. This scenario illustrates the three collisions that are associated with blunt trauma.

Newton's Second Law

Newton's second law states that force (F) equals mass (m) times acceleration (a)—that is, $F = m \times a$—in which acceleration is the change in velocity (speed) that occurs over time. This change can be positive (acceleration) or negative (deceleration). Therefore, Mass × Acceleration = Force = Mass × Deceleration.

In the example of a vehicle traveling at 30 mph, it takes approximately 3 seconds for the car to decrease its speed from 30 to 0 mph when the driver applies the brakes smoothly. The driver slows, or decelerates, at the same rate as the vehicle. But if the vehicle is stopped not by braking but by hitting a large tree and the driver is not restrained, his or her body will continue to stay in motion at 30 mph until it is stopped by an external force: in this case, by hitting the steering wheel. Although the change in the body's velocity is the same as when the vehicle was braking smoothly in 3 seconds (30 to 0 mph), that change now takes place in approximately 0.01 second. Because the period of **deceleration** is 300 times less, the average force of impact is 300 times greater. This means that the force is approximately 150 times the force of gravity. Imagine a force 150 times your body weight slamming into your chest.

Now consider the same vehicle striking the same tree, but this time, the driver is restrained with a shoulder and lap belt. The driver is essentially tied to the vehicle and stops during the same period the vehicle stops. It takes some time, although brief, to crush the front of the car and bring it to a halt. The vehicle comes to a stop in approximately 0.05 second. The change in the driver's velocity is the same (30 to 0 mph), but the longer period of deceleration results in a *g* force of only 30 times that of gravity (one *g* force is the normal acceleration due to gravity). This is still a substantial force, but it is much less than the force experienced by the unrestrained driver. More to the point, it is survivable.

In a final example, the vehicle and driver, as before, are traveling at 30 mph, and the driver is properly restrained with a 3-point belt. In this case, however, the vehicle is also equipped with an air bag. When the vehicle hits the tree and suddenly stops, the driver's upper body initially continues forward at 30 mph. The body is partially slowed by the lap and shoulder belts but is finally brought to rest by the air bag. The upper body compresses the air bag, which stops the body's forward motion in approximately 0.1 second. Thus, the air bag stretches the duration of impact by 0.05 second, buying the body even more time, and the force on the upper body decreases to approximately 15 times that of gravity.

The air bag has another advantage that, coupled with increasing the duration of impact, results in less severe injuries. The force of its impact is applied over a much larger area than the area affected by the steering wheel or the shoulder belt, shrinking the force per unit area. This point can be illustrated by an analogy. A person standing on one toe on a sheet of ice applies a concentrated load in a very small area, thus breaking the ice and falling through. If the person lies flat on the ice, he or she greatly expands the contact area and reduces the stress on the ice, making it less likely to break. The dual action of the air bag (distributing the force of impact over a greater area and increasing the duration of impact) results in less severe injuries.

Newton's Third Law

Newton's third law states that for every action, there is an equal and opposite reaction. Therefore, if you push on a door, the door pushes back (reacts) with an equal force but in the opposite direction. In the case of a dented A-pillar, the force of the driver's head was sufficient to dent the strong metal. But in patient assessment, the more important point is the reaction force of the pillar on the head. Regarding Newton's third law, the head was essentially hit by an A-pillar traveling at 30 mph. Similarly, it takes a substantial force to collapse a steering wheel. When you notice a collapsed steering wheel during scene size-up, suspect serious chest injuries, even if the driver initially has no visible signs of chest injury.

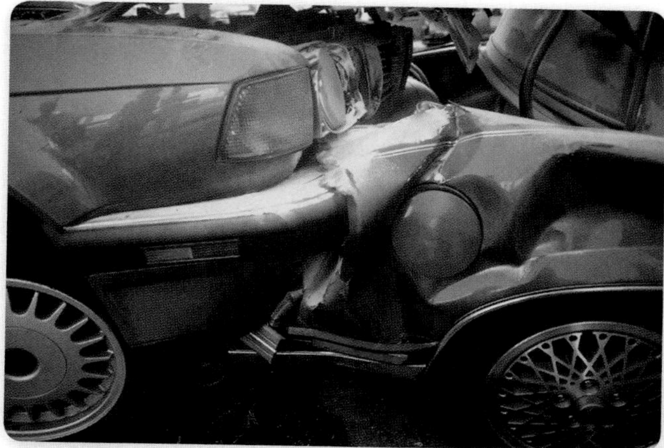

Figure 26-2 In a motor vehicle collision, the kinetic energy of the speeding vehicle is converted into the work of stopping the vehicle, usually by crushing the vehicle's exterior.

doubles. This point is even clearer when considering gunshot wounds. The speed of the bullet (high velocity compared with low velocity) has a greater effect on producing injury than the mass (size) of the bullet. This is why it is so important to report to the hospital the type of firearm that was used in a shooting. The amount of kinetic energy that is converted to do work on the body determines the severity of the injury. High-energy injuries often produce such severe damage that only immediate transport to an appropriate facility may save the patient.

Potential energy is the product of mass (weight), force of gravity, and height and is mostly associated with the energy of falling objects. It would be present in an object sitting at a height. In that case, gravity would be the *potential* source of energy that converts to kinetic energy if the object falls. A worker on a scaffold has some potential energy because he or she is some height above the ground. If the worker falls, potential energy is converted into kinetic energy. As the worker hits the ground, the kinetic energy is converted into work, that is, the work of bringing the body to a stop and thereby fracturing bones and damaging tissues.

Chemical energy is the energy released as a result of a chemical reaction and can be found in an explosive, an acid, or even from a reaction to an ingested or medically delivered agent or drug. **Thermal energy** is energy transferred from sources that are hotter than the body, such as a flame, hot water, and steam. **Electrical energy** comes in the form of high-voltage electrocution or a lightning strike. **Barometric energy** can result from sudden and radical changes in pressure, as can occur during scuba diving or flying in an unpressurized cabin.

Kinetics studies the relationships among speed, mass, direction of the force, and, for AEMTs, the physical injury caused by speed, mass, and force. Knowledge of kinetics can help you predict injury patterns found in your patient.

Mechanism of Injury Profiles

Different types of MOIs will produce many types of injuries. Some will involve an isolated body system; many will result in injury to more than one body system. Injuries sustained by trauma patients may be the result of **multisystem trauma** (injury to more than one body system), falls from heights, motor vehicle and motorcycle crashes, vehicle versus pedestrian (or bicycle or motorcycle), gunshot wounds, and stabbings. Whether one body system or more than one system is involved, maintain a high index of suspicion for serious unseen injuries. Table 26-1 lists significant MOIs that you will read about in this chapter.

Blunt and Penetrating Trauma

Traumatic injuries can be described in two separate categories: **blunt trauma** and **penetrating trauma**. Blunt trauma is the result of force (or energy transmission) to the body that causes injury primarily without anything penetrating the soft tissues or internal organs and cavities. Penetrating

Table 26-1 Significant Mechanisms of Injury

Age	Mechanisms
Adults	▪ Multiple body systems injured ▪ Ejection from a vehicle ▪ Death of another person in the same vehicle ▪ Fall from a height >20 feet (6 m) ▪ Vehicle rollover (unrestrained) ▪ High-speed (>40 mph) vehicle crash ▪ Vehicle-pedestrian collision ▪ Motorcycle crash of >20 mph ▪ Unresponsiveness or altered mental status following trauma ▪ Penetrating trauma to the head, chest, or abdomen
Children	All mechanisms in the adult list, with the following additions or modifications: ▪ Fall >10 feet (3 m) or two to three times the child's height ▪ Fall of <10 feet (3 m) with loss of consciousness ▪ Medium- to high-speed vehicle crash (≥25 mph) ▪ Bicycle crash

trauma results in injury by objects that pierce and penetrate the surface of the body and injure the underlying soft tissues, internal organs, and body cavities. Either type of trauma may occur from a variety of MOIs. It is important for you to consider unseen as well as visible, obvious injuries with either type of trauma. Damage to the underlying deeper tissues is often more substantial.

Words of Wisdom

The top five causes of death from unintentional injury in the United States are poisoning (specifically opioiod overdose), motor vehicle crashes, falls, choking and suffocation, and drowning.[3]

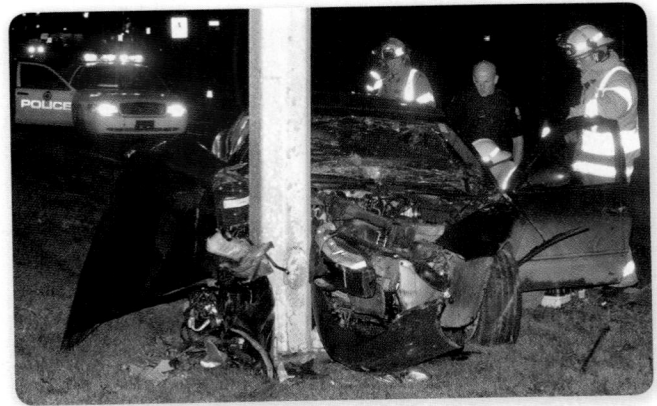

Figure 26-3 The first collision in a typical impact is that of the vehicle against another object (in this case, a utility pole). The appearance of the vehicle can provide you with critical information about the severity of the crash. The greater the damage to the vehicle, the greater the energy that was involved.

Blunt Trauma

Blunt force trauma results from an object making contact with the body. Any object (eg, a baseball bat) can cause blunt trauma if it is moving fast enough. Motor vehicle crashes and falls are two of the most common MOIs for blunt trauma. Be alert to signs of skin discoloration or reports of pain because these may be the only signs of blunt trauma. Maintain a high index of suspicion during patient assessment for hidden (internal) injuries in patients with blunt trauma.

Motor Vehicle Crashes

In 2014, according to the National Highway Traffic Safety Administration, 32,675 people were killed in police-reported motor vehicle traffic crashes, and 2.34 million people were injured.[4] That calculates to almost 90 people dying and more than 6,300 people being injured in motor vehicle crashes every day in the United States.

Motor vehicle crashes are classified traditionally as frontal (head-on), rear-end, lateral (T-bone), rollovers, and rotational (spins). The principal difference among these crash types is the direction of the force of impact; also, with spins and rollovers, there is the possibility of multiple impacts. Motor vehicle crashes typically consist of a series of three collisions. Understanding the events that occur during each collision will help you be alert for certain types of injury patterns. The three collisions in a typical impact are as follows:

1. The collision of the vehicle against another vehicle, a tree, or some other object. Damage to the vehicle is perhaps the most dramatic part of the collision, but it does not directly affect patient care, except possibly to make extrication difficult Figure 26-3. However, it does provide information about the severity of the collision and, therefore, has an indirect effect on patient care. The greater the damage to the vehicle, the greater the energy that was involved and, therefore, the greater the potential to cause injury to the patient. By assessing the vehicle that has crashed, you can often determine the MOI, which may allow you to predict what injuries may have happened to the passengers at the time of impact according to forces that acted on their bodies. When you arrive at the crash scene and perform your scene size-up, quickly inspect the severity of damage to the vehicle or vehicles. If there is substantial damage to a vehicle, your index of suspicion for the presence of life-threatening injuries should automatically increase. A great amount of force is required to crush and deform a vehicle, cause intrusion into the passenger compartment, tear seats from their mountings, and collapse steering wheels. Such damage suggests the presence of high-energy trauma and serious injury.
2. The collision of the passenger against the interior of the vehicle. Just as the kinetic energy produced by the vehicle's mass and velocity is converted into the work of bringing the vehicle to a stop, the kinetic energy produced by the passenger's mass and velocity is converted into the work of stopping his or her body Figure 26-4. Just like the obvious damage to the exterior of the vehicle, the injuries that result are often dramatic and usually immediately apparent during your scene size-up or primary survey. Common injuries include lower extremity fractures (knees into the dashboard), rib fractures (rib cage into the steering wheel), and head trauma (head into the windshield). Such injuries occur more frequently if the passenger is not restrained. But even when the passenger is restrained with a properly adjusted seat belt,

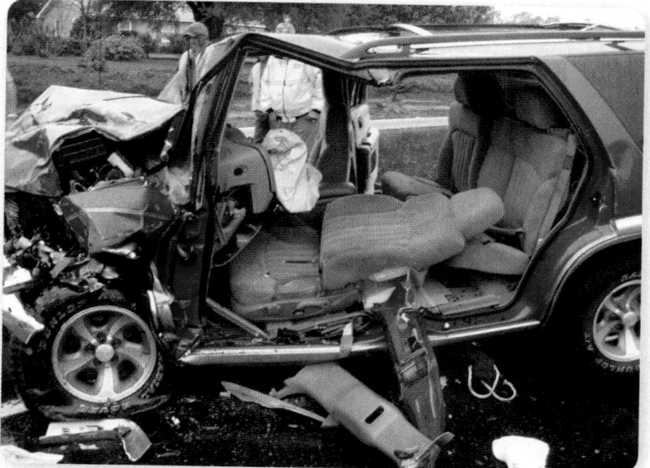

Figure 26-4 The second collision in a frontal impact is that of the passenger against the interior of the vehicle. Examining the interior of the vehicle may give you clues to hidden injuries.

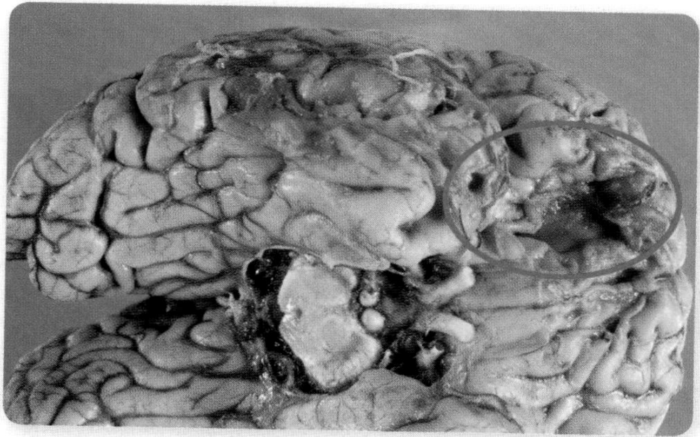

Figure 26-5 The discolored spots show injuries (contusions) in this brain.

injuries can occur, especially in lateral and rollover impacts.

3. The collision of the passenger's internal organs against the solid structures of the body. The injuries that occur during the third collision may not be as obvious as external injuries, but they are often the most life threatening. For example, as the passenger's head hits the windshield, the brain continues to move forward until it comes to rest by striking the inside of the skull. This results in compression injury (or bruising) to the anterior portion of the brain and stretching (or tearing) of the posterior portion of the brain **Figure 26-5**. Remember that for every action there is an equal and opposite reaction. As the brain strikes the front of the skull, the body begins its path of moving backward. The head falls back against the headrest and/or seat, and the brain slams into the rear of the skull. Damage is produced to both the front and rear of the brain. This type of injury is known as a

YOU are the Provider — PART 2

As you arrive on scene, you find an unidentifiable car with substantial front-end damage and a small pickup with severe rear-end damage. You immediately assign your partner to the patient in the pickup while you assess the patient in the car. You find the patient unrestrained, pulseless, and apneic, with severe facial trauma and exposed brain matter from the impact with the windshield. You tag the patient "Black" according to your triage protocols, and inform the officers that he is dead.

As you join your partner, she informs you that the patient is severely entrapped and has a Glasgow Coma Scale (GCS) score of 4 (E-1, V-2, M-1). You request that the fire department upgrade their response to a rescue assignment and also request your local flight service for aeromedical evacuation.

Recording Time: 1 Minute	
Appearance	Poor
Level of consciousness	Unresponsive, moans to pain
Airway	Patent
Breathing	8 breaths/min, shallow
Circulation	Cool, pale, and clammy

3. To which type of hospital should this patient be transported?

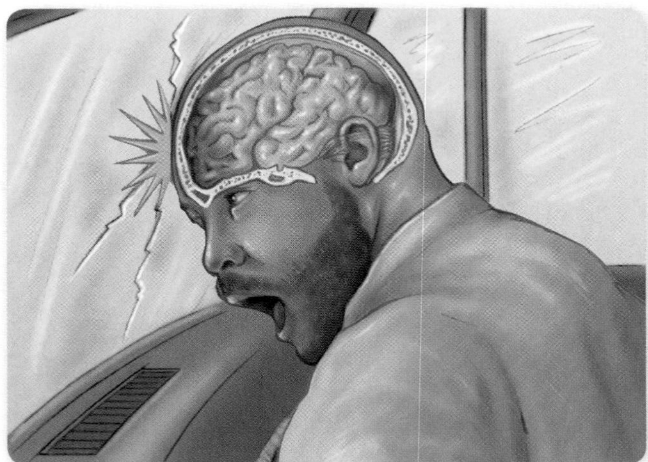

Figure 26-6 The third collision in a typical impact is that of the passenger's internal organs against the solid structures of the body. A coup-contrecoup injury occurs when the brain continues its forward motion and strikes the inside of the skull, resulting in a compression injury to the anterior portion of the brain and stretching of the posterior portion.

coup-contrecoup injury **Figure 26-6**. The same type of injury may occur on opposite sides of the brain in a lateral collision. Similarly, in the thoracic cage, the heart may slam into the sternum, occasionally rupturing the aorta and causing fatal bleeding.

Understanding the relationship among the three collisions will help you to make the connections between the amount of damage to the exterior of the vehicle and potential injury to the passenger. For example, in a high-speed crash that results in massive damage to the vehicle, you should suspect serious injuries to the passengers, even if the injuries are not readily apparent. Several potential physical problems may develop as a result of traumatic injuries. Your initial general impression of the patient and the evaluation of the MOI can help to direct lifesaving care and provide critical information to the hospital staff. Therefore, if you see a contusion on the patient's forehead and the windshield is starred and pushed out, you should strongly suspect an injury to the brain. After you inform medical control about the damage to the windshield, hospital staff can prepare for the patient by ordering a computed tomography scan of the brain. Without your input, the physician might have found the brain injury anyway, but it might not have been detected until the brain had swollen sufficiently to cause clinical signs of the injury. Whenever there is a substantial impact to the head, you should also consider the possibility of a spinal injury and take cervical spine precautions if indicated.

The amount of damage that is considered substantial varies, depending on the type of crash, but any substantial deformity of the vehicle should be enough cause for you to consider transporting the patient to a trauma center. Severe deformity of the vehicle or intrusion into the vehicle as listed below correlates to significant MOI:

- Severe deformities of the frontal part of a vehicle, with or without intrusion into the passenger compartment
- Moderate intrusions from a lateral (T-bone) type of collision
- Severe damage from the rear
- Crashes in which rotation is involved (rollovers and spins)

Words of Wisdom

When a patient has died in a vehicle, others in the vehicle may be upset by the death and unaware of their own injuries. As with all patients, be sure to assess them thoroughly.

Damage to the vehicle that was involved and information obtained during scene size-up are not the only clues to crash severity. Clearly, if one or more of the passengers is dead, you should suspect that the other passengers have sustained serious injuries, even if the injuries are not obvious. Therefore, you should focus on treating life-threatening injuries and providing rapid transport to a trauma center, because these passengers have likely experienced the same amount of force that caused the death of the other passengers. Digital photos of the crash scene may provide valuable information to the staff and treating physicians of the trauma center; however, photos should never be shared over social media. Photos containing patient images or other identifiable patient information may become part of the medical record or may need to be deleted after review by the receiving health care providers, depending on policies.

Patients should be assessed according to the area of the body that was most likely injured. Your evaluation should also be based, to some extent, on the patient's position in the vehicle, the use of seat belts, air bag deployment, and how the patient's body shifted during the crash. Drivers are typically at higher risk for serious injury than passengers because of the potential for striking the steering wheel with the chest, abdomen, or head. Front seat passengers may also be injured by striking the dashboard or windshield. **Table 26-2** describes the structural clues, body clues, and resulting injuries for different types of crashes.

Frontal Crashes. Understanding the MOI after a frontal crash first involves evaluation of the supplemental restraint system, including seat belts and air bags. You should determine whether the passenger was restrained by a full, properly applied three-point restraint. In addition, you should determine whether the air bag was deployed. Identifying the types of restraints used

Table 26-2 Mechanism of Injury: Motor Vehicle Crash

Structural Clues	Body Clues	Potential Injuries
Head-on or Frontal Impact		
Deformed front end Cracked windshield	Bruised or lacerated head or face	Brain injury Scalp, facial cuts Cervical spine injury Tracheal injury
Deformed steering column	Bruised neck Bruised chest	Sternal or rib fracture Flail chest Myocardial contusion Pericardial tamponade Pneumothorax or hemothorax Exsanguination from aortic tear
Deformed dashboard	Bruised abdomen Bruised knee, dislocated patella	Ruptured spleen, liver, bowel, diaphragm Fractured patella Dislocated knee Femoral fracture Dislocated hip
Lateral or Side Impact		
Deformed side of vehicle	Bruised shoulder	Clavicular fracture Fractured humerus Multiple rib fractures
Door smashed in	Bruised shoulder or pelvis	Fractured hip Fractured iliac wing Fractured clavicle or ribs
"B" pillar deformed	Bruised temple	Brain injury Cervical spine fracture
Broken door or window handles	Bruised or deformed arms	Contusions
Broken window glass	Dicing lacerations	Multiple lacerations
Rear-end Impact		
Posterior deformity of the vehicle	Secondary anterior injuries, especially if the patient was unrestrained	Whiplash injuries Deceleration injuries of a head-on impact
Headrest not adjusted	None detected	Bleeding, bruising, or tearing inside skull

Words of Wisdom

When you are assessing trauma incidents, MOI is a crucial element of patient history. Be alert to the extent of damage to the interior and exterior of the vehicles involved in crashes. Use these observations to paint a picture of the scene for later caregivers in verbal and written communication.

and whether air bags were deployed will help you identify injury patterns related to the supplemental restraint systems.

When properly applied, seat belts are successful in restraining the passengers in a vehicle and preventing a second collision inside the motor vehicle. According to the NHTSA, seat-belt use saved an estimated 13,941 lives in 2015.[5] In addition, they may decrease the severity of the third collision, that of the passenger's organs with the chest or abdominal wall. The protective abilities of seat belts are further enhanced by deployment of the air bags. Air bags provide the final capture point of the passengers and decrease the severity of deceleration injuries by allowing seat belts to be more compliant and by cushioning the occupant as the body slows, or decelerates.

Remember that air bags decrease injury to the chest, face, and head very effectively. However, you should still suspect that other serious injuries to the extremities (resulting from the second collision) and to internal organs (resulting from the third collision) have occurred.

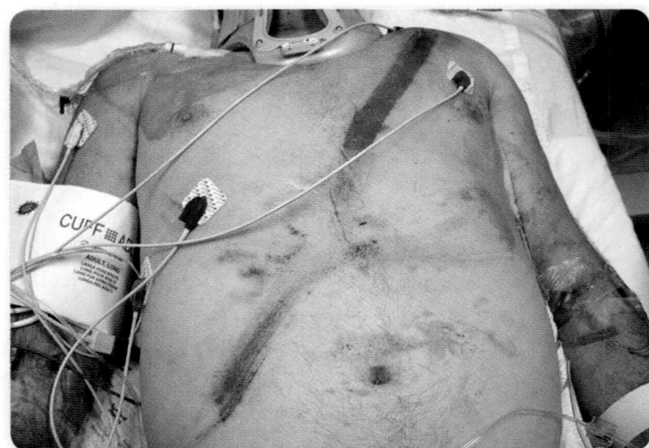

Figure 26-7 Injuries may result if the seat belt is worn too high or too low across the waist. Although less common, injuries can also result from seat belts worn in the correct position across the torso.

Safety

Never place yourself or your patient in front of an undeployed air bag. Even if the battery cables are disconnected, a charge can be held in the line, allowing the air bag to deploy at a later time and causing potentially severe injuries.

Most new motor vehicles are manufactured with air bag safety systems. These safety devices enhance the safety and survival of forward-facing occupants inside the vehicle during a crash. In an emergency braking event or crash, the air bag inflates very quickly. Because a rear-facing car seat is close to the dashboard, rapid inflation of the air bag could cause serious injury or death to an infant. All children who are shorter than 4 feet 9 inches (145 cm) should ride in the rear seat or, in the case of a pickup truck or other single-seated vehicle, the air bag should be turned off.

When you are providing care to an occupant inside a motor vehicle, it is important to remember that if the air bag did not inflate during the accident, it may deploy during extrication. If this occurs, you may be seriously injured or even killed. Extreme caution must be used when extricating a patient in a vehicle with an air bag that has not deployed.

Seat belts may also cause unseen abdominal injuries, particularly in pediatric patients. Seat belts are designed to be worn over the iliac crests of the pelvis to distribute the force over the bony surface. Hip injuries may result if seat belts are worn too low. Internal injuries can occur when the belt is worn too high, resulting in damage to abdominal organs **Figure 26-7**. Lumbar spine fractures are also possible, particularly in elderly patients.

When passengers who are riding in vehicles equipped with air bags are not restrained by seat belts, they are often thrown forward in the act of emergency braking. As a result, they come in contact with the air bag and/or the doors at the time of deployment. This MOI is also responsible for some severe injuries to children who are riding unrestrained in the front seats of vehicles, unrestrained passengers, and those sitting too close to the air bag.

In addition, some passengers may pass out before impact, and you may find them lying against the deployed air bag. When you encounter these types of situations, look for abrasions and/or traction-type injuries on the face, lower part of the neck, and chest **Figure 26-8**.

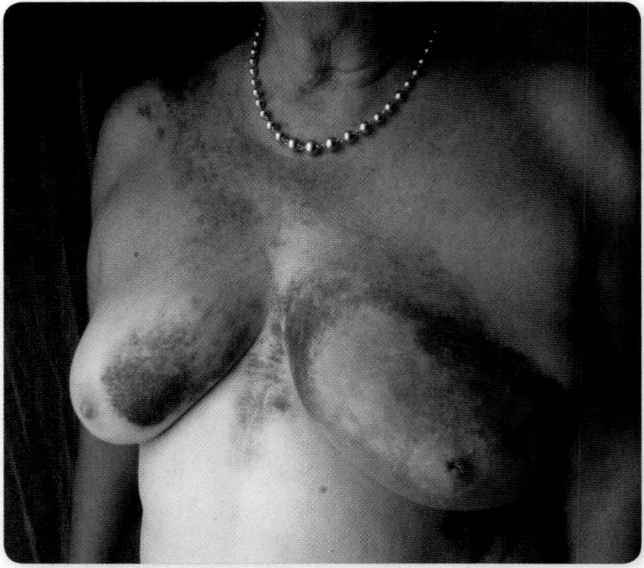

Figure 26-8 Air bags can cause injury in frontal crashes, specifically, abrasions, contusions, and traction-type injuries to the face, neck, and inner arms. This photo shows a seatbelt injury across the chest, and airbag contusions on the left breast.

Contact points are often obvious from a simple, quick evaluation of the interior of the vehicle. If there is no intrusion into the passenger compartment, you might see that an unrestrained front-seat passenger in a frontal crash has come in contact with the dashboard or instrument panel at the knees, thus transferring energy from the knees through the femur to the pelvis and hip joint **Figure 26-9A**. The chest and/or abdomen may

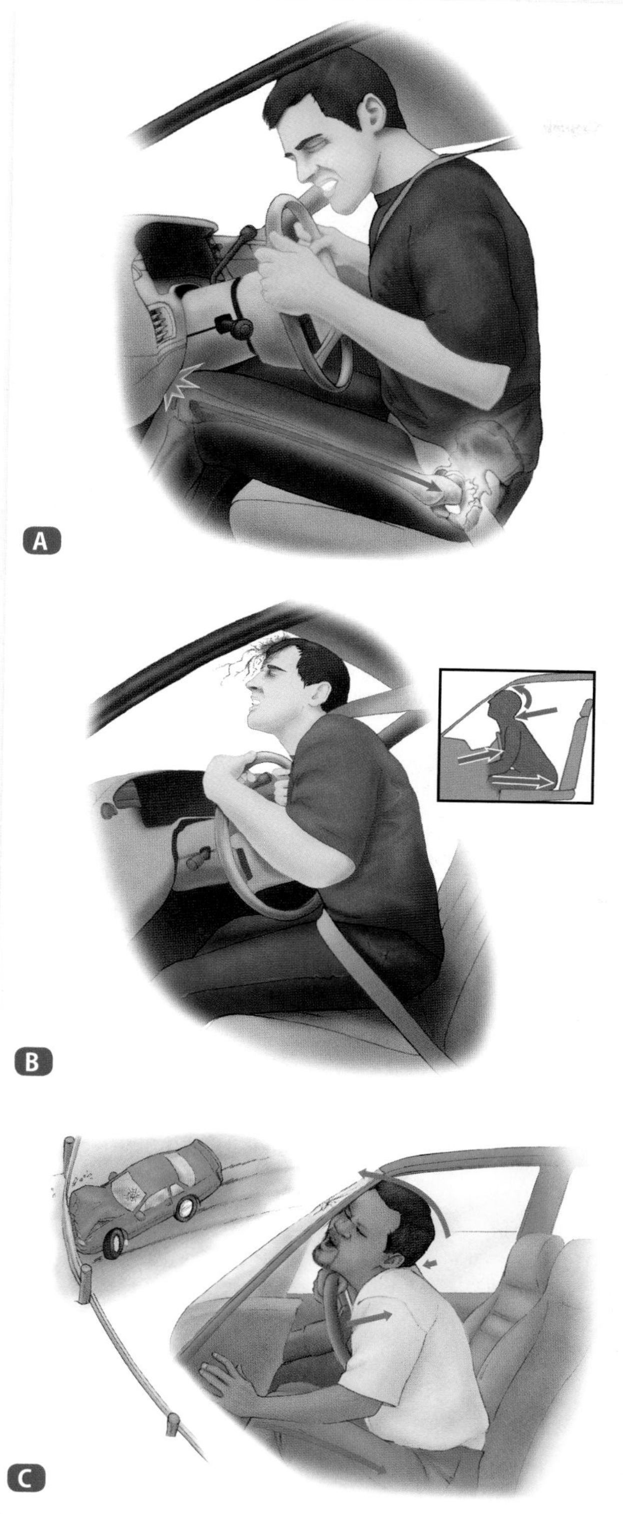

Figure 26-9 Mechanism of injury and condition of the vehicle interior suggest likely areas of injury. **A.** The knee can strike the dashboard, resulting in a hip fracture or dislocation. **B.** Serious chest and abdominal injuries can result from striking the steering wheel. **C.** Head and spinal injuries can result when the face and head strike the windshield.

also hit the steering wheel Figure 26-9B. In addition, the passenger's face often hits the steering wheel or may launch forward and up, hitting the windshield and/or the roof header in the area of the visors Figure 26-9C. Signs of most of these injuries can be found by inspecting the interior of the vehicle during extrication of the patient.

Supplemental restraint systems can also cause harm whether they are used properly or improperly. For example, some older models have seat belts that buckle automatically at the shoulder but require the passengers to buckle the lap portion; these can cause the occupant to travel down and under the shoulder strap as the body continues forward, resulting in the lower body striking the dashboard. This movement of the body can cause the lower extremities and the pelvis to crash into the dashboard because that part of the body is unrestrained. People who do not wear seat belts are at much higher risk for a number of injuries because they may be catapulted through the car or ejected from the vehicle. If a patient is unrestrained and involved in a frontal collision, he or she may be thrown up and over the steering wheel, resulting in the head hitting the windshield, roof, or rearview mirror. The chest may contact the steering column or dash, and the abdomen may also strike the steering column or dash. If the patient is driving, either femur or the pelvis may sustain substantial injury as contact is made with the bottom of the steering wheel. Finally, an unrestrained person may be ejected from the vehicle, dramatically increasing the risk of head injury, spinal cord injury, and death. Table 26-3 lists injury patterns.

Table 26-3	Frontal Collision Injury
Up-and-over pathway injuries	Head injuries Spine injuries Chest injuries ▪ Rib fractures or flail chest ▪ Pneumothorax ▪ Hemothorax ▪ Contusions ▪ Great vessel injury Vena cava Aorta Abdominal injuries ▪ Solid organs ▪ Hollow organs ▪ Diaphragm Fractured pelvis
Down-and-under pathway injuries	Posterior knee and hip dislocations Femur fractures Lower extremity fractures Pelvic and acetabular fractures

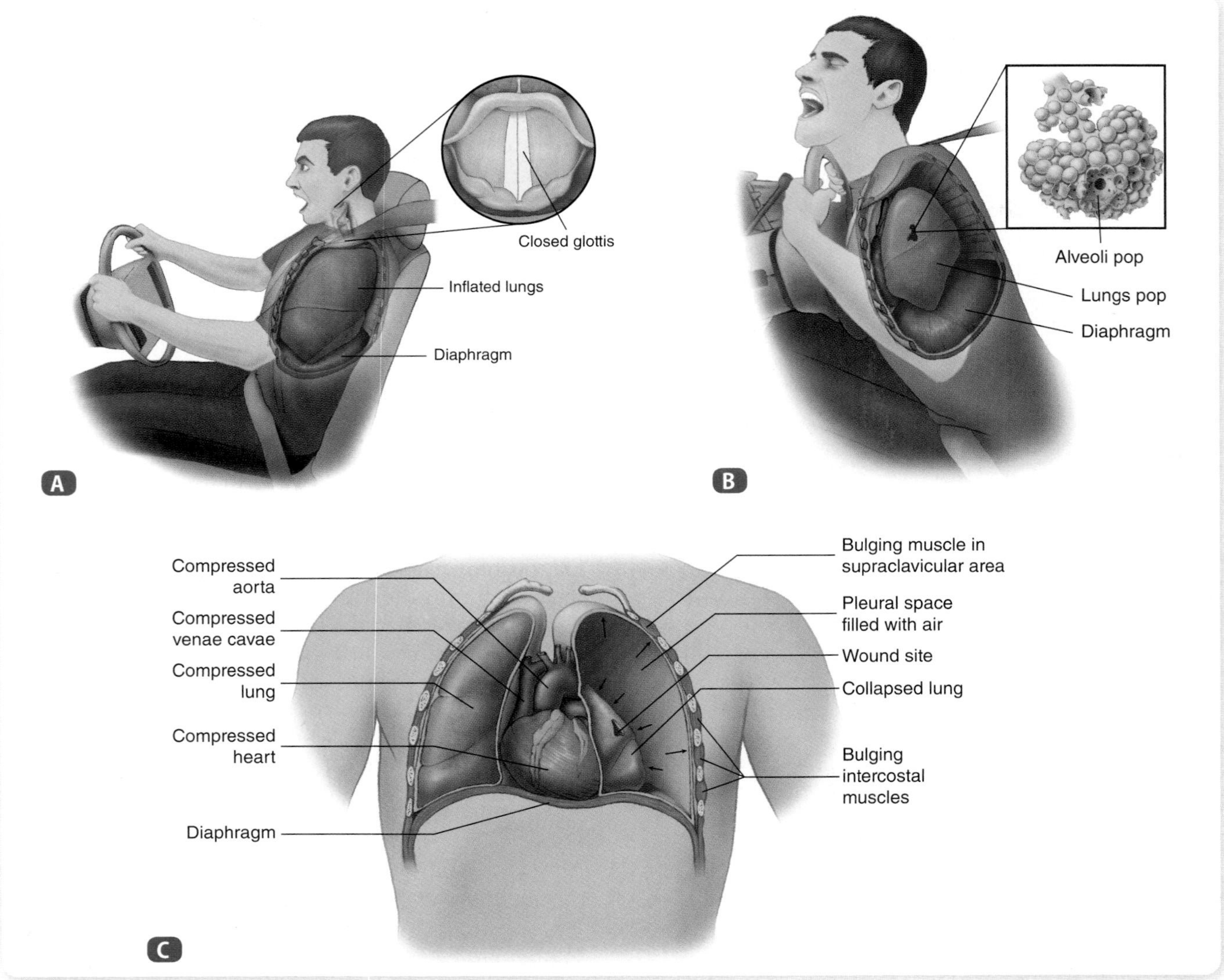

Figure 26-10 The paper-bag syndrome. **A.** The occupant takes a deep breath just before crashing, closing the glottis and filling the lungs with air. **B.** The occupant's chest hits the steering wheel, popping the alveoli in the lungs. **C.** A pneumothorax results.

Ejection is possible if the windshield does not stop the body from penetrating through it. Ejection results in second-impact injuries when the body comes in contact with the ground or objects outside of the vehicle. These injuries can be as severe as initial-impact injuries, and they increase the likelihood of great vessel damage and death. The spine absorbs energy as it is compressed between the stationary head and the moving torso, which results in injury.

A dangerous lung injury may occur if your patient reflexively takes a deep breath just before impact, hyperinflating the lungs and closing the glottis. The impact of the steering wheel can injure the lungs by generating pressures in the lungs beyond the capabilities of the lung tissue, like a "paper bag being exploded." This often results in a pneumothorax Figure 26-10. In addition, Table 26-4 lists the "ring" of chest injuries that can occur from impact with the steering wheel or dashboard.

Table 26-4 "Ring" of Chest Injuries From Impact With the Steering Wheel or Dashboard

- Facial injuries
- Soft-tissue neck trauma
- Larynx and tracheal trauma
- Fractured sternum
- Myocardial contusion
- Pericardial tamponade
- Pulmonary contusion
- Hemothorax, rib fractures
- Flail chest
- Ruptured aorta
- Intra-abdominal injuries

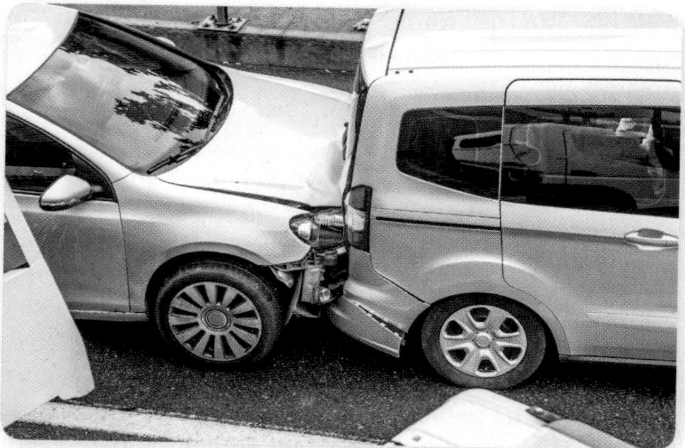

Figure 26-11 Rear-end impacts often cause whiplash-type injuries, particularly when the head and/or neck is not supported by a headrest.

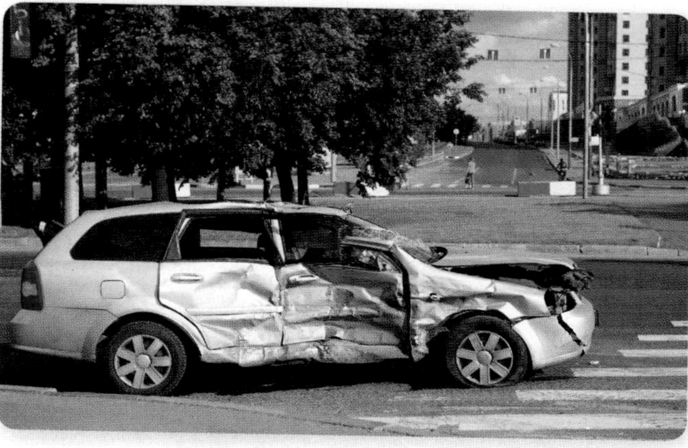

Figure 26-12 In a lateral crash, the vehicle is typically struck above its center of gravity and begins to rock away from the side of impact. This causes a type of lateral whiplash in which the passenger's shoulders and head whip toward the intruding vehicle.

Rear-End Crashes. Rear-end impacts are known to cause whiplash-type injuries, particularly when the head and/or neck is not supported by an appropriately placed headrest **Figure 26-11**. On impact, the vehicle seat pushes the body and torso forward. As the body is propelled forward, the head and neck are left behind because a headrest does not support them, and they appear to be whipped back relative to the torso. As the vehicle comes to rest, the unrestrained passenger moves forward, striking the dashboard. In this type of crash, the cervical spine and surrounding area may be injured. The cervical spine is less tolerant of damage when it is bent back. Headrests decrease extension of the head and neck during a crash and, therefore, help reduce injury. Other parts of the spine and the pelvis may also be at risk for injury. In addition, the patient may sustain an acceleration injury to the brain—that is, the third collision of the brain within the skull. Passengers in the backseat wearing only a lap belt might have a higher incidence of injuries to the thoracic and lumbar spine.

Lateral Crashes. Lateral or side impacts (commonly called T-bone crashes) are a very common cause of death associated with motor vehicle crashes. When a vehicle is struck from the side, it is typically struck above its center of gravity and begins to rock away from the side of the impact. This results in a lateral whiplash injury **Figure 26-12**. The movement is to the side, and the passenger's shoulders and head whip toward the intruding vehicle. This action may thrust the shoulder, thorax, upper extremity, and, more important, the skull, against the doorpost or the window. The patient could experience rotation of the neck, lateral flexion, or a combination of both. Because the cervical spine is relatively unstable, it has little tolerance for lateral bending.

If there is substantial intrusion into the passenger compartment, suspect lateral chest and abdomen injuries on the side of the impact, as well as possible fractures of the lower extremities, pelvis, and ribs. In addition, the organs within the abdomen are at risk because of a possible third collision. According to the *Journal of Safety Research*, lateral crashes cause approximately 25% of all severe injuries to the aorta and approximately 30% of all fatalities that occur in motor vehicle crashes.[6]

Rollover Crashes. Certain vehicles, such as large trucks and some sport utility vehicles, are more prone to rollover crashes because of their high center of gravity. Injury patterns that are commonly associated with rollover crashes differ, depending on whether the passenger was restrained or unrestrained. With the potential for multiple impacts on the body, injury patterns are difficult to predict. An unrestrained passenger may have sustained multiple strikes within the interior of the vehicle as it rolled one or more times.

The most common life-threatening event in a rollover is ejection or partial ejection of the passenger from the vehicle **Figure 26-13**. Passengers who have been ejected may have struck the interior of the vehicle many times before ejection and may have also struck objects, such as a tree, a guardrail, or the vehicle's exterior, before landing. Passengers who have been partially ejected may have struck both the interior and exterior of the vehicle and may have been sandwiched between the exterior of the vehicle and the environment as the vehicle rolled. Ejection and partial ejection are significant MOIs; in these instances, prepare to care for life-threatening injuries.

Even when restrained, passengers can sustain severe injuries during a rollover crash, although the patterns of injury tend to be more predictable, and when the restraint system is properly used, ejection from the vehicle is prevented. In a rollover, a passenger on the outboard side (the side the vehicle rolls onto) of a vehicle is at high risk for injury because of the centrifugal force (the patient is pinned against the door of the vehicle). When the roof hits the ground during a rollover, a passenger who is restrained can still move far enough toward the roof to make contact and sustain head or a spinal cord injury.

Therefore, rollover crashes are dangerous for both restrained and, to a greater degree, unrestrained passengers

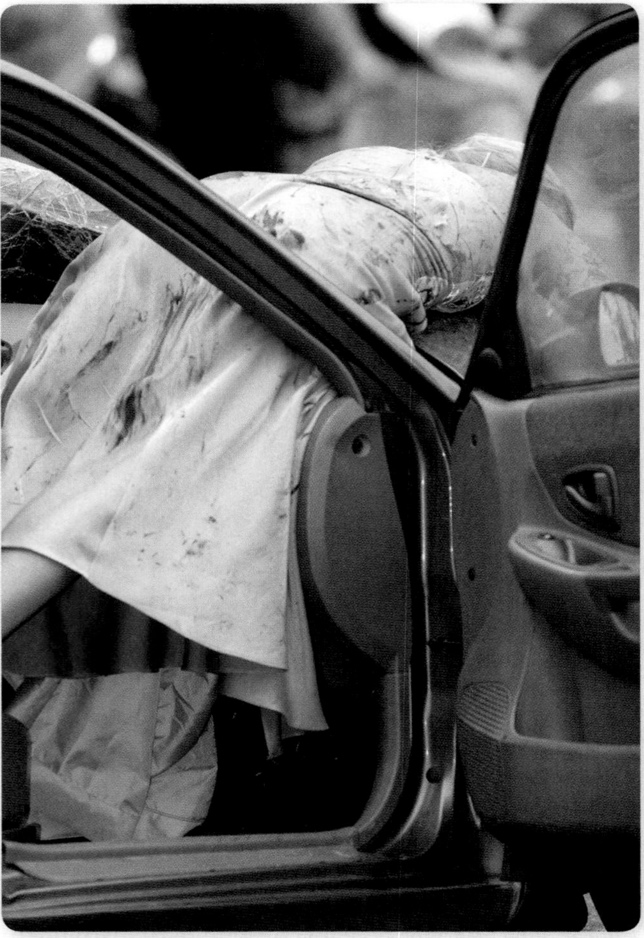

Figure 26-13 Passengers who have been ejected or partially ejected may have struck the interior of the vehicle many times before ejection.

because these crashes provide multiple opportunities for second and third collisions. The chance of death increases any time an occupant is ejected from a vehicle.

Rotational Crashes. Rotational crashes (spins) are conceptually similar to rollovers. The rotation of the vehicle as it spins provides opportunities for the vehicle to strike objects such as utility poles. Part of the vehicle stops, while the rest remains in motion. Injuries are the result of a combination of frontal and lateral impacts. For example, as a vehicle spins and strikes a pole, the passengers experience not only the rotational motion but also a lateral impact. Three-point seat belts are effective in preventing injury in angled crashes of up to 45°.

Table 26-5 summarizes how to recognize developing problems in trauma patients; many of these apply during vehicle crashes.

Vehicle-Versus-Pedestrian Crashes

In crashes involving pedestrians, there are three phases of impact. Initially the vehicle-pedestrian impact occurs, the pedestrian rotates onto the hood, and then the pedestrian rolls off onto the ground. The injury pattern depends on the height of the pedestrian and the body area facing the impact.

Vehicle-versus-pedestrian crashes often result in patients who have graphic and apparent injuries, such as broken bones; however, this type of crash can cause serious unseen injuries to underlying body systems. Therefore, you must maintain a high index of suspicion for unseen injuries. A thorough evaluation of the MOI is critical. First, estimate the speed of the vehicle that struck the patient; next, determine whether the patient ejected, what surface the patient landed on, and at what distance or whether the patient was struck and pulled under the vehicle. Evaluate the vehicle that struck the patient for structural damage that might indicate contact points with the patient and alert you to potential injuries. Multisystem trauma (multiple traumatic injuries involving more than one body system) is common after this type of event. Consider paramedic backup for any patients who have or are thought to have sustained a significant MOI; paramedic care may be needed for endotracheal intubation or cardiac arrest management.

Special Populations

As a result of smaller body structure and height, pediatric patients generally sustain more injuries to the thoracic and abdominal areas in the initial impact than do adults. Because their bones are more pliable, maintain a high index of suspicion for underlying organ damage in the absence of fractures.

Vehicle-Versus-Bicycle Crashes

In a vehicle-versus-bicycle collision, evaluate the MOI in much the same manner as vehicle-versus-pedestrian crashes. However, additional evaluation of damage to and the position of the bicycle is warranted. If the patient was wearing a helmet, inspect the helmet for damage and suspect potential injury to the head Figure 26-14. Presume that the patient has sustained an injury to the spinal column, or spinal cord, until proven otherwise at the hospital. Initiate and maintain spinal stabilization during the encounter. When practical, roll the patient onto his or her side to allow for an appropriate assessment to the posterior side of the body.

Motorcycle Crashes

In 2015, there were 4,976 motorcyclists killed in motor vehicle traffic crashes—an 8% increase from 4,594 motorcyclists killed in 2014. There were an estimated 88,000 motorcyclists injured during 2015, a 3% decrease from the 92,000 motorcyclists injured in 2014.[7]

Motorcycle collisions are especially dangerous because the rider has nothing to help protect him or her except

Table 26-5 Recognizing Developing Problems in Trauma Patients

Mechanism of Injury	Potential Injuries or Conditions	Signs and Symptoms
Blunt or penetrating trauma to the neck	Airway obstruction (from bleeding, secretions, or foreign bodies in upper or lower airway)	▪ Noisy or labored respirations ▪ Swelling of the face or neck
Substantial chest wall blunt or penetrating trauma	Breathing problems, cardiac or pulmonary contusion, pneumothorax or hemothorax, broken ribs	▪ Substantial chest pain ▪ Shortness of breath ▪ Asymmetrical chest wall movement ▪ Penetrating trauma to the chest
Substantial blunt or penetrating trauma to chest, abdomen, or groin	Hidden blood loss, damage to major vessels	▪ Bruising, redness, abrasions, or obvious trauma to the abdomen or pelvis ▪ Abdominal distention or rigidity ▪ Tenderness on gentle palpation of the pelvis
Blow to the head (blunt force trauma or fall)	Brain injury	▪ History of losing consciousness, altered mental status, inability to recall events, combativeness, or changes in speech patterns ▪ Difficulty moving extremities ▪ Severe headache, especially if accompanied by nausea and vomiting
Substantial blunt force trauma, penetrating trauma, or fall from a substantial height	Spinal injury (to bones of the spinal column or spinal cord)	▪ Severe neck or back pain ▪ Difficulty moving or feeling the extremities ▪ Loss of sensation or tingling in the extremities

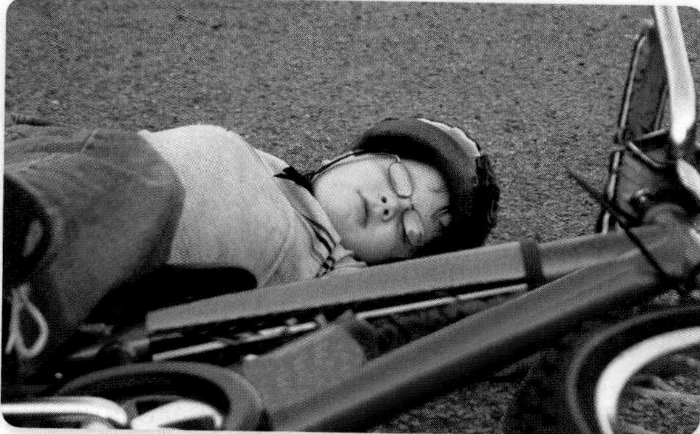

Figure 26-14 If the patient's bike helmet is damaged, suspect head and spine injuries.

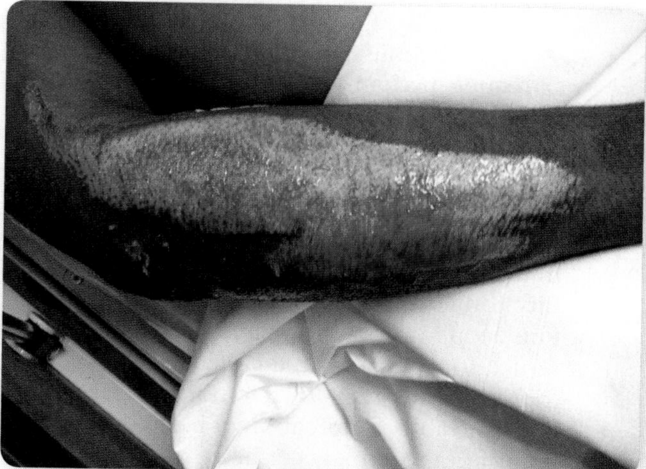

Figure 26-15 Abrasions from a motorcycle collision.

any protective devices that may be worn—that is, helmet, leather or abrasion-resistant clothing, and boots. There is no structural protection around the rider. Although helmets are designed to protect against impact forces to the head, they do not protect against cervical spine injury. Patients who have experienced a motorcycle crash should undergo cervical spine assessment and have cervical collars placed if indicated. Leather and synthetic gear worn over the body was initially designed to protect professional riders in competition, where falls tend to be controlled and result in long sliding mechanisms on hard surfaces rather than multiple collisions against road objects and other vehicles. Leather clothing protects mostly against road abrasion but offers no protection against blunt trauma from secondary impacts Figure 26-15. In a street crash, impacts occur usually against other larger vehicles or stationary objects.

When you are assessing the scene of a motorcycle crash, look for deformity of the motorcycle, the side of most damage, the distance of skid in the road, the deformity of stationary objects or other vehicles, and the extent and location of deformity in the helmet. These findings can be helpful in estimating the extent of trauma in a patient.

There are four types of motorcycle impacts.

- **Head-on crash.** The motorcycle strikes another object and stops its forward motion while the rider and parts of the motorcycle that are broken off continue their forward motion until stopped by an outside force, such as contact from the road or another opposing force from a secondary crash. Because the motorcycle's center of gravity is above the front axle, there is a forward and upward motion at the point of the impact, causing the rider to go over the handlebars. If the rider's feet remain on the pegs or pedals, then the forward and upward motion of the upper torso is restrained by the legs, producing bilateral femur or tibia fractures and severe foot injuries.
- **Angular crash.** The motorcycle strikes an object or another vehicle at an angle so that the rider sustains direct crushing injuries to the lower extremity between the object and the motorcycle. Trapped legs may be fractured and/or dislocated. This usually results in severe open, comminuted lower extremity injuries with severe neurovascular compromise, often requiring surgical amputation. Traumatic amputations are also common high-speed injuries.

  After the initial crush injury to the lower extremity, mechanisms such as those described in a head-on impact also apply. Often, the rider is propelled over the hood of the colliding vehicle. Because the impact is at an angle, severe thoracoabdominal torsion and lateral bending spine injuries can result, in addition to head injury and pelvic trauma.
- **Ejection.** The rider will travel at high speed until stopped by a stationary object, another vehicle, or contact with the road. Severe abrasion injuries (road rash) down to bone can occur. An unpredictable combination of blunt injuries can occur from secondary crashes.
- **Laying the bike down (also known as a controlled crash).** A technique used to separate the rider from the body of the motorcycle and the object to be hit is referred to as laying the bike down. It was developed by motorcycle racers and adapted by street bikers as a means of achieving a controlled crash. As a collision approaches, the motorcycle is turned flat and tipped sideways at 90° to the direction of travel so that one leg is dropped to the grass or asphalt. This slows the occupant faster than the motorcycle, allowing for the rider to become separated from the motorcycle. If properly protected with leather or synthetic abrasion-resistant gear, injuries should be limited to those sustained by rolling over the pavement and any secondary crash that may occur. When executed properly, this maneuver prevents the rider from being trapped between the bike and the object. However, a rider unable to clear the bike will continue into the vehicle, often with devastating results.

Bicycles and off-road vehicles, such as four-wheelers and snowmobiles, are capable of producing injuries similar to those from motorcycles, with a few differences. Possibly the biggest difference with injuries from off-road vehicles is that reaching the patients is often a challenge. If the traumatic event happens in a remote location, then you must make immediate decisions about issues such as what medical equipment to take to the location and how you will evacuate the patients. Also, in these types of situations patients are often not wearing helmets or other safety equipment that motorcycle riders often employ. Although bicycle riders who are hit by motor vehicles are more likely to be wearing a helmet, they will sustain injuries similar to those found in pedestrians struck by motor vehicles.

Falls

The injury potential of a fall is related to the height from which the patient fell. The greater the height of the fall, the greater the potential for injury. As mentioned earlier, any adult patient who has fallen more than 20 feet (6 m) should be considered at risk for injuries to multiple body systems. Falls from substantial heights are associated with potential for high-energy injury, and patients should be evaluated accordingly.

When falling from a height, the patient lands on the surface just as an unrestrained passenger smashes into the interior of a vehicle. The internal organs travel at the speed of the patient's body before it hits the ground and stop by smashing into the interior of the body. Again, as in a motor vehicle crash, it is these internal injuries that are the least obvious on assessment but pose the gravest threat to life. Therefore, suspect internal injuries in a patient who has fallen from a substantial height, just as you would in a patient who has been in a high-speed motor vehicle crash.

When possible, you should also identify what type of surface the patient landed on and how he or she landed. This information, which may be gleaned from the environment, the patient, and/or bystanders, may help you to predict what areas of the body might be the most seriously injured.

Patients who fall and land on their feet may have less severe internal injuries because their legs may have absorbed much of the energy of the fall **Figure 26-16**. However, as a result, they may have very serious injuries

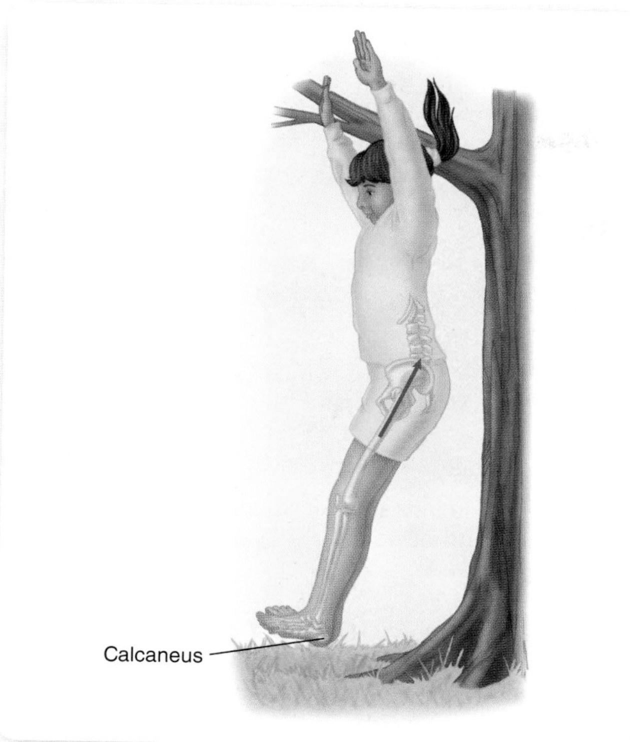

Figure 26-16 When a patient falls and lands on his or her feet, the energy is transmitted to the spine, sometimes producing a spine injury in addition to injuries to the legs and pelvis.

to the lower extremities and pelvic and spinal injuries from energy that the legs did not absorb.

Patients who fall onto their heads, as in diving accidents, will likely have serious head and/or spinal injuries. In either case, a fall from a substantial height is a serious event with great injury potential, and the patient should be evaluated thoroughly. Take the following factors into account:

- The height of the fall
- The type of surface struck
- The part of the body that hit first, followed by the path of energy displacement
- Area of the body over which the impact is distributed

Many falls, especially those sustained by older people, are not the result of high-energy trauma, even though broken bones may result. Older patients often have osteoporosis, a condition in which the musculoskeletal system can fail under relatively low stress because the bones are structurally weakened. An older patient with osteoporosis can sustain a fracture as a result of a fall from a standing position. These cases do not constitute high-energy trauma unless the patient fell from a substantial height.

Finally, always consider syncope or other underlying medical causes of the fall. If the patient's condition is stable, attempt to determine exactly what happened to cause the fall; did the person simply slip and fall or lose consciousness and then fall?

YOU are the Provider PART 3

As the fire department arrives and begins extrication, you ask the law enforcement officers to establish a landing zone for the helicopter. As you are preparing your airway equipment and intravenous (IV) supplies, you hear your partner yell that the patient has been extricated. You rapidly apply a cervical collar, place her on a long backboard, and move her to the back of the ambulance. Finding inadequate respirations, you place a dual-lumen airway device and instruct your partner to ventilate at the appropriate rate and depth. You quickly establish bilateral IV lines and rapidly infuse the first two 250-mL boluses of normal saline to increase the patient's blood pressure.

Recording Time: 14 Minutes	
Respirations	8 breaths/min, shallow; assisted at 12 breaths/min
Pulse	Unobtainable radially; 140 beats/min at carotid artery
Skin	Cool, pale, and clammy
Blood pressure	Unable to obtain via palpation
Oxygen saturation (Spo_2)	Unable to obtain
Pupils	Nonreactive

4. Does this patient meet the criteria for aeromedical evacuation?

Special Populations

To evaluate the MOI when your patient is a child, remember this: falls greater than 10 feet (3 m) or two to three times the child's height indicate a significant MOI; injuries to multiple body systems are likely in such cases. Also note that small children are top heavy so they tend to land on their head even from small falls of a minimal height.

Special Populations

Many geriatric patients are seriously injured from falls. Completely assess the older patient for all possible injuries, even from low-impact falls.

▶ Penetrating Trauma

In 2015, the CDC reported almost 35,000 deaths from firearms, which is just under the number of deaths related to motor vehicles.[8] Penetrating trauma can be classified as low energy, medium energy, or high energy. Low-energy penetrating trauma may be caused accidentally by impalement or intentionally by a knife, ice pick, or other weapon Figure 26-17.

Penetrating trauma, often the result of a gunshot or stab injury, is difficult to assess because there is often little external evidence of the actual damage. The amount of force that is applied to the body in a gunshot wound is most directly related to the caliber of the weapon and the distance of the weapon from the patient when it was fired. Point-blank and high-velocity gunshot wounds result in more significant injuries. By comparison, the force that is exerted on the patient in stab injuries is minimal, even though these injuries can still be lethal.

In some penetrating wounds, such as stab wounds, the body area that is involved can be estimated by looking at the location of entrance and the length of the weapon, if known. However, angle or direction of travel is also pertinent. In gunshot wounds, the internal organs that are injured may have no relationship to the **entrance wound** and the **exit wound**, if these wounds exist Figure 26-18. Bullets may bounce off bones or dense organs in the body, making the exact path almost impossible to determine. Some bullets are designed to tumble, flatten out, break apart, ricochet, or "mushroom" after they enter the body.

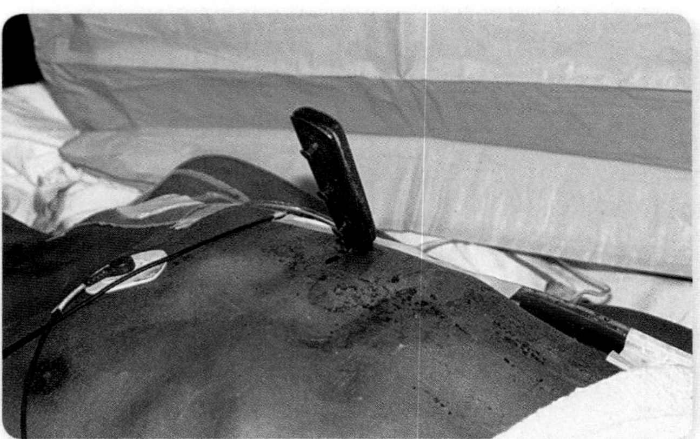

Figure 26-17 Injuries from low-energy penetrations, such as a stab wound, are caused by the sharp edges of the object moving through the body.

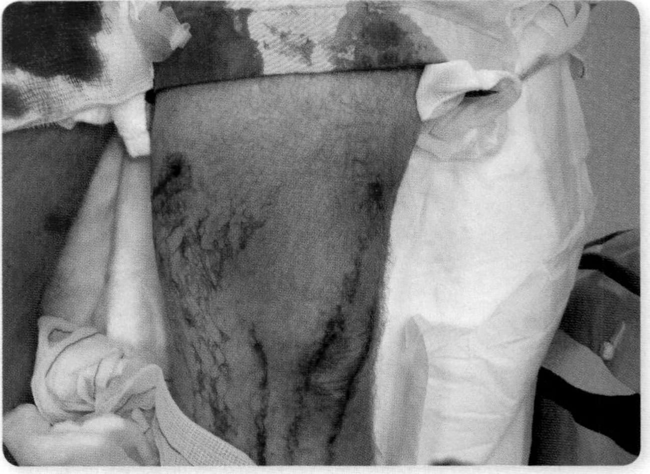

Figure 26-18 Entrance and exit wounds in the leg from a low-velocity gunshot wound.

When assessing a patient with a penetrating injury, first determine the number of penetrating injuries, and then combine that information with what you know about the potential pathway of penetrating projectiles to form an index of suspicion about unseen life-threatening injuries. Remember that you can only *estimate* the extent of the injury. For example, in some cases of assault, an assailant may have moved the weapon in a back-and-forth motion after it entered the patient.

Gunshot Wounds

The path the projectile takes is referred to as a **trajectory**. Fragmentation, especially frangible bullets that are designed to disintegrate into tiny particles on impact, will increase damage as multiple fragments increase the likelihood of multiple organs/vessels sustaining injury. Hollow point bullets expand as they enter the target in order to decrease penetration and cause more tissue damage. Full metal jacket bullets cause less damage than fragmented rounds because of their tendency to pass through the body's tissues. The bullet's speed is a major factor in the resulting injury pattern; there is often additional damage caused by the object moving inside the body but not along the suspected pathway. This phenomenon, called **cavitation**, which results from the rapid changes in tissue and fluid pressure that occur with the passage of the projectile, can result in serious injury to internal organs distant to the actual path of the bullet Figure 26-19. A temporary cavity is produced by stretching the tissue surrounding the point of impact. Permanent cavitation injury results closer to the bullet path where the pressure fluctuations are greatest and remains after the projectile has passed through the tissue.

The relationship between distance and severity of injury varies depending on the type of weapon involved, such as a rifle, pistol, or shotgun. Air resistance, often referred to as **drag**, slows the projectile, decreasing the depth of penetration and energy of the projectile and thus reducing tissue damage. Much like a boat moving through water, the bullet disrupts not only the tissues that are directly in its path but also those in its wake. Therefore, the area that is damaged by medium- and high-velocity projectiles is typically many times larger than the diameter of the projectile itself Figure 26-20. This is one reason that exit wounds are often much larger than entrance wounds. You must remain alert during assessment because patients will exhibit various signs and symptoms depending on the organ or organs struck.

As with motor vehicle crashes, the energy available for a bullet to cause damage is more a function of its speed than its mass (weight). If the mass of the bullet is doubled, the energy that is available to cause injury is doubled. If the speed (velocity) of the bullet is doubled, the energy that is available to cause injury is quadrupled. For this reason, it is important for you to try to determine the type of weapon that was used. Although it is not necessary (or always possible) for you to distinguish between medium- and high-velocity injuries, any information regarding the type of weapon that was used should be relayed to medical control. Police at the scene may be a useful source of information regarding the caliber and type of weapon. Organs injured in a gunshot wound vary depending on the pathway of the projectile. There is an entrance wound, and, if the bullet goes completely through, an exit wound. The entrance wound is characterized by a round or oval hole that is crushed inward. The rim is usually 1 to 2 mm wide and dark because of the grease or other substance on the bullet. There may be an abrasion produced by the spinning of the bullet. The size of the abrasion depends on the contact with the skin. It will be larger when the impact is at an angle. If the end of the weapon is within 4 to 6 inches from the skin, there may also be burns from the flame emitted from the barrel. In contrast, the exit wound is pushed outward and, rather than being round, may be stellate (star-shaped) or a slit.

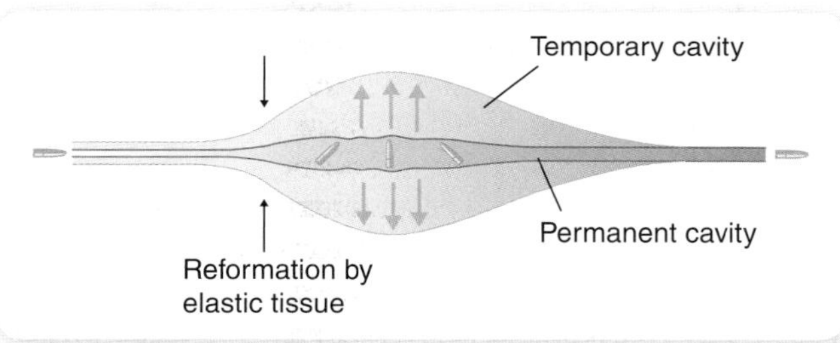

Figure 26-19 There are two types of cavitations: temporary and permanent.

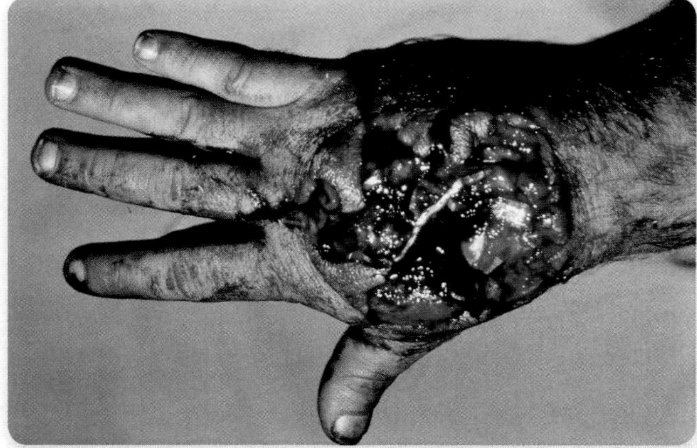

Figure 26-20 The area damaged by high-velocity projectiles such as bullets can be many times larger than the diameter of the projectile itself.

> **Words of Wisdom**
>
> A blunt object that contacts minimal surface area (such as a wooden dowel compressed against the forearm) creates damage that is similar to that of penetrating trauma but without breaking the skin.

Blast Injuries

Although most commonly associated with military conflict, **blast injuries** are also seen in civilian practice in industrial settings such as mines, shipyards, and chemical plants and, increasingly, in association with terrorist activities. They are also more common today owing to the increased use of explosives as a tool for urban terrorism and, in the United States, from methamphetamine laboratory explosions. Although civilian explosions in an industrial or mining setting used to be mostly characterized by blast injuries and burns, terrorist bombs often contain shrapnel. As an AEMT, you and other emergency medical services (EMS) and trauma services personnel should be fully educated and aware of what to expect in these scenarios. People who are injured in explosions may be injured by any of five different mechanisms, often causing multisystem trauma Figure 26-21.

▶ Categories of Blast Injuries

Primary Blast Injuries

Primary blast injuries are due entirely to the blast itself—that is, damage to the body caused by the pressure wave generated by the explosion. When an explosion occurs, a pressure wave rapidly develops; this tremendous, concentrated pressure results from air displacement and heat

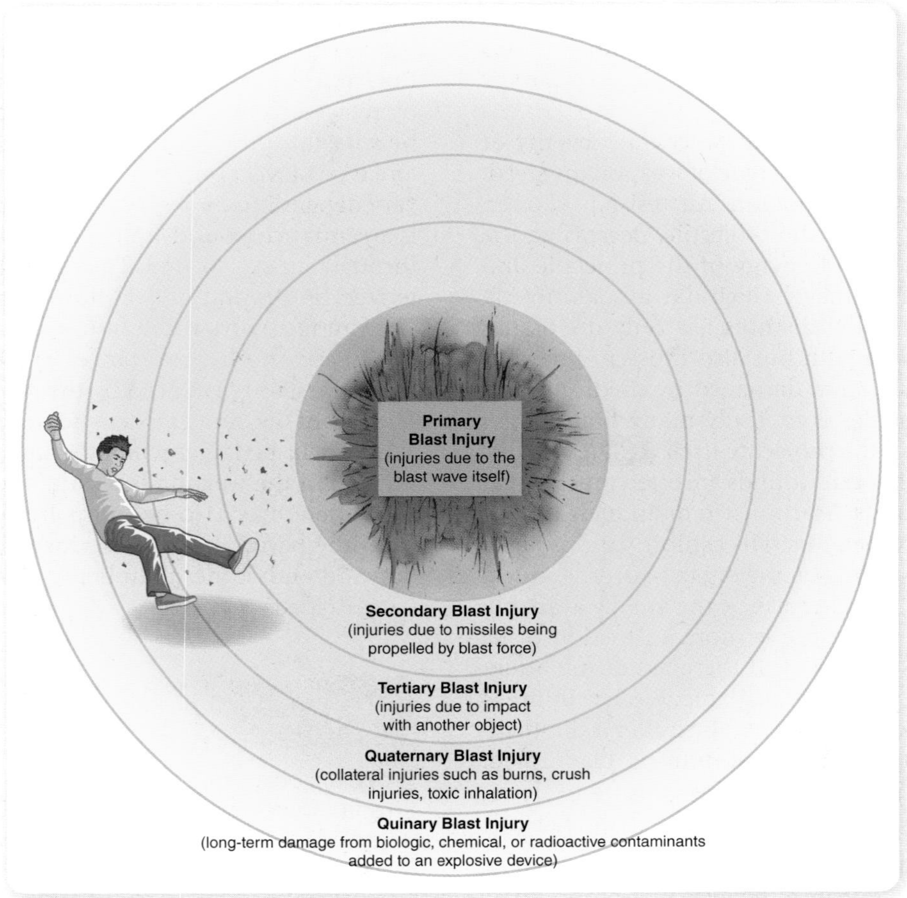

Figure 26-21 Mechanisms of blast injuries.

originating from the center of the blast. **Flash burns** are also considered part of the primary injury pattern (in addition to the overpressure). The organs generally affected by primary blast effects are the lungs, eardrums, and other compressible structures. The pressure wave damages air-filled cavities.

Proximity to the origin of the pressure wave is associated with a high risk of injury or death. Explosions from a bomb start at the center and move outward, so people closer to the device will be affected more. Explosions from fumes or dust involve an entire area, so there is no "safe" region. Underwater blasts have a threefold greater range because of the near-incompressibility of water. Explosions that occur within a confined space result in more force applied to the body.

Secondary Blast Injuries

Secondary blast injuries result from being struck by flying debris (such as shrapnel from the device or from glass or splinters) that has been set in motion by the explosion. Objects are propelled by the force of the blast and strike the person, causing injury. These objects can travel great distances and can be propelled at tremendous speeds, up to almost 3,000 mph for conventional military explosives.

A blast wind occurs as the shock wave applies force to air molecules. Although less forceful than the pressure wave, the blast wind is longer lasting and can hurl projectiles at high velocities. Projectiles present serious hazards—flying debris may cause blunt and penetrating injuries. With bombs, the casing fragments rip apart with monumental force, spreading in all directions. Structural elements can break apart and travel at high rates of speed. Nails, wood splinters, and glass shards can impale people located near the blast.

Tertiary Blast Injuries

Tertiary blast injuries occur when a person is hurled by the force of the explosion (or blast wind) against stationary, rigid objects, such as the ground or walls. Physical displacement of the body is also referred to as ground shock when the body impacts the ground. The injuries that result are numerous and result from both blunt and penetrating mechanisms. A blast wind also causes the patient's body to be hurled or thrown, causing further injury.

Quaternary (Miscellaneous) Blast Injuries

Quaternary injuries result from the miscellaneous events that occur during an explosion. For example, the heat generated during an explosion may cause burns, ranging from superficial flash burns to full-thickness burns involving the entire or large areas of the body. These injuries can include burns from hot gases or fires started by the blast, respiratory injury from inhaling toxic gases, and crush injury from the collapse of buildings. There is also a risk for entrapment that may be prolonged for days.

Quinary Blast Injuries

Quinary blast injuries are caused by biological, chemical, or radioactive contaminants that have been added to a traditional explosive device. The initial explosion disperses these materials, causing additional long-term damage through biological, chemical, or radioactive mechanisms. This type of blast injury is associated with "dirty bombs" and is of increased concern because of the threat of its use by terrorist organizations.

Most patients who survive an explosion will have some combination of the types of injuries mentioned. The discussion here will be confined to primary blast injuries because these injuries are the ones that are most easily overlooked.

Safety

Personal safety and the safety of your partner are primary. You cannot provide care for a patient if you are injured. Always carefully assess the environment from the ambulance as you are approaching the scene, and continue to survey the scene as you approach the patient. A scene is dynamic; it has the potential to change continually, and you must be aware to protect yourself. Watch for passing vehicles who may be rubbernecking, scene hazards, hostile environments, suspicious items or people, unsecured crime scenes, and suicidal patients who may become homicidal.

▶ Tissues at Risk

Organs that contain air, such as the middle ear, lung, and gastrointestinal tract, are most susceptible to barotrauma. The ear is the organ system that is most sensitive to blast injuries. The **tympanic membrane** evolved to detect minor changes in pressure and will rupture at pressures of 5 to 7 pounds per square inch above atmospheric pressure. Thus, the tympanic membranes are a sensitive indicator that you can use to help determine the possible presence of other blast injuries. The patient may report ringing in the ears, pain in the ears, or some loss of hearing, and blood may be visible in the ear canal. Dislocation of structural components of the ear, such as the ossicles conforming the inner ear, may occur. Permanent hearing loss is possible. These findings can be used to assist in triaging patients as they indicate risk of pressure injuries to the lungs.

Pulmonary blast injuries are defined as pulmonary trauma (consisting of contusions and hemorrhages) that results from short-range exposure to the detonation of explosives. When the explosion occurs in an open area, the patient's side that was toward the explosion is usually injured, but the injury can be bilateral when the victim is in a confined space. Primary blast injury is often characterized by a lack of external visible injuries and thus can go unrecognized. The patient may report tightness or pain in the chest and may cough up blood and have tachypnea or other signs of respiratory distress. Subcutaneous emphysema (crackling under the skin) can be detected over the chest using palpation, indicating air in the thorax. Pneumothorax (covered in Chapter 31, *Chest Injuries*) is a common injury and may require emergency decompression in the field by paramedics for your patient to survive. Pulmonary edema may ensue rapidly. If there is any reason to suspect lung injury in a blast victim (even just the presence of a ruptured eardrum), administer oxygen. Avoid giving oxygen under positive pressure, however (that is, by demand valve) because that may simply increase the damage to the lung. Be cautious as well with IV fluids, which may be poorly tolerated in patients with this type of lung injury and result in pulmonary edema.

One of the most concerning pulmonary blast injuries is **arterial air embolism**, which occurs on alveolar disruption with subsequent air embolization into the pulmonary vasculature. Even small air bubbles can enter a coronary artery and cause myocardial injury. Air embolisms to the cerebrovascular system can produce disturbances in vision, changes in behavior, changes in level of consciousness, and a variety of other neurologic signs.

Solid organs are relatively protected from shock wave injury but may be injured by secondary missiles or a hurled body. **Petechiae** (pinpoint hemorrhages on the skin) to large hematomas are the dominant form of pathology. Hollow organs, however, may be injured by similar mechanisms as for lung tissue. Perforation or rupture of the bowel and colon is possible. Underwater explosions result in the most severe abdominal injuries.

Neurologic injuries and head trauma are the most common causes of death from blast injuries. Concussion, intracerebral bleeding, or air embolism may occur. Bradycardia and hypotension are common after an intense pressure wave from an explosion.

Extremity injuries, including traumatic amputations, are common. Patients with traumatic amputation by post-blast wind are likely to sustain fatal injuries secondary to the blast. In the global war on terrorism, improved body armor has increased the number of survivors of blast injuries from shrapnel wounds to the torso. However, the number of severe orthopaedic and extremity injuries has increased. In addition, whereas body armor may limit or prevent shrapnel from entering the body, it also catches more energy from the blast wave, possibly resulting in the victim's being thrown backward, thus increasing the potential for spine and spinal cord injury.

Although blast injuries have usually been the domain of military surgeons, they often occur in industrial settings

Words of Wisdom

Although the prospect of assessing and treating a multisystem trauma patient may be daunting for a new AEMT, the course of care remains the same for all. Remain calm, control any major hemorrhage, and manage the ABCs (airway, breathing, and circulation). If you lose focus of what to do next, go back to the basics and reassess ABCs.

and are, unfortunately, more common today owing to the increased use of explosives as a tool for urban terrorism and, in the United States, from methamphetamine lab explosions. Although civilian blast injuries in an industrial or mining setting were mostly characterized by blast injuries and burns, terrorist bombs often have shrapnel. Modern EMS and trauma services personnel should be fully educated and aware of what to expect in these scenarios.

Multisystem Trauma

Multisystem trauma refers to the injuries of a person who has been subjected to multiple traumatic injuries involving more than one body system such as head and spinal trauma, chest and abdominal trauma, or chest and multiple extremity trauma. You must recognize patients who fit into this classification, provide rapid treatment and transportation, and alert medical control as to the nature of the patient's injuries so that the trauma center is prepared prior to your arrival. Multisystem trauma patients have high morbidity and mortality; therefore, they require teams of physicians to treat their injuries. These teams may include specialists such as neurosurgeons, thoracic surgeons, and orthopaedic surgeons.

Golden Principles of Prehospital Trauma Care

As with any EMS call, your main priority in managing multisystem trauma is to ensure your safety, the safety of your crew, and the patient. Next, you must determine the need for additional personnel or equipment, evaluate the MOI, and identify and appropriately manage life threats. After these steps have been completed, you can focus on patient care. Begin by assessing and managing the airway, including ventilatory support and high-flow oxygen while maintaining cervical spine stabilization. Ensure that basic shock therapy, such as controlling hemorrhages, stopping arterial bleeding, and keeping the patient warm, is completed. If bleeding cannot be controlled rapidly by direct pressure, consider the use of a tourniquet. If the patient is bleeding profusely, this must be controlled to ensure sufficient perfusion of organs and tissues.

After threats to the ABCs are corrected, rapidly proceed with spinal immobilization if indicated. If the patient is trapped, consider the use of rapid extrication techniques. In most patients with multisystem trauma, definitive care requires surgical intervention; therefore, on-scene time should be limited to 10 minutes or less. This is referred to as the platinum 10 minutes. During transport, obtain a SAMPLE (Signs and symptoms, Allergies, Medications, Pertinent past medical history, Last oral intake, Events leading up to the illness or injury) history, and complete a secondary assessment. Most care can be provided in transport. However, keep in mind that your patient has sustained multisystem trauma, and the order in which you usually provide treatment and care may need to be adjusted depending on the needs of the patient including maintaining a patent airway, ensuring adequate ventilation, and controlling hemorrhage. For critically injured

YOU are the Provider PART 4

While you are performing your assessment of the patient, the flight crew calls you on the radio advising that they are 10 minutes from touchdown on the scene. You acknowledge the transmission and focus on your assessment. As you are assessing the neck, you note a crackling sound on the lower portion of the neck when you palpate. Your examination findings of the chest are unremarkable, but when you palpate the abdomen, you find it rigid and distended. As you are completing the remainder of your exam, the flight crew touches down and steps into your ambulance. You provide a quick report and assist them in preparing the patient for flight. Approximately 5 minutes later, the patient is airborne, on her way to the local trauma center.

Recording Time: 20 Minutes	
Respirations	Assisted at 12 breaths/min
Pulse	120 beats/min at carotid artery, weak radially
Skin	Cool, pale, and clammy
Blood pressure	Unobtainable
Oxygen saturation (Spo_2)	Unobtainable
Pupils	Nonreactive

5. What is the crackling sound heard on the neck, and how is it caused?
6. Now that the critical patient has departed the scene, what should you do with the deceased patient?

patients, consider paramedic intercept and/or air medical transportation. Regardless of the mode of transport, ensure that the patient is transported to an appropriate facility and that the facility is notified as soon as possible. Specific standards of care regarding multisystem trauma will be addressed in detail in different chapters.

Words of Wisdom

Rapid transport decisions are needed for patients who have sustained substantial trauma. After the first 60 minutes, the body has increasing difficulty in compensating for shock and traumatic injuries. This is referred to as the Golden Hour. Because many injured patients require definitive care in less than 1 hour, this is also referred to as the Golden Period.

Words of Wisdom

Do not develop tunnel vision as you are approaching a scene. You may feel drawn to a screaming patient entrapped in a vehicle, but rushing toward a scene can result in potential injury to you if the scene is not safe. Also, gross injuries may not be life threatening. Occult injuries, such as closed chest or abdominal trauma, may have the potential for greater mortality than isolated extremity injuries.

Patient Assessment

Identifying life-threatening illnesses and injuries as soon as possible improves patient outcomes. As an AEMT, you must apply this knowledge as well as the appropriate assessment skills to assess, triage, treat, and transport patients with traumatic injuries to the most appropriate facility. The major components of patient assessment include the following:

- Scene size-up
- Primary survey
- History taking
- Secondary assessment
- Reassessment

When assessing a patient with trauma, follow the XABCDE mnemonic (eXsanguinating hemorrhage, Airway, Breathing, Circulation, Disability, and Exposure). This mnemonic adds the letter *X* to the ABCDE mnemonic for assessment. *X* represents the importance of looking for severe, exsanguinating hemorrhage first. Such hemorrhage can be addressed quickly when it is coming from an extremity. Failure to address it quickly will result in loss of total blood volume and rapid progression to death.

When you are caring for a patient who has experienced a significant MOI and is considered to be in serious or critical condition, you should rapidly perform a physical examination. Any patient who has sustained a nonsignificant MOI should receive an assessment focused on the chief complaint. The human body is divided into areas (or systems) based on body function, and its internal organs are subject to unseen injuries when force is applied to the body. For example, the brain may have bruising, the heart and lungs may have bruising or unseen bleeding, and the organs of the abdomen may have life-threatening bleeding. The following sections discuss the assessment of various body systems.

Words of Wisdom

Provide thorough documentation of the scene as well as patient assessment and care. As a prehospital provider, you are the eyes and ears of the physician. You must paint a picture for the providers who will assume care at the hospital in order for them to maintain an appropriate index of suspicion for the patient. Cameras provide an invaluable wealth of information for trauma surgeons, but patient care must not be delayed to take photos. Kinematics of trauma along with mechanisms of injury are important for trauma teams. Also remember to frequently reassess and document vital signs. Trending can be vital to direct appropriate patient care.

▶ Injuries to the Head

The brain lies well protected within the skull. However, when the head is injured from trauma, disability and unseen injury to the brain may occur. The brain itself, or the blood vessels around it, may tear or become bruised, causing bleeding. Bleeding or swelling inside the skull from brain injury is often life threatening; therefore, your assessment must include conducting frequent neurologic examinations. Neurologic assessments coupled with the patient's level of consciousness will often provide details on subtle changes in the patient's condition. Some patients will not have obvious signs or symptoms, such as changes in pupillary size and reactivity, of unseen brain injury until minutes or hours after the injury has occurred.

▶ Injuries to the Neck and Throat

The neck and throat contain many structures that are susceptible to injuries from trauma that could be serious or deadly to your patients. In this region of the human body, the trachea (or windpipe) may become torn or swell after an injury to the neck or deviate after an injury to the lungs. These types of injuries may result in an airway problem that could quickly become a serious life threat because they interfere with the patient's ability to breathe; therefore, your assessment must include frequent physical examination looking for Deformities, Contusions, Abrasions, Punctures/penetrations, Burns, Tenderness,

Lacerations, Swelling (DCAP-BTLS) in the neck region. In addition, you should assess for jugular venous distention and tracheal deviation (late sign of injury).

The neck also contains large blood vessels that supply the brain with oxygen-rich blood. When a neck injury occurs, swelling may prevent blood flow to the brain and cause injury to the central nervous system, even though the brain may not have been directly affected by the initial force that caused the injury to the neck. If a penetrating injury to the neck results in an open wound, the patient may have substantial bleeding, or air may be drawn into the circulatory system resulting in an air embolism. Always use an occlusive dressing on any open neck wound. A crushing injury to the upper part of the neck may cause the cartilage of the upper airway and larynx to fracture. This can result in the leakage of air into the soft tissue of the neck. When air is trapped in subcutaneous tissue (subcutaneous emphysema), it produces a crackling feeling when palpated, called subcutaneous crepitation. Either air in the circulation or an airway cartilage fracture may cause rapid death.

▶ Injuries to the Chest

The chest contains the heart, the lungs, and the large blood vessels of the body. When injury occurs to this area of the body, many life-threatening injuries may occur. For example, blunt trauma to the chest can fracture ribs or the sternum. When ribs are broken and the chest wall does not expand normally during breathing, this interferes with the body's ability to obtain sufficient amounts of oxygen for the cells. Bruising may occur to the heart and cause an irregular heartbeat. Depending on the severity of the trauma, the large vessels of the heart may be torn inside the chest and cause massive unseen bleeding that can quickly kill the trauma patient. In some chest injuries the lungs become bruised, thus interfering with normal oxygen exchange in the body.

Some chest injuries result in air collecting between the lung tissue and the chest wall. As air accumulates in this space, the lung tissue becomes compressed, again interfering with the body's ability to effectively exchange oxygen. This injury is called a pneumothorax. If left untreated or unrecognized, the lung tissue becomes squeezed under pressure until the heart is also squeezed, preventing a return of venous blood and thereby reducing preload. This condition is called a tension pneumothorax and is a life-threatening emergency. Bleeding develops in some patients in this portion of the chest. Instead of air collecting in this space, blood collects here and causes interference with breathing. This condition is called a hemothorax, and it also poses a threat to the patient's life.

A penetration or perforation of the integrity of the chest is called an open chest wound. As air enters the chest cavity, the natural pressure balance within the chest cavity is no longer equal. If left untreated, shock and/or death will result. Regardless of the particular injury, it is imperative that you reassess a trauma patient's chest region every 5 minutes. The assessment should include DCAP-BTLS, breath sounds, and chest rise and fall. Some patients will not have immediately obvious signs or symptoms such as absent breath sounds or respiratory difficulty.

▶ Injuries to the Abdomen

The abdomen is an area of the human body that contains many organs vital to body function. These organs also require a high amount of blood flow so they can perform the functions necessary for life. Recall that the organs of the abdomen and retroperitoneum (the space immediately behind the true abdomen) can be classified into two simple categories: solid and hollow. The solid organs include the liver, spleen, pancreas, and kidneys. The hollow organs include the stomach, large and small intestines, and urinary bladder.

When injuries from trauma occur in this region of the body, serious and life-threatening problems may occur. The solid organs may tear, lacerate, or fracture. This causes serious bleeding into the abdomen that can quickly cause death. Be alert for a trauma patient who reports abdominal pain—it may be a symptom of abdominal bleeding. Also be alert to vital signs that begin to worsen; this can be a sign of serious, unseen bleeding inside the abdomen.

When the hollow organs of the body have been injured, they may rupture and leak toxic chemicals used for digestion into the abdomen. This not only causes pain; since the contents of the intestines are not sterile, the patient also may eventually develop a life-threatening infection.

The abdomen also contains large blood vessels that supply the organs of this region and the lower extremities with oxygen-rich blood. Occasionally these vessels rupture or tear and cause serious unseen bleeding that may cause death. Some patients, particularly healthy young adults, are able to compensate longer than others for blood loss; therefore, you should always maintain a high index of suspicion when the MOI suggests injury to the abdominal region. This is best accomplished by reassessing the abdominal region using DCAP-BTLS.

Management: Transport and Destination

Caring for victims of traumatic injuries requires you to have a solid understanding of the trauma system in the United States. You need to have a good working knowledge of the resources available to you, including the most optimal methods of rapid transport and trauma centers that can best provide definitive care.

▶ Trauma Lethal Triad

Recent research has identified what has been termed the **trauma lethal triad** of hypothermia, coagulopathy (poor blood clotting), and acidosis as a major contributor to death in patients with severe traumatic bleeding[9] Figure 26-22. It has been well documented that even mildly hypothermic patients have a lower survival rate than normothermic patients. In addition, hypothermia

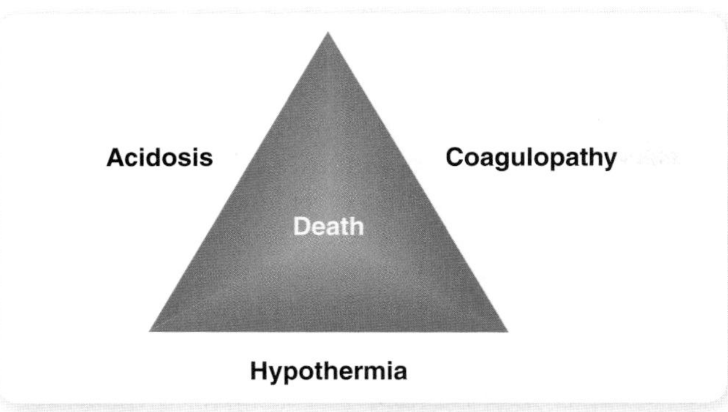

Figure 26-22 The trauma lethal triad.

contributes to coagulopathy, which also reduces survival from traumatic bleeding (if the blood cannot clot, the body cannot stop the bleeding). Any factor that interferes with blood clotting will cause more blood loss in the patient than would otherwise occur. This will result in poor perfusion and ultimately, death. Finally, acidosis (defined as a blood pH of less than 7.35) often occurs with excessive bleeding and treatments to compensate for it. For example, normal saline, which is commonly administered via bolus to treat hypotension, is acidic and can increase acidosis. Acidosis contributes to coagulopathy and complicates treatment of these patients.

How should knowledge of this lethal triad of conditions affect your treatment of trauma patients? First, you need to aggressively seek to control all bleeding to the best of your ability. Do not hesitate to use a tourniquet to stop bleeding from an extremity. Next, keep your patients warm; place blankets under them as well as on top of them, and ensure IV fluids are warmed to at least normal body temperature. Finally, minimize the volume of acidic IV fluid you administer to prevent interfering with coagulation and contributing to acidosis. If possible, monitor end-tidal carbon dioxide and ventilations to prevent respiratory acidosis, and consider calling for paramedic backup for administration of tranexamic acid (TXA), a medication that can help control internal bleeding, if local protocols allow and transport times to a trauma center may be prolonged.

▶ Scene Time

Because survival of critically injured trauma patients is time dependent, limit on-scene time to the minimum amount necessary to correct life-threatening injuries and package the patient. As mentioned, on-scene time for critically injured patients should ideally be less than 10 minutes—the platinum 10. The following criteria will help you identify a critically injured patient:

- Dangerous MOI
- Decreased level of consciousness
- Any threats to airway, breathing, or circulation

Patients who present with these criteria or who are very young or old or who have chronic illnesses should also be considered to be high risk, thus requiring rapid treatment and transport.

▶ Type of Transport

As discussed in Chapter 16, *Medical Overview*, modes of transport ultimately come in one of two categories: ground or air. When making the decision to transport by ground, several factors should be taken into consideration. Can the appropriate facility be reached within a reasonable time frame by ground transport? Ground transportation EMS units are generally staffed by emergency medical technicians, AEMTs, and paramedics. Air transportation EMS units or critical care transport units are generally staffed by critical care transport professionals such as critical care nurses and paramedics (Figure 26-23). What is the extent of injuries? If you're in a congested area, can the patient be transported to a more accessible landing zone for air medical transport?

You should be familiar with your local protocols defining indications for use of air medical transport. The Association of Air Medical Services (AAMS) and MedEvac Foundation International identify the following criteria in the white paper, *Air Medicine: Accessing the Future of Healthcare*, for the appropriate use of emergency air medical services for trauma patients.

- There is an extended period required to access or extricate a remote (eg, injured hiker, snowmobiler, or boater) or trapped patient (eg, in a crashed vehicle) that depletes the time frame to get the patient to the trauma center by ground.
- Distance to the trauma center is greater than 20 to 25 miles.
- The patient needs medical care and stabilization at the advanced life support (ALS) level, and there is no ALS-level ground ambulance service available within a reasonable time frame.
- Traffic conditions or hospital availability make it unlikely that the patient will get to a trauma center via ground ambulance within the ideal time frame for best clinical outcome.
- There are multiple patients who will overwhelm resources at the trauma centers reachable by ground within the time frame.
- EMS systems require patients to be brought to the nearest hospital for initial evaluation and stabilization, rather than bypassing those facilities and going directly to a trauma center.

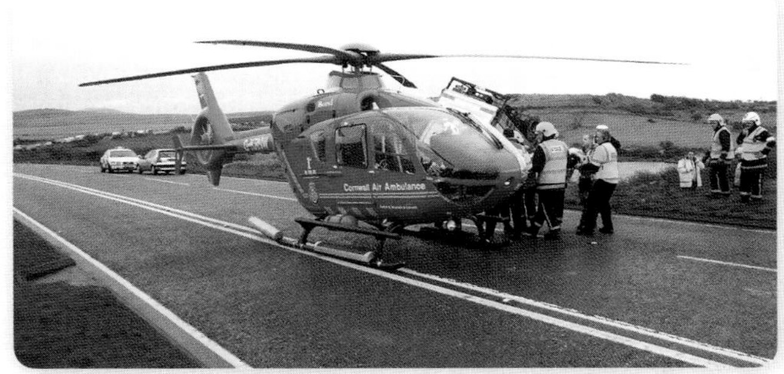

Figure 26-23 A helicopter may be used to transport patients quickly to a trauma center.

This may add delay to definitive surgical care and necessitate air transport to mitigate the effect of that delay.
- There is a multiple-casualty incident.

These recommendations serve as a guideline for local decision makers to develop more comprehensive protocols for the use of air medical transport. You should always follow your local protocols when determining what type of patient transportation is appropriate.

Destination Selection

You will often be summoned to accident scenes to transport critically ill trauma patients to definitive care. Before you even get to the scene, you should know the criteria for referral to a trauma center and what hospital resources are available in your area. It is important to transport your trauma patient to the most appropriate facility based on his or her injuries. The National Study on the Costs and Outcomes of Trauma reported a 25% decrease in mortality for severely injured adult patients who received care at a Level I trauma center compared with those treated at a lower level trauma center.[10] Trauma centers are classified into Levels I through IV, with Level I having the most resources followed by Levels II, III, and IV, respectively Table 26-6.

A Level I facility is a regional resource center and generally serves large cities or heavily populated areas.

Table 26-6 Key Elements for Trauma Centers

Level	Definition	Key Elements
Level I	A comprehensive regional resource that is a tertiary care facility; capable of providing total care for every aspect of injury—from prevention through rehabilitation	**1.** 24-hour in-house coverage by general surgeons **2.** Availability of care in specialties such as orthopaedic surgery, neurosurgery, anesthesiology, emergency medicine, radiology, internal medicine, and critical care **3.** Should also include cardiac, hand, pediatric, and microvascular surgery and hemodialysis **4.** Provides leadership in prevention, public education, and continuing education of trauma team members **5.** Committed to continued improvement through a comprehensive quality assessment program and organized research to help direct new innovations in trauma care
Level II	Able to initiate definitive care for all injured patients	**1.** 24-hour immediate coverage by general surgeons **2.** Availability of orthopaedic surgery, neurosurgery, anesthesiology, emergency medicine, radiology, and critical care **3.** Tertiary care needs such as cardiac surgery, hemodialysis, and microvascular surgery may be referred to a Level I trauma center **4.** Committed to trauma prevention and continuing education of trauma team members **5.** Provides continued improvement in trauma care through a comprehensive quality assessment program
Level III	Ability to provide prompt assessment, resuscitation, and stabilization of injured patients and emergency operations	**1.** 24-hour immediate coverage by emergency medicine physicians and prompt availability of general surgeons and anesthesiologists **2.** Program dedicated to continued improvement in trauma care through a comprehensive quality assessment program **3.** Has developed transfer agreements for patients requiring more comprehensive care at a Level I or Level II trauma center **4.** Committed to continuing education of nursing and allied health personnel or the trauma team **5.** Must be involved with prevention and have an active outreach program for its referring communities
Level IV	Ability to provide ATLS before transfer of patients to a higher level trauma center	**1.** Includes basic ED facilities to implement ATLS protocols and 24-hour laboratory coverage **2.** Transfer to higher level trauma centers follows the guidelines outlined in formal transfer agreements **3.** Committed to continued improvement of these trauma care activities through a formal quality assessment program **4.** Involved in prevention, outreach, and education within its community

Abbreviations: ATLS, Advanced Trauma Life Support; ED, emergency department

Data from: American College of Surgeons Committee on Trauma. *Resources for Optimal Care of the Injured Patient*. Chicago, IL: American College of Surgeons; 2014.

Level I facilities must be capable of providing every aspect of trauma care from prevention through rehabilitation; therefore, the facility must have adequate personnel and resources. Because of the extensive requirements, most Level I facilities are university-based teaching hospitals.

A Level II facility is typically located in areas of lower population density. Level II centers are expected to provide initial definitive care, regardless of injury severity. These facilities can be academic institutions or a public/private community facility. Because of its location and resources, a Level II trauma center may not be able to provide the same comprehensive care as a Level I trauma center. The major difference between Level I and Level II facilities is that the latter typically lack the same level of programmatic focus on trauma research and trauma prevention.

Level III facilities serve communities that do not have access to Level I or II facilities. Level III facilities provide assessment, resuscitation, emergency care, and stabilization. A Level III facility must have transfer agreements with a Level I or II trauma center and must have protocols in place to transfer patients whose needs exceed the resources of the facility.

Level IV facilities are typically found in remote outlying areas where no higher level of care is available. These facilities provide advanced trauma life support prior to transfer to a higher level trauma center. Such a facility may be a clinic urgent care facility, with or without a physician.

Although an inclusive trauma system should leave no facility without a direct link to a Level I or II facility, all facilities are expected to provide the same high quality of initial care regardless of the classification level.

Trauma centers are categorized as either adult trauma centers or pediatric trauma centers but not necessarily both. Pediatric trauma centers are not nearly as common as adult trauma centers. When transporting a pediatric trauma patient, you must be certain to transport your patient to a pediatric trauma center if there is one in your area; do not make the mistake of transporting a pediatric patient to an adult trauma center when a pediatric trauma center is available.

Words of Wisdom

Because traumatic injuries are as varied as the mechanisms that cause them, it is almost impossible for you to prepare for every possible situation that you may face during your career. In all situations, you must remain calm, complete an organized assessment, correct life-threatening injuries, and do no harm. You should never hesitate to contact paramedic backup or medical control for guidance.

It is important for you to be familiar with how the American College of Surgeons Committee on Trauma (ACS-COT) classifies trauma care. In 2011, the ACS-COT and the CDC published an updated field triage decision scheme **Figure 26-24**. These criteria are intended to help prehospital care providers recognize injured patients who are likely to benefit from transport to a trauma center compared with transport to an emergency department. It is not intended as a mass-casualty or disaster triage tool; it is only intended for individual patients.

Words of Wisdom

It is imperative that you have a strong understanding of trauma scoring systems to appropriately classify patients. The **trauma score** calculates a number from 1 to 16, with 16 being the best possible score. It accounts for the GCS score, respiratory rate, respiratory expansion, systolic blood pressure, and capillary refill. (See Chapter 10, *Patient Assessment*, for the GCS.) The GCS is an evaluation tool used to determine level of consciousness, which evaluates and assigns point values (scores) for eye opening, verbal response, and motor response; these scores are then totaled and help to effectively predict patient outcomes. Note that the lower the score, the more severe the extent of brain injury. The trauma score relates to the likelihood of patient survival. However, this scoring system does not accurately predict survivability in patients with severe head injuries because motor and verbal deficits make those criteria difficult to assess; in its place, the Revised Trauma Score, discussed next, is used.

Revised Trauma Score

The numeric scoring of trauma patients for determining the severity of their injury is common practice in the health care profession. When the various scoring systems were created, it was thought that the implementation of the scoring system would assist in rapidly identifying the severity of the patient's injuries. There are several different trauma scoring systems. The one that is the most commonly used for patients with head trauma is the **Revised Trauma Score (RTS)** because it is heavily weighted to compensate for major head injury without multisystem injury or major physiologic changes.

The RTS is a physiologic scoring system that is also used to assess the severity of a trauma patient's injuries. Objective data used to calculate the RTS include the GCS score, systolic blood pressure, and respiratory rate. In addition to assessing injury severity, the RTS has also demonstrated reliability in predicting survival in patients with severe injuries. The highest RTS a patient can receive is 12; the lowest is 0. The RTS is calculated as shown in **Table 26-7**.

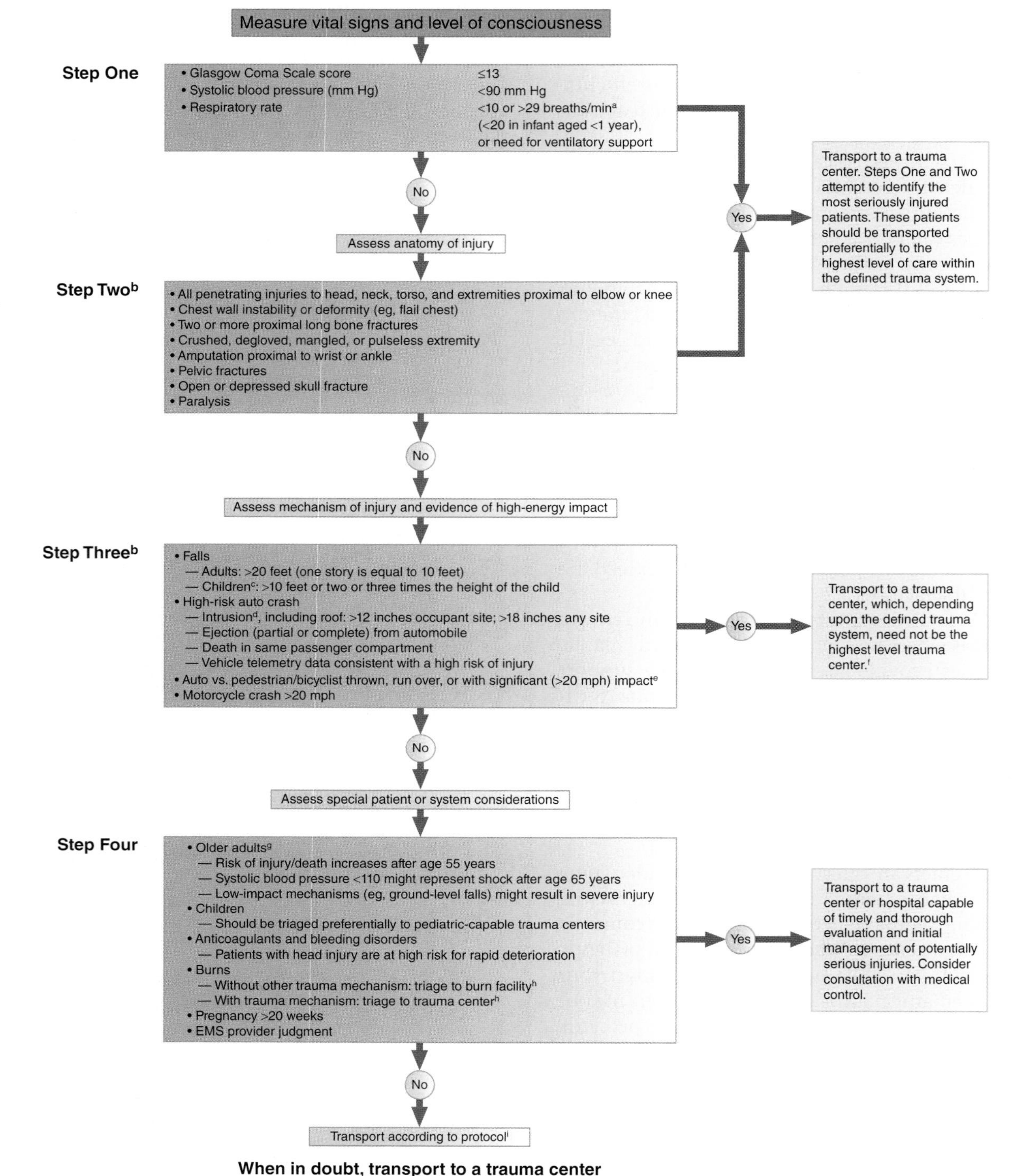

Measure vital signs and level of consciousness
Step One
• Glasgow Coma Scale score ≤13
• Systolic blood pressure (mm Hg) <90 mm Hg
• Respiratory rate <10 or >29 breaths/min[a] (<20 in infant aged <1 year), or need for ventilatory support
No
Yes
Transport to a trauma center. Steps One and Two attempt to identify the most seriously injured patients. These patients should be transported preferentially to the highest level of care within the defined trauma system.
Assess anatomy of injury
Step Two[b]
• All penetrating injuries to head, neck, torso, and extremities proximal to elbow or knee
• Chest wall instability or deformity (eg, flail chest)
• Two or more proximal long bone fractures
• Crushed, degloved, mangled, or pulseless extremity
• Amputation proximal to wrist or ankle
• Pelvic fractures
• Open or depressed skull fracture
• Paralysis
No
Assess mechanism of injury and evidence of high-energy impact
Step Three[b]
• Falls
— Adults: >20 feet (one story is equal to 10 feet)
— Children[c]: >10 feet or two or three times the height of the child
• High-risk auto crash
— Intrusion[d], including roof: >12 inches occupant site; >18 inches any site
— Ejection (partial or complete) from automobile
— Death in same passenger compartment
— Vehicle telemetry data consistent with a high risk of injury
• Auto vs. pedestrian/bicyclist thrown, run over, or with significant (>20 mph) impact[e]
• Motorcycle crash >20 mph
Yes
Transport to a trauma center, which, depending upon the defined trauma system, need not be the highest level trauma center.[f]
No
Assess special patient or system considerations
Step Four
• Older adults[g]
— Risk of injury/death increases after age 55 years
— Systolic blood pressure <110 might represent shock after age 65 years
— Low-impact mechanisms (eg, ground-level falls) might result in severe injury
• Children
— Should be triaged preferentially to pediatric-capable trauma centers
• Anticoagulants and bleeding disorders
— Patients with head injury are at high risk for rapid deterioration
• Burns
— Without other trauma mechanism: triage to burn facility[h]
— With trauma mechanism: triage to trauma center[h]
• Pregnancy >20 weeks
• EMS provider judgment
Yes
Transport to a trauma center or hospital capable of timely and thorough evaluation and initial management of potentially serious injuries. Consider consultation with medical control.
No
Transport according to protocol[i]
When in doubt, transport to a trauma center

Abbreviation: EMS, emergency medical services

[a] The upper limit of respiratory rate in infants is >29 breaths per minute to maintain a higher level of overtriage for infants.

[b] Any injury noted in Step Two or mechanism identified in Step Three triggers a "yes" response.

[c] Age <15 years.

[d] Intrusion refers to interior compartment intrusion, as opposed to deformation which refers to exterior damage.

[e] Includes pedestrians or bicyclists thrown or run over by a motor vehicle or those with estimated impact >20 mph with a motor vehicle.

[f] Local or regional protocols should be used to determine the most appropriate level of trauma center within the defined trauma system; need not be the highest-level trauma center.

[g] Age >55 years.

[h] Patients with both burns and concomitant trauma for whom the burn injury poses the greatest risk for morbidity and mortality should be transferred to a burn center. If the nonburn trauma presents a greater immediate risk, the patient may be stabilized in a trauma center and then transferred to a burn center.

[i] Patients who do not meet any of the triage criteria in Steps One through Four should be transported to the most appropriate medical facility as outlined in local EMS protocols.

Figure 26-24 2011 decision scheme for field triage of injured patients.

Data from: Centers for Disease Control and Prevention. Guidelines for field triage of injured patients: recommendations of the national expert panel on field triage, 2011. *Morbidity and Mortality Weekly Report (MMWR)*, January 13, 2012.

Table 26-7 Revised Trauma Score

Glasgow Coma Scale Score	Systolic Blood Pressure	Respiratory Rate	Value
13 to 15	>89 mm Hg	10 to 29 breaths/min	4
9 to 12	76 to 89 mm Hg	>29 breaths/min	3
6 to 8	50 to 75 mm Hg	6 to 9 breaths/min	2
4 to 5	1 to 49 mm Hg	1 to 5 breaths/min	1
3	0	0	0

YOU are the Provider SUMMARY

1. On the basis of the information provided, what are some possible injuries you may encounter?

Rear-end impacts are known to cause whiplash-type injuries, particularly when the head and/or neck is not restrained by an appropriately placed headrest. In this type of crash, the cervical spine and surrounding area may be injured. The cervical spine is less tolerant of damage when it is bent backward. Other parts of the spine and the pelvis may also be at risk for injury. In addition, the patient may sustain a deceleration injury to the brain—that is, the third collision of the brain within the skull.

2. With the understanding that patients at this scene are most likely critical, how long should you remain on-scene?

In most patients with multisystem trauma, definitive care requires surgical intervention; therefore, on-scene time should be limited to 10 minutes or less. This time frame is referred to as the platinum 10 minutes.

3. To which type of hospital should this patient be transported?

On the basis of the patient's MOI and obvious trauma, she should be transported to a Level I trauma center; however, many jurisdictions do not have readily available trauma centers. If a trauma center is not available, the patient should be transported to the closest appropriate facility, according to your protocols.

4. Does this patient meet the criteria for aeromedical evacuation?

This patient meets the criteria for aeromedical evacuation based on the suspected prolonged extrication time and the amount of time that it would take to reach the trauma center.

The Association of Air Medical Services and MedEvac Foundation International recommendations serve as a guideline for local decision makers to develop more comprehensive protocols for the use of air medical transport. Always follow your local protocols when determining what type of patient transportation is appropriate.

5. What is the crackling sound heard on the neck, and how is it caused?

A fracture of the cartilage of the upper airway and larynx can result in the leakage of air into the soft tissue of the neck (subcutaneous emphysema), producing a crackling feeling when palpated. Either air in the circulation or an airway cartilage fracture may cause rapid death.

6. Now that the critical patient has departed the scene, what should you do with the deceased patient?

Appropriate procedures for handling a deceased patient depend on your local protocols. If your jurisdictional policies and procedures require you to transport the deceased to the funeral home or medical examiner, consult with on-scene law enforcement to ensure that you are clear to commence transport. If local custom does not allow for transport of the deceased, you should approach law enforcement and ascertain if there is any additional information they need from your service or if you are clear to depart the scene. In some cases, you will be asked to remain on scene with the body until the medical examiner arrives. Understand your local protocols and laws regarding the management of deceased persons.

YOU are the Provider SUMMARY *(continued)*

EMS Patient Care Report (PCR)			
Date: 10-8-18	**Incident No.:** 20108752-2	**Nature of Call:** MVC	**Location:** 500 block of West 3rd Street

Dispatched: 1622	**En Route:** 1623	**At Scene:** 1628	**Transport:**	**At Hospital:**	**In Service:** 1728

Patient Information	
Age: Approximately 45-50 **Sex:** F **Weight (in kg [lb]):** 72 kg (160 lb)	**Allergies:** Unknown **Medications:** Unknown **Past Medical History:** Unknown **Chief Complaint:** Multisystem trauma

Vital Signs				
Time: 1629	**BP:** Not obtained	**Pulse:** Not obtained	**Respirations:** 8	**Spo_2:** Not obtained
Time: 1642	**BP:** Unable to obtain	**Pulse:** 140 carotid	**Respirations:** 12 assisted	**Spo_2:** Unable to obtain
Time: 1648	**BP:** Unable to obtain	**Pulse:** 120 carotid	**Respirations:** 12 assisted	**Spo_2:** Unable to obtain

EMS Treatment (circle all that apply)			
Oxygen @ 15 **L/min via (circle one):** **NC** **NRM** **(Bag-mask device)**	**(Assisted Ventilation:** Yes**)**	**(Airway Adjunct:** Dual-lumen airway**)**	**CPR**

Defibrillation	**Bleeding Control**	**Bandaging**	**Splinting**	**Other:**

Narrative
EMS dispatched to the 500 block of W 3rd Street for MVC. En route dispatch advises MVC is a result of high-speed police pursuit. Vehicle rear-ended another at approximately 85 to 90 miles per hour. Officers believe that patient in fleeing vehicle is deceased. On arrival triage performed. Driver in vehicle #2 tagged black based on unresponsiveness, cardiac arrest, and exposed brain matter (see PCR 20108752-1). Patient #2 found in small pickup with severe rear-end damage, unrestrained, severely entrapped with a GCS of 4 (E-1, V-2, M-1). Fire department on scene for extrication. Helicopter requested. Once patient extricated, cervical collar applied, secured on long backboard. Patient found to have decreased respirations. Dual-lumen airway inserted without difficulty, ventilated at 12 breaths/min. Bilateral 18-gauge IVs established with 250-mL bolus of normal saline x 2 infused for hypotension. Physical exam reveals subcutaneous emphysema to base of neck. Abdomen noted to be distended and rigid. On arrival of flight crew, report given. Assisted with transfer of patient into helicopter. Care released to flight crew without further incident.**End of report**

Prep Kit

▶ Ready for Review

- Mechanism of injury (MOI) is the way in which traumatic injuries occur; it describes the forces (or energy transmission) acting on the body that cause injury.
- Obtaining information about the MOI—that is, how the injuries occurred and what forces were likely involved—can be just as important as obtaining vital signs in assessing the patient. This information can help hospital staff to focus their attention on damage that may not be immediately obvious.
- Significant mechanisms of injury include ejection from a vehicle; injury to more than one body system (multisystem trauma); falls from heights, motor vehicle and motorcycle crashes, vehicle versus pedestrian (or bicycle or motorcycle), gunshot wounds, and stabbings; unresponsiveness or altered mental status following trauma; and penetrating trauma to the head, chest, or abdomen.
- Index of suspicion is an AEMT's awareness and concern for potentially serious underlying and unseen injuries. The index of suspicion should be partly based on the MOI.
- Whether one body system or more than one system is involved, maintain a high index of suspicion for serious unseen injuries.
- In every crash there are three collisions: the collision of the vehicle against another vehicle or some other object, the collision of the passenger against the interior of the car, and the collision of the passenger's internal organs against the solid structures of the body.
- There are several types of collisions, including frontal crashes, rear-end crashes, lateral crashes, rollover crashes, and rotational crashes. Each type of collision will result in certain injury patterns and may cause blunt trauma, penetrating trauma, or both. Remember to determine whether the passenger was restrained, and note whether the air bag deployed.
- In crashes involving a vehicle and a pedestrian, the pedestrian is likely to have unseen injuries. Estimate the speed of the vehicle that struck the patient. Determine whether the patient was ejected, what surface the patient landed on, and at what distance or whether the patient was struck and pulled under the vehicle. Evaluate the vehicle for structural damage that might indicate contact points with the patient.
- In a vehicle-versus-bicycle crash, evaluate the MOI as you normally would, but also evaluate damage to and the position of the bicycle. Assume spinal injury. If there is damage to the rider's helmet, suspect potential injury to the head.
- When you are assessing the scene of a motorcycle crash, note any deformity of the motorcycle, the side with the most damage, the distance of skid in the road, the deformity of stationary objects or other vehicles, and the extent and location of deformity in the helmet.
- The injury potential of a fall is related to the height from which the patient fell. The greater the height of the fall, the greater the potential for injury. Again, as in a motor vehicle crash, it is these internal injuries that are the least obvious on assessment but pose the gravest threat to life.
- Penetrating trauma is classified as low energy, medium energy, or high energy. A projectile that impacts the body may fragment and cause cavitation—additional damage caused by the object moving inside the body and not along the suspected pathway.
- You should suspect serious injuries in passengers who have been involved in a high-speed crash that results in massive damage to the vehicle. The same is true of a patient who has fallen from a substantial height, sustained a high-velocity penetrating injury, or is the victim of an explosion or blast.
- Multisystem trauma is a term that describes the injuries of a person who has been subjected to multiple traumatic injuries involving more than one body system such as head and spinal trauma, chest and abdominal trauma, or chest and multiple extremity trauma. You must recognize multisystem trauma patients and provide rapid treatment and transportation.
- Limit on-scene time to the minimum amount necessary to correct life-threatening injuries and package the patient. On-scene time for critically injured patients should be less than 10 minutes.
- The type of transport needed will vary based on the patient's condition. Options include standard

Prep Kit *(continued)*

EMS ground transport, or critical care transport, which can occur over ground or air in a specialized ambulance or helicopter, respectively.

- As an AEMT, you will need to determine the most appropriate destination for trauma patients based on local protocols. There are four levels of trauma centers in the United States: Levels I, II, III, and IV. Extensive requirements apply to Level I facilities, which must be capable of providing every aspect of trauma care from prevention through rehabilitation. Level IV facilities are typically found in remote areas where no higher level of care is available.
- Finally, it is important to be familiar with the American College of Surgeons Committee on Trauma decision scheme for field triage of injured patients.

▶ Vital Vocabulary

arterial air embolism Air bubbles in the arterial blood vessels.

barometric energy The energy that results from sudden changes in pressure as may occur in a diving accident or sudden decompression in an airplane.

blast injuries Injuries resulting from explosions; possible injuries include internal injuries resulting from the pressure wave, penetrating trauma from shrapnel or from being thrown, blunt trauma from being thrown, and burns.

blunt trauma Result of force (or energy transmission) to impact on the body that causes injury without penetrating soft tissues or internal organs and cavities.

cavitation Formation of a temporary cavity that is produced by stretching of the tissue surrounding the point of impact—for example, when speed causes a bullet to generate pressure waves, which cause damage distant from the bullet's path.

chemical energy The energy released as a result of a chemical reaction.

coup-contrecoup Occurs when the brain continues its forward motion and strikes the inside of the skull, resulting in a compression injury to the anterior portion of the brain and stretching of the posterior portion.

deceleration The slowing of an object.

drag Resistance, such as air, that slows a projectile.

electrical energy Energy delivered in the form of high voltage.

entrance wound The point at which a penetrating object enters the body.

exit wound The point at which a penetrating object leaves the body, which may or may not be in a straight line from the entry wound.

flash burns Electrothermal injuries caused by arcing of electric current.

index of suspicion The AEMT's awareness that unseen serious and/or life-threatening injuries may exist when determining the mechanism of injury.

kinetic energy The energy of a moving object.

kinetics The study of the relationship among speed, mass, vector direction, and physical injury.

mechanical energy The energy that results from motion (kinetic energy) or that is stored in an object (potential energy).

mechanism of injury (MOI) The way in which traumatic injuries occur; the forces that act on the body to cause injury.

multisystem trauma A term that describes the injuries of a person who has been subjected to multiple traumatic injuries involving more than one body system; these patients have a high level of morbidity and mortality.

penetrating trauma Injury caused by objects that pierce and penetrate the surface of the body and injure the underlying tissues, such as knives and bullets, and damage internal organs and body cavities.

petechiae Small, purple, nonblanching spots on the skin.

potential energy The product of mass (weight), gravity, and height that is converted into kinetic energy and results in injury, such as from a fall.

pulmonary blast injuries Pulmonary trauma resulting from short-range exposure to the detonation of explosives.

Revised Trauma Score (RTS) A scoring system used for patients with head trauma.

thermal energy Energy transferred from sources that are hotter than the body, such as a flame, hot water, or steam.

Prep Kit *(continued)*

trajectory The path a projectile takes after it is propelled from a weapon or explosion.

trauma lethal triad A combination of hypothermia, coagulopathy (poor blood clotting), and acidosis that is a major contributor to death in patients with severe traumatic bleeding.

trauma score A score that relates to the likelihood of patient survival of traumatic injuries with the exception of a severe head injury. It calculates a number from 1 to 16, with 16 being the best possible score taking into account the Glasgow Coma Scale score, respiratory rate, respiratory expansion, systolic blood pressure, and capillary refill.

tympanic membrane The eardrum; a thin, semitransparent membrane in the middle ear that transmits sound vibrations to the internal ear by means of auditory ossicles.

work In the context of kinematics, the product of force times distance.

▶ References

1. 10 leading causes of death by age group, United States – 2015. National Vital Statistics System, National Center for Health Statistics, Centers for Disease Control and Prevention. https://www.cdc.gov/injury/wisqars/LeadingCauses.html. Accessed September 22, 2017.
2. Injury Prevention and Control: Data and Statistics. Centers for Disease Control and Prevention website. (WISQARS). http://www.cdc.gov/injury/wisqars/overview/key_data.html. Updated September 19, 2016. Accessed October 26, 2017.
3. Top causes of unintentional injury and death in homes and communities. The National Safety Council website. http://www.nsc.org/learn/safety-knowledge/Pages/safety-at-home.aspx. Accessed November 3, 2017.
4. 2014 motor vehicle crashes: overview. National Center for Statistics and Analysis. National Highway Traffic Safety Administration website. https://crashstats.nhtsa.dot.gov/Api/Public/ViewPublication/812246. Published March 2016. Accessed October 29, 2017.
5. Seat Belts. National Highway Traffic Safety Administration website. https://www.nhtsa.gov/risky-driving/seat-belts. Accessed December 20, 2017.
6. Laberge-Nadeau C, Bellavance F, Messier S, Vézina L, Pichette F. Occupant injury severity from lateral collisions: a literature review. *J Safety Res.* 2009;40(6):427–435.
7. 2015 Summary of motor vehicle crashes (final edition). National Center for Statistics and Analysis. National Highway Traffic Safety Administration website. https://crashstats.nhtsa.dot.gov. Published October 2017. Accessed October 31, 2017.
8. 10 Leading Causes of Injury Deaths by Age Group Highlighting Unintentional Injury Deaths, United States–2015. Centers for Disease Control and Prevention website. https://www.cdc.gov/injury/images/lc-charts/leading_causes_of_injury_deaths_unintentional_injury_2015_1050w760h.gif. Accessed November 13, 2017.
9. Gerecht R. The lethal triad. Hypothermia, acidosis & coagulopathy create a deadly cycle for trauma patients. *J Emerg Med.* 2014;39(4):56-60.
10. MacKenzie EJ, Rivara FP, Jurkovich GJ, Nathens AB. The national study on the costs and outcomes of trauma. *J Trauma.* 2007;63(suppl 6):S54-S67.

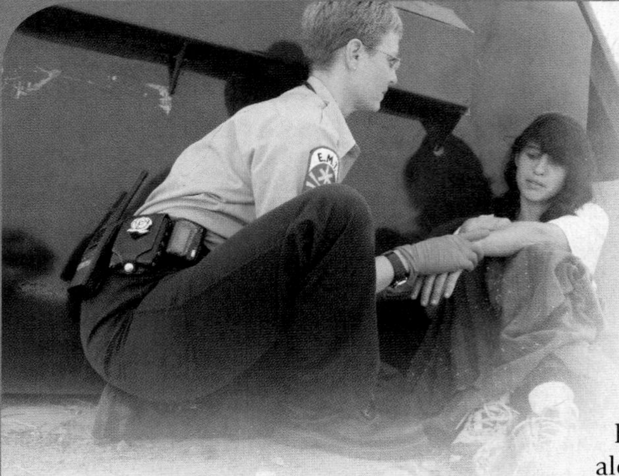

Assessment *in Action*

You arrive at a local chemical manufacturing plant for a reported explosion. You are met by the plant foreman, who states there was a flash fire and explosion caused by gasoline. He tells you that he has been able to account for all of his employees, and after inspection, only one employee has sustained injuries. As you assess the patient, you find him alert and oriented, reporting abdominal pain, a laceration to his right arm, and partial deafness in his left ear.

1. The laceration to the patient's right arm was most likely caused by which type of blast injury?

A. Primary blast injury
B. Secondary blast injury
C. Tertiary blast injury
D. Miscellaneous blast injury

2. The patient's deafness can be attributed to which type of blast injury?

A. Primary blast injury
B. Secondary blast injury
C. Tertiary blast injury
D. Miscellaneous blast injury

3. Which organs are most susceptible to injury during an explosion?

A. Liver
B. Kidney
C. Lungs
D. Ear

4. What is one of the most common causes of death from blast injuries?

A. Long bone fractures
B. Head trauma
C. Tracheal lacerations
D. Hypoxia

5. Tertiary injuries are a result of:

A. the patient striking an object.
B. a pressure wave.
C. biological, chemical, or radioactive contaminants.
D. miscellaneous events that occur during an explosion.

6. What type of energy is contained in a moving object?

A. Mass
B. Velocity
C. Kinetic energy
D. Potential energy

Assessment *in Action* *(continued)*

7. All of the following are associated with a significant MOI EXCEPT:

A. Death of an occupant in the vehicle
B. Severe deformities of the vehicle
C. Intrusion into the vehicle
D. Speed of less than 30 mph

8. In frontal collisions, there are two pathways for injuries, the up-and-over pathway and the down-and-under pathway. Which of the following injuries would most likely be a result of the down-and-under pathway?

A. Spine injuries
B. Abdominal injuries
C. Chest injuries
D. Pelvic injuries

9. Describe the three typical collisions in a crash.

10. Which factors should be taken into account when assessing a patient who fell?

CHAPTER 27

Bleeding

National EMS Education Standard Competencies

Trauma

Applies fundamental knowledge to provide basic and selected advanced emergency care and transportation based on assessment findings for an acutely injured patient.

Bleeding

Pathophysiology, assessment, and management of
- Bleeding (pp 1097-1118)
- Fluid resuscitation (Chapter 14, *Shock*)

Pathophysiology

Applies comprehensive knowledge of the pathophysiology of respiration and perfusion to patient assessment and management.

Knowledge Objectives

1. Discuss the physiology of perfusion. (pp 1095-1096)
2. Review the cardiac cycle, including the concepts of preload, afterload, and cardiac output. (pp 1096-1097)
3. Discuss the pathophysiology of external and internal bleeding. (pp 1097-1099)
4. Describe the characteristics of arterial bleeding, venous bleeding, and capillary bleeding. (pp 1097-1098)
5. Explain how to determine the nature of illness for internal bleeding, including identifying possible traumatic and nontraumatic causes. (p 1099)
6. List the signs and symptoms of internal bleeding. (p 1099)
7. List the signs and symptoms of hypovolemic shock. (p 1099)
8. Discuss the body's physiologic response to hemorrhaging. (pp 1100, 1102-1103)
9. Describe the four classes of hemorrhaging. (p 1102)
10. Describe the assessment process for patients with external and internal bleeding. (pp 1103-1107)
11. Discuss the importance of addressing life-threatening hemorrhage prior to airway and breathing concerns. (p 1104)
12. Describe what could be happening in the body when a patient with suspected internal bleeding becomes calm and still. (p 1104)
13. Discuss transport considerations for patients who are hemorrhaging. (pp 1104-1105)
14. Explain the emergency medical care of a patient with external bleeding. (pp 1107-1109)
15. Discuss situations in which a tourniquet may be used to control external bleeding. (p 1109)
16. List precautions to follow when applying a tourniquet. (p 1112)
17. Discuss the use of splints to control external bleeding. (pp 1112-1113)
18. Describe how hemostatic agents work to control severe hemorrhage. (p 1113)
19. List specific instances in which using a pneumatic antishock garment (PASG) to control bleeding may be an effective alternative. (p 1114)
20. Discuss assessment and management of bleeding from the nose, ears, and mouth. (pp 1114-1115)
21. Explain the emergency medical care of a patient with internal bleeding. (pp 1115-1117)
22. Explain how to manage hemorrhagic shock. (pp 1117-1118)

Skills Objectives

1. Demonstrate emergency medical care of the patient with external bleeding using direct pressure. (pp 1108-1109, Skill Drill 27-1)
2. Demonstrate emergency medical care of the patient with external bleeding using a commercial tourniquet. (pp 1110-1112, Skill Drill 27-2)
3. Demonstrate emergency medical care of the patient who shows signs and symptoms of internal bleeding. (pp 1115-1117, Skill Drill 27-3)

Introduction

The most current shift in trauma care takes the initial immediate focus off of airway and transfers it to circulation when there is evidence of severe external hemorrhage. Bleeding can be one of the most time-sensitive conditions you will face as an advanced emergency medical technician (AEMT).

The end goal in trauma care is to maintain perfusion. A patient with massive external hemorrhage must have his or her bleeding controlled immediately or exsanguination and death will result. In such a case, circulation takes temporary priority over airway and breathing. Addressing the airway instead of prioritizing bleeding control for severe external hemorrhage will result in ventilation and oxygenation to the lungs, but there would be inadequate blood remaining in the circulation to transport that oxygen to the tissues for perfusion, and that is a problem that cannot be corrected in the prehospital setting. A perfectly managed airway is inconsequential if the circulatory system is not able to deliver oxygen to the organs and remove accumulated waste products from them.

Bleeding can be external and obvious or internal and hidden. Either way, it is potentially dangerous, first causing weakness and, if left uncontrolled, eventually shock and death. The most common cause of shock after trauma is bleeding. This chapter begins with control of external hemorrhaging, covers recognition and management of internal hemorrhaging, and ends with transportation of patients with bleeding. Refer to Chapter 14, *Shock*, for guidelines on shock and fluid resuscitation.

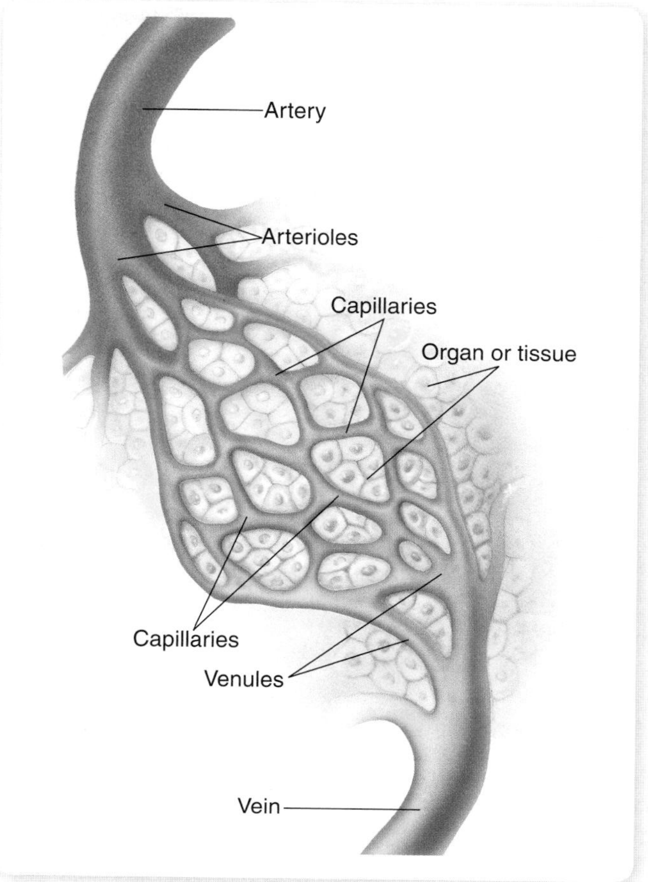

Figure 27-1 Perfusion occurs when blood circulates through tissues or an organ to provide the necessary oxygen and nutrients and remove waste products.

Physiology and Perfusion

The anatomy and physiology of the cardiovascular system was covered in Chapter 7, *The Human Body*. Recall that **perfusion** is the circulation of blood within an organ or tissue in adequate amounts to meet the cells' current needs for oxygen, nutrients, and waste removal. Blood enters an organ or tissue first through the arteries, then the arterioles, and finally the capillary beds Figure 27-1. While passing through the capillaries, the blood delivers nutrients and oxygen to the surrounding cells and picks up the wastes they have generated. Then the blood leaves the capillary beds through the venules and finally reaches the veins, which take the blood back to the heart. Oxygen and carbon dioxide exchange takes place in the lungs.

Blood must pass through the cardiovascular system at a speed that is fast enough to maintain adequate circulation throughout the body and slow enough to allow each cell time to exchange oxygen and nutrients for carbon dioxide and other waste products. Although some tissues, such as

YOU are the Provider PART 1

It is opening day of deer season, and you and your partner are dispatched to a location in the backwoods for a man who has been shot. En route to the scene, dispatch advises you that this is an accidental shooting; the patient was climbing his tree stand, slipped, and fell, causing his rifle to discharge into his left bicep. Approximately 5 minutes from the scene, dispatch advises that law enforcement is on scene requesting you to expedite because the patient is bleeding badly.

On arrival, you meet the deputy who tells you that the patient is approximately one-third to one-half mile back on a trail, and he does not look good. As your partner grabs the jump kit and a tourniquet, you radio dispatch and request a helicopter to meet you at the scene. You find the patient propped against a tree, seated in a large puddle of blood. He is holding direct pressure to the wound; however, it still appears to be bleeding.

1. What are some possible hazards in this scene?
2. Is aeromedical evacuation appropriate with this patient?

the lungs and kidneys, never rest and require a constant blood supply, most tissues require circulating blood only intermittently, especially when active. Muscles are a good example. When you sleep, they are at rest and require a minimal blood supply. However, during exercise, they need a very large blood supply. The gastrointestinal (GI) tract requires a high flow of blood after a meal. After digestion is completed, however, the GI tract functions well with only a fraction of that blood flow.

The autonomic nervous system monitors the body's needs from moment to moment and adjusts the blood flow as required. During emergencies, the autonomic nervous system automatically redirects blood away from other organs to the heart, brain, lungs, and kidneys. Thus, the cardiovascular system is dynamic, constantly adapting to changing conditions. At times, the system fails to provide sufficient circulation for every body part to perform its function. This condition is called hypoperfusion, or **shock**, which can result in death.

Safety

When you are caring for a patient who is bleeding, be sure to take necessary precautions to protect yourself from splashing or splattering. Wear appropriate protective equipment, including gloves, gown, mask, and eye protection. This equipment is especially important when arterial bleeding is present. Also remember that frequent, thorough handwashing between patients and after every run is a simple yet important protective measure.

Knowing which organs need adequate perfusion is the foundation on which your treatment of patients is based. Emergency medical care is designed to support the following systems:

- The heart (cardiovascular system)
- The brain and spinal cord (central nervous system)
- The lungs (respiratory system)
- The kidneys (renal system)

The heart requires constant perfusion or it will not function properly. The brain and spinal cord cannot be without perfusion for more than 4 to 6 minutes or the nerve cells will be permanently damaged. Remember that cells of the central nervous system do not have the capacity to regenerate. The kidneys will be permanently damaged after 45 minutes of inadequate perfusion. Skeletal muscles cannot tolerate more than 2 to 3 hours of inadequate perfusion. The GI tract can exist with limited (but not absent) perfusion for several hours. These perfusion times are based on a normal body temperature (98.6°F [37.0°C]). An organ or tissue that is considerably colder is much better able to resist damage from hypoperfusion because of a slower metabolism. As a person's metabolism decreases, so does the need for oxygen and nutrients. This also decreases the production of waste products, which can be damaging if they are not promptly removed.

Words of Wisdom

When you are treating more than one patient, it is essential to change gloves every time you alternate between patients to prevent cross-contamination.

▶ The Cardiac Cycle

The cardiac cycle is the repetitive pumping process that begins with the onset of cardiac muscle contraction and ends with the beginning of the next contraction. Myocardial contraction results in pressure changes within the cardiac chambers, causing the blood to move from areas of high pressure to areas of low pressure.

Preload is the amount of blood returned to the heart to be pumped out. It directly affects **afterload**, the pressure in the aorta or the peripheral vascular resistance (PVR), against which the left ventricle must pump blood. The greater the afterload, the harder it is for the ventricle to eject blood into the aorta. A higher afterload, therefore, reduces the stroke volume (SV), or the amount of blood ejected per contraction. To a large degree, afterload is governed by arterial blood pressure.

The cardiac cycle is connected to bleeding and shock through its relationship to blood pressure, the level of which is considered the dividing line between the stages of shock. In general terms, blood pressure is represented by the following equation:

$$\text{Blood pressure} = \text{Cardiac output (CO)} \times \text{Peripheral vascular resistance (PVR)}$$

where PVR is essentially the resistance in the vessels caused by vasoconstriction or vasodilation. Mean arterial pressure (MAP) is a measurement of arterial pressure in the vessels that perfuse the organs and indicates changes between cardiac output and PVR. It can be estimated using the following equation:

$$\text{MAP} = \text{Diastolic pressure} + 1/3 \text{ Pulse pressure}$$

The **pulse pressure** is calculated by subtracting the diastolic blood pressure (DBP) from the systolic blood pressure (SBP):

$$\text{MAP} = \text{DBP} + 1/3\ (\text{SBP} - \text{DBP})$$

Cardiac output (CO) is the amount of blood pumped through the circulatory system in 1 minute. Cardiac output is expressed in liters per minute (L/min). Cardiac output equals the stroke volume multiplied by the pulse rate:

$$\text{CO} = \text{SV} \times \text{Pulse rate}$$

Factors that influence the SV, the pulse rate, or both will affect cardiac output and, therefore, oxygen delivery (perfusion) to the tissues.

Increased venous return to the heart stretches the ventricles somewhat, resulting in increased cardiac contractility. This relationship, which was first described by the British physiologist Ernest Henry Starling, is known as the Frank-Starling mechanism or Starling law of the heart. Starling noted that if a muscle is stretched slightly before it is stimulated to contract, it will contract with greater force. Thus, if the heart is stretched, the muscle contracts more forcefully.

Although the amount of blood returning to the right atrium varies somewhat from minute to minute, a normal heart continues to pump the same percentage of blood returned, a measure called the ejection fraction. If more blood returns to the heart, the stretched heart pumps harder rather than allowing the blood to back up into the veins. As a result, more blood is pumped with each contraction, yet the ejection fraction remains unchanged: the amount of blood that is pumped increases, but so does the amount of blood returned. This relationship maintains normal cardiac function when a person changes positions, coughs, breathes, or moves.

The delivery of oxygen to the tissues is dependent on an adequate heart rate, SV, hemoglobin levels, and arterial oxygen saturation. If any of these elements is not adequate, tissues will become ischemic.

Words of Wisdom

Hematocrit blood testing measures the portion of red blood cells in whole blood. Normal hematocrit values vary, but in general are as follows:

- Men (any age): 40.7% to 50.3%
- Women (any age): 36.1% to 44.3%

If a patient's hematocrit level is out of range, the patient may have some sort of disease. Many different diseases or conditions could cause an abnormal level, resulting in anemia.

Pathophysiology

The pathophysiology of shock is covered in Chapter 14, *Shock*, but is relevant to the topic of bleeding. Review Chapter 14 for a discussion of the progression of shock and its signs and symptoms.

A **hemorrhage** is a discharge of blood from the blood vessels; it also simply means bleeding. Bleeding can range from a nicked capillary while shaving, to a severely spurting artery from a deep slash with a knife, to a ruptured spleen from being crushed against the steering column during a car crash. External bleeding (visible hemorrhaging) can often be controlled by using direct, even pressure, pressure dressings and/or splints, hemostatic dressings, tourniquets, or a pressure bandage **Figure 27-2**.

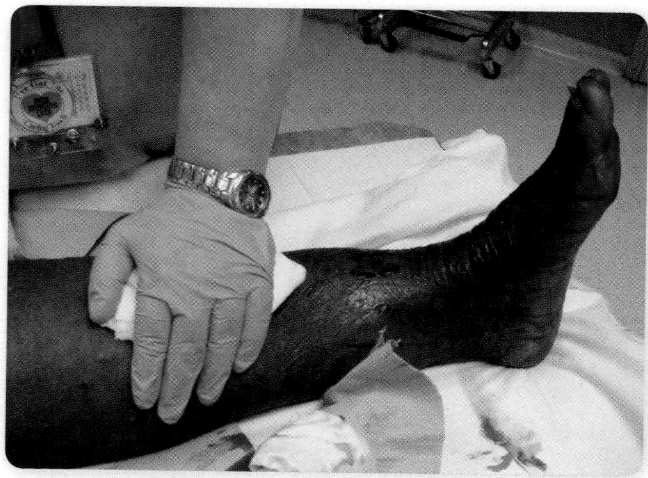

Figure 27-2 Most external bleeding can be controlled with direct pressure.

Courtesy of Rhonda Hunt.

Internal bleeding (hemorrhaging that is not visible) is usually not controlled in the prehospital setting. Because internal bleeding is not as obvious, you must rely on signs and symptoms to determine the extent and severity of the hemorrhaging.

External Hemorrhaging

External bleeding is usually a result of a break in the skin. Its extent or severity is often a function of the type of wound and the types of blood vessels that have been injured. Typically, bleeding from an open artery is bright red (high in oxygen) and spurts in time with the pulse. The pressure that causes the blood to spurt also makes this type of bleeding difficult to control. As the amount of blood circulating in the body decreases, so does the patient's blood pressure and, eventually, the arterial spurting.

Blood from an open vein is much darker (low in oxygen) and flows steadily. Because it is under less pressure, most venous blood does not spurt and is easier to manage; however, it can still be life threatening. Bleeding from damaged capillary vessels is dark red and oozes from a wound steadily but slowly. Venous and capillary bleeding is more likely to clot spontaneously than arterial blood **Figure 27-3**.

These descriptions are not infallible. For example, considerable oozing from capillaries is possible when a patient has a large abrasion (such as in the case of road rash when a cyclist slides along the pavement without protective clothing). Similarly, varicose veins on the leg can produce copious bleeding.

Arteries may spurt initially, but as the patient's blood pressure decreases, often the blood simply flows. If an artery is incised directly across, or transversely, muscle contractions will often slow or tamponade bleeding. By contrast, if the artery is cut on a bias (such as a longitudinal incision), muscular contractions may pull the wound open further, causing continual bleeding.

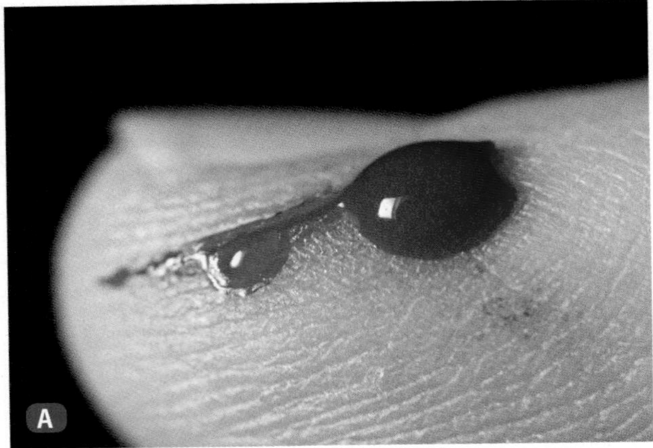

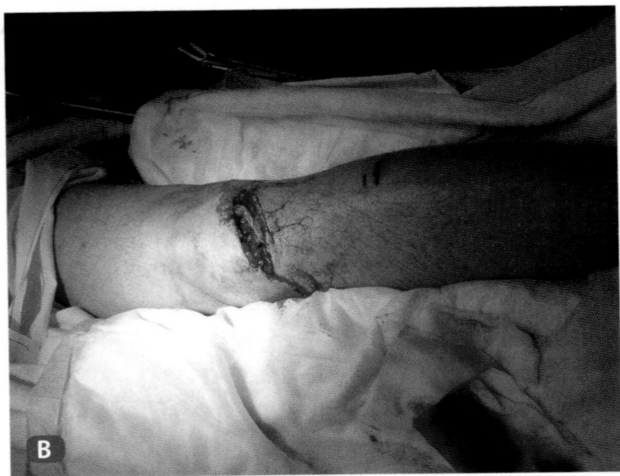

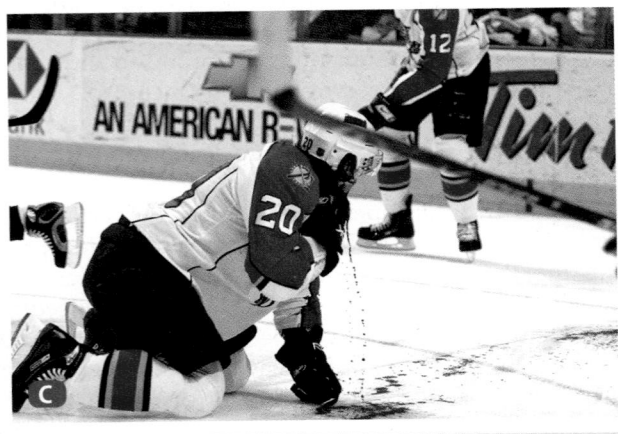

Figure 27-3 A. Bleeding from capillary vessels is dark red and oozes from the wound slowly but steadily. **B.** Venous bleeding is darker red and flows steadily. **C.** Arterial bleeding is characteristically bright red and spurts in pulses.

A: Sasha Radosavljevic/iStock/Getty; B: © E.M. Singletary, M.D. Used with permission; C: © Brian Slichta/ AP Photo.

> **Words of Wisdom**
>
> Red blood cells are approximately one-third hemoglobin, the protein that gives them their red color. Hemoglobin is responsible for the cells' ability to transport oxygen and carbon dioxide. When hemoglobin binds with oxygen, oxyhemoglobin is formed. Oxyhemoglobin is bright red. When oxygen is released, deoxyhemoglobin is formed. Deoxyhemoglobin is darker red, and blood rich in deoxyhemoglobin may appear blue when seen through blood vessels.

Some injuries that you might expect to be accompanied by considerable external bleeding do not always have serious hemorrhaging. For example, a person who falls off the platform at the train station and is run over by a train may have an amputation of one or more extremities, yet experience little bleeding because the wound was functionally cauterized by the heat of the train's wheels on the rail. Another example is a person who pulled over on the shoulder of the road and was removing the jack from his car's trunk when another motorist slammed into the rear of the car, pinning him between the two vehicles. Most likely the person's legs are severely crushed but there may be little bleeding because the legs are compressed between the vehicles.

▶ Internal Hemorrhaging

Internal bleeding as a result of trauma may appear in any portion of the body. A fracture of a small bone (such as a humerus, ankle, or tibia) produces a somewhat controlled environment in which a relatively small amount of bleeding can occur. By contrast, bleeding into the trunk (that is, thorax, abdomen, or pelvis), because of its much larger space, tends to be severe and uncontrolled. Nontraumatic internal hemorrhage often occurs in cases of GI bleeding from the upper or lower GI tract, ruptured ectopic pregnancies, ruptured aneurysms, or other conditions.

> **Words of Wisdom**
>
> Consider any patient exhibiting signs and symptoms of shock without obvious external injury to have probable internal bleeding, usually in the abdominal cavity.

You must always be alert to the possibility of internal bleeding and assess the patient for related signs and symptoms, particularly if the mechanism of injury (MOI) is severe.

Mechanism of Injury for Internal Bleeding

A high-energy MOI should increase your index of suspicion for the possibility of serious unseen injuries such as internal bleeding in the abdominal cavity. Internal bleeding is possible whenever the MOI suggests that severe forces affected the body. These forces include blunt and penetrating trauma. Internal bleeding commonly occurs as a result of falls, blast injuries, and automobile or motorcycle crashes. Remember that internal bleeding can result from penetrating trauma as well.

As you assess a patient, look for signs of injury using DCAP-BTLS (Deformities, Contusions, Abrasions,

Punctures/penetrations, Burns, Tenderness, Lacerations, and Swelling) over the chest or abdomen, including contusions, abrasions, lacerations, and other signs of injury or deformity. You should always suspect internal bleeding in a patient who has penetrating injury or blunt trauma.

Nature of Illness for Internal Bleeding

Internal bleeding is not always caused by trauma. Many illnesses can cause internal bleeding. Some of the more common causes of nontraumatic internal bleeding include bleeding ulcers, bleeding from the colon, ruptured ectopic pregnancy, and aneurysms.

Abdominal tenderness, guarding, rigidity, pain, and distention are frequent in these situations but are not always present. In older patients, dizziness, faintness, or weakness may be the first sign of nontraumatic internal bleeding. Ulcers or other GI problems may cause vomiting of blood, or bloody diarrhea or urine.

It is not as important for you to know the specific organ involved as it is to recognize that the patient is in shock and respond appropriately.

Signs and Symptoms of Internal Bleeding

The most common symptom of internal bleeding is pain. Substantial internal bleeding will generally cause swelling in the area of bleeding. Intra-abdominal bleeding will often cause pain and distention. Bruising is a sign of internal bleeding. It is most common in head, extremity, and pelvic injuries and can be a sign of substantial abdominal trauma. Bleeding into the chest may cause dyspnea in addition to tachycardia and hypotension. A bruise is also called a **contusion**, or **ecchymosis**. A **hematoma**, a mass of blood in the soft tissues beneath the skin, indicates bleeding into soft tissues and may be the result of a minor or a severe injury. Bruising or ecchymosis may not be present initially, and the only sign of severe pelvic or abdominal trauma may be redness due to impact injury, skin abrasions, or pain.

Bleeding, however slight, from any body opening is serious. It usually indicates internal bleeding that is not easy to see or control. Bright red bleeding from the mouth or rectum or blood in the urine (**hematuria**) may suggest serious internal injury or disease. Nonmenstrual vaginal bleeding is always important.

Other signs and symptoms of internal bleeding in both trauma and medical patients include the following:

- **Hematemesis**. This is vomited blood. It may be bright red or dark red, or, if the blood has been partially digested, it may look like coffee-grounds vomitus (a sign of upper GI bleeding, this is vomited blood that looks like used coffee grounds).
- **Hemoptysis**. This is bright red blood that is coughed up from the lungs by the patient.
- **Melena**. This is a black, foul-smelling, tarry stool that contains digested blood; it indicates lower GI bleeding.
- **Hematochezia**, the passage of bloody stools. If they contain bright red blood, this may indicate bleeding near the external opening of the colon. Hemorrhoids in the lower colon tend to cause hematochezia.
- **Pain, tenderness, bruising, guarding, or swelling.** These signs and symptoms may mean that a closed fracture is bleeding.
- **Broken ribs, bruises over the lower part of the chest, or a rigid, distended abdomen.** These signs and symptoms may indicate a lacerated spleen or liver. Patients with an injury to either organ may have referred pain in the right shoulder (liver) or left shoulder (spleen). You should suspect internal abdominal bleeding in a patient with referred pain.

The first sign of **hypovolemic shock** (hypoperfusion) is generally a change in mental status, such as anxiety, restlessness, or combativeness. In nontrauma patients, weakness, faintness, or dizziness on standing is another early sign. Changes in skin color or pallor (pale skin) are seen often in both trauma and medical patients. Signs of hypoperfusion suggesting internal bleeding include the following:

- Altered level of consciousness
- Tachycardia
- Weakness, fainting, or dizziness at rest
- Thirst
- Nausea and vomiting
- Cold, moist (clammy) skin
- Shallow, rapid breathing
- Dull eyes
- Slightly dilated pupils that are slow to respond to light
- Capillary refill of more than 2 seconds in infants and children
- Weak, rapid (thready) pulse
- Decreasing blood pressure (very late sign)

Patients with these signs and symptoms are at risk. Some may be in danger. Even if their bleeding stops, it could begin again at any moment. Therefore, prompt transport is necessary.

Note that blood pressure is not a reliable indicator of early shock. The body generally compensates initially, keeping blood pressure within a normal range, and sometimes the compensation causes it to rise slightly. Medications may also mask changes in vital signs. In an effort to maintain central perfusion, blood will be shunted away from the periphery and the patient will present with pale, cool, mottled skin and decreased or absent radial pulses with an increased capillary refill time.

▶ The Importance of Bleeding

For a typical adult weighing 176 pounds (80 kg), the total blood volume is approximately 10 pints (5 L). The body will not tolerate an acute blood loss of greater than 20% of this blood volume.[1,2] If the typical adult loses more than approximately 2 pints (1 L) of blood, substantial changes in vital signs occur, including increasing heart and respiratory rates and decreasing blood pressure. An isolated femur fracture can easily result in the loss of 2 pints (1 L) or more of blood in the soft tissues of the thigh.

Because infants and children have less blood volume than adults, the same effect is seen with smaller amounts of blood loss. For example, a 1-year-old child has a total blood volume of approximately 2 pints (approximately 950 mL), so substantial symptoms of blood loss will occur after only 3 to 6 ounces (100 to 200 mL) of blood loss. To put this in perspective, remember that a soft drink can contains about 11 ounces (345 mL) of liquid.

How well people compensate for blood loss is related to how rapidly they bleed. A healthy adult can comfortably donate 1 unit (1 pint [~500 mL]) of blood during 15 to 20 minutes and most can adapt well to this decrease in blood volume. However, if a similar blood loss occurs in a much shorter period, **hemorrhagic shock** may rapidly develop, a condition in which low blood volume results in inadequate perfusion and even death. The body cannot compensate for such a rapid blood loss.

You should consider bleeding to be serious if the following conditions are present:

- A significant MOI, especially when the MOI suggests that severe forces affected the abdomen, chest, or both
- Poor general appearance of the patient
- Signs and symptoms of shock (hypoperfusion)
- Substantial amount of blood loss
- Rapid blood loss
- Uncontrollable bleeding

In any situation, blood loss is a serious problem. It demands your immediate attention as soon as you have cleared the airway and managed the patient's breathing.

Physiologic Response to Hemorrhaging

Injuries and some illnesses can disrupt blood vessels and cause bleeding. On its own, bleeding tends to stop rather quickly, within approximately 10 minutes, in response to internal clotting mechanisms and exposure to air. When vessels are lacerated, blood flows rapidly from the open vessel. In response, the open ends of the vessel begin to narrow, or vasoconstrict. This reduces the amount of bleeding. Platelets aggregate at the site, plugging the hole and sealing the injured portions of the vessel. This process is called **hemostasis**. Bleeding will not stop if a clot does not form, unless the injured vessel is completely cut off from the main blood supply. Direct contact with body tissues and fluids or the external environment commonly triggers the blood's clotting factors.

Despite the efficiency of this system, it may fail in certain situations. A number of medications, including anticoagulants such as aspirin and prescription blood thinners, interfere with normal clotting. Beta blockers can also prevent vasoconstriction, resulting in excessive bleeding. With a severe injury, the damage to the vessel may be so large that a clot cannot completely block the hole. Sometimes, only part of the vessel wall is cut, preventing it from constricting. In these cases, bleeding will continue unless it is stopped by external means. Occasionally, blood loss occurs rapidly. In these cases of acute blood loss, the patient might die before the body's

YOU are the Provider — PART 2

The patient states that about 15 minutes ago, he was up approximately 14 feet above the ground in the tree stand, when he slipped and fell. When he landed, his rifle discharged into his left bicep. He is reporting pain to his obviously deformed right lower extremity, pain to his left bicep, and dizziness. As your partner attempts to obtain vital signs, you examine the wound and find a small entrance wound and a gaping wound on the posterior bicep. You determine the bleeding is arterial. You immediately apply a tourniquet. The patient denies having any other injury, stating it is only his leg and arm that hurt. You also request the local search and rescue team to be dispatched to your location to assist in extricating the patient to a safe landing zone.

Recording Time: 1 Minute	
Appearance	Anxious
Level of consciousness	Alert and oriented to person, place, time, and event
Airway	Patent
Breathing	Rapid, panting
Circulation	Weak, thready radial pulses; skin is pale

3. Does this patient require spinal immobilization?
4. How would you transport this patient one-half mile to the parking area where the helicopter could land?

Words of Wisdom

Motivated by many tragedies throughout the country, in October 2015, the White House launched the *Stop the Bleed* campaign in an attempt to train, equip, and empower bystanders to act in an emergency situation prior to the arrival of professional help[3] **Figure 27-4**. The idea is that by providing bystanders and emergency responders such as law enforcement with the skills and basic tools needed to stop uncontrolled bleeding, many lives could be saved. The principles include three key actions, as shown in the figure.

This initiative applies in not only terror attacks, but natural disasters as well.

Many agencies, including the National Security Council at the White House, the American Heart Association, American Red Cross, American College of Surgeons, Hartford Consensus, National Association of Emergency Medical Technicians, Charlotte Douglas International Airport, Johnson & Johnson, and the Harvard Kennedy School collaborated for over a year to develop this campaign.[4] The goal is to make the *Stop the Bleed* logo as recognizable as *stop, drop, and roll* and to put the materials in the hands of the public sector. In an attempt to get kits into the public, some venues have placed these materials in the same location as automated external defibrillators (AEDs). Items included in the kits range from nitrile gloves for personal protection, tourniquets, compression dressings, rolled gauze, and trauma shears. There is even the consideration of adding audio instructions to the kits, similar to that in AEDs, to provide directions for use.

The key to the success of this initiative is widespread education of the public and having kits available for use. Emergency medical services (EMS) providers can provide a vital link in this accomplishment.

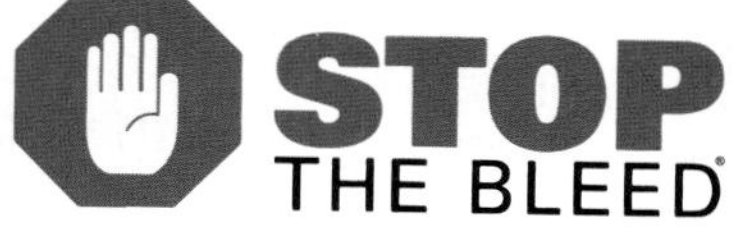

No matter how rapid the arrival of professional emergency responders, bystanders will always be first on the scene. A person who is bleeding can die from blood loss within five minutes, so it's important to quickly stop the blood loss.

Remember to be aware of your surroundings and move yourself and the injured person to safety, if necessary.

Call 911.

Bystanders can take simple steps to keep the injured alive until appropriate medical care is available. Here are three actions that you can take to help save a life:

1. Apply Pressure with Hands

EXPOSE to find where the bleeding is coming from and apply **FIRM, STEADY PRESSURE** to the bleeding site with both hands if possible.

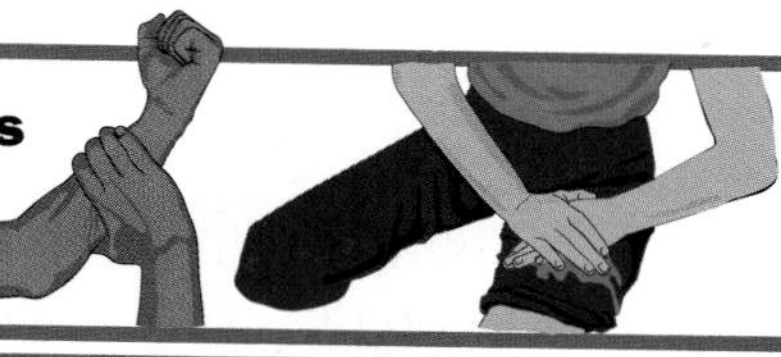

2. Apply Dressing and Press

EXPOSE to find where the bleeding is coming from and apply **FIRM, STEADY PRESSURE** to the bleeding site with bandages or clothing.

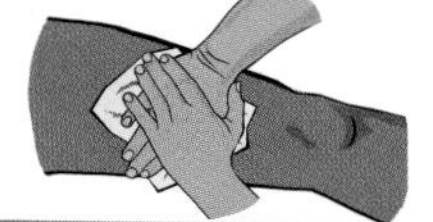

3. Apply Tourniquet(s)

If the bleeding doesn't stop, place a tourniquet as high on the extremity as possibe above the wound. The tourniquet may be applied and secured over clothing.

TIME:

PULL the strap through the buckle, **TWIST** the rod tightly, **CLIP** and **SECURE** the rod with the clasp or the Velcro strap.

If the bleeding still doesn't stop, place a second tourniquet next to the first tourniquet.

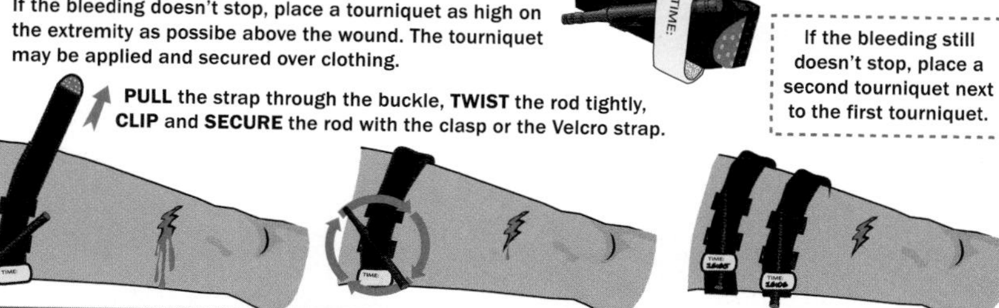

The 'Stop the Bleed' campaign was initiated by a federal interagency workgroup convened by the National Security Council Staff, The White House. The purpose of the campaign is to build national resilience by better preparing the public to save lives by raising awareness of basic actions to stop life threatening bleeding following everyday emergencies and man-made and natural disasters. Advances made by military medicine and research in hemorrhage control during the wars in Afghanistan and Iraq have informed the work of this initiative which exemplifies translation of knowledge back to the homeland to the benefit of the general public. The Department of the Defense owns the 'Stop the Bleed' logo and phrase.

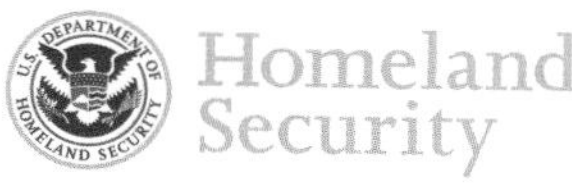

Office of Health Affairs

Figure 27-4 Three actions you can take to help save a life.

Courtesy of Department of Homeland Security "Stop the Bleed" Campaign.

> **Words of Wisdom**
>
> The American College of Surgeons, in collaboration with the medical community, representatives from governmental and nongovernmental agencies, and various emergency medical response organizations, among others, developed a national protocol to maximize survivability from active shooter and other mass-casualty incidents. These recommendations, called the Hartford Consensus, emphasize a continuum of care from initial response to definitive care that involves the seamless integration of hemorrhage control intervention.[5]
>
> An integrated active shooter response should include the critical actions contained in the acronym THREAT:
>
> - **T**hreat suppression
> - **H**emorrhage control
> - **R**apid **E**xtrication to safety
> - **A**ssessment by medical providers
> - **T**ransport to definitive care
>
> Life-threatening bleeding from extremity wounds is best controlled initially through use of tourniquets, whereas internal bleeding resulting from penetrating wounds to the chest and trunk is best addressed through immediate transport to a medical facility.

> **Words of Wisdom**
>
> Hemostasis is difficult in areas where movement is involved, such as over a joint. Movement disrupts clotting, increasing hemorrhaging. Removal of a bandage may also disrupt clotting, causing bleeding to continue.

hemostatic defenses of vasoconstriction and clotting can help. Table 27-1 shows the classes of hemorrhaging.

A small portion of the population lacks one or more of the blood's clotting factors. This condition is called **hemophilia**. There are several forms of hemophilia, most of which are hereditary and some of which are severe. Sometimes, bleeding may occur spontaneously in a person with hemophilia. Because the patient's blood does not clot, all injuries, no matter how trivial, are potentially serious. A patient with hemophilia should be transported immediately. Bleeding disorders are discussed in Chapter 21, *Endocrine and Hematologic Emergencies*.

Trauma Triad of Death

The trauma triad of death is a combination of hypothermia, coagulopathy, and acidosis that substantially increase mortality in trauma patients. These three conditions

Table 27-1 Estimated Fluid and Blood Loss for a 154-lb (70-kg) Patient

	Class I	Class II	Class III	Class IV
Blood loss (mL)	<750	750–1,500	1,500–2,000	>2,000
% Blood loss	<15	15–30	30–40	>40
Heart rate (beats/min)	Minimally elevated or normal	100–120	≥120, thready	Marked tachycardia
Systolic blood pressure	Within normal limits	Minimal or no change	Substantial drop	Substantial depression
Pulse pressure	Within normal limits	Narrow	Narrow	Very narrow
Capillary refill	Within normal limits	May be delayed	Delayed	Delayed
Respiratory rate (breaths/min)	14–20	20–24	Markedly elevated	Markedly elevated
Central nervous system/mental status	Slightly anxious	Mildly anxious	Anxious and confused	Confused and lethargic
Skin condition	Cool, pink	Cool, moist	Cold, pale, moist	Cold, pale
Urine output (mL/h)	>30	20–30	Diminished	Minimal or none
Fluid replacement	Crystalloid	Crystalloid	Crystalloid and blood	Crystalloid and blood

actually feed on one another in a positive feedback loop, rapidly worsening the patient's condition.

Even mild hypothermia can begin to inhibit the chemical reactions involved in the clotting process. **Coagulopathy**, the disruption of the body's ability to clot, can result in further hemorrhage, leading to increasing hypoperfusion. This hypoperfusion causes the cells to use anaerobic metabolism, releasing additional acidic compounds into the blood. This acidosis reduces myocardial performance, further reducing oxygen delivery and body metabolism, resulting in increased hypothermia. If this loop continues uninterrupted, the rapidly worsening shock will result in death of the trauma patient. Thus, you must seek to identify the conditions of hypothermia, coagulopathy, and acidosis in the setting of trauma and intervene where possible.

Hypothermia is often easy to identify if looked for and can be the easiest condition to treat. Trauma patients must be kept warm. This is especially true if the patient is also subjected to environmental hypothermia, such as a motor vehicle crash in cold weather. However, you must keep in mind that hypothermia in the trauma triad of death refers to the body's inability to maintain normal operating temperature. This sign may be subtle and easy to overlook.

Patient Assessment

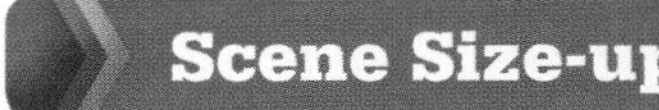

Scene Size-up

The assessment of any patient begins with a thorough scene size-up and proceeds to your general impression and primary survey. After the scene is considered safe, you will need to take the appropriate standard precautions.

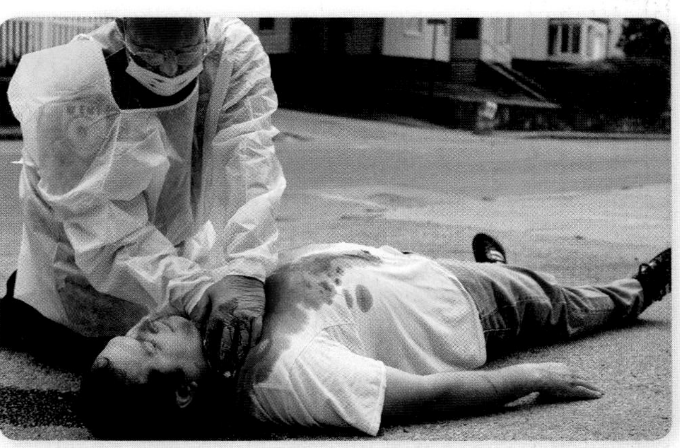

Figure 27-5 Depending on the severity of bleeding and your general impression, standard precautions will entail gloves, mask, eye shield, and, in some cases, a gown.

Depending on the severity of bleeding and your general impression, these precautions will entail gloves, mask, eye shield, and, when the patient is bloody or blood is spurting, a gown Figure 27-5.

When patients have serious external blood loss, it is often difficult to determine visually the amount of blood lost. Blood will look different on different surfaces, such as when it is absorbed in clothing or when it has been diluted when mixed in water. Attempt to determine the amount of external blood loss, but remember that this is not crucial and the presentation and assessment of the patient must direct patient care and treatment.

Determine the nature of the illness (NOI) (such as bloody emesis or bloody stool), or the MOI (such as an overturned chair). Consider the need for additional

YOU are the Provider — PART 3

After securing the tourniquet around the upper arm, you note a complete cessation of blood flow from the wound. Having taken care of the immediate life threat, you contact dispatch to obtain the estimated time of arrival of the helicopter, which is approximately 16 minutes.

Recording Time: 4 Minutes	
Respirations	32 breaths/min, rapid
Pulse	Weak and thready, 139 beats/min
Skin	Diaphoretic, cool, pale, and clammy
Blood pressure	74 mm Hg by palpation
Oxygen saturation (Spo_2)	Not obtained
Pupils	Pupils Equal, Round, and Reactive to Light and Accommodation (PERRLA)

5. What class of hemorrhaging is occurring in this patient?
6. What are the indications for a tourniquet, and when do you remove it?

resources, such as an advanced life support unit. Be sure to also consider environmental factors in your decision making. For example, caring for a sick or injured victim of a car crash on a clear, sunny day is a bit different than treating the same victim during a snowstorm. Extreme hot or cold weather can worsen a patient's overall condition.

Primary Survey

Bleeding that you can control (such as external bleeding that responds to a pressure bandage) and bleeding that you cannot control (such as a bleeding peptic ulcer) are serious emergencies. Substantial bleeding, internal or external, is an immediate life threat. As a consequence, the primary survey of the patient includes a search for life-threatening bleeding. As you approach a trauma patient, you must note important indicators that may alert you to the seriousness of the patient's condition. For example, patients with external bleeding may have blood stains on their clothing. Be aware of obvious signs of injury and distress, such as facial grimace.

Perform a rapid full-body scan of the patient. If found, life-threatening hemorrhage must be controlled *first*, even before airway and breathing. In other words, follow the XABCDE mnemonic for trauma, assessing for and managing exsanguinating hemorrhage first. If the hemorrhaging cannot be controlled in the field, all of your efforts should concentrate on attempting to control the bleeding as you rapidly transport the patient to the emergency department (ED). When life-threatening external bleeding is seen, you must also begin treatment of shock as quickly as possible. Treat the patient for shock if needed by applying oxygen, placing him or her in the proper position, improving circulation with IV fluid as needed, and maintaining a normal body temperature.

However, if the patient has minor external bleeding, you can note it and move on with the primary survey; management of this problem can wait until the patient has been properly assessed and prioritized. Do not become sidetracked by applying dressings and bandages to a patient who has much more serious problems. Non–life-threatening bleeding, such as from abrasions, can be bandaged later in your assessment as necessary.

Determine the patient's level of consciousness using the AVPU scale (Awake and alert, responsive to Verbal stimuli, responsive to Pain, Unresponsive). These indicators will help you determine whether the patient is sick or not so sick; this assists you in developing an index of suspicion for serious illness or injuries related to internal bleeding. Internal bleeding includes bleeding into any cavity or space within the body and may be severe and life threatening. Without proper assessment, internal bleeding may go undetected.

Special Populations

In older patients, dizziness, syncope, or weakness may be the first sign of nontraumatic internal hemorrhaging.

After addressing life-threatening bleeding, next manage immediate threats to life involving the airway and breathing. Consider the need for manual spinal stabilization prior to airway management. Ensure that the patient has a patent airway. If you observe bleeding from the mouth or facial areas, keep the suction unit within reach.

You must be able to quickly assess pulse rate and quality; determine the skin condition, color, and temperature; and check the capillary refill time to help establish the potential for internal bleeding and shock. Pale or gray, cool, moist skin suggests a perfusion problem.

In some instances, patients may become quiet and calm because of excessive blood loss and shock state. As mentioned, estimating the amount of blood loss by the size of a pool of blood or the amount of blood on clothing may not be accurate, especially if the patient has moved. Assessing the patient for signs of shock is a better indicator of the amount of blood loss.

Any internal bleeding must be treated promptly. The signs of internal hemorrhaging (such as discoloration, hematoma) do not always develop quickly, so you must rely on other signs and symptoms and an evaluation of the MOI to make this diagnosis. Pay close attention to patient reports of pain or tenderness, development of tachycardia, and pallor. If you suspect internal bleeding, begin management by keeping the patient warm and administering supplemental oxygen using a nonrebreathing mask at 15 L/min.

Words of Wisdom

Do not delay transport to complete an assessment, particularly when substantial bleeding is present, even if the bleeding is controlled. The assessment can be started during transport.

When making a transport decision in cases of hemorrhaging, the issue is not whether the patient will be transported, but rather how fast the transport decision should be made and where the patient should be taken for definitive care. There are a few exceptions to this rule—for example, if you are standing by at a sporting event or concert and are asked by a "walk-in" to evaluate a minor wound that has been bleeding. The decision to transport a patient with even a relatively minor wound should take into consideration factors such as the need for stitches, whether the patient has had a tetanus shot in the past 10 years, and whether the patient or his or her companion is reliable and will follow up properly; finally, the decision may depend on local protocols.

Most patients with internal or external hemorrhaging will need to be transported to a hospital for further care. Consideration for the priority of the patient and the availability of a regional trauma center should be your concerns when making a transport decision. Patients who have severe internal or external bleeding, especially if uncontrolled, will often be candidates for surgery and should be transported immediately to an appropriate facility. Patients with specific causes of bleeding such as major trauma or specific devastating wounds (such as leg amputation, glove avulsion) should be taken to a facility that is fully prepared to care for the patient. Paramedic backup or rendezvous may be needed when the patient requires advanced procedures such as endotracheal intubation, vasopressor drugs, or cardiac monitoring. In EMS systems with air medical transport available, it may be appropriate to consider this method of transportation for a patient with suspected severe internal or uncontrollable external bleeding, depending on the distance to the appropriate facility and the degree to which use of the aeromedical service can expedite arrival of the patient at the facility.

History Taking

After the primary survey is complete, investigate the chief complaint and be alert for signs or symptoms of other injuries due to the MOI and/or NOI. Internal bleeding can be found in medical and trauma patients. If the bleeding is severe, you may have identified it in the primary survey and begun treatment and rapid transport to the hospital. Carefully assess the MOI in trauma patients because it may be your best indicator that the patient has sustained an internal injury and may be bleeding. Table 27-2 lists some MOIs that can give clues about internal bleeding. In addition to evaluating the MOI, be alert for the development of shock when you suspect internal bleeding. In a responsive trauma patient who has an isolated injury with a limited MOI, consider a detailed physical exam before assessing vital signs and obtaining a history.

When you encounter a patient who is bleeding, avoid focusing solely on the bleeding. With substantial trauma, assess the entire patient, looking for the source of the problem, any preexisting illnesses, and other issues.

Gather information on the patient's chief complaint using the OPQRST (Onset, Provocation/palliation, Quality, Region/radiation, Severity, Timing) mnemonic and obtain a SAMPLE (Signs and symptoms, Allergies, Medications, Pertinent past medical history, Last oral intake, Events leading up to the illness or injury) history. Ask the patient if he or she experiences any dizziness or syncope. Are there

Table 27-2 The Mechanism of Injury: Indicators of Internal Bleeding

Mechanism of Injury	Potential Internal Bleeding Sources
Fall from a ladder striking head	Head injury or hematoma
Fall from a ladder striking extremities	Possible fractures; consider chest injury
Fall on outstretched arm	Possible broken bone or joint injury
Unrestrained driver in head-on collision (up-and-over route)	Head and neck, chest, abdomen injuries
Unrestrained driver in head-on collision (down-and-under route)	Knee, femur, hip, and pelvis injuries
Unrestrained front-seat passenger, side-impact collision with intrusion into vehicle	Humerus broken exposing the chest wall (possible flail chest); pelvis and acetabulum injuries
Unrestrained driver crushed against steering column	Chest and abdomen injuries, ruptured spleen, neck trauma
Road bike or mountain bike (over the handlebars)	Fractured clavicle, road rash, head trauma if no helmet worn
Abrupt motorcycle stop, causing rider to catapult over the handlebars	Fractured femurs, head and neck injuries
Diving into the shallow end of a swimming pool	Head and neck injuries
Assault or fight	Punching or kicking injury to chest, abdomen, and face
Blast or explosion	Injury from direct strike with debris; indirect and pressure wave in enclosed space
Child struck by car (Waddell triad)	Head trauma, chest and abdomen injuries, leg fractures
Child thrown or falls from height	Usually a headfirst impact, causing head injury

any signs and symptoms of hypovolemic shock? Ask the patient if he or she takes blood-thinning medications, because bleeding is generally more profuse and difficult to control in patients who take these; also, heart or blood pressure medications may interfere with the ability to vasoconstrict and compensate. Ask about any history of clotting insufficiency. Is there any pain, tenderness, bruising, guarding, deformity, distention, discoloration of the affected area, or swelling? These signs and symptoms may indicate internal bleeding.

Special Populations

Remember that vital signs vary depending on age. What is normal for an adult patient will not be normal for a pediatric patient. Refer to Chapter 10, *Patient Assessment*, for vital signs by age group.

Words of Wisdom

Use pulse oximetry as a diagnostic tool to help determine the patient's oxygenation. However, remember that a patient showing signs of hypoperfusion will not have an accurate pulse oximetry reading. Treat the patient, not the diagnostic tool!

Secondary Assessment

As described earlier, the secondary assessment is a detailed, comprehensive examination of the patient to uncover injuries or illness that may have been missed during the primary survey. In some cases, such as those that involve a critically injured patient or a short transport time, there may not be time to conduct a secondary assessment.

When you are performing a secondary assessment, record vital signs, complete a focused assessment of pain, and attach appropriate monitoring devices. The examination should include a systematic full-body exam. The full-body exam assesses each body system as discussed in Chapter 10, *Patient Assessment*.

Assess the respiratory system. Specifically assess the airway for patency and determine the rate and quality of respirations. In the neck, look for distended neck veins and a deviated trachea. Note, however, that these classic signs may not be present in the patient with hypovolemia. In the chest, check for paradoxical movement of the chest wall and bilateral breath sounds.

Assess the cardiovascular system, specifically the rate and quality of pulses.

Assess the neurologic system to formulate baseline data to guide further decisions. This examination should include level of consciousness, pupil size and reactivity, motor response, and sensory response.

Assess the musculoskeletal system. Perform a detailed full-body examination. Look for DCAP-BTLS to be sure that you have found all of the problems and injuries quickly. Assess all anatomic regions. When you are examining the head, be alert for raccoon eyes, Battle sign, and/or drainage of blood or fluid from the ears or nose. In the abdomen, feel all four quadrants for tenderness or rigidity. In the extremities, record the pulse and motor and sensory function.

Obtain baseline vital signs to observe the changes that may occur during treatment. In an adult, a systolic blood pressure of less than 100 mm Hg with a weak, rapid pulse should suggest to you the presence of hypoperfusion in a patient who may have substantial bleeding. Because infants and children have less blood volume than adults, the same effect is seen with smaller amounts of blood loss.

In geriatric patients, the pulse rate may not increase with early shock; therefore, if possible, try to determine the patient's normal baseline blood pressure and circulatory status.

In addition to hands-on assessment, use monitoring devices to quantify oxygenation and circulatory status. You may use a noninvasive technique to monitor blood pressure and a pulse oximeter to evaluate the effectiveness of oxygenation. Always assess the patient's blood pressure with a sphygmomanometer and stethoscope (manually) before using a noninvasive blood pressure monitor to establish a baseline blood pressure and to determine the accuracy of the noninvasive blood pressure machine.

Reassessment

Patient reassessment is an important tool to see how your patient is doing over time. Reassess the patient, especially in the areas that showed abnormal findings during the primary survey. The signs and symptoms of internal bleeding are often slow to present because of their covert nature. The reassessment is your best opportunity to determine whether your patient's condition is improving or getting worse. Assess the effectiveness of any interventions, especially tourniquets, and treatments provided to the patient.

Vital signs show how well your patient is doing internally. In all cases of severe bleeding, obtain the patient's vital signs every 5 minutes en route to the ED. Is the patient's airway still patent and breathing still adequate? Is the oxygen helping the patient to breathe easier? Is your treatment for shock resulting in better perfusion of the vital organs? Is the bandage controlling the bleeding?

In patients with severe external bleeding, it is important to recognize, estimate, and report the amount of blood loss that has occurred and how rapidly or during what period it occurred. This can be a challenge to estimate, especially if the surface the patient is on is wet or absorbs fluids or if the environment is dark. For example, you may report that approximately 1 pint (approximately 1 L) of blood was lost or that the bleeding soaked through

Special Populations

Older adult patients are more likely to take medications that interfere with normal compensatory mechanisms, such as beta blockers, calcium channel blockers, and other antidysrhythmics. The kidneys also atrophy with age and, therefore, are less responsive to fluid conservation; the blood vessels may be affected by atherosclerosis and less able to shunt blood to vital areas. In addition, other medical conditions can be exacerbated during shock states; for instance, ischemia is more likely to interfere with cardiac output in patients with a history of myocardial infarction or angina.

Pediatric patients have underdeveloped kidneys, resulting in an inability to conserve fluid similar to that of an adult. Consequently, they have a lower tolerance for volume loss. In addition, children compensate by vasoconstriction better than adults do. This factor tends to allow them to maintain a compensatory state and good blood pressure for a longer period, until the point when their vital signs collapse abruptly, possibly followed by death. They will compensate well for blood loss and then "crash" quickly. An additional complication in small children is their relatively large surface area–to–weight ratio, which means they feel cold more easily, which in turn results in coagulation difficulties.

Pregnant patients normally will have a faster pulse, greater blood volume, lower blood pressure, and nausea. Treat these patients aggressively according to the MOI and treat for shock; do not automatically assume the altered signs are a result of the pregnancy.

three trauma dressings. Report this information to hospital personnel during transport to allow the hospital to evaluate needed resources, such as the availability of surgical suites, surgeons, and other specialty providers.

With internal bleeding, describe the MOI/NOI and the signs and symptoms that make you think internal bleeding is occurring.

Your transfer report at the hospital should update hospital personnel on how your patient has responded to your care. Be sure your paperwork reflects all of the patient's injuries and the care you have provided.

Emergency Medical Care

External Hemorrhaging

Most external bleeding can be managed with direct pressure, combined with pressure dressings and/or splints, although arterial bleeding may take 5 or more minutes of direct pressure to form a clot. Military experience has proven that tourniquets can effectively and safely control hemorrhage without an increase in complications.[6] For this reason, the use of a **tourniquet** is preferred for external bleeding in an extremity that cannot be controlled with direct pressure and a pressure dressing. If a tourniquet is deemed necessary, it should be applied quickly and not released until a physician is present.

Always observe standard precautions. As with all patient care, ensure that the patient has an open airway and is breathing adequately. Whenever you suspect bleeding, either external or internal, provide high-flow oxygen and assist ventilation if needed with attention to cervical

YOU are the Provider — PART 4

Noting the vital signs, recognizing the helicopter ETA, and recognizing the seriousness of the injury, you elect to start two 18-gauge intravenous (IV) lines and administer 250-mL boluses of normal saline, checking vital signs again after each bolus until a systolic blood pressure of 80 mm Hg has been achieved. Supplemental oxygen at 15 L/min is also applied. The patient requests something for pain. You inform him that paramedics are en route and they will be able to administer pain medication soon after arrival. Just then, you see the local search and rescue team arriving.

Recording Time: 12 Minutes	
Respirations	34 breaths/min, rapid
Pulse	Weak and thready, 142 beats/min
Skin	Diaphoretic, cool, pale, and clammy
Blood pressure	76 mm Hg by palpation
Oxygen saturation (Sp_{O_2})	97% on 100% oxygen
Pupils	PERRLA

7. Why should you administer 250-mL boluses until a systolic blood pressure of 80 mm Hg is achieved?

spine control in trauma patients as indicated. To control external bleeding, follows the steps in Skill Drill 27-1.

Most instances of external bleeding can be controlled simply by applying direct local pressure to the bleeding site, including the area just proximal and distal to the injury. This method is by far the most effective way to control external bleeding. Pressure stops the flow of blood and permits normal coagulation to occur. You

Special Populations

In pregnant patients, shock leads to shunting of blood away from the fetus in an attempt to preserve the mother. The closer the maternal blood pressure is to normal, the better perfused the fetus is likely to be.

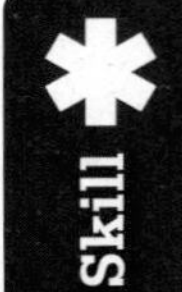

NR Skill

Skill Drill 27-1 Managing External Hemorrhage

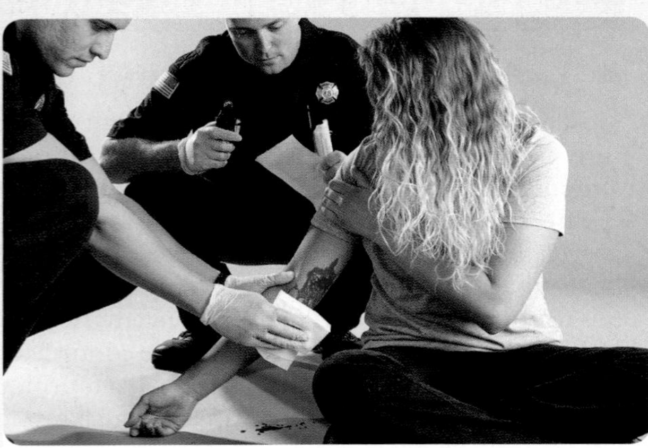

Step 1 Take standard precautions. Maintain the airway with cervical spine immobilization if the MOI suggests the possibility of spinal injury. Apply direct, even pressure over the wound with a dry, sterile dressing.

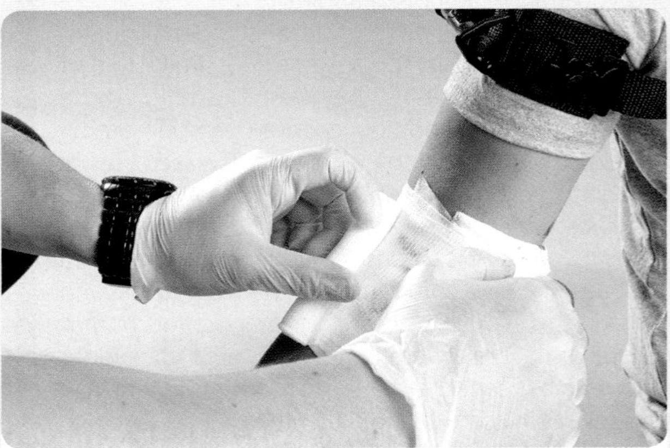

Step 2 If the bleeding stops, apply a pressure dressing and/or splint. Hold the pressure dressing in place using gauze.

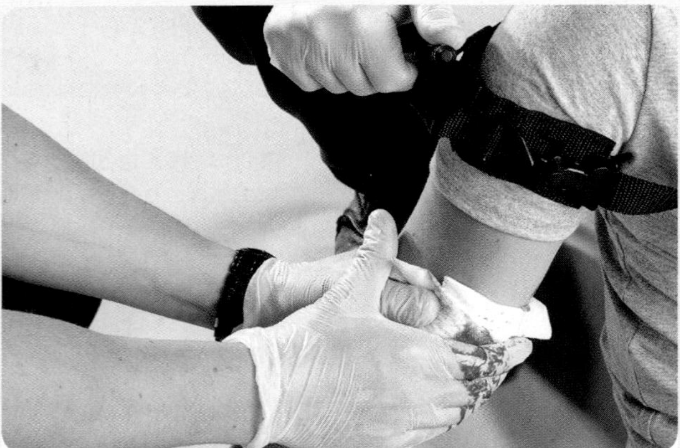

Step 3 If direct pressure does not rapidly control bleeding on an extremity injury, apply a tourniquet to the axilla or groin region of the bleeding extremity.

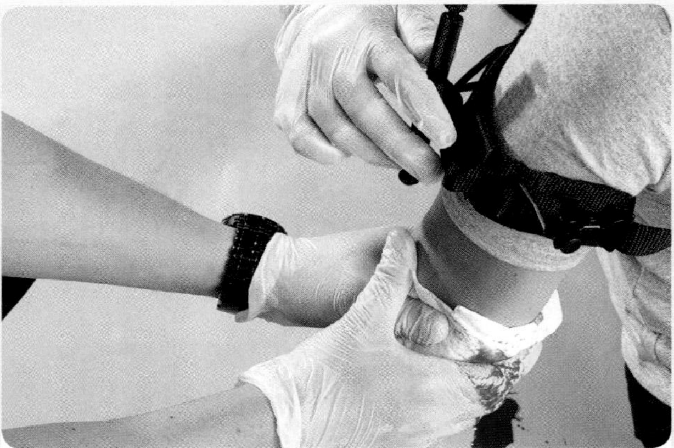

Step 4 Tighten the tourniquet until the bleeding stops. Write "TK" and the exact time (hour and minute) that you applied the tourniquet on the patient's forehead. Position the patient supine unless contraindicated. Administer oxygen as necessary. Keep the patient warm, transport promptly, monitor the serial vital signs, and watch diligently for developing shock.

may apply pressure with your gloved fingertip or hand, over the top of a sterile dressing if one is immediately available. If there is an object protruding from the wound, apply a bulky dressing to stabilize the object in place, and apply pressure as best you can without interruption until bleeding is controlled. Never remove an impaled object from a wound unless it is through the cheek and interferes with the airway, or in the chest and interferes with chest compressions.

Words of Wisdom

If an impaled object prevents transport of a patient because of its size or positioning, proper treatment includes attempting to cut through the object to create a manageable size while leaving it in place. If you determine that removal of the impaled object is mandatory in order to accomplish transport, contact medical control prior to removal of the object for direction as to how to proceed.

After you have applied a dressing and controlled the bleeding, you can create a pressure dressing to maintain the pressure by firmly wrapping a sterile, self-adhering roller bandage around the entire wound. Use 4- × 4-inch or 4- × 8-inch sterile gauze pads for small wounds and sterile universal dressings for larger wounds.

Cover the entire dressing, above and below the wound. Stretch the bandage tight enough to control bleeding. Check the distal pulse before and after applying the dressing; if you were able to palpate a distal pulse before applying the dressing, you should still be able to palpate a distal pulse on the injured extremity after applying the pressure dressing.

Bleeding will almost always stop when the pressure of the dressing exceeds arterial pressure. This will assist in controlling bleeding and helping blood to clot.

Words of Wisdom

Although it has become the standard of care to apply direct pressure initially, and then apply a tourniquet on wounds that continue to bleed, wound packing has been shown to further inhibit blood loss and increase patient survival.[7-9] Plain gauze may be used to pack open wounds, particularly those on the torso or in other areas where a tourniquet may not be applied, but there are also advantages to the use of specialized hemostatic dressings that are impregnated with various compounds to enhance hemostasis. The purpose of packing the wound is to create an *internal pressure dressing* that fills the wound cavity and applies pressure from within. Hemostatic dressings are now available over the counter and are being included in commercial bleeding control kits.

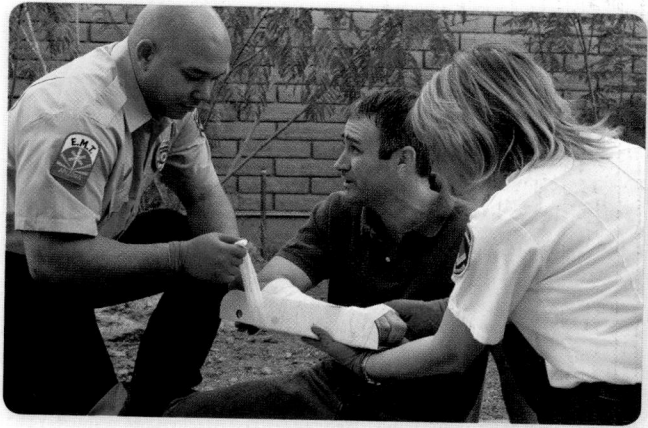

Figure 27-6 Use of a simple splint will often quickly control bleeding associated with a fracture. As long as a fracture is not immobilized, the bone ends are free to move and may continue to injure partially clotted vessels.

If direct pressure fails to immediately stop the hemorrhaging, apply a tourniquet to the groin or axilla above the site of the bleeding. If this is not possible because the bleeding is too far proximal, apply direct pressure and hold it until you arrive at the hospital.

Some of the bleeding associated with broken bones occurs because the sharp ends of the bones lacerate vessels, muscles, and other tissues. As long as a fracture remains unstable, the bone ends will move and continue to cause damage to tissues and vessels. This may also include breaking up clots that have partially formed, resulting in ongoing bleeding. Therefore, stabilizing a fracture and decreasing movement is a high priority in the prompt control of bleeding. Often, simple splints will quickly control bleeding associated with a fracture **Figure 27-6**. If the patient is unstable, however, do not waste time splinting a fracture.

After bleeding is controlled and a sterile dressing and pressure bandage have been applied, keep the patient warm and in the appropriate position. Allow the patient's condition to determine the mode of transport.

Tourniquets

A tourniquet is especially useful if a patient has severe hemorrhaging from an extremity injury below the axilla or groin and when other methods of control, such as direct pressure and pressure dressings, are ineffective or inadequate. The laceration or tear of a large artery can cause a patient to exsanguinate in as little as 2 minutes. To avoid this outcome, you must be able to apply a tourniquet in less than 20 seconds.

For many years, tourniquets were considered a last-ditch effort to be used in patients for whom the choice was between life or the limb. The consensus was that although the tourniquet could stop the bleeding, the result would be the loss of the patient's arm or leg. This belief was based on the historical use of the tourniquet—these devices were first used to stop the blood flow to the extremity prior to an amputation from battlefield injuries. In World War I, tourniquets were also used to stop bleeding from extremities. However, because of the long transport times to definitive care, the application of the tourniquet was often associated with the loss of the limb.

Since 2005, tourniquets have proven so efficient and easy to use that the US military has issued tourniquets to all field personnel.[7] A number of commercially available tourniquets are marketed, including the combat application tourniquet (CAT), the special operations forces tactical tourniquet (SOFT-T), the ratcheting medical tourniquet (RMT), and the stretch, wrap, and tuck tourniquet (SWAT-T) Figure 27-7. The CAT uses a strap and buckle system but utilizes a windlass to tighten the strap to control bleeding. The RMT uses a ratchet device to apply mechanical pressure, while the SWAT-T serves as a combination of a pressure dressing, wrap, and tourniquet.

The use of commercial tourniquets generally involves the steps in Skill Drill 27-2. A tourniquet is typically released at the hospital, but if instructed by medical control, can be released in the field in rare instances. Be aware that bleeding may rapidly return on tourniquet release, so you should be prepared to reapply it immediately, if necessary.

If a commercial tourniquet is not available, follow these steps to apply a tourniquet using a triangular bandage and a stick or rod:

1. Fold a triangular bandage until it is 4 inches (6 cm) wide and six to eight layers thick.
2. Wrap the bandage around the extremity twice. Choose an area proximal to the injury near the groin or axilla to control the bleeding.
3. Tie one knot in the bandage. Then place a stick or rod on top of the knot, and tie the ends of the bandage over the stick in a square knot.
4. Use the stick or rod as a handle, and twist it to tighten the tourniquet until the bleeding has stopped and distal pulses are no longer palpable; then stop twisting Figure 27-8.
5. Secure the stick in place, and make the wrapping neat and smooth.
6. Write "TK" (for "tourniquet") and the exact time (hour and minute) that you applied the tourniquet on the patient's forehead. Notify hospital personnel on your arrival that the patient has a tourniquet in place. Record this same information on the patient care report form.

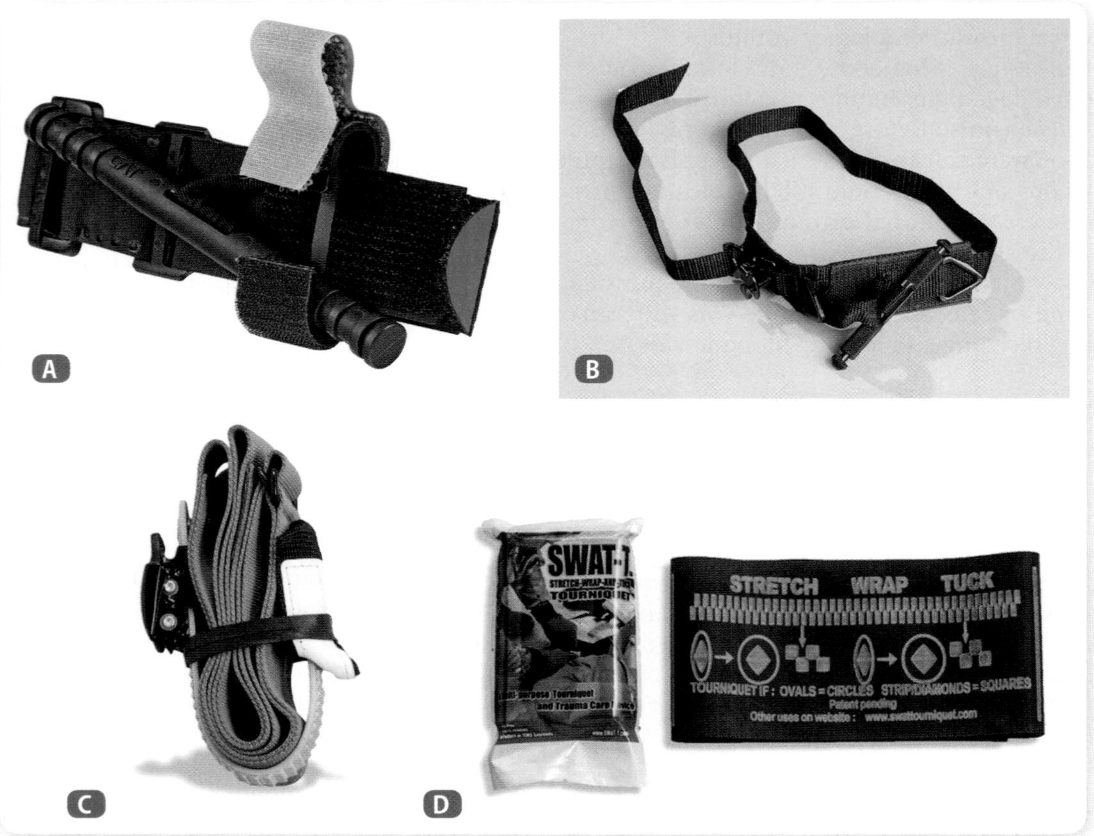

Figure 27-7 Commercially available tourniquets. **A.** The combat application tourniquet. **B.** Special operations forces tactical tourniquet. **C.** Ratcheting medical tourniquet. **D.** Stretch, wrap, and tuck tourniquet.

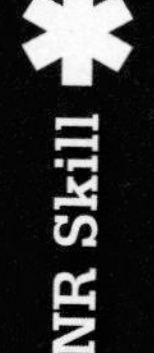

Skill Drill 27-2 Applying a Commercial Tourniquet (Combat Application Tourniquet)

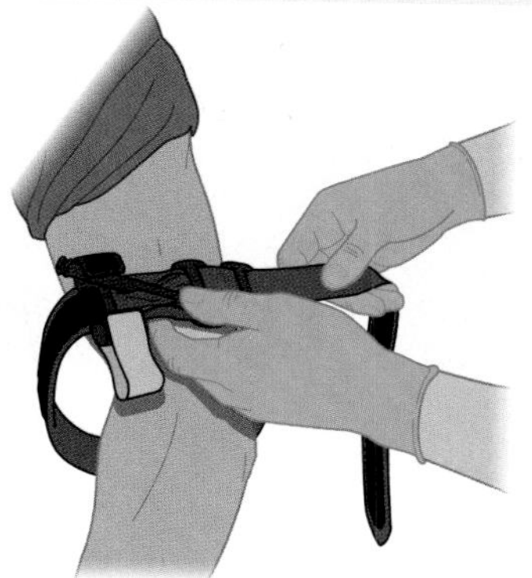

Step 1 Place the tourniquet proximal to the injury. Wrap the band around the limb and fasten it to the buckle.

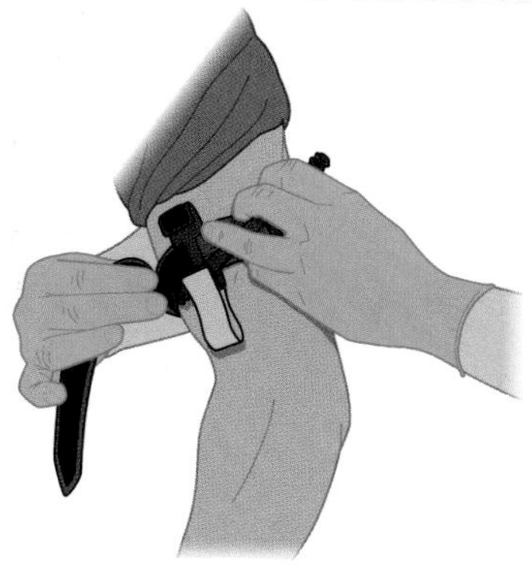

Step 2 Pull the band tightly and secure the band back on itself.

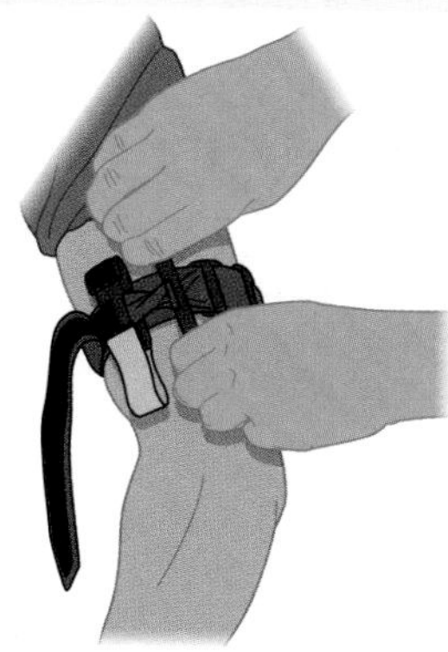

Step 3 Tighten the rod (windlass) until the bleeding stops.

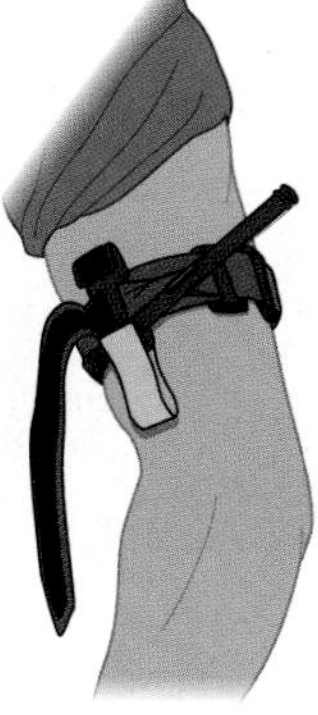

Step 4 Secure the rod inside the clip. Ensure bleeding is still controlled and assess for a distal pulse.

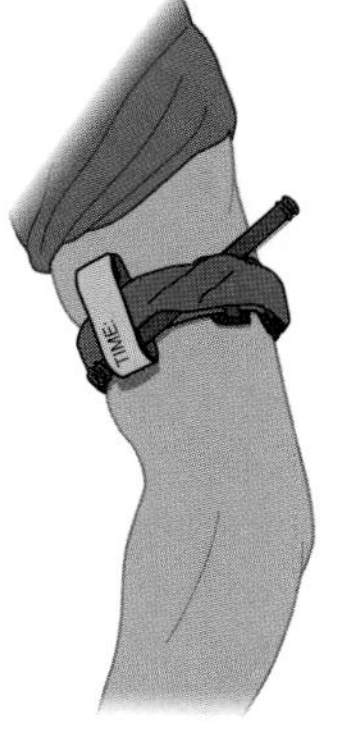

Step 5 Wrap the rest of the band through the clips. Secure the rod with the strap labeled "TK" (for "tourniquet") and the exact time (hour and minute) that you applied the tourniquet.

As a last resort, you can use a blood pressure cuff as a tourniquet—but keep in mind that blood pressure cuffs with leaks will not hold pressure. Position the cuff proximal to the bleeding point, and inflate it enough to eliminate distal pulses and stop the bleeding. Leave the cuff inflated. Monitor the gauge continuously to ensure the pressure is not gradually dropping, which could allow the bleeding to restart. You may have to clamp the tube leading from the cuff to the inflating bulb with a hemostat (a clamplike instrument used to control bleeding) to prevent loss of pressure.

As an alternative to the standard limb tourniquet, another type of tourniquet is used when the hemorrhage is inguinal or axillary. The junctional tourniquet uses a belt system to hold the device in place (either around the hips for an inguinal injury or around the chest for an axilla

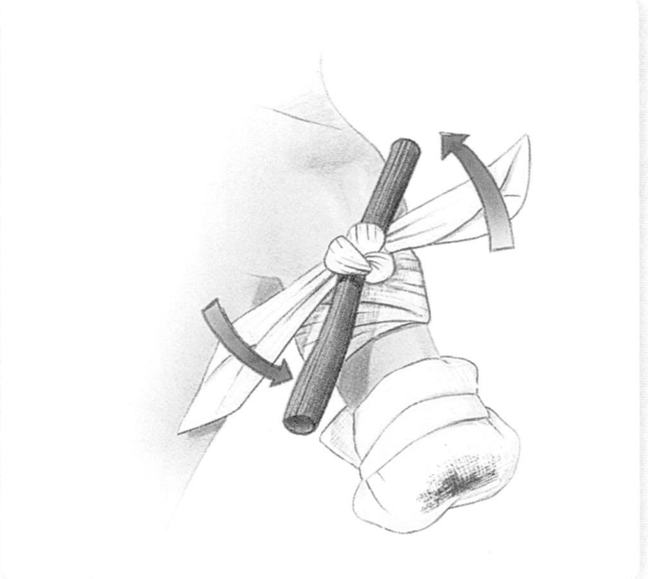

Figure 27-8 Twist the stick or rod to tighten the tourniquet until the bleeding has stopped and distal pulses are no longer palpable; then stop twisting.

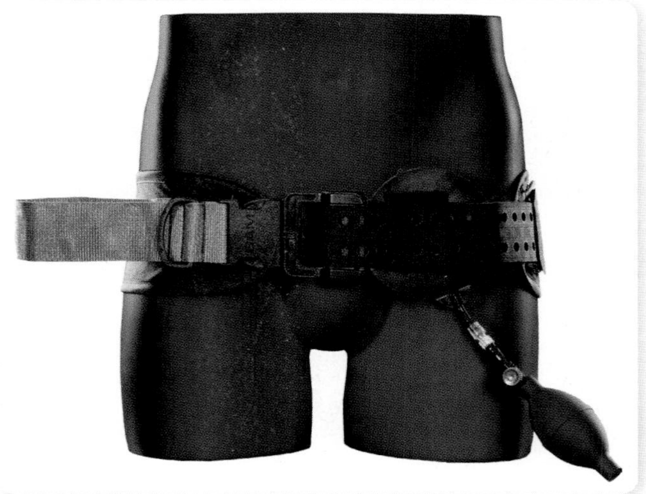

Figure 27-9 SAM junctional tourniquets can be used for inguinal or axillary hemorrhage control.

Words of Wisdom

There is no evidence that applying the tourniquet closer to the site of bleeding is preferable, and no reason to believe that normal tissue is at risk by placing the tourniquet too high. Keep in mind that there is the possibility of nerve injury by placing the tourniquets at an unsafe site, such as the proximal leg just below the knee or the proximal forearm just below the elbow, where the common peroneal nerve (leg) or the ulnar nerve (forearm) could be at risk.

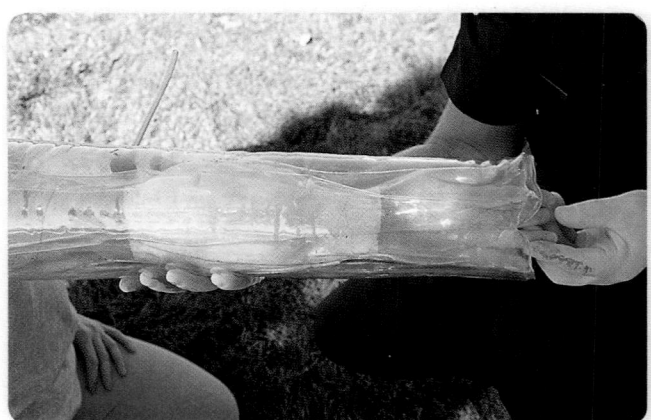

Figure 27-10 Air splints can also be used to help control bleeding because they act as a pressure bandage for the entire extremity.

injury). Using a pump, you then inflate a compression device to put pressure on the deep vessels **Figure 27-9**. The junctional tourniquet, when applied around the hips, can also be used as a pelvic immobilization device, as discussed in the next section.

Whenever you are applying a tourniquet, make sure you observe the following precautions:

- Ensure the tourniquet is proximal to the zone of injury and as close to the groin or axilla as possible.
- Use the widest bandage possible. This will protect the tissues and help with arterial compression.
- Never use wire, rope, a belt, or any other narrow material. It could cut into the patient's skin.
- Make sure the tourniquet is tightened securely.
- Never cover a tourniquet with a bandage. Leave it open and in full view.
- Inform the hospital both in your radio report and in your verbal report on arrival at the ED that a tourniquet has been applied.
- Do not loosen the tourniquet after you have applied it. Hospital personnel will loosen it when they are prepared to manage the bleeding.

Splints

Air Splints. Air splints (commonly known as pressure splints) can control the bleeding associated with severe soft-tissue injuries, such as massive or complex lacerations, or fractures **Figure 27-10**. They also immobilize the fracture itself. An air splint acts as a pressure dressing applied to an entire extremity rather than to a small, local area.

After you have applied an air splint, be sure to monitor circulation in the distal extremity. Because an air splint is typically inflated to a pressure of approximately 50 mm Hg (so you can still dent the splint with your fingertips), it would not be appropriate to use this device on a patient with arterial hemorrhage: the splint would not actually control the hemorrhage until the patient's systolic blood pressure dropped to the pressure of the splint. Use only approved, clean, or disposable valve stems when orally inflating air splints.

Rigid Splints. Rigid splints can help stabilize fractures as well as reduce pain and prevent further damage to soft-tissue injuries. After you have applied a rigid splint, be sure to monitor circulation in the distal extremity.

Traction Splints. Traction splints are designed to stabilize isolated femur fractures. When traction is applied to the ankle, countertraction is applied to the ischium and groin. This reduces the thigh muscle spasms and prevents one end of the fracture from impacting or overriding the other and realigns the limb. This not only helps to reduce pain, but also helps control hemorrhage and minimize potential vascular and neurologic complications. Be sure to pad these areas well to prevent applying excessive pressure to the soft tissue of the pelvis. After you have applied a traction splint, be sure to monitor circulation in the distal extremity.

Words of Wisdom

Research indicates that a pelvic compression device is an effective method to reduce the width of pelvic ring fractures **Figure 27-11**. Overcompression has not been identified as an issue to date. The restoration of normal pelvic diameter will assist in the control of internal bleeding resulting from the fracture, specifically an open book fracture of the pelvis.

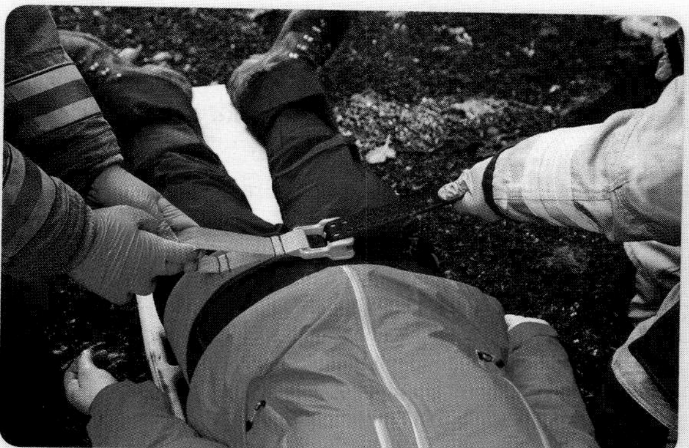

Figure 27-11 Pelvic compression devices or binders are meant to provide temporary stabilization and reduce hemorrhage from pelvic bleeding.

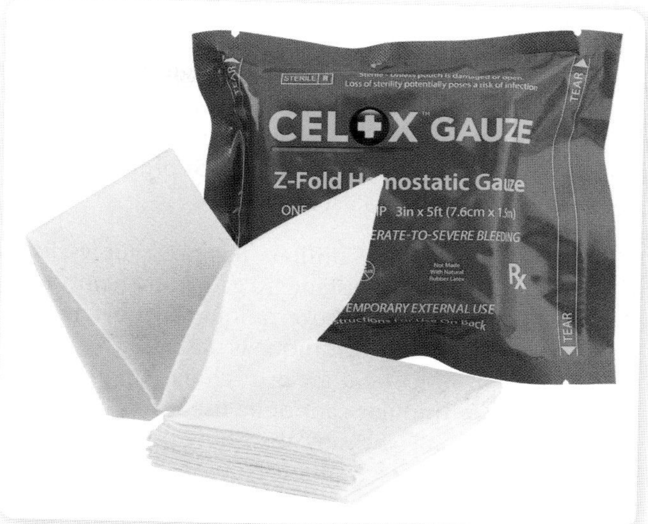

Figure 27-12 Hemostatic agents are being used by some EMS systems to control severe hemorrhage, especially in areas of the body where a tourniquet cannot be placed.

Hemostatic Agents

The military has successfully used hemostatic agents to control severe hemorrhage, especially to areas where a tourniquet cannot be placed, such as junctional wounds (inguinal and axilla) **Figure 27-12**. A **hemostatic agent** works by causing enhanced clot formation in the wound site: the agent adheres to the damaged tissue and either dehydrates the blood or undergoes a chemical reaction that stimulates the natural blood clotting cascade (ie, the intrinsic pathway). Ideally, the bleeding should be stopped in 2 minutes or less.

In general, all hemostatic agents should share a few common attributes. They should be lightweight and easy to store, carry, and deploy in emergency situations. They should be able to conform to the wound itself, allowing the agent to work where it is needed, especially at deep wound sites where direct pressure alone may not be sufficient or be difficult to apply, such as a femoral artery laceration in the groin. After application, hemostatic agents should be able to withstand the high pressure or flow of a bleeding wound, cause little or no damage to the tissues surrounding

Words of Wisdom

Hemostatic agents were primarily used in the military to promote hemostasis or, in other words, to stop profuse bleeding, but are rapidly gaining prevalence in the civilian world. These agents may consist of granules contained in a dressing. The agent absorbs the water component of blood thereby concentrating the clotting factors, activating platelets, and enhancing the coagulation cascade.

the wound site, be easy to remove from the wound, and not spread into the rest of the system as small particles. As of this writing, the prevalent agents on the market are gauzes impregnated with various proprietary clotting agents. Consult your local protocols if these agents are to be used, and seek guidance on which of these agents are approved in your EMS system.

Wound Packing. The US military has been successfully using wound packing with standard gauze and hemostatic agents for many years, and the techniques are now moving into civilian EMS.[10] The technique is particularly helpful for bleeding in junctional areas, such as the groin and axilla, where tourniquets cannot be used.

Wound packing works by absorbing liquid from the blood and helping to concentrate clotting factors, helping to transfer external direct pressure to deeper blood vessels that are the source of bleeding, and, if using hemostatic dressings, it can also chemically accelerate the clotting process.[10]

Wound packing involves taking standard initial steps to control the bleeding including direct pressure, tourniquets, and other applicable tools and techniques. Simply push the gauze into the wound with an index finger to completely and tightly pack the wound cavity. The goal is to contact the source of the bleeding if possible and to fill the cavity. If extra gauze is left over, place it on top of the wound. Hold firm, direct manual pressure on the wound for at least 3 minutes or secure the wound with a snug pressure dressing over the wound. Consult your local protocols for guidance on wound packing and the use of hemostatic agents.

Words of Wisdom

Damage control resuscitation (DCR) is a systematic approach to the treatment of the trauma patient with severe injuries. This approach begins with the prehospital care provider and continues through the ED, operating room, and intensive care unit. DCR focuses on maintaining circulating volume, controlling hemorrhage, and correcting the deadly triad of coagulopathy, acidosis, and hypothermia.

Although some tools of DCR such as blood product administration are used by only a few EMS services, many techniques including rapid assessment, minimizing the use of crystalloid fluids, patient warming, and use of tourniquets, pressure dressings, and hemostatic gauze are widely available.

Pneumatic Antishock Garment

A **pneumatic antishock garment (PASG)** is an inflatable device that covers the legs and abdomen. Historically, it was used when a patient was exhibiting signs of hypoperfusion. These devices are now rarely used, and you should always follow local protocols.

Controversies

In the 1980s, researchers began to question whether use of the military antishock trousers (MAST/PASG) and IV fluid infusion were actually effective in the treatment of shock.[11,12] At the time of this writing, the MAST/PASG is rarely applied in the treatment of hemorrhagic shock as the risks of its use likely outweigh any potential benefit based on the medical evidence available. Consult your medical director and regional protocols if you still carry the device.

The few, very specific instances in which a PASG may be used include:

- To stabilize fractures of the pelvis and bilateral femurs
- In some areas, protocols may allow PASG use to control significant internal bleeding associated with fractures of the pelvis and bilateral femurs; however, there is no evidence that this works or is safe for this indication. PASG *does not* replace the need for tourniquet use in severe extremity hemorrhage; use of PASG in these situations may be particularly dangerous.

Pulmonary edema is an absolute contraindication to the use of the PASG.

Hemorrhaging From the Nose, Ears, and Mouth

Several conditions can result in bleeding from the nose, ears, and/or mouth, including the following:

- Skull fracture
- Facial injuries, including those caused by a direct blow to the nose
- Sinusitis, infections, nose drop use and abuse, dried or cracked nasal mucosa, or other abnormalities
- High blood pressure
- Coagulation disorders
- Digital trauma (nose picking)

Epistaxis, or nosebleed, is a common emergency. Occasionally, it can cause enough of a blood loss to send a patient into shock. Keep in mind that the blood you see may be only a small part of the total blood loss. Much of the blood may pass down the throat into the stomach as the patient swallows. A person who swallows a large amount of blood may become nauseated and start vomiting the blood, which is sometimes confused with internal bleeding. Most nontraumatic nosebleeds occur from sites in the septum, the tissue dividing the nostrils.

For a nosebleed from other conditions, such as trauma directly to the nose or bleeding caused by environmental factors such as dry air, apply cold compresses to the bridge of the nose while the patient leans forward. An alternative is to roll gauze and place it under the patient's upper lip. This treatment will generate pressure on the blood supply to the nose and often works within 5 minutes. Check the patient's blood pressure and evaluate for a hypertensive emergency as the cause of epistaxis, especially in older adults. Techniques for controlling epistaxis are covered in Chapter 29, *Face and Neck Injuries*. Bleeding from the nose or ears following a head injury may indicate a skull fracture. In these cases, you should not attempt to stop the blood flow. This bleeding may be difficult to control. Applying excessive pressure to the injury may force the blood leaking through the ear or nose to collect within the head. This could increase intracranial pressure and possibly cause permanent damage. If you suspect a skull fracture, loosely cover the bleeding site with a sterile gauze pad to collect the blood and help keep contaminants away from the site. There is always a risk of infection to the brain. Apply light compression by wrapping the dressing loosely around the head Figure 27-13.

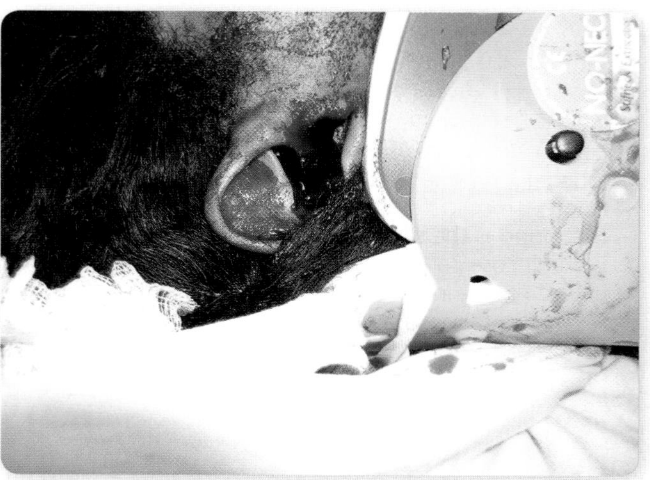

Figure 27-13 Bleeding from the ear after a head injury may indicate a skull fracture. Loosely cover the bleeding site with a sterile gauze pad, and apply light compression by wrapping the dressing loosely around the head.

Internal Hemorrhaging

Because most cases of internal bleeding are rarely fully controlled in the prehospital setting, definitive care includes rapid transport to the ED. Some treatments may be effective in the field depending on the cause of the bleeding. You can usually control internal bleeding into the extremities quite well in the field simply by splinting the extremity, usually most effectively with an air splint.

Treatment of a patient with internal hemorrhaging focuses on the treatment of shock (including prevention of hypothermia), minimizing movement of the injured or bleeding part or region, and rapid transport. Eventually, the patient will likely need a surgical procedure to stop the bleeding. Ultrasonography may be used to locate bleeding in the ED. Ultrasonography is also being used in prehospital environments, particularly the military.

YOU are the Provider — PART 5

As the search and rescue (SAR) team prepares a Stokes basket, you place a splint on the deformed right leg. You note that the patient still has a weak pulse in the leg; as expected, you are unable to find a pulse in the left upper extremity. You can hear the helicopter in the distance and advise the SAR crew that you need to get the patient moving. Taking care not to pull out the IV lines or disrupt the tourniquet, the patient is placed into the Stokes basket, secured, and carried out approximately one-half mile to the waiting helicopter. After a brief report to the flight crew including the patient's request for pain medication, the patient departs for the local trauma center, a 12-minute flight.

Recording Time: 18 Minutes	
Respirations	28 breaths/min, rapid
Pulse	Distal not obtainable, 126 beats/min centrally
Skin	Diaphoretic, cool, pale, and clammy
Blood pressure	82 mm Hg by palpation
Oxygen saturation (Spo_2)	99% on 100% oxygen
Pupils	PERRLA

8. Why was there no pulse in the left upper extremity?
9. What patient information does the flight crew need from you?

Words of Wisdom

If blood or drainage from the ears or nose contains cerebrospinal fluid (CSF), the dressing will show a staining that resembles a bull's-eye target Figure 27-14. Another method that can be used to check for CSF in the blood is the glucometer. Because the CSF has a high glucose content, the glucometer will detect this excess glucose in the blood of a normoglycemic patient.

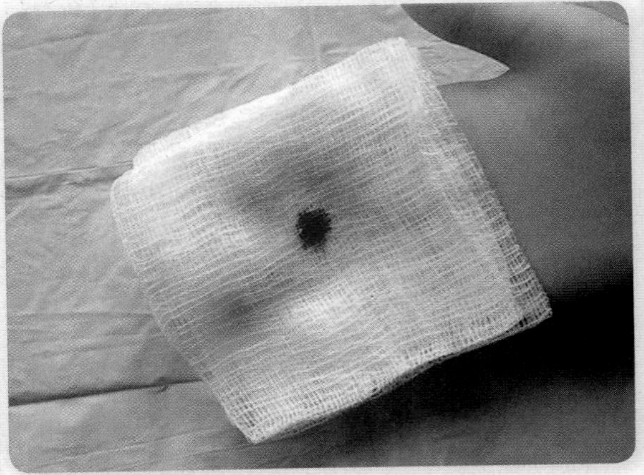

Figure 27-14 When cerebrospinal fluid is present in blood or drainage, a stain in the shape of a target or halo will appear.

Courtesy of Rhonda Hunt.

Follow the steps in Skill Drill 27-3 to care for patients with possible internal hemorrhage.

Give the patient nothing by mouth. Insert at least one 18-gauge IV catheter, and administer fluid boluses of 250 mL of normal saline or lactated Ringer solution (provided the patient's lungs are clear and the patient's condition warrants such a treatment and to a maximum of four doses before online medical consultation) without delaying patient transport. If IV access is unsuccessful or anticipated to be difficult, utilize intraosseous access, if available. Insert an IV line at the scene only if transport is delayed (eg, if the patient is pinned). Establish a second large-bore IV line if possible. Whenever possible, use warm IV fluids to prevent the patient from becoming hypothermic.

Keep the patient warm. Provide immediate transport and consider paramedic rendezvous for administration

Controversies

Some trauma surgeons prefer use of lactated Ringer solution over normal saline because lactated Ringer solution may help decrease acidosis in patients with severe hemorrhagic hypovolemia. This belief remains controversial, however, as lactated Ringer solution may also contribute to hyperkalemia in certain trauma patients.[13]

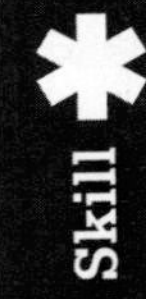

Skill Drill 27-3 Managing Internal Hemorrhage

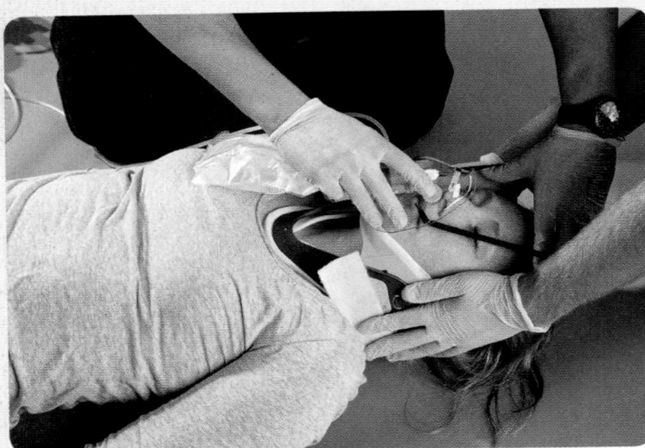

Step 1 Take standard precautions. Maintain the airway with cervical spine immobilization as indicated. Administer supplemental oxygen, and assist ventilation if necessary.

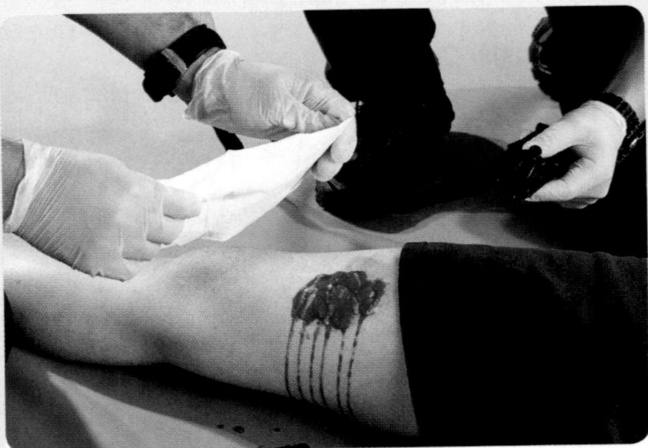

Step 2 Control all obvious external bleeding, and treat suspected internal bleeding using a splint, if possible. Apply a tourniquet for severe bleeding from an extremity that cannot be controlled with direct pressure.

Skill Drill 27-3 Managing Internal Hemorrhage *(continued)*

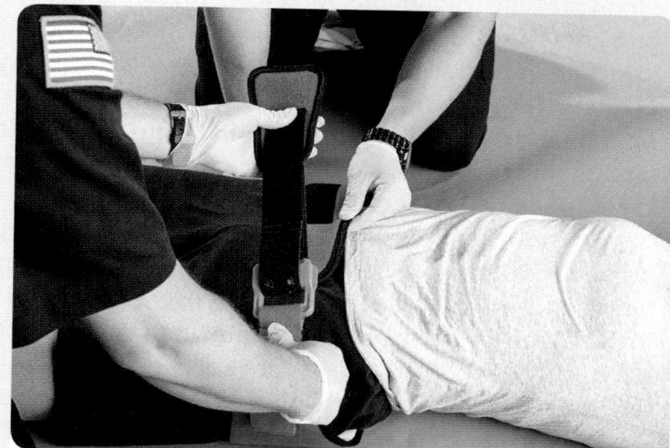

Step 3 Depending on local protocols, if a pelvic fracture is suspected, use a pelvic binder or sheets to bind the pelvic area.

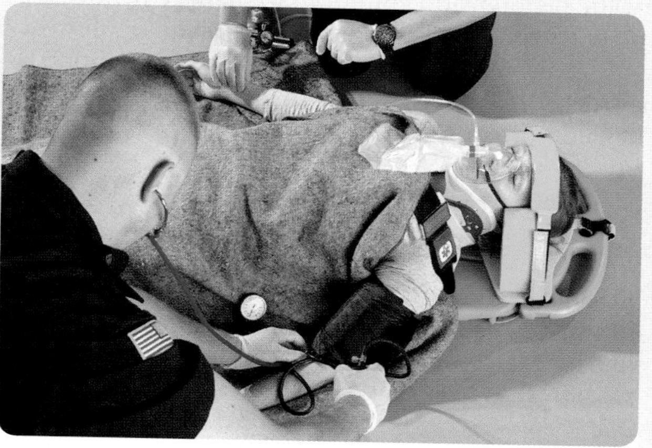

Step 4 Monitor and record vital signs at least every 5 minutes. Keep the patient warm and provide rapid transport.

of analgesics for pain. Monitor the serial vital signs, and watch diligently for developing shock en route. If the patient shows any signs of shock (hypoperfusion), transport rapidly while providing aggressive management en route. Because a patient in shock is usually emotionally upset, you should provide psychological support as well.

Words of Wisdom

Tranexamic acid (TXA) is another option for controlling internal hemorrhage.[14] TXA works by reducing fibrinolysis by inhibiting the activation of plasminogen to plasmin, which also reduces clot breakdown. Although used predominantly in the military for internal hemorrhage related to trauma, it is now widely used in the civilian sector. It should be considered early, during the assessment of airway, breathing, and circulation (ABC), for those patients presenting with signs of hemorrhagic shock. If TXA is used in your area, follow local protocols and call early for paramedic backup for administration.

▶ Management of Hemorrhagic Shock

The priorities in treating a patient in hemorrhagic shock are the same as in treating any other patient—with a focus on exsanguinating hemorrhage first (XABC). Always take standard precautions and ensure that the scene is safe. Identify and try to stop any major bleeding, and quickly evaluate the patient's hemodynamic status with a pulse check. Establish and maintain an open airway while maintaining manual stabilization if necessary, assist ventilation and use airway control adjuncts as needed, and continue to monitor the patient's breathing. Keep suction at hand to clear the mouth and pharynx if the patient vomits. Comfort, calm, and reassure the patient in the supine position. Do not allow the patient to eat or drink anything. Splint the patient on a backboard, and, unless necessary to control bleeding at the scene, splint individual extremity fractures during transport as opposed to on scene. If the patient exhibits signs or symptoms of shock, administer supplemental oxygen, keep the patient warm, and prepare for transport.

En route to the ED, insert at least one (preferably two) 18-gauge peripheral IV line, using an over-the-needle catheter. Obtain IV access at the scene only if transport of the patient is delayed. If allowed by protocol, draw blood (two red-top blood collection [Vacutainer] tubes and one purple-top tube) so that hospital personnel may obtain a hematocrit, type and cross-match, and other tests immediately on your arrival.

Unless your local protocol favors a different resuscitation fluid, administer warm isotonic crystalloids of normal saline in 250-mL increments to maintain the patient's systolic blood pressure at greater than 80 mm Hg (or greater than 90 mm Hg if there is evidence of traumatic brain injury).

Some evidence suggests that titration of systolic blood pressure to 80 to 90 mm Hg is preferred for hemorrhagic shock. This low pressure (ie, permissive hypotension) may allow the blood to clot better and not dislodge clots already formed.[15] However, you must also consider the entire patient before using permissive hypotension. In a patient with multisystem trauma and traumatic brain injury, the hypotension employed to manage hypovolemia presents severe risks and may potentially result in a lethal outcome. A retrospective observation study reported in the *Journal of Trauma* showed that a single episode of hypotension (systolic blood pressure <90 mm Hg) in patients with severe brain injury was associated with a doubling of mortality and a parallel increase in morbidity rates among survivors.[16,17] The concern is that the lower blood pressure will not provide adequate cerebral perfusion pressure. This pressure, which is the difference between the MAP and the intracranial pressure, represents the pressure gradient allowing for cerebral blood flow—and with it, oxygen and nutrients into the brain tissue. Without the oxygen and nutrients, the already damaged and delicate brain tissue will suffer secondary injury.

Do not give the patient anything by mouth because he or she is likely to vomit. Keep the patient at normal temperature, which usually means covering the patient with a blanket—patients in shock are often unable to conserve body heat effectively and are easily chilled. Monitor the level of consciousness, pulse, and blood pressure. In a patient with substantial vasoconstriction, the blood pressure sounds may be difficult to hear. If you can feel a pulse over the femoral artery but not over the radial artery, for example, the systolic blood pressure is probably between 70 and 80 mm Hg, although this technique is minimally accurate for estimating blood pressure.

Words of Wisdom

A patient's blood pressure may be the last measurable factor to change in shock. The body has several automatic mechanisms to compensate for initial blood loss and to help maintain the blood pressure. Thus, by the time you detect a decrease in the blood pressure, shock likely will be well developed. This is particularly true in infants and children, who can maintain their blood pressure until they have lost nearly one-half of their total blood volume.

YOU are the Provider SUMMARY

1. What are some possible hazards in this scene?

A scene such as a hunting accident presents multiple hazards. You are entering an area with hunters who are using firearms. If you are not properly dressed, hunters may confuse you for a deer and shoot you. Do not enter such areas without proper high-visibility clothing or without walking next to someone who is wearing such clothing. Other potential hazards with this scene include the distance you will have to walk to the patient, probably over uneven terrain, and possibly in darkness.

2. Is aeromedical evacuation appropriate with this patient?

Aeromedical evacuation is appropriate for this patient. This patient has uncontrolled arterial bleeding from a gunshot wound. On the basis of these findings and the deformed leg from the fall, this patient has a significant MOI and requires rapid transport to a trauma center.

3. Does this patient require spinal immobilization?

Yes. The patient has a significant MOI that requires spinal immobilization, although he denies having any other injuries than the ones you have located. Based on his femur fracture and the fact that he is in shock, his report of lack of spine pain should be considered unreliable, and spinal immobilization should be instituted.

4. How would you transport this patient one-half mile to the parking area where the helicopter could land?

This patient will have to be carried. On the basis of the injuries and physical findings, there is no way that this patient could or should walk. If there is a local SAR team available, they should be consulted for potential ways to extricate the patient, most likely involving a Stokes-type basket. If a SAR team is unavailable, the patient will need to be secured to a long backboard and carried out.

5. What class of hemorrhaging is occurring in this patient?

This patient is in class 3 or stage 4. At a minimum, this patient has lost 25% of his circulating blood volume, possibly upward of 40%. Prompt recognition and treatment will prevent this from resulting in death.

6. What are the indications for a tourniquet, and when do you remove it?

The indications for a tourniquet are uncontrollable arterial bleeding to an extremity. In this case, because the patient has been applying pressure for 45 minutes and the bleeding has not stopped, the best action is for EMS providers to immediately apply the tourniquet. After application, the tourniquet should not be removed in the prehospital setting.

YOU are the Provider SUMMARY *(continued)*

7. Why should you administer 250-mL boluses until a systolic blood pressure of 80 mm Hg is achieved?

Administering fluid in small increments prevents overhydration and a significant increase in blood pressure. Reassess vital signs and breath sounds after each administration and repeat until the desired goal is reached.

8. Why was there no pulse in the left upper extremity?

The application of an arterial tourniquet would prevent you from detecting a pulse in the left upper extremity. You should be able to palpate a radial pulse in the right upper extremity.

9. What patient information does the flight crew need from you?

The flight crew requires the same information from you that the ED staff does. Particularly, they need to know the MOI, initial findings, treatment (including the time of application for the tourniquet), and vital signs.

EMS Patient Care Report (PCR)

Date: 10-15-18	**Incident No.:** 3784	**Nature of Call:** Gunshot wound	**Location:** End Pyles Road, approx ½ mile back on trail

Dispatched: 0701	**En Route:** 0702	**At Scene:** 0711	**Transport:** N/A	**At Hospital:** N/A	**In Service:** 0756

Patient Information

Age: 32 **Sex:** M **Weight (in kg [lb]):** 80 kg (175 lb)	**Allergies:** No known drug allergies **Medications:** None **Past Medical History:** None **Chief Complaint:** Gunshot wound left bicep/right leg pain

Vital Signs

Time: 0715	**BP:** 74/P	**Pulse:** 139	**Respirations:** 32	**Spo_2:** Not obtained
Time: 0723	**BP:** 76/P	**Pulse:** 142	**Respirations:** 34	**Spo_2:** 97%
Time: 0729	**BP:** 82/P	**Pulse:** 126	**Respirations:** 28	**Spo_2:** 99%

EMS Treatment (circle all that apply)

Oxygen @ 15 **L/min via (circle one):** **NC** (**NRM** — circled) **Bag-mask device**	**Assisted Ventilation**	**Airway Adjunct**	**CPR**
Defibrillation	(circled) **Bleeding Control** Tourniquet: 0712	(circled) **Bandaging:** Yes	(circled) **Splinting:** Yes
Other:			

Narrative

EMS dispatched to above location for a male reporting a fall with a self-inflicted gunshot wound to the left arm. On arrival, patient found propped against tree, with large pool of blood around him. Pt states he was climbing into tree stand and fell from approximately 14 feet and his rifle discharged. Pt presents with obvious gunshot wound to left bicep, and obvious deformity to right lower leg. Tourniquet applied to left proximal humerus with cessation of bleeding at 0712. Dispatch contacted for helicopter ETA and SAR dispatch. Bilateral 18-gauge IVs established with 250-mL bolus x 4 of normal saline infusing to goal of SBP 80 mm Hg. Nonrebreathing mask applied at 15 L/min. Right leg splinted with positive distal pulse before and after. With help of SAR, patient placed inside of Stokes basket and extricated approximately ½ mile to waiting helicopter. Patient report given to flight crew. EMS remained on scene until the helicopter was safely off the ground.**End of report**

Prep Kit

Ready for Review

- Perfusion is the circulation of blood in adequate amounts to meet each cell's current needs for oxygen, nutrients, and waste removal.
- Hypoperfusion, or shock, occurs when the cardiovascular system fails to provide adequate perfusion.
- Both internal and external bleeding can cause shock. You must know how to recognize and control both.
- Signs of hypovolemic shock (hypoperfusion) include change in mental status, change in skin color or pallor, weakness, faintness, or dizziness. Key later signs include tachycardia, a weak or rapid pulse, thirst, nausea, vomiting, clammy skin, shallow or rapid breathing, dull eyes or dilated pupils, and decreasing blood pressure.
- The severity of external bleeding is often a function of the types of blood vessels that have been injured. Bleeding from an open artery is usually bright red, spurts, and is difficult to control. Blood from an open vein is much darker and flows steadily. Blood from damaged capillary vessels is dark red and oozes from a wound steadily but slowly.
- Internal bleeding may occur from trauma to any portion of the body. Bleeding into the thorax, abdomen, or pelvis tends to be severe and uncontrolled. Because internal bleeding is not as obvious, you must rely on signs and symptoms to determine the extent and severity of the bleeding.
- Signs of internal bleeding include pain, swelling, tenderness, bruised chest or abdomen, distended abdomen, guarding, hematuria, hematemesis, hemoptysis, melena, hematochezia, and broken ribs.
- The trauma triad of death is a combination of hypothermia, coagulopathy, and acidosis that substantially increases mortality in trauma patients. Closely watch for hypothermia and be sure to keep trauma patients warm.
- During the scene size-up, be sure to follow standard precautions. Depending on the severity of bleeding, this will entail wearing gloves, a mask, eye shield, and possibly a gown.
- Whether or not you can control bleeding, it is a serious emergency. During your primary survey, search for life-threatening external bleeding and control it immediately, before airway and breathing concerns.
- Patients with hemorrhage must be transported. You must determine how fast the transport decision should be made and where the patient should be taken. Consider the priority of the patient and the availability of a regional trauma center.
- Assess and promptly transport any patient who may have internal bleeding, particularly if the mechanism of injury is severe and has affected the abdomen, chest, or both.
- Methods for controlling external bleeding include direct, even pressure; pressure dressings and/or splints; and tourniquets. Most cases of external bleeding can be controlled with direct pressure to the bleeding site.
- If direct pressure fails to immediately stop the hemorrhaging, and if you are allowed by local protocol and policy, apply a tourniquet above the level of the bleeding. If a commercial tourniquet is not available, a tourniquet can be improvised with a triangular bandage and a stick or rod.
- Air splints are used to control bleeding associated with severe soft-tissue injuries or fractures. Rigid splints and traction splints are other options used in specific cases.
- Hemostatic agents and wound packing are other methods to control severe hemorrhage. Hemostatic agents cause enhanced clot formation in a wound site. Wound packing involves placing a gauze into a wound cavity to apply snug pressure to a wound.
- For a nosebleed not associated with skull fracture, apply cold compresses to the bridge of the nose while the patient leans forward. Alternatively, roll gauze and place it under the patient's upper lip. This treatment will generate pressure on the blood supply to the nose and often works within 5 minutes.
- Bleeding from the nose or ears following a head injury may indicate a skull fracture. Do not attempt to stop the blood flow. Loosely cover the bleeding site with a sterile gauze pad. Apply light compression by wrapping the dressing loosely around the head.
- If you suspect that a patient is bleeding internally or has hemorrhagic shock, maintain the airway, administer supplemental oxygen and assist ventilation as needed, keep the patient still and warm, control all obvious external bleeding, and monitor vital signs at least every 5 minutes. Establish intravenous access for fluid administration, or an intraosseous line if intravenous access is not successful. Finally, provide rapid transport.

Vital Vocabulary

afterload The pressure in the aorta against which the left ventricle must pump blood; increasing this pressure can decrease cardiac output.

cardiac output (CO) The amount of blood pumped by the heart per minute; calculated by multiplying the stroke volume by the pulse rate per minute.

Prep Kit *(continued)*

coagulopathy Any type of bleeding disorder that interferes with the activation or continuation of the clotting cascade or hemostasis.

contusion A bruise, or ecchymosis.

ecchymosis Discoloration of the skin associated with a closed wound; bruising.

epistaxis Nosebleed.

hematemesis Vomited blood.

hematochezia Passage of stools containing bright red blood, indicating lower gastrointestinal tract bleeding.

hematoma A mass of blood in the soft tissues beneath the skin.

hematuria Presence of blood in the urine.

hemophilia A congenital condition in which the patient lacks one or more of the blood's normal clotting factors.

hemoptysis Bright red blood that is coughed up by the patient.

hemorrhage A discharge of blood from the blood vessels; bleeding.

hemorrhagic shock A condition in which low blood volume due to massive internal or external bleeding results in inadequate perfusion.

hemostasis Formation of clots to plug openings in injured blood vessels and stop blood flow.

hemostatic agent Pharmacologic substances used to stop profuse bleeding and that function by absorbing the water component of blood, thereby concentrating the clotting factors, activating platelets, and enhancing the coagulation cascade.

hypovolemic shock A condition in which low blood volume, due to massive internal or external bleeding or extensive loss of body water, results in inadequate perfusion.

melena The passage of dark, tarry, foul-smelling stool, indicative of upper gastrointestinal tract bleeding.

perfusion Circulation of blood within an organ or tissue in amounts adequate to meet the cells' current needs.

pneumatic antishock garment (PASG) An inflatable device that covers the legs and abdomen; used to splint the lower extremities or pelvis, or to control bleeding in the lower extremities or pelvis.

preload The precontraction pressure in the heart, which increases as the volume of blood builds up.

pulse pressure Difference between the systolic and diastolic pressures.

shock A condition in which the circulatory system fails to provide sufficient circulation to enable every body part to perform its function; also called hypoperfusion.

tourniquet The bleeding control method used when a wound continues to bleed despite the use of direct pressure and elevation; useful if a patient is bleeding severely from a partial or complete amputation.

References

1. Guillermo G, Reines D, Wulf-Gutierrez M. Clinical review: hemorrhagic shock. *Critical Care*. 2004;8:373.
2. American College of Surgeons. *ATLS Advanced Trauma Life Support for Doctors—Student Course Manual*. Chicago, IL: American College of Surgeons; 2012.
3. Stop the Bleed. Homeland Security website. https://www.dhs.gov/stopthebleed. Updated June 16, 2017. Accessed November 13, 2017.
4. Stop the Bleeding Coalition website. https://stopthebleedingcoalition.org/. Accessed November 30, 2017.
5. American College of Surgeons. *The Hartford Consensus*. https://www.facs.org/about-acs/hartford-consensus. Accessed April 13, 2017.
6. Kragh JF Jr, Walters TJ, Baer DG, et al. Practical use of emergency tourniquets to stop bleeding in major limb trauma. *J Trauma*. 2008;64:538-550.
7. Snyder D, Tsou A, Schoelles K. *Efficacy of Prehospital Application of Tourniquets and Hemostatic Dressings to Control Traumatic External Hemorrhage.* DOT HS 811 999b. Washington, DC: National Highway Traffic Safety Administration; May 2014. https://www.ems.gov/pdf/research/Studies-and-Reports/Prehospital_Applications_Of_Tourniquest_And_Hemostatic_Dressings.pdf. Accessed April 12, 2017.
8. Bulger EM, Snyder D, Schoelles K, et al. An Evidence Based Prehospital Guideline for External Hemorrhage Control: American College of Surgeons Committee on Trauma. *Prehospital Emergency Care*. 2014;18(2):163-173.
9. Jacobs LM Jr, the Joint Committee to Create a National Policy to Enhance Survivability for Intentional Mass Casualty Shooting Events. The Hartford Consensus III: Implementation of Bleeding Control. Chicago: Bulletin of the American College of Surgeons; 2015.
10. Taillac PP, Bolleter S, Heightman AJ. Wound packing essentials for EMTs and paramedics. *J Emerg Med Serv.* 2017;42(4). http://www.jems.com/articles/print/volume-42/issue-4/features/wound -packing-essentials-for-emts-and-paramedics.html. Accessed April 26, 2017.

Prep Kit (continued)

11. Bickell WH, Pepe PE, Bailey ML, et al. Randomized trial of pneumatic antishock garments in the prehospital management of penetrating abdominal injuries. *Ann Emerg Med*. 1987;16(6):653-658.
12. Pepe PE, Bass RR, Mattox KL. Clinical trials of the pneumatic antishock garment in the urban prehospital setting. *Ann Emerg Med*. 1986;15(12):1407-1410.
13. Martini WZ, Cortez DS, Dubick MA. Comparisons of normal saline and lactated Ringer's resuscitation on hemodynamics, metabolic responses, and coagulation in pigs after severe hemorrhagic shock. *Scand J Trauma Resusc Emerg Med*. 2013;21:86.
14. Alson R, Braithwaite S. Role of TXA in Management of Traumatic Hemorrhage in the Field. https://www.itrauma.org/wp-content/uploads/2014/07/TXA-Resource-Document-FINAL-Publication-6-28-14.pdf. Accessed November 13, 2017.
15. Pape HC, Peitzman AB, Rotondo MF, Giannoudis PV. *Damage Control Management in the Polytrauma Patient*. New York, NY: Springer; 2017.
16. Chesnut RM, Marshall LF, Klauber MR, et al. The role of secondary brain injury in determining outcome from severe head injury. *J Trauma*. 1993;34(2):216-222. https://www.ncbi.nlm.nih.gov/pubmed/8459458. Accessed April 12, 2017.
17. Evidence-based EMS: permissive hypotension in trauma. EMS World website. http://www.emsworld.com/article/12163910/evidence-based-ems-permissive-hypotension-in-trauma. Accessed April 12, 2017.

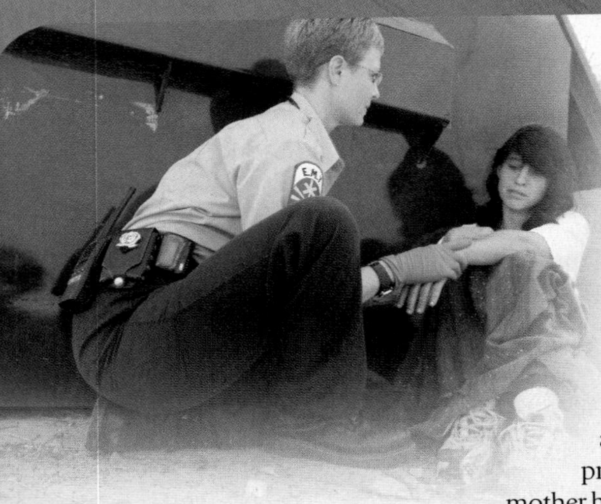

Assessment in Action

You were dispatched to a local butcher's shop for a man who cut his arm. On arrival, you find a man with an approximate 2-inch linear laceration to the medial aspect of his right forearm. He states that he cut it while trimming a roast. You note the blood to be dark and flowing steadily. On questioning the patient about his history, you learn that he takes atenolol for high blood pressure and an aspirin a day for his heart. He also tells you that his mother had some kind of "bleeding problem" and he is not sure if he has it.

1. What type of bleeding is occurring?

A. Arterial
B. Venous
C. Capillary
D. Plasma

2. The patient is an adult male. The typical adult has approximately _____ pints of blood.

A. 5
B. 10
C. 15
D. 20

Assessment *in Action* *(continued)*

3. What is the proper method to control this type of bleeding?

- **A.** Direct pressure
- **B.** Elevation
- **C.** Pressure point
- **D.** Tourniquet

4. If the bleeding continues, the patient may present with hypovolemic shock. Which of the following are early signs of hypovolemic shock?

- **A.** Rapid, weak pulse
- **B.** Rapid, strong pulse
- **C.** Warm, dry skin
- **D.** High blood pressure

5. The patient's ingestion of a beta blocker may have what effect on the bleeding?

- **A.** It can cause vasodilation and result in excessive bleeding.
- **B.** It can interfere with clotting and result in excessive bleeding.
- **C.** It can prevent vasoconstriction and result in excessive bleeding.
- **D.** It can cause vasoconstriction and result in stoppage of bleeding.

6. If bleeding continues after your attempts to control it, the next step is to use a tourniquet. If a commercial tourniquet is not available, ________ may be used instead.

- **A.** a shoe string
- **B.** wire
- **C.** a thin belt
- **D.** a blood pressure cuff

7. Which condition results when a person lacks certain clotting factors?

- **A.** Homeostasis
- **B.** Hemophilia
- **C.** Melena
- **D.** Hematochezia

8. Because his bleeding is not bright red and spurting, there is the potential for it to stop on its own. The term for platelets aggregating and sealing the injured vessel is:

- **A.** hemostasis.
- **B.** homeostasis.
- **C.** hematemesis.
- **D.** hemoptysis.

9. Discuss how to manage *epistaxis.*

10. Discuss how to manage a patient with signs of hemorrhagic shock.

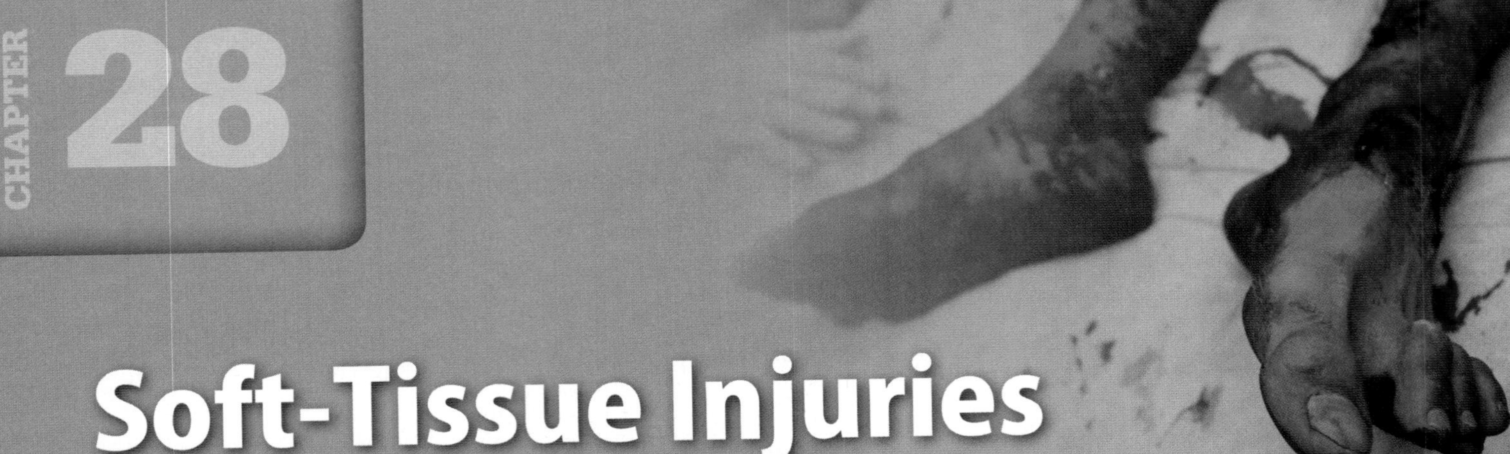

CHAPTER 28

Soft-Tissue Injuries

National EMS Education Standard Competencies

Trauma

Applies fundamental knowledge to provide basic and selected advanced emergency care and transportation based on assessment findings for an acutely injured patient.

Soft-Tissue Trauma

Recognition and management of

- Wounds (pp 1127-1131, 1134-1139)
- Burns
  - Electrical (pp 1153-1155)
  - Chemical (pp 1150-1153)
  - Thermal (pp 1149-1150)
- Chemicals in the eye and on the skin (pp 1151-1153)

Pathophysiology, assessment, and management of

- Wounds
  - Avulsions (pp 1129, 1131-1134, 1136)
  - Bite wounds (pp 1129, 1131-1134, 1136-1137)
  - Lacerations (pp 1128-1129, 1131-1136)
  - Puncture wounds (pp 1130-1137)
  - Incisions (pp 1128-1129, 1131-1136)
- Burns
  - Electrical (pp 1143-1149, 1153-1155)
  - Chemical (pp 1143-1149, 1150-1153)
  - Thermal (pp 1143-1150)
  - Radiation (pp 1143-1149, 1155)
- Crush syndrome (pp 1127-1128)

Knowledge Objectives

1. Review the anatomy and physiology of the skin. (pp 1125-1127)
2. List the functions of the skin. (p 1126)
3. Discuss the pathophysiology of soft-tissue injuries, including closed injuries, open injuries, and burns. (pp 1127-1131, 1139)
4. Describe the following types of closed soft-tissue injuries: contusion, hematoma, and crush injury. (pp 1127-1128)
5. Describe the following types of open soft-tissue injuries: abrasions, lacerations, avulsions, amputations, bite wounds, penetrating wounds, and blast injuries. (pp 1128-1131)
6. Describe the pathophysiology of wound healing. (p 1131)
7. Describe the assessment process for patients with a soft-tissue injury. (pp 1131-1134)
8. Describe the relationship between airway management and the patient with closed and open injuries. (p 1132)
9. Discuss emergency medical care of a patient with a soft-tissue injury. (pp 1134-1139)
10. List the functions of sterile dressings and bandages. (pp 1135-1136)
11. Discuss assessment and management of avulsions, amputations, bite wounds, gunshot wounds, open abdominal wounds, impaled objects, and open neck wounds. (pp 1136-1139)
12. Discuss the pathophysiology of burns, and explain the development of hypovolemic shock. (pp 1139-1140)
13. Define and give the characteristics of superficial, partial-thickness, and full-thickness burns. (pp 1140-1141)
14. Explain how the seriousness of a burn is related to its depth and extent. (pp 1142-1143)
15. Explain the steps involved in the assessment of burns. (pp 1143-1146)
16. Describe and discuss the emergency management of burns, including chemical, electrical, thermal, inhalation, and radiation burns. (pp 1147-1155)

Skills Objectives

1. Demonstrate the emergency medical care of closed soft-tissue injuries. (p 1134)
2. Demonstrate how to control bleeding in an open soft-tissue injury. (p 1134)
3. Demonstrate the emergency medical care of a patient with an open abdominal wound. (pp 1137-1138)
4. Demonstrate how to stabilize an impaled object. (p 1138, Skill Drill 28-1)
5. Demonstrate how to care for a burn. (pp 1147-1149, Skill Drill 28-2)
6. Demonstrate the emergency medical care of a patient with a chemical, electrical, thermal, inhalation, or radiation burn. (pp 1149-1155)

Introduction

The skin is the body's first line of defense against external forces and infection. Although it is relatively tough, skin is still quite susceptible to injury. Injuries to soft tissues range from simple bruises or abrasions to serious lacerations, amputations, and burns. Soft-tissue injury may result in exposure of deep structures such as blood vessels, nerves, and bones. In all cases, you must control bleeding, prevent further contamination, and protect the wound from further damage by applying dressings and bandages.

The soft tissues of the body can be injured through a variety of mechanisms. A blunt injury occurs when the energy exchange between the patient and an object is more than the tissues can tolerate, as can happen when a baseball strikes the forearm. A penetrating injury occurs when an object, such as a bullet or knife, breaks through the skin and enters the body. Burns may also result in soft-tissue injuries.

Soft-tissue trauma is a common form of injury. Death resulting from soft-tissue injury is often related to hemorrhage or infection. Uncontrolled hemorrhage can quickly result in shock and death. When the skin barrier is breached, invading pathogens—bacteria, fungi, and viruses—can cause local or systemic infection. Infection can be life or limb threatening, especially in children, older adults, and people with diabetes or other conditions that may compromise the immune system.

Preventing soft-tissue injuries and their associated complications involves simple protective actions. The use of gloves when working with abrasive materials, for example, helps prevent skin injuries. Workplace safety measures to reduce injury include use of safety devices to prevent interaction between machine parts and body parts. Teaching children to avoid (or request help when) using sharp objects also helps prevent injury.

This chapter begins with a review of anatomy and physiology. Then it divides into two parts. Closed and open injuries and their assessment and management are discussed first. Then the assessment and management of burns are discussed in a separate section because they differ from other soft-tissue injuries.

Anatomy and Physiology Review

Skin Structure and Function

The skin, or integumentary system, is the largest organ in the body. It varies in thickness, depending on a person's age and the area the skin covers. The skin of very young and very old patients is thinner than the skin of a young adult. The skin covering the scalp, back, and soles of the feet is quite thick, while the skin of the eyelids, lips, and ears is extremely thin. Thin skin is more easily damaged than thick skin.

The skin has two principal layers: the **epidermis** and the **dermis** Figure 28-1. The epidermis is the tough, external layer that forms a watertight covering for the body. The epidermis contains several layers. The cells on the surface layer of the epidermis are constantly worn away. They are replaced by cells that are pushed to the surface when new cells form in the germinal layer at the base of the epidermis.

The dermis is the inner layer of the skin that lies below the germinal cells of the epidermis. The dermis contains the hair follicles, sweat glands, and sebaceous glands. The sweat glands help cool the body by releasing sweat onto the surface of the skin through small pores, or ducts, that pass through the epidermis. Sebaceous glands produce sebum, the oily material that waterproofs the skin and keeps it supple. Sebum travels to the skin's surface along the shaft of adjacent hair follicles. Hair follicles are small organs that produce hair. There is one follicle for each hair, each connected with a sebaceous gland and a tiny muscle, the erector pili, which pulls the hair erect (appearing as goose bumps) whenever a person is cold or frightened.

Blood vessels in the dermis provide the skin with nutrients and oxygen. Small branches reach up to the

YOU are the Provider — PART 1

At 1602 hours, immediately after reporting for your shift, your ambulance is dispatched with the local fire department for a reported explosion at Lake Bronson. En route, the dispatcher reports that you have a 19-year-old man who was pouring gasoline on a barbeque when it flashed and burned him severely. Bystanders are reporting that he is burned "really badly." As you arrive on scene, you find the patient lying on the ground, moaning in pain with his clothing still smoldering on his body. You note full-thickness burns to his chest, both arms, both legs, and his groin. Miraculously, his face appears unscathed. You estimate his weight at 80 kg (178 lb).

1. How do you calculate the percentage of burned area?
2. What classification of burns does this patient have?

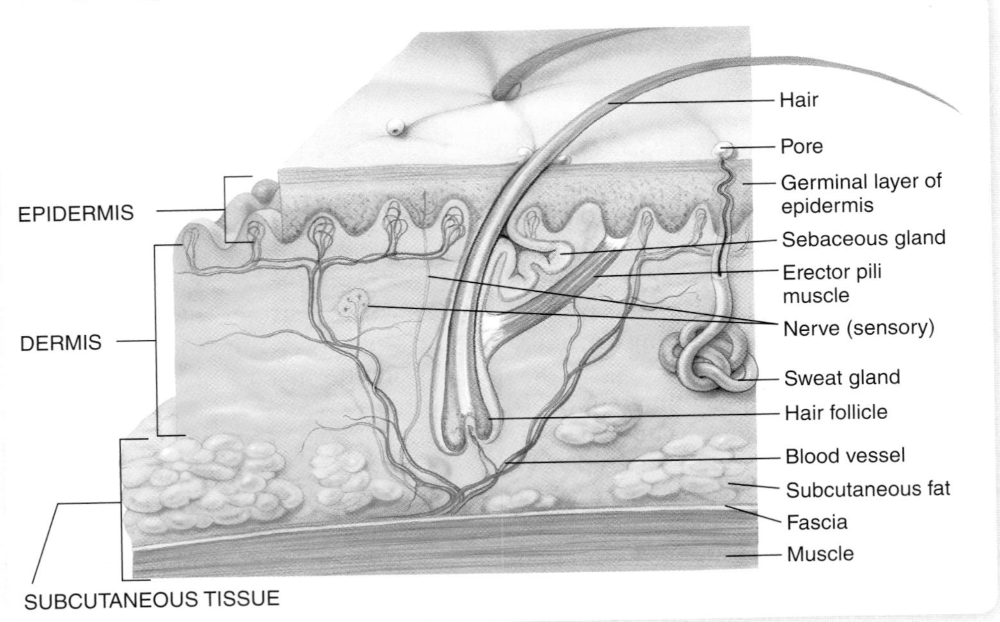

Figure 28-1 The skin comprises a tough external layer called the epidermis and a vascular inner layer called the dermis. Between the dermis and the underlying muscle and bone is a thick layer of connective tissue known as subcutaneous tissue and a layer of fascia.

germinal cells, but no blood vessels penetrate farther into the epidermis. There are also specialized nerve endings within the dermis.

The skin covers all external surfaces of the body. The various orifices in the body, including the mouth, nose, anus, and vagina, are lined with **mucous membranes**. These membranes are similar to skin in that they provide a protective barrier against invasion of harmful agents. But mucous membranes differ from skin because they secrete a watery substance that lubricates the openings. Therefore, mucous membranes are moist, while skin is dry.

The skin serves many functions. It protects the body by keeping pathogens out and fluids in. The nerves in the skin report to the brain on the environment and on many sensations. It is this nerve pathway connection that allows the body to adapt to environments through responses in the skin and surrounding tissues. The skin is also the body's major organ for regulating temperature. In a cold environment, the blood vessels in the skin constrict, diverting blood away from the skin and decreasing the amount of heat that is radiated from the body's surface. In hot environments, the vessels in the skin dilate. The skin becomes flushed or red, and heat radiates from the body's surface. Sweat glands secrete sweat, which evaporates from the skin's surface and causes a reduction in body temperature.

Any break in the skin allows potentially infectious agents to enter and increases the possibilities of infection, fluid loss, and loss of temperature control. Any one of these problems can cause serious illness and even death.

▶ Skin Tension Lines

The skin is arranged over the body structures in a manner that provides tension. This tautness varies by body region but occurs in patterns known as **tension lines**. Static tension develops over areas that have limited movement, such as the scalp. Lacerations occurring parallel to the skin tension lines may remain closed with little or no intervention. Larger wounds may be pulled open by the normal tension and require closure with sutures, staples, or biodegradable glue. Even small lacerations that lie perpendicular to the tension lines may result in a wound that remains open. Healing occurs more slowly in an open wound, and abnormal scar formation is more likely.

Dynamic tension is found in areas that lie over muscle. This tension varies according to the contraction of the underlying muscle and subsequent movement of the skin. Open injuries to dynamic tension lines interfere with

Words of Wisdom

The skin's structure includes tension lines, which make the skin become taut with movement. If the skin is cut in a direction that is perpendicular to a tension line (such as over a knee), it will be more difficult to control bleeding in that area because the tension lines will tend to pull the cut open. Splinting injuries helps address this situation and helps to control bleeding.

healing because they disrupt the clotting process and the tissue repair cycle, resulting in slowed healing and a tendency toward abnormal scar formation.

Pathophysiology of Closed and Open Injuries

Soft tissues are often injured because they are exposed to the environment. There are three types of soft-tissue injuries:

- **Closed injury**, in which soft-tissue damage occurs beneath the skin or mucous membrane but the surface remains intact.
- **Open injury**, in which there is a break in the surface of the skin or the mucous membrane, exposing deeper tissues to potential contamination.
- **Burns**, in which the soft tissue receives more energy than it can absorb without injury. The source of this energy can be thermal heat, frictional heat, toxic chemicals, electricity, or nuclear radiation.

▶ Closed Injuries

Closed soft-tissue injuries are characterized by a history of blunt trauma, pain at the site of injury, swelling beneath the skin, and discoloration. Such injuries can vary from mild to quite severe.

A **contusion**, or bruise, is an injury that causes bleeding beneath the skin but does not break the skin. Contusions result from blunt force striking the body. The epidermis remains intact, but cells within the dermis are damaged, and small blood vessels are usually torn. The depth of the injury varies, depending on the amount of energy absorbed. As fluid and blood leak into the damaged area, the patient may have swelling and pain. The buildup of blood produces a characteristic blue or black discoloration called **ecchymosis** Figure 28-2.

A **hematoma** is a pool of blood that has collected within damaged tissue or in a body cavity Figure 28-3. It occurs whenever blood vessels are damaged and bleed rapidly. It may be associated with extensive tissue damage. A hematoma can result from a soft-tissue injury, a fracture, or any injury to a large blood vessel. In severe cases, such as an aortic transection (torn aorta) or a pelvic fracture, the hematoma may contain more than 1 liter of blood.

A crushing injury occurs when substantial force is applied to the body. The extent of the damage depends on how much force is applied and how long it is applied. In addition to causing some direct soft-tissue damage, continued compression of the soft tissues cuts off circulation, producing further tissue destruction. For example, if a patient's legs are trapped under a collapsed pile of rocks, damage to the leg tissues may continue until the rocks are removed.

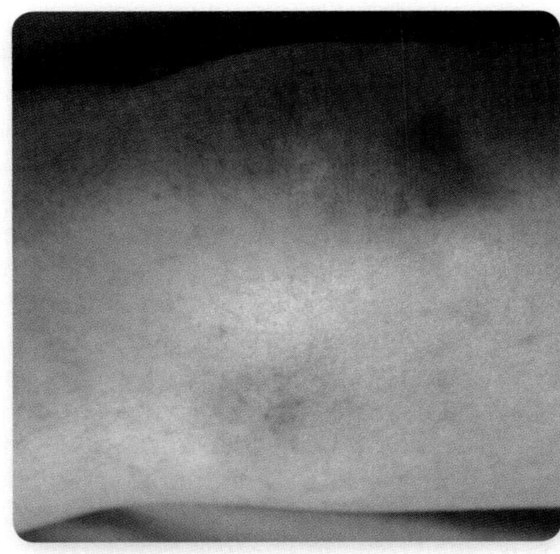

Figure 28-2 Contusions, more commonly known as bruises, occur as a result of a blunt force striking the body. The buildup of blood produces a characteristic blue or black discoloration (ecchymosis).

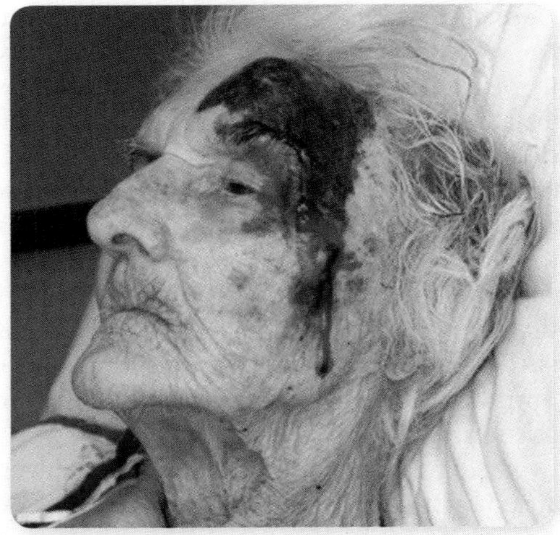

Figure 28-3 A hematoma develops whenever blood vessels are damaged and bleed substantially.

In **crush syndrome**, tissue necrosis develops and results in release of harmful products into the bloodstream when the limb is freed from entrapment. The compressing force prevents blood from returning to the injured body part; while by-products of metabolism and harmful products of tissue destruction collect in the part that is crushed. These substances are released into the body's circulation after the limb is freed and blood flow is returned. Cardiac arrest may result almost instantaneously on freeing the limb if substantial amounts of potassium are suddenly returned to circulation. Renal failure is another serious complication that may develop after the release as the kidneys attempt to filter out the harmful products associated with the degradation of dead muscle tissue (a process known as rhabdomyolysis). Life-threatening dysrhythmias may also develop as a result of the acidosis. Intravenous (IV) access should be gained prior to removal to provide a route for medication or rapid fluid replacement, and whenever possible, adequate rehydration should be achieved prior to release of compression, particularly if the victim has been trapped for several hours.

Another form of compression can result from the swelling that occurs whenever tissues are injured. The cells that are injured leak intracellular fluid into the spaces between the cells. If swelling is excessive or occurs in a confined space such as the skull, the tissue pressure will increase to dangerous levels. The pressure of the fluid may become great enough to compress the tissue and cause further damage, especially if the blood vessels become compressed, cutting off blood flow to the tissue. This condition is called **compartment syndrome**. The hallmark sign of compartment syndrome is pain out of proportion to the injury.

▶ Open Injuries

Open injuries differ from closed injuries in that the protective layer of skin is damaged. This can produce extensive bleeding. More important, a break in the protective skin layer or mucous membrane means that the wound is contaminated and may become infected. **Contamination** is the presence of infectious organisms (pathogens) or foreign bodies, such as dirt, gravel, or metal, in the wound. You must address excessive bleeding and contamination in your treatment of open soft-tissue wounds.

As an advanced emergency medical technician (AEMT), you must be prepared to manage several types of open soft-tissue wounds, including abrasions, lacerations, avulsions, amputations, penetrating wounds, bite wounds, and blast injuries.

An **abrasion** is a wound of the superficial layer of the skin, caused by friction when a body part rubs or scrapes across a rough or hard surface. An abrasion typically does not penetrate completely through the dermis, but blood may ooze from the injured capillaries in the dermis. Even though abrasions generally do not result in a considerable loss of blood volume, fluid loss may be substantial when large areas are affected. Known by a variety of names, including road rash, road burn, strawberry, and rug burn, abrasions can be extremely painful because of nerve endings located in this layer of the skin **Figure 28-4**. Even though abrasions are usually superficial, their locations may indicate possible underlying injuries. For example, you should maintain a high index of suspicion that injuries over the flank areas may be the only sign of potential kidney damage.

A **laceration** is a smooth or jagged cut caused by a sharp object or a blunt force that tears the tissue. The depth of the injury can vary, extending through the skin and subcutaneous tissue, even into the underlying muscles and adjacent nerves and blood vessels **Figure 28-5**. Lacerations and incisions may appear linear (in a line) or stellate (irregular) and may occur along with other

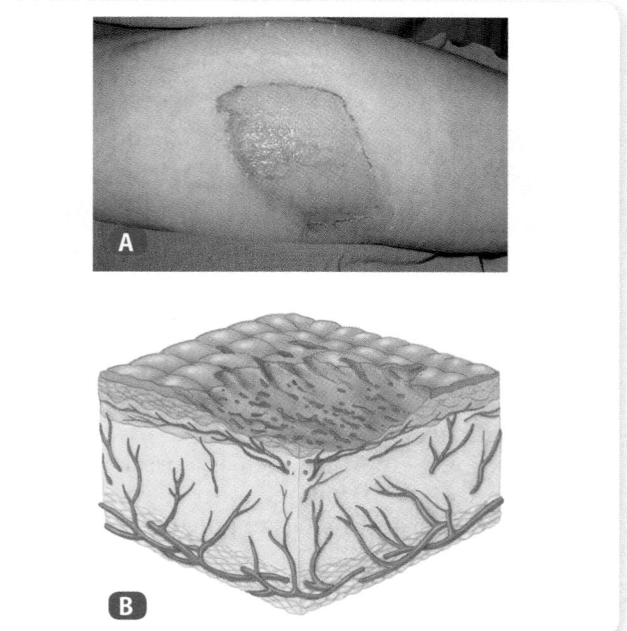

Figure 28-4 Abrasions usually do not penetrate completely through the dermis, but blood may ooze from the capillaries. These wounds are typically superficial and result from rubbing or scraping across a hard, rough surface. **(A)** shows an abrasion; **(B)** shows an anatomic illustration of an abrasion.

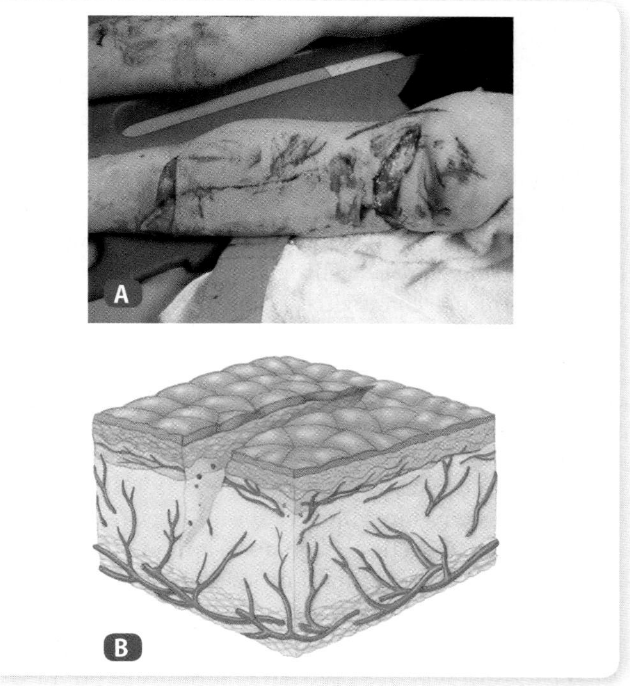

Figure 28-5 Lacerations vary in depth and can extend through the skin and subcutaneous tissue to the underlying muscles, nerves, and blood vessels. These wounds can be smooth or jagged as a result of a cut by a sharp object or a blunt force that tears the tissue. **(A)** shows laceration injuries; **(B)** illustrates the extent of damage possible.

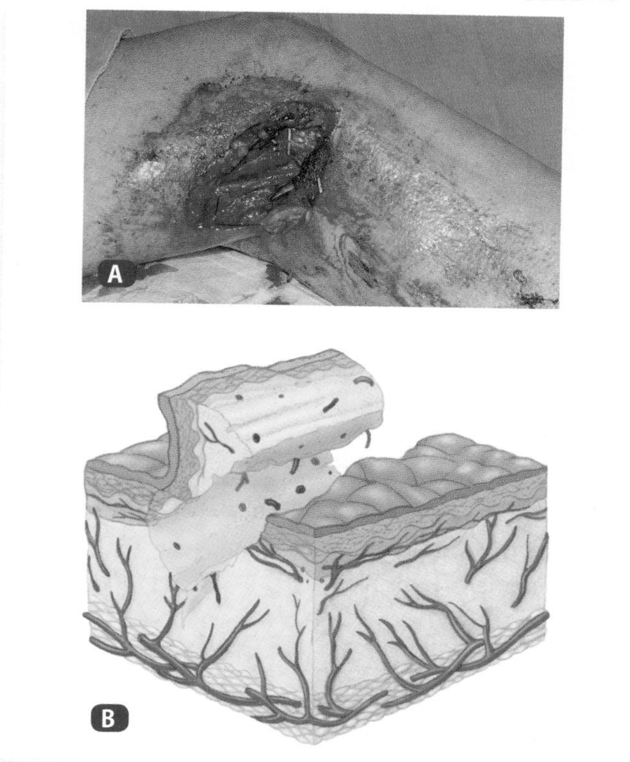

Figure 28-6 Avulsions are injuries characterized by incomplete separation of tissue with resultant flap formation. **(A)** is associated with gross contamination. **(B)** demonstrates how these injuries can be associated with substantial bleeding.

types of soft-tissue injuries. Lacerations or incisions that involve damaged arteries or veins may result in severe bleeding.

An **avulsion** is an injury that separates various layers of soft tissue (usually between the subcutaneous layer and fascia) so that they hang as a flap **Figure 28-6**. Often, there is substantial bleeding. A completely avulsed body part is considered an **amputation**. We usually think of amputations as involving the upper and lower extremities, but other body parts (eg, scalp, ear, nose, penis, and lips) may also be amputated.

Most people who are bitten by animals do not report the incident to a physician, believing that such bites are not serious. They can be very serious, however. Dogs' and cats' mouths are heavily contaminated with virulent bacteria. You should consider all such bites as contaminated and potentially infected wounds that may require antibiotics, tetanus prophylaxis, and suturing **Figure 28-7**. Occasionally, dog bites result in mangled, complex wounds that require surgical repair.

The human mouth, more so than even the dog's or cat's mouth, contains an exceptionally wide range of bacteria and viruses. For this reason, you should regard any human bite that has penetrated the skin as a serious injury. Similarly, any laceration caused by a human tooth can result in a serious, spreading infection **Figure 28-8**.

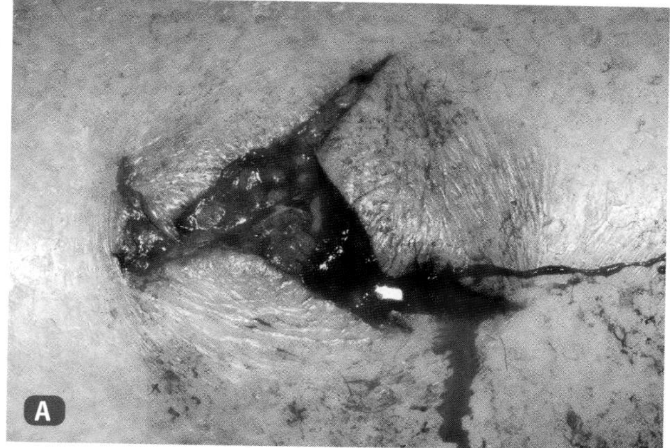

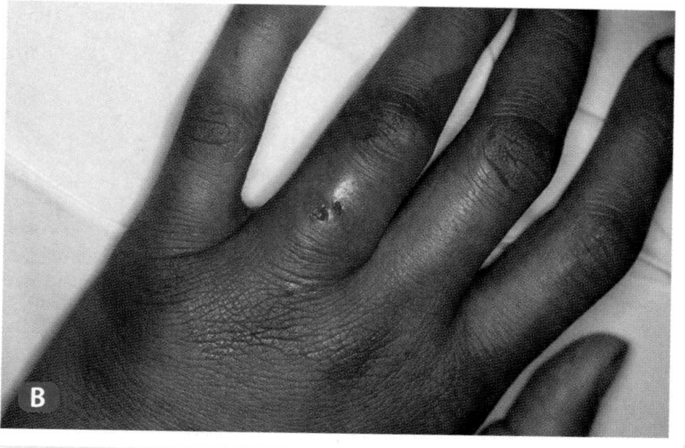

Figure 28-7 Small animal bite wounds should be examined at the hospital because these wounds are heavily contaminated with bacteria. **A.** Dog bite. **B.** Cat bite.

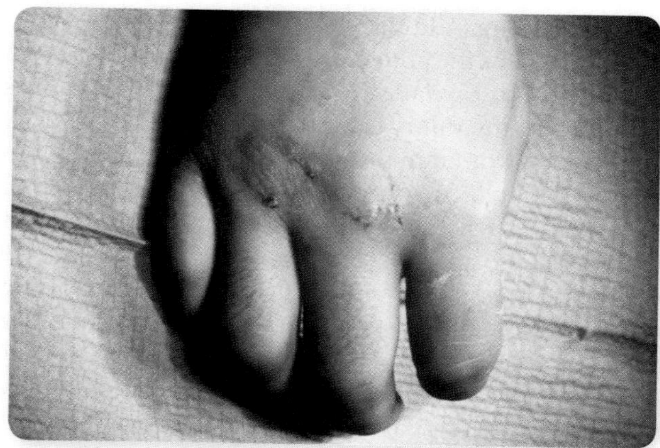

Figure 28-8 Human bites can result in infection that can spread rapidly. Patients with these injuries should be evaluated in the emergency department.

A **penetrating wound** (or puncture wound) is an injury resulting from a sharp, pointed object, such as a knife, ice pick, or splinter, or from a blunt object traveling at sufficiently high speed, such as a handgun bullet, stick, or metal rod. Objects that are small in diameter leave

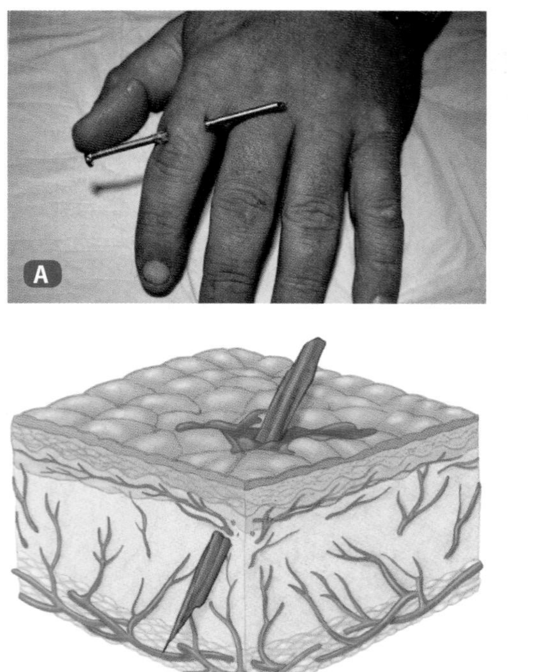

Figure 28-9 Penetrating wounds and impaled objects may cause very little external bleeding but can damage structures deep within the body. **(A)** shows a penetrating wound to the index finger. **(B)** illustrates the soft tissue structures impacted by an impaled object.

relatively small entrance wounds, so there may be little external bleeding Figure 28-9. However, these objects can damage structures deep within the body and cause unseen bleeding. Additionally, the velocity of the object greatly heightens the potential for increased tissue or organ damage due to cavitation. If the wound is to the chest or abdomen, the injury can cause rapid, fatal bleeding.

An open wound in the abdominal cavity may expose internal organs. In some cases, the organs may even protrude through the wound, an injury called an **evisceration** Figure 28-10. An open neck injury can also be life threatening; if the veins of the neck are open to the environment, they may suck in air, resulting in a condition known as **air embolism** Figure 28-11. If enough air is sucked into a blood vessel, it can actually block the flow of blood in the lungs and cause cardiac arrest.

As with closed wounds caused by crushing injuries, open wounds caused by crushing injuries may involve damaged internal organs or broken bones, as well as extensive soft-tissue damage Figure 28-12. Although external bleeding may be minimal, internal bleeding may be severe, even life threatening. The crushing force damages soft tissues, vessels, and nerves. This frequently results in a painful, swollen, deformed area.

Blast injuries, as discussed in Chapter 26, *Trauma Overview*, may also often result in multiple penetrating injuries. When a substance is detonated, a solid or liquid

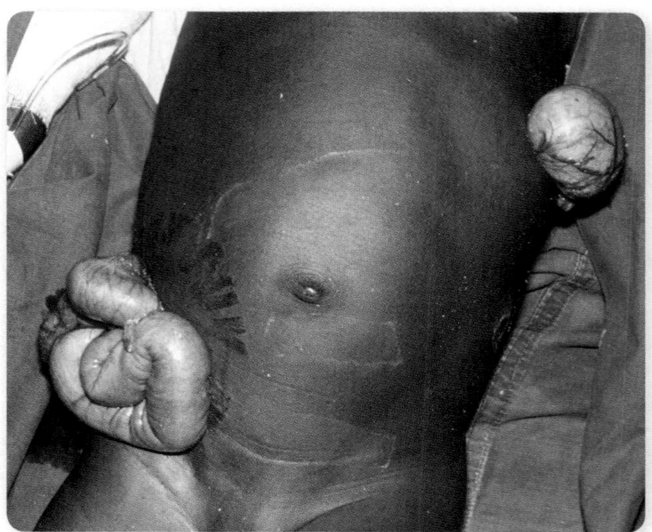

Figure 28-10 An abdominal evisceration is an open wound to the abdomen in which organs protrude through the wound.

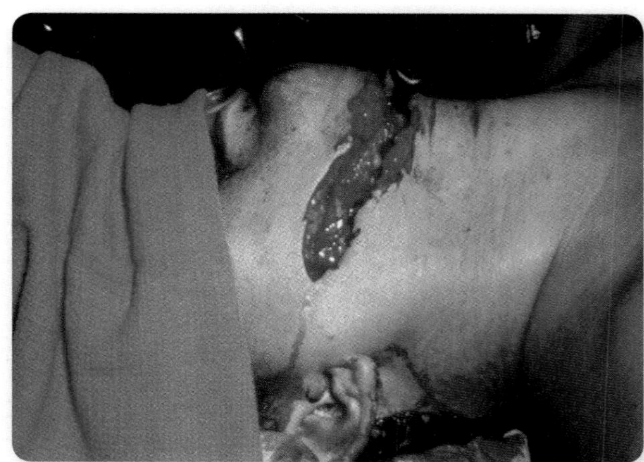

Figure 28-11 Open injuries to the neck can be very dangerous. If veins are open to the environment, they can suck in air, resulting in a potentially fatal condition called air embolism.

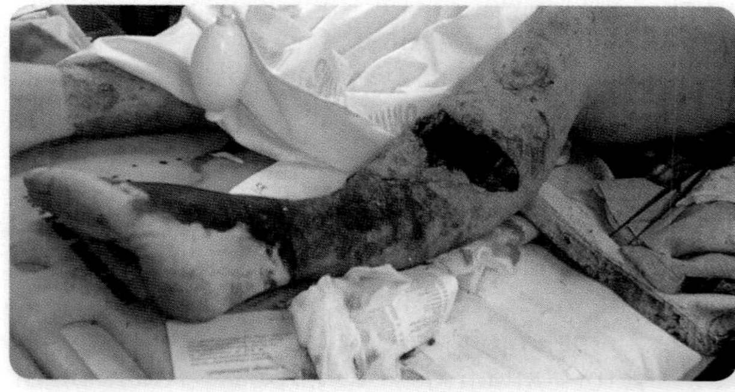

Figure 28-12 A crushing open wound is characterized by extensive tissue damage and deformity that is often accompanied by swelling and extreme pain.

is chemically converted into large volumes of gas under pressure with resultant energy release. Propellants, like gunpowder, are explosives designed to release energy relatively slowly compared with high explosives (for example, trinitrotoluene, or TNT), which are designed to detonate very quickly. Explosives such as composition C4 can create initial pressures of more than 4 million pounds per square inch. This generates a pressure pulse in the shape of a spherical blast wave that expands in all directions from the point of explosion. It is imperative for you to conduct a complete primary survey and secondary assessment to determine what type or types of injuries are sustained from a blast injury and treat appropriately.

Pathophysiology of Wound Healing

Infection

Because the skin serves as an initial barrier against microorganisms, any break in its surface can result in infection. Larger openings and deeper penetrations result in a higher level of risk for the development of an infection. Not only will there be a delay in healing from the infection, but additional complications or systemic infection can result.

Staphylococcus and *Streptococcus* bacteria account for most bacterial skin infections.[1] After pathogens have entered the body tissues, they begin to grow and multiply, although clinical signs of infection may not appear for several days. Visible clues of infection include erythema, pus, warmth, edema, and local discomfort. Red streaks adjacent to the wound indicate that the patient has developed *lymphangitis*, an inflammation of the lymph channels. More serious infections can cause systemic signs, such as fever, shaking, chills, joint pain, and hypotension.

Gangrene

Gangrene is dead tissue. It is caused when blood supply to tissue is interrupted or stopped. It can also be caused by infection and direct tissue injury. *Clostridium perfringens* is one example of an anaerobic, toxin-producing bacterium that can result in the development of gangrene. After it enters deeply into tissue, it produces a foul-smelling gas.

Diseases such as diabetes and atherosclerotic peripheral vascular disease can cause gangrene, but traumatic injuries such as burns, frostbite, and wounds can also cause it. Smokers and diabetics are more likely to develop symptoms because their peripheral vasculature is compromised.

Suspect gangrene if the patient has chronic risk factors such as diabetes and there is numbness, coolness, or swelling of an extremity. Gangrene may have a bad odor. Late signs of gangrene will be characterized by discoloration of the limb to black, blue, or red. If the gangrene is not treated, the skin will become necrotic and the infection may result in sepsis. Prompt recognition and early, aggressive hospital therapy offer the best chance for reducing morbidity and mortality.

Tetanus

Tetanus is caused by infection with an anaerobic bacterium, *Clostridium tetani* (a member of the same family that causes gangrene). This bacterium causes the body to produce a potent toxin, which results in painful muscle contractions that are strong enough to fracture bones.

Tetanus has become a rare occurrence because of the availability of a vaccine. In the United States, vaccination against tetanus is part of childhood immunization programs. A booster is needed every 10 years, although an inoculation is typically provided to patients who are injured and have not been immunized in the past 5 years. Given the severity of tetanus, you should ask injured patients about the last time they received a tetanus booster.

Muscle stiffness associated with tetanus may be noted first in the jaw ("lockjaw") and neck, with progression down the remainder of the body. Early recognition is important because conventional therapy does not result in rapid recovery.

Necrotizing Fasciitis

Fasciitis is inflammation of the fascia. The most serious form of this condition is called **necrotizing fasciitis**, "the flesh-eating disease," which involves the death of tissue from bacterial infection. Necrotizing fasciitis is caused by more than one infecting organism; often, group A streptococcus.

Look for a history of vector transmission, insect bites, or jelly fish stings. Skin at the site may be reddened and warm; additional symptoms include fever, night sweats, chills, vomiting, and diarrhea. It is important to take standard precautions and properly handle contaminated articles.

Assessment of Closed and Open Injuries

A physician should always evaluate certain wounds. The injuries in Table 28-1 require transport, even if they appear minor.

Assessing closed injuries is much more difficult than assessing open injuries. Therefore, any time you observe bruising, swelling, or deformity or the patient reports pain, the possibility of a substantial underlying injury should be considered.

Table 28-1 Conditions That Require Transport

- Compromise of:
  - Nerves
  - Vessels
  - Muscles
  - Tendons or ligaments
- Foreign body or cosmetic complications
- Heavy contamination

The assessment of an open injury is generally easier than the assessment of a closed injury because you can see the injury. Open wounds can be defined as injuries in which there is a break in the surface of the skin or the mucous membrane, exposing deeper tissues to potential contamination. You must use caution to avoid letting a patient's non–life-threatening gruesome injury distract you from recognizing another injury that is more life threatening.

Scene Size-up

As always, the first aspect to address in any scenario is safety. Ensure that you and your crew have addressed scene hazards and taken the necessary standard precautions—a minimum of gloves and eye protection. Open soft-tissue injuries can be messy. You can often identify patients with an open injury as you approach the scene; however, blood can be hidden under thick, dark clothing such as denim and leather or in the environment, such as sand, grass, or carpeting. Eye exposures may occur from splashes and droplets at a busy scene; eye protection is required when managing open injuries. Place several pairs of gloves in your pocket for easy access in case your gloves tear or there are multiple patients with bleeding. Determine the number of patients, and consider whether you need additional or specialized resources on the scene.

When evaluating the mechanism of injury (MOI), maintain a high index of suspicion for internal injuries whenever a significant MOI is present, even if external injuries appear minor. Carefully consider the forces involved as you determine the likelihood of internal damage.

Determine how many patients are involved. Diligently search for ejected patients in the case of a substantial vehicle crash, especially with rollovers.

Primary Survey

When serious trauma is present, soft-tissue injuries take a lower priority than airway control, and breathing inadequacy unless they are associated with exsanguinating hemorrhage. *Do not let soft-tissue injuries distract you from life threats that may not be readily apparent.* Rapidly determine whether threats to life are present using the XABCDE mnemonic (eXsanguinating hemorrhage, Airway, Breathing, Circulation, Disability, and Exposure). Note your general impression as you approach the patient.

If visible substantial bleeding is seen, control it quickly using appropriate methods. After you consider the MOI and form suspicions as to where bleeding may occur, expose that part of the body and treat life-threatening bleeding there as well. Patients with visible substantial bleeding or signs of substantial internal bleeding may quickly become unstable. Treatment must be directed at quickly addressing life threats and providing rapid transportation to the closest appropriate hospital.

As you begin airway assessment, perform manual immobilization if you suspect spinal injury. Check for responsiveness using the AVPU (Awake and alert, responsive to Verbal stimuli, responsive to Pain, Unresponsive) scale. Administer high-flow oxygen as needed to maintain oxygen saturation (Spo_2) at 95% or higher. Soft-tissue injuries that result in a flow of blood into the airway can also prove extremely challenging; suction as needed. Immediately correct anything that interferes with airway patency; failure to provide a patent airway can quickly result in the patient's death. Call early for paramedic assistance.

Assess the patient's breathing. Provide oxygen via nonrebreathing mask at 15 L/min or a bag-mask device and supplementary oxygen for those with inadequate oxygenation or ventilations.

Assess the circulatory status. If no pulse is present, take resuscitative measures. Closed soft-tissue injuries may not always have visible signs of bleeding, and shock may be present. Your assessment of the pulse and skin will indicate how aggressively you need to treat your patient for shock.

If substantial trauma has likely affected multiple systems, perform the 60- to 90-second rapid full-body scan to be sure that you have identified all problems and injuries. When you are done, apply a cervical collar if it is indicated.

Determine whether your patient needs immediate transport or stabilization on scene. Consider whether transport to the closest hospital is appropriate or whether the patient would be better served by transport to a trauma center that might be farther away. Reassess your priority and transport decision as needed.

History Taking

Gather information to determine how the patient was injured.

When time and patient condition permit, determine when the last tetanus booster was given. Record the information on the patient care report, and relay it during patient transfer at the hospital.

Make every attempt to obtain a SAMPLE history (Signs and symptoms, Allergies, Medications, Pertinent past medical history, Last oral intake, Events leading up to the illness or injury) from your patient. Using OPQRST (Onset, Provocation or palliation, Quality, Radiation, Severity, Time of onset) may provide some background on isolated extremity injuries. Any information you receive will be valuable if the patient becomes unresponsive.

Words of Wisdom

Patients with soft-tissue injuries will need emotional care. Patients will likely have concerns about how bruising and scarring may look later. Provide psychological support.

Ask the patient about prescribed and over-the-counter medications, paying particular attention to those that interfere with hemostasis. A higher priority should be given to patients taking warfarin or other anticoagulants.

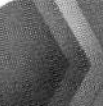

Secondary Assessment

If time allows, perform the secondary assessment to reveal injuries or medical conditions that may have been missed during the primary survey. You may need to perform it en route to the emergency department (ED).

Patients who have hidden internal injuries under a closed soft-tissue injury may have internal bleeding, and their condition may rapidly become unstable. It is important to reassess the vital signs to identify how quickly a patient's condition is changing. Signs such as tachycardia, tachypnea, low blood pressure, weak pulse, and cool, moist, and pale skin indicate hypoperfusion and imply the need for rapid transport and treatment at the hospital. Remember that soft-tissue injuries, even without a significant MOI, can cause shock. The reassessment of your patient's vital signs will give you a good understanding of how well or how poorly your patient is tolerating the injury and whether your interventions have been effective. Use monitoring devices to quantify your patient's oxygenation and circulatory status as needed.

Reassessment

Frequent reassessments of the patient's condition should be made en route to the hospital and in conjunction with any necessary interventions. A patient in stable condition should be reassessed every 15 minutes; a more serious condition warrants reexamination every 5 minutes. Reassessment includes taking and evaluating additional sets of vital signs, checking interventions, and monitoring the patient's condition.

Reassess the airway, breathing, and circulation. Are your interventions still effective? Reassessing a patient with an open soft-tissue injury is extremely important, especially if you did not personally put the bandage on the patient's injury. Frequently, other emergency care personnel may have dressed and bandaged the wound before your arrival. You may need to place additional dressings over the original dressing or bandages. Assess all bandaging frequently. If blood continues to soak through bandages, use additional methods to control bleeding. Identify and treat changes in the patient's condition.

In your communication and documentation, include a description of the MOI, the position in which you found the patient when you arrived on scene, and an estimate of the amount of blood lost. Include the location and description of any soft-tissue injuries or other wounds you have located and treated, including the size and depth

YOU are the Provider — PART 2

You quickly remove the patient's smoldering clothing to minimize the burning process, while your partner contacts dispatch and requests a paramedic intercept. By using the rule of nines, you are able to determine that the patient has severe burns over approximately 55% of his body surface area (BSA). The patient is conscious, alert, and oriented, reporting severe pain (10 on a 10-point scale) throughout his body. He denies any loss of consciousness, just requesting something for the pain. Your partner contacts dispatch again to get an estimated time of arrival of paramedics but is told that none are available.

Recording Time: 1 Minute	
Appearance	Anxious
Level of consciousness	Alert and oriented to person, place, time, and event
Airway	Patent; no stridor
Breathing	Nonlabored; 28 breaths/min
Circulation	Strong, rapid radial pulses; skin warm, dry, and pink

3. What immediate treatment is required for this patient?
4. Because this patient is complaining of pain, should you apply moist dressings to cool the burned area?

of the injuries. Provide an accurate account of how you treated these injuries. Your ability to communicate and document clearly and accurately enables the physicians and nurses at the hospital to continue quality care.

Emergency Medical Care of Closed and Open Injuries

Closed Injuries

Small contusions require no special emergency medical care. More extensive closed injuries may involve substantial swelling and bleeding beneath the skin, which could result in hypovolemic shock and be life threatening if not appropriately treated.

Severe closed injuries can also damage internal organs. The greater the amount of energy absorbed from the blunt force, the greater the risk of injury to deeper structures. Assess and manage all threats to the ABCs, and be sure to assess all patients with closed injuries for more serious hidden injuries. Remain alert for signs of shock or internal bleeding, and begin treatment of these conditions if necessary, including appropriate oxygen therapy.

Treat a closed soft-tissue injury by applying the mnemonic RICES:

- **Rest.** Help the patient rest by keeping him or her as quiet and comfortable as possible. This helps prevent pain and reduce bleeding.
- **Ice.** Apply ice or cold packs to the injured area. Cold slows bleeding by causing blood vessels to constrict, and it also reduces pain.
- **Compression.** Apply firm compression over the injured area; this compresses the blood vessels, decreasing bleeding. Compression may be manual initially but is most effectively applied with an air splint thereafter.
- **Elevate.** Elevate the injured part to a level above the heart to encourage drainage and decrease swelling.
- **Splint.** Apply a splint to an injured extremity. By preventing motion, a splint decreases bleeding. It also reduces pain by immobilizing a soft-tissue injury or an injured extremity. Splinting a fracture helps prevent ongoing soft-tissue injury associated with unstable sharp bone ends. An air splint provides a double benefit—splinting and compression, although an air splint will not control arterial bleeding.

Extremities that are painful, swollen, or deformed should be splinted. When splinting these types of injuries, remember to assess the patient's pulses and motor and sensory function before and after applying the splint. Do not forget to document the presence or absence of pulses and any changes.

In addition to using these measures to control bleeding and swelling, you should also be alert for signs of developing shock, including tachycardia, tachypnea, cool and/or clammy skin, and a later sign, hypotension. If the patient shows signs of shock, place the patient supine, initiate IV therapy, give high-flow oxygen, and provide prompt transport to the hospital.

Open Injuries

Although most open soft-tissue injuries are not serious, if not appropriately treated, many can result in substantial blood loss and even shock. By appropriately treating open soft-tissue injuries, you can minimize the common complications such as bleeding, shock, pain, and infection.

As discussed in Chapter 26, *Trauma Overview*, take standard precautions, and address life-threatening bleeding and then airway and breathing concerns. Then assess the severity of the wound. If the wound is in the chest, upper abdomen, or upper back, cover it with an **occlusive dressing**. Properly position the patient using cervical spine protection, if indicated, and cover the patient to maintain warmth.

As discussed in Chapter 27, *Bleeding*, several methods are available to control bleeding from open injuries. Start with the most commonly used; these methods include the following:

- Direct, even pressure
- Pressure dressings and/or splints
- Tourniquets

It will often be useful to combine these methods.

All open wounds are assumed to be contaminated and present a risk of infection. Although it is not always possible to use a sterile technique, you should make every effort to avoid further wound contamination. Depending on local protocol, irrigate open wounds with normal saline or sterile water to flush out gross contaminants. Chemical burns and contamination should be flushed to remove remaining chemicals. After the wound is irrigated, apply a dressing over the site. This keeps foreign material, such as hair, clothing, and dirt, out of the wound and decreases the risk of infection. To prevent the wound from drying, you may apply sterile dressings moistened with sterile saline solution, if possible, and then cover the moist dressing with a dry, sterile dressing. Finally, neatly wrap a bandage over the dressing

As with closed injuries, splinting can help control bleeding from open soft-tissue injuries as well. Splinting is covered in detail in Chapter 33, *Orthopaedic Injuries*.

Words of Wisdom

Keep in mind that a patient who is bleeding substantially from an open wound is at risk for hypovolemic shock. Be alert for this potential, and treat aggressively to reduce the risk.

▶ Dressing and Bandaging

Dressing and bandaging materials are used to cover wounds, control bleeding, and limit motion. A dressing directly covers a wound and controls bleeding, whereas a bandage keeps the dressing in place.

All wounds require dressing and bandaging. In general, dressings and bandages have three primary functions:

- To control bleeding
- To protect the wound from further damage
- To prevent further contamination and infection

There are many types of dressings and bandages Figure 28-13. You should be familiar with the function and proper application of each.

Sterile Dressings

Universal dressings, conventional 4- × 4-inch and 4- × 8-inch gauze pads, and assorted small adhesive-type dressings and soft self-adherent roller dressings are types of dressings and are used to cover most wounds. Measuring 9 × 36 inches and made of thick, absorbent material, the universal dressing is ideal for covering large open wounds. It also makes an efficient pad for rigid splints. These dressings are available in compact, commercially sterilized packages.

Gauze pads are appropriate for smaller wounds, and adhesive-type dressings are useful for minor wounds. Occlusive dressings (made of petroleum [Vaseline] gauze, aluminum foil, or plastic) prevent air and liquids from entering (or exiting) the wound. They are used to cover open chest wounds, abdominal eviscerations and penetrating wounds above the umbilicus, penetrating back wounds, and open neck injuries.

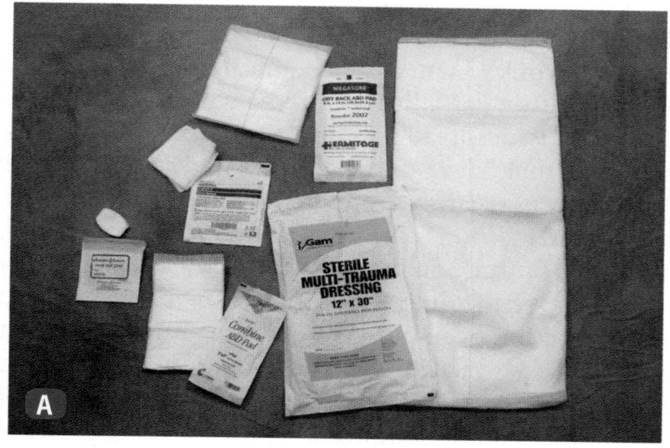

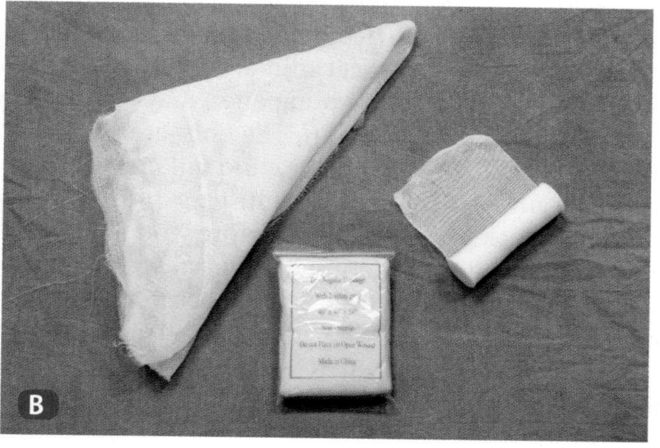

Figure 28-13 A. Many types of sterile dressings are used for covering open wounds, including universal dressings, gauze pads, adhesive dressings, and occlusive dressings. **B.** Bandages keep dressings in place and include soft roller bandages, triangular bandages, and adhesive tape. Splints may also be used to hold dressings in place.

Words of Wisdom

An occlusive dressing may be made from any material that is nonporous and airtight. For example, plastic wrap from other supplies, the foil wrapper from Vaseline gauze, and defibrillation/pacer pads can be used.

Bandages

To keep dressings in place during transport, you can use soft roller bandages, rolls of gauze, triangular bandages, or adhesive tape. Self-adherent, soft roller bandages are probably the easiest to use. They are slightly elastic, which makes them easy to apply, and you can tuck the end of the roll into a deeper layer to secure it in place. The layers adhere somewhat but should not be applied too tightly to one another.

Adhesive tape holds small dressings in place and helps to secure larger dressings. If you have a patient who has a known allergy to adhesive tape, use paper or plastic tape instead.

As discussed in Chapter 27, *Bleeding*, if an extremity wound continues to bleed despite the use of direct pressure, quickly proceed to using a tourniquet.

Complications of Improperly Applied Dressings

Improper application of dressing and bandage material can result in substantial complications. It is important for you to learn how to properly dress a wound in the laboratory, clinical, and field settings to avoid causing harm.

Hemodynamic complications include the possibility for continued bleeding. After a dressing has been placed, it should not be removed because of the risk of disrupting clot formation. If an extremity wound continues to bleed, consider the use of a tourniquet. Frequent reassessments will help prevent unchecked blood loss and hemodynamic complications. Exsanguination is a possibility when direct pressure does not stop blood loss; the same is true for an improperly applied tourniquet. If a tourniquet occludes only venous flow, bleeding may actually increase. Direct pressure is often sufficient to stop blood loss; if not, do not hesitate to apply a tourniquet to an extremity to achieve bleeding control.

Any improperly applied bandage that impairs circulation can result in additional tissue damage or even the loss of a limb. Also, tight dressings may cause pain in a patient who already has an injury. Reassess all interventions frequently. Always check the limb distal to a bandage for signs of impaired circulation or loss of sensation before, during, and after application of the bandage and frequently during transport.

► Management of Specific Wounds

Avulsion

If avulsed tissue is hanging from a small piece of skin, the circulation through the flap may be at risk. If you can, replace the avulsed flap in its original position. If an avulsion is complete, wrap the separated tissue in sterile gauze, and take it with you to the ED. This type of avulsion often presents serious infection concerns. Never remove a skin flap from an avulsion, regardless of its size.

Amputation

You can easily control the bleeding from some amputations, such as the fingers, with direct pressure and pressure dressings. If an amputation involves a large area of muscle mass, such as a thigh, there may be massive bleeding. In this situation, you should stop the bleeding, which often requires a tourniquet, and treat the patient for hypovolemic shock. Use the methods described Chapter 27, *Bleeding*.

Surgeons today can often reattach an amputated part **Figure 28-14**. However, correct prehospital care of the amputated part is vital to successful reattachment. With partial amputations, make sure to immobilize the part with bulky compression dressings and a splint to prevent further injury. Do not detach any partial amputations because this may make it impossible to reattach the part.

See Chapter 33, *Orthopaedic Injuries*, for a discussion of complete amputations and their prehospital treatment.

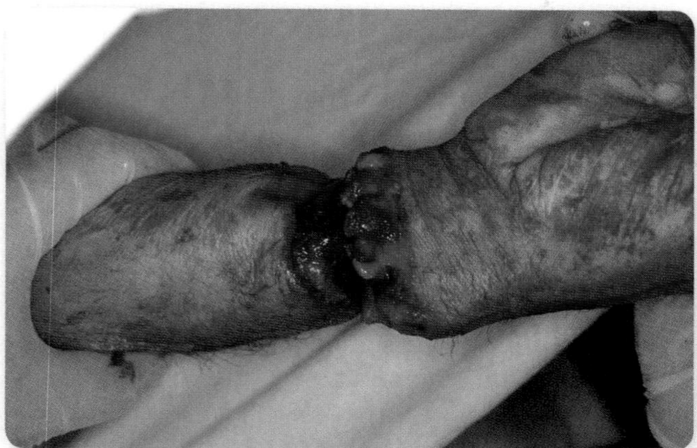

Figure 28-14 Amputated parts can often be reattached, so you should make every attempt to find the part and transport it to the emergency department along with the patient.

Words of Wisdom

Never place an amputated part directly on ice because this may cause frostbite and make reattachment impossible.

Bite Wounds

In the case of an animal bite, place a dry, sterile dressing over the wound, and promptly transport the patient to the ED. If there is gross contamination, consider irrigation of the wound with sterile water prior to dressing. If an arm or leg was injured, splint that extremity. Often, the patient will be extremely upset and frightened, a situation that calls for calm reassurance on your part.

A major concern with small animal bites is the spread of rabies, an acute, potentially fatal viral infection of the central nervous system that can affect all warm-blooded animals. Although rabies is extremely rare today, particularly with widespread inoculation of pets, it still exists. Stray dogs that have not been inoculated can be carriers of the disease, as can any mammal—squirrels, bats, foxes, skunks, and raccoons. The virus is in the saliva of a **rabid**, or infected, animal and is transmitted through biting or licking an open wound. Infection can be prevented in a person who has been bitten by such an animal only by a series of special vaccine injections that must be initiated soon after the bite. Since animals that have rabies do not always demonstrate symptoms immediately, a person's only chance to avoid the vaccine is to find the animal and turn it over to the health department for observation and/or testing. Refer to your local animal control procedures.

Children, particularly young ones, may be seriously injured or even killed by dogs. The dogs are not always vicious or rabid; sometimes, the child unknowingly provoked the animal. However, you must assume that it may turn and attack you as well. Therefore, you should not enter the scene until the animal has been secured by the police or an animal control officer. Then you may carry out the necessary emergency care and transport the child to the ED. AEMTs are required by law to report all animal bites to the appropriate authority, which is typically the ED physician.

The emergency treatment for bites, including animal and human bites, consists of the following steps:

1. Promptly control all bleeding, and apply a dry, sterile dressing.
2. Immobilize the area with a splint or bandage.
3. Provide transport to the ED for surgical cleansing of the wound and antibiotic therapy.

The AEMT is required by law to report all bites to local authorities. Follow local protocols for reporting requirements.

Penetrating Wounds

Assessing the amount of damage a puncture wound has created is difficult and should be reserved for the physician at the hospital. However, because stabbings and shootings often result in multiple penetrating injuries, you must assess patients carefully to identify all wounds. A penetrating object can pass completely through the body; therefore, you should always count the number of penetrating injuries (or holes), especially with gunshot wounds. Entrance wounds and exit wounds are difficult to distinguish in a prehospital setting, especially with the different types of ammunition available. Although entrance wounds are often smaller than exit wounds, it is better to count the number of wounds and leave the distinction between entrance and exit wounds to hospital staff Figure 28-15. However, if an entry wound or single open wound is found, look for other wounds.

Gunshot wounds have some unique characteristics that require special care. The amount of damage from a gunshot wound is directly related to the size, shape, and speed of the bullet. Thus, it is important to find out the caliber of gun that was used in the shooting, but do not let this delay patient transport. Sometimes the patient or bystanders can tell you how many rounds were fired. This information can help hospital personnel to better care for the patient. Shotgun wounds create multiple pathways of injury and create a larger surface area and volume of tissue damage. However, you should not waste valuable time trying to determine the caliber of weapon. Patient care is the first priority.

Abdominal Wounds

If internal organs are protruding through an open wound, do not touch or move the exposed organs. Cover the wound with sterile gauze compresses moistened with sterile saline solution, and secure the moist compresses in place with an occlusive dressing Figure 28-16. Because the open abdomen radiates body heat effectively and because exposed organs lose fluid rapidly, you must keep the organs moist and warm. If you do not have gauze compresses, you may use moist sterile dressings, covered and secured in place with a dry bandage and tape. Do not use any material that is adherent or loses its substance when wet, such as toilet paper, facial tissue, paper towels, or absorbent cotton. If the patient's legs and knees are uninjured, flex them to relieve pressure on the abdomen. Most patients with abdominal wounds require immediate transport to a trauma center, depending on the local protocol.

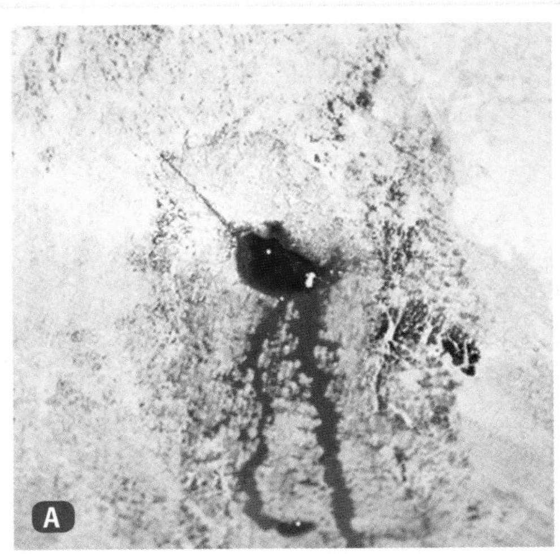

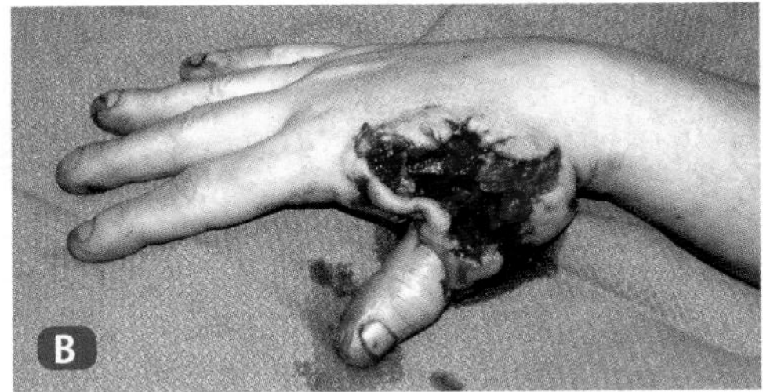

Figure 28-15 A. An entrance wound from a gunshot may have burns around the edges if the injury occurred at close range. **B.** An exit wound is often larger than an entrance wound and is associated with greater damage to surrounding skin.

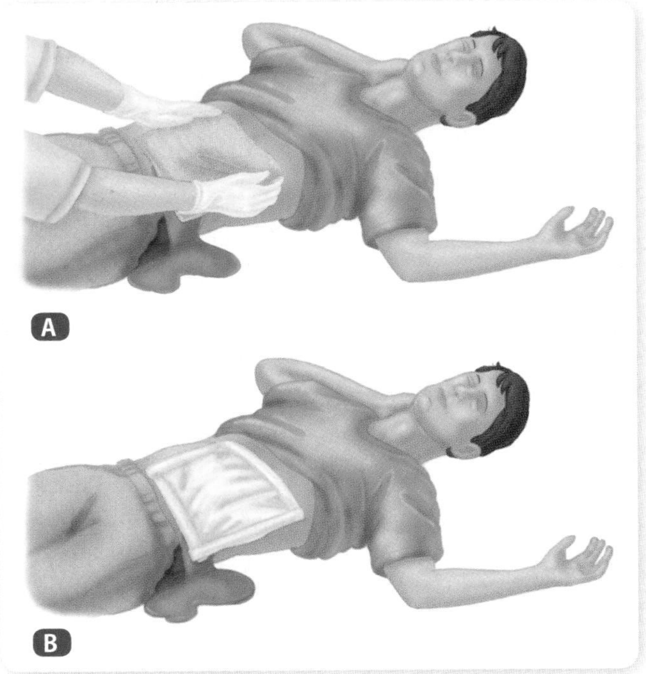

Figure 28-16 A. Cover exposed organs with sterile gauze compresses moistened with sterile saline solution. **B.** Place an occlusive dressing over the compresses, and secure it in place by taping all four sides.

Words of Wisdom

A good rule to remember is that anything normally found inside the body needs to be kept moist. Cover eviscerations with moist, sterile dressings.

Impaled Object

Occasionally, a patient will have an object, such as a knife, fishhook, wood splinter, or piece of glass, impaled in his or her body. To treat this, follow the steps in Skill Drill 28-1.

If the object is very long, cut off (shorten) the exposed portion, first securing it to minimize motion and thus internal damage and pain. After the object is secured and the bleeding is under control, provide prompt transport. Do not try to shorten an impaled object unless it is extremely cumbersome (such as a fence post impaled in the chest); any motion of the object may damage surrounding tissues.

Words of Wisdom

There are only two exceptions to the rule of not removing an impaled object: if the object is through the cheek and interferes with the airway and if the object is in the chest and interferes with chest compressions.

Skill Drill 28-1 Stabilizing an Impaled Object

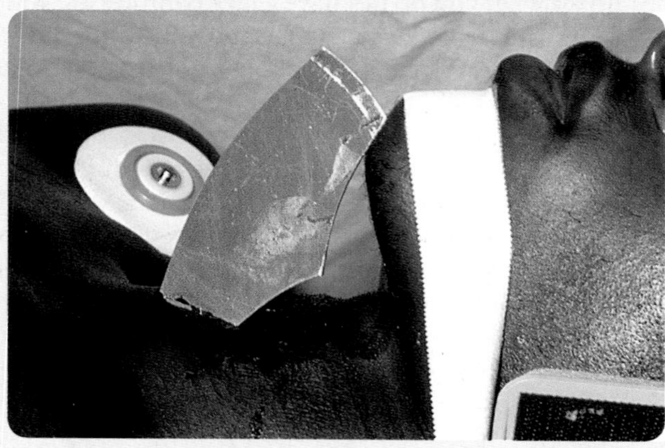

Step 1 Do not attempt to move or remove the object unless it is impaled through the cheek or mouth causing airway obstruction, or if the object is in the chest, or if the patient is pulseless and you must remove it to perform cardiopulmonary resuscitation (CPR). In most cases, a surgeon will have to remove the object; removing it in the field may cause more bleeding or damage nerves, blood vessels, or muscles within the wound. Stabilize the object in place using soft dressings, gauze, and/or tape.

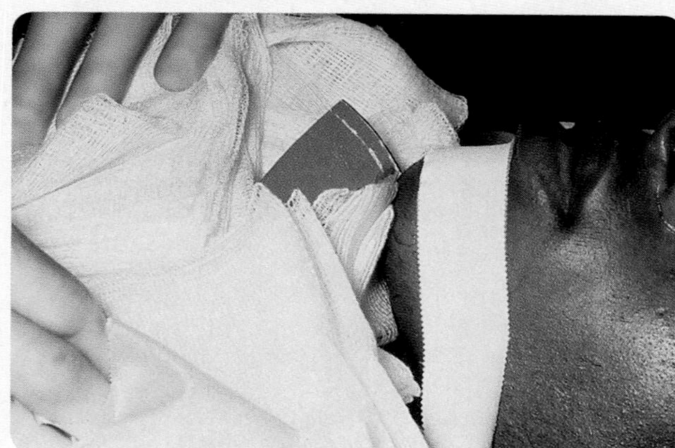

Step 2 Remove any clothing covering the injury. Control bleeding with direct pressure, and apply a bulky dressing to stabilize the object. Some combination of soft dressings, gauze, and tape may be effective, depending on the location and size of the object. To prevent further injury, manually secure the object by incorporating it into the dressing.

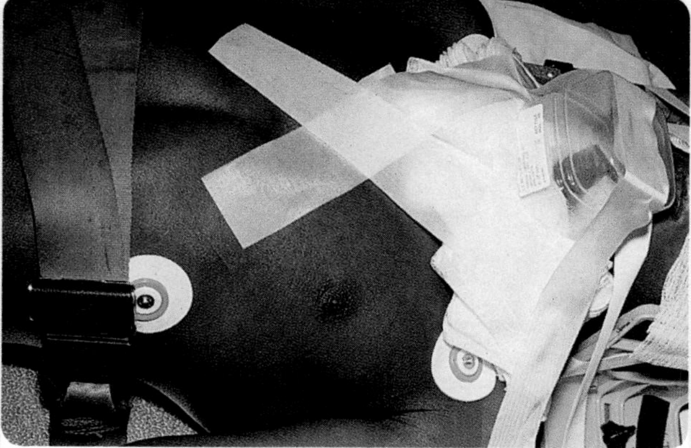

Step 3 Protect the impaled object from being bumped or moved during transport by taping a rigid item such as a plastic cup, a section of a plastic water bottle, or a supply container over the stabilized object and its bandaging.

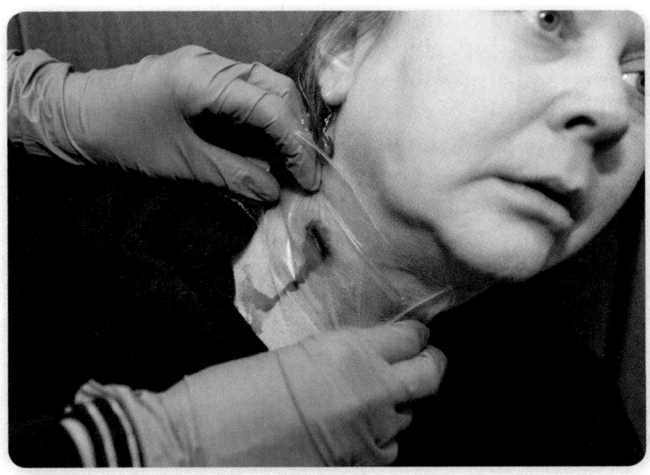

Figure 28-17 Cover neck wounds with an airtight dressing, and apply manual pressure. Do not compress both carotid arteries at the same time because this may impair circulation to the brain.

Open Neck Wounds

An open neck injury can be life threatening. If the veins of the neck are open to the environment, they may suck in air, potentially causing an air embolism and cardiac arrest. To control bleeding and prevent the possibility of an air embolism, cover the wound with an occlusive dressing. Apply manual pressure, but do not compress both carotid arteries at the same time; if you do, circulation to the brain will be impaired Figure 28-17. Secure a pressure dressing over the wound by wrapping roller gauze loosely around the neck and then firmly through the opposite axilla.

Burns

Each year in the United States, approximately 450,000 burn injuries require medical attention, and there are 3,400 fire/burn/smoke inhalation deaths.[2] Burns are also among the most serious and painful of all injuries. A burn occurs when the body, or a body part, receives more thermal, electrical, or chemical energy or is exposed to more radiation than it can absorb without injury.

▶ Pathophysiology

Burns are sometimes not simply isolated soft-tissue injuries but also systemic injuries. Initially, there is a release of catecholamines (epinephrine and norepinephrine) in response to the pain and stress of the situation. Because of overall vasoconstriction, there is a decrease in blood flow to the injured area. During the next several hours, there follows a fluid shift phase that is usually not seen in the prehospital setting. Damaged cells in the area release vasoactive substances, creating an inflammatory response and increasing capillary permeability. Massive edema is the result of fluid shifting from the intravascular space into the extravascular space. Sodium moves into the injured cells, creating even more fluid loss as osmotic pressure increases. This also causes a loss of electrolytes and may result in hypovolemia.

Tissue damage reduces the ability of the body to regulate its core temperature. Fluid seeps into the damaged area where it is exposed to surface air, causing evaporation and loss of heat. In severe burns, this can rapidly result in hypothermia.

As fluid volume decreases, less oxygen is transported to the tissues and organs, resulting in hypoxia, acidosis, and possibly anoxia. Hypovolemia causes a decrease in cardiac output, resulting in hypotension. To maintain homeostasis, the body responds with vasoconstriction in an effort to elevate blood pressure and increase perfusion to vital organs and with tachypnea to offset the metabolic acidosis and hypoxia. The burn process may result in renal failure, liver failure, dysrhythmias, and heart failure.

As the burn destroys skin, a tough leathery substance known as **eschar** is produced. Eschar is not pliable like normal skin. As edema increases, pressure is exerted on the underlying structures. A circumferential eschar around an extremity can cause circulatory compromise and may require an escharotomy—a surgical incision to relieve the pressure and restore circulation—after the patient arrives at the ED. A circumferential burn may result in compartment syndrome. The skin is unable to stretch, resulting in eventual compression and decreased or absent circulation in the tissues below. If the burn is around the thorax, tidal volume and chest excursion may be dramatically reduced by the eschar formation, resulting in ventilatory insufficiency.

▶ Hypovolemic Shock

Burns can affect the cardiovascular, respiratory, renal, gastrointestinal, hematologic, and endocrine systems. The most important systemic response to substantial burn trauma is hypovolemic shock.

Hypovolemic shock occurs because of two types of injuries: fluid loss across damaged skin and a series of volume shifts within the rest of the body. Capillaries become leaky, allowing intravascular volume to ooze out of the circulation and into the interstitial spaces. The cells of normal tissues then take in increased amounts of salt and water from the fluid around them. As blood pressure decreases, the body responds with tachycardia and vasoconstriction, which limits blood flow further and continues the shock cycle. A variety of chemical mediators are released that may cause additional damage and worsen the chain of events. Depending on the nature of the burn, coagulation disorders may cause the patient's blood either to clot more easily, resulting in emboli, or to fail to clot, causing excessive bleeding (disseminated intravascular coagulation), as discussed in Chapter 21, *Endocrine and Hematologic Emergencies*.

Hypovolemic shock involves the entire body, not just the area burned. You may have experienced sunburn over a reasonably large surface area, such as your back. In addition to the skin-related discomfort from the sunburn, you may have developed chills and nausea and felt sick as a result of the fluid shifts and electrolyte disturbances. This reaction is a mild form of burn shock. Just as in other forms of shock, these changes limit the effective distribution of oxygen and glucose to the body's tissues and hamper the circulation's ability to remove waste products from both healthy and damaged tissues. Adequate fluid resuscitation is essential to avoid the devastating consequences of burn shock.

▶ Complications of Burns

There are several complications that can result from a burn injury, all of which can be life threatening. The skin serves as a barrier between the environment and the body. When a person is burned, this barrier is destroyed; the victim is now at a high risk for infection, hypothermia, hypovolemia, and shock. Burns to the airway are of substantial importance because the loose mucosa in the hypopharynx can swell and rapidly result in complete airway obstruction. Circumferential burns of the chest can compromise breathing. Circumferential burns of an extremity can result in compartment syndrome, resulting in neurovascular compromise and irreversible damage if not appropriately treated. If you suspect any complications, consider calling for paramedic backup.

▶ Burn Zones

Historically, burn wounds have been described by three pathologic progressions, known as zones, which radiate from the central zone of greatest damage. Skin nearest the heat source suffers the most profound cellular changes. The central area of the skin that suffers the most damage is called the zone of coagulation. There is little or no blood flow to the injured tissue in this area. The peripheral area surrounding the **zone of coagulation** has decreased blood flow and inflammation; it is known as the **zone of stasis**. This area may undergo tissue necrosis within 24 to 48 hours after the injury, particularly if perfusion is compromised by burn shock. Last, the **zone of hyperemia** is the area least affected by the thermal injury. In this area, cells will typically recover in 7 to 10 days. Similar to the case with a myocardial infarction or stroke, the role of treatment is to salvage as much of the injured tissue as possible by improving perfusion and limiting the secondary changes that turn damaged tissue into dead tissue.

▶ Burn Depth

Burn formation is a progressive process: the greater the heat energy, the deeper the wound. Superficial burns may injure only the epidermis, whereas deeper burns extend into or through the dermis, subcutaneous tissue, muscle, and bone.

While evaluating the patient's burns, you must approximate the extent of the burn, or the total body surface area (TBSA) burned. The severity of burns is classified according to the depth—that is, superficial (first degree), partial thickness (second degree), and full thickness (third degree) **Figure 28-18**. You must be able to identify these:

- **Superficial burns** (first degree) involve only the top layer of skin, the epidermis. The skin turns

YOU are the Provider — PART 3

You explain to the patient that the paramedics are unavailable. You reassure him that you are doing the best you can and will get him to the hospital as quickly as possible. You and your partner lift the patient to the stretcher and secure him into the back of the ambulance. While your partner obtains vital signs and gives the patient 100% oxygen via nonrebreathing mask, you attempt to establish IV access.

Recording Time: 8 Minutes	
Respirations	Normal; 26 breaths/min
Pulse	Strong and rapid; 137 beats/min
Skin	Warm, dry, and pink
Blood pressure	102/64 mm Hg
Oxygen saturation (Spo_2)	100% oxygen via nonrebreathing mask at 15 L/min
Pupils	Pupils Equal, Round, and Reactive to Light (PERRL)

5. Should you attempt IV access through the burned area?
6. How would you calculate the amount of fluid the patient requires?

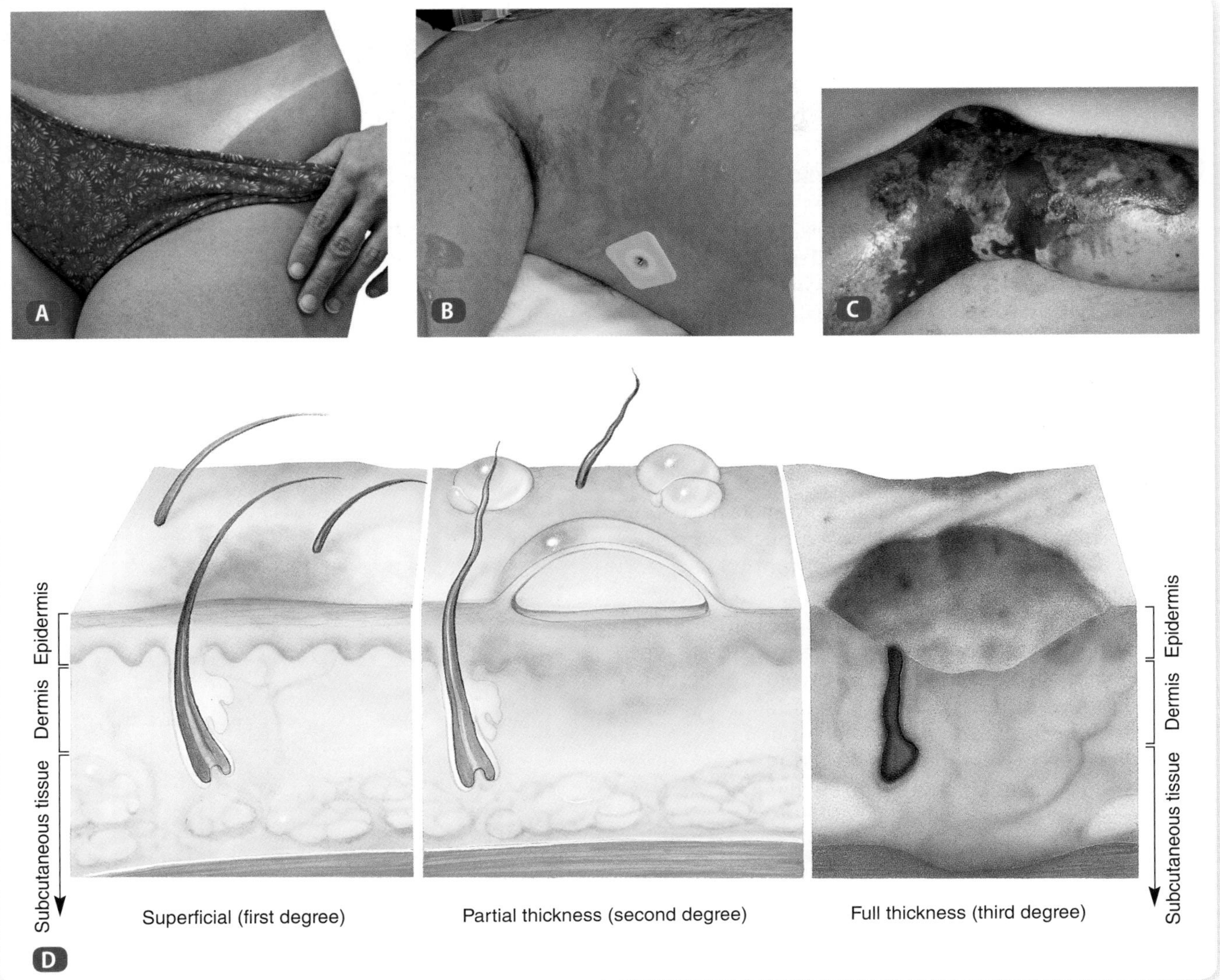

Figure 28-18 Classification of burns according to depth. **A.** Superficial, or first-degree, burns involve only the epidermis. The skin turns red but does not blister or actually burn through to the dermis. **B.** Partial-thickness, or second-degree, burns involve some of the dermis, but they do not destroy the entire thickness of the skin. The skin is mottled, white to red, and often blistered. **C.** Full-thickness, or third-degree, burns extend through all layers of the skin and may involve subcutaneous tissue and muscle. The skin is dry, leathery, and often white or charred. **D.** Illustrations of superficial, partial-thickness, and full-thickness burns, showing the extent of internal damage.

red but does not blister or actually burn through to the dermis. The burn site is painful. Sunburn is a good example of a superficial burn.

- **Partial-thickness burns** (second degree) involve the epidermis and some portion of the dermis. These burns do not destroy the entire thickness of the skin, and the subcutaneous tissue is not injured. Typically, the skin is moist, mottled, and white to red. Blisters are common. Partial-thickness burns cause intense pain.
- **Full-thickness burns** (third degree) extend through all skin layers and may involve subcutaneous layers, muscle, bone, and internal organs. The burned area is dry and leathery and may appear white, dark brown, or even charred. This rough area is known as eschar. Some full-thickness burns feel hard to the touch. Clotted blood vessels or subcutaneous tissue may be visible under the burned skin. If the nerve endings have been destroyed, a severely burned area may have no feeling. However, the surrounding, less severely burned areas may be extremely painful.

Words of Wisdom

Suspect substantial airway burns if there is singed hair within the nostrils, soot around the nose and mouth, hoarseness, or hypoxia.

Additional categories of burns exist, such as fourth-, fifth-, and sixth-degree burns, for describing deeper destruction into tissue, muscle, and bone.

A pure full-thickness burn is unusual. Severe burns are typically a combination of superficial, partial-thickness, and full-thickness burns. Superficial burns heal well without scarring. Small partial-thickness burns also heal without scarring. However, deep partial-thickness burns and all full-thickness burns are prone to scarring and may be best managed surgically.

It may be impossible to accurately estimate the depth of a particular burn. Even experienced burn specialists sometimes underestimate or, more commonly, overestimate the extent of a particular burn. Do not spend a substantial amount of time categorizing burns in the field; the hospital needs to know the approximate type of burn, and you need to generally categorize the burn to properly determine the level of care that the patient requires. These burns will look different in a few hours, as the damage evolves, and you should not waste time carefully categorizing something that will rapidly change.

Burn Severity

To assess a burn, you must consider its severity. The seriousness of a burn may influence medical control's choice of a treatment facility. Five factors will help you to determine the severity of a burn (the first two factors are the most important; after gauging these, ask yourself the remaining questions):

1. What is the depth of the burn?
2. What is the extent of the burn?
3. Are any critical areas (face, upper airway, hands, feet, genitalia) involved? Also included in critical areas are any circumferential burns, which are burns that go completely around a body part such as an arm, foot, or chest.
4. Does the patient have any preexisting medical conditions or other injuries that could be complicated by the burn injury?
5. Is the patient younger than 5 years or older than 55 years?

If the answer to any of these last three questions is yes, you should upgrade the burn's classification. Table 28-2 shows burn severity classifications.

Keep in mind that burns to the face are of particular importance because of the potential for airway involvement. In addition, burns to the hands or feet or over joints are

Table 28-2 Classification of Burn Severity

Burn Classifications	Criteria
Major burns	▪ Burns involving the hands, feet, face, major joints, or genitalia, or circumferential burns of other areas ▪ Full-thickness burns covering more than 10% of the TBSA ▪ Partial-thickness burns covering more than: • 25% of the TBSA if age 10–50 y • 20% of the TBSA if age younger than 10 y or older than 50 y ▪ Burns associated with respiratory injury (smoke inhalation or inhalation injury) ▪ Burns complicated by fractures or trauma ▪ High-voltage electrical burns ▪ Chemical burns ▪ Burns on patients younger than 5 years or older than 55 years that would be classified as moderate on young adults
Moderate burns	▪ Full-thickness burns involving 2% to 10% of the TBSA (excluding hands, feet, face, genitalia, and upper airway) ▪ Partial-thickness burns covering: • 15%–25% of the TBSA if age 10–50 y • 10%–20% of the TBSA if age younger than 10 y or older than 50 y ▪ Superficial burns covering more than 50% of the TBSA ▪ Low-voltage electrical burns ▪ Major burn characteristics absent
Minor burns	▪ Full-thickness burns covering less than 2% of the body's TBSA ▪ Partial-thickness burns covering: • Less than 15% of the TBSA if age 10–50 y • Less than 10% of the TBSA if age younger than 10 y or older than 50 y ▪ Superficial burns covering less than 50% of the TBSA ▪ Major burn characteristics absent

Abbreviation: TBSA, total body surface area

Data from: Pappas-Taffer L. Burns. In: Ferri FF, ed. *Ferri's Clinical Advisor*, 2017. Philadelphia, PA: Elsevier; 2017:219-221; and Tintinalli JE, Stapczynski JS, Ma OJ, et al. *Tintinalli's Emergency Medicine: A Comprehensive Study Guide*. 8th ed. McGraw-Hill; 2016.

also considered serious because of the potential of loss of function as a result of scarring.

▶ Burn Extent

The fastest and most universal mechanism of calculating the TBSA burned is the **rule of nines**, which is based on dividing the body into 11 sections, each representing approximately 9% of the TBSA.[3] The provider adds the portions of the body with burns to obtain the TBSA affected by the burn injury. Because our proportions change as we grow, different rules of nines apply to infants, children, and adults Figure 28-19.

Another quick way to estimate the surface area that has been burned is to use a technique known as the **rule of palms**, also called the rule of ones. This assessment uses the size of the patient's palm (including the fingers) to represent approximately 1% of the patient's TBSA. This calculation is helpful when the burn covers less than 10% of the TBSA or is irregularly shaped.

Assessment of Burns

Although a burn may be the patient's most obvious injury, you should always perform a complete assessment to determine whether there are other, more serious injuries. When you are assessing a burn, you will need to classify it to determine its severity. Assessment of a patient with burns is essentially the same as with any other trauma patient. Again, you must use caution to avoid being distracted by dramatic burn injuries and, thus, possibly overlooking other potential life threats that require treatment.

Scene Size-up

As you arrive on scene, observe the scene for hazards and threats to the safety of you and your crew, bystanders, and the patient. Ensure that the factors that resulted in the patient's burn injury do not pose a hazard to you and

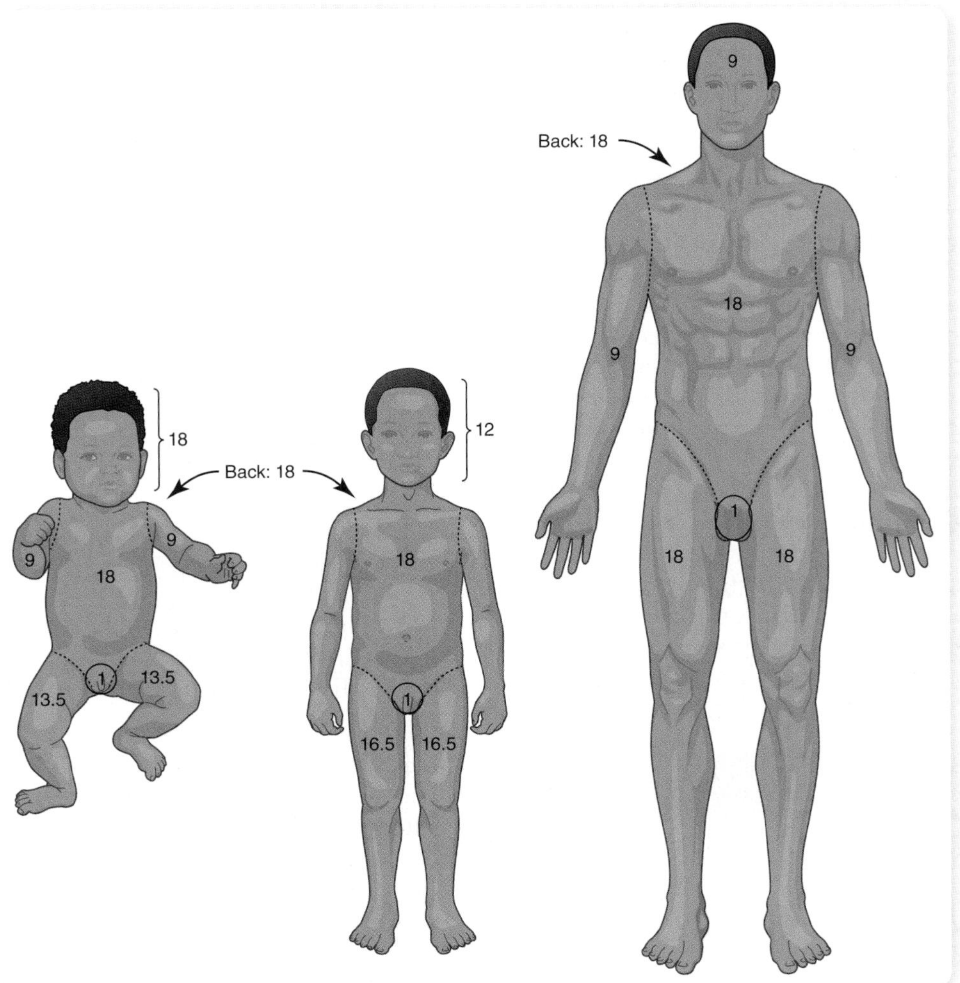

Figure 28-19 The rule of nines is a quick way to estimate the amount of surface area that has been burned. It divides the body into 11 sections, each representing approximately 9% of the total body surface area. The segments differ for infants, children, and adults.

Special Populations

Burns to children are generally considered more serious than burns to adults. This is because infants and children have more surface area relative to total body mass, which means greater fluid and heat loss. In addition, children do not tolerate burns as well as adults do. Children are also more likely to experience shock, hypothermia, and airway difficulties because of the unique differences associated with their ages and anatomy.

Some burns in infants and children result from child abuse. The classic burn resulting from deliberate immersion involves the hands and wrists, as well as the feet, lower legs, and buttocks. Similarly, burns around the genitals and multiple cigarette burns should be viewed as possible abuse. Report all suspected cases of abuse to the proper authorities (see Chapter 36, *Pediatric Emergencies*).

your crew. Is the electricity turned off? Is the chemical leak secure? Has the fire been extinguished? Is there any potential for violence?

When possible, determine the type of burn that has been sustained and the MOI. Patients with burns can be a challenge to treat physically and emotionally. It is easy to become overwhelmed by the sights, sounds, and smells of burn victims.

Assess the scene for any environmental hazards. If the patient is the victim of a lightning strike, is the weather still a threat to your safety? Wear gloves and eye protection when treating any patient with burns and gowns when serious injuries are expected. Determine the number of patients; the possibility for multiple patients increases if you are responding to a lightning strike or a vehicle crash. At vehicle crashes, ensure that there are no energized electrical lines or leaking fuel in the area where you will be working. If you determine that the power company, the fire department, or paramedic units are needed, call for additional resources early. Remember, a patient with burns may also be a trauma patient. Consider the potential for spinal injuries, inhalation injuries, and other injuries.

Primary Survey

The primary survey includes a rapid full-body scan of the patient to identify and manage life-threatening concerns and to assist with transport decisions.

As you approach a burned trauma patient, simple clues can help identify how serious the injuries are and how quickly you need to assess and treat them. A patient who greets you with a hoarse voice or is reported to have been in an enclosed space with a fire or intense heat source has indications of a significant MOI. The presence of stridor means your patient's airway is substantially swollen and can signal impending complete airway obstruction. Similarly, if the patient has singed facial hair, eyebrows, or nasal hair, your initial general impression might indicate that the patient has a potential airway and/or breathing problem. If the burn is associated with a fall, blast, or other trauma, the patient might also present with musculoskeletal injuries.

Child abuse and elder abuse are unpleasant situations to handle. Unfortunately, they are often situations that involve burns. As you enter a scene where burns are involved, be suspicious of clues that may indicate abuse.

The burned patient you encounter may have graphic injuries; however, stay focused on the primary survey. As you begin the primary survey, always consider the need for manual spinal stabilization.

Check for responsiveness using the AVPU scale. Assess a patient's mental status by asking the patient about the chief complaint. An unresponsive patient may indicate a life-threatening condition. In all patients whose level of consciousness is less than alert and oriented, administer high-flow oxygen as needed via a nonrebreathing mask or bag-mask device, and provide immediate transport to the ED.

Substantial bleeding is an immediate life threat and takes priority over airway and breathing concerns. If the patient has obvious life-threatening bleeding, it must be controlled quickly. Often, shock develops in burned patients. Treat the patient for shock as quickly as possible, according to local protocol including covering to prevent heat loss. This is important because the damaged skin has only a limited ability to regulate body temperature.

Ensure that the patient has a clear and patent airway. If the patient is unresponsive or has a substantially altered level of consciousness, consider inserting a properly sized oropharyngeal or nasopharyngeal airway.

The following are signs of airway involvement in a burn patient:

- Hoarseness
- Cough
- Stridor
- Singed nasal or facial hair
- Carbon in the sputum
- History of burn in an enclosed space

Heavy amounts of secretions and frequent coughing may also indicate a respiratory burn. A patient with signs and symptoms of airway burns can rapidly lose airway patency as a result of tissue swelling. Although rare, laryngeal edema can develop with alarming speed in burn patients, especially in infants and children. Request a paramedic rendezvous with providers capable of performing intubation or other interventions as soon as possible, and be alert to signs of impending airway closure.

Quickly assess for adequate breathing. Inspect and palpate the chest wall for DCAP-BTLS (Deformities, Contusions, Abrasions, Punctures/penetrations, Burns, Tenderness, Lacerations, Swelling). Check for clear and symmetric breath sounds, and provide high-flow oxygen or assisted ventilations using a bag-mask device as needed, depending on the level of consciousness and breathing rate and quality in your patient. Patients with burns are trauma patients. Evaluate and treat them for spinal injuries and airway problems concurrently. How you open the airway depends on whether a neck injury is suspected. Do the circumstances surrounding the MOI suggest a possible spinal injury?

Words of Wisdom

Patients with preexisting lung disease may have bronchospasm after even relatively minor exposure to smoke. These patients may respond well to inhaled beta-2 agonists.

Quickly assess the pulse rate and quality, and determine perfusion based on the patient's skin condition, color, temperature, and capillary refill time.

If the patient you are treating has an airway or breathing problem, substantial burn injuries, substantial external bleeding, or signs and symptoms of internal bleeding, consider quickly transporting the patient to the hospital for treatment. A rendezvous with paramedics may be appropriate for patients with moderate or severe burns and burns of the airway or **inhalation injury**. Paramedics can treat these patients with endotracheal intubation and analgesics for pain. These problems can progress so rapidly; immediate paramedic backup can make the difference between life and death. Provide rapid transport to the closest, most appropriate facility. If a burn center is not available, a Level I trauma center is the next-best option.

History Taking

Investigate the chief complaint or history of present illness. The first complaint in a patient with a burn injury is usually pain at the site. Next, be alert for signs or symptoms of other injuries due to the MOI.

Obtain a medical history and be alert for injury-specific signs and symptoms and any pertinent negatives, such as no pain. Typical signs of a burn are redness, swelling, blisters, or charring. Typically, symptoms include pain and/or burning at the injury site. Regardless of the type of burn injury, it is important to stop the burning process, apply dressings to prevent contamination, and treat the patient for shock.

Obtain a SAMPLE history from your patient. In addition, ask the following questions of a patient with burns:

- Are you having any difficulty breathing?
- Are you having any difficulty swallowing?
- Are you having any pain?

When you are assessing a patient with burns, check to see whether he or she has an emergency medical identification device—a wallet card, necklace, or bracelet—or ask the patient or a family member about preexisting conditions, which may increase the chances of a poor outcome. Remember that the environment, bystanders, and medical identification devices may provide important clues about your patient's condition.

Secondary Assessment

At this point, you will conduct a more detailed physical examination, or focused examination of the patient depending on the injury, to reveal any additional injuries. In some cases in which the patient is critically injured or the transport time is short, you may not have time to conduct a secondary assessment. In other cases, the secondary assessment may occur en route to the ED.

Quickly assess the patient from head to toe, looking for DCAP-BTLS to ensure that you have found all problems and injuries. Make a rough estimate, using the rule of nines, of the extent of the burned area to report to medical control. Determine what classification of burns the victim has sustained. The patient may or may not report pain depending on the amount of nerve damage. Before packaging your patient, determine the severity of the burns the victim has sustained, as described earlier. Follow your local protocols for criteria for transport to a burn center. Package the patient for transport based on your findings. Remember to immobilize your patient for spinal injuries as appropriate.

When assessing the respiratory system of a burned patient, look specifically for the following findings:

1. Soot around the mouth
2. Soot around the nose
3. Singed nasal hairs

Listen to breath sounds with a stethoscope. Breath sounds should be clear and equal bilaterally, anteriorly, and posteriorly. Determine the patient's rate and quality of respiration. Finally, assess the chest for DCAP-BTLS and asymmetric chest wall movement. Patients with burns who present with any types of airway problems should be considered critical.

If you find substantial bleeding during the secondary assessment, as always, controlling it and treating for shock are the highest treatment priorities since these are immediate life threats. Non–life-threatening bleeding, such as in abrasions, can be bandaged later in your assessment as necessary.

Assess the patient's neurologic system to formulate baseline data for further decisions on patient treatment.

Assess the musculoskeletal system by performing a detailed full-body exam if time permits. Specifically look for the following features:

- In the head, be alert for raccoon eyes, Battle sign, and/or drainage of blood or fluid from the ears or nose. Check for singed nasal or facial hair, burns or swelling of the face or ears, or burns or

swelling in the mouth. If the patient sustained electrical injury, examine the scalp for signs of entrance or exit wounds.
- In the neck, check for jugular vein distention and tracheal deviation. Be alert for patients with a stoma or tracheostomy. Also note any circumferential burns around the entire neck; these can impair breathing and circulation.
- In the chest, check for burns that encircle the entire chest, which can impair normal chest rise.
- In the abdomen, feel all four quadrants for tenderness or rigidity. If the abdomen is tender, expect internal bleeding.
- Look for burns that encircle an extremity, as they can impair circulation. If the patient sustained an electrical injury, assess thoroughly for entry or exit burn wounds. This should include the axilla and the area between digits. Record pulse and motor and sensory function.
- Examine the posterior surface of the body, as large burns or electrical exit burns may be located in this area.
- In the pelvis, check for stability.

Obtain an early set of vital signs to determine how your patient is tolerating his or her injuries while en route to the hospital. These can be obtained in the ambulance on the way to the hospital, decreasing the delay to definitive care in a patient with moderate to severe burns. Because shock is often pronounced in a burned patient, blood pressure, pulse, and skin assessment for perfusion are important vital signs to obtain.

Finally, use monitoring devices, including oxygen saturation monitors and carbon monoxide monitors when available, to quantify oxygenation and circulatory status.

Reassessment

Repeat the primary survey, and reassess the patient's vital signs. Reassess the patient's chief complaint. Reevaluate interventions and treatment you have provided to the patient, particularly those used to treat shock. Identify and treat any changes in the patient's condition.

Provide hospital personnel with a description of how the burn occurred. Many times, the ED staff can determine the appropriate diluent for chemical burns or calculate appropriate treatments for other types of burns with enough advance notice. Your report and documentation should include the extent of the burns. This should include the TBSA involved, the depth of the burn, and the location. For example, you may say 10% full-thickness burns, 15% partial-thickness burns, and 25% superficial burns to the chest, abdomen, and left lower extremity. If special areas are involved (such as the genitalia, feet, hands, face, or circumferential burns), they should be specifically mentioned and documented.

YOU are the Provider — PART 4

By using the Consensus formula, you calculate that the patient requires 8,800 mL of fluid during the first 24 hours and 4,400 mL during the first 8 hours. Seeing no readily identifiable veins in unburned areas, you establish bilateral large-bore IV lines in each antecubital fossa. With an estimated 20-minute transport time, you administer a 500-mL bolus in each IV line. You advise your partner that this patient requires emergency transport, and you begin your way to the hospital. On arrival at the ED, you give your report to the awaiting physician.

Recording Time: 12 Minutes	
Respirations	26 breaths/min; normal
Pulse	Strong and regular; 130 beats/min
Skin	Warm, dry, and pink
Blood pressure	98/58 mm Hg
Oxygen saturation (Spo_2)	100% oxygen via nonrebreathing mask at 15 L/min
Pupils	PERRL

7. What are some potential complications you may encounter with a substantial burn injury such as this?
8. Why is it important to assess for circumferential burns in patients with burn injuries?

Special Populations

Escaping from a fire can be difficult for children. Although the percentage of fatal outcomes for children younger than 5 years involved in a house fire decreased from 18% in 1980 to 6% in 2011,[4] research suggests that young children are not as effectively awakened by smoke detectors, and they are often disoriented immediately after waking. Young children are also more likely to sustain severe scald injuries. Children's thin skin and delicate respiratory structures are more easily damaged by thermal insults than are those of older children and adults.

In children, fluid resuscitation may be more challenging because of their increased body surface–to–weight ratio. Therefore, children may require more fluid per kilogram compared with adults. You may start by providing fluids based on the Consensus formula in children only to find that medical control orders additional fluids for major burns. Also, because of their relatively poor glycogen stores, children may require dextrose-containing solutions earlier than adults do. Blood glucose monitoring should be routinely performed in seriously burned children, particularly in the context of any decrease in the level of consciousness.

Burns may raise the suspicion of child abuse. Pay careful attention to the MOI, and relay this information to the hospital staff.

Approximately 1,300 older adults die of fire-related causes each year, which represents a 2.6-fold greater likelihood of fire-related deaths in this population as compared with the general population.[5] A substantial percentage of older adults smoke (more than 8.4% of US adults older than age 65 years smoke cigarettes[6]), and smoking is the leading cause of fires that result in the death of older adults. Burns from fires caused by smoking while wearing a supplementary oxygen supply are the leading sentinel event in home health care. Cooking fires represent another distinct hazard to older adults, who may be less able to smell a gas leak or a fire in the kitchen. Older adult patients are also particularly sensitive to respiratory insults. Relatively small fires can produce toxic fumes before detection or suppression devices are activated.

Older adult patients may also have poor glycogen stores, so their blood glucose levels should be checked to assess for hypoglycemia if there is any change in mental status of decreased level of consciousness. Although fluid resuscitation is important, pulmonary edema is more likely to develop in older patients. Routinely assess breath sounds in older adults who have burns.

Emergency Medical Care of Burns

The proper emergency care for a burn may increase a patient's chances of survival and decrease the risk or duration of long-term disability. Your first responsibility in caring for a patient with a burn is to stop the burning process and prevent additional injury.

While assessing a burned patient, check for traumatic injuries or other medical conditions that may be more immediately life threatening. Most patients who have been burned have normal vital signs and can communicate at first, which will make your assessment easier.

Skill Drill 28-2 presents the steps in caring for a patient with a burn.

Words of Wisdom

Remove jewelry before swelling occurs. Swelling that prevents its removal results in impaired circulation.

The goals in treating patients with burns are to stop the burning process, assess and treat breathing, support circulation (ie, supportive care for hypovolemic shock), and provide rapid transport. Because patients with burns may also have traumatic injuries, provide spinal immobilization if you suspect spinal injuries. Oxygen is mandatory for inhalation burns but is also helpful for patients with smaller burns. If the patient has signs of hypoperfusion, treat aggressively for shock, and provide rapid transport to the appropriate hospital. Cover all burns according to your local protocols. The risk of infection is extremely high and can be reduced if you cover large areas that are burned with sterile burn sheets or clean linen. Do not delay transport of a seriously injured patient to complete nonlifesaving treatments in the field, such as splinting extremity fractures. Instead, complete these types of treatments en route to the hospital.

Aggressive fluid resuscitation and general wound care may substantially increase chances of survival. Consider calling for paramedic backup for early definitive airway management (eg, endotracheal intubation) and pain

Words of Wisdom

Separate burned fingers and toes with dry, sterile gauze to prevent them from sticking together.

Words of Wisdom

To help prevent hypothermia, never apply moist dressings to any patient with more than 10% of the BSA burned unless the burning process has not been stopped.

Skill Drill 28-2 Caring for Burns

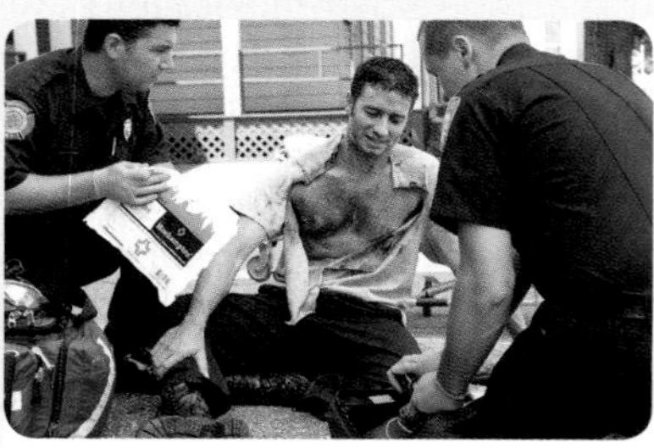

Step 1 Follow standard precautions to help prevent infection. Because a burn destroys the patient's protective skin layer, always wear gloves and eye protection when treating a burn patient. If safe to do so, move the patient away from the burning area. If any clothing is on fire, wrap the patient in a blanket or follow specific guidelines outlined by your local fire department protocol to put out the flames, and then remove any smoldering clothing and/or jewelry.

If allowed by local protocol, immerse the area in cool, sterile water or saline solution or cover with a clean, wet, cool dressing if the wound or clothing is still hot. This not only stops the burning but also relieves pain. Prolonged immersion, however, increases the risk of infection and hypothermia. For this reason, you should not keep the affected part under water for longer than 10 minutes. Moist, sterile dressings may be used if a burn covers less than 10% of the BSA. If the burning has stopped before you arrive, *do not immerse the burned part at all.* As an alternative to immersion, irrigation of the burned area until the burning stops may also be used, followed by the application of a sterile dressing.

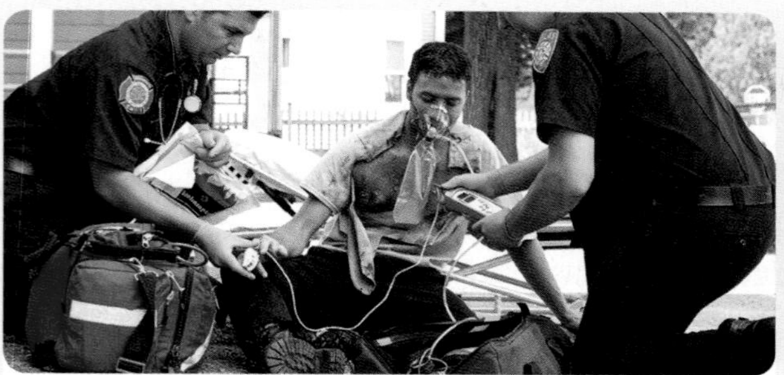

Step 2 Provide high-flow oxygen. Remember that more fire victims die of smoke inhalation than of skin burns. Respiratory distress may develop in a patient who has burns about the face or has inhaled smoke or fumes. Therefore, you should provide high-flow oxygen. Keep in mind that a patient who appears to be breathing well at first may suddenly have severe respiratory distress. Therefore, you must continue to reassess the airway for possible problems. Remember that pulse oximetry may be misleading if the patient is experiencing smoke inhalation, because of the potential for carbon monoxide poisoning.

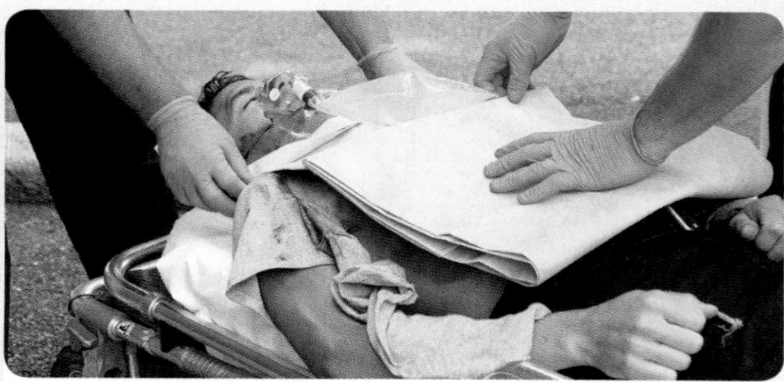

Step 3 Rapidly estimate the burn's severity. Then cover the burned area with a dry, sterile dressing to prevent further contamination. Sterile gauze is best if the area is not too large. You may cover larger areas with a clean, white sheet. Do not put anything else on the burned area. Never use ointments, lotions, or antiseptics of any kind (these products only increase the risk of infection and will have to be removed at the hospital), and do not intentionally break any blisters.

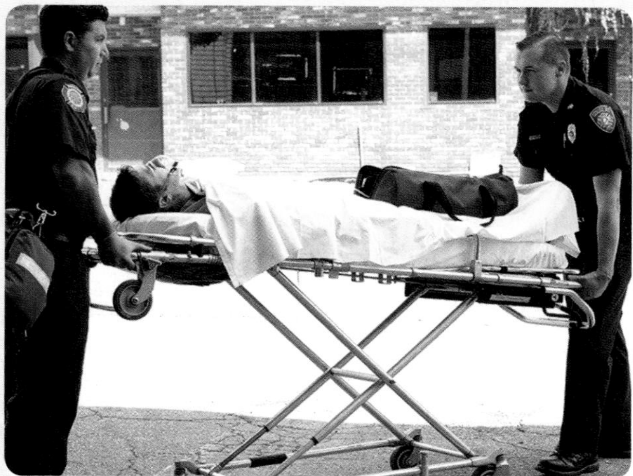

Step 4 Prepare for transport. Cover the stretcher with a burn sheet prior to placing the patient on it. Treat the patient for shock if necessary. Provide circulatory support, including establishing IV access using an isotonic crystalloid solution, proper positioning, and keeping the patient warm. An extensive burn can produce hypothermia (loss of body heat); prevent further heat loss by covering the patient with warm blankets.

Provide prompt transport by local protocol. Do not delay transport to do a prolonged assessment or to apply coverings to burns in a critically burned or injured patient. Transport to the closest, most appropriate facility in the proper mode based on the patient's condition. Provide psychological support en route.

management. Transport to the closest, most appropriate facility for definitive care.

During lengthy transport times (>1 hour), medical control may order you to administer IV fluids to the burned patient based on the **Consensus formula** (formerly known as the Parkland formula). The amount of fluids administered in the first 24 hours after injury is typically 2–4 mL of lactated Ringer solution multiplied by the patient's body weight in kilograms (kg) multiplied by the percentage of TBSA burned:

2–4 mL × Patient's weight (kg) × Percentage of body surface area burned = Total fluid in 24 hours

Thus, for a 75-kg (165-lb) patient with 45% BSA burned, the calculation is as follows, using 2 mL in the first equation and 4 mL in the second:

2 (mL) × 75 (kg) × 45 (percent TBSA)
= 6,750 mL during the first 24 hours

or

4 (mL) × 75 (kg) × 45 (percent TBSA)
= 13,500 mL during the first 24 hours

This formula further states that one-half of this amount needs to be given during the first 8 hours and the other half needs to be given over the next 16 hours in a 24-hour period.

Continuing the example using the 2-mL amount for simplicity, the patient would receive 3,375 mL during the first 8 hours (approximately 425 mL/h).

It should be noted, however, that a burned patient with signs of inadequate perfusion (ie, shock) should receive 20-mL/kg boluses of an isotonic crystalloid as needed to maintain adequate perfusion.

Even though the Consensus formula implies that burn patients need enormous amounts of fluid, remember that you should not attempt to deliver the entire initial amount in the field. The large amounts of fluid suggested by this formula often lead providers to give more fluid than necessary prior to the patient's arrival at a burn center—a phenomenon known as fluid creep. (Interestingly, the Parkland formula was devised to limit fluid overload so that burn patients would *not* develop pulmonary edema and acute respiratory distress syndrome.) Ongoing fluid resuscitation at the hospital is based on the patient's urine output and vital signs. The original Parkland formula recommended using 4 mL/kg/percentage of TBSA as a standard for calculating fluid needs in burn patients. The Consensus formula recognizes that less than that amount is appropriate for most patients and recommends starting the calculation at one-half that total amount and then adjusting fluid requirements after the patient is in the hospital based on urine output and blood chemistry analysis.

Although burn patients will need large amounts of fluid, giving it too early or too fast can result in rapidly increasing peripheral edema that may compromise the effectiveness of airway devices and vascular access and lead to compartment syndrome. It is even more important to monitor older adults and children for fluid overload during this crucial period. In short, you must administer a lot of fluid while simultaneously monitoring the patient to ensure that you are not administering too much.

▶ Specific Burns

Thermal Burns

A **thermal burn** is sometimes called trauma by fire; however, heat energy can be transmitted in a variety of ways in addition to fire. Although thermal burns are all caused by heat (as opposed to electricity, chemicals, or radiation), many different situations can cause thermal burns and pose a safety hazard to AEMTs.

Most commonly, thermal burns are caused by open flame. A **flame burn** is often a deep burn, especially if a person's clothing catches fire. The fire is fanned by running—hence the adage "stop, drop, and roll" that is taught in schools. Wrapping the patient in a blanket or other material can also smother the flame. Flame burns may also be associated with inhalation injuries.

Hot liquids produce scald injuries. A **scald burn** is most commonly seen in children, as well as adults with disabilities, but can happen to anyone, particularly while cooking. Scald burns often cover large surface areas because liquids can spread quickly. Hot liquids can soak into clothing and continue to burn until the clothing is removed. Some hot liquids, such as oil and grease, adhere to the skin, causing particularly deep scald injuries. Approximately 500,000 scald burns annually are the result of spilling hot food and beverages.[7]

Special Populations

Scalds and contact burns are sometimes associated with child or elder abuse. Burns in children, older people, and people with disabilities may be signs of abuse. Burns with formed shapes or unusual patterns and burns in atypical places such as the genitalia, buttocks, and thighs are often consistent with abuse.

Coming in contact with hot objects produces a **contact burn**. Ordinarily, reflexes protect a person from prolonged exposure to an extremely hot object, so contact burns are rarely deep unless the patient was prevented from drawing away from the hot object (eg, the patient was unconscious, intoxicated, restrained, or impaired). Prolonged contact with something that is just moderately hot can eventually result in a severe burn, however. A patient who has a stroke and falls against a household radiator, for example, may end up with severe burns.

A **steam burn** can produce a topical (scald) burn. Minor steam burns are common when uncovering the plastic wrap from microwaved food. When the plastic is peeled away, hot steam escapes directly onto a person's hand. Steam (gaseous water) can also cause airway burns. Inhalation of other hot gases may cause upper airway trauma but rarely results in burns in the lower airway. Steam is unique because the minute particles of hot water can cause substantial injury to the lower airway.

A relatively rare source of thermal burns is the flash burn produced by an explosion, which may briefly expose a person to intense heat. A common source of a flash burn occurs when the patient is lighting charcoal that has been soaked in lighter fluid, generally resulting in singed hair and superficial burns of the face and arms. Lightning strikes can also cause a flash burn. These injuries are usually minor compared with the potential for trauma from whatever caused the flash.

Inhalation Burns

According to a National Fire Protection Association report, most deaths from fires are not caused directly by burns but rather result from inhalation of toxic gases, upper airway compromise, or pulmonary injury.[8] This is generally the result of carbon monoxide or cyanide toxicity. If the patient survives the initial injury, death is usually the result of secondary infection, because the barrier of protection offered by intact skin is breached. Pathogens invade the wound shortly after the burn and may do so until the area is healed. Infection prevention is important in patients with burns.

Inhalation injuries can occur when burning takes place in enclosed spaces without ventilation. When the upper airway is exposed to excessive heat, the patient can experience rapid and serious airway compromise. The heat can be an irritant to the lungs and the airway, causing coughing, wheezing, and rapid swelling or edema of the mucosa of the upper airway tissues, often evidenced by stridor. Upper airway damage is often associated with the inhalation of superheated gases. Lower airway damage is more often associated with the inhalation of chemicals (eg, acids and aldehydes) and particulate matter. When treating a patient for inhalation injuries, you may encounter severe upper airway swelling, requiring intervention immediately after a severe burn, although this problem may not manifest itself until transport. You should consider requesting paramedic backup if the patient has signs or symptoms of edema such as stridor, a hoarse voice, singed nasal hairs, singed facial hairs, burns of the face, or carbon particles in the sputum. Application of cool mist, aerosol therapy, or humidified oxygen may help reduce some minor edema. Saline placed in a nebulizer can also provide humidified air.

Signs and symptoms of lower airway injury are usually seen later than those of the upper airway. The patient may appear unharmed only to die several hours later of pulmonary complications. It is important to maintain a high index of suspicion for any patient exposed to a burning environment.

Prehospital care of a patient with an inhalation injury is the same as for any other burned patient, with specific attention to the airway. Early recognition and treatment of a patient with an inhalation injury are key to survival. Consider calling for paramedic backup for early definitive airway treatment for a patient with an altered mental status, before edema makes such treatment virtually impossible. Prompt transport to the closest, most appropriate facility is imperative. This may include transport to a facility with access to a hyperbaric chamber for patients with suspected carbon monoxide poisoning. Patients who are hypoxic may be anxious or agitated. Provide psychological support en route.

Carbon Monoxide Intoxication

Toxins in the smoke greatly increase the risk of morbidity and mortality. As the fire uses up the oxygen in an enclosed space, the patient is left to breathe toxins such as carbon monoxide. Because carbon monoxide will bind to hemoglobin 200 times more readily than oxygen, signs of hypoxia can rapidly develop in the patient. Permanent damage to organs, including the brain, may occur if the patient is not rescued and treated promptly.

Carbon monoxide intoxication should be considered whenever a group of people in the same place all report a headache or nausea (a malfunctioning furnace or car exhaust being sucked into the air-handling system can cause carbon monoxide intoxication in groups of people). Similarly, you should be suspicious when people complain of feeling sick at home but not when they go to work or school.

Patients with severe carbon monoxide intoxication usually have an oxygen saturation level that is normal or better. For this reason, you should be suspicious of pulse oximeter readings when you are dealing with a patient who is suspected to have carbon monoxide poisoning. Devices that can measure a patient's carbon monoxide level are sometimes used in prehospital care; they allow you to find and treat low-level carbon monoxide intoxication far more readily than any other method available in the prehospital environment.

The gaseous form of cyanide is hydrogen cyanide. Hydrogen cyanide is present in the smoke of certain substances when burned, such as wood and certain plastics. It is also present in vehicle exhaust. Hydrogen cyanide is colorless and has the smell of bitter almonds; however, it can be difficult to detect at the scene of a fire. Prehospital diagnosis of hydrogen cyanide poisoning is difficult because laboratory studies are necessary. Signs and symptoms involve the central nervous, respiratory, and cardiovascular systems of the body and include faintness, anxiety, abnormal vital signs, headache, seizures, paralysis, and coma.

Chemical Burns

A chemical burn can occur whenever a toxic substance contacts the body. Strong acids or strong alkalis (bases) cause most chemical burns. Both acids and alkalis are

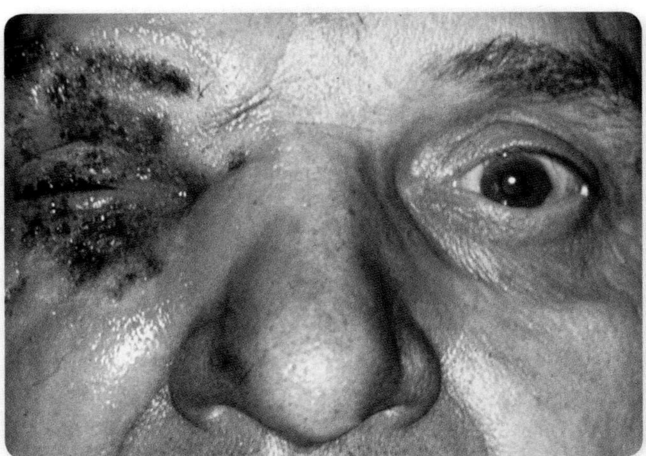

Figure 28-20 The eyes are particularly vulnerable to chemical burns.

defined as caustic and cause substantial tissue damage on contact. The eyes are particularly vulnerable to chemical burns Figure 28-20. Sometimes simply the fumes of strong chemicals can cause burns, especially to the respiratory tract.

To prevent exposure to hazardous materials, you must wear the appropriate personal protective equipment (such as gloves and eye protection) whenever you are caring for a patient with a chemical burn. Be particularly careful not to get any chemical, dry or liquid, on yourself or on your uniform; consider wearing a protective gown when this is a possibility. Remember that exposure risk is also present when you are cleaning up after the call. In cases of severe chemical burns or exposure, consider mobilization of a HazMat (hazardous materials) team, if appropriate.

Safety

Some chemicals react violently with water, which obviously precludes irrigation. Such chemicals are usually powders, so it is reasonable to brush off as much dry powder as possible. You should understand the chemical you are dealing with and the preferred method for its removal prior to initiating irrigation with water.

The severity of a chemical burn is related to several factors, including the following:

- The pH level of the agent
- The concentration of the agent
- The length of time the patient was exposed to the agent
- The volume of the agent
- The physical form of the agent

Ingestion of solid agents, such as pills, results in a longer exposure time as the offending substance travels through the digestive system. In addition, concentrated forms of some acids and alkalis generate substantial heat when diluted, resulting in thermal and caustic injury. Because industrial accidents are the most frequent types of chemical exposures, consider the MOI as well.

Treatment for chemical burns can be specific to the chemical agent. When the incident occurred in an industrial setting, ask for copies of material safety data sheets from the employer. If available, read all of the labels of the chemical agent. You may also contact poison control for assistance if you are not sure of how to respond to an incident involving a particular chemical. Do not risk exposure while attempting to gather information on the chemical.

Words of Wisdom

Many industrial sites have experts available on scene to assist with exposures.

To stop the burning process, remove any chemical from the patient. A dry chemical that is activated by contact with water may damage the skin more when it is wet than when it is dry. Therefore, always brush dry chemicals off the skin and clothing before flushing the patient with water Figure 28-21. Remove the patient's clothing, including shoes, stockings, and gloves and any jewelry or eyeglasses, because there may be small amounts of chemicals in the creases. Chemical burns are evaluated in the same manner as thermal burns when classifying depth or TBSA.

After brushing off the chemical, begin to flush the burned area with large amounts of water Figure 28-22, taking care not to contaminate uninjured areas or make the patient hypothermic. This should be integrated with your primary survey of the patient. Never direct a forceful stream of water from a hose at the patient; the extreme water pressure may mechanically injure the burned skin. Continue flooding the area with copious amounts of water for 15 to 20 minutes after the patient says the burning pain has stopped. Continue flushing the contaminated

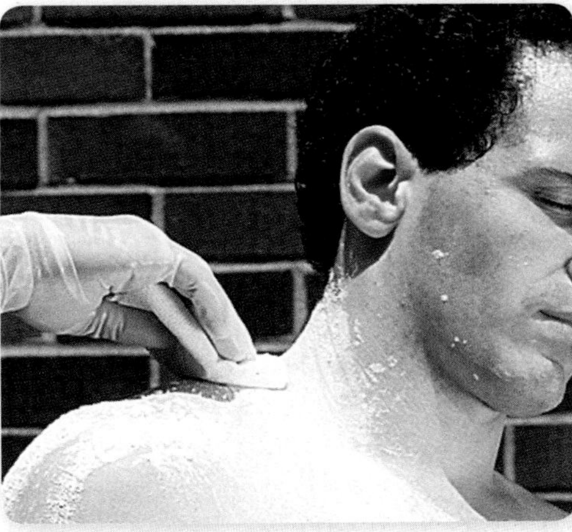

Figure 28-21 Brush off dry chemicals before you flush the burned area with water.

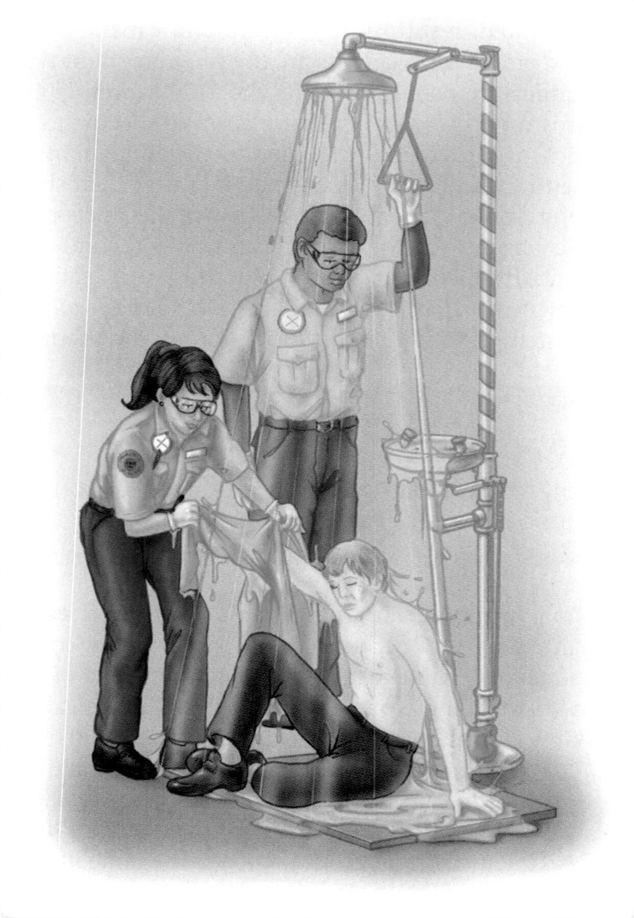

Figure 28-22 Flush the burned area with large amounts of water for 15 to 20 minutes after the patient says that the burning pain has stopped. Avoid contaminating uninjured areas.

area on the way to the hospital. Do not use any antidote or neutralizing agent. More damage may be caused by the chemical reaction of the antidote or neutralizing agent with the contaminant. Treat all chemical exposures according to local protocols.

Words of Wisdom

For a patient who has had a chemical exposure, *never* pull the patient's shirt over his or her head. This could result in chemicals being rubbed into the mouth, nose, or eyes.

Several types of chemical burns require special management techniques:

- **Dry lime.** In alkali burns caused by dry lime, combination with water will produce a highly corrosive substance. For that reason, when a patient has been in contact with dry lime, *first* remove the patient's clothing and *brush* as much lime as you can from the skin (wear gloves!). *Then* start flushing copiously with a garden hose or shower. Your intention is to completely overwhelm any damaging chemical reaction with a deluge of water.
- **Sodium metals.** Sodium metals produce considerable heat when mixed with water and may explode. Cover this type of burn with oil, which will stop the reaction by preventing the sodium from coming in contact with the atmosphere.
- **Hydrofluoric (HF) acid.** HF acid is used in drain cleaners in the home and for etching glass and plastic in industrial settings. Burns caused by HF acid that exceed 3% to 5% of the TBSA can be fatal. The patient will complain bitterly of pain (caused by the HF acid sucking calcium out of the body), and the pain will not improve even with continuous flushing—a sign that the process of tissue destruction is ongoing. Calcium gluconate gel is the preferred treatment for HF acid burns.
- **Gasoline or diesel fuel.** Because we come into contact with these chemicals almost every day, and they are present at almost all vehicle crashes, it is easy to forget the multitude of potential problems that may be caused by gasoline, kerosene, and other hydrocarbons. Prolonged contact may produce a chemical injury to the skin. This condition is managed like contact with any other chemical irritant, with the fuel being washed off as soon as possible. Most hydrocarbons are more effectively removed with a soap solution than with water alone. Hydrocarbons also stimulate gamma-aminobutyric acid receptors and can cause sleepiness and even coma. Many hydrocarbons can also cause a fire or explosion under certain circumstances.
- **Hot tar.** Burns caused by hot tar are, strictly speaking, thermal burns, not chemical burns, although they tend to be classified with chemical burns. The most important step in the prehospital phase is to immerse the affected area in cold water to dissipate the heat from the tar and speed up the hardening process. After the tar has cooled, it will not do further damage, and there is no need to try to remove it in the field.

When treating chemical burns, give particular attention to the eyes. Caustic chemicals introduced into the eyes will produce burns similar to those of thermal burns. If not removed quickly, the burning process will continue through the various layers of the eye. Chemical injuries to the eyes may be the result of acids, alkalis, mace, pepper spray, or other irritants.

If the patient's eye has been burned, hold the eyelid open (without applying pressure over the globe of the

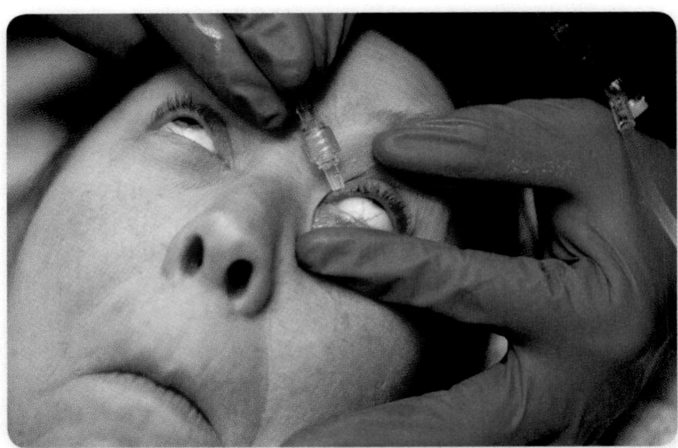

Figure 28-23 Flood the affected eye with a gentle stream of water. Holding the eyelids open is a challenging task because the patient's reflex is to keep the eye shut. Take care to prevent any of the chemical from getting into the other eye during flushing.

eye) while flooding the eye with a gentle stream of water Figure 28-23. Flush the eyes from the inside corners to the outside to prevent cross contamination. If only one eye has been affected, turn the patient's head to that side and flush. If both eyes are affected, consider hooking up a nasal cannula to a bag of saline to flush both eyes simultaneously. The prongs can be placed on the bridge of the nose to flush from the inside corners of the eyes to the outside corners. Be careful not to touch the prongs to the eye or surrounding tissue. Continue flushing the contaminated area on the way to the hospital.

Irrigate the eye for at least 5 minutes. If an alkali or a strong acid caused the burn, you should irrigate the eye for 20 minutes. After you have completed irrigation, apply a clean, dry dressing to cover the eye, and transport the patient promptly to the hospital for further care. If the irrigation can be carried out satisfactorily in the ambulance, it should be done during transport to save time.

Electrical Burns

The American Burn Association indicates that electrocution causes an average of 400 deaths and 4,400 injuries each year.[9] Electrical burns may be the result of contact with high- or low-voltage electricity. High-voltage burns may occur when utility workers make direct contact with power lines. Ordinary household current is powerful enough to cause severe burns as well as cardiac dysrhythmias.

For electricity to flow, there must be a complete circuit between the electrical source and the ground. Any substance that prevents this circuit from being completed, such as rubber, is called an insulator. Any substance that allows a current to flow through it is called a conductor. The human body, which is primarily water, is a good conductor. Thus, electrical burns occur when the body, or a part of it, completes a circuit connecting a power source to the ground Figure 28-24.

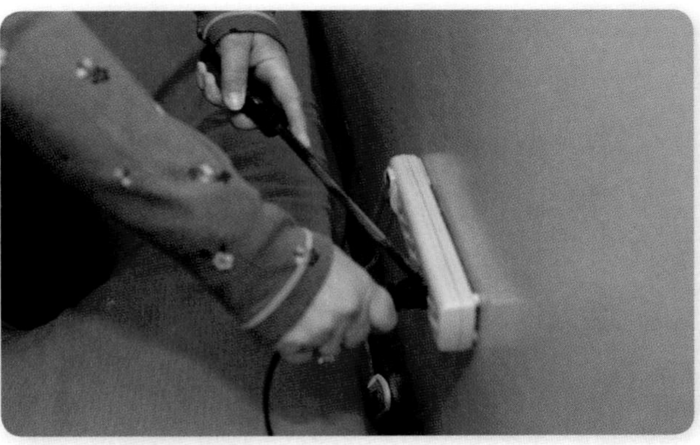

Figure 28-24 The human body is a good conductor of electricity. An electrical burn usually occurs when the body, acting as a conductor, completes a circuit.

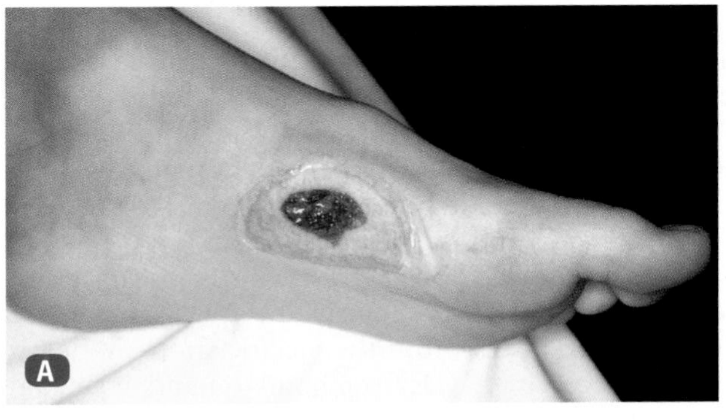

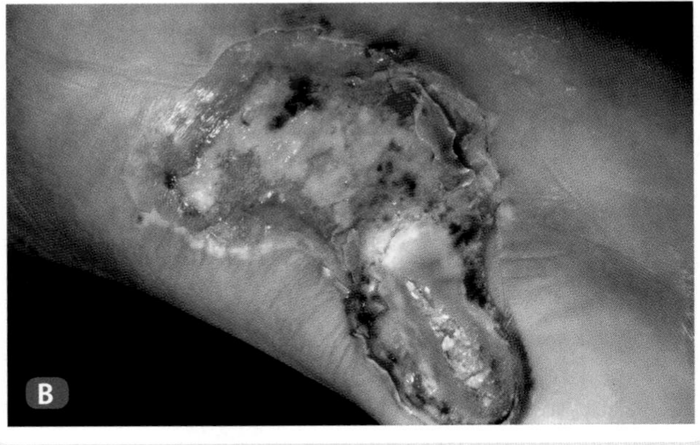

Figure 28-25 Electrical burns, like gunshot wounds, have entrance and exit wounds. **A.** An entrance wound is often quite small. **B.** The exit wound can be extensive and deep.

Heat is generated by the flow of electrical current through body tissues, resulting in direct thermal injury. Vascular injuries, renal injuries, and compartment syndrome may also result.

An electrical burn will result in two burn injuries: one where the electricity entered the body (an entrance wound) and another where it exited (an exit wound). The entrance wound may be quite small Figure 28-25A, but the exit wound can be extensive and deep Figure 28-25B. Always look for entrance *and* exit wounds.

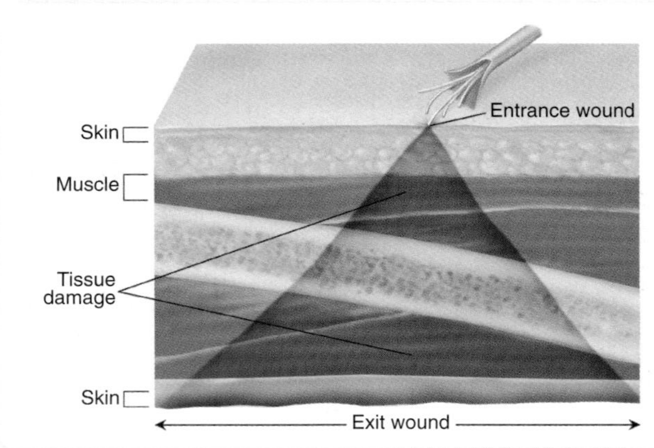

Figure 28-26 External signs of an electrical burn may be deceiving. The entrance wound may be a small burn, but the damage to deeper tissue may be massive.

There are two dangers specifically associated with electrical burns. First, there may be a large amount of deep tissue injury. Electrical burns are always more severe than the external signs indicate. The patient may have only a small burn to the skin but massive damage to the deeper tissues, organs, and the nervous system **Figure 28-26**. The force of the electrical energy can also cause fractures or joint dislocations. Second, the patient may go into cardiac or respiratory arrest from the electric shock. When the path of electricity travels from hand to hand, it generally flows through the heart, disrupting normal function of the cardiac conduction system.

Your safety is particularly important when you are called to the scene of an emergency involving electricity. Obviously, coming into direct contact with power lines can fatally injure you, but it is important to remember that touching a patient who is still in contact with a live power line or any other electrical source can be fatal to you as well. For this reason, you must never attempt to remove someone from an electrical source unless you are specifically trained to do so. Likewise, never move a downed power line unless you have the special training and equipment necessary for the job or unless you are absolutely certain that the line is not live. Notify your dispatcher to send the power company for assistance. Before even approaching someone who may still be in contact with a power line or an electrical appliance, make certain that the power is turned off. Always assume that any downed power line is live.

> **Safety**
>
> Do not try to remove someone from an electrical source or move a downed power line unless you are specifically trained and equipped to do so. Before approaching someone who may still be in contact with a power line or electrical appliance, ensure that all power is turned off.

Not all electrical injuries are the same. Determine the voltage and type of current if possible. Identify whether the injury was brief or sustained and an approximate time of contact. Note if the patient is wet or near water; this can influence the amount of energy transferred. Also ask about any loss of consciousness and any preexisting medical conditions that may exacerbate the problem and hinder effective resuscitation.

As with thermal burns, consider early definitive care of the airway if the patient is unable to maintain his or her own airway. Consider paramedic backup for early intubation of patients unable to maintain their own airway.

When assessing circulation, look for signs of hypoperfusion and assess the heart rate, specifically for regularity to detect potentially life-threatening dysrhythmias. As mentioned, cardiac dysrhythmias are common with electrical burns. If indicated, begin CPR and apply an automated external defibrillator. Although CPR may need to be quite prolonged in electrical burn cases, it has a high success rate if started promptly. Be prepared to defibrillate if necessary. If neither CPR nor defibrillation is indicated, give high-flow supplemental oxygen, and monitor the patient closely for respiratory and cardiac arrest. Establish IV access using an isotonic crystalloid solution, and administer a bolus of 250 mL, increasing up to four doses as needed, or a dose based on local protocols. This will help to maintain an adequate urine output of 1 mL/kg per hour and adequate renal perfusion.

Provide prompt transport to the closest, most appropriate facility; all electrical burns are potentially severe injuries that require further treatment in the hospital. Remember that very old and very young patients, as well as patients with preexisting conditions, are at greater risk for severe morbidity and mortality.

Taser effects. Devices such as a conducted electrical weapon (CEW) or Taser incapacitate people via electromuscular disruption. Although they are intended to offer law enforcement personnel a nonlethal option for controlling violent people, their use can create injuries that require emergency medical care. If discharged from a distance, two small darts (electrodes) that puncture the patient's skin are deployed from these weapons. Taser darts can be seen as small impaled objects, with a fishhooklike barb on the end. Although the resultant injury is typically minor, reports have cited hits to sensitive areas such as the eyes, major vessels, face, and genitalia. Even innocuous dart placement could potentially result in soft-tissue injury, bleeding, or infection, and dart removal should be done with care and while complying with the appropriate standard precautions.

Several reports of deaths in people who have been shocked with a Taser have made the use of these devices controversial.[10,11] In addition, cases exist in which people who have been covered with alcohol-based pepper spray have subsequently caught fire when an electroshock device was applied.[12] (Water-based pepper spray is typically used in the United States.) Manufacturers now recommend that such devices not be used in potentially flammable environments such as gas stations or near illicit methamphetamine-manufacturing operations.

Words of Wisdom

Lightning injuries, another type of electrical injury, are covered in Chapter 34, *Environmental Emergencies*. In patients who sustained lightning injury, it is important to remember that reverse triage applies: priority for treatment goes to patients in cardiac arrest from lightning strike because they have a good chance of successful resuscitation, even when they appear to be beyond help. Provide aggressive, continued, high-quality CPR, and apply an automated external defibrillator as soon as possible.

Radiation Burns

Radiation exposure has become more than a theoretical issue as use of radioactive materials increases in industry and medicine, and you must understand it to function effectively in the prehospital arena. Between 1944 and 2010, there were more than 400 radiation accidents worldwide involving substantial radiation exposure to more than 3,000 people.[13] More recent events in Japan (the earthquake-triggered tsunami that damaged the Fukushima Daiichi Nuclear Power Plant in March 2011) highlight that radiation accidents continue to be a threat. Other potential threats include incidents related to the use and transportation of radioactive isotopes and intentionally released radioactivity in terrorist attacks. To be effective in treating patients with radiation exposure, you must first suspect radiation and attempt to determine whether ongoing exposure exists. Increasingly, special response units are equipped with pager-sized radiation detectors, or such detection may be provided by other public safety services.

Ionizing radiation is made up of subatomic particles that contain an excess amount of energy that is emitted into the atmosphere in certain circumstances, creating radiation. These charged particles (ions) can cause damage to molecules, cells, and tissues. Any amount of ionizing radiation will produce some damage.

The three most common types of ionizing radiation are alpha, beta, and gamma. Inhalation, ingestion, and direct exposure are the three basic pathways by which people are exposed. The amount and duration of exposure affect the severity or type of health effect.

Acute exposure to radiation may result in burns and radiation sickness or radiation poisoning. Radiation sickness can cause premature aging or even death. If the dose is fatal, death usually occurs within 2 months. The symptoms of radiation sickness include nausea, weakness, hair loss, skin burns, and diminished organ function.

Radiation burns require special rescue techniques beyond the initial training of AEMTs. If not properly trained, maintain a safe distance and wait for the HazMat team to decontaminate the patient before initiating care. Follow local protocols. Establish IV access, and give fluid based on patient presentation. If there are signs of shock, give a 250-mL bolus of an isotonic crystalloid solution and reassess.

YOU are the Provider SUMMARY

1. How do you calculate the percentage of burned area?

Burns are calculated by using the rule of nines or the rule of palms. The rule of nines divides the body into sections, each of which is approximately 9% of the total surface area. The rule of palms is a quick way to estimate the surface area that has been burned. To use the rule of palms, compare the burned area with the size of the patient's palm, which is roughly equivalent to 1% of the patient's TBSA. This calculation is helpful when the burn covers less than 10% of the TBSA or is irregularly shaped.

2. What classification of burns does this patient have?

This patient's burn falls into the classification of severe burns based on the patient's full-thickness burns, including the full-thickness burns involving the genitalia. Also, the patient's burns cover more than 10% of his body's total surface area.

3. What immediate treatment is required for this patient?

Immediate treatment for this patient includes stopping the burning process by removing any still-burning materials and assessing the airway for potential burns. Because burns can be extremely painful, a paramedic intercept should be requested for narcotic pain management.

4. Because this patient is complaining of pain, should you apply moist dressings in an attempt to cool the burned area?

Moist dressings should be avoided in this patient because of the large percentage of burned area involved. Application of moist dressings may precipitate hypothermia.

YOU are the Provider SUMMARY (continued)

Instead, this patient should have his burns covered with dry, sterile dressings to reduce the introduction of bacteria into the burned area.

5. Should you attempt IV access through the burned area?

IV access is crucial in a burned patient. Attempt IV access in an unburned area first. If you are unable to locate a vein in an unburned area, it is acceptable, although not optimal, to obtain access through a burned area. Remember, there is always the option of gaining intraosseous access if there is an unburned area available.

6. How would you calculate the amount of fluid the patient requires?

Fluid replacement in a burned patient is calculated by using the Consensus formula. This formula is obtained by taking the patient's weight in kilograms multiplied by 2–4 mL multiplied by the TBSA burned. In this case, using 2 mL, it is 2 mL × 80 kg × 55%, which equals 8,800 mL of fluid that needs to be administered over the first 24 hours, with one-half that amount (4,400 mL) needing to be infused over the first 8 hours.

7. What are some potential complications you may encounter with a substantial burn injury such as this?

Some potential complications you may encounter would be a potential airway obstruction from swelling and edema, shock resulting from hypovolemia, hypothermia, and compartment syndrome.

8. Why is it important to assess for circumferential burns in patients with burn injuries?

A circumferential burn may result in compartment syndrome, in which tissues beneath the eschar are unable to stretch, resulting in compression and decreased or absent circulation. If the burn is around the thorax, tidal volume and chest excursion may be drastically reduced by the eschar formation, resulting in ventilatory insufficiency. A circumferential eschar around an extremity may require an escharotomy—a surgical incision to relieve the pressure and restore circulation—after the patient arrives at the ED.

EMS Patient Care Report (PCR)

Date: 10-6-18	**Incident No.:** 4067521733	**Nature of Call:** Explosion	**Location:** Lake Bronson		
Dispatched: 1602	**En Route:** 1604	**At Scene:** 1614	**Transport:** 1622	**At Hospital:** 1644	**In Service:** 1713

Patient Information

Age: 19 **Sex:** M **Weight (in kg [lb]):** 80 kg (178 lb)	**Allergies:** None **Medications:** None **Past Medical History:** None **Chief Complaint:** Burns/pain

Vital Signs

Time: 1615	**BP:** —	**Pulse:** —	**Respirations:** 28	**SpO_2:** —
Time: 1622	**BP:** 102/64	**Pulse:** 137	**Respirations:** 26	**SpO_2:** 100% on 15 L/min
Time: 1627	**BP:** 98/58	**Pulse:** 130	**Respirations:** 26	**SpO_2:** 100% on 15 L/min

EMS Treatment (circle all that apply)

Oxygen @ 15 **L/min via (circle one):** **NC** **(NRM)** **Bag-mask device**		**Assisted Ventilation**	**Airway Adjunct**	**CPR**
Defibrillation	**Bleeding Control**	**Bandaging**	**Splinting**	**Other:**

YOU are the Provider SUMMARY (continued)

Narrative

EMS dispatched to Lake Bronson for a reported explosion. On arrival, patient found lying on ground in severe pain. Bystanders state that patient was pouring gasoline in a barbeque when it flashed. Patient is AO×4; ABCs intact. Smoldering clothes noted on chest, removed. Full-thickness burns to chest, bilateral arms and legs, and groin. Estimated 55% total BSA burned. Paramedic intercept requested but unavailable. Patient denies any other injuries but complains of 10/10 pain. Placed patient on stretcher, secured, emergency transport to Kalispell Regional Medical Center (KRMC). En route: Bilateral 18-gauge IVs established, 500-mL LR bolus to each IV. Consensus formula calculated at 8.8 L over 24 hours. Covered patient with dry, sterile dressings. 100% oxygen at 15 L/min applied via nonrebreathing mask. On arrival at KRMC, care and report given to ED staff without incident.**End of report**

Prep Kit

▶ Ready for Review

- The soft tissues of the body can be injured through a variety of mechanisms such as blunt trauma, penetrating trauma, and burn injuries.
- Death as a result of soft-tissue injury is often related to hemorrhage or infection.
- The skin has two principal layers: the tough outer layer, called the epidermis, and the inner layer, called the dermis, which contains the hair follicles, sweat glands, and sebaceous glands.
- The functions of the skin are to keep bacteria out and water in, to report to the brain on the environment and sensations, and to regulate body temperature.
- Skin tension lines (patterns of tautness in the skin) affect wound healing.
- Concerns during wound healing include infection, gangrene, tetanus, and necrotizing fasciitis.
- Soft-tissue injuries can be subdivided into three types:
  - Closed injuries (Soft-tissue damage occurs beneath the skin or mucous membrane but the surface remains intact.)
  - Open injuries (There is a break in the surface of the skin or the mucous membrane, exposing deeper tissue to potential contamination.)
  - Burns (The soft tissue receives more energy than it can absorb without injury; the source of this energy can be thermal, frictional heat, toxic chemicals, electricity, or nuclear radiation.)
- Closed injuries include contusions, hematomas, and crushing injuries.
- Open injuries produce more extensive bleeding than closed injuries and may become infected.
- Types of open injuries include abrasions, lacerations, avulsions, amputations, bite wounds, penetrating wounds, and blast injuries.
- The assessment of an open injury is generally easier than the assessment of a closed injury because you can see the injury.
- Because skin injuries typically result in a risk of exposure to blood and other body fluids, scene size-up should include infection control procedures and standard precautions.
- Life-threatening conditions must be managed first; bleeding may not always be the most life-threatening condition. However, substantial bleeding is an immediate life threat and must be controlled quickly using appropriate methods.
- Be alert for shock in all patients with soft-tissue injury, but especially patients with closed injuries. Assess the pulse and skin to determine how aggressively you need to treat for shock.
- Soft-tissue injuries can severely compromise the airway. Immediately correct anything that interferes with airway patency.
- After the primary survey, you must make a priority decision to rapidly package and transport or to stabilize and treat on scene.

Prep Kit *(continued)*

- Closed soft-tissue injuries are characterized by a history of blunt trauma, pain at the site of injury, swelling beneath the skin, and discoloration. Treat a closed soft-tissue injury by applying the mnemonic RICES: *Rest, Ice, Compression, Elevation,* and *Splinting.*
- Dressings and bandages are designed to control bleeding, protect the wound from further damage, and prevent further contamination and infection.
- In treating open injuries, first control bleeding. Use a dry, sterile dressing, covered by a roller bandage, a second pressure dressing (if necessary), and a splint. Do not try to clean out an open wound.
- To treat avulsions, replace the avulsed flap in its original position. If an avulsion is complete, wrap the separated tissue in sterile gauze, and take it with you to the emergency department. Never remove an avulsion skin flap, regardless of the size of the flap.
- Control bleeding from amputations with pressure dressings or other methods as needed. With partial amputations, make sure to immobilize the part with bulky compression dressings and a splint to prevent further injury. Never detach partial amputations. For complete amputations, wrap the part in a sterile dressing, place it in a plastic bag, and follow your local protocols.
- Animal and human bites can result in serious infection and must be treated by a physician. Dogs and cats can carry rabies, an acute, potentially fatal viral infection present in their saliva. By law, all animal bites must be reported to the appropriate authority.
- Penetrating wounds may have entrance and exit wounds—for example, if the cause was a gun. Find out the caliber of the gun, if possible.
- If internal organs are protruding through an open wound, do not touch or move the exposed organs. Cover the wound with sterile gauze compresses moistened with sterile saline solution, and secure with an occlusive dressing.
- In the case of an impaled object, do not remove it. Stabilize it with a bulky dressing, and protect it from being moved during transport.
- An open neck injury can be life threatening. Bleeding control is crucial. Secure an occlusive dressing over the wound, and apply manual pressure.
- Although it is not always possible to use the sterile technique, you should make every effort to avoid further wound contamination. Irrigate open wounds with normal saline or sterile water to flush out contaminants.
- Burns are one of the most serious and painful of soft-tissue injuries. They can occur from heat (thermal), chemicals, electricity, and radiation.
- Burns are classified primarily by the depth and extent of the burn and the body area involved; they are superficial, partial-thickness, or full-thickness burns. The rule of nines and rule of palms can be used to estimate the surface area that has been burned.
- Although a burn may be the patient's most obvious injury, you should always perform a complete assessment to determine whether there are other, more serious injuries.
- Special emergency treatment considerations for burns include removing the patient from the burning area; removing jewelry and constrictive clothing; estimating the size of the burned area, covering it with a dry, sterile dressing; covering the stretcher with a burn sheet prior to placing the patient on it; and covering the patient with a clean blanket to prevent hypothermia.
- Be alert to signs and symptoms of inhalation injury such as difficulty breathing, stridor, and/or wheezing. Follow local protocols regarding cooling measures.
- Treat the patient for shock if necessary. Provide circulatory support, including establishing intravenous access and administering an isotonic crystalloid solution according to the Consensus formula, and proper positioning.
- There are several types of burns. A thermal burn is caused by heat, commonly an open flame. Types of thermal burns include scald burns, contact burns, steam burns, and flash burns. Follow the standard assessment and treatment process for burns.
- Inhalation burns can cause rapid and serious airway compromise, resulting in coughing, wheezing, and rapid swelling or edema of the mucosa of the upper airway tissues, often evidenced by stridor. Consider requesting paramedic backup if the patient has stridor, a hoarse voice, singed nasal hairs, singed facial hairs, burns of the face, or carbon particles in the sputum.
- A chemical burn can occur whenever a toxic substance contacts the body. You may need to wait for hazardous materials personnel before treating the patient. Wear protective equipment. A dry chemical must be brushed off the skin and clothing before flushing the patient with water. Remove the patient's clothing before flushing with water. Treat chemical burns to the eyes by flushing with copious amounts of water or a sterile saline irrigation solution. Avoid contaminating areas that were not yet exposed to the chemical, such as the other eye.
- Electrical burns can cause thermal injury, vascular injury, renal injury, compartment syndrome, and

Prep Kit *(continued)*

possible cardiac arrest. There will be an entrance and an exit wound. Do not touch power lines. Never attempt to remove someone from an electrical source unless you are specifically trained to do so. Consider paramedic backup for early intubation.

- Radiation injuries are caused by ionizing radiation emitted by certain sources. Acute exposure to radiation may result in burns and radiation sickness or radiation poisoning. Symptoms of radiation sickness include nausea, weakness, hair loss, skin burns, and/or diminished organ function. Radiation burns require special rescue techniques beyond the initial training of AEMTs.

▶ Vital Vocabulary

abrasion The loss or damage of the superficial layer of skin as a result of a body part rubbing or scraping across a rough or hard surface.

air embolism A condition resulting when veins of the neck are open to the environment and suck in air.

amputation The removal of a body part (complete avulsion).

avulsion An injury in which soft tissue is torn completely loose or is hanging as a flap.

burns Injuries in which the soft tissue receives more energy than it can absorb without injury, from thermal heat, frictional heat, toxic chemicals, electricity, or nuclear radiation.

closed injury An injury in which damage occurs beneath the skin or mucous membrane but the surface remains intact.

compartment syndrome Swelling in a confined space that produces dangerous pressure; may cut off blood flow or damage sensitive tissue.

Consensus formula A formula that recommends giving 2 to 4 mL of lactated Ringer solution for each kilogram of body weight, multiplied by the percentage of total body surface area burned during the first 24 hours following the burn; one-half of the volume is given in the first 8 hours and the other half in the next 16 hours; sometimes used to calculate fluid needs during lengthy transport times; formerly called the Parkland formula.

contact burn A burn produced by touching a hot object.

contamination The presence of infectious organisms (pathogens) or foreign bodies such as dirt, gravel, or metal in a wound.

contusion A bruise without a break in the skin.

crush syndrome A significant metabolic derangement that can result in renal failure and death. It develops when crushed extremities or other body parts remain trapped for prolonged periods.

dermis The inner layer of the skin, containing hair follicles, sweat glands, nerve endings, and sebaceous glands.

ecchymosis The discoloration associated with a closed wound; signifies bleeding.

epidermis The outer layer of skin that acts as a watertight protective covering.

eschar The thick, coagulated crust or slough of leathery skin that develops following a burn.

evisceration The displacement of organs outside the body.

fasciitis Inflammation of the fascia.

flame burn A thermal burn caused by flames touching the skin.

full-thickness burns The burns that affect all skin layers and may affect the subcutaneous layers, muscle, bone, and internal organs, leaving the area dry, leathery, and white, dark brown, or charred (eschar); formerly called a third-degree burn.

gangrene An infection commonly caused by *Clostridium perfringens*. The result is tissue destruction and gas production that may result in death.

hematoma Blood collected within the body's tissues or in a body cavity.

inhalation injury An injury to the airway as a result of breathing smoke and toxic chemicals into the lungs and airway.

laceration A smooth or jagged open wound.

mucous membranes The linings of body cavities and passages that are in direct contact with the outside environment.

necrotizing fasciitis Death of tissue from bacterial infection, caused by more than one infecting organism—most commonly, *Staphylococcus aureus* and hemolytic streptococci; this condition has a high mortality rate.

occlusive dressing A dressing made of petroleum (Vaseline) gauze, aluminum foil, or plastic that prevents air and liquids from entering or exiting a wound.

open injury An injury in which there is a break in the surface of the skin or the mucous membrane, exposing deeper tissue to potential contamination.

partial-thickness burns The burns affecting the epidermis and some portion of the dermis but not the subcutaneous tissue, characterized by blisters and skin that is white to red, moist, and mottled; formerly called a second-degree burn.

Prep Kit *(continued)*

penetrating wound An injury that penetrates the skin, resulting from a sharp, pointed object or a blunt object traveling at sufficient speed, such as a knife or a bullet.

rabid Describes an animal that is infected with rabies.

rule of nines A system that assigns percentages to sections of the body, allowing calculation of the amount of skin surface involved in the burn area.

rule of palms A system that estimates total body surface area burned by comparing the affected area with the size of the patient's palm, which is roughly equivalent to 1% of the patient's total body surface area.

scald burn A burn produced by hot liquids.

steam burn A burn that has been caused by direct exposure to hot steam exhaust, as from a broken pipe.

superficial burns The burns affecting only the epidermis, characterized by skin that is red but not blistered or actually burned through; formerly called a first-degree burn.

tension lines The pattern of tautness of the skin, which is arranged over body structures and affects how well wounds heal.

tetanus A disease caused by spores that enter the body through a puncture wound contaminated with animal feces, street dust, or soil or that can enter through contaminated street drugs.

thermal burn A burn that results from heat, usually fire.

zone of coagulation The reddened area surrounding the leathery and sometimes charred tissue that has sustained a full-thickness burn.

zone of hyperemia In a thermal burn, the area that is least affected by the burn injury; an area of increased blood flow where the body is attempting to repair injured but otherwise viable tissue.

zone of stasis The peripheral area surrounding the zone of coagulation that has decreased blood flow and inflammation; it can undergo necrosis within 24 to 48 hours after the injury, particularly if perfusion is compromised because of burn shock.

References

1. Causey WA. Staphylococcal and streptococcal infections of the skin. *Prim Care.* 1979;6(1):127-139. https://www.ncbi.nlm.nih.gov/pubmed/379890. Accessed April 17, 2017.
2. Centers for Disease Control and Prevention. Trauma statistics. National Trauma Institute website. http://nationaltraumainstitute.net/home/trauma_statistics.html. Updated February 2014. Accessed December 5, 2017.
3. Wachtel TL, Berry CC, Wachtel EE, Frank HA. The inter-rater reliability of estimating the size of burns from various burn area chart drawings. *Burns.* 2000;26(2):156.
4. Ahrens M. Characteristics of home fire victims. National Fire Protection Association website. http://www.nfpa.org/news-and-research/fire-statistics-and-reports/fire-statistics/demographics-and-victim-patterns/characteristics-of-home-fire-victims. Published October 2014. Accessed April 12, 2017.
5. US fire deaths, fire death rates, and risk of dying in a fire. US Fire Administration website. https://www.usfa.fema.gov/data/statistics/fire_death_rates.html. Accessed November 30, 2017.
6. Current cigarette smoking among adults in the United States. Centers for Disease Control and Prevention website. https://www.cdc.gov/tobacco/data_statistics/fact_sheets/adult_data/cig_smoking/index.htm. Updated December 1, 2016. Accessed November 30, 2017.
7. Safety facts on scald burns. Burn Foundation website. http://www.burnfoundation.org/programs/resource.cfm?c = 1&a = 3. Accessed April 12, 2017.
8. Hall JR. Fatal effects of fire. National Fire Protection Association website. http:// www.nfpa.org/news-and-research/fire-statistics-and-reports/fire-statistics/demographics-and-victim-patterns/fatal-effects-of-fire. Published March 2011. Accessed April 12, 2017.
9. American Burn Association. Electrical safety educator's guide. *ameriburn.org/wp-content/uploads/2017/04/electricalsafetyeducatorsguide.pdf.* Accessed December 22, 2017.
10. Reuters finds 1,005 deaths in U.S. involving Tasers, largest accounting to date. Reuters website. https://www.reuters.com/article/us-axon-taser-toll/reuters-finds-1005-deaths-in-u-s-involving-tasers-largest-accounting-to-date-idUSKCN1B21AH. August 22, 2017. Accessed January 3, 2018.
11. Thompson CW, Berman M. Improper techniques, increased risks. Washington Post website. http://www.washingtonpost.com/sf/investigative/2015/11/26/improper-techniques-increased-risks/?utm_term=.3969aab0eb4e. Published November 26, 2015. Accessed January 3, 2018.
12. Fire is a possibility when using alcohol-based pepper spray with Tasers. Police One website. https://www.policeone.com/police-products/less-lethal/articles/92573-Fire-is-a-Possibility-When-Using-Alcohol-Based-Pepper-Spray-With-Tasers/. Published October 5, 2004. Accessed April 12, 2017.
13. Turai I, Veress K. Radiation accidents: occurrence, types, consequences, medical management, and the lessons to be learned. *Cent Eur J Occup Environ Med.* 2001;7(1):3-14.

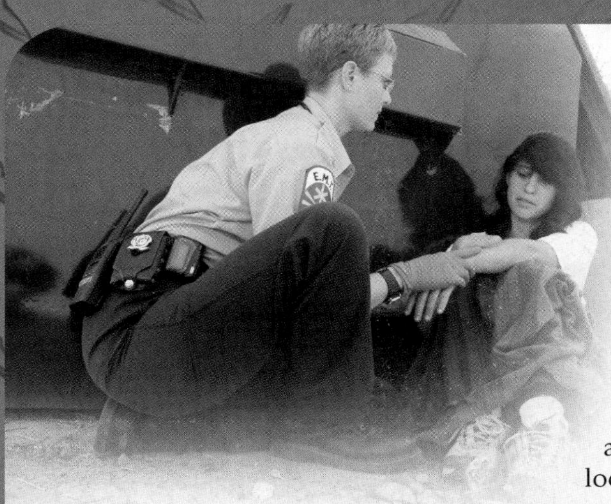

Assessment *in Action*

You are dispatched to a local automotive repair shop for a 33-year-old man who is bleeding. On arrival, you are directed to the bathroom where you find a man leaning over the sink, bleeding profusely from a laceration on his right forearm. He states that he was grinding a part and it slipped, sending his arm into the grinding wheel. There is a flap of skin hanging loosely from a small point of attachment below the laceration.

1. What type of injury does this patient have?

- **A.** Penetrating
- **B.** Blunt
- **C.** Thermal
- **D.** Crushing

2. How should you attempt to control the severe bleeding if initial attempts of direct pressure do not work?

- **A.** Splinting
- **B.** Pressure dressing
- **C.** Tourniquet
- **D.** Elevation

3. What should be done with the avulsed skin?

- **A.** Remove it completely and transport with patient.
- **B.** Place in the normal position and bandage.
- **C.** Bandage in the position found.
- **D.** Clean thoroughly and bandage.

4. After applying a dressing and bandage, a _____ may also help reduce movement and control bleeding.

- **A.** splint
- **B.** sling
- **C.** swathe
- **D.** cravat

5. A(n) ______ is blood that has collected within damaged tissue or in a body cavity.

- **A.** abrasion
- **B.** laceration
- **C.** avulsion
- **D.** hematoma

6. The _______ is the inner layer of the skin that lies below the germinal cells of the epidermis.

- **A.** dermis
- **B.** fascia
- **C.** subcutaneous fatty tissue
- **D.** erector pili

7. You treat a closed soft-tissue injury by applying the mnemonic RICES. The "I" stands for:

- **A.** immobilization.
- **B.** ice.
- **C.** injection.
- **D.** insulation.

8. If internal organs are protruding through an open wound, you should:

- **A.** attempt to replace them.
- **B.** cover with a dry dressing.
- **C.** cover with a moist dressing.
- **D.** rinse with sterile water and leave exposed.

9. Explain what happens in crush syndrome.

10. List the components for assessment of the neurologic system.

CHAPTER 29

Face and Neck Injuries

National EMS Education Standard Competencies

Medicine

Applies fundamental knowledge to provide basic and selected advanced emergency care and transportation based on assessment findings for an acutely ill patient.

Diseases of the Eyes, Ears, Nose, and Throat

Recognition and management of

- Nosebleed (pp 1184-1185)

Trauma

Applies fundamental knowledge to provide basic and selected advanced emergency care and transportation based on assessment findings for an acutely injured patient.

Head, Facial, Neck, and Spine Trauma

Recognition and management of

- Life threats (pp 1170-1171)
- Spine trauma (Chapter 30, *Head and Spine Injuries*)

Pathophysiology, assessment, and management of

- Penetrating neck trauma (pp 1188-1189)
- Laryngotracheal injuries (pp 1189-1190)
- Spine trauma (Chapter 30, *Head and Spine Injuries*)
- Facial fractures (pp 1167-1169, 1186-1187)
- Skull fractures (Chapter 30, *Head and Spine Injuries*)
- Foreign bodies in the eyes (pp 1175-1178)
- Dental trauma (pp 1169, 1187)

Knowledge Objectives

1. Review the anatomy and physiology of the head, face, and neck, including the major structures and specific landmarks that advanced emergency medical technicians must know. (pp 1163-1166)
2. Describe the factors that may cause the obstruction of the upper airway following a facial injury. (p 1166)
3. Discuss the causes and the patient care considerations related to each of the following types of facial injuries: soft-tissue injuries, nasal fractures, mandibular fractures, Le Fort fractures, orbital fractures, and zygomatic fractures. (pp 1167-1169)
4. Explain the patient assessment and management process of providing emergency medical care to the patient who has sustained facial and neck injuries. (pp 1169-1174)
5. List the steps in the emergency medical care of the patient with soft-tissue wounds of the face and neck. (pp 1174-1175)
6. List the steps in the emergency medical care of the patient with an eye injury based on the following scenarios: foreign object, impaled object, burns, lacerations, blunt trauma, closed head injuries, and blast injuries. (pp 1175-1184)
7. Describe the three different causes of burn injuries to the eye and the patient management considerations related to each cause. (pp 1177-1180)
8. List the steps in the emergency medical care of the patient with an injury of the nose. (pp 1184-1185)
9. List the steps in the emergency medical care of the patient with one of the following injuries of the ear: lacerations, avulsions, foreign body insertions, and perforation of the tympanic membrane. (pp 1185-1186)
10. List the steps in the emergency medical care of the patient with a facial fracture. (pp 1186-1187)
11. List the steps in the emergency medical care of the patient with dental and cheek injuries, including management of oropharyngeal bleeding, impaled objects, and avulsed teeth. (p 1187)
12. List the steps in the emergency medical care of the patient with an upper airway injury caused by blunt trauma. (pp 1187-1188)
13. List the steps in the emergency medical care of the patient with a penetrating injury to the neck, including management of regular and life-threatening bleeding and impaled objects. (pp 1188-1189)
14. List the steps in the emergency medical care of the patient with laryngeal injuries, including both open and occult injuries. (pp 1189-1190)
15. List the steps in the emergency medical care of the patient with muscular injuries of the neck, including both sprains and strains. (p 1190)

Skills Objectives

1. Demonstrate the care of a patient who has a penetrating eye injury. (pp 1175, 1176-1178, 1180-1181)
2. Demonstrate the removal of a foreign object from under a patient's upper eyelid. (pp 1176-1177, Skill Drill 29-1)
3. Demonstrate the stabilization of a foreign object that has been impaled in a patient's eye. (pp 1177-1178, Skill Drill 29-2)
4. Demonstrate irrigation of a patient's eye using a nasal cannula, bottle, or basin. (pp 1178-1180)
5. Demonstrate how to control bleeding from a neck injury. (pp 1188-1189, Skill Drill 29-3)

Introduction

Because the face and neck are among the most exposed regions of the body, they are frequently subjected to traumatic forces ranging from simple falls to assaults to direct blunt forces sustained in motor vehicle crashes (MVCs). Whereas other regions of the body are often covered with clothing and protective equipment, the face and neck generally do not have this same level of protection; therefore, these areas are particularly vulnerable to injury. In many cases, the injuries in this region will be some of the first you see when you arrive at the patient's side. Moreover, these injuries can be some of the most graphic. Be careful not to focus solely on these distracting injuries to avoid increasing the risk of missing other life threats.

Soft-tissue injuries and fractures to the bones of the face are common, although they vary greatly in severity. Some are potentially life threatening, and many leave disfiguring scars if not treated properly. Penetrating trauma to the neck may cause severe bleeding. An open injury may allow an air embolism to enter the circulatory system. If a hematoma forms in this area, then it may stop or slow blood flow to the brain, causing a stroke. Nevertheless, with appropriate prehospital and hospital care, even a patient with a seemingly devastating injury can have a surprisingly good outcome.

As an advanced emergency medical technician (AEMT), your objectives when treating a patient with face and neck injuries include preventing further injury (particularly to the cervical spine), managing any acute airway problems, and controlling bleeding. This chapter will first review the anatomy of the head and neck. Next, it will examine the factors that can produce upper airway obstruction. The chapter will then cover emergency medical care of soft-tissue wounds of the face, nose, and ear; facial fractures; penetrating injuries of the neck; and dental injuries.

Chapter 30, *Head and Spine Injuries*, discusses injuries specific to the head and to the spine and spinal cord, including traumatic brain injuries, skull fractures, and spine fractures. These injuries often occur in conjunction with facial trauma.

Anatomy and Physiology Review

Bones and Landmarks

The head is divided into two parts: the cranium and the face. The cranium, or skull, contains the brain. The face is composed of the eyes, ears, nose, mouth, and cheeks. The facial skeleton is composed of six major bones: the nasal bone, the two maxillae (upper jaw bones), the two zygomas (cheek bones), and the mandible (jaw bone) Figure 29-1.

YOU are the Provider — PART 1

While you and your partner are at the station, your partner remarks that he is surprised the ambulance has not been dispatched to a farming incident in the area because sugar beet harvest is in full swing. Just then, dispatch alerts you to a "machinery accident" at a beet field about 5 miles (8 km) west of town. You look at your partner with a knowing look on your face, then you begin your response. As you are responding, dispatch informs you that the fire department is also responding and that the patient is alert and oriented, with an unknown object stuck in his neck.

When you arrive on scene, you find the patient practically giving a hug to some type of farm implement. You can see a 3-foot (0.9 m) piece of round metal, approximately 0.5 inch (1 cm) in diameter, sticking out of the left side of his neck. It appears that the other end is still connected to the farm implement.

1. On the basis of the information provided to you, what are some possible injuries you may encounter?
2. What is the best way to remove the piece of metal from the machinery?

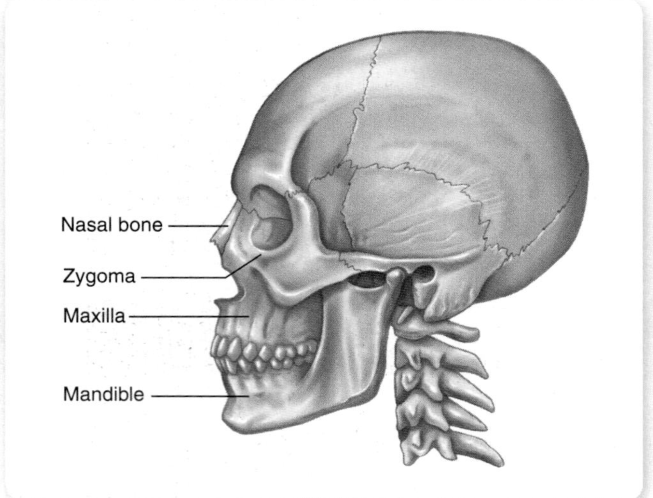

Figure 29-1 The face is composed of six bones: the nasal bone, two maxillae, two zygomas, and the mandible.

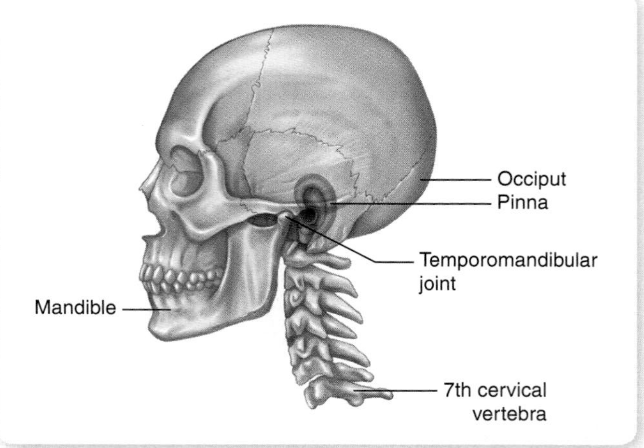

Figure 29-2 Specific landmarks of the head and neck include the pinna, the mandible, the occiput, the seventh cervical vertebra, and the temporomandibular joint.

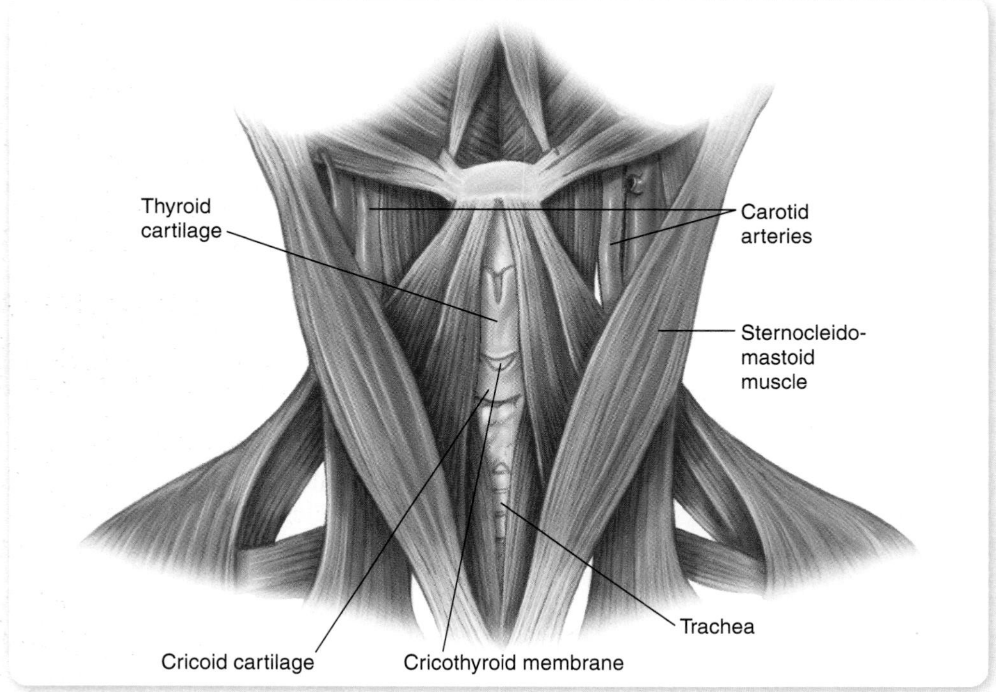

Figure 29-3 Important landmarks in the anterior region of the neck include the cricoid cartilage, the thyroid cartilage, the carotid arteries, the cricothyroid membrane, and the sternocleidomastoid muscles.

The mandible forms the jaw and chin **Figure 29-2**. Motion of the mandible occurs at the **temporomandibular joint**, which lies just in front of the ear on either side of the face. The semicircular **hyoid bone** "floats" in the superior aspect of the neck just below the mandible. Although not actually part of the face or skull, it supports and stabilizes the larynx and serves as a point of attachment for many important neck and tongue muscles.

The principal structures of the anterior region of the neck include the thyroid and cricoid cartilage, trachea, and numerous muscles and nerves **Figure 29-3**. The firm prominence in the center of the anterior surface, commonly known as the Adam's apple, is the upper part of the larynx, formed by the thyroid cartilage **Figure 29-4**. The cricoid cartilage is a firm ridge of cartilage (the only complete circular cartilage structure of the trachea) found below the thyroid cartilage. Between the thyroid cartilage and the cricoid cartilage is a thin sheet of connective tissue (fascia)—the cricothyroid membrane—that joins the two cartilages.

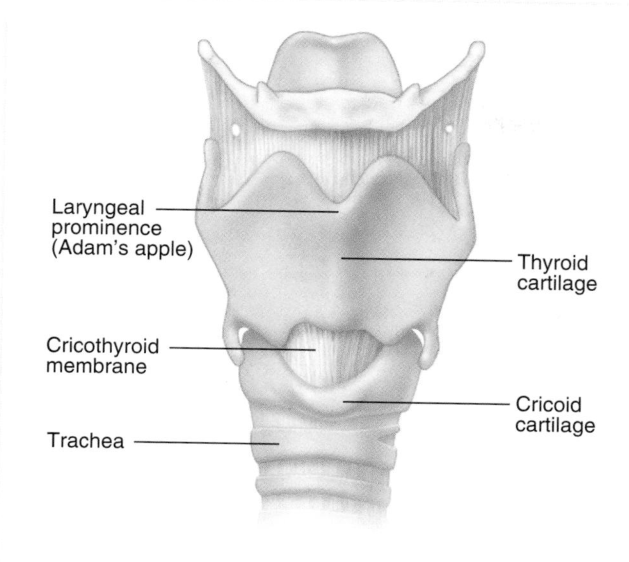

Figure 29-4 The larynx.

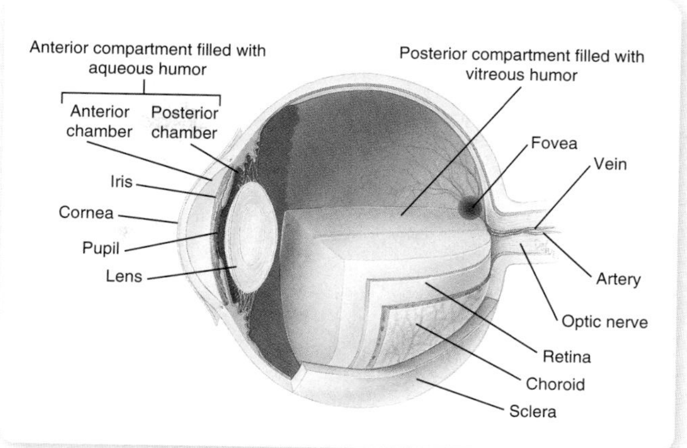

Figure 29-5 The major components of the eye.

The trachea connects the oropharynx and the larynx with the main air passages of the lungs (the bronchi). Pulsations of the carotid arteries are easily palpable in a groove approximately 0.5 inch (1 cm) lateral to the larynx. Lying immediately adjacent to these arteries, but not palpable, are the internal jugular veins and several important nerves. Lateral to these vessels and nerves lie the **sternocleidomastoid muscles**, which allow movement of the head.

A series of bony prominences, known as the spines of the cervical vertebrae, lie posteriorly, in the midline of the neck. The lower cervical spines are more prominent than the upper ones. They are more easily palpable when the neck is in flexion.

▶ The Eye

The eye is globe shaped, approximately 1 inch (2 cm) in diameter, and located within a bony socket in the skull called the orbit **Figure 29-5**. The eyes are held in place by loose connective tissue and several muscles; these muscles control the movement of the eyes. The **oculomotor nerve** innervates these muscles and carries parasympathetic nerve fibers that cause constriction of the pupil and accommodation of the lens. The **optic nerve** provides the sense of vision.

The orbit forms the base of the floor of the cranial cavity, and directly above it are the frontal lobes of the brain. Between and below the orbits are the nasal bone and the sinuses, respectively. Therefore, any severe injury to the face or head can potentially damage the eyeball or the muscles attached to the eyeball that cause the eye to move.

The eyeball, or **globe**, keeps its global shape as a result of the pressure of the fluid contained within its two chambers. The anterior chamber is filled with **aqueous humor**, a clear watery fluid. If there is a loss of aqueous humor through a penetrating injury to the eye, then it will gradually be replenished. The posterior chamber is filled with **vitreous humor**, a jellylike substance that maintains the shape of the globe. If there is a loss of vitreous humor, then it cannot be replenished, and blindness may result. The white of the eye, called the **sclera**, extends over the surface of the globe.

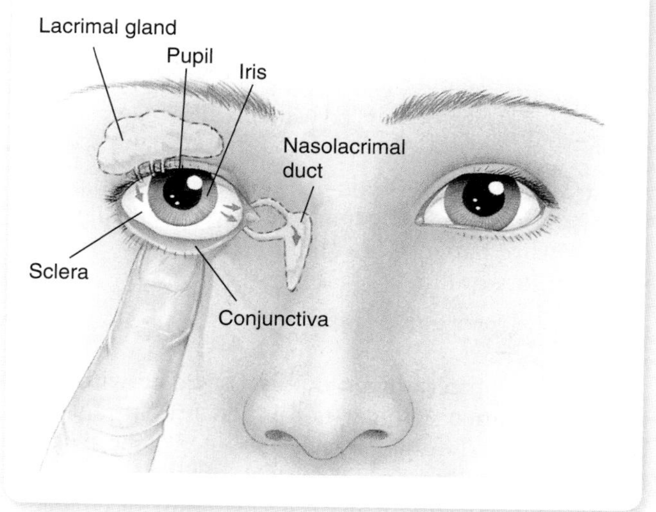

Figure 29-6 The lacrimal system consists of tear glands and ducts. Tears act as lubricants and keep the front of the eye from drying out.

The inner surface of the eyelids and the exposed surface of the eye itself, which are covered by a delicate membrane, the **conjunctiva**, are kept moist by fluid produced by the **lacrimal glands**, often called tear glands **Figure 29-6**.

The opening in the center of the iris, which allows light to move to the back of the eye, is called the **pupil**. Like the opening in a camera, the pupil becomes smaller in bright light and larger in dim light. Normally, the pupils in both

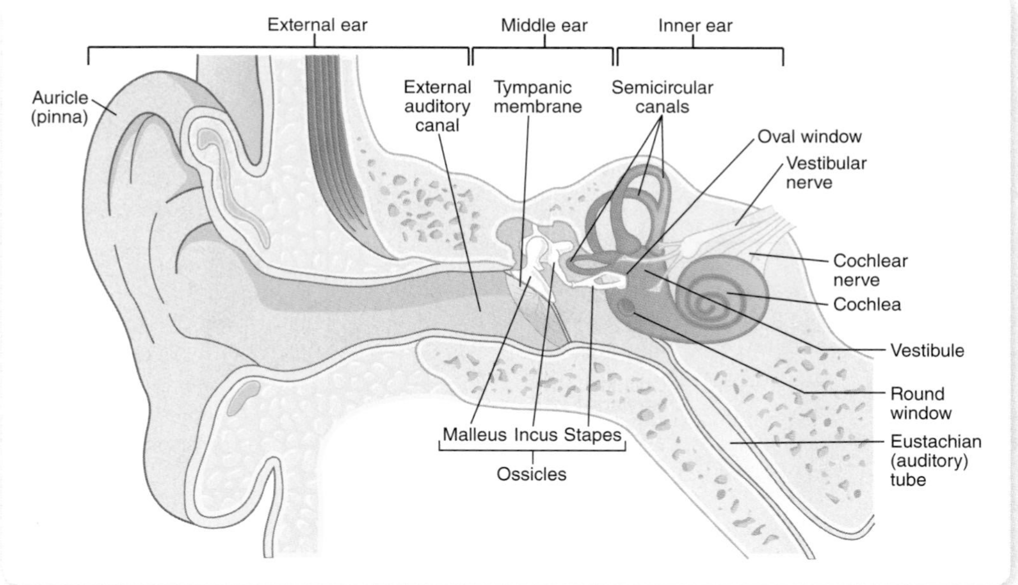

Figure 29-7 The ear has three principal parts: the external ear, composed of the pinna, external auditory canal, and tympanic membrane; the middle ear; and the inner ear, composed of bony chambers filled with fluid.

eyes are equal in size. Some people are born with pupils that are not equal (**anisocoria**); however, particularly in unresponsive patients, unequal pupil size may indicate serious injury or illness of the brain or eye.

▶ The Ear

The ear is a complex organ that is associated with hearing and balance. The ear is divided into three parts **Figure 29-7**. The external ear is composed of the **pinna**, or auricle, which is the part lying outside of the head, and the external auditory canal, which leads in toward the tympanic membrane, or eardrum. The middle ear contains three small bones (the malleus, incus, and stapes) that move in response to sound waves hitting the tympanic membrane. It is connected to the nasal cavity by the eustachian tube, which permits equalization of pressure in the middle ear when external atmospheric pressure changes. The inner ear is composed of bony chambers filled with fluid. As the head moves, so does the fluid. In response, fine nerve endings within the fluid send impulses to the brain indicating the position of the head and the rate of change of position.

Pathophysiology

Injuries of the face and neck can often lead to partial or complete obstruction of the upper airway. Several factors may contribute to the obstruction. Because the face is highly vascular, bleeding from facial injuries can be very heavy, producing large blood clots in the upper airway that can lead to complete obstruction, particularly in a patient who is not fully alert. In particular, direct injuries to the nose and mouth, the larynx, or the trachea are often the source of significant bleeding or respiratory compromise. You may need to suction the airway if you are unable to control the bleeding. In addition, the injuries may cause loosened teeth or dentures to become dislodged into the throat where they may be swallowed or aspirated. The swelling that often accompanies direct and indirect injury to the soft tissues in these areas can also contribute to airway obstruction.

The airway may also be affected when the patient's head is turned to the side, as often is done when the patient has an altered level of consciousness or is unresponsive. Other factors that interfere with normal respirations include possible injuries to the brain and/or cervical spine that may be associated with facial injuries. If the great vessels in the neck are injured, then significant bleeding and pressure on the upper airway are common; these can result in airway obstruction as well. In addition to causing massive bleeding and hemorrhagic shock, injury to any of these major vessels can produce cerebral hypoxia, infarct, air embolism, and permanent neurologic impairment.

Depending on the mechanism of injury (MOI), there may be a cervical spine injury. If there is significant impact to the face, suspect accompanying cervical spine injury and follow your agency's protocol for cervical injuries.

Special Populations

The proportionately larger amount of body surface area in the head and scalp of infants and toddlers increases the chances of injuries to the face and scalp, and a blood loss that results in this age group can quickly become significant. Consider the potential for shock and treat promptly and aggressively.

► Soft-Tissue Injuries

Soft-tissue injuries of the face and neck are very common. Because the face and neck are extremely vascular, swelling in this area from soft-tissue injuries may be more severe than in other injured parts of the body and may cause airway compromise and ventilatory insufficiency. The skin and underlying tissues in these areas have a rich blood supply, so bleeding from penetrating injuries may be heavy. Even minor soft-tissue wounds of the face and neck may bleed profusely. A blunt injury that does not break the skin may cause a break in a blood vessel wall, leading blood to collect under the skin; this is called a hematoma Figure 29-8. In some situations, a flap of skin is peeled back, or avulsed, from the underlying muscle and fascia Figure 29-9. Although open soft-tissue injuries to the face—lacerations, abrasions, and avulsions—by themselves are rarely life threatening, their presence, especially following a significant MOI, suggests the potential for more severe injuries (eg, closed head and cervical spine injuries).

Maintain a high index of suspicion when a patient presents with closed soft-tissue injuries to the face, such as contusions and hematomas. These indicators of blunt-force trauma suggest the potential for more severe underlying injuries.

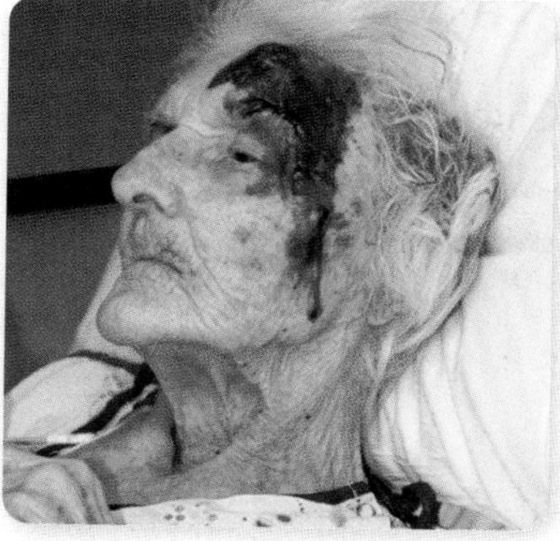

Figure 29-8 Facial hematoma.

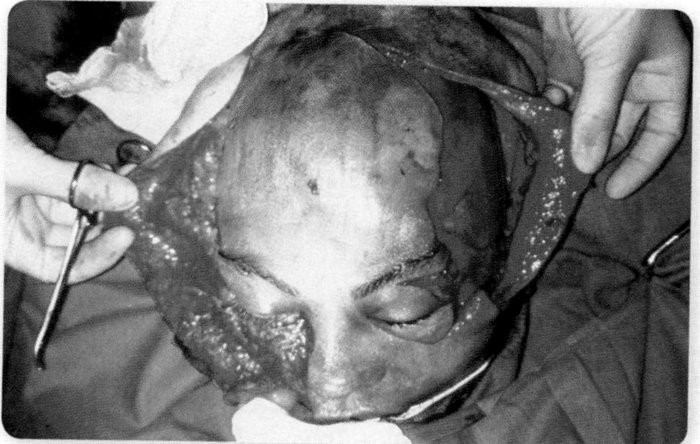

Figure 29-9 A major avulsion injury is characterized by a large flap of skin that is peeled back from the underlying muscle and tissue.

Impaled objects in the soft tissues or bones of the face may occur in association with facial trauma. Although these objects can damage facial nerves, the risk of airway compromise is of far greater consequence. This is especially true when an impaled object penetrates the cheek, because massive oropharyngeal bleeding can result in airway obstruction, aspiration, and ventilatory inadequacy. In addition, blood is a gastric irritant. Swallowing even a few tablespoons of blood can make a patient vomit, further increasing the likelihood of aspiration.

> **Words of Wisdom**
>
> Carefully assess a patient with soft-tissue injuries to the face, especially if he or she has experienced a significant mechanism of injury. Although facial lacerations and avulsions are often the most obvious and dramatic injuries, they are usually not life threatening. Do not get tunnel vision or be fooled into thinking this is the patient's only injury.

► Facial Fractures

Facial fractures commonly occur when the facial bones absorb the energy of a strong impact. The forces involved in some incidents may be massive; the magnitude of force required to fracture the maxilla (the upper jaw bone) will likely produce closed head injuries and cervical spine injuries as well. Therefore, when you assess a patient with a suspected facial fracture, protect the patient's cervical spine and monitor the patient's neurologic signs, specifically the level of consciousness.

> **Words of Wisdom**
>
> The magnitude of force required to fracture the maxilla can easily produce closed head injuries and cervical spine injuries as well!

A deep facial laceration should increase your index of suspicion that the underlying bone may have been fractured, and pain over a bone tends to support the suspicion of fracture. Other general signs and symptoms of facial fractures include ecchymosis, swelling, pain on palpation, crepitus, misalignment of the teeth, facial deformities or asymmetry, instability of the facial bones, impaired ocular movement, and visual disturbances.

Nasal Fractures

Because the nasal bones are not as structurally sound as the other bones of the face, nasal fractures are the most common facial fracture. These fractures are characterized by swelling, tenderness, and crepitus when the nasal bone is palpated. Deformity of the nose, if present, usually appears as lateral displacement of the nasal bone from its normal midline position.

Nasal fractures, like any facial fracture, are often complicated by the presence of an anterior or a posterior nosebleed (**epistaxis**), which can compromise the patient's airway.

Mandibular Fractures

Second only to nasal fractures in frequency, fractures of the mandible typically result from massive blunt-force trauma to the lower third of the face; they are particularly common following an assault injury. Because significant force is required to fracture the mandible, this structure may be fractured in more than one place and, therefore, unstable to palpation. The fracture site itself is most commonly located at the angle of the jaw.

Mandibular fractures should be suspected in patients with a history of blunt force trauma to the lower third of the face who present with dental **malocclusion** (misalignment of the teeth), numbness of the chin, and inability to open the mouth. There will likely be swelling and ecchymosis over the fracture site, and teeth may be partially or completely avulsed. As the patient moves his or her jaw to speak and answer your questions, take note of the patient's symptoms of pain, such as decreased normal range of motion. In some patients, you might elicit tenderness, for example, by palpating specific locations on the mandible such as near the joints or specific impact points. This "point tenderness" and pain on motion can identify injuries that patients might not have otherwise reported because they may be distracted by other wounds.

Temporomandibular joint dislocations may occur as a result of blunt force trauma to the lower third of the face, but this outcome is rare. Such dislocations are most often the result of exaggerated yawning or otherwise widely opening the mouth. Patients commonly feel a "pop" and then they cannot close their mouths; the mouth becomes locked in a wide-open position. The jaw muscles eventually go into spasm, causing severe pain.

Maxillary Fractures

Midfacial structures include the maxilla, zygoma, orbital floor, and nose. Maxillary fractures are most commonly associated with mechanisms that produce massive blunt facial trauma, such as MVCs, falls, and assaults. The signs include massive facial swelling, instability of the midfacial bones, malocclusion, and an elongated appearance of the patient's face.

Le Fort fractures are classified into three categories **Figure 29-10**:

- **Le Fort I fracture.** A horizontal fracture of the maxilla that separates the hard palate and lower maxilla from the remainder of the skull.
- **Le Fort II fracture.** A fracture involving the nasal bone and inferior maxilla. A Le Fort II fracture separates the nasal bone and lower maxilla from the facial skull and remainder of the cranial bones.
- **Le Fort III fracture (craniofacial disjunction).** A fracture of all midfacial bones, separating the entire midface from the cranium.

Le Fort fractures can occur as isolated fractures (Le Fort I) or in combination (Le Fort I and II), depending on the location of impact and the amount of trauma.

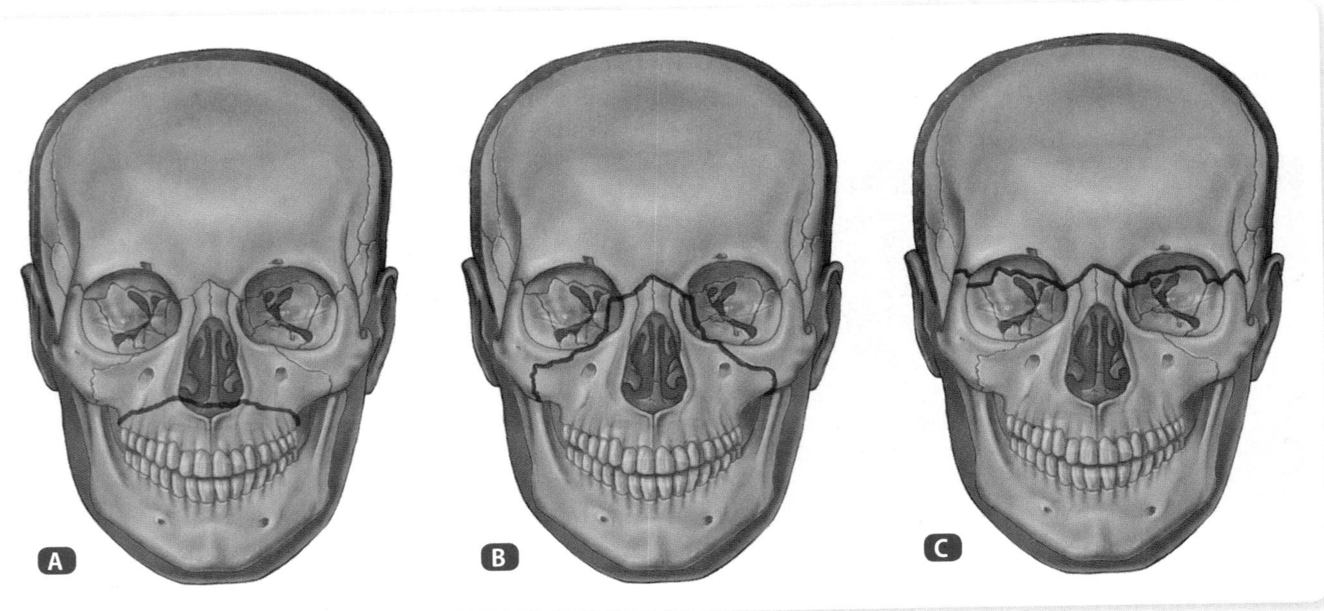

Figure 29-10 Le Fort fractures. **A.** Le Fort I. **B.** Le Fort II. **C.** Le Fort III.

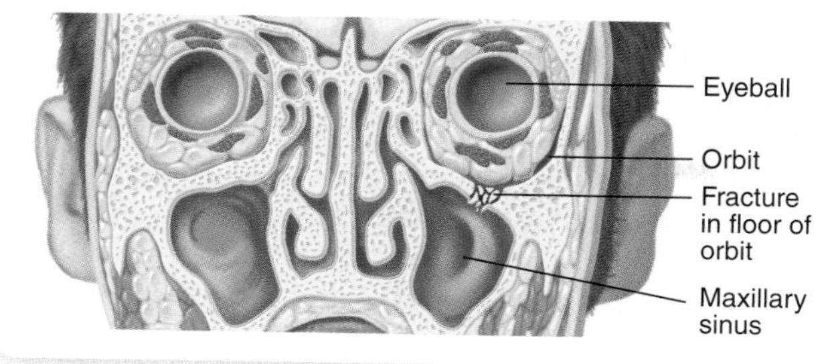

Figure 29-11 A blowout fracture of the left orbit.

Orbital Fractures

The patient with an orbital fracture, such as a **blowout fracture** Figure 29-11, may complain of double vision (**diplopia**) and lose sensation above the eyebrow or over the cheek because of associated nerve damage. Typically, this injury occurs when an object—a baseball or hockey puck, for example—strikes this region of the face during a sporting event.

The injury may cause the patient to have reduced sensation to areas that are innervated by the infraorbital nerve. The affected area extends from the tip of the nose, including the nares, and follows the margin of the maxilla, curving up to meet the temple. Also, the eyeball may retract posteriorly into the space created when the cavity is enlarged. Massive nasal discharge may occur, and vision is often impaired. Fractures of the inferior orbit are the most common type and can cause paralysis of upward gaze (the patient's injured eye will not be able to follow your finger above the midline).

Zygomatic Fractures

Fractures of the zygomatic bone (cheekbone) commonly result from blunt trauma in MVCs and assaults. When the zygomatic bone is fractured, that side of the patient's face appears flattened, and there is loss of sensation over the cheek, nose, and upper lip; paralysis of upward gaze may also be present. Other injuries and conditions commonly associated with zygomatic fractures include orbital fractures, ocular injury, and epistaxis.

Table 29-1 summarizes the characteristics of various facial fractures.

▶ Dental Injuries

Fractured and avulsed teeth are common following facial trauma. Dental injuries may be associated with mechanisms that cause severe maxillofacial trauma (eg, MVC), or they may occur in isolation (eg, a direct blow to the mouth from an assault). Always assess the patient's mouth following a facial injury, especially if your examination reveals fractured or avulsed teeth. Teeth fragments (or even whole teeth) can become an airway obstruction and should be removed immediately from the patient's mouth. In contrast, you should leave well-fitting dentures in place.

Table 29-1 Summary of Facial Fractures

Injury	Signs and Symptoms
Multiple facial bone fractures	▪ Massive facial swelling/ecchymosis ▪ Misalignment of teeth ▪ Palpable deformities and/or asymmetry ▪ Anterior or posterior epistaxis
Zygomatic and orbital fractures	▪ Loss of sensation below the orbit ▪ Flattening of the patient's cheek ▪ Paralysis of upward gaze ▪ Visual disturbances
Nasal fractures	▪ Crepitus and instability ▪ Swelling, tenderness, lateral displacement ▪ Anterior or posterior epistaxis
Maxillary (Le Fort) fractures	▪ Mobility of the facial skeleton ▪ Misalignment of teeth ▪ Facial swelling
Mandibular fractures	▪ Misalignment of teeth ▪ Mandibular instability

Patient Assessment

Scene Size-up

As you arrive on the scene, observe for hazards and threats to the safety of the crew, bystanders, and the patient. Assess the impact of hazards on patient care, and address those hazards. Assess for the potential for violence and assess for environmental hazards.

Patients who are alert and supine and have oral or facial bleeding may protect their airways by coughing, projecting the blood at you. Therefore, take standard precautions that require eye protection and a face mask. Also, put several pairs of gloves in your pocket for easy access in the event your gloves tear or you must treat multiple patients with bleeding.

Safety

Even minor facial injuries may result in copious bleeding. Always wear proper protective equipment.

If the incident involves a MVC, then you may be confronted with more than one patient in a vehicle. Determine the number of patients and consider if you need additional or specialized resources on the scene.

As you observe the scene, look for indicators of the MOI. This assessment helps you develop an early index of suspicion for underlying injuries in a patient who has sustained a significant MOI. As you put together information from dispatch and your observations of the scene, consider how the MOI produced the injuries expected. Common MOIs for face and neck injuries include MVCs, sports, falls, penetrating trauma, and blunt trauma. In MVCs, the probability of injury increases if the vehicle rolled over or came to an abrupt stop when striking an immovable object, such as a tree.

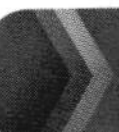

Primary Survey

The primary survey focuses on identifying and managing life-threatening concerns. *Do not let soft-tissue injuries distract you from life threats that may not be readily apparent.* Scene safety must always be first. After establishing scene safety, address any immediately obvious exsanguinating hemorrhage. Then begin the standard progression through the primary survey to include assessment and treatment of airway, breathing, and circulation.

As you approach the patient, look for important indicators to alert you to the seriousness of the patient's condition. For example, is the patient interacting with the environment or lying still, making no sounds? Assess for readily apparent life threats such as significant bleeding and signs such as changes in skin color. Combative or aggressive behavior can be a sign of a closed head injury. The general impression will help you develop an index of suspicion for serious injuries and determine your sense of urgency for medical intervention. If the patient has a potential neck or spine injury, then assign a crew member to achieve and maintain manual stabilization. Always check for responsiveness using the AVPU (Awake and alert, responsive to Verbal stimuli, responsive to Pain, Unresponsive) scale.

Ensure the patient has a clear and patent airway as soon as you arrive at the patient's side. Suction any blood, fluid, or vomit until the airway is clear. Teeth fragments (or even whole teeth) can become an airway obstruction and must be removed from the patient's mouth without delay. If the patient is unresponsive or has a significantly altered level of consciousness, then consider inserting a properly sized airway adjunct, such as an oropharyngeal airway. The use of a nasopharyngeal airway is controversial and is relatively contraindicated in the presence of midface trauma, as it is possible for it to penetrate the brain through a fracture. A nasopharyngeal airway should not be used in any patient with suspected nasal fractures or in patients with cerebrospinal fluid (CSF) or blood leakage from the nose or with any evidence of midface trauma, unless absolutely necessary. As always, be aware of and follow your local protocols.

Quickly assess for adequacy of breathing. Determine whether the patient's breathing is abnormally slow or

YOU are the Provider — PART 2

You begin your assessment of the patient and find that he is alert and oriented, and surprisingly calm, given the circumstances. He states he was attempting to free an obstruction in the piece of equipment when a tension rod broke free and impaled him in the neck. He states "it's getting hard to breathe" and that he has to "hug" the machine to keep from falling over. You instruct your partner to place the patient on a nonrebreathing mask with oxygen at 15 L/min. Fire department personnel arrive on scene, and after a brief meeting with the incident commander, he agrees with your recommendation to remove the tension rod, very carefully, from the implement. Prior to the removal, you need to attempt to secure the object in the patient's neck. You ask one of the available firefighters to maintain manual stabilization of the head.

Recording Time: 1 Minute	
Appearance	No apparent acute distress
Level of consciousness	Alert and oriented
Airway	Patent, with possible obstruction
Breathing	Difficult to assess; appears equal on both sides and adequate
Circulation	Warm, dry, and pink

3. How would you secure the tension rod to the patient?
4. Why should you be concerned about air entering the wound?

rapid, or excessively deep or shallow. An inadequate depth or rate that results in compromised breathing should prompt you to take immediate action. Advanced airway management may be needed. Assess for any injuries of the chest that may impede breathing, such as a flail segment or an open wound.

Words of Wisdom

Any patient who is having difficulty breathing should receive oxygen. If respirations are adequate, then administer oxygen as needed to maintain an oxygen saturation level of 94% or greater. However, *always treat the patient* and not a diagnostic tool. Pulse oximeters may show false readings in the presence of poor perfusion, carbon monoxide, and other circumstances.

Face and throat injuries increase the need for aggressive airway maintenance. Airway management can be especially challenging in patients with massive facial injuries. Oropharyngeal bleeding poses an immediate threat to the airway, and unstable facial bones can hinder your ability to maintain an effective mask-to-face seal for bag-mask ventilation. Still, airway and breathing take priority over soft-tissue injuries. Note the importance of suctioning and remember to reassess airway patency frequently. Call early for paramedic backup because endotracheal intubation—a paramedic skill—may be the method of choice for airway protection. If an airway cannot be established, paramedics may need to perform a surgical airway (ie, cricothyrotomy) to ventilate the patient.

Quickly palpate the pulse for rate and quality; determine the skin condition, color, and temperature; and check the capillary refill time. Significant bleeding is an immediate life threat and must be controlled quickly using the appropriate methods. Expose the patient and perform a rapid full-body scan prior to packaging the patient for transport.

Words of Wisdom

If significant trauma has likely affected multiple body systems, then expose the patient and perform a rapid exam to ensure you have found all significant injuries. A 60- to 90-second rapid full-body scan may identify factors that help you determine whether the patient requires prompt transport. Begin with the head and neck, while a partner is manually holding the head in place. When you are done, apply a cervical collar if you have not done so already and it is indicated by the patient presentation. If you identify life-threatening conditions or those that have the potential to become unstable, such as a distended abdomen or femur fracture, then the patient requires rapid and immediate transport to the closest most appropriate facility.

If the patient you are treating has an airway or a breathing problem or significant bleeding, then you must consider rapid transport to the closest, most appropriate facility. Stabilizing and maintaining the airway and breathing and controlling bleeding can be very difficult in patients with facial or neck injuries. Avoid delays in transport and consider paramedic backup or air transport if the transport time is long.

A patient with signs and symptoms of internal bleeding must be transported quickly to the appropriate hospital for surgical evaluation. Internal bleeding in face and throat injuries may compromise blood flow to the brain. Bleeding from the brain or major vessels of the throat can have a serious impact on the patient's airway. The condition of a patient with significant external bleeding or signs of significant internal bleeding may quickly become unstable. Treatment is directed at addressing immediate life threats and providing rapid transport to the closest appropriate hospital. If the patient is initially considered to be stable, then frequently reassess the patient and upgrade to rapid transport if the patient's condition worsens. Remember, any significant blow to the face or throat should increase your index of suspicion for a spinal or brain injury.

Provide rapid transport for any patient who presents with the following:

- Signs of hypoperfusion (tachycardia, tachypnea, weak pulse, pale/cool/moist skin, and/or hypotension)
- A significant MOI but in stable condition
- A poor general impression
- Any alteration in level of consciousness
- Abnormal vital signs
- Dyspnea
- Severe pain
- Isolated injuries to the eye

In some situations, surgical intervention and/or restoration of circulation to the eye will be required within 30 minutes or permanent blindness may result. Consider transporting the patient with serious, isolated eye injuries to an eye care specialty center depending on your local protocol.

In any patient with a significant MOI, maintain a high index of suspicion for internal injuries and shock, and transport the patient early. Do not wait for signs of shock to develop. Continue to maintain a high index of suspicion, and reassess your priority and transport decision as needed. Do not delay transport of a seriously injured patient, particularly one with significant bleeding even if controlled, to take the patient's history or perform a secondary assessment. Further assessment can continue during transport.

Words of Wisdom

Always consider the possibility of spinal injuries in patients with face and neck injuries.

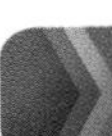

History Taking

After the life threats have been managed during the primary survey, investigate the chief complaint or history of present illness. Obtain a medical history and be alert for injury-specific signs and symptoms, as well as any pertinent negatives such as no pain or no loss of sensation.

Next, obtain a SAMPLE (Signs and symptoms, Allergies, Medications, Pertinent past medical history, Last oral intake, Events leading up to the illness or injury) history from the patient. Any information you obtain at this point will be valuable if the patient becomes unresponsive. If the patient is not responsive, then attempt to obtain the SAMPLE history from friends or family members who may be present. Otherwise, you may have to rely on your assessment and any medical alert jewelry or identification you find.

In an unresponsive patient, you will only be able to observe the signs of the patient's injuries. Any other information will need to be obtained from someone who is knowledgeable about the patient. Keep in mind the information you obtain may or may not be accurate and may be incomplete. The person providing the information may not be able to give you the actual names of the patient's medications but might be able to provide some pertinent medical history and possibly known allergies. Always document who gave you the information, and use quotation marks to indicate direct quotes.

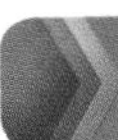

Secondary Assessment

If significant trauma has likely affected multiple systems in the patient, then start with a rapid full-body scan looking for DCAP-BTLS to confirm that you have found all life threats and injuries. When this step is completed, perform a detailed full-body exam. However, do not delay transport to complete a thorough physical examination.

Special Populations

In the geriatric population, poor skin tone and loss of body fat can produce significant soft-tissue injury in the presence of even a simple MOI. Anticoagulation therapy in older adult patients can lead to significant blood loss from minor insults. Additionally, normally trivial physical findings, such as bruises and minor lacerations, can be signs of severe underlying trauma such as traumatic brain injury.

In a responsive patient who has an isolated injury with a limited MOI, a head-to-toe exam is still necessary, but consider giving extra attention to the isolated injury, the patient's chief complaint, and the body region affected—in this case, the face and throat. Ensure your control of bleeding is maintained and note the location of the injury. Inspect open wounds for any foreign matter and stabilize impaled objects.

Special Populations

Relative to younger, healthy adults, older adult patients are at high risk for severe epistaxis following even minor facial injuries, especially patients with a history of hypertension or anticoagulant medication use (such as aspirin). This bleeding often originates in the posterior nasopharynx and may not be grossly evident during your assessment.

During the physical examination, look for swelling, deformities of the bones, contusions, and discoloration. Also gently palpate the face, looking and feeling for any abnormalities such as deformity or tenderness. Ask yourself the following questions:

1. Do the facial bones seem to be in alignment?
2. Does the nasal bone seem to deviate from the midline?
3. Note any variations from the normal facial examination; is there any facial drooping?
4. Does one eye appear to be lower than the other? If so, this is an indication of an orbital fracture.
5. Does the mandible appear to deviate toward one side or the other?

If the patient is responsive, then explain exactly what you are doing and what you are looking for. Your discovery of an abnormality may actually be an old injury that the patient can describe to you in more detail.

Assess all underlying systems. This assessment should include the neurologic system, including brain and major nerves; sensory organs, including the eyes and nose; the respiratory system, including mouth, nose, sinuses, and airway; and the circulatory system, particularly focusing on the carotid arteries and jugular veins.

When you evaluate the eyes, start on the outer aspect of the eye and work your way in toward the pupils. Examine the eye for any obvious foreign matter. The patient may relay pertinent information about this possibility to you ("I have something in my eye."). Quickly assess the patient's visual acuity—that is, the clarity of the patient's vision in each eye. Note any discoloration of the eye, bleeding in the iris area, or redness. Look for eye symmetry; asymmetry is a possible indication of a brain injury.

Look at each pupil for equal size and reaction to light. If the pupils are not symmetric, then ask the patient if he or she has had any previous eye surgeries or injuries. Previous surgery or injury, rather than brain injury, may be the root cause of the pupils not appearing the same. Cataract surgery can cause unequal pupils, but in a patient with a suspected head injury or ocular injury, anisocoria (unequal pupils in dim light) may be present. Determine whether the unequal pupils are caused by physiologic or pathologic issues. Using over-the-counter eye drops can change pupil size, and certain asthma inhalers can have the same effect if inadvertently sprayed into the eye. Brain injury, nerve disease, glaucoma, and meningitis are all possible causes of unequal pupils.

Words of Wisdom

When you treat an eye injury, remember to cover both eyes because they move consensually.

Check whether the patient has the ability to follow your finger from side to side as well as up and down, and whether he or she can read normal print. Note whether the patient reports blurry vision in either eye or a new sensitivity to light.

Assess vital signs to obtain a baseline so you can observe any changes the patient may display during treatment. A systolic blood pressure reading of less than 90 mm Hg with a weak, rapid pulse and cool, moist skin that is pale or gray should alert you to the presence of hypoperfusion in a patient who may have significant bleeding. Remember, you must be concerned with both visible bleeding and unseen bleeding inside a body cavity. With facial and throat injuries, baseline information about the rate and quality of respirations and pulse is very important, as is monitoring throughout patient care.

In addition to conducting a hands-on assessment, use monitoring devices to quantify the patient's oxygenation and circulatory status. You may also use noninvasive methods to monitor blood pressure. It is recommended that you always assess the patient's first blood pressure manually—that is, with a sphygmomanometer (blood pressure cuff) and stethoscope. Use a glucometer to assess blood glucose levels. An altered mental status in a trauma patient could be the result of hypoglycemia.

Words of Wisdom

Do not rely on diagnostic tools and forget to consider the condition of the patient. Pulse oximeters are not accurate if the patient has decreased perfusion. Treat the patient and not the device.

Reassessment

Repeat the primary survey. Reassess the patient's vital signs and chief complaint. In addition, continually reassess the adequacy of the patient's airway, breathing, and circulation. Recheck patient interventions. Are the treatments you provided for problems with the ABCs still effective? This consideration is particularly important in patients with facial or neck injuries because such injuries often affect associated systems, such as the respiratory (airway and breathing), circulatory, and nervous systems. Reassess the patient's condition at least every 5 minutes.

In your documentation, describe the MOI and the position in which you found the patient when you arrived at the scene. Document the method used to remove the patient

YOU are the Provider — PART 3

You place an occlusive dressing around the rod to reduce the chances of an air embolism, should an artery or vein be severed. After securing the dressing in place, you apply copious amounts of bulky dressings over the top of the occlusive dressing in an attempt to secure the rod as best as you can while fire department personnel begin to cut the distal end. Fire department personnel have chosen to use a hacksaw in an attempt to minimize movement to the rod and to minimize the transfer of heat. When they are approximately 80% through the rod, you note an increased amount of blood coming from the wound. You fear this may be arterial blood, so you ask fire department staff to immediately cease operations so you can assess the bleeding.

Recording Time: 8 Minutes	
Respirations	22 breaths/min; clear bilaterally
Pulse	122 beats/min
Skin	Warm, dry, and pink
Blood pressure	116/84 mm Hg
Oxygen saturation (Spo_2)	96% with oxygen at 15 L/min via nonrebreathing mask
Pupils	Pupils Equal, Round, and Reactive to Light and Accommodation (PERRLA)

5. How can you control bleeding from a neck wound?
6. Will this patient need to be immobilized with a cervical collar before transport? How will you immobilize his head?

from the vehicle, for example, "prolonged extrication." In patients with severe external bleeding, it is important to recognize, estimate, and report the amount of blood loss that has occurred and to indicate how rapidly or how much time has passed since the bleeding started. This task can be challenging, especially if the patient is lying on a wet surface or one that absorbs fluids, or if the environment is dark.

Call early to inform the hospital personnel about the various injuries involving the patient's head and neck. Specialists may need to be called to manage injuries involving the eyes, ears, teeth, mouth, sinuses, larynx, esophagus, or large vessels. These specialists are not always in the hospital, especially during the evening or night, or in smaller hospitals, so informing emergency department (ED) personnel of all injuries involving the face and throat can save valuable time.

Emergency Medical Care

Provide complete spinal immobilization to any patient with suspected spinal injuries. Spinal injuries should be suspected whenever a patient experiences significant trauma to the face or neck; the criteria for such suspicion are discussed in Chapter 30, *Head and Spine Injuries*. Maintain an open airway, be prepared to suction the patient, and consider placement of an oropharyngeal airway. Whenever you suspect significant bleeding, administer high-flow oxygen. Oxygen and airway maintenance are important for all patients with face and neck injuries. If needed, provide assisted ventilation using a bag-mask device with high-flow oxygen.

Control any significant visible bleeding. If the patient has signs of hypoperfusion, then aggressively treat him or her for shock and provide prompt transport to the closest, most appropriate facility. Do not delay transport of a seriously injured trauma patient to complete non–life-saving treatments in the field, such as splinting extremity fractures. Instead, complete these treatments en route to the hospital. If a spinal column injury is not suspected, the patient may be more comfortable and the airway may be easier to maintain in the sitting position during transport.

Gain intravenous access with one or two large-bore catheters, and give a 20-mL/kg bolus of an isotonic crystalloid solution to maintain radial pulses if signs of hypoperfusion are apparent. As discussed in Chapter 14, *Shock*, management of shock can be controversial in trauma patients. Ensure you follow local protocols, and do not delay transport in an effort to gain intravenous access on scene. Obtain vascular access en route if the patient is in unstable condition.

Assessment and Management of Specific Injuries

Soft-Tissue Injuries

All face and neck injuries are potentially serious. The emergency care of soft-tissue injuries to the face and neck must focus on protecting the airway. You should assess the ABCDEs and care for any life threats first. Remember to take standard precautions in all cases.

In the absence of life-threatening bleeding, your first step is to open and clear the airway. Securing and maintaining a patent airway is paramount. Because blood draining into the throat can produce vomiting and airway obstruction, the patient may need frequent suctioning. Take appropriate precautions if you suspect the patient has sustained a cervical spine injury; ensure you avoid moving the neck. Use the jaw-thrust maneuver to open the patient's airway, and then suction the mouth. Once you immobilize the patient in a cervical collar and on a backboard, you can turn the backboard to one side to allow any blood or vomitus to drain out of the mouth rather than allowing it to pool in the pharynx and obstruct the airway.

Although most open soft-tissue injuries are not serious, if not appropriately treated, they can lead to substantial blood loss and even shock. However, if you effectively treat open soft-tissue injuries, then you can minimize common complications such as bleeding, shock, pain, and infection. Expose all wounds, control bleeding, and be prepared to treat the patient for shock.

Control external bleeding by applying direct manual pressure with a dry, sterile dressing. Use roller gauze, wrapped around the circumference of the head, to hold a pressure dressing in place Figure 29-12. Do not apply excessive pressure if an underlying skull fracture might potentially be present. When an injury exposes the brain, eye, or other structures, cover the exposed parts with a moist, sterile dressing to protect them from further damage. When treating eye injuries, always cover both eyes. For injuries in which the skin is not broken, apply ice packs locally to help control the swelling of bruised tissues.

Treat facial lacerations and avulsions as you would any other soft-tissue injury. Control all bleeding with direct pressure, and apply sterile dressings. If you suspect the patient has an underlying facial fracture, then apply just enough pressure to control the bleeding.

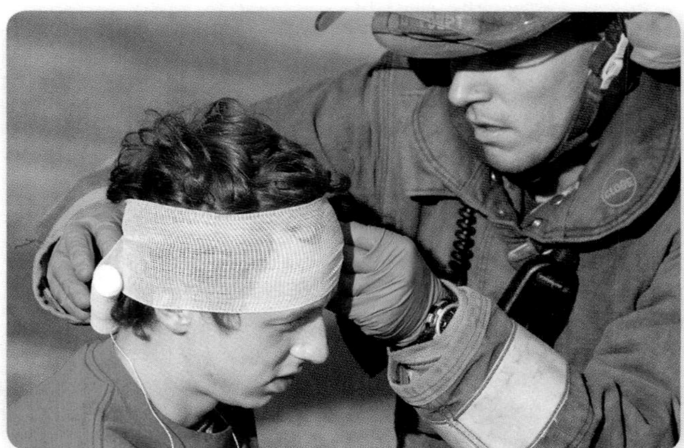

Figure 29-12 Use roller gauze, wrapped around the circumference of the head, to hold a pressure dressing in place.

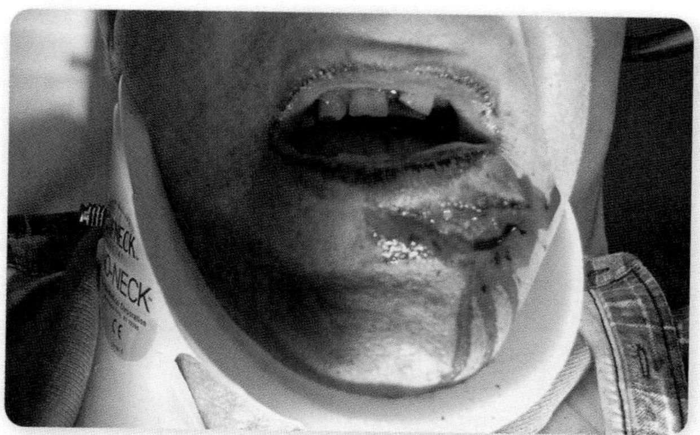

Figure 29-13 Soft-tissue injuries around the mouth can be associated with profuse bleeding inside the mouth and obstruction of the airway.

If the patient has soft-tissue injuries around the mouth, then check for bleeding inside the mouth. Broken teeth and lacerations to the tongue may cause profuse bleeding and obstruction of the upper airway Figure 29-13. Often, the patient will swallow the blood from lacerations inside the mouth, so the hemorrhage may not be apparent. You should also inspect the inside of the mouth for bleeding and hidden injuries in patients who have sustained facial trauma. Remember, patients who swallow blood are prone to vomiting.

Often, physicians will be able to graft a piece of avulsed skin back into the appropriate position. For this reason, if you find portions of avulsed skin that have become separated, if possible wrap them in a sterile dressing moistened with saline to prevent drying, place them in a plastic bag, and keep them cool. Never place tissue directly on ice—freezing will destroy the tissue and make it unusable. Deliver the bag labeled with the patient's name to the ED along with the patient. In many avulsion injuries, the skin will still be attached in a loose flap Figure 29-14. Place the flap in a position that is as close to normal as possible, and hold it in place with a dry, sterile dressing. These steps will help to increase the patient's chances of having his or her normal appearance restored.

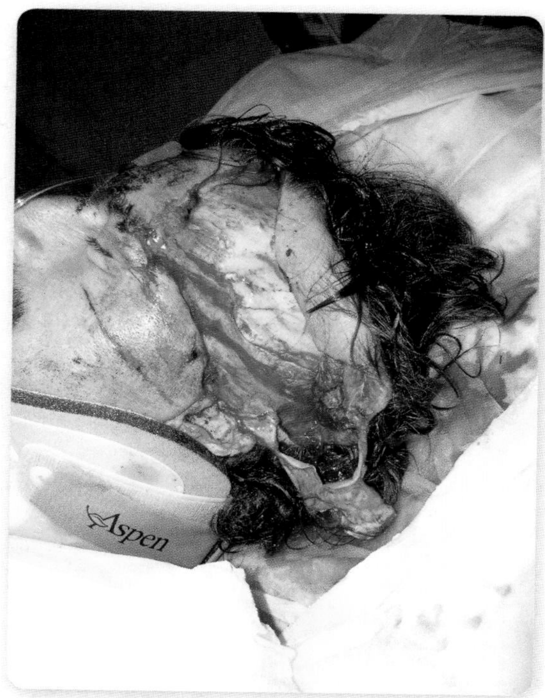

Figure 29-14 If avulsed skin is still attached, then place the flap in a position that is as close to normal as possible, and hold it in place with a dry, sterile dressing.

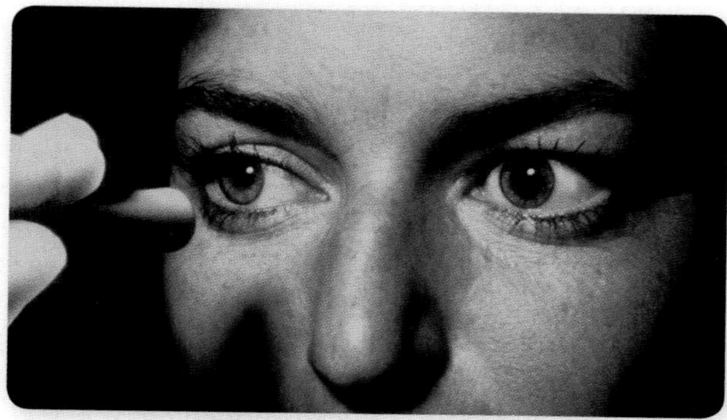

Figure 29-15 Normally, the pupils are round, equal in size, and equally reactive when exposed to light. The pupils shown here appear unequal.

▶ Injuries of the Eyes

Eye injuries are common, particularly in sports. An eye injury can produce severe, lifelong complications, including blindness. Proper emergency medical treatment will minimize pain and may very well help to prevent permanent vision loss.

In a normal, uninjured eye, the entire circle of the iris is visible. The pupils are round, usually equal in size, and react equally when exposed to light Figure 29-15. Both eyes move together in the same direction when following your moving finger. After an injury, however, pupil reaction or shape and eye movement are often disturbed. Any of these conditions should cause you to suspect an injury of the globe or its associated tissues. However, remember that abnormal pupil reactions sometimes are a sign of brain injury rather than eye injury.

Treatment starts with a thorough examination to determine the extent and nature of any damage. Always perform your examination taking standard precautions to avoid aggravating any problems. Look for specific abnormalities or conditions that may suggest the nature of the injury Figure 29-16. For example, blunt or penetrating injuries can produce swollen or lacerated eyelids. Bleeding soon after irritation or injury can result in a bright red conjunctiva. A damaged cornea quickly loses its smooth, wet appearance.

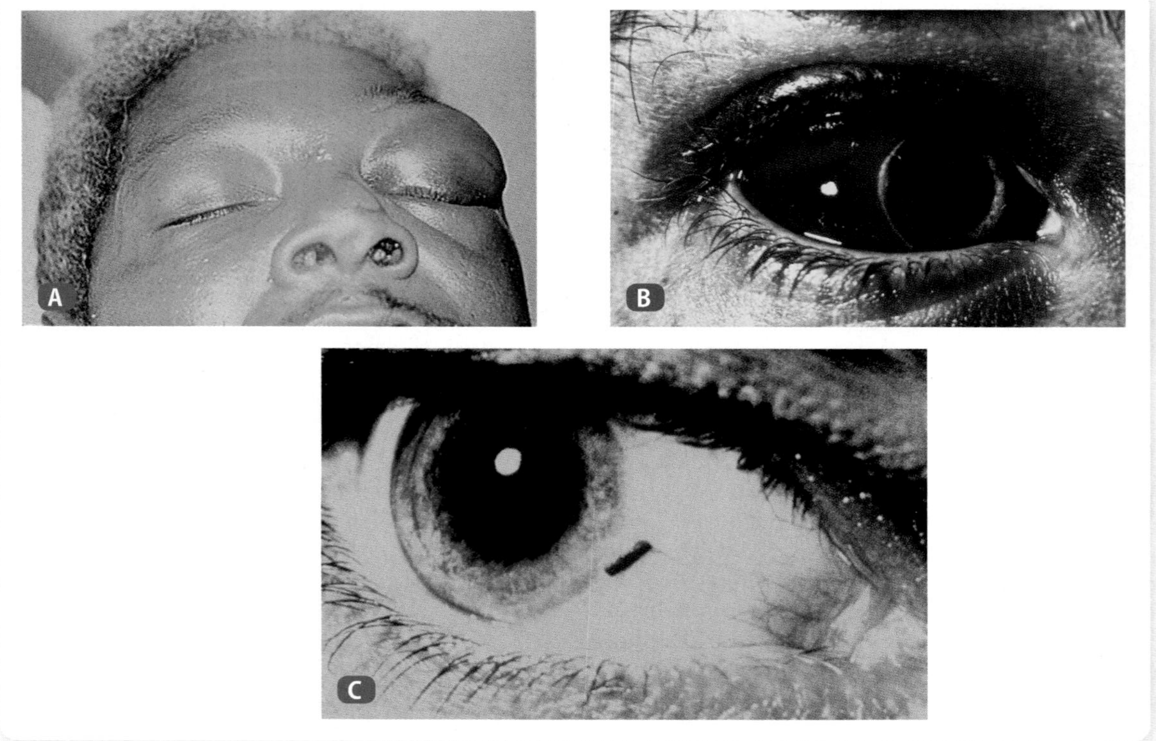

Figure 29-16 Injuries to the eyes are easily detected by swelling **(A)**, bleeding **(B)**, and the presence of foreign objects in the eye **(C)**.

Foreign Objects

Large objects are prevented from penetrating the eye by the protective orbit that surrounds it. However, moderately sized and smaller foreign objects of many different types can enter the eye and cause significant damage. Even a very small foreign object, such as a grain of sand lying on the surface of the conjunctiva, may produce severe irritation. The conjunctiva becomes inflamed and red—a condition known as **conjunctivitis**—almost immediately, and the eye begins to produce tears in an attempt to flush out the object. Irritation of the cornea or conjunctiva causes intense pain. Patients may have difficulty keeping their eyelids open, because the irritation is further aggravated by bright light.

If a small foreign object is lying on the surface of the patient's eye, you should use a normal saline solution to gently irrigate the eye. Irrigation with a sterile saline solution will frequently flush away loose, small particles. If a small bulb syringe is available, you can use it, or a nasal airway or cannula, to direct the saline into the affected eye. Always flush from the nose side of the eye toward the outside to avoid flushing material into the other eye. After it has been flushed away, a foreign body will often leave a small abrasion on the surface of the conjunctiva. For this reason, the patient may report irritation even when the particle itself is gone. It is always a good idea to transport the patient to the hospital for further assessment to ensure appropriate medical care to the affected eye.

Words of Wisdom

Large and small foreign bodies, particularly small metal fragments, can become completely embedded in the globe. The patient may not even be aware of the cause of the problem. Suspect such an injury when the patient's history includes metal work (eg, hammering, exposure to splinters, grinding, or vigorous filing) and when you observe signs of ocular injury (eg, redness, irritation, inflammation).

Gentle irrigation usually will not wash out foreign bodies that are stuck to the cornea or lying under the upper eyelid. When you examine the undersurface of the upper eyelid, pull the lid upward and forward. If you spot a foreign object on the surface of the eyelid, then try to remove it with a moist, sterile, cotton-tipped applicator, as shown in Skill Drill 29-1. Never attempt to remove a foreign body that is stuck to the cornea.

Foreign bodies ranging in size from a pencil to a sliver of metal may be impaled in the eye. These objects

Skill Drill 29-1 Removing a Foreign Object From Under the Upper Eyelid

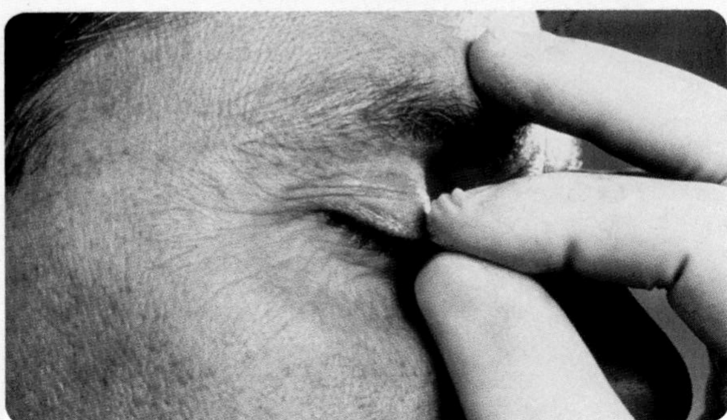

Step 1 Have the patient look down, grasp the upper lashes, and gently pull the lid away from the eyeball.

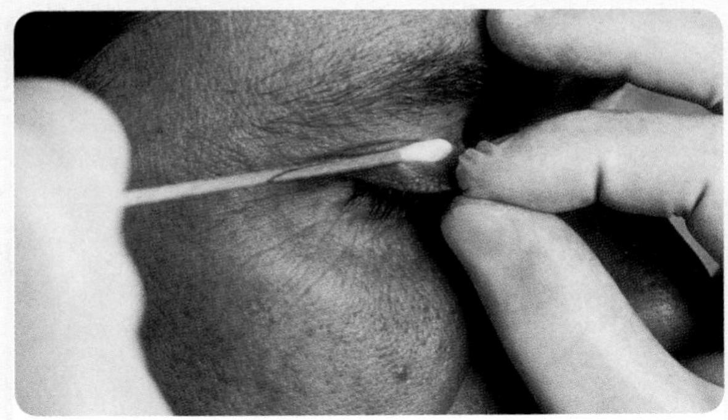

Step 2 Place a cotton-tipped applicator horizontally on the outer surface of the upper eyelid.

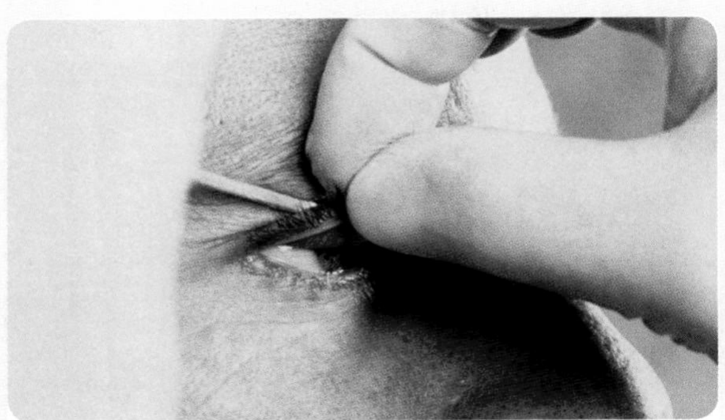

Step 3 Pull the eyelid forward and up, fold it back over the applicator and expose the undersurface of the eyelid.

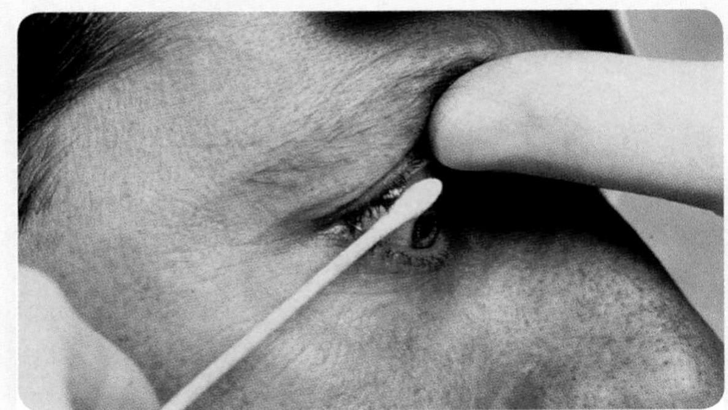

Step 4 Gently remove the foreign object from the eyelid with a moistened, sterile, cotton-tipped applicator.

must be removed by a physician. As an AEMT, your care involves stabilizing the object and preparing the patient for transport to definitive care. The greater the length of the foreign object you can see sticking out of the eye, the more important stabilization becomes in avoiding further damage. Bandage the object in place to support it. Cover the eye with a moist, sterile dressing, and then surround the object with a doughnut-shaped collar made from roller gauze or a small gauze pack. Cover the noninjured eye to prevent consensual movement and further damage of the injured eye. Follow the steps in Skill Drill 29-2.

If you see or suspect an impaled object in the eye, bandage both eyes with soft bulky dressings to prevent further injury to the affected eye. Your bandage should be loose enough to hold the eyelid closed but should not cause pressure on the eye itself. This bandaging technique prevents **sympathetic eye movement** (the movement of one eye causing both eyes to move), which may cause additional damage to the injured eye. An embedded object in the eye must be handled by an ophthalmologist on an urgent basis. X-rays and special equipment may be required to find the foreign body.

Burns of the Eye

Chemicals, heat, and light rays all can burn the delicate tissues of the eye, such as the cornea, often causing

Skill Drill 29-2 Stabilizing a Foreign Object Impaled in the Eye

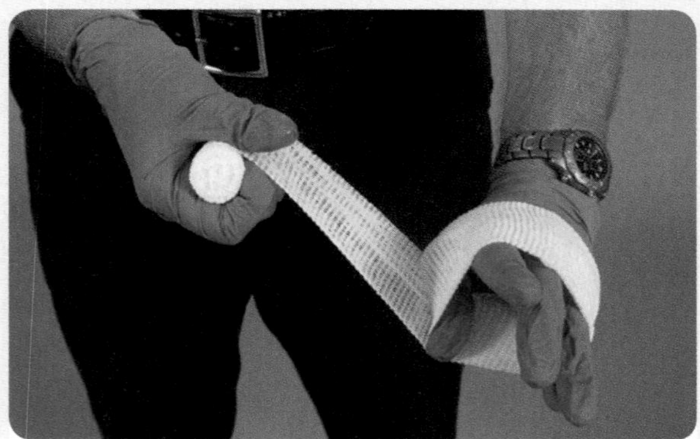

Step 1 To prepare a doughnut ring, wrap a 2-inch (5 cm) roll around your fingers and thumb seven or eight times. Adjust the diameter by spreading out your fingers or by squeezing them together.

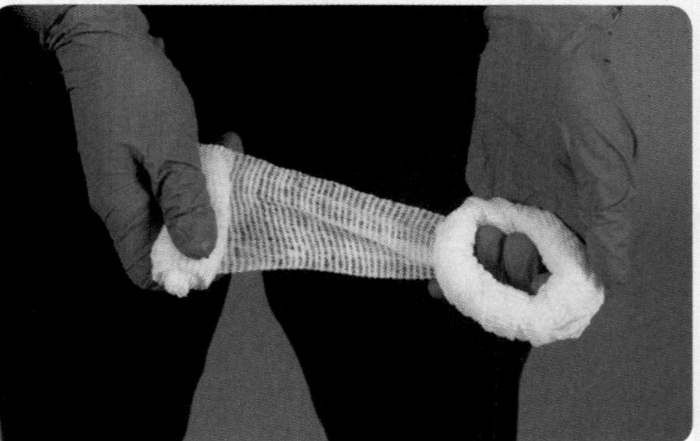

Step 2 Remove the gauze from your hand and wrap the remainder of the gauze roll radially around the ring that you have created.

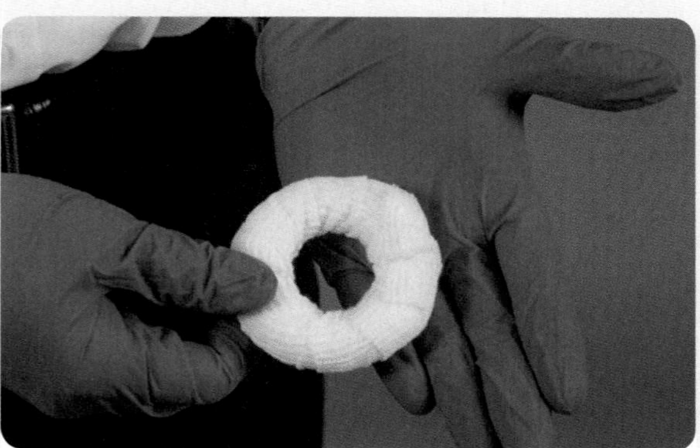

Step 3 Work around the entire ring to form a doughnut.

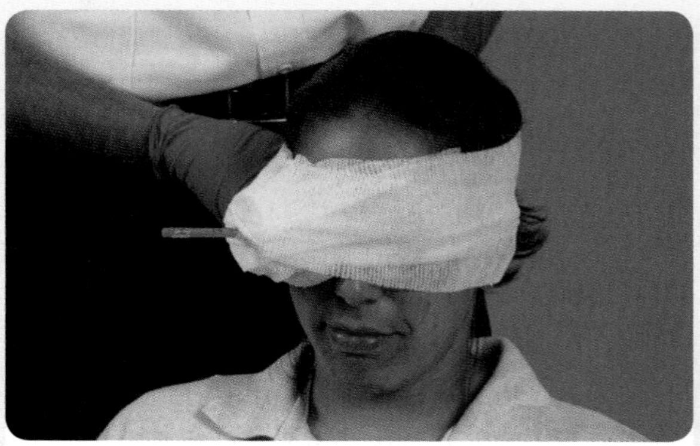

Step 4 Carefully place the ring over the eye and impaled object to stabilize the impaled object in place, and then secure it with a roller bandage.

permanent damage. Your role is to stop the burn and prevent further damage.

Chemical Burns. Chemical burns, usually caused by acid or alkaline solutions, require immediate emergency medical care Figure 29-17. Treatment consists of flushing the eye with water or a sterile saline irrigation solution. If sterile saline is not available, then you can use any clean water.

When treating a chemical burn, the idea is to direct the greatest amount of irrigating solution or water into the eye as gently as possible Figure 29-18. Because opening the eye spontaneously may cause pain, you may have to force the patient's lids open to irrigate the eye adequately. Ideally, you will use a bulb or irrigation syringe, a nasal cannula, or some other device that will allow you to control the flow; however, in some circumstances, you may have to resort to pouring water into the eye by holding the patient's head under a gently running faucet. You can even have the patient immerse his or her face in a large pan or basin of water and rapidly blink the affected eyelid. If only one eye is affected, then take care to avoid getting contaminated water into the unaffected eye.

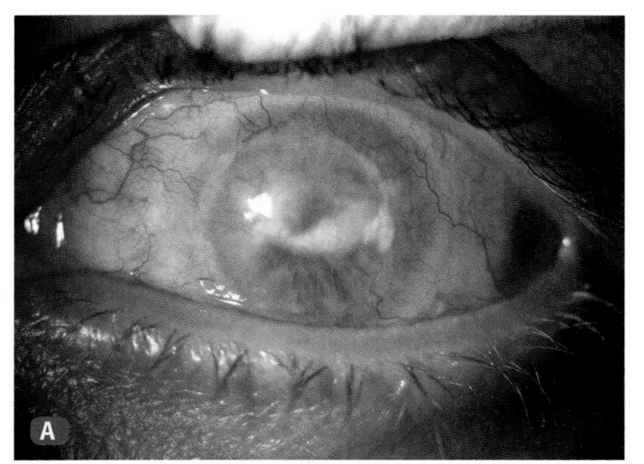

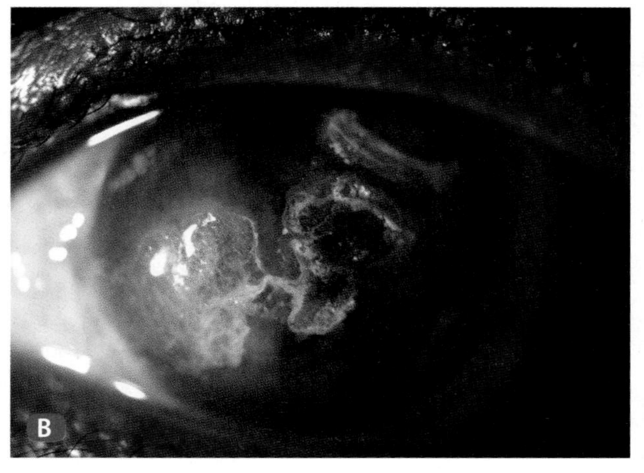

Figure 29-17 A. Chemical burns typically occur when an acid or alkali is splashed into the eye. **B.** This figure shows a chemical burn from lye, an alkaline solution. Because lye can continue to damage the eye even when it is diluted, fast action is needed.

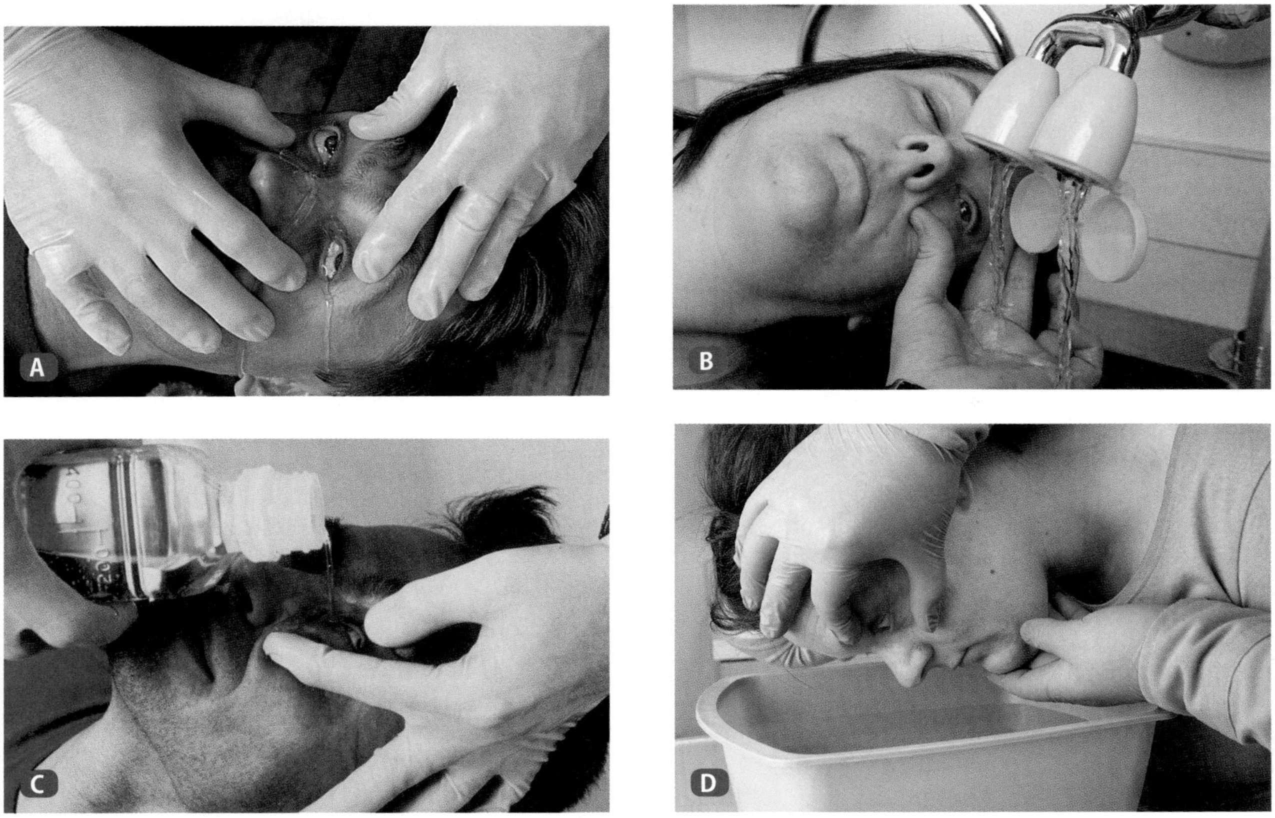

Figure 29-18 The following are four ways to effectively irrigate the eye. **A.** Nasal cannula. **B.** Shower. **C.** Bottle. **D.** Basin. Remember, you must protect the uninjured eye from the irrigating solution to prevent exposure of the unaffected eye to the substance.

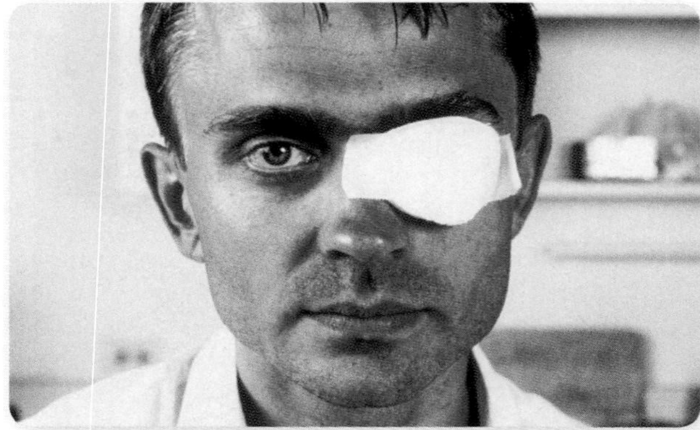

Figure 29-19 Apply a clean, dry dressing to cover the eye after you have finished irrigation.

Irrigate the eye for at least 5 minutes. Flush from the inner corner of the affected eye toward the outside corner. Never flush from the outside corner, as this technique may cause the substance to contaminate the unaffected eye. If the burn was caused by an alkali or a strong acid, then irrigate the eye continuously for 20 minutes. Follow local protocols on whether to try to irrigate while transporting or to stay on scene until flushing is complete. Strong acids and all alkaline solutions can penetrate deeply, requiring a prolonged flush. Again, always take care to protect the uninjured eye during this process.

After you have completed the irrigation, apply a clean, dry dressing to cover the eye, and transport the patient promptly to the hospital for further care Figure 29-19. If the irrigation can be carried out satisfactorily in the ambulance, it should be done during transport to save time.

Thermal Burns. When a patient is burned on the face during a fire, the eyes usually close rapidly because of the heat. This reaction is a natural reflex to protect the eye from further injury. However, the eyelids remain exposed and are frequently burned Figure 29-20. Burns of the eyelids require very specialized care. It is best to provide prompt transport for these patients without further examination. First, however, you should cover both eyes with a sterile dressing moistened with sterile saline. You may apply eye shields over the dressing.

Light Burns. Infrared rays, eclipse light (if the patient has looked directly at the sun), and laser burns all can cause significant damage to the sensory cells of the eye when rays of light become focused on the retina. Retinal injuries that are caused by exposure to extremely bright light are generally not painful but may result in permanent damage to vision.

Superficial burns of the eye can result from ultraviolet rays from an arc welding unit, light from prolonged exposure to a sunlamp, or reflected light from a bright, snow-covered area (snow blindness). Initially, this kind of burn is not painful but may become so 3 to 5 hours later, when the damaged cornea responds to the injury.

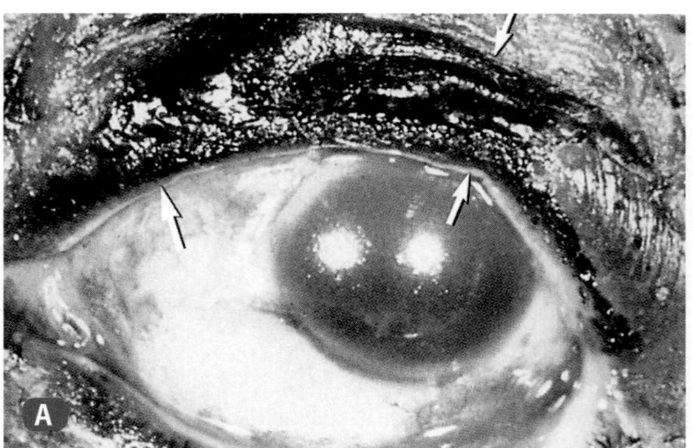

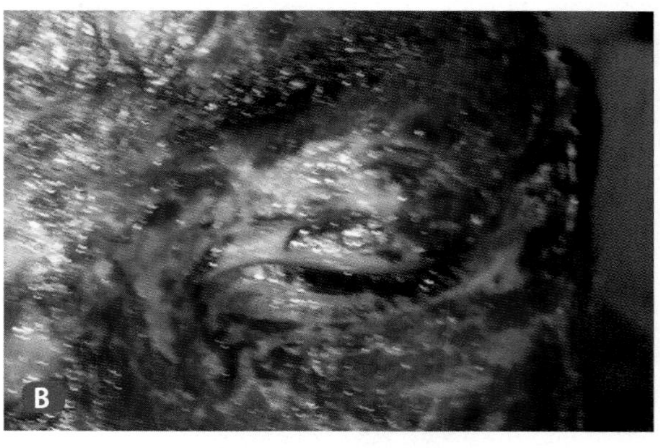

Figure 29-20 Thermal burns occasionally cause significant damage to the eyelids. **A.** Arrows show some full-thickness burns. **B.** Burns of the eyelids require immediate hospital care.

Severe conjunctivitis usually develops, with redness, swelling, and excessive tear production. You can ease the pain from these corneal burns by covering each eye with a sterile, moist pad and an eye shield. Have the patient lie down during transport to the hospital, and protect him or her from further exposure to bright light. The patient should be examined by a physician as soon as possible.

Lacerations

Lacerations of the eyelids require very careful repair to restore appearance and function. Bleeding may be heavy, but it usually can be controlled by gentle, manual pressure. If there is a laceration of the globe itself, then apply no pressure to the eye. Compression can interfere with the blood supply to the back of the eye and result in loss of vision from damage to the retina. Furthermore, pressure may squeeze the vitreous humor, iris, lens, or even the retina out of the eye and cause irreparable damage or blindness Figure 29-21.

Follow these three important guidelines in treating penetrating injuries of the eye:

1. Never exert pressure on or manipulate the injured eye (globe) in any way.

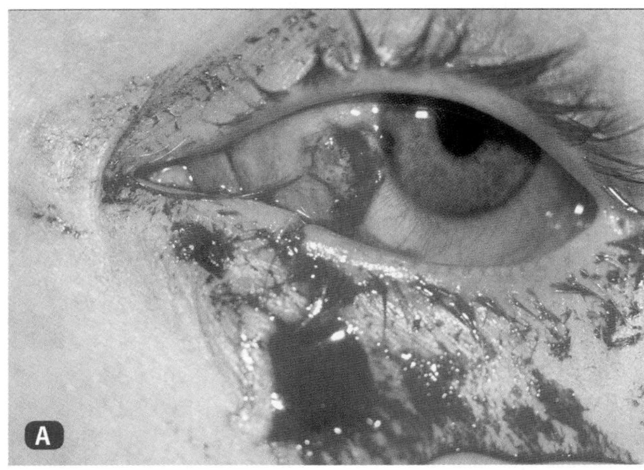

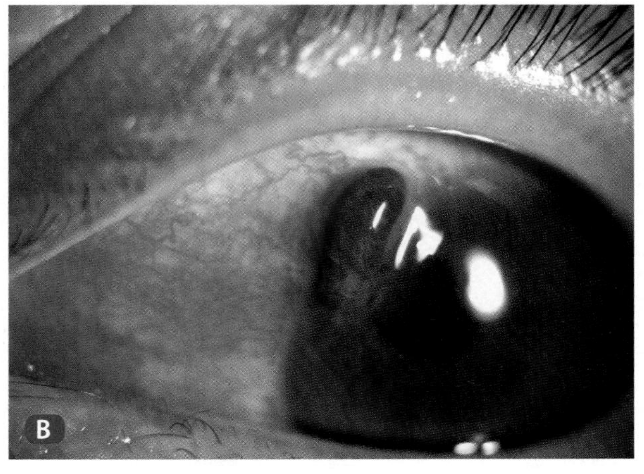

Figure 29-21 Lacerations are serious injuries that require prompt transport. **A.** Although bleeding can be heavy, never exert pressure on the eye. **B.** Pressure may squeeze the vitreous humor, iris, lens, or even the retina out of the eye.

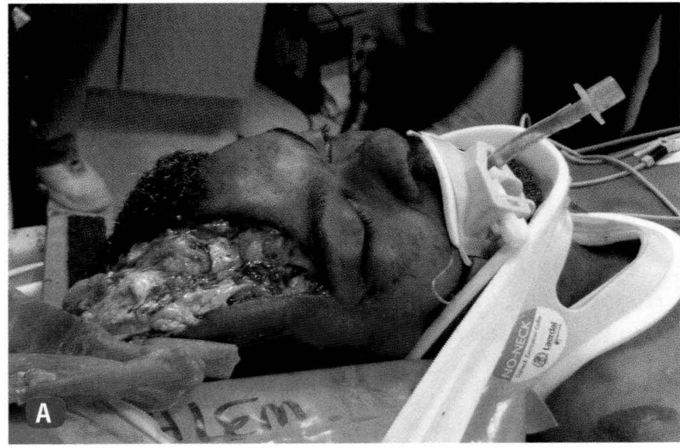

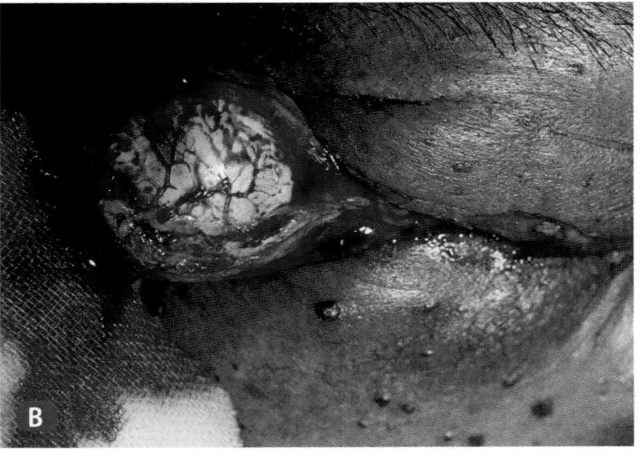

Figure 29-22 An injury that exposes the brain **(A)**, eye **(B)**, or other structures should be covered with a moist, sterile dressing to prevent further damage.

2. If part of the eyeball is exposed, gently apply a moist, sterile dressing to prevent drying.
3. Cover the injured eye with a protective metal eye shield, cup, or sterile dressing. Apply soft dressings to both eyes, and provide prompt transport to the hospital.

On rare occasions following a serious injury, the globe may be displaced (avulsed) out of its socket. Do not attempt to manipulate or reposition it in any way! Simply cover the protruding eye and stabilize it with a moist, sterile dressing Figure 29-22. Remember to cover both eyes to prevent further injury because of sympathetic eye movement. Have the patient lie in a supine position en route to the hospital to prevent further loss of fluid from the eye.

Blunt Trauma

Blunt trauma can cause a number of serious eye injuries. These range from the ordinary "black eye," characterized by bleeding into the tissue around the orbit, to a severely damaged globe Figure 29-23. You may see an injury called **hyphema**, or bleeding into the anterior chamber of the eye, that obscures part or all of the iris Figure 29-24. This injury is common in blunt trauma and may seriously impair vision. Cover the eye to protect it from further injury and transport the patient to the hospital for further medical evaluation.

Hyphema or rupture of the globe indicates that a significant amount of force was applied to the face and, therefore, may signal the presence of a spinal injury. Elevate the head of the backboard to approximately a 40° angle to decrease

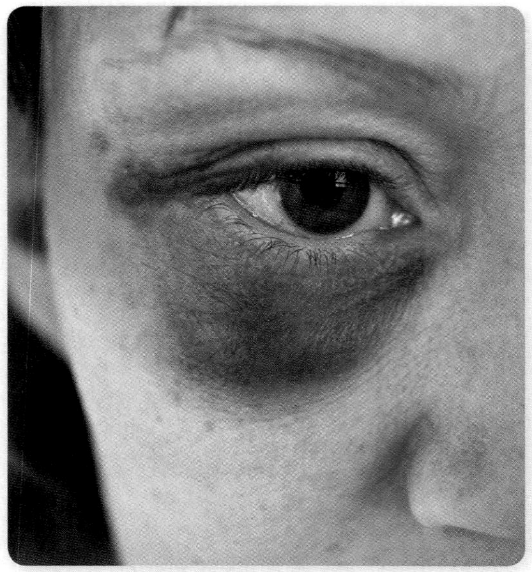

Figure 29-23 The typical "black eye" is caused by bleeding into the tissue around the orbit.

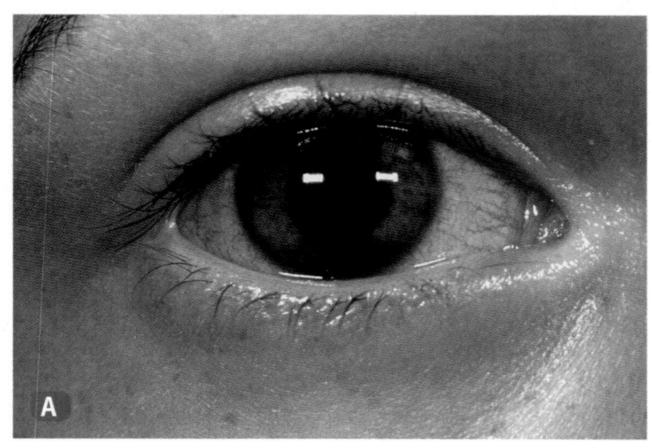

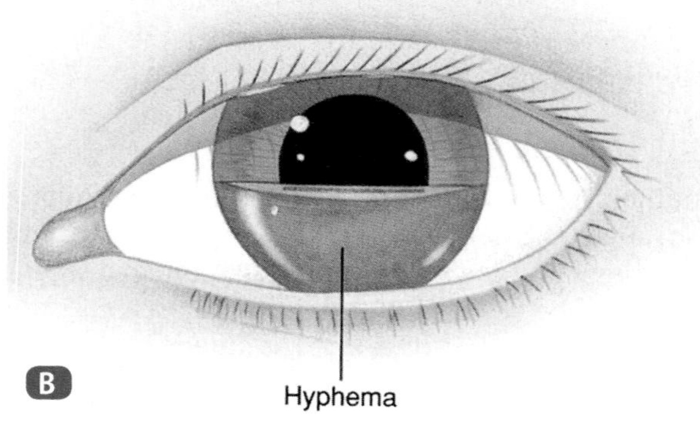

Figure 29-24 A. A hyphema, characterized by bleeding into the anterior chamber of the eye, is common following blunt trauma to the eye. This condition may seriously impair vision and should be considered a sight-threatening emergency. **B.** Illustration of hyphema.

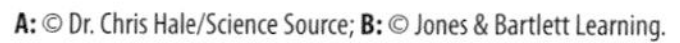

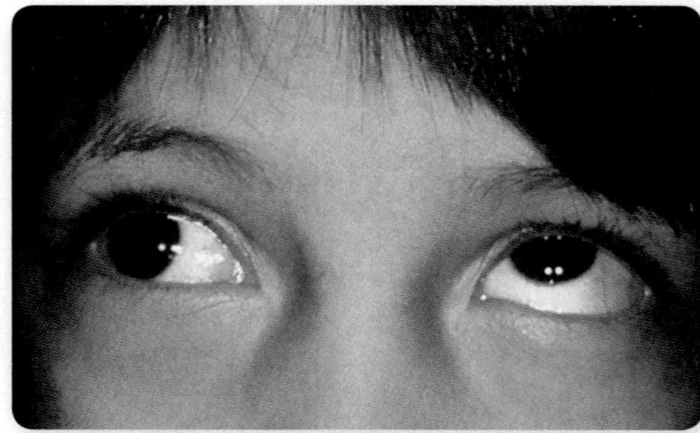

Figure 29-25 A patient with a blowout fracture may not move his or her eyes together because of muscle entrapment. Therefore, the patient sees double images of any object.

intraocular pressure (IOP), and discourage the patient from performing activities that may increase IOP (eg, coughing).

Blunt trauma can also cause a fracture of the orbit, particularly of the bones that form its floor and support the globe. Such an injury is called a blowout fracture. The fragments of fractured bone can entrap some of the muscles that control eye movement, causing double vision Figure 29-25. Any patient who reports pain, double vision, or decreased vision following a blunt injury about the eye should be placed on a stretcher and transported promptly to the ED. Protect the eye from further injury with a metal shield; cover the other eye to minimize movement on the injured side.

Another possible result of blunt eye injury is **retinal detachment**, or separation of the inner layers of the retina from the underlying choroid (the vascular membrane that nourishes the retina). This injury is often seen in sports, especially boxing. It is painless but produces flashing lights, specks, or "floaters" in the field of vision and a cloud or shade over the patient's vision. Because it can cause devastating damage to vision, retinal detachment is an ocular emergency and requires urgent medical treatment to preserve vision in the eye.

Words of Wisdom

Anisocoria—a condition in which the pupils are not of equal size—is a significant finding in patients with ocular injuries or traumatic brain injury. However, simple or physiologic anisocoria occurs in approximately 20% of the population.[1] Usually, the patient's pupils differ in size by less than 0.5 mm; however, some people have pupils that vary in size up to 1 mm.[2] This is not a clinically significant finding.

Unilateral cataract surgery may also cause unequal pupil sizes. The pupil of the eye affected by the cataract will be nonreactive to light. Remember to always consider the size of the pupils relative to each other in the context of the patient's overall condition.

Eye Injuries Following Head Injury

Abnormalities in the appearance or function of the eyes often occur following a closed head injury. Any of the following eye findings should alert you to the possibility of a head injury:

- One pupil larger than the other Figure 29-26
- The eyes do not move together or they point in different directions (**dysconjugate gaze**)
- The eyes fail to follow the movement of your finger as instructed
- Bleeding under the conjunctiva, which obscures the sclera (white portion) of the eye
- Protrusion or bulging of one eye

Record any of these observations, along with the time that you make them. With an unresponsive patient, remember to keep the eyelids closed; drying of the ocular tissues can cause permanent injury and may result in blindness. Cover the lids with moist gauze, or hold them closed with clear tape for particularly long transports. Normal tears will then keep the tissues moist.

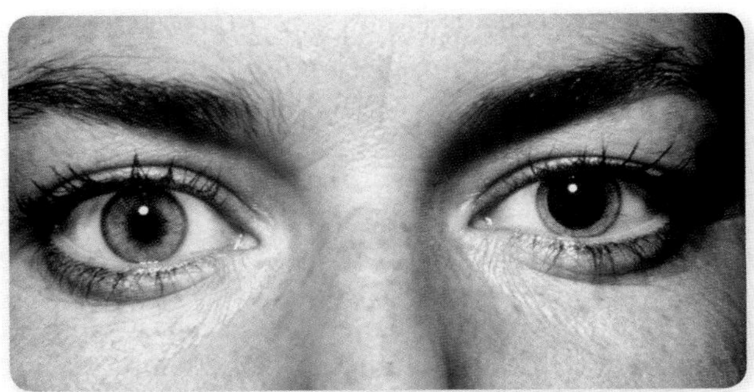

Figure 29-26 Variation of pupil size may indicate a head injury.

Blast Injuries

The signs and symptoms of blast injuries can range from severe pain and loss of vision to foreign bodies within the globe. Before responding to patients after the blast, first ensure the scene is safe.

YOU are the Provider PART 4

Finding the patient's bleeding to be venous in nature, you instruct your partner to apply mild pressure above and below the injury in an attempt to control bleeding. Once the rate of bleeding has been controlled, you advise the fire department personnel that you believe it is safe to continue operations, ensuring they are cognizant of the potential for serious injury. After the patient has been freed from the implement, you place him on a long backboard in the lateral position with the right side down and the left side up to facilitate stabilization of the impaled object. You are unable to place a cervical collar on this patient, so instead you place a large amount of padding around his neck, and stress to the patient the importance of not moving his head. He acknowledges the seriousness of the situation and assures you he has no intention of moving anything.

Once the patient is secured and placed in the back of the ambulance, you reassess the security of the object and add a few more bulky dressings as a precaution. You inform your partner that you need a rapid, but very smooth transport to the trauma center. He tells you he understands and proceeds to the trauma center approximately 12 minutes away.

While you are en route, you establish two 18-gauge IV lines with normal saline at a to keep open (TKO) rate. You remember the patient stated he was getting increasingly short of breath and you ask him how he feels now. He replies that he feels better with the oxygen mask but is concerned about the piece of steel in his neck. You discuss the possible implications of his injury with him, and he appears calm. The remainder of your examination is unremarkable.

After you arrive at the trauma center and turn over care, you complete the patient care report while your partner readies the truck for the next call.

Recording Time: 23 Minutes	
Respirations	18 breaths/min; clear bilaterally
Pulse	105 beats/min
Skin	Warm, dry, and pink
Blood pressure	124/76 mm Hg
Oxygen saturation (Spo$_2$)	95% with oxygen at 15 L/min via nonrebreathing mask
Pupils	PERRLA

7. What are some possible causes of this patient's initial shortness of breath?
8. If you do not have the tools to cut the object and free the patient, should you remove the object from his neck?

How you manage a blast injury to the eye will depend on the severity of the injury. If a foreign body is embedded within the globe, then do not attempt to remove it. Use a clean cup or similar item to protect the area. If only one eye is injured, then follow local protocol, which may include covering the other eye to eliminate sympathetic motion. Patients who experience a sudden loss or decrease of vision will need verbal instructions on which actions are taking place around them. If the patient has severe swelling or a hematoma to the eyelid, then do not attempt to force the eyelid open to examine the eye because this action increases the pressure already present within the globe.

Contact Lenses and Artificial Eyes

Small, hard contact lenses usually are tinted, making them relatively easy to see. Large, soft contact lenses are clear and can be very difficult to see. In general, you should not attempt to remove either kind of lens from a patient. You should never attempt to remove a lens from an eye that has been—or may have been—injured, because manipulating the lens can aggravate the problem. The only time when contact lenses should be removed immediately in the field is in the case of a chemical burn of the eye. In this situation, the lens can trap the chemical and make irrigation difficult.

Words of Wisdom

The only time when contact lenses should be removed immediately in the field is in the case of a chemical burn of the eye. In this situation, the lens can trap the chemical and make irrigation more difficult.

If it is necessary to remove a hard contact lens, use a small suction cup, moistening the end with saline. To remove soft lenses, place one to two drops of saline in the eye, gently pinch the lens between your gloved thumb and index finger, and lift it off the surface of the eye. Place the contact lens in a container filled with sterile saline solution to prevent damage to the contact lens. Always inform the ED staff if a patient is wearing contact lenses.

Occasionally, you may find yourself caring for a patient who is wearing an eye prosthesis (an artificial eye). Many people are surprised to find that it can be difficult to distinguish a prosthesis from a natural eye. You should suspect an eye is artificial when it does not respond to light, does not move in concert with the opposite eye, or appears different from the opposite eye. If you think a patient may have an artificial eye but you are not sure, go ahead and ask about it. Although no harm will be done if you care for an artificial eye as you would a natural one, you need to clearly understand the patient's eye function.

▶ Injuries of the Nose

Nosebleeds (epistaxis) are a common problem that can occur either spontaneously or as the result of trauma. One of the most common causes of nosebleeds is digital trauma (picking the nose with a finger). Nosebleeds are classified into two types, based on the area of the bleeding: anterior and posterior. Anterior nosebleeds usually originate from the area of the septum and bleed fairly slowly; they are usually self-limited and resolve quickly. Posterior nosebleeds are usually more severe and often cause blood to drain into the patient's throat, leading to nausea and vomiting. Trauma to the face and skull that results in a **basilar skull fracture** will often cause the posterior wall of the nasal cavity to become unstable. Attempting to place a nasopharyngeal airway in a patient with a suspected basilar skull fracture or with facial injuries is relatively contraindicated in the presence of midface trauma. As always, know and follow your local protocols.

The nose often takes the brunt of deliberate physical assaults and car crashes. Blunt injuries to the nose caused by a fist or a dashboard may be associated with fractures and soft-tissue injuries of the face, head injuries, and/or injuries to the cervical spine. Penetrating injuries to the nose can involve many mechanisms (eg, when air guns and BB pellets are fired from a close range, resulting in pellets lodging in the nasal septum and sinuses). Another type of penetrating injury to the nose is a self-inflicted one that occurs when a person attempts to insert a foreign body into the nose, such as a pencil.

When you are assessing injuries involving the nose, it helps to picture the inside of the nose itself **Figure 29-27**. The nasal cavity is divided into two sections or chambers by the nasal septum, which is made of cartilage. Each nasal chamber contains layers of bone called the **turbinates**, which are covered with a moist lining. Both chambers have a superior turbinate, a middle turbinate, and an inferior

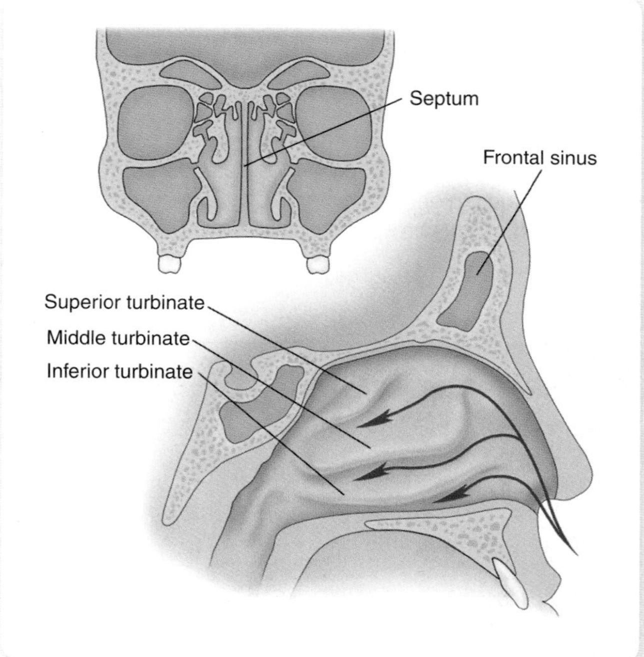

Figure 29-27 The nose has two chambers, divided by the septum. Each chamber is composed of layers of bone called turbinates. Above the nose are the frontal sinuses and, on either side, the orbit of the eye.

turbinate. As a person breathes, air moves through the nasal chambers and is humidified, warmed, and filtered as it passes over the turbinates. Directly above the nose are the frontal sinuses and, on either side, the orbit of the eye. All of these structures should be assessed for injury. In patients with severe injury, there may also be injury to the cervical spine. In addition, cerebrospinal fluid may escape down through the nose (or ears) following a fracture at the base of the skull.

Epistaxis following facial trauma can be severe and is most effectively controlled by applying direct pressure to the nares. If the patient is responsive and spinal injury is not suspected, then instruct the patient to sit up and lean forward as you pinch the nares together or press on the upper gums[3] Figure 29-28. Unresponsive patients should be positioned on their sides, unless contraindicated by a spinal injury. Proper positioning of the patient with epistaxis is important to prevent blood from draining into the throat and compromising the airway either by occlusion or by vomiting and then aspirating gastric contents.

You can control bleeding from abrasions and lacerations to the nose by applying a sterile dressing. If the patient is bleeding heavily from the nose, then you should suspect significant trauma and you must consider a cervical spine injury. The patient should not be moved if the airway can be managed in the patient's present position.

Although facial lacerations and avulsions can contribute to hemorrhagic shock, they are rarely the sole cause of this condition in adults. However, severe epistaxis can result in significant blood loss. To manage this problem, carefully assess the patient for signs of hemorrhagic shock and administer crystalloid fluid boluses intravenously as needed to maintain adequate perfusion.

▶ Injuries of the Ear

Injuries to the ear may be isolated, or they may occur in conjunction with other injuries to the head or face. Although isolated ear injuries are typically not life threatening, they can result in sensory impairment and permanent disfigurement.

Ears usually do not bleed very much. If local pressure does not control the bleeding, then you can apply a roller dressing Figure 29-29. First, however, you should place a soft, padded dressing between the back of the

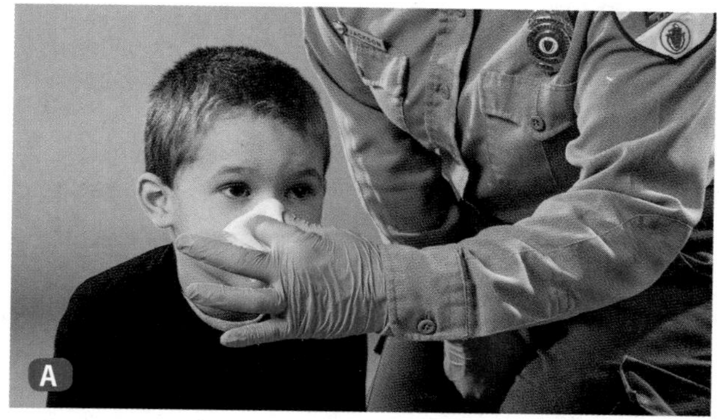

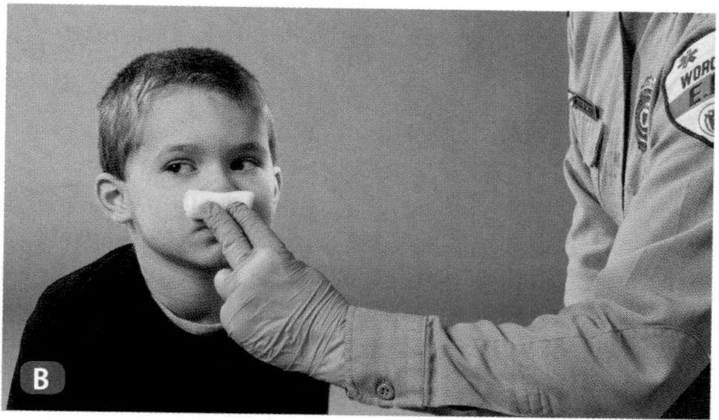

Figure 29-28 Control bleeding from the nose by one of the following methods: either pinch the nostrils together **(A)** or apply pressure on the upper gums, beneath the nose, with gloved fingers and gauze **(B)**.

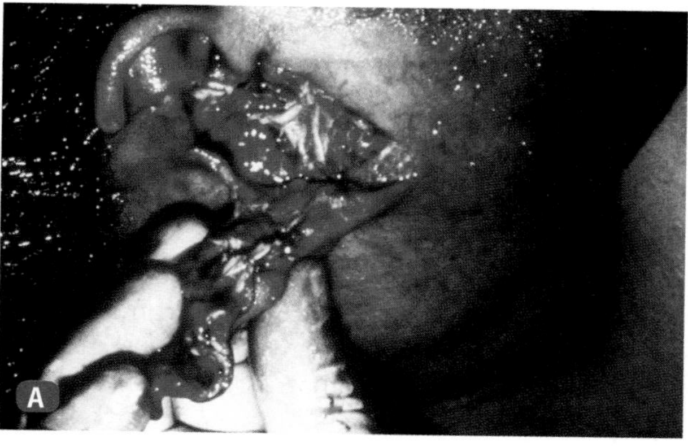

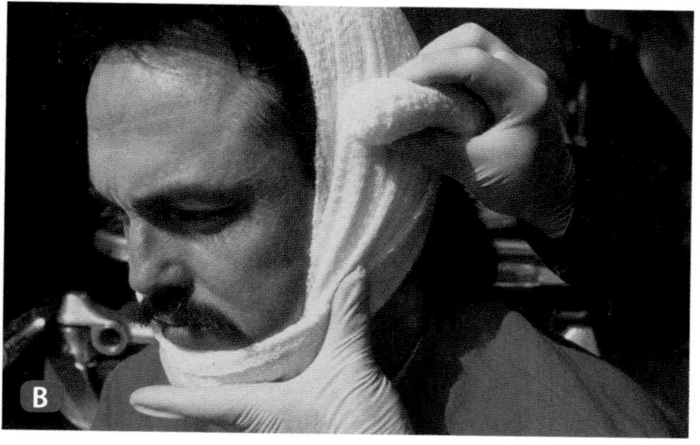

Figure 29-29 A. A major laceration of the ear. **B.** Proper treatment includes use of a soft, sterile pad behind the ear, between it and the scalp. Then wrap a roller gauze dressing around the head to include the entire ear.

ear and the scalp because bandaging the ear against the tender underlying scalp can be extremely painful for the patient. If blood or CSF drainage is noted, then apply a loose dressing over the ear—taking care *not* to stop the flow—and assess the patient for other signs of a basilar skull fracture.

If the pinna is partially avulsed, then carefully realign the ear into position and gently bandage it with sufficient padding that has been slightly moistened with normal saline. If the pinna is completely avulsed, attempt to retrieve the avulsed part, if possible, for reimplantation at the hospital. If the detached part of the ear is recovered, then treat it as any other amputation; wrap it in saline-moistened gauze, place it in a plastic bag, and place the bag in ice water. Never place an amputated part directly on ice.

Do not remove an impaled object from the ear. Instead, stabilize the object and cover the ear to prevent gross movement and minimize the risk of contamination of the inner ear.

The external auditory canal is a favorite place for children to place foreign bodies such as peanuts or candy. All such items should be removed by a physician in the ED. Never try to manipulate the foreign body because you may press it farther into the auditory canal and cause permanent damage to (perforation of) the tympanic membrane.

Perforation of the tympanic membrane (ruptured eardrum) can also result from direct blows and pressure-related injuries, such as blast injuries resulting from an explosion, or diving-related injuries that result in barotrauma to the ear. Signs and symptoms of a perforated tympanic membrane include loss of hearing and blood drainage from the ear (hemorrhagic otorrhea). Although the injury is extremely painful for the patient, the tympanic membrane typically heals spontaneously and without complication. Nevertheless, a careful assessment should be performed to detect and treat other injuries, some of which may be life threatening.

▶ Facial Fractures

Fractures of the facial bones typically result from blunt impact. For example, the patient's head may collide with a steering wheel or windshield in an automobile crash or be hit by a baseball bat or pipe in an assault. If the patient sustained a direct blow to the mouth or nose, then maintain a high index of suspicion for a facial fracture. Other clues to the possibility of fracture include bleeding in the mouth, inability to swallow or talk, absent or loose teeth, and/or loose or movable bone fragments. Patients may also report that "it doesn't feel right" when they close their jaw, signaling an irregularity of bite.

Facial fractures alone are not acute emergencies unless there is serious bleeding; however, they are an indication of significant blunt force trauma applied to that region of the body. Serious bleeding from a facial fracture can be life threatening. In addition to the danger posed by external hemorrhage, blood clots may become lodged in the upper airway and cause an obstruction Figure 29-30. Fractures around the face and mouth can also produce deformity and loose bone fragments. In most cases, plastic surgeons can repair the damage if the injuries are treated within 7 to 10 days of the injury. Ensure you remove and save loose teeth or bone fragments from the mouth; it is often possible to reimplant them Figure 29-31. Remove any loose dentures or dental bridges to protect against airway

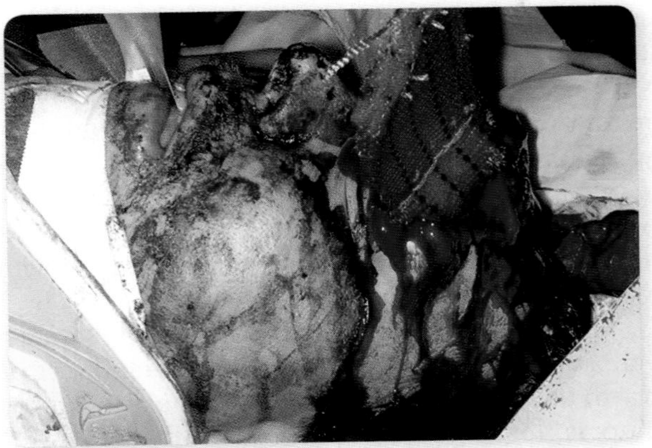

Figure 29-30 Bleeding following a crushing injury to the face can be life threatening because, in addition to the danger posed by external hemorrhage, blood clots in the airway can cause a complete obstruction.

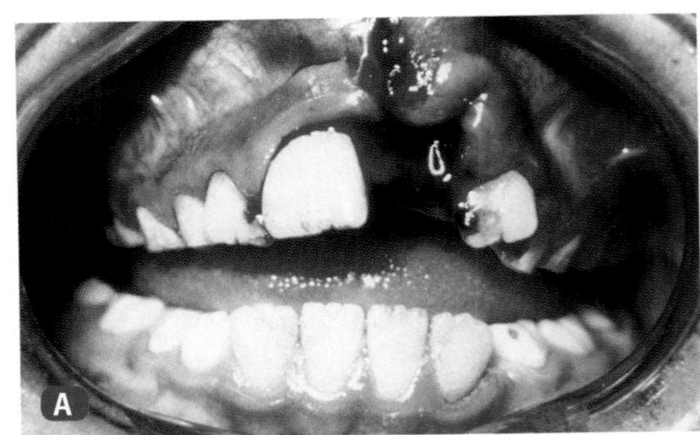

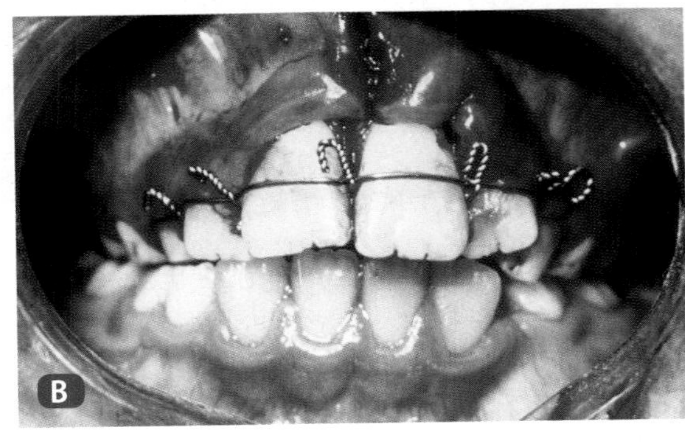

Figure 29-31 A. Save any lost teeth or bone fragments following an injury to the mouth. **B.** Even with traumatic loss of a tooth, the possibility of successful reimplantation is very good.

obstruction. The removal of dentures will affect the shape of the patient's jaw.

Another source of potential airway obstruction is swelling, which can be extreme within the first 24 hours after injury. If you notice swelling during assessment or at any time while the patient is in your care, then check for airway obstruction.

▶ Oral and Dental Injuries

Oral and dental injuries are commonly associated with trauma to the face. Blunt mechanisms typically result from MVCs or direct blows to the mouth or chin. Penetrating mechanisms often take the form of gunshot wounds, lacerations, and punctures. Dental injuries can be traumatic to a patient. Not only is the injury itself traumatic, but the patient's permanent teeth may also be lost—affecting everything from eating to smiling. Keep this in mind when providing care.

The primary risk associated with oral and dental injuries is airway compromise from oropharyngeal bleeding, occlusion by a displaced dental appliance such as a bridge or partial plate, and possibly aspiration of avulsed or fractured teeth. Any patient with significant facial trauma should be carefully assessed for injuries to the mouth and teeth. Suction the oropharynx as needed, and remove fractured tooth fragments to prevent airway compromise. Apply spinal immobilization as dictated by the MOI (a patient with significant impact to the face or mouth should be considered to have cervical spine trauma until proven otherwise).

Bleeding will occur whenever a tooth is violently displaced out of its socket; you should apply direct pressure to stop the bleeding. Patients may also swallow blood from lacerations inside the mouth, so the bleeding may not be grossly evident. Because blood irritates the gastric lining, the risks of vomiting and aspiration are significant when it is swallowed. For severe oropharyngeal bleeding in patients with inadequate ventilation, suction the airway for 15 seconds and provide ventilatory assistance for 2 minutes; continue this alternating pattern of suctioning and ventilating until the airway is cleared of blood or secured with an endotracheal tube by paramedic backup. You can also turn the backboard to the side to help clear the airway. Monitor the pulse oximeter during this process to ensure the patient does not become hypoxic.

Leave impaled objects in the face in place and appropriately stabilize them, unless they pose a threat to the airway (such as an object impaled through the cheek). When you remove an object from the cheek, carefully remove it, preferably from the same side that the object entered. Next, pack the inside of the patient's cheek with sterile gauze and apply counterpressure with a dressing and bandage firmly secured over the outside of the wound. If profuse bleeding continues, then position the patient on his or her side—while maintaining stabilization of the cervical spine—to facilitate drainage of secretions from the mouth; suction the airway as needed.

When dealing with an avulsed tooth, handle it by its crown and not by the root. Gently rinse the tooth with a sterile saline solution or water; do not use soap or chemicals, and do not scrub the tooth. When transporting the patient, bring along the tooth, place it in a special tooth storage solution, if available in your supplies, or in cold milk or sterile saline.[4,5] Do not allow the tooth to dry. Alternatively, your agency may use commercially available kits for this purpose. Be familiar with how the kit is used before you encounter a patient with dental trauma. Notify the receiving facility about the avulsed tooth, because reimplantation is recommended within 20 minutes to 1 hour after the trauma.

▶ Injuries of the Neck

The neck contains many structures that are vulnerable to injury by blunt trauma, such as from a steering wheel in a car crash, or by penetrating injury, such as a stab or gunshot wound. These structures include the upper airway, the esophagus, the carotid arteries and jugular veins, the thyroid cartilage (ie, Adam's apple), the cricoid cartilage, and the upper part of the trachea.

Any injury to the neck is serious and should be considered life threatening until proven otherwise in the ED. Blunt and penetrating mechanisms can damage both the soft tissues of the anterior part of the neck and its associated structures. In both cases, you must be alert for the possibility of cervical spine injury and airway compromise.

Blunt Injuries

Any crushing injury of the upper part of the neck is likely to involve the larynx or trachea. Examples include a collision with a steering wheel, an attempted suicide by hanging, and a clothesline injury sustained while riding a bicycle. Once the cartilages of the upper airway and larynx are fractured, they do not spring back to their normal position. This type of fracture can lead to loss of voice, difficulty swallowing, severe and sometimes fatal airway obstruction, and leakage of air into the soft tissues of the neck Figure 29-32. The presence of air in the soft tissues produces a characteristic crackling sensation called

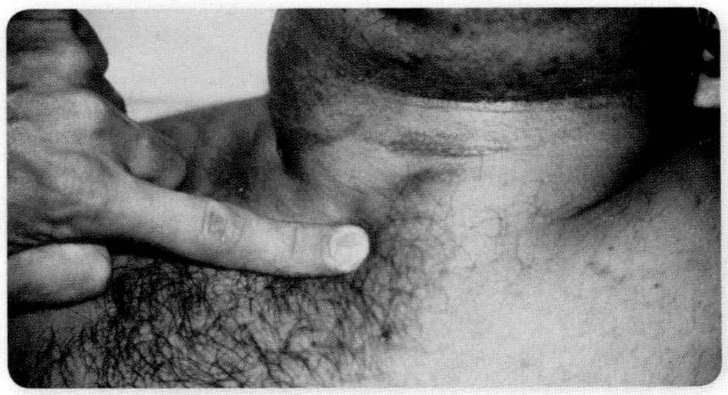

Figure 29-32 Fractures of the larynx or trachea can cause air to leak from the airway into the subcutaneous tissues. The presence of air in the soft tissues produces a crackling sensation called subcutaneous emphysema.

subcutaneous emphysema. If you feel this sensation when you palpate the neck, you should maintain the airway as best you can and provide immediate transport. Be aware that complete airway obstruction can develop very rapidly in these patients as a result of swelling or bleeding into the underlying tissues. It may be very difficult to manage the airway in patients with these injuries; therefore, paramedic support either by air or during an intercept may be necessary. Some patients will require a surgical airway at the hospital. An incident involving an injury to the throat may also have caused a cervical spinal injury; therefore, spinal immobilization may be needed.

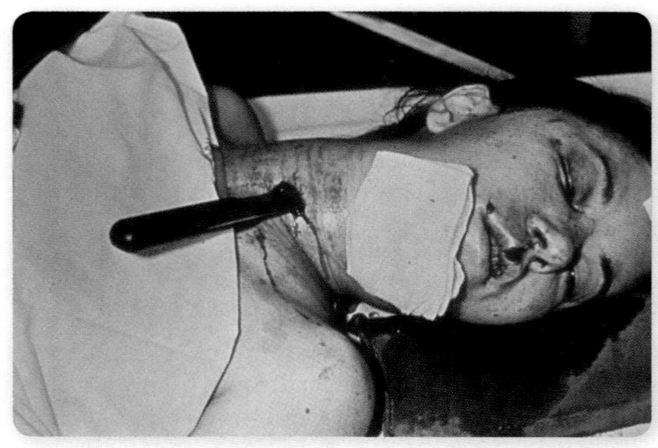

Figure 29-33 Penetrating injuries to the neck can result in profuse bleeding if a carotid artery or jugular vein is damaged.

Penetrating Injuries

The lacerations or puncture wounds produced by penetrating injuries may be superficial and involve only the fascia or fatty tissues of the neck, or they may be deep and involve injury to the larynx, trachea, esophagus, nerves, or major blood vessels. The primary threats from penetrating neck trauma are massive hemorrhage from major blood vessel disruption and airway compromise secondary to soft-tissue swelling or direct damage to the larynx or trachea.

Penetrating injuries to the neck can cause profuse bleeding from laceration of the carotid arteries or the jugular veins Figure 29-33. Injuries to the carotid and jugular vessels in the neck can cause the body to bleed out, a phenomenon also known as **exsanguination**.

A special danger associated with open neck injuries is the possibility of a fatal **air embolism**. If the jugular veins of the neck are exposed to the environment, then the veins may entrain (suck) air into the vessel and occlude the flow of blood into the lungs. A large amount of air entrained into the right atrium and right ventricle of the heart can lead to cardiac arrest. As such, immediately seal open neck wounds with an occlusive dressing. Use caution to avoid constricting the vessels and structures of the neck. Also, be alert for swelling and expanding hematomas because these conditions can turn the occlusive dressing into a constricting band.

Direct pressure over the bleeding site will control most neck bleeding. Follow the steps in Skill Drill 29-3.

Skill Drill 29-3 Controlling Bleeding From a Neck Injury

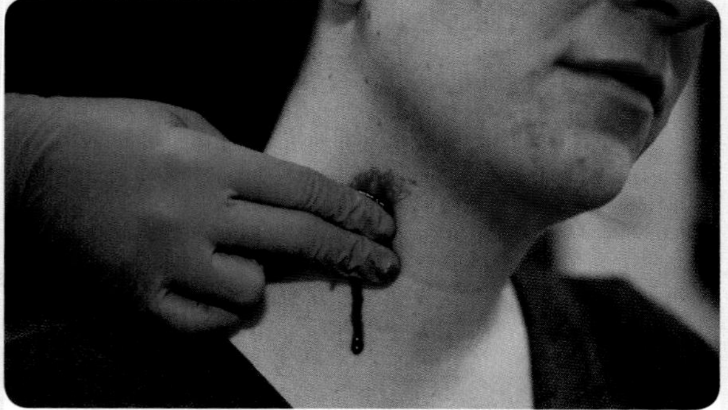

Step 1 Apply direct pressure to the bleeding site using a gloved fingertip if necessary to control bleeding.

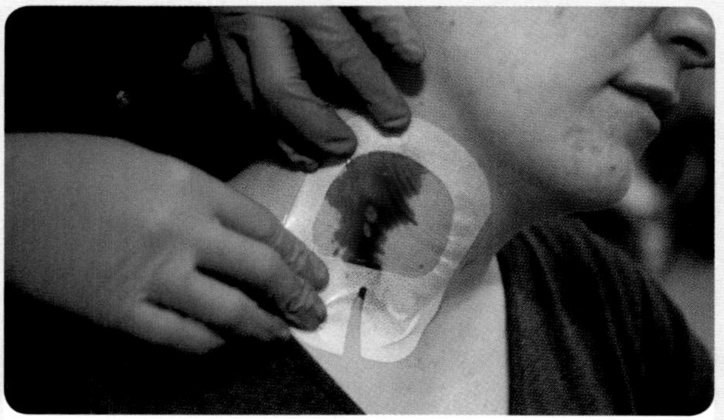

Step 2 Apply a sterile occlusive dressing to ensure air does not enter a vein or artery. Secure the dressing in place with roller gauze, adding more dressings if needed.

Words of Wisdom

Do not circumferentially wrap bandages around the neck to secure the dressing in place when controlling bleeding from a neck injury **Figure 29-34**. This practice is contraindicated and can be fatal if it impairs cerebral perfusion by occluding both carotid arteries or if it interferes with the patient's breathing. Monitor the patient's pulse for reflex bradycardia, which indicates parasympathetic nervous stimulation due to excessive pressure on the carotid artery.

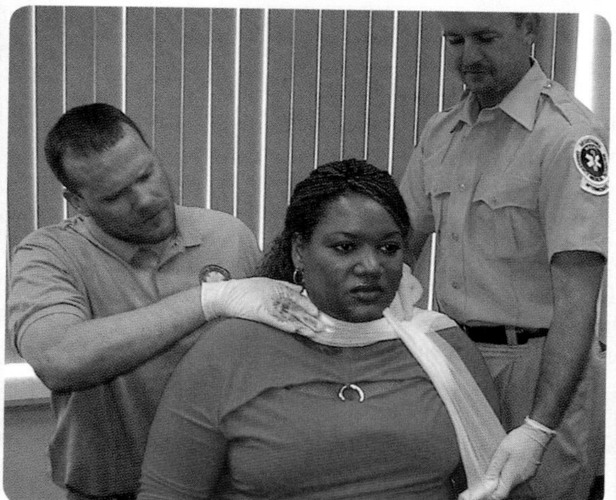

Figure 29-34 Cover open neck wounds with an occlusive dressing, and apply manual pressure to control bleeding. Secure the dressing in place by wrapping roller gauze around and under the patient's shoulder in a figure-8 pattern.

Courtesy of Rhonda Hunt.

You might find it necessary to apply pressure above *and* below the penetrating wound to control life-threatening bleeding from the carotid artery (above) and the jugular vein (below). You may also need to treat the patient for shock.

Impaled objects in the neck can present several life-threatening conditions for the patient—namely, injury to major blood vessels with massive hemorrhage; damage to the larynx, trachea, or esophagus; or injury to the cervical spine. Do not remove impaled objects. Instead, stabilize the object in place and protect it from movement. The *only* exception is if the object is obstructing the airway or impeding your ability to effectively manage the airway.

If indicated, maintain cervical spine immobilization, and with the patient fully immobilized on a backboard, provide prompt transport. Ensure the airway remains open en route, and administer high-flow oxygen. Obtain vascular access en route.

▶ Laryngeal Injuries

Blunt force trauma to the larynx can occur when an unrestrained driver strikes the steering wheel or when a snowmobile rider or off-road biker strikes a clothesline or a fixed wire strung across a property line. The larynx becomes crushed against the cervical spine, resulting in soft-tissue injury, fractures, and/or separation of the fascia that connects the thyroid and cricoid cartilages. These strangulation injuries can also be found in intentional or unintentional hangings. Whenever injury to the larynx is a possibility, you should suspect a possible cervical spine injury.

Open injuries to the larynx can occur as a result of a stabbing or penetration by a similar object. Do not remove penetrating and impaled objects unless they interfere with cardiopulmonary resuscitation. Stabilize all impaled objects if they are not obstructing the airway (see Chapter 28, *Soft-Tissue Injuries*).

Many injuries to the larynx, trachea, and esophagus are occult. They are not as obvious and dramatic as penetrating neck injuries, so you may easily overlook them. Therefore, maintain a high index of suspicion and perform a careful assessment of *any* patient with blunt trauma to the anterior part of the neck.

Significant injuries to the larynx pose an immediate risk of airway compromise because of disruption of the normal passage of air, soft-tissue swelling, or aspiration of blood. The signs and symptoms of larynx injuries include respiratory distress, hoarseness, pain, difficulty swallowing (**dysphagia**), coughing up blood (**hemoptysis**), cyanosis, pale skin, sputum in the wound, subcutaneous emphysema, bruising on the neck, structural irregularity, hematoma, or bleeding. In addition, esophageal perforation can result in **mediastinitis**, an inflammation of the mediastinum that is often due to leakage of gastric contents into the thoracic cavity. Mediastinitis has a very high mortality rate, particularly without rapid surgical treatment. Whenever injury to the anterior part of the neck (specifically the larynx) is recognized or suspected, it is prudent to ask the patient to refrain from speaking to allow the vocal cords to rest and recuperate. This will require you to ask questions that can be simply answered with a yes or no. Alternatively, you may ask the patient to write down his or her answers to your questions. Remember, if the larynx is injured, the incidence of cervical spine injury is relatively high; therefore, the patient should avoid shaking his or her head when responding.

Your primary focus when caring for a patient is always to treat the most rapidly fatal injuries. Because death following trauma to the anterior part of the neck is usually the result of airway compromise or massive bleeding, your priorities of care must be to aggressively manage the airway and control any external bleeding.

To manage a laryngeal and/or tracheal injury, provide oxygenation and ventilation, preferably with careful two-person bag-mask ventilation. Patients with injuries to the anterior part of the neck may experience concomitant maxillofacial fractures, which can make bag-mask ventilation difficult (usually because of an inadequate mask-to-face seal). Apply a cervical collar, but avoid using rigid collars because they may cause further damage to the soft tissues. Be alert to the need for frequent suctioning. Do not delay transport, because immediate surgical intervention may be the best treatment option. Call for paramedic rendezvous for advanced airway management, especially if the patient is apneic. If signs of shock are present, keep the patient warm. Establish vascular access with at least one large-bore IV line while en route to the hospital, if possible, or on scene if indicated. Infuse an isotonic crystalloid solution (such as lactated Ringer solution or normal saline) as needed to maintain adequate perfusion.

▶ Muscular Injuries

The neck, because of its relative exposure to forces both directly applied and referred, is subject to injury that does not necessarily result in specific bony injury such as fracture or dislocation. Most of these nonpenetrating injuries are typically classified as sprains and strains.

A **sprain** is a stretching or tearing of ligaments—the tough bands of fibrous tissue that connect one bone to another. In response to strains in the neck, the muscles contract as they attempt to support the neck. It is believed that this response is the result of injury to the facet joint. This injury can be difficult, if not impossible, for you to identify in the prehospital setting. As a result, maintain a high index of suspicion for cervical involvement and provide cervical spine stabilization.

A **strain** is a stretching or tearing of muscle or tendon. The most common form of cervical strain is often called **whiplash**. Whiplash can be difficult to differentiate from an unstable spine fracture or dislocation. Although whiplash is rarely life threatening, morbidity can occasionally develop in the form of persistent and chronic cervical pain, with some patients experiencing prolonged spasms and exacerbation.

Because it is difficult for you to evaluate complaints of neck pain, it is recommended that you transport patients to the ED for radiologic studies. Conduct a visual inspection for signs of soft-tissue injury, which may indicate muscular and bony involvement. If the patient is symptomatic and has pain (either with or without movement and palpation), then provide spinal immobilization.

If you suspect musculoskeletal injury to the neck, then address any airway, ventilation, and oxygenation considerations and ensure there is no major circulatory compromise. Prehospital management should focus on preventing further injury by restricting range of motion. This typically involves applying a cervical collar and placing the patient on a long backboard, scoop stretcher, or vacuum mattress, if indicated. In critical patients, it may be necessary to perform these tasks simultaneously. Whether you are applying a long backboard, scoop stretcher, or vacuum mattress, as in all splinting procedures, it is essential to check distal pulse and sensory and motor function before and after the full-body splint is applied and to document those findings in your patient care report. Regardless of MOI, patients reporting neck pain should be evaluated for occult injuries and prevention of long-term consequences.

Injury Prevention

Because face and neck injuries can be life altering and permanent, there have been many medical improvements and advancements in how these areas of the body are protected. This is especially true in the area of organized sporting events such as contact sports and other types of sports. Helmets, face shields, mouth guards, and safety eyewear help to prevent injury during activities in which the risk of being hit with objects that are in motion is proportionately high. There have also been many advances in motor vehicle safety. Better occupant safety restraints and airbags help to prevent contact with the interior of the vehicle, and improvements to the headrests, if they are used properly, are reducing the number of neck strains.

YOU are the Provider SUMMARY

1. On the basis of the information provided, what are some possible injuries you may encounter?

Penetrating injuries to the neck can cause profuse bleeding from laceration of the great vessels in the neck—the carotid arteries or the jugular veins. Injuries to the carotid and jugular vessels in the neck can cause the body to bleed out, also known as exsanguination. There is also a potential for cervical spine injury, as well as tracheal injury.

2. What is the best way to remove the piece of metal from the machinery?

There is no best way to remove this piece of metal from the machinery, and each situation is unique. If you are not familiar with different extrication methods that may be used to free the patient, then decisions made regarding extrication are best left to subject matter experts, after discussing the matter with emergency medical service providers and determining the potential risks and precautions that may need to be taken. Regardless of the method used, seek to minimize movement of the object and use methods to decrease the amount of heat generated.

3. How would you secure the tension rod to the patient?

This tension rod should be secured with large amounts of bulky dressing. Bulky dressings can be applied around the object in an attempt to create an environment that will ensure the rod does not move.

4. Why should you be concerned about air entering the wound?

If a vein has been punctured, then air may be sucked through it to the heart, causing an air embolism. The entry of a large amount of air in the right atrium and right ventricle of the heart can lead to cardiac arrest. An occlusive dressing should be applied over the entrance wound to prevent the introduction of air into the circulation.

5. How can you control bleeding from a neck wound?

Controlling bleeding from a neck wound may be difficult because direct pressure may compress arterial blood flow, creating a situation that can diminish the amount of oxygen delivered to the brain. Pressure can be applied above and below the wound, depending on whether the bleeding is arterial or venous, in an attempt to slow the bleeding, but always be cognizant of the potential for diminished blood flow to the brain. Also, ensure you use an occlusive dressing for any neck wound.

6. Will this patient need to be immobilized with a cervical collar before transport? How will you immobilize his head?

This patient has an isolated puncture injury to his neck. There is no mechanism consistent with injury to other parts of his spine. As long as he is awake and alert and able to report no back or low lumbar pain or tenderness, and as long as he is reliable based on no evidence of intoxication, traditional spinal immobilization with a backboard and collar can and should be avoided in favor of positioning in a way that facilitates stabilization of the impaled object, typically the lateral recumbent position on a backboard. However, with an object protruding from his neck, it may be difficult, if not impossible, to apply a cervical collar. If this is the case, manual stabilization can be maintained until arrival at the trauma center, or improvised materials may be applied to create a makeshift collar. *Any* neck movement could result in massive injury. Immobilize the patient to prevent further soft-tissue damage from the rod and to protect the neck from further injury. Keep suction readily available to assist in airway management.

7. What are some possible causes of this patient's initial shortness of breath?

There may be many different causes for this patient's shortness of breath. It could be a result of anxiety, shock, or potentially a fractured trachea. Signs and symptoms of a fractured trachea include respiratory distress, hoarseness, pain, difficulty swallowing (dysphagia), hemoptysis, cyanosis, pale skin, sputum in the wound, subcutaneous emphysema, bruising on the neck, structural irregularity, hematoma, and bleeding. Regardless of the cause, administer high-flow oxygen to the patient until it has been determined oxygen is no longer needed.

8. If you do not have the tools to cut the object and free the patient, should you remove the object from his neck?

If you do not have the necessary equipment or training to free the patient, extrication is best left to subject matter experts, typically, the responding fire department personnel. In the event that you do not have that option, removal is a last resort. In that case, it should be done quickly and the wound should be rapidly covered with an occlusive dressing and direct pressure applied.

YOU are the Provider SUMMARY (continued)

EMS Patient Care Report (PCR)			
Date: 9-11-18	**Incident No.:** 200989154	**Nature of Call:** Impaled object	**Location:** S. HWY 341 @ MM 27

Dispatched: 0857	**En Route:** 0900	**At Scene:** 0912	**Transport:** 1002	**At Hospital:** 1014	**In Service:** 1035

Patient Information	
Age: 19 **Sex:** M **Weight (in kg [lb]):** 99 kg (220 lb)	**Allergies:** Penicillin **Medications:** None **Past Medical History:** None **Chief Complaint:** Penetrating neck injury

Vital Signs				
Time: 0913	**BP:** Not obtained	**Pulse:** Not obtained	**Respirations:** Difficult to assess	**Spo_2:** Not obtained
Time: 0920	**BP:** 116/84	**Pulse:** 122	**Respirations:** 22	**Spo_2:** 96% on 15 L/min NRM
Time: 0935	**BP:** 124/76	**Pulse:** 105	**Respirations:** 18	**Spo_2:** 95% on 15 L/min NRM

EMS Treatment (circle all that apply)				
Oxygen @ 15 L/min via (circle one): **NC** **(NRM)** **Bag-mask device**		**Assisted Ventilation**	**Airway Adjunct**	**CPR**
Defibrillation	**(Bleeding Control:** Yes**)**	**(Bandaging:** Yes**)**	**Splinting**	**(Other:** Extrication**)**

Narrative

EMS dispatched to a residential farm for an unknown machinery accident. En route, dispatch updated information that the patient is male, with an unknown object impaled in his neck; fire department responding as well. On arrival, patient found standing with arms wrapped around farm implement, with approximately a 3-foot piece of 0.5-inch-diameter metal impaled in left side of neck. Distal end still connected to implement. Patient presents as alert and oriented × 4; ABCs intact. States he was attempting to free an obstruction when tension rod "snapped" and impaled him in the neck. Complaining of increasing shortness of breath. Administered oxygen at 15 L/min via NRM with cervical spine being held by firefighter. Occlusive dressing placed around rod, with copious amounts of bulky dressings applied for stabilization. Firefighters used hacksaw to cut rod, leaving approximately 10 inches protruding from neck. Noted an increase in visible bleeding from wound; direct pressure applied to superior and inferior vein, with bleeding being controlled. Once tension rod separated from implement, patient placed in lateral position on backboard to facilitate stabilization of rod. Patient had strong pulse, normal motor activity, and normal circulation in all 4 extremities. Unable to apply cervical collar owing to nature of injury; head immobilized with towel rolls and secured to backboard. Patient placed in back of ambulance and transported on emergency basis to trauma center. En route, 18-gauge IV line established in right AC and left AC with NS TKO in both. Patient states that he is breathing better with oxygen, and other than being scared, he has no other complaints. Physical examination is unremarkable. On arrival at trauma center, care and report given to staff without incident.**End of report**

Prep Kit

▶ Ready for Review

- The skull is divided into two large bony structures that protect the brain: the cranium and the face.
- Soft-tissue injuries and fractures of the bones of the face and neck are common and vary in severity.
- Airway compromise may be caused by heavy bleeding into the airway, swelling in and around the structures of the airway located in the face and neck, and injuries to the central nervous system that interfere with normal respiration.
- Trauma to the face can range from a broken nose to more severe injuries, including massive soft-tissue trauma, maxillofacial fractures, oral or dental trauma, and eye injuries.
- In face and neck injuries, your priorities are to prevent further injury to the cervical spine, manage the patient's airway and breathing, and control bleeding. Do not let soft-tissue injuries distract you from life threats that may not be readily apparent.
- Always check for bleeding inside the mouth, as it may produce an airway obstruction.
- Provide rapid transport for a patient with any of the following signs and symptoms: hypoperfusion, significant mechanism of injury, poor general impression, altered level of consciousness, abnormal vital signs, dyspnea, severe pain, or an isolated eye injury.
- To control heavy bleeding from soft-tissue injuries to the face, use direct pressure with a dry, sterile dressing. If brain tissue is exposed, then use a moist, sterile dressing.
- Save avulsed pieces of skin and tissue, and transport them with the patient for possible reattachment at the hospital.
- Maintain a high index of suspicion for patients with unequal pupils—this sign may indicate an illness or an injury to the brain. However, some people are born with one pupil larger than the other, so ask the patient whether he or she normally has unequal pupils.
- Foreign bodies on the surface of the eye should be irrigated gently with normal saline solution. Always flush from the region of the eye closest to the nose toward the outside, away from the midline.
- If a foreign body is stuck on the underside of the eyelid, then gently remove it with a cotton-tipped applicator. Never remove foreign bodies that are stuck to the cornea.
- Chemicals, heat, and light rays can all cause burn injury to the eyes, resulting in permanent damage. Treat chemical burns of the eye using gentle irrigation. Cover thermal eye burns and eye burns from light and transport the patient.
- If there is a laceration of the globe itself, then apply a moist, sterile dressing, and cover the injured eye with a protective metal eye shield, cup, or sterile dressing.
- Epistaxis following facial trauma can be severe. To effectively control it, apply direct pressure to the nares or apply pressure on the upper gums. Be alert to clear fluid draining from the ears or nose, as it may indicate a basilar skull fracture.
- When treating an ear injury, if local pressure does not control the bleeding, use a roller dressing. In the case of an ear avulsion, wrap the avulsed part in a moist, sterile dressing and put it in a labeled plastic bag, keep it cool, and transport it to the hospital with the patient. Never try to manipulate a foreign body that is in the ear canal.
- With dental injuries, apply direct pressure to stop the bleeding, keep the airway patent, and suction if needed. Cracked or loose teeth are possible airway obstructions. If a tooth is avulsed, then transport it with the patient, in an appropriate solution; do not let it become dry.
- If an object is impaled in the patient's cheek and bleeding from the wound is compromising the patient's airway, consider removing the impaled object, if possible. Apply direct pressure on the inside and outside of the cheek.
- Blunt and penetrating trauma to the neck can produce life-threatening injuries. Palpate the neck for signs of subcutaneous emphysema. In patients with this sign, complete airway obstruction may develop in minutes.
- If bleeding is present from a penetrating injury, then apply direct pressure over the site to control most forms of bleeding.
- Be alert to the possibility of an air embolism from an open neck injury. Place an occlusive dressing over the site, and provide direct pressure.
- Blunt force trauma can crush the larynx, resulting in soft-tissue injury, fractures, and potential spinal injury. Signs and symptoms of larynx injuries include hoarseness, pain, difficulty swallowing (dysphagia), hemoptysis, cyanosis, sputum in the wound, subcutaneous emphysema, and structural irregularity. Aggressively manage the airway, and call for paramedic rendezvous.
- If you recognize or suspect injury to the anterior part of the neck (specifically the larynx), then ask the patient to refrain from speaking to allow the vocal cords to rest and recuperate.
- In the case of a complaint of neck pain, maintain spinal immobilization and transport the patient to the ED for radiologic studies.

Prep Kit (continued)

▶ Vital Vocabulary

aqueous humor The clear, watery fluid in the anterior chamber of the globe (eyeball).

air embolism The presence of air in the veins, which can lead to cardiac arrest if it enters the heart.

anisocoria Uneven pupil size; can be naturally occurring, but also can be a sign of pathology.

basilar skull fracture Usually occurs following diffuse impact to the head (such as in falls, motor vehicle crashes); generally results from extension of a linear fracture to the base of the skull and can be difficult to diagnose with a radiograph (x-ray).

blowout fracture A fracture of the orbit or of the bones that support the floor of the orbit.

conjunctiva The delicate membrane that lines the eyelids and covers the exposed surface of the eye.

conjunctivitis Inflammation of the conjunctiva.

craniofacial disjunction A Le Fort III fracture; involves a fracture of all of the midfacial bones, thereby separating the entire midface from the cranium.

diplopia Double vision.

dysconjugate gaze Paralysis of gaze or lack of coordination between the movements of the two eyes.

dysphagia Difficulty swallowing.

epistaxis Nosebleed.

exsanguination Severe, possibly life-threatening loss of blood.

globe The eyeball.

hemoptysis Coughing up blood.

hyoid bone A bone at the base of the tongue that supports the tongue and its muscles.

hyphema Bleeding into the anterior chamber of the eye; results from direct ocular trauma.

lacrimal glands The glands that produce fluids to keep the eye moist; also called tear glands.

Le Fort fractures Maxillary fractures that are classified into three categories based on their anatomic location.

malocclusion Misalignment of the teeth.

mediastinitis Inflammation of the mediastinum that often results when gastric contents leak into the thoracic cavity after esophageal perforation.

oculomotor nerve A cranial nerve that innervates the muscles that cause motion of the eyeballs and upper eyelid.

optic nerve A cranial nerve that transmits visual information to the brain.

pinna The external, visible part of the ear.

pupil The circular opening in the middle of the iris that admits light to the back of the eye.

retinal detachment Separation of the retina from its attachments at the back of the eye.

sclera The tough, fibrous, white portion of the eye that protects the more delicate inner structures.

sprain Stretching or tearing of ligaments.

sternocleidomastoid muscles The muscles on either side of the neck that allow movement of the head.

strain Stretching or tearing of a muscle or tendon.

subcutaneous emphysema A characteristic crackling sensation felt on palpation of the skin, caused by the presence of air in soft tissues.

sympathetic eye movement The movement of both eyes in unison.

temporomandibular joint The joint formed where the mandible and cranium meet, just in front of the ear.

turbinates Layers of bone within the nasal cavity.

vitreous humor A jellylike substance found in the posterior compartment of the eye between the lens and the retina.

whiplash An injury to the neck in which hyperextension occurs as a result of the head moving abruptly forward or backward; can be difficult to differentiate from injuries that involve cervical bony structures and the spine.

▶ References

1. Eggenberger ER. Anisocoria. *Medscape.* June 16, 2016. http://emedicine.medscape.com/article/1158571-overview#a6. Retrieved February 17, 2017.
2. Anisocoria. *Medline Plus.* June 1, 2015. https://medlineplus.gov/ency/article/003314.htm. Retrieved February 17, 2017.
3. Simmen DB, Jones NS. Epistaxis. In: Flint PW, Haughey BH, Lund V, Niparko JK, Robbins T, Thomas JR, Lesperance MM, eds. *Cummings Otolaryngology*. 6th ed. Philadelphia, PA: Saunders; 2015:678-690.
4. Patil S, Dumsha T, Sydiskis R. Determining periodontal ligament (PDL) cell vitality from exarticulated teeth stored in saline or milk using fluorescein diacetate. *Int Endodontic J.* 1994; 27(1):1-5.
5. Poi W, Sonoda C, Martins C, et al. Storage media for avulsed teeth: a literature review. *Braz Dent J.* 2013;24(5):437-445.

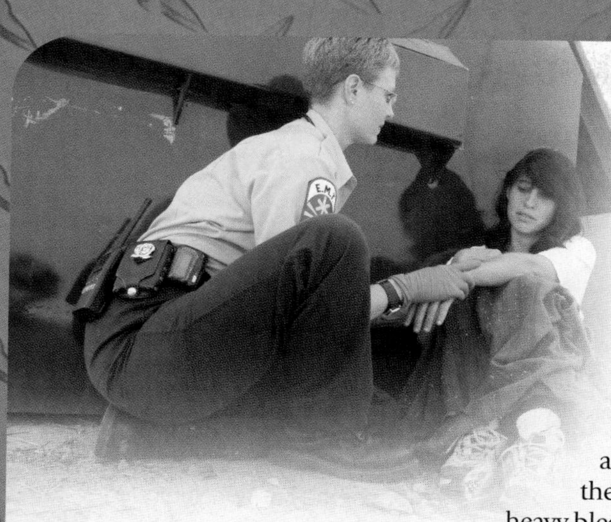

Assessment *in Action*

You arrive at the scene of a motorcycle crash to find a young male patient who was not wearing a helmet and struck a deer at a speed of approximately 35 miles per hour. He is currently unresponsive with a significant amount of facial trauma, including an elongated, flattened appearance of his face, and an apparent separation of the nasal bone and lower maxilla from the facial skull and remainder of the cranial bones. There is also heavy bleeding from an apparent puncture wound to the side of his neck.

1. Based on the patient's presentation, which of the following describes his injury?

- **A.** Le Fort I
- **B.** Le Fort II
- **C.** Le Fort III
- **D.** Le Fort IV

2. Fractures of the _____ can result in a flattened appearance of the face.

- **A.** orbits
- **B.** zygomatic bones
- **C.** maxilla
- **D.** mandible

3. If this patient also has dental malocclusion, then you should suspect a ____________ fracture.

- **A.** mandible
- **B.** maxilla
- **C.** zygomatic
- **D.** nasal

4. Because of the possible facial fracture, which type of airway adjunct should be used to help maintain an open airway?

- **A.** Nasopharyngeal airways are the only appropriate choice for possible facial fractures.
- **B.** Oropharyngeal airways are the only appropriate choice for possible facial fractures.
- **C.** You should not use an airway adjunct at all with a possible facial fracture.
- **D.** Either a nasopharyngeal airway or an oropharyngeal airway adjunct is appropriate with a possible facial fracture.

5. What is the proper method to control bleeding for this patient?

- **A.** Direct pressure
- **B.** Elevation of the head
- **C.** Pressure point
- **D.** Tourniquet

6. Patients presenting with a(n) _______ commonly report double vision.

- **A.** Le Fort fracture
- **B.** temporomandibular joint dislocation
- **C.** orbital fracture
- **D.** nasal fracture

7. Fluid draining from the ears may indicate a:

- **A.** basilar skull fracture.
- **B.** local infection.
- **C.** mandibular fracture.
- **D.** zygomatic fracture.

8. When you assess the pupils, you should inspect for size, shape, and reactivity to light. However, patients with _____ will present with unequal pupils even in the absence of injury.

- **A.** central vision
- **B.** cataracts
- **C.** peripheral vision
- **D.** anisocoria

9. Explain the difference between a neck *sprain* and a neck *strain*.

10. Explain the appropriate way to manage an impaled object in the cheek.

CHAPTER 30

Head and Spine Injuries

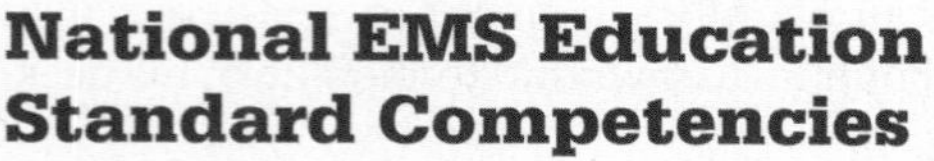

National EMS Education Standard Competencies

Trauma

Applies fundamental knowledge to provide basic and selected advanced emergency care and transportation based on assessment findings for an acutely injured patient.

Head, Facial, Neck, and Spine Trauma

Recognition and management of
- Life threats (pp 1218-1220)
- Spine trauma (pp 1213-1215, 1216-1220, 1224-1242)

Pathophysiology, assessment, and management of
- Penetrating neck trauma (Chapter 29, *Face and Neck Injuries*)
- Laryngotracheal injuries (Chapter 29, *Face and Neck Injuries*)
- Spine trauma (pp 1213-1222, 1224-1242)
- Facial fractures (Chapter 29, *Face and Neck Injuries*)
- Skull fractures (pp 1205-1207, 1215-1224)
- Foreign bodies in the eyes (Chapter 29, *Face and Neck Injuries*)
- Dental trauma (Chapter 29, *Face and Neck Injuries*)
- Laryngeotracheal injuries (Chapter 29, *Face and Neck Injuries*)

Nervous System Trauma

Pathophysiology, assessment, and management of
- Traumatic brain injury (pp 1198, 1207-1208, 1215-1224)
- Spinal cord injury (pp 1214-1222, 1224-1242)

Knowledge Objectives

1. List the major bones of the skull and spinal column and their related structures, and describe their functions as related to the nervous system. (pp 1198-1200)
2. Review the anatomy and physiology of the nervous system, including its divisions into the central nervous system (CNS) and peripheral nervous system and the structures and functions of each. (pp 1200-1204)
3. Describe the regions of the brain, including the cerebrum, diencephalon, brainstem, and the cerebellum, and their functions. (pp 1200-1202)
4. Discuss age-related variations that are required when providing emergency care to a pediatric patient who has a suspected head or spinal injury. (pp 1204, 1207, 1220, 1221, 1242)
5. List the mechanisms of injury that cause a high index of suspicion for the possibility of a head or spinal injury. (pp 1204-1205, 1207, 1213-1214)
6. Discuss the different types of head injuries, their potential mechanism of injury (MOI), and general signs and symptoms of a head injury that the advanced emergency medical technician (AEMT) should consider when performing a patient assessment. (pp 1204-1207)
7. Distinguish between the signs and symptoms of head injury and those of traumatic brain injury. (p 1205)
8. Define traumatic brain injury (TBI) and explain the difference between a primary (direct) injury and a secondary (indirect) injury, providing examples of possible mechanisms of injury that may cause each one. (pp 1207-1208)
9. Discuss the different types of brain injuries and their corresponding signs and symptoms, including increased intracranial pressure (ICP), concussion, contusion, and injuries caused by medical conditions. (pp 1208-1213)
10. Discuss the different types of injuries that may damage the cervical, thoracic, or lumbar spine, providing examples of possible mechanisms of injury that may cause each one. (pp 1213-1214)
11. Describe the steps in the patient assessment process for a person who has a suspected head or spinal injury, including specific variations that may be required as related to the type of injury. (pp 1215-1222)
12. Discuss when it would be appropriate to establish intravenous access in a patient with a head or spinal injury, including the importance of judicious fluid administration. (pp 1219, 1223-1224)

13. Describe the process of providing emergency medical care to a patient with a head injury, including the four general principles designed to protect and maintain the critical functions of the CNS. (pp 1222-1224)
14. Describe the process of providing emergency medical care to a patient with a spinal injury, including the implications of not properly caring for patients with injuries of this nature, the steps for performing manual in-line stabilization, implications for sizing and using a cervical spine immobilization device, and key symptoms that contraindicate in-line stabilization. (pp 1224-1228)
15. Describe the process of preparing patients who have suspected head or spinal injuries for transport, including the use and functions of a long backboard, short backboard, and other short spinal extrication devices to immobilize the patient's cervical and thoracic spine. (pp 1227-1239)
16. Explain the different circumstances in which a helmet should be either left on or taken off a patient with a possible head or spinal injury, and then list the steps AEMTs must follow to remove a helmet, including the alternate method for removing a football helmet. (pp 1239-1242)

Skills Objectives

1. Demonstrate how to perform a jaw-thrust maneuver on a patient with a suspected spinal injury. (p 1218)
2. Demonstrate how to perform manual in-line stabilization on a patient with a suspected spinal injury. (p 1225, Skill Drill 30-1)
3. Demonstrate how to apply a cervical collar to a patient with a suspected spinal injury. (pp 1225-1226, Skill Drill 30-2)
4. Demonstrate how to immobilize a patient with a suspected spinal injury to a long backboard. (pp 1228-1232, Skill Drill 30-3)
5. Demonstrate how to immobilize a patient with a suspected spinal injury to a scoop stretcher. (pp 1229, 1233, Skill Drill 30-4)
6. Demonstrate how to immobilize a patient with a suspected spinal injury to a vacuum mattress. (pp 1230, 1232-1236, Skill Drill 30-5)
7. Demonstrate how to immobilize a patient with a suspected spinal injury who was found in a sitting position. (pp 1233, 1237-1239, Skill Drill 30-6)
8. Demonstrate how to immobilize a patient with a suspected spinal injury to a short backboard. (pp 1233, 1237-1239)
9. Demonstrate how to remove a helmet from a patient with a suspected head or spinal injury. (pp 1239-1241, Skill Drill 30-7)
10. Demonstrate the alternate method for removal of a helmet from a patient with a suspected head or spinal injury. (pp 1240, 1242)

Introduction

The nervous system is a complex network of nerve cells that enables all parts of the body to function. It includes the brain, spinal cord, and **peripheral nervous system**, which contains several billion nerve fibers that carry information to and from all parts of the body. Because the nervous system is so vital, it is well protected. The brain lies within the skull, and the spinal cord is inside the bony spinal canal. Despite this protection, serious blows can damage the nervous system.

Terminology related to head trauma includes the following:

- **Head trauma** refers to both head injuries and traumatic brain injuries.
- **Head injury** is traumatic injury to the head that may result in injury to the scalp, head, or skull, but not including the face. The terms *head injury*

YOU are the Provider — PART 1

Your ambulance is dispatched to a local community swimming pool for a possible spinal injury. On arrival, you are met by the lifeguards who state the patient was running alongside the pool, slipped, and fell into the pool headfirst, striking his head on the bottom. They immediately took spinal precautions, placed the patient onto a floating backboard, and placed him alongside the pool. The patient has been in and out of consciousness. As you begin your assessment, you find the patient alert and oriented, reporting no feeling in his arms and legs.

1. On the basis of the information provided, what are some possible injuries you may encounter?
2. Is this patient experiencing a primary or secondary brain injury?

and *traumatic brain injury* are frequently used interchangeably. For the purposes of this chapter however, the term *head injury* will be used to describe injuries to the scalp or skull but not the brain or face.

- **Traumatic brain injury (TBI)** refers to an injury to the brain caused by an external force that may or may not result in physical, emotional, social, and vocational consequences.

These injuries, as well as spinal cord injury (SCI), will be discussed in this chapter. SCI is one of the most devastating injuries encountered by prehospital providers. TBI is a substantial cause of death and disability and is responsible for about 30% of trauma-related deaths each year.[1,2] In 2013, TBI resulted in approximately 2.8 million visits to emergency departments (EDs), was diagnosed in 282,000 hospitalizations, and contributed to 50,000 deaths.[2]

This chapter first briefly reviews the anatomy and function of the central and peripheral nervous systems and of the skeletal system, information that you will need to make an accurate assessment of injuries to these systems. It then discusses specific head and spinal injuries, including signs, symptoms, and treatment. Extrication of patients with possible spinal injuries and removal of helmets are also described.

Anatomy and Physiology Review

The nervous system is divided into two anatomic parts: the central nervous system and the peripheral nervous system Figure 30-1. The **central nervous system (CNS)** is composed of the brain and spinal cord. The peripheral nervous system conducts sensory and motor impulses to and from the skin, muscles, and other organs to the spinal cord. The brain, located within the cranial cavity, is the largest component of the CNS.

The nervous system is responsible for the generation and control of two types of activities in general: voluntary and involuntary. **Voluntary activities** are the actions that we consciously perform, in which sensory input determines the specific muscular activity—for example, reaching across the table for a salt shaker or to pass a dish. **Involuntary activities** are the actions that are not under conscious control, such as breathing; in most instances, we inhale and exhale without consciously thinking about it. Many of our body's functions occur independent of thought, or involuntarily.

The Scalp

The scalp is composed of multiple layers. The subcutaneous tissue contains the major vessels supplying the scalp. These vessels are attached to the superficial fascia. Laceration or other compromise of these vessels can result in profuse hemorrhage. Although this hemorrhage is sometimes not life threatening, it can distract you from other life-threatening injuries. At the same time, you cannot underestimate the potential for blood loss from scalp hemorrhage, particularly in patients who take blood thinners or have clotting disorders, to be rapidly lethal.

The Skull

The skull has two groups of bones: the cranium, which protects the brain, and the facial bones Figure 30-2.

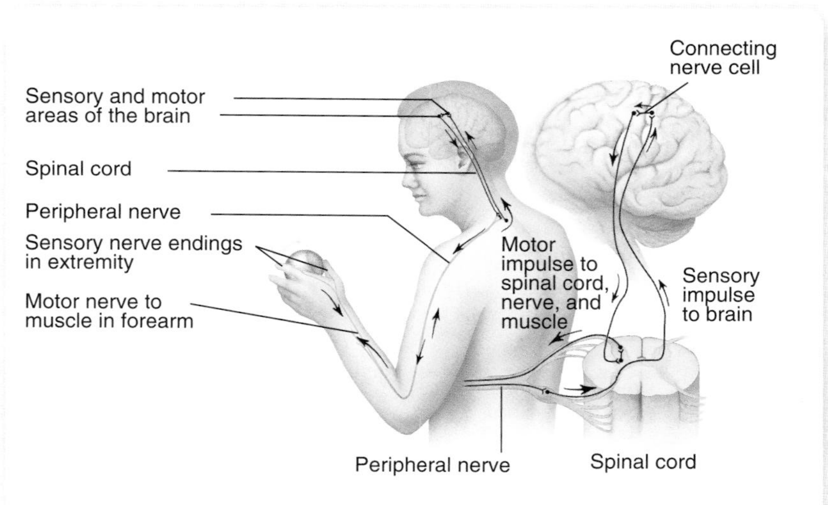

Figure 30-1 The nervous system has two anatomic components: the central nervous system (CNS) and the peripheral nervous system. The CNS is composed of the brain and the spinal cord. The peripheral nervous system is composed of nerves that conduct sensory and motor impulses to and from the skin, muscles, and other organs to the spinal cord and, eventually, the brain.

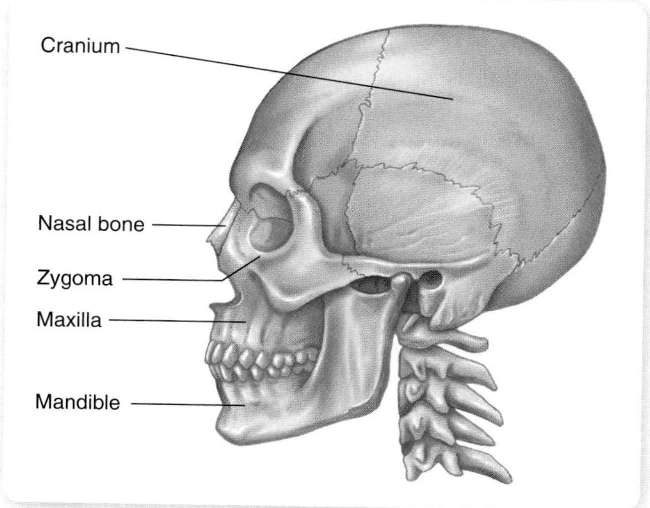

Figure 30-2 The skull has two large structures: the cranium and the face.

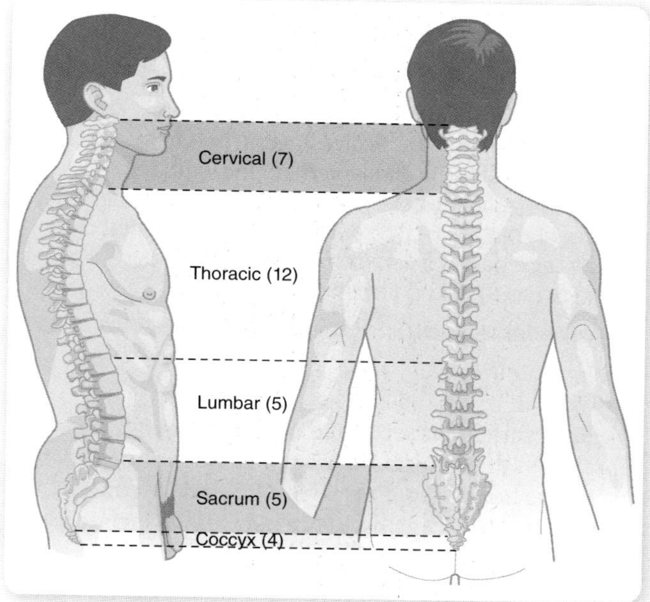

Figure 30-3 The spinal column is the body's central supporting system and consists of 33 bones divided into five sections. Each vertebra is numbered and referred to by a letter corresponding to the section of the spine where it is located plus its number. For example, the fifth thoracic vertebra is referred to as T5.

The mandible (lower jaw), the only movable facial bone, is connected to the cranium by the temporomandibular joint in front of each ear. The cranium is composed of several thick bones that fuse together to form a shell above the eyes and ears that holds and protects the brain. It is occupied by 80% brain tissue, 10% blood supply, and 10% **cerebrospinal fluid (CSF)**. The brain connects to the spinal cord through a large opening at the base of the skull called the foramen magnum.

Four major bones make up the cranium. The most posterior portion of the cranium is called the occiput. On each side of the cranium, the lateral portions are called the temples or temporal regions. Between the temporal regions and the occiput lie the parietal regions. The forehead is called the frontal region.

The face is composed of 14 bones. The upper, nonmoveable jawbones are called the maxillae, the cheekbones are called the zygomas, and the mandible is the lower, moveable portion of the jaw.

The orbit (eye socket) is made up of the frontal bone of the cranium and two facial bones: the maxilla and the zygoma. Together, these bones form a solid bony rim that protrudes around the eye to protect it. The nose mostly consists of flexible cartilage; in fact, only the proximal third of the nose is formed by bone with short bones forming the bridge of the nose.

▶ The Spine

The spine consists of 33 irregular bones (vertebrae) articulating to form the vertebral column, which is the major structural component of the axial skeleton. These skeletal components are stabilized by ligaments, joint capsules, and muscle. Together these components support and protect neural elements while allowing for fluid movement and erect stature **Figure 30-3**.

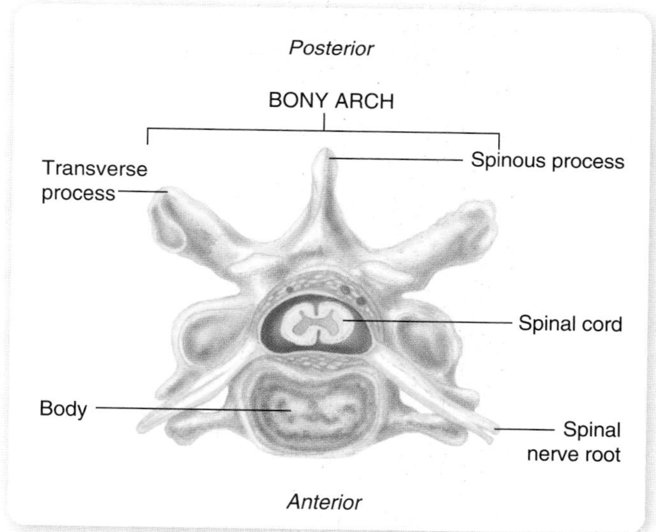

Figure 30-4 The spinal canal is formed by the vertebral body in the front (or anteriorly) and the bony arch in the back (or posteriorly).

Vertebrae are identified according to their location as cervical, thoracic, lumbar, or sacral. The **vertebral body**, the anterior weight-bearing structure, is made of bone that provides support and stability. The posterior portion of each vertebra forms a bony arch **Figure 30-4**. From one vertebra to the next, the series of arches forms a tunnel running the length of the spine. This is the spinal canal, which encases and protects the spinal cord.

> **Words of Wisdom**
>
> The lumbar spine is a common site of injury. Most of these injuries do not involve fracture or other structural disruption of the bony elements of the lumbar spine but rather involve muscle spasm and do not threaten the integrity of the spinal cord or its nerve roots. Nonetheless, low back pain is a very common problem, as well as a major cause of impairment and disability.

Each vertebra is separated and cushioned by **intervertebral disks** that limit bone wear and act as shock absorbers. As the body ages, these disks lose water content and become thinner, causing the height loss associated with aging. Stress on the vertebral column may cause a disk to herniate into the spinal canal, resulting in an injury to the spinal cord or a **nerve root injury** Figure 30-5. Nerves can also be injured at the peripheral level (anywhere in the body outside of the spinal cord); this is called **peripheral nerve injury**.

The spinal column itself is almost entirely surrounded by muscles. However, you can palpate the posterior spinous process of the vertebra. In thin people, these lie just under the skin in the midline of the back. The most prominent and most easily palpable spinous process is at the seventh cervical vertebra at the base of the neck.

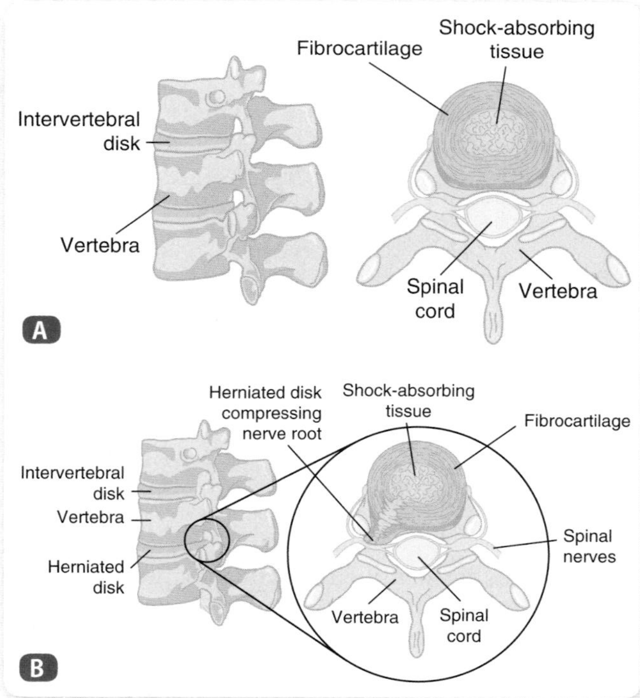

Figure 30-5 A. Normal, uninjured vertebral disk. **B.** Herniated disk.

The muscles, tendons, and ligaments that connect the vertebrae allow the spinal column a degree of flexion and extension, limited to an extent by the stabilization they must provide to the spinal column. The vertebral column can flex and extend substantially allowing motion to occur without causing injury to the spinal cord. Flexion or extension beyond what the spine is capable of tolerating at any particular level may damage structural ligaments and allow excess vertebral movement that could expose the spinal cord to injury.

▶ The Central Nervous System

The Brain

As discussed, the CNS is composed of the brain and spinal cord. The brain, which occupies 80% of the cranial vault, contains billions of neurons (nerve cells) that perform a variety of vital functions. The brain is the organ that controls the body, the center of consciousness. The major regions of the brain are the cerebrum, diencephalon (thalamus and hypothalamus), brainstem (medulla, pons, midbrain), and the cerebellum. The remaining intracranial contents include cerebral blood (12%) and CSF (8%) Figure 30-6.

The brain accounts for only 2% of total body weight, yet it is the most metabolically active and perfusion-sensitive organ in the body. The brain metabolizes 25% of the body's glucose, burning approximately 60 mg/min, and consumes 20% of the total body oxygen (45 to 50 L/min). Because the brain has no storage mechanism for oxygen or glucose, it is totally dependent on cerebral blood flow (provided by carotid and vertebral arteries) for a constant flow of both fuels. The brain will continually manipulate the physiology as needed to guarantee that a ready supply of oxygen and glucose are available. A loss of blood flow to the brain for 5 to 10 seconds will result in unresponsiveness.

The Cerebrum. The **cerebrum** contains approximately 75% of the brain's total volume. It is responsible for higher functions, such as reasoning. The cerebrum is divided into right and left hemispheres.

The largest portion of the cerebrum is the **cerebral cortex**, which regulates voluntary skeletal movement and the level of awareness. Injury to the cerebral cortex may result in paresthesia, weakness, and paralysis of the extremities. Each cerebral hemisphere is divided into anatomic areas called lobes that control specific functions Figure 30-7. The **frontal lobe** is responsible for voluntary motor action and personality traits. Injury to the frontal lobe may result in seizures or placid reactions (flat affect). (Recall that the front lobe filters the raw emotional impulses from the limbic system Figure 30-8.) The **parietal lobe** controls the somatic or voluntary sensory and motor functions for the opposite (contralateral) side of the body, as well as memory and emotions. Posteriorly, the **occipital lobe**, from which the optic nerve originates, is responsible for processing visual information. After a blow to the back of the head, a person may "see stars," which results when

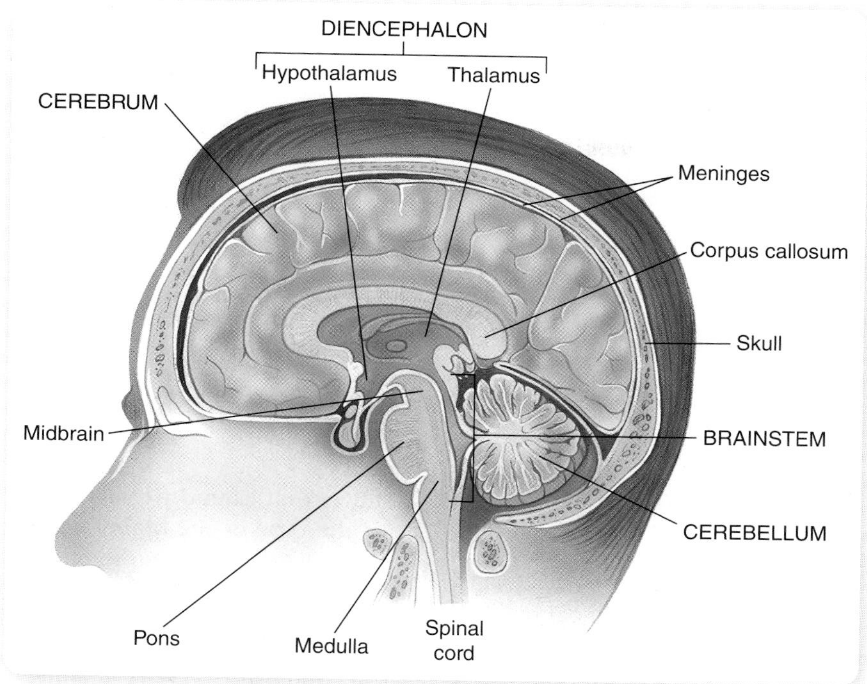

Figure 30-6 The major regions of the brain.

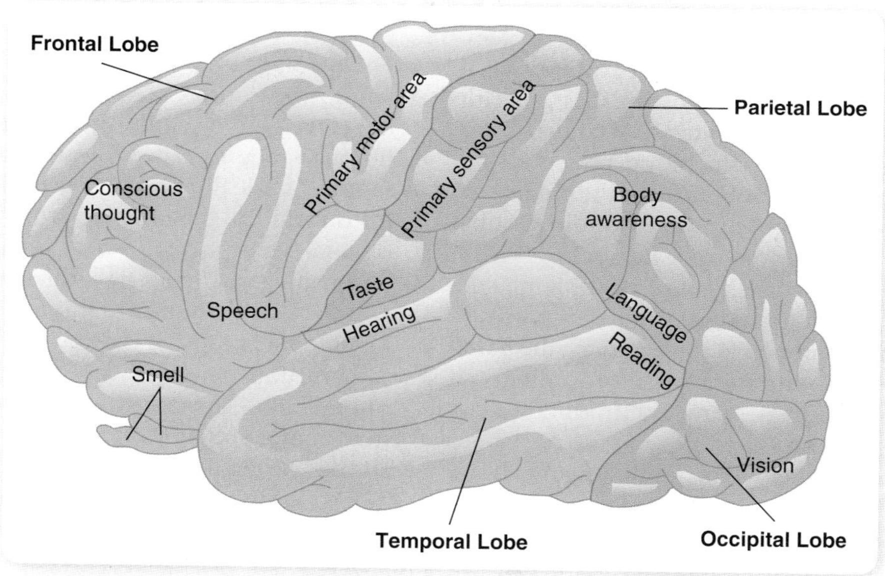

Figure 30-7 Lobes of the cerebrum.

the occipital poles (vision centers) of the brain strike the back of the skull.

The speech center is located in the **temporal lobe**. The temporal lobe also controls long-term memory, hearing, taste, and smell.

The Cerebellum. Inferior and posterior to the cerebrum lies the **cerebellum**, which coordinates body movements. It is sometimes called the "athlete's brain" because it is responsible for the maintenance of posture and equilibrium and the coordination of skilled movements.

The Brainstem. The most primitive part of the CNS, the **brainstem**, controls virtually all functions that are necessary for life, including the cardiac and respiratory systems. Deep within the cranium, the brainstem is the best-protected part of the CNS.

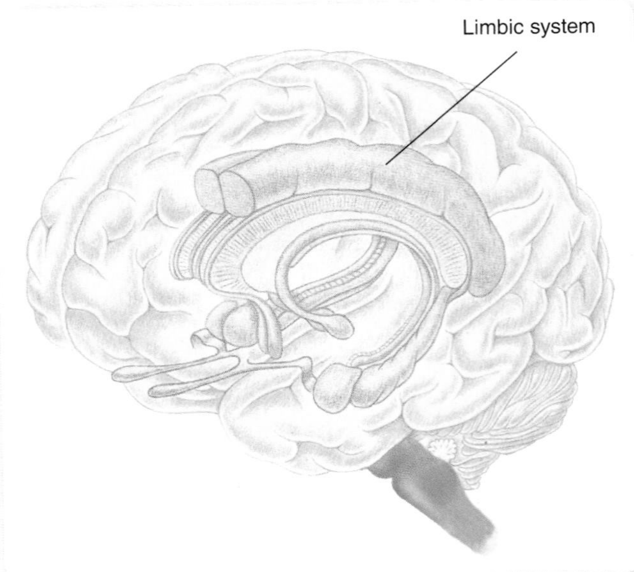

Figure 30-8 The limbic system is the seat of emotions, instincts, and other functions.

The brainstem consists of the midbrain, pons, and the medulla. It is located at the base of the brain and connects the spinal cord to the remainder of the brain. The brainstem houses many structures that are critical to the maintenance of vital functions. High in the brainstem, for example, is the **reticular activating system (RAS)**, which is responsible for maintenance of consciousness, specifically one's level of arousal. The centers that control basic but critical functions—heart rate, blood pressure, and respiration—are located in the lower part of the brainstem. Damage to this area can easily result in cardiovascular derangement, respiratory arrest, or death.

The midbrain lies immediately below the diencephalon and is the smallest region of the brainstem. Deep within the cerebrum, diencephalon, and midbrain are the **basal ganglia**, which have an important role in coordination of motor movements and posture. The midbrain also controls pupillary size and reactivity.

The **pons**, which lies below the midbrain and above the medulla, contains numerous important nerve fibers, including those for sleep, respiration, and the medullary respiratory center—the portion of the respiratory center that is in the medulla oblongata.

The inferior portion of the midbrain, the **medulla**, is continuous inferiorly with the spinal cord and serves as a conduction pathway for ascending and descending nerve tracts. It also coordinates heart rate, blood vessel diameter, breathing, swallowing, vomiting, coughing, and sneezing. The vagus nerve (tenth cranial nerve), a bundle of nerves that primarily innervates the parasympathetic nervous system, originates from the medulla.

The Spinal Cord

The spinal cord transmits nerve impulses or signals between the brain and the rest of the body. It is composed of nerve fibers that extend from the brain's nerve cells. Starting at the base of the brain, it represents the continuation of the CNS. This bundle of nerve fibers leaves the skull through a large opening at its base called the foramen magnum. The spinal cord extends from the base of the skull to approximately L2; here it terminates and forms into the **cauda equina**, a collection of individual nerve roots. In total, 31 pairs of spinal nerves arise from the different segments of the spinal cord; each pair is named according to its corresponding segment.

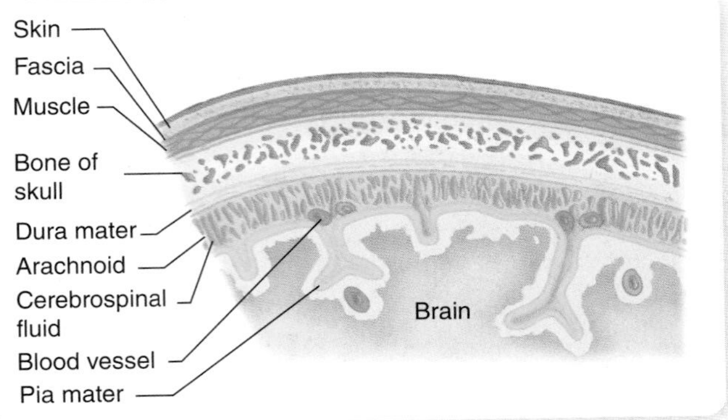

Figure 30-9 The meninges.

The Meninges

The **meninges** are protective layers that surround and enfold the entire CNS—specifically the brain and spinal cord Figure 30-9. The outermost layer is a strong, fibrous wrapping called the **dura mater** (meaning "tough mother"). The dura mater covers the entire brain, folding in to form the **tentorium**, a structure that separates the cerebral hemispheres from the cerebellum and brainstem. The meningeal arteries are located between the dura mater and the skull. Bleeding in this area results in an epidural hematoma because it is *above* the dura.

The dura mater is firmly attached to the internal wall of the skull. Just beneath the suture lines of the skull the dura mater splits into two surfaces and forms venous sinuses. When those venous sinuses are disrupted during a head injury, blood can collect beneath the dura mater to form a subdural hematoma.

The second meningeal layer is a delicate, transparent membrane called the **arachnoid**. It is so named because the blood vessels it contains resemble a spider web. The third meningeal layer, the **pia mater** ("soft mother"), is a

Words of Wisdom

A tip for remembering the names of the meningeal layers is to think of them as a "PAD" from the inside out. The innermost layer of the pad is the pia (P); the middle layer is the arachnoid (A); and the outer layer is the dura (D).

thin, translucent, highly vascular membrane that firmly adheres directly to the surface of the brain.

The meninges float in CSF, which is manufactured in the ventricles of the brain. CSF flows in the subarachnoid space, located between the pia mater and the arachnoid.

▶ The Peripheral Nervous System

Long fibers link the nerve cells to the body's various organs through openings in the bony coverings. These cables of nerve fibers make up the peripheral nervous system. The peripheral nervous system has two anatomic parts: 31 pairs of spinal nerves mentioned earlier, and 12 pairs of cranial nerves **Figure 30-10**.

The Somatic Nervous System

The part of the nervous system that regulates or controls our voluntary activities, including almost all coordinated muscular activities, is called the **somatic nervous system**. The mechanism of the somatic nervous system is simple. The brain interprets the sensory information that it receives from the peripheral nerves and responds by sending signals to the voluntary muscles.

The body functions that occur without conscious effort are regulated by the much more primitive autonomic (involuntary) nervous system. The autonomic nervous system controls the functions of many of the body's vital organs, over which the brain has no voluntary control.

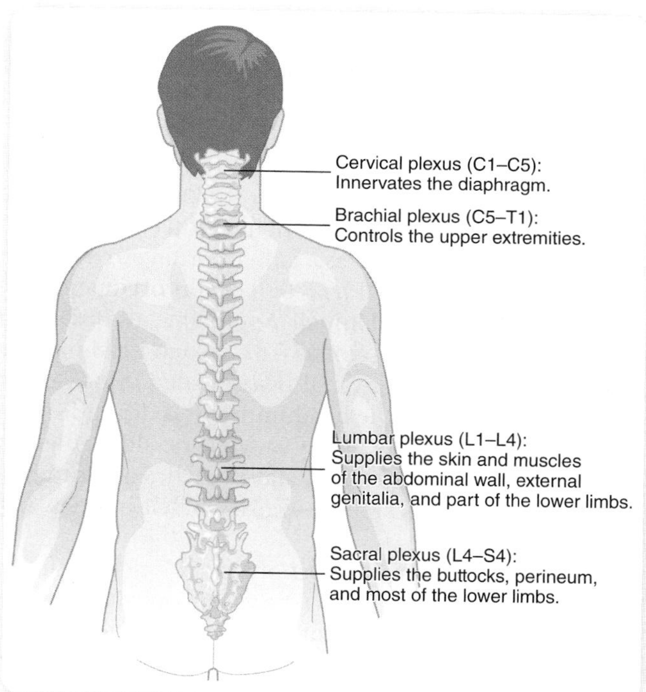
Cervical plexus (C1–C5): Innervates the diaphragm.
Brachial plexus (C5–T1): Controls the upper extremities.
Lumbar plexus (L1–L4): Supplies the skin and muscles of the abdominal wall, external genitalia, and part of the lower limbs.
Sacral plexus (L4–S4): Supplies the buttocks, perineum, and most of the lower limbs.

Figure 30-10 The peripheral nervous system is a complex network of motor and sensory nerves. The brachial plexus transmits messages to the arms, and the lumbosacral plexus transmits messages to the legs.

> **Words of Wisdom**
>
> CNS structures, whose bony enclosures protect them quite well, are also extremely fragile. Protecting them from further damage is vital to the patient's future ability to live a normal life. Lean toward caution and overprotection in assessing and treating possible brain and SCIs.

Cranial Nerves. Cranial nerves are the 12 pairs of nerves that pass through openings in the skull and transmit sensations directly to or from the brain. They primarily perform special functions in the head and face, including sight, smell, taste, hearing, and facial expressions.

Peripheral Nerves. The 31 pairs of spinal nerves conduct sensory impulses from the skin and other organs to the spinal cord. They also conduct motor impulses from the spinal cord to the muscles. Because the arms and legs have so many muscles, the spinal nerves serving the extremities are arranged in complex networks. The brachial plexus controls the arms, and the lumbosacral plexus controls the legs.

There are two major types of peripheral nerves, sensory nerves and motor nerves. The **sensory nerves**, with endings that can perceive only one type of information each (such as temperature or texture), carry information from the body to the brain via the spinal cord. The **motor nerves**, one for each muscle, carry information from the CNS to the muscles. The **connecting nerves**, found only in the brain and spinal cord, connect the sensory and motor nerves with short fibers, which allow the cells on either end to exchange messages.

By connecting the sensory and motor nerves of the limbs, the connecting nerves in the spinal cord form a reflex arc. If a sensory nerve in this arc detects an irritating stimulus, such as heat, it will bypass the brain and send a message directly to the motor nerve, causing a response such as pulling away from the heat **Figure 30-11**.

The Autonomic Nervous System

The Sympathetic Nervous System. The sensory (afferent) and motor (efferent) nerves are responsible for the somatic functions of the spinal cord and often overshadow the role of the spinal cord in the involuntary **autonomic nervous system**. The **sympathetic nervous system** is controlled by the brain's hypothalamus. Information from the brain is transmitted through the brainstem and the cervical spinal cord and then exits at the thoracic and lumbar levels of the spine to reach target structures.

Certain fibers of the sympathetic nervous system stimulate the periphery largely through alpha and beta functions. Alpha receptor stimulation induces smooth muscle contraction in blood vessels and bronchioles. Beta receptor stimulation produces relaxation of smooth muscles in blood vessels and bronchioles and has chronotropic

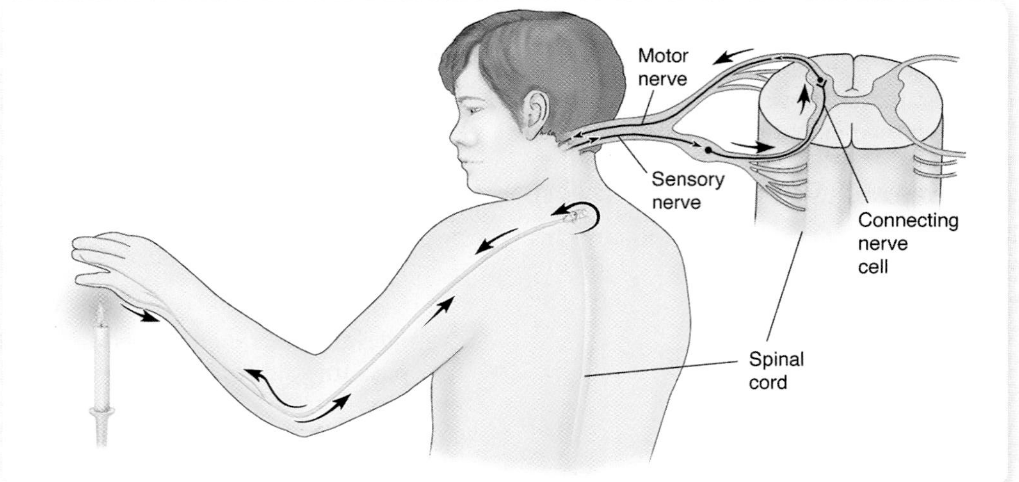

Figure 30-11 The connecting nerves in the spinal cord form a reflex arc. If a sensory nerve in this arc detects an irritating stimulus, it will bypass the brain and send a direct message to the motor nerve.

(affecting heart rate) and inotropic (affecting contractility) effects on myocardial cells. The sympathetic nervous system is also responsible for sweating, pupil dilation, and temperature regulation, as well as the shunting of blood from the periphery to the core during the fight-or-flight response.

SCI at or above the level of T6 may disrupt the flow of sympathetic communication. Loss of sympathetic stimulation can disrupt homeostasis and leave the body poorly equipped to deal with changes in its environment.

The Parasympathetic Nervous System. The **parasympathetic nervous system** is responsible for conserving energy and maintaining organ function. It includes fibers arising from the brainstem and upper spinal cord that carry signals to organs of the abdomen, heart, lungs, and the skin above the waist. The vagus nerve travels from its origin outside of the medulla to the heart via the carotid arteries; thus, vagal tone remains intact following a spine injury. Parasympathetic nerves that supply the reproductive organs, pelvis, and leg begin at the sacral level (S2 through S4). Disruption of the lower parasympathetic nerves in the sacrum results in the loss of bowel/bladder tone and sexual function.

Special Populations

In older adults, SCI can result from seemingly minor falls. Decreased bone density or osteoporosis, arthritis, and general weakening of the ligaments and musculature of the neck in older adults contribute to increased risk of SCI. For example, a fall down a small flight of stairs may be enough to cause substantial injury to the spine.

Similarly, infants and children are more susceptible to direct brain injury because their skull formation along suture lines is not complete. This flexibility of the skull may also mask injuries that may be obvious in adolescents or adult patients. A force that compresses an adult skull and readily fractures it will not necessarily fracture a pediatric skull because the sutures may allow that same force to compress the pediatric brain without causing fracture.

Pathophysiology

Head Injuries

A head injury is a traumatic insult to the head that may result in injury to soft tissue, bony structures, and/or the brain. TBI is impairment of brain function brought about by an external force, such as a fall. According to the Brain Trauma Foundation (BTF), 56,000 deaths occur annually as a result of severe head injury.[3] Approximately 30% of all traumatic deaths result from a TBI.[2] When head injuries are fatal, the cause is invariably associated injury to the brain. In addition to the head injury, and depending on the mechanism of injury (MOI), you should be alert to the fact that the patient may have sustained additional trauma such as cervical spine injuries, pelvic injuries, and chest injuries.

There are two general types of head injuries: open and closed. A **closed head injury** (the most common type) is usually associated with blunt trauma. Although the dura mater remains intact and brain tissue is not exposed to the environment, closed head injuries may result in skull fractures, focal brain injuries, or diffuse brain injuries. Furthermore, these injuries are often complicated by increased **intracranial pressure (ICP)**.

With an **open head injury**, the dura mater and cranial contents are penetrated, and brain tissue is open to the environment. Gunshot wounds—the most common penetrating MOI—have a high mortality rate, and for those who survive there is almost always substantial neurologic deficit and a decreased quality of life.

Open and closed head injuries have essentially the same signs and symptoms. Following an injury, any patient who exhibits one or more of the signs or symptoms listed in Table 30-1 should be evaluated promptly in the ED.

Table 30-1 Signs and Symptoms of Head Trauma

Head Injury
Lacerations, contusions, or hematomas to the scalp
Soft area or depression noted on palpation of the scalp
Visible skull fractures or deformities
Battle sign or raccoon eyes
CSF rhinorrhea or otorrhea
Traumatic Brain Injury
Pupillary abnormalities ▪ Unequal pupil size ▪ Sluggish or nonreactive pupils
A period of unresponsiveness
Confusion or disorientation
Repeatedly asks the same questions (perseveration)
Amnesia (retrograde and/or anterograde)
Combativeness or other abnormal behavior
Numbness or tingling in the extremities
Loss of sensation and/or motor function
Focal neurologic deficits
Seizures
Cushing triad: hypertension, bradycardia, and irregular or erratic respirations
Dizziness
Visual disturbances, blurred vision, or double vision (diplopia)
Seeing "stars" (flashes of light)
Nausea or vomiting
Posturing (decorticate and/or decerebrate)

Abbreviation: CSF, cerebrospinal fluid

Scalp Lacerations

Scalp lacerations can be minor or serious. Because both the face and the scalp have rich blood supplies, even small lacerations can quickly result in substantial blood loss Figure 30-12. This blood loss may be severe enough at times to cause hypovolemic shock, particularly in children. In any patient with multiple injuries, bleeding from scalp or facial lacerations may contribute to hypovolemia.[4] In addition, because scalp lacerations are usually the result of direct blows to the head, they often indicate deeper, more serious injuries.

Skull Fracture

Substantial force applied to the head may cause a skull fracture. As with any fracture, a skull fracture may be open or closed, depending on whether there is an overlying laceration of the scalp. Injuries from bullets or other penetrating weapons frequently result in fracture of the skull. The diagnosis of a skull fracture is usually made in the hospital with a computed tomography (CT) scan, but you should maintain a high index of suspicion that a fracture is present if the patient's head appears deformed or if there is a visible crack in the skull within a scalp laceration. Additional signs of skull fracture that you may see include ecchymosis (bruising) that develops under the eyes (**raccoon eyes**) Figure 30-13A or behind one ear over the mastoid process (**Battle sign**) Figure 30-13B. Skull fractures can be categorized into four types Figure 30-14.

Linear Skull Fractures. **Linear skull fractures** (nondisplaced skull fractures) account for most skull fractures.[5] Radiographs are required to diagnose a linear skull fracture because often there are no physical signs (such as deformity). If the brain is uninjured and there are no scalp lacerations, linear fractures are not life threatening. However, if a scalp laceration occurs in conjunction with a linear fracture—making it an open fracture—there is a risk of infection.

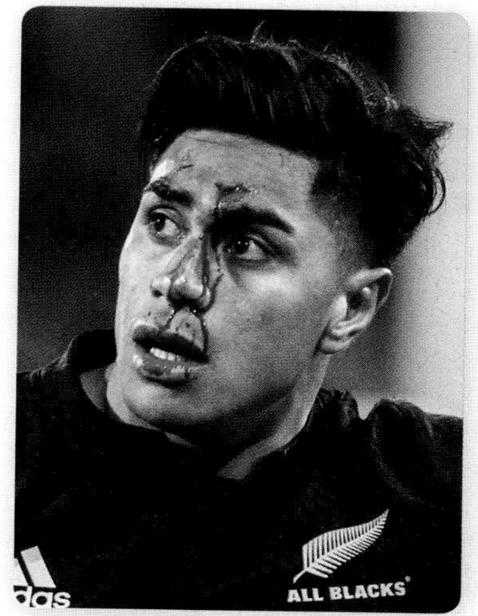

Figure 30-12 Blood loss on the face or scalp can stem from a small laceration.

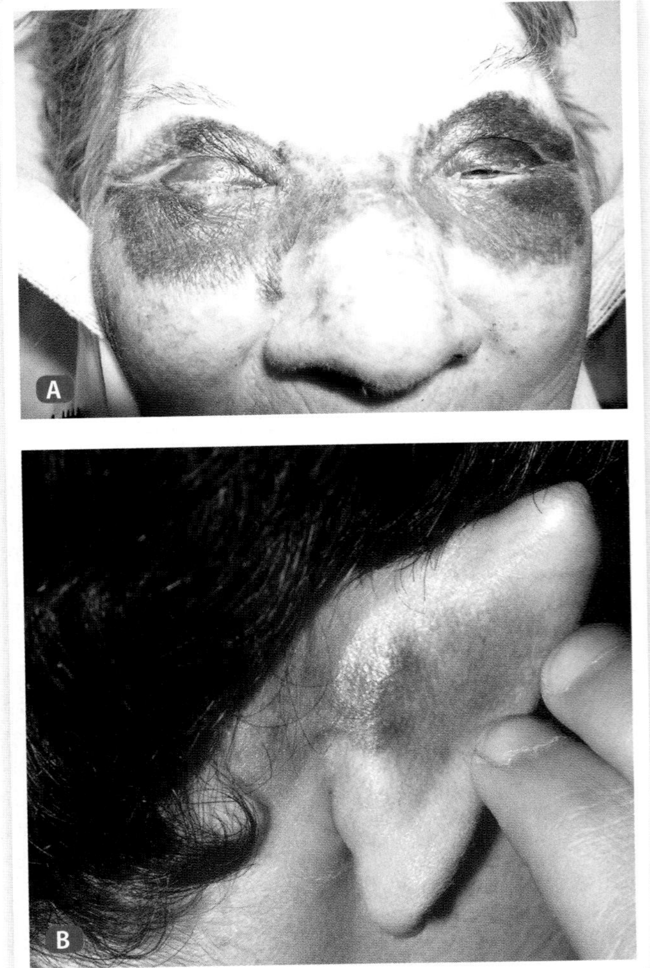

Figure 30-13 Suspect a basilar skull fracture if a head trauma patient has ecchymosis. **A.** Ecchymosis under or around the eyes (raccoon eyes). **B.** Ecchymosis behind the ear over the mastoid process (Battle sign).

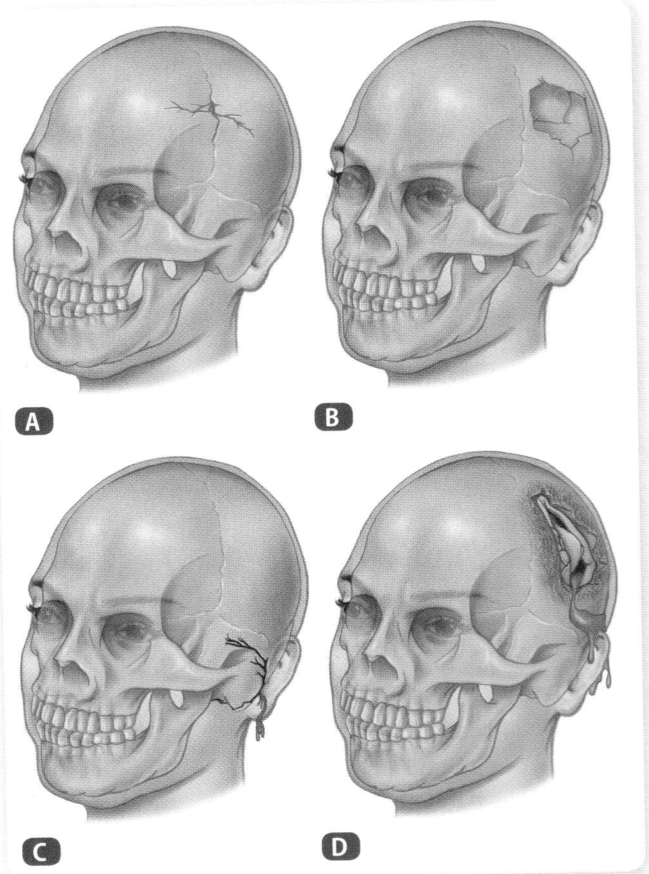

Figure 30-14 Types of skull fracture. **A.** Linear. **B.** Depressed. **C.** Basilar. **D.** Open.

Depressed Skull Fractures. **Depressed skull fracture** results from high-energy direct trauma to the head with a blunt object (such as a baseball bat to the head). The frontal and parietal regions of the skull are most susceptible to this type of fracture because the bones in these areas are relatively thin. As a consequence, bony fragments may be driven into the brain, resulting in injury. The scalp may or may not be lacerated. Patients with depressed skull fractures often present with neurologic signs (such as loss of consciousness).

Basilar Skull Fractures. **Basilar skull fracture** also is associated with high-energy trauma, but usually occurs following diffuse impact to the head (eg, falls, motor vehicle crashes). This injury generally results from extension of a linear fracture to the base of the skull and can be difficult to diagnose without CT scan.

Signs of a basilar skull fracture include CSF drainage from the ears **Figure 30-15**, which indicates rupture of the tympanic membrane and freely flowing CSF through the ear. Patients with leaking CSF are at risk for bacterial meningitis.

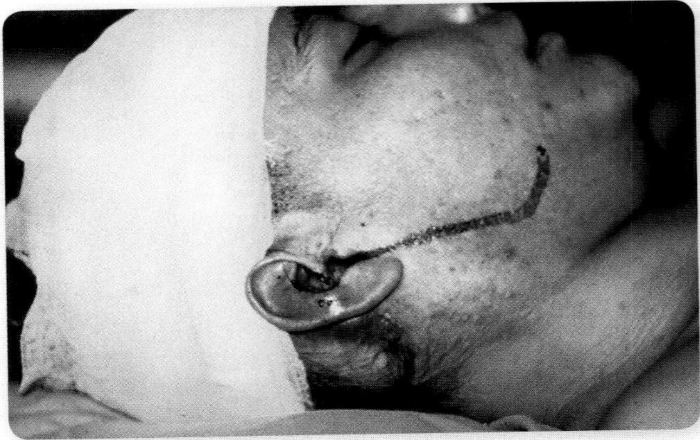

Figure 30-15 Blood draining from the ear after a head injury may contain cerebrospinal fluid and suggests a basilar skull fracture.

Other signs of a basilar skull fracture include raccoon eyes or Battle sign. Depending on the extent of the damage, raccoon eyes and Battle sign may appear relatively quickly, but in many cases, they may not appear until up to 24 hours following the injury, so their absence in the field does not rule out a basilar skull fracture.

Open Skull Fractures. Open fractures of the cranial vault result when severe forces are applied to the head and are often associated with trauma to multiple body systems. Brain tissue may be exposed to the environment, which substantially increases the risk of a bacterial infection (such as bacterial meningitis). Open cranial vault fractures have a very high mortality rate.

Traumatic Brain Injuries

TBIs can be classified into two broad categories: primary (direct) injury and secondary (indirect) injury. **Primary brain injury** is injury to the brain and its associated structures that results instantaneously from impact to the head and resultant transmission of force to brain tissue. **Secondary brain injury** is a consequence of primary injury, and results from the sequelae of the primary brain injury including **cerebral edema**, intracranial hemorrhage, increased ICP, cerebral ischemia and hypoxia, and infection. Two other significant causes of secondary brain injury that are potentially preventable in the prehospital setting are hypoxia and hypotension. According to the BTF, hypoxia and hypotension (systolic blood pressure less than 90 mm Hg) are both predictors of poor outcome in the patient with a TBI.[6] If the patient has a single incident of hypotension, regardless of the amount of time, then mortality increases from two to four times that of patients who did not experience hypotension. Hypoxia has similar effects, and the combination of hypotension and hypoxia has exponential effects on mortality. Secondary brain injury can occur anywhere from a few minutes to several days following the initial injury.

The brain can be injured directly by a penetrating object, such as a bullet, knife, or other sharp object. More commonly, such injuries occur indirectly, as a result of external forces exerted on the skull.

Consider the most common cause of brain injury, the motor vehicle crash. When the passenger's head hits the windshield on impact with a fixed object, the brain continues to move forward until it comes to an abrupt stop by striking the inside of the skull. This rapid deceleration results in compression injury (or bruising) to the anterior portion of the brain along with stretching or tearing of the posterior portion of the brain Figure 30-16.

As the brain strikes the front of the skull, the body begins its path of moving backward. The head falls back against the headrest and/or seat, and the brain slams into the rear of the skull. This type of front-and-rear injury is known as a **coup-contrecoup injury**. The same type of injury may occur on opposite sides of the brain in a lateral collision.

The injured brain starts to swell, initially because of cerebral vasodilation. An increase in cerebral edema then contributes to further brain swelling. Cerebral edema may not develop until several hours following the initial injury, however.

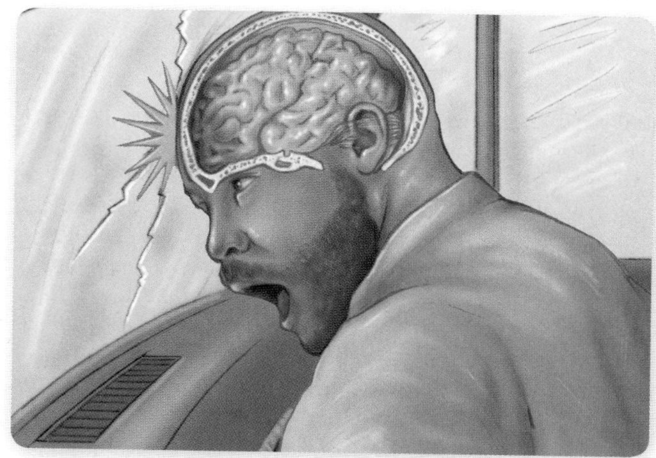

Figure 30-16 For the unrestrained person in a motor vehicle crash, the brain continues its forward motion and strikes the inside of the skull, resulting in compression injury to the anterior portion of the brain and stretching of the posterior portion.

Special Populations

A modified **Glasgow Coma Scale (GCS)** for pediatric and nonverbal patients assesses eye opening, verbal response, and motor response. The scoring indicators are the same as the GCS but the modified scale takes into consideration responses of coos and babbling, scoring these responses as oriented and appropriate.

Low oxygen levels in the blood aggravate cerebral edema. For this reason, you must make sure that the airway is open and that adequate ventilation and high-flow oxygen are given to any patient with a head injury. This is especially true if the patient is unresponsive. Do not wait for cyanosis or other obvious signs of hypoxia to develop.

However, it is important to remember that the patient should NOT be hyperventilated. The only indication for hyperventilation is signs of cerebral **herniation** such as a unilateral dilated pupil that is unresponsive to light or a decrease by 2 or more points in the GCS in a patient whose GCS score is less than 8. Even then, hyperventilation should be minimal and performed only in the context of a complete ability to monitor end-tidal carbon dioxide ($ETCO_2$) carefully. Remember that hyperventilation has the effect of decreasing cerebral blood flow! In general, patients should be ventilated at a normal, age-appropriate rate.

A common response to head injuries, especially among children with slight head injuries, is vomiting. This is usually the result of increased ICP.

As discussed earlier, the appearance of clear or pink, watery CSF from the nose, the ear, or an open scalp wound indicates that the dura and the skull have both been penetrated.

Words of Wisdom

When the brain is deprived of oxygen and carbon dioxide levels are elevated, the vessels dilate to bring more oxygenated blood to the hypoxic tissue. Increasing vessel size in an already cramped environment then increases ICP, making it even harder for blood flow to the swollen tissues. On the opposite side of the spectrum, hyperventilating will decrease vessel size, thereby diminishing blood flow and, again, diminishing oxygenation to deprived brain cells. It is important to ventilate the patient at a normal rate with high-flow oxygen while monitoring for changes in vital signs, pupils, and mental status.

It is not uncommon for a patient with a head injury to have a seizure. This is the result of excessive excitability of the brain, caused by direct injury or the accumulation of fluid within the brain (edema). Be prepared to manage seizures in all patients who have had a head injury.

Words of Wisdom

The effects of cerebral edema and increased ICP produce the signs that are collectively known as the **Cushing triad**:

- Increased blood pressure
- Decreased pulse
- Irregular respirations

Intracranial Pressure

Bleeding inside the skull increases ICP, the pressure within the cranial vault. Bleeding can occur between the skull and dura mater, beneath the dura mater but outside the brain, within the tissue of the brain itself, or into the subarachnoid space. Increased ICP squeezes the brain against the cranium.

Healthy adult ICP ranges from 5 to 15 mm Hg. An increase in ICP (such as from cerebral edema or intracranial hemorrhage) decreases cerebral perfusion pressure and cerebral blood flow. **Cerebral perfusion pressure (CPP)**, the pressure of blood flow through the brain, is the difference between the **mean arterial pressure (MAP)**, the average (or mean) pressure against the arterial wall during a cardiac cycle, and ICP (CPP = MAP − ICP). Decreasing cerebral blood flow is a potential catastrophe because the brain depends on a constant supply of blood to supply the oxygen and glucose it needs to survive.

The critical minimum threshold, or minimum CPP required to adequately perfuse the brain, is 60 mm Hg in the adult. A CPP of less than 60 mm Hg will result in cerebral ischemia, potentially resulting in permanent neurologic impairment or even death.

The body responds to a decrease in CPP by increasing MAP, resulting in cerebral vasodilation and increased cerebral blood flow; this process is called **autoregulation**. However, an increase in cerebral blood flow causes a further increase in ICP. As ICP continues to increase, CSF is forced from the cranium into the spinal cord.

The patient with increased ICP is caught in a vicious cycle. As ICP increases, cerebral blood flow increases

YOU are the Provider — PART 2

Ensuring that spinal precautions are being maintained, you quickly palpate the patient's skull and find a large hematoma on his posterior scalp. Continuing your examination, you find that the patient has no sensation or active movement in his arms or legs; the patient does have a readily palpable pulse bilaterally. You direct your partner to place a cervical collar on the patient, as you place the patient on a nonrebreathing mask at 15 L/min. After the cervical collar is secured, you strap the patient onto the long backboard and load him onto the stretcher. As you begin your vital sign assessment, you calculate his GCS and determine it to be 10. He is alert (4) and oriented (5), but has no motor function (1).

Recording Time: 1 Minute	
Appearance	Fair
Level of consciousness	Alert and oriented
Airway	Patent
Breathing	Irregular
Circulation	Warm, pink

3. What would you expect this patient's vital signs to be?
4. What are the signs and symptoms of a basilar skull fracture?

secondary to autoregulation, which results in a potentially fatal increase in ICP. Conversely, if cerebral blood flow decreases, CPP decreases as well, and the brain becomes ischemic.

ICP and CPP cannot be measured in the field, but the severity of increased ICP can be estimated based on the patient's clinical presentation. Prehospital treatment must focus on maintaining CPP (and cerebral blood flow), while preventing increased ICP as much as possible. If increased ICP is not promptly treated in a definitive care setting, cerebral herniation may occur (the brain is forced from the cranial vault).

You must closely monitor the head-injured patient for signs and symptoms of increased ICP. The exact clinical signs encountered depend on the amount of pressure inside the skull and the extent of brainstem involvement **Table 30-2**. Early signs and symptoms include vomiting (often without nausea), headache, an altered level of consciousness, and seizures.

Later, more ominous signs include hypertension (with a widening pulse pressure), bradycardia, and irregular respirations (Cushing triad), plus a unilaterally unequal and nonreactive pupil (caused by oculomotor nerve compression), coma, and posturing. **Decorticate (flexor) posturing** is characterized by flexion of the arms and extension of the legs; **decerebrate (extensor) posturing** is characterized by extension of the arms and legs **Figure 30-17**. When observed, posturing is an ominous sign and indicates substantial increase in ICP.

Focal Brain Injuries

Brain injuries are broadly classified as focal or diffuse. A **focal brain injury** is a specific, grossly observable brain injury (ie, it can be seen on a CT scan). Such injuries include cerebral contusions and intracranial hemorrhage.

Cerebral Contusion. In a **cerebral contusion**, brain tissue is bruised and damaged in a specific area. A cerebral contusion is different than a **concussion** because it involves physical damage to the brain, potentially causing greater neurologic deficits (eg, prolonged confusion, loss of consciousness). The same MOIs that cause concussions—acceleration-deceleration forces and direct blunt head trauma—also cause cerebral contusions.

The area of the brain most commonly affected by a cerebral contusion is the frontal lobe, although multiple areas of contusion can occur, especially following coup-contrecoup injuries. As with any bruise, swelling will occur. This swelling may result in increased ICP. A patient who

Table 30-2 Levels of Intracranial Pressure

Elevation Level	Clinical Indicators
Mild elevation	▪ Increased blood pressure; decreased pulse rate ▪ Pupils still reactive ▪ **Cheyne-Stokes respirations** (respirations that are fast and then become slow, with intervening periods of apnea) ▪ Patient initially attempts to localize and remove painful stimuli; this is followed by withdrawal and extension ▪ Vomiting (often without nausea) ▪ Headache ▪ Altered level of consciousness ▪ Seizures ▪ Effects usually reversible *with prompt and appropriate treatment*
Moderate elevation (indicates middle brainstem involvement)	▪ Widened pulse pressure and bradycardia ▪ Pupils are sluggish or nonreactive ▪ **Central neurogenic hyperventilation** (deep, rapid respirations; similar to Kussmaul, but without an acetone odor on breath) ▪ Decerebrate posturing ▪ Survival possible but often with some permanent neurologic deficit
Marked elevation (indicates involvement of lower portion of brainstem/medulla)	▪ Unilaterally fixed and dilated ("blown") pupil ▪ **Biot respirations** (irregular pattern, rate, and depth of breathing with intermittent periods of apnea) or absent respirations; also called ataxic respirations ▪ Flaccid response to painful stimuli ▪ Irregular pulse rate ▪ Fluctuating blood pressure; hypotension is common ▪ Most patients do not survive this level of intracranial pressure

Data from: Stiver SI, Gean AD, Manley GT. Survival with good outcome after cerebral herniation and Duret hemorrhage caused by traumatic brain injury. *J Neurosurg*. 2009;110(6):1242-1246.

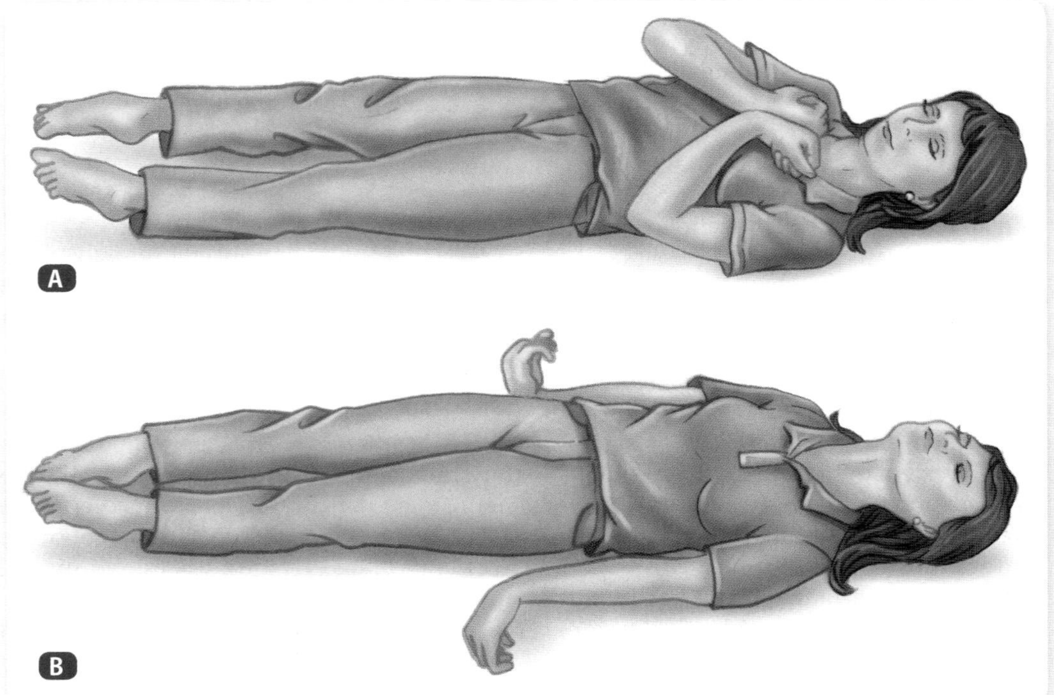

Figure 30-17 Posturing indicates substantial intracranial pressure. **A.** Decorticate (flexor) posturing. You can remember this term by thinking of the arms being pulled to the "core" of the body. **B.** Decerebrate (extensor) posturing.

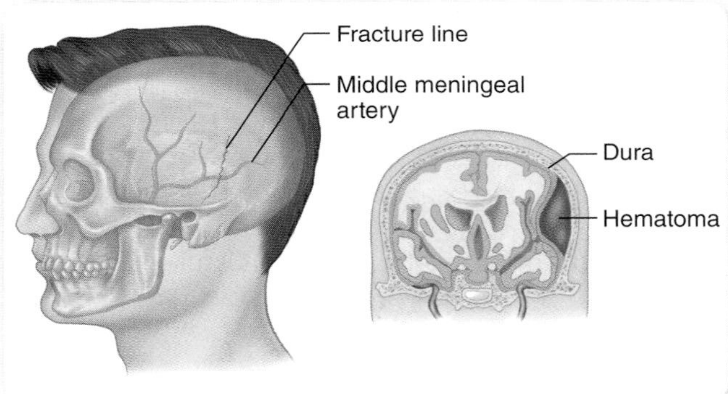

Figure 30-18 An epidural hematoma is usually the result of a blow to the head that produces a linear fracture of the temporal bone and damages the middle meningeal artery. Blood accumulates between the dura mater and the skull.

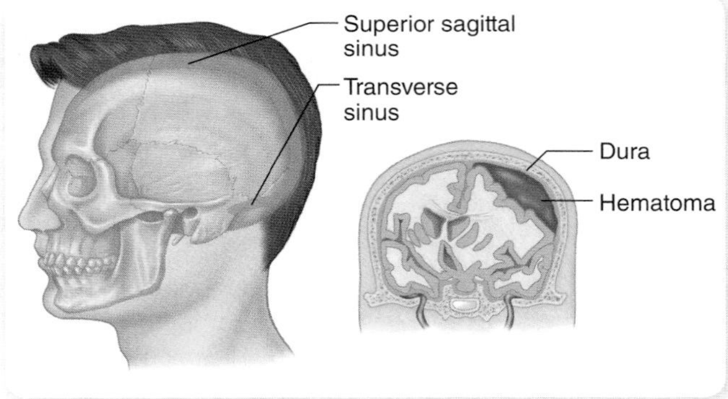

Figure 30-19 In a subdural hematoma, venous bleeding occurs beneath the dura mater but outside the brain.

has sustained a brain contusion may exhibit any or all signs of brain injury.

Epidural Hematoma. An **epidural hematoma** is an accumulation of blood between the skull and dura mater Figure 30-18. An epidural hematoma is nearly always the result of a blow to the head that produces a linear fracture of the thin temporal bone. The middle meningeal artery courses along a groove in that bone, so it is susceptible to disruption when the temporal bone is fractured.[7] In such a case, brisk arterial bleeding into the epidural space will result in rapidly progressing symptoms.

In the classic presentation, the patient loses consciousness immediately following the injury, which is then followed by a brief period of consciousness ("lucid interval"), after which the patient lapses back into unresponsiveness.[8] Meanwhile, as ICP increases, the pupil on the side of the hematoma becomes fixed and dilated. Death will follow rapidly without surgery to evacuate the hematoma.

Subdural Hematoma. A **subdural hematoma** is an accumulation of blood beneath the dura mater but outside the brain Figure 30-19. Although the exact incidence varies among studies, subdural hemorrhages are the most common intracranial hemorrhage and may or may not be associated with a skull fracture. Bleeding within the subdural space typically results from rupture of the veins that bridge the cerebral cortex and dura.

A subdural hematoma is associated with venous bleeding, so this type of hematoma—and the signs of increased ICP—typically develops more gradually than with an epidural hematoma. The patient with a subdural hematoma often experiences a fluctuating level of consciousness, focal neurologic signs (such as unilateral hemiparesis), or slurred speech.

Subdural hematomas are classified as acute (clinical signs developing within 48 hours following injury), subacute (signs developing between 2 and 14 days after the injury), or chronic (symptoms may not appear for as long as 2 weeks). Chronic subdural hematomas are more common in older adults, patients with alcoholism, patients with bleeding diatheses (such as hemophilia), and patients taking anticoagulants (such as warfarin).[9,10]

Special Populations

Older adults and those with a history of alcohol use are at higher risk for development of a subdural hematoma. This is caused by atrophy of the brain tissue that increases stretching of the bridging veins. Signs and symptoms of the condition may not occur for several hours, days, or weeks. Be sure to obtain a thorough history of any previous trauma.

Intracerebral Hematoma. An **intracerebral hematoma** involves bleeding within the brain tissue itself **Figure 30-20**. This type of injury can occur following a penetrating injury to the head or because of rapid deceleration forces.

Many small, deep intracerebral hemorrhages are associated with other brain injuries, such as diffuse axonal injury, discussed later in this chapter. After symptoms appear, the patient's condition often deteriorates quickly. Intracerebral hematomas have a high mortality rate, even if the hematoma is surgically evacuated.

Subarachnoid Hemorrhage. In a **subarachnoid hemorrhage**, bleeding occurs into the subarachnoid space, where the CSF circulates. It results in bloody CSF and signs of meningeal irritation (such as nuchal rigidity, headache). Common causes of a subarachnoid hematoma include trauma or rupture of an aneurysm or arteriovenous malformation.

Many, but not all, patients with a subarachnoid hematoma present with a sudden, severe headache.[11] As bleeding into the subarachnoid space increases, the patient experiences the signs and symptoms of increased ICP: decreased level of consciousness, pupillary changes, posturing, vomiting, and seizures. A sudden, severe subarachnoid hematoma usually results in death.[12]

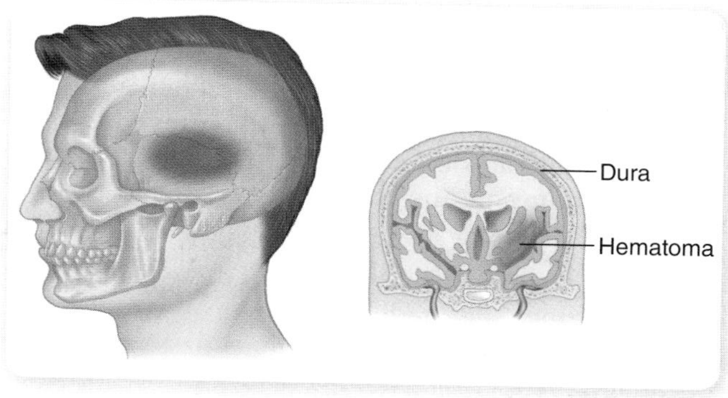

Figure 30-20 An intracerebral hematoma involves bleeding within the brain tissue itself.

People who survive often have permanent neurologic impairment.

Diffuse Brain Injuries

A **diffuse brain injury** is any injury that affects the entire brain. These injuries include cerebral concussion and DAI.

Cerebral Concussion

A blow to the head or face may cause a cerebral concussion of the brain if the brain is jarred around in the skull. This kind of mild brain injury is usually caused by rapid acceleration-deceleration forces (coup-contrecoup), such as those seen following motor vehicle crashes or falls.

Concussions are mild TBIs. A concussion injury results in cerebral dysfunction that usually resolves spontaneously and rapidly without demonstrable physical damage to the brain or permanent neurologic impairment. Loss of consciousness may occur, but in most cases, the patient remains conscious.

The exact definition of concussion continues to evolve as we learn more about this injury. The 5th International Conference on Concussion in Sport in 2016 defined concussion as a TBI induced by biomechanical forces. Common features that may be used in clinically defining a concussion include the following four items when the signs and symptoms cannot be explained by drug, alcohol, or medication use, or other injuries or comorbidities:[13]

- Concussion may be caused by either a direct blow to the head or a blow to the face, neck, or elsewhere on the body with an "impulsive" force transmitted to the head.
- Concussion typically results in the rapid onset of short-lived impairment of neurologic function that resolves spontaneously. However, in some cases, signs and symptoms may evolve over several minutes to hours.
- Concussion may result in neuropathologic changes, but the acute clinical symptoms largely reflect a functional disturbance rather than a structural injury; therefore, no abnormality is seen on standard structural neuroimaging studies.

- Concussion results in a range of clinical signs and symptoms that may or may not involve a loss of consciousness. Resolution of the clinical and cognitive features typically follows a sequential course. However, in some cases symptoms may be prolonged.

An estimated 1.6 to 3.8 million sports-related concussions occur annually, and many of these patients do not seek immediate medical treatment.[14] As a result, you may very well encounter patients days after their concussion event.

A great deal has been learned about concussions over the past several years. Researchers have exposed the damaging effects of repetitive concussions and the risk of second impact syndrome and postconcussion syndrome. You must not discount a patient with a possible concussion regardless of whether you see him or her at the time of the injury or days to weeks after the concussive event. Do not let helmet use decrease your suspicion of a concussion. Although studies have shown that helmets reduce head and facial injury and absorb energy that would otherwise act on the brain, they have not been shown to eliminate the incidence of concussions.

Athletic venues are a common site of concussions. You may be on standby for the event or be called to the event after the injury. Some youth coaches are required to take concussion training. Upper levels of play usually include athletic trainers who have undergone extensive concussion training and may have conducted a prescreening of the injured athlete that they can use for comparison.

At times, you may be the only medical professional on scene. One of the biggest questions in these situations is whether the athlete can return to play. Currently there is no diagnostic test that can reliably be used for an immediate determination of the presence of a concussion. Therefore, it is impossible to rule out a concussion in the setting of a head injury with transient neurologic symptoms. Any time a concussion is suspected, the player must be removed from play and assessed by a physician.[13] Authorizing an athlete to return to play after a potential concussion is outside the advanced emergency medical technician's (AEMT's) scope of practice. If you are faced with this decision, then consult medical direction.

If you face a situation in which a coach or parent wants to return the athlete to the game, but you think the player should not return, then explain your concerns to the coach and/or athletic trainer. Point out the signs and symptoms you observe and remind him or her of the steps in the concussion action plans developed by the National Federation of State High School Associations (NFHS) in association with the CDC's "Heads Up" program **Figure 30-21**.[15,16] Both organizations offer free concussion training on their websites.

Signs of a concussion include confusion and disorientation that may last for several minutes. **Retrograde amnesia**, a loss of memory relating to events that occurred before the injury, or **anterograde (posttraumatic) amnesia**, a loss of memory relating to events that occurred after the injury, may follow a concussion.

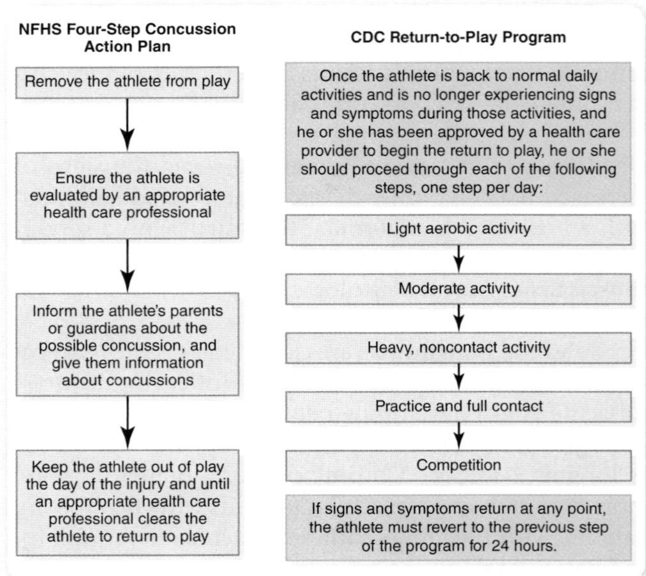

Figure 30-21 Key points of the National Federation of State High School Associations and US Centers for Disease Control concussion programs.

Data from: National Federation of State High School Associations (NFHS) Sports Medicine Advisory Committee (SMAC). Suggested guidelines for management of concussion in sports. NFHS website. https://www.nfhs.org/sports-resource-content/suggested-guidelines-for-management-of-concussion-in-sports/. Published February 16, 2017. Accessed March 24, 2017; and Centers for Disease Control and Prevention, National Center for Injury Prevention and Control, Division of Unintentional Injuries Prevention. Heads up. Managing return to activities. CDC website. http://www.cdc.gov/headsup/providers/return_to_activities.html. Updated February 8, 2016. Accessed March 24, 2017.

Usually, a concussion lasts only a short time. In fact, it has often resolved by the time you arrive. Nevertheless, you should ask about symptoms of concussion in any patient who has sustained an injury to the head; these symptoms include dizziness, weakness, or visual changes. Additional signs and symptoms you may encounter with a patient who has sustained a concussion may include nausea or vomiting, and the patient may report ringing in the ears. Slurred speech and the inability to focus may also be present. Depending on the severity of the concussion, you may also notice that the patient has a lack of coordination, has a delay of motor functions, or displays inappropriate emotional responses. Patients may also report a temporary headache and may appear to be disoriented at times.

Patients with symptoms consistent with concussion can also have more serious underlying brain injury. A CT scan is necessary to differentiate between these conditions. You should always assume that a patient with signs or symptoms of concussion has a more serious injury until proven otherwise by a CT scan at the hospital or by evaluation by a physician.

Diffuse Axonal Injury

Diffuse axonal injury (DAI) is associated with or similar to a concussion. Unlike a concussion, however, this more severe brain injury is often associated with a poor prognosis. DAI involves stretching, shearing, or tearing of nerve fibers with consequent axonal damage.[17] An **axon** is a long, slender extension of a neuron (nerve cell) that conducts electrical impulses away from the **neuronal soma** (cell body) in the brain.

DAI most often results from high-speed, rapid acceleration-deceleration forces, such as motor vehicle crashes and significant falls. The severity and, thus, the prognosis of DAI depend on the degree of damage (ie, stretching versus shearing or tearing); DAI is classified as being mild, moderate, or severe.

▶ Spine Injuries

The cervical, thoracic, and lumbar portions of the spine can be injured in a variety of ways. Compression injuries can occur as a result of a fall, regardless of whether the patient landed on his or her feet, coccyx, or, as in diving accidents, the top of the head. Motor vehicle crashes or other types of trauma can overextend, flex, or rotate the spine. Any one of these unnatural motions, as well as excessive lateral bending, can result in fractures and neurologic deficits.

Mechanism of Injury

Acute injuries of the spine are classified according to the associated mechanism, location, and stability of the injury. Vertebral fractures can occur with or without associated SCI. Stable fractures pose less risk to the spinal cord. Unstable injuries involve multiple columns of the spine and are often associated with damage to portions of the vertebrae and ligaments that directly protect the spinal cord and nerve roots. Without appropriate treatment, unstable injuries carry a higher risk of complicating SCI and progression of injury.

Flexion Injuries. **Flexion injuries** result from forward movement of the head, typically as the result of rapid deceleration (eg, in a car crash) or from a direct blow to the occiput. These forces can produce an unstable dislocation with or without an associated fracture.

Patients can also experience lateral bending, which is similar to a flexion injury. In flexion-extension, the patient's head moves from front to back and is overstretched on one side while being overcompressed on the opposite side. With lateral bending, the patient experiences the same type of injury, but from left to right rather than from front to back.

Words of Wisdom

Subluxation is an incomplete or partial dislocation that can be associated with SCI but is more commonly associated with no neurologic injury or a single nerve root injury. It is typically caused by a rotation-flexion MOI, but is possible with other mechanisms. Findings typically include pain, with or without neurologic symptoms.

Rotation With Flexion. The only area of the spine that allows for substantial rotation is C1-C2. Injuries to this area are considered unstable because of its high cervical location and scant bony and soft-tissue support. **Rotation-flexion injuries** (in which both rotation and flexion occur) often result from high acceleration forces.

Vertical Compression. **Vertical compression** forces are transmitted through vertebral bodies and directed either inferiorly through the skull or superiorly through the pelvis or feet. They typically result from a direct blow to the crown (parietal region) of the skull or rapid deceleration from a fall through the feet, legs, and pelvis. Forces transmitted through the vertebral body cause fractures, ultimately shattering and producing a "burst" or compression fracture without associated SCI **Figure 30-22**. Compression forces can cause the herniation of disks, subsequent compression on the spinal cord and nerve roots, and fragmentation into the canal.

Although most fractures resulting from these injuries are stable, primary SCI can occur when the vertebral body is shattered and fragments of bone become embedded, resulting in compression of the cord. Some compression injuries in the cervical spine can also cause serious airway compromise.

Hyperextension and Distraction. **Hyperextension** of the head and neck (extension beyond the usual range of motion) can result in fractures of bones and injury to ligaments.

Any time the spine undergoes **distraction**, or is pulled along its length, you can expect to find serious injuries to the spine. Distraction forces are the opposite of compression (axial) forces. Distraction occurs from rapid hyperextension of the skull, atlas, and axis as a unit; it results

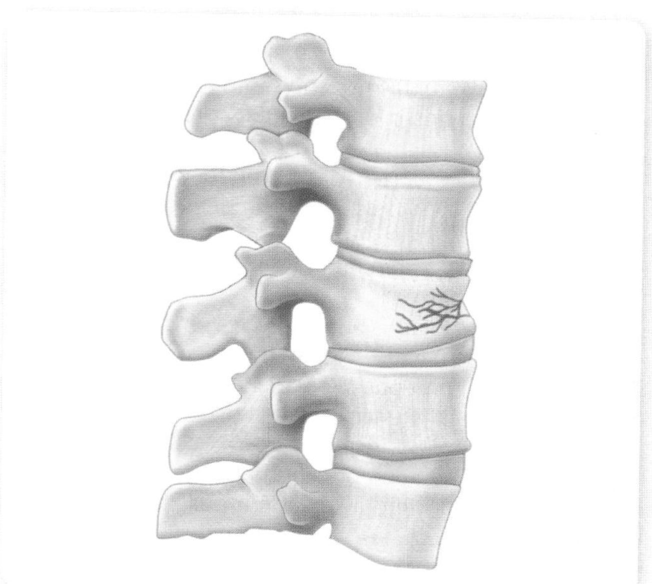

Figure 30-22 A compression fracture of the spine.

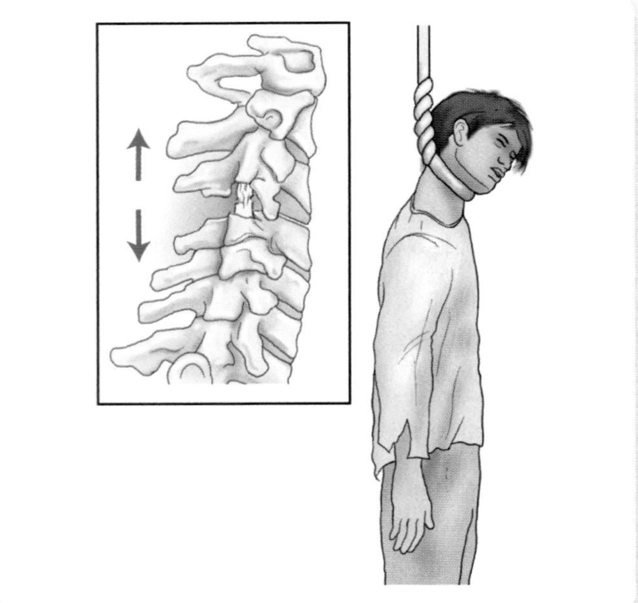

Figure 30-23 Distraction spinal injury.

when parts of the body are pulled in opposite directions Figure 30-23. Consider someone who has been hanged. The individual is moving and is jerked to a stop at one point while gravity pulls the rest of the body away from the fixed end. The result is stretching and separation of the spinal column, its ligaments, and its supporting muscles and tearing of the spinal cord. Although the type of distraction force determines the MOI, the cervical region is most vulnerable to distraction forces because it has the least support and protection.

> **Words of Wisdom**
>
> A *distracting* injury is not the same as a distraction injury. A distracting injury is an injury to another body part or system (such as a femur fracture) that causes such substantial pain and discomfort that it sufficiently distracts the patient's attention, rendering him or her unreliable. In such a case, the patient is unable to report whether there are any signs or symptoms of an occult spinal column injury.
>
> A *distraction* injury is one in which a physical distraction mechanism causes separation of spinal column elements and potential SCI. It is important to clearly recognize the difference between these two terms in evaluating patients with possible spinal column or cord injuries and when determining patients who may be safely managed without spinal immobilization.

The most classic distraction injury is a **hangman's fracture**, which, as its name implies, occurs during a hanging. In addition to distraction forces caused as the rope pulls tight, the rope causes a severe lateral force, snapping the head sideways as the spine stretches. The lateral force causes bending and fractures at the C1-C2 region, which quickly tears the spinal cord. Most hangman's fractures today occur as a result of extension and distraction from falls or motor-vehicle collisions.

Distraction or compression mechanisms rarely occur alone. Mixed mechanisms with some sort of rotation, flexion, or extension forces usually occur together. Carefully examine the incident and identify the forces that may have been involved. This information will enable you to better understand the type of injuries the patient may have sustained.

▶ Spinal Cord Injuries

Signs and symptoms of SCI are listed in Table 30-3. Note that the ability to feel or move does not rule out the possibility of a spinal injury existing.

Patients with severe spinal injury may lose sensation or experience paralysis below the suspected level of injury or be incontinent Figure 30-24. Obvious injury to the head and neck may indicate injury to the cervical spine. Injury to the shoulders, back, or abdomen may indicate injury to the thoracic or lumbar spine. Injuries of the lower extremities may indicate associated injuries of the lumbar spine or sacrum.

Injuries to the cervical area can limit the ability of the diaphragm to function fully and minimize the ability of the chest wall to fully expand. Another sign of spinal injury

Table 30-3 Signs and Symptoms of Spinal Cord Injury
Tenderness at the injury site
Pain
Obvious deformity on palpation of the spine
Soft-tissue injuries in the spinal region
Numbness, weakness, or tingling in the extremities
Inability to feel below a certain point on the body
Inability to feel the extremities
Difficulty breathing, shallow breathing
Hypotension
Loss of bladder/bowel control
Inability to maintain body temperature
Priapism (a persistent painful erection lasting more than 4 hours)

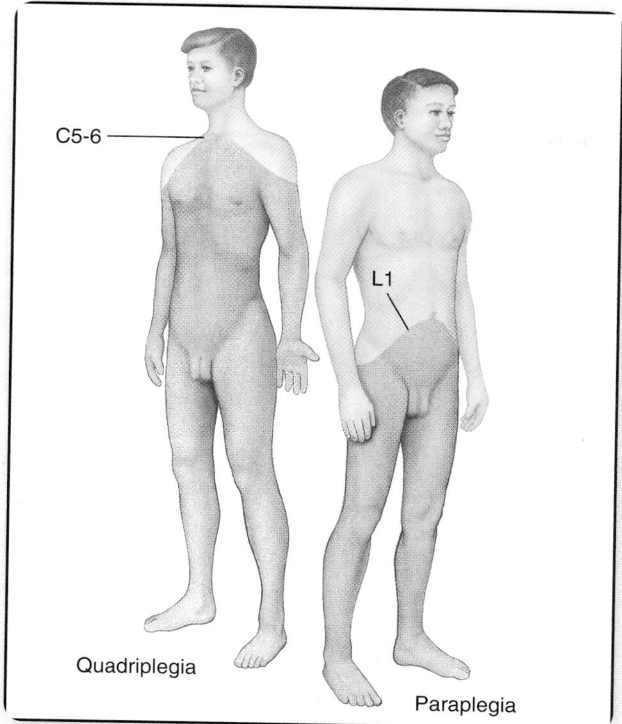

Figure 30-24 With severe spinal injuries, patients may lose sensation or experience paralysis below the suspected level of injury.

is abdominal excursion—when the patient is unable to breathe without the assistance of the abdomen.

Primary Spinal Cord Injury

Primary spinal cord injury occurs at the moment of impact. Penetrating trauma typically results in transection of neural elements that are incapable of regeneration. Blunt trauma may displace ligaments and bone fragments, resulting in compression of points of the spinal cord or an incomplete dislocation of the vertebral body. Hypoperfusion and ischemia may also result from this type of injury to the spinal vasculature. Necrosis from prolonged ischemia leads to permanent loss of function.

Spinal cord concussion is characterized by a temporary dysfunction that lasts from 24 to 48 hours. Cord concussion is considered an incomplete injury and may present in patients with simple compression fractures or in patients with no fracture at all. **Spinal cord contusion** is caused by fracture, dislocation, or direct trauma. It is associated with edema, tissue damage, and vascular leakage. Finally, cord laceration can occur when a projectile or bone enters the spinal canal. Such an injury is likely to result in hemorrhage into the cord tissue, swelling, and disruption of some portion of the cord and its associated communication pathways.

Secondary Spinal Cord Injury

Secondary spinal cord injury results from primary SCI progressing to further deterioration. These effects can be exacerbated by exposing neural elements to further hypoxemia, hypoglycemia, and hypothermia. Although some SCI may be unavoidable, you should minimize risk of further injury through stabilization, neutral alignment, and spinal immobilization. In addition, minimizing heat loss and maintaining oxygenation and perfusion are key elements in the care of a patient with a possible SCI.

Spinal Shock. **Spinal shock** refers to the temporary local neurologic condition that occurs immediately after spinal trauma. Swelling and edema of the cord begin within 30 minutes of the initial insult and can lead to a physiologic transection, mechanically disrupting all nerve conduction distal to the injury. The patient may present with varied degrees of acute spinal injury, potentially with flaccid paralysis, flaccid sphincters, and absent reflexes. Sensory function below the level of injury will be impaired, as will thermoregulation and visceral sensation below the lesion, resulting in bowel distention from a loss of peristalsis. Spinal shock usually subsides in hours to weeks, depending on the severity of injury.[18]

Neurogenic Shock. **Neurogenic shock** results from the temporary loss of autonomic function, which controls cardiovascular function, at the level of injury. Hypotension occurs because of absent or impaired peripheral vascular tone with the loss of alpha receptor stimulation; blood pools in the enlarged vascular space, causing a relative hypovolemia and making the patient extremely sensitive to sudden position changes; and cardiac preload decreases, resulting in decreased stroke volume and cardiac output. Bradycardia results as well. The adrenal gland loses its sympathetic stimulation and does not produce epinephrine or norepinephrine. Hypothermia and absence of sweating are also seen because of the loss of sympathetic stimulation. The classic case of neurogenic shock is a hypotensive, bradycardic patient whose skin is warm, flushed, and dry below the level of the spinal lesion.

Patient Assessment

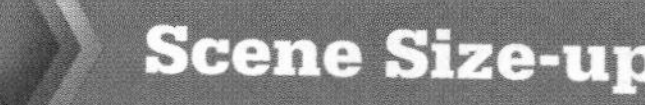

Scene Size-up

After you have taken standard precautions, the initial step of any assessment is to make a determination about scene safety and consider the need for any additional resources. Decide whether the trauma system should be activated (eg, air evacuation of the patient to a Level 1 trauma center). Also consider the need for paramedic backup.

Motor vehicle crashes, direct blows, falls from heights, assault, and sports-related injuries are common causes of head injuries and TBIs. When your patient has experienced any of these events, it should immediately increase your index of suspicion and prompt a search for signs and symptoms of these types of injuries. A damaged windshield or dented or cracked helmet indicates a major blow to the head **Figure 30-25**.

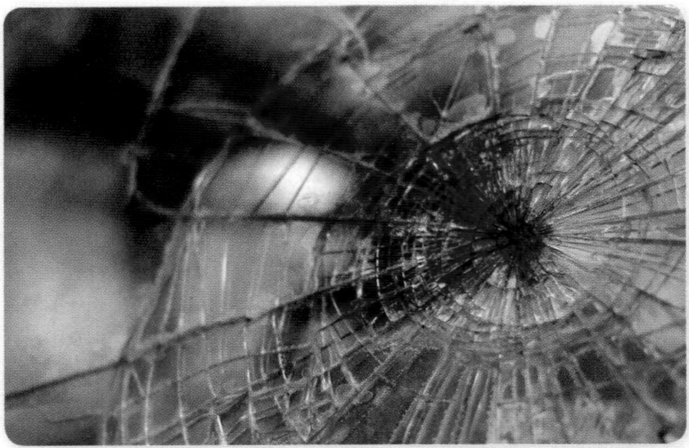

Figure 30-25 The classic "star" on the windshield after an automobile crash is an important indicator of injury. Be alert for the signs and symptoms of head and cervical spine injury.

Later in this chapter, specific indications for spinal immobilization are discussed. The decision of whether to immobilize a patient depends on your local protocols, and this decision is not usually based purely on MOI. However, the following high-risk mechanisms of injury strongly suggest the possibility of spine injury[19] and indicate that full spinal immobilization should be considered:

- High-velocity crash (greater than 40 mph) with severe vehicle damage
- Unrestrained occupant of moderate- to high-speed motor vehicle crash
- Vehicular damage with compartmental intrusion (12 inches [30 cm]) into the patient's seating space
- Fall of an adult from a height greater than 20 feet (6 m)
- Fall of a child from a height of greater than 10 feet (3 m), or a height two to three times the child's height
- Penetrating trauma near the spine
- Ejection from a moving vehicle
- Motorcycle crash of greater than 20 mph
- Auto-pedestrian or auto-bicycle crash of greater than 20 mph
- Death of occupant in the same passenger compartment
- Rollover crash (unrestrained)

Diving is also considered a high-risk MOI,[20] especially when it involves injury to the head or a witness who saw a deep dive in the shallow end of a swimming pool.

Mechanisms of uncertain risk for spinal injury include the following:

- Moderate- to low-velocity motor vehicle crash (less than 40 mph)
- Motor vehicle crash in which the patient has an isolated injury without positive assessment findings for spinal injury
- Isolated minor head injury without positive mechanism for spinal injury
- Syncopal event in which the patient was already seated or supine
- Syncopal event in which the patient was assisted to a supine position by a bystander

Words of Wisdom

The most important single sign in the evaluation of a head-injured patient is a changing level of consciousness.

Safety

Many mechanisms that cause head and spine injuries for the patient can also entail risk to emergency responders. Before you approach the patient, get the "big picture" of scene safety and take any actions necessary to ensure your own well-being. Do not rely entirely on assistance from fire or police personnel; maintain your own situational awareness of the scene from the beginning to the end of the call.

If the patient's injury is the result of an assault, be aware that the assailant may still be present. Make radio contact with an on-scene law enforcement officer, and do not enter the scene until he or she states that it is safe to do so. Remember this: the life you save may *take* your own!

Primary Survey

As you begin your primary survey of a patient with a head injury, ensure manual stabilization of the cervical spine in a neutral, in-line position. With the head and neck in a neutral position through manual stabilization, identify the level of consciousness and conduct your primary survey as described in Chapter 10, *Patient Assessment*. You may apply a cervical collar during the primary survey if your findings require it. However, take care not to skip elements of the airway, breathing, and circulation when sizing and applying a cervical collar. Avoid moving the neck unnecessarily and continue manual stabilization until you determine spinal immobilization is not indicated, or, if indicated, spinal immobilization has been applied. Application of the cervical collar is considered a treatment intervention. Failure to assess pulse, motor, and sensory function (PMS) prior to application of this medical device could potentially alter your baseline assessment. There is no way for you to know if neurovascular compromise was present prior to your intervention or if you, in fact, worsened the patient's injury.

Prior to measuring the patient for proper cervical collar size, the cervical and thoracic spine must be in a neutral position. If the patient is seated with a slouching posture, then cervical collar measurement may be inaccurate, which may not be noticed until the patient has been transferred to the backboard.

As always, the primary survey should focus on identifying and managing life-threatening concerns. Life-threatening external hemorrhaging must be treated before airway and breathing concerns; follow the XABCDE mnemonic.

It is especially important to evaluate and monitor the level of consciousness in patients with suspected head injuries, paying particular attention to any changes that may occur. As you proceed with your assessment, ask yourself these questions: Is the patient's speech clear and appropriate? Does the patient answer in a logical manner and is the patient able to make decisions? Is the patient aware of his or her current location? Is the patient alert to person, place, time, and why you are at the scene? Can the patient recall the events leading up to the incident or is there a period of memory lapse? Can the patient recall major current events? Use the AVPU scale (Awake and alert, responsive to Verbal stimuli, responsive to Pain, Unresponsive) to assess the patient's level of consciousness, and record the time.

Words of Wisdom

Any patient with substantial head injury is presumed to have a spinal column injury until proven otherwise.

If the patient is responsive, make sure you ask about the MOI and about his or her symptoms. Confused or slurred speech, repetitive questioning, or amnesia in responsive patients is a good indication of a head injury. Whereas other problems may cause similar symptoms, in the setting of trauma, assume your patient has a head injury until your assessment proves otherwise.

Reevaluate the patient and record your observations every 15 minutes if the patient's condition is stable and at least every 5 minutes if the patient's condition is unstable, until you reach the hospital.

If the patient is found unresponsive, emergency responders, family members, or bystanders may have helpful information, including knowledge of when the patient became unresponsive or what his or her previous level of consciousness was. Unresponsive patients with any trauma should be assumed to have a spinal injury. Patients with a decreased level of responsiveness on the AVPU scale (responds to verbal stimulus or responds to painful stimulus) should also be considered to have a spinal injury based on the chief complaint.

Unless the patient is absolutely clear in his or her thinking and does not have any other illnesses or injuries that may constitute a distraction, an MOI that suggests a potential spine injury should lead you to provide complete immobilization (also known as providing spinal motion restriction). Most jurisdictions are moving away from immobilizing patients based on MOI alone. However, in some jurisdictions AEMTs do not screen patients for selective immobilization; rather, patients are immobilized

YOU are the Provider PART 3

As soon as the patient is loaded into the ambulance, you obtain a baseline set of vital signs, which lead you to suspect increased ICP. Recognizing the seriousness of the patient's injuries, you establish an 18-gauge intravenous (IV) line with normal saline to keep the vein open, and initiate rapid transport to the ED. While en route to the hospital, your patient becomes unresponsive with episodes of apnea. You recalculate his GCS and determine it to be a 3. He is unresponsive (1), with no verbal (1) or motor (1) function.

Recording Time: 8 Minutes	
Respirations	26 breaths/min, Cheyne-Stokes pattern
Pulse	42 beats/min
Skin	Warm, pink
Blood pressure	216/148 mm Hg
Oxygen saturation (Spo_2)	99% on 15 L/min via nonrebreathing mask
Pupils	Pupils Equal, Round, and Reactive to Light and Accommodation

5. On the basis of your examination findings, what degree of elevated ICP does he have?
6. If this patient was unable to maintain his airway, at what rate would you initially ventilate using a bag-mask device?

based on MOI alone. Understand and follow your local protocols. Patients are not removed from backboards until they have arrived at the hospital, radiographs have been taken, and further assessments and examinations made.

Airway Management in Patients With Head or Spine Injury

While you are maintaining the head and neck in neutral alignment, clear the mouth and carefully but quickly suction if necessary. Patients with a head injury often vomit (especially children). Therefore, after opening the airway, you must be prepared to roll the patient to the side—while maintaining spinal immobilization—to prevent aspiration. If it is safe to do so, manually remove any large debris from the patient's mouth by sweeping the oropharynx with your gloved finger. Use suction to clear secretions, such as blood or thin secretions from the oropharynx. *Mortality increases substantially if aspiration occurs.*

Open the airway with the jaw-thrust maneuver if the patient is unresponsive or is otherwise unable to maintain his or her own airway spontaneously Figure 30-26. If this technique is successful, insert an oropharyngeal airway or a nasopharyngeal airway as appropriate. An intact gag reflex is a contraindication for an oropharyngeal airway because vomiting will increase the likelihood of airway compromise and increase the risk of aspiration.

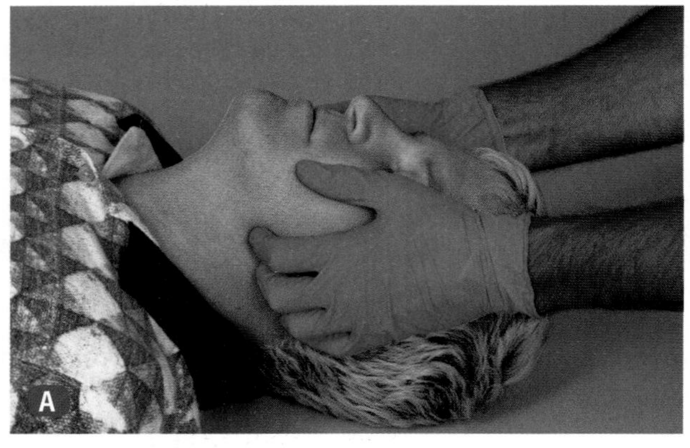

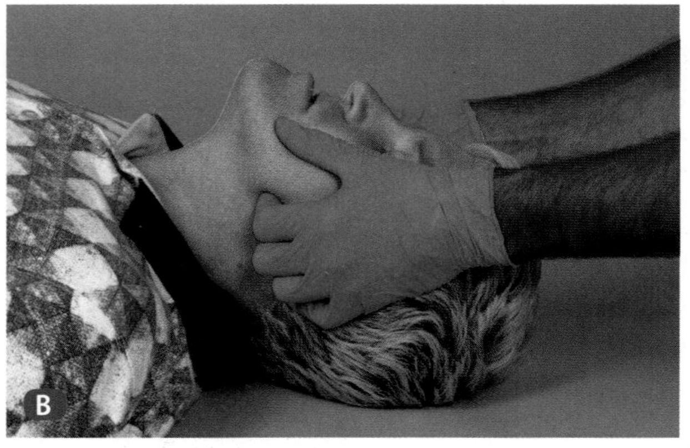

Figure 30-26 Jaw-thrust maneuver. **A.** Stabilize the neck in a neutral, in-line position. **B.** Push the angle of the lower jaw forward.

The decision to use an oropharyngeal or nasopharyngeal airway is based on the patient's ability to maintain his or her own airway, the presence of a gag reflex, and the extent of facial injuries. A nasopharyngeal airway should not be used if a basilar skull fracture is suspected or if there is nasal trauma. Review the indications and contraindications for these airway adjuncts in Chapter 11, *Airway Management*.

Be sure to monitor the airway closely and have a suctioning unit available because you will often need to clear away blood, saliva, or vomitus. With large amounts of emesis, the patient may need to be log rolled to the side and the mouth swept of secretions. When it is necessary to log roll the patient to clear the airway, roll the patient keeping the body in as straight a line as possible to restrict unnecessary spinal motion. Suctioning should be performed immediately to remove smaller amounts of secretions.

Ventilation in the Context of Head or Spine Injury

Evaluate the patient's breathing, noting the rate, depth, and symmetry of each respiration. If an SCI has paralyzed the intercostal muscles, the patient will exhibit abdominal breathing (pure use of the diaphragm to expand the chest) and may also use accessory muscles of the neck to breathe. Closely monitor the patient's oxygen saturation (Spo_2), and maintain it at 95% or higher. Cerebral edema and ICP are aggravated by hypoxia and hypercapnia; therefore, you must constantly ensure adequate oxygenation and ventilation in any patient with a head injury. Administer 100% oxygen via a nonrebreathing mask if the patient is breathing adequately (ie, adequate rate and depth [tidal volume], regular respiratory pattern). An injured brain is even less tolerant of hypoxia than a healthy one, and research has demonstrated that even brief periods of hypoxia are associated with increases in mortality.

If the respiratory center of the brain (pons, medulla) has been injured, the rate, depth, or regularity of breathing may be ineffective. Ventilation may also be impaired by concomitant chest injuries or, if the spinal cord is injured, by paralysis of some or all of the respiratory muscles. Patients with inadequate ventilation, especially if associated with a decreased level of consciousness, should receive bag-mask ventilation and 100% oxygen. Ventilate a brain-injured adult at a rate of 10 to 12 breaths/min or as determined by local protocols. *Avoid hyperventilation of brain-injured patients.* Hyperventilation causes cerebral vasoconstriction, which will shunt blood from the cranium and lower cerebral perfusion. The BTF recommends hyperventilation (20 breaths/min for adults) *only* if signs of cerebral herniation are present Table 30-4, because brief periods of hyperventilation may be beneficial. If available, $ETCO_2$ should be monitored with digital capnometry. You should ventilate the patient to maintain the $ETCO_2$—an approximation of arterial partial pressure of

Table 30-4 Signs of Cerebral Herniation

Unresponsive patient with two or more of the following:
- Asymmetric (unequal) pupils *or* bilaterally fixed and dilated pupils
- Extensor posturing *or* no motor response to physical stimuli
- Original GCS score of less than 9 that decreases by 2 or more points from the patient's best score

Abbreviation: GCS, Glasgow Coma Scale

carbon dioxide ($Paco_2$)—between 30 and 35 mm Hg.[21,22] Under no circumstances should the $ETCO_2$ be allowed to ever drop below 25 mm Hg because the subsequent vasoconstriction will increase the risk of brain death due to anoxia and cerebral ischemia.[21]

Words of Wisdom

When you assess and manage an adult with a severe head injury, remember the BTF's "90-90-9 rule":[6,23]

1. A *single* drop in the patient's oxygen saturation to less than 90% doubles his or her chance of death.[a]
2. A *single* drop in the patient's systolic blood pressure to less than 90 mm Hg substantially increases his or her chance of death.[a]
3. A *single* drop of 2 points or more in the patient's prior best GCS score of less than 9 increases his or her chance of death.

[a]The chance of death increases exponentially if both hypoxemia and hypotension occur compared with occurrences of only one of these conditions.

Words of Wisdom

Inadequate respirations with or without evidence of decreased oxygenation will require assisted ventilation with a bag-mask device with 12 to 15 L/min of supplementary oxygen flowing at 10 to 12 breaths/min. If a head injury is suspected but you do not suspect brain herniation, use $ETCO_2$ monitoring to maintain CO_2 levels at 35 to 45 mm Hg.

Circulation and Volume Resuscitation in a Patient With Head or Spine Injury

In the absence of a pulse, immediately initiate cardiopulmonary resuscitation (CPR). Control any external bleeding with direct pressure or pressure dressings. Active bleeding will cause or worsen hypoxia, as well as decrease CPP, by reducing the number of oxygen-carrying red blood cells. Volume resuscitation may be necessary in patients with absent or diminished pulses, especially if the patient has multisystem trauma with hypovolemic shock.

Assess radial pulses for presence, rate, quality, and regularity. A pulse that is too slow in the setting of a head injury can indicate a serious condition. Evaluate skin color, temperature, and moisture. Patients with substantial sensory loss from SCI may equilibrate to the surrounding environmental temperature because of the lack of input from the periphery for temperature control. In neurogenic shock, the skin is usually warm, dry, and flushed due to vasodilation and the absence of sweating. These findings should be correlated with the patient's mental status.

A single episode of hypoperfusion in a patient with a head injury can result in substantial brain damage and even death. Assess for signs and symptoms of shock and treat appropriately. Volume resuscitation may be necessary in patients with absent or diminished pulses, especially in patients with multisystem trauma with hypovolemic shock. The skull does not have enough room to accommodate large volumes of blood. As a result, an isolated closed head injury will not cause hypovolemic shock in an adult. If signs of shock are present (ie, persistent hypotension, tachycardia, diaphoresis), then carefully assess the patient for occult injuries, such as intra-abdominal or intrathoracic hemorrhage.

Early on in the primary survey, you must decide whether to complete the secondary assessment on scene or to transport the patient immediately with interventions en route. The unstable or potentially unstable patient should be transported as soon as possible to the most appropriate hospital per local trauma guidelines or online medical control instruction.

Prompt transport to a definitive care facility (ie, a trauma center) is crucial to the survival of a brain-injured patient. If available, consider air transport if your transport time will be prolonged. If you are transporting the patient by ground, do so expeditiously, yet cautiously; the use of lights and a siren could precipitate seizures and exacerbate ICP.

Many patients with severe brain injuries and increased ICP require neurosurgical intervention. The extra time it takes to move the patient from one hospital to another could mean the difference between life and death. Therefore, consider transporting the patient *directly* to a trauma center that has neurosurgical services, even if it means bypassing the nearest hospital. As always, be aware of and follow local protocols.

During transport, maintaining a patent airway and providing high-flow oxygen are paramount. In supine patients, the head should be elevated 30° to help reduce ICP if possible. Remember to maintain immobilization of the spine.

Patients who are alert and aware of the inability to move their limbs need to be offered psychological support. Remember that it can be very traumatizing for a patient to realize that he or she may now have a debilitating and life-altering injury because of an accident; therefore, you need to be careful in your choice of words. A patient may ask you difficult questions, such as "Will I be able to walk?" It is best to tell the patient that you are providing immediate care and you cannot predict the outcome.

Special Populations

Infants may lose enough blood into the skull region to produce shock, but this is not the case with the older child or the adult patient. Provide oxygen, monitor the airway, treat for shock, and provide immediate transport. A common response to head injuries, even among children with only very slight head injuries, is vomiting. This is sometimes the result of increased ICP. In managing such vomiting, you should pay particular attention to protecting the patient's airway.

History Taking

After the life threats have been managed during the primary survey, investigate the chief complaint. You should obtain a medical history and be alert for injury-specific signs and symptoms as well as any pertinent negatives such as no pain or no loss of sensation.

Using OPQRST (Onset, Provocation/palliation, Quality, Region/radiation, Severity, Timing) may provide some background on isolated extremity injuries. Does the patient have any recall of the incident? Inability to recall events is an important finding in patients with head injuries. You have the opportunity to interview the patient well in advance of the emergency physician. Any information you receive will be valuable if the patient loses consciousness.

If the patient is not responsive, attempt to obtain the history from other sources, such as friends or family members. Medical identification jewelry and cards in wallets may also provide information about the patient's medical history. Does the patient have a recent or previous history of unresponsiveness? These key indicators may lead you to suspect a developing TBI.

Make every attempt to obtain a SAMPLE (Signs and symptoms, Allergies, Medications, Pertinent past medical history, Last oral intake, Events leading up to the illness or injury) history from your patient. History may be difficult to obtain when a person is confused from a head injury or frightened from a spinal injury. Whereas the prehospital environment is an excellent place to obtain important history, do not delay rapid transport for patients who need rapid hospital intervention. Gather as much SAMPLE history as you can while preparing for transport. In less urgent situations, you should have enough time to gather a complete SAMPLE history without compromising patient care.

Words of Wisdom

Can the patient smile? An inability to smile is a sign that a cranial nerve may be injured. Part the patient's hair and inspect the scalp for bruising. Look for blood or CSF leaking from the ears, nose, or mouth and for bruising around the eyes and behind the ears.

Secondary Assessment

The secondary assessment should begin with you obtaining a complete set of baseline vital signs. Modify the physical examination of any patient with suspected SCI based on the patient's level of consciousness, reliability as a historian, and MOI. In cases of high- or intermediate-risk mechanisms, whenever possible complete the physical exam with the patient in a neutral position without any movement of the spine. Apply manual stabilization while asking the patient not to move unless specifically asked to do so. The neck and trunk must not be flexed, extended, or rotated.

Depending on the chief complaint, you may focus your physical examination on the site of injury.

Patients with moderate or severe head injuries associated with a significant MOI should receive definitive care, life-saving medical or surgical intervention at the hospital, without delay. If time allows, perform a secondary assessment to identify and treat injuries that may have been missed during the primary survey en route to the ED. Extremities can be stabilized using a long backboard and splinted individually while in the back of the ambulance as time and conditions permit.

A decreased level of consciousness is the most reliable sign of closed head injury. Monitor the patient for changes in level of consciousness, including signs of confusion, disorientation, anxiety, combativeness, and deteriorating mental status. Is the patient unresponsive or repeating questions? Experiencing seizures? Nauseated or vomiting?

Although you cannot quantify ICP (ie, you can't assign a numeric value) in the prehospital setting, you can estimate the severity of increase based on the patient's clinical presentation. You will base important treatment decisions for patients with brain injury on the presence or absence of certain key findings: posturing, hypotension or hypertension, and abnormal pupil signs.

Perform a baseline assessment using the GCS (shown in Chapter 10, *Patient Assessment*, and Chapter 19, *Neurologic Emergencies*) and record the time. Obtain a baseline GCS score and frequently (at least every 5 minutes, if possible) reassess it to capture the patient's clinical progression.

If your jurisdiction uses the Rapid Trauma Score (RTS), then the findings from the GCS will be used in determining the RTS value. See Chapter 26, *Trauma Overview*, for a discussion of this scoring system.

Document all scores and the times they were obtained on the patient care report. The physicians who treat the patient will need to know when the loss of consciousness occurred and for how long. They will want to compare their neurologic evaluation with the one you performed in the field. Always use simple, easily understood terms when reporting the level of consciousness, such as "does not remember events immediately preceding injury" or "confused about date and time." Terms such as "dazed" have different meanings to different people and should not be used in written or verbal reports.

Special Populations

When responding to an incident involving a shaken baby, you may encounter a child with an abnormal appearance but no external signs of injury. Shaken baby syndrome occurs when a caregiver violently shakes the child, often when the child is crying inconsolably, producing a severe brain injury in the child. Given that few caregivers will admit to having hurt the child, be alert for a history that is inconsistent with the clinical picture. Note whether the child has **petechial hemorrhages**. These are pinpoint red dots in the sclera of the eye and represent the rupture of tiny vessels. This finding indicates that the baby was shaken, although this finding may not be present in every case of shaken baby syndrome. Be sure to document the presence or absence of this finding; this information could be significant if law enforcement investigates the case.

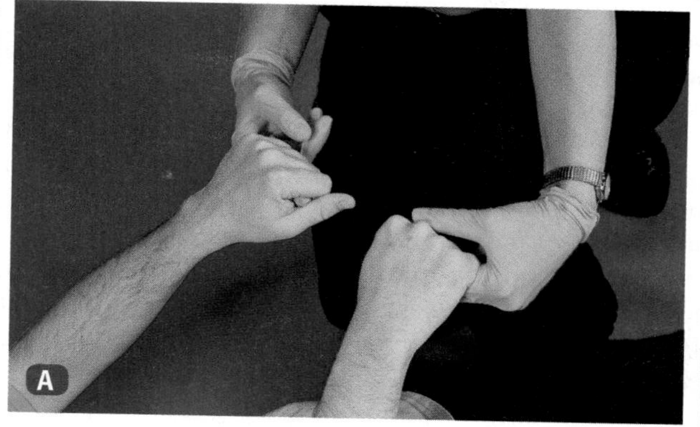

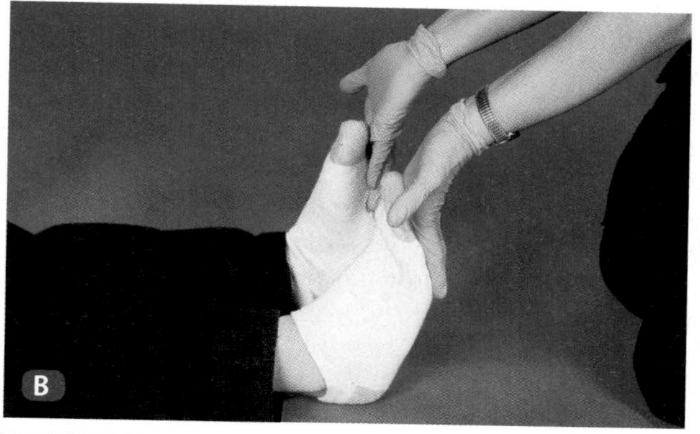

Figure 30-27 A. Assess the equality of strength of each extremity by asking the patient to squeeze your hands. **B.** Next, ask the patient to gently push each foot against your hands.

Frequently the level of consciousness will fluctuate—improving, deteriorating, and then improving again over time. On other occasions, there is a gradual, progressive deterioration in the patient's response to stimuli; this usually indicates serious brain damage that may need aggressive medical and/or surgical treatment.

To examine the spine, you will need to expose the patient for your examination. Cut away the patient's clothes to minimize motion of the spine during examination or treatment. Directly observe the back to assess for penetrating trauma. In case of potential spine injuries, the physical exam includes rapid inspection and palpation of the head, neck, chest, abdomen, pelvis, extremities, and back for injuries. Use the mnemonic DCAP-BTLS—Deformity, Contusion, Abrasion, Puncture/penetration wounds, Bruising, Tenderness, Laceration, and Swelling—to help you remember specific points. An evaluation of neurovascular integrity should include distal PMS for all four extremities Figure 30-27. Sensation may be present throughout the body. If there is impairment, note the level. You do not need to know the exact nerve impairment because this will not change your treatment.

Pain or tenderness when you palpate the spinal area is certainly a warning sign that a spinal injury may exist. Patients with spinal injuries may report constant or intermittent pain along the spinal column or in their extremities. An SCI may also produce pain independent of movement or palpation.

Evaluate the chest and abdomen for both internal and external injuries. Fractures of the ribs, sternum, clavicle, scapula, or pelvis are often associated with SCI in patients with multisystem trauma. Visualization and palpation are the mainstays of this evaluation. Remember, the physical exam in the patient with an SCI may be skewed because of decreased sensation below the level of spinal injury. Assess the chest wall visually for symmetry of chest wall movement, work of breathing, and use of accessory muscles. Auscultation to assess breath sounds may reveal a shortened inspiratory phase. Inadequate ventilation may indicate chest musculature or diaphragmatic impairment as a result of SCI.

Also, injuries to the cervical area can limit the ability of the diaphragm to function fully and minimize the ability of the chest to expand, so continue to always pay attention to managing the airway and breathing.

Use monitoring devices to quantify your patient's oxygenation and circulatory status. If available, CO_2 monitoring should be used on all patients suspected of having a head injury to ensure the patient is not hypoventilating or hyperventilating. You may also use noninvasive methods to monitor the blood pressure. It is recommended that you always assess the patient's first blood pressure manually with a sphygmomanometer (blood pressure cuff) and stethoscope.

Continually monitor the cardiovascular system for signs of shock. Neurogenic shock may require volume replacement or paramedic backup for pharmacologic management.

Examination of the gastrointestinal system may be unreliable in the presence of a neurologic deficit. First, inspect the abdomen for evidence of trauma, noting its contour. Severe gastric distention may impair respiration and result in airway compromise due to vomiting. Palpate all four quadrants for tenderness, guarding, or rigidity, but remember that patients may be insensitive to pain and may not develop a rigid abdomen because of absence of muscle tone. Lower abdominal distention with or without suprapubic tenderness may be a result of urinary retention. In men, assess the urethral meatus for evidence of blood, scrotal swelling, and scrotal ecchymosis, which may occur with pelvic fractures. Assess for priapism as well.

Look for any abnormal posturing, and assess the patient for potential long bone or other substantially distracting painful injuries that may mask a potential spine or cord injury.

After the exam is completed, cover the patient with a blanket to maintain normal body temperature. Hypothermia will impair the patient's ability to unbind oxygen from hemoglobin and increase the risk of mortality and morbidity. In colder climates, move the patient to a warmer environment, such as the ambulance, as quickly as possible without compromising the spine further.

Finally, if possible, use a glucometer to assess blood glucose level in patients who show evidence of alterations in sensation or mental status; an altered mental status may be the result of hypoglycemia.

Documentation & Communication

A single assessment of the patient's GCS score cannot reliably capture his or her clinical progression. Obtain a baseline GCS score and frequently (at least every 5 minutes if possible) reassess it in a patient with a head injury. Document all GCS scores and the times they were obtained on the patient care report. The physician will compare his or her neurologic assessment with those you performed in the field.

Words of Wisdom

Patients may experience an inability to maintain their body temperature. Always keep patients covered, even in warm weather.

Reassessment

Frequent reassessments are necessary to help you determine whether the patient is stabilizing, improving, or deteriorating. Vital signs should be monitored every 5 minutes (unstable patients) to 15 minutes (stable patients), with special attention to the patient's cardiovascular status. Be alert for hypotension without other signs of shock. The combination of hypotension with a normal or slow pulse and warm skin greatly suggests neurogenic shock. The SCI responsible for neurogenic shock also usually produces a flaccid paralysis and complete loss of sensation below the level of the injury. In contrast to neurogenic shock, hypovolemic shock is associated with pale, cold, clammy skin and tachycardia.

Check interventions such as oxygen flow and spinal immobilization to ensure that they are still effective. Repeat the physical exam and reprioritize the patient as necessary. Document suspected SCI, noting the area involved, sensation, motor function, and areas of weakness.

When providing care for patients with suspected head and spinal injuries, it is essential to maintain good communication with the destination facility. Hospitals may better prepare for seriously injured patients with more advanced warning and a description of the most serious problems found during your assessment, and additional resources can be made available when you arrive.

Your documentation should include the history you were able to obtain at the scene, your findings during your assessment, treatments you provided, and how the patient responded to them.

Words of Wisdom

The most important aspect of neurologic assessment is whether the patient's findings are changing and in what direction.

Emergency Medical Care of Head Injuries

Remember that patients with head injuries often have injuries to the cervical spine as well. Therefore, when treating a patient with a head injury, you must keep in mind the need to protect and immobilize the cervical spine at all times.

Treat the patient with a head injury according to four general principles, which are designed to protect and maintain the critical functions of the CNS:

1. Establish an adequate airway. If necessary, begin and maintain ventilation and always provide high-flow supplemental oxygen. Consult local protocols for the appropriate rate if ventilation via a bag-mask device is required.

2. Control bleeding, and provide adequate circulation to maintain cerebral perfusion. Begin CPR, if necessary. Be sure to follow standard precautions.
3. Start at least one 18-gauge intravenous (IV) line and administer an isotonic crystalloid solution as needed.
4. Assess the patient's baseline level of consciousness, and continuously monitor it.

Manage the airway and provide oxygen as indicated by patient status. Ventilate a brain-injured adult at a rate of 10 to 12 breaths/min or as determined by local protocols. Follow local protocols and medical direction regarding hyperventilation in the presence of herniation. Continue to assist ventilations or administer supplemental oxygen until the patient reaches the hospital.

As you continue to treat the patient, do not apply pressure to an open or depressed skull injury. In addition, you must assess and treat other injuries, dress and bandage open wounds as indicated in the treatment of soft-tissue injuries, splint fractures, anticipate and manage vomiting to prevent aspiration, be prepared for seizures and changes in the patient's condition, and transport the patient promptly and with extreme care.

> **Words of Wisdom**
>
> Effectively managing the airway of a brain-injured patient and ensuring adequate oxygenation and ventilation are absolutely critical to the patient's survival. Of course, severe bleeding can also result in death. Therefore, airway management and bleeding control should be performed simultaneously by you and your partner.

Shock that develops in a patient with a head injury may be the result of hypovolemia caused by bleeding from other injuries. Such patients must be transported immediately, preferably to a trauma center. Maintain the airway while you protect the patient's cervical spine, ensure adequate ventilation, administer 100% oxygen, control obvious sites of bleeding with direct pressure, place the patient supine on a long backboard, keep the patient warm, and provide immediate transport.

Establish at least one 18-gauge IV line with normal saline or lactated Ringer solution. Do not administer dextrose-containing solutions (such as 5% dextrose in water [D_5W]) because they may worsen cerebral edema. The *only* indication for administering glucose to a head-injured patient is confirmed hypoglycemia (ie, a glucometer reading of 45 mg/dL or less).

Patients with a severe closed head injury are often hypertensive—a sign of the body's autoregulatory response. Restrict your use of IV fluids for these patients to minimize cerebral edema and ICP, typically at a rate of 30 to 50 mL/h.[24] However, if hypotension develops, infuse isotonic crystalloids as needed—usually 20-mL/kg boluses or as directed by medical control—to maintain a systolic blood pressure of at least 100 mm Hg in patients with a closed TBI and a GCS score of less than 9.[25] Hypotension in a brain-injured patient can be lethal because it may decrease the CPP, with resultant cerebral ischemia, permanent brain damage, and death. You must continuously monitor the patient's blood pressure to quickly identify

YOU are the Provider — PART 4

After establishing the absence of a gag reflex, you measure and insert an appropriate-size oropharyngeal airway and begin ventilations at a rate of 10 breaths/min. You instruct your partner to contact the ED and advise them of the patient's condition and estimated time of arrival (ETA). On your arrival at the ED, you turn over care to the awaiting physician without incident.

Recording Time: 18 Minutes	
Respirations	Assisted at 10 breaths/min
Pulse	44 beats/min
Skin	Warm, pink
Blood pressure	210/144 mm Hg
Oxygen saturation (Spo_2)	100% on 15 L/min
Pupils	Left pupil dilated and nonreactive

7. At what point should you start hyperventilating the patient with a head injury?
8. What is the appropriate hospital for this patient?

any downward trend in the systolic blood pressure and respond before hypotension develops.

Do not allow the patient to become overheated. Patients with a head injury, unlike those with shock, are at risk for the development of a high body temperature (**hyperpyrexia**), which may worsen the condition of the brain. Do not cover the patient with blankets if the ambient temperature is 70°F (21°C) or higher.

If the patient has an open fracture of the skull with brain tissue oozing out, cover it lightly with a sterile dressing that has been moistened with sterile saline. Likewise, for leakage of CSF from the ears or nose, apply loose, sterile dressings just to keep the area clean. Objects impaled in the skull should be stabilized in place and protected from being jarred.

▶ Scalp Lacerations

Scalp lacerations can be minor or serious. Because both the face and the scalp have unusually rich blood supplies, even small lacerations can quickly result in substantial blood loss Figure 30-28. Scalp lacerations alone in adults rarely cause hypovolemic shock; this result is more common in children. However, bleeding from the scalp can contribute to hypovolemia in any patient, especially one with multiple injuries.[4] In addition, because scalp lacerations are usually the result of direct blows to the head, they often indicate deeper, more serious injuries.

You can almost always control bleeding from a scalp laceration by applying direct pressure over the wound. Remember to follow standard precautions. Use a dry sterile dressing, and fold any avulsions (torn skin flaps) back down onto the skin bed before applying pressure Figure 30-29A. In some cases, you will have to apply firm compression for several minutes to control the bleeding Figure 30-29B. If you suspect a skull fracture, do not apply excessive pressure to the open wound. Excessive pressure may increase the ICP or push bone fragments into the brain.

If the dressing becomes soaked, remove it and reevaluate the area where pressure is applied. Continue applying manual pressure until the bleeding is controlled, then secure the dressing in place with a soft, self-adhering roller bandage Figure 30-29C.

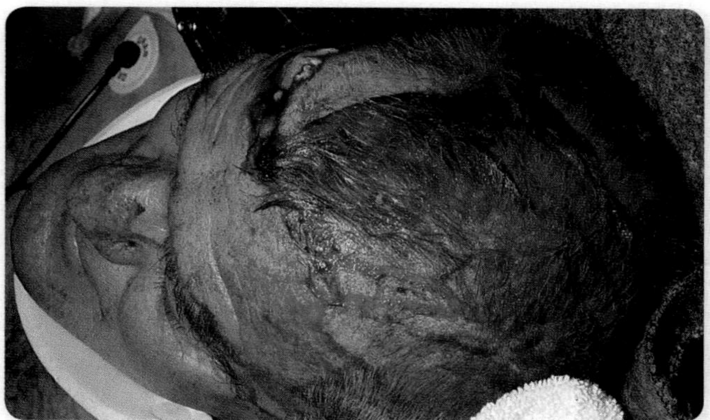

Figure 30-28 The scalp has an unusually rich blood supply; therefore, even small lacerations can result in substantial blood loss.

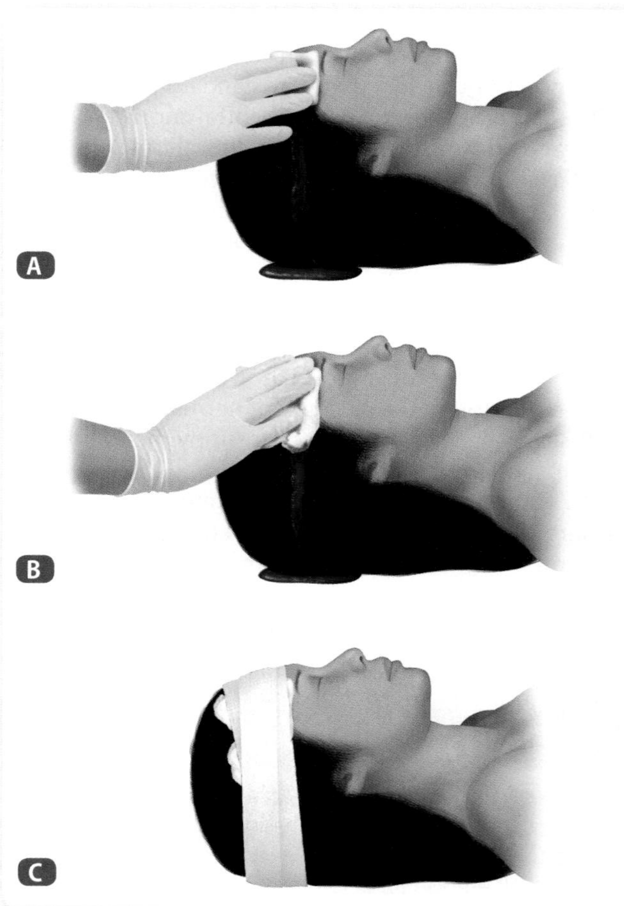

Figure 30-29 A. Use a dry sterile dressing to fold torn skin flaps back down onto the skin bed before applying pressure. **B.** If you do not suspect an open brain injury or skull fracture, apply firm compression for several minutes to control the bleeding. **C.** Secure the compression dressing in place with a soft, self-adhering roller bandage.

Emergency Medical Care of Spinal Injuries

Improper handling of a spinal injury can leave a patient permanently paralyzed, but remember that airway management always takes priority. If a patient with a spinal injury has an airway obstruction, you should perform the jaw-thrust maneuver to open the airway, as discussed earlier. After the airway is open, hold the head still, in a neutral, in-line position, until it can be fully immobilized. Assess respirations, and provide supplemental oxygen or ventilatory support as needed. Consider inserting an oropharyngeal airway. Monitor the airway closely, and have a suctioning unit available. Be prepared for any changes in the patient's condition based on your treatment.

Immobilization of the Cervical Spine

Stabilize the head and trunk so that potentially fractured bone fragments of the spine do not cause further damage. Even small movements can substantially injure the spinal cord. To perform manual in-line stabilization, follow the steps in Skill Drill 30-1.

You should never force the head into a neutral, in-line position. Do not move the head any farther if the patient reports any of the following symptoms:

- Muscle spasms in the neck
- Increased pain with movement
- Numbness, tingling, or weakness in the arms or legs
- Compromised airway or ventilations

In these situations, immobilize the patient in his or her current position.

Cervical Collars

Rigid cervical immobilization devices, or cervical collars, provide preliminary, partial support. A cervical collar should be applied to every patient who has a possible spinal injury based on MOI, history, or signs and symptoms. Keep in mind, however, that cervical collars do not fully immobilize the cervical spine. Therefore, you must be vigilant to avoid moving the cervical spine during patient transfers and supplement the immobilization using another spinal immobilization device, such as a long or short backboard or vacuum mattress when indicated.

To be effective, a rigid cervical collar must be the correct size for the patient. It should rest on the shoulder girdle and provide firm support under both sides of the mandible, without obstructing the airway or ventilation efforts in any way Figure 30-30. If you do not have an appropriate-size cervical collar, you may use a rolled towel around the patient's head. Tape the patient's head along with the towel to the backboard or vacuum mattress and provide supplemental continuous manual support Figure 30-31.

To apply a cervical collar, follow the steps in Skill Drill 30-2.

After the patient's head and neck have been manually stabilized, assess the PMS in all extremities. Then assess the cervical spine area and neck. Keep in mind that the

Skill Drill 30-1 Performing Manual In-Line Stabilization

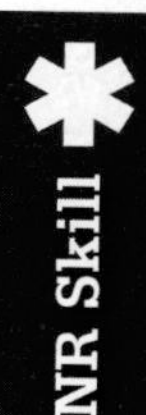

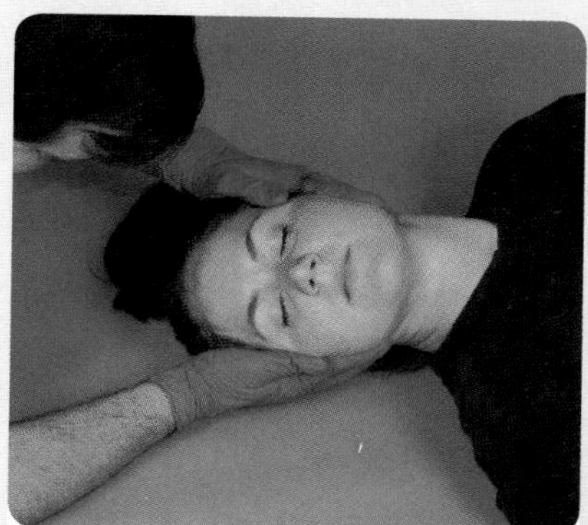

Step 1 Take standard precautions. Begin by holding or having someone firmly hold the head with both hands. Whenever possible, kneel at the head of the patient, and place your hands around the base of the skull on either side.

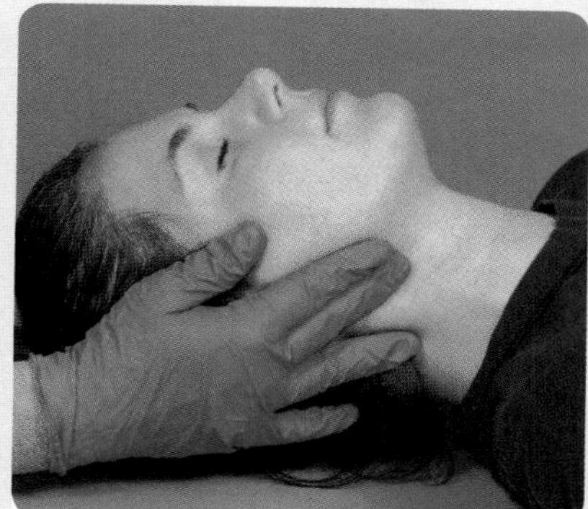

Step 2 Support the lower jaw with your index and long fingers, while you are supporting the head with your palms. Gently lift the head until the patient's eyes are looking straight ahead and the head and torso are in line. This neutral, eyes-forward position makes immobilization easier. Align the nose with the navel. Do not move the head or neck excessively, forcefully, or rapidly.

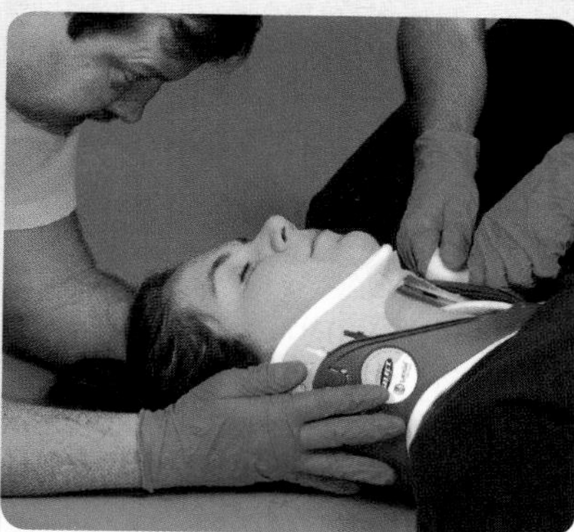

Step 3 Manually maintain this position while your partner places a rigid cervical collar around the neck to provide more stability. Do not remove your hands from the patient's head until the patient's torso and head have been secured to a backboard or other appropriate device. The patient must remain immobilized until he or she has been examined at the hospital.

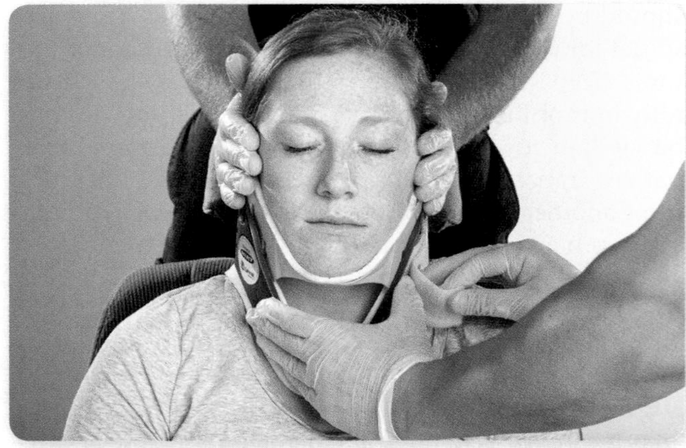

Figure 30-30 Proper fit is essential in applying a cervical collar. The collar should rest on the shoulder girdle and provide firm support under both sides of the mandible without obstructing the airway or any ventilation efforts.

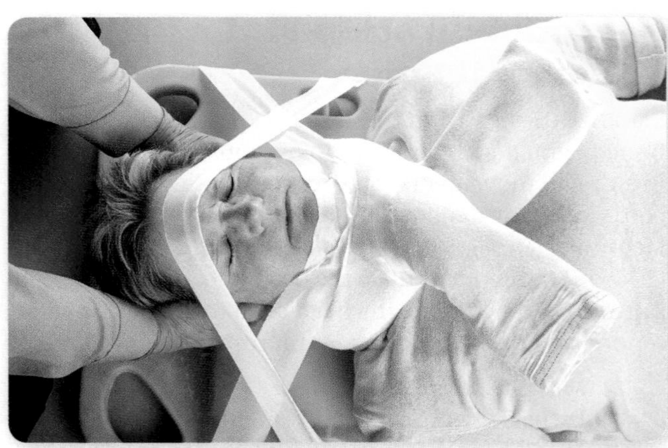

Figure 30-31 If you do not have an appropriate-size cervical collar, you may use a rolled towel around the patient's head. Tape the patient's head along with the towel to the backboard or vacuum mattress and provide supplemental continuous manual support.

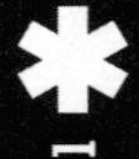

NR Skill

Skill Drill 30-2 Application of a Cervical Collar

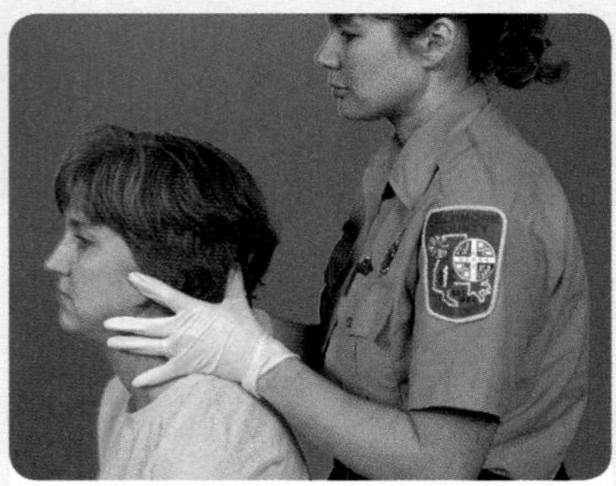

Step 1 One AEMT provides continuous manual in-line support of the head while the other prepares the collar.

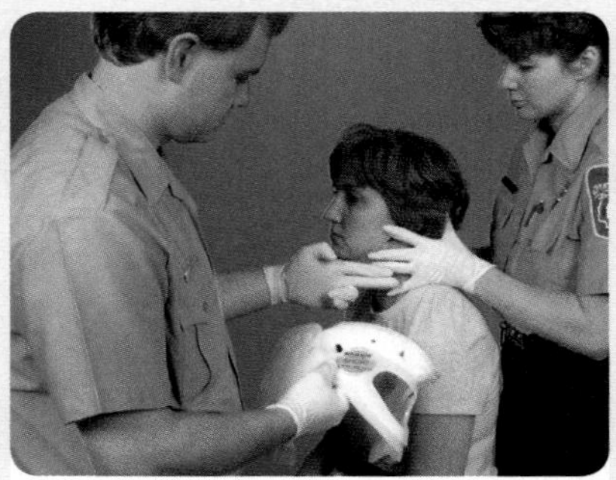

Step 2 Measure the proper collar size according to the manufacturer's specifications. It is essential that the cervical collar fits properly.

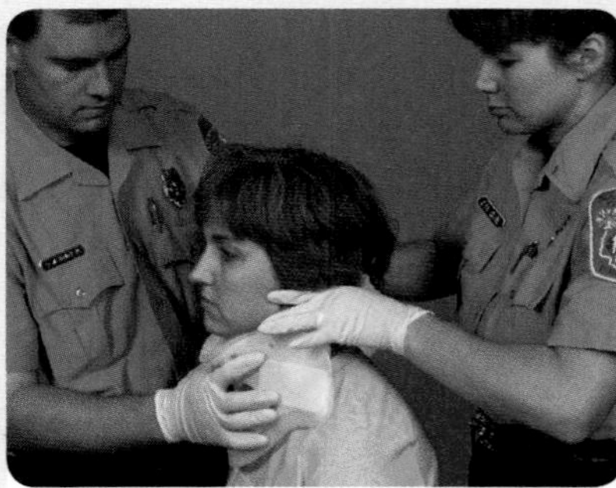

Step 3 Place the chin support snugly underneath the chin.

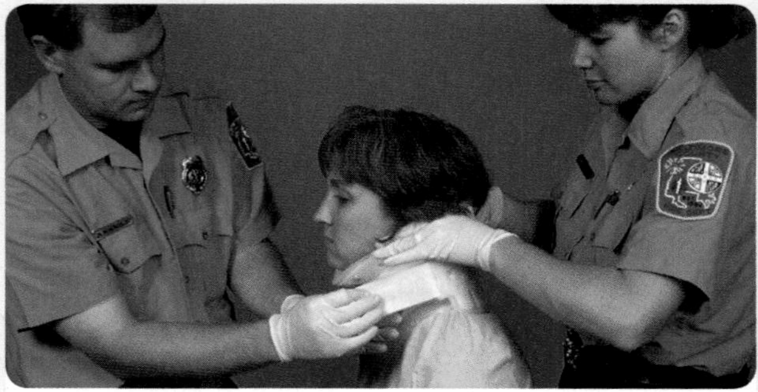

Step 4 Maintaining head stabilization and neutral neck alignment, wrap the collar around the neck, and secure the collar to the far side of the chin support.

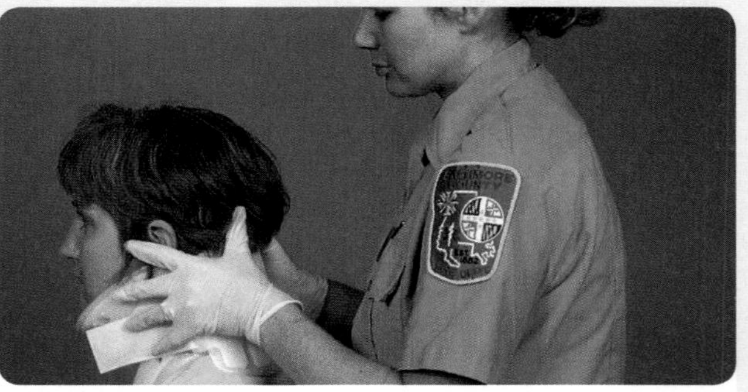

Step 5 Ensure that the collar fits properly and recheck that the patient is in a neutral, in-line position. Maintain in-line stabilization until the patient is secured to a backboard or other appropriate device.

cervical collar is used to provide increased stability to the neck. It is used in addition to, not instead of, manual cervical stabilization. An improperly fitting collar can do more harm than good. In any case, maintain manual support until the patient has been fully secured to the backboard or other appropriate immobilization device.

Words of Wisdom

Remember, applying a cervical collar is not the equivalent of performing spinal immobilization; it is a component that contributes to immobilization.

Preparation for Transport

There are several types of long backboard immobilization devices that provide full-body spinal immobilization Figure 30-32. They also provide stabilization and immobilization to the head, neck, torso, pelvis, and extremities. Long backboards can be used to immobilize patients who are found in any position (prone, sitting, supine), sometimes in conjunction with short backboards.

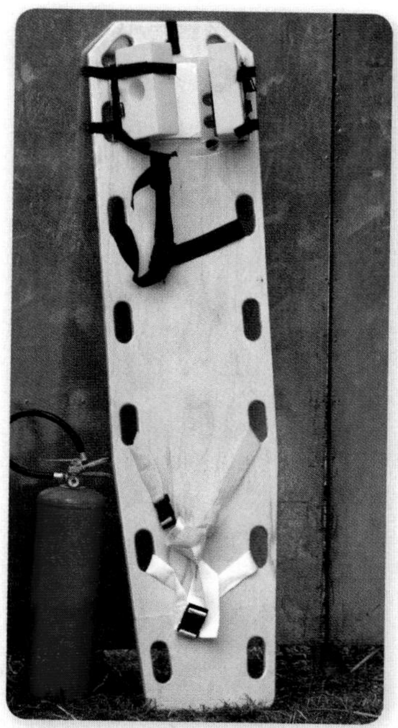

Figure 30-32 Long backboard immobilization devices allow for full-body spinal immobilization, including stabilization of the head, neck, torso, pelvis, and extremities.

Controversies

The Evolution of Spinal Care

Spinal immobilization is a controversial topic in prehospital medicine. Immobilization has been one of the most common procedures used in EMS for decades because injury to the spinal cord, especially high-level injury, is life threatening and can devastate the patient and his or her quality of life.[26]

Potential Negatives of Backboarding

It is important to remember that actions or inactions in the prehospital setting have direct consequences for the patient and the receiving facility. One study found that when immobilization procedures are used, patients spend an average total time of 54 minutes on the backboard with 33 of those minutes, on average, spent in EMS care and 21 minutes spent in the ED.[27]

Hyperextension of the cervical spine that can occur during immobilization procedures can result in neurologic deficit. Therefore, you must immobilize the patient in a neutral position. The adult patient requires 0.5 to 2 inches (1.25 to 5 cm) of padding behind the occiput to achieve a neutral position.[28] Immobilizing the patient's head directly on the backboard produces hyperextension of the cervical spine, thereby increasing the risk of neurologic deficit.

In patients immobilized for a prolonged time, pain also often develops in the occipital, sacral, and lumbar areas that they did not have before being immobilized. This can result in potentially unnecessary radiographic studies being taken, and even longer times on the backboard.[29] Padding in the lumbar region and under the patient's knees, to keep the legs slightly flexed, can reduce pain in the lumbar and sacral areas. A vacuum mattress, used either alone or with a rigid backboard, has been shown to reduce pain and neurologic deficit.

Other complications include ulcers and pressure sores, increased risk of aspiration, and respiratory compromise. Cervical collars that are applied too tightly and not reassessed for proper fit can raise ICP, which presents another risk.[30] Head injury is common in trauma, and increased ICP is associated with worse neurologic outcomes. Head injury is far more common in trauma than is cervical injury. Finally, airway management is more difficult with a cervical collar than without.

Evidence-Based Medicine

Prior practice was to immobilize everyone.[31,32] Recent publications and position statements have advocated for avoiding immobilization in a subset of patients for whom there is little potential benefit and for whom the discomfort of immobilization, the time to achieve immobilization, and the potential complications of immobilization exceed any potential advantage—in short, those for whom the risk of immobilization outweighs any potential benefits.[33]

(continued)

Controversies (continued)

Indications for cervical spine immobilization are listed in Table 30-5. Much of the impetus for change has revolved around three concerns: (1) discomfort and risk of skin breakdown associated with immobilization on a hard backboard, (2) decreased ability for a patient to protect his or her own airway when thoroughly immobilized, and (3) increased scene time associated with the immobilization process.[34-37]

An argument against immobilization has also been that it is relatively ineffective. The semantics of the discussion, including the promulgation of new terms (such as spinal motion restriction), reflects this argument. It is very true that spinal immobilization results in incomplete immobilization of the spine. It's also true that immobilization of a femur in a traction splint or immobilization of a tibia in a leg splint results in incomplete immobilization. That doesn't make it ineffective or otherwise useless. The purpose of spinal immobilization is to prevent secondary damage to the spinal cord, not to completely immobilize the spine and prevent micromotion at the site of any injury.

The published protocols (including those of the American College of Surgeons Committee on Trauma, National Association of EMS Physicians, and others) make good common sense. Patients with a low likelihood of injury based on either low-risk mechanism (eg, gunshot wounds) or reliable physical exam don't need to be immobilized. Unfortunately, trends toward decreasing the frequency of immobilization tend to flow past logic and evidence. In some cases, aggressive and potentially dangerous practices are being implemented, in which immobilization of the spine is effectively eliminated from EMS protocols and cervical collars are applied with no further immobilization of the spine instituted or even attempted. In some cases, careful processes and procedures are employed in the process of transferring patients in lieu of the traditional backboard and collar packaging. It's important to remember that the reason spinal immobilization emerged initially as a tool in EMS was that there were reported cases of patients in whom a progression of neurologic deficits developed during the course of medical care and transport, in the absence of immobilization and recognition of the potential for unstable spinal column injury.[38] We will likely never be able to know if any of those patients' neurologic injuries could have been prevented with better immobilization. The protocols and practices that followed involving the boarding and collaring of all patients with a suspicious MOI, regardless of other signs or symptoms, likely represented unnecessary treatment and may have actually resulted in some degree of harm to a few patients and some degree of discomfort to many. Although the risk of causing an unstable spinal injury in a neurologically uninjured or only partially injured patient to progress to a devastating neurologic consequence is clearly low, it remains the reason we employ spinal immobilization and other precautionary techniques in this patient population. A backboard and collar remind everyone who comes into contact with the patient that there is an unresolved question as to the presence of injury and stability of the spinal column and therefore a potential ongoing risk to the integrity of the patient's spinal cord. Failing to immobilize with a backboard and collar removes that reminder from the view of those who are not necessarily familiar with the history, MOI, or specific symptoms.

It's definitely possible to move a patient safely without use of a backboard, but it's also possible that someone will not think about the need to employ spinal precautions during a transfer and move the patient in a way that will result in permanent devastating neurologic injury. Use of a backboard and collar decreases that risk by increasing the awareness of everyone who comes into contact with the patient. It's also important to consider that between the time a patient is extricated from a vehicle and the time he or she arrives in the ED, the number of times he or she is passively moved, and the forces associated with those moves, are much greater than after arrival at the hospital. Compared to the response scene or even the back of the ambulance, the hospital is a much more controlled environment. Simply put, it's safe to remove the backboard and collar in the ED, but it's not safe to avoid applying it altogether in high-risk patients.

Remember—"first do no harm." You certainly don't want to cause injury or even unnecessary discomfort to someone when immobilization isn't necessary. But you really don't want to cause or even contribute to a permanent paraplegia or quadriplegia in someone who sustained a fracture or dislocation and had intact neurologic function prior to your involvement in his or her treatment.

Common short immobilization devices are the vest-type Figure 30-33 and the rigid short board . These devices are designed to stabilize and immobilize the head, neck, and torso. They are used to immobilize patients in noncritical condition who are found in a sitting position and have possible spinal injuries.

▶ Supine Patients

A patient who is supine can be effectively immobilized by securing him or her to a long backboard. The ideal procedure for moving a patient from the ground to a backboard is the **four-person log roll**. This procedure is recommended any time you suspect a spinal injury. In other cases, you may choose instead to slide the patient onto a backboard or use a scoop stretcher. The patient's condition, the scene, and the available resources will determine the method you choose.

You should first take the necessary standard precautions and then direct the team from a kneeling position by the patient's head so that you can maintain manual in-line stabilization. Your job is to ensure that the head,

Table 30-5 Indications for Cervical Spine Immobilization

- Appropriate patients for backboard use may include those with any of the following:
  - Blunt trauma and altered level of consciousness
  - Spinal pain or tenderness
  - Neurologic complaint (eg, numbness or motor weakness)
  - Anatomic deformity of the spine
  - High-energy MOI and any of the following:
    - Drug or alcohol intoxication
    - Inability to communicate
    - Distracting injury
- Patients for whom immobilization on a backboard is not necessary include those with all of the following:
  - Normal level of consciousness (GCS score of 15)
  - No spine tenderness or anatomic abnormality
  - No neurologic findings or complaints
  - No distracting injury
  - No intoxication
- You can maintain a degree of spinal immobilization by applying a rigid cervical collar and securing the patient to the EMS stretcher without a backboard. These measures are most appropriate for:
  - Patients who are ambulatory at the scene
  - Patients who must be transported for a long time, particularly before interfacility transfer
  - Patients for whom a backboard is not otherwise indicated
- Patients with penetrating trauma to the head, neck, or torso and no evidence of spinal injury should not be immobilized to a backboard.

Abbreviations: GCS, Glasgow Coma Scale; MOI, mechanism of injury

Data source: National Association of EMS Physicians Position Statement. EMS spinal precautions and the use of the long backboard. *Prehosp Emerg Care*. 2013;17(3):392-393.

Special Populations

As the disks between the vertebrae begin to narrow, or wear out, a decrease in height of between 2 and 3 inches may occur throughout a person's life span. A decrease in the amount of muscle mass often results in less strength, and fractures are more likely to occur because of a decrease in bone density (osteoporosis). Posture also changes as an anterior curling of the shoulders produce a condition called kyphosis (also called humpback, hunchback, or Pott curvature), making immobilization of older persons more challenging.

To immobilize kyphotic patients, several blankets and pillows or a vacuum mattress may be required to provide support to the head and upper back. Make sure that the empty spaces under the patient's knees or lumbar spine are padded as well.

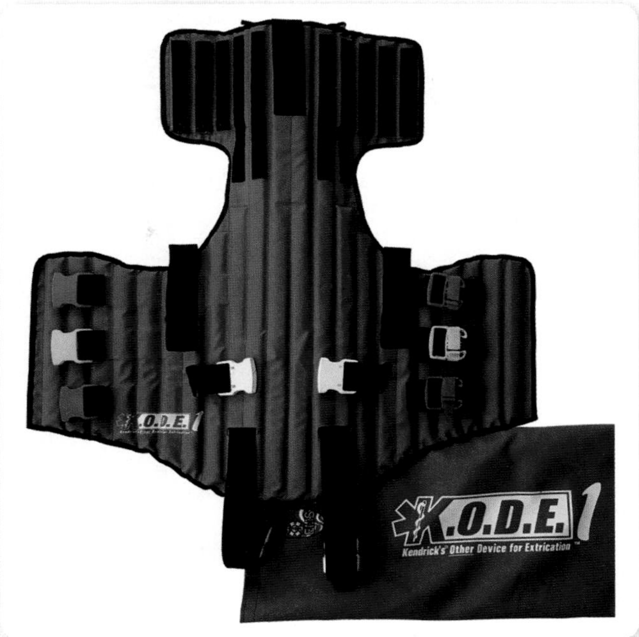

Figure 30-33 A common type of short-board immobilization device is a vest-type device.

torso, and pelvis move as a unit, with your teammates controlling the movement of the body. If necessary, you may recruit bystanders to the team, but be sure to instruct them fully before moving the patient. To secure a patient to a long backboard, follow the steps in Skill Drill 30-3.

Patients found in a prone or semiprone position must be placed in a supine position to assess airway, breathing, and circulation and to properly immobilize the spine. One rescuer should take control of the cervical spine using a crossed-hand position to roll the patient. The second rescuer should be positioned at the torso, with any additional help at the pelvis and legs. The rescuer at the head counts, and the patient should be rolled as a unit into a supine position. Assessment and immobilization should then continue as usual.

Words of Wisdom

Make sure that everyone is clear on the count *before* moving a patient. Will the count be 1, 2, 3, roll, or will the roll be performed *on* 3?

An alternative to the long backboard is the scoop stretcher. Skill Drill 30-4 summarizes how to immobilize a patient using a scoop stretcher.

Another alternative to the long backboard is to place the patient on a vacuum mattress. The vacuum mattress molds to the specific contours of the patient's body, reducing pressure point tenderness and therefore providing better comfort. The mattress also provides thermal insulation, potentially decreasing the risk of

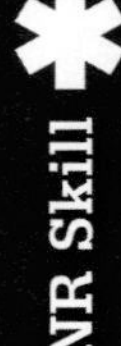

Skill Drill 30-3 Performing Spinal Immobilization of a Supine Adult Patient

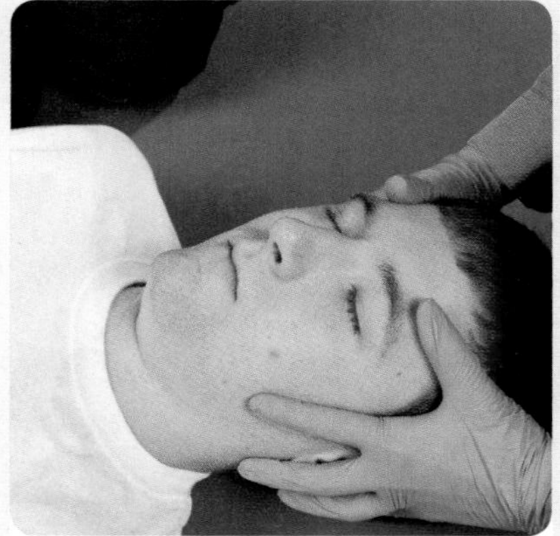

Step 1 Take standard precautions. Apply and maintain manual in-line stabilization at the patient's head, as previously discussed.

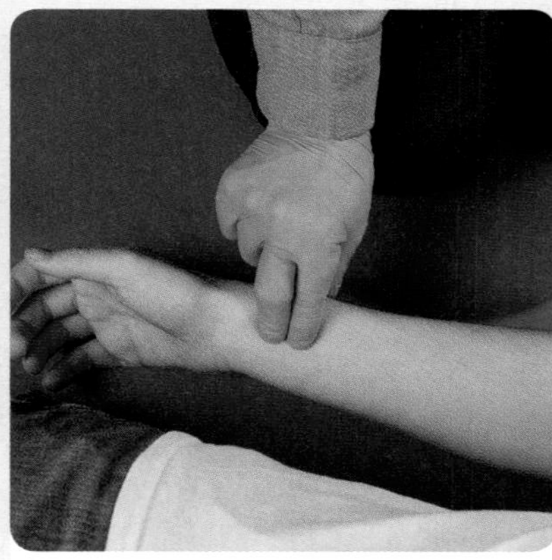

Step 2 Assess distal PMS in each extremity.

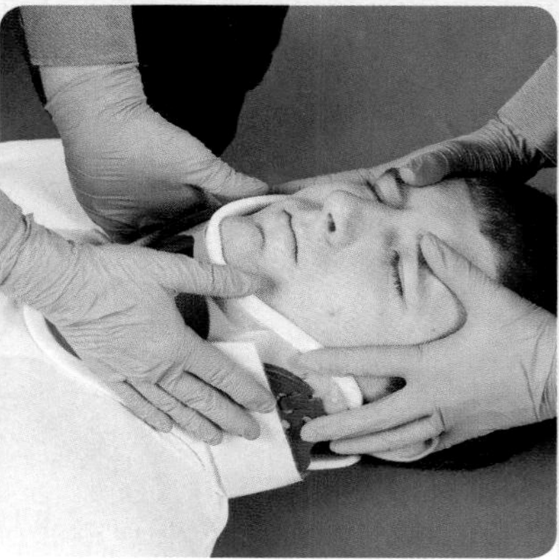

Step 3 Apply a well-fitting cervical collar as previously discussed.

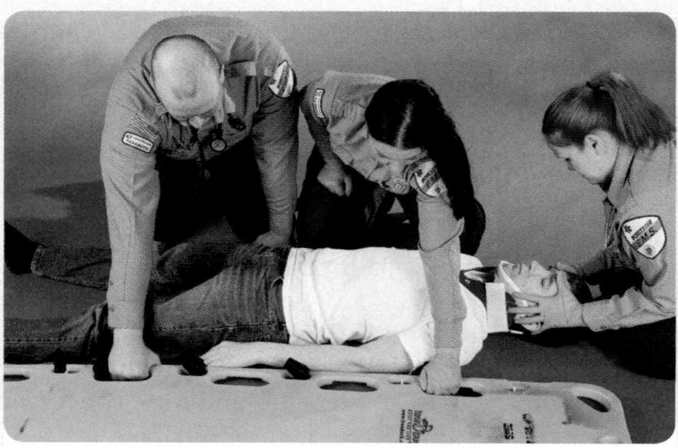

Step 4 Rescuers position the backboard or immobilization device beside the patient, kneeling on one side of the patient and placing their hands on the far side of the patient to increase their leverage. Rescuers use their body weight, shoulders, and back muscles to ensure a smooth, coordinated pull. The pull should concentrate on the heavier portions of the body.

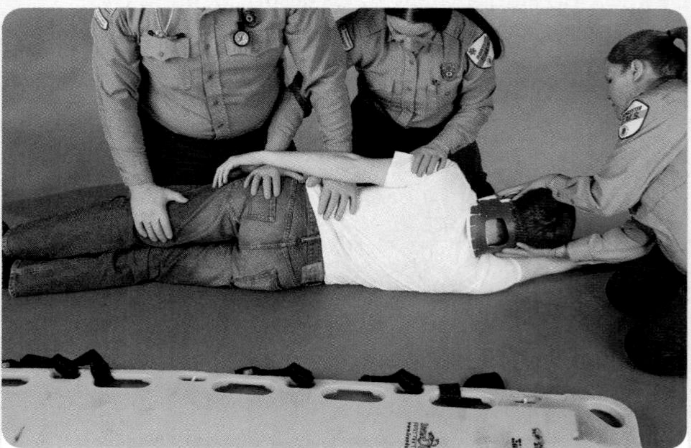

Step 5 On count/command of the person holding manual in-line stabilization, rescuers roll the patient toward themselves until the patient is balanced on his or her side. This rolling technique prevents the patient from twisting as he or she is pulled down by gravity and up by the provider. One rescuer should quickly examine the back while the patient is rolled onto the side, then slide the backboard behind and under the patient. The team should then roll the patient onto the backboard, avoiding rotation of the head, shoulders, and pelvis.

Skill Drill 30-3 Performing Spinal Immobilization of a Supine Adult Patient *(continued)*

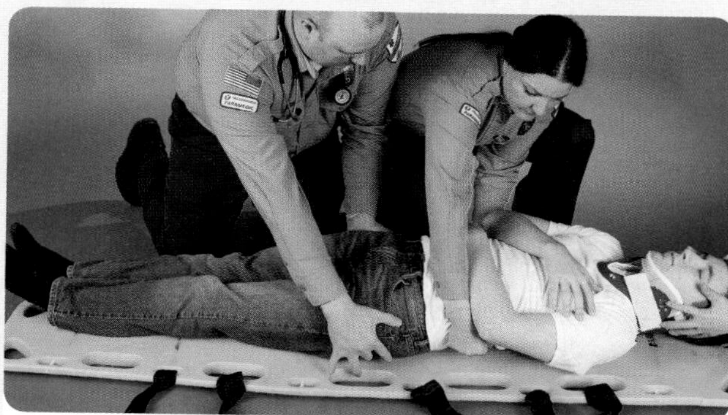

Step 6 Center the patient on the board with no lateral movement.

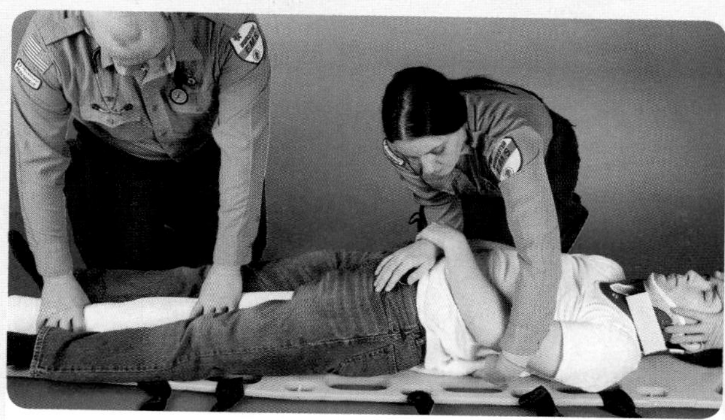

Step 7 Apply padding as necessary to fill the voids between the patient and the device. When possible, prepare blanket rolls ahead of time and have them ready to go. When you have the blankets prepared, you need only seconds to place them.

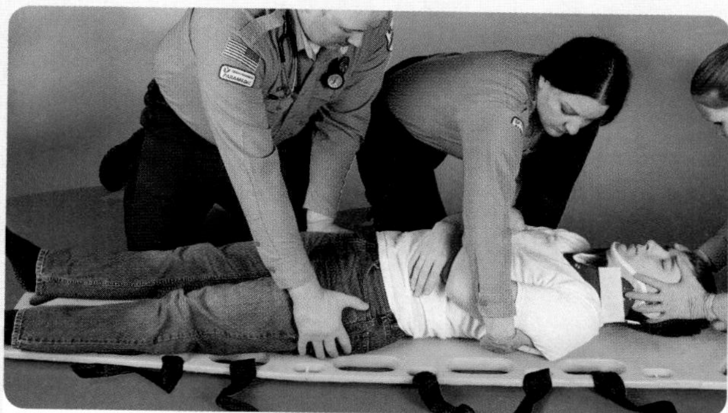

Step 8 Center the patient on the backboard.

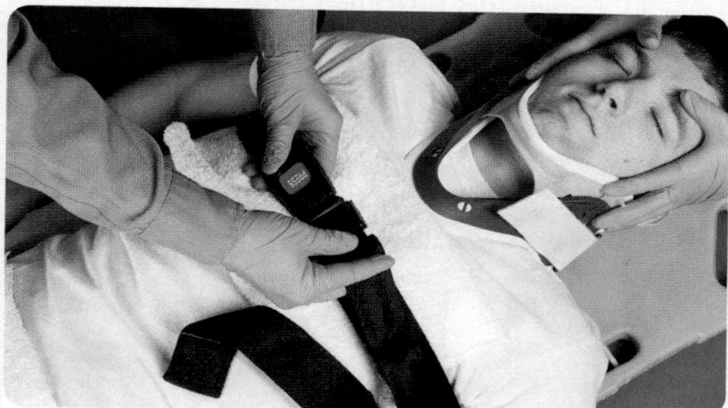

Step 9 Secure the upper torso to the backboard.

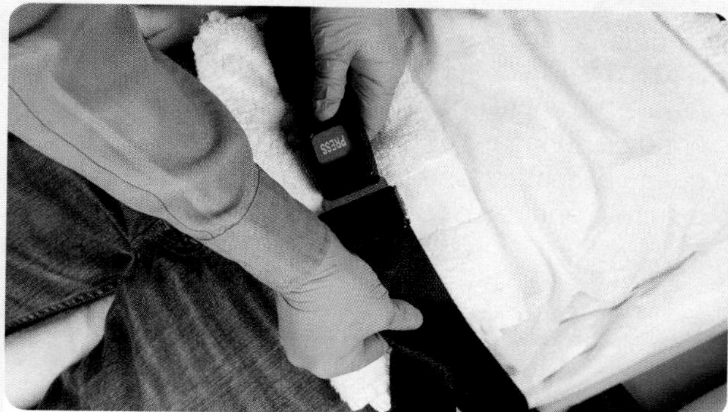

Step 10 Secure the pelvis and upper legs, using padding as needed. For the pelvis, use straps over the iliac crests and/or groin loops (leg straps).

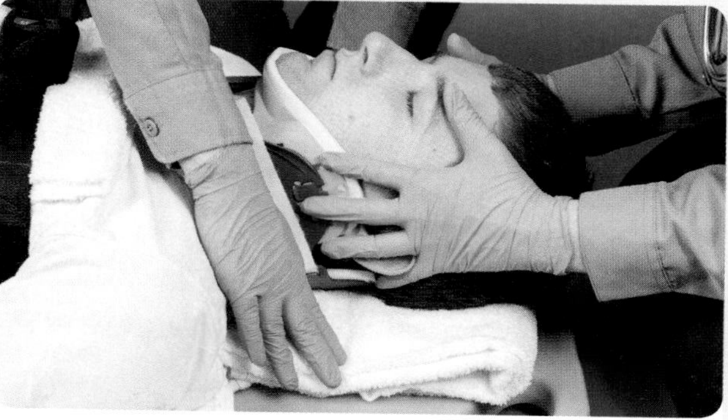

Step 11 Pad behind the patient's neck and head area as needed to maintain a neutral in-line position.

(continued)

Skill Drill 30-3 Performing Spinal Immobilization of a Supine Adult Patient *(continued)*

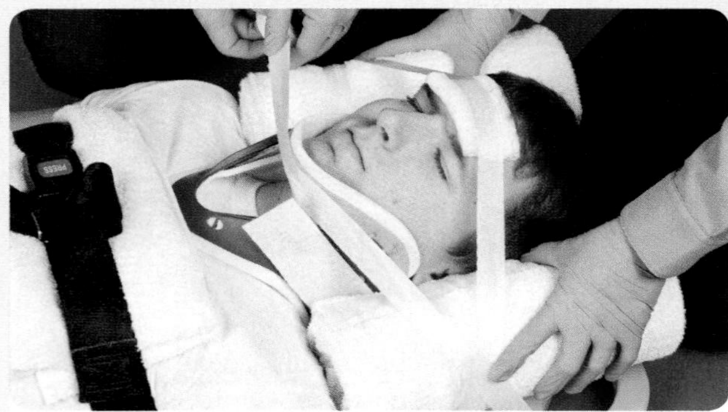

Step 12 Immobilize the head to the backboard with a commercial immobilization device per the manufacturer's instructions. Alternatively, rolled towels may be used. Secure the head to the backboard only after the entire torso has been secured. If the head is secured first and the body shifts, the spine may be compromised. Securing most of the body weight first creates better protection.

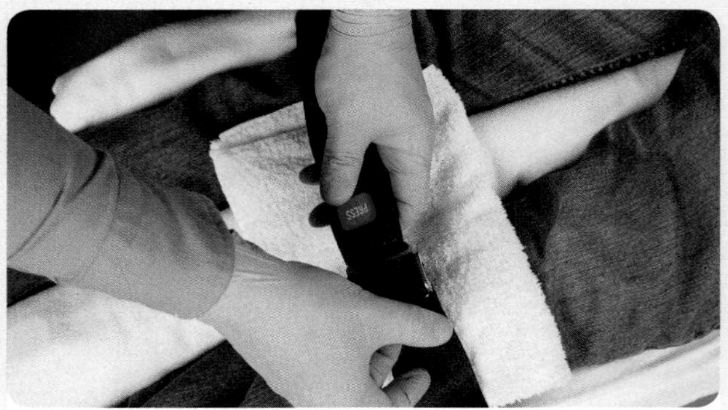

Step 13 Secure the patient's lower legs to the backboard.

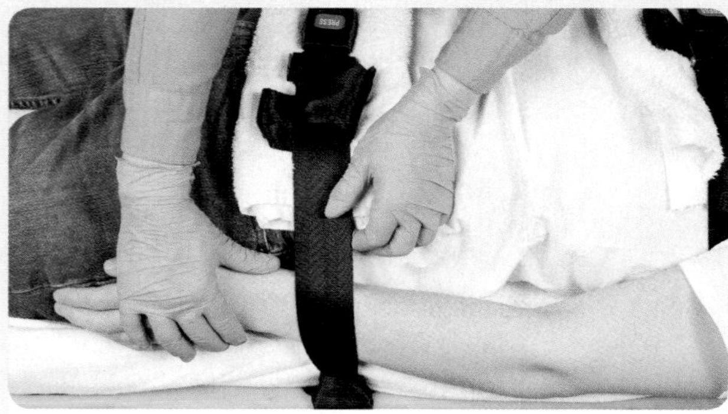

Step 14 Secure the patient's arms with a single strap.

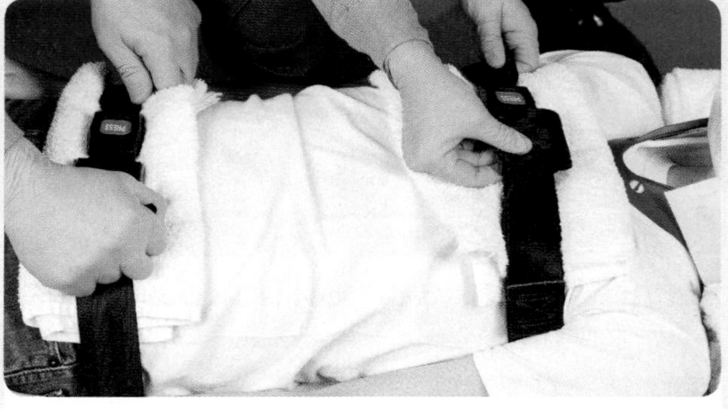

Step 15 Check and readjust straps as needed to ensure the entire body is snugly secured and will not slide during movement of the backboard or during patient transport. Reassess distal PMS in each extremity and repeat periodically.

hypothermia, and is the standard equipment used to transport patients with spinal injuries in the United Kingdom. It is an excellent alternative to a backboard for older adults or patients with abnormal curvature of the spine. A drawback to the device is its thickness, requiring careful patient movement to maintain spinal immobilization during the application procedure. The vacuum mattress cannot be used for patients who weigh more than 350 pounds (159 kilograms).

As with a backboard, a vacuum mattress can be used on a supine or sitting patient.

A patient can be moved onto the vacuum mattress with a scoop stretcher or a log roll. For the scoop stretcher method, the mattress does not need to be partially rigid.

Skill Drill 30-4 Using a Scoop Stretcher

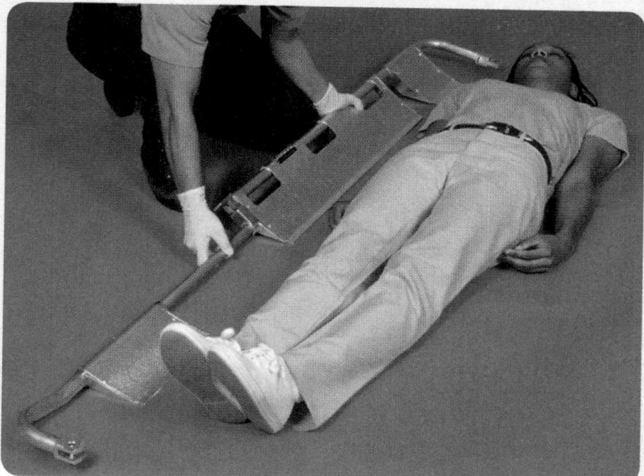

Step 1 With the scoop stretcher separated, measure the length of the scoop and adjust to the proper length.

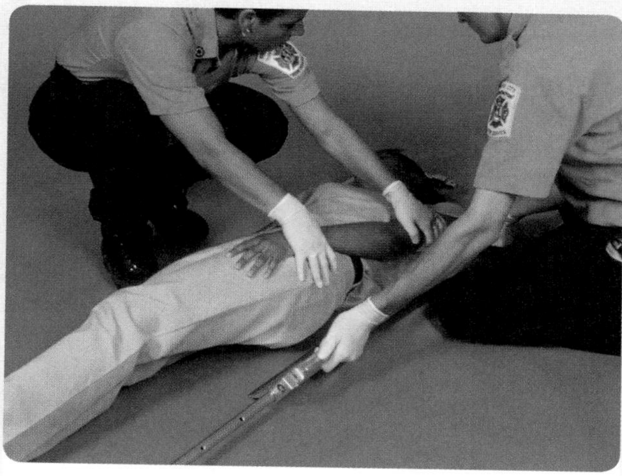

Step 2 Position the stretcher, one side at a time. Lift the patient's side slightly by pulling on the far hip and upper arm, while your partner slides the stretcher into place.

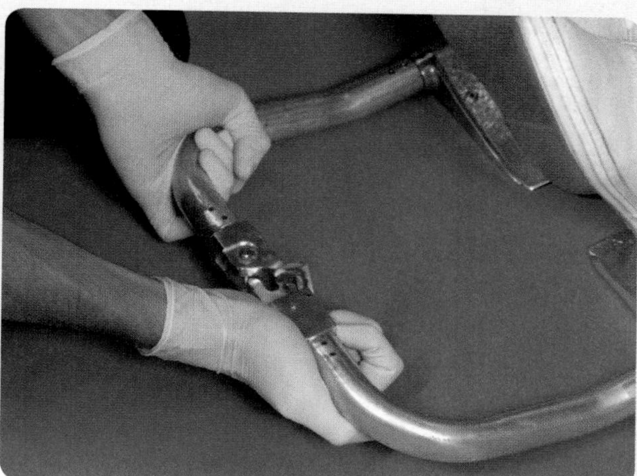

Step 3 Lock the stretcher ends together by engaging their locking mechanisms one at a time, and continue to lift the patient slightly as needed to avoid pinching the patient or your fingers.

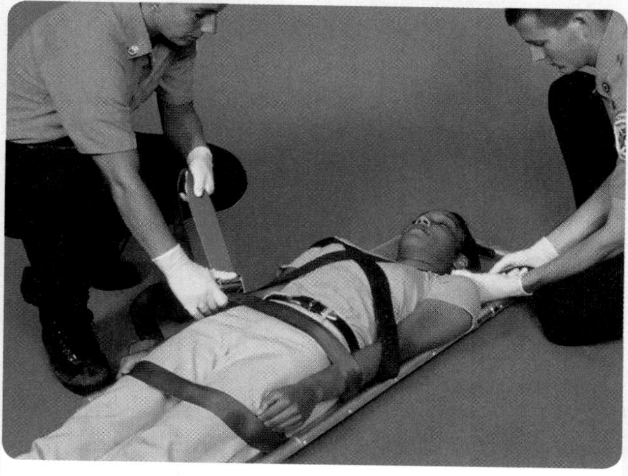

Step 4 Apply and tighten straps to secure the patient to the scoop stretcher before transferring to the stretcher.

It is important to secure the patient sufficiently but without restricting the patient's breathing. If the patient is not secured sufficiently, this can cause excessive movement, increasing the risk of subsequent SCI. Follow the steps in Skill Drill 30-5 to immobilize a patient with a vacuum mattress.

▶ Seated Patients

Some patients with a possible spinal injury will be in a sitting position, such as after an automobile crash, and reporting only isolated neck or back pain. With these patients, you should use a short backboard or a vest-style

Skill Drill 30-5 Placing a Patient on a Full-Body Vacuum Mattress

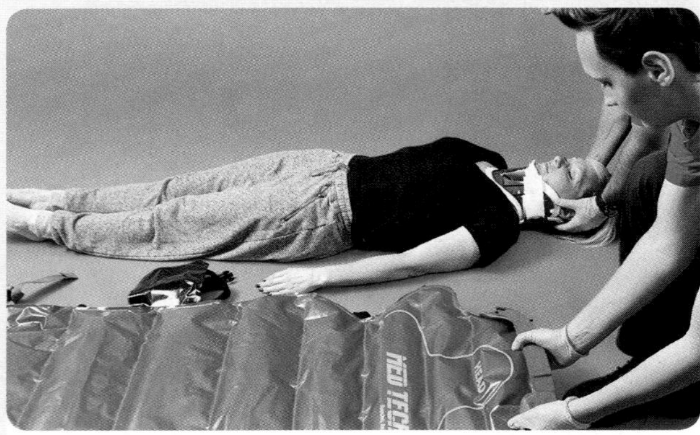

Step 1 Place the mattress on a flat surface near the patient. Make sure the head end of the mattress is at the patient's head.

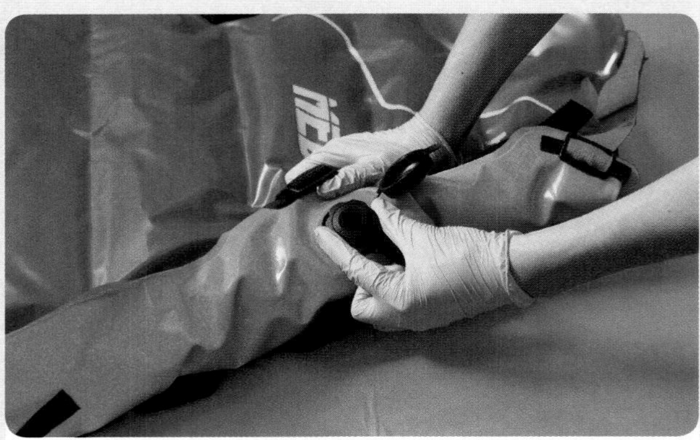

Step 2 Allow air to enter the mattress. Keep the valve stem open until the mattress is soft and pliable.

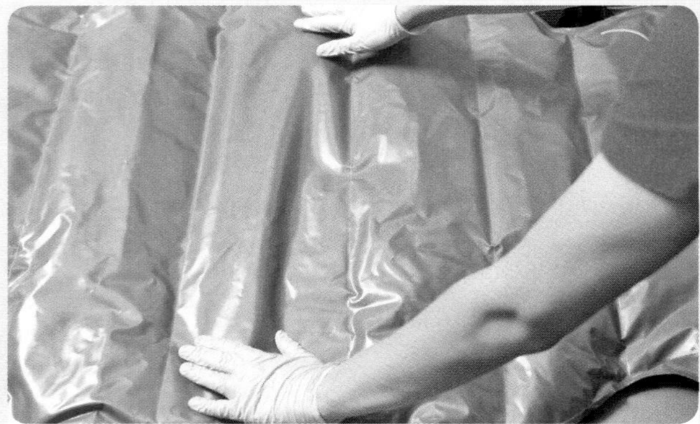

Step 3 Smooth the mattress so that it is flat and level. Remove any sharp or bulky items that may damage the mattress.

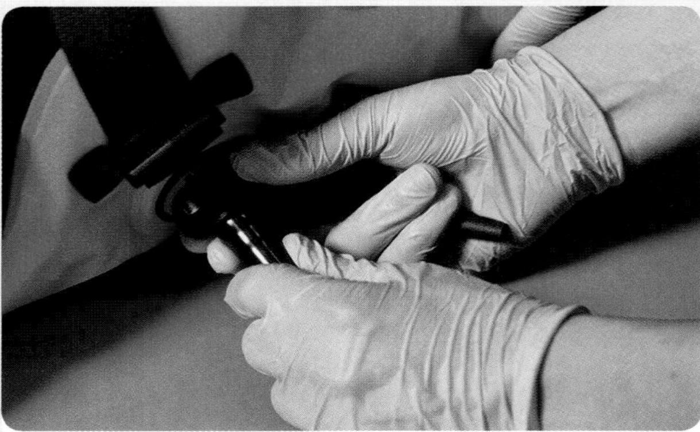

Step 4 Connect the pump to the mattress.

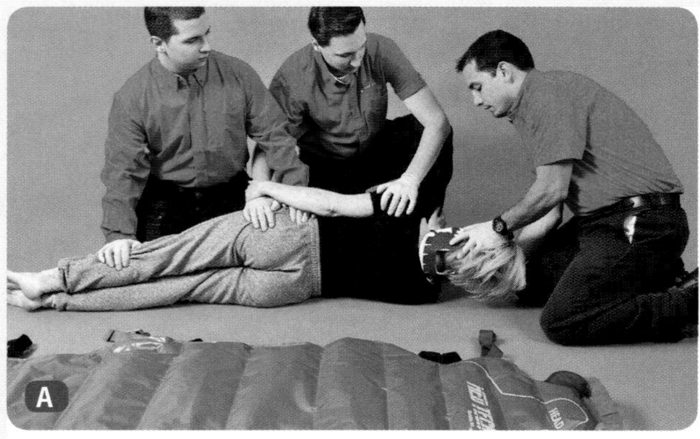

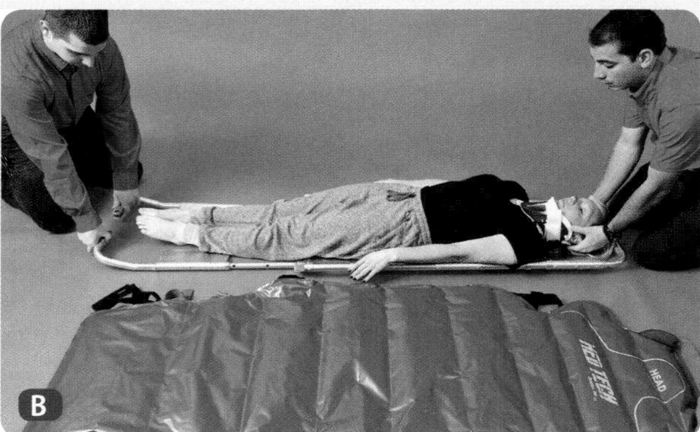

Step 5 Determine which method you will use to move the patient onto the mattress. If you use the log roll method (**A**), evacuate the mattress until it is partially rigid. (This step is not needed if using the scoop stretcher method [**B**]). The surface should be smooth and the beads should be spread out as evenly as possible.

Skill Drill 30-5 Placing a Patient on a Full-Body Vacuum Mattress *(continued)*

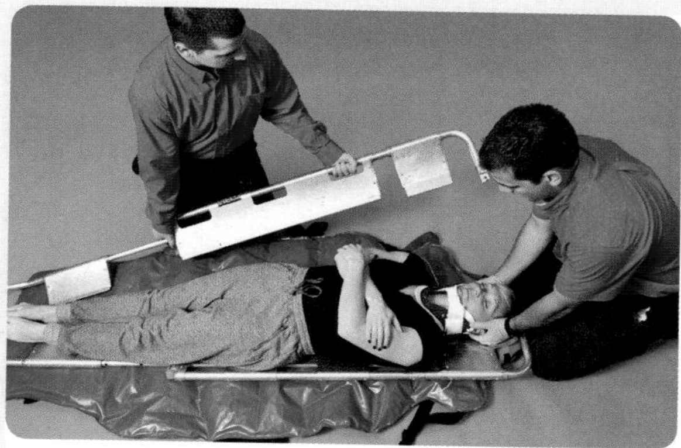

Step 6 Move the patient onto the vacuum mattress using one of the two methods: scoop stretcher or log roll. Throughout this procedure, maintain spinal alignment.

For the scoop stretcher method, the mattress does not need to be partially rigid:

a. Apply the scoop stretcher to the patient, then lift and transfer the patient onto the mattress.
b. Position the patient so his or her head is in the head area of the mattress or very close to the mattress's top edge.
c. Remove the scoop stretcher from around the patient and proceed with application of the vacuum mattress.

For the log roll method, the mattress should be partially rigid:

a. Place the mattress on a backboard or transfer device.
b. Hold the mattress in place on the backboard, and log roll the patient onto the backboard with the mattress on top of it. (The long backboard is used only for stabilization.)
c. Position the patient so his or her head is very close to the top edge.

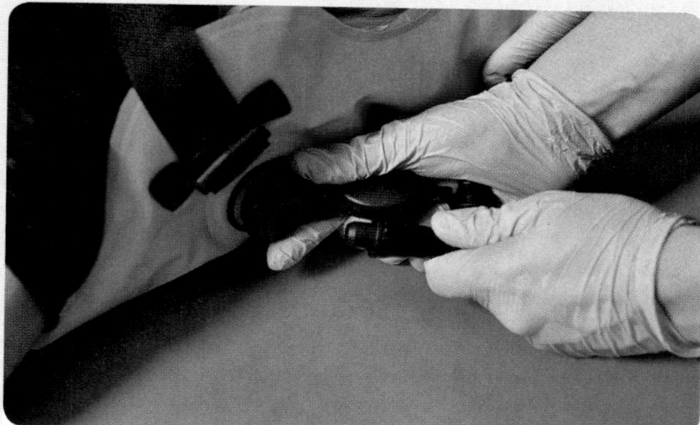

Step 7 If the vacuum mattress is partially rigid, open the valve to allow air to enter. Keep the valve open until the mattress is pliable.

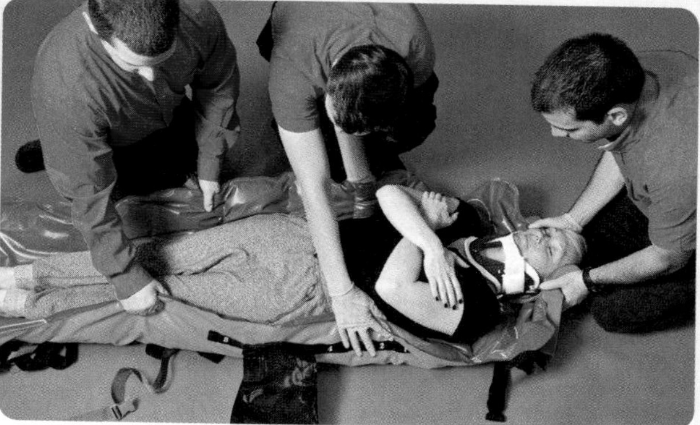

Step 8 Conform the mattress to each side of the patient's head, close to the shoulders but not the top of the head. Continue to hold these "head blocks" that you have formed, and have a second person hold up the sides of the mattress to the patient's hips until the mattress is evacuated of air completely. Always form the mattress to meet the needs of the patient. Use additional rescuers if needed. Some patients may be more comfortable with their knees slightly bent.

(continued)

Skill Drill 30-5 Placing a Patient on a Full-Body Vacuum Mattress *(continued)*

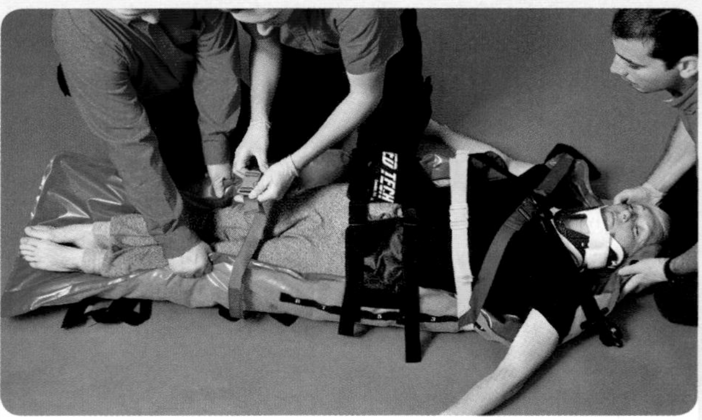

Step 9 Secure the patient's chest, hips, and legs in the mattress.

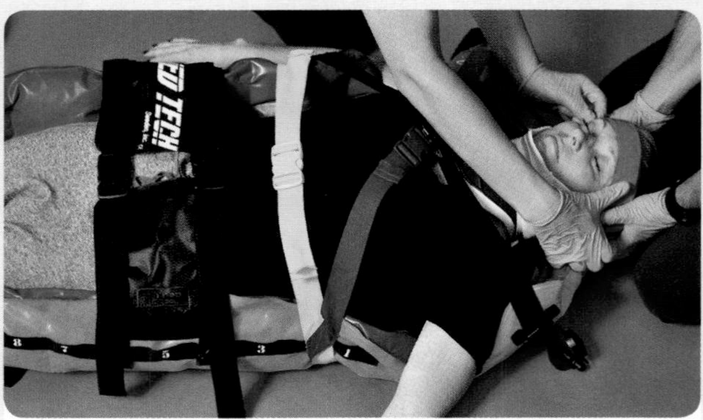

Step 10 Secure the patient's head with medical tape. Pad any voids at the top of the shoulders.

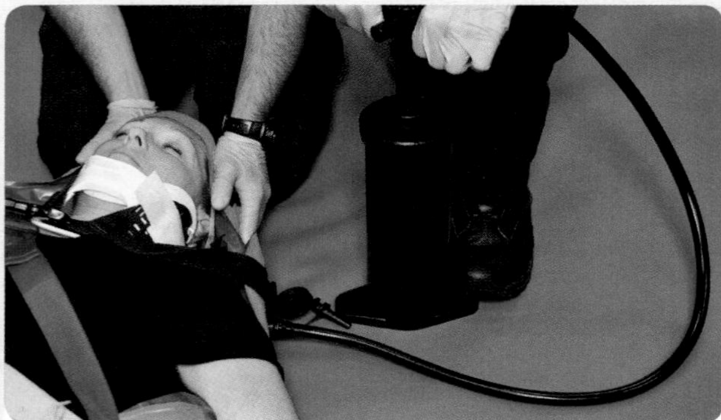

Step 11 Ensure the patient is as comfortable as possible, then evacuate the remaining air to achieve immobilization. (A portable suction unit can be used to evacuate some mattresses; see manufacturer recommendations.)

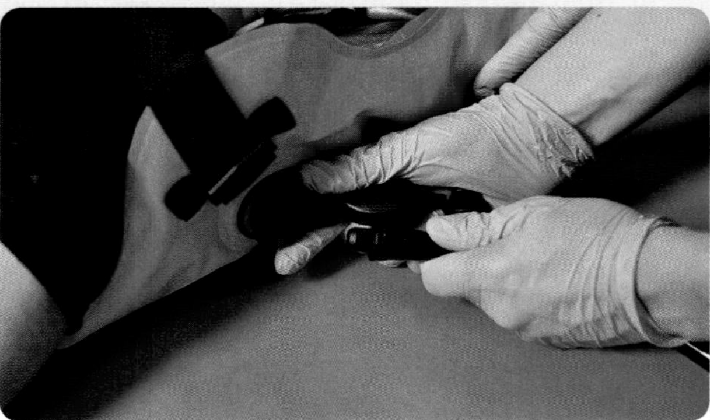

Step 12 Disconnect the vacuum pump and ensure that the valve is closed or secured so the mattress is not accidentally deflated.

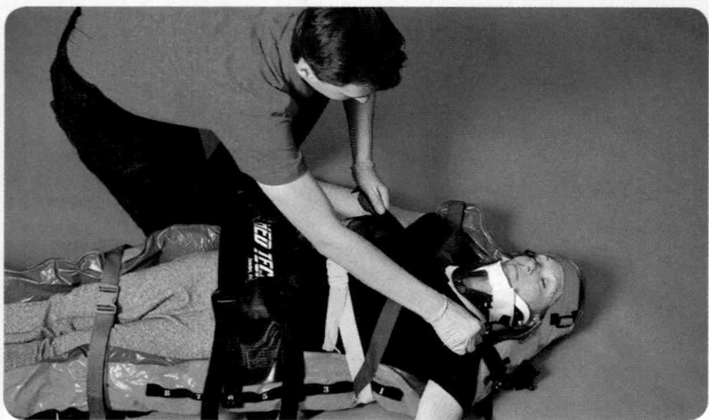

Step 13 Reassess and adjust the straps around the chest, hips, and legs.

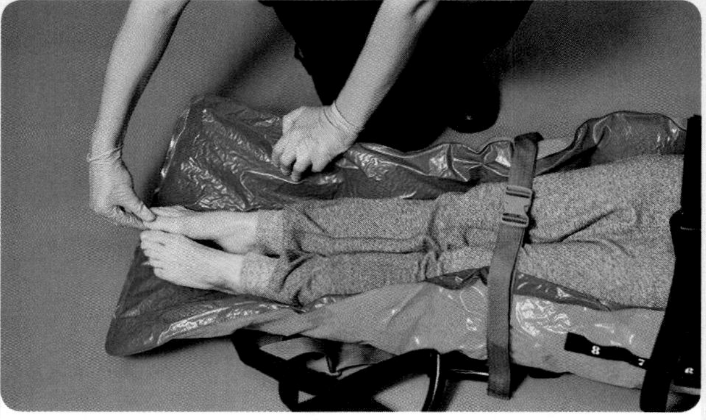

Step 14 Check the patient's neurovascular status and recheck all straps prior to lifting or moving the patient.

spinal extrication device to immobilize the cervical and thoracic spine. The short immobilization device is then secured to a long board. These short spinal immobilization devices should be used only with patients who are *stable* and do not require rapid extrication.

Special Populations

Osteoporosis in the thoracic and lumbar spine contributes to a high rate of injury in older patients. Three types of fractures are commonly encountered in the geriatric age group:

- **Compression fractures**—stable injuries that often result from minimal trauma, eg, simply bending over, rising from a chair, or sitting down forcefully.
- **Burst fractures**—unstable fractures that typically result from a high-energy MOI such as a motor vehicle crash or a fall from substantial height.
- **Seat belt–type fractures**—involve flexion and cause a fracture through the entire vertebral body and bony arch. These injuries typically result from an ejection or in people who are wearing only a lap belt without a shoulder harness.

Special Populations

When you are immobilizing a pregnant patient, tilt the backboard 15° to 20° to the left using a pillow or blankets if the size of the gravid uterus is enough to weigh heavily on the vena cava or for patient comfort. If this is not possible, manually displace the uterus to the left side.

The exceptions to this rule are situations in which you do not have time to first secure the patient to the short board, including the following situations:

- You or the patient is in danger.
- You need to gain immediate access to other patients.
- The patient's injuries justify urgent removal.

In these situations, your team should lower the patient directly onto a long backboard, using the rapid extrication technique, discussed in Chapter 6, *Lifting and Moving Patients*. Be sure that you provide manual stabilization of the cervical spine as you move the patient. Rapid extrication is indicated only in cases of life- or limb-threatening injury. In all other cases, follow the steps in Skill Drill 30-6 to immobilize a sitting patient.

Skill Drill 30-6 Performing Immobilization of a Seated Adult Patient

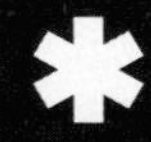

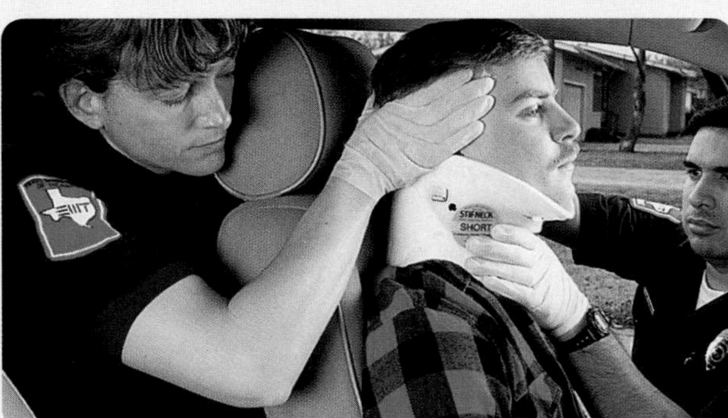

Step 1 Take standard precautions and direct another rescuer to place and maintain manual in-line stabilization of the patient's head and neck. Evaluate the patient's reliability as a historian. Assess distal PMS in each extremity.

Apply a properly sized cervical collar. Because the cervical collar does not completely immobilize the cervical spine, continue manual stabilization of the head and neck until the patient is fully immobilized and secured on a backboard.

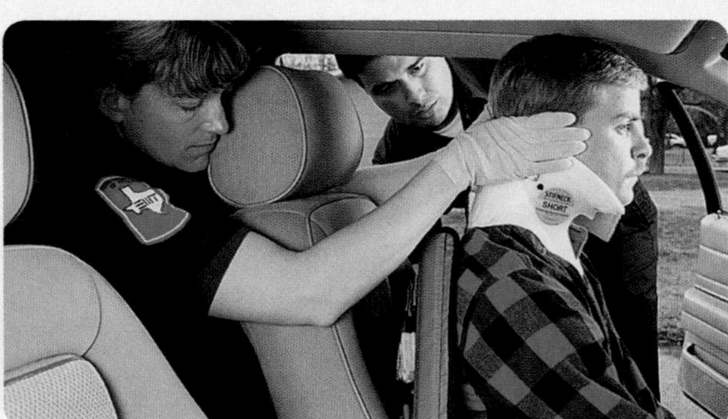

Step 2 Insert the immobilization device between the patient's upper back and the seat back.

(continued)

Skill Drill 30-6 Performing Immobilization of a Seated Adult Patient *(continued)*

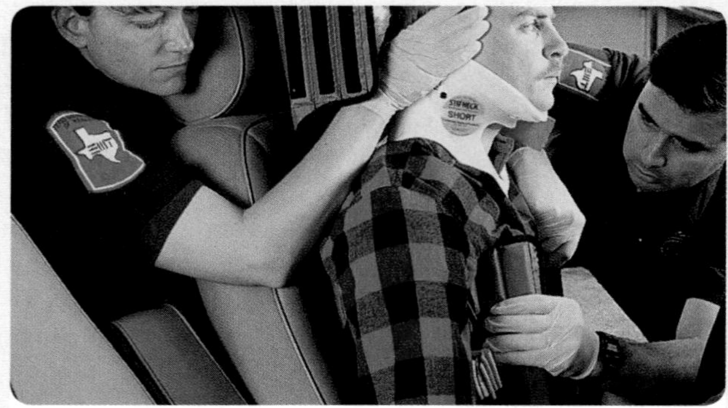

Step 3 Open the device's side flaps (if present) and position them around the patient's torso, snug under the armpits.

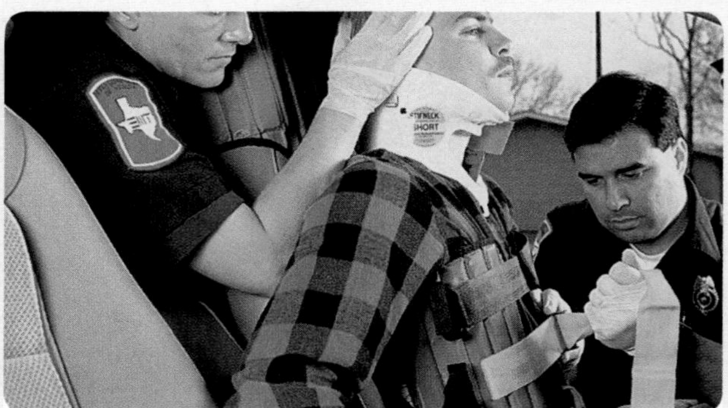

Step 4 When the device is properly positioned, secure the upper torso straps.

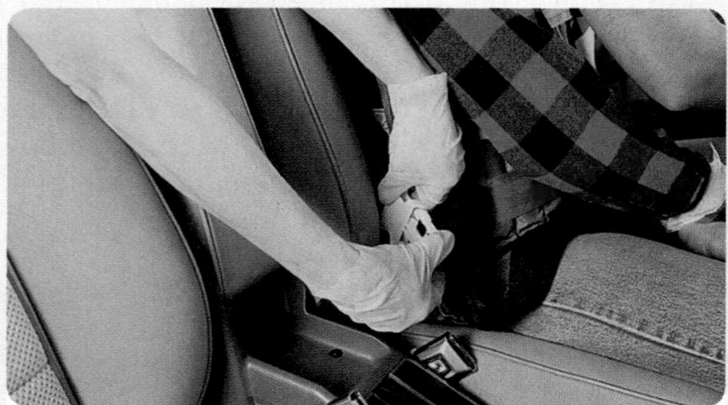

Step 5 Position and fasten both groin loops (leg straps). Pad the groin as needed. Check all torso straps and make sure they are secure. Make any necessary adjustments without excessively moving the patient.

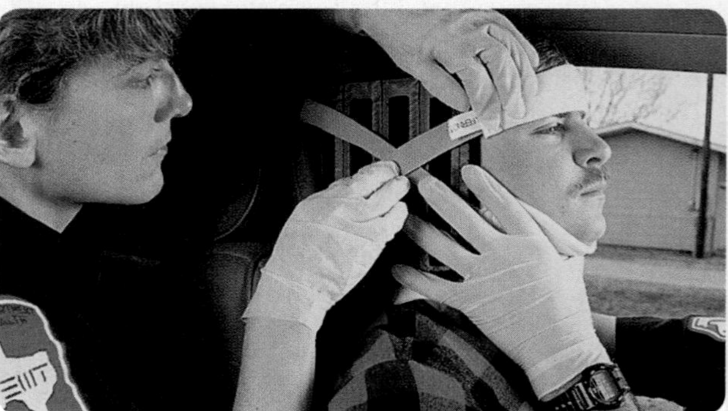

Step 6 Pad any space between the patient's head and the device. Secure the forehead strap or tape the head securely and then fasten the lower head strap around the cervical collar. Reevaluate the patient to ensure that he or she is adequately immobilized. Reassess distal PMS in each extremity.

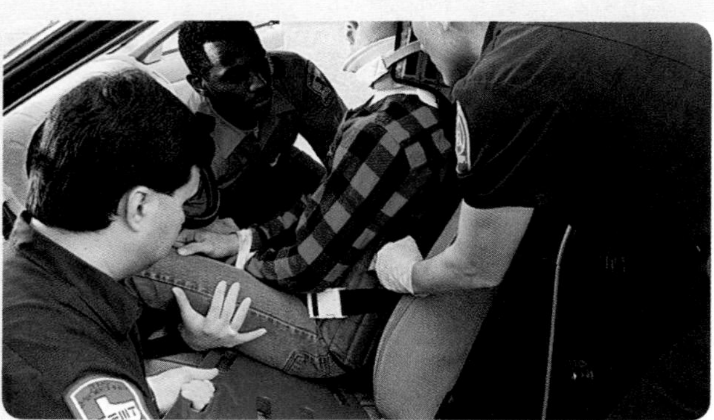

Step 7 Place a long backboard next to the patient's buttocks, perpendicular to the trunk.

Skill Drill 30-6 Performing Immobilization of a Seated Adult Patient *(continued)*

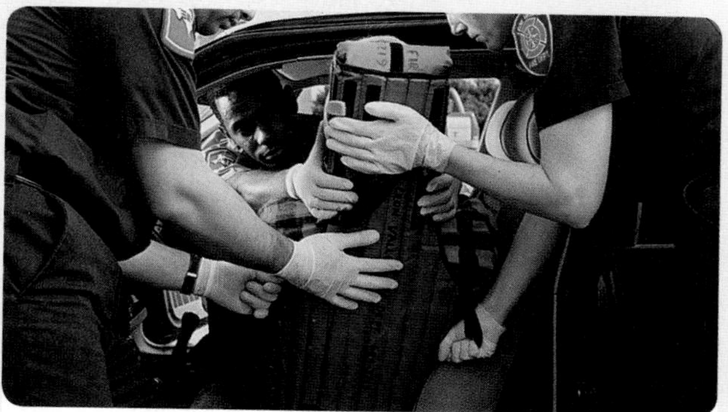

Step 8 Turn and lower the patient parallel to the long backboard and slowly lower him or her onto it. Lift the patient and the vest-type board together as a unit (without rotating the patient), and slip the long backboard under the patient and the immobilization device. Slide the patient onto the backboard as a unit using any handles that may be built into the device. Release the leg straps and loosen the chest strap to allow the legs to straighten and give the chest room to fully expand.

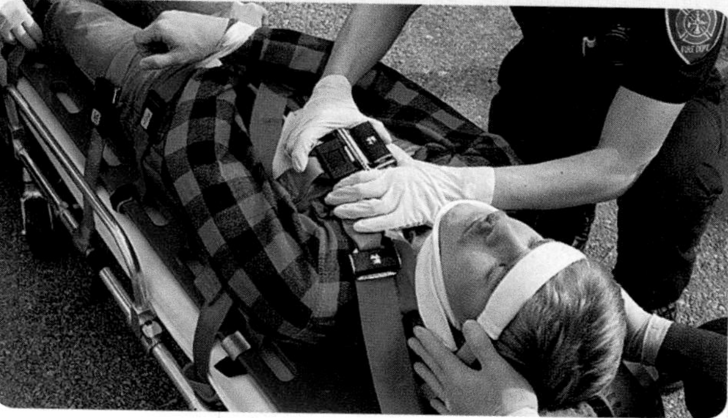

Step 9 Secure the device and the long backboard together. Do not remove the vest-type board from the patient. Reassess distal pulse and motor and sensory function in each extremity. Note your findings on the patient care report and prepare for transport.

Words of Wisdom

Ask the patient to take a deep breath before tightening the torso straps. This will ensure that breathing is not impeded by the device.

Patients Wearing Helmets

As you plan your care of a patient wearing a helmet, ask yourself the following questions:

- Is the patient's airway clear?
- Is the patient breathing adequately?
- Can you maintain the airway and assist ventilation if the helmet remains in place?
- Can the face guard be easily removed to allow access to the airway without removing the helmet?
- How well does the helmet fit?
- Can the patient's head move within the helmet?
- Can the spine be immobilized in a neutral position with the helmet on?

A helmet that fits well prevents the patient's head from moving and should be left on, as long as (1) there are no impending airway or breathing problems, (2) it does not interfere with assessment and treatment of airway or ventilation problems, and (3) you can properly immobilize the spine, which may involve padding underneath the shoulders. You should also leave the helmet on if there is any chance that removing it will further injure the patient.

Remove a helmet if (1) it is a full-face helmet, (2) it makes assessing or managing airway problems difficult and removal of a face guard to improve airway access is not possible, (3) it prevents you from properly immobilizing the spine, or (4) it allows excessive head movement.

Always remove a helmet from a patient who is in cardiac arrest.

Sports helmets are typically open in the front and may or may not include an attached face mask. The mask can be removed without affecting helmet position or function by simply removing or cutting the straps that hold it to the helmet. In this way, sports helmets allow easy access to the airway Figure 30-34. Motorcycle helmets often have a shield covering the face. This, too, can be unbuckled to allow access to the airway. If a shield cannot be removed, the helmet must be removed.

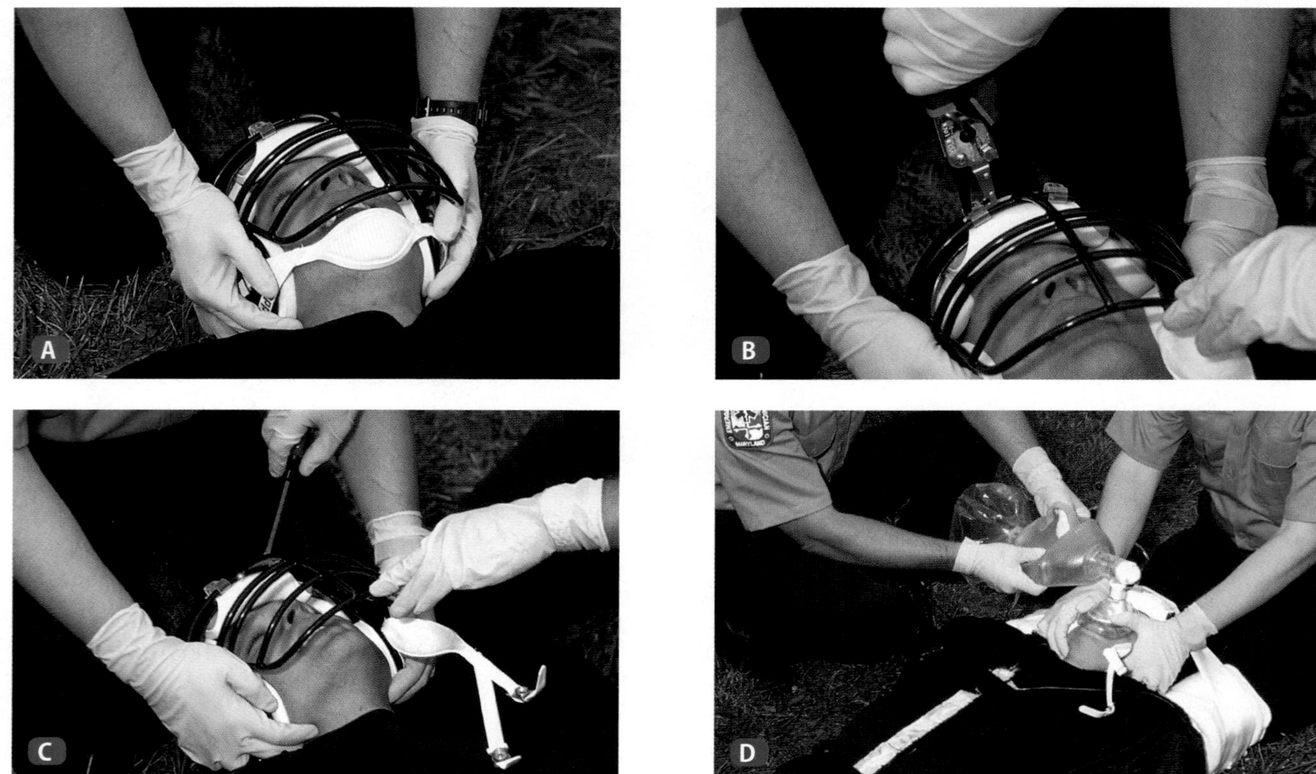

Figure 30-34 The mask on most sports helmets can be removed without affecting helmet position or function. **A.** Stabilize the patient's head and helmet. Remove the face mask in one of two ways: **B.** Use a trainer's tool designed for cutting retaining clips, or **(C)** Unscrew the retaining clips for the face mask. **D.** After the face mask is removed, the helmet can be immobilized against the backboard and a bag-mask device can be used effectively.

Words of Wisdom

Sports helmets may require the use of a specific tool to remove the face mask. Coaches or staff will have the necessary tool and will be experienced in its use.

Words of Wisdom

If a football player's helmet is removed, the shoulder pads must also be removed or padding must be placed under the head to maintain the neck in a neutral, in-line position. Likewise, if a motorcycle or other helmet is not removed, padding must be applied underneath the shoulders to maintain spinal alignment.

▶ Preferred Method

Removing a helmet is at least a two-person job; however, the technique for helmet removal depends on the actual type of helmet worn by the patient. One AEMT provides constant in-line support as the other moves; you and your partner should not move at the same time. You should first consult with medical direction, if possible, about your decision to remove a helmet. When you decide to do so, follow the steps in Skill Drill 30-7.

Remember, you do not need to remove a helmet if you can access the patient's airway, if the head is snug inside the helmet, and if the helmet can be secured to an immobilization device.

Words of Wisdom

Always take helmets to the hospital with the patient. Any damage evident on the helmet can alert physicians to areas of potential injury that may have been overlooked.

▶ Alternate Method

An alternate method for removal of football helmets has also been used. The advantage of this method is that it allows the helmet to be removed with the application of less force, therefore reducing the possibility of motion occurring at the neck. The disadvantage of this method

Skill Drill 30-7 Removing a Helmet

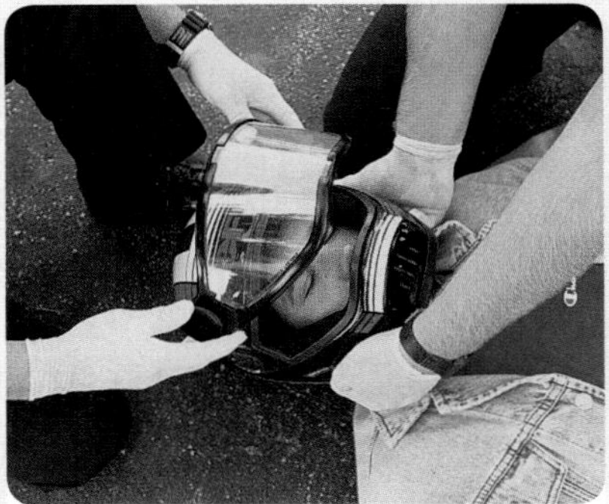

Step 1 Begin by kneeling at the patient's head. Your partner should kneel on one side of the patient, at the shoulder area. Open the face shield, if there is one, and assess the patient's airway and breathing. Remove eyeglasses if the patient is wearing them.

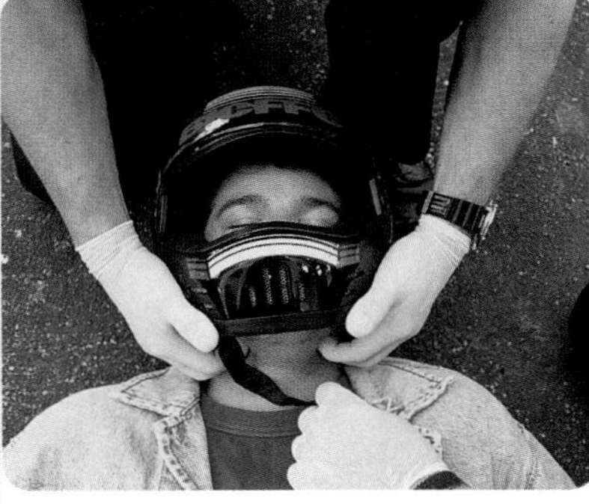

Step 2 Prevent head movement by placing your hands on either side of the helmet, with your fingers on the patient's lower jaw. After your hands are in position, your partner can loosen the face strap.

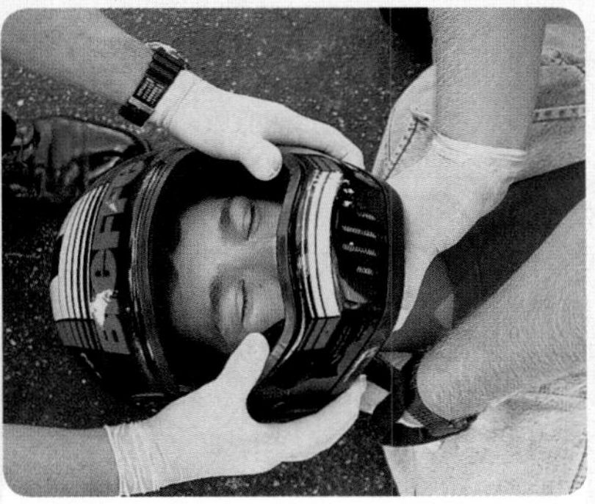

Step 3 After the strap has been loosened, your partner should place one hand on the patient's lower jaw at the angle of the lower jaw and the other behind the head at the occipital region. After your partner's hands are in position, you may pull the sides of the helmet away from the patient's head.

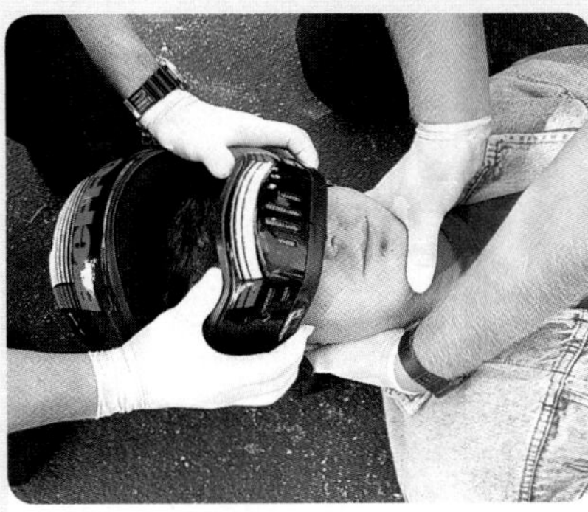

Step 4 Gently slip the helmet about halfway off the patient's head, stopping when the helmet reaches the halfway point.

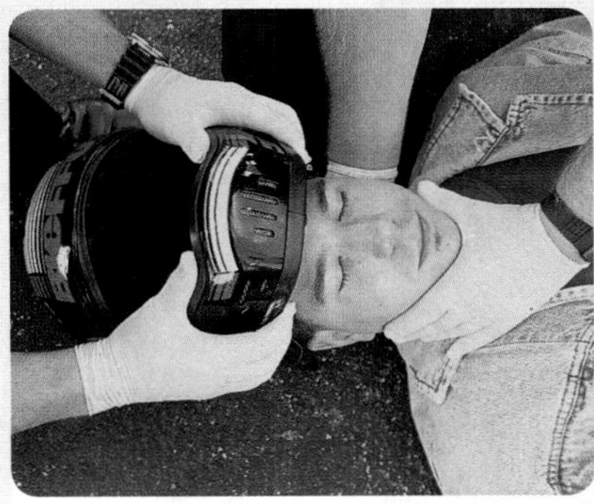

Step 5 Your partner then slides his or her hand from the occiput to the back of the head. This will prevent the head from snapping back after the helmet has been completely removed.

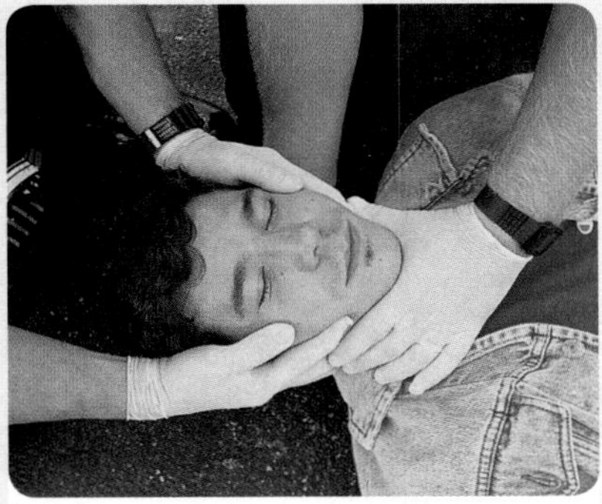

Step 6 With your partner's hand in place, remove the helmet, taking care to work over the occiput and nose, and immobilize the cervical spine. Apply a cervical collar, and then secure the patient to a long backboard. With large helmets or small patients, you may need to pad under the shoulders to prevent flexion of the neck. If shoulder pads or heavy clothing are in place, you may need to pad behind the patient's head to prevent extension of the neck.

is that it is slightly more time consuming. The first step involves removal of the chin strap. This can be cut or unsnapped carefully. Be careful during removal of the chin strap to avoid jarring the neck or head and causing excessive motion. Next, remove the face mask. The face mask is anchored to the helmet by plastic clips secured with screws. These can be removed with a screwdriver or cut with a knife. After the face mask has been removed, the jaw pads can be popped out of place. This can be accomplished with the use of a tongue depressor Figure 30-35A. You can then place your fingers inside the helmet, allowing greater control of the helmet during removal as the helmet is gently rocked back off the top of the head. The person at the side of the patient controls the head by holding the jaw with one hand and the occiput with the other Figure 30-35B. Padding is inserted behind the occiput to prevent neck extension. If the shoulder pads are in place, appropriate padding must be applied behind the head to prevent hyperextension. As with the previously described method, the person at the patient's chest is responsible for making sure that the head and neck do not move during removal of the helmet.

Remember that small children may require additional padding to maintain the neutral, in-line position. Children are not small adults. They have smaller airways and proportionally larger heads, so padding is important to maintain the airway. Pad under the shoulders to the toes, as needed, to avoid excessive neck flexion Figure 30-36. In addition, place blanket rolls between the child and the sides of an adult-size backboard to prevent the child from slipping to one side or the other Figure 30-37. Appropriate-size backboards are available for children.

Special Populations

You are likely to find infants and children who have been in motor vehicle crashes and are still in their car seats. Follow your local protocols regarding spinal immobilization techniques. See Chapter 36, *Pediatric Emergencies*, for a complete discussion on removing pediatric patients from car seats and performing spinal immobilization maneuvers.

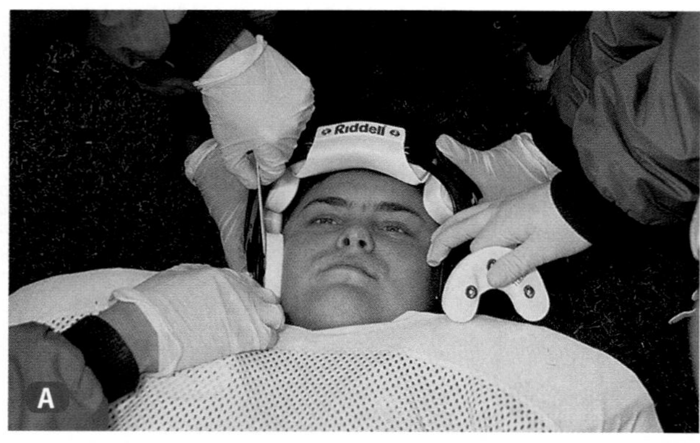

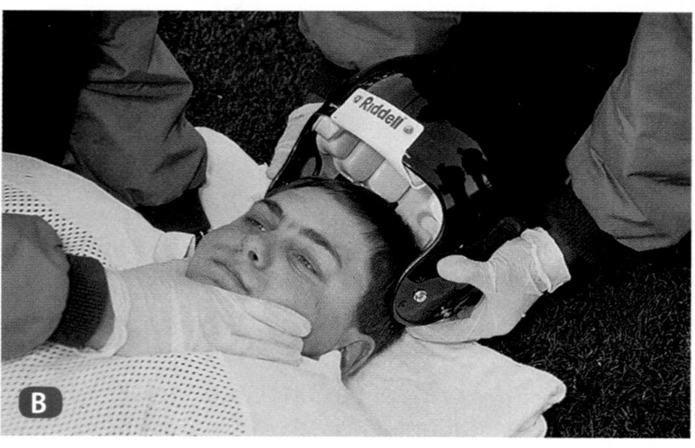

Figure 30-35 A. The jaw pads can be removed from the inside of a football helmet with the aid of a tongue depressor. **B.** Place the fingers inside the helmet, and gently rock it out of place. The person at the side controls the lower jaw with one hand and the occiput with the other. Insert padding behind the occiput to prevent neck extension.

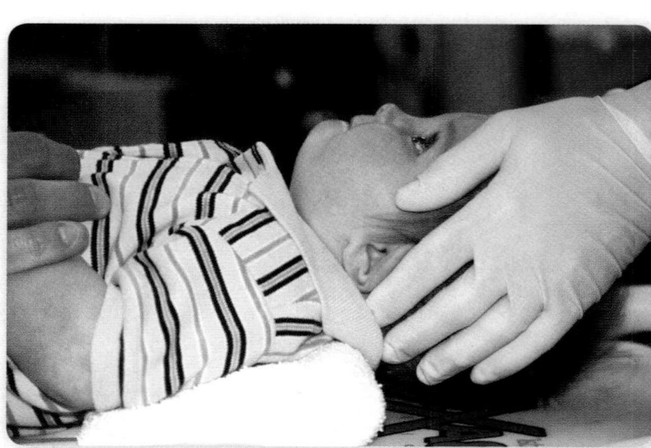

Figure 30-36 Children have proportionally larger heads than adults, so you may need to place padding under the shoulders to avoid excessive flexion of the neck.

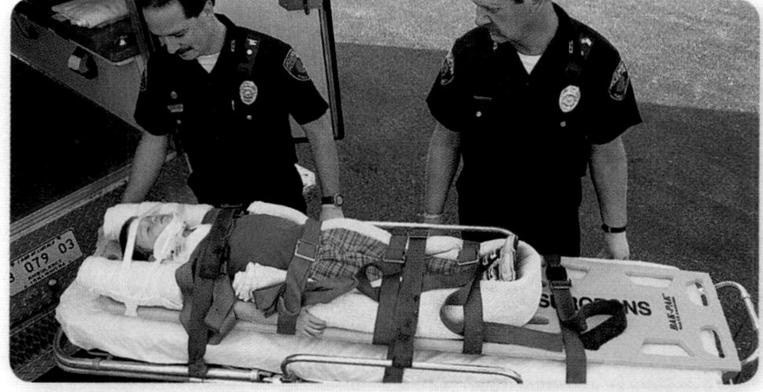

Figure 30-37 Place blanket rolls between the child and the sides of an adult-sized board to prevent the child from slipping to one side or the other.

Nontraumatic Spinal Conditions

Back pain is one of the most common physical ailments seen in EDs throughout the United States. Expenses related to back pain are high because of the extensive costs of therapy and lost wages from missed work days. Upright posture places a substantial amount of weight on the lumbar spine—specifically at L4-L5, where the natural bend in the spine's curvature changes. Therefore, most people are susceptible to injury or degenerative disease. Spinal tumors can also cause pain and debilitation. Most cases of low back pain are idiopathic (there is no known cause); making a precise diagnosis can be difficult.

When evaluating nontraumatic back pain, consider disease processes, including SCI, that can produce severely debilitating lesions Table 30-6. In the absence of trauma, assess the patient's report of low back pain with the anatomy and neurophysiology of the spine and spinal cord in mind. Pay particular attention to the patient's medications; patients with chronic back pain and tumors may be taking high dosages of narcotic agents on their own or on the advice of a physician to control their intense pain.

Pain may result from **strain** or **sprain** of paravertebral muscles and supporting ligamentous structures without substantial injury to nerve elements. Older adult patients (especially women) with a history of osteoporosis are at high risk for spontaneous compression fractures of the spine. These typically stable fractures are not associated with SCI. Tumors in the spine from a variety of metastatic carcinomas can cause pathologic spine fractures, with extension of bone fragments or the tumor itself into the spinal canal causing SCI.

Degenerative disk disease is a common entity. Over time, biomechanical and physiologic alterations of the intervertebral disk will result in loss of height and reduce the shock-absorbing effect of the disk. Substantial narrowing may result in variable segment stability.

Disk herniation may be caused by some degree of trauma in patients with preexisting disk degeneration. It typically affects men between ages 30 and 50 years, and may result from poor lifting technique. Herniation most commonly occurs at L4-L5 and L5-S1 but may also occur in C5-C6 and C6-C7. Patients will present with pain, usually with straining; they may have tenderness of the spine and often have limited range of motion. Patients may have alterations in sensation and motor functions as well. Cervical herniations may present with upper extremity pain or paresthesias that worsen with neck motion. Motor weakness may also occur as a result of spinal cord compression.

Definitive diagnosis of back pain may require multiple modalities of radiographic imaging. Prehospital management of low back pain in the absence of trauma is primarily palliative, directed at decreasing any pain or discomfort with movement.

Table 30-6 Common Causes of Low Back Pain
Muscle or ligament strains
Fractures
Osteomyelitis—bone infection
Degenerative joint/disk disease
Spondylolysis
Bursitis/synovitis
Disk herniation
Tumor

Words of Wisdom

Some patients with acute low back spasm are literally paralyzed with pain. Use a scoop stretcher to move the patient.

YOU are the Provider SUMMARY

1. On the basis of the information provided, what are some possible injuries you may encounter?

This patient may present with a multitude of injuries. Your primary concern should focus on life threats and SCIs, followed closely by TBIs. With the information provided by the lifeguards regarding the periods of unresponsiveness, you should suspect a serious TBI, which must be managed immediately to prevent worsening of the patient's condition.

2. Is this patient experiencing a primary or secondary brain injury?

This patient is most likely experiencing a primary brain injury—injury to the brain and its associated structures that results instantaneously from impact to the head. Conversely, secondary brain injury refers to injury from processes that may occur after the primary injury

3. What would you expect this patient's vital signs to be?

Vital sign findings will vary tremendously from patient to patient. However, signs of increased ICP will result in hypertension, bradycardia, and abnormal respirations. A patient with neurogenic shock will present with hypotension and normal to slow respirations and pulses. Skin will be dry and temperature will be based on the surrounding environment. If you suspect head injury, obtain multiple sets of vital signs to assist in recognizing an increase in ICP.

4. What are the signs and symptoms of a basilar skull fracture?

Signs of a basilar skull fracture include CSF drainage from the ears, which indicates rupture of the tympanic membrane and freely flowing CSF through the ear. Other signs of a basilar skull fracture include raccoon eyes or Battle sign. Depending on the extent of the damage, raccoon eyes and Battle sign may appear relatively quickly, but in many patients, they may not appear until up to 24 hours following the injury, so their absence in the field does not rule out a basilar skull fracture.

5. On the basis of your examination findings, what degree of elevated ICP does he have?

This patient is presenting with mildly elevated ICP. Mild elevation is characterized by an increase in blood pressure, decreased pulse rate, and abnormal respirations. The key finding in mild elevation is reactive pupils. Once you can recognize pupillary changes, the increased pressure has moved out of the mild category and into the moderate or severe category.

6. If this patient was unable to maintain his airway, at what rate would you initially ventilate using a bag-mask device?

Patients with cerebral edema should be ventilated at a rate of 10 breaths/min or as determined by local protocols. Hyperventilating a patient may cause vasoconstriction, further reducing oxygenation of the brain. However, if the patient exhibits late signs of increased ICP (the Cushing triad, unequal or nonreactive pupil, coma, or posturing), ventilate on the high side of a normal rate (12 to 15 breaths/min). Follow local protocols and your medical direction regarding hyperventilation in the presence of evidence of herniation.

7. At what point should you start hyperventilating the patient with a head injury?

Start hyperventilating the patient when he presents with signs of cerebral herniation. This includes unresponsiveness, the Cushing triad, unequal or nonreactive pupil, and/or posturing.

8. What is the appropriate hospital for this patient?

Many patients with severe brain injuries and increased ICP require neurosurgical intervention. The extra time it takes to move the patient from one hospital to another could mean the difference between life and death. Therefore, consider transporting the patient directly to a trauma center that has neurosurgical capabilities if it will decrease the time to surgical intervention, even if it means bypassing the nearest hospital, always taking into consideration your local protocols.

YOU are the Provider SUMMARY *(continued)*

EMS Patient Care Report (PCR)					
Date: 8-18-18	**Incident No.:** 15871	**Nature of Call:** Trauma	**Location:** YMCA Pool on Logan Ave		
Dispatched: 1325	**En Route:** 1326	**At Scene:** 1334	**Transport:** 1347	**At Hospital:** 1410	**In Service:** 1440

Patient Information	
Age: 27 **Sex:** M **Weight (in kg [lb]):** 100 kg (220 lb)	**Allergies:** No known drug allergies **Medications:** None **Past Medical History:** None **Chief Complaint:** Possible head injury

Vital Signs				
Time: 1335	**BP:** Not obtained	**Pulse:** Not obtained	**Respirations:** 30	**Spo_2:** Not obtained
Time: 1343	**BP:** 216/148	**Pulse:** 42	**Respirations:** 26	**Spo_2:** 99% on 15 L/min
Time: 1348	**BP:** 214/142	**Pulse:** 42	**Respirations:** 12 (assisted)	**Spo_2:** 99% on 15 L/min
Time: 1353	**BP:** 210/144	**Pulse:** 44	**Respirations:** 10 (assisted)	**Spo_2:** 100% on 15 L/min

EMS Treatment (circle all that apply)				
Oxygen @ 15 **L/min via (circle one):** **NC** **(NRM)** **(Bag-mask device)**		**(Assisted Ventilation:** Yes**)**	**(Airway Adjunct:** OPA**)**	**CPR**
Defibrillation	**Bleeding Control**	**Bandaging**	**Splinting**	**Other:**

Narrative
EMS dispatched to the YMCA pool for possible spinal injury. On arrival, patient found alongside of pool with lifeguards in attendance. Senior lifeguard states that patient was running alongside the pool when he slipped and fell into the pool headfirst, striking his head on the bottom. Lifeguards immediately placed the patient onto floating backboard and extricated him from the pool. They state he has been "in and out" of consciousness since the incident. Patient found AO×4, ABCs intact. Patient states that he cannot feel his arms or legs. Manual stabilization established. Physical examination reveals approximately 2-inch hematoma on posterior scalp, also noted to have no motor or sensation to bilateral arms or legs, but pulses are present. Placed patient on 15 L/min via nonrebreathing mask, cervical collar applied, and patient secured to backboard. Initial vitals as above, noted to have signs and symptoms indicative of increased ICP. GCS calculated to be 10 (alert [4], oriented [5], no motor function [1]). 18-gauge IV established to right forearm with NS TKO. Emergent transport initiated to St. Luke's trauma center ED. Approximately 6 minutes into transport, patient became unresponsive with episodes of apnea. Inserted OPA and began initial ventilations at 10 breaths/min. GCS recalculated to be 3 (unresponsive [1], no verbal [1] or motor [1] function). Report called to ED with condition and ETA. ED reports they do not have neurosurgeon today and to divert to Mercy Hospital trauma center. Divert acknowledged, with report given to Mercy trauma center ED. On arrival, care and report given to staff without incident.**End of report**

Prep Kit

▶ Ready for Review

- Important anatomic structures in the head and spine include the scalp; the skull, which includes the cranium and the face; the spinal column and its vertebrae; the brain; and the meninges.
- The brainstem houses many structures that are critical to the maintenance of vital functions, such as heart rate, blood pressure, and respiration. Damage to this area can easily result in cardiovascular derangement, respiratory arrest, or death.
- The nervous system is divided into two parts: the central nervous system and the peripheral nervous system.
- The central nervous system consists of the brain and the spinal cord. The cables of nerve fibers linking nerve cells in the brain and spinal cord to the body's organs make up the peripheral nervous system.
- The peripheral nervous system consists of spinal nerves, which conduct sensory impulses from the skin and other organs to the spinal cord and conduct motor impulses from the spinal cord to the muscles, and cranial nerves, which transmit sensations relating to sight, smell, taste, and hearing directly to the brain.
- The part of the nervous system that regulates our voluntary activities is called the somatic or voluntary nervous system.
- The much more primitive autonomic or involuntary nervous system regulates involuntary body functions. The autonomic nervous system is composed of the sympathetic and parasympathetic nervous systems, which balance each other.
- Common head injuries include skull wounds (scalp lacerations and skull fracture) and brain injuries (concussion, contusion, intracranial bleeding), typically caused by direct blows, motor vehicle crashes, falls from heights, assault, and sports injuries.
- Signs and symptoms of head injuries include lacerations, visible deformities of the skull, ecchymosis around the eyes or behind the ear, unequal pupil size and failure of the pupils to respond to light, loss of sensation and/or motor function, visual disturbances, irregular respirations, and posturing, among others.
- Types of skull fractures include linear, depressed, basilar, and open.
- Traumatic brain injuries are capable of producing physical, intellectual, emotional, social, and vocational changes. They may be classified as primary or secondary.
- Cerebral edema, seizures, vomiting, and leakage of cerebrospinal fluid are common complications of open and closed head injuries.
- Bleeding inside the skull increases intracranial pressure (ICP), the pressure within the cranial vault. In the field, the severity of increased ICP can be estimated based on the patient's clinical presentation. Prehospital treatment must focus on maintaining cerebral perfusion pressure while mitigating increased ICP as much as possible.
- If increased ICP is not promptly treated in a definitive care setting, cerebral herniation may occur, in which the brain is forced from the cranial vault.
- Early signs and symptoms of increased ICP include vomiting, headache, altered level of consciousness, and seizures. Later ominous signs include the Cushing triad plus a unilaterally unequal and nonreactive pupil, coma, and decorticate or decerebrate posturing.
- Bleeding in the brain can take the form of an epidural hematoma, subdural hematoma, intracerebral hematoma, or subarachnoid hemorrhage, depending on where the bleeding is occurring.
- A blow to the head or face may cause a concussion of the brain. A concussion injury results in cerebral dysfunction that usually resolves spontaneously and rapidly without demonstrable physical damage to the brain or permanent neurologic impairment. Signs of a concussion include confusion and disorientation. If there is any suspicion of concussion, the patient must desist from sports activity and be assessed by a physician.
- Diffuse axonal injury is a severe concussive injury to the brain resulting in physical damage to nerve fibers.
- A cerebral contusion is a bruise of brain tissue. As with any bruise, swelling will occur, which results in increased ICP.

Prep Kit *(continued)*

- Spinal injuries are categorized as primary spinal cord injury and secondary spinal cord injury. Mechanisms include flexion, rotation with flexion, vertical compression, distraction, and hyperextension. Distracting injury (different than distraction) is an important concept; an injury that causes substantial pain may distract the patient to the point that he or she does not report signs or symptoms of spinal column injury.
- Patients with head injuries often have injuries to the cervical spine as well. Therefore, when treating a patient with a head injury, you must protect and stabilize the cervical spine at all times.
- Patient assessment begins with an awareness of high-risk mechanisms that strongly suggest spine injury. If you suspect a spinal injury, keep the head in a neutral, in-line position throughout your assessment and treatment, and follow local protocols regarding further spinal immobilization procedures.
- As always, focus on addressing airway, breathing, and circulation; it is also important to prevent aspiration.
- Closely monitor the patient's oxygen saturation level and maintain it at 95% or higher. Cerebral edema and ICP are aggravated by hypoxia and hypercapnia. Ventilate a brain-injured adult at a rate of 10 to 12 breaths/min or as determined by local protocols.
- A single episode of hypoperfusion in a patient with a head injury can result in substantial brain damage and even death. Assess for signs and symptoms of shock and treat appropriately. Volume resuscitation may be necessary.
- Perform baseline and frequent reassessments of the patient's level of consciousness using the GCS or another such tool and document all values. These measurements are important to determine the patient's clinical progression.
- Prompt transport to a definitive care facility (ie, a trauma center) is crucial to the survival of a brain-injured patient.
- Cervical collars provide preliminary, partial immobilization of the spine. A patient who is supine can be further stabilized with a long backboard. Alternative methods include use of a scoop stretcher or a vacuum mattress.
- With sitting patients, you should use a short immobilization device, then secure the short device to a long board.
- A helmet that fits well prevents the patient's head from moving and should be left on, as long as it does not interfere with assessment and treatment of airway or ventilation problems and you can properly immobilize the spine. Remove a helmet if it makes assessing or managing airway problems difficult, prevents you from immobilizing the spine, or allows excessive head movement.
- Never remove a helmet if doing so will further injure the patient. Always remove a helmet if the patient is in cardiac arrest.
- Back pain is a common presenting ailment. Obtain the patient's history and perform a physical exam. Any patient with a suspected nontraumatic spinal disorder should undergo a neurologic evaluation.

▶ Vital Vocabulary

anterograde (posttraumatic) amnesia Inability to remember events after an injury.

arachnoid The middle membrane of the three meninges that enclose the brain and spinal cord.

autonomic nervous system The part of the nervous system that regulates functions that are not controlled consciously, but rather involuntarily, such as digestion and sweating.

autoregulation An increase in mean arterial pressure to compensate for decreased cerebral perfusion pressure; a compensatory physiologic response that occurs in an effort to shunt blood to the brain; manifests clinically as hypertension.

axon A long, slender extension of a neuron (nerve cell) that conducts electrical impulses away from the neuronal soma.

Prep Kit *(continued)*

basal ganglia Structures located deep within the cerebrum, diencephalon, and midbrain that have an important role in coordination of motor movements and posture.

basilar skull fracture Usually occurs following diffuse impact to the head (such as falls, motor vehicle crashes); generally results from extension of a linear fracture to the base of the skull and can be difficult to diagnose with a radiograph (x-ray imaging).

Battle sign Bruising behind an ear over the mastoid process that may indicate a skull fracture.

Biot respirations Characterized by an irregular rate, pattern, and volume of breathing with intermittent periods of apnea; also called ataxic respirations.

brainstem The part of the central nervous system that controls virtually all functions that are necessary for life, including the cardiac and respiratory systems.

cauda equina The location where the spinal cord separates; composed of nerve roots.

central nervous system (CNS) The brain and spinal cord.

central neurogenic hyperventilation Deep, rapid respirations; similar to Kussmaul, but without an acetone breath odor; commonly seen following brainstem injury.

cerebellum The part of the brain that coordinates body movements.

cerebral contusion A focal brain injury in which brain tissue is bruised and damaged in a defined area.

cerebral cortex The largest portion of the cerebrum; regulates voluntary skeletal movement and a person's level of awareness—a part of consciousness.

cerebral edema Swelling of the brain.

cerebral perfusion pressure (CPP) The pressure of blood flow through the brain; the difference between the mean arterial pressure (MAP) and intracranial pressure (ICP).

cerebrospinal fluid (CSF) Fluid produced in the ventricles of the brain that flows in the subarachnoid space and bathes the meninges.

cerebrum The largest part of the brain, comprising about 75% of the brain's total size.

Cheyne-Stokes respirations The respirations that are fast and then become slow, with intervening periods of apnea; commonly seen following brainstem injury.

closed head injury An injury in which the brain has been injured but the skin has not been broken and there is no bleeding.

concussion A temporary loss or alteration of part or all of the brain's abilities to function without actual physical damage to the brain.

connecting nerves The nerves in the brain and spinal cord that connect the motor and sensory nerves.

coup-contrecoup injury Dual impacting of the brain into the skull; coup injury occurs at the point of impact; contrecoup injury occurs on the opposite side of impact, as the brain rebounds.

Cushing triad Hypertension (with a widening pulse pressure), bradycardia, and irregular respirations; classic trio of findings associated with increased intracranial pressure.

decerebrate (extensor) posturing A posture characterized by extension of the arms and legs; indicates pressure on the brainstem and may appear in patients with severe brain trauma.

decorticate (flexor) posturing A posture characterized by flexion of the arms and extension of the legs; indicates pressure on the brainstem and may appear in patients with severe brain trauma.

depressed skull fracture A type of skull fracture that results from high-energy direct trauma to a small surface area of the head with a blunt object (such as a baseball bat to the head); commonly results in bony fragments being driven into the brain, causing injury.

diffuse axonal injury (DAI) Diffuse brain injury that is caused by stretching, shearing, or tearing of nerve fibers with subsequent axonal damage.

diffuse brain injury Any injury that affects the entire brain.

distraction The action of pulling the spine along its length.

Prep Kit *(continued)*

dura mater The outermost layer of the three meninges that enclose the brain and spinal cord; the toughest meningeal layer.

epidural hematoma An accumulation of blood between the skull and the dura mater.

flexion injuries A type of injury that results from forward movement of the head, typically as the result of rapid deceleration, such as in a motor vehicle crash, or with a direct blow to the occiput.

focal brain injury A specific, grossly observable brain injury.

four-person log roll The recommended procedure for moving a patient with a suspected spinal injury from the ground to a long backboard.

frontal lobe The portion of the brain that is important in voluntary motor actions and personality traits.

Glasgow Coma Scale (GCS) A method of evaluating the level of consciousness that uses a scoring system for neurologic responses to specific stimuli.

hangman's fracture The most classic distraction injury, which occurs when a person is hanged by the neck. Bending and fractures occur at the C1-C2 region, which quickly tear the spinal cord.

head injury A traumatic insult to the head that may result in injury to soft tissue of the scalp and bony structures of the head and skull, not including the face.

head trauma A general term that includes both head injuries and traumatic brain injuries.

herniation A process in which tissue is forced out of its normal position, such as when the brain is forced from the cranial vault, either through the foramen magnum or over the tentorium.

hyperextension Extension of a limb or other body part beyond its usual range of motion.

hyperpyrexia A high body temperature.

intervertebral disks The cushions that lie between the vertebrae.

intracerebral hematoma Bleeding within the brain tissue (parenchyma) itself; also referred to as an intraparenchymal hematoma.

intracranial pressure (ICP) The pressure within the cranial vault.

involuntary activities Actions of the body that are not under a person's conscious control.

linear skull fracture A type of skull fracture that commonly occurs in the temporal-parietal region of the skull; not associated with deformities to the skull; also referred to as a nondisplaced skull fracture.

mean arterial pressure (MAP) The average (or mean) pressure against the arterial wall during a cardiac cycle.

medulla Continuous inferiorly with the spinal cord; serves as a conduction pathway for ascending and descending nerve tracts; coordinates heart rate, blood vessel diameter, breathing, swallowing, vomiting, coughing, and sneezing.

meninges Three distinct layers of tissue that surround and protect the brain and the spinal cord within the skull and the spinal canal.

motor nerves The nerves that carry information from the central nervous system to the muscles.

nerve root injury Injury to a nerve at the level of the spinal cord.

neurogenic shock Circulatory failure caused by paralysis of the nerves that control the size of the blood vessels, resulting in widespread dilation; seen in spinal cord injuries.

neuronal soma The body of a neuron (nerve cell).

occipital lobe The portion of the brain that is responsible for the processing of visual information.

open head injury An injury to the head often caused by a penetrating object in which there may be bleeding and exposed brain tissue.

parasympathetic nervous system Subdivision of the autonomic nervous system; involved in control of involuntary, vegetative functions; mediated largely by the vagus nerve through the chemical acetylcholine.

parietal lobe The portion of the brain that is the site for reception and evaluation of most sensory information, except smell, hearing, and vision.

Prep Kit *(continued)*

peripheral nerve injury Injury to a nerve anywhere in the body outside the spinal cord.

peripheral nervous system The 31 pairs of spinal nerves and 12 pairs of cranial nerves that link the body's other organs to the central nervous system.

petechial hemorrhage A pinpoint red dot in the sclera of the eye.

pia mater The innermost and thinnest of the three meninges that enclose the brain and spinal cord; rests directly on the brain and spinal cord.

pons Lies below the midbrain and above the medulla and contains numerous important nerve fibers, including those for sleep, respiration, and the medullary respiratory center.

primary brain injury An injury to the brain and its associated structures that is a direct result of impact to the head.

primary spinal cord injury Injury to the spinal cord that is a direct result of trauma, for example transection of the spinal cord from penetrating trauma or displacement of ligaments and bone fragments, resulting in compression of the spinal cord.

raccoon eyes Bruising under the eyes that may indicate a skull fracture; also called periorbital ecchymosis.

reticular activating system (RAS) Located in the upper brainstem; responsible for maintenance of consciousness, specifically a person's level of arousal.

retrograde amnesia The inability to remember events leading up to a head injury.

rotation-flexion injuries A type of injury in which both rotation and flexion occur; typically resulting from high acceleration forces; can result in a stable unilateral facet dislocation in the cervical spine.

secondary brain injury The "after effects" of the primary injury; includes injuries caused by abnormal processes such as cerebral edema, increased intracranial pressure, cerebral ischemia and hypoxia, and infection; onset is often delayed following the primary brain injury.

secondary spinal cord injury Injury to the spinal cord, thought to be the result of multiple factors that result in a progression of inflammatory responses from primary spinal cord injury.

sensory nerves The nerves that transmit sensory input, such as touch, taste, heat, cold, and pain, from the body to the central nervous system.

somatic nervous system The part of the nervous system that regulates a person's voluntary activities, such as walking, talking, and writing.

spinal cord concussion An incomplete injury of the spinal cord in which temporary dysfunction lasts from 24 to 48 hours; may present in patients with simple compression fractures.

spinal cord contusion A bruise of the spinal cord characterized by edema, tissue damage, and vascular leakage, and caused by fracture, dislocation, or direct trauma.

spinal shock The temporary local neurologic condition that occurs immediately after spinal trauma; swelling and edema of the spinal cord begin immediately after injury, with severe pain and potential paralysis.

sprain Stretching or tearing of ligaments.

strain Stretching or tearing of muscle or tendon.

subarachnoid hemorrhage Bleeding into the subarachnoid space, where the cerebrospinal fluid circulates.

subdural hematoma An accumulation of blood beneath the dura mater but outside the brain.

subluxation A partial or incomplete dislocation.

sympathetic nervous system Subdivision of the autonomic nervous system that governs the body's fight-or-flight reactions by inducing smooth muscle contraction or relaxation of the blood vessels and bronchioles.

temporal lobe The portion of the brain that has an important role in hearing and memory.

tentorium A structure that separates the cerebral hemispheres from the cerebellum and brainstem.

traumatic brain injury (TBI) A traumatic insult to the brain capable of producing physical, intellectual, emotional, social, and vocational changes.

vertebral body Anterior weight-bearing structure in the spine made of cancellous bone and surrounded by a layer of hard, compact bone that provides support and stability.

vertical compression A type of injury typically resulting from a direct blow to the crown of the skull or rapid deceleration from a fall through the feet, legs, and pelvis, possibly causing a burst fracture or disk herniation.

voluntary activities The actions that we consciously perform, in which sensory input determines the specific muscular activity.

Prep Kit *(continued)*

▶ References

1. Rates of TBI-related emergency department visits, hospitalizations, and deaths—United States, 2001–2010. Centers for Disease Control and Prevention website. https://www.cdc.gov/traumaticbraininjury/data/rates.html. Updated January 22, 2016. Accessed March 21, 2017.
2. Traumatic brain injury and concussion. TBI: get the facts. Centers for Disease Control and Prevention website. http://www.cdc.gov/traumaticbraininjury/get_the_facts.html. Updated March 23, 2017. Accessed October 23, 2017.
3. Traumatic Brain Injury & Concussion. Centers for Disease Control and Prevention website. https://www.cdc.gov/traumaticbraininjury/. Updated July 6, 2017. Accessed October 23, 2017.
4. Turnage B, Maull K. Scalp laceration: an obvious 'occult' cause of shock. *South Med J*. 2000;93(3): 265-266.
5. Qureshi N, Harsh I, Nosko M. Skull fracture: background. Medscape website. http://emedicine.medscape.com/article/248108. Updated May 26, 2016. Accessed May 3, 2016.
6. Arabi YM, Haddad SH. Critical care management of severe traumatic brain injury in adults. *Scand J Trauma Resusc Emerg Med*. 2012;20(12).
7. Bir S, Maiti T, Ambekar S, Nanda A. Incidence, hospital costs and in-hospital mortality rates of epidural hematoma in the United States. *Clin Neurol Neurosurg*. 2015;138:99-103.
8. Smith S, Clark M, Nelson J, Heegaard W, Lufkin K, Ruiz E. Emergency department skull trephination for epidural hematoma in patients who are awake but deteriorate rapidly. *J Emerg Med*. 2010;39(3): 377-383.
9. Ducruet A, Grobelny B, Zacharia B, et al. The surgical management of chronic subdural hematoma. *Neurosurg Rev*. 2011;35(2):155-169.
10. Nayil K, Ramzan A, Sajad A, et al. Subdural hematomas: an analysis of 1181 Kashmiri patients. *World Neurosurg*. 2012;77(1):103-110.
11. Agostoni E, Zagaria M, Longoni M. Headache in subarachnoid hemorrhage and headache attributed to intracranial endovascular procedures. *Neurolog Sci*. 2015;36(suppl 1):67-70.
12. Hankey G, Nelson M. Subarachnoid haemorrhage. *Brit Med J*. 2009;339:b2874-b2874.
13. McCrory P, Meeuwisse W, Dvorak J, et al. Consensus statement on concussion in sport—the 5th international conference on concussion in sport held in Berlin, October 2016. BMJ Journals website. http://bjsm.bmj.com/content/early/2017/04/26/bjsports-2017-097699. Accessed May 23, 2017.
14. Giza C, Kutcher J, Ashwal S, et al. Summary of evidence-based guideline update: evaluation and management of concussion in sports: Report of the Guideline Development Subcommittee of the American Academy of Neurology. *Neurology*. 2013;80(24):2250-2257.
15. HEADS UP: managing return to activities. Centers for Disease Control and Prevention website. http://www.cdc.gov/headsup/providers/return_to_activities.html. Updated February 8, 2016. Accessed March 27, 2017.
16. National Federation of State High School Associations (NFHS) Sports Medicine Advisory Committee (SMAC). *Suggested Guidelines for Management of Concussion in Sports*. NFHS website https://www.nfhs.org/sports-resource-content/suggested-guidelines-for-management-of-concussion-in-sports/. February 16, 2017. Accessed March 27, 2017.
17. Johnson V, Stewart W, Smith D. Axonal pathology in traumatic brain injury. *Exp Neurol*. 2013;246:35-43.
18. Popa C, Popa F, Grigorean V, et al. Vascular dysfunctions following spinal cord injury. *J Med Life*. 2010;3(3):275-285.
19. Centers for Disease Control and Prevention. Guidelines for field triage of injured patients: recommendations of the National Expert Panel on Field Triage, 2011. *MMWR*. 2012;61(1).
20. Borius PY, Gouader I, Bousquet P, Draper L, Roux FE. Cervical spine injuries resulting from diving accidents in swimming pools: outcome of 34 patients. *Eur Spine J*. 2010;19(4):552-557.
21. Wood G, Boucher B. *PSAP-VII—Neurology and Psychiatry: Management of Acute Traumatic Brain Injury*. 7th ed. Book 10. Lenexa, KS: American College of Clinical Pharmacy; 2012.
22. Bullock R, Povlishock J. Guidelines for the management of severe traumatic brain injury. 3rd ed. *J Neurotrauma*. 2016;23(suppl 1):S1-S106.
23. Carney N, Totten AM, O'Reilly C, et al. Guidelines for the management of severe traumatic brain injury, fourth edition. *Neurosurgery*. 2016;20:1-10.

Prep Kit *(continued)*

24. Alvis-Miranda HR, Castellar-Leones SM, Moscote-Salazar LR. Intravenous fluid therapy in traumatic brain injury and decompressive craniectomy. *Bull Emerg Trauma.* 2014;2(1):3-14.
25. Brain Trauma Foundation. *Guidelines for the Management of Severe Traumatic Brain Injury.* Brain Trauma Foundation website. https://braintrauma.org/uploads/03/12/Guidelines_for_Management_of_Severe_TBI_4th_Edition.pdf. Published September 2016. Accessed March 24, 2017.
26. De Lorenzo R. A review of spinal immobilization techniques. *J Emerg Med.* 1996;14(5):603-613.
27. Cooney DR, Wallus H, Asaly M, Wojcik S. Backboard time for patients receiving spinal immobilization by emergency medical services. *Int J Emerg Med.* 2013;6:17.
28. De Lorenzo R, Olson J, Boska M. Optimal positioning for cervical immobilization. *Ann Emerg Med.* 1996;28(3):301-308.
29. Kwan I, Bunn F. Effects of prehospital spinal immobilization: a systematic review of randomized trials on healthy subjects. *Prehosp Disast Med.* 2005;20(1):47-53.
30. Sundstrøm T, Asbjørnsen H, Habiba S, Sunde GA, Wester K. Prehospital use of cervical collars in trauma patients: a critical review. *J Neurotrauma.* 2014;31(6):531-540.
31. Blackwell TH. Prehospital care. *Emerg Med Clin North Am.* 1993;11(1):1-14.
32. Hauswald M. A re-conceptualisation of acute spinal care. *Emerg Med J.* 2013;30(9):720-723.
33. White CC 4th, Domeier RM, Millin MG. Standards and Clinical Practice Committee, National Association of EMS Physicians. EMS spinal precautions and the use of the long backboard—resource document to the position statement of the National Association of EMS Physicians and the American College of Surgeons Committee on Trauma. *Prehosp Emerg Care.* 2014;18(2):306-314.
34. Barney RN, Cordell WH, Miller E. Pain associated with immobilization on rigid spine boards. *Ann Emerg Med.* 1989;18:918.
35. Lerner EB, Billittier AJ 4th, Moscati RM. The effects of neutral positioning with and without padding on spinal immobilization of healthy subjects. *Prehosp Emerg Care.* 1998;2:112-116.
36. Sheerin F, de Frein R. The occipital and sacral pressures experienced by healthy volunteers under spinal immobilization: a trial of three surfaces. *J Emerg Nurs.* 2007;33(5):447-450.
37. Jia X, Kowalski RG, Sciubba DM, Geocadin RG. Critical care of traumatic spinal cord injury. *J Intensive Care Med.* 2013;28(1):12-23.
38. Geisler WO, Wynne-Jones M, Jousse AT. Early management of the patient with trauma to the spinal cord. *Med Serv J Can.* 1966;4:512-523.

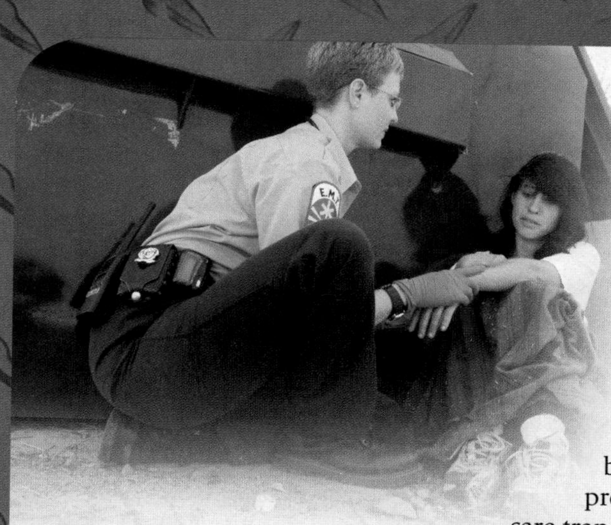

Assessment in Action

Your ambulance is dispatched to the local ED for an emergent interfacility transfer of a 71-year-old woman who slipped and fell in her house. The transferring physician has diagnosed an epidural hematoma requiring surgical evacuation. The patient is able to maintain her own airway, but has evidence of some decorticate posturing and blood pressure is increasing. You will be transporting with a critical care transport nurse.

1. An epidural hematoma is an accumulation of blood:

A. beneath the dura mater but outside the brain.
B. between the skull and the dura mater.
C. within the brain tissue itself.
D. compressing the brainstem.

2. As intracranial pressure increases, the pupil on the _____ side of her head that has the hematoma will most likely become fixed and dilated.

A. same
B. opposite
C. contralateral
D. Not applicable; differs among patients

3. With the intracranial pressure increasing, the patient is exhibiting signs of the Cushing triad. All of the following are components EXCEPT:

A. decreasing pulse.
B. irregular respirations.
C. increasing pulse.
D. increasing blood pressure.

4. The brainstem connects the spinal cord to the rest of the brain. Which of the following structures is NOT a part of the brainstem?

A. Midbrain
B. Pons
C. Medulla
D. Cerebellum

5. Which of the following structures produces cerebrospinal fluid?

A. Arachnoid and pia mater
B. Pia mater and brainstem
C. Dura mater and arachnoid
D. Dura mater and pia mater

6. In what position should this patient be transported?

A. Completely supine
B. Fully immobilized on a backboard
C. Sitting upright at a 90° angle
D. Supine with the head elevated 30°

7. Cerebral perfusion pressure is calculated by which of the following equations?

A. CPP = MAP – ICP
B. CPP = MAP + ICP
C. CPP = MAP × ICP
D. CPP = MAP/ICP

8. Patients with a TBI and increased ICP should be given fluid boluses of an isotonic crystalloid solution to maintain a systolic blood pressure of at least _____ mm Hg.

A. 80
B. 90
C. 100
D. 110

9. Explain the BTF's "90-90-9 rule."

10. When assessing a patient for possible shaken baby syndrome, the infant may present with petechial hemorrhages. Explain what these are and what they represent.

CHAPTER 31

Chest Injuries

National EMS Education Standard Competencies

Trauma

Applies fundamental knowledge to provide basic and selected advanced emergency care and transportation based on assessment findings for an acutely injured patient.

Chest Trauma

Recognition and management of

- Blunt versus penetrating mechanisms (pp 1259-1260, 1262, 1265-1279)
- Open chest wound (pp 1259, 1262, 1265-1276, 1278-1279)
- Impaled object (p 1262)

Pathophysiology, assessment, and management of

- Blunt versus penetrating mechanisms (pp 1259-1279)
- Hemothorax (pp 1273-1274)
- Pneumothorax (pp 1269-1273)
  - Open (pp 1270-1271)
  - Simple (pp 1269-1270)
  - Tension (pp 1272-1273)
- Cardiac tamponade (pp 1274-1276)
- Rib fractures (pp 1266-1267)
- Flail chest (pp 1267-1268)
- Commotio cordis (pp 1268-1269)
- Traumatic aortic disruption (pp 1277-1278)
- Pulmonary contusion (p 1274)
- Blunt cardiac injury (pp 1276-1277)
- Traumatic asphyxia (p 1279)

Knowledge Objectives

1. Review the anatomy and physiology of the thorax. (pp 1255-1258)
2. Understand the mechanics of ventilation in relation to chest injuries. (pp 1257-1258)
3. Discuss specific chest injuries, including closed versus open chest injury, blunt versus penetrating trauma, and effects on cardiac output, respiration, and ventilation. (pp 1259-1260)
4. Differentiate between a pneumothorax (open, simple, and tension) and a hemothorax. (pp 1260, 1262)
5. List general signs and symptoms of a chest injury. (pp 1260-1261)
6. Discuss the significance of various signs and symptoms of chest injury, including changes in heart rate, dyspnea, jugular vein distention, muffled heart sounds, changes in blood pressure, diaphoresis or changes in pallor, hemoptysis, and changes in mental status. (pp 1260-1263)
7. Explain the assessment process for a patient with a chest injury. (pp 1261-1265)
8. Explain the general management of a patient with a chest injury. (pp 1265-1266)
9. Explain the assessment and management of chest wall injuries, including rib fractures, flail chest, sternal fracture, clavicle fracture, and commotio cordis. (pp 1266-1269)
10. Describe the complications of rib fractures. (p 1266)
11. Describe the complications of flail chest. (p 1268)
12. Explain the assessment and management of lung injuries, including simple pneumothorax, open pneumothorax, tension pneumothorax, hemothorax, and pulmonary contusion. (pp 1269-1274)
13. Explain the complications associated with an open pneumothorax (sucking chest wound). (p 1271)
14. Explain the assessment and management of myocardial injuries, including cardiac tamponade, myocardial contusion, and myocardial rupture. (pp 1274-1277)
15. Describe the complications of cardiac tamponade. (p 1276)
16. Explain the assessment and management of vascular injuries, including traumatic aortic disruption and penetrating wounds of the great vessels. (pp 1277-1278)
17. Explain the assessment and management of other thoracic injuries, including diaphragmatic injury, esophageal injury, tracheobronchial injuries, and traumatic asphyxia. (pp 1278-1279)

Skills Objectives

1. Describe the steps to take in the assessment of a patient with a suspected chest injury. (pp 1261-1265)
2. Demonstrate the management of a patient with a sucking chest wound. (p 1271)
3. Demonstrate the management of a patient with a flail chest. (p 1268)

Courtesy of Heart Sync.

Introduction

Thoracic injuries are very common and—given the likelihood of damage to the heart, lungs, or great blood vessels—potentially very serious. Any injury that interferes with normal breathing must be treated without delay to prevent permanent damage to tissues that depend on a continuous supply of oxygen. Another major problem with chest injuries may be internal bleeding. Blood from lacerations of the thoracic organs or major blood vessels can collect in the chest cavity, compressing the lungs. Also, air can collect in the chest and prevent the lungs from expanding. As an advanced emergency medical technician (AEMT), your ability to act quickly to care for patients with these injuries can make the difference between survival and death. Prevention strategies include gun safety education, sports training, use of seat belts, and other protective measures.

Currently, thoracic trauma accounts for a significant number of serious injuries and fatalities each year. Thoracic trauma causes more than 18,000 deaths in the United States annually.[1] Only traumatic brain injuries account for more deaths among trauma victims. An estimated one in four trauma deaths is directly the result of thoracic injuries, and thoracic trauma is a contributing factor in another 25% of trauma patients who die of their injuries.[2] The mechanism producing these injuries often involves a great deal of force transmitted to the body, with motor vehicle crashes (MVCs) accounting for the majority of patients with blunt thoracic trauma.[3]

This chapter begins with a review of the anatomy of the chest and the physiology of respiration. It then describes the common signs and symptoms of thoracic injuries and the proper emergency medical treatment for specific injuries.

Anatomy and Physiology Review

▶ Anatomy Review

To understand and evaluate chest injuries in the prehospital setting, you must first understand the anatomy of the chest and the mechanism by which gases are exchanged during breathing. A quick review will help you to appreciate the logic in the emergency treatment of chest injuries and the potential complications of that treatment.

The thoracic cavity extends from the lower end of the neck to the diaphragm **Figure 31-1**. In a person who is lying down or who has just completed exhalation, the diaphragm may rise as high as the nipple line. Thus, a penetrating injury to the chest, such as a gunshot or stab wound, may also penetrate the lung and diaphragm and injure the liver or stomach. For this reason, any chest injury at or below the nipple line should be considered a thoracic injury and an abdominal injury.

The central region of the thorax is the **mediastinum**, which contains the heart, great vessels, esophagus, lymphatic channels, trachea, mainstem bronchi, and paired vagus and phrenic nerves. It encompasses all of the structures located in the center of the chest, excluding the lungs. The contents of the thorax are partially protected by the ribs, which are connected in the back to the 12 thoracic vertebrae and in the front, through the costal cartilages, to the sternum **Figure 31-2**. The muscles of

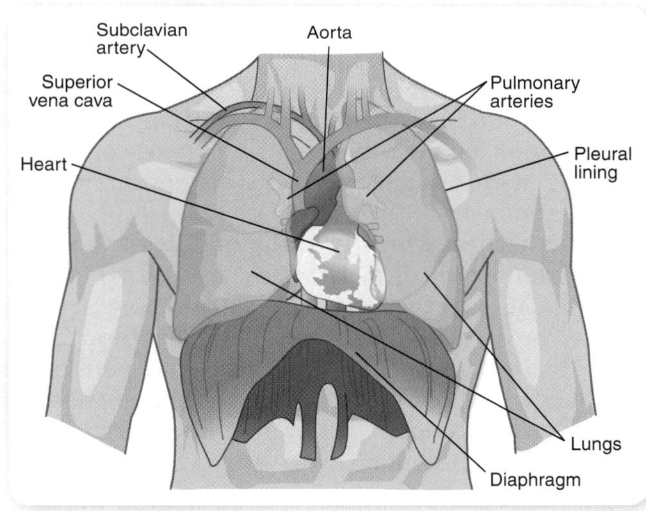

Figure 31-1 A view of the anterior aspect of the thoracic cage shows the major organs beneath the surface.

YOU are the Provider PART 1

While providing standby services to a local motocross track, you and your partner are summoned to the course for a man who landed improperly after making a large jump, crashing his dirt bike. As you and your partner are preparing to enter the track, you note another dirt bike rider coming down off of the jump, impacting your patient's chest with the front tire of his bike.

1. Should you immediately approach the patient? Is the scene safe?
2. What are some possible injuries this patient could have?

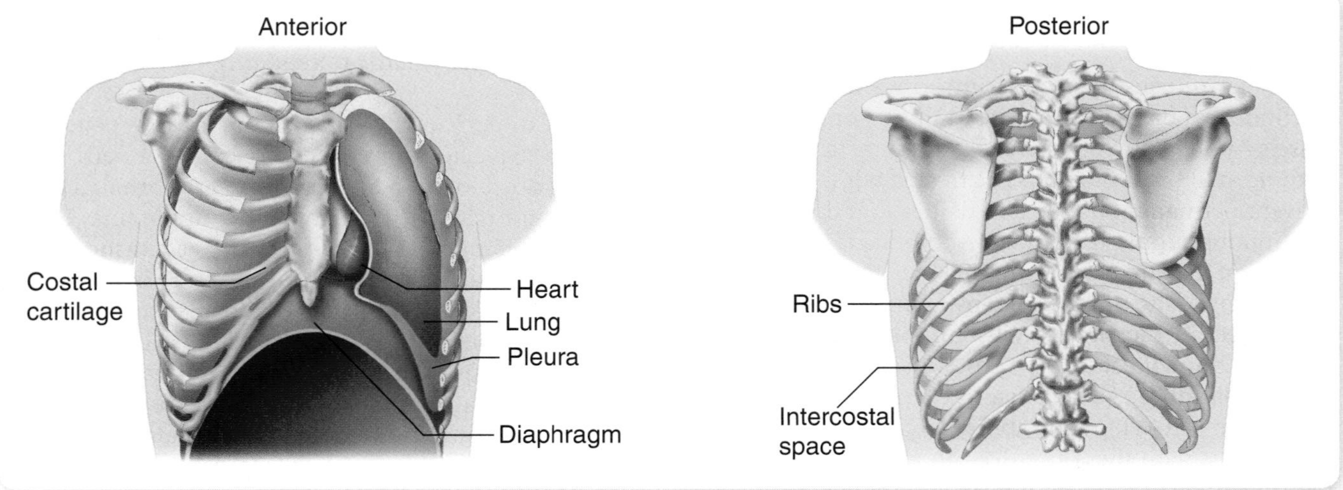

Figure 31-2 The organs within the thoracic cage are protected by the ribs, which are connected in back to the vertebrae and in the front, through the costal cartilage, to the sternum.

the thorax help protect the underlying organs and provide the necessary movement for breathing.

The intercostal muscles (located between the ribs) and the diaphragm are the primary muscles of respiration. The sternocleidomastoid muscles that provide support and movement in the neck are accessory muscles of respiration. The trapezius, rhomboids, and latissimus dorsi muscles provide the covering for the framework of the posterior thorax, and the pectoralis major surrounds the rib cage in the front.

The trachea, which is in the middle of the neck, divides at the carina (the last tracheal cartilage) into the left and right mainstem bronchi, which supply air to the lungs. The bronchi divide into the smaller bronchioles and, finally, terminate in the alveoli. The pulmonary capillaries surround the alveoli, creating an interface for gas exchange. The lungs occupy the entire thoracic cavity except the mediastinum.

The esophagus enters the thorax via the thoracic inlet and travels through the posterior of the chest, exiting through the esophageal foramen through the diaphragm. It connects the pharynx superiorly with the stomach and the abdomen. The diaphragm forms the inferior border of the thoracic cavity and the superior border of the abdominal cavity.

The nerves supplying the diaphragm (the phrenic nerves) exit the spinal cord at C3, C4, and C5. A patient whose spinal cord is injured at the C5 level or below may lose the ability to move his or her intercostal muscles, but the diaphragm will still contract. The patient will still be able to breathe because the phrenic nerves remain intact. Patients with spinal cord injuries at C3 or above can completely lose their ability to breathe spontaneously Figure 31-3.

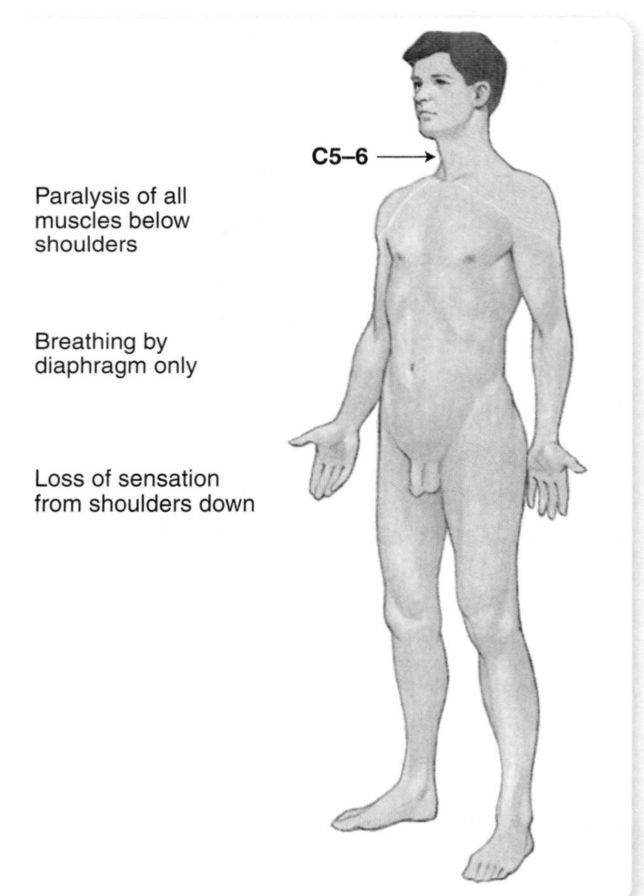

Figure 31-3 A patient who sustains a spinal cord injury at the level of C5 or below is paralyzed but can still breathe because the phrenic nerve, which controls the diaphragm, originates at the C3, C4, and C5 levels.

Words of Wisdom

Consider any injury below the nipple line to be an abdominal injury as well as a thoracic injury.

▶ Physiology Review

Ventilation occurs through expansion and contraction of the thoracic cage. Through a bellows system, the intercostal muscles between the ribs contract, elevating the rib cage and pulling the sternum forward on inhalation. At the same time, the diaphragm contracts and descends, pushing the contents of the abdomen down. The pressure inside the chest decreases, and air enters the lungs through the nose and mouth. Inspiration is an active process, whereas expiration is a passive process. On exhalation, the intercostal muscles and diaphragm relax, and the tissues move back to their normal positions. Air enters and leaves the lungs because of the changes in the intrathoracic pressure.

While *pulmonary respiration* is occurring, blood is being delivered via pulmonary circulation to the capillaries that lie adjacent to the alveoli. This blood has returned to the heart after traversing the body, delivering oxygen (O_2) to the cells, and removing cellular waste products such as carbon dioxide (CO_2). As a result, the blood entering the capillaries adjacent to the alveoli has a low O_2 concentration and a high CO_2 concentration.

The process of oxygenation includes the delivery of O_2 from the air to the blood, where it is carried to cells and tissues throughout the body. Because the air entering the alveoli contains a higher concentration of O_2 (ranging from 21% in room air to as much as 100% in a nonrebreathing mask or bag-mask device under ideal circumstances) than the blood in the nearby capillaries, the O_2 will follow its concentration gradient and enter the blood. Most of the O_2 binds to hemoglobin within the red blood cells, and the O_2 returns to the heart with the blood, where it is then pumped throughout the body.

The ability to pump blood depends on having a functional pump (the heart), an adequate volume of blood to be pumped, and a lack of resistance to the pumping mechanism (afterload)—properties that collectively determine the cardiac output. **Cardiac output** is defined as the volume of blood delivered to the body in 1 minute. It equals the heart rate (beats/min) multiplied by the stroke volume (milliliters of blood per beat). Any injury that limits the heart's pumping ability, the delivery of blood to the heart, the blood's ability to leave the heart, or the heart rate will affect cardiac output.

Ventilation is the process by which CO_2 is removed from the body. The air in the environment typically contains little CO_2 (0.033%). As a result, when air enters the alveoli, it contains little CO_2 compared with the blood in the nearby capillaries. The CO_2 diffuses down its concentration gradient, leaving the blood and entering the air within the alveoli.

As the diaphragm and the chest wall relax, positive pressure is created within the thorax. The air from which O_2 has been absorbed and into which CO_2 has been diffused is then exhaled. With each subsequent respiration (inhalation and exhalation), the process is repeated.

Even though the respiratory centers in the pons and medulla have a major role in regulating breathing, chemical changes are among the most important factors that influence the rate and depth of breathing. These chemical factors include changing levels of CO_2, O_2, and hydrogen ions in arterial blood. In respiratory physiology, **chemoreceptors** are sensors that respond to such chemical fluctuations and are located in two major body locations. Central chemoreceptors are found in the medulla, and peripheral chemoreceptors are located in the carotid and aortic bodies. Chemoreceptors closely monitor changes in CO_2 levels and stimulate breathing accordingly.

Rising levels of CO_2 are mediated mainly through influence on the central chemoreceptors of the brainstem. Carbon dioxide diffuses from the blood into the cerebrospinal fluid, where it is hydrated and forms carbonic acid. It then dissociates, freeing hydrogen and decreasing the pH of the cerebrospinal fluid. This excites the central chemoreceptors to increase the rate and depth of respirations.

$$\uparrow CO_2 + H_2O \leftrightarrow \uparrow H_2CO_3 \leftrightarrow \uparrow H^+ + HCO_3^-$$

(Increased levels of CO_2 combine with water to make carbonic acid. Carbonic acid is weak and easily dissociates, liberating hydrogen ions and decreasing the pH of the cerebrospinal fluid.)

Even though the increase in levels of CO_2 is the initial stimulus, it is the rising hydrogen ion levels that incite the central chemoreceptors into action in an attempt to maintain homeostasis by regulating hydrogen ion concentrations in the brain.

Respiratory alkalosis is the result of hyperventilation, regardless of the cause. As CO_2 levels fall, there is a reduction in circulating carbonic acid. Treatment for the classic hyperventilation syndrome focuses on restoring the normal respiratory rate to increase levels of carbon dioxide. If the hyperventilation is caused by a serious medical condition, then reducing the respiratory rate may seriously aggravate the problem **Figure 31-4**.

$$\uparrow \text{Breathing} = \downarrow CO_2 = \downarrow H_2CO_3 = \uparrow \text{pH}$$

Respiratory acidosis is always related to the body's inability to remove CO_2, and chest trauma is a common cause of respiratory acidosis. A buildup of CO_2 and the respiratory system's inability to excrete it cause the body to rely on the much slower renal system for compensation.

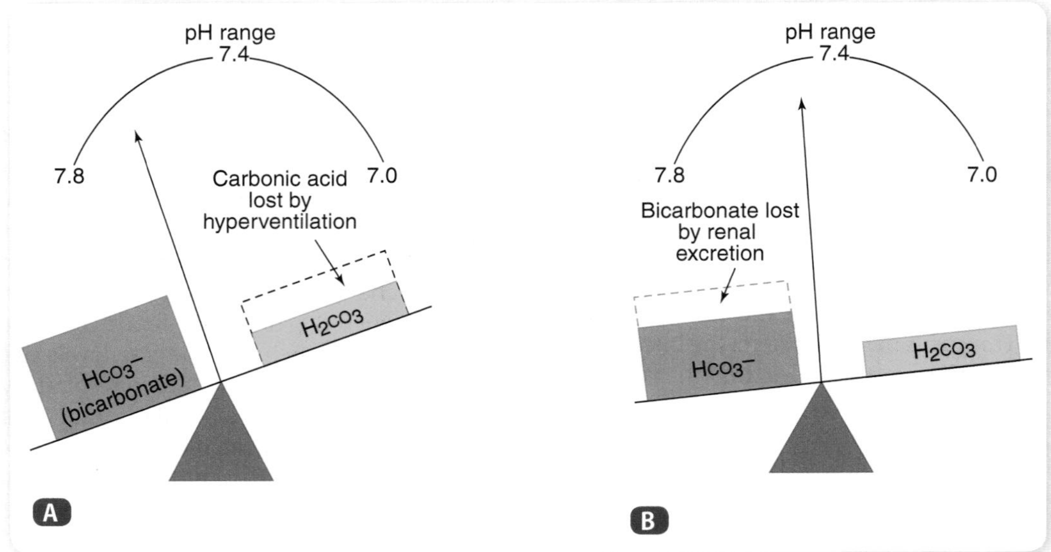

Figure 31-4 A. Derangement of acid-base balance in respiratory alkalosis. **B.** Compensation by excretion of bicarbonate.

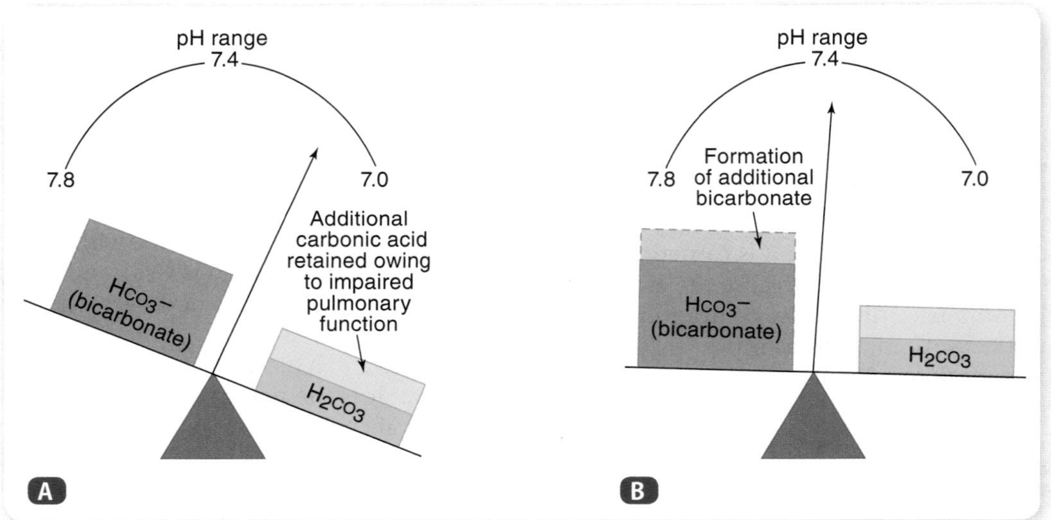

Figure 31-5 A. Derangement of acid-base balance in respiratory acidosis. **B.** Compensation by formation of additional bicarbonate.

The acidosis that results is quick, overwhelming, and usually fatal, making it impossible for the slower-acting renal system to compensate in time for the pH shift **Figure 31-5**.

$$\downarrow \text{Breathing} = \uparrow CO_2 = \uparrow H_2CO_3 = \downarrow \text{pH}$$

Changes in arterial pH can modify the respiratory rate and depth even when CO_2 and O_2 levels are normal. This occurs in metabolic imbalances. Because few hydrogen ions diffuse from the blood into the cerebrospinal fluid, there is little effect on central chemoreceptors. Ventilation changes occur in response to changes in pH detected by the peripheral chemoreceptors. A decrease in blood pH may be the result of CO_2 retention or a metabolic cause such as an increase in lactic acid. As the arterial pH falls, the respiratory system compensates by increasing the rate and depth of respirations in an attempt to eliminate CO_2 and, in turn, raise the pH level. The reverse occurs in metabolic alkalosis, in which the respiratory rate and depth decrease in an attempt to retain CO_2 and lower pH levels.

Pathophysiology

Mechanisms of injury (MOIs) in thoracic trauma can be separated into two general categories: blunt and penetrating. A thorough scene size-up will help you determine the forces involved.

Chest injuries can also be sorted into the categories of open and closed. As the name implies, a **closed chest injury** is one in which the skin overlying the injury remains intact. This type of injury is generally caused by blunt trauma, such as when a driver strikes a steering wheel in a MVC or is struck by a falling object **Figure 31-6**.

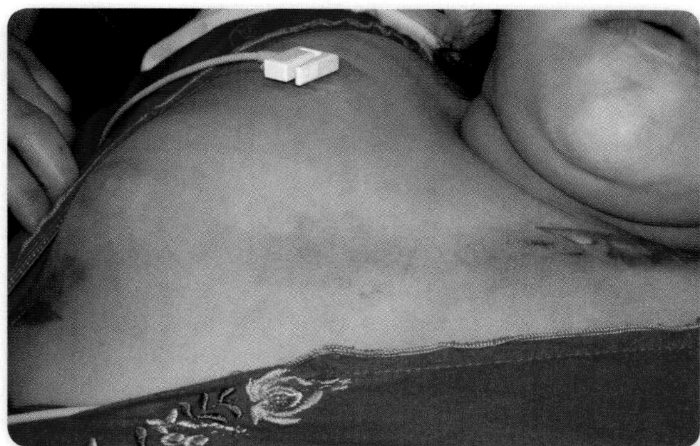

Figure 31-6 Closed injuries usually result from blunt trauma, such as when a patient strikes the steering wheel or an airbag in a motor vehicle crash or is struck by a falling object. A closed chest injury can even occur when a seat belt is worn.

The force is distributed over a large area. Visceral injuries occur from deceleration, shearing forces, compression, or rupture. In an **open chest injury**, the chest wall itself is penetrated by some object, such as a knife, a bullet, or a piece of metal **Figure 31-7**. Penetrating injuries often distribute the forces of injury over a smaller area; however, the trajectory of a bullet is often unpredictable and all thoracic structures are at risk.

In blunt trauma, a blow to the chest may fracture the ribs, the sternum, or whole areas of the chest wall; bruise the lungs and the heart; and even damage the aorta. In fact, traumatic rupture of the aorta is the second most common cause of death in MVCs, after head injury.[4] Although the skin and chest wall are not penetrated in a closed injury, broken ribs may lacerate the intrathoracic organs. Indeed,

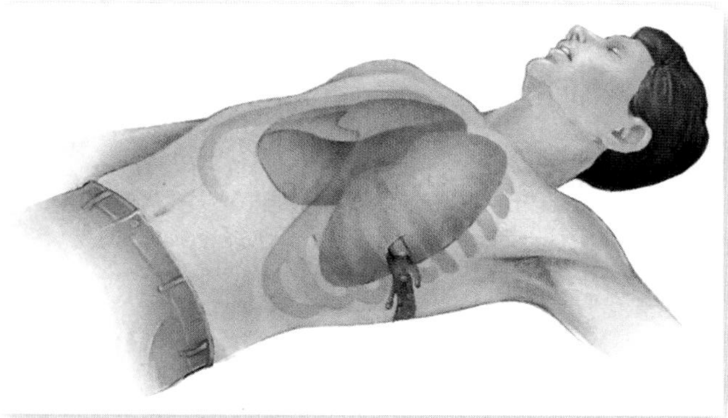

Figure 31-7 Open injuries occur when the chest wall is penetrated by some type of object.

YOU are the Provider PART 2

As you enter the track, you note that both patients are wearing personal protective equipment, including a helmet, knee and elbow pads, and a chest protector. When you reach the patients, you quickly manually stabilize the cervical spine and triage the original patient, while your partner triages the other patient. Your patient is alert, oriented, and able to recall all events. However, he has severe dyspnea and pain on palpation to the midchest area.

Recording Time: 1 Minute	
Appearance	Anxious
Level of consciousness	Alert and oriented to person, place, time, and event
Airway	Appears patent
Breathing	Shallow and rapid; increased work of breathing
Circulation	Strong radial pulse; skin warm, dry, and pink

3. Does this patient require spinal immobilization?
4. Does this patient require helmet removal?

vital organs can actually be torn from their attachment in the chest cavity without any break in the skin.

Blast injuries may be classified as blunt or penetrating. The shock wave during the primary blast compresses organs similar to blunt trauma. During the secondary phase of blast injury, objects may be thrown and penetrate the body.

Thoracic trauma may impair cardiac output, decreasing blood pressure and perfusion to vital organs. Considering the contents of the thoracic cavity, any injury to the chest has the potential to be lethal. Trauma may result in blood loss, pressure changes, vital organ damage, or any combination of these. Bleeding into the thoracic cavity significantly increases the chance of hypovolemia and hypoxia. Increased intrapleural pressures not only decrease lung volume and oxygenation but also impair the heart's ability to pump effectively. Blood in the pericardial sac compresses the heart, eventually stopping it altogether. Myocardial valve damage from trauma to the heart can disrupt ventricular filling, allowing for backflow into the atria and further decreasing cardiac output. Vascular disruption may also occur as the result of trauma. A rupture of a major vessel can lead to fatal blood loss, and even a small tear or blockage can cause lack of oxygenation and tissue ischemia. You should have a good understanding of the underlying structures of the chest because this knowledge improves your assessment abilities and may increase the patient's chance of survival.

Aside from massive blood loss, impairments in ventilatory efficiency may also be rapidly fatal. Any injury that compromises the chest bellows action decreases air exchange and subsequent oxygenation. A patient experiencing severe chest pain tends to breathe shallowly in an attempt to decrease the discomfort created by movement. This further reduces **minute volume**, the volume of air exchanged between the lungs and environment in 1 minute. Air may enter the **pleural space**, which is potential space between the visceral and parietal pleura of the lung and chest wall, respectively. This space is normally absent, as these two pleural surfaces are in direct contact in the normal, uninjured chest. In cases of pneumothorax, however, the pleural space is created and air can be introduced between the two pleural surfaces. In **hemothorax**, blood accumulates between them.

Air entering the pleural space as the result of an open or closed pneumothorax, a tracheal tear, or other damage compresses the lungs and decreases tidal volume. This problem also occurs when blood collects in the thoracic cavity and prevents full expansion of the lungs. Various injuries caused by chest trauma, such as rib fractures and diaphragmatic injury, result in fewer pressure changes and, therefore, less movement of air, which further decreases the amount of oxygen available for gas exchange.

Other complications are also capable of impairing gas exchange. **Atelectasis** is alveolar collapse that prevents the use of that portion of the lung for ventilation and oxygenation. Atelectasis significantly reduces the surface area available for gas exchange. The more alveoli that are damaged, the less gas exchange occurs. Bruised lung tissue may produce marked hypoxemia as fluid accumulates and impairs gas exchange. Disruption of the respiratory tract occurring from rupture or tearing of any of the respiratory structures prevents oxygen from reaching the alveoli, further impairing gas exchange.

▶ Signs and Symptoms of Chest Injury

Important signs and symptoms of chest injury include the following:

- Pain at the site of injury
- Pain localized at the site of injury that is aggravated by or increased with breathing
- Bruising to the chest wall
- **Crepitus** (the sensation felt when broken bone ends grind together) with palpation of the chest
- Any penetrating injury to the chest
- Dyspnea (difficulty breathing, shortness of breath)
- Hemoptysis (coughing up blood)
- Failure of one or both sides of the chest to expand normally with inspiration (asymmetric movement)
- Rapid, weak pulse and low blood pressure
- Cyanosis around the lips or fingernail beds

After a chest injury, any change in normal breathing is a particularly important sign. A healthy, uninjured adult usually breathes 12 to 20 times per minute without difficulty and without pain. Fewer than 12 breaths/min or more than 20 breaths/min may indicate inadequate breathing, especially with poor tidal volume. Patients with chest injuries often have tachypnea (rapid respirations) and shallow respirations because it hurts to take a deep breath. They may also present with bradypnea (slow respirations) and labored respirations.

In an injured patient, dyspnea (difficulty breathing) has many causes, including airway obstruction, damage to the chest wall, improper chest expansion because of the loss of normal control of breathing, or lung compression because of accumulated blood or air. Dyspnea in an injured patient indicates significant compromise of lung function; therefore, prompt, vigorous support and transport are required.

As with any other injury, pain and tenderness are common at the point of impact as a result of a bruise or fracture. The normal process of breathing usually aggravates pain. Irritation of or damage to the pleural surfaces causes a characteristic sharp or stabbing pain with each breath when these normally smooth surfaces slide on one another. This sharp pain is called pleuritic pain or pleurisy.

Hemoptysis, the spitting or coughing up of blood, usually indicates that the lung parenchyma itself or the air passages leading to the lungs have been damaged. With a laceration of the lung, blood can enter the bronchial passages and is coughed up as the patient tries to clear the airway.

The presence or absence of a pulse in a particular location varies according to the nature and extent of injury. A rapid, weak pulse and hypotension are the principal signs of hypovolemic shock, which can result from extensive bleeding from lacerated structures within the chest cavity. Shock following a chest injury may also result from insufficient oxygenation of the blood by the poorly functioning lungs. An absence of radial pulses may indicate severe hypotension. Tachycardia may be indicative of compensatory shock or hypoxemia. Bradycardia is generally an ominous sign. It may be the result of spinal damage or the final stage of shock in which the body is no longer able to compensate.

Changes in blood pressure also vary with the nature and extent of injury. Hypertension may be the result of increased sympathetic discharge, whereas hypotension is a sign of hypovolemia, relative hypovolemia (massive vasodilation), or late shock. Increased pressure on the myocardium decreases filling, resulting in a narrowed **pulse pressure** (the difference between the systolic blood pressure and the diastolic blood pressure). Loss of the peripheral pulse during inspiration suggests **pulsus paradoxus** (the systolic blood pressure drops more than 10 mm Hg during inspiration compared with expiration; also known as a paradoxical pulse) and the presence of **cardiac tamponade**. The patient may also present with hypothermia secondary to neurogenic shock if the injury involves the spinal cord.

Diaphoresis and pallor accompany peripheral vasoconstriction resulting from the sympathetic response of the autonomic nervous system to the injury. Cyanosis in a patient with a chest injury is a sign of inadequate respiration. The classic blue appearance around the lips and fingernail beds indicates that blood is not being oxygenated sufficiently. Patients with cyanosis are unable to provide a sufficient supply of oxygen to the blood through the lungs and require immediate respiratory support and high-flow supplemental oxygen.

Many of these signs and symptoms occur simultaneously. When any one of them develops as a result of a chest injury, the patient requires prompt hospital care. Remember, the principal reason for concern about a patient who has a chest injury is that his or her body has no means of storing oxygen; it is supplied and used continuously, even during sleep. Any interruption in the oxygen supply can be rapidly lethal and must be treated aggressively.

Patient Assessment

Scene Size-up

When you arrive on the scene, your first responsibility is to ensure the safety of both you and your partner. Ensure the scene is safe to enter and that you are using the appropriate personal protective equipment.

Ensure you and your crew take standard precautions and wear, at a minimum, gloves and eye protection. Put several pairs of gloves in your pocket for easy access in case your gloves tear or there are multiple patients with bleeding. Darker clothing may mask signs of bleeding, so you must remain vigilant, especially when the MOI suggests the patient may be bleeding.

A patient who has sustained a significant MOI will allow you to develop an early index of suspicion for underlying injuries. Chest injuries are common in MVCs, falls, and assaults.

After you identify the number of patients, triage those patients, and request any additional resources needed, then begin assessing your assigned patient. Consider the need for spinal immobilization.

Words of Wisdom

Patients with gunshot or stab wounds to the chest should not be fully immobilized on a backboard. Instead, rapidly move and secure the patient to the stretcher and transport in a semi-Fowler position. A cervical collar may be applied if needed based on some additional mechanism of injury. Time is critical for these patients, and they should be transported as rapidly as possible to an appropriate trauma center.

Primary Survey

As you approach the patient, you will form a general impression of the patient's condition. It is important to note the patient's level of consciousness. Responsive patients may be able to tell you their chief complaint. Note not only what they say, but also how they say it.

Difficulty speaking may indicate several problems, and chest injury is an important one. Perform a rapid exam of the patient. Look for obvious injuries, the appearance of blood, and difficulty breathing. Look for cyanosis, irregular breathing, and chest rise and fall on only one side. Observe the neck, looking for accessory muscle use while breathing; also look for extended or engorged external jugular veins. The initial general impression will help you develop an index of suspicion for serious injuries and determine your sense of urgency for medical intervention. A good question to ask yourself is "How sick is this patient?" Patients with significant chest injuries will "look" sick and are often frightened or anxious.

If no obvious problems are seen, then begin an assessment to identify life threats (assess exsanguinating hemorrhage, airway, breathing, circulation, disability, and exposure [XABCDEs]). Addressing life threats begins with assessing airway and breathing unless life-threatening uncontrolled bleeding is present. Ensure the patient has a clear and patent airway. Normal breathing should be effortless, and any deviation from this pattern should be cause for concern. How you assess and manage the airway depends a great deal on whether you suspect the patient has a spinal injury. A significant number of patients with traumatic chest injuries also have spinal injuries, and proper precautions should be taken when trauma is present. Protect the spine early in your care, even if your assessment later confirms that there is no spinal injury.

Examine the neck for the presence of penetrating wounds and the position of the trachea. Palpate and note the presence of any subcutaneous emphysema.

Once you have determined the patient has a patent airway, determine whether breathing is present and adequate. With chest injuries, begin by inspecting for DCAP-BTLS (Deformities, Contusions, Abrasions, Punctures/penetrations/paradoxical movement, Burns, Tenderness, Lacerations, and Swelling), and look for equal expansion of the chest wall. Look for retractions around the ribs, neck, and clavicles, along with other evidence of respiratory distress. Visualize the region looking for deformities, such as asymmetry of the left and right sides of the chest or shoulder girdle, which may reveal the presence of multiple rib fractures, crush injuries, or significant chest wall injury. Identify discrete areas of contusion or abrasion to help pinpoint a specific point of impact. The presence of puncture wounds or other penetrating injuries suggests an open chest injury that should be managed accordingly. Be alert for associated burns, which may alter respiratory mechanics. Palpate for tenderness to localize the injury and identify the presence of fractures. Look for lacerations and local swelling. Apply this systematic approach to patient assessment to minimize the chance of missing a significant injury.

Listen with a stethoscope to each side of the chest. Absent or decreased breath sounds on one side usually indicate significant damage to a lung, preventing it from expanding properly. Be alert to the pattern of symmetric rise and fall of the patient's chest wall. If the chest wall does not expand on each side when the patient inhales, then the chest muscles may have lost their ability to function appropriately.

Words of Wisdom

An impaled object should be removed only when it is in the cheek and interferes with breathing, or when it is in the chest and interferes with chest compressions. Otherwise, it should be stabilized in place.

Loss of muscle function may be the result of a direct injury to the chest wall, or it may be related to an injury of the nerves that control those muscles. Also, check for **paradoxical motion**, an abnormality associated with multiple fractured ribs in which one segment of the chest wall moves opposite the remainder of the chest—for example, one part moves out with expiration and in with inspiration.

If you determine the patient has penetrating trauma, then address this life threat at once. Open chest injuries may interfere with the normal mechanics of breathing and can cause the patient's condition to worsen quickly. For quick initial care, you can immediately cover any open wounds with your gloved hand, and then apply an **occlusive dressing** to all penetrating injuries to the chest. Depending on local protocol, the dressing may be taped on three sides to allow air to escape during exhalation. Administer oxygen via a nonrebreathing mask at 15 L/min. Provide positive pressure ventilations with 100% oxygen if breathing is inadequate based on the patient's level of consciousness and breathing rate and quality. Remember, positive pressure ventilation is a process of overcoming the normal physiologic functions; thus, if the patient has a pneumothorax (collapsed lung), this intervention may quickly exacerbate the injury. Be diligent with auscultation of breath sounds, and evaluate the effectiveness of your ventilatory support by looking for signs of circulation to the skin. Be aware of decreasing oxygen saturation (Spo_2) values because they may indicate hypoxia is developing. Watch for signs of an impending tension pneumothorax, such as increasingly poor compliance during ventilation.

Pay close attention to any changes in the patient's mental status. A decrease in the level of consciousness may indicate worsening of the condition or increasing hypoxia.

Assess the patient's pulse. Determine whether it is present and adequate. If the pulse is too fast or too slow, or if the skin is pale, cool, or clammy, then consider the patient to be in shock. You need to treat this condition aggressively to eliminate the cause and support the patient's circulatory system. Note that in the early stage of shock, the body compensates for blood loss by increasing the heart rate. Be alert for this change, especially if tachycardia is still present beyond a few minutes after the initial adrenaline rush from the incident or injury.

External bleeding may or may not be significant, but if it is considered life threatening, address this threat immediately. Control such bleeding with direct pressure and a bulky trauma dressing. Bleeding inside the chest can be significant and, as discussed earlier, can be a quick cause of death.

Auscultation of the heart sounds is another part of the circulatory assessment, though it may be difficult to perform in the prehospital or ambulance setting. For patients with potential intrathoracic injuries, note whether their heart sounds are easily heard or whether they are muffled. The presence of muffled heart tones is an important diagnostic clue to the presence of either a tension pneumothorax (due to the resultant mediastinal shift) or a cardiac tamponade.

After auscultation, percuss the chest and note any abnormal findings. Recall, hyperresonance is a tympanic, drum-like sound that generally indicates the presence of air. When hyperresonance is heard on percussion of the chest, this finding suggests air in the pleural space, or a pneumothorax. Conversely, hyporresonance is a dull sound that generally indicates a solid or fluid, rather than air. Therefore, when heard on percussion of the chest, hyporresonance may suggest the presence of blood, or a hemothorax.

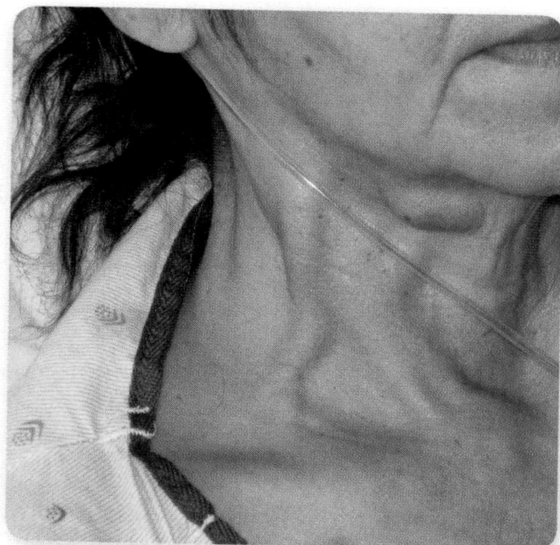

Figure 31-8 Jugular vein distention.

Note the presence of a scaphoid (hollow, boat-shaped) abdomen, which indicates the abdominal contents have shifted upward into the thoracic cage as a result of a ruptured diaphragm. If possible, then note whether bowel sounds are heard in the lower hemithorax; this also could indicate a ruptured diaphragm.

Note whether the jugular veins are distended **Figure 31-8**. **Jugular vein distention (JVD)** suggests increased intravenous pressure—perhaps resulting from a tension pneumothorax, volume overload, right-sided heart failure, or cardiac tamponade. Because true JVD is measured with the patient sitting in a 45° angle, it may be difficult to assess when spinal immobilization has been implemented. Nevertheless, a lack of JVD in the supine position in combination with other physical findings (eg, tachycardia, altered mental status, thready pulses, poor skin perfusion) may suggest a hypovolemic state.

Even if your assessment of the patient's circulatory status suggests hypovolemic shock, you should recognize that the cause may not lie within the thorax. Some patients with a combination of thoracic trauma and shock will have a significant hemorrhage within the chest, but others may experience hypovolemic shock secondary to intra-abdominal injury, neurogenic shock following a spinal cord injury, or cardiogenic shock due to myocardial infarction, for example.[5] For this reason, after you complete the primary survey, manage any immediate life-threatening conditions, and prioritize the patient, you must obtain the patient's history and perform a complete physical exam to identify other significant injuries.

Priority patients are those who have airway, breathing, and/or circulation problems. Sometimes the priority is obvious, and the decision to transport quickly is also easy. At other times, what is happening outside the body may not provide obvious clues to the seriousness of what is happening inside the body. Pay attention to subtle clues such as the appearance of the skin, level of consciousness, or a sense of impending doom in the patient. These symptoms are not as dramatic as a large gash across the chest or bubbles coming out of a wound in the chest wall, but they can be equally important indicators of a life-threatening condition. When you find signs of poor perfusion or inadequate breathing, transport quickly and perform the remainder of the assessment en route to the emergency department (ED). A delay on the scene to perform a lengthy assessment will reduce the chances of survival for your patient. With chest injuries, when in doubt, transport rapidly to a hospital. **Table 31-1** lists the "deadly dozen" chest injuries.

Table 31-1 Life-Threatening Chest Injuries

Immediately life-threatening chest injuries that must be detected and managed during the primary survey:

1. Airway obstruction
2. Bronchial disruption
3. Diaphragmatic tear
4. Esophageal injury
5. Open pneumothorax
6. Tension pneumothorax
7. Hemothorax
8. Flail chest
9. Cardiac tamponade

Potentially lethal chest injuries that may be identified during the secondary assessment:

10. Thoracic aortic dissection
11. Myocardial contusion
12. Pulmonary contusion

Data source: Yamamoto L, Schroeder C, Morley D, Beliveau C. Thoracic trauma: the deadly dozen. *Crit Care Nurs Q.* 2005;28(1):22-40. https://www.ncbi.nlm.nih.gov/pubmed/15732422. Accessed December 12, 2016.

History Taking

Depending on the severity of the injuries identified up to this point, history taking may need to be done en route to the ED.

Once you have identified and treated life threats, further investigate the chief complaint and MOI, and obtain a history of the present illness (OPQRST: Onset, Provocation, Quality, Region/radiation/referral, Severity, Timing) and a past medical history (SAMPLE: Signs and symptoms, Allergies, Medications, Pertinent past medical history, Last oral intake, Events leading up to the illness or injury). Also obtain a history of the patient's mental status and include the following information when applicable:

- Dyspnea
- Chest pain

- Associated symptoms
  - Other areas of pain or discomfort
  - Symptoms before the incident
- History of cardiorespiratory disease
- Use of restraint in an MVC
- Any medications the patient may be taking (Remember, certain medications can mask compensatory mechanisms.)

Investigate associated signs and symptoms and pertinent negatives. If the patient was assaulted with a blunt object such as a bat, then further evaluate the spinal region for injury because the force may have been transferred through the body from the point of impact. If the patient fell from a great height and is reporting chest discomfort or dyspnea, then this may distract the patient from recognizing that he or she has fractures or is bleeding from the extremities. Palpation of the chest will typically cause direct pain at the site of a fracture. When a patient reacts to the pain, make certain to verify where the pain was located in relationship to the area being touched.

Pertinent negatives when examining the chest include no associated shortness of breath, no rapid breathing, no absent or abnormal breath sounds, and no areas of deformity or abnormal movement. In a patient with a suspected spinal cord injury, equal expansion of the chest and movement of the rib cage and the diaphragm can confirm to you that there is nerve conduction to that region of the body.

Obtaining a SAMPLE history from a patient with a chest injury may not seem very important, but a basic evaluation of signs and symptoms; allergies; medications; pertinent medical history, including respiratory or cardiovascular disease; and last oral intake should be attempted if time permits. The events leading to the emergency should also be identified. Questions about the events surrounding the incident should focus on the MOI: the speed of the vehicle or height of the fall; the use of safety equipment, such as a helmet, airbag, seat belt, or life jacket; the type of weapon used; the number of penetrating wounds; and so on. A SAMPLE history can be obtained quickly in most situations and can certainly be obtained while accomplishing other tasks. However, if the patient becomes unresponsive, it will no longer be possible to obtain the information.

Secondary Assessment

During the secondary assessment, look for injuries with the potential to compromise the management of the ABCs—namely, aortic transections, great vessel injuries, bronchial disruptions, myocardial contusions, pulmonary contusions, simple pneumothoraces, rib fractures, and sternal fractures.

In a patient who has an isolated injury to the chest with a limited MOI, such as in a stabbing, focus your assessment on the isolated injury, the patient's complaint, and the body region affected. However, it is important in patients with a chest injury not to focus only on a chest wound. With significant trauma, you should quickly assess the entire patient from head to toe. While you are assessing the skin, look for ecchymosis and other evidence of trauma. Ensure wounds are identified and control of the bleeding has been established. Note the location and extent of the injury. Assess all underlying systems. Examine the anterior and posterior aspects of the chest wall, and be alert to changes in the patient's ability to maintain adequate respirations.

Repeat the rapid full-body scan looking for DCAP-BTLS to determine any changes in thoracic injuries previously discovered and to search for problems not previously found. You may have symmetrical chest rise in the primary survey only to discover that upon reassessment chest rise is unequal due to the progression of a pneumothorax. Some signs are not initially prevalent but become more pronounced as damage progresses. It is for this reason that it is necessary to reassess those areas already covered in the primary survey.

If you have not already done so, obtain a full set of vital signs—including pulse rate, blood pressure, respirations, oxygen saturation, mental status, skin condition, and pupils. Each of these is considered a sign indicating how the patient is tolerating the injuries. Consider these signs as a window to the functioning of the vital organs. This baseline set of vital signs will be used to evaluate changes in the patient's condition. Because patients with significant chest injury have the potential for life-threatening deterioration in their condition, they should be reevaluated every 5 minutes or less. This will allow you to quickly recognize changes in the vital sign numbers or trends.

If you find an accelerated pulse rate or respiratory rate, then the chest injury may be causing either a decrease in available oxygen (hypoxia) or blood loss that results in a decreased number of red blood cells that can carry oxygen (hypoxemia). The increased respiratory rate is often associated with an obvious increase in work of breathing. This can be identified by noting increased use of the accessory muscles in the face, neck, and chest to assist in the movement of air. In the later stages of injuries, the pulse rate can slow as the myocardium becomes starved for oxygen and the body is no longer able to keep up with the demands. The respiratory rate may drop as the brain becomes starved for oxygen and overloaded with carbon dioxide and other waste products. These are usually signs of impending cardiopulmonary arrest. In the case of increasing pressure on the heart from the pleural space or the pericardial space, the blood pressure may exhibit a narrowing pulse pressure as the systolic and diastolic pressures come closer together. This is a result of the inability of the heart to fill with an adequate volume of blood and contract normally.

Words of Wisdom

While pulse oximetry can evaluate the effectiveness of oxygenation, it cannot measure the amount of oxygen being consumed by a patient's cells during cellular metabolism. Measuring carbon dioxide levels is a more accurate method of determining oxygen consumption. Carbon dioxide is the by-product of aerobic cellular metabolism and reflects the amount of oxygen being consumed during the process. *Metabolism* refers to the chemical reactions that occur in the body or cells to maintain life. There are two noninvasive methods in which carbon dioxide is monitored in the field: capnometry and capnography. Capnometry typically consists of a disposable or electronic device that provides you with a means of measuring exhaled carbon dioxide. Capnography not only includes measuring exhaled carbon dioxide, it also provides a waveform based on serial measurements. Capnography can provide information about a patient's ventilatory status, circulation, and metabolism. Capnography can also serve as an indicator of chest compression effectiveness and detect return of spontaneous circulation. The provision of this information is possible because blood must circulate through the lungs for carbon dioxide to be exhaled and measured. These devices are typically used by paramedics in the prehospital setting as the gold standard for confirming endotracheal tube placement, to optimize an intubated patient's ventilatory rate, and to avoid inadvertent hyperventilation of head-injured patients, which has been linked to poor outcomes. For more information, refer to Chapter 10, *Patient Assessment*.

Using diagnostic tools—most commonly the pulse oximeter—to evaluate the effectiveness of the respiratory system is especially important with an injury or insult to the thorax because the injury can decrease the amount of available oxygen within the blood. The pulse oximeter monitors the oxygen saturation of hemoglobin by directing a beam of infrared light through the capillary beds of an area (such as a finger) between two probes. The light received after passing through the capillary bed is measured as a percentage that indicates how well the hemoglobin in the red blood cells is coated or saturated with oxygen. In normal circumstances, the hemoglobin is saturated with oxygen, and the Spo_2 is greater than 94%. However, if the patient has a decreased number of red blood cells, a damaged pump (heart), or a pulmonary contusion, less oxygen is available to be absorbed by the hemoglobin, resulting in a decreased Spo_2.

However, when there is carbon monoxide in the patient's bloodstream, the pulse oximeter may give misleading results. Carbon monoxide binds to hemoglobin with a higher affinity than oxygen. Because the oximeter can only recognize that the hemoglobin is bound to something and cannot distinguish between hemoglobin bound to carbon monoxide and hemoglobin bound to oxygen, the values produced by pulse oximetry can be misleading, potentially resulting in your undertreating the patient. In general, then, it is advisable to use the pulse oximeter on any patient with a chest injury to establish a baseline measurement and to help you recognize any downward trends that indicate the patient's condition is worsening. If you suspect carbon monoxide exposure that may be causing a falsely elevated pulse oximetry value, provide supplemental oxygen regardless of the measured Spo_2 level.

Reassessment

When you are reassessing the patient with thoracic trauma, reassess the patient's vital signs, oxygenation, circulatory status, and breath sounds. Reassess the chief complaint to identify and treat any changes in the patient's condition and recheck interventions. Reevaluate the patient every 5 minutes or less. Because the progression from pneumothorax to tension pneumothorax can occur quite rapidly, all patients with a presumptive diagnosis of a pneumothorax should be considered to be in an unstable condition and should be reassessed frequently for worsening dyspnea, tachycardia, and developing JVD. Similarly, other thoracic injuries may suggest the presence of more serious underlying pathologic conditions. Because these injuries may have been overlooked during the initial examinations, you need to maintain a high degree of suspicion during the on-scene treatment and transport of these patients.

Communicating with hospital staff early when the patient has a significant MOI to the chest can help them be prepared with appropriate equipment and personnel when you arrive. If a penetrating injury is present, then describe it in your verbal report, along with the interventions that you applied. If a flail segment is present, then hospital staff may be able to offer assistance on how to manage it. Your documentation should be complete and thorough. Describe all injuries and the treatment given. Remember, your documentation is your legal record of what happened.

Emergency Medical Care

Stabilizing the ABCs is the primary management concern for all patients, and thoracic trauma is no exception. Evaluate the patient's airway and respiratory status while maintaining cervical spine immobilization. Be prepared to suction the patient, consider placing an oropharyngeal or nasopharyngeal airway, and consider definitive airway management.

Whenever you suspect significant bleeding, administer high-flow oxygen. If needed, provide assisted ventilation using a bag-mask device with high-flow oxygen. If you find penetrating trauma to the chest wall, then place an occlusive dressing over the wound. Use caution to avoid increasing the patient's work of breathing and pain. Be prepared to provide positive pressure ventilation if the patient's respiratory efforts are not effective. If the patient has signs of hypoperfusion, then treat for shock and provide rapid transport to the appropriate hospital. Do not delay transport of a seriously injured trauma patient to complete non–life-saving treatments such as splinting extremity fractures; instead, complete these types of treatments en route to the hospital. Keep the patient warm. Maintain circulation and gain intravenous (IV) access. Establish at least one large-bore IV catheter, preferably two, and administer a 20-mL/kg bolus of an isotonic crystalloid solution to maintain adequate perfusion. With thoracic trauma, your goal is to maintain radial pulses. Titrate fluid administration to a systolic blood pressure of 80 to 90 mm Hg. Increasing blood pressure above this point may increase bleeding into the chest and worsen the patient's condition. Always follow local protocols.

Words of Wisdom

Increasing the patient's blood pressure excessively may increase bleeding, causing a more rapid deterioration of the patient's condition. For this reason, you should titrate IV fluid rates to maintain perfusion (radial pulses) without significantly raising the blood pressure.

Call for paramedic support, if available, in a timely manner if there is any suspicion of impending cardiac arrest or a potential need for chest decompression. In-hospital management may include a tube thoracostomy for a hemothorax or pericardiocentesis for cardiac tamponade. Early recognition of signs and symptoms and early transport can significantly increase your patient's chance of survival.

Pathophysiology, Assessment, and Management of Specific Emergencies

This section covers specific thoracic injuries that fall into the following categories: chest wall injuries, lung injuries, myocardial injuries, vascular injuries, and other injuries such as diaphragmatic injury, esophageal injury, tracheobronchial injuries, and traumatic asphyxia.

Special Populations

The incidence of rib fractures varies with age. The ribs of children are pliable, so the ribs may injure underlying structures without being fractured. Significant force can be transmitted directly to underlying organs in pediatric patients, causing significant blunt trauma. In older adult patients, the frail nature of the bones makes the ribs more likely to fracture.

Rib Fractures

Rib fractures are infrequent in children because of the pliability of their thoracic cage. Rib fractures occur most often in older patients, who have lost pliability and whose bones may be very brittle (for example, because of osteoporosis). Because the upper four ribs are well protected by the bony girdle of the clavicle and scapula, a fracture of one of these upper ribs is a sign of a very severe MOI. A significant force is required to cause fractures and may be indicative of other injuries. Morbidity and mortality rates increase with age, number of fractures, and location of the fractures.

A fractured rib may potentially lacerate the surface of the lung, causing a pneumothorax, tension pneumothorax, hemothorax, or hemopneumothorax. One sign of this complication is a "crackly" feeling to the skin in the area (also called subcutaneous emphysema), which indicates that air escaping from a lacerated lung is leaking into the subcutaneous layer of the chest wall. Ensure you communicate this finding to hospital personnel.

Rib fractures are most often caused by blunt trauma, with the fracture occurring at midshaft owing to the bowing effect of the ribs. Ribs four through nine are the ones most often fractured because they are thinner and poorly protected. The patient will usually present using an arm to splint the injury and with shallow respirations to decrease chest movement, thereby decreasing pain. Unfortunately, decreasing chest excursion also decreases tidal volume, minute volume, and the amount of oxygen available for gas exchange. The development of atelectasis, or collapse of the alveoli, caused by trauma also decreases the surface area for gas exchange. The result is a ventilation/perfusion mismatch. The circulatory system is intact, but the amount of lung tissue available for gas exchange has been greatly diminished. The mismatch may also occur when inadequate perfusion is present. An underlying pulmonary or cardiac contusion or an intercostal vessel injury may hinder perfusion, leading to hypoxemia that is just as severe.

When the first and second ribs are injured by severe trauma, the result may be a ruptured aorta, tracheobronchial tree injury, or vascular injury. Trauma to the left lower rib may contribute to injury of the spleen, and trauma to the right lower rib may cause liver injury. Multiple rib fractures may lead to atelectasis, hypoventilation, inadequate cough, and pneumonia. With a posterior fracture, the fifth through the ninth ribs are the most frequently injured. Owing to their location in the thorax, lower rib fractures are associated with spleen and kidney injuries. The floating ribs, because they are well protected by the strong abdominal musculature, are rarely fractured; therefore, injury to these ribs suggests a severe MOI and a strong potential for other life-threatening injuries.

Regardless of the position, any rib fracture puts the patient at risk for multiple injuries. It is imperative to maintain a high index of suspicion, even if the patient appears to have no visible injury.

Patients with one or more fractured ribs will report localized tenderness and pain on breathing, typically during inspiration. This pain is the result of the broken ends of the fractured rib rubbing against each other with each inspiration and expiration, deep breathing, and/or coughing. Patients will tend to avoid taking deep breaths, breathing rapidly and shallowly instead. They will often hold the affected portion of the rib cage in an effort to minimize the discomfort. On palpation, the patient may present with point tenderness over the site, crepitus or an audible crunch, and pain when anteroposterior pressure is applied.

Managing rib fractures focuses on managing the ABCs and evaluating the patient for other, more lethal injuries. Administer supplemental oxygen and gently splint the patient's chest wall by having the patient hold a pillow or blanket against the area; this measure may allow the patient to take deeper breaths—something that should be encouraged despite the pain. Intravenous analgesics may also assist in this regard. If permitted by medical control, then you can administer nitrous oxide.

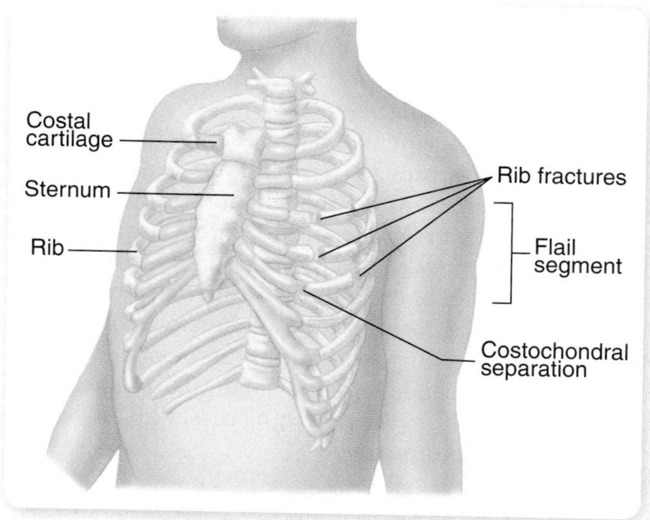

Figure 31-9 When two or more adjacent ribs are fractured in two or more places, a flail chest results. A flail segment will move paradoxically when the patient breathes.

Words of Wisdom

Considering the potential seriousness of chest injuries, always keep an automated external defibrillator (AED) ready when responding to a call for a chest injury. Be ready to apply the AED should cardiac arrest occur.

Flail Chest

Ribs may be fractured in more than one place. If two or more adjacent ribs are fractured in two or more places or if the sternum is fractured along with several ribs, then a segment of the chest wall may be detached from the rest of the thoracic cage, producing a free-floating segment **Figure 31-9**.[6] This condition is known as **flail chest**. The most common cause of a flail segment is a MVC, but it may also be caused by falls from significant heights, industrial accidents, or assault. Significant chest trauma is required to cause a flail chest. When flail chest is present, patient mortality averages 16%, often because of associated injuries.[7] Mortality also increases with advanced age, seven or more fractured ribs, three or more associated injuries, shock, and head injuries.[8]

In what is called paradoxical motion, the detached portion of the chest wall moves in the opposite direction of normal—that is, it moves in instead of out during inhalation, and it moves out instead of in during expiration. This occurs because of negative pressure that has built up in the thorax. Breathing with a flail chest can be extremely painful and often does not allow for adequate oxygenation. Paradoxical motion is usually minimal because of muscle spasm. The patient will breathe as shallowly as possible to decrease movement of the thorax and, therefore, decrease pain, but this decreases ventilation. Respiratory failure in a patient with a flail chest generally results from other associated injuries. A pulmonary contusion resulting from a flail segment will impair gas exchange, leading to hypoxia and hypercapnia.

The blunt force trauma that causes the flail segment can also produce a **pulmonary contusion**, an injury to the underlying lung tissue that inhibits the normal diffusion of O_2 and CO_2. If the blunt force that fractures the ribs drives bone fragments farther into the body, then a pneumothorax or hemothorax may result. In addition, the pain associated with the fractures may prevent the patient from taking in adequate tidal volume because he or she is consciously trying to minimize the movement of that segment of the chest. This "self-splinting" action uses the intercostal muscles and purposefully limits chest wall movement to minimize pain. Unfortunately, this action further limits the pulmonary system's ability to compensate for the injury.

Words of Wisdom

With flail chest injuries, pulmonary contusion is often the primary cause of hypoxemia.

Flail chest is a serious condition and suggests impact with a force that is significant enough to cause other serious internal damage. When flail chest is suspected, expose and examine the chest for DCAP-BTLS. Look for any chest wall contusions, signs of respiratory distress and accessory muscle use, and any paradoxical motion. The patient may also present with pleuritic chest pain and pain and splinting of the affected side. Note any areas of crepitus on palpation of the thorax. Tachypnea and tachycardia may also be present and are signs of inadequate oxygenation.

Typical management of flail chest is to first assess the need for positive pressure ventilation, then administer oxygen. If ventilations are inadequate (or the end-tidal CO_2 measurement reveals that the patient has hypercapnia), then you may use positive pressure ventilation (via a bag-mask device or continuous positive airway pressure [CPAP]) as well as positive end-expiratory pressure (PEEP) when you are assisting ventilations for the patient. In the past, treatment included splinting of the flail segment with bulky dressings; however, restricting chest wall movement is no longer recommended.

Words of Wisdom

Stabilization of a flail segment is a controversial issue. Current guidelines suggest that providing positive pressure ventilation when appropriate provides internal stabilization and increases oxygenation and ventilation for managing a pulmonary contusion. Splinting as previously recommended is of little to no value and may in fact limit ventilation. In the trauma center, some studies have shown patients may benefit from early operative stabilization that may possibly reduce further acute complications.[9] Always follow local protocols.

▶ Sternal Fracture

Sternal fracture may occur in patients experiencing blunt chest trauma—for example, when the sternum strikes the steering wheel or dashboard during deceleration. A blow significant enough to fracture the sternum causes severe hyperflexion of the thoracic cage. Isolated sternal fracture has a mortality rate that rises with additional injuries and as people age (17% mortality for persons younger than 55 years versus 27% mortality for those older than 55 years).[10] If sternal fracture is present, then myocardial or lung injury is also very likely.

Morbidity and mortality are generally the result of associated injuries.[11] Enough force to fracture the sternum may also result in pulmonary and myocardial contusions, flail chest, vascular disruption of thoracic vessels, intra-abdominal injuries, and head injuries. It is rare for the fracture to be displaced posteriorly and directly impinge on the heart or vessels.

Words of Wisdom

The sternum is a thick bone. If the thorax receives enough force to fracture the sternum, then you must assume the same force was transmitted to the heart, great vessels, lungs, and diaphragm.

When a sternal fracture is present, expect to find localized pain and tenderness over the sternum, along with crepitus on palpation. The patient's presentation or MOI may be clues to the presence of a sternal fracture. Tachypnea is a common finding, and there may be electrocardiographic changes associated with a myocardial contusion.

When you are managing a sternal fracture, you should focus on maintaining a good respiratory status and monitoring for respiratory and/or cardiovascular changes. Provide positive pressure ventilations as needed, but do not use overly aggressive ventilations that further exacerbate injuries. Establish IV access, but provide fluid sparingly (maintain radial pulses). Administer an isotonic crystalloid solution to maintain a systolic blood pressure of 80 to 90 mm Hg. Elevate the head of the long backboard to help reduce pressure in the thoracic cavity and facilitate lung expansion.

▶ Clavicle Fracture

The clavicle, or collarbone, is one of the most commonly fractured bones in the body. Fractures of the clavicle occur most often in children when they fall on an outstretched hand. They can also occur with crushing injuries of the chest. A patient with a fracture of the clavicle will report pain in the shoulder and will usually hold the arm across the front of his or her body.

Fractures of the clavicle can be splinted effectively with a sling and swathe. Information about fractures of the clavicle, scapula (shoulder blade), and acromioclavicular joint can be found in Chapter 33, *Orthopaedic Injuries*.

▶ Commotio Cordis

If the thorax receives a direct blow during the critical portion of the heart's repolarization phase, then the result may be immediate cardiac arrest. This phenomenon, termed **commotio cordis**, may occur after patients are struck in the chest with softballs, baseballs, bats, snowballs, fists, and even kicks during kickboxing. Commotio cordis is ultimately the result of the chest wall impact directly over the heart, especially directly over the left ventricle. Impacts to the chest that are not directly over the heart will not cause commotio cordis. The affected patient may present with ventricular fibrillation that responds positively to early defibrillation if provided within the first 3 minutes. For this reason, public access to defibrillators in schools and sports venues is essential.

Patients who are unresponsive, apneic, and pulseless may be experiencing commotio cordis. Many of these patients are cyanotic, and tonic-clonic (grand mal) seizures have been evident in some. Chest wall contusions and localized bruising that correspond to the site of chest impact are also indicators.

Increased awareness of this condition and preparation such as cardiopulmonary resuscitation (CPR) and AEDs being accessible at sporting events have increased survival rates from approximately 34% between 1994 and 2012 to 58% in the past 6 years.[12] Factors such as delays in CPR and AED access of more than 3 minutes may decrease survival rates significantly.[12] Advanced life support (ALS) treatments must follow standard advanced cardiovascular life support (ACLS) guidelines for sudden cardiac arrest, and treatments of the underlying rhythm must be initiated early if successful resuscitation is to occur. Public awareness, CPR, AED access, and protective gear are all necessary elements to decrease the occurrence and improve survivability of this type of event.

▶ Simple Pneumothorax

In any chest injury, damage to the heart, lungs, great vessels, and other organs in the thorax can be complicated by the accumulation of air in the pleural space. This accumulation causes a serious condition called a **pneumothorax** (commonly called a collapsed lung). In this condition, air enters through a hole in the chest wall or the surface of the lung as the patient attempts to breathe, causing the lung on that side to collapse as pressure continues to build in the pleural space **Figure 31-10**. As a result, blood that passes through the lung is not oxygenated, and hypoxia can develop. Depending on the size of the hole and the rate at which air fills the cavity, the lung may collapse in a few seconds or a few hours. The larger the hole, the more rapidly the lung will collapse. Delayed or improper treatment of a simple pneumothorax may lead to a tension pneumothorax, discussed later. Most low-velocity wounds self-seal, remedying the problem. The lungs are situated in the thoracic cavity so that at any point they are only 1 to 3 cm away from the chest wall. In a simple pneumothorax, there may only be a small accumulation of air and pulmonary function may remain adequate. The internal wound allows air to enter

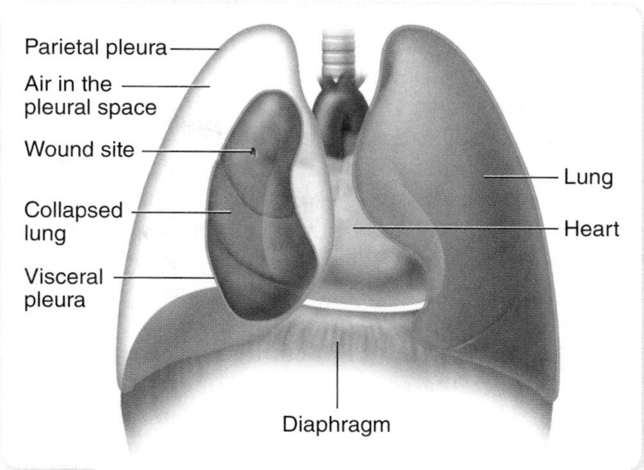

Figure 31-10 Pneumothorax occurs when air leaks into the space between the pleural surfaces from an opening in the chest wall or the surface of the lung. The lung collapses as air fills the pleural space.

YOU are the Provider — PART 3

While you are performing the primary survey on your patient, your partner tells you that the other patient was not injured and is refusing care. You ask your partner to retrieve the spinal immobilization equipment. The motocross safety official arrives, and you assign him to provide manual stabilization of the head as you begin to remove the patient's shirt to expose any possible injuries. As you remove the chest protector and shirt, you notice pain and tenderness over the sternum, with some possible crepitus as well. The patient denies having any head or neck pain, so you decide to remove his helmet to enable proper alignment on the backboard.

Recording Time: 5 Minutes	
Respirations	32 breaths/min, shallow
Pulse	Strong and regular, 120 beats/min
Skin	Warm, dry, and pink
Blood pressure	98/55 mm Hg
Oxygen saturation (Spo_2)	97% on room air
Pupils	Pupils Equal, Round, and Reactive to Light and Accommodation (PERRLA)

5. What are some possible causes of this patient's dyspnea?
6. Does this patient require rapid transport to the hospital?

the pleural space. Small tears often seal themselves, and the patient experiences only minor discomfort. However, larger tears may progress.

Some people are born with or develop weak areas on the surface of the lungs. Occasionally, such a weak area will rupture spontaneously, allowing air to leak into the pleural space. Usually this event, called **spontaneous pneumothorax**, is not related to trauma, but simply happens with normal breathing. The patient experiences sudden, sharp chest pain and increasing difficulty breathing. The affected lung collapses, losing its ability to expand normally. The amount of pneumothorax that develops varies, as does the amount of respiratory distress the patient experiences. You should suspect a spontaneous pneumothorax in a patient who experiences sudden sharp chest pain and shortness of breath without a specific known cause. Young men who are tall and thin seem to be at an increased risk for a spontaneous pneumothorax, especially if they have recently traveled by air.[13] Both a pneumothorax (an accumulation of air) and a hemothorax (an accumulation of blood) occur in 80% of all cases of penetrating chest trauma.[14]

A patient who takes a deep breath just before blunt trauma to the chest may experience the **paper bag syndrome**, or paper bag effect. On impact, the lungs rupture like a paper bag that has been blown up and popped with your hand.

If the patient is standing, then air will accumulate in the apices. You should auscultate the apices first for diminished breath sounds. If the patient is supine, then air accumulates in the anterior portion of the chest. As air accumulates, it forces the structures of the mediastinum toward the opposite side of the chest, dragging the trachea along. Although you may note the trachea tugging away from the affected side, tracheal deviation is a very late sign and is not seen in most cases. Compression of the lungs, myocardium, and great vessels cause a ventilation/perfusion mismatch because air is unable to enter the lungs and blood is unable to circulate.

The presentation and physical findings in a patient with a simple pneumothorax depend on the size of the pneumothorax and the degree of resulting pulmonary compromise. With a small pneumothorax, the patient may report only mild dyspnea and pleuritic chest pain on the affected side, and in young and fit patients, the simple pneumothorax may be well tolerated.

Patients with a simple pneumothorax may present with tachypnea and tachycardia as a result of hypoxia. If their conditions progress, respiratory distress increases and breath sounds may be decreased or absent on the affected side. Chest wall movement decreases as pressure increases, and hyperresonance can be detected with percussion. The patient may also experience dyspnea, chest pain that is referred to the shoulder or arm on the affected side, and pleuritic chest pain. The patient may also present with subcutaneous emphysema, signs of hypovolemia, or cardiac dysrhythmias.

As the pneumothorax increases in size, the degree of compromise also increases. Patients with larger pneumothoraces will report increasing dyspnea and demonstrate signs of more serious respiratory compromise and hypoxia: agitation, altered mental status, tachypnea, tachycardia, cyanosis, lowered pulse oximetry readings, pulsus paradoxus (a drop in blood pressure on inspiration greater than 10 mm Hg), and absent breath sounds on the affected side.

When pneumothorax is suspected, immediately cover any open wounds with an occlusive dressing. Maintain the ABCs. Use positive pressure ventilation sparingly because excessive pressure may result in a tension pneumothorax. The most critical intervention for these patients is conducting repeated assessments to ensure the injury has not progressed to a tension pneumothorax. If signs and symptoms show the development of a tension pneumothorax, then you may need to "burp" or remove the dressing to allow for the release of the trapped air within the thoracic cage. Most pneumothoraces result from a small pulmonary injury that seals itself off, preventing further air loss. For those that do progress, however, rapid recognition and management of this condition can be lifesaving. Call for paramedic backup for treatment of potential cardiac dysrhythmias and/or a tension pneumothorax.

Words of Wisdom

Percussion of the chest produces hyperresonance when the thorax is full of air, and hyporresonance, or dullness, when it is full of blood.

▶ Open Pneumothorax

An **open pneumothorax** occurs with penetrating trauma to the chest. Profound hypoventilation could result, and death may occur quickly if care is delayed.

With an open pneumothorax, an open injury in the chest wall allows for communication between the pleural space and the atmosphere, limiting the development of negative intrapleural pressure on inspiration and resulting in collapse of a portion of the lung. Of course, this also means the affected lung does not have the ability to ventilate. Hypoventilation results from the increased pressure and decreased lung surface area available for gas exchange to occur, and hypoxia occurs as less oxygen is available for gas exchange.

Air enters the pleural space during the inspiratory phase. Negative pressure draws air into the lungs and through the opening in the chest wall. Air may exit during the exhalation phase or may remain trapped in the pleural space. Resistance to air flow through the respiratory tract may be greater than through the open wound, resulting in an ineffective respiratory effort.

A one-way flap valve may let air in but not out, resulting in a buildup of pressure in the pleural space. Direct lung injury may be present if the lung parenchyma was penetrated. The vena cava may become kinked from swaying of the mediastinum as pressure builds, resulting in decreased preload and a subsequent decrease in cardiac output.

The presence of a defect in the chest wall or penetrating injury should be noted as the patient is exposed during the primary survey. Air motion may be detected at the site of the defect as the patient inhales and exhales. A sucking sound may be heard on inhalation as air is drawn into the thoracic cavity through the opening in the chest wall. For this reason, an open or penetrating wound to the chest wall is often called a **sucking chest wound** Figure 31-11. Tachycardia and tachypnea increase in relation to the level of respiratory distress as intrathoracic pressure increases and oxygenation decreases. Subcutaneous emphysema may also be found, along with decreased breath sounds on the affected side. The patient may also present with signs of hypovolemia and cardiac dysrhythmias.

Sucking chest wounds must be treated immediately. The injury should first be converted to a closed injury to prevent further expansion of the pneumothorax. To do so, immediately place your gloved hand over the injury and then replace that hand with an occlusive dressing or a commercial chest seal Figure 31-12. Because of the possibility that an underlying lung injury may continue to contribute to the pneumothorax, this dressing should be secured on three sides to facilitate the release of increased pressure, should it develop.

Managing an open pneumothorax is the same as managing a simple pneumothorax. When you use an occlusive dressing to seal an open chest wound, record the type of material used, whether three or four sides were sealed, and any changes noted in skin color, vital signs, breath sounds, and particularly the patient's level of respiratory distress after application of the dressing. Monitor for changes and "burp" the dressing if the patient presents with any signs of increasing distress.

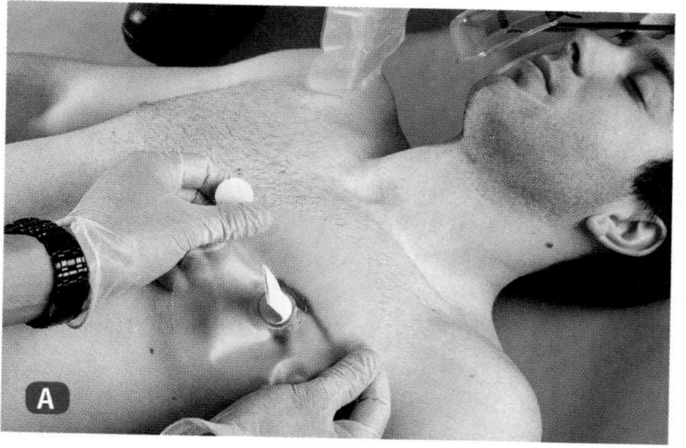

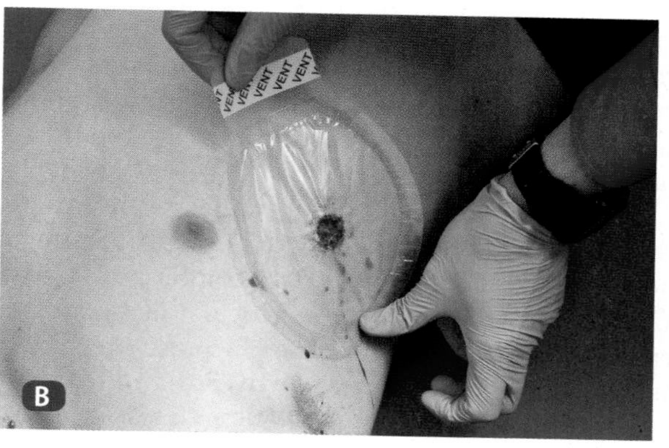

Figure 31-12 A commercial occlusive dressing may be used to seal all four sides of a sucking chest wound. **A.** An Asherman Chest Seal, which is vented. **B.** A HALO Chest Seal, which is unvented.

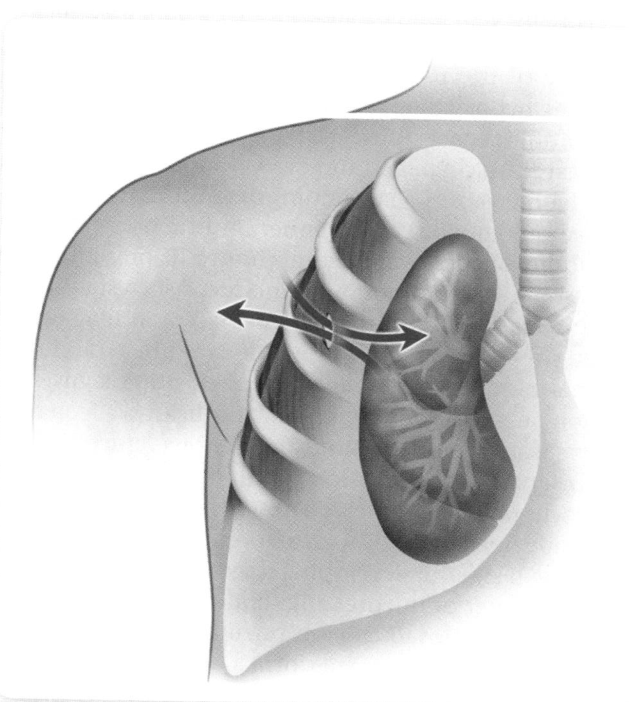

Figure 31-11 With a sucking chest wound, air passes from the outside into the pleural space and back out with each breath, creating the sucking sound.

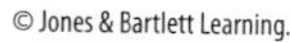

Words of Wisdom

If a patient with an open chest wound sealed with an occlusive dressing shows signs of developing tension, then raise one side of the dressing to allow air to escape. This is known as burping the dressing.

▶ Tension Pneumothorax

A **tension pneumothorax** may be the result of blunt or penetrating trauma **Figure 31-13**. This can occur when there is a significant ongoing air accumulation in the pleural space. The increase in pressure causes the collapse of the affected lung and pushes the mediastinum (the central part of the chest containing the heart and the great vessels) into the opposite pleural cavity. This prevents blood from returning through the venae cavae to the heart, decreasing cardiac output, causing shock, and ultimately leading to death.

Tension pneumothorax can result from a defect in the airway that allows for communication with the pleural space. This defect may be the result of blunt trauma in which a lung is penetrated by a fractured rib (most common), a sudden increase in intrapulmonary pressure culminating in rupture of pulmonary structures, or bronchial disruption from shearing forces, allowing air to enter the pleural space and increase the intrathoracic pressure.

The classic signs of a tension pneumothorax are an absence of breath sounds on the affected side, unequal chest rise, pulsus paradoxus, tachycardia and dysrhythmias such as progression to ventricular tachycardia and ventricular fibrillation, JVD, narrow pulse pressure, and tracheal deviation. Whereas tachycardia may not be a unique finding in the trauma patient, tension pneumothorax induces this change—not because of a hypovolemic state, but rather because of the inability of blood to easily return to the heart from the venous system. The increasing pressure within the thoracic cage leads to the accumulation of blood within the great vessels just outside the thoracic cage. As the pressure is translated into the most superficial of these veins—the jugular veins—they become distended with blood. Such JVD is usually a late sign of tension pneumothorax.

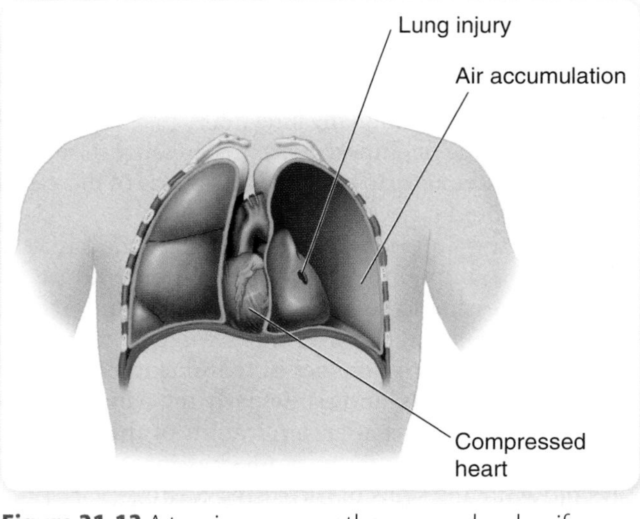

Figure 31-13 A tension pneumothorax can develop if a penetrating chest wound is bandaged tightly and air from a damaged lung cannot escape. The air then accumulates in the pleural space, eventually compressing the heart and great vessels. If a dressing sealed on four sides with no vent is used, then monitor for signs of tension pneumothorax developing and prepare to vent one side of the dressing.

During normal inspiration, the negative pressure within the chest increases blood return to the heart, thus increasing preload and, therefore, cardiac output. In tension pneumothorax, the effect on preload of inspiration is blunted because of compression on the great vessels, and a decrease in cardiac output results.

Because of the mediastinal shift caused by the increasing pressure, palpate or visualize the trachea, which may show a deviation of the trachea away from the affected side. However, this typically very late finding in a tension pneumothorax may not be present despite the rapid decompensation of the patient's clinical status. For this reason, you must be vigilant in watching for the cardiopulmonary findings associated with a tension pneumothorax and not rely on the presence of all the classic physical findings in making the diagnosis.

The accumulation of air within the pleural space decreases the lung volume and diminishes the breath sounds on the affected side when you auscultate the chest. Because air causes the loss of breath sounds on that side, the chest will be resonant (like a bell) when percussed, as opposed to the dull sensation expected with fluid or blood buildup.

A patient with a developing or early tension pneumothorax often reports pleuritic chest pain and dyspnea because of the injury and the collapsing lung. The resulting hypoxia in a patient with a developing tension pneumothorax may cause the patient to become anxious, tachycardic, tachypneic, and even cyanotic.

Hypotension—a late finding of tension pneumothorax—should not be used to either confirm or exclude the possibility of a tension pneumothorax. Its presence may suggest the pneumothorax has produced such significant pressure as to severely impede preload, or it may represent a simultaneous shock state due to other injuries. A normal blood pressure suggests when other signs of a tension pneumothorax are present, the heart is adequately compensating for the diminished venous return.

In a patient with tension pneumothorax, you should first focus on maintaining the ABCs. Inspect the chest and cover any open wounds with an occlusive or nonporous dressing. If signs of developing tension are present, then lift one corner of the dressing to allow air to escape. In the event of a closed tension pneumothorax, call early for paramedic backup to perform a needle chest decompression and for treatment of possible dysrhythmias or transport rapidly to a trauma center, depending on which is faster.

Words of Wisdom

Assessment findings in a patient experiencing a pneumothorax that is developing tension include the following:

- Unilaterally decreased or absent breath sounds
- Unequal chest rise
- Dyspnea
- Tachypnea
- Respiratory distress
- Extreme anxiety
- Cyanosis
- Bulging of the intercostal muscles
- Tachycardia
- Hypotension
- Narrowed pulse pressure
- Subcutaneous emphysema
- Jugular venous distention (JVD)
- Tracheal deviation
- Hyperresonance
- Pulsus paradoxus

Tracheal deviation and JVD are late signs and should not be used as determining factors for initiating invasive treatment. Moreover, JVD may not occur at all in patients with hypovolemia.

▶ Hemothorax

A hemothorax occurs when the potential space between the parietal and visceral pleura is violated and blood begins to accumulate within this space Figure 31-14. Although it is most commonly caused by tears of lung parenchyma, a hemothorax may sometimes result from penetrating wounds that puncture the heart or major vessels within the mediastinum or from blunt trauma with deceleration shearing of major vessels or of intercostal vessels. Rib fractures and injuries to the lung parenchyma are the most common sources of injury in cases of hemothorax. Other causes include injury to the liver, spleen, aorta, internal mammary arteries, intercostal arteries (which can lose up to 50 mL of blood per minute), and other intrathoracic vessels. The location of these injuries makes controlling the bleeding impossible in the prehospital setting; in turn, the amount of circulating blood can be greatly reduced, causing hypovolemic shock. A hemothorax is a life-threatening injury that frequently requires the urgent placement of a chest tube and/or surgery.

A **massive hemothorax** is defined as accumulation of more than 1,500 mL of blood within the pleural space. For the average adult, this amount represents a nearly 25% to 30% blood volume loss, meaning that the patient's condition has progressed to decompensated shock. Because each lung can hold up to 3,000 mL of blood, it is possible for a patient to completely bleed out into the thoracic cavity.

As blood accumulates, it causes lung collapse. The degree of respiratory insufficiency depends on the amount of blood in the pleural space. Hypoxia results from the decreased gas exchange, and hypotension and inadequate perfusion may result from the blood loss. Hypoxia and hypovolemic shock develop rapidly.

Signs and symptoms of a massive hemothorax are produced by hypovolemia and respiratory compromise. You should suspect a hemothorax if the patient has signs and symptoms of shock or decreased breath sounds on the affected side—an indication that the lung is being compressed by the blood. Expect to find tachypnea; tachycardia; dyspnea; respiratory distress; hypotension; a narrowed pulse pressure; pleuritic chest pain; pale, cool, moist skin; dullness on percussion; and decreased

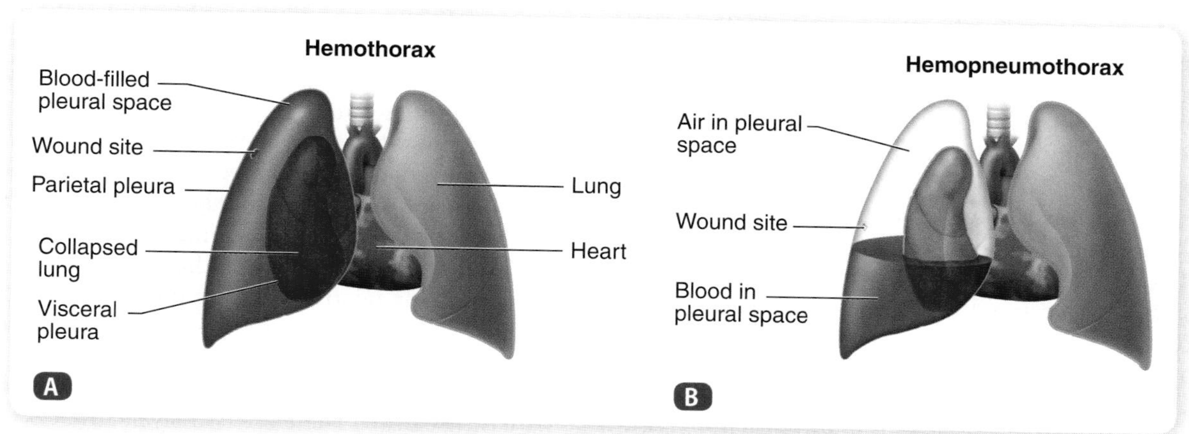

Figure 31-14 A. A hemothorax is a collection of blood in the pleural space produced by bleeding within the chest. **B.** When blood and air are present, the condition is called a hemopneumothorax.

or unequal breath sounds. Neck veins will be flat with associated hypovolemia or distended if there is increased intrathoracic pressure.

A **hemopneumothorax** is a pneumothorax with air and bleeding in the pleural space. Findings and management are the same as those for a hemothorax.

Managing the ABCs is the key consideration for patients with hemothorax. Administer oxygen and provide positive pressure ventilation as needed. If hypovolemia is present, then give a fluid bolus, while using caution so as not to increase blood pressure past the point of maintaining perfusion and further increase bleeding. Provide rapid transport.

▶ Pulmonary Contusion

In addition to fracturing ribs, any severe blunt trauma to the chest can injure the lung, leading to pulmonary contusion, or bruising of the lung parenchyma. The pulmonary alveoli may become filled with blood in such a case, and fluid may accumulate in the injured area, leaving the patient hypoxic. Lung compliance is also decreased with such injuries. Pulmonary contusion is the most common injury from blunt thoracic trauma, and it is commonly associated with a rib fracture.

Severe pulmonary contusion should always be suspected in patients with a flail chest and usually develops over a period of hours. The damage in such a case may be diffuse or localized. Bruising of the lung parenchyma may also occur with high-energy shock waves from an explosion, high-velocity missile wounds, wounds from low-velocity weapons, and rapid deceleration. Pulmonary contusions are often missed because of the high incidence of other associated injuries. To ensure you recognize them, you must maintain a high index of suspicion based on the MOI.

Although pulmonary contusion is usually caused by blunt trauma, it may also occur in scenarios involving explosions or events that create shock waves. There are three physical mechanisms for creating pulmonary contusions. The first is the implosion effect. With this mechanism, overexpansion of air in the lungs secondary to a pressure wave causes blunt trauma and results in rapid, excessive stretching and tearing of the alveoli. The second mechanism, the inertial effect, strips the alveoli from the heavier bronchial structures when the alveoli are pulled at varying rates by a pressure wave. The final mechanism is the Spalding effect, in which the liquid–gas interface, or exchange, is disrupted by a shock wave. The wave releases energy, and this differential transmission of energy causes disruption of the tissues.

Alveolar and capillary damage resulting from any of these mechanisms cause interstitial and intra-alveolar hemorrhage. It immediately leads to a loss of fluid and blood into the involved tissues, followed by white blood cell migration into the area, and, eventually, local tissue edema. This inflammation and local tissue injury and edema dilute the local surfactant in the alveoli, diminishing their compliance and causing alveolar collapse (atelectasis).The edema also reduces the delivery of oxygen across the capillary–alveolar interface, resulting in hypoxia. The hypoxia then worsens the situation by thickening the mucus produced, which may in turn lead to bronchiolar obstruction, air trapping, or an increase in physiologic dead air space and further atelectasis.

If the contusion is large, then the body attempts to compensate for its effects by vasoconstricting pulmonary blood flow and increasing cardiac output. Specifically, there is an attempt to shunt blood from the injured area and increase its delivery to pulmonary tissue that may be able to oxygenate the blood. This pulmonary shunting decreases the functional reserve capacity and leads to mixed venous blood being returned to the heart, further worsening the hypoxemia.

Hypoxia and carbon dioxide retention lead to respiratory distress, dyspnea, tachypnea, agitation, and restlessness. Because of the capillary injury and the hemorrhage into the pulmonary parenchyma, the patient may present with hemoptysis (coughing up blood). Evidence of overlying injury may include contusions, tenderness, crepitus, or paradoxical motion. Auscultation may reveal wheezes, rhonchi, rales, or diminished breath sounds in the affected area. In severe cases, cyanosis and low oxygen saturation levels may be found. The degree of respiratory compromise is directly related to the size of the area of contusion.

Treatment for pulmonary contusion is supportive. When managing a pulmonary contusion, both high-concentration oxygen and positive pressure ventilation may be used to overcome the pathologic changes described earlier. Do not overhydrate the patient as this will create an increase in pulmonary edema and bleeding. Give only small amounts of IV fluid to improve cardiac output as needed, titrating to a systolic blood pressure of 80 to 90 mm Hg.

▶ Cardiac Tamponade

In cardiac tamponade, also known as pericardial tamponade, blood or other fluid collects in the **pericardium**, the fibrous sac surrounding the heart Figure 31-15. In the context of chronic medical conditions, that fluid buildup occurs over time, and can be tolerated to a degree. In the context of acute trauma, that fluid is almost always blood and accumulates rapidly. This prevents the heart from filling during the diastolic phase, causing a decrease in the amount of blood pumped to the body and lowering the blood pressure. Ultimately, as blood accumulates within the pericardial sac, it compresses the heart until it can no longer function and cardiac arrest occurs. Cardiac tamponade is relatively uncommon and is seen more often with penetrating injuries to the heart itself than with blunt injuries to the chest.

The pericardium attaches to the great vessels at the base of the heart. There are two layers: the visceral pericardium, which forms the epicardium, and the parietal pericardium, which is regarded as the sac itself. The purpose of the pericardium is to anchor the heart, restricting excess movement and preventing kinking of the great vessels. The space between the layers can normally hold 30 to

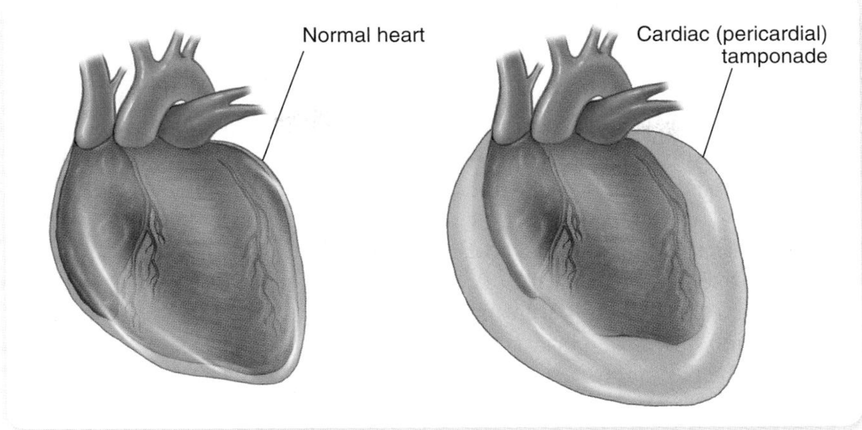

Figure 31-15 Cardiac tamponade is a potentially fatal condition in which blood builds up within the pericardial sac, causing compression of the heart's chambers and dramatically impairing its ability to pump blood to the body.

50 mL of fluid and can slowly distend with as much as 1,000 to 1,500 mL of blood or other fluid.

Accumulation of fluid over minutes to hours leads to increases in intrapericardial pressure. The more pliable structures within the pericardium—namely, the atria and the venae cavae—become compressed, which drastically reduces the preload being delivered to the heart and thereby diminishes stroke volume. The heart initially attempts to compensate for this reduction in preload by increasing the heart rate; however, this attempt to maintain cardiac output is only temporary because the continued bleeding will further restrict preload and diastolic filling. The pressure

YOU are the Provider PART 4

Your partner arrives with the spinal immobilization equipment. During your primary survey, you do not visualize any additional injuries. You secure your patient to the backboard, administer 100% oxygen via a nonrebreathing mask, and, with the assistance of track personnel, carry the patient approximately 1,000 feet (30 m) to your ambulance. On the basis of the patient's MOI and visible injuries, you elect to establish an 18-gauge IV line at a to-keep-open (TKO) rate given his blood pressure. You decide to provide rapid transport to the Level I trauma center instead of the community hospital based on the patient's injuries. Once en route, you contact the trauma center personnel and advise them of your estimated time of arrival. You establish a second 18-gauge IV line en route and set the line to a TKO rate. On arrival, you give your report to the trauma department staff and prepare your ambulance for the next call.

Recording Time: 15 Minutes	
Respirations	30 breaths/min, shallow
Pulse	Strong and regular, 136 beats/min
Skin	Warm, dry, and pink
Blood pressure	104/62 mm Hg
Oxygen saturation (Spo_2)	97% on 100% oxygen
Pupils	PERRLA

7. Would this patient meet trauma system activation and/or criteria?
8. What are some possible interventions that may be required if the patient's condition deteriorates en route to the trauma center?

within the pericardial sac will also reduce the perfusion in the myocardium, resulting in global myocardial dysfunction. The combination of these two processes leads to the development of hypotension. Fluid amounts as small as 50 mL can cause a reduction in cardiac output. Ischemic dysfunction may result in infarction. Removal of as little as 20 mL of blood may drastically improve cardiac output.

Cardiac tamponade can occur in both medical and trauma patients. In the medical setting, inflammatory processes (ie, pericarditis, uremia, myocardial infarction) lead to the slow collection of fluid within the pericardial sac and the gradual distention of the parietal pericardium. Conversely, the bleeding in the trauma patient is rapid, with blood loss from the coronary vasculature or the myocardium quickly collecting between the visceral and parietal pericardium.

The reduced cardiac output, hypoperfusion, and hypotension observed in cardiac tamponade produce the findings typical of a patient in shock: weak or absent peripheral pulses, diaphoresis, dyspnea, cyanosis, altered mental status, tachycardia, tachypnea, and agitation. Although these symptoms alone do not suggest or exclude the presence of cardiac tamponade, identifying them can flesh out the physical assessment. The classic signs of cardiac tamponade are known as Beck triad—narrowing pulse pressure, neck vein distention, and muffled heart tones—but occur only in the advanced stage. As noted earlier, heart tones can be difficult to auscultate in the often noisy prehospital setting or ambulance.

Physical findings in a patient with cardiac tamponade are not significantly different than those of a tension pneumothorax—namely, hypotension, JVD, tachycardia, altered mental status, and signs of tissue hypoperfusion. One way to differentiate between the two is to remember in cardiac tamponade, the breath sounds will be equal and the trachea will be midline because the lungs are not affected. Table 31-2 compares the physical findings of these two emergencies.

In the patient with cardiac tamponade, it is essential to assess and manage the ABCs, administering oxygen and positive pressure ventilation as needed. Inspect the chest and cover any open wounds with an occlusive dressing. Initiate large-bore IV access and provide a rapid fluid bolus to maintain systolic blood pressure at 80 to 90 mm Hg. Administering IV fluids may slow the patient's deterioration by momentarily increasing preload. Provide rapid transport and call for paramedic backup for treatment of potential dysrhythmias.

The ultimate treatment for cardiac tamponade is **pericardiocentesis**, which involves inserting a needle attached to a syringe far enough into the chest to penetrate the pericardium to withdraw fluid.

▶ Myocardial Contusion

Myocardial contusion, or bruising of the heart muscle, may occur from blunt trauma. Blunt myocardial injury results in hemorrhage with edema and fragmented myocardial fibers along with cellular injury. Vascular damage may occur, and there may be a lacerated epicardium or endocardium. The fibrinous reaction at the contusion site may lead to delayed rupture or a ventricular aneurysm. The areas of damage are well demarcated, and conduction defects may occur resulting in cardiac dysrhythmias. Right- or left-side heart failure may also be present. See Chapter 18, *Cardiovascular Emergencies*, for a review of heart failure.

As an AEMT, you must maintain a high index of suspicion for serious injury in all patients with blunt chest trauma. Clinical signs of myocardial contusion will vary based on the area of injury—affected areas may include the vessels, the myocardium, or the conduction system.

Table 31-2 Physical Findings of Cardiac Tamponade Versus Tension Pneumothorax

Physical Finding	Cardiac Tamponade	Tension Pneumothorax
Presenting sign/symptom	Shock	Respiratory distress
Neck veins	Distended	Distended
Trachea	Midline	Deviated (late sign)
Breath sounds	Equal on both sides	Decreased or absent on side of injury
Chest percussion	Normal	Hyperresonant on side of injury
Heart sounds	Muffled	Typically, normal

Associated injuries include one to three rib fractures and/or a sternal fracture. The patient may also present with sharp, retrosternal chest pain. The patient may or may not show external signs, such as bruising. Inspect the area to identify any soft-tissue or bone injury. Crackles or rales (due to pulmonary edema from left ventricular dysfunction) may be heard on auscultation. Often, the pulse rate is irregular, but life-threatening dysrhythmias such as ventricular tachycardia and ventricular fibrillation are less common.

When you are treating a patient for a myocardial contusion, stay alert for signs of heart failure and beware of the risks of administering too much fluid if these signs appear. Provide supportive care including administering oxygen, frequently assessing vital signs, and establishing IV access. Assess for JVD and pulmonary edema. Call for paramedic backup early, and carefully monitor for rapid deterioration if the patient presents with tachycardia or an irregular pulse.

▶ Myocardial Rupture

Myocardial rupture is an acute perforation of the ventricles, atria, intraventricular septum, intra-atrial septum, chordae tendineae, papillary muscles, or valves. Severe blunt force to the chest compresses the heart between the sternum and the vertebrae, which can rupture the myocardium. In penetrating trauma, a foreign object or bony fragment may be propelled into the heart, resulting in a laceration of the myocardial wall. Whether it occurs from a penetrating injury or blunt trauma, a ruptured myocardium is a life-threatening event.

Patients with myocardial rupture may present with acute pulmonary edema or signs of cardiac tamponade. They should receive supportive care and be rapidly transported to a facility where a thoracotomy can be performed.

▶ Traumatic Aortic Disruption

Rupture of the aorta (also called **traumatic aortic disruption**) and aortic dissection occur most often in blunt trauma patients as a result of MVCs and falls. Aortic rupture occurs when an aortic aneurysm (an outpouching of the aorta where the vessel's diameter exceeds 5 cm) bursts, causing massive blood loss.[15] Aortic dissection, by comparison, involves a tear in the aortic intima and the formation of a false channel in the aorta; the diversion of blood into this false channel results in poor perfusion to the organs and tissues normally supplied with blood from this source.[15] Of patients with an aortic *rupture*, only 60% survive until they arrive at the hospital; that is, 40% die in the prehospital stage.[16] Notably, fewer than one-third of patients with either type of traumatic aortic disruption survive 3 days or longer.[16] Given the body's entire blood volume passes through the aorta or great vessel, the high mortality associated with such an injury comes as no surprise. Nevertheless, some patients reached by EMS personnel can survive with prompt management including surgical intervention.

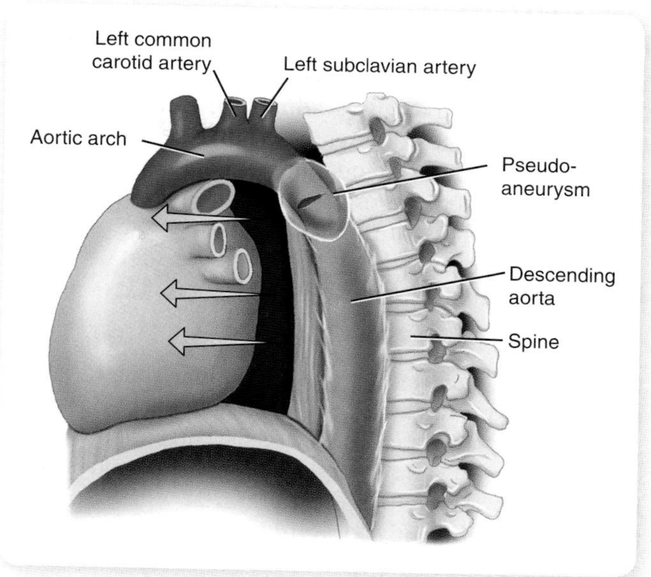

Figure 31-16 Tension from a rapid deceleration injury can cause the descending aorta to rupture at its point of attachment to the posterior thoracic wall.

The most widely accepted theory of how aortic dissection evolves holds that the aorta is injured at its fixed points due to shearing forces. The high-velocity, high-energy impacts that result in these injuries cause the aortic arch to swing forward. The resulting tension, along with rotation and torque on the area, causes the descending aorta to rupture at its point of attachment to the posterior thoracic wall **Figure 31-16**.

As shown in Figure 31-16, the aorta includes three layers—the intima, the media, and the adventitia. If the injury tears the intima, then the high pressure within the aorta allows the blood to dissect along the media. More severe injuries damage all three layers of the aorta, allowing blood to leak from the aorta into the surrounding tissues. If these tissues cannot stop the bleeding, then the patient can survive only with prompt intervention; otherwise, the injury will be rapidly fatal.

Recognizing a traumatic aortic disruption often comes from a high index of suspicion based on the MOI because a high percentage of patients have no signs of external chest trauma. Assessment findings associated with traumatic aortic disruption include retrosternal or interscapular pain described as "tearing," dyspnea, dysphagia, hoarseness or stridor, ischemic pain of the extremities, and upper extremity hypertension with absent or decreased strength of femoral pulses. Hypotension and signs of shock may present as bleeding continues.

Medical care of patients with dissection or rupture of the aorta includes completing a primary survey, maintaining the ABCs, and providing immediate transport. The patient should receive gradual IV hydration en route to treat the hypotension. Aggressive fluid administration may result in sudden changes in the intra-aortic pressure that could worsen the injury. Expedited transport to a trauma center is essential.

▶ Penetrating Wounds of the Great Vessels

Injuries to the great vessels usually are associated with injuries to the chest, abdomen, or neck. The chest contains several large blood vessels: the superior vena cava, the inferior vena cava, the pulmonary arteries, four main pulmonary veins, and the aorta, with its major branches distributing blood throughout the body. The abdominal aorta and inferior vena cava travel through the abdomen, and the carotid arteries and external jugular veins are located in the neck. Wounds to any of these vessels may be accompanied by massive hemorrhage, hypovolemic shock, cardiac tamponade, and enlarging hematomas. Frequently, blood loss is not obvious because it remains within the chest cavity. Hematomas may cause compression of any structure, including the vena cava, trachea, esophagus, great vessels, or heart. Here, particularly, immediate transport to the hospital is critical—a few minutes can mean the difference between life and death.

The management of potential injuries to the great vessels includes maintaining ABCs. Establish an IV line to provide hydration en route to the trauma center. Consider air transport if transport to a Level I trauma center may be delayed due to distance.

▶ Diaphragmatic Injury

Injuries to the diaphragm may be the result of blunt or penetrating trauma. Because the diaphragm is protected by the liver on the right side, most diaphragmatic injuries (particularly those due to blunt trauma) occur on the left side. Once the diaphragm has been injured, the healing process is inhibited by the natural pressure differences between the abdominal and thoracic cavities.

Diaphragmatic injury may be life threatening; in studies, the overall mortality for such injuries has varied widely depending on the extent of injury and treatment.[17] Injury occurs as high-pressure compression to the abdomen results in an increase in intra-abdominal pressure. Bowel obstruction and strangulation may also occur. As the diaphragm impinges on the thoracic cage, lung expansion is restricted, causing hypoventilation and hypoxia. A mediastinal shift can result in cardiac and respiratory compromise.

Injury to the diaphragm and the associated physical findings have been separated into three phases: acute, latent, and obstructive. The acute phase begins at the time of injury and ends with recovery from other injuries, which may overshadow the diaphragmatic injury, and serves to explain why more than two-thirds of these injuries are missed at the time of hospital admission.[18] In the latent phase, the patient experiences intermittent abdominal pain due to the periodic herniation or entrapment of abdominal contents in the defect. The obstructive phase occurs when any abdominal contents herniate through the defect, cutting off their blood supply (infarct) in the process.

A rare but ultimate complication of a diaphragmatic injury is the herniation of sufficient abdominal contents into the thoracic cavity. The resulting increased intrathoracic pressure both compresses the lung on the affected side and compromises circulatory function; this finding is called a tension gastrothorax.[19]

Signs and symptoms of diaphragmatic injury may be subtle. Findings include tachypnea, tachycardia, respiratory distress, dullness to percussion, scaphoid (hollow; boat-shaped) abdomen, bowel sounds in the affected hemithorax, and decreased breath sounds.

Little can be done in the prehospital environment for diaphragmatic injury. Elevate the head of the backboard or stretcher as possible to help keep abdominal contents in the abdominal cavity and provide positive pressure ventilation for hypoventilation.

Words of Wisdom

Avoid using nitrous oxide in patients with a possible diaphragmatic injury because it can greatly increase the volume of gas within entrapped viscera.

▶ Esophageal Injury

Penetrating trauma is the most frequent cause of esophageal injury. It is rare in blunt trauma, but could potentially be life threatening if undetected. Missile and knife wounds may penetrate the esophagus, or it may perforate spontaneously in violent emesis, carcinoma (cancer), or anatomic distortions produced by diverticula or gastric reflux. Damage to the esophagus is often associated with other significant injuries because of its location in the body.

Patients typically present with pain (eg, pleuritic chest pain or pain made worse by swallowing), hoarseness, dysphagia, respiratory distress, and shock. Signs of cervical esophageal perforation include local tenderness and subcutaneous emphysema. In nontraumatic causes, you may be able to detect resistance of the neck on passive motion. Such an exam is contraindicated in trauma patients. If the perforation is in the intrathoracic esophagus, then signs may include mediastinal emphysema, mediastinitis, subcutaneous emphysema (suspect associated tracheal injury), mediastinal crunch, and splinting of the chest wall.

Prehospital care for a patient with esophageal injury is supportive. Manage the patient's symptoms.

▶ Tracheobronchial Injuries

Tracheobronchial injuries are rare, occurring in fewer than 3% of chest trauma cases.[20] When they occur, they are usually the result of blunt or penetrating trauma and carry a high mortality rate.

As with aortic injuries, the site of a tracheobronchial injury is often close to a point of attachment—namely, the carina. The injury to the trachea or mainstem bronchi allows for rapid movement of air into the pleural space, resulting in a pneumothorax. As this injury progresses to a tension pneumothorax, a needle thoracentesis is often insufficient because the rate of air entry into the pleural space exceeds the rate at which the air can escape from the inserted angiocatheter. Such injury also causes severe hypoxia.

Findings associated with tracheobronchial injuries include hoarseness, tachypnea, tachycardia, massive subcutaneous emphysema, dyspnea, respiratory distress, hemoptysis, and signs of tension pneumothorax that do not respond to needle decompression.

Early recognition and rapid transport are key to managing tracheobronchial injuries. Treat the patient symptomatically, positioning appropriately and ventilating as needed. Because of the rapid loss of air into the pleural space, high ventilatory pressures should be avoided when you are providing positive pressure ventilation (bag the patient gently and slowly).

▶ Traumatic Asphyxia

Sometimes patients will experience a sudden, severe compression injury of the chest, which produces a rapid increase in intrathoracic pressure. This condition is called **traumatic asphyxia** **Figure 31-17**. Traumatic asphyxia may occur in an unrestrained driver who hits a steering wheel or a pedestrian who is compressed between a vehicle and a wall. A sudden compressional force squeezes the chest, and blood backs up into the head and neck, causing the jugular veins to engorge and capillaries to rupture.

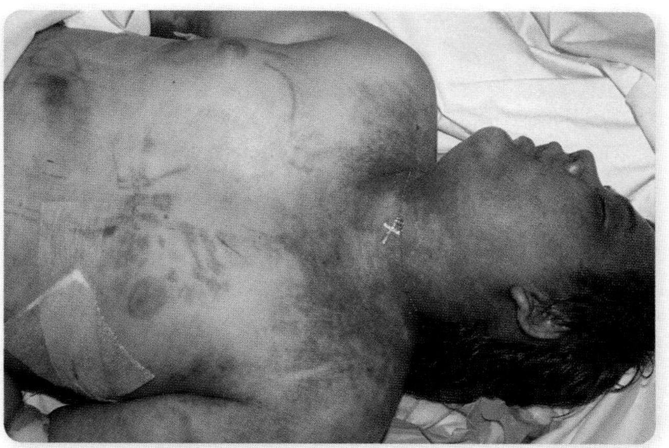

Figure 31-17 Traumatic asphyxia has a characteristic appearance.

The sudden increase in intrathoracic pressure results in the characteristic appearance of traumatic asphyxia, including distended neck veins; cyanosis in the face and upper neck, extremities, and the torso above the level of the compression; and swelling and cyanosis of the tongue and lips. Ocular hemorrhage may be mild, such as bleeding into the anterior surface of the eye (**subconjunctival hematoma**), or extremely dramatic, causing the eyes to protrude from their normal position (**exophthalmos**). The skin below the area of compression remains normal color, and hypotension occurs when the pressure is released.

Again, early recognition and rapid transport are key. Treat the patient's symptoms, position the patient appropriately, and ventilate as needed. Take cervical spine precautions, including spinal immobilization. Obtain IV access with two large-bore IV lines. Transport the patient to the nearest appropriate trauma center.

YOU are the Provider SUMMARY

1. Should you immediately approach the patient? Is the scene safe?

No, the scene is not safe, and you should not immediately approach the patient. Whenever your ambulance provides standby services at an event, it is always recommended to meet with the event representative, who will brief you on the positioning of the ambulance, access and egress routes, and any hand signals or visual clues that may direct you. The scene cannot be made safe until all of the motocross riders have stopped riding on the track. You should not enter the track until all riders have come to a stop and you are directed to enter by the event representative.

2. What are some possible injuries this patient could have?

Until proven otherwise, this patient has multisystem trauma and may present with a wide variety of injuries. You should expect both open and closed fractures, arterial bleeding, hemothorax, pneumothorax, and hemodynamic instability.

3. Does this patient require spinal immobilization?

Initially, this patient requires, at a minimum, manual stabilization of the head. A complete and thorough history and physical exam, in conjunction with your local protocols, will further direct your actions.

4. Does this patient require helmet removal?

If you are able to adequately treat and immobilize the patient with his helmet in place, then it should remain on his head. However, if the helmet interferes with the ability to administer oxygen or ventilation or to otherwise manage the airway, or it interferes with your ability to properly secure the patient to a spinal immobilization device, it should be removed using the technique described in Chapter 30, *Head and Spine Injuries*. In general, motocross helmets do not fit the head tight enough to allow effective immobilization to occur while the patient is still wearing one.

5. What are some possible causes of this patient's dyspnea?

This patient could possibly be experiencing a flail chest injury, hemothorax, pneumothorax, pulmonary contusion, myocardial contusion, cardiac tamponade, or possibly tracheobronchial disruption.

6. Does this patient require rapid transport to the hospital?

A blow significant enough to fracture the sternum causes severe hyperflexion of the thoracic cage. The patient's condition is critical. Myocardial and/or pulmonary contusion or myocardial rupture may occur with compression of the thorax. Because of these facts, rapid transport to the appropriate facility is critical.

7. Would this patient meet trauma system activation and/or criteria?

Typical trauma center criteria fall into one of three categories: anatomic, physiologic, and mechanism criteria, as discussed in Chapter 26, *Trauma Overview*. On the basis of these criteria, the patient would meet any Level I trauma center activation protocols.

8. What are some possible interventions that may be required if the patient's condition deteriorates en route to the trauma center?

The patient may require positive pressure ventilations with a bag-mask device, increased fluid boluses, and CPR. Paramedic interventions may include endotracheal intubation and needle chest decompression.

YOU are the Provider SUMMARY (continued)

EMS Patient Care Report (PCR)					
Date: 07-07-18	**Incident No.:** 20093913671		**Nature of Call:** Traumatic injury	**Location:** Glendale Motorsports	
Dispatched: —	**En Route:** —	**At Scene:** 1420	**Transport:** 1432	**At Hospital:** 1450	**In Service:** 1515
Patient Information					
Age: 24 **Sex:** M **Weight (in kg [lb]):** 82 kg (180 lb)			**Allergies:** No known drug allergies **Medications:** None **Past Medical History:** Multiple broken bones from extreme sports **Chief Complaint:** Blunt chest trauma		
Vital Signs					
Time: 1425	**BP:** 98/55	**Pulse:** 120	**Respirations:** 32	**Spo_2:** 97%	
Time: 1440	**BP:** 104/62	**Pulse:** 136	**Respirations:** 30	**Spo_2:** 97%	
Time:	**BP:**	**Pulse:**	**Respirations:**	**Spo_2:**	
EMS Treatment (circle all that apply)					
Oxygen @ 15 **L/min via (circle one):** **NC** **(NRM — circled)** **Bag-mask device**		**Assisted Ventilation**	**Airway Adjunct**	**CPR**	
Defibrillation	**Bleeding Control**	**Bandaging**	**Splinting**	**(Other — circled): ** Spinal immobilization; established two 18-gauge IV lines	
Narrative					
EMS at Glendale Motorsports for motocross race. Witnessed rider in full protective gear (helmet, knee/elbow pads, and chest protector) launch from jump approximately 15 feet in the air and land on his front tire, going headfirst over handlebars, hitting the ground in a left lateral position, ultimately coming to rest in the supine position. As we were waiting for the track official to stop the race, we witnessed another rider making the same jump, come down, and directly hit the first patient's chest. When we were directed onto the track to the patient, he presents AO×4, with a patent airway. Breathing appears labored. Manual stabilization obtained. He is able to recall all events, and states his chest hurts and it is hard to breathe. Shirt and chest protector removed, pain and tenderness noted midsternum, possible crepitus. Patient denies having any head or neck pain. Helmet removed to facilitate immobilization to backboard. Patient secured to board with pulse, motor, sensation present before and after. 100% O_2 applied via a nonrebreathing mask. Bilateral 18-gauge IV lines established both at TKO rate. Patient transported emergent to Altru Hospital with trauma activation requested en route. On arrival, care and report given to ED staff without incident. **Note: Kittson County Hospital was bypassed in lieu of Altru because of the patient meeting trauma protocols. **End of report**					

Prep Kit

▶ Ready for Review

- The thoracic cavity extends from the lower end of the neck to the diaphragm, but an injury to the chest may also injure structures in the abdomen. Always assume there are chest and abdominal injuries when managing a patient who has a chest injury.
- The thorax contains many important structures, such as the trachea and great vessels, and organs, such as the heart and lungs; therefore, chest injuries can have serious consequences, such as adverse effects on the body's ability to perform respiration and ventilation. Respiratory alkalosis and respiratory acidosis can result.
- A blow to the chest (blunt trauma) may fracture the ribs, the sternum, or whole areas of the chest wall. Compression of these structures creates other problems, including contusions of the lungs and the heart and possible damage to the aorta. Even if the skin and chest wall are intact, the contents of the thorax may be injured.
- Thoracic trauma may impair cardiac output, decreasing blood pressure and perfusion to vital organs. Bleeding into the thoracic cavity significantly increases the chance of hypovolemia and hypoxia. Significant blood loss can disrupt critical processes.
- A patient with severe chest pain tends to have shallow breathing. This further reduces minute volume—the volume of air exchanged between the lungs and environment in 1 minute. If blood collects in the thoracic cavity, then this can also prevent full expansion of the lungs.
- There are two types of chest injuries: penetrating (open) injuries and blunt (closed) injuries. Specific chest injuries can include rib fractures, flail chest, sternal fracture, clavicle fracture, commotio cordis, simple pneumothorax, open pneumothorax, tension pneumothorax, hemothorax, hemopneumothorax, pulmonary contusion, cardiac tamponade, myocardial contusion, myocardial rupture, traumatic aortic disruption, penetrating wounds of the great vessels, diaphragmatic injury, esophageal injury, tracheobronchial injuries, and traumatic asphyxia.
- Signs and symptoms of chest injury include pain at the site of injury or localized pain that worsens with breathing; bruising to the chest wall; crepitus; penetrating injury to the chest; dyspnea; hemoptysis; failure of one or both sides of the chest to expand normally with inspiration; rapid, weak pulse; low blood pressure; and cyanosis around the lips or fingernail beds.
- Note whether heart sounds are easily heard or muffled on auscultation. Muffled heart sounds are an important clue when distinguishing tension pneumothorax and cardiac tamponade.
- Jugular vein distention suggests increased intravenous pressure that can occur with a tension pneumothorax. Note that jugular vein distention must be measured with the patient in a 45° semi-Fowler position.
- If the patient's mental status permits, then ask about a history of dyspnea, chest pain, other areas of pain or discomfort, symptoms before the incident, history of cardiorespiratory disease, any medications the patient may be taking, and in a motor vehicle collision, whether restraints were used.
- Monitoring a patient's airway, breathing, and circulation (ABCs) is the primary management for all patients; this is no different for the patient with thoracic injury. Occlude open chest wounds with an occlusive dressing. Stabilize any flail segments. Administer positive pressure ventilation if indicated. Consider definitive airway management. Maintain circulation and gain intravenous (IV) access. Finally, call for additional backup if needed and provide rapid transport.
- IV fluid therapy during thoracic trauma should be closely monitored and administered according to local protocol. The goal is to maintain adequate perfusion without causing a marked increase in blood pressure.
- Any injury to the thoracic cavity may disrupt normal cardiac function. Always treat the patient based on advanced cardiac life support and local protocols. Consider aggressive airway management.
- Multiple rib fractures, with or without a fracture of the sternum, often result in flail chest, in which a portion of the chest wall is detached from the thoracic cage and moves paradoxically during respiration.
- Flail chest causes painful breathing and requires respiratory support and supplemental high-flow oxygen. External stabilization of a flail chest is not indicated. Positive pressure ventilation may be necessary in severe cases with resultant inadequate ventilator function.
- If a sternal fracture is present, then you should expect to find pain and tenderness over the sternum, and crepitus on palpation.
- If a clavicle fracture is present, then you should splint it with a sling and swathe. Clavicle fracture can lead to neurovascular compromise.
- Commotio cordis is cardiac arrest that results from a patient receiving a blow during the heart's repolarization period. Such a patient may present with ventricular fibrillation that responds positively to defibrillation provided within the first 3 minutes.
- Simple pneumothorax is the accumulation of air in the pleural space, occurring when air enters a hole in the chest wall or lung. The lung collapses as pressure builds in the pleural space. Cover open

Prep Kit *(continued)*

chest wounds with an occlusive dressing and manage the ABCs.

- Spontaneous pneumothorax can occur in people with weak areas on the surface of the lungs. The patient will experience sudden, sharp pain and shortness of breath without known cause. The most critical intervention is conducting repeated assessments to ensure the injury has not progressed to a tension pneumothorax.
- Open pneumothorax is a pneumothorax in which the pleural space is in direct contact with the atmosphere. The opening causes increased thoracic pressure and the lung collapses. Sucking sounds may be heard on inhalation; this is often called a sucking chest wound.
- Seal a sucking chest wound with an occlusive dressing. If the patient shows signs of a tension pneumothorax, then burp the dressing (raise one side of the dressing to allow air to escape).
- A tension pneumothorax can occur in a closed, blunt injury of the chest in which a fractured rib lacerates the surface of the lung or as a result of the paper bag syndrome. The classic signs of a tension pneumothorax are an absence of breath sounds on the affected side, unequal chest rise, tachycardia and dysrhythmias such as progression to ventricular tachycardia and ventricular fibrillation, jugular vein distention, narrow pulse pressure, and as a very late sign, tracheal deviation. In the event of a closed tension pneumothorax, consider calling for paramedic backup because needle chest decompression will need to be performed.
- Hemothorax is a life-threatening condition in which blood accumulates between the parietal and visceral pleura of the lung. Look for signs and symptoms of shock and decreased breath sounds on the affected side. Manage the ABCs, administer oxygen and positive pressure ventilation as needed, give a fluid bolus if needed, and provide rapid transport.
- Pulmonary contusion is bruising of the lung and may occur in conjunction with fractured ribs. Treatment is supportive. Ensure you do not overhydrate the patient because this could create increased pulmonary edema and bleeding.
- Cardiac tamponade is collection of blood in the pericardium, which prevents the heart from pumping effectively. Signs and symptoms include weak or absent peripheral pulses, diaphoresis, dyspnea, cyanosis, altered mental status, tachycardia, tachypnea, and agitation; Beck triad (narrowing pulse pressure, distended neck veins, and muffled heart sounds) occurs in the advanced state. Manage the ABCs, administer oxygen, and be cautious with positive pressure ventilation because this may cause a tension pneumothorax. Provide a rapid fluid bolus to maintain cardiac output and ensure rapid transport.
- Myocardial contusion is bruising of the heart muscle, which can lead to heart failure. Maintain a high suspicion for serious injury in patients who experience blunt chest trauma. Pulse may be irregular, but life-threatening dysrhythmias are uncommon. Limit fluids if signs of heart failure are present.
- Myocardial rupture is acute perforation of any portion of the heart. This life-threatening condition requires aggressive care of the ABCs and rapid transport.
- Traumatic aortic disruption is dissection or rupture of the aorta. Recognition often comes from a high index of suspicion based on the MOI. Assessment may reveal retrosternal or interscapular pain described as "tearing," ischemic pain of the extremities, and hoarseness or stridor, among others. Management includes maintaining the ABCs and taking care not to overhydrate and increase bleeding.
- Laceration of the large blood vessels in the chest can cause a fatal hemorrhage. Suspect this condition in any patient with a chest wound who shows signs of shock, even if you see little blood; it may be collecting within the chest cavity. Provide immediate transport—a few minutes can be the difference between life and death.
- The diaphragm can be injured when the chest is injured, but signs and symptoms can be subtle. Findings include scaphoid abdomen, dullness to percussion, and (sometimes) bowel sounds in the affected side of the thorax. Provide rapid transport.
- Esophageal injury, like many chest injuries, is a life-threatening condition. Signs may include local tenderness and subcutaneous emphysema. Provide rapid transport.
- Damage to the esophagus is often associated with other significant injuries because of its location in the body. Patients typically present with pain, hoarseness, dysphagia, respiratory distress, and shock. Prehospital care is supportive.
- Tracheobronchial injuries are rare but can be a significant cause of mortality. An injury to the trachea or mainstem bronchi allows for rapid movement of air into the pleural space, resulting in a pneumothorax. If this occurs, then the tension pneumothorax may not respond to needle chest decompression.
- Traumatic asphyxia occurs when a patient experiences sudden, severe compression injury to the chest, causing a rapid increase in intrathoracic pressure. This injury squeezes the chest, such that blood backs

Prep Kit *(continued)*

up into the head and neck, causing the appearance of distended neck veins; cyanosis in the face and upper part of the neck, extremities, and the torso above the level of the compression; swelling and cyanosis of the tongue and lips; bulging eyes; and swelling or hemorrhage of the conjunctiva. Skin below the area of compression remains normal color.

▶ Vital Vocabulary

atelectasis Alveolar collapse that prevents the use of that portion of the lung for ventilation and oxygenation.

cardiac output The amount of blood pumped by the heart per minute.

cardiac tamponade Compression of the heart caused by a buildup of blood or other fluid in the pericardial sac.

chemoreceptors Sensors that respond to chemical fluctuations such as a decreased oxygen concentration in the bloodstream.

closed chest injury An injury to the chest in which the skin is not broken, usually from blunt trauma.

commotio cordis An event in which an often fatal cardiac dysrhythmia is produced by a sudden blow to the thoracic cavity.

crepitus The sensation felt when broken bone ends grind together.

exophthalmos Bulging of the eyes.

flail chest A condition in which two or more ribs are fractured in two or more places or in association with a fracture of the sternum, so a segment of chest wall is effectively detached from the rest of the thoracic cage.

hemopneumothorax A collection of blood and air in the pleural cavity.

hemoptysis The spitting or coughing up of blood.

hemothorax A collection of blood in the pleural cavity.

jugular vein distention (JVD) A prominence of the jugular veins caused by increased volume or increased pressure within the central venous system or the thoracic cavity.

massive hemothorax An accumulation of more than 1,500 mL of blood within the pleural space.

mediastinum The central region of the thorax, which contains the heart, great vessels, esophagus, lymphatic channels, trachea, mainstem bronchi, and paired vagus and phrenic nerves.

minute volume The volume of air exchanged between the lungs and environment in 1 minute.

myocardial contusion A bruise of the heart muscle.

myocardial rupture An acute perforation of the ventricles, atria, intraventricular septum, intra-atrial septum, chordae, papillary muscles, or valves.

occlusive dressing A dressing made of gauze with petroleum jelly, aluminum foil, or plastic that prevents air and liquids from entering or exiting a wound.

open chest injury An injury to the chest in which the chest wall itself is penetrated by some external object such as a knife or bullet.

open pneumothorax An accumulation of air or gas in the pleural space, resulting from a defect or penetration into the chest wall that allows air to enter the thoracic cavity.

paper bag syndrome Rupture of the lungs that occurs as the chest meets with blunt trauma after taking a deep breath, usually during a motor vehicle crash, similar to the rupture of an air-filled paper bag.

paradoxical motion The motion of the portion of the chest wall that is detached in a flail chest; the motion—in during inhalation, out during exhalation—is the opposite of normal chest wall motion during breathing.

pericardiocentesis The ultimate treatment for cardiac tamponade, which involves inserting a needle attached to a syringe far enough into the chest to penetrate the pericardium to withdraw fluid.

pericardium The fibrous sac that surrounds the heart.

pleural space Potential space between the visceral and parietal pleura of the lung and chest wall respectively; it is normally absent, as these surfaces are usually in direct contact.

pneumothorax An accumulation of air or gas in the pleural space.

pulmonary contusion A bruise of the lung.

pulse pressure The difference between the systolic blood pressure and the diastolic blood pressure.

pulsus paradoxus A drop in the systolic blood pressure of 10 mm Hg or more; commonly seen in patients with cardiac tamponade or severe asthma.

spontaneous pneumothorax Pneumothorax that occurs when a weak area on the lung ruptures in the absence of major injury, allowing air to leak into the pleural space.

subconjunctival hematoma Bleeding into the anterior surface of the eye.

sucking chest wound An open or penetrating chest wall wound through which air passes during inspiration and expiration, creating a sucking sound.

tension pneumothorax An accumulation of air or gas in the pleural space that progressively collapses the lung with potentially fatal results.

Prep Kit *(continued)*

traumatic aortic disruption Dissection or rupture of the aorta.

traumatic asphyxia A pattern of injuries seen after a severe force is applied to the thorax, forcing blood from the great vessels and back into the head and neck.

▶ References

1. Trauma statistics. National Trauma Institute website. http://nationaltraumainstitute.org/home/trauma_statistics.html. Updated February, 2014. Accessed April 3, 2017.
2. American College of Surgeons, National Trauma Data Bank. National Trauma Data Bank 2015 annual report. https://www.facs.org/~/media/files/quality%20programs/trauma/ntdb/ntdb%20annual%20report%202015.ashx. Accessed April 3, 2017.
3. Legome E. Initial evaluation and management of blunt thoracic trauma in adults. *UpToDate*. http://www.uptodate.com/contents/initial-evaluation-and-management-of-blunt-thoracic-trauma-in-adults#H2. Accessed December 12, 2016.
4. Richens D, Field M, Neale M, Oakley C. The mechanism of injury in blunt traumatic rupture of the aorta. *Eur J Cardiothorac Surg*. 2002;21(2):288-293. http://ejcts.oxfordjournals.org/content/21/2/288.full. Accessed December 12, 2016.
5. Kauvar DS, Lefering R, Wade CE. Impact of hemorrhage on trauma outcome: an overview of epidemiology, clinical presentations, and therapeutic considerations. *J Trauma Injury Infect Crit Care*. 2006;60(6):S3-S11. http://journals.lww.com/jtrauma/Fulltext/2006/06001/Impact_of_Hemorrhage_on_Trauma_Outcome__An.2.aspx. Accessed December 12, 2016.
6. Bjerke, Scott H, MD, Flail Chest. http://emedicine.medscape.com/article/433779-overview#a6. Accessed January 5, 2017.
7. Dehghan N, de Mestral C, McKee MD, Schemitsch EH, Nathens A. Flail chest injuries: a review of outcomes and treatment practices from the National Trauma Data Bank. *J Trauma Acute Care Surg*. 2014;76(2):462-468. https://www.ncbi.nlm.nih.gov/pubmed/24458051. Accessed December 13, 2016.
8. Kilic D, Findikcioglu A, Akin S, Hatipoglu A. Factors affecting morbidity and mortality in flail chest: comparison of anterior and lateral location. *Thoracic Cardiovasc Surg*. 2011;59(1):45-48. https://www.researchgate.net/publication/49763672_Factors_Affecting_Morbidity_and_Mortality_in_Flail_Chest_Comparison_of_Anterior_and_Lateral_Location. Accessed December 13, 2016.
9. Pettiford BL, Luketich JD, Landreneau RJ. The management of flail chest. *Thorac Surg Clin*. 2007;17(1):25-33. https://www.ncbi.nlm.nih.gov/pubmed/17650694. Accessed December 13, 2016.
10. Recinos G, Inaba K, Dubose J, et al. Epidemiology of sternal fractures. *Am Surg*. 2009;75(5):401-404. https://www.ncbi.nlm.nih.gov/pubmed/19445291. Accessed December 13, 2016.
11. Khoriati AA, Rajakulasingam R, Shah R. Sternal fractures and their management. *J Emerg Trauma Shock*. 2013;6(2):113-116. https://www.ncbi.nlm.nih.gov/pubmed/23723620. Accessed December 13, 2016.
12. Maron BJ, Haas TS, Ahluwalia A, Garberich RF, Mark Estes NA III, Link MS. Increasing survival rate from commotio cordis. *Heart Rhythm J*. 2013;10(2):219-223. http://www.heartrhythmjournal.com/article/S1547-5271(12)01254-4/pdf. Accessed December 13, 2016.
13. Light RW. Primary spontaneous pneumothorax in adults. *UpToDate*. http://www.uptodate.com/contents/primary-spontaneous-pneumothorax-in-adults. Accessed December 13, 2016.
14. Sharma A, Jindal P. Principles of diagnosis and management of traumatic pneumothorax. *J Emerg Trauma Shock*. 2008;1:34-41. http://www.onlinejets.org/text.asp?2008/1/1/34/41789. Accessed December 13, 2016.
15. Thoracoaortic aneurysms and dissections: guidance for the primary care clinician. *Medscape Nurses*. February 5, 2007. http://www.medscape.org/viewarticle/551441. Accessed January 6, 2017.
16. Franzen D, Genoni M. Analysis of risk factors for death after blunt traumatic rupture of the thoracic aorta. *Emerg Med J*. 2013. http://emj.bmj.com/content/32/2/124. Accessed December 13, 2016.
17. Vilallonga R, Pastor V, Alvarez L, Charco R, Armengol M, Navarro S. Right-sided diaphragmatic rupture after blunt trauma. An unusual entity. *World J Emerg Surg*. 2011;6:3. http://wjes.biomedcentral.com/articles/10.1186/1749-7922-6-3. Accessed December 13, 2016.
18. Farboud A, Luckraz H, Butchart EG. Delayed presentation of diaphragmatic injury secondary to rib fracture. *Respir Med CME*. 2008;1(2):158-160. http://www.sciencedirect.com/science/article/pii/S1755001708000286. Accessed December 13, 2016.
19. Naess PA, Wiborg J, Kjellevold K, Gaarder C. Tension gastrothorax: acute life-threatening manifestation of late onset congenital diaphragmatic hernia (CDH) in children. *Scand J Trauma Resusc Emerg Med*. 2015;23:49.
20. Prokakis C, Koletsis EN, Dedeilias P, Fligou F, Filos K, Dougenis D. Airway trauma: a review on epidemiology, mechanisms of injury, diagnosis and treatment. *J Cardiothoracic Surg*. 2014;9:117. http://cardiothoracicsurgery.biomedcentral.com/articles/10.1186/1749-8090-9-117. Accessed December 13, 2016.

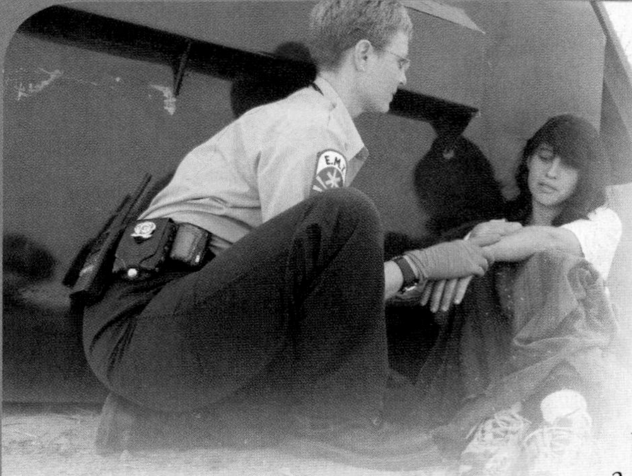

Assessment *in Action*

You are dispatched to a reported gunshot wound on a rural farm road. On arrival, you find an obviously intoxicated man with a 0.22-caliber rifle standing over a man lying prone and not moving. Law enforcement is on scene and secures the weapon. The man tells you the pair were shooting beer cans out of a tree; when his friend was placing a can on a limb, the man accidentally shot him in the back while trying to shoot the can out of his hand. The patient presents with a small entrance wound just medial to his left scapula. Your partner monitors the patient's airway while you log roll the patient and perform a rapid assessment. You note the patient has a patent airway and is breathing at a rate of 34 breaths/min, but appears cyanotic. As you prepare to auscultate breath sounds, you note a small exit wound at the fifth intercostal space just left of the sternum. You note diminished breath sounds on the left, and distended neck veins are noted.

1. On the basis of your findings, you suspect this patient has a:

A. hemopneumothorax.
B. tension pneumothorax.
C. cardiac tamponade.
D. pulmonary contusion.

2. Treatment for this condition includes all of the following EXCEPT:

A. requesting paramedic backup, if available and timely.
B. providing supportive care.
C. applying an occlusive dressing on both wounds.
D. transporting in a prone position.

3. Which of the following is a late sign of a tension pneumothorax?

A. Tachycardia
B. Anxiety
C. Hypotension
D. Dyspnea

4. Jugular vein distention is best assessed in patients in which position?

A. Supine
B. Prone
C. Semi-Fowler position
D. Fowler position

5. How should this patient's injuries be bandaged?

A. Place an occlusive dressing on the chest and nothing on the back.
B. Place an occlusive dressing on the chest and a gauze dressing on the back.
C. Place an occlusive dressing on the back and leave the chest open for reassessment.
D. Place occlusive dressings on both the chest and the back.

Assessment *in Action* *(continued)*

6. A massive hemothorax equates to an accumulation of more than 1,500 mL of blood within the pleural space. For the average adult, this amount represents a nearly _______ blood volume loss.

A. 15% to 20%
B. 20% to 25%
C. 25% to 30%
D. 30% to 35%

7. Which of the following would you find with a tension pneumothorax that you would not find with a massive hemothorax?

A. Neck vein distention
B. Hypotension
C. Tachycardia
D. Tachypnea

8. How does commotio cordis occur?

A. From a sudden compression injury that produces a rapid increase in intrathoracic pressure
B. Through a direct blow to the chest during the heart's repolarization period
C. From rupture of the aorta during high-speed deceleration
D. From high-pressure compression to the abdomen

9. What are the signs and symptoms of a massive hemothorax?

10. What is the appropriate management for a sternal fracture?

CHAPTER 32

Abdominal and Genitourinary Injuries

National EMS Education Standard Competencies

Trauma

Applies fundamental knowledge to provide basic and selected advanced emergency care and transportation based on assessment findings for an acutely injured patient.

Abdominal and Genitourinary Trauma

Recognition and management of

- Blunt versus penetrating mechanisms (pp 1292-1296, 1304-1306)
- Evisceration (pp 1296, 1306-1307)
- Impaled object (pp 1303, 1306, 1308)

Pathophysiology, assessment, and management of

- Solid and hollow organ injuries (pp 1289-1292, 1296, 1300-1306)
- Blunt versus penetrating mechanisms (pp 1292-1296, 1304-1306)
- Evisceration (pp 1296, 1306-1307)
- Injuries to the external genitalia (pp 1298-1299, 1308-1309)
- Vaginal bleeding due to trauma (p 1309)
- Sexual assault (pp 1300, 1309)
- Vascular injury (pp 1299-1301)
- Retroperitoneal injuries (pp 1291, 1297-1298, 1301, 1304-1305)

Knowledge Objectives

1. Review the anatomy and physiology of the abdomen, including the abdominal quadrants and boundaries. (pp 1289-1290)
2. Discuss the difference between hollow and solid organs. (pp 1289-1290)
3. Review the anatomy and physiology of the female and male genitourinary systems. (p 1290)
4. Describe some special considerations related to the care of pediatric patients and geriatric patients who have experienced abdominal trauma. (pp 1292, 1294, 1297)
5. Discuss closed abdominal injuries, providing examples of the mechanisms of injury that are likely to cause this type of trauma in a patient, as well as key signs and symptoms. (pp 1292-1295)
6. Discuss open abdominal injuries, including ways to distinguish low-velocity, medium-velocity, and high-velocity injuries, examples of the mechanisms of injury that would cause each, and signs and symptoms exhibited by a patient who has experienced this type of injury. (pp 1295-1296)
7. Describe the different ways hollow and solid organs of the abdomen can be injured and include the signs and symptoms a patient might exhibit, depending on the organ(s) involved. (pp 1296-1298)
8. Discuss the types of traumatic injuries that may be sustained by the organs of the male and female genitourinary systems, including the kidneys, urinary bladder, and internal and external genitalia. (pp 1298-1299)
9. Discuss the assessment of a patient who has experienced an abdominal or genitourinary injury. (pp 1300-1304)
10. Discuss special considerations related to patient privacy when assessing a patient with a genitourinary injury. (pp 1300, 1302)
11. Discuss the emergency medical care of a patient who has sustained a closed abdominal injury. (p 1305)
12. Discuss the emergency medical care of a patient who has sustained an open abdominal injury, including penetrating injuries and abdominal evisceration. (pp 1305-1307)
13. Discuss the emergency medical care of a patient who has sustained a genitourinary injury related to the kidneys, bladder, external male genitalia, female genitalia, or rectum. (pp 1307-1309)

Skills Objectives

1. Demonstrate proper emergency medical care of a patient who has experienced a blunt abdominal injury. (p 1305)
2. Demonstrate proper emergency medical care of a patient who has a penetrating abdominal injury with an impaled object. (p 1306)
3. Demonstrate how to apply a dressing to an abdominal evisceration wound. (pp 1306-1307)

Introduction

The abdomen is the lower of the two major body cavities, extending from the diaphragm to the pelvis. It contains several organs that make up the digestive, urinary, and genitourinary systems. Although any of these organs may be injured, some are better protected than others. You must know where these organs are located within the abdominal and pelvic cavities. You must also understand their functions so that when an illness or injury occurs, you can assess its seriousness.

The abdomen contains multiple organs and organ systems that are not well protected, and it is a highly vascular region. Injuries to the abdomen that go unrecognized or untreated are a leading cause of traumatic death, particularly in pediatric patients.[1] Similarly, trauma to the genitourinary system is often overlooked, despite 10% of all trauma patients having some form of genitourinary injury.[2] Given this risk, a high index of suspicion and prompt treatment are required with any abdominal or genitourinary injury.

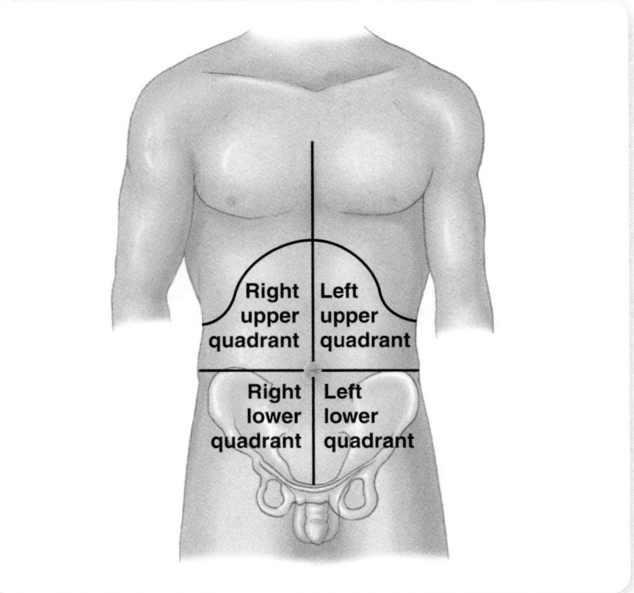

Figure 32-1 The abdomen is divided into four general quadrants.

Anatomy and Physiology Review

Abdominal Quadrants

The abdomen is divided arbitrarily into quadrants by two perpendicular lines that intersect at the umbilicus Figure 32-1. These areas are referred to as the right upper quadrant, left upper quadrant, right lower quadrant, and left lower quadrant. Remember that here, right and left refer to the patient's right and left, not yours. These quadrants provide a frame of reference for identifying and reporting abdominal signs and symptoms.

The quadrant location of bruising or pain can delineate which organs are possibly involved in a traumatic injury. Organs commonly found in the right upper quadrant are the liver, gallbladder, duodenum of the intestines, and a small portion of the pancreas. The stomach occupies most of the left upper quadrant, but shares this space with the spleen. The pancreas is mostly posterior to this region. Different portions of the intestines are located in each of the four quadrants. The left lower quadrant holds some of the large and small bowel, notably the descending colon and the left half of the transverse colon. The right lower quadrant also holds portions of the large and small intestines that include the ascending colon and the right half of the transverse colon. Also located in this region is the appendix, which can be a source of infection if it ruptures.

The diaphragm is the dividing line between the thoracic and abdominal cavities. Because the diaphragm moves its position during inspiration and expiration, in addition to other pulmonary and thoracic structures, it may be injured along with abdominal organs. For example, a patient may take a deep breath as he or she sees the traumatic force approaching, causing the diaphragm to flatten.

Hollow and Solid Organs

The abdomen contains both hollow and solid organs, any of which may be damaged. Owing to the size of the **peritoneal cavity** (the abdominal cavity) and the structures it includes, a patient could lose all of his or her circulating blood volume into this area without any visible external bleeding.

YOU are the Provider — PART 1

As you and your partner are enjoying the nice day outside your station, your ambulance is dispatched to an "ATV [all-terrain vehicle] accident, unknown further" call. As you are responding, dispatch informs you that the patient is a 32-year-old woman who hit a rock at moderate speed and possibly has a tree branch impaled in her abdomen.

1. Do you need additional resources to manage this call?
2. What are the potential injuries you may encounter?

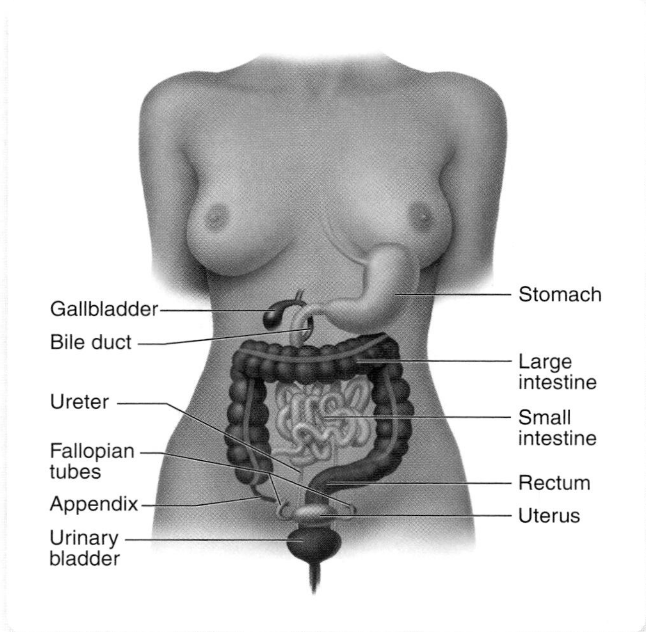

Figure 32-2 The hollow organs in the abdominal cavity are structures through which materials pass.

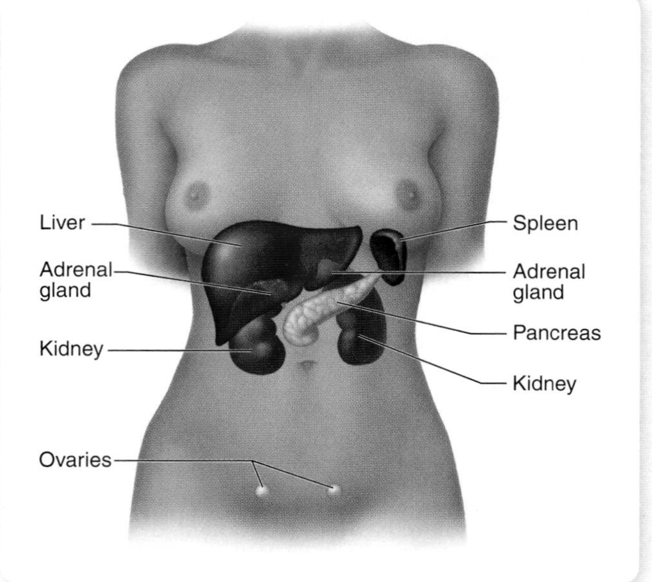

Figure 32-3 The solid organs are solid, highly vascular masses of tissue that do much of the chemical work in the body—for example, digestion, excretion, and energy production.

Hollow organs, including the stomach, gallbladder, intestines, ureters, and urinary bladder, are actually structures through which materials pass Figure 32-2. Hollow organs usually contain food that is in the process of being digested, urine that is being passed to the bladder for release, or bile. They are more resilient to blunt trauma and less likely to be injured by trauma unless they are full.

The **solid organs**, as their name suggests, are solid masses of tissue. They include the liver, spleen, pancreas, and kidneys Figure 32-3. The kidneys and great vessels (the abdominal aorta and the inferior vena cava), as well as most of the pancreas, actually lie in the retroperitoneal space, directly behind the peritoneal cavity Figure 32-4. Solid organs have a rich blood supply, so their injury can cause severe hemorrhage. Blood in the peritoneal cavity irritates tissue and fills any voids or spaces, which can make it difficult to determine the exact source of the bleeding. Unlike gastric juices and bacteria, blood within the peritoneal cavity does not provoke an inflammatory response. Therefore, the absence of pain and tenderness does not necessarily mean the absence of major bleeding in the abdomen. Abdominal pain from penetration or rupture of solid organs has a slow onset.

▶ The Genitourinary System

The genitourinary system is composed of the reproductive system and the urinary system. The urinary system controls the discharge of certain waste materials filtered from the blood by the kidneys. In the urinary system, the kidneys are solid organs; the ureters, bladder, and urethra are hollow organs.

The reproductive system controls the reproductive processes from which life is created. The male genitalia, except for the prostate gland and the seminal vesicles, lie outside the pelvic cavity. The female genitalia, except for the vulva, clitoris, and labia, are contained entirely within the pelvis. In females, conditions in the reproductive system may cause abdominal pain; such emergencies are discussed in Chapter 25, *Gynecologic Emergencies*. Refer to Chapter 7, *The Human Body*, for more information about the anatomy and physiology of the urinary and reproductive systems.

Pathophysiology

Abdominal injuries may be as obvious as loops of intestines protruding from a stab wound or as subtle as a laceration to the liver or spleen due to blunt trauma. Injuries to the abdomen are considered open or closed and can involve hollow and/or solid organs.

▶ General Pathophysiologic Concerns

Hemorrhage

Hemorrhage is a major concern in patients with abdominal trauma. It can occur when there is external or internal blood loss. When you are caring for patients with abdominal trauma, especially blunt abdominal trauma, estimating the volume of blood lost is difficult. Signs and symptoms will vary greatly depending on the volume of blood lost and the rate at which the body is losing blood. Key indicators of hemorrhagic shock will become apparent with the assessment of the neurologic and cardiovascular systems.

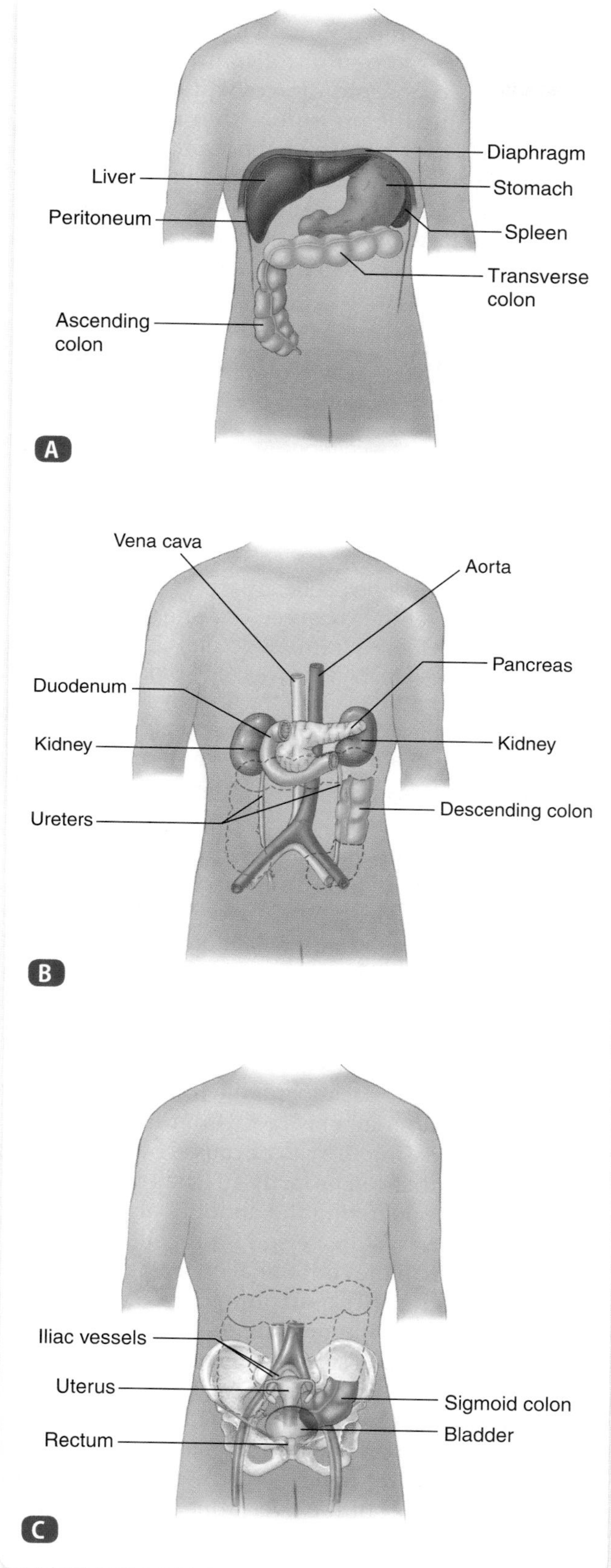

Figure 32-4 Different organs of the abdomen are contained in the peritoneum **(A)**, the retroperitoneal space **(B)**, and the pelvis **(C)**.

As hypovolemia increases, the patient will initially experience agitation and confusion. The heart compensates early for this loss by an increase in heart rate (tachycardia) and stroke volume. As hypoperfusion continues, arterial blood flow throughout the body becomes insufficient to meet the increased demands of the tissues in every organ system. If left untreated, hypoperfusion will result in anaerobic metabolism and acidosis.

Words of Wisdom

A patient may lose all of his or her circulating blood volume internally without any visible external hemorrhage. You must maintain a high index of suspicion based on the mechanism of injury (MOI) and changes in vital signs. Tachycardia is a common sign of blood loss, whether the loss is internal or external.

Peritonitis and Pneumoperitoneum

Injuries to hollow or solid organs can result in the spillage of their contents into the abdominal cavity. When the enzymes, acids, or bacteria leak from hollow organs into the peritoneal or retroperitoneal space, they cause irritation of the nerve endings. These nerve endings are found in the fascia of the surrounding tissues. As the inflammation affects deeper nerve endings (such as the endings of the afferent nerves), localized pain will result. Pain is localized if the extent of the contamination is confined; pain becomes generalized if the entire peritoneal cavity is involved.

If ruptured or lacerated organs spill their toxic contents into the peritoneal cavity, the result may be an intense, potentially life-threatening inflammatory reaction called **peritonitis**. The first signs of peritonitis are severe abdominal pain, tenderness, and muscular spasm. Later, normal bowel sounds diminish or disappear as the bowel stops functioning. A patient may feel nauseous and may vomit; the abdomen may become distended and firm to the touch. If the site of the perforation or rupture is not rapidly identified and repaired, severe infection and septic shock may develop. Patients with peritonitis generally prefer to lie very still with their legs drawn up because it hurts to move or straighten their legs. They may complain about every bump in the road during transport.

Pneumoperitoneum, or free air in the peritoneal cavity, may also occur as a result of rupture of a hollow organ, perforated peptic ulcer, recent abdominal surgery, or rupture of an abscess, among other conditions. Perforation with free air is usually very painful. Any air in the peritoneal cavity seeks the most superior space or void; thus, the location of the air can change with positioning of the patient. Pneumoperitoneum secondary to hollow organ rupture requires surgical intervention.

Special Populations

Falls are the most common MOI in geriatric patients.[3,4] In addition to the typical orthopaedic injuries that a geriatric patient sustains in a fall, the abdominal organs that have lost some elasticity over time are exposed to forces that can damage them. Specifically, the aorta, liver, and spleen are at risk of injury from falls. In addition, a geriatric patient's brittle bones can fracture in a fall, creating dangerously sharp edges that can puncture internal organs.

▶ Closed Abdominal Injuries

A **closed abdominal injury** is one in which a severe blow damages the abdomen without breaking the skin; closed abdominal injuries are also known as blunt injuries. Such a blow might come from the patient striking the handlebar of a bicycle or the steering wheel of a car Figure 32-5. Other causes of closed injuries include compression, deceleration, crush injuries, motorcycle crashes, falls, assaults, blast injuries, and pedestrian injuries.

Words of Wisdom

When considering fluid administration for a patient with the potential for internal bleeding, it is important not to overhydrate. The goal is to maintain a systolic blood pressure of 80 to 90 mm Hg to allow for perfusion but not increase bleeding. The presence of a radial pulse has been used as a proxy for a systolic blood pressure greater than 80 mm Hg, although this relationship is not well supported by scientific evidence. If systolic blood pressure is greater than 80 mm Hg, set the intravenous (IV) flow at a to-keep-open (TKO) rate to avoid exacerbating any internal bleeding.

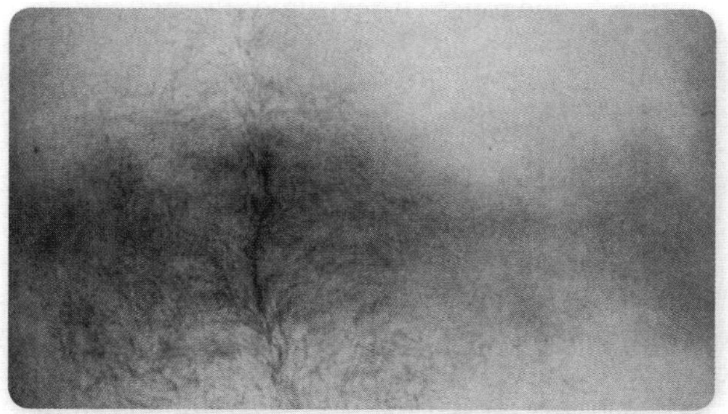

Figure 32-5 Blunt trauma to the abdomen can occur when a patient strikes the steering wheel of an automobile as a result of a crash.

Compression injuries are typically caused by a poorly placed lap belt. A compression injury can also be caused when a person is run over or rolled over by vehicles or objects. These compression forces will deform hollow organs, increasing the pressure within the abdominal cavity. This dramatic change in abdominal pressure can cause a rupture of the small intestine or diaphragm. Deceleration injuries commonly occur when a person or the vehicle in which he or she is traveling strikes a large immovable mass such as a larger vehicle, a bridge abutment, or the ground.

Special Populations

In pediatric patients, a common MOI is a motor vehicle–versus–pedestrian or motor vehicle–versus–bicycle accident. In pediatric patients, the chest and abdomen are less protected by bony structures than in adults. A pediatric patient may experience significant transfer of energy on impact. In pediatric patients, the rib cage is so flexible that the chest can be flattened almost to the spine before rib fractures occur. This extensive compression can involve not only the organs of the chest, but also the organs in the abdomen. The ribs then recoil to their normal position, and the patient is left with few outward signs that an injury has occurred.

Crush injuries are the result of external factors at the time of impact; they differ from deceleration injuries, which occur before impact. When abdominal contents are compressed between the anterior abdominal wall and the spinal column (or other structures in the rear), crushing occurs. Solid organs like the kidneys, liver, and spleen are at the greatest risk of injury from this mechanism. Direct application of crushing forces to the abdomen would come from objects like the dashboard, the front hood of a car (in a vehicle-pedestrian crash), or from falling objects. Additionally, these injuries can be caused by a restraining device that has not been properly attached or worn or by the steering wheel striking the abdominal cavity of an unrestrained driver as the person is propelled forward.

Many organs in the abdominal cavity may be injured from blunt trauma. The diaphragm, along with the abdominal wall, may sustain compression tears. The solid organs (eg, the liver and spleen) may burst, causing severe bleeding, and the hollow organs (eg, the gallbladder and intestines) may rupture on impact, spilling their contents into the abdominal cavity. Shearing may cause tears from the ligamentum teres hepatis, which extends from the liver, or an avulsion of the liver from the inferior vena cava at the hepatic veins. There may be an avulsion of the pedicle, or stem, of the spleen. Avulsion of mesenteric vessels from the aorta or vena cava, tears along the mesenteric vessels, or avulsion of vessels from the intestines may also occur, as may avulsion of the gallbladder from the liver or avulsion of a cystic duct.

Words of Wisdom

Think of bleeding into the peritoneal cavity as being similar to pouring water into a jar of rocks. Before you see the water at the top of the jar, it must fill in the spaces around the rocks. The same is true of abdominal distention—the blood must fill in the spaces around the organs before you see the swelling or distention. Reassess frequently to ensure that you note changes.

Signs and Symptoms of a Closed Injury

Patients with abdominal injuries generally have one principal complaint: pain. However, other significant injuries may mask the pain at first, and some patients may not be able to tell you about pain because they are unresponsive, such as after a head injury or drug or alcohol overdose. The most common sign of significant abdominal injury is tachycardia. The patient may also present with tachypnea and signs of agitation. It is important to note these signs early, before later signs of shock appear, such as decreased blood pressure and pale, cool, moist skin. In some cases, the abdomen may become distended from the accumulation of blood and fluid. As an advanced emergency medical technician (AEMT), you must look for other clues.

In addition to the general signs already mentioned, signs and symptoms of blunt injuries include bruises or other visible marks, whose location should guide your attention to underlying structures. Crepitus in the lower rib areas may indicate broken ribs that have the potential to puncture underlying organs. In patients with liver and spleen injuries, where there is bleeding into the peritoneal space, pain is referred to the shoulder. This finding is called the **Kehr sign** when it involves injury to the spleen and pain in the tip of the left shoulder. However, shoulder pain can be misleading, and injury to the liver or spleen could possibly be overlooked if the shoulder is also injured or if the MOI suggests that an impact or injury may have occurred in the shoulder girdle.

When a patient reports pain that is tearing and describes it as going from the abdomen posteriorly, he or she is often describing symptoms of an abdominal aneurysm that is undergoing dissection. Pain that follows the angle from the lateral part of the hip to the midline of the groin can be the result of damage to the kidneys or the ureters. Pain primarily located in the right lower quadrant can indicate an inflamed or ruptured appendix. Pain from the gallbladder due to direct injury or inflammation can be found just under the margin of the ribs on the right side or between the shoulder blades.

Determining the location of the pain or referred pain can be more difficult when the patient has voluntary or involuntary **guarding**. In guarding, the patient intentionally or unintentionally stiffens the muscles of the surface of the abdomen. Most often it is the rectus abdominis muscles (that run from the pubis to the xiphoid process) that are held tight, and the tightness can be mistaken for abdominal rigidity. This stiffening is a natural response to abdominal

YOU are the Provider PART 2

On the basis of the additional information you received from dispatch, you request that the fire department respond for assistance. On arrival at the scene, you find a 32-year-old woman who presents as alert and oriented, with an impaled tree branch in her right upper abdominal quadrant. Surprisingly, the patient is relatively calm and appears in no distress, but she is obviously anxious. She states that she was riding her ATV at approximately 20 miles per hour when it struck a large rock, and she was thrown off the ATV. She landed on some brush and became impaled on a large tree branch. The tree branch is still attached to the tree. Beyond this, she denies any injuries, other than some abdominal pain. She was not wearing a helmet or protective clothing.

Recording Time: 1 Minute	
Appearance	Anxious
Level of consciousness	Alert and oriented to person, place, time, and event
Airway	Patent
Breathing	Nonlabored
Circulation	Strong, rapid radial pulses; skin warm, dry, and pink

3. How do you remove the branch from the wound?
4. On the basis of the patient's presentation, does she require spinal immobilization?

pain; the body is attempting to splint the area to prevent unnecessary movement and to avoid further pain.

Closed abdominal injuries may initially appear as abrasions to the surface of the skin depending on the MOI, such as an assault or auto versus pedestrian accident. In some circumstances, depending on how deep in the abdomen the injury occurs, it may take several minutes to hours for the contusion or hematoma to become present on the surface. In other circumstances, these signs may never develop despite the presence of severe underlying injuries. Therefore, it is not prudent for you to rule out injury simply on the basis of the absence of these findings.

The signs of abdominal injury are usually more indicative of the specific injury than the symptoms, including firmness on palpation of the abdomen, obvious penetrating wounds, bruises, and altered vital signs such as tachycardia, tachypnea, hypotension, and shallow respirations (although these signs might not appear until later). For example, bruises in the right upper quadrant, left upper quadrant, or **flank** (region below the rib cage and above the hip), called the Grey Turner sign, might suggest an injury to the liver, spleen, or kidney, respectively Figure 32-6. Bruises around the umbilicus (**Cullen sign**) are predictive of significant internal abdominal bleeding Figure 32-7.

Words of Wisdom

Cullen sign is a black-and-blue discoloration (ecchymosis) in the umbilical region caused by peritoneal bleeding. Grey Turner sign includes ecchymosis present in the lower abdominal and flank regions. Both are caused by intra-abdominal bleeding found 12 to 24 hours after the initial injury. The presence of these signs is helpful, but their absence does not rule out life-threatening abdominal hemorrhage.

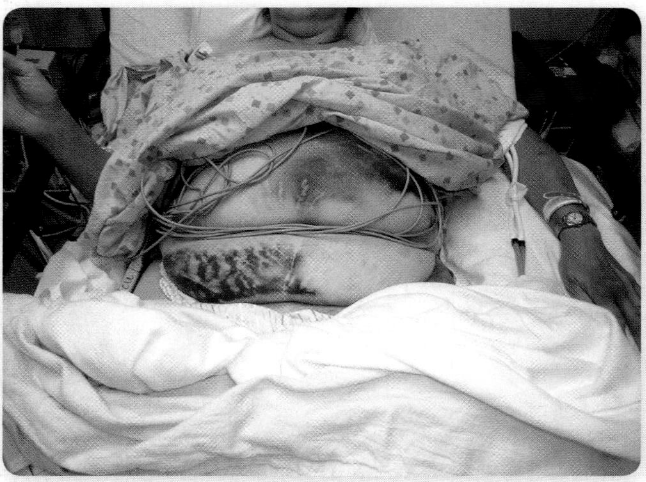

Figure 32-6 Bruises in the right upper quadrant, left upper quadrant, or flank, called Grey Turner sign, suggest an injury to the liver, spleen, or kidney, respectively.

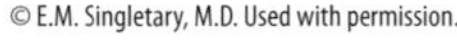

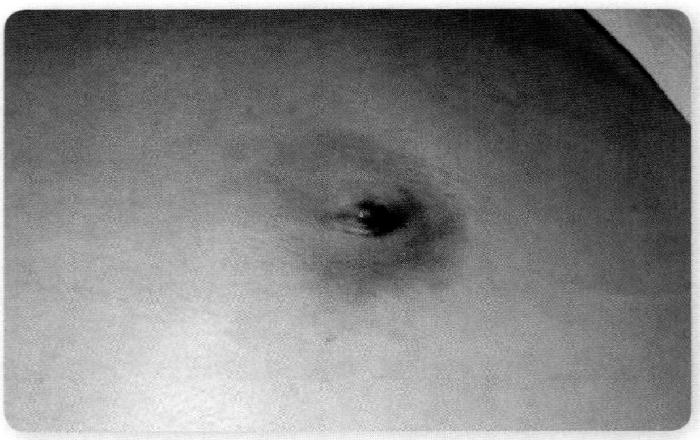

Figure 32-7 Bruises around the umbilicus, called Cullen sign, are predictive of significant internal abdominal bleeding.

Common symptoms include abdominal tenderness, particularly localized tenderness, and difficulty with movement because of pain.

Injuries From Seat Belts and Airbags

Seat belts have prevented many thousands of injuries and saved many lives, including those of people who otherwise would have been ejected during a motor vehicle crash. However, seat belts occasionally cause blunt injuries to the abdominal organs.[5] When worn properly, a seat belt lies below the anterior superior iliac spines of the pelvis and against the hip joints. If the belt lies too high, it can squeeze abdominal organs or great vessels against the spine when the car suddenly decelerates or stops Figure 32-8. Occasionally, fractures of the lumbar spine have been reported. If you are called to the scene of such an accident, keep in mind that the use of seat belts in many cases turns what could have been a fatal injury into a manageable one.

In current-model automobiles, the lap and diagonal (shoulder) safety belts are combined into a single unit so that they may not be used independently. Of course, people can still place the diagonal portion of the belt behind the back; however, this significantly reduces the effectiveness of this design. In some older cars, only lap belts or two separate belts are provided. Used alone, diagonal shoulder safety belts can cause injuries to the upper part of the trunk, such as thoracic bruising, fractured ribs, lacerated liver, or even decapitation. Far fewer head and neck injuries are seen when this belt is used in combination with a lap belt and a properly positioned headrest.

The airbag, which is standard equipment in today's vehicles, can be a genuine lifesaver. However, airbags must be used in combination with properly worn safety belts. Small children and short people who are in the front seat of the automobile may be at risk of injury when the airbag is deployed. Special attention should be used in evaluating patients when a deployed airbag is noted. Remember to inspect beneath the airbag for signs of damage to the steering wheel Figure 32-9.

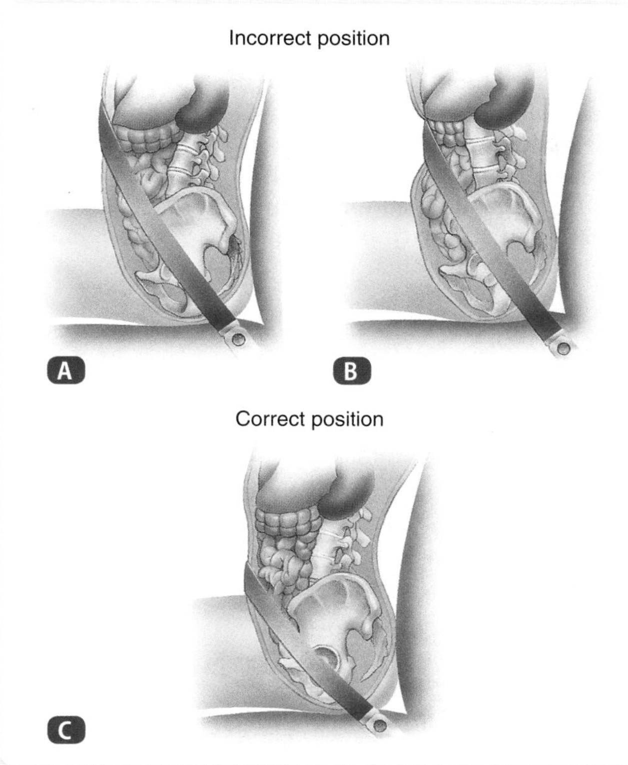

Figure 32-8 Diagrams **(A)** and **(B)** show improper positioning of lap seat belts. The proper position for a seat belt is below the anterior superior iliac spines of the pelvis and against the hip joints, as shown in diagram **(C)**.

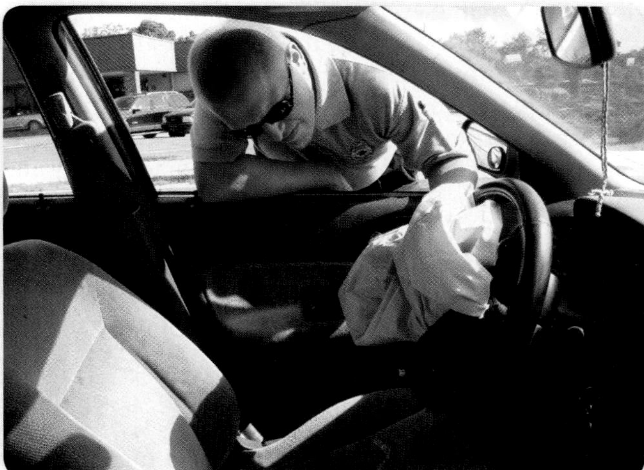

Figure 32-9 Raise a deployed air bag to note signs of damage to the steering wheel.

▶ Open Abdominal Injuries

An **open abdominal injury** is one in which a foreign object enters the abdomen and opens the peritoneal cavity to the outside (such as a stab wound or gunshot wound). Open abdominal injuries are also known as penetrating injuries. Open injuries might not go deeper than the wall of the abdomen, but the depth is often difficult to determine outside of the operating room **Figure 32-10**. Therefore, you must assume the worst—that organs have been damaged—and provide prompt transport.

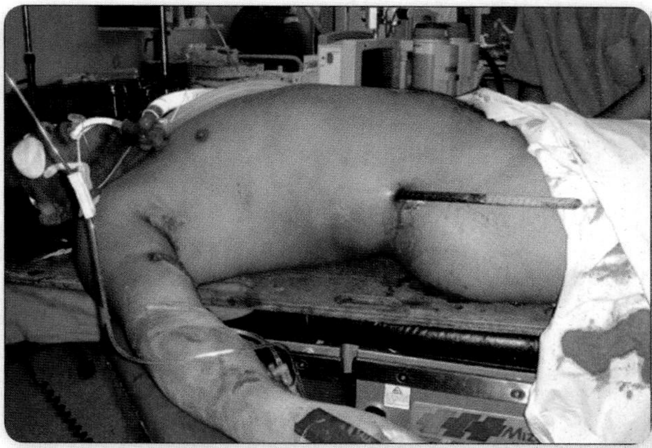

Figure 32-10 Because it is difficult to know how deep a penetrating injury is, assume organ damage and transport promptly.

When a patient has sustained a penetrating injury to the abdomen, it is important to attempt to determine the velocity of the object that penetrated the abdominal wall, because this information can help predict the amount of damage to tissue. Gunshot wounds often cause more injury than stab wounds because bullets travel deep into the body and have more kinetic energy, increasing the damage lateral to the track of the missile due to temporary cavitation. Gunshot wounds most commonly involve injury to the small bowel, colon, liver, and vascular structures. The extent of injury from gunshot wounds is less predictable than the injury caused by stab wounds, because gunshot wounds depend mostly on the characteristics of the weapon and the characteristics of the bullet.[6] In penetrating trauma from stab wounds, the liver, small bowel, diaphragm, and colon are the organs most frequently injured.[7] Don't underestimate the danger of stab wounds, however. They are often rapidly fatal.

Words of Wisdom

The extent of damage from a penetrating injury is often a function of the energy that has been imparted to the body. Remember the following equation:

$$\text{Kinetic energy} = \frac{\text{Mass}}{2} \times \text{Velocity}^2$$

or

$$KE = \frac{mv^2}{2}$$

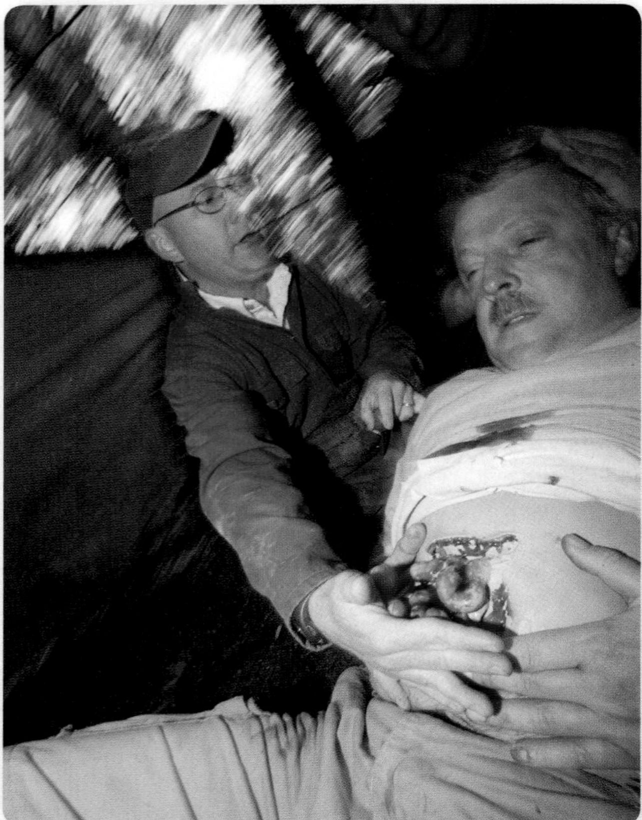

Figure 32-11 An abdominal evisceration is an open abdominal wound from which internal organs or fat protrudes.

An **evisceration** results when a penetrating wound goes all the way through the skin and muscle layer and through the fascia or the interior covering of the abdomen resulting in bowel protruding through the skin **Figure 32-11**. This visually shocking injury can be extremely painful.

Signs and Symptoms of an Open Injury

Penetrating abdominal trauma may include signs of bleeding and puncture wounds (entrance and exit wounds). Many signs and symptoms of closed abdominal wounds may also be present along with puncture wounds. A very common sign of significant abdominal injury is tachycardia because the heart is increasing its pumping action to compensate for blood loss, an early indication of compensated blood loss. Later signs include evidence of shock, such as decreased blood pressure; pale, cool, and moist skin; or changes in the patient's mental status, combined with trauma to the abdomen. In some cases, the abdomen may become distended from the accumulation of blood and fluid. Keep in mind that puncture wounds made by a hand-driven weapon (such as a knife) may create significant damage based on the direction of travel and whether the weapon was moved around inside the wound. Wounds created by medium- and high-velocity weapons can produce increased areas of damage due to areas of cavitation (cavity formation). Cavitation can produce significant bleeding, depending on the speed or velocity of the penetrating object.

If major blood vessels are cut or solid organs are lacerated, bleeding may be rapid and severe. Other signs of intra-abdominal injuries may develop slowly, particularly in penetrating wounds to hollow organs. Once such an organ is punctured and its contents are discharged into the abdominal cavity, peritonitis may develop, but this may take several hours.

Words of Wisdom

Consider any stab wound at the nipple line or below to have potential for injury to upper abdominal organs depending on direction of travel and length of the weapon. Any stab wound at the level of the umbilicus or higher may also penetrate the thoracic cavity.

▶ Injuries to Specific Structures

Injury to the Diaphragm

If the diaphragm is penetrated or ruptured, abdominal organs may be pushed upward into the thoracic cavity. Because these will displace lung tissue and vital capacity, patients will exhibit dyspnea or feel short of breath, may have abnormal respiratory sounds, and may have an abdomen with a sunken, concave anterior wall (**scaphoid abdomen**). Patients with this type of injury may require positive pressure ventilation with a bag-mask device depending on the severity of their respiratory symptoms.

Patients with a ruptured diaphragm after a motor vehicle crash may become very anxious and short of breath if placed in the supine position on a backboard. Change in position from upright to supine results in more abdominal contents spilling into the thoracic cavity and compressing the lungs, preventing the lungs from fully expanding. Thus, any injury to the diaphragm will cause signs and symptoms of ventilatory compromise. Note that diaphragmatic injuries or ruptures are not isolated incidents; patients often have associated thoracic, abdominal, head, and extremity injuries.

Injury to the Kidney

Kidneys are the most commonly injured organs of the genitourinary system.[8] AEMTs should consider trauma to these organs whenever a patient has injuries to the lower rib cage, abdomen, pelvis, or upper part of the leg. Injuries to the kidneys generally involve large forces, such as falls from height, high-speed motor vehicle crashes, or sports-related injuries.[9]

Blunt renal trauma results when the kidney becomes compressed against the lower ribs or lumbar spine (as seen in sports injuries, also known as kidney punch) and when the upper abdomen becomes compressed just below the rib cage (such as when a child is run over by a car). Contact sports such as football, soccer, hockey, boxing, and rugby are some of the more common culprits in renal injury.[10] Suspect injury to these organs with fractures of the 11th and 12th ribs or flank tenderness. A ruptured kidney will usually present with pain on inspiration in the abdomen and flank areas. The kidneys are very vascular, and kidney injury may present with blood in the urine (**hematuria**).

Penetrating renal trauma can occur with gunshot or stab wounds in the abdomen or lower chest. A high suspicion for significant injury must be maintained regardless of the site of the entry wound. Penetrating renal trauma is more likely to be associated with injury to the liver, lung, and spleen. For instance, the upward motion of stabbing may cause a renal laceration as well as a pneumothorax. A gunshot wound may result in direct injury to the kidney, but produce greater surrounding tissue destruction due to the expanding cavity created by the traveling bullet.

Injuries to the kidney rarely occur in isolation, because the kidneys lie in the well-protected retroperitoneal space, which is the area behind the true, or anterior, abdomen. Injuries confined to the retroperitoneum can be very difficult to diagnose. In general, this area is remote from physical examination, and an injury there initially does not present with signs and symptoms of peritonitis. Because the blood or other contaminants are held in the retroperitoneal space, they frequently do not cause abdominal pain, peritoneal signs, or abdominal distention.

A penetrating wound that reaches the kidneys almost always involves other organs; the same is true with blunt injuries. A blow that is forceful enough to cause significant kidney damage almost always damages other intra-abdominal organs, often fracturing ribs as well. Less significant injuries to the kidneys may result from a direct blow or even from a tackle in football **Figure 32-12**. Suspect kidney damage if the patient has a history or physical evidence of any of the following findings:

- An abrasion, laceration, contusion, or hematoma to the flank region
- A penetrating wound in the region below the rib cage and above the hip (the flank) or the upper abdomen
- Fractures on either side of the lower rib cage or of the lower thoracic or upper lumbar vertebrae

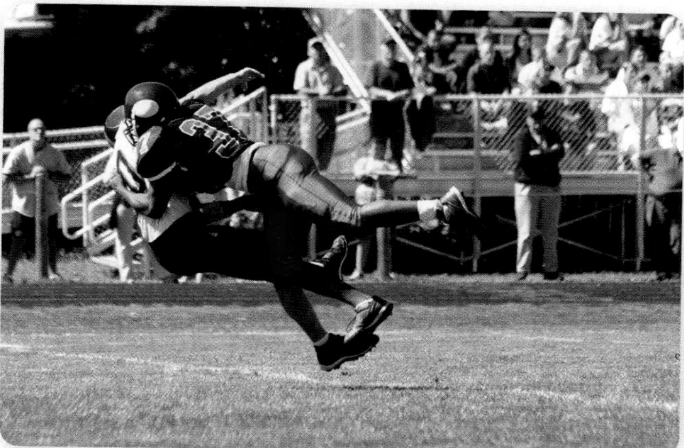

Figure 32-12 A tackle in football that results in blunt trauma to the lower rib cage or the flank can cause kidney injury.

Injury to the Liver

The liver is the largest solid organ in the abdomen and is very vascular; its penetration or rupture may quickly lead to signs of shock. Because of its size and location, the liver is the most vulnerable organ in the abdomen. The superior border of this organ can be as high as the patient's nipples, so a liver injury must be suspected in all patients who have right-side chest trauma as well as abdominal trauma. The liver may be punctured by lower right rib fractures, especially the seventh through ninth ribs. A common finding during assessment of patients with an injured liver is referred pain to the right shoulder.

Injury to the Spleen

The spleen is often injured in motor vehicle crashes, falls, and bicycle or motorcycle collisions or as the result of penetrating trauma or lower left rib fractures. It is the most commonly injured abdominal organ in blunt trauma in adults and the second most injured abdominal organ in children.[11] The potential for rupture is much higher if the spleen is enlarged from mononucleosis or other underlying disease. When the spleen ruptures, large amounts of blood spill into the peritoneum, which can ultimately cause shock and death. Unlike with trauma to the liver, penetrating trauma to the spleen does not present as much of an immediate threat of shock unless a major blood vessel supplying the organ is lacerated. Suspect spleen lacerations when fractures of the 9th through 10th ribs on the left side are present or when the patient reports left upper quadrant tenderness, hypotension, and tachycardia. It is common for the patient to report left shoulder pain, but this sign does not appear until 1 to 2 hours after the injury.

Special Populations

In pediatric patients the liver and spleen are very large in proportion to the size of the abdominal cavity and are more easily injured. The soft, flexible ribs of infants and young children do not protect these two organs very well.

Injury to the Pancreas

Because of its anatomic position, the pancreas is relatively well protected. It typically takes a high-energy force to damage this organ. Such high-energy forces are most commonly produced by penetrating trauma (eg, from a bullet) but can also be caused by blunt trauma (eg, impact with a steering wheel or handlebars from a motorcycle). Patients with pancreatic injury tend to present with vague upper and midabdominal pain that can radiate into the back. The patient may also develop peritoneal irritation hours after the injury, revealing the presence of traumatic pancreatitis. Some patients have been known to develop a form of diabetes after a severe injury to the pancreas.[12]

Injury to the Intestines and Stomach

The intestines are most commonly injured from penetrating trauma, although they can be injured from severe blunt trauma as well. When ruptured, the intestines spill their contents (which contain fecal matter and a large amount of bacteria) into the peritoneal or retroperitoneal cavities, resulting in peritonitis.

Blunt trauma to the abdominal wall most commonly causes injury to the duodenum because of its location and ligamentous attachment. This type of injury may present as back pain. The duodenum can rupture, spilling its contents into the retroperitoneum. Contamination of the retroperitoneum with duodenal contents may ultimately produce abdominal pain or fever, although symptoms will not likely develop for hours to days. Abdominal pain, nausea, and vomiting may develop, although belatedly. Because of the delayed presentation and variable symptoms, a high degree of suspicion for duodenal injury must be maintained in any abdominal trauma, but especially in high-speed deceleration crashes. A duodenal injury should be suspected in children who are thrown from a bicycle and strike their abdomen on the handlebars.

Most injuries to the stomach result from penetrating trauma; the stomach is rarely injured from blunt trauma. When rupture of the stomach does occur after blunt trauma, it is usually associated with a recent meal or inappropriate use of a seat belt. Trauma to the stomach frequently results in the spillage of acidic material into the peritoneal space, creating a chemical irritation that produces abdominal pain and peritoneal signs relatively quickly, although patients taking antacid medications may have delayed symptoms.

Trauma to the abdomen may cause injury to the small bowel, the stomach, and the large intestine. The most common cause of such trauma is impact with a seat belt in a motor vehicle collision, because the lap belt lies along the lower quadrant of the abdominal cavity. Symptoms will be caused by the spillage of contents rather than the blood loss. Rupture of the stomach causes rapid, burning epigastric pain; rigidity; and **rebound tenderness**. Small-bowel and colon injury may present with only generalized pain.

Words of Wisdom

Pain may be intense with injuries that result in rupture of the stomach or small bowel, and infection is a delayed complication that may prove fatal.

Injury to the Urinary Bladder

Bladder injuries are usually associated with pelvic fractures from motor vehicle crashes, falls from heights, and physical assaults to the lower abdomen. Injury to the urinary bladder, whether blunt or penetrating, may result in its rupture. Bladder injury should be suspected in any patient with trauma to the lower abdomen or pelvis. Blunt injuries to the lower abdomen or pelvis often cause rupture of the urinary bladder, particularly when the bladder is full and distended. A seat belt that causes contusions to the lower abdomen may also cause blunt trauma to the bladder. Sharp, bony fragments from a fracture of the pelvis often perforate the urinary bladder **Figure 32-13**. Penetrating wounds of the lower midabdomen or the perineum (the pelvic floor and associated structures that occupy the pelvic outlet) can directly involve the bladder. In males, sudden deceleration from a motor vehicle or motorcycle crash can literally shear the bladder from the urethra. Trauma to the bladder or urethra is often associated with other significant injuries.

Approximately 20% of bladder injuries occur as a result of a blow to the lower abdomen with a distended bladder.[13] If a bladder rupture results from sudden deceleration forces, such as those occurring in motor vehicle crashes, urine may be spilled into any part of the abdominal cavity, leading to intraperitoneal, extraperitoneal, or retroperitoneal rupture. When urine spills into surrounding tissues, any urine that passes through the urethra is likely to be bloody.

Injury to the External Male Genitalia

Injuries to the external male genitalia include all types of soft-tissue wounds. Although these injuries are very painful and generally a source of great concern to the patient, they are rarely life threatening. One such injury

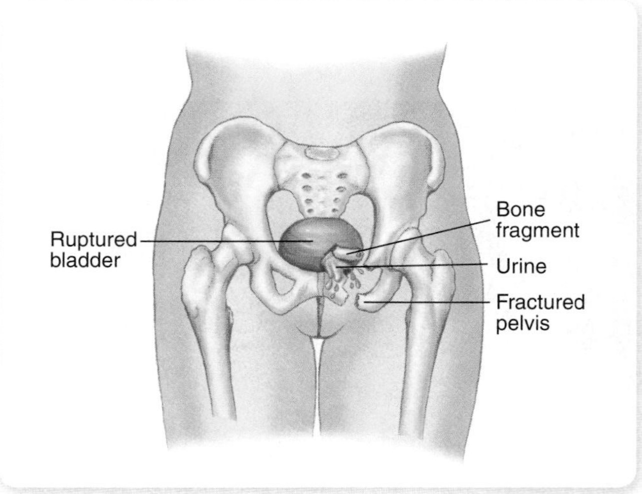

Figure 32-13 Fracture of the pelvis can result in a laceration of the bladder by the bony fragments. Urine then leaks into the pelvis.

is testicular torsion, which can occur as a result of trauma. Although it is not life threatening, it is time-sensitive and requires rapid transport. These injuries should not be given priority over other, more severe wounds.

Injuries to the Testicle or Scrotal Sac. Severe injuries to the testicles are rare because of their mobility and natural position. Although loss of fertility is the major concern when a patient sustains a testicular injury, the exact outcome depends on whether the testicle can be preserved via definitive treatment in the hospital setting.

Blunt trauma to the testicles or scrotal sac can result from motor vehicle crashes, physical assaults, or sports injuries. Blunt testicular trauma can result in simple contusions, rupture of the testicle, and, in rare cases, torsion (twisting) of the testicle. Most testicular ruptures occur in sports participants. Testicular injuries frequently present following trauma to the thighs, buttocks, penis, lower abdomen, and pelvis.

Penetrating trauma to the testicles or scrotal sac may result from stab wounds, gunshot wounds, blast wounds, or animal bites. You should have a high suspicion for other associated injuries in cases of obvious penetrating trauma.

Penis Injuries. The penis is a vital organ for both proper urination and sexual function. Injuries to the penis may result from blunt or penetrating trauma but also may arise from sexual behavior or self-mutilation. Physiologically, the penis becomes erect when blood fills the corpus cavernosa. Priapism—a painful, tender, persistent erection—can have nontraumatic causes, such as sickle cell disease.

A fractured penis may occur when an erect penis is accidentally impacted against the partner's pubic symphysis or bent too far via self-manipulation.

Penetrating trauma to the penis most often results from gunshot wounds. Self-mutilation or amputation may also be a cause. Typically, this type of injury occurs in patients with significant psychiatric disorders.

Injury to the Female Genitalia

Internal Female Genitalia. The uterus, ovaries, and fallopian tubes are subject to the same kinds of injuries as any other internal organ. However, they are rarely damaged because they are small, deep in the pelvis, and well protected by the pelvic bones. Unlike the bladder, which lies adjacent to the bony pelvis, they are usually not injured in a pelvic fracture. Penetrating trauma to the reproductive organs may result from stabbings to the lower pelvis or gunshot wounds. Because the path of a bullet cannot be predicted from the entry wound alone, any injuries to the abdomen or upper legs also may have damaged the reproductive organs.

An exception is the pregnant uterus. As pregnancy progresses, the uterus enlarges substantially and rises out of the pelvis, becoming vulnerable to penetrating and blunt injuries. These injuries can be particularly severe because the uterus has a rich blood supply during pregnancy, even though the injuries may be masked initially owing to the increased blood volume during pregnancy. You must also keep in mind that another life—that of the unborn child—is at risk. You can expect to see the signs and symptoms of shock with pregnant patients; be prepared to provide all necessary support and prompt transport. Note that contractions may begin as well. If possible, ask the patient when she is due, and report this information to hospital staff.

In the last trimester of pregnancy, the uterus is large and may obstruct the inferior vena cava, decreasing the amount of blood returning to the heart if the patient is placed in a supine position (**supine hypotensive syndrome**). As a result, blood pressure may decrease. The patient should be carefully placed on her left side so that the uterus will not lie on the vena cava. If the patient is secured to a backboard, tilt the board to the left. Care for pregnant patients is described in greater detail in Chapter 35, *Obstetrics and Neonatal Care*.

External Female Genitalia. The external female genitalia include the vulva, the clitoris, and the major and minor labia (lips) at the entrance of the vagina. Injuries to the external female genitalia can include all types of soft-tissue injuries.

In any case of trauma, it is important to attempt to determine the possibility of pregnancy. It will be important to ask the patient for the date of her last known menstrual period or if she has been sexually active. The assumption is that all women of childbearing age are possibly pregnant. This information is medically relevant because some medications and tests are harmful for a fetus, and there is the potential for another source of blood loss in the gravid uterus.

Vascular Injuries

In addition to the kidneys, the vascular structures found in the retroperitoneal space include the descending aorta (and its branches), the superior and inferior phrenic arteries, the inferior vena cava, and the mesenteric vessels. Injuries to these structures occur with both blunt and penetrating trauma, but penetrating trauma that causes injury to the great vessels of the abdomen will also be associated with injuries to multiple intra-abdominal organs. Blunt trauma can cause injuries to vascular structures in the intraperitoneal space as they are sheared from their points of attachment.

Vascular injuries are often masked by other injuries. The significance of the injury depends on how many vessels were injured and the length of time that has passed since the injury occurred. Assessment findings in a patient with vascular injuries differ depending on whether the bleeding is contained (a hematoma) or there is active hemorrhage. In active hemorrhage, the patient will present with significant hypotension, tachycardia, and shock.

The intestinal blood supply comes from the mesentery. The term *mesentery* refers to any fold of tissue that attaches an organ to the body wall. The intestinal mesentery, therefore, is a fold of tissue that contains a web of blood vessels, as well as nerves and lymphatic tissues; it connects the small intestine to the posterior of the abdominal wall. Blunt and penetrating abdominal injuries affect this vasculature, and patients with injuries to the mesentery can bleed significantly into the peritoneal cavity. A common sign of bleeding in the abdomen is rigidity, with an almost boardlike feeling to the abdomen. Occasionally you will find periumbilical bruising or ecchymosis (Cullen sign).

Sometimes a patient may have an **abdominal aortic aneurysm (AAA)** that has developed and become worse as a result of abdominal trauma. The presence of a pulsating mass near the umbilicus is indicative of an AAA. Remember to palpate *gently* when assessing the abdomen of a patient with a history of or presence of an AAA.

Rectal bleeding is a common complaint and something that you may encounter as a chief complaint or secondary to abdominal or pelvic complaints. Bleeding from the rectum may present as blood stains or blood soaking through underwear or patients may report blood in the toilet after a bowel movement or attempted bowel movement. Rectal bleeding can be caused by a sexual assault, rectal foreign bodies, hemorrhoids, colitis, or ulcers of the digestive tract. Significant rectal bleeding can occur after hemorrhoid surgery and can lead to significant blood loss and shock.

Patient Assessment

While the cause of an abdominal or genitourinary injury may be readily apparent as a result of the MOI or the visibility of a penetrating wound, the resulting damage may not be so apparent. Often, other injuries, such as a fractured bone, may be painful and distracting for the patient. The patient may not tell you about more subtle pain that could indicate an abdominal or genitourinary injury. In addition, some abdominal or genitourinary injuries develop and worsen over time, making reassessment critical.

When you are assessing a genitourinary injury, there is a potential for embarrassing the patient. This is why you need to maintain a professional presence at all times when treating these injuries. Remember to provide privacy for the patient during the assessment process. When examining the patient, expose only what is needed and then cover what has been exposed. Whenever possible, have an AEMT of the same sex as the patient perform the assessment. You will need to look for blood on the patient's underwear and inspect the external genitalia when there are complaints of pain or external signs of injury.

Scene Size-up

As with any situation, scene safety is your first consideration. Remember to follow standard precautions because these injuries often bleed profusely, and even if they do not, some blood or other body fluid is likely to be present. Eye protection is required when managing open injuries. Observe the scene for hazards and threats to your safety. If dispatch information indicates a possible assault, domestic dispute, or shooting—all of which commonly lead to abdominal injuries—be sure that law enforcement personnel have controlled the scene.

Look for indicators of the MOI, and consider early spinal precautions. This approach helps you develop an early index of suspicion for underlying injuries in a patient who has sustained a significant MOI. As you put together information from dispatch and your observations of the scene, consider the possible injuries the MOI could have produced. As you inspect a vehicle, look at the damage. Could this damage result in an abdominal injury? In the case of an assault, think about how many times the patient was struck, with what object, and where the patient was struck. Information from the scene will help to determine your index of suspicion.

If the wound is penetrating, inspect the object of penetration. Is the object's edge serrated, smooth, or jagged? Is it clean or dirty? The MOI may also provide indications of potential safety threats. For example, a knife wound may indicate the presence of a violent person.

With genitourinary injuries, be aware that the patient may avoid discussing the injury to avoid undergoing a physical examination. Also, the patient may provide an MOI that seems "less embarrassing" than the actual MOI. By maintaining a professional demeanor, respecting the patient's privacy, and maintaining the patient's dignity, you will earn the patient's trust. If the patient trusts you, you are more likely to learn the true facts behind the injury.

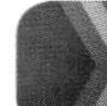

Primary Survey

Your goal during the primary survey is to evaluate the patient's airway, breathing, circulation, disability, and exposure (ABCDEs) and then immediately care for any life threats. Control any external hemorrhage, and look for indication of internal bleeding. Abdominal injuries may be overlooked in multisystem injuries, so it is important to maintain a high index of suspicion for abdominal injuries based on the MOI. The evaluation of a patient who has abdominal or genitourinary trauma must be systematic, keeping the entire patient in mind and prioritizing accordingly.

In trauma patients, life-threatening external hemorrhage must be addressed before airway or breathing concerns; follow the XABCDE mnemonic, assessing and managing exsanguinating hemorrhage immediately after establishing scene safety. Next, ensure the patient has a clear and patent airway. If a spinal injury is suspected, prevent the patient from moving by having a team member manually stabilize the patient's head and verbally remind the patient not to move. Patients may report feeling nauseous, and they may vomit. Remember to keep the airway clear of vomitus so that it is not aspirated into the lungs, especially in a patient who is unconscious or has an altered level of consciousness. Turn the patient on one side, stabilizing the spine if necessary, and try to clear any material from the throat and mouth. Note the nature of the vomitus: undigested food, blood, mucus, or bile.

You must also quickly assess the patient for adequate breathing. A distended abdomen or pain may prevent adequate inhalation. When these guarded respirations decrease the effectiveness of the patient's breathing, providing supplemental oxygen with a nonrebreathing mask will help improve oxygenation. If the patient's level of consciousness is decreased and respirations are shallow, consider supplementing respirations with a bag-mask device.

All abdominal organs have a generous blood supply, so an injury to the abdomen can be fatal because of hemorrhage. Retroperitoneal hemorrhage may be present because of damaged muscle, lacerated or avulsed kidneys, and injuries to the vessels of the supporting mesentery. If visible significant bleeding is seen, you must begin the steps necessary to control bleeding. Recall that significant bleeding is an immediate life threat and must be controlled quickly using appropriate methods, even before addressing airway and breathing concerns. In dark environments, bleeding can be difficult to see. Thick clothing may also hide bleeding. After you consider the MOI and form suspicions as to where bleeding may occur, expose that part of the body.

Evaluate the patient's pulse and skin color, temperature, and condition. If you suspect shock, treat the patient for shock according to your protocols.

Early Assessment of the Abdomen

With significant trauma, you should perform a rapid full-body scan of the patient. If the patient has been subjected to a significant MOI, a rapid full-body scan will help you to quickly identify any injuries the patient may have, not just abdominal injuries. Begin with the head, and finish with the lower extremities, moving in a systematic manner. Your goal is not to identify the extent of all the injuries, but to determine whether other injuries are present. This requires you to work quickly but thoroughly. If you find a life-threatening problem during this scan, stop and treat it immediately; otherwise, move on. The injuries you find will help you in packaging the patient for transport.

Examine the abdomen closely looking for DCAP-BTLS (Deformities, Contusions, Abrasions, Punctures/penetrations, Burns, Tenderness, Lacerations, Swelling). All of these may be signs of **hemoperitoneum**—that is, collection of blood in the abdominal cavity. Clues to intra-abdominal trauma will include symptoms of shock not proportional to obvious external evidence or estimated blood loss. During palpation, involuntary muscle guarding and reaction to sudden, jarring movements are reliable signs of peritoneal irritation. Or, you may note rebound tenderness (pain that the patient feels when pressure is released as opposed to when pressure is applied); it is characteristic of the pain associated with peritonitis.

History Taking

Once you have identified and treated life threats, you can then move on to gathering a history from the patient. If you have not yet done so, you should determine and investigate the patient's chief complaint and further investigate the MOI. You will also identify any associated signs and symptoms and pertinent negatives.

Obtain a history of the present illness using the OPQRST mnemonic (Onset, Provocation/palliation, Quality, Region/radiation, Severity, Timing), and a past medical history using the SAMPLE mnemonic (Signs and symptoms, Allergies, Medications, Pertinent past medical history, Last oral intake, Events leading up to the illness or injury) from the patient. Using OPQRST to help explain an abdominal injury may provide some helpful information, such as the description of the pain and whether the pain is radiating. If the patient is not responsive, attempt to obtain the SAMPLE history from friends or family members.

Be sure to ask whether the patient has experienced any nausea, vomiting, or diarrhea. If the patient has experienced any of these symptoms, ask how many times and during which time period. Ask about the appearance of any bowel movements and urinary output to check for any blood in the urine, black tarry stools (**melena**), or the presence of blood in the stools (**hematochezia**). This information can help to determine whether the patient has gastrointestinal bleeding. In addition, note the presence of any rectal bleeding.

The incidence of repeated or previous injury or illness involving the genitourinary system can help determine the extent of the current injury and possibly the MOI. The last intake of food and fluids is important because it can help to predict what is contained in the genitourinary system and whether the symptoms are related to the ingestion of those foods and fluids.

Words of Wisdom

Obtaining a good patient history that includes medications being taken may help to increase your index of suspicion for significant injury. For example, a patient taking a beta blocker or using a constant pacemaker will not necessarily have the increase in pulse associated with shock.

Secondary Assessment

The secondary assessment may need to be performed en route to the emergency department (ED). If you have not already done so, obtain a full set of vital signs—including pulse rate, blood pressure, respirations, oxygen saturation, mental status, skin condition, and pupils. Each of these is considered an indication of how the patient is tolerating the injuries.

Many abdominal emergencies, in addition to those that cause severe bleeding, can cause a rapid pulse and low blood pressure. Your record of vital signs, made as early as possible and periodically thereafter (every 5 minutes in a patient whom you suspect has a serious injury), will help you to identify changes in the patient's condition and be alert to signs of decompensation from blood loss. If the patient is experiencing external or internal hemorrhaging, as in the case of a stab wound or a direct blow to the abdomen, monitor the vital signs closely with a degree of suspicion and pay close attention to shifts in the vital signs. Signs such as tachycardia, tachypnea, low blood pressure, weak pulse, and cool, moist, and pale skin indicate hypoperfusion and imply the need for rapid treatment at the hospital.

In a patient who has an isolated injury to the abdomen with a limited MOI, such as in a stabbing, you should focus your assessment on the isolated injury, the patient's complaint, and the body region affected. However, usually, you will perform the physical examination on all patients with abdominal injuries in the same manner:

- Remove or loosen clothes to expose the injured regions of the body. Inspect the patient for bleeding again before removing the patient's clothing to prevent damaging any exposed tissues such as in the case of an evisceration.
- Provide privacy as needed, or wait until you are in the back of the ambulance.
- A patient without suspected spinal injury should be allowed to stay in the position of comfort—with the legs pulled up toward the abdomen. This position will relieve some of the tension on the abdomen and, therefore, provide pain relief.
- For patients with spinal injury, place padding such as blankets or pillows under the patient's knees to help alleviate tension on the abdominal wall. Keep in mind that you can worsen the spinal injury if you are too aggressive when placing these items.

Examine the entire abdomen, including all posterior, anterior, and lateral surfaces. This is a critical step when patients have an injury with an entrance wound. Examine the axillae (armpits) for entrance wounds.

When you auscultate the bowel, keep in mind that in the prehospital setting, bowel sounds can be difficult to hear, difficult to interpret, and diverse in cause. Blood, gastrointestinal contents, and urine that have spilled into the peritoneum may produce peritonitis that could result in decreased or absent abdominal sounds. Maintain a high index of suspicion, and provide early treatment for shock.

Look for the presence of contusions and abrasions, which can help localize focal points of impact and may indicate significant internal injury. Bruises or other visible marks are important clues to the cause

YOU are the Provider PART 3

Once fire department personnel arrive on scene, you consult with the officer in charge on the engine and request that the branch be cut approximately 12 inches (30 cm) from the patient, making sure that extreme care is taken to minimize movement of the branch. Your partner maintains manual stabilization of the patient's head while you apply a cervical collar. While the fire department personnel are preparing their equipment, you insert a single 18-gauge IV line.

Recording Time: 8 Minutes	
Respirations	22 breaths/min; normal
Pulse	Strong and rapid; 122 beats/min
Skin	Cool, pale, and clammy
Blood pressure	78/46 mm Hg
Oxygen saturation (Spo_2)	100% on room air
Pupils	Pupils Equal, Round, and Reactive to Light (PERRL)

5. Does this patient require a second IV line?
6. Once the tree branch is cut free from the tree, how do you secure it?

Words of Wisdom

Assess the abdomen for:

- DCAP-BTLS
- Distention
- Rigidity
- Guarding
- Rebound tenderness

and severity of any blunt injury. Steering wheels and seat belts produce characteristic patterns of bruising on the abdomen or chest. Note the presence of any burns, and manage them appropriately. Identify and treat any lacerations with appropriate dressings. Swelling may involve the abdomen globally and indicate significant intra-abdominal injury.

Next, inspect the skin of the abdomen for holes (puncture wounds) through which bullets, knives, or other missile-type foreign bodies may have passed. Keep in mind that the size of the wound does not necessarily indicate the extent of underlying injuries. If you find an entry wound, you must always check for a corresponding exit wound in the patient's back or sides. If the injury was caused by a high-velocity missile from a rifle, you may see a small, harmless-looking entrance wound with a large, gaping exit wound. Do not attempt to remove a knife or other object that is impaled in the patient. Instead, stabilize the object with bulky dressings and supportive bandaging.

The kidneys are located in the flank region of the back. Inspect and palpate this area for tenderness, bruising, swelling, and other signs of trauma. Although you may not be able to elicit pain from the specific organ, the tissues around it may exhibit symptoms of pain.

Up to this point in the patient assessment process, you may have been stabilizing the patient's spine by simply holding the head still and telling the patient not to move. If a cervical collar has not been applied, place one on the patient now before you log roll the patient to inspect the posterior part of the body and place the patient on a backboard. Penetrating trauma alone is not an indication for spinal immobilization. For example, time should not be wasted immobilizing a patient who has penetrating trauma to the head, neck, or torso.[14]

Finally, note whether the patient has hematuria (blood in the urine). This is a cardinal sign of renal and urinary tract injury, which can occur when renal or urinary vessels rupture, or when blood is able to enter the urine during glomerular filtration. Note the color of the urine: a darker brown suggests bleeding in the upper urinary tract, whereas a brighter red is most likely due to bleeding in the lower portion of the tract.

Pain Assessment

A common misconception is that patients without abdominal pain or abnormal vital signs are unlikely to have serious intra-abdominal injuries. In reality, peritonitis can take hours to days to develop. Similarly, nonspecific symptoms such as hypotension, tachycardia, and confusion may not develop until the patient has lost more than 40% of his or her circulating blood volume.[15] Always maintain a high index of suspicion in any patient who has an MOI consistent with abdominal trauma, regardless of the examination findings. Abdominal distention is a late indication of abdominal trauma. Patients must have a significant volume of blood enter the abdominal cavity to fill it and produce distention.

Words of Wisdom

Log rolling the patient onto a backboard is a valuable opportunity to examine the back for signs of injury. Instruct and position assistants to ensure your ability to inspect and palpate the back briefly while the patient is rolled onto the side.

If possible, pad the backboard before returning the patient to a supine position. This helps reduce discomfort and prevents aggravating soft-tissue injuries.

Avoid log rolling patients with an evisceration because this movement can cause more of the intestines to protrude from the wound. Instead, keep the patient in the supine position and allow him or her to flex the knees when possible to help relieve tension on the abdomen. A scoop stretcher is an option for lifting the patient in this case.

Quickly assess the patient's condition with a simple inspection, noting the manner in which he or she is lying. Movement of the body or the abdominal organs irritates the inflamed peritoneum, causing additional pain. To minimize this pain, patients may lie still, usually with the knees drawn up, and breathe using rapid and shallow breaths. For the same reason, they may contract abdominal muscles (guarding).

Assess the patient's pain. **Somatic pain** comes from skin and muscle, as well as joints, ligaments, and tendons. It is often described as sharp and localized to the area of injury. Bleeding, swelling, and cramping may exist with somatic pain. This pain usually responds well to medications such as opioids and nonsteroidal anti-inflammatory drugs. **Visceral pain** comes from organs inside the body with injury or illness. This type of pain travels from pain receptors in the nerves running throughout the body. The pain receptors transfer the information to the brain, where the pain is then perceived. Visceral pain can radiate to other locations such as the back and chest. There are three main areas where visceral pain is felt: the thorax, abdomen, and pelvis. Such pain is often described as a deep ache with cramping.

Because pain is a common symptom in abdominal and urologic ailments, it is often difficult to determine the source of the pain. Do not waste valuable time trying to determine the exact cause of the pain in the prehospital setting.

Abdominal pain together with an MOI that suggests injury to the abdomen or flank is a good indication for rapid transport. Transport to a trauma center is indicated for any patient who has an MOI that produces a high index of suspicion and who has any visible significant trauma, whether blunt or penetrating. Do not delay transport of a seriously injured trauma patient to complete non–lifesaving treatments such as splinting extremity fractures. Instead, complete these types of treatments en route to the hospital to the extent feasible.

Special Populations

Pregnant patients pose special challenges. Traumatic injuries to pregnant patients can be further complicated by the physiologic changes experienced by the patient. Some changes can mimic shock. For example, the pregnant patient's heart rate can increase by as much as 20 beats/min, blood volume can increase by as much as 50% during midpregnancy, and a pregnant woman can experience relative anemia from hemodilution (hemoglobin remains steady while fluid volume increases).[16] Due to the increase in blood flow to the uterus, the risk for massive blood loss is greatly increased with trauma to the bony pelvis. At term, the placenta/uterus can perfuse approximately 600 to 800 mL of blood per minute.

Treatment of pregnant patients should always start with the ABCs. There is a higher risk of aspiration and increase in gastric acidity. All pregnant patients should receive maximum oxygenation because of increased oxygen consumption and reduced reserve. Hypoxia can cause a 30% reduction in uterine blood flow.[17] Also, remember that if the pregnant patient is at more than 20 weeks' gestation, she should be tilted at least 15° to her left to prevent supine hypotensive syndrome, which can result from pressure on the vena cava. This may be accomplished by placing blankets or other padding material underneath the backboard. If the patient is secured to a long backboard, towel rolls can be placed under the backboard to accomplish the tilting.

Reassessment

Repeat the patient's primary survey and reassess vital signs. Reassess the interventions and treatment you have provided to the patient. Identifying trends in pain, vital signs, and the progress of treatments will help determine whether the patient's condition is improving or getting worse. Adjustments in care can be based on these objective findings.

Communicate the MOI and injuries found during your assessment, so the hospital staff will be prepared for the patient. Documentation of your assessment and the trends in vital signs is also a tremendous help to physicians in evaluating the problem when the patient arrives in the ED. Document the results of the physical examination and any pertinent negatives such as no blood loss noted in bowel movements. Also document if you passed over any step of the physical examination, such as with a patient with acute abdominal pain in whom you opted to not perform palpation. It is imperative that you be able to describe the scene in enough detail so the trauma team has a clear idea of the circumstances surrounding the event. Some services and departments now carry digital or other instant cameras that enable AEMTs to show the MOI to the trauma team.

If assault is suspected, you may have a legal requirement to inform the hospital staff of your suspicions; however, this information can wait until you have delivered the patient to the hospital and have a chance to discuss it privately with appropriate hospital personnel.

Be cautious and diligent when dealing with patients who refuse transport to the hospital after sustaining an injury to the abdomen or genitourinary system. Patients with these injuries are at high risk for complications; therefore, that information should be explained to them in great detail. Contacting medical control for assistance to convince the patient of the need for transport can be very useful. If the patient continues to refuse transport, have the patient sign a document of refusal or an "against medical advice" form.

Assessment and Management of Specific Injuries

Patients presenting with blunt injury and evidence of substantial abdominal trauma are potentially not reliable based on the distracting nature of the abdominal injury. Based on mechanism, therefore, they should undergo spinal immobilization or spinal motion restriction. If there is no suspected spinal trauma involved and the patient is reliable, the patient may be placed in a position of comfort. High-flow oxygen should also be administered. Cover the patient to maintain warmth. Consider the use of a pneumatic antishock garment (PASG) for an unstable pelvis if dictated by local protocol.[18] PASG is discussed in Chapter 27, *Bleeding*.

Most abdominal trauma requires rapid transport to the closest, most appropriate facility. Surgery is often the required definitive care for these injuries. Provide emotional and psychological support en route. For AEMT units, consider calling for paramedic mutual aid. Call your report in to the ED as soon as possible to allow for preparation for your arrival. Complete your documentation thoroughly and as soon as possible after transferring the patient to the ED.

▶ Closed/Blunt Abdominal Injuries

A patient with a blunt abdominal injury may have one or some combination of the following:

- Severe bruises of the abdominal wall
- Laceration of the liver and spleen
- Rupture of the intestine, gallbladder, or stomach
- Tears in the mesentery
- Rupture of the kidneys or avulsion of the kidneys from their supporting structures
- Rupture of the urinary bladder, especially in a patient who had a full and distended bladder at the time of injury (for example, a patient who had been drinking)
- Severe intra-abdominal hemorrhage
- Peritoneal irritation and inflammation in response to the rupture of hollow organs

If you suspect injury to the diaphragm, focus on the airway, breathing, and circulatory status of the patient. Signs and symptoms of a diaphragmatic rupture can include abdominal pain, acute respiratory distress, decreased breath sounds, abdominal sounds in the chest, subcutaneous emphysema, and a scaphoid abdomen—a sunken abdomen or an abdomen that appears empty. Examine the patient's neck and chest, paying particular attention to the trachea (tracheal deviation due to mediastinal shift), symmetry of the chest during expansion, and absence of breath sounds.

Immobilize any patient who has sustained a blunt abdominal injury when indicated by MOI and/or patient presentation. If the patient vomits, turn him or her to one side and clear the mouth and throat of vomitus. Monitor the patient's vital signs for any indication of shock, such as pallor, diaphoresis, low blood pressure, and rapid, thready pulse. If you see any of these signs, administer supplemental oxygen via a nonrebreathing mask or provide positive pressure ventilation via a bag-mask device if needed and take all the appropriate measures to treat for shock. Keep the patient warm with blankets, and provide prompt transport to the ED.

▶ Open/Penetrating Abdominal Injuries

Patients with penetrating injuries generally have obvious wounds and external bleeding Figure 32-14A. A large wound may have bowel, fat, or a fold of peritoneum protruding from it. In addition to pain, patients often report nausea and vomiting.

YOU are the Provider — PART 4

On the basis of the patient's vital signs and physical examination findings, you elect to insert a second IV line and administer four sequential 250-mL boluses of normal saline, checking the blood pressure after each bolus and stopping the boluses once systolic blood pressure exceeds 80 mm Hg. Once the fire department personnel have cut the branch free from the tree, you pad around the branch with multiple bulky dressings and roller gauze in an attempt to secure it. With the assistance of everyone on scene, you secure the patient to a long backboard and initiate rapid transport to the local Level I trauma center, approximately 9 minutes away. The remainder of the transport remains uneventful, with the patient's vital signs stabilizing with a blood pressure above 80 mm Hg systolic.

Recording Time: 14 Minutes	
Respirations	20 breaths/min; normal
Pulse	Strong and regular; 100 beats/min
Skin	Warm, dry, and pink
Blood pressure	92/60 mm Hg (after initial 250-mL fluid bolus)
Oxygen saturation (Spo_2)	100% with oxygen at 15 L/min via nonrebreathing mask
Pupils	PERRL

7. Does this patient require evaluation at a trauma center, or should she be transported to the closest facility for evaluation first?

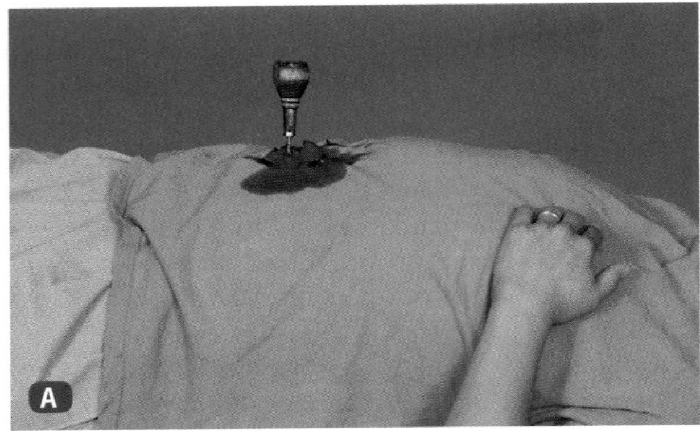

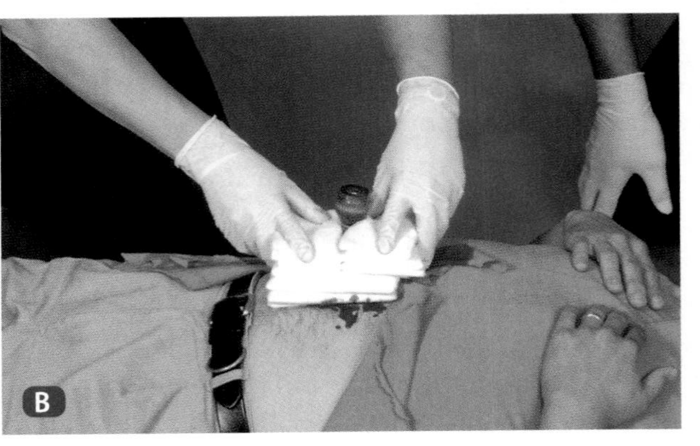

Figure 32-14 A. Penetrating injuries have obvious wounds and may also have external bleeding. **B.** If the penetrating object is still in place, use bulky dressings and a roller bandage to stabilize the object and to control bleeding.

Table 32-1 Penetrating Trauma: Velocity and Resulting Cavitation

Velocity	Type of Weapon	Cavitation
Low energy	Hand-driven weapons such as knives, scissors, and ice picks	There is minimal cavitation, and the damage is only by the cutting edge.
Medium energy	Low-velocity weapons such as handguns and low-powered firearms (such as .38 special, .45 ATC [authorization to carry]) in which the muzzle velocity is less than 1,500 feet per second	The projectile is small, and cavitation is 6 to 10 times the bullet's frontal area.
High energy	High-velocity weapons such as high-powered rifles and military high-velocity, small-caliber weapons such as M16, AK-47, which have a muzzle velocity of greater than 1,500 feet per second	Cavitation is 20 to 30 times the frontal area of the missile.

Some penetrating injuries go no deeper than the abdominal wall, but the severity of the injury can be difficult to determine. Only a surgeon can accurately assess the damage. Therefore, as you care for a patient with this type of wound, you should assume that the object has penetrated the peritoneum, entered the abdominal cavity, and possibly injured one or more organs, even if there are no immediate obvious signs. See Chapter 26, *Trauma Overview*, for further explanation of low-, medium-, and high-velocity penetrating trauma, outlined here in Table 32-1.

In caring for a patient with a penetrating wound of the abdomen, follow the general procedures previously described for care of a blunt abdominal wound, as well as the following specific steps for the penetrating wound: inspect the patient's back and sides for exit wounds, and apply a dry, sterile dressing to all open wounds.

If the penetrating object is still in place, do not remove it. Expose the wound. Then, while manually stabilizing the object in its position, apply bulky dressings around it to control external bleeding, and then secure the dressings in place with a stabilizing bandage, which will minimize movement of the object Figure 32-14B.

Words of Wisdom

The only reason to remove an impaled object is when it is through the cheek and interferes with breathing or maintaining an airway, or when it is in the chest and interferes with cardiopulmonary resuscitation.

Initiate two 18-gauge IV lines or larger or follow local protocol, and administer isotonic crystalloid solutions to deliver sequential 250-mL boluses (up to a maximum of four) or the amount needed to obtain a systolic blood pressure of 80 mm Hg. Increasing blood pressure can increase internal bleeding, so fluid should be given in a volume to maintain perfusion to vital organs.

▶ Abdominal Evisceration

During assessment of an evisceration, do not push down on the patient's abdomen. Perform only a visual assessment when there is any suspicion of this type of injury. If there is clothing close to the wound, carefully cut the clothing around the wound, leaving a border of intact cloth outside the injured area. Never pull, even gently, on any clothing stuck to or in the wound channel because this may remove even more of the organ.

When you are caring for an evisceration, never try to replace an organ that is protruding from the abdomen, whether it is a small fold of peritoneum or nearly all of the intestines. Instead, cover it with sterile gauze compresses moistened with sterile saline solution, and secure them with a dry, sterile dressing. (Protocols in some EMS systems call for an occlusive dressing over the organs, secured by trauma dressings.)

Because the open abdomen radiates body heat very effectively and because exposed organs lose fluid rapidly, you must keep the organs moist and warm. If you do not have gauze compresses, you may use moist, sterile dressings, covered and secured in place with a bandage and tape **Figure 32-15**. Do not use any material that is adherent or loses its substance when wet, such as toilet paper, facial tissue, paper towels, or absorbent cotton.

Once you have covered the extruding organ, you should provide other emergency care as necessary and provide prompt transport to the ED. Treat the patient for shock by keeping the patient warm and, if possible, placing the patient in the position dictated by local protocol for shock patients. Provide high-flow oxygen and transport according to local protocols and destination policy. Transport the patient to the highest-level trauma center available.

Words of Wisdom

Anything that is normally located within the body must be kept moist when it is outside the body. Cover eviscerated organs with sterile, moist dressings.

Kidneys

Damage to the kidneys may not be obvious on inspection of the patient. You may or may not see bruises or lacerations on the overlying skin. However, you will see signs of shock if the injury is associated with significant blood loss. Because one of the functions of the kidney is the formation of urine, another sign of kidney damage is blood in the urine (hematuria). Treat shock and associated injuries in the appropriate manner. Provide prompt transport to the hospital, monitoring the patient's vital signs carefully en route.

Urinary Bladder

Suspect a possible injury to the urinary bladder if you see blood at the urethral opening or physical signs of trauma on the lower abdomen, pelvis, or perineum. There may be blood at the tip of the penis or a stain on the patient's underwear.

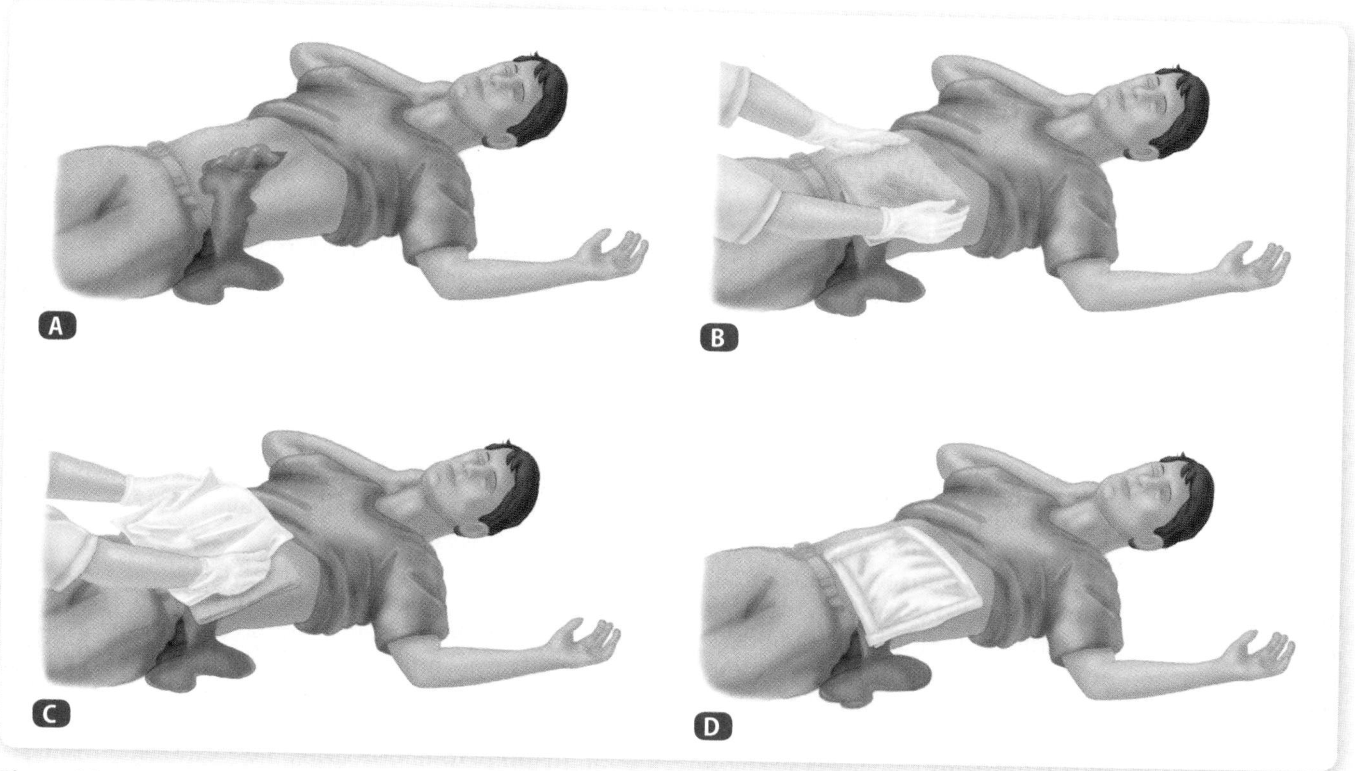

Figure 32-15 A. The open abdomen radiates body heat rapidly and must be covered. **B.** Cover the wound with moistened, sterile dressings and with an occlusive dressing, depending on local protocol. **C.** Secure the dressing with a bandage. **D.** Secure the bandage with tape.

The presence of associated injuries or of shock will dictate the urgency of transport. In most cases, provide prompt transport, and monitor the patient's vital signs en route.

▶ External Male Genitalia

A few general rules apply to the treatment of injuries involving the external male genitalia:

- These injuries are very painful. Make the patient as comfortable as possible.
- Use sterile, moist compresses to cover areas that have been stripped of skin.
- Apply direct pressure with dry, sterile gauze dressings to control bleeding.
- Never move or manipulate impaled instruments or foreign bodies in the urethra.
- If possible, always identify and take avulsed parts to the hospital with the patient; label the bag with the patient's name.

If you encounter a patient with an avulsion (tearing away) of skin of the penis, wrap the penis in a soft, sterile dressing moistened with sterile saline solution, and transport the patient promptly. Use direct pressure to control any bleeding. You should try to save and preserve the avulsed skin, but do not delay treatment or transport for more than a few minutes to do so.

Managing blood loss is your top priority in amputation of the penile shaft, whether partial or complete. You should use local pressure with a sterile dressing on the remaining stump. Never apply a constricting device to the penis to control bleeding. Surgical reconstruction of even a completely amputated penis is possible if you can locate the amputated part. Wrap it in a moist, sterile dressing; place it in a plastic bag; and transport it in a cooled container without allowing it to come in direct contact with ice.

If the connective tissue surrounding the erectile tissue in the penis is severely damaged, the shaft of the penis can be fractured or severely angled, sometimes requiring surgical repair. The injury may occur during particularly active sexual intercourse. It is associated with intense pain, bleeding into the tissues, and fear. Provide prompt transport to the ED.

Accidental laceration of the skin about the head of the penis usually occurs when the penis is erect and is associated with heavy bleeding. The injury usually appears worse than it actually is; once the penis becomes flaccid, the size of the laceration decreases. Local pressure with a sterile dressing is usually sufficient to stop the hemorrhage.

It is not uncommon for the skin of the shaft of the penis or the foreskin to get caught in the zipper of pants. If a small segment of the zipper is involved (one or two teeth), you can try to unzip the pants. If a longer segment is involved or the patient is agitated, use heavy scissors to cut the zipper out of the pants to make the patient more comfortable during transport. Explain all procedures to alert patients to reduce anxiety in an already stressful situation. Be particularly careful not to cause additional injury to the scrotum while cutting the zipper away from the penis.

Urethral injuries in men are not uncommon. Lacerations of the urethra can result from straddle injuries, pelvic fractures, or penetrating wounds of the perineum. These injuries may bleed quite severely, although this may not be evident externally. Direct pressure with a dry, sterile dressing usually controls any external hemorrhage. Because the urethra is the channel for urine, it is very important to know whether the patient can urinate and whether hematuria is present. For this reason, you should save any voided urine for later examination at the hospital. Any foreign bodies that may be protruding from the urethra will have to be removed in a surgical setting.

Avulsion of the skin of the scrotum may damage the scrotal contents. If possible, preserve the avulsed skin in a moist, sterile dressing for possible use in reconstruction. Wrap the scrotal contents or the perineal area with a sterile, moist compress, and use a local pressure dressing to control bleeding. Promptly transport the patient to the ED.

Words of Wisdom

A scrotal laceration may serve as a portal through which bacteria can enter the scrotum or perineum. The resulting infection, called Fournier gangrene, causes necrosis of the muscle and other subcutaneous tissue within the scrotum. The scrotum may feel spongy, and the accumulation of gas in the scrotal sac may produce the distinctive sounds of crepitus. The scrotal tissues will become gray-black, drainage will occur at the wound site, and fever and scrotal pain will be present. This is a true emergency, and prompt transport to the hospital is indicated. If left untreated, the infection can enter the bloodstream and can be rapidly fatal.

Testicular torsion should always be suspected when there was direct trauma to the testicles and the patient has persistent pain. Transport patients with these injuries rapidly to an ED that has ultrasound capability and an available urologist.

Direct blows to the scrotum can result in the rupture of a testicle or significant accumulation of blood around the testes. In either case, you should apply an ice pack to the scrotal area while transporting the patient.

A number of reports have described patients who have placed tight objects around the penis, testicles, or both. Inability to remove the object can result in incarceration of the organ, with tissue death being the most feared consequence. No attempt to remove the object should be made in the field. Instead, the patient should be transported to the hospital for proper evaluation and treatment, which may necessitate the use of cutting devices or aspiration of the distal edema.

▶ Female Genitalia

Lacerations, abrasions, and avulsions should be treated with moist, sterile compresses. Use local pressure to control bleeding and a diaper-type bandage to hold dressings in place. Under no circumstances should you pack or place dressings into the vagina. Leave any foreign bodies in place, and stabilize them with bandages.

Because the genitals have a rich nerve supply, injuries to them are very painful, but in general, they are not life threatening. Bleeding may be heavy, but it can usually be controlled by local compression. Contusions and other blunt injuries all require careful in-hospital evaluation. However, the urgency of the need for transport will be determined by associated injuries, the amount of hemorrhage, and the presence of shock.

If you believe your patient has been sexually assaulted, do not examine the genitalia unless obvious bleeding requires you to apply a dressing. Sexual assault is covered in detail in Chapter 25, *Gynecologic Emergencies*.

YOU are the Provider SUMMARY

1. Do you need additional resources to manage this call?

The decision to request additional resources will depend on the availability of the resources and your level of training. If you are a great distance from a trauma center and have aeromedical services available, they should also be dispatched to minimize the time to surgical care. If your ambulance is not equipped with simple extrication equipment or you do not have the necessary training to perform extrication, the fire department should be requested to perform the extrication.

2. What are the potential injuries you may encounter?

The potential injuries you may encounter will vary widely based on several factors. You may encounter a patient who is unresponsive, has multiple fractures, has an uncontrolled airway, or has a significant internal or external hemorrhage. You should be prepared to encounter a patient with significant multisystem trauma.

3. How do you remove the branch from the wound?

Do not attempt to remove the impaled object from a wound. Using extreme caution to prevent further injury, you should have the branch cut as far away from the patient as possible (but not so far as to impair transport to the hospital), and then stabilize the branch with substantial amounts of bulky dressings and roller gauze.

4. On the basis of the patient's presentation, does she require spinal immobilization?

Absolutely. The patient hit a stationary object at a moderate rate of speed and was not wearing any protective gear. Furthermore, she has an impaled object in her abdominal cavity, which may cause further unseen injuries. Finally, the shock state she is clearly experiencing makes her unreliable from the standpoint of being able to report (based on history and physical examination findings) that she has no spinal pain, no neurologic symptoms such as numbness or tingling in her extremities, no weakness on examination of her limbs, and no tenderness along her spine. All of these criteria must be present in a reliable patient to make a determination that spinal immobilization is unnecessary.

5. Does this patient require a second IV line?

This patient is presenting with signs and symptoms of shock. On the basis of your exam findings, she has a great potential for uncontrolled internal hemorrhage. She therefore requires a second IV line. The second line should be started en route to the trauma center so as not to prolong scene time.

6. Once the tree branch is cut free from the tree, how do you secure it?

The branch should be handled with care, minimizing its movement, to avoid causing secondary injuries. Multiple bulky dressings should be applied to pad around the branch to stabilize it, and roller gauze should be applied to hold the bulky dressings in place.

7. Does this patient require evaluation at a trauma center, or should she be transported to the closest facility for evaluation first?

Because this patient presented with a penetrating injury, she requires a surgical consultation. If there is a Level I or Level II trauma center available, she should be transported there, if possible. If you do not have a local trauma center, the patient should be transported to the closest appropriate facility. As always, consult your local protocols and online medical control if you are unsure of the appropriate facility.

YOU are the Provider SUMMARY (continued)

EMS Patient Care Report (PCR)					
Date: 10-4-18	**Incident No.:** 20107128131		**Nature of Call:** ATV accident	**Location:** 2 miles south of Jones Road	
Dispatched: 1312	**En Route:** 1313	**At Scene:** 1324	**Transport:** 1344	**At Hospital:** 1353	**In Service:** 1420

Patient Information	
Age: 32 **Sex:** F **Weight (in kg [lb]):** 57 kg (127 lb)	**Allergies:** None **Medications:** Birth control pills **Past Medical History:** None **Chief Complaint:** Impaled object

Vital Signs				
Time: 1332	**BP:** 78/46	**Pulse:** 122	**Respirations:** 22	**Spo_2:** 100% R/A
Time: 1338	**BP:** 92/60	**Pulse:** 100	**Respirations:** 20	**Spo_2:** 100% on 15 L
Time: 1344	**BP:** 88/62	**Pulse:** 100	**Respirations:** 20	**Spo_2:** 100% on 15 L/min
Time: 1349	**BP:** 92/64	**Pulse:** 96	**Respirations:** 18	**Spo_2:** 100% on 15 L/min

EMS Treatment (circle all that apply)				
Oxygen @ 15 **L/min via (circle one):** **NC** **(NRM)** **Bag-mask device**		**Assisted Ventilation**	**Airway Adjunct**	**CPR**
Defibrillation	**(Bleeding Control:** Yes)	**(Bandaging:** Yes)	**(Splinting:** Yes)	**Other:**

Narrative

EMS dispatched to unknown ATV accident 2 miles south of Jones Road on county road 55. En route, additional information received that patient struck a rock at moderate speed and is impaled on a tree branch. Pembina County Rural Volunteer Fire Department requested for extrication. On arrival, pt found lying on brush, AO×4, ABCs intact, with an approximately 4-foot-long, 2-inch-diameter tree branch impaling her RUQ. Pt denies any injuries other than obvious tree branch. Manual stabilization established while FD cuts branch from tree. 18-gauge IV established to left antecubital area with 250-mL bolus of normal saline given. Once free from tree, branch secured with multiple bulky dressings and roller gauze. Patient secured to long backboard with +PMS to all 4 extremities. States pain 6/10. Emergency transport initiated to Legacy Hospital per trauma criteria. En route, patient vital signs improve, still reporting 6/10 pain. On arrival at ED, care and report left with MD without incident.**End of report**

Prep Kit

▶ Ready for Review

- The abdomen is divided arbitrarily into quadrants by two perpendicular lines that intersect at the umbilicus. These areas are referred to as the right upper quadrant, left upper quadrant, right lower quadrant, and left lower quadrant. The quadrant location of bruising or pain can delineate which organs are possibly involved in a traumatic injury.
- The genitourinary system is composed of the reproductive system and the urinary system. The urinary system controls the discharge of certain waste materials filtered from the blood by the kidneys. The reproductive system controls the reproductive processes from which life is created.
- Abdominal injuries can be categorized as open (penetrating trauma) or closed (blunt force trauma). Either type of injury can result in injury to the hollow or solid organs of the abdomen and cause significant life-threatening bleeding.
- Blunt force that causes closed injuries results from an object striking the body without breaking the skin, such as being hit with a baseball bat or when the patient's body strikes the steering wheel during a motor vehicle crash.
- Penetrating injuries are most frequently caused by knives or handguns. Other mechanisms of injury such as a fall on an object can also cause penetrating trauma to the abdomen.
- Blunt and penetrating trauma cause pain, although the pain may be masked at first.
- The most common sign of significant abdominal injury is tachycardia. Later signs are those of shock: decreased blood pressure and pale, cool, moist skin.
- Injury to the solid internal organs often causes significant unseen bleeding that can be life threatening.
- Injury to the hollow organs of the abdomen may cause an intense inflammatory reaction called peritonitis as caustic digestive juices leak into the peritoneal cavity. Infection may occur over as little as several hours. Peritonitis is serious and may become life threatening.
- Seat belts occasionally cause blunt injuries to the abdominal organs, and special attention should be given when evaluating patients injured in a motor vehicle with a deployed airbag.
- Injuries to the kidneys or bladder will not have obvious external signs, but there are usually more subtle clues such as lower rib pain or a possible pelvic fracture.
- Injuries to the kidneys may be difficult to detect because of the well-protected region of the body where they are located. Be alert to bruising or a hematoma in the flank region.
- Injury to the external genitalia of male and female patients is very painful but not usually life threatening.
- Always maintain a high index of suspicion for serious intra-abdominal injury in trauma patients, particularly in a patient who exhibits signs of shock.
- To assess abdominal injuries, place the patient in a supine position, assess and record vital signs, and perform a visual inspection. Always assume that major damage has occurred to abdominal organs, even if there are no obvious signs.
- When assessing a genitourinary injury, always consider patient privacy. Be sensitive to any embarrassment, and maintain a professional presence at all times.
- Assess the abdomen for bruises or other marks that may point you toward underlying damage: a firm abdomen, difficulty moving, abdominal tenderness and guarding, obvious entry and exit wounds, and altered vital signs.
- Treat for shock as necessary, keep the airway clear of vomitus, keep the patient warm, and promptly transport him or her to the emergency department or a trauma center, if available.
- Never remove an impaled object from the abdominal region. Secure it in place with a large bulky dressing, and provide prompt transport.
- Never replace an organ that protrudes from an open injury to the abdomen (evisceration). Instead, keep the organ moist and warm. Cover the injury site with a large, sterile, moist, bulky dressing.
- Establish intravenous access, and administer fluid at a rate to maintain systolic blood pressure greater than 80 mm Hg. Attempting to return blood pressure to normal limits may increase internal bleeding.

▶ Vital Vocabulary

abdominal aortic aneurysm (AAA) A condition in which the walls of the aorta in the abdomen weaken and blood leaks into the layers of the vessel, causing it to bulge.

closed abdominal injury An injury in which there is soft-tissue damage inside the body but the skin remains intact.

Cullen sign A black-and-blue discoloration (ecchymosis) in the umbilical region caused by peritoneal bleeding.

evisceration The displacement of organs outside of the body.

flank The region below the rib cage and above the hip.

guarding Contracting the stomach muscles to minimize the pain of abdominal movement; a sign of peritonitis.

hematochezia Blood in the stool.

hematuria Blood in the urine.

Prep Kit *(continued)*

hemoperitoneum Collection of blood in the abdominal cavity.

hollow organs Structures through which materials pass, such as the stomach, gallbladder, small intestine, large intestine, ureters, and urinary bladder.

Kehr sign Left shoulder pain caused by blood in the peritoneal cavity due to rupture of the spleen.

melena Black, tarry stools.

open abdominal injury An injury in which there is a break in the surface of the skin or mucous membrane, exposing deeper tissue to potential contamination.

peritoneal cavity The abdominal cavity.

peritonitis Inflammation of the peritoneum.

pneumoperitoneum Air in the peritoneal cavity.

rebound tenderness Pain that the patient feels when pressure is released as opposed to when pressure is applied.

scaphoid abdomen Concave abdomen (sunken abdomen or an abdomen that appears empty), which is generally the result of a ruptured diaphragm.

solid organs Solid masses of tissue where much of the chemical work of the body takes place (eg, the liver, spleen, pancreas, and kidneys).

somatic pain Localized pain, usually felt deeply, which represents irritation or injury to tissue, causing activation of peripheral nerve tracts.

supine hypotensive syndrome A drop in blood pressure caused when the heavy uterus of a supine, third-trimester–pregnant patient obstructs the vena cava, lowering blood return to the heart.

visceral pain Crampy, aching pain deep within the body, the source of which is usually difficult to pinpoint; common with genitourinary problems.

▶ References

1. Saxena AK. Pediatric abdominal trauma. Medscape website. https://emedicine.medscape.com/article/1984811-overview. Updated October 5, 2017. Accessed December 8, 2017.
2. McGready JB, Breyer BN. Current epidemiology of genitourinary trauma. *Urol Clin North Am*. 2013;40(3):323-334.
3. Centers for Disease Control and Prevention, National Center for Health Statistics. All injuries. http://www.cdc.gov/nchs/fastats/injury.htm. Accessed November 23, 2016.
4. Centers for Disease Control and Prevention. Home and recreational safety: important facts about falls. http://www.cdc.gov/HomeandRecreationalSafety/Falls/adultfalls.html. Accessed November 23, 2016.
5. Greingor JL, Lazarus S. Chest and abdominal injuries caused by seat belt wearing. *South Med J*. 2006;99(4):534-535.
6. Wilson AJ. Gunshot injuries: what does a radiologist need to know? *RadioGraphics*. 1999;19(5). http://pubs.rsna.org/doi/full/10.1148/radiographics.19.5.g99se171358. Accessed November 23, 2016.
7. Characteristics of stab wounds. *Forensic medicine for medical students*. http://www.forensicmed.co.uk/wounds/sharp-force-trauma/stab-wounds/. Accessed November 23, 2016.
8. Snyder KA, Veronese VR. *Genitourinary injuries and renal management*. http://musculoskeletalkey.com/genitourinary-injuries-and-renal-management/. Accessed January 19, 2017.
9. What is kidney (renal) trauma? Urology Care Foundation. http://www.urologyhealth.org/urologic-conditions/kidney-(renal)-trauma. Accessed November 23, 2016.
10. Osterweil N. Sports-related injuries can cause isolated renal trauma. Medscape Medical News from the American Urological Association (AUA) 2014 Annual Scientific Meeting. May 27, 2014. http://www.medscape.com/viewarticle/825724. Accessed November 23, 2016.
11. Aziz A, Bota R, Ahmed M. Frequency and pattern of intra-abdominal injuries in patients with blunt abdominal trauma. *J Trauma Treat*. 2014;3:196. Accessed November 23, 2016.
12. Ahmed N, Vernick JJ. Pancreatic injury. *South Med J*. 2009;102(12):1253-1256.
13. Khadjibaev AM, Maksudkhon R, Khalilov ML. Bladder trauma: a 7 year review. *MedCrave*. 2017;5(3).
14. National Association of EMS Physicians, American College of Surgeons Committee on Trauma. EMS spinal precautions and the use of the long backboard. *Prehosp Emerg Care*. 2013;17:392-393.
15. Gutierrez G, Reines HD, Wulf-Gutierrez ME. Clinical review: hemorrhagic shock. *Crit Care*. 2004;8:373. http://ccforum.biomedcentral.com/articles/10.1186/cc2851. Accessed November 29, 2016.
16. Foley MR. Maternal cardiovascular and hemodynamic adaptations to pregnancy. *UpToDate*. November 11, 2015. http://www.uptodate.com/contents/maternal-cardiovascular-and-hemodynamic-adaptations-to-pregnancy. Accessed November 29, 2016.
17. Makowski EL, Hertz RH, Meschia G. Effects of acute maternal hypoxia and hyperoxia on the blood flow to the pregnant uterus. *Am J Obstet Gynecol*. 1973;115(5):624-631.
18. Bickell WH, Pepe PE, Bailey ML, Wyatt CH, Mattox KL. Randomized trial of pneumatic antishock garments in the prehospital management of penetrating abdominal injuries. *Ann Emerg Med*. 1987;16(6):653-658.

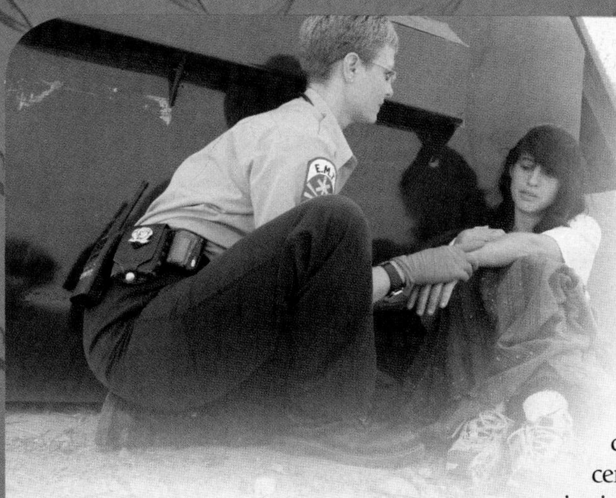

Assessment *in Action*

You are dispatched to a high-speed motor vehicle crash. On your arrival, you find an unresponsive, hypotensive man properly restrained in the driver's seat with significant bruising around the area of the lap belt. On the basis of the patient's MOI and rapid assessment, you recognize that the patient is in critical condition and must be rapidly transported to the local trauma center. Your initial set of vital signs is as follows: pulse, 136 beats/min; respirations, 16 breaths/min; and blood pressure, 76 mm Hg by palpation.

1. When worn properly, a seat belt lies below the ________ and against the hip joints.

- **A.** posterior inferior iliac spine of the pelvis
- **B.** anterior inferior iliac spine of the pelvis
- **C.** posterior superior iliac spine of the pelvis
- **D.** anterior superior iliac spine of the pelvis

2. Although the patient has an altered mental status, you may notice the presence of ______ when palpating the abdomen, which is a reliable sign of peritoneal irritation.

- **A.** guarding
- **B.** swelling
- **C.** deformity
- **D.** distention

3. Bruising in the lower abdominal area may be an indicator of internal bleeding. Which type of shock may be present?

- **A.** Cardiogenic
- **B.** Septic
- **C.** Hypovolemic
- **D.** Neurogenic

4. When abdominal organs are ruptured or lacerated, these organs spill their contents into the abdominal cavity, causing which intense inflammatory reaction?

- **A.** Peritonitis
- **B.** Pneumonitis
- **C.** Pneumothorax
- **D.** Pneumomediastinum

5. You gain IV access and decide to give a fluid bolus. The goal of fluid administration for this patient is to maintain a systolic blood pressure of at least ____ mm Hg.

- **A.** 120
- **B.** 100
- **C.** 80
- **D.** 60

6. Based on MOI and patient presentation, all of the following are indicated EXCEPT:

- **A.** spinal immobilization
- **B.** high-flow oxygen
- **C.** position of comfort
- **D.** IV fluid boluses

7. Movement of the body or the abdominal organs irritates the inflamed peritoneum, causing additional pain. To minimize this pain, patients typically prefer which position?

- **A.** Supine with the legs outward
- **B.** Fetal position with legs drawn in toward the chest
- **C.** Prone
- **D.** Variable according to each patient

8. A distended abdomen or pain may prevent adequate:

- **A.** inhalation.
- **B.** exhalation.
- **C.** circulation.
- **D.** perfusion.

9. Explain the treatment for a patient with an impaled object in the abdomen.

10. What is *Kehr sign* and what does it indicate?

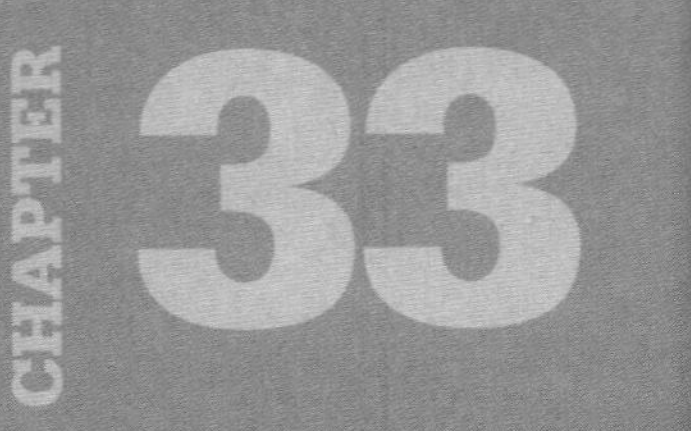

Orthopaedic Injuries

National EMS Education Standard Competencies

Trauma

Applies fundamental knowledge to provide basic and selected advanced emergency care and transportation based on assessment findings for an acutely injured patient.

Orthopaedic Trauma

Recognition and management of
- Open fractures (pp 1323-1326, 1335-1345)
- Closed fractures (pp 1323-1326, 1335-1345)
- Dislocations (pp 1326-1327, 1349-1354, 1357-1358, 1360-1364)
- Amputations (pp 1327, 1364)

Pathophysiology, assessment, and management of
- Upper and lower extremity orthopaedic trauma (pp 1321-1345, 1348-1354, 1359-1364)
- Open fractures (pp 1323-1345)
- Closed fractures (pp 1323-1345)
- Dislocations (pp 1326-1327, 1349-1354, 1357-1358, 1360-1364)
- Sprains/strains (pp 1327, 1364)
- Pelvic fractures (pp 1354-1357)
- Amputations/replantation (pp 1327, 1364)
- Compartment syndrome (p 1346)

Medicine

Applies fundamental knowledge to provide basic and selected advanced emergency care and transportation based on assessment findings for an acutely ill patient.

Nontraumatic Musculoskeletal Disorders

Anatomy, physiology, pathophysiology, assessment, and management of
- Nontraumatic fractures (pp 1321-1322)

Knowledge Objectives

1. Describe the function of the musculoskeletal system. (pp 1315-1316)
2. Review the anatomy and physiology of the musculoskeletal system. (pp 1316-1321)
3. Name the four types of forces that can cause musculoskeletal injuries. (p 1322)
4. Describe the various types of musculoskeletal injuries and the signs and symptoms of each. (pp 1323-1327)
5. Differentiate between open and closed fractures. (p 1323)
6. Describe the signs and symptoms of a dislocation, sprain, and a strain. (pp 1326-1327)
7. Explain how to assess the severity of a musculoskeletal injury. (p 1328)
8. Explain the reasons for splinting at the scene versus transporting the patient immediately. (pp 1330, 1336)
9. Explain the emergency medical care of a patient with an orthopaedic injury. (pp 1335-1345)
10. Explain the emergency medical care of a patient with a swollen, painful, deformed extremity (fracture). (pp 1335-1345)
11. Understand the need for splinting, including its principles and possible complications. (pp 1336-1337)
12. Describe the complications that can result from musculoskeletal injuries. (pp 1345-1348)
13. Recognize the characteristics of specific types of musculoskeletal injuries. (pp 1348-1364)
14. Explain the significance and the assessment and management of a patient with a pelvic fracture. (pp 1354-1357)
15. Explain the emergency medical care of the patient with an amputation. (p 1364)

Skills Objectives

1. Demonstrate the assessment of neurovascular status. (pp 1332-1334, Skill Drill 33-1)
2. Demonstrate the care of musculoskeletal injuries. (p 1335, Skill Drill 33-2)
3. Demonstrate how to apply a Hare traction splint. (pp 1339-1340, Skill Drill 33-3)
4. Demonstrate how to apply a Sager traction splint. (pp 1339-1341, Skill Drill 33-4)
5. Demonstrate how to apply a rigid splint. (pp 1341-1342, Skill Drill 33-5)

6. Demonstrate how to apply a zippered air splint. (p 1343, Skill Drill 33-6)
7. Demonstrate how to apply an unzippered air splint. (p 1343, Skill Drill 33-7)
8. Demonstrate how to apply a vacuum splint. (p 1344, Skill Drill 33-8)
9. Demonstrate how to splint the clavicle, the scapula, the shoulder, the humerus, the elbow, and the forearm. (pp 1349-1353)
10. Demonstrate how to splint the hand and wrist. (pp 1353-1354, Skill Drill 33-9)
11. Demonstrate how to care for a patient with an amputation. (p 1364)

Introduction

Musculoskeletal injuries are among the most common reasons why patients seek medical attention. Complaints related to the musculoskeletal system affect more than 126 million people in the United States, or more than one in every two adults older than 18 years.[1] More than 70% of Americans who lose workdays from health conditions report having some type of musculoskeletal impairment,[2] costing the US economy an estimated $210 billion yearly in direct and indirect costs.[3] These conditions are diagnosed in more women than men, and the incidence increases with age, with more than 70% of all people older than 65 years having a musculoskeletal disorder.[1]

Musculoskeletal injuries are often easily identified because of pain, swelling, and deformity. Although these injuries are rarely fatal, they often result in short- or long-term disability. By providing prompt assessment and treatment, such as splinting and analgesia, advanced emergency medical technicians (AEMTs) may help reduce the disability period for patients. Despite the dramatic appearance of some musculoskeletal injuries, do not focus solely on the injury without first determining that no life-threatening injuries exist. *Never forget to assess exsanguinating hemorrhage airway, breathing, circulation, disability, and exposure (XABCDEs).*

As an AEMT, you must be familiar with the basic anatomy of the musculoskeletal system. Although muscles are technically soft tissue, they are discussed in this chapter because of their close relationship with the skeleton. Therefore, the chapter begins with a review of the musculoskeletal anatomy. Various types and causes of musculoskeletal injuries in general are identified, and the assessment and treatment process for each is explained, followed by a detailed discussion of splinting. The chapter concludes with discussions on specific musculoskeletal injuries, beginning at the clavicle and ending at the feet.

Anatomy and Physiology Review

The musculoskeletal system gives the body its shape and allows for its movement. It also performs many important functions. Bones, for example, form a framework that gives the human body its shape and allows it to maintain an erect posture. *Movement* is generated because muscles are attached to bones by **tendons**. When a muscle contracts, the force generated by the muscle is transferred to a bone

YOU are the Provider — PART 1

Your ambulance is assigned standby service at a local arena for a high school rodeo event. As you are watching the rodeo, you see a young man bucked off a bull; he lands on his left side. You immediately ascertain that the bull has been secured within a gated area and that the scene is now safe for you to enter. Upon arriving at the patient's side, you note he is alert and oriented and in moderate distress. You see an obvious deformity of the left femur in the midshaft area, and a possibly unstable pelvis. Per your protocols, you ask your partner to contact dispatch and request the local flight service as you continue to assess the patient. As a precaution, you place the patient on a nonrebreathing mask and administer oxygen at 15 L/min. Upon completion of your primary survey, your partner informs you there are no helicopter or paramedic units available.

1. How should you prepare this patient for transport?
2. What should you do when advanced modes of transport are not available?

on the opposite side of the **joint** from the muscle, leading to motion. Bones also protect the more fragile organs and structures beneath them—for example, the skull protects the brain, the rib cage protects the heart and lungs, and the spinal column protects the spinal cord.

> **Words of Wisdom**
>
> To remember the meaning of *tendon*, use this: Muscles-to-bones (MTB) means muscles–tendons–bones.

Another important function of the musculoskeletal system is **hematopoiesis**—the process of generating blood cells.

Muscles

Muscles are composed of specialized cells that contract when stimulated to exert a force on a part of the body. The muscular system includes three types of muscles: cardiac, skeletal, and smooth **Figure 33-1**. Skeletal muscle is also called voluntary muscle, or striated muscle, because its contractions are largely under direct voluntary control of the brain. By maintaining a state of partial contraction, skeletal muscle allows the body to maintain its posture and to sit or stand. Because of its high metabolic rate and demand for energy and oxygen, skeletal muscle has a very rich blood supply, which causes it to bleed significantly when injured.

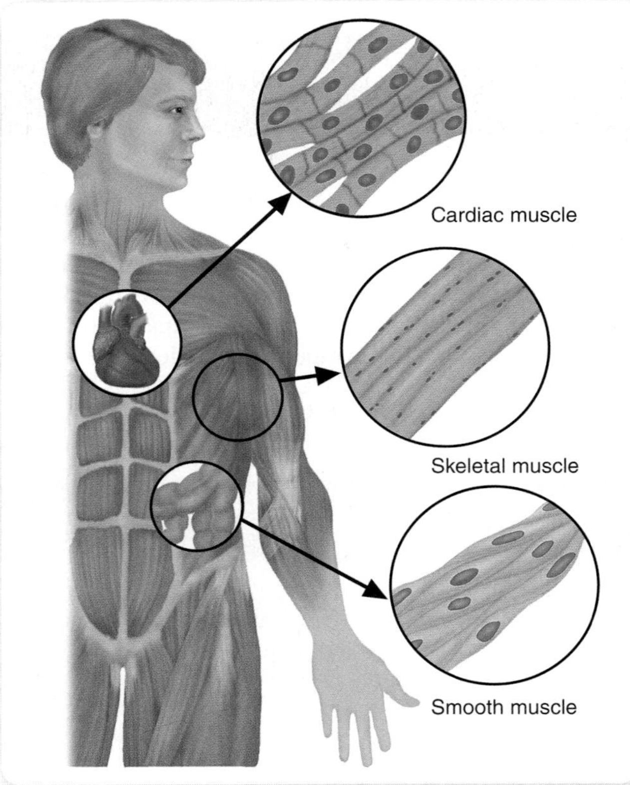

Figure 33-1 The three types of muscles are cardiac, skeletal, and smooth.

Muscle contraction requires energy. This energy is derived from the metabolism of glucose and results in the production of **lactic acid** (lactate). Lactic acid, in turn, must be converted into carbon dioxide (CO_2) and water, a process that requires oxygen. For this reason, vigorous muscular activity puts the body in a state of metabolic acidosis. Increasing the respiratory rate increases oxygen delivery to the tissues and increases the removal of CO_2 (acid) from the tissues to return the body to its normal acid-base state.

> **Words of Wisdom**
>
> Vigorous muscular activity puts the body in a state of metabolic acidosis. Increasing the respiratory rate increases oxygen delivery to the tissues and increases the removal of CO_2 (acid) from the tissues to return the body to its normal acid-base state.
>
> $$\uparrow H^+ + HCO_3^- \leftrightarrow \uparrow H_2CO_3 \leftrightarrow \uparrow CO_2 + H_2O$$

Muscle Innervation

Skeletal muscle is innervated by somatic motor neurons that transmit electrical stimuli to a muscle that cause it to contract. The combination of the muscle and the neuron that innervates it constitutes a motor unit. A motor unit that receives a signal to contract responds as forcefully as possible or does not contract at all: it is an all-or-nothing response. To generate a more forceful contraction, more neurons need to signal more muscle cells to contract, a process called recruitment.

Musculoskeletal Blood Supply

Skeletal muscle is supplied with arteries, veins, and nerves. Disease or trauma can result in the loss of a muscle's nerve supply; this, in turn, can lead to weakness and eventually atrophy, or a decrease in the size of the muscle and its inherent ability to function.

When a person has a musculoskeletal injury, the arteries that supply the injured region may also be damaged. Therefore, it is important to realize which arteries (and corresponding veins) are present in each part of the extremity **Figure 33-2**.

The blood supply in each upper extremity originates from the subclavian artery. When the subclavian artery reaches the axilla, it is referred to as the axillary artery. After giving off several branches that supply the shoulder region with blood, the artery leaves the axilla and becomes the brachial artery. After it passes through the elbow, the brachial artery divides into the radial artery and ulnar artery. In the hand, the radial and ulnar arteries form superficial and deep arcades of blood vessels that branch to form the arteries of each finger, the digital arteries.

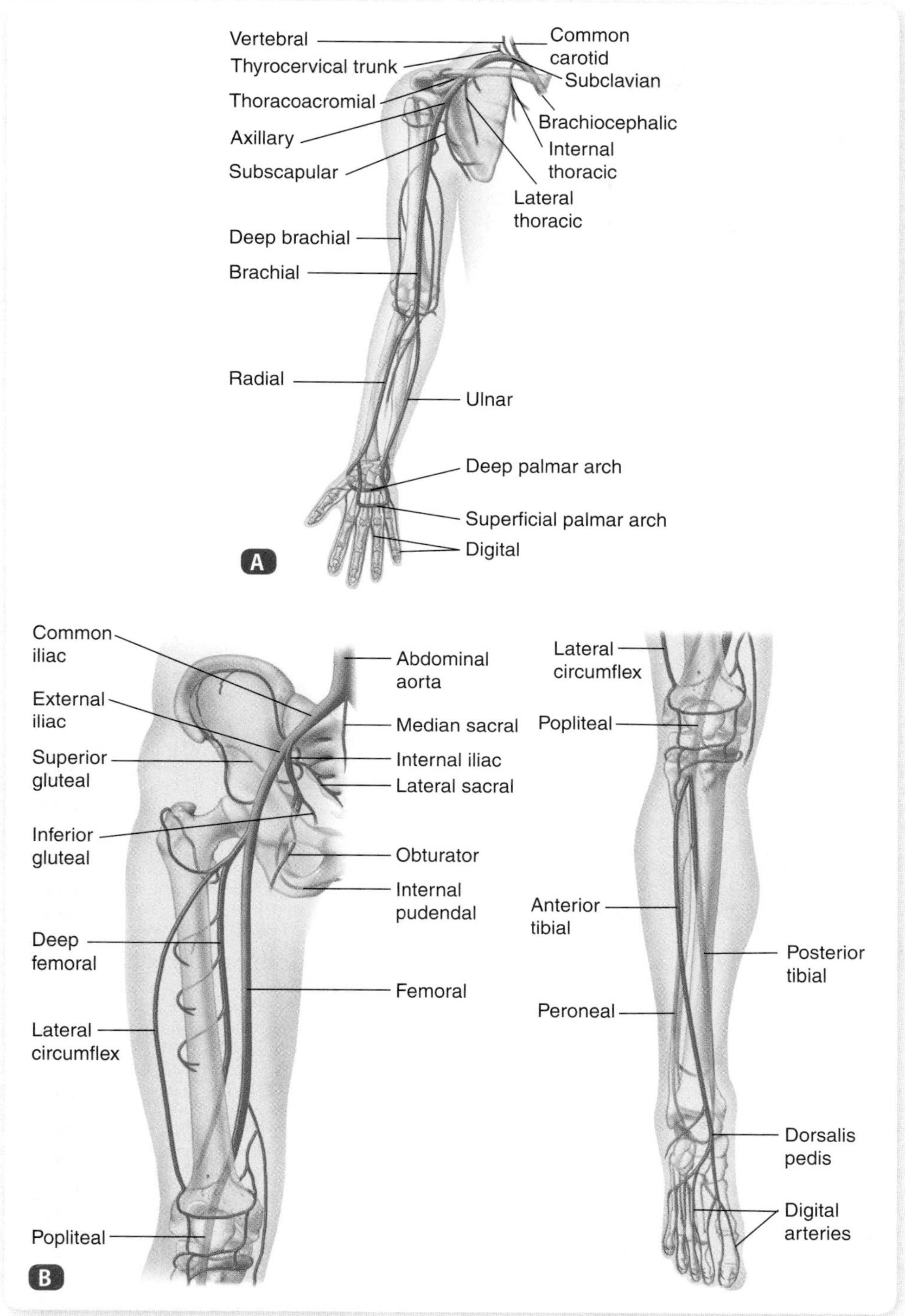

Figure 33-2 The arterial supply of the extremities. **A.** Upper extremity. **B.** Lower extremity.

In the lower extremities, the blood supply originates from the external iliac arteries. When the external iliac artery reaches the leg, it becomes the femoral artery. When it reaches the knee, the femoral artery turns medially and posteriorly and is referred to as the popliteal artery. The popliteal artery divides into the peroneal artery, the anterior tibial artery, and the posterior tibial artery. The anterior tibial artery travels along the anterior and lateral surface of the tibia until it reaches the ankle, where it proceeds along the dorsal surface of the foot toward the great toe and becomes the dorsalis pedis artery. The posterior tibial artery travels along the posterior aspect of the tibia until it reaches the ankle, where it follows a path just behind the medial malleolus until it reaches the plantar aspect of the foot. Within the foot, arcades of arteries supply the various structures with blood and give off branches that form the digital arteries of the toes.

▶ The Skeleton

The skeleton, which gives us our recognizable human form, protects our vital internal organs, and allows us to move, is made up of approximately 206 bones. It may be divided into two distinct portions: the **axial skeleton** and the **appendicular skeleton**.

The axial skeleton comprises the bones of the central part, or axis, of the body; its divisions include the vertebral column, skull, ribs, and sternum.

The appendicular skeleton is divided into the pectoral girdle, the pelvic girdle, and the bones of the upper and lower extremities. The pectoral girdle (shoulder girdle) consists of two scapulae and two clavicles **Figure 33-3**. The clavicles act as struts to keep the shoulder propped up; however, because they are both slender and very exposed, these bones are vulnerable to injury.

The upper extremity extends from the shoulder to the fingertips and is composed of the upper arm (humerus), elbow, and forearm **Figure 33-4**. The radius and ulna make up the forearm. Because these bones are arranged in parallel, when one is broken, the other is often broken as well.

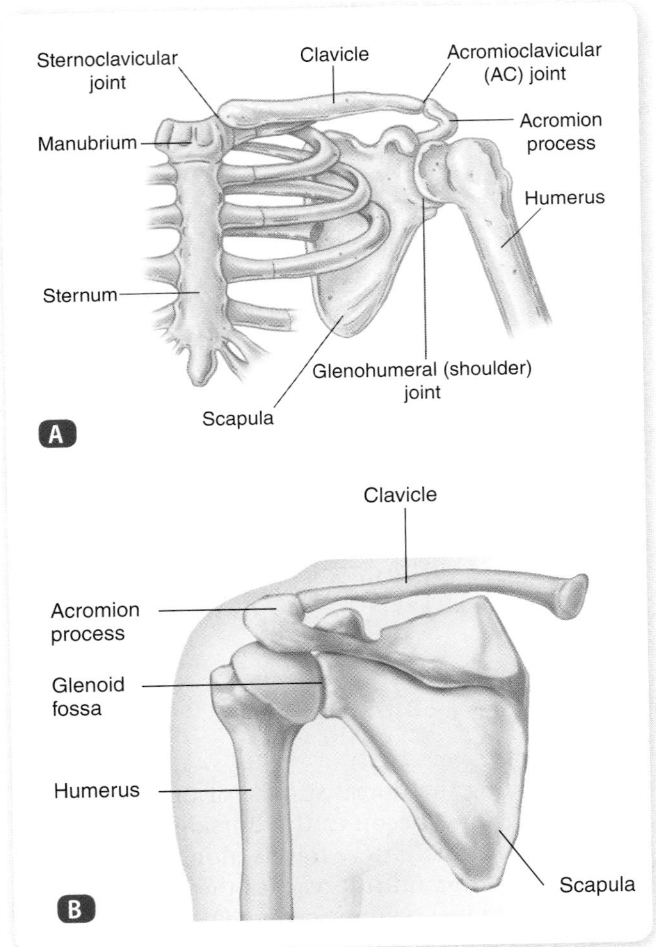

Figure 33-3 The pectoral girdle. **A.** Anterior view, including the clavicle. **B.** Posterior view, including the scapula.

The hand contains three sets of bones: wrist bones (carpals), hand bones (metacarpals), and finger bones (phalanges) **Figure 33-5**. The carpals, especially the scaphoid, are vulnerable to fracture when a person falls on an outstretched hand. Phalanges are more apt to be injured by a crush injury, such as being slammed in a car door.

The pelvis supports the body weight and protects the structures within the pelvis: the urinary bladder, rectum, and female reproductive organs. The pelvic girdle consists of three separate bones—the ischium, ilium, and

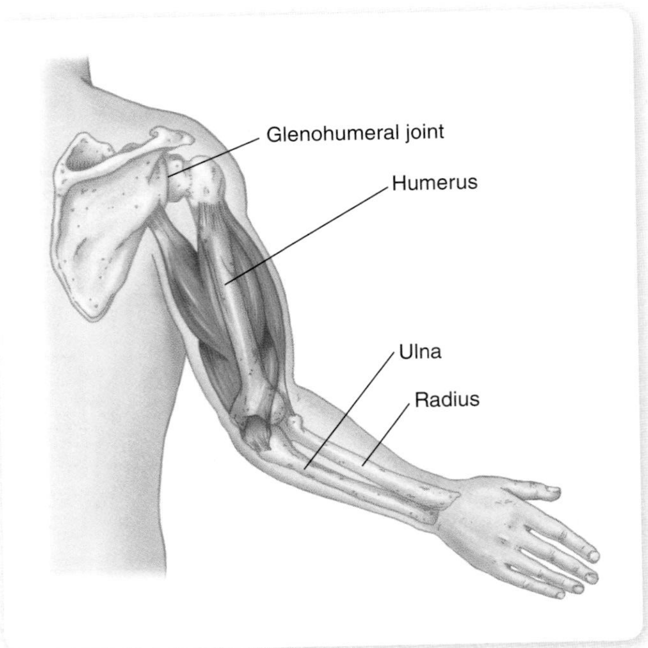

Figure 33-4 The anatomy of the arm.

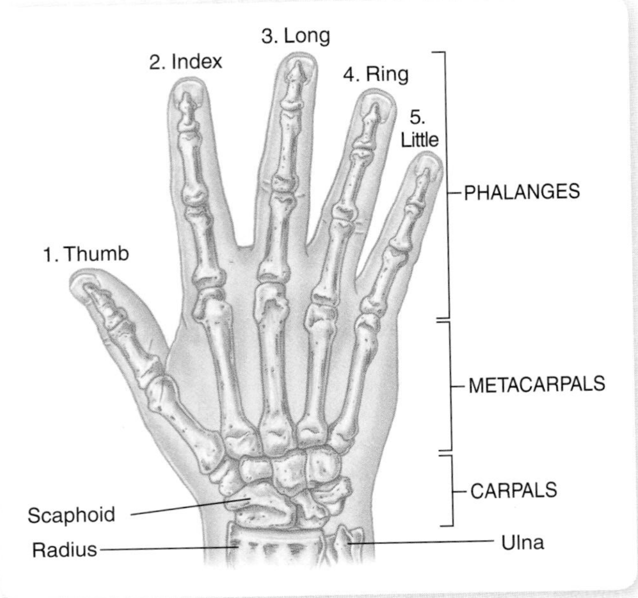

Figure 33-5 The anatomy of the wrist and hand.

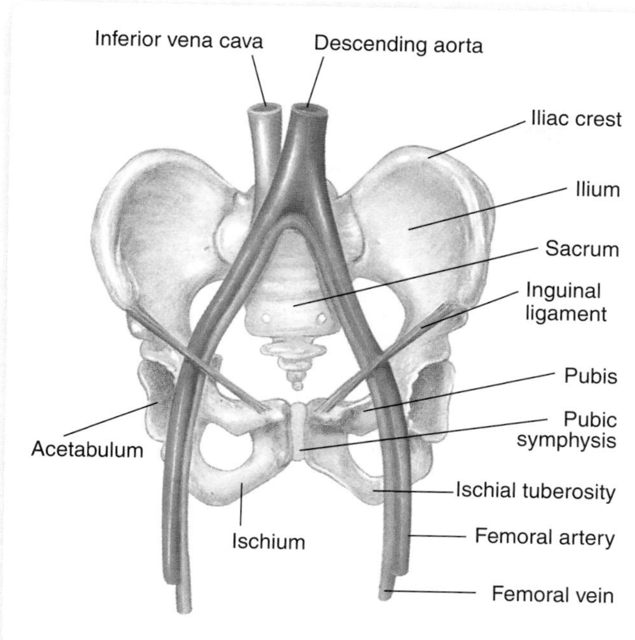

Figure 33-6 The pelvic girdle.

pubis—fused together to form the innominate (or hip) bone **Figure 33-6**. The two iliac bones are joined posteriorly by tough ligaments to the sacrum at the sacroiliac joints; the two pubic bones are connected anteriorly by equally tough ligaments at the pubic symphysis. These joints allow very little motion, so the pelvic ring is strong and stable.

Each lower extremity consists of the bones of the thigh, leg, and foot **Figure 33-7**. The femur (thigh bone) is a long, powerful bone that connects in the ball-and-socket joint of the pelvis and in the hinge joint of the knee. The femoral head is the ball-shaped part that fits into the acetabulum. It is connected to the shaft (diaphysis) of the femur by the femoral neck. The femoral neck is a common site for fractures, generally referred to as hip fractures, especially in the older adult population.

The lower leg consists of two bones, the tibia and the fibula. The tibia is vulnerable to direct blows and can be felt just beneath the skin. The fibula is an attachment point for the lateral ligaments of the knee joint; it also serves as the lateral stabilizer of the ankle joint (lateral malleolus) at its distal **articulation**.

The foot consists of three classes of bones: ankle bones (tarsals), foot bones (metatarsals), and toe bones (phalanges) **Figure 33-8**. The largest of the tarsal bones is the heel bone (calcaneus), which is subject to injury with axial loading injuries, such as when a person jumps from a height and lands on the feet.

A joint is formed wherever two bones come into contact. The sternoclavicular joint, for example, is where the sternum and the clavicle come together. Joints are held together in a tough fibrous structure known as a capsule

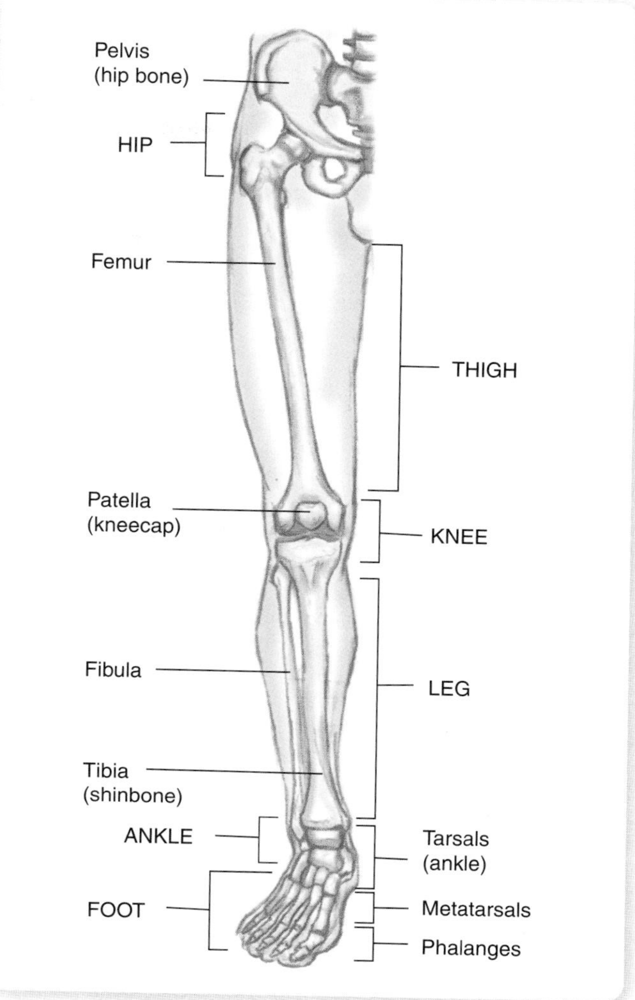

Figure 33-7 The bones of the thigh, leg, and foot.

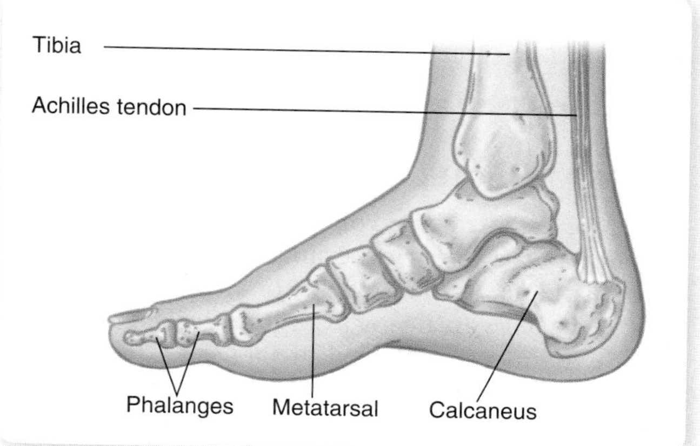

Figure 33-8 The bones of the foot and ankle.

and are bathed and lubricated by synovial fluid. The various motions that a joint may allow include flexion, extension, **abduction**, **adduction**, rotation, circumduction, pronation, and supination **Figure 33-9**.

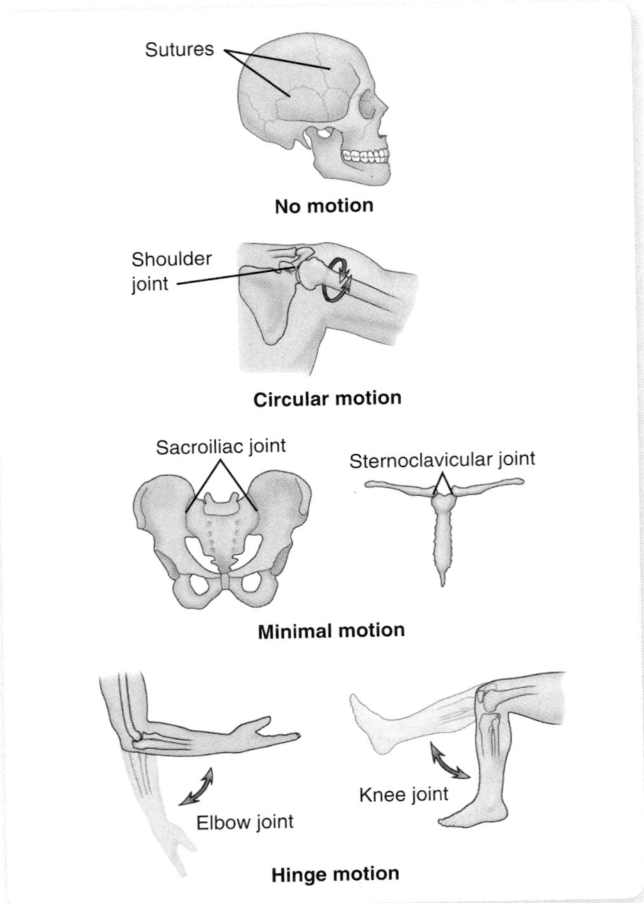

Figure 33-9 Joints in the body.

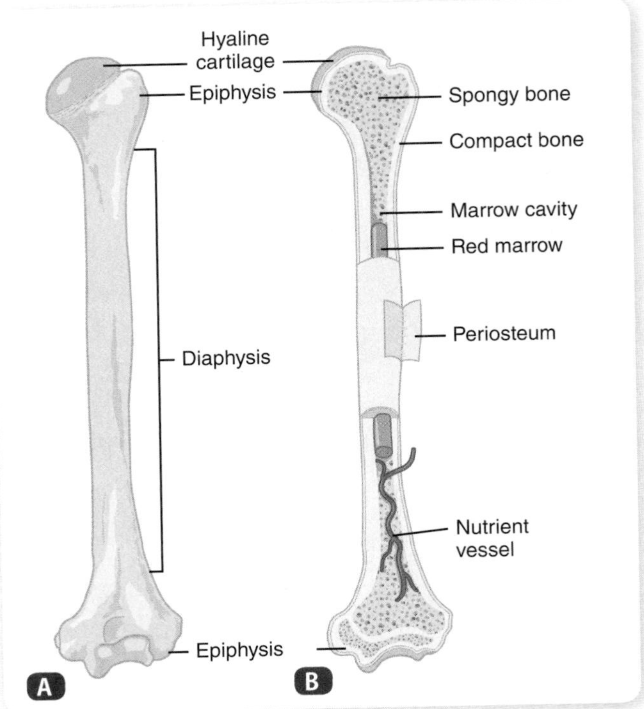

Figure 33-10 Anatomy of the long bone. **A.** The humerus. Notice the long shaft and dilated ends. **B.** Longitudinal section of the humerus showing compact bone, spongy bone, and marrow.

Special Populations

Fractures that occur through the growth (epiphyseal) plate in a bone of a child may affect the future growth of that bone.

Bone Classifications

Bones are classified based on their shapes. *Long bones* are longer than they are wide; examples include the femur, humerus, tibia, fibula, clavicle, phalanges, radius, and ulna. *Short bones* are nearly as wide as they are long; they include the metacarpals and metatarsals. *Flat bones* are thin, broad bones; they include the sternum, ribs, scapulae, and cranial bones. *Irregular bones* have complex shapes that are designed to perform specific functions, such as the bones of the vertebrae and the mandible. Sesamoid bones, or *round bones,* are generally found in tendons. The patella is the largest of the sesamoid bones.

Typical Long Bone Architecture

Long bones have several distinct regions and anatomic features **Figure 33-10**. These bones can grow to such lengths because of the presence of the growth plate, or **physis**, in children. Once a person reaches adulthood, the growth plate closes and the mature adult bone is complete. The long bone is divided into three regions: the diaphysis, the epiphysis, and the metaphysis.

The area where two bones come in contact to form a joint is covered by a thin layer of articular cartilage, a smooth, pearly white substance that acts as a cushion to protect the bones from damage and wear and allows the ends of the bones to easily glide over each other. The portion of bone that is not covered by articular cartilage is, instead, covered by the periosteum. This dense, fibrous membrane contains capillaries and cells that are important for bone repair and maintenance.

In the inner portion of the long bone, blood comes from the nutrient artery of the bone. Once it penetrates the bone's outer cortex, the artery enters the medullary canal, the hollow inner portion of the shaft that is lined by the endosteum and contains yellow (fatty) marrow in adults.

▶ Tendons, Ligaments, and Cartilage

Tendons connect skeletal muscle to bone. These flat or cordlike bands of connective tissue are white and have a glistening appearance. Tendons cross joints to create a pulling force between two bones when a muscle contracts.

Ligaments connect bone to bone and help maintain the stability of joints and determine the degree of joint motion. These inelastic bands of connective tissue have a structure similar to tendons.

Cartilage consists of fibers of collagen embedded in a gelatinous substance. This flexible connective tissue forms the smooth surface over bone ends where they articulate, provides cushioning between vertebrae, gives structure to the nose and external ear, forms the framework of the larynx and trachea, and serves as the model for the formation of the skeleton in children. Cartilage has a very limited vascular supply, and it does not heal if it is injured.

> **Special Populations**
>
> A large portion of the older adult population has joint pain that ranges from mild to debilitating. As the body ages, wear and tear creates injury and causes inflammation of the joints, resulting in arthritis, bursitis, and a host of other medical conditions.

▶ Age-Associated Changes

The musculoskeletal system, like any body system, is affected by aging. Bones age as do other tissues of the body, decreasing in density after the age of 35 years. This trend leads to a loss of height and produces changes in facial structure. In women, the decrease in bone density accelerates once menopause is reached because of the loss of estrogen, a hormone that helps promote bone formation. A significant decrease in bone density, called **osteoporosis** Figure 33-11, is associated with a higher risk of fracture. People with osteoporosis are at increased risk for incurring fractures, especially in the hip, spine, and wrist.

Aging of muscles, cartilage, and other connective tissues may also lead to degradation of joints and disk herniation. For example, the water content of the intervertebral disks decreases as a person ages, increasing the risk of disk herniation. In some joints, the cartilage may become degraded, leading to arthritis and pain; in others, the cartilage becomes calcified, leading to restricted motion. For more information about musculoskeletal differences associated with age, see Chapter 36, *Pediatric Emergencies*, and Chapter 37, *Geriatric Emergencies*.

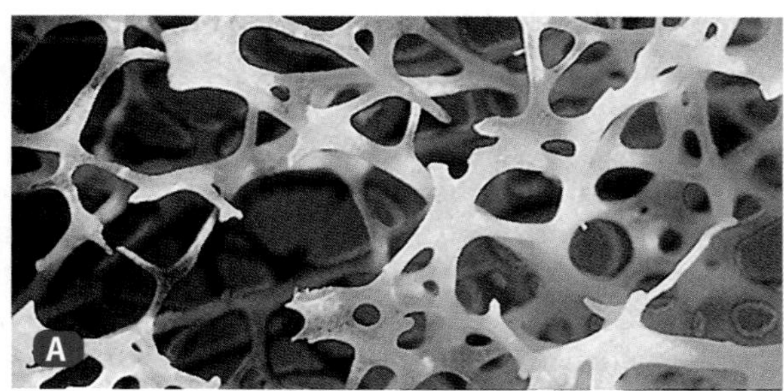

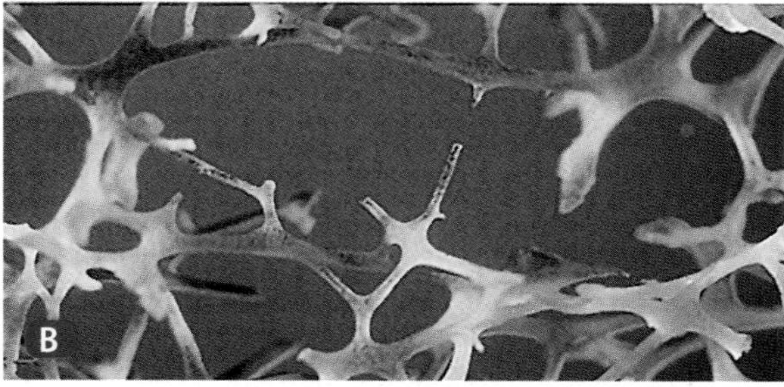

Figure 33-11 The structural difference between normal and osteoporotic bone. **A.** Normal bone in a 29-year-old woman. **B.** Osteoporotic bone in a 92-year-old woman.

> **Special Populations**
>
> Splinting an injured extremity (eg, a fractured forearm) is most optimally performed with the extremity in a straightened position. In some older adult patients, straightening the injured extremity may not be possible and may cause further injury. This is particularly true in patients with arthritis—a degenerative condition that causes a reduced range of motion in the joints. If, while attempting to straighten the extremity, the patient experiences increasing joint pain or you feel resistance, stop and splint the injured limb in the position in which it is resting.

Pathophysiology

Musculoskeletal injuries may result from both blunt and penetrating trauma. Sports injuries account for a significant number of musculoskeletal injuries: 4.5 million sports musculoskeletal injuries require medical attention in the United States each year.[4] Other common causes of these injuries include motor vehicle crashes (MVCs) and falls. Among children, intentional trauma or abuse is a common cause of fractures and musculoskeletal injuries, with one-third to one-half of all abused children experiencing fractures.[5]

In some cases, a force that might not generally cause harm to normal healthy bone produces a fracture. Such a **pathologic fracture** occurs when a medical condition (eg, metastatic cancer) causes the bone to become abnormally weak; a fracture may then occur with even minimal force. Older adults—particularly those with osteoporosis—have weaker, more brittle bones, which leaves them more susceptible to fractures than are younger people.

> **Special Populations**
>
> Assessment and treatment of pathologic fracture (also called nontraumatic facture) are the same as with any fracture, but require special consideration given the patient's history. Apply gentle force when manipulating a fracture so you do not create more harm in an already weakened area, and pad the area as needed for comfort and support. Document the patient history and ensure you include the presence or absence of any injury preceding the event.

Special Populations

Osteogenesis imperfecta, or brittle bone disease, makes people more prone to pathologic fractures. Fractures may occur from something as simple as lifting a child or leaning onto an outstretched arm. Use extreme care when handling these patients, because the most minute force may cause concomitant injury or fractures. Stress the patient history when communicating with the receiving facility.

Words of Wisdom

Injury to bones and joints is often associated with injury to the surrounding soft tissues, especially to the adjacent nerves and blood vessels. The entire affected area is known as the **zone of injury** Figure 33-12. Depending on the amount of kinetic energy that the tissues absorb from forces acting on the body, this zone may extend to a distant point. For this reason, do not be distracted by a patient's obvious injury; you must first complete a primary survey to check for life-threatening injuries. This is especially true when assessing damage from high-energy trauma.

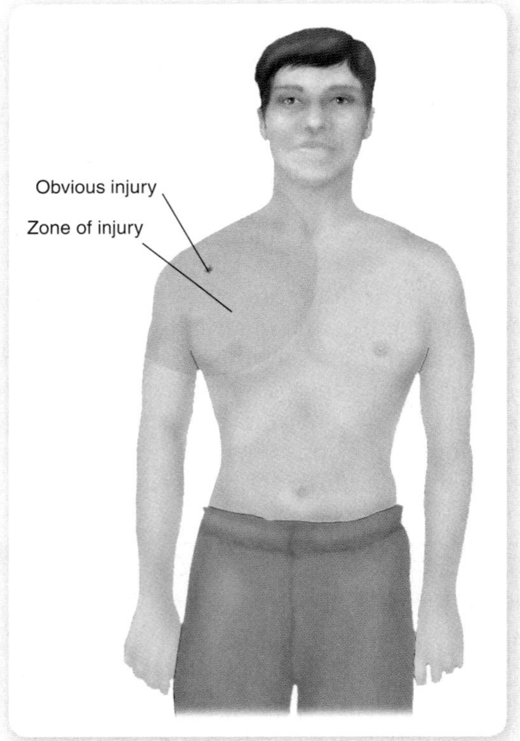

Figure 33-12 The zone of injury is the area of soft tissue, including the adjacent nerves and blood vessels, that surround the obvious injury of a bone or joint.

▶ Mechanism of Injury

Significant force is generally required to cause fractures and dislocations. This force may be applied to a limb in any of the following ways:

- Direct blows
- Indirect forces
- Twisting forces
- High-energy injuries

A direct blow fractures the bone at the point of impact. Penetrating injuries may also lead to a fracture or other musculoskeletal injury. A high-velocity injury, such as that caused by a high-power rifle, typically shatters bone and causes extensive soft-tissue damage. An impalement injury commonly causes a soft-tissue injury similar to that seen in a low-velocity penetrating injury. If the impaled object happens to strike a bone, it may cause a fracture. In any case of impalement, it is essential to stabilize the object to protect the soft tissues from further injury.

An **indirect injury** occurs when force is applied to one region of the body but causes an injury (eg, fracture, dislocation) in another region of the body. In this type of injury, the force is transmitted through the skeleton until, at some point, it reaches an area that is structurally weak in comparison with the other parts of the musculoskeletal system through which the force has traveled. For example, a hip fracture may occur when a person's knee strikes the dashboard during a MVC. In this case, the force is applied to the knee and travels proximally along the femur. When this force reaches the femoral neck, it causes the femoral neck to fracture.

Forces may be transmitted along the entire length of a bone or through several bones in series, and may cause an injury anywhere along the way. Thus, a person falling on an outstretched hand may have one or more injuries as the result of forces transmitted proximally from the point of impact: (1) fracture of the scaphoid bone of the hand (direct blow), (2) fracture of the distal ulna and radius, (3) fracture-dislocation of the elbow, (4) fracture-dislocation of the shoulder, or (5) fracture of the clavicle. When you are caring for patients who have fallen, immediately identify the point of contact and the mechanism of injury (MOI) so you decrease the chance of overlooking any associated injuries.

Twisting forces are a common cause of musculoskeletal injury and can result in fractures, sprains, and dislocations. These kinds of injuries are common in football and skiing. Typically, the distal part of the limb remains fixed, as when cleats or a ski holds the foot to the ground, while torsion develops in the proximal section of the limb; the resulting force causes tearing of tendons and ligaments and fractures of bone.

Some injuries are commonly encountered together because of the way the causative forces are transmitted; thus, if you find one, look for the others Table 33-1. Pain and swelling over the scaphoid (navicular) bone of the wrist, for example, means the patient fell hard against an outstretched hand, so he or she may have other injuries anywhere along the axis from the hand to the shoulder.

Table 33-1 Musculoskeletal Injuries That Commonly Occur Together

If You Find	Look For
Scapular fracture	Rib fracture, pulmonary contusions, pneumothorax
Scaphoid fracture	Wrist, elbow, or shoulder fracture
Pelvic fracture	Lumbosacral spine and other long bone fractures, intra-abdominal or genitourinary injury
Hip dislocation	Fracture of the acetabulum or femoral head
Femoral fracture	Dislocation of ipsilateral hip
Patellar fracture	Fracture-dislocation of ipsilateral hip
Knee dislocation	Tibial fracture; distal pulse may be absent
Calcaneal fracture	Fracture of the ankle, leg, hip, pelvis, spine, and the other calcaneus

▶ Fractures

A **fracture** is a broken bone. More precisely, it is a break in the continuity of a bone. Fractures occur when the magnitude of the force applied to a bone (a single application or an accumulation of repetitive applications) overcomes the strength of the bone. The strength of a bone may be affected by age, osteoporosis, nutritional status, and disease processes.

Types of Fractures

Fractures are classified as either open or closed. In an **open fracture**, sometimes called a **compound fracture**, a break in the overlying skin allows the fracture to be exposed to the outside environment **Figure 33-13**. In addition to having a higher risk of infection, open fractures have the potential for more blood loss than a closed fracture.

In a **closed fracture**, the skin over the fracture site remains intact **Figure 33-14**. The increased interstitial pressure within the hematoma compresses the blood vessels, limiting the size of the hematoma. In a closed femur fracture, the blood loss may exceed 1 L before enough pressure develops to tamponade the bleeding. In contrast, open fractures allow much of the blood to escape, so tamponade does not occur as readily or at all.

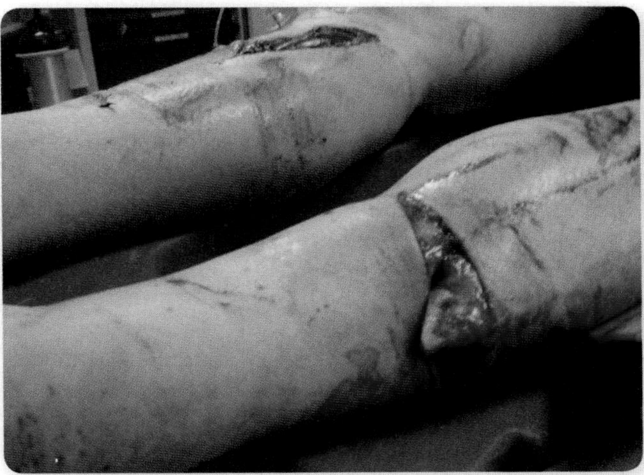

Figure 33-13 An open fracture.

Courtesy of Rhonda Hunt.

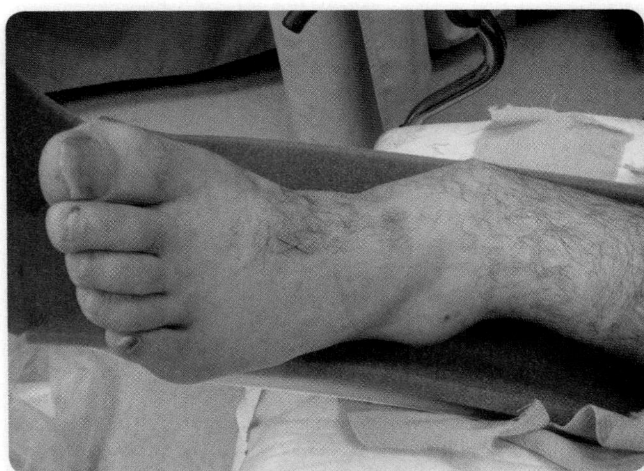

Figure 33-14 A closed fracture.

Courtesy of Rhonda Hunt.

Determining whether a fracture is open or closed is not always as easy as it sounds. With an open fracture, there is an external wound, caused either by the same blow that fractured the bone or by the broken bone ends lacerating the skin. The wound may vary in size from a very small puncture to a gaping tear that exposes bone and soft tissue. When you assess and treat patients with possible fractures or dislocations, determine whether the overlying skin is damaged. Regardless of the extent and severity of the damage to the skin, you should treat any injury that breaks the skin as a possible open fracture. Significant blood loss and a higher likelihood of infection are complications that you must try to limit; these tend to occur with open fractures.

Fractures are also described by whether the bone is moved from its normal position. **Angulation** of a fracture means that the bone is misaligned as a result of the injury and that an angle has formed between the fractured fragments. Angulation may occur in the frontal plane, sagittal plane, or both. A **nondisplaced fracture** (also known as a hairline fracture) is a simple crack of the bone that may be difficult to distinguish from a sprain or simple contusion. Radiographic examinations are required for physicians to diagnose any type of fracture, particularly a nondisplaced fracture. In a **displaced fracture** the two bone ends at the fracture are separated in at least one plane and may produce actual deformity, or distortion, of the limb by shortening, rotating, or angulating it. Often, the deformity is obvious and can be associated with crepitus. However, in some cases the deformity is minimal. Ensure you look for differences between the injured limb and the opposite uninjured limb in any patient with a suspected fracture of an extremity **Figure 33-15**.

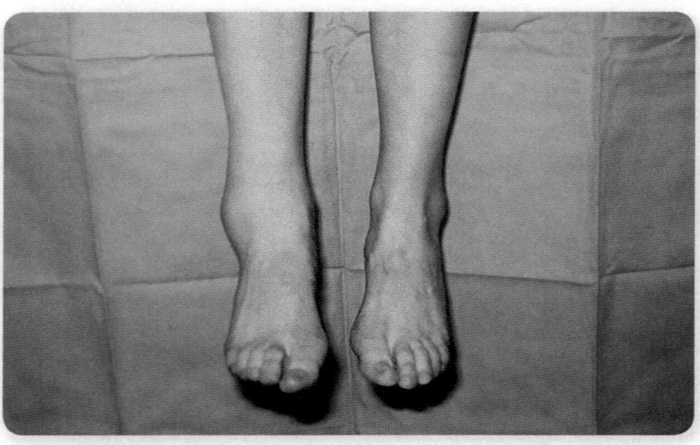

Figure 33-15 Always compare the injured limb with the uninjured limb when checking for deformity.

Medical personnel often use the following special terms to describe types of fractures **Figure 33-16**:

- **Transverse.** A fracture that occurs straight across the bone. This is usually the result of a direct blow injury.
- **Oblique.** A fracture in which the bone is broken at an angle across the bone. This is usually the result of a sharp, angled blow to the bone.
- **Spiral.** A fracture caused by a twisting or spinning force, causing a long, spiral-shaped break in the bone. This is sometimes the result of abuse in young children.
- **Comminuted.** A fracture in which the bone is broken into more than two fragments.
- **Greenstick.** An incomplete fracture that passes only partway through the shaft of a bone but may still cause substantial angulation; occurs in children.
- **Incomplete.** A fracture that does not run completely through the bone; a nondisplaced partial crack.
- **Pathologic.** A fracture of weakened or diseased bone, seen in patients with osteoporosis, infection, or cancer; often produced by minimal force.
- **Epiphyseal.** A fracture that occurs within the growth plate of a child's bone and may lead to growth abnormalities.

Signs and Symptoms of a Fracture

The primary symptom of a fracture is *pain* that is usually well localized to the fracture site. In addition, the patient may report hearing a snap or feeling a break. Signs of

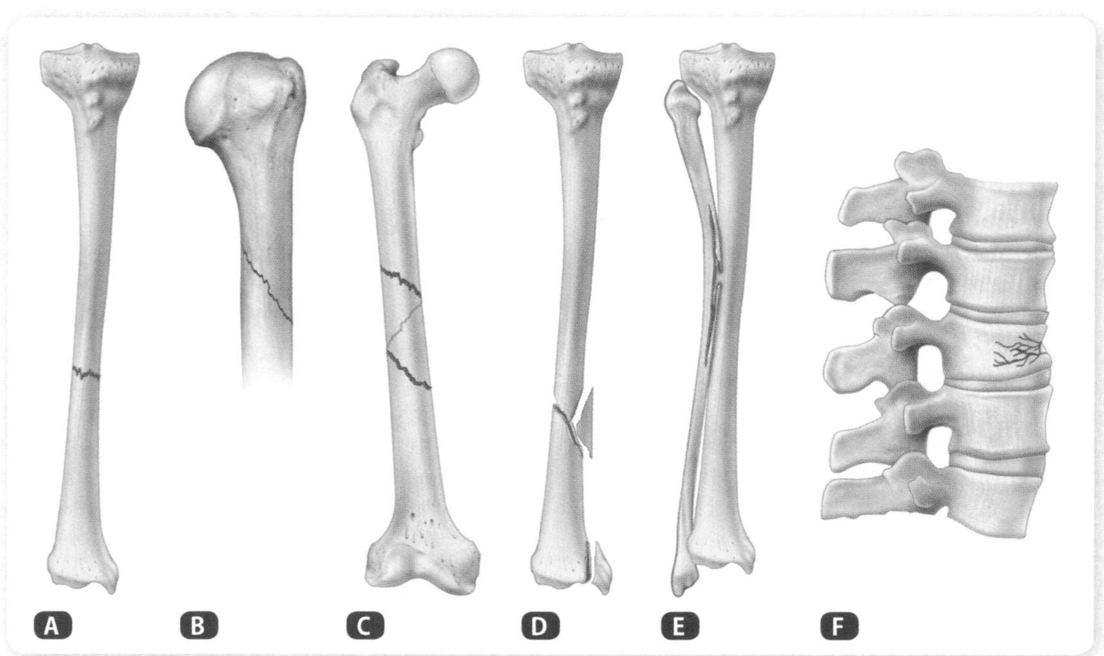

Figure 33-16 Types of fractures. **A.** Transverse fracture of the tibia. **B.** Oblique fracture of the humerus. **C.** Spiral fracture of the femur. **D.** Comminuted fracture of the tibia. **E.** Greenstick fracture of the fibula. **F.** Compression fracture of a vertebral body.

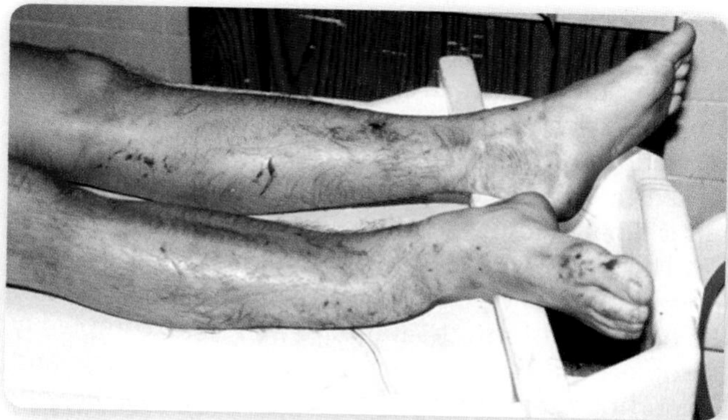

Figure 33-17 Obvious deformity should increase your index of suspicion for a fracture.

fracture detected on physical examination include the following:

- *Deformity* is one of the most reliable signs of a fracture. The limb may be found in an unnatural position or show motion at a place where there is no joint. Compare the deformed limb with the extremity on the other side **Figure 33-17**.
- *Shortening* occurs in fractures when the broken ends of a bone override each other. It is characteristic of femur fractures, for example, because the broken femur can no longer serve as a strut to oppose spasm in the powerful thigh muscles.
- Visual inspection will usually reveal *swelling* at the fracture site due to bleeding from the broken bone and the accumulation of fluid. If swelling is severe, it may mask deformity of the limb. Generalized swelling may occur several hours after injury.
- As blood infiltrates the tissues around the broken bone ends, *bruising* will become apparent **Figure 33-18**. Fractures are very often associated with **ecchymosis** (discoloration) of the surrounding soft tissues. Bruising may be present after almost any injury; it is not specific for bone or joint injuries **Figure 33-19**.
- A fractured bone is almost invariably *tender to palpation* over the fracture site. **Point tenderness** is tenderness that is sharply localized at the site of injury, found by gently palpating along the bone with the tip of one finger.
- *Pain*, along with tenderness and bruising, commonly occurs in association with fractures. Occasionally, nondisplaced fractures are not very painful, and there is minimal soft-tissue damage.
- *Guarding* and *loss of use* characterize most fractures. Guarding occurs when the muscles around the fracture contract to prevent any movement of the broken bone. Guarding is also used to describe behavior of the patient to protect the injury against movement and further discomfort. Guarding does not occur with all fractures; some patients may continue to use the injured part for some time. An inability to use the extremity is the patient's way of immobilizing it to minimize pain. The patient will try to keep a fractured bone still and will avoid putting any stress on it. Sometimes the measures a patient takes to protect a fractured bone from movement are so characteristic that you can almost know the type of fracture without examining the extremity. A patient who walks to the ambulance holding the dorsum of one wrist in the other hand, for example, very often has a Colles fracture. A patient standing with the head cocked toward a "knocked-down shoulder" probably has a fracture of the clavicle on the side to which the head is leaning.

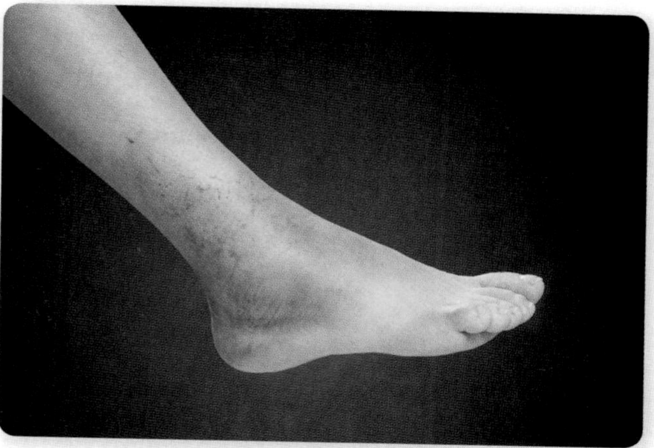

Figure 33-18 Fractures almost always have associated bruising into the surrounding soft tissue.

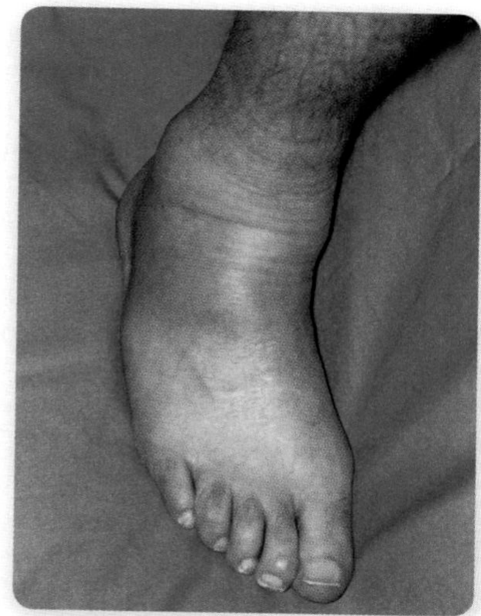

Figure 33-19 Swelling around an ankle from an injury. It is often not possible without radiographic imaging to determine whether a patient has a fracture or not.

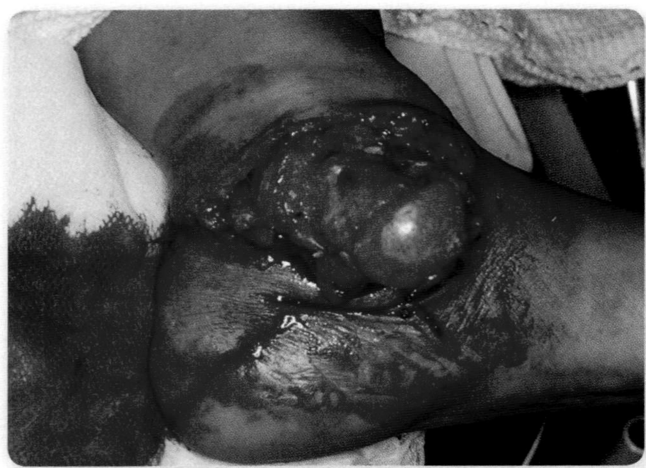

Figure 33-20 Bone ends may protrude through the skin or be visible within the wound of an open fracture.

- Palpation may reveal **crepitus**, a grating sensation, over the broken bone ends. Crepitus may be noted as an incidental finding during splinting attempts. Do *not* try to elicit this sign, because your efforts may result in further injury to the bone and surrounding soft tissues, and severe pain.
- Also called free movement, *false motion* occurs at a point in the limb where there is no joint. It is a positive indication of a fracture.
- A *locked joint* (a joint that is locked into position) is difficult and painful to move.
- In an open fracture, *exposed bone ends* may be visible in the wound **Figure 33-20**.

Words of Wisdom

Point tenderness is the most reliable indicator of an underlying fracture.

▶ Dislocations

When bones are forced beyond their normal limits, the bones that form a joint may break, or they may become displaced and the supporting ligaments and joint capsule may tear. In a **dislocation**, a bone is totally displaced from the joint. Typically, at least part of the supporting joint capsule and some of the joint's ligaments are disrupted. Dislocations occur when a body part moves beyond its normal range of motion. The dislocated bones become locked in place by muscle spasms. Evaluate the patient for obvious and significant deformity, a significant decrease in the joint's range of motion, and severe pain. In all cases of a dislocation, you should suspect a fracture until it is ruled out by radiographs.

A dislocated joint may spontaneously undergo **reduction**, or return to its normal position, before you begin your assessment. In this situation, you may suspect a dislocation based on the patient history. Often, however, the joint surfaces remain completely separated from each other. A dislocation that does not spontaneously reduce is a serious problem: the ends of the bone can become locked in a displaced position, making any attempt at motion of the joint very difficult and painful.

The partial dislocation of a joint is known as a **subluxation**. In this type of injury, the articular surfaces of the bones that form the joint are no longer completely in contact. In some cases, part of the joint capsule and supporting ligaments may be damaged. Despite the subluxation, the patient may be able to move the joint to some degree. Failure to recognize and treat a subluxation may lead to persistent joint instability and pain.

Words of Wisdom

The principal sign of a dislocation is deformity. Symptoms may include pain, a feeling of pressure over the involved joint, and a loss of motion of the joint (ie, the joint seems "frozen"). Patients with a posterior dislocation of the shoulder, for example, are unable to raise their arm, so they hold it against their side instead.

The signs and symptoms of a dislocated joint are similar to those of a fracture **Figure 33-21**:

- Marked deformity
- Swelling
- Pain that is aggravated by any attempt at movement
- Tenderness on palpation
- Virtually complete loss of normal joint motion (locked joint)
- Numbness or impaired circulation to the limb or digit

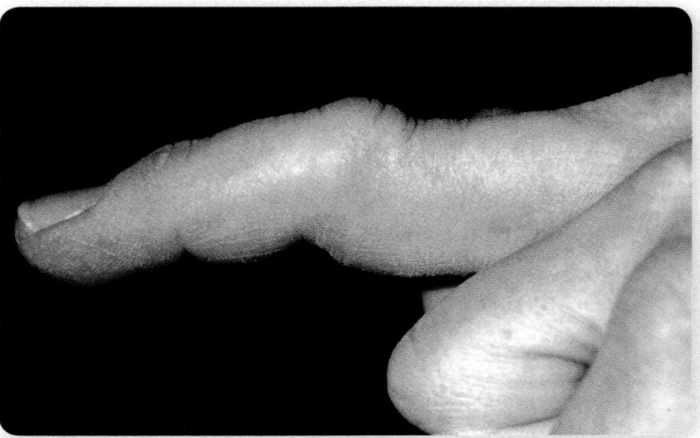

Figure 33-21 Joint dislocations, such as in this finger, are characterized by deformity, swelling, pain with any movement, tenderness, locking, and impaired circulation.

A dislocation is considered an urgent injury because of its potential to cause **neurovascular compromise** distal to the site of injury. If the dislocated bone presses on a nerve, the patient may experience numbness or weakness distally; if an artery is compressed, distal pulses may be absent (such as in a knee dislocation). For these reasons, you should always assess the patient's neurovascular status distal to the site of dislocation (check pulse and motor and sensory function [PMS]) prior to as well as after splinting.

▶ Sprains

Sprains are injuries in which ligaments are stretched or torn. They usually result from a sudden movement of a joint beyond its normal range of motion, accompanied by a temporary subluxation. Most sprains involve the ankle or the knee—most of these injuries occur after a person misjudges a step or landing. Evasive moves, such as those performed during sporting events, commonly cause sprains in athletes. The following signs and symptoms may indicate a patient has a sprain:

- Point tenderness can be elicited over the injured ligaments.
- Swelling and ecchymosis appear at the point of injury to the ligament resulting from torn blood vessels.
- Pain causes the patient to be unwilling to move or use the limb normally.
- Instability of the joint is indicated by increased motion, especially at the knee; however, this may be masked by severe swelling and guarding.

In contrast to fractures and dislocations, sprains rarely involve deformity. In these injuries, joint mobility is usually limited by pain, not by joint incongruity.

▶ Strains

A **strain** (pulled muscle) is an injury to a muscle and/or tendon that results from a violent muscle contraction or from excessive stretching. Patients typically report an immediate sharp pain and the sound of a "snap" when the muscle tears. Often no deformity is present, and only minor swelling may be noted at the site of injury, along with severe muscle weakness. Some patients may report extreme point tenderness and increased pain with passive movement of the injured extremity. The general treatment of strains is similar to field management for sprains, dislocations, and fractures.

▶ Achilles Tendon Rupture

A rupture of the Achilles tendon usually occurs in athletes older than 30 years who are involved in start-and-stop sports such as basketball or football. Recent use of certain types of antibiotics may also predispose to these injuries. The most immediate indications are pain from the heel to the calf and a sudden inability to perform **plantar flexion** of the foot. As time passes, the calf muscles begin to contract proximally and a deformity within the calf may develop. Acute management of an Achilles tendon injury includes RICE—rest, ice, compression, and elevation—and pain control. Long-term treatment may involve splinting or surgery.

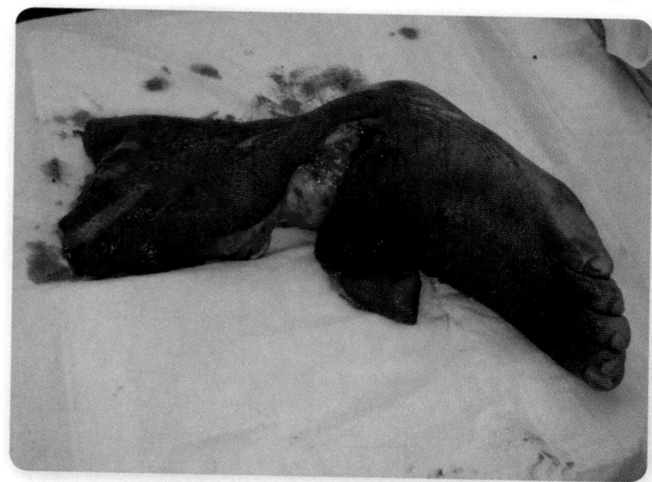

Figure 33-22 An amputation involving a leg.

Courtesy of Andrew N. Pollak, MD, FAAOS.

▶ Amputations

An **amputation** is the separation of a limb or other body part from the remainder of the body **Figure 33-22**. The amputation may be incomplete, leaving only a small segment of tissue connecting the part, or it may be complete, causing the part to be fully separated. Hemorrhage from complete or incomplete amputations can be severe and life threatening. Fractures may also be present with amputations.

> **Words of Wisdom**
>
> Lacerations can extend through skin and subcutaneous tissue, and even into the underlying muscles and adjacent nerves and blood vessels. The presence of lacerations may also be a sign of an underlying fracture.

Patient Assessment

As an AEMT, your assessments, attempts to splint, and work to stabilize the patient's condition are very important. However, when you are assessing an injured patient, *do not become distracted by visually impressive injuries!* It is essential to complete the primary survey of the patient to determine and address life threats before focusing on the extremities. Always carefully assess the MOI to try to determine the amount of kinetic energy that an injured limb has absorbed, and maintain a high index of suspicion for associated injuries. Other priorities should include identifying the injuries, preventing further harm or damage to the injured structures and surrounding tissues, supporting the injured area, and administering pain medication if necessary.

In cases of musculoskeletal injuries, patients may be classified based on the presence or absence of associated injuries:

- Life- or limb-threatening injury or condition, including life- or limb-threatening musculoskeletal trauma
- Life-threatening injuries and only simple musculoskeletal trauma
- Life- or limb-threatening musculoskeletal trauma and no other life-threatening injuries
- Isolated, non–life-threatening or non–limb-threatening injuries

You must become skilled at quickly and accurately assessing the severity of injury. The Golden Hour (or initial Golden Period) is critical not only for maintaining life, but also for preserving limbs. In an extremity with anything less than complete circulation, prolonged hypoperfusion can cause significant damage. For this reason, any suspected open fracture or vascular injury is considered a medical emergency, especially in a patient with multiple traumatic injuries.

Remember that most injuries are not critical; you can identify critical injuries by using the musculoskeletal injury grading system shown in Table 33-2.

Table 33-2	Musculoskeletal Injury Grading System
Minor injuries	▪ Minor sprains ▪ Fractures or dislocations of digits
Moderate injuries	▪ Open fractures of digits ▪ Nondisplaced long bone fractures ▪ Nondisplaced pelvic fractures ▪ Major sprains of a major joint
Serious injuries	▪ Displaced long bone fractures ▪ Multiple hand and foot fractures ▪ Open long bone fractures ▪ Displaced pelvic fractures ▪ Dislocations of major joints ▪ Multiple digit amputations ▪ Laceration of major nerves or blood vessels
Severe, life-threatening injuries (survival is probable)	▪ Multiple closed fractures ▪ Limb amputations ▪ Fractures of both long bones of the legs (bilateral femur fractures)
Critical injuries (survival is uncertain)	▪ Multiple open fractures of the limbs ▪ Suspected pelvic fractures with hemodynamic instability

YOU are the Provider PART 2

You ask your partner to retrieve the pelvic splints and spinal immobilization equipment from the ambulance while you continue to question the patient. The patient states that he remembers the entire incident and just wishes that you could "knock him out." When your partner returns with the equipment, you apply a cervical collar to the patient, then gently slide the pelvic splint underneath the patient and cinch it to the appropriate size. As you secure the splint, the patient breathes a sign of relief, saying that the pain feels a little better now. You and your partner gently place the patient onto a long backboard, move him onto your stretcher, and wheel him to the ambulance. Once the patient is in your ambulance, you establish one intravenous (IV) line and initiate a 250-mL normal saline bolus due to his circulatory status.

Recording Time: 1 Minute	
Appearance	Responsive
Level of consciousness	Alert and oriented
Airway	Patent
Breathing	22 breaths/min, nonlabored
Circulation	Cool, clammy

3. What is the potential blood loss in a femur fracture? Pelvic fracture?
4. Should this patient have a second IV line initiated?

Scene Size-up

Information from dispatch may indicate the MOI, the number of patients involved, and any first aid procedures used prior to your arrival. This will be useful information for you to think about as you travel to the scene. Remember that the information given by the dispatcher is only as accurate as the patient's or bystander's report. In addition, the situation may change prior to your arrival at the incident.

As you arrive at the scene, observe the scene for hazards. Try to identify the forces associated with the MOI. A mask, gown, and eye protection may be needed for incidents involving severe MOIs or when there is the possibility of hidden bleeding. Evaluate the need for law enforcement support, paramedic backup, or additional ambulances, and request assistance early based on your initial scene assessment.

Safety

The *first* step for *any* assessment is to ensure scene safety, use personal protective equipment, and take standard precautions!

As you observe the scene, look for indicators of the MOI. When you are assessing a patient who has experienced a significant MOI, be alert for both primary and secondary injuries. Primary injuries are a result of the MOI, whereas secondary injuries are the result of what happens after the initial injury. For example, a pedestrian who is hit by a motor vehicle may experience a primary pelvic injury, but a secondary head injury may occur when the patient rolls onto the hood of the motor vehicle.

Primary Survey

Perform a primary survey by focusing on the patient's mental status, XABCDEs, and priority. If the primary survey indicates the patient has no immediate life-threatening condition and only localized musculoskeletal trauma, then continue with history taking and a secondary assessment. If the patient has a significant MOI, then complete a rapid full-body scan on scene, and then perform a full-body exam en route to the emergency department (ED). The priorities throughout the assessment and management of musculoskeletal injuries should be to identify the injuries, prevent further harm or damage to the injured structures and surrounding tissues, and support the injured areas.

Evaluate the patient's level of consciousness and orientation. Check for responsiveness using the AVPU scale (Awake and alert, responsive to Verbal stimuli, responsive to Pain, Unresponsive). Generally, you can assess a patient's mental status by asking the patient about his or her chief complaint. If the patient is alert, the information he or she provides should help direct you to any apparent life threats. If the patient is not alert, determine whether he or she responds to verbal or painful stimuli or whether he or she is unresponsive. An unresponsive patient may indicate a life-threatening condition. Administer oxygen as needed via a nonrebreathing mask (or a bag-mask device, if indicated) to all patients whose level of consciousness is less than alert and oriented and provide immediate transport to the ED.

Perform a rapid full-body scan of the patient and ask about the MOI. Was it a direct blow, indirect force, twisting force, or high-energy injury? In many situations, the musculoskeletal complaints will be simple and usually not life threatening. In other situations, such as those with a significant MOI, patients may complain of multiple problems, only one of which involves a musculoskeletal injury. The initial interaction with the patient will provide you with a starting point and help you to distinguish simple conditions from complex injuries. If the patient was subjected to significant trauma and multiple body systems are affected, the musculoskeletal injuries may be a lower priority. Do not waste scene time on prolonged musculoskeletal assessment or splinting in such a case.

Words of Wisdom

Be mindful of scene time. Use a long backboard as a "full-body splint," and complete additional assessment and treatment of musculoskeletal injuries during transport.

Fractures and sprains usually do not create airway and breathing conditions. Other problems, such as injuries to the head, intoxication, or other related illnesses and injuries may cause inadequate breathing. Evaluate the chief complaint and MOI to help you identify whether the patient has an open airway and whether breathing is present and adequate. In a responsive patient, this step is as simple as noting whether the patient can speak normally. In an unresponsive patient, it is as simple as opening the airway to check for breathing. If a spinal injury is suspected, take the appropriate precautions and prepare for stabilization. Address musculoskeletal injuries first if there is profuse bleeding; however, even then, direct another provider if available to control bleeding while you assess the airway. Address exsanguinating hemorrhage first; very quickly afterwards, address airway and breathing concerns.

Your circulatory assessment should focus on determining whether the patient has a pulse, has adequate perfusion, or is bleeding. If the patient is alert—as are most patients with fractures and dislocations—he or she will have a pulse. If the patient is unresponsive, check for a pulse by palpating the carotid artery. Hypoperfusion (shock) and bleeding problems will most likely be your primary concern. If the skin is pale, cool, or clammy and capillary refill time is slow, treat the patient for shock immediately. Maintain a normal body temperature, and improve perfusion by administering oxygen. If musculoskeletal injuries in the extremities are suspected, at least initially stabilize them (or splint them) before you move

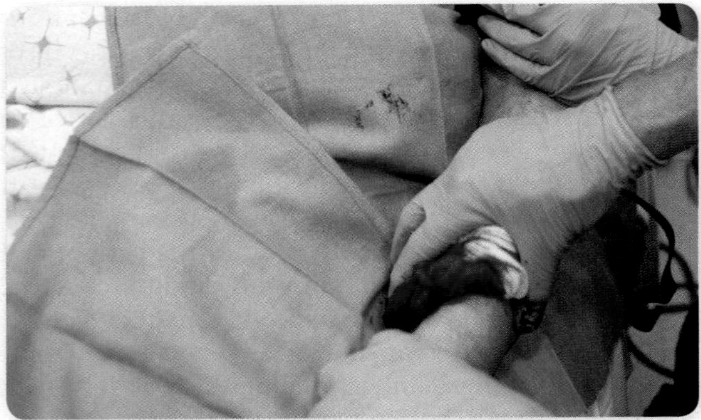

Figure 33-23 Control external bleeding with direct pressure. If this technique is not effective, apply a tourniquet.

the patient. Eliminating such injuries as a potential cause of shock may need to be done later in your assessment. Assess for pulses proximal to the injury, and note any circulatory changes before and after any manipulation as well as frequently during transport.

Fractures can break through the skin and cause external bleeding. This rupture may occur either during the initial injury or during manipulation of the extremity while preparing for splinting or transport. Careful handling of the extremity minimizes this risk. If external bleeding is present, bandage the extremity quickly to control bleeding **Figure 33-23**. Use sterile dressings to cover the wound and bone to reduce the potential for bone infection. The bandage should be secure enough to control bleeding without restricting circulation distal to the injury. Monitor bandage tightness by assessing the pulse, sensation, and movement distal to the bandage. Swelling from fractures and internal bleeding may cause bandages to become too tight. If bleeding cannot be controlled, then quickly apply a tourniquet.

If the patient has an airway or breathing condition, or significant bleeding, provide rapid transport to the closest hospital for treatment. A patient who has a significant MOI but whose condition appears otherwise stable should also be transported promptly to the closest most appropriate hospital. Patients with bilateral fractures of the long bones (humerus, femur, or tibia) have been subjected to a high amount of kinetic energy, which should dramatically increase your index of suspicion for serious occult (unseen) injuries. When a decision for rapid transport is made, use your backboard as a splinting device to splint the patient's whole body rather than individually splinting each extremity. If you take the extra time required to individually splint each of the patient's arms and legs, you may delay the prompt surgical intervention needed for other injuries when a significant MOI has occurred. Individual splints should be applied en route if the patient is stable (ie, the ABCs are stable) and time permits.

Patients with a simple MOI, such as a twisted ankle or dislocated shoulder, may be further assessed on scene. Stabilize their conditions prior to transport if no other problems exist. Handle fractures carefully while preparing the patient for transport. Gentle care is necessary to limit pain and to prevent sharp bone ends from breaking through the skin or damaging nerves and blood vessels in the extremity.

History Taking

After the life threats have been managed during the primary survey, investigate the chief complaint. Obtain a medical history and be alert for injury-specific signs and symptoms and for any pertinent negatives such as no pain or loss of sensation.

Obtain information from the patient and any bystanders who witnessed it about what led to the incident. Specifically, determine the condition of the patient immediately before the incident, the details of the incident, and the patient's position after the incident. Ask the patient for a subjective description of the injury: How did this happen? Did you hear a pop? Do you have pain? Which functional limitations do you now have? Have you had any abnormal movement or loss of movement?

Remember to obtain a SAMPLE (Signs and symptoms, Allergies, Medications, Pertinent past medical history, Last oral intake, Events leading up to the illness or injury) history for all trauma patients. How much you explore this history depends on the seriousness of the patient's condition and how quickly you need to transport the patient to the hospital.

For patients with simple fractures, dislocations, or sprains, it is easier to obtain a SAMPLE history. At the scene, you may have access to family members and others who have information about the patient's history. Try to obtain this history without delaying the time to definitive care. If time allows, complete the SAMPLE history to identify any preexisting musculoskeletal disorders and attempt to learn more about the injury. Some information obtained will be very relevant to the injury (eg, the patient is taking anticoagulant medications or has a history of osteoporosis).

The OPQRST mnemonic (Onset, Provocation/palliation, Quality, Region/radiation, Severity, Timing) is of limited use in cases of severe injury and is usually too time consuming to use when the patient's airway, breathing, circulation, and rapid transport require immediate attention. However, OPQRST may be more useful when the MOI is unclear, the patient's condition is stable, details of the injury are uncertain,

Words of Wisdom

When assessing a patient's pain, use the OPQRST mnemonic: *O*nset of the pain; *P*rovoking or Palliating factors; *Q*uality of the pain (eg, sharp, pressure, crampy); *R*egion of the pain, including its primary location and the area where pain radiates or refers; *S*everity of the pain; and *T*ime (duration) that the patient has been experiencing pain. It is also useful to have the patient quantify the severity of the pain by using a 1 to 10 pain scale or a pain scale that uses images of facial expressions (see pain scale presented in Chapter 36, *Pediatric Emergencies*).

or evaluation of the patient's pain is necessary. In a case of simple trauma, this more detailed investigation may help you and the hospital staff to better understand the specific injury.

As mentioned, a person may experience acute pain in conjunction with a musculoskeletal injury. It is useful to have the patient quantify the severity of the pain by using a 1 to 10 pain scale or a pain scale that uses images of facial expressions to assess pain.

Special Populations

Children with fractures may not want you to see, touch, or splint the injured extremity. Always be honest with children about what you are doing and whether it will hurt. Explain that splinting is necessary and sometimes painful, but that there will be less pain once the splint is in place, the fracture is stabilized, and cold packs are applied.

Secondary Assessment

The secondary assessment is a more detailed, comprehensive examination of the patient that can reveal injuries that may have been missed during the primary survey. In some cases, such as with a critically injured patient or a short transport time, you may not have time to conduct a secondary assessment. If two or more extremities are injured, treat the patient as having experienced significant trauma and provide rapid transport to the hospital. The likelihood of other, more severe injuries increases when two or more bones have been broken.

If the patient has suffered significant trauma that has likely affected multiple systems, start the secondary assessment with a full-body exam to confirm you have found all problems and injuries. Begin with the head and systematically work toward the feet. Assess the patient's head, chest, abdomen, genitalia, extremities, and back. This full-body exam will help you identify any hidden and potentially life-threatening injuries and will also help you prepare the patient for rapid transport. For example, you want to identify an unstable pelvis before you attempt to move the patient onto a backboard and secure the patient to the board.

When examining a stable patient with an isolated injury, obtain a baseline set of vital signs. Your focus can then shift to evaluating the injured extremity. One of the simplest ways to assess an extremity is to compare one side with the other, noting any discrepancy in length, position, or skin color.

Complete the secondary assessment by noting DCAP-BTLS (Deformities, Contusions, Abrasions, Punctures/penetrations, Burns, Tenderness, Lacerations, Swelling) as you observe and palpate the soft tissue from head to toe and assess the patient for limitations, such as inability to move a joint. While performing the exam, ensure you cover the **six Ps of musculoskeletal assessment**: Pain, Paralysis, **Paresthesias** (numbness or tingling), Pulselessness, Pallor (pale or delayed capillary refill in children), and Pressure. Evaluate the circulation, motor function, and abnormal sensations distal to the injury.

During the secondary assessment, ensure you consider distracting injuries; that is, the injuries that are immediately obvious. In the case of an obvious open fracture of the femur, a patient might direct you only to the site of greatest pain. Distal extremity injuries (fractures and dislocations of the feet and hands) are commonly overlooked due to a distracting injury.[6]

Assess the entire zone of injury. Remove clothing from the area and look and palpate for injuries. In musculoskeletal injuries, this zone generally extends from the joint above (proximal) to the joint below (distal), front and back. Always evaluate the joint above and below the site of injury because the injuring force may have affected these sites as well.

Inspection

Inspect for the following signs:

- Deformity, including asymmetry, angulation, shortening, and rotation
- Skin changes, including contusions, abrasions, avulsions, punctures, burns, lacerations, and bone ends
- Swelling
- Muscle spasms
- Abnormal limb positioning
- Increased or decreased range of motion
- Color changes, including pallor and cyanosis
- Bleeding, including estimating the amount of blood loss

Palpation

Palpate for tenderness, which, like contusions or abrasions, may be the only significant sign of an underlying musculoskeletal injury. In addition to palpating the injury site, palpate the regions above and below it, identifying any regions with point tenderness (those that the patient identifies as painful). Frequently reassess any tender areas to determine whether the location or severity of the pain or tenderness has changed. Although point tenderness is one of the best indicators of an injury, it may be absent in patients who are intoxicated or who have an injury to the spinal cord.

When you palpate an injured site, attempt to identify instability, deformity, abnormal joint or bone continuity, and displaced bones. Feel for crepitus, which is commonly found at the site of a fracture. Palpate distal pulses on all extremities, and pay special attention to comparing the strength of the pulses in the injured extremity with those in a normal one.

Occasionally, evidence of an arterial injury may be identified while palpating an extremity. Signs of an arterial injury include a pulsatile expanding hematoma, diminished or absent distal pulses, a palpable thrill (vibration) over the site of injury that correlates with the patient's heartbeat, and bleeding that is difficult to control.

Palpate the pelvis to identify instability and point tenderness. Apply pressure over the pubic symphysis to evaluate for tenderness and crepitus. Next, press the iliac wings toward the midline and then posteriorly. Any gross instability found during this examination should be reported to hospital personnel—it may indicate a severe pelvic injury. Do not repeatedly examine the pelvis if instability is found because the manipulations may disrupt blood clots and cause further bleeding.

The examination of the upper and lower extremities should include independently palpating the entire length of each arm and leg to identify any sites of injury. The most efficient way to accomplish this is to place your hands around the extremity and squeeze. Repeat this procedure every few centimeters until you reach the end of the extremity. When you evaluate the upper extremities, always examine the cervical spine and shoulder, because complaints within the arm may be caused by a more proximal disorder. Likewise, with the lower extremities, always conduct an examination of the pelvis and hip if the patient complains of pain in the leg.

If your assessment reveals no external signs of injury, ask the patient to carefully move each limb, and to stop immediately if a movement causes pain. Skip this step in your evaluation if the patient reports neck or back pain. Even slight movement can cause permanent damage to the spinal cord.

Neurovascular Status

Many important blood vessels and nerves lie close to bones, especially around the major joints. Therefore, any injury or deformity of a bone may be associated with vessel or nerve injury. For this reason, you must assess neurovascular function every 5 to 10 minutes during the care process, depending on the patient's condition, until the patient is at the hospital. Always recheck the patient's neurovascular function before and after you splint or otherwise manipulate the limb, as manipulation may potentially cause a bone fragment to press against or impale a nerve or vessel. Failure to restore circulation in this situation can lead to death of the limb. Always give priority to patients with impaired circulation resulting from bone fragments. To assess neurovascular status, follow the steps in Skill Drill 33-1.

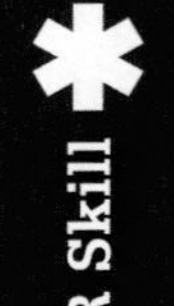

Skill Drill 33-1 Assessing Neurovascular Status

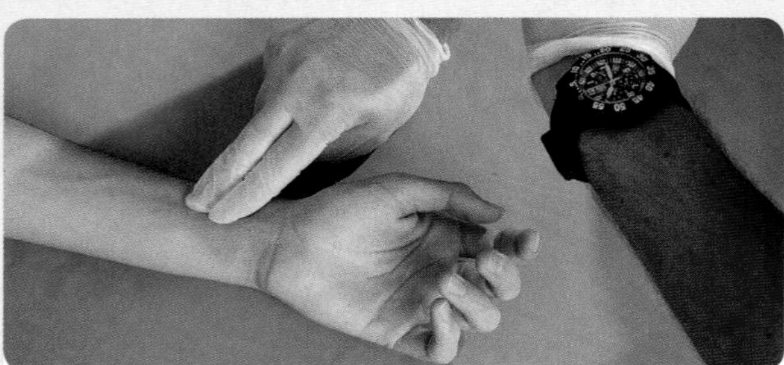

Step 1 Palpate the radial pulse in the upper extremity.

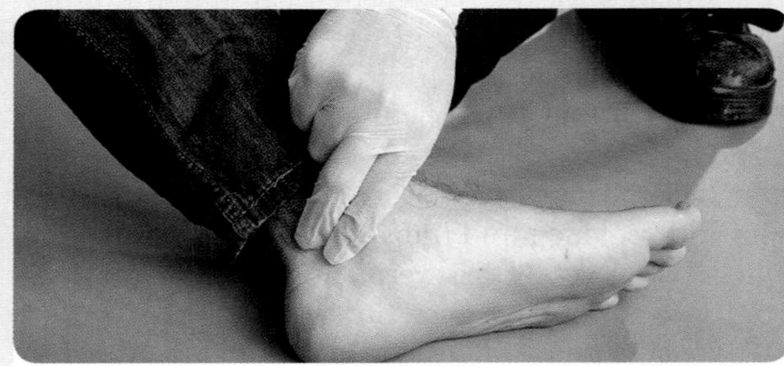

Step 2 Palpate the posterior tibial and dorsalis pedis pulses in the lower extremity.

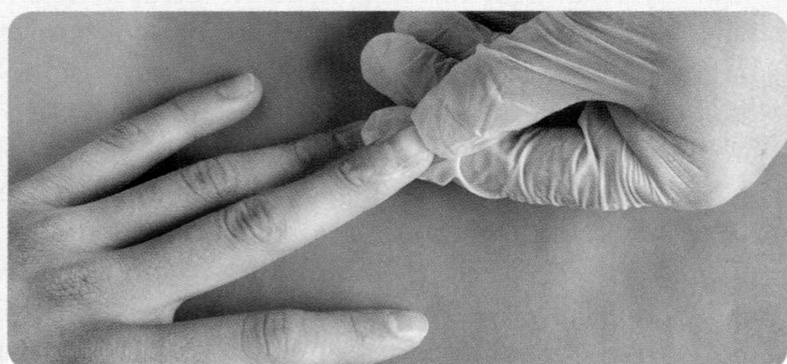

Step 3 Assess capillary refill by blanching a fingernail or toenail. If normal color does not return within 2 seconds after you release the nail, then assume circulation is impaired. This test is typically recommended for children, although it can be used in adults as well.

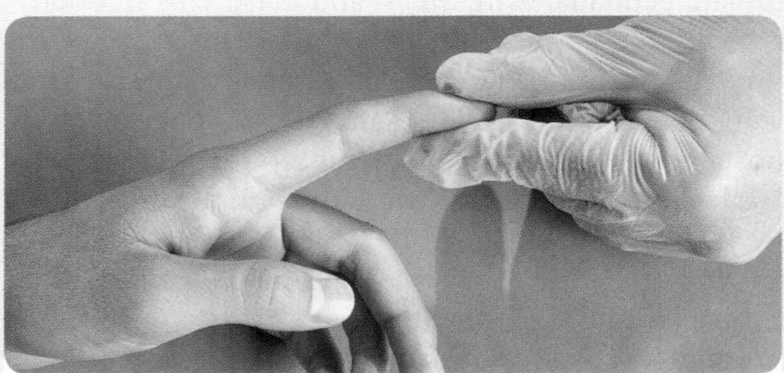

Step 4 Assess sensation in the flesh near the tip of the index finger and thumb, as well as the little finger. The patient's ability to sense a light touch in the fingers or toes distal to the site of a fracture is a good indication that the nerve supply is intact.

Skill Drill 33-1 Assessing Neurovascular Status *(continued)*

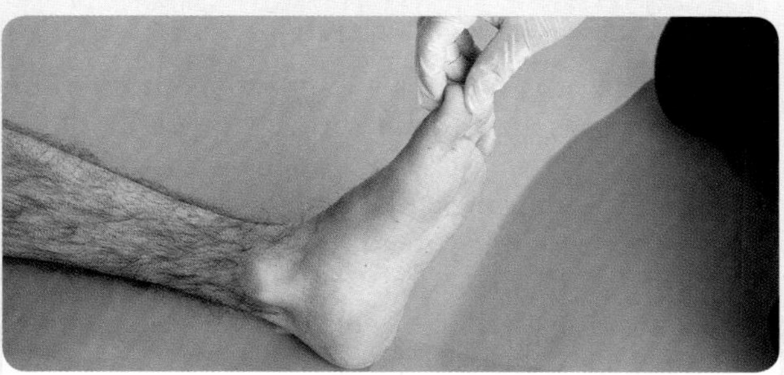

Step 5 On the foot, check sensation on the flesh near the tip of the big toe.

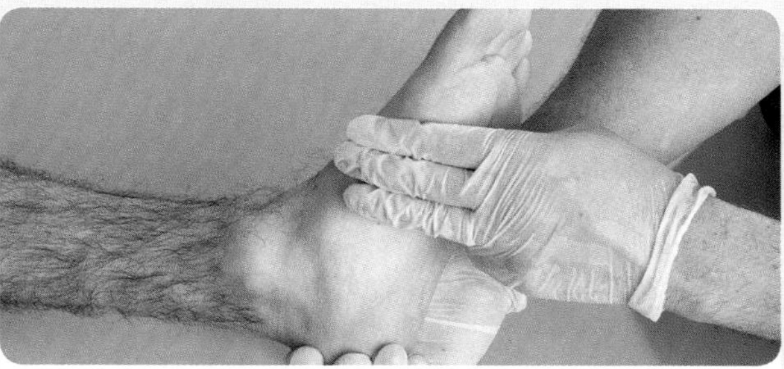

Step 6 Check sensation on the medial side of the foot.

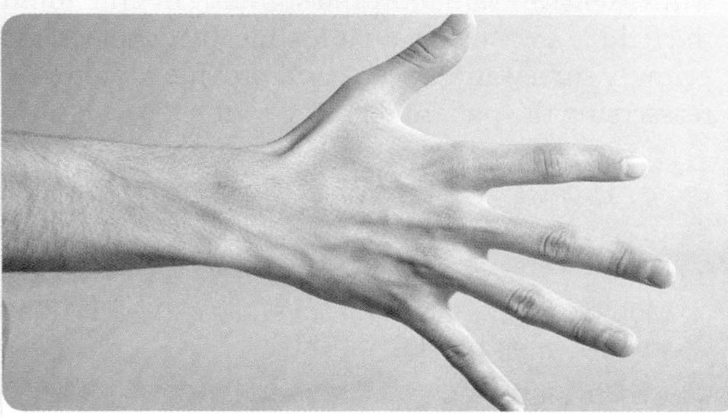

Step 7 For an upper extremity injury, evaluate motor function by asking the patient to open the hand. (Perform motor tests only if the hand or foot is not injured. Stop the test if it causes pain.)

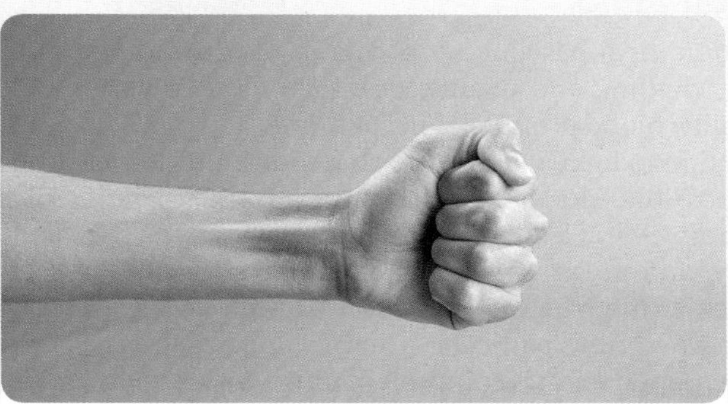

Step 8 Ask the patient to make a fist.

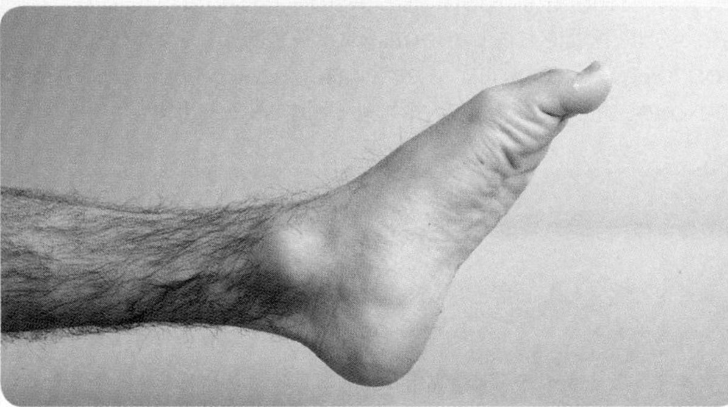

Step 9 For a lower extremity injury, ask the patient to flex the foot and toes downward.

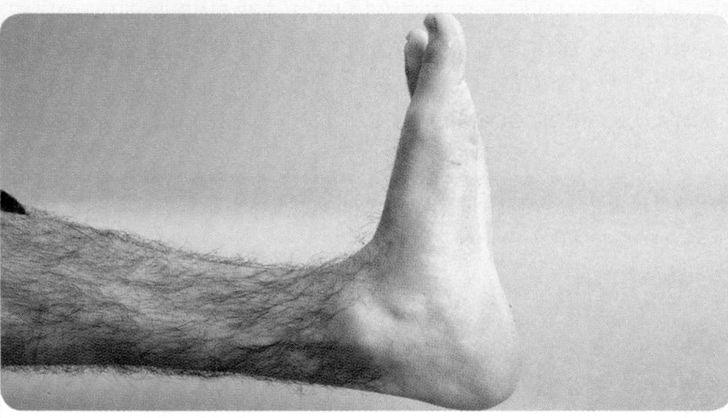

Step 10 Ask the patient to extend the foot and ankle and pull the toes and foot upward.

Because many of the steps in the detailed physical exam require patient cooperation, you will not be able to assess sensory and motor function in an unresponsive patient. Nevertheless, you can evaluate an unresponsive patient's limb for deformity, swelling, ecchymosis, false motion, and crepitus.

Words of Wisdom

Extremity injuries that impair circulation or nerve function in distal tissues are urgent situations. Patients with these injuries need careful assessment, prompt transport, and frequent reassessment of distal functions. It is also crucial to report this information in your initial radio contact with the hospital to allow personnel to prepare for prompt diagnostic evaluation and potentially surgery, which may be necessary to save the limb.

Vital Signs

Determine a baseline set of vital signs, including pulse rate, rhythm, and quality; respiratory rate, rhythm, and quality; blood pressure; skin condition; and pupil size and reaction to light. Obtain these baseline indicators as soon as possible. The patient may appear to be tolerating the injury well—at least, until you reassess these vital signs and they indicate otherwise. Trends in vital signs can indicate whether the patient's condition is improving or getting worse over time, particularly during long transports. Shock or hypoperfusion is common in musculoskeletal injuries, and the baseline information provided by the vital signs is very important in assessing for these conditions. In addition, remember to assess blood glucose levels in all patients who present with altered mental status.

Reassessment

Repeat the primary survey to ensure your interventions are working as they should. A reassessment should be performed every 5 minutes for a patient in unstable condition and every 15 minutes for a patient in stable condition.

Because trauma patients often have multiple injuries, ensure you assess their overall condition, stabilize the ABCs, and control any serious bleeding before further treating the injured area. Consider calling early for paramedic backup if needed. In a critically injured patient, you should secure the patient to a long backboard to stabilize the spine, pelvis, and extremities and provide prompt transport to a trauma center. In this situation, a secondary assessment with extensive evaluation and splinting of limb injuries in the field is a waste of valuable time. Instead, perform the primary survey at the scene and provide rapid transport, reassessing the patient en route to the ED.

Words of Wisdom

Musculoskeletal injuries are rarely an immediate threat to life. Remember the ABCs!!

YOU are the Provider — PART 3

After you have the patient situated in the back of the ambulance, you ask your partner to initiate rapid transport to the trauma center, which is approximately 45 minutes away, attempting to keep the ride as smooth as possible to minimize the patient's pain and discomfort. As you obtain the patient's baseline vital signs, you decide the patient would benefit from having a second IV line inserted because of the potential for significant blood loss. You establish a second 18-gauge IV line with normal saline TKO (to keep open). Although the patient is in a moderate amount of pain, he states the pain is bearable.

Recording Time: 14 Minutes	
Respirations	24 breaths/min, clear
Pulse	122 beats/min
Skin	Cool, pale, and clammy
Blood pressure	92/40 mm Hg
Oxygen saturation (Spo_2)	97% on 15 L/min
Pupils	Pupils Equal, Round, and Reactive to Light and Accommodation (PERRLA)

5. What are some potential complications of femur and pelvic fractures?
6. What are the considerations when using lactated Ringer solution with trauma patients?

If the patient has no life-threatening injuries, you may take extra time at the scene to stabilize any obvious injuries and perform a more thorough evaluation.

Words of Wisdom

Always splint a joint above and a joint below the injury, and assess the patient's circulation, motor function, and sensation both prior to and after splinting. Stabilize the injury in the most comfortable position that allows for maintenance of good circulation distal to the injury.

Your radio report to the hospital should include a description of the problems found during your assessment. Report problems with the patient's ABCs, open fractures, and compromised circulation that occurred before or after splinting and that may require specialized care.

In your documentation, give complete descriptions of injuries and the MOIs associated with them. It is important to assess and document the presence or absence of circulation, motor function, and sensation distal to the injury before you move an extremity, after manipulation or splinting of the injury, and on arrival at the hospital. In other words, always document the findings of a neurovascular exam, even if they are normal. When an abnormality is identified, document the specific deficit—for example, the patient was unable to extend the thumb or move the wrist. Hospital staff may later refer to your notes to compare changes to the patient's condition over time. In addition, your careful documentation may protect you from legal action if patients or their families pursue it later. Do not rely on your memory to recall details from situations; your memory is unreliable and will not hold up in a court of law.

Emergency Medical Care

Your first steps in providing care for any patient are the primary survey and stabilizing the patient's ABCs. If needed, perform a rapid full-body scan or focus on a specific injury. Remember to always take standard precautions and be alert for signs and symptoms of internal bleeding. Internal bleeding should be suspected whenever the MOI suggests that severe forces have affected the body. Consider administering nitrous oxide for pain relief as indicated by local protocols.

Follow the steps in Skill Drill 33-2 when caring for patients with musculoskeletal injuries.

Skill Drill 33-2 Caring for Musculoskeletal Injuries

NR Skill

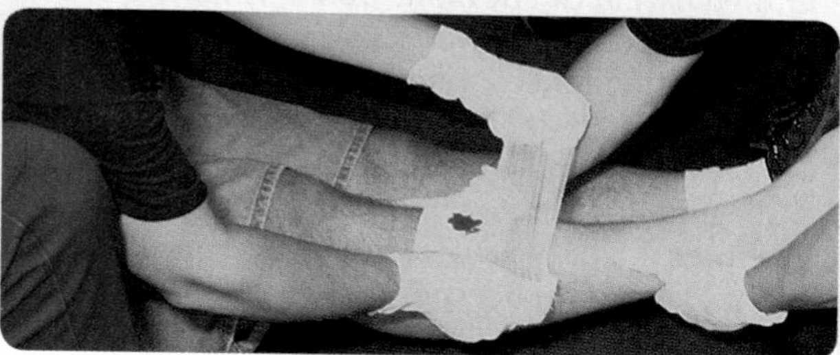

Step 1 Cover open wounds with a dry, sterile dressing, and apply direct pressure to control bleeding. Assess distal pulse and motor and sensory function. If bleeding cannot be controlled, then apply a tourniquet.

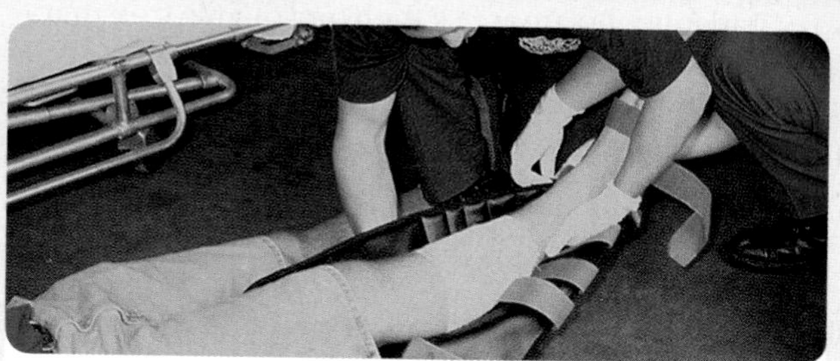

Step 2 Apply a splint, and elevate the extremity approximately 6 inches (15 cm) (slightly above the level of the heart). Assess distal pulse and motor and sensory function.

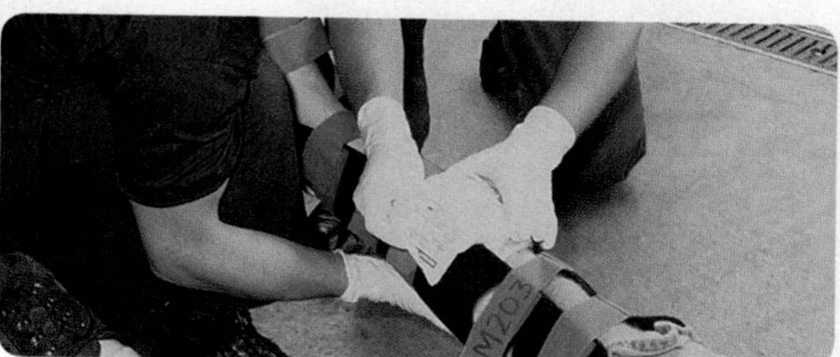

Step 3 Apply cold packs if there is swelling, but do not place them directly on the skin.

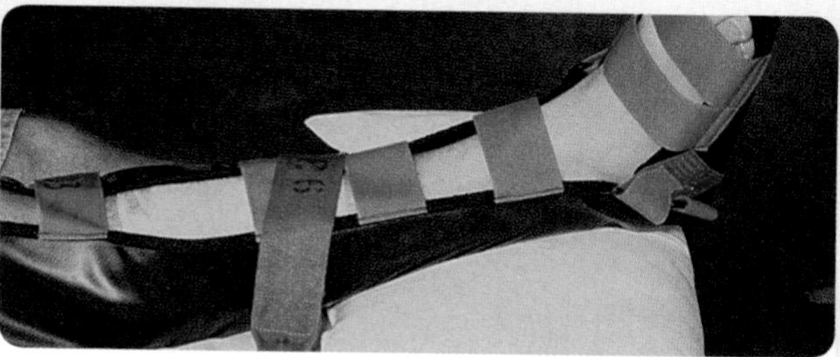

Step 4 Position the patient for transport, and secure the injured area. Consider requesting paramedic backup for additional pain management.

Words of Wisdom

Straightening or splinting an injured limb can compromise distal functions, just as the initial injury can. Record the status of distal circulation and nervous function (neurovascular status) before and after splinting. At a minimum, your written record should describe these functions before splinting, immediately after splinting, and on arrival at the hospital. Also indicate the results of reassessments en route.

▶ Volume Deficit Due to Musculoskeletal Injuries

Fractures may lead to significant blood loss from damaged blood vessels within the bone and musculature around the bone and, in some cases, from damage to large blood vessels in the region of the fracture. When you care for patients with fractures, implement interventions such as applying direct pressure, splinting, and administering intravenous fluids to prevent the development of hypotension and an unstable condition. Table 33-3 lists the potential amounts of blood loss from various fracture sites and may serve as a guideline for estimating the level of resuscitation required. The goal of prehospital management should be to keep the patient's fluid volume, vital signs, and mental status normal.

For patients who are at risk for hypovolemia from fractures, such as pelvic fractures or bilateral femur fractures, IV access should be gained and an isotonic crystalloid solution given. Administer fluids in 20-mL/kg increments to maintain blood pressure (and radial pulses) and perfusion.

▶ Cold and Heat Application

Cold packs are useful for treating patients during the initial 48 hours following an injury and are very effective at decreasing both pain and swelling. Cooling the injured area causes vasoconstriction of the blood vessels in the region and decreases the release of inflammatory mediators. As a result, swelling and inflammation are reduced when cold packs are used during the acute stage of an injury.

Conversely, heat therapy should generally be avoided during the initial 48 to 72 hours following an injury, because heat may increase pain and swelling during this period. Once the acute phase of the injury ends and clotting occurs in damaged blood vessels, heat packs are useful for increasing blood flow to the region to decrease stiffness and to promote healing. Consequently, heat packs may be beneficial for patients who report an injury that occurred several days before contacting emergency medical services (EMS).

Table 33-3 Potential Blood Loss From Fracture Sites

Fracture Site	Potential Blood Loss (mL)
Pelvis	1,500–3,000
Femur	1,000–1,500
Humerus	250–500
Tibia or fibula	250–500
Ankle	250–500
Elbow	250–500
Radius or ulna	150–250

▶ Splinting

A **splint** is a flexible or rigid device that is used to protect and maintain the position of an injured extremity Figure 33-24. Unless the patient's life is in immediate danger, you should splint all fractures, dislocations, and sprains before moving the patient. Splinting an injured extremity properly not only decreases the patient's pain, but splinting also reduces the risk of further damage to muscles, nerves, blood vessels, and skin. In addition, splinting helps to control bleeding by allowing clots to form where vessels were damaged.

A splint is simply a device to prevent motion of the injured part. It can be made from any material when you need to improvise. However, you should have an adequate supply of standard commercial splints on hand. When no splinting materials are available, the patient's arm can be bound to the chest wall, and an injured leg can be bound to the uninjured leg to provide at least temporary stability. The three major types of splints are traction splints, rigid splints, and formable splints.

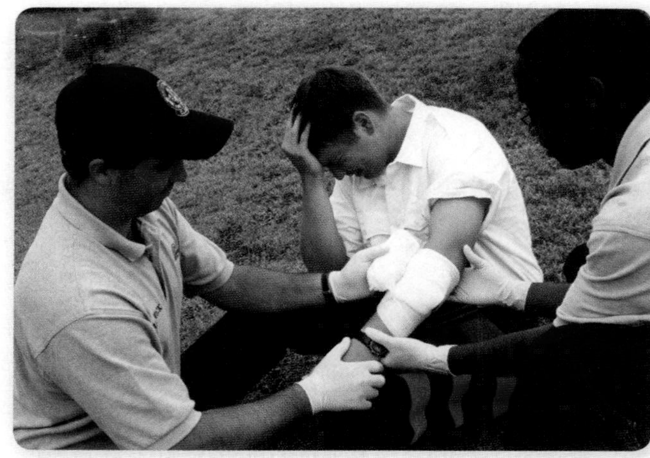

Figure 33-24 Splinting reduces pain and prevents additional damage to an injured extremity. Maintain manual support of the injured extremity during bandaging and splinting.

When a patient with multiple orthopaedic injuries must be transported immediately, you will not have time to splint each fracture one by one. Instead, the best way to stabilize multiple fractures when the patient's overall condition is critical is to splint the axial skeleton by using a long backboard and straps or an alternative device, such as a vacuum mattress. This will serve three purposes: (1) protect against a spinal injury; (2) reduce movement of the injured extremities by securing them to the board; and (3) save time at the scene.

Words of Wisdom

One of the primary indications for splinting is to prevent a closed fracture from becoming an open fracture (conversion).

Principles of Splinting

The following principles of splinting apply to most situations:

1. Remove clothing from the area of any suspected fracture or dislocation so you can inspect the extremity for DCAP-BTLS (Deformities, Contusions, Abrasions, Punctures/penetrations, Burns, Tenderness, Lacerations, Swelling). Also, remove any jewelry, as swelling may cause rings or watches to cut off circulation.
2. Assess and record the patient's neurovascular status distal to the site of the injury, including pulse, sensation, and movement. Reassess frequently en route to the hospital.
3. Cover all wounds with a dry, sterile dressing before splinting. To prevent infection following an open fracture, brush away any obvious debris on the skin surrounding an open fracture before applying the dressing. Do not enter or probe the open fracture site to retrieve debris, because this may lead to further contamination. Do not attempt to push exposed bone ends back under the skin.
4. Do not move the patient before splinting an extremity unless there is an immediate hazard to the patient or yourself.
5. For *fractures*, the splint should immobilize the bone ends and the two adjacent joints—above and below the fracture. For *dislocations*, the splint must extend along the entire length of the bone above and the entire length of the bone below the dislocated joint. Do not attempt to straighten fractures involving joints without first obtaining medical direction.
6. Pad all rigid splints to prevent local pressure and discomfort to the patient.
7. Manually support the injured site with hands placed above and below the injury to minimize movement until the splint is applied and secured.
8. If a long bone fracture is severely angulated and no pulse is present in the extremity, gently apply longitudinal traction (tension) to attempt to realign the bone and improve circulation. Use a smooth, firm grip to apply manual traction, and avoid any sudden, jerky movements of the limb. *Do not attempt to straighten fractures involving joints without first obtaining medical direction.* There is no need to straighten or manipulate the joint unless it has no distal pulse.
9. If the patient reports severe pain or is resistant to movement, discontinue applying traction, splint the joint or bone in the position of deformity, and carefully monitor the distal neurovascular status.
10. If possible, avoid covering the fingers and toes with the splint to allow for monitoring of skin color, temperature, and condition.
11. If possible, apply cold packs and elevate the splinted limb to minimize swelling.
12. Stabilize all suspected spinal injuries in a neutral, in-line position on a long backboard.
13. If the patient has signs of shock (hypoperfusion), align the limb in the normal anatomic position and provide transport.
14. When in doubt, splint.

Be aware of the hazards associated with the improper application of splints, which include the following:

- Compression of nerves, tissues, and blood vessels
- Delay in transport of a patient with a life-threatening injury
- Reduction of distal circulation
- Aggravation of the injury
- Injury to tissue, nerves, blood vessels, or muscles due to excessive movement of the bone or joint

Words of Wisdom

When treating a patient with multiple serious fractures, immediately secure the patient to a long backboard and provide rapid transport. Spending time on scene immobilizing individual non–life-threatening injuries may result in a well-splinted corpse!

Traction Splints

Applying in-line **traction** is the act of exerting a pulling force on a body structure in the direction of its normal alignment. It is the most effective way to realign a fracture of the shaft of a long bone so the limb can be splinted more effectively. Following a femur fracture, the strong muscles of the thigh go into spasm—a condition that often leads to significant pain and deformity. Traction splints provide constant pull on a fractured femur, thereby preventing the broken bone ends from overriding due to unopposed muscle contraction. In addition, these splints help maintain alignment of the fracture pieces and provide effective stabilization of the fracture site. As a result, patients are likely to experience less pain.

Traction splints also reduce blood loss. Normally, the thigh is shaped like a cylinder. In a femur fracture, the thigh is shortened and becomes spherical. The volume of a sphere can be substantially greater than that of a cylinder, so a person with an untreated femur fracture can accumulate more blood in the thigh than a person whose thigh is pulled out to length by a traction splint.

Excessive traction can be harmful to an injured limb. When applied correctly, however, traction stabilizes the bone fragments and improves the overall alignment of the limb. Do not attempt to reduce the fracture or force all the bone fragments back into alignment. This is the physician's responsibility and is outside the AEMT's scope of practice. In the field, the goals of in-line traction are as follows:

- To stabilize the fracture fragments to prevent excessive movement
- To align the limb sufficiently to allow it to be placed in a splint
- To avoid potential neurovascular compromise

The amount of pull that is required to accomplish these objectives varies, but rarely exceeds 15 pounds (7 kg). Use the least amount of force necessary. Firmly grasp the patient's foot at the end of the injured limb; once you start pulling, do not stop until the limb is fully splinted. When pulling traction for a possible femur fracture, place one hand underneath the patient's knee for support. The direction of traction pull is always along the long axis of the limb. Imagine where the normal, uninjured limb would lie, and pull gently along the line of that imaginary limb until the injured limb is in approximately that position **Figure 33-25**. Grasping the foot and the initial pull of traction usually causes some discomfort as the bone fragments move. It helps if a second person can support the injured limb directly under the site of the fracture. This initial discomfort will quickly subside, and you can then apply further, gentle traction. However, if the patient strongly resists the traction or if it causes more pain that persists, then stop and splint the limb in the deformed position.

Words of Wisdom

When you apply traction to an injured lower extremity, place one hand underneath the patient's knee to provide support for the joint and grasp under the patient's ankle with your other hand to pull traction.

Traction splints are used primarily to stabilize isolated fractures of the midshaft femur, which are characterized by pain, swelling, and deformity of the midthigh. Do not use a traction splint if the patient has a joint or lower leg injury. Several different types of lower extremity traction splints are commercially available, such as the Hare traction splint, the Sager traction splint, the Reel splint, and the Kendrick splint. Become familiar with the unique method of applying each one. (The uses of the Hare and Sager splints are described later in this section.) Consult with your local agency on which traction splint you will use in the field, and ensure you are comfortable applying this device to a patient.

Traction splints are not suitable for use on the upper extremities because the major nerves and blood vessels in the patient's axilla cannot tolerate countertraction forces. In addition, do not use traction splints in patients with any of the following conditions:

- Injuries close to or involving the knee
- Injuries of the pelvis

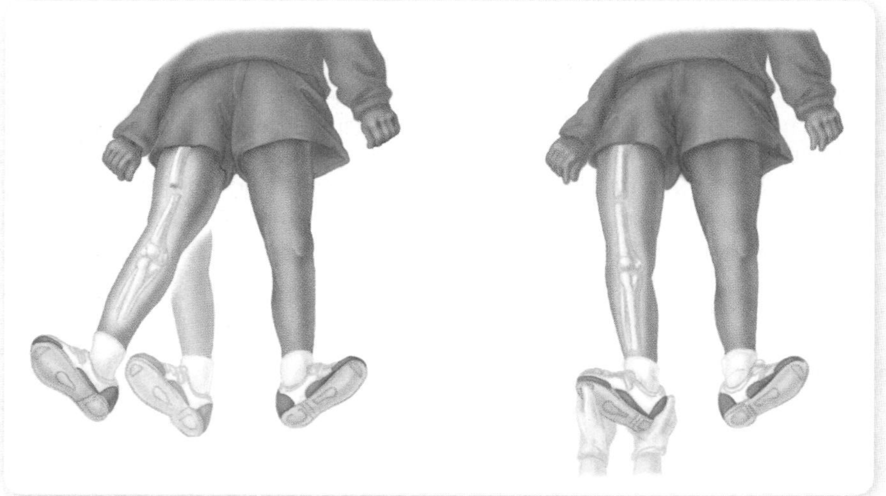

Figure 33-25 To apply traction, imagine the position where the normal uninjured limb would lie, then gently pull along that line until the injured limb is in that position. Do not release traction once you have applied it.

- Partial amputations or avulsions with bone separation
- Lower leg, foot, or ankle injury

Proper application of a traction splint requires two well-trained providers working together. To apply a Hare traction splint, follow the steps in Skill Drill 33-3. Because the Hare traction splint stabilizes the limb by producing countertraction on the ischium and in the groin, you should pad these areas well. Avoid excessive pressure on the external genitalia. Always use commercially available padded ankle hitches rather than pieces of rope, cord, or tape; such improvised hitches can sometimes be painful and can potentially obstruct circulation in the foot.

Words of Wisdom

A traction splint is *only* used for an isolated femur fracture. Do not spend valuable time on scene applying a traction splint on a critical patient—if time permits, it can be applied en route once other life threats have been addressed.

The Sager traction splint is lightweight, easy to store, and applies a measurable amount of traction. Best of all, you can apply it by yourself when necessary. To apply a Sager traction splint, follow the steps in Skill Drill 33-4.

Skill Drill 33-3 Applying a Hare Traction Splint

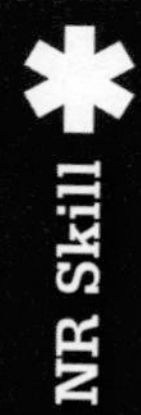

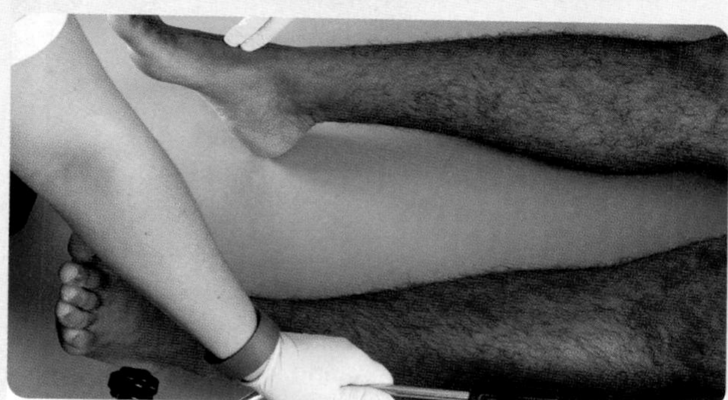

Step 1 Take standard precautions. Expose the injured limb and check the pulse and motor and sensory function. Place the splint beside the uninjured limb, adjust the splint to the proper length, and prepare the straps.

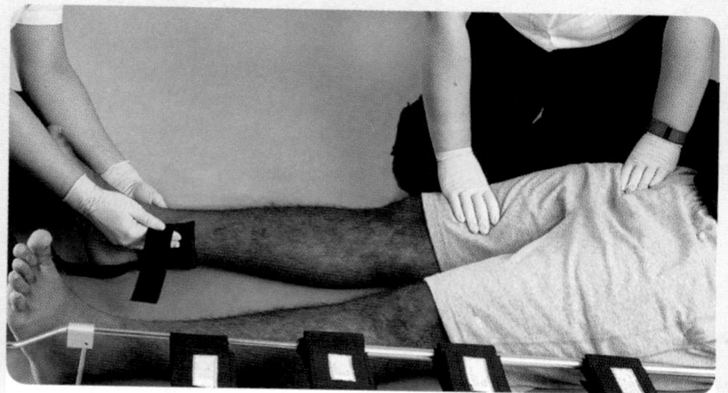

Step 2 Support the injured limb as your partner fastens the ankle hitch about the foot and ankle. Usually, the patient's shoe is removed for this procedure.

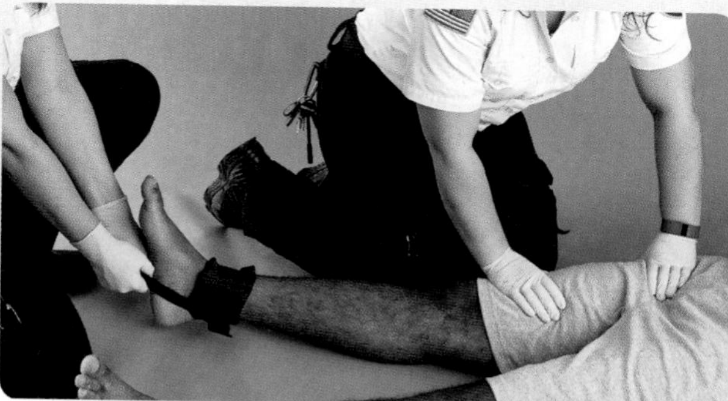

Step 3 Continue to support the limb as your partner applies gentle in-line traction to the ankle hitch and foot.

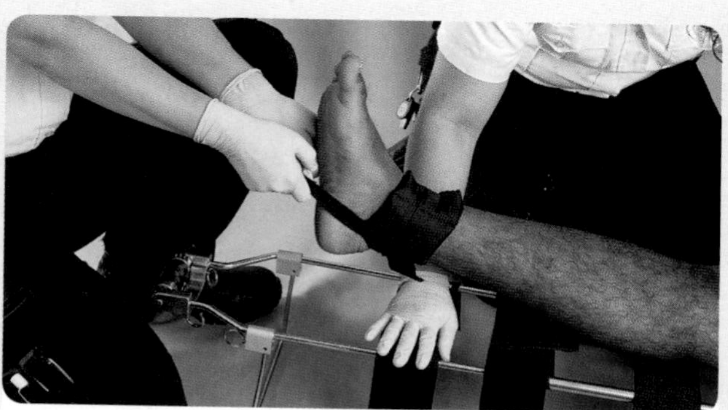

Step 4 Slide the splint into position under the injured limb until it seats against the ischial tuberosity, while your partner supports the heel and underneath the calf.

(continued)

Skill Drill 33-3 Applying a Hare Traction Splint *(continued)*

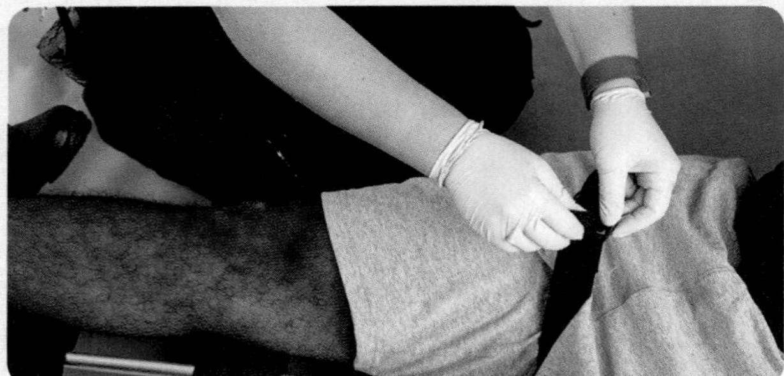

Step 5 Pad the groin and fasten the ischial strap.

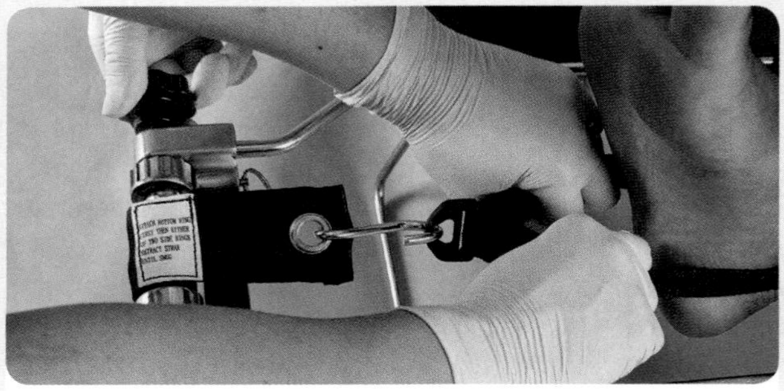

Step 6 Connect the loops of the ankle hitch to the end of the splint as your partner continues to maintain traction. Carefully tighten the ratchet to the point the splint holds adequate traction. Adequate traction has been applied when the leg is the same length as the uninjured leg or when the patient's pain is relieved.

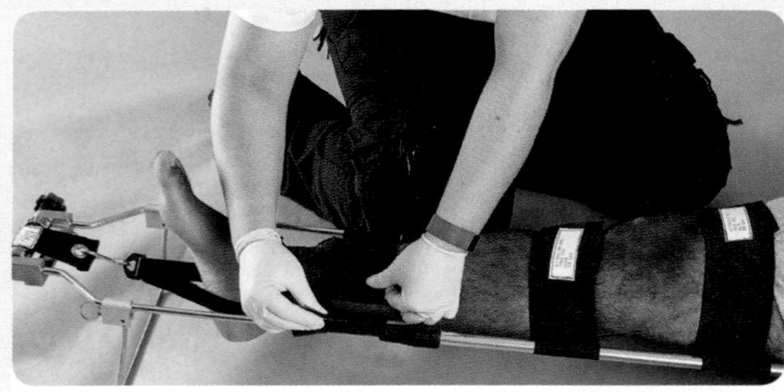

Step 7 Secure and check the support straps; take care not to place a strap over the fracture site. Reassess the patient's pulse and motor and sensory function.

Step 8 Secure the patient and splint to the backboard in a way that will prevent movement of the splint during patient movement and transport.

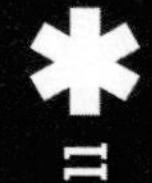

NR Skill

Skill Drill 33-4 Applying a Sager Traction Splint

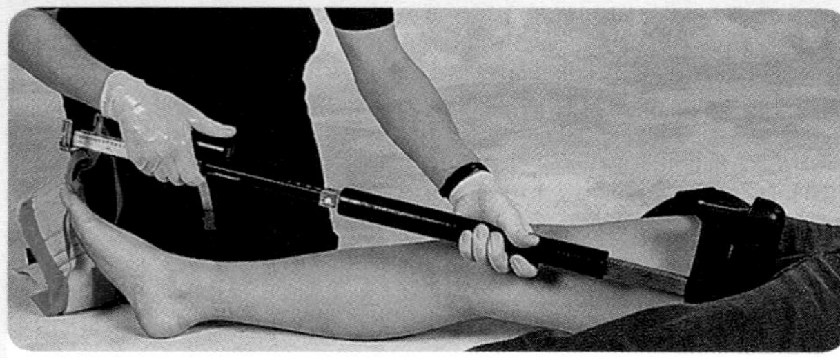

Step 1 Take standard precautions and expose the injured area. Check the patient's pulse and motor and sensory functions. Adjust the thigh strap so it lies anteriorly when secured.

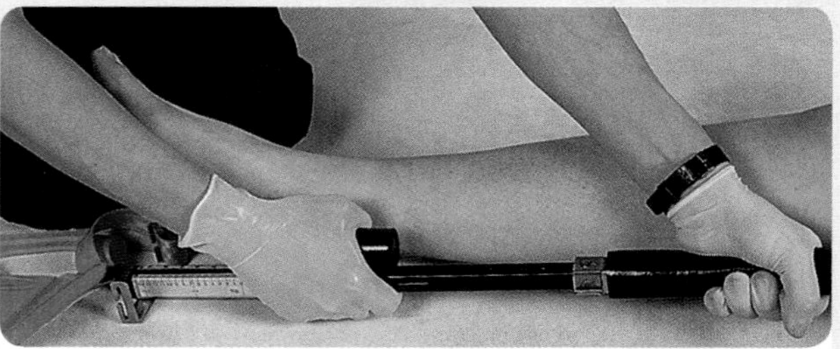

Step 2 Estimate the proper length of the splint by placing it next to the uninjured limb. Fit the ankle pads to the ankle.

Skill Drill 33-4 Applying a Sager Traction Splint *(continued)*

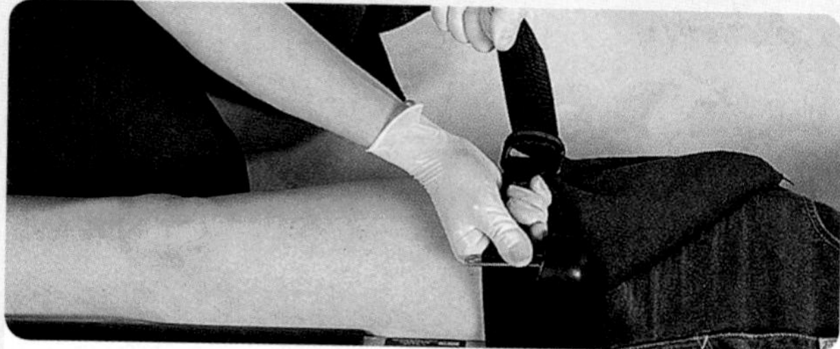

Step 3 Place the splint at the inner thigh, apply the thigh strap at the upper thigh so the perineal cushion is snug against the groin and the ischial tuberosity, and secure the splint snugly.

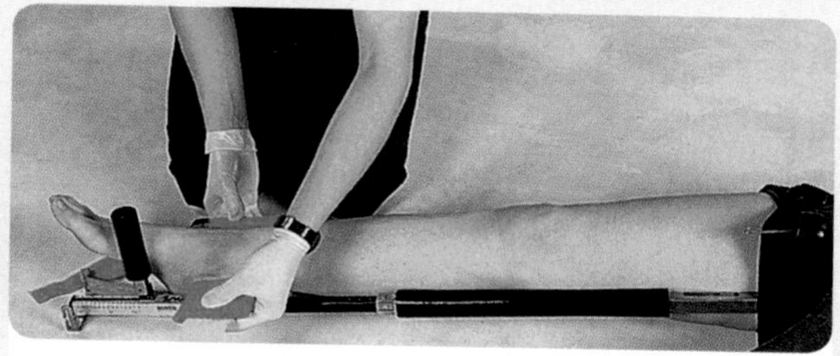

Step 4 Tighten the ankle harness just above the malleoli. Pull and secure the cable ring against the bottom of the foot.

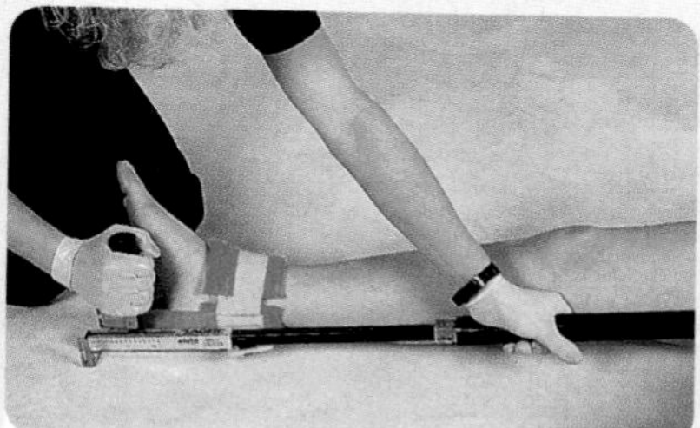

Step 5 Extend the splint's inner shaft to apply traction of approximately 10% of the patient's body weight, using a maximum of 15 pounds (7 kg).

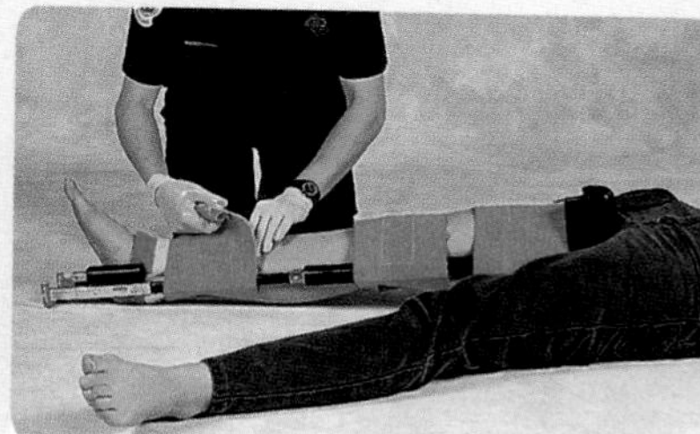

Step 6 Secure the splint with elasticized cravat bandages.

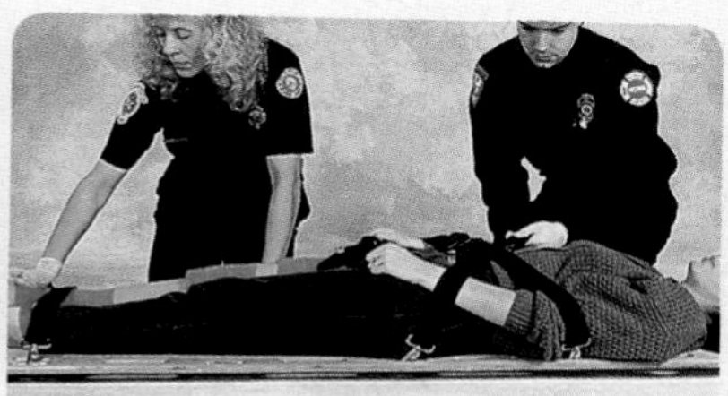

Step 7 Secure the patient to a long backboard. Reassess pulse and motor and sensory function.

Words of Wisdom

The Reel splint is a relatively new traction splint used by the military and is currently making its way into the commercial market. This splint is designed to be used on a lower extremity Figure 33-26. It provides the option to stabilize the joint or bone in the position found and, with the hinges, can be adjusted without removing the splint.

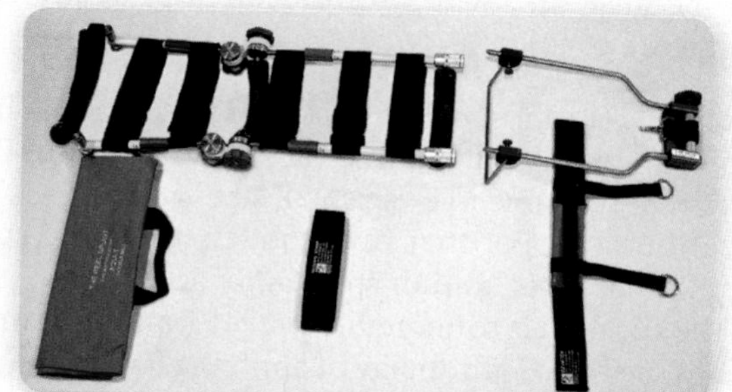

Figure 33-26 The Reel splint is being used by the military.

Rigid Splints

Rigid (nonformable) splints are made from firm material and are applied to the sides, front, and/or back of an injured extremity to prevent motion at the injury site. Common examples of rigid splints include padded board splints, molded plastic and metal splints, padded wire ladder splints, and folded cardboard splints. As always, take standard precautions. It takes two AEMTs to apply a rigid splint. Follow the steps in Skill Drill 33-5.

There are two situations in which you must splint the limb in the position of deformity: (1) when the deformity is severe, as is the case with many dislocations, and (2) when you encounter resistance or extreme pain when applying gentle traction to the fracture of a shaft of a long bone. You should only attempt to straighten an extremity if there is no pulse. If a pulse is present, it should not be manipulated, just splinted in the position found. In either situation, you should apply padded board splints to each side of the limb and secure them with soft roller bandages Figure 33-27. Most dislocations should be splinted as found, but follow local protocols. Attempts to realign or reduce dislocations can lead to more damage.

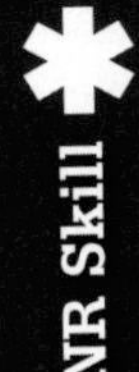

Skill Drill 33-5 Applying a Rigid Splint

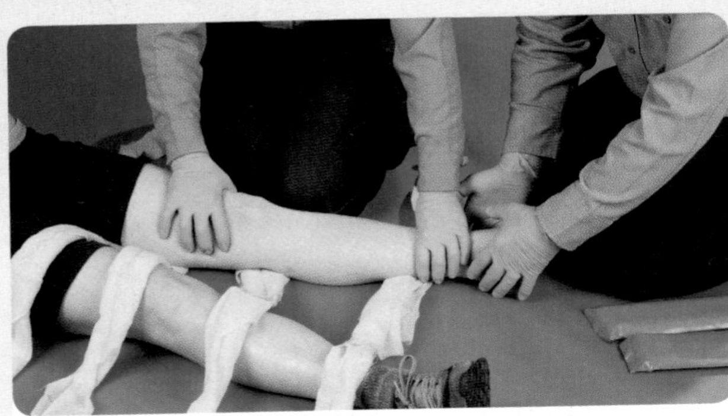

Step 1 Provide gentle support and in-line traction for the limb. Assess distal pulse and motor and sensory function.

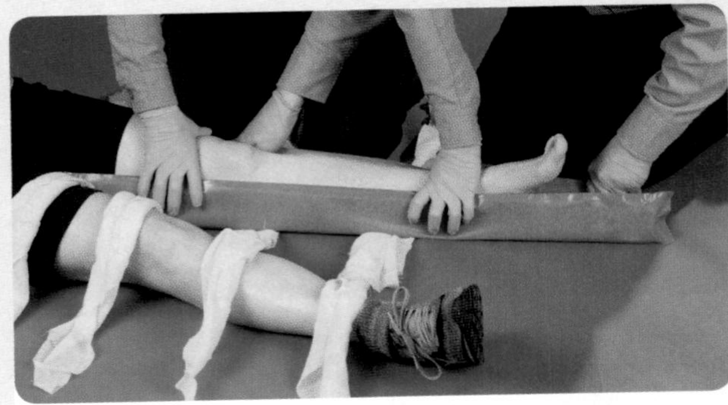

Step 2 Place the splint alongside or under the limb. Pad between the limb and the splint as needed to ensure even pressure and contact. Pad any bony prominences.

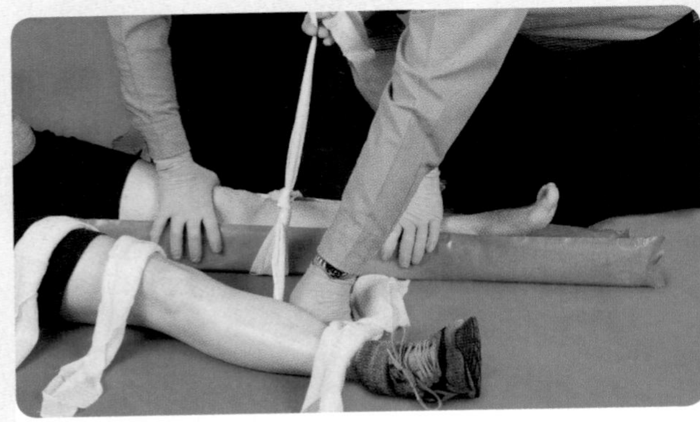

Step 3 Secure the splint to the limb with bindings.

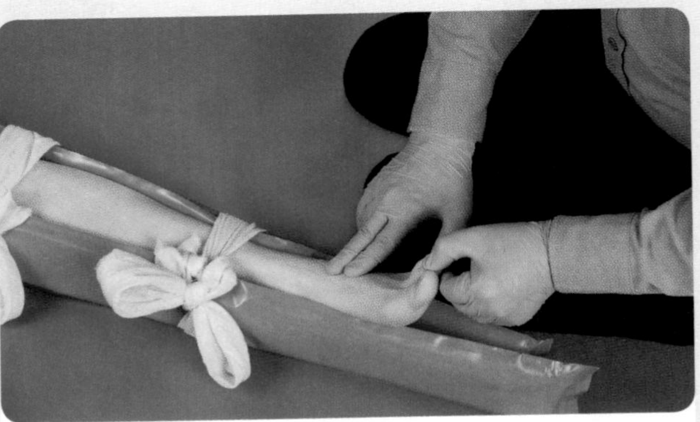

Step 4 Assess and record distal neurovascular function.

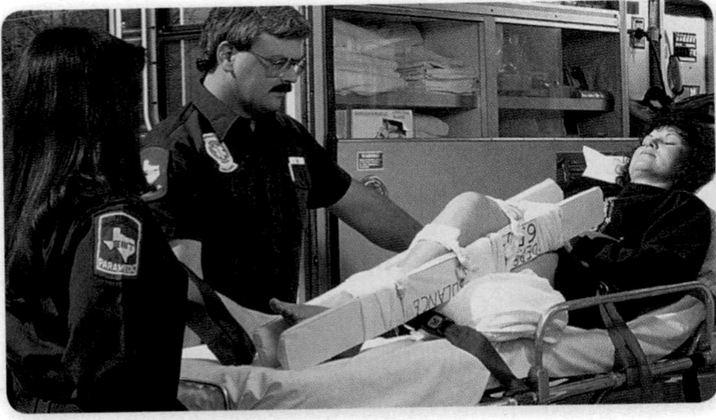

Figure 33-27 If you encounter resistance or extreme pain when applying traction to a long bone, apply padded board splints to each side of the limb, and secure them with soft roller bandages, stabilizing the limb in its deformed position.

Pneumatic Splints

Pneumatic splints are useful for stabilizing fractures involving the lower leg or forearm. They are not effective for angulated fractures or for fractures that involve a joint, because they will forcefully attempt to straighten the fracture or joint.

Air Splints. The most commonly used pneumatic splint is the precontoured, inflatable, clear plastic air splint. These devices are available in a variety of sizes and shapes, with or without a zipper that runs the length of the splint. Always inflate this kind of splint *after* applying it.

The air splint is comfortable, provides uniform contact, and has the added advantage of applying firm pressure to help control bleeding and reduce swelling. These splints should not be used on open fractures in which any sharp bone ends are exposed. All open wounds must be covered with a dressing before applying these splints.

Air splints have some drawbacks, particularly in areas prone to cold weather. The zipper can stick, clog with dirt, or freeze. Significant changes in the weather affect the pressure of the air in the splint. Therefore, carefully monitor air splints to ensure they do not lose pressure or become overinflated. Overinflation can occur when the splint is applied in a cold area and the patient is subsequently moved to a warmer area—the air inside the splint will expand as it gets warmer, possibly increasing pressure and causing pulses to cease. The same thing happens when there are changes in altitude, which can be a problem with air transport of patients. Air splints will expand in a higher altitude if the patient compartment of the aircraft is unpressurized (eg, in a helicopter). Therefore, carefully monitor the splint and let out air if the splint becomes overinflated.

The method of applying an air splint depends on whether it has a zipper. With either type (zippered or unzippered), you must first cover all wounds with a dry, sterile dressing, ensuring you take standard precautions. Inflate the splint just to the point at which finger pressure will make a slight dent in the splint's surface. For a splint that has a zipper, follow the steps in Skill Drill 33-6. If you use an unzippered or partially zippered type of air splint, follow the steps in Skill Drill 33-7.

Skill Drill 33-6 Applying a Zippered Air Splint

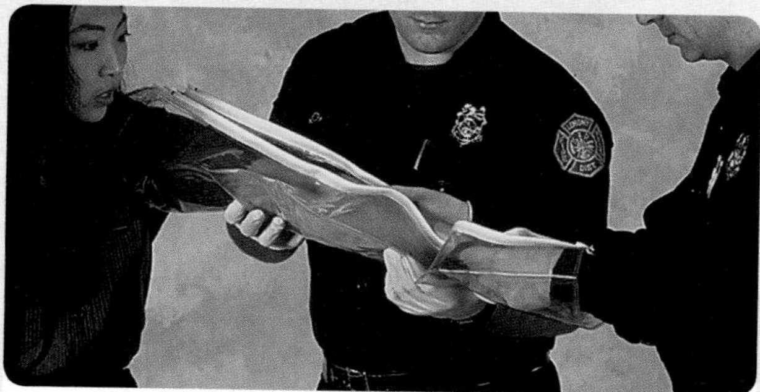

Step 1 Assess distal pulse and motor and sensory function. Cover any open wounds with a dressing. Support the injured limb and apply gentle traction as your partner applies the open, deflated splint.

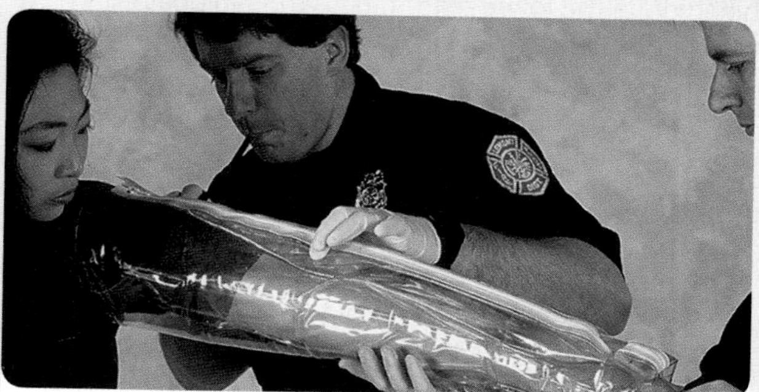

Step 2 Zip up the splint, inflate it by pump or by mouth, and test the pressure. Check and record distal neurovascular function and monitor periodically.

Skill Drill 33-7 Applying an Unzippered Air Splint

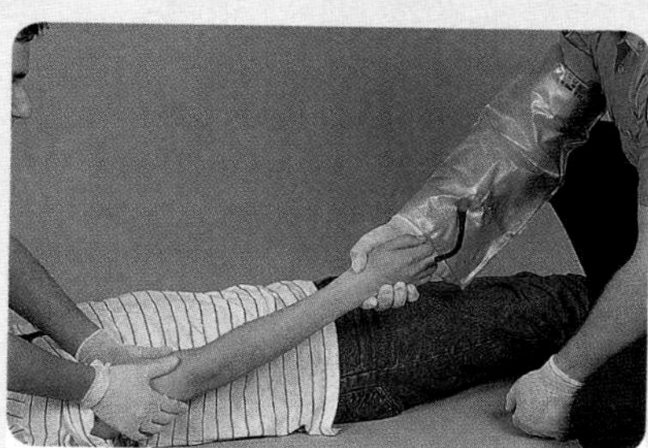

Step 1 Assess distal pulse and motor and sensory function. Have your partner support the injured limb. Place your arm through the splint to grasp the patient's hand or foot.

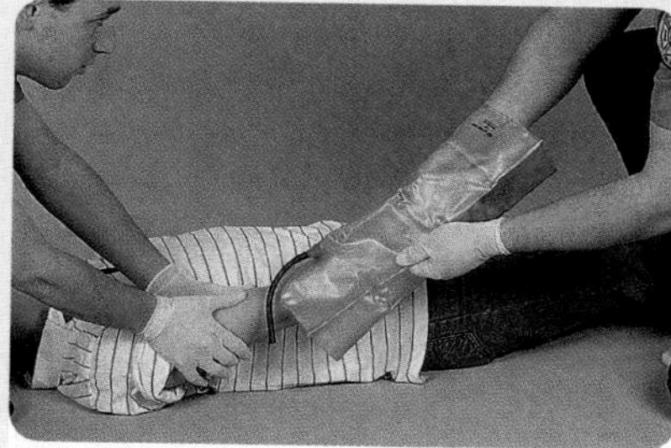

Step 2 Apply gentle traction while sliding the splint onto the injured limb.

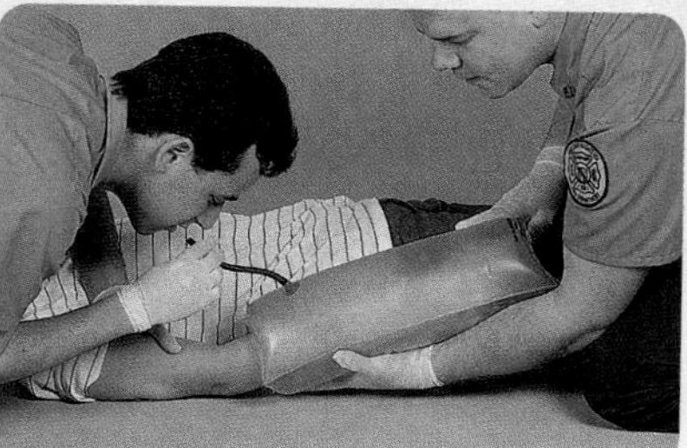

Step 3 Have your partner inflate the splint by pump or by mouth and test the pressure. Reassess distal pulse and motor and sensory function and monitor en route.

Pneumatic Antishock Garments. If a patient has injuries to the lower extremities or pelvis, you may be able to use a pneumatic antishock garment (PASG) as a splinting device, if local protocol allows. Situations in which use of a PASG is allowed vary widely by locale. Many EMS systems no longer use this device because of problems reported with its use. The PASG is contraindicated for treatment of shock but may have some value as a splinting device in rare circumstances.

Words of Wisdom

The primary use of the PASG is to stabilize pelvic fractures or bilateral femur fractures. This device may also be beneficial for applying pressure to help control bleeding in the lower extremities when injuries cover a large surface area.

Do not use the PASG if any of the following conditions exist, as the PASG may worsen or complicate the patient's condition:

- Pregnancy
- Pulmonary edema
- Acute heart failure
- Penetrating chest injuries
- Groin injuries
- Major head injuries

Consult with medical direction if you think prolonged use or use in unusual circumstances may be necessary.

If you are using the device to stabilize a possible pelvic fracture, you must inflate all compartments.

Do not remove a PASG in the field. This type of splint must be deflated gradually in the hospital under careful supervision by a physician. Before handing off the patient to hospital personnel, report the patient's blood pressure, the time you applied the PASG, and the results.

Formable Splints

Formable splints include vacuum splints, pillow splints, structural aluminum malleable (SAM) splints, a sling and swathe, and pelvic binders for pelvic fractures. Just like an air splint, a vacuum splint can be easily shaped to fit around a deformed limb. Instead of pumping in air, however, you use a hand pump to pull out the air through a valve. Follow the steps in Skill Drill 33-8 to apply a vacuum splint.

Special Populations

Because vacuum mattresses conform to the body, they may be the best choice to immobilize older adult patients who have abnormal curvatures of the spine and are suspected of having spinal column injuries.

Pelvic Binder. **Pelvic binders** are used to splint the bony pelvis to reduce hemorrhage from bone ends, venous disruption, and pain Figure 33-28. Pelvic binders are meant to provide temporary stabilization until definitive stabilization can be achieved. Generally, pelvic binders should be light, made of soft material, and easily applied by one person, and they should allow access to the abdomen, perineum, anus, and groin for examination and diagnostic testing. Because there are various manufacturers

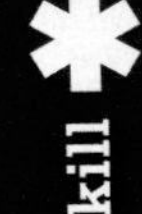

NR Skill

Skill Drill 33-8 Applying a Vacuum Splint

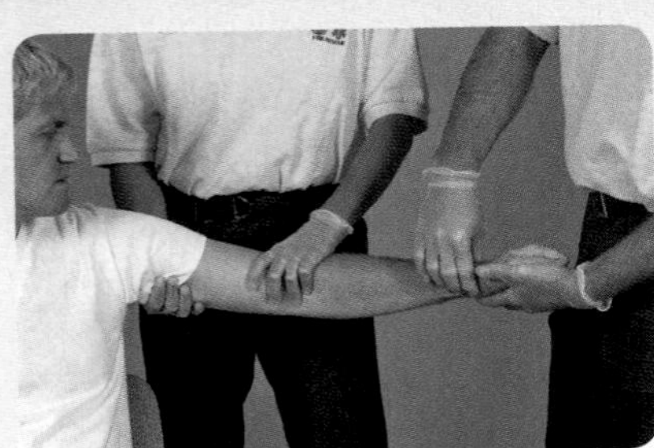

Step 1 Assess distal pulse and motor and sensory functions. Have your partner stabilize and support the injury, applying traction if needed.

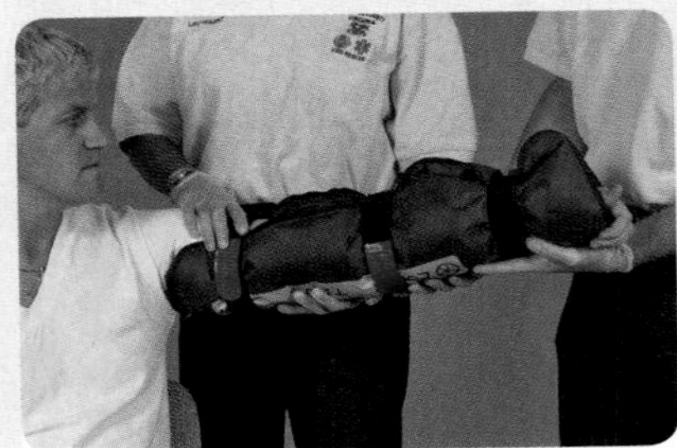

Step 2 Place the splint and wrap it around the injured limb.

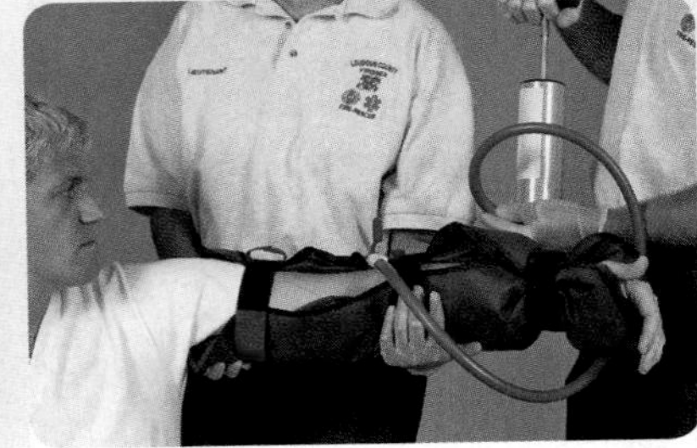

Step 3 Draw out the air from the splint through the suction valve, and then seal the valve. Reassess distal pulse and motor and sensory function.

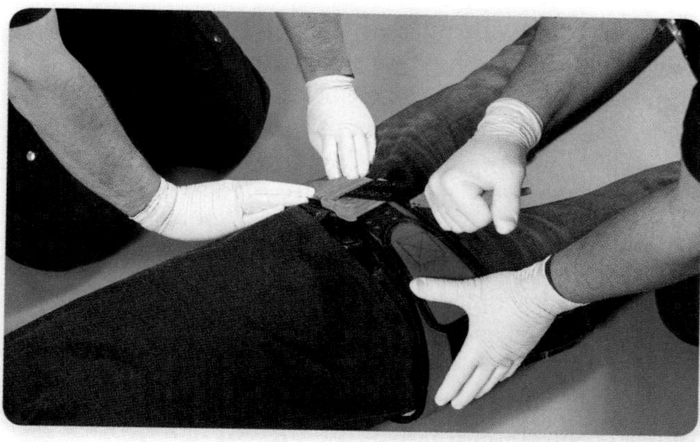

Figure 33-28 Pelvic binders are meant to provide temporary stabilization until definitive stabilization can be achieved.

of pelvic binder devices, you should be familiar with the manufacturer's instructions for your specific device.

Buddy Splinting

Buddy splinting is used to splint injuries that involve the fingers or toes. With this technique, an adjacent uninjured finger or toe serves as a splint to the injured one. To buddy splint, tape the injured digit to an uninjured one. Place a gauze pad between the digits that are taped together, and ensure the tape does not pass over joints. Ensure the tape is not so tight as to cut off circulation.

▶ Transportation

Once an injured limb is adequately splinted, the patient is ready to be transferred to a backboard or stretcher and transported.

Very few, if any, injuries justify the use of excessive speed during transport. The limb will be stable once a dressing and splint have been applied. Although a patient with a pulseless limb or possible compartment syndrome must be given a high priority, if the hospital is only a few minutes away, speeding to the ED will make no difference to the patient's eventual outcome. If the treatment facility is more than an hour away, the patient with a pulseless limb should be transported by helicopter or immediate ground transportation. If circulation in the distal limb is impaired, always consult medical direction so the proper steps can be taken quickly once the patient arrives in the ED.

Pathophysiology, Assessment, and Management of Complications of Musculoskeletal Injuries

Musculoskeletal injuries can lead to numerous complications—not just those involving the musculoskeletal system, but also systemic changes or illness. It is essential to not focus all your attention on the musculoskeletal injury; such "tunnel vision" may cause you to miss less obvious but more serious injuries.

The likelihood of developing a complication is often related to the strength of the force that caused the injury, the injury's location, and the patient's overall health. Any injury to a bone, muscle, or other musculoskeletal structure is often accompanied by bleeding. In general, the greater the force that caused the injury, the greater the hemorrhage that will be associated with it.

Special Populations

Pregnancy creates the potential for additional complications with musculoskeletal injuries, especially with a pelvic fracture. Any force significant enough to fracture the pelvis may injure the fetus or the interface between the placenta and the uterus. Aside from direct force, injuries may occur from broken bone ends penetrating the uterus. Significant bleeding may result in fetal death caused by the shunting of blood as her body attempts to protect the mother. Aggressive care of the pregnant woman, especially one with signs of shock, provides the best chance for a positive outcome for both patients.

Following a fracture, the sharp ends of the broken bone may damage muscles, blood vessels, arteries, and nerves, or the ends may penetrate the skin and produce an open fracture. A significant loss of tissue may occur at the fracture site if the muscle is severely damaged or if the bone's penetration of the skin causes a large defect. To prevent infection following an open fracture, you should brush away any obvious debris on the skin surrounding an open fracture before applying a dressing. Do not enter or probe the open fracture site to retrieve debris, because this may lead to further contamination.

Long-term disability is one of the most devastating consequences of a musculoskeletal injury. In many cases, a severely injured limb can be repaired and made to look almost normal. Unfortunately, many patients cannot return to work for long periods of time because of the extensive rehabilitation required and because of chronic pain. AEMTs have a critical role in mitigating the risk of long-term disability. By preventing further injury, reducing the risk of wound infection, minimizing pain through the application of cold and administration of analgesia, and transporting patients with musculoskeletal injuries to an appropriate medical facility, you help reduce the risk or duration of long-term disability.

▶ Peripheral Nerve and Vascular Injuries

When blood vessels are damaged following a musculoskeletal injury, the patient may experience **devascularization**—that is, the loss of blood to a part of the body. Vessel injuries may include a contusion of the vessel wall, laceration, kinking or bending, and formation of pseudoaneurysms. Additionally, neurovascular injuries can occur. The skeletal system normally protects the neurovascular structures within the limbs from injury. These critical structures typically lie deep within the limb and close to the skeleton. For example, the brachial plexus is situated within the axilla and the inner aspect of the arm, shielded from injury by the shoulder girdle. When the shoulder girdle or proximal humerus is fractured, displaced fracture fragments may lacerate or impale nerves, leading to a neurologic deficit. Neurovascular injuries are also likely to occur following a joint dislocation because the nerves and vessels in the region of a joint tend to be more securely tethered to the soft tissues and are less likely to escape injury.

Regardless of the type of vascular injury involved, it is important to assess and reassess pulses, control bleeding, and maintain adequate intravascular volume by administering intravenous (IV) fluid.

▶ Compartment Syndrome

Within a limb, groups of muscles are surrounded by an inelastic membrane called **fascia** that confines the muscles to an enclosed space, or compartment. This compartment can accommodate only a limited amount of swelling. When bleeding or swelling occurs within a compartment as the result of a fracture or severe soft-tissue injury, the pressure within the compartment rises. Pressure that is too high may impair circulation and lead to pain, sensory changes, and progressive muscle death. This condition, known as **compartment syndrome**, is one of the most devastating consequences of a musculoskeletal injury. The longer this situation persists, the greater the chance for tissue necrosis (death).

Both external and internal factors can lead to the development of compartment syndrome. External factors include a bandage, splint, cast, or PASG that is applied too tightly and restricts circulation. Internal factors can increase the amount of material within a compartment. For example, bleeding within a compartment may occur because of a fracture, dislocation, crush injury, vascular injury, soft-tissue injury, or bleeding disorder. Alternatively, fluid leakage or edema may occur secondary to ischemia with reperfusion, excessive exercise, trauma, burns, or any condition associated with the leakage of proteins and fluid from vessels into the interstitial space. A common misconception is that open fractures are safe from compartment syndrome—that is not true. Open fractures may actually have a higher risk of compartment syndrome because they are typically associated with higher-energy injuries and because the open injury typically results in inadequate decompression of the compartment to alleviate the increased swelling that results.

Compartment syndrome usually develops within 6 to 12 hours after injury. It is characterized by severe pain that is localized to the involved compartment and often described as out of proportion to the injury due to the passive stretching of the muscles from the pressure increasing in the compartment. This pain is typically not relieved with pain medication, including narcotics.

As time progresses, the affected area may feel very firm although this is an unreliable sign. Skin pallor may be apparent as well as paresthesias, such as a burning sensation, numbness, or tingling, and paralysis of the involved muscles. Another late sign of compartment syndrome is absence of distal pulses in the affected extremity. By the time the pressure within the compartment reaches the point where it totally occludes the artery passing through it, significant muscle necrosis has probably occurred.

Words of Wisdom

The potential for compartment syndrome increases dramatically with the presence of circumferential burns. Damaged tissue that is unable to expand with the increased edema within the tissues results in increasing pressures and, ultimately, compartment syndrome.

Words of Wisdom

Provide rapid transport for a patient who shows evidence of compartment syndrome. There is no treatment for this syndrome other than surgery!

If a patient has a fracture below the elbow or the knee, ask about the following: extreme pain, decreased pain sensation, pain on stretching of affected muscles, and decreased strength. These signs and symptoms may suggest the pressure within a fascial compartment is elevated—that is, compartment syndrome may be developing.

The goal of prehospital care is to deliver the patient with compartment syndrome to an emergency facility before the extremity is pulseless. Thus, management should include elevating the extremity to heart level (not above), placing ice packs over the extremity, and opening or loosening constrictive clothing and splint material. Administer oxygen and crystalloid solution as needed. Consider administering nitrous oxide for pain management as allowed by local protocols. Provide immediate transport, and frequently reassess the patient's neurovascular status during transport. Compartment syndrome must be managed surgically.

▶ Crush Syndrome

Crush syndrome occurs when a prolonged compressive force impairs muscle metabolism and circulation following the extrication or release of an entrapped limb. When muscles are crushed beyond repair, tissue necrosis develops and

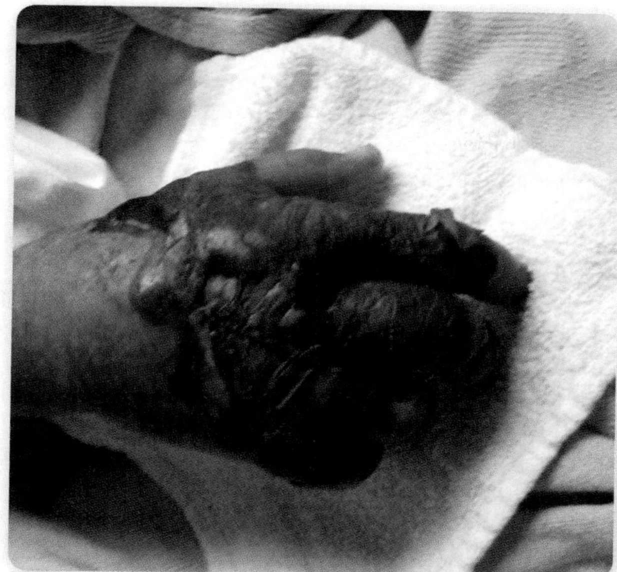

Figure 33-29 Crush injury with tissue necrosis. The patient laid on this hand for hours, resulting in injury.

Courtesy of Rhonda Hunt.

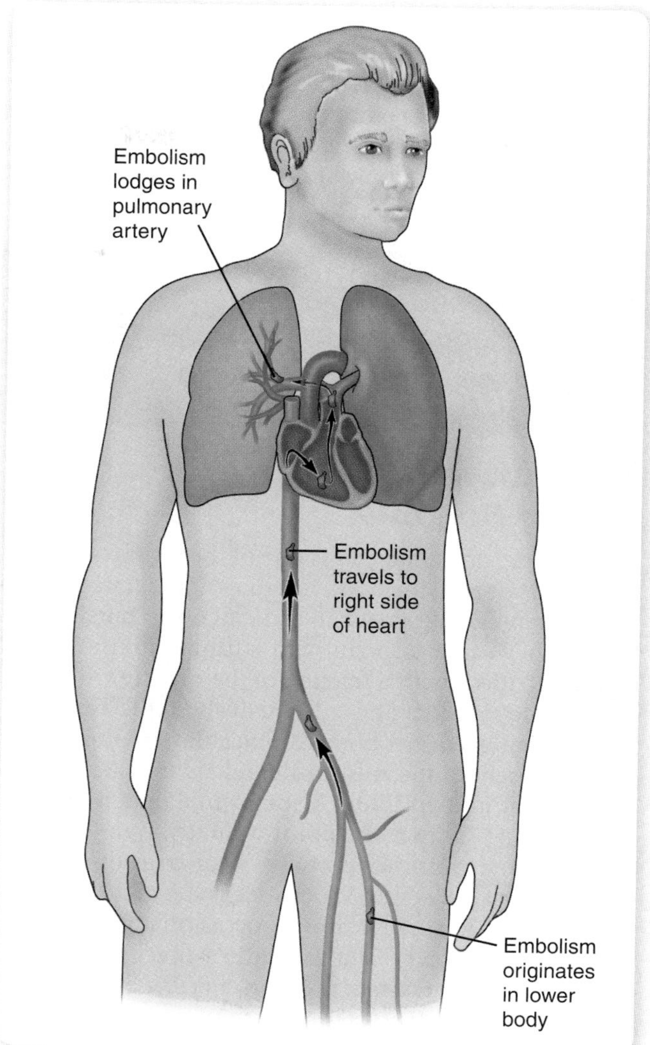

Figure 33-30 When a portion of a deep vein thrombosis dislodges, it may travel to the pulmonary arteries and inhibit blood flow from the heart to the lungs.

leads to release of harmful products, a process known as **rhabdomyolysis**. Rhabdomyolysis may also lead to compartment syndrome. This condition may arise not only in trauma patients, but also in patients who have been lying on an extremity for an extended period (4 to 6 hours of compression)—for example, when a patient who experienced a drug overdose or stroke is not found for an extended period **Figure 33-29**.

After a muscle is compressed for 4 to 6 hours, the muscle cells begin to die and release their contents into the localized vasculature. When the force compressing the region is removed, blood flow is reestablished and the material from the cells that was released into the local vasculature quickly returns to the systemic vasculature. The substances that are of primary concern during this process are lactic acid, potassium, and myoglobin. This process is likely to result in decreased blood pH (acidemia), hyperkalemia, and renal dysfunction.

Treatment of crush syndrome, which aims to prevent complications caused by toxin release, should always be performed with medical direction. Many steps must be taken *before* releasing the compressing force. As with all patients, assess the ABCs in case of suspected crush syndrome. Administer supplemental oxygen as needed, and then consider administering a bolus of crystalloid solution to increase the intravascular volume and to protect the kidneys from the forthcoming myoglobin load. Do not apply a compressive device such as a PASG.

▶ Thromboembolic Disease

Thromboembolic disease, including **deep vein thrombosis (DVT)** and **pulmonary embolism**, is a significant cause of death during the days and weeks after musculoskeletal injuries, especially injuries to the pelvis and lower extremities that lead to prolonged immobilization. Signs and symptoms of DVT include disproportionate swelling of an extremity, discomfort in an extremity that worsens with use, and warmth and erythema of the extremity. When a DVT dislodges, it may cause a pulmonary embolism—a blood clot that occludes a portion or all of the pulmonary arteries **Figure 33-30**. Signs and symptoms of a pulmonary embolism include a sudden onset of dyspnea, pleuritic chest pain, dyspnea, tachypnea, tachycardia, right-sided heart failure, shock, and, in some cases, cardiac arrest.

In addition to the risk of DVT, patients with long bone or pelvic fractures are at risk for the development of fat embolism syndrome, which occurs when fat globules are released into the bloodstream. In this condition, fat droplets become lodged in the vasculature of the lungs. Affected patients have inflammation of the vasculature of the lungs and other blood vessels where fat is deposited. Generally, symptoms appear between 12 and 72 hours after injury; they include tachycardia, dyspnea, tachypnea, pulmonary congestion, fever, petechiae, change in mental status, and organ dysfunction.

Treatment for fat embolism syndrome in the field is limited to maintaining the airway, adequate oxygenation, and intravascular volume, and rapid transport to an ED.

Pathophysiology, Assessment, and Management of Specific Injuries

Injuries of the Clavicle and Scapula

The clavicle, or collarbone, is one of the most commonly fractured bones in the body. Fractures of the clavicle occur most often in children when they fall on an outstretched hand. They can also occur with crushing injuries of the chest. A patient with a fracture of the clavicle will report pain in the shoulder and will usually hold the arm across the front of his or her body. Young children often report pain throughout the entire arm and are unwilling to use any part of injured limbs. These complaints may make it difficult to localize the point of injury, but, generally, swelling and point tenderness occur over the clavicle Figure 33-31. Because the clavicle is subcutaneous (just beneath the skin), the skin will occasionally "tent" over the fracture fragment. The clavicle lies directly over major arteries, veins, and nerves; therefore, fracture of the clavicle may lead to neurovascular compromise although this is thankfully rare.

Fractures of the scapula, or shoulder blade, occur much less frequently because this bone is well protected by many large muscles. Fractures of the scapula are almost always the result of violent, direct trauma to the back, directly over the scapula, which may also injure the thoracic cage, lungs, and heart. For this reason, you must carefully assess the patient for signs of pneumothorax, hemothorax, and rib fractures. Provide supplemental oxygen and prompt transport for patients who are having respiratory difficulty. The associated chest injuries, not the fractured scapula, pose the greatest threat of long-term disability or death.

Abrasions, contusions, and significant swelling may also occur, and the patient will often limit use of the arm because of pain at the fracture site Figure 33-32. The scapula has bony projections that may be fractured with less force.

The joint between the lateral aspect of the clavicle and the acromion process of the scapula is called the acromioclavicular (AC) joint. This joint is frequently separated during football and hockey games when a player falls and lands on the point of the shoulder, driving the scapula away from the outer end of the clavicle. This dislocation is often called an AC separation. The distal end of the clavicle will usually stick out, and the patient will report pain, including point tenderness over the AC joint Figure 33-33.

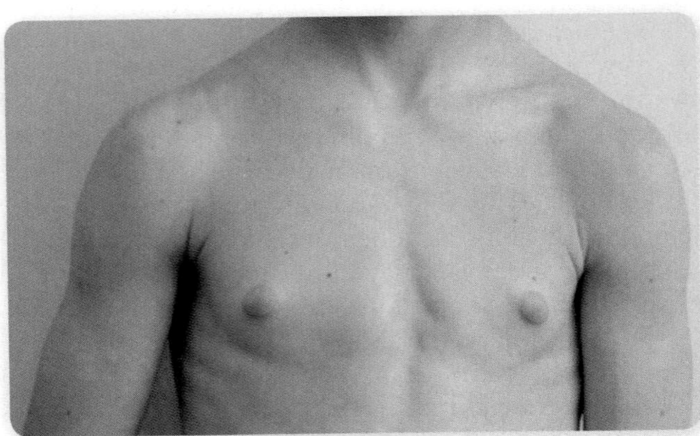

Figure 33-31 A clavicle injury is characterized by swelling, point tenderness, and "tenting" over the fracture fragment.

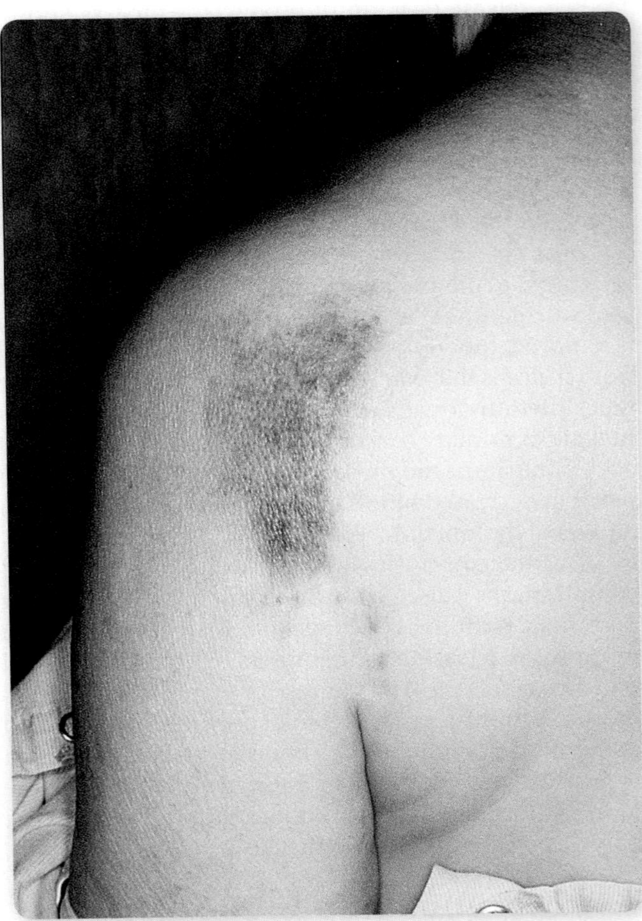

Figure 33-32 Contusions or abrasions over the scapular area may indicate a fracture.

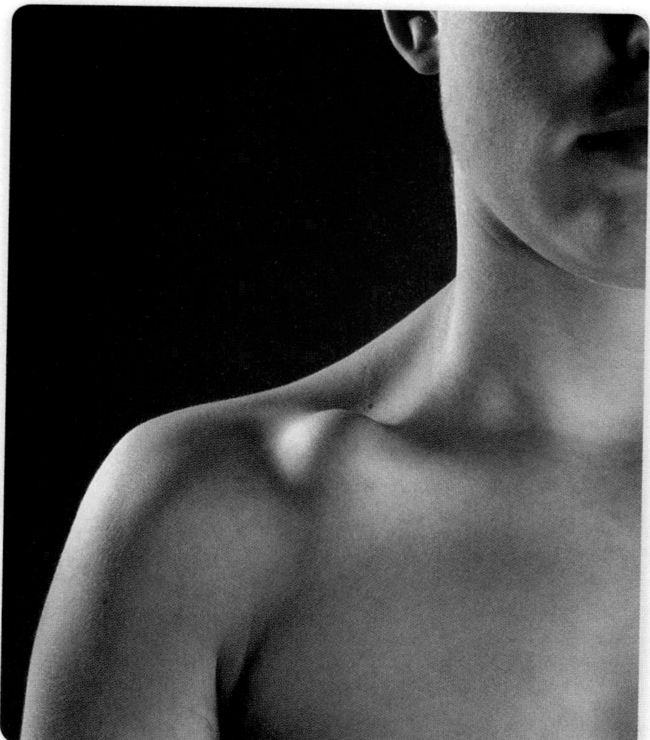

Figure 33-33 With acromioclavicular joint separations, the distal end of the clavicle often sticks out.

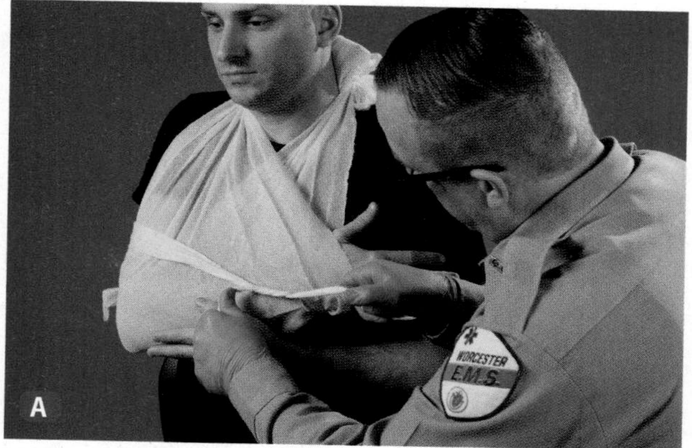

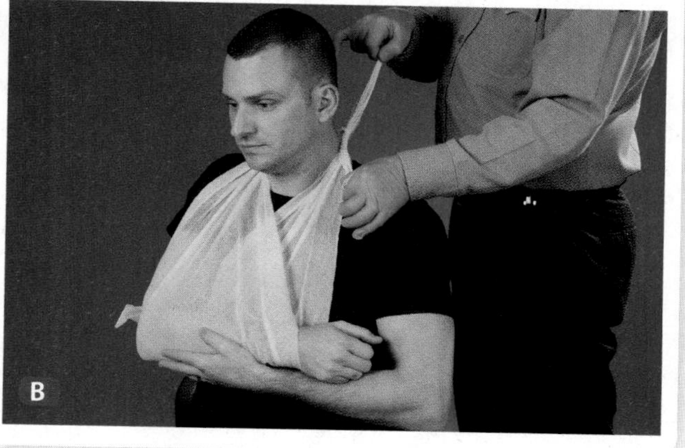

Figure 33-34 A. Apply the sling so the knot is tied to one side of the neck. **B.** Bind the arm to the chest wall with a swathe so the arm cannot swing freely. Leave the patient's fingers exposed so you can assess distal circulation.

Fractures of the clavicle and scapula and AC separations can all be effectively splinted with a sling and swathe. A **sling** is any bandage or material that helps support the weight of an injured upper extremity, relieving the downward pull of gravity on the injured site. To effectively apply a sling, use gentle upward support to the olecranon process of the ulna (at the elbow). The knot of the sling should be tied to one side of the neck so it does not press uncomfortably on the cervical spine Figure 33-34A.

To fully immobilize the shoulder region, a **swathe**—a bandage that passes completely around the chest—must be used to bind the arm to the chest wall. The swathe should be tight enough to prevent the arm from swinging freely but not so tight as to compress the chest and compromise breathing. Leave the patient's fingers exposed so you can assess neurovascular function at regular intervals Figure 33-34B.

Special Populations

A large portion of the older adult population has *osteoporosis*, or a diminished bone density, that occurs as part of the normal aging process. Women are more susceptible than men to this condition. The presence of osteoporosis increases the likelihood of fractures with even minimal trauma—for example, hip or femur fracture due to a fall from a standing position.

Commercially available shoulder immobilizers or slings provide adequate splinting for injuries of the shoulder region, as will triangular bandage slings.

Dislocation of the Shoulder

The glenohumeral joint (shoulder joint) is where the head of the humerus, the supporting bone of the upper arm, meets the glenoid fossa of the scapula. The glenoid fossa joins with the humeral head to form the glenohumeral joint. It is the most commonly dislocated large joint in the body. Often, the humeral head will dislocate anteriorly, coming to lie in front of the scapula as a result of forced abduction (away from the midline) and external rotation of the arm Figure 33-35.

Shoulder dislocations are extremely painful. The patient will guard the shoulder and try to protect it by holding the dislocated arm in a fixed position away from the chest wall Figure 33-36. The shoulder joint will usually be locked, and the shoulder will appear squared off or flattened. The humeral head will protrude anteriorly underneath the

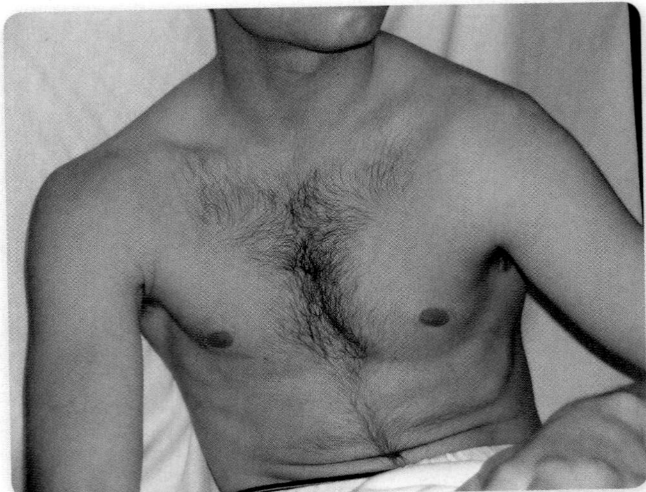

Figure 33-35 Most shoulder dislocations are anterior. Note the absence of the normal rounded appearance of the shoulder.

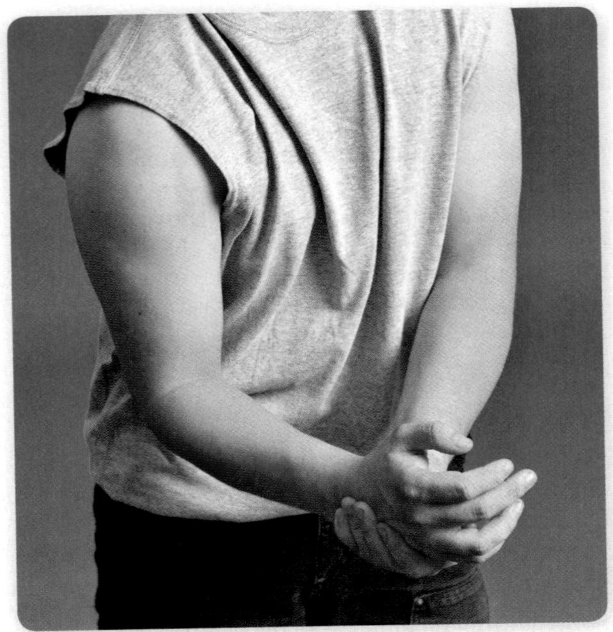

Figure 33-36 A patient with a dislocated shoulder will guard the shoulder, trying to protect it by holding the arm in a fixed position away from the chest wall.

pectoralis major on the anterior chest wall. As a result, the axillary nerve may be compressed, causing a numb patch on the outer aspect of the shoulder. Ensure you document this finding. Some patients may also report some numbness in the hand because of compromise of the nerves or the circulation.

Stabilizing an anterior shoulder dislocation is difficult because any attempt to bring in the arm toward the chest will produce pain. You must splint the joint in whatever position is most comfortable for the patient. If necessary,

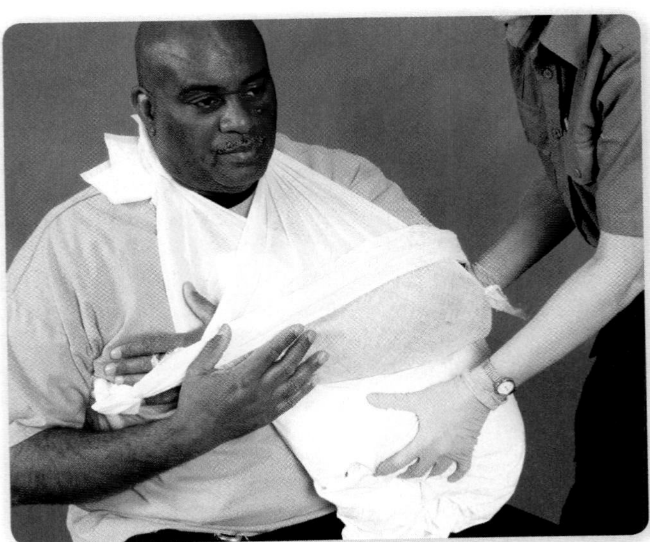

Figure 33-37 Splint the shoulder joint in a position of comfort, and place a pillow or towel between the arm and the chest wall to stabilize the arm, after which the elbow can be flexed to a 90° angle. Apply a sling; secure the arm to the chest with a swathe.

Words of Wisdom

When you are assessing a patient with a possible shoulder dislocation, position yourself behind the patient and compare the shoulders. The dislocated side is usually lower than the uninjured side.

place a pillow, rolled blankets, or rolled towels between the arm and chest to fill up the space between them **Figure 33-37**. Once the arm is stabilized in this way, the elbow can usually be flexed to a 90° angle without causing further pain. At this point, you can apply a sling to the forearm and wrist to support the weight of the arm. Finally, secure the arm in the sling to the pillow and chest with a swathe. Transport the patient in a sitting or semiseated position.

When a shoulder dislocates, it disrupts the supporting ligaments of the anterior aspect of the shoulder. Often these ligaments fail to heal properly, so the dislocation recurs. Each time a dislocation occurs, it may cause further neurovascular compromise and joint injury. In certain cases, surgical repair may be required. Some patients can reduce (set) their own dislocated shoulders. Generally, this occurs in patients who have had multiple shoulder dislocations in the past and are familiar with the maneuver necessary to achieve reduction. For first-time dislocations, this maneuver must typically be done in a hospital setting and only after radiographs have been obtained. The exception is for dislocations that occur in athletic activity where the event was witnessed by a physician and a physician is present to perform the reduction maneuver.

In addition, some wilderness EMS providers are trained in dislocation reduction maneuvers in order to facilitate allowing the patient to assist with his or her own extrication from the wilderness environment.

A shoulder will dislocate posteriorly instead of anteriorly about once in every 20 cases. Football players, especially linemen, are susceptible to this injury. Dislocations can sometimes be caused by violent seizure activity and these are also often posterior dislocations. The arm will often be locked in an adducted position (toward the midline), so it cannot be rotated. Reducing the dislocation usually requires medical supervision.

▶ Fracture of the Humerus

Fractures of the humerus may occur either proximally, in the midshaft, or distally, at the elbow. Fractures of the proximal humerus resulting from falls are common among older adults. Fractures of the midshaft occur more often in young patients, usually as the result of high-energy injury.

Examine the extremity to reveal any significant swelling, ecchymosis, gross instability of the region, and crepitus. If the force that caused the injury is severe enough, the nerves and blood vessels in the upper arm may also be damaged. Of particular concern is the radial nerve, which may be injured by the force itself or become entrapped within the fracture site. The classic sign of a radial nerve injury is wrist drop.

If the fracture is angulated, longitudinal traction may be applied to correct the deformity, but this effort should be halted if the patient's pain is too severe or if neurovascular status worsens. Once the extremity is in the desired position, apply a rigid splint that extends from the axilla to the elbow. Next, apply a sling and swathe to stabilize the arm to the chest wall Figure 33-38, and place cold packs over the fracture site to decrease the patient's pain and swelling. Note: Compartment syndrome can develop in the forearm in children with these fractures.

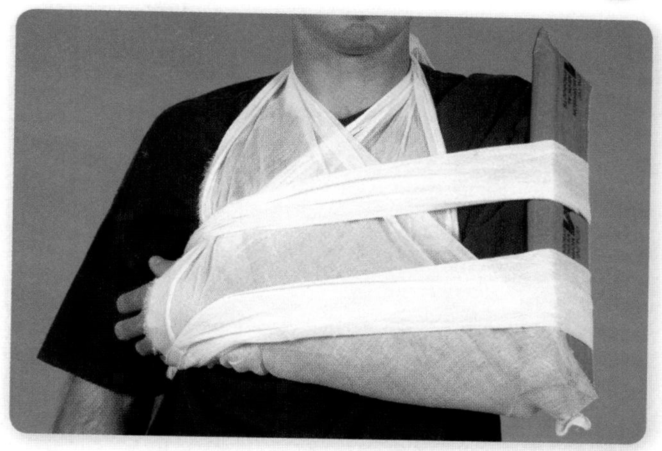

Figure 33-38 Splint a humeral shaft fracture with a sling and swathe supplemented by a padded board splint on the lateral aspect of the arm.

▶ Elbow Injuries

Fractures and dislocations often occur around the elbow, and the different types of injuries are difficult to distinguish without radiographs Table 33-4. However, they all produce similar limb deformities and require the same

Table 33-4 Types of Elbow Injuries

Type of Injury	Characteristics
Fracture of distal humerus (supracondylar or intercondylar fracture)	▪ Fracture fragments may rotate significantly, producing deformity and causing injuries to nearby vessels and nerves. ▪ Swelling occurs rapidly and is often severe. ▪ Significant potential for vessel or nerve injury.
Elbow dislocation	▪ Typically occurs in athletes; rare in young children. ▪ Ulna and radius are most often displaced posteriorly, which makes the olecranon process of the ulna much more prominent Figure 33-39. ▪ Joint is usually locked, making any attempt at motion extremely painful.
Elbow joint sprain	▪ Rare; usually diagnosed by stress radiographs. ▪ The real problem may be a hard-to-detect fracture.
Fracture of the olecranon process of the ulna	▪ Usually the result of a direct blow. ▪ Often characterized by lacerations and abrasions. ▪ Patient may be unable to extend the elbow.
Fracture of the radial head	▪ Results from a fall on an outstretched arm or a direct blow to the lateral aspect of the elbow. ▪ Attempts to rotate the elbow and wrist cause severe discomfort.

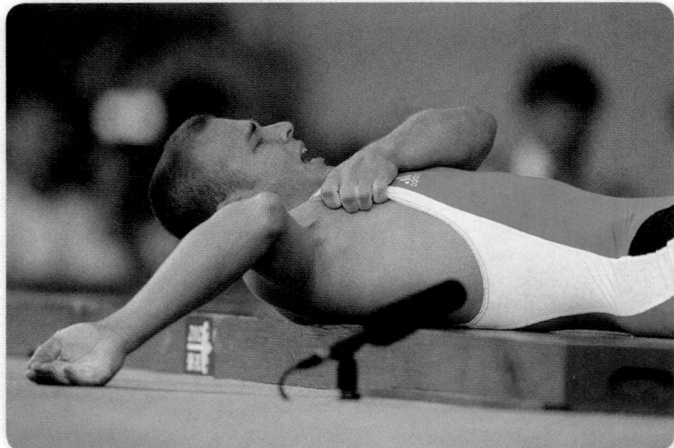

Figure 33-39 Posterior dislocation of the elbow makes the olecranon process of the ulna much more prominent.

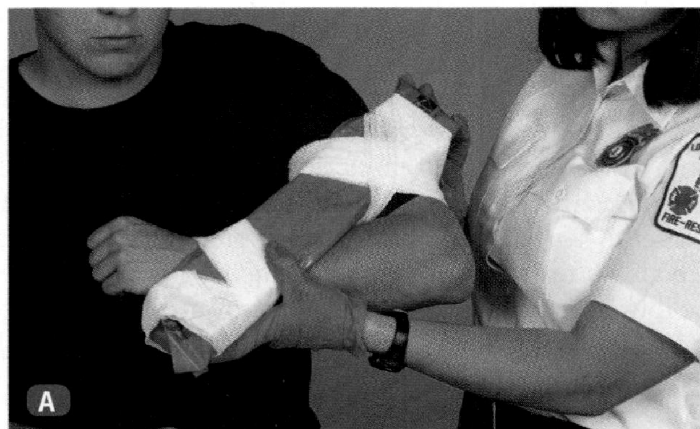

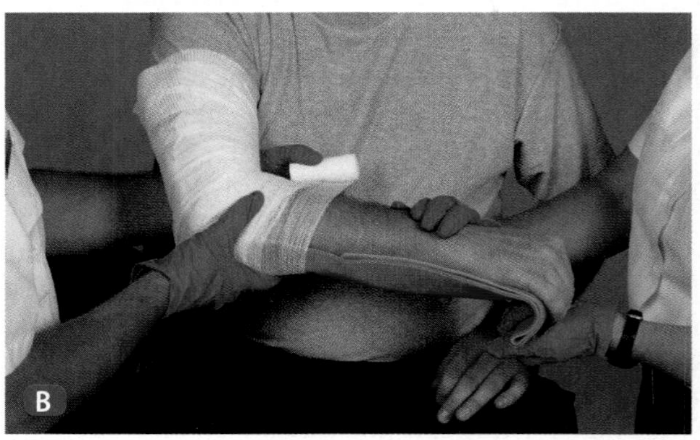

Figure 33-40 A. Two padded board splints provide adequate stabilization for an injured elbow. **B.** A structural aluminum malleable splint can be molded to the shape of the limb so you can splint it in the position in which it was found.

emergency medical care. Injuries to nerves and blood vessels are quite common in this region. Such injuries can be caused or worsened by inappropriate emergency medical care, particularly by excessive manipulation of the injured joint.

Care of Elbow Injuries

Like any joint injury, elbow injuries are serious and require careful management. Always assess distal neurovascular functions periodically in patients with elbow injuries. If you find strong pulses and good capillary refill, splint the elbow in the position in which you found it, adding a wrist sling if this seems helpful. Two padded board splints, applied to each side of the limb and secured with soft roller bandages, usually are enough to stabilize the arm Figure 33-40A. Ensure the board extends from the shoulder joint to the wrist joint, stabilizing the entire bone above and below the injured joint. Alternatively, you can mold a padded wire ladder splint or a SAM splint to the shape of the limb Figure 33-40B. If necessary, you may add further support to the limb with a pillow.

A cold, pale hand or a weak or absent pulse and poor capillary refill indicate the blood vessels have likely been injured. Further care of this patient must be dictated by a physician. Consult medical direction immediately. If you are within 15 minutes of the hospital, splint the limb in the position in which you found it and provide prompt transport. Otherwise, consult medical direction to direct you in trying to realign the limb to improve circulation in the hand.

If the limb is pulseless and significantly deformed at the elbow, then apply gentle manual traction in line with the long axis of the limb to decrease the deformity. This maneuver may restore the pulse. Excessive manipulation will only worsen the vascular problem. If no pulse returns after one attempt, splint the limb in the most comfortable position for the patient. If the pulse is restored by gentle realignment, splint the limb in whatever position allows the strongest pulse. Provide prompt transport for all patients with impaired distal circulation.

Assume any deformity in proximity to a joint in children younger than 16 years is a growth plate injury. The child should be transported and treated appropriately.

Special Populations

Epiphyseal (growth) plate injuries in children are common, especially around the wrist, elbow, knee, and ankle. Injuries tend to occur through these cartilaginous growth centers because they are inherently weaker than the surrounding bone. Because longitudinal growth of the limb is dependent on the function of the growth plate, it is extremely important to recognize the possibility of growth plate injuries, stabilize the injured limb, and transport the patient in a timely manner to an appropriate center with pediatric orthopaedic coverage. Proper functioning of the injured growth plate throughout the remainder of skeletal growth may depend on timely anatomic reduction of the fracture and close follow-up by an orthopaedic surgeon.

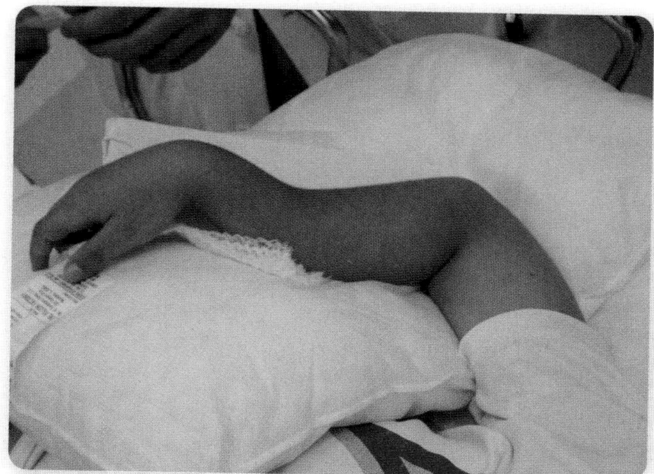

Figure 33-41 Fractures of the forearm often occur in children as a result of a fall on an outstretched hand.

▶ Fractures of the Forearm

Fractures of the shaft of the radius and ulna are common in people of all age groups, but are seen most often in children and older adults. Usually, both bones break at the same time when the injury is the result of a fall on an outstretched hand Figure 33-41. An isolated fracture of the shaft of the ulna may occur as the result of a direct blow to it—an injury known as a nightstick fracture.

Fractures of the distal radius, which are especially common in older adult patients with osteoporosis, are often known as Colles fractures. The term *silver fork deformity* is used to describe the distinctive appearance of the patient's arm Figure 33-42. In children, this fracture may occur through the growth plate Figure 33-43 and can sometimes have long-term consequences.

To stabilize fractures of the forearm or wrist, you can use a padded board, air, vacuum, or pillow splint. If the shaft of the bone has been fractured, ensure you include the elbow joint in the splint. Splinting of the elbow joint is not essential with fractures near the wrist; however, the patient will be more comfortable if you add a sling or pillow for more support. If possible, elevate the injured extremity above the heart to help alleviate swelling.

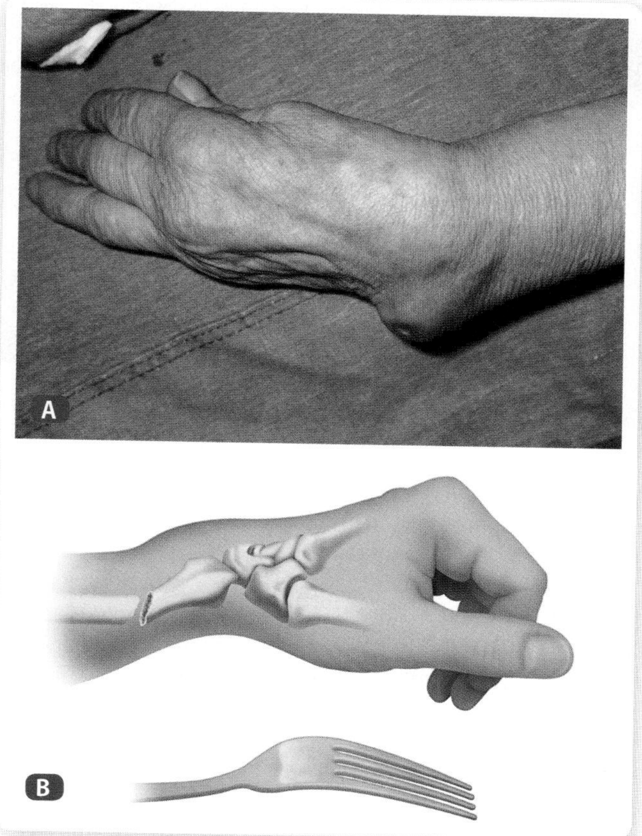

Figure 33-42 A. Fractures of the distal radius produce a characteristic silver fork deformity. **B.** An artist's illustration.

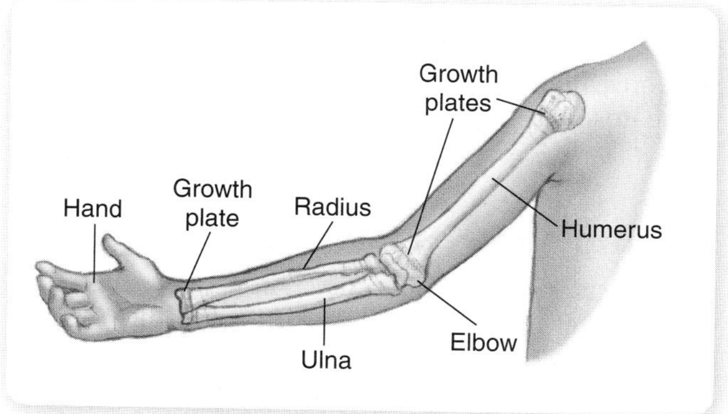

Figure 33-43 The growth plates at the ends of children's bones are easily fractured.

▶ Injuries of the Wrist and Hand

Injuries of the wrist, ranging from dislocations to sprains, must be confirmed by radiographs. Dislocations are usually associated with a fracture, resulting in a fracture-dislocation. Another common wrist injury is the isolated, nondisplaced fracture of a carpal bone, especially the scaphoid. Any questionable wrist sprain must be splinted and evaluated in the ED or an orthopaedic surgeon's office.

Hand injuries vary widely, and some have potentially serious consequences. Dislocations, fractures, lacerations, burns, and amputations occur in industrial, recreational, and home accidents. Because the fingers and hands are required to function in such intricate ways, any injury that is not treated properly may result in permanent disability and deformity. For this reason, all injuries to the hand, including simple lacerations, must be evaluated promptly by a physician. Do not attempt to "pop" a dislocated finger joint back into place.

Always take any amputated parts to the hospital with the patient. Ensure you wrap the amputated part in a dry or moist sterile dressing, depending on your local protocol, and place it in a dry plastic bag. Put the bag in

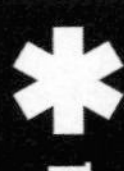

NR Skill

Skill Drill 33-9 Splinting the Hand and Wrist

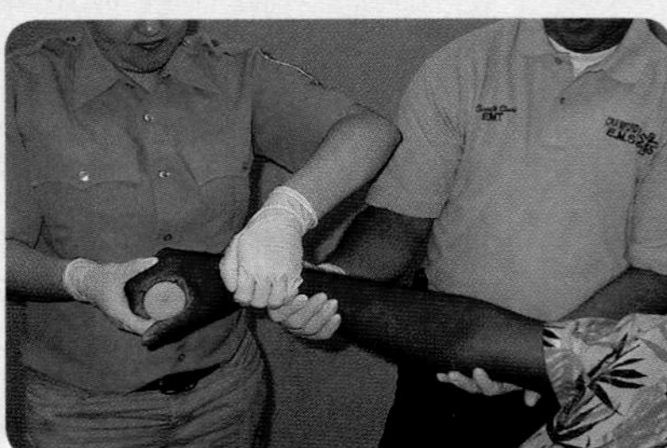

Step 1 Take standard precautions and cover open wounds with a dry, sterile dressing. Assess pulse and motor and sensory function. Support the injured limb, and move the hand into the position of function. Place a soft roller bandage in the palm of the patient's injured hand.

Step 2 Apply a padded board splint on the palmar side of the wrist, leaving the fingers exposed.

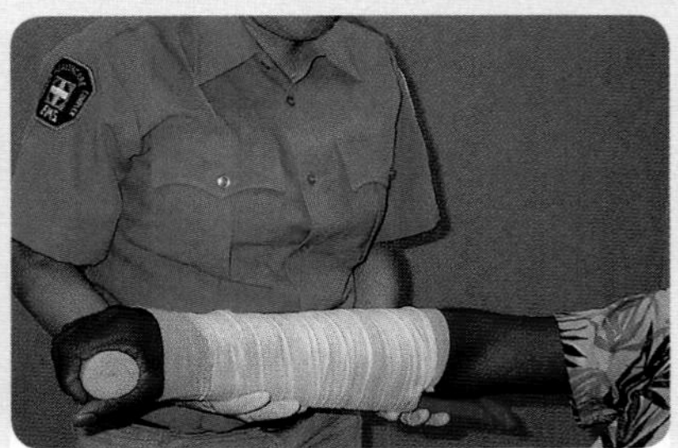

Step 3 Secure the entire length of the splint with a soft roller bandage. Apply a sling and swathe or prop the splinted hand and wrist on a pillow or on the patient's chest during transport.

a cooled container; *do not* soak the part in water or allow it to freeze.

A bulky forearm dressing makes an effective splint for any hand or wrist injury. Once the injury is splinted, apply a sling and swathe or prop the splinted hand and wrist on a pillow or on the patient's chest during transport to the hospital. To splint the hand and wrist, follow the steps in Skill Drill 33-9.

▶ Fractures of the Pelvis

Pelvic fractures are relatively uncommon injuries, accounting for fewer than 3% of all fractures.[7] Despite the low incidence, these injuries are responsible for a significant number of deaths in blunt trauma patients. The risk of death following a pelvic fracture ranges from 19% to 50% in older adult patients,[8] and from 3% to 20% overall,[7] depending on the severity of the injury; when the fracture is open, the mortality rate rises to as high as 50%.[9] Usually, death after a pelvic fracture results from massive hemorrhage caused by damage to the arteries and veins of the pelvis.

Disruptions of the pelvic ring occur secondary to high-energy trauma such as crush injuries, motorcycle crashes, and falls from a significant height. Many structures within the pelvis are at risk for injury when it is fractured—the bladder, urethra, rectum, vagina, and sacral nerve plexus. The blood vessels that are most prone to damage are the veins within the pelvis, but there may be damage to the internal or external iliac and arteries in the lumbar region. The nerves at greatest risk of injury are those in the lumbar and sacral regions and the sciatic and femoral nerves. In addition, if a woman who is pregnant experiences a pelvic fracture, her fetus may be injured.

Fractures of the pelvis may be accompanied by a life-threatening loss of blood from the laceration of blood vessels affixed to the pelvis at certain key points. Up to several liters of blood may drain into the pelvic space and the **retroperitoneal space**, which lies between the abdominal cavity and the posterior abdominal wall. The result is significant hypotension, shock, and sometimes death. Therefore, take immediate steps to treat shock, even if there is only minimal swelling. Often, there are no visible signs of bleeding with pelvic fracture until severe blood loss has occurred. Be prepared to resuscitate the patient rapidly if this becomes necessary.

Patients with pelvic ring disruptions who have a stable injury, such as a minimal lateral compression injury, may report pain in the pelvis and difficulty bearing weight. Patients with a more severe injury may show evidence of profound shock, gross pelvic instability, and diffuse pelvic and lower abdominal pain. There may also be bruising or lacerations in the perineum, scrotum, groin, suprapubic region, and flank, and hematuria (blood in the urine) or blood coming from the meatus of the penis, vagina, or rectum.

Specific types of fractures are discussed in the next sections.

Lateral Compression Pelvic Ring Disruptions

Lateral compression injuries result from an impact on the side of the body (such as being struck by a motor vehicle from the side or falling from a significant height and landing on one side of the body). The side of the pelvis that sustains the impact becomes internally rotated around the sacrum, and the actual volume within the pelvis decreases **Figure 33-44**. Although this injury does not commonly cause massive hemorrhage into the pelvis, it is often associated with injuries in other regions of the body.

Anterior–Posterior Compression Pelvic Ring Disruptions

Anterior–posterior compression pelvic ring disruptions may occur following a head-on MVC, motorcycle crash, fall, or when a pedestrian is struck head-on by a motor vehicle. The force of the impact compresses the pelvis in the anterior-to-posterior direction, causing the pubic symphysis and posterior supporting ligaments to be disrupted and tear apart. The pelvis then spreads apart and opens like a book—hence the name **open book pelvic fracture**. Such an injury has the potential for massive blood loss because the volume of the pelvis is greatly increased.

Vertical Shear

Vertical shear injuries occur when a major force is applied to the pelvis from above or below, such as when a person falls from a significant height and lands on the feet. On landing, the force is transmitted through the legs to the pelvis, leading to the complete displacement of one or both sides of the pelvis toward the head. Thus, this kind of injury has anterior and posterior components. The anterior component involves a fracture of the rami or disruption of the symphysis pubis. The posterior component involves a fracture of the ilium or sacrum or a disruption of the sacroiliac joint. The patient is likely to have significant shortening of the limb on the affected side and is at risk for massive hemorrhage into the pelvis.

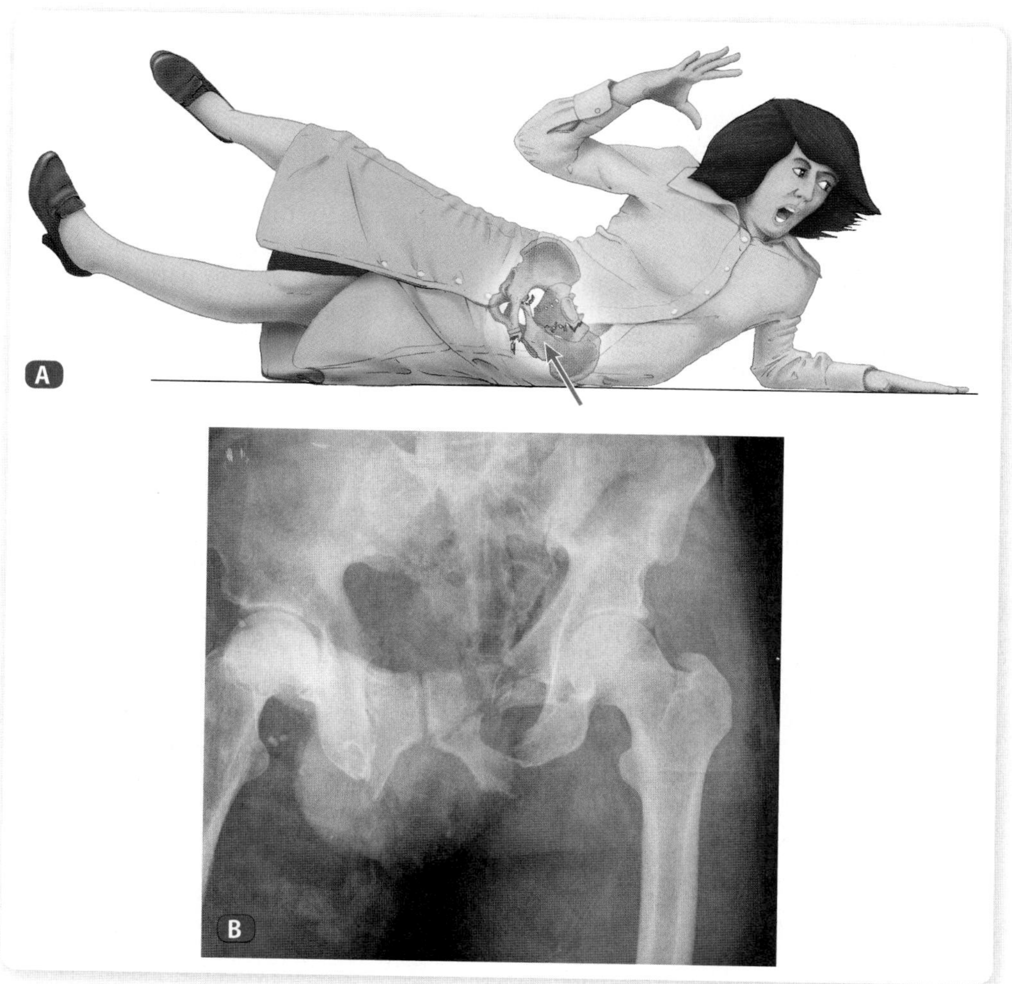

Figure 33-44 A. A lateral compression injury to the pelvis. **B.** A radiograph of a lateral compression injury.

Straddle Fracture

A **straddle fracture** occurs after a fall when a person lands in the region of the perineum and sustains bilateral fractures of the inferior and superior rami. This injury does not interfere with weight bearing, but it does carry a risk because of its associated complications, particularly those of the lower genitourinary system.

Open Pelvic Fractures

Open pelvic fractures are life-threatening injuries. Such an injury is defined by the presence of a laceration of the skin in the pelvic region, vagina, or rectum. This uncommon fracture is caused by a high-velocity injury with subsequent massive hemorrhage. Even small amounts of blood found during a vaginal or rectal exam should raise your suspicion for an open fracture.

Special Populations

A hip fracture in an older adult patient can be a debilitating and life-altering injury. In many cases, these injuries occur in the home after slipping on a throw rug, tripping over an object that extends into the walkway, or stumbling because of poor lighting. To help prevent this injury and other fall-related problems, you should point out any safety hazards in the home to the patient or a family member. It takes only a minute, and most patients and families appreciate the advice.

Care of Pelvic Fractures

You should suspect a fracture of the pelvis in any patient who has sustained a high-velocity injury and experiences discomfort in the lower back or abdomen. Because large muscle and other soft tissues cover the area, deformity or swelling may be difficult to see. The most reliable sign of fracture of the pelvis is simple tenderness on firm compression and palpation. Firm compression on the two iliac crests will produce pain at a fracture site in the pelvic ring. Assess for tenderness by taking the following steps Figure 33-45:

1. Place the palms of your hands over the lateral aspect of each iliac crest, and apply firm but gentle inward pressure on the pelvic ring.
2. With the patient lying supine, place a palm over the anterior aspect of each iliac crest, and apply firm downward pressure.
3. Use the palm of your hand to firmly but gently palpate the pubic symphysis, the firm cartilaginous joint between the two pubic bones. This area will be tender if there is injury to the anterior portion of the pelvic ring.

Once you have identified significant tenderness or any instability, further pressure on the pelvis for the purposes of examination is contraindicated as it could potentially result in worsening hemorrhage or injury by displacing fracture fragments or blood clots that have formed over bleeding veins or arteries. Do not manipulate this area during reassessments.

If there has been injury to the bladder or the urethra, the patient will have lower abdominal tenderness and may have evidence of **hematuria** (blood in the urine) or blood at the urethral opening.

Perform a primary survey, and carefully monitor the general condition of any patient you suspect has a pelvic fracture, because he or she is at high risk for hypovolemic shock.

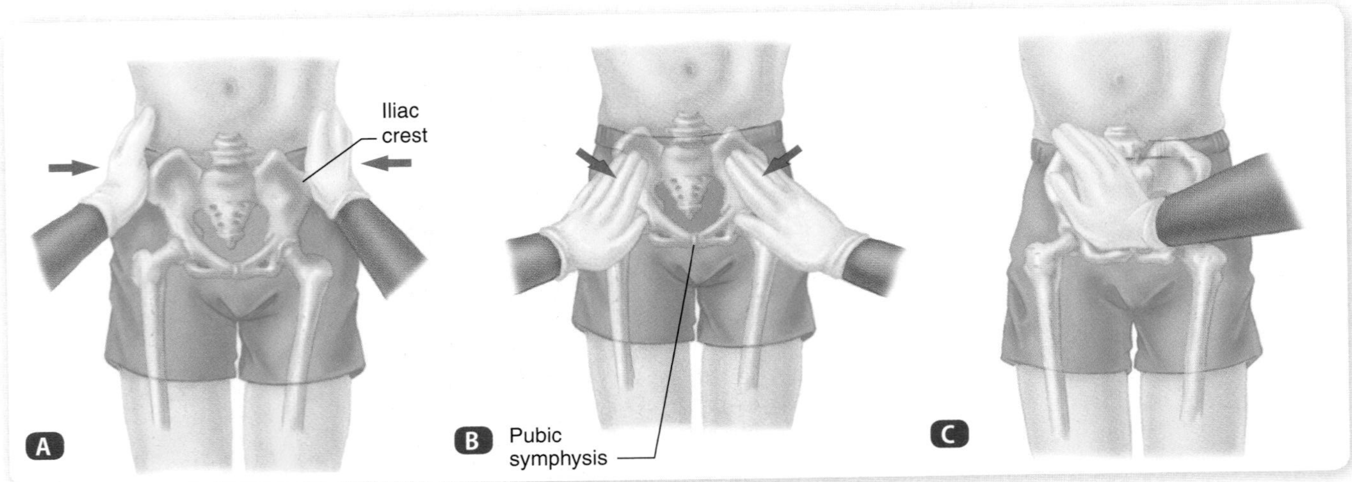

Figure 33-45 A. To assess for tenderness in the pelvic region, place your hands over the lateral aspect of each iliac crest, and gently compress the pelvis. **B.** With the patient in a supine position, place your palms over the anterior aspect of each iliac crest, and apply firm but gentle downward pressure. **C.** Palpate the pubic symphysis with the palm of your hand.

Treatment should include careful monitoring of the ABCs, spinal immobilization, and IV access with at least one (if not two) large-bore catheter. Managing a pelvic injury involves reducing the amount of bleeding and decreasing the degree of instability. It is often appropriate to seek medical direction to manage these patients, especially to determine how to best stabilize the pelvis. Methods used to accomplish this stabilization may include application of a PASG or pelvic binder or simply tying a sheet around the pelvis at the level of the femoral trochanters and pubic symphysis. This reduces the potential space within the pelvis, which may allow for tamponade of the bleeding vessels. Once immobilized on a long backboard, the patient should be rapidly transported to a trauma center, and IV fluid should be administered to maintain adequate tissue perfusion (radial pulses) yet avoid hypertension, which may increase internal hemorrhage.

Words of Wisdom

Consider ways to avoid log rolling a patient with pelvic pain. If the pain is on one side, log roll to the other side to avoid discomfort. If the pain is bilateral and time allows, use a scoop stretcher to move the patient onto a board, or simply use the scoop stretcher to immobilize the patient. Try to avoid causing unnecessary discomfort to the patient by paying attention to his or her complaints of pain and your findings in the secondary survey.

Dislocation of the Hip

The hip joint is a very stable ball-and-socket joint that is dislocated only after significant injury. Almost all dislocations of the hip are posterior; that is, the femoral head is displaced posteriorly to lie in the muscles of the buttock. Posterior dislocation of the hip most commonly occurs during MVCs in which the knee meets with a direct force, such as the dashboard, and the entire femur is driven posteriorly, dislocating the joint Figure 33-46. Thus, suspect a hip dislocation in any patient who has been in an MVC and has a contusion, laceration, or obvious fracture in the knee region. Rarely does the femoral head dislocate anteriorly; in this circumstance, the legs are suddenly and forcibly spread wide apart and locked in this position.

Posterior dislocation of the hip is frequently complicated by injury to the sciatic nerve, which is located directly behind the hip joint. The **sciatic nerve** is the most important nerve in the lower extremity; it controls the activity of muscles in the thigh and below the knee, as well as sensation in the entire leg and foot. When the head of the femur is forced out of the hip socket, it may compress or stretch the sciatic nerve, leading to partial or complete paralysis of the

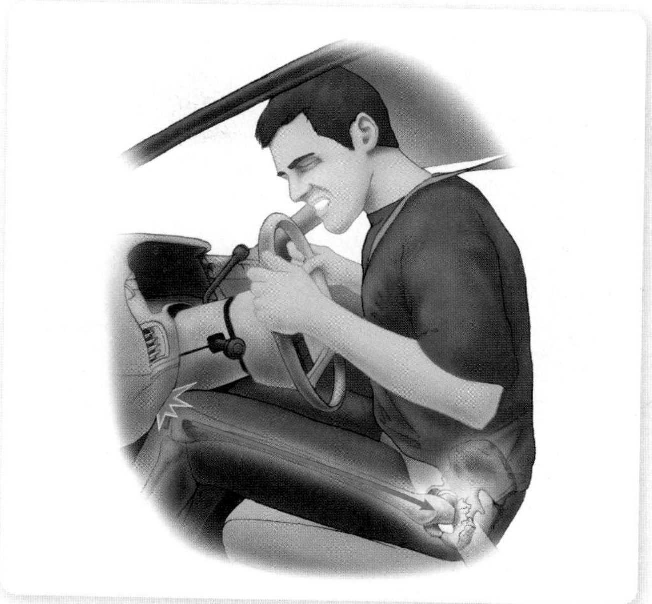

Figure 33-46 Posterior dislocation of the hip can occur as a result of the knee hitting the dashboard in a motor vehicle crash. The impact drives the femur posteriorly (see arrow), dislocating the joint.

nerve. The result is decreased sensation in the leg and foot and, frequently, weakness in the foot muscles. Generally, only the dorsiflexors—the muscles that raise the toes or foot—are involved, causing the "foot drop" that is characteristic of damage to the portion of the sciatic nerve that controls the muscles in the anterior and lateral compartments of the leg, particularly those that control ankle dorsiflexion.

Patients with a posterior dislocation of the hip typically lie with the hip joint flexed (the knee joint drawn up toward the chest) and the thigh rotated inward toward the midline of the body over the top of the opposite thigh Figure 33-47A. With the less common anterior dislocation, the limb is in the opposite position, extended straight out, rotated, and pointing away from the midline of the body.

Dislocation of the hip is associated with distinctive signs. The patient will have severe pain in the hip and will strongly resist any attempt to move the joint. The lateral and posterior aspects of the hip region will be tender on palpation. With some people who are thin, you can palpate the femoral head deep within the muscles of the buttock. Check for a sciatic nerve injury by carefully assessing sensation and motor function in the lower extremity. Occasionally, sciatic nerve function will be normal at first and then slowly diminish.

As with any other extremity injury, do not attempt to reduce the dislocated hip in the field. Splint the dislocation in the position of the deformity and place the

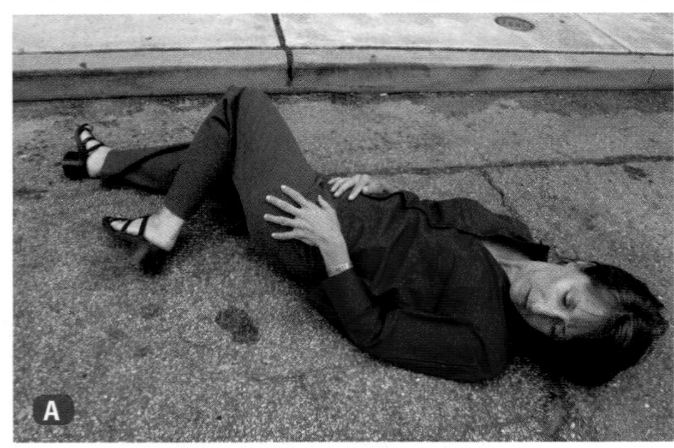

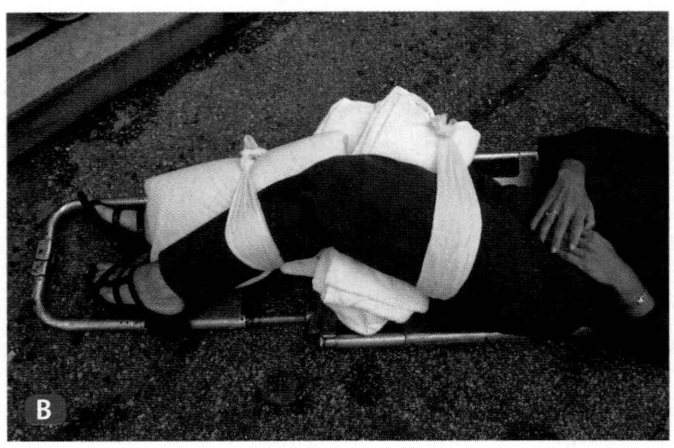

Figure 33-47 A. The usual position of a patient with a posterior dislocation of the hip. The hip joint is flexed, and the thigh is rotated inward and adducted across the midline of the body. **B.** Support the affected limb with pillows and blankets, particularly under the flexed knee. Secure the entire limb to a scoop stretcher or long backboard with long straps to prevent movement during transport.

patient supine on a scoop stretcher or long backboard. Support the affected limb with pillows and rolled blankets, particularly under the flexed knee (Figure 33-47B). Then secure the entire limb to the backboard with long straps so the hip region will not move. Provide prompt transport.

Words of Wisdom

When you find a knee injury in the victim of a motor vehicle crash, especially one in the front seat, look for posterior dislocation of the hip.

YOU are the Provider — PART 4

Approximately 35 minutes into your transport, the patient begins to report searing pain to his femoral area and numbness and tingling in his left foot. You examine the area and find that the area around his femur is very firm, and he has decreased sensation in his left foot. You know this is an important finding, so you call the trauma center and report your findings. The physician on call states it sounds as if compartment syndrome may be developing. After discussing care with the physician on call, your partner informs you that you are 8 minutes from the hospital and you begin to prepare the patient for removal from the ambulance. On arrival at the hospital, you wheel the patient into the trauma bay and turn over his care to the awaiting trauma surgeon.

Recording Time: 45 Minutes	
Respirations	22 breaths/min, clear
Pulse	127 beats/min
Skin	Cool, pale, and clammy
Blood pressure	96/44 mm Hg
Oxygen saturation (Spo_2)	98% on 15 L/min
Pupils	PERRLA

7. Which signs and symptoms may suggest compartment syndrome?
8. What should your treatment of compartment syndrome include?

▶ Fractures of the Proximal Femur

Fractures of the proximal (upper) end of the femur are among the most common fractures, especially in older adults. Although they are usually called hip fractures, they rarely involve the hip joint. Instead, the break goes through the neck of the femur, the intertrochanteric (middle) region, or across the proximal shaft of the femur (subtrochanteric fractures). Although these three fracture types occur most often in older adult patients, particularly patients with osteoporosis, they may also be seen as a result of high-energy injuries in young patients.

Patients with displaced fractures of the proximal femur display a characteristic deformity. They lie with the leg externally rotated, and the injured leg is usually shorter than the opposite, uninjured limb Figure 33-48A. When the fracture is not displaced, this deformity is not present. With any kind of hip fracture, patients typically are unable to walk or move the leg because of pain in the hip region or in the groin or inner aspect of the thigh. The hip region is usually tender on palpation, and gentle rolling of the leg will cause pain but will not do further damage. On occasion, the pain is referred to the knee, and it is not uncommon for an older adult patient with a hip fracture to complain of knee pain after a fall.

You should assess the pelvis for any soft-tissue injury and bandage appropriately. In addition, assess pulses and motor and sensory functions, looking for signs of vascular and nerve damage. Once you complete your assessment, splint the lower extremity of an older adult patient who has fallen and reports pain in the hip or the knee, even if there is no deformity, and then transport the patient to the ED.

The age of the patient and the severity of the injury will dictate how you splint the fracture. A geriatric patient with an isolated hip fracture does not require a traction splint. You can effectively immobilize such a fracture by placing the patient on a long backboard or scoop stretcher, using pillows or rolled blankets to support the injured limb in the deformed position. Then secure the injured limb carefully to the uninjured limb or to the backboard Figure 33-48B.

All patients with hip fractures may have significant blood loss. Therefore, administer oxygen as needed and frequently monitor vital signs, being alert for signs of shock. Initiate IV therapy and give a 20-mL/kg bolus of an isotonic crystalloid solution, repeating as necessary to maintain radial pulses.

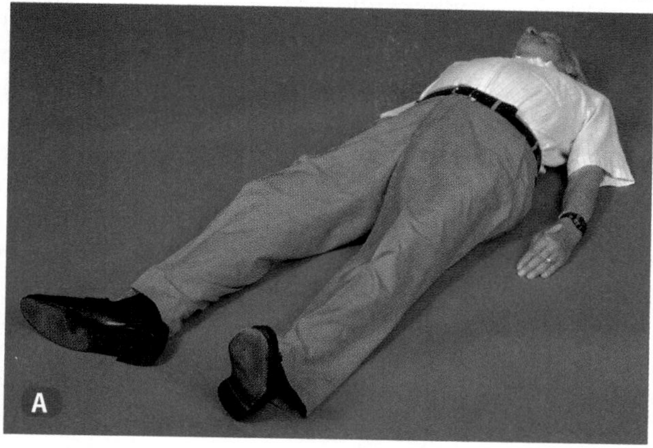

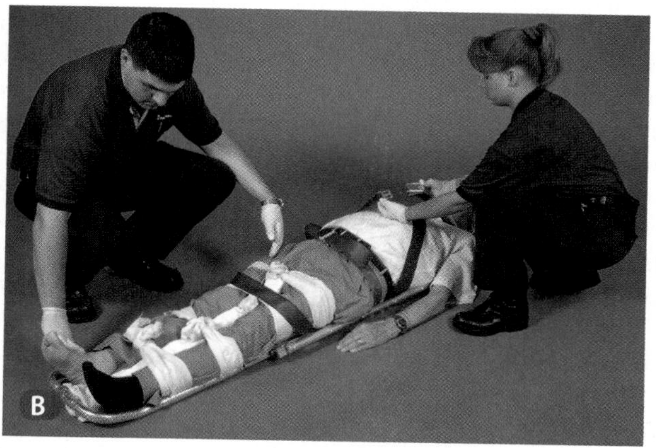

Figure 33-48 A. A patient with a fracture of the proximal femur will typically lie still with the extremity rotated, making the injured leg appear shorter than the other leg. **B.** Splint the injured leg to the uninjured leg or to the backboard, and secure the patient on a scoop stretcher or long backboard.

▶ Femoral Shaft Fractures

Fractures of the femur can occur in any part of the shaft, from the hip region to the femoral condyles just above the knee joint. Following a fracture, the quadriceps muscles begin to spasm and often produce significant deformity of the limb, with severe angulation or external rotation at the fracture site. Usually the limb shortens significantly as well. Fractures of the femoral shaft are occasionally open, and fragments of bone may protrude through the skin. As with any other open fracture, do not attempt to push the bones back into the skin.

Patients often experience significant blood loss (perhaps 500 to 1,500 mL) at the fracture site. In addition, damage to the neurovascular structures of the thigh is possible. Continue to watch for the onset of hypovolemic shock. Provide immediate transport in this situation.

Cover any wound with a dry, sterile dressing. If the foot or leg below the level of the fracture shows signs of impaired circulation (is pale, cold, or pulseless), apply gentle longitudinal traction to the deformed limb in line with the long axis of the limb. Gradually turn the leg from the deformed position to restore the limb's overall alignment. Often, this action restores or improves circulation to the foot. If it does not, the patient may have sustained a serious vascular injury and needs prompt medical attention.

Managing femoral shaft fractures includes monitoring for evidence of shock, full spinal immobilization, and establishing vascular access. Place the injured extremity in a traction splint or use a PASG to achieve stability and hemorrhage control. Because these injuries may be extremely painful, consider calling for paramedic backup to administer pain medication if it will not delay transport to a trauma center.

▶ Knee Injuries

The knee is very vulnerable to injury; therefore, many different types of injuries occur in this region. Ligament injuries, for example, range from mild sprains to complete dislocation of the joint. The patella can also dislocate. In addition, all the bony elements of the knee (distal femur, upper tibia, and patella) can fracture. Assess the patient's knee to reveal any significant pain in the knee, decreased range of motion, pain with movement and weight bearing, ecchymosis, swelling, and, in the case of displaced fractures, deformity.

Injuries of Knee Ligaments

The knee is especially susceptible to ligament injuries, which occur when abnormal bending or twisting forces are applied to this joint. Such injuries are often seen in both recreational and competitive athletes. The ligaments on the medial side of the knee are the ones that are most frequently injured, typically when the foot is fixed to the ground and a heavy object strikes the lateral aspect of the knee, such as when a football player is clipped or tackled from the side.

Dislocation of the Knee

A dislocated knee is a true emergency that may threaten the limb. When the knee is dislocated, the ligaments that provide support to it may be damaged or torn. When this happens, the proximal end of the tibia is completely displaced from its juncture with the lower end of the femur, usually producing a significant deformity. Although substantial ligament damage always occurs with a knee dislocation, the more urgent injury is to the popliteal artery, which is often lacerated or compressed by the displaced tibia. When gross deformity, severe pain, and an inability to move the joint cause you to suspect a dislocation of the knee, always check the distal circulation carefully before taking any other step. If the distal pulses are absent, contact medical direction immediately for further stabilization instructions.

The direction of dislocation refers to the position of the tibia with respect to the femur. Anterior knee dislocations, which result from extreme hyperextension of the knee, are the most common, occurring in almost half of all cases. Commonly, the anterior and posterior ligaments are damaged, but there is also a high risk of injury to the popliteal artery.

In posterior dislocations, a direct blow to the knee forces the tibia to shift posteriorly. There is also the possibility of damage to the ligaments. These dislocations are associated with the highest degree of risk to the popliteal artery.

Medial dislocations result from a direct blow to the lateral part of the leg. Because the deforming force causes the medial aspect of the knee to stretch apart, there is a high likelihood of injury to the medial ligaments. When the force is applied from the medial direction, a lateral dislocation occurs and the lateral part of the knee is stretched apart, injuring the lateral ligament. Lateral and medial dislocations happen less commonly and are less likely to injure the popliteal artery.

Patients with a knee dislocation will typically report pain in the knee and report that the knee "gave out." If the knee did not spontaneously reduce, there may be evidence of significant deformity and decreased range of motion. Complications may include limb-threatening popliteal artery disruption, injuries to the nerves, and joint instability. Do not confuse this injury with a relatively minor patella dislocation.

If adequate distal pulses are present, splint the knee in the position in which you found it, and promptly transport the patient. Do not attempt to manipulate or straighten any severe knee injury if there are good distal pulses. If the limb is straight, then apply leg splints to both sides of the limb to immobilize it Figure 33-49A. If the knee is bent and the foot has a good pulse, then splint the joint in the bent position, using parallel padded board splints secured at the hip and ankle joint to provide a stable A-frame Figure 33-49B. Secure the limb to a backboard or stretcher with pillows and straps to eliminate any motion during transport.

On rare occasions, medical direction may instruct you to realign a deformed, pulseless limb to reduce compression of the popliteal artery, thereby restoring distal circulation. You should make only one attempt to do this. First, straighten the limb by applying gentle longitudinal traction in the axis of the limb. Maintain stability until the limb is fully splinted. If manipulation significantly increases the patient's pain, do not continue. As you straighten the leg, monitor the posterior tibial pulse to see whether it returns. Splint the limb in the position in which you feel the strongest pulse. If you are unable to restore the distal pulse, then splint the limb in the position that is most comfortable for the patient, and then provide prompt transport to the hospital. Notify medical direction of the status of the distal pulse so arrangements to treat the patient can be made in advance.

Fractures About the Knee

Fractures about the knee may occur at the distal end of the femur, at the proximal end of the tibia, or in the patella. Because of local tenderness and swelling, it is easy to confuse a nondisplaced or minimally displaced fracture about the knee with a ligament injury. Likewise, a displaced fracture about the knee may produce significant deformity that makes it look like a dislocation.

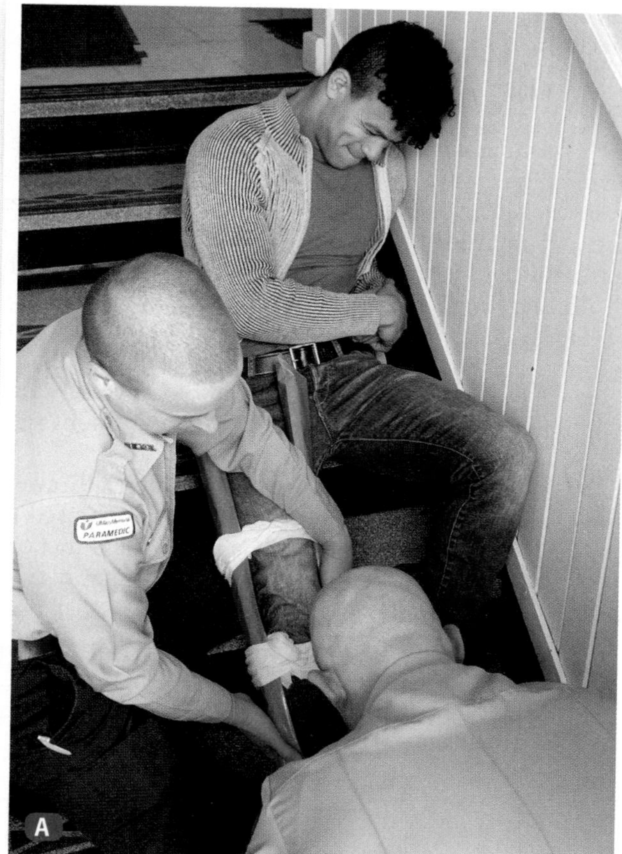

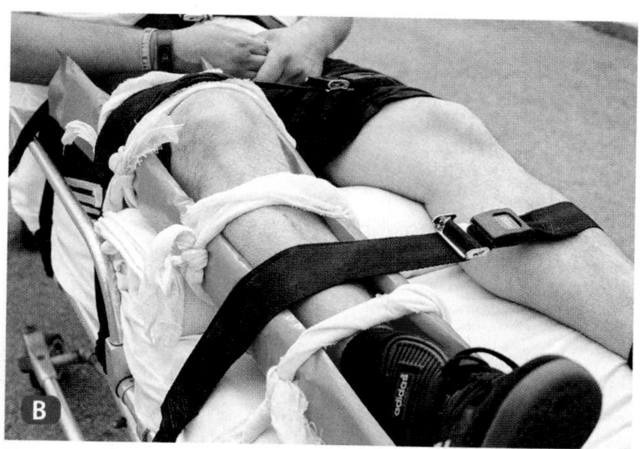

Figure 33-49 A. When the injured knee is straight, apply padded board splints extending from the hip to the ankle. **B.** If the knee is flexed and the foot has good pulses, apply padded board splints with the knee in the flexed position.

How you manage a knee fracture will depend on the position of the leg and the status of distal pulses. If the patient has a good distal pulse, then splint the extremity in the position in which it is found. If there is no distal pulse, then seek medical consultation to determine whether you should attempt manipulation before transportation. In all cases, elevate the leg to the heart level and apply cold packs. Frequent neurovascular checks are mandatory,

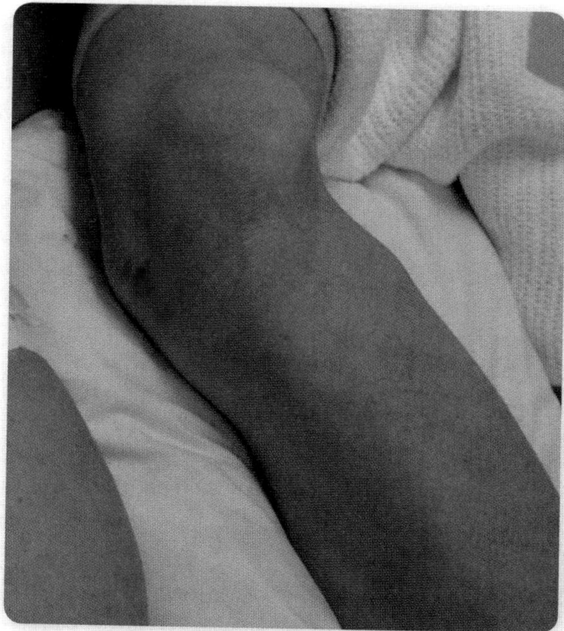

Figure 33-50 Usually, a dislocated patella displaces to the lateral side, and the knee is held in a partially flexed position.

given the high incidence of compartment syndrome and neurovascular injury in cases of knee fracture. Continue to monitor the distal neurovascular function en route to the hospital.

Dislocation of the Patella

A dislocated patella most commonly occurs in teenagers and young adults who are engaged in athletic activities. Some patients have recurrent dislocations of the patella. As with recurrent dislocation of the shoulder, minor twisting may be enough to produce the problem. The displacement of the patella produces a significant deformity in which the knee is held in a slightly flexed position and the patella is displaced to the lateral side of the knee **Figure 33-50**.

Splint the knee in the position in which you found it. Most often, this position involves the knee being flexed to a moderate degree. To immobilize the knee, apply padded board splints to the medial and lateral aspects of the joint, extending from the hip to the ankle. Use pillows to support the limb on the stretcher.

Occasionally, as you apply the splint, the patella will spontaneously return to its normal position. When this occurs, stabilize the limb as you would for any knee injury, in a padded long leg splint. The patient still needs to be transported to the ED. Report the spontaneous reduction as soon as you arrive at the hospital so the medical staff is aware of the severity of the injury.

▶ Injuries of the Tibia and Fibula

The tibia (shinbone) is the larger of the two leg bones that are responsible for supporting the major weight-bearing surface of the knee and ankle; the fibula is the smaller of them. Fractures of the shaft of the tibia or the fibula may occur at any place between the knee joint and the ankle joint. Usually both bones fracture at the same time Figure 33-51. Even a single fracture may result in severe deformity, with significant angulation or rotation. Because the tibia is located just beneath the skin, open fractures of this bone are common Figure 33-52.

Fractures of the tibia and fibula should be stabilized with a padded, rigid long leg splint or an air splint that extends from the foot to the upper thigh. Once splinted, the affected leg should be secured to the opposite leg. As with most other fractures of the shaft of long bones, you should correct a severe deformity before splinting by applying gentle longitudinal traction. The goal here is to restore a position that will take a standard splint; it is not necessary to replace the fracture fragments in their anatomic position.

Fractures of the tibia and fibula are sometimes associated with vascular injury as a result of the distorted position of the limb following injury. Realigning the limb may restore adequate blood supply to the foot. If it does not, transport the patient promptly and notify medical direction while you are en route.

Ankle Injuries

Ankle fractures usually result from sudden, forceful movements of the foot that damage the malleoli and sometimes produce dislocation (called a fracture-dislocation). In other cases, an axial load is transmitted through the foot and causes the talus (the bone of the foot that articulates with the tibia) to impact the distal tibia, leading to a fracture.

Signs and symptoms of an ankle fracture include pain, deformity, and swelling Figure 33-53. Ankle fractures may lead to damage of the nerves and blood vessels that supply the foot, the development of compartment syndrome, and chronic ankle pain and arthritis.

Stabilize ankle fractures using a commercially available splint or a pillow splint. Leave the toes exposed to allow for frequent checks of distal neurovascular function. Elevate the extremity to the heart level, and apply cold packs to reduce swelling Figure 33-54.

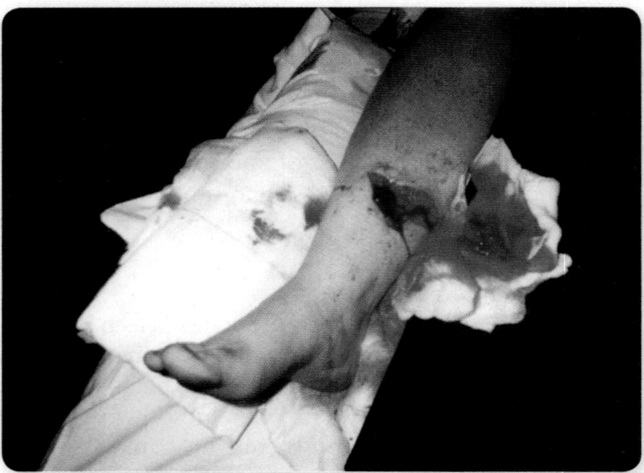

Figure 33-51 Open tibia and fibula fracture.

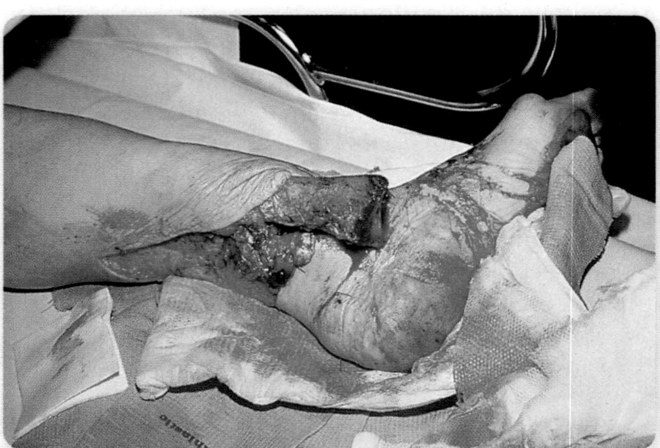

Figure 33-52 Because the tibia is so close to the skin, open fractures are common.

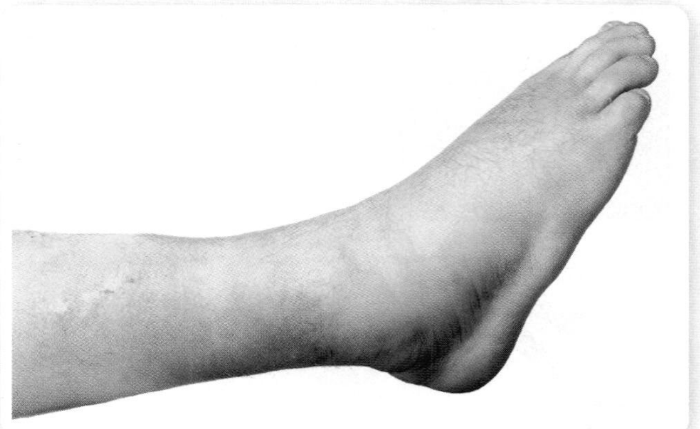

Figure 33-53 Swelling about the ankle is characteristic of both sprains and fractures.

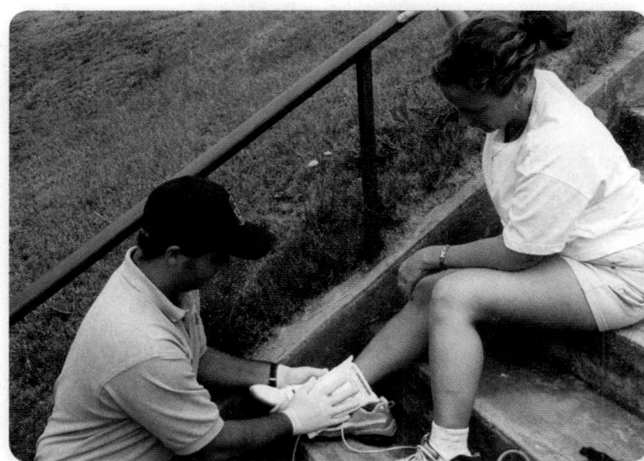

Figure 33-54 Apply cold packs to ankle injuries, and splint with the foot in the position of function. Remember to check the distal pulse.

If an ankle fracture-dislocation is associated with a pulseless foot, then medical direction may recommend that you attempt reduction. To reduce a fracture-dislocation of the ankle, first relax the calf muscle by flexing the patient's leg at the knee to allow the foot to move more freely. With the leg flexed, grasp the heel and the foot just proximal to the toes and apply gentle traction. Next, rotate the foot back into its normal position without forcing it. If this procedure is successful, reassess the distal neurovascular status and splint the extremity in the reduced position, using care not to allow the ankle to dislocate again. If you are unable to reduce the fracture-dislocation, then notify medical direction, splint the ankle in the position it was found, and provide rapid transport.

▶ Foot Injuries

Injuries to the foot can result in the fracture of one or more of the tarsals, metatarsals, or phalanges of the toes. Toe fractures are especially common.

Of the tarsal bones, the calcaneus, or heel bone, is the most frequently fractured. Injury usually occurs when the patient falls or jumps from a height and lands directly on the heel. The force of injury compresses the calcaneus, producing immediate swelling and ecchymosis. If the force of impact is great enough, such as from a fall off a roof or out of a tree, there may be other fractures as well.

Frequently, the force of injury is transmitted up the legs to the spine, producing a fracture of the lumbar spine Figure 33-55. When a patient who has jumped or fallen from a height reports heel pain, ensure you ask the patient about any back pain and carefully assess the spine for tenderness or deformity.

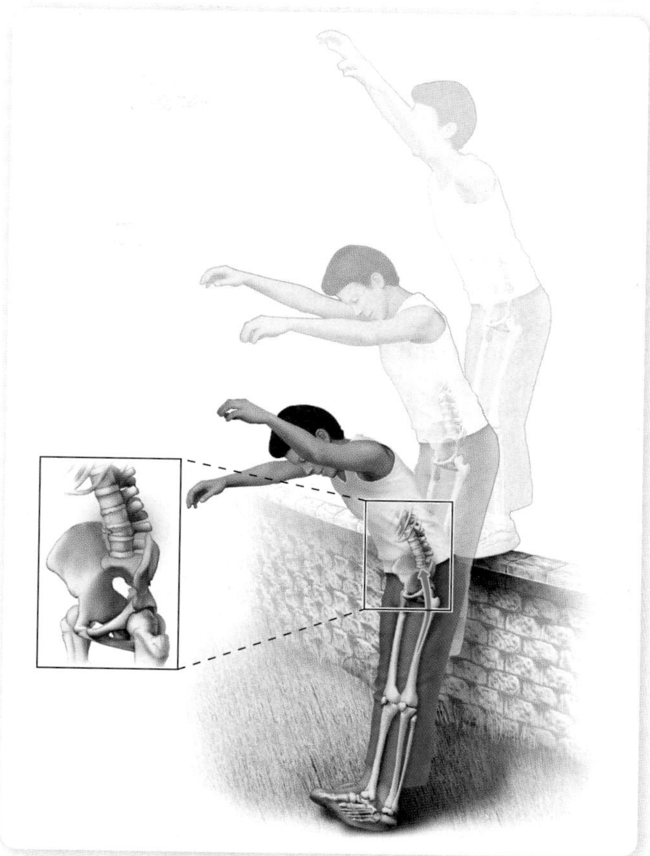

Figure 33-55 Frequently, the force of injury after a fall is transmitted up the legs to the spine, sometimes resulting in a fracture of the lumbar spine.

If you suspect that the foot is dislocated, immediately assess the patient's pulses and motor and sensory function. If pulses are present, immobilize the extremity using a commercially available splint or a pillow splint, leaving the toes exposed so you can periodically assess neurovascular function. If pulses are absent, consult medical direction and discuss reduction of the dislocation if local protocols permit.

Injuries of the foot are associated with significant swelling but rarely with gross deformity. Vascular injuries are not common. As in the hand, lacerations about the ankle and foot may damage important underlying nerves and tendons. Puncture wounds of the foot are common and may cause serious infection if not treated early. These injuries must be evaluated and treated by a physician.

To splint the foot, apply a rigid padded board splint, an air splint, or a pillow splint, stabilizing the ankle joint as well as the foot Figure 33-56. Leave the toes exposed so you can periodically assess neurovascular function.

When the patient is lying on the stretcher, elevate the foot approximately 6 inches (15 cm) to minimize swelling. All patients with lower extremity injuries should be transported in the supine position to allow for elevation of the limb. Never allow the foot and leg to dangle off the stretcher onto the floor or ground.

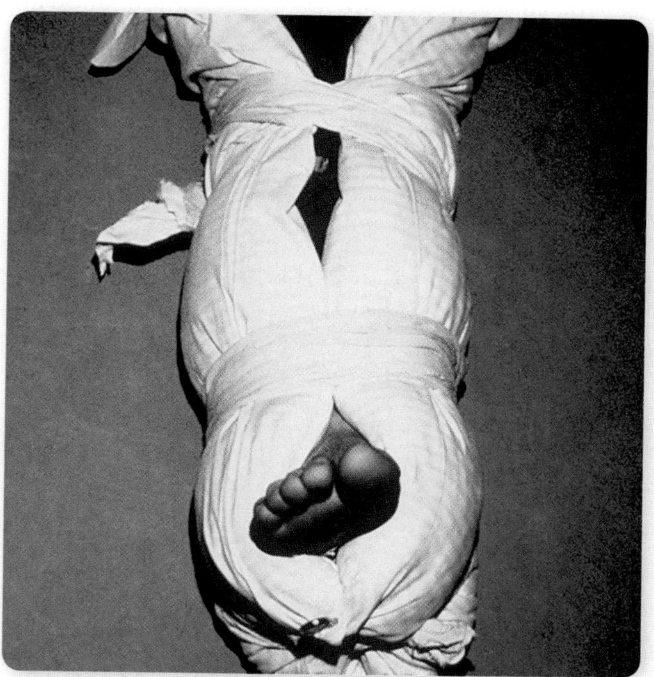

Figure 33-56 A pillow splint provides excellent stabilization of the foot and ankle.

If a patient has fallen from a height and reports heel pain, then use a long backboard to stabilize any possible spinal injury in addition to splinting the foot.

▶ Amputations

Surgeons can often reattach amputated parts. However, correct prehospital care of the amputated part is vital to successful reattachment. With partial amputations, ensure you immobilize the part with bulky compression dressings and a splint to prevent further injury. Do not sever any partial amputations, as this may complicate later reattachment.

Hemorrhage from complete or incomplete amputations can be severe and life threatening. You must control bleeding and treat for shock when dealing with amputations. Control any bleeding to the stump. If bleeding cannot be controlled, then quickly apply a **tourniquet** just above the site of the amputation. Complete traumatic amputations may not bleed much because the cut vessels may spasm, preventing the bleeding.

Make every attempt to preserve an amputated part in optimal condition to maximize the chances of it being successfully reimplanted. With a complete amputation, wrap the amputated part in a sterile dressing and place it in a plastic bag. Follow your local protocols regarding how to preserve amputated parts. In some areas, dry sterile dressings are recommended for wrapping amputated parts; in other areas, dressings moistened with sterile saline are recommended. Put the plastic bag in a cool container filled with ice water. Float the bag containing the wrapped part on a bed of ice water; do not pack it in ice, and never lay the wrapped part directly onto the ice. The goal is to keep the part cool without allowing it to freeze or for frostbite to develop. Do not warm an amputated part or place an amputated part in water. Rapidly transport the patient with the amputated part to the appropriate facility.

When the amputated part is a limb or part of a limb, notify the ED staff in advance of the type of case you are transporting and your estimated time of arrival so a surgical team can be mobilized while you are en route. Consider administering a bolus of an isotonic crystalloid solution if the patient has experienced significant blood loss or is hypotensive.

Finally, be aware of the patient's emotional stress, which can lead to psychogenic shock. Amputations are discussed in more detail in Chapter 28, *Soft-Tissue Injuries*.

▶ Sprains and Strains

Because it may be difficult to differentiate among the various types of injuries in the field, it is best to err on the side of caution and treat every severe sprain as if it were a fracture. General treatment of sprains is similar to the treatment of fractures and includes the following components (numbers 1 through 5 form the RICES mnemonic):

1. **Rest** (Immobilize or splint the injured area.)
2. **Ice** or cold pack over the injury
3. **Compression** with an elastic bandage (usually applied at the hospital once radiography rules out a fracture)
4. **Elevation**
5. **Splinting**
6. Reduced or protected weight bearing
7. Pain management as soon as practical

Strains are treated the same way as sprains.

YOU are the Provider SUMMARY

1. How should you prepare this patient for transport?

You know this patient could have a pelvic fracture and a femur fracture, so take steps to immobilize these fractures. This includes ensuring adequate and appropriate IV access and splinting. Splinting of the pelvis may be accomplished by various methods, according to local protocols, but should include applying a pelvic binder, or simply tying a sheet around the pelvis for stabilization. Failure to properly immobilize these injuries may result in significant internal bleeding for the patient as well as an increase in pain.

2. What should you do when advanced modes of transport are not available?

Transport patients in critical condition according to your local protocols. This patient requires rapid transport to a trauma center capable of orthopaedic surgery. Fractures such as these often result in severe pain, which paramedics can treat with the administration of narcotics. In this scenario, the flight crew is unavailable; likewise, no paramedics are available in the area. Treatment of this patient en route will, for the most part, be supportive.

3. What is the potential blood loss in a femur fracture? Pelvic fracture?

Blood loss from a femur fracture can be life threatening or minor, depending on the severity of the fracture and extent of pelvic displacement. Blood loss from a femur fracture can be as much as 1,000 mL to 1,500 mL; for a pelvic fracture, the loss can be 3,000 mL or more. Thus, a patient with a pelvic fracture is predisposed to hypovolemic shock as well as the potential for exsanguination.

4. Should this patient have a second IV line initiated?

This patient requires a second IV line, depending on local protocols. Given his potential for significant blood loss, rapid administration of IV fluid may be required en route as well as administration of blood products at the receiving facility. By having a second IV line in place, the AEMT can ensure the correct amount of fluid is administered to this patient in a timely manner.

5. What are some potential complications of femur and pelvic fractures?

Pelvic fractures can cause injuries to all the structures that occupy the pelvic cavity. Injuries are often seen in the urinary bladder, urethra, and rectum. Injuries to the weight-bearing area of the hip joint within the pelvis can lead to early arthritis.

Significant bleeding can result if the rich blood supply to the femur and surrounding muscle is disrupted after fracture. Shock, anemia, and injury to the sciatic nerve or the superficial femoral artery or other veins may occur.

6. What are the considerations when using lactated Ringer solution with trauma patients?

Traumatic injuries, especially crush injuries, may result in the buildup of toxins. The primary substances that are of concern are lactic acid, potassium, and myoglobin. Patients may also experience rhabdomyolysis and hyperkalemia from muscle breakdown. Because lactated Ringer solution contains potassium and other components, it is better to use normal saline if a crush injury or compartment syndrome is suspected. Remember, blood products are incompatible with lactated Ringer solution. For this reason, if you are starting an IV line on a patient with multisystem trauma whom you suspect will require a blood transfusion, always have an IV line of normal saline.

7. Which signs and symptoms may suggest compartment syndrome?

Compartment syndrome is characterized by severe pain that is localized to the involved compartment and out of proportion to the injury. This pain is typically not relieved with pain medication, including narcotics. As time progresses, the affected area may feel very firm although this is an unreliable sign. Skin pallor may be apparent as well as paresthesias (eg, burning sensation, numbness, tingling) and paralysis of the involved muscles. A very late sign of compartment syndrome is pulselessness.

8. What should your treatment of compartment syndrome include?

There is no specific treatment for compartment syndrome at the AEMT level, other than supportive care. The definitive treatment for compartment syndrome is surgical intervention, so rapid transport to the correct facility is important.

YOU are the Provider SUMMARY (continued)

EMS Patient Care Report (PCR)

Date: 8-7-18	**Incident No.:** 714	**Nature of Call:** Rodeo injury	**Location:** Running Eagle Rodeo		
Dispatched: 1605	**En Route:** 1605	**At Scene:** 1605	**Transport:** 1617	**At Hospital:** 1702	**In Service:** 1730

Patient Information

Age: 16 **Sex:** M **Weight (in kg [lb]):** 81 kg (180 lb)	**Allergies:** Penicillin **Medications:** None **Past Medical History:** None **Chief Complaint:** Multisystem trauma

Vital Signs

Time: 1606	**BP:** Not obtained	**Pulse:** Not obtained	**Respirations:** 22	**Spo_2:** Not obtained
Time: 1619	**BP:** 92/40	**Pulse:** 122	**Respirations:** 24	**Spo_2:** 97% on 15 L/min
Time: 1650	**BP:** 96/44	**Pulse:** 127	**Respirations:** 22	**Spo_2:** 98% on 15 L/min

EMS Treatment (circle all that apply)

Oxygen @ 15 **L/min via (circle one):** **NC** **(NRM)** **Bag-mask device**		**Assisted Ventilation**	**Airway Adjunct**	**CPR**
Defibrillation	**Bleeding Control**	**Bandaging**	**(Splinting:** pelvic**)**	**Other:**

Narrative

EMS assigned to stand by at Running Eagle rodeo ground for high school rodeo. Called to arena for male bucked off a bull. Patient presents AO×4, ABCs intact, obvious deformity to left leg and unstable pelvis. Requested air medical transport; not available. 15 L/min via nonrebreathing applied. Prior to movement, cervical collar and spinal immobilization applied, along with pelvic splint with some relief from pain. Placed patient on stretcher, secured, transport emergent. En route, established bilateral IVs with normal saline—one IV running wide open, one IV TKO. Approximately 35 minutes into transport, patient has signs and symptoms consistent with compartment syndrome—severe pain in his femoral area and tingling in left foot. Assessment reveals firmness in femur and decreased sensation in left foot. Contacted receiving physician, who suspects compartment syndrome and advises rapid transport. Preparation made for rapid removal of patient upon arrival at ED. On arrival, report given to receiving physician and ED staff without incident.**End of report**

Prep Kit

► Ready for Review

- Skeletal or voluntary muscle attaches to bone and forms the major muscle mass of the body. This muscle contains arteries, veins, and nerves.
- There are 206 bones of the skeleton. When these living tissues are fractured, they can produce bleeding and severe pain.
- A joint is a junction where two bones come into contact. Joints are stabilized in key areas by ligaments.
- Tendons connect skeletal muscle to bone. Ligaments connect bone to bone and help maintain the stability of joints and determine the degree of joint motion. Cartilage is a flexible connective tissue that forms a smooth surface over bone ends where they articulate.
- Age-associated changes in the musculoskeletal system include decreased bone density, degradation of joints, and disk herniation. People with osteoporosis have a higher risk of fracture.
- When a person has a musculoskeletal injury, many structures may be damaged, including muscles, bones, tendons, ligaments, cartilage, and vessels.
- A fracture is a broken bone; a dislocation is a disruption of a joint; a sprain is a stretching injury to the ligaments around a joint; and a strain is stretching of a muscle.
- A pathologic fracture, or nontraumatic fracture, occurs from a force that would usually not harm a healthy bone; however, due to a medical condition, the bone has become abnormally weak and more vulnerable to damage.
- Depending on the amount of kinetic energy absorbed by the tissues, the zone of injury may extend beyond the point of contact. Always maintain a high index of suspicion for associated fractures and other injuries.
- Fractures are classified as open or closed, and displaced or nondisplaced. Open and closed fractures are splinted in the same manner, but remember to control bleeding and apply a sterile dressing to the open extremity injury before splinting. Open fractures have a higher risk of infection.
- Other specific types of fractures include greenstick, comminuted, epiphyseal, oblique, transverse, spiral, and incomplete.
- The most common life-threatening musculoskeletal injuries are multiple fractures, open fractures with arterial bleeding, pelvic fractures, bilateral femur fractures, and limb amputations.
- Fractures and dislocations are often difficult to diagnose without a radiographic examination. You will treat these injuries similarly. Stabilize the injury with a splint, and transport the patient.
- Signs of a fracture and dislocation include pain, deformity, point tenderness, guarding, loss of use, swelling, bruising, crepitus, and false motion. Signs specific to fractures include shortening and exposed bone ends.
- Signs of a sprain (ligament injury) include swelling, ecchymosis, and instability of the joint.
- Signs of a strain (pulled muscle) include pain, but there is often no deformity and only minor swelling at the site of injury.
- Compare the unaffected extremity with the injured extremity for differences whenever possible.
- Interventions for patients with musculoskeletal injuries include addressing the ABCs; splinting; securing critical patients to a long backboard; providing prompt transport, possibly to a trauma center; and establishing intravenous (IV) access with possible administration of IV fluids.
- For each limb, your neurovascular examination should include assessment of pulse and motor and sensory function. Repeat this exam every 5 to 10 minutes.
- The principles of splinting include the following: if you suspect a fracture of the shaft of any bone, ensure the splint stabilizes the joints above and below the fracture; with injuries in and around a joint, ensure the splint immobilizes the bones above and below the injured joint; and where fracture of a long bone shaft has resulted in severe deformity, use constant, gentle, manual traction (pull) to align the limb so it can be splinted, unless this is too painful.
- There are three types of splints: traction splints, rigid splints, and formable splints.
- Neurovascular injury is a potential complication of musculoskeletal injury. Treatment is to assess and reassess pulses, control bleeding, and maintain adequate intravascular volume by administering intravenous fluid.
- Compartment syndrome is a complication of a musculoskeletal injury that occurs when bleeding or swelling leads to increased pressure within the space a muscle occupies. This pressure can impair circulation and cause pain, sensory changes, and muscle death. Compartment syndrome can occur

Prep Kit *(continued)*

in both open and closed fractures. Immediate transport is crucial.

- Crush syndrome may occur when an entrapped limb has been compressed and is then freed, causing the release of harmful products (rhabdomyolysis). Before releasing the compressing force, administer supplemental oxygen to the patient as needed and consider contacting medical direction regarding administering a bolus of crystalloid solution.
- A sling and swathe is used commonly to treat shoulder dislocations and to secure injured upper extremities to the body. Lower extremities can be secured to the unaffected limb or to a long backboard.
- Pelvic binders can be used to splint the pelvis. Another option may be to use a pneumatic antishock garment (PASG), depending on local protocols.
- Amputations may be partial or complete. Amputated parts may often be reattached by surgeons. Correct prehospital care of the amputated part is vital to successful reattachment. Never sever a partial amputation, and always control bleeding.
- Sprains and strains should be treated with rest, ice, compression, elevation, and pain management. Also, protect the limb from bearing weight.

▶ Vital Vocabulary

abduction Movement *away* from the midline of the body.

adduction Movement *toward* the midline of the body.

amputation An injury in which part of the body is completely severed.

angulation In a fracture, when each end of the fracture is not aligned in a straight line and an angle has formed between them.

appendicular skeleton The part of the skeleton comprising the upper and lower extremities.

articulation The surfaces of long bones that come in contact with other bones.

axial skeleton The part of the skeleton comprising the skull, spinal column, and rib cage.

buddy splinting Securing an injured finger or toe to an adjacent uninjured one to allow the intact digit to act as a splint.

cartilage The support structure of the skeletal system that provides cushioning between bones; it also forms the nasal septum and portions of the outer ear.

closed fracture A fracture in which the skin is not broken.

compartment syndrome An elevation of pressure within the fascial compartment, characterized by extreme pain, decreased pain sensation, pain on stretching of affected muscles, and decreased power; most frequently seen in fractures below the elbow or knee in children.

compound fracture An open fracture; a fracture beneath an open wound.

crepitus A grating or grinding sensation or sound caused by fractured bone ends or joints rubbing together.

crush syndrome Significant metabolic derangement that develops when crushed extremities or body parts remain trapped for prolonged periods; it can lead to renal failure and death.

deep vein thrombosis (DVT) The formation of a blood clot within the larger veins of an extremity, typically following a period of prolonged immobilization.

devascularization The loss of perfusion to a part of the body.

dislocation Disruption of a joint in which ligaments are damaged and the bone ends are completely displaced.

displaced fracture A fracture in which bone fragments are separated from one another and are not in anatomic alignment.

ecchymosis Bruising or discoloration associated with bleeding within or under the skin.

fascia The fiberlike connective tissue that covers arteries, veins, tendons, and ligaments.

fracture A break in the continuity of a bone.

hematopoiesis The process of generating blood cells.

hematuria Blood in the urine.

indirect injury An injury that occurs when force is applied to one region of the body but causes an injury in another area.

joint The point at which two or more bones articulate, or come together.

lactic acid A metabolic end product of the breakdown of glucose that accumulates when metabolism proceeds in the absence of oxygen.

lateral compression A force that is directed from the side toward the midline of the body.

ligaments Bands of fibrous tissue that connect bones to bones and support and strengthen the joints.

Prep Kit *(continued)*

neurovascular compromise The loss of the nerve supply, blood supply, or both to a region of the body, typically distal to a site of injury; characterized by alterations in sensation, including numbness and tingling, or by a loss or decrease of motor function; vascular compromise is indicated by weak or absent pulses, poor skin color, and cool skin.

nondisplaced fracture A simple crack in the bone that has not caused the bone to move from its normal anatomic position; also called a hairline fracture.

open book pelvic fracture A life-threatening fracture of the pelvis caused by a force that displaces one or both sides of the pelvis laterally and posteriorly.

open fracture Any break in a bone in which the overlying skin has been damaged.

osteoporosis A generalized bone disease, commonly associated with postmenopausal women but occurring in either sex, in which there is a reduction in the amount of bone mass leading to fractures after minimal trauma.

paresthesias Abnormal sensations such as burning, numbness, or tingling.

pathologic fracture A fracture that occurs in an area of abnormally weakened bone.

pelvic binders Devices used to splint the bony pelvis to reduce hemorrhage from bone ends, venous disruption, and pain.

physis The growth plate in long bones.

plantar flexion Bending of the foot toward the ground.

point tenderness Tenderness that is sharply localized at the site of the injury, found by gently palpating along the bone with the tip of one finger.

pulmonary embolism A blood clot that breaks off from a large vein and travels to the blood vessels of the lung, causing obstruction of blood flow.

reduction Repositioning of a bone to near its normal position after a fracture or dislocation.

retroperitoneal space The space between the abdominal cavity and the posterior abdominal wall, which contains the kidneys, certain large vessels, and parts of the gastrointestinal tract.

rhabdomyolysis The destruction of muscle tissue leading to a release of potassium and myoglobin.

sciatic nerve The major nerve to the lower extremity; it controls much of the muscle function in the leg and sensation in the entire leg and foot.

six Ps of musculoskeletal assessment Pain, Paralysis, Paresthesias, Pulselessness, Pallor, and Pressure.

sling A bandage or material that helps to support the weight of an injured upper extremity.

splint A flexible or rigid appliance used to protect and maintain the position of an injured extremity.

sprain A joint injury involving damage to supporting ligaments and partial or temporary dislocation of bone ends.

straddle fracture A fracture of the pelvis that results from landing on the perineal region.

strain Stretching or tearing of a muscle; also called a muscle pull.

subluxation Partial dislocation of a joint.

swathe A bandage that passes around the chest to secure an injured arm to the chest.

tendons Tough, ropelike cords of fibrous tissue that attach skeletal muscle to bones.

tourniquet A bandage or device applied to an extremity to control bleeding, used when a wound continues to bleed despite the use of direct pressure; works by compressing or constricting blood flow.

traction The act of exerting a pulling force on a body.

vertical shear The type of pelvic fracture that occurs when a massive force displaces the pelvis superiorly.

zone of injury The entire affected area in a bone or joint injury, which may include the surrounding soft tissues, especially to the adjacent nerves and blood vessels.

▶ References

1. Bone and Joint Initiative. The burden of musculoskeletal diseases in the United States: prevalence of select medical conditions. 2014. http://www.boneandjointburden.org/2014-report/ib0/prevalence-select-medical-conditions. Accessed February 25, 2017.
2. Bone and Joint Initiative. The burden of musculoskeletal diseases in the United States: lost work days and bed days. 2014. http://www.boneandjointburden.org/2014-report/id0/lost-work-days-and-bed-days. Accessed February 25, 2017.
3. Bone and Joint Initiative. The burden of musculoskeletal diseases in the United States: health care utilization and economic cost. 2014. http://www.boneandjointburden.org/2014-report/if0/health-care-utilization-and-economic-cost. Accessed February 25, 2017.

Prep Kit *(continued)*

4. Bone and Joint Initiative. By the numbers: musculoskeletal conditions. 2014. http://www.boneandjointburden.org/docs/By%20The%20Numbers%20-%20Musculoskeletal%20Conditions%20%28Big%20Picture%29_update%202-24-16.pdf. Accessed February 25, 2017.
5. Musculoskeletal Medicine for Medical Students. Child abuse fractures. February 20, 2012. http://orthopaedicsone.com/display/MSKMed/Child+Abuse+Fractures. Accessed February 26, 2017.
6. Stawicki SP, Lindsey DE. Trauma corner—missed traumatic injuries: a synopsis. *OPUS 12 Sci.* 2009;3(2):35-43.
7. Mechum CC. Pelvic fracture in emergency medicine. *Medscape.* August 20, 2015. http://emedicine.medscape.com/article/825869-overview#a6. Accessed March 1, 2017.
8. Bible JE, Kadakia RJ, Wegner A, Richards JE, Mir HR. One-year mortality after isolated pelvic fractures with posterior ring involvement in elderly patients. *Orthopedics.* 2013;36(6):760-764. http://www.healio.com/orthopedics/journals/ortho/2013-6-36-6/%7B0a42488e-67c3-4cf9-9afe-83803d576946%7D/one-year-mortality-after-isolated-pelvic-fractures-with-posterior-ring-involvement-in-elderly-patients. Accessed March 1, 2017.
9. Richardson JD, Harty J, Amin M, Flint LM. Open pelvic fractures. *J Trauma.* 1982;22(7):533-538. https://www.ncbi.nlm.nih.gov/pubmed/7097812. Accessed March 1, 2017.

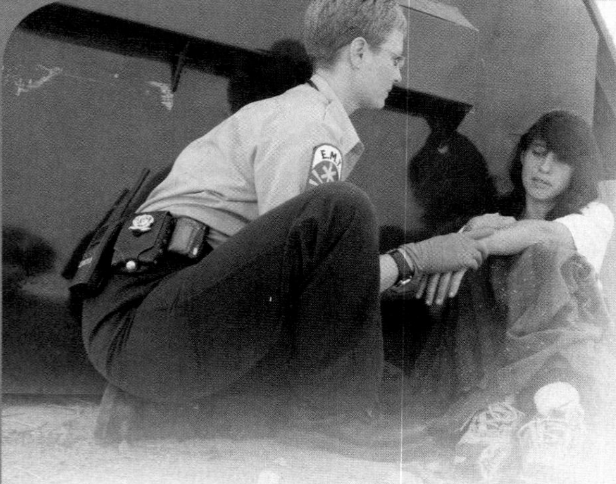

Assessment *in Action*

Your ambulance is dispatched to a local grain elevator for a male worker who has his arm stuck in an auger. On arrival, you are directed to the patient, who has now been removed from the auger. He is seated on the ground, with copious amounts of blood around him. You see a completely amputated right arm, severed in the midhumerus area.

1. How should this patient's bleeding be controlled?

- **A.** Direct pressure
- **B.** Elevation
- **C.** Tourniquet
- **D.** Pressure point

2. How should an amputated extremity be transported?

- **A.** Wrap the part, place in a plastic bag, then place in ice water.
- **B.** Wrap the part and place it on the stretcher with the patient.
- **C.** Place the part in a water bath.
- **D.** Wrap the part in hot packs to keep it warm.

Assessment in Action (continued)

3. When presented with a partial amputation, you should:
   - **A.** complete the amputation so you can properly package the part.
   - **B.** leave the partial amputation in place and submerge it in ice water.
   - **C.** place the partial amputation in the correct anatomic position and bandage it.
   - **D.** complete the amputation and apply a bandage.
4. Limb amputations are graded as:
   - **A.** minor injuries.
   - **B.** moderate injuries.
   - **C.** slight injuries.
   - **D.** severe injuries.
5. Considering the amount of blood loss, all of the following may be appropriate treatment EXCEPT:
   - **A.** spinal immobilization.
   - **B.** treating for shock.
   - **C.** rapid transport.
   - **D.** a fluid bolus.
6. Severing any partial amputations may:
   - **A.** help with bleeding control.
   - **B.** complicate later reattachment.
   - **C.** make packaging easier.
   - **D.** make reattachment easier.
7. The "C" in the RICES mnemonic stands for which term?
   - **A.** Contusion
   - **B.** Chill
   - **C.** Compression
   - **D.** Circulation
8. What is the appropriate care for pelvic injuries?
9. How do weather changes and altitude affect air splints?
10. Describe the appropriate way to splint an AC separation.

CHAPTER 34

Environmental Emergencies

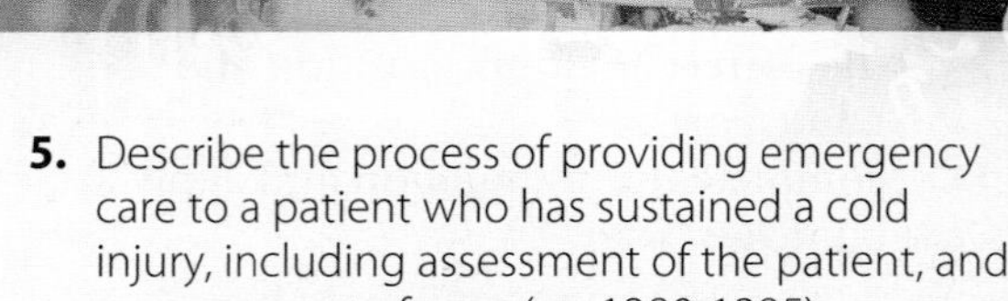

National EMS Education Standard Competencies

Trauma

Applies fundamental knowledge to provide basic and selected advanced emergency care and transportation based on assessment findings for an acutely injured patient.

Environmental Emergencies

Recognition and management of

- Submersion incidents (pp 1392-1393, 1399-1404)
- Temperature-related illness (pp 1377-1379, 1382-1388, 1390-1392)

Pathophysiology, assessment, and management of

- Near drowning (1392-1393, 1399-1404)
- Temperature-related illness (pp 1377-1392)
- Bites and envenomations (pp 1408-1415)
- Dysbarism
  - High-altitude (p 1405)
  - Diving injuries (pp 1393-1399, 1401-1403)
- Electrical injury (pp 1405-1408, and see Chapter 28, *Soft-Tissue Injuries*)
- Radiation exposure (see Chapter 28, *Soft-Tissue Injuries*)

Knowledge Objectives

1. Describe four factors that affect how a person deals with exposure to a cold or hot environment and how each one relates to emergency medical care. (pp 1374-1375)
2. Explain the five different ways a body can lose heat and ways the rate and amount of heat loss or gain can be modified in an emergency situation. (pp 1375-1377)
3. Define and discuss hypothermia, including the signs and symptoms of its four different stages and the risk factors for developing it. (pp 1377-1379)
4. Explain local cold injuries and their underlying causes. (pp 1379-1380)
5. Describe the process of providing emergency care to a patient who has sustained a cold injury, including assessment of the patient, and management of care. (pp 1380-1385)
6. Explain the importance of following regional and state protocols when rewarming a patient who is experiencing moderate or severe hypothermia. (pp 1384-1385)
7. Describe the three forms of illness that are caused by heat exposure, including their signs and symptoms, and give examples of persons who are at the greatest risk of developing one of them. (pp 1386-1388)
8. Describe the process of providing emergency care to a patient who has sustained a heat injury, including assessment of the patient, and management of care. (pp 1388-1392)
9. Define *drowning* and discuss its incidence, risk factors, and prevention. (pp 1392-1393, 1404)
10. Describe three physical laws that affect pressure in the context of diving and diving-related conditions. (pp 1393-1394)
11. Describe the three different types of diving emergencies, how they may occur, and their signs and symptoms. (pp 1395-1399)
12. List the basic rules of performing a water rescue, and discuss why rescue personnel should have a prearranged water rescue plan based on the environment in which they work. (pp 1399-1400)
13. List four conditions that may result in a spinal injury following a submersion incident and the steps for stabilizing a patient with a suspected spinal injury in the water. (pp 1400-1401)
14. Discuss recovery techniques you may need to follow when managing a patient who has been involved in a submersion incident. (pp 1401, 1404)
15. Describe the process of providing emergency care to a patient who has been involved in a drowning or diving emergency, including assessment of the patient, and management of care. (pp 1401-1404)
16. Discuss the types of dysbarism injuries that may be caused by high altitudes, including their signs and

symptoms and emergency medical treatment in the field. (p 1405)

17. Discuss lightning injuries, including their incidence, risk factors, assessment, and emergency medical treatment. (pp 1405-1408)
18. Identify the species of spiders found in the United States that may cause life-threatening injuries, and then describe the process of providing emergency care to patients who have been bitten by each type. (pp 1408-1409)
19. Discuss the emergency medical care of patients who have been stung by Hymenoptera, including steps you should follow if a patient develops a severe reaction to the sting or bite. (p 1409)
20. Identify the species of snakes found in the United States that are venomous, and then describe the process of providing emergency care to patients who have been bitten by each type and are showing signs of envenomation. (pp 1409-1413)
21. Discuss the emergency medical care of patients who have been stung by scorpions or bitten by ticks, including steps you should follow if a patient develops a severe reaction to the sting or bite. (pp 1413-1414)
22. Discuss the emergency medical care of patients who have been stung by a coelenterate or other marine animal. (pp 1414-1415)

Skills Objectives

1. Demonstrate the emergency medical treatment of local cold injuries in the field. (pp 1382, 1384-1385)
2. Demonstrate using a warm-water bath to rewarm the limb of a patient who has sustained a local cold injury. (p 1385)
3. Demonstrate how to treat a patient with heat cramps. (p 1390)
4. Demonstrate how to treat a patient with heat exhaustion. (pp 1390-1391, Skill Drill 34-1)
5. Demonstrate how to treat a patient with heatstroke. (pp 1391-1392)
6. Demonstrate how to stabilize a patient with a suspected spinal injury in the water. (pp 1400-1401, Skill Drill 34-2)
7. Demonstrate how to care for a patient who is suspected of having an air embolism or decompression sickness following a drowning or diving emergency. (p 1403)
8. Demonstrate how to care for a patient who has been bitten by a pit viper and is showing signs of envenomation. (pp 1411-1413)
9. Demonstrate how to care for a patient who has been bitten by a coral snake and is showing signs of envenomation. (pp 1412-1413)
10. Demonstrate how to care for a patient who has sustained a coelenterate envenomation. (pp 1414-1415)

Introduction

An **environmental emergency** is a medical condition caused or exacerbated by the weather, terrain, or atmospheric pressure at high altitude or underwater. Environmental factors such as temperature and atmospheric pressure can overwhelm the body's mechanisms for regulating temperature, including sweating and the radiation of body heat into the atmosphere.

A variety of medical emergencies can result, particularly in children, older people, people with chronic illnesses, and young adults who overexert themselves. These can result in mental status changes, functional changes, and, possibly, death. The environmental effect on morbidity and mortality increases with stressors that induce or exacerbate other medical or traumatic conditions.

In addition, a range of medical emergencies also arise from water recreation, which can sometimes be

YOU are the Provider — PART 1

Your ambulance is dispatched to an unresponsive man who is outside a local fast food establishment. As you proceed to your ambulance, you tell your partner that this will probably be hypothermia induced by the −20°F temperatures and 12 inches of snow on the ground. As you arrive on scene, you are greeted by law enforcement officers who state that the patient is homeless and they believe he was trying to sleep in front of the door in an effort to keep warm.

1. What are four factors that affect exposure?
2. What are five methods of heat loss?

complicated by cold temperatures. These emergencies include localized injuries and systemic illnesses.

As an advanced emergency medical technician (AEMT), you can save lives by recognizing and responding properly to these emergencies, most of which require prompt treatment in the hospital.

In this chapter, you will learn how the body regulates **core temperature**, and the ways in which body heat is lost to the environment. The various forms of heat-, cold-, and water-related emergencies are described, including how to diagnose and treat **hypothermia**, **frostbite**, and **hyperthermia**. You will also learn about pressure-related emergencies, or **dysbarism injuries**, caused by diving and high-altitude climbing; injuries caused by lightning; and envenomation, caused by bites and stings.

Factors Affecting Exposure

The body works to ensure balance between heat production and heat excretion (**thermoregulation**). A rise in core body temperature elicits responses that increase heat loss and shut off normal heat production pathways (called **thermogenesis**); a decrease in core body temperature prompts heat production and conservation and turns off normal heat-liberating pathways (called **thermolysis**) **Figure 34-1**.

There are four factors that affect how a person deals with a cold or hot environment. These can be used as prevention strategies for those who work or play in extreme environmental temperatures. They can also be useful during the assessment of your patient to determine how prepared he or she was for a cold or hot environment.

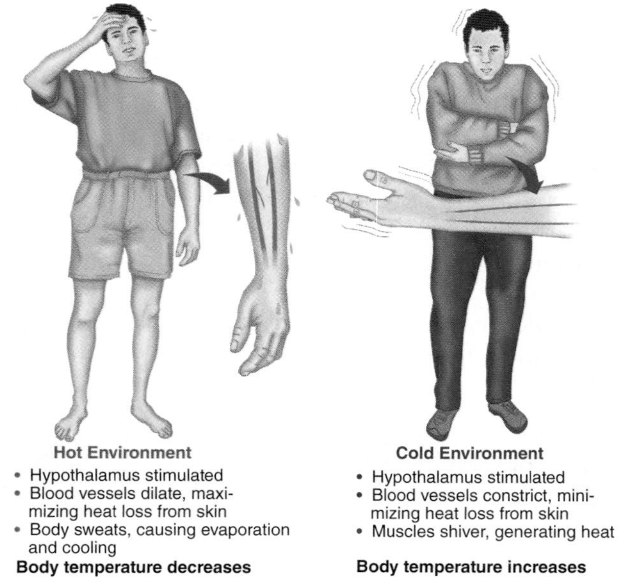

Hot Environment
• Hypothalamus stimulated
• Blood vessels dilate, maximizing heat loss from skin
• Body sweats, causing evaporation and cooling
Body temperature decreases
Cold Environment
• Hypothalamus stimulated
• Blood vessels constrict, minimizing heat loss from skin
• Muscles shiver, generating heat
Body temperature increases

Figure 34-1 Similar to a thermostat, the hypothalamus notes a rise or fall in core body temperature and elicits responses to regulate it.

A hiker prepared for a warm summer hike in the foothills will present and respond to treatment differently from a traveler stranded in a hot vehicle because the radiator boiled over. Factors affecting exposure include:

1. **Physical condition.** Patients who are already ill or in poor physical condition will not be able to tolerate extreme temperatures as well as those whose cardiovascular, metabolic, and nervous systems are all functioning well. For example, an athlete in peak physical condition performs better and is less likely to experience injury or illness than a person who is not in peak physical condition. Exertion also plays a role. Increasing your activity will generate more heat, which is beneficial in the cold but potentially problematic when it is hot.
2. **Age.** Children and older adults are more likely to experience temperature-related illness. Infants have poor thermoregulation at birth and do not have the ability to shiver and generate heat when needed until about 12 to 18 months. Their surface area–to–body mass ratio is larger, contributing to their more rapid heat loss and heat gain. When you get cold, you put on a sweater; a small child may not think to do this or may have difficulty finding and putting one on. On the other end of the spectrum, older adults lose subcutaneous tissue as they age, reducing the amount of insulation they have and their ability to tolerate temperature extremes. This is why older people often wear extra layers of clothing. Poor circulation also contributes to increased risk of frostbite. Medications can also affect an older person's body thermostat, putting him or her at increased risk for temperature-related emergencies. Finally, older patients are at high risk for falls, and lying immobile on a hot or cold surface can rapidly result in overexposure.
3. **Nutrition and hydration.** The body needs calories for its metabolism to function. Staying well hydrated provides water as a catalyst for much of this metabolism. A decrease in calorie intake or water intake increases susceptibility to heat or cold illness or injury. Calories provide fuel to burn, creating heat during the cold, and water provides sweat for **evaporation** and removing heat. Alcohol use may increase fluid loss and place the patient at greater risk for temperature-related emergencies.
4. **Environmental conditions.** Conditions such as air temperature, humidity levels, and wind can complicate or improve environmental situations. A cool breeze helps when it is hot outside, but a cold wind when it is cold outside can be uncomfortable. Extremes in temperature and humidity are not needed to produce hot

or cold injuries. Many hypothermia cases occur at temperatures between 30°F (−1°C) and 50°F (10°C). Most **heatstroke** cases occur when the temperature is 80°F (26.7°C) and the humidity is 80%; however, heat injury can also occur at moderate temperatures when there is a combination of extreme exertion and inadequate hydration.[1] Be sure to examine the environmental temperature of your patient. Older patients may turn the heat down in the winter or neglect to use air conditioning in the summer because of cost concerns. Some people may not open windows in a heat wave for fear of burglars. When evaluating your patient's condition, consider the environment and whether your patient is prepared for that situation. It may help in your treatment decisions and give you an idea about how the patient will respond to your care.

Cold Exposure

Normal body temperature must be maintained within a narrow range for the body's chemistry to work efficiently. Homeostasis, or a constant internal balance, must be maintained. If the body, or any part of it, is exposed to a cold environment, these mechanisms may be overwhelmed. Cold exposure may cause injury to individual parts of the body, such as the feet, hands, ears, or nose, or to the body as a whole. When the entire core body temperature falls because of inadequate internal heat production (thermogenesis), excess cold stress, or a combination of both, the condition is called *hypothermia*.

Because heat always travels from a warmer place to a cooler place, the body will tend to lose heat to the environment. Through thermolysis, or methods of heat loss, the body can lose heat in the following five ways:

- **Conduction** is the direct transfer of heat from a part of the body to a colder object or substance by direct contact, such as when a warm hand touches cold metal or ice, is immersed in cold water, or lies on a cold surface such as pavement. Heat passes directly from the body to the colder object. Heat can also be gained if the object or substance being touched is warm. This is why people with chronic medical problems are advised to limit time in hot tubs.
- **Convection** occurs when heat is transferred to circulating air, such as when cool air moves across the body surface. A person standing outside in windy winter weather, wearing only lightweight clothing, is losing heat to the environment mostly by convection. The **wind-chill factor** measures the chilling effect of a given temperature at a given wind speed. For example, the chilling effect of a 30°F (−1.1°C) **ambient temperature** (the temperature of the surrounding environment) with a 35-mph wind is −4°F (−20.0°C) Figure 34-2. A person can gain heat if the air moving across the person's

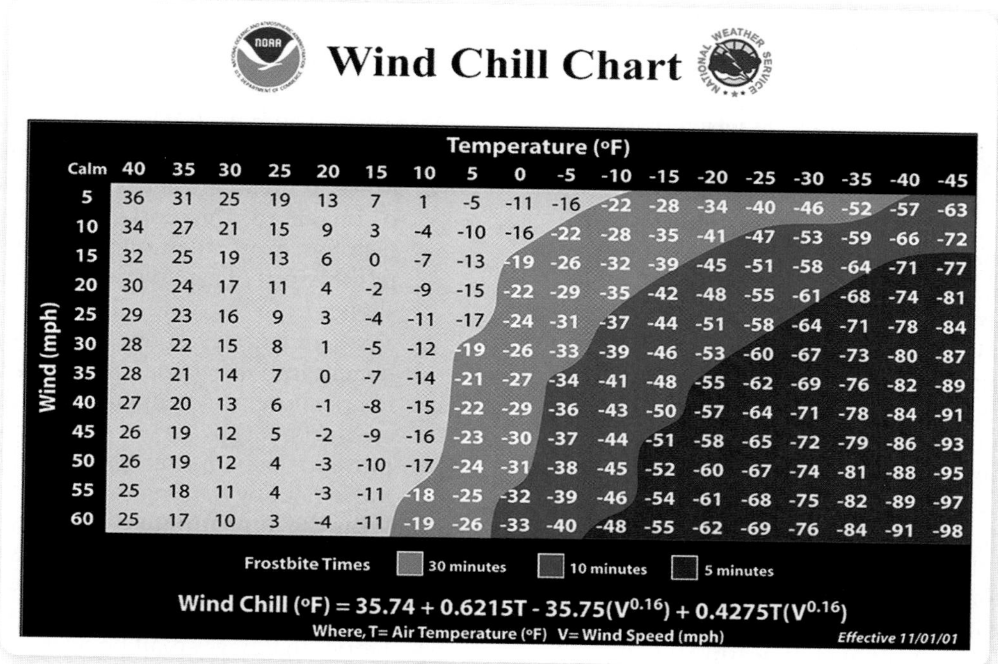

Wind Chill Chart

Temperature (°F)

Wind (mph)	Calm 40	35	30	25	20	15	10	5	0	-5	-10	-15	-20	-25	-30	-35	-40	-45
5	36	31	25	19	13	7	1	-5	-11	-16	-22	-28	-34	-40	-46	-52	-57	-63
10	34	27	21	15	9	3	-4	-10	-16	-22	-28	-35	-41	-47	-53	-59	-66	-72
15	32	25	19	13	6	0	-7	-13	-19	-26	-32	-39	-45	-51	-58	-64	-71	-77
20	30	24	17	11	4	-2	-9	-15	-22	-29	-35	-42	-48	-55	-61	-68	-74	-81
25	29	23	16	9	3	-4	-11	-17	-24	-31	-37	-44	-51	-58	-64	-71	-78	-84
30	28	22	15	8	1	-5	-12	-19	-26	-33	-39	-46	-53	-60	-67	-73	-80	-87
35	28	21	14	7	0	-7	-14	-21	-27	-34	-41	-48	-55	-62	-69	-76	-82	-89
40	27	20	13	6	-1	-8	-15	-22	-29	-36	-43	-50	-57	-64	-71	-78	-84	-91
45	26	19	12	5	-2	-9	-16	-23	-30	-37	-44	-51	-58	-65	-72	-79	-86	-93
50	26	19	12	4	-3	-10	-17	-24	-31	-38	-45	-52	-60	-67	-74	-81	-88	-95
55	25	18	11	4	-3	-11	-18	-25	-32	-39	-46	-54	-61	-68	-75	-82	-89	-97
60	25	17	10	3	-4	-11	-19	-26	-33	-40	-48	-55	-62	-69	-76	-84	-91	-98

Frostbite Times: 30 minutes; 10 minutes; 5 minutes

Wind Chill (°F) = $35.74 + 0.6215T - 35.75(V^{0.16}) + 0.4275T(V^{0.16})$

Where, T = Air Temperature (°F) V = Wind Speed (mph)

Effective 11/01/01

Figure 34-2 Wind-chill factor table.

Courtesy of the National Weather Service/NOAA.

Temperature (°F)

Relative Humidity (%)	80	82	84	86	88	90	92	94	96	98	100	102	104	106	108	110
40	80	81	83	85	88	91	94	97	101	105	109	114	119	124	130	136
45	80	82	84	87	89	93	96	100	104	109	114	119	124	130	137	
50	81	83	85	88	91	95	99	103	108	113	118	124	131	137		
55	81	84	86	89	93	97	101	106	112	117	124	130	137			
60	82	84	88	91	95	100	105	110	116	123	129	137				
65	82	85	89	93	98	103	108	114	121	128	136					
70	83	86	90	95	100	105	112	119	126	134						
75	84	88	92	97	103	109	116	124	132							
80	84	89	94	100	106	113	121	129								
85	85	90	96	102	110	117	126	135								
90	86	91	98	105	113	122	131									
95	86	93	100	108	117	127										
100	87	95	103	112	121	132										

Likelihood of Heat Disorders with Prolonged Exposure or Strenuous Activity
Caution · Extreme Caution · Danger · Extreme Danger

Figure 34-3 Heat index.

Courtesy of National Oceanic and Atmospheric Administration.

body is hotter than the temperature of the environment, such as in deserts or industrial settings like foundries, but it is more common to see rapid heat gain in spas and hot tubs where the water temperature may be well above body temperature **Figure 34-3**.

- Evaporation is the conversion of a liquid to a gas, a process that requires energy, or heat. Evaporation is the natural mechanism by which sweating cools the body. This is why swimmers coming out of the water feel a sensation of cold as the water evaporates from their skin. People who exercise vigorously in a cool environment may sweat and feel warm at first, but later, as their sweat evaporates, they can become cold.
- **Radiation** is the loss of body heat directly to colder objects in the environment by radiant energy. Radiant energy is a type of invisible light that transfers heat. Because heat always travels from a warm object to a cooler one, a person standing in a cold room will lose heat by radiation. Heat can also be gained by radiation: for example, when a person stands by a fire.
- Respiration causes body heat to be lost, as warm air in the lungs is exhaled into the atmosphere and cooler air is inhaled. In warm climates, the air temperature can be well above body temperature, causing an individual to gain heat with each breath.

The rate and amount of heat loss or gain by the body can be modified in three ways:

1. **Increase or decrease heat production.** One way for the body to increase its heat production is to increase the rate of metabolism of its cells; the body can accomplish this through shivering. In addition, people often have a natural urge to move around when they are cold. When a person is hot, he or she tends to reduce their level of activity, thus reducing heat production.
2. **Move to an area where heat loss is decreased or increased.** The most obvious ways to decrease heat loss from radiation and convection are to move out of a cold environment and seek shelter from the wind. The same holds true for a patient who is too hot. Simply moving the patient into the shade can reduce the ambient temperature (the temperature of the surrounding environment) by 10° or more. If you cannot move the patient, create shade and increase air movement by fanning the patient.
3. **Wear the appropriate clothing for the environment.** To avoid heat loss in cold environments, wear layers of clothing that provide good insulation, such as wool, down, and synthetic fabrics that have small pockets of trapped air. Protective clothing traps perspiration and prevents evaporation, which prevents cooling. Keep the head, hands, and feet covered, and

remove wet clothing if possible. Sweating without evaporation will not result in cooling. To encourage heat loss, wear lightweight, loose-fitting clothing, particularly around the head and neck.

▶ Pathophysiology

Hypothermia

Hypothermia literally means "low temperature." It occurs when the core temperature of the body—the temperature of the heart, lungs, and vital organs—falls below 95°F (35°C). The body can usually tolerate a decrease in core temperature of a few degrees. However, below this critical point, the body cannot regulate its temperature and generate body heat. Progressive loss of body heat then begins.

To protect itself against heat loss, the body normally constricts blood vessels in the skin; this results in the characteristic pale appearance of the hypothermic patient. As a secondary compensatory mechanism against heat loss, the body attempts to create additional heat by shivering, which is the active moving of many muscles to generate heat. Many body functions begin to slow down as cold exposure continues and these mechanisms are overwhelmed. Eventually, the functioning of key organs such as the heart and brain begins to slow. Untreated, this can result in coma and eventually death.

Hypothermia can develop either quickly, as when someone is immersed in cold water, or gradually, as when a person is exposed to the cold environment for several hours or more. The temperature does not have to be below freezing (less than 32°F, 0°C) for hypothermia to occur. In winter, homeless people and those whose homes lack heating may develop hypothermia at higher temperatures. Even during summer, swimmers who remain in the water for extended periods are at risk of hypothermia. Like all heat- and cold-related injuries, hypothermia is more common among geriatric, pediatric, and ill populations who are less able to adjust to temperature extremes. Also, infants and children have a relatively large body surface area in relation to mass and have less body fat than do adults. Therefore, if an infant or child is not clothed appropriately, he or she can develop hypothermia.

Patients with injuries or illness, such as burns, shock, head injury, stroke, generalized infection, injuries to the spinal cord, malnutrition, hypothyroidism, diabetes, and hypoglycemia, are more susceptible to hypothermia, as are patients who have taken certain drugs or poisons.

Alcohol is a common contributor to hypothermia.[2] It predisposes the patient to hypothermia by impairing shivering thermogenesis (decreased thermogenesis) and by promoting cutaneous vasodilation (increased thermolysis), which hinders the body's attempts to create an insulating shell around its warm core. Liver disease, which results in inadequate glycogen stores, and the subnormal nutritional status of most people with alcoholism further impair metabolic heat generation. Finally, alcohol impairs judgment, which often results in inappropriate behavior in cold conditions. Impaired thermoregulation can also occur with therapeutic use or overdoses of sedative medications, tricyclic antidepressants, and phenothiazines, primarily by interfering with central nervous system–mediated vasoconstriction.

Special Populations

Because of their small muscle mass, children may not be able to shiver as effectively as adults, and infants do not shiver at all.

Words of Wisdom

The National Institutes of Health has initiated a public awareness campaign informing the public to watch for "umbles"--fumbles (coordination and fine motor control problems), stumbles, mumbles (speech difficulty), and crumbles (incoherence, hemodynamic collapse). These behaviors are good indicators of how the cold affects the cerebral and cognitive functioning of patients in the early stages (mild) of hypothermia. Older people may simply have a flatter affect, be slightly more confused, or develop symptoms suggestive of a possible stroke, including dysarthria and ataxia.

Signs and Symptoms. Signs and symptoms of hypothermia increase in severity as the core temperature falls. Hypothermia generally progresses through four stages, as shown in Table 34-1. Although there is no clear distinction among the stages, the different signs and symptoms of each will help you estimate the severity of the hypothermia. When you assess a patient in the field, you should be able to distinguish between mild and severe hypothermia.

It is important to assess the temperature of the patient's skin close to the trunk, or core, of the body. Extremities may be cold as a result of exposure, yet the patient may be hemodynamically stable. To assess the patient's core body temperature, pull your glove back and place the back of your hand on the patient's skin at the abdomen Figure 34-4. If the skin feels cool, the patient is likely experiencing a generalized cold emergency. Rectal temperature is considered the most accurate for assessment of hypothermia, but rectal thermometers are not typically available in ambulance equipment. Oral and tympanic thermometers may be markedly off when measuring core body temperature.

If you work in a cold environment, and/or depending on local protocols, you may carry a hypothermia thermometer, which registers lower core temperatures. It must be inserted into the rectum for an accurate reading. Regular thermometers will not register the temperature of a patient who has substantial hypothermia.

Table 34-1 Characteristics of Systemic Hypothermia

Extent of hypothermia	Mild: 95°F to 90°F (35°C to 32°C)		Moderate: 90°F to 82°F (32°C to 28°C)	Severe: <82°F (28°C)
Core temperature	**95°F to 93°F (35°C to 33.9°C)**	**92°F to 89°F (33.3°C to 31.7°C)**	**88°F to 80°F (31.1°C to 26.7°C)**	**<80°F (<26.7°C)**
Signs and symptoms	Shivering, foot stamping	Loss of coordination, muscle stiffness	Coma	Apparent death
Cardiorespiratory response	Constricted blood vessels, rapid breathing	Slowing respirations, slow pulse	Weak pulse, dysrhythmias, very slow respirations	Cardiac arrest
Level of consciousness	Withdrawn	Confused, lethargic, sleepy	Unresponsive	Unresponsive

Data from: Zafren K, Giesbrecht GG, Danzl DF, et al. Wilderness Medical Society practice guidelines for the out-of-hospital evaluation and treatment of accidental hypothermia: 2014 update. *Wilderness Environ Med.* 2014;25(suppl 4):S66-S85. https://www.ncbi.nlm.nih.gov/pubmed/25498264. Accessed November 15, 2016.

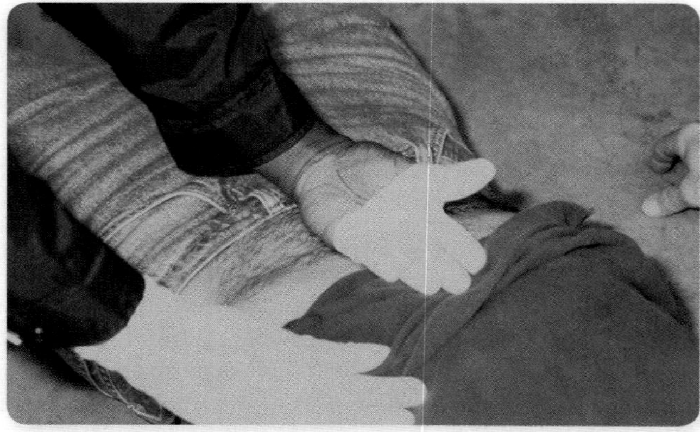

Figure 34-4 To assess a patient's core body temperature, pull back your glove and place the back of your hand on the patient's skin at the abdomen.

Mild hypothermia occurs when the core temperature is between 95°F and 93°F (35°C and 33.9°C). The patient is usually alert (may be withdrawn, anxious, or restless) and shivering in an attempt to generate more heat through muscular activity. In a further attempt to generate body heat, the patient may jump up and down and stamp his or her feet. Pulse rate and respirations are usually rapid. The skin in light-skinned people can be red but may eventually appear pale and then cyanotic. People in a cold environment may have blue lips or fingertips because of the body's constriction of blood vessels at the skin to retain heat.

Moderate hypothermia exists when the core temperature is 92°F to 89°F (33.3°C to 31.7°C). As the body compensates, the patient may present with signs and symptoms of a cold emergency while maintaining a normal core body temperature. The temperature is actually being maintained by thermogenesis. As energy stores of glycogen in the liver and muscles are exhausted, the core body temperature begins to drop. Shivering stops, and muscular activity decreases. At first, small, fine muscle activity such as coordinated finger motion ceases. Eventually, as the temperature falls further, all muscle activity stops.

As the core temperature drops toward 85°F (29.4°C), the patient becomes lethargic, usually losing the ability to continue to fight the cold. The level of consciousness decreases, and the patient may try to remove his or her own clothes as a result of altered mental status. Poor coordination and memory loss follow, along with reduced or complete loss of sensation to touch, mood changes, and impaired judgment. The patient becomes less communicative, experiences joint or muscle stiffness, and has trouble speaking. The patient begins to appear stiff or rigid.

If the core temperature continues to fall to 80°F (26.7°C), vital signs slow; the pulse becomes weaker, and respirations decrease in rate and depth or become absent altogether. Cardiac dysrhythmias may occur as a direct effect of cold as cardiac tissue becomes more irritable, or as the blood pressure decreases.

At a core temperature of less than 80°F (26.7°C), all cardiorespiratory activity may cease, pupillary reaction is slow, and the patient may appear dead.

*Never assume that a cold, pulseless patient is dead. Patients are not dead until they are **warm** and dead.* Patients may

Words of Wisdom

The stress of the cold environment, a remote terrain, a feeling of impending doom, and impaired judgment may result in suicidal tendencies in some patients with hypothermia. It is important to protect patients from harming themselves while considering your own safety at all times.

survive even severe prolonged hypothermia if proper emergency care is provided.

Local Cold Injuries

Most injuries from cold are localized to exposed parts of the body. The extremities, particularly the feet and hands, and the ears, nose, and face are especially vulnerable to cold injury Figure 34-5. When exposed parts of the body become very cold but not frozen, injuries such as **frostnip**, chilblains, or **immersion foot** (also called trench foot) can result. When the parts become frozen, the injury is called frostbite. Frostnip is reversible on rewarming (there is no blister formation, and color returns to normal), but frostbite is not.

In systemic hypothermia, blood is shunted away from the extremities to maintain the core temperature. This shunting of blood increases the risk of local cold injury to the extremities, ears, nose, and face. Thus, the patient with systemic hypothermia should also be assessed for frostbite or other local cold injury. The reverse is also true. Remember that both local and systemic cold exposure injuries can occur in the same patient.

Frostnip and Immersion Foot. After prolonged exposure to the cold, the skin may freeze while the deeper tissues are unaffected. This condition, which often affects the ears, nose, and fingers, is called frostnip. Because frostnip is usually not painful, the patient is often unaware that a cold injury has occurred. Immersion foot occurs after prolonged exposure to cold water. It is particularly common in hikers or hunters who stand for a long time in a river or lake. In both frostnip and immersion foot, the skin is pale (blanched) and cold to the touch; normal color does not return after palpation of the skin. In some cases, the skin of the foot will be wrinkled, but it can also remain soft. The patient reports loss of feeling and sensation in the affected area.

Frostbite. Frostbite is the most serious local cold injury because the tissues are actually frozen. Freezing permanently damages cells via one of two mechanisms: direct cellular damage or progressive dermal ischemia.[3,4] The presence of ice crystals within the cells may cause physical damage. The change in the water content in the cells may also cause changes in the concentration of critical electrolytes, producing permanent changes in the chemistry of the cell. When the ice thaws, further chemical changes occur in the cell, causing permanent damage or cell death, called gangrene Figure 34-6. If gangrene occurs, the dead tissue must be surgically removed, sometimes by amputation. Following less severe damage, the exposed part will become inflamed, tender to the touch, and unable to tolerate further exposure to cold.

Frostbite can be identified by the hard, waxy feel of the affected tissues Figure 34-7. The injured part feels firm to frozen as you gently touch it. If the frostbite is only skin deep, it will feel leathery or thick instead of hard. Blisters and swelling may be present. In light-skinned people with a deep injury that has thawed or partially thawed, the skin may appear red with purple and white areas, or it may be mottled and cyanotic.

As with a burn, the depth of skin damage will vary. With superficial frostbite, only the skin is frozen; with deep frostbite, the deeper tissues are frozen as well. You may not be able to tell superficial from deep frostbite in

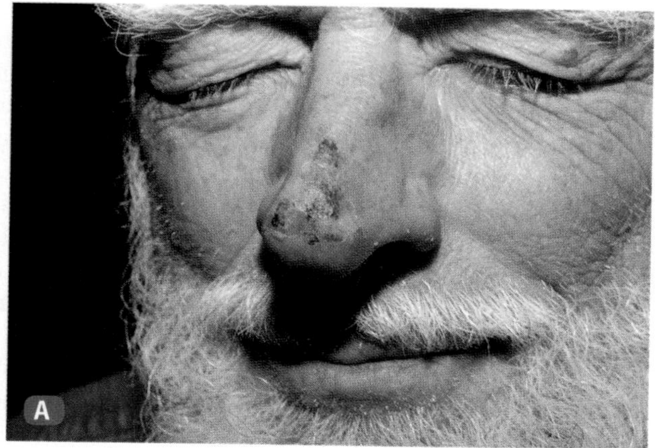

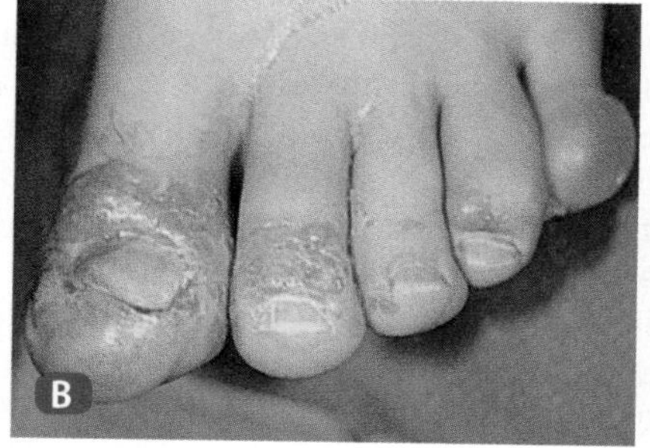

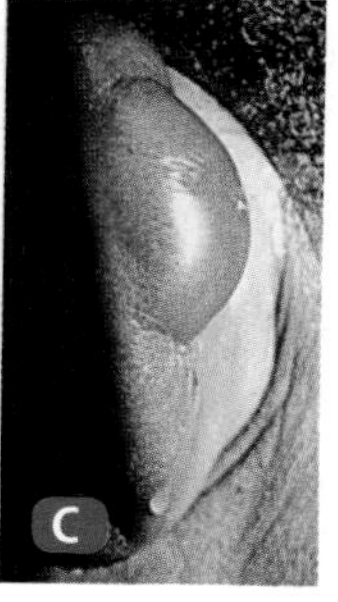

Figure 34-5 The tip of the nose **(A)**, the extremities **(B)**, and the ears **(C)** are particularly susceptible to frostbite.

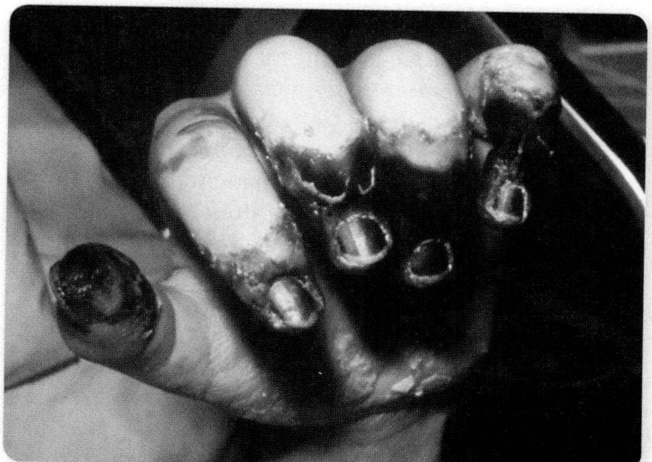

Figure 34-6 Gangrene, or permanent cell death, can occur when tissue is frozen and chemical changes occur in the cells.

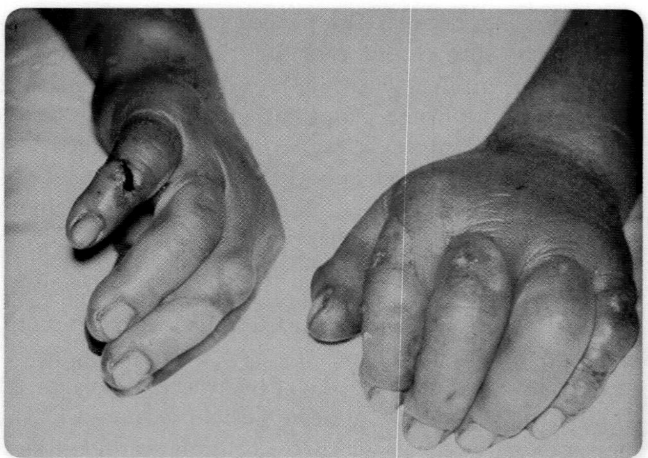

Figure 34-7 Frostbitten skin is hard and usually waxy to the touch.

the field. Even an experienced surgeon in a hospital setting may not be able to tell until several days have passed.

Assessment of Cold Injuries

Management of hypothermia in the field, regardless of the severity of the exposure, consists of stabilizing the ABCs (airway, breathing, and circulation) and preventing further heat loss. All patients who are injured are at risk for hypothermia. Keep this in mind when you are evaluating a patient with multiple injuries.

Scene Size-up

Typically, your scene assessment begins with information provided by dispatch and consideration of the environmental conditions. Air temperature, wind chill, and whether it is wet or dry are important aspects of scene size-up and will likely affect the patient.

Ensure that the scene is safe for you and other responders. Identify potential safety hazards, such as wet grass, mud, snow, or icy streets. Consider special hazards such as avalanches. Cold environments may present special problems both for you and your patient. Use appropriate standard precautions including dressing appropriately for the weather, and consider the number of patients you may have. Summon additional help, such as a search-and-rescue team, as quickly as possible.

As you observe the scene, look for indicators of the mechanism of injury (MOI). This helps you develop an early index of suspicion for underlying injuries in the patient who has sustained a significant MOI. For example, if you find a vehicle in a secluded ditch off the highway and the vehicle's roof and hood are covered with fresh snow, then you may assume that the patient was in a motor vehicle crash and has been exposed to the cold for a long period. Or the cause may be unrelated to trauma—for example, when a person becomes lost and is stranded overnight.

Primary Survey

In a cold emergency, your patient's chief complaint may be only that he or she is cold, or the cold may complicate an existing medical condition or injury. Perform a rapid full-body scan to determine whether a life threat exists, and if so, treat it. If the chief complaint is simply being cold, quickly assess the patient's core temperature by placing the back of your hand on the abdomen. Evaluate the patient's mental status quickly using the AVPU scale (*Alert* to person, place, and day; responsive to *Verbal* stimuli; responsive to *Pain*; *Unresponsive*). An altered mental status can indicate the intensity of the cold injury.

Your assessment should take into account the physiologic changes that occur as a result of hypothermia. If you believe the patient is in cardiac arrest, proceed directly to the circulation ("C") step by providing high-quality chest compressions, and address airway and breathing ("A and B") afterward. If you cannot feel a radial pulse, gently palpate for a carotid pulse, and wait for up to 60 seconds before you decide that the patient is pulseless. Some physicians disagree about performing cardiopulmonary resuscitation (CPR) on a patient with hypothermia who appears to be pulseless. Such a patient actually may be in a kind of metabolic ice box, having achieved a metabolic balance that CPR may disrupt; therefore, some recommend that CPR may be delayed or suspended in severe hypothermia to allow for evacuation of the patient from the place where he or she was found.[5] Even a pulse rate of 1 or 2 beats/min indicates cardiac activity, and cardiac activity may spontaneously recover after the body core is warmed. However, CPR, when performed correctly, will increase blood flow to the critical parts of the body. For this reason, some authorities recommend starting CPR on a patient with hypothermia and no pulse. The American Heart Association recommends that CPR be started if the patient has no detectable pulse or breathing.[6] Again, for a patient with hypothermia, this may require a prolonged pulse check of up to 60 seconds.

Perfusion will be compromised based on the severity of the cold exposure. Your assessment of the patient's skin will not be helpful in determining shock. Assume that shock is present and treat it appropriately. Bleeding may be difficult to find because of the slow-moving circulation and thick clothing. If the scene size-up, MOI, or chief complaint suggests the potential for bleeding, look for it.

After immediate circulation concerns are addressed, ensure that the patient has an adequate airway and is breathing. If your patient's breathing is slow or shallow, ventilation with a bag-mask device may be necessary. Use warmed and humidified oxygen if it is available because it helps to warm the patient from the inside out.

Words of Wisdom

Oxygen may be warmed or cooled by taping hot packs or cold packs to the oxygen tubing, respectively. This will also work for intravenous (IV) fluids.

Even mild hypothermia can have serious consequences and complications, including cardiac dysrhythmias and blood clotting abnormalities. Therefore, all patients with hypothermia require immediate transport for evaluation and treatment. Assess the scene for the safest way to quickly move your patient from the cold environment. As you package your patient for transport, work quickly, safely, and gently. Gentle transportation is necessary. Rough handling of a patient with hypothermia may cause a cold, slow, weak heart to fibrillate and the patient to lose any pulse that may have existed; exertion can also trigger dysrhythmia in a cold heart. Transport the patient with the head level or slightly down. Always transport to the closest appropriate facility. Call in your radio report as soon as possible to allow time for the receiving facility to prepare for the patient. The availability of cardiac bypass rewarming capabilities would be preferable in considering the destination. If transportation is delayed, protect the patient from further heat loss.

Words of Wisdom

Handle patients with hypothermia *very gently*. Excessive movement increases the risk of inducing ventricular fibrillation.

History Taking

After the life threats have been managed during the primary survey, investigate the chief complaint. Obtain a medical history, and be alert for injury-specific signs and symptoms as well as any pertinent negatives.

Obtaining a patient's history in these situations may be difficult. If possible, determine the duration of the exposure, the temperature to which the body part was exposed, and the wind velocity during exposure, either from the patient or bystanders. These are important factors in determining the severity of a local cold injury. Exposures may be acute (such as a demented patient who wandered out into the cold) or chronic (as in the case of a homeless person living on the street). Your SAMPLE history (Signs and symptoms, Allergies, Medications, Pertinent past medical history, Last oral intake, Events leading up to the illness or injury) can provide important information affecting both your treatment in the field and the treatment your patient will receive in the hospital. Medications your patient has taken, alcoholic beverages your patient has consumed, and underlying medical conditions may have an effect on the way cold affects the patient's metabolism. The patient's last oral intake and activity prior to the exposure will help to determine the severity of the cold injury.

You should also investigate several underlying factors:

- Exposure to wet conditions
- Inadequate insulation from cold or wind
- Restricted circulation from tight clothing or shoes or circulatory disease
- Fatigue
- Inadequate nutrition
- Alcohol or drug abuse
- Hypothermia
- Diabetes
- Cardiovascular disease
- Age

Secondary Assessment

Use the secondary assessment to uncover injuries that may have been missed during the primary survey. In some instances, such as a critically injured patient or a short transport time, you may not have time to conduct a secondary assessment.

Focus your physical examination on the severity of hypothermia, assessing the areas of the body directly affected by cold exposure, and the degree of damage. Is the whole body cold (hypothermia) or just isolated parts (frostbite)? These determinations will have important consequences for your treatment decisions. For example, shivering indicates a protective mechanism to produce more heat because the body is cold. When shivering stops and the patient remains in a cold environment, the cold injury is more severe.

Determine the degree and extent of cold injury, as well as any other injuries or conditions that may not have been initially detected. The numbing effect of cold, both on the brain and on the body, may impair your patient's ability to tell you about other injuries or illnesses. Therefore, a careful examination of your patient's entire body, with special attention to skin temperatures, textures, and **turgor**, will help you avoid missing important clues to your patient's condition.

Keep in mind that vital signs may be altered by the effects of hypothermia and can be an indicator of its severity. Respirations may be slow and shallow, resulting in low oxygen levels in the body. Low blood pressure and a slow pulse also indicate moderate to severe hypothermia. Carefully evaluate your patient for changes in mental status.

Determine a core body temperature using a hypothermia thermometer based on local protocol. Pulse oximetry will often be inaccurate because of the lack of perfusion in the extremities.

Reassessment

Repeat the primary survey. Reassess vital signs and the chief complaint. Review all treatments that have been performed. Has the patient's condition improved with the interventions? Identify and treat changes in the patient's condition. Keep a close eye on your patient's level of consciousness and vital signs. As the body rewarms, the sudden redistribution of fluids and the release of built-up chemicals can have harmful effects, including cardiac dysrhythmias. Be vigilant and monitor your patient closely, even if his or her condition appears to be improving.

Communicate all information you have gathered to the receiving facility, which may be essential in evaluating and treating your patient in the hospital. Your documentation should always include the patient's physical status, the conditions at the scene, information gathered from bystanders, and any changes in the patient's mental status during treatment and transport.

Words of Wisdom

Recording specific results of your early assessment is particularly valuable when the patient has hypothermia. If there is a question regarding the initiation of CPR, note the anatomic location where you checked the pulse and for how long you checked it. Also note the initial body temperature and the anatomic location where it was taken. These points will be important to hospital staff and will help protect you if medicolegal issues ever arise.

Emergency Medical Care for Cold Emergencies

The following are general steps to take promptly to prevent further cold injury:

1. Remove wet clothing, and keep the patient dry.
2. Prevent conduction heat loss. Move the patient away from any wet or cold surfaces, such as a car frame.
3. Insulate all exposed body parts, especially the head, by wrapping them in a blanket or any other available dry, bulky material.
4. Prevent convection heat loss by erecting a wind barrier around the patient.
5. Remove the patient from the cold environment as promptly as possible.

Figure 34-8 illustrates recommendations for prehospital care of a hypothermic patient.

In most cases, you should move the patient from the cold environment to prevent further heat loss. To prevent further damage to the feet, do not allow the patient to walk. Provide for a warm environment by removing any wet or frozen clothing. Do not remove any clothing frozen to the patient's skin. Place dry blankets over and under the patient Figure 34-9.

If available, give the patient warm, humidified oxygen. In a cold-related emergency, depending on your local and state protocols, your treatment may only include oxygen delivery (warmed and humidified if possible).

Obtain IV access, but follow local protocols for administering fluid to a patient with hypothermia. When possible,

YOU are the Provider — PART 2

On approaching the patient, you find him to be responsive to deep, painful stimuli, breathing adequately at 14 breaths/min. You also note that his clothing is soaked from the snow, but he does not appear to be shivering. You ask the police officer if he can get your stretcher, and you ask your partner to turn up the heat all the way in the patient compartment while you perform a rapid assessment of the patient.

Recording Time: 1 Minute	
Appearance	Poor
Level of consciousness	Responsive to deep painful stimuli
Airway	Patent
Breathing	Nonlabored
Circulation	Cold

3. Discuss ways to increase heat in the body.
4. What stage of hypothermia does this patient present in?

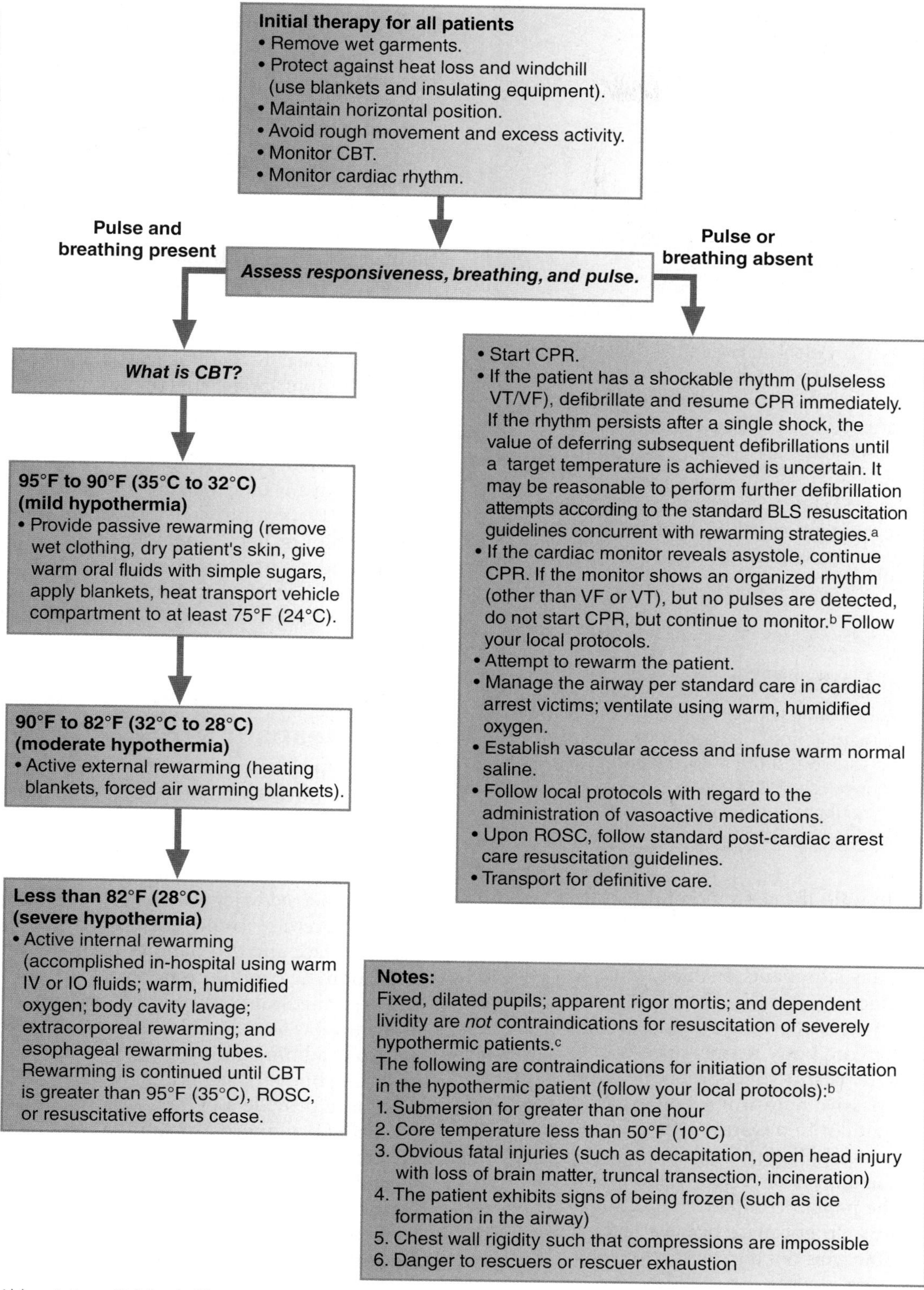

Initial therapy for all patients
• Remove wet garments.
• Protect against heat loss and windchill (use blankets and insulating equipment).
• Maintain horizontal position.
• Avoid rough movement and excess activity.
• Monitor CBT.
• Monitor cardiac rhythm.
Pulse and breathing present
Assess responsiveness, breathing, and pulse.
Pulse or breathing absent
What is CBT?
95°F to 90°F (35°C to 32°C) (mild hypothermia)
• Provide passive rewarming (remove wet clothing, dry patient's skin, give warm oral fluids with simple sugars, apply blankets, heat transport vehicle compartment to at least 75°F (24°C).
90°F to 82°F (32°C to 28°C) (moderate hypothermia)
• Active external rewarming (heating blankets, forced air warming blankets).
Less than 82°F (28°C) (severe hypothermia)
• Active internal rewarming (accomplished in-hospital using warm IV or IO fluids; warm, humidified oxygen; body cavity lavage; extracorporeal rewarming; and esophageal rewarming tubes. Rewarming is continued until CBT is greater than 95°F (35°C), ROSC, or resuscitative efforts cease.
• Start CPR.
• If the patient has a shockable rhythm (pulseless VT/VF), defibrillate and resume CPR immediately. If the rhythm persists after a single shock, the value of deferring subsequent defibrillations until a target temperature is achieved is uncertain. It may be reasonable to perform further defibrillation attempts according to the standard BLS resuscitation guidelines concurrent with rewarming strategies.[a]
• If the cardiac monitor reveals asystole, continue CPR. If the monitor shows an organized rhythm (other than VF or VT), but no pulses are detected, do not start CPR, but continue to monitor.[b] Follow your local protocols.
• Attempt to rewarm the patient.
• Manage the airway per standard care in cardiac arrest victims; ventilate using warm, humidified oxygen.
• Establish vascular access and infuse warm normal saline.
• Follow local protocols with regard to the administration of vasoactive medications.
• Upon ROSC, follow standard post-cardiac arrest care resuscitation guidelines.
• Transport for definitive care.
Notes:
Fixed, dilated pupils; apparent rigor mortis; and dependent lividity are not contraindications for resuscitation of severely hypothermic patients.[c]
The following are contraindications for initiation of resuscitation in the hypothermic patient (follow your local protocols):[b]
1. Submersion for greater than one hour
2. Core temperature less than 50°F (10°C)
3. Obvious fatal injuries (such as decapitation, open head injury with loss of brain matter, truncal transection, incineration)
4. The patient exhibits signs of being frozen (such as ice formation in the airway)
5. Chest wall rigidity such that compressions are impossible
6. Danger to rescuers or rescuer exhaustion
Abbreviations: BLS, basic life support; CBT, core body temperature; CPR, cardiopulmonary resuscitation; IO, intraosseous; IV, intravenous; ROSC, return of spontaneous circulation; VF, ventricular fibrillation; VT, ventricular tachycardia

Figure 34-8 Prehospital hypothermia treatment algorithm. Note that some of the items in the algorithm, such as cardiac monitoring and administration of vasoactive medications, are performed at the paramedic level but not by AEMTs.

Data from: [a]Web-based Integrated 2010 & 2015 American Heart Association Guidelines for Cardiopulmonary Resuscitation and Emergency Cardiovascular Care. Part 10: special circumstances of resuscitation. © 2015 American Heart Association. https://eccguidelines.heart.org/index.php/circulation/cpr-ecc-guidelines-2/part-10-special-circumstances-of-resuscitation/. Accessed May 4, 2017.
[b]Hypothermia. In: National Model EMS Clinical Guidelines. National Association of State EMS Officials. V.08-16. https://www.nasemso.org/Projects/ModelEMSClinicalGuidelines/index.asp. Accessed May 4, 2017.
[c]Zafren K, Giesbrecht GG, Danzl DF, et al. Wilderness Medical Society practice guidelines for the out-of-hospital evaluation and treatment of accidental hypothermia: 2014 update. *Wilderness Environ Med.* 2014;25(suppl 4):S66-S85.

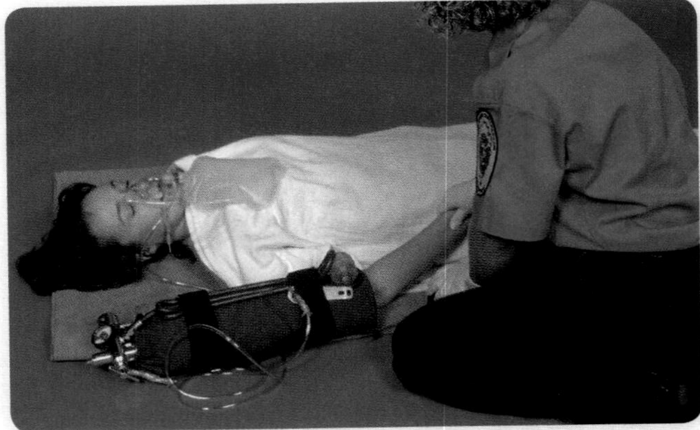

Figure 34-9 Place dry blankets over and under the patient with hypothermia; give warm, humidified oxygen, if available; assess the pulse for up to 60 seconds before considering cardiopulmonary resuscitation.

administer fluid that has been warmed so as not to further lower the core temperature. Also, check the blood glucose levels of any patient with an altered mental status or a history of diabetes.

Words of Wisdom

IV fluids may be warmed by placing them over a defroster or hanging them in front of a heater vent. If fluids are warmed, be sure to test the temperature (eg, run the fluid over your inner wrist like you would a baby's bottle) before infusing them into a patient.

Always handle the patient gently so that you do not cause any pain or further injury to the skin. Do not massage the extremities. Do not allow the patient to eat or to use any stimulants, such as coffee, tea, cola, or tobacco products.

If the patient is alert, shivering, responds appropriately, and the core body temperature is between 90°F and 95°F (32.2°C and 35°C), then the hypothermia is mild. Begin passive rewarming slowly, which includes placing the patient in a warm environment, removing wet clothing, and applying heat packs or hot water bottles to the groin, axillary, and cervical regions. Turn the heat up high in the patient compartment of the ambulance. To avoid burns, do not place heat packs directly on the skin. If possible, you can give warm fluids by mouth, as allowed by local protocols, assuming that the patient is alert and can swallow without difficulty.

Words of Wisdom

Never place hot or cold packs directly against the patient's skin. Always wrap them in a towel or cloth to prevent burning or freezing the skin, respectively.

When the patient has moderate or severe hypothermia, active rewarming is best accomplished in the emergency department (ED) utilizing aggressive strategies to introduce heat to the body's core. Such therapies might include lavage with warm fluids and rewarming blood outside the body before reintroducing it (extracorporeal rewarming). In general, rewarming should occur rapidly; however, rewarming the patient too quickly may cause a fatal cardiac dysrhythmia or other substantial complications. Also, rewarming extremities too rapidly without rewarming the core can cause vasodilation, leading to return of cold blood from the limbs and causing further cooling of the core. For this reason, local protocols may dictate the appropriate type of rewarming strategy based on the patient's body temperature.

If you cannot get the patient out of the cold immediately, move the patient out of the wind and away from contact with any object that will conduct heat away from the body. Place a protective cover on the patient and beneath him or her. Remember that most body heat is lost around the head and neck.

Regardless of the nature or severity of the cold injury, remember that even an unresponsive patient may be able to hear you.

▶ Withholding and Cessation of Resuscitative Efforts

In the field, patients with obviously lethal traumatic injuries or those so solidly frozen as to block the airway or chest compression efforts generally are dead. If submersion preceded the arrest, then successful resuscitation is unlikely, with the possible exception of people who have been submerged in icy waters. Trauma, alcohol overdose, and drug overdose could have resulted in hypothermia in the first place and can hamper resuscitation efforts. Try to factor these conditions into your treatment decisions, and seek medical control input. For example, a heroin user who was found outdoors and quickly recovers after naloxone administration requires a full set of vital signs, including body temperature.

Some providers believe that patients who appear dead after prolonged exposure to cold temperatures are not dead until "warm and dead." The effects of hypothermia may essentially protect the brain and organs if hypothermia develops quickly, a fact that is being used to successfully treat some cardiac arrest patients. Sometimes it may be impossible to know which came first—a cardiac arrest and then hypothermia or vice versa. In those situations, it is prudent to attempt resuscitation. Although a cutoff of 50°F (10°C) for possible survival of accidental hypothermia has been proposed, no compelling evidence or consensus exists that there is any single reasonable temperature below which a human cannot survive. However, there are clear physiologic signs that indicate a patient is "cold and dead" with no chance of resuscitation. The Wilderness Medical Society includes in such criteria obvious fatal injuries (such as decapitation, open head injuries with loss of brain matter, truncal transection, incineration) or a chest wall that is so stiff that compressions are not possible. It is worth noting that, according to the 2014 WMS practice guidelines, fixed, dilated pupils, apparent rigor mortis, and dependent lividity are *not* contraindications for resuscitation of severely hypothermic patients. Follow your local protocols regarding resuscitation.

▶ Emergency Medical Care of Local Cold Injuries

The emergency treatment of local cold injuries in the field should include the following steps:

1. Remove the patient from further exposure to the cold.
2. Handle the injured part gently, and protect it from further injury.
3. Administer oxygen, if this was not already done during the primary survey.
4. Remove any wet or restrictive clothing over the injured part.

If there is no chance of reinjury or if transport to the ED will be substantially delayed, consider active rewarming if local protocols allow, or contact medical control for direction. With frostnip, contact with a warm object may be all the patient needs; you can use your hands, your breath, or the patient's own body. During rewarming, the affected part will often tingle and become red in light-skinned people. With immersion foot, remove wet shoes, boots, and socks, and rewarm the foot gradually, protecting it from further cold exposure. Next, splint the extremity, and cover it loosely with a dry, sterile dressing. Never rub injured tissues, which could cause further damage. Do not reexpose the injury to the cold.

With a late or deep cold injury, such as frostbite, remove any jewelry or other potentially restrictive items from the injured part, and cover the injury loosely with a dry, sterile dressing. Do not break blisters or rub or massage the area. Do not apply heat or rewarm the part. Unlike frostnip and trench foot, rewarming of the frostbitten extremity is best accomplished under controlled circumstances in the ED. You can cause further injury to fragile tissues by attempting to rewarm a frostbitten part. Never apply something warm or hot, such as the exhaust from the ambulance engine or, even worse, an open flame. Do not allow the patient to stand or walk on a frostbitten foot. Splinting a frostbitten extremity may also help prevent secondary injury by limiting use.

Evaluate the patient's general condition for the signs or symptoms of systemic hypothermia. Support the vital functions as necessary, and transport the patient promptly to the hospital.

If prompt hospital care is unavailable and medical control instructs you to institute rewarming in the field, use a warm-water bath. Immerse the frostbitten part in water with a temperature between 102°F and 104°F (38.9°C and 40°C). Check the water temperature with a thermometer before immersing the limb, and recheck it frequently during the rewarming process. The water temperature should never exceed 105°F (40.6°C). Stir the water continuously. Ensure the frostbitten part does not rest against the side of the warm container. Keep the frostbitten part in the water until it feels warm and sensation has returned to the skin. Dress the area with dry, sterile dressings, placing them also between injured fingers or toes. Expect the patient to report severe pain. You may consider administering nitrous oxide or calling for paramedic backup to administer analgesics.

Never attempt rewarming if there is any chance that the part may freeze again before the patient reaches the hospital. Some of the most severe consequences of frostbite, including gangrene and amputation, have occurred when parts were thawed and then refrozen.

Cover the frostbitten part with soft, padded, sterile cotton dressings. If blisters have formed, do not break them. Remember, you cannot accurately predict the outcome of a case of frostbite early in its course. Even body parts that appear gangrenous may recover following proper emergency and hospital treatment.

Cold Exposure and You

As an AEMT, you are also at risk for hypothermia if you work in a cold environment. If cold-weather search-and-rescue operations are a possibility in your assigned areas, you should receive survival training and precautionary tips. You should be thoroughly familiar with local conditions. Be aware of existing and potential weather conditions, and stay abreast of changes that are forecast for the area. Make sure to wear proper clothing whenever appropriate. Your vehicle, too, must be properly equipped and maintained for a cold environment. As with so many hazards, you cannot help others if you do not practice self-protection. Never allow yourself to become a casualty!

Safety

Do not become a victim! You cannot help others if you do not protect yourself.

Heat Exposure

Normal body temperature is 98.6°F (37°C). Complicated regulatory mechanisms keep this internal temperature constant, regardless of the ambient temperature. In a hot environment or during vigorous physical activity, when the body itself produces excess heat, it will try to rid itself of the excess heat. The body does this by a process known as thermolysis. The two most efficient methods to decrease heat are sweating (and evaporation of the sweat) and dilation of peripheral blood vessels, which brings warm blood to the skin's surface (causing flushing) to increase the rate of heat radiation. In addition, of course, the person who becomes overheated can remove clothing and seek a cooler environment.

Ordinarily, the heat-regulating mechanisms of the body work very well, and people are able to tolerate substantial temperature changes. When the body is exposed to or generates more heat energy than it can lose because of inadequate thermolysis, hyperthermia can result. Hyperthermia is a high core temperature, usually 101 °F (38.3 °C) or higher.

▶ Pathophysiology

When the body's mechanisms to decrease body heat are overwhelmed and the body is unable to tolerate the excessive heat, illness develops. High air temperature can reduce the body's ability to lose heat by radiation; high humidity reduces the ability to lose heat through evaporation. Another contributing factor is vigorous exercise, during which the body can lose more than 1 L of sweat per hour, causing loss of fluid and electrolytes. Signs of thermolysis include diaphoresis, increased skin temperature, and flushing. Signs of severe heat illness include altered mentation and altered levels of consciousness. The patient may also present with signs of dehydration. Illness from heat exposure can cause the following problems:

- Heat cramps
- Heat exhaustion
- Heatstroke

All three forms of heat illness may be present in the same patient because untreated **heat exhaustion** may progress to heatstroke. Heatstroke is a life-threatening emergency.

Persons at greatest risk for heat illnesses are children; geriatric patients; people with heart disease, chronic obstructive pulmonary disease (COPD), diabetes, dehydration, and obesity; and people with limited mobility. The autonomic neuropathy in diabetes interferes with vasodilation and perspiration and may interfere with thermoregulatory input, predisposing people with diabetes to heat illnesses. Older people, newborns, and infants exhibit poor thermoregulation. Alcohol and certain drugs, including medications that dehydrate the body (such as diuretics) or decrease the ability of the body to sweat (such as antihistamines), also make a person more susceptible to heat illnesses.

Other contributing factors to heat illnesses include the length of exposure, intensity of exposure, and the environment itself. Ambient environmental conditions, such as humidity and wind, have a major role as well. This also includes indoor conditions.

Preventive measures to protect from heat emergencies include maintaining an adequate fluid intake, acclimatizing to the environment, and limiting exposure. Thirst is not an adequate indicator of dehydration.[7] People working outside in high temperatures should drink water continually to replace what is lost through perspiration. In addition, the body adapts to the environment by excreting less sodium through perspiration, although continued exposure to air conditioning blunts the body's adaptation response.[7] This sodium retention increases fluid volume in the body and decreases the chances of dehydration. Spending time outdoors in the early morning or late evening when temperatures and humidity are lower, as opposed to the middle of the day, can also decrease a patient's risk.

Words of Wisdom

Keeping yourself hydrated while on duty is very important, especially during periods of heavy exertion or when working in the heat. Drink at least 3 L of water per day and more when exertion or heat is involved. The color of urine (usually darker with dehydration) and frequency of urination correlate directly with the body's fluid level.

The following subsections discuss the major types of heat illnesses Table 34-2.

Heat Cramps

Heat cramps are painful muscle spasms that occur after vigorous exercise. They do not occur only when it is hot outdoors. They may be seen in factory workers and even well-conditioned athletes. A recent study of US college football players showed a twofold increase in sweat sodium losses in athletes susceptible to heat cramps.[8] The exact cause of heat cramps is not well understood. It is known that sweat produced during strenuous exercise, particularly in a warm environment, causes a change in the body's balance of electrolytes. The result may be a loss of essential electrolytes from the cells. Dehydration may also have a role in the development of muscle cramps. Large amounts of water can be lost from the body as a result of excessive sweating. This loss of water may affect muscles that are being stressed and cause them to spasm.

Heat cramps usually occur in the legs or abdominal muscles. When the abdominal muscles are involved, the pain and muscle spasm may be so severe that the patient appears to have an acute abdominal condition. If a patient with a sudden onset of abdominal cramps has been exercising vigorously in a hot environment, suspect heat cramps.

Heat Exhaustion

Heat exhaustion, also called heat prostration or heat collapse, is the most common illness caused by heat. It is the result of the body losing so much water and so many electrolytes through very heavy sweating that hypovolemia (fluid depletion) occurs. For sweating to be an effective

Table 34-2 Comparing Conditions Resulting From Heat Stress

Variable	Heat Cramps	Heat Exhaustion	Heatstroke
Pathophysiology	Sodium and water loss	Sodium and water loss, hypovolemia	Failure of heat-regulating mechanisms
Mental and neurologic status	Normal	Normal or mild confusion	Altered, delirium, seizures
Temperature	May be mildly elevated	Usually mildly elevated	Usually >104°F (40°C)
Skin	Cool, moist	Pale, cool, moist	Dry, hot, but sweating may persist, especially with exertional heatstroke
Muscle cramping	Severe	May or may not be present	Absent

cooling mechanism, the sweat must be able to evaporate from the body. People standing in the hot sun, particularly those wearing several layers of clothing, such as sports fans or parade watchers, may sweat profusely but experience little body cooling. High humidity will also decrease the amount of evaporation that can occur.

People working or exerting themselves in poorly ventilated areas are unable to release heat through convection. Thus, people who work or exercise vigorously and those who wear heavy clothing in a warm, humid, or poorly ventilated environment are particularly susceptible to heat exhaustion.

The signs and symptoms of heat exhaustion and those of associated hypovolemia are as follows:

- Onset while working vigorously or exercising in a hot, humid, or poorly ventilated environment and sweating heavily.
- Onset, even at rest, in the older and infant age groups in hot, humid, and poorly ventilated environments or extended time in hot, humid environments. People who are not acclimatized to the environment may also experience onset at rest.
- Cold, clammy skin with ashen pallor.
- Dry tongue and thirst.
- Dizziness, weakness, or faintness, with accompanying nausea or headache. Muscle cramping may also be present, including abdominal cramping.
- Normal vital signs, although the pulse is often rapid and the blood pressure may be low.
- Normal or slightly elevated body temperature; on rare occasions, as high as 104°F (40°C).

In heat exhaustion, there may be a subtle increase in core body temperature with some neurologic deficit. Symptoms may be solely a result of dehydration combined with overexertion. The result is orthostatic hypotension. Symptoms generally resolve with rest and supine positioning. Fluids and elevation of the legs are also beneficial. Symptoms that do not resolve with rest and positioning may be a result of the increased core body temperature and are predictive of impending heatstroke and must be treated aggressively.

Heatstroke

Heatstroke, the least common but most serious illness caused by heat exposure, occurs when the body is subjected to more heat than it can effectively remove, and normal mechanisms for getting rid of the excess heat are overwhelmed. The body temperature then rises rapidly to the level at which tissues are destroyed, with substantial neurologic deficit. Organ damage occurs in the brain, liver, and kidneys. Heatstroke is a profound emergency, with mortality rates as high as 10% in patients who receive timely treatment and 30% to 80% in patients who are untreated or who receive delayed treatment.[9]

Heatstroke can develop in patients during vigorous physical activity or when they are outdoors or in a closed, poorly ventilated, humid space. It also occurs during heat waves among people (particularly older people) who live in buildings with no air conditioning or with poor ventilation. It may also develop in children who are left unattended in a locked car on a hot day.

Many patients with heatstroke have hot, dry, flushed skin because their sweating mechanism has been overwhelmed and they are severely dehydrated. However, early in the course of heatstroke, the skin may be moist or wet because of residual sweat from earlier perspiration. For this reason, do not rule out heatstroke if the patient's skin is still moist. Keep in mind that a patient can have heat stroke even if he or she is still sweating. This presentation is often seen in endurance athletes, military personnel, or emergency providers who wear personal protective equipment, such as firefighters, SWAT (special weapons and tactics) team members, or hazmat (hazardous materials) workers. The minute someone is detected to be having a heat injury, consider that other personnel wearing similar gear or performing similar duties are likely to also have heat injury. The body temperature rises rapidly in patients with heatstroke and can rise to 106 °F (41.1 °C) or higher. As the body core temperature rises, the patient's level of consciousness falls.

Often, the first sign of heatstroke is a change in behavior. However, the patient can quickly become unresponsive. Seizure activity may also be noted. The pulse is usually rapid and strong at first, but as the patient becomes increasingly unresponsive, the pulse becomes weaker and the blood pressure falls. The respiratory rate increases because the body is attempting to compensate. One of the telltale signs you should be acutely aware of is when your patient no longer perspires, which means the body has lost its thermoregulatory mechanism. If you are perspiring in the environment, your patient should also be perspiring.

Two types of heatstroke are distinguished: classic and exertional. Classic heatstroke commonly presents in people with chronic illnesses. There is an increased core body temperature because of deficient thermoregulatory function. Predisposing conditions include age, diabetes, and other medical conditions. Hot, red, dry skin is common in these patients. Exertional heatstroke commonly presents in people who are in good general health but have an increased core body temperature because of overwhelming heat stress, which may be caused by excessive ambient temperature, excessive exertion, prolonged exposure, or poor acclimatization. Moist, pale skin is common in these patients.

Recovery from heatstroke depends on the speed with which treatment is administered, so you must be able to identify this condition quickly. Emergency treatment has one objective: get the body temperature down to normal quickly and by any means available.

Assessment of Heat Injuries

Scene Size-up

As part of your scene size-up, perform an environmental assessment. How hot is it outside? How hot is it in the room where your patient is located? How well is the patient tolerating the heat? Dispatch may report the call initially as a medical or trauma emergency. The heat illness may only be secondary. Approach the scene looking for hazards as well as clues as to what may have caused your patient's emergency. If you anticipate a prolonged scene time, protect yourself from the heat and remember to stay hydrated. Use appropriate standard precautions. Long-sleeved shirts and long pants may be uncomfortable in warm weather; however, they can help protect you from being splashed by blood or other fluids.

As you observe the scene, look for indicators of the MOI. For example, you arrive on the scene at a shopping mall to find an older man with a decreased level of consciousness inside a parked vehicle on a warm, humid, sunny day. The MOI for this patient is sitting in a warm environment under direct sunlight with no ventilation.

Heat emergencies commonly occur in the context of athletic events and practices, often with athletic trainers present. In those instances, you may find the patient submerged in a cold-water immersion bath inside the athletic training room. It is harmful to allow heat to persist for any amount of time; therefore, cooling prior to transport is indicated if facilities such as an ice bath are available. If the patient is placed in a cold-water immersion bath on your arrival, monitor the patient in the water, and assist as necessary. Do not remove the patient until the temperature has normalized to the appropriate level, between 101 °F and 102 °F (38.3 °C and 38.9 °C). Do not overcool the patient. Overcooling can result in shivering, which generates more heat. Monitor the patient closely. While you wait, consider consulting medical control or calling for paramedic intercept or backup as these patients are prone to cardiac dysrhythmias and may benefit from cardiac monitoring.

Primary Survey

As you approach your patient, observe how the patient interacts with you and the environment. A heat illness may be the primary problem or it may simply be aggravating a medical or trauma condition. Remember, prolonged heat exposure may stress the heart, causing a heart attack. Use this initial interaction to guide you in assessing for immediate life threats and related problems. Perform a rapid full-body scan, and avoid tunnel vision.

Assess the patient's mental status using the AVPU scale. Gathering clues about his or her mental status may identify the severity of your patient's condition. The more altered the patient's mental status is, the more serious the heat problem.

Assess the patient's airway and breathing, and treat any life threats, such as exsanguinating hemorrhage. Unless the patient is unresponsive, the airway should be patent. Nausea and vomiting, however, may occur. Position the patient to protect the airway as necessary. If the patient is unresponsive, be cautious how you open the airway; consider spinal precautions if trauma is a possibility. Breathing will be fast, depending on the patient's core temperature, but should otherwise be adequate. Providing oxygen to the patient will assist with the perfusion of body tissues and may decrease nausea. If your patient is unresponsive, insert an airway and provide bag-mask device ventilations according to protocol. Call early for paramedic backup if you feel a more definitive airway is needed.

Assess the patient's circulation by palpating a pulse and feeling the skin. If the pulse is adequate, assess the patient for perfusion and bleeding. Assess the patient's

Table 34-3 Skin Condition	
Skin Condition	**Indicates**
Moist, pale, cool skin	Excessive fluid and salt loss
Hot, dry skin	Body is unable to regulate core temperature
Hot, moist skin	Body is unable to regulate core temperature

skin condition carefully Table 34-3. Treat the patient aggressively for shock by removing the patient from the heat and positioning the patient as dictated by local protocol to improve circulation. If the patient is bleeding, bandage according to protocol.

If your patient has any signs of heatstroke (high temperature; red, dry skin; altered mental status; tachycardia; poor perfusion), then transport without delay to the closest appropriate facility, but begin aggressive cooling en route using whatever means are at your disposal.

History Taking

After the life threats have been managed during the primary survey, investigate the chief complaint. Obtain a medical history, and be alert for specific signs and symptoms such as the absence of perspiration, decreased level of consciousness, confusion, muscle cramping, nausea, and vomiting. Obtaining a thorough patient history of the present illness can help differentiate between a fever and a heat emergency.

Obtain a SAMPLE history, noting any activities, conditions, or medications that may predispose a patient to dehydration or heat-related problems. Patients with inadequate oral intake or who are taking diuretics may have difficulty tolerating exposure to heat. Many medications used by geriatric patients affect how well they tolerate heat. Be thorough in your questioning. Determine your patient's exposure to heat and humidity and activities prior to the onset of symptoms.

Secondary Assessment

As always, use the secondary assessment to uncover injuries that may have been missed during the primary survey, and remember that you may not have time to conduct a secondary assessment in critical patients.

If your patient is unresponsive, perform a physical examination of the entire body looking for problems or explanations of what is wrong. Obtain the patient's vital signs, including a blood glucose level, to help understand the severity of the emergency.

If the patient is alert, perform a focused assessment. Exposure to heat has substantial effects on the metabolism, muscles, and cardiovascular system. Assess the patient for muscle cramps or confusion. Examine the patient's mental status, and obtain the patient's vital signs.

Pay special attention to the patient's skin temperature, turgor, and level of moisture. Skin turgor is the ability of the skin to resist deformation. It is tested by gently pinching skin on the forearm or back of the hand; in older patients, the abdomen or chest are better locations to test. Normally the skin will quickly flatten out. If the patient is dehydrated, the skin will remain tented (poor skin turgor). Also, perform a careful neurologic examination.

Special Populations

When testing skin turgor of an older patient, remember to gently pinch the skin on the trunk of the body because the extremities normally have poor turgor.

Patients with hyperthermia will often be tachycardic and tachypneic. As long as they maintain a normal blood pressure, their bodies will compensate for the fluid loss. After their blood pressure begins to fall, it indicates they are no longer able to compensate for fluid loss and are going into shock. Your assessment of the patient's skin will help determine the severity of the emergency. For example, in heat exhaustion, the skin temperature may be normal or may even be cool and clammy; however, in heatstroke, the skin is hot.

Check the patient's temperature with a thermometer, depending on protocol. Your unit's equipment may include disposable or oral thermometers with disposable covers, or forehead scanning thermometers. Some agencies provide tympanic/ear thermometers. You may not use these devices routinely, so become familiar with how they work. Keep in mind that that oral temperature can be misleading if the patient just ingested a cool drink. In patients with a heat-related illness, monitoring of pulse oximetry is also indicated.

Reassessment

Watch your patient's condition carefully for deterioration. Any decline in level of consciousness is an ominous sign. Monitor the patient's vital signs at least every 5 minutes. Evaluate the effectiveness of your interventions. Be careful not to cause shivering when cooling down a patient who is experiencing a heat emergency. Shivering generates more heat and can occur when cooling is not monitored closely.

Inform the staff at the receiving facility early on that your patient is experiencing heatstroke because additional resources may be required. Document the weather conditions and the activities the patient was performing prior to the emergency in your patient care report.

Emergency Medical Care for Heat Emergencies

▶ Heat Cramps

Take the following steps to treat heat cramps in the field.

1. Promptly remove the patient from the hot environment, including direct sunlight, a source of radiant heat gain. Loosen any tight clothing.
2. Administer high-flow oxygen if indicated (the patient shows signs of hypoxia or respiratory distress) if this was not already done as part of the primary survey.
3. Rest the cramping muscles. Have the patient sit or lie down until the cramps subside.
4. Replace fluids by mouth if protocol allows. Use water or a diluted (half-strength) balanced electrolyte solution, such as a sports drink. In most cases, plain water is the most useful. Do not give salt tablets or solutions that have a high salt concentration. The patient already has an adequate amount of electrolytes circulating; they are just not distributed properly. With adequate rest and fluid replacement, the body will adjust the distribution of electrolytes, and the cramps will disappear.
5. Cool the patient with cool water spray or mist, and add convection to the cooling method by manually or mechanically fanning the patient.

When the heat cramps are gone, the patient may resume activity. For example, an athlete can return to play after the heat cramps have disappeared. However, heavy sweating may cause the cramps to recur. The best preventive and treatment strategy is hydration by drinking sufficient quantities of water.

If the cramps do not go away after these measures, initiate an IV line and transport the patient to the hospital. If you are uncertain that the patient's cramps were caused by the heat or you note anything out of the ordinary, contact medical control or transport the patient to the hospital.

▶ Heat Exhaustion

To treat the patient with heat exhaustion, follow the steps in Skill Drill 34-1. The treatment of heat exhaustion is aimed at removing the patient from exposure to heat and urgently reversing the increase in body temperature through active cooling efforts.

If an ice bath or similar facility is available, provide cold-water immersion to the patient if allowed per local protocol. Cold-water (ice bath) immersion is recommended for patients with a core temperature of 104°F (40°C) or an altered mental status.

Skill Drill 34-1 Treating for Heat Exhaustion

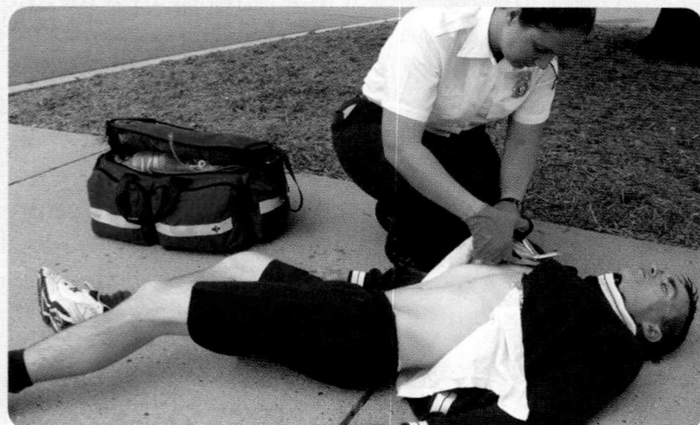

Step 1 Promptly remove the patient from the hot environment, preferably into the back of the air-conditioned ambulance. If outdoors, move out of direct sunlight. Remove any excessive layers of clothing, particularly around the head and neck.

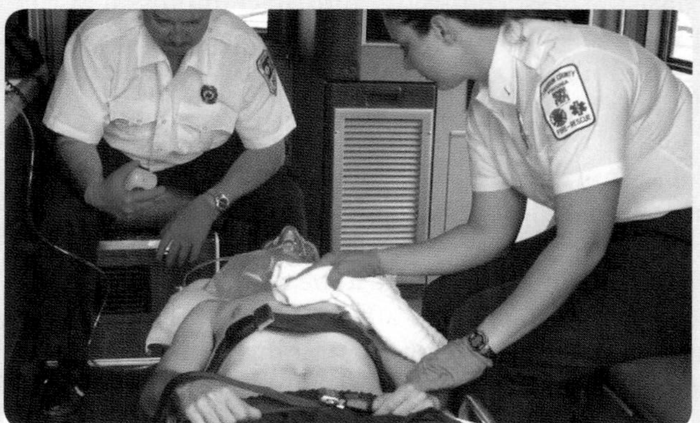

Step 2 Administer oxygen if indicated and if this was not already done as part of the primary survey. If the patient has an altered mental status, check the blood glucose level.

Cool the patient with misting and administration of ice packs to the trunk of the patient's body. Use an ice bath or similar facility if available, per local protocol. Encourage the patient to lie down. Loosen any tight clothing, and cool the patient by manually or mechanically fanning him or her.

Skill Drill 34-1 Treating for Heat Exhaustion *(continued)*

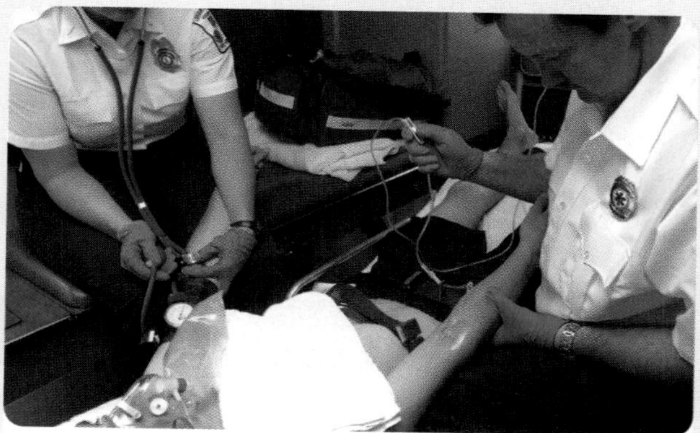

Step 3 If the patient is fully alert, encourage him or her to sit up and slowly drink up to 1 liter of water, as long as nausea does not develop. Never force fluids by mouth on a patient who is not fully alert, or allow drinking while supine, because the patient could aspirate the fluid into the lungs. If the patient does become nauseated, transport the patient on the left side to prevent aspiration.

Gain IV access, and administer normal saline fluid boluses of 20 mL/kg as needed if the patient is nauseated or unable to take fluid by mouth.

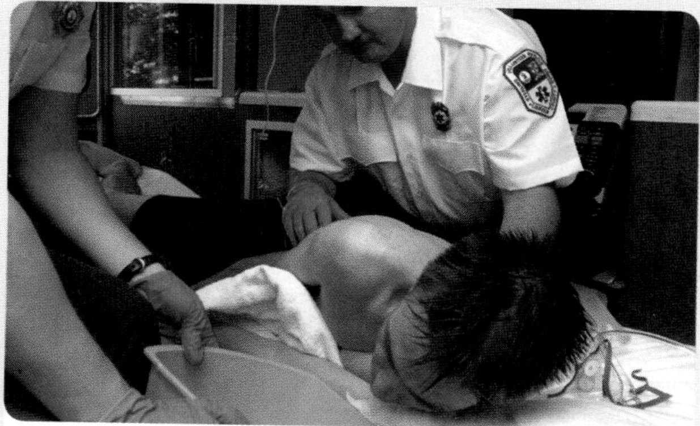

Step 4 Transport the patient on his or left her side if you think the patient may be nauseated, but make certain that the patient is secured.

In most cases, measures undertaken to cool the patient will reverse the symptoms, causing the patient to feel better within 30 minutes; however, you should prepare to transport the patient to the hospital for more aggressive treatment, especially in the following circumstances:

- The symptoms do not clear up promptly.
- The level of consciousness decreases.
- The body temperature remains elevated.
- The person is very young, older, or has any underlying medical condition, such as diabetes or cardiovascular disease.

▶ Heatstroke

Recovery from heatstroke depends on the speed with which treatment is administered, so you must be able to identify this patient quickly. As mentioned, the goal of emergency treatment is to lower the body temperature by any means available. Take the following steps when treating a patient with heatstroke:

1. Move the patient out of the hot environment and into the ambulance.
2. Set the air conditioning to maximum cooling.
3. Remove the patient's clothing.
4. Administer oxygen if indicated, if this was not already done as part of the primary survey. If needed, assist the patient's ventilations with a bag-mask device and appropriate airway adjuncts as per your protocol. Call for paramedic backup if a definitive airway is needed, but never delay transport to do so. Provide cold-water immersion in an ice bath, if possible. Cooling should begin immediately and continue en route to the hospital Figure 34-10. If it is not possible to cool en route and cold-water immersion is available at the scene, continue cold-water immersion at the scene until the core body temperature is between 101°F and 102°F (38.3°C and 38.9°C). This is the only time you should consider delaying transport for a patient with possible heatstroke. Consult medical control for advice in any instance where you are remaining on scene to provide active cooling for a patient with heatstroke prior to initiating transport.
5. Cover the patient with wet towels or sheets, or spray the patient with cool water and fan him or her to quickly evaporate the moisture on the skin.
6. Obtain IV access, and administer a 20-mL/kg bolus of an isotonic crystalloid solution, repeating as needed to maintain adequate perfusion and alleviate symptoms of dehydration.

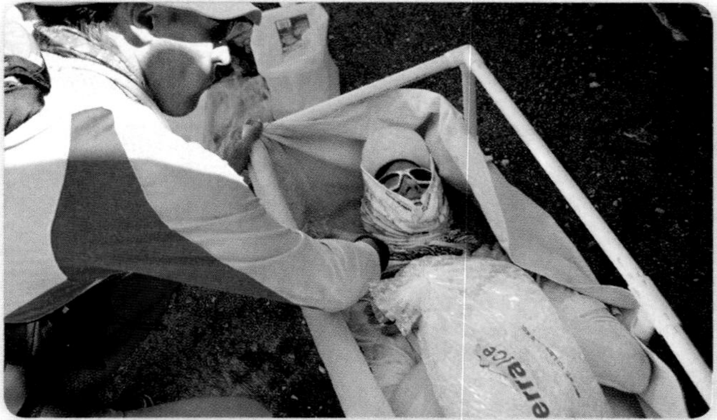

Figure 34-10 As part of the treatment of heatstroke, if consistent with local protocol, immerse the patient in an ice water bath if one is available.

7. Provide immediate transport to the hospital.
8. Notify the hospital as soon as possible so that the staff can prepare to treat the patient immediately on arrival.

Special Populations

Remember that the aging process alters the body's ability to compensate for its surroundings. Temperature-related emergencies can develop in older people over time, even in indoor environments that may not seem uncomfortable to you. Be vigilant for temperature-related illnesses.

Words of Wisdom

Do not cool a patient to the point of shivering, or you will increase rather than decrease the body temperature. Ice packs and cold-water immersion may produce reflex vasoconstriction and shivering because of the effect on peripheral thermoreceptors. Reflex hyperthermia results from overcooling, since shivering produces heat.

Water Emergencies

Drowning

Drowning is the process of experiencing respiratory impairment from **submersion** or immersion in liquid. Some agencies may still use the term *near drowning* to refer to a patient who survives, at least temporarily (24 hours), after suffocation in water or other liquids; the current term is *submersion*. Patients with submersion injury can die of secondary complications (such as pneumonia) that occur beyond 24 hours. According to the US Centers for Disease Control and Prevention (CDC), 46,419 drowning deaths were recorded between 1999 and 2010 in the United States, yielding an average of 3,868 deaths per year, or an average of approximately 10 deaths per day.[10] In the United States, drowning is the second leading cause of injury-related death among children younger than 15 years and is the leading cause of death in the age group 1 to 4 years, with 388 deaths

Special Populations

As a person ages, the body can lose the ability to respond to the environment. Older adults undergo changes in their ability to compensate for low or high ambient temperatures. For example, if the ambient temperature rises from 85°F to 94°F (29.5°C to 34.5°C), the older adult may not recognize the change or be able to compensate for it. Therefore, unless the person is accustomed to the heat, heatstroke can develop relatively quickly.

Shivering, a common effect of hypothermia, is the body's attempt to maintain heat. However, because of a decrease in muscle mass or tone, the hypothermic geriatric patient may not shiver. Furthermore, a decrease in muscle mass and body fat means that there is less insulation and protection from the cold. Because of the body's altered response to heat loss and its ability to gain heat, the health care provider might not suspect or report hypothermia. In caring for the geriatric patient in cold climates, be sure to protect the patient against unwanted heat loss. Cover all exposed areas with loose-fitting blankets. Pay particular attention to protecting the patient's head because heat loss from the head and neck is substantial.

Because of reduced circulation to the skin, heat loss via conduction, convection, and radiation is substantially lower. Additionally, the aging process alters the patient's ability to perspire; therefore, heat loss through evaporation is reduced. Because the older patient cannot disperse heat effectively, classic heatstroke can develop rapidly. Typically, the older adult will not go through an initial stage of heat exhaustion. During the summer, you should be acutely aware of the potential for heatstroke and factors that can predispose a patient to heat illness. Factors that increase the possibility of heatstroke include medications, diabetes, alcohol abuse, malnutrition, parkinsonism, hyperthyroidism, and obesity.

Both hypothermia and hyperthermia can appear in older patients in environmental settings that are subtle. These problems are commonly found when an older person has cost concerns about heating or cooling their home and thus keeps the heat turned down in the winter or does not use air conditioning in hot weather. Thermal emergencies can develop over time for older persons in these indoor urban environments that may not seem uncomfortable to you.

in 2014 alone.[11,12] Alcohol consumption, preexisting seizure disorders, geriatric patients with cardiovascular disease, and unsupervised access to water are among the major risk factors.

Drowning is often the last in a cycle of events caused by panic in the water. It can happen to anyone who is submerged in water for even a short time. Struggling toward the surface or the shore, the person becomes fatigued or exhausted, which leads him or her to sink even deeper. However, drowning also occurs in mop buckets, puddles, bathtubs, and other places where the person is not completely submerged. Small children can drown in only a few inches of water if left unattended.

Inhaling very small amounts of fresh or salt water can severely irritate the larynx, sending the muscles of the larynx and the vocal cords into spasm, called **laryngospasm**. The typical person experiences this to a mild degree when a small amount of a liquid is inhaled and the patient coughs and seems to be choking for a few seconds. This is the body's attempt at self-preservation because laryngospasm prevents more water from entering the lungs. In severe cases such as water submersion, however, the patient's lungs cannot be ventilated because substantial laryngospasm is present. Instead, progressive hypoxia occurs until the patient becomes unresponsive. At this point, the spasm relaxes, making rescue breathing possible. Of course, if the patient has not already been removed from the water, the patient may now inhale deeply, and more water may enter the lungs.

Hypothermia is also a major consideration in submersion. Heat loss is rapid, particularly if the patient is actively flailing about, which expends a lot of energy. However, hypothermia may also be beneficial. The body's **diving reflex**, discussed later, may actually slow metabolism to the point of protecting vital organs, such as the brain, heart, lungs, and kidneys. Hypoxia is always the first concern, but all submersion victims should be treated for hypothermia.

Words of Wisdom

All submersion patients should be transported for evaluation.

▶ Diving Emergencies

Most serious water-related injuries are associated with dives, with or without **SCUBA** (self-contained underwater breathing apparatus) gear. (SCUBA gear is a system that delivers air to the mouth and lungs at atmospheric pressures that increase with the depth of the dive.) Some of these injuries are related to the nature of the dive; others result from panic. Panic is not restricted to the person who is frightened by water. It can even happen to an experienced diver or swimmer.

There are more than 3.5 million recreational SCUBA divers in the United States, in addition to people engaged in diving for commercial and military purposes.[13] Medical emergencies relating to SCUBA diving techniques and equipment are becoming increasingly common.

General Pathophysiology: Physical Principles of Pressure Effects

Pressure, which is defined as force per unit area, may be expressed in several ways. The weight of air at sea level, for example, can be expressed as 14.7 pounds per square inch (psi), as 760 mm Hg, or as 1 atmosphere absolute (ATA). The latter system—measurement in ATA—is most commonly used in diving medicine. Because water is much denser than air, relatively small changes in depth produce large changes in pressure. For every 33 feet of seawater (fsw), the pressure increases 1 ATA. The depth of the dive can be used to estimate the pressure to which the diver was exposed: at sea level, the pressure is 1 ATA; at a depth of 33 fsw, the pressure is 2 ATA; at 66 fsw, it is 3 ATA; and so forth. Most SCUBA diving is done at depths between 30 and 60 fsw (2 to 3 ATA).

Liquids such as water are not compressible—that is, their volumes do not change with pressure. Because the body and its tissues are composed primarily of water, their volumes are not substantially affected by the pressure changes experienced in descent or ascent through water. Gas-filled organs are another matter, however, because gases are compressible and follow several physical laws:

- *Boyle's law* states that at a constant temperature, the volume of a gas is inversely proportional to its pressure (if you double the pressure on a gas, you halve its volume):

$$PV = k$$

where P = pressure, V = volume, and k = a constant. As a diver descends (and the pressure goes up), gas volume is reduced; as the diver ascends (pressure goes down), gas volume increases. As shown in **Figure 34-11**, this effect is most extreme near the water's surface. This law explains the **barotrauma** that can occur in gas-filled spaces in the body (including lungs, gastrointestinal tract, sinuses, and parts of the ear).

- *Dalton's law* deals with the pressures exerted by mixtures of different gases. Dalton's law states that each gas in mixture exerts the same partial pressure that it would exert if it were alone in the same volume and that the total pressure of a mixture of gases is the sum of the partial pressures of all gases in the mixture. Thus, for fresh air:

$$P_{total} = PO_2 + PCO_2 + PN_2$$

When total pressure increases, the partial pressure of each gas increases proportionally.

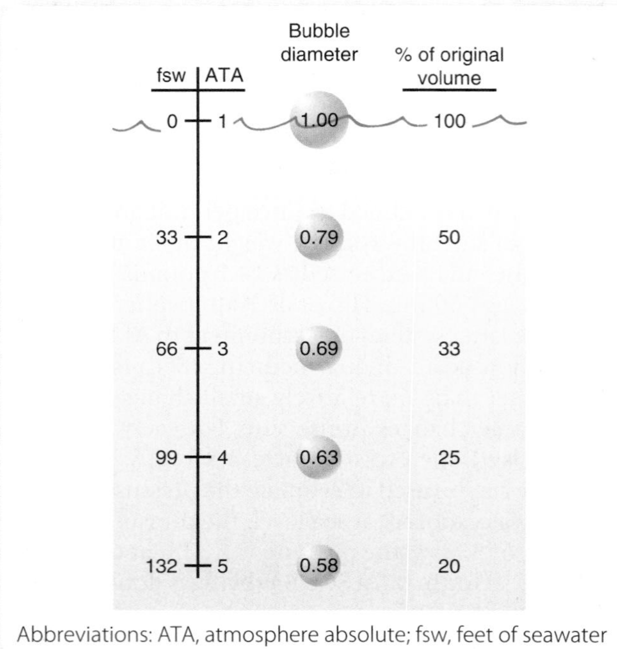

Figure 34-11 Boyle's law: As a bubble descends through water, its volume changes in inverse proportion to the ambient pressure.

This law helps explain nitrogen narcosis, oxygen toxicity, and the dangers of contamination in pressurized breathing systems. Because the relative percentage of each gas remains constant at different pressures, it also explains why pulse oximetry readings in divers with nitrogen narcosis remain unaffected.

- *Henry's law* states that the amount (concentration) of gas dissolved in a liquid is directly proportional to the partial pressure of the gas above the liquid:

$$P = kC$$

where P is partial pressure of the gas above the liquid, k is a constant, and C is concentration of gas in the liquid. A classic example of this law is when a sealed bottle that has dissolved carbon dioxide is opened. The opened bottle allows carbon dioxide to escape, lowering the partial pressure (P) of the gas. This forces the concentration of carbon dioxide in the soda to decrease as well, and the extra carbon dioxide escapes as bubbles. This law explains **decompression sickness** (the **bends**).

Fresh air is composed of about 79% nitrogen and 21% oxygen. Nitrogen is an inert fat-soluble gas (it prefers to dissolve in fatty or lipid-rich tissues including the nervous system). Nitrogen in the body follows the laws described above. Per Boyle's law, the volume of nitrogen decreases as pressure increases (during descent) and its volume increases as pressure decreases (during ascent), resulting in barotrauma. Per Dalton's law, the partial pressure of nitrogen increases as total pressure increases. Nitrogen at a high enough partial pressure becomes an anesthetic, resulting in nitrogen narcosis at depths of approximately 100 fsw.

Per Henry's law, as pressure decreases during ascent, nitrogen comes out of solution in the blood and may cause bubbles in tissue, resulting in decompression sickness, or the bends. Oxygen also follows these laws, and it can cause oxygen toxicity at depths via the same mechanism as nitrogen narcosis. However, because oxygen is taken up and metabolized by the body, oxygen does not contribute to decompression sickness. To avoid the problems listed above, commercial divers use a decompression schedule to allow gases time to equilibrate. Recreational divers usually adhere to a no-decompression limit (a table outlining safe times at various depths) so they do not have to decompress on surfacing. Use of enriched Nitrox gas, which is a gas with a lower nitrogen and a higher oxygen concentration, decreases the risk of nitrogen narcosis and decompression illness, but it increases the risk of oxygen toxicity. Dive tables and dive computers provide guidelines for divers regarding when to take decompression stops during the dive, but they are not perfect. Even if divers follow recommended tables or use the appropriate gas mixture, they may still be at risk for any type of diving injury.

Words of Wisdom

As a diver descends, the gases in the body take up less space, allowing for more gas within the body. As the diver ascends, the gas bubbles get larger, and, unless the diver continually breathes out to rid the lungs of the excess gas, gas-filled organs may rupture.

General Assessment: Diving History

It is important for you to obtain as many details as you can about the dive and the onset of the patient's symptoms. As you obtain the diving history, it is helpful to use a special form that records the following information:

- When did symptoms start (during ascent or descent)? Decompression sickness will usually manifest within the first hour of surfacing and usually within 24 hours. If the patient flew after diving, then consider decompression sickness up to 72 hours afterward. Symptoms occurring within 10 minutes of surfacing suggest **air embolism**, especially when they are accompanied by a loss of consciousness.
- What type of diving was done, and what type of equipment was used?

- What type of tank was used (compressed air or a Nitrox system [combination of nitrogen and oxygen] with distinctive yellow and green stripes on the tank or a different mixed gas)?
- Where is the diving site, and what was the water temperature?
- How many dives were made during the past 72 hours, and what were the depth, bottom time, and surface interval for each?
- Was a dive computer used?
- Were safety stops used?
- Were there any attempts at in-water decompression (considered risky)?
- Were there any dive complications?
- What were predive and postdive activities?

Descent Emergencies

Diving injuries are separated into three phases of the dive: descent, bottom, and ascent.

The major problem divers encounter during descent is barotrauma (squeeze). This injury results from a pressure imbalance between gas-filled spaces inside the body and the external atmosphere. Barotrauma can result from two different mechanisms: compression of gases within body spaces during descent or expansion of gases within those spaces during ascent (discussed later). Barotrauma can affect any gas-filled space in the body, including the sinuses, the inner and middle ears, and even teeth. Some body cavities cannot adjust to the increased external pressure of the water, resulting in severe pain. Usually, the pain caused by these problems forces the diver to return to the surface to equalize the pressures, and the problem clears up by itself. A diver who continues to report pain, particularly in the ear, after returning to the surface should be transported to the hospital. Table 34-4 summarizes the types of barotrauma.

A person who is SCUBA diving is generally protected from barotrauma by breathing compressed air that matches the pressure of the surrounding environment. Thus, as long as the air-filled cavities of the body can equilibrate freely, they will not implode. This no longer holds true if there is an obstruction, such as with a sinus or ear infection.

As the diver ascends and the ambient pressure around him or her decreases, the gases within the body's air-filled

Table 34-4 Diving Injuries (Types of Barotrauma)

Mechanisms and Pathophysiology	Body Region	Condition	Clinical Features	Treatment
During *descent:* compression of gas in closed spaces	Ear	External ear squeeze *(barotitis externa)*	Otalgia, bloody otorrhea	Keep ear canal dry; no swimming or diving until healed
		Middle ear squeeze *(barotitis media)*	Severe ear pain, tympanic membrane can rupture; emesis, vertigo, nystagmus; self-limited facial nerve palsy	Decongestants; IV antiemetic (call for paramedic backup for administration if needed); no diving until healed
		Inner ear squeeze	Tinnitus, vertigo, hearing loss; emesis, pallor, diaphoresis	Decongestants; IV antiemetics (call for paramedic backup for administration); surgical repair
	Paranasal sinuses	Sinus squeeze	Severe pain over affected sinuses and upper teeth, epistaxis	Topical and oral decongestants
	Face	Face mask squeeze	Ecchymoses and petechiae of skin beneath face mask; scleral/conjunctival hemorrhage	Cold compresses, prevent by forced exhalation through nose

(continued)

Table 34-4 Diving Injuries (Types of Barotrauma) *(continued)*

Mechanisms and Pathophysiology	Body Region	Condition	Clinical Features	Treatment
During *ascent:* expansion of gas in closed spaces	Gastrointestinal tract	"Gas in gut" *(aerogastralgia)*	Colicky belly pain, belching, flatulence; rare pneumoperitoneum	Rare reports of rupture; usually, no care needed
	Lungs	Pulmonary barotrauma "burst lung," POPS	Dyspnea, dysphagia, hoarseness, substernal pain; subcutaneous emphysema around neck; pneumothorax, syncope	100% oxygen; call for paramedic backup to decompress tension pneumothorax
		Air embolism (complication of POPS)	Altered mental status, vertigo, dizziness, seizures, dyspnea, pleuritic chest pain, sudden loss of consciousness on surfacing; sudden death	100% oxygen; transport supine, if air embolism suspected, place in left lateral recumbent position; hyperbaric therapy
Decompression sickness	Skin		Pruritus, subcutaneous emphysema, swelling, rashes	100% oxygen; observe for complications
	Joints and muscles	Bends ("pain-only bends")	Arthralgias, especially in elbows and shoulders, relieved by pressure	100% oxygen, observe
	Cerebrum		Multiple sensory and motor disturbances	100% oxygen, hyperbaric therapy; IV fluids
	Cerebellum	The "staggers"	Unsteadiness, incoordination, vertigo	100% oxygen, hyperbaric therapy; IV fluids
	Spinal cord		Paraplegia, paraparesis, bladder dysfunction (inability to void), back pain	100% oxygen, hyperbaric therapy; IV fluids
	Lungs	Venous air embolism (the "chokes")	Chest pain, cough, dyspnea, signs of pulmonary embolism	100% oxygen, hyperbaric therapy; IV fluids
Dissolved nitrogen	Central nervous system	Nitrogen narcosis ("rapture of the deep")	Symptoms like those of alcohol intoxication	Controlled ascent to shallower water
Hyperventilation before dive	Central nervous system	Shallow water blackout (in breath-hold dives)	Loss of consciousness just before reaching surface	100% oxygen; assisted breathing

Abbreviations: IV, intravenous; POPS, pulmonary overpressurization syndrome

spaces expand. Similar to barotrauma during descent, this commonly affects the ears and sinuses. In one common scenario in which a diver has used decongestants before a dive, the medication may wear off before ascent. The increased mucosal swelling allows air to become trapped in the sinuses and ears, creating a reverse squeeze in which the increasing pressure cannot equalize during ascent. Symptoms are identical to those observed during descent.

A person with a perforated tympanic membrane (ruptured eardrum) may develop a special problem while diving. If cold water enters the middle ear through a ruptured eardrum, the diver may lose his or her balance and orientation. As a result, the diver may ascend too quickly, causing further problems.

Injuries at Depth

Nitrogen narcosis ("rapture of the deep" or "narc'ed") is a state of altered mental status caused by breathing compressed nitrogen-containing air at depth. The human body does not use nitrogen for metabolism; thus, in a breathing gas mixture, nitrogen dilutes the concentration of oxygen. Nitrogen, which makes up 79% of fresh air, will also make up 79% of compressed air according to Dalton's law. When the pressure increases, the partial pressure of nitrogen increases as well. At a partial pressure of about 3.2 ATA, reached at about 100 feet, nitrogen begins to have anesthetic properties, and divers may begin to feel the effects of nitrogen narcosis. It becomes more pronounced at 150 fsw and is why sport divers should not use compressed air for dives of greater than 120 feet.

Ascent Emergencies

Most of the serious injuries associated with diving are related to ascending from the bottom and are referred to as ascent problems. These emergencies usually require aggressive resuscitation. Two particularly dangerous medical emergencies are air embolism and decompression sickness (also called the bends).

Pulmonary Overpressurization Syndrome (POPS). A more dangerous form of barotrauma can occur when divers fail to exhale during an ascent, and pressure in the lungs is increased. The lung volume of SCUBA divers who have inhaled to their total lung capacity at a depth of 33 fsw (1 ATA) doubles by the time divers reach the surface if they hold their breath during ascent. This is likely to occur in an emergency ascent, for example, when divers panic due to difficulty with their equipment and give in to the instinctive impulse to hold their breath under water. The result is one of the worst forms of barotrauma of ascent—**pulmonary overpressurization syndrome (POPS)**, also known as "burst lung." It can cause pneumothorax, mediastinal and subcutaneous emphysema, alveolar hemorrhage, and a lethal air embolism, discussed in the next section. Because the relative pressure and volume changes are greatest near the surface of the water, a small

YOU are the Provider PART 3

You find no signs of trauma on the patient, and as soon as the police officer returns with the stretcher, you gently lift the patient onto the stretcher and secure him. As soon as the patient is placed into the warmed ambulance, you instruct your partner to quickly remove all of the patient's clothing, wipe him down in an attempt to dry him, and place several blankets on top of him to try to warm his core temperature. Recognizing that this patient requires supplemental, warmed oxygen, you place him on a nonrebreathing mask at 15 L/min. You advise your partner that this patient requires rapid, but smooth, transport to the local ED.

Recording Time: 8 Minutes	
Respirations	14 breaths/min, clear
Pulse	46 beats/min, irregular
Skin	Cold
Blood pressure	Unable to obtain
Oxygen saturation (Spo_2)	95% on 15 L/min
Pupils	Pupils Equal, Round, and Reactive to Light (PERRL)

5. How can warmed, supplemental oxygen be provided to a hypothermic patient?
6. What are some potential complications of rough handling of hypothermic patients?

overpressurization—that produced by breath holding for the last 6 feet (2 m) of ascent, for example—can be sufficient to rupture alveoli. For that reason, all diving students are trained to exhale constantly as they are ascending to vent air from their lungs. People with COPD and asthma are at a slightly increased risk owing to their already altered air movement dynamics.

When alveoli rupture, the signs and symptoms depend partly on where the escaping air ends up. Most commonly, it leaks into the mediastinum and beneath the skin, causing mediastinal and subcutaneous emphysema. The patient may report a sensation of fullness in the throat, pain on swallowing (odynophagia), dyspnea, or substernal chest pain. When the patient speaks, he or she may be hoarse or have a brassy quality to the voice. Physical examination may reveal palpable subcutaneous air above the clavicles. Sometimes a crunching noise that is synchronous with the heartbeat may be audible by auscultation (called Hamman sign). Another less common result of alveolar rupture is pneumothorax; therefore, you should always look for unequal breath sounds, low pulse oximetry values, and hyperresonance on the affected side of the chest.

The prehospital treatment of a patient with pulmonary barotrauma depends—at least in terms of urgency—on whether the patient has an air embolism (discussed next). A diver with only pneumomediastinum and subcutaneous emphysema will most likely be managed symptomatically in the hospital. A pneumothorax may require needle decompression or a chest tube. In the field, provide 100% oxygen (by nonrebreathing mask; if you must bag the patient be careful—that is, do not give positive end-expiratory pressure to a patient with POPS!) because it increases oxygen's partial pressure and may decrease bubble size and speed up "off-gassing."

Air Embolism. The most dangerous, and most common, emergency in SCUBA diving is air embolism, a condition involving bubbles of air in the blood vessels. An air embolism may occur on a dive as shallow as 6 feet (2 m). The problem starts when the diver holds his or her breath during a rapid ascent. The air pressure in the lungs remains at a high level, while the external pressure on the chest decreases. As a result, the air inside the lungs expands rapidly, causing the alveoli in the lungs to rupture and forcing air into the bloodstream. The air released from this rupture can cause the following injuries:

- Air may enter the pleural space and compress the lungs (pneumothorax).
- Air may enter the mediastinum (the space within the thorax that contains the heart and great vessels), causing a condition called pneumomediastinum.
- Air may enter the bloodstream and create bubbles of air in the vessels called air emboli.

Pneumothorax and pneumomediastinum both result in pain and severe dyspnea. An air embolus will act as a plug and prevent the normal flow of blood and oxygen to a specific part of the body. The brain and spinal cord are the organs most severely affected by air embolism because they require a constant supply of oxygen.

The following are potential signs and symptoms of air embolism:

- Blotching (mottling of the skin)
- Froth (often pink or bloody) at the nose and mouth
- Severe pain in muscles, joints, or abdomen
- Dyspnea
- Localized pleuritic (sharp) chest pain
- Dizziness, nausea, and vomiting
- Dysphasia (difficulty speaking)
- Cough
- Cyanosis
- Difficulty with vision
- Paralysis and/or coma
- Irregular pulse and even cardiac arrest

Decompression Sickness. Decompression sickness, commonly called the bends, occurs when bubbles of gas, especially nitrogen, obstruct the blood vessels. This condition results from too rapid an ascent from a dive, too long of a dive at too deep a depth, or repeated dives within a short period. During the dive, nitrogen that is being breathed dissolves in the blood and tissues because it is under pressure. When the diver ascends, the external pressure is decreased, and the dissolved nitrogen forms small bubbles within the tissues. These bubbles can result in problems similar to those that occur in air embolism (blockage of tiny blood vessels, depriving parts of the body of their normal blood supply), but severe pain in certain tissues or spaces in the body is the most common problem.

The most striking symptom is abdominal and/or joint pain so severe that the patient literally doubles over or bends. Dive tables and small diving computers are available to calculate and record the proper rate of ascent from a dive, including the number and length of pauses that a diver should make (staged ascent). However, even divers who stay within these limits can experience the bends.

Even after a safe dive, decompression sickness can occur from driving a car up a mountain or flying in an unpressurized airplane that climbs too rapidly to a great height. However, the risk of this diminishes after 24 to 48 hours. The problem is exactly the same as ascent from a deep dive: a sudden decrease of external pressure on the body and release of dissolved nitrogen from the blood that forms bubbles of nitrogen gas within the blood vessels.

You may find it difficult to distinguish between air embolism and decompression sickness. In general, air embolism occurs immediately on return to the surface, whereas the symptoms of decompression sickness may not occur for several hours. The emergency treatment is the same for both. It consists of basic life support (BLS) including oxygen administration, monitoring, and transport, followed by recompression in a **hyperbaric chamber**, a chamber or a small room that is pressurized to a level higher

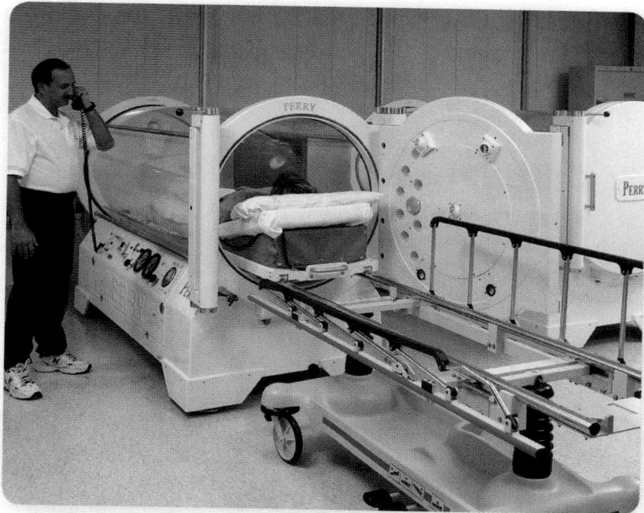

Figure 34-12 A hyperbaric chamber, usually a small room, is pressurized to a level higher than atmospheric pressure and used in the treatment of decompression sickness and air embolism.

Courtesy of Perry Baromedical Corporation.

than atmospheric pressure Figure 34-12. Recompression treatment allows the bubbles of gas to dissolve into the blood and equalizes the pressures inside and outside the lungs. After these pressures are equalized, gradual decompression can be accomplished under controlled conditions to prevent the bubbles from reforming.

Water Rescue

Before you can assess or treat a patient in water, rescue and removal from the water must occur. You must ensure the safety of rescue personnel and request additional rescue resources, as appropriate, before a water rescue can begin. If the patient is alert and still in the water, you should perform a water rescue. An old saying sums up the basic rule of water rescue: "Reach, throw, and row, and only then go." Figure 34-13 sums up the basic rule of water rescue:

1. First, try to reach for the patient.
2. If that does not work, then throw the patient a rope, a life preserver, or any floatable object that is available. For example, an inflated spare tire, rim and all, will float well enough to support two people in the water.
3. Next, use a boat if one is available.
4. Do not attempt a swimming rescue unless you are trained and experienced in the proper techniques. Even then, you should always wear a helmet and a personal flotation device Figure 34-14.

Too many well-meaning rescuers have become victims while attempting a water rescue. A panicked swimmer will make every effort to remain above water, even if this means submerging the rescuer in the process. In cold climates or

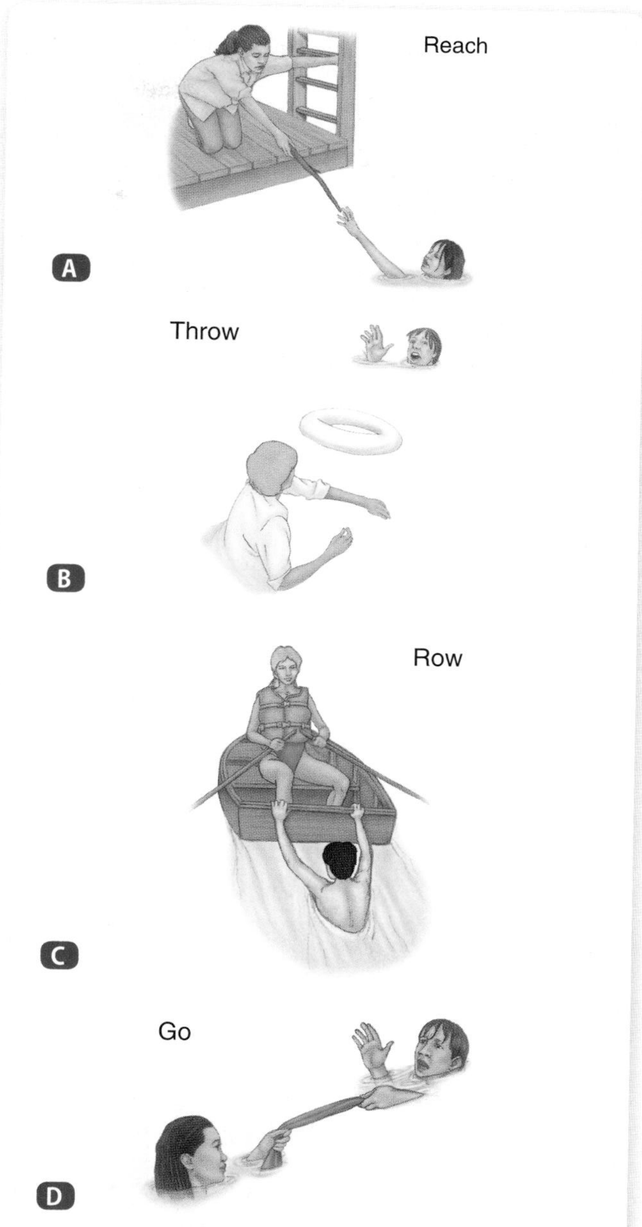

Figure 34-13 Basic rules of water rescue. **A.** Reach for the person from shore. If you cannot reach the person from shore, wade closer. **B.** If an object that floats is available, throw it to the person. **C.** Use a boat if one is available. **D.** If you must swim to the person, use a towel or board for him or her to hold onto. Do not let the person grab you.

© Jones & Bartlett Learning.

cold-water locations, rapid hypothermia is also a concern for rescuers. Be prepared for this potential event.

The steps for ice rescue are similar and may involve reaching with a pole or ladder or throwing a rope or flotation device. A victim who has fallen through the ice may also be coached into placing his or her arms out of the water and onto the ice, kicking and rolling out of the water, and crawling to safety.

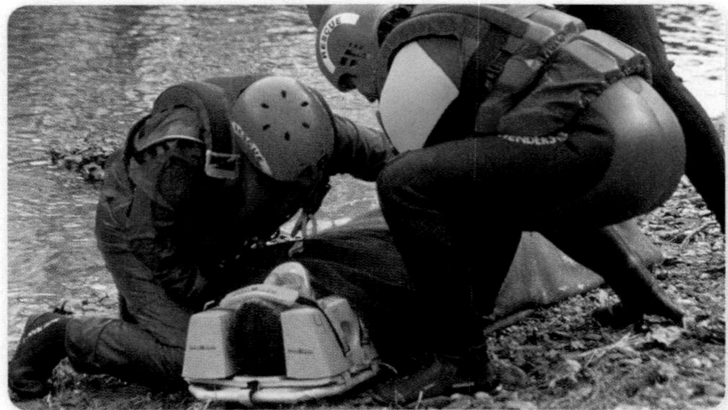

Figure 34-14 When performing a water rescue, you must be properly trained and must wear proper personal protective equipment, including a personal flotation device.

If you work in a recreation area near lakes, rivers, or the ocean, you should have a prearranged plan for water rescue. For colder areas, a plan for ice rescue is also necessary. This plan should include access to and cooperation with local providers who are trained and skilled in water rescue; these providers should help to develop the protocols for water rescue. Because the success of any water rescue depends on how rapidly the patient is removed from the water and ventilated, make sure you always have immediate access to personal flotation devices and other rescue equipment. Survival rates drastically decline the longer a victim is immersed. Cold-water drowning survival rates are somewhat higher.

Spinal Injuries in Submersion Incidents

Submersion incidents may be complicated by spinal fractures and spinal cord injuries. You must assume that spinal injury exists with the following conditions:

- The submersion has resulted from a diving mishap or fall from a substantial height.
- The patient is unresponsive, and no information is available to rule out the possibility of a neck injury.
- The patient is responsive but reports weakness, paralysis, numbness, or tingling in the arms or legs.
- You suspect the possibility of a spinal injury despite what witnesses say.

Most spinal injuries in diving incidents affect the cervical spine. When spinal injury is suspected, the neck must be protected from further injury. This means that you will have to stabilize the suspected injury while the patient is still in the water. To stabilize a suspected spinal injury in the water, follow the steps in Skill Drill 34-2.

Skill Drill 34-2 Stabilizing a Suspected Spinal Injury in the Water

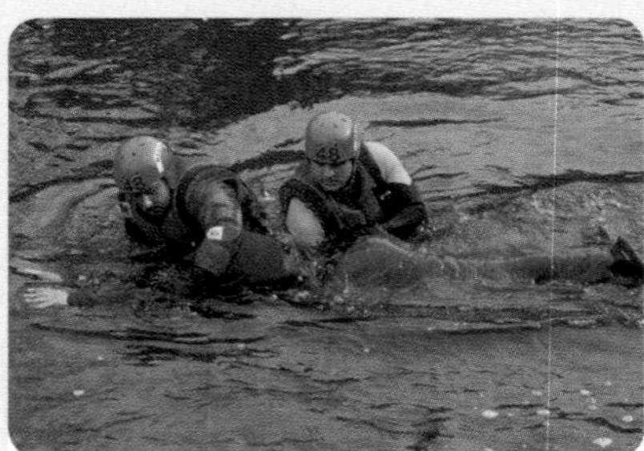

Step 1 Turn the patient supine. Two rescuers are usually required to turn the patient safely, although in some cases one rescuer will suffice. Always rotate the entire upper half of the patient's body as a single unit. Twisting only the head, for example, may aggravate any injury to the cervical spine.

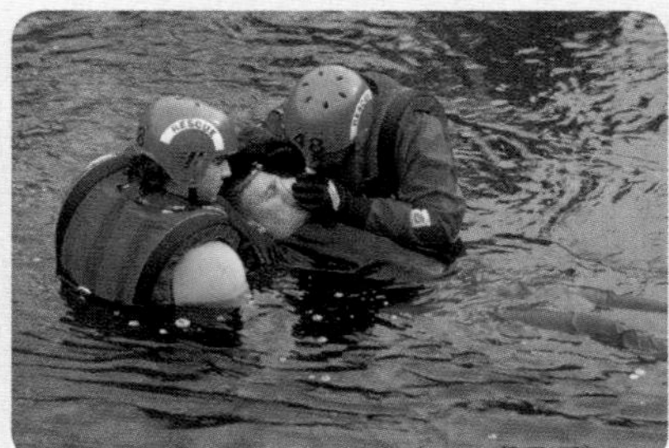

Step 2 Restore the airway and begin ventilation. Immediate ventilation is the primary treatment of all drowning patients as soon as the patient is face up in the water. Use a pocket mask if available. Have the other rescuer support the head and trunk as a unit while you open the airway and begin artificial ventilation.

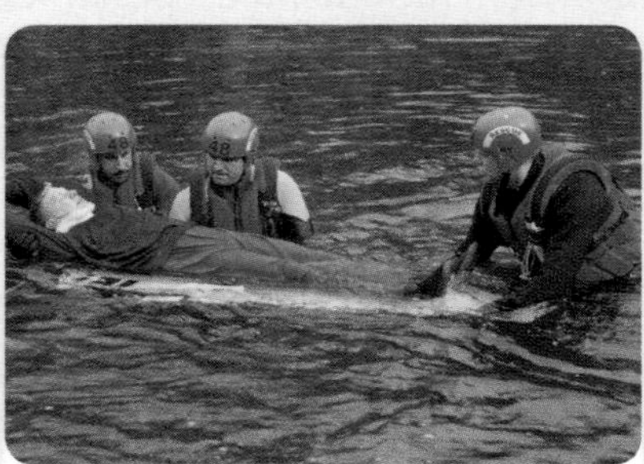

Step 3 Float a buoyant backboard under the patient as you continue ventilation.

Skill Drill 34-2 Stabilizing a Suspected Spinal Injury in the Water *(continued)*

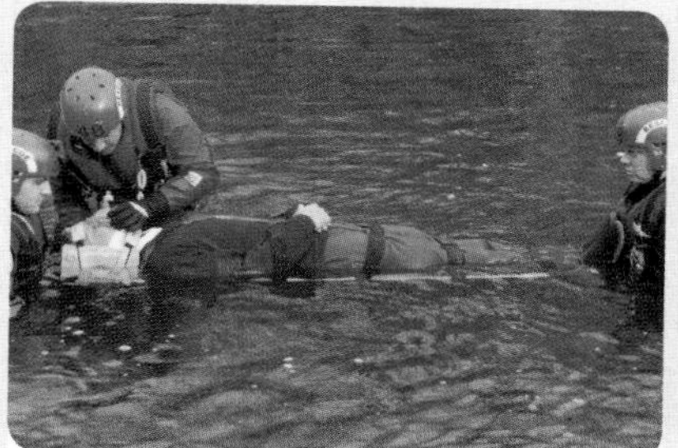

Step 4 Secure the head and trunk to the backboard to stabilize the cervical spine. Do not remove the patient from the water until this is done.

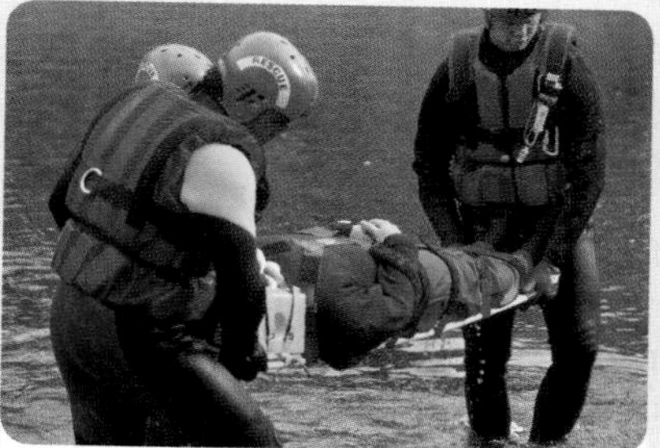

Step 5 Remove the patient from the water, on the backboard.

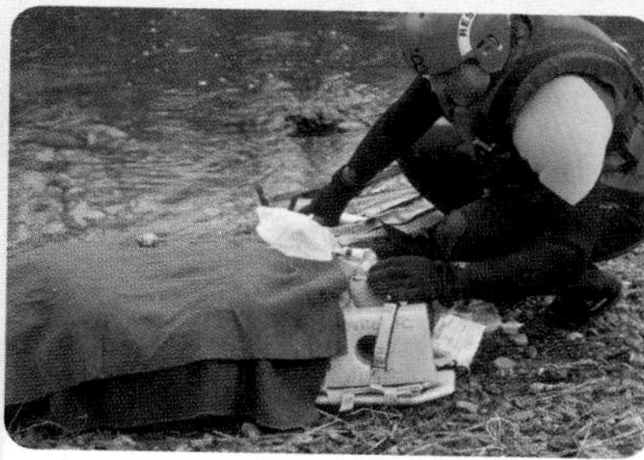

Step 6 Cover the patient with a blanket. Give oxygen if the patient is breathing spontaneously. Begin CPR if there is no pulse. Effective chest compressions are extremely difficult to perform when the patient is still in the water so remove the patient as quickly as possible. Consider paramedic backup for endotracheal intubation to maintain the airway if needed.

▶ Recovery Techniques

On occasion, you may be called to the scene of a drowning and find that the patient is not floating or visible in the water. An organized rescue effort in these circumstances calls for providers who are experienced with recovery techniques and equipment, including snorkel, mask, and SCUBA gear Figure 34-15.

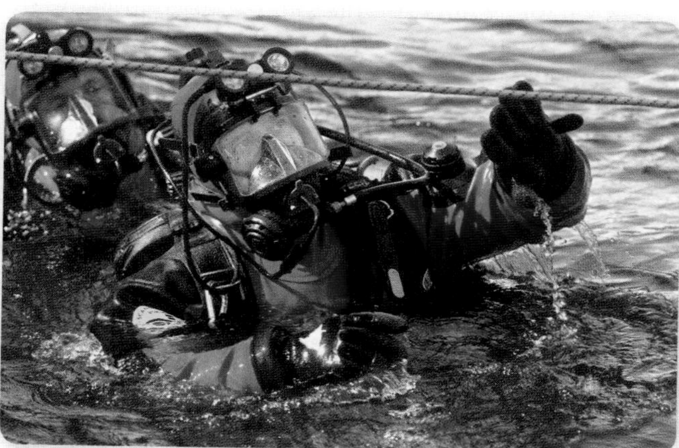

Figure 34-15 Never attempt a deep-water rescue without proper training and equipment.

Words of Wisdom

Never give up on resuscitating a cold-water drowning victim.

Patient Assessment of Drowning and Diving Emergencies

Scene Size-up

In managing water emergencies, your standard precautions should include gloves and eye protection at a minimum. Check for hazards to your crew. Never drive through moving water—a small amount can cause the vehicle to be swept away. Use extreme caution when driving through standing water. Never attempt a water rescue without proper training and equipment. Call for additional resources early.

If your patient is still in the water, look for the best, safest means of removal. This may require additional help from search and rescue teams or special extrication equipment. Trauma and spinal stabilization must be considered when the scene is a recreational setting. Check for additional patients based on where and how the emergency occurred. Finally, as you observe the scene, look for indicators of the MOI.

Primary Survey

Use your evaluation of the patient's chief complaint to guide you in your assessment of life threats, addressing exsanguinating hemorrhage first, and determine whether spinal stabilization is necessary. Pay particular attention to chest pain, dyspnea, and complaints related to sensory changes when a diving emergency is suspected. Determine the patient's level of consciousness using the AVPU scale. Be suspicious of drug and alcohol use and the effects on the patient's level of consciousness.

Standard measures should be employed for any patient found or injured while in the water. Begin with opening the airway and assessing breathing in unresponsive patients. Consider the possibility of spinal trauma, and take appropriate actions as discussed earlier. The airway may be obstructed with water. Suction according to protocol if the patient has vomited or pink, frothy secretions are found in the airway. Foam in the mouth and airway of submersion patients is mostly surfactant and debris and does not need to be cleared; it can be pushed back into the lungs during ventilation and will be reabsorbed.[14] Do not spend substantial amounts of time trying to clear foam from the airway. Provide ventilations with a bag-mask device for inadequate breathing. Use an airway adjunct to facilitate bag-mask device ventilations as necessary.

If the patient is responsive, provide high-flow oxygen with a nonrebreathing mask and if there is no risk of spinal injury, position the patient to protect the airway from aspiration in the event of vomiting. When necessary, begin artificial ventilation as soon as possible, even before the patient is removed from the water.

Obtaining and continually monitoring breath sounds in drowning patients is a key part of your assessment. Through auscultation, you may hear diminished sounds or even gurgling sounds from the water that has been inhaled. This information and any changes in the patient's breath sounds are important to relay to paramedics who may rendezvous with your unit as well as to the receiving facility.

Words of Wisdom

The patient's breathing or lack of breathing can be a determining factor in submersion time. A patient who was briefly submerged may be coughing if rescued early. The longer the patient is under water, the more water enters the lungs. Respiratory arrest occurs from prolonged submersion.

Check for a pulse. It may be difficult to find a pulse because of constriction of the peripheral blood vessels and low cardiac output resulting in cyanosis. Nevertheless, if the pulse is unmeasurable, then the patient may be in cardiac arrest. Begin CPR with chest compressions, and apply your automated external defibrillator (AED) according to BLS and the International Liaison Committee on Resuscitation (ILCOR) guidelines.

Never give up on resuscitating a cold-water drowning victim. When a person is submerged in water that is colder than body temperature, heat will be conducted from the body to the water. The resulting hypothermia can protect vital organs from the lack of oxygen. In addition, exposure to cold water will occasionally activate certain primitive reflexes, which may preserve basic body functions for prolonged periods.

Words of Wisdom

When a person dives or jumps into extremely cold water, the diving reflex (also known as the mammalian diving reflex), slowing of the heart rate caused by submersion in cold water, may cause immediate bradycardia, a slow heart rhythm.[15] Loss of consciousness and drowning may follow. However, the person may be able to survive for an extended time under water because of a lowering of the metabolic rate and decreased oxygen demand and consumption associated with hypothermia. For this reason, you should continue full resuscitation efforts no matter how long the patient has been submerged.

Evaluate the patient for adequate perfusion, and treat for shock by maintaining normal body temperature and improving circulation through positioning the patient in the position dictated by local protocol. The patient's skin may be cold to the touch. If the MOI suggests trauma, assess for bleeding and treat appropriately.

Even if resuscitation in the field appears successful, always transport patients to the hospital. Symptoms may not appear for 24 hours or more after resuscitation. Adult respiratory distress syndrome (ARDS) or renal failure may occur after resuscitation. Inhalation of any amount of fluid can result in delayed complications lasting for days or weeks. Patients with decompression sickness and air embolism must be treated in a recompression chamber. If you live in an area with a substantial amount of SCUBA diving activity, you will have transport protocols in this regard. To minimize your scene time, perform your interventions en route to the nearest ED for stabilization.

History Taking

After the life threats have been managed during the primary survey, investigate the chief complaint. Obtain a medical history, and be alert for injury-specific signs and symptoms as well as any pertinent negatives.

Obtain a SAMPLE history with special attention to the dive parameters, including depth, the length of time the patient was under water, the time of onset of symptoms, and previous diving activity. Note any physical activity, alcohol or drug consumption, and other medical conditions. All of these factors may have an effect on the diving or drowning emergency.

Secondary Assessment

If the patient is responsive, focus your physical examination on the basis of the chief complaint and the history obtained. This should include a thorough examination of the patient's lungs, including breath sounds.

Serious drowning situations typically result in an unresponsive patient. It is important to begin with a rapid full-body scan in these situations to look for hidden life threats and potential trauma, even if trauma is not suspected. A SCUBA diver with problems should be given a rapid full-body scan for indications of the bends or an air embolism. Focus on pain in the joints and the abdomen. Pay attention to whether your patient is getting adequate ventilation and oxygenation, and check for signs of hypothermia. Obtain a baseline Glasgow Coma Scale score to assess the patient's neurologic status and thinking, and be sure to reassess throughout patient care.

Time and personnel permitting, complete a detailed full-body exam en route to the hospital. A careful examination may reveal additional injuries not initially observable. Monitor the patient for respiratory, circulatory, and neurologic compromise. A careful distal circulatory, sensory, and motor function examination will be helpful in assessing the extent of the injury. Assess for peripheral pulses, skin color and discoloration, itching, pain, and paresthesia (numbness and tingling).

Check the patient's vital signs, including pulse rate, quality, and rhythm. Pulse and blood pressure may be difficult to palpate in a patient with hypothermia. Check carefully for both peripheral and central pulses, and listen over the chest for a heartbeat if pulses are weak. Check the respiratory rate, quality, and rhythm, and listen to breath sounds. Assess and document pupil size and reactivity. Also check blood glucose levels.

Although it is a valuable tool, oxygen saturation readings may produce a false low reading because of hypoperfusion of the patient's monitoring finger. Shivering also can interfere with obtaining an accurate reading because of excessive movement.

Reassessment

Repeat the primary survey. Reassess vital signs and the chief complaint. Are the airway, breathing, and circulation still adequate? Recheck patient interventions. Are your treatments still effective?

The condition of patients who have experienced submersion in water may deteriorate rapidly because of pulmonary injury, fluid shifts in the body, cerebral hypoxia, and hypothermia—call early for paramedic backup if a definitive airway is needed. Patients with pneumothorax, air embolism, or decompression sickness may decompensate quickly. Assess your patient's mental status constantly, and assess vital signs at least every 5 minutes. Pay particular attention to respirations and breath sounds.

Document the circumstances of the drowning and extrication. The receiving facility personnel will need to know how long the patient was submerged, the temperature of the water, the clarity of the water, and whether there was any possibility of cervical spine injury.

If you respond to a diving accident, the receiving facility personnel will also need a complete dive profile to properly treat your patient. This information may be available in a dive log, on a dive computer, or from the patient's diving partners. If possible, bring all of the diver's equipment to the hospital. It will be helpful in determining the cause of the accident. Be sure to document the disposition of this equipment—what happened to it and who it was left with.

Emergency Care for Drowning or Diving Emergencies

After removing the patient from the water and addressing concerns related to the ABCs and possible spinal injury, make sure that the patient is kept warm, especially after cold-water immersion. Provide blankets and protection from the environment as needed. Obtain IV access to be used as a medication route even if the patient does not need fluid resuscitation, but do not delay transport by attempting IV access.

When treating responsive patients who are suspected of having air embolism or decompression sickness, follow these accepted treatment steps:

1. Remove the patient from the water. Try to keep the patient calm.
2. Administer oxygen via nonrebreathing mask or bag-mask device assist.
3. Place the patient in a left lateral recumbent position with the head down.
4. Consider the possibility of pneumothorax, and monitor the patient's breath sounds for development of a tension pneumothorax.
5. Provide prompt transport to the ED or to the nearest recompression facility for treatment.

Injury from decompression sickness is usually reversible with proper treatment. However, if the bubbles block critical blood vessels that supply the brain or spinal cord, permanent central nervous system injury may result. Therefore, the key in emergency management of patients with these serious ascent problems is to recognize that an emergency exists and treat and transport as soon as possible.

Words of Wisdom

Do not perform manual abdominal thrusts (Heimlich maneuver) to remove water from the lungs because they may displace water from the stomach into the lungs, increasing the risk of pneumonitis and subsequent lung infections. Suction may be used to clear the airway. Early advanced airway placement is indicated if BLS airway interventions fail.

▶ Submerged Vehicle Incidents

According to the WMS, Project ALIVE, the Wilderness EMS Medical Director Course, and drowning experts, the current best evidence suggests that the safest time to escape from a submerging vehicle is immediately after it enters the water, during the initial floating phase, which usually lasts 60 seconds or less.[16] A sequence of steps has been established to ensure that occupants in a submerging vehicle prioritize egress strategies: seat belts, windows, children, out. These steps indicate that seat belts should be removed (one's own and anyone else unable to do it themselves), followed by opening or breaking windows, releasing children (oldest to youngest), then immediately exiting the vehicle.

Almost every year, deaths occur while callers are on the phone with emergency medical dispatchers because they are not instructed to immediately exit the vehicle. At least one major prehospital dispatch system has changed its protocols to address this. Many people drown in submerging vehicles without contacting 9-1-1 and without exiting the vehicle. One reason is a prevailing myth that victims in a submerging vehicle should allow the passenger compartment to fill with water before attempting egress. This action is not evidence-based and is extremely dangerous.

When arriving on the scene of an actively submerging vehicle, attempt to remove the passengers from the vehicle as quickly as possible, usually through the rear window after breaking it. Attempt this only if you have adequate training for water entry and the circumstances are reasonable from a scene safety perspective.

▶ Other Water Hazards

Pay close attention to the body temperature of a person who is rescued from cold water. Treat hypothermia caused by immersion in cold water the same way you treat hypothermia caused by cold exposure. Prevent further heat loss from contact with the ground, stretcher, or air, and transport the patient promptly.

A person swimming in shallow water may experience **breath-holding syncope**, a loss of consciousness caused by a decreased stimulus for breathing. This happens to swimmers who breathe in and out rapidly and deeply before entering the water in an effort to expand their capacity to stay underwater. Whereas this technique increases the swimmer's oxygen level, the hyperventilation involved lowers the carbon dioxide level. Because an elevated level of carbon dioxide in the blood is the strongest stimulus for breathing, the swimmer may not feel the need to breathe even after using up all the oxygen in his or her lungs. The emergency treatment for a patient with breath-holding syncope is the same as that for drowning or submersion Figure 34-16.

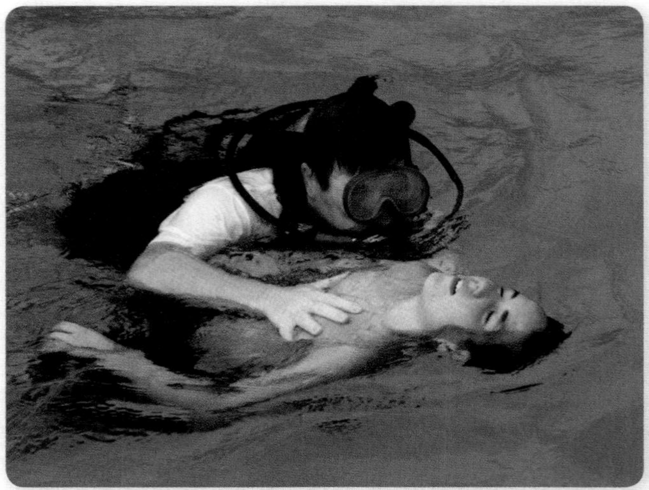

Figure 34-16 Even the best swimmer can panic and become a victim. Only properly trained personnel should attempt a rescue.

Injuries caused by boat propellers, sharp rocks, water skis, or dangerous marine life may be complicated by immersion in cold water. In these cases, remove the patient from the water, taking care to protect the spine, and administer oxygen. Apply dressings and splints if indicated, and monitor the patient closely for any signs of immersion or cold injury.

You should be aware that a child who is involved in a drowning or submersion may be the victim of child abuse. Although it may be difficult to prove, such incidents should be handled according to laws regarding suspected child abuse.

▶ Prevention

Each year, many small children drown in residential pools.[17] Appropriate precautions can prevent most immersion incidents. All pools should be surrounded by a fence that is at least 6 feet (2 m) high, with slats no farther apart than 3 inches (8 cm) and self-closing, self-locking gates. The most common problem is lack of adult supervision, even when a child is unattended for only a few seconds. Approximately 70% of all teenage and adult drownings are associated with alcohol use.[17] As a health care professional, you should be involved in public education efforts to make people aware of the hazards of swimming pools and water recreation.

High Altitude

High altitudes can cause dysbarism injuries. Dysbarism injuries are any signs and symptoms caused by the difference between the surrounding atmospheric pressure and the total gas pressure in various tissues, fluids, and cavities of the body. Altitude illnesses occur when an unacclimated person is exposed to diminished oxygen pressure in the air at high altitudes. These illnesses affect the central nervous system and pulmonary system and range from the common acute mountain sickness to the rare deaths from high-altitude cerebral edema (HACE) and high-altitude pulmonary edema (HAPE).

Acute mountain sickness is caused by diminished oxygen pressure in the air at altitudes above 5,000 feet (1.5 km), resulting in diminished oxygen in the blood (hypoxia). It strikes those who ascend too high too fast and those who have not acclimatized to high altitudes. The signs and symptoms include a headache, lightheadedness, fatigue, loss of appetite, nausea, difficulty sleeping, shortness of breath during physical exertion, and a swollen face. However, there may be other possible causes for the same symptoms, such as hypoglycemia or carbon monoxide poisoning from a camping stove.

With HAPE, fluid collects in the lungs, hindering the passage of oxygen into the bloodstream. It can occur at altitudes of 8,000 feet (2 km) or greater. The signs and symptoms include shortness of breath, cough with pink sputum, cyanosis, and a rapid pulse.

HACE usually occurs in climbers who climb above 12,000 feet. It may accompany HAPE and can quickly become life threatening. The symptoms of HACE and HAPE may overlap. The signs and symptoms include a severe, constant throbbing headache; ataxia (lack of muscle coordination and balance); extreme fatigue; vomiting; and loss of consciousness.

In the field, treatment for altitude illness consists of providing oxygen, descending from the height, and transporting the patient. If local protocols allow, continuous positive airway pressure (CPAP) may be very helpful for a patient with respiratory distress from HAPE.

Lightning Injuries

Approximately 35 people die from lightning strikes in the United States each year.[18] Those who do not die from their injuries are left with varied degrees of disability. Most lightning deaths and injuries caused by lightning occur during the summer months when people are enjoying outdoor activities, despite an approaching thunderstorm. Those most commonly struck by lightning include boaters, swimmers, and golfers. Any type of activity that exposes the person to a large, open area increases the risk of being struck by lightning.

Lightning strikes when a massive discharge of electricity occurs between two bodies that have different charges—for example, between a thundercloud and the ground. The stream of current takes the path of least resistance from

YOU are the Provider — PART 4

As you begin your transport, you establish a large-bore IV and infuse a 250-mL bolus of warmed normal saline to try to increase his blood pressure. You reassess the patient and find him responsive to deep, painful stimuli only but still able to maintain a patent airway. Your partner advises that you are about two blocks from the hospital, and you begin preparations to turn over care. After you are at the ED, you give your report to the nurse and complete your patient care report.

Recording Time: 12 Minutes	
Respirations	14 breaths/min, clear
Pulse	52 beats/min
Skin	Cold
Blood pressure	82 by palpation
Oxygen saturation (Spo_2)	97% on 15 L/min
Pupils	PERRL

7. What are the two methods of rewarming this patient?
8. Why should active rewarming not be attempted in this patient?

its origin to its destination. If any object projects above the surface of the earth that is a better conductor of electricity than the air—such as a building, a light pole, an antenna, a flagpole, or a tree—that object will "attract" the lightning bolt.

Whether lightning injures or kills depends on whether a person is in the path of the lightning discharge. The current associated with the lightning discharge travels along the ground. Although some people are injured or killed by a direct lightning strike, many victims are indirectly struck when standing near an object that has been struck by lightning, such as a tree, and the lightning spreads out from that point (splash effect).

A person need not sustain a direct hit from lightning to be injured; in fact, most victims are not struck directly. Much more commonly, the victim is splashed by lightning striking a nearby tree or other projecting object, resulting in an arc-type or flash burn that leaves a characteristic "feathering" pattern on the skin **Figure 34-17**. Ground current produced by lightning striking the ground near the victim can also cause severe injury and accounts for incidents in which there are multiple casualties in an extended area, such as on a golf course or in an open field.

Lightning carries enormous electrical power. Its energy can reach 100 *million* volts, and peak currents can be in the range of 200,000 amps. Unlike other high-voltage electric current, the electricity from lightning is *direct*—not alternating—current, and the duration of exposure is measured in milliseconds. Thus, lightning injuries tend to resemble blast injuries more than they do high-voltage injuries, with damage occurring to the tympanic membranes of the ears and air-containing internal organs. Many reports of lightning strikes indicate victims' clothes were "blown off" of their bodies. Muscle damage may occur, and the release of myoglobin from injured muscle may jeopardize the kidneys.

For the cardiovascular system, lightning acts as a cosmic defibrillator, delivering a massive direct-current countershock that depolarizes the entire heart. The heart may resume beating spontaneously shortly after the shock or after 5 cycles (30:2) or approximately 2 minutes of CPR that is started immediately. Because respiratory arrest is apt to persist in patients who have been struck by lightning, continued ventilatory support may be required. The phenomenon of someone regaining a pulse after a lightning strike and having respiratory arrest is known to result in a secondary cardiac arrest if left untreated. The central nervous system is almost invariably affected by a lightning strike. Temporary paralysis of the legs has occurred, and permanent paralysis and quadriplegia have been reported in a few cases.

During your assessment, look for not only the entrance wound but also the exit wound. The exit wound does not necessarily occur on the same side of the body. Additionally, because the duration of a lightning strike is short, skin burns are usually superficial; full-thickness (third-degree) burns are rare. Lightning injuries are categorized as being mild, moderate, or severe:

- **Mild.** Loss of consciousness, amnesia, confusion, tingling, and other nonspecific signs and symptoms. Burns, if present, are typically superficial.
- **Moderate.** Seizures, respiratory arrest, cardiac standstill (asystole) that spontaneously resolves, and superficial burns.
- **Severe.** Cardiopulmonary arrest. Because of the delay in resuscitation, often the result of remote locations, many of these patients do not survive.

Despite the unique circumstances surrounding a lightning strike, the immediate threats to life are the same as those caused by a high-voltage power line injury: airway obstruction, respiratory arrest, and cardiac arrest.

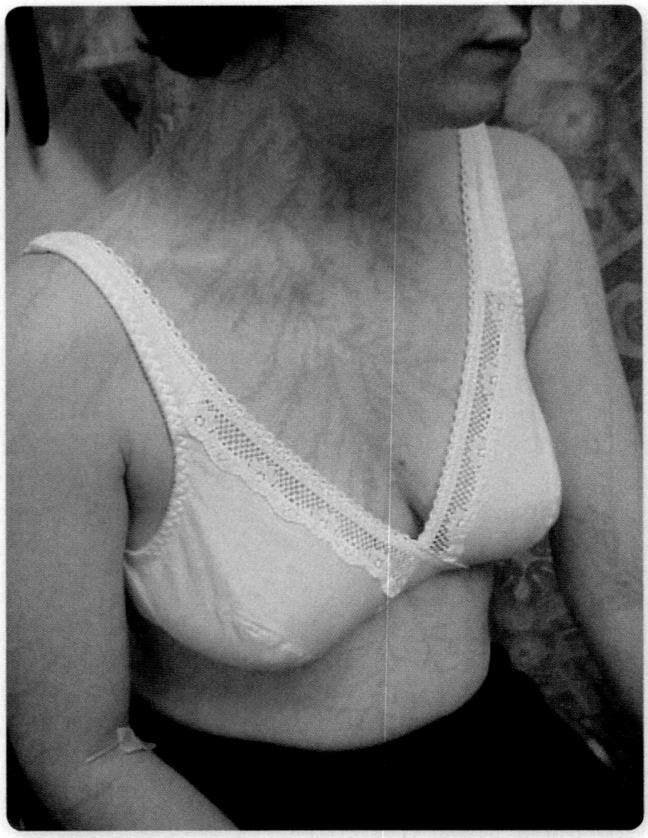

Figure 34-17 An arc-type burn resulting from a nearby lightning strike may leave a characteristic feathering pattern on the skin.

Words of Wisdom

Touching the victim of a lightning strike is not hazardous; contrary to what your grandparent may have told you, electricity does not remain within the body of a person who has been hit by lightning.

Emergency Medical Care for Lightning Injuries

When you reach the scene of a lightning strike, all the usual priorities apply, but there are two special considerations to keep in mind.

First, if the electrical storm is ongoing, your first priority is to get any patients and rescuers to a safe place, preferably indoors, or at least inside the ambulance. Lightning *can* strike twice in the same place. If you are in an open area and adequate shelter is unavailable, it is important to recognize the signs of an impending lightning strike and take immediate action to protect yourself. If you suddenly feel a tingling sensation or your hair stands on end, the area around you has become charged—a sure sign of an imminent lightning strike. Curl up in a ball and squat; make yourself as small a target as possible. If you are standing near a tree or other tall object, move away as fast as possible, preferably to a low-lying area. Lightning has an affinity for objects that project from the ground (ie, trees, fences, buildings) and that are good conductors.

Second, be aware that a lightning strike is apt to injure more than one person. Therefore, the first thing you need to do on arrival at the scene—before you leave the safety of the ambulance—is to perform a rapid size-up of the entire scene to determine the number of patients.

The process of triaging multiple victims of a lightning strike is different from the conventional triage methods used during a mass-casualty incident. When a person is struck by lightning, respiratory or cardiac arrest, if it occurs, usually occurs immediately. Those who are conscious following a lightning strike are much less likely to develop delayed respiratory or cardiac arrest; most of these people will survive. Therefore, you should focus your efforts on those who are in respiratory or cardiac arrest. This, process, called **reverse triage**, differs from conventional triage, where such patients would ordinarily be classified as deceased.

Words of Wisdom

In a lightning strike with multiple victims, priority goes to the victims who are not breathing.

After safety and triage have been addressed, you may assess and treat the patient or patients. Start CPR when necessary. Carry out the primary survey as usual. When establishing an airway, keep in mind the possibility of cervical spine injury, and do not hyperextend the neck; instead, use the jaw-thrust maneuver.

Patients with cardiac arrest caused by a lightning strike deserve aggressive, continuing CPR. The chances of a successful resuscitation in such a case are good, even when the patient appears beyond help initially and even when there is a long delay in the return of spontaneous breathing. Minimize the interruption in compressions, and push hard and fast with full chest recoil!

If severe bleeding is present, control it immediately. Because of the massive direct current shock caused by lightning, the patient experiences massive muscle spasms (tetany), which can result in fractures of long bones and spinal vertebrae. Therefore, manually stabilize the patient's head in a neutral inline position, and open the airway with the jaw-thrust maneuver. If the patient is in respiratory arrest with a pulse, begin immediate bag-mask ventilations with 100% oxygen. If the patient is in cardiac arrest, begin chest compressions immediately, then attach an AED as soon as one is available, and provide immediate defibrillation if indicated.

If you are unable to effectively ventilate the patient with a bag-mask device, insert an advanced airway device. Insert at least one large-bore IV line and provide crystalloid (ie, normal saline, lactated Ringer) fluid boluses of 20 mL/kg to treat suspected hypovolemia and to promote the excretion of myoglobin, a chemical released by injured muscle that can result in renal damage or failure.

Provide full spinal immobilization and transport the patient to the closest appropriate facility. If CPR or ventilations are not required, address other injuries (ie, splint fractures, dress and bandage burns) and provide continuous monitoring while en route to the hospital. A patient with signs and symptoms of a lightning strike but no obvious life threats should still be transported to the ED for evaluation.

Treatment of lightning injuries can be summarized as follows:

- Make sure the scene is safe. Move the victim to a safer location if necessary.
- Priority for treatment goes to patients who are not breathing.
- Perform CPR as needed. Establish an airway, and take cervical spine precautions.
- Administer supplemental oxygen.
- Insert a large-bore IV catheter and deliver an isotonic crystalloid solution wide open to keep the kidneys flushed out.
- Cover any surface burns with dry, clean dressings.
- Splint fractures.

Words of Wisdom

Cardiac arrest secondary to lightning strike can often be successfully treated with early defibrillation.

The best treatment for lightning injuries is prevention, and all health care professionals have a responsibility to educate the public in preventive measures. Clearly, the most effective precaution is to come in out of the storm, but that is not always possible. The rules in Table 34-5 can help avoid lightning injuries.

Table 34-5 Techniques to Avoid Being Struck by Lightning

Rule 1: Don't be the tallest object that is a good conductor. Stay away from the middle of fields, lakes, golf courses, and other large, open areas. If you are stuck in the middle of an open area, try to be as small as you can. Do not hold up an umbrella, golf club, or lightning rod. Do not fly a kite.
Rule 2: Don't stand under or near the tallest object that is a good conductor. Although you do not want to be in the middle of the field, you also do not want to be under the tallest tree, radio antenna, or golf umbrella.
Rule 3: Take shelter in the most substantial structure that you can to remain safe if it is hit by lightning. A large building with a lightning suppression system is the best choice. An enclosed building is better than an open one (eg, shed, lean-to). Close the shelter as much as possible. If in a vehicle, keep the windows rolled up. Lightning tends to flash over the outside of objects (and people). It can travel substantial distances through conductors, however.
Rule 4: Avoid touching good conductors during a lightning storm. Examples of good conductors include plumbing fixtures, fences, and electrical appliances, particularly those connected to wires outside (eg, telephone, TV, computer).

Bites and Envenomations

Spider Bites

Spiders are numerous and widespread in the United States. Many species of spiders can bite people, and most all of these spiders are venomous. However, only two in the United States, the female black widow spider and the brown recluse spider, are able to deliver serious, even life-threatening bites. When you care for a patient who has sustained a spider bite, be alert to the possibility that the spider may still be in the area. Remember that your safety is of paramount importance.

Black Widow Spider

The female black widow spider *(Latrodectus)* is fairly large, measuring approximately 2 inches (5 cm) long with its legs extended. It is usually black and has a distinctive, bright red-orange marking in the shape of an hourglass on its abdomen (Figure 34-18). The female is larger and more toxic than the male. Black widow spiders are found in every state except Alaska. They prefer dry, dim places around buildings, in woodpiles, and among debris.

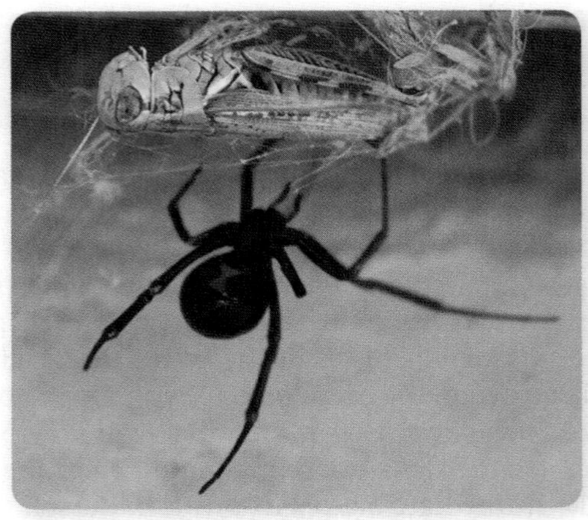

Figure 34-18 Black widow spiders are distinguished by their glossy black color and bright red-orange hourglass marking on the abdomen.

The bite of the black widow spider is sometimes overlooked. If the site becomes numb right away, the patient may not even recall being bitten. However, most black widow spider bites cause immediate localized pain and symptoms, including agonizing muscle spasms. In some cases, a bite on the abdomen causes muscle spasms so severe that the patient may be thought to have an acute abdominal condition, such as peritonitis. The main danger with this type of bite, however, comes from the fact that the black widow's venom can damage nerve tissues (it is neurotoxic). Other systemic symptoms include dizziness, sweating, nausea, vomiting, and rashes. Tightness in the chest and difficulty breathing typically develop within 24 hours, as do severe cramps, with boardlike rigidity of the abdominal muscles. Generally, these signs and symptoms subside over 48 hours.

If necessary, a physician can administer a specific **antivenin**, a serum containing antibodies that counteract the venom, but because of a high incidence of side effects, its use is reserved for severe bites, for older or extremely feeble people, and for children younger than 5 years. In children, these bites can be fatal. The severe muscle spasms are usually treated in the hospital with IV benzodiazepines such as diazepam (Valium) or lorazepam (Ativan). In general, emergency treatment for a black widow spider bite consists of BLS for the patient in respiratory distress, cleaning the bite with soap and water, and applying an ice pack to the area. Much more often, the patient will only require pain relief. Transport the patient to the ED as soon as possible for treatment. If possible, safely bring the spider to the hospital, or take a photo of the spider with a cell phone and send it to the hospital ahead of time so that it can be definitively identified.

Brown Recluse Spider

The brown recluse spider *(Loxosceles)* is dull brown and, at 1 inch (3 cm), smaller than the black widow (Figure 34-19). The short-haired body has a violin-shaped mark that is

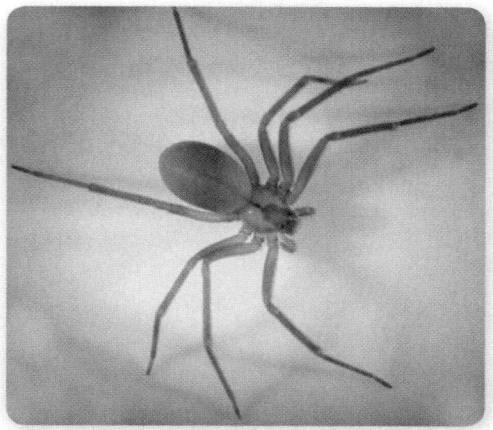

Figure 34-19 Brown recluse spiders are dull brown and have a dark, violin-shaped mark on the back.

Courtesy of Kenneth Cramer, Monmouth College.

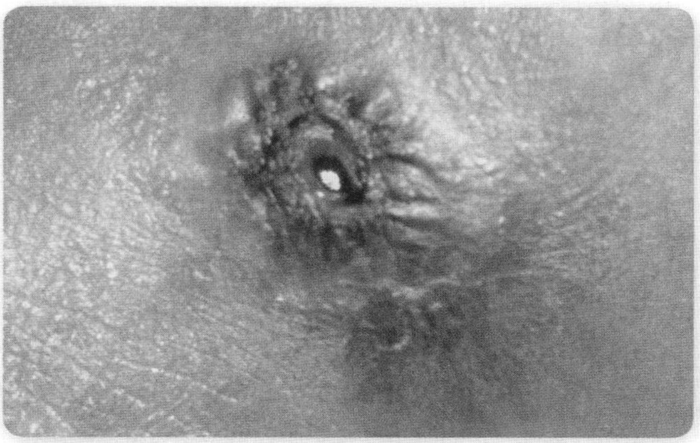

Figure 34-20 The bite of a brown recluse spider is characterized by swelling, tenderness, and a pale, mottled, cyanotic center. There may also be a small blister on the bite.

Courtesy of Department of Entomology, University of Nebraska.

brown to yellow on its back, which is why it is commonly referred to as the "fiddleback" spider. Although it lives mostly in the southern and central parts of the country, the brown recluse may be found throughout the continental United States. The spider is named for its tendency to live in dark areas—in corners of old, unused buildings, under rocks, and in woodpiles. In cooler areas, it moves indoors to closets, drawers, cellars, and clothing.

In contrast with the venom of the black widow spider, the venom of the brown recluse spider is not neurotoxic but cytotoxic; that is, it causes severe local tissue damage. Typically, the bite is not painful at first but becomes so within hours. The area becomes swollen and tender and develops a pale, mottled, cyanotic center and possibly a small blister Figure 34-20. Over the next several days, a scab of dead skin, fat, and debris will form and dig into the skin, producing a large ulcer that may not heal unless treated promptly. Transport patients with such symptoms as soon as possible.

Brown recluse spider bites rarely cause systemic symptoms and signs. When they do, provide BLS and prompt transport to the ED. Again, it is helpful if you can identify the spider and either safely bring it to the hospital with the patient, or take a picture of the spider and send it to the hospital ahead of time.

▶ Hymenoptera Stings

Typically **Hymenoptera** (bees, wasps, ants, and yellow jackets) stings are painful but are not a medical emergency. Remove the stinger and, if still present, the venom sac. This is best done by using a firm-edged item such as a credit card to scrape the stinger and sac off the skin. If you inadvertently squeeze the venom sac while trying to grasp the stinger with tweezers or forceps you will worsen the patient's exposure by increasing the amount of envenomation. After the stinger is removed, clean thoroughly with soap and water or an antiseptic solution, and treat with cool compresses and elevation.

If the patient is allergic to the venom, then anaphylaxis may occur. The signs and symptoms of anaphylaxis are flushed skin, low blood pressure, difficulty breathing usually associated with reactive airway sounds such as wheezes, or in severe cases diminished or absent breath sounds. The patient can also have swelling to the throat and tongue. This is a dire emergency and can be fatal if not recognized and treated quickly. The patient may develop hives (urticaria) near the site of envenomation or centrally on the body. If anaphylaxis develops, be prepared to administer epinephrine (via an EpiPen or similar auto-injector or subcutaneously). Also be prepared to support the airway and breathing should the patient experience substantial respiratory compromise. Chapter 22, *Immunologic Emergencies,* covers treatment of anaphylaxis.

▶ Snakebites

Snakebites are a global problem. More than 5.4 million snakebites occur annually worldwide, resulting in approximately 81,000 to 137,000 deaths.[19] Approximately 10,000 snakebites occur in the United States every year; approximately 30% of those are venomous.[20] However, fatalities from snakebites in the United States are extremely rare, at approximately five per year for the entire country.[21]

Of the approximately 115 different species of snakes in the United States, only 19 are venomous. These include the rattlesnake *(Crotalus)*, the copperhead *(Agkistrodon contortrix)*, the cottonmouth, or water moccasin *(Agkistrodon piscivorus)*, and the coral snakes *(Micrurus fulvius* and *Micruroides euryxanthus)* Figure 34-21. At least one of these poisonous species is found in every state except Alaska, Hawaii, and Maine. In general, these creatures are timid. They usually do not bite unless provoked or accidentally injured, such as when they are stepped on. There are a few exceptions to these rules. Cottonmouths are often rather aggressive, and rattlesnakes are easily

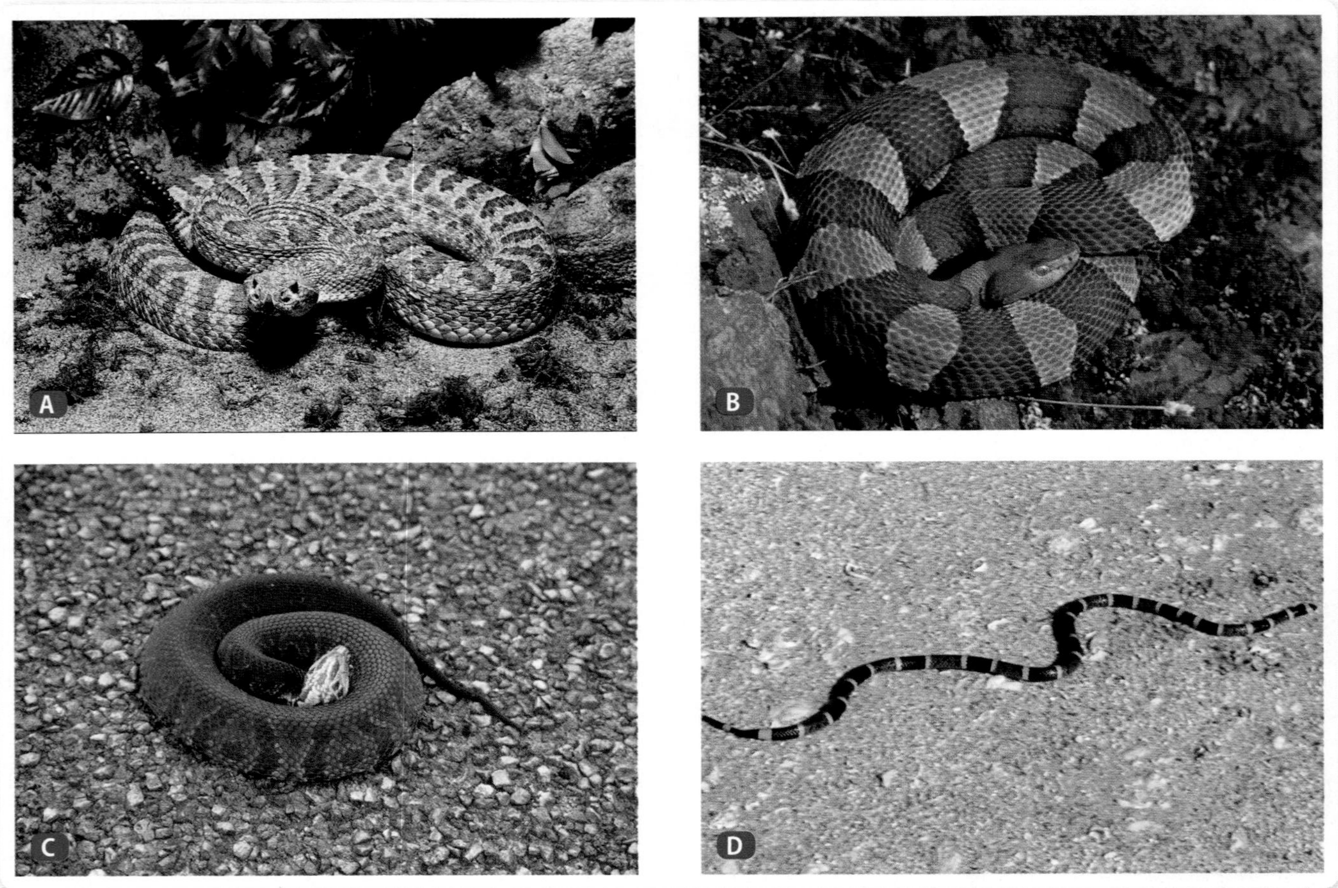

Figure 34-21 A. Rattlesnake. **B.** Copperhead. **C.** Cottonmouth. **D.** Coral snake.

A: © Photos.com/Getty; B: Courtesy of Ray Rauch/U.S. Fish & Wildlife Service; C: © SuperStock/Alamy; D: Courtesy of Luther C. Goldman/U.S. Fish & Wildlife Service.

provoked. Coral snakes, in contrast, usually bite only when they are being handled.

Most snakebites occur between April and October, when the animals are active, and tend to involve young men who have been drinking alcohol. Texas reports the largest number of bites. Other states with a major concentration of snakebites are Louisiana, Georgia, Oklahoma, North Carolina, Arkansas, West Virginia, and Mississippi. If you work in one of these areas, you should be thoroughly familiar with the emergency care of snakebites. Remember, almost any time you are caring for a patient with a snakebite, another snake, or perhaps the same one, could come along and create a second victim—you. Therefore, use extreme caution on these calls, and be sure to wear the proper protective equipment for the area.

The amount of toxin injected is directly related to toxicity, but often, there is little or no envenomation. In general, only one-third of snakebites result in substantial local or systemic injuries. Often, envenomation does not occur because the snake has recently struck another animal and temporarily exhausted its supply of venom.

With the exception of the coral snake, venomous snakes native to the United States all have hollow fangs in the roof of the mouth that inject the poison from two sacs at the back of the head. The classic appearance of the venomous snakebite, therefore, is two small puncture wounds, usually approximately 0.5 inch (1 cm) apart, with discoloration and swelling, and the patient usually reports pain surrounding the bite **Figure 34-22**. Nonpoisonous snakes can also bite, usually leaving horseshoe-shaped

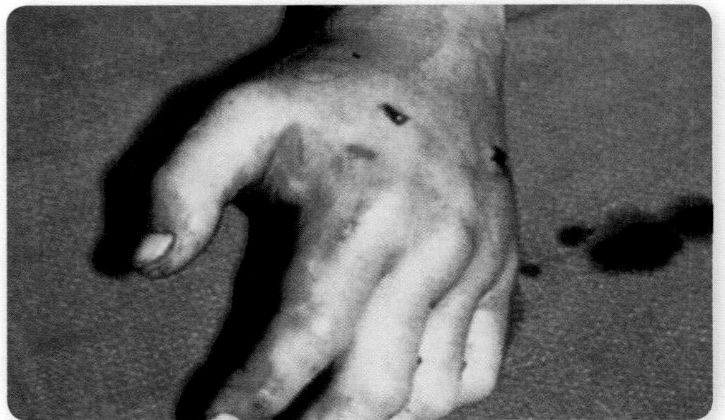

Figure 34-22 A snakebite wound from a venomous snake has characteristic markings: two small puncture wounds approximately 0.5 inch (1 cm) apart, discoloration, and swelling.

© American Academy of Orthopaedic Surgeons.

teeth marks. However, some poisonous snakes have teeth as well as fangs, making it impossible to determine the type of snake responsible for a given set of teeth marks. On the other hand, fang marks are a clear indication of a venomous snakebite.

A person who has been bitten by any venomous snake needs prompt transport. Also, notify the hospital as soon as possible if a patient has been bitten by a pit viper or coral snake. Some venoms can cause paralysis of the nervous system, and hospitals may not have appropriate antivenin on hand.

Pit Vipers

Rattlesnakes, copperheads, and cottonmouths are all pit vipers, with triangular-shaped, flat heads **Figure 34-23**. They take their name from the small pits located just behind each nostril and in front of each eye. The pit is a heat-sensing organ that allows the snake to strike accurately at any warm target, especially in the dark when it cannot see through its vertical, slitlike pupils.

The fangs of the pit viper normally lie flat against the roof of the mouth and are hinged to swing back and forth as the mouth opens. When the snake strikes, the mouth opens wide and the fangs extend; in this way, the fangs penetrate whatever the mouth strikes. The fangs are actually special hollow teeth that act similar to hypodermic needles. They are connected to a sac containing a reservoir of venom, which is attached to a poison gland. The gland itself is a specifically adapted salivary gland, which produces powerful enzymes that digest and destroy tissue. The primary purpose of the venom is to kill small animals and to start the digestive process before they are eaten.

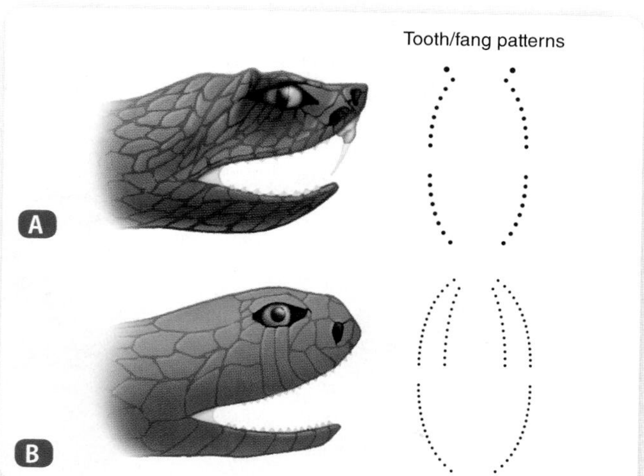

Figure 34-23 Characteristics of pit vipers and nonpoisonous snakes. **A.** Pit vipers have vertical pupils (with the exception of the coral snake, which has round pupils), a pit between the eye and the nostril, a single row of teeth, and two erectile fangs. **B.** Nonpoisonous snakes have round pupils and often a double row of upper teeth; they do not leave fang marks.

In the United States, the most common form of pit viper is the rattlesnake. Several different species of rattlesnake can be identified by the rattle on the tail. The rattle is actually numerous layers of dried skin that were shed but failed to fall off, coming to rest against a small knob on the end of the tail. When agitated or endangered, rattlesnakes shake their tails, or rattles, to warn the invader away. Rattlesnakes have many patterns of color, often with a diamond pattern. They can grow to 6 feet (2 m) or more in length.

Copperheads are smaller than rattlesnakes, usually 2 to 3 feet long (60 to 90 cm), with a red-copper color crossed with brown or red bands. These snakes typically inhabit woodpiles and abandoned dwellings, often close to areas of habitation. Although they account for most of the venomous snakebites in the eastern United States, copperhead bites are typically not fatal; however, note that the venom can cause substantial damage to tissues in the extremities.

Cottonmouths grow to approximately 4 feet (1 m) in length. Also called water moccasins, these snakes are olive or brown, with black cross-bands and a yellow undersurface. They are water snakes, with a particularly aggressive pattern of behavior. Although deaths from the bites of these snakes are rare, tissue destruction from the venom may be severe. Cottonmouths have been known to strike at their victims from the water.

The signs of envenomation by a pit viper are severe burning pain at the site of the injury, followed by swelling and, in light-skinned people, a bluish discoloration (ecchymosis) that signals bleeding under the skin. These signs are evident within 5 to 10 minutes after the bite has occurred, and they spread during the next 36 hours. In addition to destroying tissues locally, the venom of the pit viper can also interfere with the body's blood-clotting mechanisms and cause bleeding at various distant sites. This toxin affects the entire nervous system. Other systemic signs, which may or may not occur, include weakness, nausea, vomiting, vision problems, seizures, sweating, fainting, changes in level of consciousness, and shock. Patient age and size are also factors. The smaller the patient, the more severe the symptoms are likely to be with envenomation. If the patient has no local signs 1 hour after being bitten, envenomation more than likely did not occur. If swelling has occurred, use a pen to mark its edges on the skin. This will allow physicians to assess the timing and extent of the swelling with greater accuracy. Frequently measuring the circumference of the affected

Words of Wisdom

When treating the victim of a snakebite, use a marker to outline the area of swelling. This will show how much swelling has occurred between the time the patient was picked up and arrived at the ED.

extremity will allow you to determine the speed at which swelling is occurring.

Coral Snakes

The coral snake is a small reptile with a series of bright red, yellow, and black bands completely encircling the body. Many harmless snakes have similar coloring (such as the king snake), but only the coral snake has red and yellow bands next to one another, as this helpful rhyme suggests: "Red on yellow will kill a fellow; red on black, venom will lack."

A rare creature that lives in most southern states and in the Southwest, the coral snake is a relative of the cobra. It has tiny fangs and injects the venom with its teeth by a chewing motion, leaving behind one or more puncture or scratchlike wounds. Because of its small mouth and teeth and limited jaw expansion, the coral snake usually bites its victims on a small part of the body, such as a finger or toe.

Coral snake venom is a powerful toxin that causes paralysis of the nervous system (neurotoxic). Within a few hours of being bitten, a patient will exhibit bizarre behavior, followed by progressive paralysis of eye movements and respiration. Often, there are limited or no local symptoms.

Treatment of Snakebites

The steps for emergency care of a pit viper bite and a coral snakebite are similar.

In treating a snakebite from a pit viper, follow these steps:

1. Calm the patient; assure him or her that poisonous snakebites are rarely fatal. Have the patient lie supine, and explain that remaining still and calm will slow the spread of any venom through the system. Determine the approximate time of the bite, and document your time en route to a receiving facility. This time from onset to evaluation at the facility is one of the criteria used in grading the severity of the incident and in determining the amount of antivenin to be used.
2. Locate the bite area; clean it gently with soap and water or a mild antiseptic to wash away any poison left on the surface of the skin. *Do not apply ice* to the area because this will cause local vasoconstriction and push the venom farther into the bloodstream. If the patient is hypotensive, then a constricting band may be applied 4 to 6 inches above the bite site if called for by your local protocols. You should be able to slide two fingers underneath the band. Some local protocols do not allow the use of a constricting band in treating snakebites because of the potential of the venom pooling into the localized bite area. This could potentially cause greater damage to the localized area.
3. If the bite occurred on an arm or leg, consider the use of a pressure immobilization bandage of the extremity (eg, 40 to 70 mm Hg in the arms and 55 to 70 mm Hg in the legs), and then place the affected extremity below the level of the heart.
4. Be alert for an anaphylactic reaction to the venom, and treat with an epinephrine auto-injector, as appropriate.
5. Do not give anything by mouth, and be alert for vomiting.
6. If, as rarely happens, the patient was bitten on the trunk, keep him or her supine and calm and transport as quickly as possible.
7. Monitor the patient's vital signs, and mark the skin with a pen over the area that is swollen, proximal to the swelling, to note whether swelling is spreading **Figure 34-24**.
8. If signs of shock are present, place the patient supine and administer 100% oxygen. Be prepared to assist ventilations if needed. Initiate IV therapy according to local protocols.
9. If the snake has been killed, as is often the case, take it with you, or take a photo on your cell phone, so that physicians can identify it and administer the proper antivenin. Be careful in handling any snake. The fangs of a pit viper are sharp and may scratch your skin, allowing the remaining venom to penetrate.
10. Notify the hospital that you are bringing in a patient who has a snakebite; if possible, describe the snake.
11. Transport the patient promptly to the hospital.
12. Call for paramedic backup if needed.

Successful treatment for a coral snakebite, either emergency or long term, depends on positive identification of the snake and support of vital central nervous system functions, such as breathing **Figure 34-25**. Antivenin is

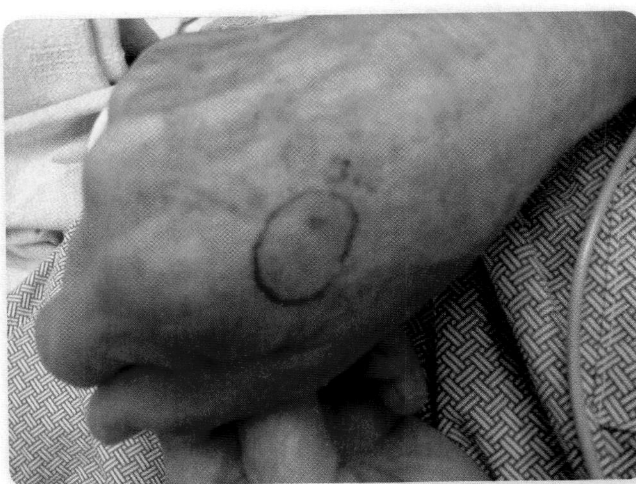

Figure 34-24 In a patient with a snakebite, mark the skin to indicate the area that is swollen.

Courtesy of Rhonda Hunt.

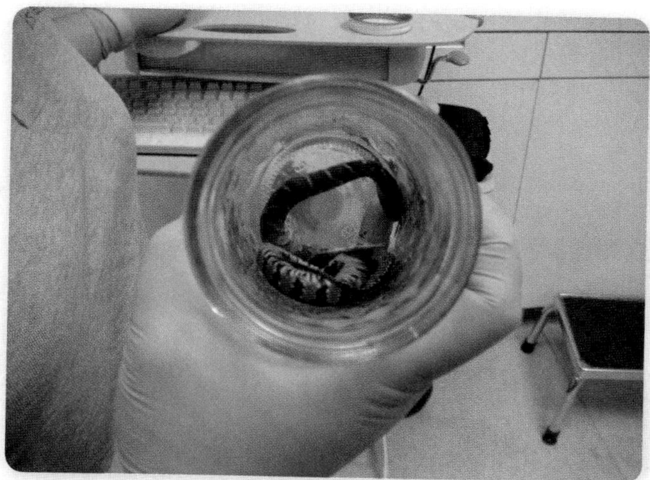

Figure 34-25 If possible, take the snake with you to the hospital for identification.

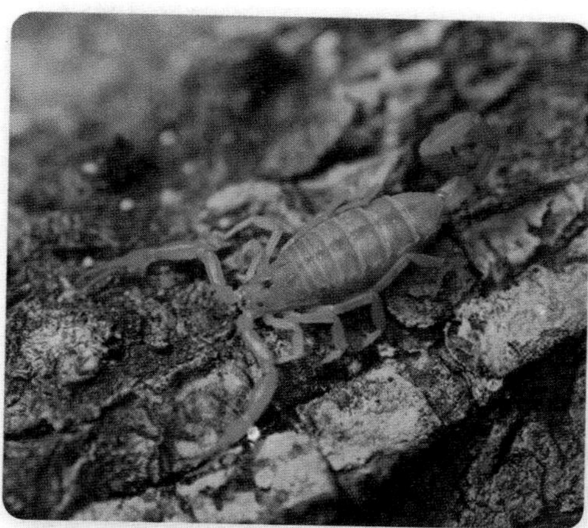

Figure 34-26 The sting of a scorpion is usually more painful than it is dangerous, causing localized swelling and discoloration.

available for coral snakebites, but most hospitals do not stock it. Therefore, you should notify the receiving hospital of the need for it as soon as possible. Follow the same steps listed for emergency care of a pit viper bite, check the patient's vital signs (particularly respirations), and continue to monitor them along with neurologic status.

If the patient shows no sign of envenomation, provide BLS as needed, place a sterile dressing over the suspected bite area, and immobilize the injury site. All patients with a suspected snakebite should be taken to the ED, whether they show signs of envenomation or not. Treat the wound as you would any deep puncture wound to prevent infection.

Words of Wisdom

Evidence of the exact source of an allergic reaction or envenomation may be scarce when you arrive, or bystanders may give you incorrect information. The cause is more likely to pose a risk to responders, and added risk to the patient, if you draw incorrect conclusions about its nature. Keep your eyes and ears open, avoid making unsupported assumptions, and be curious about things that don't quite make sense.

Safety

When treating a snakebite victim, take the snake along to the hospital for identification if it has been killed; however, if you are scratched or punctured by the fangs when handling it, you may also be envenomated. Use extreme caution.

If you work in an area where poisonous snakes are known to live, know your local protocol for handling snakebites. There may be specific hospitals where antivenin is more readily available, either in the facility or through zoos, health departments, or other services.

▶ Scorpion Stings

Scorpions are eight-legged arachnids from the biological group *Arachnida*, with a venom gland and a stinger at the end of their tail **Figure 34-26**. Scorpions live primarily in the southwestern United States and in deserts. With one exception, the sting of scorpions in the US is usually very painful but not dangerous, causing localized swelling and discoloration. The exception is the *Centruroides sculpturatus*. Although it is found naturally in Arizona and New Mexico, as well as parts of Texas, California, and Nevada, it may be kept as a pet by anyone. The venom of this particular species may produce a severe systemic reaction that brings about circulatory collapse, severe muscle contractions, excessive salivation, hypertension, seizures, and cardiac failure. Antivenin is available but must be administered by a physician. If you are called to care for a patient with a suspected sting from a *C sculpturatus* specimen, notify medical control as soon as possible. Administer BLS and provide rapid transport to the ED.

▶ Tick Bites

Found most often on brush, shrubs, trees, sand dunes, or other animals, ticks usually attach themselves directly to the skin **Figure 34-27**. Only a fraction of an inch (approximately 3 mm) long, they can easily be mistaken for a freckle, especially because their bite is not painful. Indeed, the danger with a tick bite is not usually from the bite itself but from the infecting organisms that the tick carries. The most common tickborne diseases are Lyme disease and Rocky Mountain spotted fever; however, other diseases such as ehrlichiosis and tularemia may be important locally. Tickborne diseases are spread through

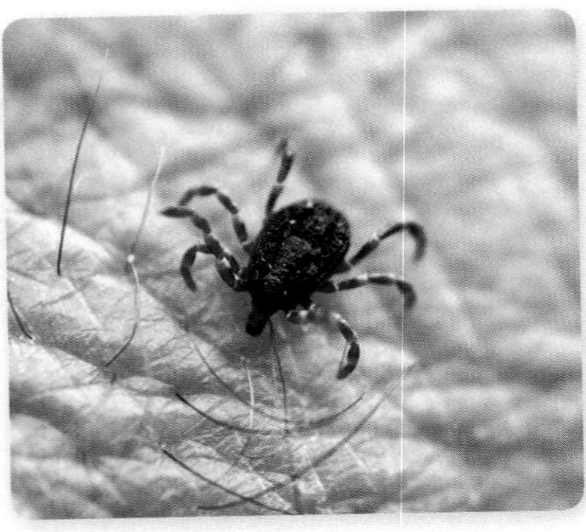

Figure 34-27 Ticks typically attach themselves directly to the skin.

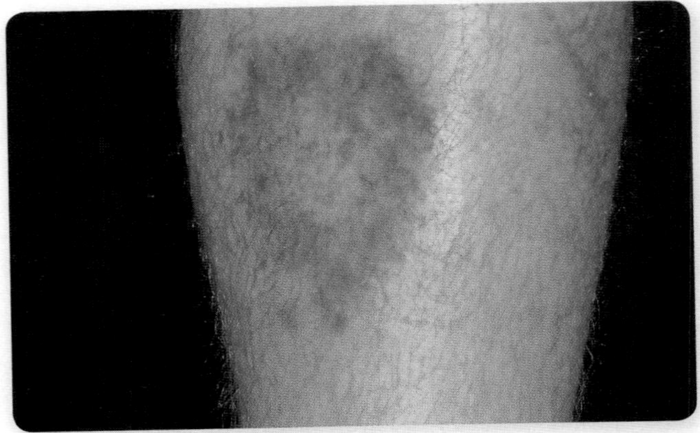

Figure 34-28 The rash associated with Lyme disease has a characteristic bull's-eye pattern.

the tick's saliva, which is injected into the skin when the tick attaches itself. The longer a tick stays embedded, the greater the chance that a disease will be transmitted.

Rocky Mountain spotted fever, which is not limited to the Rocky Mountains, occurs within 7 to 10 days after a bite by an infected tick. Its symptoms include nausea, vomiting, headache, weakness, paralysis, and possibly cardiorespiratory collapse.

Lyme disease has received extensive publicity. It was originally seen only in Connecticut. According to the CDC, Lyme disease has now been reported in all states with the exception of Hawaii.[22] It occurs most commonly in the Northeast, the Great Lakes states, and the Pacific Northwest; Pennsylvania reported the largest number of confirmed cases for 2016.[22] The first symptoms generally include fever, flulike symptoms, and a rash that may spread to several parts of the body and typically begins approximately 3 days after the bite of an infected tick. The rash may eventually resemble a target or bull's-eye pattern in one-third of patients **Figure 34-28**. After a few days or weeks, painful swelling of the joints, particularly the knees, occurs. Lyme disease may be confused with rheumatoid arthritis and, like that disease, may result in permanent disability. However, if it is recognized and treated promptly with antibiotics, the patient may recover completely.

> **Words of Wisdom**
>
> Lyme disease is often mistaken for rheumatoid arthritis, and patients infected may go for long periods without appropriate treatment. It is vital to avoid tunnel vision and obtain a complete history, especially onset of symptoms, when interviewing a patient.

Tick bites occur most commonly during the summer months, when people are out in the woods wearing little protective clothing. Transmission of the infection from tick to person takes at least 12 hours, so if you are called to remove a tick, you should proceed carefully and slowly. Do not attempt to suffocate the tick with gasoline or petroleum jelly, or burn it with a lighted match; you will only increase the risk of infection or burn the patient. Using fine tweezers, grasp the tick by the head and pull it gently but firmly straight up so that the skin is tented. Hold this position until the tick releases. Special tweezers are available for this but are unnecessary. This method will usually remove the whole tick. (Partial removal can result in infection.) Cleanse the area with antiseptic, and save the tick in a glass jar or other container so that it can be identified. Do not handle the tick with your fingers. The patient should follow up with his or her health care provider as soon as possible.

Injuries From Marine Animals

Coelenterates, including the fire coral, Portuguese man-of-war, sea wasp, sea nettles, true jellyfish, sea anemones, true coral, and soft coral, are responsible for more envenomations than any other marine animals **Figure 34-29**. The stinging cells of the coelenterate are called nematocysts, and large animals may discharge hundreds of thousands of them. In light-skinned people, envenomation causes extremely painful red lesions extending in a line from the site of the sting. Systemic symptoms include headache, dizziness, muscle cramps, and fainting.

To treat a sting from the tentacles of a jellyfish, a Portuguese man-of-war, various anemones, corals, or hydras (a type of stinging shrimp), remove the patient from the water and remove the tentacles by scraping them off with the edge of a stiff object such as a credit card. Wash the affected area with vinegar immediately if available for at least 30 seconds to help inactivate the nematocysts. Alcohol may be used but is not as effective. Limit further discharge of nematocysts by avoiding fresh water, wet sand, showers, or careless manipulation of the tentacles.

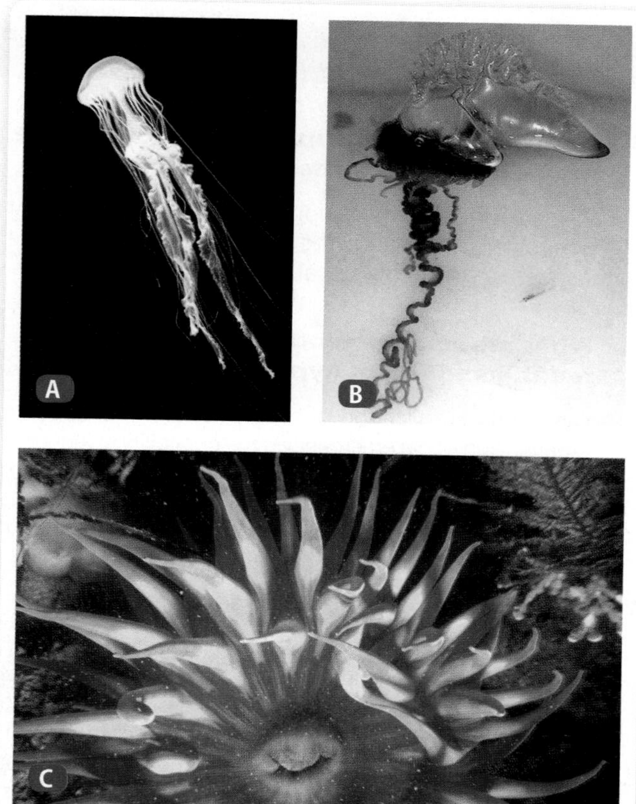

Figure 34-29 Coelenterates are responsible for many marine envenomations. **A.** Jellyfish. **B.** Portuguese man-of-war. **C.** Sea anemone.

A: © Creatas/Alamy; B: Courtesy of NOAA; C: © Photos.com/Getty.

Keep the patient calm, and reduce motion of the affected extremity. Persistent pain may respond to immersion of the area in hot water (110°F to 115°F, 43°C to 46°C) for 30 minutes. On very rare occasions, a patient may have a systemic allergic reaction to the sting of one of these animals. Treat such a patient for anaphylactic shock, and provide immediate transport to the hospital. Call for paramedic backup if needed.

Table 34-6	Common Marine Animal Envenomations
Dogfish	Scorpion fish
Dragonfish	Sea anemone
Fire coral	Sea urchins
Hydroids	Starfish
Jellyfish	Stingray
Lionfish	Stonefish
Marine snail	Tiger fish
Portuguese man-of-war	Toadfish
Ratfish	Weever fish

© Jones & Bartlett Learning.

Toxins from the spines of urchins, stingrays, and certain spiny fish such as the lionfish, scorpion fish, and stonefish are heat sensitive Table 34-6. Therefore, the best treatment for such injuries is to immobilize the affected area and soak it in hot water for 30 minutes. This will often provide dramatic relief from local pain. However, the patient still needs to be transported to the ED because he or she could develop an allergic reaction or infection, including tetanus.

If you work near the ocean, you should be familiar with the marine life in your area.

YOU are the Provider SUMMARY

1. What are four factors that affect exposure?

Four factors that affect exposure are the physical condition of the patient, the patient's age, the patient's nutrition and hydration status, and environmental conditions. Patients who are already ill or in poor physical condition may not be able to tolerate extreme temperatures as well. Patients at extremes of age (very young or older people) are more likely to experience illness as a result of temperatures. The body requires calories for metabolism, and malnourished or emaciated patients may not have the available calories to function. Finally, conditions such as air temperature, humidity, and wind can complicate environmental situations.

2. What are the five methods of heat loss?

The five methods of heat loss are conduction, convection, evaporation, radiation, and respiration. Conduction occurs when heat passes from a warmer object to a cooler object. Convection occurs when heat is transferred to circulating air, such as across the body surface. Evaporation occurs when liquids convert to a gas. Radiation is the loss of body heat directly to colder objects in the environment by radiant energy, and respiration causes body heat to be lost because warm air in the lungs is exhaled and cooler air is inhaled.

3. Discuss ways to increase heat in the body.

The body can increase heat production by increasing the rate of metabolism of the cells. Actions a person can take to increase heat are to move to an area where heat loss is decreased, such as a warmer environment, and wear layers of clothing in cold environments.

4. What stage of hypothermia does this patient present in?

This patient is in severe hypothermia, evidenced by unresponsiveness, a weak and irregular pulse, and lack of shivering.

5. How can warmed, supplemental oxygen be provided to a hypothermic patient?

You can provide warmed, supplemental oxygen to a patient by applying hot packs to the oxygen tubing to warm the inspired oxygen that the patient receives.

6. What are some potential complications of rough handling of hypothermic patients?

The main complication of rough handling of patients experiencing a cold emergency is the possibility of inducing ventricular fibrillation because of the increased irritability of the hypothermic patient's heart. Rough handling can also result in increased pain and the potential for further injury.

7. What are the two methods of rewarming this patient?

The two methods for rewarming hypothermic patients are active and passive rewarming. Passive rewarming involves placing the patient in a warm environment, removing wet clothing, and applying heat packs or hot water bottles to the groin, axillary, and cervical regions. Active rewarming is best accomplished in the ED and includes therapies such as lavage with warm fluids and rewarming blood outside the body before reintroducing it (extracorporeal rewarming).

8. Why should active rewarming not be attempted in this patient?

When a patient has moderate or severe hypothermia, active rewarming is best accomplished in the ED. Rewarming the patient too quickly may cause a fatal dysrhythmia or other substantial complications. For this reason, local protocols may dictate the appropriate type of rewarming strategies based on the patient's body temperature.

YOU are the Provider SUMMARY *(continued)*

EMS Patient Care Report (PCR)

Date: 10-12-18	**Incident No.:** 038	**Nature of Call:** Unresponsive	**Location:** 24225 NE Dresser Rd		
Dispatched: 0213	**En Route:** 0218	**At Scene:** 0229	**Transport:** 0242	**At Hospital:** 0251	**In Service:** 0310

Patient Information

Age: Approximately 45-50 **Sex:** M **Weight (in kg [lb]):** 92 kg (202 lb)	**Allergies:** Unknown **Medications:** Unknown **Past Medical History:** Unknown **Chief Complaint:** Unresponsive/hypothermia

Vital Signs

Time: 0230	**BP:** Not obtained	**Pulse:** Not obtained	**Respirations:** Nonlabored	**Spo_2:** Not obtained
Time: 0237	**BP:** Unable to obtain	**Pulse:** 46, irregular	**Respirations:** 14	**Spo_2:** 95% on 15 L/min
Time: 0241	**BP:** 82/P	**Pulse:** 52	**Respirations:** 14	**Spo_2:** 97% on 15 L/min

EMS Treatment (circle all that apply)

Oxygen @ 15 **L/min via (circle one):** **NC** **(NRM)** **Bag-mask device**		**Assisted Ventilation**	**Airway Adjunct**	**CPR**
Defibrillation	**Bleeding Control**	**Bandaging**	**Splinting**	**Other:**

Narrative

EMS dispatched to above location for unresponsive male. Temperature −20°F, heavy snow. On arrival, met by PD who states patient is a known transient who he or she believes was trying to stay warm for the evening. Patient presents responsive to deep painful stimuli, breathing 14 breaths/min. Negative shivering. Rapid assessment of patient is unremarkable, with no obvious signs of trauma. Patient secured to stretcher, loaded into ambulance. All clothing removed, patient dried. Temperature in patient compartment placed at maximum, blankets applied to patient. 15 L/min of warmed supplemental oxygen given. Emergent transport initiated. 18-gauge IV established to left forearm with bolus of normal saline infusing. Active rewarming not initiated per protocols. On arrival at ED, care and report given to ED staff without incident.**End of report**

Prep Kit

▶ Ready for Review

- An environmental emergency is a medical condition caused or exacerbated by the weather, terrain, or atmospheric pressure at high altitude or underwater.
- Cold illness can be either a local or a systemic problem.
- There are four factors that affect how a person deals with a cold or hot environment: physical condition; age; nutrition and hydration; environmental conditions.
- The body's regulatory mechanisms normally maintain body temperature within a very narrow range around 98.6°F (37°C). Body temperature is regulated by heat loss to the atmosphere via conduction, convection, evaporation, radiation, and respiration.
- The key to treating hypothermic patients is to stabilize vital functions and prevent further heat loss. Do not attempt to rewarm patients who have moderate to severe hypothermia because they are susceptible to developing dysrhythmias.
- Do not consider a patient dead until he or she is "warm and dead." Local protocol will dictate whether or not such patients receive cardiopulmonary resuscitation (CPR) or defibrillation in the field.
- Local cold injuries include frostbite, frostnip, and immersion foot. Frostbite is the most serious because tissues actually freeze. All patients with a local cold injury should be removed from the cold and protected from further exposure.
- If instructed to do so by medical control, rewarm frostbitten parts by immersing them in water at a temperature between 102°F and 104°F (38.9°C and 40°C).
- Heat illness can take three forms: heat cramps, heat exhaustion, and heatstroke.
  - Heat exhaustion is essentially a form of hypovolemic shock caused by dehydration. Body temperature can be high, and the patient may or may not still be sweating. Treatment includes removing the patient from the heat and treating for mild hypovolemic shock.
  - Heat cramps are painful muscle spasms that occur with vigorous exercise. Treatment includes removing the patient from the heat, resting the affected muscles, and replacing lost fluids.
  - Heatstroke is a life-threatening emergency, usually fatal if untreated. Patients with heatstroke are usually dry and will have high body temperatures. Often, the first sign of heatstroke is a change in behavior. Rapid lowering of the body temperature in the field is critical.
- Drowning is the process of experiencing respiratory impairment from submersion or immersion in liquid. Treatment for drowning begins with rescue and removal from the water. Immobilize and protect the patient's spine when a fall from a substantial height or suspected diving injury has occurred (or if this is a possibility). Be aware of the possibility of hypothermia.
- Diving emergencies during descent, at depth, and during ascent can occur as a result of the effects of changes in pressure. Organs in the body contain gases; the variation in the pressure of these gases with changes in atmospheric pressure and volume is described by Boyle's law, Dalton's law, and Henry's law.
- Diving emergencies include barotrauma, nitrogen narcosis, air embolism, and decompression sickness. Injuries associated with SCUBA diving may be immediately apparent or may show up hours later. Patients with air embolism or decompression sickness may have pain, paralysis, or altered mental status. Obtain a detailed diving history. Be prepared to transport such patients to a recompression facility with a hyperbaric chamber.
- High altitudes can cause dysbarism injuries, and include acute mountain sickness, high-altitude cerebral edema (HACE), and high-altitude pulmonary edema (HAPE). Field treatment includes providing oxygen, descending from the height and transporting the patient.
- Lightning injuries may cause cardiac arrest and may damage the nervous system. Ensure the safety of the patient, yourself, and your partner. Look for an entrance and an exit wound. Use the concept of reverse triage when treating patients with lightning injuries. If CPR is instituted promptly, most lightning strike victims will survive.
- Poisonous spiders include the black widow spider and the brown recluse spider; their bites are neurotoxic and cytotoxic, respectively, and can be life threatening.
- Anaphylactic reaction to Hymenoptera stings is a dire emergency and can be fatal if not recognized and treated quickly. Prompt removal of hymenopteran stingers or venom sacs can decrease toxin exposure.
- Poisonous snakes include pit vipers (rattlesnakes, copperheads, and cottonmouths) and coral snakes.
- A person who has been bitten by a pit viper needs prompt transport; clean the bite area and keep the patient quiet to slow the spread of venom.
- If a patient has been bitten by a coral snake, notify the hospital as soon as possible. Coral snake venom can cause paralysis of the nervous system, and most hospitals do not have appropriate antivenin on hand.

Prep Kit *(continued)*

- Scorpion stings can produce a severe systemic reaction. Antivenin is available but must be administered by a physician. If you suspect a scorpion sting, notify the receiving hospital as soon as possible.
- Patients who have been bitten by ticks may be infected with Rocky Mountain spotted fever or Lyme disease and should see a physician within a day or two. Remove the tick using tweezers, and save it for identification.
- Many marine envenomations may benefit from submersion in hot water to deactivate the heat-sensitive toxins. The patient still needs to be transported to the emergency department because he or she could develop an allergic reaction or infection, including tetanus.
- Always provide prompt transport to the hospital for any patient who has been bitten by a poisonous insect or animal. Remember that vital signs can deteriorate rapidly. Carefully monitor the patient's vital signs en route, especially for airway compromise.

▶ Vital Vocabulary

air embolism Air bubbles in the blood vessels.

ambient temperature The temperature of the surrounding environment.

antivenin A serum that counteracts the effect of venom from an animal or insect.

barotrauma Results from a pressure imbalance between gas-filled spaces inside the body and the external atmosphere.

bends Common name for decompression sickness.

breath-holding syncope Loss of consciousness caused by a decreased breathing stimulus.

conduction The loss of heat by direct contact (eg, when a body part comes into contact with a colder object).

convection The loss of body heat caused by air movement (eg, breeze blowing across the body).

core temperature The temperature of the central part of the body (eg, the heart, lungs, and vital organs).

decompression sickness A painful condition seen in divers who ascend too quickly, in which gas, especially nitrogen, forms bubbles in blood vessels and other tissues; also called the bends.

diving reflex Slowing of the heart rate caused by submersion in cold water.

drowning The process of experiencing respiratory impairment from submersion or immersion in liquid.

dysbarism injuries Any signs and symptoms caused by the difference between the surrounding atmospheric pressure and the total gas pressure in various tissues, fluids, and cavities of the body.

environmental emergency A medical condition caused or exacerbated by the weather, terrain, or by atmospheric pressure at high altitude or underwater.

evaporation Conversion of water or another fluid from a liquid to a gas.

frostbite Damage to tissues as the result of exposure to cold; frozen body parts.

frostnip A condition in which tissues are frozen but upon rewarming can be reversed, and deeper tissues are unaffected.

heat cramps Painful muscle spasms usually associated with vigorous activity in a hot environment.

heat exhaustion A form of heat injury in which the body loses substantial amounts of fluid and electrolytes because of heavy sweating; also called heat prostration or heat collapse.

heatstroke A life-threatening condition of severe hyperthermia caused by exposure to excessive natural or artificial heat, marked by warm, dry skin; severely altered mental status; and often irreversible coma.

Hymenoptera A family of insects that includes bees, wasps, ants, and yellow jackets.

hyperbaric chamber A chamber, usually a small room, pressurized to a level higher than atmospheric pressure.

hyperthermia A condition in which the body core temperature rises to 101 °F (38.3 °C) or higher.

hypothermia A condition in which the body core temperature falls below 95 °F (35 °C) after exposure to a cold environment.

immersion foot A condition that occurs after prolonged exposure to cold water, in which the skin of the foot is pale and cold, and there is a loss of sensation; also called trench foot.

laryngospasm A severe constriction of the larynx and vocal cords.

pulmonary overpressurization syndrome (POPS) A diving emergency that can occur during rapid ascent and can cause pneumothorax, mediastinal and subcutaneous emphysema, alveolar hemorrhage, and the lethal air embolism; also called burst lung.

radiation The transfer of heat by radiant energy—for example, heat gain from a fire.

Prep Kit (continued)

reverse triage A triage process in which efforts are focused on those who are in respiratory and cardiac arrest and different from conventional triage where such patients would be classified as deceased. Used in triaging multiple victims of a lightning strike.

SCUBA A system that delivers air to the mouth and lungs at various atmospheric pressures, increasing with the depth of the dive; stands for self-contained underwater breathing apparatus.

submersion Survival, at least temporarily, after suffocation in water or other liquids; also called near-drowning.

thermogenesis The physiologic process of heat production in the body.

thermolysis The process of heat loss; methods include conduction, convection, radiation, evaporation, and respiration.

thermoregulation The balance between heat production and heat excretion.

turgor The ability of the skin to resist deformation; tested by gently pinching skin on the forehead or back of the hand.

wind-chill factor A measurement that takes into account the temperature and wind velocity in calculating the effect of a given ambient temperature on living organisms.

▶ References

1. Roberts WO. Exertional heat stroke during a cool weather marathon: a case study. *Med Sci Sports Exerc*. 2006;38(7):1197-1203.
2. Centers for Disease Control and Prevention: Hypothermia-Related Deaths–United States. *MMWR Weekly*. 2004;53(08);172-173.
3. Heggers JP, Robson MC, Manavalen K, et al. Experimental and clinical observations on frostbite. *Ann Emerg Med*. 1987;16(9):1056-1062.
4. Hallam MJ, Cubison T, Dheansa B, Imray C. Managing frostbite. *BMJ*. 2010;341:c5864.
5. Giesbrecht GG, Danzl DF, et al. Wilderness Medical Society practice guidelines for the out-of-hospital evaluation and treatment of accidental hypothermia: 2014 update. *Wilderness Environ Med*. 2014;25(4 Suppl):S69.
6. CPR and ECC guidelines: cardiac arrest in accidental hypothermia. American Heart Association website. https://eccguidelines.heart.org/index.php/circulation/cpr-ecc-guidelines-2/part-10-special-circumstances-of-resuscitation/cardiac-arrest-in-accidental-hypothermia/. Accessed November 11, 2017.
7. Yu J, Ouyang Q, Zhu Y, et al. A comparison of the thermal adaptability of people accustomed to air-conditioned environments and naturally ventilated environments. *Indoor Air*. 2012;22(2): 110-118.
8. Stofan JR, Zachwieja JJ, Horswill CA, Murray R, Anderson SA, Eichner ER. Sweat and sodium losses in NCAA football players: a precursor to heat cramps? *Int J Sport Nutri Exerc Metab*. 2005;15:641-652.
9. Brege D. Recognizing and treating heatstroke. *Nursing Made Incredibly Easy!* 2009;7(4):13-18.
10. Xu JQ. Unintentional drowning deaths in the United States, 1999-2010. National Center for Health Statistics Data Brief, no. 149. Hyattsville, MD: National Center for Health Statistics. 2014. http://www.cdc.gov/nchs/data/databriefs/db149.pdf. Accessed November 14, 2017.
11. Sempsrott JS, Schmidt AC, Hawkins SC, Cushing TA. Drowning and submersion injuries. In: Auerbach PS, ed. *Auerbach's Wilderness Medicine*. 7th ed. Philadelphia, PA: Elsevier; 2017.
12. 10 leading causes of injury deaths by age group highlighting unintentional injury deaths, United States-2014. Centers for Disease Control and Prevention website. Available at https://www.cdc.gov/injury/images/lc-charts/leading_causes_of_injury_deaths_unintentional_injury_2014_1040w740h.gif. Accessed November 14, 2017.
13. van Hoesen KB, Lang MA. Diving medicine. In: Auerbach PS, ed. *Auerbach's Wilderness Medicine*. 7th ed. Philadelphia, PA: Elsevier; 2017.
14. Schmidt AC. Drownings present as hypoxic events. *J Emerg Med*. 2012;37(7). http://www.jems.com/articles/print/volume-37/issue-7/patient-care/drownings-present-hypoxic-events.html. Accessed March 13, 2017.
15. What is the mammalian dive reflex? Emergency Medical Paramedic website. http://www.emergencymedicalparamedic.com/what-is-the-mammalian-diving-reflex/. Accessed January 22, 2018.
16. Schmidt AC, Sempsrott JR, Hawkins SC, Arastu AS, Cushing TA, Auerbach PS. Wilderness Medical Society practice guidelines for the prevention and treatment of drowning. *Wilderness Environ Med*. 2016;27(2):236-251.
17. Unintentional Drowning: Get the Facts: Risk Factors. Centers for Disease Control and Prevention website. https://www.cdc.gov/homeandrecreationalsafety/water-safety/waterinjuries-factsheet.html. Updated April 28, 2016. Accessed January 12, 2018.
18. Lightning. Centers for Disease Control and Prevention website. https://www.cdc.gov/disasters

Prep Kit *(continued)*

/lightning/. Updated February 16, 2014. Accessed January 11, 2018.

19. Snakebite envenoming fact sheet. World Health Organization website. http://www.who.int /mediacentre/factsheets/fs337/en/. Updated September 2017. Accessed November 15, 2017.
20. Sanders L. Management of venomous snakebites in North America. emDocs website. http://www.emdocs .net/management-of-venomous-snake-bites-in -north-america/. September 11, 2015. Accessed November 15, 2017.
21. Venomous snakes. Centers for Disease Control and Prevention website. https://www.cdc.gov/niosh/ topics/snakes/default.html. Updated July 1, 2016. Accessed January 11, 2018.
22. Control and Prevention website. Lyme disease data tables: reported cases of Lyme disease by state or locality, 2006-2016. https://www.cdc.gov/lyme/stats /tables.html. Updated November 1, 2017. Accessed November 16, 2017.

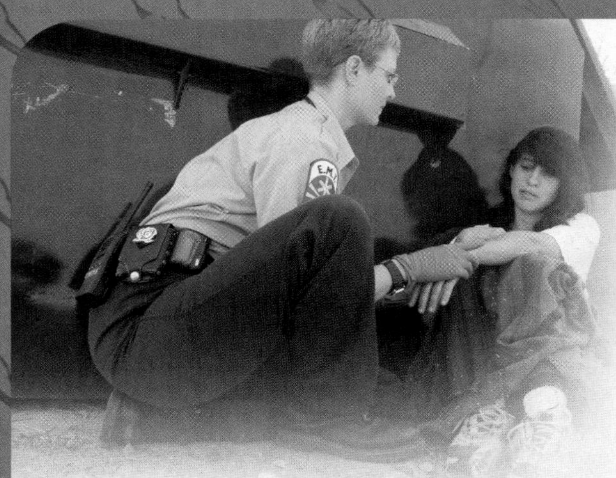

Assessment *in Action*

Your ambulance is dispatched to a remote wilderness area for a patient who was bitten by a rattlesnake. On arrival, you are met by the patient and his hunting partner, who states he was bitten in the leg by a very large rattlesnake. He reports severe pain and swelling of his left calf muscle.

1. A rattlesnake is categorized as a pit viper. Which of the following is not a pit viper?

- **A.** Copperhead
- **B.** Cottonmouth
- **C.** Coral snake
- **D.** King snake

2. Which of the following is not a characteristic of a rattlesnake?

- **A.** Round pupils
- **B.** Vertical pupils
- **C.** Two erectile fangs
- **D.** A single row of teeth

Assessment in Action (continued)

3. Which of the following is not an appropriate treatment for the bite of a rattlesnake?

A. Clean the wound with soap and water.
B. Keep the wound below the level of the heart.
C. Apply ice to the wound to reduce swelling.
D. Use a pressure immobilization bandage.

4. Which of the following is not a sign of envenomation by a pit viper?

A. Ecchymosis around the wound
B. Shock
C. Weakness
D. Hyperactivity

5. The most serious form of heat-related emergency is:

A. heat cramps.
B. heat exhaustion.
C. heatstroke.
D. hypothermia.

6. For a patient with heatstroke, IV fluid should be administered at what rate?

A. 10 mL/kg
B. 20 mL/kg
C. 250-mL bolus
D. 500-mL bolus

7. Which of the following would not make a person more susceptible to a heat illness?

A. Alcohol
B. Diuretics
C. Caffeine
D. Antihistamines

8. When diving, an air embolism can occur in as little as ______ feet of water.

A. 6
B. 10
C. 14
D. 18

9. List the *umbles* behaviors that are good indicators of how the cold affects the cerebral and cognitive functioning of patients in the early stages of (mild) hypothermia.

10. List the potential signs and symptoms of an air embolism that may occur during the ascent of a dive.

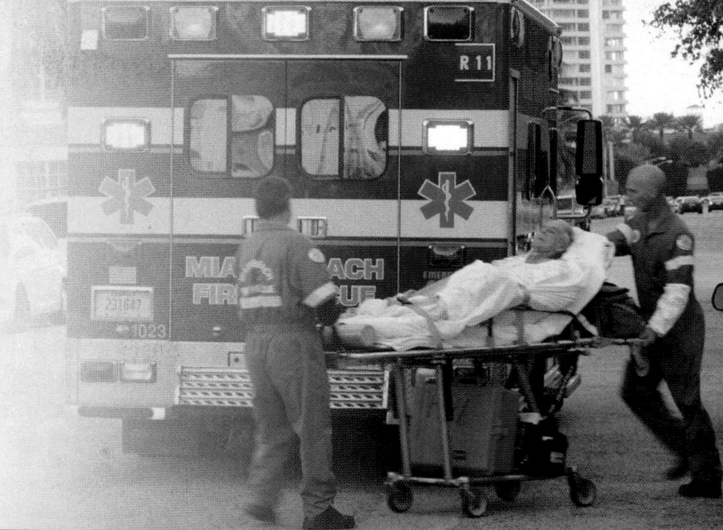

SECTION 9

Special Patient Populations

CHAPTER 35

Obstetrics and Neonatal Care

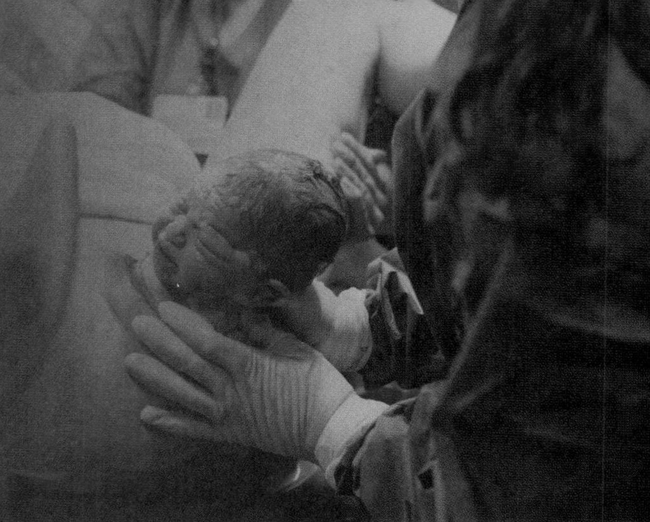

National EMS Education Standard Competencies

Special Patient Populations

Applies a fundamental knowledge of growth, development, aging, and assessment findings to provide basic and selected advanced emergency care and transportation for a patient with special needs.

Obstetrics

- Recognition and management of
  - Normal delivery (pp 1436-1440, 1442-1445)
  - Vaginal bleeding in the pregnant patient (pp 1430-1432, 1435, 1437, 1440-1441)
- Anatomy and physiology of normal pregnancy (pp 1426-1429)
- Pathophysiology of complications of pregnancy (pp 1430-1433, 1449-1450)
- Assessment of the pregnant patient (pp 1436-1440)
- Management of
  - Normal delivery (pp 1442-1445)
  - Abnormal delivery (pp 1447-1452)
    - Nuchal cord (pp 1451-1452)
    - Prolapsed cord (p 1452)
    - Breech delivery (pp 1450-1451)
  - Third-trimester bleeding (pp 1440-1441)
    - Placenta previa (pp 1431-1432)
    - Abruptio placenta (p 1431)
  - Spontaneous abortion/miscarriage (pp 1430, 1440)
  - Ectopic pregnancy (p 1441)
  - Preeclampsia/eclampsia (p 1441)

Neonatal Care

Assessment and management

- Newborn (pp 1454-1463)
- Neonatal resuscitation (pp 1457-1461)

Trauma

Applies fundamental knowledge to provide basic and selected advanced emergency care and transportation based on assessment findings for an acutely injured patient.

Special Considerations in Trauma

Recognition and management of trauma in

- Pregnant patient (pp 1433-1435)
- Pediatric patient (Chapter 36, *Pediatric Emergencies*)
- Geriatric patient (Chapter 37, *Geriatric Emergencies*)

Pathophysiology, assessment, and management of trauma in the

- Pregnant patient (pp 1433-1435)
- Pediatric patient (Chapter 36, *Pediatric Emergencies*)
- Geriatric patient (Chapter 37, *Geriatric Emergencies*)
- Cognitively impaired patient (Chapter 38, *Patients With Special Challenges*)

Knowledge Objectives

1. Review the anatomy and physiology of the female reproductive system and gestation. (pp 1426-1428)
2. Describe the normal changes that occur in the body during pregnancy. (pp 1428-1429)
3. Discuss the pathophysiology of the obstetric patient, including spontaneous abortion (miscarriage), ectopic pregnancy, hypertension, isoimmunization, gestational diabetes, placenta previa, abruptio placenta, and trauma. (pp 1430-1435)
4. Recognize the need to consider two patients—the woman and the unborn fetus—when treating a pregnant trauma patient. (pp 1434-1435)
5. List special considerations involving pregnancy in different cultures and with teenage patients. (pp 1435-1436)
6. Describe commonly used obstetric terminology. (p 1436)
7. Outline the assessment process for pregnant patients. (pp 1436-1440)
8. Describe the indications of an imminent delivery. (p 1438)
9. Discuss assessment and management of nondelivery emergencies. (pp 1440-1441)
10. Differentiate between the three stages of labor. (p 1442)
11. Explain the steps involved in normal delivery management. (pp 1442-1445)

12. Explain the necessary care of the baby as the head appears. (pp 1444-1445)
13. Discuss Apgar scores, including how and when to obtain them. (p 1446)
14. Describe the procedure followed to cut and tie the umbilical cord. (p 1446)
15. Describe delivery of the placenta. (p 1446)
16. Discuss postpartum care to provide, including addressing postpartum hemorrhage. (pp 1446-1447)
17. Explain how to manage complications of labor, including preterm labor, fetal distress, and uterine rupture. (pp 1447-1449)
18. Discuss high-risk pregnancy conditions and their prehospital management, including meconium staining, multiple gestation, cephalopelvic disproportion, intrauterine fetal death, and amniotic fluid embolism. (pp 1449-1450)
19. Discuss complications of delivery, including breech presentation, limb presentation, shoulder dystocia, nuchal cord, and prolapsed umbilical cord. (pp 1450-1452)
20. Discuss postpartum complications and their prehospital management, including uterine inversion, pulmonary embolism, and spina bifida. (pp 1452-1453)
21. Discuss the initial steps of assessment for neonates, including drying and warming, positioning, suctioning, and stimulation. (pp 1454-1456)
22. Explain how to measure essential parameters including heart rate, color, and respiratory effort. (p 1457)
23. List the steps of the algorithm for neonatal resuscitation, including key time frames for interventions. (pp 1457-1458)
24. Discuss techniques for airway management during neonatal resuscitation. (pp 1458-1460)
25. Discuss techniques for circulation support during neonatal resuscitation. (pp 1460-1461)
26. Describe vascular access considerations in the neonate. (pp 1460-1461)
27. Discuss assessment and management of specific emergencies including apnea or inadequate respiratory effort, bradycardia, hypoglycemia, and hypovolemia. (pp 1462-1463)

Skills Objectives

1. Demonstrate the procedure to assist in a normal cephalic delivery. (pp 1442-1445, Skill Drill 35-1)
2. Demonstrate care procedures of the infant as the head appears. (p 1444)
3. Demonstrate the steps to follow in postdelivery care of the infant. (p 1445)
4. Demonstrate how to cut and tie the umbilical cord. (p 1446)
5. Demonstrate how to assist in delivery of the placenta. (p 1446)
6. Demonstrate the postdelivery care of the woman. (pp 1446-1447)
7. Describe how to assist with a breech delivery in the field. (pp 1450-1451)
8. Describe how to assist with a limb presentation in the field. (p 1451)
9. List the steps of neonatal resuscitation. (pp 1457-1458)
10. Explain how to perform chest compressions on a neonate. (pp 1460-1461)

YOU are the Provider PART 1

You and your partner are dispatched to intercept with a vehicle, southbound on I-75 at mile marker 135 for a woman in labor. After you intercept with the vehicle, you find the patient in the rear of the vehicle in obvious distress. She states that they were on their way to the hospital but her contractions keep getting closer together and stronger, and she thought it best to call for an ambulance. The patient states that this is her second pregnancy and that her first baby was born at 29 weeks' gestation. She also tells you that she has a medical history of eclampsia and gestational diabetes.

You decide that the patient needs to be transported via ambulance. Your partner brings the stretcher alongside the car and you assist her onto it and load her into the ambulance. After the patient is placed inside of the ambulance, she tells you she feels a lot of pressure "down there." You turn the heat all the way up and instruct the patient to remove her undershorts. On physical exam, you do not note any crowning or discharge.

1. What stage of labor is the patient in?
2. Is this patient's medical history important?

Introduction

Most births are uneventful and require little or no medical intervention beyond basic interventions, such as suctioning, drying, and warming the baby; others, however, may be life threatening to both the woman and baby. Arriving at the scene of a woman in labor can cause anxiety and fear on the part of both the advanced emergency medical technician (AEMT) and the expecting parents. Parents usually expect to deliver their child in the controlled setting of a hospital delivery room. Unfortunately, if labor progresses quickly or other factors intervene, you may have to deliver the newborn in the field. The birthing process usually requires little help from the health care provider, only supportive care of the pregnant woman and newborn.

This chapter will describe and discuss the normal anatomic and physiologic changes that occur during pregnancy, the normal process of childbirth, and common complications. You will learn how to assess whether to proceed with delivery in the field, how to deliver a newborn, how to manage delivery complications, and how to perform neonatal resuscitation.

Anatomy and Physiology Review: The Female Reproductive System

Recall from Chapter 7, *The Human Body*, that the female reproductive system includes the ovaries, fallopian tubes, uterus, cervix, vagina, and breasts. Hormones from the pituitary gland stimulate the **ovaries** to produce oocytes, which undergo oogenesis that results in an **ovum**, or mature egg cell. An ovum is released regularly, approximately every 28 days, during the adult female's reproductive years. This egg travels through the **fallopian tubes**, hollow tubes or ducts that extend from the uterus to the region of the ovary, where fertilization normally occurs. The fallopian tubes exit into the **uterus**.

During each menstrual cycle, the lining of the uterus thickens in preparation for pregnancy. Pregnancy most frequently occurs during a certain time in the menstrual cycle, after an ovum is mature. If fertilization occurs, the fertilized ovum proceeds through the fallopian tube to implant in the uterus. If fertilization does not occur, the lining of the uterus sheds during **menstruation**.

The **vagina** is the female organ that receives the male penis during sexual intercourse. The muscular walls of the vagina are able to expand, allowing the vagina to stretch greatly during childbirth.

The female external genitalia include the vulva, the labia minora, the clitoris, the prepuce, the labia majora, and the mons pubis. The **perineum** is the area between the urethral opening and the anus. It includes skin, the external genitalia, and underlying tissues.

Figure 35-1 shows the anatomic structures of the pregnant female. The top portion of the uterus is called

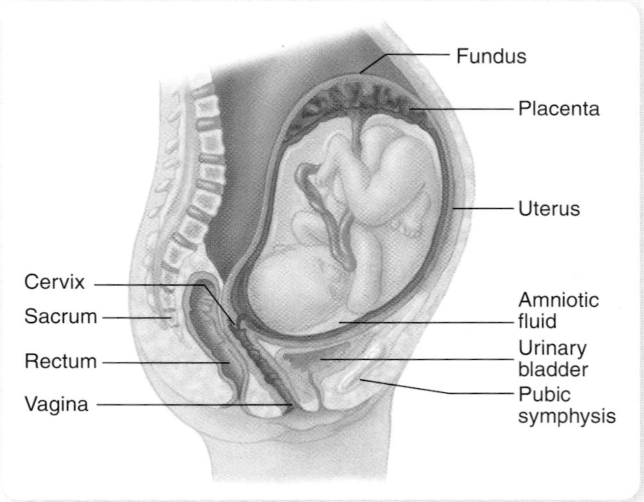

Figure 35-1 Anatomic structures of the pregnant female.

the **fundus**, and the main portion of the uterus is the body. The **cervix** is the part of the uterus that extends into the vagina. The vagina and cervix together are referred to as the **birth canal**.

Gestation

Gestation refers to the process of fetal development following fertilization of an egg. Fertilization occurs when sperm and an ovum meet, usually in the distal third of the fallopian tube. The fertilized egg, called the **zygote**, moves through the fallopian tube toward the uterus. At the same time, the zygote undergoes progressive cell divisions. When the **embryo** contains approximately 32 cells, it usually implants into the uterine wall, which has been thickened by progesterone in preparation for implantation. Implantation usually occurs approximately 7 days after fertilization. The inner group of blastocyst cells (the embryoblast) becomes the embryo; the outer group of cells (the trophoblast) becomes the **placenta** **Figure 35-2**. From the time of fertilization to the end of the ninth week, the developing embryoblast part of the blastocyst is referred to as an embryo; in the 10th week and beyond, it is referred to as a **fetus**. Approximately 3 weeks after fertilization, the placenta is formed in the uterus and merges the fetal and maternal tissue to provide nutrients to and eliminate waste products from the developing fetus.

Approximately 14 days after ovulation, the placenta begins to develop. The placenta carries out a number of crucial functions during pregnancy. The placenta serves as an early liver, taking care of the synthesis of glycogen and cholesterol, metabolizes fatty acid, and allows for the transfer of certain antibodies that protect the fetus. It also performs respiratory gas exchange, transport of nutrients, excretion of wastes, and transfer of heat. Finally, it produces necessary hormones and serves as a barrier against harmful substances in the pregnant woman's circulation.

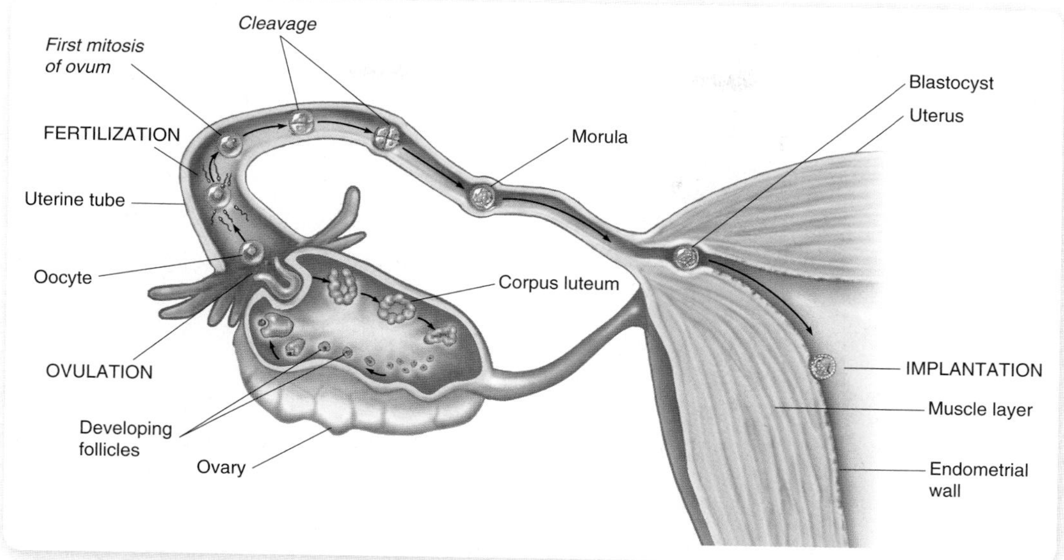

Figure 35-2 Fertilization and implantation of the embryo.

The **umbilical cord** connects the placenta to the fetus via the fetal umbilicus (navel). The cord is gray, easily compressed, and soft and pliant though structurally tough. The umbilical cord contains two arteries and one vein.

Fetal circulation differs from that of the pregnant woman. The umbilical vein carries oxygenated blood from the placenta to the fetus, while the umbilical arteries carry arteriovenous blood to the placenta. Because the fetus obtains its oxygen via the placenta, the fetal circulation bypasses the lungs until birth. A duct connects the umbilical vein and the inferior vena cava (ie, the ductus venosus), another duct connects the pulmonary artery and the aorta (ie, the **ductus arteriosus**), and an opening (ie, the **foramen ovale**) separates the right and left atria of the fetal heart. At birth, the neonate's lungs begin to function, and these arteriovenous shunts close.

Words of Wisdom

Remember: Arteries always carry blood *away* from the heart, and veins always carry blood *toward* the heart. Therefore, the umbilical arteries carry deoxygenated blood away from the heart (to the placenta). Oxygenated blood is returned to the fetus's heart via the umbilical vein.

The **amniotic sac** (also called the amniotic membranes) is a membranous bag that fills with **amniotic fluid** to protect and cushion the developing fetus. The amniotic fluid is produced by the filtration of maternal and fetal blood through blood vessels in the placenta and by excretion of fetal urine into the amniotic sac. Amniotic fluid is swallowed by the fetus and removed by the placenta, where it passes into the woman's blood. The amount of amniotic fluid reaches about 500 to 1,000 mL (1 L) at term, but this volume is constantly changing throughout the pregnancy and reduces to one-half liter by the time the fetus is at term. During labor, when the fetus descends into the birth canal, the pressure on the amniotic sac causes its rupture (**rupture of membranes**). This rupture releases the amniotic fluid that has cushioned the fetus during development. If the amniotic sac ruptures before labor occurs, the fetus is at higher risk for complications, including trauma and infection. This is called **premature rupture of membranes**.

The **gestational period** is the time that it takes for the infant to develop in utero. This process normally takes 38 weeks, with substantial developmental progress occurring each week except for the last several weeks, in which growth primarily occurs. The time of conception is calculated from the first day of the pregnant woman's last menstrual period. This dating method adds 2 weeks to the entire calculation, resulting in a standard 40 total weeks of pregnancy from conception to birth. Some normal pregnancies may last more than 40 weeks.

These 40 weeks of pregnancy form the prenatal period and are divided into three **trimesters** Figure 35-3. The first trimester extends from the last menstrual cycle through week 12 of the pregnancy. Major events in the first trimester include a positive pregnancy test result (blood or urine hCG) at 8 to 10 days, a palpable uterine fundus at the pubic symphysis at week 12, and audible fetal heart tones noted on Doppler ultrasonography. All major fetal organ systems begin to develop during the **embryonic period** (weeks 3 through 8) Figure 35-4. From the embryonic period until delivery, organ systems undergo continuing maturation and development.

The second trimester extends from week 13 through week 27. The major events are a palpable uterine fundus between the pubic symphysis and the umbilicus at week 16, the first fetal movements (quickening) at weeks 16

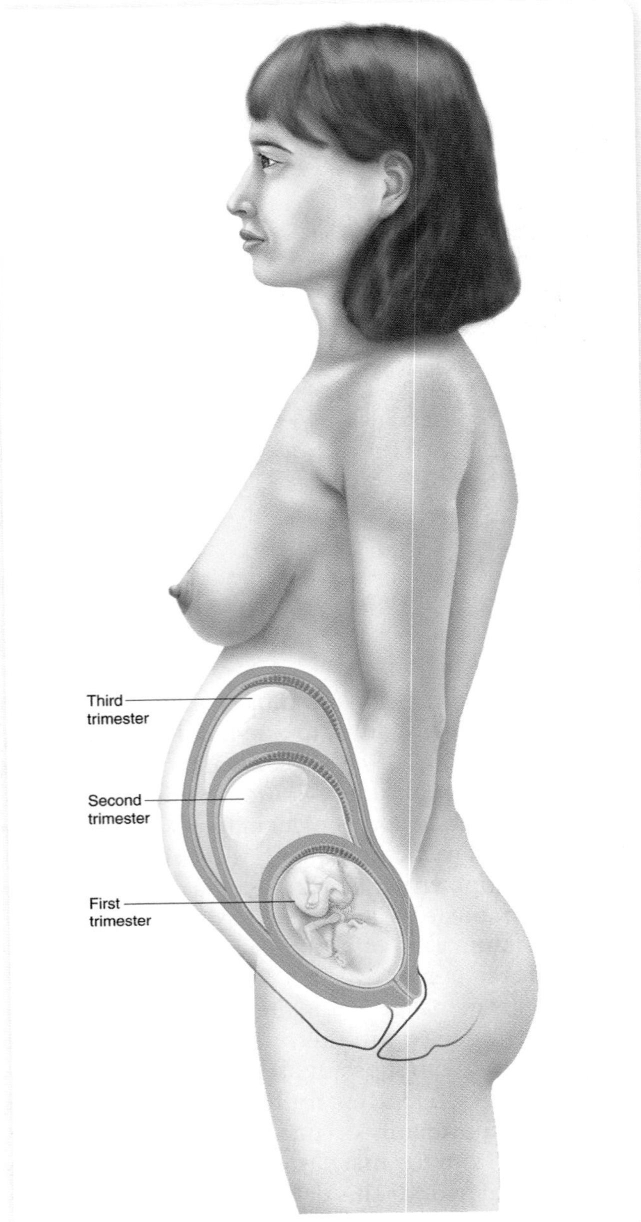

Figure 35-3 The three trimesters of pregnancy. You will usually not be able to see any physical change in a woman during the first trimester. You may be able to estimate whether the woman is in the second or third trimester.

through 18 in a woman who has had one or more previous pregnancies, and fetal heart tones that become audible with a **fetoscope** at weeks 17 through 20. In addition, female and male genitalia may be distinguished by **ultrasonography** at week 18, first fetal movements are noted in a woman's first pregnancy at weeks 18 through 20 (the woman may detect fetal movement earlier if she has been pregnant before), and the uterine fundus is palpable at the umbilicus at week 20. At weeks 25 through 27, the lungs become capable of respiration and produce surfactant, a liquid protein substance that coats the alveoli in the lungs.

The third trimester extends from week 28 until **term** (week 40). The major events of the third trimester include

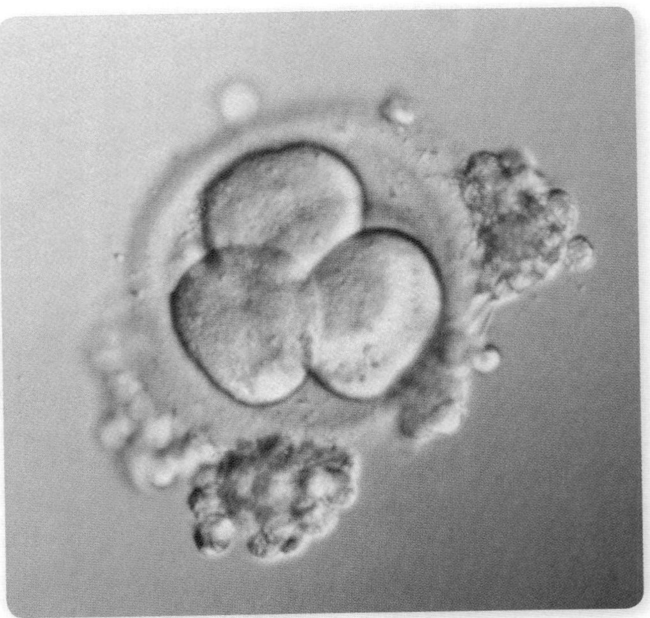

Figure 35-4 All major organ systems begin to develop during the embryonic period.

the presence of papillary light reflex in the fetus, descent of the fetal head to the pelvic inlet (lightening), and rupture of the amniotic sac. After the amniotic sac has ruptured, it is optimal that the fetus be delivered within 24 hours because of the risk of infection. At the end of the third trimester, the fetus typically weighs 7.0 to 7.5 lb (approximately 3.2 to 3.4 kg).

A **newborn** is a recently born baby and is generally considered "newborn" for the first few hours of its life. During the first 28 days of life, a baby is considered to be a **neonate**. Between the ages of 1 month and 1 year, a baby is referred to as an **infant**.

Special Populations

A newborn delivered at less than 37 completed weeks of gestation is considered **preterm**; a newborn born at 38 to 42 weeks of gestation is described as term; and a newborn born at more than 42 weeks of gestation is described as postterm (or postdates).

Normal Maternal Changes of Pregnancy

In addition to changes in the reproductive system, during pregnancy, many other body systems undergo changes to support the growing fetus.

The maternal cardiovascular system undergoes dramatic changes during pregnancy. The total blood volume increases by about 50% by 40 weeks and the red blood cells increase in number by about 30%. The heart rate elevates by 10 to 20 beats/min. Cardiac output increases by 30% to 50% more than the prepregnancy level, reaching its maximum capacity at approximately 22 weeks' gestation, and then declines to approximately 20% near term.[1] The systolic and diastolic blood pressures decrease by 10 to 15 mm Hg by the second trimester of pregnancy and return to near-normal by full term. In the second and third trimesters of pregnancy, the **gravid** (pregnant) uterus may compress the woman's inferior vena cava when she lies supine. This can substantially reduce the return of blood to the heart (preload), thereby causing a decrease in blood pressure.

The increase in red blood cells heightens the pregnant woman's need for iron, which is why most women have to take prenatal vitamins. If the woman does not take iron supplements, the fetus will rob maternal stores for its needs, resulting in anemia for the woman and possibly resulting in preterm labor or **spontaneous abortion** (miscarriage). Women who live in socioeconomically disadvantaged areas and lack access to prenatal health care, along with those who do not obtain prenatal health care, are the most likely to experience pregnancy-related anemia.

The respiratory minute volume of the patient increases by about 40% by full term to accommodate the increased blood volume and demand for oxygen from the fetus. In pregnancy, the woman's tidal volume also initially increases. After the gravid uterus has grown enough to lie against the diaphragm, the patient may not be able to fully inspire the tidal volume needed to maintain adequate minute volume. If so, the woman's respiratory rate increases to compensate for the reduced tidal volume.

Because of the increase in the amount of air that goes in and out of the lungs, the amount of carbon dioxide that the patient exhales increases. A relative respiratory alkalosis develops in the patient, which may cause dizziness and shortness of breath. Also, carbon dioxide produced by the fetus travels to the placenta and diffuses into the maternal bloodstream.

The pregnant woman often experiences gastrointestinal complaints at some time during the pregnancy. Often called morning sickness, nausea and sometimes vomiting occurs most commonly between the 8th and 14th week of pregnancy. As the uterus grows later in the pregnancy, the stomach and intestines of the woman are compressed and pushed superiorly, resulting in heartburn, a burning sensation around the epigastrium. If the patient is unresponsive and has no gag reflex, the risk of regurgitation and aspiration also increases. The peristalsis of the bowels decreases from the pressure of the uterus on the gastrointestinal tract and so digestion slows, often resulting in constipation. Decreased gastrointestinal function could also affect the absorption of medications, resulting in medications remaining in the blood longer than usual.

On average, the pregnant woman gains approximately 27 lb during a full-term pregnancy. If the patient gains substantially more weight than average, she may be at risk for several of the disorders of pregnancy that will be discussed later. Pregnant women often have edema in their lower extremities.

All of these are monitored with standard prenatal care. If the woman has not received prenatal care, the potential for complications can be increased.

YOU are the Provider — PART 2

The patient states that she is approximately 32 weeks pregnant based on her last menstrual cycle and has not had any prenatal care. You note that her contractions are approximately 1 minute in length and 1 minute apart. You obtain a set of vital signs as your partner prepares the obstetric (OB) kit. As a precaution, you establish an 18-gauge intravenous (IV) line in her right forearm with normal saline solution at a to-keep-open (TKO) rate. Just as you finish securing the IV site, the patient states that she needs to have a bowel movement "NOW!"

Recording Time: 1 Minute	
Appearance	Anxious
Level of consciousness	Alert and oriented to person, place, day, and event
Airway	Patent
Breathing	Rapid, panting
Circulation	Strong radial pulses; skin warm, dry, and pink

3. Is immediate transport of this patient warranted?
4. Does this patient need IV access at this point?

Pathophysiology During Pregnancy

Many complications can occur during the pregnancy that can threaten the health or life of both the woman and fetus. We will examine the most common of these conditions. One of the common early pregnancy emergencies that you will care for is vaginal bleeding. This can be a sign of several conditions that range from benign to life threatening.

▶ Abortion

The most common cause of vaginal bleeding during the first and second trimesters of pregnancy is spontaneous abortion or miscarriage. Most spontaneous abortions occur during the first trimester, before the placenta is fully mature. The term *abortion* does not imply any cause and simply means that the fetus is released from the uterus before 20 weeks of gestation **Figure 35-5**.

Abortions can be broadly classified as spontaneous or elective (induced). A spontaneous abortion (miscarriage) occurs naturally, and affects an estimated 10% to 25% of all pregnancies.[2] Causes may include acute or chronic illness in the pregnant woman, maternal exposure to toxic substances (illicit drugs), abnormalities in the fetus, or abnormal attachment of the placenta. In many cases, the cause of a spontaneous abortion cannot be identified.

An **elective abortion** is brought about intentionally. When you are obtaining a medical history that includes an abortion, you must be dispassionate and professional regardless of your personal convictions. You may encounter patients who are experiencing complications following an elective abortion, such as vaginal bleeding or sepsis from having parts of the fetus remaining in the uterus. You may also encounter patients who have "self-medicated" in an attempt to induce an abortion and are experiencing toxic effects of the herbal remedy as well as a threatened or progressing abortion. Herbal preparations work by making the uterus and bloodstream too toxic for the fetus to survive, which may be too toxic for the woman to survive.

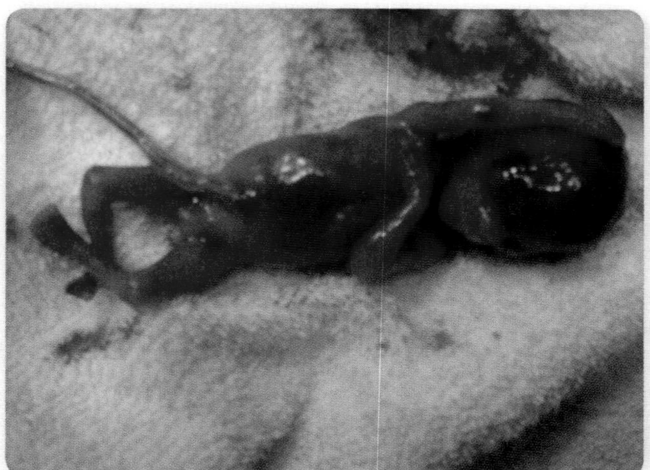

Figure 35-5 A miscarried fetus.

Courtesy of Rhonda Hunt.

A **threatened abortion** is an abortion that is impending or potentially occurring. It is generally characterized by vaginal bleeding during the first half of pregnancy, usually in the first trimester. The patient may present with abdominal discomfort or report menstrual cramps. Severe pain is rarely a presenting complaint because uterine contractions are not rhythmic. The cervix remains closed. A threatened abortion can progress to a miscarriage or abortion, or it may subside, allowing the pregnancy to go to term. The treatment for a threatened abortion is usually complete bed rest to avoid activity or fluctuations in vital signs that could further provoke an abortion. Your role in this case is usually transport and emotional support.

An **imminent abortion** is an impending or threatened spontaneous abortion that cannot be prevented. The patient will generally present with severe abdominal pain caused by strong uterine contractions. Vaginal bleeding, sometimes substantial, will be present, as well as cervical dilation because the uterus is preparing to expel the products of conception. When you are treating a patient who is experiencing a spontaneous abortion, your goals are to maintain blood pressure and prevent hypovolemia. Treatment consists of administering 250-mL boluses of normal saline, repeating as needed, to maintain a blood pressure of greater than 80 mm Hg, 100% supplemental oxygen via a nonrebreathing mask at 15 L/min, and providing emotional support with rapid transport. Be alert for signs of shock.

An **incomplete abortion** occurs when part of the products of conception are expelled but some remain in the uterus. (For example, the fetus is expelled but the placenta remains, or only part of the fetus is expelled.) Because the cervix has dilated to expel the fetus, vaginal bleeding will be present, which may be slight or substantial, but will be continuous. Be alert for signs and symptoms of shock, and start an IV line of normal saline. If products of conception are protruding from the vagina, consult medical control for instructions; gentle removal of protruding tissues may prevent or relieve signs of shock. You will most often encounter this situation when you find the patient on the toilet, having attempted a bowel movement, with the fetus in the toilet still attached to the umbilical cord hanging from the vagina. The fetus should be gently collected, and emotional support provided to the patient. Fundal massage may be beneficial in stimulating the placenta to deliver. All products of conception need to be collected and presented to the receiving facility. Do not deter the patient from viewing the fetus if she wishes, but be prepared for a strong emotional reaction. A **complete abortion** has occurred when all the products of conception have been expelled.

▶ Ectopic Pregnancy

Another cause of first-trimester bleeding is the implantation and growth of the embryo outside of the uterus. This **ectopic pregnancy** can implant in the fallopian tube, on the ovary, in the abdominal cavity or peritoneum, or in the cervix. The most common place to find an ectopic pregnancy is in the fallopian tube (tubal pregnancy). During the first trimester, the embryo grows rapidly. It quickly grows into the walls of the fallopian tube, where it causes tearing and finally ruptures the tube. As this occurs, the woman usually feels lower abdominal pain and cramping. She usually, but not always, has vaginal bleeding. Depending on where the embryo implants, the bleeding may be internal or external and may be scant or profuse. This can be a life-threatening emergency for the pregnant woman during the first trimester. The embryo will not survive and must be removed surgically to save the woman. If the fallopian tube actually ruptures, she may present to you in severe shock and possibly cardiac arrest from massive hemorrhage. Ectopic pregnancy is discussed in Chapter 25, *Gynecologic Emergencies*.

▶ Third-Trimester Bleeding

Abortion accounts for most vaginal bleeding that results in an emergency call. Any detachment of the ovum or embryo from the uterine wall will result in bleeding. The patient may report light or heavy bleeding, normally accompanied by cramping abdominal pain. She may also report the passage of tissue or clots. Vaginal bleeding is a serious sign at any stage of pregnancy, but the complications of bleeding increase as the gestation progresses.

Third-trimester bleeding presents the most dangerous hemorrhage in terms of risk to the health of the mother. This becomes even more acute as the woman approaches term. A complicating factor of third-trimester bleeding is the large volume of blood present within the pregnant woman's body and the compensatory mechanisms that are functioning as a result of pregnancy. A pregnant woman can lose a full 40% of her circulating volume before substantial signs and symptoms of hypovolemia become apparent.

▶ Bleeding and the Placenta

Major causes of substantial hemorrhage before delivery are abruptio placenta and placenta previa.

Abruptio placenta refers to a premature separation of a normally implanted placenta from the wall of the uterus **Figure 35-6**. It most commonly occurs during the last trimester of pregnancy, but can take place in the second trimester as well. Abruptio placenta affects approximately 1 of every 100 pregnancies that go to term.[3,4] Although the exact cause of abruptio placenta is unknown, hypertension, trauma, drug use, alcohol use, diabetes, and having multiple pregnancies increase the risk for this condition.[3,4]

The patient with abruptio placenta will present with a sudden onset of severe abdominal pain, often radiating into the back; there will also be decreased fetal movement and decreased fetal heart tones. The patient may report vaginal bleeding, although in some cases the blood does not emerge through the cervix and the bleeding may remain concealed within the endometrium. Physical examination may reveal signs of shock, often out of proportion to the apparent volume of blood loss. The abdomen will be tender and the uterus rigid to palpation. Other complications include severe hemorrhaging. If the hemorrhaging cannot be controlled after delivery, a hysterectomy may be necessary.

In **placenta previa**, the placenta is implanted low in the uterus and, as it grows, it partially or fully obscures the cervical canal **Figure 35-7**. This condition is the leading cause of vaginal bleeding in the second and third trimesters of pregnancy, with most problems occurring near term because the cervix begins to dilate in preparation for delivery. Maternal age and multiparity are risk factors.

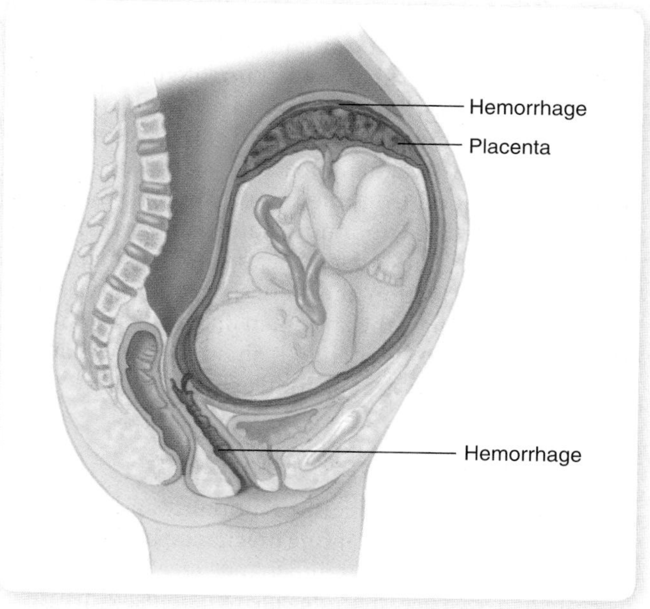

Figure 35-6 In abruptio placenta, the placenta separates prematurely from the wall of the uterus.

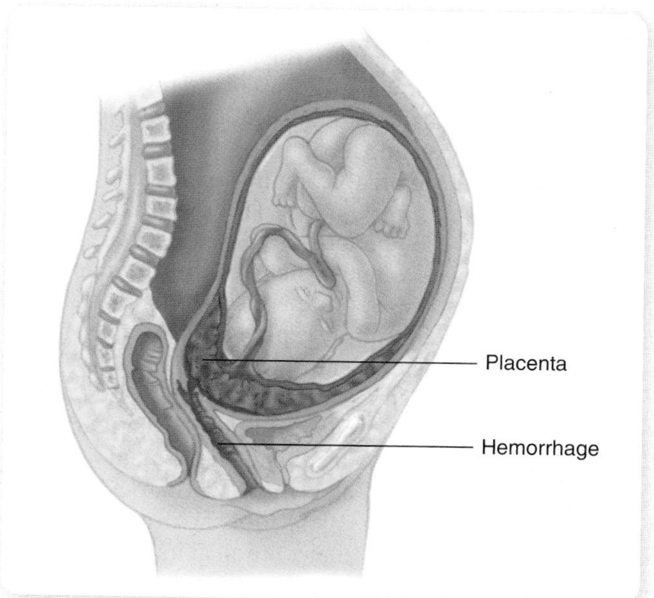

Figure 35-7 In placenta previa, the placenta develops over and covers the cervix.

Placenta previa occurs in approximately 1 of every 200 births,[5] with a maternal mortality rate of less than 1%.[6] Complications may include disseminated intravascular coagulation, hemorrhage, and low fetal birth weight.

The chief complaint of a woman with placenta previa is usually painless vaginal bleeding, with the expulsion of bright red blood from the vagina. Because the blood supply to the fetus is not immediately jeopardized, fetal movements continue and fetal heart sounds remain audible. On gentle palpation, the uterus is soft and nontender. (Do *not* try to palpate the abdomen deeply in any woman with third-trimester bleeding; if she does have placenta previa, deep palpation may induce heavy bleeding.)

Hypertensive Disorders

Hypertension is a major cause of mortality and morbidity in the pregnant woman. During pregnancy, blood pressure is usually lower than at prepregnancy levels, but women who are hypertensive or borderline hypertensive may have their hypertension exacerbated by pregnancy.

Chronic hypertension is defined as a blood pressure that is equal to or greater than 130/80 mm Hg, which existed prior to pregnancy, occurs before the 20th week of pregnancy, or continues to persist postpartum.[7] Diastolic pressures higher than 110 mm Hg place the patient at an increased risk for stroke and other cardiovascular dangers. Chronic hypertension can also retard growth and development of the fetus, impair liver and renal function, cause pulmonary edema, or progress to life-threatening tonic-clonic seizures.

Gestational hypertension (formerly known as pregnancy-induced hypertension) develops after the 20th week of pregnancy in women with previously normal blood pressures and resolves spontaneously in the postpartum period. It is more commonly experienced by women who are obese or glucose intolerant.

Preeclampsia is defined as an increase in blood pressure after the 20th week of gestation. Women younger than 18 years who are experiencing their first pregnancy, women with advanced maternal age (those who are 35 years or older), and women with risk factors of chronic hypertension, renal disease, and diabetes are all at increased risk for preeclampsia.[8] In the first trimester of pregnancy the blood pressure typically increases slightly; it decreases below the baseline during the second trimester and returns to the baseline during the third trimester. Chronic hypertension can retard growth and development of the fetus; in the woman, it can impair liver and renal function, cause pulmonary edema, or progress to life-threatening tonic-clonic seizures.

Preeclampsia is accompanied by a protein release in the urine and often by edema, particularly in the face, ankles, and hands. The protein in the urine will not typically be detected by emergency medical services (EMS) personnel, and edema can be normal for a pregnant woman.

The most important feature of preeclampsia for you to recognize is hypertension. Other symptoms include severe headache, nausea and vomiting, agitation, rapid weight gain, and visual disturbances.

Special Populations

Preeclampsia manifests after the 20th week of pregnancy, with the onset of a triad of symptoms: edema, usually of the face, ankles, and hands; gradual onset of hypertension; and protein in the urine.

Eclampsia is a seizure in a pregnant woman who has preeclampsia and no other cause for the seizure. A woman who is an epileptic and has a seizure may or may not be eclamptic. Eclampsia may occur before labor, during labor, after delivery of the newborn, or even up to several weeks following delivery (postpartum eclampsia). A woman may have only one seizure or may have continuous or multiple seizures (status epilepticus). As mentioned in Chapter 25, *Gynecologic Emergencies*, **postpartum eclampsia** usually presents within the first 24 hours after delivery, but may occur as late as 4 weeks following the birth.

Another common finding in a pregnant patient is hypotension when lying supine, called **supine hypotensive syndrome** or vena cava compression syndrome, which may be an issue when a woman is injured and must be immobilized. This happens mainly in the second and third trimesters of pregnancy when the woman lies supine (but can occur when sitting) and is a result of compression of the inferior vena cava by the weight of the gravid uterus.[9] Left uncorrected, supine hypotensive syndrome can result in substantial maternal hypotension and potentially result in fetal distress because the maternal hypotension translates into placental hypoperfusion. It generally takes 3 to 7 minutes of compression before signs and symptoms manifest, and in the majority of women, symptoms never develop. Nausea, dizziness, tachycardia, and claustrophobia are early signs, progressing to breathing difficulty and syncopal episodes. Precipitating factors may include hypovolemia, from either blood loss or dehydration.

Special Populations

Simply rolling the patient onto the left side alleviates supine hypotension. If the patient is on a long backboard, tilt the board approximately 30° to the left by propping it up, for example with blankets.

Isoimmunization (Rh Sensitization)

As mentioned in Chapter 7, *The Human Body*, Rh factor is a protein found on the red blood cells of most people. When the factor is absent, the person is said to be Rh negative. When a woman who is Rh negative becomes pregnant by a man who has the Rh factor (Rh positive) and the fetus inherits this factor, the fetal blood can pass into the woman's circulation and produce maternal antibody (isoimmunization) to the factor.

This is normally not a problem in first pregnancies, but in subsequent pregnancies, the antibody will aggressively cross the placental barrier to attack the fetal red blood cells, which the woman's body identifies as foreign proteins. This attack can result in death for the fetus or cause hemolytic disease (erythroblastosis fetalis) in a newborn. Newborns with hemolytic disease may present with jaundice, anemia, and hepatomegaly.

▶ Gestational Diabetes

Gestational diabetes mellitus is the inability to process carbohydrates during pregnancy. Increased maternal insulin production may lead to an imbalance between the supply of the woman's insulin and glucose production. The patient may be asymptomatic or may exhibit the same signs observed in patients with diabetes mellitus: polyuria, polydipsia, and polyphagia. Treatment consists of diet control and oral hypoglycemic medications. As gestational diabetes mellitus may occur early in the pregnancy, it is recommended that patients undergo a fasting glucose test as part of routine prenatal testing.

Diabetes may be markedly affected by pregnancy. As the hormones of pregnancy alter the insulin-regulating mechanisms, patients with diabetes may experience wildly fluctuating blood glucose levels, manifested as hyperglycemic or hypoglycemic episodes. Unfortunately, oral hypoglycemic agents can cross the placental barrier and affect the fetus, so women with insulin-dependent diabetes may have to adjust their daily dosing during pregnancy.

Gestational diabetes predisposes the patient to hyperglycemia or hypoglycemia. If a woman with preexisting or gestational diabetes does not control her blood glucose levels throughout her pregnancy, she may have problems during labor and delivery. The fetus may grow to a larger-than-average size and may not fit through the birth canal. Additionally, diabetes (gestational diabetes or diabetes mellitus) in a pregnant woman predisposes the newborn to hypoglycemia. Usually, gestational diabetes spontaneously resolves following delivery.

▶ Hyperemesis Gravidarum

Nearly all women experience the infamous (but normal) "morning sickness," especially during the first several weeks of pregnancy. **Hyperemesis gravidarum** is a condition of persistent nausea and vomiting during pregnancy.[10] Its prolonged vomiting results in dehydration and malnutrition, which have negative effects on the woman and fetus. The exact cause of the condition is unknown, but suspected causes include increased hormone levels (especially estrogen and human chorionic gonadotropin), stress, and changes to the gastrointestinal system. Hyperemesis gravidarum is most common in first-time pregnancies, with multiple gestations, and in women who are obese.

Symptoms include severe and persistent vomiting, in excess of three or four times daily. Vomiting is usually projectile and generally consists of bile and possibly blood. Severe nausea, pallor, and possibly jaundice may also be seen.

Prehospital treatment includes administering 100% oxygen via nonrebreathing mask, checking blood glucose level, providing an IV line of normal saline with fluid boluses as needed, and providing transport. Severe cases require hospitalization.

Special Populations

Any pregnant patient with a history of hyperemesis gravidarum who presents with hematemesis should alert you to the possibility of a Mallory-Weiss tear. This typically occurs after a prolonged or forceful bout of straining or vomiting and hyperemesis gravidarum is the most common cause in women of childbearing age.[11] Maintain the airway and provide rapid transport. Gain IV access en route.

▶ Premature Rupture of Membranes

When the amniotic sac ruptures or "opens" more than an hour before labor, it is called premature rupture of the membranes. In some instances, the sac will self-seal and heal itself, but more commonly, labor will begin within 48 hours. If the pregnancy is at or near term, there is usually no concern. However, if the pregnancy is not yet at term, there is a risk of infection. In either situation, you should provide emotional support to the patient and provide transport to the hospital.

Special Populations

If a pregnant woman is assaulted or otherwise injured, this may result in injury to the fetus, or the fetus can be harmed indirectly as a result of the woman's blood loss.

Special Considerations for Trauma and Pregnancy

Trauma is a serious complicating factor in pregnancy, partly because of the many physiologic changes that occur during pregnancy, but mostly because of the involvement of two patients—the woman and her fetus. Both patients are particularly vulnerable to trauma because of the unique features of pregnancy. The major causes of injury to pregnant women are motor vehicle crashes, falls, domestic abuse, and penetrating injuries such as gunshot wounds.

When a pregnant woman is involved in a motor vehicle crash or a similar mechanism of injury (MOI), severe hemorrhaging may occur from injuries to the pregnant uterus.

The anatomic changes during pregnancy have important implications for trauma. As the woman approaches term, her abdominal contents are compressed into the upper part of the abdomen. There is a higher incidence of abdominal injuries associated with chest trauma. Meanwhile, because the peritoneum is maximally stretched, substantial abdominal trauma may occur without peritoneal signs.

In the second and third trimesters of pregnancy, the uterus is more vulnerable to trauma. The bladder is displaced upward (superior) and forward (anterior) and is therefore at increased risk of injury, particularly from a deceleration injury. Deceleration forces may bring about abruptio placenta or **uterine rupture**.

A relative redistribution of blood volume also occurs during pregnancy, with blood flow to the pelvic region increasing tenfold. Therefore, if a pregnant woman sustains a pelvic fracture, her chances of bleeding to death are much higher than those of a nonpregnant woman. A substantial amount of blood can be lost before signs and symptoms of shock develop because other mechanisms are compensating for the loss.

Recall that a pregnant woman has an increased need for oxygen. If she should need artificial ventilation, you will have to administer supplemental oxygen at a higher minute volume than usual (she will require a slightly faster rate of ventilation). Also remember that with the gravid uterus placing pressure on the stomach, the chances of vomiting and aspiration are dramatically increased.

Pregnant women have an increased risk of falls compared with nonpregnant women. Hormonal changes "loosen" up the joints in the musculoskeletal system, and the weight of the uterus and displacement of abdominal organs can change the patient's balance.

Increases in blood volume, cardiac output, and in the resting pulse rate during pregnancy make it more difficult to interpret tachycardia. Furthermore, because of the pregnant woman's vastly expanded blood volume, other signs of hypovolemia, such as a falling blood pressure, may not be evident until she has lost as much as 40% of her blood volume. Therefore, you need to aggressively treat a pregnant woman with an MOI that indicates shock.

The muscular wall of the uterus acts as a cushion for the fetus against the direct effects of blunt trauma, but fetal injury can occur. The most common cause of fetal death from trauma is maternal death, but a woman will often survive an incident that proves fatal for the fetus. For instance, blunt trauma resulting in abruptio placenta has a good statistical outcome for pregnant women but often results in fetal death.[12]

If a pregnant woman has sustained trauma and is bleeding massively, the maternal circulation will shunt blood away from fetal circulation to maintain maternal homeostasis—maternal circulation takes precedence over the requirements of the fetus. Therefore, any injury that involves substantial maternal bleeding will threaten the life of the fetus. By the time the woman shows clinical signs of shock, fetal circulation will be so compromised that you can expect a fetal mortality rate of 70% to 80%.

Finally, not all pregnant women properly position their seat belts when in a vehicle. The lap belt should be placed under the abdomen and over the hip bones, and the shoulder belt should be positioned between the breasts. If a pregnant woman is involved in a motor vehicle crash with an improperly positioned seat belt, the seat belt can cause harm to the woman and fetus because the seat belt compresses the uterus. Shoulder restraints, by contrast, decrease the chance of uterine injury.

Words of Wisdom

When the body encounters a catastrophic event (shock) threatening the life of a pregnant woman, the fetus is treated as a parasite by the woman's body. The best hope of a positive outcome for the fetus is aggressive treatment of the woman.

Words of Wisdom

In a pregnant patient who has sustained trauma, remember to assess first for exsanguinating hemorrhage (follow the XABCDE mnemonic [eXsanguinating hemorrhage, Airway, Breathing, Circulation, Disability, Exposure]).

Assessment and Treatment of the Pregnant Trauma Patient

A pregnant woman involved in a motor vehicle crash, fall, assault, or other injury must be evaluated in the emergency department (ED). In general, what is good for the woman will be good for the fetus. For example, any effort to improve maternal perfusion will improve fetal circulation. Potential damage to the fetus cannot be adequately assessed in the field. Whereas a decreased fetal heart rate signals an emergency situation, a normal fetal heart rate does not guarantee that all is well.

In general, the prehospital management of pregnant women with abdominal trauma is the same as for nonpregnant patients. Airway, breathing, and circulation remain the highest priorities.

In addition to abdominal tenderness, the examination of an injured pregnant woman may reveal an abnormal fetal position, an easily palpated fetus, inability to palpate the top of the uterus, or vaginal bleeding.

Carefully assess a pregnant woman's abdomen and chest for seat belt marks, bruising, and obvious trauma. Maintain a high index of suspicion for internal abdominal bleeding in the woman and possible direct injury to the fetus, regardless of seat belt placement.

Remember to treat the woman aggressively if there is an index of suspicion for injury. This is your only opportunity to provide optimal care for the fetus. Assess the abdomen for rigidity and question the woman about movement of the fetus since the accident.

Remember that the likelihood of domestic abuse increases greatly during a woman's pregnancy; be suspicious for evidence of abuse.

Because the large uterus can compress the vena cava (decreasing right atrial preload), a pregnant woman should be transported to the hospital on her left side or with her right hip elevated about 6 inches (15 cm) to minimize the pressure of the vena cava depending on the degree of suspicion for spinal column injury. The fetus may be in shock before signs appear in the woman, so initiate early, aggressive fluid resuscitation.

In summary, field treatment of a pregnant trauma patient is as follows:

1. **Maintain an open airway.** A pregnant patient has an increased risk of vomiting and aspiration compared with patients who are not pregnant. Be prepared for and anticipate vomiting; keep your suction unit readily available. If the patient is unresponsive, call for paramedic backup to provide early endotracheal intubation to isolate the airway.
2. **Administer high-flow oxygen.** A pregnant woman's oxygen needs are 10% to 20% higher than normal, so provide 100% supplemental oxygen via a nonrebreathing mask if the patient is responsive.
3. **Ensure adequate ventilation.** Listen to breath sounds, and confirm that bilateral breath sounds are present. If the patient has inadequate ventilation, provide or assist ventilation with a bag-mask device and 100% oxygen. Because the uterus of a pregnant woman presses up against the diaphragm, she will be more difficult to ventilate.
4. **Assess circulation.** Control external bleeding promptly with direct pressure. Maintain a high index of suspicion for internal bleeding and shock based on the MOI because a pregnant patient will not always display typical signs and symptoms of shock. Keep the patient warm. Splint any fractures. Provide spinal immobilization if there is an indication and remember to tilt the board to the left to take pressure off the inferior vena cava.
5. **Provide IV fluids.** Start one or two IV lines of normal saline. Use large-bore catheters and macrodrip sets. Administer a bolus if signs and symptoms of hemodynamic compromise are present, with the goal of maintaining blood pressure above 80 mm Hg. Remember that a larger volume of fluid is necessary for the pregnant patient.
6. **Transport considerations.** Transport the woman on her left side (to anticipate vomiting and to avoid supine hypotensive syndrome). If she is on a backboard, tilt the backboard 30° to the left by wedging pillows beneath it. This will cause the uterus to shift, taking the weight off the inferior vena cava and improving venous return to the heart. Call early for assistance or a medical helicopter for significant MOIs or major traumatic injuries. Transport the patient to a trauma center if one is available in your area. Give early notification that you have a pregnant trauma patient in transport.

Because of the change in anatomy with the increasing size of the fetus, managing the airway becomes more challenging. There is greater pressure on the diaphragm and airways. Call early for paramedic backup for airway management and medication administration.

Finally, in any case of substantial vaginal bleeding or severe abdominal pain, quickly assess and transport the patient, support the airway, administer high-flow oxygen, place sanitary pads against the vaginal opening, position the patient on her left side, and call for paramedic backup.

If cardiac arrest occurs, provide cardiopulmonary resuscitation (CPR), beginning with chest compressions, as you would for a nonpregnant patient. The 2015 CPR and Emergency Cardiovascular Care (ECC) guidelines recommend positioning the pregnant patient experiencing cardiac arrest in a supine position while another rescuer provides manual left uterine displacement.[13] This is shown in Chapter 15, *BLS Resuscitation*. Hand placement for chest compressions in an obviously pregnant patient should be moved up the sternum, generally between the breasts. Additionally, the normal landmarks you would use for chest compressions may not be obvious in a pregnant patient in the third trimester—use the sternal notch as a guideline for hand placement (approximately 5 to 7 inches [13 to 18 cm] below the angle of Louis).

If resuscitation efforts are not effective within 5 minutes, an emergency cesarean section must be performed to save the woman and possibly the fetus. Therefore, your patient requires rapid transport and prior notification to the closest medical facility. Even if the woman has obvious mortal injuries, good CPR and ventilatory support may keep the fetus viable until a cesarean section can be performed.

Cultural Value Considerations

The United States is among the most culturally diverse nations in the world. This diversity may be a factor when you are assessing and treating an obstetric patient from a culture different from yours. Women of some cultures may have a value system that will affect their pregnancy, the choice of how they care for themselves during pregnancy, and how they have planned the childbirth process. Some cultures may not permit a male health care provider, especially in the prehospital setting, to assess or examine a female patient. Different cultures may view pregnancy differently than you do in terms of social, psychological, and emotional issues. Some may see pregnancy as a means of achieving status and recognition within the family unit, whereas others may experience a drop in self-esteem. Your responsibility is to the patient and is limited to providing care and transport. You should respect these differences and honor requests from the patients.

Teenage Pregnancy

The United States has high teenage pregnancy rates compared with other developed countries.[14] During your career, you are likely to respond to a pregnant teenager who may or may not be in labor. Adolescents present their own challenges to the EMS community in terms of physical and psychological development, even when pregnancy is not a contributing factor for a female teenager.

Pregnant teenagers may or may not know that they are pregnant or may be in denial about their pregnancy. As you begin to assess all female teenagers, you should remember that pregnancy is a possibility, as you would for any woman of childbearing age. The pregnancy itself may or may not be related to the nature of the call, but you should consider the possibility when assessing the patient, talking to the patient, obtaining a history, and providing treatment. Respect the teenager's privacy and need for independence. If possible, perform your assessment and obtain the patient's history in a location away from her parents.

Special Populations

Often, adolescents who become pregnant are frightened and neglect to tell their parents or caregivers about their pregnancy, resulting in a lack of prenatal care. It is not uncommon for pregnant adolescents to skip meals to avoid gaining excess weight in an attempt to hide the expanding waistline. Lack of medical attention, poor diet, and a lifestyle that is not conducive to pregnancy, (ie, use of recreational drugs and smoking) can result in danger to the adolescent or the fetus. Other emergencies may occur when the adolescent, without financial resources, tries "home remedies" to induce an abortion. It is important to question any female of childbearing age about the possibility of pregnancy, regardless of the chief complaint. Be sure to interview the patient in private where she will be more likely to confide in you.

Patient Assessment

In most cases, childbirth is a natural process that does not require your assistance. When childbirth is complicated by trauma or other conditions, any interventions you provide for the patient will benefit the fetus. For example, if a pregnant patient has a low pulse oximetry reading, the fetus does as well; applying oxygen to the patient also improves the oxygen level in the fetus.

Understanding certain terms unique to pregnancy will allow you to more accurately communicate the patient's obstetric history with other health care providers. **Gravida** is a term used to describe the number of times a woman has been pregnant. **Para** is a term used to describe the number of times a pregnant woman has delivered a viable newborn, one carried for more than 20 weeks' gestation. For example, if a woman has been pregnant twice, but had a miscarriage during her first pregnancy and one healthy child, she would be gravida 2, para 1. A woman who is pregnant for the first time would be gravida 1, para 0. After she delivers a viable baby, however, she then becomes gravida 1, para 1. A woman's history of pregnancy may be documented with G (gravida), P (para), and A (abortive history). For example, a woman who has had two pregnancies, one of which resulted in a viable newborn and one of which miscarried, this would be documented as G2P1A1. Some other commonly encountered obstetric terms are:

- **Primigravida**—a woman who is pregnant for the first time.
- **Primipara**—a woman who has had only one delivery.
- **Multigravida**—a woman who has been pregnant two or more times, irrespective of the outcome.
- **Nullipara**—a woman who has never delivered a viable newborn, although she may have been pregnant before.
- **Multipara**—a woman who has delivered two or more viable newborns.
- **Grand multipara**—a woman who has delivered five or more viable newborns.

Scene Size-up

As with every emergency call, your safety is the top priority when dealing with an obstetric case. Take standard precautions—gloves and eye protection are a minimum if delivery has already begun or is imminent. If the call will result in a field delivery, you should also don a mask and gown. Consider calling for additional or specialized resources.

You will also encounter pregnant patients who are not in labor, so it is important to determine the MOI or nature of illness in a pregnant patient. Because a pregnant

Safety

It is important that you always follow standard precautions to protect yourself from exposure to body fluids. There is a high potential of exposure to body fluids during childbirth.

woman's balance may be altered by the weight and size of the fetus and hormones that relax the musculature, falls and spinal immobilization must be considered.

Primary Survey

The primary survey with a pregnant patient is the same as with any patient—assess the ABCDEs (Airway, Breathing, Circulation, Disability, and Exposure), and manage life threats.

The general impression is a good across-the-room assessment that should tell you whether the patient is in active labor or if you have time to assess for imminent delivery and address other possible life threats. The chief complaint may be, "The baby is coming!" Take a moment to confirm whether the infant will be delivered in the next few minutes or whether you have time to continue to evaluate the situation. When trauma or other medical problems such as vaginal bleeding or seizures are the presenting complaint, evaluate these first and then assess the effect of these problems on the fetus. Use the AVPU (*Awake and alert*; responsive to *Verbal* stimuli; responsive to *Pain*; or *Unresponsive*) scale to determine the patient's level of consciousness.

During an uncomplicated birth, life-threatening conditions with the woman's airway and breathing are not usually an issue. In contrast, a motor vehicle crash, an assault, or any number of medical conditions in a pregnant woman may cause a life threat to exist and, sometimes, result in a complicated delivery. In these situations, assess the airway and breathing to ensure they are adequate. If needed, provide airway management and oxygen as appropriate.

Recall that normal changes in pregnancy result in increased overall blood volume, increased heart rate, and changes in blood clotting. These changes can have a substantial effect on a pregnant patient who is bleeding, regardless of the cause. Quickly assess for any potential life-threatening bleeding, and begin treatment immediately. Assess the skin for color, temperature, and condition, and check the pulse to determine whether it is too fast or too slow. If there are signs of shock, control the bleeding, give oxygen, and keep the patient warm. A minimum of one IV line should be established in preparation for a fluid bolus if needed.

If delivery is imminent, prepare to deliver at the scene. The ideal place to deliver an infant prehospitally is in the security of your ambulance or the privacy of the woman's home. The area should be warm and private with plenty of room to move around.

If the delivery is not imminent, prepare the patient for transport and perform the remainder of the assessment en route to the ED. Administer oxygen. Pregnant women in the last two trimesters of pregnancy should be transported lying in the left lateral recumbent position to displace the weight of the uterus from the superior vena cava, if possible. Although the left lateral recumbent position is an accepted treatment and transportation option, if the woman does not develop supine hypotension and is more comfortable in a supine position, it is acceptable to use a supine position. If spinal immobilization is indicated, secure the woman to the backboard and elevate the right side of the board with rolled towels or blankets to prevent supine hypotensive syndrome **Figure 35-8**. Provide rapid transport for pregnant patients who have substantial bleeding and pain, are hypertensive, are having a seizure, or have an altered mental status.

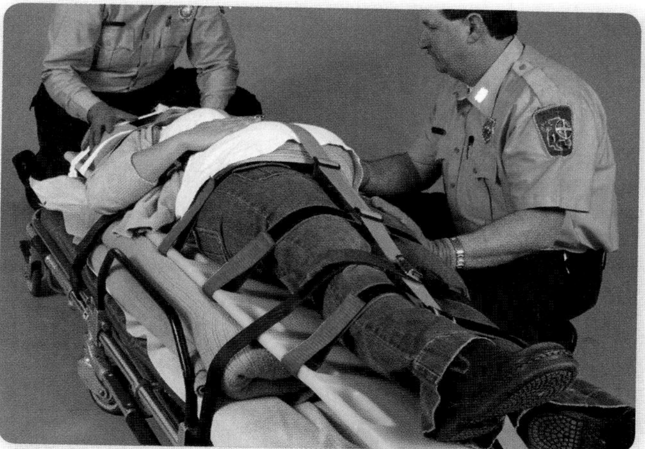

Figure 35-8 Place a blanket under the right side of the backboard to prevent supine hypotensive syndrome in pregnant patients.

Words of Wisdom

Avoid tunnel vision when assessing a woman in labor. Remember, the ABCs still come first. Do a complete assessment including SAMPLE (Signs and symptoms, Allergies, Medications, Pertinent past medical history, Last oral intake, Events leading up to the illness or injury) history, vital signs, obstetric history, and recent fetal movement.

History Taking

When you are assessing a pregnant patient, determine the patient's chief complaint, and elaborate on the chief complaint using the OPQRST (Onset, Provocation/palliation, Quality, Region/radiation, Severity, Timing) mnemonic. Specifically, you want to know if the patient is pregnant, how many times she has been pregnant (gravida), and how many times she has had a live birth (para). The first question ("Are you pregnant?") can generally be bypassed if the patient is obviously pregnant. Asking a woman who is near term if she is pregnant (the unspoken implication is that she is obese) is not a good way to develop patient trust, but, if in doubt, ask. The number of times a woman has been pregnant may also need to be clarified because some women may not count abortions or miscarriages as pregnancies. Also ask about the length of gestation and her estimated due date or date of confinement. You should also ask about fetal movement.

If the patient tells you she has abdominal pain, ask her to describe the pain; this information will help determine whether she is having contractions.

Has the woman had a baby before? Labor in a woman who is pregnant for the first time usually proceeds more slowly and takes longer (average time, 16 hours) than in subsequent pregnancies, allowing more time for transport. If the patient has already had a child, she may be able to tell you when she is about to deliver. If she believes that she is ready, examine for crowning and, if indicated, make immediate preparations for delivery.

Identifying potential complications prior to the delivery will better prepare you to treat the woman and newborn. Ask the patient whether she has experienced complications with any of her pregnancies, or whether she has had any obstetric or gynecologic complications. In addition, ask:

- Has she ever had a cesarean section? If so, is the current delivery planned for as a cesarean delivery or does the patient intend to have a vaginal birth after cesarean (VBAC)? (Complications of VBAC can include uterine rupture.[15-17])
- Is the patient currently under a physician's care?
- Has she been taking prenatal vitamins?
- When was her last visit to her physician?
- Has her physician indicated any concerns about this pregnancy?
- Has the patient recently undergone ultrasonography? If so, what were the findings? Did the ultrasonogram reveal more than one fetus or any abnormal presentations?
- Is the patient taking any current medications? Any over-the-counter drugs, recreational drugs, or herbal supplements?
- Does the patient have any allergies?

Consider delivering a newborn at the scene under the following circumstances:

- Delivery is expected within a few minutes.
- A natural disaster, bad weather, or some other type of catastrophe makes it impossible to reach the hospital.
- No transportation is available.

To determine whether delivery may occur within a few minutes, first look for **crowning**, then ask the pregnant woman the following questions:

- How many weeks pregnant are you and when are you due? (The more premature the infant, the more resuscitation and care it is likely to require. Knowing the gestational age can also help you select the correct-sized equipment for the newborn.)
- Is this your first baby?
- Are you having contractions? How far apart are the contractions? How long do the contractions last? (Contractions are timed from the beginning of one contraction until the beginning of the next. If they are less than 5 minutes apart and regular, delivery may be imminent.)
- Do you feel the urge to move your bowels? (This indicates that the fetus has entered the birth canal and is resting on top of the woman's rectum.)
- Have you had any spotting or bleeding? If so, what color was it and how much? (Be sure to take any tissue that may have been passed during the bleeding with you to the hospital for evaluation.)
- Have you had a rush of fluid from the vagina? (This indicates that the membranes have ruptured.)

Do not allow the pregnant woman to get up to go to the bathroom. Instead, reassure her that the sensation of needing to move her bowels is normal and that it means she is about to deliver.

Also consider asking the following questions:

- Have you had a complicated pregnancy in the past?
- Do you use illicit (recreational) drugs, drink alcohol, or take any medications? (Many depressant drugs and alcohol pass through the placental barrier to the fetus. If they have been recently ingested, the newborn may be born with respiratory depression and require aggressive resuscitation.)
- Have you recently undergone ultrasonography, and is there a possibility that this is a multiple birth? (Multiple births are often lower in birth weight, and if they require invasive care, you may need additional assistance for each newborn in addition to the woman.)

If the patient's water has broken, ask about the color of the fluid and whether it had an odor. If it is brown or black or has a strong odor, it may be an indication of meconium staining. **Meconium**, a thick, tarry substance, is the fetus's first bowel movement and can pass into the amniotic fluid. If meconium is present after birth, you should call early for paramedic back up who may need to perform more invasive suctioning of the newborn's trachea (discussed later in this chapter).

Secondary Assessment

Your physical exam should be based on the patient's chief complaint. Just because a woman is pregnant, you should not rule out the possibility of other emergencies such as asthma, heart attack, or allergic reactions, for example. No matter what the chief complaint, the secondary assessment should include a complete set of vital signs including pulse; respirations; skin color, temperature, and condition; blood pressure; and pulse oximetry if time permits. Also obtain fetal heart tones and heart rate. By feeling the abdomen, you can roughly palpate the fetal position as well as assess fetal movement. Pay close attention to the vital signs of both patients—the woman and the fetus. Watch for tachycardia and hypotension (which could mean hemorrhage or compression of the vena cava) or hypertension (possibly indicating preeclampsia). Compare your findings with previous blood pressure readings she may know of from prenatal visits. Hypertension, even mildly elevated blood pressure, may indicate more serious problems.

During the onset of labor, initial uterine contractions are often irregular. The woman may feel only a backache or abdominal cramping. As the labor progresses, the frequency and intensity of contractions increase. The full-term delivery usually occurs when the contractions are 1 to 2 minutes apart and last from 30 to 60 seconds. Some women may experience **Braxton-Hicks contractions**—intermittent uterine contractions that may occur every 10 to 20 minutes. They can occur any time during pregnancy but are usually seen in the third trimester. This condition is also known as false labor. Because you have no way of telling in the field if a patient's contractions are from a miscarriage or another complication of pregnancy, the patient needs to be transported to the ED. The pains of true labor are regularly spaced and increase in intensity over time. **Table 35-1** lists the characteristics of false labor and true labor.

For a pregnant patient in labor, your physical examination should focus on contractions and possible delivery. Women who are pregnant for the first time typically take longer to deliver, whereas multigravida and multipara women can deliver very quickly. Assess the length and frequency of contractions by asking the patient and by placing your hand on the abdomen. Compare what you feel with the patient's experience during each contraction. If at any point you suspect delivery is imminent, you should check for crowning. This specific assessment should be performed only when appropriate and according to local protocol. If you do not suspect an imminent delivery and the patient has other complaints unrelated to delivery, you should not visually inspect the vaginal area. Be sure to protect the woman's privacy during the physical examination.

If you see bleeding or discharge, ascertain when it started and check the abdomen for tenderness and rigidity. Normal abdomens are not rigid during pregnancy. Assessment of the serial vital signs will tell you if the woman or fetus is in distress.

Table 35-1 False Labor Versus True Labor

Parameter	True Labor	False Labor
Contractions	Regularly spaced	Irregularly spaced
Interval between contractions	Gradually shortens	Remains long
Intensity of contractions	Gradually increases	Stays the same
Effects of analgesics	Do not abolish the pain	Often abolish the pain
Cervical changes	Progressive effacement and dilation	No changes

Words of Wisdom

Deep palpation of the abdomen in any woman with third-trimester bleeding may result in massive hemorrhage if she has placenta previa.

Reassessment

As time allows, repeat the primary survey with a focus on the patient's ABCs and vaginal bleeding, particularly after delivery. Obtain another set of vital signs and compare the results with those obtained earlier. Frequent reassessment of vital signs may identify hypoperfusion from excessive blood loss as a result of delivery. Recheck interventions and treatments to see whether they were effective. Is the vaginal bleeding slowing with uterine massage? Uterine massage, discussed later in this chapter, can be used to slow vaginal bleeding after delivery. Finally, transport to an appropriate facility.

If your assessment determines that delivery is imminent, notify staff at the receiving hospital. Provide an update on the status of the woman and newborn after delivery. On the rare occasion that the delivery does not occur within 30 minutes or you determine that a complication is occurring that cannot be treated in the field, notify the hospital staff of your findings and provide rapid transport. Be sure to notify staff at the receiving hospital of all relevant information so there is time to prepare. The information you provide may help the hospital staff determine whether the patient will be seen in the ED or whether you will be asked to bring the patient directly to the labor and delivery unit.

For a pregnant patient with complaints unrelated to childbirth (such as trauma or difficulty breathing), be sure to include the pregnancy status of your patient in your radio report. The hospital staff will want to know the number of weeks of gestation, her due date, and any known complications of the pregnancy.

Thorough documentation is essential, especially the status of the newborn if delivery occurred in the field. You will have two patient care reports to complete. Obstetrics is among the most litigated specialties in medicine; this is another reason why scrupulous documentation is essential.

Assessment and Management of Nondelivery Emergencies

▶ Spontaneous Abortion

If spontaneous abortion occurs during the first half of the pregnancy, it is generally characterized by vaginal bleeding and abdominal cramping. Severe pain is rarely a presenting complaint because uterine contractions are not rhythmic, and the cervix remains closed. In the second half of pregnancy, the patient may present with severe abdominal pain caused by strong uterine contractions, substantial vaginal bleeding, and cervical dilation.

There is no specific treatment that you must provide to the patient with a suspected spontaneous abortion. The patient should receive high-flow oxygen, a large-bore IV line of an isotonic crystalloid (ie, normal saline or lactated Ringer solution) in the event fluid boluses are required for severe bleeding and shock, and transport to an appropriate hospital. You should support her emotionally, without giving false hope, and try to keep her calm.

▶ Third-Trimester Bleeding

When the patient presents with the chief complaint of vaginal bleeding in the third trimester of pregnancy, try to determine as much as possible about the nature of the bleeding by asking the following questions:

- When did the bleeding start?
- What activity was the woman engaged in at the onset (ie, was she active or at rest)?
- How much blood has been lost (how many pads soaked)?
- Is the patient experiencing abdominal pain? If so, what is the nature of the pain? Is it sharp, cramping, dull, achy?

Use the OPQRST mnemonic to elaborate on the chief complaint of pain. Rate the severity of pain on a scale of 1 to 10. During the physical examination, identify any changes in orthostatic vital signs. Orthostatic changes indicate a substantial blood loss, which may be contrary to the physical evidence of bleeding, which may be slight. Look for a positive Grey Turner sign (ecchymosis of the flanks) or Cullen sign (ecchymosis around the umbilicus), which can indicate the presence of internal bleeding.

You do not need to identify the underlying cause of the bleeding in the third trimester of pregnancy to begin treatment. Regardless of the source of hemorrhage, prehospital management is the same as follows:

1. Keep the patient in a recumbent position on her left side.
2. Administer 100% supplemental oxygen via a nonrebreathing mask at 15 L/min.

YOU are the Provider — PART 3

While assessing the patient you note the baby's head crowning and make the determination to deliver on scene. You prepare for immediate childbirth by placing the sterile drapes in their appropriate positions and reminding the woman to breathe through the contractions. Your partner calls for a second ambulance for assistance. Placing your hand gently against the baby's head to prevent an explosive delivery, the baby starts to deliver. As the baby's head emerges, you note that the umbilical cord is around the neck.

Recording Time: 6 Minutes	
Respirations	32 breaths/min, rapid
Pulse	Strong and regular, 120 beats/min
Skin	Warm, dry, and pink
Blood pressure	96/54 mm Hg
Oxygen saturation (Spo_2)	99% on room air
Pupils	Pupils Equal, Round, and Reactive to Light and Accommodation (PERRLA)

5. What are the possible complications if you do not support the baby's head?
6. How do you correct nuchal cord?

3. Provide rapid transport to a definitive care facility, notifying the facility of the patient's condition en route.
4. Start an IV line of normal saline with an 18-gauge IV catheter. Begin infusing a 250-mL bolus of fluid and then reevaluate. Continue with such boluses as indicated up to four boluses. If blood pressure has not yet reached 80 mm Hg systolic, obtain medical direction and prepare to administer additional fluid boluses. An additional IV line may be indicated.
5. Obtain baseline vital signs. Do not attempt to examine the woman internally or pack the vagina with trauma pads.
6. Use loosely placed trauma pads over the vagina in an effort to stop the flow of blood and massage the fundus.
7. If bleeding is severe and signs and symptoms of shock are present, consider calling for paramedic backup to rendezvous en route.

Words of Wisdom

When starting an IV line on a patient in labor, try to choose a site other than the antecubital fossa. If the woman bends her arm to push during labor, the flow rate is cut off.

▶ Ectopic Pregnancy

In cases of ectopic pregnancy, all the normal signs and symptoms of pregnancy are usually present. The patient is in severe pain, possibly in hypovolemic shock. The treatment of the patient with a suspected ectopic pregnancy is focused on supporting the ABCs. She should receive high-flow oxygen, at least one large-bore IV line of an isotonic crystalloid, and rapid transport to a hospital that can provide immediate surgery. If she is already in shock, she should receive 250-mL fluid boluses to maintain a minimum systolic blood pressure of 80 mm Hg and receive airway management as indicated.

▶ Preeclampsia

Preeclampsia is characterized by the following signs and symptoms:

- Headache
- Swelling in the hands, face, and feet
- Anxiety
- Nausea/vomiting

In severe preeclampsia, you may also find:

- Pulmonary edema/shortness of breath
- Confusion or other altered level of consciousness
- Visual disturbances, such as blurry vision or scotomata (seeing spots)
- Upper abdominal pain
- **Myoclonus** (hyperactive reflexes)

Preeclampsia is most life threatening to the fetus and woman if seizures occur. If you suspect preeclampsia, it is important to obtain an accurate blood pressure. You should suspect preeclampsia if the blood pressure of a woman in her second or third trimester of pregnancy is above 140 systolic or 90 diastolic.

The treatment of a woman with preeclampsia is mostly supportive. You should ensure the ABCs and try to keep the patient calm. The patient should be kept in a position of comfort and monitored closely. At a minimum, she should receive supplemental oxygen to prevent fetal distress and an IV line of an isotonic crystalloid solution at a TKO rate for medication administration if it becomes necessary.

If a seizure occurs, you must protect the patient from being injured during the seizure. Administer oxygen and maintain an open airway. You should be ready to provide suctioning or other aggressive airway maneuvers, if necessary, including calling for paramedic backup.

Words of Wisdom

If you are transporting a patient with suspected preeclampsia, be sure to keep the emergency lights and siren on the ambulance off and decrease sensory input as much as possible to avoid triggering seizure activity.

▶ Supine Hypotensive Syndrome

Supine hypotensive syndrome is most easily treated by placing the woman onto her left side, which causes the uterus to shift off of the vena cava. This simple maneuver will cause an increase in venous return, preload, and therefore cardiac output, thereby increasing maternal blood pressure and perfusion. If the patient must be immobilized on the long backboard, you should place blanket rolls or something similar under the right side of the board.

▶ Gestational Diabetes

Patients with gestational diabetes may be asymptomatic or may exhibit the same signs observed in patients with diabetes mellitus. Pregnant patients with a history of diabetes or who present with an altered mental status or seizures should have their blood glucose level checked with a glucometer. Prehospital management should include high-flow oxygen, IV fluids, and administration of dextrose if indicated by a low blood glucose reading. Patients who are hyperglycemic should receive oxygen and IV fluid therapy per local protocol. Isotonic crystalloid fluid boluses may be necessary to treat the associated dehydration. Several fluid boluses may be required because diabetic ketoacidosis is commonly associated with severe hypovolemia, and possibly even shock.

Normal Childbirth

▶ Stages of Labor

The onset of labor starts with contractions of the uterus. **Lightening** refers to the movement of the baby down into the pelvis prior to birth. Although lightening usually occurs prior to the onset of contractions, it may not happen until labor actually starts.

There are three stages of labor. The first stage begins with the onset of contractions and ends when the cervix is fully effaced and dilated.

The average length of the first stage of labor is 12 hours for a nulliparous woman and up to 8 hours for a multiparous woman. The second stage of labor is from the point of full cervical **effacement** (thinning and shortening of the cervix) and dilation (or crowning in the field) until the fetus is delivered. The average length of time for the second stage of labor is 1 to 2 hours for the nulliparous patient and 30 minutes for the multiparous patient.

The third stage of labor begins with the delivery of the newborn and ends with the delivery of the placenta. This stage takes an average of 30 minutes. Occasionally the placenta is delivered immediately after the newborn is delivered.

Special Populations

The stages of labor are:

- **Stage 1.** Begins with the onset of contractions and ends when the cervix is fully effaced and dilated (or crowning).
- **Stage 2.** From the point of full cervical effacement and dilation (or crowning) until the fetus is delivered.
- **Stage 3.** Begins with the delivery of the newborn and ends with the delivery of the placenta.

▶ Preparing for Delivery

When birth is imminent, you should prepare your equipment and position the patient for the delivery. Begin by administering oxygen as needed, if this has not already been done. If there is time, you should start a large-bore IV line of an isotonic crystalloid on the pregnant woman. IV access will be necessary if fluid boluses are needed for excessive postpartum bleeding.

After labor has begun, there is no way it can be slowed down or stopped in the field. Never attempt to hold the pregnant woman's legs together; doing so would only complicate the delivery and cause potential injury to the newborn.

If you decide to deliver the newborn at the scene, remember that you are only *assisting* the pregnant woman with the delivery. Your part is to help, guide, and support the newborn as it is born. Take standard precautions at all times. Limit distractions for yourself and for the patient. You want to appear calm and reassuring while protecting the patient's modesty. Recognize your own limitations; if you are unsure about what to do, contact medical control and provide rapid transport. If delivery must occur during transport, stop the vehicle and have your partner or partners assist with the delivery. After delivery of the newborn and any needed resuscitation have occurred, you may resume transport to the hospital.

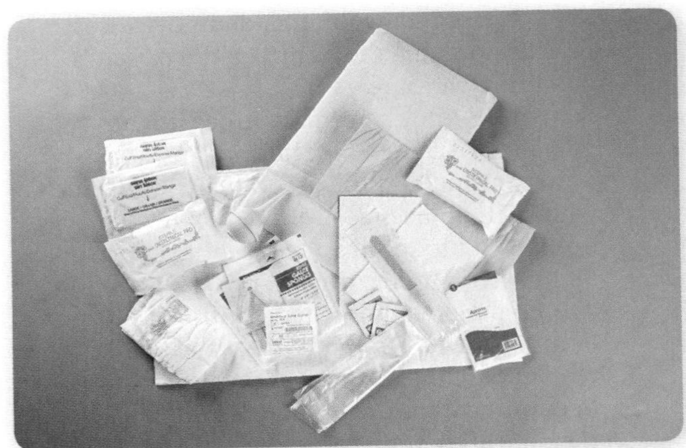

Figure 35-9 Your unit should contain a sterile obstetric kit.

Your emergency vehicle should always be equipped with one or more sterile emergency obstetric (OB) kits containing the following items Figure 35-9:

- Surgical scissors or a scalpel
- Umbilical cord clamps
- A small rubber bulb syringe
- Towels, drapes, or sheets
- 4- × 4-inch (10 × 10-cm) and/or 2- × 10-inch (5 × 25-cm) gauze sponges
- Sterile gloves
- Infant blanket
- Sanitary pads
- Plastic bag

Two items that need to be available but are not usually included in the OB kit are an infant-sized bag-mask device and goggles.

Patient Position

The patient's clothing and undergarments should be removed or pushed up to her waist. Cover her lower half with a sheet or blanket. Limit the patient's exposure and preserve her modesty as much as you can. If the emergency delivery is occurring at home, move the patient to the floor or other sturdy flat surface if she will allow it. You will find it easier to work on a firm surface padded with blankets, folded sheets, or towels rather than on a bed. Put a pillow or blankets beneath her hips to elevate them approximately 2 to 4 inches (5 to 10 cm). Support the patient's head, neck, and upper back with pillows and blankets. Have her keep her legs and hips flexed, with her feet flat on the surface beneath her and her knees spread apart, helping her to move into a semi-Fowler position Figure 35-10. If delivery is occurring in an automobile, the patient should lie across the rear seat, with one foot on the floor and the other on the seat, with the upper knee and hip bent.

Track the progression of the delivery closely at all times. You do not want an abrupt delivery, when the head pops out uncontrollably, to occur. This could result in neck injuries or other injuries to the newborn.

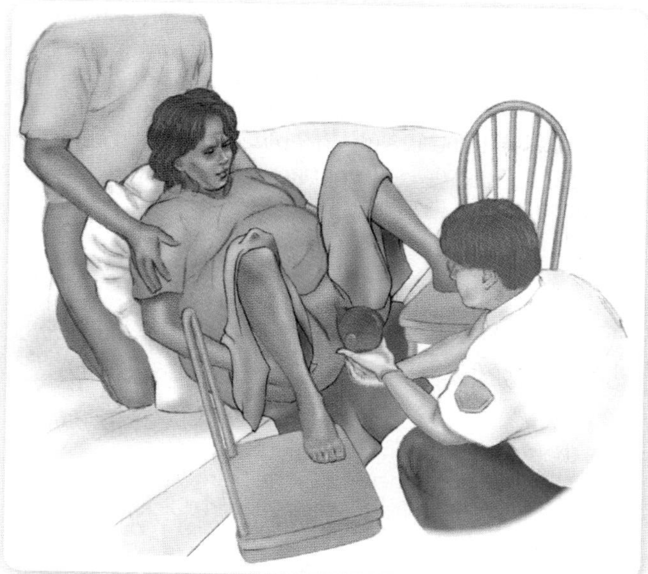

Figure 35-10 The semi-Fowler position.

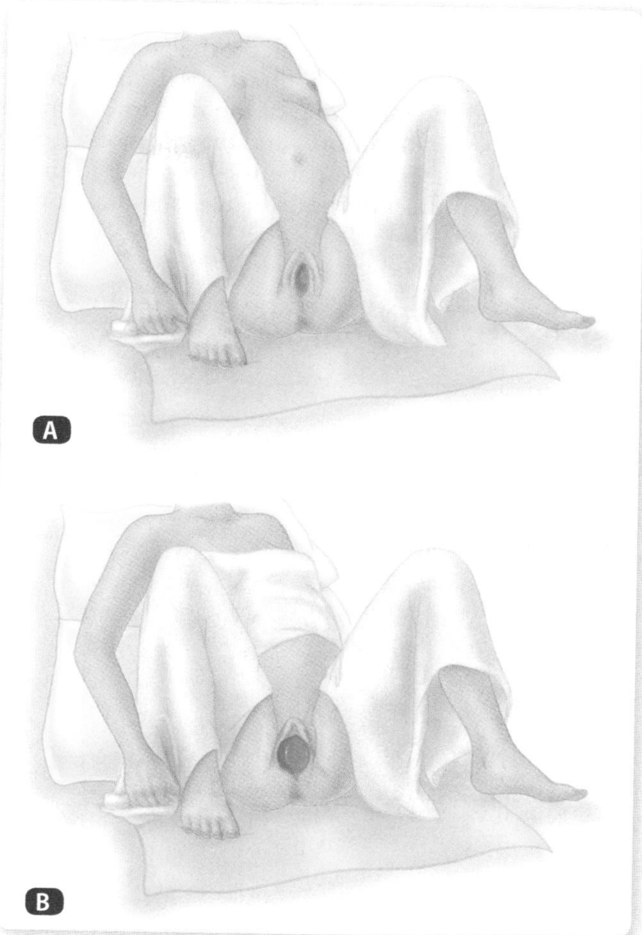

Figure 35-11 Preparing the delivery field. **A.** Place sheets or towels under the woman, elevate the woman's hips, and support her head with one or two pillows. **B.** Use sterile sheets and towels from the obstetric kit to make a clean delivery field. Place one sheet under her buttocks, drape the other over her abdomen, and place drapes over the thighs.

Preparing the Delivery Field

Take the following steps to prepare the area where the newborn will be born:

1. If there is enough time, place towels or sheets on the floor around the delivery area to help soak up the amniotic fluid that will be released when the amniotic sac ruptures and any blood that comes from the release of the mucous plug or during delivery. Determine if the amniotic sac has ruptured before you arrived.
2. Open the OB kit carefully so that its contents remain sterile (touch only the outside of the packaging).
3. Wash your hands thoroughly with a povidone-iodine or chlorhexidine scrub solution, if available.
4. Put on the sterile gloves, goggles, and gown.
5. Use the sterile sheets and towels from the OB kit to make a sterile delivery field. Place one sheet or towel under the patient's buttocks, and unfold it toward her feet Figure 35-11A. The other sheet should be draped over her abdomen and upper legs. Alternatively, you can use three sheets as follows Figure 35-11B:
   - One folded under the buttocks
   - One placed between the legs, just below the vagina
   - One placed across the abdomen

Words of Wisdom

There are only two instances when you should insert your hand inside the patient's vagina: in cases of breech delivery when the body delivers but the head is too large to fit through the pelvic inlet, and cord presentation (prolapsed umbilical cord).

▶ Delivering the Newborn

Your partner should be at the patient's head to comfort, soothe, and reassure her during the delivery. If she will allow it, administer oxygen. The patient may want to grip someone's hand. She may yell, cry, or say nothing at all. It is common for women to become nauseated during delivery, and some may vomit. If this occurs, have your partner turn the patient's head to the side so that her mouth and airway can be cleared with suction, as needed.

You must continually assess the patient for crowning. Do not allow an abrupt delivery to occur; when labor is too fast, the tissues do not have enough time to stretch, and the patient is at risk for tears in the perineal area. Position yourself so that you can see the perineal area at all times. Time the patient's contractions from the beginning of one to the beginning of the next to determine their frequency. In addition, time the duration of each contraction by feeling the patient's abdomen from the moment the contraction begins (uterus and abdomen tightening) to the moment it ends (uterus and abdomen relaxing). Remind the patient to take quick, short breaths during each contraction but not to strain or push until ready to give birth. Between contractions, encourage the patient to rest and breathe deeply through her mouth.

Skill Drill 35-1 summarizes the steps to deliver the newborn.

Skill Drill 35-1 Delivering a Newborn

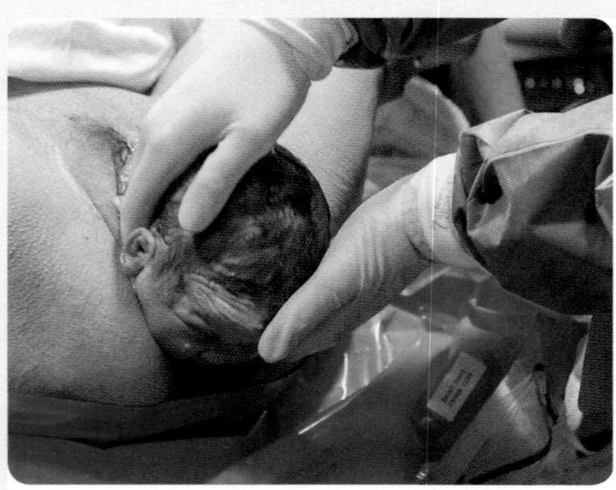

Step 1 Control the delivery. When crowning occurs, place *gentle* pressure on the newborn's head with the palm of your gloved hand to prevent the head from delivering too quickly and tearing the woman's vagina.

As the newborn's head begins to emerge from the vagina, it will start to turn. Support the head as it turns. Do *not* attempt to pull the newborn from the vagina! If the membranes cover the head after it emerges, tear the amniotic sac with your fingers or forceps to permit escape of amniotic fluid and enable the newborn to breathe.

Slip your middle finger alongside the newborn's head to check for a nuchal cord. If you find a nuchal cord, try to slip it gently over the newborn's shoulder and head. Should this maneuver fail, and if the cord is wrapped tightly around the neck, place umbilical clamps 2 inches apart and cut the cord between the clamps.

If the airway appears to be obstructed, cradle and support the newborn's head in your hand, and clear the airway by suctioning with the bulb syringe.

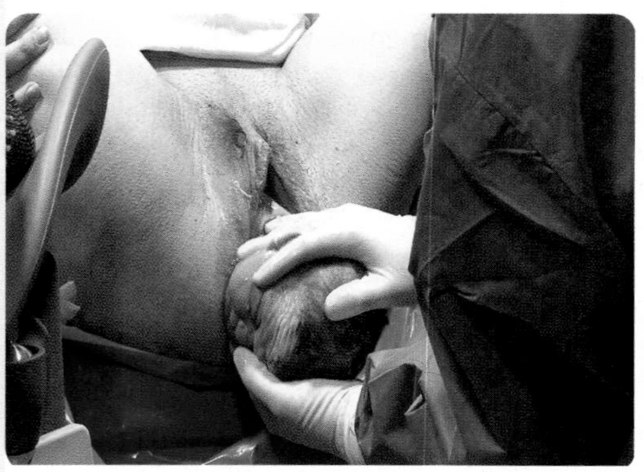

Step 2 Gently guide the head downward to allow delivery of the upper shoulder. Do not pull on the newborn to facilitate the delivery.

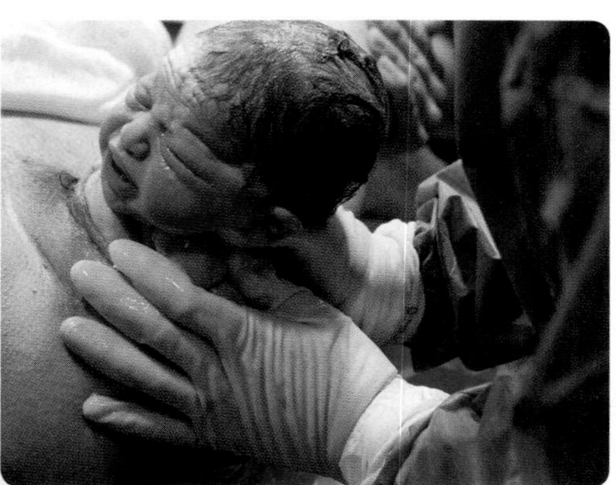

Step 3 Gently guide the head upward to allow delivery of the lower shoulder.

Skill Drill 35-1 Delivering a Newborn *(continued)*

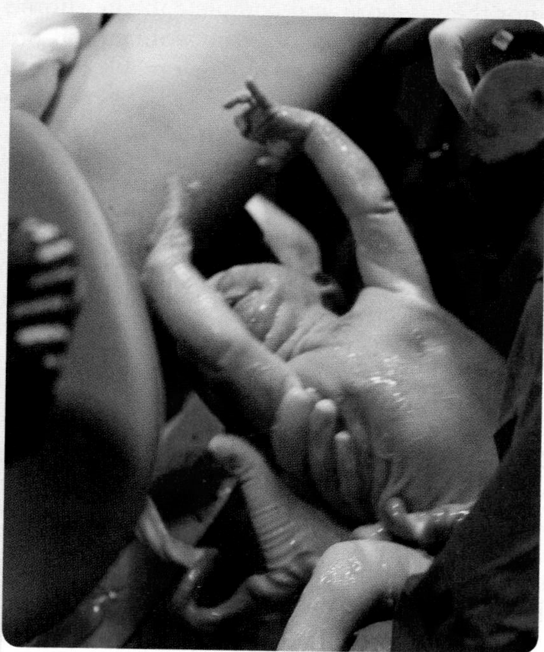

Step 4 After the shoulders are delivered, the newborn's trunk and legs will follow rapidly. Be prepared to grasp and support the newborn as it emerges. Handle the newborn firmly but carefully. Newborns will be slippery and usually covered with a harmless, white, cheesy substance called vernix caseosa.

After the newborn is delivered, maintain its body position at the same level as the vagina to prevent blood drainage from the umbilical cord.

Wipe any blood or mucus from the newborn's nose and mouth with a sterile gauze. If airway obstruction is noted, use the bulb syringe to suction the mouth and nostrils. Be sure to squeeze the bulb before inserting the tip, and only then place the tip in the newborn's mouth or nostril and release the bulb slowly. Withdraw the bulb, expel its contents into a waste container, and repeat suctioning as needed.

Dry the newborn with sterile towels (wet newborns lose heat faster than dry ones), and either wrap the newborn with a dry blanket or place skin-to-skin on the mother's abdomen to encourage breast feeding.

Record the time of birth for your patient care report.

Words of Wisdom

As a newborn delivers, you must divide your attention between two patients. Designate one member of the crew to provide primary care to each patient. Call for help early if you suspect that both patients will need special care or that one will require resuscitation.

Words of Wisdom

If there is more than one fetus, immediately call for a second EMS unit. With a normal, single birth, you will have two patients—the woman and the newborn. Multiple births will require additional assistance.

A newborn's body temperature can drop very quickly. Therefore, as soon as the entire newborn is born, dry the newborn off. Wrap the newborn immediately in a blanket or towel, and place the newborn on one side, with the head slightly lower than the rest of the body. Wrap the newborn so that only the face is exposed, making sure that the top of the head is covered. Make sure that the newborn's neck is in a neutral position to maintain an open airway. Newborns are extremely sensitive to cold, so if at all possible, you should warm the blanket or towel before you use it. Use a sterile gauze pad to gently wipe the newborn's mouth, and again suction the mouth and nose if needed. Suctioning the nose is particularly important because newborns breathe through their noses. If you prefer, you can pick up and cradle the newborn in your arm at the level of the woman's vagina while doing this, but always keep the head slightly downward to help prevent aspiration. After suctioning, keep the newborn at the same level as the woman's vagina until the umbilical cord is cut. If the newborn is higher than the vagina, blood will be siphoned back through the umbilical cord to the placenta, resulting in fetal hypovolemia.

Words of Wisdom

Keep a towel or sheet handy to wipe your hands and to help hold the newborn because he or she will be very slippery.

▶ Apgar Scoring

The **Apgar score system** (devised by Virginia Apgar, MD) is a useful means of evaluating the adequacy of a newborn's vital functions immediately after birth; such information will prove useful to those who take over the care of the newborn after your delivery. In this system, five parameters—heart rate, respiratory effort, muscle tone, reflex irritability, and color—are each given a score from 0 to 2 first at 1 minute and again at 5 minutes after birth. Most newborns are vigorous and have a total score of 7 to 10; they cough or cry within seconds of delivery and require no further resuscitation. Newborns with a score in the 4 to 6 range are moderately depressed; they may be pale or blue 1 minute after delivery, with poorly sustained respirations and flaccid muscle tone. These newborns will require resuscitation. Neonatal resuscitation is discussed in detail later in this chapter.

▶ Cutting the Umbilical Cord

After the newborn has been delivered and is breathing well, the umbilical cord can be clamped and cut because it is no longer necessary for the newborn's survival. Clamping of the cord should be delayed 30 seconds after delivery for most vigorous term and preterm (34 to 36 weeks) newborns, unless the newborn requires resuscitation.[18] The steps are as follows:

1. Handle the umbilical cord with care. It tears easily.
2. After the cord has stopped pulsating, tie or clamp the cord approximately 4 inches (10 cm) from the newborn's navel, and then place the second tie (or clamp) 2 inches (5 cm) from the first tie. Cut the cord between the two ties or clamps.
3. Examine the cut ends of the cord to be certain there is no bleeding. If the cut end attached to the newborn is bleeding, tie or clamp the cord *proximal* to the previous clamp, and examine it again (do *not* remove the first clamp). There should not be any oozing from the newborn's end of the cord.
4. After the cord is clamped and cut, wrap the newborn in a dry blanket. If the woman's condition is stable, you may give the newborn to her allowing it to rest on her chest skin-to-skin. This will give her a chance to bond and she may want to begin breastfeeding the newborn. The suckling reflex triggers the uterus to contract, which will speed the delivery of the placenta and reduce bleeding.

Words of Wisdom

A delay in clamping the umbilical cord and keeping the newborn below the placenta may allow blood to flow into the newborn, which can result in polycythemia (an abnormally high red blood cell count).

By now, the newborn should be pinkish and breathing on his or her own. You can give the newborn, wrapped in a warm blanket, to your partner, and he or she can monitor the newborn and complete the newborn's initial care. You should reassess the woman and prepare for delivery of the placenta. If the woman's condition is stable, you may give the newborn to her. She may want to begin breastfeeding the newborn.

▶ Delivery of the Placenta

The placenta is attached to the end of the umbilical cord that is coming out of the woman's vagina. As with the newborn, you need only assist with the delivery. Usually the uterus will deliver the placenta within a few minutes of the birth, although it may take as long as 30 minutes. During this time you should reassess the woman and wait for the placenta to begin to separate spontaneously. Never pull on the end of the umbilical cord in an attempt to speed delivery of the placenta. This can cause tearing of the cord, the placenta, or both, and cause serious, perhaps life-threatening, hemorrhage. If the placenta has not delivered in the time it takes to reassess the woman, and in the time it takes to prepare both her and the newborn for transport, do not delay transport just to await the delivery of the placenta.

Wrap the entire placenta and umbilical cord in a towel and place them in a plastic bag. The placenta and remaining cord must be transported to the hospital. Hospital personnel will examine them to make certain that the entire placenta has been delivered.

Words of Wisdom

Never pull on the umbilical cord. This could result in tearing or uterine inversion that can be detrimental to the woman.

▶ Postpartum Care

After delivery of the placenta and before transport, place a sterile pad or sanitary napkin over the vagina and straighten the woman's legs. You can help to slow postpartum bleeding by gently massaging the uterine fundus with a firm, circular, kneading motion Figure 35-12. The abdominal skin will be wrinkled and very soft. You should be able to feel a firm, grapefruit-sized mass in the lower abdomen; this is the fundus. As you massage it, the uterus will contract and become firmer. This may sometimes be uncomfortable for the woman. Reassure her and explain that it is necessary to help control the bleeding. If the woman chooses to breastfeed the newborn, this will also stimulate the uterus to contract. Massaging the uterus and having the newborn stimulate the woman's nipples by nursing will cause a release of **oxytocin**, a hormone produced in the posterior pituitary gland that will help to contract the uterus and

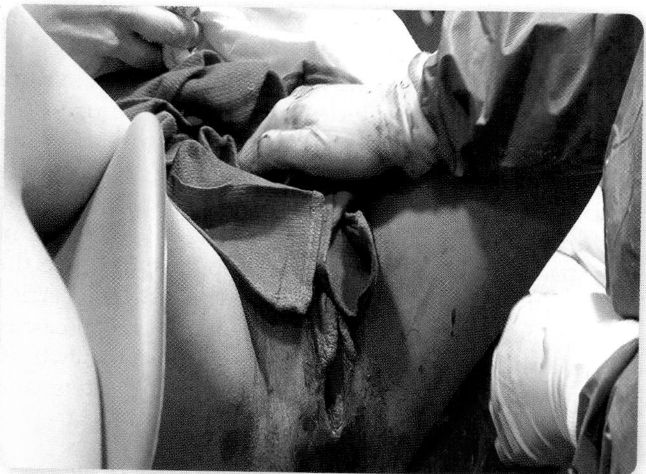

Figure 35-12 After delivery, massage the woman's abdomen in a firm, circular motion.

slow bleeding. Take a minute to congratulate the woman and thank anyone who assisted. Be sure to record the time of birth in your patient care report.

Words of Wisdom

Allowing the woman to breastfeed or firmly massaging the fundus can help the uterus to contract and diminish bleeding.

After delivery of the newborn, obtain the woman's vital signs. Monitor the woman's condition closely for postpartum hemorrhage and shock, seizure activity, or respiratory difficulty. Determine whether the vaginal discharge following delivery—lochia—is the expected normal vaginal discharge of blood and mucus. This discharge is usually red in the first few days and will decrease in amount and change to a brown color for several weeks after delivery. The average blood loss during the third stage of labor is normally approximately 0.3 pints (150 mL). Some bleeding, usually less than 500 mL, occurs before the placenta delivers.

Postpartum Hemorrhage

When blood loss exceeds 1 pint (500 mL) during the first 24 hours after giving birth, it is considered postpartum hemorrhage (bleeding after birth). Anything that interferes with the contractions of the interlacing uterine muscle fibers after delivery of the placenta may cause postpartum hemorrhage.

The following are emergency situations:

- The placenta has not delivered after 30 minutes.
- More than 500 mL of bleeding occurs before delivery of the placenta.
- Substantial bleeding occurs after the delivery of the placenta.

If any of these events occur, provide rapid transport of the woman and newborn to the hospital. Place a sterile pad or sanitary napkin over the woman's vagina to collect any blood; manage external bleeding from perineal tears with firm pressure. Never pack the vagina with dressings in an attempt to control the hemorrhage; these will only have to be removed at the hospital, and the bleeding is coming from a source that you cannot control. Treat the woman for shock according to local protocol, apply a blanket to keep her and the newborn warm, and administer oxygen and isotonic fluid boluses (250 mL) to maintain perfusion.

Complications of Labor

Occasionally you may be called to help a woman with an abnormal labor or delivery. These problems are rare, but can be life threatening for both the woman and fetus. The definitive treatment for many of these problems is a cesarean section; therefore, rapid transport to the hospital is crucial. The next sections will prepare you to provide the best care possible for patients with abnormal or complicated labors and deliveries and know when to initiate rapid transport rather than attempt delivery at the scene.

▶ Preterm Labor

Labor (uterine contractions that are regular, intense, and accompanied by effacement) that begins after the 20th week of gestation but before the 37th week is considered preterm. The threat to the unborn fetus is a premature birth. Signs and symptoms are the same as normal childbirth labor. The treatment for a woman in preterm labor is to prevent labor from occurring, thereby allowing the fetus to more fully develop and have a better chance of survival. If the pregnancy is not near term, the patient's physician may admit her to the hospital for medications, bed rest, and close monitoring. In the field, the best treatment option is a bolus of an isotonic crystalloid solution.

A newborn that delivers before 36 weeks of gestation or weighs less than 5 lb (2.25 kg) at birth is considered to be **premature**. A premature newborn is smaller and thinner than a full-term newborn, and its head is proportionately larger in comparison with the rest of its body **Figure 35-13**. The **vernix caseosa** that is found on the full-term newborn will be missing on the premature newborn or will be minimally present. There will also be less body hair. Premature newborns are often deficient of surfactant, resulting in increased alveolar surface tension. Therefore, positive pressure ventilations (PPV) may be difficult to perform. Be careful, however, and do not become overzealous while ventilating a premature newborn; doing so may result in a pneumothorax.

Any premature newborn needs special care, although as with any newborn, you should keep the premature newborn warm, dry, and positioned on the mother's chest.

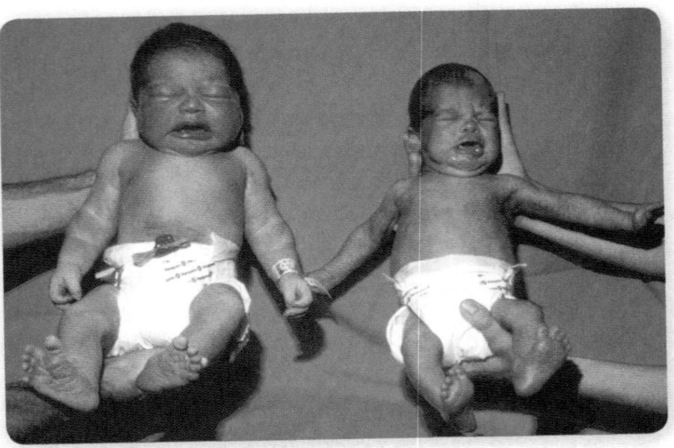

Figure 35-13 Premature newborns (at right) are smaller and thinner than full-term newborns (at left).

Keep the ambulance interior warm—between 90°F and 95°F (32.2°C and 35°C). Maintain the newborn's airway.

Administer supplemental oxygen through a tent above the newborn's head. Do *not* blast oxygen directly into the newborn's eyes. Use low flow (<4 L/min).

Prevent bleeding from the umbilical cord; a very small newborn cannot afford to lose even a small amount of blood. If the cord is oozing, apply another clamp.

Finally, prevent contamination. Premature newborns are highly susceptible to infection. Wear a surgical gown and mask, and keep bystanders at a distance, including any family members other than the mother.

You may have access to a specialized premature newborn carrier (isolette), which can be used for immediate care as well as transport. Fill the hot water bottles, and pad them well so that they do not come into direct contact with the newborn's skin. Place one on the bottom of the carrier and one on each side of the space for the newborn. After you have wrapped the newborn in a blanket and placed it inside the carrier, secure the carrier inside the vehicle. If a special carrier is not available, you must keep the premature newborn warm with additional blankets, thermal packets, and warmed patient compartments.

▶ Fetal Distress

Many conditions may cause fetal distress including hypoxia, nuchal cord, trauma, abruptio placenta, fetal developmental disabilities, and a prolapsed cord. It will be difficult for you to assess for fetal distress in the field. Most pregnant women will be acutely aware of how much or how little the fetus is moving. You should rely on the information provided by the woman—for example, if she reports that the fetus is not moving or that movement is markedly decreased. Remember that the best care for the fetus is quality care for the woman. Provide support to the woman and rapid transport.

YOU are the Provider PART 4

You feel around the baby's neck and find that the cord is loose enough to remove without clamping and cutting it. As you gently slip the umbilical cord from around the newborn's head, the body delivers, and you note the time to be 1429. The newborn is small and listless, but you do not see any signs of meconium staining. When the umbilical cord stops pulsating, you clamp and cut it. As you attempt to remember all of the steps of neonatal resuscitation, you recall that you need to "Do What Probably Seems Simple," which you recall to be Dry, Warm, Position, Stimulate, and Suction. You vigorously dry the patient remembering to change out towels frequently to ensure that the newborn remains warm. As you are warming the newborn, the second ambulance arrives and assumes care of the woman.

Newborn Assessment Recording Time: 1 Minute After Birth	
Respirations	None
Pulse	120 beats/min, regular
Skin	Central cyanosis
Blood pressure	Not obtained
Oxygen saturation (Spo_2)	Not obtained
Pupils	Not obtained

7. Why is it important to note the time of birth?
8. Why is it important to note whether there was meconium present on delivery?

Uterine Rupture

If the uterus ruptures, it will happen during labor. Patients at greatest risk are women who have had several children and those with a scar on the uterus (eg, from a previous cesarean section). Typically, you will find a woman in active labor who is reporting weakness, dizziness, and thirst. She may tell you that she initially had very strong and painful contractions, but then the contractions slackened off and she now has severe abdominal pain. The abdomen may be rigid from peritonitis. Physical examination will reveal signs of shock—sweating, tachycardia, and falling blood pressure. Substantial vaginal bleeding may or may not be obvious. One possible sign of uterine rupture is being able to palpate fetal body parts through the abdominal wall.

High-Risk Pregnancy Conditions

Meconium Staining

While in utero, the fetus passively ingests several elements—for example, lanugo (fine, downy hair), mucus, and amniotic fluid. This material is stored in the intestines and constitutes the first stool the fetus passes. This first stool (meconium) is odorless, green-black, and has a tar-like consistency. Unlike later feces, it is also sterile. In cases of fetal distress, or with the stresses of labor and delivery, the fetus may expel the meconium into the amniotic fluid; this is termed **meconium staining**. If this occurs in utero, it can be aspirated into the fetus's lungs and may result in chemical pneumonia in the newborn. Umbilical cord prolapse is one condition that can cause such fetal distress and induce meconium expulsion, if compression of the cord has occurred.

There is no way for you to ascertain whether meconium is in the amniotic fluid until the amniotic sac breaks. Normally, the amniotic fluid should be clear. A yellow tint to the amniotic fluid suggests the meconium has been in the amniotic fluid for a while. A green-black color, especially with the presence of particulate matter, indicates recent passage of meconium and is a sign of danger.

You need to be vigilant regarding the need for suctioning if meconium staining is present and the newborn is not responding normally. The viscosity of meconium can cause the newborn's airway to become partially or completely blocked, and meconium trapped in the airways will irritate the respiratory tract, further hampering the newborn's efforts to breathe.

If the newborn is vigorously moving and is not presenting with indications of needing ventilation assistance, suctioning is not recommended. Call early for paramedic backup if meconium is present. If the newborn is depressed, he or she will require tracheal suctioning through an endotracheal tube if meconium is present in the airway.

Multiple Gestation

According to the US Centers for Disease Control and Prevention, the incidence of women carrying twins reached an all-time high in 2014 and began to decline in 2015.[19] Odds are, you will have to assist in the delivery of multiple births at some point. The delivery of multiple births does not usually pose special problems, except that you have to do a few things twice (or more). Always keep a spare OB kit in your equipment.

The woman will usually know that she is carrying multiple fetuses, especially if she has had appropriate prenatal care. Consider the possibility of twins if the uterus is still large and firm after delivery of the first newborn. If you have reason to suspect there is more than one fetus, proceed as follows:

- Repeat the earlier preparations for delivery. If time permits, put on new gloves and a gown from the spare OB kit.
- Contractions will usually start again within about 10 minutes after the birth of the first newborn, and the second newborn can be expected to arrive within 45 minutes of its twin.
- Twins are usually delivered one at a time. When the first newborn is born, clamp and cut the cord approximately 30 seconds following birth and before the second newborn is delivered. Inspect *both* ends of the cord for oozing, and apply a second clamp if necessary, to prevent hemorrhage from the twin if there is a shared placenta (you will not know until the placenta delivers). Some twins share a placenta; others may have separate placentas or may share two placentas that have fused into one. Usually both newborns are delivered before the first placenta is delivered.
- Given that twins tend to be smaller than single-term newborns, pay meticulous attention to keeping them warm, well oxygenated, and in as sterile an environment as possible.
- Identify the first newborn delivered as "Baby A" by loosely tying an extra length of tape around the foot. Record the time of birth of each twin separately. With the delivery of two or more newborns, you can indicate the order of delivery by writing on a piece of tape and placing it on the blanket or towel that is wrapped around each newborn.

Cephalopelvic Disproportion

In cephalopelvic disproportion, the head of the fetus is larger than the pelvis. In most cases, a cesarean section will be required to prevent maternal and fetal distress. Before you attempt delivery in the field, ask the patient if this complication was identified during prenatal care. Cephalopelvic disproportion may cause massive hemorrhage, along with other postpartum complications.

▶ Intrauterine Fetal Death

On rare occasions, you may find yourself delivering a fetus who died in the woman's uterus before labor. Good prenatal care most often identifies a dead fetus well before delivery, but in the absence of such care, it may be totally unexpected. Complications of labor and delivery can also result in death of the fetus, with the fetus dying in utero shortly before birth. This situation will test your medical, emotional, and social abilities. Grieving parents will be emotionally distraught and will require all your professionalism and support skills.

If intrauterine infection has caused the death, you may note an extremely foul odor. The delivered newborn may have skin blisters, skin sloughing, and a dark discoloration depending on the stage of decomposition. The head will be soft and perhaps grossly deformed.

Do not attempt to resuscitate an obviously dead newborn (ie, signs of petrification are evident). However, do not confuse such a newborn with newborns who have had a cardiopulmonary arrest as a complication of the birthing process. You must attempt to resuscitate normal-appearing newborns.

▶ Amniotic Fluid Embolism

Amniotic fluid embolism is a life-threatening condition that is extremely rare and hardly ever seen in the hospital setting. Factors increasing the chance of this type of complication include maternal age greater than 35 years, eclampsia, abruptio placenta, placenta previa, uterine rupture, and fetal distress. Amniotic fluid embolism occurs when amniotic fluid and fetal cells enter the woman's pulmonary and circulatory system through the placenta via the umbilical veins. This transfer may occur owing to ruptured membranes and ruptured cervical or uterine veins. Regardless of the cause, the result is an exaggerated response from the pregnant woman's body (allergic reaction) that results in coagulopathies, cardiac and respiratory collapse, and eventually death.

Signs and symptoms include a sudden onset of respiratory distress and hypotension. Many of these patients are extremely cyanotic and have seizures. They eventually go into cardiogenic shock, become unresponsive, and may experience cardiac arrest. In patients who survive this initial reaction, coagulopathies (their blood loses the ability to clot) typically develop. Your treatment should focus on supporting the woman's vital systems (respiratory and circulatory) and providing rapid transport. Treatment for the fetus is aimed at successful resuscitation of the woman and probable cesarean section delivery in the hospital.

Complications of Delivery

▶ Breech Presentation

The presentation is the position in which a newborn is born—the part of the body that comes out first, also known as the presenting part. Most newborns are born head first, or a vertex presentation. Occasionally, the buttocks or both feet come out first. This is called a **breech presentation** Figure 35-14. There are different types of breech presentations:

- **Frank.** Hips flexed and knees extended, with the buttocks as the presenting part
- **Incomplete.** One or both hips and knees may be extended, with one or both feet as the presenting part
- **Complete.** Hips and knees both flexed, with the buttocks as the presenting part

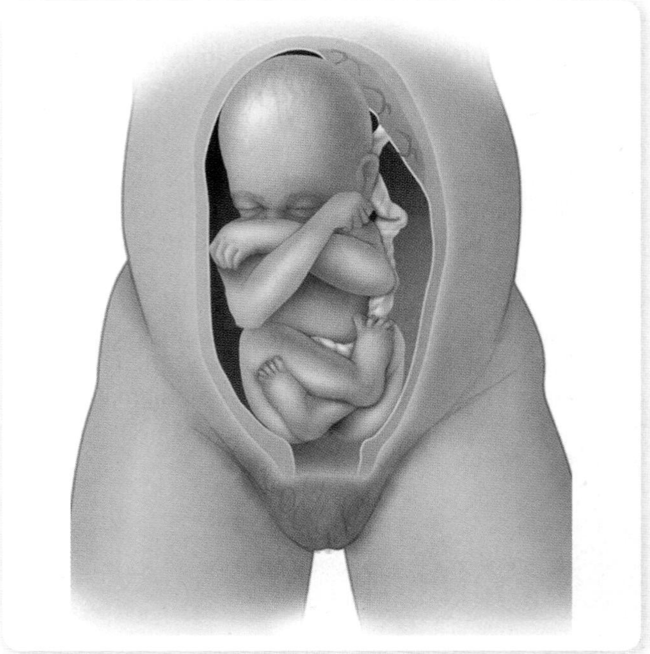

Figure 35-14 In breech presentation, the buttocks present first. Breech deliveries are usually slow, so you will often have time to transport the patient to the hospital.

With breech presentation, the newborn is at greater risk for delivery trauma. Prolapsed umbilical cords (discussed later in this section) are more common in breech deliveries. Fortunately, breech deliveries are usually slow, so there is time to get the patient to the hospital. If the newborn's buttocks have already passed through the vagina, delivery is under way, and you must prepare to assist. Call for paramedic backup if time allows. In general, if the woman does not deliver within 10 minutes of the buttocks presentation, provide rapid transport. You should have medical control guide you in this difficult situation.

The preparations for a breech delivery are the same as those for a vertex delivery:

- Position the patient, unwrap the emergency delivery kit, and place yourself and your partner as you would for a normal delivery.
- Allow the buttocks and legs to deliver spontaneously, supporting them with your hand

to prevent rapid expulsion. The buttocks will usually come out easily. Let the legs dangle on either side of your arm while you support the trunk and chest as they are delivered.

- The head is almost always facedown and should be allowed to deliver spontaneously. If the delivery of the head stalls, you must keep the newborn's airway open: Make a "V" with your gloved fingers, and place them into the vagina. You must push the walls of the vagina away from the mouth and nose of the newborn. This is a true emergency and requires rapid transport. *A breech presentation in which the head will not deliver is one of only two circumstances in which you should put your fingers into the vagina; the other is in the event of a prolapsed cord.*
- Cover the newborn's body to maintain warmth during transport.

Special Populations

Any fetus that is not delivering headfirst or buttocks first must be managed at the hospital.

▶ Limb Presentation

On rare occasions, the presenting part of the newborn is neither the head nor buttocks, but is a single arm, leg, or foot. This is called a **limb presentation** Figure 35-15. You cannot successfully deliver such a presentation in the field; these newborns must be delivered surgically in the hospital. If your patient has a limb presentation, you must transport the patient to the hospital immediately. If a limb is protruding, cover it with a sterile towel. Never try to push it back in, and never pull on it. Place the patient on her back with her head down and hips elevated. In this situation, you have two goals: (1) to prevent further trauma to the newborn that could result from the patient's continued pushing and (2) to transport the patient rapidly and safely to the hospital. Contact medical control and the receiving hospital to make certain they are prepared for your arrival. You should administer high-flow oxygen to the woman and closely monitor her condition en route.

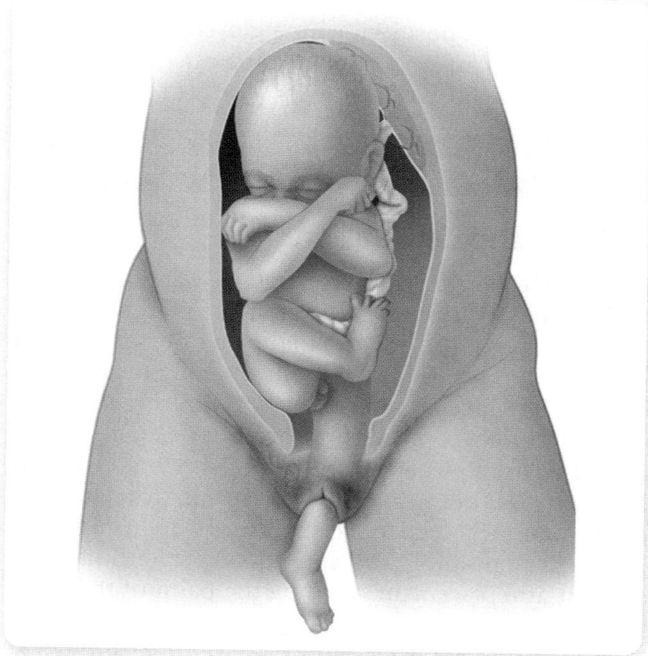

Figure 35-15 In rare instances, a newborn's limb, usually a single arm or leg, presents first. This is a serious situation, and you must provide prompt transport for hospital delivery.

▶ Shoulder Dystocia

Another complication of delivery is **shoulder dystocia** or difficulty in delivering the shoulders. Women with diabetes, large fetuses, and fetuses that are postterm are at increased risk for this complication. Shoulder dystocia occurs after the head has been delivered and the shoulder cannot get past the woman's symphysis pubis; there is either difficulty in getting it to pass or it gets "stuck" behind the pelvic bones and the fetus is unable to be delivered. This unexpected complication is a threat to the life of the fetus if it is not delivered because of the increased chance of cord compression. As time passes and the shoulders are not clearing, the fetus cannot breathe (the lungs are still inside the birth canal) and/or the cord is compressed between the fetus and the woman's tissue. The delivery needs to be completed for the fetus to breathe. The major concern for the newborn after it is born is damage to the brachial nerve plexus.

There are several maneuvers that may be attempted in an effort to widen the woman's pelvis or reposition the fetus to allow for a successful delivery. The McRoberts maneuver is one of the safest (for woman and fetus) maneuvers to use in the case of shoulder dystocia. To widen the woman's pelvis and flatten the lower back, hyperflex her legs tightly to her abdomen. It may be necessary to apply suprapubic pressure (on the woman's lower abdomen) and to *gently* pull on the fetus's head.

▶ Nuchal Cord

During delivery, the umbilical cord may potentially become wrapped around the newborn's neck—a condition called a **nuchal cord**. Nuchal cords occur in 15% to 34% of all births.[20] In most cases, a nuchal cord is not a substantial problem, but as the fetus descends during labor, cord compression may occur, causing the fetal heart rate to slow and resulting in fetal distress. A nuchal cord that is wound tightly around the neck could cause the newborn to asphyxiate.

If you observe that the umbilical cord is wrapped around the newborn's neck, slip your finger under the cord and gently attempt to slip it over the newborn's shoulder and head. If this attempt is not successful or the cord is wrapped too tightly, you must cut it before the delivery can continue. Carefully place two umbilical clamps 2 inches (5 cm) apart on the cord and carefully cut the cord between the clamps in a motion going away from (not toward) the infant.

If the cord is wrapped more than once around the neck, a rare event, you must clamp and cut only once. After you have cut the cord, unwrap it from around the neck. Handle the cord carefully; it is fragile and easily torn. If the cord does tear, severe hemorrhage can occur from the mother, newborn, or both. Fortunately, the cord is usually not wrapped around the newborn's neck and does not have to be clamped and cut until after the entire newborn has been born. However, you must always check for the presence of a nuchal cord.

Prolapsed Umbilical Cord

Prolapsed umbilical cord is a rare presentation in which the cord emerges from the uterus ahead of the newborn, for example, when the amniotic sac ruptures. With a prolapsed umbilical cord, the blood supply to the newborn may be interrupted **Figure 35-16**. As the newborn starts to exit the cervix, the cord will be pressed against the pelvis. This can slow or stop the blood supply to and from the newborn. This presentation requires surgical intervention.

Your goal in the treatment of this patient is to prevent the woman from pushing and compressing the umbilical cord. If possible, place the patient supine with her lower extremities elevated. You may also use pillows or folded sheets to accomplish this position. Alternatively, the patient may be placed in a knee-chest position—kneeling and bent forward, facedown **Figure 35-17**. Either of these positions is meant to use gravity to help keep the weight of the newborn off of the prolapsed cord.

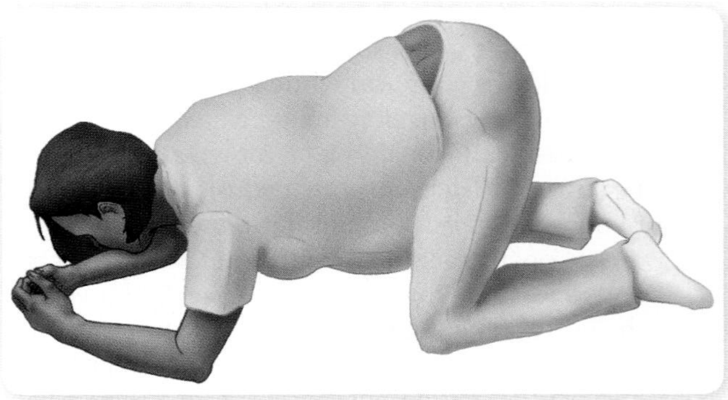

Figure 35-17 When a patient has a prolapsed cord, place her on an incline with feet higher than the head or in the kneeling position shown here. These positions help keep weight off the cord.

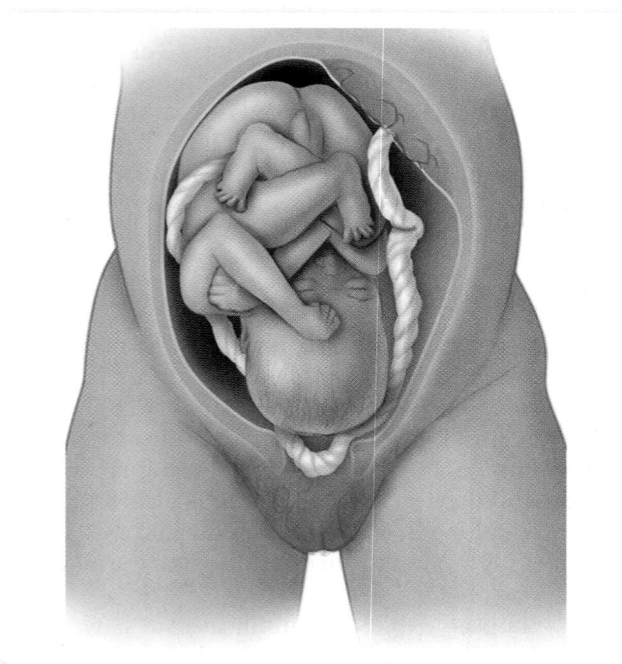

Figure 35-16 A prolapsed umbilical cord, another rare situation, is dangerous and must be cared for at the hospital.

After the patient is positioned, insert a gloved hand into the vagina and gently push the presenting part away from the umbilical cord, back into the vagina until it no longer presses on the cord. *This is one of only two situations in which you should insert your hand into the vagina (the other is breech presentation in which the head will not deliver)*. You should push with only enough pressure to keep the pulsations in the umbilical cord. You should be extremely careful because too much pressure could cause head or neck damage to the newborn.

While you maintain pressure on the presenting part, have your partner cover the exposed portion of the cord with dressings moistened in warmed normal saline. Try to maintain that position, with a gloved hand pushing the presenting part away from the cord, throughout *urgent transport* to the hospital.

Postpartum Complications

Uterine Inversion

Uterine inversion is a rare but potentially fatal complication of childbirth. In this condition, the placenta fails to detach properly and adheres to the uterine wall when it is expelled. As a result, the uterus literally turns inside out. Uterine inversion usually occurs during the third stage of labor. Its cause is not well understood, but it can result from placing excessive pressure on the uterus during fundal massage or from exerting excess traction on the umbilical cord to hasten delivery of the placenta.

If the uterus prolapses, appropriate care includes one attempt at replacement by using the palm of the hand to try to push it back inside the body. If this does not work, cover it with moist dressings and transport while providing supportive care. Never use your fingers to try to replace a prolapsed uterus because this may cause it to tear and result in massive hemorrhage. Administer 100% supplemental oxygen via a nonrebreathing mask.

Start two IV lines with normal saline, and titrate fluid administration based on the woman's vital signs. If the placenta is still attached to the uterus, do *not* attempt to remove it. Carefully monitor the patient's vital signs, and treat for shock.

▶ Pulmonary Embolism

One of the most common causes of maternal death during childbirth or postpartum is pulmonary embolism. An embolism may form from several sources, but a blood clot arising in the pelvic circulation is a frequent cause. Leakage of amniotic fluid into the maternal circulation (amniotic embolism), a clot arising from deep vein thrombosis (pregnancy-related venous thromboembolism), and an open vessel (air embolism) are examples of potential embolic processes. Should the woman experience sudden dyspnea, tachycardia, or hypotension in the postpartum state, you should suspect pulmonary embolism. The patient may report sudden, sharp chest pain, or abdominal pain, or may experience syncope. Physical examination may reveal nothing unusual except for an increased pulse rate, tachypnea, and hypotension—signs that may be mistaken for shock. Management of a postpartum embolism is the same as management of pulmonary embolism occurring in nonpregnant states: awareness/recognition, high-flow oxygen, and rapid transport.

Special Populations

Amniotic fluid embolism occurs when amniotic fluid and fetal cells enter the woman's pulmonary and circulatory system through the placenta via the umbilical veins. This may be from ruptured membranes and ruptured cervical or uterine veins. Regardless of the cause, the result is an exaggerated response from the pregnant woman's body (allergic reaction) that causes coagulopathies (the blood loses the ability to clot), cardiac and respiratory collapse, and eventually death.

Signs and symptoms include a sudden onset of respiratory distress and hypotension. Many of these patients are extremely cyanotic and have seizures. They eventually go into cardiogenic shock, become unresponsive, and may experience cardiac arrest. Treatment is aimed at supporting the respiratory and circulatory systems and providing rapid transport.

▶ Spina Bifida

Spina bifida is a developmental defect in which a portion of the spinal cord or meninges may protrude outside of the vertebrae and possibly outside of the body. This is easily seen on the newborn's back and usually occurs in the lower third of the back in the lumbar area. It is important to cover the open area of the spinal cord with a sterile, moist dressing immediately after birth to help prevent a potentially fatal infection. This treatment will have a positive effect on the newborn's outcome. However, maintenance of body temperature is important when applying moist dressings because the moisture can lower the newborn's body temperature. To prevent this, have someone hold the newborn against his or her body. Chapter 38, *Patients With Special Challenges*, discusses spina bifida in greater detail.

Neonatal Resuscitation

▶ Physiology

Following birth, the newborn will no longer be connected to the placenta; therefore, it must depend on its own lungs as the only source for oxygen intake and carbon dioxide removal. Over a matter of seconds, the lungs must therefore fill with oxygen and the pulmonary vasculature must dilate to perfuse the alveoli.

In utero (ie, in the pregnant woman's womb), a fetus receives its oxygen from the placenta **Figure 35-18**. The fetal lung is collapsed and filled with fluid, receiving only 10% of the total blood supply. As the fetus is delivered, a rapid series of events needs to occur to enable the newborn to breathe. This process is called **fetal transition**.

The first breath is triggered by mild hypoxia and hypercapnia related to partial occlusion of the umbilical cord during normal delivery. As pulmonary blood vessels continue to dilate and blood levels of oxygen increase, the ductus arteriosus constricts and blood flows preferentially into the lungs, picking up more oxygen to be transported throughout the body. (The ductus arteriosus is a small artery that connects the left pulmonary artery to the aorta and diverts blood away from the fetal lungs while in utero.)

Tactile stimulation and cold stress also promote early breathing. As the newborn's lungs become filled with air, the pulmonary vascular resistance drops, causing more blood to flow to the lungs, picking up oxygen to supply to the body.

Following fetal transition, the neonate is now breathing and oxygenating his or her own blood. As oxygen levels in the blood continue to increase, the neonate's skin turns from cyanotic to pink.

Any event that delays this decline in pulmonary pressure can result in delayed transition, hypoxia, brain injury, and, ultimately, death **Table 35-2**.

▶ Pathophysiology

When certain conditions are present, fetal transition may be delayed. Factors that predispose a newborn to have depressed respiratory function include meconium staining and recent ingestion of drugs or alcohol by the woman.

If fetal distress occurs in utero, the problem is usually caused by compromised blood flow in the placenta or umbilical cord; after delivery, the cause is usually the result of an airway or breathing problem. Clinical findings of fetal distress include the following:

- Persistent cyanosis and/or bradycardia secondary to systemic hypoxia
- Hypotension resulting from decreased coronary perfusion, decreased cardiac output, or blood loss

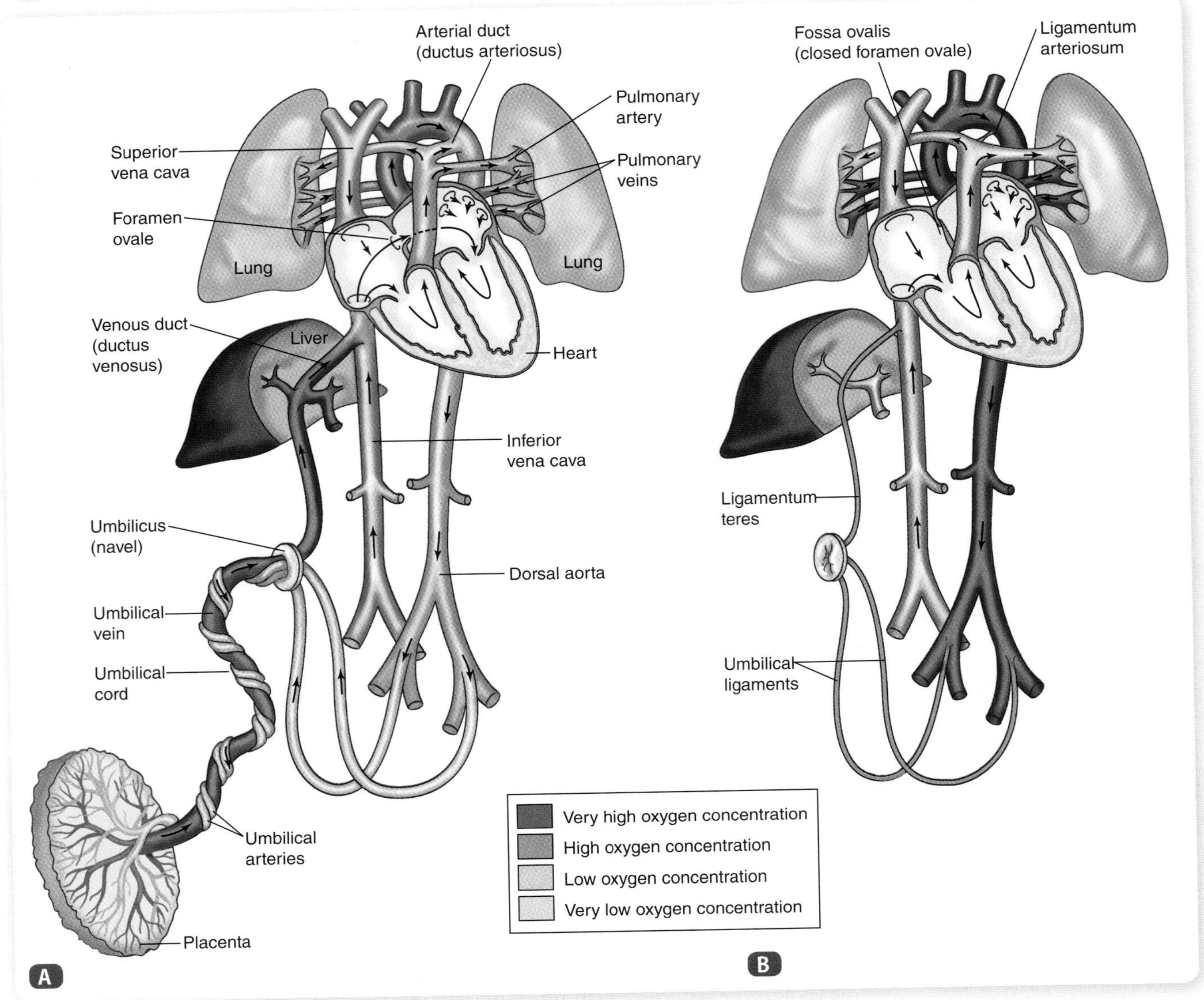

Figure 35-18 Fetal circulation. **A.** Oxygenated blood from the placenta reaches the fetus through the umbilical vein. Blood returns to the placenta via two umbilical arteries. Shunts (movements of blood from the normal path) occur at the ductus venosus, foramen ovale, and the ductus arteriosus. **B.** Fetal circulation following transition.

Table 35-2 Causes of Delayed Transition in Newborns

- Hypoxia
- Meconium staining or blood aspiration
- Acidosis
- Hypothermia
- Pneumonia
- Hypotension
- Sepsis
- Birth asphyxia
- Pulmonary hypoplasia (underdevelopment)
- Respiratory distress syndrome

- Respiratory depression or apnea caused by insufficient oxygen delivery to the brain
- Poor muscle tone from hypoxia and hypercapnia in the muscles

Respiratory distress in the newborn can occur as well and, if untreated, may result in cardiac arrest.

▶ Neonatal Assessment and Initial Steps

Initial steps are aimed at stimulating the newborn to begin spontaneous, effective breathing. They consist of drying, warming, positioning, suctioning, and stimulating the neonate. In most newborns, these initial steps are all that are required to initiate effective breathing.

Words of Wisdom

Bradycardia in a newborn is almost always the result of *hypoxia*! Provide positive pressure ventilations for a heart rate of less than 100 beats/min.

Words of Wisdom

Even during a normal delivery, the time surrounding the birth of a newborn is a very anxious and stressful time. Try to reassure the woman as you work with a distressed newborn. It is best not to separate the newborn from the woman unless you are resuscitating the newborn. Do your best to address concerns and to relieve fears.

At birth, a rapid assessment focusing on certain key elements listed in Table 35-3 will determine whether the newborn is in distress. If the answer to any of the questions is no, you must proceed with the initial steps of resuscitation and determine the need for further interventions.

Your initial rapid assessment of the newborn may be done simultaneously with any treatment interventions.

Words of Wisdom

To help remember the initial steps of neonatal resuscitation, remember the saying "Do What Probably Seems Simple," which stands for:

- **D**o: Drying
- **W**hat: Warming
- **P**robably: Positioning
- **S**eems: Suctioning
- **S**imple: Stimulation

Table 35-3 Immediate Assessment of the Newborn

- Is this term gestation?
- Is the newborn breathing or crying?
- Does the newborn have good muscle tone?

Note the time of delivery, and monitor the ABCs. In particular, assess color, tone, patency of the airway, respiratory rate, respiratory effort, and pulse rate.

YOU are the Provider PART 5

At 1 minute, you calculate the Apgar score as A = 0, P = 2, G = 0, A = 0, R = 0. You aggressively stimulate the newborn while drying, and are relieved to hear her take two gasping breaths followed by a high-pitched cry. At 5 minutes, you note the Apgar score to be 9, taking off only one point for appearance. You note the newborn's color improving and you ask the AEMT who is assisting if the woman can nurse the baby. The AEMT states that the woman is stable and you place the newborn skin-to-skin on the woman's abdomen to allow her to nurse. After ensuring that everyone is safely secured in the back of the ambulance, you instruct your partner to provide smooth transport to Memorial Hospital, which is about 3 miles away. You call in your report to the labor and delivery unit; they confirm they are awaiting your arrival. After you arrive at the hospital you turn the patients over to the labor and delivery staff and complete your patient care reports—one for each patient, while your partner readies the ambulance for the next call.

Newborn Assessment Recording Time: 5 Minutes After Birth	
Respirations	35 breaths/min
Pulse	147 beats/min, regular
Skin	Acrocyanosis
Blood pressure	Not obtained
Oxygen saturation (Spo_2)	96% on room air
Pupils	Not obtained

9. What are the components of the Apgar score, and what are the average normal scores?

Assessing skin color in newborns has several unique features. If the newborn has cyanosis, determine whether it is central or peripheral. This difference will help with decision making and treatment. A newborn who has not begun to breathe air will appear cyanotic. This is normal until effective spontaneous breathing occurs, at which time the skin usually "pinks up" rapidly. Many newborns become centrally pink but have blue hands and feet (**acrocyanosis**). This is considered normal in newborns through the first 24 to 48 hours of life and requires no therapy. If the newborn has a normal breathing pattern and a pulse rate of greater than 100 beats/min but maintains **central cyanosis** of the trunk or of the mucous membranes, provide supplemental **free-flow oxygen**. If there is no other warming source available, keep the newborn on the mother's chest and continue to manage the airway.

Crying is proof of breathing. Normally, a newborn's respiratory rate will be between 40 and 60 breaths/min. Breathing effort may be slightly irregular in normal newborns. Signs such as gasping, grunting, retractions, or nasal flaring indicate increased work of breathing and respiratory distress. Remember that respiratory distress in the newborn, if untreated, may result in cardiac arrest.

Words of Wisdom

If the newborn does not have adequate respiratory effort and a pulse above 100 beats/min within the first minute after birth, you must begin PPV. Ventilation of the newborn's lungs is the most important and effective treatment during neonatal resuscitation.[21]

The first step in caring for the newborn is to provide warmth, clear the airway if necessary, and dry and stimulate the newborn. You need to prevent hypothermia. Towels (preferably warmed) should be used for this purpose and should be present immediately following delivery. Thoroughly dry the newborn, particularly the head, which can be a source of substantial body heat loss. Remove any wet blankets, place a cap on the newborn's head, and place the newborn "skin to skin" with the mother, if possible. When responding to a call for a possible delivery, ensure that the heater in the back of the ambulance is turned on, regardless of the time of season. The hypothermic newborn will likely not respond to even the most simple and basic resuscitation measures (such as bag-mask ventilations or blow-by oxygen).

Next, position the newborn on a flat surface and ensure an open airway (sniffing position). Place a towel or blanket under the newborn's shoulders to help maintain this position **Figure 35-19**.

Words of Wisdom

In the absence of a warmer, blankets or towels may be warmed by wrapping them around chemical hot packs.

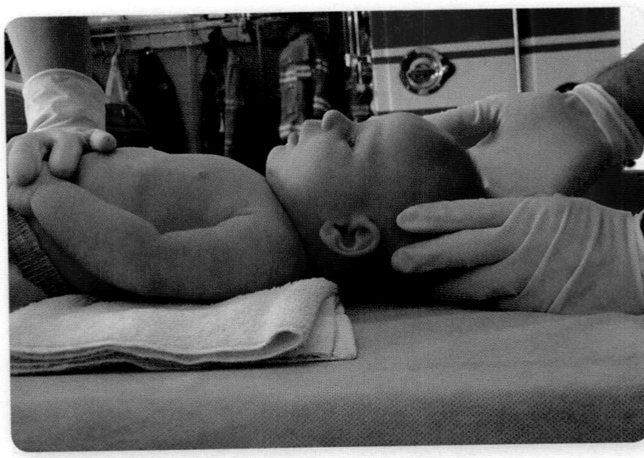

Figure 35-19 To avoid airway obstruction, it may be necessary to place a folded towel in between the newborn's shoulders.

If there are substantial oral secretions, the airway can be cleared using a bulb syringe or suction catheter. Turn the newborn's head to the side; suction the mouth before the nose to prevent aspiration. Do not suction vigorously or deeply, as this can induce a vagal response and bradycardia. After the airway is cleared, return the newborn to the sniffing position.

Drying the newborn's head and body with towels provides adequate stimulation in most cases. However, if the newborn still does not have adequate respirations, additional **tactile stimulation** may be provided *briefly* to stimulate breathing. There are only two acceptable and safe methods for providing tactile stimulation to the newborn: slapping or flicking the soles of the feet and gently rubbing the back, trunk, or extremities. Vigorous stimulation is not helpful and may result in injury to the newborn. *Never* shake a newborn.

Continued use of tactile stimulation in an apneic newborn is wasting precious time. Begin PPV with a bag-mask device and 100% oxygen immediately if brief tactile stimulation fails to initiate breathing or the heart rate is less than 100 beats/min.

As mentioned earlier, the Apgar score **Table 35-4** is the result of an objective method of quantifying the newborn's condition and helps record the condition of the newborn in the first few minutes after birth based on five signs. This score can help you determine the need for specific resuscitation measures and the effectiveness of their resuscitation efforts to facilitate the transition from fetus to newborn. The Apgar score is typically recorded at 1 and 5 minutes after birth. If the 5-minute Apgar score is less than 7, the newborn's condition should be reassessed and an additional score assigned every 5 minutes until 20 minutes after birth. If resuscitation is necessary, the Apgar score is assigned after the resuscitation.

Table 35-4 The Apgar Score

Condition	Description	Score
Appearance—skin color	Completely pink	2
	Body pink, extremities blue	1
	Centrally blue, pale	0
Pulse rate	>100	2
	<100, >0	1
	Absent	0
Grimace—irritability	Cries	2
	Grimaces	1
	No response	0
Activity—muscle tone	Active motion	2
	Some flexion of extremities	1
	Limp	0
Respiratory—effort	Strong cry	2
	Slow and irregular	1
	Absent	0

Safety

During the birth and resuscitation of the newborn, you must protect yourself from the splashing of blood and other body fluids. Minimum standard precautions include gloves, goggles or a face shield, and a gown.

▶ Algorithm for Neonatal Resuscitation

Neonatal resuscitation consists of the following sequence of steps:

1. Initial steps in stabilization (provide warmth, clear airway if necessary, dry, stimulate)
2. Positive pressure ventilation with oxygen saturation (Spo_2) monitoring
3. Chest compressions if heart rate is below 60 beats/min
4. Consider intubation (call for paramedic backup), continue chest compressions, and coordinate with positive pressure ventilation
5. If the heart rate remains below 60 beats/min, administer IV epinephrine (a paramedic skill) and consider hypovolemia or pneumothorax

The steps for neonatal resuscitation are outlined in Figure 35-20. Following the initial steps of resuscitation, the need for and extent of further resuscitation is based on the assessment of three key parameters: respiratory effort, heart rate, and color.

In newborns, bradycardia (heart rate <100 beats/min) is usually the result of hypoxia. Assess the heart rate carefully in a newborn who is not active or who requires PPV. This means either listening to the heart with a stethoscope or palpating the base of the umbilical cord Figure 34-21.

If breathing is not visible (apnea) in the newborn, immediate PPV is required. Room air is preferred when resuscitating term infants, and the addition of supplemental oxygen may not be necessary.[22]

After 30 seconds of adequate ventilations, assess the heart rate. If the heart rate is at least 100 beats/min and the newborn is breathing adequately, you can stop ventilations and assess the newborn's color. Do not suddenly stop ventilations. Instead, gradually decrease the rate and volume of ventilations to determine whether the newborn will continue to breathe adequately on his or her own. If not, continue ventilations until the newborn does. You may find that gently stimulating the newborn by flicking the soles of the feet or rubbing the torso will help maintain effective respirations.

Treat heart rates of less than 100 beats/min with PPV, even if respirations are normal. In most newborns with bradycardia, ventilation improves the heart rate to more than 100 beats/min immediately, and no further treatment is necessary.

If the heart rate is less than 60 beats/min, continue ventilation and begin chest compressions. Call for paramedic backup for advanced airway management.

Reassess the newborn after 30 seconds of PPV and chest compressions. If the heart rate is above 60 but below 100 beats/min, discontinue chest compressions and continue ventilations until the heart rate increases to more than 100 beats/min. If the heart rate remains less than 60 beats/min, continue PPV and chest compressions.

Special Populations

Indications for artificial ventilation of the newborn:

- Apnea
- Pulse rate of less than 100 beats/min
- Persisting central cyanosis despite breathing 100% oxygen

If prolonged ventilatory support or certain medications will be needed for the newborn, you should call for paramedic backup.

If central cyanosis is present, administer free-flow oxygen as described later. Continually assess the newborn's color while providing free-flow oxygen. If after 30 seconds of free-flow oxygen central cyanosis persists, perform PPV with 100% oxygen. If the cyanosis dissipates, gradually withdraw the oxygen until you are certain the newborn remains pink on room air. *Never* abruptly withdraw oxygen from any newborn.

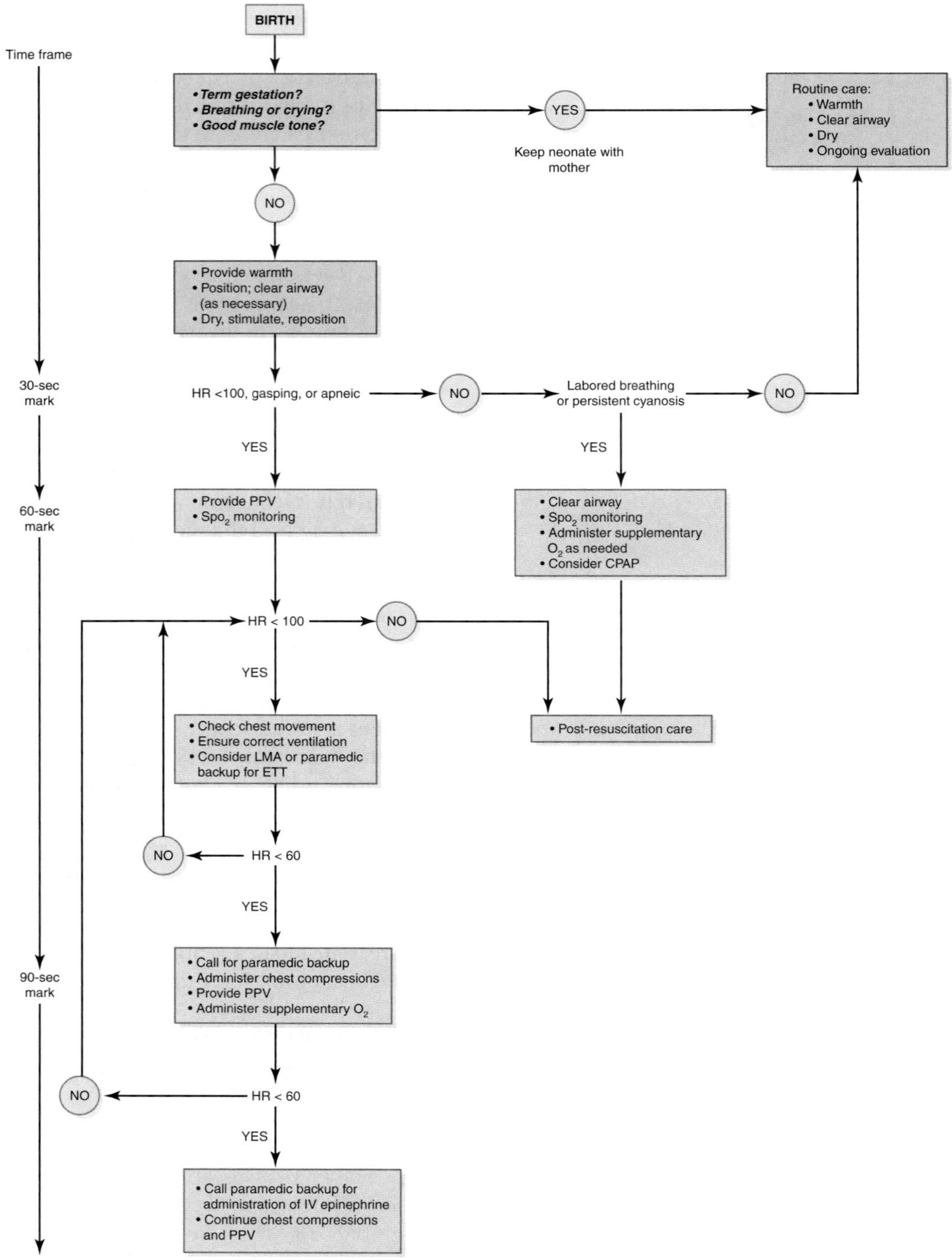

BIRTH
Time frame
• Term gestation?
• Breathing or crying?
• Good muscle tone?
YES
Keep neonate with mother
Routine care:
• Warmth
• Clear airway
• Dry
• Ongoing evaluation
NO
• Provide warmth
• Position; clear airway (as necessary)
• Dry, stimulate, reposition
30-sec mark
HR <100, gasping, or apneic
NO
Labored breathing or persistent cyanosis
NO
YES
YES
60-sec mark
• Provide PPV
• Spo_2 monitoring
• Clear airway
• Spo_2 monitoring
• Administer supplementary O_2 as needed
• Consider CPAP
HR < 100
NO
YES
• Check chest movement
• Ensure correct ventilation
• Consider LMA or paramedic backup for ETT
• Post-resuscitation care
NO
HR < 60
YES
90-sec mark
• Call for paramedic backup
• Administer chest compressions
• Provide PPV
• Administer supplementary O_2
NO
HR < 60
YES
• Call paramedic backup for administration of IV epinephrine
• Continue chest compressions and PPV

Abbreviations: CPAP, continuous positive airway pressure; ETT, endotracheal tube; HR, heart rate; IV, intravenous; LMA, laryngeal mask airway; PPV, positive pressure ventilation; SpO_2, oxygen saturation as measured by pulse oximeter

Figure 35-20 Algorithm for neonatal resuscitation.

Data from: Web-based Integrated 2015 American Heart Association Guidelines for CPR & ECC. Part 13: neonatal resuscitation. © 2015 American Heart Association, Inc.

▶ Airway Management

Free-Flow Oxygen

If a newborn is cyanotic or pale, provide supplemental oxygen. Given that 5 g/dL of deoxygenated hemoglobin is needed before clinical cyanosis becomes apparent, a severely anemic hypoxic newborn will be pale, but not cyanotic. Therefore, provide oxygen to a pale newborn until an accurate oxygen saturation reading can be obtained using a pulse oximeter. Warm and humidify the oxygen if it will be provided for more than a few minutes. If PPV is not indicated (ie, the pulse rate is greater than 100 beats/min and the newborn has adequate respiratory effort), oxygen can initially be delivered through an oxygen mask or via

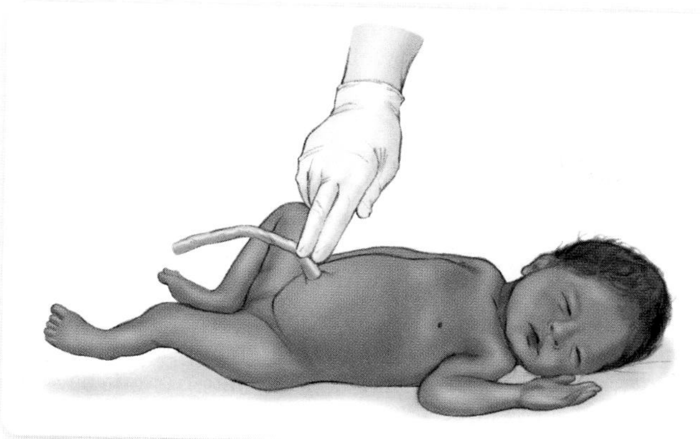

Figure 35-21 Feel for a pulse at the base of the umbilical cord.

oxygen tubing within your hand that is cupped and held close to the newborn's nose and mouth Figure 35-22. The oxygen flow rate should be set at 5 L/min. Apply free-flow oxygen directly to the newborn's face; do not blow oxygen directly into the newborn's eyes.

Bag-Mask Ventilation

Bag-mask ventilation is indicated when a newborn is apneic, has inadequate respiratory effort, or has a pulse rate of less than 100 beats/min (bradycardia) after you clear the airway of secretions, relieve obstruction from the tongue, and dry and stimulate the newborn. Signs of respiratory distress that suggest a need for bag-mask ventilation include periodic breathing, intercostal retractions (sucking in between the ribs), nasal flaring, and grunting on expiration.

Recognizing and treating respiratory distress early can reduce mortality and morbidity in newborns. In the field, you will most likely use a self-inflating bag for bag-mask ventilation. If available, always use the infant size (240 mL). Given that the breath size (tidal volume) of a newborn is only 3 to 6 mL/kg, only one-tenth of the bag's volume will be used for each breath—which explains why a larger bag can easily create problems. If a neonatal bag is not available and the newborn is in severe respiratory distress, has apnea, or has bradycardia, you can use a bag designed for adults or older children (750 mL or greater volume) as long as you carefully keep the delivered breath size appropriately small and monitor chest rise to avoid excessive volumes of delivered breaths.

When you are administering bag-mask ventilation with 100% oxygen, the face mask needs to provide an airtight seal, fitting over the newborn's mouth and nose, and extending down to the chin but not over the eyes Figure 35-23. Pressure on the eyes, such as deep suctioning, can result in a vagal response and bradycardia. The newborn needs to have a patent airway, cleared of secretions, with his or her neck slightly extended in the sniffing position Figure 35-24. The first few breaths after birth will frequently require higher pressures (possibly approximately 30 mm Hg) because the lungs are not yet expanded and are still full of fluid. To deliver these initial breaths, you may need to manually (cover with your finger) disable the spring-loaded pop-off valve (it is usually set by the manufacturer at 30 to 40 cm H_2O) Figure 35-25. Subsequent breaths should be delivered with sufficient pressure to result in visible but not excessive chest rise, with the pop-off valve on.

PPV is successful if you see both sides of the newborn's chest rise and hear breath sounds bilaterally. Use

> **Special Populations**
>
> It may be necessary to bypass the pop-off valve on a bag-mask device during the first few breaths to achieve higher inspiratory pressures in order to clear additional fluid from the alveoli.

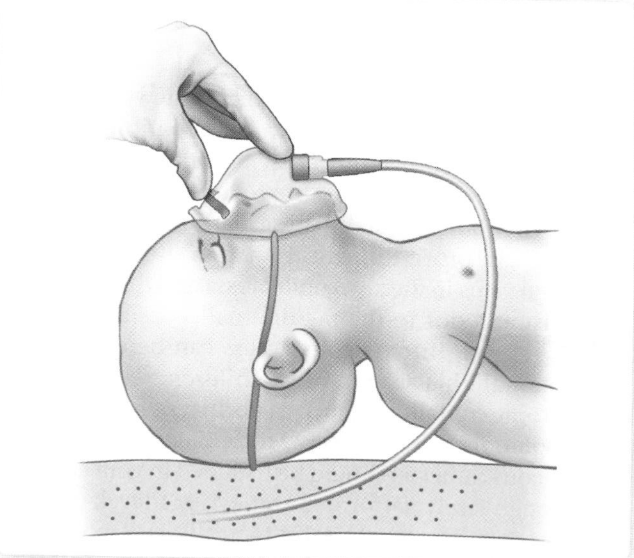

Figure 35-22 Free-flow oxygen can be delivered through an oxygen mask.

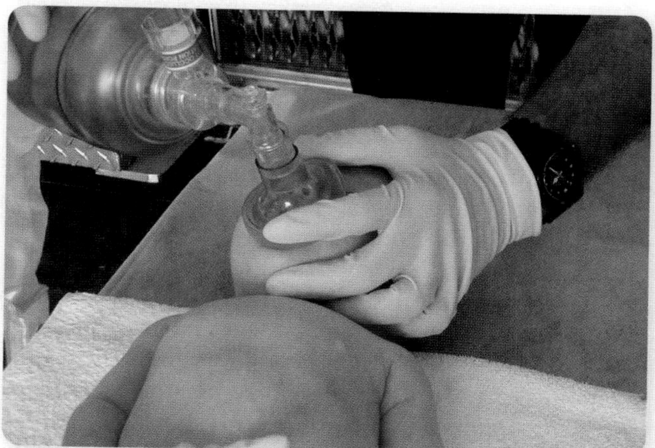

Figure 35-23 Bag-mask ventilation of the newborn. Hold the mask securely to the face with your thumb and index finger. Apply counter-pressure under the bony part of the chin with your middle finger.

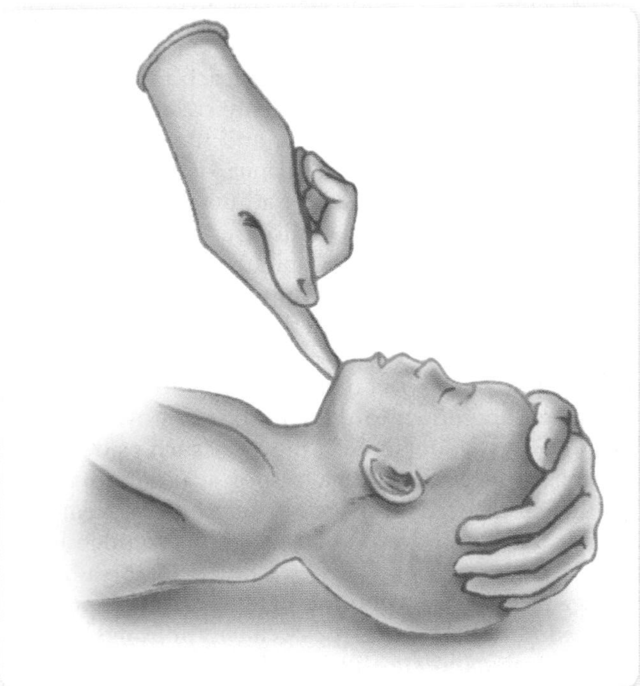

Figure 35-24 The sniffing position.

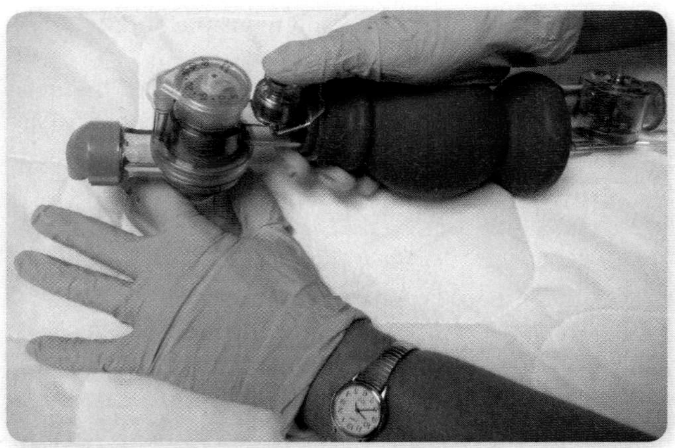

Figure 35-25 If a pop-off valve is present, occlude it to achieve higher inspiratory pressures.

caution when you are ventilating the newborn to avoid inadvertently delivering too much volume, potentially resulting in a pneumothorax.

In a newborn, it is important to provide the correct timing for ventilation at a rate of 40 to 60 breaths/min because breaths delivered at a higher rate can result in hypocapnia, air trapping, or pneumothorax. To help with the timing, count "breathe-two-three, breathe-two-three" as you ventilate: give a breath on "breathe," and release on "two-three." Continue PPV as long as the pulse rate remains at less than 100 beats/min or the newborn's respiratory effort is ineffective.

The most common reasons for ineffective bag-mask ventilations are inadequate seal of the mask on the face and incorrect head position. Other causes such as copious secretions, pneumothorax, or equipment malfunction need to be considered as well.

Words of Wisdom

Room air is preferred initially in the resuscitation of the term neonate, as hyperoxic injury may occur as a result of the free radicals produced when 100% oxygen is used. The current best practice is to initiate resuscitation with 21% oxygen (room air) and proceed for approximately 90 seconds. After 90 seconds of resuscitation efforts have elapsed with signs of hypoxia still present, providers may use an oxygen blender to administer inspired oxygen concentrations greater than 21%, targeting the desired preductal oxygen saturation for the neonate's age.[23,24] However, if an oxygen blender is not available, 100% oxygen may be administered. Regardless of the amount of oxygen initiated, the American Academy of Pediatrics recommends using a pulse oximeter to titrate the amount of oxygen delivered.[25] Bag-mask ventilation can be initiated with room air while an oxygen source is being secured.

▶ Circulation

Chest Compressions

There are two ways to perform chest compressions in the newborn. **Figure 35-26** shows chest compressions in the newborn.

Bag-mask ventilation is performed during a pause after every third compression. Avoid giving a compression and a ventilation simultaneously because one will decrease the effectiveness of the other. You should deliver compressions and ventilations in a 3:1 ratio, for a combined total of 120 "actions" per minute, 90 compressions and 30 ventilations. Keep in mind that adequate ventilation is absolutely critical to the successful resuscitation of the neonate.

Vascular Access

Vascular access is not usually needed in newborns; most problems can be corrected with oxygenation and ventilation. However, if fluid resuscitation or medications are necessary, you must be able to access the newborn's venous circulation. Establishing peripheral access in a newborn can prove difficult. IV access sites include the peripheral veins in the antecubital fossa and the saphenous veins just anterior to the medial malleolus at the ankle **Figure 35-27**. Intraosseous access can be obtained at the proximal tibia as with older children.

Isotonic crystalloids (such as normal saline or lactated Ringer solution), IV catheters (22 to 24 gauge), and pediatric intraosseous catheters should be included in your supplies.

Though rarely performed at the AEMT level, you may also carry **umbilical vein catheters (UVCs)** if your local protocols allow umbilical vein catheterization. Umbilical catheterization performed by prehospital care providers is a controversial procedure. Although this route of vascular access in experienced hands is effective and quick, the

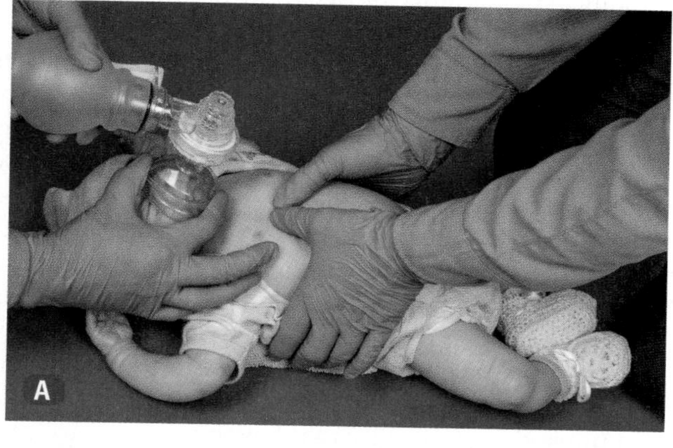

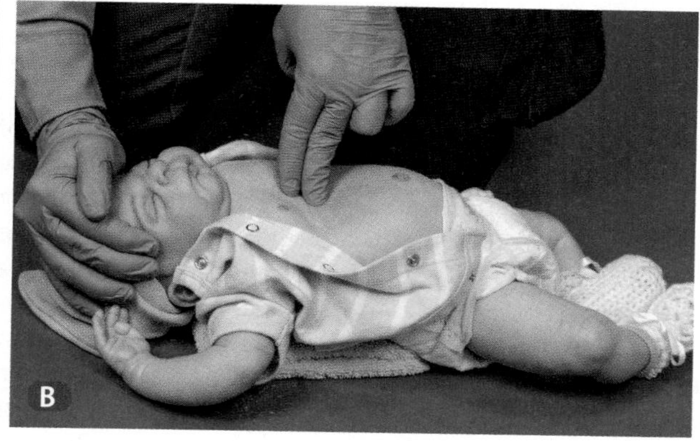

Figure 35-26 Chest compressions in the newborn. **A.** When using the thumb technique, position your thumbs side by side, placed between the xiphoid and an imaginary line drawn between the two nipples. Support the spine by encircling your fingers around the torso. **B.** When the newborn is large, use two fingers placed between the xiphoid and an imaginary line drawn between the nipples. Use the other hand to support the newborn's head.

prehospital care provider rarely needs to perform it and complications can occur.

If your EMS system uses UVCs, consider giving all medications and IV fluids this way. The umbilical vein can be catheterized using an umbilical vein line in a newborn by following these steps:

- Clean the cord with alcohol or another antiseptic. Place a sterile tie firmly, but not too tightly, around the base of the cord to control bleeding. Place a sterile drape over the site. Although the line must be placed quickly in a code situation, maintain sterile technique as much as possible.
- Prefill a sterile 3.5F to 5F umbilical vein line catheter (a comparable-size sterile feeding tube can be used in an emergency) with normal saline using a 3-mL syringe. Turn the stopcock to off toward the patient.
- Cut the cord with a scalpel below the clamp placed on the cord at birth approximately 1 to 2 cm from the skin (between the clamp and the cord tie).
- The umbilical vein is a large, thin-walled vessel usually found at the 12-o'clock position, as compared with the two thick-walled umbilical arteries usually found at the 4- and 8-o'clock positions. Insert the catheter into this vein for a distance of 2 to 4 cm (less in preterm newborns) until blood can be aspirated. If the catheter is advanced into the liver, this may result in irreversible damage. If the catheter is advanced into the heart, dysrhythmias may develop.
- Flush the catheter with 0.5 mL of normal saline and tape it in place.

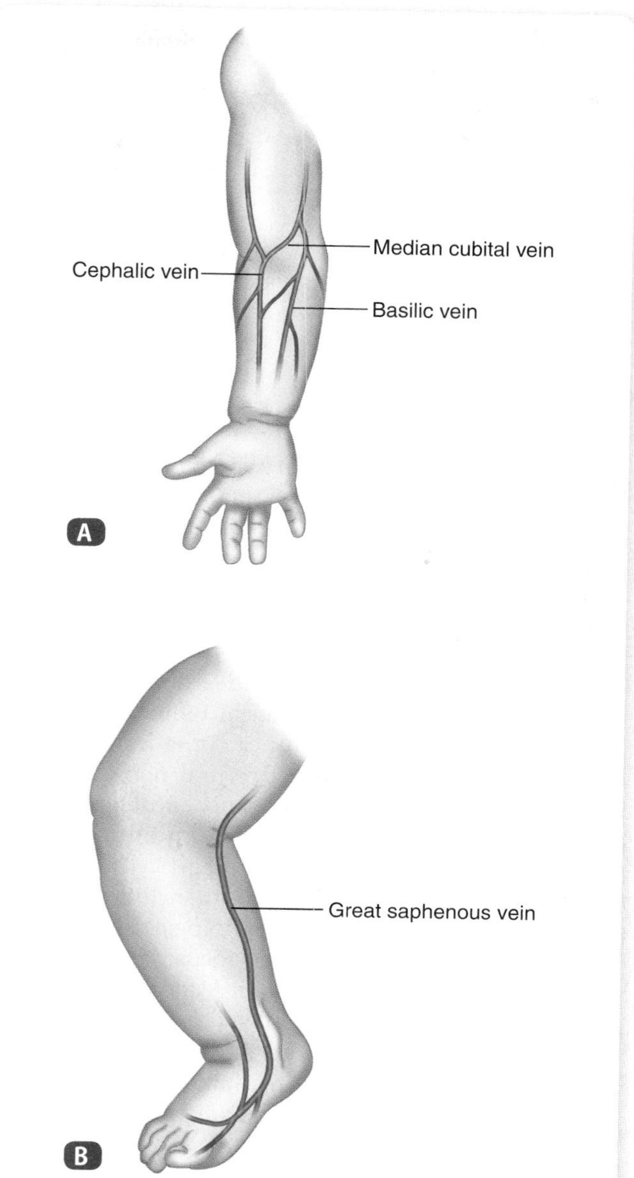

Figure 35-27 Intravenous access sites in a newborn. **A.** Peripheral veins in the antecubital fossa. **B.** Saphenous veins anterior to the medial malleolus of the ankle.

Do not place the umbilical catheter in too far, but place it to a depth where blood return is first seen. This will help keep the catheter out of the **portal venous system** and avoid complications of certain drugs entering the liver.

Pathophysiology, Assessment, and Management of Specific Conditions

Apnea

Apnea (a respiratory pause greater than or equal to 20 seconds) is common in newborns delivered before 32 weeks of gestation, but is rarely seen in the first 24 hours after delivery, even in premature newborns. If apnea does not respond to stimulation and further steps such as PPV are not taken, it can result in hypoxemia and bradycardia. Apnea often follows a period of hypoxia or hypothermia. Other causes include maternal or infant narcotic exposure, airway or respiratory muscle weakness, septicemia, prolonged or difficult labor and delivery, gastroesophageal reflux, central nervous system abnormalities including seizures, and metabolic disorders. The pathophysiology of apnea depends on the underlying etiology. Apnea of prematurity is a result of an underdeveloped central nervous system. Gastroesophageal reflux can trigger a vagal response, resulting in apnea. Drug-induced apnea frequently results from direct central nervous system depression. Regardless of the cause, a newborn with apnea needs respiratory support to minimize hypoxic brain damage and other organ damage.

Assessment of an apneic newborn includes obtaining a careful history to elicit possible etiologic risk factors and performing a physical exam that focuses on neurologic signs and symptoms or signs of infection. At birth, it is important to differentiate between **primary apnea** (apnea caused by oxygen deprivation) and **secondary apnea** (a period of gasping respirations, falling pulse rate, and falling blood pressure that occurs after primary apnea in an infant). If the newborn has experienced a relatively short period of hypoxia, he or she will have a period of rapid breathing, followed by apnea and bradycardia. At this point, the use of drying and stimulation may cause a resumption of breathing and improvement in the pulse rate. If hypoxia continues during primary apnea, the newborn will gasp and enter secondary apnea. At this point, stimulation alone will not restart the newborn's breathing. Instead, PPV by bag-mask device is required. Follow the steps for neonatal resuscitation discussed earlier in the chapter.

Bradycardia

Bradycardia in a newborn is most frequently a result of inadequate ventilation and often responds to effective PPV. Although increased intracranial pressure in older children can result in bradycardia, neonates have open fontanelles so they rarely present with increased intracranial pressure. Interventions can result in bradycardia as well as vagal stimulation from prolonged suctioning. The morbidity and mortality of bradycardia are determined by the underlying cause and how quickly it can be corrected.

Heart rate in a newborn is assessed via auscultation or by palpating the base of the umbilical cord. The algorithm for neonatal resuscitation (Figure 35-20) addresses the steps to take when an infant with a heart rate below 100 beats/min is encountered.[26] Assess the patency of the airway. If hypoxia continues, there could be persistent bradycardia. Begin chest compressions for a heart rate that is less than 60 beats/min despite at least 30 seconds of effective PPV.[27] For persistent bradycardia, call early for paramedic backup for administration of epinephrine. Focus on maintaining normothermia, and provide rapid transport to a facility that has the capacity to treat high-risk neonates.

Hypoglycemia

In the first 1 to 2 hours of life, the blood glucose level of healthy neonates may be 30 mg/dL and increase to more than 45 mg/dL 12 hours after birth.[28] In full-term or preterm newborns, hypoglycemia is a blood glucose level of less than 45 mg/dL. This condition represents an imbalance between glucose supply and utilization. Glucose levels may be low because of inadequate intake or storage or increased utilization of glucose. Most newborns remain asymptomatic until the glucose level decreases to less than 20 mg/dL for a substantial length of time. Because the brain relies on glucose as its primary fuel, hypoglycemia may result in seizures and severe, permanent brain damage. Table 35-5 lists risk factors for hypoglycemia in the newborn.

The fetus receives glucose from the mother and deposits glycogen in the liver, lung, heart, and skeletal muscle in utero. The newborn then begins to use those glycogen stores to meet glucose needs after birth; most full-term newborns will have sufficient glycogen stores to meet their glucose needs for 8 to 12 hours. Disorders related to decreased glycogen stores (small for gestational age, prematurity, postmaturity), including increased use of glucose (hypoxia, hypothermia, sepsis), or increased insulin in the fetus (newborn of a woman with diabetes, large for gestational age) place the newborn at increased risk for hypoglycemia. Frequently, stressed newborns will become hypoglycemic.

Symptoms of hypoglycemia can be quite nonspecific. They may include cyanosis, apnea, irritability, poor sucking or feeding, limpness or floppiness (hypotonia), irregular respirations, eye rolling, hypothermia, and decreased response to stimuli. These symptoms may also be associated with lethargy, tremors, twitching or seizures, and coma. Newborns may also have tachycardia, tachypnea, or vomiting.

In these cases, blood glucose measurement and administration of dextrose (10% solution) may be lifesaving in the field. Check the blood glucose level in all sick newborns (by heel stick), and evaluate the newborn's vital signs. After you establish good oxygenation,

Table 35-5 Hypoglycemia in the Newborn	
Risk Factor	**Specific Indicators**
Disorders of fetal growth and maturity	▪ Small for gestational age ▪ Smaller of discordant twins (weight difference >25% ▪ Large for gestational age ▪ Low–birth weight infant (birth weight <5.5 lb [2.5 kg])
Prematurity	▪ Less than 37 weeks of gestation or less than 5.5 lb (2.5 kg)
Disorders of maternal glucose regulation	▪ Insulin-dependent diabetic mother ▪ Gestational diabetic mother ▪ Morbid obesity in mother
Neonatal conditions with disturbed oxidative metabolism	▪ Perinatal distress (eg, 5-minute Apgar score <5) ▪ Hypoxemia due to cardiac or lung disease ▪ Shock, hypoperfusion, sepsis, cold stress
Severe anemia	▪ Pallor (in the absence of hypovolemia)
Congenital anomalies and genetic disorders	▪ Visible anatomic deformities/abnormalities

ventilation, and circulation, manage the hypoglycemia. Establish IV access as necessary. Medical control personnel may order the administration of a dextrose solution if the newborn's blood glucose level is less than 40 mg/dL. This intervention may be followed by an IV infusion of dextrose based on the newborn's gestational age. Recheck the blood glucose level in about 30 minutes. As always, maintain normal body temperature—hypothermia places additional stress on glucose demand. Warm IV fluids can assist in rewarming the newborn who is hypothermic.

▶ Hypovolemia

Newborns in shock will appear pale and have weak pulses. They may have persistent tachycardia or bradycardia, and cardiovascular function will often not improve in response to effective ventilation, chest compressions, and cardiac medications. For suspected hypovolemia in the newborn, administer 10 mL/kg of an isotonic crystalloid (such as normal saline or lactated Ringer solution) over 5 to 10 minutes. Although hypovolemia should be corrected fairly quickly, some clinicians are concerned that rapid fluid administration in a newborn may result in intracranial hemorrhage. Reassess the newborn and provide additional fluids as needed.

Words of Wisdom

Treat a hypovolemic newborn as you would an acute trauma patient with life-threatening blood loss who needs blood products. If venous access is needed because of bleeding, transport the newborn immediately and attempt IV or intraosseous access on the way to the hospital.

YOU are the Provider SUMMARY

1. What stage of labor is the patient in?

This patient is presenting in the first stage of labor, which is characterized by the onset of contractions and ends with the cervix being fully effaced and dilated. Because checking for cervical dilation is outside of the AEMT's scope of practice, the end of the first stage of labor is typically determined in the field by the presence of crowning, when the fetus's head is visible at the vaginal opening.

2. Is this patient's medical history important?

This patient has a history that should concern you. With a medical history of eclampsia, gestational diabetes, and delivering her first baby at 29 weeks of gestation, you should be thinking about the possibility of complications with this pregnancy. Because of this information, you should ensure that there is another unit that can respond to your location to assist with multiple patients.

3. Is immediate transport of this patient warranted?

Immediate transport of this patient is not warranted at this point. Even though you and your partner may feel like you need to get this patient to the hospital quickly so that she does not deliver in your ambulance, you should remain on scene and prepare for delivery. The signs of imminent delivery on this call were the frequency and

YOU are the Provider SUMMARY *(continued)*

duration of the woman's contractions, the lack of prenatal care coupled with a history of preterm delivery, and the patient's urge to have a bowel movement. All of these findings point to an imminent delivery.

4. Does this patient need IV access at this point?

Given that this patient has a history of eclampsia and preterm childbirth, it is preferable to obtain IV access sooner rather than later. After labor has progressed and delivery is imminent, there will probably not be enough time to establish IV access in the woman. If IV access can be obtained during the "calm before the storm," it will be one less thing to think about in the middle of the delivery.

5. What are the possible complications if you do not support the baby's head?

After it is obvious that the head is coming out farther with each contraction, you should place your gloved hand over the emerging bony parts of the head and exert very gentle pressure on it, decreasing the pressure slightly between contractions. This will allow the head to come out smoothly, preventing any tears to the perineum of the woman and possible trauma to the newborn.

6. How do you correct nuchal cord?

A nuchal cord is usually loose and easy to remove from around the newborn's neck; simply slip the cord gently over the newborn's head or shoulder. A nuchal cord that is wound tightly around the neck could cause the newborn to asphyxiate. It must therefore be released from the neck immediately. If you cannot slide the cord over the newborn's head, you must clamp and cut it before the delivery can continue. After you have cut the cord, unwrap it from around the neck. Handle the cord very carefully; it is fragile and easily torn. If it does tear, severe hemorrhage can occur from the woman, newborn, or both.

7. Why is it important to note the time of birth?

Recording time of birth provides you with a starting point from which to time the intervals for Apgar scores. It will ensure that the information is available and accurate for the birth certificate.

8. Why is it important to note whether there was meconium present on delivery?

Meconium causes concern because it can be aspirated into the fetus's lungs, resulting in potentially life-threatening airway issues and possibly sepsis. If meconium is present on birth, you may have to alter the sequence of initial resuscitation and perform more invasive suctioning of the newborn's trachea.

9. What are the components of the Apgar score, and what are the average normal scores?

The Apgar score quantifies a newborn's condition and response to resuscitation. This method is performed 1 and 5 minutes following birth. The Apgar score is not used to determine the need for resuscitation, what interventions are necessary, or when to use them, but rather just to assess the newborn. The components of the Apgar score include **A**ppearance, **P**ulse, **G**rimace or irritability, **A**ctivity or muscle tone, and **R**espiration. Each of the five signs is assigned a value of 2, 1, or 0. The five values are then added. Most newborns will have a score of 7 or 8 at 1 minute and a score of 8 to 10 at 5 minutes.

EMS Patient Care Report (PCR)

Date: 9-12-18	**Incident No.:** 2257A	**Nature of Call:** Active labor	**Location:** I-75 SB MM 135		
Dispatched: 1417	**En Route:** 1417	**At Scene:** 1423	**Transport:** 1458	**At Hospital:** 1504	**In Service:** 1529

Patient Information

Age: 23 **Sex:** F **Weight (in kg [lb]):** 83 kg (184 lb)	**Allergies:** No known drug allergies **Medications:** None **Past Medical History:** G2P1A0, eclampsia, gestational diabetes mellitus **Chief Complaint:** Labor

Vital Signs

Time: 1435	**BP:** 96/54	**Pulse:** 120	**Respirations:** 32	**Spo_2:** 99%
Time: 1501	**BP:** 98/60	**Pulse:** 88	**Respirations:** 18	**Spo_2:** 99%
Time:	**BP:**	**Pulse:**	**Respirations:**	**Spo_2:**

YOU are the Provider SUMMARY (continued)

EMS Treatment (circle all that apply)				
Oxygen @ _______ L/min via (circle one): NC NRM Bag-mask device		Assisted Ventilation	Airway Adjunct	CPR
Defibrillation	Bleeding Control	Bandaging	Splinting	Other: Childbirth

Narrative
EMS dispatched to southbound I-75 at mile marker 135 for a woman in labor. On arrival, found male frantically waving us down, states that his girlfriend is going to have a baby, and points to the back of the car, where audible screams can be heard. Patient found supine on rear seat, AO×4, ABCs intact. States her water broke 3 hours ago, and they were on their way to the hospital, but she doesn't think they can make it. States that the contractions are approximately 1 minute apart, lasting 1 minute each. Past medical history of gestational diabetes and eclampsia, no prenatal care this pregnancy. G2P1A0, last pregnancy 29 weeks, vaginal delivery, currently 32 weeks' gestation. Assisted patient to stretcher and placed in back of ambulance. Clothing on lower body removed. 18-gauge IV line right DH established with NS TKO. Patient complains of needing to have a bowel movement, and crowning noted. 2nd ambulance called for additional manpower. Patient prepped for imminent delivery. Baby presents with nuchal cord, easily removed by slipping over head. Cord clamped and cut. Mother appears stable, care of woman turned over to additional crew on scene while newborn is attended. **Female, Time of Birth 1429** 1 minute APGAR was "7" and repeat at 5 minutes was "9." Both patients transported to Memorial Hospital and turned over to L&D staff without incidence. See addendum from additional crew for continuing documentation on woman and second PCR for documentation of care of newborn.**End of report**

Prep Kit

Ready for Review

- Most births are uneventful and do not require substantial medical intervention.
- When ovulation occurs and a mature egg is released, it travels down the fallopian tubes toward the uterus. If sperm are present, fertilization may occur. The zygote should implant into the lining of the uterus.
- The umbilical cord connects woman and fetus through the placenta. The placenta provides nutrients and eliminates waste from the developing fetus, and acts as a barrier.
- As the fetus grows, the different structures that are recognizable begin to form. All fetal organs have formed by the eighth week of development.
- A newborn born at 38 to 42 weeks of gestation is described as term. During the first 28 days of life, a baby is considered a neonate. Between the ages of 1 month and 1 year, a baby is referred to as an infant.
- During pregnancy, the woman's body undergoes many changes to support and protect the developing fetus. Menstruation ceases, the total blood volume

Prep Kit *(continued)*

increases, the heart rate elevates, blood pressure changes, the respiratory minute volume increases, and gastrointestinal complaints such as morning sickness and heartburn can occur.

- Emergencies can occur prior to delivery. The most common cause of vaginal bleeding during the first and second trimesters of pregnancy is spontaneous abortion (miscarriage).
- Third-trimester bleeding presents the greatest danger of hemorrhage; a large volume of blood is present within the pregnant woman's body.
- Ectopic pregnancy occurs when the embryo implants in the fallopian tube, ovary, in the abdominal cavity, or the cervix. This is the most life-threatening emergency for the pregnant woman during the first trimester.
- Abruptio placenta and placenta previa are major causes of substantial hemorrhage before delivery. Do *not* try to palpate the abdomen deeply in any woman with third-trimester bleeding; if she has placenta previa, deep palpation may induce heavy bleeding.
- Hypertension may occur during pregnancy. The most common disorder is preeclampsia, an increase in blood pressure after the 20th week of gestation. Preeclampsia can result in cerebral hemorrhage or seizures.
- When a fetus has a different Rh factor than his or her mother, the antibody may attack fetal red blood cells and create complications such as hemolytic disease.
- Gestational diabetes predisposes the patient to hyperglycemia or hypoglycemia. Uncontrolled diabetes may result in problems during labor and delivery.
- Hyperemesis gravidarum is persistent nausea and vomiting during pregnancy and can result in dehydration and malnutrition. Severe cases require hospitalization.
- Trauma is a serious complicating factor in pregnancy. If a pregnant woman has sustained trauma and is bleeding massively, the maternal circulation will shunt blood away from fetal circulation to maintain maternal homeostasis. Any injury that involves substantial maternal bleeding will threaten the life of the fetus.
- Maintain a high index of suspicion for internal abdominal bleeding in pregnant patients who experienced trauma. Field treatment of pregnant trauma patients focuses on airway management, administration of high-flow oxygen, adequate ventilation, bleeding control, immobilization as needed, administration of intravenous fluids, and transport.
- Use of key obstetric terms such as *gravida* (the number of times a woman has been pregnant) and *para* (the number of times a woman has delivered a viable newborn) will facilitate communication between health care providers.
- Obtain an obstetric history from the patient, asking about any prior pregnancies, complications, prenatal care, and her current condition.
- You will have to determine whether you have time to provide transport to the hospital or attempt delivery in the field. Assist with the delivery of the newborn at the scene when delivery can be expected within a few minutes.
- Management of nondelivery emergencies includes patient positioning, administration of oxygen, intravenous fluid administration depending on the emergency, and emotional support.
- Manage bleeding by positioning the patient in a recumbent position on her left side, administering oxygen, providing rapid transport, providing intravenous fluids, placing trauma pads loosely over the vagina, and considering paramedic backup for pharmacologic treatment.
- There are three stages of labor. The first stage begins with the onset of contractions and ends when the cervix is fully effaced and dilated. The second stage is from the point of full dilation and effacement (crowning) until the newborn is delivered. The third stage is from delivery of the newborn until delivery of the placenta.
- The only times you should place a finger or hand into the vagina are to keep the walls of the vagina from compressing the newborn's airway during a facedown breech presentation or to push the newborn's head away from the umbilical cord if it is prolapsed.
- If you deliver a newborn in the field, remember that your job is to help, guide, and support the newborn during delivery. Always contact medical control for guidance if you have concerns.
- To deliver a newborn, prepare a sterile delivery field. Support the newborn's head as it emerges and feel to see if the cord is wrapped around the newborn's neck. Guide the head and upper body to help deliver the shoulders. Keep the airway open, clamp and cut the cord, and allow the woman to deliver the placenta. Dry the newborn off and wrap the newborn to maintain body heat.
- The Apgar score is designed to measure the success of resuscitation, and should be taken at 1 and 5 minutes following birth.
- After the newborn is delivered and is breathing, you will need to cut the umbilical cord. Clamping of the cord should be delayed 30 seconds after delivery in most vigorous newborns.

Prep Kit *(continued)*

- After delivery of the placenta, gently massage the uterine fundus to slow postpartum bleeding. There are many complications that can occur during labor, delivery, and postpartum. Be prepared to assess and manage emergencies by supporting the airway, breathing, and circulation; administering intravenous fluid if needed; and providing rapid transport.
- Complications of labor include preterm labor, fetal distress, and uterine rupture. Uterine rupture can occur after the mother experiences trauma; it causes substantial bleeding that may be internal, external, or both.
- High-risk pregnancy conditions include meconium staining, multiple gestation, cephalopelvic disproportion, intrauterine fetal death, and amniotic fluid embolism.
- Complications of delivery include breech and limb presentations, shoulder dystocia, nuchal cord, and prolapsed umbilical cord. Quickly transport the patient with a limb presentation or prolapsed umbilical cord to the hospital.
- Postpartum complications include uterine inversion, pulmonary embolism, and spina bifida.
- After birth, the newborn makes a transition from receiving oxygen through the umbilical cord to breathing on its own. Most newborns breathe spontaneously without any advanced interventions. In a small percentage of births, fetal distress occurs.
- Newborn resuscitation refers to the series of interventions used to stimulate spontaneous breathing. Initial steps of neonatal resuscitation include drying and warming, positioning, suctioning, and stimulating the newborn.
- Three criteria are used to assess the need for further resuscitation in newborns: heart rate, color, and respiratory effort.
- Acrocyanosis is considered normal in newborns in the first 24 go 48 hours of life and requires no therapy. If the newborn has central cyanosis, provide supplemental free-flow oxygen.
- A newborn who is not breathing or whose heart rate is less than 100 beats/min requires immediate positive pressure ventilation and 100% oxygen. After 30 seconds of adequate ventilation, if the heart rate is at least 100 beats/min and the infant is breathing adequately, you may stop ventilations and assess the newborn's color.
- If a newborn's heart rate is less than 60 beats/min, provide ventilation and begin chest compressions.
- Vascular access is not usually needed for newborns, but if required, intravenous access sites include the peripheral veins in the antecubital fossa and the saphenous vein just anterior to the medial malleolus of the ankle. Umbilical vein catheterization may be allowed in some emergency medical services systems.
- Apnea is a respiratory pause of 20 seconds or longer. If apnea does not respond to stimulation and further steps such as positive pressure ventilation are not taken, it can result in hypoxemia and bradycardia. A newborn with apnea needs respiratory support to minimize hypoxic brain damage and other organ damage.
- Bradycardia in a newborn often responds to effective positive pressure ventilation. Follow the algorithm for neonatal resuscitation when caring for a newborn with bradycardia.
- Signs of hypoglycemia in the newborn can be nonspecific. Measure blood glucose level and evaluate vital signs. If the newborn is hypoglycemic, administer 10% dextrose in water, and keep the infant warm.
- A newborn with hypovolemia may be given an isotonic crystalloid.

▶ Vital Vocabulary

abruptio placenta Premature separation of the placenta from the wall of the uterus; also called placental abruption.

acrocyanosis A decrease in the amount of oxygen delivered to the extremities. The hands and feet turn blue because of narrowing (constriction) of small arterioles (tiny arteries) toward the end of the arms and legs.

amniotic fluid The fluid produced by the filtration of maternal and fetal blood through blood vessels in the placenta and by excretion of fetal urine into the amniotic sac.

amniotic fluid embolism An extremely rare, life-threatening condition that occurs when amniotic fluid and fetal cells enter the pregnant woman's pulmonary and circulatory system through the placenta via the umbilical veins, causing an exaggerated allergic response from the woman's body.

amniotic sac The fluid-filled, baglike membrane in which the fetus develops.

Apgar score system A scoring system for assessing the status of a newborn that assigns a number value to each of the five areas of assessment.

birth canal The vagina and cervix.

Braxton-Hicks contractions Intermittent uterine contractions that may occur every 10 to 20 minutes, usually seen in the third trimester of the pregnancy, but which are not indicative of labor beginning or occurring; also known as false labor.

Prep Kit *(continued)*

breech presentation A type of abnormal delivery in which the buttocks emerge first.

central cyanosis Cyanosis to the newborn's face and trunk; indicates hypoxia.

cervix The lower third, or neck, of the uterus.

chronic hypertension A blood pressure that is equal to or greater than 130/80 mm Hg, which exists prior to pregnancy, occurs before the 20th week of pregnancy, or persists postpartum.

complete abortion The expulsion of all products of conception from the uterus.

crowning The appearance of the newborn's head at the vaginal opening during labor.

ductus arteriosus A small artery that connects the left pulmonary artery to the aorta; diverts blood away from the fetal lungs while in utero.

eclampsia Convulsions (seizures) resulting from severe hypertension in the pregnant woman.

ectopic pregnancy A pregnancy that develops outside the uterus; typically, in a fallopian tube.

effacement Thinning and shortening of the cervix; a normal process that occurs as the uterus contracts.

elective abortion Intentional expulsion of the fetus.

embryo The term used to describe the developing infant from fertilization to the end of the eighth week of gestation.

embryonic period The period of gestation between weeks 3 and 8 in which all major organ systems begin to develop.

fallopian tubes The two hollow tubes or ducts that extend from the uterus to the region of the ovary and serve as a passage for the egg and sperm.

fetal transition Process through which the fluid in the fetal lungs is replaced with air, the ductus arteriosus constricts, and the neonate begins adequate oxygenation of its own blood.

fetoscope A device used for listening to fetal heart tones.

fetus The developing, unborn infant inside the uterus; the embryo becomes the fetus at the beginning of the ninth week of gestation.

foramen ovale An opening between the two atria that is present in the fetus but usually closes shortly after birth.

free-flow oxygen Oxygen administered via oxygen tube and a cupped hand on the patient's face.

fundus The top portion of the uterus.

gestation The process of fetal development following fertilization of an egg.

gestational diabetes mellitus The condition in which progesterone (the pregnancy hormone) makes the cells resistant to insulin, resulting in the potential for hypoglycemia or hyperglycemia; typically resolves following delivery.

gestational hypertension High blood pressure that develops after the 20th week of pregnancy in women with previously normal blood pressures, and that resolves spontaneously in the postpartum period; formerly known as pregnancy-induced hypertension.

gestational period The time that it takes for a fetus to develop in utero; normally takes 38 weeks.

grand multipara A term used to describe a woman who has delivered five or more viable infants.

gravid Pregnant.

gravida A term used to describe the number of times a woman has been pregnant.

hyperemesis gravidarum A condition of persistent nausea and vomiting during pregnancy.

imminent abortion A spontaneous abortion that cannot be prevented.

incomplete abortion Expulsion of the fetus that results in some products of conception remaining in the uterus.

infant A baby from 1 month of age to 1 year of age.

lightening Movement of the fetus down into the pelvis prior to birth.

limb presentation A delivery in which the presenting part is a single arm, leg, or foot.

meconium The newborn's first bowel movement.

meconium staining The occurrence of a dark green material in the amniotic fluid that can cause lung disease in the newborn.

menstruation The period in the menstrual cycle of sloughing and discharge of the functional layer of the endometrium.

multigravida A term used to describe a woman who has been pregnant more than once.

multipara A term used to describe a woman who has delivered two or more viable infants.

myoclonus Hyperactive reflexes; occurs during severe preeclampsia.

neonate The phase of life that occurs during the first 28 days after birth.

newborn The phase of life from the first few minutes to the first hours after birth.

nuchal cord An umbilical cord that is wrapped around the newborn's neck.

nullipara A term used to describe a woman who has never delivered a viable infant.

ovaries Female glands that produce sex hormones and ova (eggs).

ovum A mature egg released by the ovary during ovulation.

Prep Kit *(continued)*

oxytocin A hormone secreted in the pituitary gland that promotes uterine contractions.

para A term used to describe the number of times a woman has delivered a viable (live) infant.

perineum The area of skin between the urethral opening and the anus.

placenta Tissue attached to the uterine wall that nourishes the fetus through the umbilical cord.

placenta previa A condition in which the placenta develops over and covers the cervix.

portal venous system Special venous drainage system that takes blood from the intestines to the liver.

postpartum eclampsia Eclampsia that occurs after a woman has delivered a newborn; can occur up to several weeks after the birth.

preeclampsia A condition during pregnancy characterized by hypertension, protein in the urine, and edema; a precursor to eclampsia.

premature A newborn that delivers before 36 weeks of gestation or weighs less than 5 lb (2.25 kg) at birth.

premature rupture of membranes Rupture of the amniotic sac prior to the onset of labor; increases risk of fetal infection or injury.

preterm Before 36 complete weeks of gestation.

primary apnea Apnea caused by oxygen deprivation; usually corrected with stimulation, such as drying or slapping the newborn's feet; typically preceded by an initial period of rapid breathing.

primigravida A woman's first pregnancy.

primipara A woman who has had only one delivery.

prolapsed umbilical cord A situation in which the umbilical cord comes out of the vagina before the newborn.

rupture of membranes The rupture of the amniotic sac, which normally occurs during labor.

secondary apnea A period of gasping respirations, falling pulse rate, and falling blood pressure that occurs after primary apnea in an infant.

shoulder dystocia A complication of delivery in which there is difficulty delivering the shoulders of a newborn; the shoulder cannot get past the woman's symphysis pubis.

spina bifida A developmental defect in which a portion of the spinal cord or meninges may protrude outside of the vertebrae and possibly even outside of the body, usually at the lower third of the spine in the lumbar area.

spontaneous abortion Delivery of the fetus and placenta by natural causes before 20 weeks of gestation; also known as miscarriage.

supine hypotensive syndrome Low blood pressure resulting from compression of the inferior vena cava by the weight of the gravid uterus when a woman is supine.

tactile stimulation Method of stimulating a newborn to breathe by flicking or slapping the soles of the feet or rubbing the lateral thorax.

term Between 38 and 42 weeks' gestation.

threatened abortion Expulsion of the fetus that is attempting to take place but has not occurred yet; usually occurs in the first trimester.

trimesters Three segments of time, each made up of approximately 3 months, that comprise the length of a pregnancy.

ultrasonography The use of a special device that uses sound waves to determine the location and shape of internal tissues and organs.

umbilical cord The conduit connecting woman to infant via the placenta; contains two arteries and one vein.

umbilical vein catheters (UVCs) Special catheters designed to be inserted into the umbilical cord.

uterine inversion A potentially fatal maternal complication of childbirth in which the placenta fails to detach properly and results in the uterus turning inside out.

uterine rupture Rupture of the uterus, usually by trauma, that can result in life-threatening hemorrhage in the woman and fetus.

uterus The muscular organ where the fetus grows, also called the womb; responsible for contractions during labor.

vagina The muscular tube that forms the lower part of the female reproductive tract; the birth canal.

vernix caseosa A white, cheesy substance that covers the fetus.

zygote A fertilized egg.

▶ References

1. Records K, Tanaka L. Physiology of pregnancy. In: Mattson S, Smith JE, eds. *Core Curriculum for Maternal Newborn Nursing*. 5th ed. St. Louis, MO: Elsevier; 2011:83-107.
2. Miscarriage: signs, symptoms, treatment, and prevention. American Pregnancy Association website. August 2016. http://americanpregnancy.org/pregnancy-complications/miscarriage/. Accessed March 31, 2017.
3. Placental abruption. March of Dimes website. January 2012. http://www.marchofdimes.org/pregnancy/placental-abruption.aspx. Accessed March 31, 2017.
4. Ananth CV, Kinzler WL. Placental abruption: clinical features and diagnosis. UpToDate website. February

Prep Kit *(continued)*

23, 2017. https://www.uptodate.com/contents/placental-abruption -clinical-features-and-diagnosis?source=search_result&search=Abruptio%20placenta%20 causes&selectedTitle=1~150#H1. Accessed March 31, 2017.

5. Placental previa. March of Dimes website. January 2012. http://www.marchofdimes.org/complications/placenta-previa.aspx. Accessed March 30, 2017.
6. Lockwood CJ, Russo-Stieglitz K. Clinical features, diagnosis, and course of placenta previa. UpToDate website. November 30, 2016. https://www.uptodate.com/contents/clinical-features-diagnosis-and-course-of-placenta-previa?source=search_result&search=placenta%20previa&selectedTitle=2~104#H14. Accessed March 31, 2017.
7. New ACC/AHA High Blood Pressure Guidelines Lower Definition of Hypertension. American College of Cardiology website. 2017. http://www.acc.org/latest-in-cardiology/articles/2017/11/08/11/47/mon-5pm-bp-guideline-aha-2017. Accessed January 30, 2018.
8. August P, Sabai BM. Preeclampsia: clinical features and diagnosis. February 2017. https://www.uptodate.com/contents/preeclampsia-clinical-features-and-diagnosis?source=search_result&search=preeclampsia&selectedTitle=1~150. Accessed March 30, 2017.
9. Kinsella SM, Lohmann G. Supine hypotensive syndrome. *Obstet Gynecol.* 1994;83(5 Pt 1):774-788.
10. American Pregnancy Association. Hyperemesis gravidarum: Signs, Symptoms and Treatment. http://americanpregnancy.org/pregnancy-complications/hyperemesis-gravidarum/. Accessed March 30, 2017.
11. Harding M. Mallory-Weiss syndrome. Patient website. https://patient.info/doctor/mallory-weiss-syndrome-pro. November 13, 2014. Accessed January 16, 2018.
12. Boisrame T, Sananes N, Fritz G, et al. Placental abruption: risk factors, management and maternal-fetal prognosis. Cohort study over 10 years. *Eur J Obstet Gynecol Reprod Biol.* 2014;179:100-104.
13. 2015 CPR & EEC guidelines. Part 10: special circumstances of resuscitation. American Heart Association website. https://eccguidelines.heart.org/index.php/circulation/cpr-ecc-guidelines-2/part-10-special-circumstances-of-resuscitation/. Accessed May 1, 2017.
14. Teen pregnancy in the United States. Centers for Disease Control and Prevention website. April 26, 2016. https://www.cdc.gov/teenpregnancy/about/. Accessed March 31, 2017.
15. Cahill AG, Waterman BM, Stamilio DM, et al. Higher maximum doses of oxytocin are associated with an unacceptably high risk for uterine rupture in patients attempting vaginal birth after cesarean delivery. *Am J Obstet Gynecol.* 2008;199(1):32.e1-5.
16. Dekker GA, Chan A, Luke CG, et al. Risk of uterine rupture in Australian women attempting vaginal birth after one prior cesarean section: a retrospective population-based cohort study. *BJOG.* 2010;117(11):1358-1365.
17. Tahseen S, Griffiths M. Vaginal birth after two caesarean sections (VBAC-2)- a systematic review with meta-analysis of success rate and adverse outcomes of VBAC-2 versus VBAC-1 and repeat (third) caesarean sections. *BJOG.* 2010;117(1):5-19.
18. Weiner GM, Zaichkin J. *Textbook of Neonatal Resuscitation (NRP).* 7th ed. Elk Grove Village, IL: American Academy of Pediatrics; 2016:36.
19. Martin JA, Hamilton BE, Osterman MJK, Driscoll AK, Mathews TJ. Births: final data for 2015. *Natl Vital Stat Rep.* 2017;66(1). https://www.cdc.gov/nchs/data/nvsr/nvsr66/nvsr66_01.pdf. Accessed May 1, 2017.
20. Henry E, Andres RL, Christensen RD. Neonatal outcomes following a tight nuchal cord. *J Perinatol.* 2013;33(3):231-234. http://www.medscape.com/viewarticle/780171_1. Accessed April 4, 2017.
21. Weiner GM, Zaichkin J. Lesson 3: initial steps of newborn care. In: *Textbook of Neonatal Resuscitation (NRP).* 7th ed. Elk Grove Village, IL: American Academy of Pediatrics; 2016:44.
22. Wyckoff MH, Aziz K, Escobedo MB, et al. Part 13: neonatal resuscitation: 2015 American Heart Association Guidelines Update for Cardiopulmonary Resuscitation and Emergency Cardiovascular Care. *Circulation.* 2015;132(suppl 2):S547.
23. Kliegman RM, Stanton BF, St. Geme JW, Schor NF. Chapter 100: delivery room emergencies. In: *Nelson Textbook of Pediatrics.* 20th ed. Philadelphia, PA: Elsevier; 2016:845.
24. Weiner GM, Zaichkin J. Lesson 3: initial steps of newborn care. In: *Textbook of Neonatal Resuscitation (NRP).* 7th ed. Elk Grove Village, IL: American Academy of Pediatrics; 2016:49.
25. Weiner GM, Zaichkin J. Lesson 3: initial steps of newborn care. In: *Textbook of Neonatal Resuscitation (NRP).* 7th ed. Elk Grove Village, IL: American Academy of Pediatrics; 2016:47.
26. Weiner GM, Zaichkin J. *Textbook of Neonatal Resuscitation (NRP).* 7th ed. Elk Grove Village, IL: American Academy of Pediatrics; 2016.
27. Weiner GM, Zaichkin J. Lesson 6: chest compressions. In: *Textbook of Neonatal Resuscitation (NRP).* 7th ed. Elk Grove Village, IL: American Academy of Pediatrics; 2016:166.
28. Adamkin DH. Postnatal glucose homeostasis in late-preterm and term infants. *Pediatrics.* 2011;127(3):575-579.

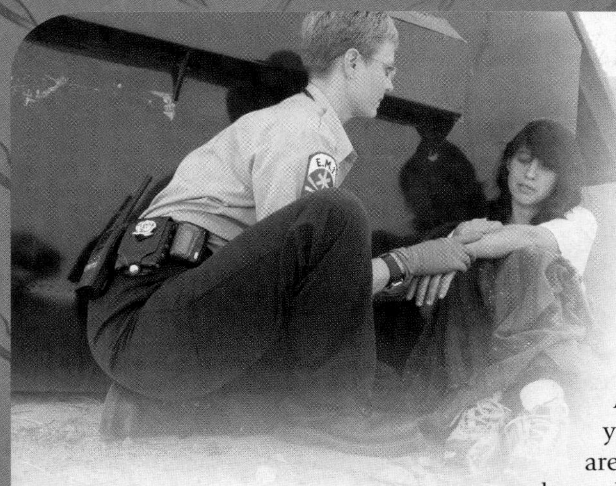

Assessment in Action

You were dispatched to assist a basic life support (BLS) crew who reportedly just performed a field delivery. On arrival, an EMT from the BLS crew hands you a reported full-term, approximately 3.8-kg child. The EMT states that the 1-minute Apgar score was 9 and the 5-minute Apgar score was 10. When you look at the newborn, you are unsure if the Apgar scores are correct because the baby looks limp and sick. You palpate a pulse and find the pulse to be 65 beats/min.

1. What is the initial treatment for a newborn with a heart rate of 65 beats/min?

- **A.** Chest compressions
- **B.** Blow-by oxygen
- **C.** Intubation
- **D.** Assisted ventilation

2. If the heart rate continues to decrease after assisted ventilations, what should you do?

- **A.** Switch to blow-by oxygen.
- **B.** Continue assisted ventilations with chest compressions.
- **C.** Continue assisted ventilations, but no chest compressions.
- **D.** Provide chest compressions only.

3. What is the compression to ventilation ratio for CPR in the newborn?

- **A.** 3:1
- **B.** 5:1
- **C.** 15:2
- **D.** 30:2

4. How often do you reassess the newborn during CPR?

- **A.** Every 5 minutes
- **B.** Every 2 minutes
- **C.** Every 1 minute
- **D.** Every 30 seconds

5. If peripheral cyanosis is present:

- **A.** provide oxygen via blow-by.
- **B.** provide positive pressure ventilations.
- **C.** initiate chest compressions.
- **D.** provide continuous positive airway pressure to improve positive end-expiratory pressure.

6. By 40 weeks of gestation, a pregnant woman's circulating blood volume has typically ______ by ____.

- **A.** increased, 25%
- **B.** decreased, 25%
- **C.** increased, 50%
- **D.** decreased, 50%

7. Which of the following is NOT a sign of preeclampsia?

- **A.** Headache
- **B.** Seizure
- **C.** Anxiety
- **D.** Nausea and vomiting

8. The Apgar score for a limp newborn who has central cyanosis, a pulse rate of 65 beats/minute, and a weak cry with slow respirations is:

- **A.** 1.
- **B.** 2.
- **C.** 3.
- **D.** 4.

9. What are the symptoms of hypoglycemia in a neonate?

10. What are the indications for providing positive pressure ventilations to the newborn?

CHAPTER 36

Pediatric Emergencies

National EMS Education Standard Competencies

Special Patient Populations

Applies a fundamental knowledge of growth, development, aging, and assessment findings to provide basic and selected advanced emergency care and transportation for a patient with special needs.

Pediatrics

Age-related assessment findings, age-related, and developmental stage related assessment and treatment modifications for pediatric-specific major diseases and/or emergencies:

- Upper airway obstruction (pp 1496-1497)
- Lower airway reactive disease (pp 1499-1501)
- Respiratory distress/failure/arrest (pp 1494-1495)
- Shock (pp 1507-1508)
- Seizures (pp 1513-1514)
- Sudden infant death syndrome (pp 1529-1531)
- Gastrointestinal disease (p 1515)

Patients With Special Challenges

Recognizing and reporting abuse and neglect (pp 1526-1528 and Chapter 37, *Geriatric Emergencies*)

Health care implications of

- Abuse (pp 1526-1528 and Chapter 37, *Geriatric Emergencies*)
- Neglect (pp 1526-1528 and Chapter 37, *Geriatric Emergencies*)
- Homelessness (Chapter 38, *Patients With Special Challenges*)
- Poverty (Chapter 38, *Patients With Special Challenges*)
- Bariatrics (Chapter 38, *Patients With Special Challenges*)
- Technology dependent (Chapter 38, *Patients With Special Challenges*)
- Hospice/terminally ill (Chapter 38, *Patients With Special Challenges*)
- Tracheostomy care/dysfunction (Chapter 38, *Patients With Special Challenges*)
- Home care (Chapter 38, *Patients With Special Challenges*)
- Sensory deficit/loss (Chapter 38, *Patients With Special Challenges*)
- Developmental disability (Chapter 38, *Patients With Special Challenges*)

Trauma

Applies fundamental knowledge to provide basic and selected advanced emergency care and transportation based on assessment findings for an acutely injured patient.

Special Considerations in Trauma

Recognition and management of trauma in

- Pregnant patient (Chapter 35, *Obstetrics and Neonatal Care*)
- Pediatric patient (pp 1520-1526)
- Geriatric patient (Chapter 37, *Geriatric Emergencies*)

Pathophysiology, assessment, and management of trauma in the

- Pregnant patient (Chapter 35, *Obstetrics and Neonatal Care*)
- Pediatric patient (pp 1520-1526)
- Geriatric patient (Chapter 37, *Geriatric Emergencies*)
- Cognitively impaired patient (Chapter 38, *Patients With Special Challenges*)

Knowledge Objectives

1. Explain some of the challenges inherent in providing emergency care to pediatric patients and why effective communication with both the patient and his or her family members is critical to a successful outcome. (pp 1474-1475)
2. Describe differences in the anatomy, physiology, and pathophysiology of the pediatric patient as compared with the adult patient and their implications for the health care provider, with a focus on the following body systems: respiratory, circulatory, nervous, musculoskeletal, gastrointestinal, and integumentary. (pp 1478-1482)
3. Describe the steps in the primary survey for providing emergency care to a pediatric patient, including the elements of the pediatric assessment

triangle (PAT), hands-on ABCDEs, transport decision considerations, and privacy issues. (pp 1483-1490)

4. Discuss the steps in the secondary assessment of a pediatric patient, describing what the advanced emergency medical technician (AEMT) should look for related to different body areas and the method of injury. (pp 1491-1492)
5. Describe the different causes of pediatric respiratory emergencies, the signs and symptoms of increased work of breathing, the difference between respiratory distress and respiratory failure, and the emergency medical care strategies used in the management of each. (pp 1494-1496)
6. List the possible causes of an upper and a lower airway obstruction in a pediatric patient and the steps in the management of foreign body airway obstruction. (pp 1496-1501)
7. List lower airway emergencies in a pediatric patient, including asthma, and possible causes, signs and symptoms, and steps in patient management. (pp 1499-1501)
8. Explain how to determine the correct size of an airway adjunct intended for a pediatric patient during an emergency. (pp 1501-1503)
9. List the different oxygen delivery device options that are available for providing oxygen to a pediatric patient, including the indications for the use of each and precautions the AEMT must take to ensure the patient's safety. (pp 1503-1505)
10. Discuss the most common causes of shock (hypoperfusion) in a pediatric patient, its signs and symptoms, and emergency medical management in the field. (pp 1507-1508)
11. Discuss the use of intravenous therapy in pediatric patients, including intraosseous access and fluid resuscitation. (pp 1508-1512)
12. Discuss the most common causes of altered mental status in a pediatric patient, its signs and symptoms, and emergency medical management in the field. (p 1513)
13. List the common causes of seizures in a pediatric patient, the different types of seizures, and their emergency medical management in the field. (pp 1513-1514)
14. List the common causes of meningitis, patient groups who are at the highest risk for contracting it, its signs and symptoms, special precautions, and emergency medical management in the field. (pp 1514-1515)
15. Discuss the types of gastrointestinal disease emergencies that might affect pediatric patients and their emergency medical management. (p 1515)
16. Discuss poisoning in pediatric patients, including common poison sources, signs and symptoms of poisoning, and its emergency medical management. (pp 1515-1516)
17. Discuss dehydration emergencies in pediatric patients, including how to gauge their severity based on key signs and symptoms, and emergency medical management. (pp 1516-1517)
18. Discuss the common causes of a fever emergency in a pediatric patient and the role of the AEMT regarding patient management. (pp 1517-1518)
19. Discuss assessment and management of a child with hypoglycemia. (pp 1518-1519)
20. Discuss assessment and management of a child with hyperglycemia. (p 1519)
21. Discuss the common causes of drowning emergencies in pediatric patients, their signs and symptoms, and emergency medical management. (pp 1519-1520)
22. Discuss the common causes of pediatric trauma emergencies and differentiate between injury patterns in adults, infants, and children. (pp 1520-1524)
23. Discuss the significance of burns in pediatric patients, their most common causes, and general guidelines an AEMT should follow when assessing patients who have sustained burns. (pp 1524-1525)
24. Explain the four triage categories used in the JumpSTART system for pediatric patients during disaster management. (p 1526)
25. Describe child abuse and neglect and its possible indicators, and then describe the medical and legal responsibilities of an AEMT when caring for a pediatric patient who is a possible victim of child abuse. (pp 1526-1528)
26. Discuss why managing posttraumatic stress is important for all health care professionals. (p 1529)
27. Discuss sudden infant death syndrome (SIDS), including its risk factors, patient assessment, and special management considerations related to the death of an infant patient. (pp 1529-1530)
28. Discuss the responsibilities of the AEMT when communicating with family or loved ones following the death of a child. (pp 1530-1531)

Skills Objectives

1. Demonstrate how to position the airway in a pediatric patient. (pp 1486-1487, Skill Drill 36-1)
2. Demonstrate how to palpate the pulse and estimate the capillary refill time in a pediatric patient. (p 1488)
3. Demonstrate how to use a length-based resuscitation tape to size equipment appropriately for a pediatric patient. (pp 1501-1502)
4. Demonstrate how to insert an oropharyngeal airway in a pediatric patient. (p 1502, Skill Drill 36-2)

5. Demonstrate how to insert a nasopharyngeal airway in a pediatric patient. (p 1503, Skill Drill 36-3)
6. Demonstrate how to administer blow-by oxygen to a pediatric patient. (p 1504)
7. Demonstrate how to apply a nasal cannula to a pediatric patient. (p 1504)
8. Demonstrate how to apply a nonrebreathing mask to a pediatric patient. (pp 1504-1505)
9. Demonstrate how to assist ventilation of an infant or child using a bag-mask device. (p 1505)
10. Demonstrate how to perform one-person bag-mask device ventilation on a pediatric patient. (pp 1505-1506, Skill Drill 36-4)
11. Demonstrate how to perform two-person bag-mask device ventilation on a pediatric patient. (p 1505)
12. Demonstrate how to obtain intraosseous access in a pediatric patient. (pp 1510-1511, Skill Drill 36-5)
13. Demonstrate how to immobilize a pediatric patient who has been involved in a trauma emergency. (pp 1521-1522, Skill Drill 36-6)
14. Demonstrate how to immobilize a pediatric patient who has been involved in a trauma emergency in a car seat. (pp 1522-1523, Skill Drill 36-7)

Introduction

Although pediatric emergencies account for a relatively small percentage (13%) of an emergency medical services (EMS) system's call volume,[1] pediatric mortality is a significant health concern in the United States. Therefore, it is important for you to learn and continually refine your pediatric skills.

It is not uncommon for the prehospital professional to experience anxiety when responding to a call involving a pediatric patient. Assessment and management of infants and children present you with unique challenges. Children differ anatomically, physically, and emotionally from adults. The injuries and illnesses that children sustain, and the children's responses to them, vary based on age or developmental level. Unlike their adult counterparts, pediatric patients, especially infants and small children, cannot provide you with the historic information that is usually easily obtained from an adult, such as events preceding the incident, what happened, medical history, and where they hurt.

In addition to caring for the sick or injured child, you must also be prepared to deal with parents or caregivers. Many times, they can provide you with the vital information that you need; other times, they may be of little assistance to you.

It is often said that children are not simply small adults—a statement that could not be more true. Unlike adults, children have special needs that require you to adjust assessment and management strategies accordingly. This chapter discusses those special needs, including anatomic and physiologic differences between children and adults, and the assessment and management of pediatric medical and trauma emergencies.

YOU are the Provider — PART 1

Your ambulance, staffed with an emergency medical responder, an emergency medical technician (EMT), and yourself, is dispatched to 424 N. Cavalier Street for an unresponsive child. On arrival, you are met by an elderly man at the front door who states that the patient is in the back bedroom. You attempt to question him as you proceed to the back of the residence, but he cannot tell you any additional information. In the back bedroom, you find an approximately 5-year-old girl lying supine on the bed; she appears to be unresponsive. You note a middle-aged woman sobbing next to her, who you are able to ascertain is the child's mother. She states that her parents were babysitting and called her about 15 minutes ago, stating that they think the child got into some of their medication. When you ask what type of medication, she states "something for diabetes."

1. What stage of growth and development is this child in, and what are some of the key milestones that you can anticipate seeing?
2. When treating an infant or pediatric patient, what is often the best source of information regarding the current condition?

Communication With the Patient and the Family

It is important to remember that when children are ill or injured, especially those with chronic illnesses, you may have multiple patients to treat rather than just one. Family members, especially the parent or primary caregiver, often need help or support when medical emergencies or problems develop. It is common for parents or caregivers to become angry and demanding when their child is sick or injured. You must realize that this anger is not directed toward you; it is a manifestation of the parents' or caregivers' fear of the situation. A calm parent usually helps to contribute to a calm child. An agitated parent usually means that the child will act the same way. You must remain compassionate, calm, and professional as you deal with pediatric patients and their families.

When possible, allow parents or caregivers to participate in the care of the child. This often helps to calm both the parent and the child, and makes the parent or caregiver feel as if he or she is making a positive contribution to the situation. If the child is not critically ill or injured, allow him or her to remain on the parent's or caregiver's lap.

Growth and Development

The growth and development of infants, toddlers, preschoolers, school-age children, and adolescents was discussed in Chapter 9, *Life Span Development*. Refer to that chapter to familiarize yourself with pediatric stages of development. Infancy and toddlerhood have their own specific phases that are discussed in detail in the next section.

▶ The Infant

Infancy is usually defined as the first year of life; the first month after birth is called the neonatal or newborn period.

0 to 2 Months

Infants younger than 2 months spend most of their time sleeping or eating. Sleep accounts for up to 18 hours a day between feeding times and parent or caregiver interactions.[2] Infants respond mainly to physical stimuli such as light, warmth, hunger, and sound. An infant should be aroused easily from a sleeping state, and it should be considered an emergency if this is not the case.

Infants at this stage have a sucking reflex for feeding. Head control is limited, but infants can turn their heads and focus on faces. Infants have poor thermoregulation, and their heads have a relatively large surface area. These factors predispose them to hypothermia, which is why parents and caregivers will often bundle infants to keep them warm.

Crying is one of the main avenues of expression during this period. Infants may cry when hungry or if they require certain needs to be met. If all obvious needs have been addressed and the infant is still inconsolable, then this could be a sign of significant illness.

Infants are not able to tell the difference between parents and strangers. Their basic needs consist of being kept warm, dry, and fed. They experience the world through their bodies. Being held, cuddled, or rocked soothes the infant. Hearing is also well developed at birth, so calm and reassuring talk is often helpful in soothing the infant.

2 to 6 Months

Infants between ages 2 and 6 months spend more time awake, are more active and social, and can recognize their caregivers. Voluntary smiles and increasing eye contact are common, and at this point in development, infants will begin to roll over. By 4 months of age, infants are able to hold their heads up.

Healthy infants in this age group will have a strong sucking reflex, active extremity movement, and a vigorous cry. They may follow a bright light or toy with their eyes or turn their heads toward a loud sound or the caregiver's voice.

The infant now has an increased awareness of what is going on around him or her and will use both hands to examine objects and explore the world. As with younger infants, persistent crying and irritability can be an indicator of serious illness. A lack of eye contact in a sick infant can also be a sign of significant illness, depressed mental status, or a delay in development.

6 to 12 Months

Most infants between 6 and 12 months of age can sit unsupported, reach for objects, sleep through the night, and are becoming more mobile—crawling and even walking. Because of this, they are exposed to more physical dangers than before. They become more aware of their surroundings and also explore their own bodies. During this stage, infants are also teething and tend to pick up anything and place it in their mouths. The risk for foreign body aspirations and poisonings from toxic substances is yet another impending danger. They also begin getting teeth and eating soft foods. Babbling is also common, and by 12 months they learn their first word.

At 6 to 12 months, infants may cry if they are separated from their parents or caregivers **Figure 36-1**. This behavior, called separation anxiety, is common among this age group.

As with the younger infants, persistent crying or irritability can be a symptom of serious illness.

Assessment of the Infant

Your assessment of an infant begins with observation of the child's appearance, **work of breathing**, and circulation. These three factors are measured using the **pediatric assessment triangle (PAT)**, which is described in detail later in this chapter.

Because infants cannot communicate their feelings or needs verbally, it is especially important to respect a parent or caregiver's perception that "something is wrong."

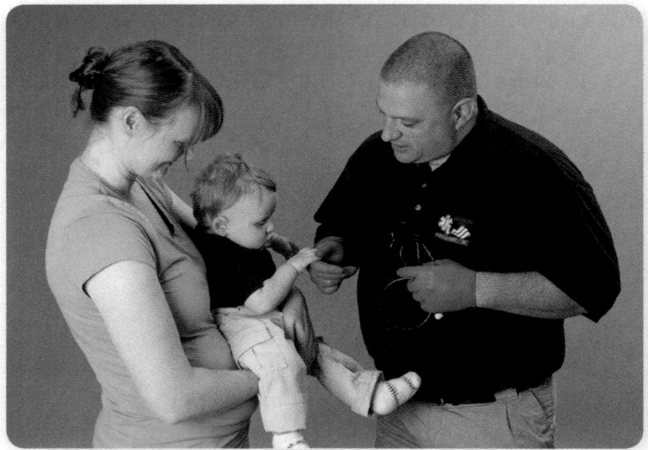

Figure 36-1 Infants are usually not afraid of strangers, but as they reach 6 months to 1 year, they may show signs that they prefer to be with their caregivers.

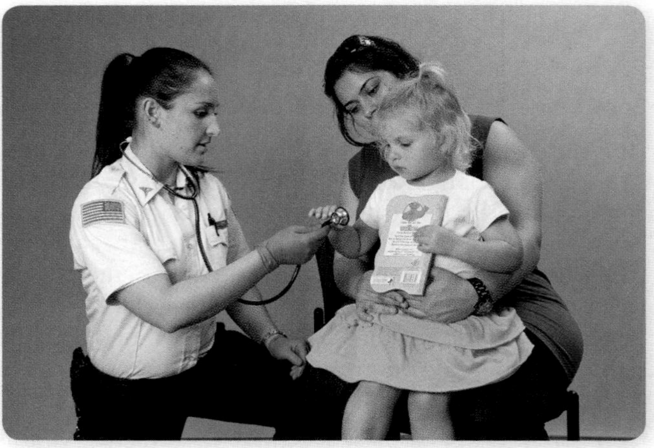

Figure 36-2 Allow a toddler to sit on the parent's or caregiver's lap during your assessment, and use a toy to distract him or her.

Nonspecific concerns about a young infant's behavior, feeding, or sleep patterns may be tip-offs to a serious underlying illness or injury. When obvious reasons for crying, such as hunger or needing to be changed, have been addressed, persistent crying can be a sign of significant illness. Although infants spend much time sleeping, they should arouse easily. Inability to arouse an infant should be considered an emergency. By age 6 months, infants should make eye contact. Lack of eye contact by infants in this age group may be a sign of significant illness or of depressed mental status or delayed development. Those infants approaching age 12 months are at risk for foreign body aspiration and poisoning because of exploration of the environment with their mouths. Crawling and walking also increase exposure to physical dangers.

Words of Wisdom

You should keep infants and young children close to their parents during your assessment to help them feel safe and to improve your ability to perform the assessment.

Consider the best location for performing your primary survey. Although separating a 2-week-old infant from a parent will not cause distress, an older infant in stable condition will be most calm in a parent's arms. Make sure that your hands and stethoscope are warm—a startled, crying infant will be difficult to examine. Be opportunistic with your examination. If the child is quiet, listen to the heart and lungs first, perhaps listening over the clothes before you expose the chest and disturb the infant. If a young infant starts crying, letting the baby suck on a pacifier or gloved finger may quiet the child enough to allow you to complete your assessment. Jingling keys or shining a penlight may distract an older infant long enough for you to finish an examination. Remember to explain each procedure to the parent or caregiver before you perform it.

The Toddler

After infancy, until about 3 years of age, a child is called a **toddler**. Toddlers experience rapid changes in growth and development.

12 to 18 Months

During this period, toddlers begin to walk and to explore their environment. They are able to open doors, drawers, boxes, and bottles. Because they are explorers by nature and are not afraid, injuries in this age group increase. At 12 to 18 months, toddlers begin to imitate the behaviors of older children and parents and may express a desire to dress like mommy or daddy. The toddler knows major body parts when you point to them and may speak four to six words. Because of a lack of molars, toddlers may not be able to fully chew their food before swallowing, leading to an increased risk of food aspiration and choking.

18 to 24 Months

The mind of the toddler develops rapidly. At the beginning of this stage, the toddler may have a vocabulary of 10 to 15 words. By age 2 years, a toddler should be able to pronounce approximately 100 words. When you point to a common object, toddlers should be able to name it. At this stage, toddlers begin to understand cause and effect with such activities as pop-up toys (jack-in-the-box) and turning on and off a light switch. The toddler's balance and gait also improve rapidly during this period. Running and climbing are two skills that develop. At this stage, toddlers tend to cling to their parents and caregivers and often have a special object such as a blanket or teddy bear that comforts them when they are separated Figure 36-2.

Assessment of the Toddler

Begin with an assessment of the toddler's interactions with the caregiver, vocalizations, and mobility, measured through the PAT. Persistent crying or irritability can be a symptom of serious illness. Remember that increased mobility in this age group increases their exposure to physical dangers and injury. There is also an increased risk of food aspiration and choking because, given a lack of molars, children may not be able to properly grind up food before swallowing. Examine a toddler in stable condition on the parent's lap and allow them to hold objects that are important to the child. Get down to the child's level, sitting or squatting for the examination. Begin your assessment with the feet and move toward the head. You may need to be creative to perform a good examination on a toddler with stranger anxiety: use a parent to lift the shirt so that you can assess the respiratory rate, or have the parent press on the abdomen to see if that appears painful. Use play and distraction techniques whenever possible—listening to a doll's chest first may buy you a few minutes of cooperation. Because of their newly found independence, toddlers may be unhappy about being restrained or held for procedures. Offer toddlers limited choices when possible because they like to be in control. If you ask yes or no questions, the answer is likely to be "No!"

Toddlers may have a hard time describing or localizing pain. Pain in the abdomen may be "My tummy hurts," and examination may reveal tenderness throughout the body. This is not because the child is trying to be difficult but because he or she cannot tell the difference. The use of visual clues and the Wong-Baker FACES pain scale, discussed later in this chapter, can be helpful with this age group.

Consider performing the more upsetting parts of the examination, such as palpating a tender abdomen or examining an injured extremity, last. Painful procedures make lasting impressions and only increase the difficulty of examining the patient. Be flexible in your approach—some toddlers will not let you complete an orderly full-body examination. Because of developmental changes, children in this age group will generally no longer require shoulder rolls to limit flexion of the neck when ventilating with a bag-mask device or performing advanced airway procedures.

▶ The Preschool-Age Child

Preschool-age children are ages 3 to 6 years **Figure 36-3**. As discussed in Chapter 9, *Life Span Development*, this age group can understand directions, be much more specific in describing their sensations, and identify painful areas when asked. The most rapid increase in language occurs at this stage and toilet training is mastered.

Preschool-age children have a rich imagination, which can make them particularly fearful about pain and change involving their bodies. They are also learning which behaviors are appropriate. Tantrums may occur when they feel they cannot control a situation or its outcomes. The risk of foreign body aspiration continues to be high at this age.

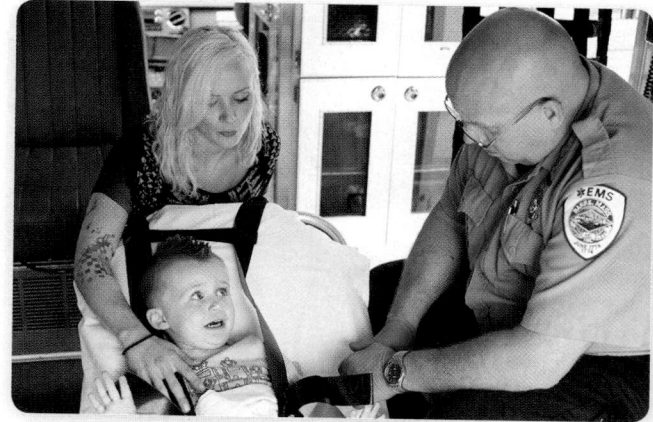

Figure 36-3 Preschool-age children have vivid imaginations, so much of the history must still be obtained from the parent or caregiver.

Assessment of the Preschooler

As you perform your assessment beginning with the PAT, take advantage of the child's curiosity and desire to cooperate. If the patient is in medically stable condition, offer to take turns with the child in listening to the heart and lungs. Let the preschooler play with or hold equipment that is safe. Respect modesty and only expose as much as is necessary to complete your examination. To help give the child some sense of control, offer simple choices and tell the child what you are going to do before you do it. Never lie to the patient; after you have lost your pediatric patient's trust, it will be difficult to regain it. Avoid yes or no questions. Set limits on behavior if the child acts out. For the most part, you should be able to talk a preschooler through an orderly full-body examination. Begin your assessment with the feet and move toward the head, similar to assessing a toddler.

> **Special Populations**
>
> Allowing a child to participate in his or her assessment and care can greatly reduce anxiety. However, you must be careful not to back yourself into a corner. Instead of asking, "Can I listen to your heart?" offer options. Explain, "I need to listen to your heart and feel your tummy. Which would you like for me to do first?" You are giving the child the ability to make decisions while not allowing them to just say, "No!"

▶ The School-Age Child

School-age children are ages 6 to 12 years and are beginning to act more like adults. They can think in concrete terms, respond sensibly to direct questions, and help take care of themselves **Figure 36-4**.

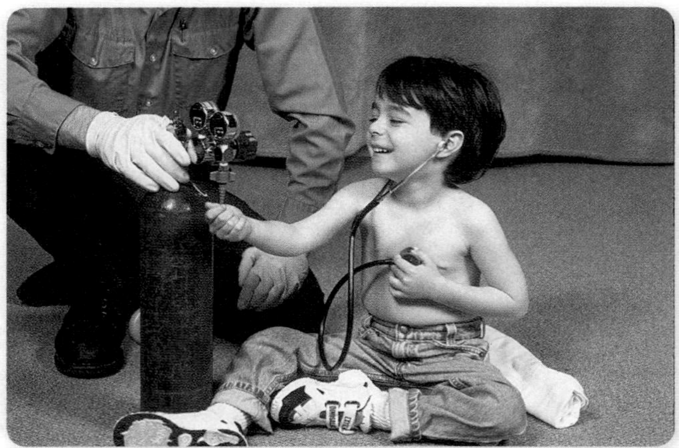

Figure 36-4 School-age children are more like adults in that they can answer your questions and help take care of themselves.

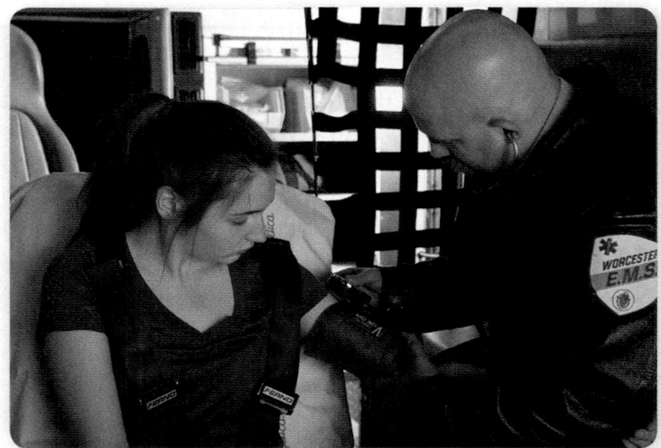

Figure 36-5 Respect the adolescent's privacy at all times; give the patient whatever information he or she requests.

School is important at this stage, and concerns about popularity and peer pressure occupy a great deal of time and energy.

Assessment of the School-Age Child

Your assessment begins to be more like an adult assessment; talk to the child, not just the parent or caregiver, while taking the medical history. This will help you gain the patient's trust. At this stage, the child is probably familiar with the process of a physical examination. This may make your job easier or more difficult, depending on whether the child's prior health care experiences have been positive or negative. Begin your assessment at the head and move toward the feet, similar to assessing an adult.

School-age children can understand the difference between emotional and physical pain. They also have concerns about the meaning of pain. Give them simple explanations about what is causing their pain and what will be done about it. Give the child appropriate choices and control whenever possible, and provide ongoing reassurance and encouragement. Respect the patient's modesty and keep them covered as much as possible during your examination. Games and conversation may distract these patients. Asking about school will often allow them to warm up to you. Ask them to describe their favorite place, their pets, or their toys. Ask the caregiver's advice in choosing the right distraction. Rewarding the school-age child after a procedure can be helpful in his or her recovery, but only reward a child for completing the procedure.

▶ The Adolescent

Adolescents are ages 12 to 18 years. They can think abstractly, participate in decision making, and discriminate between what is right and wrong. The adolescent years are when puberty begins and can be difficult. Adolescents are struggling with issues of independence, body image, sexuality, and peer pressure. Although adolescents are still children on an emotional level, this is a time of experimentation and risk-taking behaviors.

Assessment of the Adolescent

The adolescent child should be treated as an adult. During the assessment, you must address the patient. Failure to do so can result in the adolescent feeling left out of his or her own care, thus resulting in you possibly alienating the patient and making it difficult for you to get an accurate assessment or give appropriate treatment. Encourage the patient's questions and involvement. Also, provide accurate information—a teen may become alienated and uncooperative if you are suspected of misleading him or her. Address concerns and fears about the lasting effects of their injuries—especially cosmetic—and reassure them when possible. When communicating, find out what they are interested in, such as sports, books, movies, or friends, and get them talking about this.

When you perform the physical examination, respect the patient's privacy and modesty (Figure 36-5). If possible, address the adolescent without a caregiver present, especially about sensitive topics such as sexuality, self-endangerment, possible pregnancy, or drug use. Assess his or her level of pain by observing facial and body expressions as well as by asking questions. If the adolescent's friends are on scene, he or she may want them to remain during the assessment. Let the patient have as much control over the situation as is appropriate. Of course, do not let down your guard regarding scene safety.

Anatomy, Physiology, and Pathophysiology

There is no other time in our lives that our bodies are growing and changing as fast as during childhood. Newborns quickly change once outside the mother's body. Toddlers learn to walk and talk. School-age children explore the world without thought of consequences.

The anatomic and physiologic changes and differences can create difficulties with your assessment of the child if you do not understand them. You need to alter your patient care accordingly.

▶ The Respiratory System

To manage the pediatric airway effectively, you must have a thorough understanding of the anatomic and physiologic difference in the child's airway.

A child's airway is smaller in diameter and shorter in length. The tongue is proportionally larger relative to the size of the mouth and is in a more anterior location in the mouth. The child's tongue also takes up more room in the oropharynx and can easily block the airway. A child's epiglottis is a floppy, narrow, U-shaped structure that is larger than an adult's, relative to the size of the airway, and it extends at a 45° angle into the airway. The larynx is higher (at the C3 to C4 level) and is more anterior. In relation to the adult, whose airway is narrowest at the level of the vocal cords, the narrowest portion of the child's airway is at the level of the cricoid cartilage.

The opening to the trachea (glottic opening) is higher (more superior) in the neck and more anterior than in adults, the trachea is smaller in diameter, and the neck and trachea are shorter. Because of the smaller diameter of the trachea in infants, which is about the same diameter as a drinking straw, their airway is easily obstructed by secretions, blood, and swelling. The trachea, which is likened to a piece of corrugated tubing, is easily collapsible in children; therefore, when they experience respiratory distress, the trachea tends to draw into the neck; this is called **tracheal tugging**.

Figure 36-6 illustrates the major differences between pediatric and adult airways.

Infants have little use of their chest muscles to make their chests expand during inspiration; they use the diaphragm (making them belly breathers). Anything that puts pressure on the abdomen of an infant or young child can block the movement of the diaphragm and cause respiratory compromise. Young children also experience muscle fatigue much more quickly than older children, which can lead to respiratory failure if a child has had to breathe hard for long periods.

The tissues of the lungs are more fragile in a child, and the ribs are more cartilaginous, making them softer and more pliable. In addition, less overlying muscle and fat exist to protect the ribs and vital organs.

Substantial compression injuries to the chest may injure vital intrathoracic organs (such as the heart, lungs, great vessels), often without obvious signs of external injury. When assessing a sick or injured child, expect the ribs to be positioned horizontally. Rib fractures occur less frequently in children but are not uncommon following trauma or abuse.

The fragile **parenchyma** of the child's lungs makes them susceptible to barotrauma (pressure trauma), such as a pneumothorax, as the result of injury or overzealous ventilation. The respiratory muscles in a child are more immature and fatigue more quickly than an adult's; therefore, the child tends to tire more easily as a result of respiratory distress. In addition, because of the thin wall of the child's chest, breath sounds are easily transmitted to all areas of the chest, making it difficult when assessing for a chest injury (such as pneumothorax) or for correct placement of an advanced airway device.

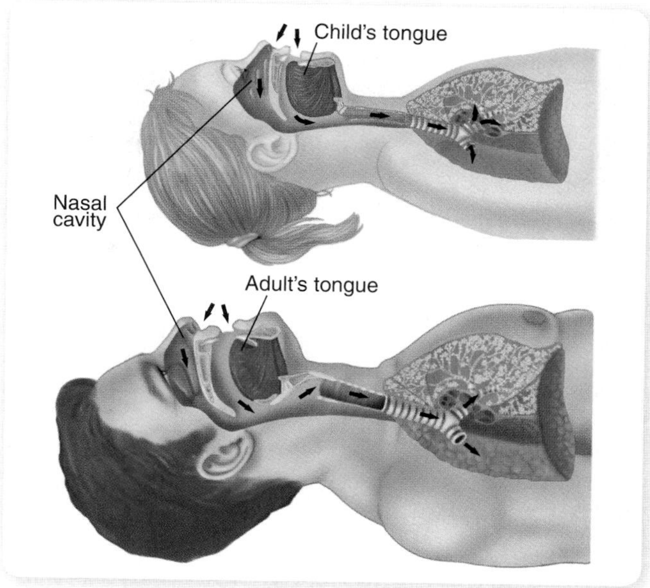

Figure 36-6 The anatomy of a child's airway differs from that of an adult's in several ways. The back of the head is larger in a child. The tongue is proportionally larger and is located more anteriorly in the mouth. The trachea is smaller in diameter and more flexible. The airway itself is lower and narrower (funnel-shaped).

The child's **mediastinum** is more mobile than an adult's. Therefore, you may see a more pronounced mediastinal shift as the result of a tension pneumothorax.

Words of Wisdom

The pediatric patient's ribs and sternum are much more pliable than those of an adult; therefore, you should expect more injuries from blunt trauma to the underlying organs and structures.

Proportionally, tidal volume in children is similar to that in adolescents and adults; however, their metabolic oxygen demand is doubled. In addition, their **functional residual capacity** is smaller, resulting in proportionally smaller oxygen reserves.

An infant needs to breathe faster than an older child **Table 36-1**. The child's lungs will grow and develop better abilities to handle the exchange of oxygen as the child ages. A respiratory rate of 30 to 60 breaths/min is

Table 36-1 Pediatric Respiratory Rates

Age	Respirations (breaths/min)
Neonate (0 to 1 month)	30 to 60
Infant (1 month to 1 year)	30 to 53
Toddler (1 to 2 years)	22 to 37
Preschool age (3 to 5 years)	20 to 28
School age (6 to 12 years)	18 to 25
Adolescent (12 to 15 years)	12 to 20

Data from: American Heart Association (AHA). Vital signs in children. In: AHA. *Pediatric Advanced Life Support*. Dallas, TX: AHA; 2015.

Table 36-2 Responsive Pediatric Pulse Rates

Age	Pulse Rate (beats/min)
Neonate (0 to 1 month)	Awake: 100 to 205 Asleep: 90 to 160
Infant (1 month to 1 year)	Awake: 100 to 180 Asleep: 90 to 160
Toddler (1 to 2 years)	Awake: 98 to 140 Asleep: 80 to 120
Preschool age (3 to 5 years)	Awake: 80 to 120 Asleep: 65 to 100
School age (6 to 12 years)	Awake: 75 to 118 Asleep: 58 to 90
Adolescent (12 to 15 years)	Awake: 60 to 100 Asleep: 50 to 90

Data from: American Heart Association (AHA). Vital signs in children. In: AHA. *Pediatric Advanced Life Support*. Dallas, TX: AHA; 2015.

normal for newborns, whereas teenagers are expected to have rates closer to the adult range (12 to 20 breaths/min). Breathing also requires the use of the chest muscles and the diaphragm.

Infants suck air in when they cry. Gastric distention, a more common and significant complication in pediatric patients, can interfere with movement of the diaphragm, resulting in hypoventilation and increased risk of regurgitation with aspiration.

Until the age of approximately 4 to 6 months, infants breathe through their nose. If the nasal passages are blocked by secretions, they may not have the intuition to open their mouths to breathe.

With the aforementioned anatomic differences, it is important for you to remember the following:

- Keep the **nares** clear in infants younger than 6 months.
- Avoid hyperextension of the child's neck; this may result in reverse hyperflexion and kinking of the trachea and may also displace the tongue posteriorly, creating an airway obstruction.
- Keep the airway clear of all secretions; even a small amount of particulate matter may result in an airway obstruction.
- Use care when managing the child's airway, such as when inserting airway adjuncts; the soft tissues are delicate and susceptible to swelling. In many cases, the child's airway can be maintained by correct positioning, thereby negating the use of airway adjuncts (that is, oral or nasal airways).

You must be aware that infants and children, especially during respiratory distress, are highly susceptible to hypoxia because of their decreased oxygen reserves, increased oxygen demand, and easily fatigued respiratory muscles. Use a larger bag if needed to ventilate a pediatric patient, but use only enough pressure to achieve visible chest rise.

▶ Cardiovascular System

It is important to know the normal pulse ranges when evaluating children (Table 36-2). Children rely mainly on their heart rate to maintain adequate cardiac output. An infant's heart rate (normally, 90 to 180 beat/min) can be 200 beats/min or more if the body needs to compensate for injury or illness. Because this is the primary method for the child's body to compensate for decreased oxygenation, you must be aware of the normal heart rate ranges when evaluating children.

Children have limited but vigorous cardiac reserves. Proportionally, they have a larger circulating blood volume compared with adults; however, their absolute blood volume is less, approximately 70 mL/kg. The ability of a child to constrict blood vessels (vasoconstriction) provides the ability to keep vital organs well perfused.

Because a child's circulating blood volume is large compared with an adult's, injured children can maintain their blood pressure for longer periods than adults, even though they are still in shock (hypoperfusion). In other words, a proportionally larger volume of blood loss must occur in the child before hypotension develops.

Suspect shock when an infant or child presents with tachycardia. **Bradycardia**, however, usually indicates severe hypoxia and must be managed aggressively. Remember that hypotension, when it occurs in a child, is an ominous sign and often indicates impending cardiopulmonary arrest.

Constriction of the blood vessels can be so profound that blood flow to the periphery of the body diminishes.

Signs of vasoconstriction can include weak peripheral (radial or pedal) pulses in the extremities, delayed capillary refill (in children younger than 6 years), and pale, cool extremities.

> **Words of Wisdom**
>
> When you are assessing a sick or injured child, be aware that bradycardia is most often the result of hypoxia; therefore, treatment is aimed at ensuring adequate oxygenation and ventilation. In addition, despite the presence of a normal blood pressure, a child, even more so than an adult, may still be in shock.

▶ The Nervous System

The nervous system develops continuously throughout childhood. The brain and spinal cord are not as well protected by the developing skull and spinal vertebrae as in adults.

Until the nervous system is fully developed, the neural tissue and vasculature are extremely fragile, easily damaged, and susceptible to bleeding from injury. Because the brain and spinal cord are less well protected than in adults, it takes less force to cause brain and spinal cord injuries in children.

Brain injuries in young children, when they occur, are frequently more devastating.

The subarachnoid space in a child is relatively smaller than that seen in an adult, providing less cushioning effect for the brain. Bruising and damage to the brain may be the result of head momentum such as that seen in "shaken baby syndrome." The pediatric brain also requires nearly twice the cerebral blood flow as the adult brain, making even minor injuries significant. This requirement increases the risk of hypoxia. Head injuries are greatly exacerbated by hypoxia and hypotension, causing ongoing damage.

Spinal cord injuries are less common in pediatric patients; however, injury to the spinal cord may occur without injury to the spinal column itself. Cervical spine injuries are more commonly ligamentous injuries.

▶ Musculoskeletal System

Bones in children are softer and more porous until adolescence. A child's softer bones make incomplete fractures (**greenstick fractures**) more likely in this population. Treat any sprain or strain as though a fracture exists, and immobilize the injury accordingly.

Injury to the **epiphyseal plate** (growth plate or physis) of the bone during its development, or inadvertent puncture of the growth plate during intraosseous (IO) cannulation (discussed later), may result in abnormalities in normal bone growth and development.

The child's head, specifically the **occiput**, is proportionally larger than an adult's. During infancy, the anterior and posterior **fontanelles** are open. The fontanelles are areas where the infant's skull bones have not fused together, thus allowing for compression of the head during the birthing process and for rapid growth of the brain. By the time the child reaches the age of approximately 18 months, both of the fontanelles have closed.

Because of their proportionally larger heads, infants and children are especially susceptible to head trauma, such as during a fall, in which gravity takes them headfirst. Infants may also experience excessive heat loss as a result of the larger size of the head.

Because of the proportionally larger occiput, special care must be taken when you are positioning the child's airway. In seriously injured children younger than 3 years, place a layer of padding under the shoulders and/or upper back to obtain a neutral position. In seriously ill children younger than 3 years, place a thin layer of padding under the occiput and a thicker layer of padding under the shoulders and/or upper back to obtain a **sniffing position**.[3]

The fontanelles are an important anatomic landmark when you are assessing a sick or injured infant. Bulging of the fontanelles suggests increased intracranial pressure; sunken fontanelles suggest dehydration. These conditions are discussed later in this chapter.

> **Words of Wisdom**
>
> Always assess the fontanelles in the infant:
>
> - Bulging = increased intracranial pressure
> - Sunken = dehydration

▶ The Gastrointestinal System

The abdominal musculature in the child is immature and provides less protection to solid, vascular organs such as the spleen and liver, both of which are proportionally larger and more vascular in children. In addition, the abdominal organs are closer to one another.

For these reasons, pediatric patients are at higher risk for splenic and hepatic injuries than adults; even seemingly insignificant forces can cause serious internal injury. Multiple organ injuries are more common.

▶ The Integumentary System

In comparison with adults, infants and children have thinner and more elastic skin, a larger body surface area-to-body mass ratio, and less subcutaneous (fatty) tissue.

The above factors contribute to the following:

- Increased risk of injury following exposure to temperature extremes
- Increased risk of hypothermia (can complicate resuscitative efforts) and dehydration
- Increased severity of burns
  - Many burns that would ordinarily be classified as minor or moderate in adults are classified as severe in children.

Special Populations

Because of their thinner skin and proportionally larger body surface area-to-body mass ratio, burns are more severe in a child and thus are a leading cause of death in the pediatric age group.

▶ Metabolic Differences

Infants and children have limited stores of glycogen and glucose, which are rapidly depleted as a result of injury or illness. Because it takes glucose to produce energy and energy is required to maintain body temperature, infants and children are highly susceptible to hypothermia. The risk of hypothermia is further increased because of the child's larger body surface area-to-body mass ratio. When you are assessing and treating a newborn (neonate), you must remain aware that these young infants lack the ability to shiver—one of the body's ways of producing heat.

Significant hypovolemia and electrolyte derangements are also more common in children as a result of severe vomiting and diarrhea.

It is critical to keep the child warm during transport and take measures to prevent the loss of body heat. To conserve body heat, be sure to cover the child's head, which because of its proportionally large size, is a source of substantial heat loss. However, newborns should not be overwarmed because this can worsen their neurologic outcomes.

Pediatric Assessment

As mentioned previously, young children will not be able to provide you with information needed to make treatment decisions (such as medical history, medications). Furthermore, children often cannot tell you where they hurt. Therefore, you must rely on a parent or caregiver to obtain as much information as you can.

Scene Size-up

Each child and situation is unique; therefore, you may have to modify your assessment of the child based on his or her age. Ensure that you have age-appropriate equipment and review age-appropriate vital signs in anticipation of potential developments. In general, however, you should follow the same general approach to patient assessment for children as you do for adults.

On the way to the scene, prepare for a pediatric scene size-up, pediatric equipment, and the age-appropriate physical assessment. If possible, collect information from dispatch such as the age and sex of the child, the location of the scene, the nature of illness, the mechanism of injury (MOI), and the chief complaint.

As with any EMS call, the scene size-up begins by ensuring that you and your partner have taken the appropriate standard precautions. On arriving at the scene, observe for any hazards or potential hazards that may pose a threat to you, your partner, or the patient. Resist the temptation to hastily approach the patient because you know it is a child. Personal safety must always remain your priority.

YOU are the Provider — PART 2

Using the PAT, you note the child's appearance to be poor, the work of breathing is substantially decreased, and circulation to the skin is poor based on the finding of cyanosis. Recognizing that this patient is on the verge of respiratory failure, you instruct your partner to insert an appropriate-size oropharyngeal airway and begin bag-mask ventilations with a child-size bag-mask device. After effective assisted ventilations have been established, you quickly place the patient onto the stretcher and into the back of the ambulance. You instruct the mother to sit in the front passenger seat for the transport.

Recording Time: 1 Minute	
Appearance	Poor
Level of consciousness	Unresponsive
Airway	Open with oropharyngeal airway
Breathing	4 breaths/min, assisted
Circulation	Cool, clammy, cyanotic

3. What is the purpose of the PAT, and what does it assess?
4. When should an oropharyngeal airway be inserted in a pediatric patient, and how is it measured?

> **Special Populations**
>
> Sick or injured children should not be separated from their parents or caregivers unless aggressive resuscitation is needed. The stress produced by separation anxiety can worsen a sick child's condition. If you need to separate the parents or caregiver and child, try to leave them within eyesight and talking distance of one another to minimize the stress of the situation.

At a traumatic scene, when the child is unable to communicate because of his or her developmental age or is unresponsive, and caregivers are not present to provide information, assume that the MOI was significant enough to cause head or neck injuries. You must not discount the possibility of child abuse. Conflicting information from the parents or caregivers, bruises or other injuries that are not consistent with the MOI described, or injuries that are not consistent with the child's age and developmental abilities should increase your index of suspicion for abuse. Observe and note the parents' or caregivers' interaction with the child. Do they appear to be appropriately concerned, angry, or indifferent? Does the child seem comforted by their presence or scared by them? Child abuse will be discussed in greater detail later in this chapter.

Primary Survey

As with the adult population, the objective of the primary survey is to identify and treat immediate or potential life threats. Perform cervical spine immobilization if the MOI is severe. Remember the need to pad under the pediatric patient's head and/or shoulder to facilitate a neutral position for airway management. Always follow local protocols.

When assessing a pediatric patient, use the PAT to form a general impression.

Pediatric Assessment Triangle

The PAT is a structured assessment tool that allows you to rapidly form a general impression of the infant's or child's condition without touching him or her. This 15- to 30-second assessment is conducted prior to the assessment of airway, breathing, circulation, disability, and exposure (ABCDEs), discussed next, and does not require touching the patient. Its intent is to provide a "first glance" assessment to identify the general category of the child's physiologic problem and to establish urgency for treatment and/or transport **Table 36-3**.

The PAT consists of three elements: appearance (muscle tone and mental status), work of breathing, and circulation to the skin **Figure 36-7**. The only equipment required for the PAT are your own eyes and ears; it does not require a stethoscope, blood pressure cuff, cardiac monitor, or pulse oximeter.

Table 36-3 Possible Physiologic States Found Using the Pediatric Assessment Triangle

- Respiratory distress
- Respiratory failure
- Cardiovascular shock
- Cardiopulmonary failure or arrest
- Isolated head injury
- Ingestion
- Other primary central nervous system abnormality
- Stable patient

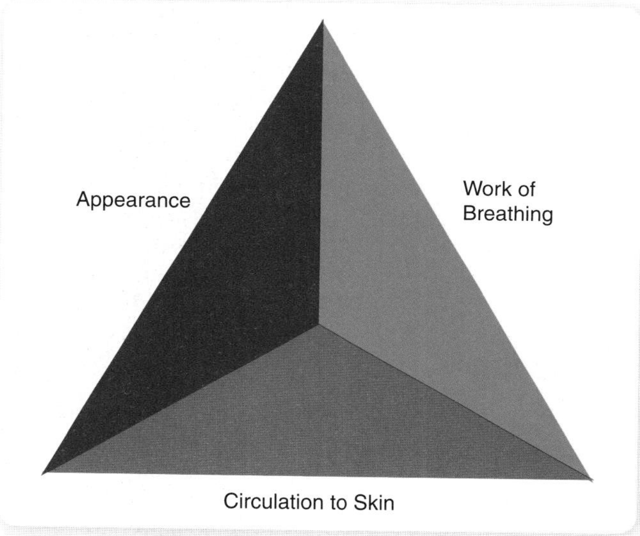

Figure 36-7 The three components of the pediatric assessment triangle include appearance, work of breathing, and circulation to the skin.

Appearance

The first element of the PAT is the child's appearance. In many cases, this is the most important factor in determining the severity of illness, the need for treatment, and the response to therapy. Appearance reflects the adequacy of ventilation, oxygenation, brain perfusion, body homeostasis, and central nervous system function. The TICLS (pronounced "tickles") mnemonic highlights the most important features of a child's appearance: Tone, Interactiveness, Consolability, Look or gaze, and Speech or cry **Table 36-4**.

To assess appearance, observe the child from a distance, allowing the child to interact with the caregiver as he or she chooses. Delay touching the patient until you have developed your general impression because the child may become agitated by your touch. Unless a child is

Table 36-4 Characteristics of Appearance: The TICLS Mnemonic

Characteristics	Features to Look For
Tone	Is the child moving or resisting examination vigorously? Does the child have good muscle tone? Or is the child limp, listless, or flaccid?
Interactiveness	How alert is the child? How readily does a person, object, or sound distract the child or draw the child's attention? Will the child reach for, grasp, and play with a toy or exam instrument, like a penlight or tongue blade? Or is the child uninterested in playing or interacting with the caregiver or AEMT?
Consolability	Can the child be consoled or comforted by the caregiver or the AEMT? Or is the child's crying or agitation unrelieved by gentle reassurance?
Look or gaze	Does the child fix his or her gaze on a face, or is there a "nobody home," glassy-eyed stare?
Speech or cry	Is the child's cry strong and spontaneous or weak or high-pitched? Is the content of speech age-appropriate or confused or garbled?

Modified from American Academy of Pediatrics. Pediatric assessment. In: Fuchs S, Klein BL, eds. *Pediatric Education for Prehospital Professionals*. Rev 3rd ed. Burlington, MA: Jones & Bartlett Learning; 2016:6.

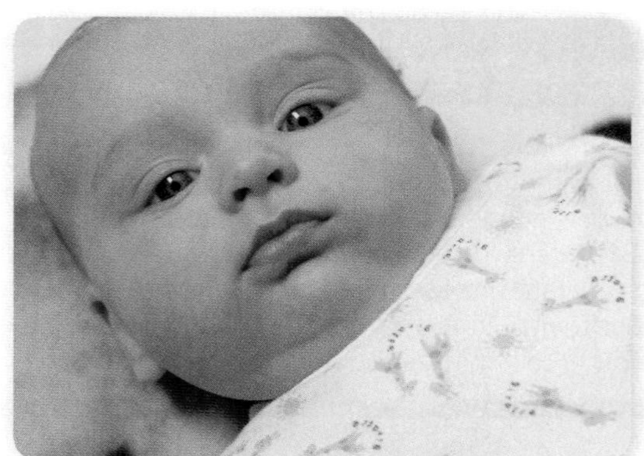

Figure 36-8 An infant or child making good eye contact is most likely not critically ill.

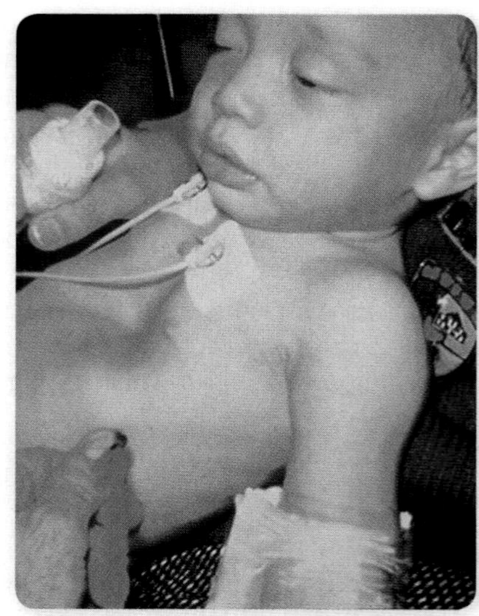

Figure 36-9 A limp child who is unable to maintain eye contact may be critically ill or injured.

Courtesy Health Resources and Services Administration, Maternal and Child Health Bureau, Emergency Medical Services for Children Program.

unresponsive or critically ill, take your time in assessing his or her general appearance by observation before you begin the hands-on assessment and obtain vital signs.

An infant or child with a normal level of consciousness will act appropriately for his or her age, exhibiting good muscle tone and maintaining good eye contact Figure 36-8. An abnormal level of consciousness is characterized by age-inappropriate behavior or interactiveness, poor muscle tone, or poor eye contact with the caregiver or with you Figure 36-9.

Work of Breathing

Observing a child's work of breathing often provides a better assessment of his or her oxygenation and ventilation status than using auscultation or assessing the respiratory rate. The work of breathing reflects the child's attempt to compensate for abnormalities in oxygenation and ventilation and is therefore a good measure for effectiveness of gas exchange. The hands-off assessment of work of breathing includes listening for abnormal airway sounds and looking for signs of increased breathing effort Table 36-5.

> **Words of Wisdom**
>
> Identifying an abnormal appearance by using the PAT is a more effective way for you to detect subtle changes in a child's level of consciousness than by using the AVPU scale (Awake and alert, responsive to Verbal stimuli, responsive to Pain, Unresponsive). Many children with mild to moderate illness or injury are "alert" on the AVPU scale, although they may have an abnormal appearance.

Table 36-5 Characteristics of Work of Breathing

Characteristic	Features to Look For
Abnormal airway sounds	Snoring, muffled or hoarse speech, stridor, grunting, or wheezing
Abnormal posturing	Sniffing position, tripod position, refusing to lie down
Accessory muscle use	Retractions of the muscles above the clavicles (supraclavicular)
Retractions	Drawing in of the muscles between the ribs (intercostal retractions) or of the sternum (substernal retractions) during inspiration
Head bobbing	The head lifts and tilts back during inspiration, then moves forward during expiration
Nasal flaring	The nares widen; usually seen during inspiration
Tachypnea	Increased respiratory rate

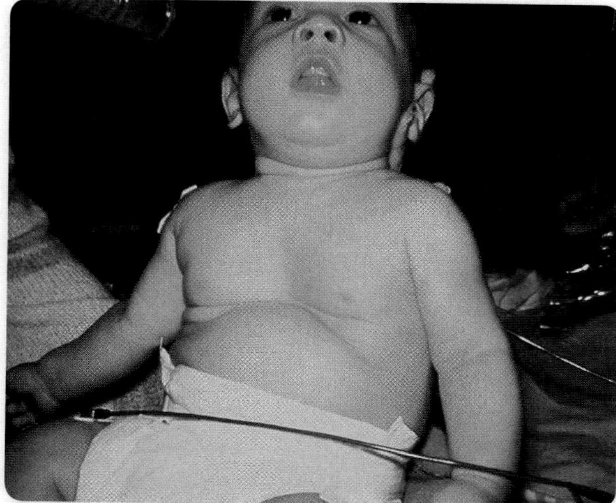

Figure 36-10 Retractions of the intercostal muscles or sternum indicate increased work of breathing.

Courtesy of Health Resources and Services Administration, Maternal and Child Health Bureau, Emergency Medical Service for Children Program.

Increased work of breathing often manifests as **tachypnea**, abnormal airway noise (**grunting** or wheezing), retractions of the intercostal muscles or sternum **Figure 36-10**, or the way the pediatric patient positions himself or herself.

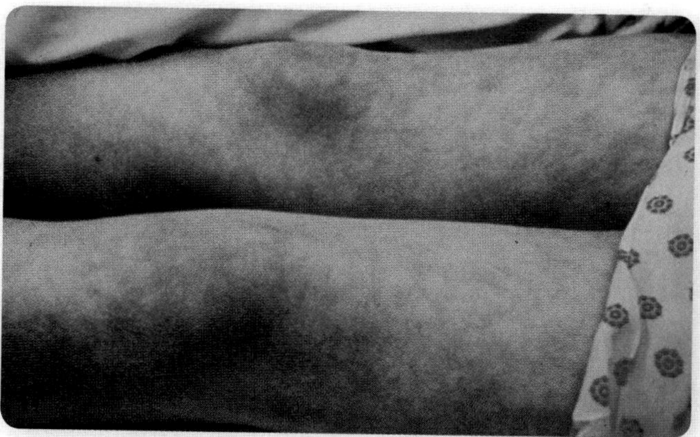

Figure 36-11 Mottling of the skin indicates poor perfusion and is the result of constriction of peripheral blood vessels.

Courtesy of Health Resources and Services Administration, Maternal and Child Health Bureau, Emergency Medical Service for Children Program.

Circulation to the Skin

The goal of rapid circulatory assessment is to determine the adequacy of cardiac output and core perfusion. When cardiac output diminishes, the body responds by shunting circulation from nonessential areas (eg, skin) toward vital organs. Therefore, circulation to the skin reflects the overall status of core circulation. The three characteristics considered when assessing the circulation are pallor, mottling, and cyanosis.

Pallor of the skin and mucous membranes may be the initial sign of poor circulation or even the only visual sign in a child with compensated shock. It indicates reflex peripheral vasoconstriction that is shunting blood toward the core. Pallor may also indicate anemia or hypoxia. Mottling is caused by constriction of peripheral blood vessels and is another sign of poor perfusion **Figure 36-11**.

Cyanosis, a bluish discoloration of the skin and mucous membranes, is the most extreme visual indicator of poor perfusion or poor oxygenation. **Acrocyanosis**, blue hands or feet in an infant younger than 2 months, is distinct from cyanosis; it is a normal finding when a young infant is cold. True cyanosis is seen in the skin and mucous membranes and is a late finding of respiratory failure or shock. *Never wait for the development of cyanosis before administering oxygen!*

Stay or Go

On the basis of the findings of the PAT, you will decide if the pediatric patient is stable or requires urgent care. If the pediatric patient is unstable, assess ABCDEs, treat any life threats, and transport the pediatric patient immediately to an appropriate facility. If the pediatric patient is stable, then you have time to continue with the remainder of the patient assessment process.

Hands-On ABCDEs

After forming your general impression of the child's condition using the PAT, perform a hands-on assessment of the child's vital functions—ABCDEs (airway, breathing, circulation, disability, and exposure)—and treat any immediate or potential threats to life. If you suspect this is a cardiac arrest, which is rare, the order is CABDE because chest compressions would be the priority. As previously discussed, your assessment of the child may require modification based on his or her age, but the overall assessment flow is essentially the same as it is for adults.

Words of Wisdom

You should use caution when opening the airway of a pediatric patient using the head tilt–chin lift maneuver. You can overextend the neck and actually close off the trachea.

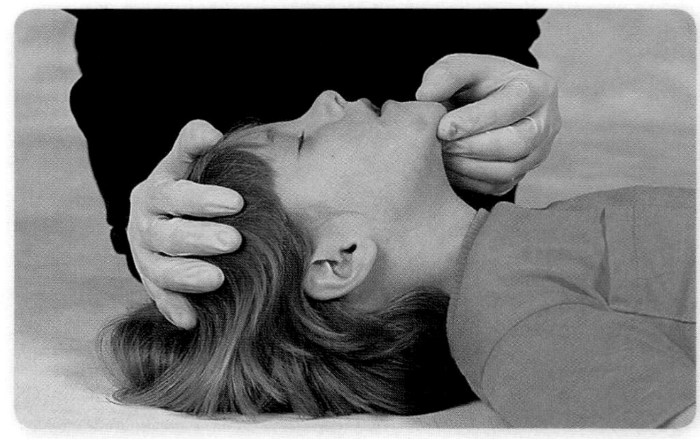

Figure 36-12 Use the head tilt–chin lift maneuver to open the airway of a pediatric patient without trauma.

Airway

If the infant or child is responsive and the airway is open, you can proceed with assessment of respiratory adequacy. However, if the child is unresponsive or has difficulty keeping the airway clear, you must ensure that the airway is properly positioned and that it is clear of mucus, vomitus, blood, and foreign bodies.

If trauma has been ruled out, open the child's airway with the head tilt–chin lift maneuver Figure 36-12. If the child has been involved in trauma or trauma is suspected, use the jaw-thrust maneuver to open the airway Figure 36-13.

Follow these steps to position the airway in a pediatric patient without trauma Skill Drill 36-1.

After the child's airway has been opened, ensure that it is clear of potential obstructions (such as mucus, blood,

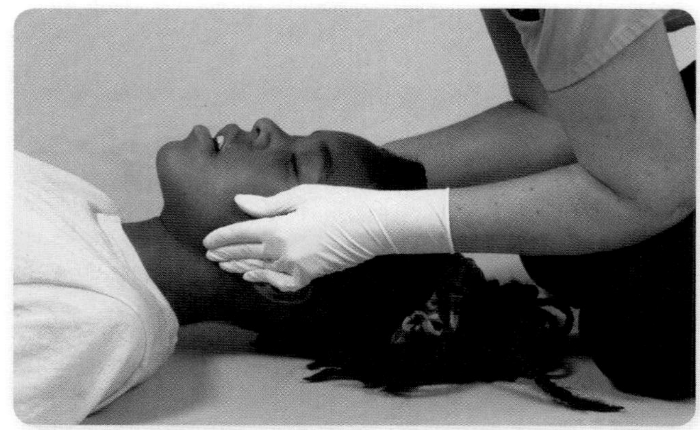

Figure 36-13 Use the jaw-thrust maneuver to open the airway in a pediatric patient with possible spinal injury.

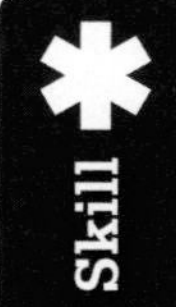

NR Skill

Skill Drill 36-1 Positioning the Airway in a Pediatric Patient

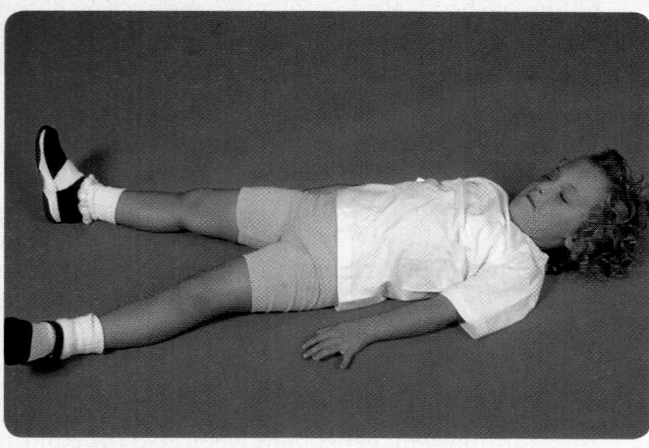

Step 1 Place the pediatric patient on a firm surface such as the ground or a short backboard or pediatric immobilization device.

Skill Drill 36-1 Positioning the Airway in a Pediatric Patient *(continued)*

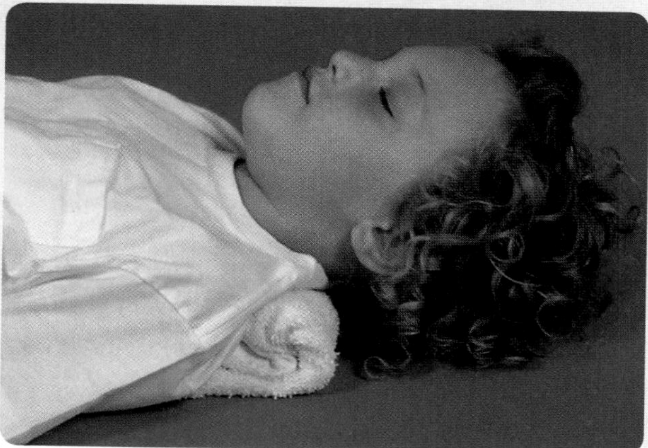

Step 2 Fold a small towel, about 1 inch (2.5 cm) thick, and place it under the pediatric patient's shoulders and back.

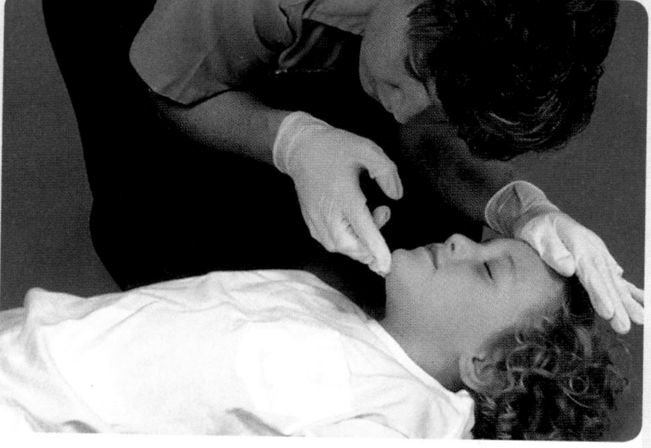

Step 3 Stabilize the forehead to limit movement of the head during transport. Use the head tilt–chin lift maneuver to open the airway.

and foreign bodies). Next, establish whether the child can maintain his or her own airway spontaneously (without the use of airway adjuncts) or whether adjuncts will be necessary to maintain airway patency. Techniques of airway management will be discussed later in this chapter.

Breathing

The breathing component of the primary survey involves calculating the respiratory rate, auscultating breath sounds, and checking pulse oximetry for oxygen saturation. Assess the child's breathing by noting the degree of air movement at the nose and mouth and determining whether the chest is rising adequately and symmetrically. Assess the respiratory rate and effort with which the pediatric patient is breathing as well.

Place both hands on the pediatric patient's chest to feel for the rise and fall of the chest wall. You will be able to count the actual respiratory rate and assess for symmetry. This assessment maneuver is especially helpful when your pediatric patient requires assisted ventilations with a bag-mask device. In infants, belly breathing is considered adequate because of the soft pliable bones of the chest and the strong muscular diaphragm.

If the child is responsive and not in need of immediate intervention (such as suctioning or assisted ventilation), assessing respirations is usually easier with the child sitting on the parent or caregiver's lap. Listen for abnormal respiratory sounds and note any signs of increased respiratory effort.

As the child begins to tire, retractions often become weak and ineffective and the accessory muscles become less prominent during breathing. **Bradypnea**, a decrease in the respiratory rate, is an ominous sign and indicates impending respiratory arrest. Do not mistake bradypnea for a sign of improvement; it usually indicates that the child's condition has deteriorated. Therefore, you must be prepared to begin ventilatory assistance.

Circulation

When you are assessing circulation, you must first control any active bleeding. Remember, infants and children can tolerate only small amounts of blood loss before circulatory compromise occurs. Also assess the pulse rate and quality, skin (color, temperature, moisture), **capillary refill time**, and blood pressure.

Pulses may be difficult to palpate if they are weak, extremely fast, or extremely slow. In infants, palpate the brachial pulse or femoral pulse. In children older than 1 year, palpate the carotid pulse Figure 36-14. Note the rate and quality of the pulse: Is it weak or strong? Is it normal, slow, or fast? Strong **central pulses** usually indicate that the child is not hypotensive; however, this does not rule out the possibility of compensated shock. Weak or absent peripheral pulses indicate decreased perfusion. Weak central pulses indicate significant hypotension and decompensated shock. The absence of a central pulse (that is, brachial or femoral in infants, carotid in older children) indicates the immediate need for cardiopulmonary resuscitation (CPR).

Tachycardia may be an early sign of hypoxia or shock, but it may also reflect less serious conditions such as fever, anxiety, pain, and excitement. Like respiratory rate and

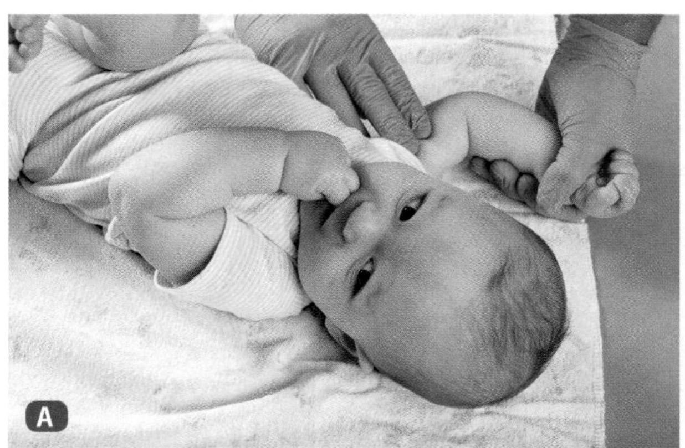

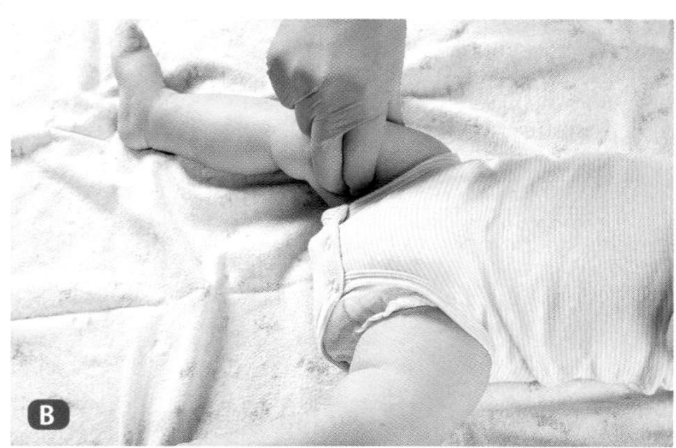

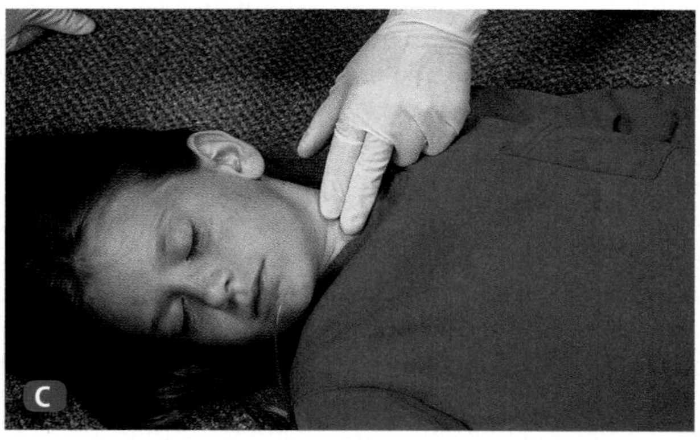

Figure 36-14 A. Palpate the brachial pulse in infants.
B. Palpate the femoral pulse as a second choice.
C. In children older than 1 year, palpate the carotid pulse.

effort, the heart rate should be interpreted within the context of the overall history, PAT, and entire primary survey.

A trend of an increasing or decreasing heart rate may be quite useful information and may suggest worsening hypoxia or shock or improvement after treatment. When hypoxia or shock becomes critical, bradycardia occurs. As with slowing respirations, bradycardia in a child is an ominous sign and often indicates impending cardiopulmonary arrest.

Feel the skin for temperature and moisture while you assess the child's pulse. Is the skin warm and dry or cold

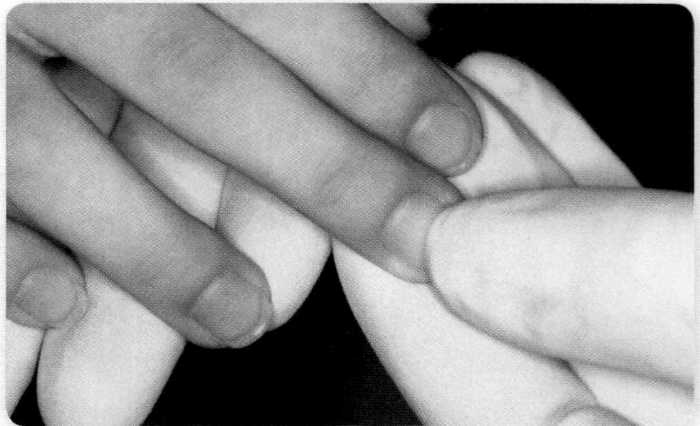

Figure 36-15 Estimate the capillary refill time by squeezing the end of a finger or toe for several seconds until the nail bed blanches. Normal color should return within 2 seconds after you let go.

and clammy? Estimate the capillary refill time by squeezing the end of a finger or toe for several seconds and then observing the return of blood to the area **Figure 36-15**. Color should return within 2 seconds after you let go. The capillary refill time is used to assess **end-organ perfusion**. It is most reliable in children younger than 6 years; however, factors such as cold temperatures may affect the capillary refill time.

Special Populations

Blood pressure is just one component of the overall assessment of pediatric patients. Determination of physiologic stability should be based on all data collected from the PAT, physical examination, and initial vital signs. Remember that compensated shock can exist in the face of adequate blood pressure.

Disability

The assessment of the pediatric patient's level of consciousness can be done using the AVPU scale or the Pediatric Glasgow Coma Scale **Table 36-6**.

Words of Wisdom

You should carry an EMS field guide or place a copy of the modified Glasgow Coma Scale on the wall of the ambulance or in the trauma kit to help you remember how to calculate this difficult formula.

Check the responses of each pupil to a direct beam of light. A normal pupil constricts after a light stimulus. Pupillary response may be abnormal in the presence of

Table 36-6 Pediatric Glasgow Coma Scale

Activity	Score	Infant	Score	Child
Eye opening	4	Open spontaneously	4	Open spontaneously
	3	Open to sound	3	Open to sound
	2	Open to pressure	2	Open to pressure
	1	No response	1	No response
Verbal	5	Coos, babbles	5	Oriented conversation
	4	Irritable cry	4	Confused conversation
	3	Cries	3	Cries
	2	Moans	2	Moans
	1	No response	1	No response
Motor	6	Normal spontaneous movement	6	Obeys verbal commands
	5	Localizes pain or pressure	5	Localizes pain or pressure
	4	Normal flexion	4	Normal flexion
	3	Abnormal flexion	3	Abnormal flexion
	2	Extension	2	Extension
	1	No response	1	No response

Modified from: Davis RJ, et al. Head and spinal cord injury. In: Rogers MC, ed. *Textbook of Pediatric Intensive Care*. Baltimore, MD: Williams & Wilkins; 1987; James H, Anas N, Perkin RM. *Brain Insults in Infants and Children*. New York, NY: Grune & Stratton; 1985; and Morray JP, Tyler DC, Jones TK, et al. Coma scale for use in brain-injured children. *Critical Care Medicine*. 1984;12:1018.

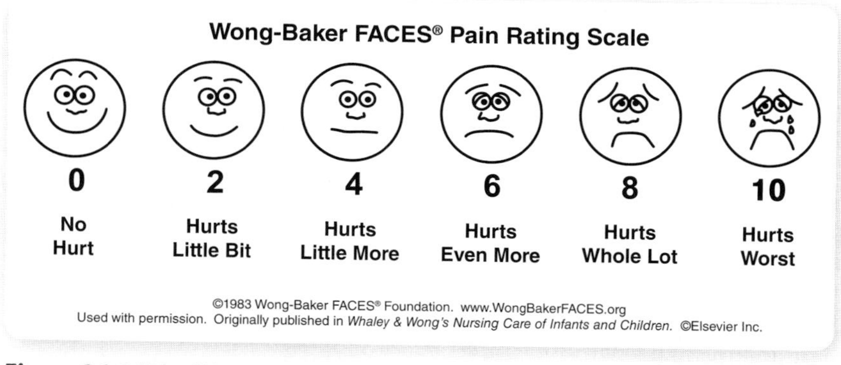

Figure 36-16 The Wong-Baker FACES scale.

drugs, ongoing seizures, hypoxia, or brain injury. Note if the pupils are dilated, constricted, reactive, or fixed.

Next, look for symmetric movement of the extremities and note any neurologic motor deficit such as the inability to move the upper or lower extremities, an inability to communicate, weakness, or difficulty walking (gait).

Pain is present with most types of injury and many illnesses. Inadequate treatment of pain has many adverse effects on the pediatric patient and the family. Pain causes significant morbidity and misery for pediatric patients and caregivers and interferes with assessment.

Assessment of pain must take into consideration the developmental age of the patient. The ability to recognize pain will improve as patients become older. For example, crying and agitation in an infant may be the result of hunger or a dirty diaper. Meanwhile, a 3-year-old child can use words to say, "My tummy really hurts." In children ages 3 years and older, pain scales using pictures of facial expressions (Wong-Baker FACES scale) may be helpful in assessing the level of pain **Figure 36-16**.

Exposure

Proper exposure of the child is necessary to complete the hands-on ABCDEs. The PAT requires that the caregiver remove part of the pediatric patient's clothing to allow careful observation of the face, chest wall, and skin. Completing the components requires further exposure, as needed, to fully evaluate physiologic functions, anatomic abnormalities, and unsuspected injuries or rashes. Be careful to avoid heat loss, especially in infants, by covering the patient as soon as possible. Keep the temperature in the ambulance high, and use blankets when necessary.

Transport Decision

After you have completed the primary survey using the hands-on ABCDEs and initiated any treatment, you must make a crucial decision: is immediate transport to the hospital indicated, or is additional assessment and treatment required at the scene? If the child is in hemodynamically stable condition, you may elect to perform a secondary assessment at the scene.

However, immediate transport is indicated if the scene is unsafe for the child or if any of the following conditions exist:

- A significant MOI (same MOIs for the adult [Chapter 26, *Trauma Overview*], in addition to the following):
  - Any fall from a height equal to or greater than a pediatric patient's height, especially with a head-first landing
  - Bicycle crash (when not wearing a helmet)
- A history compatible with a serious illness
- A physical abnormality noted during the primary survey
- A potentially serious anatomic abnormality
- Significant pain
- Level of consciousness that is not normal for the pediatric patient, altered mental status, and/or any signs or symptoms of shock

In addition to the preceding factors, you should also consider the following when making a transport decision:

- The type of clinical problem (injury versus illness)
- The expected benefits of advanced life support treatment in the field
- Local EMS system treatment and transport protocols
- Your comfort level
- Transport time to the hospital

If the child's condition is urgent, initiate immediate transport to the closest appropriate facility. Additional assessment and treatment should occur en route to the hospital.

If the child's condition is stable, perform a secondary assessment at the scene, provide additional treatment as needed, and then transport. Remember that unnecessary use of lights and siren may only increase the anxiety level of the child, parent, or caregiver.

Pediatric patients who weigh less than 40 pounds (18 kg) who do not require spinal stabilization should be transported in a car seat as long as the situation allows. Do not use the patient's car seat if there is the potential that it has been damaged. Instead, use a proper immobilization device suited to the size of the child.

To mount a car seat to the stretcher, place the head of the stretcher in an upright position. Place the seat so it is against the back of the stretcher. Secure one of the stretcher straps from the upper portion of the stretcher through the seat belt positions on the seat and strap it tightly to the stretcher. Repeat on the lower portion of the stretcher. Push the car seat into the stretcher tightly and retighten the straps.

To secure a car seat to the captain's chair, follow the seat manufacturer's instructions. Remember that pediatric patients younger than 2 years must be transported in a rear-facing position because of the lack of mature neck muscles.

In some situations, it is not appropriate to secure a pediatric patient in a car seat, for example, if the pediatric patient has to be immobilized on a long backboard or other suitable immobilization device or requires splinting that does not fit in the seat. If the patient's condition is unstable and requires airway or ventilatory support, he or she should be positioned to maximize the airway and ventilatory requirements. Pediatric patients in cardiopulmonary arrest should likewise not be placed in a car seat but on a device that can be secured to the stretcher. Follow local protocols.

History Taking

Whenever interacting with a child, parents, or caregivers, you should continue to provide emotional support.

When speaking to the child, use terminology that is appropriate for his or her age; use simple, nonmedical terms when communicating with the parent or caregiver as well. Information exchange will be more accurate and effective if the parent or caregiver understands what you are asking and saying.

Crying and fear are inherent responses of sick or injured children; therefore, you should allow them to express these feelings.

Your approach to the history will depend on the age of the patient. Historic information for an infant, toddler, or preschool-age child will need to be obtained from the parent or caregiver.

Information about sexual activity, the possibility of pregnancy, or the use of illicit drugs or alcohol should be obtained from an adolescent patient in private. Most of these patients will be reluctant to provide this information in the presence of their parents or caregivers. When asking such questions, assure the adolescent that this information is important and is needed to provide the most appropriate care.

Questioning of the parent or child about the immediate illness or injury should be based on the child's chief complaint. This, together with an evaluation of the child's medical history, may provide clues to the underlying illness or injury and other conditions that may exist.

When interviewing the parent or caregiver or older child about the chief complaint, obtain the same pertinent information you would for an adult patient. When obtaining information about the child's medical history, inquire whether the child is currently under the care of a physician, has any chronic illnesses, takes any medications on a regular basis, or has any known drug allergies.

If the parent or caregiver is unable to accompany you to the hospital, obtain a name and phone number so a staff person can call if there are questions. This might be the case when you respond to a day care facility or babysitter's location. Most day care facilities require emergency contact information, medical history, and/or a list of current prescribed medications taken by the child in case of an emergency. Care may be delayed if this information is not discovered early; however, you must never delay care of a critical patient.

Obtaining a SAMPLE history for a pediatric patient is the same as obtaining an adult's. However, the questions should be based on the pediatric patient's age and developmental stage of life.

Recall from Chapter 10, *Patient Assessment*, that the OPQRST format can help you gather additional information about a patient's history of present illness and current symptoms. As with the SAMPLE history, the questions should be based on the pediatric patient's age and developmental stage of life.

Secondary Assessment

As with the adult, a secondary assessment of the child should be performed at the scene, unless his or her condition determines immediate transport. The purpose of the secondary assessment is to obtain additional, specific information about the child's illness or injury.

A full-body exam should be performed on all children with the potential for hidden illness or injury; for example, unresponsive medical patients or trauma patients with a significant MOI. This type of examination may help to identify problems such as distended abdomen or possible fractures that were not as obvious during the primary survey.

Use the DCAP-BTLS mnemonic (Deformities, Contusions, Abrasions, Punctures/Penetrations, Burns, Tenderness, Lacerations, and Swelling) to remind you what to assess for a pediatric patient involved in a traumatic event.

A focused assessment is generally performed on patients who have sustained nonsignificant MOIs and on responsive medical patients with a specific complaint. This examination focuses on a certain area or region of the body affected by illness or injury, often determined through the chief complaint. Circumstances will determine which aspects of the physical examination will be used.

Infants, toddlers, and preschool-age children who do not have apparent life-threatening illness or injuries should be assessed starting at the feet and ending at the head; school-age children and adolescents can be assessed using the head-to-toe approach, as with adults. The extent of the physical examination will depend on the situation and may include the following:

- **Head.** The younger the infant or child, the larger the head is in proportion to the rest of the body, increasing the risk for head injury with deceleration (such as in falls or motor vehicle crashes). Look for bruising, swelling, and hematomas. Significant blood can be lost between the skull and scalp of a small infant. A tense or bulging fontanelle in an upright, noncrying infant suggests elevated intracranial pressure caused by meningitis, encephalitis, or intracranial bleeding. A sunken fontanelle suggests dehydration.
- **Pupils.** Note the size, equality, and reactivity of the pupils to light. The response of the pupils is a good indication of how well the brain is functioning, particularly when trauma has occurred.
- **Nose.** Young infants prefer to breathe through their nose, so nasal congestion with mucus can cause respiratory distress. Gentle bulb or catheter suction of the nostrils may bring relief.
- **Ears.** Look for any drainage from the ear canals. Leaking blood suggests a skull fracture. Check for bruises behind the ear or Battle sign, a late sign of skull fracture. The presence of pus may indicate an ear infection or perforation of the ear drum.
- **Mouth.** In the trauma patient, look for active bleeding and loose teeth. Note the smell of the breath. Some ingestions are associated with identifiable odors, such as hydrocarbons (eg, gasoline). Acidosis, as in diabetic ketoacidosis (DKA), may impart a fruity smell to the breath.
- **Neck.** Examine the trachea for swelling or bruising. Note if the pediatric patient cannot move his or her neck and has a high fever. This may indicate that the pediatric patient has bacterial or viral meningitis.
- **Chest.** Examine the chest for penetrating injuries, lacerations, bruises, or rashes. If the pediatric patient is injured, feel the clavicles and every rib for tenderness and/or deformity.
- **Back.** Inspect the back for lacerations, penetrating injuries, bruises, or rashes.
- **Abdomen.** Inspect the abdomen for distention. Gently palpate the abdomen and watch closely for guarding or tensing of the abdominal muscles, which may suggest infection, obstruction, or intra-abdominal injury. Note any tenderness or masses. Look for any seat belt abrasions or bruising.
- **Extremities.** Assess for symmetry. Compare both sides for color, warmth, size of joints, swelling, and tenderness. Put each joint through full range of motion while watching the eyes of the pediatric patient for signs of pain, unless there is obvious deformity of the extremity suggesting a fracture.
- **Capillary refill (in children younger than 6 years).** Normal capillary refill time should occur within 2 seconds. As discussed earlier, assess capillary refill time by blanching the

finger or toenail beds; the soles of the feet may also be used. Cold temperatures will increase capillary refill time, making it a less reliable sign.

- **Level of hydration.** Assess skin turgor, noting the presence of **tenting** (in which the skin, when pinched and pulled away slightly from the body, retracts more slowly than normal). In infants, note whether the fontanelles are sunken or flat. Ask the parent or caregiver how many diapers the infant has soiled over the past 24 hours. Determine whether the child is producing tears when crying; note the condition of the mouth. Is the oral mucosa moist or dry?

If the child's condition suggests a cardiac etiology, call early for paramedic backup.

It is important to note that some of the guidelines used to assess adult circulatory status—heart rate and blood pressure—have important limitations in children. First, normal heart rates vary with age in children. Second, blood pressure is usually not assessed in children younger than 3 years; it offers little information about the child's circulatory status and is usually difficult to obtain. In these pediatric patients, assessment of the skin is a better indication of their circulatory status.

It is important to use appropriate-size equipment when you are assessing a pediatric patient's vital signs. To obtain an accurate reading of a pediatric patient's blood pressure, you must use a cuff that covers two-thirds of the pediatric patient's upper arm. A blood pressure cuff that is too small may give you a falsely high reading, whereas a cuff that is too large may give you a falsely low reading.

Words of Wisdom

To estimate the *lower limit of normal* for the systolic blood pressure in children ages 1 to 10 years, use the following formula: (Age [in years] × 2) + 70 = Systolic blood pressure

Respiratory rates may be difficult to interpret. Rapid respiratory rates may simply reflect high fever, anxiety, pain, or excitement. Normal rates, however, may occur in a child who has been breathing rapidly with increased work of breathing for some time and is now becoming tired. Count the respirations for 30 seconds and then double that number. If the patient yawns, sighs, coughs, or talks during the 30-second period, wait a few seconds and begin again. In infants and children younger than 3 years, evaluate respirations by assessing the rise and fall of the abdomen. Assess the pulse rate by counting for at least 1 minute, noting its quality and regularity. Consider taking an **apical pulse** in infants and small children. An apical pulse is obtained by auscultating heart tones over the chest with a stethoscope.

Note that normal vital signs in pediatric patients vary with the age of the child. Remember that your approach to taking vital signs also varies with the age of the child. Be gentle, talk to the child, assess respirations and then the pulse, and assess blood pressure last Table 36-7. Warm your stethoscope on your hands or a cloth before placing it on the skin. You may also want to let the child hold the equipment or stethoscope before placing it on him or her; this may help to reduce the child's anxiety.

Table 36-7 Pediatric Blood Pressure Ranges

Age	Blood Pressure (mm Hg)
Neonate (0 to 1 month)	Systolic: 67 to 84 Diastolic: 35 to 53
Infant (1 month to 1 year)	Systolic: 72 to 104 Diastolic: 37 to 56
Toddler (1 to 2 years)	Systolic: 86 to 106 Diastolic: 42 to 63
Preschool age (3 to 5 years)	Systolic: 89 to 112 Diastolic: 46 to 72
School age (6 to 12 years)	Systolic: 97 to 120 Diastolic: 57 to 80
Adolescent (12 to 15 years)	Systolic: 110 to 131 Diastolic: 64 to 83

Data from: American Heart Association (AHA). Vital signs in children. In: AHA. *Pediatric Advanced Life Support*. Dallas, TX: AHA; 2015.

It is recommended that you always obtain the patient's first blood pressure reading manually with a sphygmomanometer (blood pressure cuff) and a stethoscope.

Evaluate pupils in a child using a small penlight. The response of pupils is a good indication of how well the brain is functioning, particularly when trauma has occurred. Be sure to compare the size of the pupils against each other.

In addition, a pulse oximeter is a valuable tool to measure the oxygen saturation in a pediatric patient with respiratory issues Figure 36-17. Also assess blood glucose levels with a glucometer.

Reassessment

Reassess the child's condition as determined by the situation; every 15 minutes for a child in stable condition and at least every 5 minutes for a child in unstable condition.

The physiologic safeguards in infants and children can decompensate with alarming unpredictability; therefore, continually monitor respiratory effort, skin color and condition, and level of consciousness or interactiveness. Frequently reassess oxygen saturation and vital signs. Repeat the primary survey and adjust your treatment accordingly.

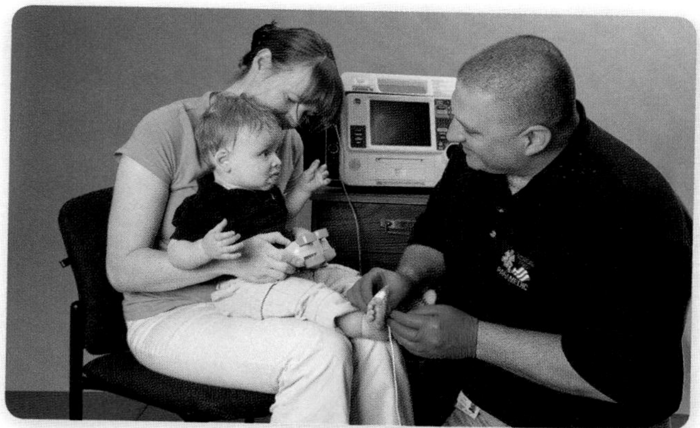

Figure 36-17 Pulse oximetry, which measures the pediatric patient's oxygen saturation, can be used to monitor the pediatric patient's status.

When you are providing interventions for a pediatric patient, you should always consider getting help from the patient's parent or caregiver during these procedures. This is especially helpful during painful procedures (such as IV therapy). It facilitates your ability to assess and treat the child, it calms the child, and it helps to alleviate anxiety in the parent or caregiver. You should build a trusting environment and attempt to not frighten the pediatric patient who is already in a state of stress. Pediatric patients can sense fear from a provider and may not be willing to let you render care.

Words of Wisdom

Perform frequent reassessment of serial vital signs, and record them on your documentation form. By recording each set of vital signs, you can visualize trends and transfer important information to the accepting physicians.

Communicate with the hospital on your findings and the interventions you used to improve the pediatric patient's condition. Be sure that all of this information is documented and given to emergency department (ED) personnel. Remember, a patient care report is a legal document and you may be called to answer questions about this report for years to come.

Pediatric Emergency Medications

In your care for pediatric patients, you may sometimes administer medications. Table 36-8 lists medications in your scope of practice at the advanced emergency medical technician (AEMT) level, for reference as you read about assessment and management of specific emergencies throughout the rest of this chapter.

Table 36-8 Pediatric Emergency Medications

Drug	Pediatric Dosage	Route
Albuterol (Proventil, Ventolin)	<20 kg: 1.25 mg/dose via handheld nebulizer or mask over 20 min. >20 kg: 2.5 mg/dose via handheld nebulizer or mask over 20 min. Repeat once in 20 min.	Inhalation
D_{25}	*Age 1 year and older:* 0.5–1 g/kg of D_{25} via slow IV/IO push. May be repeated as necessary. *Neonates and infants*: 200–500 mg/kg slow IV push (see below). May be repeated as necessary. Maximum concentration of 12.5% (vasculature extremely sensitive to high concentrations).	IV
Dextrose 10%	2.5–5.0 mL/kg If needed, it can be administered via infusion, likely with a 10% dextrose solution.	IV
EPINEPHrine[a] (Adrenalin)	Anaphylaxis and asthma: 0.01 mg/kg (0.1 mL/kg) of 1 mg/mL (1:1,000) solution subcutaneous/IM. Maximum dosage of 0.3 mg. Can be repeated every 5 minutes.	Subcutaneous/IM
Glucagon	Hypoglycemia: 1 mg IM/IN for body weight of 20 kg or greater (or age 5 years or more); 0.5 mg IM/IN if less than 20 kg or younger than 5 years.	IM

(continued)

Table 36-8 Pediatric Emergency Medications *(continued)*

Drug	Pediatric Dosage	Route
Naloxone hydrochloride (Narcan)	0.1 mg/kg IV/IO/IM for infants and children from birth to 5 years of age or 20 kg of body weight. Children older than 5 years of age or weighing more than 20 kg may be given 2.0 mg. These doses may be repeated every 2 minutes as needed to maintain opiate reversal to a maximum dose of 2 mg.	IV
Nitrous oxide	Invert the cylinder several times and have the patient inhale deeply through the demand valve or the mouthpiece. Titrate to effect.	Inhalation
Oxygen	Cardiac arrest and carbon monoxide poisoning 100%. Hypoxemia 12–15 L/min via nonrebreathing mask. Be prepared to provide positive pressure ventilations for those with inadequate respiratory effort.	Inhalation
Activated charcoal	0.5–1 g/kg PO Typical dose is 12.5–25 g up to 1 year of age and 25–50 g for ages 1–12 years.	Oral

Abbreviations: D_{25}, 25% dextrose; IM, intramuscular; IN, intranasal; IO, intraosseous; IV, intravenous; PO, per os (oral route/by mouth)
[a]As done in Chapter 12, *Principles of Pharmacology*, capital letters (tall-man lettering) is used here to prevent confusion with similar medication names.

Data sources: Hazard Vallerand A, Sanoski CA. *Davis' Drug Guide for Nurses*. 14th ed. Philadelphia, PA: FA Davis Company; 2016; Truven Health Analytics. Micromedex database. http://www.micromedexsolutions.com/. Accessed February 29, 2017; Lexi-Comp website. online.lexi.com. Accessed April 2017; American Heart Association. 2015 American Heart Association Guidelines for CPR and ECC. https://eccguidelines.heart.org/index.php/circulation/cpr-ecc-guidelines-2/. Accessed February 29, 2017; National Model EMS Clinical Guidelines. National Association of State EMS Officials. V.08-16. https://www.nasemso.org/Projects/ModelEMSClinicalGuidelines/index.asp. Accessed April 7, 2017; Society of Critical Care Medicine. Surviving Sepsis Campaign. http://www.survivingsepsis.org/Pages/default.aspx. Accessed February 29, 2017; National Association of Emergency Medical Technicians (NAEMT). Tactical Combat Casualty Care Guidelines for Medical Personnel. http://www.naemt.org/education/TCCC/guidelines_curriculum. Published June 3, 2016. Accessed February 29, 2017; Hypoglycemia/Hyperglycemia. In: *National Model EMS Clinical Guidelines*. National Association of State EMS Officials. V.08-16:58. https://www.nasemso.org/Projects/ModelEMSClinicalGuidelines/index.asp. Accessed April 7, 2017.

Assessment and Management of Respiratory Emergencies

Infants have a limited ability to compensate for respiratory insults and often expend huge amounts of energy to breathe. At times, infants are intubated to take over the work of breathing even when adequate physiologic parameters are being maintained. In older children, increasing compensatory skills develop, and juvenile patients with asthma can sometimes compensate for days, with adequate oxygen saturation, before tiring out and literally dying of fatigue.

Many infants and children with respiratory conditions have respiratory distress (difficulty breathing), some have respiratory failure (which invariably leads to decompensation), and a few are in respiratory arrest. If the child in respiratory arrest can be resuscitated before cardiac arrest occurs, survival with a return to full function is likely. Any respiratory compromise in children must be monitored closely and the child transported to the closest ED. If a pediatric-specific ED is available, consult medical direction or your local transport protocols for advice.

When you are faced with a respiratory emergency, the first step is to determine the severity of the disease: is the patient in respiratory distress, respiratory failure, or respiratory arrest? Keep the anatomic and physiologic respiratory differences in mind as you approach the child.

Respiratory distress entails increased work of breathing to maintain oxygenation and/or ventilation; that is, it is a compensated state in which increased work of breathing results in adequate pulmonary gas exchange. Signs of respiratory distress—which is classified as mild, moderate, or severe—include the following:

- Pallor or mottled color
- Irritability, anxiety, restlessness
- Respiratory rate faster than normal for age
- Retractions (suprasternal, intercostal, subcostal)
- Abdominal breathing
- Nasal flaring
- Inspiratory stridor
- Grunting
- Mild tachycardia

A patient experiencing **respiratory failure** can no longer compensate for the underlying pathologic or anatomic problem by increased work of breathing, so hypoxia and/or carbon dioxide retention occur. Signs of respiratory failure may include decreased or absent retractions caused by fatigue of the chest wall muscles, altered mental status caused by inadequate oxygenation and ventilation of the brain, and an abnormally low respiratory rate **Table 36-9**. Respiratory failure is a decompensated state, requiring urgent intervention to ensure adequate oxygenation and ventilation and prevent respiratory or

Table 36-9 Signs of Impending Respiratory Failure

Assess	Sign
Mental status	Agitation, restlessness, confusion, lethargy (VPU components of the AVPU scale)
Skin color	Central cyanosis despite oxygen administration, pallor
Respiratory rate	Tachypnea → bradypnea → apnea
Respiratory effort	Severe retractions and accessory muscle use, nasal flaring, grunting, paradoxical abdominal motion, tripod positioning
Auscultation	Stridor, wheezing, crackles, or diminished air movement
Blood oxygen saturation	Low despite supplemental oxygen administration
Pulse rate	Tachycardia → bradycardia

Abbreviation: AVPU, Awake and alert, responsive to Verbal stimuli, responsive to Pain, Unresponsive

cardiopulmonary arrest. Do not be afraid to assist ventilations at this point if you judge the tidal volume or respiratory effort to be inadequate.

Special Populations

Initiate aggressive airway management and ventilator support with a bag-mask device and supplemental oxygen as soon as possible for a child with respiratory failure.

Respiratory arrest means the patient is not breathing spontaneously. Administer immediate bag-mask ventilation with supplemental oxygen to prevent progression to cardiopulmonary arrest. Resuscitation of a child from respiratory arrest is often successful, whereas resuscitation of a child in cardiopulmonary arrest may or may not be.

Your determination of whether the patient is in respiratory distress, respiratory failure, or respiratory arrest will drive your next steps by indicating the urgency for treatment and transport. You can obtain the SAMPLE history at the scene or during transport, depending on the

Table 36-10 SAMPLE Components for Pediatric Respiratory Emergencies

Component	Features
Signs and symptoms	Shortness of breath, hoarseness, stridor, wheezing, cough, chest pain, choking, rash/hives, cyanosis
Allergies	Known medication or food allergies; smoke exposure
Medications	Names and doses of ongoing medications; recent use of corticosteroids
Past medical history	History of asthma, chronic lung disease, heart problems, prematurity; prior hospitalizations and intubation for breathing problems; history of choking or anaphylaxis; immunizations
Last oral intake	Timing of last food, including bottle or breastfeeding
Events leading to illness or injury	Fever history or recent illness; history of injury to chest; history of choking on food or object

patient's stability. Table 36-10 lists key components to ask about during a respiratory emergency.

Most pediatric patients with a primary respiratory issue will have respiratory distress and require only supportive care. Allow the child to assume a position of comfort and provide supplemental oxygen. The choice of oxygen delivery method will depend on the severity of illness and the child's developmental level. Young children may become agitated by a nasal cannula or face mask. Because crying and thrashing increase metabolic demands and oxygen consumption, you must weigh the benefits of this therapy against the potential cost. Allowing a caregiver to deliver **blow-by oxygen** to a calm toddler may be your best choice, if the child does not show signs of respiratory failure.

As a child becomes fatigued, respiratory distress may progress to respiratory failure. As part of your reassessment, electronically monitor the patient's pulse rate, respiratory rate, and oxygen saturation level. A significant change or trend in any of these variables requires prompt attention. You should also perform frequent reassessment to evaluate the effects of your treatment.

Consider the following when caring for a child with a respiratory emergency:[4]

- Give supplemental oxygen; escalate from a nasal cannula to a simple face mask to a nonrebreathing mask as needed to maintain normal oxygenation.
- Perform electrocardiographic monitoring if there are no signs of clinical improvement after treating respiratory distress.
- Establish IV access if you have clinical concerns about dehydration or if you anticipate the need to administer IV medications.
- The child's airway should be managed in the least invasive way possible. Supraglottic airway devices and intubation should be performed only if bag-mask ventilation fails.

Special Populations

Respiratory distress, respiratory failure, and respiratory arrest exist along a continuum. Intervene early to prevent progression to respiratory arrest in pediatric patients.

Upper Airway Emergencies

Airway obstructions can be caused by foreign objects, infection, or disease. For example, infections, such as pneumonia, croup, epiglottitis, and bacterial tracheitis should be considered as a possible cause of airway obstruction if a pediatric patient has congestion, fever, drooling, and cold symptoms.

Signs and symptoms that are frequently associated with an upper airway obstruction include decreased or absent breath sounds and stridor. Stridor, a high-pitched noise heard mainly on inspiration, is usually caused by swelling of the area surrounding the vocal cords or upper airway obstruction. In pediatric patients with croup, it resembles the bark of a seal.

Foreign Body Aspiration or Obstruction

Children, especially those younger than 5 years, can (and do) obstruct their airway with any object that they can fit into their mouth (such as hot dogs, balloons, grapes, or coins) Figure 36-18. In cases of trauma, a child's teeth may have been dislodged into the airway. Blood, vomitus, or other secretions can also cause mild or severe airway obstruction.

As discussed, signs and symptoms of an upper airway obstruction include decreased or absent breath sounds and stridor. In pediatric patients with croup, it resembles the bark of a seal.

YOU are the Provider — PART 3

You contact dispatch to request a paramedic intercept and are informed that there are no units available. You obtain a complete set of vital signs, including a capillary blood glucose level, which reads 26 mg/dL. Knowing that this value is extremely low, you retrieve your supplies and prepare to cannulate a vein. On the basis of the patient's size and the need for intravenous (IV) glucose, you select the largest-size catheter that you believe you can insert on the first attempt, a 22-gauge catheter. Following local protocols, you place a Volutrol onto your bag of normal saline and fill the chamber to 100 mL. You successfully establish IV access to the patient's left wrist on the first attempt. After ensuring that the line is patent and secure, you prepare your IV glucose solution. You direct your partner to initiate rapid transport to the closest hospital, which is approximately 18 minutes away. Once en route, you ensure that your other partner is continuing assisted ventilations with the bag-mask device and that there is good chest rise and fall.

Recording Time: 8 Minutes	
Respirations	20 breaths/min, assisted
Pulse	155 beats/min, regular
Skin	Warm, dry, and pink
Blood pressure	Unable to obtain
Oxygen saturation (Spo_2)	99% on 15 L/min
Pupils	Equal and sluggish

5. What are normal vital signs for a patient of this age?
6. What is the purpose of a Volutrol?
7. How should the glucose be prepared?

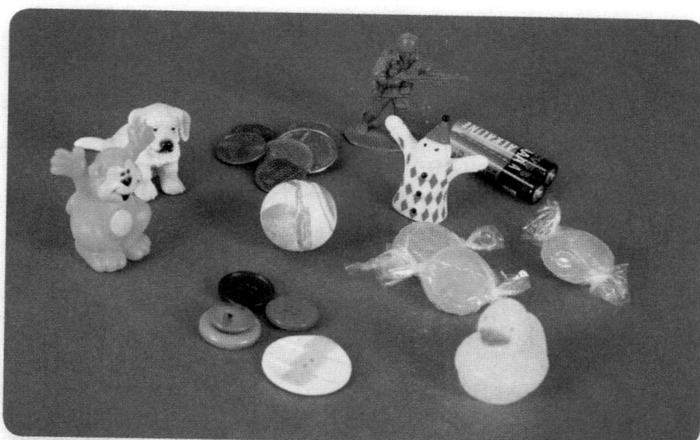

Figure 36-18 Any number of objects can obstruct a child's airway. Some of the more common ones include batteries, coins, toys, buttons, and candy.

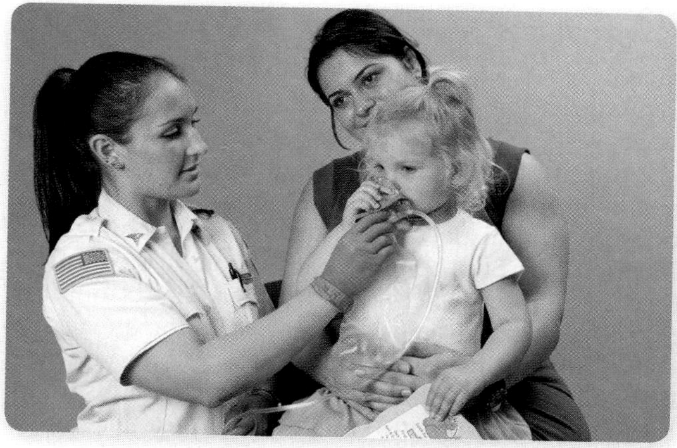

Figure 36-19 If a pediatric patient has a partial airway obstruction, do not intervene except to give supplemental oxygen. Allow the child to remain in whatever position is most comfortable during transport.

Words of Wisdom

Infants or children presenting with acute respiratory distress in the absence of fever should be suspected of having a foreign body airway obstruction.

Treatment of the pediatric patient with an airway obstruction must begin immediately. If the patient is responsive and coughing forcefully and you know for sure that there is a foreign body in the airway—that is, if someone actually saw the object go into the child's mouth—encourage the child to cough to clear the airway. If the material in the airway does not completely block the flow of air, the pediatric patient may be able to breathe adequately on his or her own without any intervention. In such cases, do not intervene except to provide supplemental oxygen **Figure 36-19**. Allow the pediatric patient to remain in whatever position is most comfortable, and monitor his or her condition during transport.

If you see signs of a severe airway obstruction, however, you must attempt to clear the airway immediately. The signs include the following:

- Ineffective cough (no sound)
- Inability to speak or cry
- Increasing respiratory difficulty, with stridor
- Cyanosis
- Loss of consciousness

If an infant is responsive with a complete airway obstruction, perform up to five back blows followed by five chest thrusts. First, position the infant facedown on your forearm. Support the infant's jaw and head with your hand. Next, use the heel of your other hand to slap the back forcefully five times (between the shoulder blades). If the airway does not clear, flip the infant onto his or her back, using your hand to support the head. Perform up to five chest thrusts in the same manner you would provide chest compressions for CPR. Repeat the process until the obstruction clears or until the infant becomes unresponsive.

If a child (older than 1 year) is responsive with a complete airway obstruction, perform abdominal thrusts (Heimlich maneuver). Continue until the obstruction clears or until the child becomes unresponsive.

If there is reason to believe that an unresponsive child has a foreign body obstruction and there are no suspected spinal injuries, open the airway using the head tilt–chin lift maneuver and look inside the mouth to see whether the obstructing object is visible. If the object is visible, try to remove it using a finger sweep motion. Never use finger sweeps if you cannot see the object because you may push it further into the airway.

Chest compressions are recommended to relieve a severe airway obstruction in an unresponsive pediatric patient. Chest compressions increase the pressure in the chest, creating an artificial cough that may force a foreign body from the airway. Chapter 15, *BLS Resuscitation*, covers clearing a foreign body obstruction in an infant and child in detail.

Special Populations

Cystic fibrosis, a genetic disease that primarily affects the respiratory and digestive systems, chronically produces copious amounts of thick mucus in the respiratory and digestive tracts, which makes patients susceptible to recurrent respiratory infections. Pediatric patients may present with tachypnea, chest pain, and crackles, although it may be difficult to separate acute exam findings from chronic disease.

Anaphylaxis

Anaphylaxis is a potentially life-threatening allergic reaction, triggered by exposure to an antigen (foreign protein). Food—especially nuts, shellfish, eggs, and milk—and beestings are among the most common causes, although anaphylaxis to antibiotics and other medications can occur as well. Exposure to the antigen stimulates the release of histamine and other vasoactive chemical mediators from white blood cells, leading to multiple organ system involvement. Onset of symptoms generally occurs immediately after the exposure and may include hives, respiratory distress, circulatory compromise, and gastrointestinal symptoms (vomiting, diarrhea, abdominal pain). See Chapter 22, *Immunologic Emergencies*, for more information about the sequence of events in anaphylaxis.

Although a child with mild anaphylaxis may experience only hives and some wheezing, a child with severe anaphylaxis may be in respiratory failure and shock when you arrive. The PAT may reveal an anxious child (many adults describe a sense of impending doom at the onset of anaphylaxis). With severe anaphylaxis, the child may be unresponsive as a result of respiratory failure and shock. He or she may have increased work of breathing due to upper airway edema or bronchospasm and poor circulation. The primary survey will usually reveal hives, with other findings potentially including swelling of the lips and oral mucosa, stridor and/or wheezing, and diminished pulses. If the child has a known allergy, the SAMPLE history may reveal recent contact with or ingestion of the potentially offending agent (including consumption of prepared foods containing traces of eggs, nuts, and milk at day care or school).

The "gold standard" treatment for anaphylaxis is epinephrine. Epinephrine's alpha-agonist effect decreases airway edema by **vasoconstriction** and improves circulation by increasing peripheral vascular resistance. Its beta agonist effect causes bronchodilation, resulting in improved oxygenation and ventilation. Epinephrine should be given by the intramuscular (IM) route at a dose of 0.01 mg/kg of the 1 mg/mL (1:1,000) solution, to a maximum dose of 0.3 mg. This dose may be repeated as necessary every 5 minutes. In addition to epinephrine, treatment of anaphylaxis should include supplemental oxygen, fluid resuscitation for shock, and bronchodilators for wheezing. Diphenhydramine (Benadryl) is also indicated for its antihistamine effect, but is not within the scope of practice of the AEMT.

Many children with a history of anaphylaxis will have been treated with IM epinephrine by a caregiver before EMS activation. Given the short half-life of this drug, the child should be transported, even if asymptomatic on your arrival.

Croup

Croup (laryngotracheobronchitis) is an infection of the upper airway below the level of the vocal cords, usually caused by a virus. The parainfluenza virus is the pathogen most commonly responsible for croup, but respiratory syncytial virus (RSV), influenza, and adenovirus have also been implicated. The virus is transmitted by respiratory secretions. Croup primarily affects children 6 months to 3 years of age, with most cases occurring in the fall and winter months.[5] The virus has an affinity for the subglottic space—the narrowest part of the pediatric airway—and causes edema and progressive airway obstruction. Turbulent airflow through the narrowed subglottic airway causes the hallmark sign of croup—stridor.

Words of Wisdom

RSV is highly contagious and spread through droplets when the pediatric patient coughs or sneezes. RSV is more common in premature infants and results in copious secretions that may require suctioning. The virus can also survive on surfaces, including hands and clothing—including on yours. The infection tends to spread rapidly through schools and in child care centers. RSV is discussed in Chapter 17, *Respiratory Emergencies*.

Most cases of croup are mild. EMS may be called when the symptoms come on abruptly, often in the middle of the night, or if symptoms cause moderate to severe respiratory distress. The PAT for a child with croup will typically reveal an alert infant or toddler who has audible stridor with activity or agitation, a barky cough, some increased work of breathing, and normal skin color. If a child with a history compatible with croup is sleepy or obtunded or has significant respiratory distress or cyanosis, be concerned about critical airway obstruction. On your primary survey, breath sounds will likely be clear over the lung fields, although you may hear stridor (originating at the level of the subglottic space). Because the pathophysiology of croup largely involves the upper airway, hypoxia is uncommon, and its presence should alert you to critical obstruction and the need for immediate treatment. The SAMPLE history usually reveals several days of cold symptoms and low-grade fever, followed by the onset of a barky cough, stridor, and trouble breathing. The cough and respiratory distress are often worse at night.

The initial management of croup is the same as for most respiratory emergencies. Allow the child to assume a position of comfort, and avoid agitating him or her. The use of humidified oxygen may be beneficial.[6,7] For patients with stridor at rest, moderate to severe respiratory distress, poor air exchange, hypoxia, or altered appearance, nebulized epinephrine is the treatment of choice. It works by causing vasoconstriction and decreasing upper airway edema. Call early for paramedic backup if nebulized epinephrine is needed.

In the case of croup and respiratory failure, assisted ventilation with bag-mask ventilation will often succeed in overcoming the upper airway obstruction. Advanced airway placement is rarely needed in croup. Children requiring medication or assisted ventilation need to be transported immediately to an appropriate treatment facility.

Words of Wisdom

DO NOT do anything to agitate a child with suspected croup or epiglottitis. Doing so could create a laryngospasm and cause closure of the airway.

Epiglottitis

Epiglottitis (supraglottitis), at one time a dreaded inflammation of the supraglottic structures (soft tissue in the area above the vocal cords), usually due to bacterial infection, is now rare in children. With the introduction of a childhood vaccine against *Haemophilus influenzae*, type B, the incidence of this life-threatening condition has decreased dramatically. Nevertheless, sporadic cases have been reported among adolescents, adults, and unimmunized children.

The classic presentation of epiglottitis is easily distinguishable using the PAT. A child with epiglottitis looks sick and will be anxious, will sit upright in the sniffing position with the chin thrust forward to allow for maximal air entry, and may be drooling because of an inability to swallow secretions. The work of breathing is increased, and pallor or cyanosis may be evident.

Stridor heard on auscultation over the neck, a muffled voice, decreased or absent breath sounds, and hypoxia are all signs of a significant airway obstruction. The SAMPLE history will reveal a sudden onset of high fever and sore throat. Because symptoms progress rapidly, children with epiglottitis are generally sick for only a few hours before they come to medical attention. Remember to ask about immunizations as part of the pertinent medical history for patients suspected of having epiglottitis.

Your goal is to get the child with epiglottitis to an appropriate hospital with a maintainable airway. Because rapidly progressive disease is associated with a risk for acute airway obstruction and respiratory arrest, you should minimize your scene time and not attempt procedures that might agitate the child. Allow the patient to assume a position of comfort, and provide supplemental oxygen only if tolerated by the patient. Do not attempt to look in the mouth because this can precipitate complete airway obstruction, and do not attempt IV access. Be prepared with a bag-mask device in the event of complete obstruction during transport and the need for assisted ventilation. Alert personnel at the receiving facility to the suspected diagnosis and the patient's condition because they will need to mobilize a team for the management of this difficult airway.

Special Populations

There are some special considerations when suctioning an infant or child's airway. Use a bulb syringe, flexible suction catheter, or rigid (tonsil-tip) suction catheter. Follow these guidelines:

- Avoid vigorous suctioning.
- Avoid upper airway stimulation; the vagal stimulation can cause bradycardia and hypoxia.
- Decrease suction negative pressure to 100 mm Hg or less.
- Suction *only* when withdrawing the catheter.
- Limit suction time to 10 seconds in children and 5 seconds in infants.
- If bradycardia occurs, stop suctioning immediately and oxygenate the child.

Lower Airway Emergencies

Signs and symptoms of a lower airway obstruction include wheezing, a whistling sound caused by air traveling through narrowed air passages within the bronchioles, and/or crackles. Crackles are caused by the flow of air through liquid, present in the air pouches and smaller airways in the lungs. They produce a crackling sound like that of blowing bubbles through a straw in a glass filled with liquid. The best way to auscultate breath sounds in a pediatric patient is to listen on both sides of the chest at the level of the armpit Figure 36-20.

Asthma

Asthma is an acute spasm and inflammation of the bronchioles in the lungs (bronchospasm) and is associated with excessive mucus production. Asthma is typically encountered in children with a preexisting history of the

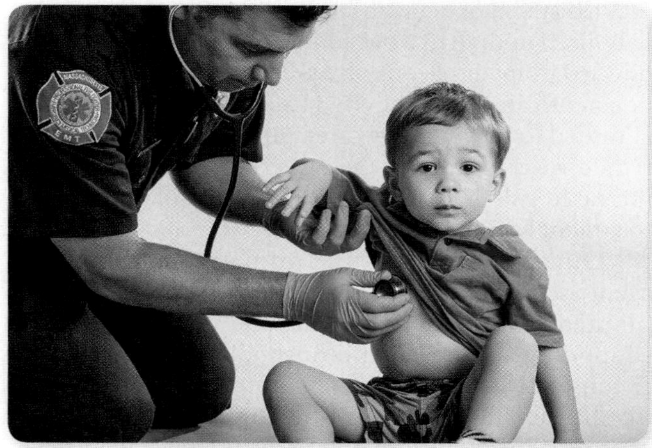

Figure 36-20 The best way to auscultate breath sounds in pediatric patients is to listen on both sides of the chest at the level of the armpit.

disease. It is a true emergency if not promptly identified and treated. According to the Centers for Disease Control and Prevention, approximately 8.6% of children (6.3 million) currently have asthma.[8] In between attacks, the child is usually asymptomatic. However, an acute attack can be caused by various triggers, including upper respiratory infections, allergies, changes in environmental temperature, smoke, physical exertion, and emotional stress.

An acute asthma attack occurs when the hyperreactive bronchioles become narrowed, causing a reduction of airflow through them. The initial response during an acute asthma attack is the result of the immune system's response to the trigger, which releases chemicals called histamines. As the attack progresses, swelling of the mucous membranes in the bronchiolar walls and mucus plugging of the bronchiolar lumen further restrict expiratory airflow. Pulmonary gas exchange is impaired, and the child becomes hypoxemic.

The signs and symptoms of an acute asthma attack vary, depending on the severity of the attack. You will typically find the child sitting up, in a preferential position, and in obvious respiratory distress. When you are evaluating breathing, you will often note a prolonged expiratory phase, indicating the child's difficulty in expelling air from his or her lungs. Wheezing is commonly heard during auscultation of the chest, usually during expiration. During a more severe asthma attack, however, wheezing may become so loud that it is audible without a stethoscope. Other signs include tachycardia, tachypnea, and agitation.

Administer oxygen by the method most tolerated by the child: a nonrebreathing mask or the blow-by technique.

During your assessment, you should determine whether the child has been prescribed a metered-dose inhaler (MDI) containing a beta-2 agonist (ie, albuterol) or other medication. If so, determine how many puffs, if any, he or she took prior to your arrival. Depending on how many, if any, puffs the child has taken from his or her MDI, you may assist him or her with the medication or administer a nebulized updraft of a beta-2 agonist such as albuterol as directed by medical control. Ask the child (if old enough) or parent/caregiver if the child has ever been intubated or admitted to the intensive care unit for his or her asthma. If the answer to either of these questions is yes, there is an increased risk that the child will need similar aggressive treatment again.

Other than oxygen, the primary pharmacologic agent used for an acute asthma attack is a beta-2 agonist. Albuterol (Ventolin, Proventil) seems to be the most commonly administered bronchodilator. Other medications, however, such as metaproterenol (Alupent), or isoetharine (Bronkosol), may be administered depending on local protocols. Albuterol (or other beta-2 agonists) is administered through a nebulizer. Always contact medical control prior to administration of any medication as well as following local protocols.

Children experiencing a prolonged asthma attack tend to tire quickly. If the child is showing signs of respiratory failure, begin assisted ventilations with a bag-mask device and 100% oxygen. If needed, bronchodilator therapy can be administered during positive pressure ventilations with a small-volume in-line nebulizer.

Endotracheal intubation may be necessary if prolonged ventilatory support is needed or if bag-mask ventilations are ineffective. Call early for paramedic backup.

Additional treatment consists of monitoring the child's oxygen saturation level and transporting promptly to the hospital. If the child's condition will allow, do not separate him or her from the parent or caregiver.

A prolonged asthma attack that is unrelieved may progress into a condition known as status asthmaticus, in which there is minimal air movement. Status asthmaticus is a dire emergency. Although the treatment for status asthmaticus is essentially the same as it is for a mild or moderate asthma attack, it is more aggressive and must be performed en route to the hospital. Many children with status asthmaticus will experience respiratory failure secondary to severe hypoxia, acidosis, and physical exhaustion, and will require assisted ventilations including advanced airway management.

Special Populations

The pediatric dose of albuterol depends on the child's weight and may need to be repeated based on the child's clinical response. The dose for albuterol is provided earlier in this chapter.

Medical control or local protocol may determine if the administration of epinephrine 1 mg/mL (1:1,000) subcutaneously in children with severe respiratory distress or failure resulting from a reactive airway disease is an option. Follow local protocols regarding the appropriate pediatric dosage.

Pneumonia

Pneumonia is a common disease process that infects the lower airway and the lung. Although it can occur at any age, in pediatric patients it is commonly seen in infants, toddlers, and preschoolers (ages 1 to 5 years). According to the World Health Organization, there are approximately 156 million new cases of pneumonia reported each year in children younger than 5 years, accounting for 16% of all deaths in children under 5 years.[9,10] In children, pneumonia is usually caused by a virus. However, as children get older, the incidence of bacterial pneumonia increases. Children with pneumonia typically have a recent history of a cough or cold, or a lower airway infection (ie, bronchitis). Pneumonia can also be caused by direct lung injuries, such as from an accidental ingestion of a chemical or a submersion incident.

Often, pediatric patients with pneumonia will present with unusually rapid breathing or will breathe with grunting or wheezing sounds. Additional signs and symptoms include nasal flaring, tachypnea, crackles, and hypothermia or fever. The patient may also exhibit unilateral diminished breath sounds. Assess the work of breathing by observing for signs of accessory muscle usage. Pneumonia in the infant population may not be tolerated as well as in the older child or adult populations because infants have an increased oxygen demand and less respiratory reserve amounts.

For a pediatric patient with suspected pneumonia, your primary treatment is supportive, consisting of monitoring the patient's airway and breathing status, and administering supplemental oxygen if required. If the child is wheezing, administer a bronchodilator if permitted by your EMS system. Vascular access is generally not indicated for children with pneumonia; however, if the child's condition warrants medication therapy, establish IV or IO access en route to the hospital. A diagnosis of pneumonia must be confirmed in the hospital setting with a chest radiograph, followed by the administration of antibiotics as the primary treatment.

Bronchiolitis

Bronchiolitis is a viral infection that results in inflammation and constriction of the bronchioles and is often caused by RSV.

Bronchiolitis occurs during the first 2 years of life and is more common in males. These infections are most widespread in the winter and early spring. Bronchioles, the tiny airways that lead to alveoli in the lungs, become inflamed, swell, and fill with mucus. The airways of infants and young children can become easily blocked.

When assessing a pediatric patient, look for signs of dehydration—infants with RSV often refuse liquids. If the RSV has progressed to bronchiolitis, shortness of breath and fever may be present.

Approach the pediatric patient with a calm demeanor and allow for a position of comfort. Treat airway and breathing problems as appropriate. Humidified oxygen is helpful if available. Be prepared to assist ventilations as needed. Call early for paramedic backup if you anticipate the need for advanced airway management.

Pertussis

Pertussis, also known as whooping cough, is a disease caused by a bacterium that is spread through respiratory droplets. As a result of vaccinations, this potentially deadly disease is less common in the United States. The typical signs and symptoms are similar to a common cold: coughing, sneezing, and a runny nose. As the disease progresses, the coughing becomes more severe and is characterized by the distinctive whoop sound heard during the inspiratory phase. In infants infected with pertussis, pneumonia or respiratory failure may develop. To treat these pediatric patients, keep the airway patent and transport the patient to the hospital. Because pertussis is contagious, follow standard precautions, including wearing a mask and eye protection.

General Assessment and Management of Respiratory Emergencies

Airway Adjuncts

In children with inadequate ventilation, regardless of the cause, you should use an airway adjunct to maintain a patent airway. Placing the adjuncts correctly starts with choosing the appropriate-size equipment Table 36-11. If an airway adjunct is not the correct size for the child's size and age, it may cause more harm than good.

Oropharyngeal Airway

An oropharyngeal (oral) airway should be used for pediatric patients who are unresponsive and in respiratory failure. However, this adjunct should not be used in responsive patients or those who have a gag reflex. In addition, this adjunct should not be used in children who have ingested a caustic (corrosive) or petroleum-based product because it may induce vomiting.

Table 36-11 Pediatric Equipment: Getting the Size Right

The best way to identify the appropriate-size equipment for a pediatric patient is to use **length-based resuscitation tape** (Broselow tape). This color-coded tool can estimate weight as well as height in pediatric patients weighing up to 75 lb (34 kg) Figure 36-21. The proper sequence for using the tape is the following:

1. Place the pediatric patient supine on a flat surface.
2. Lay the tape next to the pediatric patient with the multicolored side up.
3. Place the red end of the tape at the top of the pediatric patient's head (Red to Head).
4. Place one hand, side down, on top of the pediatric patient's head, covering the red box at the end of the tape.
5. Starting from the pediatric patient's head, run the side of your free hand down the tape.
6. Stretch the tape out the full length of the child, stopping at the heel. If the child is longer than the tape, stop here and use the appropriate adult technique.
7. Place your free hand, side down, at the bottom of the child's heel.
8. Note the color or letter block and weight range on the edge of the tape where your hand is. Say the color or letter out loud.
9. Select the appropriate-size equipment by matching the color or letter on the tape to the color or letter on the equipment.

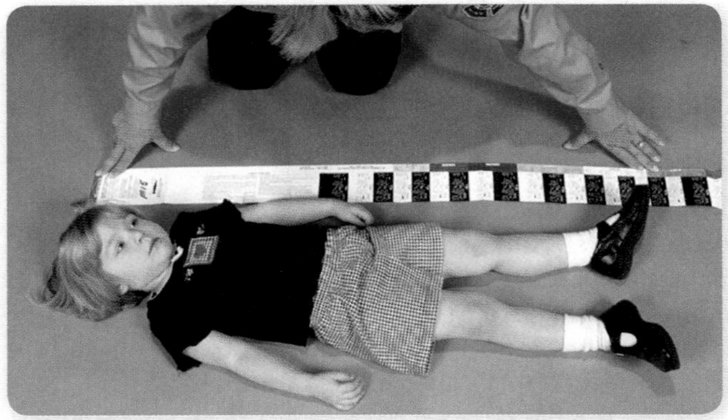

Figure 36-21 Use of a length-based resuscitation tape is the best way to identify the correct size for pediatric equipment, including basic and advanced airway devices and medication doses.

Skill Drill 36-2 shows the steps for inserting an oropharyngeal airway in a child.

If a tongue blade is not available, point the airway tip toward the roof of the mouth to depress the tongue. Gently rotate the airway into position as it passes through the mouth toward the curve of the tongue.

Take care to avoid injuring the hard palate as you insert the airway. Rough insertion can cause bleeding, which may aggravate airway problems and may even cause vomiting. Note also that if the patient's airway is too small, the tongue may be pushed back into the pharynx, obstructing the airway. If the oropharyngeal airway is too large, it may obstruct the larynx.

Nasopharyngeal Airway

In pediatric patients, the nasopharyngeal (nasal) airway is typically used for pediatric patients who are responsive.

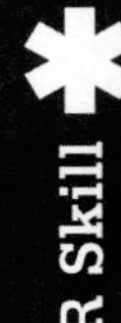

NR Skill

Skill Drill 36-2 Inserting an Oropharyngeal Airway in a Pediatric Patient

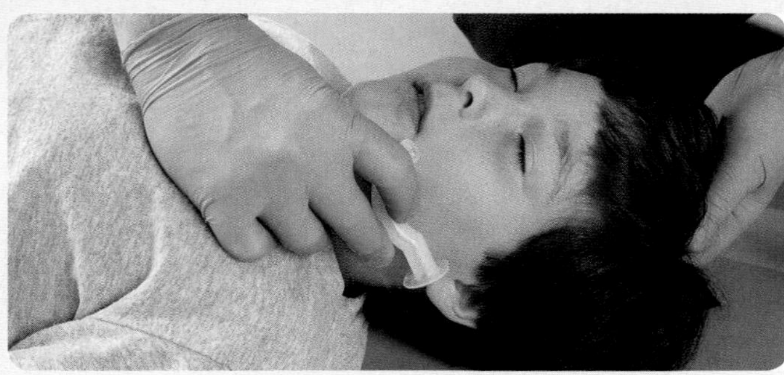

Step 1 Determine the appropriate size airway by placing the airway next to the face with the flange at the level of the central incisors and the bite block segment parallel to the hard palate. The tip of the airway should reach the angle of the jaw. Or, use a length-based resuscitation tape to determine the appropriate size airway.

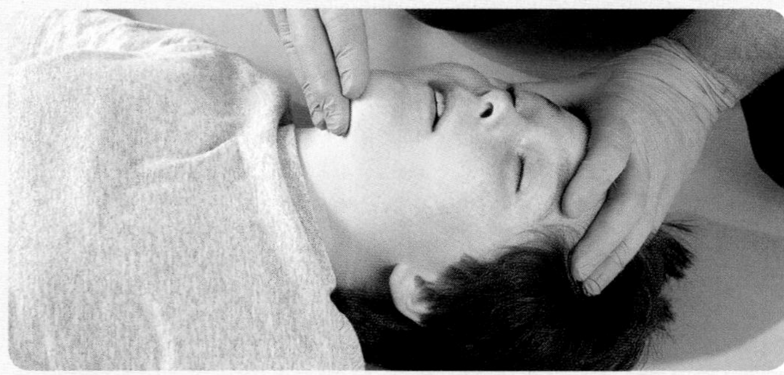

Step 2 Position the patient's airway. In medical patients, use the head tilt–chin lift maneuver, avoiding hyperextension; you may place a towel under the patient's shoulders to assist in holding the position. If the patient has a traumatic injury, use the jaw-thrust maneuver and provide manual in-line stabilization.

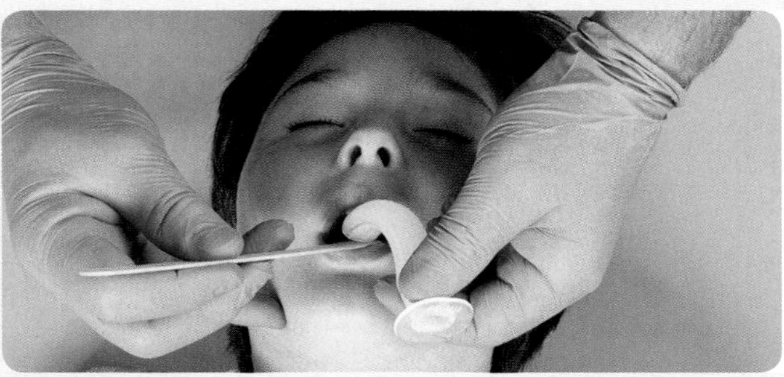

Step 3 Open the mouth by applying pressure on the chin with your thumb. Insert the airway by depressing the tongue with a tongue blade applied to the base of the tongue and inserting the airway directly over the tongue blade. Insert the airway until the flange rests against the lips. Reassess the airway after insertion.

It is well tolerated and not as likely as the oropharyngeal airway to cause vomiting. In pediatric patients, the nasopharyngeal airway is typically used in association with respiratory failure. It is rarely used in infants younger than 1 year.

A nasopharyngeal airway should not be used in patients with nasal obstruction, head trauma (possible basilar skull fracture), or facial trauma, or in patients with moderate to severe head trauma because this adjunct could increase intracranial pressure.

Follow the steps in Skill Drill 36-3 to insert a nasopharyngeal airway in a pediatric patient. Keep in mind that the external diameter of the airway should not be larger than the diameter of the naris or the child's pinkie finger, and there should be no **blanching** (turning white) of the naris after insertion. As for length, the airway should extend from the tip of the nose to the tragus of the ear. The **tragus** is the small cartilaginous projection in front of the opening of the ear.

The right naris is commonly larger than the left naris. However, if you are inserting the airway on the left side, insert the tip into the left naris upside down, with the bevel pointing toward the septum. Move the airway forward slowly approximately 1 inch (2.5 cm) until you feel a slight resistance, and then rotate the airway 180°. Reassess the airway after insertion.

Oxygen Delivery Devices

All ill or injured infants and children should receive supplemental oxygen. The method of oxygen delivery will be determined by the adequacy of the patient's breathing, or tidal volume. In treating infants and children who require supplemental oxygen, the following devices and techniques can be used:

- Blow-by oxygen at 6 L/min provides more than 21% oxygen concentration.
- Nasal cannula at 1 to 6 L/min provides 24% to 44% oxygen concentration.
- Nonrebreathing mask at 10 to 15 L/min provides up to 95% oxygen concentration (unassisted ventilations).
- Bag-mask device (with oxygen reservoir) at 15 L/min provides nearly 100% oxygen concentration (assisted ventilations).

Children need enough air to be delivered for adequate gas exchange in the lungs. Therefore, use of a nonrebreathing mask or the blow-by technique is indicated only for patients who have adequate respiratory rates and tidal volumes. **Tidal volume** is the amount of air that is delivered to the lungs in one inhalation. Because the nonrebreathing mask and blow-by technique deliver oxygen passively,

Skill Drill 36-3 Inserting a Nasopharyngeal Airway in a Pediatric Patient

NR Skill

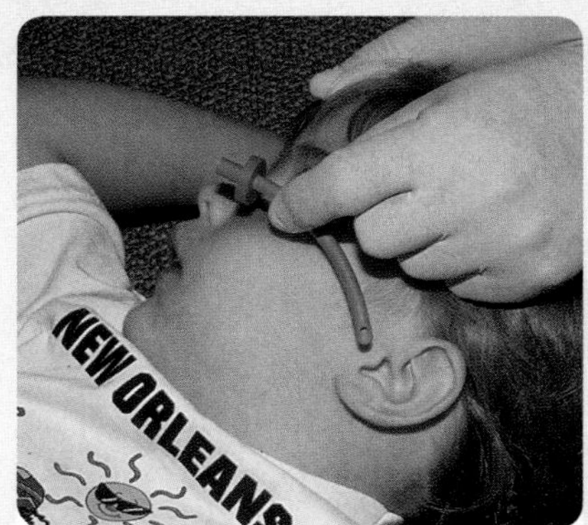

Step 1 Determine the appropriate size airway by comparing its diameter with the opening of the nostril (naris). Place the airway next to the patient's face to confirm correct length. Position the airway appropriately, using the techniques described for the oropharyngeal airway.

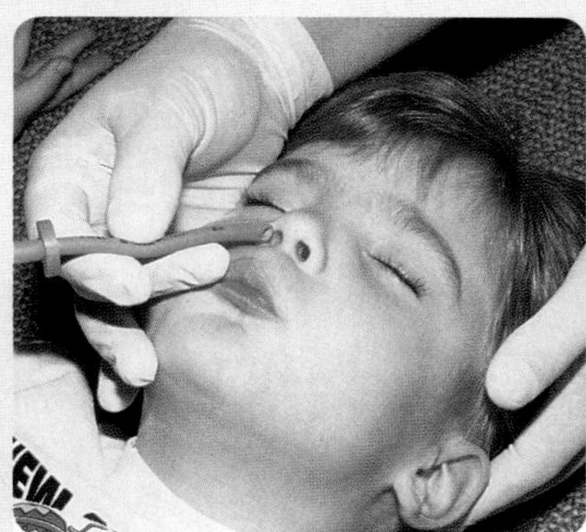

Step 2 Lubricate the airway with a water-soluble lubricant. Insert the tip into the right naris (nostril opening) with the bevel pointing toward the septum, or central divider in the nose.

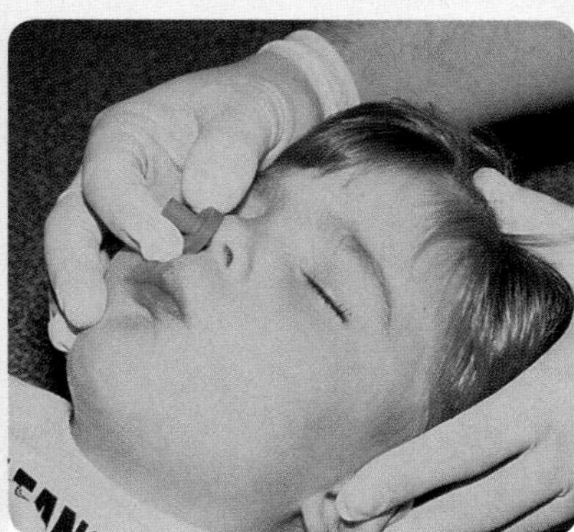

Step 3 Carefully advance the airway, following the curvature of the anatomy, until the flange rests against the outside of the nostril.

positive pressure ventilations with a bag-mask device are needed in children with inadequate breathing. Children with respirations of less than 12 breaths/min or more than 60 breaths/min, an altered level of consciousness, and/or an inadequate tidal volume should receive assisted ventilations with a bag-mask device.

Blow-by Oxygen. Blow-by oxygen does not deliver a high concentration of oxygen; however, if the child will not tolerate a nonrebreathing mask, the blow-by technique is better than no oxygen at all.

After ensuring a patent airway and maintaining proper head position, administration of oxygen via the blow-by technique may require assistance from the parent or caregiver. This method may be less frightening to a child than an air mask. In the blow-by technique, an oxygen tube is held near the infant or child's nose and mouth. Allowing a parent or caregiver to hold the device near the child's face may facilitate his or her tolerance. To administer blow-by oxygen:

1. Place oxygen tubing through a small hole in the bottom of an 8-oz (237-mL) cup **Figure 36-22**. A cup is a familiar object that is less likely to frighten young children than an oxygen mask.
2. Connect the oxygen tubing to an oxygen source set at 6 L/min.
3. Hold the cup approximately 1 to 2 inches (2 to 5 cm) away from the child's nose and mouth.

Words of Wisdom

You cannot use a nonrebreathing mask for blow-by oxygen because of the one-way valve. It will not deliver oxygen unless it is applied firmly to the child's face.

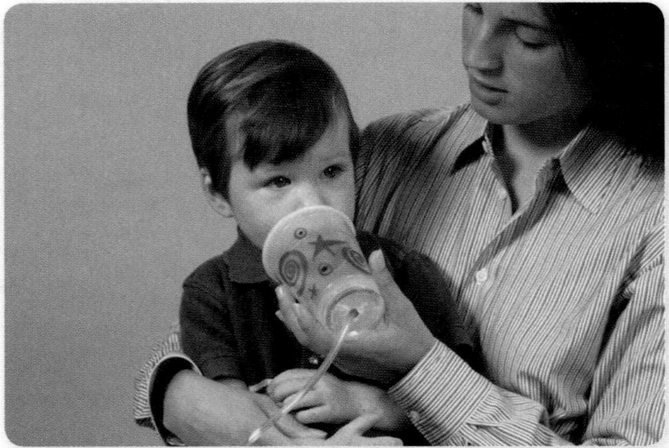

Figure 36-22 To use the blow-by technique, make a small hole in a 8-oz (237-mL) cup, or use a funnel inserted into the end of the oxygen tubing. Connect tubing to an oxygen source, and hold the cup about 1 to 2 inches (2 to 5 cm) from the child's face.

Nasal Cannula. Some pediatric patients prefer the nasal cannula whereas others find it uncomfortable. To apply a nasal cannula:

1. Choose the appropriate-size pediatric nasal cannula. The prongs should not fill the nares entirely **Figure 36-23**. If the nares blanch, select a smaller cannula.
2. Connect the tubing to an oxygen source set at 1 to 6 L/min.

Nonrebreathing Mask. A nonrebreathing mask delivers up to 95% oxygen to the patient and allows the patient to exhale all air containing carbon dioxide without rebreathing it **Figure 36-24**. To apply a nonrebreathing mask:

1. Select the appropriate-size pediatric nonrebreathing mask. The mask should extend from the bridge of the nose to the cleft of the chin.

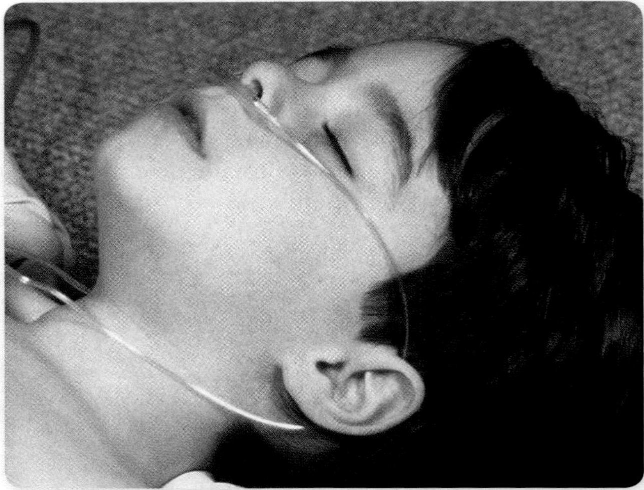

Figure 36-23 The prongs of the pediatric nasal cannula should not fill the nares entirely.

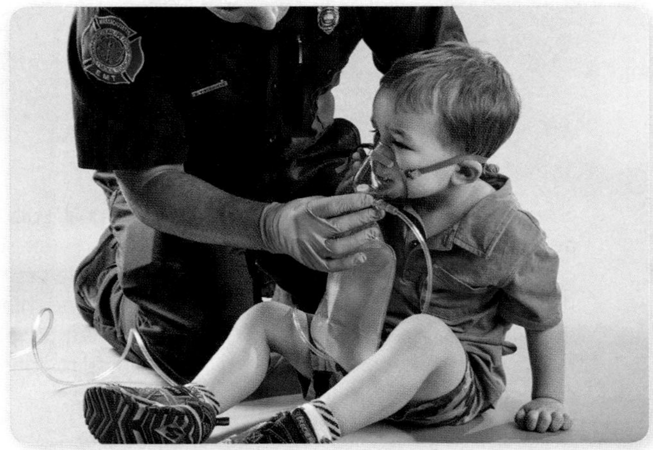

Figure 36-24 A pediatric nonrebreathing mask delivers up to 95% oxygen and allows the patient to exhale air containing carbon dioxide without rebreathing it.

2. Connect the tubing to an oxygen source set at 10 to 15 L/min.
3. Adjust the oxygen flow as needed to match the patient's respiratory rate and depth. The reservoir bag should neither deflate completely nor fill to bulging during the respiratory cycle.

Special Populations

Nasal cannulas are rarely used to administer oxygen in pediatric patients. Infants and children are usually not tolerant of the device, which causes anxiety and increased oxygen demand. Agitating an already hypoxic infant or child may exacerbate the condition.

Bag-Mask Device. Assisted ventilation with a bag-mask device is indicated for patients who have respirations that are too fast or too slow to provide adequate tidal volume of inhaled oxygen, who are unresponsive, or who do not respond in a purposeful way to painful stimuli.

Assist ventilation of an infant or child using a bag-mask device in the following way:

1. Ensure that you have the appropriate equipment in the right size. The mask should extend from the bridge of the nose to the cleft of the chin, avoiding compression of the eyes **Figure 36-25**. The mask is transparent, so you can observe for cyanosis and vomiting. In addition, mask volume should be small to decrease dead space and avoid rebreathing; however, the bag should contain at least 450 mL of air. Use an infant bag rather than a neonatal bag for infants younger than 1 year; use a pediatric bag for children older than 1 year. Older children and adolescents may need an adult bag. Make sure that there is no pop-off valve on the bag, or, if there is one, make sure that you can hold it shut as necessary to achieve visible chest rise.
2. Maintain a good seal with the mask on the face. An inadequate mask-to-face seal will result in inadequate tidal volume delivery and a decreased concentration of delivered oxygen.
3. Ventilate at the appropriate rate and volume using a slow, gentle squeeze, not a sharp, quick one. Stop squeezing and begin to release the bag as soon as the chest wall begins to rise, indicating that the lungs are filled to capacity. To keep from ventilating too rapidly, use the phrase "squeeze, release, release." Say "squeeze" as you squeeze the bag; when you see the chest start to rise, release pressure on the bag and slowly say "Release, release."

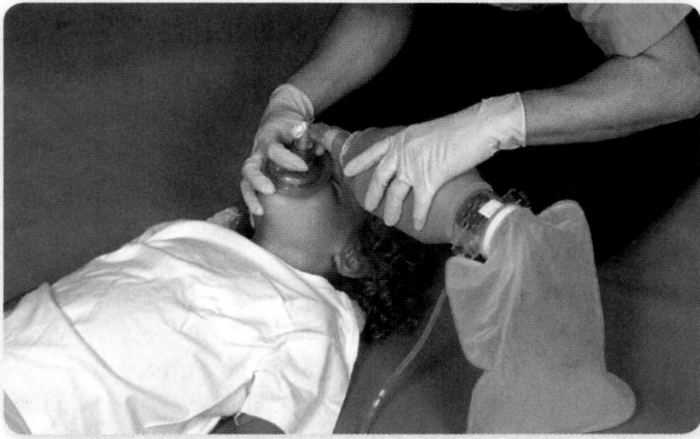

Figure 36-25 Proper mask size for bag-mask ventilation is critical. The mask should extend from the bridge of the nose to the cleft of the chin, avoiding compression of the eyes.

Errors in technique, including providing too much volume with each breath, squeezing the bag too forcefully, or ventilating at too fast a rate, can result in gastric distention or a pneumothorax. Even with the best technique, however, the patient may regurgitate and aspirate the contents of his or her stomach. An inadequate mask-to-face seal or improper head position can lead to inadequately delivered tidal volume and hypoxia.

One-Person Bag-Mask Device Ventilation. Perform one-person bag-mask ventilation in an infant or child according to the steps in **Skill Drill 36-4**. Ensure a good mask-to-face seal while maintaining the airway by forming a *C* with the thumb and index finger along the mask while the other three fingers form an *E* along the mandible. With infants and toddlers, support the jaw with only your third fingertip. Be careful not to compress the area under the chin because you may push the tongue into the back of the mouth and block the airway. Keep your fingers on the mandible.

Words of Wisdom

To use the EC clamp technique, form a *C* with the thumb and index finger along the mask while the other three fingers form an *E* along the mandible. With infants and toddlers, support the jaw with only your third fingertip. Be careful not to compress the area under the chin because you may push the tongue into the back of the mouth and block the airway. Keep fingers on the mandible.

Two-Person Bag-Mask Device Ventilation. This procedure is similar to one-person ventilation except that it requires two AEMTs, one to maintain an adequate mask-to-face seal and maintain the patient's head position and the other to ventilate the patient. This technique is usually more effective in maintaining a tight seal. Because it is not possible to perform a one-handed jaw-thrust maneuver and also maintain spinal immobilization, ventilating the trauma patient is a two-person skill.

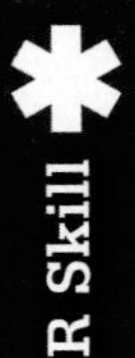

Skill Drill 36-4 One-Person Bag-Mask Device Ventilation on a Pediatric Patient

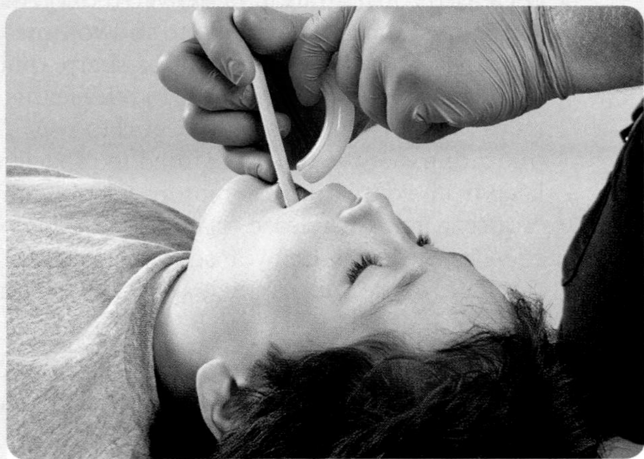

Step 1 Open the airway and insert the appropriate airway adjunct.

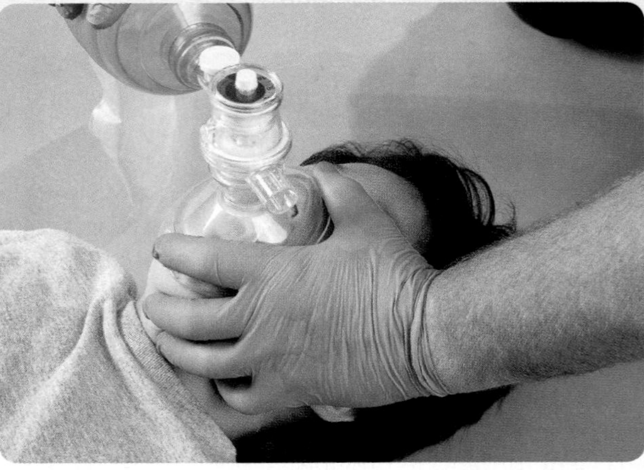

Step 2 Hold the mask on the pediatric patient's face with a one-handed head tilt–chin lift maneuver (EC clamp technique). Ensure a good mask-to-face seal while maintaining the airway.

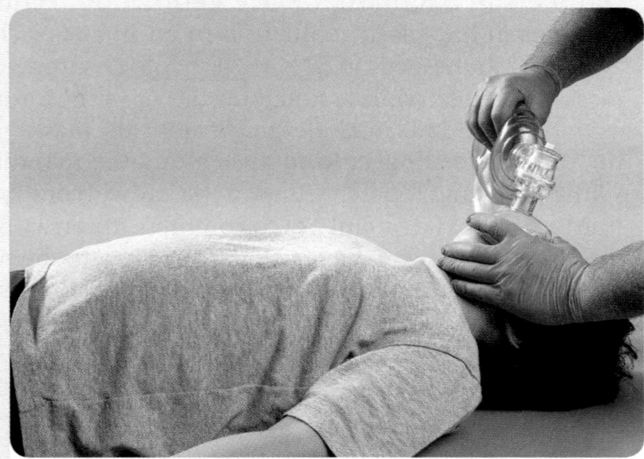

Step 3 Squeeze the bag using the correct ventilation rate of 1 breath every 3 to 5 seconds, or 12 to 20 breaths/min. Allow adequate time for exhalation.

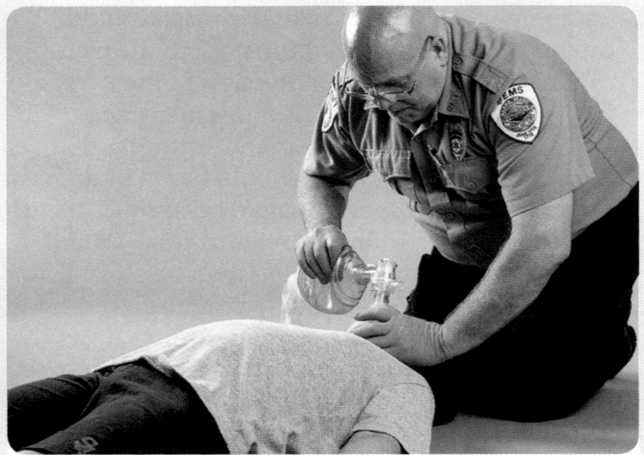

Step 4 Assess the effectiveness of the ventilation by watching for adequate bilateral rise and fall of the chest.

Cardiopulmonary Arrest

Cardiopulmonary arrest in infants and children is most often associated with respiratory failure and respiratory arrest. Children are affected differently than adults when it comes to decreasing oxygen concentrations. An adult becomes hypoxic and the heart gets irritable, and sudden cardiac death occurs from a dysrhythmia. This is often in the form of ventricular fibrillation and is the reason that an automated external defibrillator (AED) is the treatment of choice. A child, however, becomes hypoxic and the heart slows down, becoming more and more bradycardic. The heart will beat slower and become weaker with each beat until no pulse is felt. The overall survival rate from cardiac arrest in the prehospital setting in children is low, with infants having a much worse prognosis than children or adolescents. Approximately 8% of children survive.[11] Many of those who do survive have permanent brain injury as a result of the arrest. However, the survival rate from only respiratory arrest is 75% to 93%.[12] Therefore, a child who is breathing poorly with a slowing heart rate must be ventilated with high concentrations of oxygen early to try to oxygenate the heart and avoid the development of cardiac arrest. Chapter 15, *BLS Resuscitation*, covers providing CPR to pediatric patients in detail.

The signs, symptoms, and treatment of shock and cardiopulmonary arrest were discussed in other chapters. The following section will address methods of maintaining and improving circulation in the infant or child, including vascular access (IV and IO), and IV fluid resuscitation.

Assessment and Management of Circulation Emergencies

Pediatric patients have a larger proportional amount of circulating blood volume than adults, but are more dependent on the actual cardiac output than adults. A pediatric patient may actually be in a state of shock while displaying a normal blood pressure. Infants and children have less circulating blood volume than adults do, so the loss of even a small amount of fluid or blood may result in shock.

▶ Shock

Shock, as discussed in Chapter 14, *Shock*, is a condition that develops when the circulatory system is unable to deliver a sufficient amount of blood to the organs of the body. Shock can result in pediatric cardiac arrest. Although data regarding prehospital pediatric arrest are limited, just as with the adult, early recognition and prompt intervention can prevent permanent disability or death.[13]

Compared with adults, children can compensate for shock for longer periods of time, maintaining adequate perfusion because of vasoconstriction. However, when hypotension occurs, it does so quickly and unpredictably and may result in rapid deterioration to cardiopulmonary arrest.

Common causes of shock in the pediatric population include hypovolemia (from trauma or illness) and sepsis. Although less common, allergic reactions and poisonings can result in shock. Shock from a primary cardiac event is rare in infants and children.

Greater than 25% blood volume loss significantly increases the risk of shock in children.[14] Signs of shock in children are as follows:

- Tachycardia
- Poor capillary refill (>2 seconds)
- Mental status changes

For comparison, signs of shock in adults are:

- Tachycardia
- Hypotension
- Mental status changes

Blood volume loss greater than 30% to 40% significantly increases risk of shock in adults.[15]

Begin treating shock by assessing the ABCDEs, intervening immediately as required; do not wait until you have performed the complete assessment to take action. If cardiac arrest is suspected, the order becomes CABDE (compressions, airway, breathing, disability, exposure) because compressions are essential. Pediatric patients in shock often have increased respirations but do not demonstrate a decrease in blood pressure until shock is severe.

In assessing circulation, you should pay particular attention to the following:

- **Pulse.** Assess both the rate and the quality of the pulse. A weak, "thready" pulse is a sign that a problem exists. The appropriate rate depends on age; a rate of more than 160 beats/min suggests shock.
- **Skin signs.** Assess the temperature and moisture of the hands and feet. How does this compare with the temperature of the skin on the trunk of the body? Is the skin dry and warm, or cold and clammy?
- **Capillary refill time.** Does the fingertip return to its normal color within 2 seconds, or is it delayed?
- **Color.** Assess the patient's skin color. Is it pink, pale, ashen, or blue?
- **Changes.** Changes in pulse rate, skin signs, capillary refill time, and color are all important clues suggesting shock.

Blood pressure is the most difficult vital sign to measure in younger pediatric patients. The cuff must be the proper size—two-thirds the length of the upper arm. The value for normal blood pressure is also age specific. Remember that blood pressure may be normal in a patient with compensated shock. Low blood pressure is a sign of decompensated shock, requiring oxygenation, fluid administration, and immediate transport.

Part of your assessment should also include talking with the parents or caregivers to determine when the signs and symptoms first appeared and whether any of the following has occurred:

- Decrease in urine output (with infants, are there fewer than 6 to 10 wet diapers?)
- Absence of tears, even when the child is crying
- A sunken or depressed fontanelle (infant patient)
- Changes in level of consciousness and behavior

Limit your management to these simple interventions. Time should not be wasted performing field procedures. Ensure that the airway is open, prepare for artificial ventilation; control bleeding; and give supplemental oxygen by mask or blow-by method as tolerated. Continue to monitor airway and breathing. Position the pediatric patient in a position of comfort determined by local protocol. Keep the pediatric patient warm with blankets and by turning up the heat in the patient compartment. Unless it is absolutely critical, time-consuming procedures (ie, IV, IO access) should be performed en route. Establish vascular access and administer normal saline or 20-mL/kg boluses of lactated Ringer solution as needed to maintain adequate perfusion. After each fluid bolus, reassess the child; several fluid boluses are often needed in children with severe hypovolemia. Provide immediate transport to the nearest appropriate facility and continue monitoring vital signs en route. Contact paramedic backup as needed. Allow a parent or caregiver to accompany the pediatric patient whenever possible.

Special Populations

You should carefully assess any infant or child suspected of being in a state of shock. At first, the signs and symptoms may be subtle and hard to detect. A thorough assessment and history and a keen eye will enable you to recognize shock in its earliest stages.

Anaphylactic Shock

Anaphylaxis is a major allergic reaction that involves a generalized, multisystem response to an antigen (foreign substance). The airway and cardiovascular system are important sites of this potentially life-threatening reaction. Common causes are insect stings, medications, or food.

Words of Wisdom

Shock in children is most likely caused by hypovolemia. Fluid resuscitation with an isotonic crystalloid solution is the mainstay of treatment. Do not waste time with multiple IV insertion attempts when caring for a child in decompensated shock from hypovolemia. Insert an IO needle and begin fluid therapy.

A pediatric patient in anaphylactic shock will have hypoperfusion as well as additional signs such as stridor and/or wheezing, with increased work of breathing. The pediatric patient will also have an altered appearance with restlessness, agitation, and sometimes a sense of impending doom. Hives, an intensely itchy skin rash, are usually present.

Maintain the airway and administer oxygen via a route that is tolerated. If the child is stable, allow the parent or caregiver to assist in the positioning of the patient, oxygen delivery, and keeping the child calm. Increased agitation and crying, combined with an increased work of breathing, may lead to increased bronchoconstriction. Based on local protocol, assist the parent or caregiver with administering a prescribed epinephrine auto-injector, if available. Transport promptly.

If anaphylactic shock is present, administer epinephrine subcutaneously or via auto injector. Obtain IV or IO access for fluid resuscitation and administer 20 mL/kg of an isotonic crystalloid solution to maintain perfusion. Administer oxygen as needed. Call early for paramedic backup if advanced airway management is anticipated.

Special Populations

Remember, bradycardia in infants and children is almost always the result of severe hypoxia. Provide ventilatory assistance with 100% oxygen. The most common cause of tachycardia in an infant or young child is from fever, dehydration, or pain.

▶ Bleeding Disorders

Hemophilia is a congenital condition in which the patient lacks one or more of the normal clotting factors of blood. There are several forms of hemophilia, most of which are hereditary and some of which are severe. Hemophilia is found predominantly in males. Sometimes bleeding may occur spontaneously. Because the hemophiliac patient's blood does not clot, all injuries, no matter how minor, are potentially serious. Transport a child with hemophilia immediately, and do not delay tourniquet application for life-threatening hemorrhage.

▶ Intravenous Access

Although IV therapy is not performed as frequently in children as it is in adults, the technique, indications, and contraindications in the infant and child are the same as they are for adults. In addition, the same IV solutions and equipment used for adults can be used for pediatric patients (discussed in Chapter 13, *Vascular Access and Medication Administration*), with a few exceptions.

Words of Wisdom

Helpful tips for vascular access:

- Make sure all equipment is prepared and within easy reach prior to attempting IV access.
- Explain what you are doing and allow the child to see the equipment.
- Wrap the child in a blanket (or consider heat packs) to encourage vasodilation and make veins easier to feel.
- Allow the extremity to hang down and pat or rub the area.
- Take care when using a tourniquet on infants. Often, another provider holding gentle pressure around an extremity is sufficient.
- After two unsuccessful attempts, ask your partner to try.
- In a critical patient, do not waste time trying multiple IV attempts. Instead, insert an IO line.

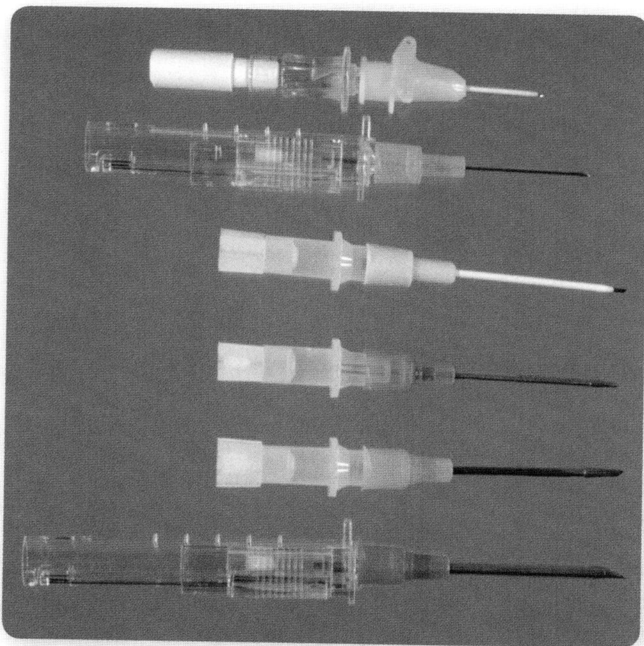

Figure 36-26 Note the difference in sizes of intravenous catheters.

Catheters

If you are using an over-the-needle catheter ("angiocath") to start a pediatric IV, the 20-, 22-, 24-, and 26-gauge catheters are best for insertion Figure 36-26. Butterfly catheters are useful for pediatric patients and can be placed in the same locations as over-the-needle catheters and in visible scalp veins in infants. However, butterfly catheters are associated with a higher rate of infiltration because a stainless steel needle lies in the vein, instead of the Teflon catheter or an over-the-needle catheter.

Administration Sets

Fluid control for pediatric patients is important. Using a special type of microdrip set called a **Volutrol** (also called Buretrol) allows you to fill the large drip chamber with a specific amount of fluid and administer only this amount to avoid fluid overload. The 100-mL calibrated drip chamber on the Volutrol can be shut off from the IV bag.

If your EMS system does not use the Volutrol, a regular microdrip administration set can be used; however, use caution when administering fluid through these administration sets.

IV Locations

When starting IV access, take both the child and the parent or caregiver into consideration. The parent can become as stressed as the child. If the condition of the child permits, take time to thoroughly explain the procedure to both the child and the parent or caregiver. When possible, allow the infant or child to sit on the parent's or caregiver's lap when starting IV access.

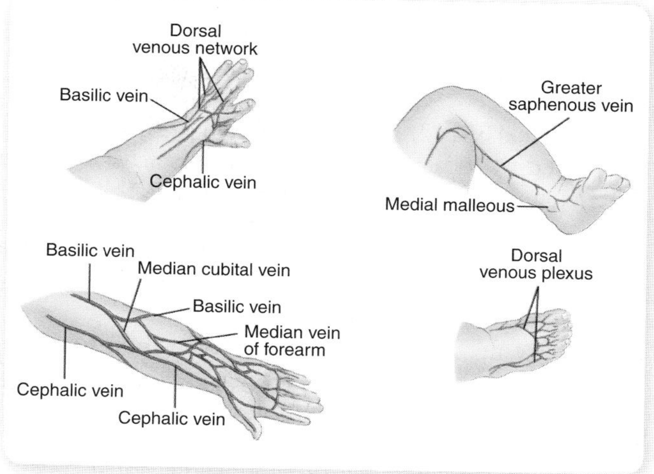

Figure 36-27 Sites for intravenous lines in infants and children are the hands, antecubital fossa, the saphenous veins at the ankle, and the feet.

The younger the child, the fewer choices you have for IV sites. Hand veins are painful and difficult to manage in younger children; however, they remain the location of choice for starting peripheral IV lines.

Protecting the IV site after it has been established is critical and is sometimes best accomplished by immobilizing the site with an arm board before cannulation. One of the better techniques for starting pediatric IV lines is to use a penlight to illuminate the veins on the back of the hand. Shine the light through the palm side of the hand to illuminate the veins on the dorsal aspect of the hand. After a suitable site is located, mark the vein with a pen so you can find the location after you turn off the penlight. Proceed with obtaining IV access, using the mark you created as a guide. Sometimes the best choice is an antecubital vein, especially if the child is critically ill or injured and needs fluid resuscitation or medication therapy. Figure 36-27 illustrates the different sites for starting IV lines in infants and children.

Special Populations

Most pediatric patients do not require prehospital IV therapy. Do not start an IV line in an infant or child unless it is absolutely necessary (for example, severe shock or hypoglycemia). Remember that unnecessarily agitating a child can exacerbate the child's condition, especially if he or she is already hypoxic.

▶ Intraosseous Access

Intraosseous (IO) infusion is used for emergency vascular access in pediatric patients as defined by protocol when immediate IV access is difficult or impossible. When placed correctly, the IO needle will rest in the **medullary canal**, the space within the bone that contains bone marrow. IO access should be attempted immediately if you are unable to obtain IV access.[16] A general guideline is to attempt IO access if IV access is not successful within three attempts *or* 90 seconds in a critically ill or injured pediatric patient as allowed by local protocols. Often these children are experiencing a life-threatening situation such as cardiac arrest, status epilepticus, or progressive shock. An IO infusion is contraindicated if a secure IV line is available or if a possible fracture exists in the same bone in which you plan to insert the IO needle.

The IO needle is usually inserted in the proximal tibia with a special IO needle Figure 36-28. Products that may be used include the FAST1, the EZ-IO, and the Bone Injection Gun (BIG). A commonly used IO catheter is the **Jamshidi needle**. This double needle, consisting of a solid-bore needle inside a sharpened hollow needle, is pushed into the bone with a screwing, twisting action. After the needle pops through the bone, the solid needle is removed, leaving the hollow steel needle in place. Standard IV tubing is then attached to this catheter.

Anything that can be administered intravenously can be administered through an IO line (such as isotonic fluids and medications). The IO lines require full and careful stabilization because they rest at a 90° angle to the bone and are easily dislodged. Stabilization is critical for these lines to maintain adequate flow. Stabilize the IO needle in the same manner that you would any impaled object. Follow the steps in Skill Drill 36-5 to establish an IO infusion in the pediatric patient. Before you begin, remember to look for any discoloration or particles floating in the IV fluid. If found, discard and choose another bag of fluid. Also, keep in mind it is possible to fracture the bone during insertion of the IO. If this happens, you should remove the IO needle and switch to the other leg.

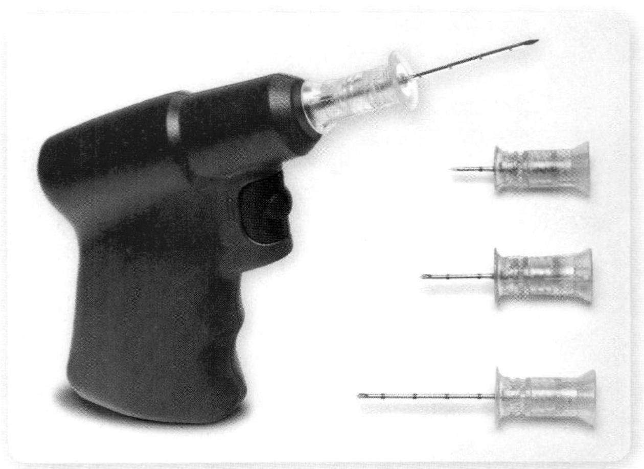

Figure 36-28 Standard pediatric intraosseous needles.

As with any invasive procedure, there are potential complications with IO infusion that you must be aware of.

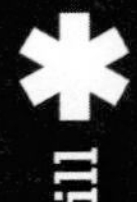

NR Skill

Skill Drill 36-5 Pediatric IO Access and Infusion

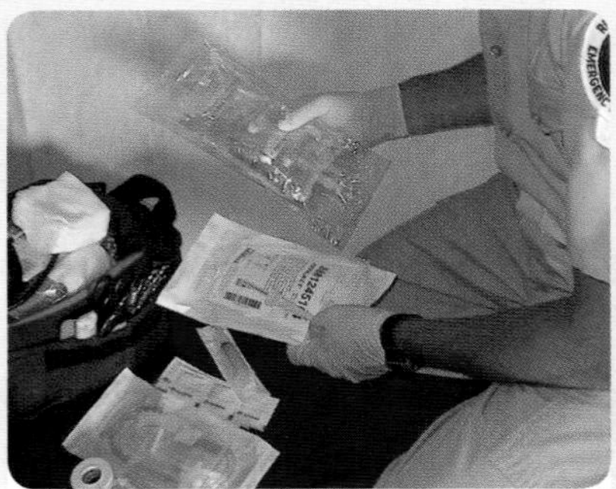

Step 1 Ensure you have selected the proper IV fluid. Check for clarity and expiration date. Select the appropriate equipment, including an IO needle, syringe, saline, and extension set. A three-way stopcock may also be used to facilitate easier fluid administration.

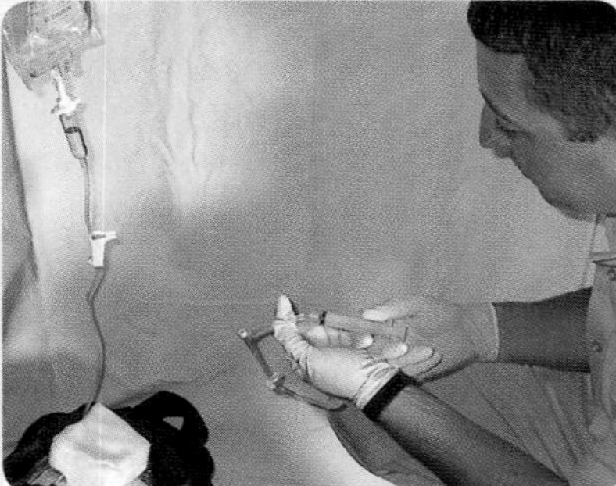

Step 2 Select the proper administration set. Connect the administration set to the bag. Prepare the administration set. Fill the drip chamber and flush the tubing. Make sure all air bubbles are removed from the tubing. Prepare the syringe and extension tubing.

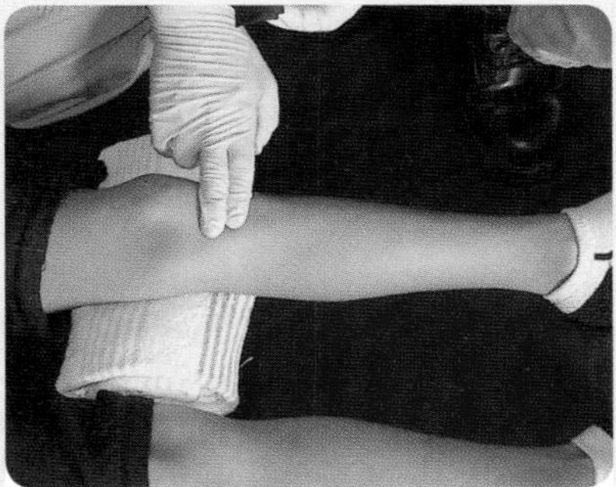

Step 3 Cut or tear the tape. Follow standard precautions (this must be done before IO puncture). Identify the proper anatomic site for IO puncture. To miss the epiphyseal (growth) plate, you should measure two fingerbreadths below the knee on the medial side of the leg.

Skill Drill 36-5 Pediatric IO Access and Infusion *(continued)*

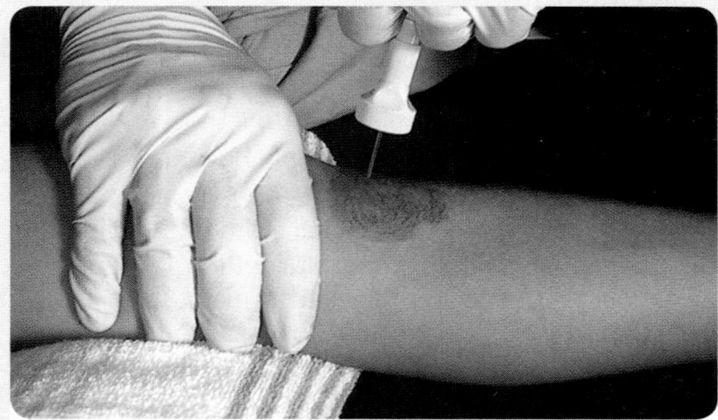

Step 4 Cleanse the site appropriately. Perform the IO puncture as follows: Stabilize the tibia. Place a folded towel underneath the knee and hold in such a manner as to keep your fingers away from the site of puncture. Insert the needle at a 90° angle to the leg. Advance the needle with a twisting motion until a "pop" is felt.

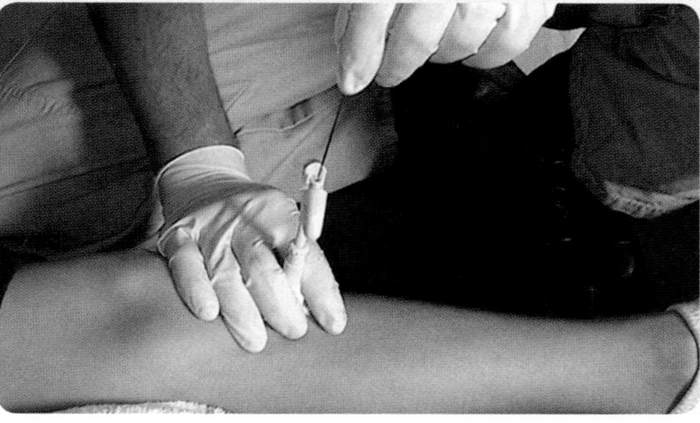

Step 5 Unscrew the cap, and remove the stylet from the needle.

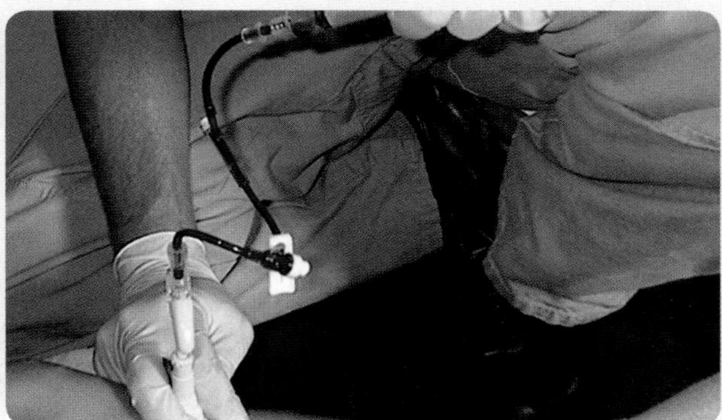

Step 6 Attach the syringe and extension set to the IO needle. Pull back on the syringe to aspirate blood and particles of bone marrow to ensure placement. Slowly inject saline to ensure proper placement of the needle. Watch for infiltration, and stop the infusion immediately if noted. Connect the administration set, and adjust the flow rate as appropriate. Fluid does not flow well through an IO needle, and boluses are given by administering the fluid using the syringe.

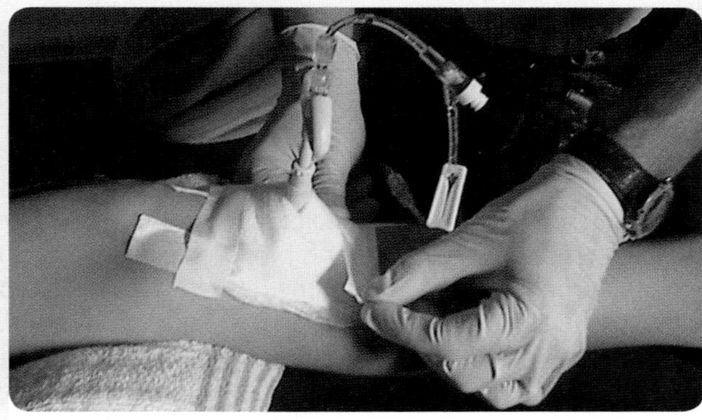

Step 7 Secure the needle with tape, and support it with a bulky dressing. Stabilize in place in the same manner that an impaled object is stabilized. Dispose of the needle in the proper container.

With proper technique, the following potential complications may be avoided:

- Compartment syndrome
- Failed infusion
- Growth plate injury
- Bone and muscle inflammation caused by infection (**osteomyelitis**)
- Skin infection
- Bony fracture

▶ Fluid Resuscitation

As previously mentioned, appropriate fluid administration in the pediatric patient is crucial; IV fluids must be administered based on the child's clinical condition. If too much fluid is administered, overload can result and cause acute left-side heart failure and pulmonary edema. Conversely, administering insufficient fluid volumes will not be effective in treating the child's condition.

> **Words of Wisdom**
>
> Remember to ask the parent or caregiver how much the child weighs and then convert the weight in pounds to kilograms. If the weight of the child is unknown, use the following formula to estimate the weight in kilograms:
>
> $$(\text{Age [in years]} \times 2) + 8 = \text{Weight in kilograms}$$
>
> When administering IV fluids, it is crucial to obtain as accurate an estimate of the child's weight as possible.

Fluid resuscitation for the infant or child in hypovolemic shock begins with an initial bolus of 20 mL/kg of an isotonic crystalloid solution (for example, normal saline, lactated Ringer solution), followed by a careful reassessment. Administer further boluses of 20 mL/kg as needed to maintain adequate perfusion.

In children who require multiple IV fluid boluses, you should carefully and frequently assess their breath sounds, noting signs of pulmonary edema (for example, rales, rhonchi).

> **Words of Wisdom**
>
> Because most cases of cardiopulmonary arrest in infants and children are related to respiratory failure, oxygen is the most common medication that you will administer to them in the prehospital setting. Most pediatric emergencies can be managed by maintaining a patent airway, administering 100% oxygen, and transporting to the hospital.

Assessment and Management of Neurologic Emergencies

There are several causes of altered mental status in children. Some of the most common causes are hypoglycemia, hypoxia, seizure, and drug or alcohol ingestion. The parent

YOU are the Provider — PART 4

After diluting dextrose 50% (D_{50}) into dextrose 10% (D_{10}), you estimate the patient's weight at 18 kg (39 lb). Your protocols state that for hypoglycemia in a child older than 1 year, the beginning dosage of D_{10} is 0.5 to 1 g/kg via slow IV push. You elect to start at the 0.5-g/kg dose, and prepare 90 mL of D_{10}. You briefly run the IV line wide open for 2 to 3 seconds to ensure patency, and then slowly administer the desired dose of dextrose. After approximately 60 seconds, you recheck the patient's blood glucose level and find that it has increased to 134 mg/dL. You also note that the patient is beginning to take gasping breaths on her own, as well as have some movement in her extremities. After confirming that the patient is now beginning to breathe adequately, you direct your partner to stop ventilations, and place the patient on a nonrebreathing mask at 15 L/min. You contact the receiving hospital and inform them of the patient's condition and your 8-minute estimated time of arrival. Approximately 4 minutes later, the patient is responsive, alert and oriented, and crying for her mother. In an effort to calm the patient, you ask your partner to pull over to the side of the road, so that you can have the mother come to the back of the ambulance. After the patient's mother is in the back of the ambulance, you ensure that she is properly secured on the bench seat, and she consoles her daughter. You then ask the driver to resume transport to the hospital, now in nonemergency mode. On your arrival at the ED, you turn over care to the awaiting nurse.

Recording Time: 24 Minutes	
Respirations	30 breaths/min
Pulse	130 beats/min
Skin	Warm, dry, and pink
Blood pressure	90 mm Hg—palpated
Oxygen saturation (Spo_2)	99% on 15 L/min
Pupils	Pupils Equal, Round, and Reactive to Light and Accommodation (PERRLA)

8. What are the indications and contraindications for dextrose administration in pediatric patients?
9. If this patient should require IV fluid, how much fluid should she receive?

or caregiver is an important resource for you when you are gathering information regarding the baseline neurologic status of the pediatric patient. A child with altered mental status may appear sleepy, lethargic, combative, or even unresponsive to tactile stimulus. Be diligent about assessing and managing the airway because pediatric patients may be susceptible to airway obstructions from their large tongues.

Altered Mental Status

People who are aware of themselves and their surroundings are said to be responsive. Nonverbal infants may demonstrate responsiveness by following a person's face or an object (tracking), by babbling and cooing, or by crying. Infants and children may exhibit an altered mental status in many ways, including lack of response to vocal commands and pain, combative behavior, confusion, thrashing about, drifting into and out of an alert state, or a change in the pitch and nature of their cry.

The mnemonic AEIOU-TIPS, discussed in Chapter 19, *Neurologic Emergencies*, reflects the major causes of altered mental status.

Words of Wisdom

Always check the glucose level in any patient with an altered mental status.

The signs and symptoms of altered mental status vary widely from simple confusion to coma. Management of altered mental status focuses on the ABCs and transport. If the pediatric patient's level of consciousness is low, then the child may not be able to protect his or her airway. Ensure a patent airway and adequate breathing through a nonrebreathing mask or a bag-mask device. Pediatric patients with an altered level of consciousness may have inadequate breathing despite spontaneous respiratory effort, based on an inadequate respiratory rate or inadequate tidal volume. Transport to the hospital.

Seizures

A seizure is the result of disorganized electrical activity in the brain. It can be frightening to witness a seizure in a pediatric patient. Therefore, it is important to reassure the family and to approach assessment and management in a calm, step-by-step manner. Common causes of seizures in children include:

- Child abuse
- Electrolyte imbalance
- Fever
- Hypoglycemia (low blood glucose level)
- Infection
- Ingestion
- Hypoxia
- Medications
- Poisoning
- Seizure disorder
- Recreational drug use
- Head trauma
- Idiopathic (no cause can be found)

Seizures in children may appear in several different ways, depending on the age of the child. Seizures in infants can be extremely subtle, consisting only of an abnormal gaze, sucking motions, or "bicycling" motions. In older children, seizures are more obvious and typically consist of repetitive muscle contractions and unresponsiveness.

After a seizure has stopped, the patient's muscles relax, becoming almost flaccid, or floppy, and the breathing becomes labored (fast and deep). This is the postictal state. The longer and more intense the seizure is, the longer it will take for this imbalance to correct itself. Likewise, longer and more severe seizures will result in longer postictal unresponsiveness and confusion. When the pediatric patient regains a normal level of consciousness, the postictal state is over.

Seizures that continue every few minutes without regaining consciousness or last longer than 30 minutes are referred to as status epilepticus. Recurring or prolonged seizures should be considered potentially life-threatening situations in which pediatric patients need emergency medical care. If the pediatric patient remains unresponsive or continues to seize, protect the pediatric patient from harming himself or herself and call for paramedic backup. These pediatric patients need advanced airway management and medication to stop the seizure.

Securing and protecting the airway are your priorities. Position the head to open the airway. Clear the mouth with suction. Consider placing the pediatric patient in the recovery position if the child is actively vomiting and suction is inadequate to control the airway **Figure 36-29**. Provide 100% oxygen by nonrebreathing mask or blow-by method. If there are no signs of improvement, begin bag-mask device ventilation with

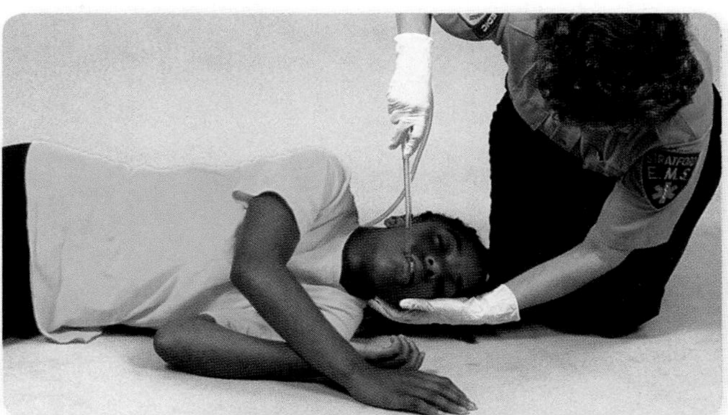

Figure 36-29 In a child having a seizure, position the head to open the airway and clear the airway with suction. Consider placing the patient in the recovery position if the patient is actively vomiting and suction is inadequate to control the airway.

appropriate-size equipment with supplemental oxygen. Transport the pediatric patient to the appropriate facility.

Febrile Seizures

Febrile seizures are caused by an abrupt rise in body temperature and occur in approximately 2% to 4% of children younger than 5 years.[17] Most pediatric seizures are caused by fever alone, which is why they are called febrile seizures.

These seizures typically occur on the first day of a febrile illness, are characterized by generalized **tonic-clonic seizure** activity, and last less than 15 minutes with a short postictal phase or none at all. The seizures may be a sign of a more serious problem, such as meningitis. Obtain a history from the caregivers because these children may have had a febrile seizure in the past.

> **Words of Wisdom**
>
> A febrile seizure is caused by an abrupt rise in body temperature. It is not necessarily how high the fever gets, but how quickly it gets there.

If you are called to care for a child who has had a febrile seizure, you often will find that the patient is awake, alert, and fully interactive when you arrive. Keep in mind that a persistent fever can result in another seizure. Carefully assess the ABCDEs, begin cooling measures with tepid (not cold) water, and provide prompt transport; all children with febrile seizures need to be seen in the hospital setting **Figure 36-30**.

Establish IV or IO access and obtain a blood glucose reading, and administer glucose if the child is hypoglycemic.

▶ Meningitis

Meningitis is an inflammation of the tissues, called the meninges, that cover the spinal cord and brain. It is caused by an infection by bacteria, viruses, fungi, or parasites. If left untreated, meningitis can result in permanent brain damage or death. The ability to recognize a patient who may have meningitis is an important skill for AEMTs to have.

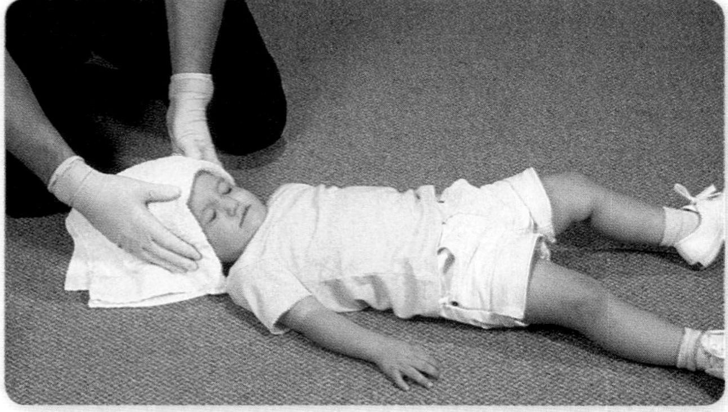

Figure 36-30 Following a febrile seizure, carefully assess the child's airway, breathing, circulation, disability, and exposure (ABCDEs). Then begin cooling measures and prepare the child for transport.

Meningitis can occur in both children and adults, but some people are at greater risk than others, as follows:[18,19]

- Males
- Newborn infants
- Geriatric patients
- Those with a prior history of meningitis
- Those living in crowded conditions such as in camps, day care centers, schools, and college dormitories
- Children who have not received proper immunizations
- Those with compromised immune systems (such as HIV/AIDS or cancer) or a nonfunctioning spleen
- Those who have sustained head trauma or undergone brain surgery
- Those with shunts, pins, or other foreign bodies within their brain or spinal cord

At especially high risk are children with a ventriculoperitoneal (VP) shunt. VP shunts drain excess fluids from around the brain into the abdomen. These children with special needs have tubing that can usually be seen and felt just under the scalp.

The signs and symptoms of meningitis vary, depending on the age of the patient. Fever, headache, and altered level of consciousness are common symptoms of meningitis in patients of all ages. Changes in level of consciousness can range from a mild or severe headache to confusion, lethargy, and/or an inability to understand commands or interact appropriately. The child may also experience a seizure, which may be a first sign of meningitis. Infants younger than 2 to 3 months can have apnea, cyanosis, fever, a distinct high-pitched cry, or hypothermia.

In describing children with meningitis, physicians often use the term *meningeal irritation* or *meningeal signs* to describe pain that accompanies movement. Bending the neck forward or back increases the tension within the spinal canal and stretches the meninges, causing a great deal of pain (**nuchal rigidity**). This results in the characteristic stiff neck of children with meningitis, who will often refuse to move their neck, lift their legs, or curl into a "C" position, even if coached to do so. One sign of meningitis in an infant is increasing irritability, especially when being handled. Another sign is a bulging fontanelle without crying.

One form of meningitis deserves special attention. ***Neisseria meningitidis*** is a bacterium that causes a rapid onset of meningitis symptoms, often leading to shock and death. Children with *N meningitidis* typically have small, pinpoint, cherry-red spots or a larger purple or black rash **Figure 36-31**. This rash may be on part of the face or body. These children are at serious risk of sepsis, shock, and death.

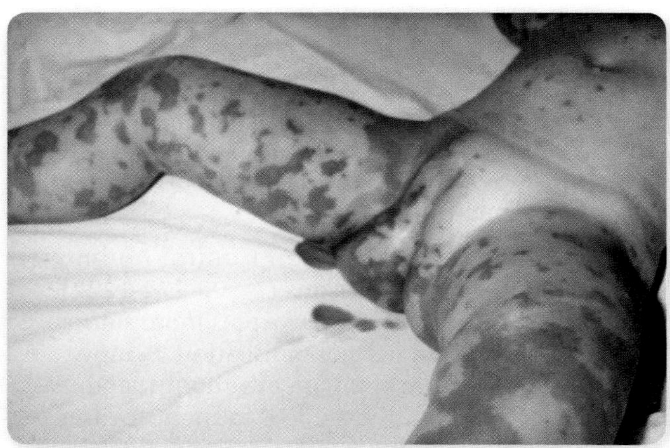

Figure 36-31 Children with *Neisseria meningitidis* typically have small, pinpoint, cherry-red spots or a larger purple or black rash.

Courtesy of Ronald Dieckmann, MD.

All patients with possible meningitis should be considered highly contagious. Therefore, follow standard precautions whenever you suspect meningitis and follow up with the hospital to learn the patient's final diagnosis. If you have been exposed to saliva and respiratory secretions from a child with *N meningitidis*, you should receive antibiotics to protect yourself and others from the bacteria. This is particularly true if you managed the patient's airway. If you were not in close contact with the pediatric patient or his or her respiratory secretions, you do not need treatment.

Provide these pediatric patients with supplemental oxygen and assist with ventilations if necessary. Reassess the child's vital signs frequently as you transport the patient to the highest level of service available. If the patient's vital signs are unstable, obtain vascular access and administer IV fluids as needed to maintain adequate perfusion.

Safety Tips

Some forms of meningitis are highly contagious. Use standard precautions whenever you suspect meningitis, including mask and eye protection when there is coughing, sneezing, or any other possibility of contact with the patient's respiratory secretions. Local protocols may also call for putting a mask on the patient.

Assessment and Management of Gastrointestinal Emergencies

As with any injury or complaint in the abdominal region, the signs and symptoms of a gastrointestinal emergency may be vague in nature. The abdominal wall muscles are not as developed, which leaves this region more susceptible to injury. Pediatric patients may not be able to pinpoint the exact site where the pain or discomfort originates, but will have complaints of diffuse tenderness. Never take a complaint of abdominal pain and discomfort lightly because a large amount of bleeding may occur within the abdominal cavity without any outward signs of shock. Remember that liver and splenic injuries are common in this age group and may result in life-threatening emergencies. The pediatric patient needs to be monitored for signs and symptoms of shock, which include an altered mental status; pale, cool skin; tachypnea; tachycardia; and bradycardia (late sign).

A common source of gastrointestinal upset is the ingestion of certain foods, such as milk or ice cream (lactose intolerance), or unknown substances. In most cases, you will be faced with a pediatric patient who is experiencing abdominal discomfort with nausea, vomiting, and/or diarrhea. This can become a concern because both vomiting and diarrhea can cause dehydration in children.

Appendicitis is also common in pediatric patients, and if untreated can result in peritonitis (inflammation of the peritoneum, which lines the abdominal cavity) or shock. Pediatric patients with appendicitis will typically present with a fever and pain on palpation of the right lower abdominal quadrant. Rebound tenderness is a common sign associated with appendicitis. Remember that constipation also can be a cause of abdominal pain in children. If you suspect appendicitis, immediately transport the pediatric patient to the hospital for further evaluation.

Because the pediatric population is sensitive to fluid loss, obtain a thorough history from the parent or primary caregiver. In particular, ask questions such as:

- How many wet diapers has the child had today?
- Is your child tolerating liquids, and is he or she able to keep them down?
- How many times has your child had diarrhea and for how long?
- Are tears present when your child cries?

These questions can help to determine just how dehydrated the pediatric patient may be. If the pediatric patient is dehydrated, transport to the hospital for further care.

Assessment and Management of Toxicologic Emergencies

Poisoning is common among children. It can occur by ingesting, inhaling, injecting, or absorbing a toxic substance. Common sources of poisoning in children include:

- Alcohol
- Aspirin, acetaminophen
- Household cleaning products (such as bleach and furniture polish)
- Houseplants
- Iron
- Prescription medications

- Illicit (street) drugs (such as crack, cocaine, or phencyclidine [PCP])
- Vitamins

The signs and symptoms of poisoning vary widely, depending on the substance and the age and weight of the child. The pediatric patient may appear normal at first, even in serious cases, or he or she may be confused, sleepy, or unresponsive.

Infants may be poisoned as a result of being fed a harmful substance by a sibling, parent, or caregiver, or as a result of child abuse. Infants can be exposed to drugs and poisons left on floors and carpeting. They can also be exposed in a room or automobile in which harmful and illicit drugs such as cigarettes, crack, cocaine, or PCP are being smoked. Toddlers are curious and often ingest poisons when they find them in the home or garage Figure 36-32. For example, some people store petroleum products in soda bottles. Toddlers may believe the substance to be soda. Adolescents are more likely to have ingested alcohol and street drugs while at parties or during a suicide attempt.

After you have completed your primary survey and addressed any immediate life threats, you should ask the caregiver the following questions:

- What is the substance(s) involved?
- Approximately how much of the substance was ingested or involved in the exposure (eg, number of pills, amount of liquid)?
- What time did the incident occur?

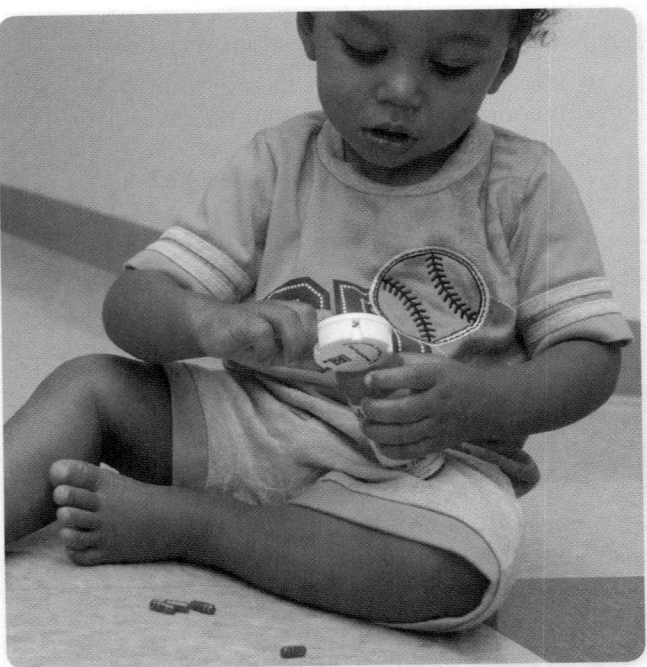

Figure 36-32 A curious child will try to taste or swallow almost any substance. A common victim of accidental ingestion of dangerous compounds is the unwatched toddler.

- Has the child vomited?
- How much does the child weigh?
- Are there any changes in behavior or level of consciousness?
- Was there any choking or coughing after the exposure? (These can be signs of airway involvement.)

Contact the national Poison Control hotline for assistance in identifying poisons (1-800-222-1222). To treat a pediatric patient exposed to a poisonous substance, first perform an external decontamination. Remove tablets or fragments from the patient's mouth, and wash or brush poison from the skin. Treatment focuses on support: maintaining the pediatric patient's ABCs and monitoring breathing. Provide oxygen and perform ventilations if necessary. If the patient demonstrates signs and symptoms of shock, position the child supine, keep the child warm, and transport promptly to the nearest appropriate hospital.

In some cases, you will give activated charcoal to pediatric patients who have ingested poison, if approved by medical control or local protocol. Activated charcoal is not indicated for pediatric patients who have ingested an acid, an alkali, or a petroleum product; who have a decreased level of consciousness and cannot protect their airway; or who are unable to swallow. If local protocol permits, you will likely carry plastic bottles of premixed suspension, each containing up to 50 g of activated charcoal. Some common trade names for the suspension form are Insta-Char, Actidose, and LiquiChar. The usual dose for a child is 0.5 to 1 g of activated charcoal per kilogram of body weight. The usual pediatric dose is 12.5 to 25 g for small children and 25 to 50 g for larger children.[20] Chapter 23, *Toxicology*, discusses the administration of activated charcoal in detail.

Words of Wisdom

Have the American Association of Poison Control Centers number (1-800-222-1222) handy for suspected poisonings.[21] This free service is available 24 hours a day, 7 days a week.

Assessment and Management of Dehydration Emergencies

Dehydration occurs when fluid losses are greater than fluid intake. The most common cause of dehydration in children is vomiting and diarrhea. If left untreated, dehydration can lead to shock and eventually death. Infants and children are at greater risk than adults for dehydration because their fluid reserves are smaller than those in adults. Life-threatening dehydration can overcome an infant in a matter of hours.

Table 36-12 Vital Signs and Symptoms of Dehydration

	Mild Dehydration	Moderate Dehydration	Severe Dehydration
Pulse	Normal	Increased	Increased; >160 beats/min is sign of impending shock in pediatric patients, except newborns
Level of activity	Normal or slowed	Slowed	Variable, weak to unresponsive
Urine output	Decreased	Decreased	No output
Skin	Normal	Cool, mottled; poor turgor	Cool, clammy; poor turgor; delayed capillary refill time
Mouth	Decreased saliva	Dry mucous membranes	Dry mucous membranes
Eyes	Normal	No tears	Sunken eyes
Anterior fontanelle	Normal to sunken	Sunken	Extremely sunken
Level of consciousness	Normal	Altered	Altered; lethargic
Blood pressure	Normal	Normal	Normal to low

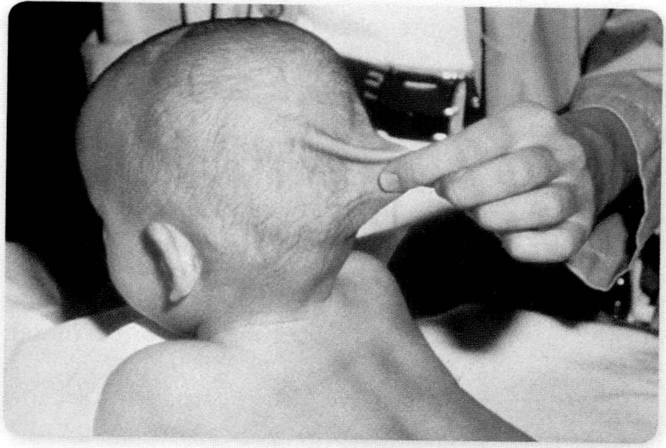

Figure 36-33 An infant with dehydration may exhibit tenting or poor skin turgor.

Courtesy of Ronald Dieckmann, M.D.

Dehydration can be mild, moderate, or severe. The severity of the dehydration can be gauged by looking at several clues **Table 36-12**. For example, an infant with mild dehydration may have dry lips and gums, decreased saliva, and fewer wet diapers throughout the day. As the dehydration grows more severe, the lips and gums may become dry, the eyes may look sunken, and the infant may be sleepy and/or irritable, refusing bottles. The skin may be loose and have no elasticity; this is called poor skin turgor **Figure 36-33**. Also, infants may have sunken fontanelles.

Young children can compensate for fluid losses by decreasing blood flow to the extremities and directing blood flow to vital organs such as the brain and heart. Children who are moderately to severely dehydrated may have mottled, cool, clammy skin and delayed capillary response time. Respirations will usually be increased. Be aware that blood pressure may remain within a normal range while the pediatric patient is in shock, because the compensatory mechanisms are still in place.

Emergency medical care should include careful attention while assessing the ABCDEs and obtaining baseline vital signs. All pediatric patients with signs and symptoms of moderate to severe dehydration should be transported to the ED for further evaluation and treatment.

Assessment and Management of Fever Emergencies

Fever is a common reason parents or caregivers call 9-1-1. Simply defined, fever is an increase in body temperature, usually in response to an infection. Body temperatures of 100.4°F (38°C) or higher are considered to be abnormal. Fevers have many causes and are rarely life-threatening events. However, do not underestimate the potential seriousness of fevers, such as those that occur in conjunction with a rash, which is a sign of a serious illness such as meningitis. Common causes of a fever in pediatric patients include the following:

- Infection, such as pneumonia, meningitis, or urinary tract infection
- Status epilepticus
- Neoplasm (cancer)
- Drug ingestion (aspirin)

Table 36-13 Pediatric Normal Temperatures

Age	Temperature (°F)
Neonate (0 to 1 month)	98° to 100° (37° to 38°C)
Infant (1 month to 1 year)	96.8° to 99.6° (36° to 37.5°C)
Toddler (1 to 2 years)	96.8° to 99.6° (36° to 37.5°C)
Preschool age (3 to 5 years)	98.6° (37°C)
School age (6 to 12 years)	98.6° (37°C)
Adolescent (12 to 15 years)	98.6° (37°C)

Data from: American Heart Association (AHA). Vital signs in children. In: AHA. *Pediatric Advanced Life Support*. Dallas, TX: AHA; 2015.

- Collagen vascular disease, including arthritis and systemic lupus erythematosus (rash across the nose)
- High environmental temperature

Note that there are other conditions in which the body temperature increases that are not a fever. Hyperthermia differs from fever in that it is an increase in body temperature caused by an inability of the body to cool itself. Hyperthermia is typically seen in warm environments, such as a closed car on a hot day.

An accurate body temperature is an important vital sign for pediatric patients Table 36-13. A rectal temperature is the most accurate for infants to toddlers. Older children will be able to follow directions if placing a thermometer under the tongue or under the arm.

A fever can have several causes, such as a viral or a bacterial infection. Depending on the source of infection, the pediatric patient may present with additional signs of respiratory distress, shock, a stiff neck, a rash, skin that is hot to the touch, flushed cheeks, seizures, sensitivity to light, and bulging fontanelles in an infant. Assess the patient for other signs and symptoms such as nausea, vomiting, diarrhea, decreased feedings, and headache.

A pediatric patient with a fever may require only minimal interventions in the field. Provide immediate transport and manage the patient's ABCs. Follow standard precautions if you suspect that the patient may have a communicable disease such as meningitis.

Special Populations

Do not induce shivering in a child with fever, which may in turn increase body temperature.

Unless associated with shock or severe dehydration, IV therapy is generally not necessary in a child with fever.

Assessment and Management of Hypoglycemia Emergencies

Hypoglycemia is defined as an abnormally low blood glucose level. Infants and children have limited stores of glucose, which can be quickly depleted in times of illness, injury, or stress. You must recognize that hypoglycemia is a life-threatening emergency that requires immediate treatment. If hypoglycemia is unrecognized or treatment is delayed, permanent brain damage or death can result.

Words of Wisdom

Although hypoglycemia is more common in children with diabetes, physical exertion, illness, or injury can result in hypoglycemia in children without diabetes. Remember to assess blood glucose levels in all ill or injured children with an altered mental status or bizarre behavior.

General signs and symptoms of hypoglycemia include hunger, malaise, tachycardia, tachypnea, diaphoresis, and tremors. The severity of the patient's clinical presentation depends on how low the blood glucose level has dropped. You should obtain a blood glucose reading in any infant or child that you suspect is hypoglycemic. Normal blood glucose levels range from 80 to 120 mg/dL.

In children with a known history of diabetes, ask the parent or caregiver the following questions. Allow the child to answer the questions if he or she is old enough and understands what you are asking:

1. Have you taken your insulin today? If so, what was the dosage?
2. Has your medication recently changed?
3. When was the last time that you ate? What did you eat?
4. Have you been playing outside or otherwise exerting yourself?

Management of hypoglycemia begins by administering 100% oxygen or assisted ventilation if needed. Monitor vital signs closely. Treat the symptomatic child with glucose if his or her blood glucose reading is less than 80 mg/dL.

If the child is responsive and alert enough to swallow, administer oral glucose as allowed by local protocol. If, however, the child has an altered mental status or is otherwise incapable of swallowing, administer IV glucose in the following doses:

- For age 1 year and older, administer 0.5 to 1 g/kg of D_{25} via slow IV/IO push. This dose may be repeated as necessary.
- For infants and neonates, administer 200 to 500 mg/kg slow IV/IO push (see below). This dose may be repeated as necessary. Do not exceed a maximum concentration of 12.5% (vasculature extremely sensitive to high concentrations).
- D_{10} may be given in place of D_{25}. Administer 0.5 to 1 g/kg slow IV/IO push. This dose may be repeated as necessary.

If an IV line cannot be established, insert an IO needle. If vascular access (IV or IO) is not available, medical control may order the administration of 1 mg of glucagon via IM injection.

Repeat a blood glucose reading 10 to 15 minutes following the administration of glucose. If the patient is still symptomatic and his or her blood glucose reading remains below 80 mg/dL, repeat the glucose as needed.

Words of Wisdom

Use the following guide to dilute D_{50} (0.5 g/mL) for pediatric use:

- D_{50} to D_{25}
  - D_{50} is supplied in an ampule with 25 g of dextrose in 50 mL of water. Push out 25 mL of the D_{50} and draw 25 mL of normal saline (NS) into the ampule, agitating to mix. (Mix 1 part D_{50} with 1 part NS, for a result of 12.5 g in 50 mL.)
- D_{50} to D_{10}
  - Draw 4 mL of D_{50} into a 20-mL syringe. Draw 16 mL of NS into the same syringe, agitating to mix. (Mix 1 part D_{50} with 4 parts NS, for a result of 2 g in 20 mL.)
- D_{25} to D_{10}
  - Use the prepared D_{25} in 50 mL as discussed above. Push out 40 mL of the D_{25} and draw 40 mL of NS into the ampule, agitating to mix, for a result of 5 g in 50 mL.

Assessment and Management of Hyperglycemia Emergencies

Hyperglycemia is an abnormally high blood glucose level. It can either be the presenting problem in a child with new-onset diabetes mellitus or it may occur as a complication in a child with a known history of diabetes. If not recognized or promptly treated, hyperglycemia can result in severe dehydration and DKA, both of which are potentially life threatening.

During your assessment of the child with suspected hyperglycemia, you will typically find that a dose of insulin was missed, a greater proportion of food was eaten compared with the dose of insulin, or the insulin pump malfunctioned.

Like hypoglycemia, the signs and symptoms of hyperglycemia depend on how high the blood glucose level is. During your assessment, ask the same questions of the child or parent as you did for suspected hypoglycemia.

Management of hyperglycemia begins by administering 100% oxygen or assisted ventilation if needed. Monitor vital signs closely. Obtain IV access and administer 20-mL/kg boluses of normal saline or lactated Ringer solution as needed to maintain adequate perfusion. Children with hyperglycemia and DKA are often severely dehydrated.

Closely monitor the patient's ABCs and be prepared to adjust your treatment accordingly. The patient with DKA desperately needs insulin; however, this is not a drug that is administered in the prehospital setting. Therefore, immediate transport to the closest appropriate facility is critical.

If you are unable to obtain IV access, insert an IO needle. If the patient's respiratory status deteriorates, call for paramedic backup.

Words of Wisdom

If you are unable to determine whether a child with an altered mental status has hypoglycemia or hyperglycemia (ie, glucometer failure), administer glucose. If the child is experiencing DKA, the extra glucose likely will not cause further harm. However, if he or she is hypoglycemic, the glucose could save his or her life.

Assessment and Management of Drowning Emergencies

Drowning is the number one cause of unintentional death among children ages 1 to 4 in the United States.[22] At this age, children often fall into swimming pools and lakes, but many drown in bathtubs and even buckets of water. Older adolescents, who account for the most drownings after toddlers, drown when swimming or boating; alcohol is frequently a factor.

As discussed in Chapter 34, *Environmental Emergencies*, the principal cause of injury in a drowning incident is lack of oxygen. Even a few minutes (or less) without oxygen affects the heart, lungs, and brain, causing life-threatening problems such as cardiac arrest, respiratory failure, and coma. Submersion in icy water can rob the body of heat, causing hypothermia. Although a few patients subjected to submersion hypothermia have survived long periods in cardiac arrest in icy water, most people in this situation die. Diving into the water, of course, increases the risk of neck and spinal cord injuries.

Signs and symptoms of a drowning patient will vary based on the type and length of submersion. These pediatric patients may present with coughing; choking; airway obstruction; difficulty breathing; altered mental status; seizure activity; unresponsiveness; fast, slow, or no pulse noted; pale, cyanotic skin; and abdominal distention from ingestion of fluids.

Safety is critical when dealing with a submersion emergency. In submersion situations, always take steps to ensure your own safety when rescuing the patient from the water. Do not become a victim yourself! After the pediatric patient is successfully removed from the water, assess and manage the ABCs and contact a paramedic crew to intervene if needed. Administer oxygen at 100% via a nonrebreathing mask or bag-mask device if assisted ventilations are required. Be prepared to apply suction, given that these patients often vomit. If trauma is suspected, apply a cervical collar and place the child on a backboard. Pad all open spaces under the pediatric patient before securing the patient onto the backboard. If the pediatric patient is unresponsive and in cardiopulmonary arrest, perform CPR beginning with chest compressions.

Safety Tips

Before using an automated external defibrillator (AED) on a pulseless drowning patient, ensure that the patient is dried off first. Use extreme caution when operating an AED in this situation.

Pediatric Trauma Emergencies and Management

Trauma is the number one cause of death of children in the United States.[23] As an AEMT, you will frequently treat injured children; therefore, you must have a thorough understanding of how trauma affects them. The quality of care in the first few minutes after a child has been injured can have an enormous effect on that child's chances for complete recovery.

Infants and toddlers are most commonly hurt as a result of unintentional suffocation, drowning, falls, or abuse.[22] According to the Centers for Disease Control and Prevention, automobile crashes, including those involving bicycles and pedestrians, are the most significant threat to the well-being of children ages 5 years and older.[24] Other common causes of traumatic injury and death include falls, gunshot wounds, blunt injuries, and sports activities.

▶ Psychologic Differences

Children are less mature psychologically than adults; therefore, they are often injured because of their undeveloped judgment and their lack of experience. For example, children are more likely than adults to cross the street without looking for oncoming traffic. As a result, children are more likely than adults to be struck by motor vehicles. Children and adolescents are also more likely to sustain injuries from diving into shallow water because they forget to check the depth of the water before they dive. In such situations, always assume that the child has serious head and neck injuries.

▶ Physical Differences

Children are smaller than adults; therefore, when they are hurt in the same type of crash as an adult, the location of their injuries may differ from those in an adult. For example, the bumper of a motor vehicle will strike an adult pedestrian in the lower leg, whereas that same bumper will strike a child in the pelvis. In a crash involving sudden deceleration, an adult might injure a ligament in the knee; in that same accident, a child might injure the bones in the leg.

The younger the child, the more flexible the bone structures are to trauma. Children's bones and soft tissues are less well developed than those of adults; therefore, the force of an injury affects these structures somewhat differently than it does in an adult. Because a child's head is proportionately larger than an adult's, it exerts greater stress on the neck structures during a deceleration injury. Because of these anatomic differences, you should always carefully assess children for head and neck injuries.

Words of Wisdom

The XABCDE mnemonic reminds us that the first critical step for any trauma patient is controlling eXsanguinating hemorrhage. The use of tourniquets is especially effective for extremity hemorrhage. Shortly after the active shooter incident at Sandy Hook Elementary School that occurred on December 14, 2012 in Newtown, Connecticut, the American College of Surgeons (ACS) convened a committee of representatives from many organizations to create a national policy to enhance survivability. This effort was based on autopsy reports that many children at Sandy Hook died of extremity hemorrhage that could have been successfully controlled with the placement of tourniquets. The nationwide *Stop the Bleed* campaign (see *Chapter 27, Bleeding*) is another result that came about as an outcome of the committee findings.

▶ Injury Patterns

Although you are not responsible for diagnosing injuries in children, your ability to recognize and report serious injuries will provide critical information to hospital staff. For this reason, it is important for you to understand the special physical and psychologic characteristics of children and what makes them more likely to have certain kinds of injuries.

Vehicle Collisions

Children playing or riding a bicycle can dart out in front of motor vehicles without looking. In such a situation, the driver may have little time to slow down or stop to prevent hitting the child. The area of greatest injury varies, depending on the size of the child and the height of the bumper at the time of impact. When vehicles slow down at the moment of impact, the bumper dips slightly, causing the point of impact with the child to be lowered. The exact area that is struck depends on the child's height and the final position of the bumper at the time of impact. Children who are injured in these situations often sustain high-energy injuries to the head, spine, abdomen, pelvis, or legs. In addition to differences in size and anatomy, children will often turn toward an oncoming vehicle when they see it approaching and, therefore, sustain different injuries than an adult who turns away.

▶ Injuries to Specific Body Systems

Head Injuries

Head injuries are common in children. This is because the size of a child's head, in relation to the body, is larger than that of an adult. An infant also has a softer, thinner skull, which may result in injury to the underlying brain tissues. The scalp and facial vessels can bleed easily and may cause a great deal of blood loss if the bleeding is not controlled.

The signs and symptoms of head injury in a child are similar to those in an adult, but there are some important differences. Nausea and vomiting are common signs and symptoms of head injury in children; however, it is easy to mistake these for an abdominal injury or illness. You should suspect a serious head injury in any child who experiences nausea and vomiting after a traumatic event. Pediatric patients are managed in the same manner as adults. Chapter 30, *Head and Spine Injuries*, discusses head injuries in detail.

Immobilization. Spinal immobilization is necessary for all children who have possible head or spinal injuries after a traumatic event.

To immobilize a pediatric patient on a short backboard or pediatric immobilization device, follow the steps in Skill Drill 36-6.

Immobilization can be difficult to perform because of the child's body proportions. Young children require padding under the torso to maintain a neutral position. At approximately 8 to 10 years of age, children no longer require padding underneath the torso to create a neutral position.

Skill Drill 36-6 Immobilizing a Pediatric Patient

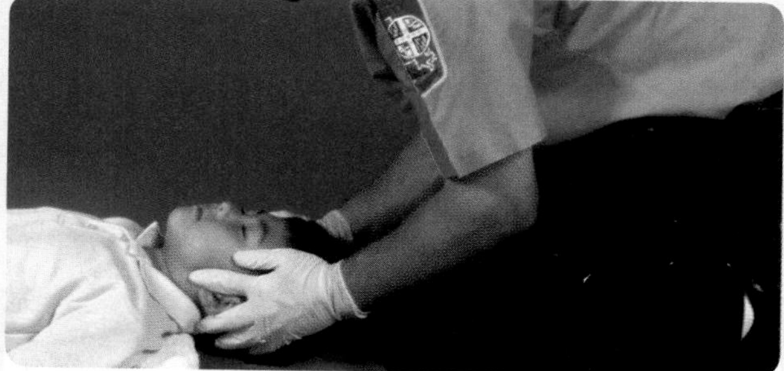

Step 1 Maintain the child's head in a neutral position by placing a towel under the torso, from the shoulders to the hips.

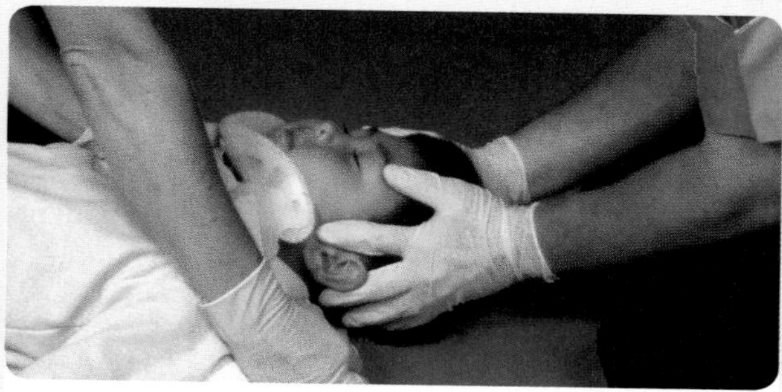

Step 2 Apply an appropriate-size cervical collar.

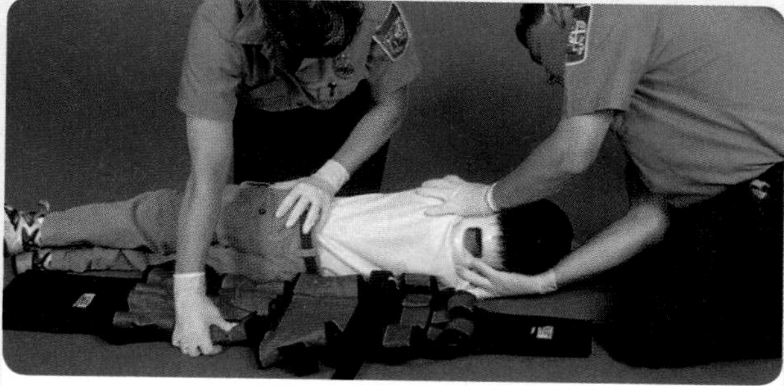

Step 3 Log roll the child onto the short backboard or pediatric immobilization device.

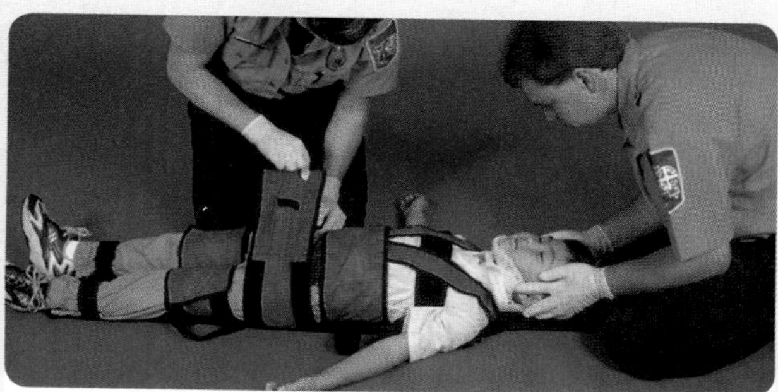

Step 4 Secure the pediatric patient's torso to the short backboard or pediatric immobilization device first.

(continued)

Skill Drill 36-6 Immobilizing a Pediatric Patient *(continued)*

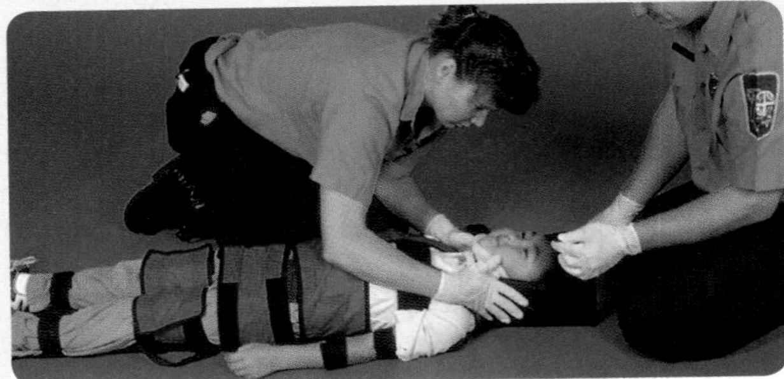

Step 5 Secure the child's head to the short backboard or pediatric immobilization device.

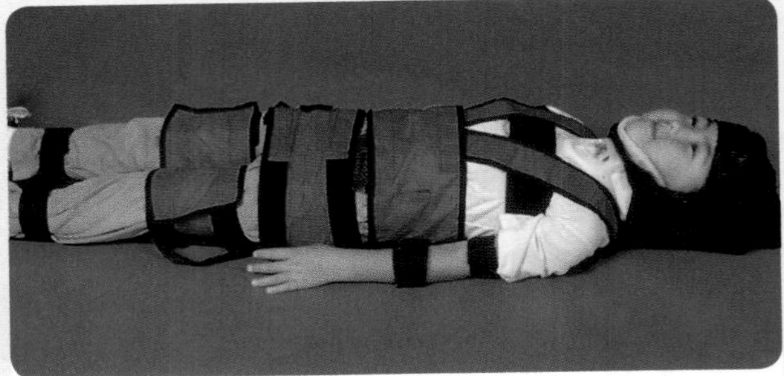

Step 6 Ensure that the child is strapped in properly.

Instead, they can simply lie supine on the backboard. However, another complication may occur if a child is put onto an adult-size backboard. Because a child's body is narrower than an adult's, padding will be required along the sides so that the child can be properly secured on an adult-size backboard. If using an adult-size backboard, make sure to slide the child all the way up to the head of the backboard.

Many infants and children will be in a car seat when you approach them. There are two methods of transportation that are determined by the severity of the pediatric patient's condition. If the pediatric patient has stable vital signs, minimal injury, and the car seat is visibly undamaged, the patient may be left in the seat. Ensure that the patient is secured within the seat and the seat is secured in the ambulance for transportation. If the pediatric patient is unstable, has injuries other than minor ones, or the car seat is visibly damaged, the child must be removed from the car seat and immobilized on a short backboard or pediatric immobilization device prior to transport.

Ideally, a cervical collar would be used when immobilizing an infant or toddler; however, an appropriate-size cervical collar may not be available. In this case, place rolled towels on either side of the head to prevent side-to-side movement. Do not place a towel in the shape of an upside-down "U" over the pediatric patient's head; this may press down on the head and compromise the airway and spinal cord. The steps for removing a pediatric patient from a car seat and immobilizing him or her on a short backboard or pediatric immobilization device are shown in Skill Drill 36-7.

Skill Drill 36-7 Immobilizing a Patient Found in a Car Seat

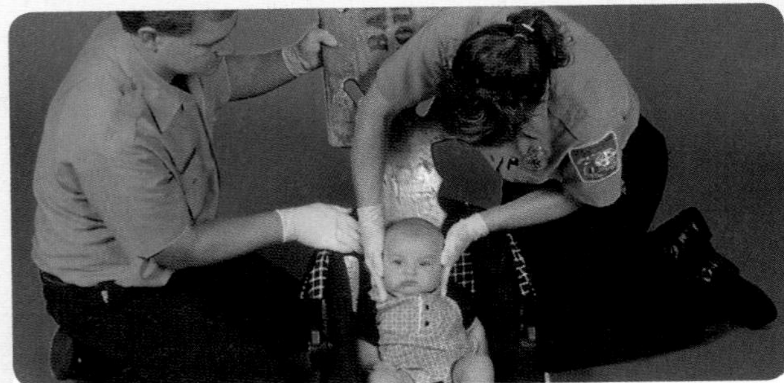

Step 1 Carefully stabilize the patient's head in a neutral position. Leave all car seat straps in place.

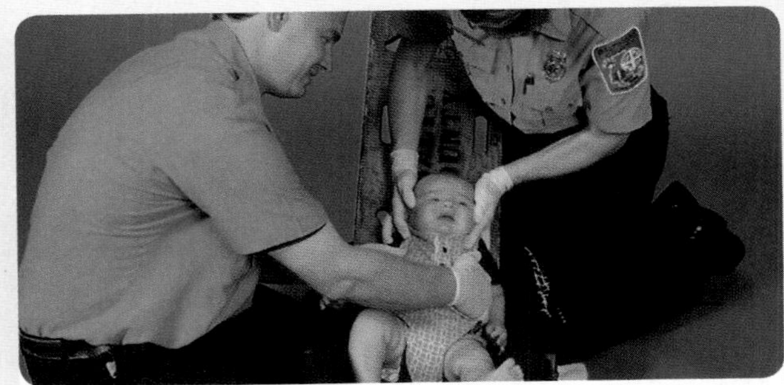

Step 2 Lay the car seat down into a reclined position on a hard surface. Position a short backboard or pediatric immobilization device between the patient and the surface on which the patient is resting.

Skill Drill 36-7 Immobilizing a Patient Found in a Car Seat *(continued)*

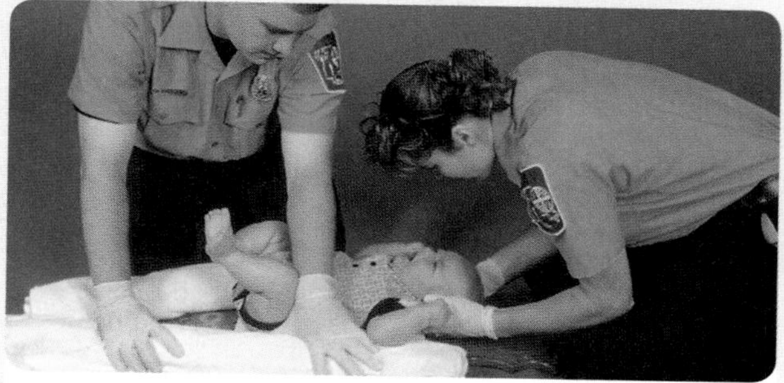

Step 3 Slide the patient into position on the short backboard or pediatric immobilization device. Remove the patient and device from the car seat as one unit.

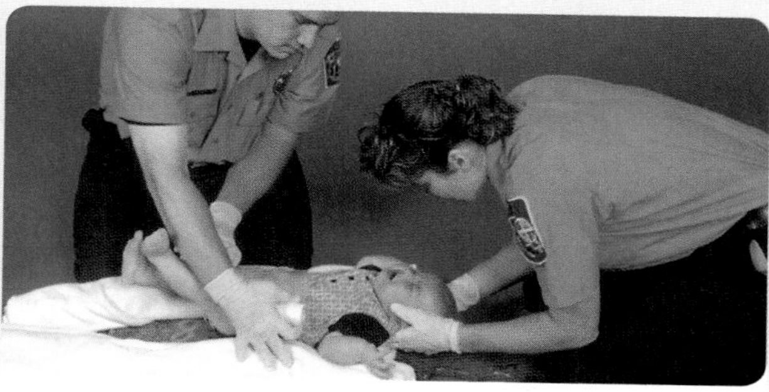

Step 4 Place a towel under the back, from the shoulders to the hips, to ensure neutral head position.

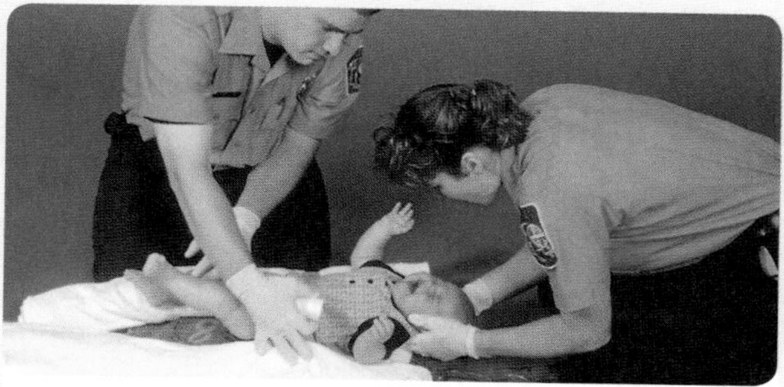

Step 5 Secure the torso first and place padding to fill any voids.

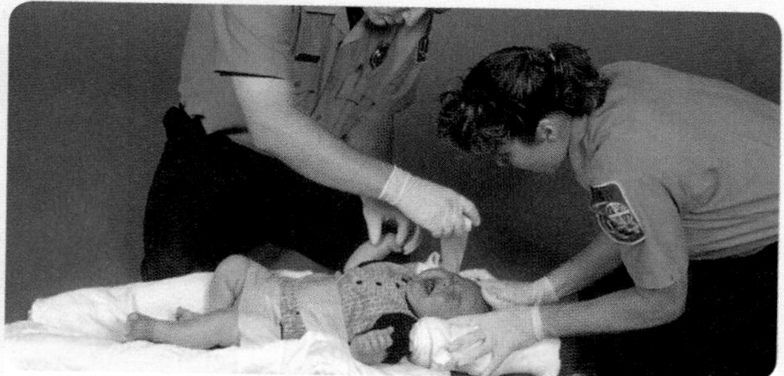

Step 6 Secure the patient's head to the short backboard or pediatric immobilization device.

Chest Injuries

Chest injuries in children are usually the result of blunt trauma rather than penetrating objects. Remember that children have extremely soft, flexible ribs that can be substantially compressed without breaking. Keep this in mind as you assess a child who has sustained high-energy blunt trauma to the chest. Although there may be no external sign of injury such as broken ribs, contusions, or bleeding, there may be significant injuries within the chest Figure 36-34. Pediatric patients with chest injuries are managed in the same manner as adults. Chapter 31, *Chest Injuries,* discusses the treatment of chest injuries in detail.

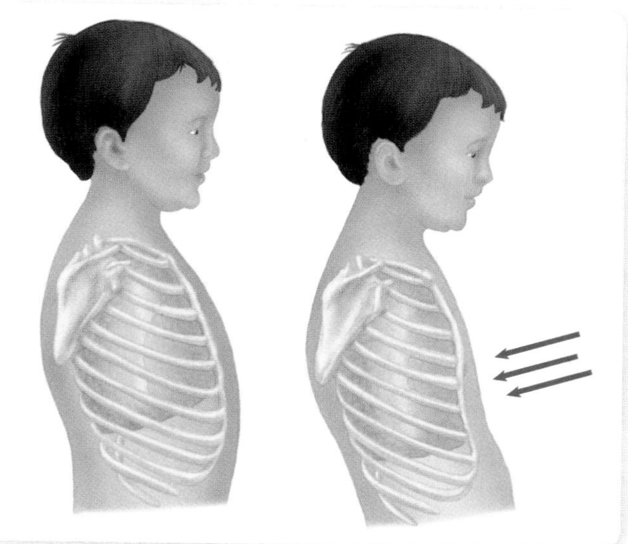

Figure 36-34 A child's ribs are softer and more flexible than an adult's. As a result, the ribs may compress the lungs and heart if there is blunt trauma, causing serious injury with no obvious external damage.

Abdominal Injuries

Abdominal injuries are common in children. Remember, though, that children can compensate for substantial blood loss better than adults without signs or symptoms of shock developing Figure 36-35. Children can also have a serious injury without early external evidence of a problem. All children with abdominal injuries should be monitored for signs and symptoms of shock, including a weak, rapid pulse; cold, clammy skin; decreased

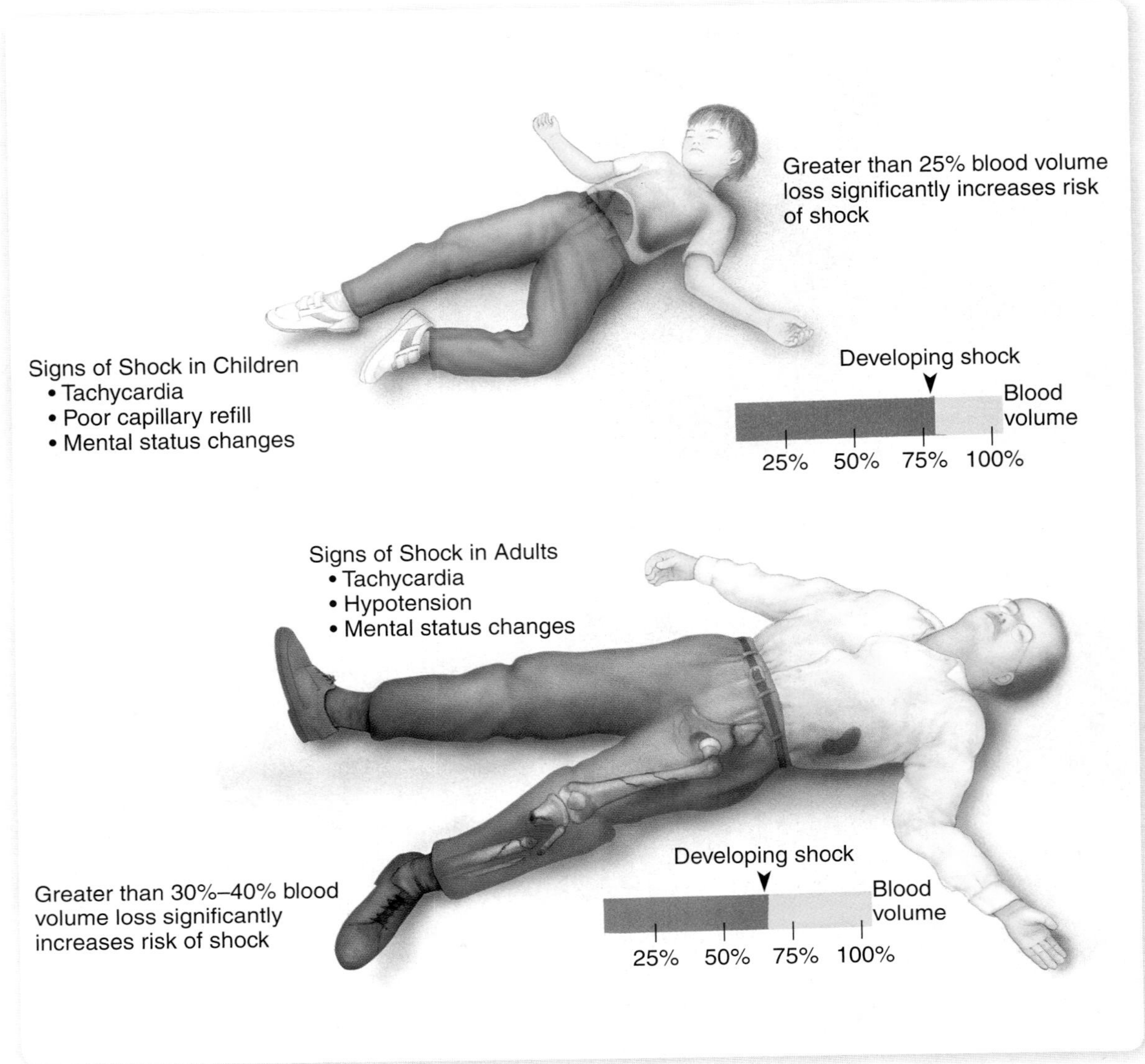

Figure 36-35 All children with abdominal injuries should be monitored closely for signs of shock. Although children may compensate for significant blood loss better than adults, shock develops in children after proportionally smaller blood losses.

capillary refill (an early sign); confusion; and decreased systolic blood pressure (a late sign). Even in the absence of signs and symptoms of shock, or with only a few signs and symptoms, you should remain cautious about the possibility of internal injuries.

Pediatric patients with abdominal injuries are treated in the same manner as adults. Chapter 32, *Abdominal and Genitourinary Injuries*, discusses abdominal injuries in detail. If the patient shows signs and symptoms of shock, prevent hypothermia by keeping the patient warm with blankets. If the patient has bradycardia, ventilate. Monitor the patient's condition during transport.

▶ Injuries of the Extremities

Children have immature bones with active growth centers. Growth of long bones occurs from the ends at specialized growth plates. These growth plates, or epiphyseal plates, are potential weak spots in the bone and are often injured as a result of trauma. In general, children's bones bend more easily than those of an adult. As a result, incomplete or greenstick fractures can occur.

Extremity injuries in children are generally managed in the same manner as those in adults. Painful, deformed limbs with evidence of broken bones should be splinted. Specific splinting equipment, such as a traction splint for fractures of the femur, should be used only if it fits the child. Do not attempt to use adult immobilization devices on a child unless the child is large enough to properly fit in the device. Chapter 33, *Orthopaedic Injuries*, discusses extremity injuries.

▶ Burns

Burns to children are generally considered more serious than burns to adults. This is because infants and

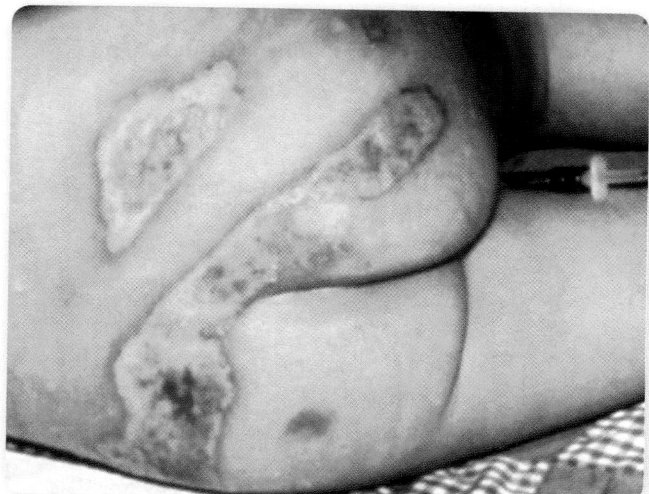

Figure 36-36 The most common burns in children involve exposure to hot surfaces. This child's buttocks were placed against a hot heating grate.

children have more body surface area relative to their total body mass, which means greater fluid and heat loss. In addition, children do not tolerate burns as well as adults do. Hypothermia is more likely to develop, and children may go into shock and experience airway problems because of the unique differences related to age and anatomy.

Children can be burned in a variety of ways. The most common incidents involve exposure to hot substances such as scalding water in a bathtub, or hot items on a stove, or exposure to caustic substances such as cleaning solvents or paint thinners **Figure 36-36**. You should suspect possible internal injuries from chemical ingestion when you see a child who has burns around the face and mouth.

One common problem following burn injuries in children is infection. Burned skin cannot resist infection as effectively as normal skin can. For this reason, sterile techniques should be used in handling the skin of children with burn wounds, if possible.

Table 36-14 provides some general guidelines to follow in assessing a child who has been burned. These guidelines may help you to determine which children should be treated primarily at specialized burn centers. Always consider the possibility of abuse in any burn situation.

Treat a pediatric burn patient as you would an adult burn patient. Chapter 28, *Soft-Tissue Injuries*, discusses burn care in detail. Obtain vascular access, preferably in a nonburned area, and administer 20-mL/kg boluses of normal saline or lactated Ringer solution if the child is in shock. Keep the patient warm. If the patient has bradycardia, ventilate. Reassess the child's condition and administer additional IV fluids as needed.

Insert an IO catheter if you are unable to obtain IV access after three tries or 90 seconds, as determined by local protocols.

Table 36-14 Severity of Burns in Pediatric Patients

Severity of Burn	Body Area Involved
Minor	Partial-thickness burns involving less than 10% of the body surface
Moderate	Partial-thickness burns involving 10% to 20% of the body surface
Critical	Any full-thickness burn Any partial-thickness burn involving more than 20% of the body surface Any burn involving the hands, feet, face, airway, or genitalia

▶ Fluid Management

Circulatory compromise is less common in children than in adults as the result of trauma; therefore, airway management and ventilatory support take priority over management of circulation. Consider the following when you are establishing vascular access in the injured child:

- Large-bore IV catheters should be inserted into a large peripheral vein whenever possible.
- Because definitive care can only be provided at the hospital, never delay transport for the purpose of starting an IV line; this procedure should be performed en route to the hospital.
- To maintain perfusion in a child, administer an initial bolus of 20 mL/kg using an isotonic crystalloid solution (ie, normal saline, lactated Ringer solution).
  - Frequently reassess the child's vital signs and provide additional IV fluid boluses of 20 mL/kg if no improvement is noted following the initial bolus.
  - If the child's condition does not improve following two boluses of an isotonic crystalloid, blood loss is likely severe and will probably need surgical intervention. Provide rapid transport with continuous monitoring of the child en route.

If IV access cannot be obtained within three attempts *or* 90 seconds, insert an IO needle to gain access to the vascular system.

▶ Pain Management

The first step in pain management is recognizing the patient is in pain. Some patients will be nonverbal or have a limited vocabulary. Look for visual clues and use the Wong-Baker FACES pain scale (see Figure 36-16).

When dealing with pediatric pain management issues, you are limited to the following interventions: positioning, ice packs, extremity elevation, and nitrous oxide administration as allowed by local protocols. These interventions will decrease the pain and swelling to the site of an injury. However, additional interventions (medications) from a paramedic provider may be necessary. Another important tool is simple kindness and providing emotional support to the patient and the parent or caregiver. This act alone can decrease anxiety and allow for a more soothing environment for all involved. Children can sense fear and frustration from adults, so it is important to maintain a calm, professional, and trusting relationship with your patient and the family during the course of treatment.

Disaster Management

The JumpSTART triage system was developed for pediatric patients because the original START triage system did not account for the developmental and physiologic differences in children Figure 36-37. This system is intended for pediatric patients younger than age 8 years or who appear to weigh less than 100 pounds (45 kg). Because infants and children may not be able to walk or follow commands during a disaster event, they must be considered for immediate delivery to the treatment area.

There are four triage categories in the JumpSTART system, designated by colors corresponding to different levels of urgency for treatment. Decision points include: able to walk (except in infants); presence of spontaneous breathing; respirations of less than 15 or greater than 45 breaths/min; palpable peripheral pulse; and appropriate response to painful stimuli on the AVPU scale.

Pediatric patients who are able to walk are designated as the third or minor priority (green tag), meaning they are not in immediate need of treatment. Those patients breathing spontaneously, with a peripheral pulse and appropriately responsive to painful stimuli, are considered second priority (yellow tag). Their treatment and transport can be delayed. Pediatric patients who are apneic and responsive to positioning or rescue breathing; who are in respiratory failure; who are breathing but pulseless; or who are inappropriately responsive to painful stimuli, are considered highest priority (red tag). Pediatric patients who are both apneic and pulseless, or who are apneic and unresponsive to rescue breathing are considered deceased or expectant deceased (black tag).

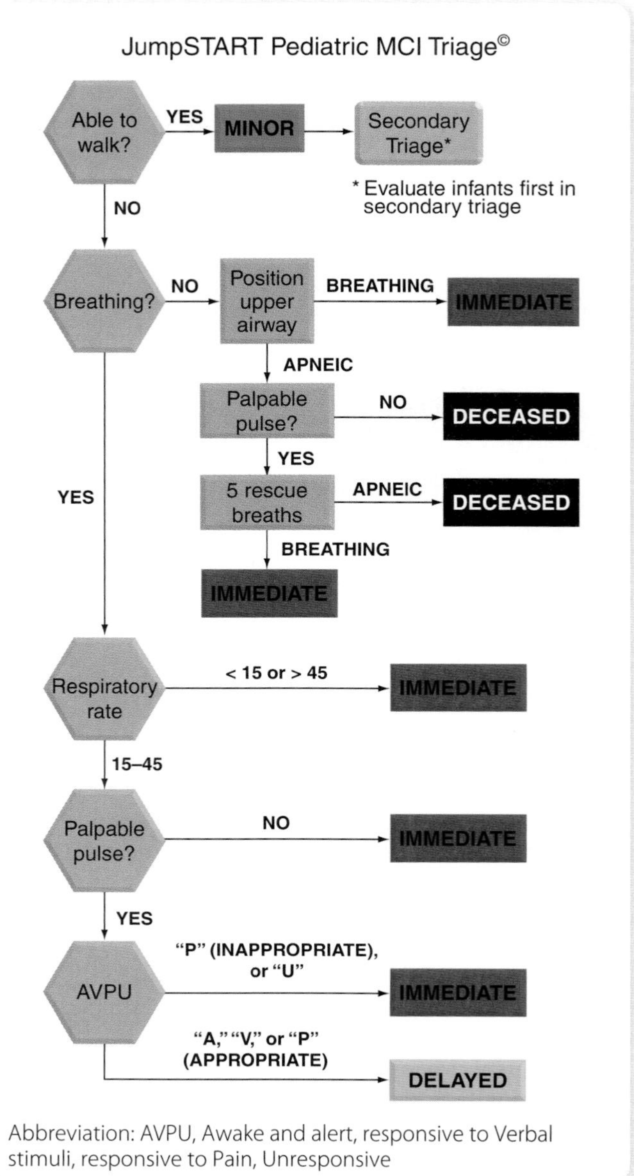

Figure 36-37 The JumpSTART triage system.

Child Abuse and Neglect

The term **child abuse** means any improper or excessive action that injures or otherwise harms a child or infant; it includes physical abuse, sexual abuse, neglect, and emotional abuse. The intentional injury of a child, whether physical or emotional, is not rare in our society. According to the Department of Health and Human Services, nearly 1 million cases of child abuse are reported to child protection agencies annually.[25] The number of patients has increased 3.8% since 2011.[26] Many of these children sustain life-threatening injuries, and some die. If suspected child abuse is not reported, the child is likely to be abused again and again, perhaps sustaining permanent injuries or even death. Therefore, you must be aware of the signs of child abuse and neglect, and of your responsibility to report suspected abuse to law enforcement or child protection agencies.

Signs of Abuse

As an AEMT, you will be called to homes because of a reported injury to a child. Child abuse occurs in every socioeconomic status, so be aware of the patient's surroundings and document your findings objectively. AEMTs are often called to testify in abuse cases, so it is essential to record all findings, including any statements made by parents or caregivers or others on the scene. If you suspect that physical or sexual abuse is involved, ask yourself the following questions:

- Is the injury typical for the developmental level of the child?
- Is the method of injury reported by the parent or caregiver consistent with the child's injuries?
- Is the parent or caregiver behaving appropriately (concerned about the child's well-being)?
- Is there evidence of drinking or drug use at the scene?
- Was there a delay in seeking care for the child?
- Is there a good relationship between the child and the parent or caregiver?
- Does the child have multiple injuries at different stages of healing?
- Does the child have any unusual marks or bruises that may have been caused by cigarettes, heating grates, or branding injuries?
- Does the child have several types of injuries, such as burns, fractures, and bruises?
- Does the child have any burns on the hands or feet that involve a glove distribution (marks that encircle a hand or foot in a pattern that looks like a glove)?
- Is there an unexplained decreased level of consciousness?
- Is the child clean and an appropriate weight for his or her age?
- Is there any rectal or vaginal bleeding?
- What does the home look like? Clean or dirty? Is it warm or cold? Is there adequate food?

Your assessment in the field will allow a better assessment by the medical staff later. An easy way to remember these is the mnemonic CHILD ABUSE shown in Table 36-15.

As you assess the pediatric patient, look for and pay particular attention to the following signs Figure 36-38.

Table 36-15	CHILD ABUSE Mnemonic for Assessing Possible Child Abuse
C Consistency of the injury with the child's developmental age	
H History inconsistent with injury	
I Inappropriate parental concerns	
L Lack of supervision	
D Delay in seeking care	
A Affect (of the parent or caregiver and the child in relation to the caregiver)	
B Bruises of varying ages	
U Unusual injury patterns	
S Suspicious circumstances	
E Environmental clues	

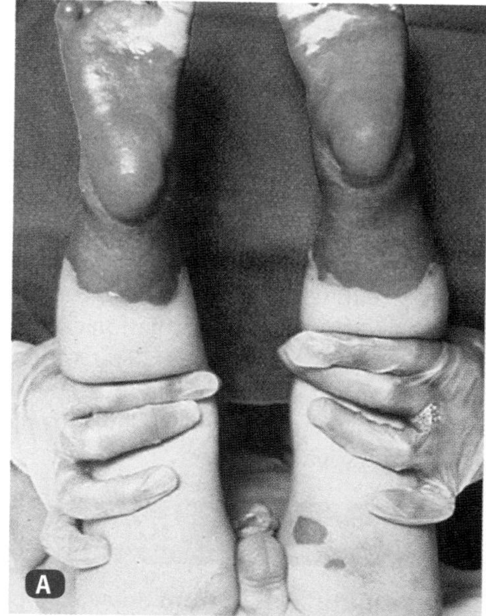

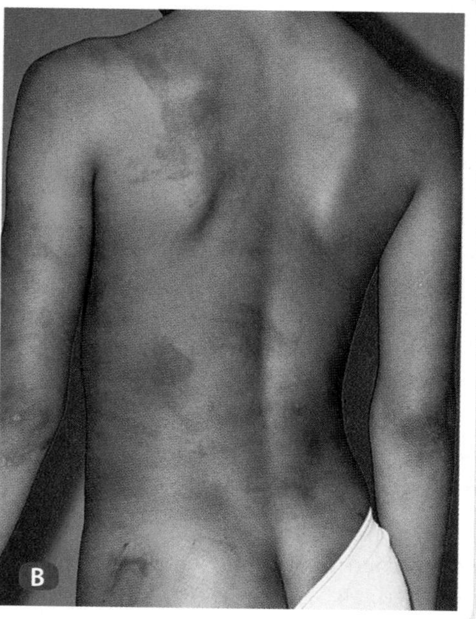

Figure 36-38 Signs of child abuse. **A.** A scald injury. **B.** Multiple injuries at different stages of healing.

Courtesy of Ronald Dieckmann, M.D.

Bruises

Observe the color and location of any bruises. New bruises are pink or red. Over time, bruises turn blue, then green, then yellow-brown and faded. Note the location. Bruises to the back, buttocks, ears, or face are suspicious and are usually inflicted by someone else.

Burns

Burns to the penis, testicles, vagina, or buttocks are usually inflicted by someone else, as are burns that encircle a hand or foot to look like a glove. You should suspect abuse if the child has cigarette burns or grid pattern burns.

Fractures

Fractures of the humerus or femur do not normally occur without major trauma, such as a fall from a high place or a motor vehicle crash. Falls from bed are not usually associated with fractures. You should maintain some index of suspicion if an infant or young child sustains a femur fracture or a complete fracture of any bone.

Shaken Baby Syndrome

Infants may sustain life-threatening head trauma by being shaken or struck on the head, a life-threatening condition called **shaken baby syndrome**. With this condition, there is bleeding within the head and damage to the cervical spine as a result of intentional, forceful shaking. The infant will be found unresponsive, often without evidence of external trauma. The call for help may be for an infant who has stopped breathing or is unresponsive. The infant may appear to be in cardiopulmonary arrest, but what has likely occurred is that the shaking tore blood vessels in the brain, resulting in bleeding around the brain. The pressure from the blood results in increased cranial pressure, leading to coma and/or death.

Neglect

Neglect is refusal or failure on the part of the parent or caregiver to provide life necessities, such as food, water, clothing, shelter, personal hygiene, medicine, comfort, and personal safety.

Children who are neglected are often dirty or too thin or appear developmentally delayed because of lack of stimulation. You may observe such children when you are making calls for unrelated problems. Report all cases of suspicious neglect.

▶ Symptoms and Other Indicators of Abuse

An abused child may appear withdrawn, fearful, or hostile. Be particularly concerned if the child refuses to discuss how an injury occurred. Occasionally, the parent or caregiver will reveal a history of several "accidents." Be alert for conflicting stories or a marked lack of concern from the parents or caregiver. Remember, the abuser may be a parent, caregiver, relative, or friend of the family. Sometimes the abuser is an acquaintance of a single parent.

AEMTs in all states must report all cases of suspected abuse, even if the ED fails to do so. Most states have special forms for reporting. Supervisors are generally forbidden from interfering with the reporting of suspected abuse, even if they disagree with the assessment. You do not have to prove that there has been abuse. Law enforcement and child protection agencies are mandated to investigate all reported cases. Take all necessary precautions to protect yourself, your team, and the pediatric patient involved in this situation.

▶ Sexual Abuse

Children of any age and either sex can be subjected to sexual abuse. According to the Department of Health and Human Services, approximately 8.3% of child abuse cases reported are sexual abuse.[26] Among children, the most likely victims of rape and sexual assault are females aged 16 to 19 years.[27] However, males and younger children may be victims as well. This type of abuse is often the result of long-standing abuse by relatives.

Your assessment of a child who has been sexually abused should be limited to determining the type of dressing any injuries require. Sometimes, a sexually abused child is also beaten. Therefore, treat any bruises or fractures as well. Do not examine the genitalia of a young child unless there is evidence of bleeding or there is an injury that must be treated.

In addition, if you suspect that a child has been subjected to sexual abuse, do not allow the child to wash, urinate, or defecate before a physician completes an examination. Although this step can be difficult for the patient, it is important to preserve evidence. If possible, ensure that an AEMT or police officer of the same gender remains with the child, unless locating one will delay transport.

You must maintain professional composure the entire time you are assessing and caring for a sexually abused child. Assume a concerned, caring demeanor, and shield the child from onlookers and curious bystanders. Obtain as much information as possible from the child and any witnesses. The child may be hysterical or unwilling to say anything at all, especially if the abuser is a relative or family friend. You are in the best position to obtain the most accurate firsthand information about the incident. Therefore, record any information carefully and completely on the patient care report. Transport all children who are victims of sexual assault. Sexual abuse of a child is a crime. Cooperate fully with law enforcement officials in their investigations.

Death of a Child

The death of a child from any cause poses special challenges for EMS personnel. In addition to any medical treatment the child may require, you must be prepared to offer the family a high level of support and understanding as they begin the grieving process. First, the family may want you to initiate resuscitation efforts, which may or may not conflict with your EMS protocols. If the child is clearly deceased and, under protocol, can be declared dead in the field, but the family is so distraught that they insist that resuscitation efforts be made, initiate CPR and transport the child.

Again, coping with the death of a child can be highly stressful for health care professionals. You may find yourself with unexpected feelings of pain and loss. It is helpful to take some time before going back on the job to work through your feelings and to talk about the event with your EMS colleagues. Be alert for signs of posttraumatic stress in yourself and others: nightmares, restlessness, difficulty sleeping, lack of appetite, or a constant need for food, and the like. Consider the need for professional help if these signs or symptoms continue. Some EMS programs have found it helpful to have critical incident stress management (CISM) protocols and defusing and debriefing teams available for traumatic incidents. For more information about defusing, debriefing, and CISM programs, see Chapter 2, *Workforce Safety and Wellness*.

Although you may experience the death of a child as a failure, your skill at coping with this kind of emotional event can be a great comfort to the family, helping them to accept their loss and begin the long process of grieving.

Words of Wisdom

Some EMS systems arrange for home visits after the death of a child so that EMS providers and family members can come to some sort of closure together. This also gives the family an opportunity to ask any remaining questions about the event. However, you need special training for such visits. This can be a session with a trained counselor or a group discussion with your colleagues or the entire health care team.

▶ Sudden Infant Death Syndrome

The unexpected death of an infant or young child is called **sudden infant death syndrome (SIDS)** when, after a complete autopsy, the cause of death remains unexplained. SIDS is the leading cause of death in infants 1 to 12 months old; approximately 1,600 infants die of SIDS annually.[28]

Although it is impossible to predict SIDS, there are several known risk factors:[29]

- Mother smoked during pregnancy or anyone smokes around the infant
- Low birth weight
- The baby is placed on his or her stomach in a crib or on soft surfaces with loose bedding

Deaths as the result of SIDS can occur at any time of the day; however, these children are often discovered in the morning when the parents or caregivers go in to check on the infant. If you are the first provider at the scene of suspected SIDS, you will face three tasks: assessment of the scene, assessment and management of the patient, and communication and support of the family.

Scene Assessment

Carefully inspect the environment, following local protocols, noting the condition of the scene where the caregivers found the infant or young child. Your assessment of the scene should concentrate on the following:

- Signs of illness, including medications, humidifiers, or thermometers
- The general condition of the house
- Signs of poor hygiene
- Family interaction. Do not allow yourself to be judgmental about family interactions at this time. Note and report any behavior that is clearly not within the acceptable range, such as physical and verbal abuse.
- The site where the child was discovered. Note all items in the child's crib or bed, including pillows, stuffed animals, toys, and small objects.

Assessment and Management of SIDS

SIDS is a diagnosis of exclusion. All other potential causes must first be ruled out, a process that may take physicians a lot of time. An infant who has been a victim of SIDS will be pale or blue, not breathing, pulseless, and unresponsive. Other causes for such a condition include the following:

- Accidental suffocation or strangulation in bed
- Overwhelming infection
- Child abuse
- Airway obstruction from a foreign object or as a result of infection
- Meningitis
- Accidental or intentional poisoning
- Hypoglycemia (low blood glucose level)
- Congenital metabolic defects

Regardless of the cause, assessment and management of the infant remain the same. Remember that what you find in assessing the infant and the scene may provide important diagnostic information.

Begin with an assessment of the ABCDEs and provide interventions as necessary. Depending on how much time has passed since the child was discovered, he or she may show signs of postmortem changes. These include stiffening of the body, called rigor mortis, and dependent lividity, which is the pooling of blood in the lower parts of the body or those that are in contact with the floor or bed.

If the child shows such signs, call medical control. In some EMS systems, a victim of SIDS may be declared dead on the scene. Deciding whether to start CPR on a child who shows clear signs of rigor mortis or dependent lividity can be difficult. Family members may consider anything less as withholding critical care. In this situation, the best course of action may be to initiate CPR, beginning with chest compressions, and transport the patient and the family to the nearest ED, where the family can receive more extensive support (follow local protocols). If there is no evidence of postmortem changes, begin CPR immediately. Chapter 15, *BLS Resuscitation*, covers providing CPR to pediatric patients in detail.

As you assess the infant, pay special attention to any marks or bruises on the child before performing any procedures, including CPR. Also note any intervention such as CPR that was done by the parents before you arrived.

Communication and Support of the Family

The extent of your interaction with the family will depend, to some degree, on the number of providers available at the scene. Always introduce yourself to the child's parents or caregivers and ask the child's name, date of birth, and medical history. If and when the decision is made to start or stop resuscitation efforts, inform the family immediately. Find a place for family members where they can watch resuscitation without being in the way. Do not, in any case, speculate on the cause of the child's death. The family will want to see the child and should be asked whether they want to hold the child and say good-bye. Parents or caregivers may be experiencing strong feelings of denial.

Remember that each individual and each culture expresses grief in a different way, some more visibly than others. Some will require intervention; others will not. Most parents or caregivers feel directly or indirectly responsible for the death of a child and may express this immediately; this does not mean that they actually are responsible. Although you should keep the possibility of abuse or neglect in mind, your role is not that of investigator. Any further inquiry is the responsibility of law enforcement.

Part of your job at this point is to allow the family to express their grief in ways that may differ from your own cultural, religious, and personal practices. Provide support in whatever ways you can Table 36-16.

Table 36-16 How You Can Help the Family of a Deceased Child

When arriving on site:	Introduce yourself quickly. Speak to family members at eye level, maintaining good eye contact with them. Obtain a brief history. When possible, one provider should stay with the family. Ask the child's name and refer to the child by that name.
If resuscitation is attempted:	Give brief, frequent updates and explanations. Allow family members to stay within viewing distance if they wish. Allow family members to accompany the child to the hospital when possible.
If no resuscitation is performed:	Sit down with the family. Inform the family immediately. Explain why no resuscitation will be attempted. Offer to arrange for religious support, including baptism or last rites.
Beginning the grieving process:	Cover the child in a blanket. Learn and use the child's name. Allow the family to express emotions; be nonjudgmental. Offer to call other family members. Give brief explanations and answers. Acknowledge the family's feelings ("I know this is devastating for you"). Use the word "dead" or "died" when informing the family of the child's death. Explain to the family that the cause of death is still unknown. Allow time for questions.
Do:	Tell the family how sorry you are. Tell the family whom they can call if they have questions later. Give written instructions and referrals.
Do Not:	Say, "You have other children," or "You can have other children." Attempt to answer the question "Why did this happen?" Try to tell the family that they will feel better with time. Use euphemisms such as "passed away" or "gone." Say, "I know how you feel," even if you have experienced a similar event.

Parents often have questions that you should be prepared to answer: Why did this happen? How did this happen? Let them know that their concerns will be addressed but that answers are not immediately available Table 36-17. Always use the child's name in speaking to family members. If possible, allow the family to spend time with the child and to ride in the ambulance to the hospital.

▶ Brief Resolved Unexplained Event

Infants who are not breathing and are cyanotic and unresponsive when found by their families sometimes resume breathing and color with stimulation. These children have had what is called a **brief resolved unexplained event (BRUE)**, called "near-miss SIDS" in the past. In addition to cyanosis and apnea, a classic BRUE is characterized by a distinct change in muscle tone (limpness) and choking or gagging. After the event, a child may appear healthy and show no signs of illness or distress. Nevertheless, you must complete a careful assessment and provide immediate transport to the ED.

Pay strict attention to management of the airway. Assess the infant's history and, if possible, the environment. Allow caregivers to ride in the ambulance. If asked, explain that you cannot say what caused the event and that this is something that the physician will have to determine at the hospital.

Table 36-17 Common Questions Following Death of a Child
Q: Was there pain? **A:** This often can be answered by a simple "No." If you are uncertain, you may give an indirect answer such as "We really don't know what patients feel in these circumstances."
Q: What did the child die of? **A:** Do not answer this question; you would probably be guessing.
Q: Why did this happen? **A:** Do not attempt to answer this question either because the answer depends on one's own individual philosophy or religion. "I wish I had an answer for you" is usually the most appropriate response.
Q: What happens now? **A:** This question usually concerns the next few minutes or the next hour. If you know, you should give the family a general idea of what will happen. For example, if there is no history of illness, you can say, "A medical examination will be done, and then [the child's name] will be taken to the mortuary."

YOU are the Provider — SUMMARY

1. What stage of growth and development is this child in, and what are some of the key milestones that you can anticipate seeing?

This 5-year-old child is categorized as a preschool-aged child. When they are responsive, you should expect children of this age range to use simple language effectively and have a lively imagination. Also, they can understand directions, are able to be specific in describing their sensations, and identify painful areas when asked.

2. When treating an infant or pediatric patient, what is often the best source of information regarding the current condition?

Depending on the age of the pediatric patient and his or her level of responsiveness, he or she may or may not be able to provide you with information needed to make treatment decisions. Furthermore, younger children often cannot tell you where they hurt. Therefore, you must rely on a parent or caregiver to obtain as much information as you can.

3. What is the purpose of the PAT, and what does it assess?

The PAT is a structured assessment tool that allows you to rapidly form a general impression of the patient's condition without touching him or her. It is intended to provide a "first glance" assessment to help you identify the general category of the child's physiologic problem and to establish the urgency for treatment and/or transport. The PAT assesses three elements: appearance, work of breathing, and circulation to the skin.

4. When should an oropharyngeal airway be inserted in a pediatric patient, and how is it measured?

An oropharyngeal airway should be inserted in the pediatric patient any time the patient is unresponsive and cannot maintain his or her own airway spontaneously. The oropharyngeal airway is measured from the corner of the patient's mouth to the earlobe (on the same side) or by using a length-based resuscitation tape to measure the patient.

5. What are normal vital signs for a patient of this age?

"Normal" vital signs are going to vary depending on the state of the child and the techniques used to obtain them. After ensuring that you are using appropriate-size equipment, and explaining to the patient step-by-step what you are going to do, the generally accepted respiratory rate for a preschool-aged child is 20 to 28 breaths/min, the pulse should be between 65 and 120 beats/min, and the systolic blood pressure should be between 89 and 112 mm Hg. It is important to remember that blood pressure should not be obtained in children younger than 3 years in the prehospital setting.

6. What is the purpose of a Volutrol?

A Volutrol is a special type of macrodrip set that allows you to fill the large drip chamber with a specific amount of fluid and administer only that amount. The 100-mL drip chamber on the Volutrol can be isolated from the IV bag, preventing fluid overload.

7. How should the glucose be prepared?

Glucose administration in pediatric patients age 1 year and older should be accomplished with D_{25} or D_{10} instead of D_{50}. Because of the thickness of D_{50}, there is a greater potential of extravasation, and subsequent tissue necrosis. If your service does not routinely stock D_{25}, it can be easily made from D_{50}. To make D_{25}, you should replace 25 mL of the D_{50}-prefilled syringe with 25 mL of normal saline (NS), resulting in a concentration of D_{25}. To make D_{10}, you should draw 4 mL from the D_{50}-prefilled syringe into a 20-mL syringe and add an additional 16 mL of NS.

8. What are the indications and contraindications for dextrose administration in pediatric patients?

The indications for dextrose administration in pediatric patients are the same as with adult patients, to include symptomatic bradycardia, altered level of consciousness for unknown reasons, unresponsiveness with unknown patient history, and a coma of unknown etiology.

Contraindications for dextrose administration include the presence of increased intracranial pressure or possible intracranial bleeding.

9. If this patient should require IV fluid, how much fluid should she receive?

Fluid resuscitation for this patient should begin with an initial bolus of 20 mL/kg, which is a 360-mL bolus for this patient because she weighs 18 kg (39 lb), followed by careful reassessment. Additional fluid boluses of 20 mL/kg may be administered as needed to maintain adequate perfusion.

YOU are the Provider SUMMARY *(continued)*

EMS Patient Care Report (PCR)					
Date: 10-7-18	**Incident No.:** 0103	**Nature of Call:** Unresponsive	**Location:** 424 N. Cavalier Street		
Dispatched: 1255	**En Route:** 1302	**At Scene:** 1309	**Transport:** 1318	**At Hospital:** 1335	**In Service:** 1400
Patient Information					
Age: 5 **Sex:** F **Weight (in kg [lb]):** 18 kg (39 lb)			**Allergies:** None **Medications:** None **Past Medical History:** None **Chief Complaint:** Unresponsive, possible overdose		
Vital Signs					
Time: 1310	**BP:** Not obtained	**Pulse:** Not obtained	**Respirations:** 4-A	**Spo_2:** Not obtained	
Time: 1317	**BP:** Unable to obtain	**Pulse:** 155	**Respirations:** 20-A	**Spo_2:** 99% on 15 L/min	
Time: 1333	**BP:** 90/P	**Pulse:** 130	**Respirations:** 30	**Spo_2:** 99% on 15 L/min	
EMS Treatment (circle all that apply)					
Oxygen @ 15 **L/min via (circle one):** NC (**NRM**) (**Bag-mask device**)		(**Assisted Ventilation:** Yes)	(**Airway Adjunct:** OPA)	**CPR**	
Defibrillation	**Bleeding Control**	**Bandaging**	**Splinting**	(**Other:** Medication administration)	
Narrative					

EMS dispatched to above location for unresponsive child. Met at door of residence by elderly man who directs us to patient found in back bedroom. Patient found supine on bed, unresponsive, with agonal respirations. Mother states that patient possibly got into some diabetes medication in the house. Airway established with OPA and ventilations assisted via bag-mask device with oxygen. PAT – poor. Once ventilations established, patient placed on stretcher, secured, and placed in back of ambulance. Dispatch contacted for paramedic transport, advised no units available. Vital signs as above, blood glucose obtained at 26 mg/dL. IV established with 22-gauge catheter on Volutrol. Emergency transport initiated. Verified patency, administered 90 mL D_{10}. On recheck of blood glucose level, found to be 134 mg/dL with patient beginning to breathe more effectively, with some purposeful movement. Patient placed on 15 L/min via NRB. Patient crying for mother. Transport stopped, mother secured in back of ambulance to calm patient. Transport resumed non emergency. On arrival at ED, patient acting appropriate for age, in no acute distress. Care and report given to ED staff without incident.**End of report**

Prep Kit

▶ Ready for Review

- Children are not only smaller than adults and more vulnerable, they are also anatomically, physiologically, and psychologically different from adults in some important ways.
- General rules for caring for pediatric patients of all ages include appearing confident, being calm, remaining honest, and keeping parents or caregivers together with the pediatric patient as much as possible.
- Infancy is the first year of life. If possible, allow the parent or caregiver to hold the infant during the assessment.
- The toddler is 1 to 3 years of age. Toddlers may experience stranger anxiety but may be able to be distracted by a special object (blanket) or toy.
- Preschool-age children are 3 to 6 years of age. Preschool-age children can understand directions and can identify painful areas when questioned. Tell these children what you are going to do before you do it. This action can help prevent the development of frightening fantasies.
- School-age children are 6 to 12 years of age. These children are familiar with the physical examination process. Talk about their interests to distract them during a procedure.
- Adolescents are 12 to 18 years of age. Respect the adolescent's modesty. Remember that even though this age group is physically similar to adults, adolescents are still children on an emotional level.
- The growing bodies of the pediatric patient create some special considerations.
- The tongue is large relative to other structures, so it poses a higher risk of airway obstruction than in an adult.
- An infant breathes faster than an older child. Breathing requires the use of chest muscles and the diaphragm.
- The airway in a child has a smaller diameter than the airway in an adult and is therefore more easily obstructed.
- A rapid heart beat and blood vessel constriction help pediatric patients to compensate for decreased perfusion.
- Children's internal organs are not as insulated by fat as in adults and may be injured more severely. Also, children have less circulating blood than adults, so although they exhibit the signs of shock more slowly they go into shock more quickly, with less blood loss.
- Children's bones are more flexible and bend more with injury; the ends of the long bones, where growth occurs, are weaker and may be injured more easily.
- Because a young child might not be able to speak, your assessment of his or her condition must be based in large part on what you can see and hear yourself. Families may be helpful in providing vital information about an accident or illness.
- Use the pediatric assessment triangle to obtain a general impression of the infant or child. Use the AVPU scale or the Pediatric Glasgow Coma Scale to assess a pediatric patient's level of consciousness.
- You will need to carry special sizes of airway equipment for pediatric patients. Use a length-based resuscitation tape to help determine the appropriate size of equipment for children.
- The three keys to successful use of the bag-mask device in a child are: (1) have the appropriate equipment in the right size; (2) maintain a good face-to-mask seal; and (3) ventilate at the appropriate rate and volume.
- You must intervene immediately if bradycardia develops in a child in respiratory distress, providing oxygenation and assisted ventilations if they become necessary.
- Signs of shock in children are tachycardia, poor capillary refill time, and mental status changes. You must be extremely alert for signs of shock in pediatric patients because they can decompensate rapidly.
- Appropriate fluid administration in the pediatric patient is crucial; intravenous (IV) fluids must be administered based on the child's clinical condition.
- IV therapy is not performed as frequently in children as it is in adults, but the technique, indications, and contraindications in the infant and child are the same as they are for adults.
- Fluid control for pediatric patients is important. Using a special type of microdrip set allows you to administer a specific amount of fluid.
- When possible, allow the infant or child to sit on the parent or caregiver's lap when starting the IV line.
- Intraosseous (IO) infusion is used for emergency vascular access in pediatric patients as defined by protocol when immediate IV access is difficult or impossible. As a general guideline, an IO insertion should be attempted if you are unable to obtain IV access within three attempts *or* 90 seconds or based on local protocols in a critically ill or injured pediatric patient.

Prep Kit *(continued)*

- An IO infusion is contraindicated if a secure IV line is available or if a possible fracture exists in the same bone in which you plan to insert the IO needle.
- Establish vascular access in any infant or child in shock; administer 20-mL/kg boluses of normal saline or lactated Ringer solution as needed to maintain adequate perfusion.
- Febrile seizures may be a sign of a more serious problem such as meningitis.
- The most common cause of dehydration in children is vomiting and diarrhea. Life-threatening diarrhea can develop in an infant in hours.
- Fever is a common reason why parents or caregivers call 9-1-1. A body temperature of 100.4°F (38°C) or higher is considered to be abnormal.
- Manage hypoglycemia in a pediatric patient in the same way you would in an adult, treating the symptomatic child with glucose if his or her blood glucose level is less than 80 mg/dL. Use pediatric IV glucose dosages based on the patient's age.
- Trauma is the number one killer of children in the United States.
- Note and report any signs of abuse or neglect when assessing a pediatric patient, such as bruises in different stages of healing, burn patterns, fractures, developmental delay, or emotional indicators (withdrawn, afraid, hostile).
- If you suspect sexual abuse, limit your assessment to determining the type of dressing any injuries require. Do not allow the child to wash, urinate, or defecate before a physician completes an examination.
- A victim of sudden infant death syndrome (SIDS) will be pale or blue, not breathing, and unresponsive. He or she may show signs of postmortem changes, including rigor mortis and dependent lividity; if so, call medical control to report the situation.
- Carefully inspect the environment where a SIDS victim was found, looking for signs of illness, abusive family interactions, and objects in the child's crib.
- Provide support for the family in whatever way you can, but do not make judgmental statements.
- Any death of a child is stressful for family members and for health care providers. In dealing with the family, acknowledge their feelings, keep any instructions short and simple, use the child's name, and maintain eye contact.
- Be prepared to respond to philosophical as well as medical questions, in most cases by indicating concern and understanding; do not be specific about the cause of death.
- Be alert for signs of posttraumatic stress in yourself and others after dealing with the death of a child. It can help to talk about the event and your feelings with your EMS colleagues.

▶ Vital Vocabulary

acrocyanosis Blue hands or feet that can occur at any age; may be benign in infants younger than 2 months.

adolescents People between 12 and 18 years of age.

apical pulse Obtained by auscultating heart tones over the chest with a stethoscope.

blanching Turning white.

blow-by oxygen A method of delivering oxygen by holding a face mask or similar device near the infant or child's face; used when a nonrebreathing mask is not tolerated.

bradycardia A slow heart rate; less than 80 beats/min in children; less than 100 beats/min in infants.

bradypnea Slow respiratory rate; ominous sign in a child; indicates impending respiratory arrest.

brief resolved unexplained event (BRUE) An event that causes unresponsiveness, cyanosis, and apnea in an infant, who then resumes breathing with stimulation.

capillary refill time The amount of time that it takes for blood to return to the capillary bed after applying pressure to the skin or nail bed; indicates the status of end-organ perfusion; reliable in children younger than 6 years.

central pulses Pulses that are closest to the core (central) part of the body where the vital organs are located.

child abuse Any improper or excessive action that injures or otherwise harms a child or infant; includes physical abuse, sexual abuse, neglect, and emotional abuse.

croup Infection of the airway below the level of the vocal cords, usually caused by a virus; also referred to as laryngotracheobronchitis.

end-organ perfusion The status of perfusion to the vital organs of the body; determined by assessing capillary refill time.

epiglottitis An acute bacterial infection that results in rapid swelling of the epiglottis and surrounding tissues; also referred to as acute supraglottic laryngitis.

epiphyseal plate The growth plate of the bone; responsible for normal bone growth and development.

Prep Kit *(continued)*

febrile seizures Seizures relating to fever.

fontanelles Areas where the infant's skull has not fused together; usually disappear at approximately 18 months of age.

functional residual capacity The volume of air remaining in the lungs following exhalation; also referred to as oxygen reserve.

greenstick fracture An incomplete fracture of a bone; seen in children, whose bones are pliable and may not completely fracture.

grunting An "uh" sound heard during exhalation; reflects the child's attempt to keep the alveoli open; a sign of increased work of breathing.

infancy The first year of life.

intraosseous (IO) infusion Method of delivering fluids or medications into the medullary canal of the bone; used when intravenous access cannot be quickly obtained.

Jamshidi needle A double needle, consisting of a solid-bore needle inside a sharpened hollow needle; used to access the medullary canal for intraosseous infusion.

length-based resuscitation tape A tape used to estimate an infant or child's weight on the basis of length; appropriate drug doses and equipment sizes are listed on the tape; one type is called a Broselow tape.

mediastinum The space in between the lungs that contains the trachea, heart, great vessels, and a portion of the esophagus.

medullary canal The space within the bone that contains bone marrow.

meningitis Inflammation of the meninges that cover the spinal cord and the brain.

nares The external openings of the nostrils.

neglect Refusal or failure on the part of the caregiver to provide life necessities.

Neisseria meningitidis A form of bacterial meningitis characterized by rapid onset of symptoms, often leading to shock and death.

nuchal rigidity A stiff or painful neck; commonly associated with meningitis.

occiput The posterior (back) aspect of the head.

osteomyelitis Infection of the bone and muscle; a potential complication of intraosseous infusion.

parenchyma The tissue of an organ itself.

pediatric assessment triangle (PAT) A structured assessment tool that allows you to rapidly form a general impression of the infant or child without touching him or her; consists of assessing appearance, work of breathing, and circulation to the skin.

pertussis An airborne bacterial infection that affects primarily children younger than 6 years; patients will be feverish and exhibit a "whoop" sound on inspiration after a coughing attack; highly contagious through droplet infection; also called whooping cough.

preschool age Between 3 and 6 years of age.

respiratory arrest The absence of respirations with detectable cardiac activity.

respiratory distress A clinical state characterized by increased respiratory rate, effort, and work of breathing.

respiratory failure A clinical state of inadequate oxygenation, ventilation, or both.

school age Between 6 and 12 years of age.

septum A central divider, such as the nasal septum.

shaken baby syndrome Bleeding within the head and damage to the cervical spine as a result of intentional, forceful shaking of an infant or small child.

sniffing position Optimum head position for the uninjured child who requires airway management.

sudden infant death syndrome (SIDS) Unexpected death of an infant or young child that remains unexplained after a complete autopsy.

tachypnea Increased respiratory rate.

tenting A sign of dehydration in which the skin slowly retracts after being pinched and pulled away slightly from the body.

tidal volume The amount of air that is delivered to the lungs in one inhalation.

toddler A child between 1 and 3 years of age.

tonic-clonic seizure A type of seizure that features rhythmic back-and-forth motion of an extremity and body stiffness.

tracheal tugging Pulling of the trachea into the neck during inspiration; a sign of increased work of breathing.

tragus The small cartilaginous projection in front of the opening of the ear.

vasoconstriction Narrowing of the diameter of a blood vessel.

Volutrol A special type of microdrip set; allows you to fill a large drip chamber with a specific amount of fluid to avoid fluid overload.

Prep Kit *(continued)*

work of breathing An indicator of oxygenation and ventilation. Work of breathing reflects the child's attempt to compensate for hypoxia.

▶ References

1. Shah MN, Cushman JT, Davis CO, et al. The epidemiology of emergency medical services use by children: an analysis of the National Hospital Ambulatory Medical Care Survey. *Prehosp Emerg Care*. 2008;12:269. https://www.uptodate.com/contents/prehospital-pediatrics-and-emergency-medical-services-ems?source=search_result&search=pediatric%20emergencies&selectedTitle=6~150. Accessed February 13, 2017.
2. Anders TF, Sadeh A, Appareddy V. Normal sleep in neonates and children. In: Ferber R, Kryger M (eds). *Principles and Practice of Sleep Medicine in the Child*. Philadelphia, PA: W.B. Saunders; 1995:7. https://www.uptodate.com/contents/sleep-physiology-in-children?source=machineLearning&search=infants%20sleep&selectedTitle=3~150§ionRank=1&anchor=H4#H4. Accessed February 24, 2017.
3. Tomek S. How to manage the pediatric airway. EMSWorld website. http://www.emsworld.com/article/10476091/pediatric-airway-management. December 7, 2011. Accessed September 5, 2017.
4. National Association of State EMS Officials. *National Model EMS Clinical Guidelines*. V.11.14. Croup (p.108). https://nasemso.org/Projects/ModelEMSClinicalGuidelines/documents/National-Model-EMS-Clinical-Guidelines-23Oct2014.pdf. Accessed April 17, 2017.
5. Woods CR. Croup: Approach to management. January 2017. Available: https://www.uptodate.com/contents/croup-approach-to-management?source=search_result&search=croup&selectedTitle=1~62. Accessed February 27, 2017.
6. Defendi GL. Croup treatment & management. Medscape website. http://emedicine.medscape.com/article/962972-treatment. Updated September 27, 2016. Accessed September 5, 2017.
7. Moore M, Little P. Humidified air inhalation for treating croup: a systematic review and meta-analysis. *Family Practice*. 2007;24(4):295–301.
8. Centers for Disease Control and Prevention. Asthma. https://www.cdc.gov/nchs/fastats/asthma.htm. Accessed February 27, 2017.
9. Barson WJ. Pneumonia in children: epidemiology, pathogenesis, and etiology. https://www.uptodate.com/contents/pneumonia-in-children-epidemiology-pathogenesis-and-etiology?source=see_link. Accessed February 27, 2016.
10. World Health Organization. Pneumonia. September 2016. http://www.who.int/mediacentre/factsheets/fs331/en/. Accessed February 27, 2017.
11. Atkins DL, Berger S, Duff JP, Gonzales JC, Hunt EA, Joyner BL, Meaney PA, Niles DE, Samson RA, Schexnayder SM. Part 11: pediatric basic life support and cardiopulmonary resuscitation quality: 2015 American Heart Association Guidelines Update for Cardiopulmonary Resuscitation and Emergency Cardiovascular Care. *Circulation*. 2015;132(suppl 2):S519–S525.
12. Bardella IJ. Pediatric advanced life support: a review of the AHA recommendations. Oct. 15, 1999. http://www.aafp.org/afp/1999/1015/p1743.html. Accessed September 5, 2017.
13. Sahu S, Kishore K, Lata K. Better outcome after pediatric resuscitation is still a dilemma. *J Emerg Trauma Shock*. 2010; 3(3):243–250. https://www.ncbi.nlm.nih.gov/pmc/articles/PMC2938489/. Accessed September 5, 2017.
14. Pomerantz WJ. Hypovolemic shock in children: initial evaluation and management. In: UpToDate, Post TW (Ed), UpToDate, Waltham, MA. https://www.uptodate.com/contents/hypovolemic-shock-in-children-initial-evaluation-and-management?source=see_link. Accessed March 2, 2017.
15. Colwell C. Initial evaluation and treatment of shock in adult trauma. In: UpToDate, Post TW (ed), UpToDate, Waltham, MA. https://www.uptodate.com/contents/initial-evaluation-and-management-of-shock-in-adult-trauma?source=see_link§ionName=PATHOPHYSIOLOGY%20AND%20CLASSIFICATION&anchor=H2#H2. Accessed March 2, 2017.
16. American Heart Association (AHA). *Pediatric Advanced Life Support*. Dallas, TX: AHA; 2015.
17. Millicap JJ. Clinical features and evaluation of febrile seizures. In: UpToDate, Post TW (ed), UpToDate, Waltham, MA. https://www.uptodate.com/contents/clinical-features-and-evaluation-of-febrile-seizures?source=search_result&search=febrile%20seizures&selectedTitle=1~130. Accessed March 2, 2017.
18. Bacterial meningitis - risk factors. Centers for Disease Control and Prevention website. https://www.cdc.gov/meningitis/bacterial.html. Updated January 25, 2017. Accessed September 6, 2017.
19. Meningitis – what increases your risk. WebMD website. http://www.webmd.com/children/vaccines/tc/meningitis-what-increases-your-risk. Accessed September 6, 2017.

Prep Kit *(continued)*

20. Drugs and supplements: charcoal, activated (oral route). Mayo Clinic website. http://www.mayoclinic.org/drugs-supplements/charcoal-activated-oral-route/proper-use/drg-20070087. Updated March 1, 2017. Accessed September 6, 2017.
21. American Association of Poison Control Centers website. http://www.aapcc.org/. Accessed March 2, 2017.
22. Centers for Disease Control and Prevention. 10 Leading Causes of Injury Deaths By Age Group Highlighting Unintentional Injury Deaths, United States–2014. https://www.cdc.gov/injury/images/lc-charts/leading_causes_of_injury_deaths_unintentional_injury_2014_1040w740h.gif. Accessed March 2, 2017.
23. 10 leading causes of death by age group, United States – 2015. National Vital Statistics System, National Center for Health Statistics, Centers for Disease Control and Prevention. https://www.cdc.gov/injury/wisqars/LeadingCauses.html. Accessed September 22, 2017.
24. CDC childhood injury report. Centers for Disease Control and Prevention website. https://www.cdc.gov/safechild/child_injury_data.html. Updated December 23, 2015. Accessed September 6, 2017.
25. Boos SC. Physical child abuse: recognition. UpToDate website. https://www.uptodate.com/contents/physical-child-abuse-recognition?source=search_result&search=child%20abuse&selectedTitle=1~150#H706482144. Updated February 15, 2017. Accessed September 6, 2017.
26. Department of Health and Human Services. Children's Bureau. Child Maltreatment 2015. https://www.acf.hhs.gov/cb/resource/child-maltreatment-2015. Accessed February 13, 2017.
27. Victims of sexual violence: statistics. RAINN website. https://www.rainn.org/statistics/victims-sexual-violence. Accessed September 6, 2017.
28. About SUID and SIDS. Centers for Disease Control and Prevention website. https://www.cdc.gov/sids/aboutsuidandsids.htm. Updated February 1, 2017. Accessed September 6, 2017.
29. U.S. Department of Health and Human Services. Known risk factors for SIDS and other sleep-related causes of infant death. Safe to Sleep website. https://www.nichd.nih.gov/sts/about/risk/Pages/factors.aspx. Accessed September 6, 2017.

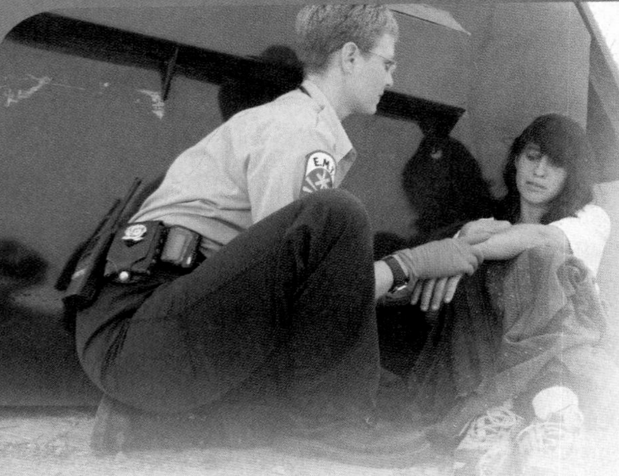

Assessment *in Action*

Your ambulance is dispatched to a local residence for a child with a possible leg fracture. On arrival, you are greeted by the mother's boyfriend who states the child fell from the countertop. Your examination reveals a frightened 6-year-old boy with an obviously deformed left lower leg. When you ask him what happened, he just looks at the mother's boyfriend.

1. Which of the following is not consistent with a suspicion of child abuse?

A. History inconsistent with injury
B. Lack of supervision
C. Urgency in seeking care
D. Inappropriate parental concerns

2. In the mnemonic for assessing possible child abuse, the "D" stands for:

A. deformities.
B. delay in seeking care.
C. defecation.
D. distal injuries.

Assessment in Action *(continued)*

3. The abused child may appear as all of the following except:

- **A.** relieved.
- **B.** withdrawn.
- **C.** hostile.
- **D.** fearful.

4. A deformity in bones of children this age is particularly concerning because of the potential damage that may occur to the:

- **A.** pubic symphysis.
- **B.** epiphyseal plates.
- **C.** ego.
- **D.** skin.

5. An appropriate pulse rate for a child of this age who is awake is ____ beats/min.

- **A.** 32
- **B.** 58
- **C.** 74
- **D.** 100

6. A brief resolved unexplained event (BRUE) includes which of the following?

- **A.** Cyanosis
- **B.** Tachypnea
- **C.** Vigorous activity
- **D.** Cooing

7. A child of this age can think in _____ terms, respond sensibly to direct questions, and help take care of himself or herself.

- **A.** concrete
- **B.** abstract
- **C.** simple
- **D.** vague

8. ________ is a common cause of shock in children and occurs with blood volume loss.

- **A.** Anaphylactic shock
- **B.** Hypovolemic shock
- **C.** Cardiogenic shock
- **D.** Neurogenic shock

9. What is the Pediatric Assessment Triangle?

10. List the signs of a severe airway obstruction.

CHAPTER 37

Geriatric Emergencies

National EMS Education Standard Competencies

Special Patient Populations

Applies a fundamental knowledge of growth, development, aging, and assessment findings to provide basic and selected advanced emergency care and transportation for a patient with special needs.

Geriatrics

- Impact of age-related changes on assessment and care (pp 1554-1560)
- Changes associated with aging, psychosocial aspects of aging, and age-related assessment and treatment modifications for the major or common geriatric diseases and/or emergencies
  - Cardiovascular diseases (pp 1546-1547, 1562-1565)
  - Respiratory diseases (pp 1545-1546, 1561-1562)
  - Neurologic diseases (pp1547-1549, 1565-1566)
  - Endocrine diseases (pp 1552, 1566-1568)
  - Alzheimer disease (pp 1549-1550)
  - Dementia (p 1549)
- Fluid resuscitation in the elderly (p 1561)

Patients With Special Challenges

- Recognizing and reporting abuse and neglect (pp 1576-1578 and Chapter 36, *Pediatric Emergencies*)

Health care implications of

- Abuse (pp 1576-1578 and Chapter 36, *Pediatric Emergencies*)
- Neglect (pp 1576-1578 and Chapter 36, *Pediatric Emergencies*)
- Homelessness (Chapter 38, *Patients With Special Challenges*)
- Poverty (Chapter 38, *Patients With Special Challenges*)
- Bariatrics (Chapter 38, *Patients With Special Challenges*)
- Technology dependent (Chapter 38, *Patients With Special Challenges*)
- Hospice/terminally ill (Chapter 35, *Patients With Special Challenges*)
- Tracheostomy care/dysfunction (Chapter 38, *Patients With Special Challenges*)
- Home care (Chapter 38, *Patients With Special Challenges*)
- Sensory deficit/loss (Chapter 38, *Patients With Special Challenges*)
- Developmental disability (Chapter 38, *Patients With Special Challenges*)

Trauma

Applies fundamental knowledge to provide basic and selected advanced emergency care and transportation based on assessment findings for an acutely injured patient.

Special Considerations in Trauma

Recognition and management of trauma in the

- Geriatric patient (pp 1572-1576)

Pathophysiology, assessment, and management of trauma in the

- Geriatric patient (pp 1573-1576)

Knowledge Objectives

1. Define the term *geriatrics*. (p 1541)
2. Discuss the economic impact of aging, independent and dependent living, advance directives, and end-of-life care. (pp 1542-1543)
3. Discuss generational considerations when communicating with geriatric patients and their families. (pp 1543-1544)
4. Discuss how to respond to nursing or skilled care facilities. (p 1544)
5. Explain the leading causes of death among geriatric patients. (p 1545)
6. Discuss the normal physiologic changes that occur in various body systems as people age. (pp 1545-1554)
7. Describe the pathophysiology of common conditions affecting geriatric patients. (pp 1545-1554)
8. Discuss psychiatric emergencies in the older population. (p 1550)

9. Define polypharmacy, and explain the toxicity issues that can result. (p 1554)
10. Know the potential implications of a patient taking multiple medications. (p 1554)
11. Discuss special considerations when performing the patient assessment process on a geriatric patient with a medical condition. (pp 1554-1560)
12. Explain the GEMS diamond (Geriatric patients, Environmental assessment, Medical assessment, and Social assessment) and its role in the assessment and care of the geriatric patient. (pp 1556-1557)
13. Discuss emergency medical care of a geriatric patient including fluid resuscitation. (pp 1560-1561)
14. Discuss assessment and management of common conditions and injuries affecting geriatric patients, including respiratory, cardiovascular, neurologic, endocrine, gastrointestinal, renal, and toxicologic emergencies. (pp 1561-1571)
15. Explain special considerations for a geriatric patient who has experienced trauma, including performing the patient assessment process on a geriatric patient with a traumatic injury. (pp 1572-1576)
16. Discuss elder abuse and neglect, and its implications in assessment and management of the patient. (pp 1576-1578)

Skills Objectives

There are no skills objectives for this chapter.

Introduction

Geriatrics is the assessment and treatment of disease and/or injury in someone 65 years or older. Prevention and management of disease and disability in later life are becoming more important as a result of an aging society **Figure 37-1**. For some time, emergency medical services (EMS) education approached the treatment of geriatric patients with the same considerations as those for younger adults. Now this has changed.

A decline in our body systems starts in our late 20s and progresses slowly throughout our life span. Think of yourself and subtle changes you have seen as a result of aging. Perhaps you have noticed a slight deficit in eyesight or hearing, or difficulty in doing activities you had no problem doing 10 years ago. The reality is that we all age, and older persons will continue to become a larger percentage of the population.

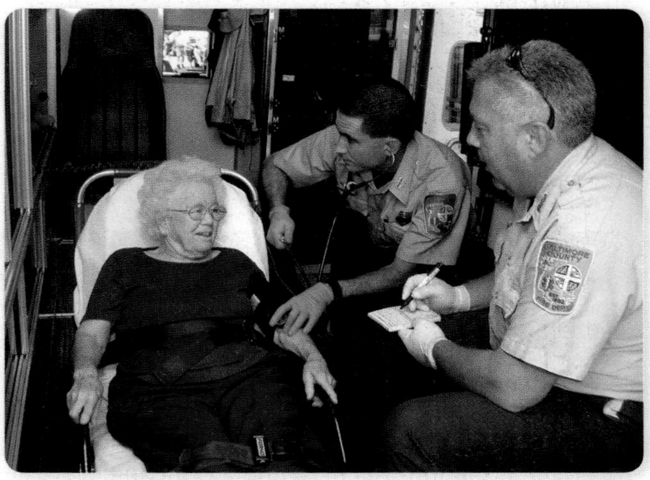

Figure 37-1 Working with geriatric patients is a large part of being an EMS provider.

YOU are the Provider PART 1

Your ambulance is dispatched to a local apartment complex for an unknown medical problem. On your arrival, you are greeted at the door by a distraught middle-aged woman who states she came over to check on her elderly father, and he was not acting normally. As you approach the patient, he informs you that his name is Darwin Feakes and that he is 82 years old, but he appears slightly confused about anything else. His daughter tells you that he has been getting progressively "senile" over several years, has numerous medical problems, takes numerous medications, and that he has lived by himself since her mother died last year.

1. What are some possible causes of confusion in geriatric patients?
2. Does this patient present with any risk factors that could affect his mortality?

According to the 2015 US Census estimates, more than 44.6 million Americans are age 65 years and older—a 13.2% increase from the 2010 Census.[1] Why is the number so large? Remember that people today are living longer than they did 15 to 20 years ago. Advances in medical care and preventive measures have been instrumental in this increased longevity. These calls may be challenging because the classic presentation of medical conditions common in younger patients may not be seen in older patients. For example, an acute myocardial infarction (MI) may present in an atypical fashion in an older patient; nonspecific symptoms such as weakness, dizziness, or nausea are not uncommon. Some older patients may not experience chest pain or pressure (ie, a silent MI). An aging body can mask serious medical conditions. Older patients frequently have chronic medical problems and may be taking numerous medications for their illnesses. Providing effective treatment for this increasing number of patients will require you to understand the issues related to aging and modify some of your assessment and treatment approaches.

We should respect the wealth of knowledge that older patients have to offer. In many countries, older people are treated with reverence. In many other cultures, older people are seen as a valuable resource of history. In Japan, there is a "Respect for the Aged Day." This same degree of respect may not be shared by many people in the United States, but as an advanced emergency medical technician (AEMT), you must remember to treat every patient the way you would want your loved ones to be treated.

General Considerations

The Economic Impact of Aging

As an AEMT, you need to be aware of the economic impact of aging. Many older people today did not have the benefit of retirement planning. The Social Security Administration reports that the four major sources of income for older people are social security, income from assets, pensions, and earnings.[2] For most older people, Social Security is the major source of income.[3] For many older people, this is their *only* source of income, forcing them to prioritize their needs on a monthly basis. Older people may not seek medical assistance because of the concern over cost.

The cost of prescriptions for older persons may cause some patients to either skip days of their medication or cut their dosage in half. The average annual prescription spending per person older than 65 years was $18,424 in 2010.[4] Therefore, many older people who have reached retirement age continue to be a part of the workforce to supplement their limited income.

> **Words of Wisdom**
>
> By halving medications, a 30-day supply of medications turns into a 60-day supply. Stress the importance of taking medications in the strength prescribed. Take the time to familiarize yourself with programs that may help to pay for medications for those who cannot afford them.

Independent and Dependent Living

Not all geriatric patients you are called to assist will be living in a nursing home. Many older patients are able to live independently. You may also encounter a senior citizen who is the primary caregiver for his or her parent or parents. Often, these patients will be in the same home in which they grew up. Be aware that many of these same patients have a fear that if you take them to the hospital, they will never see their home again.

Most healthy older adults strive to live independently. They may believe that they are able to care for themselves and handle **activities of daily living (ADLs)** such as tooth brushing, showering, and dressing. When one of the adults becomes ill and can no longer take care of himself or herself, that person becomes dependent on others in the home. Someone else in the home may become a caregiver. Many older couples or friends and family who live together can provide basic assistance for each other; however, some older patients do not have family or friends to assist them. They are totally dependent on themselves, may attempt to do everything on their own, and may not seek available assistance. Patients who become isolated from outside social events are susceptible to self-abuse or alcohol or medication abuse.

What happens when an individual is unable to care for himself or herself? For financial reasons or previous experience, the family may decide to provide care to the older patient in the home. They may seek the help of a visiting nurse agency. Outsiders, as well as the AEMT, may believe the patient can receive better care in a dependent care facility. You need to remember that families have their reasons for wanting an older patient to stay in a familiar home environment. Sometimes older patients refuse to accept that they need assistance and may not be aware of the danger in insisting on caring for themselves. The care of an older patient may fall on a spouse or family members who may have additional medical problems themselves. You may respond to a home or facility for a patient only to find out that the caregiver is actually more in need of care than the patient. The stress of caring for a chronically ill person can become overwhelming. Caregivers may neglect their own health care and/or social needs. Caregivers may be afraid to leave the house, may limit social interactions, and may need help coping with stress.

Dependent living (sometimes known as residential care) has many different levels of assistance. The level is based on two factors. One level of care is based on the needs of the person, while the other level of care is based on restrictions that are placed on the person. Dependent care can range from the least restrictive retirement community to the structured skilled nursing facility to specialty care facilities for patients with dementia or Alzheimer disease.

Advance Directives and End-of-Life Care

Mentally competent adults and emancipated minors have the right to consent to or decline treatment. To prepare for the possibility that they become mentally incompetent, many people today are making use of advance directives. As discussed in Chapter 3, *Medical, Legal, and Ethical Issues,* advance directives are legal documents that specify the desired medical treatment for a competent patient, should he or she become unable to make decisions. An advance directive is also commonly called a living will.

Advance directives may take the form of do not resuscitate (DNR) orders, sometimes called do not attempt resuscitation (DNAR) orders. DNR orders give you permission not to attempt resuscitation for a patient in cardiac arrest. Even in the presence of a DNR order, you are still obligated to provide supportive measures that may include oxygen delivery, pain relief, and comfort when you can. DNR does not mean do not treat. Learn and become familiar with your state laws regarding this issue.

You may also encounter an end-of-life document known as Physician Orders for Life-Sustaining Treatment (POLST). Although similar to a DNR, the POLST is more expansive and encourages physicians to speak with patients with a terminal illness and create specific orders to be followed at the end of life. A DNR generally applies to patients who are in cardiac arrest, whereas POLST may apply to patients with such conditions as impending pulmonary failure who are not in cardiac arrest.

In the absence of an advance directive or DNR, some patients may have a durable power of attorney for health care or a health care proxy, a named surrogate to make decisions for them regarding their health care in the event they are incapacitated and unable to make decisions themselves. Be sure to follow your service's protocol when faced with any advance directive. For more information about consent, advance directives, and durable power of attorneys for health care, see Chapter 3, *Medical, Legal, and Ethical Issues.*

You will inevitably be involved with end-of-life care for patients. Many communities have nursing home facilities (residential facilities with health care), **hospice** services (homes provided for the terminally ill), and home health care programs (patients are treated in their homes). If these programs exist in your community, consider how you or your service might collaborate on providing quality care for a person at the end of life.

Communicating With Older Patients and Spouses

Communication is the key to a productive encounter with a patient. Consider your own personal communication skills. Does the patient understand what you are saying, asking, or doing? When the patient is sitting in a chair, bend down or position yourself at the patient's level to speak directly to the patient, allowing the patient to see your face. Maintaining eye contact and speaking in a steady tone will assist you in communicating with the patient. You may be required to repeat a question or statement when it appears that the patient does not comprehend what you are asking or saying. Ask as many open-ended questions as possible and use closed-ended questions to clarify points.

Avoid being overly familiar with the patient, and do not use first names or nicknames unless the patient asks you to. Avoid being judgmental. You must be able to gain your patient's confidence, which is best accomplished by treating the patient with respect, taking a slow, deliberate approach, and explaining what you are doing. Be sure to have one provider obtain the patient's history, one question at a time, providing as much privacy as possible **Figure 37-2**. After interviewing the patient, ask family members or caregivers to clarify what you just learned from the patient. Past medical conditions can provide information about the patient's current problem. Older patients often have more than one chronic condition, and the symptoms of one disease may make the assessment of another more difficult. Do not assume that just because a patient is older, he or she is unable to communicate, and do not assume an altered mental status is *normal*.

An AEMT may encounter a geriatric couple who has been together for many years with no immediate family. In times of crisis, the patient is cared for, and the spouse may be forgotten. If the spouse cannot drive, there may be no way for him or her to get to the hospital. Depending on circumstances, it may also be difficult for the spouse to contact the hospital or follow up on the loved one's progress. You can help by simply asking a bystander, firefighter, police officer, or anyone who is not directly caring for the patient to help the spouse into the passenger seat

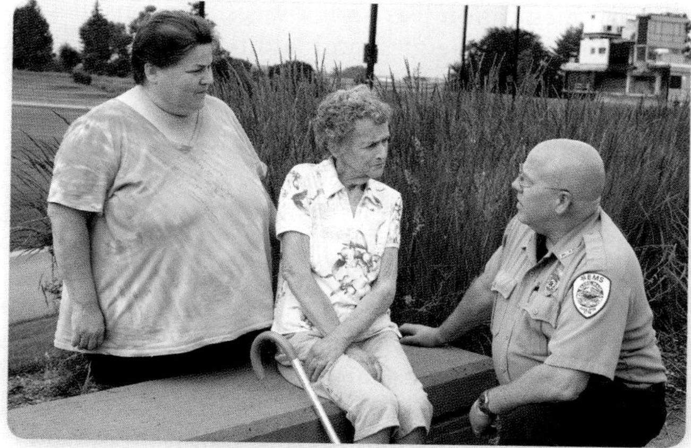

Figure 37-2 A slow, deliberate approach to the patient history, with one AEMT asking the questions, is generally the best strategy in assessing an older patient.

of the ambulance and to fasten the seat belt so that when you are ready to go, the spouse is ready also.

For more information about communicating with older patients, see Chapter 4, *Communications and Documentation*.

Words of Wisdom

When communicating with an older patient, choose appropriate terminology or describe conditions to eliminate confusion. For example, when asked about patient history, an older patient may say, "I have sugar and high blood." These terms are often used in place of *diabetes* and *hypertension* if the patient is not familiar with the appropriate terminology.

Response to Nursing and Skilled Care Facilities

Nursing homes or skilled care facilities are common locations in which the AEMT will encounter an older patient. Before you provide transport for the patient, you should find out the following critical information from the nursing staff:

- What is the patient's chief complaint today?
- What is the patient's admitting diagnosis? In other words, what is the initial problem that led to admission to the facility?

To determine the nature of the problem, you will usually have to compare the patient's present condition with his or her condition before the onset of the symptoms. Ask the staff about the patient's mobility, ADLs, and ability to speak. This will help to establish the patient's baseline condition and determine whether today's behavior differs.

Many facilities that are transferring patients will include a transfer record containing the patient's medical history, medication lists and dosages, previous diagnoses, vital signs, allergies, and additional information. These records provide you, as well as other health care providers who will be involved in the care of the patient, with essential information and will save time, especially when the patient cannot speak for himself or herself. Be sure to obtain this essential record before leaving for the hospital and relay it to the hospital staff when giving your report.

Infection control needs to be a high priority for AEMTs when visiting these facilities. You not only need to protect yourself, but you also need to inhibit the spread of pathogens from patient to patient. Good handwashing and standard precautions can inhibit the spread of infectious pathogens to people who already have compromised immune systems. An infection in an older patient can lead to life-threatening sepsis. Infections such as **methicillin-resistant *Staphylococcus aureus* (MRSA)** are common among people who are living in close quarters such as nursing homes. The organism can be found in decubitus ulcers (bed sores), on feeding tubes, and on indwelling urinary catheters. The symptoms of MRSA depend on the type of infection. The bacteria can cause mild infections on the skin or invade the bloodstream, lungs, or the urinary tract. MRSA is primarily spread by broken skin–to-skin contact but is also acquired by touching objects that have the bacteria on them.

Similarly, many infections in hospitals are caused by vancomycin-resistant enterococci. Enterococci are bacteria that are normally present in the human intestines and the female genital tract. Under the right circumstances, these bacteria can cause infection. Some of the enterococci have become resistant to the antibiotic commonly used to treat these infections, which is vancomycin.

The **respiratory syncytial virus** causes an infection of the upper and lower respiratory tracts. Although more typically seen in children, the virus can also cause serious illness in geriatric persons, especially in those with lung disease or weakened immune systems. The symptoms are similar to those of the common cold but can be more severe and last longer. The virus is highly contagious and is found in discharges from the nose and throat of an infected person. Respiratory syncytial virus is also transmitted by direct contact with droplets from coughs or sneezes and by touching a contaminated surface.

MRSA and respiratory syncytial virus infections can be life threatening, especially in an immunocompromised patient. Look for "isolation" signs or ask about contagious disease when you approach a patient. Be sure to wear appropriate personal protective equipment and decontaminate your ambulance and diagnostic equipment after contact with nursing home residents if there is a history of infectious disease or if the patient shows signs and symptoms of a potentially infectious disease. Be sure to document the infection control issue; advise the receiving facility; and, depending on local protocol, report any infectious disease to your company or the local health department.

Clostridium difficile is a bacterium responsible for the most common cause of hospital-acquired infectious diarrhea and regularly causes sporadic cases of diarrhea in nursing homes. The bacterium normally grows in the intestines. Antibiotic use may account for the rapid increase in toxic strains that ultimately cause illness. Health care workers may carry this bacterium following contact with contaminated feces. It can also be found on environmental surfaces like furniture, floors, toilets, sinks, and bedding. The symptoms from the resultant colitis can range from minor diarrhea to a life-threatening inflammation of the colon.

You should also be cognizant of potential airborne pathogens. Something as simple as a cold or flu virus could result in a life-threatening pneumonia for a compromised older adult. Be sure to wear a mask if you have an upper respiratory infection, and mask the patient if he or she has one.

Words of Wisdom

There is much you can do to assist with end-of-life care, beginning with demonstrating a caring and concerned attitude and approach.

Leading Causes of Death

The leading cause of death in older people is heart disease, followed by cancer, chronic low respiratory disease, stroke, Alzheimer disease, diabetes, trauma, and pneumonia.[5] Contrary to popular belief, people do not die of "old age." The aging physiology of older people makes them more vulnerable than younger people to the effects of disease and injury. In addition, acute illness and trauma are more likely to involve organ systems beyond those initially involved. For example, an older person who has fallen and fractured a hip may develop pneumonia during recovery because of a weakened immune system. Table 37-1 lists the risk factors that affect mortality in older patients.

Anatomy, Physiology, and Pathophysiology

As people get older, their anatomy and physiology change. In general, a 65-year-old person cannot expect to have the same degree of physical performance as when he or she was 30 years old. Organ systems begin to deteriorate, the heart muscle thickens, the arteries become less elastic, valves degenerate, and maximum vital capacity of the lungs may decline. However, the aging process does not necessarily mean that a person will experience disease.

Table 37-1 Risk Factors Affecting Mortality in Geriatric Patients
Age older than 75 years
Living alone
Recent death of a spouse or significant other
Recent hospitalization
Incontinence (inability to hold urine or feces)
Immobility
Unsound mind

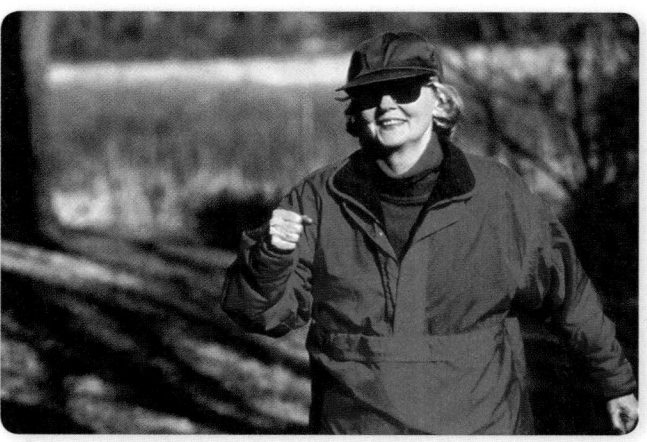

Figure 37-3 Older people can continue to stay fit and active.

Courtesy of the National Cancer Institute.

Common stereotypes about older persons include the presence of mental confusion, illness, a sedentary lifestyle, and immobility. Although these perceptions are common, they are usually far from the truth. Older persons can continue to stay fit and active even though they will not be able to perform at the same level as they did in their youth Figure 37-3. Most older people lead very active lives, participating in sports and in the community, and they are generally healthy despite the aging process. As body systems age, they undergo several important changes, for example:

- Motor nerves begin to deteriorate; reaction time decreases.
- Blood pressure steadily increases.
- Ability to maintain normal body temperature decreases.
- Muscles become less flexible and strength declines.
- Oxygen/carbon dioxide exchange in the lungs and at the cellular level declines, and the body fatigues at a faster rate than when younger.
- Metabolism rate decreases; weight gain may result.

Changes in other body systems are outlined in the following sections.

▶ Changes in the Respiratory System

A person's respiratory capacity undergoes substantial reductions with age for several reasons. As a person ages, the alveoli become enlarged, but their elasticity decreases, making it harder to expel the used air in an older person's lung tissue. This lack of elasticity, caused by a decrease in pulmonary surfactant, results in a decreased ability to exchange oxygen and carbon dioxide, which further causes an increase in residual volume (the amount of air left in the lungs at the end of a maximal exhalation). The body's receptors that monitor the changes in oxygen and carbon dioxide slow with age, which causes lower pulse oximetry (Spo_2) readings even in healthy people. Thus, although the total amount of air in the lungs does not change with age, the proportion of that air used in gas exchange progressively declines. Airflow, which depends largely on airway size and resistance, also deteriorates somewhat with age.

Meanwhile, changes in the distribution of blood flow within the lungs result in a declining partial pressure of oxygen in arterial blood (Pao_2). As the aging process takes place, a decline in Pao_2 can have a substantial effect on the patient's ability to maintain homeostasis. Furthermore, the respiratory drive becomes dulled as a person ages because of decreased sensitivity to changes in arterial blood gases or decreased central nervous system (CNS) response to such changes. Consequently, older people have a slower reaction to hypoxemia and hypercapnia.

Another important change is that calcification tends to make the chest wall stiffer. Other musculoskeletal changes, such as **kyphosis** (outward curvature of the thoracic spine; also called hunchback), may also affect pulmonary function by limiting lung volume and maximal inspiratory pressure. In addition, the lung's defense mechanisms become less effective as a natural consequence of aging. The cough and gag reflexes decrease with age, increasing the risk of aspiration. Furthermore, the ciliary mechanisms that normally help remove bronchial secretions are markedly slowed. A decrease in the number of cilia that line the bronchial tree lessens the ability to cough and therefore increases the chances of infections such as pneumonia.

Finally, with aging, decreases occur in the size and strength of the respiratory muscles. Therefore, a patient who is having trouble breathing may not be able to compensate as well with accessory muscles as a younger person would. This means there is an increased likelihood of an airway obstruction from either secretions or food particles.

Although tobacco abuse seems to be decreasing among older patients, chronic lower respiratory disease and pneumonia remain in the top causes of geriatric deaths.[5] In fact, one of the most common causes of death in older patients is infection with *Pneumococcus* bacteria.

Pneumonia is an infection of the lungs that may be bacterial or fungal in origin. Those most at risk include anyone who already has a preexisting chronic disease of the lungs, those in institutions such as nursing homes, patients with chronic obstructive pulmonary disease (COPD) and cancer, immunocompromised patients, and those who have inhaled toxins or aspirated.

Another condition that can cause respiratory distress in older people is a **pulmonary embolism**. Pulmonary embolism is a condition that causes a sudden blockage of an artery by a venous clot. Clots develop in the veins of the legs or pelvis and then break off and embolize (move) through the pulmonary artery or one of its branches, where they lodge. This potentially life-threatening condition can present as another disease. A patient with a pulmonary embolism will generally complain of symptoms of chest pain; thus, the pulmonary embolism can be confused with a cardiac, lung, or musculoskeletal problem. Risk factors for a pulmonary embolism include recent surgery (especially in a lower extremity), history of blood clots, obesity, cancer, recent long-distance travel, and sedentary behavior, especially after surgery. Other conditions that render the patient bedridden also increase the risk of a pulmonary embolism.

▶ Changes in the Cardiovascular System

A variety of changes occur in the cardiovascular system as a person grows older that decrease the efficiency of the system. Specifically, the heart hypertrophies (enlarges) with age, probably in response to the chronically increased afterload imposed by stiffened blood vessels. Bigger is not better, however. Over time, cardiac output declines, mostly as a result of a decreasing stroke volume. (Cardiac output, which is the amount of blood pumped from the heart in 1 minute, is a measure of the workload of the heart.) Normally, an increased demand on the cardiovascular system is compensated for by increasing the heart rate, increasing the contraction of the heart, and constricting the blood vessels to nonvital organs to shunt blood to vital organs. However, aging decreases a person's ability to increase the heart rate, increase cardiac contraction strength, and constrict blood vessels (called **vasoconstriction**) because the vessels are stiffer.

Also, over time, it is normal that the electrical conduction system will show signs of wear. The cells of the sinoatrial node (the heart's primary pacemaker) will decrease in number and in function;[6] therefore, dysrhythmias may begin to develop.

Some changes in cardiovascular performance are probably not a direct consequence of aging, but rather reflect the deconditioning effect of a sedentary lifestyle. Whether because of other disabilities (such as arthritis) or for psychological reasons, many people tend to limit physical activity as they grow older. The bodybuilder's slogan, "Use it or lose it," applies just as much to the cardiac muscle as to the biceps.

Many older patients are at risk for **atherosclerosis**, an accumulation of fatty material in the arteries **Figure 37-4**. Major complications of atherosclerosis include MI and stroke. The presence of **arteriosclerosis**, a disease that causes the arteries to thicken, harden, and calcify, increases the risk of stroke, heart disease, hypertension, and bowel infarction.

Older people are also at an increased risk for an **aneurysm**, a weakening in the wall of a blood vessel (usually an artery), resulting in an area of dilation or "ballooning" of the vessel. Severe blood loss occurs when an aneurysm ruptures.

Abdominal aortic aneurysm (AAA) is one of the most rapidly fatal conditions. In 2014, 9,863 deaths were primarily caused by AAA.[7] Major risk factors for AAA include age greater than 60 years, male sex, smoking, hypertension, and a family history of AAA.

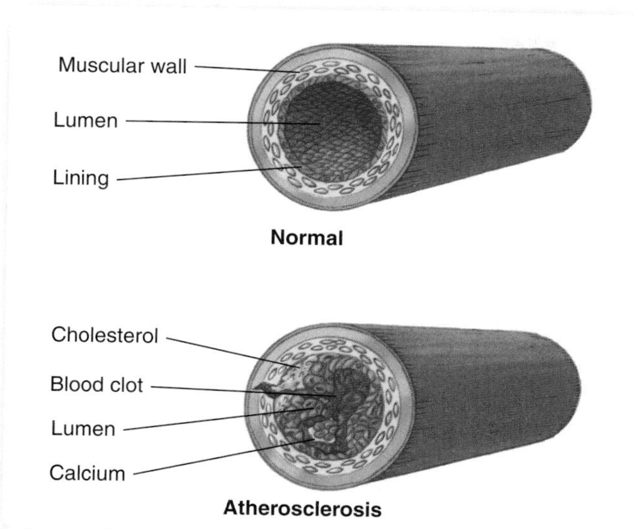

Figure 37-4 Atherosclerosis, the buildup of fatty plaque on arterial walls, may progress to the point that the plaque occludes the artery.

With an AAA, the walls of the aorta weaken and blood begins to leak into the layers of the vessel, causing the aorta to bulge like a bubble on a tire. If enough blood is lost into the vessel wall itself, shock occurs. If the wall bursts, it rapidly leads to fatal blood loss. If the aneurysm is detected early, there is a chance to repair the vessel before rupture and fatal blood loss occur.

A patient with an AAA most commonly reports abdominal pain radiating through to the back with occasional flank pain. If the AAA becomes large enough, it can be felt as a pulsating mass just above and slightly to the left of the umbilicus during your physical examination. Occasionally, the AAA causes a decrease in blood flow to one of the legs, and the patient complains of some discomfort in the affected extremity. Assessment may also reveal diminished or absent pulses in the extremity. Evidence of shock as a result of blood loss is common. Because of a decrease in blood volume and decreased blood flow to the brain, the patient may experience **syncope** (fainting).

▶ Changes in the Nervous System

Aging produces changes in the nervous system that are reflected in the neurologic examination. By age 80 years, a 10% to 20% reduction in brain weight can result in increased risk of head trauma owing to a larger area in the skull in which the brain can move during injury.[8] The human brain has an enormous reserve capacity, and having a smaller, lighter brain does not generally interfere with the mental capabilities of productive older people.

Short-term memory impairment, a decrease in the ability to perform psychomotor skills, and slower reflex times are all normal in the aging process. Because of deterioration of the nervous system and its control over various functions, you may see changes in the rate and depth of respirations, heart rate, blood pressure, hunger, thirst, and temperature. This decline may make assessment of the older patient challenging. Because of these changes, your patient may have slower responses to questioning or may request that you repeat a question.

Undeniably, the performance of most sense organs declines with increasing age. Hearing begins to decline around 40 years of age. At 50 years of age, vision and tactile senses decrease. Taste senses begin to change around 60 years of age, although the ability to smell does not begin to diminish until 70 years of age. Sense of body position (**proprioception**) also becomes impaired with age. Proprioception enables us to maintain postural stability by using a variety of receptors in the joints and information provided by the eyes. As these mechanisms fail with age, people become less steady on their feet, and the tendency to fall increases markedly.

Vision

As people age, the pupils begin to lose the ability to handle changes in light and require more time to adjust. Decreases in visual acuity are common in older people, even without disease processes. Aging affects an older person's ability to differentiate color, and tear production also decreases. Light changes and the increase in glare can cause problems of visual acuity and depth perception. Night vision becomes impaired. These changes can make driving and walking more hazardous, which can increase the risk of falls and affect an older person's independence.

The two most common causes of visual disturbances in older people are cataracts and glaucoma. A **cataract**, clouding of the lenses or their surrounding membranes, may interfere with vision and make it difficult for an older patient to distinguish colors and see clearly, increasing the likelihood of falls, accidents, and mistakes in taking medications. Cataracts are a result of hardening of the lenses over time. The lenses eventually become opaque, which prevents light and images from being transmitted to the rear of the eye. Patients with cataracts may complain of blurred vision, double vision, spots, and/or ghost images. Surgical treatment may be required to gain vision. By contrast, **glaucoma** is caused by an increase in intraocular pressure severe enough to damage the optic nerve, potentially resulting in permanent loss of peripheral and central vision. Treatment of glaucoma consists of oral medications and eye drops.

Macular degeneration, a condition that is common in persons with diabetes, is a disease that causes vision loss in the central part of the visual field. The macula in the retina of the eye is responsible for detailed vision such as reading. This disease may cause small or large items to seem different than they really are. Color perception can also vary within both eyes. Patients with macular degeneration have the ability to see outlines of objects but the center portion of the object may appear as a dark spot.

Retinal detachment is another problem in older patients. This is a disorder in which the retina peels away from the underlying support tissue and can result in vision loss and blindness.

Words of Wisdom

When you are treating a patient with a visual impairment, always stay in direct contact with the patient. Allow him or her to rest a hand on your arm or leg for comfort. Also explain any procedures in advance so that your patient is not taken by surprise.

Hearing

Approximately 25% of patients between 65 and 74 years of age have a disabling hearing loss. It increases to nearly 50% in those who are 75 years and older.[9] Changes to the ear can also cause problems with balance, increasing the risk of falls.

Changes in the inner ear make hearing high-frequency sounds difficult—muffled sounds are sometimes not even heard. For this reason, increasing the volume of your voice may not make it any easier for the patient to hear your words. To compensate for the hearing deficits, many older patients are prescribed hearing-assistance devices (eg, hearing aids). Although these devices may not return hearing to normal levels, they can increase your ability to communicate with the patient, so consider assisting the patient inserting his or her hearing device. Many audiologists have brochures to help patients with these devices. It would be beneficial for you to read this same information and obtain additional training about inserting a hearing aid.

A common cause of hearing impairment in geriatric patients is **presbycusis**, a progressive hearing loss, particularly in the high frequencies, along with a lessened ability to discriminate between a particular sound and background noise. Patients who lose the ability to interpret speech experience a decreased ability to communicate, which may result in isolation and depression.

For many older people, physiologic changes make it difficult to produce speech that is loud enough, clear, and well-spaced. Weakness, paralysis, poor hearing, or brain damage can impair a person's ability to produce speech.

Words of Wisdom

Always position yourself so that you are on the "good" side of the patient with a hearing deficit. Because hearing deficits usually involve the loss of high-frequency sounds, yelling in the patient's ear will only serve to further distort the patient's hearing.

Taste

Changes in appetite may occur because taste buds decrease in number as a person ages. Remaining taste buds also begin to shrink.[10] Although these changes are gradual, the salty and sweet sensation appears to be among the first to diminish. A patient with diminished taste may not be able to discern fresh food from spoiled food. Older people commonly add large amounts of salt to their food in an attempt to improve its taste, but this could be dangerous for a patient with a history of hypertension.

Touch

The sense of touch decreases from loss of specialized nerve fibers. This loss, in conjunction with the slowing of the peripheral nervous system, can result in a delayed reflex reaction when an older person touches something hot, causing a burn. Alterations in pain perception can result in patients not calling EMS when needed. A syncopal episode or tightness in the chest may not be viewed as a sign of an impending heart attack. Despite these changes, the touch of a provider's hand may be comforting and reassuring and should be considered in your assessment. Many older patients may grasp your hand as a means for comfort or during severe pain episodes.

Smell

The sense of smell is among the last to diminish in older patients. However, factors such as upper respiratory infections (ie, the common cold), to which older persons are more susceptible, can affect the sense of smell.

Disorders Affecting Mental Status

Delirium. **Delirium** is a change in mental status that is marked by the inability to focus, think logically, and maintain attention. Acute anxiety may be present in addition to the other symptoms. Usually, memory remains mostly intact. Delirium is commonly marked by an acute or recent onset (generally within minutes, hours, or days) and is a "red flag"—a serious, potentially life-threatening problem—for some type of new health problem. Signs and symptoms of delirium include disorganized thoughts, inattention, memory loss, disorientation, hallucinations, delusions, or changes in level of consciousness. You may also see changes in pupillary response, motor tests, blood pressure, and breath sounds.

Delirium may be caused by tumors, fever, urinary tract infections (UTIs), bowel obstructions, dehydration, cardiovascular disease, hyperglycemia, hypoglycemia, nutritional deficiencies, psychiatric disorders such as depression, environmental emergencies, or drug, alcohol, or sedative intoxication or withdrawal. Delirium can be present from metabolic causes as well. Any time a patient has an acute onset of delirious behavior, you should rapidly assess the patient for the following four conditions:

- Hypoxia
- Hypovolemia

- Hypothermia
- Hypoglycemia

Any of these four conditions, if left unrecognized or untreated, may be rapidly fatal. Delirium is short in its onset and usually correctable if identified early.

Words of Wisdom

Dementia and delirium are different disorders, yet they both present with alterations in mental status. Dementia is a chronic problem (ie, Alzheimer disease), whereas delirium is an acute problem (ie, hypoglycemia). Because both delirium and dementia can present in a similar manner, it is important to determine the patient's baseline mental status.

Dementia. **Dementia** is the slow onset of progressive disorientation, shortened attention span, and loss of cognitive function. It is a chronic, generally irreversible condition that causes progressive loss of cognitive abilities, psychomotor skills, and social skills. Dementia develops slowly over a period of years rather than a few days. Causes include Alzheimer disease, genetic factors, various forms of encephalitis, a history of working with metals or organic or airborne toxins, and cerebrovascular accidents (strokes). The patient's history and determination of function in the recent past are key factors in determining the difference between delirium and dementia. A patient with dementia may be experiencing a delirious event. Delirium is caused by emergent problems; dementia is not.

Signs and symptoms of dementia take months to years to become apparent and may include short-term memory loss or shortened attention span, jargon aphasia (talking nonsense), hallucinations, confusion, disorientation, inability to perform ADLs, difficulty in learning and retaining new information, and personality changes such as social withdrawal or inappropriate behavior. Patients with dementia will often be angry and uncooperative. Dementia is not synonymous with delirium, however, and a patient with dementia can also have delirium.

Safety

Be alert when dealing with any patient exhibiting an altered mental status, even if it is normal for that patient. Some patients with dementia, Alzheimer disease, or other illnesses can become extremely violent, posing a danger to family as well as rescuers.

Neurodegenerative Diseases

Alzheimer Disease. Alzheimer disease is believed to be caused by the death of neurons in the brain. The disease begins gradually, with a person having difficulty performing routine tasks and/or forgetting recent events. As the disease advances, personality changes, impaired judgment, and an impaired ability to communicate thoughts or ideas become

YOU are the Provider — PART 2

As you perform your physical exam on the patient, you note that he is cold to the touch, has delayed capillary refill, and has a thready radial pulse. The patient states that he has been vomiting up "foul" smelling emesis for the last 4 days, that he is weaker than usual, and that he gets extremely dizzy when he stands up. He asks to use the bathroom before transport and as you assist him to the standing position, you note that his radial pulse disappears and that he becomes extremely pale.

Recording Time: 1 Minute	
Appearance	Pale, poor general impression
Level of consciousness	Alert and oriented to person, place, time, and event, but slow to respond
Airway	Patent
Breathing	Nonlabored
Circulation	Prior to taking orthostatic vital signs: thready, slow radial pulses; skin cool, pale, and clammy

3. Does this patient require immediate transport?
4. On the basis of the patient's presentation, what do you suspect is happening?

more prominent. In 2017, approximately 5.5 million Americans were living with Alzheimer dementia; of those, approximately 5.3 million were 65 years and older and approximately 200,000 were younger than 65 years of age (known as early-onset Alzheimer).[11]

In Alzheimer disease, symptoms may present as confusion (lack of familiarity with surroundings), changes in personality or judgment, and extreme difficulty with daily activities, such as feeding, bathing, and bowel and bladder control.

Parkinson Disease. Parkinson disease involves the nerve cells in the motor area of the brain and is caused by the insufficient formation and action of dopamine, a neurotransmitter that carries messages. It is a chronic and progressive disorder that worsens over time. In 2017, almost 1 million Americans were living with Parkinson disease.[12]

Parkinson disease may present as dyskinesia (involuntary movements or tremors affecting one or both sides of the body), dementia, depression, autonomic dysfunction (bladder and gastrointestinal [GI] problems), and postural instability (loss of reflexes or inability to "right oneself"). The involuntary movements or tremors appear to increase during times of stress and normally can be seen when a patient is sitting still.

Depression and Suicide

Late life can be a time of fulfillment and satisfaction, but for some older adults, later life is characterized by physical pain, psychological distress, doubts about the importance of life's accomplishments, financial concerns, loss of loved ones, dissatisfaction with living conditions, and seemingly unbearable disability. When these factors lead to hopelessness about the possibility for positive change in their lives, depression and, unfortunately, even suicide are possible outcomes. You are often the first health care professional to have contact with older adults who are depressed.

Depression is not part of normal aging, but rather a medical disease. It is treatable with medication and therapy; however, if depression goes unrecognized or untreated, it is associated with a high suicide rate in the geriatric population.[13] Depression in older patients can mimic the effects of many other medical problems (such as dementia). Risk factors for depression in older people include a history of depression, chronic disease, and loss (function, independence, or significant others). Approximately 40% of older adults residing in skilled nursing facilities are affected.[14] Depression may be difficult to recognize in older people because many do not want to complain about feeling sad, worthless, or unwanted.

Unlike a normal experience of sadness, grief, or loss, depression is extreme and persistent and can interfere substantially with an older adult's ability to function. It is impossible to predict which older adults will have depression, but substance abuse, isolation, prescription medication use, and chronic medical conditions all may contribute to the onset of substantial depression.[15] Treatment of severe depression in older adults usually consists of psychological counseling, medication, or a combination of both. For many older adults, simply reestablishing relationships with the community or with family is enough to lessen the severity of the illness.

Older adults may not pursue medical treatment for psychological issues. Many older adults do not seek care and also frequently deny the problem when asked about it. It is vital that all members of the health care team be aware of these issues and take appropriate steps to ensure patient safety and well-being.

▶ Changes in the Musculoskeletal System

Aging is associated with a widespread decrease in bone mass in men and women, especially among postmenopausal women. Bones become more brittle and tend to break more easily. Narrowing of the intervertebral disks and compression fractures of the vertebrae contribute to a decrease in height as a person ages, along with changes in posture. Joints lose their flexibility naturally with age, and may be further impaired by arthritic changes. A decrease in the amount of muscle mass often results in less strength.

Changes in physical abilities can affect older adults' confidence in their mobility. Muscle mass decreases throughout the body, with an accompanying decrease in muscle strength. Muscle fibers become smaller and fewer, motor neurons decline in number, and strength declines. The ligaments and cartilage of the joints lose their elasticity. Cartilage also goes through degenerative changes with aging, contributing to arthritis. From an AEMT's perspective, the changes in the musculoskeletal system most often translate into fractures incurred as the result of falls.

Posture also changes as flexion at the neck and an anterior curling of the spine produce a condition called kyphosis (also called humpback, hunchback, or a Pott curvature) **Figure 37-5**, making immobilization of older persons more challenging.

Osteoporosis, a condition that affects women to a greater extent than men, is characterized by a decrease in bone mass resulting in reduction in bone strength and greater susceptibility to fracture. The extent of bone loss that a person undergoes is influenced by numerous factors, including genetics, smoking, level of activity, diet, alcohol consumption, hormonal factors, and body weight. The most rapid loss of bone occurs in women during the years following menopause, and many perimenopausal women use hormone replacement therapy to help reduce bone loss. Calcium and vitamin D supplementation is another treatment of the condition, and many other medications are available to improve bone strength. Older people should remain active and engage in a low-impact exercise program to maintain bone and muscle strength.

Osteoarthritis is a progressive disease of the joints that destroys cartilage, promotes the formation of bone

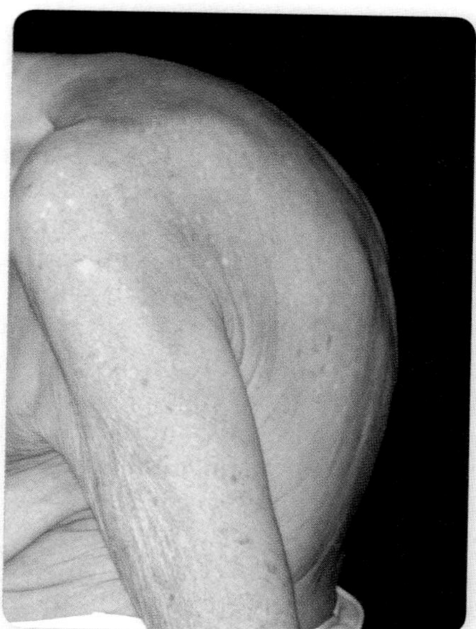

Figure 37-5 Kyphosis, which can occur with aging, is a condition in which the spine has excessive forward curvature. This may lead to the shoulders being positioned forward.

spurs in joints, and results in joint stiffness. This type of arthritis is thought to result from "wear and tear" and, in some cases, from repetitive trauma to the joints. It affects a substantial portion of the population older than 65 years. Typically, osteoarthritis affects several joints of the body, most commonly those in the hands, knees, hips, and spine. Patients report pain and stiffness that gets worse with exertion. The end result is often substantial disability and disfigurement. Patients are typically treated with anti-inflammatory medications and physical therapy to improve the range of motion.

▶ Changes in the Gastrointestinal System

The process of digestion begins in the mouth, which is also where aging-related changes in the digestive system may first be noted. A decrease in the number of taste buds and changes in olfactory receptors may diminish an older person's senses of taste and smell, which may also interfere with the enjoyment of food. The consequent decrease in appetite may result in malnutrition. Other changes in the mouth include a reduction in the volume of saliva, with a resulting dryness of the mouth making it harder to chew and begin to digest foods. Dental loss is not a normal result of the aging process, but rather the result of disease of the teeth and gums; nevertheless, dental loss is widespread in the geriatric population and contributes to nutritional and digestive problems.

Like oral secretions, hydrochloric acid in the stomach decreases, further inhibiting digestion as a person ages—although enough acid is still present to produce ulcers under certain conditions. Changes in gastric motility also occur, which may result in slower gastric emptying—a factor of some importance when assessing the risk of aspiration.

Function of the small and large bowel changes little as a result of aging, although the incidence of certain diseases involving the bowel (such as diverticulosis) increases as a person grows older. Slowing of the movement of food through the digestive tract may also result in constipation.

In the liver, there are changes in hepatic enzyme systems, with some systems declining in activity and others increasing. Notably, the activity of the enzyme systems concerned with the detoxification of drugs and alcohol declines as a person ages.

A cause of abdominal pain and shock is GI bleeding, which can occur for a variety of reasons, ranging from infection to ruptured varices to regular use of nonsteroidal anti-inflammatory drugs (NSAIDs) or alcohol to cancer of the stomach or esophagus. GI bleeding is usually heralded by vomiting of blood or material that looks like coffee grounds, called **hematemesis**. Bleeding that travels through the lower digestive tract usually manifests as black or tarry stools, called **melena**, whereas red blood in the stool usually means a local source of bleeding, such as hemorrhoids. A patient with GI bleeding may experience weakness, dizziness, dyspepsia, or syncope. A patient may also present with hepatomegaly (enlarged liver), jaundice, and agitation. Bleeding into the GI system can be life threatening because of the potential for blood loss and shock.

Bowel obstructions occur frequently in the geriatric population. The GI tract slows with aging and the patient can experience problems having bowel movements. Straining while attempting to have a bowel movement can stimulate the vagus nerve, resulting in vasovagal syncope, in which the heart rate drops dramatically and the patient becomes dizzy or passes out. The patient's condition will usually be stable on your arrival, but transport is required to rule out other causes of the syncopal episode. Another reason for bowel obstruction in older patients is the use of narcotic analgesics, which also decrease GI function.

Geriatric patients are at risk for dehydration as a result of diarrhea. Drug-related diarrhea and associated nausea and vomiting usually occur after a new medication is initiated or after a change in dosage. Infectious agents such as viruses and bacteria can cause acute diarrhea, which, if it lasts less than 4 weeks, is considered an illness. Chronic diarrhea is defined as lasting longer than the 4-week period.

Geriatric patients are at risk for food poisoning, also known as bacterial gastroenteritis, due to existing medical conditions such as dementia. Symptoms of *Salmonella* poisoning usually begin within 12 to 72 hours of eating and may last 2 to 3 days. *S aureus* will have a more rapid onset, usually within 2 to 8 hours, and the symptoms are typically more severe.

In addition, patients with lactose intolerance, constipation, reaction to certain cancer medications and treatments, and bowel obstructions may present with nausea, vomiting, or diarrhea.

▶ Changes in the Renal System

Age is associated with changes in the kidneys as well. The kidneys are responsible for maintaining the body's fluid and electrolyte balance and have important roles in maintaining the body's long-term acid-base balance and eliminating drugs from the body. As the body ages, the kidney loses functioning nephron units, which translates into a lesser ability to effectively filter wastes. Also, renal blood flow decreases by as much as 50% as a person ages.

Although the kidneys of an older person may be capable of addressing day-to-day demands, they may not be able to meet unusual challenges, such as those imposed by illness. Therefore, acute illness in older patients is often accompanied by derangements in fluid and electrolyte balance. Aging kidneys, for example, respond sluggishly to sodium deficiency. An older patient may lose a great deal of sodium before the kidneys halt urinary sodium excretion, a problem that is exacerbated by the markedly decreased thirst mechanism in older people. The net result may be a rapid development of severe dehydration.

Conversely, older patients are at considerable risk of overhydration if they are exposed to large sodium loads (such as from intravenous (IV) saline solutions or heavily salted foods). The aging kidney is less able to excrete a large sodium load because of its lower glomerular filtration rate, making the patient vulnerable to acute volume overload.

The same factors that reduce an older person's ability to handle sodium also affect the body's ability to handle potassium. Thus, older patients are susceptible to hyperkalemia, which can become serious—even lethal—if the patient becomes acidotic or if the potassium load is increased from any source.

Urinary incontinence (involuntary loss of urine) can have a substantial social and emotional effect, but relatively few people admit to the problem and even fewer seek treatment. Incontinence can result in skin irritation, skin breakdown, and UTIs. As people age, bladder capacity decreases. Therefore, an older person may find it difficult to postpone voiding or may have involuntary bladder contractions. Two major types of incontinence are distinguished: stress and urge. Stress incontinence occurs during activities such as coughing, laughing, sneezing, lifting, and exercise. Urge incontinence is triggered by hot or cold fluids, running water, and even thinking about going to the bathroom. Treatment of incontinence consists of medications, physical therapy, and, possibly, surgery.

The opposite of incontinence is urinary retention or difficulty urinating. Patients may have difficulty voiding or absence of voiding as a result of many medical causes. In men, enlargement of the prostate (benign prostatic hypertrophy) can place pressure on the urethra, making voiding difficult. Bladder and urinary tract infections can also cause inflammation. In severe cases of urinary retention, patients may have acute or chronic renal failure.

▶ Changes in the Endocrine System

Hormone levels and the production of hormones change as we age. Diabetes develops when the body cannot oxidize complex carbohydrates (sugars) as a result of impaired pancreatic activity—namely, impaired production of insulin by the beta cells. With diabetes, more glucose is present in the blood than the body can handle. Geriatric patients with diabetes are at increased risk for hypoglycemia for several reasons: medications, inadequate or irregular dietary intake, inability to recognize the warning signs because of cognitive problems, and/or blunted warning signs. Delirium may be the only indication of hypoglycemia in an older patient.

The most common risk factor for this disease is having more than one chronic disease, and many older people with diabetes also have hypertension, heart disease, and stroke. Symptoms of an elevated blood glucose level (that is, hyperglycemia) include fatigue, poor wound healing, blurred vision, and frequent infections. Other symptoms of diabetes include the three Ps: polyuria, polydipsia, and polyphagia. Prevention of type 2 diabetes is aimed at changes in lifestyle that include dietary restrictions, exercise, and controlling obesity.

Hyperosmolar hyperglycemic syndrome (HHS), also called hyperosmolar nonketotic coma (HONK) or hyperosmolar hyperglycemic nonketotic coma, is a metabolic derangement that occurs principally in patients with type 2 diabetes;[16-19] however, approximately 20% of patients with HHS do not have a prior diagnosis of diabetes.[20] This condition is characterized by hyperglycemia, hyperosmolarity, and an absence of significant ketosis; it is similar to diabetic ketoacidosis (DKA) in type 1 diabetes.

Physical changes noted during the assessment of the HHS patient are primarily a result of excessive dehydration and hyperglycemia. Glucose levels are greater than 600 mg/dL. Warm, flushed skin with poor skin turgor and pale, dry oral mucosa are common findings. The tongue may be furrowed as well. In extreme cases of dehydration, the patient may present with tachycardia, hypotension, and signs of shock.

Thyroid abnormalities also increase with aging. Many older patients remain asymptomatic, and the disease is diagnosed only when a routine blood test reveals a thyroid problem. With hypothyroidism, for example, the signs and symptoms may match those seen with normal aging: cold intolerance, constipation, dry skin, weakness, and so on. For acute-onset hyperthyroidism (thyrotoxicosis), the presentation can be blunted; although tachycardia is generally present, older patients may experience less tremor, anxiety, or hyperactive reflexes than younger patients do. Atrial fibrillation is more likely to be induced by an overactive thyroid gland in a geriatric patient. A smaller percentage of older hyperthyroid patients present with symptoms opposite those expected: weakness, lethargy, and depression.

▶ Changes in the Immune System

Because nearly every function of the immune system is affected by aging, older persons are more susceptible to infection and secondary complications than are younger people. Chronic conditions such as diabetes, dementia, malnutrition, and cardiovascular disease place older people at greater risk of serious infection.

Older persons manifest infections differently. Although fever is often present with minor illness in young people, fever in older persons usually indicates a serious infection. However, not all older adults with a serious infection have a fever, owing to the decreased ability of the aging immune system to initiate a fever.

Sepsis occurs when an infection develops in the patient (which may be caused by bacteria, viruses, or fungi) and microorganisms or their toxic products enter the bloodstream. Sepsis may affect a part of (local) or the entire (systemic) body. The degree of sepsis can vary, from such a common occurrence as a dental abscess to the more severe sepsis, which affects more than one of the body's organs or systems. Septic shock occurs when hypoperfusion occurs following severe systemic infection. The signs and symptoms of septic shock may be fever, respiratory distress, increased pulse rate, generalized weakness, and hypotension. Site-specific infections may allow other signs and symptoms to be present. A patient with a UTI may have a foul odor associated with the urine and sometimes pain on urinating or cloudy urine. Pneumonia is the leading cause of death from infection in Americans older than 65 years.[5] Patients may develop infections through their lungs, through a urinary catheter, or even through IV access.

▶ Changes in the Integumentary System

Collagen (the substance that makes skin strong) and elastin (the substance that makes the skin pliable) decrease as people age. This makes the skin wrinkled, thinner, less elastic, and more susceptible to injury.

Because the elasticity of the skin has declined, bruising becomes more common because the peripheral blood vessels cannot constrict and stop the bleeding as quickly. This causes a greater number of bruises as well as large hematomas from minimal trauma. The healing process takes longer as people age because of a decrease in the blood flow to the capillaries.

The blood vessels that supply the skin also provide less oxygenated blood at the cellular level. As a result of the skin's lower metabolism, epidermal cells develop more slowly and do not replace outgoing cells as quickly as with younger skin. Older patients, therefore, are at higher risk for secondary infection after the skin breaks, for skin tumors, and for fungal or viral infections of the skin.

In addition, as a person ages, the sebaceous glands produce less oil, making the skin drier. Sweat gland activity also decreases, hindering the ability to sweat and to regulate heat. Subcutaneous fat also becomes thinner. For these two reasons, you may often see geriatric patients wearing multiple layers of clothing.

Pressure Ulcers

The thinning of subcutaneous fat makes bedsores or pressure ulcers more common in an older, bedridden patient. These sores, also called **decubitus ulcers**, form when a person lies in the same position for too long, causing decreased blood flow to an area of already thin skin, which results in tissue death and the development of a pressure ulcer. Therefore, persons confined to a bed or stationary position need special care and a regular regimen of documented position changes every 1 to 2 hours.

Possible risk factors include brain or spinal cord injury, neuromuscular disorders, and nutritional problems. These ulcers are exacerbated by fecal and urinary incontinence, particularly when the patient is exposed to saturated materials for a prolonged time. You should be particularly aware of pressure ulcers during spinal immobilization and ensure that padding is adequate throughout the posterior. Pressure ulcers are most commonly located on the lower legs, sacrum, greater trochanter, and the glutes.

Pressure ulcers can be classified as follows:

- **Stage 1.** A persistent area of skin redness (without a break in the skin) that does not disappear when pressure is relieved Figure 37-6.
- **Stage 2.** A partial thickness of skin is lost and may appear as an abrasion, blister, or shallow crater.

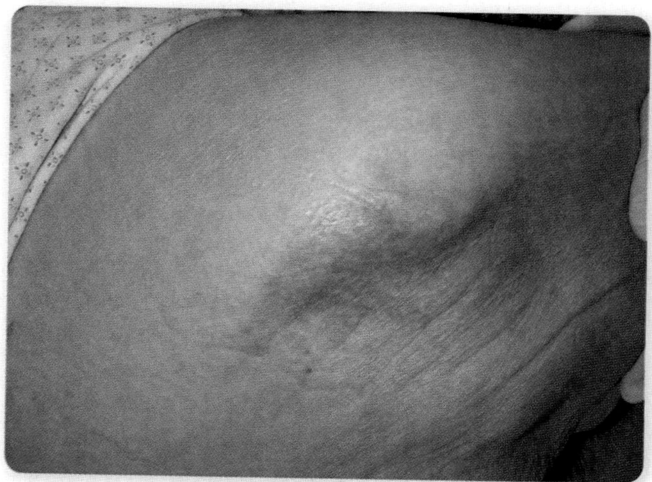

Figure 37-6 A decubitus ulcer. This sore is in stage 1, meaning it is in the early stages of development.

- **Stage 3.** A full thickness of skin is lost, exposing the subcutaneous tissues; presents as a deep crater with or without undermining adjacent tissue.
- **Stage 4.** Full thickness of skin and subcutaneous tissues are lost, exposing muscle or bone.

Prehospital treatment for pressure ulcers is mostly basic life support care. However, ulcers that remain untreated can evolve into a source of substantial infection and potentially result in sepsis. When you observe pressure ulcers that suggest infection in a patient, you should monitor the patient's body temperature and vital signs, administer oxygen, establish an IV line, and consider administration of a fluid bolus.

▶ Homeostatic and Other Changes

Homeostasis is the process by which the body maintains a constant internal environment. Many homeostatic mechanisms work on a feedback principle, much like the thermostat in a house—that is, a change in the internal environment feeds back to the control system to induce a corrective response. For example, when the body temperature starts to rise, temperature sensors are activated, which in turn activate compensatory responses. Cutaneous blood vessels dilate, and excess heat is transferred from the body to the environment.

With aging, a progressive loss of these homeostatic capabilities occurs. Therefore, a specific illness or injury in older adults is more likely to result in generalized deterioration. For example, the thirst mechanism that ordinarily protects a person from dehydration becomes depressed in older adults. Likewise, temperature-regulating mechanisms tend to become disordered, which, when combined with integumentary changes makes older patients more vulnerable to environmental stresses such as heat exhaustion and accidental hypothermia after relatively minor exposures. A defect in temperature regulation also may account for the absence of a febrile response to illness in some older adults. Infections that would ordinarily produce high fever, such as pneumococcal pneumonia, may produce only a low-grade or no fever in older adults.

The regulatory system that manages the blood glucose level similarly becomes impaired with increasing age, such that an elevated blood glucose level occurs quite commonly in older patients. Ordinarily, moderate hyperglycemia does no harm, but overly aggressive treatment of this problem may produce damaging hypoglycemia.

Words of Wisdom

A specific illness or injury in an older person is more likely to result in generalized deterioration.

Toxicology

Several pathophysiologic changes cause older people to be susceptible to toxicity. These include decreased kidney function, altered GI absorption, and decreased vascular flow in the liver, which alters metabolism and excretion. The kidneys undergo many changes with age. Decreased liver function makes it harder for the liver to detoxify the blood and eliminate substances such as medications and alcohol. These metabolic issues also can make it difficult for physicians to determine the appropriate dosage for new medications.

The use of medications by older people accounts for 34% of prescribed medications and 30% of the over-the-counter (OTC) medication use.[21] Typical OTC medicines used by older people include aspirin, antacids, cough syrups, and decongestants. Many people believe OTC medications cannot be dangerous, but these medications can have negative effects when mixed with each other and/or with herbal substances, alcohol, and prescription medications.

Older patients are often prescribed multiple medications. **Polypharmacy**, or the use of multiple medications by one patient, is a common finding in geriatric patients. The use of medications by people aged 65 years and older accounts for more than one-third of the prescribed medications in the United States even though they only comprise 13% of the population. The introduction of integrated health systems and computerized databases have helped to greatly reduce the incidence of multiple prescriptions of the same medication from varying physicians or hospitals. Of course, this does not affect samples that may be given to the patient for a trial period.

Medication interactions and noncompliance with instructions for taking prescribed drugs are common and may contribute to the patient's symptoms or problem. Medication noncompliance may occur because of financial challenges; inability to open containers; or impaired cognitive, vision, and hearing ability. If you suspect medication noncompliance, you should check prescription dates and the number of pills available.

The geriatric population is more likely to have cases of polypharmacy because older people are affected most by the process of aging. Physiologic factors known to be true about the hepatic and renal functions of excretion and metabolism of medications can change in the face of multiple prescriptions being consumed at once. Always be mindful of this issue when obtaining the patient's medication history.

Assessment of Geriatric Medical Emergencies

Any time you assess a patient, start with the same basic approach: scene size-up, primary survey, history taking, secondary assessment, and reassessment. Assessing an older patient is no different; however, there are some issues that may require you to modify your approach to the primary survey or become more aware of some conditions that may affect older patients.

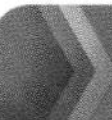

Scene Size-up

Begin by ensuring scene safety. Will you need assistance? How many patients do you have? Have you taken proper standard precautions?

When you first arrive at a patient's residence, look for important clues to determine not only your safety, but also that of the patient. The environment will provide a great deal of important information if you know where to look and what to look for.

The general condition of the home will give you some important information. Are there hazards, such as steep stairs, missing or loose handrails, or other things that could cause a fall? Is it evident that the person may be having difficulty keeping the house clean? Is there evidence of adequate food, water, heat, lighting, and ventilation? Are there many pill bottles around, indicating treatment for multiple diseases? Does someone else live there who can help to answer your questions? These are important scene clues that can provide a wealth of information before you even make contact with the patient.

In a nursing home or residential care facility, you will need to locate the patient's room and find a staff member who may be able to explain why you were called. The presence of a hospital bed, oxygen tanks, or therapeutic devices can give you a clue to the patient's medical history.

The nature of illness (NOI) may be difficult to determine in older people who may have an altered mental status or dementia. Often it is someone other than the patient who called, so you must ask the family member, caregiver, or bystander why he or she called. Multiple and chronic disease processes may also complicate the determination of the NOI. Reports from an older person may be vague, such as weakness, dizziness, or fatigue. These could indicate a more serious problem and require more assessment. You may need to ask specifically what is different *today* or specifically why the person called to distinguish acute versus chronic problems. Chest pain, shortness of breath, and an altered level of consciousness should always be considered serious. You also may find that the patient's problem is a symptom of something more serious. For example, sudden changes in the ability to talk could indicate a stroke, or the need to sleep on five pillows could suggest early heart failure.

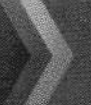

Primary Survey

The sequence of the primary survey is the same for pediatric, adult, and geriatric patients. However, you should not make any assumptions about an older patient's level of consciousness. Never assume that an altered mental status is normal. Always compare the patient's current level of consciousness or ability to function with the level or ability before the problem began. You may have to rely on a family member or caregiver to determine the patient's baseline level of consciousness.

Words of Wisdom

Remember that routine medications may mask signs and symptoms. A good understanding of the NOI/mechanism of injury, along with a high index of suspicion and an in-depth patient history, should guide your assessment and subsequent care. For example, many patients take beta blockers that prevent the normal sympathetic response of raising pulse and respirations and mask the changes that would be expected from certain conditions (such as a tachycardic response to severe blood loss).

The general impression is an important aspect of all patient assessment. As you approach the patient, you should be able to tell if the patient is generally in stable or unstable condition. You will use this information to help you with your further assessment. Use the AVPU scale (Awake and alert, responsive to Verbal stimuli, responsive to Pain, Unresponsive) to determine the patient's level of consciousness.

Anatomic changes that occur as a person ages predispose geriatric patients to airway problems. Aging and disease can compromise a patient's ability to protect his or her airway with loss of a gag reflex and normal swallowing mechanisms. Changes in level of consciousness, dementia, and weakness or paralysis resulting from stroke can cause airway obstruction or aspiration. Ensure that the patient's airway is open and is not obstructed by dentures, vomitus, fluids, or blood. Suction may be necessary.

Anatomic changes with aging also affect a person's ability to breathe effectively. Increased chest wall stiffness, brittle bones, weakening of the airway musculature, and decreased muscle mass contribute to breathing problems. Loss of mechanisms that protect the upper airway, like cough and gag reflexes, cause a decreased ability to clear secretions. A decrease in the number of cilia that line the bronchial tree results in the inability of the patient to remove material from the lung, which can cause infection. In some patients, the alveoli are damaged, and a lack of elasticity results in a decreased ability to exchange oxygen and carbon dioxide. Superimposed on the physiologic changes are the chronic respiratory diseases common in older people that affect the ability of the patient to breathe effectively. Airway and breathing issues should be treated with oxygen as soon as possible.

Poor perfusion is a serious issue in an older adult. People who normally live with compromised circulation have little in the way of reserves during a circulatory crisis. Physiologic changes may negatively affect circulation.

Less responsive nerve stimulation may lower the rate and strength of the heart's contractions, so lower heart rates and weaker and irregular pulses are common in geriatric patients. Vascular changes and circulatory compromise might make it difficult to feel a radial pulse on an older patient. If choosing an alternative pulse point like the carotid, press gently. Another option is to listen to the apical pulse right over the heart. The pulse may be irregular because of common heart rhythm problems. Apply supplemental oxygen as needed for an Spo_2 below 94%.

Patient assessment is more complicated in an older adult, and multiple problems can exist. Any problems that compromise airway, breathing, or circulation should result in transportation of the patient on a priority basis. Priority patients include those who have any of the following:

- A poor general impression
- Airway or breathing problems
- Acute altered level of consciousness
- Shock
- Any severe pain
- Uncontrolled bleeding

Older people do not have the reserves that younger people do, and they will easily decompensate. Even a general report of weakness and dizziness can be an indication of something more serious like a heart problem. Consider paramedic rendezvous and provide immediate treatment and transport to the closest, most appropriate facility.

Many acronyms are used in the prehospital setting to help you remember steps in your assessment and treatment. The GEMS diamond (the components of which are Geriatric, Environmental, Medical, and Social assessments) was created to help providers recall key themes when caring for geriatric patients Table 37-2.

The "G" of the GEMS diamond calls on you to recognize that the patient is a geriatric patient. In such a case, your thought process needs to be geared to the possible problems of an aging patient.

The "E" of the GEMS diamond stands for an environmental assessment. Preventive care is important for an older patient, who may not carefully study the environment or may not realize where risks exist. For example, if you walk into a room and trip over a rug, you should mention it to bring potential hazards to the patient's attention. Assessment of the environment can help give clues regarding the patient's condition. Are there hazardous conditions? Preventive interventions for geriatric patients include reviewing the home environment to ensure that safe and livable conditions exist, providing information on preventing falls, and making referrals to appropriate social services agencies when needed.

The "M" of the GEMS diamond stands for medical assessment. Older patients tend to have a variety of medical problems and may be taking numerous prescription, OTC, and herbal medications. Obtaining a thorough medical history is important in older patients.

The "S" stands for social assessment. Numerous social agencies are readily available to help the older patient. Many agencies can provide assistance to our older population, but they must be made aware of the need. Older people may be too proud to ask for help, may not want others to know they need assistance, or may be wary of a financial cost. Consider obtaining information pamphlets about some of the agencies for older people in your area. If you have these brochures with you and encounter a person in need, you can provide this valuable information. Social agencies that deal with the older population will be able to provide a listing of their services

History Taking

It is often said that 80% of a medical diagnosis is based on the patient's history. In addition to clearing the airway and managing the ABCs (airway, breathing, and circulation), obtaining a thorough history is one of the most important things you can do. An inaccurate or inadequate history can lead to an incorrect field impression, which may result in an inappropriate treatment plan.

To obtain an accurate history, patience and good communication skills are essential. An older patient's diminished sight, hearing, and speaking ability may hamper communications. If possible, take a few moments to have the patient put in his or her dentures or hearing aid or, if necessary, assist the patient in doing any of these things. All of these items can help the patient to communicate with you more effectively.

Words of Wisdom

Remember that patients' medications are a vital part of their history. Don't forget to include any OTC medications or herbal remedies in the history.

An older patient can have multiple problems, or the primary issue can be caused by a secondary problem. Many patients will only reveal a lesser problem during questions asked in your assessment. Additionally, they may not consider the secondary problem to be important. You will have to play the role of detective many times to determine the actual problem. The more facts and information that you can obtain from the patient and bystanders or caregivers, the more informed your treatment decision will be.

The patient who is in respiratory distress may not report shortness of breath, but may report feeling dizzy. Are the two problems related? A patient who is hypoxic will report being dizzy. Often a syncopal episode is the only indication of a cardiac dysrhythmia. Older patients can develop a tolerance to their diseases. Many have been able to modify their lifestyles to their diseases. In addition, some older patients do not want to bother anyone. This mindset causes a delay in seeking help and may exacerbate the patient's condition.

Table 37-2 The GEMS diamond

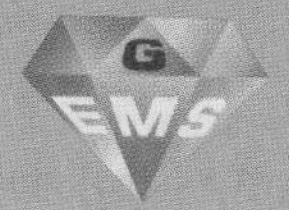

G Geriatric Patients

- Present atypically.
- Deserve respect.
- Experience normal changes with age.

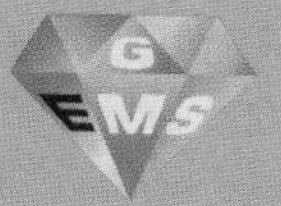

E Environmental Assessment

- Check the physical condition of the patient's home: Is the exterior of the home in need of repair? Is the home secure?
- Check for hazardous conditions that may be present (eg, poor wiring, rotted floors, unventilated gas heaters, clutter that prevents adequate egress).
- Are smoke detectors present and working?
- Is the home too hot or too cold?
- Is there an odor of feces or urine in the home?
- Is bedding soiled or urine soaked?
- Are pets well cared for?
- Is food present in the home? Is it adequate and unspoiled?
- Are liquor bottles present? If so, are they empty?
- Are there burn patterns on the walls, cabinets, or floors?
- Are there unsecured throw rugs that could result in falls?
- If the patient has a disability, are appropriate assistive devices (eg, a wheelchair or walker) present and in adequate condition?
- Does the patient have access to a telephone?
- Are medications prescribed to someone else, expired, unmarked, or from many physicians?
- If living with others, is the patient confined to one part of the home?
- If the patient is residing in a nursing facility, does the care appear to be adequate to meet the patient's needs?

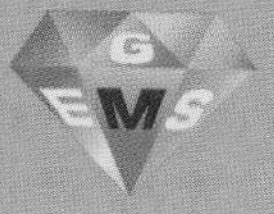

M Medical Assessment

- Older patients tend to have a variety of medical problems, making their assessment complex. Keep this consideration in mind in all cases—both trauma and medical. A trauma patient may have an underlying medical condition that could have caused or may be exacerbated by the injury.
- Obtaining a medical history is important in older patients, regardless of the chief complaint.
- Perform a primary survey.
- Perform a reassessment.

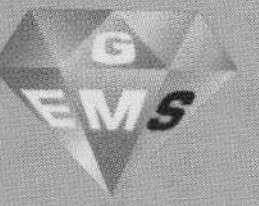

S Social Assessment

- Assess activities of daily living (eating, dressing, bathing, toileting).
- Are these activities being provided for the patient? If so, by whom?
- Are there delays in obtaining food, medication, or toileting? The patient may complain of such a delay, or the environment may suggest a problem.
- Does the patient have regular visits from family members, live with family members, or live with a spouse?
- If in an institutional setting, is the patient able to feed himself or herself? If not, is food still sitting on the food tray? Has the patient been lying in his or her own urine or feces for prolonged periods?
- Does the patient have a social network? Does the patient have a mechanism to interact socially with others on a daily basis?

When a patient's chief complaint seems trivial, it may be necessary to go through a standard list of screening questions to confirm that you are not missing important pieces of information. In such a review of systems, the questions are designed to evaluate the functions of the body's major organ systems. In the field, you do not have sufficient time to conduct a complete review of all systems, but a few well-chosen questions can provide you with a great deal of information about the function of the patient's more important systems:

- Cardiovascular
  - Have you had any pain or discomfort in your chest? When?
  - Have you had any pain in your left arm or jaw?
  - Have you noticed any fluttering in your chest or fast heartbeats?
- Respiratory
  - Are you ever short of breath? When?
  - Have you had a cough lately? Is it painful and, if productive, what color?
  - What position have you been sleeping in? (Recall that patients with heart failure may find themselves sleeping in an upright position in bed, with pillows behind their back, or in a reclining chair.)
- Neurologic
  - Can you explain the reason for calling 9-1-1?
  - Have you had any dizzy spells? Have you fainted?
  - Have you had any trouble speaking?
  - Have you had headaches recently?
  - Have you noticed any unusual weakness or odd sensations in your arms or legs?
- Gastrointestinal
  - Have there been any changes in your appetite lately?
  - Have you gained or lost any weight?
  - Have there been any changes in your bowel movements?
  - Have you had any nausea or vomiting?
- Genitourinary
  - Do you have any pain or difficulty urinating?
  - Have you noticed any change in the color of your urine?
  - Have you noticed any changes in the frequency of urination?

If any of these screening questions yields a positive answer, follow up with further questions. For example, if the patient states that he has been coughing lately, find out whether he is bringing up sputum and, if so, what the sputum looks like (eg, is there blood in the sputum?).

Getting an accurate SAMPLE history (Signs and symptoms, Allergies, Medications, Pertinent past medical history, Last oral intake, Events leading up to the illness or injury) can be complicated, especially in a patient who has an altered mental status. You may have to depend on a relative or caregiver to help you in collecting a SAMPLE history including allergies to food and medications.

The last meal is particularly important in a patient with diabetes, but lack of nutrition can have a negative effect on any patient. A history of last oral intake can indicate that the patient may be dehydrated. Last, what is the event that prompted the call? Again, it is advantageous to provide transport to a facility that "knows" the patient's medical history if the patient's condition and other factors allow as long as that facility has the capability to handle the patient's current problem.

Most important, you should obtain the most detailed history possible of the patient's medications, because medications account for a substantial percentage of medical problems in older people. A medication history should include all medications, not just prescription drugs, because many people do not think to mention common OTC preparations such as aspirin, antacid tablets, and herbal medicines. Ask the patient to list the medications by name, and determine the dosing and frequency for each one. Also, inquire about medications that are prescribed but not taken (eg, because of cost issues or side effects) and medications that may have been provided by other sources (eg, a spouse's medication). Obtain the patient's permission to take medications to the hospital, and then collect them all—prescription and nonprescription—and include the information in your documentation. If the patient cannot tell you where the medicines are stored, check the bathroom medicine cabinet, the bedside table, the kitchen table and counters, and the refrigerator.

Many older patients will have a written list of their medication names and dosages. Some agencies have provided medication lists for older patients to use. Some of these are known as the Envelope of Life or Vial of Life and are placed in the refrigerator **Figure 37-7**. A sticker or magnet that is affixed to the refrigerator or front door will alert EMS providers that there is important patient information available, such as the patient's medical history, current medications, and allergies.

Some patients may not recall the actual name of their medications and may refer to them by color or what they are prescribed for: "I take the little blue one for my heart at night and the pink one for my blood pressure twice a day." This information may also help determine pertinent past history. The opposite end of the spectrum is possible when a patient hands you a shopping bag full of medications. Many of the bottles may be empty or outdated, and there may be numerous medications from different physicians or hospitals. Assess compliance by checking the fill dates on the bottles. This tool may help you to determine if the patient has been taking his or her medications regularly.

There are many commercially available medication reminders and containers. The most common is the weekly pill box. This box is divided into days of the week. The patient (or another responsible party) fills the box with

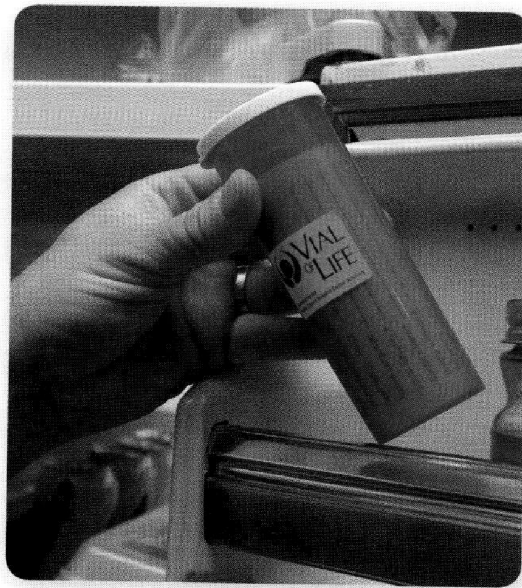

Figure 37-7 Medication containers such as the Vial of Life can be provided to older patients to keep track of medical information.

the medication for the week, separated into the 7 days. Many older patients rely on this pill box to recall if they have taken their medication for the day. You can be aware of the patient's medication compliance by checking the box. Many patients will leave open those days in which they have taken their medication. It is important to find out who fills the box and on what day it is normally filled. There are also electronic versions of the same device that will emit a beeping sound when it is time to take the medication.

Obtaining a history from an older patient requires patience. You must be prepared to listen, often for an extended period. But your listening will be rewarded—not only by helping you discover the patient's problem, but also by allowing you to provide part of the solution to the problem. Listening is a demonstration of caring, and your caring can mean a great deal to a lonely or frightened older person.

Dizziness or Weakness. Obtaining an accurate history of a patient complaining of dizziness or weakness is often difficult with an older patient. This problem can be caused by a cardiac problem, infections with the inner ear, hypotension, or hypertension. During your assessment, it is important to check the patient's pulse and motor and sensory function in all extremities as the patient may be experiencing a stroke. Ask the patient if the weakness, dizziness, or both are always present or if they only occur during certain activity.

Fever. You may be called for a patient who has a fever. This is the body's immune response to combat an infection. Consider the circumstances surrounding the fever. Is the patient unresponsive or does the patient have an altered mental status? Is the patient septic? When was the fever first noticed?

Pain. The OPQRST mnemonic (Onset, Provocation/palliation, Quality, Region/radiation, Severity, Timing) will help you understand more about the patient's pain. Remember that as the body ages, pain sensation changes. Many older patients live with pain on a daily basis. ADLs are often modified because of the pain. Consider the current weather when assessing a patient's pain; many patients experience an exacerbation of pain when the weather changes. Is the pain of an acute onset, or has it been developing over a period of days or weeks? Were OTC medications used? If so, did they help to alleviate the pain?

Words of Wisdom

If a patient tells you that his or her pain is chronic, determine if its onset was slow and progressive or acute. The patient may have experienced an acute onset of pain 1 week ago; however, because the pain worsened, EMS was called. Many patients will interpret an acute onset of gradually worsening pain as being "chronic."

Secondary Assessment

Be aware that the sensation of pain may be diminished in an older patient, leading you to underestimate the severity of his or her condition. This diminished sensation is associated with the aging nervous system. The incidence of "silent" MIs (heart attacks) without the typical symptom of chest pain is greater in older patients, and these are often associated with a dire prognosis.[22]

During the physical exam, protect the patient's modesty at all times. Inspection and palpation can be hampered by multiple layers of clothing; remove only the clothing that is necessary for an accurate assessment, and cover the patient when you are finished. Older people are more susceptible to hypothermia than are younger people. Be sure to keep the patient warm and maintain body temperature.

Words of Wisdom

Unless you have a true emergency situation, take care when removing an older patient's clothing for assessment. Use scissors wisely—this may be the only sweater, coat, or undergarment belonging to that person.

Vital signs may be different in older people because of the physiologic changes that come with aging, chronic disease, and the effects of medications. The heart rate should be in the normal adult range but may be compromised by medications such as beta blockers. These medications keep the heart rate low and prevent the tachycardia that might be typically seen in dehydration or shock. Weaker and irregular pulses are common in older patients. The pulse may be irregular secondary to atrial fibrillation. Circulatory compromise may make it difficult to feel a radial pulse on an older patient, and other pulse points may need to be considered.

Blood pressure tends to be higher in older people. A geriatric patient who has a blood pressure in a normal adult range could be hypotensive. Hypertension could signal impending stroke. Try to confirm if the patient has missed taking any medications for hypertension.

Capillary refill is not a good assessment tool in older adults because of skin changes and reduced circulation to the skin.

The respiratory rate should be in the same range as in a younger adult, but remember that chest rise will be compromised by increased chest wall stiffness. Be sure to auscultate breath sounds to listen for crackles associated with pulmonary edema, rhonchi associated with pneumonia, and wheezes associated with asthma.

Careful interpretation of Spo_2 data is necessary in older adults because the pulse oximetry device requires adequate perfusion to get an accurate reading. Older adults may have poor circulation, vasoconstriction, hypotension, hypothermia, lack of red blood cells, or carbon monoxide poisoning that could result in an inaccurate reading. Adhesive probes, if available and in local protocol, might help confirm accuracy of the data if poor peripheral perfusion is a concern.

Try to determine the patient's normal blood pressure. The baseline blood pressure obtained for this patient and any change from the patient's normal baseline can alert you to a potential problem.

Reassessment

Reassess the geriatric patient often because the condition of an older adult may deteriorate quickly. Repeat the primary survey. Reassess the vital signs. Reassess the patient's problem. Recheck interventions. Identify and treat changes in the patient's condition.

Communicate all findings and interventions provided to emergency department (ED) personnel. Document all history, medications, assessment, and intervention information and leave a copy of your documentation with the ED as well.

Emergency Medical Care

Typical interventions include positioning, oxygenation, administration of glucose, and psychological support. In specific cases, you may also assist with nitroglycerin, aspirin, or inhalers. An older patient reporting shortness of breath will want to sit up or assume the tripod position. Accommodations to these requests should be made except in cases in which you need to manage the patient's airway. The patient's position may be maintaining a patent

YOU are the Provider — PART 3

You immediately assist the patient back to the supine position once you note that he is demonstrating signs of orthostatic hypotension when standing. Your partner then leaves to get the stretcher and bring it to the bathroom door. Given this patient's confusion, you elect to check his blood glucose level. You discover that the patient's blood glucose level is normal. Suspecting substantial GI bleeding, you place the patient on 15 L/min of oxygen via a nonrebreathing mask, establish an 18-gauge IV line to his left antecubital fossa vein, and administer a 250-mL bolus of normal saline. While you are waiting for your partner to arrive with the stretcher, you obtain a complete set of vital signs, then review his medications, which his daughter has handed to you. You note bottles of warfarin (Coumadin), atenolol (Tenormin), metformin (Glucophage), and aspirin.

Recording Time: 6 Minutes	
Respirations	26 breaths/min, normal
Pulse	Slow and thready, 52 beats/min
Skin	Cool, pale, and clammy
Blood pressure	72/36 mm Hg
Oxygen saturation (Spo_2)	96% on room air
Pupils	Pupils Equal, Round, and Reactive to Light and Accommodation (PERRLA)

5. Does this patient require a second IV line?
6. What is the significance of the medications that the patient is taking?

airway. Forcing a patient supine who is short of breath may result in respiratory failure or arrest. Allow the patient to maintain a position of comfort, unless the patient is unable to maintain it. Assist ventilation as needed.

Administration of oxygen may be a useful therapy for many geriatric problems, including vague reports of weakness or dizziness, particularly if the Spo_2 level indicates hypoxia. When administering oxygen, be mindful of monitoring the level of consciousness in a patient with COPD. Be prepared to ventilate if the patient's hypoxic drive becomes inadequate.

Other interventions include administration of glucose in a patient with diabetes who has altered mental status and a manageable airway. In a patient with a cardiac history, consider assisting with the patient's nitroglycerin if he or she is having chest pain, or assist a patient with medication for asthma when the patient is experiencing shortness of breath.

Last, and critically important in older adults, is providing emotional support. An older person is often fearful of what may be happening and that he or she may never return home from the hospital. Listen to your patient, respond to your patient, and provide reassurance.

Fluid Resuscitation in Geriatric Patients

Fluid resuscitation in an older person can be challenging. Because geriatric patients often have chronic hypertension, baseline values for blood pressure may be higher than those of other adults. Because of decreases in circulation along with atherosclerosis and arteriosclerosis, increased blood pressure may assist the body in achieving end organ perfusion. An older patient may actually be in shock with systolic pressures of greater than 100 mm Hg.

Modest amounts of blood loss can quickly result in shock in a geriatric patient because of the patient's inability to adapt and compensate quickly. Reduced blood volume, possible anemia, and medications such as beta blockers also may interfere with coping mechanisms. Large volumes of fluid may result in circulatory overload and pulmonary edema. Monitor breath sounds frequently when providing fluid resuscitation. Introducing fluid into the system of a geriatric patient can produce electrolyte alterations and hemodilution. Diluting the blood will decrease its ability to carry oxygen and result in hypoxia as well as making clotting mechanisms less effective. Use fluid sparingly; you can always add more, but cannot easily take fluid out.

Words of Wisdom

Remember that the skin of the older patient tends to be very fragile. Try tying the tourniquet loosely or not using one at all when trying to gain IV access. Pull the skin taunt to avoid "wrinkling" and be alert for the potential for excessive bleeding from attempts. For critical patients, do not hesitate to use the intraosseous route when gaining IV access is difficult.

Assessment and Management of Respiratory Emergencies

Shortness of Breath

Many of your older patient contacts will involve a patient reporting respiratory distress, either acutely or chronically. Remember that, in addition to the shortness of breath, another condition may be an underlying cause. Obtaining an accurate pertinent medical and prescribed medication history may help you determine the etiology of the problem (ie, respiratory versus cardiac). If the patient has a history of pedal edema, discomfort of the chest, and hypertension, the cause may be cardiac related. A productive cough and signs of emphysema point toward a respiratory condition.

Patients in respiratory distress should not be overwhelmed with questions. A bystander or family member may be able to answer your questions. It is important to find out whether the patient has a history of respiratory problems and what, if any, medications he or she is taking.

Patients experiencing respiratory distress should receive supplemental oxygen as soon as possible and be observed for signs of inadequate breathing, which would necessitate assisted ventilations. Nonrebreathing masks can be intimidating to an older patient; they may want to remove the mask to answer your questions. If you remove the patient's glasses, replace them once you have applied the mask. If the patient cannot tolerate a nonrebreathing mask, use a nasal cannula. Some older patients with COPD may be on home oxygen. Many of these patients will medicate themselves. Medications taken prior to your arrival may affect your treatment, so gather this important information, if possible.

Words of Wisdom

Apply oxygen to patients experiencing dyspnea prior to asking questions.

Asthma

Asthma is a common disease among older adults. Onset can occur in old age with presenting symptoms of shortness of breath (especially with effort), chronic or nocturnal cough, and wheezing. Patients with asthma that is worsened by exertion may find that they are more susceptible to asthma attacks as they age.

Management of asthma in the geriatric population is similar to management in other age groups, although when asthma and cardiac disease coexist, the administration of

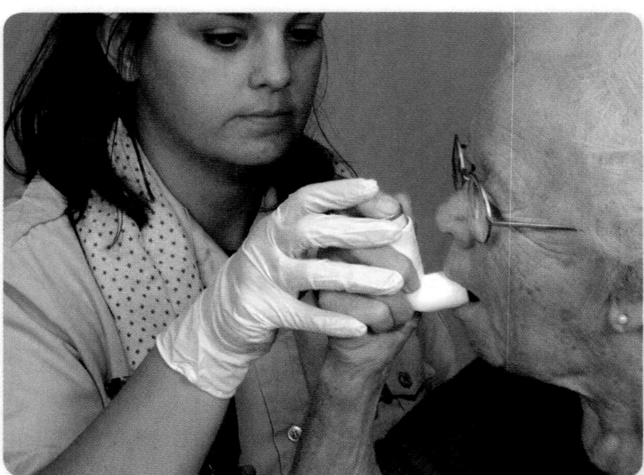

Figure 37-8 A patient having an asthma attack may have a bronchodilator medication in a metered-dose inhaler. An older patient may need assistance with the use of an inhaler.

preferred beta-adrenergic agents for asthma may exacerbate cardiac symptoms. Asthma clinical practice guidelines are the same for younger and older patients Figure 37-8. On rare occasions, epinephrine may be indicated for a life-threatening asthma exacerbation. See Chapter 17, *Respiratory Emergencies*, for more information about asthma.

▶ Pneumonia

Older patients with pneumonia often do not have the classic presentation of chills, fever, and productive cough. Instead, these symptoms are often supplanted by acute confusion (delirium), normal temperature, and a minimal to absent cough. The patient will often have flulike symptoms: exertional dyspnea, chest pain or discomfort, nausea and vomiting, muscle aches and pains, weight loss, wheezing, headache, and confusion.

The patient may exhibit signs of dehydration including poor skin turgor, furrowed tongue, dry mucosa, tachycardia, and hypotension. He or she may be pale, with hot, dry skin caused by dehydration and an elevated temperature. Breath sounds range from diminished to wheezing, crackles, or rhonchi, and the chest may be dull to percussion. Assess for orthostatic changes and monitor oxygen saturation.

Prehospital treatment is supportive and includes oxygen to relieve dyspnea with appropriate adjuncts and IV access and fluid as indicated. The patient may benefit from application of continuous positive airway pressure (CPAP). Reassure the patient and keep the patient warm without overheating and increasing his or her temperature. The receiving facility staff will determine whether antibiotics are necessary.

▶ Pulmonary Embolism

Many pulmonary emboli are silent or present with tachypnea alone—that is, the classic triad of a sudden onset of dyspnea, chest pain, and hemoptysis is often altered or absent. If you suspect a pulmonary embolus, check for swelling, erythema, and warmth or tenderness of the lower leg; all are signs of a deep venous thrombosis, which is a common cause of pulmonary embolus. If deep venous thrombosis might be present, handle the leg gently and monitor the patient for respiratory changes.

Other symptoms associated with an embolism include syncope, fatigue, fever, anxiety, and/or cardiac arrest. The patient may present with tachycardia, wheezes, crackles, diminished breath sounds on the affected side, low oxygen saturation, and/or hypotension.

Prehospital treatment is largely supportive after ensuring that airway and ventilation are adequate. Rapid transport with oxygen and a position of comfort are the best treatment. Because aggressive airway management may be needed, call early for paramedic backup. Reassess the patient frequently during transport.

Assessment and Management of Cardiovascular Emergencies

As in all prehospital emergencies, health care providers must prioritize the patient's airway, breathing, and circulatory status during cardiovascular emergencies. Use the appropriate oxygen delivery device and airway adjunct consistent with the patient's condition. Remember to reassess the patient often.

Remember the changes that occur with aging or with ingestion of certain medications when you are assessing a geriatric patient. You may note peripheral edema that is chronic or changes in circulation strength and rate. The skin may be pale and diaphoretic and breath sounds may be decreased or unusual. The next sections discuss specific cardiovascular emergencies and their assessment and treatment.

▶ Syncope

You should always assume that syncope, or fainting, in an older person is a life-threatening problem until proven otherwise. Syncope is the result of a temporary interruption of blood flow to the brain. Syncope has many causes, some more serious than others. Regardless, an older person who has experienced a loss of consciousness should be transported to the hospital and examined to determine the cause. Table 37-3 shows some of the causes of syncope in an older patient.

▶ Chest Pain

As mentioned previously, older patients may experience and present with chest pain differently than the general population. An older person experiencing an MI may only report dyspnea, weakness, or syncope, or there may be no associated pain. Remember that the pain threshold of older patients may be different. The OPQRST mnemonic

Table 37-3 Possible Causes of Syncope in an Older Patient

Cause	Mechanism
Cardiac dysrhythmias/ myocardial infarction	The heart is beating too fast or too slow, the cardiac output drops, and blood flow to the brain is interrupted. A myocardial infarction can also cause syncope.
Vascular and volume	Medication interactions can cause venous pooling and **vasodilation** (widening of a blood vessel), resulting in a decrease in blood pressure and inadequate blood flow to the brain. Another cause of syncope can be a decrease in blood volume because of hidden bleeding from a condition such as a leaking aortic aneurysm.
Neurologic	A transient ischemic attack or a "small stroke" can sometimes cause syncope.

Table 37-4 Common Signs and Symptoms of MI in an Older Patient

Signs/ Symptoms	Potential Causes
Dyspnea	Dyspnea, the feeling of shortness of breath or difficulty in breathing, is a common symptom in older people and is commonly associated with an MI. Dyspnea is often combined with other symptoms, such as nausea, weakness, and sweating. In older persons, chest pain is often not present, but dyspnea on exertion is noted.
Generalized weakness	Generalized weakness (malaise) can be caused by many things. However, you should suspect an MI in a patient with a sudden onset of weakness. Weakness is often associated with sweating.
Syncope/ confusion/ altered mental status	Syncope can have many causes, and in older people, none of these causes should be presumed to be minor. Syncope often has a cardiac cause. Altered mental status is usually a signal of poor blood supply to the brain, often from a cardiac dysrhythmia and MI.

Abbreviation: MI, myocardial infarction

for pain in the older patient is important. If the patient has a history of angina, determine if this episode is different from previous events. Is the patient taking the medication that is prescribed for the condition? Often, the patient will not use the term *pain*, but may use the word *discomfort* or *fluttering*.

Instead of asking about pain, say, "Describe to me exactly how you feel." The patient may respond negatively about any pain, but may be experiencing tightness or fullness in the chest, dyspnea, palpitations, or other symptoms.

Prehospital treatment for chest pain remains essentially unchanged in older patients, albeit with extra precautions because of the increased potential for medication side effects. Nitroglycerin may produce more hypotension in older patients than in younger patients or may react adversely with long-term medications. Aspirin may increase bleeding in a patient who is already taking anticoagulants. Additional treatments by prehospital providers should include close monitoring of fluids and avoidance of excessive fluid overload.

▶ Myocardial Infarction

The classic symptoms of an MI, or heart attack, are often not present in older people. Some experience silent MIs, in which the usual chest pain is not present. Table 37-4 shows signs and symptoms that are commonly noted in older patients who are experiencing an MI. The patient may also complain of epigastric or abdominal pain along with nausea, vomiting, and weakness. Treatment of MI is discussed in Chapter 18, *Cardiovascular Emergencies*.

Words of Wisdom

If the patient is hypotensive and is wearing a nitroglycerin patch, remove it. The patient's issue could be caused by too much of this medication.

▶ Heart Failure

People 65 years and older are in a high-risk group for heart failure.[23] Cardiovascular diseases are the most common reason for hospitalization in the geriatric population.[24] Heart failure increases with age because of the associated risk factors, such as hypertension and coronary artery disease. Other risk factors for heart failure include sex, ethnicity, family history and genetics, long-term alcohol abuse, and multiple medical conditions—coronary artery disease, emphysema, hyperthyroidism, thiamine (vitamin B) deficiency, and human immunodeficiency virus infection, among others.[23,25] As with acute coronary syndrome, prevention is aimed at lifestyle changes: cessation of tobacco use, eating a healthy diet, control of blood glucose levels (in patients with diabetes), exercise, weight control, and control of hypertension.

Acute exacerbation of heart failure results in pulmonary edema that decreases the ability of the lungs to exchange gases. It may present with dyspnea or orthopnea. Because of the decreased oxygenation of all organ systems including the brain, mental status changes may also be seen in acute exacerbation of heart failure, including a sensation of air hunger, or the perception that the person cannot take deep enough breaths to get enough air. Peripheral edema may also indicate worsening heart failure, although in the absence of other more serious symptoms, it may also be the result of any number of other circulatory, integumentary, or infectious conditions.

You should pay close attention to the position in which the patient with heart failure is found. When assessing for peripheral edema, the ankles are the logical site for evaluation. Because edema is likely to be formed in the lowest point to the ground on the patient's body, those patients who are confined to bed may present instead with **sacral edema**, edema that presents around the sacral region of the spinal column.

The presentation of heart failure in an older person can be masked by symptoms and signs symbolic of old age and shared by several chronic diseases—for example, dyspnea on exertion, easy fatigability (especially with left-side heart failure), confusion, crackles on lung exam, orthopnea, dry cough progressing to productive cough, and dependent peripheral edema in right-side heart failure. Acute exacerbations of heart failure are often related to poor diet, medication noncompliance, onset of dysrhythmias such as atrial fibrillation, or acute myocardial ischemia.

Prehospital treatment is unchanged from that of younger patients, although greater consideration is given to becoming familiar with the patient's medications and their implications for your proposed treatment. End-tidal carbon dioxide ($ETCO_2$) should be evaluated immediately and monitored throughout transport. Additional treatments by prehospital providers should include close monitoring of fluids and avoidance of excessive fluid overload, consideration of CPAP, and potential use of anticoagulation therapy in patients with atrial dysrhythmias to prevent thromboembolism.

Heart failure may also be exacerbated by fluid imbalances, particularly when overhydration occurs. Because the weakened and less-effective heart is not able to adequately pump normal vascular volumes, an increase in volume within the vascular system may stress the heart further. IV fluids should be administered judiciously in patients with heart failure because even slight changes can result in substantial negative outcomes, and achieving an appropriate balance of fluid and electrolyte administration may be complicated when both dehydration and heart failure are present.

▶ Dysrhythmias

Rhythm disturbances (dysrhythmias) of the heart occur when the electrical system controlling the heartbeat experiences an interruption or malfunction. These irregularities cause heartbeats that are too fast, too slow, irregular, or absent. Many people experience an occasional or harmless dysrhythmia that they may describe as a skipping, fluttering, or fast heartbeat. Dysrhythmias in older people are generally a result of age-related changes in the heart, existing cardiac disease, adverse drug effects, or a combination of these factors.

Atrial fibrillation (coming from the atria), which is the most common dysrhythmia among older people, increases the risk of stroke and heart failure. The fibrillating atria allow stasis of the blood, thereby encouraging clot formation and increasing the chances that a clot fragment might travel to the brain and cause a stroke. Most of the blood in the atria enters the ventricles when the valves open, with about 20% being kicked in by contraction of the atria. The aging heart may function adequately when the preload provided by the atria ends up in the ventricles; however, when that 20% remains in the atria, new signs or symptoms of heart failure may develop or stable heart failure may decompensate.

Bradycardias are also more common in older people. The aging conduction system may produce sinus dysrhythmias such as sick sinus syndrome and atrioventricular blocks. Medications such as beta blockers or calcium-channel blockers can cause excessive slowing of the heart. Even seemingly benign conditions, such as constipation, can result in bradycardia, particularly when the patient strains to have a bowel movement. Persistent bradycardias are often addressed with an internal pacemaker.

▶ Hypertension

More than one-half of all older persons are hypertensive.[26] Most have isolated systolic hypertension resulting from a loss of arterial elasticity. Controlling systolic and/or diastolic hypertension in older people helps prevent strokes and MIs. Geriatric hypertensive emergencies require a controlled decline in blood pressure that often cannot be achieved in the field. Prompt transport is essential for these patients.

▶ Aneurysms

The incidence of aneurysm increases with age. An aneurysm is a weakness in any artery that produces a balloon defect, weakening the arterial wall. This weakness may be congenital (present at birth) or acquired. In the latter case, hypertension, atherosclerotic disease, and obesity are contributing factors to development of this defect. Life-threatening aneurysms can develop in the brain, chest, or abdomen. A new headache or a change in chronic headache patterns, for example, may signal early cerebral bleeding from an aneurysm. Frequently, however, the first manifestation is a sudden, devastating stroke. Use of anticoagulants for the management of cardiac disease increases the negative effects of an aneurysm by increasing the amount of time necessary for bleeding to stop. Preventive measures—proper diet, exercise, smoking cessation, and cholesterol control—aim to control the risk factors associated with hypertension and atherosclerotic diseases.

Thoracic aneurysms generally remain asymptomatic until they become large or rupture. Early symptoms may be related to compression by the aneurysm, such as difficulty swallowing or hoarseness from laryngeal nerve pressure. AAAs present typically with abdominal pain or possibly only with back pain. Asymptomatic thoracic and abdominal aneurysms that do not exceed a certain size and are not expanding are generally treated without surgery but are reassessed on a regular schedule. In an older patient with back pain, examine the chest and abdomen carefully. The treatment of abdominal emergencies is surgical, so early recognition, assessment, stabilization, and rapid transport to an appropriate medical facility are essential.

▶ Traumatic Aortic Disruption

Traumatic aortic disruption or aortic dissection occurs when the inside wall of the artery becomes torn and allows blood to collect between the arterial wall layers. It may occur with trauma or sustained hypertension, particularly when an AAA is present. Dissection weakens the arterial wall, making it susceptible to rupture. A thoracic dissection, for example, can produce chest pain that is difficult to differentiate from cardiac ischemia. Therefore, it is helpful to obtain blood pressure readings in both arms in all patients with chest pain. A systolic blood pressure difference of 15 mm Hg or higher suggests a thoracic dissection.

Assessment and Management of Neurologic and Endocrine Emergencies

In any patient with delirium, assess for recent changes in the patient's level of consciousness or orientation. Specifically, look for an acute onset of anxiety, an inability to think logically or maintain attention, and an inability to focus. Also assess for changes in vital signs, temperature (indicating infection), glucose level, and medications—all frequent causes of delirium. Use the DELIRIUMS mnemonic to identify other causes of delirium:

- Drugs or toxins
- Emotional (psychiatric)/electrolyte imbalance
- Low PaO_2 (carbon monoxide poisoning, COPD, heart failure, acute coronary syndrome, pneumonia)
- Infection (pneumonia, UTI, sepsis)
- Retention of stool or urine
- Ictal (seizures)
- Undernutrition or underhydration
- Metabolism (thyroid or endocrine, electrolytes, kidneys)
- Subdural hematoma

Treatment of patients with delirium is mostly supportive. Monitor vital signs, including breath sounds. Use airway adjuncts if the patient is unable to maintain his or her airway, and obtain IV access to use as a fluid resuscitation route if needed.

▶ Stroke

Stroke (cerebrovascular accident) is a leading cause of death in older people.[5] The likelihood of experiencing a stroke becomes greater as a person gets older. The major risk factors include hypertension, diabetes, cardiac diseases (such as coronary heart disease, cardiomyopathy, heart failure, and atrial fibrillation), smoking, personal or family history of stroke or transient ischemic attack (TIA), and brain aneurysms.[27] Also of consideration are alcohol and illegal drug use, obesity, stress, high cholesterol levels, an unhealthy diet, and the use of NSAIDs.[27]

Signs and symptoms of stroke include acute altered level of consciousness; numbness, weakness, or paralysis on one side of the body; slurred speech; difficulty speaking (aphasia); visual disturbances; headache and dizziness; incontinence; and, in the worst cases, seizure.

Hemorrhagic strokes, in which a ruptured vessel causes bleeding into the brain, are less common and more likely to be fatal. Ischemic strokes occur when a clot blocks the flow of blood to a portion of the brain. Brain tissue distal to this clot is deprived of oxygen and will die if the clot is not removed.

Effective prehospital acute stroke care includes early recognition, discovery of conditions that mimic strokes (such as hypoglycemia or hypoxia), and timely transport to the most appropriate facility. Use a stroke assessment tool as appropriate, accounting for the patient's history when you are evaluating the components of the scale. An older person with severe arthritis may not move as well on one side, or damage from a previous stroke may make his or her speech difficult to assess. Always ask family or caregivers for information that may help you identify deviations from the patient's normal pattern of behavior or activity.

The treatment goal is to salvage as much of the surrounding brain tissue as possible. Many communities now have stroke centers that specialize in fast, effective treatment of stroke. Determining the onset of the symptoms of stroke is important. If the symptoms occurred within the past few hours, the patient will be a candidate for stroke center therapy and has a higher chance for recovery. See Chapter 19, *Neurologic Emergencies*, for information on assessment and treatment of stroke patients.

▶ Transient Ischemic Attack

TIAs, also called ministrokes, entail a temporary disturbance of blood supply to the brain that results in a sudden, temporary decrease in brain function. The symptoms are the same as those for a stroke but generally last less than 24 hours; they are warning signs of a future stroke. Although a TIA results in no lasting damage to the brain, the gravity of this condition should not be minimized in the field. Because of the short amount of time that you often have with your patient, you most likely will not be able to determine whether the patient is experiencing a stroke or a TIA; therefore, any patient experiencing stroke-like symptoms should be treated as though he or she is having a stroke. Furthermore, patients who report a history of previous TIAs should be considered at a much higher risk of having a stroke instead of another TIA.

Neuropathy

Your patient could be experiencing a **neuropathy**, a disorder of the nerves of the peripheral nervous system in which function and structure of the peripheral motor, sensory, and autonomic neurons are impaired. Symptoms depend on whether the nerves affected are motor, sensory, or autonomic and where the nerves are located.

- **Motor nerves:** muscle weakness, cramps, spasms, loss of balance, and loss of coordination
- **Sensory nerves:** tingling, numbness, itching, and pain; burning, freezing, or extreme sensitivity to touch
- **Autonomic nerves:** affect involuntary functions that could include changes in blood pressure and heart rate, constipation, bladder and sexual dysfunction

Neuropathies are treated with medication and other therapies not available in a field setting. You should make your patient as comfortable as possible and transport.

Altered Mental Status

Altered mental status is a symptom, not a disease. Consequently, the assessment and subsequent management of its numerous causes are complicated. Confused or disoriented patients make poor historians. In addition, they may be unable to speak and follow commands, making assessment extremely difficult. Always consider head injury (medical or traumatic), tumors, emotional disorders, eye or ear problems, heart rhythm disturbances, dementia, medications, fluid balance changes (such as blood loss), respiratory disorders (such as hypoxia), endocrine changes (such as blood glucose level fluctuations), hyperthermia or hypothermia, and infection. Most important, prehospital providers need to consider neurologic causes (such as Alzheimer disease, Huntington disease, and Parkinson disease) and endocrine changes (such as diabetes).

An altered mental status is not normal. You need to rapidly determine if this patient requires immediate transport. When you are assessing a patient with signs of altered mental status, it is important to determine the onset of symptoms. Ascertain what is normal for this patient and whether the patient has a pertinent history that may be attributed to the problem. If the patient has diabetes, have the appropriate medications been taken? Is it possible the patient may have taken the wrong medication or taken alcohol with medications? Because of cost concerns, many older patients will try medications that are not prescribed for them. They may be taking a medication that is prescribed for a spouse who has a similar problem, or worse, a completely different problem.

Potential causes of altered mental status can be remembered using the VITAMINS C & D mnemonic:

- Vascular: stroke, brain, embolism
- Inflammation: inflammation of the blood vessels in the brain
- Toxins: carbon monoxide poisoning
- Trauma: concussion, intracerebral hemorrhage
- Tumors: primary brain tumor, or metastasis (developed elsewhere and spread to the brain)
- Autoimmune: production of immune system components against a normal structure in the body
- Metabolic: liver or renal failure, hypoglycemia, hyperglycemia, hypothyroidism or hyperthyroidism, HHS
- Infection: meningitis, encephalitis
- Narcotics and other drugs: many possibilities, with a higher chance of mental status changes if preexisting CNS disease exists
- Systemic: sepsis, hypoxia
- Congenital: seizures
- Degenerative: Alzheimer disease and other dementias, Parkinson disease

Diabetic Disorders

Among people older than 65 years, one of every four in the United States has diabetes—primarily type 2 diabetes (formerly called adult-onset, or non–insulin-dependent diabetes mellitus).[28] Type 1 diabetes has historically been referred to as insulin-dependent diabetes mellitus or juvenile diabetes, because it generally affects children. Many normal changes of aging contribute to the development of diabetes. The most common risk factor for this disease is having more than one chronic disease, and many older people with diabetes also have hypertension, heart disease, and stroke. Other risk factors for diabetes include a family history of diabetes, genetics, age, diet, obesity, and a sedentary lifestyle. Management of diabetes is complicated when other acute diseases are present, particularly infections; because older adults are more likely to have several comorbid disorders, management is especially complicated for them.

In the emergency setting, diabetes can result in two life-threatening conditions: hypoglycemia and hyperglycemia. Normal blood glucose levels range from approximately 70 to 120 mg/dL. Hypoglycemia occurs when blood glucose levels drop below the normal range, and hyperglycemia occurs when blood glucose levels exceed 120 mg/dL.

Geriatric patients with diabetes are at increased risk for hypoglycemia for several reasons: confusion about medication doses or usage, inadequate or irregular dietary intake, inability to recognize the warning signs because of cognitive problems, and/or blunted warning signs. Delirium may be the only indication of hypoglycemia in a geriatric patient. Other symptoms include mental status changes and confusion, diaphoresis, and decreased respiratory effort.

Symptoms of an elevated blood glucose level (hyperglycemia) include fatigue, poor wound healing, blurred vision, and frequent infections. Other symptoms of chronic hyperglycemia include the three Ps: polyuria (excessive urine output), polydipsia (excessive thirst), and polyphagia (excessive eating). New-onset diabetes in geriatric patients is often a mild progression that produces no symptoms.

Assessment of hyperglycemia and hypoglycemia is complicated by many of the changes associated with aging. Particularly, changes in peripheral vascular function make assessment of skin condition for key signs of hypoglycemia much more difficult because many older patients may be paler and cooler at baseline. Diaphoresis may also be less prominent as a result of changes in regulatory mechanisms and secretory functions of the skin. Baseline alterations of mentation may also be confused with acute mental status changes that are related to either hyperglycemia or hypoglycemia.

You should ensure that all vital signs, including blood pressure, blood glucose levels, temperature, and distal pulses, are assessed every 15 minutes and monitored for changes. Capnography, if available, should be used throughout the transport to monitor $ETCO_2$ as well as ventilatory status. Whereas Spo_2 is a valuable tool, poor perfusion may make it difficult to obtain an Spo_2 reading.

Treatment of diabetic emergencies in geriatric patients is no different than treatment in other populations, although care with fluid resuscitation and electrolyte balance is particularly important. Prevention of type 2 diabetes is aimed at lifestyle changes that include dietary restrictions, exercise, and controlling obesity. Long-term management may include limiting of carbohydrate intake and the use of insulin and oral antihyperglycemic agents. Diabetes management also focuses on preventing many of the devastating systemic effects of the disease, including aggressive wound management, frequent screening for impaired renal function, and management of pain associated with neuropathy.

Hyperosmolar Hyperglycemic Syndrome

Older people with diabetes and consistently high blood glucose levels are more susceptible to HHS/HONK than DKA. DKA is a life-threatening condition that is associated predominantly with type 1 diabetes (patients who have this condition tend to be young—teenagers and young adults). See Chapter 21, *Endocrine and Hematologic Emergencies*, for more information on this condition.

The most frequent cause for HHS/HONK is infection. Other potential risk factors include hypothermia, hyperthermia, cardiac disease, pancreatitis, and stroke. The patient is likely to present with hyperglycemia that is generally greater than 600 mg/dL and has acute confusion with dehydration, although signs of dehydration may be altered in older adults Table 37-5. With HHS/HONK, hyperglycemia and hyperosmolarity result in osmotic diuresis and an osmotic shift of fluid to the intravascular space, resulting in further intracellular dehydration. Signs and symptoms include dizziness, confusion, altered mental status, and polydipsia.

Table 37-5 Signs of Dehydration in Older Adults

- Dry tongue
- Longitudinal furrows in the tongue
- Dry mucous membranes
- Weak upper body musculature
- Confusion
- Difficulty in speech
- Sunken eyes

Prehospital treatment of HHS in younger and older patients is the same; however, the systems of older patients may be less tolerant of aggressive fluid therapy. Airway management is the top priority. Use appropriate airway adjuncts and consider calling for paramedic backup if endotracheal intubation is indicated. Spinal motion restriction should be used for all unresponsive patients found down, unless witnesses can validate that no fall occurred. Treat for shock as indicated. Large-bore IV access should be gained as soon as possible, but do not delay transport while initiating the IV line. Also, obtain a blood glucose level as soon as possible.

A 20-mL/kg bolus of 0.9% normal saline is appropriate for nearly all adults who are clinically dehydrated. In patients with a history of heart failure and/or renal insufficiency, give fluid sparingly and auscultate breath sounds frequently. If the glucose level is less than 70 mg/dL and the patient is symptomatic, administer supplemental dextrose either orally or intravenously depending on level of consciousness and local protocols, as soon as possible.

▶ Thyroid Disorders

Thyroid abnormalities increase with aging. Many older patients remain asymptomatic, and the disease is diagnosed only when a routine blood test reveals a thyroid problem. Adult hypothyroidism (*myxedema*) is manifested by a general slowing of the body's metabolic processes as a result of the reduction or absence of thyroid hormone. With hypothyroidism, the signs and symptoms may match those seen with normal aging: cold intolerance, constipation, dry skin, weakness, and weight gain. Prior thyroidectomy is also more common in geriatric patients, who typically take synthetic thyroid hormones.

With acute-onset hyperthyroidism (thyrotoxicosis), the presentation can be blunted in older people; although tachycardia is generally present, older patients may experience less tremor, anxiety, or hyperactive reflexes than do younger patients. Atrial fibrillation is more likely to be induced by an overactive thyroid gland in a geriatric patient. A smaller percentage of older patients with hyperthyroidism present with symptoms opposite of those expected: weakness, lethargy, and depression.

Patients with hyperthyroidism or hypothyroidism are likely to require supplemental oxygen. Hypoglycemia may need correction with supplemental dextrose. Hypothyroid conditions may result in diminished respiratory effort that may require positive pressure ventilation.

Continued decrease of hormone levels may result in myxedema coma, an extreme manifestation of hypothyroidism that is accompanied by physiologic decompensation. Myxedema coma is more likely in women than in men and occurs primarily in the geriatric population.[29] See Chapter 21, *Endocrine and Hematologic Emergencies*, for more information on these conditions.

Assessment and Management of Gastrointestinal Emergencies

A number of life-threatening abdominal problems are common in older patients. Remember that internal bleeding may be a cause of the patient's abdominal problem, which can result in shock and death.

Abdominal Pain

Constipation is a frequent and substantial problem in older people. Although it can cause acute abdominal pain, it should not be the initial condition suspected when a patient experiences such discomfort. Instead, causes with high mortality, such as bleeding from an acute abdominal aneurysm or dead bowel from mesenteric ischemia, should be investigated first. In your assessment of a gastric emergency, ask the patient about food and fluid intake, history of abdominal issues, current bowel and bladder habits, and medications and supplements before proceeding with a physical exam.

The geriatric patient who reports abdominal pain may be among the most frustrating patients because it will be difficult to determine the cause of the pain. Many older patients presenting with abdominal pain will require hospital admission, and some will need surgical intervention. The history of acute versus chronic pain may help in your assessment, and the mnemonic OPQRST for pain may help you determine what is happening to your patient. There are numerous causes of acute abdominal pain in the geriatric population, including inflammation, infection, and ischemic disorders. The patient may have a difficult time localizing the pain and describing whether or not the pain is radiating or referred. Symptoms are often vague and manifest only as diffuse abdominal pain with no

YOU are the Provider — PART 4

Your partner arrives with the stretcher. You place the patient on the stretcher and secure him with all straps. After the stretcher is secured inside the ambulance, you instruct your partner to drive emergently to the local hospital, approximately 12 minutes away. En route to the hospital, you elect to administer a second 250-mL fluid bolus to increase the patient's blood pressure based on persistent hypotension. Approximately 6 minutes from the hospital, the patient vomits what appears to be 200 mL of coffee ground–looking emesis. You ensure that the airway is clear, carefully position the patient on his left side, and call your report in to the ED. On arrival at the hospital, you turn over care to the waiting ED staff without further incident.

Recording Time: 20 Minutes	
Respirations	26 breaths/min, normal
Pulse	Slow and thready, 68 beats/min
Skin	Cool, pale, and clammy
Blood pressure	78/42 mm Hg
Oxygen saturation (Spo_2)	100% on 15 L/min via a nonrebreathing mask
Pupils	PERRLA

7. What are the potential hazards of the patient vomiting?
8. Why should lactated Ringer solution be avoided in this patient?

particular point of origin. Abdominal and gastric problems often require surgical treatment, so early recognition and rapid transport for definitive hospital care are the best practice. If you suspect an AAA, treat the patient for shock if evident and provide prompt transport to the hospital.

▶ Gastrointestinal Bleeding

GI bleeding also becomes more common with age, and it is almost always the result of either physiologic changes that lead to an increased likelihood of bleeding systemically or pathologic processes that specifically affect the digestive system. Several normal changes of aging increase the time needed to obtain hemostasis, including decreased vascular tone and thinning of various epithelial tissues. Decreased rates of peristalsis also increase the likelihood that irritating substances will damage the gastric lining. Older patients are also more likely to take medications that alter coagulation, including warfarin, aspirin, and heparin. Pathologic processes within the GI system that are sometimes responsible for bleeding include ulcers and varices; cancers of the stomach, esophagus, colon, and rectum; diverticulitis; cirrhosis; and bowel obstructions.

Although the source of GI bleeding may vary, the signs and symptoms vary more by the location where the bleeding is noted. Bleeding from the esophagus is most commonly associated with varices and alcohol abuse; the patient will present with violent vomiting of emesis that contains almost no food and a large quantity of bright red, uncoagulated blood. Bleeding from the stomach may produce either red or darker coffee-ground emesis, and it is most commonly associated with peptic ulcer disease. Bloody stool usually indicates bleeding from the lower GI system, although blood from the stomach may be digested and appear as dark, tarry stool. Bright red blood in the stool usually comes from the large intestine or rectum and may be caused by diverticulitis, large bowel obstructions, anal fissures, or hemorrhoids. In general, the darker the blood, the longer it has been in the body, and, therefore, the further the distance between the site of bleeding and the portal of exit.

Upper GI hemorrhage occurs when bleeding occurs from the esophagus, stomach, or duodenum. When severe, this condition is a true medical emergency that must be recognized and assessed quickly. Not only are older people more susceptible to upper GI bleeding, they often need urgent surgery and also are at a greater risk of complications and death.

It is not possible to determine the cause of upper GI bleeding without an endoscopic examination (inspection of the inside of a hollow organ or body cavity) of the esophagus, stomach, and duodenum. However, obtaining a thorough history can provide you with clues to the cause. Regular use of NSAIDs or alcohol may result in bleeding from irritation of the lining of the stomach or from ulcers (a hollowing out or disintegration of tissue) in the stomach or duodenum. Forceful vomiting can cause tears in the esophagus that result in bleeding. Cirrhosis of the liver from long-term alcohol use or chronic infectious hepatitis may cause enlargement of the veins (varices) in the esophagus. These varices can rupture and result in massive bleeding. Stomach cancer or esophageal cancer can also produce upper GI bleeding. Recent weight loss or difficulty swallowing would raise the suspicion of cancer as the source of bleeding.

Lower GI hemorrhage primarily describes bleeding from the colon and rectum and should never simply be attributed to hemorrhoids. Colon polyps and colon cancer are also possible causes, among others. Minor lower GI bleeding is characterized by small amounts of red blood covering formed brown stools or scant amounts of red blood noticed on the toilet paper. Severe lower GI bleeding is characterized by passing significant amounts of red blood or maroon-colored stools.

Assessment should begin with identifying risk factors such as a history of previous lower GI bleeding, symptoms or signs suggestive of colon cancer, recent constipation or diarrhea, and use of medications such as blood thinners. Treat for shock. Severe lower GI bleeding requires immediate transportation to the nearest ED.

Some signs and symptoms of GI bleeding are associated with hypovolemia that occurs from the blood loss. These include agitation, dizziness, syncope, hypotension, and changes in mental status. Others may be associated with the disease processes that caused the bleeding, including jaundice, hepatomegaly, constipation or diarrhea, pain with voiding, nausea, and abdominal pain.

When you arrive at the scene, it is more important for you to be able to assess the severity of the bleeding than to determine the cause of bleeding. Slower bleeding is characterized by emesis with coffee grounds appearance. With minor bleeding, the pulse rate and systolic blood pressure are normal. Brisk bleeding presents with hematemesis (vomiting red blood) or melena (black, tarlike stools). Note that melena, not pain, is the most common presenting symptom of GI bleeding. Prehospital treatment is supportive.

Regardless of the cause of GI bleeding, treatment should be focused on recognition and management of hypovolemic shock and transport to a facility capable of providing definitive care; many patients with GI bleeding may require surgery to repair the site of injury or disease. Be cautious in fluid resuscitation and bear in mind that the older adult's compensatory mechanisms may be altered because of normal aging processes. Finally, keep in mind that these patients may be on blood-thinning medications (eg, warfarin) that prevent them from forming clots following major injuries.

▶ Nausea, Vomiting, and Diarrhea

Nausea, vomiting, and diarrhea need to be investigated to determine the underlying cause. These issues may be attributed to conditions inside or outside the GI tract. If an older patient is complaining only of nausea, this does not mean that vomiting and/or diarrhea will not soon follow. Remember that nausea may be an older patient's problem during a cardiac episode. There are many possible causes of GI issues. During the assessment of the patient, determining the onset may provide a clue to possible causes. Viral gastroenteritis, which your patient may self-diagnose as stomach flu, is a common finding.

During your assessment of the patient who reports having nausea, vomiting, or diarrhea, remember to ask the color associated with the vomiting and/or diarrhea. Take note in your environmental assessment if there are basins or waste baskets near the patient, and look inside to see any abnormal emesis or if it appears to be blood tinged. Bright red bleeding is not normal and must be noted in your report. As discussed, bloody emesis or diarrhea is a clinically important finding and may indicate serious GI bleeding.

Prepare for episodes of vomiting while assessing your patient and also during transport; ensure standard precautions and have your suction ready. Many patients are unable to provide you any warning prior to vomiting.

▶ Bowel Obstruction

Large bowel obstructions in older people are likely to be caused by cancer, impacted stool, or sigmoid volvulus. In addition, small bowel obstruction secondary to gallstones increases substantially with age. With one or more episodes of cholecystitis (inflammation of the gallbladder), the gallbladder adheres to the small bowel and, over time, creates an opening, or fistula. The stone(s) or stones drop into the bowel and produce the obstruction. The large and small intestines are at risk for obstruction from adhesions due to previous surgery or infection or when a segment of bowel is forced into a fascial defect (hernia) in the abdominal wall.

▶ Biliary Diseases

Along with implications for small bowel obstructions, biliary diseases, including cirrhosis, hepatitis, and cholecystitis, may also present independently in older patients. Signs and symptoms of biliary disease include jaundice, fever, right upper quadrant pain with possible radiation to the upper back or shoulder, and vomiting or nausea. Jaundice may be more profound in paler patients because less melanin is present to interfere with visibility of bilirubin. Although these diseases cause fever, this response may be repressed in older patients. Pain sensation may be altered, as well, resulting in unusual referral paths or the absence of abdominal pain.

Pain management may be indicated for patients with acute cholecystitis; however, be cautious in administering opiates to older patients because their ability to compensate for cardiovascular and respiratory changes that may accompany these medications will be decreased.

▶ Peptic Ulcer Disease

Older patients are more likely than younger ones to have stomach or duodenal ulcers (peptic ulcer disease). The main risk factors for peptic ulcers are regular use of NSAIDs and infection with *Helicobacter pylori* (an ulcer-associated bacterium of the stomach), both of which are more common in older patients. Other medications have also been implicated in ulcer formation. Social factors, such as high-stress professions, and certain personality types have also been associated with ulcer formation. The main symptom of peptic ulcer disease is dyspepsia (gnawing, burning pain in the upper abdomen), which usually improves immediately after eating but returns several hours later. Other causes of dyspepsia include acid reflux, gastritis, and gastric cancer. Be aware that symptoms of chest pain due to dyspepsia and chest pain due to cardiac disease or acute MI are easily confused, especially in older patients with altered pain sensation.

Assessment and Management of Renal Emergencies

Although the kidneys of an older person may be capable of dealing with day-to-day demands, they may not be able to meet unusual challenges, such as those imposed by illness.

▶ Urinary Tract Infections

UTIs are common in the older adult population.[30] UTIs usually develop in the lower urinary tract (urethra and bladder) when normal flora (the bacteria that naturally populate the skin) enter the urethra and grow. Although UTIs are usually more common in women due to the relatively short urethra and its proximity to the vagina and rectum, an increase in UTIs is seen in men older than 50 years because of obstruction of the urethra by the prostate. Common risk factors include diabetes, prostatitis, cystocele (prolapse of the bladder into the vagina), urethrocele (prolapse of the urethra into the vagina), kidney obstruction, and indwelling urinary catheters.

While you are performing a physical assessment, you may notice a fever, shortness of breath, GI symptoms, neurologic symptoms, poor urinary output, increased urinary frequency, and hematuria. These patients will report painful urination, frequent urges to urinate, and difficulty urinating. You should evaluate the patient's indwelling catheter, if applicable, for sediment, opacity, color, or presence of blood. A strong odor may be present. Later signs and symptoms may include hypotension, tachycardia, diaphoresis, and pale skin.

▶ Renal Failure

Renal failure results from a decrease in the rate of filtration through the glomeruli, causing toxins to accumulate in the blood. If the kidneys are no longer able to excrete waste, concentrate urine, and control electrolytes, pH, or blood pressure, then renal failure develops. Risk factors for chronic renal failure include diabetes, cardiac disease, pyelonephritis, hypertension, autoimmune disorders, glomerulonephritis, and polypharmacy. Chronic renal failure may require lifelong hemodialysis or kidney transplantation. Hemodialysis is a process in which patients are attached to a hemodialysis machine for 3 to 4 hours three times per week so that the patient's blood can be filtered through the machine and waste can be removed.

Although dialysis treatments are generally considered to be basic life support nonemergency transport, if a patient misses a treatment, the situation can become an ALS emergency. Signs and symptoms of such an emergency include hypertension, headache, anxiety, fatigue, anorexia, vomiting, increased dark urination, altered mental status, and seizures. All vital signs should be monitored regularly; however, you should not obtain blood pressure readings on the same arm that has a fistula. Breath sounds should be monitored. The patient should be transported to a hospital that has hemodialysis capabilities. IV fluids should be administered to assist circulation as necessary.

Special Populations

The best dose of a drug for an older patient is the lowest dose that will achieve a therapeutic effect.

Assessment and Management of Toxicologic Emergencies

The most common therapeutic error in cases of reported poison exposure occurs when a patient inadvertently takes or is given medication twice, which is called "double dosing." Essentially, medications are poisons with beneficial side effects. Noncompliance of medication (not taking the medication in the prescribed dose) also may cause an emergency, as discussed earlier.

Another factor contributing to the toxic effects of drugs in older people is alterations in pharmacokinetics related to aging (that is, the absorption, distribution, metabolism, and excretion of drugs). Decreases in kidney function and GI absorption further increase susceptibility to toxicity. Pharmacokinetics may also be influenced by diet, smoking, alcohol consumption, and use of other drugs. Medications such as digoxin that depend on the liver and kidney for metabolism and excretion are particularly likely to accumulate to toxic levels in older patients. With most medications, we know little about the optimal dosage for older people because almost all clinical trials to establish the safe dosages of medications are performed in young populations. For the most part, dosages for older people need to be reduced compared with those for younger patients. ("Start low, go slow.")

Although almost any medication can produce toxic effects in an older person, certain medications and classes of drugs are implicated more often than others. Typically, toxic effects present with psychiatric symptoms (such as hallucinations, paranoia, delusions, agitation, and psychosis) and cognitive impairment (such as delirium, confusion, disorientation, amnesia, stupor, and coma) Figure 37-9.

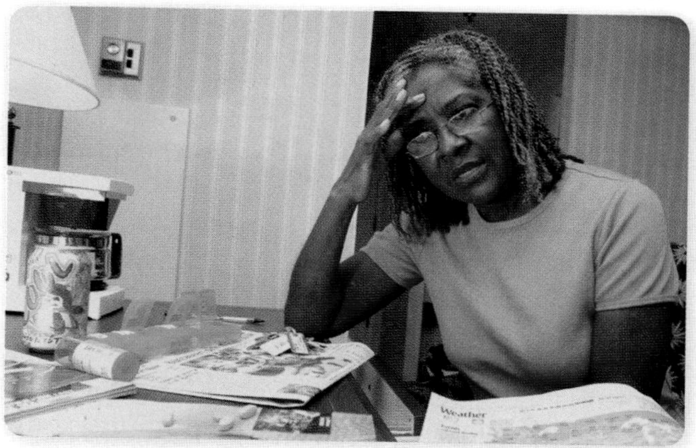

Figure 37-9 The toxic effects of drugs may initially manifest in the form of confusion.

Drug and Alcohol Abuse

Many geriatric patients see multiple physicians for various disorders that may include pain management and/or require sedation. Some states have instituted a statewide system to control and monitor scheduled medication distribution, which is then used by all pharmacies in the state. These measures help prevent the same medications being prescribed by multiple physicians. However, it does not prevent taking subsequent doses of the same medication.

Substance abuse among older adults is often in response to a life-changing event such as the loss of a spouse, declining health, or low self-esteem. The prevalence of alcohol and drug misuse among older people is also attributable to the multiplicity of medications that are prescribed for them and their heightened vulnerability to abuse owing to the effects of aging. Decreased body mass and total body water means higher concentrations of blood alcohol compared with consumption of the same amount of alcohol by younger adults; at the same time, the combination of digestive, renal, and hepatic system changes results in slower elimination of alcohol from the older adult's body.

As the geriatric population continues to grow and experiences even more chronic disabilities, the likelihood of substance abuse–related problems in this group will increase. Recognizing substance abuse in older people can be difficult. If they have engaged in this behavior for a long time, it may be well hidden from—or even accepted by—family and friends. Because substance abuse can complicate your field assessment and treatment, it is important to ask about this issue.

Geriatric Trauma Emergencies and Management

Unintentional injury is the seventh leading cause of death in people age 65 years and older in the United States.[5] Several factors place an older person at higher risk of trauma than a younger person such as slower reflexes, visual and hearing deficits, equilibrium disorders, and an overall reduction in agility. In particular, changes in the body's homeostatic compensatory mechanisms combined with the effects of aging on body systems and any preexisting conditions usually add up to less favorable outcomes in trauma situations. Compensation in trauma is successful when an increased pulse rate, increased respirations, and adequate vasoconstriction make up for trauma-related blood loss. In contrast, reduced cardiac reserve, decreased respiratory function, impaired renal activity, and ineffective vasoconstriction may result in unsuccessful recovery from traumatic situations. Furthermore, an older adult is more likely to sustain a serious injury in a trauma situation because stiffened blood vessels and fragile tissues tear more readily, and brittle, demineralized bone is more vulnerable to fracture. A decreased ability to thermoregulate and a limited tolerance of thermal extremes also make a geriatric patient more susceptible to hypothermia.[31]

Most geriatric trauma cases involve falls or motor vehicle crashes. Although most falls do not produce serious injury, they do result in increased mortality in geriatric patients—a trend that is directly related to the patient's age, preexisting disease processes, and complications related to the trauma. Falls are associated with a higher incidence of anxiety and depression, a loss of confidence, and postfall syndrome. In postfall syndrome, geriatric patients develop a lack of confidence and anxiety about potential falls.

Words of Wisdom

Compensatory mechanism changes + aging systems + preexisting conditions = bad outcomes.

Falls among older adults are divided between those resulting from extrinsic (external) causes, such as tripping on a loose rug or slipping on ice, and those resulting from intrinsic (internal) causes, such as a dizzy spell or a syncopal attack **Table 37-6**. The risk of falls increases in people with preexisting gait abnormalities (such as from neurologic or musculoskeletal impairment) and cognitive impairment. Older patients with osteoporosis have lower-density bones, so even a sudden, awkward turn may fracture a bone.

When you are treating a patient who has fallen, you need to obtain a careful history. Although the patient often attributes the fall to an accidental cause ("I must have tripped over the rug."), meticulous questioning often reveals a period of dizziness or palpitations just before the fall, suggesting a different cause.

Table 37-6 Causes of Falls in Older Adults

Cause	Clues That Suggest This Cause
Extrinsic (mechanical)	Obvious environmental hazard at the scene, such as poor lighting, scatter rugs, uneven sidewalk, or ice or another slippery surface
Intrinsic (internal causes)	Sudden fall; patient found on the ground somewhat confused, often temporarily paralyzed and unable to get up; no premonitory symptoms
Postural (orthostatic) hypotension	Fall when getting up from a recumbent or sitting position (Check medications the patient is taking, and ask about occult blood loss, such as presence of black stools. Measure blood pressure in recumbent and sitting positions.)
Dizziness or syncope	Marked bradycardia or tachydysrhythmias
Stroke	Other characteristic signs of stroke, such as hemiparesis, hemiplegia, or aphasia
Fracture	Patient reports feeling something snap before falling—this is extremely rare and often associated with preexisting bone abnormality such as a tumor or prior fracture.

Home safety assessments by EMS—during a routine visit or as part of an outreach program—may reduce fall incidence. Components of this assessment should include clear pathways to and from the bathroom, handrails in bathtubs and on steps, no loose rugs or other objects on the floor, wheelchair ramps with grip tape, and caregivers who are trained to lift and move patients.

After falls, motor vehicle crashes are the second leading cause of accidental death from injury among older adults.[32] An older patient is far more likely than a younger patient to be fatally injured in a motor vehicle crash,[33] even though excessive speed is rarely a causative factor in the older age group. Impaired vision, errors in judgment, and underlying medical conditions contribute to the higher risk. Impairments in vision and hearing, along with diminished agility, also contribute to pedestrian deaths involving older adults.

▶ Pathophysiology of Trauma

Consider the aging body's decreasing ability to isolate simple trauma when you are assessing and caring for an older patient. An isolated hip fracture in a healthy 25-year-old is rarely associated with systemic decline. However, the same injury in an 85-year-old patient can produce a systemic effect that results in deterioration, shock, and life-threatening hypoxia or multiple end-organ system failure, a dangerous condition in which the body tissues and cells do not have enough oxygen.

Although an injury may be considered isolated and not alarming in most adults, an older patient's overall physical condition may decrease the body's ability to compensate for the effects of even simple injuries. Younger patients have the capability to increase their heart rate, constrict their blood vessels, and breathe faster and deeper to compensate for injuries. The aging body has a heart that can no longer beat as fast, vessels that cannot constrict as well because of atherosclerosis, and lungs that do not exchange oxygen as well.

Older patients have reduced stroke volume along with potential dysrhythmias, decreased respiratory function, and a decrease in chest wall compliance as well as a decrease in ciliary action to remove secretions, impaired renal activity, ineffective vasoconstriction, and a reduction in neuron mass and velocity of impulses. These factors make it more difficult for an older patient to recover from a traumatic situation.

As the brain shrinks, there is a higher risk of cerebral bleeding following head trauma. Because brain tissue atrophies with age, older persons are more likely to sustain closed head injuries, such as subdural hematomas, in trauma situations. These hematomas can go unnoticed because the blood has a void to fill before it can produce pressure in the skull and, therefore, signs of head trauma. Geriatric female patients may have decreased bone mass and strength from osteoporosis, a generalized bone disease that is commonly associated with postmenopausal women; this can increase the likelihood of fractures, especially in the hip. In all older patients, the spine stiffens as a result of atrophy of intervertebral disks, and the vertebrae become brittle. Therefore, compression fractures of the spine also are more likely to occur in older patients.

Burns are a substantial risk of morbidity and mortality in older adults because of physiologic and pathophysiologic changes. Older people are more likely to experience burns because of altered mental status, inattention, and a compromised neurologic status. The risk of mortality is increased when preexisting medical conditions are present, the immune system is weakened, and fluid replacement is complicated by renal compromise. When you are assessing a burn patient, you need to monitor the patient's hydration status by assessing current vital signs, mucous membranes, and urine output, which is typically 50 to 60 mL/h or 0.5 to 1.0 mL/kg/h for adults.

There is higher mortality from penetrating trauma in older adults, especially in the case of gunshot wounds. Penetrating trauma can easily cause serious internal bleeding. An older patient's limited physiologic reserves and more subtle presentation can affect proper management and transportation options.

Internal temperature regulation is slowed in older adults and continues to slow with increasing age. The body's ability to recognize fluctuations in temperature becomes delayed owing to a slowed endocrine system. Heat gain or loss in response to environmental changes is delayed by atherosclerotic vessels, slowed circulation, and decreased sweat production in the skin. In addition, thermoregulation can be adversely affected by chronic disease, medications, and alcohol use, all of which are more frequent in older adults.

Not surprisingly, approximately one-half of all deaths from hypothermia occur in older adults, and most indoor hypothermia deaths involve geriatric patients.[34] Although living in an area with typically harsh winters is a risk factor, hypothermia can develop at temperatures above freezing when an older person is exposed to them for a prolonged period.

Providers should be aware of environmental emergencies during extreme heat and cold, particularly in lower socioeconomic areas that may not have sufficient heat or air conditioning. Managing such events may require public awareness and preplanning. You may have to keep the ambulance's patient compartment at a temperature that is higher than normal, and perhaps uncomfortable for you, to adequately maintain the geriatric patient's temperature.

Trauma in older adults can also be caused by abuse. Abuse comes in many forms and may include physical assault. Be aware of the environment and conditions that a patient lives in, and take note of soft-tissue injuries that cannot be explained by the person's lifestyle and physical condition. Patients may be reluctant to talk about it. If you have any doubt that abuse is a consideration, submit an elder abuse report. Elder abuse is discussed in more detail later in this chapter.

▶ Assessment of Geriatric Trauma

Scene Size-up

Trauma to an older person can be more debilitating than trauma to a younger person. Consider what may happen to the patient following trauma: bone fractures, recovery, and a possible nursing home stay. Was there an underlying medical

Words of Wisdom

When you respond to a motor vehicle crash, be alert to the possibility that a medical emergency may have caused the accident, especially in single-vehicle crashes with no apparent cause.

cause that led to the traumatic event? Did the patient have a syncope episode before the fall or the motor vehicle crash?

As with all scenes, ensure your own safety first. Take standard precautions. Consider the number of patients, especially in the case of a motor vehicle crash. Determine if you need additional or specialized resources.

In an older person, decreased muscle mass in the abdomen can mask abdominal trauma. Consider the mechanism of injury and maintain a high index of suspicion.

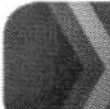

Primary Survey

During the primary survey, address life threats. Determine whether this is a priority patient and to which facility he or she will be transported. The decision that the patient has a potentially critical or life-threatening condition would limit on-scene treatment to that which is absolutely necessary for patient stabilization. Be conservative in your thinking. A geriatric patient who sustained a minor fall could have intracranial bleeding, especially if the patient drinks alcohol or is taking blood thinners. It is recommended that older trauma patients be transported to a trauma center regardless of the severity of obvious injuries.

The general impression is an important aspect of all patient assessment. As you approach the patient, you should be able to tell if he or she is generally in stable or unstable condition. You will use this information to help you with your further assessment. The GEMS diamond, discussed earlier in the chapter, is also useful in the assessment of a geriatric trauma patient. Determining neurologic status may be difficult if you do not know the patient's baseline status. Try to get information from someone familiar with the patient, if possible. Use the AVPU mnemonic and the Glasgow Coma Scale to determine mental status. An important consideration with any patient is the inability to remember the event.

If the patient is talking to you, the airway is patent. Patients who have noisy respirations have airway compromise. Older patients may have a diminished ability to cough, so suctioning is important. Suction any blood or foreign material. Dentures should be left in place as long as they fit well because they provide shape and stability for the mouth, creating a better seal when ventilating a patient with a mask. However, loose dentures may create an airway obstruction. It is more difficult to ventilate a patient with no teeth.

In an unresponsive patient, open the airway with a modified jaw-thrust maneuver. Use an oropharyngeal or nasopharyngeal airway as appropriate, and ventilate with a bag-mask device if the patient's respiratory effort is inadequate or absent. Any curvature of the patient's spine will require padding to keep the patient supine and the airway open.

Breathing problems caused by trauma can be made worse by preexisting respiratory disease and the compromised respiratory effort that comes with aging. Remember that minor chest trauma can cause lung injury. Perform a thorough respiratory assessment and physical assessment of the chest, and treat accordingly. Monitor Spo_2 and maintain a high index of suspicion in a patient with chest trauma that can cause underlying lung injury. Keep suction readily available and wrap patients warmly to prevent hypothermia.

Manage any external bleeding immediately. Be suspicious of signs and symptoms of internal bleeding. The bodies of older people do not compensate for blood loss as well as the bodies of younger people do, and older patients can more easily go into shock. A head injury with minimal mechanism can cause cerebral bleeding. Drinking alcohol and taking anticoagulant medications can worsen internal bleeding or make external bleeding more difficult to control. Also, remember that patients who were hypertensive prior to injury may have a normal blood pressure when they are actually in shock.

History Taking

When you are assessing a geriatric trauma patient, look for family members or bystanders who may be able to provide information about the patient's history. Because of alterations in mentation, an older patient may be a poor historian.

When called for a medical alert activation, find out if it is an inactivity alarm or a distress alarm. Consider who has a key to gain entry to check on the patient. Many times this may be the person who calls for assistance. Consider these factors if you have to force entry to check on the welfare of a patient. Responsibilities vary according to jurisdiction regarding who is allowed to force entry. Find out what laws and policies exist within your EMS system.

Medications taken for various medical conditions may affect coping mechanisms. Do not lower your index of suspicion when vital signs do not change as anticipated based on suspected injuries. Remember, changes in vital signs may be delayed in older patients. A lack of change may also be due to medications that the patient is taking.

Assessment of Falls. When you are assessing a patient who experienced a fall, always consider what factors may have contributed to the event **Figure 37-10**. Did the patient wake up in the middle of the night to go to the bathroom and trip? Did the patient miss a step because of visual impairment? Many older patients will be able to tell you how many steps they have in their home. Counting the stairs as they ascend or descend may help them be more aware and in control of their body mechanics. Did the patient trip over a loose item such as a rug? Patients with walking assist devices also are susceptible to falls.

Try to determine how long the patient has been on the ground. Use your keen sense of awareness to investigate the surroundings and the potential mechanism of injury, especially if the patient is unable to recall the events that may have caused the fall. If you are called early in the morning and the previous night's dinner is still on the table, the patient may have fallen 12 to 16 hours earlier. Look for other clues such as mail and newspapers building up outside. Also consider the neighbors; although they can be a valuable source of information, you must be careful to maintain the patient's privacy.

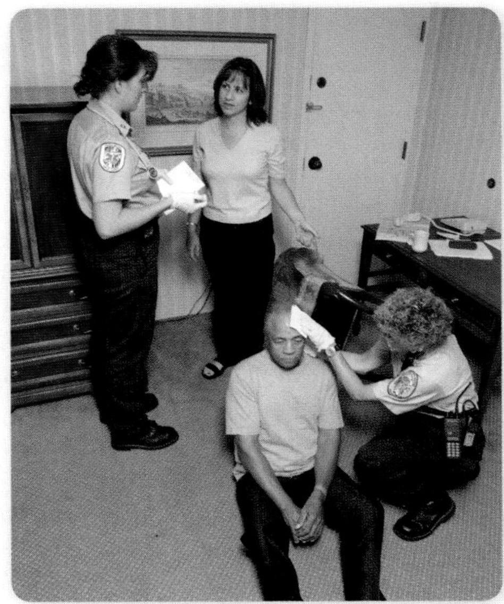

Figure 37-10 When you are assessing a patient for a fall, look for clues about what may have caused or contributed to the event.

Attempt to determine why the fall occurred. As mentioned, medical conditions such as syncope (fainting), a cardiac rhythm disturbance, or a medication interaction may lead to a fall that causes injury to the patient. Sometimes, a recent history of starting or stopping blood pressure medication is enough to cause a patient to become dizzy and fall. Look for clues from the patient, bystanders, and the environment. Although the trauma that the patient sustains from the fall can be serious, you should also consider that if a medical condition caused the fall, it could exacerbate, or be exacerbated by, the injury.

Secondary Assessment

The physical examination should be performed on a geriatric trauma patient in the same manner as for any adult but with consideration of the higher likelihood of damage from trauma. Remember that any head injury can be life threatening in an older adult. When you are examining the chest, consider that breathing may be impaired as part of the normal aging process. Check breath sounds, and look to see if there is any evidence of pacemakers or previous cardiac surgery. Even though it may appear that the patient has only experienced trauma, keep in mind that this does not mean he or she may not also be having medical problems. When you are assessing the abdomen, remember that older patients have a flaccid abdominal wall and may not present with pain and rigidity in the abdomen when trauma has been sustained. Decreased muscle size in the abdomen may mask abdominal trauma. Look for bruising and other evidence of trauma. Injury to the liver or spleen may present with diffuse abdominal pain, or pain may refer to the left shoulder.

Assess the pulse, blood pressure, and skin signs. Capillary refill is unreliable in older people because of compromised circulation. Remember that some older people take beta blockers, which will inhibit their heart from becoming tachycardic as you would expect in shock. Even a heart rate in normal ranges may be high for someone taking beta blockers. Try to determine if the patient's blood pressure is normal for him or her. Remember that an older patient may have what appears to be a normal blood pressure but may still be in shock.

Reassessment

Reassessment of the primary survey, level of consciousness, vital signs, and interventions should be performed and documented as with any patient, but remember that a geriatric patient has a higher likelihood of decompensating after trauma. Be prepared.

▶ Management of Geriatric Trauma

Broken bones are common and should be splinted in a manner appropriate to the injury. Because of the amount of flexion that occurs in the spinal column, hips, and knees of older patients, effective application of conventional splints and backboards to immobilize them may be difficult or impossible unless a large amount of padding is used. What is considered a normal anatomic position for children and adults is often abnormal for geriatric trauma patients. Do not try to force a patient with pronounced joint flexion or kyphosis into a normal anatomic position; this can be very painful and may cause further harm. Some devices, such as traction splints, simply do not work on patients with flexed hips and knees and should never be used to treat hip fractures. Splinting devices such as vacuum mattresses that conform to body contours may be a good choice for immobilization in these cases **Figure 37-11**. In hip and pelvic fractures, avoid log rolling the patient because you risk causing more damage and increased pain. When immobilization is indicated, patients with kyphosis will require padding. In general, padding should be done for comfort and to help decrease the likelihood of decubitus ulcer formation.

Additional treatment will depend on the patient's specific injuries, although there are a few general principles to keep in mind:

- Use caution inserting IV catheters and administering isotonic solutions. It is easy to overload an older person with sodium, and you must balance that risk with the need to maintain adequate perfusion pressure. Use small boluses, and reassess the patient frequently, especially for signs of pulmonary edema.
- Take steps to preserve temperature in geriatric trauma patients. Regulation of temperature is slowed in older adults, and the blood in cold patients does not clot as well.

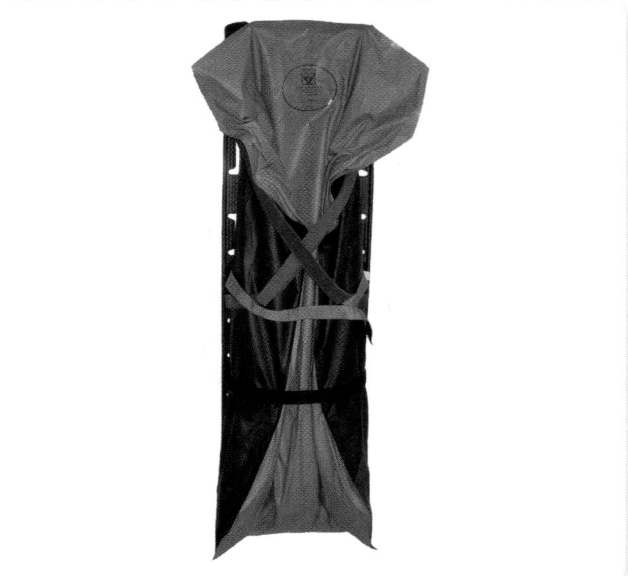

Figure 37-11 Vacuum mattresses that conform to body contours are a good choice for immobilizing older patients.

- Frail geriatric patients may not do well with a traction splint for a femoral fracture. If possible, place the patient on a well-padded backboard and buttress him or her well with pillows secured firmly in place.
- Immobilize the cervical spine before transporting the patient. If a backboard is used, pad it generously, because the skin of an older person may be damaged by the direct trauma of the pressure and the decrease in blood flow. Target areas where the bone is near the surface, from top to bottom: occiput, scapula, spinous processes, elbows, sacrum, and heels. A pressure ulcer can develop in as little as 45 minutes and can have devastating consequences.

Special Populations

Remember that older adults do not have the mechanisms that help keep them warm. Provide blankets and heat to prevent hypothermia.

Communication with older adults can be challenging in any situation, but it can become even more complicated when the patient is in pain, or is experiencing fear from trauma. Older people also tend to fear that a trauma may end their mobility and independence. Remember to provide psychological support, as well as medical treatment. Document assessment, treatment, and reassessment, including any changes in the patient's status.

Elder Abuse and Neglect

Reports of abuse, neglect, and other related problems among the nation's geriatric population are on the rise. **Elder abuse** is defined as any action or inaction on the part of an older person's family member, caregiver, or other associated person who takes advantage of the older person's person (for example, physical abuse), property, or emotional state **Table 37-7**. **Neglect** is the failure to provide needed care, services, or supervision.

The prevalence of elder abuse is not fully known for several reasons, including the following:

- Elder abuse is a problem that has been largely hidden from society.
- The definitions of abuse and neglect among older people vary.
- Victims of elder abuse are often hesitant to report the problem to law enforcement agencies or human and social welfare personnel.
- Elder abuse is most commonly seen as financial abuse, which may not be as visibly obvious.[35]

An older adult who is being abused by his or her relative or caregiver may feel ashamed or guilty. The abused person may feel shame, anger, or guilt (or all three). If the abuser is a family member, the abused person may fear retribution or anger from other family members for reporting the abuse to an outside agency. If the abuser is not a family member, the abused older person may be afraid to report the abuse for fear of no longer receiving care.

The physical and emotional signs of abuse, such as rape, spouse beating, or nutritional deprivation, are often overlooked or inaccurately identified. Older women are particularly unlikely to report incidents of sexual assault to

Table 37-7 Categories of Elder Abuse

Category	Examples
Physical	▪ Assault ▪ Neglect or abandonment ▪ Dietary (malnutrition) ▪ Poor maintenance of home ▪ Poor personal hygiene ▪ Sexual assault
Psychological	▪ Benign neglect ▪ Verbal ▪ Treating the person in a demeaning way ▪ Deprivation of sensory stimulation
Financial	▪ Theft of valuables ▪ Embezzlement

law enforcement agencies. Patients with sensory deficits, senility, and other forms of altered mental status, such as drug-induced depression, may not be able to report abuse.

The abused person is often frail with multiple chronic medical conditions, has dementia, and may have an impaired sleep cycle, sleepwalking, and periodically shout at others. The person may be incontinent and is generally dependent on others for ADLs.

Abusers of older people are sometimes products of child abuse, and the abuse that is inflicted on the person may be retaliatory. Most abusers are not trained in the particular care that the older person requires and have little relief time from the constant care demands of their own family. The stress associated with this situation may contribute to abusive behavior.

The abuser may also have marked fatigue, be unemployed and/or have financial difficulties, or be a substance abuser. With a careful eye, you can recognize the clues to these stressful situations and help guide the family toward programs in the community that are geared to helping the whole family. Programs such as adult day care, meals on wheels, or many local individualized programs help to decrease the stress put on the family, thus decreasing the chance of abuse.

Abuse is not restricted to the home; environments such as nursing homes, convalescent homes, and continuing care centers (assisted-living facilities) are also sites where older people sustain physical, psychological, financial, or pharmacologic abuse. Often, care providers in these environments consider older people to be management problems or categorize them as obstinate and undesirable patients.

▶ Signs of Physical Abuse

Signs of abuse may be obvious or subtle. Inflicted bruises are usually found on the buttocks and lower back, genitals and inner thighs, cheeks or earlobes, neck, upper lip, and inside the mouth. Pressure bruises caused by the human hand may be identified by oval grab marks, pinch marks, or handprints. Human bites are typically inflicted on the upper extremities and can cause lacerations and infection. You should inspect the patient's ears for indications of twisting, pulling, or pinching or evidence of frequent trauma to the external ears. You should also investigate multiple bruises in various states of healing by questioning the patient and reviewing the patient's ADLs.

Burns are a common form of abuse. If you see burns, especially cigarette burns or physical marks that indicate that certain parts of the patient's body have been scalded systematically, you must suspect abuse. Typical abuse from burns are caused by contact with cigarettes, matches, heated metal, forced immersion in hot liquids, chemicals, and electrical power sources.

It may be difficult to see a failure to thrive in an older patient who has been abused. You should observe the patient's weight and try to determine whether the patient appears undernourished or has been unable to gain weight in the current environment. Does the patient have a ravenous appetite? Has medication been withheld? Is money being withheld so the patient cannot buy food or medicine? You should also check for signs of neglect, such as evidence of a lack of hygiene, poor dental hygiene, poor temperature regulation, or lack of reasonable amenities in the home.

You must regard injuries to the genitals or rectum with no reported trauma as evidence of sexual abuse in any patient. Geriatric patients with an altered mental status may never be able to report sexual abuse. In addition, many women do not report cases of sexual abuse because of fear, shame, and a desire to forget the incident.

▶ Assessment and Management of Elder Abuse

While you are assessing the patient, try to obtain an explanation of what happened. You should suspect abuse when answers to questions about what caused the injury are concealed or avoided.

You must also suspect abuse when you are given unbelievable answers. Be suspicious if you think, "Does this make sense?" or "Do I really believe this story?" while reviewing the patient's history. As an AEMT, you may be the first health care provider to observe the signs of possible abuse. Information that may be important in assessing possible abuse includes the following:

- Caregiver apathy about the patient's condition
- Overly defensive reaction by caregiver to your questions
- Caregiver does not allow patient to answer questions
- Repeated visits to the ED or clinic
- A history of being accident prone
- Soft-tissue injuries
- Unbelievable, vague, or inconsistent explanations of injuries
- Psychosomatic issues
- Chronic pain without medical explanation
- Self-destructive behavior
- Eating and sleep disorders
- Depression or a lack of energy
- A history of substance and/or sexual abuse

In addition to the lifesaving care that you can provide the patient, your examination of the patient can help to reduce further trauma from abuse through its very identification. Repeated abuse can lead to a high risk of death.

If the patient is in stable condition but the situation is unsafe, see if the patient will accept transportation to the hospital. If the patient refuses transport, see if he or she will accept help from the local **adult protective services (APS)**. In some cases, patients may be hesitant to go with EMS personnel because of fear of caregiver retaliation. If the situation is immediately unsafe, notify law enforcement personnel and remain with the patient only if the scene remains safe to do so.

Consult local authorities, but in general, you should assume that you have the same obligation to report suspected elder abuse as you do suspected child abuse. Notify receiving hospital personnel of your concerns, report to the proper authorities based on local protocols, and factually document your findings. If you are in doubt, err on the side of caution and make a report. Note that it is not your responsibility to prove that the abuse occurred, only to report your findings according to protocols.

YOU are the Provider SUMMARY

1. What are some possible causes of confusion in geriatric patients?

Causes of confusion in geriatric patients include the common causes in patients of younger age, as well as delirium, dementia, and Alzheimer disease. Dementia develops slowly over a period of years rather than a few days. Alzheimer disease begins gradually with difficulty performing routine tasks and/or forgetting recent events. As it advances, personality changes, impaired judgment, and impaired ability to communicate thoughts or ideas become more prominent. Based on the information provided by the daughter, this patient is most likely experiencing a form of dementia.

2. Does this patient present with any risk factors that could affect his mortality?

Yes. Of the risk factors that affect mortality in older patients, this patient has the following: age older than 75 years, living alone, recent death of a spouse, and altered mental status. In older people who live alone, potential is increased for incorrect medication doses, which could result in inadvertent underdosing or overdosing.

3. Does this patient require immediate transport?

This patient requires immediate transport to the closest appropriate facility, because he is presenting with signs and symptoms consistent with hypovolemic shock. This patient is confused, is slow to respond, has thready radial pulses, and his skin is cool, pale, and clammy. He warrants aggressive treatment for shock.

4. On the basis of the patient's presentation, what do you suspect is happening?

On the basis of clinical interpretation, the patient is experiencing GI bleeding that requires immediate treatment and transport. The patient stated he has been vomiting "foul" smelling emesis; it can further be assumed that he is experiencing upper GI tract bleeding.

5. Does this patient require a second IV line?

This patient would potentially benefit from a second IV line because of profound hypotension and signs and symptoms of shock. A second IV access is valuable for fluid administration and to have a secondary access point should the first IV line become infiltrated or dislodged. Never delay transport to obtain a second IV line, however. It is more important to get the patient to definitive care rapidly.

6. What is the significance of the medications that the patient is taking?

This patient is taking Coumadin, Tenormin, and Glucophage. Coumadin is a blood thinner, which in the presence of GI bleeding can exacerbate the condition, resulting in increased bleeding and delayed clotting times. Tenormin is a beta blocker that slows down the heart rate. The fact that this patient is taking Tenormin needs to be considered when interpreting the patient's heart rate. Normally, you would expect a patient in shock to present with tachycardia. In this case, however, Tenormin would cause the patient's heart rate to be lower; even in shock, the patient could have a normal blood pressure or even be bradycardic. Glucophage is an antidiabetic medication that should indicate that the patient has a history of diabetes. Because this patient was confused and taking Glucophage, it was wise to check his blood glucose level. Even though the shock explains the confusion, he could also be hypoglycemic based on his vomiting. With a careful evaluation of the patient's medications, you will be able to gain insight into the patient's present condition.

7. What are the potential hazards of the patient vomiting?

The biggest potential hazard of vomiting is aspiration. Treatment for this patient should include proper positioning and rapid transport.

8. Why should lactated Ringer solution be avoided in this patient?

Because of changes in the renal system of geriatric patients, they are susceptible to hyperkalemia. Although administering lactated Ringer solution to a younger patient may not appreciably increase potassium levels, the same amount of fluid may increase a geriatric patient's already elevated potassium level to become lethal.

YOU are the Provider SUMMARY *(continued)*

EMS Patient Care Report (PCR)

Date: 10-5-18	**Incident No.:** 20108256440	**Nature of Call:** Unknown medical	**Location:** 414 Hilltop Drive		
Dispatched: 0842	**En Route:** 0843	**At Scene:** 0850	**Transport:** 0902	**At Hospital:** 0914	**In Service:** 0933

Patient Information

Age: 82 **Sex:** M **Weight (in kg [lb]):** 114 kg (250 lb)	**Allergies:** Tetracaine **Medications:** Tenormin, Coumadin, Glucophage, aspirin **Past Medical History:** Atrial fibrillation, type 2 diabetes **Chief Complaint:** GI bleeding

Vital Signs

Time: 0856	**BP:** 72/36	**Pulse:** 52	**Respirations:** 26	**Spo_2:** 96% on room air
Time: 0902	**BP:** 74/40	**Pulse:** 58	**Respirations:** 26	**Spo_2:** 98% on 15 L/min
Time: 0910	**BP:** 78/42	**Pulse:** 68	**Respirations:** 26	**Spo_2:** 100% on 15 L/min

EMS Treatment (circle all that apply)

Oxygen @ 15 **L/min via (circle one):** **NC** (**NRM** — circled) **Bag-mask device**	**Assisted Ventilation**	**Airway Adjunct**	**CPR**
Defibrillation / **Bleeding Control**	**Bandaging**	**Splinting**	**Other:**

Narrative

EMS dispatched to unknown medical problem. On arrival, find daughter who states her father "isn't acting normal." Patient is alert, slightly confused, and slow to answer questions. Patient states that he has been vomiting "foul" smelling emesis × 4 days and is weak and dizzy. Patient is cold to touch, 4-second capillary refill, and a thready, slow radial pulse. Checked pt's blood glucose level, which was normal (116 mg/dL). While assisting patient to a standing position to use the bathroom prior to transport, he becomes pale and radial pulse is absent when in standing position. Patient assisted back to supine position. 18-gauge IV line established to left AC with two normal saline boluses infusing. Initial vital signs as above. Patient placed on stretcher and secured in ambulance. Emergent transport initiated to Oschner Hospital. En route—second 250-mL bolus infusing due to persistent hypotension. Approximately 6 minutes from Oschner ED, patient vomits approximately 200 mL of coffee-ground-looking emesis. Suctioned airway and repositioned patient to left lateral position. On arrival at Oschner, care and report left with ED RN without incident.**End of report**

Prep Kit

▶ Ready for Review

- Treatment of older patients can present you with many challenges that are not encountered with younger patients that may be difficult.
- It is important to understand social and economic factors that can affect geriatric patients including the economic impact of aging and independent and dependent living.
- Advanced emergency medical technicians (AEMTs) should be aware of advance directives such as do not resuscitate orders, as well as end-of-life care and considerations.
- Good communication techniques are important when working with older patients. Position yourself at the patient's level, look the patient in the eye, and remember to ask open-ended questions.
- The aging process is accompanied by changes in physiologic function. The decrease in the functional capacity of various organ systems can affect the way in which the patient responds to illness.
- A person's respiratory capacity undergoes substantial reductions with age because of decreases in the elasticity of the lungs and in the size and strength of the respiratory muscles, stiffening in the chest wall, and musculoskeletal changes.
- Within the cardiovascular system, changes include hypertrophy (enlargement) of the heart, arteriosclerosis (the stiffening of vessel walls), and deterioration of the electric conduction system of the heart.
- Changes in the nervous system result in a decrease in sensory function, as evidenced by visual changes (glaucoma and cataracts are common) and hearing loss.
- Changes in the endocrine system may result in diabetes and thyroid abnormalities in older patients.
- The gastrointestinal (GI) system changes as appetite decreases, digestion becomes more difficult as a result of a reduction in saliva, and dental loss contributes to digestive problems. Slow movement through the digestive system and use of narcotic pain medications may result in constipation.
- Geriatric patients may experience renal system changes. Although the kidneys of an older adult may be capable of dealing with day-to-day demands, they may not be able to meet unusual challenges, such as those imposed by illness. Therefore, acute illness in older adults is often accompanied by derangements in fluid and electrolyte balance.
- Aging is associated with a widespread decrease in bone mass in men and women, but especially among postmenopausal women. Bones become more brittle and tend to break more easily.
- Within the integumentary system, the skin wrinkles and thins, elastin and collagen decrease, and the sebaceous glands produce less oil, making the skin drier. In addition, the skin does not replace itself as quickly. This combination places older adults at higher risk for skin injury and complications.
- The ability of a geriatric person to regulate temperature is decreased, resulting in increased cases of heat and cold illness.
- The health problems of older people are quantitatively and qualitatively different from those of younger people. The special problems of older people require special approaches.
- Heart disease is the leading cause of death among older adults in the United States, along with cancer, stroke, chronic obstructive pulmonary disease, pneumonia, diabetes, and trauma.
- Abdominal problems are common in older patients and extremely difficult to assess. Abdominal aortic aneurysm and GI bleeding are serious emergencies and require rapid transport.
- In older adults, delirium often replaces or confounds the typical presentation caused by a medical problem, an adverse medication effect, or drug withdrawal.
- Unlike delirium, dementia is a disease that produces irreversible brain failure. Alzheimer disease is a neurologic cause of dementia.
- Older patients with diabetes whose blood glucose levels tend to be high are susceptible to hyperosmolar hyperglycemic nonketotic (HHNK) coma. The most frequent cause for HHNK is infection. Presentation is likely to be acute confusion with dehydration.
- The GEMS diamond is a valuable assessment tool to help providers recall key considerations for geriatric patients.
- Although assessment of the older patient involves the same basic approach as with any other patient, you may have to take a slower approach to the older patient. To perform an adequate assessment will require patience, but it is time well spent.
- The injury or medical condition may be worse than indicated by the existing signs and symptoms, and the injuries and conditions that are found will

Prep Kit *(continued)*

have a more profound effect than they would in a younger patient.

- In addition to the critical needs that an underlying medical problem may cause, the older patient's condition is more unstable than a younger patient's and has an increased possibility for sudden, rapid deterioration.
- When a patient's chief complaint seems trivial, it may be necessary to go through a review of systems to confirm that you are not missing important pieces of information. Follow up with further questions when you determine more information is necessary.
- You must obtain an accurate history of the patient, be compassionate, and communicate your findings effectively. Be an advocate for your patients.
- The secondary assessment of older patients can be difficult. Poor cooperation and easy fatigability may require that you keep manipulations of the patient to a minimum. You may have to remove many layers of clothing from an older adult patient to perform an adequate exam.
- The AEMT must try to obtain an accurate list of medications and dosages, because many geriatric patients take multiple medications and are particularly susceptible to adverse drug reactions.
- Several factors place an older person at higher risk of trauma than a younger person: slower reflexes, visual and hearing deficits, equilibrium disorders, and an overall reduction in agility.
- Most geriatric trauma cases involve falls or motor vehicle crashes. Falls are evenly divided between those resulting from extrinsic (external) causes, such as tripping on a loose rug or slipping on ice, and those resulting from intrinsic (internal) causes, such as a dizzy spell or a syncopal attack.
- The prevalence of elder abuse is not fully known because many patients do not report it. Abusers are often family members who must care for the older person in addition to caring for their own spouses and children.
- Elder abuse also occurs in nursing, convalescent, and continuing care centers. Elder abuse can be gruesome, vulgar, and barbaric; however, your responsibility is to provide potentially lifesaving care to the patient and try to reduce additional abuse through identification of the problem.
- The duty that we owe to our older population should be no less than we would expect in our own golden years.

▶ Vital Vocabulary

abdominal aortic aneurysm (AAA) A condition in which the walls of the aorta in the abdomen weaken and blood leaks into the layers of the vessel, causing it to bulge.

activities of daily living (ADLs) Activities of daily living include cooking and caring for oneself, bathing, housework, and personal hygiene as well as toilet activities.

adult protective services (APS) An organization that investigates cases involving abuse and neglect and provides case management services in some cases.

aneurysm A weakening in the wall of a blood vessel, usually an artery.

arteriosclerosis A disease that is characterized by hardening, thickening, and calcification of the arterial walls.

atherosclerosis The most common form of arteriosclerosis in which fatty material is deposited and accumulates in the innermost layer of medium- and large-size arteries.

cataract Clouding of the lens of the eye or its surrounding transparent membrane.

decubitus ulcers Ulcers that occur when pressure is applied to body tissue, resulting in a lack of perfusion and ultimately necrosis.

delirium An acute change in mental status marked by the inability to focus, think logically, and maintain attention.

dementia The slow onset of progressive disorientation, shortened attention span, and loss of cognitive function.

dependent living A type of care in which a person receives assistance based on his or her needs or restrictions; can range from the least restrictive retirement community to the structured skilled nursing facility and dementia/Alzheimer disease specialty care facilities. Sometimes known as residential.

elder abuse Any action or inaction on the part of a family member, caregiver, or other associated person

Prep Kit *(continued)*

that takes advantage of the older adult's person, property, or emotional state; also called parent battering.

geriatrics The assessment and treatment of disease in someone 65 years or older.

glaucoma A disease of the eye caused by an increase in intraocular pressure; when severe enough, this may damage the optic nerve and potentially cause permanent loss of vision.

hematemesis Vomited blood, which may be bright red or dark, or if the blood has been partially digested, may look like coffee grounds.

homeostasis A tendency to constancy or stability in the body's internal environment.

hospice An organization that provides end-of-life care to patients with terminal illnesses and their families.

hyperosmolar hyperglycemic syndrome (HHS) A metabolic derangement that occurs principally in patients with type 2 diabetes; it is characterized by hyperglycemia, hyperosmolarity, and an absence of significant ketosis. Also called hyperosmolar nonketotic coma (HONK).

kyphosis A condition in which the back becomes hunched over due to an abnormal curvature of the spine.

macular degeneration Deterioration of the central portion of the retina.

melena Black, tarry stools caused by digested blood that has traveled through the digestive tract.

methicillin-resistant *Staphylococcus aureus* (MRSA) A bacterium that causes infections in different parts of the body and is often resistant to commonly used antibiotics; can be found on the skin, in surgical wounds, and in the bloodstream, lungs, and urinary tract.

neglect The failure to provide needed care, services, or supervision.

neuropathy A group of conditions in which the nerves leaving the spinal cord are damaged, resulting in distortion of signals to or from the brain.

osteoporosis A generalized bone disease, commonly associated with postmenopausal women, in which there is a reduction in the amount of bone mass resulting in increased susceptibility to fractures after minimal trauma in either sex.

polypharmacy Simultaneous use of many medications.

presbycusis An age-related condition of the ear that produces progressive bilateral hearing loss that is most noted at higher frequencies.

proprioception The ability to perceive the position and movement of one's body or limbs.

pulmonary embolism A condition that causes a sudden blockage of the pulmonary artery by a venous clot.

respiratory syncytial virus A highly contagious virus that causes an infection of the upper and lower respiratory system.

sacral edema Swelling that presents around the sacral region of the spinal column.

syncope Fainting, often caused by an interruption of blood flow to the brain.

vasodilation Widening of a blood vessel.

vasoconstriction Narrowing of a blood vessel.

▶ References

1. Population 65 years and over in the United States: 2011-2015. American community survey 5-year estimates. American Fact Finder, United States Census Bureau website. https://factfinder.census.gov/faces/tableservices/jsf/pages/productview.xhtml?pid=ACS_15_5YR_S0103&prodType=table. Accessed April 7, 2017.
2. Income of the Population 55 or Older, 2014. Social Security Administration. SSA Publication No. 13-11871. April 2016. https://www.ssa.gov/policy/docs/statcomps/income_pop55/. Accessed September 22, 2017.
3. Wu, KB. Fact Sheet: Sources of Income for Older Americans, 2012. AARP Public Policy Institute. Washington, DC. Fact Sheet 296, December, 2013.
4. Leatherby L. Medical spending among the U.S. elderly. https://journalistsresource.org/studies/government/health-care/elderly-medical-spending-medicare. Updated February 22, 2016. Accessed September 22, 2017.
5. 10 Leading Causes of Death by Age Group, United States – 2015. Centers for Disease Control and Prevention. https://www.cdc.gov/injury/wisqars/LeadingCauses.html. Accessed September 22, 2017.
6. Upadhyaya RC. Cardiovascular function. In: Meiner SE, ed. *Gerontologic Nursing*. 5th ed. Maryland Heights, MO: Mosby; 2015:388-421.
7. Aortic Aneurysm Fact Sheet. Centers for Disease Control and Prevention website. https://www.cdc.gov/dhdsp/data_statistics/fact_sheets/fs_aortic_aneurysm.htm. Updated June 16, 2016. Accessed September 22, 2017.
8. Balter M. The incredible shrinking human brain. Science website. http://www.sciencemag.org/news/2011/07/incredible-shrinking-human-brain. Published July 25, 2011. Accessed April 25, 2017.

Prep Kit *(continued)*

9. Quick Statistics About Hearing. National Institutes on Deafness and Other Communication Disorders website. https://www.nidcd.nih.gov/health/statistics/quick-statistics-hearing. Accessed October 9, 2017.
10. Aging Changes in the Senses. MedLinePlus website. https://medlineplus.gov/ency/article/004013.htm. Updated October 3, 2017. Accessed October 9, 2017.
11. 2017 Alzheimer's Disease Facts and Figures. Alzheimer's Association website. http://www.alz.org/facts/#prevalence. Accessed October 9, 2017.
12. What is Parkinson's Disease? Parkinson's Disease Foundation website. http://www.pdf.org/about_pd. Accessed October 9, 2017.
13. Conwell Y, Van Orden K, Caine ED. Suicide in older adults. *Psychiatr Clin North Am*. 2012;34(2):451-468.
14. Sollitto M. Does Moving Into a Nursing Home Cause Depression? AgingCare.com. https://www.agingcare.com/articles/nursing-home-depression-147347.htm. Accessed October 9, 2017.
15. Geriatric Depression (Depression in Older Adults). Healthline website. https://www.healthline.com/health/depression/elderly#Causes2. Accessed October 9, 2017.
16. Diabetic hyperglycemic hyperosmolar syndrome. U.S. National Library of Medicine Medline website. https://medlineplus.gov/ency/article/000304.htm. Updated April 4, 2017. Accessed May 1, 2017.
17. Crandall J, Shamoon H. Diabetes mellitus. In: Goldman L, Schafer AI, eds. *Goldman-Cecil Medicine*. 25th ed. Philadelphia, PA: Saunders; 2016:1527-1548.
18. Cydulka RK, Maloney GE. Diabetes mellitus and disorders of glucose homeostasis. In: Marx JA, Hockberger RS, Walls RM, eds. *Rosen's Emergency Medicine*. 8th ed. Philadelphia, PA: Saunders; 2014:1652-1666.
19. Whitlatch HB. Hyperosmolar hyperglycemic syndrome. In: Ferri FF, ed. *Ferri's Clinical Advisor 2017*. Philadelphia, PA: Elsevier; 2017:632-633.
20. Pasquel FJ, Umpierrez GE. Hyperosmolar hyperglycemic state: a historic review of the clinical presentation, diagnosis, and treatment. *Diabetes Care*. 2014;37(11):3124–3131.
21. Fact Sheet: Prescription Medications Use by Older Adults. Medscape website. http://www.medscape.com/viewarticle/501879. Accessed October 9, 2017.
22. Gregoratos G. Clinical manifestations of acute myocardial infarction in older patients. *Am J Geriatr Cardiol*. 2001;10(6):345-347.
23. Who Is at Risk for Heart Failure? National Heart, Lung, and Blood Institute website. https://www.nhlbi.nih.gov/health/health-topics/topics/hf/atrisk. Updated June 22, 2015. Accessed May 3, 2017.
24. Mattison M. Hospital management of older adults. UpToDate website. https://www.uptodate.com/contents/hospital-management-of-older-adults. Updated October 4, 2017. Accessed October 9, 2017.
25. Vigen R, Maddox TM, Allen LA. Aging of the United States population: impact on heart failure. *Curr Heart Fail Rep*. 2012;9(4):369-374.
26. National Center for Chronic Disease Prevention and Health Promotion, Division for Heart Disease and Stroke Prevention. High blood pressure facts. Centers for Disease Control and Prevention website. https://www.cdc.gov/bloodpressure/facts.htm. Updated November 30, 2016. Accessed March 2, 2017.
27. Who Is at Risk for a Stroke? National Heart, Lung, and Blood Institute website. https://www.nhlbi.nih.gov/health/health-topics/topics/stroke/atrisk. Accessed October 9, 2017.
28. Gupta S. Type 2 diabetes and the elderly. Everyday Health website. http://www.everydayhealth.com/sanjay-gupta/type-2-diabetes-and-the-elderly/. Updated October 10, 2013. Accessed March 2, 2017.
29. Wall CR. Myxedema coma: diagnosis and treatment. *Am Fam Physician*. 2000;62(11):2485-2490.
30. Rowe TA, Mehta MJ. Urinary tract infection in older adults. *Aging Health*. 2013;9(5). https://www.ncbi.nlm.nih.gov/pmc/articles/PMC3878051/. Accessed April 2, 2017.
31. Blatteis CM. Age-dependent changes in temperature regulation – a mini review. *Gerontology*. 212;58(4):289-295.
32. 10 Leading Causes of Injury Deaths by Age Group Highlighting Unintentional Injury Deaths, United States – 2015. Centers for Disease Control and Prevention. https://www.cdc.gov/injury/wisqars/LeadingCauses.html. Accessed September 27, 2017.
33. Yee WY, Cameron PA, Bailey MJ. Road traffic injuries in the elderly. *Emerg Med J*. 2006;23(1):42-46.
34. Hypothermia. University of Maryland Medical Center website. http://umm.edu/health/medical/altmed/condition/hypothermia. Reviewed May 26, 2014. Accessed April 3, 2017.
35. Elder Abuse Facts. National Council on Aging website. https://www.ncoa.org/public-policy-action/elder-justice/elder-abuse-facts/. Accessed October 9, 2017.

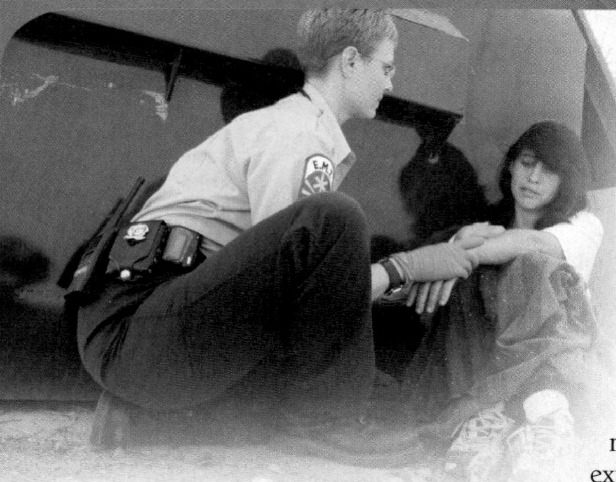

Assessment *in Action*

You are dispatched to an elderly woman who has fallen at a local church. On arrival, you find a 92-year-old woman who is alert and oriented and complaining of pain in her left hip. She states she was exiting the church when she tripped on the door's threshold. On physical exam, you note obvious shortening of the left leg, accompanied by external rotation. The patient's vital signs are as follows: blood pressure, 178/94 mm Hg; pulse, 104 beats/min, regular; respirations, 16 breaths/min with crackles in the lower bases bilaterally. Left pedal pulse is present, and capillary refill time is normal. She has a history of hypertension, heart failure, asthma, and diabetes, and her medications include metoprolol, furosemide, albuterol, and insulin.

1. Of the medications the patient is taking, which one might interfere with her body's attempt to compensate for blood loss from her injury?

A. Metoprolol
B. Furosemide
C. Albuterol
D. Insulin

2. Which of the following factors does NOT place an older person at higher risk of trauma than a younger person?

A. Slower reflexes
B. Equilibrium disorders
C. Visual deficits
D. Hypertension

3. Which of the following disease processes likely contributed to this patient's fracture?

A. Organic brain syndrome
B. Osteoarthritis
C. Osteoporosis
D. Peripheral neuropathy

4. This patient's fall can be attributed to which type of cause?

A. Intrinsic
B. Extrinsic
C. Stroke
D. Pathologic

5. Proper immobilization of this patient entails which type of immobilization?

A. Traction splint, vacuum mattress, and extra padding
B. Vacuum mattress and traction splint
C. Traction splint and extra padding
D. Vacuum mattress and extra padding

6. It would benefit the patient to have a(n) __________ to ensure that her wishes are followed regarding the type of treatment she receives.

A. power of attorney
B. advance directive
C. DNR order
D. DNAR order

Assessment in Action (continued)

7. Less responsive nerve stimulation may __________ the rate and strength of the heart's contractions.

- **A.** increase
- **B.** decrease
- **C.** initially increase, followed by a decrease
- **D.** initially decrease, followed by an increase

8. What term indicates the simultaneous use of many medications?

- **A.** Inattentiveness
- **B.** Drug seeking
- **C.** Overdosing
- **D.** Polypharmacy

9. List 7 signs of dehydration in an older patient.

10. What is the difference between *dementia* and *delirium*?

CHAPTER 38

Patients With Special Challenges

National EMS Education Standard Competencies

Special Patient Populations

Applies a fundamental knowledge of growth, development, aging, and assessment findings to provide basic and selected advanced emergency care and transportation for a patient with special needs.

Patients With Special Challenges

Recognizing and reporting abuse and neglect (Chapter 36, *Pediatric Emergencies*, and Chapter 37, *Geriatric Emergencies*)

Healthcare implications of

- Abuse (Chapter 36, *Pediatric Emergencies*, and Chapter 37, *Geriatric Emergencies*)
- Neglect (Chapter 36, *Pediatric Emergencies*, and Chapter 37, *Geriatric Emergencies*)
- Homelessness (p 1607)
- Poverty (p 1607)
- Bariatrics (pp 1597-1598)
- Technology dependent (pp 1598-1605)
- Hospice/terminally ill (p 1606)
- Tracheostomy care/dysfunction (pp 1598-1600)
- Home care (p 1606)
- Sensory deficit/loss (pp 1590-1592)
- Developmental disability (pp 1587-1590)

Trauma

Applies fundamental knowledge to provide basic and selected advanced emergency care and transportation based on assessment findings for an acutely injured patient.

Special Considerations in Trauma

Recognition and management of trauma in

- Pregnant patient (Chapter 35, *Obstetrics and Neonatal Care*)
- Pediatric patient (Chapter 36, *Pediatric Emergencies*)
- Geriatric patient (Chapter 37, *Geriatric Emergencies*)

Pathophysiology, assessment, and management of trauma in the

- Pregnant patient (Chapter 35, *Obstetrics and Neonatal Care*)
- Pediatric patient (Chapter 36, *Pediatric Emergencies*)
- Geriatric patient (Chapter 37, *Geriatric Emergencies*)
- Cognitively impaired patient (p 1605)

Knowledge Objectives

1. List examples of patients with special needs whom advanced emergency medical technicians (AEMTs) may encounter during an emergency. (p 1587)
2. Describe how to interact with patients with special needs, based on the nature of their impairment. (pp 1588, 1590-1593, 1598, 1602, 1605-1606)
3. Discuss the special patient care considerations that may be required when providing emergency medical care to patients with developmental disabilities, including patients with autism spectrum disorder, Down syndrome, and prior brain injuries. (pp 1588-1590)
4. Describe different types of visual impairments and the special patient care considerations that may be required when providing emergency medical care for these patients depending on the level of their disability. (pp 1590-1591)
5. Describe different types of hearing impairments and the special patient care considerations that may be required when providing emergency medical care for these patients, including tips for effective communication. (pp 1591-1592)
6. Describe the four types of hearing aids that may be worn by patients, including troubleshooting strategies that may help to fix a hearing aid that is not working. (pp 1592-1593)
7. Discuss the special patient care considerations that may be required when providing emergency medical care to patients who have the following conditions:
   - Cerebral palsy (pp 1592-1594)
   - Cystic fibrosis (p 1594)
   - Multiple sclerosis (p 1594)
   - Muscular dystrophy (p 1595)
   - Spina bifida (p 1595)
   - Paralysis (pp 1595-1596)
8. Define obesity and bariatrics. (p 1597)
9. Discuss the special patient care considerations that may be required when providing

emergency medical care to bariatric patients, including the best way to move a patient with obesity. (pp 1597-1598)

10. Discuss the special patient care considerations that may be required when providing emergency medical care to patients who rely on a form of medical technology assistance, including the following:
    - Tracheostomy tube (pp 1598-1599)
    - Mechanical ventilator (p 1601)
    - Apnea monitor (pp 1601-1602)
    - Internal cardiac pacemaker (p 1602)
    - Left ventricular assist device (p 1602)
    - External defibrillator vest (p 1602)
    - Intra-aortic balloon pump (p 1603)
    - Central venous catheter (p 1603)
    - Gastrostomy tube (pp 1603-1604)
    - Shunt (pp 1604-1605)
    - Vagus nerve stimulator (p 1605)
    - Colostomy, ileostomy, or urostomy bag (p 1605)
11. Describe the assessment and management process for patients with special needs. (p 1605)
12. Describe home care, the types of patients it serves, and the services it encompasses. (p 1606)
13. Discuss hospice and palliative care. (p 1606)
14. Explain the responsibilities of AEMTs when responding to calls for terminally ill patients who have do not resuscitate orders. (p 1606)
15. Discuss the issues of poverty and homelessness in the United States, including the negative effects on a person's health, and the role of AEMTs as patient advocates. (p 1607)

Skills Objectives

1. Demonstrate different strategies to communicate effectively with a patient who is hard of hearing or deaf. (pp 1591-1592)
2. Explain how to suction and clean a tracheostomy. (p 1600, Skill Drill 38-1)

Introduction

A number of children and adults live with chronic diseases and injuries. Thanks to advances in medicine and medical technology, many people with these diseases and injuries live at home or in other environments outside the hospital setting. As an advanced emergency medical technician (AEMT), you should be familiar with the special needs created by chronic diseases and injuries.

Some examples of patients with special needs include the following:

- Children who were born prematurely and who have associated respiratory conditions
- Infants or small children with congenital heart disease
- Patients with neurologic disease (occasionally caused by hypoxemia at the time of birth, as with cerebral palsy)
- Patients with congenital or acquired diseases resulting in altered body function that requires medical assistance for breathing, eating, urination, or bowel function
- Patients with sensory deficits such as hearing or visual impairments
- Geriatric patients with chronic diseases requiring visitation from a home health care service

You may be called on to treat children and adults who are living at home who depend on mechanical ventilators, intravenous (IV) pumps, or other devices to maintain their lives. You should assess and care for patients with special needs the same way you care for your other patients, although you may adapt your approach to communication depending on the patient's special needs. Your priority is to manage airway, breathing, and circulation (ABCs). Incorporate the patient, family members, and/or caregivers into your process, and solve problems as a group. Remember your ultimate goal: to give the patient the best emergency medical care possible, in the most efficient way, and still accommodate for his or her individual needs.

Developmental Disability

A **developmental disability** refers to insufficient development of the brain, resulting in some level of dysfunction or impairment. Developmental disabilities can include intellectual, hearing, or vision impairment. As the term implies, the disability appears during a person's development—that is, during infancy, childhood, or adolescence.

Intellectual disability results in the inability to learn and socially adapt at a normal developmental rate. An intellectual disability may be caused by genetic factors, congenital infections, complications at birth, malnutrition, or environmental factors. Prenatal drug or alcohol use may also cause intellectual disability, such as fetal alcohol syndrome. Other causes that may occur after birth include traumatic brain injury and poisoning (eg, from lead or other toxins).

A person with a slight intellectual impairment may appear slow to understand or have a limited vocabulary and might behave immaturely in comparison with their peers. People with severe intellectual disabilities may not have the ability to care for themselves, communicate, understand, or respond to their surroundings.

Speaking to patients and family members will give you a good idea of how well the patient can understand you and how the patient will interact with you. Family or friends of the patient may also be able to supply additional medical information regarding the patient.

Some patients with disabilities may have difficulty adjusting to change or a break in routine, so an emergency call that generates a roomful of strangers can be overwhelming. An anxious patient may have difficulty interacting with you. Make every effort to respect the patient's wishes and concerns; take as much time as necessary to calmly and clearly explain the treatment the patient is about to receive.

▶ Autism Spectrum Disorder

Autism and **autism spectrum disorder (ASD)** are general terms used to describe a complex disorder that varies greatly in signs and symptoms. Autism is a pervasive developmental disorder characterized by impairment of social interaction. Other characteristics can include severe behavioral problems, repetitive motor activities, and verbal and nonverbal language impairment. The spectrum of disability is wide. Some children with autism will grow up to be independent, whereas others will be unable to care for themselves.

Patients with autism do not use or understand nonverbal means of communication, such as gestures. They frequently have difficulty making eye-to-eye contact and resist encouragement to do so. They have extreme difficulty with complex tasks that require many steps and do best with simple, one-step directions, such as "Please put on your shoes." Some patients with autism tend to become confused during long conversations and have trouble answering open-ended questions (for example, "What sorts of things do you enjoy doing?"). They might talk in robotic or monotone speech patterns and sometimes repeat phrases over and over again. Many patients with autism confuse pronouns and will say "you" when they mean "I," as in, "You are going to the hospital," when they mean, "I am going to the hospital." A small percentage of patients with autism do not speak at all, but instead rely on actions such as pulling parents and caregivers around by the hand to get their needs met.

No simple explanation exists as to why autism develops in children. According to the US Centers for Disease Control and Prevention (CDC), approximately 1 in every 68 American children is diagnosed with autism. The prevalence in boys is five times the prevalence in girls.[1] Autism is typically diagnosed by age 3. The parents or caregivers often report unique, repetitive behaviors (hand flapping, twirling objects) or isolated abnormal behaviors. Many children with autism receive special instruction and care in school-based settings, but this was not always the case in the past. It is likely that some older adults with autism have never been diagnosed and, therefore, have never received any assistance.

Patients with autism generally have medical needs similar to those of their peers without autism. Rely on parents or caregivers for information, and involve them in the treatment of the patient. As with any patient, explain what you are going to do before you do it. Move slowly, stay calm, and show the patient what to expect by demonstrating the exam on a parent or caregiver first.

▶ Down Syndrome

Down syndrome is characterized by a genetic chromosomal defect that can occur during fetal development, resulting in mild to severe intellectual impairment **Figure 38-1**. The normal human somatic cell contains 23 pairs of chromosomes. In most cases, Down syndrome, also known as trisomy 21, occurs when the two 21st chromosomes fail to separate, so that the ovum or sperm contains 24 chromosomes. When an ovum or sperm with an extra chromosome 21 combines with a normal cell from the other parent, an embryo with 3 copies of chromosome 21 is formed. The extra copy of chromosome 21 disrupts the normal course of development.

According to the CDC, approximately 6,000 babies are born with Down syndrome in the United States each year. Increased maternal age (older than 35 years) and a family history of Down syndrome are known risk factors for this condition. A variety of physical abnormalities are

YOU are the Provider — PART 1

Your ambulance is dispatched to a local group home for a man having a seizure. Based on previous responses to this location, you are aware that the residents all have some type of disability and often require complex management. As you arrive on scene, you are directed to the dining area where you find Gary. You know from previous encounters that he has Down syndrome and often experiences seizures. Presently the patient is not having a seizure and appears to be breathing adequately, but he remains in a postictal state. The on-duty caregiver states that Gary had a tonic-clonic seizure, lasting approximately 90 seconds, and it resolved on its own.

1. What abnormalities are associated with Down syndrome?
2. What type of medical complications may patients with Down syndrome experience?

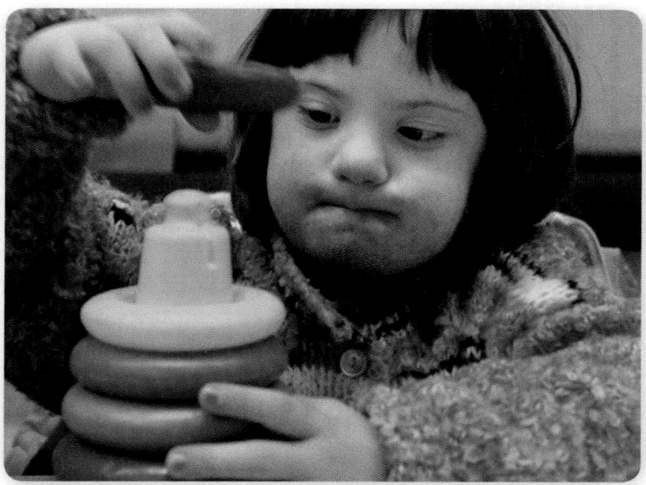

Figure 38-1 A child with Down syndrome.

associated with Down syndrome: a round head with a flat occiput; an enlarged, protruding tongue; slanted, wide-set eyes; folded skin on either side of the nose, covering the inner corners of the eye; short, wide hands; a small face and features; congenital heart defects; thyroid problems; and hearing and vision problems.[2] People with Down syndrome usually do not have all of these signs, but a diagnosis can be made rapidly at birth because a combination of signs can be seen. Depending on their level of intellectual disability, people with Down syndrome may lead relatively independent lives. They may be employed, vote, and get involved in their communities.

People with Down syndrome are at increased risk for medical complications, including those that affect the cardiovascular, sensory, endocrine, musculoskeletal, dental, gastrointestinal, and hematologic systems, as well as neurologic development. Approximately 50% of children born with Down syndrome have congenital heart defects present at birth.[3] People with Down syndrome may also have instability of the cervical spine. This can be a cause of injury in children when they participate in contact sports without having undergone proper screening.

Emergency treatment for patients with Down syndrome should therefore include airway management, supplemental oxygen, and IV access. In patients with heart failure, administer diuretics with judicious fluid resuscitation only if necessary.

Because people with Down syndrome often have large tongues and small oral and nasal cavities, bag-mask ventilation can be challenging. Misalignment of the teeth and other dental anomalies may be present. The enlarged tongue and dental anomalies can lead to speech abnormalities as well. In the case of airway obstruction, a jaw-thrust maneuver may be all that is needed to clear the airway. In an unresponsive patient, the jaw-thrust maneuver or a nasopharyngeal (nasal) airway may be necessary. Call for paramedic backup early if you suspect the need for advanced airway management.

Many people with Down syndrome have epilepsy. Most of the seizures are tonic-clonic. Patient management is the same as with other patients with seizures. Chapter 19, *Neurologic Emergencies*, discusses the emergency management of seizures in detail.

YOU are the Provider PART 2

You ask the caregiver about the patient's medical history, and she states he has a developmental disability. Even though Gary is 37 years old, he has the mental capacity of a 6-year-old. She also states he has a central venous catheter and a gastrostomy tube. You approach the patient and find that he has a patent airway and is breathing adequately. However, owing to the postictal state, you instruct your partner to administer oxygen with a nonrebreathing mask. You attempt to communicate with the patient, but he remains nonverbal. You ask the caregiver whether this is normal for him, and she states "No, he can usually answer simple questions."

Recording Time: 1 Minute	
Appearance	Fair
Level of consciousness	Decreased
Airway	Patent
Breathing	12 breaths/min
Circulation	Warm, dry, and pink

3. How should you interact with a patient with Down syndrome?
4. How should you incorporate the caregiver into your treatment?

▶ Patient Interaction

It is normal to feel somewhat uncomfortable when initiating contact with a patient with a disability, especially if you have not encountered such situations frequently. The best plan of action is to treat the patient as you would any other patient.

Approach a patient in a calm and friendly manner, watching him or her for signs of increased anxiety or fear. Remember, you are a stranger and are approaching with a group of people. The patient may not understand your uniform or realize that you and your team are there to help. It may be helpful to have your team members wait until you can establish a rapport with the patient. You can then introduce the team members, explain what they are going to do, and slowly bring them forward.

Begin interacting with the patient by introducing yourself, shaking the patient's hand if he or she will allow it. Converse with the patient as you normally would. For example, say, "Your mother called us. She says you're not feeling well today, and we're here to help you feel better. My friend John is going to take your blood pressure." Allow the patient to see and touch your equipment before you use it. Move slowly but deliberately, explaining beforehand what you are going to do, just like you would with any other patient.

Watch carefully for signs of fear or reluctance from the patient. Do your best to soothe the patient's anxiety and/or discomfort as you work through your assessment and treatment plan. Make sure you are at eye level with the patient. If the patient is sitting, then kneel or sit down. By initially establishing trust and communication, you will have much better luck successfully executing your treatment plan.

Brain Injury

A patient with a prior brain injury may be difficult to assess and treat. Chapter 30, *Head and Spine Injuries*, discusses head injuries and traumatic brain injuries in detail. Patients with brain injuries may face a complex array of challenges related to the injury. In such cases, obtaining a complete medical history from the patient, family, and friends will be helpful. You will need to tailor your interaction with patients with brain injuries to their specific abilities. Take the time to speak with the patient and family to establish what is considered normal for the patient; for example, determine whether the patient has cognitive, sensory, communication, motor, behavioral, or psychological deficits.

When you care for a patient with a prior brain injury, talk in a calm, soothing tone, and watch the patient closely for signs of anxiety or aggression. In some cases, the patient may need to be specially positioned or restrained to ensure your safety and the safety of the patient. Although not all people with brain injuries have physical impairments, do not expect the patient to walk to the ambulance or stretcher. As always, treat the patient with respect, use his or her name, explain procedures, and reassure the patient throughout the process.

Sensory Disabilities

▶ Visual Impairment

Visual impairments may result from a multitude of causes—a congenital defect, disease, injury, infection (eg, the cytomegalovirus), or degeneration of the eyeball, optic nerve, or nerve pathway (eg, with aging). The degree of visual impairment may range from partial to total. Some patients have a loss of peripheral or central vision; others can distinguish light from dark or discern general shapes.

Visual impairments may be difficult to recognize. During your scene size-up, look for signs that indicate the person is visually impaired, such as the presence of eyeglasses, a cane, or a service animal **Figure 38-2**. Immediately introduce yourself when you enter the room. Have your team members introduce themselves so the patient can identify their voices and locations. In addition, retrieve any visual aids (eg, eyeglasses) and give them to your patient to make the interaction more comfortable for him or her.

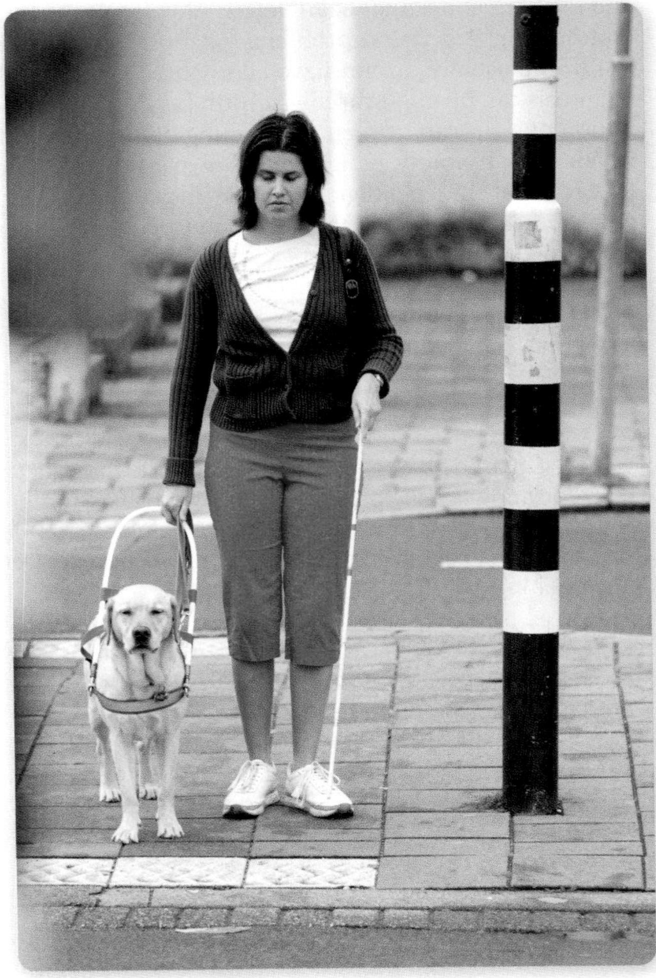

Figure 38-2 A service dog is easily identified by its special harness.

A visually impaired person may feel vulnerable, especially during the chaos of an incident scene. He or she may have learned to use other senses such as hearing, touch, and smell to compensate for the loss of sight, and the sounds and smells of the scene may be disorienting. Remember to tell the patient what is happening, identify noises, and describe the situation and surroundings, especially if you must move the patient.

Words of Wisdom

Service animals are not classified as pets and should, by law, be allowed to stay with a visually impaired patient unless it is a critical situation or the animal is out of control. Review the Service Animals section in the Americans with Disabilities Act for further information.

Some patients use a cane or walker. Even if the person will be carried out on your gurney, do not forget to take the patient's cane or walker. Unless it is a critical situation, the service animal can remain with the patient and will provide reassurance for the patient and prevent delays in transport; however, in some cases, you may need to make arrangements for the care or accompaniment of the animal. A friend or animal control officer can be helpful in this situation.

An ambulatory patient may be led by a light touch on the arm or elbow. You may also allow the patient to rest his or her hand on your shoulder, as this may enhance the patient's sense of balance and security while moving. You may also ask the patient which method he or she prefers to use while traveling to the ambulance. Patients should be gently guided but never pulled or pushed. Communicate about obstacles in advance. Statements such as, "You're approaching the stairs. We're going to take five steps down," will allow the patient to anticipate and navigate the obstacles safely.

Words of Wisdom

Allow a visually impaired patient to stay in contact with you by keeping one hand on the patient or allowing the patient to hold onto you.

▶ Hearing Impairment

Hearing impairment may range from a slight hearing loss to total deafness. Some patients may have difficulty with pitch, volume, and speaking distinctly. Some patients learn to speak even though they have never heard sounds. Others may have heard speech and learned to talk but have since sustained partial or total hearing loss, leading them to speak too loudly. Parkinson disease and other disease processes may cause the patient to slur words, speak very slowly, or speak in a monotone.

The two most common forms of hearing loss are known as sensorineural deafness and conductive hearing loss. **Sensorineural deafness**, or nerve damage, is the most common hearing loss you will encounter in the field. Sensorineural deafness may be caused by a lesion or damage of the inner ear. Older adults will have some degree of sensorineural hearing loss because of advanced age. **Conductive hearing loss** is caused by a faulty transmission of sound waves, which can occur when a person has an accumulation of wax within the ear canal or a perforated eardrum.

During your scene size-up, look for clues that a person could be hard of hearing or deaf, including the presence of hearing aids, poor pronunciation of words, and failure to respond to your presence or questions. Check to make sure the hearing aid is in place. Most people who are hard of hearing have learned to read body language, such as hand gestures and lip movement. Therefore, face the patient while communicating so he or she can see your mouth; do not exaggerate your lip movements or look away. Position yourself approximately 18 inches (46 cm) directly in front of the patient. Because patients who are hard of hearing typically have more difficulty hearing higher-frequency sounds, never shout if the patient seems to have difficulty hearing you; instead, try lowering the pitch of your voice.

Ask the patient, "How would you like to communicate with me?" American Sign Language may be his or her preferred method of communication **Figure 38-3**. An interpreter, family member, or friend may be able to interpret. If an interpreter is not readily available, then call your receiving facility early on to request one. Ideally, an interpreter will arrive before you begin your assessment. Other patients may prefer written communication or communication of concepts or procedures with gestures or pictures.

Here are some helpful tips for working with patients who are hard of hearing or deaf:

- If indoors, then adjust the lighting so the patient can see you.
- Face the patient and speak slowly and distinctly. The patient may want to read your lips.
- Change speakers. Given that 80% of hearing loss is related to an inability to hear high-pitched sounds, look for a team member with a low-pitched voice.
- Provide paper and a pencil so you may write your questions and the patient may write his or her responses.
- Have only one person ask interview questions, to avoid confusing the patient.
- Try the "reverse stethoscope" technique: put the earpieces of your stethoscope in the patient's ear and speak softly into the diaphragm of the stethoscope to amplify your voice.

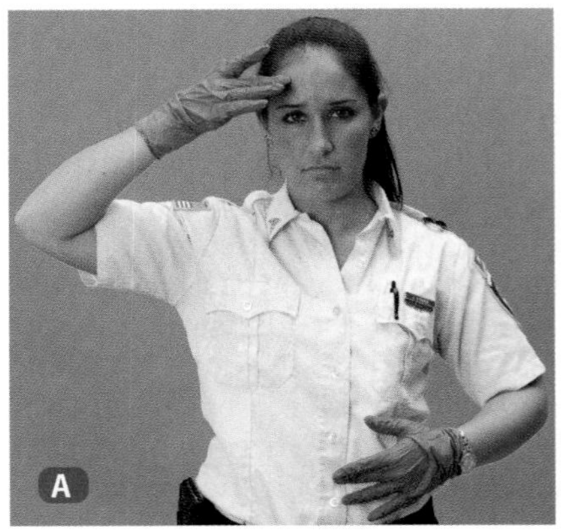
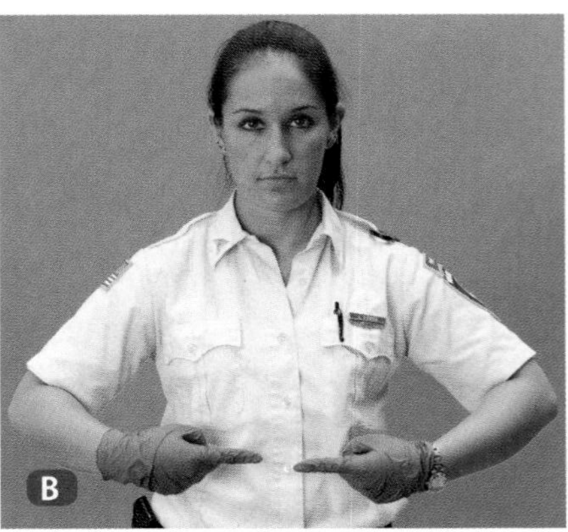
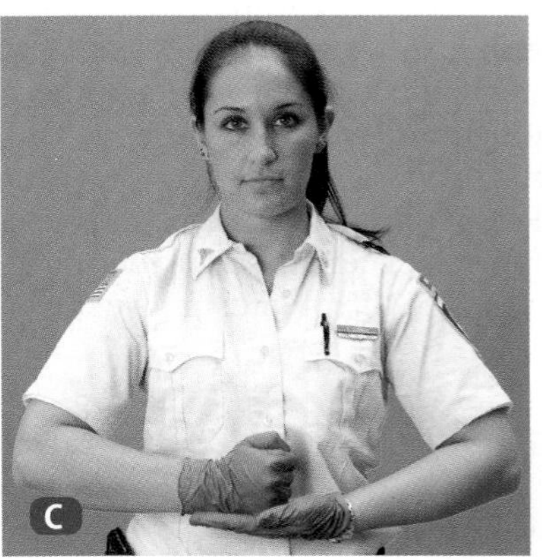

Figure 38-3 Consider learning common terms in American Sign Language related to illness and injury. **A.** Sick. **B.** Hurt. **C.** Help.

Words of Wisdom

Some patients who are hard of hearing are sensitive to loud noises close to their ears. Remember to use a normal tone of voice when speaking to these patients.

Words of Wisdom

When you care for a patient who is hard of hearing, one communication solution is to place the ear pieces of your stethoscope into the patient's ears while you speak softly into the diaphragm of the stethoscope.

Hearing Aids

A hearing aid is essentially a device that makes sound louder. Hearing aids cannot restore damaged hearing to normal, but they do improve hearing and listening ability. Four types of hearing aids are available Figure 38-4:

- **Behind-the-ear.** The working parts are contained in a plastic case that rests behind the ear.
- **Conventional body.** This older style is generally used by people with profound hearing loss. This type fits within the ear.
- **In-the-canal and completely in-the-canal.** These hearing aids are contained in a tiny case that fits partly or completely into the ear canal.
- **In-the-ear.** All parts are contained in a shell that fits in the outer part of the ear.

Implantable hearing aids are also an option for patients with less profound hearing loss. It is preferable to have the patient insert his or her own hearing aid. Provide assistance if needed. To insert a hearing aid, follow the natural shape of the ear. The device needs to fit snugly without forcing. If you hear a whistling sound after the device is inserted and turned on, then the hearing aid may not be in far enough to create a seal, or the volume may be too loud. Try repositioning the hearing aid, or remove it and turn down the volume. If you cannot insert the hearing aid after two tries, then put it in its box, take it with you, and document the transport and transfer of hearing aids to hospital personnel. Never try to clean hearing aids, and do not get them wet.

If a patient's hearing aid is inserted correctly but is still not working, then try troubleshooting the problem. First, make sure the hearing aid is turned on. Next, try a fresh battery, and check the tubing to make sure it is not twisted or bent. Check the switch to make sure it is set on M (microphone), not T (telephone). For a conventional body–type hearing aid, try a spare cord; the old one may be broken or shorted. Finally, check the ear mold to make sure it is not clogged with earwax.

Physical Disabilities

▶ Cerebral Palsy

Cerebral palsy is a term for a group of disorders characterized by poorly controlled body movement Figure 38-5. This disorder results from developmental brain defects in utero, traumatic brain injury at birth or in early childhood, oxygen deprivation at birth, or from infection, such as meningitis, during the neonatal period or infancy. There may also be a genetic cause. Patients with cerebral palsy can have symptoms that range from mild to severe, involving spastic movements of their limbs and inability to maintain proper posture.

Cerebral palsy is also associated with other conditions such as visual and hearing impairments, difficulty communicating, epilepsy (seizures), and intellectual disabilities.

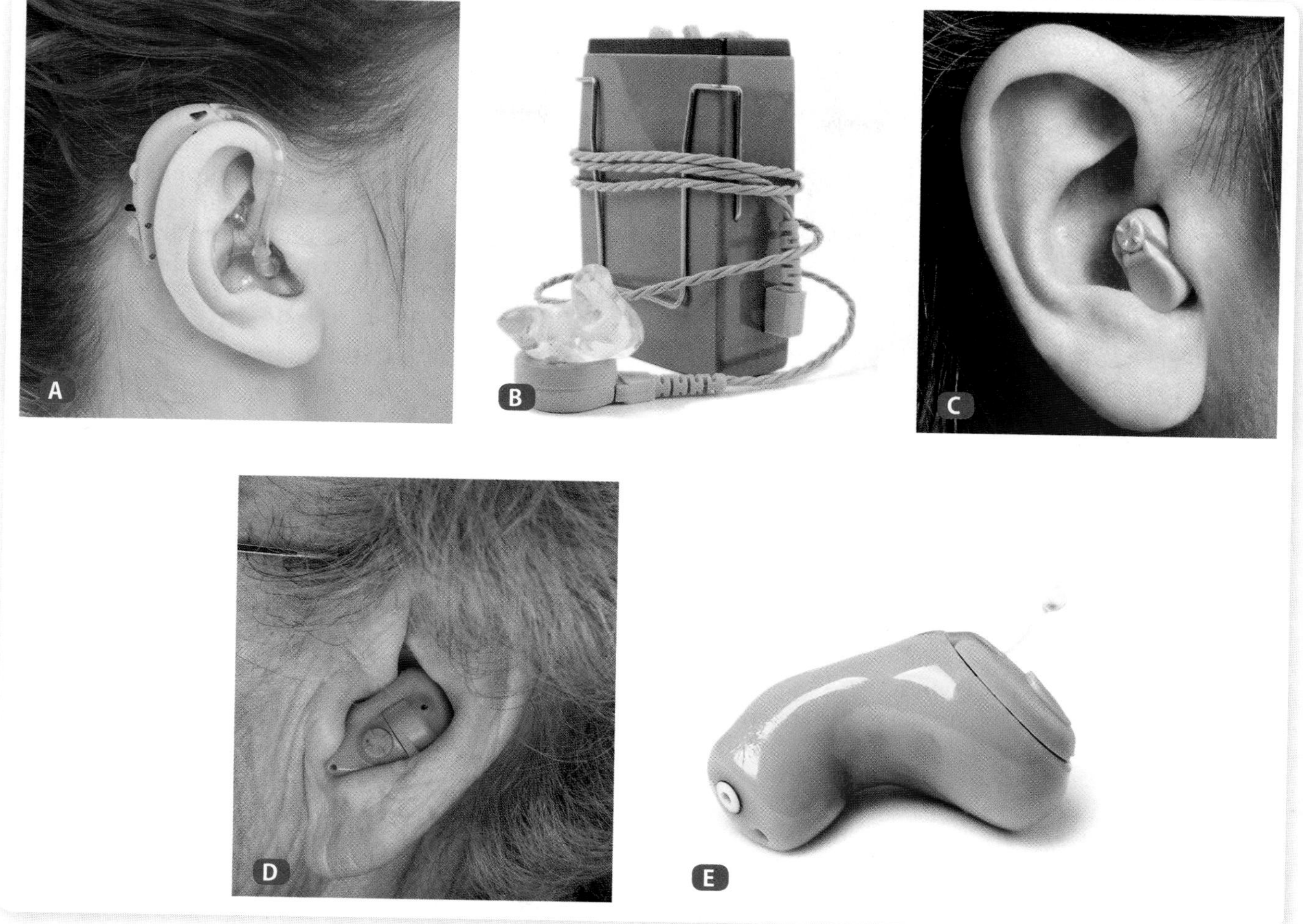

Figure 38-4 Different types of hearing aids. **A.** Behind-the-ear. **B.** Conventional body. **C.** In-the-canal. **D.** In-the-ear. **E.** Completely in-the-canal.

A: © Piotr Marcinski/Shutterstock; B: © Stine Lise Nielsen/Shutterstock; C: © Steve Hamblin/Alamy; D: © Terry Smith Images/Alamy; E: © Jiri Hera/Shutterstock.

Some people with cerebral palsy are able to learn to walk with assistive devices, whereas others need support even to sit and cannot stand, walk, or speak. If the person is able to speak, then grimacing and uncontrolled movement may make speaking difficult and the person's speech hard to understand. To cope with ordinary tasks, many people with cerebral palsy use computerized household controls and speaking aids. Motorized wheelchairs may be controlled with a joystick or mouth control. Specially shaped chairs and pillows may be custom built to facilitate the person's comfort and ease movement. Toys may also be adapted to allow for learning and play. In addition, computers may be specially configured to aid the person with speech simulation and provide the ability to perform household tasks, such as temperature control and lighting.

As with all patients, assessing the ABCDEs (airway, breathing, circulation, disability, and exposure) is of the utmost importance. Closely observe the airway status of a patient with cerebral palsy because the patient may have increased production of secretions and **dysphagia**, or difficult swallowing, requiring aggressive suctioning to clear the airway.

When you care for a patient with cerebral palsy, note the following:

- Do not assume that all patients with cerebral palsy have an intellectual disability. Although 50% have some intellectual disability, many people with cerebral palsy have a normal intelligence quotient or only slight intellectual impairment.[4]
- Limbs are often underdeveloped and are prone to injury (eg, a fall from a wheelchair).
- Patients who have the ability to walk may have an unsteady gait and are prone to falls.
- If the patient has a specially made pillow or chair (as many pediatric patients do), the patient may prefer to use it during transport. Remember to pad the patient to ensure his or her comfort, and never force a patient's extremities into any position.

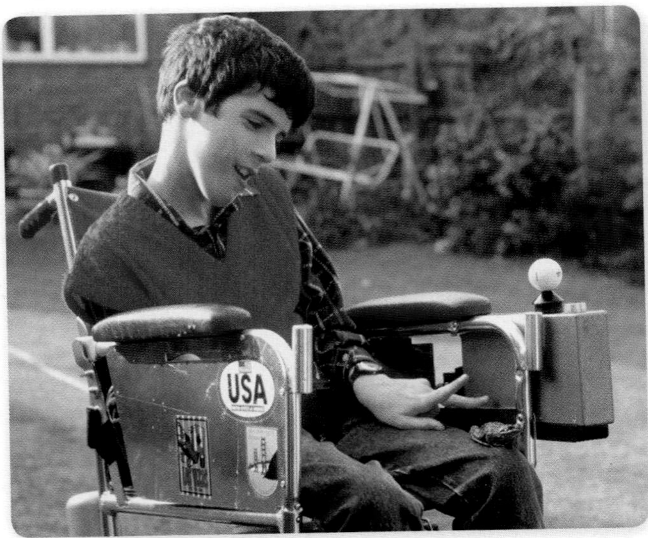

Figure 38-5 A person with cerebral palsy.

- Whenever possible, transport walkers or wheelchairs with the patient.
- About 25% to 35% of children with cerebral palsy have epilepsy, according to the Epilepsy Foundation.[5] Be prepared to treat the patient during a seizure if one occurs, and keep a suctioning unit available.

▶ Cystic Fibrosis

Infants and young children may be diagnosed with **cystic fibrosis (CF)** (mucoviscidosis), a genetic disorder that is characterized by increased production of mucus in the lungs and digestive system. CF is caused by a defective recessive gene, inherited from each parent, which disrupts the normal function of cells that make up the sweat glands in the skin and that also line the lungs and the digestive and reproductive systems. The end result is that the mucus becomes thick, sticky, and hard to move. The mucus holds germs, causing the lungs to become infected. The increased mucus impairs respiration, disrupts digestion of food, predisposes the patient to repeated lung infections, and may become a life-threatening emergency in severe situations.

Patients with CF are prone to the development of venous thrombosis. Pulmonary manifestations include pneumonia, pneumothorax, cough, respiratory distress, and respiratory failure. Malnutrition and a poor growth rate are not uncommon symptoms; in some cases, a child with CF may fail to thrive. Mild cases can go undetected until after a patient reaches adulthood. CF often causes death in childhood because of chronic pneumonia secondary to the very thick pathologic mucus in the airway. Because of advances in treatment, the life expectancy for CF patients improves each year.

Patients with CF receive frequent or continuous treatment with antibiotics. Medical devices promoting lung function and removal of mucus may also be used by patients with CF. Patients may be on intermittent or continuous home oxygen, and a significant number of patients with CF await or receive lung transplants to prolong and improve the quality of life. You may encounter patients with CF who may have minimal to profound respiratory or gastrointestinal compromise from this disorder. Treatment is supportive. Maintain the airway, providing oxygen and suction as needed. Humidified oxygen, if available, may help thin mucus and improve respirations.

▶ Multiple Sclerosis

Multiple sclerosis (MS) is a severe, incurable, degenerative disorder involving the central nervous system (brain and spinal cord). Immune cells within the body attack the myelin sheath of certain nerve fibers, ultimately destroying nerve fibers and preventing nerve transmission to other body tissues. It is not entirely clear what causes MS, although some sources describe a connection between genetic predisposition, environmental factors, and possibly nutrition or exposure to a particular virus. According to the National Institute of Neurological Disorders and Stroke, this disease strikes women in their 20s to 40s two to three times more often than men. Approximately 350,000 Americans have MS, some with serious handicaps.[6]

Patients typically present with conditions related to muscle coordination, muscle tone, altered sensation, and altered gait. These patients report periods of varied improvement followed by relapse and progression of the disease. A vast array of signs and symptoms related to neurologic function are possible with MS. Patients may develop problems with the musculoskeletal system such as clumsiness and ataxia, constipation or bladder incontinence, fatigue, decreased sexual performance, extremities that feel heavy or weak, altered sensations (dizziness or vertigo), numbness or tingling in parts of the body, cognitive impairment, disruption of speech or swallowing, and visual impairment. Skin breakdown may result from immobility or poor positioning. Severe manifestations of the disease may render patients bedridden and incontinent. Symptoms can present in many different combinations and last anywhere from several days to months, often interrupted by periods of absent or reduced symptoms. Life expectancy may be normal, but profound symptoms may cause significant disability or impairment depending on the severity of the disease process.

MS is managed with medications, physical therapy, and counseling. No specific emergency medical services (EMS) treatment for MS exists. Allow additional time for assessment due to cognitive or communication barriers. Because of the disease process, the patient may lack feeling, so the physical exam findings may be difficult to interpret. Other supportive measures include IV hydration, analgesic or muscle-relaxing medications, careful patient positioning, and assisted ventilation when indicated.

Muscular Dystrophy

Muscular dystrophy is a broad term that describes a category of incurable genetic diseases that cause a slow, progressive degeneration of the muscle fibers. In many cases, the destroyed fibers are replaced by adipose (fat) or connective tissue.

Children may present with obvious facial muscle changes, altered gait, delayed psychomotor developmental milestones, and changes in posture. Severe manifestations of certain specific diseases in this group include cardiomyopathy, cognitive impairment, and respiratory compromise. An infant may show obvious signs of muscular dystrophy at birth or have an onset as late as adulthood. In severe cases, profound symptoms or death from muscular dystrophy may occur in children and teenagers. Death typically occurs secondary to cardiac or respiratory dysfunction associated with the disease.

According to the CDC, Duchenne muscular dystrophy (DMD), the most common type of muscular dystrophy, is caused by a sex-linked recessive gene that chiefly affects males (1 in every 3,500 to 6,000 male births in the United States).[7] This disorder is characterized by enlarged heart muscle tissue (dilated cardiomyopathy), heart dysrhythmias, scoliosis (abnormal curvature) of the spine, and gait disturbances. Children with DMD often require the use of a wheelchair by age 15 years.[8]

EMS treatment is primarily limited to careful positioning, supportive treatment, and assisted ventilation in severe cases. Smaller or younger children with muscular dystrophy are typically relatively easy to examine or transport. Larger children or adults may require additional assistance during movement to or from an ambulance.

Spina Bifida

Spina bifida, also known as myelomeningocele, is a birth defect caused by the incomplete closure of the spinal column during embryonic or fetal development, resulting in an exposed portion of the spinal cord **Figure 38-6**. The opening can be surgically closed, but the child is often left with spinal and neurologic damage. To reduce the occurrences of such disabling birth defects, pregnant women are advised to take vitamin B9 (folic acid). Unfortunately, spina bifida is still one of the most common disabling birth defects in the United States. According to the CDC, one in 2,858 children are born with this defect.[9] Some patients with spina bifida also have hydrocephalus, which requires the placement of a shunt to drain excessive amounts of cerebrospinal fluid (CSF) from the brain.[10]

Be aware that some patients with spina bifida will have partial or full paralysis of the lower extremities and loss of bowel and bladder control; they might also have an extreme allergy to latex products. A supply of latex-free products should be kept on the ambulance to avoid a severe anaphylactic reaction in patients with spina bifida.

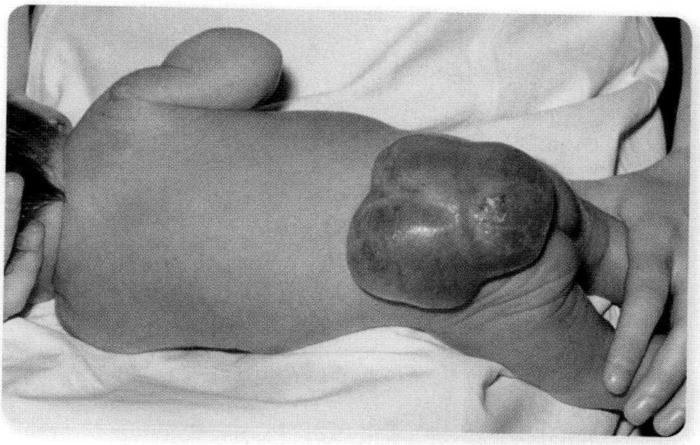

Figure 38-6 Spina bifida is one of the most common disabling birth defects in the United States.

Patients with spina bifida will benefit from the same considerations that you offer when you treat a patient with paralysis or a patient who has difficulty moving. Ask patients how it is best to move them before you transport them. Remember to rule out a fall or other event that may have caused an injury. Check carefully for injuries because patients may not be able to feel them—or the pain of an infiltrated IV solution, for that matter. Also, be aware that patients may have urinary catheters or other aids in place.

Paralysis

Paralysis is the inability to voluntarily move one or more body parts. It may be caused by cerebrovascular accident (stroke), trauma, or birth defects.

Several types of paralysis exist, including:

- **Hemiplegia**: Paralysis of one side of the body, possibly from a stroke or head injury
- **Paraplegia**: Paralysis of the lower part of the body, possibly from thoracic or lumbar spinal injury or spina bifida
- **Quadriplegia**: Paralysis of all four extremities and the trunk, possibly from a cervical spine injury

Dysphagia, caused by a partial paralysis of the esophagus, is the inability to swallow. Patients with dysphagia may easily choke or aspirate food and drink, leading to the need for emergency airway interventions. Paralysis of the respiratory muscles causes patients to be completely dependent on a mechanical ventilator or similar device. Interruption of assisted ventilation for even brief periods may have devastating consequences.

Decubitus ulcers (pressure ulcers) are a constant threat for those with paralysis. Patients require frequent mechanical or caregiver assistance to change position. Tissue perfusion to the coccyx region and over bony prominences becomes compromised when external pressure is applied to these areas for a short or long period, as occurs often with bedridden patients. Infection related to pressure ulcers is a significant cause of mortality in these patients.

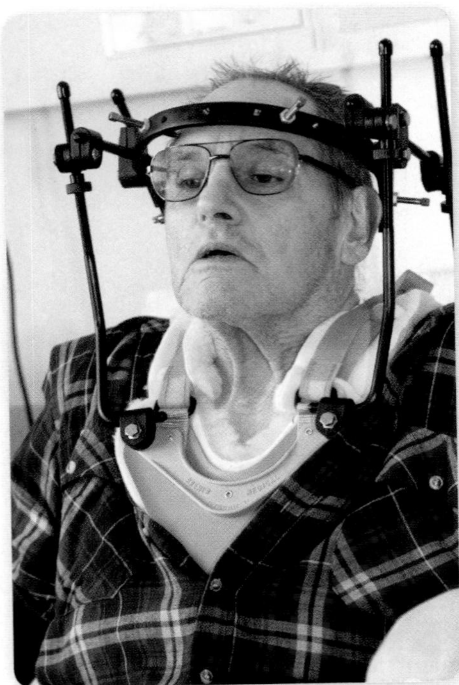

Figure 38-7 A halo ring/vest combination used for spinal stabilization after initial management of significant fracture or dislocation is shown here.

Patients who have paralysis related to spinal cord injury are at risk for a life-threatening condition known as autonomic dysreflexia. A stressor within the body—sometimes as simple as a full bladder, constipation, or pain—triggers a large release of catecholamines (epinephrine and norepinephrine) from the autonomic nervous system. This release causes vasodilation above the level of the spinal cord injury, as well as massive arterial vasoconstriction. The patient's blood pressure can become dangerously high.

External devices such as halo vests (also called halo rings) are used to immobilize the spine following initial management of significant fractures or dislocations Figure 38-7. These devices require additional consideration and coordination while you are moving these patients. Halo vests have substantial weight. It is necessary to support the halo vest without applying any force to it during patient movement. In the event of cardiac arrest, you will typically find an Allen wrench (hex key) attached to the anterior chest portion of the vest for removal only to perform external cardiac compressions. As an AEMT, do not otherwise attempt to reposition or adjust the halo vest.

Words of Wisdom

Do not hesitate to call for additional assistance when transporting a patient with a halo vest, home ventilator, or other piece of equipment that may be bulky and require extra hands to load.

Patients with paralysis are particularly susceptible to environmental extremes. It is often impossible for these patients to regulate perfusion to the skin. Fluctuations of the autonomic nervous system place patients at risk for hypothermia and (particularly) hyperthermia.

Paralysis does not always entail a loss of sensation. In some cases, the patient will have normal sensation or hyperesthesia (increased sensitivity) that may cause the patient to interpret touch as pain in the affected area. Some male patients with a severe spinal cord injury will present with priapism (a prolonged penile erection) unrelated to sexual arousal. Depending on the pattern of sensation loss, the priapism may be associated with discomfort for the patient. For a patient with priapism, maintain his privacy and continue to provide supportive care.

Scheduled urinary catheterization is required for many patients with paralysis. Urinary infection, urinary reflux, and autonomic dysreflexia are all possible if patients do not regularly empty the bladder.

Total lifting assistance is typically required for patients with quadriplegia. These patients may or may not need a tracheostomy tube, indwelling urinary catheter, colostomy, or ventilator. You may need to request additional lifting assistance or specialty consultation regarding the ventilator or a similar device.

Words of Wisdom

Patients with significant paralysis have the potential to create challenges for EMS providers. Remember to ask for help and know your equipment!

Patients who have partial or total loss of sensation in the affected limbs cannot tell you when you are hurting them. Take great care to use a gentle touch, especially when lifting or moving a patient with paralysis. Ask the patient or caregiver how to best move them before you transport them. Because paralyzed limbs lack muscle tone, provide IV access and medication on the nonaffected side whenever possible. Check IV sites frequently for infiltration, especially after medication administration.

Safety Tips

It takes planning and coordination to move a patient with paralysis without dislodging or compromising his or her extra equipment. You may need to recruit more team members so that you can efficiently move the patient without causing further complications. Strategically placed padding or pillows may help keep the patient more comfortable during transport.

Bariatric Patients

Obesity is a complex condition in which a person has an excessive amount of body fat. It is the result of an imbalance between calories consumed and calories used. The study of **bariatrics** examines the causes, prevention, and treatment of obesity. The solution to the obesity problem may sound relatively simple—reestablish the caloric balance—but unfortunately, the causes of obesity are not fully understood. Oftentimes, this condition may be attributed to low basal metabolic rate or genetic predisposition.

According to the Mayo Clinic, the term *obese* is used when someone is 30% or more over his or her ideal body weight.[11] This is a good general guideline, except in cases where body weight does not correlate to excess fat, for example, in very muscular people. In severe obesity (also called extreme or morbid obesity), the person is two or three times over the ideal weight. The patient's general quality of life is often negatively affected, and the extra weight can cause a variety of health problems, such as diabetes, hypertension, heart disease, and stroke. Patients with obesity are also prone to mobility difficulties, physical injuries, and a variety of musculoskeletal conditions.

Special Populations

Avoid placing a patient with obesity in the supine position. The excessive weight makes it difficult for the chest to expand. If the patient requires spinal immobilization, then use blankets or other padding to elevate the head from the backboard to facilitate breathing.

Clinical Concerns for the Patient With Obesity

Routine procedures for patients with obesity can be extremely complicated. Airway procedures are made more difficult by a larger tongue, larger head size, and limited neck mobility associated with obesity. Bag-mask ventilation may be ineffective with patients who are in a supine position. Bag-mask ventilation may also become difficult because of poor mask seal or increased resistance due to excess body tissue on the chest wall and abdomen. To perform airway and ventilation procedures, you may need to place the patient in a semi-Fowler position or, if he or she is on a backboard, with the head raised to facilitate optimal chest expansion.

Peripheral IV access is often problematic in patients with obesity. IV attempts are often unsuccessful in extremities and a large neck mass may obscure landmarks for external jugular IV line placement. Many conventional intramuscular (IM) needles will not be able to reach the IM space through excess adipose tissue. Auscultation of heart, lung, or bowel sounds may be more difficult through extra abdominal and chest wall mass. You may also have difficulty determining extent of injury when palpating a particular area due to the excess tissue. If you are unable to determine whether a specific injury exists (ie, a fracture),

YOU are the Provider **PART 3**

You place the patient onto the stretcher and move him into the ambulance. Once in the back of the ambulance, the patient gradually becomes more alert and oriented. You ask your partner to obtain a baseline set of vital signs, and you begin to establish IV access.

Recording Time: 10 Minutes	
Respirations	20 breaths/min
Pulse	104 beats/min; regular
Skin	Warm, dry, and pink
Blood pressure	108/86 mm Hg
Oxygen saturation (Spo_2)	99% on 15 L/min
Pupils	Pupils Equal, Round, and Reactive to Light and Accommodation (PERRLA)

5. This patient has a central venous catheter already in place. Should you insert another IV line or use the central line?
6. What is the purpose of the patient's gastrostomy tube?

then treat the patient as if you could actually feel crepitus (a grating or grinding sensation made when two pieces of broken bone are rubbed together).

Special Populations

As an AEMT, you need to advocate for EMS equipment that is capable of safely transporting bariatric patients. Some EMS systems use ambulances with special winches, stretchers, and ramps that allow safe loading and unloading of bariatric patients. Even simple items such as larger blood pressure cuffs, longer injection or intraosseous (IO) needles, or special cervical collars may dramatically improve your ability to provide patient care.

▶ Interaction With Patients With Obesity

People with obesity are often ridiculed publicly and sometimes subjected to discrimination. Patients with obesity may be embarrassed by their condition or fearful of ridicule as a result of past experiences. Some of the negative interactions may have occurred with an insensitive health care professional. As with any patient, work hard to put the patient at ease. Determine the patient's chief complaint, and then communicate your plan to help. Many patients with severe obesity have a complex and extensive medical history, so mastering the art of conducting a patient interview will serve you well in your interactions with patients with obesity.

If transport is necessary, plan early for extra help, and do not be afraid to call for more help or specialized equipment. In particular, send a member of your team to find the easiest and safest exit to use. Remember, everyone's safety is at stake! You do not want to risk dropping the patient or injuring a team member by trying to lift too much weight. Patient moves, no matter how simple they may seem, become far more complex with a patient with obesity.

Special Populations

As with older adults and pediatric patients, be alert for the possibility of abuse and neglect when treating patients with special needs.

▶ Interaction With Patients With Morbid Obesity

Patients with morbid obesity may overcome mobility difficulties by pulling, rocking, or rolling into a position. The constant strain on their body's structures may leave them with chronic joint injuries or osteoarthritis. When you move a patient with morbid obesity, follow these tips:

- Treat the patient with dignity and respect.
- Ask your patient how best to move him or her before attempting to do so.
- Avoid trying to lift the patient by only one limb, which would risk injury to overtaxed joints.
- Coordinate and communicate all moves to all team members before starting to lift.
- If the move becomes uncontrolled at any point, then stop, reposition, and resume.
- Look for pinch or pressure points from equipment because they could cause significant soft-tissue injuries or a deep venous thrombosis.
- Very large patients will often have difficulty breathing when lying supine. When safe and appropriate to do so, transport patients with the head of the stretcher elevated.
- Many manufacturers now make specialized equipment for patients with morbid obesity, and some areas have specially equipped bariatric ambulances. Become familiar with the resources available in your area.
- Plan egress routes to accommodate large patients, equipment, and the lifting crew members. Remember: Do no harm!
- Notify the receiving facility early to allow special arrangements to be made before your arrival to accommodate the patient's needs.

Words of Wisdom

When transporting a patient with obesity, be sure to alert the receiving facility in advance if special accommodations, equipment, or other resources may be needed.

Patients With Medical Technology Assistance

▶ Tracheostomy Tubes

A **tracheostomy tube** is a plastic tube used to facilitate breathing. The tube is placed in a tracheal **stoma**, or surgical opening in the neck, and provides a path between the anterior part of the neck and the trachea. The tube can be temporary or permanent and passes from the neck directly into the major airways (Figure 38-8).

A **laryngectomy** is a surgical procedure in which the larynx is removed, usually because of cancer. The trachea is then curved anteriorly and sewn to tissues of the neck. Bag-mask ventilation through the nose and mouth is

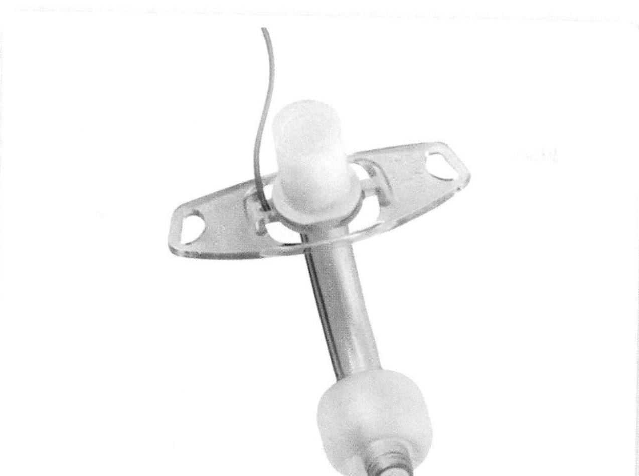

Figure 38-8 Some patients require a tracheostomy tube to breathe.

ineffective for a patient with a laryngectomy, and you must be careful not to introduce liquids into the stoma. Most patients with a stoma use a stoma cover to act as a filter and prevent mucus from being coughed onto others. A patient with a laryngectomy cannot produce normal speech and must learn to swallow and regurgitate air from the stomach or use an assistive device.

Special Populations

If you are transporting a child with a tracheostomy in a standard car seat, then avoid using seats with a tray or shield. The tray or shield could come into contact with the tracheostomy and injure the child or block the airway.

Patients with a tracheostomy tube include those who depend on home automatic ventilators and those who have chronic pulmonary conditions. Because these tubes are foreign to the respiratory tract, the body reacts by building up secretions in or around the tube. The tubes are prone to obstruction by mucous plugs or foreign bodies. Routine care that is provided by caregivers includes keeping the inner cannula, as well as the outer cannula, of the tracheostomy tube clean and dry and suctioning any secretions. The outer cannula should be changed as needed.

An obstruction of the tracheostomy tube is a life-threatening emergency. Airway management is your first priority. Blood or air may be leaking around the tube, which usually happens with new tracheostomies, and the tube can become loose or dislodged. A useful mnemonic in these situations is DOPE Table 38-1. The DOPE mnemonic can help you remember the possible causes of an airway obstruction and correct the problem. Failure to clear an obstructed tracheostomy tube could lead to cardiopulmonary arrest.

Table 38-1 DOPE Mnemonic

D Displaced, dislodged, or damaged tube
O Obstructed tube (secretions, blood, mucus, vomitus)
P Pneumothorax
E Equipment failure (kinked tubing, ventilator malfunction, empty oxygen supply)

It is important to assess for airway patency in all patients, but it is especially important in patients with artificial airways. The basic airway techniques of opening, repositioning, and clearing (especially suctioning) the airway are the most critical steps in improving airway clearance and patency, thereby improving oxygenation and ventilation.

Assess the flow of oxygen, and ensure sufficient oxygen is available in the patient's oxygen system. If you are uncertain about the oxygen flow, then transfer the patient to the flowmeter attached to the main oxygen cylinder in the ambulance.

Words of Wisdom

If a tracheostomy tube becomes plugged, then you can ventilate the patient by deflating the cuff, covering the nose and mouth with a mask, and using the bag-mask device. If you are unable to ventilate the patient through the tracheostomy tube, then plug the tracheostomy stoma and attempt to ventilate the patient in the traditional manner with a bag-mask device.

Occasionally, the opening around the tracheostomy tube may become infected. To suction and clean a tracheostomy tube, follow the steps given here Skill Drill 38-1.

Special Populations

For cost reasons, home care patients often reuse their suction catheters. If the catheters do not have visible contamination and have been stored in a clean manner, then they are acceptable for use.

Skill Drill 38-1 Suctioning and Cleaning a Tracheostomy Tube

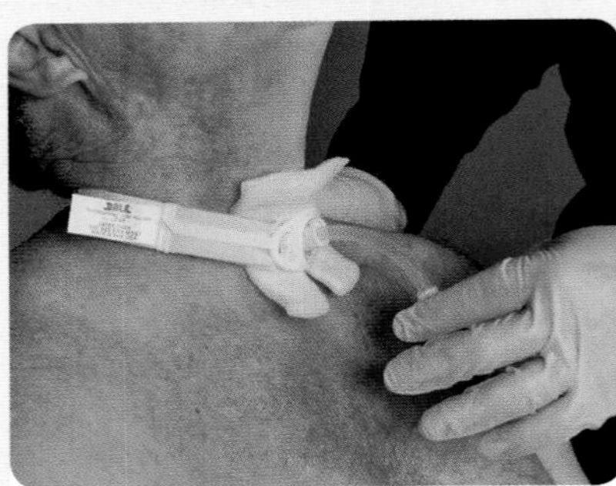

Step 1 Wash your hands, and apply a mask, goggles, and clean nonlatex gloves. Remove the inner cannula, and place the device to soak in the proper solution. If the caregiver is not available, then use a mixture of one-half hydrogen peroxide and one-half water. Placing the cannula in plain water is acceptable in short-term situations. (With one-piece tracheostomy tubes, this step is unnecessary.) If the patient is dependent on a ventilator, then have a replacement cannula immediately available.

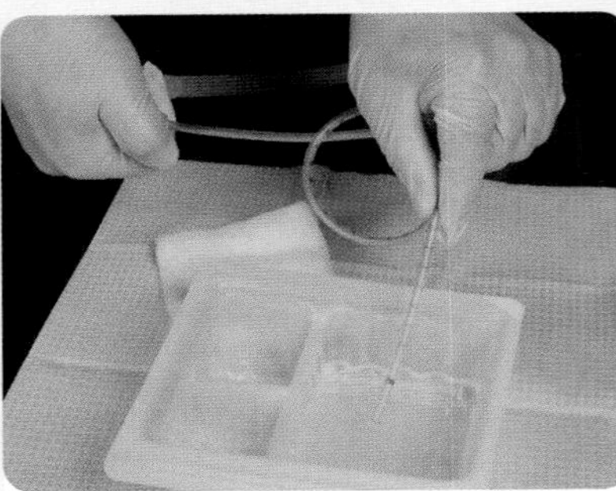

Step 2 Attach the catheter to negative pressure. Check the suction, and clear the catheter by drawing up a small amount of saline.

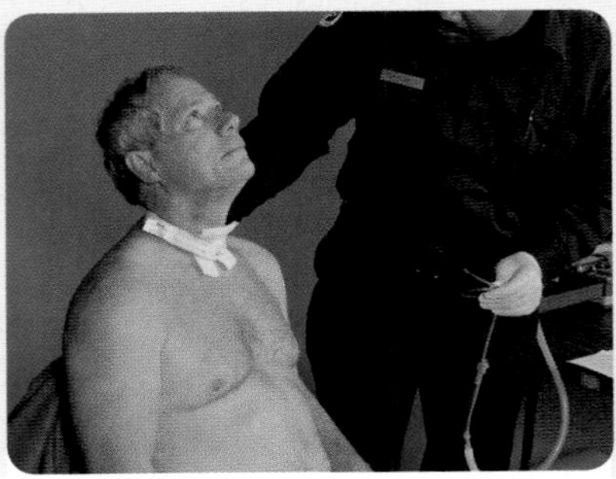

Step 3 Have the patient take a deep breath or preoxygenate him or her using the ventilator.

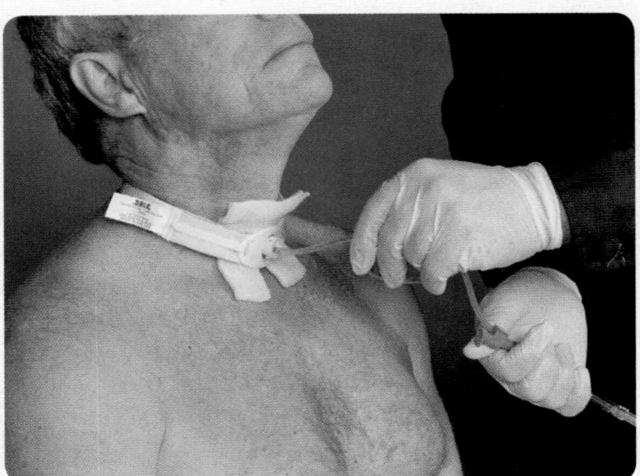

Step 4 Insert the catheter into the trachea without suction. Apply intermittent suction while removing the catheter. Repeat as necessary. Keep the patient well oxygenated during the procedure.

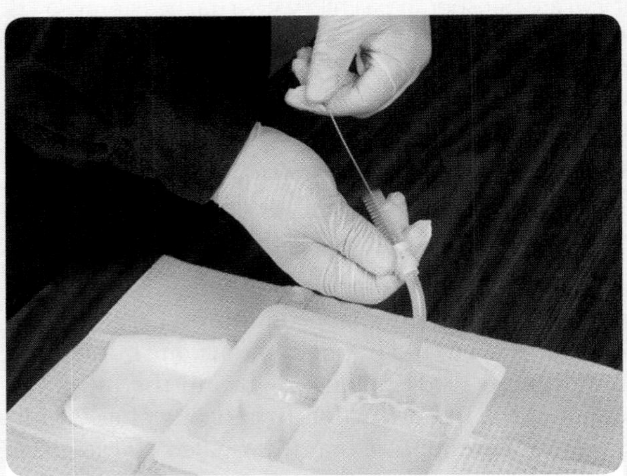

Step 5 Clean the inner cannula with the tracheostomy brush. Rinse, replace, and lock it into place. (Omit this step for a one-piece tracheostomy tube.) Remove your gloves, and wash your hands. Document the procedure and assessment.

▶ Mechanical Ventilators

A mechanical ventilator, also called a respirator, mechanically delivers air to the lungs Figure 38-9. Patients who require a mechanical ventilator at home cannot breathe without assistance. Patients requiring a mechanical ventilator may or may not have an underlying respiratory drive because of a congenital defect or a chronic lung disease process. Other patients may have a traumatic brain injury, muscular dystrophy, or another disease process that weakens their ability to breathe and requires a permanent tracheostomy and mechanical ventilator.

If a patient is using a ventilator when you arrive, then assess the patient's chest for synchronous movement with the ventilator. If you have any doubt about ventilator function, then do not be afraid to disconnect the ventilator and begin bag-mask ventilation. To do this, remove the mask from a bag-mask device and directly attach the bag and valve to the tracheostomy tube, which will allow you to ventilate directly through the tracheostomy. Remember, a patient with a tracheostomy does not breathe through his or her mouth and nose. Therefore, you cannot use a face mask or nasal cannula to treat the patient. A tracheostomy collar is an oxygen delivery device designed specifically for patients with tracheostomies. The collar covers the tracheostomy stoma and has a strap that goes around the neck. Tracheostomy collars are usually available in intensive care units, where many patients have tracheostomies, and may not be available in a prehospital setting. If you do not have a tracheostomy collar, then you can improvise by placing a face mask over the stoma Figure 38-10. Even though the mask is shaped to fit the face, you can usually achieve an adequate fit over the patient's neck by adjusting the strap.

Patients using home mechanical ventilators require assisted ventilation throughout transport. Remember that the patient's caregivers will know how the mechanical ventilator works and will be of great help to you in attaching the bag and valve from a bag-mask device to the tracheostomy tube in preparation for transport. Avoid adjusting home ventilator settings unless you are specifically credentialed to work with the particular device. Again, solicit the help of the patient, family, and caregivers.

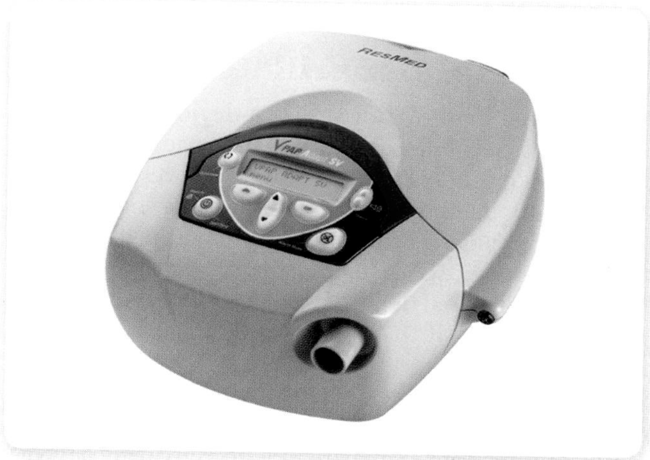

Figure 38-9 A home ventilator.

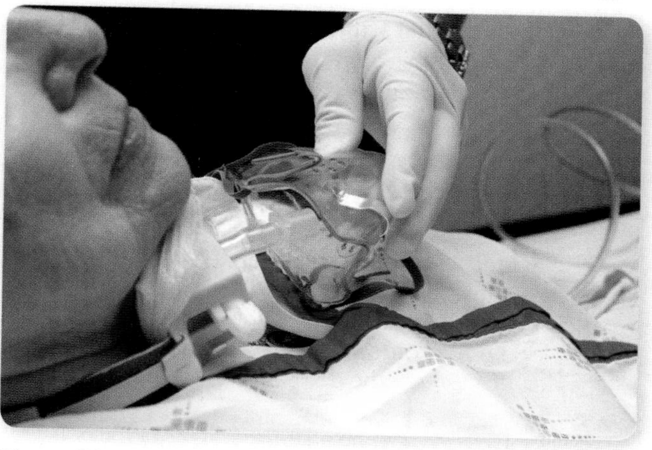

Figure 38-10 If you do not have a tracheostomy collar, then use a face mask instead.

▶ Apnea Monitors

When you care for infants with special challenges, you may come across an apnea monitor. The apnea monitor is typically used when an infant is born prematurely, has severe gastroesophageal reflux that causes choking episodes, has experienced an apparent life-threatening event, or if a family history of sudden infant death syndrome (SIDS) exists. Chapter 36, *Pediatric Emergencies*, discusses SIDS and apparent life-threatening events in detail. Because the central nervous system is not mature in pediatric patients with special challenges, the apnea monitor is used for 2 weeks to 2 months after birth to monitor the respiratory system. A typical episode of apnea may last only approximately 15 to 20 seconds, during periods of sleep. The apnea monitor is designed to sound an alarm if the infant experiences bradycardia or if an episode of apnea occurs.

The apnea monitor is attached with electrodes or a belt wrapped around the infant's chest or stomach. A pulse oximeter may also be used, which measures the oxygenation of the infant's hemoglobin. The apnea monitor will provide a pulse oximetry reading that will assist you in assessing the patient's respiratory status.

The parents or caregivers of pediatric patients with special challenges will be a useful resource to obtain a patient history and the events leading to the call for assistance. Parents and caregivers become very knowledgeable regarding the use of apnea monitors and may be able to provide you and your partner with a computerized printout to share with paramedics or emergency department (ED) personnel. If possible, take the apnea monitor to the receiving hospital with the pediatric patient so that it may be evaluated and any stored information may be retrieved for further analysis.

Words of Wisdom

False alarms are common with apnea monitors and may be caused by movement, loose lead wires, or improperly placed electrodes. When in doubt, follow your local EMS protocols and have the family contact the manufacturer of the device.

▶ Internal Cardiac Pacemakers

An internal cardiac pacemaker is a device implanted under the patient's skin to regulate the heart rate. These devices are typically placed on the nondominant side of the patient's chest so that normal activities are not hindered. In patients who are small or extremely thin, the device may be implanted in the abdomen. In some cases, the pacemaker may also include an automated implanted cardioverter-defibrillator, which monitors the patient's heart rhythm and is able detect and shock certain cardiac dysrhythmias.

Never place defibrillator paddles or pacing patches directly over the implanted device. When you obtain the patient's history during the patient assessment process, you may find it helpful to obtain specific information for the hospital staff, such as the type of cardiac pacemaker Table 38-2.

Table 38-2 Questions for Patients With Pacemakers or Implanted Defibrillators

Pacemakers
▪ What type of heart disorder do you have? ▪ How long has this device been implanted? ▪ What is your normal baseline rhythm and heart rate? ▪ Is your heart completely dependent on the pacemaker device?
Defibrillators
▪ At what heart rate will the defibrillator fire? ▪ How many times has the defibrillator shocked you?

▶ Left Ventricular Assist Devices

A left ventricular assist device (LVAD) is a special piece of medical equipment that takes over the function of one or both heart ventricles. These types of devices are either used as a bridge to heart transplantation while a donor heart is being located or as a permanent solution for patients who do not qualify for a transplant. In addition to the multiple LVAD devices available for adult patients with heart failure, there is one approved LVAD designed for children aged 5 to 16 years. It may be difficult to palpate a pulse in patients who use an LVAD. In such cases, assess perfusion by noting the level of consciousness, skin color, temperature, moisture, and blood pressure.

If you encounter a patient with an LVAD, you will primarily provide support measures and basic care while using the caregiver as a resource during transport. The patient should have a "go bag" that must always be transported with him or her. Risk factors associated with the implantation of an LVAD include excessive bleeding following the operation, infection, blood clots leading to strokes, and acute heart failure. Although medical equipment failure is rare in these cases, be prepared to provide cardiopulmonary resuscitation (CPR) if the situation arises. Keep in mind that the LVAD may be functioning in the absence of a palpable pulse. If you encounter a patient with this device, then contact medical control or follow your local protocols. Understand that CPR could dislodge the device or its connections. Notify paramedics as soon as possible so that other supportive measures may be initiated.

Words of Wisdom

The manufacturers of special equipment such as an LVAD often include a 1-800 number to call for information specific to patient care. Patients and family members typically carry identification cards with necessary phone numbers and may be able to share this information with you.

▶ External Defibrillator Vest

The external defibrillator vest is a device with built-in monitoring electrodes and defibrillation pads. It is worn by the patient under his or her clothing. The vest is attached to a monitor that provides alerts and voice prompts when it recognizes a dangerous rhythm and before it delivers a shock. The device uses high-energy shocks similar to an automated external defibrillator (AED), so avoid contact with the patient if the device warns that it is about to deliver a shock.

If the patient is in cardiac arrest, then the vest should remain in place while you perform CPR unless it interferes with compressions. Any patient who is wearing a device that has already delivered a shock should be transported to the hospital for further evaluation.

▶ Intra-Aortic Balloon Pumps

As an AEMT, you may assist with transport of patients being treated with an intra-aortic balloon pump (IABP) Figure 38-11. IABPs are used to decrease cardiac workload and augment perfusion in patients with cardiogenic shock, structural abnormalities in the heart, myocardial infarction, or following cardiac surgery. You would never be solely responsible for care of a patient with an IABP. It is conceivable, however, that you could accompany a critical care transport team or other health care provider who is responsible for managing the IABP during interfacility transport of a patient.

IABPs consist of a relatively large machine, connective tubing, monitor cables, and the balloon catheter itself. A cylindrical balloon is inserted through the femoral artery and placed in the aorta, just outside the heart. Tubing connects the balloon catheter to the machine. Monitor leads from the machine are connected to the patient. Movement of both the patient and IABP machine requires careful planning and coordination among members of the transport team.

The balloon is inflated and actively deflated at precise times during the cardiac cycle. During diastole (relaxation of the heart), the balloon inflates, pushing blood forward into systemic circulation. During systole (contraction of the heart), the balloon actively deflates, creating a brief vacuum, and reducing cardiac afterload. This process decreases myocardial oxygen demand, reduces cardiac workload, and improves systemic circulation.

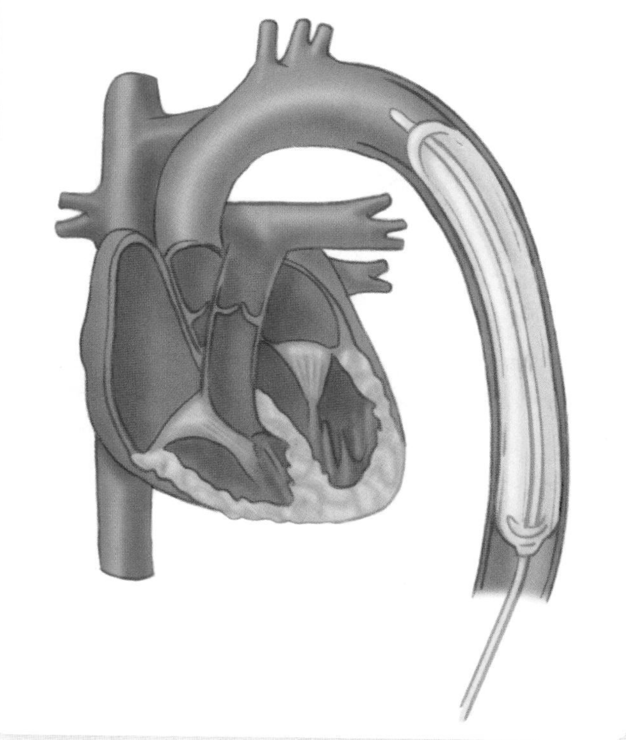

Figure 38-11 Intra-aortic balloon pump inflation.

Illustration from source material by Datascope Corp. and Maquet Cardiovascular. Used with permission.

The IABP is bulky and often difficult to move and secure in an ambulance. The transport team must use additional straps to prevent the machine from injuring the patient and/or providers in the event of an ambulance crash. The transport team also needs to take care when handling and securing the connective tubing between the machine and balloon catheter. Accidental removal of the balloon catheter often creates a life-threatening emergency for the patient.

▶ Central Venous Catheters

A central venous catheter, or central line—a venous access device with the tip of the catheter in the vena cava—is used for many types of home care patients, including patients receiving chemotherapy, long-term antibiotic therapy, pain management, total parenteral nutrition, high-concentration glucose solutions, and hemodialysis Figure 38-12. Central venous catheters are often located in the chest, upper arm, or subclavicular area.

These devices place the patient at increased risk for cardiovascular complications, including anticoagulation, embolus formation, stasis, air embolus, and obstructed or malfunctioning devices.

Problems associated with central venous catheters may include broken lines, infections around the lines, clotted lines, and bleeding around the line or from the tubing attached to the line. If bleeding occurs, then apply direct pressure to the tubing and provide prompt transport to the hospital.

Inspect and secure all external devices before moving the patient, especially when preparing for transport.

▶ Gastrostomy Tubes

Gastrostomy tubes are sometimes referred to as gastric tubes or G-tubes. A gastric tube may be placed when the patient cannot ingest fluids, food, or medications by mouth Figure 38-13. Tubes may be inserted through the nose or mouth into the stomach (using nasogastric or orogastric tubes).

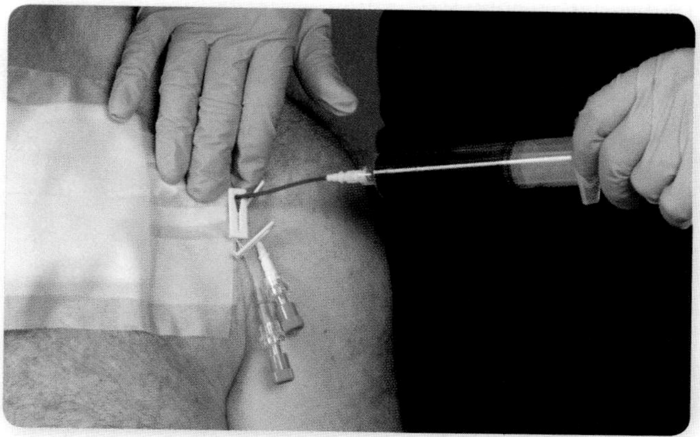

Figure 38-12 Patients who require frequent intravenous medications may have a central line in place.

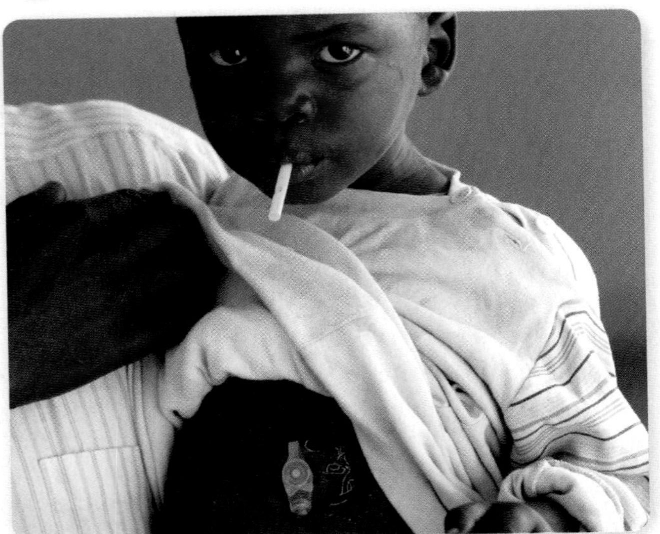

Figure 38-13 Gastric tubes may be placed through the skin into the stomach for children or adults who cannot adequately be fed by mouth.

In some cases, a gastric tube may be placed surgically through the abdominal wall. Gastric tubes are typically sutured in place and may become dislodged during the patient's normal daily activity. If such a situation arises, then immediately stop the flow of any fluids being infused through the tube. Assess the patient for signs or symptoms of bleeding into the stomach such as vague abdominal discomfort, nausea, vomiting (especially emesis with a "coffee-ground" appearance [old blood]), and blood in emesis.

Patients who have a gastric tube in place may still be at increased risk for aspiration. Always have suction readily available to clear any materials from the patient's mouth and prevent airway problems. Stop the flow of fluids if signs of aspiration are present. To minimize the risk of regurgitation and aspiration, transport the patient while sitting or lying on the right side with the head elevated 30 degrees. Give supplemental oxygen if the patient has any difficulty breathing.

Patients with diabetes who receive insulin and gastric tube feedings may develop hypoglycemia quickly if the gastric tube feedings are discontinued for any reason. Be alert for an altered mental status or a change in the baseline behavior of your patient. Unless the gastric tube is dysfunctional, dislodged, or partially dislodged, continue the tube feeding and transport the pump with you.

▶ Shunts

Some patients with chronic neurologic conditions may have shunts in place. For example, patients with hydrocephalus will have a shunt. In the case of hydrocephalus, **shunts** are tubes that extend from the brain down to the abdomen or heart to drain excess CSF that may accumulate around the brain.

A few different types of shunts exist, such as a ventricular peritoneum shunt and a ventricular atrium shunt. A ventricular peritoneum shunt drains excess fluid from the ventricles of the brain into the peritoneum of the abdomen. A ventricular atrium shunt drains excess fluid from the ventricles of the brain into the right atrium of the heart. These shunts keep pressure in the skull from building up.

During the assessment of a patient with a shunt, you will likely feel a device beneath the skin on the side of the head, behind the ear. The device is a fluid reservoir, and

YOU are the Provider — PART 4

Approximately 3 minutes from the hospital, you note that Gary is now fully awake and oriented to his normal status. You ask him about the events surrounding the seizure, but he states that he does not know. On your arrival at the ED, you turn over care to the awaiting staff.

Recording Time: 15 Minutes	
Respirations	20 breaths/min
Pulse	96 beats/min
Skin	Warm, dry, and pink
Blood pressure	124/86 mm Hg
Oxygen saturation (Spo_2)	99% on 15 L/min
Pupils	PERRLA

7. In which position should you transport this patient?
8. What are the most common causes of developmental disabilities?

the presence of the device should alert you to the possibility that the patient has an underlying shunt. Should the shunt become dysfunctional, the patient could be predisposed to respiratory arrest.

If a shunt becomes blocked or infected, then changes in mental status and respiratory arrest may occur. Infections of shunts may occur within the first 2 months after the insertion. A blocked shunt may also present as a medical emergency. If the shunt is unable to drain properly, then intracranial pressure may increase and the patient will experience an altered mental status and other signs of increased intracranial pressure.

The signs that a patient is in distress include bulging fontanelles (in infants), headache, projectile vomiting, altered mental status, irritability, high-pitched cry, fever, nausea, difficulty with coordination (walking), blurred vision, seizures, redness along the shunt track, bradycardia, and heart dysrhythmias. Emergency medical care includes airway management and artificial ventilation during transport.

▶ Vagus Nerve Stimulators

According to the Epilepsy Foundation, approximately 150,000 patients are diagnosed with epilepsy each year in the United States.[12] Vagus nerve stimulation is a form of treatment used for seizures that are not controlled with anti epileptic medications or if the patient is not a good candidate for brain surgery. Vagus nerve stimulators stimulate the vagus nerve at predetermined intervals to prevent seizure activity. These devices are used in conjunction with medication to reduce the frequency of seizures. They are not meant to replace medications and are not currently used in children under 12 years. Further studies are being done regarding the effectiveness for seizure disorders. The device, which is about the size of a silver dollar, is surgically implanted under the patient's skin. The stimulator can last for up to 6 years or until the battery runs out. If you encounter a patient with this device, then contact medical control or follow your local protocols.

▶ Colostomies, Ileostomies, and Urostomies

A **colostomy** is a surgical opening between the colon and the surface of the body for the purpose of providing drainage of the bowel. An **ileostomy** is a surgical opening between the ileum (part of the small intestine) and the surface of the body to provide drainage of the bowel. The surgical opening is referred to as a stoma. Feces are expelled and collected into a clear external bag or pouch, which is emptied or changed frequently.

If you encounter a patient with a colostomy or ileostomy bag, then assess for signs and symptoms of dehydration if the patient reports diarrhea or vomiting. The area around the stoma is prone to infection, so patients and caregivers must be diligent with daily hygiene. Signs of infection include redness, warm skin around the stoma, and tenderness with palpation over the colostomy or ileostomy site.

A **urostomy** is a surgical procedure which connects the urinary system to the surface of the skin, allowing urine to drain through a stoma in the abdominal wall instead of through the urethra. For example, a patient who has had his or her bladder removed due to cancer requires a urostomy.

Contact medical control, or follow your local protocols for the care of a patient with a colostomy, ileostomy, or urostomy bag.

Words of Wisdom

Signs of potential failure of a gastrointestinal or genitourinary device in the home care setting include abdominal pain or distention, decreased or absent bowel sounds, bladder distention, dysuria, and changes in urinary output or color.

Patient Assessment Guidelines

Interaction with the caregiver of a child or adult with special challenges will be an important part of the patient assessment process. The parents, caregivers, or home health care staff members have become experts on the illness or disability and are trained to use and troubleshoot problems with medical equipment on a daily basis. Assess the patient's baseline vital signs and note any allergies (eg, to medications or latex), medications, and other pertinent medical history. You must first determine the patient's normal baseline status before an assessment of the current condition can be made. It is often helpful to ask, "What is different today?"

Although a patient with special needs may not be able to communicate easily, even patients who cannot speak well or do not speak English may be able to say important words or phrases. Find out how much the patient can speak. Use short, simple questions and simple words whenever possible. Avoid difficult medical terms, and point to specific parts of the body as you ask questions.

Special Populations

A traumatic event can be especially frightening for patients with special needs, as well as challenging for the provider. Attempt to calm the patient; try to determine if he or she has sight, hearing, or communication problems that could affect assessment. If possible, have a caregiver present during any examination and for patient history.

Home Care

Home care occurs within a patient's home environment. Patients requiring home services represent a spectrum of special health care needs. Patients might be infants or older people, patients with chronic illnesses, or patients with developmental disabilities. Home care services are commonly needed among patients older than 65 years.

Services offered by home care agencies include, but are not limited to, meal delivery, house cleaning, laundry, yard maintenance, physical therapy, and personal care, including bathing and wound care. Oftentimes, EMS is called to a residence when a home care provider has found the patient injured or has recognized a change in the patient's health status. Home care personnel are an important resource for you when you are obtaining the patient's baseline health status and the history of the present illness or condition. Home care personnel are usually familiar with the patient's surroundings and can obtain any health care documentation or medications that need to be transported with the patient to the hospital.

Words of Wisdom

Prehospital providers often find it most difficult to work with patients who are in the acceptance stage of the dying process because the patient appears to have given up. Allow the patient to do as much as possible for himself or herself. Talk with the patient or caregiver so that you are aware of what the patient expects from your treatment.

Hospice Care and Terminally Ill Patients

Unfortunately, some illnesses cannot be cured. As health care providers, you and your team will often be called on to assist a patient who has a terminal illness. The patient may be receiving hospice care at a hospice facility or at home. Hospice care provides comfort care or palliative care (pain medications) during a person's last days. Comfort care and palliative care improve the patient's quality of life before death, allowing the patient to be with family and friends.

Terminally ill patients include patients with illnesses such as cancer, heart and lung failure, end-stage Alzheimer disease, and acquired immunodeficiency syndrome. Many family members who care for chronically ill patients are medically knowledgeable and are often your best source of information and care guidelines.

Terminally ill patients usually need only supportive care. The person may have a displaced urinary catheter or need intervention in a pain crisis. Because terminally ill patients may use a complex array of pain medications, transdermal patches, or self-administered pain management devices, you may need to consult medical direction for guidance in their care.

If you are called to a facility that provides hospice care, then you will need to follow your local protocols, the patient's wishes, or legal documents such as a do not resuscitate (DNR) order. Other legal documents that a terminally ill patient may have include a living will and a durable power of attorney, as discussed in Chapter 3, *Medical, Legal, and Ethical Issues*. Although these orders require you to withhold life-sustaining treatment in the event of cardiac or respiratory arrest, they do not mean that you should not give any treatment; patients should receive pain medication, supplemental oxygen therapy, nutrition, and hydration as needed based on assessment.

Even if a DNR order is in place, family members may not understand what to do and they may not be ready to face the death of a loved one. In such cases, obtain a thorough history and compassionately discuss the patient's wishes. Ask to review the DNR order, and contact medical control.

If you are called to a scene in which death is imminent, then the actions you take will have a lasting impact on the family. This is a time when compassion, understanding, and sensitivity are most needed. Some scenes may be chaotic. The family may be having a difficult time coping with the situation, and they may act out with anger and hostility. Treat everyone with compassion and understanding. The other members of your team may be able to separate the people present and speak with them individually to defuse intense emotions and restore order to the situation.

Ascertain the family's wishes about having the patient remain in the home versus transport to the hospital. If a family member requests to accompany the patient, then he or she should be allowed to do so. If the family wants the patient to remain at home, then this request should be honored provided it is in accordance with your local or state protocol.

Local protocols for handling the death of a patient vary, so learn your local or state regulations. The protocols identify whether the coroner needs to be called to report the death and, if so, who is responsible for contacting the coroner. Also determine whether a pronouncement of death is required and, if so, who is responsible for the determination.

Words of Wisdom

A terminally ill patient has the following rights:

- The right to know the truth
- The right to confidentiality and privacy
- The right to consent to treatment
- The right to determine the disposition of his or her body

Poverty and Homelessness

According to a US Bureau of the Census report, 14.8% of the US population lived in poverty in 2014.[13] People who live in poverty are unable to provide for all of their basic needs such as housing, food, child care, health insurance, and medication. An impoverished person or family may have housing but may go without food or medication to pay for that housing. Disease prevention strategies such as dental care, good nutrition, and exercise are likely absent, which increases the probability of disease in people who live in poverty.

Homelessness occurs when people are unable to acquire and/or maintain affordable housing. According to the National Alliance to End Homelessness, nearly 600,000 people experience homelessness on any given night in the United States.[14] The homeless population includes people with mental illnesses, prior brain trauma, survivors of domestic violence, people with addiction disorders, and impoverished families. You may be called to care for a person who has experienced sexual or physical assault, mental health emergencies, overdose, respiratory illness, heat- or cold-related illness, and wound or skin infections.

Part of your job as an AEMT is to be an advocate for patient rights and appropriate care. Your job is to provide emergency medical care and transport patients to the appropriate facility. Remember that under the Emergency Medical Treatment and Active Labor Act, all health care facilities *must* provide a medical assessment and required treatment, regardless of the patient's ability to pay. You can also be an advocate by becoming familiar with the social services resources within your community so you can refer patients to these lifelines.

The evolution of Mobile Integrated Healthcare and Community Paramedicine (MIH-CP) will benefit many patient populations, including patients with special challenges.[15] As EMS agencies around the country continue to implement these new positions, patients with low-acuity (nonemergency) conditions may be able to be assessed and treated on scene without transport. In addition, EMS roles may expand to include providing telephone advice to 9-1-1 callers, preventive care, chronic disease management, and postdischarge follow-up.

YOU are the Provider SUMMARY

1. What abnormalities are associated with Down syndrome?

Down syndrome is caused by a genetic chromosomal defect that can occur during fetal development. Known risk factors for Down syndrome include an increased maternal age and a family history of Down syndrome. A variety of abnormalities are associated with Down syndrome, including a round head with a flat occiput; an enlarged, protruding tongue; slanted and wide-set eyes; congenital heart defects; thyroid problems; vision and hearing problems, and instability of the cervical spine.

2. What type of medical complications may patients with Down syndrome experience?

Patients with Down syndrome are at an increased risk for medical complications including those that affect cardiovascular, sensory, endocrine, musculoskeletal, gastrointestinal, and hematologic systems, as well as neurologic development. Because people with Down syndrome often have large tongues and small oral and nasal cavities, insertion of advanced airways may be difficult. Patients may also have misalignment of teeth and other dental abnormalities. The enlarged tongue and dental anomalies can lead to speech abnormalities as well.

3. How should you interact with a patient with Down syndrome?

It is normal to feel somewhat uncomfortable when initiating contact with a patient with a disability. The best plan of action is to treat the patient as you would any other patient.

4. How should you incorporate the caregiver into your treatment?

Interaction with the caregiver of a patient with special needs is an important part of the patient assessment process. Always speak with the caregiver or family members; they have become experts on the illness or disability.

5. This patient has a central venous catheter already in place. Should you insert another IV line or use the central line?

In most areas, AEMTs are prohibited from using the already established central line. This prohibition exists largely because of the increased rate of infection when central lines are accessed by prehospital providers. The only time that you should manipulate a central line is when it becomes broken and bleeding occurs. If bleeding occurs, then apply direct pressure to the tubing and provide prompt transport to the hospital.

6. What is the purpose of the patient's gastrostomy tube?

The purpose of gastrostomy tubes are for the feeding of patients who cannot ingest fluids, food, or medication by mouth. Typically, these tubes are inserted through the nose or mouth and into the stomach. In some patients, a gastric tube may be placed surgically. Occasionally these tubes may become dislodged during daily activity. If this happens, then you should assess the patient for signs or symptoms of bleeding into the stomach such as vague abdominal discomfort, nausea, vomiting, and hematemesis.

YOU are the Provider SUMMARY (continued)

7. In which position should you transport this patient?

Transport this patient in the position of comfort. In the presence of a gastric tube, transport the patient while he or she is sitting or lying on the right side with the head elevated 30°. This position will minimize the chance of aspiration.

8. What are the most common causes of developmental disabilities?

A developmental disability may be caused by genetic factors, congenital infections, complications at birth, malnutrition, or environmental factors. Prenatal drug or alcohol use may also cause disability, as in fetal alcohol syndrome. Postnatal causes may include traumatic brain injury or poisoning (such as with lead or other toxins).

EMS Patient Care Report (PCR)					
Date: 7-17-18	**Incident No.:** 189433		**Nature of Call:** Seizure	**Location:** Shining Star Living	
Dispatched: 0915	**En Route:** 0917	**At Scene:** 0923	**Transport:** 0934	**At Hospital:** 0945	**In Service:** 0958

Patient Information	
Age: 37 **Sex:** M **Weight (in kg [lb]):** 80 kg (175 lb)	**Allergies:** Codeine, penicillin **Medications:** Phenytoin, fosphenytoin, lorazepam, amiodarone **Past Medical History:** Down syndrome, mental retardation, epilepsy **Chief Complaint:** Seizure activity

Vital Signs				
Time: 0924	**BP:** Not obtained	**Pulse:** Not obtained	**Respirations:** 12	**Spo_2:** Not obtained
Time: 0934	**BP:** 108/86	**Pulse:** 104	**Respirations:** 20	**Spo_2:** 99% on 15 L/min
Time: 0939	**BP:** 124/86	**Pulse:** 96	**Respirations:** 20	**Spo_2:** 99% on 15 L/min

EMS Treatment (circle all that apply)				
Oxygen @ 15 **L/min via (circle one):** **NC** **(NRM)** **Bag-mask device**		**Assisted Ventilation**	**Airway Adjunct**	**CPR**
Defibrillation	**Bleeding Control**	**Bandaging**	**Splinting**	**Other:**

Narrative
EMS dispatched to above location for seizure. Upon arrival, directed to dining room for patient well known to EMS, who had experienced a seizure. Per caregiver, patient had tonic-clonic seizure lasting approximately 90 seconds, ending approximately 2 minutes before our arrival. Caregiver states that patient has Down syndrome and epilepsy. She also states that he has decreased mental capacity and has a G-tube and central line in place. Physical exam of the patient reveals postictal state with ABCs intact. Oxygen via nonrebreathing mask given at 15 L/min. Patient placed on stretcher, secured, and loaded into ambulance. Transport on nonemergency basis to ED. En route: Vitals as above. 20-gauge saline lock established to right forearm. Approximately 3 minutes from ED, patient is alert and oriented to normal status. When asked about events, pt states, "I don't know." Upon arrival, care and report given to staff without incident.**End of report**

Prep Kit

▶ Ready for Review

- As medicine and medical technology continue to improve, the number of children and adults living with chronic diseases or injuries continues to grow. Assess and care for patients with special needs in the same manner as all other patients.
- You may find children and adults who are living at home who depend on mechanical ventilators, intravenous pumps, or other medical devices to maintain their lives.
- Developmental disability is caused by insufficient development of the brain, resulting in the inability to learn and socially adapt at a normal developmental rate.
- Developmental disabilities include autism spectrum disorder and Down syndrome.
- A patient may have a sensory disability, such as a visual or hearing impairment. Look for signs, such as the presence of eyeglasses, a service animal, hearing aids, or failure to respond to questions.
- Cerebral palsy is a physical disability associated with other conditions such as visual and hearing impairments, difficulty communicating, epilepsy, and intellectual disabilities. Patients may also have an unsteady gait and may require the assistance of a wheelchair or walker.
- Cystic fibrosis is a genetic physical disability characterized by increased production of mucus in the lungs and digestive tract. Pulmonary manifestations include pneumonia, pneumothorax, cough, respiratory distress, and respiratory failure.
- Patients with multiple sclerosis experience an incurable, degenerative breakdown of the central nervous system.
- Muscular dystrophy is a genetic disease characterized by the slow, progressive degeneration of muscle fibers.
- Patients with spina bifida will have either partial or full paralysis of the lower extremities, loss of bowel and bladder control, and an extreme allergy to latex products.
- Several types of paralysis exist, including hemiplegia, paraplegia, and quadriplegia. Paralysis may be caused by cerebrovascular accident (stroke), trauma, or birth defects.
- Patients with obesity may be embarrassed by their condition or fearful of ridicule. If transport is necessary, then plan early for extra help. Identify the easiest and safest exit.
- Patients who depend on home automatic ventilators or who have chronic pulmonary medical conditions may breathe through a tracheostomy tube.
- Patients who require a mechanical ventilator at home cannot breathe without assistance. If the ventilator malfunctions, then disconnect the mechanical ventilator and begin ventilations with a tracheostomy collar or by placing a bag-mask device over the stoma.
- Certain infants may require an apnea monitor. The apnea monitor is designed to sound an alarm if the infant experiences bradycardia or if apnea occurs.
- An internal cardiac pacemaker is a device implanted under the patient's skin to regulate the heart rate.
- A left ventricular assist device (LVAD) is special medical equipment that takes over the function of one or both heart ventricles. LVADs are used as either a bridge to transplantation while a donor heart is being located or as a permanent solution for patients who do not qualify for a transplant.
- An external defibrillator vest provides alerts and voice prompts when it recognizes a dangerous rhythm and before it delivers a shock.
- Intra-aortic balloon pumps decrease cardiac workload and augment perfusion.
- A central venous catheter is used for many types of home care patients, including patients receiving chemotherapy, long-term antibiotic therapy or pain management, total parenteral nutrition, high-concentration glucose solutions, and hemodialysis.
- Gastrostomy tubes are placed directly into the stomach for feeding in patients who cannot ingest fluids, food, or medication by mouth. These tubes may be inserted through the nose or mouth or placed through the abdominal wall surgically.
- Hydrocephalus shunts are tubes that extend from the brain to the abdomen or heart to drain excess cerebrospinal fluid that may accumulate around the brain.
- A colostomy or ileostomy is a surgical procedure that creates an opening from the small or large intestine to the surface of the body to eliminate waste products. Feces are expelled and collected into a clear external bag or pouch. A urostomy allows for the elimination of urine.
- You and your team may be called on to assist a patient who is terminally ill. Terminally ill patients may be in a hospice facility or at home.
- All health care facilities *must* provide a medical assessment and required treatment, regardless of the patient's ability to pay under the Emergency Medical Treatment and Active Labor Act.

Prep Kit *(continued)*

▶ Vital Vocabulary

autism spectrum disorder (ASD) A group of complex disorders of brain development, characterized by impairment of social interaction; may include severe behavioral problems, repetitive motor activities, and impairment in verbal and nonverbal skills.

bariatrics The study of the causes, prevention, and treatment of obesity.

cerebral palsy A group of disorders characterized by poorly controlled body movement.

colostomy The surgical procedure to create an opening (stoma) between the colon and the surface of the body to provide drainage of the bowel.

conductive hearing loss Hearing loss caused by a faulty transmission of sound waves.

cystic fibrosis (CF) A genetic disorder that is characterized by increased production of mucus in the lungs and digestive system; also called mucoviscidosis.

developmental disability Insufficient development of the brain, resulting in some level of dysfunction or impairment.

Down syndrome A genetic chromosomal defect that can occur during fetal development and that results in intellectual impairment and certain physical characteristics, such as a round head with a flat occiput and slanted, wide-set eyes.

dysphagia Difficulty swallowing.

hemiplegia Paralysis of one side of the body, possibly from a stroke or head injury.

ileostomy The procedure to create an opening (stoma) between the ileum (part of the small intestine) and the surface of the body to provide drainage of the bowel.

laryngectomy A surgical procedure in which the larynx is removed.

multiple sclerosis (MS) A severe, incurable degenerative disorder involving the central nervous system (brain and spinal cord).

muscular dystrophy A category of incurable genetic diseases that cause a slow, progressive degeneration of the muscle fibers.

obesity A complex condition in which a person has an excessive amount of body fat; the result of an imbalance between calories consumed and calories used.

paraplegia Paralysis of the lower part of the body, possibly from thoracic or lumbar spinal injury or spina bifida.

quadriplegia Paralysis of all four extremities and the trunk, possibly from a cervical spine injury.

sensorineural deafness A permanent lack of hearing caused by a lesion or damage of the inner ear.

shunts In cases of hydrocephalus, the tubes that drain excess cerebrospinal fluid from the brain to another part of the body outside of the brain, such as the abdomen; lowers pressure in the brain.

spina bifida A development defect in which a portion of the spinal cord or meninges may protrude outside of the vertebrae and possibly even outside of the body, usually at the lower third of the spine in the lumbar area; also called myelomeningocele.

stoma A surgical opening through the skin and into an organ or other structure, such as into the trachea.

tracheostomy tube A plastic tube used to facilitate breathing. The tube is placed within the tracheostomy site (stoma).

urostomy The procedure to create an opening (stoma) between the urinary system and the surface of the skin, allowing urine to drain through a stoma in the abdominal wall instead of through the urethra.

▶ References

1. Autism spectrum disorder: data and statistics. Centers for Disease Control and Prevention website. http://www.cdc.gov/ncbddd/autism/data.html. Accessed July 14, 2016.
2. Birth defects: Down syndrome: data and statistics. Centers for Disease Control and Prevention website. http://www.cdc.gov/ncbddd/birthdefects/down syndrome/data.html. Accessed July 14, 2016.
3. Facts about Down syndrome. National Association for Down syndrome website. http://www.cdc.gov/ncbddd/birthdefects/downsyndrome.html. Accessed July 14, 2016.
4. How does cerebral palsy affect people? Cerebral Palsy Alliance. https://www.cerebralpalsy.org.au/what-is-cerebral-palsy/how-cerebral-palsy-affects-people/. Accessed November 17, 2016.
5. Wheless JW, Sirven JI. When it's more than just seizures. Epilepsy Foundation website. http://www.epilepsy.com/learn/seizures-youth/about-kids/when-its-more-just-seizures. Accessed August 31, 2016.
6. Multiple sclerosis: hope through research. National Institute for Neurologic Disorders and Stroke website. http://www.ninds.nih.gov/disorders/multiple_sclerosis/detail_multiple_sclerosis.htm. Accessed July 14, 2016.
7. Muscular Dystrophy: hope through research. National Institute of Neurologic Disorders and

Prep Kit *(continued)*

Stroke website. http://www.ninds.nih.gov/disorders/md/detail_md.htm. Accessed July 14, 2016.

8. Muscular Dystrophy, MD STARnet data and statistics. Centers for Disease Control and Prevention website. http://www.cdc.gov/ncbddd/musculardystrophy/data.html. Accessed July 14, 2016.
9. Birth defects: data and statistics. Centers for Disease Control and Prevention website. http://www.cdc.gov/ncbddd/birthdefects/data.html. Accessed July 14, 2016.
10. Sgouros S. Spina bifida, hydrocephalus, and shunts. Medscape website. http://emedicine.medscape.com/article/937979-overview. Updated October 12, 2015. Accessed July 14, 2016.
11. Mayo Clinic Staff. Diseases and conditions: obesity. Mayo Clinic website. http://www.mayoclinic.org/diseases-conditions/obesity/basics/symptoms/con-20014834. Updated July 10, 2015. Accessed July 14, 2016.
12. Shafer PO. Epilepsy statistics. Epilepsy Foundation website. http://www.epilepsy.com/learn/epilepsy-statistics. Accessed July 14, 2016.
13. Income, poverty and health insurance coverage in the United States: 2014 [news release]. Suitland, MD: United States Census Bureau; September 16, 2015. http://census.gov/newsroom/press-releases/2015/cb15-157.html. Accessed July 14, 2016.
14. Snapshot of homelessness. National Alliance to End Homelessness website. http://www.endhomelessness.org/pages/snapshot_of_homelessness. Accessed July 14, 2016.
15. What is MIH-CP? National Association of Emergency Medical Technicians website. http://www.naemt.org/MIH-CP/WhatisMIH-CP.aspx. Accessed July 14, 2016.

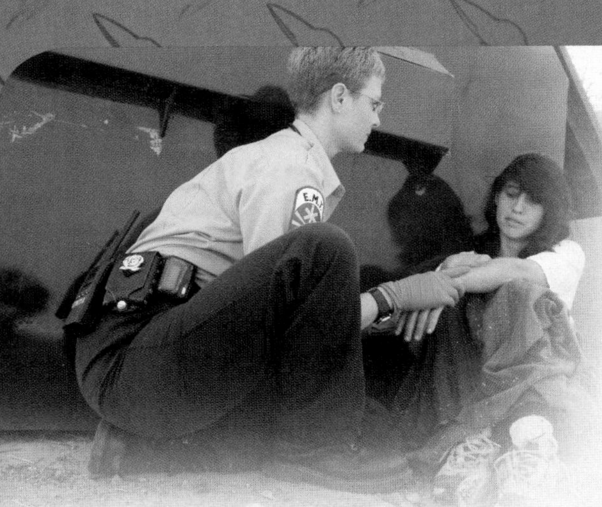

Assessment *in Action*

Your ambulance is dispatched to a local residence for a woman with shortness of breath. You recognize the address and know this patient has a history of cerebral palsy. She is a long-term, ventilator-dependent patient with a tracheostomy tube in place.

1. When you treat a patient with a tracheostomy, the DOPE mnemonic can help you remember the possible causes of an airway obstruction and correct the problem. The *D* in DOPE stands for all of the following EXCEPT:

A. dirty tube.
B. dislodged tube.
C. damaged tube.
D. displaced tube.

2. After taking standard precautions and performing a scene size-up, how should you begin your assessment?

A. Begin bag-mask ventilation.
B. Adjust the ventilator settings.
C. Call for paramedic backup.
D. Note whether the patient's chest has synchronous movement with the ventilator.

Assessment *in Action* *(continued)*

3. A tracheostomy may be temporary or permanent and pass from the neck directly into the:

A. oropharynx.
B. esophagus.
C. major airways.
D. terminal airways.

4. If her tracheostomy is plugged, then what is the best way to ventilate this patient?

A. Perform mouth-to-stoma ventilation.
B. Deflate the cuff, cover the nose and mouth with a mask, and use the bag-mask device.
C. Clean the tube, reinsert it, and coach the patient.
D. Ventilation of a patient with a tracheostomy is not possible in the prehospital environment.

5. Which of the following factors is NOT a common cause of cerebral palsy?

A. Congenital heart defect
B. Infection, such as meningitis
C. Developmental brain defects in utero
D. Traumatic brain injury at birth

6. Patients with cerebral palsy who have the ability to walk may have an ataxic or unsteady gait and are prone to:

A. fractures.
B. vertigo.
C. visual disturbances.
D. falls.

7. The airway of patients with cerebral palsy should be closely monitored because the patient may have increased production of secretions and ___________, requiring aggressive suctioning to clear the airway.

A. dysarthria
B. dysphagia
C. dysphonia
D. dysplasia

8. Autism is ______ times greater in ______ and is usually diagnosed by 3 years of age.

A. 2, females
B. 2, males
C. 5, females
D. 5, males

9. You arrive on scene to find a patient with severe obesity who needs to be transported. He is too large for you and your partner to lift. How will you handle this situation?

10. Intellectual disability results in the inability to learn and socially adapt at a normal developmental rate. What are some of the causes of an intellectual disability?

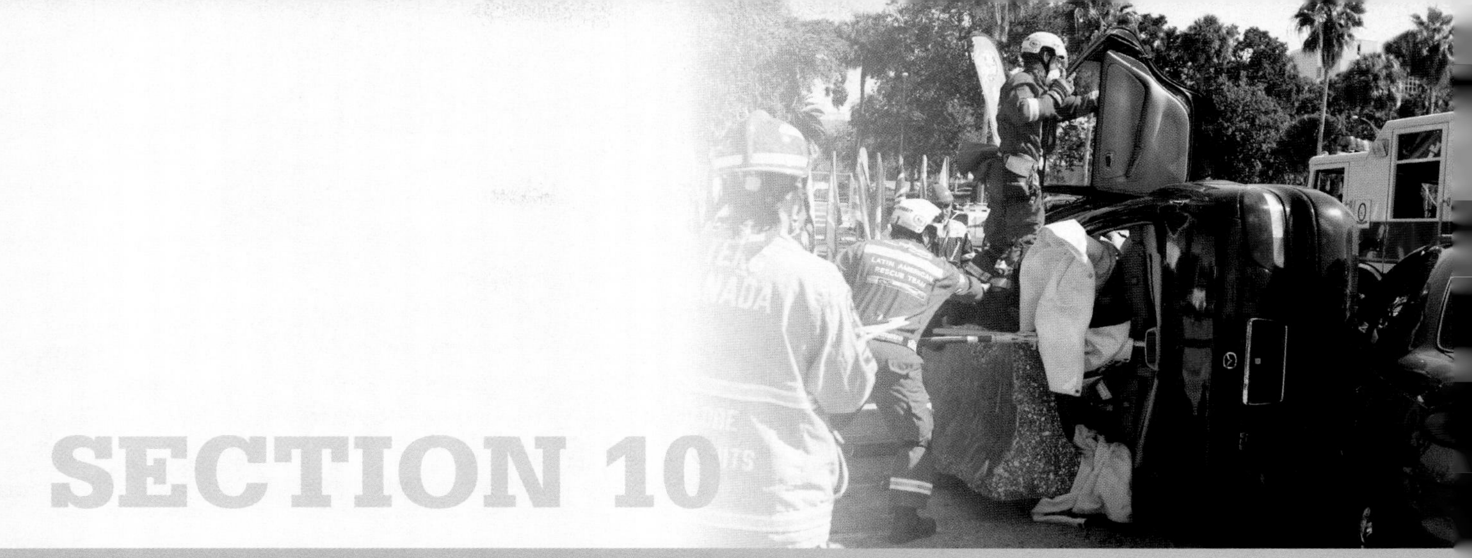

SECTION 10

EMS Operations

CHAPTER 39

Transport Operations

National EMS Education Standard Competencies

EMS Operations

Knowledge of operational roles and responsibilities to ensure patient, public, and personnel safety.

Principles of Safely Operating a Ground Ambulance

- Risks and responsibilities of emergency response (pp 1617-1618, 1623-1638)
- Risks and responsibilities of transport (pp 1627-1628, 1630-1638)

Air Medical

- Safe air medical operations (pp 1638-1643)
- Criteria for utilizing air medical response (pp 1639-1640)

Medicine

Applies fundamental knowledge to provide basic and selected advanced emergency care and transportation based on assessment findings for an acutely ill patient.

Infectious Diseases

Awareness of

- A patient who may have an infectious disease (p 1629)
- How to decontaminate equipment after treating a patient (pp 1629-1630)

Assessment and management of

- How to decontaminate the ambulance and equipment after treating a patient (pp 1629-1630)

Knowledge Objectives

1. Describe the nine phases of an ambulance call, including examples of key tasks that advanced emergency medical technicians (AEMTs) perform during each phase. (pp 1617-1630)
2. Describe the medical equipment carried on an ambulance, including examples of supplies that are included in each main category of the ambulance equipment checklist. (pp 1617-1622)
3. Provide examples of the safety and operations equipment carried on an ambulance, including how each item might be used by AEMTs in an emergency. (pp 1623-1624)
4. Explain the importance of performing regular vehicle inspections. (pp 1623-1624)
5. List the specific parts of an ambulance that should be inspected daily. (pp 1623-1624)
6. Describe the minimum information that should be gathered by the emergency medical services (EMS) dispatcher for every emergency call. (pp 1624-1625)
7. Provide examples of some high-risk situations and hazards that may affect the operation of the ambulance and the safety of its passengers during both pretransport and transport. (pp 1625-1627)
8. Discuss specific considerations that are required for ensuring scene safety, including personal safety, patient safety, and traffic control. (pp 1625-1627)
9. Describe the key elements related to patient information that must be included in the patient care report upon patient delivery to the hospital. (p 1628)
10. Summarize the tasks that must be completed by AEMTs at the completion of an ambulance call. (pp 1628-1630)
11. Define the terms cleaning, disinfection, high-level disinfection, and sterilization. (p 1629)
12. Discuss the guidelines for driving an ambulance safely and defensively, including key steps EMS personnel can take to improve safety while en route to the scene, the hospital, and the station. (pp 1630-1638)
13. Describe the elements that dictate the use of emergency warning lights and siren to the scene and to the hospital and the factors required to perform a risk-benefit analysis regarding the use of these devices. (pp 1632-1633)
14. Give examples of the specific, limited privileges that are provided to emergency vehicle drivers by most state laws and regulations. (p 1637)
15. Explain why using police escorts and crossing intersections pose additional risks to EMS

personnel during transport, including the special considerations related to each. (pp 1637-1638)

16. Describe the capabilities, protocols, and methods for air medical operations. (pp 1638-1639)
17. Describe key scene safety considerations when preparing for the medical evacuation of a patient by helicopter, including establishing a landing zone, mitigating onsite hazards, and approaching the aircraft. (pp 1639-1643)

Skills Objectives

1. Demonstrate how to perform a daily inspection of an ambulance. (pp 1623-1624)
2. Demonstrate how to clean and disinfect the ambulance and equipment during the postrun phase. (pp 1629-1630)
3. Demonstrate how to use defensive ambulance driving techniques. (pp 1630-1638)
4. Demonstrate how to operate safely around an air ambulance. (pp 1641-1643)

Introduction

During the late 1700s, Napoleon Bonaparte commissioned one of the most advanced professional emergency medical patient care systems in the world. At that time, horse-drawn ambulances were already in use in major cities throughout the United States **Figure 39-1**. American hospitals initiated professional ambulance services during the late 1860s. Ambulance attendants traveled with limited medical supplies, including brandy, a few tourniquets, assorted bandages and sponges, basic splinting materials, and blankets.

Today's ambulances have come a long way since the first horse-drawn ambulances of the 1700s. Modern ambulances are stocked with standard medical supplies. Many are equipped with state-of-the-art technology, including defibrillators and monitors that can transmit information directly to the emergency department (ED), blood and oxygen testing equipment, automatic ventilators, automated cardiopulmonary resuscitation (CPR) machines, global positioning systems (GPS), mobile data terminals (MDTs), and computer-aided dispatch consoles. Even when you follow all safety guidelines, today's emphasis on technology places you in great danger while driving to calls. Although technology can aid in tasks such as directing the route and mode of response of the ambulance, it is also distracting. Therefore, the use of technology potentially increases your risk for crashes.

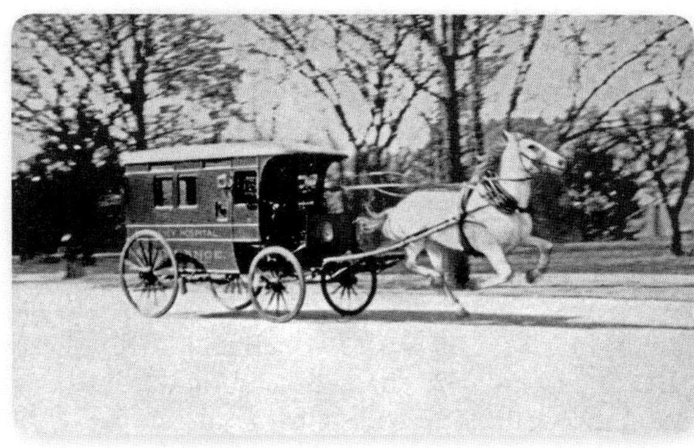

Figure 39-1 Horse-drawn ambulances were used in major cities throughout the United States beginning in the late 1700s.

This chapter discusses ambulance design and how to equip and maintain an ambulance. It focuses on the techniques and judgment that you will need to learn to drive an ambulance or ambulance service vehicle, which include parking considerations, emergency vehicle control and operation, the effects of weather on driving, and common hazards that are encountered while driving an ambulance. Finally, it describes how to work safely with air ambulances.

YOU are the Provider — PART 1

At 2100 hours, your ambulance is dispatched to a standby for a structure fire with possible entrapment. En route to the call, you note that your partner is driving aggressively through city traffic and motorists are slamming on their brakes in front of you. To avoid causing a collision, you advise him to leave more room between the ambulance and other vehicles you are approaching. He slows down and you arrive on scene 5 minutes after you were dispatched.

1. What are the nine phases of an ambulance call?
2. Which of the nine phases of an ambulance call is the most important?
3. What are some potential distractions that may be found inside of the ambulance?

> **Words of Wisdom**
>
> Anything can be a distraction while driving. It is imperative that you work with your partner to eliminate the need for the driver to take his or her attention off the road. For example, the provider in the passenger seat should operate the GPS so the driver can focus on driving.

Emergency Vehicle Design

An **ambulance** is a specialized vehicle that is used for treating and transporting sick and injured patients to a hospital. The first motor-powered ambulance was introduced in the late 1800s. For many decades after that, a hearse was the vehicle that was most often used as an ambulance, because it was the only vehicle with room enough for a person to lie down. Few supplies were carried onboard, and little space was available for attendants.

The hearse-ambulance has gone the way of its horse-drawn predecessor. Modern ambulances are designed according to strict government regulations based on the National Fire Protection Association's *Standard for Automotive Ambulances,* otherwise known as NFPA 1917.[1] The standards themselves are based in large part on suggestions from the ambulance industry, including emergency medical services (EMS) personnel. One of the most significant developments in ambulance design has been the enlargement of the patient compartment. Another development is the use of specialized **first-responder vehicles**, which allow firefighters, law enforcement officers, and other providers to respond initially to the scene with EMS equipment and to treat the sick and injured until an ambulance arrives.

The modern ambulance is a vehicle for emergency medical care that has the following features:

- A driver's compartment (cab)
- A patient compartment that can accommodate two EMS providers and usually two supine patients (one patient on the stretcher, and one patient on the bench or area designed with swivel seats to accommodate a long backboard) positioned so at least one of the patients can receive CPR during transport
- Equipment and supplies used to provide emergency medical care at the scene and during transport, to safeguard personnel and patients from hazardous conditions, and to carry out basic extrication procedures
- Two-way radio communications so ambulance personnel can speak with the dispatcher, the hospital, public safety authorities, and online medical control
- Design and construction that ensure maximum safety and comfort. For example, the **chassis** is the structural framework of the ambulance.

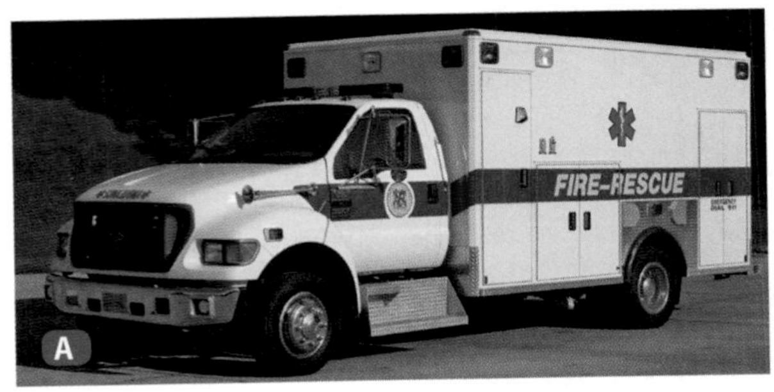

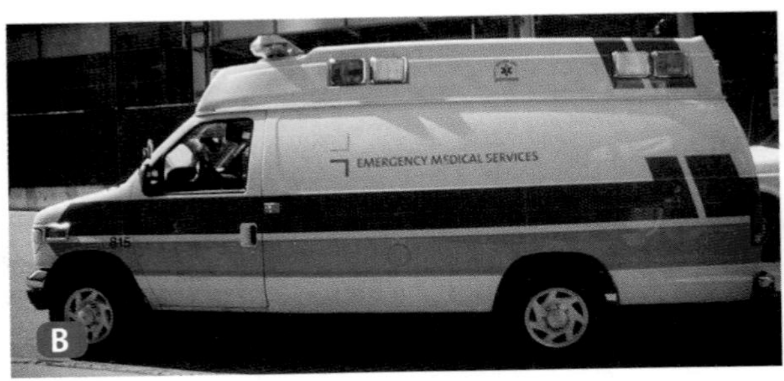

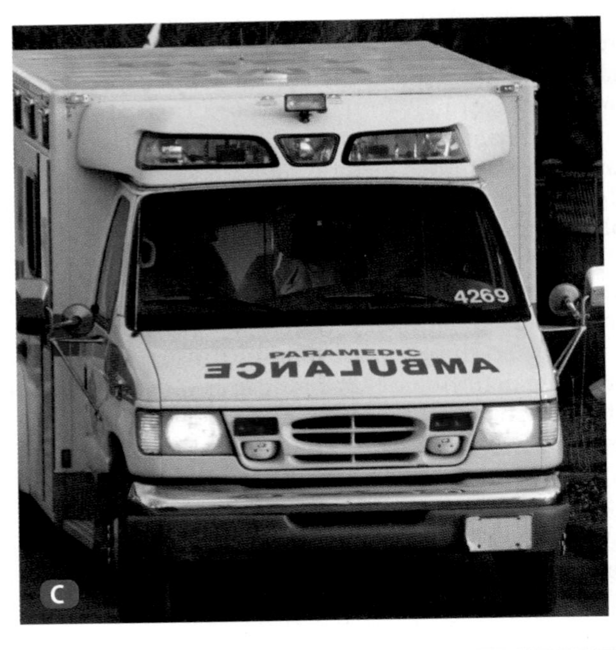

Figure 39-2 A. The conventional, truck cab-chassis has a modular ambulance body that can be transferred to a newer chassis (type I). **B.** The standard van ambulance has a forward-control integral cab body (type II). **C.** The specialty van ambulance has a cab that is mounted on a cutaway van chassis (type III).

A: © Jones & Bartlett Learning. Courtesy of MIEMSS; B: Courtesy of Captain David Jackson, Saginaw Township Fire Department; C: © Kevin Norris/Shutterstock.

Each state establishes its own standards for licensing or certifying ambulances; however, most states use the federal specifications (NFPA 1917) that cover three types of basic ambulance designs **Figure 39-2** **Table 39-1**.

Table 39-1 Basic Ambulance Designs

Type I	Conventional, truck cab-chassis with a modular ambulance body that can be transferred to a newer chassis as needed
Type II	Standard van, forward-control integral cab-body ambulance
Type III	Specialty van cab with a modular ambulance body that is mounted on a cutaway van chassis

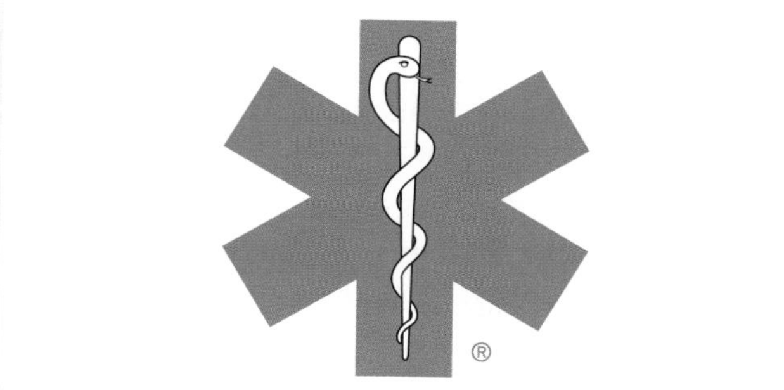

Figure 39-3 The Star of Life.

Courtesy of National Highway Traffic Safety Administration.

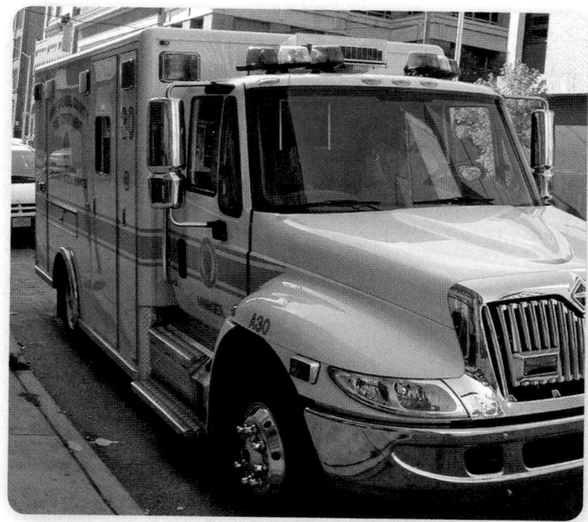

Figure 39-4 Emergency warning lights and public address systems are necessary on licensed or certified ambulances.

The six-pointed **Star of Life** emblem Figure 39-3 identifies vehicles as ambulances. It is often affixed to the sides, rear, and roof of the ambulance. Local or state regulatory authorities determine what emblems may be displayed on the side of an ambulance. Figure 39-4 illustrates some of the required features of a licensed or certified ambulance.

Table 39-2 Phases of an Ambulance Call

1. Preparation for the call
2. Dispatch
3. En route to the scene
4. Arrival at the scene
5. Transfer of the patient to the ambulance
6. En route to the receiving facility (transport)
7. Arrival at the receiving facility (delivery)
8. En route to the station
9. Postrun

Phases of an Ambulance Call

An ambulance call has three main phases divided as follows: prior to the scene (preparation, dispatch, en route); at the scene (arrival at the scene, transfer of patient to ambulance, transport to receiving facility); and after the scene (arrival at receiving facility, en route to station, postrun). These are shown in Table 39-2. These nine phases address the ambulance and its team, and their roles in a response to a medical emergency. The details of patient care are not included in these nine phases.

Preparation for the Call

An important part of preparing for the call is to ensure that equipment and supplies are in the proper place and ready for use and that the ambulance is in good working order with adequate fluid levels, fuel, and tire pressure. Some services have special personnel to stock and clean the ambulances. Items that are missing or that do not work are of no use to you or the patient. Furthermore, many EMS items have never been rigorously tested under field conditions and could turn out to be expensive mistakes. For this reason, new equipment should be placed on an ambulance only after approval by the medical director. Additionally, you must receive proper instruction on the use and care of any new piece of equipment before using it in the field. As a general rule, the more complex a piece of equipment is and the harder it is to learn to use, the more likely it is to malfunction during an emergency.

Equipment and supplies should be durable and, to the extent possible, standardized. This makes it easy to quickly exchange equipment with other ambulances or with the ED, thus, saving time during patient transfer.

Store equipment and supplies in the ambulance according to how urgently and how often they are used Figure 39-5. Give priority to items that are needed to care for life-threatening conditions, including equipment

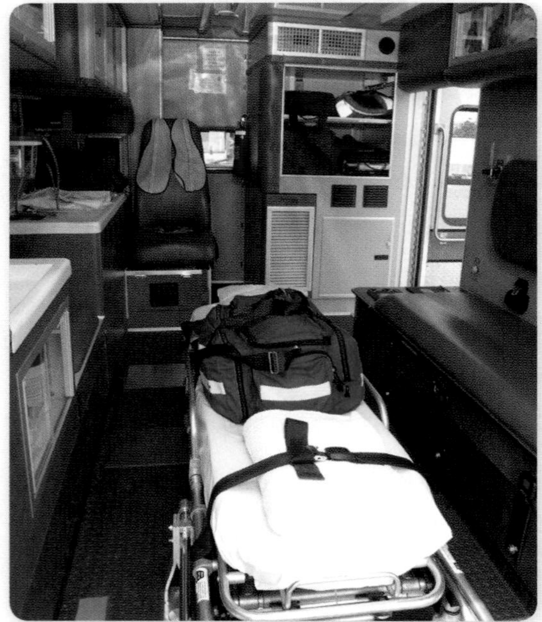

Figure 39-5 Store equipment and supplies in the ambulance according to how urgently and how often they are used.

for airway management, artificial ventilation, and oxygen delivery. Place these items within easy reach of the head of the primary stretcher. Place items for cardiac care, control of external bleeding, and monitoring of blood pressure at the side of the stretcher. Make sure batteries are fresh and equipment is functioning properly. For example, the most common cause of a malfunctioning automatic external defibrillator (AED) is a dead battery.

Storage cabinets and kits should open easily. They should also close securely so they do not fly open while the ambulance is in motion. Cabinet doors and drawers should be transparent so you can quickly identify the contents inside; if they are not transparent, then clearly label each storage container.

Medical Equipment

As an advanced emergency medical technician (AEMT), you have access to a large variety of medical equipment and supplies, far more than can be described here. Certain items on the ambulance must be available at all times, as dictated by state and jurisdictional requirements.

Basic Supplies. Table 39-3 lists the common supplies carried on ambulances. These supplies include basic items such as disposable gloves and sharps containers, airway and ventilation equipment, basic wound care supplies, splinting supplies, childbirth supplies, an AED, patient transfer equipment, medications, and other supplies such as a snakebite kit or regional supplies.

Airway and Ventilation Equipment. The ambulance should carry the following equipment for airway management:

- Oropharyngeal airways for adults, children, and infants
- Nasopharyngeal airways for adults and children
- Equipment for advanced airway procedures, if your service is authorized by state regulations and the medical director to perform these

It is important that the ambulance carry two portable artificial ventilation devices that operate independently of an oxygen supply: one for use in the ambulance and

Table 39-3 Ambulance Equipment Checklist

Basic Supplies
Pillows and pillowcases
Sterile sheets
Blankets
Towels
Disposable emesis bags or basins
Boxes of disposable tissue
Bedpan (optional)
Urinals (one each for men and women; optional)
Blood pressure cuffs (pediatric, adult, large adult)
Stethoscope
Disposable drinking cups
Unbreakable container of water
Wet wipes
Chemical cold/hot packs
Sterile irrigation fluid
Restraining devices
Plastic bags for waste or severed parts
Hypoallergenic nitrile, vinyl, or other disposable hypoallergenic gloves (various sizes)
Sharps container
Set of hearing protectors
Airway and Ventilation Equipment
Infection control kits (goggles, masks, waterproof gowns)
Oropharyngeal airways and nasopharyngeal airways of various sizes

Table 39-3 Ambulance Equipment Checklist *(continued)*

Advanced airway supplies, if local protocol permits (laryngeal mask airway, Combitube, King airways), with secondary placement confirmation devices
Bag-mask devices (adult, child, and infant)
Mounted suction unit and a portable suction unit
Assorted oxygen delivery devices (adult and pediatric)
Oxygen supply units (both portable and installed)
Disposable humidifier (for mounted oxygen system)
Basic Wound Care Supplies
Trauma shears
Sterile sheets
Sterile burn sheets
Adhesive tape in several widths
Self-adhering, soft roller bandages, 4 in. × 5 yd (10 cm × 5 m)
Self-adhering, soft roller bandages, 2 in. × 5 yd (5 cm × 5 m)
Sterile dressings, gauze, 4 in. × 4 in. (10 cm × 10 cm)
Sterile dressings, abdominal or laparotomy pads, usually 6 in. × 9 in. (15 cm × 23 cm) or 8 in. × 10 in. (20 cm × 25 cm)
Sterile universal trauma dressings, usually 10 in. × 36 in. (25 cm × 91 cm), folded into 9 in. × 10 in. (23 cm × 25 cm) packages
Sterile, occlusive, nonadherent dressings (aluminum foil sterilized in original package)
Occlusive dressings, or chest seals
Assortment of adhesive bandages
Tourniquets
Splinting Supplies
Adult-size traction splint
Child-size traction splint
A variety of arm and leg splints, such as inflatable, vacuum, cardboard, plastic, foam-covered wire-ladder or aluminum alloy, or padded board (the number and type of splints should be determined by state regulations and your medical director)
A variety of triangular bandages and roller bandages
Short backboard/short immobilization device
Long backboard
Cervical collars in an adjustable size or a variety of sizes
Head immobilization devices
Childbirth Supplies
Emergency obstetric kit, including: ▪ Surgical scissors ▪ Hemostats or special cord clamps ▪ Umbilical tape or sterilized cord ▪ Small rubber bulb syringe ▪ Towels ▪ Gauze sponges ▪ Sterile gloves ▪ Sanitary napkins ▪ Plastic bag ▪ Baby blanket ▪ Baby stocking cap
Automated External Defibrillator
Semiautomated defibrillation equipment
Patient Transfer Equipment
Wheeled ambulance stretcher
Wheeled stair chair
Other devices also carried on ambulances include:
Scoop stretcher
Portable/folding stretcher
Flexible stretcher
Transfer tarp or slide board
Basket stretcher
Medications and Other Supplies
Activated charcoal
Drinkable water and cups
Oral glucose
Oxygen
Supplies for irrigating the skin and eyes
Aspirin and epinephrine (in some areas)
DuoDote or other regional equipment, depending on the area and local protocol
Portable radio or cell phone

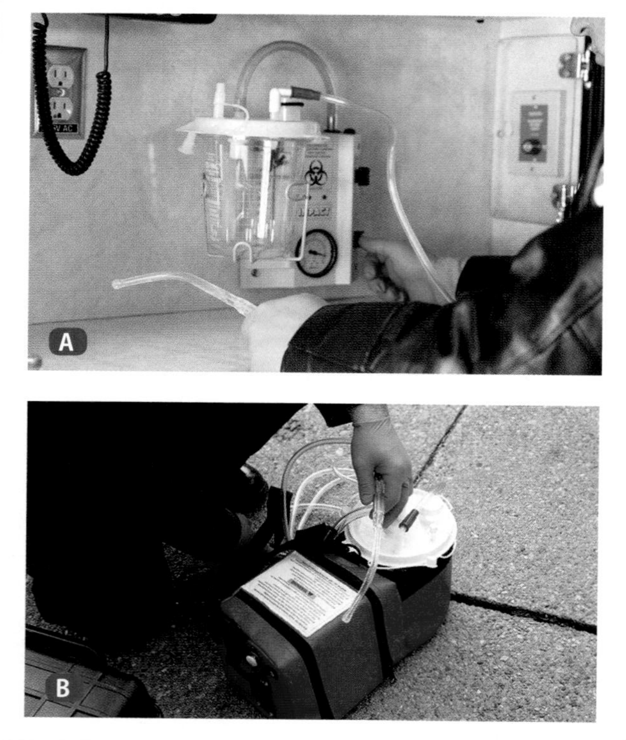

Figure 39-6 The ambulance should carry both a mounted suctioning unit **(A)** and a portable suctioning unit **(B)**.

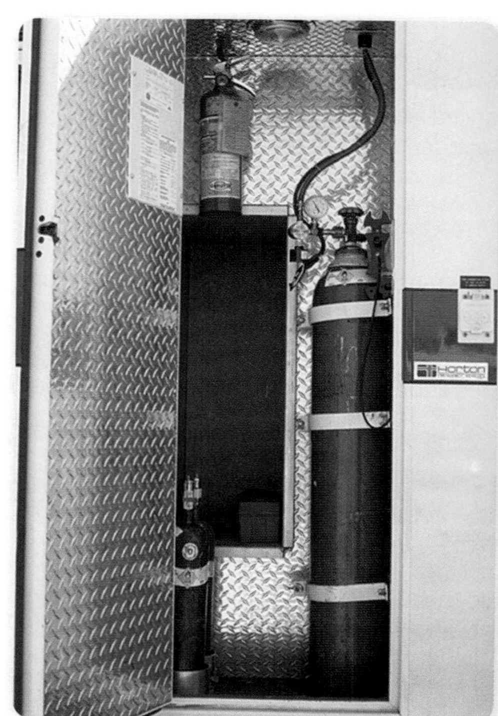

Figure 39-7 An oxygen unit with a capacity of 3,000 L of oxygen should be mounted in the ambulance.

one for use outside the ambulance or as a spare. These devices include disposable pocket masks and bag-mask devices. Bag-mask devices capable of oxygen enrichment and, when attached to an oxygen supply with the oxygen reservoir in place, able to supply almost 100% oxygen should also be carried. Masks for these devices come in a variety of sizes, from neonatal to adult, and are necessary materials to carry on the ambulance. Oxygen-powered devices are also available to provide ventilation to a patient, but these may quickly deplete available oxygen sources. Follow local guidelines in identifying the specific ventilation equipment carried on the ambulance.

The ambulance should carry both portable and mounted suctioning units **Figure 39-6**. These units must be powerful enough to provide an airflow of 30 L/min at the end of the tube and a vacuum of 300 mm Hg when the tube is clamped. The suctioning force must be adjustable for use on infants and children. The suctioning units should include large-bore, nonkinking suction tubing and semirigid tips. The installed unit should include a suction yoke, an unbreakable collection canister, suction catheters, water for rinsing the suction tips, and suction tubing. All of these components must be easily accessible when you are sitting at the head of the stretcher. The suction tubing must reach the patient's airway, regardless of the patient's position. All components of the suctioning unit must be disposable or made of material that is easily cleaned and **decontaminated**.

The ambulance should carry at least two oxygen supply units: one portable and one mounted onboard the vehicle. The portable unit should be located near a door or in the jump kit, for easy use outside the ambulance. It should have a minimum capacity of 500 L of oxygen and be equipped with a yoke, pressure gauge, flowmeter, oxygen supply tubing, nonrebreathing mask, and nasal cannula. This unit must be able to deliver oxygen at a variable rate between 1 and 15 L/min. At least one additional portable 500-L cylinder should be kept on the ambulance. Many services equip the backup cylinder with its own yoke, gauge, regulator, and tubing so that it can be used for a second patient.

The mounted oxygen unit should have a capacity of 3,000 L of oxygen **Figure 39-7**. It should also be equipped with visible flowmeters that are capable of delivering 1 to 15 L/min and that are accessible when you are at the head of the stretcher. Oxygen masks, with and without nonrebreathing bags, should be transparent, disposable, and available in sizes for adults, children, and infants.

Ambulance services that often transport patients on runs lasting longer than 1 hour should consider using a disposable, single-use humidifier for the mounted oxygen system, which reduces the patient's risk of infection. On runs of less than 1 hour, humidification is usually unnecessary.

CPR Equipment. A **CPR board** provides a firm surface under the patient's torso so you can give effective chest compressions **Figure 39-8A**. It also assists in establishing an appropriate degree of head tilt **Figure 39-8B**. Only a few ambulances across the country carry this item. If you do not have a CPR board, then you can place a backboard or short backboard

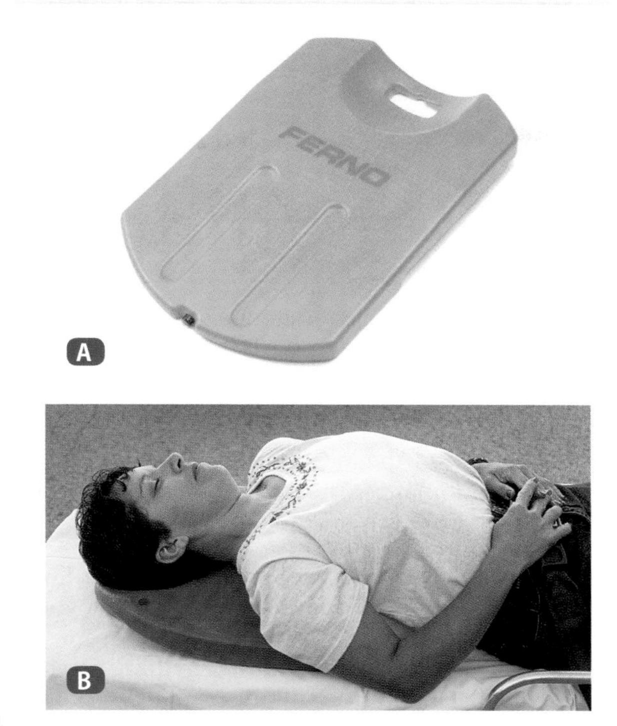

Figure 39-8 A. A cardiopulmonary resuscitation (CPR) board may be carried on the ambulance. **B.** A patient on a CPR board has the appropriate degree of head tilt for effective artificial ventilation.

A: Courtesy of Ferno Washington, Inc.; B: © Jones & Bartlett Learning. Courtesy of MIEMSS.

under the patient on the stretcher. Use a tightly rolled sheet or towel to raise the patient's shoulders 3 inches (8 cm) to 4 inches (10 cm); this technique will also keep the patient's head in a position of maximum backward tilt and keep the shoulders and chest in a straight position. Do not use this roll to hyperextend the neck if you suspect a spinal injury.

Mechanical devices that operate on compressed gas and deliver chest compressions and ventilations are also available.

Basic Wound Care Supplies. Basic supplies for dressing open wounds should be included on the ambulance. These supplies include a pair of trauma shears; sterile sheets; sterile burn sheets; adhesive tape in several widths; self-adhering, soft roller bandages; sterile dressings; gauze; abdominal or laparotomy pads; sterile universal trauma dressings; sterile, occlusive, nonadherent dressings (aluminum foil sterilized in original package); an assortment of adhesive bandages; and tourniquets.

Splinting Supplies. Examples of supplies for splinting fractures and dislocations that may be carried on ambulances are shown in Figure 39-9. These supplies include both an adult-size and a child-size traction splint; a variety of arm and leg splints, such as inflatable, vacuum, cardboard, plastic, foam wire-ladder, or padded board; a variety of triangular bandages and roller bandages; a short backboard; a backboard; head immobilization devices; and cervical collars in either an adjustable size or a variety of sizes.

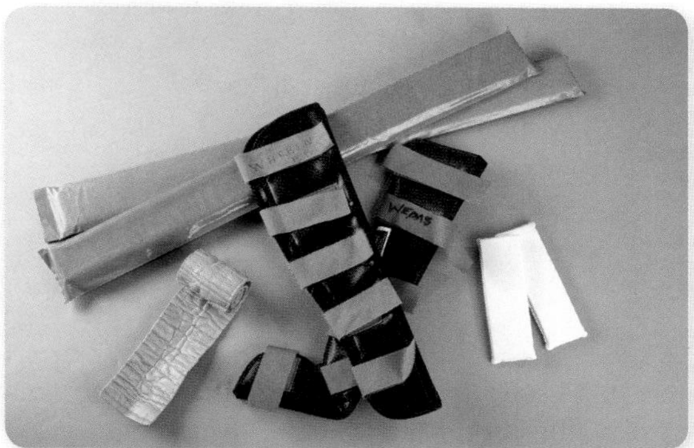

Figure 39-9 Supplies for splinting fractures and dislocations should be carried on the ambulance.

© Jones & Bartlett Learning.

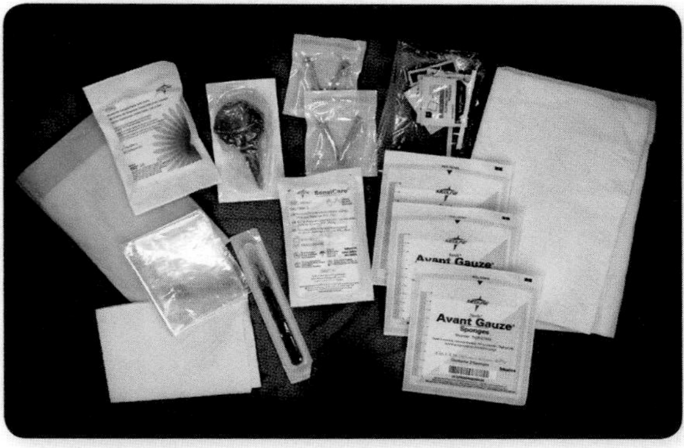

Figure 39-10 A sterile emergency obstetric kit must be carried on the ambulance.

© Mark C. Ide.

Childbirth Supplies. You must carry at least one sterile emergency obstetric kit Figure 39-10 that includes the supplies listed in Table 39-3, including a pair of surgical scissors, hemostats or special cord clamps, umbilical tape or sterilized cord, a small rubber bulb syringe, towels, gauze sponges, pairs of sterile gloves, plastic wrap, sanitary napkins, a plastic bag, a baby stocking cap, and a baby blanket.

AED. Semiautomated defibrillation equipment or manual monitor/defibrillators that have automated external defibrillation capability, as permitted by regulations and the local medical director, should always be carried on the ambulance Figure 39-11.

Patient Transfer Equipment. Each ambulance should carry the following patient transfer equipment:

- A primary wheeled ambulance stretcher
- A wheeled stair chair for use in narrow spaces
- A backboard
- A short backboard or short immobilization device

You should be able to tilt the head of the stretcher upward to at least a 60-degree angle semisitting position. Stretchers must be provided with fasteners to secure them firmly to the floor or side of the ambulance during transport. Stretcher restraints should be capable of holding the stretcher in place in case the vehicle rolls over. Make

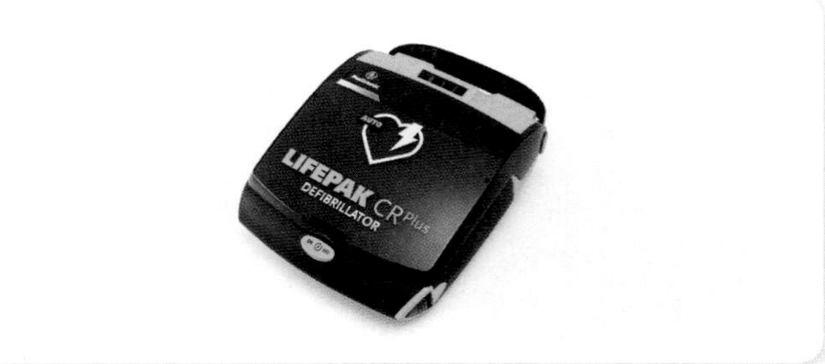

Figure 39-11 Every ambulance should carry an automated external defibrillator.

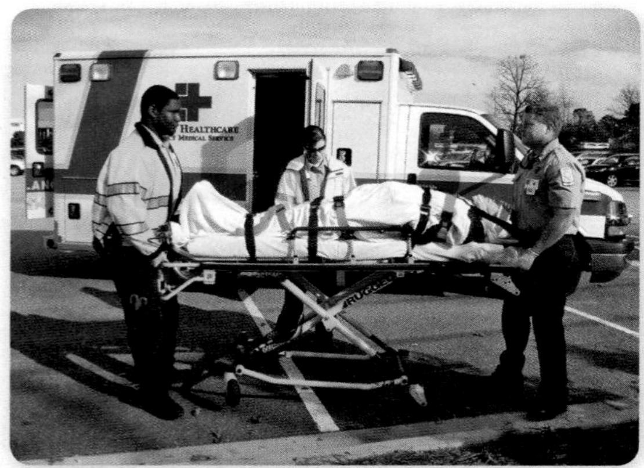

Figure 39-12 The wheeled ambulance stretcher should be locked into place at an appropriate height.

certain that the wheeled stretcher is properly locked into position, because injuries can occur to the patient and you if the stretcher becomes loose while the ambulance is in motion Figure 39-12. Make sure there are at least two restraining devices for the patient, such as deceleration or stopping straps over the shoulders, to prevent the patient from continuing to move forward in case the ambulance suddenly slows or stops. Regardless of the equipment used, it is important to perform proper lifting techniques to avoid injuries. Chapter 6, *Lifting and Moving*, discusses the proper lifting and moving of patients.

Words of Wisdom

You can move the patient to the ambulance in different ways, depending on the injury or illness. It is easier and safer to have some patients walk to the ambulance, rather than trying to use a stretcher. For patients with spinal injuries, the use of a backboard or other immobilization device is advised. If you do not suspect any spinal injuries, then transport patients with respiratory conditions in a sitting position to allow for optimal comfort and safety.

Medications. It is important that the ambulance carry valid and appropriate medications. Be certain that you have the telephone number and radio frequency of online medical control or the local poison control center with you on the ambulance. The back of your clipboard is a good place to keep this information.

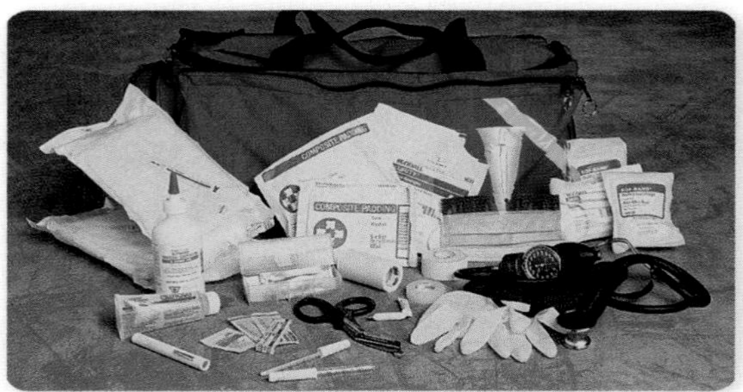

Figure 39-13 A portable jump kit should contain practically anything you will need during the first 5 minutes with the patient.

The Jump Kit. The ambulance must be equipped with a portable, durable, and waterproof jump kit that you can carry to the patient Figure 39-13. Think of the **jump kit** as the "5-minute kit," containing anything you might need in the first 5 minutes with the patient except for the semiautomated external defibrillator, possibly the oxygen cylinder, and portable suctioning unit. The jump kit must be easy to open and secure. Table 39-4 lists the items that are typically contained in a jump kit.

Table 39-4 Items Carried in a Jump Kit

- Nitrile, vinyl, or other disposable gloves
- Face shield or mask with goggles
- Triangular bandages
- Pair of trauma shears
- Adhesive tape in various widths
- Universal trauma dressings
- Self-adhering soft roller bandages, 4 in. × 5 yd (10 cm × 5 m) and 2 in. × 5 yd (5 cm × 5 m)
- Oropharyngeal airways in adult, child, and infant sizes[a]
- Bag-mask device with masks for adults, children, and infants[b]
- Blood pressure cuff
- Stethoscope
- Penlight
- Sterile gauze dressings, 4 in. × 4 in. (10 cm × 10 cm)
- Sterile dressings (abdominal pads), 6 in. × 9 in. (15 cm × 23 cm) or 8 in. × 10 in. (20 cm × 25 cm)
- Adhesive strips
- Oral glucose
- Activated charcoal
- Other medications as allowed by local protocols
- Intravenous supplies (administration set, bag of fluid)[c]

[a, b] These items might be carried in a separate airway kit, along with the portable oxygen cylinder.
[c] Medications are carried in a separate drug box and depend on local protocols for the AEMT level; therefore, specific medications are not listed here.

Safety and Operations Equipment

In addition to medical equipment, a properly stocked ambulance carries several kinds of equipment for responder safety, rescue operations, and locating emergency scenes. To do the job effectively, EMS personnel will need the following equipment:

- Personal protective equipment (PPE) that meets the standards of the American National Standards Institute (ANSI)
- Equipment for work areas
- Preplanning and navigation guides
- Extrication equipment

Personal Safety Equipment. Along with your ANSI Class 2 reflective vest, always carry PPE that allows you to work safely in a limited variety of hazardous or contaminated situations. These situations include the edges of a structural fire or explosion, vehicle extrication incidents, and in crowds. The equipment should protect you from exposure to blood and other potentially infectious body fluids. Note that you will not be equipped to face all hazardous materials (hazmat) and other exposure situations that you may encounter; this is the job of specially trained hazmat technicians and response teams. Your PPE might include the following:

- Face shields
- Gowns, shoe covers, caps
- Turnout gear
- Helmets with face shields or safety goggles
- Safety shoes or boots

Equipment for Work Areas. A weatherproof compartment that you can reach from outside the patient compartment should hold equipment for safeguarding patients and responders, controlling traffic and bystanders, and illuminating work areas **Figure 39-14**. The following items are recommended:

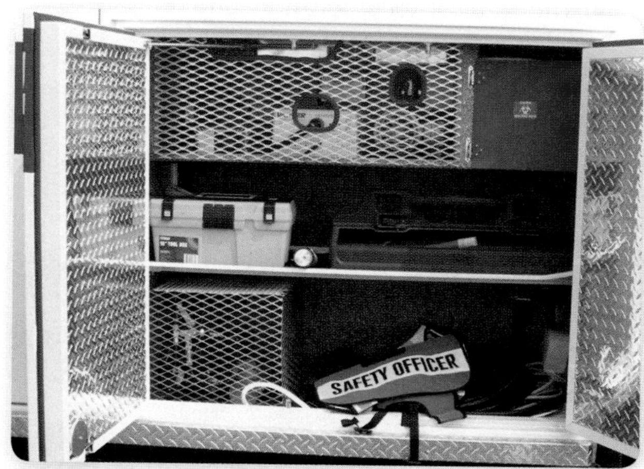

Figure 39-14 The ambulance should have a weatherproof compartment that can be reached from outside the patient compartment. It should hold equipment for safeguarding patients and responders, controlling traffic and bystanders, and illuminating work areas.

- Warning devices that flash intermittently or have reflectors (road flares are not acceptable because they can pose an additional hazard, such as ignition of flammable liquids or gases)
- Two high-intensity, rechargeable halogen flashlights (20,000 candlepower) of the stand-up type
- Fire extinguisher, dry chemical, type ABC (5-pound [2-kg] minimum)
- Hard hats or helmets with face shields or safety goggles
- Portable floodlights

Preplanning and Navigation Guides. GPS devices and MDTs are standard equipment in modern ambulances. Store the addresses of area hospitals, nursing homes, and other key locations for easy access. Enter the address of the hospital into the GPS device before initiating transport to the hospital. Remember that if you are driving the vehicle, never turn your attention away from the road to use a device of any type. Make sure you also have detailed street and area maps in the driver's compartment of the ambulance, along with directions to key locations. Become familiar with the roads and traffic patterns in your town or city so you can plan alternative routes to frequent destinations. Pay particular attention to ways around frequently raised bridges, congested traffic, or blocked railroad crossings. Often, switching to an alternative route will save more time than driving faster. Also, be familiar with special facilities within your regional operating area—such as other medical facilities, airports, arenas and stadiums, and chemical or research facilities—that might pose unusual challenges (staging areas may be predefined for emergency operations).

Extrication Equipment. A weatherproof compartment outside the patient compartment should contain equipment that is needed for basic extrication, even if an extrication and rescue unit is readily available. **Table 39-5** lists the items that may be included in the compartment.

If rescue and extrication services are not readily available, then additional equipment may be needed. See Chapter 40, *Vehicle Extrication, Special Rescue, and Hazardous Materials,* for more information.

Personnel

Every ambulance must be staffed with at least one EMS provider in the patient compartment whenever a patient is being transported; two EMS providers are strongly recommended. Some services may operate with a civilian (non-EMS) driver and a single EMS provider in the patient compartment.

Daily Inspections

Being fully prepared means you and your team must inspect both the ambulance and equipment daily to ensure all items are in proper working order. The ambulance inspection should include the following:

- Fuel level
- Oil level
- Transmission fluid level

Table 39-5	Basic Extrication Equipment

- 12-in. (30-cm) wrench, adjustable, open-end
- 12-in. (30-cm) screwdriver, standard square bar
- 8-in. (20-cm) screwdriver, #2 Phillips head
- Hacksaw with 12-in. (30-cm) carbide wire blades
- Vise-grip pliers, 10 in. (25 cm)
- 5-lb hammer with 15-in. (38-cm) handle
- Fire ax with 24-in. (61-cm) handle
- Wrecking bar with 24-in. (61-cm) handle (may be a combination tool with a hammer and ax)
- 51-in. (130-cm) crowbar, pinch point
- Bolt cutter with 1-in. to 1.25-in. (3-cm) jaw opening
- Folding shovel, pointed blade
- Tin snips, double action, 8 in. (20 cm) minimum
- Gauntlets, reinforced, leather covering past midforearm, one pair per team member
- Rescue blanket
- Ropes, 5,400-lb (2,449-kg) tensile strength in 50-ft (15-m) lengths in protective bags
- Mastic knife (able to cut seat belt webbing)
- Spring-loaded center punch
- Roll of duct tape (for application to window prior to center punch use)
- Pruning saw
- Heavy-duty shoring (cribbing) blocks, 2 in. × 4 in. (5 cm × 10 cm) and 4 in. × 4 in. (10 cm × 10 cm), various lengths

- Engine cooling system and fluid levels
- Batteries
- Brake fluid
- Engine belts
- Wheels and tires, including the spare, if available. Check inflation pressure and look for signs of unusual or uneven wear.
- All interior and exterior lights
- Windshield wipers and fluid
- Horn
- Siren
- Air conditioners and heaters
- Ventilation system
- Doors. Make sure they open, close, latch, and lock properly.
- Communication systems, vehicle and portable
- All windows and mirrors. Check for cleanliness and position.

Check all medical equipment and supplies daily, including all the oxygen supplies, the jump kit, splints, dressings and bandages, backboards and other immobilization equipment, and the emergency obstetrics kit. Is the equipment functioning properly? Are the supplies clean? Are enough supplies available? Perform checks of all battery-operated equipment each day according to the manufacturer's guidelines, including the AED. Rotate the batteries according to an established schedule and the manufacturer's guidelines.

Words of Wisdom

Because the mechanical aspects of emergency work such as driving and moving patients strongly impact your safety and that of others, your service should have specific procedures for daily inspections. Following them protects you physically, and documenting your compliance is an important legal protection. As discussed in Chapter 4, *Communications and Documentation*, these procedures should call for dating and either signing or initialing the check sheets and for storing them in a secure location.

Safety Precautions

A final part of the preparation phase is reviewing safety precautions. Follow these precautions, which include standard traffic safety rules and regulations, on every call. Check safety devices, such as the seat belts in the cab and patient compartment, to ensure they are in proper working order.

▶ Dispatch

The dispatch center must be easy to access and in service 24 hours a day **Figure 39-15**. It may be operated by the local EMS agency or by a shared service that also covers law enforcement and the fire department. The dispatch center might serve only one jurisdiction, such as a single city or town, or it might be an area or regional center serving several communities or an entire county. In either case, it should be staffed by trained personnel who are familiar with the agencies they are dispatching and the geography of the service area. For every emergency call, the dispatcher should gather and record the following minimum information:

- The nature of the call
- The name, present location, and callback telephone number of the caller

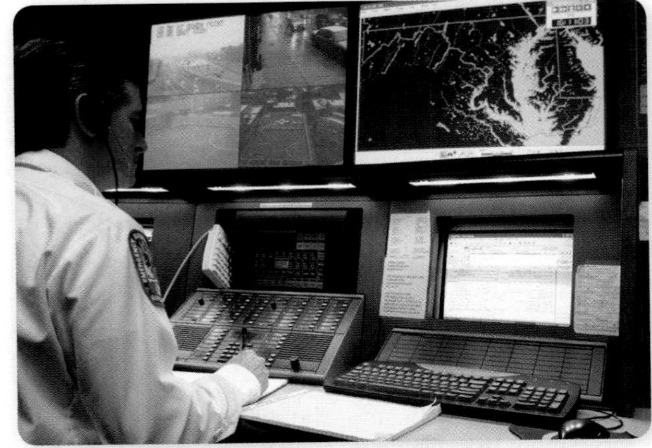

Figure 39-15 The dispatcher is the key communications link throughout all nine phases of the ambulance run.

- The location of the patient(s)
- The number of patients and some idea of the severity of their conditions
- Any other special challenges or pertinent information about hazards or weather conditions

Words of Wisdom

During the dispatch phase, it is important for the AEMT to clarify all information received and ask for additional information as needed. For example, if a call is dispatched for a possible cardiac arrest and the information is not given, the AEMT should ask if CPR is in progress.

Many areas implement emergency medical dispatch, a sophisticated system that allows the dispatcher to provide the caller with instructions for patient care before the ambulance arrives. The emergency medical dispatcher follows a set of guidelines to determine the type of information given and then guides the caller through basic care such as bleeding control or CPR.

▶ En Route to the Scene

In many ways, the en route or response phase of the call is the most dangerous for responders. Crashes that involve emergency vehicles cause many serious injuries among EMS personnel. (Techniques to make vehicle operation safer will be discussed later in this chapter.) As you and your partner prepare to respond to the scene, make sure you fasten your seat belts and shoulder harnesses before you move the ambulance. At this point, inform dispatch that your unit is responding and confirm the nature and location of the call. This is also an excellent time to ask for any other available information about the location. For example, you might learn that the patient is located on the third floor or that the best door to use is around the side of the house.

While en route, your team should prepare to assess and care for the patient. Review dispatch information about the nature of the call and the location of the patient. Assign specific initial duties and scene management tasks to each team member, and decide what type of equipment to take initially. Depending on your operation procedures, you may also decide which stretcher to bring to the patient.

▶ Arrival at the Scene

On arrival at the incident, perform a scene size-up. After you complete your scene size-up, report to dispatch the nature of the incident (if this is part of your local protocols). If additional units are en route, then provide dispatch with your size-up information to help determine whether the additional units should continue to the scene. For example, if you determine the patient is potentially violent during your scene size-up, then law enforcement personnel should continue to the incident scene.

If you are the first responder to arrive on the scene of a mass-casualty incident (MCI), then inform dispatch that you have arrived and give a brief report of what you see. Quickly estimate the number of patients and report the need for additional units, such as a heavy rescue unit

YOU are the Provider PART 2

On arrival you see members of the fire department fighting a fully engulfed structure fire. Law enforcement is also on scene directing traffic around the incident. After making contact with the incident commander, you stage your ambulance in the designated area. Suddenly, you hear a shout. You see several firefighters carrying an adult man out of the structure. They place him in a safe area and return to the fire because of the potential for additional victims. The patient has obvious burns to his face, chest, and arms, and you note the following findings:

Recording Time: 1 Minute	
Appearance	Poor; blisters on his face
Level of consciousness	Unresponsive
Airway	Soot around his mouth; singed nasal hair
Breathing	Slow and shallow
Circulation	Weak, rapid radial pulses

4. While en route, how should you prepare to assess and care for the patient?
5. What equipment do you need to carry to the patient's side?

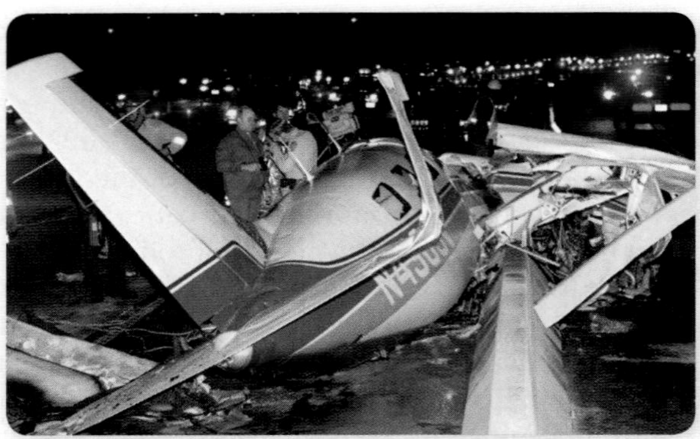

Figure 39-16 If you are the first responder to arrive on the scene of a mass-casualty incident, then report to dispatch and ask for additional units, such as rescue or hazmat units, as needed.

or a hazmat team Figure 39-16. Do not enter the scene if any safety hazards are present. If safety hazards are present at the scene, then move the patient out of danger before you begin care. Emergency moves are discussed in Chapter 6, *Lifting and Moving Patients*.

Immediately size up the scene by using the following guidelines:

- Look for safety hazards to yourself, your partner, bystanders, and your patient(s).
- Evaluate the need for additional units or other assistance.
- Determine the mechanism of injury (MOI) in trauma patients or the nature of the illness in medical patients.
- Evaluate the need to immobilize the spine.
- Take standard precautions. The type of emergency medical care that you expect to give will dictate the PPE you wear.

If you are not the first responder to arrive at the scene of an MCI, then locate and communicate with the designated incident commander Figure 39-17. As discussed in Chapter 41, *Incident Management*, MCIs involve complex organization of personnel under the incident command system. In this system, you may be assigned a specific role by the incident commander, such as beginning the triage process, assisting in treating patients, or loading patients for transportation to the hospital.

Safe Parking at a Crash Scene

In assessing the situation, you must decide where to park the ambulance. Pick a position that will allow for efficient traffic control and flow around a crash scene. Do not park alongside the scene, because you may block the movement of other emergency vehicles and/or impede your own exit. Instead, park in front of or behind the scene, depending on whether other responders have arrived. If other responders such as firefighters or law enforcement officers are on scene, then they should position their vehicles about 100 feet (30 m) past the scene, whereas

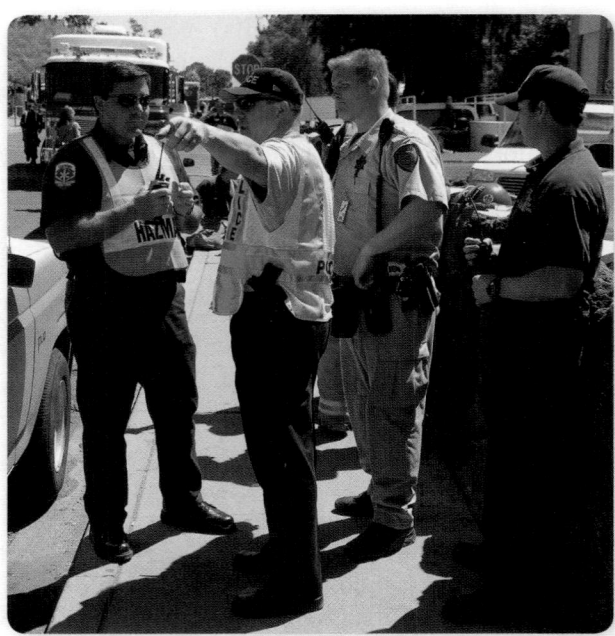

Figure 39-17 At a mass-casualty incident, follow the instructions from the incident commander. Your assigned role may include assisting with triage, treating patients, or loading patients for transportation to the hospital.

you should park the ambulance about 100 feet (30 m) before the scene. If you are the first responder to arrive, then park about 100 feet (30 m) past the scene on the same side of the road Figure 39-18. Use the ambulance to create a barrier between operations at the scene and oncoming traffic. It is best to park uphill and/or upwind of the scene if smoke or hazmat are present. Be sure to set the parking brake. Always leave on the emergency warning lights, but turn off your headlights to avoid impairing the vision of motorists in oncoming traffic. Use extra caution if you must park on a hill or curve or at night. Assume that someone may collide with your vehicle and strike personnel on the scene.

Words of Wisdom

When you park at a scene at night, leave on the emergency warning lights but turn off your headlights. Utilize parking lights to prevent impairing the vision of motorists in oncoming traffic.

Stay away from any fires, explosive hazards, downed wires, and structures that might collapse. If your ambulance is blocking part of the roadway, then leave on the emergency warning lights. If your ambulance has them, then leave on only the flashing yellow lights. Some motorists tend to drive toward emergency vehicles with flashing red or red and white lights. Within these safety guidelines, try to park your ambulance as close to the scene as possible to

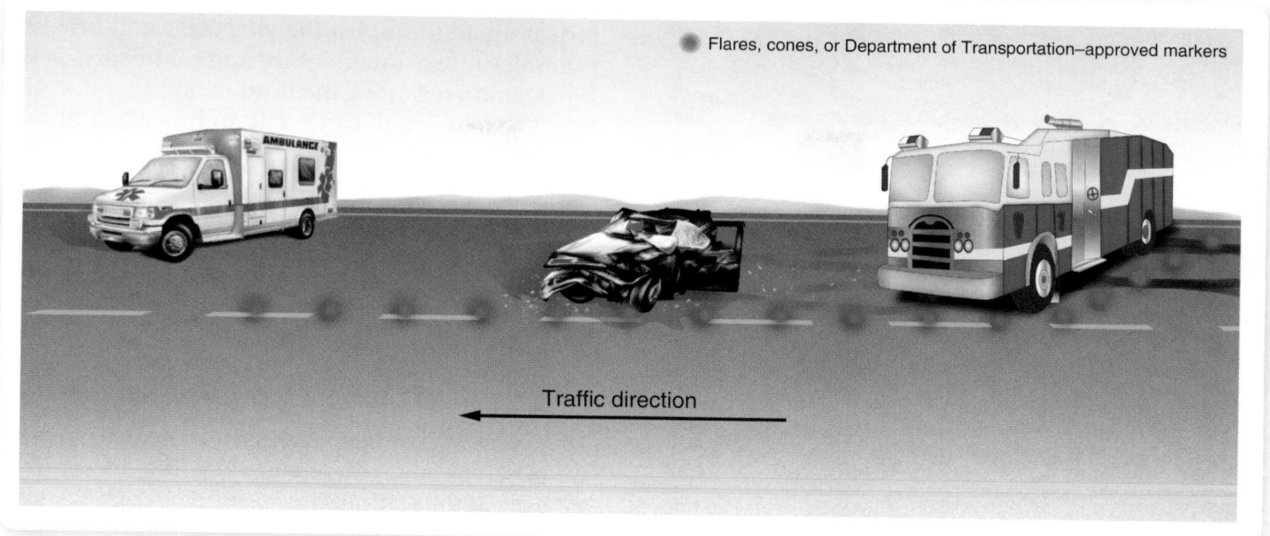

Figure 39-18 Park the ambulance about 100 feet (30 m) away from the scene on the same side of the road.

facilitate emergency medical care. If necessary, then you can temporarily block traffic to unload equipment and to load patients quickly and safely. Do not block traffic any longer than is absolutely necessary. Finally, lock all doors when leaving the ambulance and ensure the designated driver has the keys.

Traffic Control at a Crash Scene

After ensuring your own safety, your first responsibility at a crash scene is to care for the patients. Only after all the patients have been treated and the emergency situation is under control should you be concerned with restoring the flow of traffic. If the police do not arrive quickly at the scene, then you might need to temporarily provide traffic control.

The main objectives of traffic control are to warn other motorists, to prevent additional crashes, and to ensure an orderly traffic flow so emergency medical care of the injured is not interrupted. Under ordinary circumstances, traffic control is difficult. A crash or disaster scene presents serious additional challenges. Passing motorists often slow down and stare, paying little attention to the roadway in front of them. Some curiosity seekers may park down the road and return on foot, creating still other hazards. As soon as possible, place appropriate warning devices, such as reflectors, on both sides of the crash.

▶ Transfer of the Patient to the Ambulance

Many patients have said that one of the most frightening parts of being suddenly ill or injured is the ambulance ride to the hospital. A patient who is already anxious may be made more so by a fast, bumpy ride with a siren blaring. Sometimes, such a ride is truly lifesaving. However, in most cases, excessive speed is unnecessary and dangerous and may prevent the provider in the back of the ambulance from rendering appropriate care. It is necessary that the patient be safely transported to an appropriate medical care facility in the shortest practical time. Speed is no substitute for common sense and defensive driving techniques. In almost every case, you will provide life-saving care right where you find the patient, before moving the patient to the ambulance. You may then begin less critical measures, such as bandaging and splinting. Next, package the patient for transport by securing him or her to a device such as a backboard, a scoop stretcher, or the wheeled ambulance stretcher. Finally, move to the ambulance and properly lift the patient into the patient compartment.

No matter how careful the ambulance driver may be, riding to the hospital while lying down on a stretcher can be uncomfortable and even dangerous. Be sure to secure the patient with at least three straps across the body Figure 39-19. Use deceleration or stopping straps over the shoulders to prevent the patient from continuing to move forward in case the ambulance suddenly slows or stops. This step is especially important if the patient is lying flat or secured to a backboard.

▶ En Route to the Receiving Facility (Transport)

Inform dispatch when you are ready to leave with the patient. Report the number of patients you have and the name of the receiving hospital. Even though you have already assessed and treated the patient, continue to monitor the patient's condition en route. These ongoing assessments may reveal changes in the patient's vital signs and overall condition. Recheck the patient's vital signs en route. The frequency of checking vital signs depends on the situation, but checking them every 15 minutes for a stable patient and every 5 minutes for an unstable

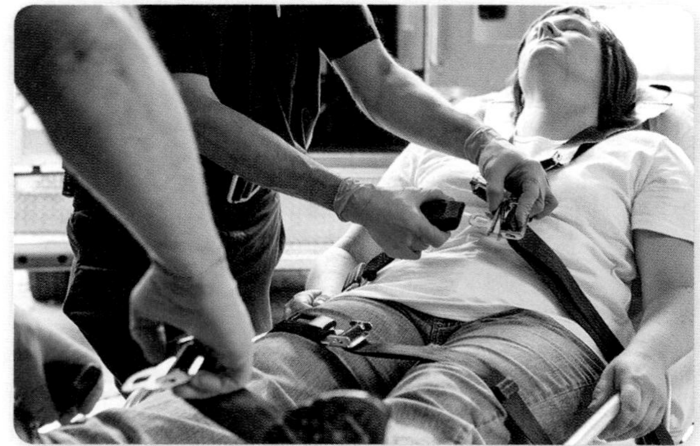

Figure 39-19 Secure the patient appropriately to ensure his or her safety during transport.

patient is a practice that many services use. In addition, it is important to continually reassess the patient's clinical situation and record and address new conditions and the patient's responses to earlier treatment.

At this time, also contact the receiving hospital. Inform medical control about your patient(s) and the nature of the problem(s). Depending on the number of AEMTs on your team and how much emergency medical care the patient needs, you might also want to begin working on your patient care report (PCR) while en route.

Finally, and most importantly, do not abandon the patient emotionally. Do not become so involved in paperwork and reassessments that you ignore the patient's fears. You are there to help the patient, so use this time to reassure him or her. Some patients, such as very young or older people, may benefit from added attention during transport. Be aware of your patient's level of need.

▶ Arrival at the Receiving Facility (Delivery)

Inform dispatch as soon as you arrive at the hospital. Then follow these four steps to transfer the patient to the receiving hospital:

1. Report your arrival to the triage nurse or other arrival personnel.
2. Physically transfer the patient from the stretcher to the bed directed for your patient.
3. Present a complete verbal report at the bedside to the nurse or physician who is taking over the patient's care.
4. Complete a detailed PCR, obtain the required signatures, and leave a copy with an appropriate staff member. Electronic reports are commonly used. Your service should have a method for printing or sending electronic reports as well as obtaining electronic signatures.

The PCR should include a summary of the history of the patient's current illness or injury with pertinent positives and negatives, the MOI, and findings on your arrival. In addition, list the vital signs and briefly mention relevant past medical or surgical history, as well as information regarding medication and allergies. Also, be sure to include any treatment and its effect during the prehospital setting.

While at the hospital, you may be able to restock any items that were used during the run, such as oxygen masks or dressings and bandages Figure 39-20. Remember, though, that your priority is transfer of the patient and patient information to the hospital staff. Restocking the ambulance comes second.

▶ En Route to the Station

After you leave the hospital, inform dispatch whether you are in service and where you are going. As soon as you are back at the station, do the following:

- Clean and disinfect the ambulance and any equipment that was used, if you did not do so before leaving the hospital Figure 39-21.
- Restock any supplies you did not get at the hospital.

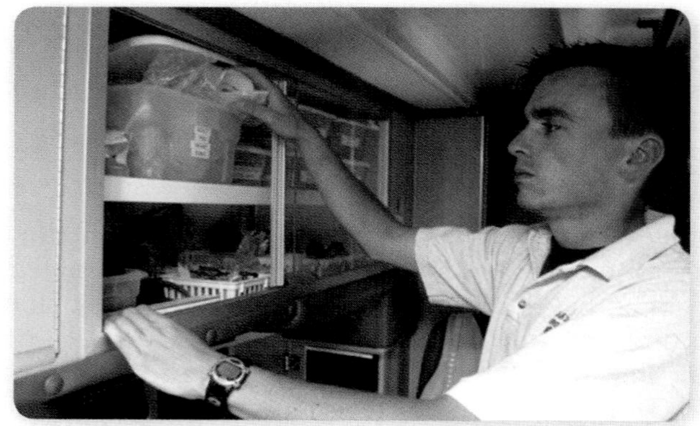

Figure 39-20 After transferring the patient and relating patient information to the hospital staff, you should restock any items that were used during the run.

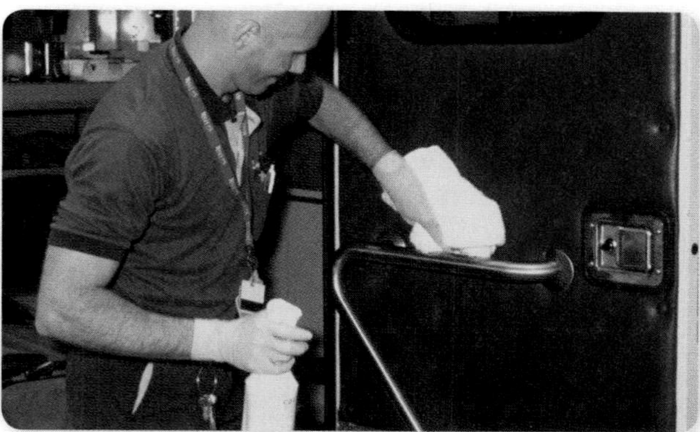

Figure 39-21 Clean and disinfect the ambulance and equipment at the station if you did not do so at the hospital.

▶ Postrun

During the postrun phase, complete and file any additional reports and again inform dispatch of the status, location, and availability of the unit.

Each team member is responsible for maintaining the ambulance so that it is safe and available on a moment's notice. As discussed previously, this responsibility means you should perform routine inspections. Use a written checklist to document any needed repairs or the replacement of equipment and supplies.

Ambulance Cleaning and Disinfection

One way to protect patients is by complying with work restriction guidelines: Reporting for work when you have a sore throat or the flu is not in the best interests of your patients or your coworkers.

Another way to protect patients from nosocomial infections is to keep the ambulance interior and its equipment clean and disinfected.

It is important that you know the meanings of the following terms:

- **Cleaning**. The process of removing dirt, dust, blood, or other visible contaminants from a surface or equipment.
- **Disinfection**. The killing of pathogenic agents by directly applying a chemical made for that purpose to a surface or equipment.
- **High-level disinfection**. The killing of pathogenic agents by the use of potent means of disinfection.
- **Sterilization**. A process, such as the use of heat, which removes all microbial contamination.

When you are cleaning equipment, select cleaning solutions to fit the equipment category:

- **Critical equipment:** items that come in contact with mucous membranes, such as; laryngoscope blades and surgical forceps, endotracheal tubes, Combitubes. High-level disinfection—that is, use of EPA-registered chemical "sterilants"—is the minimum level for this equipment.
- **Semicritical equipment:** items that come in direct contact with intact skin; stethoscopes, blood pressure cuffs, splints, pneumatic antishock garments. Clean with solutions that have a label claiming to kill HBV. Bleach and water at 1:100 dilution fits this requirement.
- **Noncritical equipment:** cleaning surfaces, floors, ambulance seats, work surfaces. EPA-registered hospital-grade cleaner or bleach and water mixture is effective for this equipment.

General cleaning routines need to be listed in the department's Exposure Control Plan. A basic rule is to do the following after every call:

1. Strip used linens from the stretcher immediately after use, and place them in a plastic bag or in the designated receptacle in the emergency department.
2. In an appropriate receptacle, discard all disposable equipment used for care of the patient that meets your state's definition of medical waste. Most items will be considered general trash.
3. Wash contaminated areas with soap and water. For disinfection to be effective, cleaning must be done first.
4. Disinfect all nondisposable equipment used in the care of the patient. For example, disassemble the bag-mask device and place the components in a liquid sterilization solution as recommended by the manufacturer.
5. Clean the stretcher with an EPA-registered germicidal/virucidal solution or bleach and water at 1:100 dilution.
6. If any spillage or other contamination occurred in the ambulance, clean it up with the same germicidal/virucidal or bleach/water solution.
7. Create a schedule for routine full cleaning for the vehicle, as required by the Exposure Control Plan. Name the brands of solution to be used.
8. Have a written policy/procedure for cleaning each piece of equipment. Refer to the manufacturer's recommendations as a guide.

A basic rule is to ensure that the following 12 steps are taken after every call:

1. Immediately strip used linens from the stretcher after use, and place them in a plastic bag or in the designated receptacle in the ED.
2. Discard in an appropriate receptacle all disposable equipment used for care of the patient that meets the definition of medical waste as dictated by your state. Most items will be considered general trash. Discard disposable equipment that is bloody or contaminated by body fluids in a biohazard container approved by the Occupational Safety and Health Administration (OSHA). Discard noncontaminated disposable equipment used for care of the patient according to OSHA and local guidelines.
3. Wash all contaminated areas with soap and water. Scrub blood, vomitus, and other substances from the floors, walls, and ceilings with soap and water. For disinfection to be effective, you must first clean the ambulance. (You can use a 10% solution of bleach in water to clean the ambulance after any contamination.)
4. Disinfect all reusable equipment used in the care of the patient. For example, properly clean and disinfect stethoscopes, blood pressure cuffs, and pulse oximetry probes.
5. Clean the stretcher with either a germicidal/virucidal solution registered by the Environmental

Protection Agency, or bleach and water at 1:100 dilution.

6. Clean up any spillage or other contamination that occurred in the ambulance, with the same germicidal/virucidal or bleach/water solution.
7. Clean the outside of the ambulance as needed.
8. Replace or repair broken or damaged equipment without delay.
9. Replace any other equipment or supplies that were used.
10. Refuel the ambulance if the fuel tank is below required reserves. Check the oil level each time the ambulance is refueled.
11. Create a schedule for routine full cleaning of the vehicle.
12. Have a written policy or procedure for cleaning each piece of equipment. Refer to the manufacturer's recommendations as a guide.

Safety Tips

Remember to assess for the following hazards while operating an ambulance:

- Downed power lines
- Leaking fuels or fluids
- Smoke or fire
- Broken glass
- Trapped or ejected patients
- MOI

Before leaving the scene:

- Ensure that hazards have been addressed.
- Ensure that all equipment has been properly stored or disposed of.
- Ensure that the scene has been turned over to the appropriate authority (law enforcement, fire department, etc).

Defensive Ambulance Driving Techniques

According to the National Highway Traffic Safety Administration, approximately 4,500 motor vehicle crashes involving an ambulance occurred every year between 1992 and 2011. Of these crashes, 65% resulted in damage to property only; 34% resulted in one or more injuries; and 1% resulted in one or more fatalities.[2] These statistics show the significant impact of traffic crashes on pedestrians, motorists, ambulance passengers, and EMS personnel. Learning how to properly operate the ambulance is just as important as learning how to care for patients when you arrive on the scene. As you will learn, ambulances do not handle the same as personal vehicles. Ambulances require a longer braking time and stopping distance. In addition, the weight of the ambulance is unevenly distributed, which makes it more prone to roll over. These factors greatly increase the chance that a crash may occur. An ambulance that is involved in a crash delays patient care at a minimum, and may take the lives of the EMS providers, other motorists, or pedestrians at worst. The following section is provided to introduce you to safe driving techniques; however, you cannot become a proficient and safe ambulance driver without specialized training and practice. You are strongly encouraged to participate in an emergency driving program, such as the NAEMT EMS Vehicle Operator Safety (EVOS) course, designed for the EMS vehicle operator, and those offered through your EMS organization, before operating an emergency vehicle.

Driver Characteristics

Not everyone who drives a motor vehicle is qualified to drive an ambulance. In some states, you must successfully complete an approved emergency vehicle operations course before you are allowed to drive the ambulance on emergency calls. In any state, due diligence and caution are important characteristics, as are a positive attitude about your ability and tolerance of other motorists.

One basic requirement is physical fitness. Many crashes occur as a result of physical impairment of the driver. Do not drive if you are taking medications that may cause drowsiness or slow your reaction times. These medications include cold remedies, analgesics, and tranquilizers. Of course, never drive or provide emergency medical care after drinking alcohol. Fatigue can also play a prominent role in crashes, so it is imperative to get as much rest as possible during free times. Driving alone may also be a factor during long transports.

Another requirement is emotional fitness. Do not take emotions lightly. A person's personality can change once he or she is behind a steering wheel. Emotional maturity and stability are closely related to the ability to operate under stress. In addition to knowing exactly what to do, you must be able to do it under difficult conditions.

Having the proper attitude is very important. Never get behind the wheel of an ambulance thinking that you can drive in any manner that pleases you. Great responsibility is placed on the driver of an ambulance.

In addition to training and experience, the good judgment and knowledge that you need to drive an ambulance require practice. Remember, even the best drivers can benefit from practice.

Safe Driving Practices

The first rule of safe driving in an ambulance is that speed does not save lives; good emergency medical care does. The second rule is that the driver and all passengers must wear seat belts and shoulder restraints at all times. These devices are the most important items of safety equipment on every ambulance.

Words of Wisdom

Speed does not save lives; good emergency medical care does! Your partner cannot provide adequate patient care if all he or she can do is hang on. Drive carefully and call out upcoming movements such as "Sharp turn to the left," or "Railroad tracks."

Learn how your ambulance responds to **acceleration** (increasing speed), cornering, and **deceleration** (decreasing speed) under various conditions. For example, disc booster brakes make braking more efficient but increase sway. When you drive an ambulance on a multilane highway, stay in the far left (passing) lane whenever possible. This tactic allows other motorists to move over to the right when they see or hear the ambulance approach.

Table 39-6 lists additional guidelines to follow when you are en route to a call.

Use of Safety Restraints

Standard operating procedures should mandate that everyone in the ambulance use seat belts, not just the patient. Wear restraints en route to the scene and whenever you are not performing direct patient care. Remember to properly restrain the patient. Do not transport children on the stretcher unless they are properly restrained. It is not advisable to use adult seat belts for children. Many pediatric transport devices are available; use them when appropriate.

Studies show that fewer than half of all AEMTs wear seat belts while the ambulance is in emergency mode, and few AEMTs wear lap belts in the rear compartment while patient care is being rendered. If you must remove your seat belt to care for the patient, then fasten it again as soon as possible. As mentioned previously, unrestrained or improperly restrained patients and medical equipment (especially portable oxygen tanks) may become airborne during a crash and place you and your patient at an additional risk. Secure all equipment and cabinets, as well as the patient and any passengers accompanying the patient.

Excessive Speed

Even in extreme life-and-death emergencies, excessive speed is not indicated. In most instances, if you properly assess and immobilize the patient at the scene, then excessive speed during transport is unnecessary and undesirable. Regardless of the situation, never travel at a speed that is unsafe for the given road conditions.

Excessive speed, in addition to being unnecessary, does not increase a patient's chance of survival. More often, using excessive speed while driving to and from the scene has resulted in crashes in which the AEMT, the patient, and occupants of other vehicles are killed. It also makes it very difficult for the AEMT attending to the patient to be able to provide emergency medical care because of the rough ride typically created by the excessive speed and maneuvering. Excessive speed also reduces the

YOU are the Provider — PART 3

As you perform your primary survey of the patient, you note his respirations are slow and shallow and he has blisters on his chest and arms. The skin in unburned areas is pink. You direct your partner to begin positive pressure ventilations while you complete your assessment. Because of the extent of his burns and obvious airway compromise, the decision is made to transport this patient via air ambulance. Law enforcement personnel establish a safe landing zone in the parking lot of a local elementary school. You and your partner load the patient into the ambulance to continue treatment and await the arrival of the helicopter.

Recording Time: 8 Minutes	
Respirations	6 breaths/min, shallow
Pulse	124 beats/min, thready
Skin	Burns to the face, chest, and arms
Blood pressure	96/52 mm Hg
Oxygen saturation (Spo_2)	86% on room air
Pupils	Equal but sluggish to respond

6. What are some advantages of using an air ambulance?
7. What are some disadvantages of using an air ambulance?
8. What factors must you take into consideration when creating a landing zone?

Table 39-6 Guidelines for Safe Ambulance Driving

1. Select the shortest and least congested route to the scene at the time of the dispatch.
2. Avoid routes with heavy traffic congestion; know alternative routes to each hospital during rush hours.
3. Avoid one-way streets; they may become clogged. Do not drive against the flow of traffic on a one-way street unless absolutely necessary.
4. Watch carefully for bystanders as you approach the scene. Curiosity seekers rarely move out of the way.
5. Park the ambulance in a safe place after you arrive at the scene. If you park facing into traffic, turn off your headlights so that they do not impair the vision of oncoming motorists unless your headlights are needed to illuminate the scene. If the ambulance is blocking part of the road, then leave on your emergency warning lights to alert oncoming motorists; otherwise, turn them off.
6. Drive within the speed limit while transporting patients, except in the rare extreme emergency.
7. Go with the flow of the traffic.
8. Always exercise due regard for people and property.
9. Always drive defensively.
10. Always maintain a safe following distance. Use the "4-second rule": stay at least 4 seconds behind another vehicle in the same lane.
11. Maintain an open space in the lane next to you as an escape route in case the vehicle in front of you stops suddenly.
12. Use your siren if you turn on the emergency warning lights.
13. Always assume that other motorists will not hear the siren or see your emergency warning lights.

driver's reaction time and increases the time and distance needed to stop the ambulance. Although many state laws allow emergency vehicles to travel beyond the posted speed limits in emergencies, these laws offer little or no protection against prosecution should the driver become involved in a crash. The legal ramifications of driving an emergency vehicle will be covered later in this section.

Siren Risk-Benefit Analysis

Whether responding to a call or transporting a patient from the scene to the hospital, the decision to activate the emergency warning lights and siren will depend on several factors such as local protocols, the patient's condition, and the anticipated clinical outcome of the patient. Some local protocols require that all responders to the scene use their emergency warning lights and sirens, whereas other EMS systems incorporate response modes based on the information received from dispatch. Regardless of your jurisdictional requirements, as the driver of the ambulance, you need to evaluate the risk versus the benefit of your response mode. Numerous studies have been done to determine whether the emergency warning lights and siren save time getting to the patient or getting the patient from the scene to the hospital. The findings of these studies show that only minimal time is saved.

Three basic principles govern the use of the warning lights and siren on an ambulance:

1. The unit, to the best of your knowledge, must be on a true emergency call.
2. Audible and visual warning devices must be used simultaneously.
3. The unit must be operated with due regard for the safety of all others, on and off the roadway.

As an AEMT, you also need to take into account the patient's condition before activating the emergency warning lights and siren. For example, patients who have experienced a seizure may have another seizure as a result of the rapid flash pattern of the emergency lighting. In cases such as this, it may be preferable to transport your patient without activating the emergency warning lights and siren in an effort to minimize external stimuli and to avoid making your patient's condition worse. If you have to use the siren, then warn the patient before you turn it on. Be especially mindful not to increase the speed of the ambulance just because the siren is in use.

The siren may also have a psychological effect on motorists. Recognizing this will help you become aware of your or other motorists' tendencies to drive faster in the presence of a siren. Although a siren signifies a request for motorists to yield the right-of-way, motorists do not always yield.

Never assume that your emergency warning lights and siren will allow you to drive through a congested area without stopping or slowing down. Slow down to ensure that all drivers are stopping as you approach an intersection, and proceed with due caution. Consider using a different siren tone as you approach an intersection. Remember, the siren is a request that other drivers yield the right-of-way to you; it does not guarantee they will.

Driver Anticipation

As an ambulance driver, never assume that motorists and pedestrians will yield the right-of-way. Always assume that people cannot hear the siren and/or PA system or see the ambulance until proven otherwise by their actions. Motorists may indeed pull over to the nearest curb and stop or drive as close to the curb as possible, but you cannot take this behavior for granted. At any time, a motorist might stop suddenly in front of the ambulance or pull in front of you. These actions may result in a collision. Whenever a motorist yields the right-of-way to you, attempt to establish eye contact with him or her to confirm you have been seen.

It is often difficult for motorists to hear instructions called out over the PA system, especially when their windows are closed. The PA system may make the situation worse because motorists may hesitate or make unexpected moves so that they can hear or follow instructions. Moreover, when you issue commands to motorists and pedestrians over the PA system, they are now distracted from the business of driving. With this said, you should not use the PA system often, if at all, while you drive the ambulance.

Most important, always drive defensively. Never assume what another motorist will do unless you get a clear visual signal. Even then, be prepared to take defensive action in the case of a misunderstanding, panic, or careless driving on the part of the other motorist. Aggressive ambulance driving—such as cutting off other vehicles—may also cause anxiety or irrational behavior in other motorists, because you may not allow enough time for them to respond to your vehicle.

Safety Tips

When multiple agencies respond to the same emergency, responders may choose the same route of travel. In such instances, be extremely cautious at intersections and side streets. Aside from the fact that personal vehicles are now virtually soundproof, a motorist may be distracted by the first emergency vehicle and may not see another vehicle coming behind the first. If you must travel behind a fire truck or law enforcement vehicle, then make sure you leave plenty of distance between your vehicles and use a different siren tone.

The Cushion of Safety

To operate an ambulance safely, maintain a safe following distance from the vehicles in front of you and try to avoid being tailgated from behind. Also ensure that the **blind spots** in your mirrors do not prevent you from seeing vehicles or pedestrians on either side of the ambulance. When you follow these steps, you are maintaining a **cushion of safety**. To ensure that you have enough reaction time and stopping distance from the vehicle in front of you, follow at a safe distance, allowing the motorist enough time to move over to the right. If the motorist does not move, then you need to allow for enough time to avoid colliding with the vehicle. This means driving about 4 seconds behind a vehicle traveling at an average speed (remember the 4-second rule).

While operating in emergency mode, tailgaters may follow your vehicle dangerously closely in congested areas simply to use your ambulance to get through traffic. If you stop the ambulance suddenly, then the tailgating vehicle could collide with the rear of the ambulance, possibly causing you to lose control and strike other vehicles or pedestrians. Always scan your rearview and side mirrors for vehicles that are following too closely.

If you are being tailgated, then never speed up to create more distance. The tailgater may, in turn, increase his or her speed to continue to follow you through traffic, thereby decreasing your cushion of safety and reaction time. Slamming on your brakes to scare the other motorist usually does not work either and may cause a collision. You can have your dispatcher contact the local police to let them know that someone is driving recklessly behind you.

Never, under any circumstance, get out of the ambulance to confront a driver. This action will only delay your response to the scene or transport of the patient and can lead to a dangerous situation. It is also unprofessional for you to become involved in a verbal argument with any member of the public and may lead to disciplinary actions or termination, depending on the conduct regulations of your service.

Finally, be aware of three blind spots around the ambulance that you cannot see with the side or rearview mirrors:

1. The rearview mirror itself creates a blind spot, obstructing the view ahead and preventing you from seeing pedestrians or vehicles. To eliminate this blind spot, lean forward in your seat so that the mirror does not obstruct the view, especially when making turns at intersections.
2. You cannot fully see the rear of the vehicle through the rearview mirror; therefore, it is a blind spot. Because of the configuration of modern ambulances and the relative height of the vehicle, the rearview mirror generally gives you only a view of the patient compartment at best and is not intended to be used for alerting the driver of a vehicle behind the ambulance.

Because of this blind spot, many crashes occur when the ambulance is backing up. It is highly recommended—and required in many jurisdictions—that you use a **spotter** to help you back up the ambulance (discussed later in this chapter). Rear-facing cameras are also helpful and much more common; however, cameras do not replace the assistance of a spotter if one is available.

3. Often you cannot see the side of the ambulance through the side-view mirrors at a certain angle. You may be unable to see an entire vehicle in the side mirrors, even though the vehicle is right next to the ambulance. To eliminate this problem, many EMS agencies place small, rounded mirrors on the side mirrors to assist you in visualizing this blind spot. However, if these mirrors are unavailable, then you need to lean forward or backward in the seat to eliminate the blind spot. This technique is especially important to use when shifting lanes or making turns.

Frequently scan your mirrors for any new hazards to maintain your cushion of safety; however, keep in mind that your mirrors can give you a misleading view and may block pedestrians or vehicles. Adjust your position in the driver's seat to avoid blind spots in your mirrors. Always use a spotter who you can see from the driver's side mirror.

Safety Tips

Ambulance crashes that kill EMS providers, patients, or occupants of other vehicles are disturbingly common. Many of them could be prevented by the driver of the ambulance. Attending thoroughly to your own driving skills, driving according to established standards, and dealing with any obvious deficiencies in your partner's driving skills are all crucial to your safety on the job.

Emergency Vehicle Control

As the driver of an ambulance, you have only two ways to control the vehicle: by changing its direction or changing its speed. Either maneuver requires a continuous rolling contact between the surface of the tires and the surface of the road. Two factors are involved in this contact. The first is the **coefficient of friction**, which is a measure of the grip of the tires on the road; **friction** is resistance to the motion of one body against another. The second factor is the **footprint** of the tire, or the area of contact between the tire and surface of the road. On the typical ambulance, the footprint is about 8 inches (20 cm) long and as wide as the tire.

The grip of the tire on the road may vary widely on different parts of the same road, depending on the condition of the surface, the age of the road, and the weather. Unpaved roadways may also present a challenge, especially in inclement weather. The grip of the tire also varies according to its tread design and wear. As a driver, you must constantly evaluate the road surface. Ask yourself: At a given speed, how much frictional force can the tires apply before the ambulance becomes unstable? This evaluation is especially important while cornering, in which additional centrifugal force is acting on the vehicle.

Words of Wisdom

Centrifugal force is the tendency for objects to be pulled outward when rotating around a center. Vehicles are subject to this force when making a turn. If you must brake on a turn, then brake gently while making the turn.

Vehicle Size and Distance Judgment

The length and width of the ambulance are critical factors in maneuvering, driving, and parking it. These factors are especially important with type I and type III ambulances, which are wider than they look from behind the steering wheel. To brake and pass effectively, you must know the width and length of your vehicle. As mentioned previously, crashes often occur when the driver is backing up the ambulance. To avoid any incidents, always use a spotter outside the ambulance as a guide when you are backing up. The size and weight of the ambulance also greatly influence braking and stopping distances. Good peripheral vision and depth perception will help you to judge distances, but they are no substitute for intensive training, experience, and frequent evaluation of the vehicle.

Road Positioning and Cornering

Road position means the position of the vehicle on the roadway relative to the inside or outside edge of the paved surface. To corner efficiently, you must know the present position of the ambulance and its projected path. The aim is to take the corner at the speed that will put you in the proper road position as you exit the curve Figure 39-22. The apex of the turn through a curve is the point at which the ambulance is closest to the inside edge of the curve. If you reach the apex early in the curve, then the ambulance will be forced toward the outside of the roadway as it exits the curve. If you reach the apex late in the curve, then the ambulance will tend to stay on the inside of the roadway; this tactic helps you to keep the ambulance in the proper lane and allows room for error if you enter the turn too fast.

Controlled Acceleration and Braking

Recall that the chassis is the structural framework of a vehicle. The **chassis set** is the transfer of weight (center

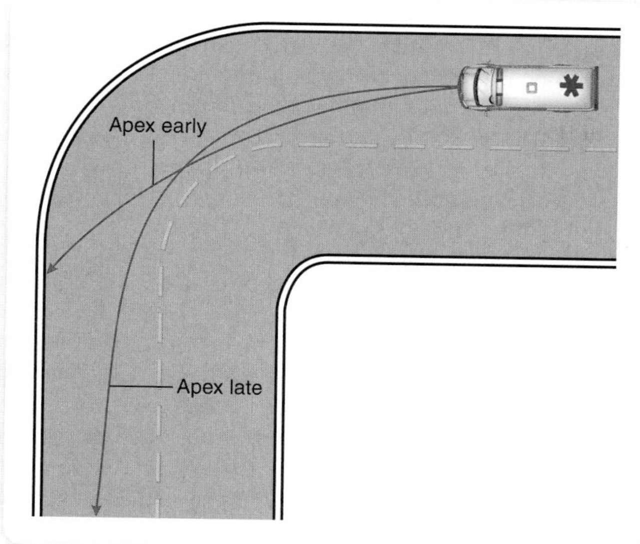

Figure 39-22 To keep the ambulance in the proper lane on a curve, you must know the present position and projected path of the vehicle, and take the corner at the correct speed.

of mass) to different points on the chassis. Basically, the weight of a vehicle is concentrated over one of three points on the chassis: (1) the front wheels, (2) the rear wheels, or (3) the center between the front and rear wheels. The transfer of weight from one point to another is caused by either acceleration or deceleration. When a vehicle accelerates, the weight is transferred to the rear. As a result, the front wheels have some loss of traction, which means that your ability to steer is reduced. A vehicle has a tendency to travel in a straight line. When braking, the opposite shift in weight occurs; this factor is why the rear end of the vehicle tends to slide to the outside of a curve when cornering.

Controlled Acceleration. Controlled acceleration is the use of acceleration to control the vehicle. Acceleration is most efficient when the vehicle is traveling in a straight line, because the force of linear acceleration is equally distributed to the rear wheels. If you accelerate in a curve or during a turn, however, then you force the vehicle to the outside of the curve. If acceleration in this direction becomes excessive, then the vehicle may drift out of control and become unstable. Therefore, accelerate as you come out of a curve to provide stability to the vehicle.

Controlled Braking. Controlled braking is the use of the brakes to control the vehicle. Brakes not only control the movement of the vehicle, causing it to slow or stop, but they also help to control its direction. The safest, most efficient method of braking is to brake while the vehicle is traveling in a straight line. Braking during a turn causes a loss of efficiency. You might not notice this effect at low speed, but it becomes more apparent at higher speeds. Applying the brakes while cornering is not an effective way to slow the vehicle and may actually cause it to skid or spin.

Each vehicle has a different braking action. With experience and practice, you will develop a sense of the proper brake pressure. For example, the brakes on types I and III ambulances have a heavier feel than the brakes on a type II ambulance. Braking on a diesel-powered unit will be different from braking on a gasoline-powered unit, even if the two units are identically equipped. Certain heavy vehicles use air brakes, which have yet another feel. Get to know each vehicle you drive, and be sure you understand its braking characteristics and the appropriate downshifting techniques.

Words of Wisdom

Take your foot off the accelerator when you enter a curve, allowing the ambulance to coast into it, and accelerate as you exit the curve to provide the greatest stability to the vehicle.

Words of Wisdom

Hold the steering wheel with your hands placed outside of the steering wheel in the "9" and "3" positions.[3] This technique allows you to turn the wheel without removing either hand; one hand pulls while the other slides so that they remain parallel. Your hands should not pass the twelve-o'clock or six-o'clock positions. Let the hand that was pulling start to slide, and use the opposite hand to pull, which will keep both hands on the steering wheel at all times.

Backing Up the Ambulance

Backing up a vehicle is the most common source of vehicle damage and may result in costly repairs. Most EMS agencies have established a policy regarding this process. If possible, then avoid situations in which the ambulance will have to be backed up. If it must be done, then remember to follow these rules:

- Use a spotter to guide you.
- Agree on hand signals to use with the spotter before you place the ambulance in reverse. Some people have different ideas of which gesture means "Stop."
- Keep your spotter in view at all times. If you lose sight of the spotter, then immediately stop until he or she is back in your line of sight.
- Keep your window rolled down when in motion. This practice may allow you to hear people warning you of unseen dangers.

- Walk around the ambulance before getting behind the wheel and look up as well as down. Objects on the ground may not be visible after you start backing up.
- Use audible warning devices whenever the ambulance is in motion.

Weather and Road Conditions

Although most ambulance crashes occur on clear days with dry roads, certain conditions can limit your ability to control your vehicle. Remember, ambulances do not handle the same as personal vehicles. These differences, in addition to adverse environmental conditions, greatly increase the chance that a crash may occur. Therefore, be constantly alert to changing weather and road conditions. Whether traveling to or coming from an emergency, modify your speed according to road conditions. Take warnings of ice or hazardous conditions seriously, and be prepared to take an alternative route, if necessary. During a major disaster, all public safety and emergency services should be coordinated. If you encounter unexpected traffic congestion, then notify the dispatcher so other emergency vehicles can select alternative routes.

Even the most careful drivers will occasionally encounter unexpected situations that may require special driving skills. However, if you drive at a speed that is appropriate for the weather and road conditions and maintain an adequate cushion of safety, then you will minimize these situations. Therefore, it is safer if you decrease speed in weather situations involving fog, rain, snow, or ice. The following are examples of adverse conditions that require you to decrease speed, increase following distance, and be alert.

Hydroplaning. On a wet road, a tire usually displaces the water on the road surface and stays in direct contact with the road. However, at speeds of greater than 30 miles per hour (mph), tires may be lifted off the road as water builds up underneath; the vehicle may then feel as if it is floating. This condition is known as **hydroplaning**. At higher speeds on wet roadways, the front wheels may actually be riding on a sheet of water, robbing the driver of control of the vehicle. If hydroplaning occurs, then gradually slow down without slamming on the brakes.

Water on the Roadway. Wet brakes will not slow the vehicle as efficiently as dry brakes will, and the vehicle may pull to one side or the other. If at all possible, then avoid driving through large pools of standing water; often, you cannot tell how deep they are. If you must drive through standing water, then slow down and turn on the windshield wipers. After driving out of the water, lightly tap the brakes several times until they are dry. If the vehicle is equipped with antilock brakes, then apply a steady, light pressure to dry the brakes. Avoid driving through moving water at all times.

Decreased Visibility. The presence of fog, smog, snow, or heavy rain indicates that you must slow down. Warn the vehicles behind you by turning on your emergency warning lights. At night, use only low headlight beams for maximum visibility without reflection. Always use headlights during the day to increase your visibility to other drivers. Also, watch carefully for stopped or slow-moving vehicles.

Ice and Slippery Surfaces. A light mist on an oily, dusty road can be just as slippery as a patch of ice. Good all-weather tires and an appropriate speed will significantly reduce traction problems. If you are in an area that often has snowy or icy conditions, then consider using studded snow tires or tire chains, if they are permitted by law. Be especially careful on bridges and overpasses when temperatures are close to freezing. These road surfaces will freeze much faster than surrounding road surfaces because they lack the warming effect of the ground underneath.

Words of Wisdom

Although preventing skids and sliding is ideal, you are likely to skid or slide occasionally, especially if you live in climates with ice and snow. Your training should include the technique for correcting slides during turns. If you are likely to drive on ice and snow, then practice control maneuvers until they become automatic. Practice at low speeds in open areas with no danger of collisions. Remember that four-wheel-drive and front-wheel-drive vehicles function differently than rear-wheel-drive vehicles when sliding. It is also important to remember that although four-wheel-drive vehicles have better traction for acceleration in slippery conditions, they do not stop any faster than two-wheel-drive vehicles do.

Safety Tips

If possible, then avoid these distractions while driving:

- Mobile data terminals
- GPS devices
- Mobile two-way radios
- Mobile phones
- Visual and audible devices (emergency warning lights and siren)
- Vehicle stereo
- Wireless devices
- Eating and/or drinking

Fatigue

Fatigue has many causes, such as stress, working the night shift, and lack of quality sleep in accordance with your body's circadian rhythms. As a result of fatigue, operating a large vehicle, such as an ambulance, creates a considerable risk. You must be able to recognize when you are fatigued. Do not be ashamed to admit it to yourself, your partner, or your supervisor. If you are feeling fatigued, then you should be placed out of service for the remainder of the shift or until the fatigue has passed and you feel capable of operating the vehicle safely.

Special Populations

When you approach a school bus that is stopped, stop and turn off your siren. Wait until the bus driver turns off the flashing lights and disengages the stop signal arm before cautiously proceeding. Children are unpredictable and may run into your path of travel when scared or confused by the siren.

Laws and Regulations

Regulations regarding vehicle operations vary among states and by city, but some regulations are the same regardless of location. Drivers of emergency vehicles have certain limited privileges in every state. However, these privileges do not lessen their liability in a crash. In fact, in most cases, the driver is presumed to be guilty if a crash occurs while the ambulance is operating with emergency warning lights and siren. Motor vehicle crashes comprise a large number of lawsuits against EMS personnel and systems.

While on an emergency call, emergency vehicles typically are exempt from usual vehicle operations. If you are on an emergency call and are using your emergency warning lights and siren, then you may be allowed to take the following actions:

- Park or stand in an otherwise illegal location
- Proceed through a red traffic light or stop sign after stopping at the intersection
- Drive faster than the posted speed limit
- Drive against the flow of traffic on a one-way street or make a turn that is normally illegal
- Travel left of center to make an otherwise illegal pass

Remember, these exemptions vary by state and local jurisdiction. Check your local statutes for regulations in your area.

An emergency vehicle is never allowed to pass a school bus that has stopped to load or unload children and is displaying its flashing red lights or stop signal arm. If you approach a school bus that has its lights flashing, then stop before reaching the bus and turn off your siren. Next, wait for the bus driver to make sure the children are safe, close the bus door, and turn off the flashing lights. Only then may you carefully proceed past the stopped school bus.

Right-of-Way Privileges. A right-of-way privilege is just that: a privilege. State motor vehicle statutes or codes often grant the operator of an emergency vehicle the right to disregard the rules of the road when responding to an emergency. However, in doing so, the operator of an emergency vehicle must not endanger people or property under any circumstances.

Consider this case: An ambulance is approaching an intersection that is controlled by a four-way stop sign. The ambulance, with its emergency warning lights and siren turned on, proceeds through the intersection without slowing or stopping and collides with a vehicle coming from its right. Did the operator of the ambulance act appropriately by going through the intersection in this manner?

Right-of-way privileges for ambulances vary from state to state. Some states allow you to proceed through a red light or stop sign after you stop and make sure it is safe to continue. Other states allow you to proceed through a controlled intersection with so-called due regard, using flashing lights and siren. Due regard means that you may proceed only if you consider the safety of all people who are using the highway. If you fail to use due regard, then your service might be sued. If you are found to be at fault, then you may personally have to pay punitive damages or face civil and/or criminal sanctions.

Learn your local right-of-way privileges. Exercise them only when it is absolutely necessary for the patient's well-being. The use of emergency warning lights and siren is a matter of state and local practice and protocol.

Safety Tips

Always pass on the left, even if it means traveling into oncoming traffic. This action should only be done when you are driving in emergency mode with emergency warning lights and siren activated.

Use of Escorts. Using a police escort is an extremely dangerous practice. As discussed previously, when other motorists hear a siren and see a police vehicle passing, they might assume that the police vehicle is the only emergency vehicle and might not expect the ambulance. The only time an escort is justified is when you are in unfamiliar territory and truly need a guide. In such cases, alert motorists that a second unit is approaching by using a siren tone that is different from the police vehicle. Be prepared to stop if needed. If you are being guided, then follow at a safe distance. Do not assume nearby traffic will be aware of your presence. Exercise extreme caution when following another emergency vehicle, particularly when approaching an intersection.

Intersection Hazards. Intersection crashes are the most common and usually the most serious type of crash in which ambulances are involved. Always be alert and careful when approaching an intersection. If you are on an urgent call and cannot wait for the traffic light to change, then come to a momentary stop at the traffic light and look around for other motorists and pedestrians before proceeding into the intersection.

Motorists who "time the traffic lights" present a serious hazard. You may arrive at an intersection while the light is green. At the same time, a motorist who is timing the lights on the cross street arrives at the intersection. The motorist has a red light but knows that it is about to turn green and is expecting to go through. The stage is now set for a serious collision.

Highways. When you are responding to an emergency call and you must travel on the highway, shut down your emergency warning lights and siren until you have reached the far left lane. Shutting down your emergency warning devices minimizes the possibility of confusion for motorists who might not know what to do or where to go. Remember to travel in the far left lane whenever possible, which allows the ambulance to safely pass vehicles while still leaving a cushion of safety on the left side of the ambulance in case of emergency or unexpected obstacles.

When you exit the highway, follow the same procedures as when you entered the highway: turn off all emergency devices, move onto the off-ramp, and then reactivate the emergency warning lights and siren if necessary.

Unpaved Roadways. When you are required to drive the ambulance on an unpaved roadway, you must take special care. Unpaved roadways often have uneven surfaces, as well as large potholes. While responding on this type of roadway, operate the vehicle at a lower speed and maintain a firm grip on the steering wheel in an effort to maintain complete control of the ambulance at all times.

School Zones. When you respond through a school zone with your emergency warning lights turned on, it is important to remember that the lights and siren tend to attract children to the roadway and create a potential hazard. In many states, it is unlawful for an emergency vehicle to exceed the speed limit in school zones regardless of the condition of the patient.

Air Medical Operations

Air ambulances are used to evacuate medical and trauma patients. They land at or near the scene and transport patients to trauma facilities every day in many areas. They may also be used for search and rescue operations.

The two basic types of air medical units are fixed-wing aircraft and rotary-wing aircraft, otherwise known as helicopters Figure 39-23. Fixed-wing aircraft are generally used for interhospital patient transfers over distances greater than 100 to 150 miles (161 to 241 km). For shorter distances, ground transport or rotary-wing aircraft are more efficient.

Specially trained medical flight crews accompany all air ambulance flights. This section will focus on the rotary-wing aircraft. Your role in fixed-wing aircraft transfers will probably be limited to providing ground transport for the patient and medical flight crew between the hospital and the airport.

Rotary-wing aircraft have become an important tool in providing emergency medical care. The survival rates in

YOU are the Provider PART 4

After the helicopter has safely landed, you are met by the flight crew. You recently completed an orientation course for the local flight service, and you know it likes to have the patient packaged completely prior to its arrival. You proceed to give an extensive report of your findings. After the flight crew has examined the patient, they elect to secure the airway with an endotracheal tube with the assistance of medications to temporarily sedate and paralyze the patient. After they have confirmed tube placement by both physical exam and capnography, you accompany them to the helicopter with the patient on the stretcher. As you approach the rotor arc, a flight crew member escorts you to the side of the helicopter and you quickly load the patient in. When you have completed loading the patient, a flight crew member escorts you back out of the rotor arc, and you proceed back to your ambulance to perform a quick decontamination of the unit. Shortly thereafter, the helicopter lifts off and proceeds to the burn center.

Recording Time: 14 Minutes	
Respirations	6 breaths/min (unassisted)
Pulse	130 beats/min; thready
Skin	Burns to face, chest, and arms
Blood pressure	90/50 mm Hg
Oxygen saturation (Spo_2)	95% on 100% oxygen via bag-mask device
Pupils	Equal but sluggish to respond

9. What is the most important rule when working around helicopters on an emergency scene?
10. Who has ultimate control of the aircraft when on an emergency scene?

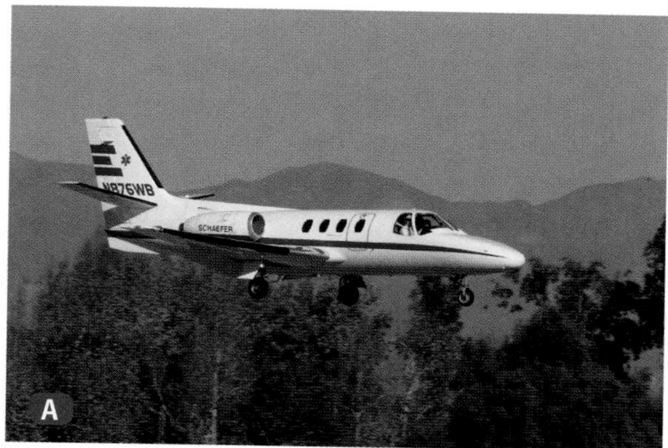

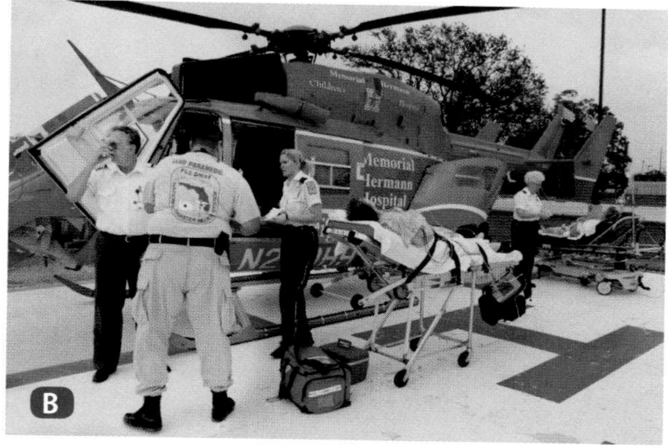

Figure 39-23 A. Fixed-wing aircraft are generally used to transfer patients from one hospital to another over distances greater than 100 to 150 miles (161 to 241 km). **B.** A rotary-wing aircraft, or helicopter, is used to help provide emergency medical care to patients who need to be transported quickly over shorter distances.

trauma patients are directly related to the time that elapses between injury and definitive treatment. Most helicopters that are used for emergency medical operations fly well in excess of 100 mph in a straight line, without road or traffic hazards. The crew may include flight paramedics, flight nurses, specialty providers such as respiratory therapists, and/or physicians. Air medical transport—especially the use of helicopters—has done much to speed up the transfer of patients from the trauma scene to definitive care. This mode of transport presents certain risks, however, and it is only appropriate in certain circumstances. You must consider several factors before calling for an air ambulance. Does the patient's condition warrant the risk of using air medical transport? Will use of the air ambulance save the patient time in getting to definitive care once all other factors are considered?

▶ Advantages of Using Air Ambulances

Air ambulances have an advantage over ground transport in that they reduce transport time and may help the patient receive definitive treatment within the Golden Hour (sometimes called the Golden Period). The decision to use rotary-wing transport should be made as early in the call as possible. If, after the patient assessment, it is determined that the helicopter is not needed, then it can always be returned to service. Some districts have local protocols that permit the automatic dispatch of a helicopter.

You need to weigh several factors to determine whether ordering a helicopter is appropriate. First, consider the time needed to start the engine of the aircraft, load personnel and gear, and travel to the scene (sometimes located a great distance away). After the helicopter arrives at the scene, time must be allotted to land the aircraft, transfer the patient to the flight crew, package the patient for air transport, and load the patient into the helicopter. Especially in metropolitan areas, it can be difficult to justify use of the helicopter. Severe traffic congestion or prolonged extrication times may sometimes make the use of a helicopter appropriate in urban areas. However, the use of an air ambulance is warranted if the transport time to the hospital by ground ambulance is too long considering the patient's condition. Use of an air ambulance may be warranted if the patient has a spinal injury and the terrain over which the patient must be carried is very rough. Even though the patient is stabilized, ground transport in a vehicle that is bouncing on the road could further injure the patient. As the AEMT on scene, you are the best judge of the patient's transportation needs. Table 39-7 summarizes the advantages and disadvantages of using an air ambulance.

▶ Disadvantages of Using Air Ambulances

The disadvantages of an air ambulance include interior space limitations, altitude limitations, and high cost. Patients in cardiac arrest or those who appear to be in precardiac arrest should be transported by ground ambulance. It is difficult to treat a patient in cardiac arrest in the helicopter because of the small cabin size.

In addition, air ambulances are usually restricted to flying under certain visual flight rules, so anything that interferes with visibility, such as adverse weather conditions, can make it too dangerous to fly. The terrain, such as uneven ground and loose objects such as rocks or debris, may also make it difficult to land the helicopter safely.

▶ Medical Evacuation Operations

A medical evacuation is commonly known as a **medevac** and is generally performed exclusively by helicopters. Most rural and suburban EMS jurisdictions and many urban systems have the capability to perform helicopter medevacs or have a mutual aid agreement with another agency, such as a police or hospital-based medevac service, to provide such service. Familiarize yourself with the medevac capabilities, protocols, and procedures of your particular EMS agency. Consider the following general guidelines before initiating a medevac operation.

Table 39-7 Advantages and Disadvantages of Using Rotary-Wing Aircraft (Helicopter)

Advantages of Using an Air Ambulance	Disadvantages of Using an Air Ambulance
Availability of specialized skills or equipment	Weather conditions
Possibility of rapid transport (typically between 130 and 150 mph)	Altitude limitations
Possibility of access to remote areas	Airspeed limitations
Availability of helicopter hospital helipads	Aircraft cabin size
	Terrain
	High cost
	Patient's condition (certain conditions may not be able to be treated within the confines of a helicopter; also, certain conditions may be worsened by altitude change)

Calling for a Medevac

Every agency has specific criteria for the type of patient who may receive medevac and how and when to call for a medevac. You must be familiar with the particular criteria used in your agency. These basic guidelines will help you to understand the process better.

- **Why call for a medevac?** The transport time to the hospital by ground ambulance is too long considering the patient's condition. Road, traffic, or environmental conditions limit or completely prohibit the use of a ground ambulance. The patient requires advanced emergency medical care that you are unable to provide. The presence of multiple patients will overwhelm resources at the hospital reachable by ground transport. (In this case, the helicopter may respond directly to the scene or it may be called to the hospital to transfer a patient to another facility with the capacity to provide definitive care.)
- **Who receives a medevac?** Patients with time-dependent injuries or illnesses may require a medevac. They are widely used for patients suspected of having a stroke, heart attack, or serious spinal cord injury, such as injuries sustained in a motor vehicle crash or while diving into a pool or horseback riding. Serious conditions that may require the use of helicopter medevacs may be found in remote areas and involve scuba diving accidents, near-drownings, or skiing and wilderness accidents. Other patients who may warrant the use of medevac are trauma patients and candidates for limb replantation (for amputations), a burn center, a hyperbaric chamber, or a venomous bite center.
- **Whom do you call?** Generally your dispatcher must be notified first. In some regions, after the medevac has been initiated, the ground EMS crew may be able to communicate with the flight crew on a specially designated radio frequency. If available, then it is important to keep this frequency clear of chatter and lengthy communications. You may be asked to give a brief presentation or update on the patient's condition. In this case, gather your thoughts and speak clearly and concisely, avoiding information that is not pertinent. Another important topic of communication between the ground and flight EMS crews will be where to land the helicopter. This topic will be covered later in this chapter.

Medevac Issues

As discussed, you must consider several important factors while making the decision to request medevac. These factors include weather, environment or terrain, altitude, airspeed limitations, cabin size, and cost. Typically, helicopters are unable to operate in severe weather such as thunderstorms, blizzards, and heavy rain. The environment may pose a risk as well. In mountainous or desert terrain, too many hazards may be present in the immediate vicinity to safely land the helicopter in the desired location.

As the elevation increases, the air thins, making it more difficult for pilots and patients to breathe. Because of this danger, helicopters have a maximum limit on flight elevations. Most helicopter services are limited to flying at 10,000 feet above sea level. This limitation could create a problem if your patient is located at 13,500 feet above sea level. It is important to remember that medevac helicopters are not jets, and it takes time for them to arrive on the scene, because of limitations in airspeed.

Because of the confined space of the helicopter cabin, helicopters are limited in the number of patients that can be safely transported and by the size of the patient that they can safely transport. Although a helicopter may be able to lift off with a 500-pound (227-kg) patient, it may be impossible to safely fit and secure the patient into the cabin area because of his or her size and girth.

Typical medevac flights are much more expensive than ground transport by ambulance. However, the level of care may be higher and the overall transport time may be shorter in the helicopter. Do not base the decision to request a medevac on the perceived ability of the patient to pay the medical bill, but rather on the medical necessity.

Establishing a Landing Zone

Although a helicopter can fly straight up and down, such movement is the most dangerous mode of operation. The safest and most effective way to land and take off is similar to that used by fixed-wing aircraft. Landing at a slight angle allows for safer operations. Takeoff combines a gradual lift and forward motion to travel up and out on a slight angle.

An important part of conducting a medevac is choosing the best location. Establishing a landing zone is the responsibility of the ground EMS crew. This process involves more than simply looking for a clear space. Be prepared to take action to make certain that the flight crew is able to land and take off safely. Actions to take and considerations to include when selecting and establishing a landing zone include the following:

- Ensure the area is a hard or grassy level surface that ideally measures 100 feet × 100 feet (30 m × 30 m) and no less than 60 feet × 60 feet (18 m × 18 m). If the landing zone is not level, then notify the flight crew of the steepness and direction of the slope.
- Ensure the area is clear of any loose debris that could become airborne and strike the helicopter or the patient and flight crew. Loose debris includes branches, trash bins, flares, caution tape, and medical equipment and supplies.
- Examine the immediate area for any overhead hazards such as power lines or telephone cables, antennas, and tall or leaning trees. Immediately relay the presence of these hazards to the flight crew because an alternative landing zone may be required. The flight crew may request that the hazard be marked or illuminated by weighted cones or that an emergency vehicle with its lights turned on be positioned next to or under the potential hazard.
- To mark the landing zone, use weighted cones or position emergency vehicles at the corners of the landing zone with headlights facing inward to form an X on the ground. This procedure is essential during night landings. Never use caution tape to mark the site. The use of flares is also not recommended, because not only can they become airborne, but they also have the potential to start a fire or cause an explosion.
- Move all nonessential people and vehicles to a safe distance outside of the landing zone.
- If the wind is strong, then radio to the flight crew the direction of the wind. The flight crew may request that you improvise some form of wind directional device to aid the crew's approach.

> **Safety Tips**
>
> Do not shine spotlights, flashlights, or any other lights in the air to help the helicopter pilot in command; the light beams may temporarily blind the pilot. Instead, direct light beams toward the ground at the landing site.

Landing Zone Safety and Patient Transfer

Be familiar with the capabilities, protocols, and methods for accessing helicopters in your area. Helicopter services provide training for AEMTs in ground operations and safety. Interactions with flight personnel should be comprehensive. Patients should be packaged prior to arrival of the air ambulance and an extensive report given to the flight crew for transfer of care. The following discussion is an introduction to safe medevac operations and is not intended to be substituted for the more extensive courses available locally.

Helicopter safety is nothing more than good common sense, along with a constant awareness of the need for personal safety. The types of helicopters that are used for medical operations vary, but the dangers are the same. If you are familiar with the way helicopters work and follow the pilot's instructions, then you will minimize these dangers. Be sure to do nothing near the helicopter and go only where the pilot or flight crew directs you.

The most important rule is to keep a safe distance from the aircraft whenever it is on the ground and "hot," which means when the main and tail rotors are spinning. The rotor blades will usually remain spinning because the flight crew does not generally expect to remain on the ground for a long time. This means that you should stay outside the perimeter of the landing zone unless directed by the pilot or a member of the flight crew to come to the aircraft. Usually, the flight crew will come to you carrying the crew's own equipment and will not require any assistance inside the landing zone. If you are asked to enter the landing zone, then stay away from the tail rotor; the tips of its blades move so rapidly that they appear invisible. With the possible exception of a rear-loading aircraft, always approach a helicopter from the front, even if it is not running, and approach only after the pilot signals it is clear to do so. If you must move from one side of the helicopter to another, then go around the front. Never duck under the body, the tail boom, or the rear section of the helicopter; the pilot cannot see you

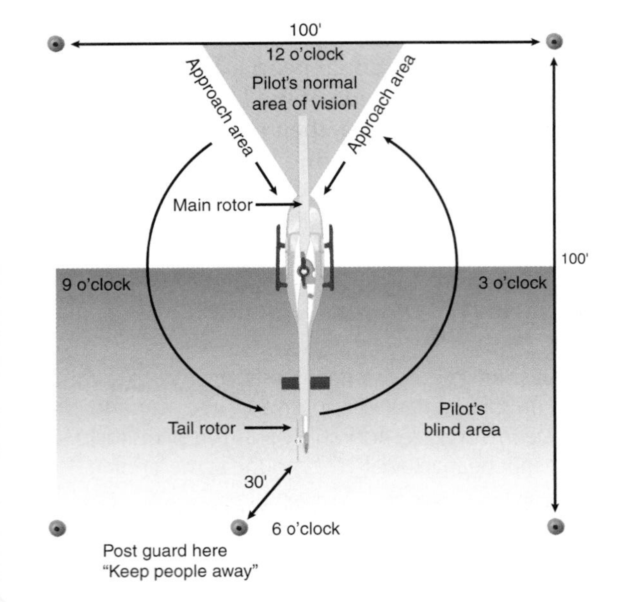

Figure 39-24 Approach a helicopter between the ten-o'clock and two-o'clock positions as the pilot faces forward.

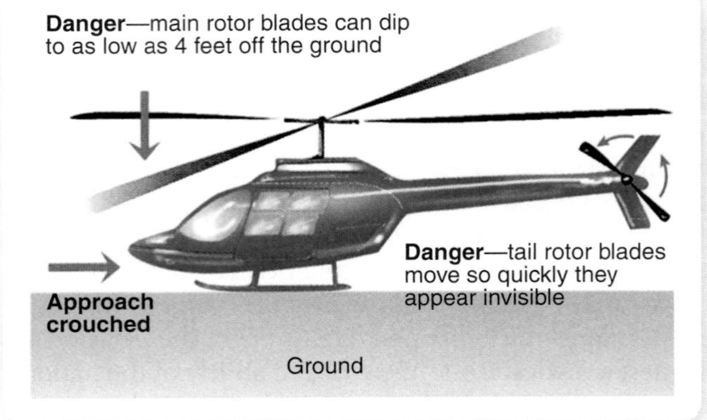

Figure 39-25 The main rotor blade of the helicopter is flexible and may dip as low as 4 feet (1 m) off the ground.

in these areas. The proper approach area is between the ten-o'clock and two-o'clock positions as the pilot faces forward **Figure 39-24**.

Another area of concern is the height of the main rotor blade. On many aircraft, it is flexible and may dip as low as 4 feet (1 m) off the ground **Figure 39-25**. When you approach the aircraft, walk in a crouched position. Wind gusts can alter the blade height without warning, so protect your equipment as you carry it under the blades. Air turbulence created by the rotor blades can blow off hats and loose equipment. These objects, in turn, can become a danger to the aircraft and personnel in the area.

When you accompany a flight crew member, follow directions exactly. Never try to open any aircraft door or move equipment unless instructed by a flight crew member. When told to approach the aircraft, use extreme caution and pay constant attention to hazards.

Keep the following guidelines in mind when operating at a landing zone:

- Familiarize yourself with the helicopter hand signals used within your jurisdiction **Figure 39-26**.
- Do not approach the helicopter unless instructed and accompanied by the flight crew.

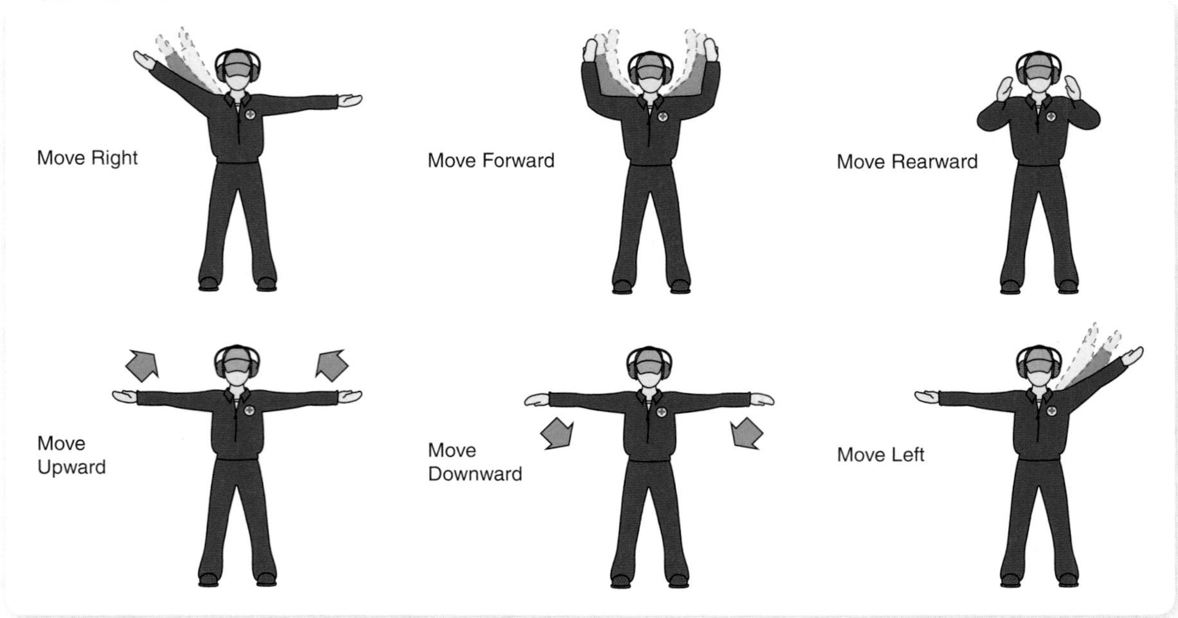

Figure 39-26 Some examples of helicopter hand signals. Be familiar with those used within your jurisdiction.

- Ensure all patient care equipment, including oxygen tanks, cervical collars, and head immobilizers, is properly secured to the stretcher and that the patient is fastened as well. Any loose articles or belongings such as hats, coats, or bags that belong to the patient or flight crew should not be brought into the landing zone and will likely need to be transported to the hospital by ground.
- Be aware some helicopters may load patients from the side, whereas others have rear-loading doors. Regardless of where the patient is being loaded, always approach the aircraft from the front unless otherwise instructed by the flight crew. It is very important that the pilot be able to see anyone who comes under the rotors. Always take the same path when exiting away from the helicopter, moving the patient headfirst.
- Smoking, open flames, and flares are prohibited within 50 feet (15 m) of the aircraft at all times.
- Wear eye protection during approach and takeoff.

Safety Tips

Pay close attention to directions by the flight crew when approaching the aircraft.

Communicating With Other Agencies

When you interact with other agencies, communication issues are always a possibility. Medevacs are no exception. Whereas the typical EMS system has its specific and well-defined jurisdiction, medevacs respond to service requests throughout a large, multijurisdictional area. Because of this large area with numerous jurisdictions, the medevac interacts with many services on a multitude of different radio frequencies.

To prevent any miscommunication, when the request is made for a medevac response, the request should include a ground contact radio channel (typically a preestablished mutual aid channel), as well as a call sign of the unit that the medevac should make contact with.

Special Considerations

Night Landings

Nighttime operations are considerably more hazardous than daytime operations because of the darkness. The pilot will generally fly over the area at least twice at varying altitudes with the lights of the helicopter turned on to identify potential obstacles and overhead wires, which can be hard to see. Do not shine spotlights, flashlights, or any other lights in the air to help the pilot; they may temporarily blind the pilot. Instead, direct low-intensity headlights or lanterns toward the ground at the landing site from opposite corners to form an X at the center of the landing zone. Turn off all headlights or lanterns that are facing in the direction of the aircraft after it has landed. After the helicopter has landed, do not aim lights near the aircraft. Always make certain the flight crew is aware of any overhead hazards or obstructions, and illuminate these if possible.

Landing on Uneven Ground

If the helicopter must land on a grade, then extra caution is advised. The main rotor blade will be closer to the ground on the uphill side. In this situation, approach the aircraft only from the downhill side or as directed by the flight crew **Figure 39-27**. Do not move the patient to the helicopter until the flight crew has signaled that the crew is ready to receive you. A flight crew member will direct and assist you in loading the patient.

Medevacs at Hazmat Incidents

Immediately notify the flight crew of the presence of hazmat at the scene. The helicopter generates tremendous wind and may easily spread any hazmat vapors present. Always consult the flight crew and incident commander about the best approach and distance from the scene for a medevac. The landing zone should be established upwind and uphill from the hazmat scene. Any patients who have been exposed to a hazmat must be properly decontaminated before they can be loaded into the aircraft. For proper procedures at hazmat incidents, refer to Chapter 41, *Incident Management*.

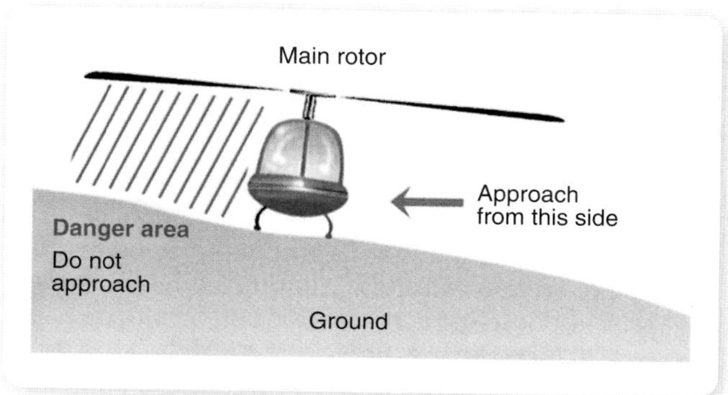

Figure 39-27 Approach a helicopter only on a grade from the downhill side.

YOU are the Provider SUMMARY

1. What are the nine phases of an ambulance call?

The nine phases of an ambulance call are as follows: preparation for the call, dispatch, en route to the scene, arrival at the scene, transfer of the patient to the ambulance, en route to the receiving facility (transport), arrival at the receiving facility (delivery), en route to the station, and postrun. During the preparation phase, ensure that the ambulance and its contents are prepared and you are both mentally and physically prepared. During the dispatch phase, obtain important information regarding the medical or traumatic emergency. En route to the call, pay careful attention to the roadways and other potential hazards. After you arrive on scene, perform a scene size-up and take standard precautions. During the transfer phase, move your patient onto your stretcher and place the patient in the back of the ambulance. During the transport phase, transfer the patient to the appropriate facility as safely and comfortably as possible. During the delivery phase, turn over care of the patient to the emergency department staff. During the en route phase, depart from the facility and return to your assigned quarters, or remain available for another call. Finally, during the postrun phase, complete all documentation and clean and sanitize the ambulance.

2. Which of the nine phases of an ambulance call is the most important?

Each phase of an ambulance call is equally important and must be safely completed before you move on to the next phase. Failure to safely complete a phase will likely result in a negative outcome for the patient.

3. What are some potential distractions that may be found inside of the ambulance?

Some ambulances have mobile dispatch terminals (MDT) and global positioning systems (GPS) that assist you in determining the location of the call. However, these devices, along with listening to the stereo, talking on a mobile phone, and eating or drinking, create additional driving hazards. While the ambulance is in motion, focus on driving and anticipating roadway hazards while your partner operates the MDT, GPS, portable radios, or siren. Minimizing the potential distractions to the driver allows for a safer response and minimizes the potential for mishaps.

4. While en route, how should you prepare to assess and care for the patient?

Review dispatch information about the nature of the call and the location of the patient. Assign specific initial duties and scene management tasks to each team member, and decide what type of equipment to take initially. Depending on your operation procedures, you may also decide which stretcher to bring to the patient.

5. What equipment do you need to carry to the patient's side?

You will only need to carry your jump kit to the patient's side. The ambulance must be equipped with a portable, durable, and waterproof jump kit that you can carry to the patient. Think of the jump kit as the "5-minute kit," containing anything you might need in the first 5 minutes with the patient except for the semiautomated external defibrillator, possibly the oxygen cylinder, and the portable suctioning unit. The jump kit must be easy to open and secure.

6. What are some advantages of using an air ambulance?

Air ambulances have an advantage over ground transport in that they reduce transport time and may help the patient receive definitive treatment within the Golden Hour (sometimes called the Golden Period). The use of an air ambulance is warranted if the transport time to the hospital by ground ambulance is too long considering the patient's condition. Use of an air ambulance may be warranted if the patient has a spinal injury and the terrain over which the patient must be carried is very rough.

7. What are some disadvantages of using an air ambulance?

When deciding whether to request an air ambulance, you need to weigh several factors. First, consider the time needed to start the aircraft, load personnel and gear, travel to the scene, land the helicopter, and transfer the patient to the flight crew. Consider the weather; anything that interferes with visibility can make it too dangerous to fly. The terrain also may make it difficult to land the helicopter safely. Finally, consider whether a safe landing zone is available; uneven ground and loose objects may impact the ability of the aircraft to land safely.

8. What factors must you take into consideration when creating a landing zone?

Actions to take and considerations to include when selecting and establishing a landing zone include the following:

- Select a hard or grassy level surface that ideally measures 100 feet × 100 feet (30 m × 30 m) and no less than 60 feet × 60 feet (18 m × 18 m).
- Clear the area of any loose debris that could become airborne and strike the helicopter or the patient and flight crew.
- Survey the immediate area for any overhead hazards such as power lines or telephone cables, antennas, and tall or leaning trees.
- To mark the landing site, use weighted cones or position emergency vehicles at the corners of the landing zone with headlights facing inward to form an X.

YOU are the Provider SUMMARY (continued)

- Make sure that all nonessential people and vehicles are moved to a safe distance outside of the landing zone.
- If the wind is strong, then radio the direction of the wind to the flight crew.

9. What is the most important rule when working around helicopters on an emergency scene?

Keep a safe distance from the aircraft whenever it is on the ground and "hot," which means when the tail rotor is spinning. Most of the time, the rotor blades will remain running because the flight crew does not generally expect to remain on the ground for a long time. Stay outside the landing zone perimeter unless directed by the pilot or a member of the flight crew to approach the aircraft. If you are asked to enter the landing zone, then stay away from the tail rotor; the tips of its blades move so rapidly that they are invisible. Never approach the helicopter from the rear, even if it is not running. If you must move from one side of the helicopter to another, then go around the front. Never duck under the body, the tail boom, or the rear section of the helicopter; the pilot cannot see you in these areas.

10. Who has ultimate control of the aircraft when on an emergency scene?

Regardless of the type of incident or the qualifications of the flight crew, the ultimate control of the aircraft rests solely on the pilot in command. The pilot in command makes the final decisions on all facets of aircraft operations.

EMS Patient Care Report (PCR)					
Date: 9-9-18	**Incident No.:** 10-9511		**Nature of Call:** Burns	**Location:** 4785 Meadowlark Cir.	
Dispatched: 2100	**En Route:** 2101	**At Scene:** 2105	**Transport:** N/A	**At Hospital:** N/A	**In Service:** 2145
Patient Information					
Age: 50 **Sex:** M **Weight (in kg [lb]):** 61 kg (135 lb)			**Allergies:** Unknown **Medications:** Unknown **Past Medical History:** Unknown **Chief Complaint:** Burns to face, chest, arms		
Vital Signs					
Time: 2106	**BP:** Not obtained	**Pulse:** Rapid, weak	**Respirations:** 6	**Spo_2:** Not obtained	
Time: 2113	**BP:** 96/52	**Pulse:** 124	**Respirations:** 6	**Spo_2:** 86% on R/A	
Time: 2119	**BP:** 90/50	**Pulse:** 130	**Respirations:** 6	**Spo_2:** 95% on O_2	
EMS Treatment (circle all that apply)					
Oxygen @ 15 **L/min via (circle one):** **NC** **NRM** **Bag-mask device** (circled)	**Assisted Ventilation** (circled)	**Airway Adjunct**	**CPR**		
Defibrillation	**Bleeding Control**	**Bandaging**	**Splinting**	**Other:**	
Narrative					
Dispatched to stand by at a structure fire. Fire department removed 50-year-old male from burning structure. Patient was unresponsive with partial-thickness (2nd-degree) burns to his face, chest, and arms. Patient presented with soot around his mouth and singed nasal hairs. Respirations were slow and shallow, and radial pulses were rapid and thready. Ventilations assisted with bag-mask device and 100% oxygen. Advised dispatch to call for air transport of patient. Landing zone established by law enforcement, and patient was transported to designated site by ambulance where emergency medical care was provided until the helicopter arrived. Upon arrival of flight crew, report given. Due to risk of airway compromise from inhalation injury, flight crew elected to manage airway with rapid sequence induction plus intubation prior to transport. Crew was assisted in loading patient into helicopter. Patient transported by flight crew to burn center.**End of report**					

Prep Kit

▶ Ready for Review

- Modern ambulances are designed according to strict governmental regulations based on national standards.
- The six-pointed Star of Life emblem identifies vehicles as ambulances. It is often affixed to the sides, rear, and roof of the ambulance. Local or state regulatory authorities determine what emblems may be displayed on the side of an ambulance.
- An ambulance call has nine phases: preparation for the call, dispatch, en route to the scene, arrival at the scene, transfer of the patient to the ambulance, en route to the receiving facility (transport), arrival at the receiving facility (delivery), en route to the station, and postrun.
- Specific patient care supplies should be carried on the ambulance, including basic medical equipment, airway management equipment and ventilation devices, suctioning equipment, oxygen delivery equipment, cardiopulmonary resuscitation equipment, basic wound care supplies, splinting supplies, childbirth supplies, and appropriate medications. An automated external defibrillator, as permitted by medical control, should always be carried on the ambulance. A jump kit, patient transfer equipment, nonmedical supplies, and initial extrication and rescue equipment are also needed.
- Every ambulance must be staffed with at least one emergency medical services (EMS) provider in the patient compartment whenever a patient is being transported. However, two EMS providers are strongly recommended. Some services may operate with a civilian (non-EMT) driver and a single EMS provider in the patient compartment.
- Check all medical equipment and supplies at least daily, including all the oxygen supplies, the jump kit, splints, dressings and bandages, backboards and other immobilization equipment, and the emergency obstetric kit.
- During the postrun phase, complete and file any additional reports and inform dispatch of the status, location, and availability of the unit. Perform a routine inspection to ensure that the ambulance is ready to respond to the next call.
- Learning how to properly operate your vehicle is just as important as learning how to care for patients when you arrive on the scene.
  - The first rule of safe driving in an emergency vehicle is that speed does not save lives; good emergency medical care does.
  - The second rule is that the driver and all passengers must wear seat belts and shoulder restraints at all times.
- Drivers must be qualified to drive the ambulance, must be physically and emotionally fit, and must have the proper attitude. The driver must know and follow safe driving practices, including wearing a seat belt, using an appropriate speed, using the emergency warning lights and siren appropriately, and maintaining a cushion of safety.
- Air ambulances are used to evacuate medical and trauma patients.
- The two basic types of air medical units are fixed-wing aircraft (airplanes) and rotary-wing aircraft (helicopters).
  - Fixed-wing aircraft generally are used for inter-hospital patient transfers over distances greater than 100 to 150 miles (161 to 241 km).
  - Rotary-wing aircraft are more efficient for shorter distances.
- A medical evacuation is commonly known as a medevac and is generally performed exclusively by helicopters.
- You must follow certain safety rules when working around landing zones and helicopters. Familiarize yourself with these guidelines before working any call involving air transport.

Prep Kit *(continued)*

▶ Vital Vocabulary

acceleration Increase speed.

air ambulances Fixed-wing aircraft (airplanes) and rotary-wing aircraft (helicopters) that have been modified for emergency medical care; used to evacuate and transport patients with life-threatening injuries to treatment facilities.

ambulance A specialized vehicle for treating and transporting sick and injured patients.

blind spots Areas of the road that are blocked from the driver's sight by his or her own vehicle or mirrors.

cleaning The process of removing dirt, dust, blood, or other visible contaminants from a surface.

chassis The structural framework of the ambulance.

chassis set The transfer of weight (center of mass) to different points on the chassis.

coefficient of friction A measure of the grip of the tires on the road.

CPR board A device that provides a firm surface under the patient's torso.

cushion of safety A defensive driving technique used to keep a safe distance between the ambulance and other vehicles on any side of the ambulance.

deceleration Decrease speed.

decontaminated To have removed or neutralized radiation, chemical, or other hazardous material from clothing, equipment, vehicles, and personnel.

disinfection The killing of pathogenic agents by direct application of chemicals.

first-responder vehicles Specialized vehicles used to transport emergency medical services equipment and personnel to the scenes of medical emergencies.

footprint The area of contact between the tire and the surface of the road.

friction The resistance to the motion of one body against another.

high-level disinfection The killing of pathogenic agents by using potent means of disinfection.

hydroplaning A condition in which the tires of a vehicle may be lifted off the road surface as water builds up under them, making the vehicle feel as though it is floating.

jump kit A portable kit containing items that are used in the initial care of the patient.

medevac Medical evacuation of a patient by helicopter.

spotter A person who assists a driver in backing up an ambulance to compensate for blind spots at the rear of the vehicle.

Star of Life The six-pointed star that identifies vehicles that meet federal specifications as licensed or certified ambulances.

sterilization A process, such as heating, that removes microbial contamination.

▶ References

1. National Fire Protection Association. *NFPA 1917, Standard for Automotive Ambulances.* www.nfpa.org. Accessed October 12, 2016.
2. The National Highway Traffic Safety Administration. *The National Highway Traffic Safety Administration and Ground Ambulance Crashes, April 2014.* https://www.naemt.org/Files/HealthSafety/2014%20NHTSA%20Ground%20Amublance%20Crash%20Data.pdf. Accessed June 24, 2016.
3. The National Highway Traffic Safety Administration. *Using Efficient Steering Techniques.* www.safercar.gov/parents/TeenDriving/pdf-teen/steeringtechniques.pdf. Accessed October 12, 2016.

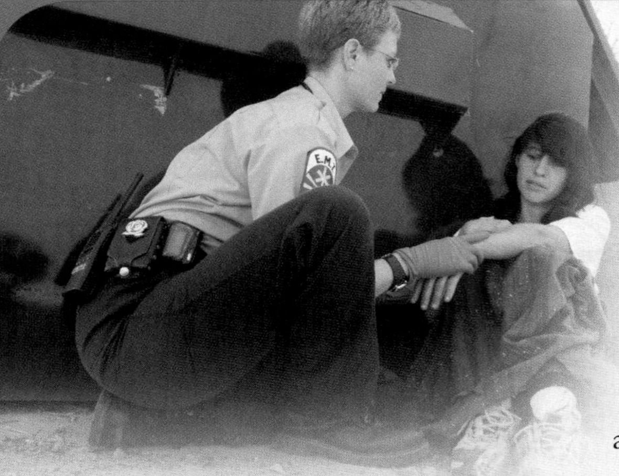

Assessment in Action

You and your paramedic partner are treating a cardiac patient in critical condition. After loading him into the ambulance and assisting with immediate care, you leave to drive to the hospital. Because of the nature of the patient's condition, your partner asks that you use the emergency warning lights and siren.

1. The use of emergency warning lights and siren depend on the following factors, EXCEPT:

A. local protocols.
B. the patient's condition.
C. time of day.
D. anticipated clinical outcome of the patient.

2. Which of the following terms describes keeping a safe distance between your vehicle and the one in front of you, checking for tailgaters behind your ambulance, and staying aware of vehicles potentially hiding in your blind spots?

A. Blind spot
B. Cushion of safety
C. Spotter
D. Hot zone

3. If you are on an emergency call and you are using your emergency warning lights and siren, then you may be allowed to take the following actions, EXCEPT:

A. park or stand in an otherwise illegal location.
B. drive faster than the posted speed limit.
C. drive against the flow of traffic on a one-way street.
D. proceed through an intersection without slowing.

4. When may an emergency vehicle proceed around a school bus that has stopped to load or unload children?

A. Only after coming to a stop and making eye contact with the bus driver
B. Only after all children have reached the sidewalk
C. As soon as the school bus door is closed
D. You may not proceed past a stopped school bus

5. The two ways to control an ambulance are either to change its direction or to change its:

A. weight.
B. speed.
C. height.
D. tire width.

6. What is the most common location for ambulance crashes?

A. Urban areas
B. Hilly terrain
C. Areas of road construction
D. Intersections

7. The recommended site for establishing a landing zone should be a hard or grassy level surface that measures no less than:

A. 40 feet × 40 feet (12 m × 12 m).
B. 60 feet × 60 feet (18 m × 18 m).
C. 80 feet × 80 feet (24 m × 24 m).
D. 100 feet × 100 feet (30 m × 30 m).

Assessment *in Action* *(continued)*

8. All of the following basic principles govern the use of emergency warning lights and siren, EXCEPT:

A. Local protocols
B. The unit must be on a true emergency call to the best of your knowledge.
C. The unit must be operated with due regard for the safety of all others, on and off the roadway.
D. Both audible and visual warning devices must be used simultaneously.

9. What are the disadvantages of using an air ambulance to transport a patient?

10. During air medical operations, emergency medical services providers often assist in loading patients into the aircraft. What are the special considerations to keep in mind when approaching a helicopter?

CHAPTER 40

Vehicle Extrication, Special Rescue, and Hazardous Materials

National EMS Education Standard Competencies

EMS Operations

Knowledge of operational roles and responsibilities to ensure patient, public, and personnel safety.

Vehicle Extrication

- Safe vehicle extrication (pp 1651-1659)
- Use of simple hand tools (p 1657)

Hazardous Materials Awareness

- Risks and responsibilities of operating in a cold zone at a hazardous material or other special incident. (pp 1659-1664, 1674-1678)

Knowledge Objectives

1. Explain the responsibilities of advanced emergency medical technicians (AEMTs) in patient rescue and extrication. (pp 1651-1659)
2. Compare the terms extrication and entrapment. (p 1651)
3. Discuss how to ensure safety at the scene of a rescue incident, including scene size-up and the selection of the proper personal protective equipment and additional necessary gear. (pp 1651-1653)
4. List the ten phases of extrication and the role of AEMTs during each one. (pp 1652-1659)
5. Discuss the situational awareness factors AEMTs must use to ensure safety at the site of a vehicle extrication. (pp 1652-1653)
6. Name some vehicle safety system components that may be hazardous to both AEMTs and patients following a motor vehicle crash; include how AEMTs can mitigate these dangers. (p 1654)
7. Explain the different factors that must be considered before attempting to gain access to the patient during an incident that requires extrication. (pp 1655-1656)
8. Discuss patient care considerations related to assisting with rapid extrication, providing emergency care to a trapped patient, and removing and transferring a patient. (pp 1656-1659)
9. Contrast simple access and complex access in vehicle extrication. (p 1657)
10. Discuss situations that would require special technical rescue teams and AEMTs role in these situations. (pp 1659-1660)
11. Describe tactical situations and the techniques used to stay safe at these incidents. (pp 1660-1661)
12. Describe some of the unique aspects of responding to a hazardous materials (hazmat) incident. (p 1663)
13. Know the entry-level training or experience requirements identified by the Hazardous Waste Operations and Emergency Response (HAZWOPER) regulation for AEMTs responding to a hazmat incident. (p 1663)
14. Describe the types of containers used to store hazardous materials. (pp 1664-1665)
15. Discuss the specific reference materials AEMTs can use to recognize a hazmat incident. (pp 1669, 1671-1673)
16. Explain the role of AEMTs during a hazmat incident before and after the hazmat team arrives and the precautions required to ensure the safety of civilians and responders. (pp 1674-1678)
17. Name the three control zones established at a hazmat incident, the characteristics of each zone, and the personnel who work within each one. (pp 1674-1676)
18. Describe the four levels of personal protective equipment required at a hazmat incident to protect responders from injury and contamination. (pp 1676-1677)
19. Explain patient care at a hazmat incident; include the special requirements that are necessary for those patients who require immediate treatment and transport prior to full decontamination. (pp 1677-1678)

Skills Objectives

1. Using an example, demonstrate how to correctly identify the US Department of Transportation's labels, placards, and markings used to designate hazardous materials. (pp 1667-1670)
2. Demonstrate the ability to use a variety of reference materials to identify a hazardous material. (pp 1669, 1671-1673)

Introduction

Rescue involves many different processes and environments, including vehicle, water, trench, tactical, and hazardous materials rescue. These kinds of rescues require training beyond the level of the advanced emergency medical technician (AEMT). For example, a motor vehicle crash (MVC) in which a fuel tank has ruptured creates a hazardous and potentially disastrous situation that requires the help of vehicle extrication and hazardous materials (hazmat) teams. Or, you may find yourself on the scene with a gunman who has begun to fire on people and is still at large. These incidents pose an increased risk to you and require the assistance of specialized law enforcement teams.

There is always a chance that you may be the first emergency unit to arrive at the scene, and your initial actions may determine how efficiently the rescue is completed. This chapter begins with a brief discussion of safety at the scene of a rescue incident, followed by the basic concepts of patient rescue and extrication, and the hazards associated with responding to a hazmat incident.

Safety

You must always be prepared, mentally and physically, for any incident that requires rescue or **extrication** (the removal of a patient from entrapment or from a dangerous situation or position). The most important part of your preparation is to think about your safety and the safety of your team. Safety begins with the proper mind-set and the proper personal protective equipment ([PPE] discussed later in this chapter).

The equipment that you use and the gear that you wear will depend on the situation you expect to encounter, as well as what you observe during your scene size-up **Figure 40-1**. Such protective gear may include turnout gear, a helmet, hearing protection, and a fire extinguisher. However, the importance of wearing blood- and fluid-impermeable gloves at all times during patient contact cannot be emphasized enough. If you are involved in an extrication, then wear a pair of leather gloves over your disposable gloves to protect yourself from injury when handling ropes, tools, broken glass, hot or cold objects, or sharp metal.

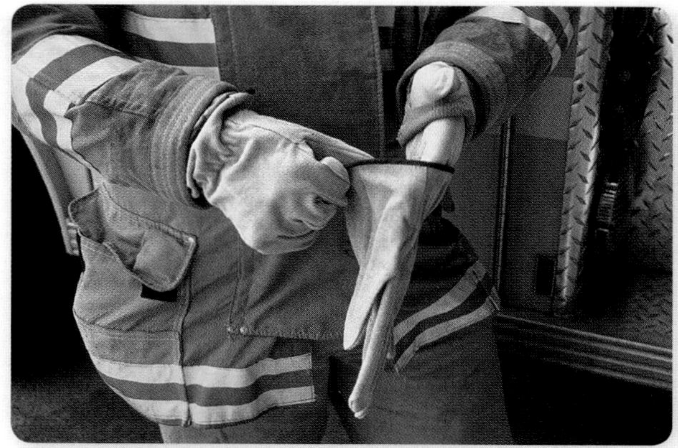

Figure 40-1 Proper protective equipment varies depending on the situation.

Fundamentals of Extrication

During all phases of rescue, your primary concern is safety, and your primary role is to provide emergency medical care and prevent further injury to the patient. You will provide care as extrication goes on around you unless this proves to be too dangerous for you or the patient. AEMTs may also be responsible for providing simple extrication when tools are not required. As discussed, extrication or disentanglement is the removal of a patient from entrapment or from a dangerous situation or position. **Entrapment** is a condition in which a person is caught within a closed area with no way out or has a limb or body part trapped. In the context of this chapter, in many cases, extrication refers to the removal of a patient from a wrecked vehicle. However, the same principles and concepts apply to other situations, such as removal of a patient from a collapsed building or from a trench.

There are 10 phases to the extrication process **Table 40-1**. Many are similar to the phases of an ambulance call (discussed in Chapter 39, *Transport Operations*). Each phase is discussed, with emphasis on the phases in which you will participate.

YOU are the Provider PART 1

Your ambulance is dispatched to a MVC on a rural road. On arrival, you are met by the incident commander (IC) who states his firefighters are attempting to gain access to the patient, who is trapped in the vehicle. As you approach the vehicle, you note that it is sitting on its roof, with massive damage to both sides of the vehicle, indicating it has rolled several times.

1. What are some hazards you may encounter with vehicle safety systems?
2. How should this vehicle be stabilized?

Table 40-1 Ten Phases of Extrication

1. Preparation
2. En route to the scene
3. Arrival and scene size-up
4. Hazard control
5. Support operations
6. Gaining access
7. Emergency medical care
8. Removal of the patient
9. Transfer of the patient
10. Termination

Safety Tips

During vehicle extrication, never position yourself between a patient and airbags! Even if the battery cables have been cut, there may still be enough of a charge left in the line to deploy an airbag, injuring you and the patient.

▶ Preparation

Preparing for an incident requiring extrication involves pre-incident training with rescue personnel for the various types of rescue situations your team might face. Some are discussed later in this chapter. Just as you must check the equipment carried on the ambulance, rescue personnel must also routinely check the extrication tools and their response vehicle to ensure its proper operation. Such preparations reduce the possibility of equipment failure at an emergency scene.

▶ En Route to the Scene

The procedures and safety precautions similar to those discussed in the phases of an ambulance call are used when responding to a rescue call.

▶ Arrival and Scene Size-up

Situational awareness allows you to recognize and understand potential threats and react proactively to avoid negative consequences **Figure 40-2**. If you are the first to arrive on scene, then position the unit in a safe location that does not add a hazard to the scene and that also helps to protect the scene. If you are not the first to arrive, then choose a location that will allow safe access to the scene while leaving yourself a way out. Do not park in an area where you will be blocked in. If law enforcement or fire units have blocked the roadway, then position your unit so the back of the ambulance is pointing toward the scene to facilitate patient transport.

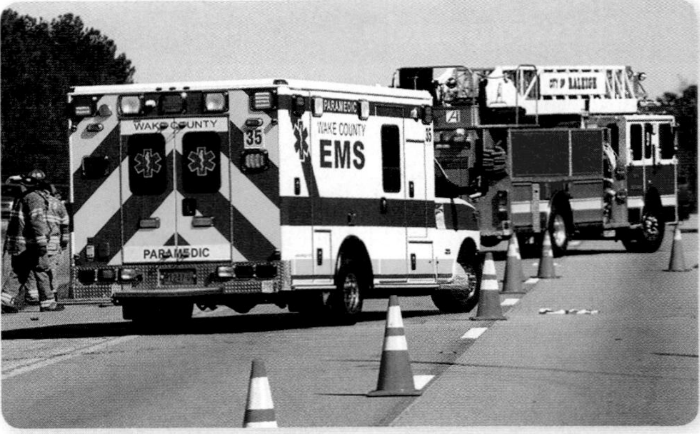

Figure 40-2 Assess the scene for any possible hazards and proactively manage them.

When you are on the scene of an MVC, use only essential warning lights. Too many lights can distract or confuse motorists. Many emergency responders have been injured on scenes when they were struck by passing vehicles. (Some local protocols require providers to reduce or turn off emergency lighting after the scene is secured; this may reduce the risk of a secondary crash.) If law enforcement is not on scene, then designate a traffic control person until law enforcement arrives. Before exiting your vehicle, check for any vehicles that might cause injury to you. Do not assume motorists will always heed the warning lights.

Safety Tips

Wear a high-visibility reflective safety vest so you will be seen by fellow responders and motorists.

In the context of extrication, scene **size-up** is the ongoing process of information gathering and scene evaluation to determine appropriate strategies and tactics to manage an emergency, while paying attention to such hazards as downed power lines, leaking fluids, fire, and broken glass. One of the important responsibilities of scene size-up is to determine what, if any, additional resources you will need. These resources may include additional emergency medical services (EMS) units and personnel. If you are first on the scene, then you may need to initiate a rescue response or call for extrication equipment, fire service personnel and equipment, law enforcement, or specialized crews such as hazmat and utility departments.

A 360° walk around the scene will allow you to evaluate the hazards and consider potential injuries and determine the number of patients. If there is a large group of patients, then implement local mass-casualty incident protocols as necessary. During your walk, look for the following:

- Downed power lines
- Leaking fuel or other substances
- Smoke or fire
- Broken glass
- The mechanism of injury

- Trapped or ejected patients
- The number of patients and vehicles involved

This assessment can be performed in a matter of seconds, but is the most important step in protecting yourself and your crew.

On the scene of an MVC, it is important to note the physical damage to the structure of the vehicle(s). For example, a bent steering wheel is a mechanism of injury for significant face and/or thoracic trauma. Imprints in the dashboard, which are usually the result of the knees striking it, indicate the potential for serious lower extremity injuries such as hip dislocations and fractures. Always lift up deployed airbags to see if there is deformity to the steering wheel or dashboard, which indicates the patient struck the structure after the airbag deflated. Determine if the patient was restrained or not. An unrestrained patient may have contact injuries as well as secondary injuries. If the unrestrained patient is thrown forward, then he or she may strike the windshield with the head, resulting in a spider web pattern of shattered glass and possible head, face, or neck injuries. Include any findings in your documentation and maintain a high index of suspicion, even if the patient does not present with significant obvious injuries.

Evaluate the need for additional resources such as:

- Extrication equipment
- Fire suppression
- Law enforcement
- Hazmat units
- Utility companies
- Advanced life support unit(s)
- Aeromedical transport

Look for leaked fuel and other flammable substances. Motor vehicles carry a variety of fuels and lubricants that pose a fire hazard. Some postcrash fires are started when sparks created during the crash ignite leaked fuel. A short in a vehicle's electrical system or a damaged battery may also cause a postcrash fire. These fires may trap the occupants of the vehicle and require fire suppression.

Environmental conditions can lead to unique hazards at a crash scene. Crashes that occur in rain, sleet, or snow, for example, present an added hazard for rescue personnel and patients. Crashes that occur on hills are harder to handle than those that occur on level ground. Uneven terrain increases the potential for vehicles to roll over, requiring vehicles to be stabilized prior to gaining access.

Some crash scenes may present threats of violence. Intoxicated people or people who are upset with other motorists may pose a threat to you or to other people present at the scene. Be alert for weapons that civilians are carrying in vehicles.

Safety Tips

The conditions responsible for an MVC may also cause other motorists to lose control of their vehicles and injure you. Maintain your situational awareness at all times.

Report to the IC (discussed later in the chapter) as soon as you arrive at a scene. Under the incident command system (described in Chapter 41, *Incident Management*), the rescue operations are integrated as a separate group. You are a member of this group, and will provide care for the patient(s) when approved by the IC. You will coordinate your efforts with the rescue team and law enforcement and communicate with members of the rescue team throughout the extrication process.

Stay focused. The rescue team is responsible for properly securing and stabilizing the scene or the vehicle, providing safe entrance and **access** to patients (the ability to reach the patient), extricating patients, ensuring patients are properly protected during extrication or other rescue activities, and providing adequate room so patients can be properly removed. You are responsible for assessing and providing immediate medical care, triage and assigning priority to patients, packaging the patient, providing additional assessment and care as needed once the patient has been removed, and providing transport to the emergency department (ED).

Hazard Control

A variety of hazards may be present at a vehicle extrication scene. Law enforcement is responsible for traffic control and direction, maintaining order at the scene, investigating the crash or crime scene, and establishing and maintaining perimeters so that bystanders are kept at a safe distance and out of the way of rescuers. Firefighters are responsible for extinguishing any fire, preventing additional ignition, ensuring that the scene is safe, and washing down any spilled fuel.

Downed power lines are a common hazard at vehicle crash scenes. Never attempt to move downed power lines. If power lines are touching or located in proximity to a vehicle involved in the crash, then instruct patients to remain in their vehicles until power is shut off by a utility company representative. If you are not the first at the scene, then there will be a protected area designated as the **safe zone**. Unless you are directed otherwise, you and the ambulance should remain in the safe zone, outside of the danger zone Figure 40-3. A **danger zone** is an area where people can be exposed to hazards such as electric wires, sharp metal edges, broken glass, toxic substances, radiation, or ignition or explosion of hazardous materials.

Sometimes, an extrication scene is further complicated by the presence of **hazardous materials**. A hazardous material is any substance that is toxic, poisonous, radioactive, flammable, or explosive and can cause injury or death with exposure. In addition to posing a threat to you and others at the immediate scene, hazardous materials may pose a threat to a much larger area and population. Whenever there is a possibility that a hazardous material is involved, you must follow a number of additional special procedures. These procedures are discussed later in this chapter.

Bystanders and family members can also create hazards. If they are allowed to get too close, they are at risk of injury and may also interfere with the overall management of the

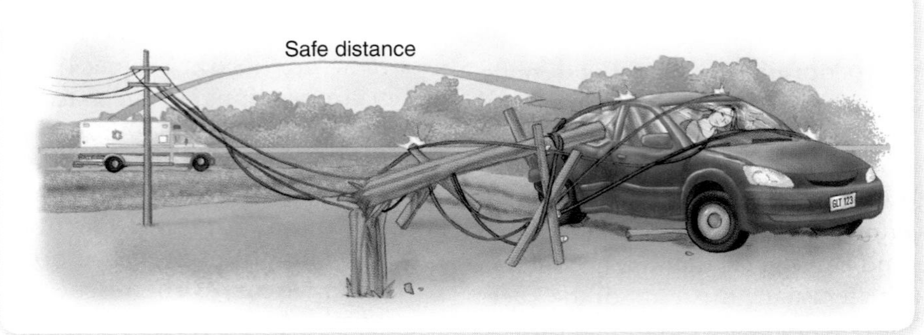

Figure 40-3 Unless you are directed otherwise, remain outside the danger zone.

incident. For these reasons, the danger zone is off-limits to bystanders. Help to set up and enforce this zone. If you arrive before the rescue team, then coordinate crowd control with law enforcement officials.

Words of Wisdom

Managing a difficult bystander may prove especially challenging when he or she claims to have medical credentials. If a physician who is not trained in EMS attempts to intervene, inform medical control immediately. Communication between medical control and the physician may reduce the risk of confrontation.

On the scene of a MVC, the actual vehicle can be a hazard. An unstable vehicle on its side or roof can be a danger to you. Rescue personnel can stabilize the vehicle with a variety of jacks or cribbing (wooden blocks). Prior to attempting to gain access to a vehicle involved in a crash, ensure the vehicle is in "park" with the parking brake set and the ignition turned off. Both battery cables should be disconnected, negative side first, to minimize the possibility of sparks or fire. Other hazards include vehicles with headrests that deploy in the event of a crash and vehicles that are already on fire or are leaking fuel. Do not approach a vehicle that is on fire or leaking fuel without proper turnout gear, and never use flares around these vehicles.

Safety Tips

"Rolling" methamphetamine laboratories are common on the highways today. Look for telltale signs such as large or older vehicles with paint peeling around the trunk area, accompanied by unusual odors. Use extreme caution when approaching these vehicles because there is the potential for an explosion and/or release of toxic gases.

Vehicle Safety Systems

A variety of safety systems are included in modern vehicles. Although many of these devices are useful when the vehicle is in motion, they can become hazards after the vehicle has been involved in a crash.

Shock-absorbing bumpers provide vehicle protection from low-speed impact. Following a front- or rear-end crash, the shock absorbers within these bumpers may be compressed or "loaded." Avoid standing directly in front of such bumpers, and always approach vehicles from the side, because the shock absorbers can release and injure your knees and legs.

Manufacturers are mandated to incorporate supplemental restraint systems such as airbags and seat belt pretentioners into their vehicles. Airbags fill with a nonharmful gas on impact and quickly deflate after the crash. Airbags are located in the steering wheel and the dashboard in front of the passenger, and they deploy when the vehicle is struck from the front or rear. Additional bags may be present to protect the driver and passengers from side impacts. These bags may be located in the doors or seats. Airbags will normally deploy and deflate before you arrive on the scene. However, airbags have inflated and caused injury while EMS providers were providing patient care. Use caution when working in damaged vehicles in which airbags have not inflated. Maintain at least a 5-inch (13-cm) clearance around side-impact airbags that have not deployed, a 10-inch (25-cm) clearance around driver-side airbags that have not deployed, and 20-inch (50-cm) clearance around passenger-side airbags that have not deployed.

Some airbag manufacturers used powder-like lubricants such as cornstarch or talcum powder to aid in deployment and lubricate the fabric of the airbag.[1] You may notice a haze similar to smoke inside vehicles in which these airbags have deployed. Although nontoxic, the appropriate protective gear, including eye protection, will reduce the potential for irritation from these substances.

Seat belt pretensioners tighten the seat belt when sensors are triggered. They are chambers of combustible gas with explosive igniter material that force the piston in the chamber to be driven upward at a high speed. Damage to this chamber can result in injury to the patient or rescuers.

Words of Wisdom

A vehicle crash scene can present many hazards to emergency medical responders (EMRs) and patients, including fuel spills that pose fire and explosion risks, downed power lines that pose electrical hazards, broken glass and torn metal, and exposure to potentially infectious body fluids. Your safety at every type of emergency scene begins with, and depends on, your scene size-up. What you see at the scene helps you determine which PPE to use and whether to call for additional or specialized assistance.

Alternative Fuel Vehicles

Today, with advances in automotive technology, EMS responders should keep in mind that some vehicles on the road are powered by an alternative fuel. An **alternative fuel vehicle** is a vehicle that uses anything other than a petroleum-based motor fuel (gasoline or diesel fuel) to propel a motorized vehicle.[2] These vehicles may be powered by alternative fuels such as propane, natural gas, methanol, or hydrogen. Other alternative fuel vehicles may be powered by electricity (battery electric vehicles) or a combination of electricity and fuel (hybrid electric vehicles).

Alternative fuel vehicles are usually identified by markings on the vehicle. You should not approach these vehicles without proper PPE. Toxic fumes and vapors from battery electric or hybrid electric vehicle batteries can be carried in smoke or steam. Do not approach the vehicle if you detect an unusual odor, and retreat if you experience burning in your eyes or throat until the scene is safe. If they have not been notified previously, then call dispatch to request additional assistance from the fire department and/or hazmat team.

Although each type of electric drive vehicle (hybrid/electric vehicle or pure battery electric vehicle) has its own unique features, one feature is common throughout—the need for properly trained responders to disconnect the high-voltage battery pack to prevent electrical shock or further fire or explosion Figure 40-4.

The batteries may not be located in the engine compartment, but in other areas, such as the trunk or under the seats. Furthermore, there also may be more than one battery present. You must remain vigilant and be aware of their inherent dangers. Electric drive vehicle batteries have a higher voltage than traditional automotive batteries, and it may take up to 10 minutes for a high-voltage system to de-energize after the main battery is turned off. Avoid contact with high-voltage wires (typically orange) and components throughout the rescue Figure 40-5.[3]

Support Operations

Support operations include lighting the scene, establishing tool and equipment staging areas, and marking helicopter landing zones. Fire and rescue personnel will work together on these functions.

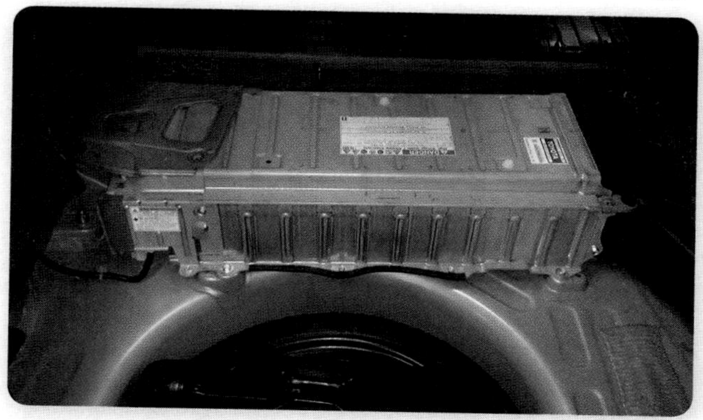

Figure 40-4 The battery pack installed in a Toyota Prius.

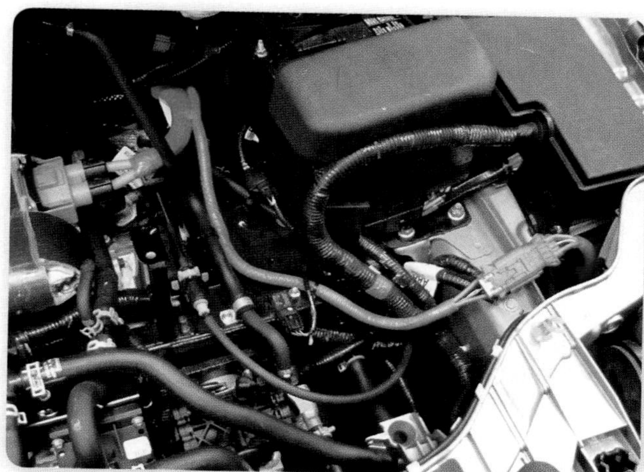

Figure 40-5 High-voltage wiring.

Safety Tips

A fire fueled by ethanol or methanol burns bright blue and can be very difficult to see on a clear day. Methanol burns without smoke, and therefore may seem to burn with an invisible flame in bright light.

Gaining Access

A crucial phase of extrication is gaining access to the patient. Never attempt to gain access to the patient or enter the vehicle until you are sure any hazards have been identified and properly controlled or eliminated. When there is an IC present, you will be authorized to enter only when these considerations have been met.

The exact way to gain access depends on many factors, including the terrain and the weather. It is up to you to identify the safest, most efficient way to gain access Figure 40-6. Darkness, uneven terrain, tall grass, shrubbery, or wreckage may make patients hard to find. Multiple vehicles with multiple patients may be involved. If this is the case, then you should locate and rapidly triage

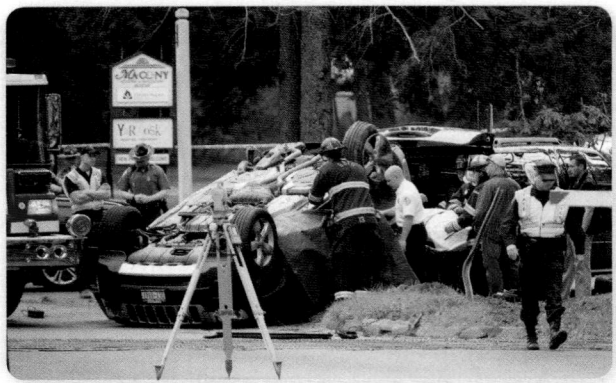

Figure 40-6 Identify the safest, most efficient way to gain access.

Words of Wisdom

Tips for Managing Alternative Fuel Vehicle Hazards

- Look for markings specific to alternative fuel vehicles, and call early for assistance.
- Do not use flares to mark off the incident scene; use nonsparking markers such as cones.
- Determine if the vehicle is stable and ensure all hazards are identified and controlled or eliminated.
- Be aware of the potential for toxic vapors, gases, or fumes even if no fire is present. Also remember that during daylight hours it may be very difficult to see flames from a fire fueled by methanol or ethanol.
- Avoid contact with any fluids leaking from the vehicle.
- Determine if the high-voltage battery pack has been disconnected on electric drive vehicles.
- Call for hazmat teams as soon as possible, and set up a safety zone around the perimeter to keep bystanders and responders safe.

each patient to determine who needs urgent care. This step is important before you proceed with any treatment and patient packaging. Take these factors into account during your scene size-up. Remember, scene size-up is a continuing process, because the situation often changes. As a result, you may need to change your plans for gaining access and providing treatment.

To determine the exact location and position of the patient, you and your team should consider the following questions:

- Is the patient in a vehicle or in some other structure?
- Is the vehicle or structure severely damaged?
- What hazards exist that pose a risk to the patient and responders?
- In what position is the vehicle? On what type of surface? Is the vehicle stable or is it likely to roll over?

Also consider the patient's injuries and their severity. You may have to change your course of action as you learn more about the patient's condition. For example, do not try to access the patient until you are sure the vehicle is stable and hazards have been identified and deemed safe. Hazards might include electrical or gas lines. Decide if you will need additional resources such as extrication equipment or a hazmat team, fire department, law enforcement, utility company, or air transport. Notify the dispatcher.

What should you do if you have to remove a patient quickly because the environment is threatening or you need to perform cardiopulmonary resuscitation (CPR)? CPR is not effective when the patient is in a sitting position or lying on the soft seat of a vehicle. In these instances, you and your team may have to use the rapid extrication technique (discussed in Chapter 6, *Lifting and Moving Patients*) to move a patient from a sitting position inside a vehicle to a supine position on a long backboard. A team of responders who are experienced in using this technique should be able to perform rapid extrication in 1 minute or less. Use the rapid extrication technique only as a last resort.

While you are gaining access to the patient and during extrication, make sure the patient remains safe. Always talk to the patient and describe what you are going to do before you do it and as you are doing it, even if you think the patient is unresponsive Figure 40-7. In many instances, you or your partner may be providing cervical spine immobilization or other care during extrication. EMS personnel should wear proper protective gear while in the working area. During vehicle extrication, both you and the patient should be covered by a thick, fire-resistant canvas or blanket for protection from broken glass, flying particles, tools, or other hazards during any cutting or forceful extrication maneuvers. A backboard may also be used as a protective

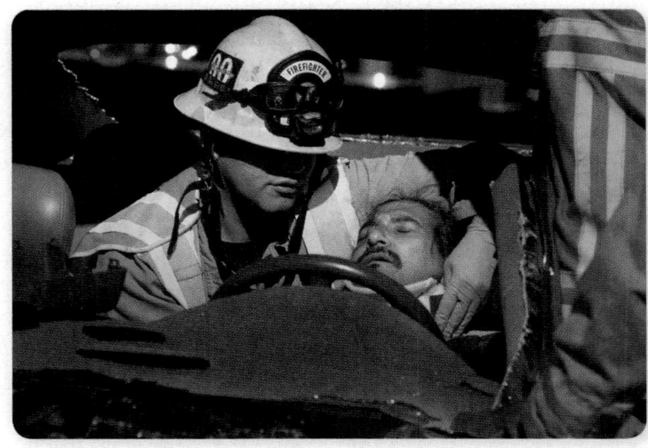

Figure 40-7 Always explain to the patient why you are there and what you are doing.

shield. Keep heat, noise, and force to a minimum. Use only what is necessary to extricate the patient safely.

Removing a patient from the vehicle can be an intensive process for the rescue team, requiring much time and equipment. It is generally a multistep process that requires stabilizing the vehicle, gaining access to the patient to initiate care, and then disentangling the patient from the wreckage. It is a coordinated effort between the caregivers and those performing the extrication. Constant communication is a must.

Words of Wisdom

Remember: Try before you pry!

Simple Access

Your first step is **simple access**; accessing the patient as quickly and simply as possible without using any tools or force. While motor vehicles are built for easy entry and exit, it may be necessary to use tools or other forcible entry methods during vehicle extrication.

Although the rescue team is responsible for providing the entrance you need to gain access to the patient, there will be some situations when the rescue team has not yet arrived and delayed access to the patient could be life threatening. During a vehicle extrication, simple hand tools, such as hammers, center punches (to break side or rear windows), pry bars, come-alongs, and hacksaws, are usually stored on the ambulance for you to use. Whenever possible, you should first try to unlock the doors or open the windows (or ask the patient to perform these actions). Try to open every door to gain access before you break any windows or use other methods of forced entry **Figure 40-8**. Enter through the doors when there is no danger to the patient.

When accessing the patient, look for potential hazards such as undeployed airbags and seat belt pretensioners.

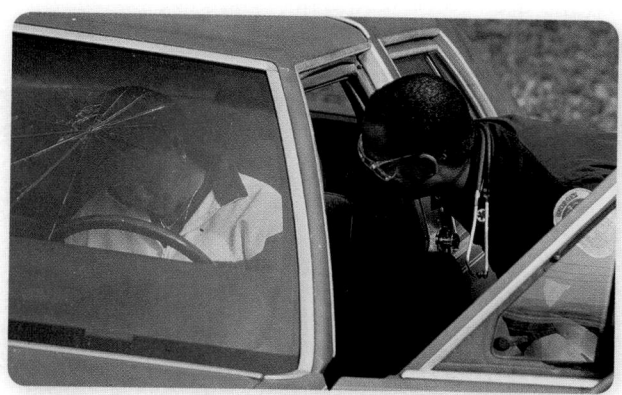

Figure 40-8 Try to open every door to gain access before you use forced entry.

Complex Access

Complex access requires special training and the use of special tools and equipment during vehicle extrication, such as pneumatic and/or hydraulic devices, to break windows or perform other forcible means of entry. The advanced extrication skills typically performed by a rescue team rather than EMS providers include the following:

- Brake and gas pedal displacement
- Dashboard roll-up
- Door removal
- Roof opening and removal
- Seat displacement
- Steering column displacement
- Steering wheel cutting

Emergency Care

Providing medical care to a patient who is trapped in a vehicle is principally the same as providing care to any other patient. Unless there is an immediate threat of fire, explosion, or other danger, once you gain entrance and access to the patient and ensure scene safety, perform a primary assessment and perform any critical interventions before further extrication begins, as follows:

1. Provide manual stabilization to protect the cervical spine, as needed.
2. Open the airway.
3. Provide high-flow oxygen.
4. Assist or provide for adequate ventilation.
5. Control any significant external bleeding.
6. Treat all critical injuries.

If the patient has obvious, life-threatening external hemorrhage, then address it first (even before airway and breathing) and control it quickly.

Safety Tips

Place a rigid backboard between the windshield and the patient during vehicle extrication to help protect the patient and you while glass is broken and metal is cut.

Good communication among team members and clear leadership are essential to ensure safe, efficient provision of proper emergency care. Although your input at the scene is important, one member of your team must be clearly in charge. The team leader's assessment of the patient and the situation will dictate the way in which medical care, packaging, and transport will proceed (Crew Resource Management is discussed in detail in Chapter 15, *BLS Resuscitation*). Customarily, the senior medical person is responsible for this role. If no IC is present, then follow local guidelines. (Chapter 41, *Incident Management*, discusses this in more detail.)

A lack of identifiable leadership at the scene hinders the rescue effort and patient care. Leaders should be identified as part of a larger incident command system. They should be medically trained and qualified to judge the priorities of patient care, and they must also be experienced in extrication.

▶ Removal of the Patient

In the case of a vehicle extrication, work with rescue personnel to coordinate the best route for removal. Whereas one accident may require removal of the patient through the driver's door, a similar crash may require complete removal of the vehicle's roof. Removing a patient from a motor vehicle is an intensive, multistep process in terms of the number of rescuers involved, the equipment used, and the effort required to prevent further injury or harm.

As a part of your assessment, participate in the preparation for patient removal. Determine how urgently the patient must be extricated, where you should be positioned to best protect the patient during extrication, and, once the patient has been freed, how you will best move the patient from the patient's current location onto the backboard and onto the stretcher. Carefully examine exposed areas of the limb or other parts of the patient to determine the extent of injury and whether there is a possibility of internal bleeding. If possible, evaluate sensation in trapped areas to determine whether increased pain indicates that an object is pressing on or impaled in the patient during extrication.

During this time, the rescue team is assessing exactly how the patient is trapped and determining the safest, easiest way to extricate him or her. Your input is essential so the patient's injuries are considered as the rescue team plans a move that protects the patient from further harm. Reevaluate whether the patient needs to be immediately removed by using manual stabilization and the rapid extrication technique, or whether the patient's condition and the scene allow for immobilization using an extrication vest or short backboard before he or she is moved further. If one of these devices is used, then remember to *always move the patient and not the device*. In most cases, it is impractical and difficult to properly apply extremity splints while inside a vehicle. Extremity injuries can generally be rapidly supported and immobilized while the patient is being removed by securing an injured arm to the body and, if a leg is injured, securing one leg to the other. This will be adequate management until the patient is secured to the backboard or time allows for a more detailed assessment and splinting of each injury.

Once the extrication plan has been devised and everyone understands what will be done, you should determine how best to protect the patient. For example, often you or your partner will be placed in a vehicle alongside the patient to monitor his or her condition and well-being as the vehicle is being forcibly cut, bent, or disassembled. Wear proper protective clothing, and protect the patient from harm.

Naturally, your safety and that of the patient are paramount during this process. Extrication is often extremely noisy, and appropriate hearing protection should be worn by you and the patient. Make sure you communicate effectively with the patient and with the rescue team so you can let the rescue team know immediately if it is necessary for them to stop.

YOU are the Provider — PART 2

The firefighter in charge of extrication informs you that this is a hybrid electric vehicle, and all batteries have been disconnected. He also states the patient is currently pinned by his legs in the overturned vehicle, and that it will take approximately 15 to 20 minutes to remove the patient. You ask if it is possible to get into the rear seat of the vehicle in an attempt to maintain spinal precautions; however, the firefighter tells you that one of his men is already in the rear of the vehicle immobilizing the patient's cervical spine. Because most of the extrication efforts are taking place on the driver's side, you proceed to the passenger side to attempt to speak with the patient. The patient is alert and oriented. He reports he is unable to feel his legs. He pleads with you to get him out. You note the patient is still wearing his seat belt and that the driver's side airbag has deployed.

Recording Time: 1 Minute	
Appearance	Fair
Level of consciousness	Conscious and alert
Airway	Patent
Breathing	Clear and equal, 20 breaths/min
Circulation	Warm, dry, and pink

3. What are the hazards that may present with hybrid electric vehicles?
4. What are the differences between simple access and complex access?

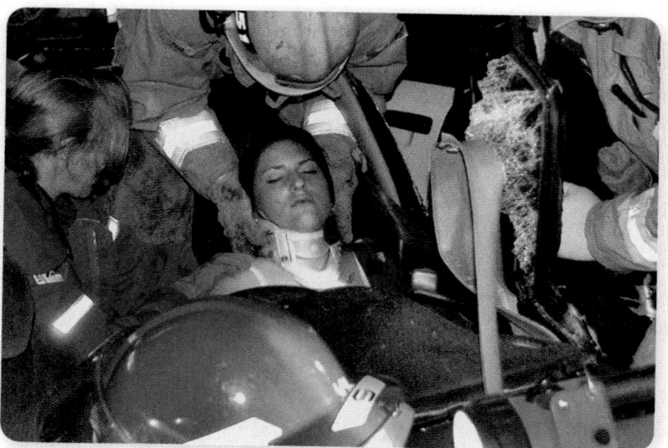

Figure 40-9 Once the patient has been accessed, rapidly assess the patient and ensure the spine is manually stabilized. Apply a cervical collar if this was not previously done.

Transfer of the Patient

Once the patient has been freed, rapidly assess any other patients who were previously inaccessible, and perform a complete primary assessment. Ensure the spine is manually stabilized, and apply a cervical collar if this was not previously done **Figure 40-9**.

Move the patient in a series of smooth, slow, controlled steps, with designated stops to allow for repositioning and adjustments. Ensure there are sufficient personnel to perform the move without causing further injury to the patient. One person should be in charge of the move and plan and verbalize the exact steps and pathway that you will follow in moving the patient from sitting in the vehicle to lying supine on the backboard or stretcher.

Choose a path that requires the least manipulation of the patient or equipment. Once you are sure that everyone understands the steps and is ready, you can move the patient safely. Move only on the team leader's command and move the patient as a unit. While moving the patient, continue to protect him or her from any hazards.

Once the patient has been placed on the stretcher, continue with any additional assessment and treatment that was deferred. If it is extremely cold or hot, raining, or snowing, then load the stretcher and patient into the climate-controlled ambulance before continuing assessment and treatment. If the patient's condition requires you to initiate transport without further delay, then provide only the additional medical care that is essential or necessary to package the patient. Perform the remaining steps while you are en route to the hospital.

Termination

Termination involves returning the emergency units to service. For rescue units, this may be a time-consuming process. All equipment used on the scene, including hydraulic, electric, and hand tools, must be checked before the vehicle is reloaded. Whereas some tools require only generalized cleaning, others may need refueling and checking of the various fluid levels.

You are required to check the ambulance thoroughly, replacing used supplies and decontaminating the unit as required by bloodborne pathogen standards.

Finally, rescue units and medical units are required to complete all necessary reports.

Specialized Rescue Situations

On most calls, you can drive the ambulance to or within a short distance of the patient's location and, with simple or complex access, you can reach and treat the patient. However, in some situations, the patient can be reached only by teams that are trained in making special technical rescues. Specialized skills of these teams include the following:

- Special weapons and tactics (SWAT)
- Missing person search and rescue
- Technical rope rescue (low- and high-angle rescue)
- Mountain-, rock-, and ice-climbing rescue
- Cross-field and trail rescue (park rangers)
- Water and small craft rescue
- White water rescue
- Dive rescue
- Cave rescue
- Confined space rescue
- Ski slope and cross-country or trail snow rescue (ski patrol)
- Lost person search and rescue
- Structural collapse rescue
- Trench rescue
- Mine rescue

Technical rescue situations may contain hidden dangers, and special technical skills and equipment are needed for personnel to safely enter and move around. It is not safe to include any personnel who do not have the necessary special training and experience in such a rescue. A **technical rescue group** is made up of people from one or more departments in a region who are trained and on call for certain types of technical rescues. Many members of a technical rescue group are also trained as EMRs, emergency medical technicians (EMTs), AEMTs, or paramedics so they can provide the necessary immediate care when they can safely reach the patient.

> **Words of Wisdom**
>
> Even when the technical rescue group includes a paramedic or physician, generally only essential simple care is provided until the group members can bring the patient to the nearest safe and stable setting, known as the staging area.

If a technical rescue group is necessary but is not present when you arrive, then immediately check with the **incident commander (IC)** to make sure the group has been summoned and is en route to your location. The IC is the individual who has overall command of the incident in

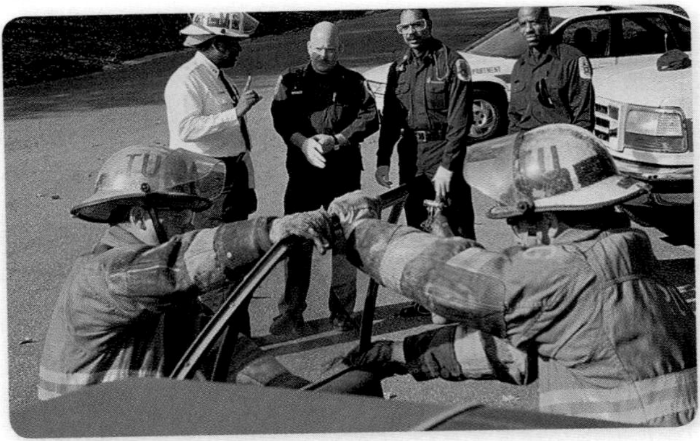

Figure 40-10 The incident commander is the person who has overall command of the scene.

the field Figure 40-10. If no IC is present, then follow local guidelines. (Chapter 41, *Incident Management*, discusses this in more detail.)

When you arrive at a scene where a technical rescue is already in progress, you will usually be met by a member of the technical rescue group and directed or led to the staging area. If the staging area is some distance from the road, then you may need to leave the ambulance on the road. If it is impractical to use a stretcher, then bring a backboard and/or basket stretcher or similar rescue stretcher to carry the patient back to the waiting ambulance. Take all of the jump kits and other equipment you may need to treat and immobilize the patient at the staging area.

As soon as the technical rescue group brings the patient to the staging area, perform a primary assessment and, after providing the treatment indicated, package the patient without delay. Although you are responsible for the patient's care, it usually requires a cooperative effort by the technical rescue group and EMS personnel to carry the patient to the waiting ambulance. Consider using air medical transport if the patient will need to be carried or transported a great distance.

▶ Tactical Emergency Medical Support

A steady increase in violence throughout the country has resulted in AEMTs taking precautions to ensure personal safety. A **tactical situation** is a hostage, robbery, or other situation in which armed conflict occurs. An **active shooter** is a gunman who has begun to fire on people and is still at large. These scenes are especially tense because someone who appears to be a released hostage could, in fact, be the perpetrator or an accomplice. These incidents pose an increased risk to you and require the use of specialized law enforcement tactical units or the **special weapons and tactics (SWAT) team.**

EMS providers who respond to a tactical situation must prepare, plan, and train for these complex and difficult, violent incidents and need to know how to stay safe. Turn off lights and siren when you are nearing the scene, and do not use outside radio speakers. Know the difference between cover and concealment, and the difference between objects that provide cover and those that provide concealment. **Cover** refers to impenetrable barriers, such as trees, utility poles, mail collection boxes, dumpsters, vehicles, and depressions in the ground. Tall grass, shrubbery, and dark shadows that limit your visibility to someone are considered areas of **concealment**. When cover is not readily available, use concealment to provide protection. Remember, people are going to need your help; do not do anything that could get you or your partner injured.

As an AEMT, you must take direction from law enforcement personnel on the scene and you may even be instructed as to *whom* to treat and *when* a victim can be treated. This is not your normal triage situation because law enforcement has absolute control of the scene, and they may dictate that you initiate or withhold treatment not based on medical necessity, but rather on public safety. Carefully document any requests or demands you receive that deviate from your local protocols. This includes being instructed to withhold treatment or being prevented from treating a patient who clearly requires emergency medical care. While law enforcement personnel are charged with public safety, and they discharge that duty to the fullest of their extent, you may encounter situations when you feel your medical ethics are being compromised. However, the time to dispute the ethics of what is being asked of you is not while there is an active shooter at large. Refer any serious matters to your on-scene supervisor, or if one is not on scene yet, contact your dispatcher only if time permits. Otherwise, it is a crime scene, and you *must* follow the directives of law enforcement personnel until the scene has been secured.

Words of Wisdom

During a mass shooting or active shooter situation, law enforcement is the lead agency. You must follow their instructions at all times for the safety of you, your partner, and the public.

Determine the location of the command post, where command, coordination, control, and communication are centralized, and report to the IC for instructions. The command post is usually located in an area that cannot be seen by the suspect and is out of range of possible gunfire. Remain in this area and do not roam around. Nearby areas may be visible to the suspect, and you could be injured. The IC will need to identify the specific location of the incident and determine a safe location (staging area) where you can meet SWAT team members or tactical EMS providers, who will bring the patient to you for treatment and transport to a medical facility. The IC should also determine a safe route to this meeting point.

Words of Wisdom

Consider having a training session with your local police department on how to assess a police officer who has been shot. Specifically, address how to remove full-body armor and the officer's duty belt. The protocol for who removes the officer's weapons, and how, should be established before an incident occurs.

To save valuable time in critical situations, designate primary and secondary helicopter landing zones if your region uses aeromedical evacuation. The closest hospital, burn center, and trauma center should be identified. The route of travel to these facilities should also be noted. Many of these measures are incorporated into the operational plan used by tactical EMS providers. If tactical EMS providers are used in your jurisdiction, then coordinate with them on your arrival at the command post.

Words of Wisdom

Tips for Responding to a Tactical Situation

- Turn off lights and siren as you approach the scene.
- Do not turn on the vehicle's outside speakers. Turn down the volume of any radios that you are carrying.
- Do not look around the sides or over the top of any building or structure that may be serving to provide cover.
- When exiting the ambulance, stay low, and remain near the side of the vehicle unless you are directed to another place of safety. Utilize cover or concealment techniques as necessary.
- Request direction from the IC.
- Stand by at the staging area to treat and package injured patients after the SWAT team, tactical EMS providers, or law enforcement officers have evacuated them.
- Leave only after the IC has verified that it is safe for the ambulance to move.
- Follow the specific route indicated by the IC or law enforcement officer when you are exiting the scene. Proceed slowly for a good distance from the incident perimeter before turning on your emergency lights and siren.

Tactical Medicine

Owing to the high potential for injuries during tactical situations, many communities have incorporated tactical medicine into their SWAT teams. **Tactical medicine** is emergency medical care provided by specially trained EMTs, AEMTs, paramedics, nurses, and even physicians during a tactical situation. In most jurisdictions, tactical EMS providers care for law enforcement teams making tactical entry into violent situations; however, these specially trained responders can also provide care for barricaded patients, patients being held hostage, and other special operations in which a provider without special training might not be able to work. Tactical medicine is a crucial link in providing medical care in hostile situations.

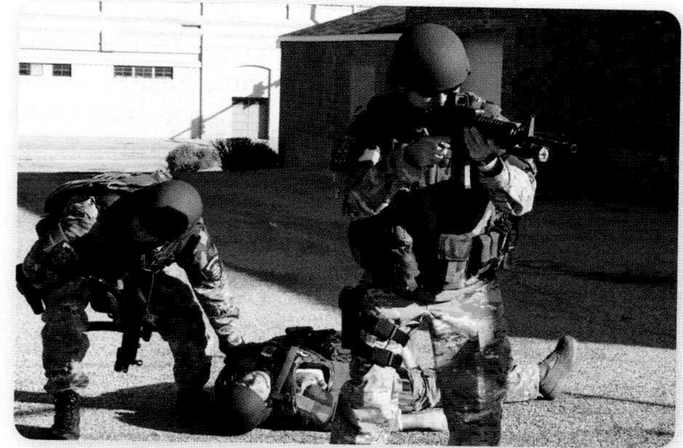

Figure 40-11 Tactical EMS providers move a downed officer; only the most basic medical care is provided in an unsecured area.

Training in this evolving EMS subspecialty is widely available from reputable training centers. The training goes well beyond the practices seen in standard emergency medical care. Thus, the techniques used may not seem appropriate or adequate. For example, spinal immobilization is not used within an unsecured area where gunfire is a risk because the time and manpower necessary to completely secure a victim to a backboard may expose them to injury or death from gunfire **Figure 40-11**. Such altered standards of care are similar to those used by military EMS providers on the battlefield and are not used in "standard" situations encountered by AEMTs.

Search and Rescue

When someone is lost in the outdoors and a search effort is initiated, an ambulance is usually summoned to the incident command post (location of the IC) or the staging area. Each search team is organized to include a member who is trained at the EMR, EMT, or AEMT level, carrying the essential equipment to provide essential, immediate care. Your role, and that of the other AEMTs who arrived with the ambulance, is to stand by at the command post or staging area until the missing person or people have been found.

As soon as you arrive at the scene and have been briefed on the situation, you should isolate and prepare the equipment you will need to carry to the patient's location; this will save time once the patient has been found or if a member of the search team is injured. Leave the prepared carry-in equipment, including a backboard and other equipment you will need to immobilize the patient, in the back of the ambulance until the patient has been found. If the ambulance should need to be relocated, then the equipment will not need to be reloaded and will not be left behind. You will usually be given a portable radio that is tuned to the search frequency so you can monitor the progress of the search and communicate with and be contacted by those in charge of the search operation.

Sometimes, you may be asked to stay with relatives of the missing person who are at the scene. Find out from relatives whether the missing person has any medical history that may need to be addressed, and pass this information on to those who are in charge of the search. Unless you have been instructed otherwise, only the IC should communicate any news or progress of the search to the family. For this reason, ensure your radio is set at a discreet volume.

Once the missing person has been found, you will be guided by search personnel to that location or a prearranged intersecting point where the patient will be carried, which allows you to begin treatment more quickly. Ensure the carry-in equipment is evenly distributed among personnel and that the pace is such that all can easily stay together. Also, consider relocating the ambulance or, if available, driving a four-wheel drive, all-terrain vehicle, or snowmobile to decrease the time and effort needed to reach and carry out the patient. As with other technical rescues, although EMS will assume the responsibility for patient care once they are at the patient's side, a cooperative effort between the EMS and search teams is necessary to safely carry the patient to the staging area and waiting ambulance.

Words of Wisdom

Never leave your ambulance to assist in the search for a missing person. Once found, he or she will be brought to you (or you will be brought to the individual) for care. Leaving your post may lead to a delay in care for the individual.

▶ Trench Rescue

Trench rescue refers to rescue for incidents involving cave-ins and collapses. Owing to the physical forces involved, many of these incidents have poor outcomes for victims. Trench collapses usually involve large areas of falling dirt that weigh approximately 100 pounds per cubic foot (1,600 kg per cubic meter). Victims with thousands of pounds of dirt resting on their chests cannot fully expand their lungs and may become hypoxic.

The risk of a secondary collapse during the rescue operation is of concern to rescue personnel and to the AEMTs. Safety measures can reduce the potential for injury from this and other hazards. When arriving at the scene of a cave-in or trench collapse, response vehicles should be parked at least 500 feet (152 m) from the scene. Because vibration is a primary cause of secondary collapse, turn off all vehicles, including on-scene construction equipment. In addition, divert all road traffic from the 500-foot safety area. Other hazards include exposed or downed electric wires and broken gas or water lines. In addition, construction equipment at the collapse site may be unstable and could fall into the cave-in or trench site.

Any witnesses to the incident should be identified. They may be valuable in providing information on the number of victims and their location within the collapsed area. Anyone who is not trapped should be assisted from the area. At no time should medical or rescue personnel enter a trench deeper than 4 feet (1 m) without proper shoring (temporary supports to prevent collapse) in place.

During the extrication of any survivors from a cave-in or trench collapse site, trained medical personnel will provide most medical care. Be prepared to receive patients once they have been extricated from the site.

▶ Structure Fires

In most areas, an ambulance is dispatched with the fire department apparatus to any structure fire, whether or not any injuries are reported. A fire in a house, apartment building, office, school, plant, warehouse, or other building is considered a structure fire. When responding to a major fire scene, you should determine whether, because of the fire, any special route will be necessary. Once you arrive at the scene, you should ask the IC where the ambulance should be parked. It is essential that the ambulance be parked far enough away from the fire to be safe from the flames or a collapsing building. Ensure the ambulance does not block or hinder other arriving equipment or become blocked in by other equipment or hose lines. However, the ambulance should be close enough to be visible and easily accessible for patients. The fire officer who is the IC will determine this location.

Safety Tips

Hazards such as fire, infectious disease, and electricity are not the only risks to your safety during an emergency response. Some calls will involve violence against rescuers. This may be a formal tactical situation or a "simple" call involving assault, possible alcohol or drug abuse, and/or a domestic dispute. Your training, your attitude when responding to calls, and your daily EMS procedures should take these risks into account.

Your next step is to determine whether there are any injured patients at the scene or whether you have been called to stand by. A number of ambulances may be dispatched to a major fire to ensure one or more units will always remain immediately available at the scene if others leave to transport the injured.

As with other technical rescue situations, search and rescue in a burning building requires special training and equipment. Search and rescue is performed by teams of firefighters wearing full turnout gear and a **self-contained**

breathing apparatus (SCBA) and carrying tools and fully charged hose lines. These teams will bring patients out of the burning building to the area where the ambulance is staged. Therefore, unless you are instructed otherwise, always stay with the ambulance. Do not leave even after the fire is extinguished, in case a firefighter becomes injured during salvage and overhaul. The ambulance should leave the scene only if transporting a patient or if the IC has released it.

Introduction to Hazardous Materials

A hazardous material is any material that poses an unreasonable risk of damage or injury to people, property, or the environment if it is not properly controlled during handling, storage, manufacture, processing, packaging, use and disposal, and transportation. Your training has taught you that rapid response to the scene of a crash can save lives. However, when you arrive at the scene of a possible hazmat incident, you must first step back and assess the situation. This can be very stressful for you, particularly if you can see a patient. However, rushing into an unsafe scene can have catastrophic results. If you are overcome by a hazardous substance, not only will patients suffer because you will be unable to assist them, but you will also place a strain on the system because you will require emergency care.

Because of the unique aspects of responding to and working at a **hazardous materials (hazmat) incident**, the Occupational Safety and Health Administration (OSHA) has published a set of guidelines known as Hazardous Waste Operations and Emergency Response (HAZWOPER). All providers, including AEMTs, must meet specific additional training requirements before becoming involved in hazmat incidents. These training requirements are published in 1910.120(q)(6)(i)—First Responder Awareness Level. This text does not include the skills and information necessary to meet those requirements. You need to check with your agency for information about specific awareness level training.

On the basis of the HAZWOPER regulation, first responders at the awareness level should have sufficient training or experience to objectively demonstrate competency in the following areas:

- An understanding of what hazardous substances are and the associated risks
- An understanding of the potential outcomes of an incident
- The ability to recognize the presence of hazardous substances
- The ability to identify the hazardous substances, if possible
- An understanding of the role of the first responder awareness individual in the emergency response plan
- The ability to determine the need for additional resources and to notify the communication center

Recognizing a Hazardous Material

Recognizing a hazmat incident, determining the identity of the material(s), and understanding the hazards involved often require some detective work. Train yourself to take the time to look at the whole scene so you can identify the crucial visual indicators and consider this information with what is known about the problem.

Hazardous materials may be involved in any of the following situations (Figure 40-12):

- A truck or train crash in which a substance is leaking from a tank truck or railroad tank car
- A leak, fire, or other emergency at an industrial plant, refinery, or other complex where chemicals or explosives are produced, used, or stored

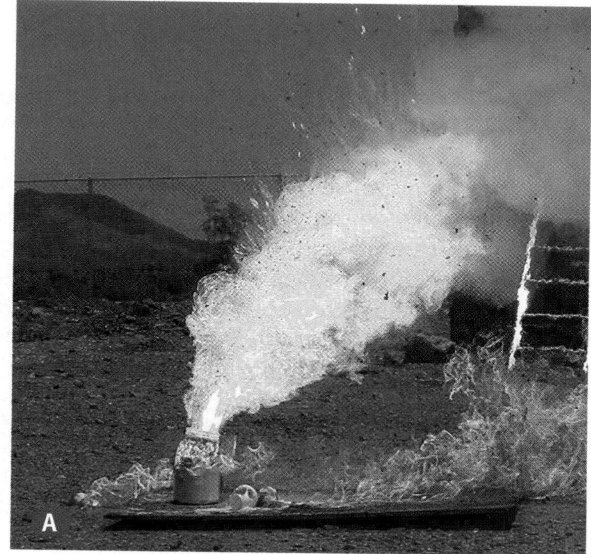

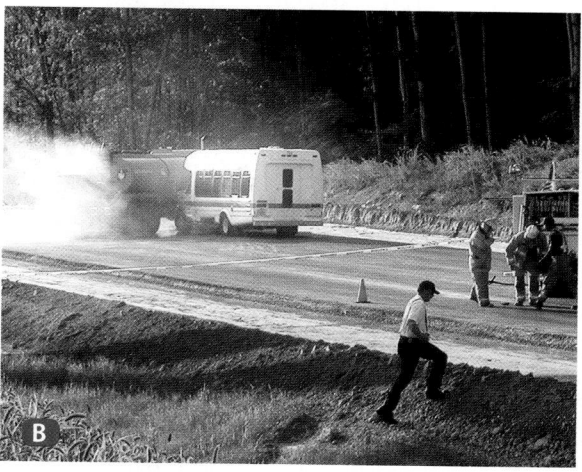

Figure 40-12 Two examples of hazardous materials incidents.

A: Courtesy of Rob L. Jackson/US Marines; B: Courtesy of George Roarty/Virginia Department of Emergency Management.

- A leak or rupture of an underground natural gas pipe
- Deterioration of underground fuel tanks and/or seepage of oil or gasoline into the environment
- Buildup of methane or other by-products of waste decomposition in sewers or sewage-processing plants
- An MVC in which a gas tank has ruptured

Initially, it is important to approach the scene from a safe location and direction. Start with the traditional rules of staying uphill and upwind. It may also be wise to use binoculars and view the scene from a safe distance. Be sure to question anyone involved in the incident—a wealth of information may be available to you if you ask the right person. Take enough time to assess the scene and interpret other clues such as discolored pavement, dead grass or animals, visible vapors or puddles, or labels that may help identify the presence of a hazardous material. Once you have a basic idea of what happened or determine that danger may be present, you can begin to formulate a plan for addressing the incident.

▶ Occupancy and Location

A wide variety of chemicals are stored in warehouses, hospitals, laboratories, industrial complexes, residential garages, bowling alleys, home improvement centers, garden supply stores, restaurants, and scores of other facilities or businesses in your response area. So many different chemicals exist in so many different locations that you could encounter almost anything during any type of emergency situation. The location and type of building are two good indicators of the possible presence of a hazardous material. For example, a warehouse is more likely than a school to have materials that could be hazardous.

Safety Tips

When responding to a potential hazmat incident, use the *rule of thumb* method of response until the scene can be deemed safe. Hold your arm straight in front of you with your fist closed and your thumb up. Close one eye. Your thumb should completely block your view of the scene. If you can see any portion of the scene around your thumb, then you are too close!!

▶ Senses

Another way to detect the presence of hazardous materials is to use your senses, although this technique must be used carefully to avoid exposure. The senses that can be safely used are those of sight and sound. Initially, the farther you are from the incident, the safer you will be. Using any of your senses that bring you in proximity to the chemical should be done with caution or avoided. When it comes to hazmat incidents, "leading with your nose" is not a good tactic—but using binoculars from a distance is.

Clues that are seen or heard may provide warning information from a distance, enabling you to take precautionary steps. The presence of vapor clouds or hazmat placards or labels at the scene, for example, is a signal to yourself and others to move to a place of safety; the sound of an alarm from a toxic gas sensor in a chemical storage room or laboratory may also serve as a warning to retreat. Some highly vaporous and odorous chemicals—chlorine and ammonia, for example—may be detected by smell a long way from the actual point of release.

▶ Containers

In basic terms, a **container** is any vessel or receptacle that holds a material. Often the container type, size, and material of construction provide important clues about the nature of the substance inside. Nevertheless, do not rely solely on the type of container when making a determination about hazardous materials.

Red phosphorus from a drug laboratory, for example, might be found in an unmarked plastic container. In this case, there may not be legitimate markings to alert you to the possible contents. Gasoline or waste solvents may be stored in 55-gallon (208-L) steel drums. Sulfuric acid, at 97% concentration, could be found in a polyethylene drum that might be colored black, red, white, or blue. In most cases, there is no correlation between the color of the drum and the possible contents. The same sulfuric acid might also be found in a 1-gallon (3.8-L) amber glass container. Steel or polyethylene drums, bags, high-pressure gas cylinders, railroad tank cars, plastic buckets, aboveground and underground storage tanks, cargo tanks, and pipelines are all representative examples of how hazardous materials are packaged, stored, and shipped **Figure 40-13**.

Some very recognizable chemical containers, such as 55-gallon (208-L) drums and compressed gas cylinders, can be found in almost every type of manufacturing facility. Materials stored in a cardboard drum are usually in solid form. Stainless steel containers hold particularly dangerous

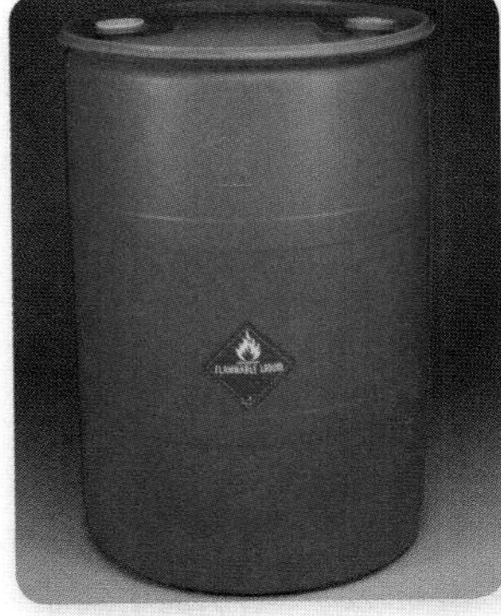

Figure 40-13 Drums may be constructed of many different types of materials, including cardboard, polyethylene, and stainless steel. The drum shown here is made of polyethylene.

Courtesy of EMD Chemicals, Inc.

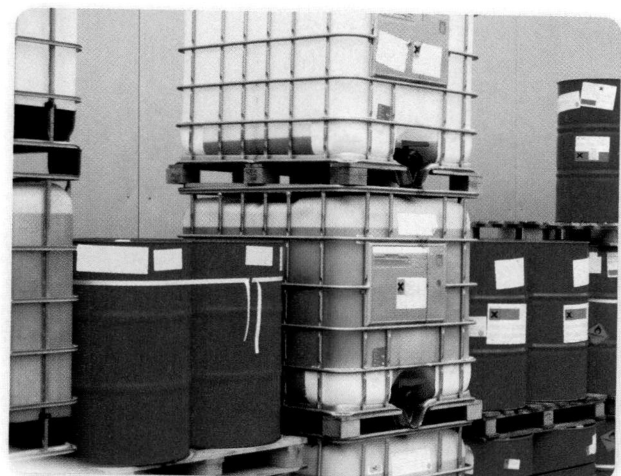

Figure 40-14 A series of chemical storage containers.

chemicals, and cold liquids are kept in containers designed to maintain the appropriate temperature Figure 40-14.

One way to distinguish containers is to divide them into two categories based on their capacity: bulk and nonbulk storage containers.

Container Volume

Bulk storage containers include fixed tanks, highway cargo tanks, rail tank cars, totes, and intermodal tanks. In general, bulk storage containers are found in buildings that rely on and need to store large quantities of a particular chemical. Most manufacturing facilities have at least one type of bulk storage container. Often these bulk storage containers are surrounded by a supplementary containment system to help control an accidental release. **Secondary containment** is an engineered method to control spilled or released product if the main containment vessel fails. A 5,000-gallon (18,927-L) vertical storage tank, for example, may be surrounded by a series of short walls that form a catch basin around the tank.

Safety Tips

When you consider locations for possible hazmat incidents, do not limit your thinking. You may be surprised at how many different kinds of containers you may find in your area.

Large-volume horizontal tanks are also common. When stored above ground, these tanks are referred to as aboveground storage tanks; if they are placed underground, they are known as underground storage tanks. These tanks can hold a few hundred gallons to several million gallons of product and are usually made of aluminum, steel, or plastic.

YOU are the Provider PART 3

Knowing that extrication is going to be prolonged and that the patient is in a critical situation, you discuss the possibility of a helicopter request with the IC. He agrees with your request; you proceed to contact dispatch to request that a helicopter be sent to the scene. Once dispatch has informed you the helicopter is en route with an approximately 10-minute ETA, you inform the IC of the need to establish a safe landing zone. He advises you that he will have his firefighters establish a landing zone that measures 100 feet × 100 feet, approximately 200 yards (183 m) from the vehicle. You proceed back to the patient's side and begin a limited assessment. He states he does not believe that he experienced a loss of consciousness and that he has no pain, only a lack of feeling in his legs, which are trapped by the steering column. You are able to slide in through the broken passenger window and place the patient on oxygen at 15 L/min via a nonrebreathing mask. You obtain the following vital signs:

Recording Time: 5 Minutes	
Respirations	20 breaths/min, irregular
Pulse	105 beats/min, regular
Skin	Warm, dry, and pink
Blood pressure	110/76 mm Hg
Oxygen saturation (Spo_2)	99% on 15 L/min
Pupils	Pupils Equal, Round, and Reactive to Light and Accommodation (PERRLA)

5. What should you do as the patient is being extricated from the vehicle?
6. How does rapid extrication differ from other methods of patient removal?

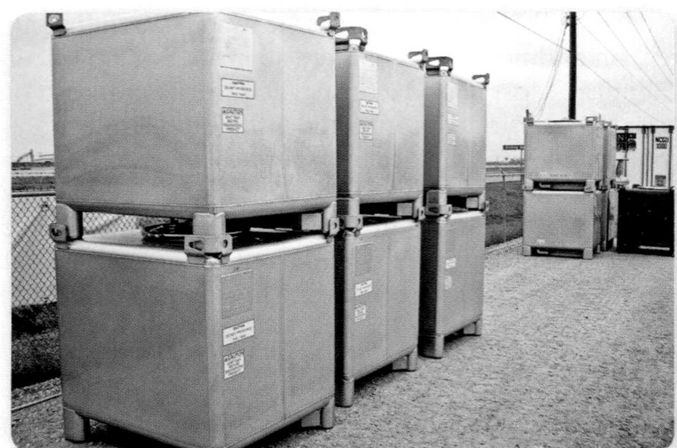

Figure 40-15 A tote is a commonly encountered bulk storage vessel.

Courtesy of Tank Service, Inc.

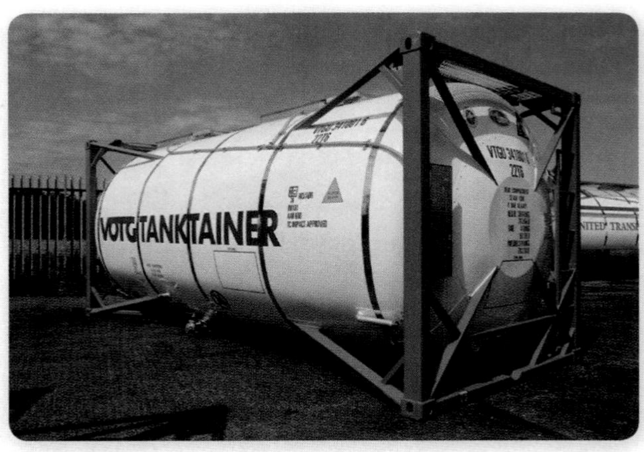

Figure 40-16 An intermodal tank.

Courtesy of UBH International Ltd.

Another commonly encountered bulk storage vessel is the tote, also referred to as an intermediate bulk container. Totes have capacities ranging from 119 gallons to 703 gallons (450 to 2,661 L); the most common sizes are 350 and 550 gallons (1,325 and 2,082 L). These portable plastic tanks are surrounded by a stainless steel web that adds both structural stability and protection to the container. They can contain any type of chemical, including flammable liquids, corrosives, food-grade liquids, or oxidizers **Figure 40-15**.

Shipping and storing totes can be hazardous. These containers are often stacked atop one another and moved with a forklift, and a mishap with the loading or moving process can compromise the tote. Because totes have no secondary containment system, any leak has the potential to create a large puddle. In addition, the steel webbing around the tote makes it difficult to access and patch leaks.

Intermodal tanks are both shipping and storage vessels. They hold between 5,000 and 6,000 gallons (18,927 and 22,712 L) of product and can be pressurized or nonpressurized. Intermodal tanks can also be used to ship and store gaseous substances that have been chilled until they liquefy, such as liquid nitrogen. In most cases, an intermodal tank is shipped to a facility where it is stored and used and then returned to the shipper for refilling. Intermodal tanks can be shipped by all methods of transportation—air, sea, and land **Figure 40-16**.

Nonbulk Storage Vessels

Essentially, **nonbulk storage vessels** are all types of containers other than bulk containers. Nonbulk storage vessels can hold a few ounces to 119 gallons (450 L) of product and include vessels such as drums, bags, compressed gas cylinders, cryogenic containers, and more. Nonbulk storage vessels hold commonly used commercial and industrial chemicals such as solvents, industrial cleaners, and compounds. This section describes the most common types of nonbulk storage vessels.

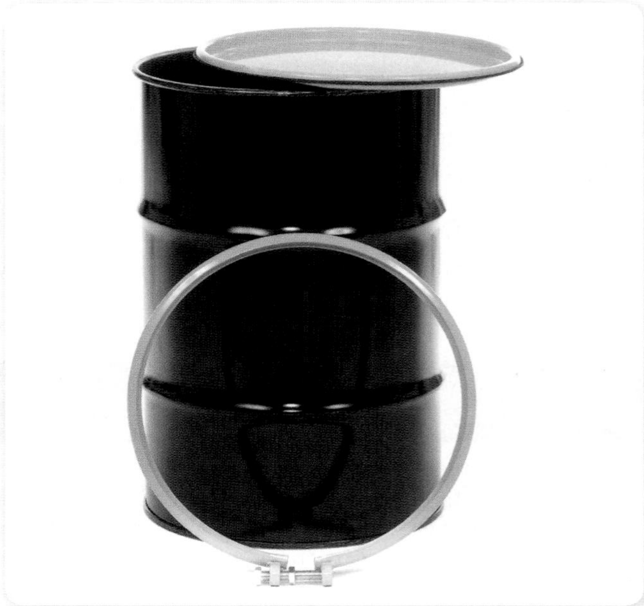

Figure 40-17 An open-head drum has a lid that is fastened with a ring that is tightened with a clasp or a nut-and-bolt assembly.

Courtesy of Globalindustrial.com.

Drums. **Drums** are easily recognizable, barrel-like containers **Figure 40-17**. They are used to store a wide variety of substances, including food-grade materials, corrosives, flammable liquids, and grease. Drums may be constructed of low-carbon steel, polyethylene, cardboard, stainless steel, nickel, or other materials. Generally, the nature of the chemical dictates the construction of the storage drum. Steel utility drums, for example, hold flammable liquids, cleaning fluids, oil, and other noncorrosive chemicals. Polyethylene drums are used for corrosives such as acids, bases, oxidizers, and other materials that cannot be stored in steel containers. Cardboard drums hold solid materials such as soap flakes, sodium hydroxide pellets, and food-grade materials. Stainless steel or other heavy-duty drums generally hold materials too aggressive (ie, too reactive) for either plain steel or polyethylene.

Bags. Bags are commonly used to store solids and powders such as cement powder, sand, pesticides, soda ash, and slaked lime. Storage bags may be constructed of plastic, paper, or plastic-lined paper. Bags come in different sizes and weights, depending on their contents.

Pesticide bags must be labeled with specific information. You can learn a great deal from the label, including the following details:

- Name of the product
- Active ingredients
- Hazard statement
- The total amount of product in the container
- The manufacturer's name and address
- The Environmental Protection Agency (EPA) registration number, which provides proof that the product was registered with the EPA
- The EPA establishment number, which shows where the product was manufactured
- Signal words to indicate the relative toxicity of the material:
    - Danger—Poison: Highly toxic by all routes of entry
    - Danger: Severe eye damage or skin irritation
    - Warning: Moderately toxic
    - Caution: Minor toxicity and minor eye damage or skin irritation
- Practical first aid treatment description
- Directions for use
- Agricultural use requirements
- Precautionary statements such as mixing directions or potential environmental hazards
- Storage and disposal information
- Classification statement on who may use the product

In addition, every pesticide label must carry the statement, "Keep out of reach of children."

Carboys. Some corrosives and other types of chemicals are transported and stored in vessels called **carboys** Figure 40-18. A carboy is a glass, plastic, or steel container that holds 5 to 15 gallons (19 to 57 L) of product. Glass carboys are often placed in a protective wood, foam, fiberglass, or steel box to help prevent breakage. For example, nitric acid, sulfuric acid, and other strong acids are often transported and stored in thick glass carboys protected by a wooden or polystyrene (Styrofoam) crate to shield the glass container from damage during normal shipping.

Cylinders. Several types of **cylinders** are used to hold liquids and gases. Uninsulated compressed gas cylinders are used to store substances such as nitrogen, argon, helium, and oxygen. They come in a range of sizes. As an AEMT, you are very familiar with the shape of a cylinder: it holds the oxygen for your patients.

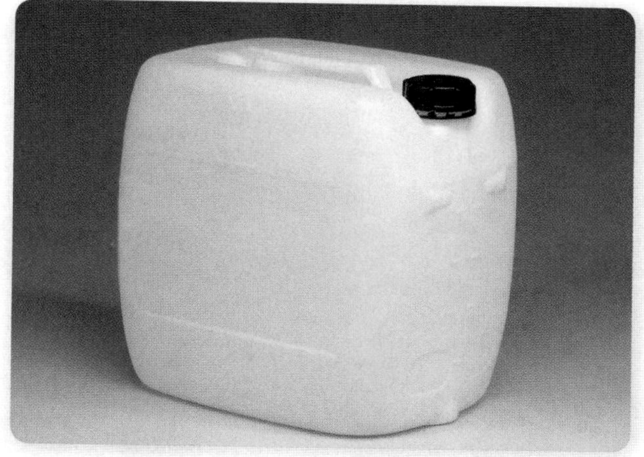

Figure 40-18 A carboy is used to transport and store corrosive chemicals.

Courtesy of EMD Chemicals, Inc.

Transportation and Facility Markings

The Department of Transportation Marking System

The presence of labels, placards, and other markings on packages, boxes, and containers can often enable you to identify a released chemical. When used correctly, marking systems indicate the presence of a hazardous material from a safe distance and provide clues about the substance.

The US Department of Transportation (DOT) marking system is an identification system characterized by labels, placards, and markings Figure 40-19.

This marking system is used when materials are being transported from one location to another in the United States. The same marking system is also used in Canada and Mexico.

Placards are diamond-shaped indicators (10.75 inches [27 cm] per side) that are placed on all four sides of highway transport vehicles, railroad tank cars, and other forms of transportation carrying hazardous materials Figure 40-20. Labels are smaller versions (4 inches [10 cm] per side) of placards; they are placed on the four sides of individual boxes and smaller packages being transported.

Placards, labels, and markings are intended to give a general idea of the hazard inside a particular container or cargo tank. A placard identifies the broad hazard class (flammable, poison, corrosive) to which the material inside belongs. A label on a box inside a delivery truck, for example, relates only to the potential hazard inside that particular package.

Other Considerations. The DOT system does not require all chemical shipments be marked with placards or labels. In most cases, the package or cargo tank must contain a certain amount of hazardous material before a placard is required.

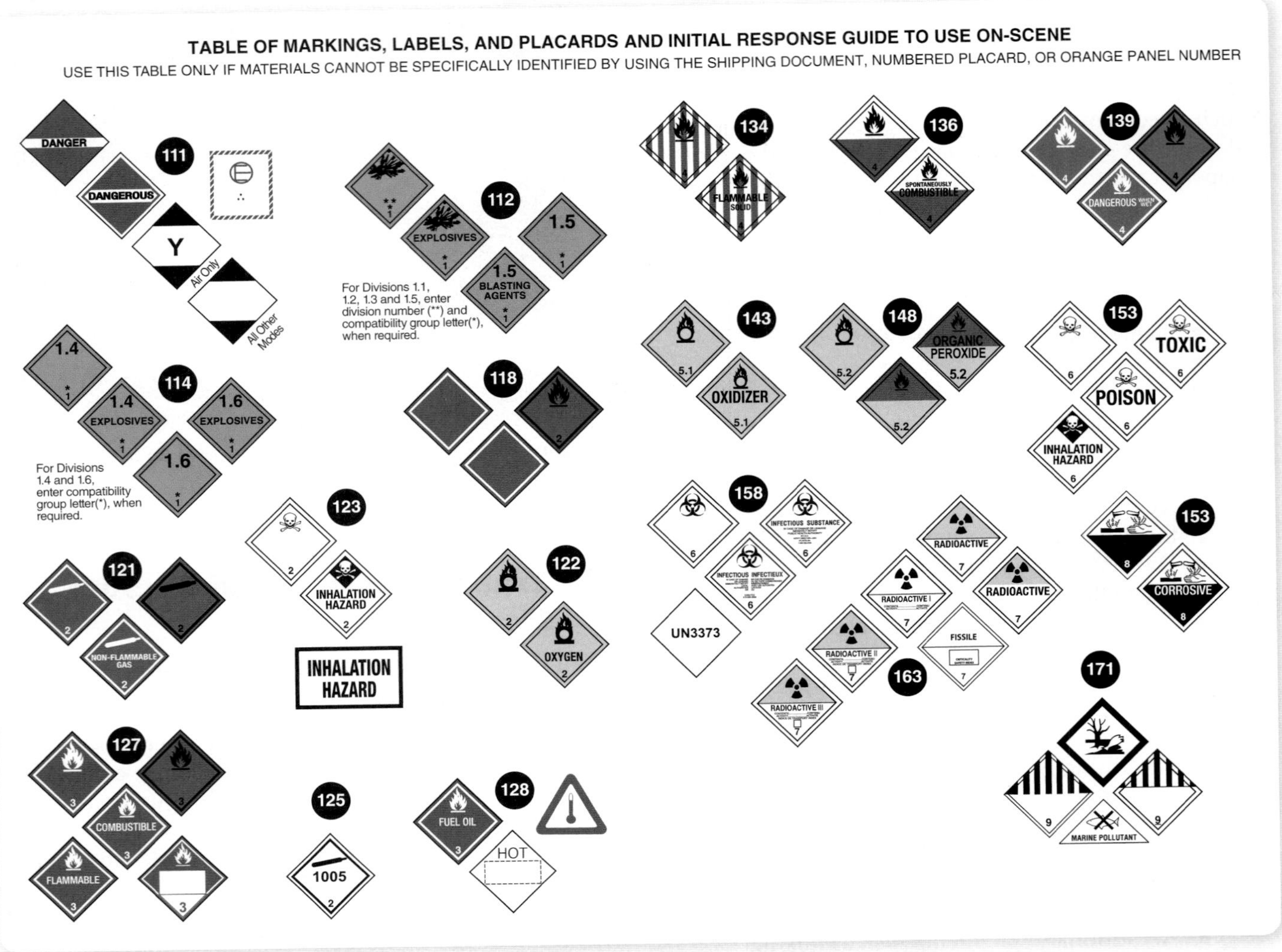

TABLE OF MARKINGS, LABELS, AND PLACARDS AND INITIAL RESPONSE GUIDE TO USE ON-SCENE

USE THIS TABLE ONLY IF MATERIALS CANNOT BE SPECIFICALLY IDENTIFIED BY USING THE SHIPPING DOCUMENT, NUMBERED PLACARD, OR ORANGE PANEL NUMBER

For Divisions 1.1, 1.2, 1.3 and 1.5, enter division number (**) and compatibility group letter(*), when required.

For Divisions 1.4 and 1.6, enter compatibility group letter(*), when required.

Figure 40-19 The US Department of Transportation uses labels, placards, and markings (such as these found in the *Emergency Response Guidebook*) to give a general idea of the hazard inside a particular container or cargo tank.

Courtesy of the US Department of Transportation.

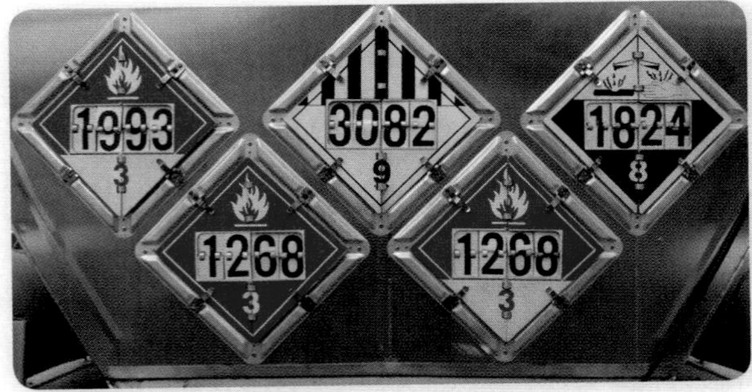

Figure 40-20 A placard is a large diamond-shaped indicator that is placed on all sides of transport vehicles that carry hazardous materials.

For example, the "1,000-pound rule" applies to blasting agents, flammable and nonflammable gases, flammable/combustible liquids, flammable solids, air-reactive solids, oxidizers and organic peroxides, poison solids, corrosives, and miscellaneous (class 9) materials. Placards are required for these materials only when the shipment weighs more than 1,000 pounds (454 kg).[4] Commercial package delivery services often carry small amounts of hazardous materials that fall below that weight limit. The vehicle exterior will not display placards to warn you of the danger.

Conversely, some chemicals are so hazardous that shipping any amount of them requires the use of labels or

Words of Wisdom

To accurately compare and contrast the DOT marking system and NFPA 704 system, remember this important difference:

- The DOT hazardous materials marking system is used when materials are being transported from one location to another.
- The NFPA 704 hazard identification system is designed for fixed-facility use.

placards. These materials include explosives, poison gases, water-reactive solids, and high-level radioactive substances. A four-digit United Nations number may be required on some placards. This number identifies the specific material being shipped; a list of United Nations numbers is included in the Emergency Response Guidebook.[5]

The National Fire Protection System 704 Marking System

The National Fire Protection Association (NFPA) 704 standard, *Standard System for the Identification of the Hazards of Materials for Emergency Response*, classifies hazardous materials for fixed facilities that store hazardous materials.[6] The standard uses a diamond-shaped symbol that is broken into four smaller diamonds, and each division is color-coded to represent a particular property or characteristic of a substance or a group of substances Figure 40-21. The three basic principles of the symbol are designated as they relate to hazards: health (blue), flammability (red), and instability/reactivity (yellow). The degree of severity or hazard for each principle is indicated using a numerical rating of 0 (no hazard) to 4 (severe risk) Table 40-2. For your safety, know the type and degree of health, fire, and reactive hazard protection you need to operate safely near these substances before you enter the scene. All health hazard levels, with the exception of 0, require respiratory and chemical protective gear. This equipment is not standard on most ambulances and requires specialized training.

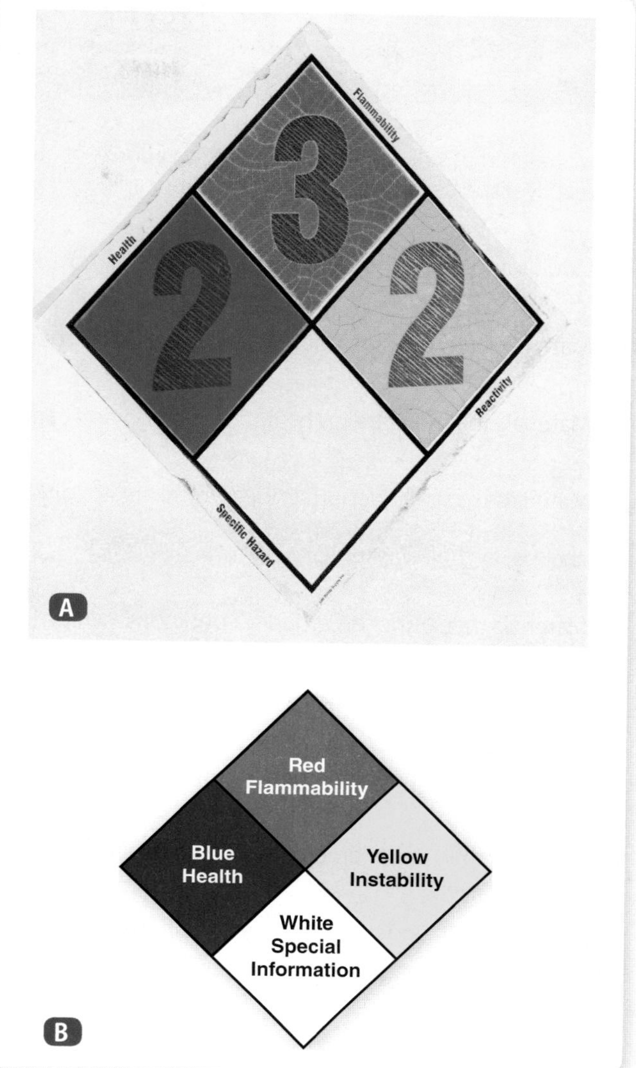

Figure 40-21 A. Example of a placard using the NFPA 704 hazard identification system that is used for fixed-facility use. **B.** Each color used in the diamond represents a particular property or characteristic.

▶ References

Numerous reference materials are available to the responder, including the DOT's *Emergency Response Guidebook (ERG)*, SDS, shipping papers, and more. The following sections describe some of these resources. Other references include Jones & Bartlett Learning's *Fire and EMS Officer Field Guide, Second Edition* and Informed's *NIMS Incident Command System Field Guide, Third Edition*.

The Emergency Response Guidebook

The DOT's ***Emergency Response Guidebook*** offers a certain amount of guidance for responders operating at a hazmat incident Figure 40-22. This guide is updated every 3 to 4 years and provides information on approximately 4,000 chemicals. The US DOT and the Secretariat of Communications and Transportation of Mexico, along with Transport Canada, jointly developed the *ERG*. You can download a free copy of the ERG via the Pipeline and Hazardous Materials Safety Administration website. A mobile app is also available.

Safety Data Sheets

A common source of information about a particular chemical is the **safety data sheet (SDS)** specific to that substance Figure 40-23.[7] Safety data sheets (SDSs) were called material safety data sheets (MSDSs) before OSHA implemented the United Nation's Globally Harmonized System of Classification and Labeling of Chemicals (GHS) in 2012. According to the DOT, the GHS system is an international guideline that aims to harmonize the classification and labeling systems for all sectors involved in the life cycle of a chemical. This includes production, storage, transport, workplace use, consumer use, and presence in the environment. The terms SDS and MSDS are used interchangeably; however, SDSs have a structured format and require information that MSDSs were not required to have. SDSs also include the use of nine recently introduced GHS symbols (to see the symbols, refer to the latest version of the *ERG*). Essentially, SDSs are designed to provide basic information about the chemical makeup of a substance, the potential hazards it presents, appropriate first aid in the event of an exposure, and other pertinent data for safe

Table 40-2 Hazard Levels in the NFPA Hazard Identification System

Flammability Hazards (Red Diamond)	
4	Materials that will rapidly or completely vaporize at atmospheric pressure and normal ambient temperature, or that are readily dispersed in air and that will burn readily.
3	Liquids and solids that can be ignited under almost all ambient temperature conditions.
2	Materials that must be moderately heated or exposed to relatively high ambient temperatures before ignition can occur.
1	Materials that must be preheated before ignition can occur.
0	Materials that will not burn under typical fire conditions.
Health Hazards (Blue Diamond)	
4	Materials that, under emergency conditions, can be lethal.
3	Materials that, under emergency conditions, can cause serious or permanent injury.
2	Materials that, under emergency conditions, can cause temporary incapacitation or residual injury.
1	Materials that, under emergency conditions, can cause significant irritation.
0	Materials that, under emergency conditions, would offer no hazard beyond that of ordinary combustible material.
Instability Hazards (Yellow Diamond)	
4	Materials that in themselves are readily capable of detonation or of explosive decomposition or reaction at normal temperatures and pressures.
3	Materials that in themselves are capable of detonation or explosive decomposition or explosive reaction but require a strong initiating source or that must be heated under confinement before initiation.
2	Materials that readily undergo violent chemical change at elevated temperatures and pressures.
1	Materials that will not burn. Materials that are normally stable, but can become unstable at elevated temperatures and pressures.
0	Materials that in themselves are normally stable, even under fire exposure conditions, and are not reactive with water.
Special Hazards (White Diamond)	
ACID	Acid
ALK	Alkali
COR	Corrosive
OX	Oxidizer
W	Reacts with water

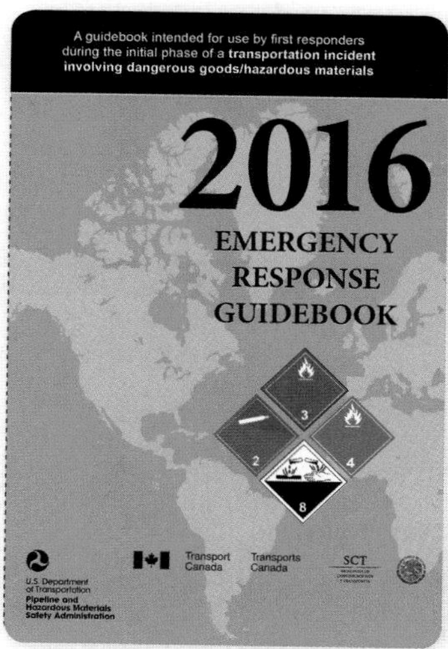

Figure 40-22 *The Emergency Response Guidebook* is a reference tool used as a base for your initial actions at a hazardous materials incident.

Courtesy of the US Department of Transportation.

handling of the material for both workers and emergency personnel. SDSs have a 16-part format and may include the following details:[8]

1. Identification
2. Hazard(s) identification
3. Composition/information on ingredients
4. First aid measures
5. Firefighting measures
6. Accidental release measures
7. Handling and storage
8. Exposure controls/personal protection
9. Physical and chemical properties
10. Stability and reactivity
11. Toxicologic information
12. Ecologic information
13. Disposal considerations
14. Transport information
15. Regulatory information
16. Other information

All facilities that use or store chemicals are required by law to have an SDS on file for each chemical used or stored in the facility. Many sites, but especially those that stock many different chemicals, may keep this information archived on a computer database. Although SDSs are not a definitive response tool, they are a key piece of the puzzle and the key to preventing exposures and accidents. SDSs can also be obtained from the transporting vehicle.

YOU are the Provider — PART 4

After approximately 10 minutes, the fire department has removed the driver's side door and freed the patient's legs from under the steering column, allowing you unrestricted access to the patient. You move to the driver's side and quickly apply a cervical collar on the patient, while instructing the firefighter in the backseat to maintain manual stabilization. You slide a long backboard under the patient's head and explain to the patient, as well as the firefighters, that you are going to remove the seat belt, gently slide the patient onto the backboard, and secure him. Once everyone in attendance has agreed with your method for extrication, you quickly remove the seat belt and lower the patient onto the waiting backboard where he is properly secured. You perform another rapid scan and find no visible trauma; however, the patient remains without motor or sensation to his lower extremities. With the assistance of the firefighters, you quickly carry the patient to the stretcher and place him in the back of the ambulance, awaiting the flight crew. Once inside the back of the ambulance, you establish intravenous (IV) access and infuse fluids at a to-keep-open (TKO) rate. Once the helicopter has arrived at the scene, you provide a report to the flight paramedic and assist in loading the patient into the helicopter. After the helicopter has departed the scene, you go back to the overturned vehicle and look for any equipment that you may have left behind.

Recording Time: 14 Minutes	
Respirations	20 breaths/min
Pulse	92 beats/min
Skin	Warm, dry, and pink
Blood pressure	110/70 mm Hg
Oxygen saturation (Spo_2)	99% on 15 L/min
Pupils	PERRLA

7. What is the last phase of extrication?

Nitrogen, refrigerated liquid

Safety Data Sheet P-4630

This SDS conforms to U.S. Code of Federal Regulations 29 CFR 1910.1200, Hazard Communication.

Date of issue : 01/01/1979 Revision date : 10/21/2016 Supersedes : 10/03/2014

SECTION: 1. Product and company identification

1.1. Product identifier

Product form	:	Substance
Name	:	Nitrogen, refrigerated liquid
CAS No	:	7727-37-9
Formula	:	N2
Other means of identification	:	Nitrogen (cryogenic liquid), Nitrogen, Medipure Liquid Nitrogen

1.2. Relevant identified uses of the substance or mixture and uses advised against

Use of the substance/mixture : Medical applications
Industrial use
Food applications

1.3. Details of the supplier of the safety data sheet

XYZ Chemical, Inc.
10 Main Street
Anytown, NY 01234-5678 - USA
T 1-800-555-4321
www.xyzchemical.com

1.4. Emergency telephone number

Emergency number : Onsite Emergency: 1-800-555-0011

CHEMTREC, 24hr/day 7days/week
— Within USA: 1-800-424-9300, Outside USA: 001-703-527-3887
(collect calls accepted, Contract 17729)

SECTION 2: Hazard identification

2.1. Classification of the substance or mixture

GHS-US classification

Refrigerated liquefied gas H281

2.2. Label elements

GHS-US labeling

Hazard pictograms (GHS-US) :

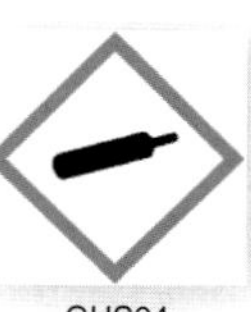

GHS04

Signal word (GHS-US) : WARNING

Hazard statements (GHS-US) : H281 - CONTAINS REFRIGERATED GAS; MAY CAUSE CRYOGENIC BURNS OR INJURY
OSHA-H01 - MAY DISPLACE OXYGEN AND CAUSE RAPID SUFFOCATION

Precautionary statements (GHS-US) : P202 - Do not handle until all safety precautions have been read and understood
P271+P403 - Use and store only outdoors or in a well-ventilated place
P282 - Wear cold insulating gloves/face shield/eye protection.
CGA-PG05 - Use a back flow preventive device in the piping
CGA-PG24 - DO NOT change or force fit connections
CGA-PG06 - Close valve after each use and when empty
CGA-PG23 - Always keep container in upright position

2.3. Other hazards

Other hazards not contributing to the classification : Asphyxiant in high concentrations
Contact with liquid may cause cold burns/frostbite

EN (English US) SDS ID : P-4630 1/9

Figure 40-23 An example of a safety data sheet for liquid nitrogen.

STRAIGHT BILL OF LADING
ORIGINAL - NOT NEGOTIABLE

BOL/Reference No.
RSI82715

CARRIER: NORFOLK SOUTHERN

Date: 12/23/2008

Shipper: RSI LOGISTICS, INC (OKEMOS, MI US)

The property described below, in apparent good order, except as noted (contents and condition of packages unknown), marked, consigned, and destined as indicated below, which said carrier (the word carrier being understood throughout this contract as meaning any person or corporation in possession of the property under the contract) agrees to carry to its usual place of delivery at said destination, if on itsroute, otherwise to deliver to another carrier on the route to said destination. It is mutually agreed, as to each carrier of all or any said property, that every service to be performed hereunder shall be subject to all the terms and conditions of the Uniform Domestic Straight Bill of Lading set forth (1) in Official, Southern, Western and Illinois Freight Classification in effect on the date hereof, if this is a rail or a rail-water shipment, or (2) in the applicable motor carrier classification or tariff if this is a motor carrier shipment.

Shipper hereby certifies that he is familiar with all the terms and conditions or the said bill of lading, including those on the back thereof, set forth in the classification or tariff which governs the transportation of this shipment, and the said terms and conditions are hereby agreed to by the shipper and accepted for himself and his assigns.

Consignee Information: CONSIGNEE DEER PARK, TX Address: City: DEER PARK, TX US	
Route: NS-ESTL-BNSF	
Origin Switch Route:	
Destination Switch Route: HUSTN-PTRA	Rail Car No: GATX290861

For assistance in any transportation emergency involving chemicals, phone CHEMTREC, day or night, Toll Free 1-800-424-9300

DESCRIPTION		*WEIGHT
ONE TANK CAR	Contains: Methyl Esters STCC#2899415 BIODIESEL-15, Biodiesel Sales Order Contract No: RSI82715 Sales Order Contract No: AAT122308-4 Purchase Order Contract No: AAT122308-4	(Sub. To Correction) 204400 Lbs.

SEAL NUMBERS:

Gross

Tare

Net

Weighed By: ______________

If charges are to be prepaid, write or stamp here, "To be Prepaid"
Prepaid

Subject to Section 7 of the conditions of applicable bill of lading, if this shipment is to be delivered to the consignee without recourse on the consignor, the consignor shall sign the following statement:: *The carrier shall not make delivery of this shipment without payment of freight and all other lawful charges.*

Not In Effect

* This is to certify that the above named materials are properly classified, described, packaged, marked, and labeled, and are in proper condition for transportation, according to the applicable regulations of the Department of Transportation.

Figure 40-24 A bill of lading or freight bill.

Courtesy of RSI Logistics.

Shipping Papers

Shipping papers are required whenever materials are transported from one place to another. They include the names and addresses of the shipper and the receiver, identify the material being shipped, and specify the quantity and weight of each part of the shipment. Shipping papers for road and highway transportation are called **bills of lading** or **freight bills** and are located in the cab of the vehicle **Figure 40-24**. Drivers transporting chemicals are required by law to have a set of shipping papers on their person or within easy reach inside the cab at all times.

CHEMTREC

Located in Falls Church, VA, the **Chemical Transportation Emergency Center (CHEMTREC),** now operated by the American Chemistry Council, is a clearinghouse of technical chemical information. Since 1971, this public service hotline has served as an invaluable information resource for first responders of all disciplines to help mitigate incidents involving hazardous materials. The toll-free number for CHEMTREC is 1-800-262-8200. CHEMTREC has the ability to provide you with technical chemical information via telephone, fax, or other electronic media. It also offers a phone conferencing service to connect you with thousands of shippers, subject matter experts, and chemical manufacturers.

When you call CHEMTREC, have the following basic information ready:

- The name of the materials involved in the incident (if known)
- Name of the caller and callback telephone number
- Description of incident and actions taken
- Shipper or manufacturer of the chemical (if known)
- Container type and number of containers
- Railcar or vehicle markings or numbers
- The shipping carrier's name
- Recipient of material
- Location, time, weather at the scene

When you are speaking with CHEMTREC personnel, spell out all chemical names; if using a third party, such as a dispatcher, it is vital that you confirm all spellings to avoid misunderstandings. One number or letter out of place could throw off all subsequent research. When in doubt, be sure to obtain clarification.

Identification of Hazardous Materials

Unfortunately, even with all of these resources, identifying materials can still be difficult. Little consistency is used on labels and placards, and sometimes dishonest transporters will not label containers or vessels appropriately. The laws and regulations that cover labeling of packages and transport vehicles can also be misleading. As discussed previously, in most cases, the package or tank must contain a certain amount of a hazardous material before a placard is required. For example, because of the small quantities of hazardous materials that are involved, a truck carrying 99 pounds (45 kg) of hazmat No. 1 and 99 pounds (45 kg) of both hazmat No. 2 and hazmat No. 3 may not be required by law to display any labels or placards. The truck may show only a "Please drive carefully" placard, implying that it carries no hazardous materials. Therefore, a crash involving this truck is a serious situation, but you would not necessarily know this if you relied on labels and placards. Always maintain a high index of suspicion when approaching the scene of a truck or train tanker incident.

Some substances are not hazardous; however, when mixed with another substance, they may become highly toxic. There may not be regulations against carrying such substances together on one truck or railroad car (or adjacent tank cars). The driver of a commercial truck and the conductor of a train, however, must carry shipping papers that identify what is being transported in their care. These shipping papers may be your first clue that there is a possible hazmat incident; however, depending on the nature of the incident, the papers may not be available to you.

In the event of a leak or spill, a hazmat incident is often indicated by the presence of the following:

- A visible cloud or strange-looking smoke resulting from the escaping substance
- A leak or spill from a tank, container, truck, or railroad car with or without hazmat placards or labels
- An unusual, strong, noxious (harmful), harsh odor in the area

To indicate the presence of normally odorless toxic gases or fluids during a leak or spill, manufacturers may add a substance that produces a strong noxious odor. However, a large number of hazardous gases and fluids are essentially odorless (or do not have a distinctive unpleasant smell) even when a substantial leak or spill has occurred. In some incidents, a large number of people are exposed and may be injured or killed before the presence of a hazmat incident is identified. If you approach a scene where more than one person has collapsed or is unresponsive or in respiratory distress, then assume there has been a hazmat leak or spill and that it is unsafe to enter the area.

It is important for you to understand the potential danger of hazardous materials and know how to operate safely at a hazmat incident. If you do not follow the proper safety measures, then you and many others could end up needlessly injured or dead. Your safety and that of your team, the other responders, and the public must be your most important concern.

There will be times when the ambulance is the first to arrive at the scene. If, as you approach the scene, you see any signs that suggest a hazmat incident has occurred, then stop at a safe distance and park upwind or uphill from the incident. After rapidly sizing up the scene, call for a hazmat team. If you do not recognize the danger until you are too close, then leave the area immediately. Once you have reached a safe place, rapidly assess the situation and provide as much information as possible when calling for the hazmat team, including your specific location, the size and shape of the containers of the hazardous material, and what you have observed and have been told has occurred. Do not reenter the scene, and do not leave the area until you have been cleared by the hazmat team, or you may contribute to the situation by spreading hazardous materials. Finally, do not allow civilians to enter the scene, if possible. No one should enter the area without the proper protective equipment, respiratory protection, or training.

Above all, avoid all contact with the material!

Hazmat Scene Operations

Once you have recognized the incident as one involving hazardous materials and have called for the hazmat team, focus your efforts on activities that will ensure the safety and survival of the greatest number of people. Use the ambulance's public address system to alert people who are near the scene and direct them to move to a location where they will be sufficiently far from danger. With the aid of others on your team, set up a perimeter to stop traffic and people from entering the area.

Safety Tips

Safety considerations at hazmat scenes differ considerably from those involved in emergency response in general. A hazmat scene requires you to have an even higher degree of alertness than usual to avoid entering a dangerous environment and to help others avoid it. There is also a need to prevent the spread of contamination to yourself and your ambulance. Understanding these two concepts is a good start toward safe operations in the presence of hazardous materials.

Establishing Control Zones

Managing a hazmat incident by setting control zones and limiting access to the incident site helps reduce the number of civilians and responders who may be exposed to the released substance. **Control zones** are established at a hazmat incident based on the chemical and physical properties of the released material, the environmental factors at the time of the release, and the general layout of the scene. Of course, isolating a city block in the busy downtown area of a large city presents far different challenges than isolating the area around a rolled-over cargo tank on an interstate highway. Each situation is different, requiring flexibility and thoughtfulness. Securing access to the incident helps ensure no one accidentally enters a contaminated area.

If the incident takes place inside a structure, then the best place to control access is at the normal points of ingress and egress (entry and exit)—doors. Once the doors are secured so that no unauthorized personnel can enter, appropriately trained emergency response crews can begin to isolate other areas as appropriate.

The same concept applies to outdoor incidents. The goal is to secure logical access points around the hazard. Begin by controlling intersections, on and off ramps, service roads, and other access routes to the scene. Police officers should assist by diverting traffic at a safe distance outside the hazard area. They should block off streets, close intersections, and redirect traffic as needed.

During a long-term incident, highway department or public works department employees may be called upon to set up traffic barriers. Whatever methods or devices are used to restrict access, they should not limit or prevent a rapid withdrawal of responders from the area.

It is not uncommon to set large control zones at the onset of an incident, only to discover that the zones may have been established too liberally. At the same time, control zones should not be defined too narrowly **Figure 40-25**. As the IC gets more information about the specifics of the chemical or material involved, the control zones may be expanded or reduced. Ideally, the control zones will be established in the right place, geographically, the first time. Wind shifts are a common reason why control zones are modified during the incident. If there is a prevailing wind pattern in your area, then factor that information into your decision-making process when it comes to control zones.

Typically, control zones at hazmat incidents are labeled as *hot, warm,* or *cold*. You may also discover that other terms are used, such as *exclusionary zone* (hot zone), *contamination reduction zone* (warm zone), and *outer perimeter* (cold zone). In any case, make sure you understand the terminology used in your jurisdiction. Be prepared to discover that different jurisdictions may use terminology and setup procedures unlike the ones used in your agency. As long as you understand the concepts behind the actions and remember that safety is the main focus, the act of setting up and naming zones can remain flexible.

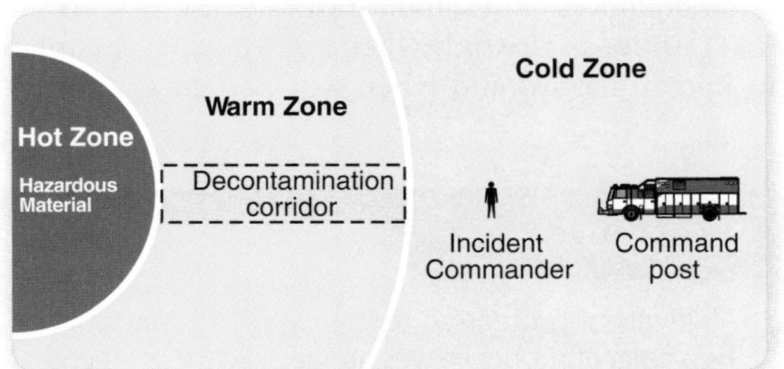

Figure 40-25 Control zones spread outward from the center of a hazardous materials incident.

The **hot zone** is the area immediately surrounding the release, which is also the most contaminated area. Its boundaries should be set large enough that adverse effects from the released substance will not affect people outside of the hot zone. An incident involving a gaseous substance or a vapor, for example, may require a larger hot zone than one involving a solid or nonvolatile liquid leak. In some cases, atmospheric monitoring, plume modeling, or reference sources such as the *ERG* may prove useful in helping to establish the parameters of a hot zone. Specially trained responders, in accordance with their level of training, should be tasked with using these tools. Keep in mind that the physical characteristics of the released substance will significantly affect the size and layout of the hot zone. In addition, all specially trained responders entering the hot zone should avoid contact with the product to the greatest extent possible—an important goal that should be clearly understood by those entering the hot zone. Adhering to this policy makes the job of decontamination easier and reduces the risk of cross-contamination.

Personnel accountability is important, so access into the hot zone must be limited to only the people necessary to control the incident. All personnel and equipment must be decontaminated when they leave the hot zone. This practice ensures that contamination is not inadvertently spread to "clean" areas of the scene.

The **warm zone** is where personnel and equipment transition into and out of the hot zone. It contains control points for access to the hot zone as well as the decontamination area. Only the minimal number of personnel and the equipment necessary to perform decontamination, or support those operating in the hot zone, should be permitted in the warm zone.

A patient's skin and clothing may contain hazardous material, so the **decontamination area** is set up in the warm zone. The decontamination area is the designated area where contaminants are removed before an individual can go to another area. **Decontamination** is the process of removing or neutralizing and properly disposing of hazardous materials from equipment, patients, and rescue personnel. The decontamination area must include special containers for contaminated clothing and special bags to isolate each patient's personal effects safely until they can be decontaminated **Figure 40-26**. The area will also contain a number of special facilities to thoroughly wash and rinse patients and backboards. The water that is used must be captured and delivered into special sealable containers.

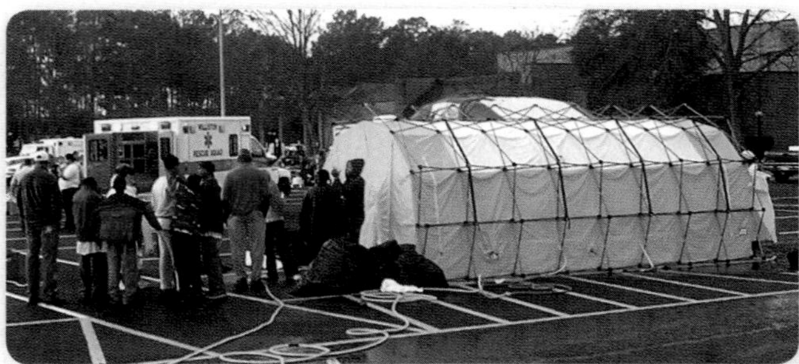

Figure 40-26 Patients should be decontaminated before they are taken to treatment areas.

© Tim Dominick/The State/MCT/Getty.

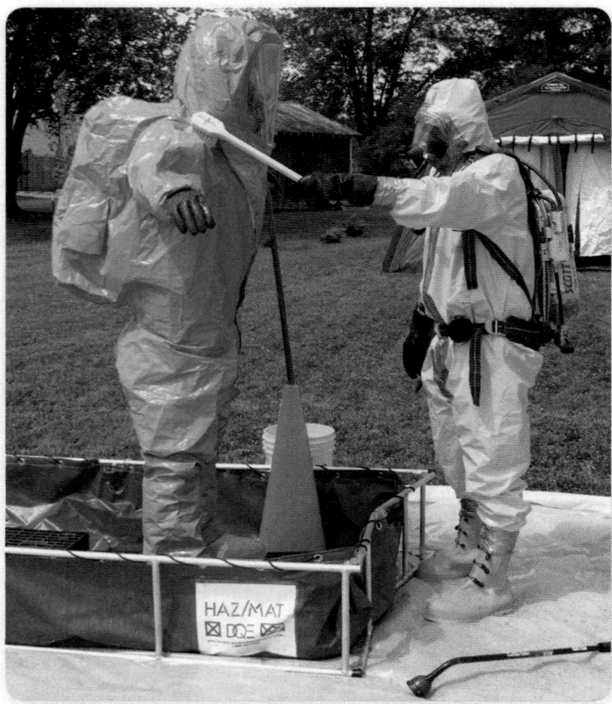

Figure 40-27 The decontamination zone is where firefighters' and hazmat team members' outer protective gear is rinsed and washed before removal.

Courtesy of Airman 1st Class Scherrie Gates/US Air Force.

Anyone who leaves the hot zone must pass through the decontamination area. Firefighters' and hazmat team members' outer protective gear is rinsed and washed in the decontamination area before it is removed **Figure 40-27**. To prevent needless contact and transmission of splash or residues, different personnel are used in the decontamination and treatment areas. Do not move into the decontamination area unless you are properly trained and equipped. Wait for the patients to be brought to you.

Beyond the warm zone is the **cold zone**. The cold zone is a safe area where personnel do not need to wear any special protective clothing for safe operation. Personnel staging, the command post, EMS providers, and the area for medical monitoring, support, and/or treatment after decontamination are all located in the cold zone.

> **Safety Tips**
>
> As an AEMT, your job is to report to a designated area outside of the hot and warm zones and provide triage, treatment, transport, or rehabilitation when hazmat team members bring patients to you.

Personal Protective Equipment Level

Personal protective equipment (PPE) levels indicate the amount and type of protective gear needed to prevent injury from a particular substance. Chemical protective clothing is rated for its effectiveness in several different ways. The EPA defines levels of protection using an alphabetic system **Figure 40-28**.[9]

Level A protection requires a fully encapsulated chemical-resistant garment that completely envelops the wearer and the respiratory apparatus, gloves, boots, and communications equipment. Use Level A protection when the hazardous material identified requires the highest level of skin, respiratory, and eye protection.

Level B protection requires chemical-resistant clothing, boots, gloves, and SCBA. The kind of gloves and boots worn depends on the chemical identified. Use this type of PPE when the type and atmospheric concentration of the hazardous material identified require a high level of respiratory protection but less skin protection is needed. The defining piece of equipment with Level B protection is an SCBA or some other type of supplied-air respirator (a respirator that obtains its air through a hose from a remote source such as a compressor or storage cylinder).

Level C protection requires standard work clothing plus chemical-protective clothing and gloves. Use respiratory protection that filters all inhaled outside air. Level C protection is appropriate when the type of airborne substance is known, its concentration is measured, the criteria for using air-purifying respirators are met, and skin and eye exposure is unlikely.

Level D protection is the lowest level of protection. This level of protection typically requires coveralls, work shoes, hard hat, gloves, and standard work clothing such as an AEMT uniform. Use only when the atmosphere contains no known hazard and when work functions preclude

> **Safety Tips**
>
> All levels of protection require you to wear gloves. Two pairs of rubber gloves are needed for protection in case one pair must be removed because of heavy contamination.

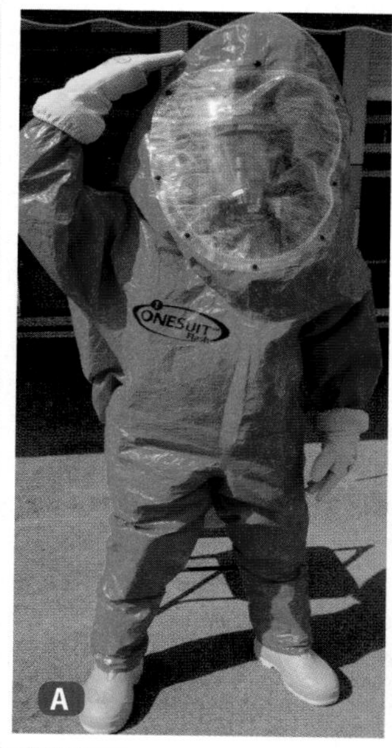
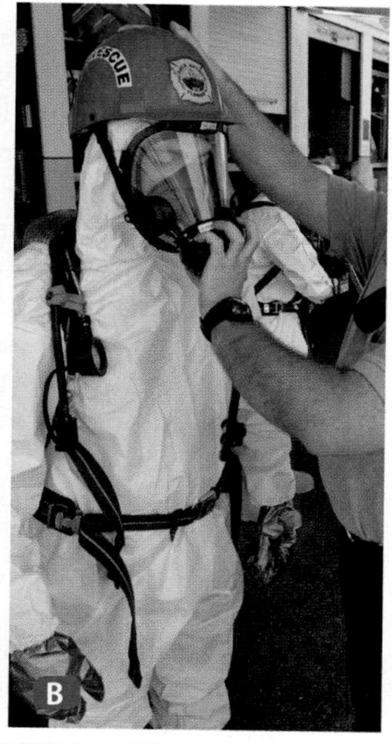
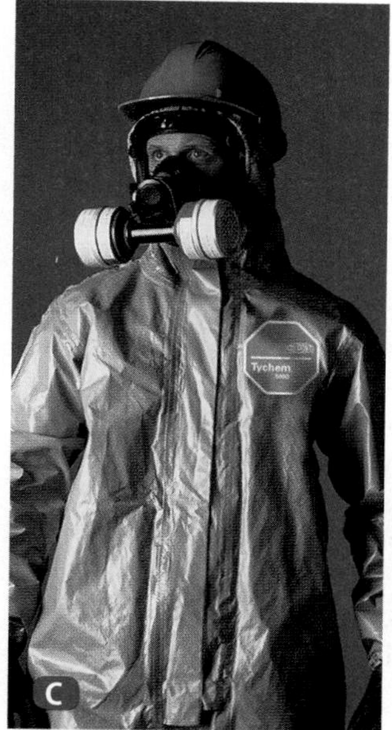
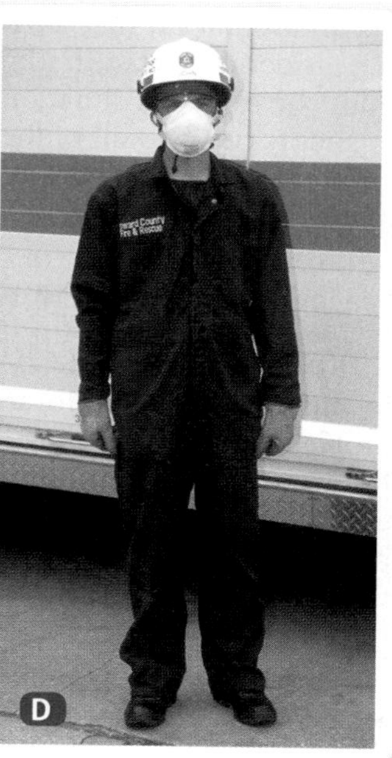

Figure 40-28 Four levels of protection. **A.** Level A protection. **B.** Level B protection. **C.** Level C protection. **D.** Level D protection.

splashes, immersion, or the potential for unexpected inhalation or contact with hazardous levels of chemicals. Use Level D protection only for nuisance contamination (such as dust); it should not be worn on any site where respiratory or skin hazards are known to exist.

▶ Caring for Patients at a Hazmat Incident

Generally, hazmat team members who are trained in prehospital emergency care will initiate emergency medical care for patients who have been exposed to a hazardous material. However, because of the dangers, time constraints, and bulky protective gear that team members wear, it is practical only to provide the simplest assessment and essential care in the hazard zone and the decontamination area. In addition, to avoid entrapment and spread of contaminants, no bandages or splints are applied—except pressure dressings that are needed to control bleeding—until the "clean" (decontaminated) patient has been moved to the treatment area. Therefore, when you are providing care in the treatment area, assess and treat the patient in the same way as you would a patient who has not been previously assessed or treated.

Your care of patients at a hazmat incident must address the following:

- Any trauma that has resulted from other related mechanisms, such as vehicle crash, fire, or explosion
- The injury and harm that have resulted from exposure to the toxic hazardous substance

Most serious injuries and deaths from hazardous materials result from airway and breathing problems. Therefore, maintain the airway, and, if the patient appears to be in distress, then give oxygen at 12 to 15 L/min with a nonrebreathing mask. Monitor the patient's breathing at all times. If you see signs that indicate respiratory distress is increasing, then you may need to provide assisted ventilation with a bag-mask device and high-flow oxygen.

Treat the patient's injuries in the same way that you would treat any injury. There are few specific antidotes or treatments for exposure to most hazardous materials. Different people may respond differently to contact with the same hazardous material. Therefore, your treatment for the patient's exposure to the toxic substance should focus mainly on supportive care and initiating transport to the hospital. If antidotes or other special treatments need to be initiated in the field, then medical control will order and relay them to the officer in charge of EMS operations at the scene. If any special treatment or advanced care, other than medications within the scope of practice of an AEMT and IV fluids, is needed, then paramedics or other advanced personnel will be sent to work with you in the treatment area.

Special Care

In some cases, before the decontamination area has been completely set up, the hazmat team will find one or two patients who need immediate treatment and transport without further delay if they are to survive. Even after the decontamination area is set up and functioning, some patients may have such respiratory distress or other critical condition that the time necessary for full decontamination may prove fatal. If additional delay for proper decontamination seems life threatening in nontoxic exposure situations, then it may be necessary to simply cut away all of the patient's clothing and do a rapid rinse to remove the majority of the contaminating matter before transport.

If you are treating and transporting a patient who has not been fully and properly decontaminated, then increase the amount of protective clothing you wear, including the use of SCBA. At the least, this should include two pairs of gloves, goggles or a face shield, a protective coat, respiratory protection, and a disposable fluid-impervious apron or similar outfit. Many hazmat teams carry light, easy-to-use, disposable, fluid-impervious protective suits for such a purpose. Remember, however, transporting a contaminated patient merely increases the scope of the event. The decision to transport even one patient with critical injuries rests with the IC, who bases his or her decision on recommendations made by the hazmat team.

To make decontaminating the ambulance easier, tape the cabinet doors shut. Any equipment kits, monitors, and other items that will not be used en route should be removed from the patient compartment and placed in the front of the ambulance or in outside compartments. Before loading the patient, turn on the power vent ceiling fan and patient compartment air-conditioning unit fan. Unless the weather is too severe, the windows in the driver's area and sliding side windows in the patient compartment should also be partially opened to prevent creating a "closed box" inside the ambulance and to ensure it is properly ventilated for the safety of the patient and your team members.

When you leave the scene, inform the hospital that you are transporting a critically injured patient who has not been fully decontaminated at the scene. This will allow the hospital to prepare to receive the patient. Many EDs have decontamination facilities and trained personnel for such an event. You may be diverted to a facility with these capabilities if the receiving hospital is not so equipped. On arrival, one AEMT enters the ED and, after giving hospital staff the report and advising them again of the incomplete decontamination, obtains directions before the patient is unloaded and brought in. If there are enough ambulances at a hazmat scene, then one ambulance may be isolated and used only to transport such patients. Remember, the ambulance needs to be decontaminated before transporting another patient.

YOU are the Provider — SUMMARY

1. What are some hazards you may encounter with vehicle safety systems?

Some of the hazards that you may encounter at a crash scene include shock-absorbing bumpers that may become compressed and be under extreme pressures and could "explode," injuring your knees and legs if you are standing in front of them. Airbags fill with a nonharmful gas when the devices deploy and are normally deflated upon arrival of emergency medical services; however, there may be instances where the airbag has not deployed prior to your arrival. The possibility of unexpected deployment has the potential to seriously injury anyone around the airbag. If you gain access to a patient via the front passenger seat and notice the airbag has not deployed, then you should exit the vehicle and seek alternative access. However, if alternative access is not possible, then use extreme caution and maintain a minimum clearance of 20 inches (50-cm) around passenger-side undeployed airbags, 10 inches (25 cm) around undeployed driver airbags, and 5 inches (13 cm) around side-impact undeployed airbags.

2. How should this vehicle be stabilized?

Unstable vehicles are typically stabilized by the fire department. However, in instances where the fire department is not yet at the scene, it may be necessary for you to stabilize the vehicle. Vehicles can be stabilized with a variety of jacks or cribbing, or any available material that may be present around the scene. Prior to attempting to gain access to a vehicle involved in a crash, ensure the vehicle is in "park" with the parking brake set and the ignition turned off. The battery should also be disconnected, negative side first, to minimize the possibility of sparks or fire.

YOU are the Provider SUMMARY *(continued)*

3. What are the hazards that may present with hybrid electric vehicles?

Hybrid electric vehicles have unique features; however, one common feature requires you to disconnect the high-voltage battery to prevent electrical shock, fire, or explosion. In many alternative fuel vehicles, the batteries are not located in the engine compartment, but in other areas, such as in the trunk or under the seats. It is also important for you to remember that in hybrid electric vehicles, there may be more than one battery present.

4. What are the differences between simple access and complex access?

Simple access is an attempt to get to the patient as quickly and simply as possible. Typically, this is accomplished by unlocking doors or opening the windows. Simple hand tools, such as hammers, center punches, pry bars, come-alongs, and hacksaws should be available on the ambulance for you to use.

Complex access requires the use of specialized tools and training, typically provided by the local fire department with the jurisdictional requirements for extrication.

5. What should you do as the patient is being extricated from the vehicle?

During the extrication process, your input is essential so the patient's injuries are considered as the rescue team plans a move that is quick and effective, but also protects the patient from further harm. Personal protection for both yourself and the patient is paramount. You and the patient should wear the appropriate personal protective equipment, as the situation permits. Finally, everyone inside of the vehicle should be covered by a protective blanket that will provide protection from flying glass, metal, or other hazards during the extrication process.

6. How does rapid extrication differ from other methods of patient removal?

Rapid extrication involves manually stabilizing the patient's head and, in most cases, moving the patient from a seated position in a vehicle to a supine position on a backboard, generally in 1 minute or less. The only resources and equipment needed are a cervical collar, a backboard, and adequate manpower.

The main difference between the rapid extrication technique and other methods of patient removal is that it is fast and requires minimal preparation of the patient in the vehicle before the patient is removed.

7. What is the last phase of extrication?

The last phase of extrication is termination. Termination involves returning the emergency units to service. For rescue units, this process may be quite involved. All equipment used on the scene, including hydraulic, electrical, and hand tools, must be checked before reloading them on the apparatus. Whereas some tools require only generalized cleaning, others may need refueling and checking of the various fluid levels.

You will also be required to check the ambulance thoroughly, replacing used supplies and conforming to cleaning needs required by bloodborne pathogen standards.

Finally, rescue units and medical units will be required to complete all necessary reports.

YOU are the Provider SUMMARY *(continued)*

EMS Patient Care Report (PCR)					
Date: 10-3-18	**Incident No.:** 0103		**Nature of Call:** MVC	**Location:** 4 miles W on 464th Street	
Dispatched: 0712	**En Route:** 0713	**At Scene:** 0725	**Transport:** N/A	**At Hospital:** N/A	**In Service:** 0755

Patient Information	
Age: 27 **Sex:** M **Weight (in kg [lb]):** 70 kg (156 lb)	**Allergies:** None **Medications:** None **Past Medical History:** None **Chief Complaint:** Lower extremity paralysis

Vital Signs				
Time: 0726	**BP:** Not obtained	**Pulse:** Not obtained	**Respirations:** 20	**Spo_2:** Not obtained
Time: 0730	**BP:** 110/76	**Pulse:** 105	**Respirations:** 20	**Spo_2:** 99%
Time: 0739	**BP:** 110/70	**Pulse:** 92	**Respirations:** 20	**Spo_2:** 99%

EMS Treatment (circle all that apply)				
Oxygen @ 15 **L/min via (circle one):** **NC** **(NRM)** **Bag-mask device**		**Assisted Ventilation**	**Airway Adjunct**	**CPR**
Defibrillation	**Bleeding Control**	(**Bandaging:** Spinal immobilization)	**Splinting**	(**Other:** Extrication)

Narrative

EMS dispatched to above location for MVC. On arrival, incident command states patient is heavily entrapped from rollover crash. Vehicle is found sitting on roof, massive damage noted to both sides of smaller passenger car. Extrication supervisor states vehicle is hybrid electric vehicle and all batteries have been disconnected. He further states the patient is pinned by his legs, extrication should take 15 to 20 minutes, and one of his firefighters is in the backseat immobilizing the patient's spine. Proceeded to passenger side of vehicle to patient. Patient is alert and oriented × 4, ABCs intact, complaining of lack of sensation to his legs. Discussed helicopter request with IC, who agreed. Dispatch contacted, requested helicopter response. Landing zone established by fire department personnel. Nonrebreathing mask applied at 15 L/min. At 0739, access to the patient via driver's side is secured. Cervical collar applied, and patient placed on long backboard and secured. Patient placed on stretcher, and into back of ambulance. 14-gauge IV established to patient's left wrist, TKO. On arrival of flight crew, report given to flight paramedic. Patient loaded into helicopter, EMS returned to service.**End of report**

Prep Kit

▶ Ready for Review

- Safety during special rescue situations such as vehicle extrication or trench rescue begins with the proper mindset and the proper personal protective equipment.
- During all phases of rescue, your primary concern is safety, and your primary role is to provide emergency medical care and prevent further injury to the patient.
- The ten phases of extrication are:
  - Preparation
  - En route to the scene
  - Arrival and scene size-up
  - Hazard control
  - Support operations
  - Gaining access
  - Emergency medical care
  - Removal of the patient
  - Transfer of the patient
  - Termination
- During scene size-up, while you are paying attention to potential hazards, identify the safest, most efficient way to access the patient. Determine what, if any, additional resources will be needed.
- A variety of hazards may be present at the extrication scene. Potential hazards include downed electrical lines, hazardous materials, traffic, bystanders, and other vehicles, including electric drive vehicle with high-voltage batteries.
- Do not approach an electric or alternative fuel vehicle without proper turnout gear, including self-contained breathing apparatus. Keep in mind a fire from methanol or ethanol may be hard to see.
- Vehicle safety systems, such as shock-absorbing bumpers and airbags, protect your patients but also have the potential to injure rescuers.
- You and the ambulance should remain outside of the danger zone, which is an area where people can be exposed to sharp metal edges, broken glass, toxic substances, lethal rays, or ignition or explosion of hazardous materials.
- A critical phase of extrication is gaining access to the patient. Do not attempt to gain access to the patient until you are sure the scene is safe and that any hazards have been identified and either properly controlled or eliminated. Ensure the patient remains safe during extrication, and extrication efforts must be well coordinated.
- Unless there is immediate danger, during a vehicle extrication, perform a primary assessment of a patient while he or she is still in the vehicle. Immobilize the cervical spine before moving the patient from the vehicle.
- If a special rescue team is needed, inform the dispatcher.
- When a scene calls for a search or for specialized rescue, you may have to call for a technical rescue group, or you may find one already at work when you arrive. Your interaction and cooperation with this group, and with an incident commander (IC) when one has been designated, are important to a smooth rescue.
- You will be involved to some degree in the logistics of patient movement and patient care.
- Tactical situations are best handled directly by special weapons and tactics teams. Your role will often largely consist of remaining out of danger, cooperating with the IC, and remaining ready to care for any patients that are brought to you.
- You may be summoned to a lost person search and rescue. In this situation, your role is to stand by at the command post or the staging area until the lost person or people have been found.
- Trench rescue refers to cave-ins and collapses. Collapses usually involve large areas of falling dirt. The risk of a secondary collapse during the rescue operation is of concern to rescue personnel and to the AEMTs. Ensure vehicles are parked at least 500 feet (152 m) from the scene and are turned off.
- At structure fires, determine whether a special route is necessary, ask the IC where the ambulance should be parked, and ensure the ambulance will not block or hinder other arriving equipment or become blocked in by other equipment or hose lines. Also, the ambulance should leave the scene only if transporting a patient or if the IC has released it.
- When you arrive at the scene of a hazmat incident, first step back and assess the situation. This can be very stressful, particularly if you see a patient.
- The presence of labels, placards, and other markings on buildings, packages, boxes, and containers can enable you to identify a released substance.
  - The US Department of Transportation hazardous materials marking system is used when materials are being transported from one location to another.
  - The NFPA 704 hazard identification system is designed for fixed-facility use.
- Valuable resources for determining what the hazardous material is and what you should do are the *Emergency Response Guidebook*, safety data sheets, and the Chemical Transportation Emergency Center.
- As an EMS provider wearing the lowest level of protection (level D), you will remain in the cold zone, or the safe area.

Prep Kit (continued)

► Vital Vocabulary

access Gaining entry to an enclosed area and reaching a patient.

active shooter A gunman who has begun to fire on people and is still at large.

alternative fuel vehicle A vehicle that uses anything other than a petroleum-based motor fuel (gasoline or diesel) to propel a motorized vehicle.

bills of lading The shipping papers used for transport of chemicals over roads and highways; also referred to as freight bills.

bulk storage containers Any container other than nonbulky storage containers such as fixed tanks, highway cargo tanks, rail tank cars, totes, and intermodal tanks. These are typically found in manufacturing facilities and are often surrounded by a secondary containment system to help control an accidental release.

carboys Glass, plastic, or steel containers, ranging in volume from 5 to 15 gallons (19 to 57 L).

Chemical Transportation Emergency Center (CHEMTREC) An agency that assists emergency responders in identifying and handling hazardous materials incidents.

cold zone A safe area at a hazardous materials incident for the agencies involved in the operations. The incident commander, the command post, EMS providers, and other support functions necessary to control the incident should be located in this zone. Also referred to as the clean zone or the support zone.

complex access Entry that requires special tools and training and includes the use of force.

concealment The use of objects to limit a person's visibility of you.

container Any vessel or receptacle that holds material, including storage vessels, pipelines, and packaging.

control zones Areas at a hazardous materials incident that are designated as hot, warm, or cold, based on safety issues and the degree of hazard found there.

cover The tactical use of an impenetrable barrier for protection.

cylinders Portable, compressed gas containers used to hold liquids and gases such as nitrogen, argon, helium, and oxygen. They have a range of sizes and internal pressures.

danger zone An area where people can be exposed to hazards such as electric wires, sharp metal edges, broken glass, toxic substances, radiation, or ignition or explosion of hazardous materials.

decontamination The process of removing or neutralizing and properly disposing of hazardous materials from equipment, patients, and responders.

decontamination area The designated area in a hazardous materials incident where all patients and responders must be decontaminated before going to another area.

drums Barrel-like containers used to store a wide variety of substances, including food-grade materials, corrosives, flammable liquids, and grease. May be constructed of low-carbon steel, polyethylene, cardboard, stainless steel, nickel, or other materials.

Emergency Response Guidebook A preliminary action guide for first responders operating at a hazardous materials incident in coordination with the US Department of Transportation's (DOT) labels and placards marking system. Jointly developed by the DOT, the Secretariat of Communications and Transportation of Mexico, and Transport Canada.

entrapment To be caught (trapped) within a vehicle, room, or other confined space with no way out, or to have a limb or other body part trapped.

extrication Removal of a patient from entrapment or a dangerous situation or position, such as removal from a wrecked vehicle, industrial incident, or building collapse.

freight bills The shipping papers used for transport of chemicals along roads and highways; also referred to as bills of lading.

hazardous materials Any substances that are toxic, poisonous, radioactive, flammable, or explosive and cause injury or death with exposure.

hazardous materials (hazmat) incident An incident in which a hazardous material is no longer properly contained and isolated.

hot zone The area immediately surrounding a hazardous materials spill or incident site that endangers life and health. All personnel working in this zone must wear appropriate protective clothing and equipment. Entry requires approval by the incident commander or other designated officer.

incident commander (IC) The individual who has overall command of the incident in the field.

intermodal tanks Shipping and storage vessels that can be either pressurized or nonpressurized.

level A protection Personal protective equipment used for protection against vapors, gases, mists, and even dusts. The highest level of protection, it is an encapsulating suit that includes a self-contained breathing apparatus.

Prep Kit *(continued)*

level B protection Personal protective equipment used when the type and atmospheric concentration of substances require a high level of respiratory protection but less skin protection. The kinds of gloves and boots worn depend on the identified chemical.

level C protection Personal protective equipment used when the type of airborne substance is known, the concentration is measured, the criteria for using an air-purifying respirator are met, and skin and eye exposure is unlikely. This ensemble consists of standard work clothing with the addition of chemical-protective clothing, chemically resistant gloves, and a form of respiratory protection.

level D protection Personal protective equipment used when the atmosphere contains no known hazard, and work functions preclude splashes, immersion, or the potential for unexpected inhalation of or contact with hazardous levels of chemicals. This is the lowest level of protection and is primarily a work uniform that includes coveralls.

nonbulk storage vessels Any container other than bulk storage containers such as drums, bags, compressed gas cylinders, and cryogenic containers. These hold commonly used commercial and industrial chemicals such as solvents, industrial cleaners, and compounds.

personal protective equipment (PPE) levels Indicate the amount and type of protective equipment that an individual needs to avoid injury during contact with a hazardous material.

placards Signage required to be placed on all four sides of highway transport vehicles, railroad tank cars, and other forms of hazardous materials transportation; the sign identifies the hazardous contents of the vehicle, using a standardization system with 10¾-inch (27-cm) diamond-shaped indicators.

safe zone An area of protection providing safety from the danger zone (hot zone).

safety data sheet (SDS) A form provided by manufacturers and compounders (blenders) of chemicals, containing information about chemical composition, physical and chemical properties, health and safety hazards, emergency response, and waste disposal of a specific material; this term has replaced material safety data sheet.

secondary containment An engineered method to control spilled or released product if the main containment vessel fails.

self-contained breathing apparatus (SCBA) Respirator with independent air supply used by firefighters to enter toxic and otherwise dangerous atmospheres.

simple access Access that is easily achieved without the use of tools or force.

situational awareness Knowledge and understanding of your surroundings and the ability to recognize potential risks to the safety of the patient or the EMS team.

size-up The ongoing process of information gathering and scene evaluation to determine appropriate strategies and tactics to manage an emergency.

special weapons and tactics (SWAT) team A specialized law enforcement tactical unit.

tactical medicine Emergency medical care provided by specially trained emergency medical responders, advanced emergency medical technicians, paramedics, nurses, and even physicians during a tactical situation.

tactical situation A hostage, robbery, or other situation in which armed conflict is threatened or shots have been fired and the threat of violence remains.

technical rescue group A team of emergency responders from one or more departments in a region who are trained and on call for certain types of technical rescue.

technical rescue situation A rescue that requires special technical skills and equipment in one of many specialized rescue areas, such as technical rope rescue, cave rescue, and dive rescue.

warm zone The area located between the hot zone and the cold zone at a hazardous materials incident. The decontamination corridor is located in the warm zone.

▶ References

1. National Highway Traffic Safety Administration. US Department of Transportation. Air bag deployment. http://www.safercar.gov/Vehicle+Shoppers/Air+Bags/Air+Bag+Deployment. Accessed August 15, 2016.
2. VanGelder KT, *CDX Automotive: Fundamentals of Automotive Technology: Principles and Practice*. Burlington, MA. Jones & Bartlett Learning, 2014:1814.
3. Long RT, Blum A, Bress T, et al. Best practices for emergency response to incidents involving electric vehicles battery hazards: a report on full-scale testing results. The Fire Protection Research Foundation. http://energy.gov/sites/prod/files/2014/02/f8/final_report_nfpa.pdf. Published June 2013. Accessed August 16, 2016.
4. United States Department of Transportation. Pipeline and Hazardous Materials Safety Administration. Hazardous materials transportation placarding requirements. http://www.phmsa.dot.gov/staticfiles/PHMSA/Hazmat/digipak/pdfs/presentation/Placarding_Requirements(04-07).pdf. Accessed August 24, 2016.

Prep Kit (continued)

5. United States Department of Transportation. Pipeline and Hazardous Materials Safety Administration. *2016 Emergency Response Guidebook.* http://phmsa.dot.gov/staticfiles/PHMSA/DownloadableFiles/Files/Hazmat/ERG2016.pdf. Accessed August 24, 2016.
6. National Fire Protection Association. *NFPA 704, Standard System for the Identification of the Hazards of Materials for Emergency Response.* www.NFPA.org. Accessed August 24, 2016.
7. United States Department of Labor. Occupational Safety and Health Administration. Hazard communication standard: safety data sheets. https://www.osha.gov/Publications/OSHA3514.html. Revised 2012. Accessed August 24, 2016.
8. United States Department of Labor. Occupational Safety and Health Administration. Hazard communication safety data sheets. https://www.osha.gov/Publications/HazComm_QuickCard_SafetyData.html. Accessed September 1, 2016.
9. Environmental Protection Agency. Personal protective equipment. https://www.epa.gov/emergency-response/personal-protective-equipment. Updated March 9, 2016. Accessed August 14, 2016.

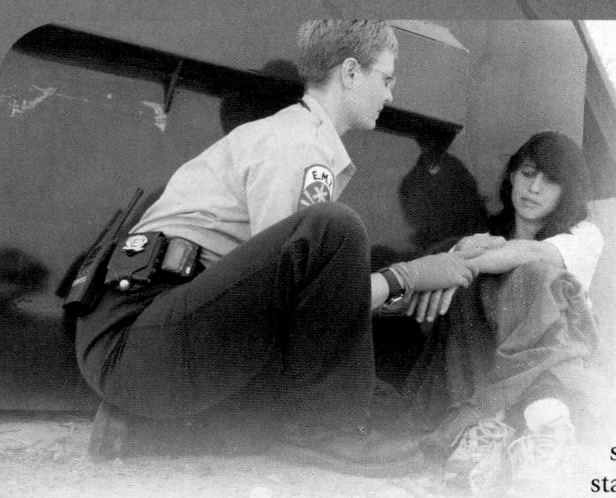

Assessment in Action

You and your partner respond to a hostage situation with the local SWAT team. On arrival, you are met by the IC. You are told the hostage has been released unharmed and the negotiator is trying to talk the perpetrator into surrendering. While he does not anticipate any difficulties in taking the person into custody, it is the team's policy to have an ambulance staged approximately 2 blocks away, ready to respond if needed.

1. When called to a tactical situation you should do all of the following EXCEPT:

A. determine the staging area.
B. identify the location of the incident.
C. establish a safe route into and out of the scene.
D. choose one member to enter with the tactical team.

2. In tactical situations, standards of care may:

A. be altered.
B. stay the same.
C. allow emergency medical services to operate beyond their scope of practice.
D. limit the AEMT's scope of practice.

3. Once your ambulance has arrived at the scene of a tactical call, you should:

A. report to the IC for instructions.
B. park near the command post and leave lights flashing.
C. turn the volume up on your portable radio.
D. do a walkthrough and examine the perimeter.

4. Which of the following is an example of concealment?

A. Trees
B. Dark shadows
C. Dumpsters
D. Vehicles

Assessment in Action *(continued)*

5. When arriving at the scene of a trench collapse, the ambulance should be parked a minimum of ____ feet away from the scene.

   A. 125
   B. 250
   C. 500
   D. 750

6. Older, large vehicles with paint peeling around the trunk area, accompanied by unusual odors, may be an indicator of:

   A. poor vehicle maintenance.
   B. leaded gasoline usage.
   C. a portable methamphetamine laboratory.
   D. living near salt water.

7. As you arrive at the scene of a missing person search and rescue, after meeting with the IC, you should:

   A. isolate and prepare needed equipment.
   B. join the search and rescue efforts.
   C. brief the media.
   D. contact family members to come to the scene.

8. What is a tactical emergency medical services responder?

9. What is the proper positioning of the ambulance when you arrive on scene at motor vehicle extrication?

CHAPTER 41

Incident Management

National EMS Education Standard Competencies

EMS Operations

Knowledge of operational roles and responsibilities to ensure patient, public, and personnel safety.

Incident Management

- Establish and work within the incident management system. (pp 1688-1695)

Multiple Casualty Incidents

- Triage principles (pp 1696-1698)
- Resource management (pp 1688-1692)
- Triage (pp 1696-1699)
  - Performing (pp 1696-1699)
  - Retriage (p 1696)
  - Destination decisions (p 1699)
  - Posttraumatic and cumulative stress (pp 1694, 1701)

Knowledge Objectives

1. Describe the National Incident Management System (NIMS) and its major components. (pp 1687-1688)
2. Describe the purpose of the incident command system (ICS) and its organizational structure. (pp 1688-1691)
3. Explain the role of emergency medical services (EMS) response within the ICS. (pp 1691-1692)
4. Describe how the ICS assists EMS in ensuring both personal safety and the safety of bystanders, health care professionals, and patients during an emergency. (p 1692)
5. Describe your role as an advanced emergency medical technician (AEMT) in establishing command under the ICS. (p 1692)
6. Describe the purpose of medical incident command within the ICS and its organizational structure. (pp 1692-1695)
7. Describe the specific conditions that would define a situation as a mass-casualty incident (MCI); include examples. (p 1695)
8. Describe what occurs during primary and secondary triage, how the four triage categories are assigned to patients on the scene, and how destination decisions regarding triaged patients are made. (pp 1696-1699)
9. Describe how to perform the START and JumpSTART triage methods. (pp 1698-1699)
10. Explain how a disaster differs from an MCI. (p 1700)
11. Describe the role of the AEMT during a disaster operation. (pp 1700-1701)

Skills Objectives

1. Demonstrate how to perform triage based on a fictitious scenario that involves a mass-casualty incident. (pp 1696-1699)

Introduction

Some of the most challenging situations you will encounter are disasters and **mass-casualty incidents (MCIs)**. In this text, a **disaster** refers to any situation that overwhelms your resources. For example, you may find a large number of patients, a lack of specialized equipment, and/or inadequate help. For example, an incident with two critical patients can constitute a disaster if only one emergency medical services (EMS) unit is available to respond. Bus or train crashes are obvious examples of MCIs.

A **multiple-casualty incident** refers to any situation with more than one patient, but which will not overwhelm available resources. There is no set numerical cutoff at which a multiple-casualty incident becomes a mass-casualty incident. Rather, a mass-casualty incident is declared when the number of patients and severity of injuries presenting at a given time or place suggest that available community resources could be overwhelmed, therefore requiring assistance per mutual aid response, discussed later in this chapter. For the purposes of this text, the term mass-casualty incident (MCI) is used throughout.

When you respond to any incident with a large number of patients, you must use a systematic approach to manage the incident most efficiently. By learning to use the principles of the incident command system (ICS), you will be able to make the best use of your resources. As an advanced emergency medical technician (AEMT), you will typically be assigned to work within the EMS/medical branch under an ICS, but you may be asked to function in other areas, which will be discussed later in this chapter. The National Incident Management System (NIMS) was developed to promote more efficient coordination between emergency responders at the regional, state, and national levels. To reduce on-scene problems and to increase your efficiency, you need a solid understanding of the basics of the NIMS. You may also access training courses through the Federal Emergency Management System (FEMA) website.[1] These courses include ICS-100, Introduction to the Incident Command System and FEMA IS-700, National Incident Management System, An Introduction.

Words of Wisdom

A multiple-vehicle pileup on an interstate may constitute a small-scale MCI. The series of terrorist attacks on September 11, 2001 are examples of MCIs on a much larger scale.

National Incident Management System

In 2004, the Department of Homeland Security implemented the **National Incident Management System (NIMS)**. The NIMS provides a consistent, nationwide approach to incident management, enabling federal, state, and local governments, private-sector and nongovernmental organizations, and all other organizations who assume a role in emergency management to work together effectively and efficiently. The NIMS is used to prepare for, prevent, respond to, and recover from domestic incidents, regardless of cause, size, or complexity, including acts of catastrophic terrorism and hazardous materials (hazmat) incidents.

Two important underlying principles of the NIMS are flexibility and standardization. The organizational structure must be flexible enough to be rapidly adapted for use in any situation. The NIMS provides standardization in terminology, resource classification, personnel training, certification, and more. Another important feature of the NIMS is the concept of interoperability, which refers to the ability of agencies of different types or from different jurisdictions to communicate with each other. Major incidents require the involvement and coordination of multiple jurisdictions, agencies, and emergency response disciplines.

The five major NIMS components are as follows:[2]

1. **Preparedness.** The NIMS establishes measures for all responders to incorporate into their systems to prepare for their responses to all incidents at any time, including procedures and protocols, licensure, and equipment certification.

YOU are the Provider — PART 1

As you are preparing to sit down for lunch with the rest of the firefighters from your station, the radio squawks, "Engines 21-1, 21-2, 21-4, Tower 21-1, 24-1, Tender 33-5, Heavy Rescue 22-3, Medic 21-1, 22-1, and Chief 21 respond to 152 Main Street for a building collapse. Multiple casualties reported. Time out 1214." Everyone looks at each other, then proceeds expeditiously to his or her apparatus. As you advise dispatch that your unit is responding, Chief 21 advises that he is at the scene of a commercial office building collapse with multiple injuries. Chief 21 will be assuming command with the command post located at the corner of Main Street and 1st Avenue. He also advises that the staging area will be located at 1st Avenue and 1st Street.

1. What is the NIMS?
2. Why is NIMS helpful to all emergency responders?

2. **Communications and information management.** Effective communications, information management, and sharing are critical aspects of domestic incident management. The NIMS communications and information systems enable the essential functions needed to provide interoperability.
3. **Resource management.** The NIMS sets up mechanisms to describe, inventory, track, and dispatch resources before, during, and after an incident. The NIMS also defines standard procedures to recover equipment used during the incident.
4. **Command and management.** The NIMS standardizes incident management for all hazards and across all levels of government. The NIMS standard incident command structures are based on three key constructs: ICS, multiagency coordination systems, and public information systems.
5. **Ongoing management and maintenance.** The multijurisdictional, multidisciplinary NIMS Integration Center (NIC) provides strategic direction for and oversight of the NIMS. It supports routine maintenance and continuous improvement of the system in the long term, including research and development of supporting technologies.

Incident Command System

The **incident command system (ICS)** is an important component of the NIMS. Developed in the 1970s and pioneered by the fire service, the ICS is a standardized, on-scene emergency management model specifically designed to provide for an integrated organizational structure that reflects the complexity and demands of an incident.[3] (Some agencies refer to the incident command system as the incident management system.) The purpose of the ICS is to enhance command, control, and communication abilities; ensure responder and public safety; achieve incident management goals; ensure the efficient use of resources; and treat patients during an emergency.

Words of Wisdom

Using the ICS gives you a modular organizational structure that can be applied to all hazards. ICS is activated for incidents ranging from a single vehicle crash with one patient to a natural gas pipeline explosion involving multiple communities and multiple patients.

The ICS is designed to avoid duplication of effort and **freelancing**, in which individual units or different organizations make independent and often inefficient decisions about the next appropriate action. Follow your local standard operating procedures for establishing the ICS.

One of the organizing principles of the ICS is limiting the **span of control** of any one individual. This principle refers to keeping the supervisor/worker ratio at one supervisor for three to seven workers. A supervisor who has more than seven people reporting to him or her is exceeding an effective span of control and needs to divide tasks and delegate the supervision of some tasks to another person.

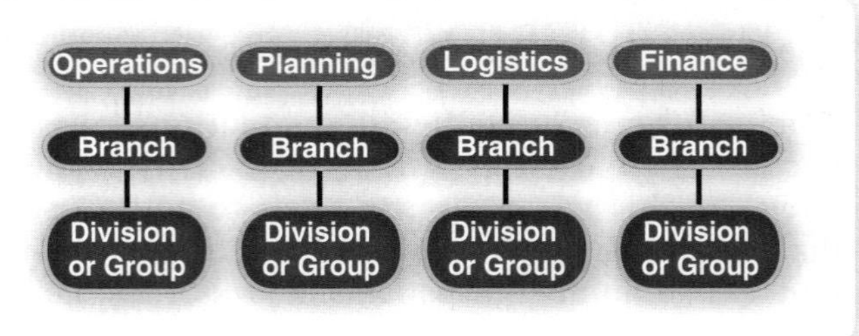

Figure 41-1 The incident command system organizational structure may include sections, branches, divisions, and groups.

The organizational levels may include sections, branches, divisions, and groups as follows **Figure 41-1**:

- **Sections** are responsible for a major functional area such as finance, logistics, planning, or operations.
- **Branches** are managed by the branch director and may be functional or geographic in nature. Branches tend to be established when span of control is a problem, such as at larger incidents, where more oversight may be needed. Branches are in charge of activity directly related to the section (eg, fire, law enforcement, EMS, operations, etc).
- **Divisions** and **groups** serve to align resources and/or crews under one supervisor. Divisions usually refer to crews working in the same geographic area. Groups usually refer to crews working in the same functional area, but possibly in different locations.

Generally speaking, the larger the incident, the more divisions there will be. A small incident may require support only from the fire department, EMS, and law enforcement. By contrast, a large incident will require many agencies to work together.

In some regions, emergency operations centers may exist. The centers are usually operated by the city, state, or federal government. These centers will usually be activated only in a large catastrophic event that may go on for days, involves hundreds of patients, and taxes the entire system.

Emergency responders who assume a role in incident management should use the ICS. Find out from your service if one exists, who is in charge, how it is activated, and what your expected role will be.

Incident Command System Roles and Responsibilities

Many roles are defined in the ICS. The general staff includes **command**, finance and administration, logistics,

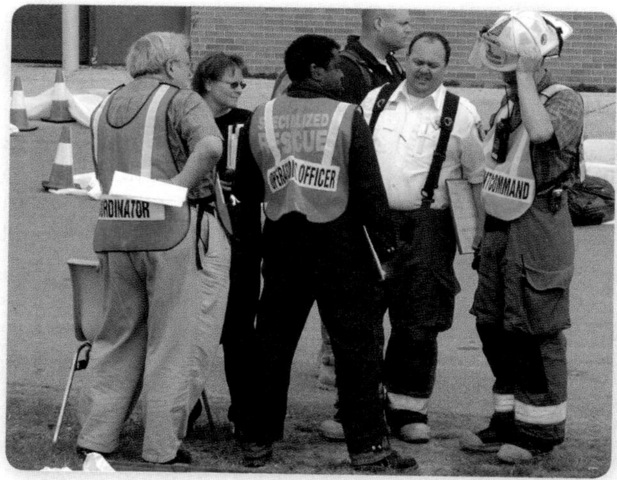

Figure 41-2 The incident commander at a mass-casualty incident oversees the incident and develops a plan for the response.

Courtesy of Captain David Jackson, Saginaw Township Fire Department.

operations, and planning personnel. It is important for you to understand the specific duties of each section and how they work to coordinate the response. Command functions may include a public information officer, safety officer, and liaison officer.

Command

The **incident commander (IC)** is the person in charge of the overall incident. The IC will assess the incident, establish the strategic objectives and priorities, and develop a plan to manage the incident Figure 41-2. The number of command duties the IC takes on often varies by the size of the incident. Small incidents often mean the IC will do it all. In an incident of medium size or complexity, the IC may delegate some functions but retain others. For example, at a motor vehicle crash with multiple patients, the IC may designate a safety officer but maintain responsibility for the other command functions. In a complex situation, the IC may appoint team members to all of the command roles.

A large-scale incident, such as a hazmat spill, requires a multiagency or multijurisdiction response and a **unified command system**. In this case, plans are drawn up in advance by all cooperating agencies that assume a shared responsibility for decision making. The response plan should designate the lead and support agencies in several kinds of incidents. (For example, the hazmat team will take the lead in a chemical leak. However, the medical team might take the lead in a multivehicle crash.) Agencies that share a border should train often with each other to ensure that a unified command system will function well and that communication among the responders is well established before a real incident occurs.

A **single command system** is one in which one person is in charge, even if multiple agencies respond. It is generally used during incidents in which one agency has the majority of responsibility for incident management. Ideally, it is used for short-duration, limited incidents that require the services of a single agency.

Your IC should be on or near the scene, where he or she can easily communicate with all emergency responders operating at the scene. It is important that you know who the IC is, how to communicate with him or her, and where the **command post** is located. If the incident is very large, then you will report to a supervisor working under the IC. (Remember the rule of span of control.) To make the IC easily identifiable, some type of garment is worn, such as a brightly colored vest labeled with the word COMMAND. If the command post is set up in a vehicle, then it should be well marked, and you should know its location. Make sure that your supervisor or the IC knows of any plans or operations before they are initiated.

Communication is particularly important if a transfer of command takes place. Because an incident can rapidly change in size and complexity, an IC may turn over command to someone with more experience in a critical area. This change, or transfer of command, must take place in an orderly manner and, if possible, face-to-face. In extreme situations, it could be done by phone, radio, or email, although these methods are not recommended. Your agency should have standard operating procedures that govern the transfer of command. Make certain to follow the standard operating procedures. When an incident draws to a close and the command structure is no longer necessary, a **termination of command** should take place. Your agency should implement **demobilization** procedures as the situation deescalates or comes to an end. Demobilization is the process of directing responders to return to their facilities when their work at an incident has finished.

Finance and Administration

The **finance and administration** section is responsible for documenting all expenditures at an incident, including the expenditures for materials and supplies, and documenting personnel hours. Finance and administration personnel are not usually needed at smaller incidents, but at larger incidents they are necessary. Ultimately, the information gathered is reported at meetings of the general staff. Responding agencies and organizations may be eligible for some types of reimbursement after the incident, and efficient finance and administration personnel will help your agency to succeed in the reimbursement process. Finance and administration personnel should be trained in the process of assessing expenditures with an eye to reimbursement long before an actual incident.

The various functions within the finance and administration section include: (1) the time unit, (2) the procurement unit, (3) the compensation/claims unit, and (4) the cost unit. The time unit is responsible for ensuring the daily recording of personnel time and equipment use. The procurement unit deals with all matters concerning vendor contracts. The compensation and claims unit has two major purposes: dealing with claims as a result of the incident and injury compensation. Finally, the cost unit is responsible for collecting, analyzing, and reporting the costs related to an incident.

Logistics

The **logistics** section is responsible for communications equipment, facilities, food and water, fuel, lighting, and medical equipment and supplies for patients and emergency responders. Local standard operating procedures will list the medical equipment needed for the incident, depending on the type of incident. Logistics personnel are trained to find food, shelter, and health care for you and the other responders at the scene. In a large incident, it is often necessary for many people to handle logistics, even though only one person (section chief) will report to the IC.

Operations

At a very large or complex incident, the IC will appoint an **operations** section chief, who is responsible for managing the tactical operations usually handled by the IC on routine EMS calls. This arrangement frees the IC to coordinate with other agencies and the media, engage in strategic planning, and ensure that logistics are functioning effectively. The operations section chief will supervise the people working at the scene of the incident, who will be assigned to branches, divisions, and groups. Operations personnel often have experience in management within EMS.

Planning

The **planning** section solves problems as they arise during the incident. Planners analyze, investigate, and obtain data; develop objectives for the incident; select a strategy to meet the objectives; and determine the resources needed to execute a plan.[4] They need to work closely with the operations, finance, and, especially, logistics sections. Planners can and should call on technical experts to help with the planning process. They document their decisions and what they learned from the incident and also set out a course for demobilizing the response when necessary.

Another important function of the planning section is the development of an **incident action plan**, which is the central tool for planning during a response to a disaster. The incident action plan is prepared by the planning section chief with input from the appropriate sections and units of the incident command team. It should be written at the outset of the response and revised continually throughout the response. For smaller, readily controlled incidents, a written plan may not be necessary and the IC may deliver the plan verbally. Larger, more complex incidents will require a formal incident action plan to coordinate activities. The level of detail required in an incident action plan will vary according to the size and complexity of the response.

Words of Wisdom

The size and scale of the incident will dictate the number of roles assigned by the IC.

Command Staff

Three important positions that help the general staff (all staff described previously) and the IC are the safety officer, the public information officer, and the liaison officer. The **safety officer** monitors the scene for conditions or operations that may present a hazard to responders and patients. The safety officer may need to work with environmental health and hazmat specialists. The importance of the safety officer cannot be underestimated—he or she has the authority to stop an emergency operation whenever a responder is in danger. A safety officer should remove hazards to EMS personnel and patients before the hazards cause injury.

The **public information officer (PIO)** provides the public and media with clear and understandable information. A wise PIO positions his or her headquarters well away from the incident command post and, most important, away from the incident, to minimize distractions. Also, the PIO must keep the media safe and from becoming part of the incident. The designated PIO may work in cooperation with PIOs from other agencies in a **joint information center (JIC)**. In some circumstances, the PIO/JIC may be responsible for distributing a message designed to help a situation, prevent panic, and provide evacuation directions.

The **liaison officer** relays information and concerns among command, the general staff, and other agencies. If an agency is not represented in the command structure, then questions and input should be given through the liaison officer.

YOU are the Provider — PART 2

You arrive at the staging area shortly after a lieutenant from Engine 21-4 has been designated as the staging supervisor. The IC directs your unit to assume the role of triage, as the rescue crews bring the patients into the triage area. As soon as you establish a triage area, you are immediately bombarded with seven patients.

3. What is the function of the staging supervisor?
4. What is the function of the triage supervisor?

▶ Communications and Information Management

Communications has historically been the weak point at most major incidents. To minimize the effects of communications problems, it is recommended that communications be integrated so that all agencies involved can communicate quickly and effortlessly via radios. Communications allow for accountability throughout the incident, as well as instant communications between recipients. As always, and more so during a large incident, it is important to maintain professionalism on all radio communications, and remember to communicate clearly and concisely using clear text (no 10-codes).

▶ Mobilization and Deployment

When an incident has been declared and the need for additional resources has been identified, a request is made for additional resources. After a request is made, these resources are mobilized and deployed to the scene. To minimize the potential for freelancing, wait until the request is made before you depart for the scene.

Check-in at the Incident

On arrival at an incident, first check in with the IC at the command post, base, staging area, or other location designated by the IC. If the incident is large in size or complexity, then remember you will be assigned to a supervisor working under the IC.[5] Check-in allows for personnel tracking throughout the incident and also ensures that costs, pay, and reimbursement can be calculated accurately.

Initial Incident Briefing

After the check-in process is complete, report to your supervisor for an initial briefing that will allow you to get information regarding the incident, as well as your specific job functions and responsibilities.

Incident Record Keeping

Record keeping is important for financial reasons and for documentation purposes. If a large piece of equipment becomes inoperable, then it may be possible for the agency to be reimbursed for replacement costs. Record keeping also allows for tracking of time spent on the incident for reimbursement purposes.

Accountability

Because of the large number of responders at a large incident, accountability is important. Accountability means keeping your supervisor advised of your location, actions, and completed tasks. It also includes advising your supervisor of the tasks that you have been unable to complete and what tools you need to complete them.

Incident Demobilization

After the incident has been stabilized and all of the hazards mitigated, the IC will determine which resources are needed or not needed and when to begin demobilization. This process allows for a prompt return of resources to their parent organizations to be placed back in service.

EMS Response Within the Incident Command System

▶ Preparedness

Preparedness involves the decisions made and basic planning done before an incident occurs. Every state is at risk for natural disasters, such as hurricanes, tornadoes, earthquakes, and wildfires. Therefore, preparedness in a given area involves anticipating the most likely natural disasters for the area, among other disasters.

Your EMS agency should have written disaster plans that you are regularly trained to carry out. A copy of the disaster plan should be kept in each EMS vehicle. EMS facilities should have disaster supplies for at least a 72-hour period of self-sufficiency. Your EMS service should have **mutual aid response** agreements with neighboring EMS systems to respond when local resources are insufficient to handle response. All groups with mutual aid response agreements should practice using the plans frequently. EMS systems should share a list of resources with each other so they will know early on what they can access. Also, your local EMS systems should develop an assistance program for the families of EMS providers. If EMS providers have concerns about their families during a disaster, then their effectiveness on the job could be diminished.

Safety Tips

You should have a personal disaster plan for your family. Families need to be prepared and know what to expect should you be required to respond to a disaster. You should also be up-to-date on immunizations for influenza, hepatitis A and B, and tetanus.

▶ Scene Size-up

Remember that scene size-up starts with dispatch. If dispatch information indicates a possible unsafe scene, then stay away from the scene or get only close enough to make an assessment without putting yourself in harm's way. When you arrive first on the scene of an incident, you will make an initial assessment and some preliminary decisions. The scene size-up will be driven by three basic questions that you must ask yourself:

- *What do I have?*
- *What resources do I need?*
- *What do I need to do?*

These questions have a symbiotic relationship. The answer from one helps answer the others, and each answer represents a piece to the puzzle. Work as a team when you answer these questions because overlooking just one safety issue early on can start a chain reaction of problems.

What Do I Have?

Start with scene safety. First, assess the scene for hazards. Warn all other responders about hazmat, fuel spills, electrical hazards, or other safety concerns as soon as possible. Confirm the incident location.

Establish whether the incident is open or closed. An **open incident** is one that is not yet contained; there may be patients who have yet to be located and the situation may be ongoing, producing yet more patients. A **closed incident** is one that is contained and in which all casualties are accounted for. However, as with any situation, a closed incident may quickly become an open incident as situations change.

Estimate the number of casualties. Immediately provide a brief incident report to dispatch. An example of such a report would be: "AEMT unit number one arriving on scene, multiple vehicles involved, full road blockage, no apparent hazards at this time, AEMT unit number one is assuming command."

What Resources Do I Need?

Decide what resources are needed. You may need more EMS responders, ambulances, or other forms of transportation. If extrication is required, then a rescue unit and fire department response may be needed. If hazmat are present, then request a hazmat team immediately. Many large EMS systems deploy specialized MCI units or mobile emergency room vehicles that are able to treat dozens of patients on the scene **Figure 41-3**.

What Do I Need to Do?

Keep the following priorities in mind:

- Safety
- Incident stabilization
- Preservation of property and the environment

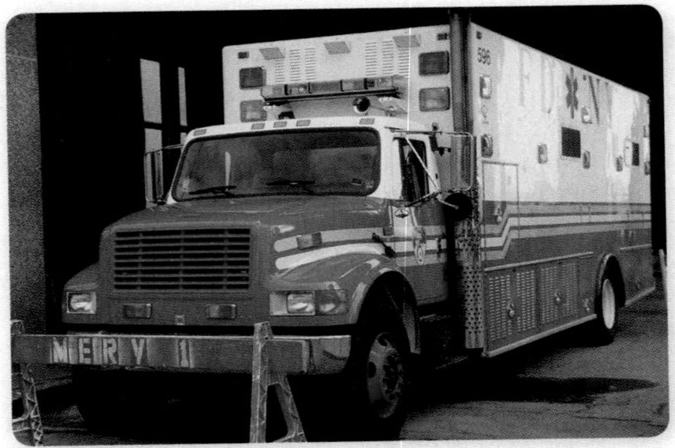

Figure 41-3 This mobile emergency room is staffed by EMTs, AEMTs, paramedics, and physicians who are able to provide advanced life support to multiple patients simultaneously on the scene of a mass-casualty incident.

You need to consider these priorities in the order they are given. Safety is paramount. Safety includes your life, your partner's life, and other responders' lives. Then, consider the safety of the patient and any bystanders. This concept will be difficult for anyone dedicated to saving lives, but it is important to put yourself and your partner first—you have the skills, and bystanders usually do not; the situation can worsen if you become a patient yourself. Often, if a responder is injured, then other responders will focus on "their own," removing available resources from the incident.

You may have to initially work to isolate or stabilize the incident before providing emergency medical care to injured people—this is another difficult concept for all emergency workers. Remember, you cannot help the injured if the scene is unstable. An unstable scene can lead to an injured AEMT.

▶ Establishing Command

After you have performed a good scene size-up and answered the three basic questions, command should be established by the most senior official, notification to other responders should go out, and necessary resources should be requested. A command system ensures that resources are effectively and efficiently coordinated. Command must be established early, preferably by the first-arriving, most experienced public safety official. These officials may include police, fire, or EMS personnel.

▶ Communications

As discussed earlier, communications is often the key challenge at an MCI or a disaster. The infrastructure may be damaged, or communications capabilities may be overwhelmed. If possible, then, use face-to-face communication to limit radio traffic. Some organizations responding to a disaster might not know how to use a radio. If you communicate via radio, then do not use 10-codes or signals. Most communications problems should be worked out before a disaster happens by designating channels strictly for command during a disaster. Whatever form of communications equipment is used, it must be reliable, durable, and field-tested. Be sure that backups are in place if the primary communications system does not work. Some regions have mobile self-contained communications centers, whereas others use local radio groups such as ham radio operators to assist with communications. Most important, your plan should include a "Plan B" in case of communications failure.

Medical Incident Command

What has traditionally been referred to as **medical incident command** is more commonly known as the medical (or EMS) branch of the ICS **Figure 41-4**. At incidents that have a significant medical factor, the IC should appoint someone as the medical branch director. This person will supervise the primary roles of the medical branch—**triage**,

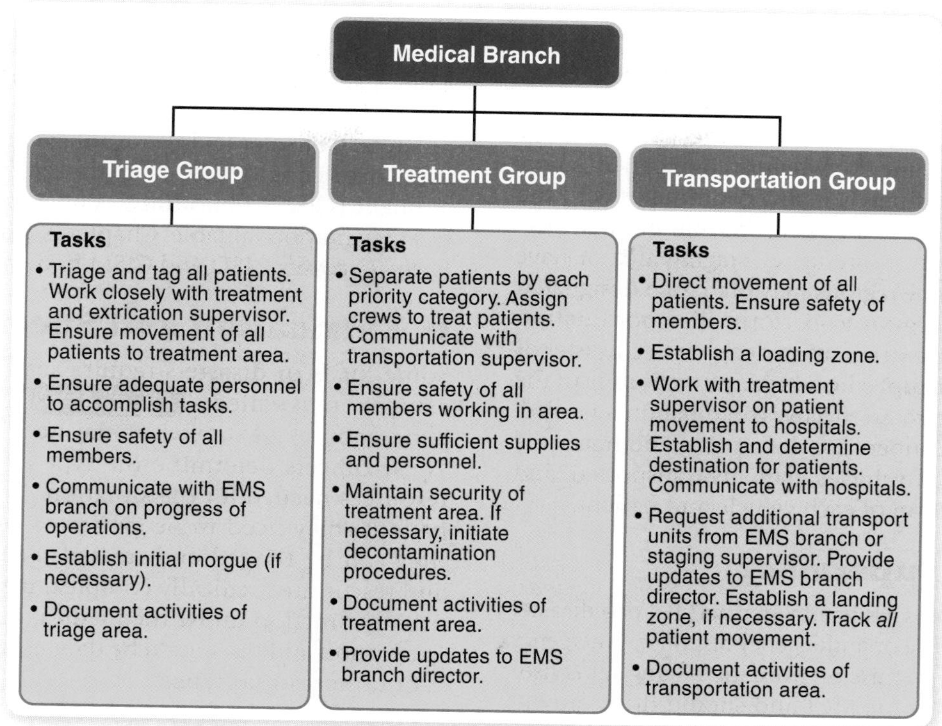

Figure 41-4 Components of the medical branch within the incident command system.

treatment, and transport of injured people. Triage simply means *to sort* your patients based on the severity of their injuries (discussed later in this chapter). The medical branch director should help ensure that EMS units responding to the scene are working within the ICS, each medical group receives a clear assignment before beginning work at the scene, and personnel remain with their vehicles in the staging area until they are assigned their duties. Depending on the scale of the incident, EMS may be a branch within the operations section or may fall under the logistics section as a unit.

▶ Triage Supervisor

The **triage supervisor** is ultimately in charge of counting and prioritizing patients. During large incidents, a number of triage personnel may be needed Figure 41-5. The primary duty of the triage group is to ensure that every patient receives an initial assessment of his or her condition. AEMTs doing triage will help move patients to the appropriate treatment sector. One of the most difficult parts of being a triage supervisor is that you must not begin treatment until all patients are triaged, or you will compromise your triage efforts.

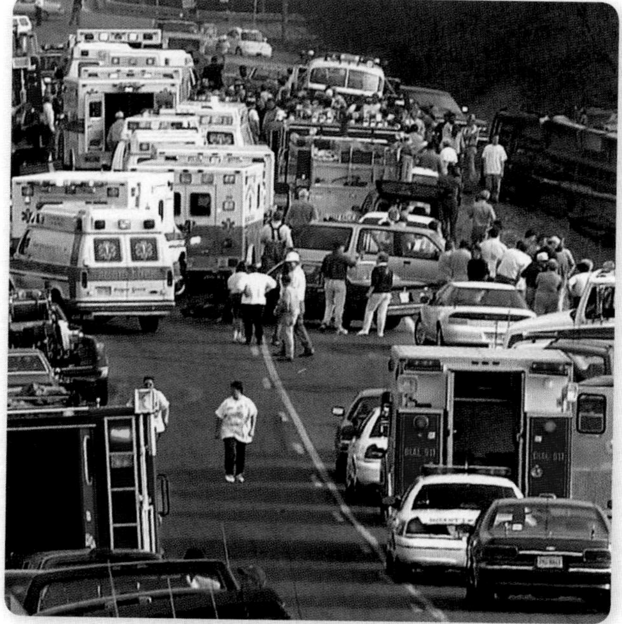

Figure 41-5 Mass-casualty incidents require triage.

▶ Treatment Supervisor

The **treatment supervisor** will locate and set up the **treatment area** with a tier for each priority of patient. The treatment supervisor ensures that secondary triage of patients is performed and that adequate patient care is given as resources allow. The treatment supervisor also assists with moving patients to the **transportation area**. While the treatment supervisor supervises the responders, he or she must communicate with the medical branch director to request sufficient quantities of supplies, including bandages, burn supplies, airway and respiratory supplies, and patient packaging equipment.

▶ Transportation Supervisor

The key role of the **transportation supervisor** is to coordinate the transportation and distribution of patients to appropriate receiving hospitals and help to ensure that hospitals do not become overwhelmed by a patient surge. The transportation supervisor also coordinates with the incident commander to help ensure that enough personnel and ambulances are in the staging area or have been requested. Some regions may plan for a designated hospital within a region to perform the coordination between hospitals on destination decisions. A disaster or an MCI typically disrupts the everyday functioning of the regional trauma system, so effective coordination is needed. The transportation supervisor documents and tracks the number of transport vehicles, patients transported, and the facility destination of each vehicle and patient.

▶ Staging Supervisor

A **staging supervisor** is assigned when an MCI or a disaster requires a multivehicle or multiagency response. Emergency vehicles must have permission from the staging supervisor to enter the scene of the MCI and should drive only in the directed area. The staging area should be established away from the scene so that the parked vehicles are not in the way. The staging supervisor locates an area to stage equipment and responders, tracks unit arrivals, and releases vehicles and supplies when ordered by incident command. The staging supervisor plans for efficient access to and exit from the disaster site and prevents traffic congestion among responding vehicles.

▶ Physicians on Scene

In an MCI or disaster, some areas have plans in place for physicians to be sent to the scene. Sometimes, even without a plan, the enormity of the situation may require physicians to be on scene. Emergency physicians, especially, will have the ability to make difficult triage decisions. They also provide secondary triage decisions in the treatment area, deciding which priority patients are to be transported first. Physicians can provide on-scene medical direction for AEMTs, and they can provide medical care in the treatment area as appropriate.

▶ Rehabilitation Supervisor

In disasters or MCIs that will last for extended periods, a rehabilitation section for the responders should be established. The **rehabilitation supervisor** establishes an area that provides protection for responders from the elements and the situation. The **rehabilitation area** should be located away from exhaust fumes and crowds (especially members of the media) and out of view of the scene itself. The rehabilitation area is where a responder's needs for rest, fluids, food, and protection from the elements are met. The rehabilitation supervisor must also monitor responders for signs of physical and/or emotional stress, including posttraumatic stress disorder (a delayed stress reaction to a prior incident) or cumulative stress (prolonged or excessive stress). These signs may include fatigue, altered thinking patterns, and complete collapse. Remember that all EMS personnel must be aware of signs of stress. Consider taking advantage of critical incident stress debriefing (CISD) or critical incident stress management (CISM) opportunities after an incident if you feel they may be valuable. Chapter 2, *Workforce Safety and Wellness*, covers CISD and CISM in detail.

▶ Extrication and Special Rescue

Some MCIs or disasters require search and rescue or extrication of patients **Figure 41-6**. An **extrication supervisor** or **rescue supervisor** may need to be appointed. These officers determine the type of equipment and resources needed for the situation. In some incidents, patients may need to be extricated or rescued before they can be triaged and treated. Because extrication and rescue are medically complex, the supervisors will usually function under the medical branch of the ICS. Extrication and rescue can be dangerous, so team safety is of utmost importance.

▶ Morgue Supervisor

Some MCIs or disasters will result in many dead patients. The **morgue supervisor** works with area medical examiners, coroners, disaster mortuary assistance teams, and law enforcement agencies to coordinate removal of the bodies and even, possibly, body parts. The morgue supervisor should attempt to leave the dead patients in the location found, if possible, until a removal and storage plan can be determined. The location of patients may help in the identification of the dead patients in mass-fatality

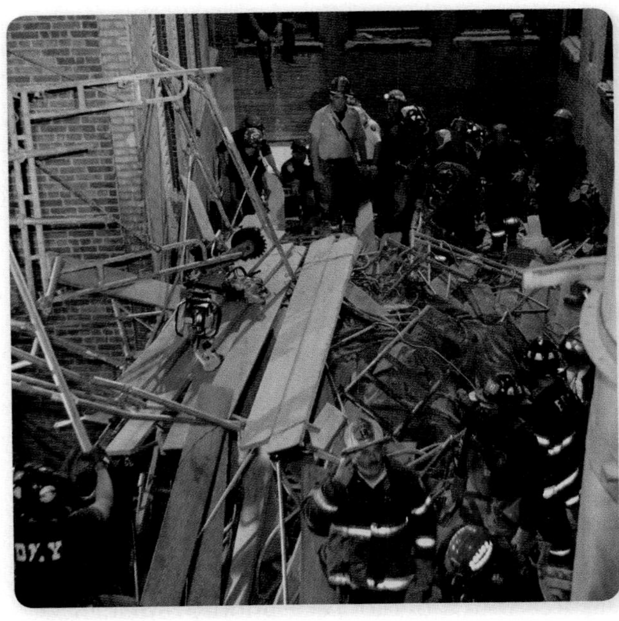

Figure 41-6 Some disasters will involve search and rescue or extrication.

situations, or there may be crime scene considerations. If it is determined that a morgue area is needed, then the morgue supervisor should ensure that the morgue area is out of view of the living patients and other responders because the psychological impact could worsen the situation. In addition, the morgue area should be secured from the public to prevent theft of any personal effects of the dead patients.

Mass-Casualty Incidents

As discussed previously, an MCI refers to any call that could overwhelm available community resources, and require a mutual aid response **Figure 41-7**. Disasters certainly qualify as MCIs, but many other causes of MCIs are far more common than disasters and are usually much smaller in scope. **Figure 41-8** is a diagram of a residential building fire confined to one apartment that may only produce one patient but that has the potential to generate dozens of patients from among the responders and residents. Loss of power to a hospital or nursing home with ventilator-dependent and nonambulatory patients is considered an MCI, although no one is injured. By using the ICS and the NIMS and understanding the various roles and responsibilities of each position, the responders and/or IC can manage the incident in a smooth, organized manner.

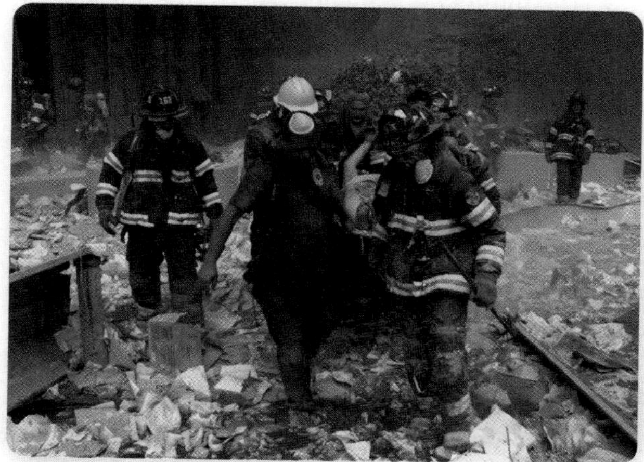

Figure 41-7 In large mass-casualty incidents, such as the terrorist attacks on September 11, 2001, mutual aid may be necessary from a large number of additional jurisdictions.

All EMS systems have different protocols for when to declare an MCI and/or initiate the ICS; however, as the AEMT, ask yourself the following questions when considering whether the call is an MCI:

- *How many seriously injured or ill patients can I effectively treat and transport in the ambulance? One? Two?*
- *What happens when I have multiple patients to manage?*
- *How long will it take for additional help to arrive?*
- *What happens if the number of patients exceeds the number of available ambulances?*

Obviously, you and your team cannot treat and transport all injured patients at the same time. At an MCI, you will often experience an increased demand for equipment and personnel. For example, you may realize that you are the only ambulance crew currently at the scene with a wait of 15 or more minutes before the next ambulance arrives. Never leave the scene to transport patients if other sick or wounded patients are still present. This action would leave patients at the scene without medical care and can be considered

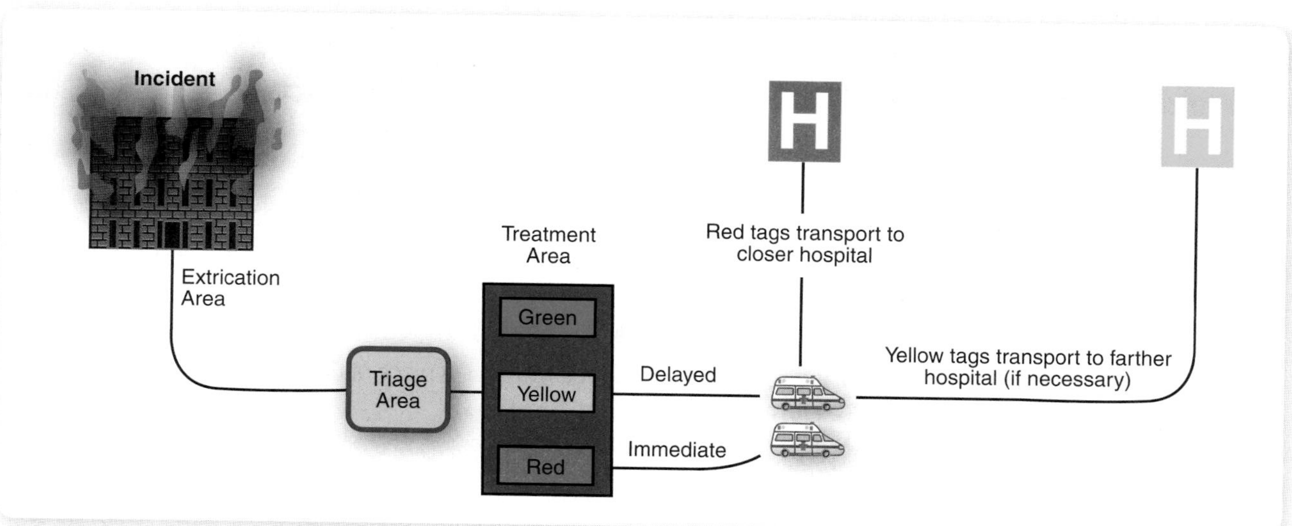

Figure 41-8 Diagram of a mass-casualty incident. The incident command system established at the scene of a building fire may look similar to this diagram.

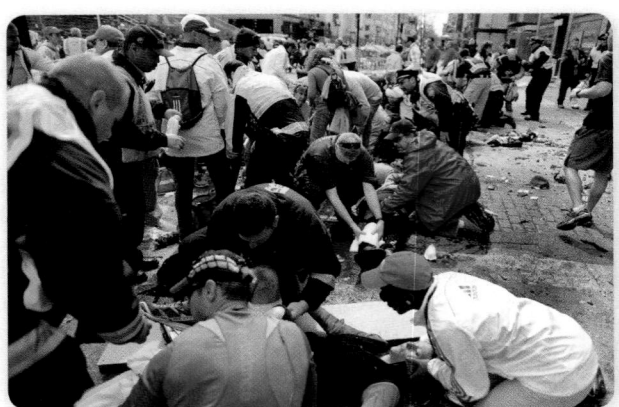

Figure 41-9 Mass-casualty incidents require additional ambulances and EMS providers from the immediate region.

abandonment. If multiple patients are present and not enough resources are available to handle them without abandoning patients, you should declare an MCI (at least for the present time), request additional resources, and initiate the ICS and triage procedures (described next) Figure 41-9. Although this process may cause some delay in initiating treatment to all patients, it will not adversely affect the patient care. Always follow your local protocol.

Triage

As discussed previously, triage is the sorting of patients based on the severity of their injuries. The goal of doing the greatest good for the greatest number means that the triage assessment is brief and the patient condition categories are basic. **Primary triage** is the initial triage done in the field, allowing you to quickly and accurately categorize the patient's condition and transport needs, whereas **secondary triage** (or re-triage) is done as patients are brought to the treatment area. During primary triage, patients are briefly assessed and then identified in some way, such as by attaching a triage tag or triage tape (discussed next). The main information needed on the tag is a unique number and a triage category. Rapid and accurate triage will help bring order to the chaos of the MCI scene and allow the most critical patients to be transported first. After the primary triage, the triage supervisor should communicate the following information to the medical branch director:

- The total number of patients
- The number of patients in each of the triage categories
- Recommendations for extrication and movement of patients to the treatment area
- Resources needed to complete triage and begin movement of patients

When the primary triage has been completed, secondary triage can occur, allowing you to reassess all remaining patients and to upgrade the triage category, if necessary. In smaller MCI events, this step may not be necessary if enough resources have arrived on the scene.

Triage Categories

The four common triage categories can be remembered using the mnemonic IDME, which stands for Immediate (red), Delayed (yellow), Minor or Minimal (green; hold), and Expectant (black; likely to die or dead) Table 41-1. IDME is the order of priority for treatment and transport of the patients at an MCI.

YOU are the Provider — PART 3

Patient No. 1 is a middle-aged woman who states she was in the lobby speaking with the receptionist when the building collapsed. She is alert and oriented, reporting a 2-inch (5-cm) laceration to her head, which appears to be venous. She keeps asking where her baby is.

Patient No. 2 is a middle-aged woman who is unresponsive but breathing adequately. You see what appears to be an abdominal evisceration.

Patient No. 3 is an older man who is screaming in pain. You note an obviously deformed left femur.

Patient No. 4 is a young adult man who has a large bruise on his right arm where a piece of the building struck him. He is able to move the arm and reports normal sensation throughout.

Patient No. 5 is a young adult man who is lying motionless on the ground. He is unresponsive and not breathing; you are unsure whether he has a pulse.

Patient No. 6 is a 7-month-old boy who is crying inconsolably. You see bruising in the abdominal area.

Patient No. 7 is a middle-aged woman who is lying motionless on the ground. You are able to hear snoring respirations at a rate of about 7 breaths/min.

5. Which triage category should be assigned to each of these patients?
6. Which patient should be transported first?

Table 41-1 Triage Priorities

Triage Category	Typical Injuries
Red tag: first priority (immediate) Patients who need immediate care and transport; treat these patients first, and transport as soon as possible.	▪ Airway and breathing compromise ▪ Uncontrolled or severe bleeding ▪ Severe medical emergencies ▪ Signs of shock (hypoperfusion) ▪ Severe burns ▪ Open chest or abdominal injuries
Yellow tag: second priority (delayed) Patients whose treatment and transport can be temporarily delayed.	▪ Burns without airway compromise ▪ Major or multiple bone or joint injuries ▪ Back injuries with or without spinal cord damage
Green tag: third priority, minimal (walking wounded) Patients who require minimal or no treatment and transport can be delayed until last.	▪ Minor fractures ▪ Minor soft-tissue injuries
Black tag: fourth priority (expectant) Patients who are already dead or have little chance for survival; treat salvageable patients before treating these patients.	▪ Obvious death ▪ Obviously nonsurvivable injury, such as major open brain trauma ▪ Respiratory arrest (if limited resources) ▪ Cardiac arrest

Immediate (red-tag) patients are your first priority. They need immediate care and transport. They usually have problems with the airway, breathing, and circulation; head trauma; or signs and symptoms of shock.

Delayed (yellow-tag) patients are the second priority and need treatment and transport, but it can be delayed. Patients usually have multiple injuries to bones or joints, including back injuries with or without spinal cord injury.

Minimal (green-tag) patients are the third priority. Patients may require no field treatment or only minimal treatment. In some parts of the world, this is the hold category. These patients are the "walking wounded" at the scene. If they have any apparent injuries, then they are usually soft-tissue injuries such as contusions, abrasions, and lacerations.

The last priority is the expectant (black-tag) patients who are dead or whose injuries are so severe that they have, at best, a minimal chance of survival. This category may include patients who are in cardiac arrest or who have an open head injury, for example. If you have limited resources, then this category may also include patients in respiratory arrest. Patients in this category receive treatment and transport only after patients in the other three categories have received care.

▶ Triage Tags

Whatever triage system is used, it is vital that a patient has a tag or some type of label. Tagging patients early assists in tracking them and can help keep an accurate record of their condition. Triage tags should be weatherproof and easily read Figure 41-10. The patient tags or tape should be color-coded and should clearly show the category of

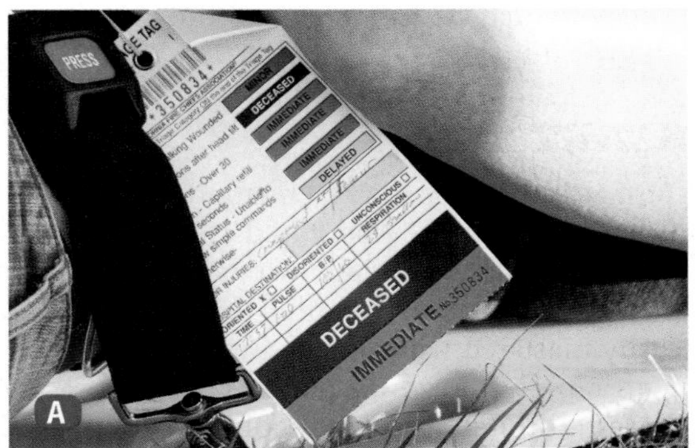

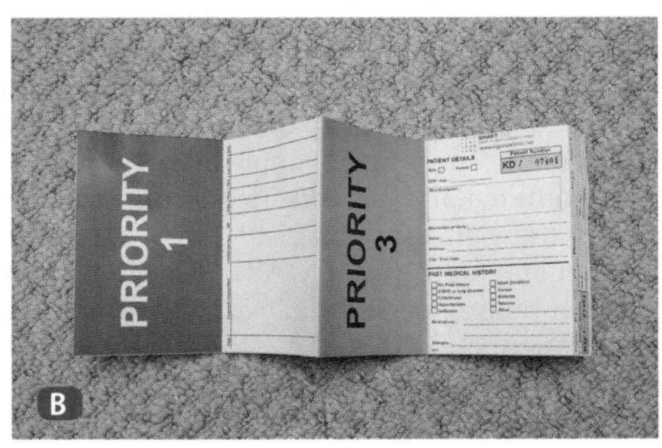

Figure 41-10 Triage tags. **A.** A START triage tag is ripped to the level of severity. **B.** A SMART triage tag folds to the level of severity.

A: © Nancy G Fire Photography/Nancy Greifenhagen/Alamy; B: Courtesy of Richard Pilbery.

the patients. The use of symbols, numbers, and colors to indicate the triage categories is important in case some responders are color-blind.

The tags will become part of the patient's medical record. Most have a tear-off receipt with a number correlating with the number on the tag. When torn off by the transportation officer, the receipt will assist him or her in tracking the patient. If the patient is unresponsive and cannot be identified at the scene, then the tag will be an identifier for tracking purposes. Some areas use digital photography to assist in identifying patients later. The photograph is catalogued with the patient's tag number, and the patient's location is tracked with this information. When family members are brought to crisis centers to help locate loved ones, the photographs may be of assistance. This technique has been used effectively in Europe and Israel with Polaroid or digital photographs. Another way of tracking and accounting for patients is to issue only 20 to 25 cards or tags at a time with a scorecard to mark how patients are triaged and their priority. When the responders return for more tags, the scorecard will provide a patient count to help command and the staff to develop a plan to respond and ensure that appropriate resources are either available or summoned. Whatever labeling system is used during triage, it is imperative for the transportation officer to be able to identify which patient was transported by which unit and to which destination, and the priority of the patient's condition.

▶ START Triage

START triage is one of the easiest methods of triage. START stands for Simple Triage And Rapid Treatment. The staff members at Hoag Memorial Hospital, Newport Beach, CA, are responsible for developing this method of triage. It is easily mastered with practice and will give you the ability to rapidly categorize patients at an MCI. START triage uses a limited assessment of the patient's ability to walk, respiratory status, hemodynamic status (pulse), and neurologic status.

The first step of the START triage system is performed on arrival at the scene by calling out to patients at the incident site, "If you can hear my voice and are able to walk . . ." and then directing patients to an easily identifiable landmark. The injured people in this group are the walking wounded and are considered minimal (green) priority, or third-priority, patients.

The second step in the START process is directed toward nonwalking patients. Move to the first nonambulatory patient and assess the respiratory status. If the patient is not breathing, then open the airway by using a simple manual maneuver. A patient who still does not begin to breathe is triaged as expectant (black). If the patient begins to breathe, then tag him or her as immediate (red), place in the recovery position, and move on to the next patient.

If the patient is breathing, then make a quick estimation of the respiratory rate. A patient who is breathing faster than 30 breaths/min or slower than 10 breaths/min is triaged as an immediate priority (red). If the patient is breathing at a rate of 10 to 29 breaths/min, then move to the next step in the START process.

The next step is to assess the hemodynamic status of the patient by checking for bilateral radial pulses. An absent radial pulse implies the patient is hypotensive; tag him or her as an immediate priority. If the radial pulse is present, then proceed to the next step.

The final assessment in START triage is to assess the patient's neurologic status, which simply means to assess the patient's ability to follow simple commands, such as "Show me three fingers." This assessment establishes that the patient can understand and follow commands. A patient who is unresponsive or cannot follow simple commands is an immediate priority (red). A patient who complies with a simple command should be triaged in the delayed category (yellow).

▶ JumpSTART Triage for Pediatric Patients

Lou Romig, MD, recognized that the START triage system does not take into account the physiologic and developmental differences of pediatric patients. She developed the **JumpSTART triage** system for pediatric patients. JumpSTART is intended for use in children younger than 8 years or who appear to weigh less than 100 pounds (45 kg). As in START, the JumpSTART system begins by identifying the walking wounded. Infants or children not developed enough to walk or follow commands (including children with special needs) should be taken to the treatment area as soon as possible for secondary triage. This action assists in getting children who cannot take care of their own basic needs into the hands of a health care provider. There are several differences within the respiratory status assessment compared with that in START. First, if you find that a pediatric patient is not breathing, then immediately check the pulse. If the patient has no pulse, then label the patient as expectant (black). If the patient is not breathing but has a pulse, then open the airway with a manual maneuver. If the patient does not begin to breathe, then give five rescue breaths and check respirations again. A child who does not begin to breathe should be labeled as expectant. The primary reason for this difference is that the most common cause of cardiac arrest in children is respiratory arrest.

The next step of the JumpSTART process is to assess the approximate rate of respirations. A patient who is breathing fewer than 15 breaths/min or more than 45 breaths/min is tagged as an immediate priority (red), and then you move on to the next patient. If the respirations are within the range of 15 to 45 breaths/min, then assess the patient further.

Just like in START, the next assessment in JumpSTART triage is also the hemodynamic status of the patient. You are simply checking for a distal pulse. This pulse does not need to be the brachial pulse; assess the pulse that you feel the most competent and comfortable checking. If you note an absence of a distal pulse, then label the child as an immediate priority (red) and move to the next patient. If the child has a distal pulse, then move on to the next assessment.

Words of Wisdom

Another triage method is the Sort, Assess, Lifesaving interventions, and Treatment and/or Transport (SALT) triage system. This triage system begins with a global sorting of patients. This method identifies the patients who are able to understand verbal instructions and are therefore likely to have good systemic perfusion. Patients who can walk are asked to move to a designated area and are assigned as last priority.[6] This is an attempt to decrease the number of patients leaving the scene and overwhelming local hospital resources before EMS can begin to move the highest priority patients. After those patients have been identified and moved, each remaining patient is assessed individually and life-saving interventions are performed.

The SALT triage method differs from other triage methods in its life-saving intervention steps, which include bleeding control, opening the airway, two rescue breaths for children, needle decompression for tension pneumothorax, and auto-injector antidotes. These interventions may be all that is needed to upgrade the patient's condition on the SALT triage scale. The final step is treatment and/or transport.

The final assessment is for neurologic status. Because of the developmental differences in children, their responses will vary. For JumpSTART, a modified AVPU scale (Awake and alert, responsive to Verbal stimuli, responsive to Pain, Unresponsive) is used. A child who is unresponsive, responds to pain by posturing or with incomprehensible sounds, or is unable to localize pain is tagged as an immediate priority (red). A child who responds to pain by localizing it or withdrawing from it or is alert is considered a delayed-priority patient (yellow).

▶ Special Considerations in Triage

A few special situations can occur in triage. Patients who are hysterical and disruptive to rescue efforts may need to be handled as an immediate priority (red) and transported out of the MCI or disaster site, even if they are not seriously injured. Panic breeds panic, and this type of behavior could have a detrimental impact on other patients and on the responders.

A responder who becomes sick or injured during the rescue effort should be handled as an immediate priority (red) and be transported off the site as soon as possible to avoid negative impact to the morale of remaining responders.

Hazmat and weapons of mass destruction incidents force the hazmat team to identify patients as either contaminated or decontaminated before the regular triage process. Contamination by chemicals or biologic weapons in a treatment area, a hospital, or trauma center could obstruct all systems and organizations coping with the MCI or disaster. Bear in mind that some incidents may require multiple triage areas or teams because the patients are located far apart.

▶ Destination Decisions

All patients triaged as immediate (red) or delayed (yellow) should preferably be transported by either ground ambulance or air ambulance, if available, to the most appropriate facility. In extremely large situations, a bus may transport the walking wounded. If a bus is used to transport minimal-priority patients, then it is strongly suggested that they be transported to a hospital or clinic distant from the MCI or disaster site to avoid overwhelming the local area hospital resources. Refer to the Centers for Disease Control and Prevention 2011 decision scheme for field triage of injured patients presented in Chapter 26, *Trauma Overview*. If a bus is used, plan for at least one responder to ride on the bus and to have an ambulance follow the bus. If the condition of a minimal-priority patient worsens, then the patient could be moved to the ambulance and transported to a closer facility. The responder can stay with the minimal-priority patients until their arrival at the designated hospital. Any worsening of a patient's condition must be relayed to the receiving hospital as soon as possible in whatever manner the incident dictates.

Immediate-priority patients should be transported two at a time until all are transported from the site. Then patients in the delayed category can be transported two or three at a time until all are at a hospital. Finally, the walking wounded are transported. Expectant patients who are still alive would receive treatment and transport at this time. Dead patients are handled or transported according to the standing operating procedure for the area.

It is important to remember that during an MCI or disaster, local hospitals may have their resources overwhelmed. Early notification to receiving facilities will allow for the hospitals to increase staffing and move patients within their facility as required. Typically, EMS agencies will know the surge capacity of a hospital, which will tell the agency how many patients of each category the hospital is able to safely handle and care for.

Words of Wisdom

Urban Search and Rescue teams (USARs) and Disaster Medical Assistance Teams (DMATs) may be mobilized in the event of a natural disaster or mass-casualty incident. USARs typically provide rescue and initial medical stabilization to patients entrapped in confined spaces, such as from a structural collapse. DMATs provide medical care during an incident; they include providers such as physicians, paramedics, nurses, AEMTs, and EMTs who work at a federal level. DMATs arrive with sufficient supplies and equipment to provide care for at least 72 hours or until further aid arrives or the situation is resolved.

Disaster Management

A disaster is a widespread event that disrupts functions and resources of a community and threatens lives and property. Many disasters may not involve personal injuries, such as droughts causing widespread crop damage. On the other hand, many disasters such as floods, fires, and hurricanes will result in widespread injuries. Unlike an MCI, which generally lasts no longer than a few hours, emergency responders will generally be on the scene of a disaster for days to weeks and sometimes months (as in the events in New Orleans, Louisiana following Hurricane Katrina in 2005) Figure 41-11. Although you can "declare" an MCI as an AEMT, only an elected official can formally declare a disaster.

As an AEMT, your role in a disaster is to respond when requested and to report to the IC for assigned tasks. In a disaster with an overwhelming number of casualties,

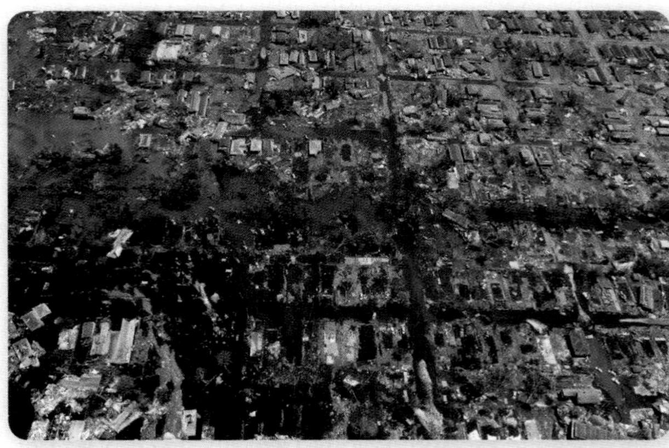

Figure 41-11 Hurricane Katrina flooded nearly 80% of New Orleans, Louisiana.[7]

YOU are the Provider — PART 4

As soon as you have finished triaging the patients that had been brought to your triage area, additional ambulance personnel arrive to assist you in treatment. You advise the IC of your triage findings and he advises you to assume the role of transportation officer, while the other crews are beginning their treatment. Knowing that your area hospitals have a trauma treatment plan for mass-casualty situations, you contact the three local hospitals to ascertain the number of critical patients they can accept. Each hospital states that they can accept two "reds" and one "yellow." You direct the first ambulance to transport one "red" and one "yellow" patient, the second ambulance to transport one "red" and one "green" patient, and the third ambulance to transport one "red" patient and the remaining "green" patients. The incident commander advises you that all the patients have been accounted for, and that you will not be receiving any additional patients. You acknowledge the information and proceed to the expectant patient.

Recording Time: 34 Minutes	
Respirations	Absent
Pulse	Absent
Skin	Cool, pale, and clammy
Blood pressure	Unobtainable
Oxygen saturation (Spo_2)	Unobtainable
Pupils	Fixed and dilated

7. What factors should you consider when determining the appropriate transport destination?
8. Should you re-triage the expectant patient at this point?

area hospitals may decide that they cannot treat all patients at their facilities. In this case, they may mobilize medical and nursing teams with equipment and set up a **casualty collection area** at a facility near the scene, such as a warehouse. Once at the casualty collection area, the teams can perform triage, provide emergency medical care, and transport patients to the hospital on a priority basis.

If a casualty collection area is established, then it will be coordinated through the ICS in the same way as all other branches and areas of the operation. This step is usually done only in a major disaster such as an earthquake, when transportation to a hospital facility is either impossible or involves prolonged delays. It may take several hours to establish a casualty collection area.

Words of Wisdom

Mass-casualty incidents and disasters take a physical and emotional toll on emergency responders. Make certain that you are medically evaluated if you have been injured, come into contact with any hazardous substance, or inhale any dust, fumes, or smoke. Often the health effects of such exposures do not manifest for years and are difficult to link back to a particular event. Also be aware of the signs of stress in yourself and in your coworkers. Consider taking advantage of CISM or CISD opportunities after an incident.

YOU are the Provider SUMMARY

1. What is the NIMS?

Although most incidents are handled at the local level, the president of the United States directed the Secretary of Homeland Security to implement the National Incident Management System (NIMS) in March 2004. Major incidents require the involvement and coordination of multiple jurisdictions, functional agencies, and emergency response disciplines. The NIMS provides a consistent nationwide template to enable federal, state, and local governments, as well as private-sector and nongovernmental organizations, to work together effectively and efficiently. Two important underlying principles of the NIMS are flexibility and standardization. The organizational structure must be flexible enough to be rapidly adapted for use in any situation. The NIMS provides standardization in terminology, resource classification, personnel training, certification, and more. Another important feature of the NIMS is the concept of interoperability, which refers to the ability of agencies of different types or from different jurisdictions to communicate with each other.

2. Why is NIMS helpful to all emergency responders?

Even on calls involving a single patient and no need for additional support, the implementation of NIMS is helpful to identify the roles and responsibilities of each crew member, particularly if the incident escalates. The structure of NIMS enables a single authority to have overall responsibility to manage the incident.

3. What is the function of the staging supervisor?

The staging supervisor locates an area to stage equipment and responders, tracks unit arrivals, and releases vehicles and supplies when ordered by incident command. This person plans for efficient access to and exit from the disaster site and prevents traffic congestion among responding vehicles.

4. What is the function of the triage supervisor?

The primary duty of the triage supervisor is to ensure that every patient receives a preliminary assessment of his or her condition. Advanced emergency medical technicians who perform triage will help move patients to the appropriate treatment sector. One of the most difficult aspects of being a triage supervisor is that you must not begin treatment until all patients are triaged, or you will compromise your triage efforts.

5. Which triage category should be assigned to each of these patients?

Patient No. 1 should be triaged as "green" or minimal because she is alert and oriented, with a venous laceration to her head, which does not appear to be life threatening.

Patient No. 2 should be triaged as "red" or immediate. This patient requires immediate treatment and transport because of her open abdominal injury and unresponsiveness.

Patient No. 3 should be triaged as "yellow" or delayed because of his obvious femur fracture. This patient requires treatment and transportation; however, it can be delayed for a short period until the immediate patients are treated.

Patient No. 4 should be triaged as "green" or minimal based on his minor injuries. This patient requires minimal or no treatment and transport can be delayed until last.

Patient No. 5 should be triaged as "black" or expectant. This patient is already dead or has little chance of survival.

Patient No. 6 should be triaged as "red" or immediate. On the basis of the JumpSTART triage system for pediatric patients, the patient is automatically placed into the immediate category because he is unable to walk or follow commands.

Patient No. 7 should be triaged as "red" or immediate. This patient requires immediate treatment and transport due to her unresponsiveness and airway and breathing difficulties.

YOU are the Provider SUMMARY (continued)

6. Which patient should be transported first?

All "red" or immediate patients should be transported prior to any of the other patients. However, with limited resources, it may be appropriate to transport multiple patients in the same ambulance. If you are transporting multiple patients, then you should only transport one "red" patient at a time, accompanied by either a "yellow" or "green" patient, so the provider in the back of the ambulance is not overwhelmed.

7. What factors should you consider when determining the appropriate transport destination?

During a mass-casualty incident (MCI), remember that the resources of local hospitals may be overwhelmed as well. The staff must now prepare for a potentially large number of MCI patients in addition to the patients they are currently treating.

As soon as you declare an MCI, notify local hospitals, apprise them of the situation, and determine their surge capacity; this information will tell you how many patients of each category they are able to safely and effectively care for. It will also allow for the hospitals to increase their staffing and, if needed, move patients within their facility.

8. Should you re-triage the expectant patient at this point?

As soon as all patients have been triaged, and as resources allow, the patients should undergo a continual re-triage to determine if their category needs to be upgraded or if a patient has died.

Patient No. 1

Triage Tag
No. 8732251

(Move the Walking Wounded) [circled]	MINIMAL
No respirations after head tilt	EXPECTANT
☐ Respirations–over 30 or less than 10	IMMEDIATE
☐ Perfusion–capillary refill over 2 seconds	IMMEDIATE
☐ Mental status–unable to follow simple commands	IMMEDIATE
Otherwise	DELAYED

MAJOR INJURIES: None
HOSPITAL DESTINATION: South Jones
(ORIENTED) ×☒4 DISORIENTED ☐ UNRESPONSIVE ☐

TIME	PULSE	B/P	RESPIRATION
N/A	N/A	N/A	N/A
N/A	N/A	N/A	N/A

PERSONAL INFORMATION:
NAME: SUSAN THOMPSON
MALE ☐ FEMALE ☒ AGE: 43 WEIGHT: 125 lb
MEDICAL COMPLAINTS/HISTORY
2-inch (5 cm) laceration to forehead. No medical history.

EXPECTANT No 8732251
IMMEDIATE No 8732251
DELAYED No 8732251
MINIMAL No 8732251

Patient No. 2

Triage Tag
No. 8732252

Move the Walking Wounded	MINIMAL
No respirations after head tilt	EXPECTANT
☐ Respirations–over 30 or less than 10	IMMEDIATE
☐ Perfusion–capillary refill over 2 seconds	IMMEDIATE
☒ Mental status–unable to follow simple commands	IMMEDIATE
Otherwise	DELAYED

MAJOR INJURIES: Abdominal evisceration
HOSPITAL DESTINATION: South Jones
ORIENTED ×☐ DISORIENTED ☐ UNRESPONSIVE ☒

TIME	PULSE	B/P	RESPIRATION
N/A	N/A	N/A	N/A
N/A	N/A	N/A	N/A

PERSONAL INFORMATION:
NAME: Not available
MALE ☐ FEMALE ☒ AGE: Mids 30s WEIGHT: Est. 147 lb (67 kg)
MEDICAL COMPLAINTS/HISTORY
Unresponsive, abdominal evisceration

EXPECTANT No 8732252
IMMEDIATE No 8732252

Note: In this style of triage tag, colored rows are torn off at perforations so the bottom-most color remaining on the tag designates the patient's category.

YOU are the Provider SUMMARY (continued)

Patient No. 3

Triage Tag
No. 8732253

Move the Walking Wounded	MINIMAL
No respirations after head tilt	EXPECTANT
☐ Respirations–over 30 or less than 10	IMMEDIATE
☐ Perfusion–capillary refill over 2 seconds	IMMEDIATE
☐ Mental status–unable to follow simple commands	IMMEDIATE
(Otherwise)	DELAYED

MAJOR INJURIES: Femur fracture
HOSPITAL DESTINATION: University
(ORIENTED) × 4 DISORIENTED ☐ UNRESPONSIVE ☐

TIME	PULSE	B/P	RESPIRATION
N/A	N/A	N/A	N/A
N/A	N/A	N/A	N/A

PERSONAL INFORMATION:
NAME: Gary Helland
MALE ☒ FEMALE ☐ AGE: 83 WEIGHT: 228 lb (103 kg)
MEDICAL COMPLAINTS/HISTORY
Severe pain, left femur deformity

EXPECTANT No 8732253
IMMEDIATE No 8732253
DELAYED No 8732253

Patient No. 4

Triage Tag
No. 8732254

(Move the Walking Wounded)	MINIMAL
No respirations after head tilt	EXPECTANT
☐ Respirations–over 30 or less than 10	IMMEDIATE
☐ Perfusion–capillary refill over 2 seconds	IMMEDIATE
☐ Mental status–unable to follow simple commands	IMMEDIATE
Otherwise	DELAYED

MAJOR INJURIES: None
HOSPITAL DESTINATION: University
(ORIENTED) × 4 DISORIENTED ☐ UNRESPONSIVE ☐

TIME	PULSE	B/P	RESPIRATION
N/A	N/A	N/A	N/A
N/A	N/A	N/A	N/A

PERSONAL INFORMATION:
NAME: Larry Pryzbyla
MALE ☒ FEMALE ☐ AGE: 27 WEIGHT: 180 lb (82 kg)
MEDICAL COMPLAINTS/HISTORY
Large bruise to right arm

EXPECTANT No 8732254
IMMEDIATE No 8732254
DELAYED No 8732254
MINIMAL No 8732254

YOU are the Provider SUMMARY *(continued)*

Patient No. 5

Triage Tag
No. 8732255

Move the Walking Wounded	MINIMAL
(No respirations after head tilt)	EXPECTANT
☐ Respirations–over 30 or less than 10	IMMEDIATE
☐ Perfusion–capillary refill over 2 seconds	IMMEDIATE
☐ Mental status–unable to follow simple commands	IMMEDIATE
Otherwise	DELAYED

MAJOR INJURIES: Cardiac arrest
HOSPITAL DESTINATION: No transport
ORIENTED ×☐ DISORIENTED ☐ UNRESPONSIVE ☒

TIME	PULSE	B/P	RESPIRATION
N/A	N/A	N/A	N/A
N/A	N/A	N/A	N/A

PERSONAL INFORMATION:
NAME: Not available
MALE ☒ FEMALE ☐ AGE: Mid 20s WEIGHT: Est. 150 lb (68 kg)
MEDICAL COMPLAINTS/HISTORY
Pulseless and apneic

EXPECTANT No 8732255

Patient No. 6

Triage Tag
No. 8732256

Move the Walking Wounded	MINIMAL
No respirations after head tilt	EXPECTANT
☐ Respirations–over 30 or less than 10	IMMEDIATE
☐ Perfusion–capillary refill over 2 seconds	IMMEDIATE
☒ Mental status–unable to follow simple commands	IMMEDIATE
Otherwise	DELAYED

MAJOR INJURIES: None
HOSPITAL DESTINATION: Baptist
(ORIENTED) ×4 DISORIENTED ☐ UNRESPONSIVE ☐

TIME	PULSE	B/P	RESPIRATION
N/A	N/A	N/A	N/A
N/A	N/A	N/A	N/A

PERSONAL INFORMATION:
NAME: John Thompson
MALE ☒ FEMALE ☐ AGE: 7 mo WEIGHT: 17 lb (8 kg)
MEDICAL COMPLAINTS/HISTORY
Inconsolable

EXPECTANT No 8732256

IMMEDIATE No 8732256

YOU are the Provider SUMMARY *(continued)*

Patient No. 7

Triage Tag
No. 8732257

Move the Walking Wounded	MINIMAL
No respirations after head tilt	EXPECTANT
☐ Respirations–over 30 or less than 10	IMMEDIATE
☐ Perfusion–capillary refill over 2 seconds	IMMEDIATE
☒ Mental status–unable to follow simple commands	IMMEDIATE
Otherwise	DELAYED

MAJOR INJURIES: Unresponsive
HOSPITAL DESTINATION: Baptist
ORIENTED ☐ DISORIENTED ☐ UNRESPONSIVE ☒

TIME	PULSE	B/P	RESPIRATION
N/A	N/A	N/A	N/A
N/A	N/A	N/A	N/A

PERSONAL INFORMATION:
NAME: Not available
MALE ☐ FEMALE ☒ AGE: Mid 40s WEIGHT: Est. 95 lb (43 kg)
MEDICAL COMPLAINTS/HISTORY
Unresponsive

EXPECTANT No 8732257

IMMEDIATE No 8732257

Prep Kit

▶ Ready for Review

- The National Incident Management System (NIMS) provides a consistent nationwide template to enable federal, state, and local governments, as well as private-sector and nongovernmental organizations, to work together effectively and efficiently. The NIMS is used to prepare for, prevent, respond to, and recover from domestic incidents, regardless of cause, size, or complexity, including acts of catastrophic terrorism and hazardous materials incidents.
- The five major NIMS components are preparedness, communications and information management, resource management, command and management, and ongoing management and maintenance.
- The purpose of the incident command system is to enhance command, control, and communications abilities, ensure responder and public safety, achieve incident management goals, ensure the efficient use of resources, and treat patients.

Prep Kit (continued)

- Preparedness involves the decisions made and basic planning done before an incident occurs.
- Your agency should have written disaster plans that you are regularly trained to carry out.
- At incidents that have a significant medical factor, the incident commander should appoint someone as the medical branch director. This person will supervise the primary roles of the medical group: triage, treatment, and transport of the injured.
- A mass-casualty incident refers to any call that could overwhelm available resources, or which could require a mutual aid response.
- The goal of triage is to do the greatest good for the greatest number. This means that the triage assessment is brief and the patient condition categories are basic.
- The four basic triage categories can be recalled using the mnemonic IDME:
  - Immediate (red)
  - Delayed (yellow)
  - Minor or Minimal (green; hold)
  - Expectant (black; likely to die or dead)
- A disaster is a widespread event that disrupts functions and resources of a community and threatens lives and property.
- Many disasters, such as a drought that causes widespread crop damage, may not involve personal injuries.

▶ Vital Vocabulary

casualty collection area An area set up by physicians, nurses, and other hospital staff near a major disaster or mass-casualty incident scene where patients can receive further triage and medical care.

closed incident An incident that is contained; all casualties are accounted for.

command In incident command, the position(s) that oversees the incident, establishes the objectives and priorities, and develops a response plan; functions may include a public information officer, safety officer, and liaison officer.

command post The designated field command center where the incident commander and support staff are located.

demobilization The process of directing responders to return to their facilities when their work at an incident has finished.

disaster A widespread event that disrupts community resources and functions, in turn threatening public safety, citizens' lives, and property.

extrication supervisor In incident command, the person appointed to determine the type of equipment and resources needed for a situation involving extrication or special rescue; also called the rescue supervisor.

finance and administration In incident command, the section responsible for accounting of all expenditures.

freelancing When individual units or different organizations make independent and often inefficient decisions about the next appropriate action.

incident action plan An oral or written plan stating general objectives reflecting the overall strategy for managing an incident.

incident commander (IC) The overall leader of the incident command system to whom commanders or leaders of incident command system divisions report.

incident command system (ICS) An on-scene emergency management model specifically designed to provide for an integrated organizational structure that reflects the complexity and demands of an incident. (Some agencies refer to the incident command system as the incident management system.)

joint information center (JIC) An area designated by the incident commander, or a designee, in which public information officers from multiple agencies distribute information about the incident.

JumpSTART triage A sorting system for pediatric patients younger than 8 years or weighing less than 100 pounds (45 kg); the system is modified for infants because they cannot ambulate on their own.

liaison officer In incident command, the person who relays information and concerns among command, the general staff, and other agencies.

logistics In incident command, the section that procures and stockpiles equipment and supplies during an incident.

mass-casualty incident (MCI) An emergency situation that can place great demand on the equipment or personnel of the EMS system or has the potential to overwhelm available resources.

medical incident command In incident command, the position responsible for the triage, treatment, and transport of injured people; also known as the medical or emergency medical services branch of the incident command system.

morgue supervisor In incident command, the person who works with area medical examiners, coroners, and law enforcement agencies to coordinate the disposition of dead patients.

Prep Kit *(continued)*

multiple-casualty incident Any situation with more than one patient, but which will not overwhelm available resources.

mutual aid response An agreement between neighboring emergency medical services systems to respond to mass-casualty incidents or disasters in each other's region when local resources are insufficient to handle the response.

National Incident Management System (NIMS) A Department of Homeland Security system designed to enable federal, state, and local governments, private-sector and nongovernmental organizations, and all other organizations who assume a role in emergency management to effectively and efficiently prepare for, prevent, respond to, and recover from domestic incidents, regardless of cause, size, or complexity, including acts of catastrophic terrorism and hazardous materials incidents.

open incident An incident that is not yet contained; there may be patients who have yet to be located and the situation may be ongoing, producing more patients.

operations In incident command, the section that carries out the orders of the incident commander to help resolve the incident.

planning In incident command, the section that ultimately produces a plan to resolve any incident.

primary triage A type of patient sorting used to rapidly categorize patients; the focus is on speed in locating all patients and determining an initial priority as their conditions warrant.

public information officer (PIO) In incident command, the person who keeps the public informed and relays information to the press.

rehabilitation area The area that provides protection and treatment to all personnel working at an emergency; here, workers are medically monitored and receive any needed care as they enter and leave the scene.

rehabilitation supervisor In incident command, the person who establishes an area that provides protection for responders from the elements and the situation.

rescue supervisor In incident command, the person appointed to determine the type of equipment and resources needed for a situation involving extrication or special rescue; also called the extrication supervisor.

safety officer In incident command, the person who monitors the scene for conditions or operations that may present a hazard to responders and patients; he or she may stop an operation when responder safety is an issue.

secondary triage A type of patient sorting used in the treatment area that involves re-triage of patients.

single command system A command system in which one person is in charge, generally used with small incidents that involve only one responding agency or one jurisdiction.

span of control In incident command, the subordinate positions under the commander's direction to which the workload is distributed; the ideal supervisor/worker ratio is one supervisor for three to seven workers.

staging supervisor In incident command, the person who locates an area to stage equipment and personnel and tracks unit arrival and deployment from the staging area.

START triage A patient sorting process that stands for Simple Triage And Rapid Treatment and uses a limited assessment of the patient's ability to walk, respiratory status, hemodynamic status, and neurologic status.

termination of command The end of the incident command structure when an incident draws to a close and the command structure is no longer necessary.

transportation area The area in a mass-casualty incident where ambulances and crews are organized to transport patients from the treatment area to receiving hospitals.

transportation supervisor In incident command, the person in charge of the transportation sector in a mass-casualty incident who assigns patients from the treatment area to awaiting ambulances in the transportation area.

treatment area The location in a mass-casualty incident where patients are brought after being triaged and assigned a priority, where they are reassessed, treated, and monitored until transport to the hospital.

treatment supervisor In incident command, the person, usually a physician, who is in charge of and directs emergency medical services providers at the treatment area in a mass-casualty incident.

triage The process of sorting patients based on the severity of injury and medical need to establish treatment and transportation priorities.

triage supervisor In incident command, the person in charge of the incident command triage sector who directs the sorting of patients into triage categories in a mass-casualty incident.

Prep Kit (continued)

unified command system A command system used in larger incidents in which there is a multiagency response or multiple jurisdictions are involved.

► References

1. National Incident Management Systems (NIMS). United States Department of Homeland Security website. Federal Emergency Management Agency. https://training.fema.gov/nims/. Accessed August 24, 2016.
2. National Incident Management System (NIMS) fact sheet. Federal Emergency Management Agency website. http://www.fema.gov/pdf/emergency/nims/NIMSFactSheet.pdf. Accessed August 17, 2016.
3. NIMS and the incident command system. Federal Emergency Management Agency website. http://www.fema.gov/txt/nims/nims_ics_position_paper.txt. Accessed August 24, 2016.
4. Incident command system review material. Federal Emergency Management Agency website. http://training.fema.gov/emiweb/is/icsresource/assets/reviewmaterials.pdf. Accessed November 15, 2016.
5. Operational templates and guidance for EMS mass incident deployment. Federal Emergency Management Agency website. United States Fire Administration; June 2012. https://www.usfa.fema.gov/downloads/pdf/publications/templates_guidance_ems_mass_incident_deployment.pdf. Accessed August 24, 2016.
6. SALT mass casualty triage algorithm. United States Department of Health and Human Services website. Chemical Hazards Emergency Medical Management. https://chemm.nlm.nih.gov/salttriage.htm. Accessed August 24, 2016.
7. Plyer, Allison. The Data Center. *Facts for Features: Katrina Impact.* http://www.datacenterresearch.org/data-resources/katrina/facts-for-impact/. Accessed November 15, 2016.

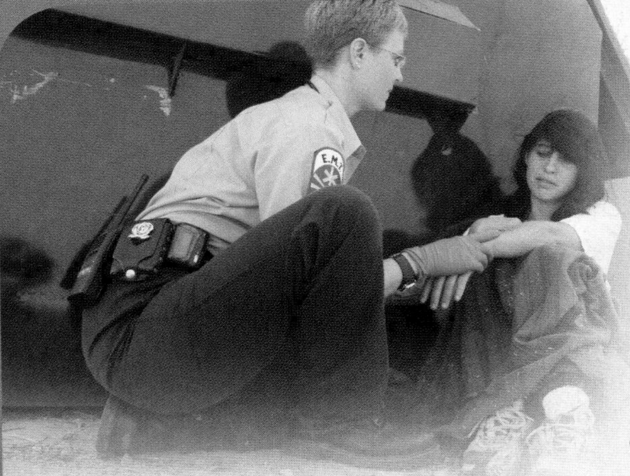

Assessment in Action

Your ambulance is dispatched to a local stadium for an explosion during a football game. The primary device was located on the side of the home team underneath the bleachers. Dispatch advises that over 500 tickets were sold for the game. Both law enforcement and the local fire department have been dispatched.

1. Communications is often an issue during a mass-casualty incident (MCI) or disaster. All of the following statements are correct, EXCEPT:

A. If possible, use face-to-face communication to limit radio traffic.
B. Some organizations responding to a disaster might not know how to use a radio.
C. If you communicate via radio, then use 10-codes or signals.
D. Be sure backups are in place if the primary communications system does not work.

2. Because of the size of this incident, local resources are insufficient to handle the response. Your service should have _______________ agreements with neighboring organizations to respond.

A. mutual aid response
B. emergency assistance
C. MCI
D. disaster

Assessment *in Action* *(continued)*

3. Because this incident may require search and rescue or the extrication of patients, a ____________ may need to be appointed.

A. staging supervisor
B. treatment supervisor
C. triage supervisor
D. rescue supervisor

4. The ____________ will work with area medical examiners, coroners, disaster mortuary assistance teams, and law enforcement agencies to coordinate removal of the bodies and even, possibly, body parts.

A. extrication supervisor
B. morgue supervisor
C. rescue supervisor
D. transportation supervisor

5. The public information officer:

A. relays information and concerns among command, the general staff, and other agencies.
B. provides the public and media with clear and understandable information.
C. monitors the scene for conditions or operations that may present a hazard to responders or patients.
D. is the person in charge of the overall incident.

6. A key role of the ________________ is to communicate with the area hospitals to determine where to transport the patients.

A. staging supervisor
B. rehabilitation supervisor
C. transportation supervisor
D. treatment supervisor

7. The ________________ is ultimately in charge of counting and prioritizing patients.

A. triage supervisor
B. staging supervisor
C. treatment supervisor
D. rehabilitation supervisor

8. A responder who becomes sick or injured during the rescue effort should be handled as a(n) ____________ and be transported off the site as soon as possible to avoid negative impact to the morale of remaining responders.

A. immediate priority (red)
B. delayed priority (yellow)
C. minimal priority (green)
D. expectant priority (black)

9. When you arrive first on the scene of an incident, you will make an initial assessment and some preliminary decisions. What three basic questions will drive the scene size-up?

10. Describe the four categories of triage.

CHAPTER 42

Terrorism Response and Disaster Management

National EMS Education Standard Competencies

EMS Operations

Knowledge of operational roles and responsibilities to ensure patient, public, and personnel safety.

Mass-Casualty Incidents Due to Terrorism and Disaster

- Risks and responsibilities of operating on the scene of a natural or man-made disaster. (pp 1713-1715, 1726-1727, 1730)

Knowledge Objectives

1. Describe international terrorism and domestic terrorism, and include some examples of incidents that have been caused by each one. (p 1711)
2. List examples of four different types of goals that commonly motivate terrorist groups to stage a terrorist attack. (pp 1711-1712)
3. Describe weapons of mass destruction (WMDs), and include examples of the five categories of weapons that are considered WMDs. (pp 1712-1713)
4. Describe how the National Terrorism Advisory System relates to your daily activities as an advanced emergency medical technician (AEMT) and your ability to respond to and survive a terrorist attack. (pp 1713-1714)
5. Describe key observations you must make on each call to assist in the determination of whether an incident is related to terrorism. (p 1714)
6. Describe the critical response actions you must perform at a suspected terrorist event related to establishing and reassessing scene safety, personnel protection, notification procedures, and establishing command. (pp 1714-1715)
7. Discuss the history of chemical agents, the four main classifications, routes of exposure, effects on the patient, and patient care. (pp 1715-1721)
8. Discuss three categories of biologic agents, the routes of exposure, effects on the patient, and patient care. (pp 1721-1727)
9. Explain the role of emergency medical services in relation to syndromic surveillance and points of distribution during a biologic event. (pp 1726-1727)
10. Describe the history of nuclear/radiologic devices, sources of radiologic materials and dispersal devices, medical management of the patient, and protective measures to take during a nuclear/radiologic incident. (pp 1727-1730)
11. Describe the mechanisms of injury caused by incendiary and explosive devices, including the types and severity of blast injuries. (pp 1730-1731)

Skills Objectives

1. Demonstrate the steps you can take to establish and reassess scene safety based on a scenario of a terrorist event. (pp 1714-1715)
2. Demonstrate how to manage a patient who has been exposed to a chemical agent. (pp 1717, 1720-1721)
3. Demonstrate the use of the DuoDote Auto-Injector and/or the Antidote Treatment Nerve Agent Auto-Injector. (p 1719)

Introduction

The increase in terrorist activity in the United States makes it possible that you may be called on to respond to a terrorist event during your career. International terrorists and domestic groups have increased their targeting of civilian populations with acts of terror. Furthermore, groups and individuals with alleged ties to terrorist organizations may seek to carry out so-called copycat attacks. The question is not whether terrorists will strike again, but rather when and where they will strike. You must be mentally and physically prepared for the possibility of a terrorist event. It is imperative that all emergency medical services (EMS) providers attend specialized training sessions to learn as much as possible about not only caring for survivors of such attacks, but also how to remain safe while doing so.

The use of weapons of mass destruction (WMDs), also known as weapons of mass casualty (WMCs), further complicates the management of the terrorist incident and places you in greater danger. Although it is difficult to plan and anticipate a response to many terrorist events, several key principles apply to every response. This chapter describes types of terrorist events, personnel safety, and patient management and gives you tools to prepare to respond to these events. You will learn the signs, symptoms, and treatment of patients who have been exposed to nuclear, chemical, or biologic agents or an explosive attack. At the end of this chapter, you will be able to answer the following key questions:

- What are my initial actions?
- Whom should I notify, and what should I tell them?
- What type of additional resources do I require?
- How should I proceed to address the needs of the patients?
- How should I ensure the safety of myself, my partner, and the patients?
- What is the clinical presentation of a patient exposed to a WMD?
- How do I assess and treat a patient exposed to a WMD?
- How do I avoid becoming contaminated or cross-contaminated with a WMD agent?

What Is Terrorism?

No one is quite sure who the first terrorist was, but terrorist forces have been at work since early civilizations. Today, terrorists pose a threat to nations and cultures everywhere. International terrorism has brought a new fear into the lives of many American citizens. The US Department of Justice defines both **international terrorism** and **domestic terrorism** with these points:

- Involves violent acts or acts dangerous to human life that violate federal or state law
- Appears to be intended (i) to intimidate or coerce a civilian population; (ii) to influence the policy of a government by intimidation or coercion; or (iii) to affect the conduct of a government by mass destruction, assassination, or kidnapping

One difference between the two types of terrorism is location. International terrorism (also known as cross-border terrorism) occurs primarily outside the territorial jurisdiction of the United States, whereas domestic terrorism occurs primarily within the territorial jurisdiction of the United States.[1]

Modern-day terrorism is common in the Middle East, where terrorist groups have frequently attacked civilian populations. In Central and South America, political terrorist groups target oil resources as a means to instill fear. In the United States, domestic terrorists have struck multiple times in previous years. The mass shooting at an Orlando, Florida nightclub in 2016 and the Boston Marathon bombing in 2013 are examples **Figure 42-1**. Terrorist organizations are generally categorized based on their beliefs and goals. Only a small percentage of groups actually turn toward terrorism as a means to achieve their goals, such as the following:

1. **Violent religious/doomsday cults.** These groups are especially dangerous because they often seek apocalyptic violence or mass murder as a means to their ends. They see other religions or "nonbelievers" as worthy targets for death, and part of their apocalyptic doctrine is to eradicate or cleanse a region (or the entire earth) of those who do not practice their faith.
2. **Extremist political groups.** They may include violent separatist groups and those who seek political, religious, economic, and social freedom **Figure 42-2**.

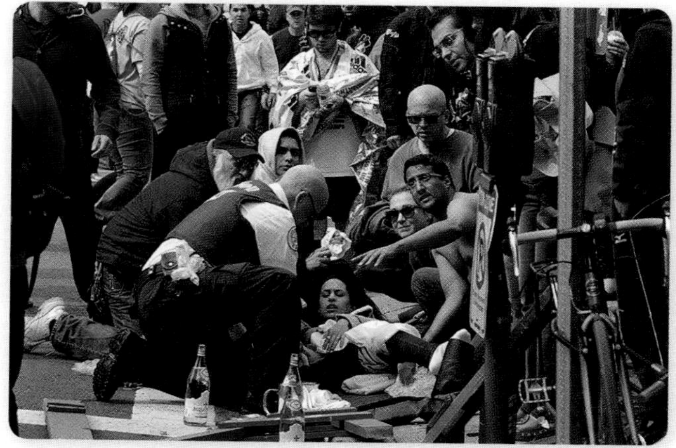

Figure 42-1 The bombings at the Boston Marathon in 2013 are a recent example of domestic terrorism.

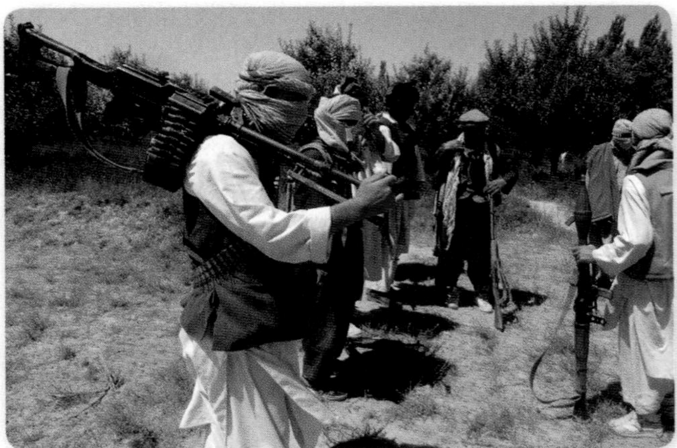

Figure 42-2 Militant groups in Afghanistan, Iraq, Syria, and Nigeria have been associated with terrorism.

3. **Cyber terrorists.** They attack a population's technological infrastructure as a means to draw attention to their cause (power grid, Internet, intranet, telecommunications).[2]
4. **Single-issue groups.** These include antiabortion groups, animal rights groups, anarchists, racists, and even ecoterrorists who threaten or use violence as a means to advance their cause.

Most terrorist attacks require the coordination of multiple terrorists or "actors" working together. For example, 19 hijackers worked together to commit the worst act of terrorism in American history on September 11, 2001 Figure 42-3. At least four terrorists worked together to commit the London Subway bombings on July 7, 2005. However, in a few instances a single terrorist has struck with devastating results. Terrorists who acted alone carried out each of the Atlanta abortion clinic attacks in 1996 and the 1996 Summer Olympics attack.

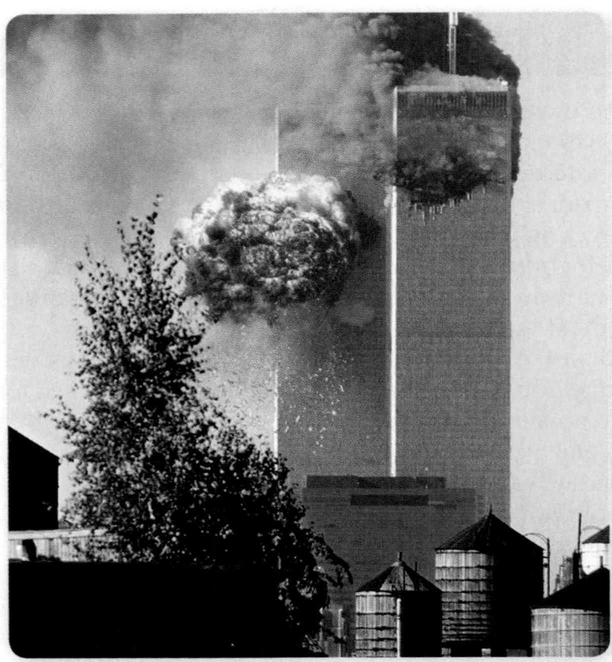

Figure 42-3 The September 11, 2001, attacks on the World Trade Center in New York City accounted for the majority of the deaths caused by terrorists in 2001.

Weapons of Mass Destruction

A **weapon of mass destruction (WMD)**, or **weapon of mass casualty (WMC)**, is any agent designed to bring about mass death, casualties, and/or massive damage to property and infrastructure (bridges, tunnels, airports, and seaports). To help remember the different kinds of WMDs, use the following two mnemonics: **B-NICE** (Biologic, Nuclear, Incendiary, Chemical, and Explosive weapons) and **CBRNE** (Chemical, Biologic, Radiologic, Nuclear, and Explosive weapons).

To date, terrorist groups have favored tactics that use explosive devices, such as truck bombs or pedestrian suicide bombers. Many previous terrorist attempts to use either chemical or biologic weapons to their full capacity have been unsuccessful. Nonetheless, as an advanced emergency medical technician (AEMT), you must understand the destructive potential of WMDs.

The motives and tactics of the new-age terrorist groups have begun to change. As with the doomsday cults, many terrorist groups participate in indiscriminate killing. This doctrine of total carnage makes the use of WMDs highly desirable. WMDs are relatively easy to obtain or create and are specifically geared toward killing large numbers of people. Had such techniques

YOU are the Provider — PART 1

Your ambulance, along with the local fire department and law enforcement, is dispatched to a suspected terrorist incident. During a ceremony to honor war veterans, a moving truck sped through the crowd and struck the wall of a building. On impact, the front of the cab exploded. The front of the truck is crumpled and smoke is coming from the engine. Several patients are visible from your unit.

1. Given the situation, what are some unique concerns about this incident?
2. Is it safe for you to enter the scene? What should be done first?

been used during the 1995 Aum Shinrikyo attack on the Tokyo subway, for example, tens of thousands of casualties may have resulted. With the fall of the former Soviet Union, the technology and expertise to produce WMDs may be available to terrorist groups with sufficient funding. Moreover, the technical instructions for making WMDs can be found readily on the Internet; in fact, they have even been published on terrorist group websites.

Words of Wisdom

Chemical warfare may consist of agents in the form of a liquid, gas, or solid.

▶ Chemical Terrorism/Warfare

Chemical agents are manufactured substances that can have devastating effects on living organisms. They can be produced in liquid, gas, or solid form depending on the desired route of exposure and dissemination technique. Developed during World War I (WWI), these agents have been implicated in thousands of deaths since being introduced on the battlefield and have been used to terrorize civilian populations. These agents consist of the following types:

- Vesicants (blister agents)
- Respiratory agents (choking agents)
- Nerve agents
- Metabolic agents (cyanides)

▶ Biologic Terrorism/Warfare

Biologic agents are organisms that cause disease. They are generally found in nature; for terrorist use, however, they are cultivated, synthesized, and mutated in a laboratory. The **weaponization** of biologic agents is performed to artificially maximize the target population's exposure to the germ, thereby exposing the greatest number of people and achieving the desired result.

The primary types of biologic agents that you may come into contact with during a biologic event include the following:

- Viruses
- Bacteria
- Toxins

▶ Radiologic/Nuclear Terrorism

Only two incidents involving the use of a nuclear device are publicly known. During World War II (WWII), the cities of Hiroshima and Nagasaki in Japan were devastated when they were targeted with nuclear bombs. The awesome destructive power demonstrated by the attack ended WWII and has since served as a deterrent to nuclear war.

Some nations hold close ties with terrorist groups (known as **state-sponsored terrorism**) and have obtained some degree of nuclear capability.

It is also possible for a terrorist to secure radioactive materials or waste to perpetrate an act of terror. Compared with a nuclear weapon, these materials are far easier for a determined terrorist to acquire and require less expertise to use. The difficulties in developing a nuclear weapon are well documented. Radioactive materials, however, can cause widespread panic and civil disturbances. This topic will be covered later in this chapter.

Words of Wisdom

When you respond to a terrorist event, the basic foundations of patient care remain the same; however, the treatment can and will vary. Terrorist events can produce a single casualty, hundreds of casualties, or even thousands of casualties. In all cases, remember situational awareness. What you may do in one situation may not be appropriate for another situation. During large-scale terrorist events, it is important to perform triage and base your patient care on available resources.

Recognizing a Terrorist Event (Indicators)

Most acts of terror are **covert**, which means that the public safety community generally has no prior knowledge of the time, location, or nature of the attack. This element of surprise makes responding to an event more complex. You must constantly be aware of your surroundings and understand the possible risks for terrorism associated with certain locations, at certain times. It is therefore important that you know the current threat level issued by the federal government through the Department of Homeland Security (DHS).

In April 2011, the color-coded Homeland Security Advisory System was replaced by the National Terrorism Advisory System (NTAS). Alerts from the NTAS contain a summary of the threat and the actions that first responders, government agencies, and the public can take to maintain safety. On the basis of threat information, take appropriate actions and precautions while continuing to perform daily duties and respond to calls. The DHS has not issued specific recommendations for EMS personnel to follow in response to the alert system. Follow your local protocols, policies, and procedures.

It is your responsibility to make sure you are aware of information sent out by the NTAS at the start of your workday. Daily newspapers, television news programs, and multiple websites (including the DHS website) all give up-to-date information. Many EMS organizations are starting to display the NTAS on boards where it can be seen by staff when they arrive for a shift.

An understanding and awareness of the current threat level is only the beginning of responding safely to calls. When you are on duty, you must be able to make appropriate decisions regarding the potential for a terrorist event. In determining the potential for a terrorist attack, make the following observations on every call:

- **Type of location.** Is the location a monument, infrastructure, government building, or a specific type of location such as a temple? Is a large gathering of people present? Is a special event taking place?
- **Type of call.** Has an explosion or suspicious device been reported nearby? Does the call come into dispatch as someone having unexplained coughing and difficulty breathing? Are there reports of people fleeing the scene?
- **Number of patients.** Are multiple patients reporting similar signs and symptoms? (This is probably the single most important clue that a terrorist attack or an incident involving a WMD has occurred.)
- **Patients' statements.** This is probably the second-best indication of a terrorist or WMD event. If the patients fleeing the scene are giving statements such as, "Everyone is passing out," "There was a loud explosion," or "There are a lot of people shaking on the ground," then something is occurring that you do not want to rush into, whether or not it is a terrorist event.
- **Preincident indicators.** Has a recent increase in violent political activism occurred? Are you aware of any credible threats made against the location, gathering, or occasion?

▶ Response Actions

Once you suspect that a terrorist event has occurred or a WMD has been used, you must take action to ensure you will be safe and be in the proper position to help the community.

Scene Safety

Ensure the scene is safe. Remember to stage your vehicle a safe distance (usually 1 to 2 blocks) from the incident, and wait for law enforcement personnel to advise you that the scene has been made secure. If you have any doubt that it may be unsafe, then do not enter. When dealing with a WMD scene, it is safe to assume that you will not be able to enter where the event has occurred—nor do you want to. The best location for staging is upwind and uphill from the incident. Wait for assistance from those who are trained in assessing and managing WMD scenes. Expect that a perimeter will be created, usually by law

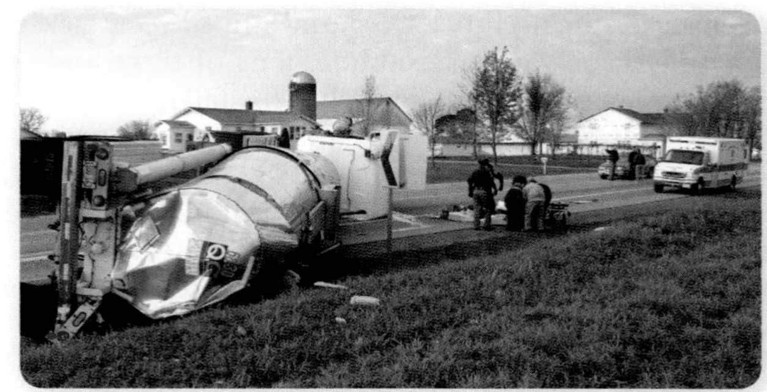

Figure 42-4 Park your vehicle at a safe location.

enforcement personnel, in an effort to isolate the scene, prevent further contamination of evidence, and protect responders and the public from further danger. Also remember the following rules:

- Failure to park your vehicle at a safe location can place you and your partner in danger **Figure 42-4**. It is important to always make an escape plan beforehand, in case the scene becomes unsafe.
- If your vehicle is blocked in by other emergency vehicles or damaged by a secondary device or event (discussed later in this chapter), then you will be unable to provide patients with transportation or escape yourself.

Responder Safety (Personnel Protection)

The best form of protection from a WMD agent is to prevent yourself from coming into contact with the agent. The greatest threats facing you in a WMD attack are contamination and **cross-contamination**. Contamination with an agent occurs when you have direct contact with the WMD or are exposed to it. Cross-contamination occurs when you come into contact with a contaminated person who has not yet been decontaminated.

Words of Wisdom

One of the easiest ways to distinguish between a nonterrorist and a terrorist mass-casualty event is whether the intentional use of a WMD affects multiple people. These patients will generally exhibit the same signs and symptoms. It is highly unlikely for more than one person to experience a seizure at any given time. It is not uncommon to find multiple patients who report difficulty breathing at the scene of a fire. However, the same report in the subway at rush hour, when no smell of smoke has been reported, is certainly cause for suspicion. In these cases, use good judgment and resist the urge to rush in and help, especially when the situation involves multiple patients and an unknown cause.

Notification Procedures

If you suspect a terrorist or WMD event has taken place, then notify the dispatcher, provided that communications function properly. Vital information needs to be communicated effectively if you are to receive the appropriate assistance (see Chapter 4, *Communications and Documentation*, for information on effective communication). Inform dispatch of the nature of the event, any additional resources that may be required, the estimated number of patients, and the upwind or optimal route of approach.

It is extremely important to establish a staging area, where other units will converge. Be mindful of access and exit routes when you direct units to respond to a location. For example, it is unwise to have units respond to the front entrance of a hotel or apartment building that has had an explosion (see information on vehicle positioning in Chapter 39, *Transport Operations*). Last, only trained responders in the proper personal protective equipment (PPE) are equipped to handle the WMD incident. These specialized units—traditionally hazardous materials (hazmat) teams—must be requested as early as possible because of the time required to assemble and dispatch the team and equipment. Many jurisdictions share hazmat teams, and the team may have to travel a long distance to reach the location of the event. It is always better to be safe than sorry; call the team early, and the outcome of the call will be more favorable.

Finally, keep in mind that more than one type of device or agent may be present (discussed next).

Words of Wisdom

On September 11, 2001, communications in New York City were severely affected by the collapse of the World Trade Center. The primary communications repeater was situated on top of one of the towers. In addition, excess radio traffic made transmitting and receiving messages extremely difficult. Not only were radio communications affected, but also most mobile phones and the majority of radio and television stations were disabled. The lesson learned from this event is to have multiple backups to ensure your ability to communicate with your dispatcher. In the event of a terrorist or WMD event, refrain from using the radio unless you have something important to transmit. If you do transmit, then gather your thoughts and speak as calmly as possible, avoiding unnecessary chatter. Remember that others may be unable to call for help while you are transmitting.

Establishing Command

The first provider to arrive on the scene must begin to sort out the chaos and define his or her responsibilities under the incident command system (ICS). As the first person on scene, you may need to establish command until additional personnel arrive. Depending on the circumstances and stage of the operation, you and other AEMTs may function as medical branch directors, triage supervisors, treatment supervisors, transportation supervisors, logistic officers, or command and general staff. If the initial ICS is already in place, then immediately seek out the medical staging officer to receive your assignment. Chapter 41, *Incident Management*, discusses how to work within the ICS and the National Incident Management System.

Reassessing Scene Safety

Terrorists have been known to plant additional explosives that are set to explode after the initial bomb. This type of **secondary device** is intended primarily to injure responders and to secure media coverage because the media generally arrive on scene just after the initial response. Secondary devices may include various types of electronic equipment, such as a mobile phone that is designed to detonate when a call is answered. Do not rely on others to secure your safety. It is your responsibility to constantly assess and reassess the scene for safety. It is easy to overlook a suspicious package lying on the floor while you are treating casualties. Stay alert. Something as subtle as a change in the wind direction during a gas attack or an increase in the number of contaminated patients can place you in danger. Never become so involved with the tasks you are performing that you do not look around and make sure that the scene remains safe.

Words of Wisdom

If you are called on to treat a suspected criminal or suspected terrorist, then it is important that this patient receive the same emergency medical care as your other patients. Although it may be difficult for you to treat the patient because of ethical or moral reasons, remember that you are not the judge or jury. It is up to the legal system to prove someone guilty in a court of law.

Chemical Agents

Modern-day chemical weapons were first developed during WWI and WWII. During the Cold War, many of these agents were perfected and stockpiled. Although the United States has long renounced the use of chemical weapons, many nations still develop and stockpile them. These agents are deadly and pose a threat if they are acquired by terrorists.

Chemical weapons have several classifications. The properties or characteristics of an agent can be described as liquid, gas, or solid material. **Persistency** and **volatility** are terms used to describe how long the agent will stay on a surface before it evaporates. Persistent or nonvolatile agents can remain on a surface for long periods, usually longer than 24 hours. Nonpersistent or volatile agents evaporate relatively fast when left on a surface in the optimal temperature range. An agent that is described as highly persistent can remain in the environment for weeks to months, whereas an agent that is highly volatile will turn from liquid to gas (evaporate) within minutes to seconds.

Route of exposure is how the chemical agent most effectively enters the body. Chemical agents can have either a vapor or contact hazard. Agents with a **vapor hazard** enter the body through the respiratory tract in the form of vapors. Agents with a **contact hazard** (or skin hazard) give off very little vapor or no vapors and enter the body through the skin.

▶ Vesicants (Blister Agents)

The primary route of exposure of blister agents, or **vesicants**, is the skin (contact); however, if vesicants are left on the skin or clothing long enough, they produce vapors that can enter the respiratory tract. Vesicants cause burn-like blisters to form on the patient's skin and in the respiratory tract. The vesicant agents consist of sulfur mustard (H), lewisite (L), and phosgene oxime (CX) (the symbols H, L, and CX are military designations for these chemicals). The vesicants usually cause the most damage to damp or moist areas of the body, such as the armpits, groin, and respiratory tract. Signs of vesicant exposure on the skin include the following:

- Skin irritation, burning, and reddening
- Immediate, intense skin pain (with L and CX)
- Formation of large blisters
- Gray discoloration of skin (a sign of permanent damage seen with L and CX)
- Swollen and closed or irritated eyes
- Permanent eye injury (including blindness)

If vapors were inhaled, then the patient may experience the following signs and symptoms:

- Hoarseness and stridor
- Severe cough
- Hemoptysis (coughing up blood)
- Severe dyspnea

Sulfur mustard (H) (commonly known as mustard gas) is a brown-yellow, oily substance that is generally considered very persistent. When released, H has the distinct smell of garlic or mustard and is quickly absorbed into the skin and/or mucous membranes. As the agent is absorbed into the skin, it begins an irreversible process of damage to the cells. Absorption through the skin or mucous membranes usually occurs within seconds, and damage to the underlying cells takes place within 1 to 2 minutes.

Mustard gas is considered a **mutagen**, which means that it mutates, damages, and changes the structures of cells. Eventually, cellular death will occur. On the surface, the patient will generally not produce any signs or symptoms until 4 to 6 hours after exposure (depending on concentration and amount of exposure) Figure 42-5.

The patient will experience a progressive reddening of the affected area, which will gradually develop into large blisters. These blisters are similar in shape and appearance to those associated with thermal second-degree burns. The fluid within the blisters does not contain any of the agent; however, the skin covering the area is considered to be contaminated until decontamination by trained personnel has been performed.

Mustard gas also attacks vulnerable cells within the bone marrow and depletes the body's ability to reproduce white blood cells. As with other burns, the primary

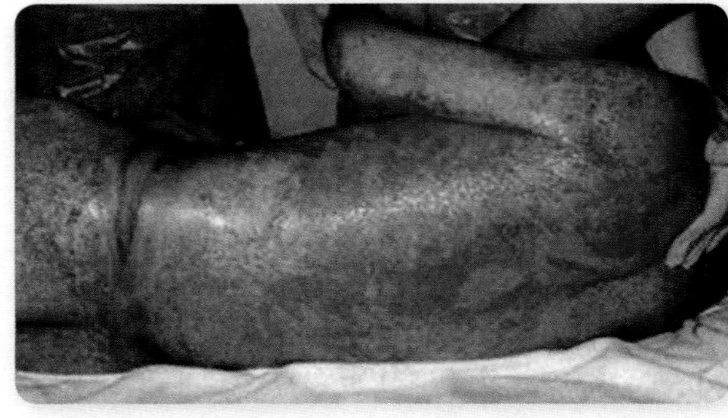

Figure 42-5 Skin damage resulting from exposure to sulfur mustard (H).

Courtesy of Dr. Saeed Keshavarz/RCCI, Research Center of Chemical Injuries/IRAN.

YOU are the Provider PART 2

When the emergency call was dispatched, you requested additional EMS units to respond to the scene. The firefighters and two deputies approach the cab of the truck to assess the potential for fire and to determine the status of the driver. The driver is slumped over the steering wheel and is wearing a vest with wires protruding from the pockets. The wires appear to be burned through and the man has obvious burns to his face and arms. The truck is stable and the firefighters determine that no threat of fire is apparent.

3. As an AEMT, what level of knowledge should you possess regarding terrorism and WMDs?
4. What is a secondary device or event?
5. Does the potential for a secondary device exist at this scene?

complication associated with vesicant blisters is secondary infection. If the patient survives the initial direct injury from the agent, then the depletion of the white blood cells leaves the patient with a decreased resistance to infections. Although sulfur mustard is regarded as persistent, it releases enough vapors when dispersed to be inhaled. This release creates upper and lower airway compromise. The result is damage and swelling of the airways. The airway compromise makes the patient's condition far more serious.

Lewisite (L) and **phosgene oxime (CX)** produce blister wounds similar to those caused by mustard gas. These agents are highly volatile and have a rapid onset of symptoms, as opposed to the delayed onset seen with mustard gas. These agents produce immediate intense pain and discomfort when contact is made. The patient's skin may have a gray discoloration at the contaminated site. Although tissue damage also occurs with exposure to L and CX, they do not cause the secondary cellular injury that is associated with mustard gas.

Vesicant Agent Treatment

No antidotes for H or CX exposure are available. British antilewisite is the antidote for agent L; however, it is not carried by civilian EMS personnel. Ensure the patient has been decontaminated before you initiate treatment. The patient may require prompt airway support if any agent has been inhaled, but this intervention should not occur until after decontamination. Gain intravenous (IV) access and initiate transport as soon as possible. Generally, burn centers are best equipped to handle the wounds and subsequent infections produced by vesicants. Follow your local protocols when deciding the transport destination.

▶ Respiratory Agents (Choking Agents)

The respiratory agents are gases that cause immediate harm to the people exposed to them. The primary route of exposure for these agents is through the respiratory tract, which makes them an inhalation or vapor hazard. Once inside the lungs, they damage the lung tissue and fluid leaks into the lungs. These agents produce respiratory-related symptoms such as dyspnea, tachypnea, and pulmonary edema because of the inability for air exchange.

Chlorine (Cl) was the first chemical agent ever used in warfare. It has a distinct odor of bleach and creates a green haze when released as a gas. Initially it produces upper airway irritation and a choking sensation. The patient may later experience the following signs and symptoms:

- Shortness of breath
- Chest tightness
- Hoarseness and stridor as a result of upper airway constriction
- Gasping and coughing

With serious exposures, patients may experience pulmonary edema, complete airway constriction, and death. The fumes from a mixture of household bleach and ammonia create an acid gas that produces similar effects to those of Cl. According to the American Association of Poison Control Centers, human exposure involving household cleaning substances was the third most frequently reported exposure in 2014.[3]

Do not confuse **phosgene** with phosgene oxime (a vesicant discussed earlier in this chapter). Not only has phosgene been produced for chemical warfare, but also it is a product of combustion. It might be produced in a fire involving other chemicals, such as at a textile factory, or as a result of metalwork or burning Freon (a liquid chemical used in refrigeration). Therefore, you may encounter a person who has been exposed to this gas during the course of a normal call or at the scene of a fire. Phosgene is a very potent agent that has a delayed onset of symptoms, usually hours. Unlike chlorine, when phosgene enters the body, it generally does not produce severe irritation that would possibly cause the patient to leave the area or hold his or her breath. In fact, the odor produced by the chemical is similar to that of freshly mowed grass or hay. As a result, a high quantity of the gas may enter the body unnoticed. Initially, a mild exposure may include the following signs and symptoms:

- Nausea
- Chest tightness
- Severe cough
- Dyspnea on exertion

The patient with a severe exposure may present with dyspnea at rest and excessive pulmonary edema. (The patient will actually expel large amounts of fluid from the pulmonary edema in the lungs.) The pulmonary edema may be so severe that the patient continually coughs up white or pink-tinged fluid. A severe exposure produces such large amounts of fluid in the lungs that the patient may develop hypovolemia and subsequently hypotension.

Respiratory Agent Treatment

The best initial treatment for any patient who has been exposed to a respiratory agent is to remove the patient from the contaminated atmosphere. This step should be done by trained personnel in the proper PPE. Aggressively manage the airway, breathing, and circulation (ABCs), paying particular attention to oxygenation, ventilation, and suctioning if required. Do not allow the patient to be active because this will worsen the condition. No antidotes to counteract the respiratory agents are available. Your primary goals for prehospital emergency medical care are to manage the ABCs, gain IV access, allow the patient to rest in a position of comfort with the head elevated, and initiate prompt transport. If the patient's condition does not improve with basic airway support, then consider requesting an advanced life support intercept. Continuous positive airway pressure may benefit some of these patients, but others will require more advanced airway management.

Nerve Agents

The **nerve agents** are among the most deadly chemicals developed. They are classified as WMDs. Nerve agents are not readily available to the general public and are extremely toxic and rapidly fatal with any route of exposure. Designed to kill large numbers of people with small quantities, nerve agents can cause cardiac arrest within seconds to minutes of exposure. Nerve agents, discovered while in search of a superior pesticide, are a class of chemical called organophosphates, which are found in household bug sprays, agricultural pesticides, and some industrial chemicals, at far lower strengths than in nerve agents. Organophosphates block an essential enzyme in the nervous system, causing the body's organs to become overstimulated and burn out.

G agents came from the early nerve agents, the G-series, which were developed by German scientists (hence the G) in the period after WWI and during WWII. The three G-series agents are all designed with the same basic chemical structure with slight variations to produce different properties. The two variations of these agents are lethality and volatility. The following G agents are listed from high volatility to low volatility:

- **Sarin (GB)**. Highly volatile colorless and odorless liquid. Turns from liquid to gas within seconds to minutes at room temperature. Highly lethal, with an **LD_{50}** of about 1 drop, depending on the purity. The LD_{50} is the standard measurement that represents the amount that will kill 50% of people who are exposed to this level.[4] GB is primarily a vapor hazard, with the respiratory tract as the main route of exposure. This agent is especially dangerous in enclosed environments such as office buildings, shopping malls, and subway cars. When this agent comes into contact with the skin, it is quickly absorbed and evaporates. When GB is on clothing, it has the effect of **off-gassing**, which means that the vapors are continuously released over time (like perfume). Off-gassing contaminates the patient and the patient's clothing.
- **Soman (GD)**. Twice as persistent as GB and five times as lethal. It has a fruity odor as a result of the type of alcohol used in the agent and generally has no color. This agent is both a contact and an inhalation hazard that can enter the body through skin absorption and through the respiratory tract. A unique additive in GD causes it to bind to the cells that it attacks faster than any other agent. This irreversible binding is called **aging**, which makes it more difficult to treat patients who have been exposed to GD.
- **Tabun (GA)**. Approximately half as lethal as GB and 36 times more persistent. Under the proper conditions it will remain present for several days. It also has a fruity smell and an appearance similar to GB. The components used to manufacture GA are easy to acquire, and the agent is easy to manufacture, which make it unique. GA is both a contact and an inhalation hazard that can enter the body through skin absorption and through the respiratory tract.
- **V agent (VX)**. Clear, oily agent that has no odor and looks like baby oil. VX was developed by the British after WWII and has chemical properties similar to the G-series agents. The difference is that VX is more than 100 times more lethal than GB and is extremely persistent (Figure 42-6). In fact, VX is so persistent that given the proper conditions, it will remain relatively unchanged for weeks to months. These properties make VX primarily a contact hazard because it lets off very little vapor. It is easily absorbed into the skin, and the oily residue that remains on the skin's surface is extremely difficult to decontaminate.

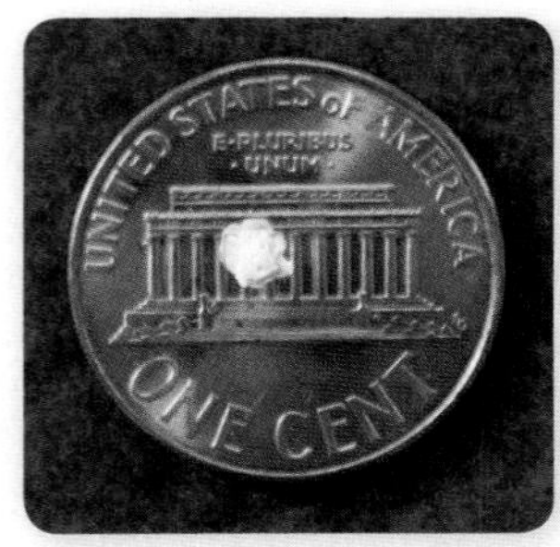

Figure 42-6 VX is the most toxic chemical ever created. The dot on the penny demonstrates the amount needed to achieve the lethal dose.

Nerve agents all produce similar symptoms but have varying routes of exposure. Nerve agents differ slightly in lethal concentration or dose and also differ in volatility. Some agents are designed to quickly become a gas (nonpersistent or highly volatile), whereas others remain liquid for a time (persistent or nonvolatile). These agents have been used successfully in warfare. After the nerve agent enters the body through skin contact or through the respiratory system, the patient will begin to exhibit a pattern of predictable symptoms. Like all chemical agents, the severity of the patient's symptoms will depend on the route of exposure of the agent and the amount of exposure. The resulting symptoms are described using the military mnemonic SLUDGEM and the medical mnemonic DUMBELS (Table 42-1). The DUMBELS mnemonic is more useful to you as an AEMT because it lists the more dangerous symptoms associated with exposure to nerve agents.

Only a handful of medical conditions are associated with the bilateral, excessively constricted (pinpoint) pupils (**miosis**) seen with nerve agent exposure. (Miosis is seen quickly in a patient with vapor exposure, but miosis may occur later after an isolated skin exposure. In some

Table 42-1 Symptoms of Exposure to Nerve Agents

Military Mnemonic: SLUDGEM	Medical Mnemonic: DUMBELS (all age groups)
Salivation, **S**weating	**D**iarrhea
Lacrimation (excessive tearing of the eyes)	**U**rination
Urination	**M**iosis (pinpoint pupils), **M**uscle weakness
Defecation	**B**radycardia, **B**ronchospasm, **B**ronchorrhea (discharge of mucus from the lungs)
Gastric upset and cramps	**E**mesis
Emesis	**L**acrimation (excessive tearing of the eyes)
Muscle twitching/**M**iosis (pinpoint pupils)	**S**eizures, **S**alivation, **S**weating

cases, the patient may have sustained both vapor and skin exposure.) Conditions such as a stroke (cerebrovascular accident), direct light to both eyes, and a drug overdose all can cause bilateral constricted pupils. Therefore, assess the patient for all of the signs and symptoms associated with SLUDGEM/DUMBELS to determine whether the patient has been exposed to a nerve agent.

Miosis is the most common symptom of nerve agent exposure and can remain for days to weeks. This symptom, along with the others listed in Table 42-1, will help you recognize exposure to a nerve agent early. The seizures that are associated with nerve agent exposure are unlike those found in patients with a history of seizure. The seizure will continue until the patient dies or until treatment is given with a nerve agent antidote kit.

Nerve Agent Treatment

Fatalities from severe nerve agent exposure occur as a result of respiratory complications, which lead to respiratory arrest. After the patient has been decontaminated, be prepared to treat aggressively. You can greatly increase the patient's chances of survival simply by providing airway and ventilatory support. As with all emergencies, securing the ABCs is the best and most important treatment that you can provide. Often in patients exposed to these agents, seizures will begin and will not stop. These patients will require administration of nerve agent antidote kits in addition to support of the ABCs.

Medical treatment for nerve agent exposure may include the **DuoDote Auto-Injector**. The DuoDote kit contains 2.1 mg of atropine and 600 mg of pralidoxime chloride (2-PAM) and is delivered as a single dose through one needle. Atropine is used to block the nerve agent from affecting the body. However, because the nerve agent may remain in the body for long periods, 2-PAM is used to eliminate the agent from the body. Many of the symptoms described in the DUMBELS mnemonic will be reversed with the use of atropine. These medications are delivered using the same technique as the EpiPen autoinjector; however, many doses may need to be administered to see these results. The military form of this combination injector is the **Antidote Treatment Nerve Agent Auto-Injector (ATNAA)**.

Words of Wisdom

On March 20, 1995, members of Aum Shinrikyo, a Japanese cult, released sarin (GB) in the Tokyo subway. The first arriving medical responders were met with chaos as hundreds and then thousands of people fled the subway system. Many were contaminated and showed signs and symptoms of nerve agent exposure. In the end, more than 5,000 people sought medical care for exposure to GB, and 12 people died. None of the EMS personnel wore protective clothing, and most became cross-contaminated. Remember, you can avoid becoming exposed. Do not become a patient!

In some regions, AEMTs may carry the DuoDote kit on the unit and will be called on to administer the antidotes to themselves or their patients. Remember that you need to properly dispose of activated antidote kits into a sharps container. If your service carries a nerve agent antidote, then refer to your local protocols for dose and use information.

Table 42-2 provides a brief comparison of nerve agents.

Table 42-2 Nerve Agents

Name	Military Designation	Odor	Special Features	Onset of Symptoms	Volatility	Route of Exposure
Tabun	GA	Fruity	Easy to manufacture	Immediate	Low	Skin contact and vapor hazard
Sarin	GB	None (if pure) or strong	Will off-gas while on patient's clothing	Immediate	High	Primarily respiratory vapor hazard; extremely lethal if skin contact is made
Soman	GD	Fruity	Ages rapidly, making it difficult to treat	Immediate	Moderate	Contact with skin; minimal vapor hazard
V agent	VX	None	Most lethal chemical agent; difficult to decontaminate	Immediate	Very low	Contact with skin; no vapor hazard (unless aerosolized)

▶ Metabolic Agents (Cyanides)

Hydrogen cyanide (AC) and cyanogen chloride (CK) are both agents that affect the body's ability to use oxygen. **Cyanide** is a colorless gas that has an odor similar to almonds. The effects of the cyanides begin on the cellular level and are rapidly seen at the organ and system levels. Besides the nerve agents, metabolic agents are the only chemical weapons known to kill within seconds to minutes. Unlike nerve agents, however, these deadly gases are commonly found in many industrial settings. Cyanides are produced in massive quantities throughout the United States every year for industrial uses such as gold and silver mining, photography, and plastics processing. They are often present in fires associated with textile and plastic factories. In fact, cyanide is naturally found in the pits of many fruits in very low doses. AC and CK share many of the same symptoms. In low doses, these chemicals are associated with dizziness, light-headedness, headache, and vomiting. Higher doses will produce symptoms that include the following:

- Shortness of breath and gasping respirations
- Respiratory distress or arrest
- Tachypnea
- Flushed skin
- Tachycardia
- Altered mental status
- Seizures
- Coma
- Apnea
- Cardiac arrest

The symptoms associated with the inhalation of a large amount of cyanide will all appear within several minutes. Death is likely unless the patient is treated promptly.

Safety Tips

As previously mentioned, the basic chemical ingredient in nerve agents is organophosphate. This common chemical is used in lesser concentrations for insecticides. Although industrial chemicals do not possess sufficient lethality to be effective WMDs, they are easy to acquire, inexpensive, and would have similar effects to the nerve agents. Agricultural aircraft (ie, crop-duster planes) could be used to disseminate these chemicals. Be cautious when responding to calls where insecticide equipment is stored and used, such as a farm or supply store that sells these products. The symptoms and medical management of patients with organophosphate insecticide poisoning are identical to those of the nerve agents.

Cyanide Agent Treatment

Cyanide binds with the body's cells, preventing oxygen from being used. Several medications act as antidotes, but most services do not carry them. After trained personnel wearing the proper PPE have removed the patient from the source of exposure, all of the patient's clothes must be removed to prevent off-gassing in the ambulance—even if no liquid contamination has occurred. Trained and protected personnel must decontaminate any patients who may have been exposed to liquid contamination before you can initiate treatment. Then support the patient's ABCs and gain IV access. Mild effects of cyanide exposure will generally resolve by simply removing the patient from the source of contamination and administering supplemental oxygen. Severe exposure, however, will

Table 42-3 Chemical Agents

Name	Military Designations	Odor	Lethality	Onset of Symptoms	Volatility	Primary Route of Exposure
Nerve agents	Tabun (GA) Sarin (GB) Soman (GD) V agent (VX)	Fruity or none	Most lethal chemical agents; can kill within minutes; effects are reversible with antidotes	Immediate	Moderate (GA, GD) Very high (GB) Low (VX)	GA: both GB: vapor hazard GD: both VX: contact hazard
Vesicants	Mustard (H) Lewisite (L) Phosgene oxime (CX)	Garlic (H) Geranium (L)	Causes large blisters to form; may severely damage upper airway if vapors are inhaled; severe, intense pain and gray skin discoloration (L and CX)	Delayed (H) Immediate (L, CX)	Very low (H, L) Moderate (CX)	Primarily contact, with some vapor hazard
Respiratory agents	Chlorine (Cl) Phosgene (CG)	Bleach Cut grass (CG)	Causes irritation choking (Cl); severe pulmonary edema (CG)	Immediate (Cl) Delayed (CG)	Very high	Vapor hazard
Cyanide agents	Hydrogen cyanide (AC) Cyanogen chloride (CK)	Almonds (AC) Irritating (CK)	Highly lethal chemical gases; can kill within minutes; effects are reversible with antidotes	Immediate	Very high	Vapor hazard

require aggressive oxygenation and perhaps ventilation with supplemental oxygen. Always use a bag-mask device or oxygen-powered ventilator device to ventilate a patient who has been exposed to a metabolic agent. The agent can easily be passed on from the patient to you through mouth-to-mouth or mouth-to-mask ventilations. If no antidote is available, then initiate transport immediately.

Table 42-3 summarizes the chemical agents. The odors of the particular chemicals are provided for informational purposes only. The sense of smell is a poor tool to use to determine whether a chemical agent is present. Many people are unable to smell the agents, and the odor could be derived from another source. This information is useful to you if you receive reports from people who claimed to smell bleach or garlic, for example. Never enter a potentially hazardous area using your sense of smell to determine whether a chemical agent is present.

Biologic Agents

Biologic agents pose many difficult issues when used as a WMD. Biologic agents can be almost completely undetectable. Also, most of the diseases caused by these agents will be similar to other minor illnesses commonly seen by EMS providers.

Biologic agents are grouped as viruses, bacteria, and neurotoxins and may be spread in various ways. **Dissemination** is the means by which a terrorist will spread the agent—for example, poisoning the water supply or aerosolizing the agent into the air or ventilation system of a building. A **disease vector** is an animal that spreads disease, once infected, to another animal. For example, bubonic plague can be spread by infected rats, smallpox by infected people, and the Zika virus or West Nile virus by infected mosquitoes. How easily the disease is able to spread from one human to another human is called communicability. Some diseases, such as those caused by human immunodeficiency virus (HIV), are difficult to spread by routine contact. Therefore, communicability is considered low. In other instances when communicability is high, such as with smallpox, the person is considered **contagious**. Typically, routine standard precautions are enough to prevent contamination from contagious biologic organisms.

Words of Wisdom

Always make sure that your patients have been thoroughly decontaminated by trained personnel before you come into contact with them. Chemical agents are primarily a vapor hazard, and all of the patient's clothing must be removed prior to you providing treatment to prevent off-gassing to you. Finally, never perform mouth-to-mouth or mouth-to-mask ventilation on a patient with a chemical agent exposure. Many of the vapors may linger in the patient's airway, and cross-contamination may occur.

Incubation period describes the time between the person becoming exposed to the agent and the appearance of the first symptom(s). It is important to understand that although your patient may not exhibit signs or symptoms, he or she may be contagious.

Be aware of when you should suspect the use of biologic agents. If the agent is in the form of a powder, such as in the October 2001 attacks involving letters laced with anthrax powder appearing in the US mail, the incident must be handled by hazmat specialists. Patients who come into direct contact with the biologic agent need to be decontaminated before you initiate treatment.

▶ Viruses

Viruses are germs that require a living host to multiply and survive. A virus is a simple organism and cannot thrive outside of a host (living body). Once in the body, the virus invades healthy cells and replicates itself to spread through the host. As the virus spreads, so does the disease that it carries. Viruses move from host to host by direct methods, such as through respiratory droplets or vectors. A *vector* is any agent that acts as a carrier or transporter.

Viral agents that may be released during a biologic terrorist event pose an extraordinary problem for health care providers, especially those in EMS. Although some viral agents do have vaccines, no treatment is available for a viral infection other than certain antiviral medications. Because of this characteristic, the following viruses have the potential to be used as agents of terrorism.

Smallpox

Smallpox is a highly contagious disease. Take all forms of standard precautions to prevent cross-contamination. You will greatly reduce this risk simply by wearing exam gloves, a high-efficiency particulate air respirator, and eye protection. According to the World Health Organization, the last natural case of smallpox in the world was seen in 1977.[5] Before the rash and blisters show, the illness will start with a high fever and body aches and headaches. The patient's temperature is usually in the range of 101 °F to 104 °F (38.3 °C to 40 °C).

An easy, quick way to differentiate the smallpox rash from other skin disorders is to observe the size, shape, and location of the lesions. In smallpox, all the lesions are identical in development. In other skin disorders, the lesions will be in various stages of healing and development. Smallpox blisters begin on the face and extremities and eventually move toward the chest and abdomen. The disease is in its most contagious phase when the blisters begin to form Figure 42-7. Unprotected contact with these blisters will promote transmission of the disease Table 42-4. A vaccine exists to prevent smallpox; however, it has been linked to medical complications and,

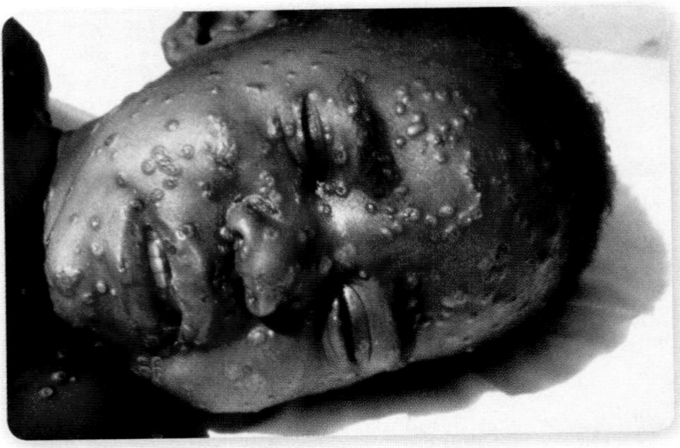

Figure 42-7 In smallpox, all the lesions are identical in development. In other skin disorders, the lesions will be in various stages of healing and development.

Courtesy of CDC.

Table 42-4 Characteristics of Smallpox

Dissemination	Aerosolized for warfare or use in a terrorist attack
Communicability	High from infected people or items (such as blankets used by infected patients); person-to-person transmission possible
Route of exposure	Inhalation of airborne droplets (cough) or direct skin contact with blisters
Signs and symptoms	Severe fever, malaise, body aches, headaches, small blisters on the skin, bleeding of the skin and mucous membranes; incubation period is 10 to 12 d; duration of the illness is approximately 4 wk
Medical management	Standard precautions; no specific treatment; provide supportive care (ABCs)

Abbreviation: ABCs, airway, breathing, and circulation

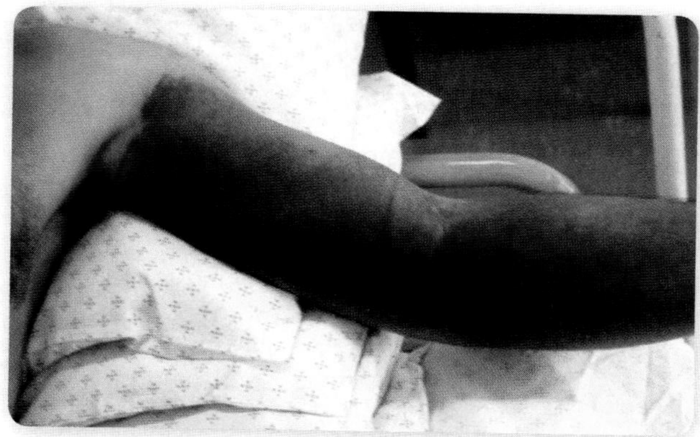

Figure 42-8 Viral hemorrhagic fevers cause the blood vessels and tissues to seep blood, resulting in ecchymosis (bruising), hemoptysis (coughing up blood), and blood in the patient's stool. Notice the severe discoloration in this patient with Crimean-Congo hemorrhagic fever, indicating internal bleeding.

Courtesy of Professor Robert Swanepoel/National Institute for Communicable Disease, South Africa.

in rare cases, death. Should an outbreak occur, the US government has enough vaccine to vaccinate every person in the United States.

Viral Hemorrhagic Fevers

Viral hemorrhagic fevers (VHFs) consist of a group of diseases caused by viruses that include the Ebola, Rift Valley, Marburg, and yellow fever viruses, among others. This group of viruses causes the blood in the body to seep out from the tissues and blood vessels Figure 42-8. Initially, the patient will have flulike symptoms, progressing to more serious symptoms such as internal and external hemorrhaging. Outbreaks are not uncommon in Africa and South America. Outbreaks in the United States, however, are extremely rare. Take all standard precautions when treating people with these illnesses. Mortality rates very depending on the strain of virus, the patient's age and health condition, and the availability of a modern health care system Table 42-5.

Table 42-5	Characteristics of Viral Hemorrhagic Fevers
Dissemination	Direct contact with an infected person's body fluids; can also be aerosolized for use in a terrorist attack
Communicability	Moderate from person to person or contaminated items
Route of exposure	Direct contact with an infected person's body fluids
Signs and symptoms	Sudden onset of fever, weakness, muscle pain, headache, and sore throat; all followed by vomiting and, as the virus runs its course, internal and external bleeding
Medical management	Standard precautions; no specific treatment for viral hemorrhagic fever; provide supportive care (ABCs) and treatment for shock and hypotension, if present

Abbreviation: ABCs, airway, breathing, and circulation

YOU are the Provider PART 3

You initiate triage of the patients who were injured by the truck. Four patients need treatment and transport. Additional units arrive on scene and take over the care of these patients. A firefighter approaches and tells you the man in the truck is unresponsive but appears to be breathing.

Recording Time: 1 Minute	
Appearance	Poor
Level of consciousness	Unresponsive
Airway	Appears patent from a distance
Breathing	Appears slow from a distance
Circulation	Unknown, with obvious burns on the face and arms

6. How should you proceed with your assessment of this patient?
7. Does the information about the terrorist threat affect your assessment of this patient?

▶ Bacteria

Unlike viruses, **bacteria** do not require a host to multiply and live. Bacteria are much more complex and larger than viruses and can grow up to 100 times larger than the largest virus. Bacteria contain all the cellular structures of a normal cell and are completely self-sufficient. Most bacterial infections can be treated with antibiotics.

> **Words of Wisdom**
>
> Because humans are acceptable hosts and vectors for many viruses and bacteria, it is important for you to take standard precautions at all times. If you fail to take standard precautions, then you may not only become a host for a virus, but you may spread it as well. Remember, a virus spreads from person to person to survive, and many infectious diseases present like common colds.

Most bacterial infections will generally begin with flulike symptoms, which can make it difficult for health care providers to identify whether the cause is a biologic attack or a natural epidemic.

Anthrax (Pulmonary and Cutaneous)

Anthrax (*Bacillus anthracis*) is caused by a deadly bacterium that lies dormant in a spore (protective shell). When exposed to the optimal temperature and moisture, the germ is released from the spore. The routes of exposure for anthrax bacteria are inhalation, cutaneous, and gastrointestinal (from consuming food that contains spores) **Figure 42-9**. The inhalational form, or pulmonary anthrax, is the most deadly and often presents as a severe cold. Pulmonary anthrax is associated with an 80% or higher death rate if untreated.[6] Antibiotics can be used to treat anthrax successfully. A vaccine to prevent anthrax infections is available. **Table 42-6** lists characteristics of anthrax.

Table 42-6 Characteristics of Anthrax

Dissemination	Aerosolized
Communicability	Only in the cutaneous form (rare)
Route of exposure	Through inhalation of spore, skin contact with spore, or direct contact with skin wound (cutaneous), or through ingestion
Signs and symptoms	Flulike symptoms, fever, respiratory distress with tachycardia, shock, pulmonary edema, and respiratory failure after 3 to 5 d of flulike symptoms
Medical management	Pulmonary: Standard precautions, oxygen, ventilatory support if in pulmonary edema or respiratory failure, and transport Cutaneous: Standard precautions, apply dry sterile dressing to prevent accidental contact with wound and fluids

Plague (Bubonic and Pneumonic)

The 14th-century plague that ravaged Asia, the Middle East, and finally Europe (the Black Death) killed an estimated 33 to 42 million people. Later on, in the early 19th century, almost 20 million people in India and China died due to plague. The plague's natural vectors are infected rodents and fleas. When a person is bitten by an infected flea or comes into contact with an infected rodent (or the waste of the rodent), the person can contract bubonic plague.

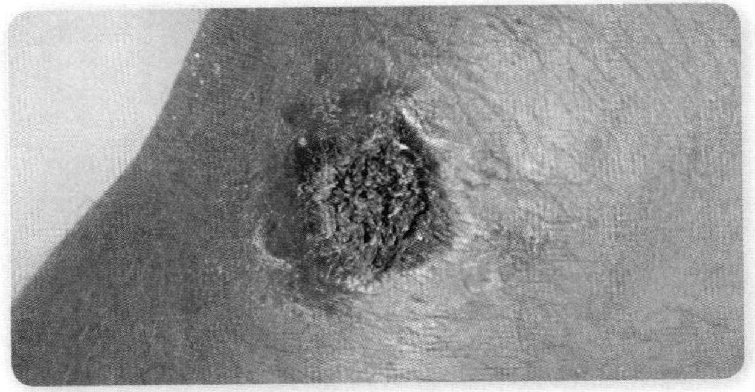

Figure 42-9 Cutaneous anthrax.

Bubonic plague infects the **lymphatic system** (a passive circulatory system in the body that bathes the tissues in lymph and works with the immune system). When this occurs, the patient's **lymph nodes** (area of the lymphatic system where infection-fighting cells are housed) become infected and grow. The glands of the nodes will grow large (up to the size of a tennis ball) and round, forming **buboes** **Figure 42-10**. If left untreated, then the infection may spread through the body, leading to sepsis and possibly death. Bubonic plague is not contagious and is not likely to be seen in a bioterrorist incident.

Pneumonic plague (also known as plague pneumonia) is a lung infection that results from inhalation of plague bacteria. This form of the disease is contagious and has a much higher death rate than the bubonic form **Table 42-7**.

▶ Neurotoxins

Neurotoxins are the most deadly substances known to humans. The strongest neurotoxin is 15,000 times more lethal than VX and 100,000 times more lethal than GB.

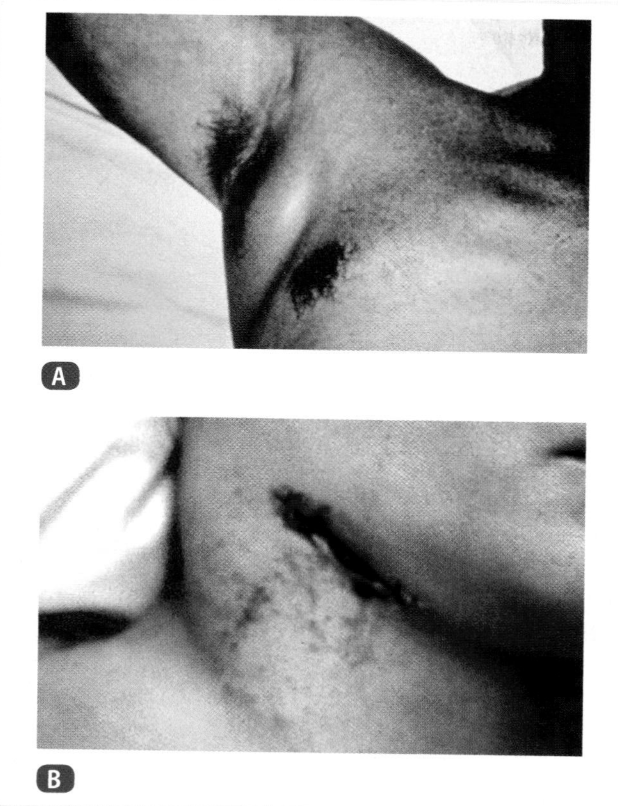

Figure 42-10 A. Plague buboe at lymph node under arm. **B.** Plague buboe at lymph node on neck.

A: Courtesy of James H. Steele/CDC; **B:** Courtesy of CDC.

Table 42-7 Characteristics of Plague

Dissemination	Aerosolized
Communicability	Bubonic: low, only from contact with fluid in buboes Pneumonic: high, from person to person
Route of exposure	Ingestion, inhalation, or cutaneous
Signs and symptoms	Fever, headache, muscle pain and tenderness, pneumonia, shortness of breath, extreme lymph node pain and enlargement (bubonic)
Medical management	Standard precautions, provide supportive care (ABCs), oxygen if indicated, and transport

Abbreviation: ABCs, airway, breathing, and circulation

These toxins are produced from plants, marine animals, molds, and bacteria. The route of exposure for these toxins is through ingestion, inhalation from aerosols, or injection. Unlike viruses and bacteria, neurotoxins are not contagious and have a faster onset of symptoms. Although these biologic toxins have immense destructive potential, they have not been used successfully as a WMD.

Table 42-8 Characteristics of Botulinum Toxin

Dissemination	Aerosolized, food supply sabotage, or injection
Communicability	None
Route of exposure	Ingestion, inhalation
Signs and symptoms	Dry mouth, intestinal obstruction, urinary retention, constipation, nausea and vomiting, abnormal pupil dilation, blurred vision, double vision, drooping eyelids, difficulty swallowing, difficulty speaking, and respiratory failure as the result of paralysis
Medical management	Provide supportive care (ABCs), oxygen, and transport; provide ventilatory support in case of paralysis of the respiratory muscles; vaccine is available

Abbreviation: ABCs, airway, breathing, and circulation

Botulinum Toxin

The most potent neurotoxin is **botulinum**, which is produced by bacteria. When introduced into the body, this neurotoxin affects the ability of the nervous system to function. Voluntary muscle control diminishes as the toxin spreads. Eventually the toxin causes muscle paralysis that begins at the head and face and travels downward throughout the body. The patient's accessory muscles and diaphragm will become paralyzed, and the patient will go into respiratory arrest Table 42-8.

Ricin

Although not as deadly as botulinum, **ricin** is still five times more lethal than VX. This toxin is derived from mash that is left from the castor bean Figure 42-11. When introduced into the body, ricin causes pulmonary edema and respiratory and circulatory failure leading to death Table 42-9.

The clinical picture depends on the route of exposure. Ricin is stable and extremely toxic by many routes of exposure, including inhalation. It is likely that 1 to 3 mg of ricin can kill an adult, and the ingestion of one seed can most likely kill a child. Although all parts of

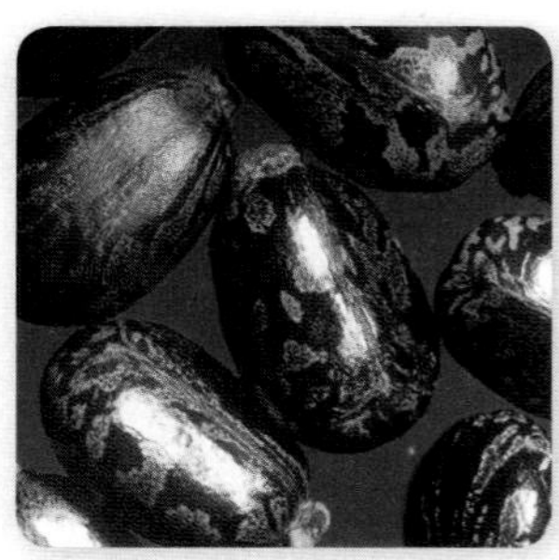

Figure 42-11 These seemingly harmless castor beans contain the key ingredient for ricin, one of the most potent toxins known to humans.

Courtesy of Brian Prechtel/USDA.

Table 42-9	Characteristics of Ricin
Dissemination	Released into indoor or outdoor air (aerosolized); food and water contamination
Communicability	None
Route of exposure	Inhalation, ingestion, injection
Signs and symptoms	Inhaled: cough, difficulty breathing, chest tightness, nausea, muscle aches, pulmonary edema, and hypoxia Ingested: nausea and vomiting, internal bleeding, and death Injection: no signs except swelling at the injection site and death
Medical management	Provide supportive care (ABCs); no treatment or vaccine available

Abbreviation: ABCs, airway, breathing, and circulation

the castor bean are poisonous, it is the seeds that are the most toxic. Castor bean ingestion causes a rapid onset of nausea, vomiting, abdominal cramps, and severe diarrhea, followed by vascular collapse. Death usually occurs on the third day in the absence of appropriate medical intervention.

Ricin is least toxic by the oral route. This is probably a result of poor absorption in the gastrointestinal tract, some digestion in the gut, and, possibly, some expulsion of the agent as caused by the rapid onset of vomiting. Ingestion causes local hemorrhage and necrosis of the liver, spleen, kidneys, and gastrointestinal tract. Signs and symptoms of ricin ingestion appear 4 to 8 hours after exposure, as follows:

- Fever
- Chills
- Headache
- Muscle aches
- Nausea
- Vomiting
- Diarrhea
- Severe abdominal cramping
- Dehydration
- Gastrointestinal bleeding
- Necrosis of the liver, spleen, kidneys, and gastrointestinal tract

Inhalation of ricin causes nonspecific weakness, cough, fever, hypothermia, and hypotension. Symptoms occur about 4 to 8 hours after inhalation, depending on the inhaled dose. The onset of profuse sweating some hours later signifies the termination of the symptoms. Signs and symptoms of ricin inhalation are as follows:

- Fever
- Chills
- Nausea
- Local irritation of eyes, nose, and throat
- Profuse sweating
- Headache
- Muscle aches
- Nonproductive cough
- Chest pain
- Dyspnea
- Pulmonary edema
- Severe lung inflammation
- Cyanosis
- Seizures
- Respiratory failure

Treatment is supportive and includes both respiratory support and cardiovascular support as needed. Early intubation and ventilation, combined with treatment of pulmonary edema, are appropriate. IV fluids and electrolyte replacement are useful for treating the dehydration caused by profound vomiting and diarrhea.

Table 42-10 summarizes the biologic agents.

▶ Roles of the AEMT During a Biologic Event

Syndromic Surveillance

Syndromic surveillance is the monitoring, usually by local or state health departments, of patients presenting to emergency departments and alternative care facilities, the recording of EMS call volume, and the use of over-the-counter medications. Patients with signs and symptoms that resemble influenza are particularly important to monitor. Local and state health departments monitor for an unusual influx of patients with these

Table 42-10 Biologic Agents

Disease	Transmission Person to Person	Incubation Period	Duration of Illness	Lethality (approximate case fatality rates)
Pulmonary anthrax	No	1 to 6 d	3 to 5 d (usually fatal if untreated)	High
Pneumonic plague	High	2 to 3 d	1 to 6 d (usually fatal)	High unless treated within 12 to 24 h
Smallpox	High	7 to 17 d (average, 12 d)	4 wk	High to moderate
Viral hemorrhagic fever	Moderate	4 to 21 d	Death within 7 to 16 d	High to moderate, depending on type of fever
Botulinum poisoning	No	1 to 5 d	Death within 24 to 72 h; lasts months if patient does not die	High without respiratory support
Ricin poisoning	No	18 to 24 h	Death within 10 to 12 d if ingested	High

symptoms in hopes of discovering an outbreak early. The role of EMS in syndromic surveillance is valuable in the overall tracking of a biologic terrorist event or infectious disease outbreak. Quality assurance personnel and dispatch operations need to be aware of an unusual number of calls from patients with unexplainable symptoms coming from a particular region or community (known as symptom clusters).

Words of Wisdom

In a mass-casualty incident, it is important to frequently communicate with your patient. Remember, your patient is probably scared and does not know what is going on. By explaining to your patient any delays that are occurring, as well as the actions you are taking, you may alleviate the patient's fears. Also, provide your patient with protection (eg, building materials, backboards, or tarps) in an effort to protect the patient from further harm.

Points of Distribution (Strategic National Stockpile)

Points of distribution (PODs) are existing facilities that are established for the mass distribution of antibiotics, chemical antidotes, antitoxins, vaccinations, and other medications and supplies during an emergency. These supplies may be released in deliveries known as "push packs" by the US Centers for Disease Control and Prevention (CDC) Strategic National Stockpile. These push packages have a delivery time of 12 hours anywhere in the country. In some regions, local and state municipalities have started to stockpile their own supplies to reduce the time delay.

Emergency medical technicians, AEMTs, and paramedics may be called on to assist in the delivery of the medications to the public (depending on local emergency management planning). Your role may include triage, treatment of seriously ill patients, and patient transport to the hospital. Most plans for PODs include at least one ambulance on standby for the transport of seriously ill patients.

Radiologic/Nuclear Devices

▶ What Is Radiation?

Ionizing radiation is energy that is emitted in the form of rays, or particles. This energy can be found in **radioactive material**, such as rocks and metals. Radioactive material is any material that emits radiation. This material is unstable, and it attempts to stabilize itself by changing its structure in a natural process called **decay**. While the substance decays, it gives off radiation until it stabilizes. The process of radioactive decay can take anywhere from minutes to billions of years; meanwhile, the substance remains radioactive.

The energy that is emitted from a strong radiologic source is **alpha radiation**, **beta radiation**, **gamma (x-ray) radiation**, or **neutron radiation**. Alpha is the least harmful penetrating type of radiation and cannot move through most objects. In fact, a sheet of paper or the body's skin easily stops it. Beta radiation is slightly more penetrating than alpha and requires a layer of clothing to stop it. Gamma rays are far faster and stronger than alpha and beta rays. These rays easily penetrate through the human body and require lead or several inches of concrete to prevent penetration. Neutron particles are among the most powerful forms of radiation. Neutrons easily penetrate through lead and require several feet of concrete to stop them Figure 42-12.

▶ Sources of Radiologic Material

Thousands of radioactive materials are found on the earth. These materials are generally used for purposes that benefit humankind, such as medicine, killing germs in food (irradiation), and construction work. After radiologic material has been used for its purpose, the remaining material is called radiologic waste. Radiologic waste remains radioactive but has no more usefulness. Radioactive materials can be found at the following locations:

- Hospitals and other health care facilities with radiology departments
- Colleges and universities
- Chemical and industrial sites
- Nuclear power plants

Not all radioactive material is tightly guarded. Radiologic waste is often not guarded at all, which makes the use of radioactive material appealing to terrorists.

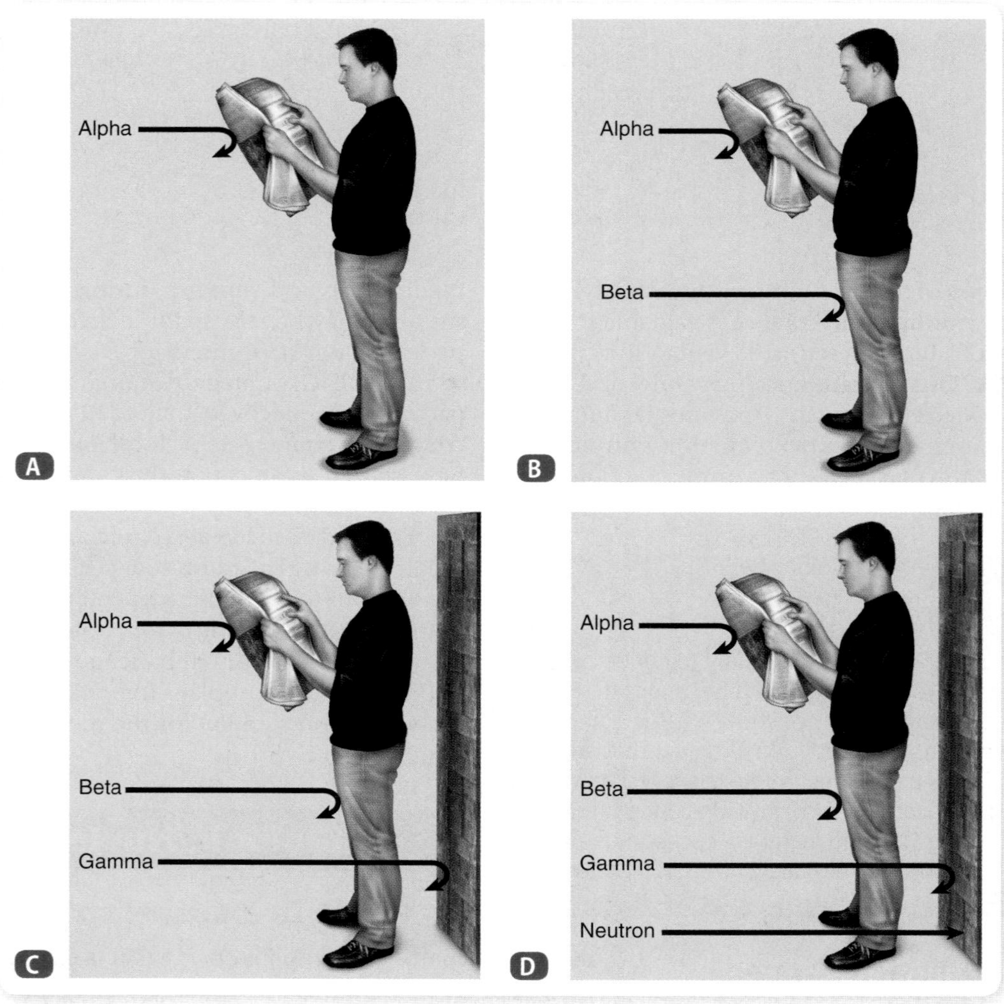

Figure 42-12 The penetrating potential of radiation. **A.** Alpha. **B.** Beta. **C.** Gamma. **D.** Neutron.

▶ Radiologic Dispersal Devices

A **radiologic dispersal device (RDD)** is any container that is designed to disperse radioactive material using explosive material. This process would generally require the use of a bomb, hence the nickname "**dirty bomb**." A dirty bomb has the potential to injure people with not only the radioactive material, but also the explosive material used to deliver it. The mere thought of an RDD creates fear in a population, and so the ultimate goal of some terrorists—fear—is accomplished. In reality, however, the destructive capability of a dirty bomb is limited to the explosives that are attached to it. Therefore, if the explosive is sufficient to kill 10 people without radioactive material, then it will also kill 10 people with the radioactive material added. Long-term injuries and illness may be associated with the use of an RDD, yet not much more than the bomb by itself would create. In short, the dirty bomb is an ineffective WMD.

▶ Nuclear Energy

Nuclear energy is artificially made by altering (splitting) radioactive atoms. The result is an immense amount of energy that usually takes the form of heat. Nuclear material is used in medicine, weapons, naval vessels, and power plants. Nuclear material gives off all forms of radiation, including neutrons (the most deadly type). Like radioactive material, when nuclear material is no longer useful, it becomes waste that is still radioactive.

▶ Nuclear Weapons

As mentioned previously, the destructive energy of a nuclear explosion is unlike any other weapon in the world. That is why nuclear weapons, such as missiles or bombs, are kept only in secure facilities throughout the world. Some nations have ties to terrorists and have actively attempted to build nuclear weapons. Yet the ability of these nations to deliver a nuclear weapon is incomplete. The threat of complete mutual annihilation is an effective deterrent. Therefore, the likelihood of a nuclear attack is extremely remote.

Unfortunately, however, because of the collapse of the former Soviet Union, the whereabouts of many small nuclear devices are unknown. These small, suitcase-sized nuclear weapons are called **Special Atomic Demolition Munitions (SADM)**. The SADM, or "suitcase nuke," was designed to destroy individual targets, such as important buildings, bridges, tunnels, and large ships. According to one report on the safety and security of Russia's nuclear arsenal, an estimated 84 Russian SADMs are missing as of the late 1990s.[7] No other information or updates on the whereabouts of these devices have been made public.

▶ Symptomatology

Patients who have been exposed to a known or suspected source of excessive radiation may have acute radiation toxicity or radiation sickness. The effects of radiation exposure will vary depending on the amount of radiation that a person receives and the route of exposure.

YOU are the Provider — PART 4

The bomb squad has finished its assessment of the vest the man is wearing and the vehicle itself, and found no remaining threat in or around the vehicle. Firefighters extricate the patient from the truck and place him on a long backboard. A rapid trauma assessment shows slow and shallow respirations, second-degree burns to his face and arms, and a rigid abdomen. He is ventilated with a bag-mask device and 100% oxygen and packaged for transport.

Recording Time: 8 Minutes	
Respirations	6 breaths/min
Pulse	122 beats/min, weak and thready
Skin	Pale and cool; burns to face and arms
Blood pressure	88/54 mm Hg
Oxygen saturation (Spo_2)	89% on room air
Pupils	Pupils Equal, Round, and Reactive to Light and Accommodation (PERRLA)

8. What potential injuries might you anticipate as a result of the explosion?
9. Do you need to take any special decontamination measures after this call?

Table 42-11	Common Signs of Acute Radiation Toxicity
Low exposure	Nausea, vomiting, diarrhea, dizziness, headache
Moderate exposure	First-degree burns, hair loss, compromised immune system (death of white blood cells), and cancer
Severe exposure	Second- and third-degree burns, cancer, and death

Radiation can be introduced into the body by all routes of exposure as well as through the body (irradiation). The patient can inhale radioactive dust from nuclear fallout or from a dirty bomb or have radioactive liquid absorbed into the body through the skin. Once inside the body, the radiation source will irradiate the person from within rather than from an external source (such as radiograph equipment). Some common signs of acute radiation toxicity are listed in Table 42-11. Additional injuries will occur with a nuclear blast such as thermal and blast trauma, trauma from flying objects, and eye injuries.

Medical Management

Being exposed to a radiation source does not make a patient contaminated or radioactive. However, when patients have a radioactive source on their bodies (such as debris from a dirty bomb), they are contaminated and must be initially cared for by a hazmat responder. After the patient is decontaminated and no threat to you exists, you may begin treatment with the ABCs and treat the patient for any burns or trauma. As always, wear appropriate PPE. Use plastic bags to secure any body fluids obtained from the patient. Place all body fluids in containers and properly dispose of them with other potentially radioactive waste.

Protective Measures

No suits or protective gear can completely shield you from radiation. The people who work in high-risk areas wear some protection like lead-lined suits; however, this equipment is not available to AEMTs. The best ways to protect yourself from the effects of radiation are to use time and distance and shield yourself using buildings and walls for protection. Do not enter a hazmat area unless you are trained as a hazmat responder and have proper training in the use of self-contained breathing apparatus.

- **Time.** Radiation has a cumulative effect on the body. The less time that you are exposed to the source, the less the effects will be. If you realize that the patient is near a radiation source, then leave the area immediately.
- **Distance.** Radiation is limited as to how far it can travel. Depending on the type of radiation, often moving only a few feet is enough to remove you from immediate danger. Alpha radiation cannot travel more than a few inches but gamma rays can travel hundreds or thousands of feet. Take this into account when responding to a nuclear or radiologic incident, and make certain that responders are stationed far enough from the incident.
- **Shielding.** As discussed earlier, the path of all radiation can be stopped by a specific object. It will be impossible for you to recognize the type of radiation being emitted or even from which direction it is coming. Therefore, always assume that you are dealing with the strongest form of radiation and use concrete shielding (such as buildings or walls) between yourself and the incident. The importance of shielding cannot be overemphasized.

Incendiary and Explosive Devices

Incendiary and explosive devices come in various shapes and sizes. Incendiary devices are weapons used to start fires. Terrorists use flamethrowers, chemicals, Molotov cocktails, or other explosive devices for this purpose. Although you are not required to recognize all of the possible types of explosive devices (including improvised explosive devices), it is important for you to be able to identify an object you believe is a potential device, notify the proper authorities, and safely evacuate the area. Always remember that the possibility of a secondary device exists when you respond to the scene of an incendiary or explosive device call.

Mechanisms of Injury

The type and severity of wounds sustained from incendiary and explosive devices primarily depend on the patient's distance from the epicenter of the explosion. Patients close to the epicenter of the explosion are likely to suffer from all wound-causing agents of the munitions. Patients who are farther away from the epicenter are likely to experience a combination of blast injuries from the explosion and penetrating trauma injuries from primary and secondary projectiles created by the explosion.

The five types of blast injuries are as follows:

- **Primary blast injury.** Caused solely by the direct effects of the pressure wave on the body. The injury from the primary blast is seen almost exclusively in the hollow organs of the body—the lungs, intestines, and inner ears. An injury to the lungs causes the greatest morbidity and mortality.

- **Secondary blast injury**. Penetrating or nonpenetrating injury that results from being struck by flying debris, such as ordnance projectiles or secondary missiles, that has been set in motion by the explosion. Objects are propelled by the force of the blast and strike the person, causing injury.
- **Tertiary blast injury**. Injury that results from whole-body displacement and subsequent traumatic impact with environmental objects (eg, trees, buildings, and vehicles). Other indirect effects include toxic effects from the inhalation of combustion gases.
- **Quaternary blast injury**. Any other injury caused by a blast, including toxic inhalation of combustible gases (carbon monoxide, cyanide, etc); flash burns, crush injuries, respiratory injuries, and medical emergencies sustained while fleeing the scene (eg, a myocardial infarction); or mental health conditions (eg, posttraumatic stress disorder, even without the presence of any other injuries).
- **Quinary blast injury**. Injuries caused by exposure to toxic materials associated with radiation (dirty bombs), bacteria, and/or chemicals resulting in contamination of tissues, or by exposure to foreign bodies that have the potential to transmit disease. Signs and symptoms are related to the type of agent.[8]

Words of Wisdom

A phenomenon known as "human remains shrapnel" is also a part of the quinary phase. This finding is often seen in suicide bombings in which a bone fragment from the assailant pierces the skin of a patient. Treatment of the patient is based on presentation: impaled object, open fracture, laceration, etc. However, penetration of the skin by allogeneic fragments (those coming from another individual) also carry the risk of transmission of bloodborne diseases such as HIV or hepatitis B. Always wear appropriate PPE and notify hospital staff of the potential for exposure.

The Physics of an Explosion

When a substance is detonated, a solid or liquid is chemically converted into large volumes of gas under high pressure with resultant explosive energy release. Propellants, such as gunpowder, are explosives designed to release energy relatively slowly compared with high-energy explosives, which are designed to detonate quickly. This detonation generates a pressure pulse in the shape of a spherical blast wave that expands in all directions from the point of explosion. Flying debris and high winds commonly cause conventional blunt and penetrating trauma.

Tissues at Risk

Hollow organs such as the middle ear, lung, and gastrointestinal tract are most susceptible to pressure changes. The junction between tissues of different densities and exposed tissues such as the head and neck are prone to injury as well. The ear is the organ system most sensitive to blast injuries. The patient may report ringing or pain in the ears or some loss of hearing, and blood may be visible in the ear canal. Permanent hearing loss is possible.

Primary **pulmonary blast injuries** occur as contusions and hemorrhages in the lungs. According to the CDC, **blast lung** (a severe pulmonary contusion, bleeding, or swelling with damage to the blood vessels and alveoli or a combination of any or all) is the most common cause of death in people who survive the initial explosion. Blast lung is characterized by the clinical triad of apnea, bradycardia, and hypotension.[9] When the explosion occurs in an open space, the patient's side that is toward the explosion is usually injured, but the injury can be bilateral when the patient is located in a confined space. The patient may report tightness or pain in the chest and may cough up blood and have tachypnea or other signs of respiratory distress. Subcutaneous emphysema (crackling under the skin) over the chest may be palpated, indicating the presence of air in the thorax. Pneumothorax is common and may require emergency decompression.

Solid organs are relatively protected from shock-wave injury but may be injured by secondary missiles or a hurled body. Hollow organs, however, may be injured by similar mechanisms as are lung tissue. Petechiae, or pinpoint hemorrhages that show up on the skin, to large hematomas are the most visible sign.

Neurologic injuries and head trauma are common causes of death from blast injuries. Subarachnoid (beneath the arachnoid layer covering the brain) and subdural (beneath the outermost covering of the brain) hematomas are often seen. Permanent or transient neurologic deficits may be secondary to concussion, intracerebral bleeding, or air embolism. Instant but transient unresponsiveness, with or without retrograde amnesia, may be initiated not only by head trauma, but also by cardiovascular conditions. Bradycardia and hypotension are common after an intense pressure wave from an explosion. This is a vagal nerve–mediated form of cardiogenic shock without compensatory vasoconstriction (for example, vasovagal syncope).

Extremity injuries, including traumatic amputations, are common and often accompanied by other significant injuries. Patients with traumatic amputation are likely to sustain fatal injuries secondary to the blast.

YOU are the Provider SUMMARY

1. **Given the situation, what are some unique concerns about this incident?**

   This incident presents a variety of concerns for you as an AEMT. Scene safety and situational awareness are paramount. You need to take special precautions with regard to vehicle positioning to protect yourself, patients, and bystanders from further injury. Because smoke is coming from the cab of the truck, be aware of the potential for fire and possible explosions. Also, because the truck is carrying an unknown load, the potential for a secondary event exists.

2. **Is it safe for you to enter the scene? What should be done first?**

   Because of the potential for fire and explosion, the scene is not safe for you to enter at the present time. You should position the ambulance back far enough from the scene until the fire department and law enforcement have removed the threats. However, if other patients are located a safe distance away from the scene, then you can start triage and treatment of these patients.

3. **As an AEMT, what level of knowledge should you possess regarding terrorism and WMDs?**

   You are not expected to be an expert in terrorism and WMDs. However, you are expected to be aware of the various types of threats—just like any other citizen—and recognize certain indicators of terrorism when responding to an incident. Always maintain a high index of suspicion and stay alert.

4. **What is a secondary device or event?**

   A secondary device is an additional explosive that is set to detonate after the initial bomb. Such devices are intended primarily to injure responders and to secure media coverage because the media generally arrive on scene just after the initial response. Secondary devices may include various types of electronic equipment, such as a mobile phone that is designed to detonate when a call is answered.

5. **Does the potential for a secondary device exist at this scene?**

   At scenes of terrorist activity, the potential for secondary devices always exists. This incident was an intentional attack on a group of people, and the driver of the truck was wearing an obvious explosive device. Until qualified responders declare the scene safe, you should remain at a safe distance and proceed with emergency medical care of the other patients as needed.

6. **How should you proceed with your assessment of this patient?**

   After the other patients have been turned over to the additional responding units, you are free to attend to the last patient—the truck driver. Do not approach the truck until scene safety is assured. Perform your assessment as you would with any other patient, with particular attention to scene safety.

7. **Does the information about the terrorist threat affect your assessment of this patient?**

   Because no other assailants have been found, you can proceed with your assessment after the scene is deemed safe by qualified responders. The fact that this was a terrorist event does not change your assessment of this patient. Remain alert for any potential secondary devices and remember that if this patient becomes responsive, then he may be violent.

8. **What potential injuries might you anticipate as a result of the explosion?**

   Injuries seen during the primary phase of a blast include those that affect gas-filled organs. Because the patient was wearing an explosive vest, he was close to the blast. Potential injuries include damage to the lungs, ruptured tympanic membranes, and other gas-filled organs. He also has burns to the face and arms.

9. **Do you need to take any special decontamination measures after this call?**

   In this case, the patient and the vehicle were thoroughly evaluated before you assessed him and decontamination was deemed unnecessary, so you do not need to take any special decontamination measures beyond your regular measures after a call. If the patient had sustained possible contamination due to an agent he may have been transporting, then you would need to decontaminate anything that came into contact with the patient, including the ambulance, any equipment, and yourself. Decontamination must occur prior to putting the ambulance back into service and prior to delivering the patient to the hospital.

YOU are the Provider SUMMARY *(continued)*

EMS Patient Care Report (PCR)

Date: 10-6-18	**Incident No.:** 20108412	**Nature of Call:** MVC and multiple pedestrian injuries	**Location:** 107 Veterans Blvd

Dispatched: 1204	**En Route:** 1205	**At Scene:** 1209	**Transport:** 1320	**At Hospital:** 1337	**In Service:** 1619

Patient Information

Age: Unknown **Sex:** M **Weight (in kg [lb]):** 102 kg (224 lb)	**Allergies:** Unknown **Medications:** Unknown **Past Medical History:** Unknown **Chief Complaint:** Altered mental status and burns to face and arms

Vital Signs

Time: 1308	**BP:** Not obtained	**Pulse:** Not obtained	**Respirations:** Slow	**Spo_2:** Not obtained
Time: 1315	**BP:** 88/54	**Pulse:** 122	**Respirations:** 6	**Spo_2:** 89% on room air
Time:	**BP:**	**Pulse:**	**Respirations:**	**Spo_2:**

EMS Treatment (circle all that apply)

Oxygen @ ______ L/min via (circle one): **NC** **NRM** **Bag-mask device** (circled)		**Assisted Ventilation** (circled)	**Airway Adjunct:** Oral (circled)	**CPR**
Defibrillation	**Bleeding Control**	**Bandaging**	**Splinting**	**Other:**

Narrative

EMS dispatched to above location for report of MVC—truck vs pedestrians then struck brick building. Upon arrival found 4 pedestrians with obvious injuries and a moving truck with damage to front situated against brick wall of building. Smoke noted to be coming from truck engine. Attended pedestrian patients until turned over to additional units. Delayed care of driver of truck due to safety concerns. After scene was deemed safe by FD and law enforcement special unit, approached truck to find male patient sitting in driver's seat, apparently unresponsive with slow respirations. Patient was extricated by FD. Exposed and performed rapid trauma assessment—findings of second-degree burns to face and arms and rigid abdomen. 100% oxygen provided via bag-mask device with oral adjunct in place, burns covered with sterile sheet and patient packaged for transport. Transported emergency to trauma center. Upon arrival at ED report given to trauma team without incident. Law enforcement also standing by at ED.**End of report**

Prep Kit

▶ Ready for Review

- As a result of the increase in terrorist activity, it is possible that you, the AEMT, could witness a terrorist event. You must be mentally and physically prepared for the possibility of a terrorist event.
- Types of groups that tend to use terrorism include violent religious groups/doomsday cults, extremist political groups, technology terrorists, and single-issue groups.
- A weapon of mass destruction (WMD) is any agent designed to bring about mass death, casualties, and/or massive damage to property and infrastructure (bridges, tunnels, airports, and seaports).
- Use the following two mnemonics to help you remember the different kinds of WMDs: B-NICE (Biologic, Nuclear, Incendiary, Chemical, and Explosive weapons) and CBRNE (Chemical, Biologic, Radiologic, Nuclear, and Explosive weapons).
- Indicators that may give you clues as to whether the emergency is the result of a terrorist attack include the type of location, type of call, number of patients, patients' statements, and preincident indicators.
- If you suspect that a terrorist or a WMD event has occurred, then ensure the scene is safe. If you have any doubt that it may not be safe, then do not enter. Wait for assistance.
- Terrorists may set secondary devices that are designed to explode after the initial bomb, thus injuring responders and securing media coverage. Constantly assess and reassess the scene for safety.
- Chemical agents are manufactured substances that can have devastating effects on living organisms. They include vesicants (blister agents), respiratory agents, nerve agents, and metabolic agents.
- The route of exposure is how the agent most effectively enters the body.
- Biologic agents are organisms that cause disease. They include viruses such as smallpox and those that cause viral hemorrhagic fevers, bacteria such as those that cause anthrax and plague, and neurotoxins such as botulinum toxin and ricin.
- Radiologic or nuclear weapons can create a massive amount of destruction.
- Explosive and incendiary devices come in various shapes and sizes. It is important to be able to identify an object you believe is a potential device and notify the proper authorities, while safely evacuating the area.

▶ Vital Vocabulary

aging The process by which the temporary bond between the organophosphate and acetylcholinesterase undergoes hydrolysis, resulting in a permanent covalent bond.

alpha radiation A type of energy that is emitted from a strong radiologic source; it is the least harmful penetrating type of radiation and cannot travel more than a few inches or through most objects.

anthrax A disease caused by deadly bacteria (*Bacillus anthracis*) that lie dormant in a spore (protective shell); the germ is released from the spore when exposed to the optimal temperature and moisture. The routes of entry are inhalation, cutaneous, and gastrointestinal (from consuming food that contains spores).

Antidote Treatment Nerve Agent Auto-Injector (ATNAA) The military form of a nerve agent antidote kit containing atropine and pralidoxime chloride; delivered as a single dose through one needle.

bacteria Single-cell microorganisms that rapidly reproduce by binary fission; some can form spores (encysted variants) when environmental conditions are harsh.

beta radiation A type of energy that is emitted from a strong radiologic source; is slightly more penetrating than alpha radiation and requires a layer of clothing to stop it.

blast lung A severe pulmonary contusion, bleeding, or swelling with damage to the blood vessels and alveoli, or a combination of any or all of these.

B-NICE A mnemonic to recall the types of weapons of mass destruction: Biologic, Nuclear, Incendiary, Chemical, and Explosive; see also *CBRNE*.

botulinum Produced by bacteria; when introduced into the body, this most potent of neurotoxins affects the ability of the nervous system to function and causes botulism.

buboes Enlarged lymph nodes (up to the size of a tennis ball) that are characteristic in people infected with the bubonic plague.

bubonic plague Bacterial infection that affects the lymphatic system; it is transmitted by infected rodents and fleas and characterized by acute malaise, fever,

Prep Kit (continued)

and the formation of tender, enlarged, inflamed lymph nodes that appear as lesions. Also called the Black Death.

CBRNE A mnemonic used to recall the types of weapons of mass destruction: Chemical, Biologic, Radiologic, Nuclear, and Explosive; see also *B-NICE*.

chlorine (Cl) The first chemical agent ever used in warfare; it has a distinct odor of bleach and creates a green haze when released as a gas. Initially it produces upper airway irritation and a choking sensation.

contact hazard The danger posed by an agent whose primary route of exposure is through the skin; also called a skin hazard.

contagious An infectious disease that can be transmitted to another; communicable.

covert An act in which the public safety community generally has no prior knowledge of the time, location, or nature of the attack.

cross-contamination Occurs when a person is contaminated by an agent as a result of coming into contact with another contaminated person.

cyanide A colorless gas that affects the body's ability to use oxygen; it has an odor similar to almonds. The effects begin on the cellular level and are rapidly seen at the organ and system levels.

decay A natural process in which a material that is unstable attempts to stabilize itself by changing its structure.

dirty bomb Any container that is designed to disperse radioactive material; see also *radiologic dispersal device*.

disease vector An animal that spreads a disease, once infected, to another animal.

dissemination The means by which a terrorist will spread an agent, such as by poisoning the water supply or aerosolizing the agent into the air or ventilation system of a building.

domestic terrorism Terrorism that is carried out by people in their own country.

DuoDote Auto-Injector A nerve agent antidote kit containing atropine and pralidoxime chloride; delivered as a single dose through one needle.

G agents Early nerve agents that were developed by German scientists in the period after World War I and into World War II: sarin, soman, and tabun.

gamma (x-ray) radiation A type of energy that is emitted from a strong radiologic source that is far faster and has more energy than alpha and beta radiation. These rays easily penetrate through the human body and require lead or several inches of concrete to prevent penetration.

incubation period The time between when a person is exposed to an agent to when symptoms first appear.

international terrorism Terrorism that is carried out by people in a country other than their own; also known as cross-border terrorism.

ionizing radiation Energy that is emitted in the form of rays or particles.

LD_{50} The standard measure of the dose amount of an agent or substance that will kill 50% of a population who are exposed to this level.

lewisite (L) A vesicant that has a rapid onset of symptoms and produces immediate, intense pain and discomfort on contact; British antilewisite is the antidote.

lymph nodes The area of the lymphatic system where infection-fighting cells are housed.

lymphatic system A passive circulatory system in the body that transports a plasmalike liquid called lymph, a thin fluid that bathes the tissues of the body.

miosis Excessively constricted (pinpoint) pupil; often bilateral after exposure to nerve agents.

mutagen A substance that mutates, damages, and changes the structures of the body's cells.

nerve agents A class of chemical called organophosphates; they function by blocking an essential enzyme in the nervous system, which causes the body's organs to become overstimulated and burn out.

neurotoxins Biologic agents that are the most deadly substances known to humans; they include botulinum toxin and ricin.

neutron radiation The type of energy that is emitted from a strong radiologic source, involving particles that are among the most powerful forms of radiation; the particles easily penetrate through lead and require several feet of concrete to stop them.

off-gassing The release of an agent after exposure, such as from a person's clothes that have been exposed to the agent.

persistency Describes how long a chemical agent will stay on a surface before it evaporates.

Prep Kit *(continued)*

phosgene A very potent respiratory agent that is a product of combustion; it has a delayed onset of symptoms, usually hours.

phosgene oxime (CX) A vesicant that has a rapid onset of symptoms and produces immediate, intense pain and discomfort on contact.

pneumonic plague A lung infection, also known as plague pneumonia, that is the result of inhalation of plague-causing bacteria.

points of distribution (PODs) Existing facilities used as mass distribution sites for antibiotics, chemical antidotes, antitoxins, vaccinations, and other medications and supplies during an emergency.

primary blast injury Injuries caused by an explosive pressure wave on the hollow organs of the body.

pulmonary blast injuries Pulmonary trauma resulting from short-range exposure to the detonation of high-energy explosives.

quaternary blast injury A blast injury that falls into one of the following categories: burns, crush injuries, toxic inhalation, medical emergencies, or mental health disorders.

quinary blast injury Injuries caused by exposure to toxic materials associated with radiation, bacteria, and/or chemicals resulting in contamination of tissues, or by foreign bodies that have the potential to transmit disease.

radioactive material Any material that emits radiation.

radiologic dispersal device (RDD) Any container that is designed to disperse radioactive material; see also *dirty bomb*.

ricin A neurotoxin derived from mash that is left from the castor bean; causes pulmonary edema and respiratory and circulatory failure leading to death.

route of exposure The manner by which a toxic substance enters the body.

sarin (GB) A nerve agent that is one of the G agents; a highly volatile, colorless, and odorless liquid that turns from liquid to gas within seconds to minutes at room temperature.

secondary blast injury A penetrating or nonpenetrating injury caused by ordnance projectiles or secondary missiles.

secondary device An explosive used by terrorists that is set to explode after the initial bomb; it is intended primarily to injure responders and to secure media coverage.

smallpox A highly contagious disease; it is most contagious when blisters begin to form.

soman (GD) A nerve agent that is one of the G agents; twice as persistent as sarin and five times as lethal; it has a fruity odor, as a result of the type of alcohol used in the agent; and is a contact and an inhalation hazard that can enter the body through skin absorption and through the respiratory tract.

Special Atomic Demolition Munitions (SADM) Small, suitcase-sized nuclear weapons that were designed to destroy individual targets, such as important buildings, bridges, tunnels, and large ships.

state-sponsored terrorism Terrorism that is funded and/or supported by nations that hold close ties with terrorist groups.

sulfur mustard (H) A vesicant also known as mustard gas; it is a brown-yellow, oily substance that is generally considered very persistent; has the distinct smell of garlic or mustard; and, when released, is quickly absorbed into the skin and/or mucous membranes and begins an irreversible process of damaging the cells.

syndromic surveillance The monitoring, usually by local or state health departments, of patients presenting to emergency departments and alternative care facilities, the recording of EMS call volume, and the use of over-the-counter medications.

tabun (GA) A nerve agent that is one of the G agents; is 36 times more persistent than sarin and approximately half as lethal; has a fruity smell; and is unique because the components used to manufacture the agent are easy to acquire and the agent is easy to manufacture.

tertiary blast injury An injury from whole-body displacement and subsequent traumatic impact with environmental objects.

V agent (VX) One of the G agents; it is a clear, oily agent that has no odor and looks like baby oil; more than 100 times more lethal than sarin and is extremely persistent.

vapor hazard The danger posed by an agent that enters the body through the respiratory tract.

vesicants Blister agents; the primary route of exposure for this agent is through the skin.

viral hemorrhagic fevers (VHFs) A group of diseases caused by viruses that include the Ebola, Rift Valley, and yellow fever viruses, among others. This group of viruses causes the blood in the body to seep out from the tissues and blood vessels.

Prep Kit *(continued)*

viruses Germs that require a living host to multiply and survive.

volatility Describes how long a chemical agent will stay on a surface before it evaporates.

weapon of mass casualty (WMC) Any agent designed to bring about mass death, casualties, and/or massive damage to property and infrastructure (bridges, tunnels, airports, and seaports); also known as a weapon of mass destruction.

weapon of mass destruction (WMD) Any agent designed to bring about mass death, casualties, and/or massive damage to property and infrastructure (bridges, tunnels, airports, and seaports); also known as a weapon of mass casualty.

weaponization The creation of a weapon from a biologic agent generally found in nature and that causes disease; the agent is cultivated, synthesized, and/or mutated to maximize the target population's exposure to the germ.

▶ References

1. Definitions of terrorism in US code. Federal Bureau of Investigation website. https://www.fbi.gov/about-us/investigate/terrorism/terrorism-definition. Accessed August 30, 2016.
2. Cyber crime. Federal Bureau of Investigation website. https://www.fbi.gov/about-us/investigate/cyber. Accessed August 30, 2016.
3. Mowry JB, Spyker DA, Brooks DE, et al. 2014 Annual Report of the American Association of Poison Control Centers' National Poison Data System (NPDS): 32nd Annual Report. *Clinical Toxicology*. 2015;53(10):962-1147.
4. US Environmental Protection Agency. Agriculture 101. https://www.epa.gov/sites/production/files/2015-07/documents/ag_101_agriculture_us_epa_0.pdf. Accessed November 16, 2016.
5. Frequently asked questions and answers on smallpox. World Health Organization website. http://www.who.int/csr/disease/smallpox/faq/en/Updated June 28, 2016. Accessed November 2, 2016.
6. US Food and Drug Administration. *Vaccines, Blood and Biologics: Anthrax*. http://www.fda.gov/Biologics BloodVaccines/Vaccines/ucm061751.htm. Accessed November 17, 2016.
7. Russian roulette: a report on the safety and security of Russia's nuclear arsenal. Frontline Online website. http://www.pbs.org/wgbh/pages/frontline/shows/russia/suitcase/. Published February 1999. Accessed September 21, 2016.
8. National Association of Emergency Medical Technicians. *Prehospital Trauma Life Support*. 8th ed. Boston, MA: Jones & Bartlett Learning; 2016.
9. Explosions and blast injuries. Centers for Disease Control and Prevention website. http://www.cdc.gov/masstrauma/preparedness/primer.pdf. Accessed September 21, 2016.

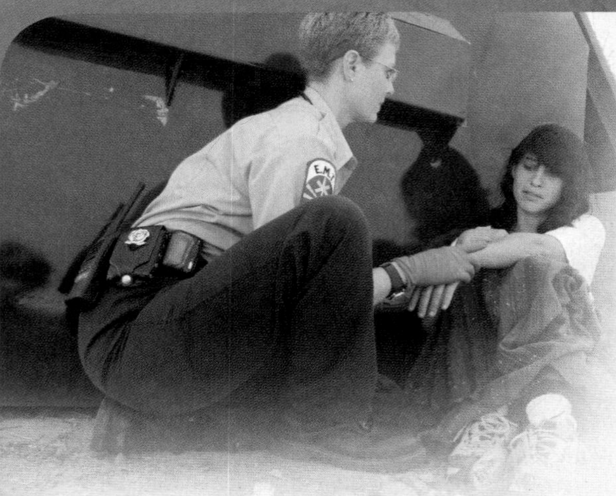

Assessment in Action

Your ambulance is the ninth ambulance dispatched to a reported terrorism incident involving nonaerosolized VX, a nerve agent. The incident commander advises that 39 patients have been triaged, and you are to report to the treatment sector to transport one "red" patient.

1. VX gas is an oily substance that has which characteristic odor?

A. Bitter almonds
B. Dandelions
C. Gasoline
D. No odor

2. The mnemonic DUMBELS is used to describe common nerve agent symptoms. The "M" stands for which of the following symptoms?

A. Minor signs and symptoms
B. Miosis
C. Mastication
D. Malfeasance

3. As you are transporting the patient to the hospital, he experiences a seizure. What is your next course of treatment?

A. Administer naloxone (Narcan) IV.
B. Administer an epinephrine auto-injector.
C. Administer a DuoDote Auto-Injector.
D. Administer epinephrine IV.

4. When do patients who have been exposed to nerve agents often develop signs and symptoms?

A. Immediately
B. After 2 to 4 hours
C. After 1 to 2 days
D. Up to weeks afterward

5. The difference between VX and GB is that VX is ______ times more lethal than GB and is extremely persistent.

A. 10
B. 100
C. 1000
D. 10,000

6. All of the following are true characteristics of VX EXCEPT:

A. it will remain relatively unchanged for weeks to months.
B. it is easily absorbed into the skin.
C. it has an oily residue.
D. it is a vapor hazard.

7. ________ are germs that require a living host to multiply and survive.

A. Disease vectors
B. Bacteria
C. Viruses
D. Neurotoxins

8. _______ is the monitoring of patients presenting to emergency departments and alternative care facilities, the recording of EMS call volume, and the use of over-the-counter medications.

A. Community surveillance
B. Syndromic surveillance
C. Medical monitoring
D. Invasion of privacy

Assessment *in Action* *(continued)*

9. The three best measures to take to protect yourself from radiation include time, distance, and which other component?

A. Protective clothing
B. Shielding
C. Age
D. Shelter

10. List the five types of blast injuries and differentiate among each.

11. What is a dirty bomb?

Glossary

abandonment Unilateral termination of emergency medical care by the AEMT without the patient's consent and without making provisions for transferring care to another medical professional with the skills and training necessary to meet the needs of the patient.

abdomen The body cavity that contains the major organs of digestion and excretion. It is located below the diaphragm and above the pelvis.

abdominal aortic aneurysm (AAA) A condition in which the walls of the aorta in the abdomen weaken and blood leaks into the layers of the vessel, causing it to bulge.

abdominal-thrust maneuver The preferred method to dislodge a severe airway obstruction in adults and children; also called the Heimlich maneuver.

abduction Movement of a limb *away* from the midline of the body.

ABO system The antigen classification given to blood.

abortion Delivery of the fetus and placenta before 20 weeks' gestation; a spontaneous abortion is called a miscarriage.

abrasion The loss or damage of the superficial layer of skin as a result of a body part rubbing or scraping across a rough or hard surface.

abruptio placenta Premature separation of the placenta from the wall of the uterus; also called placental abruption.

absence seizures The seizures that may be characterized by a brief lapse of attention in which the patient may stare and does not respond; formerly known as a petit mal seizure.

absorption In pharmacology, the process by which medications travel through body tissues until they reach the bloodstream; in allergic reactions, when foreign material is deposited on and moves into the skin.

acceleration Increase speed.

access Gaining entry to an enclosed area and reaching a patient.

access port A sealed hub on an administration set designed for sterile access to the intravenous fluid.

accessory muscles The secondary muscles of respiration that include the neck muscles (sternocleidomastoids), the chest pectoralis major muscles, and the abdominal muscles.

acetabulum The depression on the lateral pelvis where its three component bones join, in which the femoral head fits snugly.

acid A substance that increases the concentration of hydrogen ions in a solution.

acidosis A pathologic condition that results from the accumulation of acids in the body; an increase in extracellular H^+ ions; a blood pH of less than 7.35.

acquired immunity The immunity that occurs when the body is exposed to a foreign substance, antigen, or disease, and produces antibodies to the invader.

acquired immunodeficiency syndrome (AIDS) The end-stage disease process caused by the human immunodeficiency virus (HIV). A person with this disease process is extremely vulnerable to numerous infections.

acrocyanosis A decrease in the amount of oxygen delivered to the extremities. The hands and feet turn blue because of narrowing (constriction) of small arterioles (tiny arteries) toward the end of the arms and legs; can occur at any age; may be benign in infants younger than 2 months.

acromioclavicular (AC) separation One or more torn ligaments in the acromioclavicular joint, resulting in a separated shoulder.

acromion process The tip of the shoulder and the site of attachment for the clavicle and various shoulder muscles.

action The expected therapeutic effect of a medication on the body.

activation Mediators of inflammation trigger the appearance of molecules known as selectins and integrins on the surfaces of endothelial cells and polymorphonuclear neutrophils, respectively.

active compression-decompression CPR A technique that involves compressing the chest and then actively pulling it back up to its neutral position or beyond (decompression); may increase the amount of blood that returns to the heart and, thus, the amount of blood ejected from the heart during the compression phase.

active shooter A gunman who has begun to fire on people and is still at large.

active transport A method used to move compounds across a cell membrane to create or maintain an imbalance of charges.

activities of daily living (ADLs) The basic activities a person usually accomplishes during a normal day, such as eating, dressing, and washing.

acute abdomen A condition of sudden onset of pain within the abdomen, usually indicating peritonitis; demands immediate medical or surgical treatment.

acute chest syndrome A vaso-occlusive crisis that can be associated with pneumonia; common signs and symptoms include chest pain, fever, and cough.

acute coronary syndrome (ACS) A term used to describe a group of symptoms caused by myocardial ischemia; includes angina and myocardial infarction.

acute kidney injury A sudden decrease in filtration through the glomeruli of the kidneys.

acute myocardial infarction (AMI) Heart attack; death of heart muscle following obstruction of blood flow to it. Acute in this context means new or happening right now.

acute stress reactions Reactions to stress that occur during a stressful situation.

adduction Movement of a limb *toward* the midline of the body.

adenosine triphosphate (ATP) The nucleotide involved in energy metabolism; used to store energy.

adhesion The attachment of polymorphonuclear neutrophils to endothelial cells, mediated by selectins and integrins.

administration set Tubing that connects to the intravenous bag access port and the catheter to deliver the intravenous fluid.

adolescent A person age 12 to 18 years.

adrenal cortex The outer layer of the adrenal gland; it produces hormones that are important in regulating the water-and-salt balance of the body.

adrenal glands Endocrine glands located on top of the kidneys that release adrenaline when stimulated by the sympathetic nervous system.

adrenaline Hormone produced by the adrenal glands that mediates the "fight-or-flight" response of the sympathetic nervous system; also called epinephrine.

adrenergic Pertaining to nerves that release the neurotransmitter norepinephrine or noradrenaline; also pertains to the receptors acted on by norepinephrine.

adrenocorticotropic hormone (ACTH) Hormone that targets the adrenal cortex to secrete cortisol (a glucocorticoid).

adult protective services (APS) An organization that investigates cases involving abuse and neglect and provides case management services in some cases.

advance directive Written documentation that specifies medical treatment for a competent patient should the patient become unable to make decisions; see also *health care directive*.

advanced emergency medical technician (AEMT) An individual trained in specific aspects of advanced life support, such as intravenous therapy and administration of certain emergency medications.

advanced life support (ALS) Advanced life-saving procedures used to treat medical conditions, such as cardiac monitoring, administration of intravenous fluids and medications, and the use of advanced airway adjuncts. EMTs and AEMTs may be trained in some of these areas.

adventitious breath sounds Abnormal breath sounds that include crackles, rhonchi, wheezes, stridor, and pleural friction rubs.

aerobic metabolism The metabolism that takes place in the presence of oxygen.

affect The outward expression of a person's inner feelings (happy, sad, angry, fearful, withdrawn).

afterload The pressure in the aorta against which the left ventricle must pump blood; increasing this pressure can decrease cardiac output.

aging The process by which the temporary bond between an organophosphate and acetylcholinesterase undergoes hydrolysis, resulting in a permanent covalent bond.

agitated delirium An acute confrontational state characterized by global impairment of thinking, perception, judgment, and memory; also called excited delirium or exhaustive mania.

agonal gasps Occasional gasps that are ineffective attempts at breathing, occurring after the heart has stopped.

agonist A substance that mimics the actions of a specific neurotransmitter or hormone by binding to the specific receptor of the naturally occurring substance.

agoraphobia Literally, "fear of the marketplace"; fear of entering a public place from which escape may be impeded.

agranulocytes Leukocytes that lack granules.

air ambulances Fixed-wing aircraft (airplanes) and rotary-wing aircraft (helicopters) that have been modified for emergency medical care; used to evacuate and transport patients with life-threatening injuries to treatment facilities.

air embolism The presence of air in the venous circulation, which forms a gas bubble that can block the outflow of blood from the right ventricle to the lung; can lead to cardiac arrest, shock, or other life-threatening complications.

airborne transmission The spread of an infectious agent via droplets or dust.

airway The upper airway tract or the passage above the larynx, which includes the nose, mouth, and throat, and the lower airway, which includes the trachea and lungs. Also used to refer to devices used to open and maintain a patient's airway.

alcoholic ketoacidosis The metabolic acidotic state that manifests because of the inadequate nutritional habits associated with chronic alcohol abuse. The liver and body experience inadequate fuel reserves of glycogen and, thus, have to switch to fatty acid metabolism.

alcoholism A state of physical and psychological addiction to ethanol.

alkalosis A pathologic condition resulting from the accumulation of bases in the body; a decrease in extracellular H^+ ions; a blood pH greater than 7.45.

allergen A substance that causes an allergic reaction.

allergic reaction The body's exaggerated immune response to an internal or a surface antigen.

allergy A hypersensitivity reaction to the presence of an agent (allergen) that is intrinsically harmless.

alpha cells Cells located in the islets of Langerhans that secrete glucagon.

alpha effects Stimulation of alpha receptors that results in vasoconstriction.

alpha radiation A type of energy that is emitted from a strong radiologic source; it is the least harmful penetrating type of radiation and cannot travel more than a few inches or through most objects.

altered mental status Any deviation from alert and oriented to person, place, time, and event, or any deviation from a patient's normal baseline mental status; may signal disease in the central nervous system or other contributing factors.

alternative fuel vehicle A vehicle that uses anything other than a petroleum-based motor fuel (gasoline or diesel) to propel a motorized vehicle.

alveolar ducts Ducts formed from division of the respiratory bronchioles in the lower airway; each duct ends in clusters known as alveoli.

alveolar minute volume The volume of air moved through the lungs in 1 minute minus the dead space; calculated by multiplying tidal volume (minus dead space) and respiratory rate.

alveolar ventilation The volume of air that reaches the alveoli. It is determined by subtracting the amount of dead space air from the tidal volume.

alveoli The air sacs of the lungs in which the exchange of oxygen and carbon dioxide takes place.

alveolocapillary membrane The very thin membrane, consisting of only one cell layer, that lies between the alveolus and capillary, through which respiratory exchange between the alveolus and the blood vessels occurs.

ambient temperature The temperature of the surrounding environment.

ambulance A specialized vehicle for treating and transporting sick and injured patients.

amenorrhea Absence of menstruation.

American Standard System A safety system for oxygen cylinders larger than size E, designed to prevent the accidental attachment of a regulator to a cylinder containing the wrong type of gas.

Americans with Disabilities Act Comprehensive legislation that is designed to protect people with disabilities against discrimination.

amniotic fluid The fluid produced by the filtration of maternal and fetal blood through blood vessels in the placenta and by excretion of fetal urine into the amniotic sac.

amniotic fluid embolism An extremely rare, life-threatening condition that occurs when amniotic fluid and fetal cells enter the pregnant woman's pulmonary and circulatory system through the placenta via the umbilical veins, causing an exaggerated allergic response from the woman's body.

amniotic sac The fluid-filled, baglike membrane in which the fetus develops.

amphetamines A class of drugs that increase alertness and excitation (stimulants); includes methamphetamine (crank or ice), methylenedioxyamphetamine (MDA, Adam), and methylenedioxymethamphetamine (MDMA, Eve, Ecstasy).

ampules Small glass containers that are sealed and the contents sterilized.

amputation An injury in which part of the body is completely severed; complete avulsion.

anaerobic metabolism The metabolism that takes place in the absence of oxygen; the principal product is lactic acid.

analgesics A classification for medications that relieve pain or induce analgesia.

anaphylactic shock Severe shock caused by an allergic reaction; a severe hypersensitivity reaction that involves bronchoconstriction and cardiovascular collapse.

anaphylactoid reaction An extreme allergic response that does not involve immunoglobulin E (IgE) antibody mediation. The exact mechanism is unknown, but an anaphylactoid event may occur without the patient being previously exposed to the offending agent.

anaphylaxis An extreme, life-threatening, systemic allergic reaction to foreign protein or other substances, which may include shock and respiratory failure.

anatomic position The position of reference, in which the patient stands facing you, arms at the side, with the palms of the hands facing forward.

anatomy The study of the structure of an organism and its parts.

anemia A lower-than-normal hemoglobin or red blood cell level.

aneurysm A swelling or enlargement of a part of an artery, resulting from weakening of the arterial wall.

angina pectoris Transient (short-lived) chest discomfort caused by partial or temporary blockage of blood flow to the heart muscle.

angioedema Recurrent large areas of subcutaneous edema of sudden onset, often around the eyes and lips and usually disappearing within 24 hours, which is seen mainly in young women, frequently as a result of allergy to food or drugs.

angiogenesis The growth of new blood vessels.

angiotensin-converting enzyme (ACE) inhibitors Medications that suppress the conversion of angiotensin I to angiotensin II.

angulation In a fracture, when each end of the fracture is not aligned in a straight line and an angle has formed between them.

anion An ion that contains an overall negative charge.

anisocoria Uneven pupil size; can be naturally occurring, but also can be a sign of pathology.

anoxia An absence of oxygen.

antagonist Something that counteracts the action of something else; a drug of this type has an affinity for a cell receptor and, when it binds to that receptor, the cell is prevented from responding.

antecubital The anterior aspect of the elbow.

anterior The front surface of the body; the side facing you in the anatomic position.

anterograde (posttraumatic) amnesia Inability to remember events after an injury.

anteroposterior axis The axis that runs perpendicular to the coronal plane.

anthrax A disease caused by deadly bacteria (*Bacillus anthracis*) that lie dormant in a spore (protective shell); the germ is released from the spore when exposed to the optimal temperature and moisture. The routes of entry are inhalation, cutaneous, and gastrointestinal (from consuming food that contains spores).

antibody A protein secreted by certain immune cells that bind antigens to make them more visible to the immune system; an immunoglobulin.

anticholinergic Of or pertaining to blockage of acetylcholine receptors, resulting in inhibition of transmission of parasympathetic nerve impulses.

anticoagulant drugs The medications used to prevent intravascular thrombosis by preventing blood coagulation in the vascular system.

anticonvulsant medications The medications used to treat seizures, which are believed to work by inhibiting the influx of sodium into cells.

Antidote Treatment Nerve Agent Auto-Injector (ATNAA) The military form of a nerve agent antidote kit containing atropine and pralidoxime chloride; delivered as a single dose through one needle.

antidysrhythmic medications The medications used to treat and prevent cardiac rhythm disorders.

antigen An agent that, when taken into the body, stimulates the formation of specific protective proteins called antibodies.

antihypertensives The medications used to control blood pressure.

antiplatelet agents The medications that interfere with the collection of platelets.

antivenin A serum that counteracts the effect of venom from an animal or insect.

antonyms Pairs of word roots, prefixes, or suffixes that have opposite meanings.

anuria A complete halt in the production of urine.

anus The outlet of the rectum.

anxiety disorders Mental disorders in which the dominant mood is fear and apprehension.

anxious-avoidant attachment An insecure attachment observed in infants who are repeatedly rejected. Children develop an isolated lifestyle that does not depend on the support and care of others.

aorta The main artery that receives blood from the left ventricle and delivers it to all the other arteries that carry blood to the tissues of the body.

aortic aneurysm A weakness in the wall of the aorta that makes it susceptible to rupture.

aortic arch One of the three described portions of the aorta; the section of the aorta between the ascending and descending portions that gives rise to the right brachiocephalic (innominate), left common carotid, and left subclavian arteries.

aortic valve The one-way, semilunar valve that lies between the left ventricle and the aorta; keeps blood from flowing back into the left ventricle after the left ventricle ejects its blood into the aorta and is one of four heart valves.

apex (plural apices or apexes) The pointed extremity of a conical structure.

Apgar score system A scoring system for assessing the status of a newborn that assigns a number value to each of the five areas of assessment.

aphasia The inability to understand or produce speech.

apical pulse Obtained by auscultating heart tones over the chest with a stethoscope.

aplastic crisis A condition in which the body stops producing red blood cells; typically caused by infection.

apnea Absence of breathing; periods of not breathing.

apoptosis Normal, genetically programmed cell death.

appendicitis Inflammation of the appendix.

appendicular skeleton The portion of the skeletal system that comprises the arms, legs, pelvis, and shoulder girdle.

appendix A small, tubular structure that is attached to the lower border of the cecum in the lower right quadrant of the abdomen.

applied ethics The manner in which principles of ethics are incorporated into professional conduct.

aqueous humor The clear, watery fluid in the anterior chamber of the globe (eyeball).

arachnoid The middle membrane of the three meninges that enclose the brain and spinal cord.

areolar glands The glands that produce secretions that protect the nipple and areola during nursing.

arterial air embolism Air bubbles in the arterial blood vessels.

arterial rupture The rupture of an artery. Involvement of a cerebral artery may contribute to interruption of cerebral blood flow.

arteries Vessels of the circulatory system that carry oxygenated blood away from the heart.

arterioles The smallest branches of arteries leading to the vast network of capillaries.

arteriosclerosis The thickening of the arterial walls that results in a loss of elasticity and concomitant reduction in blood flow.

articulation (joint) The surfaces of long bones that come in contact with other bones.

artifact A tracing on an electrocardiogram that is the result of interference, such as patient movement, rather than the heart's electrical activity.

ascending aorta The first of three portions of the aorta; originates from the left ventricle and gives rise to two branches, the right and left main coronary arteries.

ascites The accumulation of serous fluid in the peritoneal cavity, typically signaling liver failure.

aseptic technique A method of cleansing used to prevent contamination of a site when performing an invasive procedure, such as inserting an intravenous line.

aspiration The inhalation of liquid or solid matter into the lungs through the trachea, typically as a result of an incompetent gag reflex or overaggressive resuscitation technique; may occur when the patient is unable to maintain his or her own airway and blood or fluid is present in the mouth.

assault Unlawfully placing a patient in fear of immediate bodily harm.

asthma A chronic inflammatory lower airway condition resulting in intermittent wheezing and excess mucus production; muscle spasm in the small air passageways and excess mucus result in airway obstruction.

asymmetric chest wall movement Unequal movement of the two sides of the chest; indicates decreased airflow into one lung.

asystole Complete absence of heart electrical activity.

ataxia A staggered walk or gait caused by injury to the brain or spinal cord.

ataxic respirations Irregular, ineffective respirations that may or may not have an identifiable pattern.

atelectasis A condition of airless or collapsed alveoli that causes pulmonary shunting, ventilation-perfusion mismatching, and possibly hypoxemia.

atherosclerosis A disorder in which cholesterol and possibly calcium build up inside the walls of blood vessels, forming plaque, which eventually leads to partial or complete blockage of blood flow; a plaque can become a site where blood clots can form, detach, and travel elsewhere in the circulatory system (embolize); the most common form of arteriosclerosis.

atlanto-occipital joint The location where the atlas articulates with the occipital condyles.

atlas The first cervical vertebra (C1), which provides support for the head.

atopic An allergic tendency.

atrioventricular (AV) node The site located in the right atrium adjacent to the septum that is responsible for transiently slowing electrical conduction.

atrioventricular valves The two valves through which blood flows from the atria to the ventricles.

atrium One of two (right and left) upper chambers of the heart.

atrophy A decrease in cell size due to a loss of subcellular components.

auditory ossicles The bones that function in hearing and are located deep within cavities of the temporal bone.

aura Sensations experienced before an attack occurs; common in seizures and migraine headaches.

auscultation A method of listening to sounds within an organ with a stethoscope.

autism spectrum disorder (ASD) A group of complex disorders of brain development, characterized by impairment of social interaction; may include severe behavioral problems, repetitive motor activities, and impairment in verbal and nonverbal skills.

autoantibodies Antibodies directed against the person's own proteins.

autoimmunity The production of antibodies or T cells that work against the tissues of a person's body, producing autoimmune disease or a hypersensitivity reaction.

automated external defibrillator A device that detects treatable life-threatening cardiac dysrhythmias (ventricular fibrillation and ventricular tachycardia) and delivers the appropriate electrical shock to the patient.

automatic transport ventilator (ATV) A mechanical ventilator that is used to ventilate intubated patients during transport; has settings for the tidal volume and ventilatory rate.

automaticity The ability of cardiac cells to generate an impulse to contract even when there is no external nervous stimulus.

autonomic nervous system (ANS) The part of the nervous system that regulates functions that are not controlled consciously, but rather involuntarily, such as heart rate, blood pressure, digestion, and sweating.

autoregulation An increase in mean arterial pressure to compensate for decreased cerebral perfusion pressure; a compensatory physiologic response that occurs in an effort to shunt blood to the brain; manifests clinically as hypertension.

AVPU scale A mnemonic to describe the method of assessing the level of consciousness by determining whether the patient is Awake and alert, responsive to Verbal stimuli or Pain, or Unresponsive; used principally early in the assessment process.

avulsion An injury in which soft tissue is torn completely loose or is hanging as a flap.

axial skeleton The part of the skeleton comprising the skull, spinal column, and rib cage.

axillary vein The vein that is formed from the combination of the basilic and cephalic veins; it drains into the subclavian vein.

axis The second cervical vertebra (C2); the point that allows the head to turn.

axon A long, slender extension of a neuron (nerve cell) that conducts electrical impulses away from the neuronal soma.

backboard A long, flat board made of rigid rectangular material that is used to provide support to a patient who is suspected of having a hip, pelvic, spinal, or lower extremity injury; also called a long backboard, spine board, trauma board, and longboard.

bacteria Single-cell microorganisms that rapidly reproduce by binary fission; some can form spores (encysted variants) when environmental conditions are harsh.

bacterial vaginosis An overgrowth of bacteria in the vagina, characterized by itching, burning, or pain, and possibly a "fishy" smelling discharge.

bag-mask device A device with a face mask attached to a ventilation bag containing a reservoir and connected to oxygen; delivers more than 90% supplemental oxygen.

ball-and-socket joint A joint that allows internal and external rotation, as well as bending.

barbiturates Any medications of a group of barbituric acid derivatives that act as central nervous system depressants and are used as sedatives or hypnotics; potent sedative-hypnotics historically used as sleep aids, as antianxiety drugs, and as part of the regimen for seizure control.

bariatrics A branch of medicine concerned with the management (prevention or control) of obesity and allied diseases.

barometric energy The energy that results from sudden changes in pressure as may occur in a diving accident or sudden decompression in an airplane.

baroreceptors Receptors in the blood vessels, kidneys, brain, and heart that respond to changes in pressure in the heart or main arteries to help maintain homeostasis.

barotrauma Results from a pressure imbalance between gas-filled spaces inside the body and the external atmosphere.

barrier device A protective item, such as a pocket mask with a valve, that limits exposure to a patient's body fluids.

basal ganglia Structures located deep within the cerebrum, diencephalon, and midbrain that have an important role in coordination of motor movements and posture.

base A substance that decreases the concentration of hydrogen ions.

base station Any radio hardware containing a transmitter and receiver that is located in a fixed place.

basic life support (BLS) Noninvasive emergency life-saving care used to treat medical conditions, including airway obstruction, respiratory arrest, and cardiac arrest.

basilar skull fracture Usually occurs following diffuse impact to the head (such as in falls, motor vehicle crashes); generally results from extension of a linear fracture to the base of the skull and can be difficult to diagnose with a radiograph (x-ray imaging).

basilic vein One of the two major veins of the arm; it combines with the cephalic vein to form the axillary vein.

basket stretcher A rigid stretcher commonly used in technical and water rescues that surrounds and supports the patient yet allows water to drain through holes in the bottom; also called a Stokes litter.

basophils White blood cells that work to produce chemical mediators during an immune response.

battery Unlawfully touching a patient or providing emergency medical care without consent.

Battle sign Bruising behind an ear over the mastoid process that may indicate a skull fracture.

behavior How a person functions or acts in response to his or her environment.

behavioral crisis The point at which a person's reactions to events interfere with activities of daily living; a behavioral crisis becomes a psychiatric emergency when it causes a major life interruption, such as attempted suicide.

bends Common name for decompression sickness.

benign prostate hypertrophy (BPH) Age-related nonmalignant (noncancerous) enlargement of the prostate gland.

benzodiazepines Sedative-hypnotic drugs that provide muscle relaxation and mild sedation, commonly used to treat anxiety, seizures, and alcohol withdrawal; includes drugs such as diazepam (Valium) and midazolam (Versed).

beta blocker A common class of cardiac drugs that blocks beta effects, causing a decrease in the workload of the heart by reducing the speed of contraction, as well as reducing blood pressure.

beta cells Cells located in the islets of Langerhans that secrete insulin.

beta effects Stimulation of beta receptors that results in inotropic, dromotropic, and chronotropic states.

beta radiation A type of energy that is emitted from a strong radiologic source; is slightly more penetrating than alpha radiation and requires a layer of clothing to stop it.

biceps The large muscle that covers the front of the humerus.

bilateral In anatomy, a body part or condition that appears on both sides of the midline.

bile ducts The ducts that convey bile between the liver and the intestine.

bilevel positive airway pressure (BPAP) A form of noninvasive positive pressure ventilation that delivers two pressures (a higher inspiratory positive airway pressure and a lower expiratory positive airway pressure).

bilirubin A waste product of red blood cell destruction that undergoes further metabolism in the liver.

bills of lading The shipping papers used for transport of chemicals over roads and highways; also referred to as freight bills.

bioavailability The rate at and extent to which an active drug enters the general circulation, permitting access to the site of action.

bioethics The study of ethics related to issues that arise in health care.

Biot respirations Characterized by an irregular rate, pattern, and volume of breathing with intermittent periods of apnea; also called ataxic respirations.

biotransformation The chemical alteration that a substance undergoes in the body.

bipolar mood disorder A disorder in which a person alternates between mania and depression.

birth canal The vagina and cervix.

blanching Turning white.

blast injuries Injuries resulting from explosions; possible injuries include internal injuries resulting from the pressure wave, penetrating trauma from shrapnel or from being thrown, blunt trauma from being thrown, and burns.

blast lung A severe pulmonary contusion, bleeding, or swelling with damage to the blood vessels and alveoli, or a combination of any or all of these.

blind spots Areas of the road that are blocked from the driver's sight by his or her own vehicle or mirrors.

blood The fluid that is pumped by the heart through the arteries, veins, and capillaries and consists of plasma and formed elements or cells, such as red blood cells, white blood cells, and platelets.

blood pressure The pressure that the blood exerts against the walls of the arteries as it passes through them.

bloodborne pathogens Pathogenic microorganisms that are present in human blood and can cause disease in humans. These pathogens include, but are not limited to, hepatitis B virus and human immunodeficiency virus (HIV).

blow-by oxygen A method of delivering oxygen by holding a face mask or similar device near the infant or child's face; used when a nonrebreathing mask is not tolerated.

blowout fracture A fracture of the orbit or of the bones that support the floor of the orbit.

blunt trauma Result of force (or energy transmission) to impact on the body that causes injury without penetrating soft tissues or internal organs and cavities.

B-NICE A mnemonic to recall the types of weapons of mass destruction: Biologic, Nuclear, Incendiary, Chemical, and Explosive; see also *CBRNE*.

Boerhaave syndrome Forceful vomiting that results in a tear in the esophagus that extends entirely through the esophageal wall, creating a hole.

bolus A term used to describe "in one mass"; in medication administration, a single dose given by the intravenous route; may be a small or large quantity of the drug.

bonding The formation of a close, personal relationship.

Bone Injection Gun (BIG) A spring-loaded device that is used for inserting an intraosseous needle into the proximal tibia in adult and pediatric patients.

bone marrow A substance that manufactures most red blood cells.

botulinum Produced by bacteria; when introduced into the body, this most potent of neurotoxins affects the ability of the nervous system to function and causes botulism.

botulism Poisoning characterized by severe muscle paralysis and usually caused by eating food containing botulinum toxin.

Bourdon-gauge flowmeter An oxygen flowmeter that is commonly used because it is not affected by gravity and can be placed in any position.

brachial artery The major vessel in the upper extremity that supplies blood to the arm.

bradycardia A slow heart rate; less than 60 beats/min in adults; less than 80 beats/min in children; and less than 100 beats/min in infants.

bradypnea Slow respiratory rate; ominous sign in a child; indicates impending respiratory arrest.

brain The controlling organ of the body and center of consciousness; functions include perception, control of reactions to the environment, emotional responses, and judgment.

brainstem The area of the brain between the spinal cord and cerebrum, surrounded by the cerebellum; controls functions that are necessary for life, such as respiration and cardiac system functions.

Braxton-Hicks contractions Intermittent uterine contractions that may occur every 10 to 20 minutes, usually seen in the third trimester of the pregnancy, but which are not indicative of labor beginning or occurring; also known as false labor.

breach of confidentiality Disclosure of medical information without proper authorization.

breach of duty Occurs when a person accused of negligence fails to act as another person with similar training would act under the same or similar circumstances.

breath sounds An indication of air movement in the lungs, usually assessed with a stethoscope.

breath-holding syncope Loss of consciousness caused by a decreased breathing stimulus.

breech presentation A type of abnormal delivery in which the buttocks emerge first.

brief resolved unexplained event (BRUE) An event that causes unresponsiveness, cyanosis, and apnea in an infant, who then resumes breathing with stimulation.

bronchial breath sounds Normal breath sounds made by air moving through the bronchi.

bronchioles Fine subdivisions of the bronchi made of smooth muscle that give rise to the alveolar ducts.

bronchiolitis Inflammation of the bronchioles that usually occurs in children younger than 2 years and is often caused by the respiratory syncytial virus.

bronchospasm Constriction of the airway passages of the lungs that accompanies muscle spasms.

bronchovesicular sounds Soft, breezy, and low-pitched normal breath sounds found at the midclavicular line.

bruit An abnormal "whooshinglike" sound indicating turbulent blood flow within a blood vessel.

buboes Enlarged lymph nodes (up to the size of a tennis ball) that are characteristic in people infected with the bubonic plague.

bubonic plague Bacterial infection that affects the lymphatic system; it is transmitted by infected rodents and fleas and characterized by acute malaise, fever, and the formation of tender, enlarged, inflamed lymph nodes that appear as lesions. Also called the Black Death.

buccal A medication route in which the medication is placed between the cheek and gums, where it is absorbed into the bloodstream.

buddy splinting Securing an injured finger or toe to an adjacent uninjured one to allow the intact digit to act as a splint.

buffer A substance or group of substances that controls the hydrogen levels in a solution.

buffer system Fast-acting defenses for acid-base changes, providing almost immediate protection against changes in the hydrogen ion concentration of extracellular fluid.

bulk storage containers Any container other than nonbulky storage containers such as fixed tanks, highway cargo tanks, rail tank cars, totes, and intermodal tanks. These are typically found in manufacturing facilities and are often surrounded by a secondary containment system to help control an accidental release.

bundle of His Part of the conduction system of the heart; a continuation of the atrioventricular node.

burnout A state of exhaustion of physical or emotional strength, which may be a consequence of chronic, unrelieved stress.

burns Injuries in which the soft tissue receives more energy than it can absorb without injury, from thermal heat, frictional heat, toxic chemicals, electricity, or nuclear radiation.

bursa A small fluid-filled sac located between a tendon and a bone that cushions and protects the joint.

butterfly catheters Rigid, hollow, venous cannulation devices identified by plastic "wings" that act as anchoring points for securing the catheter.

calcitonin A hormone produced by the parafollicular cells of the thyroid gland that is important in the regulation of calcium levels in the body.

calcium channel blockers The medications that suppress dysrhythmias, provide more oxygen to the heart via coronary artery dilation, and reduce peripheral vascular resistance.

cancellous bone A type of bone that consists of a lacy network of bony rods called trabeculae.

cannulation The insertion of a hollow tube into a vein to allow for fluid flow.

capillaries Microscopic, thin-walled blood vessels between the arterioles and venules through which oxygen, carbon dioxide, nutrients, and waste products are exchanged between body tissues and the blood.

capillary beds The terminal ends of the vascular system where fluids, food, and wastes are exchanged between the vascular system and the cells of the body.

capillary refill A test that evaluates distal circulatory system function by squeezing (blanching) blood from an area such as a nail bed and watching the speed of its return after releasing the pressure.

capillary refill time The amount of time that it takes for blood to return to the capillary bed after applying pressure to the skin or nail bed; indicates the status of end-organ perfusion; reliable in children younger than 6 years.

capnographer A device that attaches between the endotracheal tube and ventilation device; provides graphic information about the presence of exhaled carbon dioxide.

capnography A noninvasive method that can quickly and efficiently provide information on a patient's ventilatory status, circulation, and metabolism; effectively measures the concentration of carbon dioxide in expired air over time.

capnometer A device that performs the same function and attaches in the same way as a capnographer but provides a digital reading of the exhaled carbon dioxide.

capnometry The use of a capnometer, a device that measures the amount of expired carbon dioxide.

carbon dioxide (CO_2) A component that typically makes up 0.3% of air at sea level; also a waste product exhaled during expiration by the respiratory system.

carbon dioxide retention A condition characterized by a chronically high level of carbon dioxide in blood as the result of a respiratory disease.

carbon monoxide (CO) An odorless, highly poisonous gas that results from the incomplete oxidation of carbon during combustion.

carboys Glass, plastic, or steel containers, ranging in volume from 5 to 15 gallons (19 to 57 L).

cardiac arrest A state in which the heart fails to generate an effective and detectable blood flow; pulses are not palpable in cardiac arrest, even if muscular and electrical activity continues in the heart.

cardiac cycle The repetitive pumping process that begins with the onset of cardiac muscle contraction and ends just before the beginning of the next contraction.

cardiac glycosides A classification of medications that naturally occur in plant substances and that block certain ionic pumps in the membranes of heart cells, which indirectly increases calcium concentrations; an example is digoxin.

cardiac muscle The heart muscle.

cardiac output (CO) The amount of blood pumped by the heart per minute; calculated by multiplying the stroke volume by the pulse rate per minute.

cardiac tamponade Compression of the heart caused by a buildup of blood or other fluid in the pericardial sac.

cardiogenic shock Shock caused by inadequate function of the heart, or pump failure; caused by loss of 40% or more of the functioning myocardium; the heart is no longer able to circulate sufficient blood to maintain adequate oxygen delivery; can be a severe complication of a large acute myocardial infarction, as well as other conditions.

cardiopulmonary resuscitation (CPR) The combination of chest compressions and rescue breathing used to establish adequate ventilation and circulation in a patient who is not breathing and has no pulse.

carina Point at which the trachea bifurcates (divides) into the left and right mainstem bronchi.

carotid artery The major artery that supplies blood to the head and brain.

carpometacarpal joint The joint between the wrist and the metacarpal bones; the thumb joint.

carpopedal spasm A contorted position of the hand or foot in which the fingers or toes flex in a clawlike manner; may result from hyperventilation or hypocalcemia.

cartilage The support structure of the skeletal system that provides cushioning between bones; also forms the nasal septum and portions of the outer ear.

casualty collection area An area set up by physicians, nurses, and other hospital staff near a major disaster or mass-casualty incident scene where patients can receive further triage and medical care.

cataract Clouding of the lens of the eye or its surrounding transparent membrane.

catecholamines Hormones produced by the adrenal medulla (epinephrine and norepinephrine) that assist the body in coping with physical and emotional stress by increasing the heart and respiratory rates and the blood pressure.

catheter A flexible, hollow structure that delivers fluid.

catheter shear A free-floating segment of a catheter in the circulatory system, created if the needle slices through the catheter while it is being inserted.

cation An ion that contains an overall positive charge.

cauda equina The location where the spinal cord separates; composed of nerve roots.

caustics Chemicals that are acids or alkalis; they cause direct chemical injury to the tissues they contact.

cavitation Formation of a temporary cavity that is produced by stretching of the tissue surrounding the point of impact—for example, when speed causes a bullet to generate pressure waves, which cause damage distant from the bullet's path.

CBRNE A mnemonic used to recall the types of weapons of mass destruction: Chemical, Biologic, Radiologic, Nuclear, and Explosive; see also *B-NICE*.

cecum The first part of the large intestine, into which the ileum opens.

cell-mediated immunity The immune process by which T-cell lymphocytes recognize antigens and then secrete cytokines (specifically lymphokines) that attract other cells or stimulate the production of cytotoxic cells that kill the infected cells.

cell membrane The cell wall; the cell membrane is selectively permeable.

cell phone A low-power portable radio that communicates through an interconnected series of repeater stations called cells.

cellular immunity The immunity provided by special white blood cells called T cells that attack and destroy invaders.

cellular perfusion The ability of a cell to take in oxygen and remove carbon dioxide.

cellular respiration A biochemical process resulting in the production of energy in the form of adenosine triphosphate.

Centers for Disease Control and Prevention (CDC) The primary federal agency that conducts and supports public health activities in the United States; part of the US Department of Health and Human Services.

central cyanosis Cyanosis to the newborn's face and trunk; indicates hypoxia.

central nervous system (CNS) The brain and spinal cord.

central neurogenic hyperventilation Deep, rapid respirations; similar to Kussmaul, but without an acetone breath odor; commonly seen following brainstem injury.

central pulses Pulses that are closest to the core (central) part of the body where the vital organs are located.

central shock A type of shock caused by central pump failure, including cardiogenic shock and obstructive shock.

central vision The visualization of objects directly in front of you.

cerebellum One of the three major subdivisions of the brain, sometimes called the little brain; coordinates the various activities of the brain, particularly fine body movements.

cerebral contusion A focal brain injury in which brain tissue is bruised and damaged in a defined area.

cerebral cortex The largest portion of the cerebrum; regulates voluntary skeletal movement and a person's level of awareness—a part of consciousness.

cerebral edema Swelling of the brain.

cerebral embolism Obstruction of a cerebral artery caused by a clot that was formed elsewhere in the body and traveled to the brain.

cerebral palsy A group of disorders characterized by poorly controlled body movement.

cerebral perfusion pressure (CPP) The pressure of blood flow through the brain; the difference between the mean arterial pressure (MAP) and intracranial pressure (ICP).

cerebrospinal fluid (CSF) Fluid produced in the ventricles of the brain that flows in the subarachnoid space and bathes the meninges.

cerebrovascular accident (CVA) Interruption of blood flow to the brain that results in the loss of brain function; also referred to as a stroke or brain attack.

cerebrum The largest part of the three subdivisions of the brain, sometimes called the gray matter; made up of several lobes that control movement, hearing, balance, speech, visual perception, emotions, and personality.

certification A process in which a person, an institution, or a program is evaluated and recognized as meeting certain predetermined standards to provide safe and ethical patient care.

cervical spine The portion of the spinal column consisting of the first seven vertebrae that lie in the neck.

cervix The lower third, or neck, of the uterus.

chancroid A highly contagious sexually transmitted disease caused by the bacteria *Haemophilus ducreyi*, which causes painful sores (ulcers), usually of the genitals.

channel An assigned frequency or frequencies that are used to carry voice and/or data communications.

chassis The structural framework of the ambulance.

chassis set The transfer of weight (center of mass) to different points on the chassis.

chemical energy The energy released as a result of a chemical reaction.

chemical mediators Chemicals that work to cause the immune or allergic response—for example, histamines.

chemical name Precise description of a drug's chemical composition and molecular structure.

chemical suicide A method of suicide that involves mixing certain household chemicals in an enclosed space to create toxic gases, such as hydrogen sulfide and hydrogen cyanide, as the chemicals combine; also called detergent suicide.

Chemical Transportation Emergency Center (CHEMTREC) An agency that assists emergency responders in identifying and handling hazardous materials incidents.

chemoreceptors Receptors in the blood vessels, kidneys, brain, and heart that respond to changes in chemical composition of the blood to help maintain homeostasis.

chemotaxins Components of the activated complement system that attract leukocytes from the circulation to help fight infections.

chemotaxis The movement of additional white blood cells to an area of inflammation in response to the release of chemical mediators, such as neutrophils, injured tissue, and monocytes.

chest compression fraction The total percentage of time during a resuscitation attempt in which active chest compressions are being performed.

Cheyne-Stokes respirations The respirations that are fast and then become slow, with intervening periods of apnea; commonly seen following brainstem injury.

chief complaint The reason a patient called for emergency medical services; also, the patient's response to questions such as "What's wrong?" or "What happened?"

child abuse Any improper or excessive action that injures or otherwise harms a child or infant; includes physical abuse, sexual abuse, neglect, and emotional abuse.

chlamydia A sexually transmitted disease caused by the bacterium *Chlamydia trachomatis*.

chlorine (Cl) The first chemical agent ever used in warfare; it has a distinct odor of bleach and creates a green haze when released as a gas. Initially it produces upper airway irritation and a choking sensation.

cholecystitis Inflammation of the gallbladder.

cholinergic Fibers in the parasympathetic nervous system that release a chemical called acetylcholine.

chordae tendineae Thin bands of fibrous tissue that attach to the valves in the heart and prevent them from inverting, preventing regurgitation of blood through the valves from the ventricles to the atria.

choroid plexus Specialized cells within hollow areas in the ventricles of the brain that produce cerebrospinal fluid.

chromosomes Structures formed from condensed fibers and protein of deoxyribonucleic acid; they are threadlike and are contained within the nucleus of the cells.

chronic bronchitis Irritation and inflammation of the major lung passageways, from either infectious disease or irritants such as smoke.

chronic hypertension A blood pressure that is equal to or greater than 130/80 mm Hg, which exists prior to pregnancy, occurs before the 20th week of pregnancy, or persists postpartum.

chronic kidney disease Progressive and irreversible inadequate kidney function as a result of permanent loss of nephrons.

chronic obstructive pulmonary disease (COPD) A slow, progressive, degenerative, irreversible disease of the airway that causes destructive changes in the alveoli and bronchioles in the lungs.

chronotropic effect Affecting the rate of contraction of the heart.

chronotropic state Related to the control of the heart's rate of contraction.

chyme The name of the substance that leaves the stomach; a combination of eaten foods with added stomach acids.

circulatory system The complex arrangement of connected tubes, including the arteries, arterioles, capillaries, venules, and veins, that moves blood, oxygen, nutrients, carbon dioxide, and cellular waste throughout the body.

circumflex coronary artery One of the two branches of the left main coronary artery.

circumstantial thinking Situation in which the patient includes many irrelevant details in his or her account of things.

civil lawsuit An action instituted by a person or entity against another person or entity.

clavicle The collarbone; it is lateral to the sternum and anterior to the scapula.

cleaning The process of removing dirt, dust, blood, or other visible contaminants from a surface.

clitoris Located in the anterior margin of the vestibule and partially hidden by the labia minora, it contains erectile tissue that becomes engorged with blood as a result of sexual excitement.

clonic phase Seizure movement marked by repetitive muscle contractions and relaxations in rapid succession.

closed abdominal injury An injury in which there is soft-tissue damage inside the body but the skin remains intact.

closed chest injury An injury to the chest in which the skin is not broken, usually from blunt trauma.

closed fracture A fracture in which the skin is not broken.

closed head injury An injury in which the brain has been injured but the skin has not been broken and there is no bleeding.

closed incident An incident that is contained; all casualties are accounted for.

closed injury An injury in which damage occurs beneath the skin or mucous membrane but the surface remains intact.

closed-ended questions Questions that can be answered in short or single-word responses.

clotting factors Substances in the blood that are necessary for clotting; also called coagulation factors.

coagulation system The system that forms blood clots in the body and facilitates repairs to the vascular tree.

coagulopathy Any type of bleeding disorder that interferes with the activation or continuation of the clotting cascade or hemostasis.

Cobra perilaryngeal airway (CobraPLA) A supraglottic airway device with a shape that allows the device to slide easily along the hard palate and to hold the soft tissue away from the laryngeal inlet.

coccyx The last three to five vertebrae of the spine; the tailbone.

coefficient of friction A measure of the grip of the tires on the road.

cold zone A safe area at a hazardous materials incident for the agencies involved in the operations. The incident commander, the command post, EMS providers, and other support functions necessary to control the incident should be located in this zone. Also referred to as the clean zone or the support zone.

colic Acute, intermittent, cramping abdominal pain.

colloid solution A type of intravenous solution that contains compounds that are too large to pass out of the capillary membranes and therefore remain in the vascular compartment; for example, used to help reduce edema.

colorimetric carbon dioxide detector A device that attaches between the endotracheal tube and ventilation device; uses special paper that should turn from purple to yellow during exhalation, indicating the presence of exhaled carbon dioxide.

colorimetric devices End-tidal carbon dioxide detectors that use a chemical reaction to detect the amount of carbon dioxide present in expired gases.

colostomy The surgical procedure to create an opening (stoma) between the colon and the surface of the body to provide drainage of the bowel.

coma A state in which a person does not respond to either verbal or painful stimuli.

combining form A word root followed by a vowel.

combining vowel The vowel used to combine two word roots or a word root and a prefix or suffix.

Combitube A dual-lumen airway device that is inserted blindly; permits ventilation of the patient whether the tube is placed in the esophagus or the trachea.

command In incident command, the position(s) that oversees the incident, establishes the objectives and priorities, and develops a response plan; functions may include a public information officer, safety officer, and liaison officer.

command post The designated field command center where the incident commander and support staff are located.

common cold A viral infection usually associated with swollen nasal mucous membranes and the production of fluid from the sinuses.

commotio cordis An event in which an often fatal cardiac dysrhythmia is produced by a sudden blow to the thoracic cavity.

communicable disease A disease that can be spread from one person or species to another.

communication The transmission of information to another person—verbally or through body language.

community paramedicine A health care model in which experienced paramedics receive advanced training to allow them to provide additional services in the prehospital environment, such as health evaluations, monitoring of chronic illnesses or conditions, and patient advocacy.

compartment syndrome An elevation of pressure within the fascial compartment, characterized by extreme pain, decreased pain sensation, pain on stretching of affected muscles, and decreased power; most frequently seen in fractures below the elbow or knee in children.

compensated shock The early stage of shock, in which the body can still compensate for blood loss; also called nonprogressive shock.

compensatory damages Compensation awarded in a civil lawsuit that is intended to restore the plaintiff to the same condition that he or she was in prior to the incident.

competent Able to make rational decisions about personal well-being.

complement system A group of plasma proteins whose function is to do one of three things: attract leukocytes to sites of inflammation, activate leukocytes, and directly destroy cells.

complete abortion The expulsion of all products of conception from the uterus.

complex access Entry that requires special tools and training and includes the use of force.

complex partial seizures The seizures that involve subtle changes in the level of consciousness that may include confusion, reduced alertness, hallucinations, and inability to speak.

compound fracture An open fracture; a fracture beneath an open wound.

compound word A word containing more than one word root.

compulsions Repetitive actions carried out to relieve the anxiety of obsessive thoughts.

computer-aided dispatch (CAD) Linked dispatch center computer consoles and vehicle-mounted mobile data terminals in which a computer collects and manages the call information and makes recommendations for which emergency medical services unit is closest based on existing dispatch policy.

concealment The use of objects to limit a person's visibility of you.

concentration The total weight of a drug contained in a specific volume of liquid.

concentration gradient The natural tendency for substances to flow from an area of higher concentration to an area of lower concentration, either within the cell or outside the cell.

concussion A temporary loss or alteration of part or all of the brain's abilities to function without actual physical damage to the brain.

conduction The loss of heat by direct contact (eg, when a body part comes into contact with a colder object).

conduction system A group of complex electrical tissues within the heart that initiate and transmit stimuli that result in contractions of myocardial tissue.

conductive hearing loss Hearing loss caused by a faulty transmission of sound waves.

conductivity The ability of the cardiac cells to conduct electrical impulses.

confabulation The invention of experiences to cover gaps in memory, seen in patients with certain organic brain syndromes.

conjunctiva The delicate membrane that lines the eyelids and covers the anterior exposed surface of the eye.

conjunctivitis Inflammation of the conjunctiva.

connecting nerves The nerves in the brain and spinal cord that connect the motor and sensory nerves.

Consensus formula A formula that recommends giving 2 to 4 mL of lactated Ringer solution for each kilogram of body weight, multiplied by the percentage of total body surface area burned during the first 24 hours following the burn; one-half of the volume is given in the first 8 hours and the other half in the next 16 hours; sometimes used to calculate fluid needs during lengthy transport times; formerly called the Parkland formula.

consent Permission to render emergency medical care.

contact burn A burn produced by touching a hot object.

contact hazard The danger posed by an agent whose primary route of exposure is through the skin; also called a skin hazard.

contagious An infectious disease that can be transmitted to another; communicable.

container Any vessel or receptacle that holds material, including storage vessels, pipelines, and packaging.

contaminated stick The puncturing of an emergency care provider's skin with a catheter that was used on a patient.

contamination The presence of infectious organisms (pathogens) or foreign bodies such as dirt, gravel, or metal in a wound.

continuous positive airway pressure (CPAP) A method of ventilation used primarily in the treatment of critically ill patients with respiratory distress; can prevent the need for endotracheal intubation.

continuous quality improvement (CQI) A system of internal and external reviews and audits of all aspects of an emergency medical services system.

contractility The strength of heart muscle contraction.

contraindications Situations in which a medication should not be given because it would not help or may actually harm a patient.

contralateral On the opposite side of the body.

control zones Areas at a hazardous materials incident that are designated as hot, warm, or cold, based on safety issues and the degree of hazard found there.

contusion A bruise without a break in the skin; ecchymosis.

convection The loss of body heat caused by air movement (eg, breeze blowing across the body).

conventional reasoning A type of reasoning in which a child looks for approval from peers and society.

core temperature The temperature of the central part of the body (eg, the heart, lungs, and vital organs).

cornea The transparent tissue layer in front of the pupil and iris of the eye.

coronal plane An imaginary plane in which the body is cut into front and back portions.

coronary arteries Arteries that arise from the aorta shortly after it leaves the left ventricle and supply the heart with oxygen and nutrients.

coronary artery disease The condition that results when atherosclerosis or arteriosclerosis is present in the arterial walls.

coronary sinus The end of the great cardiac vein that collects blood returning from the walls of the heart.

corpus luteum The remnants of an unfertilized ovum that are sloughed during menstruation.

corticosteroids Any of several steroids secreted by the adrenal gland.

cortisol Hormone that stimulates most body cells to increase their energy production.

coup-contrecoup injury Occurs when the brain continues its forward motion and strikes the inside of the skull, resulting in a compression injury to the anterior portion of the brain and stretching of the posterior portion.

cover The tactical use of an impenetrable barrier for protection.

covert An act in which the public safety community generally has no prior knowledge of the time, location, or nature of the attack.

CPR board A device that provides a firm surface under the patient's torso.

crackles Crackling, moist breath sounds signaling fluid in the smaller air passages of the lungs; formerly called rales.

cranial nerves The 12 pairs of nerves that arise from the base of the brain.

cranial vault The bones that encase and protect the brain, including the parietal, temporal, frontal, occipital, sphenoid, and ethmoid bones.

craniofacial disjunction A Le Fort III fracture; involves a fracture of all of the midfacial bones, thereby separating the entire midface from the cranium.

cranium The area of the head above the ears and eyes; the skull. The cranium contains the brain.

credentialing An established process to determine the qualifications necessary to be allowed to practice a particular profession, or to function as an organization.

crenation Shrinkage of a cell that results when too much water leaves the cell through osmosis.

crepitus A grating or grinding sensation caused by fractured bone ends or joints rubbing together; also, air bubbles under the skin that produce a crackling sound or crinkly feeling.

crew resource management (CRM) A way for team members to work together with the team leader to develop and maintain a shared understanding of the emergency situation; to collaborate and communicate, fulfill their roles and responsibilities, and achieve the shared goal of the best possible patient outcome.

cribriform plate A horizontal bone perforated with numerous foramina for the passage of the olfactory nerve filaments from the nasal cavity.

cricoid cartilage A firm ridge of cartilage that forms the lower part of the larynx.

cricothyroid membrane A thin sheet of fascia that connects the thyroid and cricoid cartilages that make up the larynx.

criminal prosecution An action instituted by the government against a person for violation of criminal law.

crista galli A prominent bony ridge in the center of the anterior fossa to which the meninges are attached.

critical incident stress management (CISM) A process that confronts the responses to critical incidents and defuses them, directing the emergency services personnel toward physical and emotional equilibrium.

Crohn disease Inflammation of the ileum and possibly other portions of the gastrointestinal tract, in which the immune system attacks portions of the intestinal walls, causing them to become scarred, narrowed, stiff, and weakened.

cross section The product of slicing an object crosswise, perpendicular to its long axis.

cross-contamination Occurs when a person is contaminated by an agent as a result of coming into contact with another contaminated person.

cross-tolerance A tolerance to a particular drug that crosses over to other drugs in the same class.

croup An infectious disease of the upper respiratory system, usually caused by a virus, that may cause partial airway obstruction and is characterized by a barking cough; usually seen in children; also referred to as laryngotracheobronchitis.

crowning The appearance of the newborn's head at the vaginal opening during labor.

crush syndrome Significant metabolic derangement that develops when crushed extremities or body parts remain trapped for prolonged periods; it can lead to renal failure and death.

crystalloid solution A type of intravenous solution that contains compounds that quickly disassociate in solution and can cross membranes; considered the best choice for prehospital care of injured patients who need fluids to replace lost body fluid.

Cullen sign A black-and-blue discoloration (ecchymosis) in the umbilical region caused by peritoneal bleeding.

cultural imposition When one person imposes his or her beliefs, values, and practices on another because he or she believes his or her ideals are superior.

cumulative effect Action of increased intensity after administration of several doses of a drug.

cumulative stress reactions Exposure to prolonged or excessive stress.

Cushing triad Hypertension (with a widening pulse pressure), bradycardia, and irregular respirations; classic trio of findings associated with increased intracranial pressure.

cushion of safety A defensive driving technique used to keep a safe distance between the ambulance and other vehicles on any side of the ambulance.

cyanide A colorless gas that affects the body's ability to use oxygen; it has an odor similar to almonds. The effects begin on the cellular level and are rapidly seen at the organ and system levels.

cyanosis A blue-gray skin color that is caused by a reduced level of oxygen in the blood.

cylinders Portable, compressed gas containers used to hold liquids and gases such as nitrogen, argon, helium, and oxygen. They have a range of sizes and internal pressures.

cystic fibrosis (CF) A genetic disorder of the endocrine system that makes it difficult for chloride to move through the cells; characterized by increased production of mucus in the lungs and digestive system; also called mucoviscidosis.

cystitis Another name for urinary tract infection.

cytokines The products of cells that affect the function of other cells.

cytomegalovirus (CMV) A herpesvirus that can produce the symptoms of prolonged high fever, chills, headache, malaise, extreme fatigue, and an enlarged spleen.

D_5W An intravenous solution made up of 5% dextrose in water.

damages Compensation for injury; awarded by a court.

danger zone An area where people can be exposed to hazards such as electric wires, sharp metal edges, broken glass, toxic substances, radiation, or ignition or explosion of hazardous materials.

DCAP-BTLS A mnemonic for assessment in which each area of the body is evaluated for Deformities, Contusions,

Abrasions, Punctures/penetrations, Burns, Tenderness, Lacerations, and Swelling.

dead space Any portion of the airway that does contain air and cannot participate in gas exchange, such as the trachea and bronchi.

decay A natural process in which a material that is unstable attempts to stabilize itself by changing its structure.

deceleration The slowing of an object.

decerebrate (extensor) posturing A posture characterized by extension of the arms and legs, in which the arms rotate in a palms-down manner and the toes point; indicates pressure on the brainstem and may appear in patients with severe brain trauma.

decision-making capacity The ability to understand and process information and make a choice regarding appropriate medical care.

decompensated shock The late stage of shock when blood pressure is falling; also called progressive shock.

decompression sickness A painful condition seen in divers who ascend too quickly, in which gas, especially nitrogen, forms bubbles in blood vessels and other tissues; also called the bends.

decontaminated To have removed or neutralized radiation, chemical, or other hazardous material from clothing, equipment, vehicles, and personnel.

decontamination The process of removing or neutralizing and properly disposing of hazardous materials from equipment, patients, and responders.

decontamination area The designated area in a hazardous materials incident where all patients and responders must be decontaminated before going to another area.

decorticate (flexor) posturing A posture characterized by flexion of the arms and extension of the legs, in which the arms flex and curl toward the chest, the wrists flex, and the toes point; indicates pressure on the brainstem and may appear in patients with severe brain trauma.

decubitus ulcers Ulcers that occur when pressure is applied to body tissue, resulting in a lack of perfusion and ultimately necrosis.

dedicated line A special telephone line that is used for specific point-to-point communications; also known as a hotline.

deep Farther inside the body and away from the skin.

deep fascia A dense layer of fibrous tissue below the subcutaneous tissue; composed of tough bands of tissue that surround muscles and other internal structures.

deep vein thrombosis (DVT) The formation of a blood clot within the larger veins of an extremity, typically following a period of prolonged immobilization.

defamation The communication of false information about a person that is damaging to that person's reputation or standing in the community.

defendant In a civil lawsuit, the person against whom a legal action is brought.

defibrillate To shock a fibrillating (chaotically beating) heart with specialized electrical current in an attempt to restore a normal rhythmic beat.

delayed stress reactions Reactions to stress that occur after a stressful situation.

delirium An acute change in mental status marked by the inability to focus, think logically, and maintain attention.

delirium tremens (DTs) A severe withdrawal syndrome seen in people with alcoholism who are deprived of ethyl alcohol, which is characterized by restlessness, fever, sweating, disorientation, agitation, and seizures; it can be fatal if untreated.

delusions Fixed beliefs that are not shared by others of a person's culture or background and that cannot be changed by reasonable argument; false beliefs.

dementia The slow onset of progressive disorientation, shortened attention span, and loss of cognitive function.

demobilization The process of directing responders to return to their facilities when their work at an incident has finished.

dependent edema Swelling in the part of the body closest to the ground, caused by collection of fluid in the tissues; a possible sign of congestive heart failure.

dependent lividity Blood settling to the lowest point of the body, causing discoloration of the skin; a definitive sign of death.

dependent living A type of care in which a person receives assistance based on his or her needs or restrictions; can range from the least restrictive retirement community to the structured skilled nursing facility and dementia/Alzheimer disease specialty care facilities. Sometimes known as residential.

depolarization The rapid movement of electrolytes across a cell membrane that changes the cell's overall charge. This rapid shifting of electrolytes and cellular charges is the main catalyst for muscle contractions and neural transmissions.

depositions Verbal statements from parties and witnesses taken under oath.

depressants Agents used to slow brain activity.

depressed skull fracture A type of skull fracture that results from high-energy direct trauma to a small surface area of the head with a blunt object (such as a baseball bat to the head); commonly results in bony fragments being driven into the brain, causing injury.

depression A mental health disorder characterized by a persistent mood of sadness, despair, and discouragement.

dermatome An area of the skin supplied by a specific sensory spinal nerve.

dermis The inner layer of the skin, containing hair follicles, sweat glands, sebaceous glands, nerve endings, and blood vessels.

descending aorta One of the three portions of the aorta, it is the longest portion and extends through the thorax and abdomen into the pelvis.

designated officer The person in the department who is charged with the responsibility of managing exposures and infection control issues.

desired dose The amount of a drug that the physician orders for a patient; the drug order.

devascularization The loss of perfusion to a part of the body.

developmental disability Insufficient development of the brain, resulting in some level of dysfunction or impairment.

diabetes mellitus A metabolic disorder in which the ability to metabolize carbohydrates (sugars) is impaired due to a lack of insulin.

diabetic ketoacidosis (DKA) A form of acidosis in uncontrolled diabetes in which certain acids accumulate when insulin is not available.

diamond carry A carrying technique in which one provider is located at the head end of the stretcher or backboard, one at the foot end, and one at each side of the patient; each of the two providers at the sides uses one hand to support the stretcher or backboard so that all are able to face forward as they walk.

diapedesis A process whereby leukocytes leave blood vessels to move toward tissue where they are needed most.

diaphoretic Characterized by light or profuse sweating.

diaphragm A muscular dome that forms the undersurface of the thorax, separating the chest from the abdominal cavity. Contraction of the diaphragm (and the chest wall muscles) brings air into the lungs. Relaxation allows air to be expelled from the lungs.

diaphysis The shaft of a long bone.

diastole The relaxation phase of the heart, when the ventricles are filling with blood.

diastolic pressure The pressure that remains in the arteries during the relaxing phase of the cycle of the heart (diastole) when the left ventricle is at rest.

dieffenbachia A common houseplant that resembles "elephant ears"; its ingestion leads to burns of the mouth and tongue and, possibly, paralysis of the vocal cords and nausea and vomiting. In severe cases, ingestion may cause edema of the tongue and larynx, leading to airway compromise.

diencephalon Portion of the brain between the brainstem and cerebrum; contains the epithalamus, the thalamus, the hypothalamus, and the subthalamus.

diffuse axonal injury (DAI) Diffuse brain injury that is caused by stretching, shearing, or tearing of nerve fibers with subsequent axonal damage.

diffuse brain injury Any injury that affects the entire brain.

diffuse pain Pain that is not identified as being specific to a single location but is spread out over an area of the body or felt all over the body.

diffusion The movement of solutes (molecules) from an area of higher concentration to an area of lower concentration.

digestion The processing of food that nourishes the individual cells of the body.

digital radio The transmission of information via radio waves using native digital (computer) data or analog (voice) signals that have been converted to a digital signal and compressed.

diphtheria An infectious disease in which a membrane lining the pharynx is formed that can severely obstruct passage of air into the larynx.

diplopia Double vision.

direct carry method A nonurgent move that is a method for moving a patient from a bed to a stretcher, in which a stretcher is positioned next to the bed and two providers move the patient.

direct contact Exposure to or transmission of a communicable disease from one person to another by physical contact.

direct ground lift A lifting technique that is used for patients who are found lying supine on the ground with no suspected spinal injury.

dirty bomb Any container that is designed to disperse radioactive material; see also *radiologic dispersal device*.

disaster A widespread event that disrupts community resources and functions, in turn threatening public safety, citizens' lives, and property.

discovery The phase of a civil lawsuit where the plaintiff and defense obtain information from each other that will enable the attorneys to have a better understanding of the case and that will assist them in negotiating a possible settlement or in preparing for trial; includes depositions, interrogatories, and demands for production of records.

disease vector An animal that spreads a disease, once infected, to another animal.

disequilibrium syndrome A condition characterized by nausea, vomiting, headache, and confusion, which results when, as a consequence of dialysis, water initially shifts from the bloodstream into the cerebrospinal fluid, mildly increasing intracranial pressure.

disinfection The killing of pathogenic agents by direct application of chemicals.

dislocation Disruption of a joint in which ligaments are damaged and the bone ends are completely displaced.

disorganization A condition in which a person is characterized by uncontrolled and disconnected thought, is usually incoherent or rambling in speech, and may or may not be oriented to person and place.

disorientation A condition in which a person may be confused about his or her identity, the location, and the time of day; one of the ways in which various conditions such as schizophrenia or organic brain syndrome may present.

displaced fracture A fracture in which bone fragments are separated from one another and are not in anatomic alignment.

dissecting aneurysm A condition in which the inner layers of an artery, such as the aorta, become separated, allowing blood (at high pressures) to flow between the layers.

disseminated intravascular coagulation (DIC) A condition that begins with widespread activation of the clotting cascade, which depletes the clotting factors and platelets, and eventually results in uncontrolled hemorrhage.

dissemination The means by which a terrorist will spread an agent, such as by poisoning the water supply or aerosolizing the agent into the air or ventilation system of a building.

distal Farther from the trunk and nearer to the free end of the extremity.

distraction The action of pulling the spine along its length.

distributive shock The type of shock caused by widespread dilation of the resistance vessels (small arterioles), the capacitance vessels (small venules), or both.

diuretic medications The medications designed to promote elimination of excess salt and water by the kidneys.

diverticulitis Inflammation of a diverticulum, usually in the colon, creating abdominal discomfort; a *diverticulum* is an abnormal pouch or sac.

diving reflex Slowing of the heart rate caused by submersion in cold water.

documentation The recorded portion of the AEMT's patient interaction, either written or electronic; it becomes part of the patient's permanent medical record.

domestic terrorism Terrorism that is carried out by people in their own country.

do not resuscitate (DNR) order Written documentation by a physician giving permission to medical personnel not to attempt resuscitation in the event of cardiac arrest.

dorsal The posterior surface of the body, including the back of the hand.

dorsal respiratory group (DRG) A portion of the medulla oblongata where the primary respiratory pacemaker is found.

dorsalis pedis artery The artery on the anterior surface of the foot between the first and second metatarsals.

dose The amount of medication given on the basis of the patient's size and age.

Down syndrome A genetic chromosomal defect that can occur during fetal development and that results in intellectual impairment and certain physical characteristics, such as a round head with a flat occiput and slanted, wide-set eyes.

drag Resistance, such as air, that slows a projectile.

draw sheet method A nonurgent move that is a method for moving a patient from a bed onto a stretcher using a sheet on which the patient is lying.

drip chamber The area of the administration set where fluid accumulates so that the tubing remains filled with fluid.

drip rate Number of drops per minute.

drip set Another name for an administration set.

dromotropic Affecting the velocity of conduction in the heart.

dromotropic state Related to the control of the heart's conduction rate.

drowning The process of experiencing respiratory impairment from submersion or immersion in liquid.

drug A substance that has some therapeutic effect (such as reducing inflammation, fighting bacteria, or producing euphoria) when given in the appropriate circumstances and in the appropriate dose.

drug abuse Any use of drugs that causes physical, psychological, economic, legal, or social harm to the user or others affected by the user's behavior.

drug addiction A chronic disorder characterized by the compulsive use of a substance that results in physical, psychological, or social harm to the user who continues to use the substance despite the harm.

drug antagonism A decrease in the action of a drug by the administration of another drug.

drug dependence A psychological and sometimes physical state resulting from continued use of a substance, characterized by a compulsion to take the drug on a continuous or periodic basis to experience its effects or to avoid the discomfort of its absence.

drug reconstitution Injecting sterile water (or saline) from one vial into another vial containing a powdered form of the drug.

drugs Chemical agents used in the diagnosis, treatment, and prevention of disease.

drums Barrellike containers used to store a wide variety of substances, including food-grade materials, corrosives, flammable liquids, and grease. May be constructed of low-carbon steel, polyethylene, cardboard, stainless steel, nickel, or other materials.

ductus arteriosus A small artery that connects the left pulmonary artery to the aorta; diverts blood away from the fetal lungs while in utero.

DuoDote Auto-Injector A nerve agent antidote kit containing atropine and pralidoxime chloride; delivered as a single dose through one needle.

duplex The ability to transmit and receive simultaneously.

dura mater The outermost layer of the three meninges that enclose the brain and spinal cord; the toughest meningeal layer.

durable power of attorney for health care A type of advance directive executed by a competent adult that appoints another individual to make medical treatment decisions on his or her behalf in the event that the person making the appointment has a loss of decision-making capacity; see also *health care proxy*.

duration of action The amount of time a medication concentration can be expected to remain above the minimum level needed to provide the intended action.

duty A medicolegal term relating to certain personnel who either by statute or by function have a responsibility to provide patient care.

dysarthria The inability to pronounce speech clearly, often due to loss of the nerves or brain cells that control the small muscles in the larynx.

dysbarism injuries Any signs and symptoms caused by the difference between the surrounding atmospheric pressure and the total gas pressure in various tissues, fluids, and cavities of the body.

dysconjugate gaze Paralysis of gaze or lack of coordination between the movements of the two eyes.

dysmenorrhea Painful menstruation.

dysphagia Pain, discomfort, or difficulty in swallowing.

dysplasia An alteration in the size, shape, and organization of cells.

dyspnea Shortness of breath or difficulty breathing.

dysrhythmia An irregular or abnormal heart rhythm.

early adult A young adult age 19 to 40 years.

ecchymosis Bruising or discoloration associated with bleeding within or under the skin.

echolalia Meaningless echoing of the interviewer's words by the patient.

eclampsia Convulsions (seizures) resulting from severe hypertension in the pregnant woman.

ectopic pregnancy A pregnancy that develops outside the uterus, typically in a fallopian tube.

edema The presence of abnormally large amounts of fluid between cells in body tissues, causing swelling of the affected area.

effacement Thinning and shortening of the cervix; a normal process that occurs as the uterus contracts.

ejection fraction The portion of the blood ejected from the ventricle during systole.

elder abuse Any action or inaction on the part of a family member, caregiver, or other associated person that takes advantage of the older adult's person, property, or emotional state; also called parent battering.

elective abortion Intentional expulsion of the fetus.

electrical energy Energy delivered in the form of high voltage.

electrolytes Charged atoms or compounds that result from the loss or gain of an electron. These are ions that the body uses to perform certain critical metabolic processes.

emancipated minor A person who is under the legal age in a given state (age 18 years in most cases) but, because of other circumstances, is legally considered an adult.

embolus A blood clot or other substance in the circulatory system that breaks free from its site of origin and obstructs blood flow in a distant blood vessel.

embryo The term used to describe the developing infant from fertilization to the end of the 8th week of gestation.

embryonic period The period of gestation between weeks 3 and 8 in which all major organ systems begin to develop.

emergency A serious situation, such as injury or illness, that threatens the life or welfare of a person or group of people and requires immediate intervention.

emergency doctrine The principle of law that permits a health care provider to treat a patient in an emergency situation when the patient is incapable of granting consent because he or she is unresponsive, delusional, exhibiting an altered mental status as a result of drug or alcohol use, or is otherwise physically unable to give expressed consent; see also *implied consent*.

emergency medical care Immediate care or treatment.

emergency medical dispatch (EMD) A system that assists dispatchers in selecting appropriate units to respond to a particular call for assistance and provides callers with vital instructions until the arrival of emergency medical services crews.

emergency medical dispatcher (EMD) A specifically trained member of the emergency medical services team who receives information, makes decisions about resource allocation, and relays that information in an organized manner during the emergency.

emergency medical responder (EMR) The first trained person, such as a police officer, firefighter, lifeguard, or other rescuer, to arrive at the scene of an emergency to provide initial medical assistance.

emergency medical services (EMS) A multidisciplinary system that represents the combined efforts of several professionals and agencies to provide prehospital emergency care to sick and injured people.

emergency medical technician (EMT) An individual trained in basic emergency medical care skills, including automated external defibrillation, use of a definitive airway adjunct, and assisting patients with certain medications.

Emergency Medical Treatment and Active Labor Act (EMTALA) A federal law enacted to combat the practice of patient dumping and that pays particular attention to the practice of sending women in labor to distant hospitals; prevents emergency department staff from denying medical screening or stabilizing treatment, or inappropriately transferring a patient whose condition is not stable to another hospital.

emergency move A move in which the patient is dragged or pulled from a dangerous scene before a primary survey and care are provided.

Emergency Response Guidebook A preliminary action guide for first responders operating at a hazardous materials incident in coordination with the US Department of Transportation's (DOT) labels and placards marking system. Jointly developed by the DOT, the Secretariat of Communications and Transportation of Mexico, and Transport Canada.

emesis Vomiting.

emphysema A disease of the lungs in which there is extreme dilation and eventual destruction of pulmonary alveoli with poor exchange of oxygen and carbon dioxide; it is one form of chronic obstructive pulmonary disease.

encoded A message is put into a code before it is transmitted.

endocardium The thin membrane lining the inside of the heart.

endocrine glands Glands that secrete or release chemicals that are used inside the body.

endocrine system The complex message and control system that integrates many body functions, including the release of hormones.

endometriosis A condition in which endometrial tissue grows outside the uterus.

endometritis An inflammation of the endometrium that often is associated with a bacterial infection.

endometrium The innermost layer of the uterine wall.

end-organ perfusion The status of perfusion to the vital organs of the body; determined by assessing capillary refill time.

endosteum A layer that lines the inner surfaces of bone.

end-stage renal disease (ESRD) A condition in which the kidneys have lost all ability to function, and toxic waste materials build up in the patient's blood; occurs after acute or chronic kidney disease.

end-tidal carbon dioxide ($ETCO_2$) The partial pressure or maximal concentration of carbon dioxide at the end of an exhaled breath.

end-tidal carbon dioxide ($ETCO_2$) monitor A detection device for monitoring the amount of carbon dioxide in exhaled air that can be used to adjust oxygen administration or ventilations.

enhanced 9-1-1 An emergency communications system that collects information about 9-1-1 calls from the telephone network, such as the telephone number and location of the caller, and displays this information on the dispatcher's computer terminal.

enteral Drugs that are administered along any portion of the gastrointestinal tract, including the oral and rectal routes.

enteral medications Medications that are given through a portion of the gastrointestinal tract.

entrance wound The point at which a penetrating object enters the body.

entrapment To be caught (trapped) within a vehicle, room, or other confined space with no way out, or to have a limb or other body part trapped.

envenomation The act of injecting venom.

environmental emergency A medical condition caused or exacerbated by the weather, terrain, or atmospheric pressure at high altitude or underwater.

enzymes Substances designed to speed up the rate of specific biochemical reactions.

eosinophils Leukocytes that may play a role following infection in various areas in the body.

epicardium The layer of the serous pericardium that lies closely against the heart; also called the visceral pericardium.

epidemic A situation in which new cases of a disease in a human population substantially exceed the number expected based on recent experience.

epidermis The outer layer of skin, which is made up of cells that are sealed together to form a watertight protective covering for the body.

epididymitis An infection that causes inflammation of the epididymis along the posterior border of the testis; a possible complication of male urinary tract infection.

epidural hematoma An accumulation of blood between the skull and the dura mater.

epiglottis A thin, leaf-shaped valve that allows air to pass into the trachea but prevents food and liquid from entering.

epiglottitis An acute bacterial infection that results in rapid swelling of the epiglottis and surrounding tissues; may cause upper airway obstruction; also referred to as acute supraglottic laryngitis.

epinephrine A substance produced by the body (commonly called adrenaline), and a drug produced by pharmaceutical companies that increases pulse rate and blood pressure; the drug of choice for treating an anaphylactic reaction.

epiphyseal plate The growth plate of the bone; responsible for normal bone growth and development during childhood.

epiphyses The growth plates of a long bone; also called the epiphyseal plates.

epistaxis Nosebleed.

eponym The name of a disease, device, procedure, or drug that is based on the person who invented, discovered, or first described it.

erythropoiesis The process by which red blood cells are made.

eschar The thick, coagulated crust or slough of leathery skin that develops following a burn.

esophageal varices A condition in which the amount of pressure within the blood vessels surrounding the esophagus increases, causing blood to back up into the portal vessels and ultimately causing the capillary network of the esophagus to leak.

esophagitis Inflammation of the lining of the esophagus.

esophagus A collapsible tube that extends from the pharynx to the stomach; contractions of the muscle in the wall of the esophagus propel food and liquids through it to the stomach.

estrogen A hormone released from the ovaries that stimulates the uterine lining during the menstrual cycle.

ethics The philosophy of right and wrong, of moral duties, and of ideal professional behavior.

ethnocentrism When a person considers his or her own cultural values as more important when interacting with people of a different culture.

evaporation Conversion of water or another fluid from a liquid to a gas.

evisceration The displacement of organs outside of the body.

excitability A property of cardiac cells that provides the cells with the ability to respond to electrical impulses.

excretion The elimination of waste products from the body.

exhalation The part of the breathing process in which the diaphragm and the intercostal muscles relax, forcing air out of the lungs.

exit wound The point at which a penetrating object leaves the body, which may or may not be in a straight line from the entry wound.

exocrine gland A gland that excretes chemicals for elimination.

exophthalmos Bulging of the eyes.

expiration The process of moving air out of the lungs.

expiratory reserve volume The amount of air that can be exhaled following a normal exhalation.

exposure A situation in which a person has had contact with blood, body fluids, tissues, or airborne particles in a manner that suggests disease transmission may occur.

expressed consent A type of consent in which a patient gives verbal or nonverbal authorization for provision of emergency medical care or transport.

exsanguination Severe, possibly life-threatening loss of blood.

extension The straightening of a joint.

external jugular IV lines Intravenous catheters established in the jugular veins of the neck.

external respiration The exchange of gases between the lungs and the blood cells in the pulmonary capillaries; also called pulmonary respiration.

external rotation Rotating an extremity at its joint away from the midline.

extracellular fluid (ECF) Fluid outside of the cell, in which most of the body's supply of sodium is contained.

extrapyramidal symptoms A wide array of symptoms such as involuntary movements, tremors, rigidity, muscle contractions, restlessness, and changes in breathing and heart rate, usually as a result of taking antipsychotic drugs.

extremity lift A lifting technique that is used for patients who are supine or in a sitting position on the ground with no suspected extremity or spinal injuries.

extrication Removal of a patient from entrapment or a dangerous situation or position, such as removal from a wrecked vehicle, industrial incident, or building collapse.

extrication supervisor In incident command, the person appointed to determine the type of equipment and resources needed for a situation involving extrication or special rescue; also called the rescue supervisor.

EZ-IO A handheld, battery-powered driver to which a special intraosseous needle is attached; used for insertion of the intraosseous needle into the proximal tibia of children and adults.

facilitated diffusion Process whereby a carrier molecule moves substances in or out of cells from areas of higher to lower concentration.

fallopian tubes The two hollow tubes or ducts that extend from the uterus to the region of the ovary and serve as a passage for the egg and sperm.

false imprisonment The confinement of a person without legal authority or the person's consent that lasts for an appreciable period.

fascia The fiberlike connective tissue that covers arteries, veins, tendons, and ligaments.

fasciitis Inflammation of the fascia.

FAST devices (First Access for Shock Trauma) Manual sternal intraosseous devices used in patients age 12 years and older; include an infusion tube, subcutaneous portal, an introducer, a target/strain relief patch, and a protective dome.

febrile seizures The seizures that result from sudden high fever, particularly in children.

Federal Communications Commission (FCC) The federal agency that has jurisdiction over interstate and international telephone and telegraph services and satellite communications, all of which may involve EMS activity.

femoral arteries The principal arteries of the thigh; continuation of the external iliac arteries. These supply blood to the lower abdominal wall, external genitalia, and legs; can be palpated in the groin area.

femoral head The proximal end of the femur, articulating with the acetabulum to form the hip joint.

femoral vein A continuation of the saphenous vein that drains into the external iliac vein.

femur The thighbone; the longest and one of the strongest bones in the body.

fetal transition Process through which the fluid in the fetal lungs is replaced with air, the ductus arteriosus constricts, and the neonate begins adequate oxygenation of its own blood.

fetoscope A device used for listening to fetal heart tones.

fetus The developing, unborn infant inside the uterus; the embryo becomes the fetus at the beginning of the 9th week of gestation.

fibrin A whitish, filamentous protein formed by the action of thrombin on fibrinogen; the protein that polymerizes (bonds) to form the fibrous component of a blood clot.

fibrinolysis cascade The breakdown of fibrin in blood clots and the prevention of the polymerization of fibrin into new clots.

fibrinolytic agent Medication that dissolves blood clots after they have already formed; promotes the digestion of fibrin.

fibula The long bone on the posterior surface of the lower leg.

Fick principle States that the movement and use of oxygen in the body is dependent on adequate concentration of inspired oxygen (FIO_2 [fraction of inspired oxygen]), appropriate movement of oxygen across the alveolar-capillary membrane into the arterial bloodstream, adequate number of red blood cells to carry the oxygen, proper tissue perfusion, and efficient off-loading of oxygen at the tissue level.

filtration A type of diffusion in which water carries dissolved compounds across the cell membrane; commonly used by the kidneys to clean blood.

finance and administration In incident command, the section responsible for the accounting of all expenditures.

first-responder vehicles Specialized vehicles used to transport emergency medical services equipment and personnel to the scenes of medical emergencies.

flail chest A condition in which two or more ribs are fractured in two or more places or in association with a fracture of the sternum, so a segment of chest wall is effectively detached from the rest of the thoracic cage.

flame burn A thermal burn caused by flames touching the skin.

flank The region below the rib cage and above the hip.

flash burns Electrothermal injuries caused by arcing of electric current.

flash chamber The area of a catheter that fills with blood to help indicate when a vein is cannulated.

flat affect The absence of emotion; appearing to feel no emotion at all.

flexible stretcher A stretcher that is a rigid carrying device when secured around a patient but can be folded or rolled when not in use.

flexion The bending of a joint.

flexion injuries A type of injury that results from forward movement of the head, typically as the result of rapid deceleration, such as in a motor vehicle crash, or with a direct blow to the occiput.

flight of ideas Accelerated thinking in which the mind skips very rapidly from one thought to the next.

fluid balance The process of maintaining homeostasis through equal intake and output of fluids.

focal brain injury A specific, grossly observable brain injury.

focal pain Pain that is easily identified as being specific to a single location of the body.

focused assessment A type of physical assessment typically performed on patients who have sustained nonsignificant mechanisms of injury or on responsive medical patients. This type of exam is based on the chief complaint and focuses on one body system or part.

follicle-stimulating hormone A hormone released from the pituitary gland at roughly monthly intervals that helps to stimulate one oocyte to undergo cell division.

fontanelles Areas where the neonate's or infant's skull bones have not fused together; usually disappear at approximately 18 months of age.

foodborne transmission The contamination of food or water with an organism that can cause disease.

footprint The area of contact between the tire and the surface of the road.

foramen magnum A large opening at the base of the skull through which the brain connects to the spinal cord.

foramen ovale An opening between the two atria that is present in the fetus but usually closes shortly after birth.

foramina Small openings, perforations, or orifices in the bones of the cranial vault.

forcible restraint The act of physically subduing a patient to prevent harm.

fossa ovalis A depression between the right and left atria that indicates where the foramen ovale had been located in the fetus.

four-person log roll The recommended procedure for moving a patient with a suspected spinal injury from the ground to a long backboard.

Fowler position A sitting position, with the head elevated at a 90° angle (sitting straight upright).

fracture A break in the continuity of a bone.

free radicals A molecule that is missing one electron in its outer shell.

free-flow oxygen Oxygen administered via oxygen tube and a cupped hand on the patient's face.

freelancing When individual units or different organizations make independent and often inefficient decisions about the next appropriate action.

freight bills The shipping papers used for transport of chemicals along roads and highways; also referred to as bills of lading.

frequency The number of cycles (oscillations) per second of a radio signal.

friction The resistance to the motion of one body against another.

frontal lobe The portion of the brain that is important in voluntary motor actions and personality traits.

frostbite Damage to tissues as the result of exposure to cold; frozen body parts.

frostnip A condition in which tissues are frozen but on rewarming can be reversed, and deeper tissues are unaffected.

full-body exam A systematic head-to-toe exam that is performed during the secondary assessment of a patient who has sustained a significant mechanism of injury, is unresponsive, or is in critical condition.

full-thickness burns The burns that affect all skin layers and may affect the subcutaneous layers, muscle, bone, and internal organs, leaving the area dry, leathery, and white, dark brown, or charred (eschar); formerly called a third-degree burn.

functional disorder A disorder in which there is no known physiologic reason for the abnormal functioning of an organ or organ system.

functional residual capacity The volume of air remaining in the lungs following exhalation; also referred to as oxygen reserve.

fundus The uppermost part of the uterus, farthest from the cervical opening.

G agents Early nerve agents that were developed by German scientists in the period after World War I and into World War II: sarin, soman, and tabun.

gag reflex A normal reflex mechanism that causes retching; activated by touching the soft palate or the back of the throat.

gallbladder A sac on the undersurface of the liver that collects bile from the liver and discharges it into the duodenum through the common bile duct.

gamma (x-ray) radiation A type of energy that is emitted from a strong radiologic source that is far faster and has more energy than alpha and beta radiation. These rays easily penetrate through the human body and require lead or several inches of concrete to prevent penetration.

gamma-hydroxybutyrate (GHB) A sedative and central nervous system depressant.

gangrene An infection commonly caused by *Clostridium perfringens*. The result is tissue destruction and gas production that may result in death.

gastric distention A condition in which air fills the stomach, often as a result of high volume and pressure during artificial ventilation.

gastritis Inflammation of the stomach.

gastroenteritis A family of conditions resulting in diarrhea, nausea, and vomiting; some have infectious causes.

gastroesophageal reflux disease (GERD) A condition in which the sphincter between the esophagus and the stomach opens, allowing stomach acid to move superiorly; can cause a burning sensation within the chest (heartburn); also called acid reflux disease.

gauge In the medication administration sense, the interior diameter of a catheter or needle.

gel A semiliquid substance that is administered orally through capsules or plastic tubes.

general adaptation syndrome The body's response to stress that begins with an alarm response, followed by a stage of reaction and resistance, and then recovery or, if the stress is prolonged, exhaustion.

general impression The overall initial impression that determines the priority for patient care; based on the patient's surroundings, the mechanism of injury, nature of the illness, signs and symptoms, and the chief complaint.

generalized anxiety disorder (GAD) A disorder in which a person worries about everything for no particular reason, or the worrying is unproductive and the person cannot decide what to do about an upcoming situation.

generic name The original chemical name of a medication (in contrast with one of its trade names); not capitalized.

genital herpes An infection of the genitals, buttocks, or anal area caused by herpes simplex virus, which may cause sores of the genitals, mouth, or lips.

genital system The reproductive system in males and females.

geriatrics The assessment and treatment of disease in someone 65 years or older.

germinal layer The deepest layer of the epidermis where new skin cells are formed.

gestation The process of fetal development following fertilization of an egg.

gestational diabetes Diabetes that develops during pregnancy in women who did not have diabetes before pregnancy.

gestational diabetes mellitus The condition in which progesterone (the pregnancy hormone) makes the cells resistant to insulin, resulting in the potential for hypoglycemia or hyperglycemia; typically resolves following delivery.

gestational hypertension High blood pressure that develops after the 20th week of pregnancy in women with previously normal blood pressures and that resolves spontaneously in the postpartum period; formerly known as pregnancy-induced hypertension.

gestational period The time that it takes for a fetus to develop in utero; normally takes 38 weeks.

glands Cells or organs that selectively remove, concentrate, or alter materials in the blood and then secrete them back into the body.

Glasgow Coma Scale (GCS) A method of evaluating the level of consciousness that uses a scoring system for neurologic responses to specific stimuli.

glaucoma A disease of the eye caused by an increase in intraocular pressure; when severe enough, this may damage the optic nerve and potentially cause permanent loss of vision.

glenoid fossa The part of the scapula that forms the socket in the ball-and-socket joint of the shoulder.

globe The eyeball.

glottic opening The narrowest portion of the adult's airway; space between the vocal cords.

glucagon The hormone released from the alpha cells in the islets of Langerhans that converts glycogen to glucose when the body's blood glucose level drops.

gluconeogenesis A process that stimulates both the liver and the kidneys to produce glucose from noncarbohydrate molecules.

glucose One of the basic sugars; it is the primary fuel, along with oxygen, for cellular metabolism.

glycogen A long polymer from which glucose is converted in the liver (animal starch).

glycogenolysis The process by which glycogen is broken down and converted to glucose; facilitated by glucagon.

glycolysis The conversion of glucose into energy via metabolic pathways.

Golden Hour The time from injury to definitive care, during which treatment of shock and traumatic injuries should occur because survival potential is best; sometimes called the Golden Period.

gonads The reproductive glands.

gonorrhea A sexually transmitted disease caused by *Neisseria gonorrhoeae*.

Good Samaritan laws Statutory provisions enacted by many states to protect citizens from liability for errors and omissions in giving good faith emergency medical care, unless there is wanton, gross, or willful negligence.

governmental immunity Legal doctrine that can protect an emergency medical services provider from being sued or that may limit the amount of the monetary judgment that the plaintiff may recover; generally applies only to emergency medical services systems that are operated by municipalities or other government entities.

grand multipara A term used to describe a woman who has delivered five or more viable infants.

granulocytes Leukocytes that have large cytoplasmic granules that are easily seen with a simple light microscope.

gravid Pregnant.

gravida A term used to describe the number of times a woman has been pregnant.

greater trochanter A bony prominence on the proximal lateral side of the thigh, just below the hip joint.

greenstick fracture An incomplete fracture of a bone; seen in children, whose bones are pliable and may not completely fracture.

gross negligence Conduct that constitutes a willful or reckless disregard for a duty or standard of care.

growth plates Structures located on either end of an infant's long bone, which aid in lengthening bones as the child grows; also known as epiphyseal plates.

grunting An "uh" sound heard during exhalation; reflects the child's attempt to keep the alveoli open; a sign of increased work of breathing.

gtt A measurement that indicates number of drops.

guarding Involuntary muscle contractions (spasm) of the abdominal wall to minimize the pain of abdominal movement and protect the inflamed abdomen; a sign of peritonitis.

Guillain-Barré syndrome A disease of unknown cause characterized by progressive paralysis moving from the feet to the head (ascending paralysis); if paralysis reaches the diaphragm, the patient may require respiratory support.

habituation The situation in which there is a physical tolerance and psychological dependence on a drug or drugs.

half-life The time required by the body, tissue, or organ to metabolize or inactivate one-half of the amount of a substance taken in; an important consideration in determining the proper dose of drug and frequency of administration.

hallucinations Sense perceptions not founded on objective reality; false perceptions.

hallucinogen An agent that produces false perceptions in any one of the five senses.

hangman's fracture The most classic distraction injury, which occurs when a person is hanged by the neck. Bending and fractures occur at the C1-C2 region, which quickly tear the spinal cord.

hapten A substance that normally does not stimulate an immune response but can be combined with an antigen and at a later point initiate an antibody response.

hazardous materials Any substances that are toxic, poisonous, radioactive, flammable, or explosive and cause injury or death with exposure.

hazardous materials (hazmat) incident An incident in which a hazardous material is no longer properly contained and isolated.

head injury A traumatic insult to the head that may result in injury to soft tissue of the scalp and bony structures of the head and skull, not including the face.

head tilt–chin lift maneuver A combination of two movements to open the airway by tilting the forehead back and lifting the chin; used for nontrauma patients.

head trauma A general term that includes both head injuries and traumatic brain injuries.

health care directive A written document that specifies medical treatment for a competent patient, should he or she become unable to make decisions; see also *advance directive*.

health care proxy A type of advance directive executed by a competent adult that appoints another individual to make medical treatment decisions on his or her behalf in the event that the person making the appointment loses decision-making capacity; see also *durable power of attorney for health care*.

Health Insurance Portability and Accountability Act (HIPAA) The law enacted in 1996 that provides for criminal sanctions as well as for civil penalties for releasing a patient's protected health information in a way not authorized by the patient.

heart A hollow muscular organ that pumps blood throughout the body.

heart failure A disorder in which the heart loses part of its ability to effectively pump blood, usually as a result of damage to the heart muscle and usually resulting in a backup of fluid into the lungs.

heat cramps Painful muscle spasms usually associated with vigorous activity in a hot environment.

heat exhaustion A form of heat injury in which the body loses substantial amounts of fluid and electrolytes because of heavy sweating; also called heat prostration or heat collapse.

heatstroke A life-threatening condition of severe hyperthermia caused by exposure to excessive natural or artificial heat, marked by warm, dry skin; severely altered mental status; and often irreversible coma.

helper T cells A type of T lymphocyte that is involved in cell-mediated and antibody-mediated immune responses. It secretes cytokines that stimulate the B cells and other T cells.

hematemesis Vomit with blood; can either look like coffee grounds, indicating the presence of partially digested blood, or contain bright-red blood, indicating active bleeding.

hematochezia The passage of stools containing bright red blood, indicating lower gastrointestinal tract bleeding.

hematologic disorder Any disorder of the blood.

hematology The study and prevention of blood-related disorders.

hematoma An accumulation of blood in the tissues or in a body cavity.

hematopoiesis The process of generating blood cells.

hematopoietic system The system that includes all blood components and the organs involved in their development and production.

hematuria The presence of blood in the urine.

hemiparesis Weakness on one side of the body.

hemiplegia Paralysis of one side of the body, possibly from a stroke or head injury.

hemochromatosis An inherited disease in which the body absorbs more iron than it needs and stores it in the liver, kidneys, and pancreas.

hemoglobin An iron-containing protein within red blood cells that has the ability to combine with oxygen; carries 97% of oxygen.

hemolytic anemia A disease characterized by increased destruction of the red blood cells. It can occur from an Rh factor reaction (primarily in Rh-positive neonates born to sensitized Rh-negative mothers), exposure to chemicals, or a disorder of the immune system.

hemolytic crisis A rapid destruction of red blood cells that occurs faster than the body's ability to create new cells.

hemolytic disorders Disorders relating to the breakdown of red blood cells.

hemoperitoneum Collection of blood in the abdominal cavity.

hemophilia A congenital abnormality in which the body is unable to produce clots due to a lack of normal clotting factors, resulting in uncontrollable bleeding.

hemopneumothorax A collection of blood and air in the pleural cavity.

hemoptysis The spitting or coughing up of blood.

hemorrhage A discharge of blood from the blood vessels; bleeding.

hemorrhagic shock A condition in which low blood volume due to massive internal or external bleeding results in inadequate perfusion.

hemorrhagic stroke One of the two main types of stroke; occurs as a result of bleeding inside the brain.

hemostasis Formation of clots to plug openings in injured blood vessels and stop blood flow; the body's natural blood-clotting mechanism.

hemostatic agent Pharmacologic substances used to stop profuse bleeding and that function by absorbing the water component of blood, thereby concentrating the clotting factors, activating platelets, and enhancing the coagulation cascade.

hemostatic disorders Bleeding and clotting abnormalities.

hemothorax A collection of blood in the pleural cavity.

heparin A substance found in large amounts in basophils that inhibits blood clotting.

hepatic portal system A specialized part of the venous system that drains blood from the stomach, intestines, and spleen.

hepatic veins The veins into which blood empties after liver cells in the sinusoids of the liver extract nutrients, filter the blood, and metabolize various drugs.

hepatitis Inflammation of the liver, usually caused by a viral infection, that causes fever, loss of appetite, jaundice, fatigue, and altered liver function.

Hering-Breuer reflex The protective nervous system mechanism that terminates inhalation and prevents lung overexpansion.

hernia The protrusion of a loop of an organ or tissue through an abnormal body opening.

herniation A process in which tissue is forced out of its normal position, such as when the brain is forced from the cranial vault, either through the foramen magnum or over the tentorium.

herpes simplex A common virus caused by human herpes viruses 1 and 2, characterized by small blisters whose location depends on the type of virus. Type 2 results in blisters on the genital area, while type 1 results in blisters on nongenital areas.

high-level disinfection The killing of pathogenic agents by using potent means of disinfection.

hilum The point of entry for the bronchi, vessels, and nerves into each lung.

hinge joints Joints that can bend and straighten but cannot rotate; they restrict motion to one plane.

histamine Chemical substance released by the immune system in allergic reactions that is responsible for many of the symptoms of anaphylaxis, such as vasodilation; increases vascular permeability and tissue inflammation; found in large amounts in basophils.

history taking A step within the patient assessment process that provides detail about the patient's chief complaint and an account of the patient's signs and symptoms.

hollow organs Structures through which materials pass, such as the stomach, gallbladder, small intestine, large intestine, ureters, and urinary bladder.

homeostasis A tendency to constancy or stability in the body's internal environment; the balance of all systems of the body.

homonyms Words that sound alike but are spelled differently and have different meanings.

horizontal axis The axis that runs perpendicular to the sagittal plane; also called the mediolateral axis.

hormones Substances formed in specialized organs or glands and carried to another organ or group of cells in the same organism; these regulate many body functions, including metabolism, growth, and body temperature.

hospice An organization that provides end-of-life care to patients with terminal illnesses and their families.

host The organism or person that is attacked by the infecting agent.

hot zone The area immediately surrounding a hazardous materials spill or incident site that endangers life and health. All personnel working in this zone must wear appropriate protective clothing and equipment. Entry requires approval by the incident commander or other designated officer.

human chorionic gonadotropin (hCG) A hormone that stimulates the corpus luteum to produce progesterone during the first eight weeks of gestation.

human immunodeficiency virus (HIV) The virus that causes infection and ultimately causes acquired immunodeficiency syndrome (AIDS), which damages the cells in the body's immune system so that the body is unable to fight infection or certain cancers.

human papillomavirus (HPV) The most common sexually transmitted disease, caused by a virus, which may cause no symptoms or cause multiple growths in the genital areas.

humerus The supporting bone of the upper arm.

humoral immunity A type of immunity in which B cell lymphocytes produce antibodies called immunoglobulins, which recognize a specific antigen and then react with it.

hydrocarbons Compounds made up of hydrogen and carbon atoms; they are frequently obtained from the distillation of petroleum.

hydroplaning A condition in which the tires of a vehicle may be lifted off the road surface as water builds up under them, making the vehicle feel as though it is floating.

hydrostatic pressure The pressure of water against the walls of its container.

hymen A fold of mucous membrane that partially covers the entrance to the vagina.

hymenoptera A family of insects that includes bees, wasps, ants, and yellow jackets.

hyoid bone A bone at the base of the tongue that supports the tongue and its muscles.

hyperbaric chamber A chamber, usually a small room, pressurized to a level higher than atmospheric pressure.

hypercalcemia An elevated blood calcium level.

hypercapnia Increased carbon dioxide level in the bloodstream.

hypercholesterolemia An elevated blood cholesterol level.

hyperemesis gravidarum A condition of persistent nausea and vomiting during pregnancy.

hyperextension Extension of a limb or other body part beyond its usual range of motion.

hyperflexion Flexion beyond the normal range of motion.

hyperglycemia Abnormally high glucose level in the blood.

hyperglycemic crisis Unresponsiveness caused by dehydration, a very high blood glucose level, and ketoacidosis.

hyperkalemia An elevated serum potassium level.

hypermagnesemia An increased serum magnesium level.

hypernatremia A serum sodium level greater than or equal to 143 mEq/L.

hyperosmolar hyperglycemic syndrome (HHS) A metabolic derangement that occurs principally in patients with type 2 diabetes; it is characterized by hyperglycemia, hyperosmolarity, and an absence of significant ketosis. Also called hyperosmolar nonketotic coma (HONK).

hyperosmolar nonketotic coma (HONK) Condition characterized by severe hyperglycemia, hyperosmolality, and dehydration but no ketoacidosis; also called hyperosmolar hyperglycemic nonketotic coma (HHNC) or HONK/HHNC.

hyperoxia An excess of oxygen.

hyperphosphatemia An elevated serum phosphate level.

hyperplasia An increase in the actual number of cells in an organ or tissue, usually resulting in an increase in the size of the organ or tissue.

hyperpyrexia A high body temperature.

hypersensitivity Abnormal sensitivity; a condition in which the body manifests an exaggerated response to the stimulus of a foreign agent.

hypertension Blood pressure that is higher than the normal range.

hypertensive emergency An emergency situation created by excessively high blood pressure, which can lead to serious complications such as stroke or aneurysm.

hyperthermia A condition in which the body core temperature rises to 101 °F (38.3 °C) or higher.

hypertonic Concentration of solute is higher compared with another solution.

hypertonic solution A solution that has a greater concentration of sodium than does the cell; the increased extracellular osmotic pressure can draw water out of the cell and cause it to collapse.

hypertrophy An increase in the size of the cells as a result of synthesis of more subcellular components, resulting in an increase in tissue and organ size.

hyperventilation Rapid or deep breathing that lowers the blood carbon dioxide level below normal; may lead to increased intrathoracic pressure, decreased venous return, and hypotension when associated with bag-mask device use.

hyperventilation syndrome (panic attack) A syndrome that occurs in the absence of other physical problems and whose symptoms include anxiety, dizziness, numbness, tingling of the hands and feet, and dyspnea despite rapid breathing.

hyphema Bleeding into the anterior chamber of the eye; results from direct ocular trauma.

hypocalcemia A decreased serum calcium level.

hypoglycemia Abnormally low glucose level in the blood.

hypoglycemic crisis Unresponsiveness or altered mental status in a patient with diabetes caused by significant hypoglycemia; usually the result of excessive exercise or activity, failure to eat after a routine dose of insulin, or an inadvertent overdose of insulin.

hypokalemia A decreased serum potassium level.

hypomagnesemia A decreased serum magnesium level.

hyponatremia A serum sodium level that is less than or equal to 135 mEq/L.

hypoperfusion A condition that occurs when the level of tissue perfusion decreases below that needed to maintain normal cellular functions.

hypophosphatemia A decreased serum phosphate level.

hypotension Blood pressure that is lower than the normal range.

hypothalamic-pituitary-adrenal axis A major part of the neuroendocrine system that controls reactions to stress. It is the mechanism for a set of interactions among glands, hormones, and parts of the midbrain that mediate the general adaptation syndrome.

hypothalamus The basal part of the diencephalons; it regulates the function of the pituitary gland.

hypothermia A condition in which the internal core body temperature falls below 95°F (35°C), usually as a result of prolonged exposure to cool or freezing temperatures.

hypotonic A lower concentration of sodium in a solution than exists in the cell; the increased intracellular osmotic pressure lets water flow into the cell, causing it to swell and possibly burst.

hypotonic solution A solution that has a lower concentration of sodium than the cell does; the increased intracellular osmotic pressure lets water flow into the cell, causing it to swell and possibly burst.

hypoventilation The movement of inadequate volumes of air into the lungs.

hypovolemic shock A condition in which low blood volume, due to massive internal or external bleeding or extensive loss of body water, results in inadequate perfusion.

hypoxemia A deficiency of oxygen in arterial blood.

hypoxia A dangerous condition in which the body's tissues and cells do not have enough oxygen.

hypoxic drive A backup system that controls respirations by sensing when the oxygen level in the blood falls.

iatrogenic response An adverse condition induced in a patient by the treatment given.

idiopathic Of no known cause.

idiosyncrasy An abnormal sensitivity or reaction to a drug or other substance that is peculiar to an individual.

idiosyncratic reaction A peculiar or individual response to a drug or medication through unusual susceptibility.

i-gel A supraglottic airway device that uses a noninflatable, gellike mask to isolate the larynx and facilitate ventilation.

ileostomy The procedure to create an opening (stoma) between the ileum (part of the small intestine) and the surface of the body to provide drainage of the bowel.

ileus Paralysis of the bowel, arising from any one of several causes; it stops the contractions that normally move material through the intestine.

ilium One of three bones that fuse to form the pelvic ring.

illicit In relation to drugs, illegal drugs such as marijuana, cocaine, and lysergic acid diethylamide.

immersion foot A condition that occurs after prolonged exposure to cold water, in which the skin of the foot is pale and cold, and there is a loss of sensation; also called trench foot.

imminent abortion A spontaneous abortion that cannot be prevented.

immune The body's ability to protect itself from acquiring a disease.

immune response The body's defense reaction to any substance that is recognized as foreign.

immune system The body system that includes all of the structures and processes designed to mount a defense against foreign substances and disease-causing agents.

immunity In medicine, the body's ability to protect itself from acquiring a disease; in a legal context, legal protection from penalties that could normally be incurred under the law.

immunodeficiency An abnormal condition in which some part of the body's immune system is inadequate, and, consequently, resistance to infectious disease is decreased.

immunogen An antigen that is capable of generating an immune response.

immunoglobulins Antibodies secreted by the B cells.

immunosuppressant medications The medications intended to inhibit the body's ability to attack the "foreign" transplanted organ or, in the case of autoimmune diseases, the medications that inhibit the body's attack on itself.

impedance threshold device (ITD) A valve device placed between the endotracheal tube and a bag-mask device that limits the amount of air entering the lungs during the recoil phase between chest compressions.

implied consent A type of consent in which a patient who is unable to give consent (because he or she is unresponsive, delusional, exhibiting an altered mental status as a result of drug or alcohol use, or is otherwise physically unable to give expressed consent) is given treatment under the legal assumption that he or she would want treatment; see also *emergency doctrine*.

in loco parentis Latin phrase meaning "in the place of the parent" that refers to the legal responsibility of a person or organization to take on some of the functions and responsibilities of a parent or legal guardian on the behalf of a minor.

inappropriate affect Emotion that is out of synch with the situation (for example, wearing a waxy smile while discussing a parent's death).

incidence The number of new cases of a disease in a population.

incident action plan An oral or written plan stating general objectives reflecting the overall strategy for managing an incident.

incident commander (IC) The overall leader of the incident command system to whom commanders or leaders of incident command system divisions report.

incident command system (ICS) An on-scene emergency management model specifically designed to provide for an integrated organizational structure that reflects the complexity and demands of an incident, including disasters and mass-casualty incidents. Also called the incident management system.

incomplete abortion Expulsion of the fetus that results in some products of conception remaining in the uterus.

incontinence Loss of bowel and bladder control; can be due to a generalized seizure and to other conditions.

incubation period The time between when a person is exposed to an agent to when symptoms first appear.

index of suspicion Awareness that unseen serious and/or life-threatening injuries may exist when determining the mechanism of injury.

indications Therapeutic uses for a specific medication.

indirect contact Exposure to or transmission of infection from one person to another by contact with a contaminated object.

indirect injury An injury that occurs when force is applied to one region of the body but causes an injury in another area.

infancy The first year of life.

infant A young child age 1 month to 1 year.

infarcted cells The cells that die as a result of loss of blood flow.

infection The abnormal invasion of a host or host tissues by organisms such as bacteria, viruses, or parasites, with or without signs or symptoms of disease.

infection control Procedures to reduce transmission of infection among patients and health care personnel.

infectious disease A medical condition that is caused by the growth and spread of small, harmful organisms within the body.

inferior Below what is indicated; closer to the feet.

inferior vena cava One of the two largest veins in the body; carries blood from the lower extremities and the pelvic and the abdominal organs to the heart.

infiltration The escape of fluid into the surrounding tissue.

inflammatory response A reaction by tissues of the body to irritation or injury, characterized by pain, swelling, redness, and heat.

influenza (flu) type A A virus that has crossed the animal/human barrier and has infected humans, recently reaching a pandemic level with the H1N1 strain.

informed consent Permission for treatment given by a competent patient after the potential risks, benefits, and alternatives to treatment have been explained.

ingestion Eating or drinking materials for absorption through the gastrointestinal tract.

inhalation The active, muscular part of breathing that draws air into the airway and lungs; a medication delivery route; in allergic reactions, breathing in foreign substances through the respiratory system.

inhalation injury An injury to the airway as a result of breathing smoke and toxic chemicals into the lungs and airway.

injection In allergic reactions, piercing of the skin, followed by deposition of foreign material into the skin.

inotropic Affecting the contractility of muscle tissue, especially cardiac muscle.

inotropic state Related to the strength of the heart's contraction.

inspiration The process of moving air into the lungs.

inspiratory reserve volume The amount of air that can be inhaled after a normal inhalation; the amount of air that can be inhaled in addition to the normal tidal volume.

inspiratory/expiratory (I/E) ratio An expression for comparing the length of inspiration with that of expiration, normally 1:2, meaning that expiration is twice as long as inspiration (not measured in seconds).

insulin A hormone produced by the islets of Langerhans (an exocrine gland in the pancreas) that enables sugar in the blood to enter the cells of the body; used in synthetic form to treat and control diabetes mellitus.

integumentary system The largest organ system in the body, consisting of the skin and accessory structures (eg, hair, nails, glands).

intended effect The effect that a medication is expected to have on the body.

interatrial septum A membrane that separates the right and left atria.

interference A direct biochemical interaction between two drugs.

interferon A protein produced by cells in response to viral invasion that is released into the bloodstream or intercellular fluid to induce healthy cells to manufacture an enzyme that counters the infection.

interleukins Chemical substances that attract white blood cells to the sites of injury and bacterial invasions.

intermodal tanks Shipping and storage vessels that can be either pressurized or nonpressurized.

internal respiration The exchange of gases between the blood cells and the tissues.

internal rotation Rotating the anterior surface of an extremity toward the midline.

internal shunt Also called an arteriovenous fistula, this device is an artificial connection between a vein and an artery, usually in the forearm or upper arm.

international terrorism Terrorism that is carried out by people in a country other than their own; also known as cross-border terrorism.

interoperable communications system A communications system that uses a voice-over-Internet-protocol (VoIP) technology to allow multiple agencies to communicate and transmit data.

interrogatories Written questions that the defense and plaintiff send to one another.

interstitial Water between the vascular system and the surrounding cells (for example, between the membranes of two cells located outside the vascular compartment in the body).

interstitial fluid The fluid located outside of the blood vessels in the spaces between the body's cells.

interstitial space The space in between the cells.

interventricular septum A thick wall that separates the right and left ventricles.

intervertebral disks The cushions that lie between the vertebrae.

intracellular fluid (ICF) Fluid within cells in which most of the body's supply of potassium is contained.

intracerebral hematoma Bleeding within the brain tissue (parenchyma) itself; also referred to as an intraparenchymal hematoma.

intracranial pressure (ICP) The pressure within the cranial vault; normally 0 to 15 mm Hg in adults.

intramuscular (IM) Into a muscle; a medication delivery route.

intranasal (IN) A delivery route in which a medication is pushed through a specialized atomizer device, called a mucosal atomizer device, into the naris.

intraosseous (IO) Into the bone; a medication delivery route.

intraosseous (IO) infusion A technique of administering fluids, blood and blood products, and medications into the intraosseous space of a long bone, usually the proximal tibia; used when intravenous access cannot be quickly obtained.

intraosseous space The spongy cancellous bone of the epiphyses and the medullary cavity of the diaphysis, collectively.

intrapulmonary shunting Bypassing of oxygen-poor blood past nonfunctional alveoli to the left side of the heart.

intravascular The water portion of the circulatory system surrounding the blood cells (for example, in the heart, arteries, or veins).

intravascular fluid (plasma) The noncellular portion of blood found within the blood vessels; also called plasma.

intravenous (IV) Into a vein; a medication delivery route.

intravenous (IV) therapy The delivery of a medication directly into a vein.

involuntary activities Actions of the body that are not under a person's conscious control.

involuntary muscle A muscle over which a person has no conscious control. It is found in many automatic regulating systems of the body.

ionic concentration The amount of charged particles found in a particular area.

ionizing radiation Energy that is emitted in the form of rays or particles.

ions Charged atoms or compounds that result from the loss or gain of an electron.

ipsilateral On the same side of the body.

iris The muscle and surrounding tissue behind the cornea that dilate and constrict the pupil, regulating the amount of light that enters the eye; pigment in this tissue gives the eye its color.

irreversible shock The final stage of shock, resulting in death.

irritable bowel syndrome (IBS) A condition in which patients have abdominal pain and changes in their bowel habits; generally, the pain must be present for at least 3 days in 1 month for at least 3 months to be considered this disease.

ischemia A lack of oxygen that deprives tissues of necessary nutrients, resulting from partial or complete blockage of blood flow; potentially reversible because permanent injury has not yet occurred.

ischemic cells Cells that receive enough blood after an event, such as a cerebrovascular accident, to stay alive but not enough to function properly.

ischemic stroke One of the two main types of stroke; occurs when blood flow to a particular part of the brain is cut off by a blockage (for example, a clot) inside a blood vessel.

ischium One of three bones that fuse to form the pelvic ring.

islets of Langerhans Structures found in the pancreas that are composed of four types of cells; one type, the beta cell, is responsible for the production of insulin.

isoimmunity The formation of antibodies or T cells that are directed against antigens or another person's cells.

isolette A device used to transport a neonate in an ambulance; also called an incubator.

isotonic The same concentration of sodium in a solution as in the cell. In this case, water does not shift, and no change in cell shape occurs.

isotonic solution A solution that has the same concentration of sodium as does the cell. In this case, water does not shift, and no change in cell shape occurs.

Jamshidi needle A double needle, consisting of a solid-bore needle inside a sharpened hollow needle; used to access the medullary canal for intraosseous infusion.

jaundice Yellow skin or sclera caused by liver disease or dysfunction.

jaw-thrust maneuver Technique to open the airway by placing the fingers behind the angle of the jaw and bringing the jaw forward; used for patients who may have a cervical spine injury.

joint (articulation) The point at which two or more bones articulate, or come into contact.

joint capsule The fibrous sac that encloses a joint.

joint information center (JIC) An area designated by the incident commander, or a designee, in which public information officers from multiple agencies distribute information about the incident.

jugular vein distention (JVD) A prominence of the jugular veins caused by increased volume or increased pressure within the central venous system or the thoracic cavity.

jugular veins The two main veins that drain the head and neck.

jump kit A portable kit containing items that are used in the initial care of the patient.

JumpSTART triage A sorting system for pediatric patients younger than 8 years or weighing less than 100 pounds (45 kg); the system is modified for infants because they cannot ambulate on their own.

Kehr sign Left shoulder pain caused by blood in the peritoneal cavity due to rupture of the spleen.

ketoacidosis An acidotic state created by the production of ketones via fat metabolism.

ketonemia Excess amounts of ketone bodies in the blood.

ketones Acidic by-products of fat metabolism.

kidnapping The seizing, confining, abducting, or carrying away of a person by force, including transporting a competent adult for medical treatment without his or her consent.

kidney stones Solid crystalline masses formed in the kidney, resulting from an excess of insoluble salts or uric acid crystallizing in the urine; these masses may become trapped anywhere along the urinary tract.

kidneys Two retroperitoneal organs that excrete the end products of metabolism as urine and regulate the body's salt and water content.

killer T cells The cells released during a type IV allergic reaction that kill antigen-bearing target cells.

kinetic energy The energy of a moving object.

kinetics The study of the relationship among speed, mass, vector direction, and physical injury.

King LT airway A single-lumen airway that is blindly inserted into the esophagus; when properly placed in the esophagus, one cuff seals the esophagus, and the other seals the oropharynx.

kinin system A group of polypeptides that mediate inflammatory responses by stimulating visceral smooth muscle and relaxing vascular smooth muscle to produce vasodilation.

Kussmaul respirations Deep, rapid breathing; the result of an accumulation of certain acids when insulin is not available in the body.

kyphosis A condition in which the back becomes hunched over due to an abnormal curvature of the spine.

labia majora Two prominent, rounded folds of skin lateral to the labia minora of the female external genitalia.

labia minora A pair of skin folds in the female external genitalia that border the vestibule.

labored breathing Breathing that requires greater than normal effort; may be slower or faster than normal and characterized by grunting, stridor, and use of accessory muscles; occurs when air movement is impaired.

laceration A smooth or jagged open wound.

lacrimal glands The glands that produce fluids to keep the eye moist; also called tear glands.

lactated Ringer solution A sterile crystalloid isotonic intravenous solution of specified amounts of calcium chloride, potassium chloride, sodium chloride, and sodium lactate in water.

lactic acid A metabolic end product of the breakdown of glucose that accumulates when metabolism proceeds in the absence of oxygen.

lactic acidosis Anaerobic cellular respiration due to hypoperfusion of tissues and organs.

landline Communications system linked by wires, usually in reference to a conventional telephone system.

large intestine The portion of the digestive tube that encircles the abdomen around the small bowel, consisting of the cecum, the colon, and the rectum. It helps regulate water balance and eliminate solid waste.

laryngeal mask airway (LMA) An airway device that is inserted into the mouth blindly and comes to rest at the glottic opening. A flexible cuff is inflated, creating an almost airtight seal.

laryngectomy A surgical procedure in which the larynx is removed.

laryngospasm The spasmodic contraction of the vocal cords, accompanied by an enfolding of the arytenoid and aryepiglottic folds.

larynx A complex structure formed by the epiglottis, thyroid cartilage, cricoid cartilage, arytenoid cartilage, corniculate cartilage, and cuneiform cartilage; the voice box.

lateral In anatomy, parts of the body that lie farther from the midline.

lateral compression A force that is directed from the side toward the midline of the body.

lateral malleolus An enlargement of the distal end of the fibula, which forms the lateral wall of the ankle joint.

LD_{50} The standard measure of the dose amount of an agent or substance that will kill 50% of a population who are exposed to this level.

Le Fort fractures Maxillary fractures that are classified into three categories based on their anatomic location.

left anterior descending (LAD) artery One of the two branches of the left main coronary artery that is the largest and shortest of the myocardial blood vessels; this vessel and the circumflex coronary arteries supply blood to the left ventricle and other areas.

length-based resuscitation tape A tape used to estimate an infant or child's weight on the basis of length; appropriate drug doses and equipment sizes are listed on the tape; one type is called a Broselow tape.

lens The transparent part of the eye through which images are focused on the retina.

leukocytosis An elevated white blood cell count, often due to inflammation.

leukopenia A reduction in the number of white blood cells.

leukotrienes Arachidonic acid metabolites that function as chemical mediators of inflammation; released by the immune system in allergic reactions; also known as slow-reacting substances of anaphylaxis.

level A protection Personal protective equipment used for protection against vapors, gases, mists, and even dusts. The highest level of protection, it is an encapsulating suit that includes a self-contained breathing apparatus.

level B protection Personal protective equipment used when the type and atmospheric concentration of substances require a high level of respiratory protection but less skin protection.

The kinds of gloves and boots worn depend on the identified chemical.

level C protection Personal protective equipment used when the type of airborne substance is known, the concentration is measured, the criteria for using an air-purifying respirator are met, and skin and eye exposure is unlikely. This ensemble consists of standard work clothing with the addition of chemical-protective clothing, chemically resistant gloves, and a form of respiratory protection.

level D protection Personal protective equipment used when the atmosphere contains no known hazard, and work functions preclude splashes, immersion, or the potential for unexpected inhalation of or contact with hazardous levels of chemicals. This is the lowest level of protection and is primarily a work uniform that includes coveralls.

lewisite (L) A vesicant that has a rapid onset of symptoms and produces immediate, intense pain and discomfort on contact; British antilewisite is the antidote.

liaison officer In incident command, the person who relays information and concerns among command, the general staff, and other agencies.

libel False and damaging information about a person that is communicated in writing.

licensure The process whereby a competent authority, usually the state, allows people to perform a regulated job, trade, or profession.

licit In relation to drugs, legalized drugs such as coffee, alcohol, and tobacco.

life expectancy The average number of years a person can be expected to live.

ligament A band of fibrous tissue that connects bones to bones; supports and strengthens a joint.

lightening Movement of the fetus down into the pelvis prior to birth.

limb presentation A delivery in which the presenting part is a single arm, leg, or foot.

limbic system Structures within the cerebrum and diencephalon that influence emotions, motivation, mood, and sensations of pain and pleasure.

linear skull fracture A type of skull fracture that commonly occurs in the temporal-parietal region of the skull; not associated with deformities to the skull; also referred to as a nondisplaced skull fracture.

lipolysis The metabolism (breakdown or destruction) of stored fat that has been released into the circulation.

lithium The cornerstone drug for the treatment of bipolar disorder.

liver A large solid organ that lies in the right upper quadrant immediately below the diaphragm; it produces bile, stores glucose for immediate use by the body, and produces many substances that help regulate immune responses.

load-distributing band (LDB) A circumferential chest compression device composed of a constricting band and backboard that is either electrically or pneumatically driven to compress the heart by putting inward pressure on the thorax.

local reaction A mild or moderate allergic reaction that the body limits to a specific area after being exposed to a foreign substance.

logistics In incident command, the section that procures and stockpiles equipment and supplies during an incident.

longitudinal axis The axis that runs perpendicular to the transverse plane.

longitudinal section The view of an object cut along its long axis.

loosening of associations A situation in which the logical connection between one idea and the next becomes obscure, at least to the listener.

lumbar spine The lower part of the back, formed by the lowest five nonfused vertebrae; also called the dorsal spine.

lumen The inside diameter of an artery or other hollow structure.

lung compliance The ability of the alveoli to fully expand when air is drawn in during inhalation.

lungs The two primary organs of breathing.

luteinizing hormone A hormone released from the pituitary gland at roughly monthly intervals that helps to stimulate one oocyte to undergo cell division.

lymph A thin, plasmalike liquid formed from interstitial or extracellular fluid that bathes the tissues of the body.

lymph nodes Round or bean-shaped structures interspersed along the course of the lymph vessels, where infection fighting cells are housed, and which filter the lymph and serve as a source of lymphocytes.

lymph vessels Thin-walled vessels through which lymph circulates through the body; they travel close to the major veins.

lymphatic system A passive circulatory system in the body that transports a plasmalike liquid called lymph, a thin fluid that bathes the tissues of the body.

lymphocytes The smallest of the agranulocytes, they originate in the bone marrow but migrate through the blood to the lymphatic tissues.

lymphokines Cytokines released by lymphocytes, including many of the interleukins, gamma interferon, tumor necrosis factor beta, and chemokines.

lysis The process of disintegration, breakdown, or rupturing of cells caused by either the presence of certain enzymes, or from excess water entering the cell through osmosis.

macrodrip set An administration set named for the large orifice between the piercing spike and the drip chamber; allows for rapid fluid flow into the vascular system.

macrophages Cells that are responsible for protecting the body against infection.

macular degeneration Deterioration of the central portion of the retina.

mainstem bronchi The part of the lower airway below the larynx through which air enters the lungs.

malfeasance An unauthorized act committed outside the scope of medical practice as defined by law.

Mallory-Weiss tear A tear in the mucous membrane, or inner lining, where the esophagus and the stomach meet, causing severe bleeding and potentially death.

malocclusion Misalignment of the teeth.

mammary glands The organs of milk production in the breasts.

mandible The bone of the lower jaw.

mania A mental disorder characterized by abnormally exaggerated happiness, joy, or euphoria with hyperactivity, insomnia, and grandiose ideas.

manic-depressive illness A bipolar disorder in which mood fluctuates between depression and mania. The alterations in mood are usually episodic and recurrent.

manually triggered ventilation (MTV) device A fixed flow rate ventilation device that delivers a breath every time its button is pushed; also referred to as a flow-restricted, oxygen-powered ventilation device.

manubrium The upper fourth of the sternum.

margination The loss of fluid from the blood vessels into the tissue, causing the blood left in the vessels to have increased viscosity, which in turn slows the flow of blood and produces stasis.

marijuana The dried leaves and flower buds of the *Cannabis sativa* plant, which are smoked to achieve a high.

mass-casualty incident (MCI) An emergency situation that can place great demand on the equipment or personnel of the EMS system or has the potential to overwhelm available resources.

massive hemothorax An accumulation of more than 1,500 mL of blood within the pleural space.

mast cells Cells located in the tissues that release chemical mediators in response to an antigen-antibody reaction.

mastoid process A prominent bony mass at the base of the skull behind the ear.

maxillae The upper jawbones that assist in the formation of the orbit, the nasal cavity, and the palate and hold the upper teeth.

mean arterial pressure (MAP) The average pressure against the arterial wall during a cardiac cycle; generally considered to be the same as blood pressure.

mechanical energy The energy that results from motion (kinetic energy) or that is stored in an object (potential energy).

mechanical piston device A device that depresses the sternum via a compressed gas-powered or electric-powered plunger mounted on a backboard.

mechanism of action The way in which a medication produces the intended response.

mechanism of injury (MOI) The forces, or energy transmission, applied to the body that cause injury; the way in which traumatic injuries occur.

meconium The newborn's first bowel movement.

meconium staining The occurrence of a dark green material in the amniotic fluid that can cause lung disease in the newborn.

MED channels Very high-frequency and ultra high-frequency channels that the Federal Communications Commission has designated exclusively for EMS use.

medevac Medical evacuation of a patient by helicopter.

medial In anatomy, parts of the body that lie closer to the midline.

medial malleolus The distal end of the tibia, which forms the medial side of the ankle joint.

mediastinitis Inflammation of the mediastinum that often results when gastric contents leak into the thoracic cavity after esophageal perforation.

mediastinum The space between the lungs, in the center of the chest, that contains the heart, trachea, large blood vessels, mainstem bronchi, part of the esophagus, lymphatic channels, and paired vagus and phrenic nerves.

medical ambiguity Uncertainty regarding the specific cause of the patient's condition.

medical control Physician instructions given directly by radio or cell phone (online/direct) or indirectly by protocol/guidelines (off-line or indirect), as authorized by the medical director of the service program.

medical director The physician who authorizes or delegates to the provider the authority to perform health care in the field.

medical emergencies Emergencies caused by illnesses or conditions, not by an outside force.

medical incident command In incident command, the position responsible for the triage, treatment, and transport of injured people; also known as the medical or emergency medical services branch of the incident command system.

medical necessity A standard used by Medicare to determine whether a patient's condition requires ambulance transport in a particular situation.

medication A chemical substance that is used to treat or prevent disease or relieve pain.

medication interaction A situation in which the effects of one medication alter the response of another medication.

medicolegal A term relating to medical jurisprudence (law) or forensic medicine.

medulla Continuous inferiorly with the spinal cord; serves as a conduction pathway for ascending and descending nerve tracts; coordinates heart rate, blood vessel diameter, breathing, swallowing, vomiting, coughing, and sneezing.

medulla oblongata Nerve tissue that is continuous inferiorly with the spinal cord; serves as a conduction pathway for ascending and descending nerve tracts; coordinates heart rate, blood vessel diameter, breathing, swallowing, vomiting, coughing, and sneezing.

medullary cavity An internal cavity that contains bone marrow.

meiosis A type of cell division that occurs in the production of eggs and sperm.

melena Black, tarry, foul-smelling stools caused by digested blood that has traveled through the digestive tract; caused by upper gastrointestinal bleeding.

membrane attack complex Molecules that insert themselves into the bacterial membrane, leading to weakened areas in the membrane.

menarche The initial onset of menstruation occurring during puberty; the first menstrual cycle.

meninges A set of three tough membranes, the dura mater, arachnoid, and pia mater, that enclose and protect the entire brain and spinal cord within the skull and the spinal canal.

meningitis An inflammation of the meningeal coverings of the brain and spinal cord; it is usually caused by a virus or a bacterium.

meningococcal meningitis An inflammation of the meningeal coverings of the brain and spinal cord; can be highly contagious.

menopause The cessation of the menstrual cycle and ovarian function.

menstrual cycle A cycle lasting approximately 28 days in which physiologic changes occur in the uterus and associated reproductive organs.

menstruation The period in the menstrual cycle of sloughing and discharge of the functional layer of the endometrium; occurs approximately every 28 days.

mental disorder An illness with psychological or behavioral symptoms and/or impairment in functioning, caused by a social, psychological, genetic, physical, chemical, or biologic disturbance; may also be referred to as a psychiatric disorder.

metabolic Relating to the breakdown of ingested foodstuffs into smaller and smaller molecules and atoms that are used as energy sources for cellular function.

metabolic acidosis A pathologic condition characterized by a blood pH of less than 7.35 and caused by accumulation of acids in the body from a metabolic cause.

metabolic alkalosis A pathologic condition characterized by a blood pH of greater than 7.45 and caused by an accumulation of bases in the body from a metabolic cause.

metabolism The chemical processes that provide the cells with energy from nutrients.

metacarpal bones The bones that form the hand.

metaplasia A reversible, cellular adaptation in which one adult cell type is replaced by another adult cell type.

metered-dose inhaler (MDI) A miniature spray canister used to direct medications through the mouth to be inhaled into the lungs.

methamphetamine A highly addictive drug in the amphetamine family.

methicillin-resistant *Staphylococcus aureus* (MRSA) A bacterium that can cause infections in different parts of the body and is often resistant to commonly used antibiotics; it is transmitted by different routes, including the respiratory route, and can be found on the skin, in surgical wounds, and in the bloodstream, lungs, and urinary tract.

metric system A decimal system based on tens for the measurement of length, weight, and volume.

microangiopathy Microscopic deterioration of vessel walls caused primarily by adherence of blood lipids to vessel walls.

microdrip set An administration set named for the small orifice between the piercing spike and the drip chamber; allows for carefully controlled fluid flow and is ideally suited for medication administration.

midbrain The part of the brain that is responsible for helping to regulate the level of consciousness.

middle adult An adult age 41 to 60 years.

midsagittal plane (midline) An imaginary vertical line drawn from the middle of the forehead through the nose and the umbilicus (navel) to the floor.

mild airway obstruction A condition in which an obstruction leaves the patient able to exchange some air, but also causes some degree of respiratory distress.

minute volume The amount of air moved in and out of the respiratory tract (minus the dead space) per minute; determined by the tidal volume multiplied by the respiratory rate. Also called minute ventilation.

miosis Excessively constricted (pinpoint) pupil; often bilateral after exposure to nerve agents.

misfeasance Appropriate act performed in an improper manner, such as a medication administered at the wrong dose.

mitral valve The valve in the heart that separates the left atrium from the left ventricle.

mobile data terminal (MDT) A small computer terminal inside an ambulance that directly receives data from the dispatch center.

Mobile Integrated Healthcare (MIH) A system of delivering health care services within the community, rather than at a physician's office or a hospital, with an integrated team of health care professionals.

mobile radio A radio that is mounted inside a vehicle and used to communicate with dispatch or medical control; it operates at lower power than a base station (20 to 50 watts) and is assigned to a specific radio frequency band.

monoamine oxidase inhibitors (MAOIs) Psychiatric medication used primarily to treat atypical depression by increasing norepinephrine and serotonin levels in the central nervous system.

monocytes Agranulocytes that migrate out of the blood and into the tissues in response to an infection.

mons pubis The pad of fatty tissue and coarse skin that lies over the female pubic symphysis.

mood disorders Disorders in which the disturbance of mood is accompanied by full or partial manic or depressive syndrome.

morality A code of conduct that can be defined by society, religion, or a person, affecting character, conduct, and conscience.

morbid obesity An excessively unhealthy accumulation of body fat, defined as a body mass index of greater than or equal to 40 kg/m^2.

morbidity Number of nonfatally injured or disabled people; usually expressed as a rate, meaning the number of nonfatal injuries in a certain population in a given time period divided by the size of the population.

morgue supervisor In incident command, the person who works with area medical examiners, coroners, and law enforcement agencies to coordinate the disposition of dead patients.

Moro reflex An infant reflex in which, when an infant is caught off guard, the infant opens his or her arms wide, spreads the fingers, and seems to grab at things.

mortality The quality of being mortal; number of deaths from a disease in a given population.

motor nerves Nerves that carry information from the central nervous system to the muscles of the body.

mucosal atomizer device (MAD) A device that attaches to the end of a syringe that is used to spray (atomize) certain medications via the intranasal route.

mucous membranes The lining of body cavities and passages that communicate directly or indirectly with the environment outside the body.

mucus The opaque, sticky secretion of the mucous membranes that lubricates the body openings.

multigravida A term used to describe a woman who has been pregnant more than once.

multilumen airway device A type of airway device with a single long tube that can be used for esophageal obturation or endotracheal tube ventilation, depending on where it comes to rest following blind positioning.

multipara A term used to describe a woman who has delivered two or more viable infants.

multiple sclerosis (MS) A severe, incurable degenerative disorder involving the central nervous system (brain and spinal cord).

multiple-casualty incident Any situation with more than one patient, but which will not overwhelm available resources.

multiple-organ dysfunction syndrome (MODS) A progressive condition that occurs after severe illness or injury, usually characterized by combined failure of two or more organs or organ systems not affected by the patient's initial illness or injury, along with some clotting mechanisms.

multiplex Simultaneous transmission of multiple data streams, most often voice and electrocardiographic signals, in either or both directions over the same frequency.

multisystem trauma A term that describes the injuries of a person who has been subjected to multiple traumatic injuries involving more than one body system; these patients have a high level of morbidity and mortality.

murmur An abnormal heart sound, heard as a "whooshing-like" sound, indicating turbulent blood flow within the heart.

muscarinic cholinergic antagonists Medications that block acetylcholine exclusively at the muscarinic receptors; an example is atropine.

muscular dystrophy A category of incurable genetic diseases that cause a slow, progressive degeneration of the muscle fibers.

musculoskeletal system The bones and voluntary muscles of the body.

mutagen A substance that mutates, damages, and changes the structures of the body's cells.

mutism The absence of speech.

mutual aid response An agreement between neighboring emergency medical services systems to respond to mass-casualty incidents or disasters in each other's region when local resources are insufficient to handle the response.

myelin An insulating layer, or sheath, made up of fatty substances and protein that form around the nerves.

myocardial contractility The ability of the heart muscle to contract.

myocardial contusion A bruise of the heart muscle.

myocardial infarction Blockage of the arteries that supply oxygen to the heart, resulting in death to a portion of the myocardium.

myocardial rupture An acute perforation of the ventricles, atria, intraventricular septum, intra-atrial septum, chordae, papillary muscles, or valves.

myocardium The heart muscle.

myoclonus Hyperactive reflexes; occurs during severe preeclampsia.

myoglobin A pigment synthesized in the muscles to give skeletal muscles their red-brown color.

myometrium A thick smooth muscle that forms the middle layer of the uterine wall.

narcotic A generic term for opiates and opioids; a drug that acts as a central nervous system depressant and produces insensibility or stupor.

nares The external openings of the nostrils.

nasal cannula An oxygen-delivery device in which oxygen flows through two small, tubelike prongs that fit into the patient's nostrils.

nasal cavity The chamber inside the nose that lies between the floor of the cranium and the roof of the mouth.

nasal flaring Widening of the nostrils, indicating that an airway obstruction is present.

nasal septum The separation between the right and left nostrils.

nasopharyngeal (nasal) airway An airway adjunct inserted into the nostril of a responsive patient who is not able to maintain a natural airway.

nasopharynx The part of the pharynx that lies above the level of the roof of the mouth, or palate.

National EMS Scope of Practice Model A document created by the National Highway Traffic Safety Administration that outlines the skills performed by various emergency medical services providers.

National Incident Management System (NIMS) A Department of Homeland Security system designed to enable federal, state, and local governments, private-sector and nongovernmental organizations, and all other organizations who assume a role in emergency management to effectively and efficiently prepare for, prevent, respond to, and recover from domestic incidents, regardless of cause, size, or complexity, including acts of catastrophic terrorism and hazardous materials incidents.

natural immunity A nonspecific cellular and humoral response that operates as the body's first line of defense against pathogens; this develops as part of being exposed to an antigen and developing antibodies; also called native immunity.

nature of illness (NOI) The general type of illness a patient is experiencing.

nebulizer A device for producing a fine spray or mist that is used to deliver inhaled medications.

necrosis The death of tissue, usually caused by a cessation of the blood supply.

necrotizing fasciitis Death of tissue from bacterial infection, caused by more than one infecting organism—most commonly, *Staphylococcus aureus* and hemolytic streptococci; this condition has a high mortality rate.

negative pressure ventilation Drawing of air into the lungs; airflow from a region of higher pressure (outside the body) to a region of lower pressure (the lungs); occurs during normal (unassisted) breathing.

neglect Refusal or failure on the part of the caregiver to provide life necessities, such as needed care, services, or supervision.

negligence Failure to provide the same care that a person with similar training would provide.

negligence per se A theory that may be used when the conduct of the person being sued is alleged to have occurred in clear violation of a statute.

Neisseria meningitidis A form of bacterial meningitis characterized by rapid onset of symptoms, often leading to shock and death.

neologisms Invented words that have meaning only to their inventor.

neonate A newborn age birth to 1 month.

neoplasm A mass of tissue produced by abnormal cell growth and division that may be malignant (cancerous) or benign; a tumor.

nephrons The structural and functional units of the kidney that form urine; composed of the glomerulus, the glomerular (Bowman) capsule, the proximal convoluted tubule, loop of Henle, and the distal convoluted tubule.

nerve agents A class of chemical called organophosphates; they function by blocking an essential enzyme in the nervous system, which causes the body's organs to become overstimulated and burn out.

nerve root injury Injury to a nerve at the level of the spinal cord.

nervous system The system that controls virtually all activities of the body, both voluntary and involuntary.

neurogenic shock Circulatory failure caused by paralysis of the nerves that control the size of the blood vessels, resulting in widespread vasodilation and loss of sympathetic nervous system tone; seen in patients with spinal cord injuries.

neuronal soma The body of a neuron (nerve cell).

neuropathy A group of conditions in which the nerves leaving the spinal cord are damaged, resulting in distortion of signals to or from the brain.

neurotic disorders A collection of mental disorders without psychotic symptoms and lacking the intense psychopathology of other mood disorders; includes anxiety disorders, phobias, and panic disorder.

neurotoxins Biologic agents that are the most deadly substances known to humans; they include botulinum toxin and ricin.

neurotransmitters The chemicals produced by the body that stimulate electrical reactions in adjacent neurons.

neurovascular compromise The loss of the nerve supply, blood supply, or both to a region of the body, typically distal to a site of injury; characterized by alterations in sensation, including numbness and tingling, or by a loss or decrease of motor function; vascular compromise is indicated by weak or absent pulses, poor skin color, and cool skin.

neutron radiation The type of energy that is emitted from a strong radiologic source, involving particles that are among the most powerful forms of radiation; the particles easily penetrate through lead and require several feet of concrete to stop them.

neutrophils One of the three types of granulocytes; they have multilobed nuclei that resemble a string of baseballs held together by a thin strand of thread; they destroy bacteria, antigen-antibody complexes, and foreign matter.

New Intraosseous (NIO) device A spring-loaded device that contains neither drill nor battery, used for inserting an intraosseous needle into the proximal tibia of an adult patient.

newborn The phase of life from the first few minutes to the first hours after birth.

noise Anything that dampens or obscures the true meaning of a message.

nonbarbiturate hypnotics Medications designed to sedate without the side effects of a barbiturate.

nonbulk storage vessels Any container other than bulk storage containers such as drums, bags, compressed gas cylinders, and cryogenic containers. These hold commonly used commercial and industrial chemicals such as solvents, industrial cleaners, and compounds.

nondisplaced fracture A simple crack in the bone that has not caused the bone to move from its normal anatomic position; also called a hairline fracture.

nonfeasance Failure to perform a required or expected act.

nonhemorrhagic shock Shock that occurs as a result of fluid loss contained within the body, such as in dehydration, burn injury, crush injury, and anaphylaxis.

nonopioid analgesics Medications designed to relieve pain without the side effects of opioids.

nonrebreathing mask A combination mask and reservoir bag system that is the preferred way to give oxygen in the prehospital setting; delivers up to 90% inspired oxygen.

nonsteroidal anti-inflammatory drugs (NSAIDs) Medications with analgesic and fever-reducing properties.

norepinephrine A neurotransmitter and drug sometimes used in the treatment of shock; produces vasoconstriction through its alpha-stimulator properties.

normal saline 0.9% sodium chloride; an isotonic crystalloid.

nosocomial Hospital acquired.

nuchal cord An umbilical cord that is wrapped around the newborn's neck.

nuchal rigidity A stiff or painful neck; commonly associated with meningitis.

nullipara A term used to describe a woman who has never delivered a viable infant.

obesity A complex condition in which a person has an excessive amount of body fat; the result of an imbalance between calories consumed and calories used; defined as a body mass index of greater than or equal to 30 kg/m^2.

objective information Information that you observe and that is measurable, such as a patient's blood pressure.

obstructive shock Shock that occurs when there is a block to blood flow in the heart or great vessels, causing an insufficient blood supply to the body's tissues.

occipital lobe The portion of the brain that is responsible for the processing of visual information.

occiput The posterior (back) aspect of the head.

occlusion Blockage, usually of a tubular structure such as a blood vessel.

occlusive dressing A dressing made of gauze with petroleum jelly, aluminum foil, or plastic that prevents air and liquids from entering or exiting a wound.

Occupational Safety and Health Administration (OSHA) The federal regulatory compliance agency that develops, publishes, and enforces guidelines concerning safety in the workplace.

oculomotor nerve The cranial nerve (III) that innervates the muscles that cause motion of the eyeballs and upper eyelid.

off-gassing The release of an agent after exposure, such as from a person's clothes that have been exposed to the agent.

official name Drug name assigned by the *United States Pharmacopeia* (*USP*), generally the generic name followed by "USP."

older adult An adult age 61 years or older.

olfactory nerve The cranial nerve (I) for smell.

oliguria A decrease in urine output to the extent that total urine output drops to less than 500 mL per day.

oncotic pressure The pressure of water to move, typically into the capillary, as the result of the presence of plasma proteins.

onset of action The time needed for the concentration of the medication at the target tissue to reach the minimum effective level.

oocytes Female sex cells; the precursors to a mature egg.

oogenesis The maturation process that results in production of an ovum, or egg.

open abdominal injury An injury in which there is a break in the surface of the skin or mucous membrane, exposing deeper tissue to potential contamination.

open book pelvic fracture A life-threatening fracture of the pelvis caused by a force that displaces one or both sides of the pelvis laterally and posteriorly.

open chest injury An injury to the chest in which the chest wall itself is penetrated by some external object such as a knife or bullet.

open fracture Any break in a bone in which the overlying skin has been damaged.

open head injury An injury to the head often caused by a penetrating object in which there may be bleeding and exposed brain tissue.

open incident An incident that is not yet contained; there may be patients who have yet to be located and the situation may be ongoing, producing more patients.

open injury An injury in which there is a break in the surface of the skin or the mucous membrane, exposing deeper tissue to potential contamination.

open pneumothorax An accumulation of air or gas in the pleural space, resulting from a defect or penetration into the chest wall that allows air to enter the thoracic cavity.

open-ended questions Questions for which the patient must provide detail to give an answer.

operations In incident command, the section that carries out the orders of the incident commander to help resolve the incident.

opiate Any of the various alkaloids derived from the opium or poppy plant.

opioid A synthetic narcotic not derived from opium.

opioid agonist-antagonists Medications designed to relieve pain without the side effects of opioids.

opioid agonists Chemicals that are similar to or derived from the opium plant.

opioid antagonists A classification of medications that reverses the effects of opioid drugs.

OPQRST A mnemonic used in evaluating a patient's pain: Onset, Provocation/palliation, Quality, Region/radiation, Severity, and Timing of pain.

opsonization The process by which an antibody coats an antigen to facilitate its recognition by immune cells.

optic nerve Either of the second cranial nerves that enter the eyeball posteriorly, through the optic foramen, which transmit visual information to the brain.

oral By mouth; a medication delivery route.

oral glucose A simple sugar that is readily absorbed by the bloodstream; it is carried on the EMS unit.

orbit The eye socket, made up of the maxilla and zygoma.

orchitis A complication of a male urinary tract infection in which one or both testes become infected, enlarged, and tender, causing pain and swelling in the scrotum.

organic brain syndrome Temporary or permanent dysfunction of the brain, caused by a disturbance in the physical or physiologic functioning of brain tissue.

organophosphates A class of chemicals found in many insecticides used in agriculture and in the home.

orientation The mental status of a patient as measured by memory of person (name), place (current location), time (current year, month, and approximate date), and event (what happened).

oropharyngeal (oral) airway An airway adjunct inserted into the mouth to keep the tongue from blocking the upper airway and to make suctioning the airway easier.

oropharynx A tubular structure that extends vertically from the back of the mouth to the esophagus and trachea.

orthopnea Severe dyspnea experienced when lying down that is relieved by a change in position, such as sitting up or standing.

orthostatic hypotension Symptomatic drop in blood pressure related to the patient's body position, detected by measuring pulse and blood pressure while the patient is lying supine, sitting up, and standing. An increase in pulse rate and a decrease in blood pressure in any one of these positions is considered a positive sign for this condition.

orthostatic vital signs Assessing vital signs in two different patient positions (for example, in the supine and sitting or standing positions) to determine the degree of hypotension; also known as the tilt test.

osmolarity The ability to influence the movement of water across a semipermeable membrane.

osmosis The movement of a solvent (fluid), such as water, from an area of lower solute concentration to one of higher concentration through a selectively permeable membrane to equalize concentrations of a solute on both sides of the membrane.

osmotic pressure Pressure created against the cell wall by the presence of water.

osteogenesis imperfecta A congenital bone disease that results in fragile bones.

osteomyelitis Inflammation of the bone and muscle caused by infection; a potential complication of intraosseous infusion.

osteoporosis A generalized bone disease, commonly associated with postmenopausal women but occurring in either sex, in which there is a reduction in the amount of bone mass, resulting in increased susceptibility to fractures after minimal trauma.

ovaries Female, almond-shaped glands that lie on either side of the pelvic cavity and produce sex hormones and ova (eggs).

overdose Consumption of an excessive quantity of a drug that, when taken or administered, can have toxic or lethal consequences.

over-the-counter (OTC) medications Medications that may be purchased directly by a patient without a prescription.

over-the-needle catheters The prehospital standard for intravenous cannulation, these consist of a hollow tube over a laser-sharpened steel needle; also referred to as an angiocath.

overweight An unhealthy accumulation of body fat, defined as a body mass index of 25 to 29.9 kg/m^2.

ovulation The release of a mature egg (ovum) into the fallopian tube from the ovary.

ovum A mature egg released by the ovary during ovulation.

oxygen saturation (Spo_2) The measure of the percentage of oxygen molecules that are bound to hemoglobin in arterial blood.

oxygen toxicity A condition of excessive oxygen consumption resulting in cellular and tissue damage.

oxygenation The process of delivering oxygen to the blood by diffusion from the alveoli following inhalation into the lungs.

oxytocin A hormone secreted in the pituitary gland that promotes uterine contractions.

packaging The act of preparing a patient for movement as a unit by means of a backboard or similar immobilization device.

paging The use of a radio signal and a voice or digital message that is transmitted to pagers ("beepers") or desktop monitor radios.

palmar The position in which the palm of the hand is facing forward when in the anatomic position.

palmar grasp An infant reflex that occurs when something is placed in the infant's palm; the infant grasps the object.

palpate To examine by touch.

pancreas A flat, solid organ that can also be considered a gland, that lies below the liver and the stomach; it is a major source of digestive enzymes delivered into the duodenum, and produces the hormone insulin; considered both an endocrine gland and an exocrine gland.

pancreatitis Inflammation of the pancreas.

pandemic An outbreak of a disease that occurs on a global scale.

panic disorder A disorder characterized by sudden, usually unexpected, and overwhelming feelings of fear and dread, accompanied by a variety of other symptoms produced by a massive activation of the autonomic nervous system.

paper bag syndrome Rupture of the lungs that occurs as the chest meets with blunt trauma after taking a deep breath, usually during a motor vehicle crash, similar to the rupture of an air-filled paper bag.

papillary muscles Specialized muscles that attach the ventricles to the cusps of the valves by muscular strands called chordae tendineae.

para A term used to describe the number of times a woman has delivered a viable (live) infant.

paradoxical motion The inward movement of the chest during inhalation and outward movement during exhalation; the opposite of normal chest wall movement during breathing; occurs in a flail chest.

paramedic An individual extensively trained in advanced life support, including endotracheal intubation, emergency pharmacology, cardiac monitoring, and other advanced assessment and treatment skills.

paranasal sinuses The sinuses, or hollowed sections of bone in the front of the head, which are lined with mucous membrane and drain into the nasal cavity.

paraplegia Paralysis of the lower part of the body, possibly from thoracic or lumbar spinal injury or spina bifida.

parasympathetic nervous system A subdivision of the autonomic nervous system, involved in control of involuntary, vegetative functions, mediated largely by the vagus nerve through the chemical acetylcholine; the part of the autonomic nervous system that relaxes the body.

parasympatholytics Drugs that block the actions of the parasympathetic nervous system; also known as anticholinergics.

parasympathomimetics Drugs that produce the same effects as those of the parasympathetic nervous system; also known as cholinergics.

parathyroid glands Four glands that are embedded in the posterior portion of each lobe of the thyroid; they produce and secrete parathyroid hormone.

parathyroid hormone Hormone produced and secreted by the parathyroid glands; it maintains normal levels of calcium in the blood and normal neuromuscular function.

parenchyma The tissue of an organ itself.

parenteral Drug administration through any route other than through the gastrointestinal tract; includes intravenous, intraosseous, subcutaneous, intramuscular, sublingual, buccal, transcutaneous, intranasal, and inhalation.

parenteral medications Medications that are given through any route other than through the gastrointestinal tract.

paresthesias Abnormal sensations such as burning, numbness, or tingling.

parietal lobe The portion of the brain that is the site for reception and evaluation of most sensory information, except smell, hearing, and vision.

parietal pleura The thin membrane that lines the pleural chest cavity.

partial laryngectomy Surgical removal of a portion of the larynx.

partial pressure The term used to describe the amount of gas in air or dissolved in fluid, such as blood.

partial pressure of carbon dioxide ($Paco_2$) A measurement of the amount of carbon dioxide in the blood.

partial pressure of oxygen (Pao_2) A measurement of the amount of oxygen in the blood.

partial rebreathing mask A mask that is similar to a nonrebreathing mask except there is no one-way valve between the mask and the reservoir; therefore, patients rebreathe a small amount of their exhaled air.

partial seizures The seizures affecting a limited portion of the brain.

partial-thickness burns The burns affecting the epidermis and some portion of the dermis but not the subcutaneous tissue, characterized by blisters and skin that is white to red, moist, and mottled; formerly called a second-degree burn.

patella The kneecap; a specialized bone that lies within the tendon of the quadriceps muscle.

patent Open, clear of obstruction.

pathogen A microorganism that is capable of causing disease in a susceptible host.

pathologic fracture A fracture that occurs in an area of abnormally weakened bone.

pathophysiology The study of the physiology of altered functioning in the presence of disease.

patient autonomy The right of a patient to make informed choices regarding his or her health care.

patient care report (PCR) The legal document used to record all patient care activities. This report has direct patient care functions as well as administrative and quality control functions. PCRs are also known as prehospital care reports.

peak In a pharmacologic context, the point of maximum effect of a drug.

pedal edema Swelling of the feet and ankles caused by collection of fluid in the tissues; a possible sign of congestive heart failure.

pediatric assessment triangle (PAT) A structured assessment tool that allows you to rapidly form a general impression of the infant or child without touching him or her; consists of assessing appearance, work of breathing, and circulation to the skin.

pelvic binders Devices used to splint the bony pelvis to reduce hemorrhage from bone ends, venous disruption, and pain.

pelvic inflammatory disease (PID) An infection of the female upper organs of reproduction, specifically the uterus, ovaries, and fallopian tubes.

pelvis The attachment of the lower extremities to the body, consisting of the sacrum and two pelvic bones.

penetrating trauma Injury caused by objects that pierce and penetrate the surface of the body and injure the underlying tissues, such as knives and bullets, and damage internal organs and body cavities.

penetrating wound An injury that penetrates the skin, resulting from a sharp, pointed object or a blunt object traveling at sufficient speed, such as a knife or a bullet.

Penrose drain A type of surgical drain; can be used as a constricting band.

perfusion The circulation of oxygenated blood within an organ or tissue in adequate amounts to meet the cells' current needs.

pericardial fluid A serous fluid that fills the space between the visceral pericardium and the parietal pericardium and helps to reduce friction.

pericardial sac A thick, fibrous membrane that surrounds the heart. Also called the pericardium.

pericardial tamponade The impairment of diastolic filling of the right ventricle due to significant amounts of fluid in the pericardial sac surrounding the heart, leading to a decrease in the cardiac output.

pericardiocentesis The ultimate treatment for cardiac tamponade, which involves inserting a needle attached to a syringe far enough into the chest to penetrate the pericardium to withdraw fluid.

pericardium A thick, fibrous membrane that surrounds the heart. Also called the pericardial sac.

perineum The area of skin between the scrotum and the anus in males, and the vagina and the anus in females.

periosteum A double layer of connective tissue that lines the outer surface of the bone.

peripheral nerve injury Injury to a nerve anywhere in the body outside the spinal cord.

peripheral nervous system (PNS) The 31 pairs of spinal nerves and 12 pairs of cranial nerves that link the body's other organs to the central nervous system; these may be sensory, motor, or connecting nerves.

peripheral shock Shock caused by peripheral circulatory abnormalities; includes hypovolemic shock and distributive shock.

peripheral vision Visualization of lateral objects while looking forward.

peristalsis The wavelike contraction of smooth muscle by which the ureters or other tubular organs propel their contents.

peritoneal cavity The abdominal cavity.

peritoneum The membrane lining the abdominal cavity (parietal peritoneum) and covering the abdominal organs (visceral peritoneum).

peritonitis Inflammation of the peritoneum.

perseveration Repeating the same idea over and over again.

persistency Describes how long a chemical agent will stay on a surface before it evaporates.

personal protective equipment (PPE) Equipment that blocks exposure to a pathogen or a hazardous material.

personal protective equipment (PPE) levels Indicate the amount and type of protective equipment that an individual needs to avoid injury during contact with a hazardous material.

pertinent negatives Expected signs or symptoms with negative findings that warrant no care or intervention.

pertussis An airborne bacterial infection that affects primarily children younger than 6 years; patients will be feverish and exhibit a "whoop" sound on inspiration after a coughing attack; highly contagious through droplet infection; also called whooping cough.

petechiae Small, purple, nonblanching spots on the skin.

petechial hemorrhage A pinpoint red dot in the sclera of the eye.

pH The measure of acidity or alkalinity of a solution.

phagocytes The cells that engulf and consume foreign material such as microorganisms and debris.

phalanges The small bones of the digits of the fingers and toes.

pharmacodynamics The study of drugs and their actions on living organisms.

pharmacokinetics The study of the metabolism and action of drugs with a particular emphasis on the time required for absorption, duration of action, distribution in the body, and method of excretion.

pharmacology The study of the properties and effects of medications.

phobias Obsessive, irrational fears of specific things or situations, such as fear of heights, fear of open places, fear of confined spaces, or fear of certain animals.

phosgene A very potent respiratory agent that is a product of combustion; it has a delayed onset of symptoms, usually hours.

phosgene oxime (CX) A vesicant that has a rapid onset of symptoms and produces immediate, intense pain and discomfort on contact.

phospholipid bilayer The cell membrane's double layer, consisting of a hydrophilic outer layer composed of phosphate groups, and a hydrophobic inner layer made up of lipids, or fatty acids. It is this structure and composition that allows the cell membrane to have selective permeability.

phrenic nerves The nerves that innervate the diaphragm; necessary for adequate breathing.

physical dependence A physiologic state of adaptation to a drug, usually characterized by tolerance to the drug's effects and a withdrawal syndrome if use of the drug is stopped, especially abruptly.

physiology The study of the body functions of the living organism.

physis The growth plate in long bones.

pia mater The innermost and thinnest of the three meninges that enclose the brain and spinal cord; it rests directly on the brain and spinal cord.

piercing spike The hard, sharpened plastic spike on the end of the administration set designed to pierce the sterile membrane of the intravenous bag.

pin-indexing system A system established for portable cylinders to ensure that a regulator is not connected to a cylinder containing the wrong type of gas.

pinna The external, visible part of the ear.

pituitary gland An endocrine gland, located in the sella turcica of the brain, responsible for directly or indirectly affecting all body functions.

placards Signage required to be placed on all four sides of highway transport vehicles, railroad tank cars, and other forms of hazardous materials transportation; the sign identifies the hazardous contents of the vehicle, using a standardization system with 10¾-inch (27-cm) diamond-shaped indicators.

placenta Tissue attached to the uterine wall that nourishes the fetus through the umbilical cord.

placenta previa A condition in which the placenta develops over and partially or completely covers the cervix.

plaintiff In a civil lawsuit, the person who brings a legal action against another person.

planning In incident command, the section that ultimately produces a plan to resolve any incident.

plantar The sole or bottom surface of the foot.

plantar flexion Bending of the foot toward the ground.

plasma A sticky, yellow fluid made mostly of water, but also electrolytes, clotting factors, and glucose, that is a component of blood that carries the blood cells, formed elements, and nutrients and transports cellular waste material to the organs of excretion.

plasmin An enzyme that dissolves the fibrin in blood clots.

platelets Tiny, disk-shaped elements that are much smaller than the cells; they are essential in the initial formation of a blood clot, the mechanism that stops bleeding.

pleura The serous membrane covering the lungs and lining the thoracic cavity, completely enclosing a potential space known as the pleural space.

pleural cavity The potential space between the visceral and parietal pleura.

pleural effusion A collection of fluid between the lung and chest wall that may compress the lung.

pleural friction rub A squeaking or grating sound that occurs when the pleural linings rub together, which may be heard on inspiration, expiration, or both; commonly caused by inflammation of the pleura.

pleural space The potential space between the visceral and parietal pleura of the lung and chest wall respectively; it is normally absent, as these surfaces are usually in direct contact.

pleuritic chest pain Sharp, stabbing pain in the chest that is worsened by a deep breath or other chest wall movement; often caused by inflammation or irritation of the pleura.

pneumatic antishock garment (PASG) An inflatable device that covers the legs and abdomen; used to splint the lower extremities or pelvis, or to control bleeding in the lower extremities or pelvis.

pneumonia An infectious disease of the lung that damages lung tissue.

pneumonic plague A lung infection, also known as plague pneumonia, that is the result of inhalation of plague-causing bacteria.

pneumonitis Lung inflammation from an irritant, such as a chemical, dust, or radiation, or from aspiration, such as aspiration of gastric contents.

pneumoperitoneum Air in the peritoneal cavity.

pneumotaxic (pontine) center A portion of the pons that assists in creating shorter, faster respirations.

pneumothorax A partial or complete accumulation of air in the pleural space.

point tenderness Tenderness that is sharply localized at the site of the injury, found by gently palpating along the bone with the tip of one finger.

points of distribution (PODs) Existing facilities used as mass distribution sites for antibiotics, chemical antidotes, antitoxins, vaccinations, and other medications and supplies during an emergency.

poison A substance whose chemical action could damage structures or impair function when it is introduced into the body.

polydipsia Excessive thirst persisting for long periods despite reasonable fluid intake; often the result of excessive urination.

polymorphonuclear neutrophils (PMNs) The type of white blood cells formed by bone marrow tissue that have a nucleus consisting of several parts or lobes connected by fine strands.

polyphagia Excessive eating; in diabetes, the inability to use glucose properly can cause a sense of hunger.

polypharmacy The simultaneous use of many medications by the same patient.

polyuria The passage of an unusually large volume of urine in a given period; in diabetes, this can result from wasting of glucose in the urine.

pons An organ that lies below the midbrain and above the medulla and contains numerous important nerve fibers, including those for sleep, respiration, and the medullary respiratory center.

popliteal artery A continuation of the femoral artery at the knee.

portable radio A handheld two-way radio with a limited range and low power (1 to 5 watts).

portable stretcher A stretcher with a strong, rectangular, tubular metal frame and rigid fabric stretched across it.

portal vein The blood vessel that transports blood from the gastrointestinal tract to the liver.

portal venous system Special venous drainage system that takes blood from the intestines to the liver.

positive end-expiratory pressure (PEEP) Mechanical maintenance of pressure in the airway at the end of expiration to increase the volume of gas remaining in the lungs.

postconventional reasoning A type of reasoning in which a child bases decisions on his or her conscience.

posterior In anatomy, the back surface of the body; the side away from you in the standard anatomic position.

posterior tibial artery The artery just behind the medial malleolus; supplies blood to the foot.

postictal state The period following a seizure that lasts between 5 and 30 minutes, characterized by labored respirations and some degree of altered mental status.

postpartum eclampsia Eclampsia that occurs after a woman has delivered a newborn; can occur up to several weeks after the birth.

posttraumatic stress disorder (PTSD) A delayed stress reaction to a prior incident, characterized by the reliving of the stress and nightmares of the original situation. Often the result of one or more unresolved issues concerning the incident, and may relate to an incident that involved physical harm or the threat of physical harm.

potassium channel blockers Medications that increase the contractility of the heart and work against the reentry of blocked impulses.

potential energy The product of mass (weight), gravity, and height that is converted into kinetic energy and results in injury, such as from a fall.

potentiation Enhancement of the action of a drug by the administration of another drug.

power grip A technique in which the stretcher or backboard is gripped by inserting each hand under the handle with the palm facing up and the thumb extended, fully supporting the underside of the handle on the curved palm with the fingers and thumb.

power lift A lifting technique in which the AEMT's back is held upright, with legs bent, and the patient is lifted when the AEMT straightens the legs to raise the upper body and arms.

prearrival instructions Instructions provided by the emergency medical dispatcher to an emergency caller to care for life-threatening emergencies until help arrives.

precedence Basing current action on lessons, rules, or guidelines derived from previous similar experiences.

preconventional reasoning A type of reasoning in which a child acts almost purely to avoid punishment or to get what he or she wants.

prediabetes A condition identified in people who have certain risk factors associated with type 2 diabetes and exists when blood glucose levels or hemoglobin A1c levels are above normal levels, yet not high enough to be diagnosed as diabetes.

preeclampsia A condition during pregnancy characterized by hypertension, protein in the urine, and edema; a precursor to eclampsia.

prefix The word part that appears before a word root, changing the meaning of the term.

preload The precontraction pressure in the heart, which increases as the volume of blood builds up when returned to the heart (venous return); directly affects afterload.

premature A newborn that delivers before 36 weeks of gestation or weighs less than 5 lb (2.25 kg) at birth.

premature rupture of membranes Rupture of the amniotic sac prior to the onset of labor; increases risk of fetal infection or injury.

premenstrual syndrome (PMS) A cluster of all or some of the troubling symptoms that occur during a woman's menstrual phase that can include fluid retention, breast pain and tenderness, headache, severe cramping, and emotional changes, including agitation, irritability, depression, and anger.

prepuce A structure in the female external genitalia that is formed where the labia minora unite over the clitoris.

presbycusis An age-related condition of the ear that produces progressive bilateral hearing loss that is most noted at higher frequencies.

preschooler A child age 3 to 6 years.

prescription medications Medications that are distributed to patients only by pharmacists according to a physician's order.

pressure infuser device A sleeve that is placed around a bag of intravenous solution and inflated to force fluid to flow into the tubing.

pressure of speech Speech in which words seem to tumble out under immense emotional pressure.

pressure point A point where a blood vessel lies near a bone.

preterm Before 36 complete weeks of gestation.

prevalence The number of cases of a disease in a specific population within a given period.

priapism A painful, tender, and persistent erection of the penis; can result from spinal cord injury, use of erectile dysfunction drugs, or sickle cell disease.

primary apnea Apnea caused by oxygen deprivation; usually corrected with stimulation, such as drying or slapping the newborn's feet; typically preceded by an initial period of rapid breathing.

primary blast injury Injuries caused by an explosive pressure wave on the hollow organs of the body.

primary brain injury An injury to the brain and its associated structures that is a direct result of impact to the head.

primary prevention Efforts to prevent an injury or illness from ever occurring.

primary response The first encounter with the foreign substance that initiates the immune response.

primary service area (PSA) The designated area in which an emergency medical services agency is responsible for the provision of prehospital emergency care and transportation to the hospital.

primary spinal cord injury Injury to the spinal cord that is a direct result of trauma, for example, transection of the spinal cord from penetrating trauma or displacement of ligaments and bone fragments, resulting in compression of the spinal cord.

primary survey A step within the patient assessment process that identifies and initiates treatment of immediate and potential life threats.

primary triage A type of patient sorting used to rapidly categorize patients; the focus is on speed in locating all patients and determining an initial priority as their conditions warrant.

primigravida A woman's first pregnancy.

primipara A woman who has had only one delivery.

progesterone A hormone released from the ovaries that stimulates the uterine lining during the menstrual cycle in preparation for implantation of a fertilized egg.

prolapsed umbilical cord A situation in which the umbilical cord comes out of the vagina before the newborn.

pronation The act of rotating the forearms in a palms-down manner.

prone Lying flat, face down.

proprioception The ability to perceive the position and movement of one's body or limbs.

prostaglandins A group of lipids that act as chemical messengers.

prostate gland A small gland that surrounds the male urethra where it emerges from the urinary bladder; it secretes a fluid that is part of the ejaculatory fluid.

protected health information (PHI) Any information about health status, provision of health care, or payment for health care that can be linked to an individual. This information is interpreted rather broadly and includes any part of a patient's medical record or payment history.

protocols Precise and detailed plans for a regimen of therapy (for example, advanced cardiac life support algorithms).

proxemics The study of space between people and its effects on communication.

proximal Closer to the trunk.

proximate cause The specific reason that an injury occurred; one of the items that must be proven in order for an AEMT to be held liable for negligence.

pruritus Itching.

psychogenic A symptom or illness that is caused by mental factors as opposed to physical ones.

psychogenic shock Shock caused by a sudden, temporary reduction in blood supply to the brain that causes fainting (syncope).

psychological dependence The emotional state of craving a drug to maintain a feeling of well-being.

psychosis A mental disorder characterized by the loss of contact with reality.

pubic symphysis A hard bony and cartilaginous prominence found at the midline in the lowermost portion of the abdomen where the two halves of the pelvic ring are joined by cartilage at a joint with minimal motion.

pubis One of three bones that fuse to form the pelvic ring.

public health Focused on examining the health needs of entire populations with the goal of preventing health problems.

public information officer (PIO) In incident command, the person who keeps the public informed and relays information to the press.

public safety access point A call center staffed by trained personnel who are responsible for managing requests for police, firefighting, and ambulance services.

pulmonary artery The major artery leading from the right ventricle of the heart to the lungs; it carries oxygen-poor blood.

pulmonary blast injuries Pulmonary trauma resulting from short-range exposure to the detonation of high-energy explosives.

pulmonary circulation The flow of blood from the right ventricle through the pulmonary arteries and all of their branches and capillaries in the lungs and back to the left atrium through the venules and pulmonary veins; also called the lesser circulation.

pulmonary contusion A bruise of the lung.

pulmonary edema A buildup of fluid in the lungs, usually as a result of left-side heart failure.

pulmonary embolism A blood clot that breaks off from a large vein and travels to the blood vessels of the lung, causing obstruction of blood flow.

pulmonary embolus A blood clot trapped within the pulmonary circulation.

pulmonary overpressurization syndrome (POPS) A diving emergency that can occur during rapid ascent and can cause pneumothorax, mediastinal and subcutaneous emphysema, alveolar hemorrhage, and the lethal air embolism; also called burst lung.

pulmonary veins The four veins that return oxygenated blood from the lungs to the left atrium of the heart.

pulmonic valve The semilunar valve that regulates blood flow between the right ventricle and the pulmonary artery.

pulse The wave of pressure created as the heart contracts and forces blood out of the left ventricle and into the major arteries.

pulse oximetry An assessment tool that measures oxygen saturation of hemoglobin in the capillary beds.

pulse pressure The difference between the systolic blood pressure and the diastolic blood pressure.

pulsus paradoxus A drop in the systolic blood pressure of 10 mm Hg or more; commonly seen in patients with cardiac tamponade or severe asthma.

punitive damages Compensation that is sometimes awarded in a civil lawsuit when the conduct of the defendant was intentional or constituted a reckless disregard for the safety of the public.

pupil The circular opening in the middle of the iris that admits light to the back of the eye.

purulent Full of pus; having the character of pus.

putrefaction Decomposition of body tissues; a definitive sign of death.

pyelonephritis Inflammation of the kidney and renal pelvis.

pyrogens Chemicals or proteins that travel to the brain and affect the hypothalamus and stimulate a rise in the body's core temperature.

quadrants The four sections of the abdominal cavity shown by two imaginary lines intersecting at the umbilicus, dividing the abdomen into four equal areas.

quadriplegia Paralysis of all four extremities and the trunk, possibly from a cervical spine injury.

quality control The responsibility of the medical director to ensure the appropriate medical care standards are met by providers on each call.

quaternary blast injury A blast injury that falls into one of the following categories: burns, crush injuries, toxic inhalation, medical emergencies, or mental health disorders.

quinary blast injury Injuries caused by exposure to toxic materials associated with radiation, bacteria, and/or chemicals resulting in contamination of tissues, or by foreign bodies that have the potential to transmit disease.

rabid Describes an animal that is infected with rabies.

raccoon eyes Bruising under the eyes that may indicate a skull fracture; also called periorbital ecchymosis.

radiating pain An area of the body from which the origin of pain or discomfort may travel.

radiation The transfer of heat by radiant energy—for example, heat gain from a fire.

radioactive material Any material that emits radiation.

radiologic dispersal device (RDD) Any container that is designed to disperse radioactive material; see also *dirty bomb*.

radius The bone on the thumb side of the forearm.

range of motion The full distance that a joint can be moved.

rape Sexual intercourse inflicted forcibly on another person, against that person's will.

rapid extrication technique A technique to move a patient from a sitting position inside a vehicle to supine on a backboard in less than 1 minute when conditions do not allow for standard immobilization.

rapid full-body scan A thorough 60- to 90-second review of the patient's body to identify injuries that must be managed or protected immediately; conducted during the primary survey.

rapport A trusting relationship that you build with your patient.

reassessment A step within the patient assessment process that is performed at regular intervals during the assessment process to identify and treat changes in a patient's condition. A patient in unstable condition should be reassessed every 5 minutes, whereas a patient in stable condition should be reassessed every 15 minutes.

rebound tenderness Pain that the patient feels when pressure is released as opposed to when pressure is applied; characteristic of appendicitis; suggestive of a serious and potentially life-threatening condition.

receptor A specialized area in tissue that initiates certain actions after specific stimulation.

reciprocity The recognition by one state of another state's licensure, allowing a health care professional from another state to practice in the new state.

recovery position A side-lying position used to maintain a clear airway in unresponsive patients who are breathing adequately and do not have suspected injuries to the spine, hips, or pelvis.

rectal Through the rectum.

rectum The lowermost end of the colon.

red blood cells (RBCs) The formed elements in the blood that contain hemoglobin and are responsible for carrying oxygen to the tissues; also called erythrocytes.

reduction Repositioning of a bone to near its normal position after a fracture or dislocation.

referred pain Pain in two separate locations of the body, without a "trail" of pain between the two locations, or pain in an area of the body that is not the source of the pain.

refractory Describes a disease or condition that does not respond to treatment.

rehabilitation area The area that provides protection and treatment to all personnel working at an emergency; here, workers are medically monitored and receive any needed care as they enter and leave the scene.

rehabilitation supervisor In incident command, the person who establishes an area that provides protection for responders from the elements and the situation.

renal dialysis A technique for "filtering" the blood of its toxic wastes, removing excess fluids, and restoring the normal balance of electrolytes.

renal pelvis A cone-shaped collecting area that connects the ureter and the kidney.

renin-angiotensin system System located in the kidney that helps to regulate fluid balance and blood pressure.

repeater A special base station radio that receives messages and signals on one frequency and then automatically retransmits them on a second frequency.

res ipsa loquitur Theory of negligence that assumes an injury can only occur when a negligent act occurs.

rescue supervisor In incident command, the person appointed to determine the type of equipment and resources needed for a situation involving extrication or special rescue; also called the extrication supervisor.

residual volume The air that remains in the lungs after maximal expiration.

respiration The inhaling and exhaling of air; the physiologic process that exchanges carbon dioxide from fresh air; also, the exchange of gases that occurs at the pulmonary and cellular levels.

respiratory acidosis A pathologic condition characterized by a blood pH of less than 7.35 and caused by accumulation of acids in the body from a respiratory cause such as inadequate ventilation.

respiratory alkalosis A pathologic condition characterized by a blood pH of greater than 7.45 and caused by an accumulation of bases in the body from a respiratory cause such as overaggressive ventilation.

respiratory arrest The absence of respirations with detectable cardiac activity.

respiratory distress A clinical state characterized by increased respiratory rate, effort, and/or work of breathing.

respiratory failure A clinical state of inadequate oxygenation, ventilation, or both.

respiratory rate The number of ventilatory cycles in a unit of time, usually 1 minute; also known as the ventilation rate.

respiratory syncytial virus (RSV) A virus that causes an infection of the lungs and breathing passages; can result in other serious illnesses that affect the lungs or heart, such as bronchiolitis and pneumonia; highly contagious and spread through droplets.

respiratory system All the structures of the body that contribute to the process of breathing, consisting of the upper and lower airways and their component parts.

responsiveness The way in which a patient responds to external stimuli, including verbal stimuli (sound), tactile stimuli (touch), and painful stimuli.

reticular activating system (RAS) Located in the upper brainstem; responsible for maintenance of consciousness, specifically a person's level of arousal.

retina The light-sensitive area of the eye where images are projected; a layer of cells at the back of the eye that changes the light image into electrical impulses, which are carried by the optic nerve to the brain.

retinal detachment Separation of the retina from its attachments at the back of the eye.

retractions Movements in which the skin pulls in around the ribs during inspiration; the drawing in of the intercostal muscles and the muscles above the clavicles that can occur in respiratory distress.

retrograde amnesia The inability to remember events leading up to a head injury.

retroperitoneal space The space between the abdominal cavity and the posterior abdominal wall, which contains the kidneys, certain large vessels, and parts of the gastrointestinal tract.

retroperitoneum The space behind the peritoneum.

return of spontaneous circulation (ROSC) The return of a pulse and effective blood flow to the body in a patient who previously was in cardiac arrest.

reverse triage A triage process in which efforts are focused on those who are in respiratory and cardiac arrest and different from conventional triage where such patients would be classified as deceased. Used in triaging multiple victims of a lightning strike.

Revised Trauma Score (RTS) A scoring system used for patients with head trauma.

Rh factor An antigen found on the red blood cells of most people; in pregnancy, a woman's body can create antibodies against this, which can be problematic to future pregnancies.

rhabdomyolysis The destruction of muscle tissue leading to a release of potassium and myoglobin.

rhonchi Coarse, low-pitched, rattling breath sounds heard in patients with chronic mucus in the upper airways.

ricin A neurotoxin derived from mash that is left from the castor bean; causes pulmonary edema and respiratory and circulatory failure leading to death.

rigor mortis Stiffening of the body muscles caused by chemical changes within muscle tissue; a definitive sign of death.

rooting reflex An infant reflex that occurs when something touches an infant's cheek; the infant instinctively turns his or her head toward the touch.

rotation-flexion injuries A type of injury in which both rotation and flexion occur; typically resulting from high acceleration forces; can result in a stable unilateral facet dislocation in the cervical spine.

route of exposure The manner by which a toxic substance enters the body.

rule of nines A system that assigns percentages to sections of the body, allowing calculation of the amount of skin surface involved in the burn area.

rule of palms A system that estimates total body surface area burned by comparing the affected area with the size of the patient's palm, which is roughly equivalent to 1% of the patient's total body surface area.

rupture of membranes The rupture of the amniotic sac, which normally occurs during labor.

sacral edema Swelling that presents around the sacral region of the spinal column.

sacroiliac joints The connection points between the pelvis and the vertebral column.

sacrum One of three bones that make up the pelvic ring; consists of five fused sacral vertebrae.

saddle joint Two saddle-shaped articulating surfaces oriented at right angles to each other so that complementary surfaces articulate with each other, such as in the thumb.

safe zone An area of protection providing safety from the danger zone (hot zone).

safety data sheet (SDS) A form provided by manufacturers and compounders (blenders) of chemicals, containing information about chemical composition, physical and chemical properties, health and safety hazards, emergency response, and waste disposal of a specific material; this term has replaced material safety data sheet.

safety officer In incident command, the person who monitors the scene for conditions or operations that may present a hazard to responders and patients; he or she may stop an operation when responder safety is an issue.

sagittal (lateral) plane A plane of the body that passes vertically from front to back, dividing the body into left and right portions.

salicylates Aspirinlike drugs.

saline lock A type of intravenous access device that allows an active intravenous site to be maintained without having to run fluids through the vein, also called a buff cap or intermittent site.

salivary glands The glands that produce saliva to keep the mouth and pharynx moist.

SAMPLE history A brief history of a patient's condition to determine signs and symptoms, allergies, medications, pertinent past history, last oral intake, and events leading up to the illness or injury.

saphenous vein The longest vein in the body, it drains the leg, thigh, and dorsum of the foot.

sarin (GB) A nerve agent that is one of the G agents; a highly volatile, colorless, and odorless liquid that turns from liquid to gas within seconds to minutes at room temperature.

scald burn A burn produced by hot liquids.

scalp The thick skin covering the cranium, which usually bears hair.

scanner A radio receiver that searches or "scans" across several frequencies until the message is completed; the process is then repeated.

scaphoid abdomen Concave abdomen (sunken abdomen or an abdomen that appears empty), which is generally the result of a ruptured diaphragm.

scapula The shoulder blade.

scene size-up A step within the patient assessment process that involves a quick assessment of the scene and the surroundings to provide information about scene safety and the mechanism of injury or nature of the illness before you enter and begin patient care.

schizophrenia A complex, difficult-to-identify mental disorder with typical onset occurring during early adulthood. Dysfunctional symptoms typically become more prominent over time and include delusions, hallucinations, apathy, mutism, flat affect, a lack of interest in pleasure, erratic speech, emotional responses, and motor behavior.

school age A child age 6 to 12 years.

sciatic nerve The major nerve to the lower extremity; it controls much of the muscle function in the leg and sensation in the entire leg and foot.

sclera The tough, fibrous, white portion of the eye that protects the more delicate inner structures.

sclerosis The hardening of a vein from scar tissue after repeated cannulation.

scoop stretcher A stretcher that is designed to be split into two or four sections that can be fitted around a patient who is lying on the ground or other relatively flat surface; also called an orthopaedic stretcher.

scope of practice Most commonly defined by state law; outlines the emergency medical care that the AEMT is able to provide to the patient.

SCUBA A system that delivers air to the mouth and lungs at various atmospheric pressures, increasing with the depth of the dive; stands for self-contained underwater breathing apparatus.

sebaceous glands Glands that produce an oily substance called sebum, which discharges along the shafts of the hairs.

secondary apnea A period of gasping respirations, falling pulse rate, and falling blood pressure that occurs after primary apnea in an infant.

secondary assessment A step within the patient assessment process in which a systematic physical exam of the patient is performed. The exam may be a full-body exam or an assessment that focuses on a certain area or region of the body, often determined through the chief complaint.

secondary blast injury A penetrating or nonpenetrating injury caused by ordnance projectiles or secondary missiles.

secondary brain injury The "after effects" of the primary injury; includes injuries caused by abnormal processes such as cerebral edema, increased intracranial pressure, cerebral ischemia and hypoxia, and infection; onset is often delayed following the primary brain injury.

secondary bronchi Airway passages in the lungs that are formed from the division of the right and left mainstem bronchi.

secondary containment An engineered method to control spilled or released product if the main containment vessel fails.

secondary device An explosive used by terrorists that is set to explode after the initial bomb; it is intended primarily to injure responders and to secure media coverage.

secondary prevention Efforts to limit the effects of an injury or illness that you cannot completely prevent.

secondary response The body's reaction when it is exposed to an antigen for which it already has antibodies, in which it responds by killing the invading substance.

secondary spinal cord injury Injury to the spinal cord, thought to be the result of multiple factors that result in a progression of inflammatory responses from primary spinal cord injury.

secondary triage A type of patient sorting used in the treatment area that involves re-triage of patients.

secure attachment A bond between an infant and his or her parent or caregiver in which the infant understands that his or her parents or caregivers will be responsive to his or her needs and take care of him or her when he or she needs help.

sedative-hypnotic A drug used to reduce anxiety, calm agitated patients, and help produce drowsiness and sleep; a central nervous system depressant.

seizures Episodes often characterized by generalized, uncoordinated muscular activity associated with loss of consciousness; a convulsion.

selective permeability The ability of the cell membrane to selectively allow compounds into the cell based on the cell's current needs.

selective serotonin reuptake inhibitors (SSRIs) A class of antidepressants that inhibit the reuptake of serotonin.

self-contained breathing apparatus (SCBA) Respirator with independent air supply used by firefighters to enter toxic and otherwise dangerous atmospheres.

semen Seminal fluid ejaculated from the penis and containing sperm.

semilunar valves The two valves, the aortic and pulmonic valves, that divide the heart from the aorta and pulmonary arteries.

seminal vesicles Storage sacs for sperm and seminal fluid, which empty into the urethra at the prostate.

semipermeable Property of the cell membrane that describes the ability to allow certain elements to pass through while not allowing others to do so.

sensitivity The ability of the body to recognize a foreign substance the next time it is encountered.

sensitization Developing a sensitivity to a substance that initially caused no allergic reaction.

sensorineural deafness A permanent lack of hearing caused by a lesion or damage of the inner ear.

sensory nerves The nerves that transmit sensory input, such as touch, taste, heat, cold, and pain, from the body to the central nervous system.

separation anxiety An infant behavior that peaks between age 10 and 18 months. The child may exhibit clingy behavior and fear of unfamiliar places and people.

sepsis The spread of an infection from its initial site into the bloodstream.

septic shock The type of shock that occurs as a result of widespread infection, usually bacterial; untreated, the result is multiple organ dysfunction syndrome and often death.

septum A central divider, such as the nasal septum.

serotonin A vasoactive amine that increases vascular permeability to cause vasodilation.

serum sickness A condition in which antigen-antibody complexes formed in the bloodstream deposit in sites around the body, most notably in the kidney, with resultant inflammatory reactions.

severe acute respiratory syndrome (SARS) A potentially life-threatening viral infection that usually starts with flulike symptoms.

severe airway obstruction Occurs when a foreign body completely obstructs the patient's airway. Patients cannot breathe, talk, or cough.

sexual assault An attack against a person that is sexual in nature, the most of common of which is rape.

shaken baby syndrome Bleeding within the head and damage to the cervical spine as a result of intentional, forceful shaking of an infant or small child.

shallow respirations Respirations characterized by little movement of the chest wall (reduced tidal volume) or poor chest excursion.

shock A condition in which the circulatory system fails to provide sufficient circulation to enable every body part to perform its function; also called hypoperfusion.

shoulder dystocia A complication of delivery in which there is difficulty delivering the shoulders of a newborn; the shoulder cannot get past the woman's symphysis pubis.

shoulder girdle The proximal portion of the upper extremity, made up of the clavicle, the scapula, and the humerus.

shunt A passageway that allows fluid to move from one part of the body to another or to a dialysis machine; in cases of hydrocephalus, a tube that drains excess cerebrospinal fluid from the brain to another part of the body outside of the brain, such as the abdomen; lowers pressure in the brain.

sickle cell disease A hereditary disease that causes normal, round red blood cells to become oblong or sickle shaped.

side effects Any effects of a medication other than the desired ones.

sign Objective finding that can be seen, heard, felt, smelled, or measured (eg, a laceration or the patient's blood pressure) when assessing a patient to establish illness or injury.

simple access Access that is easily achieved without the use of tools or force.

simple partial seizures The seizures involving movement of one part of the body or altered sensations in one part of the body; the movement may stay in one body part or spread from one part to another in a wave.

simple phobia A fear that is focused on one class of objects (eg, mice, spiders, dogs) or situations (eg, high places, darkness, flying).

simplex Single-frequency radio; transmissions can occur in either direction but not simultaneously in both; when one party transmits, the other can only receive, and the party that is transmitting is unable to receive.

single command system A command system in which one person is in charge, generally used with small incidents that involve only one responding agency or one jurisdiction.

sinoatrial (SA) node The normal site of the origin of electrical impulses; located high in the right atrium, it is the heart's natural pacemaker.

sinusitis An inflammation of the paranasal sinuses.

situational awareness Knowledge and understanding of one's surroundings and the ability to recognize potential risks to the safety of the patient or the emergency medical services team.

six Ps of musculoskeletal assessment Pain, Paralysis, Paresthesias, Pulselessness, Pallor, and Pressure.

size-up The ongoing process of information gathering and scene evaluation to determine appropriate strategies and tactics to manage an emergency.

skeletal muscle Muscle that is attached to bones and usually crosses at least one joint; striated, or voluntary, muscle.

skeleton The framework that gives the body its recognizable form; also designed to allow motion of the body and protection of vital organs.

skull The structure at the top of the axial skeleton that houses the brain and consists of the 28 bones that comprise the auditory ossicles, the cranium, and the face.

slander False and damaging information about a person that is communicated by the spoken word.

sling A bandage or material that helps to support the weight of an injured upper extremity.

small intestine The portion of the digestive tube between the stomach and the cecum, consisting of the duodenum, jejunum, and ileum.

smallpox A highly contagious disease; it is most contagious when blisters begin to form.

small-volume nebulizer A respiratory device that holds liquid medicine that is turned into a fine mist. The patient inhales the medication into the airways and lungs as a treatment for conditions like asthma.

smooth muscle Involuntary muscle; it constitutes the bulk of the gastrointestinal tract and is present in nearly every organ to regulate automatic activity.

sniffing position An upright position in which the patient's head and chin are thrust slightly forward to keep the airway open; the optimum head position for the uninjured child who requires airway management.

sodium channel blockers Antidysrhythmic medications that slow conduction through the heart.

sodium/potassium (Na^+/K^+) pump The mechanism by which the cell brings in two potassium (K^+) ions and releases three sodium (Na^+) ions.

solid organs Solid masses of tissue where much of the chemical work of the body takes place (eg, the liver, spleen, pancreas, and kidneys).

solute A particle, such as salt, that is dissolved in a solvent.

solution A liquid mixture that cannot be separated by filtering or allowing the mixture to stand.

soman (GD) A nerve agent that is one of the G agents; twice as persistent as sarin and five times as lethal; it has a fruity odor, as a result of the type of alcohol used in the agent; and is a contact and an inhalation hazard that can enter the body through skin absorption and through the respiratory tract.

somatic nervous system The part of the nervous system that regulates a person's voluntary activities, such as walking, talking, and writing.

somatic pain Localized pain, usually felt deeply, which represents irritation or injury to tissue, causing activation of peripheral nerve tracts.

spacer A device that collects medication as it is released from the canister of a metered-dose inhaler, allowing more medication to be delivered to the lungs and less to be lost to the environment.

span of control In incident command, the subordinate positions under the commander's direction to which the workload is distributed; the ideal supervisor/worker ratio is one supervisor for three to seven workers.

Special Atomic Demolition Munitions (SADM) Small, suitcase-sized nuclear weapons that were designed to destroy individual targets, such as important buildings, bridges, tunnels, and large ships.

special weapons and tactics (SWAT) team A specialized law enforcement tactical unit.

sphincters Circular muscles that surround and, by contracting, constrict a duct, tube, or opening. Examples are found within the rectum, bladder, and blood vessels.

sphygmomanometer A device used to measure blood pressure.

spice An illicit drug consisting of a blend of synthetic cannabinoids; it can produce short- and long-term psychotic effects.

spina bifida A developmental defect in which a portion of the spinal cord or meninges may protrude outside of the vertebrae and possibly even outside of the body, usually at the lower third of the spine in the lumbar area.

spinal cord An extension of the brain, composed of virtually all nerves carrying messages between the brain and the rest of the body. It lies inside of and is protected by the spinal canal.

spinal cord concussion An incomplete injury of the spinal cord in which temporary dysfunction lasts from 24 to 48 hours; may present in patients with simple compression fractures.

spinal cord contusion A bruise of the spinal cord characterized by edema, tissue damage, and vascular leakage, and caused by fracture, dislocation, or direct trauma.

spinal shock The temporary local neurologic condition that occurs immediately after spinal trauma; swelling and edema of the spinal cord begin immediately after injury, with severe pain and potential paralysis.

splenic sequestration crisis An acute, painful enlargement of the spleen caused by sickle cell disease.

splint A flexible or rigid appliance used to protect and maintain the position of an injured extremity.

spontaneous abortion Delivery of the fetus and placenta by natural causes before 20 weeks of gestation; also known as miscarriage.

spontaneous pneumothorax Pneumothorax that occurs when a weak area on the lung ruptures in the absence of major injury, allowing air to leak into the pleural space.

spontaneous respirations Breathing that occurs without assistance.

spotter A person who assists a driver in backing up an ambulance to compensate for blind spots at the rear of the vehicle.

sprain A joint injury involving damage to supporting ligaments (stretching or tearing) and partial or temporary dislocation of bone ends.

staging supervisor In incident command, the person who locates an area to stage equipment and personnel and tracks unit arrival and deployment from the staging area.

stair chair A lightweight folding device that is used to carry a conscious, seated patient up or down stairs.

standard of care Written, accepted levels of emergency medical care expected by reason of training and profession; written by legal or professional organizations so that patients are not exposed to unreasonable risk or harm.

standard precautions Protective measures that have traditionally been developed and recommended by the Centers for Disease Control and Prevention for use in dealing with objects, blood, body fluids, and other potential exposure risks of communicable disease.

standing orders Written documents, signed by the EMS system's medical director, that outline specific directions, permissions, and sometimes prohibitions regarding patient care; also called protocols.

Star of Life The six-pointed star that identifies vehicles that meet federal specifications as licensed or certified ambulances.

Starling law A principle that states that if a muscle is stretched slightly before stimulation to contract, the muscle will contract harder; describes how increased venous return to the heart stretches the ventricles and allows for increased cardiac contractility.

START triage A patient sorting process that stands for Simple Triage And Rapid Treatment and uses a limited assessment of the patient's ability to walk, respiratory status, hemodynamic status, and neurologic status.

state-sponsored terrorism Terrorism that is funded and/or supported by nations that hold close ties with terrorist groups.

status asthmaticus A prolonged exacerbation of asthma that does not respond to conventional therapy.

status epilepticus A condition in which seizures recur every few minutes without a lucid interval or last more than 4 or 5 minutes.

statute of limitations The number of years after an incident during which a lawsuit can be filed.

steam burn A burn that has been caused by direct exposure to hot steam exhaust, as from a broken pipe.

steatorrhea Foamy, fatty stools associated with liver failure or gallbladder problems.

stem cell A type of cell that can develop into other types of cell in the body; this type of cell retains the ability to divide repeatedly without specializing and allows for continual growth and renewal.

stereotyped movements Repetitive movements that do not appear to serve any purpose.

sterilization A process, such as heating, that removes microbial contamination.

sternocleidomastoid muscles The muscles on either side of the neck that allow movement of the head.

sternum The breastbone.

stimulants Medications or chemicals that temporarily enhance central nervous system and sympathetic nervous system functioning and produce an excited state.

stoma A surgical opening in the body that connects an internal structure to the skin, such as in the neck to connect the trachea directly to the skin.

straddle fracture A fracture of the pelvis that results from landing on the perineal region.

strain Stretching or tearing of a muscle or tendon; also called a muscle pull.

strangulation Complete obstruction of blood circulation in a given organ as a result of compression or entrapment; an emergency situation causing death of tissue.

stratum corneal layer The outermost or dead layer of the skin.

striated muscle Muscle that is attached to bones and usually crosses at least one joint; also called skeletal or voluntary muscle.

stridor A harsh, high-pitched breath sound, generally heard during inspiration, that is caused by partial blockage or narrowing of the upper airway; may be audible without a stethoscope.

stroke A loss of brain function in certain brain cells that do not get enough oxygen during a cerebrovascular accident. Usually caused by obstruction of the blood vessels in the brain that feed oxygen to the brain cells.

stroke volume (SV) The volume of blood pumped forward from the left ventricle into the aorta with each ventricular contraction.

subarachnoid hemorrhage A hemorrhage into the subarachnoid space between the arachnoid membrane and the pia mater, where the cerebrospinal fluid circulates.

subarachnoid space The space located between the pia mater and the arachnoid membrane.

subclavian artery The proximal part of the main artery of the arm, which supplies the brain, neck, anterior chest wall, and shoulder.

subclavian veins The proximal part of the main veins of the arm, which unite with the internal jugular veins.

subconjunctival hematoma Bleeding into the anterior surface of the eye.

subcutaneous Into the tissue between the skin and muscle; a medication delivery route.

subcutaneous emphysema A characteristic crackling sensation felt on palpation of the skin, caused by the presence of air in soft tissues.

subcutaneous injection Injection into the tissue between the skin and muscle; a medication delivery route.

subcutaneous tissue Tissue, largely fat, that lies directly under the dermis and serves as an insulator of the body.

subdural hematoma An accumulation of blood beneath the dura mater but outside the brain.

subjective information Information that is told to you but that cannot be seen, such as the symptoms a patient describes.

sublingual (SL) Under the tongue; a medication delivery route.

subluxation A partial or incomplete dislocation of a joint.

submersion Survival, at least temporarily, after suffocation in water or other liquids; also called near drowning.

sucking chest wound An open or penetrating chest wall wound through which air passes during inspiration and expiration, creating a sucking sound.

sucking reflex An infant reflex in which the infant starts sucking when his or her lips are stroked.

suction catheter A hollow, cylindrical device used to remove fluids and secretions from the airway.

sudden infant death syndrome (SIDS) Unexpected death of an infant or young child that remains unexplained after a complete autopsy.

suffix The word part that comes after the word root, at the end of the term.

sulfur mustard (H) A vesicant also known as mustard gas; it is a brown-yellow, oily substance that is generally considered very persistent; has the distinct smell of garlic or mustard; and, when released, is quickly absorbed into the skin and/or mucous membranes and begins an irreversible process of damaging the cells.

summation effect Increased effect that may occur when two drugs that have the same or similar action are given together.

superficial Closer to or on the surface of the skin.

superficial burns The burns affecting only the epidermis, characterized by skin that is red but not blistered or actually burned through; formerly called a first-degree burn.

superior Above what is indicated; closer to the head.

superior vena cava One of the two largest veins in the body; carries blood from the upper extremities, head, neck, and chest into the heart.

supination Turning the palms upward (toward the sky).

supine Lying face up.

supine hypotensive syndrome A drop in blood pressure caused when the heavy uterus of a supine, third-trimester–pregnant patient obstructs the vena cava, lowering blood return to the heart.

surfactant A liquid protein substance that coats the alveoli in the lungs, decreases alveolar surface tension, and keeps the alveoli expanded, allowing for easy expansion and recoil of the alveoli; a low level in a premature baby contributes to respiratory distress syndrome.

suspension A mixture of ground particles that are distributed evenly throughout a liquid but do not dissolve.

sutures Attachment points in the skull where the cranial bones join together.

swathe A bandage that passes around the chest to secure an injured arm to the chest.

sweat glands The glands that secrete sweat, located in the dermal layer of the skin.

sympathetic blocking agents An antihypertensive medication that decreases cardiac output and renin secretions.

sympathetic eye movement The movement of both eyes in unison.

sympathetic nervous system Subdivision of the autonomic nervous system that governs the body's fight-or-flight reactions by inducing smooth muscle contraction or relaxation of the blood vessels and bronchioles; responsible for the body's response to shock and stress.

sympatholytics Drugs that block the actions of the sympathetic nervous system.

sympathomimetics Drugs that produce the same effects as the hormones of the sympathetic nervous system.

symphysis A type of joint that has grown together forming a very stable connection.

symptom Subjective findings that the patient feels, for example, what he or she tells a provider during assessment, but that can be identified only by the patient.

synapse The gap between nerve cells across which nervous stimuli are transmitted.

syncopal episode Fainting; brief loss of consciousness caused by transiently inadequate blood flow to the brain.

syncope The temporary loss of consciousness and postural tone caused by diminished cerebral blood flow.

syndromic surveillance The monitoring, usually by local or state health departments, of patients presenting to emergency departments and alternative care facilities, the recording of EMS call volume, and the use of over-the-counter medications.

synergism The action of two substances such as drugs, in which the total effects are greater than the sum of the independent effects of the two substances.

synonyms Pairs of word roots, prefixes, or suffixes that have the same or almost the same meaning.

synovial fluid The small amount of liquid within a joint used as lubrication.

synovial membrane The lining of a joint that secretes synovial fluid into the joint space.

syphilis A sexually transmitted disease caused by the bacterium *Treponema pallidum*, which manifests in three stages—primary, secondary, and tertiary—and is transmitted through direct contact with open sores.

systemic circulation The circulatory system in the body that is responsible for blood flow in all areas of the body, except for areas covered by the pulmonary circulation (blood flow from the right side of the heart to the lungs and back to the left side of the heart).

systemic complications Moderate to severe allergic reaction affecting the systems of the body.

systemic reaction A reaction that occurs throughout the body, possibly affecting multiple body systems.

systemic vascular resistance (SVR) The resistance that blood must overcome to be able to move within the blood vessels; related to the amount of dilation or constriction in the blood vessel.

systole The contraction, or period of contraction, of the heart, especially that of the ventricles.

systolic pressure The increased pressure in an artery with each contraction of the ventricles (systole).

tabun (GA) A nerve agent that is one of the G agents; is 36 times more persistent than sarin and approximately one-half as lethal; has a fruity smell; and is unique because the components used to manufacture the agent are easy to acquire and the agent is easy to manufacture.

tachycardia A rapid heart rate of more than 100 beats per minute.

tachypnea Rapid respiratory rate.

tactical medicine Emergency medical care provided by specifically trained emergency medical responders, AEMTs, paramedics, nurses, and even physicians during a tactical situation.

tactical situation A hostage, robbery, or other situation in which armed conflict is threatened or shots have been fired and the threat of violence remains.

tactile stimulation Method of stimulating a newborn to breathe by flicking or slapping the soles of the feet or rubbing the lateral thorax.

tangential thinking Leaving the current topic in midconversation to talk about something else, inhibiting interpersonal communication.

technical rescue group A team of emergency responders from one or more departments in a region who are trained and on call for certain types of technical rescue.

technical rescue situation A rescue that requires special technical skills and equipment in one of many specialized rescue areas, such as technical rope rescue, cave rescue, and dive rescue.

telemetry A process in which electronic signals are converted into coded, audible signals; these signals can then be transmitted by radio or telephone to a receiver with a decoder at the hospital.

temporal lobe The portion of the brain that has an important role in hearing and memory.

temporomandibular joint (TMJ) The joint where the mandible meets with the temporal bone of the cranium just in front of each ear.

tendon A tough, ropelike cord of fibrous tissue that attaches skeletal muscle to bone.

tension lines The pattern of tautness of the skin, which is arranged over body structures and affects how well wounds heal.

tension pneumothorax An accumulation of air or gas in the pleural space that progressively collapses the lung with potentially fatal results.

tenting A sign of dehydration in which the skin slowly retracts after being pinched and pulled away slightly from the body.

tentorium A structure that separates the cerebral hemispheres from the cerebellum and brainstem.

teratogenic Poses a risk to the normal development or health of the unborn fetus.

term Between 38 and 42 weeks' gestation.

terminal drop hypothesis A theory that a person's mental function declines in the last 5 years preceding death.

termination of action The amount of time after the concentration of a medication falls below the minimum effective level until it is eliminated from the body.

termination of command The end of the incident command structure when an incident draws to a close and the command structure is no longer necessary.

tertiary blast injury An injury from whole-body displacement and subsequent traumatic impact with environmental objects.

tertiary bronchi Airway passages in the lungs that are formed from branching of the secondary bronchi.

testes The male reproductive organs that produce sperm and secrete male hormones; also called testicles.

testicular torsion Twisting of the testicle on the spermatic cord, from which it is suspended; associated with scrotal pain and swelling and is a medical emergency.

tetanus A disease caused by spores that enter the body through a puncture wound contaminated with animal feces, street dust, or soil or that can enter through contaminated street drugs.

thalamus Structure of the diencephalon that is the sensory switchboard of the brain, through which almost all signals travel on their way in or out of the brain.

therapeutic communication Verbal and nonverbal communication techniques that encourage patients to express their feelings and to achieve a positive relationship.

therapeutic index The difference between the minimum effective concentration and the toxic level of a drug.

therapeutic threshold The minimum concentration of a drug necessary to cause the desired response.

thermal burn A burn that results from heat, usually fire.

thermal energy Energy transferred from sources that are hotter than the body, such as a flame, hot water, or steam.

thermogenesis The physiologic process of heat production in the body.

thermolysis The process of heat loss; methods include conduction, convection, radiation, evaporation, and respiration.

thermoregulation The balance between heat production and heat excretion.

third spacing The shifting of fluid into the tissues, creating edema.

thoracic duct One of two great lymph vessels; it empties into the superior vena cava.

thoracic spine The 12 vertebrae that lie between the cervical vertebrae and the lumbar vertebrae. One pair of ribs is attached to each of the thoracic vertebrae.

thorax The chest cavity that contains the heart, lungs, esophagus, and great vessels.

thought broadcasting The belief that thoughts are broadcast aloud and can be heard by others.

thought insertion The belief that thoughts are being thrust into one's mind by another person.

thought withdrawal The belief that thoughts are being removed from one's mind.

threatened abortion Expulsion of the fetus that is attempting to take place but has not occurred yet; usually occurs in the first trimester.

thrombin An enzyme that causes the conversion of fibrinogen to fibrin, which binds to the platelet plug, forming the final mature clot.

thrombocytopenia A reduction in the number of platelets.

thrombocytosis A condition in which the body produces too many platelets.

thromboembolism A blood clot that has formed within a blood vessel and is floating within the bloodstream.

thrombophilia A tendency toward the development of blood clots as a result of an abnormality of the system of coagulation.

thrombophlebitis Inflammation of a vein.

thrombosis A blood clot, either in the arterial or venous system.

thrombus In neurologic emergencies, the local clotting of blood in the cerebral arteries that may result in the interruption of cerebral blood flow and subsequent stroke.

thyroid cartilage A firm prominence of cartilage that forms the upper part of the larynx; the Adam's apple.

thyroid gland A large endocrine gland that is located at the base of the neck and produces and excretes hormones that influence growth, development, and metabolism.

thyroid storm A rare, life-threatening condition that may occur in patients with thyrotoxicosis. The condition is usually triggered by a stressful event or increased volume of thyroid hormones in the circulation.

thyroid-stimulating hormone Hormone that stimulates the release of thyroid hormone from the thyroid gland.

tibia The shin bone, the larger of the two bones of the lower leg.

tidal volume The amount of air (in milliliters) that is moved into or out of the lungs during one relaxed breath; approximately 500 mL for an adult.

tissue plasminogen activator (t-PA) A major component in the fibrinolytic system, in which clots that have already formed are lysed or disrupted, converting plasminogen to plasmin.

toddler A child between 1 and 3 years of age.

tolerance Physiologic adaptation to the effects of a drug, such that increasingly larger doses of the drug are required to achieve the same effect.

tongue-jaw lift maneuver A method of opening the airway for suctioning or inserting an oral airway; involves grasping the incisors or gums and lifting the jaw.

tonic phase In a seizure, the steady, rigid muscle contractions with no relaxation.

tonic-clonic seizures The seizures characterized by severe twitching of all of the body's muscles and body stiffness; may last several minutes or more; formerly known as a grand mal seizure.

tonicity The osmotic pressure of a solution, based on the relationship between sodium and water inside and outside the cell, that takes advantage of chemical and osmotic properties to move water to areas of higher sodium concentration.

tonsil-tip catheter A suction catheter with a large, semirigid suction tip, recommended for suctioning the pharynx; also called Yankauer tip.

topical medications Lotions, creams, and ointments that are applied to the surface of the skin and affect only that area; a medication delivery route.

topographic anatomy Superficial landmarks of the body that serve as guides to the structures that lie beneath them.

tort A wrongful act that gives rise to a civil lawsuit.

total laryngectomy Surgical removal of the entire larynx.

tourniquet A bandage or device applied to an extremity to control bleeding, used when a wound continues to bleed despite the use of direct pressure; works by compressing or constricting blood flow.

toxicity The risk that a substance will pose a health hazard to an individual or organism.

toxicologic emergencies Medical emergencies caused by toxic agents such as poisons.

toxicology The study of toxic or poisonous substances.

toxidrome The syndromelike symptoms of a poisonous agent.

toxin A poison or harmful substance produced by bacteria, animals, or plants.

trabeculae Bony rods that form the lacy network in cancellous bones and are oriented to increase weight-bearing capacity of long bones.

trachea The windpipe; the main conduit for air passing to and from the lungs.

tracheal tugging Pulling of the trachea into the neck during inspiration; a sign of increased work of breathing.

tracheostomy Surgical creation of a hole in the trachea.

tracheostomy tube A tube inserted through the hole created by a tracheostomy, used to facilitate breathing.

traction The act of exerting a pulling force on a body.

trade name The brand name that a manufacturer gives a medication; capitalized.

tragus The small cartilaginous projection in front of the opening of the ear.

trajectory The path a projectile takes after it is propelled from a weapon or explosion.

transcutaneous Through the skin; a medication delivery route; also called transdermal.

transient ischemic attack (TIA) A disorder of the brain in which brain cells temporarily stop working because of insufficient oxygen, causing strokelike symptoms that resolve completely within 24 hours of onset.

transmigration (diapedesis) The polymorphonuclear neutrophils permeate through the vessel wall, moving into the interstitial space.

transmission The way in which an infectious disease is spread: contact, airborne, by vehicles, or by vectors.

transportation area The area in a mass-casualty incident where ambulances and crews are organized to transport patients from the treatment area to receiving hospitals.

transportation supervisor In incident command, the person in charge of the transportation sector in a mass-casualty incident who assigns patients from the treatment area to awaiting ambulances in the transportation area.

transverse (axial) plane An imaginary plane passing horizontally through the body at the waist, dividing it into top and bottom halves.

trauma emergencies Emergencies that are the result of physical forces applied to the body; injuries.

trauma lethal triad A combination of hypothermia, coagulopathy (poor blood clotting), and acidosis that is a major contributor to death in patients with severe traumatic bleeding.

trauma score A score that relates to the likelihood of patient survival of traumatic injuries with the exception of a severe head injury. It calculates a number from 1 to 16, with 16 being the best possible score taking into account the Glasgow Coma Scale score, respiratory rate, respiratory expansion, systolic blood pressure, and capillary refill.

traumatic aortic disruption Dissection or rupture of the aorta.

traumatic asphyxia A pattern of injuries seen after a severe force is applied to the thorax, forcing blood from the great vessels and back into the head and neck.

traumatic brain injury (TBI) A traumatic insult to the brain capable of producing physical, intellectual, emotional, social, and vocational changes.

treatment area The location in a mass-casualty incident where patients are brought after being triaged and assigned a priority, where they are reassessed, treated, and monitored until transport to the hospital.

treatment supervisor In incident command, the person, usually a physician, who is in charge of and directs emergency medical services providers at the treatment area in a mass-casualty incident.

triage The process of sorting patients based on the severity of injury and medical need to establish treatment and transportation priorities.

triage supervisor In incident command, the person in charge of the incident command triage sector who directs the sorting of patients into triage categories in a mass-casualty incident.

triceps The muscle in the back of the upper arm.

trichomoniasis A parasitic infection.

tricuspid valve The heart valve that separates the right atrium from the right ventricle.

tricyclic antidepressants (TCAs) A group of drugs used to treat severe depression and manage pain; even minimal dosing errors with these agents can cause toxic results.

trimesters Three segments of time, each made up of approximately 3 months, that comprise the length of a pregnancy.

tripod position An upright position in which the patient leans forward onto two arms stretched forward and thrusts the head and chin forward.

trismus The involuntary contraction of the mouth resulting in clenched teeth; occurs during seizures and head injuries.

trocar A solid boring needle.

trunked radios Computerized sharing of radio frequencies by multiple units, agencies, or systems.

trust and mistrust Refers to a stage of development from birth to approximately 18 months of age, when infants gain trust of their parents or caregivers if their world is planned, organized, and routine.

tuberculosis A chronic bacterial disease, caused by *Mycobacterium tuberculosis,* that usually affects the lungs but also can affect other organs such as the brain and kidneys; it is spread by cough and can lie dormant in a person's lungs for decades and then reactivate.

tunica adventitia The outer layer of tissue of a blood vessel wall, composed of elastic and fibrous connective tissue.

tunica intima The smooth, thin, inner lining of a blood vessel.

tunica media The middle and thickest layer of tissue of a blood vessel wall, composed of elastic tissue and smooth muscle cells that allow the vessel to expand or contract in response to changes in blood pressure and tissue demand.

turbinates Bony shelves that extend from the lateral walls of the nose into the nasal passageway; increase the surface area of the nasal mucosa, improving filtration, warming, and humidification of inhaled air.

turgor The ability of the skin to resist deformation; tested by gently pinching skin on the forehead or back of the hand.

two- to three-word dyspnea A severe breathing condition in which a patient can speak only two to three words at a time without pausing to take a breath.

tympanic membrane The eardrum; a thin, semitransparent membrane in the middle ear that transmits sound vibrations to the internal ear by means of auditory ossicles.

type 1 diabetes The type of diabetic disease that usually starts in childhood and requires insulin for proper treatment and control.

type 2 diabetes The type of diabetic disease that usually starts later in life and often can be controlled through diet and oral medications.

ulcerative colitis Generalized inflammation of the inner lining of the colon that results in a weakened, dilated rectum, making it susceptible to infection and bleeding.

ulcers Abrasions of the stomach or small intestine.

ulna The inner bone of the forearm, on the side opposite the thumb.

ultrahigh-frequency (UHF) band Radio frequencies between 300 and 3,000 MHz.

ultrasonography The use of a special device that uses sound waves to determine the location and shape of internal tissues and organs.

umbilical cord The conduit connecting woman to infant via the placenta; contains two arteries and one vein.

umbilical vein catheters (UVCs) Special catheters designed to be inserted into the umbilical cord.

unified command system A command system used in larger incidents in which there is a multiagency response or multiple jurisdictions are involved.

unilateral Occurring or appearing on only one side of the body.

unintended effects Actions that are undesirable but pose little risk to the patient.

untoward effects Actions that can be harmful to the patient.

uremia The presence of excessive amounts of urea and other waste products in the blood; severe renal failure resulting in the buildup of waste products within the blood; eventually impairs brain function.

uremic frost A powdery buildup of uric acid, especially on the face.

ureter A small, hollow tube that carries urine from the kidneys to the bladder.

urethra The canal that conveys the discharge of urine, extending from the urinary bladder to the outside of the body.

urinary bladder A sac behind the pubic symphysis made of smooth muscle that collects and stores urine.

urinary retention Incomplete emptying of the bladder or a complete lack of ability to empty the bladder.

urinary system The organs that control the discharge of certain waste materials filtered from the blood and excreted as urine.

urinary tract infections (UTIs) Infections, usually of the lower urinary tract (urethra and bladder), which occur when normal flora bacteria or other bacteria enter the urethra and grow.

urostomy The procedure to create an opening (stoma) between the urinary system and the surface of the skin, allowing urine to drain through a stoma in the abdominal wall instead of through the urethra.

urticaria Small areas of generalized itching and/or burning that appear as multiple raised areas on the skin; hives. May be one of the warning signs of impending anaphylaxis.

uterine inversion A potentially fatal maternal complication of childbirth in which the placenta fails to detach properly and results in the uterus turning inside out.

uterine rupture Rupture of the uterus, usually by trauma, that can result in life-threatening hemorrhage in the woman and fetus.

uterus The muscular, inverted pear–shaped organ that lies situated between the urinary bladder and the rectum, where the fetus grows, also called the womb; responsible for contractions during labor.

V agent (VX) One of the G agents; it is a clear, oily agent that has no odor and looks like baby oil; more than 100 times more lethal than sarin and is extremely persistent.

vagina The muscular tube that forms the lower part of the female reproductive tract; connects the uterus with the vulva (the external female genitalia); also called the birth canal.

vaginal orifice Opening of the vagina.

vaginal yeast infection An infection caused by the fungus *Candida albicans*, in which fungi overpopulate the vagina.

vagus nerve The cranial nerve (X) that provides motor functions to the soft palate, pharynx, and larynx and carries taste bud fibers from the posterior tongue, sensory fibers from the inferior pharynx, larynx, thoracic, and abdominal organs, and parasympathetic fibers to thoracic and abdominal organs.

vapor hazard The danger posed by an agent that enters the body through the respiratory tract.

varicose veins Veins on the leg that are large, twisted, and ropelike and can cause pain, swelling, or itching.

vasa deferentia The spermatic duct of the testicles; also called vas deferens.

vasculitis An inflammation of the blood vessels.

vasoactive amines Substances such as histamine and serotonin that increase vascular permeability.

vasoconstriction Narrowing of the diameter of a blood vessel.

vasodilation Widening of a blood vessel.

vasodilator medications The medications that work on the smooth muscles of the arterioles and/or the veins.

vasodilatory shock A type of shock related to relaxation of the blood vessels, allowing blood to pool and impairing circulation.

vaso-occlusive crisis Ischemia and pain caused by sickle-shaped red blood cells that obstruct blood flow to a portion of the body.

vasovagal reaction A reaction consisting of precordial distress, anxiety, nausea, and sometimes syncope.

vector-borne transmission The use of an animal or insects to spread an organism from one person or place to another.

veins The blood vessels that transport unoxygenated blood back to the heart.

venous sinuses Spaces between the membranes surrounding the brain that are the primary means of venous drainage from the brain.

venous thrombosis The development of a stationary blood clot in the venous circulation.

ventilation The exchange of air between the lungs and the air of the environment, spontaneously by the patient or with assistance.

ventral The anterior surface of the body.

ventral respiratory group (VRG) A portion of the medulla oblongata that is responsible for modulating breathing during speech.

ventricle In the context of the circulatory system, one of two lower chambers of the heart; in the context of the neurologic system, hollow storage areas in the brain.

ventricular fibrillation (VF) Disorganized, ineffective twitching of the ventricles, resulting in no blood flow and a state of cardiac arrest.

ventricular tachycardia (VT) Rapid heart rhythm in which the electrical impulse begins in the ventricle (instead of the atrium), which may result in inadequate blood flow and eventually deteriorate into cardiac arrest.

venules Very small, thin-walled vessels.

vernix caseosa A white, cheesy substance that covers the fetus.

vertebrae The 33 bones that make up the spinal column.

vertebral body Anterior weight-bearing structure in the spine made of cancellous bone and surrounded by a layer of hard, compact bone that provides support and stability.

vertebral column The spine or primary support structure of the body that houses the spinal cord and the peripheral nerves.

vertical compression A type of injury typically resulting from a direct blow to the crown of the skull or rapid deceleration from a fall through the feet, legs, and pelvis, possibly causing a burst fracture or disk herniation.

vertical shear The type of pelvic fracture that occurs when a massive force displaces the pelvis superiorly.

very high-frequency (VHF) band Radio frequencies between 30 and 300 MHz; the VHF spectrum is further divided into high and low bands.

vesicants Blister agents; the primary route of exposure for this agent is through the skin.

vesicular breath sounds Fine and faint normal breath sounds noted in the lateral wall of the chest, made by air moving in and out of the smaller bronchioles and alveoli.

vestibule Small space at the beginning of an opening.

vials Small glass bottles for medications; may contain single or multiple doses.

viral hemorrhagic fevers (VHFs) A group of diseases caused by viruses that include the Ebola, Rift Valley, and yellow fever viruses, among others. This group of viruses causes the blood in the body to seep out from the tissues and blood vessels.

virulence A measure of the disease-causing ability of a microorganism.

viruses Germs that require a living host to multiply and survive.

visceral pain Crampy, aching pain deep within the body, the source of which is usually difficult to pinpoint; common with genitourinary problems.

visceral pleura The thin membrane that covers the lungs.

vital capacity The amount of air that can be forcibly expelled from the lungs after breathing in as deeply as possible.

vital signs Clinical measurements that indicate the current state of the body and how well it is functioning.

vitreous humor A jellylike substance found in the posterior compartment of the eye between the lens and the retina.

volatility Describes how long a chemical agent will stay on a surface before it evaporates.

volume on hand The amount of fluid you have on hand, such as the amount of fluid in an intravenous bag or the amount of fluid in a vial of medication.

voluntary activities The actions that we consciously perform, in which sensory input determines the specific muscular activity.

voluntary muscle Muscle that is under direct voluntary control of the brain and can be contracted or relaxed at will; skeletal, or striated, muscle.

Volutrol A special type of microdrip set; allows you to fill a large drip chamber with a specific amount of fluid to avoid fluid overload.

$\dot{V}/\dot{Q}$ mismatch A measurement that examines how much gas is being moved effectively and how much blood is gaining access to the alveoli.

vulva The visible female external genitalia; also called the pudendum.

warm zone The area located between the hot zone and the cold zone at a hazardous materials incident. The decontamination corridor is located in the warm zone.

weapon of mass casualty (WMC) Any agent designed to bring about mass death, casualties, and/or massive damage to property and infrastructure (bridges, tunnels, airports, and seaports); also known as a weapon of mass destruction.

weapon of mass destruction (WMD) Any agent designed to bring about mass death, casualties, and/or massive damage to property and infrastructure (bridges, tunnels, airports, and seaports); also known as a weapon of mass casualty.

weaponization The creation of a weapon from a biologic agent generally found in nature and that causes disease; the agent is cultivated, synthesized, and/or mutated to maximize the target population's exposure to the germ.

wheal A raised, swollen, well-defined area on the skin resulting from an insect bite or allergic reaction.

wheeled ambulance stretcher A specifically designed stretcher that can be rolled along the ground. A collapsible undercarriage allows it to be loaded into the ambulance; also called an ambulance stretcher.

wheezing A high-pitched, whistling breath sound that is most prominent on expiration, and which suggests an obstruction or narrowing of the lower airways; occurs in asthma and bronchiolitis.

whiplash An injury to the neck in which hyperextension occurs as a result of the head moving abruptly forward or backward; can be difficult to differentiate from injuries that involve cervical bony structures and the spine.

white blood cells (WBCs) Blood cells that have a role in the body's immune defense mechanisms; they provide immunity, fight infection, and remove dead cells; also called leukocytes.

wind-chill factor A measurement that takes into account the temperature and wind velocity in calculating the effect of a given ambient temperature on living organisms.

withdrawal syndrome A predictable set of signs and symptoms, usually involving altered central nervous system activity, that occurs after the abrupt cessation of a drug or after rapidly decreasing the usual dosage of a drug.

word root The foundation of a word; establishes the basic meaning of a word.

work In the context of kinematics, the product of force times distance.

work of breathing An indicator of oxygenation and ventilation. Work of breathing reflects the child's attempt to compensate for hypoxia.

xanthines A classification of medications that affect the respiratory smooth muscle and that relax bronchiole smooth muscles, stimulate cardiac muscle, and stimulate the central nervous system.

xiphoid process The narrow, cartilaginous lower tip of the sternum.

Zika A type of virus that is transmitted by the *Aedes aegypti* mosquito in which the majority of infected persons are asymptomatic; transmission can occur from an infected mother to her fetus, and from an infected male to his sexual partners.

zone of coagulation The reddened area surrounding the leathery and sometimes charred tissue that has sustained a full-thickness burn.

zone of hyperemia In a thermal burn, the area that is least affected by the burn injury; an area of increased blood flow where the body is attempting to repair injured but otherwise viable tissue.

zone of injury The entire affected area in a bone or joint injury, which may include the surrounding soft tissues, especially to the adjacent nerves and blood vessels.

zone of stasis The peripheral area surrounding the zone of coagulation that has decreased blood flow and inflammation; it can undergo necrosis within 24 to 48 hours after the injury, particularly if perfusion is compromised because of burn shock.

zygoma The quadrangular bone of the cheek, articulating with the frontal bone, the maxillae, the zygomatic processes of the temporal bone, and the great wings of the sphenoid bone.

zygote A fertilized egg.

Index

Note: Numbers followed by *f* indicate figure and *t* indicate table respectively.

B

C

D

F

H

I

J

K

L

M

N

O

T